MW00723559

Dear Ingenix Customer:

Enclosed is the new *ICD-10-CM: A Preview of the Structure and Conventions of ICD-10-CM*.

This book provides the entire pre-release draft of the ICD-10-CM code set as written by the World Health Organization (WHO) and National Center for Health Statistics (NCHS). These are the codes that are expected to replace the current ICD-9-CM system for medical documentation and reimbursement pending legislative approval. Our new ICD-10-CM code book will help you get a head start with training programs and system conversion.

Features and benefits include:

- **Official preface:** Official preface provide by National Center for Health Statistics (NCHS) as guidance concerning this pre-release draft of ICD-10-CM.

- **ICD-10-CM conventions:** Explanation of the conventions used in ICD-10-CM.

- **Index:** Official index to the tabular sections and the index to the External Causes section.

- **Neoplasm table:** This is the first look at the neoplasm table within ICD-10-CM.

- **Complete set of ICD-10-CM codes:** All 21 chapters — Infectious and Parasitic Diseases through Injuries, including External Causes and Reasons for Visit.

The codes in ICD-10-CM are not currently valid for any purpose or use. Testing of ICD-10-CM will occur using this pre-release version. It is anticipated that updates and corrections to this draft will be made by NCHS prior to implementation of ICD-10-CM.

There is not yet an anticipated implementation date for the ICD-10-CM. Implementation will be based on the process for adoption of standards under the Health Insurance Portability and Accountability Act of 1996 (HIPAA). There will be a two- year implementation window once the final notice to implement has been published in the *Federal Register*.

Thank you for choosing to be an Ingenix subscriber. If you have any questions about your *ICD-10-CM; A Preview of the Structure and Conventions of ICD-10-CM* — or about any Ingenix publication — please call our customer service department, toll free at (800) INGENIX (464-3649).

Cordially,

Elizabeth Bordne

Vice President, Publisher

Although this draft of ICD-10-CM is available, the codes in ICD-10-CM are not currently valid for any purpose or use. Furthermore, there is not yet an anticipated implementation date for ICD-10-CM. Updates to this draft are anticipated prior to implementation of ICD-10-CM.

ICD•10•CM: A Preview of the Structure and Conventions of ICD-10-CM

May 2002

ingenix

St. Anthony Publishing / Medicode

Publisher's Notice

ICD•10•CM DRAFT is designed to be an accurate and authoritative source regarding coding and every reasonable effort has been made to ensure accuracy and completeness of the content. However, Ingenix, Inc. makes no guarantee, warranty, or representation that this publication is accurate, complete, or without errors. It is understood that Ingenix, Inc. is not rendering any legal or other professional services or advice in this publication and that Ingenix, Inc. bears no liability for any results or consequences that may arise from the use of this book. Please address all correspondence to:

Ingenix Publishing Group
2525 Lake Park Blvd.
West Valley City, UT 84120

Acknowledgments

Elizabeth Boudrie, *Vice President, Publisher*
Lynn Speirs, *Senior Director, Publishing Services Group*
Sheri Poe Bernard, CPC, *Director, Essential Regulatory Products*
Anita Hart, RHIA, CCS, CCS-P, *Product Manager*
Catherine Hopkins, CPC, *Clinical/Technical Editor*
Kimberli Turner, *Project Editor*
Jean Parkinson, *Project Editor*
Jennifer Spetsas, *Project Editor*
Kerrie Hornsby, *Desktop Publishing Manager*
Greg Kemp, *Destop Publisher*

Copyright

First edition copyright ©2002 Ingenix, Inc.

First printing, October 2002

Printed in the United States of America.

ISBN 1-56329-947-X

Sheri Poe Bernard, CPC
Director of Essential Regulatory Products

Ms. Bernard has contributed to the development of coding products for Ingenix for more than 10 years, and her areas of expertise include ICD-9-CM and ICD-10 coding systems. A member of the National Advisory Board of the American Academy of Professional Coders, Ms. Bernard chairs its committee on ICD-10, and is a nationally-recognized speaker on ICD-10 coding systems. Prior to joining Ingenix, Ms. Bernard was a journalist specializing in business and medical writing and editing.

Anita C. Hart, RHIA, CCS, CCS-P
Product Manager

Ms. Hart's experience includes 15 years conducting and publishing research in clinical medicine and human genetics for Yale University, Massachusetts General Hospital, and Massachusetts Institute of Technology. In addition, she has supervised medical records management, health information management, coding and reimbursement, and workers' compensation issues as the office manager for a physical therapy rehabilitation clinic. Ms. Hart is an expert in facility coding, reimbursement systems, and compliance issues and is the Product Manager for the ICD-9-CM and DRG product lines.

Catherine A. Hopkins, CPC
Clinical/Technical Editor

Ms. Hopkins has 17 years experience in the health care field. Her experience includes six years as office manager and senior coding specialist for a large multi-specialty practice. Ms. Hopkins has written several coding manuals and newsletters and has taught seminars on CPT, HCPCS Level II, and ICD-9-CM coding. She also serves as technical support for various software products.

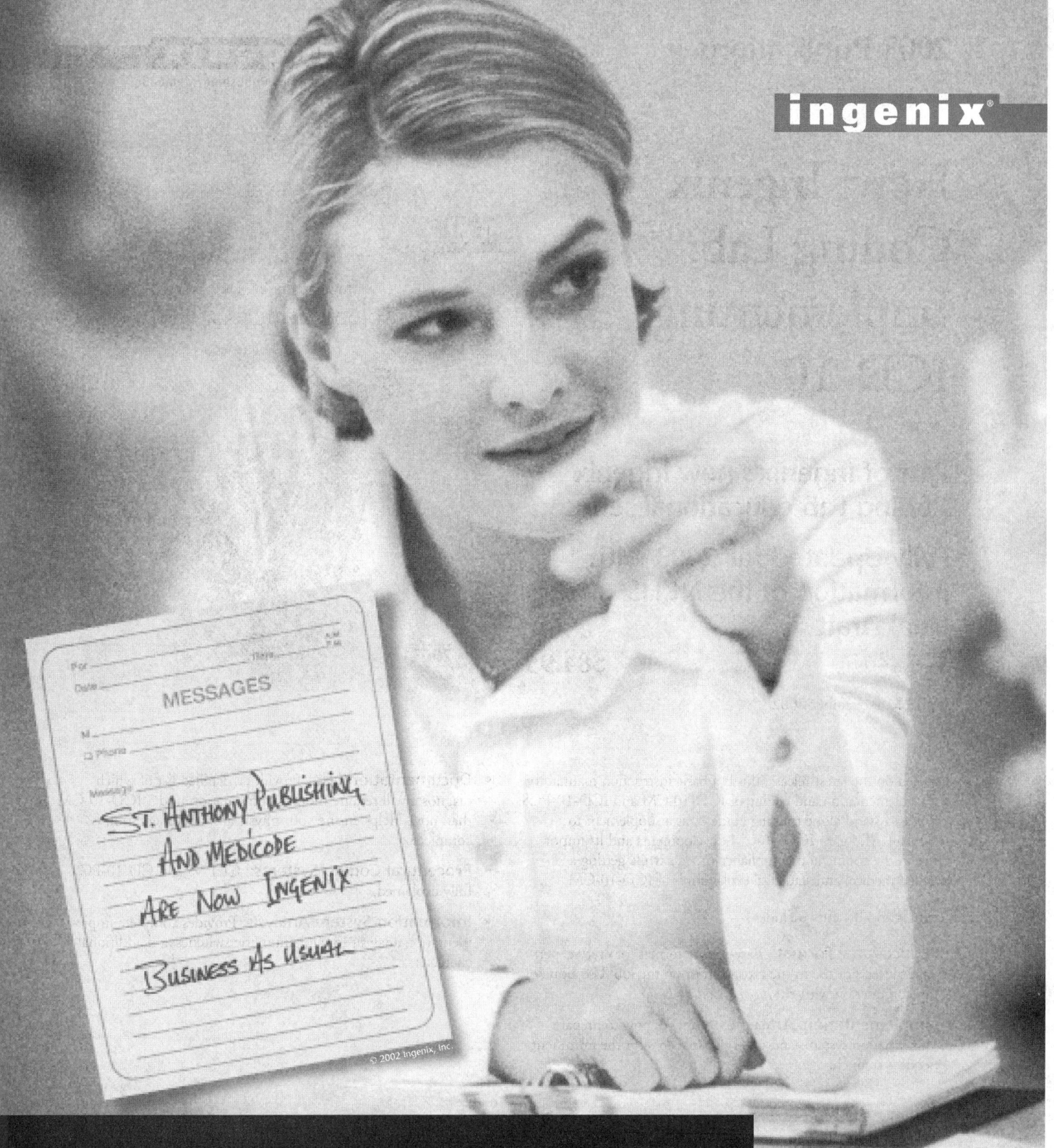

ingenix®

MESSAGES

St. Anthony Publishing
And Medicode
Are Now Ingenix

Business As Usual

© 2002 Ingenix, Inc.

Same dependability with a different name.

St. Anthony Publishing and Medicode are taking on the name of their parent company, Ingenix—one of the industry's largest health care information companies. As Ingenix, we'll continue to lead the industry with a comprehensive array of coding, reimbursement and compliance intelligence. With more than 110 titles, we'll continue to serve the industry with published materials, the latest updates and federally mandated revisions. Delivered to you in a variety of formats such as books, audio seminars, newsletters, updateable binders, email updates, CD-ROMS and the Web. Ingenix. Well into the Future.

For more information, contact us at 1-877- INGENIX or visit us at www.ingenixonline.com.

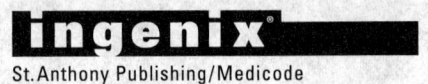

New! Ingenix Coding Lab: Implementing ICD-10

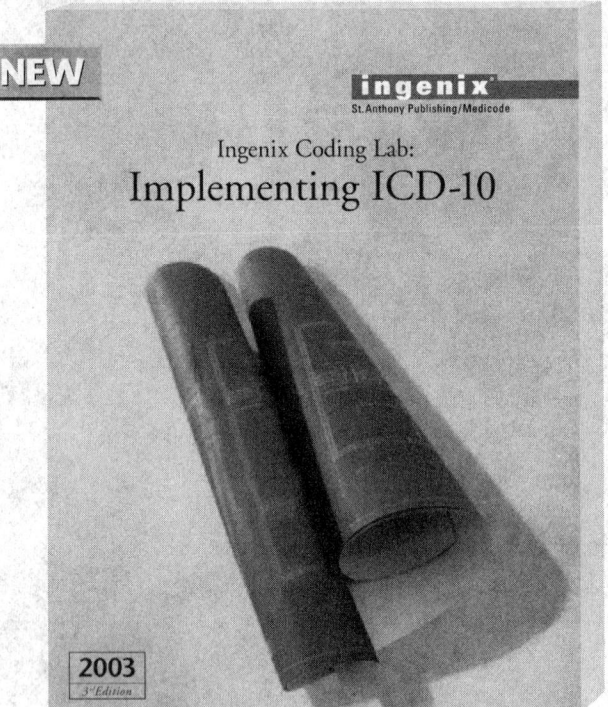

Part of Ingenix's new Ingenix Coding Lab educational series

Fully Updated for 2003 with Information of the NCHS' Final Draft

Item No.: 3299   Softbound, 8.5 x 11"   **$84.95**

Available: November 2002

Based on the latest release, this is a basic instruction manual for implementation and coding of ICD-10-CM and ICD-10-PCS. Use it as a stand-alone training guide or as a supplement to ICD-10-CM. Learn ICD-10-CM developments and its importance in the coding and compliance process while getting a detailed medical and statistical explanation of ICD-10-CM.

Features and Benefits Include:

- **Educational Format:** Easy-to-Use format for every experience level. For use in the classroom or on the job. Use alone or in conjunction with *the Ingenix Coding Lab*.

- **Implementation Strategies:** Teaches how to prepare information systems and other departments for the imminent code system change.

- **Documentation List:** Provides a detailed list of which diagnoses will require more documentation under ICD-10-CM than now. Helps ensure your physicians' documentation is complete.

- **Procedural Coding Systems:** CPT®-5 and CD-10-PCS fully explained.

- **Information System Analysis:** Provides complete implementation analysis for alphanumeric switches and additional characters.

CPT is a registered trademark of the American Medical Association.

Call Toll-Free 1.877.INGENIX (1.877.464.3649) or Shop Online at www.IngenixOnLine.com
Also Available from your Medical Bookstore or Distributor

060102

2003 Publications

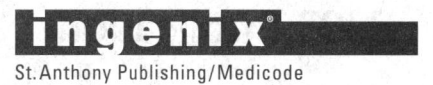

2003 ICD-9-CM Code Books for Physicians Volumes 1 & 2

ICD-9-CM Professional for Physicians, Vols. 1 & 2

Softbound
ISBN: 1-56329-872-4   Item No. 3650 **$64.95**
Available: September 2002

Compact
ISBN: 1-56329-873-2   Item No. 3661 **$64.95**
Available: September 2002

ICD-9-CM Expert for Physicians, Vols. 1 & 2

Spiral
ISBN: 1-56329-874-0   Item No. 3652 **$84.95**
Available: September 2002

Updateable Binder
ISBN: 1-56329-875-9   Item No. 3534 **$144.95**

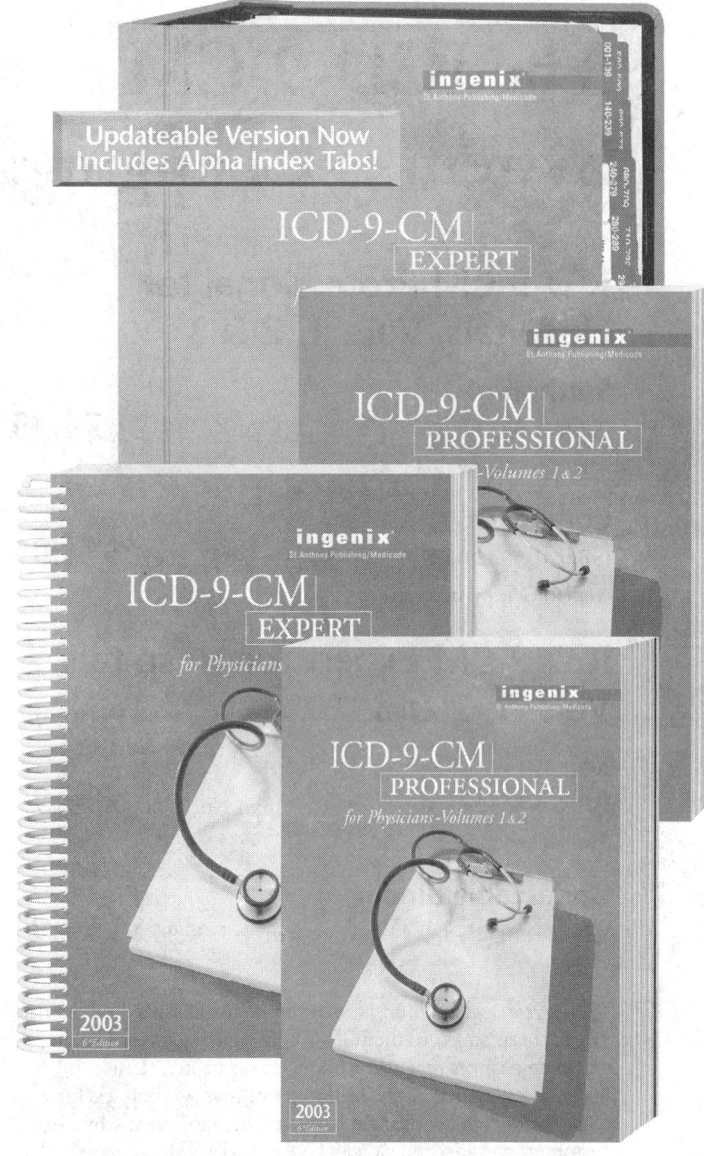

Our page design, featuring intuitive symbols, exclusive color-coding, and additional resources provides a new approach to pertinent coding and reimbursement information. New codes and changes to the ICD-9-CM make our 2003 code books a must buy! Order today and keep current on all changes!

Professional and Expert Editions of ICD-9-CM for Physicians Feature:

- New and Revised Code Symbols
- Fourth-and Fifth-digit Requirement Alerts
- Complete Official Coding Guidelines
- Age and Sex Edits
- Clinically Oriented Definitions and Illustrations
- Medicare as Secondary Payer Indicators

- Manifestation Code Alerts
- "Other" and "Unspecified" Diagnosis Alerts
- Symbols Identifying V Codes Designated for only Primary or only Secondary Diagnosis Use

Expert **Editions Also Include These Enhancements:**

- Special Reports Via E-mail.
- Code Tables--Complex coding issues are simplified in coding tables, as developed for I-9 Express
- Valid Three-digit Category List

The *Expert* Updateable Binder Subscriptions Feature:

- Money Saving Update Service
- Three Updates per Year [October (full text), January and July]

Call Toll-Free 1.877.INGENIX (464.3649) or Shop Online at www.IngenixOnline.com

Also Available from your Medical Bookstore or Distributor

060102

2003 Publications

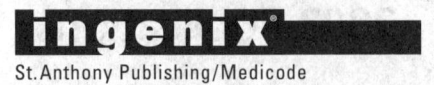

St.Anthony Publishing/Medicode

The ICD-9-CM System is Changing!

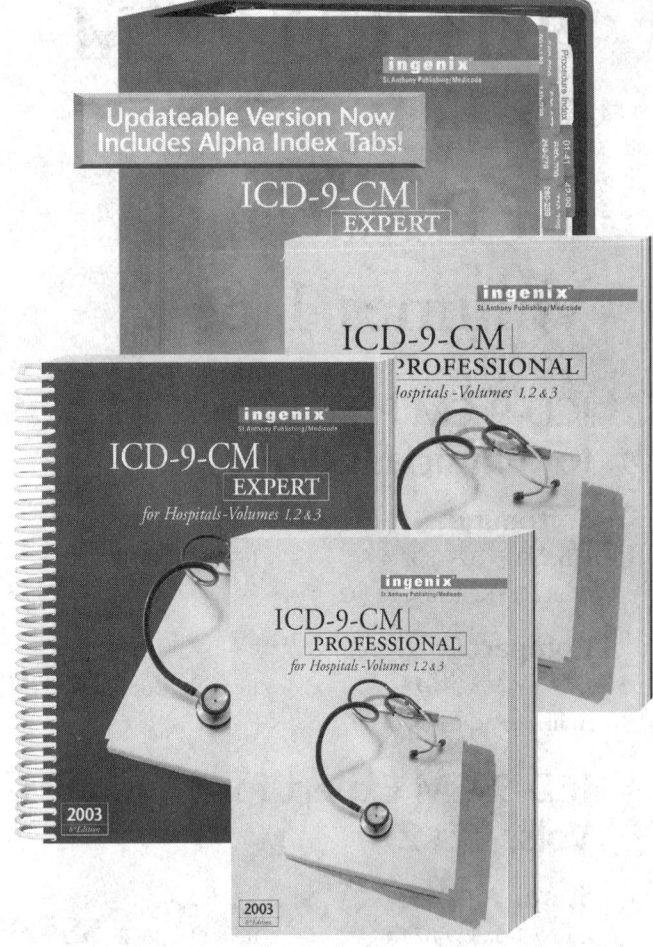

Updateable Version Now Includes Alpha Index Tabs!

ICD-9-CM Professional for Hospitals, Vols. 1, 2 & 3

Softbound
ISBN: 1-56329-876-7   Item No. 3654 **$74.95**
Available: September 2002

Compact
ISBN: 1-56329-877-5   Item No. 3662 **$74.95**
Available: September 2002

ICD-9-CM Expert for Hospitals, Vols. 1, 2 & 3

Spiral
ISBN: 1-56329-878-3   Item No. 3656 **$94.95**
Available: September 2002

Updateable Binder
ISBN: 1-56329-879-1   Item No. 3539 **$154.95**

This year, a chapter on New Technologies and Medical Services has been added to the ICD-9-CM code books for Hospitals, and code changes that affect nearly every chapter! Last year, our newly designed pages, featuring intuitive symbols, exclusive color-coding, and additional resources, demonstrated why our customers consider these codes books the BEST!

Professional and Expert editions of ICD-9-CM for Hospitals Feature:

- New and Revised Code Symbols
- Fourth-and Fifth-digit Requirement Alerts
- Complete Official Coding Guidelines
- AHA's *Coding Clinic for ICD-9-CM* References
- Illustrations and Definitions
- Age and Sex Edits
- Nonspecific and Unacceptable Primary Diagnosis Alerts
- Medicare as Secondary Payer Indicators
- Manifestation Code Alerts

- Complex Diagnosis and Major Complication Alerts
- HIV Major Related Diagnosis Alerts
- CC Principal Diagnosis Exclusion List
- CC Diagnosis Symbol
- Crucial Medicare Procedure Code Edits

Expert Editions Also Include These Enhancements:

- Special Reports Via E-mail.
- Complete Principal Diagnosis/MDC/DRG Listing
- Pharmacological List
- CC Code List
- Valid Three-digit Code List

The Expert Updateable Binder Subscriptions Feature:

- Money Saving Update Service
- Three Updates per Year [October (full text), January and July]

Call Toll-Free 1.877.INGENIX (464.3649) or Shop Online at www.IngenixOnline.com

Also Available from your Medical Bookstore or Distributor

060102

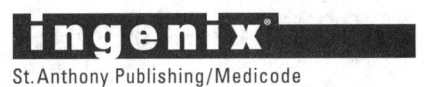

St. Anthony Publishing/Medicode

An Exceptional Code Book! An Exceptional Year for ICD-9-CM!

2003 ICD-9-CM Expert for Home Health Services, Nursing Facilities & Hospices, Volumes 1, 2 & 3

Softbound

ISBN: 1-56329-880-5   Item No. 3658 **$129.95**

Available: September 2002

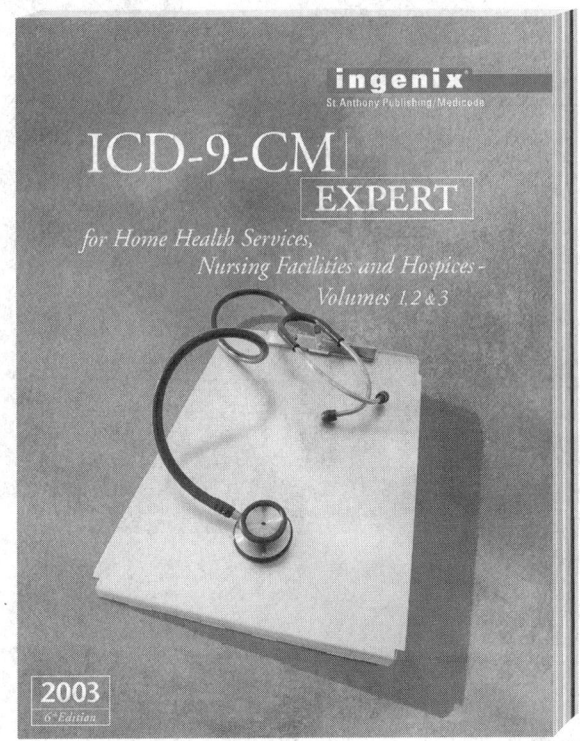

In the healthcare marketplace, this is the only ICD-9-CM code book designed specifically for the needs of the home health, nursing home, and hospice coder. This enhanced code book now includes features that will take the coder to the next level of coding. Code quickly and accurately using this resource filled with important alerts and references specific to each facility type. No other code book exists that explains each prospective payment system in detail or that can serve as a reference for specific coding guidelines.

Inside You Will Find:

- **New Chapter in Volume 3 for New Technologies and Medical Services**

- Illustrations and Definitions

- **Exclusive**—E-mail delivered Special Reports

- Additional Digit Requirement Alerts in the Index and the Tabular Sections

- "10 Steps to Correct Coding" Tutorial

- Excerpts from the Home Health Agency Prospective Payment System (HHA PPS) and Symbols Identifying Clinical Dimension Diagnoses

- Medicare Home Health Manual Section on Coverage Qualifications

- Explanation of the SNF Prospective Payment System (SNF PPS) and Color-coding Indicating ICD-9-CM Codes Associated with Specific RUG-III Categories

- Color-coding and Criteria for Acceptable Non-cancer Diagnoses for Hospice Coverage

- Complete Official Coding Guidelines, Including LTC Guidelines

- Symbols Identifying V Codes Designated for only Primary or only Secondary Diagnosis Use

Call Toll-Free 1.877.INGENIX (464.3649) or Shop Online at www.IngenixOnline.com

Also Available from your Medical Bookstore or Distributor

060102

2003 Publications

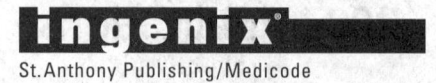
St. Anthony Publishing/Medicode

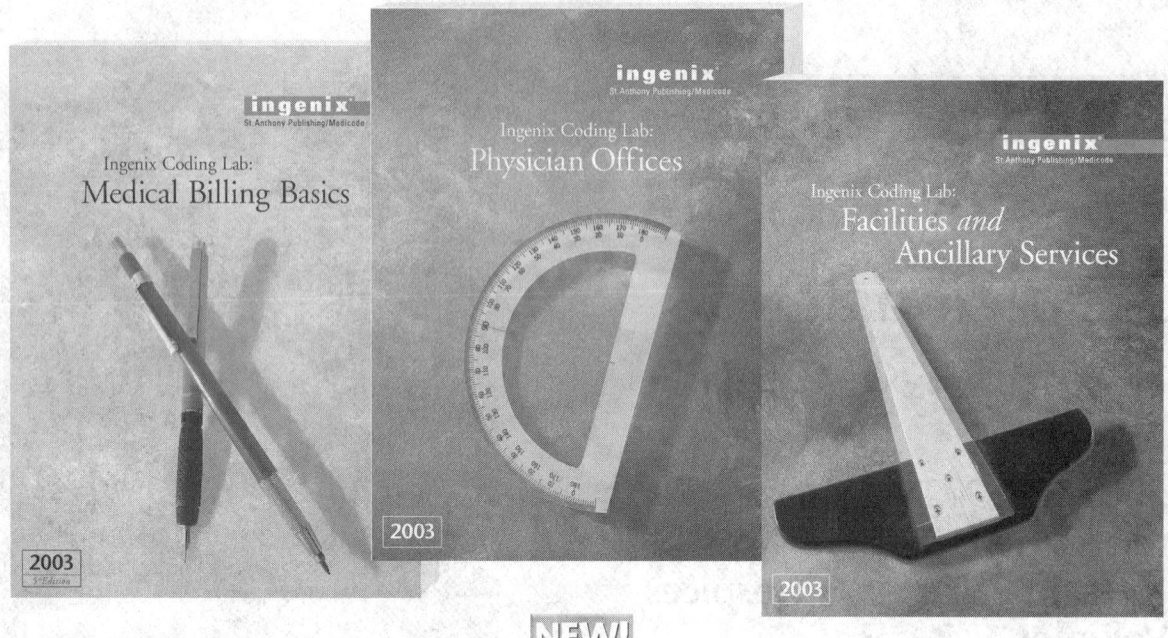

NEW!

A New Coder's Training System

These comprehensive education modules help beginning and advanced coders in the office, the facility, or the classroom. Designed to allow you to understand and master the skills needed to be an effective coder, each module includes a CD containing a student workbook and a teacher's guide, along with a three-month subscription to the popular *Code It Fast* look-up program.

All Books Include:

- **Student Workbook on CD**—Student workbook helps you convert information in the book to hands-on experience

- **Teacher's Guide on CD**—Teacher's guide helps instructors and managers tutor and challenge their students

- **Three-month Code It Fast CD**—*Code it Fast* look-up CD includes the latest ICD-9-CM, HCPCS, and CPT® codes

- **Complex Coding Scenarios**—Complex coding scenarios help assure fast and accurate physician reimbursement through example

NEW! Ingenix Coding Lab: Medical Billing Basics

Complete Foundation for Coding and Billing—Broad overview of coding, payers, and the reimbursement process for the entry-level coder or billing professional
ISBN: 1-56329-921-6   Item No. 5772 **$74.95**
Available: December 2002

NEW! Ingenix Coding Lab: Physician Offices

Complete Foundation for Physician Coding and Billing—Broad overview of physician reimbursement process for the coder or billing professional
ISBN: 1-56329-908-9   Item No. 3268 **$74.95**
Available: December 2002

NEW! Ingenix Coding Lab: Facilities and Ancillary Services

Complete Foundation for Facility Coding and Billing—Broad overview of facility reimbursement process for the coder or billing professional
ISBN: 1-56329-920-8   Item No. 3227 **$99.95**
Available: December 2002

CPT is a registered trademark of the American Medical Association

Call Toll-Free 1.877.INGENIX (464.3649) or Shop Online at www.IngenixOnLine.com
Also Available from your Medical Bookstore or Distributor

060102

2003 Publications

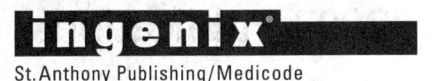

St. Anthony Publishing/Medicode

Introducing a NEW HIPAA Reference Just for Facilities!

HIPAA Facility Desk Reference—2003

ISBN: 1-56329-962-7   Item No. 2010 **$99.95**

Available: June 2002

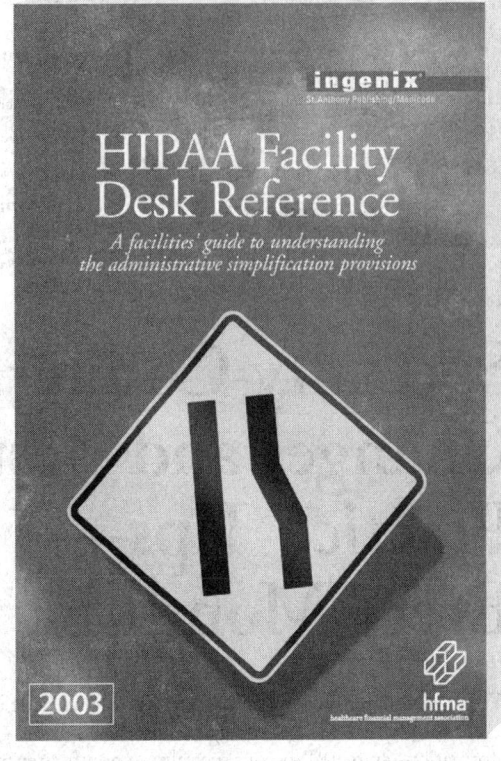

NEW

Several important HIPAA regulatory deadlines for facilities occur in 2002 and 2003. Complying with the HIPAA transactions and privacy and security requirements will be an arduous task for all facilities. Facilities must be prepared!

The *HIPAA Facility Desk Reference* walks facilities through the components of HIPAA compliance—transactions, privacy and security, and identifiers. It provides a comprehensive but concise analysis of all HIPAA provisions

- **Inexpensive, Compact, Thorough Desk Reference.** Just the right size—without being overwhelming. Ideal for training. Gives your HIPAA task force a central reference for planning and discussion.

- **Easy-to-Follow Organization of HIPAA Issues.** Now facilities have an easy-to-read but comprehensive overview of a very complex regulatory initiative.

- **Comprehensive Review of All HIPAA Provisions— Including Privacy, Security, Transactions and Code Sets, and Unique Identifiers.** Shows how the regulatory provisions affect day-to-day business, and notes the penalties for non-compliance.

- **Latest Transactions and Privacy Rule Changes.** Get help with responding to Medicare's Transaction Rule Compliance Plan; know how the March changes to privacy affect your preparations for HIPAA compliance

- **Easy-to-Use Key Term Alert Symbols, HIPAA Dictionary and FAQs.** Makes key information easy to read and remember.

- **Earn 5 CEUS from AAPC.**

- **Co-published with HFMA.** Legal and IT authors are members of the Healthcare Financial Management Association's (HFMA) HIPAA Task Force.

Call Toll-Free 1.877.INGENIX (464.3649) or Shop Online at www.IngenixOnline.com

Also Available from your Medical Bookstore or Distributor

060102

2003 Publications

ingenix®
St. Anthony Publishing/Medicode

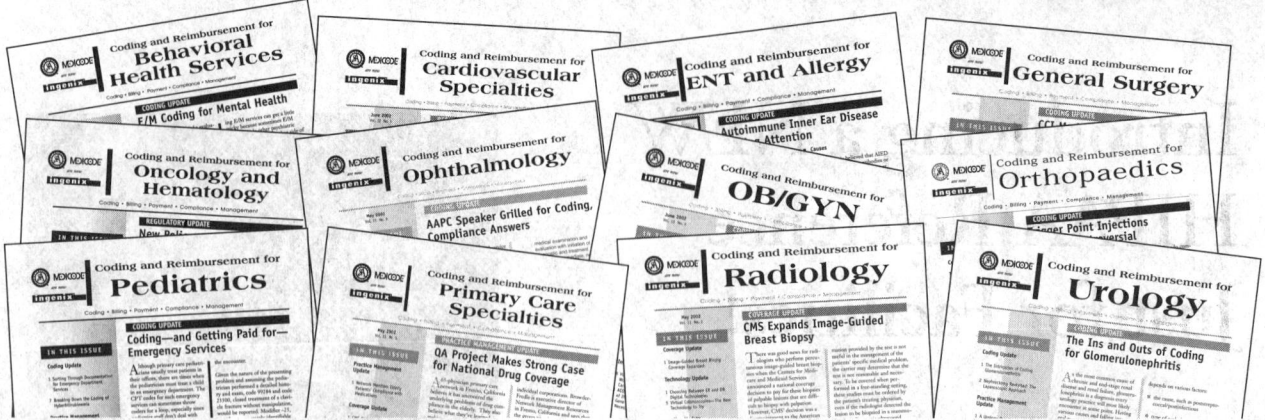

Specialty Coding Changes and Best Practice Tips— Every Month

Our newsletters are a great companion to your code book. Your practice will get timely, concise, and reliable information—targeted to your specialty—month after month.

Inside each of our specialty newsletters you'll find:

- **Expert Advice.** You'll get the help you need to code more accurately—reducing delays and denials.

- **Questions and Answers.** You'll get answers to difficult coding questions—without hiring consultants or spending hours on research.

- **Timely Coverage of Regulatory Decisions.** Our experts keep you on top of complicated government regulations and tell you how they will impact your practice.

$179.95 /year, per title

Newsletter	Item No.
Coding and Reimbursement for:	
Behavioral Health Services	6543
Cardiovascular Specialties	6542
ENT & Allergy	4276
General Surgery	4277
Oncology & Hematology	4278
Ophthalmology	4053
Ob/Gyn	4091
Orthopaedics	4097
Pediatrics	4270
Primary Care Specialties	4034
Radiology	4114
Urology	4279

Practical Guidance on HIPAA and E-Health for the Physician Practice

News, analysis, innovative strategies, case studies, and practical "how-to" articles to help you implement the administrative simplification provisions under HIPAA and related e-health technologies. Your subscription includes:

- **HIPAA News.** The latest information on HIPAA regulations and deadlines.

- **E-health Updates.** Solid information on how your practice can prepare for technology enhancements and security requirements—and even profit!

- **Practical Articles.** Strategies for upgrading computer systems, designing a workflow that protects privacy, evaluating hardware and software, and other HIPAA-related operational challenges.

- **Legislative Analysis.** Interviews with legal analysts in the field.

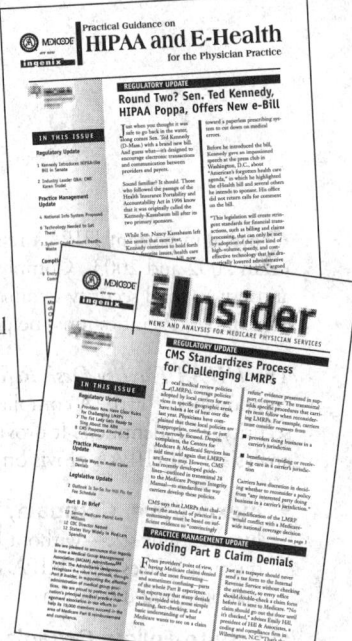

Item No. 4231 **$269.95** (12 issues annually)

Part B Insider

With *Part B Insider*, you will receive clear and current coverage of the changing Part B regulatory, compliance, and legal environment. *Part B Insider* is your guide to:

- **News.** Stay informed of new and proposed regulations, coding and billing guidelines, judicial decisions, compliance developments, and more.

- **Impact.** Learn how these developments will affect your organization—and your bottom line.

- **Action.** Discover practical ways to implement the new policies and procedures.

Item No. 4272 **$349.95** (24 issues annually)

Call Toll-Free 1.800.INGENIX (464.3649) or Shop Online at www.IngenixOnLine.com

Also Available from your Medical Bookstore or Distributor

020917

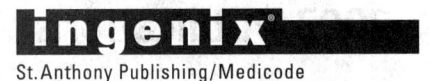

ingenix
St. Anthony Publishing/Medicode

Put the HIPAA Pieces Together!

HIPAA Desk Reference

ISBN: 1-56329-916-X   Item No. 4335 **$99.95**

Available: October 2002

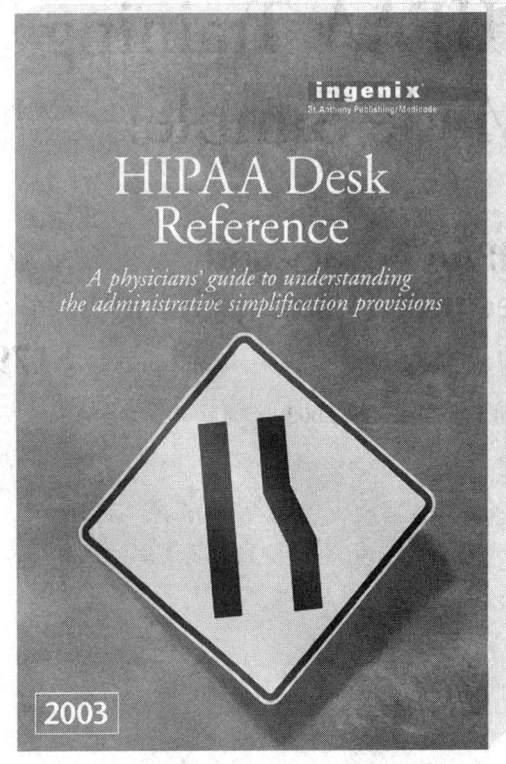

HIPAA Desk Reference is a straightforward, practical, and easy-to-use reference that provides a fundamental understanding of all the HIPAA provisions. This product will break the regulation down into targeted and manageable components, allowing users to improve their knowledge of the regulations and assist in the development of critical assessment questions. An excellent tool for:

- Office Managers
- Compliance Officers
- Physicians
- Department Managers
- Vendors working with medical practices who are responsible for storing or transmitting patient information

- **Updated Provisions.** Complete update of any changes to provisions.

- **Provision-specific Case Studies.** Provide user with examples of issues others are having problems with.

- **Alert Icons.** Icons alert users to helpful tips in HIPAA education.

- **HIPAA History.** Provides an overview of what HIPAA is and why it is now a major regulation that will change the way patient information is handled.

- **Comprehensive Review of All HIPAA Provisions: Security, Privacy, Transaction and Code Sets, and Unique Identifier.** Each provision is separated out into its own chapter, providing a compete review of the provision, identifying how the provision affects day-to-day business, and listing penalties for noncompliance.

- **HIPAA Timeline.** Identifies current status of each provision and its implementation date.

- **Key Term Alert Symbol.** Pinpoints and defines critical terms within the text that help in the comprehension of key issues specific to each provision. Each term is defined in a sidebar.

- **HIPAA Dictionary.** Complete listing of important HIPAA terms, buzzwords, and acronyms.

- **Frequently Asked Questions (FAQs).** We've done the research to provide answers to your most pressing questions to help in the education of your entire staff.

- **HIPAA Web Resources.** Comprehensive listing of government and commercial Web sites.

- **Continuing Education Units (CEUs).** Earn 3 CEUs through AAPC.

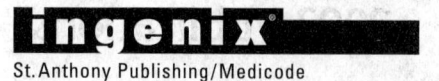

St. Anthony Publishing/Medicode

HIPAA Training Made Simple!

HIPAA Privacy and Security Training Guide

ISBN: 1-56329-925-9   Item No. 2928 **$179.95**

Available: November 2002

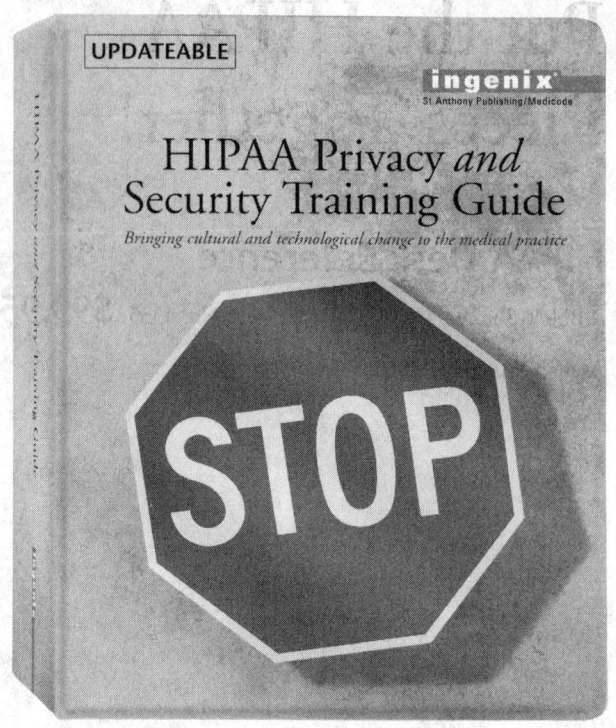

One of the most effective HIPAA privacy and security training guides available. This product is designed to help medical practices implement an internal training program.

- **Policy to Procedure Crosswalk Training Template.** Helps users organize policies and procedure in a summary format to aid in the training process.

- **PowerPoint Training Presentation.** Provides users with the foundation to develop their internal training presentation.

- **Assessment Templates.** Helps users identify and record problem areas that must be addressed during training.

- **Comprehensive Review of the Privacy and Security Provisions.**

- **HIPAA Glossary.** Complete listing of the most up-to-date acronyms, terms and web resources.

- **Walks Through the Complete Flow of Patient Information.** From front office management to submitting the claim (electronically or not), helps the user clearly identify key areas that must be addressed and are affected by HIPAA.

2003 Publications

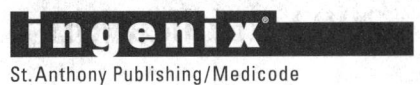

St. Anthony Publishing/Medicode

Step-by-step Guidance for HIPAA Implementation

HIPAA Assessment and Implementation Manual

ISBN: 1-56329-924-0   Item No. 3183 **$229.95**

Available: June 2002

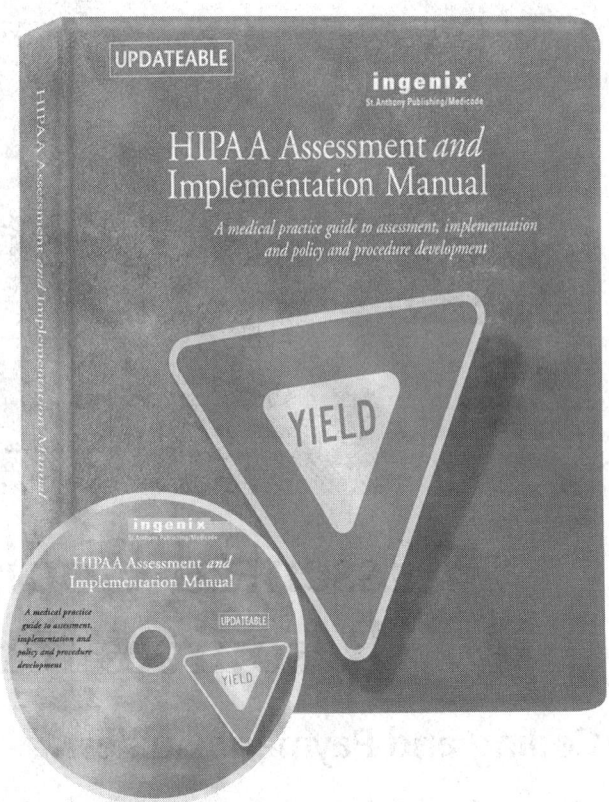

HIPAA Assessment and Implementation Manual is designed to help users put into effect HIPAA provisions using an easy and systematic process. This manual is designed to assist the user with assessing the impact of HIPAA on business as well as helping establish a HIPAA project plan. *HIPAA Assessment and Implementation Manual* also contains valuable information helping you evaluate business associates and current contracts, integrate HIPAA compliance into current structures, and develop policies and procedures.

- **Assessment and Implementation Guidance for Each Provision.** Each provision has a separate chapter dedicated to focusing on issues specific to that provision, allowing users to perform comprehensive and accurate assessments that lead to successful implementation.

- **Easy-to-use and Printable Templates.** The templates contained in this manual are designed to help the user assess current HIPAA readiness and transfer their findings into an action plan.

- **Free Updates.** These updates help keep you up to date with changes to HIPAA policies as they occur and alert you to additional changes under consideration.

- **Policy and Procedure Development Guidance and Templates.** Each provision chapter has guidelines for developing effective policies and procedures.

- **Guidance for Evaluating Business Associates.** Know what defines a business associate and what such associates are accountable for.

- **HIPAA Compliance Integration.** Helps you to incorporate HIPAA compliance efforts into your current compliance structure.

- **Free "E" Book Included.** Forms, templates, and official regulations included for easy lookup and printing.

Call Toll-Free 1.877.INGENIX (464.3649) or Shop Online at www.IngenixOnline.com

Also Available from your Medical Bookstore or Distributor

060102

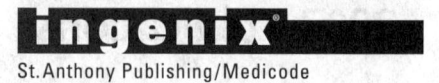
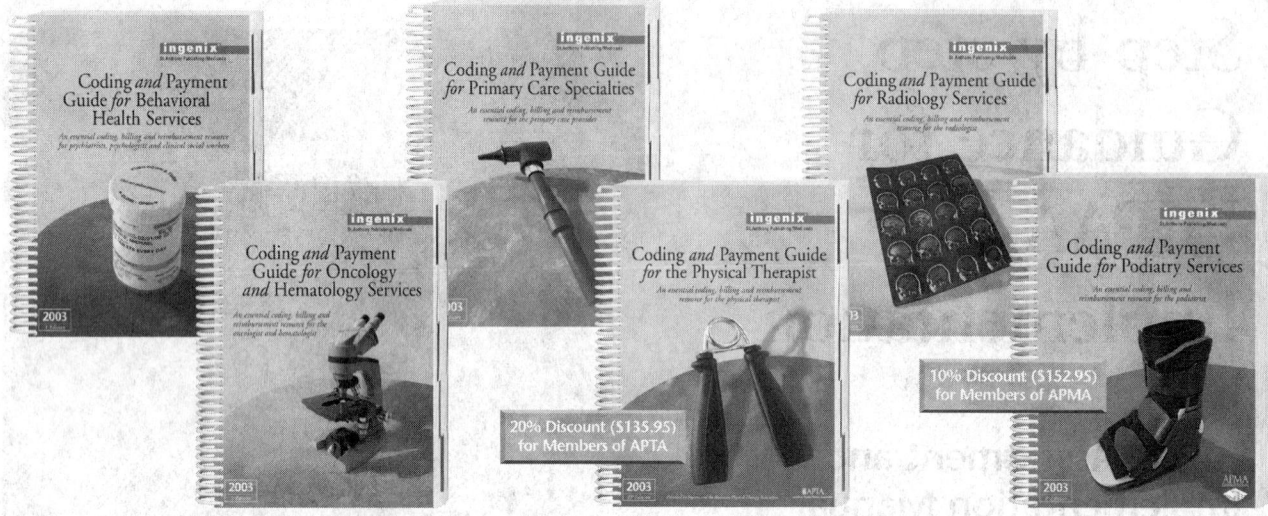

Essential Coding and Payment Resources for Your Specialty

Coding and Payment Guides

The *2003 Coding and Payment Guides* focus exclusively on coding, documentation, and reimbursement issues from A to Z for 6 different specialties. These valuable resources link coding and clinical information so you can code more accurately and get full, prompt reimbursement.

- **ICD-9-CM Codes with Icons.** Allow the user to identify the most accurate application of ICD-9-CM codes.
- **Updated with 2003 Codes.** Allows for fast and easy coding of your claims by giving you Physicians' Current Procedural Terminology (CPT®), ICD-9-CM, and HCPCS Level II codes specific to your specialty.
- **NEW—Medicare Information.** Contains *Medicare Carriers Manual* and *Coverage Issues Manual* information specific to your specialty, now linked to CPT® and HCPCS Level II codes.

- **Maintaining Medical Documentation.** Outlines how to maintain complete medical documentation and ensure compliance with third-party payers' requirements.
- **Definitions and Guidelines Specific to Your Specialty.** Help you understand diagnostic conditions.
- **National Correct Coding Initiative (NCCI) Edits.** An appendix provides listings of NCCI edits for your specialty (included in all except the *Coding and Payment Guide for the Physical Therapist*—please see the American Physical Therapy Association for the latest NCCI edits).

$169.95 each   4 to 5 CEUs from AAPC

ISBN No.	Acronym	Item Description	Item No.	Available
1-56329-841-4	SYCH	Coding and Payment Guide for Behavioral Health Services	4351	January 2003
1-56329-840-6	SONC	Coding and Payment Guide for Oncology and Hematology Services	4352	January 2003
1-56329-836-8	SPT	Coding and Payment Guide for the Physical Therapist	4353	December 2002
1-56329-837-6	SPOD	Coding and Payment Guide for Podiatry Services	4354	December 2002
1-56329-839-2	SPC	Coding and Payment Guide for Primary Care Specialties	4355	December 2002
1-56329-838-4	SRA	Coding and Payment Guide for Radiology Services	4356	December 2002

CPT is a registered trademark of the American Medical Association

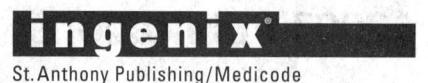

St. Anthony Publishing/Medicode

Take the Mystery Out of Medicare Coverage and Issuing ABNs

Complete Guide to Medicare Coverage Issues

Item No. 3036 **$279.95**
*Call for CD multi-user pricing

Available: Now

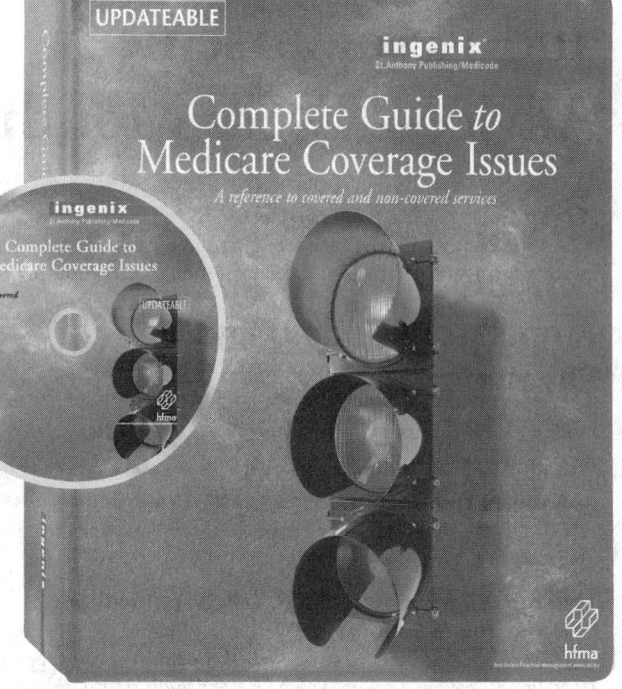

Know exactly which services and items Medicare will pay for, and which it won't, before you submit a claim.

This one-of-a-kind, updateable guide details Medicare's national coverage policies using CMS's official source documents. For any site of service, know what Medicare will and will not cover before submitting claims. Your subscription includes a CD-ROM with the full text of the manual and a newsletter with information about new and existing Medicare coverage for both Part A and Part B services.

- **New — Now Includes Pending National Decisions.**
  You'll have pending decisions available in one resource to help you and your staff manage all national coverage issues affecting Part A and Part B services.

- **Exclusive — Color-coded Coverage Prompts.**
  Know at a glance whether an item or procedure has restricted coverage, enabling you to make accurate coverage decisions promptly and submit bills correctly the first time. Helps prevent costly denials and claim resubmissions. Provides guidance regarding proper documentation for medical necessity, and helps you know when to issue an advance beneficiary notice for noncovered services. Also helps health plans understand Medicare coverage policies.

- **Fully Indexed.** Easily locate a specific item or service.

- **Updates and Coverage Alert Newsletter.** Keep you up to date on all new national Medicare coverage policies and revisions to existing policies.

- **Full Text of Manual on CD-ROM in PDF Format.**
  Electronic solution for researching national coverage decisions and medical necessity issues. Allows you to find key coverage issues and/or specific items and services with the click of a mouse. Other easy-to-use features include hypertext links and electronic bookmarks to take you quickly to the sections of the manual that you use the most.

- **Physicians' Current Procedural Terminology (CPT®) Codes and HCPCS Codes Assigned to National Issues.**
  Helps you identify coverage issues by CPT® or HCPCS code. Includes coverage issues pertaining to medical equipment, devices, procedures, clinical trials, and more!

- **Co-published with HFMA.**

- **Earn 5 CEUS from AAPC.**

CPT is a registered trademark of the American Medical Association

Call Toll-Free 1.877.INGENIX (464.3649) or Shop Online at www.IngenixOnline.com
Also Available from your Medical Bookstore or Distributor

060102

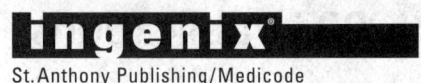

St. Anthony Publishing/Medicode

Get Expert Coding and Reimbursement Advice—Every Month

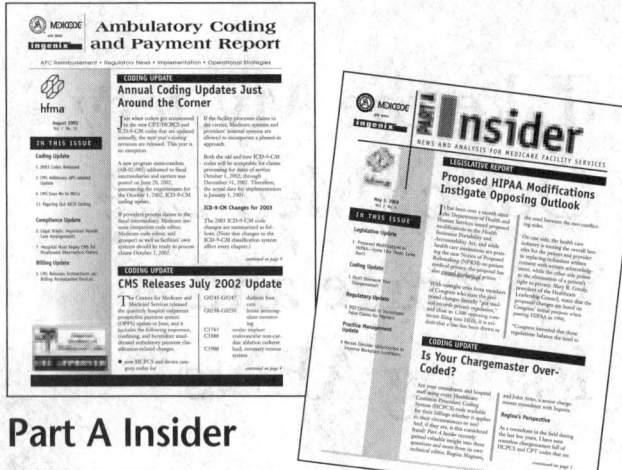

Our newsletters are a great companion to your code book. Your facility will get timely, concise, and reliable information—targeted to your specialty—month after month.

Ambulatory Coding and Payment Report

Inside each 16-page issue of *Ambulatory Coding and Payment Report*, you'll find:

- **Answers You Need to Manage APC Operations Effectively**. We'll help you prevent costly billing mistakes and collect and manage essential data properly.

- **Improve Coding Accuracy to Get Every Medicare Dollar You're Entitled To**. We'll help you train your staff on correct coding so you can avoid medical necessity denials, support additional payment where appropriate, and audit your outpatient claims for costly mistakes.

- **Stay Abreast of New Developments as APC Implementation Moves Forward**. A regular Q&A column will clarify specific operational and coding issues and give you an opportunity to ask your own questions.

Item No. 2428 **$249.95**

Clinical Coding and Reimbursement

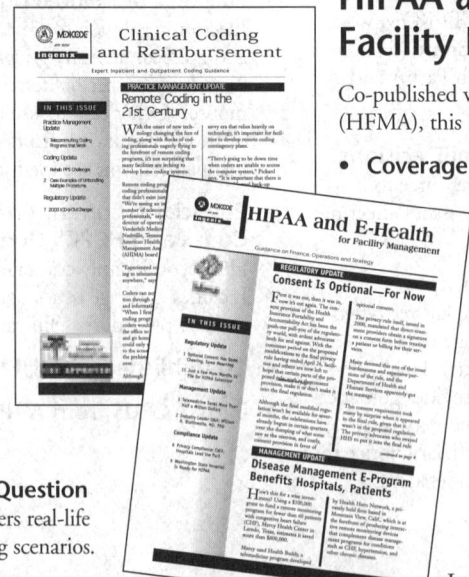

Inside each monthly issue of *Clinical Coding and Reimbursement*, you'll find:

- **In-Depth Clinical Analysis of Diseases and Procedures**. So you can choose the right code the first time. Use to train your staff!

- **Up-To-Date News on ICD-9-CM, CPT®, and HCPCS Coding Systems and Reimbursement Methodologies**. Keeps you current so you receive the appropriate reimbursement.

- **Actual Case Studies and "Question and Answer" Column**. Offers real-life solutions to your difficult coding scenarios.

Item No. 4031 **$179.95**

Part A Insider

Part A Insider is a bi-weekly publication—co-published with the Healthcare Financial Management Association (HFMA)—designed to help give you the news and analysis you need to plan, implement, and survive the regulatory, compliance, billing, and legal changes affecting your facility.

Inside *Part A Insider*, you'll find:

- **Regulatory Updates**. PPS for outpatient (APCs), inpatient, SNFs, HHA, and inpatient rehab; Medicare coverage issues that affect billing and reimbursement; HIPAA regulations and implementation, and more.

- **Compliance Updates**. OIG's advisory opinions, annual work-plan initiatives, high risk areas, audit reports, and more.

- **Billing Updates**. HCFA-1450/UB-92 and Medicare billing policy changes; common problem billing areas; correct coding and other Medicare edits.

Item No. 4281 **$349.95**

HIPAA and E-Health for Facility Management

Co-published with the Healthcare Financial Management Association (HFMA), this 12-page monthly newsletter provides:

- **Coverage on HIPAA Regulations**. Concise and to the point. Know what the latest provisions, developments, and delays are and how they affect your facility.

- **Strategies and Guidance**. Learn what's working and what's not for your colleagues through consultant interviews, guest authors, and case studies.

- **E-health Tools and Technology Updates**. Evaluate the need for EDI, electronic patient records, and point-of-care advancements.

- **HIPAA and E-health Links**. Utilize hard-to-find information from sources like digests, listservs, Web sites, white papers, and more.

Item #2431 **$299.95**

CPT is a registered trademark of the American Medical Association.

Call Toll-Free 1.800.INGENIX (464.3649) or Shop Online at www.IngenixOnLine.com

Also Available from your Medical Bookstore or Distributor

020916

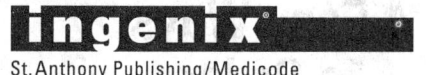

8 Out of 10 Surveyed Coders Prefer *Coders' Desk Reference*

Coders' Desk Reference

ISBN: 156329-854-6   Item No. 5762 **$119.95**
Available: December 2002

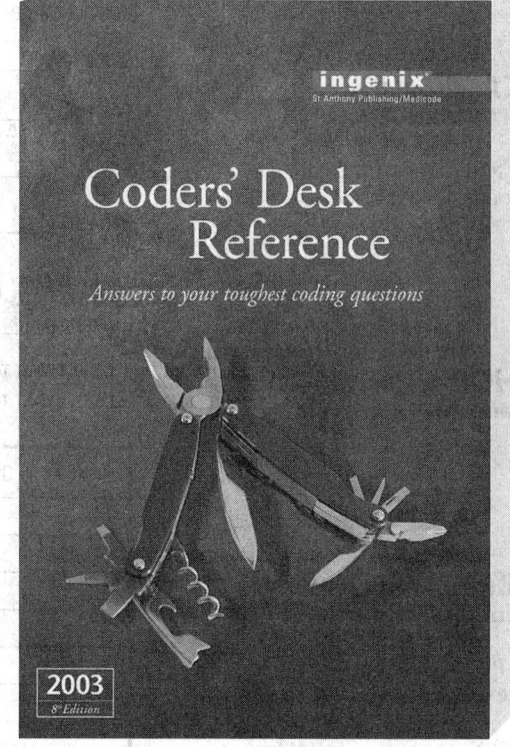

No matter how much experience you have using ICD-9-CM, Physicians' Current Procedural Terminology (CPT®), and HCPCS Level II codes, there are always tough questions that hold up the billing process. And because billing errors can result in fines, you can't afford to guess. Now you can get easy-to-understand answers to your coding questions without leaving your desk, with the 2003 *Coders' Desk Reference*.

- **NEW—Updated with 2003 CPT® Codes.** Includes accurate descriptions for more than 7,000 CPT® procedures, plus an anesthesia crosswalk and an E/M chapter.

- **More Than 6,000 Lay Descriptions of Procedures and Tests.** Improve your coding accuracy by consulting these easy-to-understand explanations of procedures.

- **Update on the CPT®-5 Project.** Keep current on changes to the CPT® codes and guidelines.

- **ICD-10-CM and ICD-10-PCS Preparation.** Learn how each will affect you and discover ways to make the transitions as smooth as possible.

- **CPT® "New," "Changed," and "Grammatically Changed" Icons from the Previous Year.** Official CPT® headings and subheadings denoting anatomical and procedural sections help users determine the codes associated with lay descriptions.

- **Earn 5 CEUs from AAPC.**

CPT is a registered trademark of the American Medical Association

Call Toll-Free 1.877.INGENIX (464.3649) or Shop Online at www.IngenixOnline.com

Also Available from your Medical Bookstore or Distributor

060102

4 Easy Ways to Order

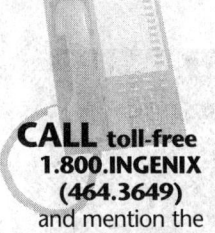

**CALL toll-free
1.800.INGENIX
(464.3649)**
and mention the
Source Code: FOBA3

**SHOP on line at
www.IngenixOnline.com**

**MAIL this form with
payment and/or purchase
order to:**
PO Box 27116
Salt Lake City, UT 84127-0116

FAX this order form with
credit card information and /or
purchase order to 801.982.4033

Customer Service Hours
7:00am to 5:00pm MT
9:00am to 7:00pm ET

100% Money Back Guarantee

If our merchandise* ever fails to meet
your expectations, please contact our
Customer Service Department toll-free
at 1.800.INGENIX (464.3649) for an
immediate response. We will resolve
any concern without hesitation.

*Software: Credit will be granted for
unopened packages only.

No. of Items	Fee
Shipping and Handling	
1	$9.95
2-4	$11.95
5-7	$14.95
8-10	$19.95
11+	Call

PUBLICATION ORDER AND FAX FORM   FOBA3

Customer No._____   Contact No._____

Purchase Order No._____   Source Code_____
(Attach copy of Purchase Order)

Contact Name _____   Title_____

Company_____

Address _____
(no P.O. Boxes, please)

City_____   State_____ Zip_____

Phone (____)_____   Fax (____)_____
(in case we have questions about your order)

IMPORTANT: E-MAIL REQUIRED FOR ORDER CONFIRMATION AND SELECT PRODUCT DELIVERY.
E-mail _____

❏ YES, I WANT TO RECEIVE SPECIAL REPORTS AND INFORMATION VIA E-MAIL.
❏ YES, I WANT TO RECEIVE NEW PRODUCT ANNOUNCEMENTS VIA E-MAIL.

Item #	Qty	Item Description	Price	Total
4025	1	(SAMPLE) DRG Guidebook	$89.95	$89.95
			Sub Total	
	TX, UT, OH, and VA residents please add applicable sales tax			
	Shipping & handling (see chart)			
	(11 plus items, foreign and Canadian orders, please call for shipping costs)			
	Total enclosed			

Payment Options

❏ Check enclosed. (Make payable to Ingenix, Inc.)

❏ Charge my: ❏ MasterCard ❏ VISA ❏ AMEX ❏ Discover

Card # I I I I I I I I I I I I I I I I Exp. Date: I I I I
                                                          MM YR

❏ Bill Me P.O.#_____

Signature _____

©2002 Ingenix, Inc. All prices subject to change without notice.   FOBA3
                                                                           020601

ICD-10-CM Official Preface DRAFT
May 2002

Introduction

This pre-release draft of the International Classification of Diseases, 10th revision, Clinical Modification (ICD-10-CM) has been developed by the United States Government in recognition of its responsibility to promulgate this classification throughout the United States for morbidity coding. The International Classification of Diseases, 10th Revision, published by the World Health Organization (WHO) is the foundation for ICD-10-CM and continues to be the classification employed in cause-of-death coding in the United States. The ICD-10-CM is comparable with the ICD-10.The WHO Collaborating Center for the Family of International Classifications in North America, housed at NCHS, has responsibility for the implementation of ICD and serves as a liaison between the WHO fulfilling international obligations for comparable classifications and the national health data needs of the United States. The historical background of the International Classification of Diseases, 10th Revision appears in the WHO publication. ICD-10-CM is a clinical modification of the World Health Organizations' International Classification of Diseases, 10th Revision (ICD-10). The term clinical is used to emphasize the modification 's intent: to serve as a useful tool in the area of classification of morbidity data for indexing of medical records, medical care review, and ambulatory and other medical care programs, as well as for basic health statistics. To describe the clinical picture of the patient the codes must be more precise than those needed only for statistical groupings and trend analysis.

Characteristics of ICD-10-CM

ICD-10-CM far exceeds its predecessors in the number of codes provided. The disease classification has been expanded to include health-related conditions and to provide greater specificity at the sixth digit level and with a seventh digit extension. Guidance for the use of this classification can be found in the Official Coding and Reporting guidelines section of ICD-10-CM (www.cdc.gov/nchs/icd9.htm). The ICD-10 is copyrighted by the World Health Organization (WHO) and reproduced by permission for United States Government purposes.

ICD-10-CM Instructional Notes and Conventions

The following appear in the disease tabular list, unless otherwise noted.

ICD-10-CM Conventions

The ICD-10-CM alphabetic index and disease tabular sections have certain abbreviations, punctuation and other conventions. Proper use of the conventions will lead to efficient and accurate coding.

Abbreviations

NEC   Not elsewhere classified

This abbreviation is used when the ICD-10-CM system does not provide a code specific for the patient's condition.

NOS   Not otherwise specified

This abbreviation is the equivalent of 'unspecified' and is used only when the coder lacks the information necessary to code to a more specific subcategory.

Other Conventions

[ ]   Brackets in the tabular section enclose synonyms, alternative terminology or explanatory phrases:

A05.2   Foodborne Clostridium perfringens [Clostridium welchii] intoxication

[ ]   Slanted brackets in the alphabetic index indicate mandatory coding of etiology and manifestation. The codes with in the slanted brackets are called manifestation codes and may never be used alone or as the primary/principal diagnosis (i.e., sequenced first). This convention indicates a mandatory dual coding situation.

Disorder (of) — *see also* Disease
bladder N32.9
in schistosomiasis B65.0 *[N33]*

( )   Parentheses enclose supplementary words that may be present in the narrative description of a disease. They appear in both the tabular list and alphabetic index:

S70.229   Blister (nonthermal), unspecified hip

Febricula (continued) (simple) R50.9

:   Colons are used in Excludes and Includes notes in the tabular list after an incomplete phrase that needs one or more of the terms that follow in order to make it assignable to a given category:

I41   Myocarditis in diseases classified elsewhere
Excludes1:   myocarditis (in):
diphtheritic (A36.81)
gonococcal (A54.83)

Boldface

Boldface type is used for all codes and titles in the tabular list and for all main terms in the alphabetic index to diseases.

Instructional Notes

These notes appear only in the Tabular List of Diseases:

Includes:

An includes note further defines or clarifies the content of the chapter, subchapter, category, subcategory, or subclassification. The includes note in the example below applies only to category K42.

K42   Umbilical hernia
Includes: paraumbilical hernia

Excludes:

There are three types of excludes notes and each is numbered accordingly. Examples and explanations are given below for each type.

Excludes1:

L26   Exfoliative dermatitis
Excludes1:   Ritter's disease (L00)

Conditions following the term "Excludes1" are not classified to the chapter, subchapter, category, subcategory, or specific subclassification code under which it is found. The note also may provide the location of the excluded diagnosis.

Excludes2:

K62   Other diseases of anus and rectum
Excludes2:   fecal incontinence (R15)

Conditions following the term "Excludes2", may be reported additionally, if present, with the chapter, subchapter, category, subcategory, or specific subclassification code under which it is found. The note may also provide the location of the additional diagnosis.

Excludes3:

A41   Other septicemia
Excludes3:   septicemia (due to) (in):
actinomycotic (A42.7)
anthrax (A22.7)
candidal (B37.7)

Conditions following the term "Excludes3" are combination codes and may be more appropriate to report rather than the chapter, subchapter, category, subcategory, or specific subclassification code under which it is found. The note may also provide the location of the combination diagnosis.

Use additional code:

This instruction signals the coder that an additional code should be used if the information is available to provide a more complete picture of that diagnosis.

F94.1   Reactive attachment disorder of childhood
Use additional code to identify any associated failure to thrive or growth retardation

Code first underlying disease:

This instruction is used in those categories not intended for primary/principal tabulation of disease. These codes, called manifestation codes, may never be used alone or indicated as the primary/principal diagnosis (i.e., sequenced first). They must always be preceded by another code. The instruction "Code first underlying disease" is usually followed by the code or codes for the most common underlying disease (etiology). Record the code for the etiology or origin of the disease, and then record the manifestation code in the next position.

N33   Bladder disorders in diseases classified elsewhere
Code first underlying disease, such as:
schistosomiasis (B65.0-B65.9)

Use additional morphology codes:

This instruction signals the coder that an additional code from the Morphology of Neoplasms table should be reported. The morphology code numbers consist of five digits. The first four identify the histological type of neoplasm and the fifth indicates its behavior.

C81   Hodgkin's disease
Use additional morphology codes M9650-M9660 with behavior code /3
The fifth digit behavior codes are:
/0   Benign
/1   Uncertain whether benign or malignant
/2   Carcinoma in situ
Intraepithelial
Noninfiltrating
Noninvasive
/3   Malignant, primary site
/6   Malignant, metastatic site
Secondary site
/9   Malignant, uncertain whether primary or metastatic site

©2002 Ingenix, Inc.

A

Aarskog's syndrome Q87.1

Abandonment — *see* Maltreatment, abandonment

Abasia (-astasia) (hysterical) F44.4

Abderhalden-Kaufmann-Lignac syndrome (cystinosis) E72.04

Abdomen, abdominal — *see also* condition
  acute R10.0
  angina K55.1
  convulsive equivalent — *see* Epilepsy, specified NEC
  muscle deficiency syndrome Q79.4

Abdominalgia — *see* Pain, abdominal

Abduction contracture, hip or other joint — *see* Contraction, joint

Aberrant (congenital) — *see also* Malposition, congenital
  adrenal gland Q89.1
  artery (peripheral) Q27.8
    basilar NEC Q28.1
    cerebral Q28.3
    coronary Q24.5
    digestive system Q27.8
    eye Q15.8
    lower limb Q27.8
    precerebral Q28.1
    pulmonary Q25.7
    renal Q27.2
    retina Q14.1
    specified site NEC Q27.8
    subclavian Q27.8
    upper limb Q27.8
    vertebral Q28.1
  breast Q83.8
  endocrine gland NEC Q89.2
  hepatic duct Q44.5
  pancreas Q45.3
  parathyroid gland Q89.2
  pituitary gland Q89.2
  sebaceous glands, mucous membrane, mouth, congenital Q38.6
  spleen Q89.09
  subclavian artery Q27.8
  thymus (gland) Q89.2
  thyroid gland Q89.2
  vein (peripheral) NEC Q27.8
    cerebral Q28.3
    digestive system Q27.8
    lower limb Q27.8
    precerebral Q28.1
    specified site NEC Q27.8
    upper limb Q27.8

Aberration
  distantial — *see* Disturbance, visual
  mental F99

Abetalipoproteinemia E78.6

Abiotrophy R68.8

Ablatio, ablation
  placentae — *see* Disorder, placenta, abruptio
  retinae — *see* Detachment, retina
  uterus Z90.71

Ablepharia, ablepharon Q10.3

Abnormal, abnormality, abnormalities — *see also* Anomaly
  acid-base balance (mixed) E87.4
    fetus — *see* Distress, fetal
  albumin R77.0
  alphafetoprotein R77.2
  alveolar ridge K08.9
  amnion, amniotic fluid O41.90
    first trimester O41.91
    second trimester O41.92
    third trimester O41.93
  anatomical relationship Q89.9
  apertures, congenital, diaphragm Q79.1
  auditory perception H93.299
    bilateral H93.293
    diplacusis — *see* Diplacusis
    hyperacusis — *see* Hyperacusis
    left H93.292
    recruitment — *see* Recruitment, auditory
    right H93.291
    threshold shift — *see* Shift, auditory threshold

Abnormal, abnormality, abnormalities — *see also* Anomaly — *continued*
  autosomes Q99.9
    fragile site Q95.5
  basal metabolic rate R94.8
  biosynthesis, testicular androgen E29.1
  blood-gas level R79.81
  blood level (of)
    cobalt R79.0
    copper R79.0
    iron R79.0
    lithium R78.89
    magnesium R79.0
    mineral NEC R79.0
    zinc R79.0
  blood pressure
    elevated R03.0
    low reading (nonspecific) R03.1
  bowel sounds R19.15
    absent R19.11
    hyperactive R19.12
  breathing R06.9
  caloric test R94.1
  cerebrospinal fluid R83.9
    cytology R83.6
    drug level R83.2
    enzyme level R83.0
    histology R83.7
    immunology R83.4
    microbiology R83.5
    nonmedicinal level R83.3
    specified type NEC R83.8
  cervix (acquired) (congenital), in pregnancy or childbirth — *see* category O34.4
    causing obstructed labor O65.5
  chemistry, blood R79.9
    drugs — *see* Findings, abnormal, in blood
    gas level R79.81
    minerals R79.0
    pancytopenia R79.1
    specified NEC R79.89
    PTT R79.2
    toxins — *see* Findings, abnormal, in blood
  chest sounds (friction) (rales) R09.89
  chorion O41.90
    first trimester O41.91
    second trimester O41.92
    third trimester O41.93
  chromosome, chromosomal Q99.9
    with more than three X chromosomes, female Q97.1
    analysis result R89.8
      bronchial washings R84.8
      cerebrospinal fluid R83.8
      cervix uteri R87.8
      nasal secretions R84.8
      nipple discharge R89.8
      peritoneal fluid R85.8
      pleural fluid R84.8
      prostatic secretions R86.8
      saliva R85.8
      seminal fluid R86.8
      sputum R84.8
      synovial fluid R89.8
      throat scrapings R84.8
      vagina R87.8
      vulva R87.8
      wound secretions R89.8
    dicentric replacement Q93.2
    fetal (suspected), affecting management of pregnancy O35.1
    ring replacement Q93.2
    sex Q99.8
      female phenotype Q97.9
        specified NEC Q97.8
      male phenotype Q98.9
        specified NEC Q98.8
      structural male Q98.6
    specified NEC Q99.8
  clinical findings NEC R68.8
  coagulation D68.9
    newborn, transient P61.6
  communication — *see* Fistula
  conjunctiva, vascular H11.419
    bilateral H11.413
    left H11.412
    right H11.411

Abnormal, abnormality, abnormalities — *see also* Anomaly — *continued*
  coronary artery Q24.5
  cortisol-binding globulin E27.8
  course, eustachian tube Q17.8
  dark adaptation curve H53.61
  dentofacial NEC — *see* Anomaly, dentofacial
  development, developmental Q89.9
    central nervous system Q07.9
  diagnostic imaging
    abdomen, abdominal region NEC R93.5
    biliary tract R93.2
    breast R92.8
    central nervous system NEC R90.8
    cerebrovascular R90.8
    coronary circulation R93.1
    digestive tract NEC R93.3
    gastrointestinal (tract) R93.3
    genitourinary organs R93.8
    head R93.0
    heart R93.1
    intrathoracic organ NEC R93.8
    limbs R93.6
    liver R93.2
    lung (field) R91
    musculoskeletal system NEC R93.7
    retroperitoneum R93.5
    sites specified NEC R93.8
    skin and subcutaneous tissue R93.8
    skull R93.0
    urinary organs R93.4
  direction, teeth M26.3
  ear ossicles, acquired NEC H74.399
    ankylosis — *see* Ankylosis, ear ossicles
    bilateral H74.393
    discontinuity — *see* Discontinuity, ossicles, ear
    left H74.392
    partial loss — *see* Loss, ossicles, ear (partial)
    right H74.391
  Ebstein Q22.5
  echocardiogram R93.1
  echoencephalogram R90.8
  echogram — *see* Abnormal, diagnostic imaging
  electrocardiogram (ECG) (EKG) R94.3
  electroencephalogram (EEG) R94.0
  electrolyte — *see* Imbalance, electrolyte
  electromyogram (EMG) R94.1
  electro-oculogram (EOG) R94.1
  electrophysiological intracardiac studies R94.3
  electroretinogram (ERG) R94.1
  erythrocytes
    congenital, with perinatal jaundice D58.9
  feces (color) (contents) (mucus) R19.5
  fetus, fetal
    acid-base balance, complicating labor and delivery O68
    affecting management of pregnancy O35.9
    causing disproportion O33.7
      with obstructed labor O66.3
    heart rate — *see* Distress, fetal
  finding
    antenatal screening, mother O28.9
      biochemical NEC O28.1
      chromosomal NEC O28.5
      cytological NEC O28.2
      genetic NEC O28.5
      hematological NEC O28.0
      radiological NEC O28.4
      specified NEC O28.8
    specimen — *see* Abnormal, specimen
    ultrasonic NEC O28.3
  fluid
    amniotic — *see* Abnormal, specimen, specified
    cerebrospinal — *see* Abnormal, cerebrospinal fluid
    peritoneal — *see* Abnormal, specimen, digestive organs
    pleural — *see* Abnormal, specimen, respiratory organs
    synovial — *see* Abnormal, specimen, specified
    thorax (bronchial washings) (pleural fluid) — *see* Abnormal, specimen, respiratory organs

Abnormal, abnormality, abnormalities — *see also* Anomaly — *continued*
- fluid — *continued*
  - vaginal — *see* Abnormal, specimen, female genital organs
- forces of labor O62.9
  - specified type NEC O62.8
- form
  - teeth K00.2
  - uterus — *see* Anomaly, uterus
- function studies
  - bladder R94.8
  - brain R94.0
  - cardiovascular R94.3
  - endocrine NEC R94.7
  - kidney R94.4
  - liver R94.5
  - nervous system
    - central R94.0
    - peripheral R94.1
  - pancreas R94.8
  - placenta R94.8
  - pulmonary R94.2
  - special senses R94.1
  - spleen R94.8
  - thyroid R94.6
- gait — *see* Gait
  - hysterical F44.4
- gastrin secretion E16.4
- globulin R77.1
  - cortisol-binding E27.8
  - thyroid-binding E07.89
- glomerular, minor — *see* N00-N07 with fourth character .0
- glucagon secretion E16.3
- glucose tolerance (test) R73.0
- gravitational (G) forces or states (effect of) T75.81
- hair (color) (shaft) L67.9
  - specified NEC L67.8
- hard tissue formation in pulp (dental) K04.3
- head movement R25.0
- heart
  - rate R00.9
    - fetus — *see* Distress, fetal
  - shadow R93.1
  - sounds NEC R01.2
- hemoglobin (disease) (*see also* Disease, hemoglobin) D58.2
  - trait — *see* Trait, hemoglobin, abnormal
- histology NEC R89.7
- immunological findings R89.4
  - in serum R76.9
    - specified NEC R76.89
- increase in appetite R63.2
- involuntary movement — *see* Abnormal, movement, involuntary
- jaw closure M26.5
- karyotype R89.8
- knee jerk R29.2
- labor NEC O62.9
- leukocyte (cell) (differential) NEC R72.8
- loss of
  - height R29.890
  - weight R63.4
- mammogram R92.8
  - microcalcification R92.0
- Mantoux test R76.1
- membranes (fetal) complicating pregnancy O41.90
  - first trimester O41.91
  - second trimester O41.92
  - third trimester O41.93
- movement (disorder) — *see also* Disorder, movement
  - head R25.0
  - involuntary R25.9
    - fasciculation R25.3
    - of head R25.0
    - spasm R25.2
    - specified type NEC R25.8
    - tremor R25.1
- myoglobin (Aberdeen) (Annapolis) R89.7
- organs or tissues of pelvis NOS in pregnancy or childbirth O34.90
  - causing obstructed labor O65.5
  - first trimester O34.91

Abnormal, abnormality, abnormalities — *see also* Anomaly — *continued*
- organs or tissues of pelvis NOS in pregnancy or childbirth — *continued*
  - second trimester O34.92
  - third trimester O34.93
- palmar creases Q82.8
- Papanicolaou (smear)
  - bronchial washings R84.6
  - cerebrospinal fluid R83.6
  - cervix R87.6
  - nasal secretions R84.6
  - nipple discharge R89.6
  - peritoneal fluid R85.6
  - pleural fluid R84.6
  - prostatic secretions R86.6
  - saliva R85.6
  - seminal fluid R86.6
  - sites NEC R89.6
  - sputum R84.6
  - synovial fluid R89.6
  - throat scrapings R84.6
  - vagina R87.6
  - vulva R87.6
  - wound secretions R89.6
- parturition — *see* Delivery, complicated
- plantar reflex R29.2
- pelvis (bony) — *see* Deformity, pelvis
- percussion, chest (tympany) R09.89
- perineum in pregnancy and childbirth — *see* Abnormal, vulva in pregnancy and childbirth
- periods (grossly) — *see* Menstruation
- phonocardiogram R94.3
- placenta NOS O43.109
  - circumvallate O43.119
    - first trimester O43.111
    - second trimester O43.112
    - third trimester O43.113
  - first trimester O43.101
  - second trimester O43.102
  - specified type NEC O43.199
    - first trimester O43.191
    - second trimester O43.192
    - third trimester O43.193
  - third trimester O43.103
  - velamentous cord insertion O43.129
    - first trimester O43.121
    - second trimester O43.122
    - third trimester O43.123
- plasma
  - protein R77.9
    - specified NEC R77.8
  - viscosity R70.1
- pleural (folds) Q34.0
- position — *see* Malposition
- posture R29.3
- presentation (fetus) — *see* Presentation, fetal, abnormal
- product of conception O02.9
  - specified type NEC O02.8
- pulmonary
  - artery, congenital Q25.7
  - function, newborn P28.8
  - test results R94.2
  - ventilation, newborn P28.8
- pulsations in neck R00.2
- pupillary H21.569
  - bilateral H21.563
  - function (reaction) (reflex) — *see* Anomaly, pupil, function
  - left H21.562
  - right H21.561
- radiological examination — *see* Abnormal, diagnostic imaging
- red blood cell(s) (morphology) (volume) R71.8
- reflex — *see* Reflex
- renal function test R94.4
- response to nerve stimulation R94.1
- retinal correspondence H53.31
- rhythm, heart — *see also* Arrhythmia
  - fetus — *see* Distress, fetal
- saliva — *see* Abnormal, specimen, digestive organs
- scan
  - kidney R94.4
  - liver R94.5

Abnormal, abnormality, abnormalities — *see also* Anomaly — *continued*
- scan — *continued*
  - thyroid R94.6
- secretion
  - gastrin E16.4
  - glucagon E16.3
- semen, seminal fluid — *see* Abnormal, specimen, male genital organs
- serum level (of)
  - acid phosphatase R74.8
  - alkaline phosphatase R74.8
  - amylase R74.8
  - enzymes R74.9
    - specified NEC R74.8
  - lipase R74.8
  - triacylglycerol lipase R74.8
- shape
  - gravid uterus — *see* Anomaly, uterus
- sinus venosus Q21.1
- size, tooth, teeth K00.2
- spacing, tooth, teeth M26.3
- specimen
  - cervix uteri — *see* Abnormal, specimen, female genital organs
  - digestive organs (peritoneal fluid) (saliva) R85.9
    - cytology R85.6
    - drug level R85.2
    - enzyme level R85.0
    - histology R85.7
    - hormones R85.1
    - immunology R85.4
    - microbiology R85.5
    - nonmedicinal level R85.3
    - specified type NEC R85.8
  - female genital organs (secretions) (smears) R87.9
    - cytology R87.6
    - drug level R87.2
    - enzyme level R87.0
    - histology R87.7
    - hormones R87.1
    - immunology R87.4
    - microbiology R87.5
    - nonmedicinal level R87.3
    - specified type NEC R87.8
  - male genital organs (prostatic secretions) (semen) R86.9
    - cytology R86.6
    - drug level R86.2
    - enzyme level R86.0
    - histology R86.7
    - hormones R86.1
    - immunology R86.4
    - microbiology R86.5
    - nonmedicinal level R86.3
    - specified type NEC R86.8
  - nipple discharge — *see* Abnormal, specimen, specified
  - respiratory organs (bronchial washings) (nasal secretions) (pleural fluid) (sputum) R84.9
    - cytology R84.6
    - drug level R84.2
    - enzyme level R84.0
    - histology R84.7
    - immunology R84.4
    - microbiology R84.5
    - nonmedicinal level R84.3
    - specified type NEC R84.8
  - specified fluid, organ, system and tissue NOS R89.9
    - cytology R89.6
    - drug level R89.2
    - enzyme level R89.0
    - histology R89.7
    - hormones R89.1
    - immunology R89.4
    - microbiology R89.5
    - nonmedicinal level R89.3
    - specified type NEC R89.8
  - synovial fluid — *see* Abnormal, specimen, specified

©2002 Ingenix, Inc.

Abnormal, abnormality, abnormalities — *see also* Anomaly — *continued*
  specimen — *continued*
    thorax (bronchial washings) (pleural fluids) — *see* Abnormal, specimen, respiratory organs
    vagina (secretion) (smear) — *see* Abnormal, specimen, female genital organs
    vulva (secretion) (smear) — *see* Abnormal, specimen, female genital organs
    wound secretion — *see* Abnormal, specimen, specified
    spermatozoa — *see* Abnormal, specimen, male genital organs
  sputum (amount) (color) (odor) R09.3
  stool (color) (contents) (mucus) R19.5
    bloody K92.1
  synchondrosis Q78.8
  thermography — *see* Abnormal, diagnostic imaging
  thyroid-binding globulin E07.89
  tooth, teeth (form) (size) K00.2
  toxicology (findings) R78.9
  transport protein E88.09
  ultrasound results — *see* Abnormal, diagnostic imaging
  umbilical cord complicating delivery O69.9
  urination NEC R39.19
  urine (constituents) R82.90
    bile R82.2
    cytological examination R82.8
    drugs R82.5
    fat R82.0
    glucose R81
    heavy metals R82.6
    hemoglobin R82.3
    histological examination R82.8
    ketones R82.4
    microbiological examination (culture) R82.7
    myoglobin R82.1
    positive culture R82.7
    protein — *see* Proteinuria
    specified substance NEC R82.99
      chromoabnormality NEC R82.91
    substances nonmedical R82.6
  uterine hemorrhage — *see* Hemorrhage, uterus
  uterus (acquired) (congenital) in pregnancy or childbirth — *see* category O34.5
    causing obstructed labor O65.5
  vagina (acquired) (congenital) in pregnancy or childbirth — *see* category O34.6
    causing obstructed labor O65.5
  vectorcardiogram R94.3
  visually evoked potential (VEP) R94.1
  vulva (acquired) (congenital) in pregnancy or childbirth — *see* category O34.7
    causing obstructed labor O65.5
  white blood cells NEC R72.8
  weight
    gain R63.5
    loss R63.4
  X-ray examination — *see* Abnormal, diagnostic imaging

Abnormity (any organ or part) — *see* Anomaly

Abocclusion M26.2

ABO
  hemolytic disease (fetus or newborn) P55.1
  incompatibility reaction T80.3

Abolition, language R48.8

Aborter, habitual or recurrent
  without current pregnancy N96
  care in current pregnancy O26.20
    first trimester O26.21
    second trimester O26.22
    third trimester O26.23
  current abortion — *see* categories O03-O06

Abortion (complete) O03.9
  with retained products of conception — *see* Abortion, incomplete
  accidental — *see* Abortion, spontaneous
  attempted (by non-physician) (failed) (induced) O07.9
    by physician O07.4
      complicated (by) O07.30
        afibrinogenemia O07.1
        cardiac arrest O07.39

Abortion — *continued*
  attempted — *continued*
    by physician — *continued*
      complicated (by) — *continued*
        chemical damage of pelvic organ(s) O07.39
        circulatory collapse O07.39
        defibrination syndrome O07.1
        electrolyte imbalance O07.39
        embolism (amniotic fluid) (blood clot) (pulmonary) (septic) O07.2
        endometritis O07.0
        genital tract and pelvic infection O07.0
        hemorrhage (delayed) (excessive) O07.1
        infection
          genital tract or pelvic O07.0
          urinary tract O07.39
        intravascular coagulation O07.1
        laceration of pelvic organ(s) O07.39
        metabolic disorder O07.39
        oliguria O07.39
        oophoritis O07.0
        parametritis O07.0
        pelvic peritonitis O07.0
        perforation of pelvic organ(s) O07.39
        renal failure or shutdown O07.39
        salpingitis or salpingo-oophoritis O07.0
        sepsis O07.0
        septic shock O07.0
        septicemia O07.0
        shock O07.39
          septic O07.0
        specified condition NEC O07.39
        tubular necrosis (renal) O07.39
        uremia O07.39
        urinary infection O07.39
        venous complication NEC O07.39
          embolism O07.2
  complicated (by) O07.80
    afibrinogenemia O07.6
    cardiac arrest O07.89
    chemical damage of pelvic organ(s) O07.89
    circulatory collapse O07.89
    defibrination syndrome O07.6
    electrolyte imbalance O07.89
    embolism (amniotic fluid) (blood clot) (pulmonary) (septic) O07.7
    endometritis O07.5
    genital tract and pelvic infection O07.5
    hemorrhage (delayed) (excessive) O07.6
    infection
      genital tract or pelvic O07.5
      urinary tract O07.89
    intravascular coagulation O07.6
    laceration of pelvic organ(s) O07.89
    metabolic disorder O07.89
    oliguria O07.89
    oophoritis O07.5
    parametritis O07.5
    pelvic peritonitis O07.5
    perforation of pelvic organ(s) O07.89
    renal failure or shutdown O07.89
    salpingitis or salpingo-oophoritis O07.5
    sepsis O07.5
    septic shock O07.5
    septicemia O07.5
    shock O07.89
      septic O07.5
    specified condition NEC O07.89
    tubular necrosis (renal) O07.89
    uremia O07.89
    urinary infection O07.89
    venous complication NEC O07.89
      embolism O07.7
  complicated (by) O03.80
    afibrinogenemia O03.6
    cardiac arrest O03.89
    chemical damage of pelvic organ(s) O03.89
    circulatory collapse O03.89
    defibrination syndrome O03.6
    electrolyte imbalance O03.89
    embolism (amniotic fluid) (blood clot) (pulmonary) (septic) O03.7

Abortion — *continued*
  complicated (by) — *continued*
    endometritis O03.5
    genital tract and pelvic infection O03.5
    hemorrhage (delayed) (excessive) O03.6
    infection
      genital tract or pelvic O03.5
      urinary tract O03.89
    intravascular coagulation O03.6
    laceration of pelvic organ(s) O03.89
    metabolic disorder O03.89
    oliguria O03.89
    oophoritis O03.5
    parametritis O03.5
    pelvic peritonitis O03.5
    perforation of pelvic organ(s) O03.89
    renal failure or shutdown O03.89
    salpingitis or salpingo-oophoritis O03.5
    sepsis O03.5
    septic shock O03.5
    septicemia O03.5
    shock O03.89
      septic O03.5
    specified condition NEC O03.89
    tubular necrosis (renal) O03.89
    uremia O03.89
    urinary infection O03.89
    venous complication NEC O03.89
      embolism O03.7
  failed — *see* Abortion, attempted
  fetus or newborn P96.8
  following threatened abortion –*see* Abortion, spontaneous
  habitual or recurrent N96
    with current abortion — *see* categories O03-O06
    without current pregnancy N96
    care in current pregnancy O26.20
      first trimester O26.21
      second trimester O26.22
      third trimester O26.23
  incomplete — *see also* Abortion, attempted
    spontaneous O03.4
      complicated (by) O03.30
        afibrinogenemia O03.1
        cardiac arrest O03.39
        chemical damage of pelvic organ(s) O03.39
        circulatory collapse O03.39
        defibrination syndrome O03.1
        electrolyte imbalance O03.39
        embolism (amniotic fluid) (blood clot) (pulmonary) (septic) O03.2
        endometritis O03.0
        genital tract and pelvic infection O03.0
        hemorrhage (delayed) (excessive) O03.1
        infection
          genital tract or pelvic O03.0
          urinary tract O03.39
        intravascular coagulation O03.1
        laceration of pelvic organ(s) O03.39
        metabolic disorder O03.39
        oliguria O03.39
        oophoritis O03.0
        parametritis O03.0
        pelvic peritonitis O03.0
        perforation of pelvic organ(s) O03.39
        renal failure or shutdown O03.39
        salpingitis or salpingo-oophoritis O03.0
        sepsis O03.0
        septic shock O03.0
        septicemia O03.0
        shock O03.39
          septic O03.0
        specified condition NEC O03.39
        tubular necrosis (renal) O03.39
        uremia O03.39
        urinary infection O03.39
        venous complication NEC O03.39
          embolism O03.2
  induced (by)
    non-physician
      complicated (by) O05.80
        afibrinogenemia O05.6
        cardiac arrest O05.89

Abortion — *continued*
  induced (by) — *continued*
    non-physician — *continued*
      complicated (by) — *continued*
        chemical damage of pelvic organ(s) O05.89
        circulatory collapse O05.89
        defibrination syndrome O05.6
        electrolyte imbalance O05.89
        embolism (amniotic fluid) (blood clot) (pulmonary) (septic) O05.7
        endometritis O05.5
        genital tract and pelvic infection O05.5
        hemorrhage (delayed) (excessive) O05.6
        infection
          genital tract or pelvic O05.5
          urinary tract O05.89
        intravascular coagulation O05.6
        laceration of pelvic organ(s) O05.89
        metabolic disorder O05.89
        oliguria O05.89
        oophoritis O05.5
        parametritis O05.5
        pelvic peritonitis O05.5
        perforation of pelvic organ(s) O05.89
        renal failure or shutdown O05.89
        salpingitis or salpingo-oophoritis O05.5
        sepsis O05.5
        septic shock O05.5
        septicemia O05.5
        shock O05.89
          septic O05.5
        specified condition NEC O05.89
        tubular necrosis (renal) O05.89
        uremia O05.89
        urinary infection O05.89
        venous complication NEC O05.89
          embolism O05.7
    uncomplicated Z33.1
    physician
      complicated (by) O04.80
        afibrinogenemia O04.6
        cardiac arrest O04.89
        chemical damage of pelvic organ(s) O04.89
        circulatory collapse O04.89
        defibrination syndrome O04.6
        electrolyte imbalance O04.89
        embolism (amniotic fluid) (blood clot) (pulmonary) (septic) O04.7
        endometritis O04.5
        genital tract and pelvic infection O04.5
        hemorrhage (delayed) (excessive) O04.6
        infection
          genital tract or pelvic O04.5
          urinary tract O04.89
        intravascular coagulation O04.6
        laceration of pelvic organ(s) O04.89
        metabolic disorder O04.89
        oliguria O04.89
        oophoritis O04.5
        parametritis O04.5
        pelvic peritonitis O04.5
        perforation of pelvic organ(s) O04.89
        renal failure or shutdown O04.89
        salpingitis or salpingo-oophoritis O04.5
        sepsis O04.5
        septic shock O04.5
        septicemia O04.5
        shock O04.89
          septic O04.5
        specified condition NEC O04.89
        tubular necrosis (renal) O04.89
        uremia O04.89
        urinary infection O04.89
        venous complication NEC O04.89
          embolism O04.7
      uncomplicated Z33.2
      complicated (by) O06.80
        afibrinogenemia O06.6
        cardiac arrest O06.89
        chemical damage of pelvic organ(s) O06.89
        circulatory collapse O06.89

Abortion — *continued*
  induced (by) — *continued*
    physician — *continued*
      defibrination syndrome O06.6
      electrolyte imbalance O06.89
      embolism (amniotic fluid) (blood clot) (pulmonary) (septic) O06.7
      endometritis O06.5
      genital tract and pelvic infection O06.5
      hemorrhage (delayed) (excessive) O06.6
      infection
        genital tract or pelvic O06.5
        urinary tract O06.89
      intravascular coagulation O06.6
      laceration of pelvic organ(s) O06.89
      metabolic disorder O06.89
      oliguria O06.89
      oophoritis O06.5
      parametritis O06.5
      pelvic peritonitis O06.5
      perforation of pelvic organ(s) O06.89
      renal failure or shutdown O06.89
      salpingitis or salpingo-oophoritis O06.5
      sepsis O06.5
      septic shock O06.5
      septicemia O06.5
      shock O06.89
        septic O06.5
      specified condition NEC O06.89
      tubular necrosis (renal) O06.89
      uremia O06.89
      urinary infection O06.89
      venous complication NEC O06.89
        embolism O06.7
    fetus P96.8
    uncomplicated Z33.2
  missed O02.1
  operative — *see* Abortion, induced (by), physician
  self-induced — *see* Abortion, induced (by), non-physician
  spontaneous (complete) O03.9
    complicated (by) O03.80
      afibrinogenemia O03.6
      cardiac arrest O03.89
      chemical damage of pelvic organ(s) O03.89
      circulatory collapse O03.89
      defibrination syndrome O03.6
      electrolyte imbalance O03.89
      embolism (amniotic fluid) (blood clot) (pulmonary) (septic) O03.7
      endometritis O03.5
      genital tract and pelvic infection O03.5
      hemorrhage (delayed) (excessive) O03.6
      infection
        genital tract or pelvic O03.5
        urinary tract O03.89
      intravascular coagulation O03.6
      laceration of pelvic organ(s) O03.89
      metabolic disorder O03.89
      oliguria O03.89
      oophoritis O03.5
      parametritis O03.5
      pelvic peritonitis O03.5
      perforation of pelvic organ(s) O03.89
      renal failure or shutdown O03.89
      salpingitis or salpingo-oophoritis O03.5
      sepsis O03.5
      septic shock O03.5
      septicemia O03.5
      shock O03.89
        septic O03.5
      specified condition NEC O03.89
      tubular necrosis (renal) O03.89
      uremia O03.89
      urinary infection O03.89
      venous complication NEC O03.89
        embolism O03.7
    incomplete O03.4
      complicated (by) O03.30
        afibrinogenemia O03.1
        cardiac arrest O03.39
        chemical damage of pelvic organ(s) O03.39
        circulatory collapse O03.39

Abortion — *continued*
  spontaneous — *continued*
    incomplete — *continued*
      complicated (by) — *continued*
        defibrination syndrome O03.1
        electrolyte imbalance O03.39
        embolism (amniotic fluid) (blood clot) (pulmonary) (septic) O03.2
        endometritis O03.0
        genital tract and pelvic infection O03.0
        hemorrhage (delayed) (excessive) O03.1
        infection
          genital tract or pelvic O03.0
          urinary tract O03.39
        intravascular coagulation O03.1
        laceration of pelvic organ(s) O03.39
        metabolic disorder O03.39
        oliguria O03.39
        oophoritis O03.0
        parametritis O03.0
        pelvic peritonitis O03.0
        perforation of pelvic organ(s) O03.39
        renal failure or shutdown O03.39
        salpingitis or salpingo-oophoritis O03.0
        sepsis O03.0
        septic shock O03.0
        septicemia O03.0
        shock O03.39
          septic O03.0
        specified condition NEC O03.39
        tubular necrosis (renal) O03.39
        uremia O03.39
        urinary infection O03.39
        venous complication NEC O03.39
          embolism O03.2
      threatened O20.0
    therapeutic — *see* Abortion, induced (by), physician
    fetus P96.8
    threatened (spontaneous) O20.0
    tubal O00.1
Abortus fever A23.9
Aboulomania F60.7
Abrami's disease D59.8
Abramov-Fiedler myocarditis (acute isolated myocarditis) I40.1
Abrasion
  abdomen, abdominal (wall) S30.811
  alveolar process S00.512
  ankle S90.519
    left S90.512
    right S90.511
  antecubital space — *see* Abrasion, elbow
  anus S30.817
  arm (upper) S40.819
    left S40.812
    right S40.811
  auditory canal — *see* Abrasion, ear
  auricle — *see* Abrasion, ear
  axilla — *see* Abrasion, arm
  back, lower S30.810
  breast S20.119
    left S20.112
    right S20.111
  brow S00.81
  buttock S30.810
  calf — *see* Abrasion, leg
  canthus — *see* Abrasion, eyelid
  cheek S00.81
    internal S00.512
  chest wall — *see* Abrasion, thorax
  chin S00.81
  clitoris S30.814
  cornea S05.00
    left S05.02
    right S05.01
  costal region — *see* Abrasion, thorax
  dental K03.1
  digit(s)
    foot — *see* Abrasion, toe
    hand — *see* Abrasion, finger
  ear S00.419
    left S00.412
    right S00.411

©2002 Ingenix, Inc.

Abrasion — *continued*
  elbow S50.319
    left S50.312
    right S50.311
  epididymis S30.813
  epigastric region S30.811
  epiglottis S10.11
  esophagus (thoracic) S27.818
    cervical S10.11
  eyebrow — *see* Abrasion, eyelid
  eyelid S00.219
    left S00.212
    right S00.211
  face S00.81
  finger(s) S60.419
    index S60.418
      left S60.411
      right S60.410
    little S60.418
      left S60.417
      right S60.416
    middle S60.418
      left S60.413
      right S60.412
    ring S60.418
      left S60.415
      right S60.414
  flank S30.811
  foot (except toe(s) alone) S90.819
    left S90.812
    right S90.811
    toe — *see* Abrasion, toe
  forearm S50.819
    elbow only — *see* Abrasion, elbow
    left S50.812
    right S50.811
  forehead S00.81
  genital organs, external
    female S30.816
    male S30.815
  groin S30.811
  gum S00.512
  hand S60.519
    left S60.512
    right S60.511
  head S00.91
    ear — *see* Abrasion, ear
    eyelid — *see* Abrasion, eyelid
    lip S00.511
    nose S00.31
    oral cavity S00.512
    scalp S00.01
    specified site NEC S00.81
  heel — *see* Abrasion, foot
  hip S70.219
    left S70.212
    right S70.211
  inguinal region S30.811
  interscapular region S20.419
  jaw S00.81
  knee S80.219
    left S80.212
    right S80.211
  labium (majus) (minus) S30.814
  larynx S10.11
  leg (lower) S80.819
    knee — *see* Abrasion, knee
    left S80.812
    right S80.811
    upper — *see* Abrasion, thigh
  lip S00.511
  lower back S30.810
  lumbar region S30.810
  malar region S00.81
  mammary — *see* Abrasion, breast
  mastoid region S00.81
  mouth S00.512
  nail
    finger — *see* Abrasion, finger
    toe — *see* Abrasion, toe
  nape S10.81
  nasal S00.31
  neck S10.91
    specified site NEC S10.81
    throat S10.11
  nose S00.31
  occipital region S00.01

Abrasion — *continued*
  oral cavity S00.512
  orbital region — *see* Abrasion, eyelid
  palate S00.512
  palm — *see* Abrasion, hand
  parietal region S00.01
  pelvis S30.810
  penis S30.812
  perineum
    female S30.814
    male S30.810
  periocular area — *see* Abrasion, eyelid
  phalanges
    finger — *see* Abrasion, finger
    toe — *see* Abrasion, toe
  pharynx S10.11
  pinna — *see* Abrasion, ear
  popliteal space — *see* Abrasion, knee
  prepuce S30.812
  pubic region S30.810
  pudendum
    female S30.816
    male S30.815
  sacral region S30.810
  scalp S00.01
  scapular region — *see* Abrasion, shoulder
  scrotum S30.813
  shin — *see* Abrasion, leg
  shoulder S40.219
    left S40.212
    right S40.211
  sternal region S20.319
  submaxillary region S00.81
  submental region S00.81
  subungual
    finger(s) — *see* Abrasion, finger
    toe(s) — *see* Abrasion, toe
  supraclavicular fossa S10.81
  supraorbital S00.81
  temple S00.81
  temporal region S00.81
  testis S30.813
  thigh S70.319
    left S70.312
    right S70.311
  thorax, thoracic (wall) S20.91
    back S20.419
      left S20.412
      right S20.411
    front S20.319
      left S20.312
      right S20.311
  throat S10.11
  thumb S60.319
    left S60.312
    right S60.311
  toe(s) (lesser) S90.416
    great S90.413
      left S90.412
      right S90.411
    left S90.415
    right S90.414
  tongue S00.512
  tooth, teeth (dentifrice) (habitual) (hard tissues) (occupational) (ritual) (traditional) K03.1
  trachea S10.11
  tunica vaginalis S30.813
  tympanum, tympanic membrane — *see* Abrasion, ear
  uvula S00.512
  vagina S30.814
  vocal cords S10.11
  vulva S30.814
  wrist S60.819
    left S60.812
    right S60.811

Abrism — *see* Poisoning, food, noxious, plant

Abruptio placentae — *see* Disorder, placenta, abruptio

Abruption, placenta — *see* Disorder, placenta, abruptio

Abscess (connective tissue) (embolic) (fistulous) (infective) (metastatic) (multiple) (pernicious) (pyogenic) (septic) L02.91
  with
    diverticular disease (intestine) K57.80
      with bleeding K57.81

Abscess — *continued*
  with — *continued*
    diverticular disease — *continued*
      large intestine K57.20
        with
          bleeding K57.21
          small intestine K57.40
            with bleeding K57.41
      small intestine K57.00
        with
          bleeding K57.01
          large intestine K57.40
            with bleeding K57.41
    lymphangitis – code by site under Abscess
  abdomen, abdominal
    cavity K65.0
    wall L02.211
  abdominopelvic K65.0
  accessory sinus — *see* Sinusitis
  adrenal (capsule) (gland) E27.8
  alveolar K04.7
    with sinus K04.6
  amebic A06.4
    brain (and liver or lung abscess) A06.6
    genitourinary tract A06.82
    liver (without mention of brain or lung abscess) A06.4
    lung (and liver) (without mention of brain abscess) A06.5
    specified site NEC A06.89
    spleen A06.89
  anerobic A48.0
  ankle — *see* Abscess, lower limb
  anorectal K61.2
  antecubital space — *see* Abscess, upper limb
  antrum (chronic) (Highmore) — *see* Sinusitis, maxillary
  anus K61.0
  apical (tooth) K04.7
    with sinus (alveolar) K04.6
  appendix K35.1
  areola (acute) (chronic) (nonpuerperal) N61
    puerperal, postpartum or gestational — *see* Infection, nipple
  arm (any part) — *see* Abscess, upper limb
  artery (wall) I77.2
  atheromatous I77.2
  auricle, ear — *see* Abscess, ear, external
  axilla (region) L02.419
    left L02.412
    lymph gland or node L04.2
    right L02.411
  back (any part, except buttock) L02.212
  Bartholin's gland N75.1
    with
      abortion — *see* Abortion, by type, complicated by, sepsis
      ectopic or molar pregnancy O08.0
    following ectopic or molar pregnancy O08.0
  Bezold's — *see* Mastoiditis, acute
  bilharziasis B65.1
  bladder (wall) — *see* Cystitis, specified type NEC
  bone (subperiosteal) — *see also* Osteomyelitis, specified type NEC
    accessory sinus (chronic) — *see* Sinusitis
    chronic or old — *see* Osteomyelitis, chronic
    jaw (lower) (upper) M27.2
    mastoid — *see* Mastoiditis, acute, subperiosteal
    petrous — *see* Petrositis
    spinal (tuberculous) A18.01
      nontuberculous — *see* Osteomyelitis, vertebra
  bowel K63.0
  brain (any part) (cystic) (otogenic) G06.0
    amebic (with abscess of any other site) A06.6
    gonococcal A54.82
    pheomycotic (chromomycotic) B43.1
    tuberculous A17.81
  breast (acute) (chronic) (nonpuerperal) N61
    newborn P39.0
    puerperal, postpartum, gestational — *see* Mastitis, obstetric, purulent
  broad ligament N73.2
    acute N73.0

Abscess — *continued*
  broad ligament — *continued*
    chronic N73.1
  Brodie's (localized) (chronic) — *see*
    Osteomyelitis, specified NEC
  bronchi J98.0
  buccal cavity K12.2
  bulbourethral gland N34.0
  bursa M71.00
    ankle M71.079
      left M71.072
      right M71.071
    elbow M71.029
      left M71.022
      right M71.021
    foot M71.079
      left M71.072
      right M71.071
    hand M71.049
      left M71.042
      right M71.041
    hip M71.059
      left M71.052
      right M71.051
    knee M71.069
      left M71.062
      right M71.061
    multiple sites M71.09
    pharyngeal J39.1
    shoulder M71.019
      left M71.012
      right M71.011
    specified site NEC M71.08
    wrist M71.039
      left M71.032
      right M71.031
  buttock L02.31
  canthus — *see* Blepharoconjunctivitis
  cartilage — *see* Disorder, cartilage, specified
    type NEC
  cecum K35.1
  cerebellum, cerebellar G06.0
    sequelae G09
  cerebral (embolic) G06.0
    sequelae G09
  cervical (meaning neck) L02.11
    lymph gland or node L04.0
  cervix (stump) (uteri) — *see* Cervicitis
  cheek (external) L02.01
    inner K12.2
  chest J86.9
    with fistula J86.0
    wall L02.213
  chin L02.01
  choroid — *see* Inflammation, chorioretinal
  circumtonsillar J36
  cold (lung) (tuberculous) — *see also*
    Tuberculosis, abscess, lung
    articular — *see* Tuberculosis, joint
  colon (wall) K63.0
  colostomy K94.02
  conjunctiva — *see* Conjunctivitis, acute
  cornea H16.319
    bilateral H16.313
    left H16.312
    right H16.311
  corpus
    cavernosum N48.21
    luteum — *see* Oophoritis
  Cowper's gland N34.0
  cranium G06.0
  Crohn's disease — *see* Enteritis, regional
  cul-de-sac (Douglas') (posterior) — *see*
    Peritonitis, pelvic, female
  cutaneous — *see* Abscess, by site
  dental K04.7
    with sinus (alveolar) K04.6
  dentoalveolar K04.7
    with sinus K04.6
  diaphragm, diaphragmatic K65.0
  Douglas' cul-de-sac or pouch — *see* Peritonitis,
    pelvic, female
  Dubois A50.59
  ear (middle) — *see also* Otitis, media,
    suppurative
    acute — *see* Otitis, media, suppurative,
      acute

Abscess — *continued*
  ear — *see also* Otitis, media, suppurative —
    continued
    external H60.00
      bilateral H60.03
      left H60.02
      right H60.01
  entamebic — *see* Abscess, amebic
  enterostomy K94.12
  epididymis N45.4
  epidural G06.2
    brain G06.0
    spinal cord G06.1
  epiglottis J38.7
  epiploon, epiploic K65.0
  erysipelatous — *see* Erysipelas
  esophagus K20
  ethmoid (bone) (chronic) (sinus) J32.2
  external auditory canal — *see* Abscess, ear,
    external
  extradural G06.2
    brain G06.0
      sequelae G09
    spinal cord G06.1
  extraperitoneal K65.0
  eye — *see* Endophthalmitis, purulent
  eyelid H00.039
    left H00.036
      lower H00.035
      upper H00.034
    right H00.033
      lower H00.032
      upper H00.031
  face (any part, except ear, eye and nose) L02.01
  fallopian tube — *see* Salpingitis
  fascia M72.52
  fauces J39.1
  fecal K63.0
  femoral (region) — *see* Abscess, lower limb
  filaria, filarial — *see* Infestation, filarial
  finger (any) — *see also* Abscess, hand
    nail — *see* Cellulitis, finger
  foot L02.619
    left L02.612
    right L02.611
  forehead L02.01
  frontal sinus (chronic) J32.1
  gallbladder K81.0
  genital organ or tract
    female (external) N76.4
      following ectopic or molar pregnancy
        O08.0
    male N49.9
      multiple sites N49.8
      specified NEC N49.8
  gingival K05.2
  gland, glandular (lymph) (acute) — *see*
    Lymphadenitis, acute
  gluteal (region) L02.31
  gonorrheal — *see* Gonococcus
  groin L02.214
  gum K05.2
  hand L02.519
    left L02.512
    right L02.511
  head NEC L02.811
    face (any part, except ear, eye and nose)
      L02.01
  heart — *see* Carditis
  heel — *see* Abscess, foot
  helminthic — *see* Infestation, helminth
  hepatic (cholangitic) (hematogenic)
    (lymphogenic) (pylephlebitic) K75.0
    amebic A06.4
  hip (region) — *see* Abscess, lower limb
  ileocecal K35.1
  ileostomy (bud) K94.12
  iliac (region) L02.214
    fossa K35.1
  infraclavicular (fossa) — *see* Abscess, upper
    limb
  inguinal (region) L02.214
    lymph gland or node L04.1
  intestine, intestinal NEC K63.0
    rectal K61.1
  intra-abdominal — *see also* Abscess,
    peritoneum K65.0

Abscess — *continued*
  intra-abdominal — *see also* Abscess,
    peritoneum — *continued*
    postoperative T81.4
    retroperitoneal K68.11
  intracranial G06.0
  intramammary — *see* Abscess, breast
  intraorbital — *see* Abscess, orbit
  intraperitoneal K65.0
  intrasphincteric (anus) K61.4
  intraspinal G06.1
  intratonsillar J36
  ischiorectal (fossa) K61.3
  jaw (bone) (lower) (upper) M27.2
  joint — *see* Arthritis, pyogenic or pyemic
    spine (tuberculous)
      nontuberculous — *see* Spondylopathy,
        infective
  kidney N15.1
    with calculus N20.0
      with hydronephrosis N13.6
    complicating pregnancy O23.00
      first trimester O23.01
      second trimester O23.02
      third trimester O23.03
    puerperal (postpartum) O86.21
  knee — *see also* Abscess, lower limb
    joint M00.9
  labium (majus) (minus) N76.4
    complicating pregnancy O23.50
      first trimester O23.51
      second trimester O23.52
      third trimester O23.53
    puerperal (postpartum) O86.1
  lacrimal
    caruncle — *see* Inflammation, lacrimal,
      passages, acute
    gland — *see* Dacryoadenitis
    passages (duct) (sac) — *see* Inflammation,
      lacrimal, passages, acute
  lacunar N34.0
  larynx J38.7
  lateral (alveolar) K04.7
    with sinus K04.6
  leg (any part) — *see* Abscess, lower limb
  lens H27.8
  lingual K14.0
    tonsil J36
  lip K13.0
  Littre's gland N34.0
  liver (cholangitic) (hematogenic) (lymphogenic)
    (pylephlebitic) (pyogenic) K75.0
    amebic (due to Entamoeba histolytica)
      (dysenteric) (tropical) A06.4
      with
        brain abscess (and liver or lung
          abscess) A06.6
        lung abscess A06.5
  loin (region) L02.211
  lower limb L02.419
    left L02.416
    right L02.415
  lumbar (tuberculous) A18.01
    nontuberculous L02.212
  lung (miliary) (putrid) J85.2
    with pneumonia J85.1
      due to specified organism (*see*
        Pneumonia, in (due to))
    amebic (with liver abscess) A06.5
      with
        brain abscess A06.6
        pneumonia A06.5
  lymph, lymphatic, gland or node (acute) — *see*
    also Lymphadenitis, acute
    mesentery I88.0
  malar M27.2
  mammary gland — *see* Abscess, breast
  marginal, anus K61.0
  mastoid — *see* Mastoiditis, acute
  maxilla, maxillary M27.2
    molar (tooth) K04.7
      with sinus K04.6
    premolar K04.7
    sinus (chronic) J32.0
  mediastinum J85.3
  meibomian gland — *see* Hordeolum
  meninges G06.2

©2002 Ingenix, Inc.

Abscess — *continued*
mesentery, mesenteric K65.0
mesosalpinx — *see* Salpingitis
mons pubis L02.215
mouth (floor) K12.2
muscle — *see* Myositis, infective
myocardium I40.0
nabothian (follicle) — *see* Cervicitis
nasal J32.9
nasopharyngeal J39.1
navel L02.216
  newborn P38
neck (region) L02.11
  lymph gland or node L04.0
nephritic — *see* Abscess, kidney
nipple N61
  associated with
    lactation O91.03
    pregnancy (gestational) O91.019
     first trimester O91.011
     second trimester O91.012
     third trimester O91.013
    puerperium O91.02
nose (external) (fossa) (septum) J34.0
  sinus (chronic) — *see* Sinusitis
omentum K65.0
operative wound T81.4
orbit, orbital — *see* Cellulitis, orbit
otogenic G06.0
ovary, ovarian (corpus luteum) — *see*
  Oophoritis
oviduct — *see* Oophoritis
palate (soft) K12.2
  hard M27.2
palmar (space) — *see* Abscess, hand
pancreas (duct) K85.0
paradontal K05.2
parafrenal N48.21
parametric, parametrium N73.2
  acute N73.0
  chronic N73.1
paranephric N15.1
parapancreatic K85.0
parapharyngeal J39.0
pararectal K61.1
parasinus — *see* Sinusitis
paraumbilical, newborn P38
parauterine (*see also* Disease, pelvis,
  inflammatory) N73.2
paravaginal — *see* Vaginitis
parietal region (scalp) L02.811
parodontal K05.2
parotid (duct) (gland) K11.3
  region K12.2
pectoral (region) L02.213
pelvis, pelvic
  female — *see* Disease, pelvis, inflammatory
  male, peritoneal K65.0
penis N48.21
  gonococcal (accessory gland) (periurethral)
    A54.1
perianal K61.0
periapical K04.7
  with sinus (alveolar) K04.6
periappendicular K35.1
pericardial I30.1
pericecal K35.1
pericemental K05.2
pericholecystic — *see* Cholecystitis, acute
pericoronal K05.2
peridental K05.2
perimetric (*see also* Disease, pelvis,
  inflammatory) N73.2
perinephric, perinephritic — *see* Abscess,
  kidney
perineum, perineal (superficial) L02.215
  urethra N34.0
periodontal (parietal) K05.2
  apical K04.7
periosteum, periosteal — *see also*
  Osteomyelitis, specified type NEC
  with osteomyelitis — *see also* Osteomyelitis,
    specified type NEC
    acute — *see* Osteomyelitis, acute
    chronic — *see* Osteomyelitis, chronic
peripharyngeal J39.0

Abscess — *continued*
peripleuritic J86.9
  with fistula J86.0
periprostatic N41.2
perirectal K61.1
perirenal (tissue) — *see* Abscess, kidney
perisinuous (nose) — *see* Sinusitis
peritoneum, peritoneal (perforated) (ruptured)
  K65.0
  with appendicitis K35.1
  following ectopic or molar pregnancy O08.0
  pelvic
    female — *see* Peritonitis, pelvic, female
    male K65.0
  postoperative T81.4
  puerperal, postpartum, childbirth O85
  tuberculous A18.31
peritonsillar J36
perityphlic K35.1
periureteral N28.89
periurethral N34.0
  gonococcal (accessory gland) (periurethral)
    A54.1
periuterine (*see also* Disease, pelvis,
  inflammatory) N73.2
perivesical — *see* Cystitis, specified type NEC
petrous bone — *see* Petrositis
phagedenic NOS L02.91
  chancroid A57
pharynx, pharyngeal (lateral) J39.1
pilonidal L05.01
pituitary (gland) E23.6
pleura J86.9
  with fistula J86.0
popliteal — *see* Abscess, lower limb
postcecal K35.1
postlaryngeal J38.7
postnasal J34.0
postoperative (any site) T81.4
postpharyngeal J39.0
posttonsillar J36
post-typhoid A01.09
pouch of Douglas — *see* Peritonitis, pelvic,
  female
premammary — *see* Abscess, breast
prepatellar — *see* Abscess, lower limb
prostate N41.2
  gonococcal (acute) (chronic) A54.23
psoas, nontuberculous M60.08
puerperal – code by site under Puerperal,
  abscess
pulmonary — *see* Abscess, lung
pulp, pulpal (dental) K04.0
rectovaginal septum K63.0
rectovesical — *see* Cystitis, specified type NEC
rectum K61.1
renal — *see* Abscess, kidney
retina — *see* Inflammation, chorioretinal
retrobulbar — *see* Abscess, orbit
retrocecal K65.0
retrolaryngeal J38.7
retromammary — *see* Abscess, breast
retroperitoneal K68.19
retropharyngeal J39.0
retrouterine — *see* Peritonitis, pelvic, female
retrovesical — *see* Cystitis, specified type NEC
root, tooth K04.7
  with sinus (alveolar) K04.6
round ligament (*see also* Disease, pelvis,
  inflammatory) N73.2
rupture (spontaneous) NOS L02.91
sacrum (tuberculous) A18.01
  nontuberculous M46.28
salivary (duct) (gland) K11.3
scalp (any part) L02.811
scapular — *see* Osteomyelitis, specified type
  NEC
sclera — *see* Scleritis
scrofulous (tuberculous) A18.2
scrotum N49.2
seminal vesicle N49.0
septal, dental K04.7
  with sinus (alveolar) K04.6
serous — *see* Periostitis
shoulder (region) — *see* Abscess, upper limb
sigmoid K63.0

Abscess — *continued*
sinus (accessory) (chronic) (nasal) — *see also*
  Sinusitis
  intracranial venous (any) G06.0
Skene's duct or gland N34.0
skin — *see* Abscess, by site
specified site NEC L02.818
spermatic cord N49.1
sphenoidal (sinus) (chronic) J32.3
spinal cord (any part) (staphylococcal) G06.1
  tuberculous A17.81
spine (column) (tuberculous) A18.01
  epidural G06.1
  nontuberculous — *see* Osteomyelitis,
    vertebra
spleen D73.3
  amebic A06.89
stitch T81.4
subarachnoid G06.2
  brain G06.0
  spinal cord G06.1
subareolar — *see* Abscess, breast
subcecal K35.1
subcutaneous — *see also* Abscess, by site
  pheomycotic (chromomycotic) B43.2
subdiaphragmatic K65.0
subdural G06.2
  brain G06.0
    sequelae G09
  spinal cord G06.1
subgaleal L02.811
subhepatic K65.0
sublingual K12.2
  gland K11.3
submammary — *see* Abscess, breast
submandibular (region) (space) (triangle) K12.2
  gland K11.3
submaxillary (region) L02.01
  gland K11.3
submental L02.01
  gland K11.3
subperiosteal — *see* Osteomyelitis, specified
  type NEC
subphrenic K65.0
  postoperative T81.4
suburethral N34.0
sudoriparous L75.8
supraclavicular (fossa) — *see* Abscess, upper
  limb
suprapelvic, acute N73.0
suprarenal (capsule) (gland) E27.8
sweat gland L74.8
tear duct — *see* Inflammation, lacrimal,
  passages, acute
temple L02.01
temporal region L02.01
temporosphenoidal G06.0
tendon (sheath) M65.00
  ankle M65.079
    left M65.072
    right M65.071
  foot M65.079
    left M65.072
    right M65.071
  forearm M65.039
    left M65.032
    right M65.031
  hand M65.049
    left M65.042
    right M65.041
  lower leg M65.069
    left M65.062
    right M65.061
  pelvic region M65.059
    left M65.052
    right M65.051
  shoulder region M65.019
    left M65.012
    right M65.011
  specified site NEC M65.08
  thigh M65.059
    left M65.052
    right M65.051
  upper arm M65.029
    left M65.022
    right M65.021

Abscess — continued
testis N45.4
thigh — see Abscess, lower limb
thorax J86.9
    with fistula J86.0
throat J39.1
thumb — see also Abscess, hand
    nail — see Cellulitis, finger
thymus (gland) E32.1
thyroid (gland) E06.0
toe (any) — see also Abscess, foot
    nail — see Cellulitis, toe
tongue (staphylococcal) K14.0
tonsil(s) (lingual) J36
tonsillopharyngeal J36
tooth, teeth (root) K04.7
    with sinus (alveolar) K04.6
    supporting structures NEC K05.2
trachea J39.8
trunk L02.219
    abdominal wall L02.211
    back L02.212
    chest wall L02.213
    groin L02.214
    perineum L02.215
    umbilicus L02.216
tubal — see Salpingitis
tuberculous — see Tuberculosis, abscess
tubo-ovarian — see Salpingo-oophoritis
tunica vaginalis N49.1
umbilicus L02.216
    newborn P38
upper
    limb L02.419
        axilla L02.419
            left L02.412
            right L02.411
        left L02.414
        right L02.413
    respiratory J39.8
urethral (gland) N34.0
urinary N34.0
uterus, uterine (wall) — see also Endometritis
    ligament (see also Disease, pelvis,
        inflammatory) N73.2
    neck — see Cervicitis
uvula K12.2
vagina (wall) — see Vaginitis
vaginorectal — see Vaginitis
vas deferens N49.1
vermiform appendix K35.1
vertebra (column) (tuberculous) A18.01
    nontuberculous — see Osteomyelitis,
        vertebra
vesical — see Cystitis, specified type NEC
vesico-uterine pouch — see Peritonitis, pelvic,
    female
vitreous (humor) — see Endophthalmitis,
    purulent
vocal cord J38.3
von Bezold's — see Mastoiditis, acute
vulva N76.4
    complicating pregnancy O23.50
        first trimester O23.51
        second trimester O23.52
        third trimester O23.53
    puerperal (postpartum) O86.1
vulvovaginal gland N75.1
web space — see Abscess, hand
wound T81.4
wrist — see Abscess, upper limb

Absence (organ or part) (complete or partial)
adrenal (gland) (congenital) Q89.1
    acquired E89.6
albumin in blood E88.09
alimentary tract (congenital) Q45.8
    upper Q40.8
alveolar process (acquired) — see Anomaly,
    alveolar
ankle (acquired) Z89.449
    left Z89.442
    right Z89.441
anus (congenital) Q42.3
    with fistula Q42.2
aorta (congenital) Q25.4
appendix, congenital Q42.8

Absence — continued
arm (acquired) Z89.209
    above elbow Z89.229
        congenital (with hand present) — see
            Agenesis, arm, with hand present
            and hand — see Agenesis, forearm,
                and hand
        left Z89.222
        right Z89.221
    below elbow Z89.219
        congenital (with hand present) — see
            Agenesis, arm, with hand present
            and hand — see Agenesis, forearm,
                and hand
        left Z89.212
        right Z89.211
    congenital — see Defect, reduction, upper
        limb
    left Z89.202
    right Z89.201
    shoulder Z89.239
        congenital (with hand present) — see
            Agenesis, arm, with hand present
        left Z89.232
        right Z89.231
artery (congenital) (peripheral) Q27.8
    brain Q28.3
    coronary Q24.5
    pulmonary Q25.7
    specified NEC Q27.8
    umbilical Q27.0
atrial septum (congenital) Q21.1
auditory canal (congenital) (external) Q16.1
auricle (ear), congenital Q16.0
bile, biliary duct, congenital Q44.5
bladder (acquired) Z90.6
    congenital Q64.5
bowel sounds R19.11
brain Q00.0
    part of Q04.3
breast(s) (acquired) Z90.1
    congenital Q83.8
broad ligament Q50.6
bronchus (congenital) Q32.8
canaliculus lacrimalis, congenital Q10.4
cerebellum (vermis) Q04.3
cervix (acquired) Z90.71
    congenital Q51.5
chin, congenital Q18.8
cilia (congenital) Q10.3
    acquired — see Madarosis
clitoris (congenital) Q52.6
coccyx, congenital Q76.49
cold sense R20.8
congenital
    lumen — see Atresia
    organ or site NEC — see Agenesis
    septum — see Imperfect, closure
corpus callosum Q04.0
cricoid cartilage, congenital Q31.8
diaphragm (with hernia), congenital Q79.1
digestive organ(s) or tract, congenital Q45.8
    acquired NEC Z90.4
    upper Q40.8
ductus arteriosus Q28.8
duodenum (acquired) Z90.4
    congenital Q41.0
ear, congenital Q16.9
    acquired — see category H93.8
    auricle Q16.0
    external Q16.0
    inner Q16.5
    lobe, lobule Q17.8
    middle, except ossicles Q16.4
        ossicles Q16.3
    ossicles Q16.3
ejaculatory duct (congenital) Q55.4
endocrine gland (congenital) NEC Q89.2
    acquired E89.9
epididymis (congenital) Q55.4
    acquired Z90.79
epiglottis, congenital Q31.8
epileptic NEC — see Epilepsy, petit mal
erythropoiesis, congenital D61.4
esophagus (congenital) Q39.8
extremity (partial) Z90.4
eustachian tube (congenital) Q16.2

Absence — continued
extremity (acquired) Z89.9
    congenital Q73.0
    lower (above knee) Z89.619
        below knee Z89.50
            left Z89.52
            right Z89.51
        left Z89.612
        right Z89.611
    upper — see Absence, arm
eye (acquired) Z90.01
    congenital Q11.1
    muscle (congenital) Q10.3
eyeball (acquired) Z90.01
eyelid (fold) (congenital) Q10.3
    acquired Z90.01
face, specified part NEC Q18.8
fallopian tube(s) (acquired) Z90.79
    congenital Q50.6
family member (causing problem in home)
    Z63.3
femur, congenital — see Defect, reduction,
    lower limb, longitudinal, femur
fibrinogen (congenital) D68.2
    acquired D65
finger(s) (acquired) Z89.029
    congenital — see Agenesis, hand
    left Z89.022
    right Z89.021
foot (acquired) Z89.439
    congenital — see Agenesis, foot
    left Z89.432
    right Z89.431
forearm (acquired) — see Absence, arm, below
    elbow
gallbladder (acquired) Z90.4
    congenital Q44.0
gamma globulin in blood D80.1
    hereditary D80.0
genital organs
    acquired (female) (male) Z90.79
    female, congenital Q52.8
        external Q52.71
        internal NEC Q52.8
    male, congenital Q55.8
genitourinary organs, congenital NEC
    female Q52.8
    male Q55.8
globe (acquired) Z90.01
    congenital Q11.1
glottis, congenital Q31.8
hand and wrist (acquired) Z89.119
    congenital — see Agenesis, hand
    left Z89.112
    right Z89.111
head, part (acquired) NEC Z90.09
heat sense R20.8
hip Z89.629
    left Z89.622
    right Z89.621
hymen (congenital) Q52.4
ileum (acquired) Z90.4
    congenital Q41.2
immunoglobulin, isolated NEC D80.3
    IgA D80.2
    IgG D80.3
    IgM D80.4
incus (acquired) — see Loss, ossicles, ear
    congenital Q16.3
inner ear, congenital Q16.5
intestine (acquired) (small) Z90.4
    congenital Q41.9
        specified NEC Q41.8
    large Z90.4
        congenital Q42.9
            specified NEC Q42.8
iris, congenital Q13.1
jejunum (acquired) Z90.4
    congenital Q41.1
joint, congenital NEC Q74.8
kidney(s) (acquired) Z90.5
    congenital Q60.2
        bilateral Q60.1
        unilateral Q60.0
labyrinth, membranous Q16.5
larynx (congenital) Q31.8
    acquired Z90.02

                                                                    ©2002 Ingenix, Inc.

Abuse — *continued*
  drug NEC — *continued*
    analgesics (non-prescribed) (over the counter) F55.8
    antacids F55.0
    antidepressants — *see* Abuse, drug, psychoactive NEC
    anxiolytics — *see* Abuse, drug, sedative
    barbiturates — *see* Abuse, drug, sedative
    caffeine — *see* Abuse, drug, stimulant NEC
    cannabis F12.10
      with
        anxiety disorder F12.180
        intoxication F12.129
          with
            delirium F12.121
            perceptual disturbance F12.122
          uncomplicated F12.120
        other specified disorder F12.188
        psychosis F12.159
          delusions F12.150
          hallucinations F12.151
        unspecified disorder F12.19
    cocaine F14.10
      with
        anxiety disorder F14.180
        intoxication F14.129
          with
            delirium F14.121
            perceptual disturbance F14.122
          uncomplicated F14.120
        mood disorder F14.14
        other specified disorder F14.188
        psychosis F14.159
          delusions F14.150
          hallucinations F14.151
        sexual dysfunction F14.181
        sleep disorder F14.182
        unspecified disorder F14.19
    counseling and surveillance Z71.51
    hallucinogen F16.10
      with
        anxiety disorder F16.180
        flashbacks F16.183
        intoxication F16.129
          with
            delirium F16.121
            perceptual disturbance F16.122
          uncomplicated F16.120
        mood disorder F16.14
        other specified disorder F16.188
        perception disorder, persisting F16.183
        psychosis F16.159
          delusions F16.150
          hallucinations F16.151
        unspecified disorder F16.19
    hashish — *see* Abuse, drug, cannabis
    herbal or folk remedies F55.1
    hormones F55.3
    hypnotics — *see* Abuse, drug, sedative
    inhalant F18.10
      with
        anxiety disorder F18.180
        dementia, persisting F18.17
        intoxication F18.129
          with delirium F18.121
          uncomplicated F18.120
        mood disorder F18.14
        other specified disorder F18.188
        psychosis F18.159
          delusions F18.150
          hallucinations F18.151
        unspecified disorder F18.19
    laxatives F55.2
    LSD — *see* Abuse, drug, hallucinogen
    marihuana — *see* Abuse, drug, cannabis
    morphine type (opioids) — *see* Abuse, drug, opioid
    opioid F11.10
      with
        intoxication F11.129
          with
            delirium F11.121
            perceptual disturbance F11.122
          uncomplicated F11.120

Abuse — *continued*
  drug NEC — *continued*
    opioid — *continued*
      with — *continued*
        mood disorder F11.14
        other specified disorder F11.188
        psychosis F11.159
          delusions F11.150
          hallucinations F11.151
        sexual dysfunction F11.181
        sleep disorder F11.182
        unspecified disorder F11.19
    PCP (phencyclidine) (or related substance) — *see* Abuse, drug, psychoactive NEC
    psychoactive NEC F19.10
      with
        amnestic disorder F19.16
        anxiety disorder F19.180
        dementia F19.17
        intoxication F19.129
          with
            delirium F19.121
            perceptual disturbance F19.122
          uncomplicated F19.120
        mood disorder F19.14
        other specified disorder F19.188
        psychosis F19.159
          delusions F19.150
          hallucinations F19.151
        sexual dysfunction F19.181
        sleep disorder F19.182
        unspecified disorder F19.19
    rehabilitation measures Z51.89
    sedative, hypnotic or anxiolytic F13.10
      with
        anxiety disorder F13.180
        intoxication F13.129
          with delirium F13.121
          uncomplicated F13.120
        mood disorder F13.14
        other specified disorder F13.188
        psychosis F13.159
          delusions F13.150
          hallucinations F13.151
        sexual dysfunction F13.181
        sleep disorder F13.182
        unspecified disorder F13.19
    solvent — *see* Abuse, drug, inhalant
    steroids F55.3
    stimulant NEC F15.10
      with
        anxiety disorder F15.180
        intoxication F15.129
          with
            delirium F15.121
            perceptual disturbance F15.122
          uncomplicated F15.120
        mood disorder F15.14
        other specified disorder F15.188
        psychosis F15.159
          delusions F15.150
          hallucinations F15.151
        sexual dysfunction F15.181
        sleep disorder F15.182
        unspecified disorder F15.19
    tranquilizers — *see* Abuse, drug, sedative
    vitamins F55.4
  hallucinogens — *see* Abuse, drug, hallucinogen
  hashish — *see* Abuse, drug, cannabis
  herbal or folk remedies F55.1
  hormones F55.3
  hypnotic — *see* Abuse, drug, sedative
  inhalant — *see* Abuse, drug, inhalant
  laxatives F55.2
  LSD — *see* Abuse, drug, hallucinogen
  marihuana — *see* Abuse, drug, cannabis
  morphine type (opioids) — *see* Abuse, drug, opioid
  non-psychoactive substance NEC F55.8
    antacids F55.0
    folk remedies F55.1
    herbal remedies F55.1
    hormones F55.3
    laxatives F55.2
    steroids F55.3
    vitamins F55.4

Abuse — *continued*
  opioids — *see* Abuse, drug, opioid
  PCP (phencyclidine) (or related substance) — *see* Abuse, drug, psychoactive NEC
  physical (adult) (child) — *see* Maltreatment, physical abuse
  psychoactive substance — *see* Abuse, drug, psychoactive NEC
  psychological (adult) (child) — *see* Maltreatment. psychological abuse
  sedative — *see* Abuse, drug, sedative
  sexual — *see* Maltreatment, sexual abuse
  solvent — *see* Abuse, drug, inhalant
  steroids F55.3
  vitamins F55.4
Acalculia R48.8
  developmental F81.2
Acanthamebiasis (with) B60.10
  conjunctiva B60.12
  keratoconjunctivitis B60.13
  meningoencephalitis B60.11
  other specified B60.19
Acanthocephaliasis B83.8
Acanthocheilonemiasis B74.4
Acanthocytosis E78.6
Acantholysis L11.9
Acanthosis (acquired) (nigricans) L83
  benign Q82.8
  tongue K14.8
  congenital Q82.8
  seborrheic L82.1
    inflamed L82.0
  tongue K14.3
Acapnia E87.3
Acarbia E87.2
Acardia, acardius Q89.8
Acardiacus amorphus Q89.8
Acardiotrophia I51.4
Acariasis B88.0
  scabies B86
Acarodermatitis (urticarioides) B88.0
Acarophobia F40.218
Acatalasemia, acatalasia E80.3
Accelerated atrioventricular conduction I45.6
Accentuation of personality traits (type A) Z73.1
Accessory (congenital)
  adrenal gland Q89.1
  anus Q43.4
  appendix Q43.4
  atrioventricular conduction I45.6
  auditory ossicles Q16.3
  auricle (ear) Q17.0
  biliary duct or passage Q44.5
  bladder Q64.79
  blood vessels NEC Q27.9
    coronary Q24.5
  bone NEC Q79.8
  breast tissue, axilla Q83.1
  carpal bones Q74.0
  cecum Q43.4
  chromosome(s) NEC (nonsex) Q92.9
    with complex rearrangements NEC Q92.5
    seen only at prometaphase Q92.8
    partial Q92.9
    sex
      female phenotype Q97.8
    13 — *see* Trisomy, 13
    18 — *see* Trisomy, 18
    21 — *see* Trisomy, 21
  coronary artery Q24.5
  cusp(s), heart valve NEC Q24.8
    pulmonary Q22.3
  cystic duct Q44.5
  digit(s) Q69.9
  ear (auricle) (lobe) Q17.0
  endocrine gland NEC Q89.2
  eye muscle Q10.3
  eyelid Q10.3
  face bone(s) Q75.8
  fallopian tube (fimbria) (ostium) Q50.6
  finger(s) Q69.0
  foreskin N47.8
  frontonasal process Q75.8
  gallbladder Q44.1

©2002 Ingenix, Inc.

Accessory — *continued*
  genital organ(s)
    female Q52.8
      external Q52.79
      internal NEC Q52.8
    male Q55.8
  genitourinary organs NEC Q89.8
    female Q52.8
    male Q55.8
  hallux Q69.2
  heart Q24.8
    valve NEC Q24.8
      pulmonary Q22.3
  hepatic ducts Q44.5
  hymen Q52.4
  intestine (large) (small) Q43.4
  kidney Q63.0
  lacrimal canal Q10.6
  leaflet, heart valve NEC Q24.8
  ligament, broad Q50.6
  liver Q44.7
    duct Q44.5
  lobule (ear) Q17.0
  lung (lobe) Q33.1
  muscle Q79.8
  navicular of carpus Q74.0
  nervous system, part NEC Q07.8
  nipple Q83.3
  nose Q30.8
  organ or site not listed — *see* Anomaly, by site
  ovary Q50.31
  oviduct Q50.6
  pancreas Q45.3
  parathyroid gland Q89.2
  parotid gland (and duct) Q38.4
  pituitary gland Q89.2
  preauricular appendage Q17.0
  prepuce N47.8
  renal arteries (multiple) Q27.2
  rib Q76.6
    cervical Q76.5
  roots (teeth) K00.2
  salivary gland Q38.4
  sesamoid bones Q74.8
    foot Q74.2
    hand Q74.0
  skin tags Q82.8
  spleen Q89.09
  sternum Q76.7
  submaxillary gland Q38.4
  tarsal bones Q74.2
  teeth, tooth K00.1
    causing crowding M26.3
  tendon Q79.8
  thumb Q69.1
  thymus gland Q89.2
  thyroid gland Q89.2
  toes Q69.2
  tongue Q38.3
  tooth, teeth K00.1
    causing crowding M26.3
  tragus Q17.0
  ureter Q62.5
  urethra Q64.79
  urinary organ or tract NEC Q64.8
  uterus Q51.2
  vagina Q52.1
  valve, heart NEC Q24.8
    pulmonary Q22.2
  vertebra Q76.49
  vocal cords Q31.8
  vulva Q52.79

Accident
  birth — *see* Birth, injury
  cardiac — *see* Infarct, myocardium
  cardiovascular I51.6
  cerebral I64
  cerebrovascular I64
    hemorrhagic — *see* Hemorrhage,
      intracranial, intracerebral
    old — *see* Sequelae (of), stroke NOS
  coronary — *see* Infarct, myocardium
  craniovascular I64
  vascular, brain I64

Accidental *see* condition

Accommodation (disorder) (*see also* condition)
  hysterical paralysis of F44.89

Accommodation (*see also* condition) — *continued*
  insufficiency of H52.4
  paresis — *see* Paresis, of accommodation
  spasm — *see* Spasm, of accommodation

Accouchement — *see* Delivery

Accreta placenta (with hemorrhage) O72.0
  without hemorrhage O73.0

Accretio cordis (nonrheumatic) I31.0

Accretions, tooth, teeth K03.6

Acculturation difficulty Z60.3

Accumulation secretion, prostate N42.89

Acephalia, acephalism, acephalus, acephaly
  Q00.0

Acephalobrachia monster Q89.8

Acephalochirus monster Q89.8

Acephalogaster Q89.8

Acephalostomus monster Q89.8

Acephalothorax Q89.8

Acerophobia F40.298

Acetonemia R79.89
  in Type I diabetes E10.10
    with coma E10.11

Acetonuria R82.4

Achalasia (cardia) (esophagus) K22.0
  congenital Q39.5
  pylorus Q40.0
  sphincteral NEC K59.8

Ache(s) — *see* Pain

Acheilia Q38.6

Achillobursitis — *see* Tendinitis, Achilles

Achillodynia — *see* Tendinitis, Achilles

Achlorhydria, achlorhydric (neurogenic) K31.83
  anemia D50.8
  diarrhea K31.83
  psychogenic F45.8
  secondary to vagotomy K91.1

Achluophobia F40.228

Acholia K82.8

Acholuric jaundice (familial) (splenomegalic) —
  see also Spherocytosis
  acquired D59.8

Achondrogenesis Q77.0

Achondroplasia Q77.4

Achroma, cutis L80

Achromat(ism), achromatopsia (acquired)
  (congenital) H53.51

Achromia, congenital — *see* Albinism

Achromia parasitica B36.0

Achylia gastrica K31.89
  psychogenic F45.8

Acid
  burn — *see* Corrosion
  deficiency
    amide nicotinic E52
      ascorbic E54
      folic E53.8
      nicotinic E52
      pantothenic E53.8
  intoxication E87.2
  peptic disease K30
  phosphatase deficiency E83.39
  stomach K30
    psychogenic F45.8

Acidemia E87.2
  argininosuccinic E72.22
  fetal — *see* Distress, fetal
  isovaleric E71.110
  methylmalonic E71.120
  pipecolic E71.39
  propionic E71.121

Acidity, gastric (high) K30
  psychogenic F45.8

Acidocytopenia — *see* Agranulocytosis

Acidocytosis D72.1

Acidopenia — *see* Agranulocytosis

Acidosis (lactic) (respiratory) E87.2
  fetal — *see* Distress, fetal
  intrauterine — *see* Distress, fetal
  in Type I diabetes E10.10
    with coma E10.11

Acidosis — *continued*
  kidney, tubular N25.8
  lactic E87.2
  metabolic NEC E87.2
    with respiratory acidosis E87.4
    late, of newborn P74.0
  newborn P84
  renal (hyperchloremic) (tubular) N25.8
  respiratory E87.2
    complicated by
      metabolic
        acidosis E87.4
        alkalosis E87.4

Aciduria
  argininosuccinic E72.22
  glutaric (type I) E72.3
    type II E71.313
  orotic (congenital) (hereditary) (pyrimidine-
    deficiency) E79.8
    anemia D53.0

Acladiosis (skin) B36.0

Aclasis, diaphyseal Q78.6

Acleistocardia Q21.1

Aclusion — *see* Anomaly, dentofacial,
  malocclusion

Acne L70.9
  artificialis L70.8
  atrophica L70.2
  cachecticorum (Hebra) L70.8
  conglobata L70.1
  cystic L70.0
  decalvans L66.2
  excoriée des jeunes filles L70.5
  frontalis L70.2
  indurata L70.0
  infantile L70.4
  keloid L73.0
  lupoid L70.2
  necrotic, necrotica (miliaris) L70.2
  nodular L70.0
  occupational L70.8
  picker's L70.5
  pustular L70.0
  rodens L70.2
  rosacea L71.9
  specified NEC L70.8
  tropica L70.3
  varioliformis L70.2
  vulgaris L70.0

Acnitis (primary) A18.4

Acosta's disease T70.29

Acoustic — *see* condition

Acousticophobia F40.298

Acquired (*see also* condition)
  immunodeficiency syndrome (AIDS) B20

Acrania Q00.0

Acroasphyxia, chronic I73.8

Acrobystitis N47.7

Acrocephalopolysyndactyly Q87.0

Acrocephalosyndactyly Q87.0

Acrocephaly Q75.0

Acrochondrohyperplasia — *see* Syndrome,
  Marfan's

Acrocyanosis I73.8
  newborn P28.2

Acrodermatitis L30.8
  atrophicans (chronica) L90.4
  continua (Hallopeau) L40.2
  enteropathica (hereditary) E83.2
  Hallopeau's L40.2
  infantile papular L44.4
  perstans L40.2
  pustulosa continua L40.2
  recalcitrant pustular L40.2

Acrodynia — *see* Poisoning, mercury

Acromegaly, acromegalia E22.0

Acromelalgia I73.8

Acromicria, acromikria Q79.8

Acronyx L60.0

Acropachy, thyroid — *see* Thyrotoxicosis

Acroparesthesia (simple) (vasomotor) I73.8

Acropathy, thyroid — *see* Thyrotoxicosis

Acrophobia F40.241
Acroposthitis N47.7
Acroscleriasis, acroscleroderma, acrosclerosis
— see Sclerosis, systemic
Acrosphacelus I96
Acrospiroma, eccrine (M8402/0) — see
Neoplasm, skin, benign
Acrostealgia — see Osteochondropathy
Acrotrophodynia — see Immersion
ACTH ectopic syndrome E24.3
Actinic — see condition
Actinobacillosis, actinobacillus A28.8
mallei A24.0
muris A25.1
Actinomyces israelii (infection) — see
Actinomycosis
Actinomycetoma (foot) B47.1
Actinomycosis, actinomycotic A42.9
with pneumonia A42.0
abdominal A42.1
cervicofacial A42.2
cutaneous A42.89
gastrointestinal A42.1
pulmonary A42.0
septicemia A42.7
specified site NEC A42.89
Actinoneuritis G62.8
Action, heart
disorder I49.9
irregular I49.9
psychogenic F45.8
Active — see condition
Acute — see also condition
abdomen R10.0
gallbladder — see Cholecystitis, acute
Acyanotic heart disease (congenital) Q24.9
Acystia Q64.5
Adair-Dighton syndrome (brittle bones and blue
sclera, deafness) Q78.0
Adamantinoblastoma (M9310/0) — see
Ameloblastoma
Adamantinoma (M9310/0) D16.5
jaw (bone) (lower) D16.5
upper D16.4
long bones (M9261/3) C40.90
left C40.92
lower limb C40.20
left C40.22
right C40.21
right C40.91
upper limb C40.00
left C40.02
right C40.01
malignant (M9310/3) C41.1
jaw (bone) (lower) C41.1
upper C41.0
mandible D16.5
tibial (M9261/3) C40.20
left C40.22
right C40.21
Adamantoblastoma (M9310/0) — see
Ameloblastoma
Adams-Stokes (-Morgagni) disease or syndrome
I45.9
Adaption reaction — see Disorder, adjustment
Addiction (see also Dependence) F19.20
alcohol, alcoholic (ethyl) (methyl) (wood)
(without remission) F10.20
with remission F10.21
affecting fetus or newborn P04.3
complicating
childbirth O99.314
pregnancy O99.313
first trimester O99.310
second trimester O99.311
third trimester O99.312
puerperium O99.315
suspected damage to fetus affecting
management of pregnancy O35.4
drug — see Dependence, drug
ethyl alcohol (without remission) F10.20
with remission F10.21

Addiction (see also Dependence) — continued
heroin — see Dependence, drug, opioid
methyl alcohol (without remission) F10.20
with remission F10.21
methylated spirit (without remission) F10.20
with remission F10.21
morphine(-like substances) — see Dependence,
drug, opioid
nicotine — see Dependence, drug, nicotine
opium and opioids — see Dependence, drug,
opioid
tobacco — see Dependence, drug, nicotine
Addisonian crisis E27.2
Addison's
anemia (pernicious) D51.0
disease (bronze) or syndrome E27.1
tuberculous A18.7
keloid L94.0
Addison-Biermer anemia (pernicious) D51.0
Addison-Schilder complex E71.428
Additional — see also Accessory
chromosome(s) Q99.8
sex — see Abnormal, chromosome, sex
21 — see Trisomy, 21
Adduction contracture, hip or other joint — see
Contraction, joint
Adenitis — see also Lymphadenitis
acute, unspecified site L04.9
axillary I88.9
acute L04.2
chronic or subacute I88.1
Bartholin's gland N75.8
bulbourethral gland — see Urethritis
cervical I88.9
acute L04.0
chronic or subacute I88.1
chancroid (Hemophilus ducreyi) A57
chronic, unspecified site I88.1
Cowper's gland — see Urethritis
due to Pasteurella multocida (p. septica) A28.0
epidemic, acute B27.09
gangrenous L04.9
gonorrheal NEC A54.89
groin I88.9
acute L04.1
chronic or subacute I88.1
infectious (acute) (epidemic) B27.09
inguinal I88.9
acute L04.1
chronic or subacute I88.1
lymph gland or node, except mesenteric I88.9
acute — see Lymphadenitis, acute
chronic or subacute I88.1
mesenteric (acute) (chronic) (nonspecific)
(subacute) I88.0
parotid gland (suppurative) — see Sialoadenitis
salivary gland (any) (suppurative) — see
Sialoadenitis
scrofulous (tuberculous) A18.2
Skene's duct or gland — see Urethritis
strumous, tuberculous A18.2
subacute, unspecified site I88.1
sublingual gland (suppurative) — see
Sialoadenitis
submandibular gland (suppurative) — see
Sialoadenitis
submaxillary gland (suppurative) — see
Sialoadenitis
tuberculous — see Tuberculosis, lymph gland
urethral gland — see Urethritis
Wharton's duct (suppurative) — see
Sialoadenitis
Adenoacanthoma (M8570/3) — see Neoplasm,
malignant
Adenoameloblastoma (M9300/0) D16.5
upper jaw (bone) D16.4
Adenocarcinoid (tumor) (M8245/3) — see
Neoplasm, malignant
Adenocarcinoma (M8140/3) — see also
Neoplasm, malignant
with
apocrine metaplasia (M8573/3)
cartilaginous (and osseous) metaplasia
(M8571/3)

Adenocarcinoma — see also Neoplasm,
malignant — continued
with — continued
osseous (and cartilaginous) metaplasia
(M8571/3)
spindle cell metaplasia (M8572/3)
squamous metaplasia (M8570/3)
acidophil (M8280/3)
specified site — see Neoplasm, malignant
unspecified site C75.1
acinar (M8550/3)
acinic cell (M8550/3)
adrenal cortical (M8370/3) C74.00
left C74.02
right C74.01
alveolar (M8251/3) — see Neoplasm, lung,
malignant
and
carcinoid, combined (M8244/3)
epidermoid carcinoma, mixed (M8560/3)
squamous cell carcinoma, mixed (M8560/3)
apocrine (M8401/3)
breast — see Neoplasm, breast, malignant
in situ (M8401/2)
breast (female) D05.70
male D05.75
specified site NEC — see Neoplasm, skin,
in situ
unspecified site D04.9
specified site NEC — see Neoplasm, skin,
malignant
unspecified site C44.9
basal cell (M8147/3)
specified site — see Neoplasm, malignant
unspecified site C08.9
basophil (M8300/3)
specified site — see Neoplasm, malignant
unspecified site C75.1
bile duct type (M8160/3) C22.1
liver C22.1
specified site NEC — see Neoplasm,
malignant
unspecified site C22.1
bronchiolar (M8250/3) — see Neoplasm, lung,
malignant
bronchioloalveolar (M8250/3) — see Neoplasm,
lung, malignant
ceruminous (M8420/3) C44.20
left ear C44.22
right ear C44.21
chromophobe (M8270/3)
specified site — see Neoplasm, malignant
unspecified site C75.1
clear cell (mesonephroid) (M8310/3)
colloid (M8480/3)
cylindroid (M8200/3)
diffuse type (M8145/3)
specified site — see Neoplasm, malignant
unspecified site C16.9
duct (M8500/3)
infiltrating (M8500/3)
with Paget's disease (M8541/3) — see
Neoplasm, breast, malignant
specified site — see Neoplasm, malignant
unspecified site (female) C50.90
male C50.95
embryonal (M9070/3)
endometrioid (M8380/3)
specified site — see Neoplasm, malignant
unspecified site
female C56.9
male C61
eosinophil (M8280/3)
specified site — see Neoplasm, malignant
unspecified site C75.1
follicular (M8330/3)
with papillary (M8340/3) C73
moderately differentiated (M8332/3) C73
specified site — see Neoplasm, malignant
trabecular (M8332/3) C73
unspecified site C73
well differentiated (M8331/3) C73
gelatinous (M8480/3)
granular cell (M8320/3)
Hurthle cell (M8290/3) C73

Adenocarcinoma — *see also* Neoplasm, malignant — *continued*
in
  adenomatous
    polyp (M8210/3)
      multiple (M8221/3)
    polyposis coli (M8220/3) C18.9
  polyp (adenomatous) (M8210/3)
    multiple (M8221/3)
  polypoid adenoma (M8210/3)
  tubular adenoma (M8210/3)
  tubulovillous adenoma (M8263/3)
  villous adenoma (M8261/3)
infiltrating duct (M8500/3)
  with Paget's disease (M8541/3) — *see* Neoplasm, breast, malignant
  specified site — *see* Neoplasm, malignant
  unspecified site (female) C50.90
    male C50.95
inflammatory (M8530/3)
  specified site — *see* Neoplasm, malignant
  unspecified site (female) C50.90
    male C50.95
intestinal type (M8144/3)
  specified site — *see* Neoplasm, malignant
  unspecified site C16.9
intracystic papillary (M8504/3)
intraductal (M8500/2)
  breast (female) D05.10
    male D05.15
  noninfiltrating (M8500/2)
    breast (female) D05.10
      male D05.15
    papillary (M8503/2)
      with invasion (M8503/3)
        specified site — *see* Neoplasm, malignant
        unspecified site (female) C50.90
          male C50.95
      breast (female) D05.10
        male D05.15
      specified site NEC — *see* Neoplasm, in situ
      unspecified site (female) D05.10
        male D05.15
    specified site NEC — *see* Neoplasm, in situ
    unspecified site (female) D05.10
      male D05.15
  papillary (M8503/2)
    with invasion (M8503/3)
      specified site — *see* Neoplasm, malignant
      unspecified site (female) C50.90
        male C50.95
    breast (female) D05.10
      male D05.15
    specified site — *see* Neoplasm, in situ
    unspecified site (female) D05.10
      male D05.15
  specified site NEC — *see* Neoplasm, in situ
  unspecified site (female) D05.10
    male D05.15
islet cell (M8150/3)
  with exocrine, mixed (M8154/3)
    specified site — *see* Neoplasm, malignant
    unspecified site C25.9
  pancreas C25.4
  specified site NEC — *see* Neoplasm, malignant
  unspecified site C25.4
lobular (M8520/3)
  in situ (M8520/2)
    breast (female) D05.00
      male D05.05
    specified site NEC — *see* Neoplasm, in situ
    unspecified site (female) D05.00
      male D05.05
  specified site — *see* Neoplasm, malignant
  unspecified site (female) C50.90
    male C50.95
medullary (M8510/3)
mesonephric (M9110/3)
mixed cell (M8323/3)
mucinous (M8480/3)

Adenocarcinoma — *see also* Neoplasm, malignant — *continued*
mucin-producing (M8481/3)
mucin-secreting (M8481/3)
mucoid (M8480/3) — *see also* Neoplasm, malignant
  cell (M8300/3)
    specified site — *see* Neoplasm, malignant
    unspecified site C75.1
mucous (M8480/3)
nonencapsulated sclerosing (M8350/3) C73
oncocytic (M8290/3)
oxyphilic (M8290/3)
papillary (M8260/3)
  with follicular (M8340/3) C73
  follicular variant (M8340/3) C73
  intraductal (noninfiltrating) (M8503/2)
    with invasion (M8503/3)
      specified site — *see* Neoplasm, malignant
      unspecified site (female) C50.90
        male C50.95
    breast (female) D05.10
      male D05.15
    specified site NEC — *see* Neoplasm, in situ
    unspecified site D05.10
      male D05.15
  serous (M8460/3)
    specified site — *see* Neoplasm, malignant
    unspecified site C56.9
papillocystic (M8450/3)
  specified site — *see* Neoplasm, malignant
  unspecified site C56.9
pseudomucinous (M8470/3)
  specified site — *see* Neoplasm, malignant
  unspecified site C56.9
renal-cell (M8312/3) C64.9
  left C64.1
  right C64.0
scirrhous (M8141/3)
sebaceous (M8410/3) — *see* Neoplasm, skin, malignant
serous (M8441/3) — *see also* Neoplasm, malignant
  papillary (M8460/3)
    specified site — *see* Neoplasm, malignant
    unspecified site C56.9
signet ring cell (M8490/3)
superficial spreading (M8143/3)
sweat gland (M8400/3) — *see* Neoplasm, skin, malignant
trabecular (M8190/3)
tubular (M8211/3)
villous (M8262/3)
water-clear cell (M8322/3) C75.0

Adenocarcinoma-in-situ (M8140/2) — *see also* Neoplasm, in situ
breast (female) D05.90
  male D05.95
in
  adenoma (polypoid) (tubular) (M8210/2)
    tubulovillous (M8263/2)
    villous (M8261/2)
  polyp, adenomatous (M8210/2)

Adenofibroma (M9013/0)
clear cell (M8313/0) — *see* Neoplasm, benign
endometrioid (M8381/0) D27.9
  borderline malignancy (M8381/1) D39.10
  malignant (M8381/3) C56.9
    left side C56.1
    right side C56.0
mucinous (M9015/0)
  specified site — *see* Neoplasm, benign
  unspecified site D27.9
papillary (M9013/0)
  specified site — *see* Neoplasm, benign
  unspecified site D27.9
prostate — *see* Hyperplasia, prostate
serous (M9014/0)
  specified site — *see* Neoplasm, benign
  unspecified site D27.9
specified site — *see* Neoplasm, benign
unspecified site D27.9

Adenofibrosis
breast — *see* Fibroadenosis, breast
endometrioid N80.0
Adenoiditis (chronic) J35.02
with tonsillitis J35.03
acute J03.90
  recurrent J03.91
  specified organism NEC J03.80
    recurrent J03.81
  staphylococcal J03.80
    recurrent J03.81
  streptococcal J03.00
    recurrent J03.01

Adenoids — *see* condition

Adenolipoma (M8324/0) — *see* Neoplasm, benign

Adenolipomatosis, Launois-Bensaude E88.8

Adenolymphoma (M8561/0)
specified site — *see* Neoplasm, benign
unspecified site D11.9

Adenoma (M8140/0) — *see also* Neoplasm, benign
acidophil (M8280/0)
  specified site — *see* Neoplasm, benign
  unspecified site D35.2
acidophil-basophil, mixed (M8281/0)
  specified site — *see* Neoplasm, benign
  unspecified site D35.2
acinar (cell) (M8550/0)
acinic cell (M8550/0)
adrenal (cortical) (M8370/0) D35.00
  clear cell (M8373/0) D35.00
  compact cell (M8371/0) D35.00
  glomerulosa cell (M8374/0) D35.00
  heavily pigmented variant (M8372/0) D35.00
  mixed cell (M8375/0) D35.00
alpha-cell (M8152/0)
  pancreas D13.7
  specified site NEC — *see* Neoplasm, benign
  unspecified site D13.7
alveolar (M8251/0) D14.30
apocrine (M8401/0)
  breast (female) D24.00
    left D24.02
    male D24.10
      left D24.12
      right D24.11
    right D24.01
  specified site NEC — *see* Neoplasm, skin, benign
  unspecified site D23.9
basal cell (M8147/0) D11.9
basophil (M8300/0)
  specified site — *see* Neoplasm, benign
  unspecified site D35.2
basophil-acidophil, mixed (M8281/0)
  specified site — *see* Neoplasm, benign
  unspecified site D35.2
beta-cell (M8151/0)
  pancreas D13.7
  specified site NEC — *see* Neoplasm, benign
  unspecified site D13.7
bile duct (M8160/0) D13.4
  common D13.5
  extrahepatic D13.5
  intrahepatic D13.4
  specified site NEC — *see* Neoplasm, benign
  unspecified site D13.4
black (M8372/0) D35.00
bronchial (M8140/1) D38.1
  carcinoid type (M8240/3) — *see* Neoplasm, lung, malignant
  cylindroid type (M8200/3) — *see* Neoplasm, lung, malignant
ceruminous (M8420/0) D23.20
  left ear D23.22
  right ear D23.21
chief cell (M8321/0) D35.1
chromophobe (M8270/0)
  specified site — *see* Neoplasm, benign
  unspecified site D35.2
clear cell (M8310/0)
colloid (M8334/0)
  specified site — *see* Neoplasm, benign
  unspecified site D04
duct (M8503/0)

Adenoma — *see also* Neoplasm, benign — *continued*
 eccrine, papillary (M8202/0) — *see* Neoplasm, skin, benign
 embryonal (M8191/0)
 endocrine, multiple (M8360/1)
  single specified site — *see* Neoplasm, uncertain behavior
  two or more specified sites D44.8
  unspecified site D44.8
 endometrioid (M8380/0) — *see also* Neoplasm, benign
  borderline malignancy (M8380/1) — *see* Neoplasm, uncertain behavior
 eosinophil (M8280/0)
  specified site — *see* Neoplasm, benign
  unspecified site D35.2
 fetal (M8333/0)
  specified site — *see* Neoplasm, benign
  unspecified site D34
 follicular (M8330/0)
  specified site — *see* Neoplasm, benign
  unspecified site D34
 hepatocellular (M8170/0) D13.4
 Hurthle cell (M8290/0) D34
 intracystic papillary (M8504/0)
 islet cell (M8150/0)
  pancreas D13.7
  specified site NEC — *see* Neoplasm, benign
  unspecified site D13.7
 liver cell (M8170/0) D13.4
 macrofollicular (M8334/0)
  specified site — *see* Neoplasm, benign
  unspecified site D34
 malignant, malignum (M8140/3) — *see* Neoplasm, malignant
 mesonephric (M9110/0)
 microcystic (M8202/0)
  pancreas D13.7
  specified site NEC — *see* Neoplasm, benign
  unspecified site D13.7
 microfollicular (M8333/0)
  specified site — *see* Neoplasm, benign
  unspecified site D34
 mixed cell (M8323/0)
 monomorphic (M8146/0)
 mucinous (M8480/0)
 mucoid cell (M8300/0)
  specified site — *see* Neoplasm, benign
  unspecified site D35.2
 multiple endocrine (M8360/1)
  single specified site — *see* Neoplasm, uncertain behavior
  two or more specified sites D44.8
  unspecified site D44.8
 nipple (female) (M8506/0) D24.00
  left D24.02
  male D24.10
   left D24.12
   right D24.11
  right D24.01
 oncocytic (M8290/0)
 oxyphilic (M8290/0)
 papillary (M8260/0) — *see also* Neoplasm, benign
  eccrine (M8408/0) — *see* Neoplasm, skin, benign
  intracystic (M8504/0)
 papillotubular (M8263/0)
 Pick's tubular (M8640/0)
  specified site — *see* Neoplasm, benign
  unspecified site
   female D27.9
   male D29.20
 pleomorphic (M8940/0)
  carcinoma in (M8941/3) — *see* Neoplasm, salivary gland, malignant
  specified site — *see* Neoplasm, malignant
  unspecified site C08.9
 polypoid (M8210/0) — *see also* Neoplasm, benign
  adenocarcinoma in (M8210/3) — *see* Neoplasm, malignant
  adenocarcinoma in situ (M8210/2) — *see* Neoplasm, in situ
 prostate — *see* Hyperplasia, prostate, localized
 rete cell (M8390/0) D29.20

Adenoma — *see also* Neoplasm, benign — *continued*
 sebaceous (M8410/0) — *see* Neoplasm, skin, benign
 Sertoli cell (M8640/0)
  specified site — *see* Neoplasm, benign
  unspecified site
   female D27.9
   male D29.20
 skin appendage (M8390/0) — *see* Neoplasm, skin, benign
 sudoriferous gland (M8400/0) — *see* Neoplasm, skin, benign
 sweat gland (M8400/0) — *see* Neoplasm, skin, benign
 testicular (M8640/0)
  specified site — *see* Neoplasm, benign
  unspecified site
   female D27.9
   male D29.20
 trabecular (M8190/0)
 tubular (M8211/0) — *see also* Neoplasm, benign
  adenocarcinoma in (M8210/3) — *see* Neoplasm, malignant
  adenocarcinoma in situ (M8210/2) — *see* Neoplasm, in situ
  Pick's (M8640/0)
   specified site — *see* Neoplasm, benign
   unspecified site
    female D27.9
    male D29.20
 tubulovillous (M8263/0) — *see also* Neoplasm, benign
  adenocarcinoma in (M8263/3) — *see* Neoplasm, malignant
  adenocarcinoma in situ (M8263/2) — *see* Neoplasm, in situ
 villoglandular (M8263/0)
 villous (M8261/1) — *see* Neoplasm, uncertain behavior
  adenocarcinoma in (M8261/3) — *see* Neoplasm, malignant
  adenocarcinoma in situ (M8261/2) — *see* Neoplasm, in situ
 water-clear cell (M8322/0) D35.1
 wolffian duct (M9110/0)

Adenomatosis (M8220/0)
 endocrine (multiple) (M8360/1)
  single specified site — *see* Neoplasm, uncertain behavior
  two or more specified sites D44.8
  unspecified site D44.8
 erosive of nipple (female) (M8506/0) D24.00
  left D24.02
  male D24.10
   left D24.12
   right D24.11
  right D24.01
 pluriendocrine (M8360/1) — *see* Adenomatosis, endocrine
 pulmonary (M8250/1) D38.1
  malignant (M8250/3) — *see* Neoplasm, lung, malignant
 specified site — *see* Neoplasm, benign
 unspecified site D12.6

Adenomatous
 goiter (nontoxic) E04.9
  with hyperthyroidism — *see* Hyperthyroidism, with, goiter, nodular
  toxic — *see* Hyperthyroidism, with, goiter, nodular

Adenomyoma (M8932/0) — *see also* Neoplasm, benign
 prostate — *see* Hyperplasia, prostate

Adenomyometritis N80.0

Adenomyosis N80.0

Adenopathy (lymph gland) R59.9
 generalized R59.1
 inguinal R59.0
 localized R59.0
 mediastinal R59.0
 mesentery R59.0
 syphilitic (secondary) A51.49

Adenopathy — *continued*
 tracheobronchial R59.0
  tuberculous A15.4
   primary (progressive) A15.7
 tuberculous — *see also* Tuberculosis, lymph gland
  tracheobronchial A15.4
   primary (progressive) A15.7

Adenosalpingitis — *see* Salpingitis

Adenosarcoma (M8933/3) — *see* Neoplasm, malignant

Adenosclerosis I88.8

Adenosis (sclerosing) breast — *see* Fibroadenosis, breast

Adenovirus, as cause of disease classified elsewhere B97.0

Adentia (complete) (partial) — *see* Absence, teeth

Adherent — *see also* Adhesions
 labia (minora) N90.8
 pericardium (nonrheumatic) I31.0
  rheumatic I09.2
 placenta (with hemorrhage) O72.0
  without hemorrhage O73.0
 prepuce, newborn N47.0
 scar (skin) L90.5
 tendon in scar L90.5

Adhesions, adhesive (postinfective) K66.0
 with intestinal obstruction K56.5
 abdominal (wall) — *see* Adhesions, peritoneum
 amnion to fetus — *see* category O41.8
 appendix K38.8
 bile duct (common) (hepatic) K83.8
 bladder (sphincter) N32.8
 bowel — *see* Adhesions, peritoneum
 cardiac I31.0
  rheumatic I09.2
 cecum — *see* Adhesions, peritoneum
 cervicovaginal N88.1
  congenital Q52.8
  postpartal O90.8
   old N88.1
 cervix N88.1
 ciliary body NEC — *see* Adhesions, iris
 clitoris N90.8
 colon — *see* Adhesions, peritoneum
 common duct K83.8
 congenital — *see also* Anomaly, by site
  fingers — *see* Syndactylism, complex, fingers
  omental, anomalous Q43.3
  peritoneal Q43.3
  toes Q70.2
  tongue (to gum or roof of mouth) Q38.3
 conjunctiva (acquired) H11.219
  bilateral H11.213
  congenital Q15.8
  left H11.212
  right H11.211
 cystic duct K82.8
 diaphragm — *see* Adhesions, peritoneum
 due to foreign body — *see* Foreign body
 duodenum — *see* Adhesions, peritoneum
 epididymis N50.8
 epidural — *see* Adhesions, meninges
 epiglottis J38.7
 eyelid H02.59
 female pelvis N73.6
 gallbladder K82.8
 globe H44.89
 heart I31.0
  rheumatic I09.2
 ileocecal (coil) — *see* Adhesions, peritoneum
 ileum — *see* Adhesions, peritoneum
 intestine — *see also* Adhesions, peritoneum
  with obstruction K56.5
 intra-abdominal — *see* Adhesions, peritoneum
 iris H21.509
  anterior H21.519
   bilateral H21.513
   left H21.512
   right H21.511
  bilateral H21.503
  goniosynechiae H21.529
   bilateral H21.523
   left H21.522
   right H21.521
  left H21.502

©2002 Ingenix, Inc.

Adhesions, adhesive — *continued*
  iris — *continued*
    posterior H21.549
      bilateral H21.543
      left H21.542
      right H21.541
    right H21.501
    to corneal graft T85.89
  joint — *see also* Derangement, joint, specified
      type NEC
    temporomandibular M26.61
  labium (majus) (minus), congenital Q52.5
  liver — *see* Adhesions, peritoneum
  lung J98.4
  mediastinum J98.5
  meninges (cerebral) (spinal) G96.1
    congenital Q07.8
    tuberculous (cerebral) (spinal) A17.0
  mesenteric — *see* Adhesions, peritoneum
  nasal (septum) (to turbinates) J34.8
  ocular muscle — *see* Strabismus, mechanical
  omentum — *see* Adhesions, peritoneum
  ovary N73.6
    congenital (to cecum, kidney or omentum)
        Q50.39
  paraovarian N73.6
  pelvic (peritoneal)
    female N73.6
      postprocedural N99.4
    male — *see* Adhesions, peritoneum
    postpartal (old) N73.6
    tuberculous A18.17
  penis to scrotum (congenital) Q55.8
  periappendiceal — *see also* Adhesions,
      peritoneum
  pericardium (nonrheumatic) I31.0
    focal I31.8
    rheumatic I09.2
    tuberculous A18.84
  pericholecystic K82.8
  perigastric — *see* Adhesions, peritoneum
  periovarian N73.6
  periprostatic N42.89
  perirectal — *see* Adhesions, peritoneum
  perirenal N28.89
  peritoneum, peritoneal (postoperative) K66.0
    with obstruction (intestinal) K56.5
    congenital Q43.3
    pelvic, female N73.6
      postprocedural N99.4
    postpartal, pelvic N73.6
    to uterus N73.6
  peritubal N73.6
  periureteral N28.89
  periuterine N73.6
  perivesical N32.8
  perivesicular (seminal vesicle) N50.8
  pleura, pleuritic J94.8
    tuberculous NEC A15.6
  pleuropericardial J94.8
  postoperative (gastrointestinal tract) K66.0
    with obstruction K91.3
    due to foreign body accidentally left in
        wound — *see* Foreign body,
        accidentally left during a procedure
    pelvic peritoneal N99.4
    urethra — *see* Stricture, urethra,
        postprocedural
    vagina N99.2
  postpartal, old (vulva or perineum) N90.8
  preputial, prepuce N47.5
  pulmonary J98.4
  pylorus — *see* Adhesions, peritoneum
  sciatic nerve — *see* Lesion, nerve, sciatic
  seminal vesicle N50.8
  shoulder (joint) — *see* Capsulitis, adhesive
  sigmoid flexure — *see* Adhesions, peritoneum
  spermatic cord (acquired) N50.8
    congenital Q55.4
  spinal canal G96.1
  stomach — *see* Adhesions, peritoneum
  subscapular — *see* Capsulitis, adhesive
  temporomandibular M26.61
  tendinitis — *see also* Tenosynovitis, specified
      type NEC
    shoulder — *see* Capsulitis, adhesive
  testis N44.8

Adhesions, adhesive — *continued*
  tongue, congenital (to gum or roof of mouth)
      Q38.3
    acquired K14.8
  trachea J39.8
  tubo-ovarian N73.6
  tunica vaginalis N44.8
  uterus N73.6
    internal N85.6
    to abdominal wall N73.6
  vagina (chronic) N89.5
    postoperative N99.2
  vitreous H43.89
  vulva N90.8
Adiaspiromycosis B48.8
Adie(-Holmes) pupil or syndrome — *see*
    Anomaly, pupil, function, tonic pupil
Adiponecrosis neonatorum P83.8
Adiposis — *see also* Obesity
  cerebralis E23.6
  dolorosa E88.2
Adiposity — *see also* Obesity
  heart — *see* Degeneration, myocardial
  localized E65
Adiposogenital dystrophy E23.6
Adjustment
  disorder — *see* Disorder, adjustment
  implanted device — *see* Management (of)
  prosthesis, external — *see* Fitting
  reaction — *see* Disorder, adjustment
Administration, prophylactic chemotherapy
    Z51.89
Admission (for)
  adjustment (of)
    artificial
      arm Z44.009
        complete Z44.019
          left Z44.012
          right Z44.011
        left Z44.002
        partial Z44.029
          left Z44.022
          right Z44.021
        right Z44.001
      eye Z44.2
      leg Z44.109
        complete Z44.119
          left Z44.111
          right Z44.111
        left Z44.102
        partial Z44.129
          left Z44.122
          right Z44.121
        right Z44.101
    brain neuropacemaker Z46.2
      implanted Z45.42
    breast
      implant Z41.1
      prosthesis Z44.3
    colostomy belt Z46.8
    contact lenses Z46.0
    cystostomy device Z46.6
    dental prosthesis Z46.3
    device NEC
      abdominal Z46.8
      implanted Z45.9
        cardiac Z45.09
          defibrillator Z45.02
          pacemaker Z45.018
            pulse generator Z45.010
        hearing device Z45.328
          bone conduction Z45.320
          cochlear Z45.321
        infusion pump Z45.1
        nervous system Z45.49
          CSF drainage Z45.41
          hearing device — *see* Admission,
              adjustment, device,
              implanted, hearing device
          neuropacemaker Z45.42
          visual substitution Z45.31
        specified NEC Z45.8
        vascular access Z45.2
        visual substitution Z45.31

Admission (for) — *continued*
  adjustment (of) — *continued*
    device NEC — *continued*
      nervous system Z46.2
        implanted — *see* Admission,
            adjustment, device, implanted,
            nervous system
      orthodontic Z46.4
      prosthetic Z44.9
        arm — *see* Admission, adjustment,
            artificial, arm
        breast Z44.3
        dental Z46.3
        eye Z44.2
        leg — *see* Admission, adjustment,
            artificial, leg
        specified type NEC Z44.8
      substitution
        auditory Z46.2
          implanted — *see* Admission,
              adjustment, device,
              implanted, hearing device
        nervous system Z46.2
          implanted — *see* Admission,
              adjustment, device,
              implanted, nervous system
        visual Z46.2
          implanted Z45.31
      urinary Z46.6
    hearing aid Z46.1
      implanted — *see* Admission, adjustment,
          device, implanted, hearing device
    ileostomy device Z46.8
    intestinal appliance or device NEC Z46.8
    neuropacemaker (brain) (peripheral nerve)
        (spinal cord) Z46.2
      implanted Z45.42
    orthodontic device Z46.4
    orthopedic (brace) (cast) (device) (shoes)
        Z46.8
    pacemaker
      cardiac Z45.018
        pulse generator Z45.010
      nervous system Z46.2
        implanted Z45.42
    prosthesis Z44.9
      arm — *see* Admission, adjustment,
          artificial, arm
      breast Z44.3
      dental Z46.3
      eye Z44.2
      leg — *see* Admission, adjustment,
          artificial, leg
      specified NEC Z44.8
    spectacles Z46.0
  aftercare (*see also* Aftercare) Z51.9
    dialysis (extracorporeal) (renal) Z51.89
    postpartum
      immediately after delivery Z39.0
      routine follow-up Z39.2
    postradiation Z51.0
    radiation therapy Z51.0
  attention to artificial opening (of) Z43.9
    artificial vagina Z43.7
    colostomy Z43.3
    cystostomy Z43.5
    enterostomy Z43.4
    gastrostomy Z43.1
    ileostomy Z43.2
    jejunostomy Z43.4
    nephrostomy Z43.6
    specified site NEC Z43.8
      intestinal tract Z43.4
      urinary tract Z43.6
    tracheostomy Z43.0
    ureterostomy Z43.6
    urethrostomy Z43.6
  breast augmentation or reduction Z41.1
  change of
    dressing Z48.0
    neuropacemaker device (brain) (peripheral
        nerve) (spinal cord) Z46.2
      implanted Z45.42
    surgical dressing Z48.0
  checkup only Z00.010
    with abnormal findings Z00.011

Admission (for) — *continued*
  circumcision, ritual or routine (in absence of diagnosis) Z41.2
  clinical research investigation Z00.6
  contraceptive management Z30.9
  convalescence Z76.8
  cosmetic surgery NEC Z41.1
  counseling (*see also* Counseling)
    dietary Z71.3
    HIV Z71.7
    human immunodeficiency virus Z71.7
    nonattending third party Z71.0
    procreative management Z31.6
  desensitization to allergens Z51.89
  dietary surveillance and counseling Z71.3
  ear piercing Z41.3
  elective surgery Z41.9
    breast augmentation or reduction Z41.1
    circumcision, ritual or routine Z41.2
    cosmetic NEC Z41.1
    ear piercing Z41.3
    face lift Z41.1
    hair transplant Z41.1
    plastic cosmetic NEC Z41.1
    specified type NEC Z41.8
  examination (*see also* Examination) at health care facility Z00.010
    with abnormal findings Z00.011
    allergy Z01.8
    clinical research investigation Z00.6
    dental Z01.20
      with abnormal findings Z01.21
    developmental testing (child) (infant) Z00.10
      with abnormal findings Z00.11
    donor (potential) Z00.5
    ear Z01.10
      with abnormal findings Z01.11
    eye Z01.00
      with abnormal findings Z01.01
    general, specified reason NEC Z00.5
    health supervision (child) (infant) Z00.10
      with abnormal findings Z00.11
    hearing Z01.10
      with abnormal findings Z01.11
    laboratory Z00.020
      with abnormal findings Z00.021
    postpartum checkup Z39.2
    pregnancy (possible) (unconfirmed) Z32.0
    psychiatric (general) Z00.8
      requested by authority Z04.6
    radiological NEC Z00.030
      with abnormal findings Z00.031
    skin hypersensitivity Z01.8
    vision Z01.00
      with abnormal findings Z01.01
    well baby and child care Z00.10
      with abnormal findings Z00.11
  face lift, cosmetic reason Z41.1
  fitting (of)
    artificial
      arm — *see* Admission, adjustment, artificial, arm
      eye Z44.2
      leg — *see* Admission, adjustment, artificial, leg
    brain neuropacemaker Z46.2
      implanted Z45.42
    breast
      implant Z41.1
      prosthesis Z44.3
    colostomy belt Z46.8
    contact lenses Z46.0
    cystostomy device Z46.6
    dental prosthesis Z46.3
    device NEC
      abdominal Z46.8
      nervous system Z46.2
        implanted-*see* Admission, adjustment, device, implanted, nervous system
      orthodontic Z46.4
      prosthetic Z44.9
        breast Z44.3
        dental Z46.3
        eye Z44.2

Admission (for) — *continued*
  fitting (of) — *continued*
    device NEC — *continued*
      substitution
        auditory Z46.2
          implanted — *see* Admission, adjustment, device, implanted, hearing device
        nervous system Z46.2
          implanted — *see* Admission, adjustment, device, implanted, nervous system
        visual Z46.2
          implanted Z45.31
    hearing aid Z46.1
    ileostomy device Z46.8
    intestinal appliance or device NEC Z46.8
    neuropacemaker (brain) (peripheral nerve) (spinal cord) Z46.2
      implanted Z45.42
    orthodontic device Z46.4
    orthopedic device (brace) (cast) (shoes) Z46.8
    prosthesis Z44.9
      arm — *see* Admission, adjustment, artificial, arm
      breast Z44.3
      dental Z46.3
      eye Z44.2
      leg — *see* Admission, adjustment, artificial, leg
      specified type NEC Z44.8
    spectacles Z46.0
  follow-up examination Z09
  hair transplant for cosmetic reason Z41.1
  intrauterine device management Z30.44
    initial prescription Z30.014
  isolation Z51.89
  issue of
    medical certificate NEC Z02.79
      for disability determination Z02.71
    repeat prescription NEC Z76.0
  mental health evaluation Z00.8
    requested by authority Z04.6
  observation — *see* Observation
  Papanicolaou smear, cervix Z12.4
    for suspected malignant neoplasm Z12.4
    no disease found Z03.8
  plastic surgery, cosmetic NEC Z41.1
  postpartum observation
    immediately after delivery Z39.0
    routine follow-up Z39.2
  poststerilization (for restoration) Z31.0
    aftercare Z31.42
  procreative management Z31.9
  prophylactic (measure) Z51.89
    administration of prophylactic drug Z51.89
    organ removal Z40.00
      breast Z40.01
      ovary Z40.02
      specified organ NEC Z40.09
      testes Z40.09
  psychiatric examination (general) Z00.8
    requested by authority Z04.6
  radiation management Z51.0
  radiotherapy Z51.0
  rehabilitation (orthoptic) (speech) Z51.89
  removal of
    cystostomy catheter Z43.5
    device
      intrauterine contraceptive Z30.44
    dressing Z48.0
    intrauterine contraceptive device Z30.44
    neuropacemaker (brain) (peripheral nerve) (spinal cord) Z46.2
      implanted Z45.42
    surgical dressing Z48.0
    sutures Z48.0
    ureteral stent Z46.6
  restoration of organ continuity (poststerilization) Z31.0
    aftercare Z31.42
  sensitivity test—*see also* Test, skin
    allergy NEC Z01.8
    Mantoux Z11.1
  speech therapy Z51.89

Admission (for) — *continued*
  therapy
    blood transfusion, without reported diagnosis Z51.89
    orthoptic Z51.89
    radiation Z51.0
    speech Z51.89
  tuboplasty following previous sterilization Z31.0
    aftercare Z31.42
  vaccination, prophylactic Z23
    immune sera (gamma globulin) Z51.89
  vasoplasty following previous sterilization Z31.0
    aftercare Z31.42
  vision examination Z01.00
    with abnormal findings Z01.01
  waiting period for admission to other facility Z75.1
  well baby and child care Z00.10
    with abnormal findings Z00.11
  x-ray of chest
    for suspected tuberculosis Z03.8
    routine Z00.030
      with abnormal findings Z00.031

Adnexitis (suppurative) — *see* Salpingo-oophoritis

Adolescent X-linked adrenoleukodystrophy E71.421

Adrenal (gland) — *see* condition

Adrenalism, tuberculous A18.7

Adrenalitis, adrenitis E27.8
  autoimmune E27.1
  meningococcal, hemorrhagic A39.1

Adrenarche, premature E27.0

Adrenocortical syndrome — *see* Cushing's syndrome

Adrenogenital syndrome E25.9
  acquired E25.8
  congenital E25.0
  salt loss E25.0

Adrenogenitalism, congenital E25.0

Adrenoleukodystrophy E71.429
  neonatal E71.411
  X-linked E71.429
    adolescent E71.421
    adrenomyeloneuropathy E71.422
    childhood cerebral E71.420
    other specified E71.429

Adrenomyeloneuropathy E71.422

Adventitious bursa — *see* Bursopathy, specified type NEC

Advice — *see* Counselling

Adynamia (episodica) (hereditary) (periodic) G72.3

Aeration lung imperfect, newborn — *see* Atelectasis

Aerobullosis T70.3

Aerocele — *see* Embolism, air

Aerodermectasia
  subcutaneous (traumatic) T79.7

Aerodontalgia T70.29

Aeroembolism T70.3

Aerogenes capsulatus infection A48.0

Aero-otitis media T70.0

Aerophagy, aerophagia (psychogenic) F45.8

Aerophobia F40.228

Aerosinusitis T70.1

Aerotitis T70.0

Affection — *see* Disease

Afibrinogenemia (*see also* Defect, coagulation) D68.89
  acquired D65
  congenital D68.2
  in abortion — *see* Abortion, by type, complicated by, afibrinogenemia
  puerperal O72.3

African
  sleeping sickness B56.9
  tick fever A68.1
  trypanosomiasis B56.9
    gambian B56.0
    rhodesian B56.1

Aftercare (*see also* Care) Z51.9
  blood transfusion without reported diagnosis Z51.89

©2002 Ingenix, Inc.

Agenesis — *continued*
  thyroid (gland) E03.1
    cartilage Q31.8
  tibia — *see* Defect, reduction, lower limb, longitudinal, tibia
  tibiofibular — *see* Defect, reduction, lower limb, specified type NEC
  toe (and foot) (complete) (partial) — *see* Agenesis, foot
  tongue Q38.3
  trachea (cartilage) Q32.1
  ulna — *see* Defect, reduction, upper limb, longitudinal, ulna
  upper limb — *see* Agenesis, arm
  ureter Q62.4
  urethra Q64.5
  urinary tract NEC Q64.8
  uterus Q51.0
  uvula Q38.5
  vagina Q52.0
  vas deferens Q55.4
  vein(s) (peripheral) Q27.9
    brain Q28.3
    great NEC Q26.8
    portal Q26.5
  vena cava (inferior) (superior) Q26.8
  vermis of cerebellum Q04.3
  vertebra Q76.49
  vulva Q52.71
Ageusia R43.2
Agitated — *see* condition
Agitation R45.1
Aglossia (congenital) Q38.3
Aglossia-adactylia syndrome Q87.0
Aglycogenosis E74.00
Agnosia (body image) (other senses) (tactile) (visual) R48.1
  developmental F88
  verbal R48.1
    auditory R48.1
      developmental F80.2
    developmental F80.2
Agoraphobia F40.00
  with panic disorder F40.01
  without panic disorder F40.02
Agrammatism R48.8
Agranulocytopenia — *see* Agranulocytosis
Agranulocytosis (angina) (chronic) (cyclical) (genetic) (infantile) (periodic) (pernicious) D70.9
  congenital D70.0
  cytoreductive cancer chemotherapy sequela D70.1
  drug-induced D70.2
    due to cytoreductive cancer chemotherapy D70.1
  secondary D70.3
    drug-induced D70.2
      due to cytoreductive cancer chemotherapy D70.1
Agraphia (absolute) R48.8
  with alexia R48.0
  developmental F81.81
Ague (dumb) — *see* Malaria
Agyria Q04.3
Ahumada-del Castillo syndrome E23.0
Aichomophobia F40.298
AIDS (related complex) B20
Ailment heart — *see* Disease, heart
Ailurophobia F40.218
Ainhum (disease) L94.6
Air
  anterior mediastinum J98.2
  compressed, disease T70.3
  conditioner lung or pneumonitis J67.7
  embolism (artery) (cerebral) (any site) T79.0
    with ectopic or molar pregnancy O08.2
    due to implanted device NEC — *see* Complications, by site and type, specified NEC
    following
      ectopic or molar pregnancy O08.2

Air — *continued*
  embolism — *continued*
    following — *continued*
      infusion, therapeutic injection or transfusion T80.0
    in pregnancy, childbirth or puerperium — *see* Embolism, obstetric
    traumatic T79.0
  hunger, psychogenic F45.8
  pollution Z58.1
    occupational NEC Z57.39
      dust Z57.2
      tobacco smoke Z57.31
  rarefied, effects of — *see* Effect, adverse, high altitude
  sickness T75.3
Airplane sickness T75.3
Akathisia, treatment-induced G21.1
Akinesia R29.898
Akinetic mutism R41.89
Akureyri's disease G93.3
Alactasia, congenital E73.0
Alagille's syndrome Q44.7
Alastrim B03
Albers-Schönberg syndrome Q78.2
Albert's syndrome — *see* Tendinitis, Achilles
Albinism, albino E70.30
  with hematologic abnormality E70.339
    Chediak-Higashi syndrome E70.330
    Hermansky-Pudlak syndrome E70.331
    other specified E70.338
  I E70.320
  II E70.321
  ocular E70.319
    autosomal recessive E70.311
    other specified E70.318
    X-linked E70.310
  oculocutaneous E70.329
    other specified E70.328
    tyrosinase (ty) negative E70.320
    tyrosinase (ty) positive E70.321
  other specified E70.39
Albinismus E70.30
Albright (-McCune) (-Sternberg) syndrome Q78.1
Albuminous — *see* condition
Albuminuria, albuminuric (acute) (chronic) (subacute) — *see also* Proteinuria
  complicating pregnancy — *see* Proteinuria, gestational
    with
      gestational hypertension — *see* Pre-eclampsia
      pre-existing hypertension — *see* Hypertension, complicating pregnancy, pre-existing with proteinuria
  gestational — *see* Proteinuria, gestational
    with
      gestational hypertension — *see* Pre-eclampsia
      pre-existing hypertension — *see* Hypertension, complicating pregnancy, pre-existing with proteinuria
  orthostatic R80.2
  postural R80.2
  pre-eclamptic — *see* Pre-eclampsia
  scarlatinal A38.8
Albuminurophobia F40.298
Alcaptonuria E70.29
Alcohol, alcoholic, alcohol-induced
  addiction (without remission) F10.20
    with remission F10.21
  amnestic disorder, persisting F10.96
    with dependence F10.26
  brain syndrome, chronic F10.97
    with dependence F10.27
  cardiopathy I42.6
  counseling and surveillance Z71.41
    family member Z71.42

Alcohol, alcoholic, alcohol-induced — *continued*
  delirium (acute) (tremens) (withdrawal) F10.231
    with intoxication F10.921
    in
      abuse F10.121
      dependence F10.221
  dementia F10.97
    with dependence F10.27
  deterioration F10.97
    with dependence F10.27
  detoxification therapy Z51.89
  hallucinosis (acute) F10.951
    in
      abuse F10.151
      dependence F10.251
  insanity F10.959
  intoxication (acute) (without dependence) F10.129
    with
      delirium F10.121
      dependence F10.229
        with delirium F10.221
  jealousy F10.959
  Korsakoff's, Korsakov's, Korsakow's F10.26
  liver K70.9
    acute — *see* Disease, liver, alcoholic, hepatitis
  mania (acute) (chronic) F10.959
  paranoia, paranoid (type) psychosis F10.950
  pellagra E52
  poisoning, accidental (acute) NEC T51.91
    administered with intent to harm by another person T51.93
    self T51.92
    circumstances undetermined T51.94
    specified type of alcohol — *see* Table of Drugs and Chemicals
  psychosis — *see* Psychosis, alcoholic
  rehabilitation measures Z51.89
  use, uncomplicated
    complicating
      childbirth O99.314
      pregnancy O99.313
        first trimester O99.310
        second trimester O99.311
        third trimester O99.312
      puerperium O99.315
  withdrawal (without convulsions) F10.239
    with delirium F10.231
Alcoholism (chronic) (without remission) F10.20
  with
    psychosis — *see* Psychosis, alcoholic
    remission F10.21
  affecting fetus or newborn P04.3
  complicating
    childbirth O99.314
    pregnancy O99.313
      first trimester O99.310
      second trimester O99.311
      third trimester O99.312
    puerperium O99.315
  Korsakov's F10.96
    with dependence F10.26
  suspected damage to fetus affecting management of pregnancy O35.4
Alder (-Reilly) anomaly or syndrome (leukocyte granulation) D72.0
Aldosteronism — *see* Hyperaldosteronism
Aldosteronoma (M8370/1) D44.10
Aldrich (-Wiskott) syndrome (eczema-thrombocytopenia) D82.0
Alektorophobia F40.218
Aleppo boil B55.1
Aleukemic — *see* condition
Aleukia
  congenital D70.0
  hemorrhagica D61.9
    congenital D61.0
  splenica D73.1
Alexia R48.0
  developmental F81.0
  secondary to organic lesion R48.0

©2002 Ingenix, Inc.

Algoneurodystrophy M89.00
  ankle M89.079
    left M89.072
    right M89.071
  foot M89.079
    left M89.072
    right M89.071
  forearm M89.039
    left M89.032
    right M89.031
  hand M89.049
    left M89.042
    right M89.041
  lower leg M89.069
    left M89.062
    right M89.061
  multiple sites M89.09
  shoulder M89.019
    left M89.012
    right M89.011
  specified site NEC M89.08
  thigh M89.059
    left M89.052
    right M89.051
  upper arm M89.029
    left M89.022
    right M89.021
Algophobia F40.298
Alienation, mental — see Psychosis
Alkalemia E87.3
Alkalosis E87.3
  metabolic E87.3
    with respiratory acidosis E87.4
  respiratory E87.3
Alkaptonuria E70.29
Allen-Masters syndrome N83.8
Allergy, allergic (reaction) T78.4
  air-borne substance NEC (rhinitis) J30.8
  alveolitis (extrinsic) J67.9
    due to
      Aspergillus clavatus J67.4
      Cryptostroma corticale J67.5
      organisms (fungal, thermophilic
        actinomycete) growing in ventilation
        (air conditioning) systems J67.7
    specified type NEC J67.8
  anaphylactic shock T80.5
  angioneurotic edema T78.3
  animal (dander) (epidermal) (hair) (rhinitis)
    J30.8
  bee sting (anaphylactic shock) — see Toxicity,
    venom, arthropod, bee
  biological — see Allergy, drug
  colitis K52.2
  dander (animal) (rhinitis) J30.8
  dandruff (rhinitis) J30.8
  dermatitis — see Dermatitis, contact, allergic
  diathesis — see History, allergy
  drug, medicament & biological (any) (correct
    substance properly administered)
    (external) (internal) T88.7
    wrong substance given or taken NEC (by
      accident) T50.901
      administered with intent to harm by
        another person T50.903
        self T50.902
      circumstances undetermined T50.904
      specified drug or substance — see Table
        of Drugs and Chemicals
  due to pollen J30.1
  dust (house) (stock) (rhinitis) J30.8
    with asthma — see Asthma, allergic
      extrinsic
  eczema — see Dermatitis, contact, allergic
  epidermal (animal) (rhinitis) J30.8
  feathers (rhinitis) J30.8
  food (any) (ingested) NEC T78.1
    anaphylactic shock — see Shock,
      anaphylactic, food
    dermatitis — see Dermatitis, due to, food
    dietary counselling and surveillance Z71.3
    in contact with skin L23.6
    rhinitis J30.5
    status (without reaction) Z91.018
      eggs Z91.012
      milk products Z91.011

Allergy, allergic — continued
  food NEC — continued
    status — continued
      peanuts Z91.010
      seafood Z91.013
      specified NEC Z91.018
  gastrointestinal K52.2
  grain J30.1
  grass (hay fever) (pollen) J30.1
    asthma — see Asthma, allergic extrinsic
  hair (animal) (rhinitis) J30.8
  history (of) — see History, allergy
  horse serum — see Allergy, serum
  inhalant (rhinitis) J30.8
    pollen J30.1
  kapok (rhinitis) J30.8
  medicine — see Allergy, drug
  nasal, seasonal due to pollen J30.1
  pneumonia J82
  pollen (any) (hay fever) J30.1
    asthma — see Asthma, allergic extrinsic
  primrose J30.1
  primula J30.1
  purpura D69.0
  ragweed (hay fever) (pollen) J30.1
    asthma — see Asthma, allergic extrinsic
  rose J30.1
  Senecio jacobae (pollen) J30.1
  serum (prophylactic) (therapeutic) T80.6
    anaphylactic shock T80.5
  shock (anaphylactic) T78.2
    due to
      adverse effect of correct medicinal
        substance properly administered
        T88.6
      serum or immunization T80.5
        anaphylactic T80.5
  tree (any) (hay fever) (pollen) J30.1
    asthma — see Asthma, allergic extrinsic
  upper respiratory J30.9
  urticaria L50.0
  vaccine — see Allergy, serum
Allescheriasis B48.2
Alligator skin disease Q80.9
Allocheiria, allochiria R20.8
Almeida's disease — see Paracoccidioidomycosis
Alopecia (hereditaria) (prematura) (seborrheica)
  L65.9
  androgenic L64.9
    drug-induced L64.0
    specified NEC L64.8
  areata L63.9
    ophiasis L63.2
    specified NEC L63.8
    totalis L63.0
    universalis L63.1
  cicatricial L66.9
    specified NEC L66.8
  circumscripta L63.9
  congenital, congenitalis Q84.0
  due to cytotoxic drugs NEC L65.8
  mucinosa L65.2
  postinfective NEC L65.8
  postpartum L65.0
  specific (syphilitic) A51.32
  specified NEC L65.8
  syphilitic (secondary) A51.32
  totalis (capitis) L63.0
  universalis (entire body) L63.1
  X-ray L58.1
Alpers' disease G31.81
Alpine sickness T70.29
Alport's syndrome — see Syndrome, Alport's
Altered
  awareness, transient R40.4
  pattern of family relationships affecting child
    Z61.2
Alternating — see condition
Altitude, high (effects) — see Effect, adverse,
  high altitude
Aluminosis (of lung) J63.0
Alveolitis
  allergic (extrinsic) — see Pneumonitis,
    hypersensitivity

Alveolitis — continued
  due to
    Aspergillus clavatus J67.4
    Cryptostroma corticale J67.6
  fibrosing (cryptogenic) (idiopathic) J84.1
  jaw M27.3
  sicca dolorosa M27.3
Alveolus, alveolar — see condition
Alymphocytosis D72.8
  thymic (with immunodeficiency) D82.1
Alymphoplasia, thymic D82.1
Alzheimer's disease or sclerosis — see Disease,
  Alzheimer's
Amastia (with nipple present) Q83.8
  with absent nipple Q83.0
Amathophobia F40.228
Amaurosis (acquired) (congenital) — see also
  Blindness
  fugax G45.3
  hysterical F44.6
  Leber's congenital H35.50
  uremic — see Uremia
Amaurotic idiocy (infantile) (juvenile) (late) E75.4
Amaxophobia F40.248
Ambiguous genitalia Q56.4
Amblyopia (congenital) (ex anopsia) (partial)
  (suppression) H53.009
  anisometropic — see Amblyopia, refractive
  bilateral H53.003
  deprivation H53.019
    bilateral H53.013
    left H53.012
    right H53.011
  hysterical F44.6
  left H53.002
  nocturnal — see also Blindness, night
    vitamin A deficiency E50.5
  refractive H53.029
    bilateral H53.023
    left H53.022
    right H53.021
  right H53.001
  strabismic H53.039
    bilateral H53.033
    left H53.032
    right H53.031
  tobacco H53.8
  toxic NEC H53.8
  uremic — see Uremia
Ameba, amebic (histolytica) — see also Amebiasis
  abscess (liver) A06.4
Amebiasis A06.9
  with abscess — see Abscess, amebic
  acute A06.0
  chronic (intestine) A06.1
    with abscess — see Abscess, amebic
  cutaneous A06.7
  cutis A06.7
  cystitis A06.81
  genitourinary tract NEC A06.82
  hepatic — see Abscess, liver, amebic
  intestine A06.0
  nondysenteric colitis A06.2
  skin A06.7
  specified site NEC A06.89
Ameboma (of intestine) A06.3
Amelia Q73.0
  lower limb — see Agenesis, leg
  upper limb — see Agenesis, arm
Ameloblastoma (M9310/0) D16.5
  jaw (bone) (lower) D16.5
    upper D16.4
  long bones (M9261/3) C40.90
    left C40.92
    lower limb C40.20
      left C40.22
      right C40.21
    right C40.91
    upper limb C40.00
      left C40.02
      right C40.01
  malignant (M9310/3) C41.1
    jaw (bone) (lower) C41.1
      upper C41.0

Ameloblastoma — *continued*
  mandible D16.5
  tibial (M9261/3) C40.20
    left C40.22
    right C40.21
Amelogenesis imperfecta K00.5
  nonhereditaria (segmentalis) K00.4
Amenorrhea N91.2
  hyperhormonal E28.8
  primary N91.0
  secondary N91.1
Amentia — *see also* Retardation, mental
  Meynert's (nonalcoholic) F04
American
  leishmaniasis B55.2
  mountain tick fever A93.2
Ametropia — *see* Disorder, refraction
Amianthosis J61
Amimia R48.8
Amino-acid disorder E72.9
  anemia D53.0
Aminoacidopathy E72.9
Aminoaciduria E72.9
Amnes(t)ic syndrome (post-traumatic) F04
  induced by
    alcohol F10.96
      with dependence F10.26
    psychoactive NEC F19.96
      with
        abuse F19.16
        dependence F19.26
    sedative F13.96
      with dependence F13.26
Amnesia R41.3
  anterograde R41.1
  auditory R48.8
  dissociative F44.0
  hysterical F44.0
  postictal in epilepsy — *see* Epilepsy
  psychogenic F44.0
  retrograde R41.2
  transient global G45.4
Amniocentesis screening Z36
Amnion, amniotic — *see* condition
Amnionitis complicating pregnancy O41.109
  first trimester O41.101
  second trimester O41.102
  third trimester O41.103
Amok F68.8
Amoral traits F60.89
Ampulla
  lower esophagus K22.8
  phrenic K22.8
Amputation — *see also* Absence, by site, acquired
  cervix (uteri) Z90.71
    in pregnancy or childbirth — *see* Abnormal, cervix, in pregnancy or childbirth
  neuroma (postoperative) (traumatic) — *see* Complications, amputation stump, neuroma
  stump (surgical)
    abnormal, painful, or with complication (late) — *see* Complications, amputation stump
    healed or old NOS Z89.9
  traumatic (complete) (partial)
    arm (upper) (complete) S48.919
      at
        elbow S58.019
          left S58.012
          partial S58.029
            left S58.022
            right S58.021
          right S58.011
        shoulder joint (complete) S48.019
          left S48.012
          partial S48.029
            left S48.022
            right S48.021
          right S48.011
      between
        elbow and wrist (complete) S58.119
          left S58.112

Amputation — *see also* Absence, by site, acquired — *continued*
  traumatic — *continued*
    arm — *continued*
      between — *continued*
        elbow and wrist — *continued*
          partial S58.129
            left S58.122
            right S58.121
          right S58.111
        shoulder and elbow (complete) S48.119
          left S48.112
          partial S48.129
            left S48.122
            right S48.121
          right S48.111
      left S48.912
        partial S48.929
          left S48.922
          right S48.921
        right S48.911
    breast (complete) S28.219
      left S28.212
      partial S28.229
        left S28.222
        right S28.221
      right S28.211
    clitoris (complete) S38.211
      partial S38.212
    ear (complete) S08.119
      left S08.112
      partial S08.129
        left S08.122
        right S08.121
      right S08.111
    finger (complete) (metacarpophalangeal) S68.119
      index S68.118
        left S68.111
        right S68.110
      little S68.118
        left S68.117
        right S68.116
      middle S68.118
        left S68.113
        right S68.112
      partial S68.129
        index S68.128
          left S68.121
          right S68.120
        little S68.128
          left S68.127
          right S68.126
        middle S68.128
          left S68.123
          right S68.122
        ring S68.128
          left S68.125
          right S68.124
      ring S68.118
        left S68.115
        right S68.114
      thumb — *see* Amputation, traumatic, thumb
      transphalangeal (complete) S68.619
        index S68.618
          left S68.611
          right S68.610
        little S68.618
          left S68.617
          right S68.616
        middle S68.618
          left S68.613
          right S68.612
        partial S68.629
          index S68.628
            left S68.621
            right S68.620
          little S68.628
            left S68.627
            right S68.626
          middle S68.628
            left S68.623
            right S68.622

Amputation — *see also* Absence, by site, acquired — *continued*
  traumatic — *continued*
    finger — *continued*
      transphalangeal — *continued*
        partial — *continued*
          ring S68.628
            left S68.625
            right S68.624
        ring S68.618
          left S68.615
          right S68.614
    foot (complete) S98.919
      at ankle level S98.019
        left S98.012
        partial S98.029
          left S98.022
          right S98.021
        right S98.011
      left S98.912
      midfoot S98.319
        left S98.312
        partial S98.329
          left S98.322
          right S98.321
        right S98.311
      partial S98.929
        left S98.922
        right S98.921
      right S98.911
      toe — *see* Amputation, traumatic, toe
    forearm (complete) S58.919
      at elbow level (complete) S58.019
        left S58.012
        partial S58.029
          left S58.022
          right S58.021
        right S58.011
      between elbow and wrist (complete) S58.119
        left S58.112
        partial S58.129
          left S58.122
          right S58.121
        right S58.111
      left S58.912
      partial S58.929
        left S58.922
        right S58.921
      right S58.911
    genital organ(s) (external)
      female (complete) S38.211
        partial S38.212
      male
        penis (complete) S38.221
          partial S38.222
        scrotum (complete) S38.231
          partial S38.232
        testes (complete) S38.231
          partial S38.232
    hand (complete) (wrist level) S68.419
      finger(s) alone — *see* Amputation, traumatic, finger
      left S68.412
      partial S68.429
        left S68.422
        right S68.421
      right S68.411
      thumb alone — *see* Amputation, traumatic, thumb
      transmetacarpal (complete) S68.719
        left S68.712
        partial S68.729
          left S68.722
          right S68.721
        right S68.711
    head
      ear — *see* Amputation, traumatic, ear
      nose (partial) S08.812
        complete S08.811
      part S08.89
      scalp S08.0
    hip (and thigh) (complete) S78.919
      at hip joint (complete) S78.019
        left S78.012

Amputation — *see also* Absence, by site, acquired
— *continued*
  traumatic — *continued*
    hip — *continued*
      at hip joint — *continued*
        partial S78.029
          left S78.022
          right S78.021
        right S78.011
      between hip and knee (complete) S78.119
        left S78.112
        partial S78.129
          left S78.122
          right S78.121
        right S78.111
      left S78.912
      partial S78.929
        left S78.922
        right S78.921
      right S78.911
    labium (majus) (minus) (complete) S38.211
      partial S38.212
    leg (lower) S88.919
      at knee level S88.019
        left S88.012
        partial S88.029
          left S88.022
          right S88.021
        right S88.011
      between knee and ankle S88.119
        left S88.112
        partial S88.129
          left S88.122
          right S88.121
        right S88.111
      left S88.912
      partial S88.929
        left S88.922
        right S88.921
      right S88.911
    nose (partial) S08.812
      complete S08.811
    penis (complete) S38.221
      partial S38.222
    scrotum (complete) S38.231
      partial S38.232
    shoulder — *see* Amputation, traumatic, arm
      at shoulder joint — *see* Amputation,
        traumatic, arm, at shoulder joint
    testes (complete) S38.231
      partial S38.232
    thigh — *see* Amputation, traumatic, hip
    thorax, part of S28.1
      breast — *see* Amputation, traumatic,
        breast
    thumb (complete) (metacarpophalangeal)
      S68.019
      left S68.012
      partial S68.029
        left S68.022
        right S68.021
      right S68.011
      transphalangeal (complete) S68.519
        left S68.512
        partial S68.529
          left S68.522
          right S68.521
        right S68.511
    toe (lesser) S98.139
      great S98.119
        left S98.112
        partial S98.129
          left S98.122
          right S98.121
        right S98.111
      left S98.132
      more than one S98.219
        left S98.212
        partial S98.229
          left S98.222
          right S98.221
        right S98.211
      partial S98.149
        left S98.142
        right S98.141
      right S98.131

Amputation — *see also* Absence, by site, acquired
— *continued*
  traumatic — *continued*
    vulva (complete) S38.211
      partial S38.212
Amputee (bilateral) (old) Z89.9
Amsterdam dwarfism Q87.1
Amusia R48.8
  developmental F80.8
Amyelencephalus, amyelencephaly Q00.0
Amyelia Q06.0
Amygdalitis — *see* Tonsillitis
Amygdalolith J35.8
Amyloid heart (disease) E85 [I43]
Amyloidosis (familial) (generalized) (genetic)
  (hemodialysis-associated) (localized)
  (neuropathic heredofamilial) (non-
  neuropathic heredofamilial) (organ limited)
  (Portuguese) (primary) (secondary systemic)
  E85
  with lung involvement E85 [J99]
  heart E85 [I43]
  liver E85 [K77]
  pulmonary E85 [J99]
  skin (lichen) (macular) E85 [L99]
  specified NEC E85
  subglottic E85 [J99]
Amylopectinosis (brancher enzyme deficiency)
  E74.03
Amylophagia — *see* Pica
Amyoplasia congenita Q79.8
Amyotonia M62.89
  congenita G70.2
Amyotrophia, amyotrophy, amyotrophic G71.8
  congenita Q79.8
  diabetic — *see* Diabetes, amyotrophy
  lateral sclerosis G12.21
  neuralgic G54.5
  spinal progressive G12.21
Anacidity, gastric K31.83
  psychogenic F45.8
Anaerosis of newborn P28.8
Analbuminemia E88.09
Analgesia — *see* Anesthesia
Analphalipoproteinemia E78.6
Anaphylactic
  purpura D69.0
  shock or reaction — *see* Shock, anaphylactic
Anaphylactoid shock or reaction — *see* Shock,
  anaphylactic
Anaphylaxis — *see* Shock, anaphylactic
Anaplasia cervix — *see* Dysplasia, cervix
Anarthria R47.1
Anasarca R60.1
  cardiac — *see* Failure, heart, congestive
  fetus or newborn P83.2
  lung J18.2
  nutritional E43
  pulmonary J18.2
  renal N04.9
Anastomosis
  aneurysmal — *see* Aneurysm
  arteriovenous ruptured brain I60.8
  intestinal K63.8
    complicated NEC K91.89
      involving urinary tract N99.89
  retinal and choroidal vessels (congenital) Q14.8
Anatomical narrow angle H40.0
Ancylostoma, ancylostomiasis (braziliense)
  (caninum) (ceylanicum) (duodenale) B76.0
  Necator americanus B76.1
Andersen's disease (glycogen storage) E74.09
Anderson-Fabry disease E75.21
Andes disease T70.29
Andrews' disease (bacterid) L08.0
Androblastoma (M8630/1)
  benign (M8630/0)
    specified site — *see* Neoplasm, benign
    unspecified site
      female D27.9
      male D29.20

Androblastoma — *continued*
  malignant (M8630/3)
    specified site — *see* Neoplasm, malignant
    unspecified site
      female C56.9
      male C62.90
  specified site — *see* Neoplasm, uncertain
    behavior
  tubular (M8640/0)
    with lipid storage (M8641/0)
      specified site — *see* Neoplasm, benign
      unspecified site
        female D27.9
        male D29.20
    specified site — *see* Neoplasm, benign
    unspecified site
      female D27.9
      male D29.20
  unspecified site
    female D39.10
    male D40.10
Androgen resistance syndrome E34.5
Android pelvis Q74.2
  with disproportion (fetopelvic) O33.3
    causing obstructed labor O65.2
Androphobia F40.290
Anectasis, pulmonary (newborn or fetus) — *see*
  Atelectasis
Anemia (childhood) (essential) (general)
  (hemoglobin deficiency) (infantile) (primary)
  (profound) D64.9
  with
    disorder of
      anaerobic glycolysis D55.2
      pentose phosphate pathway D55.1
    koilonychia D50.9
  achlorhydric D50.8
  achrestic D53.1
  Addison(-Biermer) (pernicious) D51.0
  agranulocytic — *see* Agranulocytosis
  amino-acid-deficiency D53.0
  aplastic D61.9
    congenital D61.4
    constitutional D61.0
    drug-induced D61.1
    due to
      drugs D61.1
      external agents NEC D61.2
      infection D61.2
      radiation D61.2
    idiopathic D61.3
    red cell (pure) D60.9
      chronic D60.0
      congenital D61.4
      specified type NEC D60.8
      transient D60.1
    specified type NEC D61.8
    toxic D61.2
  aregenerative
    congenital D61.4
  asiderotic D50.9
  atypical (primary) D64.9
  Baghdad spring D55.0
  Balantidium coli A07.0
  Biermer's (pernicious) D51.0
  blood loss (chronic) D50.0
    acute D62
  bothriocephalus B70.0 [D63.8]
  brickmaker's B76.9 [D63.8]
  cerebral I67.8
  chlorotic D50.8
  chronic simple D53.9
  chronica congenita aregenerativa D61.4
  combined system disease NEC D51.0 [G32.0]
    due to dietary vitamin B12 deficiency D51.3
      [G32.0]
  complicating pregnancy, childbirth or
    puerperium — *see* Anemia, obstetric
  congenital P61.4
    aplastic D61.4
    due to isoimmunization NOS P55.9
    dyserythropoietic, dyshematopoietic D64.4
    following fetal blood loss P61.3
    Heinz body D58.2
    hereditary hemolytic NOS D58.9
    pernicious D51.0

Anemia — *continued*
  congenital — *continued*
    spherocytic D58.0
  Cooley's (erythroblastic) D56.1
  cytogenic D51.0
  deficiency D53.9
    2, 3 diphosphoglycurate mutase D55.2
    2, 3 PG D55.2
    6 phosphogluconate dehydrogenase D55.1
    6-PGD D55.1
    amino-acid D53.0
    combined B12 and folate D53.1
    enzyme D55.9
      drug-induced (hemolytic) D59.2
      glucose-6-phosphate dehydrogenase
        (G6PD) D55.0
      glycolytic D55.2
      nucleotide metabolism D55.3
      related to hexose monophosphate (HMP)
        shunt pathway NEC D55.1
      specified type NEC D55.8
    erythrocytic glutathione D55.1
    folate D52.9
      dietary D52.0
      drug-induced D52.1
    folic acid D52.9
      dietary D52.0
      drug-induced D52.1
    G SH D55.1
    GGS-R D55.1
    glucose-6-phosphate dehydrogenase D55.0
    glutathione reductase D55.1
    glyceraldehyde phosphate dehydrogenase
      D55.2
    G6PD D55.0
    hexokinase D55.2
    iron D50.9
      secondary to blood loss (chronic) D50.0
    nutritional D53.9
      with
        poor iron absorption D50.8
        specified deficiency NEC D53.8
    phosphofructo-aldolase D55.2
    phosphoglycerate kinase D55.2
    PK D55.2
    protein D53.0
    pyruvate kinase D55.2
    transcobalamin II D51.2
    triose-phosphate isomerase D55.2
    vitamin B12 NOS D51.9
      dietary D51.3
      due to
        intrinsic factor deficiency D51.0
        selective vitamin B12 malabsorption
          with proteinuria D51.1
      pernicious D51.0
      specified type NEC D51.8
  Diamond-Blackfan (congenital hypoplastic)
    D61.4
  dibothriocephalus B70.0 *[D63.8]*
  dimorphic D53.1
  diphasic D53.1
  Diphyllobothrium (Dibothriocephalus) B70.0
    [D63.8]
  drepanocytic — *see* Disease, sicklecell
  due to
    blood loss (chronic) D50.0
      acute D62
    deficiency
      amino-acid D53.0
      copper D53.8
      folate (folic acid) D52.9
        dietary D52.0
        drug-induced D52.1
      molybdenum D53.8
      protein D53.0
      zinc D53.8
    dietary vitamin B12 deficiency D51.3
    disorder of
      glutathione metabolism D55.1
      nucleotide metabolism D55.3
    end stage renal disease N18.0 *[D63.1]*
    enzyme disorder D55.9
    fetal blood loss P61.3
    fish tapeworm (D.latum) infestation B70.0
      [D63.8]

Anemia — *continued*
  due to — *continued*
    hemorrhage (chronic) D50.0
      acute D62
    impaired absorption D50.9
    loss of blood (chronic) D50.0
      acute D62
    myxedema E03.9 *[D63.8]*
    Necator americanus B76.1 *[D63.8]*
    prematurity P61.2
    selective vitamin B12 malabsorption with
      proteinuria D51.1
    transcobalamin II deficiency D51.2
  Dyke-Young type (secondary) (symptomatic)
    D59.8
  dyserythropoietic (congenital) D64.4
  dyshematopoietic (congenital) D64.4
  Egyptian B76.9 *[D63.8]*
  elliptocytosis — *see* Elliptocytosis
  enzyme-deficiency, drug-induced D59.2
  epidemic (*see also* Ancylostomiasis) B76.9
    [D63.8]
  erythroblastic
    familial D56.1
    fetus or newborn (*see also* Disease,
      hemolytic) P55.9
    of childhood D56.1
  erythrocytic glutathione deficiency D55.1
  Faber's (achlorhydric anemia) D50.9
  factitious (self-induced blood letting) D50.0
  familial erythroblastic D56.1
  Fanconi's (congenital pancytopenia) D61.0
  favism D55.0
  fetus or newborn P61.4
    due to
      AB0 (antibodies, isoimmunization,
        maternal/fetal incompatibility)
        P55.1
      Rh (antibodies, isoimmunization,
        maternal/fetal incompatibility)
        P55.0
    following fetal blood loss P61.3
  fish tapeworm (D. latum) infestation B70.0
    [D63.8]
  folate (folic acid) deficiency D52.9
  glucose-6-phosphate dehydrogenase (G6PD)
    deficiency D55.0
  glutathione-reductase deficiency D55.1
  goat's milk D52.0
  granulocytic — *see* Agranulocytosis
  Heinz body, congenital D58.2
  hemolytic D58.9
    acquired D59.9
      with hemoglobinuria NEC D59.6
      autoimmune NEC D59.1
      infectious D59.4
      specified type NEC D59.8
      toxic D59.4
    acute D59.9
      due to enzyme deficiency specified type
        NEC D55.8
      fetus or newborn (*see also* Disease,
        hemolytic) P55.9
      Lederer's D59.1
    autoimmune D59.1
      drug-induced D59.0
      chronic D59.9
        idiopathic D59.9
    cold type (secondary) (symptomatic) D59.1
    congenital (spherocytic) — *see* Spherocytosis
    due to
      cardiac conditions D59.4
      drugs (nonautoimmune) D59.2
        autoimmune D59.0
      enzyme disorder D55.9
        drug-induced D59.2
      presence of shunt or other internal
        prosthetic device D59.4
    familial D58.9
    hereditary D58.9
      due to enzyme disorder D55.9
        specified type NEC D55.8
      specified type NEC D58.8
    idiopathic (chronic) D59.9
    mechanical D59.4
    microangiopathic D59.4

Anemia — *continued*
  hemolytic — *continued*
    nonautoimmune D59.4
      drug-induced D59.2
    nonspherocytic
      congenital or hereditary NEC D55.8
        glucose-6-phosphate dehydrogenase
          deficiency D55.0
        pyruvate kinase deficiency D55.2
      type
        I D55.1
        II D55.2
      type
        I D55.1
        II D55.2
    secondary D59.4
      autoimmune D59.1
    specified (hereditary) type NEC D58.8
    Stransky-Regala type (*see also*
      Hemoglobinopathy) D58.8
    symptomatic D59.4
      autoimmune D59.1
    toxic D59.4
    warm type (secondary) (symptomatic) D59.1
  hemorrhagic (chronic) D50.0
    acute D62
  Herrick's (*see also* Disease, sickle-cell) D57.1
  hexokinase deficiency D55.2
  hookworm B76.9 *[D63.8]*
  hypochromic (idiopathic) (microcytic)
    (normoblastic) D50.9
    due to blood loss (chronic) D50.0
      acute D62
    familial sex-linked D64.0
    pyridoxine-responsive D64.3
    sideroblastic, sex-linked D64.0
  hypoplasia, red blood cells D61.9
    congenital or familial D61.4
  hypoplastic (idiopathic) D61.9
    congenital or familial (of childhood) D61.4
  hypoproliferative (refractive) D61.9
  idiopathic D64.9
    aplastic D61.3
    hemolytic, chronic D59.9
  in
    end stage renal disease N18.0 *[D63.1]*
    failure, renal N18.9 *[D63.1]*
    neoplastic disease (*see also* Neoplasm)
      D49.9 *[D63.0]*
  intertropical (*see also* Ancylostomiasis) B76.9
    [D63.8]
  iron deficiency D50.9
    secondary to blood loss (chronic) D50.0
      acute D62
    specified type NEC D50.8
  Joseph-Diamond-Blackfan (congenital
    hypoplastic) D61.4
  Lederer's (hemolytic) D59.1
  leukoerythroblastic D64.8
  macrocytic D53.9
    nutritional D52.0
    of or complicating pregnancy — *see* Anemia,
      obstetric
    tropical D52.8
  malarial (*see also* Malaria) B54 *[D63.8]*
  malignant (progressive) D51.0
  malnutrition D53.9
  marsh (*see also* Malaria) B54 *[D63.8]*
  Mediterranean D56.9
  megaloblastic D53.1
    combined B12 and folate deficiency D53.1
    hereditary D51.1
    nutritional D52.0
    of or complicating pregnancy — *see* Anemia,
      obstetric
    orotic aciduria D53.0
    refractory D53.1
    specified type NEC D53.1
  megalocytic D53.1
  microcytic (hypochromic) D50.9
    due to blood loss (chronic) D50.0
      acute D62
    familial D56.8
  microelliptopoikilocytic (Rietti-GreppiMicheli)
    D56.9
  miner's B76.9 *[D63.8]*
  myelodysplastic (M9989/1) D46.9

                                                    ©2002 Ingenix, Inc.

Anemia — *continued*
  myelofibrosis D64.8
  myelogenous D64.8
  myelopathic D64.8
  myelophthisic D64.8
  myeloproliferative (M9960/1) D47.7
  newborn P61.4
    posthemorrhagic (fetal) P61.3
  nonspherocytic hemolytic — *see* Anemia,
    hemolytic, nonspherocytic
  normocytic (infectional) D64.9
    due to blood loss (chronic) D50.0
      acute D62
    myelophthisic D61.9
  nutritional (deficiency) D53.9
    with
      poor iron absorption D50.8
      specified deficiency NEC D53.8
    megaloblastic D52.0
  obstetric complicating
    childbirth O99.02
    pregnancy O99.019
      first trimester O99.011
      second trimester O99.012
      third trimester O99.013
    puerperium O99.03
  of prematurity P61.2
  orotaciduric (congenital) (hereditary) D53.0
  osteosclerotic D64.8
  ovalocytosis (hereditary) — *see* Elliptocytosis
  paludal (*see also* Malaria) B54 [D63.8]
  pernicious (congenital) (malignant) (progressive)
    D51.0
    of or complicating pregnancy — *see* Anemia,
      obstetric
  pleochromic D64.8
    of sprue D52.8
  posthemorrhagic (chronic) D50.0
    acute D62
    newborn P61.3
  pressure D64.8
  progressive D64.9
    malignant D51.0
    pernicious D51.0
  protein-deficiency D53.0
  pseudoleukemica infantum D64.8
  puerperal — *see* Anemia, obstetric
  pure red cell D60.9
    congenital D61.4
  pyridoxine-responsive D64.3
  pyruvate kinase deficiency D55.2
  refractory (M9980/1) D46.4
    with
      excess of blasts (M9983/1) D46.2
        with transformation (M9984/1) D46.3
      hemochromatosis (M9982/1) D46.1
      sideroblasts (M9982/1) D46.1
    megaloblastic D53.1
    sideroblastic (M9982/1) D46.1
    sideropenic D50.8
    without sideroblasts (M9981/1) D46.0
  Rietti-Greppi-Micheli D56.9
  scorbutic D53.2
  secondary to
    blood loss (chronic) D50.0
      acute D62
    hemorrhage (chronic) D50.0
      acute D62
  semiplastic D61.8
  septic D64.8
  sickle-cell D57.1
    with crisis D57.0
  sideroblastic D64.3
    hereditary D64.0
    hypochromic, sex-linked D64.0
    pyridoxine-responsive NEC D64.3
    secondary (due to)
      disease D64.1
      drugs and toxins D64.2
    specified type NEC D64.3
  sideropenic (refractory) D50.9
    due to blood loss (chronic) D50.0
      acute D62
  simple chronic D53.9
  specified type NEC D64.8
  spherocytic (hereditary) — *see* Spherocytosis
  splenic D64.8

Anemia — *continued*
  splenomegalic D64.8
  stomatocytosis D58.8
  syphilitic (acquired) (late) A52.79 [D63.8]
  target cell D64.8
  thalassemia D56.9
  thrombocytopenic — *see* Thrombocytopenia
  toxic D61.2
  tropical B76.9 [D63.8]
    macrocytic D52.8
  tuberculous A18.89 [D63.8]
  vegan D51.3
  vitamin
    B6-responsive D64.3
    B12 deficiency (dietary) pernicious D51.0
  von Jaksch's D64.8
  Witts' (achlorhydric anemia) D50.8

Anencephalus, anencephaly Q00.0
  fetus (suspected), affecting management of
    pregnancy O35.0

Anemophobia F40.228

Anergasia — *see* Psychosis, organic

Anesthesia, anesthetic R20.0
  complication or reaction NEC (*see also*
    Complications, anesthesia) T88.5
    due to
      correct substance properly administered
        T88.5
      overdose or wrong substance given
        T41.41
        administered with intent to harm by
          another person T41.43
          self T41.42
        circumstances undetermined T41.44
        general anesthesia (by accident) NEC
          T41.201
          administered with intent to harm
            by
            another person T41.203
            self T41.202
          circumstances undetermined
            T41.204
        gas NEC — *see* category T41.0
        intravenous NEC — *see* category
          T41.1
        local anesthesia NEC — *see* category
          T41.3
        specified anesthetic — *see* Table of
          Drugs and Chemicals
  cornea H18.819
    bilateral H18.813
    left H18.812
    right H18.811
  death from
    correct substance properly administered
      T88.2
    during delivery O74.8
    in pregnancy — *see* Complications,
      anesthesia, in, pregnancy
    overdose or wrong substance given (by
      accident) T41.41
      administered with intent to harm by
        another person T41.43
        self T41.42
      circumstances undetermined T41.44
      general anesthesia (by accident) NEC
        T41.201
        administered with intent to harm by
          another person T41.203
          self T41.202
        circumstances undetermined T41.204
        gas NEC — *see* category T41.0
        intravenous NEC — *see* category T41.1
      local anesthesia NEC — *see* category
        T41.3
      specified anesthetic — *see* Table of Drugs
        and Chemicals
    postpartum, puerperal O89.8
  dissociative F44.6
  functional (hysterical) F44.6
  hyperesthetic, thalamic G93.8
  hysterical F44.6
  local skin lesion R20.0
  sexual (psychogenic) F52.1

Anesthesia, anesthetic — *continued*
  shock (due to) T88.2
    correct substance properly administered
      T88.2
    overdose or wrong substance given (by
      accident) T41.41
      administered with intent to harm by
        another person T41.43
        self T41.42
      circumstances undetermined T41.44
      general anesthesia (by accident) NEC
        T41.201
        administered with intent to harm by
          another person T41.203
          self T41.202
        circumstances undetermined T41.204
        gas NEC — *see* category T41.0
        intravenous NEC — *see* category T41.1
      local anesthesia NEC — *see* category
        T41.3
      specified anesthetic — *see* Table of Drugs
        and Chemicals
  skin R20.0
  testicular N50.9

Anetoderma (maculosum) (of) L90.8
  Jadassohn-Pellizzari L90.2
  Schweniger-Buzzi L90.1

Aneurin deficiency E51.9

Aneurysm (anastomotic) (artery) (cirsoid) (diffuse)
  (false) (fusiform) (multiple) (saccular) I72.9
  abdominal (aorta) I71.4
    dissecting (ruptured) I71.02
    ruptured I71.3
    syphilitic A52.01
  aorta, aortic (nonsyphilitic) I71.9
    abdominal I71.4
      dissecting I71.02
      ruptured I71.3
    arch I71.2
      ruptured I71.1
    arteriosclerotic I71.9
      ruptured I71.8
    ascending I71.2
      ruptured I71.1
    congenital Q25.4
    descending I71.9
      abdominal I71.4
        ruptured I71.3
      ruptured I71.8
      thoracic I71.2
        ruptured I71.1
    dissecting (ruptured) I71.00
      abdominal I71.02
      thoracic I71.01
      thoracoabdominal I71.03
    ruptured I71.8
    sinus, congenital Q25.4
    syphilitic A52.01
    thoracic I71.2
      dissecting I71.01
      ruptured I71.1
    thoracoabdominal I71.6
      dissecting I71.03
      ruptured I71.5
    thorax, thoracic (arch) I71.2
      ruptured I71.1
    transverse I71.2
      ruptured I71.1
    valve (heart) (*see also* Endocarditis, aortic)
      I35.8
  arteriosclerotic I72.9
    cerebral I67.1
      ruptured — *see* Hemorrhage, intracranial,
        subarachnoid
  arteriovenous (congenital) (peripheral) --*see*
    also Malformation, arteriovenous
    acquired I77.0
      brain I67.1
      coronary I25.4
      pulmonary I28.0
    brain Q28.2
      ruptured I60.8
    peripheral — *see* Malformation,
      arteriovenous, peripheral
    precerebral vessels Q28.0

Aneurysm — *continued*
arteriovenous — *see also* Malformation, arteriovenous — *continued*
  specified site NEC — *see also* Malformation, arteriovenous
    acquired I77.0
    traumatic (complication) (early) T14.90
basal — *see* Aneurysm, brain
berry (congenital) (nonruptured) I67.1
  ruptured I60.7
brain I67.1
  arteriosclerotic I67.1
    ruptured — *see* Hemorrhage, intracranial, subarachnoid
  arteriovenous (congenital) (nonruptured) Q28.2
    acquired I67.1
      ruptured I60.8
    ruptured I60.8
  berry (congenital) (nonruptured) I67.1
    ruptured (see also Hemorrhage, intracranial, subarachnoid) I60.7
  congenital Q28.3
    ruptured I60.7
  meninges I67.1
    ruptured I60.8
  miliary (congenital) (nonruptured) I67.1
    ruptured (see also Hemorrhage, intracranial, subarachnoid) I60.7
  mycotic I33.0
    ruptured — *see* Hemorrhage, intracranial, subarachnoid
  syphilitic (hemorrhage) A52.05
cardiac (false) (see also Aneurysm, heart) I25.3
carotid artery (common) (external) I72.0
  internal (intracranial) I67.1
    extracranial portion I72.0
    ruptured into brain I60.0
  syphilitic A52.09
    intracranial A52.05
cavernous sinus I67.1
  arteriovenous (congenital) (nonruptured) Q28.3
    ruptured I60.8
central nervous system, syphilitic A52.05
cerebral — *see* Aneurysm, brain
chest — *see* Aneurysm, thorax
circle of Willis I67.1
  congenital Q28.3
    ruptured I60.6
  ruptured I60.6
common iliac artery I72.3
congenital (peripheral) Q27.8
  brain Q28.3
    ruptured — *see* Hemorrhage, intracranial, subarachnoid
  coronary Q24.5
  digestive system Q27.8
  lower limb Q27.8
  pulmonary Q25.7
  retina Q14.1
  specified site NEC Q27.8
  upper limb Q27.8
conjunctiva — *see* Abnormality, conjunctiva, vascular
conus arteriosus — *see* Aneurysm, heart
coronary (arteriosclerotic) (artery) I25.4
  arteriovenous, congenital Q24.5
  congenital Q24.5
  ruptured — *see* Infarct, myocardium
  syphilitic A52.06
  vein I25.8
cylindroid (aorta) I71.9
  ruptured I71.8
  syphilitic A52.01
dissecting I72.9
  aorta (ruptured) I71.00
    abdominal I71.02
    thoracic I71.01
    thoracoabdominal I71.03
  syphilitic A52.01
ductus arteriosus Q25.0
endocardial, infective (any valve) I33.0
femoral (artery) (ruptured) I72.4
heart (wall) (chronic or with a stated duration of over 4 weeks) I25.3

Aneurysm — *continued*
heart — *continued*
  acute or with a stated duration of 4 weeks or less I21.9
  valve — *see* Endocarditis
iliac (common) (artery) (ruptured) I72.3
infective I72.9
  endocardial (any valve) I33.0
innominate (nonsyphilitic) I72.8
  syphilitic A52.09
interauricular septum — *see* Aneurysm, heart
interventricular septum — *see* Aneurysm, heart
intrathoracic (nonsyphilitic) I71.2
  ruptured I71.1
  syphilitic A52.01
lower limb I72.4
lung (pulmonary artery) I28.1
mediastinal (nonsyphilitic) I72.8
  syphilitic A52.09
miliary (congenital) I67.1
  ruptured — *see* Hemorrhage, intracerebral, subarachnoid, intracranial
mitral (heart) (valve) I34.8
mural — *see* Aneurysm, heart
mycotic I72.9
  endocardial (any valve) I33.0
  ruptured, brain — *see* Hemorrhage, intracerebral, subarachnoid
myocardium — *see* Aneurysm, heart
neck I72.0
patent ductus arteriosus Q25.0
peripheral NEC I72.8
  congenital Q27.8
    digestive system Q27.8
    lower limb Q27.8
    specified site NEC Q27.8
    upper limb Q27.8
popliteal (artery) (ruptured) I72.4
precerebral, congenital (nonruptured) Q28.1
pulmonary I28.1
  arteriovenous Q25.7
    acquired I28.0
  syphilitic A52.09
  valve (heart) — *see* Endocarditis, pulmonary
racemose (peripheral) I72.9
  congenital — *see* Aneurysm, congenital
radial I72.1
Rasmussen's NEC A15.0
renal (artery) I72.2
retina — *see also* Disorder, retina, microaneurysms
  congenital Q14.1
  diabetic — *see* Diabetes, microaneurysms, retinal
sinus of Valsalva Q25.4
spinal (cord) I72.8
  syphilitic (hemorrhage) A52.09
splenic I72.8
subclavian (artery) (ruptured) I72.8
  syphilitic A52.09
syphilitic (aorta) A52.01
  central nervous system A52.05
  congenital (late) A50.54 [I79.0]
  spine, spinal A52.09
thoracoabdominal (aorta) I71.6
  dissecting I71.03
  ruptured I71.5
  syphilitic A52.01
thorax, thoracic (aorta) (arch) (nonsyphilitic) I71.2
  dissecting (ruptured) I71.01
  ruptured I71.1
  syphilitic A52.01
traumatic (complication) (early), specified site — *see* Injury, blood vessel
tricuspid (heart) (valve) I07.8
ulnar I72.1
upper limb (ruptured) I72.1
valve, valvular — *see* Endocarditis
venous — *see also* Varix I86.8
  congenital Q27.8
    digestive system Q27.8
    lower limb Q27.8
    specified site NEC Q27.8
    upper limb Q27.8
ventricle — *see* Aneurysm, heart
Anger R45.4

Angiectasis, angiectopia I99.8
Angiitis I77.6
  allergic granulomatous M30.1
  hypersensitivity M31.0
  necrotizing M31.9
    specified NEC M31.8
  nervous system, granulomatous I67.7
Angina (attack) (cardiac) (chest) (heart) (pectoris) (syndrome) (vasomotor) I20.9
  with documented spasm I20.1
    in atherosclerotic heart disease I25.13
  abdominal K55.1
  accelerated — *see* Angina, unstable
  agranulocytic — *see* Agranulocytosis
  angiospastic — *see* Angina, with documented spasm
  aphthous B08.5
  crescendo — *see* Angina, unstable
  croupous J05.0
  cruris I70.9
  de novo effort — *see* Angina, unstable
  decubitus I20.0
    in atherosclerotic heart disease I25.11
  diphtheritic, membranous A36.0
  exudative, chronic J37.0
  following acute myocardial infarction I23.7
  gangrenous diphtheritic A36.0
  in atherosclerotic heart disease I25.11
  initial — *see* Angina, unstable
  intestinal K55.1
  Ludovici K12.2
  Ludwig's K12.2
  malignant diphtheritic A36.0
  membranous J05.0
    diphtheritic A36.0
    Vincent's A69.1
  mesenteric K55.1
  monocytic — *see* Mononucleosis, infectious
  of effort — *see* Angina, specified NEC
  phlegmonous J36
    diphtheritic A36.0
  post-infarctional I23.7
  pre-infarctional — *see* Angina, unstable
  Prinzmetal — *see* Angina, with documented spasm
  progressive — *see* Angina, unstable
  pseudomembranous A69.1
  pultaceous, diphtheritic A36.0
  septic J02.0
  spasm-induced — *see* Angina, with documented spasm
  specified NEC I20.8
    in atherosclerotic heart disease I25.19
  stable I20.9
    in atherosclerotic heart disease I25.11
  stenocardia — *see* Angina, specified NEC
  stridulous, diphtheritic A36.2
  tonsil J36
  trachealis J05.0
  unstable I20.0
    in atherosclerotic heart disease I25.12
  variant — *see* Angina, with documented spasm
  Vincent's A69.1
  worsening effort — *see* Angina, unstable
Angioblastoma (M9161/1) — *see* Neoplasm, connective tissue, uncertain behavior
Angiocholecystitis — *see* Cholecystitis, acute
Angiocholitis — *see* Cholecystitis, acute
Angiodysgenesis spinalis G95.19
Angiodysplasia (cecum) (colon) (intestine) K55.20
  with bleeding K55.21
  stomach K31.81
    with bleeding K31.82
Angioedema (allergic) (any site) (with urticaria) T78.3
  hereditary D84.1
Angioendothelioma (M9130/1) — *see* Neoplasm, uncertain behavior
  benign (M9130/0) D18.00
    intra-abdominal D18.03
    intracranial D18.02
    skin D18.01
    specified site NEC D18.09
  bone (M9130/3) — *see* Neoplasm, bone, malignant

©2002 Ingenix, Inc.

Angioendothelioma — see Neoplasm, uncertain
  behavior — continued
    Ewing's (M9260/3) — see Neoplasm, bone,
      malignant
Angioendotheliomatosis (M9712/3) C85.70
Angiofibroma (M9160/0) — see also Neoplasm,
  benign
  juvenile (M9160/0)
    specified site — see Neoplasm, benign
    unspecified site D10.6
Angiohemophilia (A) (B) D68.0
Angioid streaks (choroid) (macula) (retina)
  H35.33
Angiokeratoma (M9141/0) — see Neoplasm, skin,
  benign
  corporis diffusum E75.21
Angioleiomyoma (M8894/0) — see Neoplasm,
  connective tissue, benign
Angiolipoma (M8861/0) — see also Lipoma
  infiltrating (M8856/0) — see Lipoma
Angioma (M9120/0) — see also Hemangioma, by
  site
  capillary I78.1
  hemorrhagicum hereditaria I78.0
  intra-abdominal D18.03
  intracranial D18.02
  malignant (M9120/3) — see Neoplasm,
    connective tissue, malignant
  placenta — see Abnormal, placenta, specified
    type NEC
  plexiform (M9131/0) D18.00
    intra-abdominal D18.03
    intracranial D18.02
    skin D18.01
    specified site NEC D18.09
  senile I78.1
  serpiginosum L81.7
  skin D18.01
  specified site NEC D18.09
  spider I78.1
  stellate I78.1
Angiomatosis Q82.8
  bacillary A79.8
  encephalotrigeminal Q85.8
  hemorrhagic familial I78.0
  hereditary familial I78.0
  liver K76.4
Angiomyolipoma (M8860/0) — see Lipoma
Angiomyoliposarcoma (M8860/3) — see
  Neoplasm, connective tissue, malignant
Angiomyoma (M8894/0) — see Neoplasm,
  connective tissue, benign
Angiomyosarcoma (M8894/3) — see Neoplasm,
  connective tissue, malignant
Angiomyxoma (M8841/1) — see Neoplasm,
  connective tissue, uncertain behavior
Angioneurosis F45.8
Angioneurotic edema (allergic) (any site) (with
    urticaria) T78.3
  hereditary D84.1
Angiopathia, angiopathy I99.9
  cerebral I67.9
    amyloid E85 [I68.1]
  diabetic (peripheral) — see Diabetes,
    angiopathy
  peripheral I73.9
    diabetic — see Diabetes, angiopathy
    specified type NEC I73.8
  retinae syphilitica A52.05
  retinalis (juvenilis)
    diabetic — see Diabetes, retinopathy
    proliferative — see Retinopathy, proliferative
Angiosarcoma (M9120/3) — see also Neoplasm,
  connective tissue, malignant
  liver C22.3
Angiosclerosis — see Arteriosclerosis
Angiospasm (peripheral) (traumatic) (vessel) I73.9
  brachial plexus G54.0
  cerebral G45.9
  cervical plexus G54.2
  nerve
    arm — see Mononeuropathy, upper limb
      axillary G54.0

Angiospasm — continued
  nerve — continued
    arm — see Mononeuropathy, upper limb —
      continued
        median — see Lesion, nerve, median
        ulnar — see Lesion, nerve, ulnar
    axillary G54.0
    leg — see Mononeuropathy, lower limb
    median — see Lesion, nerve, median
    plantar — see Lesion, nerve, plantar
    ulnar — see Lesion, nerve, ulnar
Angiospastic disease or edema I73.9
Angiostrongyliasis
  due to
    Parastrongylus
      cantonensis B83.2
      costaricensis B81.3
    intestinal B81.3
Anguillulosis — see Strongyloidiasis
Angulation
  cecum — see Obstruction, intestine
  coccyx (acquired) — see also category M43.8
    congenital NEC Q76.49
  femur (acquired) — see also Deformity, limb,
    specified type NEC, thigh
    congenital Q74.2
  intestine (large) (small) — see Obstruction,
    intestine
  sacrum (acquired) — see also category M43.8
    congenital NEC Q76.49
  sigmoid (flexure) — see Obstruction, intestine
  spine — see Dorsopathy, deforming, specified
    NEC
  tibia (acquired) — see also Deformity, limb,
    specified type NEC, lower leg
    congenital Q74.2
  ureter N13.5
    with infection N13.6
  wrist (acquired) — see also Deformity, limb,
    specified type NEC, forearm
    congenital Q74.0
Angulus infectiosus (lips) K13.0
Anhedonia (sexual) F52.0
Anhidrosis L74.4
Anhydration, anhydremia E86.0
  with
    hypernatremia E87.0
    hyponatremia E87.1
Anhydremia E86.0
  with
    hypernatremia E87.0
    hyponatremia E87.1
Anidrosis L74.4
Aniridia (congenital) Q13.1
Anisakiasis (infection) (infestation) B81.0
Anisakis larvae infestation B81.0
Aniseikonia H52.32
Anisocoria (pupil) H57.09
  congenital Q13.2
Anisocytosis R71.8
Anisometropia (congenital) H52.31
Ankle — see condition
Ankyloblepharon (eyelid) (acquired) — see also
  Blepharophimosis
  filiforme (adnatum) (congenital) Q10.3
  total Q10.3
Ankyloglossia Q38.1
Ankylosis (fibrous) (osseous) (joint) M24.60
  ankle M24.673
    left M24.672
    right M24.671
  cricoarytenoid (cartilage) (joint) (larynx) J38.7
  dental K03.5
  ear ossicles H74.319
    bilateral H74.313
    left H74.312
    right H74.311
  elbow M24.629
    left M24.622
    right M24.621
  foot M24.676
    left M24.675
    right M24.674

Ankylosis — continued
  hand M24.649
    left M24.642
    right M24.641
  hip M24.659
    left M24.652
    right M24.651
  incostapedial joint (infectional) — see
    Ankylosis, ear ossicles
  jaw (temporomandibular) M26.61
  knee M24.669
    left M24.662
    right M24.661
  lumbosacral (joint) M43.27
  postoperative (status) Z98.1
  produced by surgical fusion Z98.1
  sacro-iliac (joint) M43.28
  shoulder M24.619
    left M24.612
    right M24.611
  spine (joint) — see also Fusion, spine
    spondylitic — see Spondylitis, ankylosing
  surgical Z98.1
  temporomandibular M26.61
  tooth, teeth (hard tissues) K03.5
  wrist M24.639
    left M24.632
    right M24.631
Ankylostoma — see Ancylostoma
Ankylostomiasis — see Ancylostomiasis
Ankylurethria — see Stricture, urethra
Annular — see also condition
  detachment, cervix N88.8
  organ or site, congenital NEC — see Distortion
  pancreas (congenital) Q45.1
Anodontia (complete) (partial) (vera) K00.0
  with abnormal spacing M26.3
  acquired K08.1
    causing malocclusion M26.3
Anomaly, anomalous (congenital) (unspecified
    type) Q89.9
  abdominal wall NEC Q79.59
  acoustic nerve Q07.8
  adrenal (gland) Q89.1
  Alder (-Reilly) (leukocyte granulation) D72.0
  alimentary tract Q45.9
    upper Q40.9
  alveolar M26.70
    hyperplasia M26.79
      mandibular M26.72
      maxillary M26.71
    hypoplasia M26.79
      mandibular M26.74
      maxillary M26.73
    ridge (process) M26.79
    specified NEC M26.79
  ankle (joint) Q74.2
  anus Q43.9
  aorta (arch) NEC Q25.4
    coarctation (preductal) (postductal) Q25.1
  aortic cusp or valve Q23.9
  appendix Q43.8
  apple peel syndrome Q41.1
  aqueduct of Sylvius Q03.0
    with spina bifida — see Spina bifida, with
      hydrocephalus
  arm Q74.0
  arteriovenous NEC
    coronary Q24.5
  artery (peripheral) Q27.9
    basilar NEC Q28.1
    cerebral Q28.3
    coronary Q24.5
    digestive system Q27.8
    eye Q15.8
    great Q25.9
      specified NEC Q25.8
    lower limb Q27.8
    peripheral Q27.9
      specified NEC Q27.8
    pulmonary NEC Q25.7
    renal Q27.2
    retina Q14.1
    specified site NEC Q27.8
    subclavian Q27.8
    umbilical Q27.0

Anomaly, anomalous — *continued*
  artery — *continued*
    upper limb Q27.8
    vertebral NEC Q28.1
  aryteno-epiglottic folds Q31.8
  atrial
    bands or folds Q20.8
    septa Q21.1
  atrioventricular
    excitation I45.6
    septum Q21.0
  auditory canal Q17.8
  auricle
    ear Q17.8
      causing impairment of hearing Q16.9
    heart Q20.8
  Axenfeld's Q15.0
  back Q89.9
  band
    atrial Q20.8
    heart Q24.8
    ventricular Q24.8
  Bartholin's duct Q38.4
  biliary duct or passage Q44.5
  bladder Q64.70
    absence Q64.5
    diverticulum Q64.6
    exstrophy Q64.10
      cloacal Q64.12
      extroversion Q64.19
      specified type NEC Q64.19
      supravesical fissure Q64.11
    neck obstruction Q64.31
    specified type NEC Q64.79
  bone Q79.9
    arm Q74.0
    face Q75.9
    leg Q74.2
    pelvic girdle Q74.2
    shoulder girdle Q74.0
    skull Q75.9
      with
        anencephaly Q00.0
        encephalocele — *see* Encephalocele
        hydrocephalus Q03.9
          with spina bifida — *see* Spina
            bifida, by site, with
            hydrocephalus
        microcephaly Q02
  brain (multiple) Q04.9
    vessel Q28.3
  breast Q83.9
  broad ligament Q50.6
  bronchus Q32.8
  bulbus cordis Q21.9
  bursa Q79.9
  canal of Nuck Q52.4
  canthus Q10.3
  capillary Q27.9
  cardiac Q24.9
    chambers Q20.9
      specified NEC Q20.8
    septal closure Q21.9
      specified NEC Q21.8
    valve NEC Q24.8
      pulmonary Q22.3
  cardiovascular system Q28.8
  carpus Q74.0
  caruncle, lacrimal Q10.6
  cascade stomach Q40.2
  cauda equina Q06.3
  cecum Q43.9
  cerebral Q04.9
    vessels Q28.3
  cervix Q51.9
    in pregnancy or childbirth — *see* category
      O34.4
      causing obstructed labor O65.5
  Chédiak-Higashi(-Steinbrinck) (congenital
    gigantism of peroxidase granules)
    E70.330
  cheek Q18.9
  chest wall Q67.8
    bones Q76.9
  chin Q18.9
  chordae tendineae Q24.8

Anomaly, anomalous — *continued*
  choroid Q14.3
    plexus Q07.8
  chromosomes, chromosomal Q99.9
    D(1) — *see* condition, chromosome 13
    E(3) — *see* condition, chromosome 18
    G — *see* condition, chromosome 21
    sex
      female phenotype Q97.8
      gonadal dysgenesis (pure) Q56.1
      Klinefelter's Q98.4
      male phenotype Q98.9
      Turner's Q96.9
    specified NEC Q99.8
  cilia Q10.3
  circulatory system Q28.9
  clavicle Q74.0
  clitoris Q52.6
  coccyx Q76.49
  colon Q43.9
  common duct Q44.5
  communication
    coronary artery Q24.5
    left ventricle with right atrium Q21.0
  concha (ear) Q17.3
  connection
    portal vein Q26.5
    pulmonary venous Q26.4
      partial Q26.3
      total Q26.2
    renal artery with kidney Q27.2
  cornea (shape) Q13.4
  coronary artery or vein Q24.5
  cranium — *see* Anomaly, skull
  cricoid cartilage Q31.8
  cystic duct Q44.5
  dental
    alveolar — *see* Anomaly, alveolar
    arch relationship M26.2
  dentofacial M26.9
    alveolar — *see* Anomaly, alveolar
    dental arch relationship M26.2
    functional M26.5
    jaw-cranial base relationship M26.10
      asymmetry M26.12
        maxillary M26.11
      specified type NEC M26.19
    jaw size M26.00
      macrogenia M26.05
      mandibular
        hyperplasia M26.03
        hypoplasia M26.04
      maxillary
        hyperplasia M26.01
        hypoplasia M26.02
      microgenia M26.06
      specified type NEC M26.09
    malocclusion M26.4
      dental arch relationship M26.2
      jaw-cranial base relationship — *see*
        Anomaly, dentofacial, jaw-cranial
        base relationship
      jaw size — *see* Anomaly, dentofacial, jaw
        size
    specified type NEC M26.8
    temporomandibular joint M26.60
      adhesions M26.61
      ankylosis M26.61
      arthralgia M26.62
      articular disc M26.63
      specified type NEC M26.69
    tooth position M26.3
  dermatoglyphic Q82.8
  diaphragm (apertures) NEC Q79.1
  digestive organ(s) or tract Q45.9
    lower Q43.9
    upper Q40.9
  distribution, coronary artery Q24.5
  ductus
    arteriosus Q25.0
    botalli Q25.0
  duodenum Q43.9
  dura (brain) Q04.9
    spinal cord Q06.9
  ear (external) Q17.9
    causing impairment of hearing Q16.0
    inner Q16.5

Anomaly, anomalous — *continued*
  ear — *continued*
    middle (causing impairment of hearing)
      Q16.4
    ossicles Q16.3
  Ebstein's (heart) (tricuspid valve) Q22.5
  ectodermal Q82.9
  Eisenmenger's (ventricular septal defect) Q21.0
  ejaculatory duct Q55.4
  elbow Q74.0
  endocrine gland NEC Q89.2
  epididymis Q55.4
  epiglottis Q31.8
  esophagus Q39.9
  eustachian tube Q17.8
  eye Q15.9
    anterior segment Q13.9
    posterior segment Q14.9
    ptosis (eyelid) Q10.0
    specified NEC Q15.8
  eyebrow Q18.8
  eyelid Q10.3
    ptosis Q10.0
  face Q18.9
    bone(s) Q75.9
  fallopian tube Q50.6
  fascia Q79.9
  femur NEC Q74.2
  fibula NEC Q74.2
  finger Q74.0
  fixation, intestine Q43.3
  flexion (joint) NOS Q74.9
    hip or thigh Q65.8
  foot NEC Q74.2
    varus (congenital) Q66.3
  foramen
    Botalli Q21.1
    ovale Q21.1
  forearm Q74.0
  forehead Q75.8
  form, teeth K00.2
  fovea centralis Q14.1
  frontal bone — *see* Anomaly, skull
  gallbladder (position) (shape) (size) Q44.1
  Gartner's duct Q50.6
  gastrointestinal tract Q45.9
  genitalia, genital organ(s) or system
    female Q52.9
      external Q52.70
      internal NOS Q52.9
    male Q55.9
      hydrocele P83.5
      specified NEC Q55.8
  genitourinary NEC
    female Q52.9
    male Q55.9
  Gerbode Q21.0
  glottis Q31.8
  granulation or granulocyte, genetic
    (constitutional) (leukocyte) D72.0
  gum Q38.6
  gyri Q07.9
  hair Q84.2
  hand Q74.0
  hard tissue formation in pulp K04.3
  head — *see* Anomaly, skull
  heart Q24.9
    auricle Q20.8
    bands or folds Q24.8
    fibroelastosis cordis I42.4
    obstructive NEC Q22.6
    patent ductus arteriosus (Botalli) Q25.0
    septum Q21.9
      auricular Q21.1
      interatrial Q21.1
      interventricular Q21.0
        with pulmonary stenosis or atresia,
          dextraposition of aorta and
          hypertrophy of right ventricle
          Q21.3
      specified NEC Q21.8
      ventricular Q21.0
        with pulmonary stenosis or atresia,
          dextraposition of aorta and
          hypertrophy of right ventricle
          Q21.3

    ©2002 Ingenix, Inc.

Anomaly, anomalous — *continued*
 heart — *continued*
  tetralogy of Fallot Q21.3
  valve NEC Q24.8
   aortic
    bicuspid valve Q23.1
    insufficiency Q23.1
    stenosis Q23.0
     subaortic Q24.2
   mitral
    insufficiency Q23.3
    stenosis Q23.2
   pulmonary Q22.3
    atresia Q22.0
    insufficiency Q22.2
    stenosis Q22.1
     infundibular Q24.3
     subvalvular Q24.3
   tricuspid
    atresia Q22.4
    stenosis Q22.4
  ventricle Q20.8
 heel NEC Q74.2
 Hegglin's D72.0
 hemianencephaly Q00.0
 hemicephaly Q00.0
 hemicrania Q00.0
 hepatic duct Q44.5
 hip NEC Q74.2
 hourglass stomach Q40.2
 humerus Q74.0
 hydatid of Morgagni
  female Q52.8
  male Q55.4
 hymen Q52.4
 hypersegmentation of neutrophils, hereditary D72.0
 hypophyseal Q89.2
 ileocecal (coil) (valve) Q43.9
 ileum Q43.9
 ilium NEC Q74.2
 integument Q84.9
  specified NEC Q84.8
 intervertebral cartilage or disc Q76.49
 intestine (large) (small) Q43.9
  with anomalous adhesions, fixation or malrotation Q43.3
 iris Q13.2
 ischium NEC Q74.2
 jaw — *see* Anomaly, dentofacial
  alveolar — *see* Anomaly, alveolar
 jaw-cranial base relationship — *see* Anomaly, dentofacial, jaw-cranial base relationship
 jejunum Q43.8
 joint Q74.9
  specified NEC Q74.8
 Jordan's D72.0
 kidney(s) (calyx) (pelvis) Q63.9
  artery Q27.2
  specified NEC Q63.8
 Klippel-Feil (brevicollis) Q76.1
 knee Q74.1
 labium (majus) (minus) Q52.70
 labyrinth, membranous Q16.5
 lacrimal apparatus or duct Q10.6
 larynx, laryngeal (muscle) Q31.9
  web(bed) Q31.0
 lens Q12.9
 leucocytes, genetic D72.0
  granulation (constitutional) D72.0
 lid (fold) Q10.3
 ligament Q79.9
  broad Q50.6
  round Q52.8
 limb Q74.9
  lower NEC Q74.2
   reduction deformity — *see* Defect, reduction, lower limb
  upper Q74.0
 lip Q38.0
 liver Q44.7
  duct Q44.5
 lower limb NEC Q74.2
 lumbosacral (joint) (region) Q76.49
  kyphosis — *see* Kyphosis, congenital
  lordosis — *see* Lordosis, congenital
 lung (fissure) (lobe) Q33.9

Anomaly, anomalous — *continued*
 mandible — *see* Anomaly, dentofacial
 maxilla — *see* Anomaly, dentofacial
 May (-Hegglin) D72.0
 meatus urinarius NEC Q64.79
 meningeal bands or folds Q07.9
  constriction of Q07.8
  spinal Q06.9
 meninges Q07.9
  cerebral Q04.8
  spinal Q06.9
 meningocele Q05.9
 mesentery Q45.9
 metacarpus Q74.0
 metatarsus NEC Q74.2
 middle ear Q16.4
  ossicles Q16.3
 mitral (leaflets) (valve) Q23.9
  insufficiency Q23.3
  specified NEC Q23.8
  stenosis Q23.2
 mouth Q38.6
 multiple NEC Q89.7
 muscle Q79.9
  eyelid Q10.3
 musculoskeletal system, except limbs Q79.9
 myocardium Q24.8
 nail Q84.6
 narrowness, eyelid Q10.3
 nasal sinus (wall) Q30.9
 neck (any part) Q18.9
 nerve Q07.9
  acoustic Q07.8
  optic Q07.9
 nervous system (central) Q07.9
 nipple Q83.9
 nose, nasal (bones) (cartilage) (septum) (sinus) Q30.9
  specified NEC Q30.8
 ocular muscle Q15.8
 omphalomesenteric duct Q43.0
 opening, pulmonary veins Q26.4
 optic
  disc Q14.2
  nerve Q07.8
 opticociliary vessels Q13.2
 orbit (eye) Q10.7
 organ Q89.9
  of Corti Q16.5
 origin
  artery
   innominate Q25.8
   pulmonary Q25.7
   renal Q27.2
   subclavian Q25.8
 osseous meatus (ear) Q16.1
 ovary Q50.39
 oviduct Q50.6
 palate (hard) (soft) NEC Q38.5
 pancreas or pancreatic duct Q45.3
 papillary muscles Q24.8
 parathyroid gland Q89.2
 paraurethral ducts Q64.79
 parotid (gland) Q38.4
 patella Q74.1
 Pelger-Huët (hereditary hyposegmentation) D72.0
 pelvic girdle NEC Q74.2
 pelvis (bony) NEC Q74.2
  rachitic E64.3
 penis (glans) Q55.69
 pericardium Q24.8
 peripheral vascular system Q27.9
 Peter's Q13.4
 pharynx Q38.8
 pigmentation L81.9
  congenital Q82.8
 pituitary (gland) Q89.2
 pleural (folds) Q34.0
 portal vein Q26.5
  connection Q26.5
 position, tooth, teeth M26.3
 precerebral vessel Q28.1
 prepuce Q55.69
 prostate Q55.4
 pulmonary Q33.9
  artery NEC Q25.7

Anomaly, anomalous — *continued*
 pulmonary — *continued*
  valve Q22.3
   atresia Q22.0
   insufficiency Q22.2
   specified type NEC Q22.2
   stenosis Q22.1
    infundibular Q24.3
    subvalvular Q24.3
  venous connection Q26.4
   partial Q26.3
   total Q26.2
 pupil Q13.2
  function H57.00
   anisocoria H57.02
   Argyll Robertson pupil H57.01
   miosis H57.03
   mydriasis H57.04
   specified type NEC H57.09
   tonic pupil H57.059
    bilateral H57.053
    left H57.052
    right H57.051
 pylorus Q40.3
 radius Q74.0
 rectum Q43.9
 reduction (extremity) (limb)
  femur (longitudinal) — *see* Defect, reduction, lower limb, longitudinal, femur
  fibula (longitudinal) — *see* Defect, reduction, lower limb, longitudinal, fibula
  lower limb — *see* Defect, reduction, lower limb
  radius (longitudinal) — *see* Defect, reduction, upper limb, longitudinal, radius
  tibia (longitudinal) — *see* Defect, reduction, lower limb, longitudinal, tibia
  ulna (longitudinal) — *see* Defect, reduction, upper limb, longitudinal, ulna
  upper limb — *see* Defect, reduction, upper limb
 refraction — *see* Disorder, refraction
 renal Q63.9
  artery Q27.2
  pelvis Q63.9
   specified NEC Q63.8
 respiratory system Q34.9
  specified NEC Q34.8
 retina Q14.1
 rib Q76.6
  cervical Q76.5
 Rieger's Q13.81
 rotation — *see* Malrotation
  hip or thigh Q65.8
 round ligament Q52.8
 sacroiliac (joint) NEC Q74.2
 sacrum NEC Q76.49
  kyphosis — *see* Kyphosis, congenital
  lordosis — *see* Lordosis, congenital
 saddle nose, syphilitic A50.57
 salivary duct or gland Q38.4
 scapula Q74.0
 scrotum — *see* Malformation, testis and scrotum
 sebaceous gland Q82.9
 seminal vesicles Q55.4
 sense organs NEC Q07.8
 sex chromosomes NEC — *see also* Anomaly, chromosomes
  female phenotype Q97.8
  male phenotype Q98.9
 shoulder (girdle) (joint) Q74.0
 sigmoid (flexure) Q43.9
 simian crease Q82.8
 sinus of Valsalva Q25.4
 skeleton generalized Q78.9
 skin (appendage) Q82.9
 skull Q75.9
  with
   anencephaly Q00.0
   encephalocele — *see* Encephalocele
   hydrocephalus Q03.9
    with spina bifida — *see* Spina bifida, by site, with hydrocephalus
   microcephaly Q02
 specified organ or site NEC Q89.8

Anomaly, anomalous — *continued*
  spermatic cord Q55.4
  spine, spinal NEC Q76.49
    column NEC Q76.49
      kyphosis — *see* Kyphosis, congenital
      lordosis — *see* Lordosis, congenital
    cord Q06.9
    nerve root Q07.8
  spleen Q89.09
    agenesis Q89.01
  stenonian duct Q38.4
  sternum NEC Q76.7
  stomach Q40.3
  submaxillary gland Q38.4
  tarsus NEC Q74.2
  tendon Q79.9
  testis — *see* Malformation, testis and scrotum
  thigh NEC Q74.2
  thorax (wall) Q67.8
    bony Q76.9
  throat Q38.8
  thumb Q74.0
  thymus gland Q89.2
  thyroid (gland) Q89.2
    cartilage Q31.8
  tibia NEC Q74.2
    saber A50.56
  toe Q74.2
  tongue Q38.3
  tooth, teeth K00.9
    eruption K00.6
    position M26.3
    spacing M26.3
  trachea (cartilage) Q32.1
  tragus Q17.9
  tricuspid (leaflet) (valve) Q22.9
    atresia or stenosis Q22.4
    Ebstein's Q22.5
  Uhl's (hypoplasia of myocardium, right ventricle) Q24.8
  ulna Q74.0
  umbilical artery Q27.0
  union
    cricoid cartilage and thyroid cartilage Q31.8
    thyroid cartilage and hyoid bone Q31.8
    trachea with larynx Q31.8
  upper limb Q74.0
  urachus Q64.4
  ureter Q62.8
    obstructive NEC Q62.39
      cecoureterocele Q62.32
      orthotopic ureterocele Q62.31
  urethra Q64.70
    absence Q64.5
    double Q64.74
    fistula to rectum Q64.73
    obstructive Q64.39
      stricture Q64.32
    prolapse Q64.71
    specified type NEC Q64.79
  urinary tract Q64.9
  uterus Q51.9
    with only one functioning horn Q51.8
    in pregnancy or childbirth NEC — *see* category O34.0
      causing obstructed labor O65.5
  uvula Q38.5
  vagina Q52.4
  valleculae Q31.8
  valve (heart) NEC Q24.8
    coronary sinus Q24.5
    inferior vena cava Q24.8
    pulmonary Q22.3
    sinus coronario Q24.5
    venae cavae inferioris Q24.8
  vas deferens Q55.4
  vascular Q27.9
    brain Q28.3
    ring Q25.4
  vein(s) (peripheral) Q27.9
    brain Q28.3
    cerebral Q28.3
    coronary Q24.5
    great Q26.9
      specified NEC Q26.8
  vena cava (inferior) (superior) Q26.9
  venous return Q26.8

Anomaly, anomalous — *continued*
  ventricular
    bands or folds Q24.8
    septa Q21.0
  vertebra Q76.49
    kyphosis — *see* Kyphosis, congenital
    lordosis — *see* Lordosis, congenital
  vesicourethral orifice Q64.79
  vessel(s) Q27.9
    optic papilla Q14.2
    precerebral Q28.1
  vitelline duct Q43.0
  vitreous body or humor Q14.0
  vulva Q52.70
  wrist (joint) Q74.0
Anomia R48.8
Anonychia (congenital) Q84.3
  acquired L60.8
Anophthalmos, anophthalmus (congenital) (globe) Q11.1
  acquired Z90.01
Anorchia, anorchism, anorchidism Q55.0
Anorexia R63.0
  hysterical F44.89
  nervosa F50.00
    atypical F50.9
    binge-eating type F50.2
      with purging F50.02
    restricting type F50.01
Anorgasmy, psychogenic (female) F52.31
  male F52.32
Anosmia R43.0
  hysterical F44.6
  postinfectional J39.8
Anosognosia R41.89
Anosteoplasia Q78.9
Anovulatory cycle N97.0
Anoxemia R09.0
  newborn P28.9
Anoxia (pathological) R09.0
  altitude T70.20
  cerebral G93.1
    complicating
      anesthesia (general) (local) or other sedation
        in labor and delivery O74.3
        in pregnancy — *see* Complications, anesthesia, in, pregnancy, central nervous system
        postpartum, puerperal O89.2
      delivery (cesarean) (instrumental) O75.4
      during a procedure G97.81
      newborn P28.9
      resulting from a procedure G97.82
    due to
      drowning T75.1
      high altitude T70.20
  heart — *see* Insufficiency, coronary
  intrauterine — *see* Hypoxia, intrauterine
  myocardial — *see* Insufficiency, coronary
  newborn P84
  spinal cord G95.11
  systemic (by suffocation) (low content in atmosphere) — *see* Asphyxia, traumatic
Anteflexion — *see* Anteversion
Antenatal
  care (normal pregnancy) Z34.90
    first
      pregnancy Z34.00
        first trimester Z34.01
        second trimester Z34.02
        third trimester Z34.03
      trimester Z34.91
    high risk pregnancy O09.90
      assisted reproductive technology O09.819
        first trimester O09.811
        second trimester O09.812
        third trimester O09.813
      elderly
        multigravida O09.529
          first trimester O09.521
          second trimester O09.522
          third trimester O09.523

Antenatal — *continued*
  care — *continued*
    high risk pregnancy — *continued*
      elderly — *continued*
        primigravida O09.519
          first trimester O09.511
          second trimester O09.512
          third trimester O09.513
      first trimester O09.91
      grand multiparity O09.40
        first trimester O09.41
        second trimester O09.42
        third trimester O09.43
      history of
        ectopic pregnancy O09.10
          first trimester O09.11
          second trimester O09.12
          third trimester O09.13
        infertility O09.00
          first trimester O09.01
          second trimester O09.02
          third trimester O09.03
        insufficient prenatal care O09.30
          first trimester O09.31
          second trimester O09.32
          third trimester O09.33
        molar pregnancy O09.10
          first trimester O09.11
          second trimester O09.12
          third trimester O09.13
        neonatal death — *see* category O09.2
        specified obstetric problem NEC — *see* category O09.2
        stillbirth — *see* category O09.2
      second trimester O09.92
      social problems O09.70
        first trimester O09.71
        second trimester O09.72
        third trimester O09.73
      specified risk NEC O09.899
        first trimester O09.891
        second trimester O09.892
        third trimester O09.893
      third trimester O09.93
      young
        multigravida O09.629
          first trimester O09.621
          second trimester O09.622
          third trimester O09.623
        primigravida O09.619
          first trimester O09.611
          second trimester O09.612
          third trimester O09.613
    second trimester Z34.92
    subsequent Z34.80
      first trimester Z34.81
      second trimester Z34.82
      third trimester Z34.83
    third trimester Z34.93
  screening Z36
Antepartum — *see* condition
Anterior — *see* condition
Antero-occlusion M26.2
Anteversion
  cervix — *see* Anteversion, uterus
  femur (neck), congenital Q65.8
  uterus, uterine (cervix) (postinfectional) (postpartal, old) N85.4
    congenital Q51.8
    in pregnancy or childbirth — *see* Abnormal, uterus in pregnancy or childbirth
      causing obstructed labor O65.5
Anthophobia F40.228
Anthracosilicosis J60
Anthracosis (lung) (occupational) J60
  lingua K14.3
Anthrax A22.9
  with pneumonia A22.1
  cerebral A22.8
  colitis A22.2
  cutaneous A22.0
  gastrointestinal A22.2
  inhalation A22.1
  intestinal A22.2
  meningitis A22.8

©2002 Ingenix, Inc.

Anthrax — *continued*
  pulmonary A22.1
  respiratory A22.1
  septicemia A22.7
  specified manifestation NEC A22.8
Anthropoid pelvis Q74.2
  with disproportion (fetopelvic) O33.0
Anthropophobia F40.10
  generalized F40.11
Antibodies, maternal (blood group) — *see*
  Isoimmunization, affecting management of
  pregnancy
  anti-D — *see* Isoimmunization, affecting
    management of pregnancy, Rh
  fetus or newborn P55.0
Anticoagulant, circulating D68.3
  drug-induced D68.5
Antidiuretic hormone syndrome E22.2
Antimonial cholera — *see* Poisoning, antimony
Antisocial personality F60.2
Antithrombinemia — *see* Circulating
  anticoagulants
Antithromboplastinemia — *see* Circulating
  anticoagulants
Antithromboplastinogenemia — *see* Circulating
  anticoagulants
Antitoxin complication or reaction — *see*
  Complications, vaccination
Antlophobia F40.228
Antritis — *see* Sinusitis, maxillary
Antrum, antral — *see* condition
Anuria R34
  calculous (impacted) (recurrent) — *see*
    Calculus, urinary
  following ectopic or molar pregnancy O08.4
  newborn P96.0
  postprocedural N99.0
  postrenal N13.8
  sulfonamide
    correct substance properly administered
      R34
    overdose or wrong substance given or taken
      — *see* category T37.0
  traumatic (following crushing) T79.5
Anus, anal — *see* condition
Anusitis K62.8
Anxiety F41.9
  depression F41.8
  episodic paroxysmal F41.0
  generalized F41.1
  hysteria F41.8
  neurosis F41.1
  panic type F41.0
  reaction F41.1
  separation, abnormal (of childhood) F93.0
  specified NEC F41.8
  state F41.1
Aorta, aortic — *see* condition
Aortectasia I71.9
Aortitis (nonsyphilitic) (calcific) I77.6
  arteriosclerotic I70.0
  Doehle-Heller A52.02
  luetic A52.02
  rheumatic — *see* Endocarditis, acute,
    rheumatic
  specific (syphilitic) A52.02
  syphilitic A52.02
    congenital A50.54 [I79.1]
Apathetic thyroid storm — *see* Thyrotoxicosis
Apathy R45.3
Apeirophobia F40.228
Apepsia K30
  psychogenic F45.8
Aperistalsis, esophagus K22.0
Apertognathia M26.2
Apert's syndrome Q87.0
Aphagia R13.0
  psychogenic F50.9
Aphakia (acquired) (postoperative) H27.00
  bilateral H27.03
  congenital Q12.3

Aphakia — *continued*
  left H27.02
  right H27.01
Aphasia (amnestic) (global) (nominal) (semantic)
  (syntactic) R47.01
  acquired, with epilepsy (Landau-Kleffner
    syndrome) F80.3
  auditory F80.1
  developmental (receptive type) F80.2
    expressive type F80.1
    Wernicke's F80.2
  following
    cerebrovascular disease I69.920
      cerebral infarction I69.320
      intracerebral hemorrhage I69.120
      nontraumatic intracranial hemorrhage
        NEC I69.220
      specified disease NEC I69.820
      stroke NOS I69.420
      subarachnoid hemorrhage I69.020
  progressive isolated G31.0
  sensory F80.2
  syphilis, tertiary A52.19
  uremic N19
  Wernicke's (developmental) F80.2
Aphonia (organic) R49.1
  hysterical F44.4
  psychogenic F44.4
Aphthae, aphthous — *see also* condition
  Bednar's K12.0
  cachectic K14.0
  epizootic B08.8
  oral K12.0
  stomatitis K12.0
  ulcer (oral) (recurrent) K12.0
  fever B08.8
  oral (recurrent) K12.0
  stomatitis (major) (minor) K12.0
  thrush B37.0
  ulcer (oral) (recurrent) K12.0
    genital organ(s) NEC
      female N76.6
      male N50.8
    larynx J38.7
Apical — *see* condition
Apiphobia F40.218
Aplasia — *see also* Agenesis
  abdominal muscle syndrome Q79.4
  alveolar process (acquired) — *see* Anomaly,
    alveolar
    congenital Q38.6
  aorta (congenital) Q25.4
  axialis extracorticalis (congenita) E75.29
  bone marrow (myeloid) D61.9
    congenital D61.4
  brain Q00.0
    part of Q04.3
  bronchus Q32.8
  cementum K00.4
  cerebellum Q04.3
  cervix (congenital) Q51.5
  congenital pure red cell D61.4
  corpus callosum Q04.0
  cutis congenita Q84.8
  erythrocyte congenital D61.4
  extracortical axial E75.29
  eye Q11.1
  fovea centralis (congenital) Q14.1
  gallbladder, congenital Q44.0
  iris Q13.1
  labyrinth, membranous Q16.5
  limb (congenital) Q73.8
    lower — *see* Defect, reduction, lower limb
    upper — *see* Agenesis, arm
  lung, congenital (bilateral) (unilateral) Q33.3
  pancreas Q45.0
  parathyroid-thymic D82.1
  Pelizaeus-Merzbacher E75.29
  penis Q55.5
  prostate Q55.4
  red cell (pure) (with thymoma) D60.9
    chronic D60.0
    congenital D61.4
    hereditary D61.0
    of infants D61.4
    primary D61.4

Aplasia — *see also* Agenesis — *continued*
  red cell — *continued*
    specified type NEC D60.8
    transient D60.1
  round ligament Q52.8
  skin Q84.8
  spermatic cord Q55.4
  spleen Q89.01
  testicle Q55.0
  thymic, with immunodeficiency D82.1
  thyroid (congenital) (with myxedema) E03.1
  uterus Q51.0
  ventral horn cell Q06.1
Apnea, apneic (spells) R06.81
  newborn NEC P28.4
    sleep (primary) P28.3
  sleep G47.30
    central G47.31
    mixed G47.33
    obstructive G47.32
Apneumatosis, newborn P28.0
Apocrine metaplasia (breast) — *see* Dysplasia,
  mammary, specified type NEC
Apophysitis (bone) — *see also* Osteochondropathy
  calcaneus M92.8
  juvenile M92.9
Apoplectiform convulsions (cerebral ischemia)
  I67.8
Apoplexia, apoplexy, apoplectic I64
  adrenal A39.1
  attack I64
  basilar I64
  brain I64
  bulbar I64
  capillary I64
  cerebral I64
  chorea I64
  congestive I64
  embolic I63.4
  fit I64
  heart (auricle) (ventricle) — *see* Infarct,
    myocardium
  heat T67.0
  hemiplegia I64
  hemorrhagic (stroke) — *see* Hemorrhage,
    intracranial
  ingravescent I64
  meninges, hemorrhagic — *see* Hemorrhage,
    intracranial, subarachnoid
  pancreatitis K85.8
  progressive I64
  sanguineous I64
  seizure I64
  serous I64
  stroke I64
  thrombotic I63.3
  uremic N18.8 [I68.8]
Appearance
  bizarre R46.1
  specified NEC R46.89
  very low level of personal hygiene R46.0
Appendage
  intestine (epiploic) Q43.8
  preauricular Q17.0
  testicular (organ of Morgagni) Q55.4
Appendicitis (pneumococcal) (retrocecal) K37
  with
    perforation, peritonitis, or rupture K35.0
    peritoneal abscess K35.1
      with peritonitis K35.0
  acute (catarrhal) (fulminating) (gangrenous)
    (obstructive) (retrocecal) (suppurative)
    K35.9
    with
      perforation, peritonitis, or rupture K35.0
      peritoneal abscess K35.1
        with peritonitis K35.0
  amebic A06.89
  chronic (recurrent) K36
  exacerbation — *see* Appendicitis, acute
  gangrenous — *see* Appendicitis, acute
  healed (obliterative) K36
  interval K36
  neurogenic K36
  obstructive K36
  recurrent K36

Appendicitis — *continued*
  relapsing K36
  subacute (adhesive) K36
  subsiding K36
  suppurative — *see* Appendicitis, acute
  tuberculous A18.32

Appendix, appendicular — *see also* condition
  epididymus Q55.4
  Morgagni
    female Q52.8
    male Q55.4
  testis Q55.4

Appendicopathia oxyurica B80

Appetite
  depraved — *see* Pica
  excessive R63.2
  lack or loss (*see also* Anorexia) R63.0
    nonorganic origin — *see* Disorder, eating
    psychogenic F50.8
  perverted (hysterical) — *see* Pica

Apple peel syndrome Q41.1

Apprehension state F41.1

Apprehensiveness, abnormal F41.9

Approximal wear K03.0

Apraxia (classic) (ideational) (ideokinetic)
  (ideomotor) (motor) (verbal) R48.2
  following
    cerebrovascular disease I69.990
      cerebral infarction I69.390
      intracerebral hemorrhage I69.190
      nontraumatic intracranial hemorrhage
        NEC I69.290
      specified disease NEC I69.890
      stroke NOS I69.490
      subarachnoid hemorrhage I69.090
  oculomotor, congenital H51.8

Aptyalism K11.7

Apudoma (M8248/1) — *see* Neoplasm, uncertain
  behavior

Arabicum elephantiasis — *see* Infestation, filarial

Arachnidism — *see* Venom, bite, spider

Arachnitis — *see* Meningitis

Arachnodactyly — *see* Syndrome, Marfan's

Arachnoiditis (acute) (adhesive) (basal) (brain)
  (cerebrospinal) — *see* Meningitis

Arachnophobia F40.210

Araneism — *see* Venom, bite, spider

Arboencephalitis, Australian A83.4

Arborization block (heart) I45.5

ARC (AIDS-related complex) B20

Arches — *see* condition

Areola — *see* condition

Arcuatus uterus Q51.8

Arcus (cornea) senilis — *see* Degeneration,
  cornea, senile

Arc-welder's lung J63.4

Areflexia R29.2

Areola — *see* condition

Argentaffinoma (M8241/1) — *see also* Neoplasm,
  uncertain behavior
  malignant (M8241/3) — *see* Neoplasm,
    malignant
  syndrome E34.0

Argininemia E72.21

Arginosuccinic aciduria E72.22

Argyll Robertson phenomenon, pupil or
  syndrome (syphilitic) A52.19
  atypical H57.09
  nonsyphilitic H57.09

Argyria, argyriasis NEC — *see also* Poisoning,
  silver
  conjunctival — *see* Deposit, conjunctiva
  from drug or medicament
    correct substance properly administered
      L81.8
    overdose or wrong substance given or taken
      — *see* category T37.8

Argyrosis, conjunctival — *see* Deposit,
  conjunctiva

Arhinencephaly Q04.1

Ariboflavinosis E53.0

Arm — *see* condition

Arnold-Chiari disease, obstruction or syndrome
  (type II) Q07.00
  with
    hydrocephalus Q07.02
      with spina bifida Q07.03
    spina bifida Q07.01
      with hydrocephalus Q07.03
  type III — *see* Encephalocele
  type IV Q04.8

Aromatic amino-acid metabolism disorder
  E70.9
  specified NEC E70.8

Arrest, arrested
  active phase of labor O62.1
  any plane in pelvis
    complicating delivery O66.9
  cardiac I46.9
    complicating
      abortion — *see* Abortion, by type,
        complicated by, cardiac arrest
      anesthesia (general) (local) or other
        sedation
        correct substance properly
          administered I46.8
        in labor and delivery O74.2
        in pregnancy — *see* Complications,
          anesthesia, in, pregnancy,
          cardiac
        overdose or wrong substance given —
          see also Anesthesia,
          complication, due to, overdose
          specified anesthetic — *see* Table of
            Drugs and Chemicals
        postpartum, puerperal O89.1
      delivery (cesarean) (instrumental) O75.4
      surgery T81.89
    due to
      cardiac condition I46.2
      specified condition NEC I46.8
    newborn P29.1
    postoperative I97.89
      long term effect of cardiac surgery I97.1
      obstetric procedure O75.4
  cardiorespiratory — *see* Arrest, cardiac
  circulatory — *see* Arrest, cardiac
  deep transverse O64.0
  development or growth
    bone — *see* Disorder, bone, development or
      growth
    child R62.50
    fetus — *see* Slow, fetal growth
      affecting management of pregnancy —
        see category O36.5
    tracheal rings Q32.1
  epiphyseal
    complete
      femur M89.159
        distal
          left M89.156
          right M89.155
        proximal
          left M89.152
          right M89.151
      humerus M89.129
        distal
          left M89.126
          right M89.125
        proximal
          left M89.122
          right M89.121
      tibia M89.169
        distal
          left M89.165
          right M89.164
        proximal
          left M89.161
          right M89.160
      ulna M89.139
        left distal M89.132
        right distal M89.131
      forearm M89.139
      specified NEC M89.138
      ulna — *see* Arrest, epiphyseal, by type,
        ulna

Arrest, arrested — *continued*
  epiphyseal — *continued*
    lower leg M89.169
      specified NEC M89.168
      tibia — *see* Arrest, epiphyseal, by type,
        tibia
    partial
      femur M89.159
        distal
          left M89.158
          right M89.157
        proximal
          left M89.154
          right M89.153
      humerus M89.129
        distal
          left M89.128
          right M89.127
        proximal
          left M89.124
          right M89.123
      tibia M89.169
        distal
          left M89.167
          right M89.166
        proximal
          left M89.163
          right M89.162
      ulna M89.139
        left distal M89.134
        right distal M89.133
    specified NEC M89.18
  granulopoiesis — *see* Agranulocytosis
  heart — *see* Arrest, cardiac
  legal, anxiety concerning Z65.3
  physeal — *see* Arrest, epiphyseal
  respiratory R09.2
    newborn P28.5
  sinus I45.5
  spermatogenesis (complete) — *see* Azoospermia
    incomplete — *see* Oligospermia
  transverse (deep) O64.0

Arrhenoblastoma (M8630/1)
  benign (M8630/0)
    specified site — *see* Neoplasm, benign
    unspecified site
      female D27.9
      male D29.20
  malignant (M8630/3)
    specified site — *see* Neoplasm, malignant
    unspecified site
      female C56.9
      male C62.90
  specified site — *see* Neoplasm, uncertain
    behavior
  unspecified site
    female D39.10
    male D40.10

Arrhythmia (auricle) (cardiac) (juvenile) (nodal)
  (reflex) (sinus) (supraventricular) (transitory)
  (ventricle) I49.9
  block I45.9
  extrasystolic I49.4
  newborn P29.1
    occurring before birth P03.819
      before onset of labor P03.810
      during labor P03.811
  psychogenic F45.8
  specified NEC I49.8
  vagal R55
  ventricular re-entry I47.0

Arrillaga-Ayerza syndrome (pulmonary sclerosis
  with pulmonary hypertension) I27.0

Arsenical pigmentation L81.8
  from drug or medicament — *see* Table of drugs
    and medicaments

Arsenism — *see* Poisoning, arsenic

Arterial — *see* condition

Arteriofibrosis — *see* Arteriosclerosis

Arteriolar sclerosis — *see* Arteriosclerosis

Arteriolith — *see* Arteriosclerosis

Arteriolitis I77.6
  necrotizing, kidney I77.5
  renal — *see* Hypertension, kidney

Arteriolosclerosis — *see* Arteriosclerosis

©2002 Ingenix, Inc.

Arterionephrosclerosis — *see* Hypertension, kidney

Arteriopathy I77.9

Arteriosclerosis, arteriosclerotic (diffuse) (obliterans) (of) (senile) (with calcification) I70.90

  aorta I70.0

  arteries of extremities — *see* Arteriosclerosis, extremities

  basilar I65.1

  brain I67.2

  bypass graft

    coronary — *see* Disease, heart, ischemic, atherosclerotic, coronary artery bypass graft

    extremities — *see* Arteriosclerosis, extremities, bypass graft

  cardiac — *see* Disease, heart, ischemic, atherosclerotic

  cardiopathy — *see* Disease, heart, ischemic, atherosclerotic

  cardiorenal — *see* Hypertension, cardiorenal

  cardiovascular — *see* Disease, heart, ischemic, atherosclerotic

  carotid I65.2

  central nervous system I67.2

  cerebral I67.2

  cerebrovascular I67.2

  coronary (artery) — *see* Disease, heart, ischemic, atherosclerotic

  extremities (native arteries) I70.209

    bypass graft I70.309

      autologous vein graft I70.409

        leg I70.409

          with

            gangrene (and intermittent claudication, rest pain and ulcer) I70.469

            intermittent claudication I70.419

            rest pain (and intermittent claudication) I70.429

          bilateral I70.403

           with

            gangrene (and intermittent claudication, rest pain and ulcer) I70.463

            intermittent claudication I70.413

            rest pain (and intermittent claudication) I70.423

            specified type NEC I70.493

          left I70.402

           with

            gangrene (and intermittent claudication, rest pain and ulcer) I70.462

            intermittent claudication I70.412

            rest pain (and intermittent claudication) I70.422

            ulceration (and intermittent claudication and rest pain) I70.449

              ankle I70.443

              calf I70.442

              foot site NEC I70.445

              heel I70.444

              lower leg NEC I70.448

              midfoot I70.444

              thigh I70.441

            specified type NEC I70.492

          right I70.401

           with

            gangrene (and intermittent claudication, rest pain and ulcer) I70.461

            intermittent claudication I70.411

            rest pain (and intermittent claudication) I70.421

            ulceration (and intermittent claudication and rest pain) I70.439

              ankle I70.433

              calf I70.432

              foot site NEC I70.435

extremities — *continued*

  bypass graft — *continued*

    autologous vein graft — *continued*

      leg — *continued*

        right — *continued*

          with — *continued*

            ulceration — *continued*

              heel I70.434

              lower leg NEC I70.438

              midfoot I70.434

              thigh I70.431

            specified type NEC I70.491

          specified type NEC I70.499

      specified NEC I70.408

        with

          gangrene (and intermittent claudication, rest pain and ulcer) I70.468

          intermittent claudication I70.418

          rest pain (and intermittent claudication) I70.428

          ulceration (and intermittent claudication and rest pain) I70.45

          specified type NEC I70.498

    leg I70.309

      with

        gangrene (and intermittent claudication, rest pain and ulcer) I70.369

        intermittent claudication I70.319

        rest pain (and intermittent claudication) I70.329

      bilateral I70.303

        with

          gangrene (and intermittent claudication, rest pain and ulcer) I70.363

          intermittent claudication I70.313

          rest pain (and intermittent claudication) I70.323

          specified type NEC I70.393

      left I70.302

        with

          gangrene (and intermittent claudication, rest pain and ulcer) I70.362

          intermittent claudication I70.312

          rest pain (and intermittent claudication) I70.322

          ulceration (and intermittent claudication and rest pain) I70.349

            ankle I70.343

            calf I70.342

            foot site NEC I70.345

            heel I70.344

            lower leg NEC I70.348

            midfoot I70.344

            thigh I70.341

          specified type NEC I70.392

      right I70.301

        with

          gangrene (and intermittent claudication, rest pain and ulcer) I70.361

          intermittent claudication I70.311

          rest pain (and intermittent claudication) I70.321

          ulceration (and intermittent claudication and rest pain) I70.339

            ankle I70.333

            calf I70.332

            foot site NEC I70.335

            heel I70.334

            lower leg NEC I70.338

            midfoot I70.334

            thigh I70.331

        specified type NEC I70.391

      specified type NEC I70.399

extremities — *continued*

  bypass graft — *continued*

    nonautologous biological graft I70.509

      leg I70.509

        with

          gangrene (and intermittent claudication, rest pain and ulcer) I70.569

          intermittent claudication I70.519

          rest pain (and intermittent claudication) I70.529

      bilateral I70.503

        with

          gangrene (and intermittent claudication, rest pain and ulcer) I70.563

          intermittent claudication I70.513

          rest pain (and intermittent claudication) I70.523

          specified type NEC I70.593

      left I70.502

        with

          gangrene (and intermittent claudication, rest pain and ulcer) I70.562

          intermittent claudication I70.512

          rest pain (and intermittent claudication) I70.522

          ulceration (and intermittent claudication and rest pain) I70.549

            ankle I70.543

            calf I70.542

            foot site NEC I70.545

            heel I70.544

            lower leg NEC I70.548

            midfoot I70.544

            thigh I70.541

          specified type NEC I70.592

      right I70.501

        with

          gangrene (and intermittent claudication, rest pain and ulcer) I70.561

          intermittent claudication I70.511

          rest pain (and intermittent claudication) I70.521

          ulceration (and intermittent claudication and rest pain) I70.539

            ankle I70.533

            calf I70.532

            foot site NEC I70.535

            heel I70.534

            lower leg NEC I70.538

            midfoot I70.534

            thigh I70.531

          specified type NEC I70.591

      specified type NEC I70.599

    specified NEC I70.508

      with

        gangrene (and intermittent claudication, rest pain and ulcer) I70.568

        intermittent claudication I70.518

        rest pain (and intermittent claudication) I70.528

        ulceration (and intermittent claudication and rest pain) I70.55

        specified type NEC I70.598

    nonbiological graft I70.609

      leg I70.609

        with

          gangrene (and intermittent claudication, rest pain and ulcer) I70.669

          intermittent claudication I70.619

          rest pain (and intermittent claudication) I70.629

Arteriosclerosis, arteriosclerotic — *continued*
  extremities — *continued*
    bypass graft — *continued*
      nonbiological graft — *continued*
        leg — *continued*
          bilateral I70.603
            with
              gangrene (and intermittent claudication, rest pain and ulcer) I70.663
              intermittent claudication I70.613
              rest pain (and intermittent claudication) I70.623
            specified type NEC I70.693
          left I70.602
            with
              gangrene (and intermittent claudication, rest pain and ulcer) I70.662
              intermittent claudication I70.612
              rest pain (and intermittent claudication) I70.622
              ulceration (and intermittent claudication and rest pain) I70.649
                ankle I70.643
                calf I70.642
                foot site NEC I70.645
                heel I70.644
                lower leg NEC I70.648
                midfoot I70.644
                thigh I70.641
            specified type NEC I70.692
          right I70.601
            with
              gangrene (and intermittent claudication, rest pain and ulcer) I70.661
              intermittent claudication I70.611
              rest pain (and intermittent claudication) I70.621
              ulceration (and intermittent claudication and rest pain) I70.639
                ankle I70.633
                calf I70.632
                foot site NEC I70.635
                heel I70.634
                lower leg NEC I70.638
                midfoot I70.634
                thigh I70.631
            specified type NEC I70.691
        specified type NEC I70.699
      specified NEC I70.608
        with
          gangrene (and intermittent claudication, rest pain and ulcer) I70.668
          intermittent claudication I70.618
          rest pain (and intermittent claudication) I70.628
          ulceration (and intermittent claudication and rest pain) I70.65
        specified type NEC I70.698
      specified graft NEC I70.709
        leg I70.709
          with
            gangrene (and intermittent claudication, rest pain and ulcer) I70.769
            intermittent claudication I70.719
            rest pain (and intermittent claudication) I70.729
          bilateral I70.703
            with
              gangrene (and intermittent claudication, rest pain and ulcer) I70.763
              intermittent claudication I70.713
              rest pain (and intermittent claudication) I70.723

Arteriosclerosis, arteriosclerotic — *continued*
  extremities — *continued*
    bypass graft — *continued*
      specified graft NEC — *continued*
        leg — *continued*
          bilateral — *continued*
            specified type NEC I70.793
          left I70.702
            with
              gangrene (and intermittent claudication, rest pain and ulcer) I70.762
              intermittent claudication I70.712
              rest pain (and intermittent claudication) I70.722
              ulceration (and intermittent claudication and rest pain) I70.749
                ankle I70.743
                calf I70.742
                foot site NEC I70.745
                heel I70.744
                lower leg NEC I70.748
                midfoot I70.744
                thigh I70.741
            specified type NEC I70.792
          right I70.701
            with
              gangrene (and intermittent claudication, rest pain and ulcer) I70.761
              intermittent claudication I70.711
              rest pain (and intermittent claudication) I70.721
              ulceration (and intermittent claudication and rest pain) I70.739
                ankle I70.733
                calf I70.732
                foot site NEC I70.735
                heel I70.734
                lower leg NEC I70.738
                midfoot I70.734
                thigh I70.731
            specified type NEC I70.791
        specified type NEC I70.799
      specified NEC I70.708
        with
          gangrene (and intermittent claudication, rest pain and ulcer) I70.768
          intermittent claudication I70.718
          rest pain (and intermittent claudication) I70.728
          ulceration (and intermittent claudication and rest pain) I70.75
        specified type NEC I70.798
      specified NEC I70.308
        with
          gangrene (and intermittent claudication, rest pain and ulcer) I70.368
          intermittent claudication I70.318
          rest pain (and intermittent claudication) I70.328
          ulceration (and intermittent claudication and rest pain) I70.35
        specified type NEC I70.398
      leg I70.209
        with
          gangrene (and intermittent claudication, rest pain and ulcer) I70.269
          intermittent claudication I70.219
          rest pain (and intermittent claudication) I70.229
        bilateral I70.203
          with
            gangrene (and intermittent claudication, rest pain and ulcer) I70.263

Arteriosclerosis, arteriosclerotic — *continued*
  extremities — *continued*
    leg — *continued*
      bilateral — *continued*
        with — *continued*
          intermittent claudication I70.213
          rest pain (and intermittent claudication) I70.223
          specified type NEC I70.293
        left I70.202
          with
            gangrene (and intermittent claudication, rest pain and ulcer) I70.262
            intermittent claudication I70.212
            rest pain (and intermittent claudication) I70.222
            ulceration (and intermittent claudication and rest pain) I70.249
              ankle I70.243
              calf I70.242
              foot site NEC I70.245
              heel I70.244
              lower leg NEC I70.248
              midfoot I70.244
              thigh I70.241
          specified type NEC I70.292
        right I70.201
          with
            gangrene (and intermittent claudication, rest pain and ulcer) I70.261
            intermittent claudication I70.211
            rest pain (and intermittent claudication) I70.221
            ulceration (and intermittent claudication and rest pain) I70.239
              ankle I70.233
              calf I70.232
              foot site NEC I70.235
              heel I70.234
              lower leg NEC I70.238
              midfoot I70.234
              thigh I70.231
          specified type NEC I70.291
        specified type NEC I70.299
      specified site NEC I70.208
        with
          gangrene (and intermittent claudication, rest pain and ulcer) I70.268
          intermittent claudication I70.218
          rest pain (and intermittent claudication) I70.228
          ulceration (and intermittent claudication and rest pain) I70.25
        specified type NEC I70.298
  generalized I70.91
  heart (disease) — *see* Disease, heart, ischemic, atherosclerotic
  kidney — *see* Hypertension, kidney
  medial — *see* Arteriosclerosis, extremities
  mesenteric (artery) K55.1
  Mönckeberg's — *see* Arteriosclerosis, extremities
  myocarditis I51.4
  peripheral (of extremities) — *see* Arteriosclerosis, extremities
  precerebral I65.9
    specified artery NEC I65.8
  pulmonary (idiopathic) I27.0
  renal (arterioles) — *see also* Hypertension, kidney
    artery I70.1
  retina (vascular) I70.8
  specified artery NEC I70.8
  spinal (cord) G95.19
  vertebral (artery) I67.2
Arteriospasm I73.9
Arteriovenous — *see* condition
Arteritis I77.6
  allergic M31.0

©2002 Ingenix, Inc.

Arteritis — *continued*
  aorta (nonsyphilitic) I77.6
    syphilitic A52.02
  aortic arch M31.4
  brachiocephalic M31.4
  brain I67.7
    syphilitic A52.04
  cerebral I67.7
    in systemic lupus erythematosus M32.19
    listerial A32.89
    syphilitic A52.04
    tuberculous A18.89
  coronary (artery) I25.8
    rheumatic I01.8
      chronic I09.89
    syphilitic A52.06
  cranial (left) (right), giant cell M31.6
  deformans — *see* Arteriosclerosis
  giant cell NEC M31.6
    with polymyalgia rheumatica M31.5
  necrosing or necrotizing M31.9
    specified NEC M31.8
  nodosa M30.0
  obliterans — *see* Arteriosclerosis
  pulmonary I28.8
  rheumatic — *see* Fever, rheumatic
  senile — *see* Arteriosclerosis
  suppurative I77.2
  syphilitic (general) A52.09
    brain A52.04
    coronary A52.06
    spinal A52.09
  temporal, giant cell M31.6
  young female aortic arch syndrome M31.4

Artery, arterial — *see also* condition
  single umbilical Q27.0

Arthralgia (allergic) — *see also* Pain, joint
  in caisson disease T70.3
  psychogenic F45.4
  temporomandibular M26.62

Arthritis, arthritic (acute) (chronic) (nonpyogenic)
  (subacute) M19.90
  allergic — *see* Arthritis, specified form NEC
  ankylosing (crippling) (spine) — *see also*
    Spondylitis, ankylosing
    sites other than spine — *see* Arthritis,
      specified form NEC
  atrophic — *see also* Arthrosis
    spine — *see* Spondylitis, ankylosing
  back — *see* Spondylopathy, inflammatory
  blennorrhagic (gonococcal) A54.42
  Charcôt's — *see* Arthropathy, neuropathic
    diabetic — *see* Diabetes, arthropathy,
      neuropathic
    syringomyelic G95.0
  chylous (filarial) B74.9 (*see also* category M01)
  climacteric (any site) NEC — *see* Arthritis,
    specified form NEC
  crystal(-induced) — *see* Arthritis, in, crystals
  deformans — *see* Arthrosis
  degenerative — *see* Osteoarthrosis
  due to or associated with
    acromegaly E22.0
    brucellosis — *see* Brucellosis
    caisson disease T70.3
    diabetes — *see* Diabetes, arthropathy
    dracontiasis B72 (*see also* category M01)
    enteritis NEC
      regional — *see* Enteritis, regional
    erysipelas A46
    erythema
      epidemic A25.1
      nodosum L52
    filariasis NOS B74.9
    glanders A24.0
    helminthiasis B83.9 (*see also* category M01)
    hemophilia D66
    Henoch (-Schölein) purpura D69.0
    hypersensitivity reaction T78.4
    infectious disease NEC B89 (*see also*
      category M01)
    leprosy (*see also* Leprosy) A30.9 (*see also*
      category M01)
    Lyme disease A69.23
    mycobacteria A31.8
    parasitic disease NEC B89 (*see also* category
      M01)

Arthritis, arthritic — *continued*
  due to or associated with — *continued*
    paratyphoid fever (*see also* Fever,
      paratyphoid) A01.4 (*see also* category
      M01)
    rat bite fever A25.1
    regional enteritis — *see* Enteritis, regional
    respiratory disorder NOS J98.9
    serum sickness T80.6
    syringomyelia G95.0
    typhoid fever A01.04
  epidemic erythema A25.1
  febrile — *see* Fever, rheumatic
  gonococcal A54.42
  gouty (acute) — *see* Gout, idiopathic
  in (due to)
    acromegaly (*see also* category M14.8) E22.0
    amyloidosis (*see also* category M14.8) E85
    bacterial disease A49.9 (*see also* category
      M01)
    Behçet's syndrome M35.2
    caisson disease (*see also* category M14.8)
      T70.3
    coliform bacilli (Escherichia coli) — *see*
      Arthritis, in, pyogenic organism NEC
    colitis, ulcerative K51.95 *[M07.60]*
    Crohn's disease K50.95 *[M07.60]*
    crystals M11.9
      dicalcium phosphate — *see* Arthritis, in,
        crystals, specified type NEC
      pyrophosphate — *see* Arthritis, in,
        crystals, specified type NEC
      specified type NEC M11.80
      ankle M11.879
        left M11.872
        right M11.871
      elbow M11.829
        left M11.822
        right M11.821
      foot joint M11.879
        left M11.872
        right M11.871
      hand joint M11.849
        left M11.842
        right M11.841
      hip M11.859
        left M11.852
        right M11.851
      knee M11.869
        left M11.862
        right M11.861
      multiple site M11.89
      shoulder M11.819
        left M11.812
        right M11.811
      specified joint NEC M11.88
      wrist M11.839
        left M11.832
        right M11.831
    dermatoarthritis, lipoid E78.81
    dracontiasis (dracunculiasis) B72 (*see also*
      category M01)
    endocrine disorder NEC (*see also* category
      M14.8) E34.9
    enteritis, infectious NEC A09 (*see also*
      category M01)
      regional K50.95 *[M07.60]*
      specified organism NEC A08.5 (*see also*
        category M01)
    erythema
      multiforme (*see also* category M14.8)
        L51.9
      nodosum (*see also* category M14.8) L52
    gastrointestinal condition NEC K63.9
      [M02.80]
      ankle K63.9 *[M02.879]*
      elbow K63.9 *[M02.829]*
      foot joint K63.9 *[M02.879]*
      hand joint K63.9 *[M02.849]*
      hip K63.9 *[M02.859]*
      knee K63.9 *[M02.869]*
      multiple site K63.9 *[M02.89]*
      shoulder K63.9 *[M02.819]*
      specified joint NEC K63.9 *[M02.88]*
      wrist K63.9 *[M02.839]*
    gout — *see* Gout, idiopathic

Arthritis, arthritic — *continued*
  in — *continued*
    Hemophilus influenzae B96.3 *[M00.80]*
    helminthiasis NEC B83.9 (*see also* category
      M01)
    hematological disorder NEC D75.9 *[M36.3]*
    hemochromatosis (*see also* category M14.8)
      E83.11
    hemoglobinopathy NEC D58.2 *[M36.3]*
    hemophilia NEC D66 *[M36.2]*
    Henoch(-Schönlein) purpura D69.0 *[M36.4]*
    hyperparathyroidism NEC (*see also* category
      M14.8) E21.3
    hypersensitivity reaction NEC T78.4 *[M36.4]*
    hypogammaglobulinemia (*see also* category
      M14.8) D80.1
    hypothyroidism NEC (*see also* category
      M14.8) E03.9
    infection — *see* Arthritis, pyogenic or pyemic
    infectious disease NEC B99 (*see also*
      category M01)
    leprosy A30.9 (*see also* category M01)
    leukemia NEC (M9800/3) C95.90 *[M36.1]*
    lipoid dermatoarthritis E78.81
    Lyme disease A69.23
    Mediterranean fever, familial (*see also*
      category M14.8) E85
    Meningococcus A39.83
    metabolic disorder NEC (*see also* category
      M14.8) E88.9
    multiple myelomatosis (M9732/3) C90.00
      [M36.1]
    mumps B26.85
    mycosis NEC B49 (*see also* category M01)
    myelomatosis (multiple) (M9732/3) C90.00
      [M36.1]
    neurological disorder NEC G98.0
    ochronosis (*see also* category M14.8) E70.29
    O'nyong-nyong A92.1 (*see also* category
      M01)
    parasitic disease NEC B89 (*see also* category
      M01)
    paratyphoid fever A01.4 (*see also* category
      M01)
    Pseudomonas — *see* Arthritis, pyogenic,
      bacterial NEC
    psoriasis L40.50
    pyogenic organism NEC — *see* Arthritis,
      pyogenic, bacterial NEC
    regional enteritis K50.95 *[M07.60]*
      ankle K50.95 *[M07.679]*
      elbow K50.95 *[M07.629]*
      foot joint K50.95 *[M07.679]*
      hand joint K50.95 *[M07.649]*
      hip K50.95 *[M07.659]*
      knee K50.95 *[M07.669]*
      multiple site K50.95 *[M07.69]*
      shoulder K50.95 *[M07.619]*
      specified joint NEC K50.95 *[M07.68]*
      wrist K50.95 *[M07.639]*
    Reiter's disease — *see* Reiter's disease
    respiratory disorder NEC (*see also* category
      M14.8) J98.9
    reticulosis, malignant (M9713/3) (*see also*
      category M14.8) C85.70
    rubella B06.82
    Salmonella (arizonae) (cholerae-suis)
      (enteritidis) (typhimurium) A02.23
    sarcoidosis D86.86
    specified bacteria NEC — *see* Arthritis,
      pyogenic, bacterial NEC
    sporotrichosis B42.82
    syringomyelia G95.0
    thalassemia NEC D56.9 *[M36.3]*
    tuberculosis — *see* Tuberculosis, arthritis
    typhoid fever A01.04
    ulcerative colitis K51.95 *[M07.612.80]*
    urethritis, Reiter's — *see* Reiter's disease
    viral disease NEC B34.9 (*see also* category
      M01)
  infectious or infective — *see also* Arthritis,
    pyogenic or pyemic
    spine — *see* Spondylopathy, infective
  juvenile M08.90
    with systemic onset — *see* Still's disease
    ankle M08.979
      left M08.972

Arthritis, arthritic — *continued*
- juvenile — *continued*
  - ankle — *continued*
    - right M08.971
  - elbow M08.929
    - left M08.922
    - right M08.921
  - foot joint M08.979
    - left M08.972
    - right M08.971
  - hand joint M08.949
    - left M08.942
    - right M08.941
  - hip M08.959
    - left M08.952
    - right M08.951
  - in (due to)
    - Crohn's disease K50.95 [M08.90]
      - ankle K50.95 [M08.979]
      - elbow K50.95 [M08.929]
      - foot joint K50.95 [M08.979]
      - hand joint K50.95 [M08.949]
      - hip K50.95 [M08.959]
      - knee K50.95 [M08.969]
      - multiple site K50.95 [M08.99]
      - shoulder K50.95 [M08.919]
      - specified joint NEC K50.95 [M08.98]
      - wrist K50.95 [M08.939]
    - psoriasis L40.54
    - regional enteritis K50.95 [M08.90]
    - ulcerative colitis K51.95 [M08.90]
  - knee M08.969
    - left M08.962
    - right M08.961
  - multiple site M08.99
  - pauciarticular M08.40
    - ankle M08.479
      - left M08.472
      - right M08.471
    - elbow M08.429
      - left M08.422
      - right M08.421
    - foot joint M08.479
      - left M08.472
      - right M08.471
    - hand joint M08.449
      - left M08.442
      - right M08.441
    - hip M08.459
      - left M08.452
      - right M08.451
    - knee M08.469
      - left M08.462
      - right M08.461
    - shoulder M08.419
      - left M08.412
      - right M08.411
    - specified joint NEC M08.48
    - wrist M08.439
      - left M08.432
      - right M08.431
  - rheumatoid — *see* Arthritis, rheumatoid, juvenile
  - shoulder M08.919
    - left M08.912
    - right M08.911
  - vertebra M08.98
  - specified type NEC M08.80
    - ankle M08.879
      - left M08.872
      - right M08.871
    - elbow M08.829
      - left M08.822
      - right M08.821
    - foot joint M08.879
      - left M08.872
      - right M08.871
    - hand joint M08.849
      - left M08.842
      - right M08.841
    - hip M08.859
      - left M08.852
      - right M08.851
    - knee M08.869
      - left M08.862
      - right M08.861

Arthritis, arthritic — *continued*
- juvenile — *continued*
  - specified type NEC — *continued*
    - multiple site M08.89
    - shoulder M08.819
      - left M08.812
      - right M08.811
    - specified joint NEC M08.88
    - wrist M08.839
      - left M08.832
      - right M08.831
  - wrist M08.939
    - left M08.932
    - right M08.931
- meningococcal A39.83
- menopausal (any site) NEC — *see* Arthritis, specified form NEC
- mutilans (psoriatic) L40.52
- mycotic NEC B49 (*see also* category M01)
- neuropathic (Charcot) — *see* Arthropathy, neuropathic
  - diabetic — *see* Diabetes, arthropathy, neuropathic
  - nonsyphilitic NEC G98.0
  - syringomyelic G95.0
- ochronotic (*see also* category M14.8) E70.29
- palindromic (any site) *see* Rheumatism, palindromic
- pneumococcal M00.10
  - ankle M00.179
    - left M00.172
    - right M00.171
  - elbow M00.129
    - left M00.122
    - right M00.121
  - foot joint — *see* Arthritis, pneumococcal, ankle
  - hand joint M00.149
    - left M00.142
    - right M00.141
  - hip M00.159
    - left M00.152
    - right M00.151
  - knee M00.169
    - left M00.162
    - right M00.161
  - multiple site M00.19
  - shoulder M00.119
    - left M00.112
    - right M00.111
  - vertebra M00.18
  - wrist M00.139
    - left M00.132
    - right M00.131
- postdysenteric — *see* Arthropathy, postdysenteric
- postmeningococcal A39.84
- postrheumatic, chronic — *see* Arthropathy, postrheumatic, chronic
- primary progressive — *see also* Arthritis, specified form NEC
  - spine — *see* Spondylitis, ankylosing
- psoriatic L40.50
- purulent (any site) — *see* Arthritis, pyogenic or pyemic
- pyogenic or pyemic M00.9
  - bacterial NEC M00.80
    - ankle M00.879
      - left M00.872
      - right M00.871
    - elbow M00.829
      - left M00.822
      - right M00.821
    - foot joint — *see* Arthritis, bacterial NEC, ankle
    - hand joint M00.849
      - left M00.842
      - right M00.841
    - hip M00.859
      - left M00.852
      - right M00.851
    - knee M00.869
      - left M00.862
      - right M00.861
    - multiple site M00.89

Arthritis, arthritic — *continued*
- pyogenic or pyemic — *continued*
  - bacterial NEC — *continued*
    - shoulder M00.819
      - left M00.812
      - right M00.811
    - vertebra M00.88
    - wrist M00.839
      - left M00.832
      - right M00.831
  - pneumococcal — *see* Arthritis, pneumococcal
  - staphylococcal — *see* Arthritis, staphylococcal
  - streptococcal — *see* Arthritis, streptococcal NEC
  - pneumococcal — *see* Arthritis, pneumococcal
- rheumatic — *see also* Arthritis, rheumatoid
  - acute or subacute — *see* Fever, rheumatic
- rheumatoid M06.9
  - with
    - carditis — *see* Rheumatoid, carditis
    - endocarditis — *see* Rheumatoid, carditis
    - heart involvement NEC — *see* Rheumatoid, carditis
    - lung involvement — *see* Rheumatoid, lung
    - myocarditis — *see* Rheumatoid, carditis
    - myopathy — *see* Rheumatoid, myopathy
    - pericarditis — *see* Rheumatoid, carditis
    - polyneuropathy — *see* Rheumatoid, polyneuropathy
    - rheumatoid factor — *see* Arthritis, rheumatoid, seropositive
    - splenoadenomegaly and leukopenia — *see* Felty's syndrome
    - vasculitis — *see* Rheumatoid, vasculitis
    - visceral involvement NEC — *see* Rheumatoid, arthritis, with involvement of organs NEC
  - juvenile (with or without rheumatoid factor) M08.00
    - ankle M08.079
      - left M08.072
      - right M08.071
    - elbow M08.029
      - left M08.022
      - right M08.021
    - foot joint M08.079
      - left M08.072
      - right M08.071
    - hand joint M08.049
      - left M08.042
      - right M08.041
    - hip M08.059
      - left M08.052
      - right M08.051
    - knee M08.069
      - left M08.062
      - right M08.061
    - multiple site M08.09
    - shoulder M08.019
      - left M08.012
      - right M08.011
    - vertebra M08.08
    - wrist M08.039
      - left M08.032
      - right M08.031
  - seronegative M06.00
    - ankle M06.079
      - left M06.072
      - right M06.071
    - elbow M06.029
      - left M06.022
      - right M06.021
    - foot joint M06.079
      - left M06.072
      - right M06.071
    - hand joint M06.049
      - left M06.042
      - right M06.041
    - hip M06.059
      - left M06.052
      - right M06.051

©2002 Ingenix, Inc.

Arthritis, arthritic — *continued*
  rheumatoid — *continued*
    seronegative — *continued*
      knee M06.069
        left M06.062
        right M06.061
      multiple site M06.09
      shoulder M06.019
        left M06.012
        right M06.011
      vertebra M06.08
      wrist M06.039
        left M06.032
        right M06.031
    seropositive M05.9
      without organ involvement M05.70
        ankle M05.779
          left M05.772
          right M05.771
        elbow M05.729
          left M05.722
          right M05.721
        foot joint M05.779
          left M05.772
          right M05.771
        hand joint M05.749
          left M05.742
          right M05.741
        hip M05.759
          left M05.752
          right M05.751
        knee M05.769
          left M05.762
          right M05.761
        multiple site M05.79
        shoulder M05.719
          left M05.712
          right M05.711
        vertebra — *see* Spondylitis, ankylosing
        wrist M05.739
          left M05.732
          right M05.731
  specified type NEC M06.80
    ankle M06.879
      left M06.872
      right M06.871
    elbow M06.829
      left M06.822
      right M06.821
    foot joint M06.879
      left M06.872
      right M06.871
    hand joint M06.849
      left M06.842
      right M06.841
    hip M06.859
      left M06.852
      right M06.851
    knee M06.869
      left M06.862
      right M06.861
    multiple site M06.89
    shoulder M06.819
      left M06.812
      right M06.811
    vertebra M06.88
    wrist M06.839
      left M06.832
      right M06.831
  spine — *see* Spondylitis, ankylosing
  rubella B06.82
  scorbutic (*see also* category M14.8) E54
  senile or senescent — *see* Arthrosis
  septic — *see* Arthritis, pyogenic or pyemic
  serum (nontherapeutic) (therapeutic) — *see*
    Arthropathy, postimmunization
  specified form NEC M13.80
    ankle M13.879
      left M13.872
      right M13.871
    elbow M13.829
      left M13.822
      right M13.821

Arthritis, arthritic — *continued*
  specified form NEC — *continued*
    foot joint M13.879
      left M13.872
      right M13.871
    hand joint M13.849
      left M13.842
      right M13.841
    hip M13.859
      left M13.852
      right M13.851
    knee M13.869
      left M13.862
      right M13.861
    multiple site M13.89
    shoulder M13.819
      left M13.812
      right M13.811
    specified joint NEC M13.88
    wrist M13.839
      left M13.832
      right M13.831
  spine — *see also* Spondylopathy, inflammatory
    infectious or infective NEC — *see*
      Spondylopathy, infective
    Marie-Strümpell — *see* Spondylitis,
      ankylosing
    pyogenic — *see* Spondylopathy, infective
    rheumatoid — *see* Spondylitis, ankylosing
    traumatic (old) — *see* Spondylopathy,
      traumatic
    tuberculous A18.01
  staphylococcal M00.00
    ankle M00.079
      left M00.072
      right M00.071
    elbow M00.029
      left M00.022
      right M00.021
    foot joint — *see* Arthritis, staphylococcal,
      ankle
    hand joint M00.049
      left M00.042
      right M00.041
    hip M00.059
      left M00.052
      right M00.051
    knee M00.069
      left M00.062
      right M00.061
    multiple site M00.09
    shoulder M00.019
      left M00.012
      right M00.011
    vertebra M00.08
    wrist M00.039
      left M00.032
      right M00.031
  streptococcal NEC M00.20
    ankle M00.279
      left M00.272
      right M00.271
    elbow M00.229
      left M00.222
      right M00.221
    foot joint — *see* Arthritis, streptococcal,
      ankle
    hand joint M00.249
      left M00.242
      right M00.241
    hip M00.259
      left M00.252
      right M00.251
    knee M00.269
      left M00.262
      right M00.261
    multiple site M00.29
    shoulder M00.219
      left M00.212
      right M00.211
    vertebra M00.28
    wrist M00.239
      left M00.232
      right M00.231
  suppurative — *see* Arthritis, pyogenic or
    pyemic

Arthritis, arthritic — *continued*
  syphilitic (late) A52.16
    congenital A50.55 [M12.80]
  syphilitica deformans (Charcot) A52.16
  temporomandibular M26.69
  toxic of menopause (any site) — *see* Arthritis,
    specified form NEC
  transient — *see* Arthropathy, specified form
    NEC
  traumatic (chronic) — *see* Arthropathy,
    traumatic
  tuberculous A18.02
    spine A18.01
  uratic — *see* Gout, idiopathic
  urethritica (Reiter's) — *see* Reiter's disease
  vertebral — *see* Spondylopathy, inflammatory
  villous (any site) — *see* Arthropathy, specified
    form NEC

Arthrocele — *see* Effusion, joint

Arthrodesis status Z98.1

Arthrodynia — *see also* Pain, joint
  psychogenic F45.4

Arthrofibrosis, joint — *see* Ankylosis

Arthrodysplasia Q74.9

Arthrogryposis (congenital) Q68.8
  multiplex congenita Q74.3

Arthrokatadysis M24.7

Arthropathy — *see also* Arthritis
  Charcôt's — *see* Arthropathy, neuropathic
    diabetic — *see* Diabetes, arthropathy,
      neuropathic
    syringomyelic G95.0
  cricoarytenoid J38.7
  crystal(-induced) — *see* Arthritis, in, crystals
  diabetic NEC — *see* Diabetes, arthropathy
  distal interphalangeal, psoriatic L40.51
  enteropathic M07.60
    ankle M07.679
      left M07.672
      right M07.671
    elbow M07.629
      left M07.622
      right M07.621
    foot joint M07.679
      left M07.672
      right M07.671
    hand joint M07.649
      left M07.642
      right M07.641
    hip M07.659
      left M07.652
      right M07.651
    knee M07.669
      left M07.662
      right M07.661
    multiple site M07.69
    shoulder M07.619
      left M07.612
      right M07.611
    vertebra M07.68
    wrist M07.639
      left M07.632
      right M07.631
  following intestinal bypass M02.00
    ankle M02.079
      left M02.072
      right M02.071
    elbow M02.029
      left M02.022
      right M02.021
    foot joint M02.079
      left M02.072
      right M02.071
    hand joint M02.049
      left M02.042
      right M02.041
    hip M02.059
      left M02.052
      right M02.051
    knee M02.069
      left M02.062
      right M02.061
    multiple site M02.09
    shoulder M02.019
      left M02.012

Arthropathy — *see also* Arthritis — *continued*
following intestinal bypass — *continued*
shoulder — *continued*
right M02.011
vertebra M02.08
wrist M02.039
left M02.032
right M02.031
gouty — *see also* Gout, idiopathic
in (due to)
Lesch-Nyhan syndrome (*see also* category M14.8) E79.1
sickle-cell disorders (*see also* category M14.8) D57.8
hemophilic NEC D66 [*M36.2*]
in (due to)
hyperparathyroidism NEC (*see also* category M14.8) E21.3
metabolic disease NOS (*see also* category M14.8) E88.9
in (due to)
acromegaly (*see also* category M14.8) E22.0
amyloidosis (*see also* category M14.8) E85
blood disorder NOS D75.9 [*M36.3*]
Crohn's disease K50.95 [*M07.60*]
diabetes — *see* Diabetes, arthropathy
endocrine disease NOS (*see also* category M14.8) E34.9
enteropathic NOS K52.9 [*M07.60*]
erythema
multiforme (*see also* category M14.8) L51.9
nodosum (*see also* category M14.8) L52
hemochromatosis (*see also* category M14.8) E83.11
hemoglobinopathy NEC D58.2 [*M36.3*]
hemophilia NEC D66 [*M36.2*]
Henoch-Schönlein purpura D69.0 [*M36.4*]
hyperthyroidism (*see also* category M14.8) E05.90
hypothyroidism (*see also* category M14.8) E03.9
infective endocarditis I33.0 [*M12.80*]
leukemia NEC (M9800/3) C95.90 [*M36.1*]
malignant histiocytosis (M9720/3) C96.1 [*M36.1*]
metabolic disease NOS (*see also* category M14.8) E88.9
multiple myeloma (M9732/3) C90.00 [*M36.1*]
neoplastic disease NOS (*see also* Neoplasm) D49.9 [*M36.1*]
nutritional deficiency (*see also* category M14.8) E63.9
psoriasis NOS L40.50
regional enteritis K50.95 [*M07.60*]
sarcoidosis D86.86
syphilis (late) A52.77
congenital A50.55 [*M12.80*]
thyrotoxicosis (*see also* category M14.8) E05.90
ulcerative colitis K51.95 [*M07.60*]
viral hepatitis (postinfectious) NEC B19.9 [*M12.80*]
Whipple's disease (*see also* category M14.8) K90.81
Jaccoud — *see* Arthropathy, postrheumatic, chronic
juvenile — *see* Arthritis, juvenile
mutilans (psoriatic) L40.52
neuropathic (Charcot) M14.60
ankle M14.679
left M14.672
right M14.671
diabetic — *see* Diabetes, arthropathy, neuropathic
elbow M14.629
left M14.622
right M14.621
foot joint M14.679
left M14.672
right M14.671
hand joint M14.649
left M14.642
right M14.641

Arthropathy — *see also* Arthritis — *continued*
neuropathic — *continued*
hip M14.659
left M14.652
right M14.651
knee M14.669
left M14.662
right M14.661
multiple site M14.69
nonsyphilitic NEC G98.0
shoulder M14.619
left M14.612
right M14.611
syringomyelic G95.0
vertebra M14.68
wrist M14.639
left M14.632
right M14.631
osteopulmonary — *see* Osteoarthropathy, hypertrophic, specified NEC
postdysenteric M02.10
ankle M02.179
left M02.172
right M02.171
elbow M02.129
left M02.122
right M02.121
foot joint M02.179
left M02.172
right M02.171
hand joint M02.149
left M02.142
right M02.141
hip M02.159
left M02.152
right M02.151
knee M02.169
left M02.162
right M02.161
multiple site M02.19
shoulder M02.119
left M02.112
right M02.111
vertebra M02.18
wrist M02.139
left M02.132
right M02.131
postimmunization M02.20
ankle M02.279
left M02.272
right M02.271
elbow M02.229
left M02.222
right M02.221
foot joint M02.279
left M02.272
right M02.271
hand joint M02.249
left M02.242
right M02.241
hip M02.259
left M02.252
right M02.251
knee M02.269
left M02.262
right M02.261
multiple site M02.29
shoulder M02.219
left M02.212
right M02.211
vertebra M02.28
wrist M02.239
left M02.232
right M02.231
postinfectious NEC B99 [*M12.80*]
in (due to)
enteritis due to Yersinia enterocolitica A04.6 [*M12.80*]
syphilis A52.77
viral hepatitis NEC B19.9 [*M12.80*]
postrheumatic, chronic (Jaccoud) M12.00
ankle M12.079
left M12.072
right M12.071
elbow M12.029
left M12.022

Arthropathy — *see also* Arthritis — *continued*
postrheumatic, chronic — *continued*
elbow — *continued*
right M12.021
foot joint M12.079
left M12.072
right M12.071
hand joint M12.049
left M12.042
right M12.041
hip M12.059
left M12.052
right M12.051
knee M12.069
left M12.062
right M12.061
multiple site M12.09
shoulder M12.019
left M12.012
right M12.011
specified joint NEC M12.08
wrist M12.039
left M12.032
right M12.031
psoriatic NEC L40.59
interphalangeal, distal L40.51
reactive M02.9
in (due to)
infective endocarditis I33.0 [*M02.9*]
specified type NEC M02.80
ankle M02.879
left M02.872
right M02.871
elbow M02.829
left M02.822
right M02.821
foot joint M02.879
left M02.872
right M02.871
hand joint M02.849
left M02.842
right M02.841
hip M02.859
left M02.852
right M02.851
knee M02.869
left M02.862
right M02.861
multiple site M02.89
shoulder M02.819
left M02.812
right M02.811
vertebra M02.88
wrist M02.839
left M02.832
right M02.831
specified form NEC M12.80
ankle M12.879
left M12.872
right M12.871
elbow M12.829
left M12.822
right M12.821
foot joint M12.879
left M12.872
right M12.871
hand joint M12.849
left M12.842
right M12.841
hip M12.859
left M12.852
right M12.851
knee M12.869
left M12.862
right M12.861
multiple site M12.89
shoulder M12.819
left M12.812
right M12.811
specified joint NEC M12.88
wrist M12.839
left M12.832
right M12.831
syringomyelic G95.0
tabes dorsalis A52.16
tabetic A52.16

©2002 Ingenix, Inc.

Arthropathy — *see also* Arthritis — *continued*
  transient — *see* Arthropathy, specified form
    NEC
  traumatic M12.50
    ankle M12.579
      left M12.572
      right M12.571
    elbow M12.529
      left M12.522
      right M12.521
    foot joint M12.579
      left M12.572
      right M12.571
    hand joint M12.549
      left M12.542
      right M12.541
    hip M12.559
      left M12.552
      right M12.551
    knee M12.569
      left M12.562
      right M12.561
    multiple site M12.59
    shoulder M12.519
      left M12.512
      right M12.511
    specified joint NEC M12.58
    wrist M12.539
      left M12.532
      right M12.531
Arthropyosis — *see* Arthritis, pyogenic or pyemic
Arthrosis (deformans) (degenerative) (localized)
    M19.90
  erosive M15.4
  first carpometacarpal joint M18.9
    post-traumatic (unilateral) M18.30
      bilateral M18.2
      left M18.32
      right M18.31
    primary (unilateral) M18.10
      bilateral M18.0
      left M18.12
      right M18.11
    secondary NEC (unilateral) M18.50
      bilateral M18.4
      left M18.52
      right M18.51
  generalized
    primary M15.0
  hip — *see* Coxarthrosis
  interphalangeal distal M15.1
  joint NEC
  post-traumatic — *see* Arthrosis, posttraumatic
    NEC
    primary — *see* Arthrosis, primary NEC
    secondary NEC — *see* Arthrosis, secondary
      NEC
  juxtaphalangeal distal M15.2
  knee — *see* Gonarthrosis
  polyarticular M15.9
  post-traumatic NEC M19.92
    ankle M19.179
      left M19.172
      right M19.171
    elbow M19.129
      left M19.122
      right M19.121
    foot joint M19.179
      left M19.172
      right M19.171
    hand joint M19.149
      first carpometacarpal joint M18.30
        bilateral M18.2
        left M18.32
        right M18.31
      left M19.142
      right M19.141
    hip M16.50
      bilateral M16.4
      left M16.52
      right M16.51
    knee M17.30
      bilateral M17.2
      left M17.32
      right M17.31

Arthrosis — *continued*
  post-traumatic NEC — *continued*
    shoulder M19.119
      left M19.112
      right M19.111
    wrist M19.139
      left M19.132
      right M19.131
  primary M19.91
    ankle M19.079
      left M19.072
      right M19.071
    elbow M19.029
      left M19.022
      right M19.021
    foot joint M19.079
      left M19.072
      right M19.071
    hand joint M19.049
      first carpometacarpal joint M18.10
        bilateral M18.0
        left M18.12
        right M18.11
      left M19.042
      right M19.041
    hip M16.10
      bilateral M16.0
      left M16.12
      right M16.11
    knee M17.10
      bilateral M17.0
      left M17.12
      right M17.11
    shoulder M19.019
      left M19.012
      right M19.011
    spine — *see* Spondylosis
    wrist M19.039
      left M19.032
      right M19.031
  secondary M19.93
    ankle M19.279
      left M19.272
      right M19.271
    elbow M19.229
      left M19.222
      right M19.221
    foot joint M19.279
      left M19.272
      right M19.271
    hand joint M19.249
      first carpometacarpal joint M18.50
        bilateral M18.4
        left M18.52
        right M18.51
      left M19.242
      right M19.241
    hip M16.7
      bilateral M16.6
    knee M17.5
      bilateral M17.4
    multiple M15.3
    shoulder M19.219
      left M19.212
      right M19.211
    spine — *see* Spondylosis
    wrist M19.239
      left M19.232
      right M19.231
  spine — *see* Spondylosis
Arthus' phenomenon or reaction T78.4
  due to
    correct substance properly administered
      T88.7
    overdose or wrong substance given or taken
      (by accident) T50.901
      administered with intent to harm by
        another person T50.903
        self T50.902
      circumstances undetermined T50.904
      specified drug — *see* Table of Drugs and
        Chemicals
    serum T80.6
Articular — *see* condition

Artificial
  insemination complication — *see*
    Complications, artificial, fertilization
  menopause (states) (symptoms) (syndrome)
    N95.3
  opening status (functioning) (without
      complication) Z43.9
    anus (colostomy) Z93.3
    colostomy Z93.3
    cystostomy Z93.50
      appendico-vesicostomy Z93.52
      cutaneous Z93.51
      specified NEC Z93.59
    enterostomy Z93.4
    gastrostomy Z93.1
    ileostomy Z93.2
    intestinal tract NEC Z93.4
    jejunostomy Z93.4
    nephrostomy Z93.6
    specified site NEC Z93.8
    tracheostomy Z93.0
    ureterostomy Z93.6
    urethrostomy Z93.6
    urinary tract NEC Z93.6
    vagina Z93.8
    vagina status Z93.8
Arytenoid — *see* condition
Asbestosis (occupational) J61
Ascariasis B77.9
  with
    complications NEC B77.89
    intestinal complications B77.0
    pneumonia, pneumonitis B77.81
Ascaridosis, ascaridiasis — *see* Ascariasis
Ascaris (infection) (infestation) (lumbricoides) —
    see Ascariasis
Ascending — *see* condition
Aschoff's bodies — *see* Myocarditis, rheumatic
Ascites (abdominal) R18
  cardiac I50.0
  chylous (nonfilarial) I89.8
    filarial — *see* Infestation, filarial
  due to
    cirrhosis, alcoholic K70.31
    hepatitis
      alcoholic K70.11
      chronic active K71.51
    S. japonicum B65.2
  fetal, causing obstructed labor (mother) O66.3
  heart I50.0
  malignant C78.6
  pseudochylous R18
  syphilitic A52.74
  tuberculous A18.31
Aseptic — *see* condition
Asherman's syndrome N85.6
Asialia K11.7
Asiatic cholera — *see* Cholera
Askin's tumor (M8803/3) — *see* Neoplasm,
    connective tissue, malignant
Asocial personality F60.2
Asomatognosia R41.4
Aspartylglucosaminuria E77.1
Asperger's disease or syndrome F84.5
Aspergilloma — *see* Aspergillosis
Aspergillosis (with pneumonia) B44.9
  bronchopulmonary, allergic B44.81
  disseminated B44.7
  generalized B44.7
  pulmonary NEC B44.1
    allergic B44.81
    invasive B44.0
  specified NEC B44.89
  tonsillar B44.2
Aspergillus (flavus) (fumigatus) (infection)
    (terreus) — *see* Aspergillosis
Aspermatogenesis — *see* Azoospermia
Aspermia (testis) — *see* Azoospermia
Asphyxia, asphyxiation (by) R09.0
  antenatal P84
  birth P84

Astrocytoma — *continued*
  gemistocytic — *continued*
    unspecified site C71.9
  juvenile (M9421/3)
    specified site — *see* Neoplasm, malignant
    unspecified site C71.9
  pilocytic (M9421/3)
    specified site — *see* Neoplasm, malignant
    unspecified site C71.9
  piloid (M9421/3)
    specified site — *see* Neoplasm, malignant
    unspecified site C71.9
  protoplasmic (M9410/3)
    specified site — *see* Neoplasm, malignant
    unspecified site C71.9
  specified site NEC — *see* Neoplasm, malignant
  subependymal (M9383/1) D43.2
    giant cell (M9384/1)
      specified site — *see* Neoplasm, uncertain behavior
      unspecified site D43.2
    specified site — *see* Neoplasm, uncertain behavior
    unspecified site D43.2
  unspecified site C71.9
Astroglioma (M9400/3)
  specified site — *see* Neoplasm, malignant
  unspecified site C71.9
Asymbolia R48.8
Asymmetry — *see also* Distortion
  face Q67.0
  jaw (lower) — *see* Anomaly, dentofacial, jaw-cranial base relationship, asymmetry
  pelvis with disproportion (fetopelvic) O33.0
    causing obstructed labor O65.0
Asynergia, asynergy R27.8
  ventricular I51.8
Asystole (heart) — *see* Arrest, cardiac
Ataxia, ataxy, ataxic R27.0
  acute R27.8
  brain (hereditary) G11.9
  cerebellar (hereditary) G11.9
    with defective DNA repair G11.3
    alcoholic G31.2
    early-onset G11.1
    in
      alcoholism G31.2
      myxedema E03.9 [G13.8]
      neoplastic disease (*see also* Neoplasm) D49.9 [G13.1]
    late-onset (Marie's) G11.2
  cerebral (hereditary) G11.9
  congenital nonprogressive G11.0
  family, familial — *see* Ataxia, hereditary
  Friedreich's (heredofamilial) (cerebellar) (spinal) G11.1
  gait R26.0
    hysterical F44.4
  general R27.8
  hereditary G11.9
    with neuropathy G60.2
    cerebellar — *see* Ataxia, cerebellar
    spastic G11.4
    specified NEC G11.8
    spinal (Friedreich's) G11.1
  heredofamilial — *see* Ataxia, hereditary
  Hunt's G11.1
  hysterical F44.4
  locomotor (progressive) (syphilitic) (partial) (spastic) A52.11
    diabetic — *see* Diabetes, ataxia
  Marie's (cerebellar) (heredofamilial) (lateonset) G11.2
  nonorganic origin F44.4
  nonprogressive, congenital G11.0
  psychogenic F44.4
  Roussy-Lévy G60.0
  Sanger-Brown's (hereditary) G11.2
  spastic hereditary G11.4
  spinal
    hereditary (Friedreich's) G11.1
    progressive (syphilitic) A52.11
  spinocerebellar, X-linked recessive G11.1
  telangiectasia (Louis-Bar) G11.3
Ataxia-telangiectasia (Louis-Bar) G11.3

Atelectasis (massive) (partial) (pressure) (pulmonary) J98.11
  fetus or newborn P28.10
    due to resorption P28.11
    partial P28.19
    primary P28.0
    secondary P28.19
  primary (newborn) P28.0
  tuberculous — *see* Tuberculosis, pulmonary
Atelocardia Q24.9
Atelomyelia Q06.1
Atheroma, atheromatous (*see also* Arteriosclerosis) I70.90
  aorta, aortic I70.0
    valve (*see also* Endocarditis, aortic) I35.8
  aorto-iliac I70.0
  artery — *see* Arteriosclerosis
  basilar (artery) I67.2
  carotid (artery) (common) (internal) I67.2
  cerebral (arteries) I67.2
  coronary (artery) — *see* Disease, heart, ischemic, atherosclerotic
  degeneration — *see* Arteriosclerosis
  heart, cardiac — *see* Disease, heart, ischemic, atherosclerotic
  mitral (valve) I34.8
  myocardium, myocardial — *see* Disease, heart, ischemic, atherosclerotic
  pulmonary valve (heart) (*see also* Endocarditis, pulmonary) I37.8
  tricuspid (heart) (valve) I36.8
  valve, valvular — *see* Endocarditis
  vertebral (artery) I67.2
Atheromatosis — *see* Arteriosclerosis
Atherosclerosis — *see also* Arteriosclerosis
  coronary — *see* Disease, heart, ischemic, atherosclerotic
Athetosis (acquired) R25.8
  bilateral (congenital) G80.3
  congenital (bilateral) (double) G80.3
  double (congenital) G80.3
  unilateral R25.8
Athlete's
  foot B35.3
  heart I51.7
Athrepsia E41
Athyrea (acquired) — *see also* Hypothyroidism
  congenital E03.1
Atonia, atony, atonic
  bladder (sphincter) (neurogenic) N31.2
  capillary I78.8
  cecum K59.8
    psychogenic F45.8
  colon — *see* Atony, intestine
  congenital P94.2
  esophagus K22.8
  intestine K59.8
    psychogenic F45.8
  stomach K31.89
    neurotic or psychogenic F45.8
  uterus, during labor O62.2
Atopy — *see* History, allergy
Atransferrinemia, congenital E88.09
Atresia, atretic
  alimentary organ or tract NEC Q45.8
    upper Q40.8
  ani, anus, anal (canal) Q42.3
    with fistula Q42.2
  aorta (arch) (ring) Q25.2
  aortic (orifice) (valve) Q23.0
    arch Q25.2
    congenital with hypoplasia of ascending aorta and defective development of left ventricle (with mitral stenosis) Q23.4
    in hypoplastic left heart syndrome Q23.4
  aqueduct of Sylvius Q03.0
    with spina bifida — *see* Spina bifida, with hydrocephalus
  artery NEC Q27.8
    cerebral Q28.3
    coronary Q24.5
    digestive system Q27.8
    eye Q15.0
    lower limb Q27.8
    pulmonary Q25.5

Atresia, atretic — *continued*
  artery NEC — *continued*
    specified site NEC Q27.8
    umbilical Q27.0
    upper limb Q27.8
  auditory canal (external) Q16.1
  bile duct (common) (congenital) (hepatic) Q44.2
    acquired — *see* Obstruction, bile duct
  bladder (neck) Q64.39
    obstruction Q64.31
  bronchus Q32.8
  cecum Q42.8
  cervix (acquired) N88.2
    congenital Q51.8
    in pregnancy or childbirth — *see* Anomaly, cervix, in pregnancy or childbirth
      causing obstructed labor O65.5
  choana Q30.0
  colon Q42.9
    specified NEC Q42.8
  common duct Q44.2
  cricoid cartilage Q31.8
  cystic duct Q44.2
    acquired K82.8
      with obstruction K82.0
  digestive organs NEC Q45.8
  duodenum Q41.0
  ear canal Q16.1
  ejaculatory duct Q55.4
  epiglottis Q31.8
  esophagus Q39.0
    with tracheoesophageal fistula Q39.1
  eustachian tube Q17.8
  fallopian tube (congenital) Q50.6
    acquired N97.1
  follicular cyst N83.0
  foramen of
    Luschka Q03.1
      with spina bifida — *see* Spina bifida, with hydrocephalus
    Magendie Q03.1
      with spina bifida — *see* Spina bifida, with hydrocephalus
  gallbladder Q44.1
  genital organ
    external
      female Q52.79
      male Q55.8
    internal
      female Q52.8
      male Q55.8
  glottis Q31.8
  gullet Q39.0
    with tracheoesophageal fistula Q39.1
  heart valve NEC Q24.8
    pulmonary Q22.0
    tricuspid Q22.4
  hymen Q52.4
    acquired (postinfective) N89.6
  ileum Q41.2
  intestine (small) Q41.9
    large Q42.9
      specified NEC Q42.8
  iris, filtration angle Q15.0
  jejunum Q41.1
  lacrimal apparatus Q10.4
  larynx Q31.8
  meatus urinarius Q64.33
  mitral valve Q23.2
    in hypoplastic left heart syndrome Q23.4
  nares (anterior) (posterior) Q30.0
  nasopharynx Q34.8
  nose, nostril Q30.0
    acquired J34.8
  oesophagus Q39.0
    with tracheoesophageal fistula Q39.1
  organ or site NEC Q89.8
  osseous meatus (ear) Q16.1
  oviduct (congenital) Q50.6
    acquired N97.1
  parotid duct Q38.4
    acquired K11.8
  pulmonary (artery) Q25.5
    valve Q22.0
  pulmonic Q22.0
  pupil Q13.2

Atresia, atretic — continued
rectum Q42.1
  with fistula Q42.0
salivary duct Q38.4
  acquired K11.8
sublingual duct Q38.4
  acquired K11.8
submandibular duct Q38.4
  acquired K11.8
submaxillary duct Q38.4
  acquired K11.8
thyroid cartilage Q31.8
trachea Q32.1
tricuspid valve Q22.4
ureter Q62.10
  pelvic junction Q62.11
  vesical orifice Q62.12
ureteropelvic junction Q62.11
ureterovesical orifice Q62.12
urethra (valvular) Q64.39
  stricture Q64.32
urinary tract NEC Q64.8
uterus Q51.8
  acquired N85.8
vagina (congenital) Q52.4
  acquired (postinfectional) (senile) N89.5
vas deferens Q55.3
vascular NEC Q27.8
  cerebral Q28.3
  digestive system Q27.8
  lower limb Q27.8
  specified site NEC Q27.8
  upper limb Q27.8
vein NEC Q27.8
  digestive system Q27.8
  great Q26.8
  lower limb Q27.8
  portal Q26.5
  pulmonary Q26.3
  specified site NEC Q27.8
  upper limb Q27.8
vena cava (inferior) (superior) Q26.8
vesicourethral orifice Q64.31
vulva Q52.79
  acquired N90.5
Atrichia, atrichosis — see Alopecia
Atrophia — see also Atrophy
cutis senilis L90.8
  due to radiation L57.8
gyrata of choroid and retina H31.23
senilis R54
  dermatological L90.8
    due to radiation (nonionizing) (solar) L57.8
unguium L60.3
  congenita Q84.6
Atrophie blanche (en plaque) (de Milian) L95.0
Atrophoderma, atrophodermia (of) L90.9
diffusum (idiopathic) L90.4
maculatum L90.8
  et striatum L90.8
    due to syphilis A52.79
  syphilitic A51.39
neuriticum L90.8
Pasini and Pierini L90.3
pigmentosum Q82.1
reticulatum symmetricum faciei L66.4
senile L90.8
  due to radiation (nonionizing) (solar) L57.8
vermiculata (cheeks) L66.4
Atrophy, atrophic (of)
adrenal (capsule) (gland) E27.4
  primary E27.1
alveolar process or ridge (edentulous) K08.2
appendix K38.8
arteriosclerotic — see Arteriosclerosis
bile duct (common) (hepatic) K83.8
bladder N32.8
  neurogenic N31.8
blanche (en plaque) (of Milian) L95.0
bone (senile) NEC — see also Disorder, bone, specified type NEC
  due to
    tabes dorsalis (neurogenic) A52.11

Atrophy, atrophic — continued
brain (cortex) (progressive) G31.9
  circumscribed G31.0
    dementia in G31.0 [F02]
  presenile dementia G31.89 [F02]
  senile NEC G31.1
breast N64.2
  obstetric — see Disorder, breast, specified type NEC
buccal cavity K13.7
cardiac — see Degeneration, myocardial
cartilage (infectional) (joint) — see Disorder, cartilage, specified NEC
cerebellar — see Atrophy, brain
cerebral — see Atrophy, brain
cervix (mucosa) (senile) (uteri) N88.8
  menopausal N95.8
Charcot-Marie-Tooth G60.0
choroid (central) (macular) (myopic) (retina) H31.100
  bilateral H31.103
  diffuse secondary H31.129
    bilateral H31.123
    left H31.122
    right H31.121
  gyrate H31.23
  left H31.102
  right H31.101
  senile H31.119
    bilateral H31.113
    left H31.112
    right H31.111
ciliary body — see Atrophy, iris
conjunctiva (senile) H11.89
corpus cavernosum N48.89
cortical — see Atrophy, brain
cystic duct K82.8
Déjérine-Thomas G23.8
disuse NEC — see Atrophy, muscle
Duchenne-Aran G12.21
ear — see category H93.8
edentulous alveolar ridge K08.2
endometrium (senile) N85.8
  cervix N88.8
enteric K63.8
epididymis N50.8
eyeball — see Disorder, globe, degenerated condition, atrophy
eyelid (senile) — see Disorder, eyelid, degenerative
facial (skin) L90.9
fallopian tube (senile) N83.32
  with ovary N83.33
fascioscapulohumeral (LandouzyDéjérine) G71.0
fatty, thymus (gland) E32.8
gallbladder K82.8
gastric K29.40
  with bleeding K29.41
gastrointestinal K63.8
glandular I89.8
globe H44.529
  bilateral H44.523
  left H44.522
  right H44.521
gum K06.0
hair L67.8
heart (brown) — see Degeneration, myocardial
hemifacial Q67.4
  Romberg G51.8
infantile E41
  paralysis, acute — see Poliomyelitis, paralytic
intestine K63.8
iris (essential) (progressive) H21.269
  bilateral H21.263
  left H21.262
  right H21.261
  specified NEC H21.29
kidney (senile) (terminal) (see also Sclerosis, renal) N26.1
  with hypertension — see Hypertension, kidney
  congenital or infantile Q60.5
    bilateral Q60.4
    unilateral Q60.3
  hydronephrotic — see Hydronephrosis

Atrophy, atrophic — continued
lacrimal gland (primary) H04.149
  bilateral H04.143
  left H04.142
  right H04.141
  secondary H04.159
    bilateral H04.153
    left H04.152
    right H04.151
Landouzy-Déjérine G71.0
laryngitis, infective J37.0
larynx J38.7
Leber's optic (hereditary) H47.22
lip K13.0
liver (yellow) K72.90
  with coma K72.91
  acute, subacute K72.00
    with coma K72.01
  chronic K72.10
    with coma K72.11
lung (senile) J98.4
macular (dermatological) L90.8
  syphilitic, skin A51.39
    striated A52.79
muscle, muscular (diffuse) (general) (idiopathic) (primary) M62.50
  ankle M62.579
    left M62.572
    right M62.571
  Duchenne-Aran G12.21
  foot M62.579
    left M62.572
    right M62.571
  forearm M62.539
    left M62.532
    right M62.531
  hand M62.549
    left M62.542
    right M62.541
  infantile spinal G12.0
  lower leg M62.569
    left M62.562
    right M62.561
  multiple sites M62.59
  myelopathic — see Atrophy, muscle, spinal
  myotonic G71.1
  neuritic G58.9
  neuropathic (peroneal) (progressive) G60.0
  pelvic region M62.559
    left M62.552
    right M62.551
  peroneal G60.0
  progressive (spinal) (bulbar) G12.21
    adult G12.1
    infantile (spinal) G12.0
    spinal G12.9
      adult G12.1
      infantile G12.0
  pseudohypertrophic G71.0
  shoulder region M62.519
    left M62.512
    right M62.511
  specified site NEC M62.58
  spinal G12.9
    Aran-Duchenne G12.9
    adult form G12.1
    childhood form, type II G12.1
    distal G12.1
    hereditary NEC G12.1
    infantile, type I (Werdnig-Hoffmann) G12.0
    juvenile form, type III (KugelbergWelander) G12.1
    progressive G12.21
    scapuloperoneal form G12.1
    specified NEC G12.8
    syphilitic A52.78
  thigh M62.559
    left M62.552
    right M62.551
  upper arm M62.529
    left M62.522
    right M62.521
myocardium — see Degeneration, myocardial
myometrium (senile) N85.8
  cervix N88.8
myopathic NEC — see Atrophy, muscle

Atrophy, atrophic — *continued*
  myotonia G71.1
  nail L60.3
  nasopharynx J31.1
  nerve — *see also* Disorder, nerve
    abducens — *see* Strabismus, paralytic, sixth nerve
    accessory G52.8
    acoustic or auditory — *see* category H93.3
    cranial G52.9
      eighth (auditory) — *see* category H93.3
      eleventh (accessory) G52.8
      fifth (trigeminal) G50.8
      first (olfactory) G52.0
      fourth (trochlear) — *see* Strabismus, paralytic, fourth nerve
      second (optic) H47.20
      sixth (abducens) — *see* Strabismus, paralytic, sixth nerve
      tenth (pneumogastric) (vagus) G52.2
      third (oculomotor) — *see* Strabismus, paralytic, third nerve
      twelfth (hypoglossal) G52.3
    hypoglossal G52.3
    oculomotor — *see* Strabismus, paralytic, third nerve
    olfactory G52.0
    optic (papillomacular bundle)
      syphilitic (late) A52.15
      congenital A50.44
    pneumogastric G52.2
    trigeminal G50.8
    trochlear — *see* Strabismus, paralytic, fourth nerve
    vagus (pneumogastric) G52.2
  neurogenic, bone, tabetic A52.11
  nutritional E41
  old age R54
  olivopontocerebellar G23.8
  optic (nerve) H47.20
    glaucomatous H47.239
      bilateral H47.233
      left H47.232
      right H47.231
    hereditary H47.22
    syphilitic (late) A52.15
      congenital A50.44
    primary H47.219
      bilateral H47.213
      left H47.212
      right H47.211
    specified type NEC H47.299
      bilateral H47.293
      left H47.292
      right H47.291
  orbit H05.319
    bilateral H05.313
    left H05.312
    right H05.311
  ovary (senile) N83.31
    with fallopian tube N83.33
  oviduct (senile) — *see* Atrophy, fallopian tube
  palsy, diffuse (progressive) G12.22
  pancreas (duct) (senile) K86.8
  parotid gland K11.0
  penis N48.89
  pharynx J39.2
  pluriglandular E31.8
    autoimmune E31.0
  polyarthritis M15.9
  prostate N42.89
  pseudohypertrophic (muscle) G71.0
  renal (*see also* Sclerosis, renal) N26.1
  retina, retinal (postinfectional) H35.89
  rhinitis J31.0
  salivary gland K11.0
  scar L90.5
  sclerosis, lobar (of brain) G31.0
    dementia in G31.0 [F02]
  scrotum N50.8
  seminal vesicle N50.8
  senile R54
    due to radiation (nonionizing) (solar) L57.8
  skin (patches) (spots) L90.9
    degenerative (senile) L90.8
    due to radiation (nonionizing) (solar) L57.8
    senile L90.8

Atrophy, atrophic — *continued*
  spermatic cord N50.8
  spinal (acute) (cord) G95.89
    muscular — *see* Atrophy, muscle, spinal
    paralysis G12.20
      acute — *see* Poliomyelitis, paralytic
      meaning progressive muscular atrophy G12.21
  spine (column) — *see* Spondylopathy, specified NEC
  spleen (senile) D73.0
  stomach K29.40
    with bleeding K29.41
  striate (skin) L90.6
    syphilitic A52.79
  subcutaneous L90.9
  sublingual gland K11.0
  submandibular gland K11.0
  submaxillary gland K11.0
  Sudeck's — *see* Algoneurodystrophy
  suprarenal (capsule) (gland) E27.4
    primary E27.1
  systemic affecting central nervous system in
      myxedema E03.9 [G13.8]
      neoplastic disease (*see also* Neoplasm) D49.9 [G13.1]
  tarso-orbital fascia, congenital Q10.3
  testis N50.0
  thenar, partial — *see* Syndrome, carpal tunnel
  thymus (fatty) E32.8
  thyroid (gland) (acquired) E03.4
    with cretinism E03.1
    congenital (with myxedema) E03.1
  tongue (senile) K14.8
    papillae K14.4
  trachea J39.8
  tunica vaginalis N50.8
  turbinate J34.8
  tympanic membrane (nonflaccid) H73.829
    bilateral H73.823
    flaccid H73.819
      bilateral H73.813
      left H73.812
      right H73.811
    left H73.822
    right H73.821
  upper respiratory tract J39.8
  uterus, uterine (senile) N85.8
    cervix N88.8
    due to radiation (intended effect) N85.8
      adverse effect or misadventure N99.89
  vagina (senile) N95.2
  vas deferens N50.8
  vascular I99.8
  vertebra (senile) — *see* Spondylopathy, specified NEC
  vulva (senile) N90.5
  Werdnig-Hoffmann G12.0
  yellow — *see* Failure, hepatic

Attack
  Adams-Stokes I45.9
  akinetic — *see* Epilepsy, generalized
  angina — *see* Angina
  apoplectic I64
  atonic — *see* Epilepsy, generalized
  bilious R11.1
  cardiovascular I51.6
  cataleptic — *see* Catalepsy
  cerebral I64
  coronary — *see* Infarct, myocardium
  cyanotic, newborn P28.2
  drop NEC R55
  epileptic — *see* Epilepsy
  epileptiform R56.8
  heart — *see* infarct, myocardium
  hemiplegia I64
  hysterical F44.9
  jacksonian — *see* Epilepsy, focal
  myocardium, myocardial — *see* Infarct, myocardium
  myoclonic — *see* Epilepsy, generalized
  panic F41.0
  paralysis I64
  paroxysmal R56.8
  psychomotor — *see* Epilepsy, focal, with, complex partial seizures

Attack — *continued*
  salaam — *see* Epilepsy, generalized, specified NEC
  schizophreniform, brief F23
  sensory and motor R56.8
  Stokes-Adams I45.9
  syncope R55
  transient ischemic (TIA) G45.9
    specified NEC G45.8
  unconsciousness R55
    hysterical F44.89
  vasomotor R55
  vasovagal (paroxysmal) (idiopathic) R55

Attention (to)
  artificial
    opening (of) Z43.9
      digestive tract NEC Z43.4
        colon Z43.3
        ilium Z43.2
        stomach Z43.1
      specified NEC Z43.8
      trachea Z43.0
      urinary tract NEC Z43.6
        cystostomy Z43.5
        nephrostomy Z43.6
        ureterostomy Z43.6
        urethrostomy Z43.6
      vagina Z43.7
    colostomy Z43.3
    cystostomy Z43.5
  deficit disorder or syndrome F98.8
    with hyperactivity — *see* Disorder, attention-deficit hyperactivity
  gastrostomy Z43.1
  ileostomy Z43.2
  jejunostomy Z43.4
  nephrostomy Z43.6
  surgical dressings Z48.0
  sutures Z48.0
  tracheostomy Z43.0
  ureterostomy Z43.6
  urethrostomy Z43.6

Attrition
  gum K06.0
  tooth, teeth (excessive) (hard tissues) K03.0

Atypical, atypism — *see also* condition
  endometrium N85.9
    hyperplasia (adenomatous) N85.1
  parenting situation Z60.1

Auditory — *see* condition

Aujeszky's disease B33.8

Aura, jacksonian — *see* Epilepsy, focal

Aurantiasis, cutis E67.1

Auricle, auricular — *see also* condition
  cervical Q18.2

Auriculotemporal syndrome G50.8

Austin Flint murmur (aortic insufficiency) I35.1

Australian
  Q fever A78
  X disease A83.4

Autism, autistic (childhood) (infantile) F84.0
  atypical F84.9

Autodigestion R68.8

Autoerythrocyte sensitization (syndrome) D69.2

Autographism L50.3

Autoimmune
  disease (systemic) M35.9
  thyroiditis E06.3

Autointoxication R68.8

Automatism G93.8
  epileptic — *see* Epilepsy, focal, with, complex partial seizures
  paroxysmal, idiopathic — *see* Epilepsy, focal, with, complex partial seizures

Autonomic, autonomous
  bladder (neurogenic) N31.2
  hysteria seizure F44.5

Autosensitivity, erythrocyte D69.2

Autosensitization, cutaneous L30.2

Autosome — *see* condition by chromosome involved

Autotopagnosia R48.1

Autotoxemia R68.8

Autumn — *see* condition
Avellis' syndrome G46.8
Aversion, sexual F52.1
Aviator's
  disease or sickness — *see* Effect, adverse, high altitude
  ear T70.0
Avitaminosis (multiple) (*see also* Deficiency, vitamin) E56.9
  B E53.9
    with
      beriberi E51.11
      pellagra E52
  B2 E53.0
  B6 E53.1
  B12 E53.8
  D E55.9
    with rickets E55.0
  G E53.0
  K E56.1
  nicotinic acid E52
Avulsion (traumatic)
  blood vessel — *see* Injury, blood vessel
  bone — *see* Fracture, by site
  cartilage — *see also* Dislocation, by site
    symphyseal (inner), complicating delivery O71.6
  external site other than limb — *see* Wound, open, by site
  eye S05.70
    left S05.72
    right S05.71
  head (intracranial)
    external site NEC S08.89
    scalp S08.0
  internal organ or site — *see* Injury, by site
  joint — *see also* Dislocation, by site
    capsule — *see* Sprain, by site
  kidney S37.069
    left S37.062
    right S37.061
  ligament — *see* Sprain, by site
  limb — *see also* Amputation, traumatic, by site
    skin and subcutaneous tissue — *see* Wound, open, by site
  muscle — *see* Injury, muscle
  nerve (root) — *see* Injury, nerve
  scalp S08.0
  skin and subcutaneous tissue — *see* Wound, open, by site
  spleen S36.032
  symphyseal cartilage (inner), complicating delivery O71.6
  tendon — *see* Injury, muscle
  tooth S03.2
Awareness of heart beat R00.2
Axenfeld's
  anomaly or syndrome Q15.0
  degeneration (calcareous) Q13.4
Axilla, axillary — *see also* condition
  breast Q83.1
Axonotmesis — *see* Injury, nerve
Ayerza's disease or syndrome (pulmonary artery sclerosis with pulmonary hypertension) I27.0
Azoospermia (organic) N46.01
  due to
    drug therapy N46.021
    efferent duct obstruction N46.023
    infection N46.022
    radiation N46.024
    specified cause NEC N46.029
    systemic disease N46.025
Azotemia R79.89
  meaning uremia N19
Aztec ear Q17.3
Azygos
  continuation inferior vena cava Q26.8
  lobe (lung) Q33.1

B

Baastrup's disease — *see* Kissing spine
Babesiosis B60.0

Babington's disease (familial hemorrhagic telangiectasia) I78.0
Babinski's syndrome A52.79
Baby
  crying constantly R68.11
  floppy (syndrome) P94.2
Bacillary — *see* condition
Bacilluria N39.0
Bacillus — *see also* Infection, bacillus
  abortus infection A23.1
  anthracis infection A22.9
  coli infection B96.2
  Flexner's A03.1
  fragilis, as cause of disease classified elsewhere B96.6
  mallei infection A24.0
  Shiga's A03.0
  suipestifer infection — *see* Infection, salmonella
Back — *see* condition
Backache (postural) — *see also* Dorsalgia
  psychogenic F45.4
  sacroiliac M53.3
  specified NEC — *see* Dorsalgia, specified NEC
Backflow — *see* Reflux
Backward reading (dyslexia) F81.0
Bacteremia R78.81
  with sepsis — *see* Septicemia
  MAC A31.2
  meningococcal — *see* Meningococcemia
Bactericholia — *see* Cholecystitis, acute
Bacterid, bacteride (pustular) L40.3
Bacterium, bacteria, bacterial (*see also* condition)
  agent NEC, as cause of disease classified elsewhere B96.89
  in blood — *see* Bacteremia
  in urine — *see* Bacteriuria
Bacteriuria, bacteruria N39.0
  asymptomatic N39.0
    in pregnancy O23.40
      first trimester O23.41
      second trimester O23.42
      third trimester O23.43
    puerperal (postpartum) O86.20
Bad
  heart — *see* Disease, heart
  trip — *see* Disorder, drug-related, hallucinogen
Baelz's disease (cheilitis glandularis apostematosa) K13.0
Baerensprung's disease (eczema marginatum) B35.6
Bagasse disease or pneumonitis J67.1
Bagassosis J67.1
Baker's cyst — *see* Cyst, Baker's
Bakwin-Krida syndrome (craniometaphyseal dysplasia) Q78.5
Balanitis (circinata) (erosiva) (gangrenosa) (phagedenic) (vulgaris) N48.1
  amebic A06.82
  candidal B37.42
  due to Haemophilus ducreyi A57
  gonococcal (acute) (chronic) A54.09
  venereal NEC A64.1
  xerotica obliterans N48.0
Balanoposthitis N47.6
  gonococcal (acute) (chronic) A54.09
  ulcerative (specific) A63.8
Balanorrhagia — *see* Balanitis
Balantidiasis, balantidiosis A07.0
Bald tongue K14.4
Baldness — *see also* Alopecia
  male-pattern — *see* Alopecia, androgenic
Balkan grippe A78
Ballantyne (-Runge) syndrome (postmaturity) P08.2
Balloon disease — *see* Effect, adverse, high altitude
Balo's disease (concentric sclerosis) G37.5
Bamberger-Marie disease — *see* Osteoarthropathy, hypertrophic, specified type NEC

Bancroft's filariasis B74.0
Band(s)
  adhesive — *see* Adhesions, peritoneum
  anomalous or congenital — *see also* Anomaly, by site
    heart (atrial) (ventricular) Q24.8
    intestine Q43.3
    omentum Q43.3
  cervix N88.1
  constricting, congenital Q79.8
  gallbladder (congenital) Q44.1
  intestinal (adhesive) — *see* Adhesions, peritoneum
  obstructive
    intestine K56.5
    peritoneum K56.5
  periappendiceal, congenital Q43.3
  peritoneal (adhesive) — *see* Adhesions, peritoneum
  uterus N73.6
    internal N85.6
  vagina N89.5
Bandl's ring (contraction), complicating delivery O62.4
Bangkok hemorrhagic fever A91
Bang's disease (brucella abortus) A23.1
Bankruptcy, anxiety concerning Z59.8
Bannister's disease T78.3
  hereditary D84.1
Banti's disease or syndrome (with cirrhosis) (with portal hypertension) K76.6
Bar, median, prostate — *see* Hyperplasia, prostate
Barcoo disease or rot — *see* Ulcer, skin
Barlow's disease E54
Barodontalgia T70.29
Baron Münchausen syndrome — *see* Disorder, factitious
Barosinusitis T70.1
Barotitis T70.0
Barotrauma T70.29
  odontalgia T70.29
  otitic T70.0
  sinus T70.1
Barraquer (-Simons) disease or syndrome (progressive lipodystrophy) E88.1
Barré-Guillain disease or syndrome G61.0
Barré-Liéou syndrome (posterior cervical sympathetic) M53.0
Barrel chest M95.4
Barrett's ulcer or syndrome (chronic peptic ulcer of esophagus) K22.1
Bársony (-Polgár) (-Teschendorf) syndrome (corkscrew esophagus) K22.4
Bartholinitis (suppurating) N75.8
  gonococcal (acute) (chronic) (with abscess) A54.1
Barth syndrome E78.71
Bartonellosis A44.9
  cutaneous A44.1
  mucocutaneous A44.1
  specified NEC A44.8
  systemic A44.0
Barton's fracture S52.569
  left S52.562
  right S52.561
Bartter's syndrome E26.8
Basal — *see* condition
Basan's (hidrotic) ectodermal dysplasia Q82.4
Baseball finger — *see* Dislocation, finger
Basedow's disease (exophthalmic goiter) — *see* Hyperthyroidism, with, goiter
Basic — *see* condition
Basilar — *see* condition
Bason's (hidrotic) ectodermal dysplasia Q82.4
Basopenia — *see* Agranulocytosis
Basophilia D75.8
Basophilism (cortico-adrenal) (Cushing's) (pituitary) E24.0
Bassen-Kornzweig disease or syndrome E78.6

©2002 Ingenix, Inc.

Bat ear Q17.5
Bateman's
  disease B08.1
  purpura (senile) D69.2
Bathing cramp T75.1
Bathophobia F40.248
Batten (-Mayou) disease E75.4
  retina E75.4 *[H36]*
Batten-Steinert syndrome G71.1
Battered — *see* Maltreatment
Battey Mycobacterium infection A31.0
Battle exhaustion F43.0
Battledore placenta — *see* Abnormal, placenta, specified type NEC
Baumgarten-Cruveilhier cirrhosis, disease or syndrome K74.6
Bauxite fibrosis (of lung) J63.1
Bayle's disease (general paresis) A52.17
Bazin's disease (primary) (tuberculous) A18.4
Beach ear — *see* Swimmer's, ear
Beaded hair (congenital) Q84.1
Béal conjunctivitis or syndrome B30.2
Beard's disease (neurasthenia) F48.8
Beat(s)
  atrial, premature I49.1
  ectopic I49.4
  elbow — *see* Bursitis, elbow
  escaped, heart I49.4
  hand — *see* Bursitis, hand
  knee — *see* Bursitis, knee
  premature I49.4
    atrial I49.1
    auricular I49.1
    supraventricular I49.1
Beau's
  disease or syndrome — *see* Degeneration, myocardial
  lines (transverse furrows on fingernails) L60.4
Bechterev's syndrome — *see* Spondylitis, ankylosing
Beck's syndrome (anterior spinal artery occlusion) I65.8
Becker's
  cardiomyopathy I42.8
  disease (idiopathic mural endomyocardial disease) I42.3
  dystrophy G71.0
  pigmented hairy nevus (M8720/0) D22.5
Beckwith-Wiedemann syndrome Q87.3
Bedclothes, asphyxiation or suffocation by — *see* Asphyxia, traumatic, due to, mechanical, trapped
Bedfast, requiring health care provider Z74.0
Bednar's
  aphthae K12.0
  tumor (M8833/3) — *see* Neoplasm, malignant
Bedsore — *see* Decubitus
Bedwetting — *see* Enuresis
Bee sting (with allergic or anaphylactic shock) — *see* Toxicity, venom, arthropod, bee
Begbie's disease (exophthalmic goiter) — *see* Hyperthyroidism, with, goiter
Beer drinker's heart (disease) I42.6
Behavior
  antisocial
    adult Z72.811
    child or adolescent Z72.810
  disorder, disturbance — *see* Disorder, conduct
  disruptive — *see* Disorder, conduct
  inexplicable R46.2
  marked evasiveness R46.5
  obsessive-compulsive R46.81
  overactivity R46.3
  poor responsiveness R46.4
  self-damaging (life-style) Z72.89
  slowness R46.4
  specified NEC R46.89
  strange (and inexplicable) R46.2
  suspiciousness R46.5
  type A pattern Z73.1

Behavior — *continued*
  undue concern or preoccupation with stressful events R46.6
  verbosity and circumstantial detail obscuring reason for contact R46.7
Behçet's disease or syndrome M35.2
Behr's disease — *see* Degeneration, macula
Beigel's disease or morbus (white piedra) B36.2
Bejel A65
Bekhterev's syndrome — *see* Spondylitis, ankylosing
Belching — *see* Eructation
Bell's
  mania F30.8
  palsy, paralysis G51.0
    infant or newborn P11.3
  spasm G51.3
Bence Jones albuminuria or proteinuria NEC R80.3
Bends T70.3
Benedikt's paralysis or syndrome G46.3
Benign (*see also* condition)
  prostatic hyperplasia — *see* Hyperplasia, prostate
Bennett's fracture (displaced) S62.213
  left S62.212
    nondisplaced S62.216
      left S62.215
      right S62.214
  right S62.211
Benson's disease — *see* Deposit, crystalline
Bent
  back (hysterical) F44.4
  nose M95.0
    congenital Q67.4
Bereavement (uncomplicated) Z63.4
Bergeron's disease (hysterical chorea) F44.4
Berger's disease — *see* Nephropathy, IgA
Beriberi (dry) E51.11
  heart (disease) E51.12
  polyneuropathy E51.11
  wet E51.12
    involving circulatory system E51.11
Berlin's disease or edema (traumatic) S05.80
  left S05.82
  right S05.81
Berlock (berloque) dermatitis L56.2
Bernard-Horner syndrome G90.2
Bernard-Soulier disease or thrombopathia D69.1
Bernhardt(-Roth) disease — *see* Mononeuropathy, lower limb, meralgia paresthetica
Bernheim's syndrome — *see* Failure, heart, congestive
Bertielliasis B71.8
Berylliosis (lung) J63.2
Besnier-Boeck (-Schaumann) disease — *see* Sarcoidosis
Besnier's
  lupus pernio D86.3
  prurigo L20.0
Best's disease H35.50
Beta-mercaptolactate-cysteine disulfiduria E72.09
Betalipoproteinemia, broad or floating E78.2
Betting and gambling Z72.6
  pathological (compulsive) F63.0
Bezoar T18.9
  intestine T18.3
  stomach T18.2
Bezold's abscess — *see* Mastoiditis, acute
Bianchi's syndrome R48.8
Bicornate or bicornis uterus Q51.3
  in pregnancy or childbirth — *see* Anomaly, uterus, in pregnancy or childbirth
    causing obstructed labor O65.5
Bicuspid aortic valve Q23.1
Biedl-Bardet syndrome Q87.89

Bielschowsky (-Jansky) disease E75.4
Biermer's (pernicious) **anemia or disease** D51.0
Biett's disease L93.0
Bifid (congenital)
  apex, heart Q24.8
  clitoris Q52.6
  kidney Q63.8
  nose Q30.2
  patella Q74.1
  scrotum Q55.29
  toe NEC Q74.2
  tongue Q38.3
  ureter Q62.8
  uterus Q51.3
  uvula Q35.7
Biforis uterus (suprasimplex) Q51.3
Bifurcation (congenital)
  gallbladder Q44.1
  kidney pelvis Q63.8
  renal pelvis Q63.8
  rib Q76.6
  tongue, congenital Q38.3
  trachea Q32.1
  ureter Q62.8
  urethra Q64.74
  vertebra Q76.49
Big spleen syndrome D73.1
Bigeminal pulse R00.8
Bilateral — *see* condition
Bile
  duct — *see* condition
  pigments in urine R82.2
Bilharziasis — *see also* Schistosomiasis
  chyluria B65.0
  cutaneous B65.3
  galacturia B65.0
  hematochyluria B65.0
  intestinal B65.1
  lipemia B65.9
  lipuria B65.9
  oriental B65.2
  piarhemia B65.9
  pulmonary NOS B65.9 *[J99]*
    pneumonia B65.9 *[J17]*
  tropical hematuria B65.0
  vesical B65.0
Biliary — *see* condition
Bilious (attack) R11.1
  with vomiting R11.0
Bilirubin metabolism disorder E80.7
  specified NEC E80.6
Bilirubinemia, familial nonhemolytic E80.4
Bilirubinuria R82.2
Biliuria R82.2
Bilocular stomach K31.2
Binswanger's disease I67.3
Biparta, bipartite
  carpal scaphoid Q74.0
  patella Q74.1
  vagina Q52.1
Bird
  face Q75.8
  fancier's disease or lung J67.2
Birth
  complications in mother — *see* Delivery, complicated
    affecting fetus P03.9
  compression during NOS P15.9
  defect — *see* Anomaly
  immature (less than 37 completed weeks) — *see* Preterm infant, newborn
    extremely (less than 28 completed weeks) — *see* Immaturity, extreme
  inattention, at or after — *see* Maltreatment, child, neglect
  injury NOS P15.9
    basal ganglia P11.1
    brachial plexus NEC P14.3
    brain (compression) (pressure) P11.2
    central nervous system NOS P11.9
    cerebellum P11.1
    cerebral hemorrhage P10.1
    external genitalia P15.5

Birth — *continued*
  injury NOS — *continued*
    eye P15.3
    face P15.4
    fracture
      bone P13.9
        specified NEC P13.8
      clavicle P13.4
      femur P13.2
      humerus P13.3
      long bone, except femur P13.3
      radius and ulna P13.3
      skull P13.0
      spine P11.5
      tibia and fibula P13.3
    intracranial P11.2
      laceration or hemorrhage P10.9
        specified NEC P10.8
    intraventricular hemorrhage P10.2
    laceration
      brain P10.1
      by scalpel P15.8
      peripheral nerve P14.9
    liver P15.0
    meninges
      brain P11.1
      spinal cord P11.5
    nerve
      brachial plexus P14.3
      cranial NEC (except facial) P11.4
      facial P11.3
      peripheral P14.9
      phrenic (paralysis) P14.2
    paralysis
      facial nerve P11.3
      spinal P11.5
    penis P15.5
    rupture
      spinal cord P11.5
    scalp P12.9
    scalpel wound P15.8
    scrotum P15.5
    skull NEC P13.1
      fracture P13.0
    specified type NEC P15.8
    spinal cord P11.5
    spine P11.5
    spleen P15.1
    sternomastoid (hematoma) P15.2
    subarachnoid hemorrhage P10.3
    subcutaneous fat necrosis P15.6
    subdural hemorrhage P10.0
    tentorial tear P10.4
    testes P15.5
    vulva P15.5
  lack of care, at or after — *see* Maltreatment, child, neglect
  neglect, at or after — *see* Maltreatment, child, neglect
  palsy or paralysis, newborn, NOS (birth injury) P14.9
  post-term (42 weeks or more) P08.2
  premature (infant) — *see* Preterm infant, newborn
  shock, newborn P96.8
  trauma — *see* Birth, injury
  weight
    low (2499 grams or less) — *see* Low, birthweight
      extremely (999 grams or less) — *see* Low, birthweight, extreme
    4500 grams or more P08.0
Birthmark Q82.5
Bisalbuminemia E88.09
Biskra's button B55.1
Bite(s) (animal) (human)
  abdomen, abdominal S31.95
    wall S31.159
      with penetration into peritoneal cavity S31.659
      epigastric region S31.152
        with penetration into peritoneal cavity S31.652

Bite(s) — *continued*
  abdomen, abdominal — *continued*
    wall — *continued*
      left
        lower quadrant S31.154
          with penetration into peritoneal cavity S31.654
        upper quadrant S31.151
          with penetration into peritoneal cavity S31.651
        periumbilic region S31.155
          with penetration into peritoneal cavity S31.655
      right
        lower quadrant S31.153
          with penetration into peritoneal cavity S31.653
        upper quadrant S31.150
          with penetration into peritoneal cavity S31.650
      superficial NEC S30.871
        insect S30.861
    alveolar (process) — *see* Bite, oral cavity
  amphibian (venomous) — *see* Venom, bite, amphibian
  animal — *see also* Bite, by site
    venomous — *see* Venom
  ankle S91.059
    with fracture of ankle S91.069
      left S91.062
      right S91.061
    left S91.052
    right S91.051
    superficial NEC S90.579
      insect S90.569
        left S90.562
        right S90.561
      left S90.572
      right S90.571
  antecubital space — *see* Bite, elbow
  anus S31.835
    superficial NEC S30.877
      insect S30.867
  arm (upper) S41.159
    left S41.152
    lower — *see* Bite, forearm
    right S41.151
    superficial NEC S40.879
      insect S40.869
        left S40.862
        right S40.861
      left S40.872
      right S40.871
  arthropod NEC — *see* Venom, bite, arthropod
  auditory canal (external) (meatus) — *see* Bite, ear
  auricle, ear — *see* Bite, ear
  axilla — *see* Bite, arm
  back — *see also* Bite, thorax, back
    lower S31.050
      with penetration into retroperitoneal space S31.051
      superficial NEC S30.870
        insect S30.860
  breast S21.059
    left S21.052
    right S21.051
    superficial NEC S20.179
      insect S20.169
        left S20.162
        right S20.161
      left S20.172
      right S20.171
  brow — *see* Bite, head, specified site NEC
  buttock S31.805
    left S31.825
    right S31.815
    superficial NEC S30.870
      insect S30.860
  calf — *see* Bite, leg
  canaliculus lacrimalis — *see* Bite, eyelid
  canthus, eye — *see* Bite, eyelid
  centipede — *see* Toxicity, venom, arthropod, centipede
  cheek (external) S01.459
    left S01.452
    right S01.451

Bite(s) — *continued*
  cheek — *continued*
    superficial NEC S00.87
      insect S00.86
    internal — *see* Bite, oral cavity
  chest wall — *see* Bite, thorax
  chigger B88.0
  chin — *see* Bite, head, specified site NEC
  clitoris — *see* Bite, vulva
  costal region — *see* Bite, thorax
  digit(s)
    hand — *see* Bite, finger
    toe — *see* Bite, toe
  ear (canal) (external) S01.359
    left S01.352
    right S01.351
    superficial NEC S00.479
      insect S00.469
        left S00.462
        right S00.461
      left S00.472
      right S00.471
  elbow S51.059
    with fracture of elbow S51.069
      left S51.062
      right S51.061
    left S51.052
    right S51.051
    superficial NEC S50.379
      insect S50.369
        left S50.362
        right S50.361
      left S50.372
      right S50.371
  epididymis — *see* Bite, testis
  epigastric region — *see* Bite, abdomen
  epiglottis — *see* Bite, neck, specified site NEC
  esophagus, cervical S11.25
    superficial NEC S10.17
      insect S10.16
  eyebrow — *see* Bite, eyelid
  eyelid S01.159
    left S01.152
    right S01.151
    superficial NEC S00.279
      insect S00.269
        left S00.262
        right S00.261
      left S00.272
      right S00.271
  face NEC — *see* Bite, head, specified site NEC
  finger(s) S61.259
    with
      damage to nail S61.359
        with fracture S61.369
      fracture S61.269
    index S61.258
      with
        damage to nail S61.358
          with fracture S61.368
        fracture S61.268
      left S61.251
        with
          damage to nail S61.351
            with fracture S61.361
          fracture S61.261
      right S61.250
        with
          damage to nail S61.350
            with fracture S61.360
          fracture S61.260
      superficial NEC S60.478
        insect S60.468
          left S60.461
          right S60.460
        left S60.471
        right S60.470
    little S61.258
      with
        damage to nail S61.358
          with fracture S61.368
        fracture S61.268
      left S61.257
        with
          damage to nail S61.357
            with fracture S61.367

©2002 Ingenix, Inc.

Bite(s) — *continued*
  finger(s) — *continued*
    little — *continued*
      left — *continued*
        with — *continued*
          fracture S61.267
        right S61.256
          with
            damage to nail S61.356
              with fracture S61.366
            fracture S61.266
        superficial NEC S60.478
          insect S60.468
            left S60.467
            right S60.466
          left S60.477
          right S60.476
    middle S61.258
      with
        damage to nail S61.358
          with fracture S61.368
        fracture S61.268
      left S61.253
        with
          damage to nail S61.353
            with fracture S61.363
          fracture S61.263
      right S61.252
        with
          damage to nail S61.352
            with fracture S61.362
          fracture S61.262
      superficial NEC S60.478
        insect S60.468
          left S60.463
          right S60.462
        left S60.473
        right S60.472
    ring S61.258
      with
        damage to nail S61.358
          with fracture S61.368
        fracture S61.268
      left S61.255
        with
          damage to nail S61.355
            with fracture S61.365
          fracture S61.265
      right S61.254
        with
          damage to nail S61.354
            with fracture S61.364
          fracture S61.264
      superficial NEC S60.478
        insect S60.468
          left S60.465
          right S60.464
        left S60.475
        right S60.474
    superficial NEC S60.479
      insect S60.469
    thumb — *see* Bite, thumb
  flank — *see* Bite, abdomen, wall
  flea — *see* Bite, insect, by site
  foot (except toe(s) alone) S91.359
    left S91.352
    right S91.351
    superficial NEC S90.879
      insect S90.869
        left S90.862
        right S90.861
      left S90.872
      right S90.871
    toe — *see* Bite, toe
  forearm S51.859
    with fracture of radius and ulna S51.869
      left S51.862
      right S51.861
    elbow only — *see* Bite, elbow
    left S51.852
    right S51.851
    superficial NEC S50.879
      insect S50.869
        left S50.862
        right S50.861

Bite(s) — *continued*
  forearm — *continued*
    superficial NEC — *continued*
      left S50.872
      right S50.871
  forehead — *see* Bite, head, specified site NEC
  genital organs, external
    female S31.552
      superficial NEC S30.876
        insect S30.866
      vagina and vulva — *see* Bite, vulva
    male S31.551
      penis — *see* Bite, penis
      scrotum — *see* Bite, scrotum
      superficial NEC S30.875
        insect S30.865
      testes — *see* Bite, testis
  groin — *see* Bite, abdomen, wall
  gum — *see* Bite, oral cavity
  hand S61.459
    with fracture S61.469
      left S61.462
      right S61.461
    finger — *see* Bite, finger
    left S61.452
    right S61.451
    superficial NEC S60.579
      insect S60.569
        left S60.562
        right S60.561
      left S60.572
      right S60.571
    thumb — *see* Bite, thumb
  head S01.95
    cheek — *see* Bite, cheek
    ear — *see* Bite, ear
    eyelid — *see* Bite, eyelid
    lip — *see* Bite, lip
    nose — *see* Bite, nose
    oral cavity — *see* Bite, oral cavity
    scalp — *see* Bite, scalp
    specified site NEC S01.85
      superficial NEC S00.87
        insect S00.86
    superficial NEC S00.97
      insect S00.96
    temporomandibular area — *see* Bite, cheek
  heel — *see* Bite, foot
  hip S71.059
    left S71.052
    right S71.051
    superficial NEC S70.279
      insect S70.269
        left S70.262
        right S70.261
      left S70.272
      right S70.271
  hymen S31.45
  hypochondrium — *see* Bite, abdomen, wall
  hypogastric region — *see* Bite, abdomen, wall
  inguinal region — *see* Bite, abdomen, wall
  insect — *see* Bite, insect, by site
  instep — *see* Bite, foot
  interscapular region — *see* Bite, thorax, back
  jaw — *see* Bite, head, specified site NEC
  knee S81.059
    left S81.052
    right S81.051
    superficial NEC S80.279
      insect S80.269
        left S80.262
        right S80.261
      left S80.272
      right S80.271
  labium (majus) (minus) — *see* Bite, vulva
  lacrimal duct — *see* Bite, eyelid
  larynx S11.015
    superficial NEC S10.17
      insect S10.16
  leg (lower) S81.859
    ankle — *see* Bite, ankle
    foot — *see* Bite, foot
    knee — *see* Bite, knee
    left S81.852
    right S81.851

Bite(s) — *continued*
  leg — *continued*
    superficial NEC S80.879
      insect S80.869
        left S80.862
        right S80.861
      left S80.872
      right S80.871
    toe — *see* Bite, toe
    upper — *see* Bite, thigh
  lip S01.551
    superficial NEC S00.571
      insect S00.561
  lizard (venomous) — *see* Venom, bite, reptile
  loin — *see* Bite, abdomen, wall
  lower back — *see* Bite, back, lower
  lumbar region — *see* Bite, back, lower
  malar region — *see* Bite, head, specified site NEC
  mammary — *see* Bite, breast
  marine animals (venomous) — *see* Toxicity, venom, marine animal
  mastoid region — *see* Bite, head, specified site NEC
  mouth — *see* Bite, oral cavity
  nail
    finger — *see* Bite, finger
    toe — *see* Bite, toe
  nape — *see* Bite, neck, specified site NEC
  nasal (septum) (sinus) — *see* Bite, nose
  nasopharynx — *see* Bite, head, specified site NEC
  neck S11.95
    involving
      cervical esophagus — *see* Bite, esophagus, cervical
      larynx — *see* Bite, larynx
      pharynx — *see* Bite, pharynx
      thyroid gland S11.15
      trachea — *see* Bite, trachea
    specified site NEC S11.85
      superficial NEC S10.87
        insect S10.86
    superficial NEC S10.97
      insect S10.96
    throat S11.85
      superficial NEC S10.17
        insect S10.16
  nose (septum) (sinus) S01.25
    superficial NEC S00.37
      insect S00.36
  occipital region — *see* Bite, scalp
  oral cavity S01.552
    superficial NEC S00.572
      insect S00.562
  orbital region — *see* Bite, eyelid
  palate — *see* Bite, oral cavity
  palm — *see* Bite, hand
  parietal region — *see* Bite, scalp
  pelvis S31.050
    with penetration into retroperitoneal space S31.051
    superficial NEC S30.870
      insect S30.860
  penis S31.25
    superficial NEC S30.872
      insect S30.862
  perineum
    female — *see* Bite, vulva
    male — *see* Bite, pelvis
  periocular area (with or without lacrimal passages) — *see* Bite, eyelid
  phalanges
    finger — *see* Bite, finger
    toe — *see* Bite, toe
  pharynx S11.25
    superficial NEC S10.17
      insect S10.16
  pinna — *see* Bite, ear
  poisonous — *see* Venom
  popliteal space — *see* Bite, knee
  prepuce — *see* Bite, penis
  pubic region — *see* Bite, abdomen, wall
  pudendum
    female — *see* Bite, vulva
    male — *see* Bite, pelvis
  rectovaginal septum — *see* Bite, vulva

Bite(s) — continued
  red bug B88.0
  reptile NEC — see also Venom, bite, reptile
    nonvenomous — see Bite, by site
    snake — see Venom, bite, snake
  sacral region — see Bite, back, lower
  sacroiliac region — see Bite, back, lower
  salivary gland — see Bite, oral cavity
  scalp S01.05
    superficial NEC S00.07
      insect S00.06
  scapular region — see Bite, shoulder
  scrotum S31.35
    superficial NEC S30.873
      insect S30.863
  sea-snake (venomous) — see Toxicity, venom,
    snake, sea snake
  shin — see Bite, leg
  shoulder S41.059
    left S41.052
    right S41.051
    superficial NEC S40.279
      insect S40.269
        left S40.262
        right S40.261
      left S40.272
      right S40.271
  snake — see also Venom, bite, snake
    nonvenomous — see Bite, by site
  spermatic cord — see Bite, testis
  spider (venomous) — see Venom, bite, spider
    nonvenomous — see Bite, insect, by site
  sternal region — see Bite, thorax, front
  submaxillary region — see Bite, head, specified
    site NEC
  submental region — see Bite, head, specified
    site NEC
  subungual
    finger(s) — see Bite, finger
    toe — see Bite, toe
  superficial — see Bite, superficial, by site
  supraclavicular fossa S11.85
  supraorbital — see Bite, head, specified site
    NEC
  temple, temporal region — see Bite, head,
    specified site NEC
  temporomandibular area — see Bite, cheek
  testis S31.35
    superficial NEC S30.873
      insect S30.863
  thigh S71.159
    left S71.152
    right S71.151
    superficial NEC S70.379
      insect S70.369
        left S70.362
        right S70.361
      left S70.372
      right S70.371
  thorax, thoracic (wall) S21.95
    back S21.259
      left S21.252
      right S21.251
    breast — see Bite, breast
    front S21.159
      left S21.152
      right S21.151
    superficial NEC S20.97
      back S20.479
        left S20.472
        right S20.471
      front S20.379
        left S20.372
        right S20.371
      insect S20.96
        back S20.469
          left S20.462
          right S20.461
        front S20.369
          left S20.362
          right S20.361
  throat — see Bite, neck, throat
  thumb S61.059
    with
      damage to nail S61.159
        with fracture S61.169
      fracture S61.069

Bite(s) — continued
  thumb — continued
    left S61.052
      with
        damage to nail S61.152
          with fracture S61.162
        fracture S61.062
    right S61.051
      with
        damage to nail S61.151
          with fracture S61.161
        fracture S61.061
    superficial NEC S60.379
      insect S60.369
        left S60.362
        right S60.361
      left S60.372
      right S60.371
  thyroid S11.15
    superficial NEC S10.87
      insect S10.86
  toe(s) S91.159
    with
      damage to nail S91.259
        with fracture S91.269
      fracture S91.169
    great S91.153
      with
        damage to nail S91.253
          with fracture S91.263
        fracture S91.163
      left S91.152
        with
          damage to nail S91.252
            with fracture S91.262
          fracture S91.162
      right S91.151
        with
          damage to nail S91.251
            with fracture S91.261
          fracture S91.161
    lesser S91.156
      with
        damage to nail S91.256
          with fracture S91.266
        fracture S91.166
      left S91.155
        with
          damage to nail S91.255
            with fracture S91.265
          fracture S91.165
      right S91.154
        with
          damage to nail S91.254
            with fracture S91.264
          fracture S91.164
    superficial NEC S90.476
      great S90.473
        left S90.472
        right S90.471
      insect S90.466
        great S90.463
          left S90.462
          right S90.461
        left S90.465
        right S90.464
      left S90.475
      right S90.474
  tongue S01.552
  trachea S11.025
    superficial NEC S10.17
      insect S10.16
  tunica vaginalis — see Bite, testis
  tympanum, tympanic membrane — see Bite,
    ear
  umbilical region S31.155
  uvula — see Bite, oral cavity
  vagina — see Bite, vulva
  venomous — see Venom
  vocal cords S11.035
    superficial NEC S10.17
      insect S10.16
  vulva S31.45
    superficial NEC S30.874
      insect S30.864

Bite(s) — continued
  wrist S61.559
    with fracture S61.569
      left S61.562
      right S61.561
    left S61.552
    right S61.551
    superficial NEC S60.879
      insect S60.869
        left S60.862
        right S60.861
      left S60.872
      right S60.871
Biting, cheek or lip K13.1
Biventricular failure (heart) I50.9
Björck (-Thorson) syndrome (malignant
  carcinoid) E34.0
Black
  death A20.9
  eye S00.10
    left S00.12
    right S00.11
  hairy tongue K14.3
  lung (disease) J60
Blackfan-Diamond (congenital hypoplastic)
  anemia or syndrome D61.4
Blackhead L70.0
Blackout R55
Bladder — see condition
Blast (air) (hydraulic) (immersion) (underwater)
  blindness S05.80
    left S05.82
    right S05.81
  injury T14.90
    abdomen or thorax — see Injury, by site
    ear (acoustic nerve trauma) — see Injury,
      nerve, acoustic, specified type NEC
    syndrome NEC T70.8
Blastoma (M8000/3) — see Neoplasm, malignant
  pulmonary (M8972/3) — see Neoplasm, lung,
    malignant
Blastomycosis, blastomycotic B40.9
  Brazilian — see Paracoccidioidomycosis
  cutaneous B40.3
  disseminated B40.7
  European — see Cryptococcosis
  generalized B40.7
  keloidal B48.0
  North American B40.9
  primary pulmonary B40.0
  pulmonary B40.2
    acute B40.0
    chronic B40.1
  skin B40.3
  South American — see Paracoccidioidomycosis
  specified NEC B40.89
Bleb(s) R23.8
  emphysematous (lung) (solitary) J43.9
  lung (ruptured) J43.9
    congenital — see Atelectasis
    fetus or newborn P25.8
  subpleural (emphysematous) J43.9
Bleeder (familial) (hereditary) — see Hemophilia
Bleeding — see also Hemorrhage
  anal K62.5
  anovulatory N97.0
  atonic, following delivery O72.1
  capillary I78.8
    puerperal O72.2
  contact (postcoital) N93.0
  due to uterine subinvolution N85.3
  ear — see Otorrhagia
  excessive, associated with menopausal onset
    N92.4
  familial — see Defect, coagulation
  following intercourse N93.0
  gastrointestinal K92.0
  hemorrhoids NEC — see Hemorrhoids, by type,
    bleeding
  intermenstrual (regular) N92.3
    irregular N92.1
  intraoperative — see Hemorrhage,
    intraoperative
  irregular N92.6
  menopausal N92.4

Bleeding — *see also* Hemorrhage — *continued*
  nipple N64.5
  nose R04.0
  ovulation N92.3
  postclimacteric N95.0
  postcoital N93.0
  postmenopausal N95.0
    following induced menopause N95.3
  postoperative — *see* Hemorrhage, postoperative
  preclimacteric N92.4
  puberty (excessive, with onset of menstrual
    periods) N92.2
  rectum, rectal K62.5
    newborn P54.2
  tendencies — *see* Defect, coagulation
  throat R04.1
  tooth socket (post-extraction) K91.65
  umbilical stump P51.9
  uterus, uterine NEC N92.6
    climacteric N92.4
    dysfunctional of functional N93.8
    menopausal N92.4
    preclimacteric or premenopausal N92.4
    unrelated to menstrual cycle N93.9
  vagina, vaginal (abnormal) N93.9
    dysfunctional or functional N93.8
    newborn P54.6
  vicarious N94.8

Blennorrhagia, blennorrhagic — *see* Gonorrhea
Blennorrhea (acute) (chronic) — *see also*
    Gonorrhea
  alveolaris K05.3
  inclusion (neonatal) (newborn) P39.1
  lower genitourinary tract (gonococcal) A54.00
  neonatorum (gonococcal ophthalmia) A54.31

Blepharelosis — *see* Entropion
Blepharitis (angularis) (ciliaris) (eyelid) (marginal)
    (nonulcerative) H01.009
  herpes zoster B02.39
  left H01.006
    lower H01.005
    upper H01.004
  right H01.003
    lower H01.002
    upper H01.001
  squamous H01.029
    left H01.026
      lower H01.025
      upper H01.024
    right H01.023
      lower H01.022
      upper H01.021
  ulcerative H01.019
    left H01.016
      lower H01.015
      upper H01.014
    right H01.013
      lower H01.012
      upper H01.011

Blepharochalasis H02.30
  congenital Q10.0
  left H02.36
    lower H02.35
    upper H02.34
  right H02.33
    lower H02.32
    upper H02.31

Blepharoclonus H02.59
Blepharoconjunctivitis H10.509
  angular H10.529
    bilateral H10.523
    left H10.522
    right H10.521
  bilateral H10.503
  contact H10.539
    bilateral H10.533
    left H10.532
    right H10.531
  left H10.502
  ligneous H10.519
    bilateral H10.513
    left H10.512
    right H10.511
  right H10.501

Blepharophimosis (eyelid) H02.529
  congenital Q10.3
  left H02.526
    lower H02.525
    upper H02.524
  right H02.523
    lower H02.522
    upper H02.521

Blepharoptosis H02.409
  congenital Q10.0
  left H02.406
    upper H02.404
  mechanical H02.419
    left H02.416
      upper H02.414
    right H02.413
      upper H02.411
  myogenic H02.429
    left H02.426
      upper H02.424
    right H02.423
      upper H02.421
  neurogenic H02.439
    left H02.436
      upper H02.434
    right H02.433
      upper H02.431
  paralytic H02.439
    left H02.436
      upper H02.434
    right H02.433
      upper H02.431
  right H02.403
    upper H02.401

Blepharopyorrhea, gonococcal A54.39
Blepharospasm G24.5
Blighted ovum O02.0
Blind — *see also* Blindness
  bronchus (congenital) Q32.8
  loop syndrome K90.2
    congenital Q43.8
  sac, fallopian tube (congenital) Q50.6
  spot, enlarged — *see* Defect, visual field,
    localized, scotoma, blind spot area
  tract or tube, congenital NEC — *see* Atresia, by
    site
Blindness (acquired) (congenital) (both eyes)
    H54.0
  blast S05.80
    left S05.82
    right S05.81
  color — *see* Deficiency, color vision
  concussion S05.80
    left S05.82
    right S05.81
  cortical H47.619
    left brain H47.612
    right brain H47.611
  day H53.11
  due to injury (current episode) S05.90
    left S05.92
    right S05.91
  sequelae – code to injury with terminal
    extension of p
  eclipse (total) — *see* Retinopathy, solar
  emotional (hysterical) F44.6
  hysterical F44.6
  legal (both eyes) (USA definition) H54.8
  mind R48.8
  night H53.60
    abnormal dark adaptation curve H53.61
    acquired H53.62
    congenital H53.63
    specified type NEC H53.69
    vitamin A deficiency E50.5
  one eye (other eye normal) H54.40
    left (normal vision on right) H54.42
      low vision on right H54.12
    low vision, other eye H54.10
    right (normal vision on left) H54.41
      low vision on left H54.11
  psychic R48.8
  river B73.01
  snow — *see* Photokeratitis
  sun, solar — *see* Retinopathy, solar

Blindness — *continued*
  transient — *see* Disturbance, vision, subjective,
    loss, transient
  traumatic (current episode) S05.90
    left S05.92
    right S05.91
  uremic N19
  word (developmental) F81.0
    acquired R48.0
    secondary to organic lesion R48.0

Blister (nonthermal)
  abdominal wall S30.821
  alveolar process S00.522
  ankle S90.529
    left S90.522
    right S90.521
  antecubital space — *see* Blister, elbow
  anus S30.827
  arm (upper) S40.829
    left S40.822
    right S40.821
  auditory canal — *see* Blister, ear
  auricle — *see* Blister, ear
  axilla — *see* Blister, arm
  back, lower S30.820
  beetle dermatitis L24.8
  breast S20.129
    left S20.122
    right S20.121
  brow S00.82
  calf — *see* Blister, leg
  canthus — *see* Blister, eyelid
  cheek S00.82
    internal S00.522
  chest wall — *see* Blister, thorax
  chin S00.82
  costal region — *see* Blister, thorax
  digit(s)
    foot — *see* Blister, toe
    hand — *see* Blister, finger
  due to burn — *see* Burn, by site, second degree
  ear S00.429
    left S00.422
    right S00.421
  elbow S50.329
    left S50.322
    right S50.321
  epiglottis S10.12
  esophagus, cervical S10.12
  eyebrow — *see* Blister, eyelid
  eyelid S00.229
    left S00.222
    right S00.221
  face S00.82
  fever B00.1
  finger(s) S60.429
    index S60.428
      left S60.421
      right S60.420
    little S60.428
      left S60.427
      right S60.426
    middle S60.428
      left S60.423
      right S60.422
    ring S60.428
      left S60.425
      right S60.424
  foot (except toe(s) alone) S90.829
    left S90.822
    right S90.821
    toe — *see* Blister, toe
  forearm S50.829
    elbow only — *see* Blister, elbow
    left S50.822
    right S50.821
  forehead S00.82
  genital organ
    female S30.826
    male S30.825
  gum S00.522
  hand S60.529
    left S60.522
    right S60.521
  head S00.92
    ear — *see* Blister, ear
    eyelid — *see* Blister, eyelid

Blister — *continued*
  head — *continued*
    lip S00.521
    nose S00.32
    oral cavity S00.522
    scalp S00.02
    specified site NEC S00.82
  heel — *see* Blister, foot
  hip S70.229
    left S70.222
    right S70.221
  interscapular region S20.429
  jaw S00.82
  knee S80.229
    left S80.222
    right S80.221
  larynx S10.12
  leg (lower) S80.829
    knee — *see* Blister, knee
    left S80.822
    right S80.821
    upper — *see* Blister, thigh
  lip S00.521
  malar region S00.82
  mammary — *see* Blister, breast
  mastoid region S00.82
  mouth S00.522
  multiple, skin, nontraumatic R23.8
  nail
    finger — *see* Blister, finger
    toe — *see* Blister, toe
  nasal S00.32
  neck S10.92
    specified site NEC S10.82
    throat S10.12
  nose S00.32
  occipital region S00.02
  oral cavity S00.522
  orbital region — *see* Blister, eyelid
  palate S00.522
  palm — *see* Blister, hand
  parietal region S00.02
  pelvis S30.820
  penis S30.822
  periocular area — *see* Blister, eyelid
  phalanges
    finger — *see* Blister, finger
    toe — *see* Blister, toe
  pharynx S10.12
  pinna — *see* Blister, ear
  popliteal space — *see* Blister, knee
  scalp S00.02
  scapular region — *see* Blister, shoulder
  scrotum S30.823
  shin — *see* Blister, leg
  shoulder S40.229
    left S40.222
    right S40.221
  sternal region S20.329
  submaxillary region S00.82
  submental region S00.82
  subungual
    finger(s) — *see* Blister, finger
    toe(s) — *see* Blister, toe
  supraclavicular fossa S10.82
  supraorbital S00.82
  temple S00.82
  temporal region S00.82
  testis S30.823
  thermal — *see* Burn, second degree, by site
  thigh S70.329
    left S70.322
    right S70.321
  thorax, thoracic (wall) S20.92
    back S20.429
      left S20.422
      right S20.421
    front S20.329
      left S20.322
      right S20.321
  throat S10.12
  thumb S60.329
    left S60.322
    right S60.321
  toe(s) S90.426
    great S90.423
      left S90.422

Blister — *continued*
  toe(s) — *continued*
    great — *continued*
      right S90.421
    left S90.425
    right S90.424
  tongue S00.522
  trachea S10.12
  tympanum, tympanic membrane — *see* Blister, ear
  upper arm — *see* Blister, arm (upper)
  uvula S00.522
  vagina S30.824
  vocal cords S10.12
  vulva S30.824
  wrist S60.829
    left S60.822
    right S60.821
Bloating R14.0
Bloch-Sulzberger disease or syndrome Q82.3
Block
  alveolocapillary J84.1
  arborization (heart) I45.5
  arrhythmic I45.9
  atrioventricular (incomplete) (partial) I44.30
    with atrioventricular dissociation I44.2
    complete I44.2
      congenital Q24.6
    congenital Q24.6
    first degree I44.0
    second degree (types I and II) I44.1
    specified NEC I44.39
    third degree I44.2
    types I and II I44.1
  auriculoventricular — *see* Block, atrioventricular
  bifascicular (cardiac) I45.2
  bundle-branch (complete) (false) (incomplete) I45.4
    bilateral I45.2
    left I44.7
      with right bundle branch block I45.2
      hemiblock I44.6
        anterior I44.4
        posterior I44.5
      incomplete
        with right bundle branch block I45.2
    right I45.1
      with
        left bundle branch block I45.2
        left fascicular block I45.2
    Wilson's type I45.1
  cardiac I45.9
  conduction I45.9
    complete I44.2
  fascicular (left) I44.6
    anterior I44.4
    posterior I44.5
    right I45.0
  foramen Magendie (acquired) G91.1
    congenital Q03.1
      with spina bifida — *see* Spina bifida, by site, with hydrocephalus
  heart I45.9
    bundle branch
      bilateral I45.2
    complete (atrioventricular) I44.2
    congenital Q24.6
    first degree (atrioventricular) I44.0
    second degree (atrioventricular) I44.1
    specified type NEC I45.5
    third degree (atrioventricular) I44.2
  hepatic vein I82.0
  intraventricular (nonspecific) I45.4
    bundle branch
      bilateral I45.2
  kidney — *see* Failure, renal
    postcystoscopic or postprocedural N99.0
  Mobitz (types I and II) I44.1
  myocardial — *see* Block, heart
  nodal I45.5
  organ or site, congenital NEC — *see* Atresia, by site
  portal (vein) I81
  second degree (types I and II) I44.1
  sinoatrial I45.5
  sinoauricular I45.5

Block — *continued*
  third degree I44.2
  trifascicular I45.3
  tubal N97.1
  vein NOS I82.9
  Wenckebach (types I and II) I44.1
Blockage — *see* Obstruction
Blocq's disease F44.4
Blood
  constituents, abnormal R78.9
  disease D75.9
  donor — *see* Donor, blood
  dyscrasia D75.9
    with
      abortion — *see* Abortion, by type with excessive hemorrhage
      ectopic pregnancy O08.1
      molar pregnancy O08.1
    fetus or newborn P61.9
    following ectopic or molar pregnancy O08.1
    puerperal, postpartum O72.3
  flukes NEC — *see* Schistosomiasis
  in
    feces — *see* Melena
    urine — *see* Hematuria
  mole O02.0
  poisoning — *see* Septicemia
  pressure
    decreased, due to shock following injury T79.4
    examination only Z01.30
    fluctuating I99.8
    high — *see* Hypertension
      incidental reading, without diagnosis of hypertension R03.0
    low — *see also* Hypotension
      incidental reading, without diagnosis of hypotension R03.1
  spitting — *see* Hemoptysis
  staining cornea — *see* Pigmentation, cornea, stromal
  transfusion
    without reported diagnosis Z51.89
    reaction or complication — *see* Complications, transfusion
  type
    A (Rh positive) Z67.10
      Rh negative Z67.11
    AB (Rh positive) Z67.30
      Rh negative Z67.31
    B (Rh positive) Z67.20
      Rh negative Z67.21
    O (Rh positive) Z67.40
      Rh negative Z67.41
    Rh (positive) Z67.90
      negative Z67.91
  vessel rupture — *see* Hemorrhage
  vomiting — *see* Hematemesis
Blood-forming organs, disease D75.9
Bloodgood's disease — *see* Mastopathy, cystic
Bloom (-Machacek) (-Torre) syndrome Q82.8
Blount's disease or osteochondrosis — *see* Osteochondrosis, juvenile, tibia
Blue
  baby Q24.9
  diaper syndrome E72.09
  dome cyst (breast) — *see* Cyst, breast
  dot cataract Q12.0
  nevus (M8780/0) D22.9
  sclera Q13.5
    with fragility of bone and deafness Q78.0
Blueness — *see* Cyanosis
Blues, postpartal O90.6
Blurring, visual H53.8
Blushing (abnormal) (excessive) R23.2
Boarder, hospital NEC Z76.4
  accompanying sick person Z76.3
  healthy infant or child Z76.2
  foundling Z76.1
Bockhart's impetigo L01.02
Bodechtel-Guttman disease (subacute sclerosing panencephalitis) A81.1
Boder-Sedgwick syndrome (ataxia-telangiectasia) G11.3

©2002 Ingenix, Inc.

Body, bodies
　Aschoff's — *see* Myocarditis, rheumatic
　asteroid, vitreous — *see* Deposit, crystalline
　cytoid (retina) — *see* Occlusion, artery, retina
　drusen (degenerative) (macula) (retinal) — *see also* Degeneration, macula, drusen
　optic disc — *see* Drusen, optic disc
　foreign — *see* Foreign body
　loose
　　joint, except knee — *see* Loose, body, joint
　　knee M23.40
　　　left M23.42
　　　right M23.41
　　sheath, tendon — *see* Disorder, tendon, specified type NEC
　Mooser's A75.2
　rice — *see also* Loose, body, joint
　　knee M23.40
　　　left M23.42
　　　right M23.41
　rocking F98.4
Boeck's
　disease or sarcoid — *see* Sarcoidosis
　lupoid (miliary) D86.3
Boerhaave's syndrome (spontaneous esophageal rupture) K22.3
Boggy
　cervix N88.8
　uterus N85.8
Boil — *see also* Furuncle, by site
　Aleppo B55.1
　Baghdad B55.1
　Delhi B55.1
　lacrimal
　　gland — *see* Dacryoadenitis
　　passages (duct) (sac) — *see* Inflammation, lacrimal, passages, acute
　Natal B55.1
　orbit, orbital — *see* Abscess, orbit
　tropical B55.1
Bold hives — *see* Urticaria
Bombé, iris — *see* Membrane, pupillary
Bone — *see* condition
Bonnevie-Ullrich syndrome Q87.1
Bonnier's syndrome — *see* category H81.8
Bonvale dam fever T73.3
Bony block of joint — *see* Ankylosis
Borderline pelvis, with obstruction during labor O65.1
Borna disease A83.9
Bornholm disease B33.0
Boston exanthem A88.0
Botalli, ductus (patent) (persistent) Q25.0
Bothriocephalus latus infestation B70.0
Botulism (foodborne intoxication) A05.1
　infant A05.1
　wound A48.8
Bouba — *see* Yaws
Bouchard's nodes (with arthropathy) M15.2
Bouffée délirante F23
Bouillaud's disease or syndrome (rheumatic heart disease) I01.9
Bourneville's disease Q85.1
Boutonniere deformity (finger) — *see* Deformity, finger, boutonniere
Bouveret (-Hoffmann) syndrome (paroxysmal tachycardia) I47.9
Bovine heart — *see* Hypertrophy, cardiac
Bowel — *see* condition
Bowen's
　dermatosis (precancerous) (M8081/2) — *see* Neoplasm, skin, in situ
　disease (M8081/2) — *see* Neoplasm, skin, in situ
　epithelioma (M8081/2) — *see* Neoplasm, skin, in situ
　type
　　epidermoid carcinoma-in-situ (M8081/2) — *see* Neoplasm, skin, in situ
　　intraepidermal squamous cell carcinoma (M8081/2) — *see* Neoplasm, skin, in situ

Bowing
　femur — *see also* Deformity, limb, specified type NEC, thigh
　　congenital Q68.3
　fibula — *see also* Deformity, limb, specified type NEC, lower leg
　　congenital Q68.4
　forearm — *see* Deformity, limb, specified type NEC, forearm
　leg(s), long bones, congenital Q68.5
　radius — *see* Deformity, limb, specified type NEC, forearm
　tibia — *see also* Deformity, limb, specified type NEC, lower leg
　　congenital Q68.4
Bowleg(s) (acquired) — *see also* Deformity, varus, knee
　congenital Q68.5
　rachitic E64.3
Boyd's dysentery A03.2
Brachial — *see* condition
Brachycardia R00.1
Brachycephaly Q75.0
Bradley's disease A08.1
Bradyarrhythmia, cardiac I49.8
Bradycardia (any type) (vagal) R00.1
　chronic (sinus) I49.5
　fetal — *see* Distress, fetal
　reflex G90.0
　sinoatrial, chronic (with (paroxysmal) tachycardia) I49.5
　sinus (with (paroxysmal) tachycardia) (chronic) (persistent) (severe) I49.5
　tachycardia syndrome I49.5
Bradypnea R06.89
Bradytachycardia I49.5
Brailsford's disease or osteochondrosis — *see* Osteochondrosis, juvenile, radius
Brain — *see also* condition
　death G93.8
　syndrome — *see* Syndrome, brain
Branched-chain amino-acid disorder E71.2
Branchial — *see* condition
　cartilage, congenital Q18.2
Branchiogenic remnant (in neck) Q18.0
Brash (water) R12
Bravais-jacksonian epilepsy — *see* Epilepsy, focal
Brazilian leishmaniasis B55.2
Break, retina (without detachment) H33.309
　with retinal detachment — *see* Detachment, retina
　bilateral H33.303
　horseshoe tear H33.319
　　bilateral H33.313
　　left H33.312
　　right H33.311
　left H33.302
　multiple H33.339
　　bilateral H33.333
　　left H33.332
　　right H33.331
　right H33.301
　round hole H33.329
　　bilateral H33.323
　　left H33.322
　　right H33.321
Breakdown
　device, graft or implant (*see also* Complications, by site and type, mechanical) T85.618
　　arterial graft NEC — *see* Complication, cardiovascular device, mechanical, vascular
　　breast (implant) T85.41
　　catheter NEC T85.618
　　　cystostomy T83.010
　　　dialysis (renal) T82.41
　　　　intraperitoneal T85.611
　　　infusion NEC T82.514
　　　　spinal (epidural) (subdural) T85.610
　　　urinary (indwelling) T83.018

Breakdown — *continued*
　device, graft or implant (*see also* Complications, by site and type, mechanical) — *continued*
　　electronic (electrode) (pulse generator) (stimulator)
　　　bone T84.310
　　　cardiac T82.119
　　　　electrode T82.110
　　　　pulse generator T82.111
　　　　specified type NEC T82.118
　　　nervous system — *see* Complication, prosthetic device, mechanical, electronic nervous system stimulator
　　　urinary — *see* Complication, genitourinary, device, urinary, mechanical
　　fixation, internal (orthopedic) NEC — *see* Complication, fixation device, mechanical
　　gastrointestinal — *see* Complications, prosthetic device, mechanical, gastrointestinal device
　　genital NEC T83.418
　　　intrauterine contraceptive device T83.31
　　　penile prosthesis T83.410
　　heart NEC — *see* Complication, cardiovascular device, mechanical
　　joint prosthesis — *see* Complications, joint prosthesis, mechanical
　　ocular NEC — *see* Complications, prosthetic device, mechanical, ocular device
　　orthopedic NEC — *see* Complication, orthopedic, device, mechanical
　　specified NEC T85.618
　　sutures, permanent T85.612
　　　used in bone repair — *see* Complications, fixation device, internal (orthopedic), mechanical
　　urinary NEC — *see also* Complication, genitourinary, device, urinary, mechanical
　　　graft T83.21
　　vascular NEC — *see* Complication, cardiovascular device, mechanical
　　ventricular intracranial shunt T85.01
　nervous F48.8
　perineum O90.1
Breast — *see* condition
Breath
　foul R19.6
　holder, child R06.89
　holding spell R06.89
　shortness R06.02
Breathing
　exercises Z51.89
　labored — *see* Hyperventilation
　mouth R06.5
　periodic R06.3
Breathlessness R06.81
Breda's disease — *see* Yaws
Breech presentation (mother) O32.1
　causing obstructed labor O64.1
　footling O32.8
　　causing obstructed labor O64.8
　incomplete O32.8
　　causing obstructed labor O64.8
Breisky's disease N90.4
Brennemann's syndrome I88.0
Brenner
　tumor (benign) (M9000/0) D27.9
　　borderline malignancy (M9000/1) D39.10
　　　left ovary D39.12
　　　right ovary D39.11
　　left ovary D27.1
　　malignant (M9000/3) C56
　　proliferating (M9000/1) D39.10
　　　left ovary D39.12
　　　right ovary D39.11
　　right ovary D27.0
Bretonneau's disease or angina A36.0
Breus' mole O02.0
Brevicollis Q76.49

Brickmakers' anemia B76.9

Bridge, myocardial Q24.5

Bright's disease — see also Nephritis
arteriosclerotic — see Hypertension, kidney

Brill (-Zinsser) disease (recrudescent typhus)
A75.1
flea-borne A75.2
louse-borne A75.1

Brill-Symmers' disease (M9690/3) C82.90

Brion-Kayser disease — see Fever, parathyroid

Briquet's disorder or syndrome F45.0

Brissaud's
infantilism or dwarfism E23.0
motor-verbal tic F95.2

Brittle
bones disease Q78.0
nails L60.3
congenital Q84.6

Broad — see also condition
beta disease E78.2
ligament laceration syndrome N83.8
Broador floating-betalipoproteinemia E78.2

Brock's syndrome (atelectasis due to enlarged
lymph nodes) J98.19

Brocq-Duhring disease (dermatitis herpetiformis)
L13.0

Brodie's abscess or disease — see Osteomyelitis,
specified type NEC

Broken
arches — see also Deformity, limb, flat foot
congenital Q66.5
arm (meaning upper limb) — see Fracture, arm
back — see Fracture, vertebra
bone — see Fracture
implant or internal device — see Complications,
by site and type, mechanical
leg (meaning lower limb) — see Fracture, leg
nose S02.2
tooth, teeth — see Fracture, tooth

Bromhidrosis, bromidrosis L75.0

Bromidism, bromism
acute
correct substance properly administered
G92
overdose or wrong substance given or taken
— see category T42.6
chronic (dependence) F13.20
correct substance properly administered G92

Bromidrosiphobia F40.298

Bronchi, bronchial — see condition

Bronchiectasis (cylindrical) (diffuse) (fusiform)
(localized) (saccular) J47.9
with
acute exacerbation J47.1
lower respiratory infection J47.0
congenital Q33.4
tuberculous NEC — see Tuberculosis,
pulmonary

Bronchiolectasis — see Bronchiectasis

Bronchiolitis (acute) (infective) (subacute) J21.9
with
bronchospasm or obstruction J21.9
influenza, flu or grippe J10.1
chemical (chronic) J68.4
acute J68.0
chronic (fibrosing) (obliterative) J44.9
due to
external agent — see Bronchitis, acute, due
to
respiratory syncytial virus J21.0
specified organism NEC J21.8
fibrosa obliterans J44.9
influenzal J10.1
obliterative (chronic) (subacute) J44.9
due to fumes or vapors J68.4
due to chemicals, gases, fumes or vapors
(inhalation) J68.4

Bronchitis (diffuse) (fibrinous) (hypostatic)
(infective) (inflammatory) (membranous)
(with tracheitis) J40
with
influenza, flu or grippe J10.1
obstruction (airway) (lung) J44.9

Bronchitis — continued
with — continued
tracheitis (15 years of age and above) J40
acute or subacute J20.9
chronic J42
under 15 years of age J20.9
acute or subacute (with bronchospasm or
obstruction) J20.9
chemical (due to gases, fumes or vapors)
J68.0
due to
fumes or vapors J68.0
Haemophilus influenzae J20.1
Mycoplasma pneumoniae J20.0
radiation J70.0
specified organism NEC J20.8
Streptococcus J20.2
virus
coxsackie J20.3
echovirus J20.7
parainfluenzae J20.4
respiratory syncytial J20.5
rhinovirus J20.6
viral NEC J20.8
allergic (acute) J45.00
with
acute exacerbation J45.01
status asthmaticus J45.02
arachidic T17.528
aspiration (due to fumes or vapors) J68.0
asthmatic — see also Asthma
chronic J44.9
capillary — see Pneumonia, broncho
caseous (tuberculous) A15.5
Castellani's A69.8
catarrhal (15 years of age and above) J40
acute — see Bronchitis, acute
chronic J41.0
under 15 years of age J20.9
chemical (acute) (subacute) J68.0
chronic J68.4
due to fumes or vapors J68.0
chronic J68.4
chronic J42
with
airways obstruction J44.9
tracheitis (chronic) J42
asthmatic (obstructive) J44.9
catarrhal J41.0
chemical (due to fumes or vapors) J68.4
due to
chemicals, gases, fumes or vapors
(inhalation) J68.4
radiation J70.1
tobacco smoking J41.0
emphysematous J44.9
mucopurulent J41.1
non-obstructive J41.0
obliterans J44.9
obstructive J44.9
purulent J41.1
simple J41.0
croupous — see Bronchitis, acute
due to gases, fumes or vapors (chemical) J68.0
emphysematous (obstructive) J44.9
exudative — see Bronchitis, acute
fetid J41.1
grippal J10.1
in those under 15 years age — see Bronchitis,
acute
chronic — see Bronchitis, chronic
influenzal J10.1
mixed simple and mucopurulent J41.8
moulder's J62.8
mucopurulent (chronic) (recurrent) J41.1
acute or subacute J20.9
simple (mixed) J41.8
obliterans (chronic) J44.9
obstructive (chronic) (diffuse) J44.9
pituitous J41.1
pneumococcal, acute or subacute J20.2
pseudomembranous, acute or subacute — see
Bronchitis, acute
purulent (chronic) (recurrent) J41.1
acute or subacute — see Bronchitis, acute
putrid J41.1
senile (chronic) J42

Bronchitis — continued
septic, acute or subacute — see Bronchitis,
acute
simple and mucopurulent (mixed) J41.8
smokers' J41.0
spirochetal NEC A69.8
subacute — see Bronchitis, acute
suppurative (chronic) J41.1
acute or subacute — see Bronchitis, acute
tuberculous A15.5
under 15 years of age — see Bronchitis, acute
chronic — see Bronchitis, chronic
viral NEC, acute or subacute (see also
Bronchitis, acute) J20.8

Bronchoalveolitis J18.0

Bronchoaspergillosis B44.1

Bronchocele meaning goiter E04.0

Broncholithiasis J98.0
tuberculous NEC A15.5

Bronchomalacia J98.0
congenital Q32.2

Bronchomycosis NOS B49 [J99]
candidal B37.1

Bronchopleuropneumonia — see Pneumonia,
broncho

Bronchopneumonia — see Pneumonia, broncho

Bronchopneumonitis — see Pneumonia, broncho

Bronchopulmonary — see condition

Bronchopulmonitis — see Pneumonia, broncho

Bronchorrhagia (see Hemoptysis)

Bronchorrhea J98.0
acute J20.9
chronic (infective) (purulent) J42

Bronchospasm J98.0
with
bronchiolitis, acute J21.9
bronchitis, acute (conditions in J20) — see
Bronchitis, acute
due to external agent — see condition,
respiratory, acute, due to

Bronchospirochetosis A69.8
Castellani A69.8

Bronchostenosis J98.0

Bronchus — see condition

Brontophobia F40.220

Bronze baby syndrome P83.8

Brooke's tumor (M8100/0) — see Neoplasm,
skin, benign

Brown enamel of teeth (hereditary) K00.5

Brown's sheath syndrome
left H50.612
right H50.611

Brown-Séquard disease, paralysis or syndrome
G83.81

Bruce septicemia A23.0

Brucella, brucellosis (infection) A23.9
abortus A23.1
canis A23.3
dermatitis A23.9
melitensis A23.0
mixed A23.8
septicemia A23.9
melitensis A23.0
specified NEC A23.8
suis A23.2

Bruck-de Lange disease Q87.1

Bruck's disease — see Deformity, limb

Brugsch's syndrome Q82.8

Bruise (skin surface intact) — see also Contusion
with
open wound — see Wound, open
fetus or newborn P54.5
internal organ — see Injury, by site
scalp, due to birth injury, newborn P12.3
umbilical cord O69.5

Bruit (arterial) R09.89
cardiac R01.1

Brush burn — see Abrasion, by site

Bruton's X-linked agammaglobulinemia D80.0

Bruxism F45.8

Bubbly lung syndrome P27.0

©2002 Ingenix, Inc.

Bubo I88.8
  blennorrhagic (gonococcal) A54.89
  chancroidal A57
  climatic A55
  due to Haemophilus ducreyi A57
  gonococcal A54.89
  indolent (nonspecific) I88.8
  inguinal (nonspecific) I88.8
    chancroidal A57
    climatic A55
    due to H. ducreyi A57
    infective I88.8
    venereal
      female A64.4
      male A64.2
  scrofulous (tuberculous) A18.2
  soft chancre A57
  suppurating — see Lymphadenitis, acute
  syphilitic (primary) A51.0
    congenital A50.07
  tropical A55
  venereal
    female A64.4
    male A64.2
  virulent (chancroidal) A57
Bubonic plague A20.0
Bubonocele — see Hernia, inguinal
Buccal — see condition
Buchanan's disease or osteochondrosis M91.0
Buchem's syndrome (hyperostosis corticalis) M85.2
Bucket-handle fracture or tear (semilunar cartilage) — see Tear, meniscus
Budd-Chiari syndrome (hepatic vein thrombosis) I82.0
Budgerigar fancier's disease or lung J67.2
Buerger's disease (thromboangiitis obliterans) I73.1
Bulbar — see condition
Bulbus cordis (left ventricle) (persistent) Q21.8
Bulimia (nervosa) F50.2
  atypical F50.9
  normal weight F50.9
Bulky
  stools R19.5
  uterus N85.2
Bulla(e) R23.8
  lung (emphysematous) (solitary) J43.9
    fetus or newborn P25.8
Bullet wound — see also Wound, open
  fracture — code as Fracture, by site
  internal organ — see Injury, by site
Bundle
  branch block (complete) (false) (incomplete) — see Block, bundle-branch
  of His — see condition
Bunion — see Deformity, toe, hallux valgus
Buphthalmia, buphthalmos (congenital) Q15.0
Burdwan fever B55.0
Bürger-Grütz disease or syndrome E78.3
Buried roots K08.3
Burke's syndrome K86.8
Burkitt's
  cell leukemia (M9826/3) C91.00
    in remission C91.01
  lymphoma (malignant) (M9687/3) C83.70
    nodes (of)
      arm C83.74
      axilla C83.74
      head, face and neck C83.71
      inguinal C83.75
      intra-abdominal C83.73
      intrapelvic C83.76
      intrathoracic C83.72
      leg C83.75
      multiple sites C83.78
    small noncleaved, diffuse (M9687/3) C83.70
    spleen C83.77
    undifferentiated (M9687/3) C83.70
  tumor (M9687/3) C83.70
  type
    acute lymphoblastic leukemia (M9826/3) C91.00

Burkitt's — continued
  type — continued
    acute lymphoblastic — continued
      in remission C91.01
    undifferentiated (M9687/3) C83.70
Burn (electricity) (flame) (hot gas, liquid or hot object) (radiation) (steam) (thermal) T30.0
  abdomen, abdominal (muscle) (wall) T21.02
    first degree T21.12
    second degree T21.22
    third degree T21.32
  above elbow T22.039
    first degree T22.139
      left T22.032
        first degree T22.132
        second degree T22.232
        third degree T22.332
      right T22.031
        first degree T22.131
        second degree T22.231
        third degree T22.331
    second degree T22.239
    third degree T22.339
  acid (caustic) (external) (internal) — see Corrosion, by site
  alimentary tract NEC T28.2
    esophagus T28.1
    mouth T28.0
    pharynx T28.0
  alkaline (caustic) (external) (internal) — see Corrosion, by site
  ankle T25.019
    first degree T25.119
      left T25.012
        first degree T25.112
        second degree T25.212
        third degree T25.312
    multiple with foot — see Burn, lower, limb, multiple, ankle and foot
      right T25.011
        first degree T25.111
        second degree T25.211
        third degree T25.311
    second degree T25.219
    third degree T25.319
  anus — see Burn, buttock
  arm (lower) (upper) — see Burn, upper, limb
  axilla T22.049
    first degree T22.149
      left T22.042
        first degree T22.142
        second degree T22.242
        third degree T22.342
      right T22.041
        first degree T22.141
        second degree T22.241
        third degree T22.341
    second degree T22.249
    third degree T22.349
  back (lower) T21.04
    first degree T21.14
    second degree T21.24
    third degree T21.34
    upper T21.03
      first degree T21.13
      second degree T21.23
      third degree T21.33
  blisters — code as Burn, second degree, by site
  breast(s) — see Burn, chest wall
  buttock(s) T21.05
    first degree T21.15
    second degree T21.25
    third degree T21.35
  calf T24.039
    first degree T24.139
      left T24.032
        first degree T24.132
        second degree T24.232
        third degree T24.332
      right T24.031
        first degree T24.131
        second degree T24.231
        third degree T24.331
    second degree T24.239
    third degree T24.339
  canthus (eye) — see Burn, eyelid

Burn — continued
  caustic acid or alkaline — see Corrosion, by site
  cervix T28.3
  cheek T20.06
    first degree T20.16
    second degree T20.26
    third degree T20.36
  chemical (acids) (alkalines) (caustics) (external) (internal) — see Corrosion, by site
  chest wall T21.01
    first degree T21.11
    second degree T21.21
    third degree T21.31
  chin T20.03
    first degree T20.13
    second degree T20.23
    third degree T20.33
  colon T28.2
  conjunctiva (and cornea) — see Burn, cornea
  cornea (and conjunctiva) T26.10
    chemical — see Corrosion, cornea
    left T26.12
    right T26.11
  corrosion (external) (internal) — see Corrosion, by site
  deep necrosis of underlying tissue – code as Burn, third degree, by site
  dorsum of hand T23.069
    first degree T23.169
      left T23.062
        first degree T23.162
        second degree T23.262
        third degree T23.362
      right T23.061
        first degree T23.161
        second degree T23.261
        third degree T23.361
    second degree T23.269
    third degree T23.369
  due to ingested chemical agent — see Corrosion, by site
  ear (auricle) (external) (canal) T20.01
    first degree T20.11
    second degree T20.21
    third degree T20.31
  elbow T22.029
    first degree T22.129
      left T22.022
        first degree T22.122
        second degree T22.222
        third degree T22.322
      right T22.021
        first degree T22.121
        second degree T22.221
        third degree T22.321
    second degree T22.229
    third degree T22.329
  entire body T29
  epidermal loss – code as Burn, second degree, by site
  erythema, erythematous – code as Burn, first degree, by site
  esophagus T28.1
  extremity — see Burn, limb
  eye(s) and adnexa T26.40
    with resulting rupture and destruction of eyeball T26.20
      left T26.22
      right T26.21
    conjunctival sac — see Burn, cornea
    cornea — see Burn, cornea
    left T26.42
    lid — see Burn, eyelid
    periocular area — see Burn eyelid
    right T26.41
    specified site NEC T26.30
      left T26.32
      right T26.31
  eyeball — see Burn, eye
  eyelid(s) T26.00
    chemical — see Corrosion, eyelid
    left T26.02
    right T26.01
  face — see Burn, head
  finger T23.029
    first degree T23.129

Burn — *continued*
  finger — *continued*
    left T23.022
      first degree T23.122
      second degree T23.222
      third degree T23.322
    multiple sites (without thumb) T23.039
      with thumb T23.049
        first degree T23.149
        left T23.042
          first degree T23.142
          second degree T23.242
          third degree T23.342
        right T23.041
          first degree T23.141
          second degree T23.241
          third degree T23.341
        second degree T23.249
        third degree T23.349
    first degree T23.139
    left T23.032
      first degree T23.132
      second degree T23.232
      third degree T23.332
    right T23.031
      first degree T23.131
      second degree T23.231
      third degree T23.331
    second degree T23.239
    third degree T23.339
    right T23.021
      first degree T23.121
      second degree T23.221
      third degree T23.321
    second degree T23.229
    third degree T23.329
  flank — *see* Burn, abdominal wall
  foot T25.029
    first degree T25.129
    left T25.022
      first degree T25.122
      second degree T25.222
      third degree T25.322
    multiple with ankle — *see* Burn, lower, limb, multiple, ankle and foot
    right T25.021
      first degree T25.121
      second degree T25.221
      third degree T25.321
    second degree T25.229
    third degree T25.329
  forearm T22.019
    first degree T22.119
    left T22.012
      first degree T22.112
      second degree T22.212
      third degree T22.312
    right T22.011
      first degree T22.111
      second degree T22.211
      third degree T22.311
    second degree T22.219
    third degree T22.319
  forehead T20.06
    first degree T20.16
    second degree T20.26
    third degree T20.36
  fourth degree – code as Burn, third degree, by site
  friction — *see* Burn, by site
  from swallowing caustic or corrosive substance NEC — *see* Corrosion, by site
  full thickness skin loss – code as Burn, third degree, by site
  gastrointestinal tract NEC T28.2
    from swallowing caustic or corrosive substance T28.7
  genital organs
    external
      female T21.07
        first degree T21.17
        second degree T21.27
        third degree T21.37
      male T21.06
        first degree T21.16
        second degree T21.26

Burn — *continued*
  genital organs — *continued*
    external — *continued*
      male — *continued*
        third degree T21.36
    internal T28.3
      from caustic or corrosive substance T28.8
  groin — *see* Burn, abdominal wall
  hand(s) T23.009
    back — *see* Burn, dorsum of hand
    finger — *see* Burn, finger
    first degree T23.109
    left T23.002
      first degree T23.102
      second degree T23.202
      third degree T23.302
    multiple sites with wrist T23.099
      first degree T23.199
      left T23.092
        first degree T23.192
        second degree T23.292
        third degree T23.392
      right T23.091
        first degree T23.191
        second degree T23.291
        third degree T23.391
      second degree T23.299
      third degree T23.399
    palm — *see* Burn, palm
    right T23.001
      first degree T23.101
      second degree T23.201
      third degree T23.301
    second degree T23.209
    third degree T23.309
    thumb — *see* Burn, thumb
  head (and face) (and neck) T20.00
    cheek — *see* Burn, cheek
    chin — *see* Burn, chin
    ear — *see* Burn, ear
    eye(s) only — *see* Burn, eye
    first degree T20.10
    forehead — *see* Burn, forehead
    lip — *see* Burn, lip
    multiple sites T20.09
      first degree T20.19
      second degree T20.29
      third degree T20.39
    neck — *see* Burn, neck
    nose — *see* Burn, nose
    scalp — *see* Burn, scalp
    second degree T20.20
    third degree T20.30
  hip(s) — *see* Burn, lower, limb
  infected T79.3
  inhalation — *see* Burn, respiratory tract
    caustic or corrosive substance (fumes) — *see* Corrosion, respiratory tract
  internal organ(s) T28.40
    alimentary tract T28.2
      esophagus T28.1
    eardrum T28.41
    esophagus T28.1
    from caustic or corrosive substance (swallowing) NEC — *see* Corrosion, by site
    genitourinary T28.3
    mouth T28.0
    pharynx T28.0
    respiratory tract — *see* Burn, respiratory tract
    specified organ NEC T28.49
  interscapular region — *see* Burn, back, upper
  intestine (large) (small) T28.2
  knee T24.029
    first degree T24.129
    left T24.022
      first degree T24.122
      second degree T24.222
      third degree T24.322
    right T24.021
      first degree T24.121
      second degree T24.221
      third degree T24.321
    second degree T24.229
    third degree T24.329

Burn — *continued*
  labium (majus) (minus) — *see* Burn, genital organs, external, female
  lacrimal apparatus, duct, gland or sac — *see* Burn, eye, specified site NEC
  larynx T27.0
    with lung T27.1
  leg(s) (lower) (upper) — *see* Burn, lower, limb
  lightning — *see* Burn, by site
  limb(s)
    lower (except ankle or foot alone) — *see* Burn, lower, limb
    upper — *see* Burn, upper limb
  lip(s) T20.02
    first degree T20.12
    second degree T20.22
    third degree T20.32
  lower
    back — *see* Burn, back
    limb T24.000
      ankle — *see* Burn, ankle
      calf — *see* Burn, calf
      first degree T24.109
      foot — *see* Burn, foot
      knee — *see* Burn, knee
      left T24.002
        first degree T24.102
        second degree T24.202
        third degree T24.302
      multiple sites, except ankle and foot T24.099
        ankle and foot T25.099
          first degree T25.199
          left T25.092
            first degree T25.192
            second degree T25.292
            third degree T25.392
          right T25.091
            first degree T25.191
            second degree T25.291
            third degree T25.391
          second degree T25.299
          third degree T25.399
        first degree T24.199
        left T24.092
          first degree T24.192
          second degree T24.292
          third degree T24.392
        right T24.091
          first degree T24.191
          second degree T24.291
          third degree T24.391
        second degree T24.299
        third degree T24.399
      right T24.001
        first degree T24.101
        second degree T24.201
        third degree T24.301
      second degree T24.209
      hip — *see* Burn, thigh
      thigh — *see* Burn, thigh
      third degree T24.309
      toe — *see* Burn, toe
  lung (with larynx and trachea) T27.1
  mouth T28.0
  multiple body regions T29
  neck T20.07
    first degree T20.17
    second degree T20.27
    third degree T20.37
  nose (septum) T20.04
    first degree T20.14
    second degree T20.24
    third degree T20.34
  ocular adnexa — *see* Burn, eye
  orbit region — *see* Burn, eyelid
  palm T23.059
    first degree T23.159
    left T23.052
      first degree T23.152
      second degree T23.252
      third degree T23.352
    right T23.051
      first degree T23.151
      second degree T23.251
      third degree T23.351

©2002 Ingenix, Inc.

Burn — *continued*
  palm — *continued*
    second degree T23.259
    third degree T23.359
  partial thickness – code as Burn, unspecified degree, by site
  pelvis — *see* Burn, trunk
  penis — *see* Burn, genital organs, external, male
  perineum
    female — *see* Burn, genital organs, external, female
    male — *see* Burn, genital organs, external, male
  periocular area — *see* Burn, eyelid
  pharynx T28.0
  rectum T28.2
  respiratory tract T27.3
    larynx — *see* Burn, larynx
    specified part NEC T27.2
    trachea — *see* Burn, trachea
  sac, lacrimal — *see* Burn, eye, specified site NEC
  scalp T20.05
    first degree T20.15
    second degree T20.25
    third degree T20.35
  scapular region T22.069
    first degree T22.169
    left T22.062
      first degree T22.162
      second degree T22.262
      third degree T22.362
    right T22.061
      first degree T22.161
      second degree T22.261
      third degree T22.361
    second degree T22.269
    third degree T22.369
  sclera — *see* Burn, eye, specified site NEC
  scrotum — *see* Burn, genital organs, external, male
  shoulder T22.059
    first degree T22.159
    left T22.052
      first degree T22.152
      second degree T22.252
      third degree T22.352
    right T22.051
      first degree T22.151
      second degree T22.251
      third degree T22.351
    second degree T22.259
    third degree T22.359
  stomach T28.2
  temple — *see* Burn, head
  testis — *see* Burn, genital organs, external, male
  thigh T24.019
    first degree T24.119
    left T24.012
      first degree T24.112
      second degree T24.212
      third degree T24.312
    right T24.011
      first degree T24.111
      second degree T24.211
      third degree T24.311
    second degree T24.219
    third degree T24.319
  thorax (external) — *see* Burn, trunk
  throat (meaning pharynx) T28.0
  thumb(s) T23.019
    first degree T23.119
    left T23.012
      first degree T23.112
      second degree T23.212
      third degree T23.312
    multiple sites with fingers T23.049
      first degree T23.149
      left T23.042
        first degree T23.142
        second degree T23.242
        third degree T23.342
      right T23.041
        first degree T23.141
        second degree T23.241

Burn — *continued*
  thumb(s) — *continued*
    multiple sites with fingers — *continued*
      right — *continued*
        third degree T23.341
      second degree T23.249
      third degree T23.349
    right T23.011
      first degree T23.111
      second degree T23.211
      third degree T23.311
    second degree T23.219
    third degree T23.319
  toe T25.039
    first degree T25.139
    left T25.032
      first degree T25.132
      second degree T25.232
      third degree T25.332
    right T25.031
      first degree T25.131
      second degree T25.231
      third degree T25.331
    second degree T25.239
    third degree T25.339
  tongue T28.0
  tonsil(s) T28.0
  total body T29
  trachea T27.0
    with lung T27.1
  trunk T21.00
    abdominal wall — *see* Burn, abdominal wall
    anus — *see* Burn, buttock
    axilla — *see* Burn, upper limb
    back — *see* Burn, back
    breast — *see* Burn, chest wall
    buttock — *see* Burn, buttock
    chest wall — *see* Burn, chest wall
    first degree T21.10
    flank — *see* Burn, abdominal wall
    genital
      female — *see* Burn, genital organs, external, female
      male — *see* Burn, genital organs, external, male
    groin — *see* Burn, abdominal wall
    interscapular region — *see* Burn, back, upper
    labia — *see* Burn, genital organs, external, female
    lower back — *see* Burn, back
    penis — *see* Burn, genital organs, external, male
    perineum
      female — *see* Burn, genital organs, external, female
      male — *see* Burn, genital organs, external, male
    scapula region — *see* Burn, scapular region
    scrotum — *see* Burn, genital organs, external, male
    second degree T21.20
    specified site NEC T21.09
      first degree T21.19
      second degree T21.29
      third degree T21.39
    testes — *see* Burn, genital organs, external, male
    third degree T21.30
    upper back — *see* Burn, back, upper
    vulva — *see* Burn, genital organs, external, female
  unspecified site with extent of body surface involved specified
    less than 10 percent T31.0
    10-19 percent (0-9 percent third degree) T31.10
      with 10-19 percent third degree T31.11
    20-29 percent (0-9 percent third degree) T31.20
      with
        10-19 percent third degree T31.21
        20-29 percent third degree T31.22

Burn — *continued*
  unspecified site with extent of body surface involved specified — *continued*
    30-39 percent (0-9 percent third degree) T31.30
      with
        10-19 percent third degree T31.31
        20-29 percent third degree T31.32
        30-39 percent third degree T31.33
    40-49 percent (0-9 percent third degree) T31.40
      with
        10-19 percent third degree T31.41
        20-29 percent third degree T31.42
        30-39 percent third degree T31.43
        40-49 percent third degree T31.44
    50-59 percent (0-9 percent third degree) T31.50
      with
        10-19 percent third degree T31.51
        20-29 percent third degree T31.52
        30-39 percent third degree T31.53
        40-49 percent third degree T31.54
        50-59 percent third degree T31.55
    60-69 percent (0-9 percent third degree) T31.60
      with
        10-19 percent third degree T31.61
        20-29 percent third degree T31.62
        30-39 percent third degree T31.63
        40-49 percent third degree T31.64
        50-59 percent third degree T31.65
        60-69 percent third degree T31.66
    70-79 percent (0-9 percent third degree) T31.70
      with
        10-19 percent third degree T31.71
        20-29 percent third degree T31.72
        30-39 percent third degree T31.73
        40-49 percent third degree T31.74
        50-59 percent third degree T31.75
        60-69 percent third degree T31.76
        70-79 percent third degree T31.77
    80-89 percent (0-9 percent third degree) T31.80
      with
        10-19 percent third degree T31.81
        20-29 percent third degree T31.82
        30-39 percent third degree T31.83
        40-49 percent third degree T31.84
        50-59 percent third degree T31.85
        60-69 percent third degree T31.86
        70-79 percent third degree T31.87
        80-89 percent third degree T31.88
    90 percent or more (0-9 percent third degree) T31.90
      with
        10-19 percent third degree T31.91
        20-29 percent third degree T31.92
        30-39 percent third degree T31.93
        40-49 percent third degree T31.94
        50-59 percent third degree T31.95
        60-69 percent third degree T31.96
        70-79 percent third degree T31.97
        80-89 percent third degree T31.98
        90-99 percent third degree T31.99
  upper limb T22.00
    above elbow — *see* Burn, above elbow
    axilla — *see* Burn, axilla
    elbow — *see* Burn, elbow
    first degree T22.10
    forearm — *see* Burn, forearm
    hand — *see* Burn, hand
    interscapular region — *see* Burn, back, upper
    multiple sites T22.099
      first degree T22.199
      left T22.092
        first degree T22.192
        second degree T22.292
        third degree T22.392
      right T22.091
        first degree T22.191
        second degree T22.291
        third degree T22.391
      second degree T22.299

Burn — continued
  upper limb — continued
    multiple sites — continued
      third degree T22.399
    second degree T22.20
    scapular region — see Burn, scapular region
    shoulder — see Burn, shoulder
    third degree T22.30
    wrist — see Burn, wrist
  uterus T28.3
  vagina T28.3
  vulva — see Burn, genital organs, external,
    female
  wrist T23.079
    first degree T23.179
    left T23.072
      first degree T23.172
      second degree T23.272
      third degree T23.372
    multiple sites with hand T23.099
      first degree T23.199
      left T23.092
        first degree T23.192
        second degree T23.292
        third degree T23.392
      right T23.091
        first degree T23.191
        second degree T23.291
        third degree T23.391
      second degree T23.299
      third degree T23.399
    right T23.071
      first degree T23.171
      second degree T23.271
      third degree T23.371
    second degree T23.279
    third degree T23.379

Burnett's syndrome E83.59

Burning
  feet syndrome E53.9
  sensation R20.8
  tongue K14.6

Burn-out (state) Z73.0

Burns' disease or osteochondrosis — see
  Osteochondrosis, juvenile, ulna

Bursa — see condition

Bursitis M71.9
  Achilles — see Tendinitis, Achilles
  adhesive — see Bursitis, specified NEC
  ankle — see Enthesopathy, lower limb, ankle,
    specified type NEC
  calcaneal — see Enthesopathy, foot, specified
    type NEC
  collateral ligament, tibial — see Bursitis, tibial
    collateral
  due to use, overuse, pressure — see also
    Disorder, soft tissue, due to use, specified
    type NEC
    specified NEC — see Disorder, soft tissue,
      due to use, specified NEC
  Duplay's — see Tendinitis, calcific, shoulder
  elbow NEC M70.30
    left M70.32
    olecranon M70.20
      left M70.22
      right M70.21
    right M70.31
  finger — see Disorder, soft tissue, due to use,
    specified type NEC, hand
  foot — see Enthesopathy, foot, specified type
    NEC
  gonococcal A54.49
  gouty — see Gout, idiopathic
  hand M70.10
    left M70.12
    right M70.11
  hip NEC M70.70
    left M70.72
    right M70.71
    trochanteric M70.60
      left M70.62
      right M70.61
  infective NEC M71.10
    abscess — see Abscess, bursa
    ankle M71.170
      left M71.172

Bursitis — continued
  infective NEC — continued
    ankle — continued
      right M71.171
    elbow M71.129
      left M71.122
      right M71.121
    foot M71.179
      left M71.172
      right M71.171
    hand M71.149
      left M71.142
      right M71.141
    hip M71.159
      left M71.152
      right M71.151
    knee M71.169
      left M71.162
      right M71.161
    multiple sites M71.19
    shoulder M71.119
      left M71.112
      right M71.111
    specified site NEC M71.18
    wrist M71.139
      left M71.132
      right M71.131
  ischial — see Bursitis, hip
  knee NEC M70.50
    left M70.52
    prepatellar M70.40
      left M70.42
      right M70.41
    right M70.51
  occupational NEC — see also Disorder, soft
    tissue, due to, use
  olecranon — see Bursitis, elbow, olecranon
  pharyngeal J39.1
  popliteal — see Bursitis, knee
  prepatellar M70.40
    left M70.42
    right M70.41
  radiohumeral M77.8
  rheumatoid M06.20
    ankle M06.279
      left M06.272
      right M06.271
    elbow M06.229
      left M06.222
      right M06.221
    foot joint M06.279
      left M06.272
      right M06.271
    hand joint M06.249
      left M06.242
      right M06.241
    hip M06.259
      left M06.252
      right M06.251
    knee M06.269
      left M06.262
      right M06.261
    multiple site M06.29
    shoulder M06.219
      left M06.212
      right M06.211
    vertebra M06.28
    wrist M06.239
      left M06.232
      right M06.231
  scapulohumeral — see Bursitis, shoulder
  semimembranous muscle (knee) — see
    Bursitis, knee
  shoulder M75.50
    adhesive — see Capsulitis, adhesive
    left M75.52
    right M75.51
  specified NEC M71.50
    ankle M71.579
      left M71.572
      right M71.571
    due to use, overuse or pressure — see
      Disorder, soft tissue, due to, use
    elbow M71.529
      left M71.522
      right M71.521

Bursitis — continued
  specified NEC — continued
    foot M71.579
      left M71.572
      right M71.571
    hand M71.549
      left M71.542
      right M71.541
    hip M71.559
      left M71.552
      right M71.551
    knee M71.569
      left M71.562
      right M71.561
    shoulder — see Bursitis, shoulder
    specified site NEC M71.58
    tibial collateral M76.40
      left M76.42
      right M76.41
    wrist M71.539
      left M71.532
      right M71.531
  subacromial — see Bursitis, shoulder
  subcoracoid — see Bursitis, shoulder
  subdeltoid — see Bursitis, shoulder
  syphilitic A52.78
  Thornwaldt, Tornwaldt J39.2
  tibial collateral — see Bursitis, tibial collateral
  toe — see Enthesopathy, foot, specified type
    NEC
  trochanteric (area) — see Bursitis, hip,
    trochanteric
  wrist — see Bursitis, hand

Bursopathy M71.9
  specified type NEC M71.80
    ankle M71.879
      left M71.872
      right M71.871
    elbow M71.829
      left M71.822
      right M71.821
    foot M71.879
      left M71.872
      right M71.871
    hand M71.849
      left M71.842
      right M71.841
    hip M71.859
      left M71.852
      right M71.851
    knee M71.869
      left M71.862
      right M71.861
    multiple sites M71.89
    shoulder M71.819
      left M71.812
      right M71.811
    specified site NEC M71.88
    wrist M71.839
      left M71.832
      right M71.831

Burst stitches or sutures (complication of
  surgery) T81.3

Buruli ulcer A31.1

Bury's disease L95.1

Buschke's
  disease B45.3
  scleredema — see Sclerosis, systemic

Busse-Buschke disease B45.3

Buttock — see condition

Button
  Biskra B55.1
  Delhi B55.1
  oriental B55.1

Buttonhole deformity (finger) — see Deformity,
  finger, boutonniere

Bwamba fever A92.8

Byssinosis J66.0

Bywaters' syndrome T79.5

C

Cachexia R64
cancerous (M8000/3) C80
cardiac — *see* Disease, heart
dehydration E86.0
with
hypernatremia E87.0
hyponatremia E87.1
due to malnutrition E41
exophthalmic — *see* Hyperthyroidism
heart — *see* Disease, heart
hypophyseal E23.0
hypopituitary E23.0
lead — *see* Poisoning, lead
malignant (M8000/3) C80
marsh — *see* Malaria
nervous F48.8
old age R54
paludal — *see* Malaria
pituitary E23.0
renal N28.9
saturnine — *see* Poisoning, lead
senile R54
Simmonds' E23.0
splenica D73.0
strumipriva E03.4
tuberculous NEC — *see* Tuberculosis

Café, au lait spots L81.3

Caffey's syndrome Q78.8

Caisson disease T70.3

Cake kidney Q63.1

Caked breast (puerperal, postpartum) O92.7

Calabar swelling B74.3

Calcaneal spur — *see* Spur, bone, calcaneal

Calcaneo-apophysitis M92.8

Calcareous — *see* condition

Calcicosis J62.8

Calciferol (vitamin D) **deficiency** E55.9
with rickets E55.0

Calcification
adrenal (capsule) (gland) E27.4
tuberculous B90.8 [E35]
aorta I70.0
artery (annular) — *see* Arteriosclerosis
auricle (ear) — *see* Disorder, pinna, specified
type NEC
basal ganglia G23.8
bladder N32.8
due to Schistosoma hematobium B65.0
brain (cortex) — *see* Calcification, cerebral
bronchus J98.0
bursa M71.40
ankle M71.479
left M71.472
right M71.471
elbow M71.429
left M71.422
right M71.421
foot M71.479
left M71.472
right M71.471
hand M71.449
left M71.442
right M71.441
hip M71.459
left M71.452
right M71.451
knee M71.469
left M71.462
right M71.461
multiple sites M71.49
shoulder M75.30
left M75.32
right M75.31
specified site NEC M71.48
wrist M71.439
left M71.432
right M71.431
cardiac — *see* Degeneration, myocardial
cerebral (cortex) G93.8
artery I67.2
cervix (uteri) N88.8
choroid plexus G93.8
conjunctiva — *see* Concretion, conjunctiva

Calcification — *continued*
corpora cavernosa (penis) N48.89
cortex (brain) — *see* Calcification, cerebral
dental pulp (nodular) K04.2
dentinal papilla K00.4
fallopian tube N83.8
falx cerebri G96.1
gallbladder K82.8
general E83.59
heart — *see also* Degeneration, myocardial
valve — *see* Endocarditis
intervertebral cartilage or disc (postinfective) —
see Disorder, disc, specified NEC
intracranial — *see* Calcification, cerebral
joint — *see* Disorder, joint, specified type NEC
kidney N28.89
tuberculous B90.8 [N29]
larynx (senile) J38.7
lens — *see* Cataract, specified NEC
lung (active) (postinfectional) J98.4
tuberculous B90.9
lymph gland or node (postinfectional) I89.8
tuberculous (*see also* Tuberculosis, lymph
gland) B90.8
massive (paraplegic) — *see* Myositis, ossificans,
in, quadriplegia
medial — *see* Arteriosclerosis, extremities
meninges (cerebral) (spinal) G96.1
metastatic E83.59
Mönckeberg's — *see* Arteriosclerosis,
extremities
muscle M61.9
due to burns — *see* Myositis, ossificans, in,
burns
paralytic — *see* Myositis, ossificans, in,
quadriplegia
specified type NEC M61.40
ankle M61.479
left M61.472
right M61.471
foot M61.479
left M61.472
right M61.471
forearm M61.439
left M61.432
right M61.431
hand M61.449
left M61.442
right M61.441
lower leg M61.469
left M61.462
right M61.461
multiple sites M61.49
pelvic region M61.459
left M61.452
right M61.451
shoulder region M61.419
left M61.412
right M61.411
specified site NEC M61.48
thigh M61.459
left M61.452
right M61.451
upper arm M61.429
left M61.422
right M61.421
myocardium, myocardial — *see* Degeneration,
myocardial
ovary N83.8
pancreas K86.8
penis N48.89
periarticular — *see* Disorder, joint, specified
type NEC
pericardium (*see also* Pericarditis) I31.1
pineal gland E34.8
pleura J94.8
postinfectional J94.8
tuberculous NEC B90.9
pulpal (dental) (nodular) K04.2
sclera H15.89
spleen D73.8
subcutaneous L94.2
suprarenal (capsule) (gland) E27.4
tendon (sheath) — *see also* Tenosynovitis,
specified type NEC
with bursitis, synovitis or tenosynovitis —
see Tendinitis, calcific

Calcification — *continued*
uterus N85.8
trachea J39.8
ureter N28.89
uterus N85.8
vitreous — *see* Deposit, crystalline

Calcified — *see* Calcification

Calcinosis (interstitial) (tumoral) (universalis)
E83.59
with Raynaud's phenomenon, esophageal
dysfunction, sclerodactyly, telangiectasia
(CREST syndrome) M34.1
circumscripta (skin) L94.2
cutis L94.2

Calcium
deposits — *see* Calcification, by site
metabolism disorder E83.50
salts or soaps in vitreous — *see* Deposit,
crystalline

Calciuria R82.99

Calculi — *see* Calculus

Calculosis, intrahepatic — *see* Calculus, bile
duct

Calculus, calculi, calculous
ampulla of Vater — *see* Calculus, bile duct
anuria (impacted) (recurrent) N20.0
appendix K38.1
bile duct (common) (hepatic) K80.50
with
calculus of gallbladder — *see* Calculus,
gallbladder and bile duct
cholangitis K80.30
with
cholecystitis — *see* Calculus, bile
duct, with cholecystitis
obstruction K80.31
acute K80.32
with
chronic cholangitis K80.36
with obstruction K80.37
obstruction K80.33
chronic K80.34
with
acute cholangitis K80.36
with obstruction K80.37
obstruction K80.35
cholecystitis (with cholangitis) K80.40
with obstruction K80.41
acute K80.42
with
chronic cholecystitis K80.46
with obstruction K80.47
obstruction K80.43
chronic K80.44
with
acute cholecystitis K80.46
with obstruction K80.47
obstruction K80.45
obstruction K80.51
biliary — *see also* Calculus, gallbladder
specified NEC K80.80
with obstruction K80.81
bilirubin, multiple — *see* Calculus, gallbladder
bladder (encysted) (impacted) (urinary)
(diverticulum) N21.0
bronchus J98.0
calyx (kidney) (renal) — *see* Calculus, kidney
cholesterol (pure) (solitary) — *see* Calculus,
gallbladder
common duct (bile) — *see* Calculus, bile duct
conjunctiva — *see* Concretion, conjunctiva
cystic N21.0
duct — *see* Calculus, gallbladder
dental (subgingival) (supragingival) K03.6
diverticulum
bladder N21.0
kidney N20.0
epididymis N50.8
gallbladder K80.20
with
bile duct calculus — *see* Calculus,
gallbladder and bile duct
cholecystitis
with obstruction K80.11

Calculus, calculi, calculous — *continued*
gallbladder — *continued*
  with — *continued*
    cholecystitis — *continued*
      acute K80.00
        with
          chronic cholecystitis K80.12
            with obstruction K80.13
          obstruction K80.01
      chronic K80.10
        with
          acute cholecystitis K80.12
            with obstruction K80.13
          obstruction K80.11
      specified NEC K80.18
        with obstruction K80.19
      obstruction K80.21
  gallbladder and bile duct K80.70
    with
      cholecystitis K80.60
        with obstruction K80.61
      acute K80.62
        with
          chronic cholecystitis K80.66
            with obstruction K80.67
          obstruction K80.63
      chronic K80.64
        with
          acute cholecystitis K80.66
            with obstruction K80.67
          obstruction K80.65
      obstruction K80.71
  hepatic (duct) — *see* Calculus, bile duct
  ileal conduit N21.8
  intestinal (impaction) (obstruction) K56.4
  kidney (impacted) (multiple) (pelvis) (recurrent) (staghorn) N20.0
    with calculus, ureter N20.2
    congenital Q63.8
  lacrimal passages — *see* Dacryolith
  liver (impacted) — *see* Calculus, bile duct
  lung J98.4
  nephritic (impacted) (recurrent) — *see* Calculus, kidney
  nose J34.8
  pancreas (duct) K86.8
  parotid duct or gland K11.5
  pelvis, encysted — *see* Calculus, kidney
  prostate N42.0
  pulmonary J98.4
  pyelitis (impacted) (recurrent) N20.9
    with hydronephrosis N13.2
  pyelonephritis (impacted) (recurrent) N20.9
    with hydronephrosis N13.2
  renal (impacted) (recurrent) — *see* Calculus, kidney
  salivary (duct) (gland) K11.5
  seminal vesicle N50.8
  staghorn — *see* Calculus, kidney
  Stensen's duct K11.5
  stomach K31.89
  sublingual duct or gland K11.5
    congenital Q38.4
  submandibular duct, gland or region K11.5
  submaxillary duct, gland or region K11.5
  suburethral N21.8
  tonsil J35.8
  tooth, teeth (subgingival) (supragingival) K03.6
  tunica vaginalis N50.8
  ureter (impacted) (recurrent) N20.1
    with calculus, kidney N20.2
      with hydronephrosis N13.2
        with infection N13.6
  urethra (impacted) N21.1
  urinary (duct) (impacted) (passage) (tract) N20.9
    with hydronephrosis N13.2
      with infection N13.6
    in (due to)
      lower N21.9
        specified NEC N21.8
  vagina N89.8
  vesical (impacted) N21.0
  Wharton's duct K11.5
  xanthine E79.8 [N22]
Calicectasis N28.89

California
  disease B38.9
  encephalitis A83.5
Caligo cornea — *see* Opacity, cornea, central
Callositas, callosity (infected) L84
Callus (infected) L84
  bone — *see* Osteophyte
  excessive, following fracture – code as Sequelae of fracture
Calorie deficiency or malnutrition (*see also* Malnutrition) E46
Calvé-Perthes disease — *see* Legg-Calve-Perthes disease
Calvé's disease — *see* Osteochondrosis, juvenile, spine
Calvities — *see* Alopecia, androgenic
Cameroon fever — *see* Malaria
Camptocormia (hysterical) F44.4
Camurati-Engelmann syndrome Q78.3
Canal — *see also* condition
  atrioventricular common Q21.2
Canaliculitis (lacrimal) (acute) (subacute) H04.339
  Actinomyces A42.89
  bilateral H04.333
  chronic H04.429
    bilateral H04.423
    left H04.422
    right H04.421
  left H04.332
  right H04.331
Canavan's disease E75.29
Canceled procedure (surgical) Z53.9
  because of
    contraindication Z53.09
      smoking Z53.01
    left AMA Z53.21
    patient's decision Z53.20
      for reasons of belief or group pressure Z53.1
    specified reason NEC Z53.29
  specified reason NEC Z53.8
Cancer (M8000/3) — *see also* Neoplasm, malignant
  bile duct type (M8160/3), liver C22.1
  blood — *see* Leukemia
  hepatocellular (M8170/3) C22.0
Cancer(o)phobia F45.29
Cancerous (M8000/3) — *see* Neoplasm, malignant
Cancrum oris A69.0
Candidiasis, candidal B37.9
  balanitis B37.42
  bronchitis B37.1
  cheilitis B37.83
  congenital P37.5
  cystitis B37.41
  disseminated B37.89
  endocarditis B37.6
  enteritis B37.82
  esophagitis B37.81
  intertrigo B37.2
  lung B37.1
  meningitis B37.5
  mouth B37.0
  nails B37.2
  neonatal P37.5
  onychia B37.2
  oral B37.0
  osteomyelitis B37.89
  otitis externa B37.84
  paronychia B37.2
  perionyxis B37.2
  pneumonia B37.1
  proctitis B37.82
  pulmonary B37.1
  pyelonephritis B37.49
  septicemia B37.7
  skin B37.2
  specified site NEC B37.89
  stomatitis B37.0
  systemic B37.89
  urethritis B37.41
  urogenital site NEC B37.49

Candidiasis, candidal — *continued*
  vagina B37.3
  vulva B37.3
  vulvovaginitis B37.3
Candidid L30.2
Candidosis — *see* Candidiasis
Candiru infection or infestation B88.8
Canities (premature) L67.1
  congenital Q84.2
Canker (mouth) (sore) K12.0
  rash A38.9
Cannabinosis J66.2
Canton fever A75.9
Cantrell's syndrome Q87.89
Capillariasis (intestinal) B81.1
  hepatic B83.8
Capillary — *see* condition
Caplan's syndrome — *see* Rheumatoid, lung
Capsule — *see* condition
Capsulitis (joint) — *see also* Enthesopathy
  adhesive (shoulder) M75.00
    left M75.02
    right M75.01
  hepatic K65.8
  labyrinthine — *see* Otosclerosis, specified NEC
  thyroid E06.9
Caput
  crepitus Q75.8
  medusae I86.8
  succedaneum P12.81
Car sickness T75.3
Carapata (disease) A68.0
Carate — *see* Pinta
Carbon lung J60
Carboxyhemoglobinemia — *see* Poisoning, carbon monoxide
Carbuncle L02.93
  abdominal wall L02.231
  anus K61.0
  auditory canal, external — *see* Abscess, ear, external
  auricle ear — *see* Abscess, ear, external
  axilla L02.439
    left L02.432
    right L02.431
  back (any part) L02.232
  breast N61
  buttock L02.33
  cheek (external) L02.03
  chest wall L02.233
  chin L02.03
  corpus cavernosum N48.21
  ear (any part) (external) (middle) — *see* Abscess, ear, external
  external auditory canal — *see* Abscess, ear, external
  eyelid — *see* Abscess, eyelid
  face NEC L02.03
  femoral (region) — *see* Carbuncle, lower limb
  finger — *see* Carbuncle, hand
  flank L02.231
  foot L02.639
    left L02.632
    right L02.631
  forehead L02.03
  genital — *see* Abscess, genital
  gluteal (region) L02.33
  groin L02.234
  hand L02.539
    left L02.532
    right L02.531
  head NEC L02.831
  heel — *see* Carbuncle, foot
  hip — *see* Carbuncle, lower limb
  kidney — *see* Abscess, kidney
  knee — *see* Carbuncle, lower limb
  labium (majus) (minus) N76.4
  lacrimal
    gland — *see* Dacryoadenitis
    passages (duct) (sac) — *see* Inflammation, lacrimal, passages, acute
  leg — *see* Carbuncle, lower limb
  lower limb L02.439
    left L02.436

©2002 Ingenix, Inc.

Carbuncle — *continued*
    lower limb — *continued*
        right L02.435
    malignant A22.0
    multiple sites L02.93
    navel L02.236
    neck L02.13
    nose (external) (septum) J34.0
    orbit, orbital — *see* Abscess, orbit
    palmar (space) — *see* Carbuncle, hand
    partes posteriores L02.33
    pectoral region L02.233
    penis N48.21
    perineum L02.235
    pinna — *see* Abscess, ear, external
    popliteal — *see* Carbuncle, lower limb
    scalp L02.831
    seminal vesicle N49.0
    shoulder — *see* Carbuncle, upper limb
    specified site NEC L02.838
    temple (region) L02.03
    thumb — *see* Carbuncle, hand
    toe — *see* Carbuncle, foot
    trunk L02.239
        abdominal wall L02.231
        back L02.232
        chest wall L02.233
        groin L02.234
        perineum L02.235
        umbilicus L02.236
    umbilicus L02.236
    upper limb L02.439
        left L02.434
        right L02.433
    urethra N34.0
    vulva N76.4

Carbunculus — *see* Carbuncle

Carcinoid (tumor) (M8240/3) — *see also*
        Neoplasm, malignant
    with struma ovarii (M9091/1) D39.10
    appendix (M8240/1) D37.3
    argentaffin (M8241/1) — *see* Neoplasm,
            uncertain behavior
        malignant (M8241/3) — *see* Neoplasm,
            malignant
    benign (M8240/0) — *see* Neoplasm, benign
    composite (M8244/3) — *see* Neoplasm,
            malignant
    goblet cell (M8243/3) — *see* Neoplasm,
            malignant
        specified site — *see* Neoplasm, malignant
        unspecified site C18.1
    malignant (M8240/3) — *see* Neoplasm,
            malignant
    mucinous (M8243/3)
        specified site — *see* Neoplasm, malignant
        unspecified site C18.1
    strumal (M9091/1) D39.10
    syndrome (intestinal) (metastatic) E34.0
    type bronchial adenoma (M8240/3) — *see*
            Neoplasm, lung, malignant

Carcinoidosis E34.0

Carcinoma (M8010/3) — *see also* Neoplasm,
        malignant
    with
        apocrine metaplasia (M8573/3)
        cartilaginous (and osseous) metaplasia
            (M8571/3)
        osseous (and cartilaginous) metaplasia
            (M8571/3)
        productive fibrosis (M8141/3)
        spindle cell metaplasia (M8572/3)
        squamous metaplasia (M8570/3)
    acidophil (M8280/3)
        specified site — *see* Neoplasm, malignant
        unspecified site C75.1
    acidophil-basophil, mixed (M8281/3)
        specified site — *see* Neoplasm, malignant
        unspecified site C75.1
    acinar (cell) (M8550/3)
    acinic cell (M8550/3)
    adenocystic (M8200/3)
    adenoid
        cystic (M8200/3)
        squamous cell (M8075/3)
    adenosquamous (M8560/3)

Carcinoma — *see also* Neoplasm, malignant —
        continued
    adnexal (skin) (M8390/3) — *see* Neoplasm,
            skin, malignant
    adrenal cortical (M8370/3) C74.00
        left C74.02
        right C74.01
    alveolar (M8251/3) — *see* Neoplasm, lung,
            malignant
        cell (M8250/3) — *see* Neoplasm, lung,
            malignant
    ameloblastic (M9270/3) C41.1
        upper jaw (bone) C41.0
    anaplastic type (M8021/3)
    apocrine (M8401/3)
        breast — *see* Neoplasm, breast, malignant
        specified site NEC — *see* Neoplasm, skin,
            malignant
        unspecified site C44.9
    basal cell (pigmented) (M8090/3) — *see also*
            Neoplasm, skin, malignant
        fibro-epithelial (M8093/3) — *see* Neoplasm,
            skin, malignant
        morphea (M8092/3) — *see* Neoplasm, skin,
            malignant
        multicentric (M8091/3) — *see* Neoplasm,
            skin, malignant
    basaloid (M8123/3)
    basal-squamous cell, mixed (M8094/3) — *see*
            Neoplasm, skin, malignant
    basophil (M8300/3)
        specified site — *see* Neoplasm, malignant
        unspecified site C75.1
    basophil-acidophil, mixed (M8281/3)
        specified site — *see* Neoplasm, malignant
        unspecified site C75.1
    basosquamous (M8094/3) — *see* Neoplasm,
            skin, malignant
    bile duct (M8160/3)
        with hepatocellular, mixed (M8180/3) C22.0
        liver C22.1
        specified site NEC — *see* Neoplasm,
            malignant
        unspecified site C22.1
    branchial or branchiogenic C10.4
    bronchial or bronchogenic — *see* Neoplasm,
            lung, malignant
    bronchiolar (M8250/3) — *see* Neoplasm, lung,
            malignant
    bronchioloalveolar (M8250/3) — *see* Neoplasm,
            lung, malignant
    C cell (M8510/3)
        specified site — *see* Neoplasm, malignant
        unspecified site C73
    ceruminous (M8420/3) C44.20
        left ear C44.22
        right ear C44.21
    chorionic (M9100/3)
        specified site — *see* Neoplasm, malignant
        unspecified site
            female C58
            male C62.90
    chromophobe (M8270/3)
        specified site — *see* Neoplasm, malignant
        unspecified site C75.1
    clear cell (mesonephroid) (M8310/3)
    cloacogenic (M8124/3)
        specified site — *see* Neoplasm, malignant
        unspecified site C21.2
    colloid (M8480/3)
    cribriform (M8201/3)
    cylindroid (M8200/3)
    diffuse type (M8145/3)
        specified site — *see* Neoplasm, malignant
        unspecified site C16.9
    duct (cell) (M8500/3)
        with Paget's disease (M8541/3) — *see*
            Neoplasm, breast, malignant
        infiltrating (M8500/3)
            with lobular carcinoma (in situ)
                (M8522/3)
            specified site — *see* Neoplasm,
                malignant
            unspecified site (female) C50.90
                male C50.95
        specified site — *see* Neoplasm, malignant

Carcinoma — *see also* Neoplasm, malignant —
        continued
    duct — *continued*
        infiltrating — *continued*
            unspecified site (female) C50.90
                male C50.95
        ductal (M8500/3)
            with lobular (M8522/3)
                specified site — *see* Neoplasm, malignant
                unspecified site (female) C50.90
                    male C50.95
        ductular, infiltrating (M8521/3)
            specified site — *see* Neoplasm, malignant
            unspecified site (female) C50.90
                male C50.95
        embryonal (M9070/3)
            with teratoma, mixed (M9081/3)
            combined with choriocarcinoma (M9101/3)
            infantile type (M9071/3)
            liver C22.7
            polyembryonal type (M9072/3)
        endometrioid (M8380/3)
            specified site — *see* Neoplasm, malignant
            unspecified site
                female C56.9
                male C61
        eosinophil (M8280/3)
            specified site — *see* Neoplasm, malignant
            unspecified site C75.1
        epidermoid (M8070/3) — *see also* Carcinoma,
                squamous cell
            with adenocarcinoma, mixed (M8560/3)
            in situ, Bowen's type (M8081/2) — *see*
                Neoplasm, skin, in situ
            keratinizing (M8071/3)
            large cell, nonkeratinizing (M8072/3)
            small cell, nonkeratinizing (M8073/3)
            spindle cell (M8074/3)
            verrucous (M8501/3)
        epithelial-myoepithelial (M8562/3)
        fibroepithelial, basal cell (M8093/3) — *see*
                Neoplasm, skin, malignant
        follicular (M8330/3)
            with papillary (mixed) (M8340/3) C73
            moderately differentiated (M8332/3) C73
            pure follicle (M8331/3) C73
            specified site — *see* Neoplasm, malignant
            trabecular (M8332/3) C73
            unspecified site C73
            well differentiated (M8331/3) C73
        gelatinous (M8480/3)
        giant cell (M8031/3)
            with spindle cell (M8030/3)
        glycogen-rich (M8315/3) — *see* Neoplasm,
                breast, malignant
        granular cell (M8320/3)
        granulosa cell (M8620/3) C56.9
            left side C56.1
            right side C56.0
        hepatic cell (M8170/3) C22.0
        hepatocellular (M8170/3) C22.0
            with bile duct, mixed (M8180/3) C22.0
            fibrolamellar (M8171/3) C22.0
        hepatocholangiolitic (M8180/3) C22.0
        Hurthle cell (M8290/3) C73
        hypernephroid (M8311/3)
        in
            adenomatous
                polyp (M8210/3)
                polyposis coli (M8220/3) C18.9
            pleomorphic adenoma (M8941/3) — *see*
                Neoplasm, salivary glands, malignant
            polyp (M8210/3)
            polypoid adenoma (M8210/3)
            situ (M8010/2) — *see* Carcinoma-in-situ
            tubular adenoma (M8210/3)
            villous adenoma (M8261/3)
        infiltrating
            duct (M8500/3)
                with lobular (M8522/3)
                    specified site — *see* Neoplasm,
                        malignant
                    unspecified site (female) C50.90
                        male C50.95
                with Paget's disease (M8541/3) — *see*
                    Neoplasm, breast, malignant
                specified site — *see* Neoplasm, malignant

Carcinoma — *see also* Neoplasm, malignant — *continued*
 infiltrating — *continued*
  duct — *continued*
   unspecified site (female) C50.90
    male C50.95
   ductural (M8521/3)
    specified site — *see* Neoplasm, malignant
    unspecified site (female) C50.90
     male C50.95
   lobular (M8520/3)
    specified site — *see* Neoplasm, malignant
    unspecified site (female) C50.90
     male C50.95
 inflammatory (M8530/3)
  specified site — *see* Neoplasm, malignant
  unspecified site (female) C50.90
   male C50.95
 intestinal type (M8144/3)
  specified site — *see* Neoplasm, malignant
  unspecified site C16.9
 intracystic (M8504/3)
  noninfiltrating (M8504/2) — *see* Neoplasm, in situ
 intraductal (noninfiltrating) (M8500/2)
  with Paget's disease (M8543/3) — *see* Neoplasm, breast, malignant
  breast (female) D05.10
   male D05.15
  papillary (M8503/2)
   with invasion (M8503/3)
    specified site — *see* Neoplasm, malignant
    unspecified site (female) C50.90
     male C50.95
   breast (female) D05.10
    male D05.15
   specified site NEC — *see* Neoplasm, in situ
   unspecified site (female) D05.10
    male D05.15
  specified site NEC — *see* Neoplasm, in situ
  unspecified site (female) D05.10
   male D05.15
 intraepidermal (M8070/2) — *see* Neoplasm, in situ
  squamous cell, Bowen's type (M8081/2) — *see* Neoplasm, skin, in situ
 intraepithelial (M8010/2) — *see* Neoplasm, in situ
  squamous cell (M8070/2) — *see* Neoplasm, in situ
 intraosseous (M9270/3) C41.1
  upper jaw (bone) C41.0
 islet cell (M8150/3)
  with exocrine, mixed (M8154/3)
   specified site — *see* Neoplasm, malignant
   unspecified site C25.9
  pancreas C25.4
  specified site NEC — *see* Neoplasm, malignant
  unspecified site C25.4
 juvenile, breast (M8502/3) — *see* Neoplasm, breast, malignant
 Kulchitsky's cell (carcinoid tumor of intestine) E34.0
 large cell (M8012/3)
  small cell (M8045/3)
   specified site — *see* Neoplasm, malignant
   unspecified site C34.90
  squamous cell (M8070/3)
   keratinizing (M8071/3)
   nonkeratinizing (M8072/3)
 Leydig cell (testis) (M8650/3)
  specified site — *see* Neoplasm, malignant
  unspecified site
   female C56.9
   male C62.90
 lipid-rich (female) (M8314/3) C50.90
  male C50.95
 liver cell (M8170/3) C22.0
 lobular (infiltrating) (M8520/3)
  with intraductal (M8522/3)
   specified site — *see* Neoplasm, malignant
   unspecified site (female) C50.90
    male C50.95

Carcinoma — *see also* Neoplasm, malignant — *continued*
 lobular — *continued*
  noninfiltrating (M8520/2)
   breast (female) D05.00
    male D05.05
   specified site NEC — *see* Neoplasm, in situ
   unspecified site (female) D05.00
    male D05.05
  specified site — *see* Neoplasm, malignant
  unspecified site (female) C50.90
   male C50.95
 lymphoepithelial (M8082/3)
 medullary (M8510/3)
  with
   amyloid stroma (M8511/3)
    specified site — *see* Neoplasm, malignant
    unspecified site C73
   lymphoid stroma (M8512/3)
    specified site — *see* Neoplasm, malignant
    unspecified site (female) C50.90
     male C50.95
 Merkel cell (M8247/3) — *see* Neoplasm, skin, malignant
 mesometanephric (M9110/3)
 mesonephric (M9110/3)
 metastatic (M8010/6) — *see* Neoplasm, secondary
 metatypical (M8095/3) — *see* Neoplasm, skin, malignant
 morphea, basal cell (M8092/3) — *see* Neoplasm, skin, malignant
 mucinous (M8480/3)
 mucin-producing (M8481/3)
 mucin-secreting (M8481/3)
 mucoepidermoid (M8430/3)
 mucoid (M8480/3)
  cell (M8300/3)
   specified site — *see* Neoplasm, malignant
   unspecified site C75.1
 mucous (M8480/3)
 myoepithelial-epithelial (M8562/3)
 neuroendocrine (M8246/3)
 nonencapsulated sclerosing (M8350/3) C73
 noninfiltrating (M8010/2)
  intracystic (M8504/2) — *see* Neoplasm, in situ
  intraductal (M8500/2)
   breast (female) D05.10
    male D05.15
   papillary (M8503/2)
    breast (female) D05.10
     male D05.15
    specified site NEC — *see* Neoplasm, in situ
    unspecified site (female) D05.10
     male D05.15
   specified site — *see* Neoplasm, in situ
   unspecified site (female) D05.10
    male D05.15
  lobular (M8520/2)
   breast (female) D05.00
    male D05.05
   specified site NEC — *see* Neoplasm, in situ
   unspecified site (female) D05.00
    male D05.05
 oat cell (M8042/3)
  specified site — *see* Neoplasm, malignant
  unspecified site C34.90
 odontogenic (M9270/3) C41.1
  upper jaw (bone) C41.0
 oncocytic (M8290/3)
 oxyphilic (M8290/3)
 papillary (M8050/3)
  with follicular (mixed) (M8340/3) C73
  epidermoid (M8052/3)
  follicular variant (M8340/3) C73
  intraductal (noninfiltrating) (M8503/2)
   with invasion (M8503/3)
    specified site — *see* Neoplasm, malignant
    unspecified site (female) C50.90
     male C50.95

Carcinoma — *see also* Neoplasm, malignant — *continued*
 papillary — *continued*
  intraductal — *continued*
   breast (female) D05.10
    male D05.15
   specified site NEC — *see* Neoplasm, in situ
   unspecified site (female) D05.10
    male D05.15
  serous (M8460/3)
   specified site — *see* Neoplasm, malignant
   surface (M8461/3)
    specified site — *see* Neoplasm, malignant
    unspecified site C56.9
   unspecified site C56.9
  squamous cell (M8052/3)
  transitional cell (M8130/3)
 papillocystic (M0450/3)
  specified site — *see* Neoplasm, malignant
  unspecified site C56.9
 parafollicular cell (M8510/3)
  specified site — *see* Neoplasm, malignant
  unspecified site C73
 pilomatrix (M8110/3) — *see* Neoplasm, skin, malignant
 pleomorphic (M8022/3)
 polygonal cell (M8034/3)
 pseudoglandular, squamous cell (M8075/3)
 pseudomucinous (M8470/3)
  specified site — *see* Neoplasm, malignant
  unspecified site C56.9
 pseudosarcomatous (M8033/3)
 renal cell (M8312/3) C64.9
  left C64.1
  right C64.0
 reserve cell (M8041/3)
 round cell (M8041/3)
 Schmincke (M8082/3) — *see* Neoplasm, nasopharynx, malignant
 Schneiderian (M8121/3)
  specified site — *see* Neoplasm, malignant
  unspecified site C30.0
 scirrhous (M8141/3)
 sebaceous (M8410/3) — *see* Neoplasm, skin, malignant
 secondary (M8010/6) — *see* Neoplasm, secondary
 secretory, breast (M8502/3) — *see* Neoplasm, breast, malignant
 serous (M8441/3)
  papillary (M8460/3)
   specified site — *see* Neoplasm, malignant
   unspecified site C56.9
  surface, papillary (M8461/3)
   specified site — *see* Neoplasm, malignant
   unspecified site C56.9
 Sertoli cell (M8640/3)
  specified site — *see* Neoplasm, malignant
  unspecified site C62.90
   female C56.9
   male C62.90
 signet ring cell (M8490/3)
  metastatic (M8490/6) — *see* Neoplasm, secondary
 simplex (M8231/3)
 skin appendage (M8390/3) — *see* Neoplasm, skin, malignant
 small cell (M8041/3)
  fusiform cell (M8043/3)
   specified site — *see* Neoplasm, malignant
   unspecified site C34.90
  intermediate cell (M8044/3)
   specified site — *see* Neoplasm, malignant
   unspecified site C34.90
  large cell (M8045/3)
   specified site — *see* Neoplasm, malignant
   unspecified site C34.90
  squamous cell, nonkeratinizing (M8073/3)
 solid (M8230/3)
  with amyloid stroma (M8511/3)
   specified site — *see* Neoplasm, malignant
   unspecified site C73
 spheroidal cell (M8010/3)
 spindle cell (M8032/3)
  with giant cell (M8030/3)

©2002 Ingenix, Inc.

Carcinoma — *see also* Neoplasm, malignant — *continued*
spinous cell (M8070/3)
squamous (cell) (M8070/3)
with adenocarcinoma, mixed (M8560/3)
adenoid (M8075/3)
keratinizing, large cell (M8071/3)
large cell, nonkeratinizing (M8072/3)
metastatic (M8070/6) — *see* Neoplasm, secondary
microinvasive (M8076/3)
specified site — *see* Neoplasm, malignant
unspecified site C53.9
nonkeratinizing (large cell) (M8072/3)
papillary (M8052/3)
pseudoglandular (M8075/3)
small cell, nonkeratinizing (M8073/3)
spindle cell (M8074/3)
verrucous (M8051/3)
superficial spreading (M8143/3)
sweat gland (M8400/3) — *see* Neoplasm, skin, malignant
theca cell (M8600/3) C56.9
left side C56.1
right side C56.0
thymic (M8580/3) C37
trabecular (M8190/3)
transitional (cell) (M8120/3)
papillary (M8130/3)
spindle cell (M8122/3)
tubular (M8211/3)
undifferentiated (M8020/3)
urothelial (M8120/3)
verrucous (epidermoid) (squamous cell) (M8051/3)
villous (M8262/3)
water-clear cell (M8322/3) C75.0
wolffian duct (M9110/3)
Carcinoma-in-situ (M8010/2) — *see also* Neoplasm, in situ
breast NOS (female) D05.90
left D05.92
male D05.95
left D05.94
right D05.93
right D05.91
specified type NEC (female) D05.70
left D05.72
male D05.75
left D05.74
right D05.73
right D05.71
epidermoid (M8070/2) — *see also* Neoplasm, in situ
with questionable stromal invasion (M8076/2)
cervix D06.9
specified site NEC — *see* Neoplasm, in situ
unspecified site D06.9
Bowen's type (M8081/2) — *see* Neoplasm, skin, in situ
in
adenomatous polyp (M8210/2)
polyp NEC (M8210/2)
intraductal (M8500/2)
breast (female) D05.10
left D05.12
male D05.15
left D05.14
right D05.13
right D05.11
specified site NEC — *see* Neoplasm, in situ
unspecified site (female) D05.10
male D05.15
lobular (M8520/2)
with
infiltrating duct (M8522/3)
breast (female) C50.90
male C50.95
specified site NEC — *see* Neoplasm, malignant
unspecified site (female) C50.90
male C50.95
intraductal (M8522/2)
breast (female) D05.70
male D05.75

Carcinoma-in-situ — *see also* Neoplasm, in situ — *continued*
lobular — *continued*
with — *continued*
intraductal — *continued*
specified site NEC — *see* Neoplasm, in situ
unspecified site (female) D05.70
male D05.75
breast (female) D05.00
left D05.02
male D05.05
left D05.04
right D05.03
right D05.01
specified site NEC — *see* Neoplasm, in situ
unspecified site (female) D05.00
male D05.05
papillary (M8050/2) — *see* Neoplasm, in situ
squamous cell (M8070/2) — *see also* Neoplasm, in situ
with questionable stromal invasion (M8076/2)
cervix D06.9
specified site NEC — *see* Neoplasm, in situ
unspecified site D06.9
transitional cell (M8120/2) — *see* Neoplasm, in situ
Carcinomaphobia F45.29
Carcinomatosis
peritonei (M8010/6) C78.6
specified site NEC (M8010/3) — *see* Neoplasm, malignant
unspecified site (M8010/6) C80
Carcinosarcoma (M8980/3) — *see* Neoplasm, malignant
embryonal (M8981/3) — *see* Neoplasm, malignant
Cardia, cardial — *see* condition
Cardiac — *see also* condition
death, sudden — *see* Arrest, cardiac
pacemaker
in situ Z95.0
management or adjustment Z45.018
tamponade I31.9
Cardialgia — *see* Pain, precordial
Cardiectasis — *see* Hypertrophy, cardiac
Cardiochalasia K21.9
Cardiomalacia I51.5
Cardiomegalia glycogenica diffusa E74.02 *[I43]*
Cardiomegaly — *see also* Hypertrophy, cardiac
congenital Q24.8
glycogen E74.02 *[I43]*
idiopathic I51.7
Cardiomyoliposis I51.5
Cardiomyopathy (congestive) (constrictive) (familial) (idiopathic) I42.9
alcoholic I42.6
amyloid E85 *[I43]*
arteriosclerotic — *see* Disease, heart, ischemic, atherosclerotic
beriberi E51.12
cobalt-beer I42.6
complicating
childbirth O99.42
pregnancy O99.419
first trimester O99.411
second trimester O99.412
third trimester O99.413
puerperium O99.43
congenital I42.4
dilated I42.0
due to
alcohol I42.6
beriberi E51.12
cardiac glycogenosis E74.02 *[I43]*
drugs I42.7
Friedreich's ataxia G11.1
external agents NEC I42.7
myotonia atrophica G71.1
progressive muscular dystrophy G71.0
glycogen storage E74.02 *[I43]*
hypertensive — *see* Hypertension, heart

Cardiomyopathy — *continued*
hypertrophic (nonobstructive) I42.2
obstructive I42.1
congenital Q24.8
in
Chagas' disease (chronic) B57.2
acute B57.0
sarcoidosis D86.85
ischemic I25.5
metabolic E88.9 *[I43]*
thyrotoxic E05.90 *[I43]*
with thyroid storm E05.91 *[I43]*
nutritional E63.9 *[I43]*
beriberi E51.12
obscure of Africa I42.8
postpartum O90.3
restrictive NEC I42.5
rheumatic I09.0
secondary I42.9
thyrotoxic E05.90 *[I43]*
with thyroid storm E05.91 *[I43]*
toxic NEC I42.7
tuberculous A18.84
viral B33.24
Cardionephritis — *see* Hypertension, cardiorenal
Cardionephropathy — *see* Hypertension, cardiorenal
Cardionephrosis — *see* Hypertension, cardiorenal
Cardiopathia nigra I27.0
Cardiopathy (*see also* Disease, heart) I51.9
idiopathic I42.9
mucopolysaccharidosis E76.3 *[I52]*
Cardiopericarditis — *see* Pericarditis
Cardiophobia F45.29
Cardiorenal — *see* condition
Cardiorrhexis — *see* Infarct, myocardium
Cardiosclerosis — *see* Disease, heart, ischemic, atherosclerotic
Cardiosis — *see* Disease, heart
Cardiospasm (esophagus) (reflex) (stomach) K22.0
congenital (without mention of megaesophagus) Q40.2
with megaesophagus Q39.5
Cardiostenosis — *see* Disease, heart
Cardiosymphysis I31.0
Cardiovascular — *see* condition
Carditis (acute) (bacterial) (chronic) (subacute) I51.8
meningococcal A39.50
rheumatic — *see* Disease, heart, rheumatic
rheumatoid — *see* Rheumatoid, carditis
viral B33.20
Care (of) (for) (following)
child (routine) Z76.2
convalescent Z76.8
family member (handicapped) (sick)
creating problem for family Z63.6
provided away from home for holiday relief Z75.5
unavailable, due to
absence (person rendering care) (sufferer) Z74.2
inability (any reason) of person rendering care Z74.2
foundling Z76.1
holiday relief Z75.5
improper — *see* Maltreatment
lack of (at or after birth) (infant) — *see* Maltreatment, child, neglect
lactating mother Z39.1
orthodontic Z51.89
palliative Z51.5
postpartum
immediately after delivery Z39.0
routine follow-up Z39.2
pregnancy — *see* Maternal care
prenatal
first pregnancy — *see* Antenatal, care, first, pregnancy
high risk pregnancy — *see* Antenatal, care, high risk pregnancy
preparatory, for subsequent treatment Z51.89
respite Z75.5

Care — *continued*
  unavailable, due to
    absence of person rendering care Z74.2
    inability (any reason) of person rendering
      care Z74.2
  well-baby Z76.2
Caries
  bone NEC A18.03
  cementum K02.2
    arrested K02.3
    specified NEC K02.8
  dental K02.9
    arrested K02.3
    cementum K02.2
    dentine K02.1
    enamel only K02.0
    odontoclasia K02.4
    specified type NEC K02.8
  dentin (acute) (chronic) K02.1
  enamel (acute) (chronic, incipient) K02.0
  external meatus — *see* Disorder, ear, external,
    specified type NEC
  hip (tuberculous) A18.02
  initial K02.0
  knee (tuberculous) A18.02
  labyrinth — *see* category H83.8
  limb NEC (tuberculous) A18.03
  mastoid process (chronic) — *see* Mastoiditis,
    chronic
    tuberculous A18.03
  middle ear — *see* category H74.8
  nose (tuberculous) A18.03
  orbit (tuberculous) A18.03
  ossicles, ear — *see* Abnormal, ear ossicles
  petrous bone — *see* Petrositis
  sacrum (tuberculous) A18.01
  spine, spinal (column) (tuberculous) A18.01
  syphilitic A52.77
    congenital (early) A50.02 [M90.80]
  tooth, teeth — *see* Caries, dental
  tuberculous A18.03
  vertebra (column) (tuberculous) A18.01
Carious teeth — *see* Caries, dental
Carneous mole O02.0
Carnitine insufficiency E71.320
Carotid body or sinus syndrome G90.0
Carotidynia G90.0
Carotinemia (dietary) E67.1
Carotinosis (cutis) (skin) E67.1
Carpal tunnel syndrome — *see* Syndrome, carpal
  tunnel
Carpenter's syndrome Q87.0
Carpopedal spasm — *see* Tetany
Carr-Barr-Plunkett syndrome Q97.1
Carrier (suspected) **of**
  amebiasis Z22.1
  bacterial disease NEC Z22.39
    diphtheria Z22.2
    intestinal infectious NEC Z22.1
      typhoid Z22.0
    meningococcal Z22.31
    sexually transmitted Z22.4
    specified NEC Z22.39
    staphylococcal Z22.32
    streptococcal Z22.338
      group B Z22.330
    typhoid Z22.0
  cholera Z22.1
  diphtheria Z22.2
  gastrointestinal pathogens NEC Z22.1
  gonorrhea Z22.4
  HAA (hepatitis Australian-antigen) Z22.59
  HB(c)(s)-AG Z22.51
  hepatitis (viral) Z22.50
    Australia-antigen (HAA) Z22.59
    B surface antigen (HBsAg) Z22.51
      with acute delta-(super)infection B17.0
    C Z22.52
    specified NEC Z22.59
  human T-cell lymphotropic virus type-1 (HTLV-
    1) infection Z22.6
  infectious organism Z22.9
    specified NEC Z22.8
  meningococci Z22.31

Carrier (suspected) **of** — *continued*
  Salmonella typhosa Z22.0
  serum hepatitis — *see* Carrier, hepatitis
  staphylococci Z22.32
  streptococci Z22.338
    group B Z22.330
  syphilis Z22.4
  typhoid Z22.0
  venereal disease NEC Z22.4
Carrion's disease A44.0
Carter's relapsing fever (Asiatic) A68.1
Cartilage — *see* condition
Caruncle (inflamed)
  conjunctiva (acute) — *see* Conjunctivitis, acute
  labium (majus) (minus) N90.8
  lacrimal — *see* Inflammation, lacrimal,
    passages
  myrtiform N89.8
  urethral (benign) N36.2
Cascade stomach K31.2
Caseation lymphatic gland (tuberculous) A18.2
Cassidy (-Scholte) syndrome (malignant
  carcinoid) E34.0
Castellani's disease A69.8
Castration, traumatic, male S38.231
Casts in urine R82.99
Cat
  cry syndrome Q93.4
  ear Q17.3
Catabolism, senile R54
Catalepsy (hysterical) F44.2
  schizophrenic F20.2
Cataplexy (idiopathic) G47.4
Cataract (cortical) (immature) (incipient) H26.9
  with
    neovascularization — *see* Cataract,
      complicated
  age-related — *see* Cataract, senile
  anterior
    and posterior axial embryonal Q12.0
    pyramidal Q12.0
  associated with
    galactosemia E74.21 [H28]
    myotonic disorders G71.1 [H28]
  blue Q12.0
  central Q12.0
  cerulean Q12.0
  complicated H26.20
    with
      neovascularization H26.219
        bilateral H26.213
        left H26.212
        right H26.211
      ocular disorder H26.229
        bilateral H26.223
        left H26.222
        right H26.221
      glaucomatous flecks H26.239
        bilateral H26.233
        left H26.232
        right H26.231
  congenital Q12.0
  coraliform Q12.0
  coronary Q12.0
  crystalline Q12.0
  diabetic — *see* Diabetes, cataract
  drug-induced H26.30
    bilateral H26.33
    left H26.32
    right H26.31
  due to
    ocular disorder — *see* Cataract, complicated
    radiation H26.8
  electric H26.8
  glass-blower's H26.8
  heat ray H26.8
  heterochromic — *see* Cataract, complicated
  in (due to)
    chronic iridocyclitis — *see* Cataract,
      complicated
    diabetes — *see* Diabetes, cataract
    endocrine disease E34.9 [H28]
    eye disease — *see* Cataract, complicated
    hypoparathyroidism E20.9 [H28]

Cataract — *continued*
  in — *continued*
    malnutrition-dehydration E46 [H28]
    metabolic disease E88.9 [H28]
    myotonic disorders G71.1 [H28]
    nutritional disease E63.9 [H28]
  infantile — *see* Cataract, presenile
  irradiational — *see* Cataract, specified NEC
  juvenile — *see* Cataract, presenile
  malnutrition-dehydration E46 [H28]
  morgagnian — *see* Cataract, senile, morgagnian
    type
  myotonic G71.1 [H28]
  myxedema E03.9 [H28]
  nuclear
    embryonal Q12.0
    sclerosis — *see* Cataract, senile, nuclear
  presenile H26.009
    bilateral H26.003
    combined forms H26.009
      bilateral H26.063
      left H26.062
      right H26.061
    cortical H26.019
      bilateral H26.013
      left H26.012
      right H26.011
    lamellar — *see* Cataract, presenile, cortical
    left H26.002
    nuclear H26.039
      bilateral H26.033
      left H26.032
      right H26.031
    right H26.001
    specified NEC H26.09
    subcapsular polar (anterior) H26.049
      bilateral H26.043
      left H26.042
      posterior H26.059
        bilateral H26.053
        left H26.052
        right H26.051
      right H26.041
    zonular — *see* Cataract, presenile, cortical
  secondary H26.40
    Soemmering's ring H26.419
      bilateral H26.413
      left H26.412
      right H26.411
    specified NEC H26.499
      bilateral H26.493
      left H26.492
      right H26.491
    to eye disease — *see* Cataract, complicated
  senile H25.9
    brunescens — *see* Cataract, senile, nuclear
    combined forms H25.819
      bilateral H25.813
      left H25.812
      right H25.811
    coronary — *see* Cataract, senile, incipient
    cortical H25.019
      bilateral H25.013
      left H25.012
      right H25.011
    hypermature — *see* Cataract, senile,
      morgagnian type
    incipient (mature) (total) H25.099
      bilateral H25.093
      cortical — *see* Cataract, senile, cortical
      left H25.092
      right H25.091
      subcapsular — *see* Cataract, senile,
        subcapsular
    morgagnian type (hypermature) H25.20
      bilateral H25.23
      left H25.22
      right H25.21
    nuclear (sclerosis) H25.10
      bilateral H25.13
      left H25.12
      right H25.11
    polar subcapsular (anterior) (posterior) —
      see Cataract, senile, subcapsular
    punctate — *see* Cataract, senile, incipient
    specified NEC H25.89

Cataract — *continued*
  senile — *continued*
    subcapsular polar (anterior) H25.039
      bilateral H25.033
      left H25.032
      posterior H25.049
        bilateral H25.043
        left H25.042
        right H25.041
      right H25.031
  snowflake — *see* Diabetes, cataract
  specified NEC H26.8
  toxic — *see* Cataract, drug-induced
  traumatic H26.109
    bilateral H26.103
    left H26.102
    localized H26.119
      bilateral H26.113
      left H26.112
      right H26.111
    partially resolved H26.129
      bilateral H26.123
      left H26.122
      right H26.121
    right H26.101
    total H26.139
      bilateral H26.133
      left H26.132
      right H26.131
  zonular (perinuclear) Q12.0
Cataracta — *see also* Cataract
  brunescens — *see* Cataract, senile, nuclear
  centralis pulverulenta Q12.0
  cerulea Q12.0
  complicata — *see* Cataract, complicated
  congenita Q12.0
  coralliformis Q12.0
  coronaria Q12.0
  diabetic — *see* Diabetes, cataract
  membranacea
    accreta — *see* Cataract, secondary
    congenita Q12.0
  nigra — *see* Cataract, senile, nuclear
  sunflower — *see* Cataract, complicated
Catarrh, catarrhal (acute) (febrile) (infectious) (inflammation) (*see also* condition) J00
  bronchial — *see* Bronchitis
  chest — *see* Bronchitis
  chronic J31.0
  due to congenital syphilis A50.03
  enteric — *see* Enteritis
  eustachian H68.009
  fauces — *see* Pharyngitis
  gastrointestinal — *see* Enteritis
  gingivitis K05.0
  hay — *see* Fever, hay
  intestinal — *see* Enteritis
  larynx, chronic J37.0
  liver B15.9
    with hepatic coma B15.0
  lung — *see* Bronchitis
  middle ear, chronic — *see* Otitis, media, nonsuppurative, chronic, serous
  mouth K12.1
  nasal (chronic) — *see* Rhinitis
  nasobronchial J31.1
  nasopharyngeal (chronic) J31.1
    acute J00
  pulmonary — *see* Bronchitis
  spring (eye) (vernal) — *see* Conjunctivitis, acute, atopic
  summer (hay) — *see* Fever, hay
  throat J31.2
  tubotympanal — *see also* Otitis, media, nonsuppurative
    chronic — *see* Otitis, media, nonsuppurative, chronic, serous
Catastrophe, cerebral I64
Catatonia (schizophrenic) F20.2
Cat-scratch — *see also* Abrasion
  disease or fever A28.1
Cauda equina — *see* condition
Caul over face (causing asphyxia) P28.9
Cauliflower ear M95.10
  left M95.12
  right M95.11

Causalgia (upper limb) G56.40
  left G56.42
  lower limb G57.70
    left G57.72
    right G57.71
  right G56.41
Cause
  external, general effects T75.89
  not stated (morbidity) R69
  unknown (morbidity) R69
Caustic burn — *see* Corrosion, by site
Cavare's disease (familial periodic paralysis) G72.3
Cave-in, injury
  crushing (severe) T14.90
  suffocation — *see* Asphyxia, traumatic, due to low oxygen, due to cave-in
Cavernitis (penis) N48.29
Cavernositis N48.29
Cavernous — *see* condition
Cavitation of lung — *see also* Tuberculosis, pulmonary
  nontuberculous J98.4
Cavity
  lung — *see* Cavitation of lung
  optic papilla Q14.2
  pulmonary — *see* Cavitation of lung
Cavovarus foot, congenital Q66.1
Cavus foot (congenital) Q66.7
  acquired — *see* Deformity, limb, foot, specified NEC
Cazenave's disease L10.2
Cecitis K52.9
  with perforation, peritonitis, or rupture K65.8
Cecum — *see* condition
Celiac
  artery compression syndrome I77.4
  disease K90.0
  infantilism K90.0
Cell(s), cellular — *see also* condition
  in urine R82.99
Cellulitis (diffuse) (phlegmonous) (septic) (suppurative) L03.90
  abdominal wall L03.311
  anaerobic A48.0
  ankle — *see* Cellulitis, lower limb
  anus K61.0
  arm — *see* Cellulitis, upper limb
  auricle (ear) — *see* Cellulitis, ear
  axilla L03.119
    left L03.112
    right L03.111
  back (any part) L03.312
  broad ligament
    acute N73.0
  buttock L03.317
  cervical (meaning neck) L03.221
  cervix (uteri) — *see* Cervicitis
  cheek (external) L03.211
    internal K12.2
  chest wall L03.313
  chronic L03.90
  clostridial A48.0
  corpus cavernosum N48.22
  digit
    finger — *see* Cellulitis, finger
    toe — *see* Cellulitis, toe
  Douglas' cul-de-sac or pouch
    acute N73.0
  drainage site (following operation) T81.4
  ear (external) H60.10
    bilateral H60.13
    left H60.12
    right H60.11
  eosinophilic (granulomatous) L98.3
  erysipelatous — *see* Erysipelas
  external auditory canal — *see* Cellulitis, ear
  eyelid — *see* Abscess, eyelid
  face NEC L03.211
  finger (intrathecal) (periosteal) (subcutaneous) (subcuticular) L03.019
    left L03.012
    right L03.011
  foot — *see* Cellulitis, lower limb

Cellulitis — *continued*
  gangrenous — *see* Gangrene
  genital organ NEC
    female (external) N76.4
    male N49.9
      multiple sites N49.8
      specified NEC N49.8
  gluteal (region) L03.317
  gonococcal A54.89
  groin L03.314
  hand — *see* Cellulitis, upper limb
  head NEC L03.811
    face (any part, except ear, eye and nose) L03.211
  heel — *see* Cellulitis, lower limb
  hip — *see* Cellulitis, lower limb
  jaw (region) L03.211
  knee — *see* Cellulitis, lower limb
  labium (majus) (minus) — *see* Vulvitis
  lacrimal passages — *see* Inflammation, lacrimal, passages
  larynx J38.7
  leg — *see* Cellulitis, lower limb
  lip K13.0
  lower limb L03.119
    left L03.116
    right L03.115
    toe — *see* Cellulitis, toe
  mouth (floor) K12.2
  multiple sites, so stated L03.90
  nasopharynx J39.1
  navel L03.316
    newborn P38
  neck (region) L03.221
  nose (septum) (external) J34.0
  orbit, orbital H05.019
    bilateral H05.013
    left H05.012
    right H05.011
  palate (soft) K12.2
  pectoral (region) L03.313
  pelvis, pelvic (chronic)
    female (*see also* Disease, pelvis, inflammatory) N73.2
      acute N73.0
    following ectopic or molar pregnancy O08.0
    male K65.0
  penis N48.22
  perineal, perineum L03.315
  perirectal K61.1
  peritonsillar J36
  periurethral N34.0
  periuterine (*see also* Disease, pelvis, inflammatory) N73.2
    acute N73.0
  pharynx J39.1
  rectum K61.1
  retroperitoneal K65.0
  round ligament
    acute N73.0
  scalp (any part) L03.811
  scrotum N49.2
  seminal vesicle N49.0
  shoulder — *see* Cellulitis, upper limb
  specified site NEC L03.818
  submandibular (region) (space) (triangle) K12.2
    gland K11.3
  submaxillary (region) K12.2
    gland K11.3
  thigh — *see* Cellulitis, lower limb
  thumb (intrathecal) (periosteal) (subcutaneous) (subcuticular) — *see* Cellulitis, finger
  toe (intrathecal) (periosteal) (subcutaneous) (subcuticular) L03.039
    left L03.032
    right L03.031
  tonsil J36
  trunk L03.319
    abdominal wall L03.311
    back (any part) L03.312
    buttock L03.317
    chest wall L03.313
    groin L03.314
    perineal, perineum L03.315
    umbilicus L03.316
  tuberculous (primary) A18.4
  umbilicus L03.316
    newborn P38

Cellulitis — *continued*
  upper limb L03.119
    axilla — *see* Cellulitis, axilla
    finger — *see* Cellulitis, finger
      left L03.114
      right L03.113
      thumb — *see* Cellulitis, finger
  vaccinal T88.0
  vocal cord J38.3
  vulva — *see* Vulvitis
  wrist — *see* Cellulitis, upper limb
Cementoblastoma, benign (M9273/0) D16.5
  upper jaw (bone) D16.4
Cementoma (M9272/0) D16.5
  gigantiform (M9275/0) D16.5
    upper jaw (bone) D16.4
  upper jaw (bone) D16.4
Cementoperiostitis K05.3
Cementosis K03.4
Cephalematocele, cephal(o)**hematocele**
  fetus or newborn P52.8
    birth injury P10.8
  traumatic — *see* Hematoma, brain
Cephalematoma, cephalhematoma (calcified)
  fetus or newborn (birth injury) P12.0
  traumatic — *see* Hematoma, brain
Cephalgia, cephalalgia — *see* Headache
Cephalic — *see* condition
Cephalitis — *see* Encephalitis
Cephalocele — *see* Encephalocele
Cephalomenia N94.8
Cephalopelvic — *see* condition
Cerclage (with cervical incompetence) **in**
    pregnancy — *see* Incompetence, cervix, in
    pregnancy
Cerebellitis — *see* Encephalitis
Cerebellum, cerebellar — *see* condition
Cerebral — *see* condition
Cerebritis — *see* Encephalitis
Cerebro-hepato-renal syndrome Q87.89
Cerebromalacia — *see* Softening, brain
Cerebroside lipidosis E75.22
Cerebrospasticity (congenital) G80.0
Cerebrospinal — *see* condition
Cerebrum — *see* condition
Ceroid-lipofuscinosis, neuronal E75.4
Cerumen (accumulation) (impacted) H61.20
  left H61.22
    with right H61.23
  right H61.21
    with left H61.23
Cervical — *see also* condition
  auricle Q18.2
  dysplasia in pregnancy — *see* Abnormal, cervix,
    in pregnancy or childbirth
  erosion in pregnancy — *see* Abnormal, cervix,
    in pregnancy or childbirth
  fibrosis in pregnancy — *see* Abnormal, cervix,
    in pregnancy or childbirth
  fusion syndrome Q76.1
  rib Q76.5
Cervicalgia M54.2
Cervicitis (acute) (chronic) (nonvenereal) (senile
    (atrophic) (subacute) (with ulceration) N72
  with
    abortion — *see* Abortion, by type
      complicated by genital tract and pelvic
      infection
    ectopic pregnancy O08.0
    molar pregnancy O08.0
  chlamydial A56.09
  complicating pregnancy O23.50
    first trimester O23.51
    second trimester O23.52
    third trimester O23.53
  following ectopic or molar pregnancy O08.0
  gonococcal A54.03
  herpesviral A60.03
  puerperal (postpartum) O86.1
  syphilitic A52.76
  trichomonal A59.09
  tuberculous A18.16

Cervicocolpitis (emphysematosa) (*see also*
    Cervicitis) N72
Cervix — *see* condition
Cesarean operation or section previous,
    affecting management of pregnancy
    O34.21
Céstan (-Chenais) **paralysis or syndrome** G46.3
Céstan-Raymond syndrome I65.8
Cestode infestation B71.9
  specified type NEC B71.8
Cestodiasis B71.9
Chabert's disease A22.9
Chacaleh E53.8
Chafing L30.4
Chagas' (-Mazza) disease (chronic) B57.2
  with
    cardiovascular involvement NEC B57.2
    digestive system involvement B57.30
      megacolon B57.32
      megaesophagus B57.31
      other specified B57.39
    megacolon B57.32
    megaesophagus B57.31
    myocarditis B57.2
    nervous system involvement B57.40
      meningitis B57.41
      meningoencephalitis B57.42
      other specified B57.49
    specified organ involvement NEC B57.5
  acute (with) B57.1
    cardiovascular NEC B57.0
    myocarditis B57.0
Chagres fever B50.9
Chairfast, requiring health care provider Z74.0
Chalasia (cardiac sphincter) K21.9
Chalazion H00.19
  left H00.16
    lower H00.15
    upper H00.14
  right H00.13
    lower H00.12
    upper H00.11
Chalcosis — *see also* Disorder, globe,
    degenerative, chalcosis
  cornea — *see* Deposit, cornea
  crystalline lens — *see* Cataract, complicated
  retina H35.89
Chalicosis (pulmonum) J62.8
Chancre (any genital site) (hard) (hunterian)
    (mixed) (primary) (seronegative) (seropositive)
    (syphilitic) A51.0
  congenital A50.07
  conjunctiva NEC A51.2
  Ducrey's A57
  extragenital A51.2
  eyelid A51.2
  lip A51.2
  nipple A51.2
  Nisbet's A57
  of
    carate A67.0
    pinta A67.0
    yaws A66.0
  palate, soft A51.2
  phagedenic A57
  simple A57
  soft A57
    bubo A57
    palate A51.2
  urethra A51.0
  yaws A66.0
Chancroid (anus) (genital) (penis) (perineum)
    (rectum) (urethra) (vulva) A57
Chandler's disease (osteochondritis dissecans,
    hip) — *see* Osteochondritis, dissecans, hip
Change(s) (of) — *see also* Removal
  arteriosclerotic — *see* Arteriosclerosis
  bone — *see also* Disorder, bone
    diabetic — *see* Diabetes, bone change
  bowel habit R19.4
  cardiorenal (vascular) — *see* Hypertension,
    cardiorenal
  cardiovascular — *see* Disease, cardiovascular

Change(s) — *see also* Removal — *continued*
  circulatory I99.9
  cognitive (mild) (organic) due to or secondary to
    general medical condition F06.8
  color, tooth, teeth
    during formation K00.8
    posteruptive K03.7
  contraceptive device Z30.44
  corneal membrane H18.30
    Bowman's membrane fold or rupture
      H18.319
        bilateral H18.313
        left H18.312
        right H18.311
    Descemet's membrane
      fold H18.329
        bilateral H18.323
        left H18.322
        right H18.321
      rupture H18.339
        bilateral H18.333
        left H18.332
        right H18.331
  coronary — *see* Disease, heart, ischemic
  degenerative, spine or vertebra — *see*
    Spondylosis
  dental pulp, regressive K04.2
  dressing Z48.0
  heart — *see* Disease, heart
  hip joint — *see* Derangement, joint, hip
  hyperplastic larynx J38.7
  hypertrophic
    nasal sinus J34.8
    turbinate, nasal J34.3
    upper respiratory tract J39.8
  indwelling catheter Z46.6
  inflammatory — *see also* Inflammation
    sacroiliac M46.1
  job, anxiety concerning Z56.1
  joint — *see* Derangement, joint
  life — *see* Menopause
  malignant (M8000/3) – code as primary
    malignant neoplasm of the site of the
    lesion
  mental F99
  minimal (glomerular) (*see also* N00-N07 with
    fourth character .0) N05.0
  myocardium, myocardial — *see* Degeneration,
    myocardial
  of life — *see* Menopause
  pacemaker Z45.018
    pulse generator Z45.010
  personality (enduring) F68.8
    due to (secondary to)
      general medical condition F07.0
    secondary (nonspecific) F60.89
  regressive, dental pulp K04.2
  renal — *see* Disease, renal
  retina H35.9
    myopic — *see* Disorder, globe, degenerative,
      myopia
  sacroiliac joint M53.3
  senile (*see also* condition) R54
  sensory R20.8
  skin R23.9
    acute, due to ultraviolet radiation L56.9
      specified NEC L56.8
    chronic, due to nonionizing radiation L57.9
      specified NEC L57.8
    cyanosis R23.0
    flushing R23.2
    pallor R23.1
    petechiae R23.3
    specified change NEC R23.8
    swelling — *see* Mass, localized
    texture R23.4
  suture Z48.0
  trophic
    arm — *see* Mononeuropathy, upper limb
    leg — *see* Mononeuropathy, lower limb
  vascular I99.9
  vasomotor I73.9
  voice R49.9
    psychogenic F44.4
    specified NEC R49.8
Changing sleep-work schedule, affecting sleep
  F51.22

©2002 Ingenix, Inc.

Changuinola fever A93.1

Chapping skin T69.8

Charcot-Marie-Tooth disease, paralysis or syndrome G60.0

Charcôt's
arthropathy — *see* Arthropathy, neuropathic
cirrhosis K74.3
disease (tabetic arthropathy) A52.16
joint (disease) (tabetic) A52.16
diabetic — *see* Diabetes, arthropathy, neuropathic
syringomyelic G95.0
syndrome (intermittent claudication) I73.9

Charley-horse (quadriceps) S76.119
left S76.112
muscle, except quadriceps — *see* Sprain
right S76.111

Charlouis' disease — *see* Yaws

Cheadle's disease E54

Checking (of)
cardiac pacemaker (battery) (electrode(s)) Z45.018
pulse generator Z45.010
device
contraceptive Z30.44

Check-up
health (routine) Z00.010
with abnormal findings Z00.011
infant (not sick) Z00.10
pregnancy (normal)
first — *see* Antenatal, care, first, pregnancy
high risk — *see* Antenatal, care, high risk pregnancy

Chédiak-Higashi (-Steinbrinck) syndrome (congenital gigantism of peroxidase granules) E70.330

Cheek — *see* condition

Cheese itch B88.0

Cheese-washer's lung J67.8

Cheese-worker's lung J67.8

Cheilitis (acute) (angular) (catarrhal) (chronic) (exfoliative) (gangrenous) (glandular) (infectional) (suppurative) (ulcerative) (vesicular) K13.0
actinic (due to sun) L56.8
other than from sun L59.8
candidal B37.83

Cheilodynia K13.0

Cheiloschisis — *see* Cleft, lip

Cheilosis (angular) K13.0
with pellagra E52 [K93]
due to
vitamin B2 (riboflavin) deficiency E53.0 [K93]

Cheiromegaly M79.8

Cheiropompholyx L30.1

Cheloid — *see* Keloid

Chemical burn — *see* Corrosion, by site

Chemodectoma (M8693/1) — *see* Paraganglioma, nonchromaffin

Chemoprophylaxis Z51.89

Chemosis, conjunctiva — *see* Edema, conjunctiva

Chemotherapy (session) (for) Z51.89
cancer Z51.1
maternal, affecting fetus or newborn P04.1
convalescence Z76.8
neoplasm Z51.1

Cherubism M27.8

Chest — *see* condition

Cheyne-Stokes breathing (respiration) R06.3

Chiari's
disease or syndrome (hepatic vein thrombosis) I82.0
malformation
type I G93.5
type II — *see* Spina bifida
net Q24.8

Chicago disease B40.9

Chickenpox — *see* Varicella

Chiclero ulcer or sore B55.1

Chigger (infestation) B88.0

Chignon (disease) B36.8
fetus or newborn (from vacuum extraction) (birth injury) P12.1

Chilaiditi's syndrome (subphrenic displacement, colon) Q43.3

Chilblain(s) (lupus) T69.1

Child behavior causing concern Z63.8

Childbirth (mother) (*see also* Delivery) O80

Childhood
cerebral X-linked adrenoleukodystrophy E71.420
period of rapid growth Z00.2

Chill(s) R68.8
with fever R50.0
congestive in malarial regions B54
septic — *see* Septicemia

Chilomastigiasis A07.8

Chimera 46,XX/46,XY Q99.0

Chin — *see* condition

Chinese dysentery A03.9

Chionophobia F40.228

Chitral fever A93.1

Chlamydia, chlamydial A74.9
cervicitis A56.09
conjunctivitis A74.0
cystitis A56.01
endometritis A56.11
epididymitis A56.19
female
pelvic inflammatory disease A56.11
pelviperitonitis A56.11
orchitis A56.19
peritonitis A74.81
pharyngitis A56.4
proctitis A56.3
psittaci (infection) A70
salpingitis A56.11
sexually-transmitted infection NEC A56.8
specified NEC A74.89
urethritis A56.01
vulvovaginitis A56.02

Chlamydiosis — *see* Chlamydia

Chloasma (skin) (idiopathic) (symptomatic) L81.1
eyelid H02.719
hyperthyroid E05.90 [H02.719]
with thyroid storm E05.91 [H02.719]
left H02.716
lower H02.715
upper H02.714
right H02.713
lower H02.712
upper H02.711

Chloroma (M9930/3) C92.30

Chlorosis D50.9
Egyptian B76.9 [D63.8]
miner's B76.9 [D63.8]

Chlorotic anemia D50.9

Chocolate cyst (ovary) N80.1

Choked
disc or disk — *see* Papilledema
on food, phlegm, or vomitus NOS — *see* Asphyxia, food
while vomiting NOS — *see* Asphyxia, food

Chokes (resulting from bends) T70.3

Choking sensation R06.89

Cholangiectasis K83.8

Cholangiocarcinoma (M8160/3)
with hepatocellular carcinoma, combined (M8180/3) C22.0
liver C22.1
specified site NEC — *see* Neoplasm, malignant
unspecified site C22.1

Cholangiohepatitis K83.8
due to fluke infestation B66.1

Cholangiohepatoma (M8180/3) C22.0

Cholangiolitis (acute) (chronic) (extrahepatic) (gangrenous) (intrahepatic) K83.0
paratyphoidal — *see* Fever, paratyphoid
typhoidal A01.09

Cholangioma (M8160/0) D13.4
malignant (M8160/3) — *see* Cholangiocarcinoma

Cholangitis (ascending) (primary) (recurrent) (sclerosing) (secondary) (stenosing) (suppurative) K83.0
with calculus, bile duct — *see* Calculus, bile duct, with cholangitis
chronic nonsuppurative destructive K74.3

Cholecystectasia K82.8

Cholecystitis K81.9
with
calculus, stones in
bile duct (common) (hepatic) — *see* Calculus, bile duct, with cholecystitis
cystic duct — *see* Calculus, gallbladder, with cholecystitis
gallbladder — *see* Calculus, gallbladder, with cholecystitis
choledocholithiasis — *see* Calculus, bile duct, with cholecystitis
cholelithiasis — *see* Calculus, gallbladder, with cholecystitis
acute (emphysematous) (gangrenous) (suppurative) K81.0
with
calculus, stones in
cystic duct — *see* Calculus, gallbladder, with cholecystitis, acute
gallbladder — *see* Calculus, gallbladder, with cholecystitis, acute
choledocholithiasis — *see* Calculus, bile duct, with cholecystitis, acute
cholelithiasis — *see* Calculus, gallbladder, with cholecystitis, acute
chronic cholecystitis K81.2
with gallbladder calculus K80.12
with obstruction K80.13
chronic K81.1
with acute cholecystitis K81.2
with gallbladder calculus K80.12
with obstruction K80.13
emphysematous (acute) — *see* Cholecystitis, acute
gangrenous — *see* Cholecystitis, acute
paratyphoidal, current A01.4
suppurative — *see* Cholecystitis, acute
typhoidal A01.09

Cholecystolithiasis — *see* Calculus, gallbladder

Choledochitis (suppurative) K83.0

Choledocholith — *see* Calculus, bile duct

Choledocholithiasis (common duct) (hepatic duct) — *see* Calculus, bile duct
cystic — *see* Calculus, gallbladder
typhoidal A01.09

Cholelithiasis (cystic duct) (gallbladder) (impacted) (multiple) — *see* Calculus, gallbladder
bile duct (common) (hepatic) — *see* Calculus, bile duct
hepatic duct — *see* Calculus, bile duct
specified NEC K80.80
with obstruction K80.81

Cholemia — *see also* Jaundice
familial (simple) (congenital) E80.4
Gilbert's E80.4

Choleperitoneum, choleperitonitis K65.8

Cholera (Asiatic) (epidemic) (malignant) A00.9
antimonial — *see* Poisoning, antimony
classical A00.0
due to Vibrio cholerae 01 A00.9
biovar cholerae A00.0
biovar eltor A00.1
el tor A00.1
el tor A00.1
vaccination, prophylactic Z23

Cholerine — *see* Cholera

Cholestasis NEC K83.1
with hepatocyte injury K71.0
pure K71.0

Cholesteatoma (ear) (middle) (with reaction)
H71.90
attic H71.00
bilateral H71.03
left H71.02
right H71.01
bilateral H71.93
external ear (canal) H60.40
bilateral H60.43
left H60.42
right H60.41
left H71.92
mastoid H71.20
bilateral H71.23
left H71.22
right H71.21
postmastoidectomy cavity (recurrent) — see
Complications, postmastoidectomy,
recurrent cholesteatoma
recurrent (postmastoidectomy) — see
Complications, postmastoidectomy,
recurrent cholesteatoma
right H71.91
tympanum H71.10
bilateral H71.13
left H71.12
right H71.11
Cholesteatosis, diffuse H71.30
bilateral H71.33
left H71.32
right H71.31
Cholesteremia E78.0
Cholesterin in vitreous — see Deposit,
crystalline
Cholesterol
deposit
retina H35.89
vitreous — see Deposit, crystalline
imbibition of gallbladder K82.4
Cholesterolemia (essential) (familial) (hereditary)
(pure) E78.0
Cholesterolosis, cholesterosis (gallbladder)
K82.4
cerebrotendinous E75.5
Cholocolic fistula K82.3
Choluria R82.2
Chondritis (purulent) — see Disorder, cartilage,
specified NEC
costal (Tietze's) M94.0
patella, posttraumatic — see Chondromalacia,
patella
tuberculous NEC A18.02
intervertebral A18.01
Chondroblastoma (M9230/0) — see also
Neoplasm, bone, benign
malignant (M9230/3) — see Neoplasm, bone,
malignant
Chondrocalcinosis M11.20
ankle M11.279
left M11.272
right M11.271
elbow M11.229
left M11.222
right M11.221
familial M11.10
ankle M11.179
left M11.172
right M11.171
elbow M11.129
left M11.122
right M11.121
foot joint M11.179
left M11.172
right M11.171
hand joint M11.149
left M11.142
right M11.141
hip M11.159
left M11.152
right M11.151
knee M11.169
left M11.162
right M11.161
multiple site M11.19

Chondrocalcinosis — continued
familial — continued
shoulder M11.119
left M11.112
right M11.111
specified joint NEC M11.18
wrist M11.139
left M11.132
right M11.131
foot joint M11.279
left M11.272
right M11.271
hand joint M11.249
left M11.242
right M11.241
hip M11.259
left M11.252
right M11.251
knee M11.269
left M11.262
right M11.261
multiple site M11.29
shoulder M11.219
left M11.212
right M11.211
specified joint NEC M11.28
specified type NEC M11.20
ankle M11.279
left M11.272
right M11.271
elbow M11.229
left M11.222
right M11.221
foot joint M11.279
left M11.272
right M11.271
hand joint M11.249
left M11.242
right M11.241
hip M11.259
left M11.252
right M11.251
knee M11.269
left M11.262
right M11.261
multiple site M11.29
shoulder M11.219
left M11.212
right M11.211
specified joint NEC M11.28
wrist M11.239
left M11.232
right M11.231
wrist M11.239
left M11.232
right M11.231
Chondrodermatitis nodularis helicis or
anthelicis — see Perichondritis, ear
Chondrodysplasia Q78.9
with hemangioma Q78.4
calcificans congenita Q77.3
fetalis Q77.4
punctata Q77.3
Chondrodystrophy, chondrodystrophia (familial)
(fetalis) (hypoplastic) Q78.9
calcificans congenita Q77.3
punctata Q77.3
Chondroectodermal dysplasia Q77.6
Chondrogenesis imperfecta Q77.4
Chondrolysis
hip M94.359
left M94.352
right M94.351
Chondroma (M9220/0) — see also Neoplasm,
cartilage, benign
juxtacortical (M9221/0) — see Neoplasm, bone,
benign
periosteal (M9221/0) — see Neoplasm, bone,
benign
Chondromalacia (systemic) M94.20
acromioclavicular joint M94.219
left M94.212
right M94.211
ankle M94.279
left M94.272

Chondromalacia — continued
ankle — continued
right M94.271
elbow M94.229
left M94.222
right M94.221
foot joint M94.279
left M94.272
right M94.271
glenohumeral joint M94.219
left M94.212
right M94.211
hand joint M94.249
left M94.242
right M94.241
hip M94.259
left M94.252
right M94.251
knee M94.269
left M94.262
patella — see Chondromalacia, patella
right M94.261
multiple sites M94.29
patella M22.40
left M22.42
right M22.41
rib M94.28
sacroiliac joint M94.259
shoulder M94.219
left M94.212
right M94.211
sternoclavicular joint M94.219
left M94.212
right M94.211
vertebral joint M94.28
wrist M94.239
left M94.232
right M94.231
Chondromatosis (M9220/1) — see also
Neoplasm, cartilage, uncertain behavior
internal Q78.4
Chondromyxosarcoma (M9220/3) — see
Neoplasm, cartilage, malignant
Chondro-osteodysplasia (Morquio-Brailsford
type) E76.219
Chondro-osteodystrophy E76.29
Chondro-osteoma (M9210/0) — see Neoplasm,
bone, benign
Chondropathia tuberosa — see Disorder,
cartilage, specified type NEC
Chondrosarcoma (M9220/3) — see Neoplasm,
cartilage, malignant
juxtacortical (M9221/3) — see Neoplasm, bone,
malignant
mesenchymal (M9240/3) — see Neoplasm,
connective tissue, malignant
myxoid (M9231/3) — see Neoplasm, cartilage,
malignant
Chordee (nonvenereal) N48.89
congenital Q54.4
gonococcal A54.09
Chorditis (fibrinous) (nodosa) (tuberosa) J38.2
Chordoma (M9370/3) — see also Neoplasm,
malignant
Chorea (chronic) (gravis) (posthemiplegic) (senile)
(spasmodic) G25.5
with
heart involvement I02.0
active or acute (conditions in I01-) I02.0
rheumatic I02.9
with valvular disorder I02.0
rheumatic heart disease (chronic) (inactive)
(quiescent) – code to rheumatic heart
condition involved
apoplectic I64
drug-induced G25.4
habit F95.8
hereditary G10
Huntington's G10
hysterical F44.4
minor I02.9
with heart involvement I02.0
progressive G25.5
hereditary G10

©2002 Ingenix, Inc.

Chorea — *continued*
rheumatic (chronic) I02.9
with heart involvement I02.0
Sydenham's I02.9
with heart involvement — *see* Chorea, with rheumatic heart disease
nonrheumatic G25.5
Choreoathetosis (paroxysmal) G25.5
Chorioadenoma (destruens) (M9100/1) D39.2
Chorioamnionitis O41.129
first trimester O41.121
second trimester O41.122
third trimester O41.123
Chorioangioma (M9120/0) D26.7
Choriocarcinoma (M9100/3)
combined with
embryonal carcinoma (M9101/3) — *see* Neoplasm, malignant
other germ cell elements (M9101/3) — *see* Neoplasm, malignant
teratoma (M9101/3) — *see* Neoplasm, malignant
specified site — *see* Neoplasm, malignant
unspecified site
female C58
male C62.90
Chorioencephalitis (acute) (lymphocytic) (serous) A87.2
Chorioepithelioma (M9100/3) — *see* Choriocarcinoma
Choriomeningitis (acute) (lymphocytic) (serous) A87.2
Chorionepithelioma (M9100/3) — *see* Choriocarcinoma
Chorioretinitis — *see also* Inflammation, chorioretinal
disseminated — *see also* Inflammation, chorioretinal, disseminated
in neurosyphilis A52.19
focal — *see also* Inflammation, chorioretinal, focal
Egyptian B76.9 [D63.8]
histoplasmic B39.9 [H32]
in (due to)
histoplasmosis B39.9 [H32]
syphilis (secondary) A51.43
late A52.71
toxoplasmosis (acquired) B58.01
congenital (active) P37.1 [H32]
tuberculosis A18.53
juxtapapillary, juxtapapillaris — *see* Inflammation, chorioretinal, focal, juxtapapillary
leprous A30.9 [H32]
miner's B76.9 [D63.8]
progressive myopia (degeneration) — *see* Disorder, globe, degenerative, myopia
syphilitic (secondary) A51.43
congenital (early) A50.01 [H32]
late A50.32
late A52.71
tuberculous A18.53
Chorioretinopathy, central serous H35.719
bilateral H35.713
left H35.712
right H35.711
Choroid — *see* condition
Choroideremia H31.21
Choroiditis — *see* Chorioretinitis
Choroidopathy — *see* Disorder, choroid
Choroidoretinitis — *see* Chorioretinitis
Choroidoretinopathy, central serous — *see* Chorioretinopathy, central serous
Christian-Weber disease M35.6
Christmas disease D67
Chromaffinoma (M8700/0) — *see also* Neoplasm, benign
malignant (M8700/3) — *see* Neoplasm, malignant
Chromatopsia — *see* Deficiency, color vision
Chromhidrosis, chromidrosis L75.1
Chromoblastomycosis — *see* Chromomycosis
Chromoconversion R82.91

Chromomycosis B43.9
brain abscess B43.1
cerebral B43.1
cutaneous B43.0
skin B43.0
specified NEC B43.8
subcutaneous abscess or cyst B43.0
Chromophytosis B36.0
Chromosome — *see* condition by chromosome involved
D(1) — *see* condition, chromosome 13
E(3) — *see* condition, chromosome 18
G — *see* condition, chromosome 21
Chromotrichomycosis B36.8
Chronic — *see* condition
Churg-Strauss syndrome M30.1
Chyle cyst, mesentery I89.8
Chylocele (nonfilarial) I89.8
filarial (*see also* Infestation, filarial) B74.9 [N51]
tunica vaginalis N50.8
filarial (*see also* Infestation, filarial) B74.9 [N51]
Chylomicronemia (fasting) (with hyperprebetalipoproteinemia) E78.3
Chylopericardium I31.3
acute I30.9
Chylothorax (nonfilarial) I89.8
filarial (*see also* Infestation, filarial) B74.9 [J91]
Chylous — *see* condition
Chyluria (nonfilarial) R82.0
due to
bilharziasis B65.0
Brugia (malayi) B74.1
timori B74.2
schistosomiasis (bilharziasis) B65.0
Wuchereria (bancrofti) B74.0
filarial — *see* Infestation, filarial
Cicatricial (deformity) — *see* Cicatrix
Cicatrix (adherent) (contracted) (painful) (vicious) (*see also* Scar) L90.5
adenoid (and tonsil) J35.8
alveolar process M26.79
anus K62.8
auricle — *see* Disorder, pinna, specified type NEC
bile duct (common) (hepatic) K83.8
bladder N32.8
bone — *see* Disorder, bone, specified type NEC
brain G93.8
cervix (postoperative) (postpartal) N88.1
common duct K83.8
cornea H17.9
tuberculous A18.59
duodenum (bulb), obstructive K31.5
esophagus K22.2
eyelid — *see* Disorder, eyelid function
hypopharynx J39.2
lacrimal passages — *see* Obstruction, lacrimal
larynx J38.7
lung J98.4
middle ear — *see* category H74.8
mouth K13.7
muscle M62.89
with contracture — *see* Contraction, muscle NEC
nasopharynx J39.2
palate (soft) K13.7
penis N48.89
pharynx J39.2
prostate N42.89
rectum K62.8
retina — *see* Scar, chorioretinal
semilunar cartilage — *see* Derangement, meniscus
seminal vesicle N50.8
skin L90.5
infected L08.89
postinfective L90.5
tuberculous B90.8
specified site NEC L90.5
throat J39.2
tongue K14.8
tonsil (and adenoid) J35.8
trachea J39.8
tuberculous NEC B90.9

Cicatrix (*see also* Scar) — *continued*
urethra N36.8
uterus N85.8
vagina N89.8
postoperative N99.2
vocal cord J38.3
wrist, constricting (annular) L90.5
CIN — *see* Neoplasia, intraepithelial, cervix
Cinchonism
correct substance properly administered — *see* Deafness, ototoxic
overdose or wrong substance given or taken — *see* category T37.2
Circle of Willis — *see* condition
Circular — *see* condition
Circulating anticoagulants D68.3
due to drugs D68.5
following childbirth O72.3
Circulation
collateral, any site I99.8
defective (lower extremity) I99.8
congenital Q28.9
embryonic Q28.9
failure (peripheral) R57.9
fetus or newborn P29.8
fetal, persistent P29.3
heart, incomplete Q28.9
Circulatory system — *see* condition
Circulus senilis (cornea) — *see* Degeneration, cornea, senile
Circumcision (in absence of medical indication) (ritual) (routine) Z41.2
Circumscribed — *see* condition
Circumvallate placenta — *see* Abnormal, placenta, circumvallate
Cirrhosis, cirrhotic (dietary) (liver) (nodular) (periportal) (posthepatitic) (septal) (trabecular) K74.6
alcoholic K70.30
with ascites K70.31
atrophic — *see* Cirrhosis, liver
Baumgarten-Cruveilhier K74.6
biliary (cholangiolitic) (cholangitic) (hypertrophic) (obstructive) (pericholangiolitic) K74.5
due to
Clonorchiasis B66.1
flukes B66.3
primary K74.3
secondary K74.4
cardiac (of liver) K76.1
Charcôt's K74.3
cholangiolitic, cholangitic, cholostatic (primary) K74.3
congestive K76.1
Cruveilhier-Baumgarten K74.6
cryptogenic — *see* Cirrhosis, liver
due to
hepatolenticular degeneration E83.01
Wilson's disease E83.01
xanthomatosis E78.2
fatty K76.0
alcoholic K70.0
Hanot's (hypertrophic) K74.3
hepatic — *see* Cirrhosis, liver
hypertrophic K74.3
Indian childhood K74.6
kidney — *see* Sclerosis, renal
Laennec's K74.6
alcoholic K70.30
with ascites K70.31
liver (chronic) (hepatolienal) (hypertrophic) (nodular) (splenomegalic) K74.6
alcoholic K70.30
with ascites K70.31
fatty K70.0
congenital P78.81
syphilitic A52.74
lung (chronic) — *see* Fibrosis, lung
macronodular K74.6
alcoholic K70.30
with ascites K70.31
micronodular K74.6
alcoholic K70.30
with ascites K70.31

Cold — *continued*
on lung — *see* Bronchitis
rose J30.1
sensitivity, auto-immune D59.1
virus J00
Coldsore B00.1
Colibacillosis A49.8
as the cause of other disease B96.2
generalized A41.50
Colic (bilious) (infantile) (intestinal) (recurrent)
(spasmodic) R10.83
abdomen R10.83
psychogenic F45.8
appendix, appendicular K38.8
bile duct — *see* Calculus, bile duct
biliary — *see* Calculus, bile duct
common duct — *see* Calculus, bile duct
cystic duct — *see* Calculus, gallbladder
Devonshire NEC — *see* Poisoning, lead
flatulent R14.3
gallbladder — *see* Calculus, gallbladder
gallstone — *see* Calculus, gallbladder
gallbladder or cystic duct — *see* Calculus,
gallbladder
hepatic (duct) — *see* Calculus, bile duct
hysterical F45.8
kidney N23
lead NEC — *see* Poisoning, lead
mucous K58.9
with diarrhea K58.0
psychogenic F54
nephritic N23
painter's NEC — *see* Poisoning, lead
pancreas K86.8
psychogenic F45.8
renal N23
saturnine NEC — *see* Poisoning, lead
ureter N23
urethral N36.8
due to calculus N21.1
uterus NEC N94.8
menstrual — *see* Dysmenorrhea
worm NOS B83.9
Colicystitis — *see* Cystitis
Colitis (acute) (catarrhal) (chronic) (noninfective)
(hemorrhagic) (*see also* Enteritis) K52.9
allergic K52.2
amebic (acute) (*see also* Amebiasis) A06.0
nondysenteric A06.2
anthrax A22.2
bacillary — *see* Infection, Shigella
balantidial A07.0
coccidial A07.3
cystica superficialis K52.8
dietary counseling and surveillance (for) Z71.3
dietetic K52.2
due to radiation K52.0
food hypersensitivity K52.2
giardial A07.1
granulomatous — *see* Enteritis, regional, large
intestine
infectious — *see* Enteritis, infectious
ischemic K55.9
acute (fulminant) (subacute) K55.0
chronic K55.1
due to mesenteric artery insufficiency K55.1
fulminant (acute) K55.0
membranous
psychogenic F54
mucous — *see* Syndrome, irritable, bowel
psychogenic F54
noninfective K52.9
specified NEC K52.8
polyposa — *see* Pseudopolyposis of colon
presumed noninfective K52.9
protozoal A07.9
pseudomucinous — *see* Syndrome, irritable,
bowel
regional — *see* Enteritis, regional, large
intestine
segmental — *see* Enteritis, regional, large
intestine
septic — *see* Enteritis, infectious
spastic K58.9
with diarrhea K58.0
psychogenic F54

Colitis (*see also* Enteritis) — *continued*
staphylococcal A04.8
foodborne A05.0
subacute ischemic K55.0
thrombonulcerative K55.0
toxic K52.1
transmural — *see* Enteritis, regional, large
intestine
trichomonal A07.8
tuberculous (ulcerative) A18.32
ulcerative (chronic) K51.95
with
complication K51.90
abscess K51.94
fistula K51.93
obstruction K51.92
rectal bleeding K51.91
specified complication NEC K51.99
enterocolitis — *see* Enterocolitis, ulcerative
ileocolitis — *see* Ileocolitis, ulcerative
mucosal proctocolitis — *see* Proctocolitis,
mucosal
proctitis — *see* Proctitis, ulcerative
pseudopolyposis — *see* Pseudopolyposis of
colon
psychogenic F54
rectosigmoiditis — *see* Rectosigmoiditis,
ulcerative
specified type NOS K51.85
with
complication K51.80
abscess K51.84
fistula K51.83
obstruction K51.82
rectal bleeding K51.81
specified complication NEC K51.89
Collagenosis, collagen disease (nonvascular)
(vascular) M35.9
cardiovascular I42.8
reactive perforating L87.1
specified NEC M35.8
Collapse R55
adrenal E27.2
cardiorenal I13.2
cardiorespiratory R57.0
cardiovascular R57.0
newborn P29.8
circulatory (peripheral) R57.9
during or after labor and delivery O75.1
fetus or newborn P29.8
following ectopic or molar pregnancy O08.3
during or after labor and delivery O75.1
external ear canal — *see* Stenosis, external ear
canal
general R55
heart — *see* Disease, heart
heat T67.1
hysterical F44.89
labyrinth, membranous (congenital) Q16.5
lung (massive) (*see also* Atelectasis) J98.19
pressure due to anesthesia (general) (local)
or other sedation T88.2
during labor and delivery O74.1
in pregnancy — *see* Complications,
anesthesia, in, pregnancy,
pulmonary
postpartum, puerperal O89.09
myocardial — *see* Disease, heart
nervous F48.8
neurocirculatory F45.8
nose M95.0
postoperative (cardiovascular) T81.1
pulmonary (*see also* Atelectasis) J98.19
fetus or newborn — *see* Atelectasis
trachea J39.8
tracheobronchial J98.0
valvular — *see* Endocarditis
vascular (peripheral) R57.9
cerebral I64
during or after labor and delivery O75.1
fetus or newborn P29.8
following ectopic or molar pregnancy O08.3
vertebra M48.50
cervical region M48.52
cervicothoracic region M48.53

Collapse — *continued*
vertebra — *continued*
in (due to)
metastasis (M8000/6) — *see* Collapse,
vertebra, in, specified disease NEC
osteoporosis (*see also* Osteoporosis)
M80.88 [M48.50]
cervical region M80.88 *[M48.62]*
cervicothoracic region M80.88 *[M48.63]*
lumbar region M80.88 *[M48.66]*
lumbosacral region M80.88 *[M48.67]*
multiple sites M80.88 *[M48.69]*
occipito-atlanto-axial region M80.88
[M48.61]
sacrococcygeal region M80.88 *[M48.68]*
thoracic region M80.88 *[M48.64]*
thoracolumbar region M80.88 *[M48.65]*
specified disease NEC M48.50
cervical region M48.52
cervicothoracic region M48.53
lumbar region M48.56
lumbosacral region M48.57
occipito-atlanto-axial region M48.51
sacrococcygeal region M48.58
thoracic region M48.54
thoracolumbar region M48.55
lumbar region M48.56
lumbosacral region M48.57
occipito-atlanto-axial region M48.51
sacrococcygeal region M48.58
thoracic region M48.54
thoracolumbar region M48.55
Collateral — *see also* condition
circulation (venous) I87.8
dilation, veins I87.8
Colles' fracture S52.539
left S52.532
right S52.531
Collet (-Sicard) syndrome G52.7
Collier's asthma or lung J60
Collodion baby Q80.2
Colloid nodule (of thyroid) (cystic) E04.1
Coloboma (iris) Q13.0
eyelid Q10.3
fundus Q14.8
lens Q12.2
optic disc (congenital) Q14.2
acquired H47.319
bilateral H47.313
left H47.312
right H47.311
Coloenteritis — *see* Enteritis
Colon — *see* condition
Coloptosis K63.4
Color blindness — *see* Deficiency, color vision
Colostomy
attention to Z43.3
fitting or adjustment Z46.8
malfunctioning K94.03
status Z93.3
Colpitis (acute) — *see* Vaginitis
Colpocele N81.5
Colpocystitis — *see* Vaginitis
Colpospasm N94.2
Column, spinal, vertebral — *see* condition
Coma R40.20
with
motor response (none) R40.231
abnormal R40.233
extension R40.232
flexion withdrawal R40.234
localizes pain R40.235
obeys commands R40.236
opening of eyes (never) R40.211
in response to
pain R40.212
sound R40.213
spontaneous R40.214
verbal response (none) R40.221
confused conversation R40.224

Coma — *continued*
  with — *continued*
    verbal response — *continued*
      inappropriate words R40.223
      incomprehensible words R40.222
      oriented R40.225
  apoplectic I64
  eclamptic — *see* Eclampsia
  epileptic — *see* Epilepsy
  hepatic — *see* Failure, hepatic, by type, with
    coma
  hyperglycemic (diabetic) — *see* Diabetes, coma
  hyperosmolar (diabetic) — *see* Diabetes, coma
  hypoglycemic (diabetic) — *see* Diabetes, coma,
    hypoglycemic
    nondiabetic E15
  in diabetes — *see* Diabetes, coma
  insulin-induced — *see* Coma, hypoglycemic
  myxedematous E03.5
  newborn P91.5
  persistent vegetative state R40.3
  prediabetic — *see* Diabetes, hyperosmolarity
  uremic N19

Comatose — *see* Coma

Combat fatigue F43.0

Combined — *see* condition

Comedo, comedones (giant) L70.0

Comedocarcinoma (M8501/3) — *see also*
  Neoplasm, breast, malignant
  noninfiltrating (M8501/2)
    breast (female) D05.70
      male D05.75
    specified site — *see* Neoplasm, in situ
    unspecified site (female) D05.70
      male D05.75

Comedomastitis — *see* Ectasia, mammary duct

Comminuted fracture – code as Fracture, closed

Common
  arterial trunk Q20.0
  atrioventricular canal Q21.2
  atrium Q21.1
  cold (head) J00
    vaccination, prophylactic Z23
  truncus (arteriosus) Q20.0
  variable immunodeficiency — *see*
    Immunodeficiency, common variable
  ventricle Q20.4

Commotio, commotion (current)
  brain — *see* Injury, intracranial, concussion
  cerebri — *see* Injury, intracranial, concussion
  retinae S05.80
    left S05.82
    right S05.81
  spinal cord — *see* Injury, spinal cord, by region
  spinalis — *see* Injury, spinal cord, by region

Communication
  between
    base of aorta and pulmonary artery Q21.4
    left ventricle and right atrium Q20.5
    pericardial sac and pleural sac Q34.8
    pulmonary artery and pulmonary vein,
      congenital Q25.7
    congenital between uterus and digestive or
      urinary tract Q51.7

Compensation
  failure — *see* Disease, heart
  neurosis, psychoneurosis — *see* Disorder,
    factitious

Complaint — *see also* Disease
  bowel, functional K59.9
    psychogenic F45.8
  intestine, functional K59.9
    psychogenic F45.8
  kidney — *see* Disease, renal
  miners' J60

Complete — *see* condition

Complex
  Addison-Schilder E71.428f
  cardiorenal — *see* Hypertension, cardiorenal
  Costen's M26.69
  disseminated mycobacterium
    aviumintracellulare (DMAC) A31.2
  ego-dystonic homosexuality F66
  Eisenmenger's (ventricular septal defect) Q21.0
  homosexual, ego-dystonic F66

Complex — *continued*
  hypersexual F52.8
  jumped process, spine — *see* Dislocation,
    vertebra
  primary, tuberculous A15.7
  Schilder-Addison E71.428
  subluxation (vertebral) M99.19
    abdomen M99.19
    acromioclavicular M99.17
    cervical region M99.11
    cervicothoracic M99.11
    costochondral M99.18
    costovertebral M99.18
    head region M99.10
    hip M99.15
    lower extremity M99.16
    lumbar region M99.13
    lumbosacral M99.13
    occipitocervical M99.10
    pelvic region M99.15
    pubic M99.15
    rib cage M99.18
    sacral region M99.14
    sacrococcygeal M99.14
    sacroiliac M99.14
    specified NEC M99.19
    sternochondral M99.18
    sternoclavicular M99.17
    thoracic region M99.12
    thoracolumbar M99.12
    upper extremity M99.17
  Taussig-Bing (transposition, aorta and
    overriding pulmonary artery) Q20.1

Complications (from) (of)
  accidental puncture or laceration
    operative site during procedure on the
      circulatory system I97.51
      digestive system K91.71
      ear H95.31
      endocrine system E36.11
      eye and adnexa H59.41
      genitourinary system N99.71
      mastoid H95.31
      musculoskeletal system M96.821
      nervous system G97.41
      respiratory system J95.71
      skin L76.11
      spleen D78.11
      subcutaneous tissue L76.11
    site NEC during procedure on the
      circulatory system I97.52
      digestive system K91.72
      ear H95.32
      endocrine system E36.12
      genitourinary system N99.72
      mastoid H95.32
      musculoskeletal system M96.822
      nervous system G97.42
      respiratory system J95.72
      skin L76.12
      spleen D78.12
  amputation stump (surgical) (late) NEC T87.9
    infection or inflammation T87.40
      lower limb
        left T87.44
        right T87.43
      upper limb
        left T87.42
        right T87.41
    necrosis T87.50
      lower limb
        left T87.54
        right T87.53
      upper limb
        left T87.52
        right T87.51
    neuroma T87.30
      lower limb
        left T87.34
        right T87.33
      upper limb
        left T87.32
        right T87.31
    specified type NEC T87.8

Complications — *continued*
  anastomosis (and bypass) — *see also*
    Complications, prosthetic device or
    implant
    intestinal (internal) NEC K91.89
      involving urinary tract N99.89
    urinary tract (involving intestinal tract)
      N99.89
    vascular — *see* Complications,
      cardiovascular device or implant
  anesthesia, anesthetic (*see also* Anesthesia,
    complication) T88.5
    brain, postpartum, puerperal O89.2
    cardiac
      in
        labor and delivery O74.2
        pregnancy — *see* Complications,
          anesthesia, in, pregnancy,
          cardiac
      postpartum, puerperal O89.1
    central nervous system
      in
        labor and delivery O74.3
        pregnancy — *see* Complications,
          anesthesia, in, pregnancy,
          central nervous system
      postpartum, puerperal O89.2
    difficult or failed intubation T88.4
    in pregnancy — *see* Complications,
      anesthesia, in, pregnancy, failed
      intubation
    hyperthermia, malignant T88.3
    hypothermia T88.5
    in
      abortion — *see* Abortion
      labor and delivery O74.9
        specified NEC O74.8
      postpartum, puerperal O89.9
        specified NEC O89.8
      pregnancy O29.90
        cardiac O29.10
          first trimester O29.11
          second trimester O29.12
          third trimester O29.13
        central nervous system O29.20
          first trimester O29.21
          second trimester O29.22
          third trimester O29.23
        failed intubation O29.60
          first trimester O29.61
          second trimester O29.62
          third trimester O29.63
        first trimester O29.91
        pulmonary O29.00
          first trimester O29.01
          second trimester O29.02
          third trimester O29.03
        second trimester O29.92
        specified NEC — *see* category O29.8
        spinal
          headache O29.40
            first trimester O29.41
            second trimester O29.42
            third trimester O29.43
          specified NEC O29.50
            first trimester O29.51
            second trimester O29.52
            third trimester O29.53
        third trimester O29.93
        toxic reaction to local O29.30
          first trimester O29.31
          second trimester O29.32
          third trimester O29.33
    intubation failure T88.4
    malignant hyperthermia T88.3
    pulmonary
      in
        labor and delivery O74.1
        pregnancy — *see* Complications,
          anesthesia, in, pregnancy,
          pulmonary
      postpartum, puerperal O89.09
    shock T88.2

Complications — *continued*
anesthesia, anesthetic (*see also* Anesthesia, complication) — *continued*
  spinal and epidural
    in
      labor and delivery NEC O74.6
        headache O74.5
      pregnancy — *see* Complications, anesthesia, in, pregnancy, spinal
    postpartum, puerperal NEC O89.5
      headache O89.4
anti-reflux device — *see* Complications, esophageal anti-reflux device
aortic (bifurcation) graft — *see* Complications, graft, vascular
aortocoronary (bypass) graft — *see* Complications, coronary artery (bypass) graft
aortofemoral (bypass) graft — *see* Complications, graft, vascular
arteriovenous
  fistula, surgically created T82.9
    embolism T82.818
    fibrosis T82.828
    hemorrhage T82.838
    infection or inflammation T82.7
    mechanical
      breakdown T82.510
      displacement T82.520
      leakage T82.530
      malposition T82.520
      obstruction T82.590
      perforation T82.590
      protrusion T82.590
    pain T82.848
    specified type NEC T82.898
    stenosis T82.858
    thrombosis T82.868
  shunt, surgically created T82.9
    embolism T82.818
    fibrosis T82.828
    hemorrhage T82.838
    infection or inflammation T82.7
    mechanical
      breakdown T82.511
      displacement T82.521
      leakage T82.531
      malposition T82.521
      obstruction T82.591
      perforation T82.591
      protrusion T82.591
    pain T82.848
    specified type NEC T82.898
    stenosis T82.858
    thrombosis T82.868
arthroplasty — *see* Complications, joint prosthesis
artificial
  fertilization or insemination N98.9
    attempted introduction (of)
      embryo in embryo transfer N98.3
      ovum following in vitro fertilization N98.2
    hyperstimulation of ovaries N98.1
    infection N98.0
    specified NEC N98.8
  heart T82.9
    embolism T82.817
    fibrosis T82.827
    hemorrhage T82.837
    infection or inflammation T82.7
    mechanical
      breakdown T82.512
      displacement T82.522
      leakage T82.532
      malposition T82.522
      obstruction T82.592
      perforation T82.592
      protrusion T82.592
    pain T82.847
    specified type NEC T82.897
    stenosis T82.857
    thrombosis T82.867

Complications — *continued*
artificial — *continued*
  opening
    cecostomy — *see* Complications, colostomy
    colostomy — *see* Complications, colostomy
    cystostomy — *see* Complications, cystostomy
    enterostomy — *see* Complications, enterostomy
    gastrostomy — *see* Complications, gastrostomy
    ileostomy — *see* Complications, enterostomy
    jejunostomy — *see* Complications, enterostomy
    nephrostomy — *see* Complications, stoma, urinary tract
    tracheostomy — *see* Complications, tracheostomy
    ureterostomy — *see* Complications, stoma, urinary tract
    urethrostomy — *see* Complications, stoma, urinary tract
balloon implant or device
  gastrointestinal T85.89
    embolism T85.81
    fibrosis T85.82
    hemorrhage T85.83
    infection and inflammation T85.79
    pain T85.84
    specified type NEC T85.89
    stenosis T85.85
    thrombosis T85.86
  vascular (counterpulsation) T82.9
    embolism T82.818
    fibrosis T82.828
    hemorrhage T82.838
    infection or inflammation T82.7
    mechanical
      breakdown T82.513
      displacement T82.523
      leakage T82.533
      malposition T82.523
      obstruction T82.593
      perforation T82.593
      protrusion T82.593
    pain T82.848
    specified type NEC T82.898
    stenosis T82.858
    thrombosis T82.868
bile duct implant (prosthetic) T85.89
  embolism T85.81
  fibrosis T85.82
  hemorrhage T85.83
  infection and inflammation T85.79
  mechanical
    breakdown T85.510
    displacement T85.520
    malfunction T85.510
    malposition T85.520
    obstruction T85.590
    perforation T85.590
    protrusion T85.590
    specified NEC T85.590
  pain T85.84
  specified type NEC T85.89
  stenosis T85.85
  thrombosis T85.86
bladder device (auxiliary) — *see* Complications, genitourinary, device or implant, urinary system
bleeding (postoperative) — *see also* Hemorrhage, postoperative
  intraoperative — *see* Hemorrhage, intraoperative
blood vessel graft — *see* Complications, graft, vascular
bone
  device NEC T84.9
    embolism T84.81
    fibrosis T84.82
    hemorrhage T84.83
    infection or inflammation T84.7

Complications — *continued*
bone — *continued*
  device NEC — *continued*
    mechanical
      breakdown T84.318
      displacement T84.328
      malposition T84.328
      obstruction T84.398
      perforation T84.398
      protrusion T84.398
    pain T84.84
    specified type NEC T84.89
    stenosis T84.85
    thrombosis T84.86
  graft — *see* Complications, graft, bone
  growth stimulator (electrode) — *see* Complications, electronic stimulator device, bone
  marrow transplant — *see* Complications, transplant, bone, marrow
brain neurostimulator (electrode) — *see* Complications, electronic stimulator device, brain
breast implant (prosthetic) T85.89
  embolism T85.81
  fibrosis T85.82
  hemorrhage T85.83
  infection and inflammation T85.79
  mechanical
    breakdown T85.41
    displacement T85.42
    leakage T85.43
    malposition T85.42
    obstruction T85.49
    perforation T85.49
    protrusion T85.49
    specified NEC T85.49
  pain T85.84
  specified type NEC T85.89
  stenosis T85.85
  thrombosis T85.86
bypass — *see also* Complications, prosthetic device or implant
  aortocoronary — *see* Complications, coronary artery (bypass) graft
  arterial — *see also* Complications, graft, vascular
    extremity — *see* Complications, extremity artery (bypass) graft
  cardiac — *see also* Disease, heart
    device, implant or graft T82.9
      embolism T82.817
      fibrosis T82.827
      hemorrhage T82.837
      infection or inflammation T82.7
        valve prosthesis T82.6
      mechanical
        breakdown T82.519
          specified device NEC T82.518
        displacement T82.529
          specified device NEC T82.528
        leakage T82.539
          specified device NEC T82.538
        malposition T82.529
          specified device NEC T82.528
        obstruction T82.599
          specified device NEC T82.598
        perforation T82.599
          specified device NEC T82.598
        protrusion T82.599
          specified device NEC T82.598
      pain T82.847
      specified type NEC T82.897
      stenosis T82.857
      thrombosis T82.867
cardiorenal I13.2
cardiovascular device, graft or implant T82.9
  arteriovenous
    fistula, artificial — *see* Complication, arteriovenous, fistula, surgically created
    shunt — *see* Complication, arteriovenous, shunt, surgically created
  aortic graft — *see* Complications, graft, vascular

Complications — *continued*
  cardiovascular device, graft or implant — *continued*
    artificial heart — *see* Complication, artificial, heart
    balloon (counterpulsation) device — *see* Complication, balloon implant, vascular
    carotid artery graft — *see* Complications, graft, vascular
    coronary bypass graft — *see* Complication, coronary artery (bypass) graft
    dialysis catheter (vascular) — *see* Complication, catheter, dialysis
    electronic T82.9
      electrode T82.9
        embolism T82.817
        fibrosis T82.827
        hemorrhage T82.837
        infection T82.7
        mechanical
          breakdown T82.110
          displacement T82.120
          leakage T82.190
          obstruction T82.190
          perforation T82.190
          protrusion T82.190
          specified type NEC T82.190
        pain T82.847
        specified NEC T82.897
        stenosis T82.857
        thrombosis T82.867
      embolism T82.817
      fibrosis T82.827
      hemorrhage T82.837
      infection T82.7
      mechanical
        breakdown T82.119
        displacement T82.129
        leakage T82.199
        obstruction T82.199
        perforation T82.199
        protrusion T82.199
        specified type NEC T82.199
      pain T82.847
      pulse generator T82.9
        embolism T82.817
        fibrosis T82.827
        hemorrhage T82.837
        infection T82.7
        mechanical
          breakdown T82.111
          displacement T82.121
          leakage T82.191
          obstruction T82.191
          perforation T82.191
          protrusion T82.191
          specified type NEC T82.191
        pain T82.847
        specified NEC T82.897
        stenosis T82.857
        thrombosis T82.867
      specified condition NEC T82.897
      specified device NEC T82.9
        embolism T82.817
        fibrosis T82.827
        hemorrhage T82.837
        infection T82.7
        mechanical
          breakdown T82.118
          displacement T82.128
          leakage T82.198
          obstruction T82.198
          perforation T82.198
          protrusion T82.198
          specified type NEC T82.198
        pain T82.847
        specified NEC T82.897
        stenosis T82.857
        thrombosis T82.867
      stenosis T82.857
      thrombosis T82.867
    extremity artery graft — *see* Complication, extremity artery (bypass) graft
    femoral artery graft — *see* Complication, extremity artery (bypass) graft

Complications — *continued*
  cardiovascular device, graft or implant — *continued*
    heart-lung transplant — *see* Complication, transplant, heart, with lung
    heart
      transplant — *see* Complication, transplant, heart
      valve — *see* Complication, prosthetic device, heart valve
      graft — *see* Complication, heart, valve, graft
    infection or inflammation T82.7
    umbrella device — *see* Complication, umbrella device, vascular
    vascular graft (or anastomosis) — *see* Complication, graft, vascular
  carotid artery (bypass) graft — *see* Complications, graft, vascular
  catheter (device) NEC — *see also* Complications, prosthetic device or implant
    cystostomy T83.89
      embolism T83.81
      fibrosis T83.82
      hemorrhage T83.83
      infection and inflammation T83.59
      mechanical
        breakdown T83.010
        displacement T83.020
        leakage T83.030
        malposition T83.020
        obstruction T83.090
        perforation T83.090
        protrusion T83.090
        specified NEC T83.090
      pain T83.84
      specified type NEC T83.89
      stenosis T83.85
      thrombosis T83.86
    dialysis (vascular) T82.9
      embolism T82.818
      fibrosis T82.828
      hemorrhage T82.838
      infection and inflammation T82.7
      intraperitoneal — *see* Complications, catheter, intraperitoneal
      mechanical
        breakdown T82.41
        displacement T82.42
        leakage T82.43
        malposition T82.42
        obstruction T82.49
        perforation T82.49
        protrusion T82.49
      pain T82.848
      specified type NEC T82.898
      stenosis T82.858
      thrombosis T82.868
    epidural infusion T85.89
      embolism T85.81
      fibrosis T85.82
      hemorrhage T85.83
      infection and inflammation T85.79
      mechanical
        breakdown T85.610
        displacement T85.620
        leakage T85.630
        malfunction T85.610
        malposition T85.620
        obstruction T85.690
        perforation T85.690
        protrusion T85.690
        specified NEC T85.690
      pain T85.84
      specified type NEC T85.89
      stenosis T85.85
      thrombosis T85.86
    intraperitoneal dialysis T85.89
      embolism T85.81
      fibrosis T85.82
      hemorrhage T85.83
      infection and inflammation T85.71
      mechanical
        breakdown T85.611
        displacement T85.621

Complications — *continued*
  catheter NEC — *see also* Complications, prosthetic device or implant — *continued*
    intraperitoneal dialysis — *continued*
      mechanical — *continued*
        leakage T85.631
        malfunction T85.611
        malposition T85.621
        obstruction T85.691
        perforation T85.691
        protrusion T85.691
        specified NEC T85.691
      pain T85.84
      specified type NEC T85.89
      stenosis T85.85
      thrombosis T85.86
    intravenous infusion T82.9
      embolism T82.818
      fibrosis T82.828
      hemorrhage T82.838
      infection or inflammation T82.7
      mechanical
        breakdown T82.514
        displacement T82.524
        leakage T82.534
        malposition T82.524
        obstruction T82.594
        perforation T82.594
        protrusion T82.594
      pain T82.848
      specified type NEC T82.898
      stenosis T82.858
      thrombosis T82.868
    subdural infusion T85.89
      embolism T85.81
      fibrosis T85.82
      hemorrhage T85.83
      infection and inflammation T85.79
      mechanical
        breakdown T85.610
        displacement T85.620
        leakage T85.630
        malfunction T85.610
        malposition T85.620
        obstruction T85.690
        perforation T85.690
        protrusion T85.690
        specified NEC T85.690
      pain T85.84
      specified type NEC T85.89
      stenosis T85.85
      thrombosis T85.86
    urethral, indwelling T83.89
      embolism T83.81
      fibrosis T83.82
      hemorrhage T83.83
      infection and inflammation T83.51
      mechanical
        breakdown T83.018
        displacement T83.021
        leakage T83.031
        malposition T83.021
        obstruction T83.091
        perforation T83.091
        protrusion T83.091
        specified NEC T83.091
      pain T83.84
      specified type NEC T83.89
      stenosis T83.85
      thrombosis T83.86
    urinary (indwelling) — *see* Complications, catheter, urethral, indwelling
  cecostomy (stoma) — *see* Complications, colostomy
  cesarean section wound NEC O90.8
    disruption O90.0
    hematoma O90.2
    infection (following delivery) O86.0
  chin implant (prosthetic) — *see* Complication, prosthetic device or implant, specified NEC
  circulatory system I99.8
    intraoperative I97.90

©2002 Ingenix, Inc.

Complications — *continued*
 circulatory system — *continued*
  postprocedural I97.91
   following cardiac surgery (failure)
     (insufficiency) I97.1
    in the immediate postoperative period
      T81.89
    postcardiotomy syndrome I97.0
   lymphedema after mastectomy I97.2
   hypertension I97.3
   specified NEC I97.89
  procedure I97.91
   hematoma (operative site)
     (postprocedural) I97.47
    due to accidental laceration I97.51
    intraoperative I97.43
     due to accidental laceration I97.51
     site NEC (postprocedural) I97.48
      due to accidental laceration I97.52
     intraoperative I97.44
      due to accidental laceration
        I97.52
   hemorrhage (intraoperative) (operative
     site) I97.418
    due to accidental laceration I97.51
    during cardiac
     bypass I97.411
     catheterization I97.410
    postprocedural I97.45
     due to accidental laceration I97.51
     site NEC (intraoperative) I97.42
      due to accidental laceration I97.52
      postprocedural I97.46
       due to accidental laceration
         I97.52
   laceration, accidental (operative site)
     I97.51
    site NEC I97.52
   puncture, accidental (operative site)
     I97.51
    site NEC I97.52
   specified NEC (postprocedural) I97.89
    intraoperative I97.81
  colostomy (stoma) K94.00
   hemorrhage K94.01
   infection K94.02
   malfunction K94.03
   mechanical K94.03
   specified complication NEC K94.09
  contraceptive device, intrauterine — *see*
    Complications, intrauterine, contraceptive
    device
  cord (umbilical) — *see* Complications, umbilical
    cord
  corneal graft — *see* Complications, graft,
    cornea
  coronary artery (bypass) graft T82.9
   atherosclerosis I25.700
    with angina pectoris I25.709
     with documented spasm I25.702
     specified type NEC I25.708
     unstable I25.701
    autologous (vein) graft I25.710
     with angina pectoris I25.719
      with documented spasm I25.712
      specified type NEC I25.718
      unstable I25.711
    artery I25.720
     with angina pectoris I25.729
      with documented spasm I25.722
      specified type NEC I25.728
      unstable I25.721
    nonautologous biological graft I25.730
     with angina pectoris I25.739
      with documented spasm I25.732
      specified type NEC I25.738
      unstable I25.731
    specified graft NEC I25.790
     with angina pectoris I25.799
      with documented spasm I25.792
      specified type NEC I25.798
      unstable I25.791
   embolism T82.818
   fibrosis T82.828
   hemorrhage T82.838
   infection and inflammation T82.7

Complications — *continued*
 coronary artery graft — *continued*
  mechanical T82.290
   breakdown T82.210
   displacement T82.220
   leakage T82.230
   malposition T82.280
   obstruction T82.280
   perforation T82.280
   protrusion T82.280
  pain T82.848
  specified type NEC T82.898
  stenosis T82.858
  thrombosis T82.868
 counterpulsation device (balloon), intraaortic —
   see Complications, balloon implant,
   vascular
 cystostomy (stoma) N99.519
  catheter — *see* Complications, catheter,
    cystostomy
  hemorrhage N99.510
  infection N99.511
  malfunction N99.512
  specified type NEC N99.518
 delivery (*see also* Complications, obstetric)
   O75.9
  procedure (instrumental) (manual) (surgical)
    O75.4
  specified NEC O75.89
 dialysis (peritoneal) (renal) — *see also*
   Complications, infusion
  catheter (vascular) — *see* Complication,
    catheter, dialysis
   peritoneal, intraperitoneal — *see*
     Complications, catheter,
     intraperitoneal
 dorsal column (spinal) neurostimulator — *see*
   Complications, electronic stimulator
   device, spinal cord
 ear — *see also* Disorder, ear
  intraoperative H95.919
   hematoma — *see* Complications, ear,
     procedure, hematoma,
     intraoperative
   hemorrhage — *see* Complications, ear,
     procedure, hemorrhage
   laceration — *see* Complications, ear,
     procedure, laceration
   left H95.912
   right H95.911
   specified NEC H95.829
    left H95.822
    right H95.821
  postoperative H95.999
   external ear canal stenosis H95.819
    bilateral H95.813
    left H95.812
    right H95.811
   hematoma — *see* Complications, ear,
     procedure, hematoma
   hemorrhage — *see* Complications, ear,
     procedure, hemorrhage,
     postprocedural
   laceration — *see* Complications, ear,
     procedure, laceration
   left H95.992
   postmastoidectomy — *see* Complications,
     postmastoidectomy
   right H95.991
   specified NEC H95.899
    left H95.892
    right H95.891
  procedure H95.999
   hematoma (postprocedural) H95.27
    due to accidental laceration H95.31
    intraoperative H95.23
     due to accidental laceration H95.31
   hemorrhage (intraoperative) H95.21
    due to accidental laceration H95.31
    postprocedural H95.25
     due to accidental laceration H95.31
   laceration, accidental H95.31
   puncture, accidental H95.31
 ectopic pregnancy O08.9
  damage to pelvic organs O08.6
  embolism O08.2

Complications — *continued*
 ectopic pregnancy — *continued*
  genital infection O08.0
  hemorrhage (delayed) (excessive) O08.1
  metabolic disorder O08.5
  renal failure O08.4
  shock O08.3
  specified type NEC O08.0
  venous complication NEC O08.7
 electronic stimulator device
  bladder (urinary) — *see* Complications,
    electronic stimulator device, urinary
  bone T84.89
   breakdown T84.310
   displacement T84.320
   embolism T84.81
   fibrosis T84.82
   hemorrhage T84.83
   infection or inflammation T84.7
   malfunction T84.310
   malposition T84.320
   mechanical NEC T84.390
   obstruction T84.390
   pain T84.84
   perforation T84.390
   protrusion T84.390
   specified type NEC T84.89
   stenosis T84.85
   thrombosis T84.86
  brain T85.89
   embolism T85.81
   fibrosis T85.82
   hemorrhage T85.83
   infection and inflammation T85.79
   mechanical
    breakdown T85.110
    displacement T85.120
    leakage T85.190
    malposition T85.120
    obstruction T85.190
    perforation T85.190
    protrusion T85.190
    specified NEC T85.190
   pain T85.84
   specified type NEC T85.89
   stenosis T85.85
   thrombosis T85.86
  cardiac (defibrillator) (pacemaker) — *see*
    Complications, cardiovascular device
    or implant, electronic
  muscle T84.89
   breakdown T84.418
   displacement T84.428
   embolism T84.81
   fibrosis T84.82
   hemorrhage T84.83
   infection or inflammation T84.7
   mechanical NEC T84.498
   pain T84.84
   specified type NEC T84.89
   stenosis T84.85
   thrombosis T84.86
  nervous system T85.9
   brain — *see* Complications, electronic
     stimulator device, brain
   embolism T85.81
   fibrosis T85.82
   hemorrhage T85.83
   infection and inflammation T85.79
   mechanical
    breakdown T85.118
    displacement T85.128
    leakage T85.199
    malposition T85.128
    obstruction T85.199
    perforation T85.199
    protrusion T85.199
    specified NEC T85.199
   pain T85.84
   peripheral nerve — *see* Complications,
     electronic stimulator device,
     peripheral nerve
   specified type NEC T85.89
   spinal cord — *see* Complications,
     electronic stimulator device, spinal
     cord

Complications — continued
electronic stimulator device — continued
  nervous system — continued
    stenosis T85.85
    thrombosis T85.86
  peripheral nerve T85.89
    embolism T85.81
    fibrosis T85.82
    hemorrhage T85.83
    infection and inflammation T85.79
    mechanical
      breakdown T85.111
      displacement T85.121
      leakage T85.191
      malposition T85.121
      obstruction T85.191
      perforation T85.191
      protrusion T85.191
      specified NEC T85.191
    pain T85.04
    specified type NEC T85.89
    stenosis T85.85
    thrombosis T85.86
  spinal cord T85.89
    embolism T85.81
    fibrosis T85.82
    hemorrhage T85.83
    infection and inflammation T85.79
    mechanical
      breakdown T85.112
      displacement T85.122
      leakage T85.192
      malposition T85.122
      obstruction T85.192
      perforation T85.192
      protrusion T85.192
      specified NEC T85.192
    pain T85.84
    specified type NEC T85.89
    stenosis T85.85
    thrombosis T85.86
  urinary T83.9
    embolism T83.81
    fibrosis T83.82
    hemorrhage T83.83
    infection and inflammation T83.59
    mechanical
      breakdown T83.110
      displacement T83.120
      malposition T83.120
      perforation T83.190
      protrusion T83.190
      specified NEC T83.190
    pain T83.84
    specified type NEC T83.89
    stenosis T83.85
    thrombosis T83.86
electroshock therapy T88.9
  specified NEC T88.8
endocrine E34.9
  postprocedural E89.9
    adrenal hypofunction E89.6
    hypoinsulinemia E89.1
    hypoparathyroidism E89.2
    hypopituitarism E89.3
    hypothyroidism E89.0
    ovarian failure E89.4
    specified NEC E89.8
    testicular hypofunction E89.5
  procedure
    hematoma (operative site)
      (postprocedural) E36.07
      due to accidental laceration E36.11
      intraoperative E36.03
        due to accidental laceration E36.11
      site NEC (postprocedural) E36.08
        due to accidental laceration E36.12
        intraoperative E36.04
          due to accidental laceration
          E36.12
    hemorrhage (intraoperative) (operative
      site) E36.01
      due to accidental laceration E36.11
      postprocedural E36.05
        due to accidental laceration E36.11

Complications — continued
endocrine — continued
  procedure — continued
    hemorrhage — continued
      site NEC E36.02
        due to accidental laceration E36.12
        postprocedural E36.06
          due to accidental laceration
          E36.12
    laceration, accidental (operative site)
      E36.11
      site NEC E36.12
    puncture, accidental (operative site)
      E36.11
      site NEC E36.12
    specified complication NEC
      (postprocedural) E36.89
      intraoperative E36.81
enterostomy (stoma) K94.10
  hemorrhage K94.11
  infection K94.12
  malfunction K94.13
  mechanical K94.13
  specified complication NEC K94.19
episiotomy, disruption O90.1
esophageal anti-reflux device T85.89
  embolism T85.81
  fibrosis T85.82
  hemorrhage T85.83
  infection and inflammation T85.79
  mechanical
    breakdown T85.511
    displacement T85.521
    malfunction T85.511
    malposition T85.521
    obstruction T85.591
    perforation T85.591
    protrusion T85.591
    specified NEC T85.591
  pain T85.84
  specified type NEC T85.89
  stenosis T85.85
  thrombosis T85.86
extracorporeal circulation T80.9
extremity artery (bypass) graft T82.9
  arteriosclerosis — see Arteriosclerosis,
    extremities, bypass graft
  embolism T82.818
  fibrosis T82.828
  hemorrhage T82.838
  infection and inflammation T82.7
  mechanical
    breakdown T82.318
      femoral artery T82.312
    displacement T82.328
      femoral artery T82.322
    leakage T82.338
      femoral artery T82.332
    malposition T82.328
      femoral artery T82.322
    obstruction T82.398
      femoral artery T82.392
    perforation T82.398
      femoral artery T82.392
    protrusion T82.398
      femoral artery T82.392
  pain T82.848
  specified type NEC T82.898
  stenosis T82.858
  thrombosis T82.868
eye H57.9
  corneal graft — see Complications, graft,
    cornea
  implant (prosthetic) T85.89
    embolism T85.81
    fibrosis T85.82
    hemorrhage T85.83
    infection and inflammation T85.79
    mechanical
      breakdown T85.318
      displacement T85.328
      leakage T85.398
      malposition T85.328
      obstruction T85.398
      perforation T85.308
      protrusion T85.398

Complications — continued
eye — continued
  implant — continued
    mechanical — continued
      specified NEC T85.398
    pain T85.84
    specified type NEC T85.89
    stenosis T85.85
    thrombosis T85.86
  intraocular lens — see Complications,
    intraocular lens
  intraoperative H59.90
    specified type NEC H59.88
  orbital prosthesis — see Complications,
    orbital prosthesis
  postoperative H59.91
    cataract surgery H59.91
      cystoid macular edema H59.20
        bilateral H59.23
        left H59.22
        right H59.21
      lens fragments H59.10
        bilateral H59.13
        left H59.12
        right H59.11
      vitreous touch H59.00
        bilateral H59.03
        left H59.02
        right H59.01
    retinal detachment surgery H59.91
      chorioretinal scars H59.819
        bilateral H59.813
        left H59.812
        right H59.811
    specified NEC H59.89
  procedure H59.91
    cataract surgery H59.91
      cystoid macular edema H59.20
        bilateral H59.23
        left H59.22
        right H59.21
      lens fragments H59.10
        bilateral H59.13
        left H59.12
        right H59.11
      vitreous touch H59.00
        bilateral H59.03
        left H59.02
        right H59.01
    hematoma (operative site)
      (postprocedural) H59.37
      due to accidental laceration H59.41
      intraoperative H59.33
        due to accidental laceration H59.41
      site NEC (postprocedural) H59.38
        due to accidental laceration H59.42
        intraoperative H59.34
          due to accidental laceration
          H59.42
    hemorrhage (intraoperative) (operative
      site) H59.31
      due to accidental laceration H59.41
      postprocedural H59.35
        due to accidental laceration H59.41
      site NEC H59.32
        due to accidental laceration H59.42
        postprocedural H59.36
          due to accidental laceration
          H59.42
    laceration, accidental (operative site)
      H59.41
      site NEC H59.42
    puncture, accidental H59.41
      site NEC H59.42
    retinal detachment surgery H59.91
      chorioretinal scars H59.819
        bilateral H59.813
        left H59.812
        right H59.811
    specified complication NEC H59.89
female genital N94.9
  device, implant or graft NEC — see
    Complications, genitourinary, device or
    implant, genital tract

Complications — *continued*
  femoral artery (bypass) graft — *see*
    Complication, extremity artery (bypass)
    graft
  fixation device, internal (orthopedic) T84.9
    infection and inflammation T84.60
      arm T84.619
        humerus
          left T84.611
          right T84.610
        radius
          left T84.613
          right T84.612
        ulna
          left T84.615
          right T84.614
      leg T84.629
        femur
          left T84.621
          right T84.620
        fibula
          left T84.625
          right T84.624
        tibia
          left T84.623
          right T84.622
      specified site NEC T84.69
      spine T84.63
    mechanical
      breakdown
        limb T84.119
          carpal T84.210
          femur
            left T84.115
            right T84.114
          fibula
            left T84.117
            right T84.116
          humerus
            left T84.111
            right T84.110
          metacarpal T84.210
          metatarsal T84.213
          phalanx
            foot T84.213
            hand T84.210
          radius
            left T84.113
            right T84.112
          tarsal T84.213
          ulna
            left T84.113
            right T84.112
          tibia
            left T84.117
            right T84.116
        specified bone NEC T84.218
        spine T84.216
      displacement
        limb T84.129
          carpal T84.220
          femur
            left T84.125
            right T84.124
          fibula
            left T84.127
            right T84.126
          humerus
            left T84.121
            right T84.120
          metacarpal T84.220
          metatarsal T84.223
          phalanx
            foot T84.223
            hand T84.220
          radius
            left T84.123
            right T84.122
          tarsal T84.223
          ulna
            left T84.123
            right T84.122
          tibia
            left T04.127
            right T84.126

Complications — *continued*
  fixation device, internal — *continued*
    mechanical — *continued*
      displacement — *continued*
        specified bone NEC T84.228
        spine T84.226
      malposition — *see* Complications, fixation
        device, internal, mechanical,
        displacement
      obstruction — *see* Complications, fixation
        device, internal, mechanical,
        specified type NEC
      perforation — *see* Complications, fixation
        device, internal, mechanical,
        specified type NEC
      protrusion — *see* Complications, fixation
        device, internal, mechanical,
        specified type NEC
      specified type NEC
        limb T84.199
          carpal T84.290
          femur
            left T84.195
            right T84.194
          fibula
            left T84.197
            right T84.196
          humerus
            left T84.191
            right T84.190
          metacarpal T84.290
          metatarsal T84.293
          phalanx
            foot T84.293
            hand T84.290
          radius
            left T84.193
            right T84.192
          tarsal T84.293
          tibia
            left T84.197
            right T84.196
          ulna
            left T84.193
            right T84.192
        specified bone NEC T84.298
        vertebra T84.296
      specified type NEC T84.89
        embolism T84.81
        fibrosis T84.82
        hemorrhage T84.83
        pain T84.84
        specified complication NEC T84.89
        stenosis T84.85
        thrombosis T84.86
  following
    acute myocardial infarction NEC I23.8
      angina I23.7
      atrial
        septal defect I23.1
        thrombosis I23.6
      cardiac wall rupture I23.3
      chordae tendinae rupture I23.4
      hemopericardium I23.0
      papillary muscle rupture I23.5
      specified NEC I23.8
      ventricular
        septal defect I23.2
        thrombosis I23.6
    ectopic or molar pregnancy O08.9
      cardiac arrest O08.81
      specified type NEC O08.89
  gastrointestinal K92.9
    bile duct prosthesis — *see* Complications,
      bile duct implant
    esophageal anti-reflux device — *see*
      Complications, esophageal anti-reflux
      device
    postoperative (*see also* Complications, by
      type and site) K91.9
      colostomy — *see* Complications,
        colostomy
      dumping syndrome K91.1
      enterostomy — *see* Complications
        enterostomy

Complications — *continued*
  gastrointestinal — *continued*
    postoperative (*see also* Complications, by
      type and site) — *continued*
      gastrostomy — *see* Complications,
        gastrostomy
      malabsorption NEC K91.2
      obstruction K91.3
      postcholecystectomy syndrome K91.5
      specified NEC K91.89
      vomiting after GI surgery K91.0
    procedure
      hematoma (operative site)
        (postprocedural) K91.67
        due to accidental laceration K91.71
        intraoperative K91.63
          due to accidental laceration K91.71
        site NEC (postprocedural) K91.68
          due to accidental laceration K91.72
          intraoperative K91.64
            due to accidental laceration
              K91.72
      hemorrhage (operative site)
        (intraoperative) K91.61
        due to accidental laceration K91.71
        postprocedural K91.65
          due to accidental laceration K91.71
        site NEC (intraoperative) K91.62
          due to accidental laceration K91.72
          postprocedural K91.66
            due to accidental laceration
              K91.72
      laceration, accidental (operative site)
        K91.71
        site NEC K91.72
      puncture, accidental (operative site)
        K91.71
        site NEC K91.72
      specified complication NEC
        (postprocedural) K91.89
    prosthetic device or implant
      bile duct prosthesis — *see* Complications,
        bile duct implant
      esophageal anti-reflux device — *see*
        Complications, esophageal anti-
        reflux device
      specified type NEC
        embolism T85.81
        fibrosis T85.82
        hemorrhage T85.83
        mechanical
          breakdown T85.518
          displacement T85.528
          malfunction T85.518
          malposition T85.528
          obstruction T85.598
          perforation T85.598
          protrusion T85.598
          specified NEC T85.598
        pain T85.84
        specified complication NEC T85.89
        stenosis T85.85
        thrombosis T85.86
  gastrostomy (stoma) K94.20
    hemorrhage K94.21
    infection K94.22
    malfunction K94.23
    mechanical K94.23
    specified complication NEC K94.29
  genitourinary
    device or implant T83.9
      genital tract T83.9
        infection or inflammation T83.6
        intrauterine contraceptive device —
          see Complications, intrauterine,
          contraceptive device
        mechanical — *see* Complications, by
          device, mechanical
        penile prosthesis — *see* Complications,
          prosthetic device, penile
        specified type NEC T83.89
          embolism T83.81
          fibrosis T83.82
          hemorrhage T83.83
          pain T83.84
          specified complication NEC T83.89

Complications — *continued*
  genitourinary — *continued*
    device or implant — *continued*
      genital tract — *continued*
        specified type NEC — *continued*
          stenosis T83.85
          thrombosis T83.86
      urinary system T83.9
        cystostomy catheter — *see*
            Complication, catheter,
            cystostomy
        electronic stimulator — *see*
            Complications, electronic
            stimulator device, urinary
        indwelling urethral catheter — *see*
            Complications, catheter,
            urethral, indwelling
        infection or inflammation T83.59
          indwelling urinary catheter T83.51
        kidney transplant — *see* Complication,
            transplant, kidney
        organ graft — *see* Complication, graft,
            urinary organ
        specified type NEC T83.89
          embolism T83.81
          fibrosis T83.82
          hemorrhage T83.83
          mechanical T83.198
            breakdown T83.118
            displacement T83.128
            malfunction T83.118
            malposition T83.128
            obstruction T83.198
            perforation T83.198
            protrusion T83.198
            specified NEC T83.198
          pain T83.84
          specified complication NEC T83.89
          stenosis T83.85
          thrombosis T83.86
        sphincter implant — *see*
            Complications, implant, urinary
            sphincter
    postprocedural NOS N99.9
      pelvic peritoneal adhesions N99.4
      renal failure N99.0
      specified NEC N99.89
      stoma — *see* Complications, stoma,
          urinary tract
      urethral stricture — *see* Stricture,
          urethra, postprocedural
    vaginal
      adhesions N99.2
      vault prolapse N99.3
  graft (bypass) (patch) — *see also* Complications,
      prosthetic device or implant
    aorta — *see* Complications, graft, vascular
    arterial — *see* Complication, graft, vascular
    bone T86.839
      failure T86.831
      infection T86.832
      mechanical T84.318
        breakdown T84.318
        displacement T84.328
        protrusion T84.398
        specified type NEC T84.398
      rejection T86.830
      specified type NEC T86.838
    carotid artery — *see* Complications, graft,
        vascular
    cornea T86.849
      failure T86.841
      infection T86.842
      mechanical T85.318
        breakdown T85.318
        displacement T85.328
        protrusion T85.398
        specified type NEC T85.398
      rejection T86.840
      specified type NEC T86.848
    coronary (artery) — *see* Complication,
        coronary artery (bypass) graft
    extremity artery — *see* Complication,
        extremity artery (bypass) graft
    femoral artery (bypass) — *see* Complication,
        extremity artery (bypass) graft

Complications — *continued*
  graft — *see also* Complications, prosthetic
      device or implant — *continued*
    genital organ or tract — *see* Complications,
        genitourinary, device or implant,
        genital tract
    muscle T84.9
      breakdown T84.410
      displacement T84.420
      embolism T84.81
      fibrosis T84.82
      hemorrhage T84.83
      infection and inflammation T84.7
      mechanical NEC T84.490
      pain T84.84
      specified type NEC T84.89
      stenosis T84.85
      thrombosis T84.86
    nerve — *see* Complication, prosthetic device
        or implant, specified NEC
    skin — *see* Complications, prosthetic device
        or implant, skin graft
    tendon T84.89
      breakdown T84.410
      displacement T84.420
      embolism T84.81
      fibrosis T84.82
      hemorrhage T84.83
      infection and inflammation T84.7
      mechanical NEC T84.490
      pain T84.84
      specified type NEC T84.89
      stenosis T84.85
      thrombosis T84.86
    urinary organ T83.89
      embolism T83.81
      fibrosis T83.82
      hemorrhage T83.83
      infection and inflammation T83.59
        indwelling urinary catheter T83.51
      mechanical
        breakdown T83.21
        displacement T83.22
        leakage T83.23
        malposition T83.22
        obstruction T83.29
        perforation T83.29
        protrusion T83.29
        specified NEC T83.29
      pain T83.84
      specified type NEC T83.89
      stenosis T83.85
      thrombosis T83.86
    vascular T82.9
      coronary artery — *see* Complication,
          coronary artery (bypass) graft
      embolism T82.818
      extremity artery — *see* Complication,
          extremity artery (bypass) graft
      femoral artery — *see* Complication,
          extremity artery (bypass) graft
      fibrosis T82.828
      hemorrhage T82.838
      mechanical
        breakdown T82.319
          aorta (bifurcation) T82.310
          carotid artery T82.311
          specified vessel NEC T82.318
        displacement T82.329
          aorta (bifurcation) T82.320
          carotid artery T82.321
          specified vessel NEC T82.328
        leakage T82.339
          aorta (bifurcation) T82.330
          carotid artery T82.331
          specified vessel NEC T82.338
        malposition T82.329
          aorta (bifurcation) T82.320
          carotid artery T82.321
          specified vessel NEC T82.328
        obstruction T82.399
          aorta (bifurcation) T82.390
          carotid artery T82.391
          specified vessel NEC T82.398
        perforation T82.399
          aorta (bifurcation) T82.390

Complications — *continued*
  graft — *see also* Complications, prosthetic
      device or implant — *continued*
    vascular — *continued*
      mechanical — *continued*
        perforation — *continued*
          carotid artery T82.391
          specified vessel NEC T82.398
        protrusion T82.399
          aorta (bifurcation) T82.390
          carotid artery T82.391
          specified vessel NEC T82.398
      pain T82.848
      specified complication NEC T82.898
      stenosis T82.858
      thrombosis T82.868
  heart I51.9
    following acute myocardial infarction — *see*
        Complications, following, acute
        myocardial infarction
    postoperative — *see* Complications,
        circulatory system
    transplant — *see* Complication, transplant,
        heart
      and lung(s) — *see* Complications,
          transplant, heart, with lung
    valve
      graft T82.9
        embolism T82.817
        fibrosis T82.827
        hemorrhage T82.837
        infection and inflammation T82.7
        mechanical T82.291
          breakdown T82.211
          displacement T82.221
          leakage T82.231
          malposition T82.281
          obstruction T82.281
          perforation T82.281
          protrusion T82.281
        pain T82.847
        specified type NEC T82.897
        stenosis T82.857
        thrombosis T82.867
      prosthesis T82.9
        breakdown T82.01
        displacement T82.02
        embolism T82.817
        fibrosis T82.827
        hemorrhage T82.837
        infection or inflammation T82.6
        leakage T82.03
        obstruction T82.09
        pain T82.847
        perforation T82.09
        protrusion T82.09
        specified type NEC T82.897
          mechanical T82.09
        stenosis T82.857
        thrombosis T82.867
    hematoma
      operative site associated with procedure on
        circulatory system (postprocedural)
            I97.47
          due to accidental laceration I97.51
          intraoperative I97.43
            due to accidental laceration I97.51
        digestive system (postprocedural) K91.67
          due to accidental laceration K91.71
          intraoperative K91.63
            due to accidental laceration K91.71
        ear (postoperative) H95.27
          due to accidental laceration H95.31
          intraoperative H95.23
            due to accidental laceration H95.31
        endocrine system (postoperative) E36.07
          due to accidental laceration E36.11
          intraoperative E36.03
            due to accidental laceration E36.11
        eye (postoperative) H59.37
          due to accidental laceration H59.41
          intraoperative H59.33
            due to accidental laceration H59.41

 ©2002 Ingenix, Inc.

Complications — *continued*
  musculoskeletal system — *continued*
    procedure — *continued*
      puncture, accidental M96.821
        with hemorrhage M96.811
      specified complication NEC M96.89
  nephrostomy (stoma) — *see* Complications,
    stoma, urinary tract, external NEC
  nervous system G98.8
    central G96.9
    device, implant or graft — *see also*
      Complication, prosthetic device or
      implant, specified NEC
      electronic stimulator (electrode(s)) — *see*
        Complications, electronic stimulator
        device
      ventricular shunt — *see* Complications,
        ventricular shunt
    electronic stimulator (electrode(s)) — *see*
      Complications, electronic stimulator
      device
    postprocedural G97.9
      intracranial hypotension G97.2
      specified NEC G97.82
      spinal fluid leak G97.0
    procedure
      hematoma (operative site)
        (postprocedural) G97.37
        due to accidental laceration G97.41
        intraoperative G97.33
          due to accidental laceration G97.41
        site NEC (postprocedural) G97.38
          due to accidental laceration G97.42
          intraoperative G97.34
            due to accidental laceration
              G97.42
      hemorrhage (operative site)
        (intraoperative) G97.31
        due to accidental laceration G97.41
        postprocedural G97.35
          due to accidental laceration G97.41
        site NEC G97.32
          due to accidental laceration G97.42
          postprocedural G97.36
            due to accidental laceration
              G97.42
      laceration, accidental (operative site)
        G97.41
        site NEC G97.42
      puncture, accidental (operative site)
        G97.41
        site NEC G97.42
      specified complication NEC
        (postprocedural) G97.82
        intraoperative G97.81
      spinal puncture G97.1
        spinal fluid leak G97.0
  nonabsorbable (permanent) sutures — *see*
    Complication, sutures, permanent
  obstetric O75.9
    procedure (instrumental) (manual) (surgical)
      specified NEC O75.4
    specified NEC O75.89
    surgical wound NEC O90.8
      hematoma O90.2
      infection O86.0
  ocular lens implant — *see* Complications,
    intraocular lens
  orbital prosthesis T85.89
    embolism T85.81
    fibrosis T85.82
    hemorrhage T85.83
    infection and inflammation T85.79
    mechanical
      breakdown
        left T85.311
        right T85.310
      displacement
        left T85.321
        right T85.320
      malposition
        left T85.321
        right T85.320
      obstruction
        left T85.391
        right T85.390

Complications — *continued*
  orbital prosthesis — *continued*
    mechanical — *continued*
      perforation
        left T85.391
        right T85.390
      protrusion
        left T85.391
        right T85.390
      specified NEC
        left T85.391
        right T85.390
    pain T85.84
    specified type NEC T85.89
    stenosis T85.85
    thrombosis T85.86
  organ or tissue transplant (partial) (total) — *see*
    Complications, transplant
  orthopedic — *see also* Disorder, soft tissue
    device or implant T84.9
      bone
        device or implant — *see* Complication,
          bone, device NEC
        graft — *see* Complication, graft, bone
      breakdown T84.418
      displacement T84.428
      electronic bone stimulator — *see*
        Complications, electronic stimulator
        device, bone
      embolism T84.81
      fibrosis T84.82
      fixation device — *see* Complication,
        fixation device, internal
      hemorrhage T84.83
      infection or inflammation T84.7
      joint prosthesis — *see* Complication, joint
        prosthesis, internal
      malfunction T84.418
      malposition T84.428
      mechanical NEC T84.498
      muscle graft — *see* Complications, graft,
        muscle
      obstruction T84.498
      pain T84.84
      perforation T84.498
      protrusion T84.498
      specified complication NEC T84.89
      stenosis T84.85
      tendon graft — *see* Complications, graft,
        tendon
      thrombosis T84.86
    fracture (following insertion of device) — *see*
      Fracture, following insertion of
      orthopedic implant, joint prosthesis or
      bone plate
    marrow transplant T86.00
      graft vs host disease T86.01
      specified type NEC T86.09
    postprocedural M96.9
      fracture — *see* Fracture, following
        insertion of orthopedic implant,
        joint prosthesis or bone plate
      postlaminectomy syndrome NEC M96.1
        kyphosis M96.3
        lordosis M96.4
      postradiation
        kyphosis M96.2
        scoliosis M96.5
      pseudarthrosis post-fusion M96.0
      specified type NEC M96.89
    pacemaker (cardiac) — *see* Complications,
      cardiovascular device or implant,
      electronic
    pancreas transplant — *see* Complications,
      transplant, pancreas
    penile prosthesis (implant) — *see*
      Complications, prosthetic device, penile
  perfusion NEC T80.9
  perineal repair (obstetrical) NEC O90.8
    disruption O90.1
    hematoma O90.2
    infection (following delivery) O86.0
  phototherapy T88.9
    specified NEC T88.8
  postmastoidectomy NEC H95.199
    bilateral H95.193

Complications — *continued*
  postmastoidectomy NEC — *continued*
    cyst, mucosal H95.139
      bilateral H95.133
      left H95.132
      right H95.131
    granulation H95.129
      bilateral H95.123
      left H95.122
      right H95.121
    inflammation, chronic H95.119
      bilateral H95.113
      left H95.112
      right H95.111
    left H95.192
    recurrent cholesteatoma H95.00
      bilateral H95.03
      left H95.02
      right H95.01
    right H95.191
  postoperative — *see also* Complications,
    surgical procedure T81.9
    circulatory — *see* Complications, circulatory
      system
    ear — *see* Complications, ear
    endocrine — *see* Complications, endocrine
    eye — *see* Complications, eye
    lumbar puncture G97.1
      cerebrospinal fluid leak G97.0
    nervous system (central) (peripheral) — *see*
      Complications, nervous system
    respiratory system — *see* Complications,
      respiratory system
    specified NEC T81.89
  postprocedural — *see* Complications,
    postoperative
  pregnancy NEC — *see* Pregnancy, complicated
    by
  prosthetic device or implant T85.9
    bile duct — *see* Complications, bile duct
      implant
    breast — *see* Complications, breast implant
    cardiac and vascular NEC — *see*
      Complications, cardiovascular device
      or implant
    corneal transplant — *see* Complications,
      graft, cornea
    electronic nervous system stimulator — *see*
      Complications, electronic stimulator
      device
    epidural infusion catheter — *see*
      Complications, catheter, epidural
    esophageal anti-reflux device — *see*
      Complications, esophageal anti-reflux
      device
    genital organ or tract — *see* Complications,
      genitourinary, device or implant,
      genital tract
    heart valve — *see* Complications, heart,
      valve, prosthesis
    infection or inflammation T85.79
      intestine transplant T86.892
      liver transplant T86.43
      lung transplant T86.812
      pancreas transplant T86.892
      skin graft T86.822
    intraocular lens — *see* Complications,
      intraocular lens
    intraperitoneal (dialysis) catheter — *see*
      Complications, catheter,
      intraperitoneal
    joint — *see* Complications, joint prosthesis,
      internal
    mechanical NEC T85.698
      dialysis catheter (vascular) — *see also*
        Complication, catheter, dialysis,
        mechanical
      peritoneal — *see* Complication,
        catheter, intraperitoneal,
        mechanical
      gastrointestinal device T85.598
      ocular device T85.398
      subdural (infusion) catheter T85.690
      suture, permanent T85.692
        that for bone repair — *see*
          Complications, fixation device,
          internal (orthopedic), mechanical

Complications — *continued*
  prosthetic device or implant — *continued*
    mechanical NEC — *continued*
      ventricular shunt
        breakdown T85.01
        displacement T85.02
        leakage T85.03
        malposition T85.02
        obstruction T85.09
        perforation T85.09
        protrusion T85.09
        specified NEC T85.09
    orbital — *see* Complications, orbital
        prosthesis
    penile T83.89
      embolism T83.81
      fibrosis T83.82
      hemorrhage T83.83
      infection and inflammation T83.6
      mechanical
        breakdown T83.410
        displacement T83.420
        leakage T83.490
        malposition T83.420
        obstruction T83.490
        perforation T83.490
        protrusion T83.490
        specified NEC T83.490
      pain T83.84
      specified type NEC T83.89
      stenosis T83.85
      thrombosis T83.86
    skin graft T86.829
      artificial skin or decellularized allodermis
        embolism T85.81
        fibrosis T85.82
        hemorrhage T85.83
        infection and inflammation T85.79
        mechanical
          breakdown T85.613
          displacement T85.623
          malfunction T85.613
          malposition T85.623
          obstruction T85.693
          perforation T85.693
          protrusion T85.693
          specified NEC T85.693
        pain T85.84
        specified type NEC T85.89
        stenosis T85.85
        thrombosis T85.86
      failure T86.821
      infection T86.822
      rejection T86.820
      specified NEC T86.828
    specified NEC T85.89
      embolism T85.81
      fibrosis T85.82
      hemorrhage T85.83
      infection and inflammation T85.79
      mechanical
        breakdown T85.618
        displacement T85.628
        leakage T85.638
        malfunction T85.618
        malposition T85.628
        obstruction T85.698
        perforation T85.698
        protrusion T85.698
        specified NEC T85.698
      pain T85.84
      specified type NEC T85.89
      stenosis T85.85
      thrombosis T85.86
    subdural infusion catheter — *see*
        Complications, catheter, subdural
    sutures — *see* Complications, sutures
    urinary organ or tract NEC — *see*
        Complications, genitourinary, device or
        implant, urinary system
    vascular — *see* Complications,
        cardiovascular device or implant
    ventricular shunt — *see* Complications,
        ventricular shunt (device)
  puerperium — *see* Puerperal

Complications — *continued*
  puncture, spinal G97.1
    cerebrospinal fluid leak G97.0
    headache or reaction G97.1
  pyelogram N99.89
  radiation T66
  radiotherapy NEC T66
    kyphosis M96.2
    scoliosis M96.5
  reattached
    extremity (infection) (rejection)
      lower T87.10
        left T87.12
        right T87.11
      upper T87.00
        left T87.02
        right T87.01
    specified body part NEC T87.2
  reimplant NEC — *see also* Complications,
      prosthetic device or implant
    limb (infection) (rejection) — *see*
        Complications, reattached, extremity
    organ (partial) (total) — *see* Complications,
        transplant
    prosthetic device NEC — *see* Complications,
        prosthetic device
  renal N28.9
    allograft — *see* Complications, transplant,
        kidney
    dialysis — *see* Complications, dialysis
  respiratory system J98.9
    device, implant or graft — *see* Complication,
        prosthetic device or implant, specified
        NEC
    lung transplant — *see* Complications,
        prosthetic device or implant, lung
        transplant
    postoperative J95.9
      Mendelson's syndrome (chemical
          pneumonitis) J95.4
      pneumothorax J95.81
      pulmonary insufficiency (acute) (after
          nonthoracic surgery) J95.2
        chronic J95.3
        following thoracic surgery J95.1
      respiratory failure J95.82
      specified NEC J95.89
      subglottic stenosis J95.5
      tracheostomy complication — *see*
          Complications, tracheostomy
    procedure J95.9
      hematoma (operative site)
          (postprocedural) J95.67
        due to accidental laceration J95.71
        intraoperative J95.63
          due to accidental laceration J95.71
        site NEC (postprocedural) J95.68
          due to accidental laceration J95.72
          intraoperative J95.64
            due to accidental laceration
                J95.72
      hemorrhage (operative site)
          (intraoperative) J95.61
        due to accidental laceration J95.71
        postprocedural J95.65
          due to accidental laceration J95.71
        site NEC (intraoperative) J95.62
          due to accidental laceration J95.72
          postprocedural J95.66
            due to accidental laceration
                J95.72
      laceration, accidental (operative site)
          J95.71
        site NEC J95.72
      post-tracheostomy — *see* Complications,
          tracheostomy
      puncture, accidental (operative site)
          J95.71
        site NEC J95.72
      specified complication NEC J95.89
    therapy T81.89
  sedation during labor and delivery O74.9
    affecting fetus or newborn P04.0
    cardiac O74.2
    central nervous system O74.3
    pulmonary NEC O74.1

Complications — *continued*
  shunt — *see also* Complications, prosthetic
      device or implant
    arteriovenous — *see* Complications,
        arteriovenous, shunt
    ventricular (communicating) — *see*
        Complications, ventricular shunt
  skin
    graft T86.829
      failure T86.821
      infection T86.822
      rejection T86.820
      specified type NEC T86.828
    procedure
      hematoma (operative site)
          (postprocedural) L76.07
        due to accidental laceration L76.11
        intraoperative L76.03
          due to accidental laceration L76.11
        site NEC (postprocedural) L76.08
          due to accidental laceration L76.12
          intraoperative L76.04
            due to accidental laceration
                L76.12
      hemorrhage (operative site)
          (intraoperative) L76.01
        due to accidental laceration L76.11
        postprocedural L76.05
          due to accidental laceration L76.11
        site NEC (intraoperative) L76.02
          due to accidental laceration L76.12
          postprocedural L76.06
            due to accidental laceration
                L76.12
      laceration, accidental (operative site)
          L76.11
        site NEC L76.12
      puncture, accidental (operative site)
          L76.11
        site NEC L76.12
      specified complication NEC L76.8
  spinal
    anesthesia — *see* Complications, anesthesia,
        spinal
    catheter (epidural) (subdural) — *see*
        Complications, catheter
    puncture or tap G97.1
      cerebrospinal fluid leak G97.0
      headache or reaction G97.1
  spleen D73.9
    procedure
      hematoma (postprocedural) D78.07
        with accidental puncture D78.11
        intraoperative D78.03
          with accidental puncture D78.11
      hemorrhage (intraoperative) D78.01
        with accidental puncture D78.11
        postprocedural D78.05
          with accidental puncture D78.11
      laceration, accidental D78.11
      puncture, accidental D78.11
      specified complication NEC
          (postoperative) D78.89
        intraoperative D78.81
  stent
    bile duct — *see* Complications, bile duct
        prosthesis
    urinary T83.89
      embolism T83.81
      fibrosis T83.82
      hemorrhage T83.83
      infection and inflammation T83.59
      mechanical
        breakdown T83.112
        displacement T83.122
        leakage T83.192
        malposition T83.122
        obstruction T83.192
        perforation T83.192
        protrusion T83.192
        specified NEC T83.192
      pain T83.84
      specified type NEC T83.89
      stenosis T83.85
      thrombosis T83.86

©2002 Ingenix, Inc.

Complications — *continued*
  stoma
    digestive tract K94.00
      colostomy — *see* Complications, colostomy
      enterostomy — *see* Complications, enterostomy
      gastrostomy — *see* Complications, gastrostomy
    urinary tract N99.539
      cystostomy — *see* Complications, cystostomy
      external NOS N99.529
        hemorrhage N99.520
        infection N99.521
        malfunction N99.522
        specified type NEC N99.528
      hemorrhage N99.530
      infection N99.531
      malfunction N99.532
      specified type NEC N99.538
  surgical material, nonabsorbable — *see* Complication, suture, permanent
  surgical procedure (on) T81.9
    accidental puncture or laceration at operative site during procedure on
      circulatory system I97.51
      digestive system K91.71
      ear H95.31
      endocrine system E36.11
      eye and adnexa H59.41
      genitourinary system N99.71
      mastoid process H95.31
      musculoskeletal system M96.821
      nervous system G97.41
      respiratory system J95.71
      skin L76.11
      spleen D78.11
      subcutaneous tissue L76.11
    amputation stump (late) — *see* Complications, amputation stump
    anoxic brain damage T88.5
    burst stitches or sutures T81.3
    cardiac — *see* Complications, circulatory system
    cholesteatoma, recurrent — *see* Complications, postmastoidectomy, recurrent cholesteatoma
    circulatory (early) — *see* Complications, circulatory system
    dehiscence (of wound) T81.3
      cesarean section O90.0
      episiotomy O90.1
    digestive system — *see* Complications, gastrointestinal
    disruption of wound (internal) T81.3
      cesarean section O90.0
      episiotomy O90.1
    dumping syndrome (postgastrectomy) K91.1
    ear — *see* Complications, ear
    elephantiasis or lymphedema I97.89
      postmastectomy I97.2
    emphysema (surgical) T81.82
    endocrine — *see* Complications, endocrine
    evisceration T81.3
    eye — *see* Complications, eye
    fistula (persistent postoperative) T81.83
    foreign body inadvertently left in wound (sponge) (suture) (swab) — *see* Foreign body, accidentally left during a procedure
    gastrointestinal — *see* Complications, gastrointestinal
    genitourinary N99.9
      specified NEC N99.89
    hematoma — *see* Complications, hematoma
    hemorrhage — *see* Complications, hemorrhage associated with procedure
    hepatic failure K91.81
    hyperglycemia (postpancreatectomy) E89.1
    hypoinsulinemia (postpancreatectomy) E89.1
    hypoparathyroidism (postparathyroidectomy) E89.2
    hypopituitarism (posthypophysectomy) E89.3
    hypothyroidism (post-thyroidectomy) E89.0

Complications — *continued*
  surgical procedure — *continued*
    intestinal obstruction K91.3
    intracranial hypotension following ventricular shunting (ventriculostomy) G97.2
    lymphedema I97.89
      postmastectomy I97.2
    malabsorption (postsurgical) NEC K91.2
      osteoporosis — *see* Osteoporosis, postsurgical malabsorption
    mastoidectomy cavity NEC — *see* Complications, postmastoidectomy
    metabolic E89.9
      specified NEC E89.8
    musculoskeletal — *see* Complications, musculoskeletal system
    nervous system (central) (peripheral) — *see* Complications, nervous system
    ovarian failure E89.4
    peripheral vascular T81.7
    postcardiotomy syndrome I97.0
    postcholecystectomy syndrome K91.5
    postcommissurotomy syndrome I97.0
    postgastrectomy dumping syndrome K91.1
    postlaminectomy syndrome NEC M96.1
      kyphosis M96.3
    postmastectomy lymphedema syndrome I97.2
    postmastoidectomy cholesteatoma — *see* Complications, postmastoidectomy, recurrent cholesteatoma
    postvagotomy syndrome K91.1
    postvalvulotomy syndrome I97.0
    pulmonary insufficiency (acute) J95.2
      chronic J95.3
      following thoracic surgery J95.1
    reattached body part — *see* Complications, reattached
    respiratory — *see* Complications, respiratory system
    shock (endotoxic) (hypovolemic) (septic) T81.1
    specified NEC T81.89
    spleen (postoperative) D78.89
      intraoperative D78.81
    stitch abscess T81.4
    subglottic stenosis (postsurgical) J95.5
    testicular hypofunction E89.5
    transplant — *see* Complications, organ or tissue transplant
    urinary N99.9
      specified NEC N99.89
    vaginal vault prolapse (posthysterectomy) N99.3
    vascular (peripheral) T81.7
    vitreous (touch) syndrome — *see* Complication, eye, postoperative, cataract surgery, vitreous touch
    wound infection T81.4
  suture, permanent (wire) NEC T85.89
    with repair of bone — *see* Complications, fixation device, internal
    embolism T85.81
    fibrosis T85.82
    hemorrhage T85.83
    infection and inflammation T85.79
    mechanical
      breakdown T85.612
      displacement T85.622
      malfunction T85.612
      malposition T85.622
      obstruction T85.692
      perforation T85.692
      protrusion T85.692
      specified NEC T85.692
    pain T85.84
    specified type NEC T85.89
    stenosis T85.85
    thrombosis T85.86
  tracheostomy J95.00
    hemorrhage J95.01
    infection J95.02
    malfunction J95.03
    mechanical J95.03
    obstruction J95.03
    sepsis J95.02

Complications — *continued*
  tracheostomy — *continued*
    specified type NEC J95.09
    tracheo-esophageal fistula J95.04
  transfusion (blood) (lymphocytes) (plasma) T80.9
    embolism T80.1
      air T80.0
    hemolysis T80.8
    incompatibility reaction (ABO) (blood group) T80.3
      Rh (factor) T80.4
    infection T80.2
    reaction NEC T80.8
    sepsis T80.2
    shock T80.8
    thromboembolism, thrombus T80.1
  transplant T86.90
    bone T86.839
      failure T86.831
      infection T86.832
      marrow T86.00
        graft vs host disease T86.01
        specified type NEC T86.09
      mechanical T84.318
      rejection T86.830
      specified type NEC T86.839
    cornea T86.849
      failure T86.841
      infection T86.842
      rejection T86.840
      specified type NEC T86.848
    failure T86.92
    heart T86.20
      with lung T86.30
        failure T86.32
        infection T86.33
        rejection T86.31
        specified type NEC T86.39
      failure T86.22
      infection T86.23
      rejection T86.21
      specified type NEC T86.29
    infection T86.93
    intestine T86.859
      failure T86.851
      infection T86.852
      rejection T86.850
      specified type NEC T86.858
    kidney T86.10
      failure T86.12
      infection T86.13
      rejection T86.11
      specified type NEC T86.19
    liver T86.40
      failure T86.42
      infection T86.43
      rejection T86.41
      specified type NEC T86.49
    lung T86.819
      with heart T86.30
        failure T86.32
        infection T86.33
        rejection T86.31
        specified type NEC T86.39
      failure T86.811
      infection T86.812
      rejection T86.810
      specified type NEC T86.818
    pancreas T86.899
      failure T86.891
      infection T86.892
      rejection T86.890
      specified type NEC T86.898
    rejection T86.91
    skin T86.829
      failure T86.821
      infection T86.822
      rejection T86.820
      specified type NEC T86.828
    specified
      tissue T86.899
        failure T86.891
        infection T86.892
        rejection T86.890
        specified type NEC T86.898

Complications — continued
  transplant — continued
    specified — continued
      type NEC T86.99
  trauma (early) T79.9
    specified NEC T79.8
  ultrasound therapy NEC T88.9
  umbilical cord NEC
    complicating delivery O69.9
      specified NEC O69.8
  umbrella device, vascular T82.9
    embolism T82.818
    fibrosis T82.828
    hemorrhage T82.838
    infection or inflammation T82.7
    mechanical
      breakdown T82.515
      displacement T82.525
      leakage T82.535
      malposition T82.525
      obstruction T82.595
      perforation T82.595
      protrusion T82.595
    pain T82.848
    specified type NEC T82.898
    stenosis T82.858
    thrombosis T82.868
  urethral catheter — see Complications, catheter, urethral, indwelling
  vaccination T88.1
    anaphylaxis NEC T80.5
    arthropathy — see Arthropathy, postimmunization
    cellulitis T88.0
    encephalitis or encephalomyelitis G04.0
    infection (general) (local) NEC T88.0
    meningitis G03.8
    myelitis G04.0
    protein sickness T80.6
    rash T88.1
    reaction (allergic) T88.1
      Herxheimer's T78.2
      serum T80.6
    sepsis, septicemia T88.0
    serum intoxication, sickness, rash, or other serum reaction NEC T80.6
      anaphylactic shock T80.5
    shock (allergic) (anaphylactic) T80.5
    vaccinia (generalized) (localized) T88.1
  vas deferens device or implant — see Complications, genitourinary, device or implant, genital tract
  vascular I99.9
    device or implant T82.9
      embolism T82.818
      fibrosis T82.828
      hemorrhage T82.838
      infection or inflammation T82.7
      mechanical
        breakdown T82.519
          specified device NEC T82.518
        displacement T82.529
          specified device NEC T82.528
        leakage T82.539
          specified device NEC T82.538
        malposition T82.529
          specified device NEC T82.528
        obstruction T82.599
          specified device NEC T82.598
        perforation T82.599
          specified device NEC T82.598
        protrusion T82.599
          specified device NEC T82.598
      pain T82.848
      specified type NEC T82.898
      stenosis T82.858
      thrombosis T82.868
    dialysis catheter — see Complication, catheter, dialysis
    graft T82.9
      coronary artery — see Complication, coronary artery (bypass) graft
      embolism T82.818
      extremity artery — see Complication, extremity artery (bypass) graft

Complications — continued
  vascular — continued
    graft — continued
      femoral artery — see Complication, extremity artery (bypass) graft
      fibrosis T82.828
      hemorrhage T82.838
      mechanical
        breakdown T82.319
          aorta (bifurcation) T82.310
          carotid artery T82.311
          specified vessel NEC T82.318
        displacement T82.329
          aorta (bifurcation) T82.320
          carotid artery T82.321
          specified vessel NEC T82.328
        leakage T82.339
          aorta (bifurcation) T82.330
          carotid artery T82.331
          specified vessel NEC T82.338
        malposition T82.329
          aorta (bifurcation) T82.320
          carotid artery T82.321
          specified vessel NEC T82.328
        obstruction T82.399
          aorta (bifurcation) T82.390
          carotid artery T82.391
          specified vessel NEC T82.398
        perforation T82.399
          aorta (bifurcation) T82.390
          carotid artery T82.391
          specified vessel NEC T82.398
        protrusion T82.399
          aorta (bifurcation) T82.390
          carotid artery T82.391
          specified vessel NEC T82.398
      pain T82.848
      specified complication NEC T82.898
      stenosis T82.858
      thrombosis T82.868
    following infusion, therapeutic injection or transfusion T80.1
    postoperative — see Complications, postoperative, circulatory
    vena cava device (filter) (sieve) (umbrella) — see Complications, umbrella device, vascular
  ventilation therapy NEC T81.81
  ventricular (communicating) shunt (device) T85.89
    embolism T85.81
    fibrosis T85.82
    hemorrhage T85.83
    infection and inflammation T85.79
    mechanical
      breakdown T85.01
      displacement T85.02
      leakage T85.03
      malposition T85.02
      obstruction T85.09
      perforation T85.09
      protrusion T85.09
      specified NEC T85.09
    pain T85.84
    specified type NEC T85.89
    stenosis T85.85
    thrombosis T85.86
  wire suture, permanent (implanted) — see Complications, suture, permanent

Compressed air disease T70.3
Compression
  with injury – code by Nature of injury
  artery I77.1
    celiac, syndrome I77.4
  brachial plexus G54.0
  brain (stem) G93.5
    due to
      contusion (diffuse) — see Injury, intracranial, diffuse
        focal — see Injury, intracranial, focal
      injury NEC — see Injury, intracranial, diffuse
    traumatic — see Injury, intracranial, diffuse
  bronchus J98.0
  cauda equina G83.4
  celiac (artery) (axis) I77.4
  cerebral — see Compression, brain

Compression — continued
  cervical plexus G54.2
  cord
    spinal — see Compression, spinal
    umbilical — see Compression, umbilical cord
  cranial nerve G52.9
    eighth — see category H93.3
    eleventh G52.8
    fifth G50.8
    first G52.0
    fourth — see Strabismus, paralytic, fourth nerve
    ninth G52.1
    second — see Disorder, nerve, optic
    seventh G52.8
    sixth — see Strabismus, paralytic, sixth nerve
    tenth G52.2
    third G52.8
    twelfth G52.3
  diver's squeeze T70.3
  during birth (fetus or newborn) P15.9
  esophagus K22.2
  eustachian tube — see Obstruction, eustachian tube, cartilaginous
  facies Q67.1
  fracture — see Fracture
  heart — see Disease, heart
  intestine — see Obstruction, intestine
  laryngeal nerve, recurrent J38.7
  lumbosacral plexus G54.1
  lung J98.4
  lymphatic vessel I89.0
  medulla — see Compression, brain
  nerve (see also Disorder, nerve) G58.9
    arm NEC — see Mononeuropathy, upper limb
    axillary G54.0
    cranial — see Compression, cranial nerve
    leg NEC — see Mononeuropathy, lower limb
    median (in carpal tunnel) — see Syndrome, carpal tunnel
    optic — see Disorder, nerve, optic
    plantar — see Lesion, nerve, plantar
    posterior tibial (in tarsal tunnel) — see Syndrome, tarsal tunnel
    root or plexus NOS (in) G54.9
      intervertebral disc disorder NEC — see Disorder, disc, with, radiculopathy
        with myelopathy — see Disorder, disc, with, myelopathy
      neoplastic disease (see also Neoplasm) D49.9 *[G55]*
      spondylosis — see Spondylosis, with radiculopathy
    sciatic (acute) — see Lesion, nerve, sciatic
    sympathetic G90.8
    traumatic — see Injury, nerve
    ulnar — see Lesion, nerve, ulnar
    upper extremity NEC — see Mononeuropathy, upper limb
  spinal (cord) G95.2
    by displacement of intervertebral disc NEC — see also Disorder, disc, with, myelopathy
    nerve root NOS G54.9
      due to displacement of intervertebral disc NEC — see Disorder, disc, with, radiculopathy
        with myelopathy — see Disorder, disc, with, myelopathy
    spondylogenic (cervical) (lumbar, lumbosacral) (thoracic) — see Spondylosis, with myelopathy NEC
      anterior — see Syndrome, anterior, spinal artery, compression
    traumatic -see Injury, spinal cord, by region
  subcostal nerve (syndrome) — see Mononeuropathy, upper limb, specified NEC
  sympathetic nerve NEC G90.8
  syndrome T79.5
  trachea J39.8
  ulnar nerve (by scar tissue) — see Lesion, nerve, ulnar

©2002 Ingenix, Inc.

Compression — *continued*
umbilical cord
complicating delivery O69.2
cord around neck O69.1
prolapse O69.0
specified NEC O69.2
ureter N13.5
vein I87.1
vena cava (inferior) (superior) I87.1

Compulsion, compulsive
gambling F63.0
neurosis F42
personality F60.5
states F42
swearing F42
in Gilles de la Tourette's syndrome F95.2
tics and spasms F95.9

Concato's disease (pericardial polyserositis)
A19.9
nontubercular I31.1
pleural — *see* Pleurisy, with effusion

Concavity chest wall M95.4

Concealed penis Q55.69

Concern (normal) **about sick person in family**
Z63.6

Concrescence (teeth) K00.2

Concretio cordis I31.1
rheumatic I09.2

Concretion — *see also* Calculus
appendicular K38.1
canaliculus — *see* Dacryolith
clitoris N90.8
conjunctiva H11.129
bilateral H11.123
left H11.122
right H11.121
eyelid — *see* Disorder, eyelid, specified type
NEC
lacrimal passages — *see* Dacryolith
prepuce (male) N47.8
salivary gland (any) K11.5
seminal vesicle N50.8
tonsil J35.8

Concussion (brain) (cerebral) (current) S06.01
with
intracranial injury – code to specific injury
loss of consciousness S06.00
brief (< 1 hour) S06.02
minor (1-6 hours) S06.03
blast (air) (hydraulic) (immersion) (underwater)
abdomen or thorax — *see* Injury, blast, by
site
brain S06.01
with loss of consciousness S06.00
brief (< 1 hour) S06.02
minor (1-6 hours) S06.03
ear with acoustic nerve injury — *see* Injury,
nerve, acoustic, specified type NEC
cauda equina S34.3
conus medullaris S34.139
ocular S05.80
left S05.82
right S05.81
spinal (cord)
cervical S14.0
lumbar S34.01
sacral S34.02
thoracic S24.0
syndrome F07.81

Condition — *see* Disease

Conduct disorder — *see* Disorder, conduct

Condyloma A63.0
acuminatum A63.0
gonorrheal A54.09
latum A51.31
syphilitic A51.31
congenital A50.07
venereal, syphilitic A51.31

Conflagration — *see also* Burn
asphyxia (by inhalation of smoke, gases, fumes
or vapors) — *see* Table of Drugs and
Chemicals

Conflict (with) — *see also* Discord
family Z73.9

Conflict — *see also* Discord — *continued*
marital Z63.0
involving divorce or estrangement Z63.5
social role NEC Z73.5

Confluent — *see* condition

Confusion, confused R41.0
epileptic F05
mental state (psychogenic) F44.89
psychogenic F44.89
reactive (from emotional stress, psychological
trauma) F44.89

Congelation T69.9

Congenital — *see also* condition
aortic septum Q25.4
intrinsic factor deficiency D51.0
malformation — *see* Anomaly

Congestion (chronic) (passive)
asphyxia, newborn P28.9
bladder N32.8
bowel K63.8
brain G93.8
breast N64.5
bronchial J98.0
catarrhal J31.0
chest — *see* Edema, lung
chill, malarial — *see* Malaria
circulatory NEC I99.8
duodenum K31.89
eye — *see* Hyperemia, conjunctiva
facial, due to birth injury P15.4
general R68.8
glottis J37.0
heart — *see* Failure, heart, congestive
hepatic K76.1
hypostatic (lung) — *see* Edema, lung
intestine K63.8
kidney N28.89
labyrinth — *see* category H83.8
larynx J37.0
liver K76.1
lung (chronic) (hypostatic) — *see also* Edema,
lung
active or acute — *see* Pneumonia
malaria, malarial — *see* Malaria
nasal R09.81
orbit, orbital — *see also* Exophthalmos
inflammatory (chronic) — *see* Inflammation,
orbit
ovary N83.8
pancreas K86.8
pelvic, female N94.8
pleural J94.8
prostate (active) N42.1
pulmonary — *see* Congestion, lung
renal N28.89
retina H35.81
seminal vesicle N50.1
spinal cord G95.19
spleen (chronic) D73.2
stomach K31.89
trachea — *see* Tracheitis
urethra N36.8
uterus N85.8
with subinvolution N85.3
venous (passive) I87.8
viscera R68.8

Congestive — *see* Congestion

Conical
cervix (hypertrophic elongation) N88.4
cornea — *see* Keratoconus
teeth K00.2

Conjoined twins Q89.4

Conjugal maladjustment Z63.0
involving divorce or estrangement Z63.5

Conjunctiva — *see* condition

Conjunctivitis (staphylococcal) (streptococcal)
NOS H10.9
Acanthamoeba B60.12
acute H10.30
atopic H10.10
bilateral H10.13
left H10.12
right H10.11
bilateral H10.33
left H10.32

Conjunctivitis NOS — *continued*
acute — *continued*
right H10.31
mucopurulent H10.029
bilateral H10.023
follicular H10.019
bilateral H10.013
left H10.012
right H10.011
left H10.022
right H10.021
pseudomembranous H10.229
bilateral H10.223
left H10.222
right H10.221
serous except viral H10.239
bilateral H10.233
left H10.232
right H10.231
viral — *see* Conjunctivitis, viral
toxic H10.219
bilateral H10.213
left H10.212
right H10.211
adenoviral (acute) (follicular) B30.1
allergic (acute) — *see* Conjunctivitis, acute,
atopic
chronic H10.45
vernal H10.44
anaphylactic — *see* Conjunctivitis, acute,
atopic
Apollo B30.3
atopic (acute) — *see* Conjunctivitis, acute,
atopic
Béal's B30.2
blennorrhagic (gonococcal) (neonatorum)
A54.31
chlamydial A74.0
due to trachoma A07.0
neonatal P39.1
chronic (nodosa) (petrificans) (phlyctenular)
H10.409
allergic H10.45
vernal H10.44
bilateral H10.403
follicular H10.439
bilateral H10.433
left H10.432
right H10.431
giant papillary H10.419
bilateral H10.413
left H10.412
right H10.411
left H10.402
right H10.401
simple H10.429
bilateral H10.423
left H10.422
right H10.421
vernal H10.44
coxsackievirus 24 B30.3
diphtheritic A36.86
due to
dust — *see* Conjunctivitis, acute, atopic
filariasis B74.3
mucocutaneous leishmaniasis B55.2
enterovirus type 70 (hemorrhagic) B30.3
epidemic (viral) B30.9
hemorrhagic B30.3
gonococcal (neonatorum) A54.31
granular (trachomatous) A71.1
late effect B94.0
hemorrhagic (acute) (epidemic) B30.3
herpes zoster B02.31
in (due to)
Acanthamoeba B60.12
adenovirus (acute) (follicular) B30.1
Chlamydia A74.0
coxsackievirus 24 B30.3
diphtheria A36.86
enterovirus type 70 (hemorrhagic) B30.3
filariasis B74.9
gonococci A54.31
herpes (simplex) virus B00.53
infectious disease NEC B99 *[H13]*
meningococci A39.89
mucocutaneous leishmaniasis B55.2

©2002 Ingenix, Inc.

Constriction — *see also* Stricture — *continued*
external — *continued*
thumb S60.349
left S60.342
right S60.341
toe(s) (lesser) S90.446
great S90.443
left S90.442
right S90.441
left S90.445
right S90.444
tongue S00.542
trachea S10.14
tunica vaginalis S30.843
uvula S00.542
vagina S30.844
vulva S30.844
wrist S60.849
left S60.842
right S60.841
gallbladder — *see* Obstruction, gallbladder
intestine — *see* Obstruction, intestine
larynx J38.6
congenital Q31.9
specified NEC Q31.8
subglottic Q31.1
organ or site, congenital NEC — *see* Atresia, by site
prepuce (acquired) (congenital) N47.1
pylorus (adult hypertrophic) K31.1
congenital or infantile Q40.0
newborn Q40.0
ring dystocia (uterus) O62.4
spastic — *see also* Spasm
ureter N13.5
ureter N13.5
with infection N13.6
urethra — *see* Stricture, urethra
visual field (peripheral) (functional) — *see* Defect, visual field
Constrictive — *see* condition
Consultation
medical — *see* Counseling, medical
religious Z71.81
specified reason NEC Z71.89
spiritual Z71.81
without complaint or sickness Z71.9
feared complaint unfounded Z71.1
specified reason NEC Z71.89
Consumption — *see* Tuberculosis
Contact (with)
acariasis Z20.7
AIDS virus Z20.6
cholera Z20.0
communicable disease Z20.9
sexually-transmitted Z20.2
specified NEC Z20.8
viral NEC Z20.8
German measles Z20.4
gonorrhea Z20.2
HIV Z20.6
HTLV-III/LAV Z20.6
human immunodeficiency virus (HIV) Z20.6
infection
human immunodeficiency virus (HIV) Z20.6
intestinal Z20.0
sexually-transmitted Z20.2
specified NEC Z20.8
infestation (parasitic) NEC Z20.7
intestinal infectious disease Z20.0
parasitic disease Z20.7
pediculosis Z20.7
poliomyelitis Z20.8
rabies Z20.3
rubella Z20.4
sexually-transmitted disease Z20.2
smallpox (laboratory) Z20.8
syphilis Z20.2
tuberculosis Z20.1
venereal disease Z20.2
viral disease NEC Z20.8
viral hepatitis Z20.5
Contamination, food — *see* Intoxication, foodborne

Contraception, contraceptive
advice Z30.09
counseling Z30.09
device (intrauterine) (in situ) Z97.5
causing menorrhagia T83.83
checking Z30.44
complications — *see* Complications, intrauterine, contraceptive device
in place Z97.5
initial prescription Z30.014
reinsertion Z30.44
removal Z30.44
initial prescription Z30.019
injectable Z30.013
intrauterine device Z30.014
pills Z30.011
specified type NEC Z30.018
subdermal implantable Z30.012
maintenance Z30.40
examination Z30.8
injectable Z30.43
intrauterine device Z30.44
pills Z30.41
specified type NEC Z30.49
subdermal implantable Z30.42
management Z30.9
specified NEC Z30.8
post-coital Z30.6
prescription Z30.019
repeat Z30.40
sterilization Z30.2
surveillance (drug) — *see* Contraception, maintenance
Contraction, contracture, contracted
Achilles tendon — *see also* Short, tendon, Achilles
congenital Q66.8
amputation stump (surgical) (flexion) (late) T87.8
anus K59.8
bile duct (common) (hepatic) K83.8
bladder N32.8
neck or sphincter N32.0
bowel, cecum, colon or intestine, any part — *see* Obstruction, intestine
bronchial J98.0
burn (old) — *see* Cicatrix
cervix — *see* Stricture, cervix
cicatricial — *see* Cicatrix
conjunctiva, trachomatous, active A71.1
late effect B94.0
Dupuytren's M72.0
eyelid — *see* Disorder, eyelid function
fascia (lata) (postural) M72.8
Dupuytren's M72.0
palmar M72.0
plantar M72.2
finger NEC — *see also* Deformity, finger
congenital Q68.8
joint — *see* Contraction, joint, hand
flaccid — *see* Contraction, paralytic
gallbladder K82.0
heart valve — *see* Endocarditis
hip — *see* Contraction, joint, hip
hourglass
bladder N32.8
congenital Q64.79
gallbladder K82.0
congenital Q44.1
stomach K31.89
congenital Q40.2
psychogenic F45.8
uterus (complicating delivery) O62.4
hysterical F44.4
internal os — *see* Stricture, cervix
joint (abduction) (acquired) (adduction) (flexion) (rotation) M24.50
ankle M24.573
left M24.572
right M24.571
congenital NEC Q68.8
hip Q65.8
elbow M24.529
left M24.522
right M24.521
foot joint M24.576
left M24.575

Contraction, contracture, contracted — *continued*
joint — *continued*
foot joint — *continued*
right M24.574
hand joint M24.549
left M24.542
right M24.541
hip M24.559
congenital Q65.8
left M24.552
right M24.551
hysterical F44.4
knee M24.569
left M24.562
right M24.561
shoulder M24.519
left M24.512
right M24.511
specified joint NEC M24.58
wrist M24.539
left M24.532
right M24.531
kidney (granular) (secondary) N26.9
congenital Q63.8
hydronephritic — *see* Hydronephrosis Page N26.2
pyelonephritic — *see* Pyelitis, chronic
tuberculous A18.11
ligament — *see also* Disorder, ligament
congenital Q79.8
muscle (postinfective) (postural) NEC M62.40
with contracture of joint — *see* Contraction, joint
ankle M62.479
left M62.472
right M62.471
congenital Q79.8
sternocleidomastoid Q68.0
extraocular — *see* Strabismus
eye (extrinsic) — *see* Strabismus
foot M62.479
left M62.472
right M62.471
forearm M62.439
left M62.432
right M62.431
hand M62.449
left M62.442
right M62.441
hysterical F44.4
ischemic (Volkmann's) T79.6
lower leg M62.469
left M62.462
right M62.461
multiple sites M62.49
pelvic region M62.459
left M62.452
right M62.451
posttraumatic — *see* Strabismus, paralytic
psychogenic F45.8
conversion reaction F44.4
shoulder region M62.419
left M62.412
right M62.411
specified site NEC M62.48
thigh M62.459
left M62.452
right M62.451
upper arm M62.429
left M62.422
right M62.421
neck — *see* Torticollis
ocular muscle — *see* Strabismus
organ or site, congenital NEC — *see* Atresia, by site
outlet (pelvis) — *see* Contraction, pelvis
palmar fascia M72.0
paralytic
joint — *see* Contraction, joint
muscle — *see also* Contraction, muscle NEC
ocular — *see* Strabismus, paralytic
pelvis (acquired) (general) M95.5
with disproportion (fetopelvic) O33.1
causing obstructed labor O65.1
inlet O33.2
mid-cavity O33.3

Contraction, contracture, contracted —
continued
  pelvis — *continued*
    with disproportion — *continued*
      outlet O33.3
  plantar fascia M72.2
  premature
    atrium I49.1
    auriculoventricular I49.4
    heart I49.4
    junctional I49.2
    supraventricular I49.1
    ventricular I49.3
  prostate N42.89
  pylorus NEC — *see also* Pylorospasm
    psychogenic F45.8
  rectum, rectal (sphincter) K59.8
  ring (Bandl's) (complicating delivery) O62.4
  scar — *see* Cicatrix
  spine — *see* Dorsopathy, deforming
  sternocleidomastoid (muscle), congenital Q68.0
  stomach K31.89
    hourglass K31.89
      congenital Q40.2
      psychogenic F45.8
    psychogenic F45.8
  tendon (sheath) M67.10
    with contracture of joint — *see* Contraction, joint
    Achilles — *see* Short, tendon, Achilles
    ankle M67.179
      Achilles — *see* Short, tendon, Achilles
      left M67.172
      right M67.171
    foot M67.179
      left M67.172
      right M67.171
    forearm M67.139
      left M67.132
      right M67.131
    hand M67.149
      left M67.142
      right M67.141
    lower leg M67.169
      left M67.162
      right M67.161
    multiple sites M67.19
    neck M67.18
    pelvic region M67.159
      left M67.152
      right M67.151
    shoulder region M67.119
      left M67.112
      right M67.111
    thigh M67.159
      left M67.152
      right M67.151
    thorax M67.18
    trunk M67.18
    upper arm M67.129
      left M67.122
      right M67.121
  toe — *see* Deformity, toe, specified NEC
  ureterovesical orifice (postinfectional) N13.5
    with infection N13.6
  urethra — *see also* Stricture, urethra
    orifice N32.0
  uterus N85.8
    abnormal NEC O62.9
    clonic (complicating delivery) O62.4
    dyscoordinate (complicating delivery) O62.4
    hourglass (complicating delivery) O62.4
    hypertonic O62.4
    hypotonic NEC O62.2
    inadequate
      primary O62.0
      secondary O62.1
    incoordinate (complicating delivery) O62.4
    poor O62.2
    tetanic (complicating delivery) O62.4
  vagina (outlet) N89.5
  vesical N32.8
    neck or urethral orifice N32.0
  visual field — *see* Defect, visual field, generalized
  Volkmann's (ischemic) T79.6

Contusion (skin surface intact)
  abdomen, abdominal (muscle) (wall) S30.1
  adnexa, eye NEC S05.80
    left S05.82
    right S05.81
  adrenal gland S37.812
  alveolar process S00.532
  ankle S90.00
    left S90.02
    right S90.01
  antecubital space — *see* Contusion, forearm
  anus S30.3
  arm (upper) S40.029
    left S40.022
    lower (with elbow) — *see* Contusion, forearm
    right S40.021
  auditory canal — *see* Contusion, ear
  auricle — *see* Contusion, ear
  axilla — *see* Contusion, arm, upper
  back — *see also* Contusion, thorax, back
    lower S30.0
  bile duct S36.13
  bladder S37.22
  bone NEC T14.90
  brain (diffuse) — *see* Injury, intracranial, diffuse
    focal — *see* Injury, intracranial, focal
  brainstem S06.381
    with loss of consciousness S06.389
      brief (<1 hour) S06.382
      minor (1-6 hours) S06.383
      moderate (6-24 hours) S06.384
      prolonged (>24 hours) S06.385
      without return to consciousness S06.386
  breast S20.00
    left S20.02
    right S20.01
  broad ligament S37.892
  brow S00.83
  buttock S30.0
  canthus, eye S00.10
    left S00.12
    right S00.11
  cauda equina (spine) S34.3
  cerebellar, traumatic S06.371
    with loss of consciousness S06.379
      brief (<1 hour) S06.372
      minor (1-6 hours) S06.373
      moderate (6-24 hours) S06.374
      prolonged (>24 hours) S06.375
      without return to consciousness S06.376
  cerebral S06.331
    with loss of consciousness S06.339
      brief (<1 hour) S06.332
      minor (1-6 hours) S06.333
      moderate (6-24 hours) S06.334
      prolonged (>24 hours) S06.335
      without return to consciousness S06.336
    left side S06.321
      with loss of consciousness S06.329
        brief (<1 hour) S06.322
        minor (1-6 hours) S06.323
        moderate (6-24 hours) S06.324
        prolonged (>24 hours) S06.325
        without return to consciousness S06.326
    right side S06.311
      with loss of consciousness S06.319
        brief (<1 hour) S06.312
        minor (1-6 hours) S06.313
        moderate (6-24 hours) S06.314
        prolonged (>24 hours) S06.315
        without return to consciousness S06.316
  cheek S00.83
    internal S00.532
  chest (wall) — *see* Contusion, thorax
  chin S00.83
  clitoris S30.23
  colon — *see* Injury, intestine, large, contusion
  common bile duct S36.13
  conjunctiva S05.10
    with foreign body (in conjunctival sac) — *see* Foreign body, conjunctival sac

Contusion — *continued*
  conjunctiva — *continued*
    left S05.12
    right S05.11
  conus medullaris (spine) S34.139
  cornea — *see* Contusion, eyeball
    with foreign body — *see* Foreign body, cornea
  corpus cavernosum S30.21
  cortex (brain) (cerebral) — *see* Injury, intracranial, diffuse
    focal — *see* Injury, intracranial, focal
  costal region — *see* Contusion, thorax
  cystic duct S36.13
  diaphragm S27.802
  duodenum S36.420
  ear S00.439
    left S00.432
    right S00.431
  elbow S50.00
    with forearm — *see* Contusion, forearm
    left S50.02
    right S50.01
  epididymis S30.22
  epigastric region S30.1
  epiglottis S10.0
  esophagus (thoracic) S27.812
    cervical S10.0
  eyeball S05.10
    left S05.12
    right S05.11
  eyebrow S00.10
    left S00.12
    right S00.11
  eyelid (and periocular area) S00.10
    left S00.12
    right S00.11
  face NEC S00.83
  fallopian tube S37.529
    bilateral S37.522
    unilateral S37.521
  femoral triangle S30.1
  fetus or newborn P54.5
  finger(s) S60.00
    with damage to nail (matrix) S60.10
    index S60.029
      with damage to nail S60.129
      left S60.022
        with damage to nail S60.122
      right S60.021
        with damage to nail S60.121
    little S60.059
      with damage to nail S60.159
      left S60.052
        with damage to nail S60.152
      right S60.051
        with damage to nail S60.151
    middle S60.039
      with damage to nail S60.139
      left S60.032
        with damage to nail S60.132
      right S60.031
        with damage to nail S60.131
    ring S60.049
      with damage to nail S60.149
      left S60.042
        with damage to nail S60.142
      right S60.041
        with damage to nail S60.141
    thumb — *see* Contusion, thumb
  flank S30.1
  foot (except toe(s) alone) S90.30
    left S90.32
    right S90.31
    toe — *see* Contusion, toe
  forearm S50.10
    elbow only — *see* Contusion, elbow
    left S50.12
    right S50.11
  forehead S00.83
  gallbladder S36.122
  genital organs, external
    female S30.202
    male S30.201
  globe (eye) — *see* Contusion, eyeball
  groin S30.1
  gum S00.532

©2002 Ingenix, Inc.

Convulsions — *continued*
  reflex R25.8
  scarlatinal A38.8
  tetanus, tetanic — *see* Tetanus
  thymic E32.8
  uremic N19
Convulsive — *see also* Convulsions
  equivalent, abdominal — *see* Epilepsy, specified NEC
Cooley's anemia D56.1
Coolie itch B76.9
Cooper's
  disease — *see* Mastopathy, cystic
  hernia — *see* Hernia, abdomen, specified site NEC
Copra itch B88.0
Coprolith or coprostasis K56.4
Coprophagy F50.8
Coprophobia F40.298
Coproporphyria, hereditary E80.29
Cor
  biloculare Q20.8
  bovis, bovinum — *see* Hypertrophy, cardiac
  pulmonale (chronic) I27.9
   acute I26.0
  triatriatum, triatrium Q24.2
  triloculare Q20.8
   biatrium Q20.4
   biventriculare Q21.1
Corbus' disease (gangrenous balanitis) N48.1
Cord — *see also* condition
  around neck (tightly) (with compression) complicating delivery O69.1
  bladder G95.89
   tabetic A52.19
Cordis ectopia Q24.8
Corditis (spermatic) N49.1
Corectopia Q13.2
Cori's disease (glycogen storage) E74.03
Corkhandler's disease or lung J67.3
Corkscrew esophagus K22.4
Corkworker's disease or lung J67.3
Corn (infected) L84
Cornea — *see also* condition
  donor Z52.5
  plana Q13.4
Cornelia de Lange syndrome Q87.1
Cornu cutaneum L85.8
Cornual gestation or pregnancy O00.8
Coronary (artery) — *see* condition
Coronavirus, as cause of disease classified elsewhere B97.2
Corpora — *see also* condition
  amylacea, prostate N42.89
  cavernosa — *see* condition
Corpulence — *see* Obesity
Corpus — *see* condition
Corrected transposition Q20.5
Corrosion (injury) (acid) (caustic) (chemical) (lime) (external) (internal) T30.4
  abdomen, abdominal (muscle) (wall) T21.42
   first degree T21.52
   second degree T21.62
   third degree T21.72
  above elbow T22.439
   first degree T22.539
   left T22.432
    first degree T22.532
    second degree T22.632
    third degree T22.732
   right T22.431
    first degree T22.531
    second degree T22.631
    third degree T22.731
   second degree T22.639
   third degree T22.739
  alimentary tract NEC T28.7
  ankle T25.419
   first degree T25.519
   left T25.412
    first degree T25.512

Corrosion — *continued*
  ankle — *continued*
   left — *continued*
    second degree T25.612
    third degree T25.712
   multiple with foot — *see* Corrosion, lower, limb, multiple, ankle and foot
   right T25.411
    first degree T25.511
    second degree T25.611
    third degree T25.711
   second degree T25.619
   third degree T25.719
  anus — *see* Corrosion, buttock
  arm(s) (meaning upper limb(s)) — *see* Corrosion, upper limb
  axilla T22.449
   first degree T22.549
   left T22.442
    first degree T22.542
    second degree T22.642
    third degree T22.742
   right T22.441
    first degree T22.541
    second degree T22.641
    third degree T22.741
   second degree T22.649
   third degree T22.749
  back (lower) T21.44
   first degree T21.54
   second degree T21.64
   third degree T21.74
   upper T21.43
    first degree T21.53
    second degree T21.63
    third degree T21.73
  blisters – code as Corrosion, second degree, by site
  breast(s) — *see* Corrosion, chest wall
  buttock(s) T21.45
   first degree T21.55
   second degree T21.65
   third degree T21.75
  calf T24.439
   first degree T24.539
   left T24.432
    first degree T24.532
    second degree T24.632
    third degree T24.732
   right T24.431
    first degree T24.531
    second degree T24.631
    third degree T24.731
   second degree T24.639
   third degree T24.739
  canthus (eye) — *see* Corrosion, eyelid
  cervix T28.8
  cheek T20.46
   first degree T20.56
   second degree T20.66
   third degree T20.76
  chest wall T21.41
   first degree T21.51
   second degree T21.61
   third degree T21.71
  chin T20.43
   first degree T20.53
   second degree T20.63
   third degree T20.73
  colon T28.7
  conjunctiva (and cornea) — *see* Corrosion, cornea
  cornea (and conjunctiva) T26.60
   left T26.62
   right T26.61
  deep necrosis of underlying tissue – code as Corrosion, third degree, by site
  dorsum of hand T23.469
   first degree T23.569
   left T23.462
    first degree T23.562
    second degree T23.662
    third degree T23.762
   right T23.461
    first degree T23.561
    second degree T23.661
    third degree T23.761

Corrosion — *continued*
  dorsum of hand — *continued*
   second degree T23.669
   third degree T23.769
  ear (auricle) (external) (canal) T20.41
   drum T28.91
   first degree T20.51
   second degree T20.61
   third degree T20.71
  elbow T22.429
   first degree T22.529
   left T22.422
    first degree T22.522
    second degree T22.622
    third degree T22.722
   right T22.421
    first degree T22.521
    second degree T22.621
    third degree T22.721
   second degree T22.629
   third degree T22.729
  entire body — *see* Corrosion, multiple body regions
  epidermal loss – code as Corrosion, second degree, by site
  epiglottis T27.4
  erythema, erythematous – code as Corrosion, first degree, by site
  esophagus T28.6
  extremity — *see* Corrosion, limb
  eye(s) and adnexa T26.90
   with resulting rupture and destruction of eyeball T26.70
    left T26.72
    right T26.71
   conjunctival sac — *see* Corrosion, cornea
   cornea — *see* Corrosion, cornea
   left T26.92
   lid — *see* Corrosion, eyelid
   periocular area — *see* Corrosion eyelid
   right T26.91
   specified site NEC T26.80
    left T26.82
    right T26.81
  eyeball — *see* Corrosion, eye
  eyelid(s) T26.50
   left T26.52
   right T26.51
  face — *see* Corrosion, head
  finger T23.429
   first degree T23.529
   left T23.422
    first degree T23.522
    second degree T23.622
    third degree T23.722
   multiple sites (without thumb) T23.439
    with thumb T23.449
     first degree T23.549
     left T23.442
      first degree T23.542
      second degree T23.642
      third degree T23.742
     right T23.441
      first degree T23.541
      second degree T23.641
      third degree T23.741
    second degree T23.649
    third degree T23.749
   first degree T23.539
   left T23.432
    first degree T23.532
    second degree T23.632
    third degree T23.732
   right T23.431
    first degree T23.531
    second degree T23.631
    third degree T23.731
   second degree T23.639
   third degree T23.739
   right T23.421
    first degree T23.521
    second degree T23.621
    third degree T23.721
   second degree T23.629
   third degree T23.729
  flank — *see* Corrosion, abdomen

©2002 Ingenix, Inc.

Corrosion — *continued*
- foot T25.429
  - first degree T25.529
  - left T25.422
    - first degree T25.522
    - second degree T25.622
    - third degree T25.722
  - multiple with ankle — *see* Corrosion, lower, limb, multiple, ankle and foot
  - right T25.421
    - first degree T25.521
    - second degree T25.621
    - third degree T25.721
  - second degree T25.629
  - third degree T25.729
- forearm T22.419
  - first degree T22.519
  - left T22.412
    - first degree T22.512
    - second degree T22.612
    - third degree T22.712
  - right T22.411
    - first degree T22.511
    - second degree T22.611
    - third degree T22.711
  - second degree T22.619
  - third degree T22.719
- forehead T20.46
  - first degree T20.56
  - second degree T20.66
  - third degree T20.76
- fourth degree – code as Corrosion, third degree, by site
- full thickness skin loss – code as Corrosion, third degree, by site
- gastrointestinal tract NEC T28.7
- genital organs
  - external
    - female T21.47
      - first degree T21.57
      - second degree T21.67
      - third degree T21.77
    - male T21.46
      - first degree T21.56
      - second degree T21.66
      - third degree T21.76
  - internal T28.7
    - from caustic or corrosive substance T28.8
- groin — *see* Corrosion, abdominal wall
- hand(s) T23.409
  - back — *see* Corrosion, dorsum of hand
  - finger — *see* Corrosion, finger
  - first degree T23.509
  - left T23.402
    - first degree T23.502
    - second degree T23.602
    - third degree T23.702
  - multiple sites with wrist T23.499
    - first degree T23.599
    - left T23.492
      - first degree T23.592
      - second degree T23.692
      - third degree T23.792
    - right T23.491
      - first degree T23.591
      - second degree T23.691
      - third degree T23.791
    - second degree T23.699
    - third degree T23.799
  - palm — *see* Corrosion, palm
  - right T23.401
    - first degree T23.501
    - second degree T23.601
    - third degree T23.701
  - second degree T23.609
  - third degree T23.709
  - thumb — *see* Corrosion, thumb
- head (and face) (and neck) T20.40
  - cheek — *see* Corrosion, cheek
  - chin — *see* Corrosion, chin
  - ear — *see* Corrosion, ear
  - eye(s) only — *see* Corrosion, eye
  - first degree T20.50
  - forehead — *see* Corrosion, forehead
  - lip — *see* Corrosion, lip
  - multiple sites T20.49
    - first degree T20.59

Corrosion — *continued*
- head — *continued*
  - multiple sites — *continued*
    - second degree T20.69
    - third degree T20.79
  - neck — *see* Corrosion, neck
  - nose — *see* Corrosion, nose
  - scalp — *see* Corrosion, scalp
  - second degree T20.60
  - third degree T20.70
- hip(s) — *see* Corrosion, lower, limb
- inhalation — *see* Corrosion, respiratory tract
- internal organ(s) T28.90
  - alimentary tract T28.7
    - esophagus T28.6
  - esophagus T28.6
  - from caustic or corrosive substance (swallowing) NEC — *see* Corrosion, by site
  - genitourinary T28.8
  - mouth T28.5
  - pharynx T28.5
  - specified organ NEC T28.99
- interscapular region — *see* Corrosion, back, upper
- intestine (large) (small) T28.7
- knee T24.429
  - first degree T24.529
  - left T24.422
    - first degree T24.522
    - second degree T24.622
    - third degree T24.722
  - right T24.421
    - first degree T24.521
    - second degree T24.621
    - third degree T24.721
  - second degree T24.629
  - third degree T24.729
- labium (majus) (minus) — *see* Corrosion, genital organs, external, female
- lacrimal apparatus, duct, gland or sac — *see* Corrosion, eye, specified site NEC
- larynx T27.4
  - with lung T27.5
- leg(s) (meaning lower limb(s)) — *see* Corrosion, lower limb
- limb(s)
  - lower — *see* Corrosion, lower, limb
  - upper — *see* Corrosion, upper limb
- lip(s) T20.42
  - first degree T20.52
  - second degree T20.62
  - third degree T20.72
- lower
  - back — *see* Corrosion, back
  - limb T24.409
    - ankle — *see* Corrosion, ankle
    - calf — *see* Corrosion, calf
    - first degree T24.509
    - foot — *see* Corrosion, foot
    - knee — *see* Corrosion, knee
    - left T24.402
      - first degree T24.502
      - second degree T24.602
      - third degree T24.702
    - multiple sites, except ankle and foot T24.499
      - ankle and foot T25.499
        - first degree T25.599
        - left T25.492
          - first degree T25.592
          - second degree T25.692
          - third degree T25.792
        - right T25.491
          - first degree T25.591
          - second degree T25.691
          - third degree T25.791
        - second degree T25.699
        - third degree T25.799
      - first degree T24.599
      - left T24.492
        - first degree T24.592
        - second degree T24.692
        - third degree T24.792
      - right T24.491
        - first degree T24.591
        - second degree T24.691

Corrosion — *continued*
- lower — *continued*
  - limb — *continued*
    - multiple sites, except ankle and foot — *continued*
      - right — *continued*
        - third degree T24.791
      - second degree T24.699
      - third degree T24.799
    - right T24.401
      - first degree T24.501
      - second degree T24.601
      - third degree T24.701
    - second degree T24.609
    - hip — *see* Corrosion, thigh
    - thigh — *see* Corrosion, thigh
    - third degree T24.709
- lung (with larynx and trachea) T27.5
- mouth T28.5
- multiple body regions T29
- neck T20.47
  - first degree T20.57
  - second degree T20.67
  - third degree T20.77
- nose (septum) T20.44
  - first degree T20.54
  - second degree T20.64
  - third degree T20.74
- ocular adnexa — *see* Corrosion, eye
- orbit region — *see* Corrosion, eyelid
- palm T23.459
  - first degree T23.559
  - left T23.452
    - first degree T23.552
    - second degree T23.652
    - third degree T23.752
  - right T23.451
    - first degree T23.551
    - second degree T23.651
    - third degree T23.751
  - second degree T23.659
  - third degree T23.759
- partial thickness – code as Corrosion, unspecified degree, by site
- pelvis — *see* Corrosion, trunk
- penis — *see* Corrosion, genital organs, external, male
- perineum
  - female — *see* Corrosion, genital organs, external, female
  - male — *see* Corrosion, genital organs, external, male
- periocular area — *see* Corrosion, eyelid
- pharynx T28.5
- rectum T28.7
- respiratory tract T27.7
  - larynx — *see* Corrosion, larynx
  - specified part NEC T27.6
  - trachea — *see* Corrosion, larynx
- sac, lacrimal — *see* Corrosion, eye, specified site NEC
- scalp T20.45
  - first degree T20.55
  - second degree T20.65
  - third degree T20.75
- scapular region T22.469
  - first degree T22.569
  - left T22.462
    - first degree T22.562
    - second degree T22.662
    - third degree T22.762
  - right T22.461
    - first degree T22.561
    - second degree T22.661
    - third degree T22.761
  - second degree T22.669
  - third degree T22.769
- sclera — *see* Corrosion, eye, specified site NEC
- scrotum — *see* Corrosion, genital organs, external, male
- shoulder T22.459
  - first degree T22.559
  - left T22.452
    - first degree T22.552
    - second degree T22.652
    - third degree T22.752
  - right T22.451

Corrosion — *continued*
 shoulder — *continued*
  right — *continued*
   first degree T22.551
   second degree T22.651
   third degree T22.751
  second degree T22.659
  third degree T22.759
 stomach T28.7
 temple — *see* Corrosion, head
 testis — *see* Corrosion, genital organs, external, male
 thigh T24.419
  first degree T24.519
  left T24.412
   first degree T24.512
   second degree T24.612
   third degree T24.712
  right T24.411
   first degree T24.511
   second degree T24.611
   third degree T24.711
  second degree T24.619
  third degree T24.719
 thorax (external) — *see* Corrosion, trunk
 throat (meaning pharynx) T28.5
 thumb(s) T23.419
  first degree T23.519
  left T23.412
   first degree T23.512
   second degree T23.612
   third degree T23.712
  multiple sites with fingers T23.449
   first degree T23.549
   left T23.442
    first degree T23.542
    second degree T23.642
    third degree T23.742
   right T23.441
    first degree T23.541
    second degree T23.641
    third degree T23.741
   second degree T23.649
   third degree T23.749
  right T23.411
   first degree T23.511
   second degree T23.611
   third degree T23.711
  second degree T23.619
  third degree T23.719
 toe T25.439
  first degree T25.539
  left T25.432
   first degree T25.532
   second degree T25.632
   third degree T25.732
  right T25.431
   first degree T25.531
   second degree T25.631
   third degree T25.731
  second degree T25.639
  third degree T25.739
 tongue T28.5
 tonsil(s) T28.5
 total body — *see* Corrosion, multiple body regions
 trachea T27.4
  with lung T27.5
 trunk T21.40
  abdominal wall — *see* Corrosion, abdominal wall
  anus — *see* Corrosion, buttock
  axilla — *see* Corrosion, upper limb
  back — *see* Corrosion, back
  breast — *see* Corrosion, chest wall
  buttock — *see* Corrosion, buttock
  chest wall — *see* Corrosion, chest wall
  first degree T21.50
  flank — *see* Corrosion, abdominal wall
  genital
   female — *see* Corrosion, genital organs, external, female
   male — *see* Corrosion, genital organs, external, male
  groin — *see* Corrosion, abdominal wall
  interscapular region — *see* Corrosion, back, upper

Corrosion — *continued*
 trunk — *continued*
  labia — *see* Corrosion, genital organs, external, female
  lower back — *see* Corrosion, back
  penis — *see* Corrosion, genital organs, external, male
  perineum
   female — *see* Corrosion, genital organs, external, female
   male — *see* Corrosion, genital organs, external, male
  scapular region — *see* Corrosion, upper limb
  scrotum — *see* Corrosion, genital organs, external, male
  shoulder — *see* Corrosion, upper limb
  second degree T21.60
  specified site NEC T21.49
   first degree T21.59
   second degree T21.69
   third degree T21.79
  testes — *see* Corrosion, genital organs, external, male
  third degree T21.70
  upper back — *see* Corrosion, back, upper
  vagina T28.8
  vulva — *see* Corrosion, genital organs, external, female
 unspecified site with extent of body surface involved specified
  less than 10 percent T32.0
  10-19 percent (0-9 percent third degree) T32.10
   with 10-19 percent third degree T32.11
  20-29 percent (0-9 percent third degree) T32.20
   with
    10-19 percent third degree T32.21
    20-29 percent third degree T32.22
  30-39 percent (0-9 percent third degree) T32.30
   with
    10-19 percent third degree T32.31
    20-29 percent third degree T32.32
    30-39 percent third degree T32.33
  40-49 percent (0-9 percent third degree) T32.40
   with
    10-19 percent third degree T32.41
    20-29 percent third degree T32.42
    30-39 percent third degree T32.43
    40-49 percent third degree T32.44
  50-59 percent (0-9 percent third degree) T32.50
   with
    10-19 percent third degree T32.51
    20-29 percent third degree T32.52
    30-39 percent third degree T32.53
    40-49 percent third degree T32.54
    50-59 percent third degree T32.55
  60-69 percent (0-9 percent third degree) T32.60
   with
    10-19 percent third degree T32.61
    20-29 percent third degree T32.62
    30-39 percent third degree T32.63
    40-49 percent third degree T32.64
    50-59 percent third degree T32.65
    60-69 percent third degree T32.66
  70-79 percent (0-9 percent third degree) T32.70
   with
    10-19 percent third degree T32.71
    20-29 percent third degree T32.72
    30-39 percent third degree T32.73
    40-49 percent third degree T32.74
    50-59 percent third degree T32.75
    60-69 percent third degree T32.76
    70-79 percent third degree T32.77
  80-89 percent (0-9 percent third degree) T32.80
   with
    10-19 percent third degree T32.81
    20-29 percent third degree T32.82
    30-39 percent third degree T32.83
    40-49 percent third degree T32.84

Corrosion — *continued*
 unspecified site with extent of body surface involved specified — *continued*
  80-89 percent — *continued*
   with — *continued*
    50-59 percent third degree T32.85
    60-69 percent third degree T32.86
    70-79 percent third degree T32.87
    80-89 percent third degree T32.88
  90 percent or more (0-9 percent third degree) T32.90
   with
    10-19 percent third degree T32.91
    20-29 percent third degree T32.92
    30-39 percent third degree T32.93
    40-49 percent third degree T32.94
    50-59 percent third degree T32.95
    60-69 percent third degree T32.96
    70-79 percent third degree T32.97
    80-89 percent third degree T32.98
    90-99 percent third degree T32.99
 upper limb (axilla) (scapular region) T22.40
  above elbow — *see* Corrosion, above elbow
  axilla — *see* Corrosion, axilla
  elbow — *see* Corrosion, elbow
  first degree T22.50
  forearm — *see* Corrosion, forearm
  hand — *see* Corrosion, hand
  interscapular region — *see* Corrosion, back, upper
  multiple sites T22.499
   first degree T22.599
   left T22.492
    first degree T22.592
    second degree T22.692
    third degree T22.792
   right T22.491
    first degree T22.591
    second degree T22.691
    third degree T22.791
   second degree T22.699
   third degree T22.799
  scapular region — *see* Corrosion, scapular region
  second degree T22.60
  shoulder — *see* Corrosion, shoulder
  third degree T22.70
  wrist — *see* Corrosion, hand
 uterus T28.8
 vagina T28.8
 vulva — *see* Corrosion, genital organs, external, female
 wrist T23.479
  first degree T23.579
  left T23.472
   first degree T23.572
   second degree T23.672
   third degree T23.772
  multiple sites with hand T23.499
   first degree T23.599
   left T23.492
    first degree T23.592
    second degree T23.692
    third degree T23.792
   right T23.491
    first degree T23.591
    second degree T23.691
    third degree T23.791
   second degree T23.699
   third degree T23.799
  right T23.471
   first degree T23.571
   second degree T23.671
   third degree T23.771
  second degree T23.679
  third degree T23.779

Corrosive burn — *see* Corrosion

Corsican fever — *see* Malaria

Cortical — *see* condition

Cortico-adrenal — *see* condition

Coryza (acute) J00
 with grippe or influenza J10.1
 syphilitic
  congenital (chronic) A50.05

Costen's syndrome or complex M26.69

©2002 Ingenix, Inc.

Costiveness — *see* Constipation
Costochondritis M94.0
Cotard's syndrome F22
Cot death R99
Cotton wool spots (retinal) H35.81
Cotungo's disease — *see* Sciatica
Cough (affected) (chronic) (epidemic) (nervous) R05
  with hemorrhage — *see* Hemoptysis
  bronchial R05
    with grippe or influenza J10.1
  functional F45.8
  hysterical F45.8
  laryngeal, spasmodic R05
  psychogenic F45.8
  smokers' J41.0
  tea taster's B49
Counseling Z71.9
  alcohol abuser Z71.41
    family Z71.42
  child abuse (parental) (perpetrator) Z69.02
    nonparental (perpetrator) Z69.04
      victim Z69.03
    victim Z69.01
  consanguinity Z71.89
  contraceptive Z30.09
  dietary Z71.3
  drug abuser Z71.51
    family member Z71.52
  family Z71.89
  for non-attending third party Z71.0
    related to sexual behavior or orientation Z70.2
  genetic Z31.5
  health (advice) (education) (instruction) — *see* Counseling, medical
  human immunodeficiency virus (HIV) Z71.7
  impotence Z70.1
  medical (for) Z71.9
    boarding school resident Z59.3
    condition not demonstrated Z71.1
    consanguinity Z71.89
    feared complaint and no disease found Z71.1
    human immunodeficiency virus (HIV) Z71.7
    institutional resident Z59.3
    on behalf of another Z71.0
      related to sexual behavior or orientation Z70.2
    person living alone Z60.2
    specified reason NEC Z71.89
  procreative Z31.6
  promiscuity Z70.1
  sex, sexual (related to) Z70.9
    attitude(s) Z70.0
    behavior or orientation Z70.1
    combined concerns Z70.3
    non-responsiveness Z70.1
    on behalf of third party Z70.2
    specified reason NEC Z70.8
  specified reason NEC Z71.89
  spousal abuse (perpetrator) Z69.12
    victim Z69.11
  substance abuse Z71.89
    alcohol Z71.41
    drug Z71.51
    tobacco Z71.6
    tobacco use Z71.6
Coupled rhythm R00.8
Couvelaire syndrome or uterus (complicating delivery) — *see* Disorder, placenta, abruptio
Cowperitis — *see* Urethritis
Cowper's gland — *see* condition
Cowpox B08.0
  due to vaccination T88.1
Coxa
  magna M91.40
    left M91.42
    right M91.41
  plana M91.20
    left M91.22
    right M91.21
  valga (acquired) — *see also* Deformity, limb, specified type NEC, thigh
    congenital Q65.8

Coxa — *continued*
  valga — *see also* Deformity, limb, specified type NEC, thigh — *continued*
    late effect of rickets E64.3
  vara (acquired) — *see also* Deformity, limb, specified type NEC, thigh
    congenital Q65.8
    late effect of rickets E64.3
Coxalgia, coxalgic (nontuberculous) — *see also* Pain, joint, hip
  tuberculous A18.02
Coxarthrosis M16.9
  dysplastic (unilateral) M16.30
    bilateral M16.2
    left M16.32
    right M16.31
  post-traumatic (unilateral) M16.50
    bilateral M16.4
    left M16.52
    right M16.51
  primary (unilateral) M16.10
    bilateral M16.0
    left M16.12
    right M16.11
  secondary NEC (unilateral) M16.7
    bilateral M16.6
Coxitis — *see* Monoarthritis, hip
Coxsackie (virus) (infection) B34.1
  as cause of disease classified elsewhere B97.11
  carditis B33.20
  central nervous system NEC A88.8
  endocarditis B33.21
  enteritis A08.3
  meningitis (aseptic) A87.0
  myocarditis B33.22
  pericarditis B33.23
  pharyngitis B08.5
  pleurodynia B33.0
  specific disease NEC B33.8
Crabs, meaning pubic lice B85.3
Cracked nipple N64.0
  associated with
    lactation O92.13
    pregnancy O92.119
      first trimester O92.111
      second trimester O92.112
      third trimester O92.113
    puerperium O92.12
Cradle cap L21.0
Craft neurosis F48.8
Cramp(s) R25.2
  abdominal — *see* Pain, abdominal
  bathing T75.1
  colic R10.83
    psychogenic F45.8
  due to immersion T75.1
  fireman T67.2
  heat T67.2
  immersion T75.1
  intestinal — *see* Pain, abdominal
    psychogenic F45.8
  limb (lower) (upper) NEC R25.2
  linotypist's F48.8
    organic G25.8
  muscle (limb) (general) R25.2
    due to immersion T75.1
    psychogenic F45.8
  occupational (hand) F48.8
    organic G25.8
  salt-depletion E87.1
  stoker's T67.2
  swimmer's T75.1
  telegrapher's F48.8
    organic G25.8
  typist's F48.8
    organic G25.8
  uterus N94.8
    menstrual — *see* Dysmenorrhea
  writer's F48.8
    organic G25.8
Cranial — *see* condition
Craniocleidodysostosis Q74.0
Craniofenestria (skull) Q75.8
Craniolacunia (skull) Q75.8
Craniopagus Q89.4

Craniopathy, metabolic M85.2
Craniopharyngeal — *see* condition
Craniopharyngioma (M9350/1) D44.4
Craniorachischisis (totalis) Q00.1
Cranioschisis Q75.8
Craniostenosis Q75.0
Craniosynostosis Q75.0
Craniotabes (cause unknown) M83.8
  neonatal P96.3
  rachitic E64.3
  syphilitic A50.56
Cranium — *see* condition
Craw-craw — *see* Onchocerciasis
Creaking joint — *see* Derangement, joint, specified type NEC
Creeping
  eruption B76.9
  palsy or paralysis G12.22
Crenated tongue K14.8
Creotoxism A05.9
Crepitus
  caput Q75.8
  joint — *see* Derangement, joint, specified type NEC
Crescent or conus choroid, congenital Q14.3
CREST syndrome M34.1
Cretin, cretinism (congenital) (endemic) (nongoitrous) (sporadic) E00.9
  pelvis
    with disproportion (fetopelvic) O33.0
      causing obstructed labor O65.0
  type
    hypothyroid E00.1
    mixed E00.2
    myxedematous E00.1
    neurological E00.0
Creutzfeldt-Jakob disease or syndrome A81.0
  with dementia A81.0 *[F02]*
Crib death R99
Cri-du-chat syndrome Q93.4
Crigler-Najjar disease or syndrome E80.5
Crime, victim of Z65.4
Crimean hemorrhagic fever A98.0
Criminalism F60.2
Crisis
  abdomen R10.0
  acute reaction F43.0
  addisonian E27.2
  adrenal (cortical) E27.2
  brain, cerebral I64
  celiac K90.0
  Dietl's N13.8
  emotional — *see also* Disorder, adjustment
    acute reaction to stress F43.0
    specific to childhood and adolescence F93.8
  glaucomatocyclitic — *see* Glaucoma, secondary, inflammation
  heart — *see* Failure, heart
  nitritoid
    correct substance properly administered I95.2
    overdose or wrong substance given or taken — *see* category T37.8
  oculogyric H51.8
    psychogenic F45.8
  Pel's (tabetic) A52.11
  psychosexual identity F64.2
  renal N28.0
  sickle-cell D57.0
  state (acute reaction) F43.0
  tabetic A52.11
  thyroid— *see* Thyrotoxicosis with thyroid storm
  thyrotoxic— *see* Thyrotoxicosis with thyroid storm
Crocq's disease (acrocyanosis) I73.8
Crohn's disease — *see* Enteritis, regional
Crooked septum, nasal J34.2
Cross syndrome E70.328
Crossbite (anterior) (posterior) M26.2
Cross-eye — *see* Strabismus

Croup, croupous (catarrhal) (infectious) (inflammatory) (nondiphtheritic) J05.0
  bronchial J20.9
  diphtheritic A36.2
  false J38.5
  spasmodic J38.5
    diphtheritic A36.2
  stridulous J38.5
    diphtheritic A36.2
Crouzon's disease Q75.1
Crowding, tooth, teeth M26.3
CRST syndrome M34.1
Cruchet's disease A85.8
Cruelty in children — see also Disorder, conduct
Crural ulcer — see Ulcer, lower limb
Crush, crushed, crushing T14.90
  abdomen S38.1
  ankle S97.00
    left S97.02
    right S97.01
  arm (upper) (and shoulder) S47.9
    left S47.2
    right S47.1
  axilla — see Crush, arm
  back, lower S38.1
  buttock S38.1
  cheek S07.0
  chest S28.0
  cranium S07.1
  ear S07.0
  elbow S57.00
    left S57.02
    right S57.01
  extremity
    lower
      ankle — see Crush, ankle
      below knee — see Crush, leg
      foot — see Crush, foot
      hip — see Crush, hip
      knee — see Crush, knee
      thigh — see Crush, thigh
      toe — see Crush, toe
    upper
      below elbow S67.90
        left S67.92
        right S67.91
      elbow — see Crush, elbow
      finger — see Crush, finger
      forearm — see Crush, forearm
      hand — see Crush, hand
      thumb — see Crush, thumb
      upper arm — see Crush, arm
      wrist — see Crush, wrist
  face S07.0
  finger(s) S67.10
    with hand (and wrist) — see Crush, hand, specified site NEC
    index S67.198
      left S67.191
      right S67.190
    little S67.198
      left S67.197
      right S67.196
    middle S67.198
      left S67.193
      right S67.192
    ring S67.198
      left S67.195
      right S67.194
    thumb — see Crush, thumb
  foot S97.80
    left S97.82
    right S97.81
    toe — see Crush, toe
  forearm S57.80
    left S57.82
    right S57.81
  genitalia, external
    female S38.002
      vagina S38.03
      vulva S38.03
    male S38.001
      penis S38.01
      scrotum S38.02
      testis S38.02

Crush, crushed, crushing — continued
  hand (except fingers alone) S67.20
    with wrist S67.40
      left S67.42
      right S67.41
    left S67.22
    right S67.21
  head S07.9
    specified NEC S07.8
  heel — see Crush, foot
  hip S77.00
    with thigh S77.20
    left S77.02
      with thigh S77.22
    right S77.01
      with thigh S77.21
  internal organ (abdomen, chest, or pelvis) T14.90
  knee S87.00
    left S87.02
    right S87.01
  labium (majus) (minus) S38.03
  larynx S17.0
  leg (lower) S87.80
    knee — see Crush, knee
    left S87.82
    right S87.81
  lip S07.0
  lower
    back S38.1
    leg — see Crush, leg
  neck S17.9
  nerve — see Injury, nerve
  nose S07.0
  pelvis S38.1
  penis S38.01
  scalp S07.8
  scapular region — see Crush, arm
  scrotum S38.02
  severe, unspecified site T14.90
  shoulder (and upper arm) — see Crush, arm
  skull S07.1
  syndrome (complication of trauma) T79.5
  testis S38.02
  thigh S77.10
    with hip S77.20
    left S77.12
      with thigh S77.22
    right S77.11
      with thigh S77.21
  throat S17.8
  thumb S67.00
    with hand (and wrist) — see Crush, hand, specified site NEC
    left S67.02
    right S67.01
  toe(s) S97.109
    great S97.119
      left S97.112
      right S97.111
    left S97.102
    lesser S97.129
      left S97.122
      right S97.121
    right S97.101
  trachea S17.0
  vagina S38.03
  vulva S38.03
  wrist S67.30
    with hand S67.40
      left S67.42
      right S67.41
    left S67.32
    right S67.31
Crusta lactea L21.0
Crusts R23.4
Crutch paralysis — see Injury, brachial plexus
Cruveilhier-Baumgarten cirrhosis, disease or syndrome K76.6
Cruveilhier's atrophy or disease G12.8
Cryoglobulinemia (essential) (idiopathic) (mixed) (primary) (purpura) (secondary) (vasculitis) D89.1
  with lung involvement D89.1 [J99]
Cryptitis (anal) (rectal) K62.8

Cryptococcosis, cryptococcus (infection) (neoformans) B45.9
  bone B45.3
  cerebral B45.1
  cutaneous B45.2
  disseminated B45.7
  generalized B45.7
  meningitis B45.1
  meningocerebralis B45.1
  osseous B45.3
  pulmonary B45.0
  skin B45.2
  specified NEC B45.8
Cryptopapillitis (anus) K62.8
Cryptophthalmos Q11.2
  syndrome Q87.0
Cryptorchid, cryptorchism, cryptorchidism Q53.9
  bilateral Q53.20
    abdominal Q53.21
    perineal Q53.22
  unilateral Q53.10
    abdominal Q53.11
    perineal Q53.12
Cryptosporidiosis A07.2
Cryptostromosis J67.6
Crystalluria R82.99
Cubitus
  congenital Q68.1
  valgus (acquired) — see also Deformity, limb, specified type NEC, upper arm
    late effect of rickets E64.3
  varus (acquired) — see also Deformity, limb, specified type NEC, upper arm
    late effect of rickets E64.3
Cultural deprivation or shock Z60.3
Curling esophagus K22.4
Curling's ulcer — see Ulcer, peptic, acute
Curschmann (-Batten) (-Steinert) disease or syndrome G71.1
Curse, Ondine's — see Apnea, sleep
Curvature
  organ or site, congenital NEC — see Distortion
  penis (lateral) Q55.61
  Pott's (spinal) A18.01
  radius, idiopathic, progressive (congenital) Q74.0
  spine (acquired) (angular) (idiopathic) (incorrect) (postural) — see Dorsopathy, deforming
    congenital Q67.5
    due to or associated with
      Charcot-Marie-Tooth disease (see also category M49.8) G60.0
      osteitis
        deformans M88.88
        fibrosa cystica (see also category M49.8) E21.0
      tuberculosis (Pott's curvature) A18.01
    late effect of rickets (see also category M49.8) E64.3
    tuberculous A18.01
Cushingoid due to steroid therapy
  correct substance properly administered E24.2
  overdose or wrong substance given or taken — see category T38.0
Cushing's
  syndrome or disease E24.9
    drug-induced E24.2
    iatrogenic E24.2
    pituitary-dependent E24.0
    specified NEC E24.8
  ulcer — see Ulcer, peptic, acute
Cusp, Carabelli — see Excludes note K00.2
Cut (external) — see also Laceration
  muscle — see Injury, muscle
Cutaneous — see also condition
  hemorrhage R23.3
  larva migrans B76.9
Cutis — see also condition
  hyperelastica Q82.8
    acquired L57.4
  laxa (hyperelastica) — see Dermatolysis
  marmorata R23.8

Cutis — *see also* condition — *continued*
  osteosis L94.2
  pendula — *see* Dermatolysis
  rhomboidalis nuchae L57.2
  verticis gyrata Q82.8
    acquired L91.8
Cyanosis R23.0
  due to
    patent foramen botalli Q21.1
    persistent foramen ovale Q21.1
  enterogenous D74.8
  paroxysmal digital — *see* Raynaud's disease
    with gangrene I73.01
  retina, retinal H35.89
Cyanotic heart disease I24.9
  congenital Q24.9
Cycle
  anovulatory N97.0
  menstrual, irregular N92.6
Cyclencephaly Q04.9
Cyclical vomiting R11.3
  with nausea R11.0
  psychogenic F50.8
Cyclitis (*see also* Iridocyclitis) H20.9
  chronic — *see* Iridocyclitis, chronic
  Fuchs' heterochromic H20.819
    bilateral H20.813
    left H20.812
    right H20.811
  granulomatous — *see* Iridocyclitis, chronic
  lens-induced — *see* Iridocyclitis, lens-induced
  posterior H30.20
    bilateral H30.23
    left H30.22
    right H30.21
Cycloid personality F34.0
Cyclophoria H50.54
Cyclopia, cyclops Q87.0
Cyclopism Q87.0
Cyclosporiasis A07.4
Cyclothymia F34.0
Cyclothymic personality F34.0
Cyclotropia
  left H50.432
  right H50.431
Cylindroma (M8200/3) — *see also* Neoplasm, malignant
  eccrine dermal (M8200/0) — *see* Neoplasm, skin, benign
  skin (M8200/0) — *see* Neoplasm, skin, benign
Cylindruria R82.99
Cynanche
  diphtheritic A36.2
  tonsillaris J36
Cynophobia F40.218
Cynorexia R63.2
Cyphosis — *see* Kyphosis
Cyprus fever — *see* Brucellosis
Cyst (colloid) (mucous) (simple) (retention)
  adenoid (infected) J35.8
  adrenal gland E27.8
    congenital Q89.1
  air, lung J98.4
  allantoic Q64.4
  alveolar process (jaw bone) M27.40
  amnion, amniotic — *see* category O41.8
  anterior
    chamber (eye) — *see* Cyst, iris
    nasopalatine K09.1
  antrum J34.1
  anus K62.8
  apical (tooth) (periodontal) K04.8
  appendix K38.8
  arachnoid, brain (acquired) G93.0
    congenital Q04.6
  arytenoid J38.7
  Baker's M71.20
    left M71.22
    right M71.21
    ruptured M66.0
    tuberculous A18.02
  Bartholin's gland N75.0
  bile duct (common) (hepatic) K83.5

Cyst — *continued*
  bladder (multiple) (trigone) N32.8
  blue dome (breast) — *see* Cyst, breast
  bone (local) NEC M85.60
    aneurysmal M85.50
      ankle M85.579
        left M85.572
        right M85.571
      foot M85.579
        left M85.572
        right M85.571
      forearm M85.539
        left M85.532
        right M85.531
      hand M85.549
        left M85.542
        right M85.541
      jaw M27.49
      lower leg M85.569
        left M85.562
        right M85.561
      multiple site M85.59
      neck M85.58
      rib M85.58
      shoulder M85.519
        left M85.512
        right M85.511
      skull M85.58
      specified site NEC M85.58
      thigh M85.559
        left M85.552
        right M85.551
      toe M85.579
        left M85.572
        right M85.571
      upper arm M85.529
        left M85.522
        right M85.521
      vertebra M85.58
    solitary M85.40
      ankle M85.479
        left M85.472
        right M85.471
      fibula M85.469
        left M85.462
        right M85.461
      foot M85.479
        left M85.472
        right M85.471
      hand M85.449
        left M85.442
        right M85.441
      humerus M85.429
        left M85.422
        right M85.421
      jaw M27.49
      neck M85.48
      pelvis M85.459
        left M85.452
        right M85.451
      radius M85.439
        left M85.432
        right M85.431
      rib M85.48
      shoulder M85.419
        left M85.412
        right M85.411
      skull M85.48
      specified site NEC M85.48
      tibia M85.469
        left M85.462
        right M85.461
      toe M85.479
        left M85.472
        right M85.471
      ulna M85.439
        left M85.432
        right M85.431
      vertebra M85.48
    specified type NEC M85.60
      ankle M85.679
        left M85.672
        right M85.671
      foot M85.679
        left M85.672
        right M85.671

Cyst — *continued*
  bone NEC — *continued*
    specified type NEC — *continued*
      forearm M85.639
        left M85.632
        right M85.631
      hand M85.649
        left M85.642
        right M85.641
      jaw M27.40
        developmental (nonodontogenic) K09.1
        odontogenic K09.0
      latent M27.0
      lower leg M85.669
        left M85.662
        right M85.661
      multiple site M85.69
      neck M85.68
      rib M85.68
      shoulder M85.619
        left M85.612
        right M85.611
      skull M85.68
      specified site NEC M85.68
      thigh M85.659
        left M85.652
        right M85.651
      toe M85.679
        left M85.672
        right M85.671
      upper arm M85.629
        left M85.622
        right M85.621
      vertebra M85.68
  brain (acquired) G93.0
    congenital Q04.6
    hydatid B67.99 *[G94]*
    third ventricle (colloid), congenital Q04.6
  branchial (cleft) Q18.0
  branchiogenic Q18.0
  breast (benign) (blue dome) (female) (pedunculated) (solitary) N60.00
    left N60.02
    male N60.05
      left N60.04
      right N60.03
    right N60.01
    involution — *see* Dysplasia, mammary, specified type NEC
    sebaceous– *see* Dysplasia, mammary, specified type NEC
  broad ligament (benign) N83.8
  bronchogenic (mediastinal) (sequestration) J98.4
    congenital Q33.0
  buccal K09.8
  bulbourethral gland N36.8
  bursa, bursal NEC M71.30
    with rupture — *see* Rupture, synovium
    ankle M71.379
      left M71.372
      right M71.371
    elbow M71.329
      left M71.322
      right M71.321
    foot M71.379
      left M71.372
      right M71.371
    hand M71.349
      left M71.342
      right M71.341
    hip M71.359
      left M71.352
      right M71.351
    multiple sites M71.39
    pharyngeal J39.2
    popliteal space — *see* Cyst, Baker's
    shoulder M71.319
      left M71.312
      right M71.311
    specified site NEC M71.38
    wrist M71.339
      left M71.332
      right M71.331
  calcifying odontogenic (M9301/0) D16.5
    upper jaw (bone) D16.4

Cyst — *continued*
canal of Nuck (female) N94.8
  congenital Q52.4
canthus — *see* Cyst, conjunctiva
carcinomatous (M8010/3) — *see* Neoplasm, malignant
cauda equina G95.89
cavum septi pellucidi — *see* Cyst, brain
celomic (pericardium) Q24.8
cerebellopontine (angle) — *see* Cyst, brain
cerebellum — *see* Cyst, brain
cerebral — *see* Cyst, brain
cervical lateral Q18.1
cervix NEC N88.8
  embryonic Q51.6
  nabothian N88.8
chiasmal optic NEC — *see* Disorder, optic, chiasm
chocolate (ovary) N80.1
choledochus, congenital Q44.4
chorion — *see* category O41.8
choroid plexus G93.0
ciliary body — *see* Cyst, iris
clitoris N90.7
colon K63.8
common (bile) duct K83.5
congenital NEC Q89.8
  adrenal gland Q89.1
  epiglottis Q31.8
  esophagus Q39.8
  fallopian tube Q50.4
  kidney Q61.00
    more than one Q61.02
      specified as polycystic Q61.3
        adult type Q61.2
        infantile type Q61.19
          collecting duct dilation Q61.11
    solitary Q61.01
  larynx Q31.8
  liver Q44.6
  lung Q33.0
  mediastinum Q34.1
  ovary Q50.1
  oviduct Q50.4
  periurethral (tissue) Q64.79
  prepuce Q55.69
  salivary gland (any) Q38.4
  sublingual Q38.6
  submaxillary gland Q38.6
  thymus (gland) Q89.2
  tongue Q38.3
  ureterovesical orifice Q62.8
  vulva Q52.79
conjunctiva H11.449
  bilateral H11.443
  left H11.442
  right H11.441
cornea H18.89
corpora quadrigemina G93.0
corpus
  albicans N83.29
  luteum (hemorrhagic) (ruptured) N83.1
Cowper's gland (benign) (infected) N36.8
cranial meninges G93.0
craniobuccal pouch E23.6
craniopharyngeal pouch E23.6
cystic duct K82.8
Cysticercus — *see* Cysticercosis
Dandy-Walker Q03.1
  with spina bifida — *see* Spina bifida
dental (root) K04.8
  developmental K09.0
  eruption K09.0
  primordial K09.0
dentigerous (mandible) (maxilla) K09.0
dermoid (M9084/0) — *see also* Neoplasm, benign
  with malignant transformation (M9084/3) C56.9
    left side C56.1
    right side C56.0
  implantation
    external area or site (skin) NEC L72.0
    iris — *see* Cyst, iris, implantation
    vagina N89.8
    vulva N90.7
  mouth K09.8

Cyst — *continued*
dermoid — *see also* Neoplasm, benign — *continued*
  oral soft tissue K09.8
  sacrococcygeal — *see* Cyst, pilonidal
developmental K09.1
  odontogenic K09.0
  oral region (nonodontogenic) K09.1
  ovary, ovarian Q50.1
dura (cerebral) G93.0
  spinal G96.1
ear (external) Q18.1
echinococcal — *see* Echinococcus
embryonic
  cervix uteri Q51.6
  fallopian tube Q50.4
  vagina Q51.6
endometrium, endometrial (uterus) N85.8
  ectopic — *see* Endometriosis
enterogenous Q43.8
epidermal, epidermoid (inclusion) (*see also* Cyst, skin) L72.0
  mouth K09.8
  oral soft tissue K09.8
epididymis N50.8
epiglottis J38.7
epiphysis cerebri E34.8
epithelial (inclusion) L72.0
epoophoron Q50.5
eruption K09.0
esophagus K22.8
ethmoid sinus J34.1
external female genital organs NEC N90.7
eye NEC H57.8
  congenital Q15.8
eyelid (sebaceous) H02.829
  infected — *see* Hordeolum
  left H02.826
    lower H02.825
    upper H02.824
  right H02.823
    lower H02.822
    upper H02.821
fallopian tube N83.8
fimbrial (twisted) Q50.4
fissural (oral region) K09.1
follicle (graafian) (hemorrhagic) N83.0
  nabothian N88.8
follicular (atretic) (hemorrhagic) (ovarian) N83.0
  dentigerous K09.0
  odontogenic K09.0
  skin L72.9
    specified NEC L72.8
frontal sinus J34.1
gallbladder K82.8
ganglion — *see* Ganglion
Gartner's duct Q50.5
gingiva K09.0
gland of Moll — *see* Cyst, eyelid
globulomaxillary K09.1
graafian follicle (hemorrhagic) N83.0
granulosal lutein (hemorrhagic) N83.1
hemangiomatous (M9120/0) D18.00
  intra-abdominal D18.03
  intracranial D18.02
  skin D18.01
  specified site NEC D18.09
hydatid (*see also* Echinococcus) B67.90
  brain B67.99 *[G94]*
  liver (*see also* Cyst, liver, hydatid) B67.8
  lung NEC B67.99 *[J99]*
  Morgagni
    female Q52.8
    male Q55.4
  specified site NEC B67.99
hymen N89.8
  embryonic Q52.4
hypopharynx J39.2
hypophysis, hypophyseal (duct) (recurrent) E23.6
  cerebri E23.6
implantation (dermoid)
  external area or site (skin) NEC L72.0
  iris — *see* Cyst, iris, implantation
  vagina N89.8
  vulva N90.7
incisive canal K09.1

Cyst — *continued*
inclusion (epidermal) (epithelial) (epidermoid) (squamous) L72.0
  not of skin – code under Cyst, by site
intestine (large) (small) K63.8
intracranial — *see* Cyst, brain
intraligamentous — *see also* Disorder, ligament
  knee — *see* Derangement, knee
intrasellar E23.6
iris H21.309
  exudative H21.319
    bilateral H21.313
    left H21.312
    right H21.311
  idiopathic H21.309
    bilateral H21.303
    left H21.302
    right H21.301
  implantation H21.329
    bilateral H21.323
    left H21.322
    right H21.321
  parasitic H21.339
    bilateral H21.333
    left H21.332
    right H21.331
  pars plana (primary) H21.349
    bilateral H21.343
    exudative H21.359
      bilateral H21.353
      left H21.352
      right H21.351
    left H21.342
    right H21.341
jaw (bone) (aneurysmal) (hemorrhagic) (traumatic) M27.40
  developmental (odontogenic) K09.0
  fissural K09.1
joint NEC — *see* Disorder, joint, specified type NEC
kidney (congenital) (single) Q61.00
  acquired N28.1
  calyceal — *see* Hydronephrosis
  more than one Q61.02
    specified as polycystic Q61.3
      adult type Q61.2
      infantile type Q61.19
        collecting duct dilation Q61.11
  pyelogenic — *see* Hydronephrosis
  simple N28.1
  solitary Q61.01
    acquired N28.1
labium (majus) (minus) N90.7
  sebaceous N90.7
lacrimal — *see also* Disorder, lacrimal system, specified NEC
  gland H04.139
    bilateral H04.133
    left H04.132
    right H04.131
  passages or sac — *see* Disorder, lacrimal system, specified NEC
larynx J38.7
lateral periodontal K09.0
lens H27.8
  congenital Q12.8
lip (gland) K13.0
liver K76.8
  congenital Q44.6
  hydatid B67.8
    granulosus B67.0
    multilocularis B67.5
lung J98.4
  congenital Q33.0
  giant bullous J43.9
lutein N83.1
lymphangiomatous (M9173/0) D18.1
lymphoepithelial, oral soft tissue K09.8
macula — *see* Degeneration, macula, hole
malignant (M8000/3) — *see* Neoplasm, malignant
mammary gland — *see* Cyst, breast
mandible M27.40
  dentigerous K09.0
  radicular K04.8
maxilla M27.40
  dentigerous K09.0

©2002 Ingenix, Inc.

Cyst — *continued*
- maxilla — *continued*
  - radicular K04.8
- medial, face and neck Q18.8
- median
  - anterior maxillary K09.1
  - palatal K09.1
- mediastinum, congenital Q34.1
- meibomian (gland) — *see* Chalazion
  - infected — *see* Hordeolum
- membrane, brain G93.0
- meninges (cerebral) G93.0
  - spinal G96.1
- meniscus, knee — *see* Derangement, knee, meniscus, cystic
- mesentery, mesenteric K66.8
  - chyle I89.8
- mesonephric duct
  - female Q52.8
  - male Q55.4
- milk N64.8
- Morgagni (hydatid)
  - female Q52.8
  - male Q55.4
- mouth K09.8
- muellerian duct Q50.4
- multilocular (ovary) (M8000/1) D39.10
  - benign (M8000/0) — *see* Neoplasm, benign
- myometrium N85.8
- nabothian (follicle) (ruptured) N88.8
- nasoalveolar K09.8
- nasolabial K09.8
- nasopalatine (anterior) (duct) K09.1
- nasopharynx J39.2
- neoplastic (M8000/1) — *see also* Neoplasm, uncertain behavior
  - benign (M8000/0) — *see* Neoplasm, benign
- nervous system NEC G96.8
- neuroenteric (congenital) Q06.8
- nipple — *see* Cyst, breast
- nose (turbinates) J34.1
  - sinus J34.1
- odontogenic, developmental K09.0
- omentum (lesser) K66.8
  - congenital Q45.8
- ora serrata — *see* Cyst, retina, ora serrata
- oral
  - region K09.9
    - developmental (nonodontogenic) K09.1
    - specified NEC K09.8
  - soft tissue K09.9
    - specified NEC K09.8
- orbit H05.819
  - bilateral H05.813
  - left H05.812
  - right H05.811
- ovary, ovarian (twisted) N83.20
  - adherent N83.20
  - chocolate N80.1
  - corpus
    - albicans N83.29
    - luteum (hemorrhagic) N83.1
  - dermoid (M9084/0) D27.9
  - developmental Q50.1
  - due to failure of involution NEC N83.20
  - endometrial N80.1
  - follicular (graafian) (hemorrhagic) N83.0
  - hemorrhagic N83.20
  - in pregnancy or childbirth — *see* category O34.8
    - with obstructed labor O65.5
  - multilocular (M8000/1) D39.10
  - pseudomucinous (M8470/0) D27.9
  - retention N83.29
  - serous N83.20
  - specified NEC N83.29
  - theca lutein (hemorrhagic) N83.1
  - tuberculous A18.18
- oviduct N83.8
- palate (median) (fissural) K09.1
- palatine papilla (jaw) K09.1
- pancreas, pancreatic (hemorrhagic) (true) K86.2
  - congenital Q45.2
  - false K86.3
- paramesonephric duct Q50.4
- paranephric N28.1
- paraphysis, cerebri, congenital Q04.6

Cyst — *continued*
- parasitic B89
- parathyroid (gland) E21.4
- paratubal N83.8
- paraurethral duct N36.8
- paroophoron Q50.5
- parotid gland K11.6
- parovarian Q50.5
- pelvis, female N94.8
  - in pregnancy or childbirth — *see* category O34.8
    - causing obstructed labor O65.5
- penis (sebaceous) N48.89
- periapical K04.8
- pericardial, congenital Q24.8
  - acquired (secondary) I31.8
- pericoronal K09.0
- periodontal K04.8
  - lateral K09.0
- peripelvic (lymphatic) N28.1
- peritoneum K66.8
  - chylous I89.8
- periventricular, acquired, newborn P91.1
- pharynx (wall) J39.2
- pilar L72.1
- pilonidal (infected) (rectum) L05.91
  - with abscess L05.01
  - malignant (M9084/3) C44.5
- pituitary (duct) (gland) E23.6
- placenta (amniotic) — *see* Abnormal, placenta, specified type NEC
- pleura J94.8
- popliteal — *see* Cyst, Baker's
- porencephalic Q04.6
  - acquired G93.0
- postanal (infected) — *see* Cyst, pilonidal
- postmastoidectomy cavity (mucosal) — *see* Complications, postmastoidectomy, cyst
- preauricular Q18.1
- prepuce N47.4
  - congenital Q55.69
- primordial (jaw) K09.0
- prostate N42.89
- pseudomucinous (ovary) (M8470/0) D27.9
- pupillary, miotic H21.279
  - bilateral H21.273
  - left H21.272
  - right H21.271
- radicular (residual) K04.8
- radiculodental K04.8
- ranular K11.8
- Rathke's pouch E23.6
- rectum (epithelium) (mucous) K62.8
- renal (congenital) — *see* Cyst, kidney
- residual (radicular) K04.8
- retention (ovary) N83.29
  - salivary gland K11.6
- retina H33.199
  - bilateral H33.193
  - left H33.192
  - ora serrata H33.119
    - bilateral H33.113
    - left H33.112
    - right H33.111
  - parasitic H33.129
    - bilateral H33.123
    - left H33.122
    - right H33.121
  - right H33.191
- retroperitoneal K68.9
- sacrococcygeal (dermoid) — *see* Cyst, pilonidal
- salivary gland or duct (mucous extravasation or retention) K11.6
- Sampson's N80.1
- sclera H15.89
- scrotum L72.9
  - sebaceous L72.1
- sebaceous (duct) (gland) L72.1
  - breast — *see* Dysplasia, mammary, specified type NEC
  - eyelid — *see* Cyst, eyelid
  - genital organ NEC
    - female N94.8
    - male N50.8
  - scrotum L72.1
- semilunar cartilage (knee) (multiple) — *see* Derangement, knee, meniscus, cystic

Cyst — *continued*
- seminal vesicle N50.8
- serous (ovary) N83.20
- sinus (accessory) (nasal) J34.1
- Skene's gland N36.8
- skin L72.9
  - breast — *see* Dysplasia, mammary, specified type NEC
  - epidermal, epidermoid L72.0
  - epithelial L72.0
  - eyelid — *see* Cyst, eyelid
  - genital organ NEC
    - female N90.7
    - male N50.8
  - inclusion L72.0
  - scrotum L72.9
  - sebaceous L72.1
  - sweat gland or duct L74.8
- solitary
  - bone — *see* Cyst, bone, solitary
  - jaw M27.40
  - kidney N28.1
- spermatic cord N50.8
- sphenoid sinus J34.1
- spinal meninges G96.1
- spleen NEC D73.4
  - congenital Q89.09
  - hydatid (*see also* Echinococcus) B67.99 [D77]
- Stafne's M27.0
- subarachnoid intrasellar R93.0
- subcutaneous, pheomycotic (chromomycotic) B43.2
- subdural (cerebral) G93.0
  - spinal cord G96.1
- sublingual gland K11.6
- submandibular gland K11.6
- submaxillary gland K11.6
- suburethral N36.8
- suprarenal gland E27.8
- suprasellar — *see* Cyst, brain
- sweat gland or duct L74.8
- synovial — *see also* Cyst, bursa
  - ruptured *see* Rupture, synovium
- tarsal — *see* Chalazion
- tendon (sheath) — *see* Disorder, tendon, specified type NEC
- testis N44.2
  - tunica albuginea N44.1
- theca lutein (ovary) N83.1
- Thornwaldt's J39.2
- thymus (gland) E32.8
- thyroglossal duct (infected) (persistent) Q89.2
- thyrolingual duct (infected) (persistent) Q89.2
- thyroid (gland) E04.1
- tongue K14.8
- tonsil J35.8
- tooth — *see* Cyst, dental
- Tornwaldt's J39.2
- trichilemmal L72.1
- trichodermal L72.1
- tubal (fallopian) N83.8
  - inflammatory — *see* Salpingitis, chronic
- tubo-ovarian N83.8
  - inflammatory N70.13
- tunica
  - albuginea testis N44.1
  - vaginalis N50.8
- turbinate (nose) J34.1
- Tyson's gland N48.89
- urachus, congenital Q64.4
- ureter N28.89
- ureterovesical orifice N28.89
- urethra, urethral (gland) N36.8
- uterine ligament N83.8
- uterus (body) (corpus) (recurrent) N85.8
  - embryonic Q51.8
  - cervix Q51.6
- vagina, vaginal (implantation) (inclusion) (squamous cell) (wall) N89.8
  - embryonic Q52.4
- vallecula, vallecular (epiglottis) J38.7
- vesical (orifice) N32.8
- vitreous body H43.89
- vulva (implantation) (inclusion) N90.7
  - congenital Q52.79
  - sebaceous gland N90.7
- vulvovaginal gland N90.7

Cyst — *continued*
 wolffian
  female Q52.8
  male Q55.4
Cystadenocarcinoma (M8440/3) — *see also*
 Neoplasm, malignant
 bile duct (M8161/3) C22.1
 endometrioid (M8380/3) — *see* Neoplasm,
  malignant
  specified site — *see* Neoplasm, malignant
  unspecified site
   female C56.9
   male C61
 mucinous (M8470/3)
  papillary (M8471/3)
   specified site — *see* Neoplasm, malignant
   unspecified site C56.9
  specified site — *see* Neoplasm, malignant
  unspecified site C56.9
 papillary (M8450/3)
  mucinous (M8471/3)
   specified site — *see* Neoplasm, malignant
   unspecified site C56.9
  pseudomucinous (M8471/3)
   specified site — *see* Neoplasm, malignant
   unspecified site C56.9
  serous (M8460/3)
   specified site — *see* Neoplasm, malignant
   unspecified site C56.9
  specified site — *see* Neoplasm, malignant
  unspecified site C56.9
 pseudomucinous (M8470/3)
  papillary (M8471/3)
   specified site — *see* Neoplasm, malignant
   unspecified site C56.9
  specified site — *see* Neoplasm, malignant
  unspecified site C56.9
 serous (M8441/3)
  papillary (M8460/3)
   specified site — *see* Neoplasm, malignant
   unspecified site C56.9
  specified site — *see* Neoplasm, malignant
  unspecified site C56.9
Cystadenofibroma (M9013/0)
 clear cell (M8313/0) — *see* Neoplasm, benign
 endometrioid (M8381/0) D27.9
  borderline malignancy (M8381/1) D39.10
   left ovary D39.12
   right ovary D39.11
  malignant (M8381/3) C56.9
   left side C56.1
   right side C56.0
 mucinous (M9015/0)
  specified site — *see* Neoplasm, benign
  unspecified site D27.9
 serous (M9014/0)
  specified site — *see* Neoplasm, benign
  unspecified site D27.9
 specified site — *see* Neoplasm, benign
 unspecified site D27.9
Cystadenoma (M8440/0) — *see also* Neoplasm,
 benign
 bile duct (M8161/0) D13.4
 endometrioid (M8380/0) — *see also* Neoplasm,
  benign
  borderline malignancy (M8380/1) — *see*
   Neoplasm, uncertain behavior
 malignant (M8440/3) — *see* Neoplasm,
  malignant
 mucinous (M8470/0)
  borderline malignancy (M8472/1)
   ovary (M8472/3) C56.9
    left side C56.1
    right side C56.0
   specified site NEC — *see* Neoplasm,
    uncertain behavior
   unspecified site C56.9
  papillary (M8471/0)
   borderline malignancy (M8473/1)
    ovary (M8473/3) C56.9
     left side C56.1
     right side C56.0
    specified site NEC — *see* Neoplasm,
     uncertain behavior
    unspecified site C56.9
   specified site — *see* Neoplasm, benign

Cystadenoma — *see also* Neoplasm, benign —
 continued
 mucinous — *continued*
  papillary — *continued*
   unspecified site D27.9
  specified site — *see* Neoplasm, benign
  unspecified site D27.9
 papillary (M8450/0)
  borderline malignancy (M8451/1)
   ovary (M8451/3) C56.9
    left side C56.1
    right side C56.0
   specified site NEC — *see* Neoplasm,
    uncertain behavior
   unspecified site C56.9
  lymphomatosum (M8561/0)
   specified site — *see* Neoplasm, benign
   unspecified site D11.9
  mucinous (M8471/0)
   borderline malignancy (M8473/1)
    ovary (M8473/3) C56.9
     left side C56.1
     right side C56.0
    specified site NEC — *see* Neoplasm,
     uncertain behavior
    unspecified site C56.9
   specified site — *see* Neoplasm, benign
   unspecified site D27.9
  pseudomucinous (M8471/0)
   borderline malignancy (M8473/1)
    ovary (M8473/3) C56.9
     left side C56.1
     right side C56.0
    specified site NEC — *see* Neoplasm,
     uncertain behavior
    unspecified site C56.9
   specified site — *see* Neoplasm, benign
   unspecified site D27.9
  serous (M8460/0)
   borderline malignancy (M8462/1)
    ovary (M8462/3) C56.9
     left side C56.1
     right side C56.0
    specified site NEC — *see* Neoplasm,
     uncertain behavior
    unspecified site C56.9
   specified site — *see* Neoplasm, benign
   unspecified site D27.9
  specified site — *see* Neoplasm, benign
  unspecified site D27.9
 pseudomucinous (M8470/0)
  borderline malignancy (M8472/1)
   ovary (M8472/3) C56.9
    left side C56.1
    right side C56.0
   specified site NEC — *see* Neoplasm,
    uncertain behavior
   unspecified site C56.9
  papillary (M8471/0)
   borderline malignancy (M8473/1)
    ovary (M8473/3) C56.9
     left side C56.1
     right side C56.0
    specified site NEC — *see* Neoplasm,
     uncertain behavior
    unspecified site C56.9
   specified site — *see* Neoplasm, benign
   unspecified site D27.9
  specified site — *see* Neoplasm, benign
  unspecified site D27.9
 serous (M8441/0)
  borderline malignancy (M8442/1)
   ovary (M8442/3) C56.9
    left side C56.1
    right side C56.0
   specified site NEC — *see* Neoplasm,
    uncertain behavior
   unspecified site C56.9
  papillary (M8460/0)
   borderline malignancy (M8462/1)
    ovary (M8462/3) C56.9
     left side C56.1
     right side C56.0
    specified site NEC — *see* Neoplasm,
     uncertain behavior
    unspecified site C56.9

Cystadenoma — *see also* Neoplasm, benign —
 continued
 serous — *continued*
  papillary — *continued*
   specified site — *see* Neoplasm, benign
   unspecified site D27.9
  specified site — *see* Neoplasm, benign
  unspecified site D27.9
Cystathionine synthase deficiency E72.11
Cystathioninemia E72.19
Cystathioninuria E72.19
Cystic — *see also* condition
 breast (chronic) — *see* Mastopathy, cystic
 corpora lutea (hemorrhagic) N83.1
 duct — *see* condition
 eyeball (congenital) Q11.0
 fibrosis — *see* Fibrosis, cystic
 kidney (congenital) Q61.3
  adult type Q61.2
  infantile type Q61.19
   collecting duct dilatation Q61.11
  medullary Q61.5
 liver, congenital Q44.6
 lung disease J98.4
  congenital Q33.0
 mastitis, chronic — *see* Mastopathy, cystic
 medullary, kidney Q61.5
 meniscus — *see* Derangement, knee, meniscus,
  cystic
 ovary N83.20
Cysticercosis, cysticerciasis B69.9
 with
  epileptiform fits B69.0
  myositis B69.81
 brain B69.0
 central nervous system B69.0
 cerebral B69.0
 ocular B69.1
 specified NEC B69.89
Cysticercus cellulose infestation — *see*
 Cysticercosis
Cystinosis (malignant) E72.04
Cystinuria E72.01
Cystitis (exudative) (hemorrhagic) (septic)
 (suppurative) N30.90
 with
  fibrosis — *see* Cystitis, chronic, interstitial
  hematuria N30.91
  leukoplakia — *see* Cystitis, chronic,
   interstitial
  malakoplakia — *see* Cystitis, chronic,
   interstitial
  metaplasia — *see* Cystitis, chronic,
   interstitial
  prostatitis N41.3
 acute N30.00
  with hematuria N30.01
  of trigone N30.30
   with hematuria N30.31
 allergic — *see* Cystitis, specified type NEC
 amebic A06.81
 bilharzial B65.9
 blennorrhagic (gonococcal) A54.01
 bullous — *see* Cystitis, specified type NEC
 calculous N21.0
 chlamydial A56.01
 chronic N30.20
  with hematuria N30.21
  interstitial N30.10
   with hematuria N30.11
  of trigone N30.30
   with hematuria N30.31
  specified NEC N30.20
   with hematuria N30.21
 complicating pregnancy O23.10
  first trimester O23.11
  second trimester O23.12
  third trimester O23.13
 cystic(a) — *see* Cystitis, specified type NEC
 diphtheritic A36.85
 echinococcal
  granulosus B67.2
  multilocularis B67.69
 emphysematous — *see* Cystitis, specified type
  NEC
 encysted — *see* Cystitis, specified type NEC

Cystitis — continued
  eosinophilic — see Cystitis, specified type NEC
  follicular — see Cystitis, of trigone
  gangrenous — see Cystitis, specified type NEC
  glandularis — see Cystitis, specified type NEC
  gonococcal A54.01
  incrusted — see Cystitis, specified type NEC
  interstitial (chronic) — see Cystitis, chronic, interstitial
  irradiation N30.40
    with hematuria N30.41
  irritation — see Cystitis, specified type NEC
  malignant — see Cystitis, specified type NEC
  of trigone N30.30
    with hematuria N30.31
  panmural — see Cystitis, chronic, interstitial
  polyposa — see Cystitis, specified type NEC
  prostatic N41.3
  puerperal (postpartum) O86.22
  radiation — see Cystitis, irradiation
  specified type NEC N30.80
    with hematuria N30.81
  subacute — see Cystitis, chronic
  submucous — see Cystitis, chronic, interstitial
  syphilitic (late) A52.76
  trichomonal A59.03
  tuberculous A18.12
  ulcerative — see Cystitis, chronic, interstitial
  venereal NEC (nongonococcal) A64.0

Cystocele (-urethrocele)
  female N81.1
    with prolapse of uterus — see Prolapse, uterus
    in pregnancy or childbirth — see category O34.8
      causing obstructed labor O65.5
  male N32.8

Cystolithiasis N21.0

Cystoma (M8440/0) — see also Neoplasm, benign
  endometrial, ovary N80.1
  mucinous (M8470/0)
    specified site — see Neoplasm, benign
    unspecified site D27.9
  serous (M8441/0)
    specified site — see Neoplasm, benign
    unspecified site D27.9
  simple (ovary) N83.29

Cystoplegia N31.2

Cystoptosis N32.8

Cystopyelitis — see Pyelonephritis

Cystorrhagia N32.8

Cystosarcoma phyllodes (female) (M9020/1) D48.60
  benign (female) (M9020/0) D24.00
    left D24.02
    male D24.10
      left D24.12
      right D24.11
    right D24.01
  male D48.65
  malignant (M9020/3) — see Neoplasm, breast, malignant

Cystostomy
  attention to Z43.5
  complication — see Complications, cystostomy
  status Z93.50
    appendico-vesicostomy Z93.52
    cutaneous Z93.51
    specified NEC Z93.59

Cystourethritis — see Urethritis

Cystourethrocele — see also Cystocele
  female N81.1
    with uterine prolapse — see Prolapse, uterus
  male N32.8

Cytomegalic inclusion disease
  congenital P35.1

Cytomegalovirus infection B25.9
  maternal, (suspected) damage to fetus affecting management of pregnancy O35.3

Cytomycosis (reticuloendothelial) B39.4

Cytotoxic drug, maternal, affecting fetus or newborn P04.1

Czerny's disease (periodic hydrarthrosis of the knee) — see Effusion, joint, knee

---

D

Daae (-Finsen) disease (epidemic pleurodynia) B33.0

Da Costa's syndrome F45.8

Dabney's grip B33.0

Dacryoadenitis, dacryadenitis H04.009
  acute H04.019
    bilateral H04.013
    left H04.012
    right H04.011
  bilateral H04.003
  chronic H04.029
    bilateral H04.023
    left H04.022
    right H04.021
  left H04.002
  right H04.001

Dacryocystitis H04.309
  acute H04.329
    bilateral H04.323
    left H04.322
    right H04.321
  bilateral H04.303
  chronic H04.419
    bilateral H04.413
    left H04.412
    right H04.411
  left H04.302
  neonatal P39.1
  phlegmonous H04.319
    bilateral H04.313
    left H04.312
    right H04.311
  right H04.301
  syphilitic A52.71
    congenital (early) A50.01
  trachomatous, active A71.1
    late effect B94.0

Dacryocystoblenorrhea — see Inflammation, lacrimal, passages, chronic

Dacryocystocele — see Disorder, lacrimal system, changes

Dacryolith, dacryolithiasis H04.519
  bilateral H04.513
  left H04.512
  right H04.511

Dacryoma — see Disorder, lacrimal system, changes

Dacryopericystitis — see Dacryocystitis

Dacryops H04.119
  bilateral H04.113
  left H04.112
  right H04.111

Dacryostenosis — see also Stenosis, lacrimal
  congenital Q10.5

Dactylitis L08.9
  bone — see Osteomyelitis
  syphilitic A52.77
  tuberculous A18.03

Dactylolysis spontanea (ainhum) L94.6

Dactylosymphysis Q70.9
  fingers — see Syndactylism, complex, fingers
  toes Q70.2

Damage
  arteriosclerotic — see Arteriosclerosis
  brain (nontraumatic) G93.9
    anoxic, hypoxic G93.1
      resulting from a procedure G97.82
    child NOS G80.9
    due to birth injury P11.2
  cardiorenal (vascular) — see Hypertension, cardiorenal
  cerebral NEC — see Damage, brain
  coccyx, complicating delivery O71.6
  coronary — see Disease, heart, ischemic
  eye, birth injury P15.3
  liver (nontraumatic) K76.9
    alcoholic K70.9
    due to drugs — see Disease, liver, toxic
    toxic — see Disease, liver, toxic
  myocardium I51.6
  pelvic
    joint or ligament, during delivery O71.6

Damage — continued
  pelvic — continued
    organ NEC
      during delivery O71.5
      following ectopic or molar pregnancy O08.6
  renal — see Disease, renal
  subendocardium, subendocardial — see Degeneration, myocardial
  vascular I99.9

Dana-Putnam syndrome (subacute combined sclerosis with pernicious anemia) — see Degeneration, combined

Danbolt (-Closs) syndrome (acrodermatitis enteropathica) L08.89

Dandruff L21.0

Dandy-Walker syndrome Q03.1
  with spina bifida — see Spina bifida

Danlos' syndrome Q79.6

Darier (-White) disease (congenital) Q82.8
  meaning erythema annulare centrifugum L53.1

Darier-Roussy sarcoid D86.3

Darling's disease or histoplasmosis B39.4

Darwin's tubercle Q17.8

Dawson's (inclusion body) **encephalitis** A81.1

De Beurmann (-Gougerot) disease B42.1

De la Tourette's syndrome F95.2

De Lange's syndrome Q87.1

De Morgan's spots (senile angiomas) I78.1

De Quervain's
  disease (tendon sheath) M65.4
  thyroiditis (subacute granulomatous thyroiditis) E06.1

De Toni-Fanconi (-Debré) syndrome E72.09
  with cystinosis E72.04

Dead
  fetus, retained (mother) O36.4
    early pregnancy O02.1
  labyrinth — see category H83.2
  ovum, retained O02.0

Deaf and dumb NEC H91.3

Deafmutism (acquired) (congenital) NEC H91.3
  hysterical F44.6
  syphilitic, congenital (see also category H94.8) A50.09

Deafness (acquired) (complete) (hereditary) (high frequency) (low frequency) (partial) H91.90
  with blue sclera and fragility of bone Q78.0
  auditory fatigue — see Deafness, specified type NEC
  aviation T70.0
    nerve injury — see Injury, nerve, acoustic, specified type NEC
  bilateral H91.93
  boilermaker's — see category H83.3
  central — see Deafness, sensorineural
  conductive H90.2
    and sensorineural, mixed H90.8
      bilateral H90.6
      left H90.72
      right H90.71
    bilateral H90.0
    left H90.12
    right H90.11
  congenital — see also Deafness, sensorineural
    with blue sclera and fragility of bone Q78.0
  due to toxic agents — see Deafness, ototoxic
  emotional (hysterical) F44.6
  functional (hysterical) F44.6
  hysterical F44.6
  left H91.92
  mental R48.8
  mixed conductive and sensorineural H90.8
    bilateral H90.6
    left H90.72
    right H90.71
  nerve — see Deafness, sensorineural
  neural — see Deafness, sensorineural
  noise-induced — see also category H83.3
    nerve injury — see Injury, nerve, acoustic, specified type NEC
  nonspeaking H91.3
  ototoxic — see category H91.0

Defect, defective — *continued*
  reduction — *continued*
    limb — *continued*
      lower — *continued*
        right Q72.91
        specified type NEC Q72.80
          bilateral Q72.83
          left Q72.82
          right Q72.81
      specified type NEC Q73.8
      upper Q71.90
        absence — *see* Agenesis, arm
          forearm — *see* Agenesis, forearm
          hand — *see* Agenesis, hand
        bilateral Q71.93
        left Q71.92
        lobster-claw hand Q71.60
          bilateral Q71.63
          left Q71.62
          right Q71.61
        longitudinal
          radius Q71.40
            bilateral Q71.43
            left Q71.42
            right Q71.41
          ulna Q71.50
            bilateral Q71.53
            left Q71.52
            right Q71.51
        right Q71.91
        specified type NEC Q71.80
          bilateral Q71.83
          left Q71.82
          right Q71.81
  renal pelvis Q63.8
    obstructive Q62.39
  respiratory system, congenital Q34.9
  retinal nerve bundle fibers H35.89
  septal (heart) NOS Q21.9
    acquired (atrial) (auricular) (ventricular) (old)
      I51.0
    atrial Q21.1
      concurrent with acute myocardial
        infarction — *see* Infarct,
        myocardium
      following acute myocardial infarction
        (current complication) I23.1
    ventricular — *see also* Defect, ventricular
      septal Q21.0
  sinus venosus Q21.1
  speech R47.9
    developmental F80.9
    specified NEC R47.89
  Taussig-Bing (aortic transposition and
    overriding pulmonary artery) Q20.1
  teeth, wedge K03.1
  vascular (local) I99.9
    congenital Q27.9
  ventricular septal Q21.0
    concurrent with acute myocardial infarction
      — *see* Infarct, myocardium
    following acute myocardial infarction
      (current complication) I23.2
    in tetralogy of Fallot Q21.3
  vision NEC H54.7
  visual field H53.40
    bilateral
      heteronymous H53.47
      homonymous H53.46
    generalized contraction H53.489
      bilateral H53.483
      left H53.482
      right H53.481
    localized
      arcuate H53.439
        bilateral H53.433
        left H53.432
        right H53.431
      scotoma (central area) H53.419
        bilateral H53.413
        blind spot area H53.429
          bilateral H53.423
          left H53.422
          right H53.421
        left H53.412
        right H53.411

Defect, defective — *continued*
  visual field — *continued*
    localized — *continued*
      sector H53.439
        bilateral H53.433
        left H53.432
        right H53.431
      specified type NEC H53.459
        bilateral H53.453
        left H53.452
        right H53.451
  voice R49.9
    specified NEC R49.8
  wedge, tooth, teeth (abrasion) K03.1

Deferentitis N49.1
  gonorrheal (acute) (chronic) A54.23

Defibrination (syndrome) D65
  antepartum — *see* Hemorrhage, antepartum,
    with coagulation defect, disseminated
    intravascular coagulation
  fetus or newborn P60
  following ectopic or molar pregnancy O08.1
  intrapartum O67.0
  postpartum O72.3

Deficiency, deficient
  3B hydroxysteroid dehydrogenase E25.0
  5-alpha reductase (with male
    pseudohermaphroditism) E29.1
  11 hydroxylase E25.0
  21 hydroxylase E25.0
  abdominal muscle syndrome Q79.4
  accelerator globulin (Ac G) (blood) D68.2
  AC globulin (congenital) (hereditary) D68.2
    acquired D68.4
  acid phosphatase E83.39
  activating factor (blood) D68.2
  adenosine deaminase (ADA) D81.3
  aldolase (hereditary) E74.19
  alpha-1-antitrypsin E88.01
  amino-acids E72.9
  anemia — *see* Anemia
  aneurin E51.9
  antibody with
    hyperimmunoglobulinemia D80.6
    near-normal immunoglobins D80.6
  antidiuretic hormone E23.2
  anti-hemophilic
    factor (A) D66
      B D67
      C D68.1
    globulin (AHG) NEC D66
  ascorbic acid E54
  attention (disorder) (syndrome) F98.8
    with hyperactivity — *see* Disorder, attention-
      deficit hyperactivity
  autoprothrombin
    I D68.2
    II D67
    C D68.2
  beta-glucuronidase E76.29
  biotin E53.8
  biotin-dependent carboxylase D81.819
  biotinidase D81.810
  brancher enzyme (amylopectinosis) E74.03
  calciferol E55.9
    with
      adult osteomalacia M83.8
      rickets — *see* Rickets
  calcium (dietary) E58
  calorie, severe E43
    with marasmus E41
    and kwashiorkor E42
  cardiac — *see* Insufficiency, myocardial
  carnitine (palmityltransferase) R82.1
    muscle E71.328
    secondary E71.322
  carotene E50.9
  central nervous system G96.8
  ceruloplasmin (Wilson) E83.01
  choline E53.8
  Christmas factor D67
  chromium E61.4
  clotting (blood) (*see also* Deficiency, coagulation
    factor) D68.9
  clotting factor NEC (hereditary) (*see also*
    Deficiency, factor) D68.2

Deficiency, deficient — *continued*
  coagulation NOS D68.9
    with
      ectopic pregnancy O08.1
      molar pregnancy O08.1
    acquired (any) D68.4
    antepartum hemorrhage — *see* Hemorrhage,
      antepartum, with coagulation defect
    clotting factor NEC (*see also* Deficiency,
      factor) D68.2
    due to
      hyperprothrombinemia D68.4
      liver disease D68.4
      vitamin K deficiency D68.4
    newborn, transient P61.6
    postpartum O72.3
    specified NEC D68.2
  color vision H53.50
    achromatopsia H53.51
    acquired H53.52
    deuteranomaly H53.53
    protanomaly H53.54
    specified type NEC H53.59
    tritanomaly H53.55
  contact factor D68.2
  copper (nutritional) E61.0
  corticoadrenal E27.4
    primary E27.1
  craniofacial axis Q75.0
  cyanocobalamin E53.8
  C1 esterase inhibitor (C1-INH) D84.1
  debrancher enzyme (limit dextrinosis) E74.03
  dehydrogenase
    long chain/very long chain acyl CoA
      E71.310
    medium chain acyl CoA E71.311
    short chain acyl CoA E71.312
  diet E63.9
  disaccharidase E73.9
  edema — *see* Malnutrition, severe
  endocrine E34.9
  energy-supply — *see* Malnutrition
  enzymes, circulating NEC E88.09
  ergosterol E55.9
    with
      adult osteomalacia M83.8
      rickets — *see* Rickets
  essential fatty acid (EFA) E63.0
  factor — *see also* Deficiency, coagulation
    Hageman D68.2
    I (congenital) (hereditary) D68.2
    II (congenital) (hereditary) D68.2
    IX (congenital) (functional) (hereditary) (with
      functional defect) D67
    multiple (congenital) D68.89
      acquired D68.4
    V (congenital) (hereditary) D68.2
    VII (congenital) (hereditary) D68.2
    VIII (congenital) (functional) (hereditary)
      (with functional defect) D66
      with vascular defect D68.0
    X (congenital) (hereditary) D68.2
    XI (congenital) (hereditary) D68.1
    XII (congenital) (hereditary) D68.2
    XIII (congenital) (hereditary) D68.2
  femoral, proximal focal (congenital) — *see*
    Defect, reduction, lower limb,
    longitudinal, femur
  fibrin-stabilizing factor (congenital) (hereditary)
    D68.2
    acquired D68.4
  fibrinase D68.2
  fibrinogen (congenital) (hereditary) D68.2
    acquired D65
  folate E53.8
  folic acid E53.8
  foreskin N47.3
  fructokinase E74.11
  fructose 1,6-diphosphatase E74.19
  fructose-1-phosphate aldolase E74.19
  galactokinase E74.29
  galactose-1-phosphate uridyl transferase
    E74.29
  gammaglobulin in blood D80.1
    hereditary D80.0
  glass factor D68.2
  glucose-6-phosphatase E74.01

Deficiency, deficient — continued
glucose-6-phosphate dehydrogenase anemia D55.0
glucuronyl transferase E80.5
glycogen synthetase E74.09
gonadotropin (isolated) E23.0
growth hormone (idiopathic) (isolated) E23.0
Hageman factor D68.2
hemoglobin D64.9
hepatophosphorylase E74.09
homogentisate 1,2-dioxygenase E70.29
hormone
 anterior pituitary (partial) NEC E23.0
 growth E23.0
 growth (isolated) E23.0
 pituitary E23.0
 testicular E29.1
hypoxanthine-(guanine)-phosphoribosyltransferase (HGPRT) (total H-PRT) E79.1
immunity D84.9
 cell-mediated D84.8
 with thrombocytopenia and eczema D82.0
 combined D81.9
 humoral D80.9
 IgA (secretory) D80.2
 IgG D80.3
 IgM D80.4
immuno — see Immunodeficiency
immunoglobulin, selective
 A (IgA) D80.2
 G (IgG) (subclasses) D80.3
 M (IgM) D80.4
inositol (B complex) E53.8
intrinsic
 factor (congenital) D51.0
 sphincter N36.42
 with urethral hypermobility N36.43
iodine E61.8
 congenital syndrome — see Syndrome, iodine-deficiency, congenital
iron E61.1
 anemia D50.9
kalium E87.6
kappa-light chain D80.8
labile factor (congenital) (hereditary) D68.2
 acquired D68.4
lacrimal fluid (acquired) — see also Syndrome, dry eye
 congenital Q10.6
lactase
 congenital E73.0
 secondary E73.1
Laki-Lorand factor D68.2
lecithin cholesterol acyltransferase E78.6
lipocaic K86.8
lipoprotein (familial) (high density) E78.6
liver phosphorylase E74.09
lysosomal (-1, 4 glucosidase E74.02
magnesium E61.2
major histocompatibility complex
 class I D81.6
 class II D81.7
manganese E61.3
menadione (vitamin K) E56.1
 newborn P53
mental (familial) (hereditary) — see Retardation, mental
methylenetetrahydrofolate reductase E72.12
mineral NEC E61.8
molybdenum (nutritional) E61.5
moral F60.2
multiple nutrient elements E61.7
muscle
 carnitine (palmityltransferase) E71.328
 phosphofructokinase E74.09
myoadenylate deaminase E79.2
myocardial — see Insufficiency, myocardial
myophosphorylase E74.04
NADH diaphorase or reductase (congenital) D74.0
NADH-methemoglobin reductase (congenital) D74.0
natrium E87.1
niacin(amide) (-tryptophan) E52
nicotinamide E52

Deficiency, deficient — continued
nicotinic acid E52
number of teeth — see Anodontia
nutrient element E61.9
 multiple E61.7
 specified NEC E61.8
nutrition, nutritional E63.9
 sequelae — see Sequelae, nutritional deficiency
 specified NEC E63.8
ornithine transcarbamylase E72.4
ovarian E28.3
oxygen — see Anoxia
pantothenic acid E53.8
parathyroid (gland) E20.9
perineum (female) N81.8
phenylalanine hydroxylase E70.1
phosphoenol pyruvate carboxykinase E74.4
phosphofructokinase E74.19
phosphorylase kinase, liver E74.09
pituitary hormone (isolated) E23.0
placenta — see Insufficiency, placental
plasma thromboplastin
 antecedent (PTA) D68.1
 component (PTC) D67
platelet NEC D69.1
 constitutional D68.0
polyglandular E31.8
 autoimmune E31.0
potassium (K) E87.6
prepuce N47.3
proaccelerin (congenital) (hereditary) D68.2
 acquired D68.4
proconvertin factor (congenital) (hereditary) D68.2
 acquired D68.4
protein — see also Malnutrition
 anemia D53.0
prothrombin (congenital) (hereditary) D68.2
 acquired D68.4
Prower factor D68.2
pseudocholinesterase E88.09
psychobiological F60.7
PTA (plasma thromboplastin antecedent) D68.1
PTC (plasma thromboplastin component) D67
purine nucleoside phosphorylase (PNP) D81.5
pyracin (alpha) (beta) E53.1
pyridoxal E53.1
pyridoxamine E53.1
pyridoxine (derivatives) E53.1
pyruvate
 carboxylase E74.4
 dehydrogenase E74.4
riboflavin (vitamin B2) E53.0
salt E87.1
secretion
 ovary E28.3
 salivary gland (any) K11.7
 urine R34
selenium (dietary) E59
serum antitrypsin, familial E88.01
sodium (Na) E87.1
SPCA (factor VII) D68.2
sphincter, intrinsic N36.42
 with urethral hypermobility N36.43
stable factor (congenital) (hereditary) D68.2
 acquired D68.4
Stuart-Prower (factor X) D68.2
sucrase E74.39
sulfatase E75.29
sulfite oxidase E72.19
thiamin, thiaminic (chloride) E51.9
 beriberi (dry) E51.11
 wet E51.12
thrombokinase D68.2
 newborn P53
thyroid (gland) — see Hypothyroidism
tocopherol E56.0
tooth bud K00.0
transcobalamine II (anemia) D51.2
vanadium E61.6
vascular I99.9
vasopressin E23.2
viosterol — see Deficiency, calciferol

Deficiency, deficient — continued
vitamin (multiple) NOS E56.9
 A E50.9
 with
 Bitot's spot (corneal) E50.1
 follicular keratosis E50.8
 keratomalacia E50.4
 manifestations NEC E50.8
 night blindness E50.5
 scar of cornea, xerophthalmic E50.6
 xeroderma E50.8
 xerophthalmia E50.7
 xerosis
 conjunctival E50.0
 and Bitot's spot E50.1
 cornea E50.2
 and ulceration E50.3
 sequelae E64.1
 B (complex) NOS E53.9
 with
 beriberi (dry) E51.11
 wet E51.12
 pellagra E52
 B1 NOS E51.9
 beriberi (dry) E51.11
 with circulatory system manifestations E51.11
 wet E51.12
 B12 E53.8
 B2 (riboflavin) E53.0
 B6 E53.1
 C E54
 sequelae E64.2
 D E55.9
 with
 adult osteomalacia M83.8
 rickets — see Rickets
 25-hydroxylase E83.32
 E E56.0
 folic acid E53.8
 G E53.0
 group B E53.9
 specified NEC E53.8
 H (biotin) E53.8
 K E56.1
 of newborn P53
 nicotinic E52
 P E56.8
 PP (pellagra-preventing) E52
 specified NEC E56.8
 thiamin E51.9
 beriberi — see Beriberi
zinc, dietary E60

Deficit — see also Deficiency
cognitive
 following
 cerebrovascular disease I69.91
 cerebral infarction I69.31
 intracerebral hemorrhage I69.11
 nontraumatic intracranial hemorrhage NEC I69.21
 specified disease NEC I69.81
 stroke NOS I69.41
 subarachnoid hemorrhage I69.01
neurologic due to cerebrovascular lesion I64
oxygen R09.0

Deficit attention — see Attention, deficit

Deflection
radius — see Deformity, limb, specified type NEC, forearm
septum (acquired) (nasal) (nose) J34.2
spine — see Curvature, spine
turbinate (nose) J34.2

Defluvium
capillorum — see Alopecia
ciliorum — see Madarosis
unguium L60.8

Deformity Q89.9
abdomen, congenital Q89.9
abdominal wall
 acquired M95.8
 congenital Q79.59
acquired (unspecified site) M95.9
adrenal gland Q89.1
alimentary tract, congenital Q45.9
 upper Q40.9

©2002 Ingenix, Inc.

Deformity — *continued*
- ankle (joint) (acquired) — *see also* Deformity, limb, lower leg
  - abduction — *see* Contraction, joint, ankle
  - congenital Q68.8
  - contraction — *see* Contraction, joint, ankle
  - specified type NEC — *see* Deformity, limb, foot, specified NEC
- anus (acquired) K62.8
  - congenital Q43.9
- aorta (arch) (congenital) Q25.4
  - acquired I77.8
- aortic
  - arch, acquired I77.8
  - cusp or valve (congenital) Q23.8
    - acquired (*see also* Endocarditis, aortic) I35.8
- arm (acquired) (upper) — *see also* Deformity, limb, upper arm
  - congenital Q68.8
  - forearm — *see* Deformity, limb, forearm
- artery (congenital) (peripheral) NOS Q27.9
  - acquired I77.8
  - coronary (acquired) I25.9
    - congenital Q24.5
  - umbilical Q27.0
- atrial septal Q21.1
- auditory canal (external) (congenital) — *see also* Malformation, ear, external
  - acquired — *see* Disorder, ear, external, specified type NEC
- auricle
  - ear (congenital) — *see also* Malformation, ear, external
    - acquired — *see* Disorder, pinna, deformity
- back — *see* Dorsopathy, deforming
- bile duct (common) (congenital) (hepatic) Q44.5
  - acquired K83.8
- biliary duct or passage (congenital) Q44.5
  - acquired K83.8
- bladder (neck) (trigone) (sphincter) (acquired) N32.8
  - congenital Q64.79
- bone (acquired) NOS M95.9
  - congenital Q79.9
  - turbinate M95.0
- brain (congenital) Q04.9
  - acquired G93.8
  - reduction Q04.3
- breast (acquired) N64.8
  - congenital Q83.9
- bronchus (congenital) Q32.8
  - acquired NEC J98.0
- bursa, congenital Q79.9
- canaliculi (lacrimalis) (acquired) — *see also* Disorder, lacrimal system, changes
  - congenital Q10.6
- canthus, acquired — *see* Disorder, eyelid, specified type NEC
- capillary (acquired) I78.8
- caruncle, lacrimal (acquired) — *see also* Disorder, lacrimal system, changes
  - congenital Q10.6
- cascade, stomach K31.2
- cecum (congenital) Q43.9
  - acquired K63.8
- cerebral, acquired G93.8
  - congenital Q04.9
- cervix (uterus) (acquired) NEC N88.8
  - congenital Q51.9
- cheek (acquired) M95.2
  - congenital Q18.9
- chest (acquired) (wall) M95.4
  - congenital Q67.8
  - late effect or rickets E64.3
- chin (acquired) M95.2
  - congenital Q18.9
- choroid (congenital) Q14.3
  - acquired H31.8
  - plexus Q07.8
    - acquired G96.1
- cicatricial — *see* Cicatrix
- cilia, acquired — *see* Disorder, eyelid, specified type NEC

Deformity — *continued*
- clavicle (acquired) — *see also* Deformity, limb, specified type NEC, upper limb
  - congenital Q68.8
- clitoris (congenital) Q52.6
  - acquired N90.8
- clubfoot — *see* Clubfoot
- coccyx (acquired) — *see* category M43.8
- colon (congenital) Q43.9
  - acquired K63.8
- concha (ear), congenital — *see also* Malformation, ear, external
  - acquired — *see* Disorder, pinna, deformity
- cornea H18.70
  - congenital Q13.4
  - descemetocele — *see* Descemetocele
  - ectasia — *see* Ectasia, cornea
  - staphyloma — *see* Staphyloma, cornea
- coronary artery (acquired) I25.9
  - congenital Q24.5
- cranium (acquired) — *see* Deformity, skull
- cricoid cartilage (congenital) Q31.8
  - acquired J38.7
- cystic duct (congenital) Q44.5
  - acquired K82.8
- Dandy-Walker Q03.1
  - with spina bifida — *see* Spina bifida
- diaphragm (congenital) Q79.1
  - acquired J98.6
- digestive organ NOS Q45.9
- ductus arteriosus Q25.0
- duodenal bulb K31.89
- duodenum (congenital) Q43.9
  - acquired K31.89
- dura — *see* Deformity, meninges
- ear (acquired) — *see also* Disorder, pinna, deformity
  - congenital (external) Q17.9
    - internal Q16.5
    - middle Q16.4
      - ossicles Q16.3
    - ossicles Q16.3
- ectodermal (congenital) NEC Q84.9
- ejaculatory duct (congenital) Q55.4
  - acquired N50.8
- elbow (joint) (acquired) — *see also* Deformity, limb, upper arm
  - congenital Q68.8
  - contraction — *see* Contraction, joint, elbow
- endocrine gland NEC Q89.2
- epididymis (congenital) Q55.4
  - acquired N50.8
  - torsion N44.01
- epiglottis (congenital) Q31.8
  - acquired J38.7
- esophagus (congenital) Q39.9
  - acquired K22.8
- eustachian tube (congenital) NEC Q17.8
- eye, congenital Q15.9
- eyebrow (congenital) Q18.8
- eyelid (acquired) — *see also* Disorder, eyelid, specified type NEC
  - congenital Q10.3
- face (acquired) M95.2
  - congenital Q18.9
- fallopian tube, acquired N83.8
- femur (acquired) — *see* Deformity, limb, specified type NEC, thigh
- fetal
  - with fetopelvic disproportion O33.7
  - causing obstructed labor O66.3
- finger (acquired) M20.009
  - boutonniere M20.029
    - left M20.022
    - right M20.021
  - congenital Q68.8
  - flexion contracture — *see* Contraction, joint, hand
  - left M20.002
  - mallet finger M20.019
    - left M20.012
    - right M20.011
  - right M20.001
  - specified NEC M20.099
    - left M20.092
    - right M20.091

Deformity — *continued*
- finger — *continued*
  - swan-neck M20.039
    - left M20.032
    - right M20.031
  - flexion (joint) (acquired) — *see also* Deformity, limb, flexion
    - congenital NOS Q74.9
    - hip Q65.9
  - foot (acquired) — *see also* Deformity, limb, lower leg
    - cavovarus (congenital) Q66.1
    - congenital NOS Q66.9
      - specified type NEC Q66.8
    - specified type NEC — *see* Deformity, limb, foot, specified NEC
    - valgus (congenital) Q66.6
      - acquired — *see* Deformity, valgus, ankle
    - varus (congenital) NEC Q66.3
      - acquired — *see* Deformity, varus, ankle
  - forearm (acquired) — *see also* Deformity, limb, forearm
    - congenital Q68.8
  - forehead (acquired) M95.2
    - congenital Q75.8
  - frontal bone (acquired) M95.2
    - congenital Q75.8
  - gallbladder (congenital) Q44.1
    - acquired K82.8
  - gastrointestinal tract (congenital) NOS Q45.9
    - acquired K63.8
  - genitalia, genital organ(s) or system NEC
    - female (congenital) Q52.9
      - acquired N94.8
      - external Q52.70
    - male (congenital) Q55.9
      - acquired N50.8
  - globe (eye) (congenital) Q15.8
    - acquired H44.89
  - gum, acquired NEC K06.8
  - hand (acquired) — *see* Deformity, limb, forearm
    - congenital Q68.1
  - head (acquired) M95.2
    - congenital Q75.8
  - heart (congenital) Q24.9
    - septum Q21.9
      - auricular Q21.1
      - ventricular Q21.0
    - valve (congenital) NEC Q24.8
      - acquired — *see* Endocarditis
  - heel (acquired) — *see* Deformity, foot
  - hepatic duct (congenital) Q44.5
    - acquired K83.8
  - hip (joint) (acquired) — *see also* Deformity, limb, thigh
    - congenital Q65.9
    - due to (previous) juvenile osteochondrosis — *see* Coxa, plana
    - flexion — *see* Contraction, joint, hip
  - hourglass — *see* Contraction, hourglass
  - humerus (acquired) — *see also* Deformity, limb, specified type NEC, upper arm
    - congenital Q74.0
  - hypophyseal (congenital) Q89.2
  - ileocecal (coil) (valve) (acquired) K63.8
    - congenital Q43.9
  - ileum (congenital) Q43.9
    - acquired K63.8
  - ilium (acquired) M95.5
    - congenital Q74.2
  - integument (congenital) Q84.9
  - intervertebral cartilage or disc (acquired) — *see* Disorder, disc, specified NEC
  - intestine (large) (small) (congenital) NOS Q43.9
    - acquired K63.8
  - intrinsic minus or plus (hand) — *see* Deformity, limb, specified type NEC, forearm
  - iris H21.8
    - congenital Q13.2
  - ischium (acquired) M95.5
    - congenital Q74.2
  - jaw (acquired) (congenital) M26.9
  - joint (acquired) NEC M21.90
    - congenital Q68.8
  - kidney(s) (calyx) (pelvis) (congenital) Q63.9
    - acquired N28.89

Deformity — continued
kidney(s — continued
  artery (congenital) Q27.2
    acquired I77.8
Klippel-Feil (brevicollis) Q76.1
knee (acquired) NEC — see also Deformity,
    limb, lower leg
  congenital Q68.2
labium (majus) (minus) (congenital) Q52.79
  acquired N90.8
lacrimal passages or duct (congenital) NEC
    Q10.6
  acquired — see Disorder, lacrimal system,
    changes
larynx (muscle) (congenital) Q31.8
  acquired J38.7
  web (glottic) Q31.0
leg (upper) (acquired) NEC — see also
    Deformity, limb, thigh
  congenital Q68.8
  lower leg — see Deformity, limb, lower leg
lens (acquired) H27.8
  congenital Q12.9
lid (fold) (acquired) — see also Disorder, eyelid,
    specified type NEC
  congenital Q10.3
ligament (acquired) — see Disorder, ligament
  congenital Q79.9
limb (acquired) M21.90
  clawfoot M21.539
    left M21.532
    right M21.531
  clawhand M21.519
    left M21.512
    right M21.511
  clubfoot M21.549
    left M21.542
    right M21.541
  clubhand M21.529
    left M21.522
    right M21.521
  congenital, except reduction deformity Q74.9
  flat foot M21.40
    left M21.42
    right M21.41
  flexion M21.20
    ankle M21.279
      left M21.272
      right M21.271
    elbow M21.229
      left M21.222
      right M21.221
    finger M21.249
      left M21.242
      right M21.241
    hip M21.259
      left M21.252
      right M21.251
    knee M21.269
      left M21.262
      right M21.261
    shoulder M21.219
      left M21.212
      right M21.211
    toe M21.279
      left M21.272
      right M21.271
    wrist M21.239
      left M21.232
      right M21.231
  foot
    claw — see Deformity, limb, clawfoot
    club — see Deformity, limb, clubfoot
    drop M21.379
      left M21.372
      right M21.371
    flat — see Deformity, limb, flat foot
    specified NEC M21.60
      left M21.62
      right M21.61
  forearm M21.939
    left M21.932
    right M21.931
  hand M21.949
    left M21.942
    right M21.941

Deformity — continued
limb — continued
  lower leg M21.969
    left M21.962
    right M21.961
  specified type NEC M21.80
    forearm M21.839
      left M21.832
      right M21.831
    lower leg M21.869
      left M21.862
      right M21.861
    thigh M21.859
      left M21.852
      right M21.851
    upper arm M21.829
      left M21.822
      right M21.821
  thigh M21.959
    left M21.952
    right M21.951
  unequal length M21.70
    short site is
      femur M21.759
        left M21.752
        right M21.751
      fibula M21.769
        left M21.764
        right M21.763
      humerus M21.729
        left M21.722
        right M21.721
      radius M21.739
        left M21.734
        right M21.733
      tibia M21.769
        left M21.762
        right M21.761
      ulna M21.739
        left M21.732
        right M21.731
  upper arm M21.929
    left M21.922
    right M21.921
  valgus — see Deformity, valgus
  varus — see Deformity, varus
  wrist drop M21.339
    left M21.332
    right M21.331
lip (acquired) NEC K13.0
  congenital Q38.0
liver (congenital) Q44.7
  acquired K76.8
lumbosacral (congenital) (joint) (region) Q76.49
  acquired — see category M43.8
  kyphosis — see Kyphosis, congenital
  lordosis — see Lordosis, congenital
lung (congenital) Q33.9
  acquired J98.4
lymphatic system, congenital Q89.9
Madelung's (radius) Q74.0
mandible (acquired) (congenital) M26.9
maxilla (acquired) (congenital) M26.9
meninges or membrane (congenital) Q07.9
  cerebral Q04.8
    acquired G96.1
  spinal cord (congenital) G96.1
    acquired G96.1
metacarpus (acquired) — see Deformity, limb,
    forearm
  congenital Q74.0
metatarsus (acquired) — see Deformity, foot
  congenital Q66.9
middle ear (congenital) Q16.4
  ossicles Q16.3
mitral (leaflets) (valve) I05.8
  Ebstein's Q22.5
  parachute Q23.2
  stenosis, congenital Q23.2
mouth (acquired) K13.7
  congenital Q38.6
multiple, congenital NEC Q89.7
muscle (acquired) M62.89
  congenital Q79.9
    sternocleidomastoid Q68.0
musculoskeletal system (acquired) M95.9
  congenital Q79.9

Deformity — continued
musculoskeletal system — continued
  specified NEC M95.8
nail (acquired) L60.8
  congenital Q84.6
nasal — see Deformity, nose
neck (acquired) M95.3
  congenital Q18.9
    sternocleidomastoid Q68.0
nervous system (congenital) Q07.9
nipple (congenital) Q83.9
  acquired N64.8
nose (acquired) (cartilage) M95.0
  bone (turbinate) M95.0
  congenital Q30.9
    bent or squashed Q67.4
  saddle M95.0
    syphilitic A50.57
  septum (acquired) J34.2
    congenital Q30.8
  sinus (wall) (congenital) Q30.8
    acquired M95.0
  syphilitic (congenital) A50.57
    late A52.73
ocular muscle (congenital) Q10.3
  acquired — see Strabismus, mechanical
oesophagus (congenital) Q39.9
  acquired K22.8
opticociliary vessels (congenital) Q13.2
orbit (eye) (acquired) H05.30
  atrophy — see Atrophy, orbit
  congenital Q10.7
  due to
    bone disease NEC H05.329
      bilateral H05.323
      left H05.322
      right H05.321
    trauma or surgery H05.339
      bilateral H05.333
      left H05.332
      right H05.331
  enlargement — see Enlargement, orbit
  exostosis — see Exostosis, orbit
organ of Corti (congenital) Q16.5
ovary (congenital) Q50.39
  acquired N83.8
oviduct, acquired N83.8
palate (congenital) Q38.5
  acquired M27.8
  cleft (congenital) — see Cleft, palate
pancreas (congenital) Q45.3
  acquired K86.8
parathyroid (gland) Q89.2
parotid (gland) (congenital) Q38.4
  acquired K11.8
patella (acquired) — see Disorder, patella,
    specified NEC
pelvis, pelvic (acquired) (bony) M95.5
  with disproportion (fetopelvic) O33.0
    causing obstructed labor O65.0
  congenital Q74.2
  rachitic (late effect) E64.3
penis (glans) (congenital) Q55.69
  acquired N48.89
pericardium (congenital) Q24.8
  acquired — see Pericarditis
pharynx (congenital) Q38.8
  acquired J39.2
pinna, acquired — see also Disorder, pinna,
    deformity
  congenital Q17.9
pituitary (congenital) Q89.2
posture — see Dorsopathy, deforming
prepuce (congenital) Q55.69
  acquired N47.8
prostate (congenital) Q55.4
  acquired N42.89
pupil (congenital) Q13.2
  acquired — see Abnormality, pupillary
pylorus (congenital) Q40.3
  acquired K31.89
rachitic (acquired), old or healed E64.3
radius (acquired) — see also Deformity, limb,
    forearm
  congenital Q68.8
rectum (congenital) Q43.9
  acquired K62.8

Deformity — *continued*
　reduction (extremity) (limb), congenital (*see also* condition and site) Q73.8
　　brain Q04.3
　　lower — *see* Defect, reduction, lower limb
　　upper — *see* Defect, reduction, upper limb
　renal — *see* Deformity, kidney
　respiratory system (congenital) Q34.9
　rib (acquired) M95.4
　　congenital Q76.6
　　　cervical Q76.5
　rotation (joint) (acquired) *see* Deformity, limb, specified site NEC
　　congenital Q74.9
　　hip — *see* Deformity, limb, specified type NEC, thigh
　　congenital Q65.8
　sacroiliac joint (congenital) Q74.2
　　acquired — *see* category M43.8
　sacrum (acquired) — *see* category M43.8
　saddle
　　back — *see* Lordosis
　　nose M95.0
　　　syphilitic A50.57
　salivary gland or duct (congenital) Q38.4
　　acquired K11.8
　scapula (acquired) — *see also* Deformity, limb, specified type NEC, upper limb
　　congenital Q68.8
　scrotum (congenital) — *see also* Malformation, testis and scrotum
　　acquired N50.8
　seminal vesicles (congenital) Q55.4
　　acquired N50.8
　septum, nasal (acquired) J34.2
　shoulder (joint) (acquired) — *see* Deformity, limb, upper arm
　　congenital Q74.0
　　contraction — *see* Contraction, joint, shoulder
　sigmoid (flexure) (congenital) Q43.9
　　acquired K63.8
　skin (congenital) Q82.9
　skull (acquired) M95.2
　　congenital Q75.8
　　　with
　　　　anencephaly Q00.0
　　　　encephalocele — *see* Encephalocele
　　　　hydrocephalus Q03.9
　　　　　with spina bifida — *see* Spina bifida, by site, with hydrocephalus
　　　　microcephaly Q02
　soft parts, organs or tissues (of pelvis)
　　in pregnancy or childbirth NEC — *see* category O34.8
　　　causing obstructed labor O65.5
　spermatic cord (congenital) Q55.4
　　acquired N50.8
　　torsion — *see* Torsion, spermatic cord
　spinal — *see* Dorsopathy, deforming
　　column (acquired) — *see* Dorsopathy, deforming
　　congenital Q67.5
　　cord (congenital) Q06.9
　　　acquired G95.89
　　nerve root (congenital) Q07.9
　spine (acquired) — *see also* Dorsopathy, deforming
　　congenital Q67.5
　　rachitic (*see also* category M49.8) E64.3
　　specified NEC — *see* Dorsopathy, deforming, specified NEC
　spleen
　　acquired D73.8
　　congenital Q89.09
　Sprengel's (congenital) Q74.0
　sternocleidomastoid (muscle), congenital Q68.0
　sternum (acquired) M95.4
　　congenital NEC Q76.7
　stomach (congenital) Q40.3
　　acquired K31.89
　submandibular gland (congenital) Q38.4
　submaxillary gland (congenital) Q38.4
　　acquired K11.8
　talipes — *see* Talipes

Deformity — *continued*
　testis (congenital) — *see also* Malformation, testis and scrotum
　　acquired N44.8
　　　torsion — *see* Torsion, testis
　thigh (acquired) — *see also* Deformity, limb, thigh
　　congenital NEC Q68.8
　thorax (acquired) (wall) M95.4
　　congenital Q67.8
　　sequelae of rickets E64.3
　thumb (acquired) — *see also* Deformity, finger
　　congenital NEC Q68.8
　thymus (tissue) (congenital) Q89.2
　thyroid (gland) (congenital) Q89.2
　　cartilage Q31.8
　　　acquired J38.7
　tibia (acquired) — *see also* Deformity, limb, specified type NEC, lower leg
　　congenital NEC Q68.8
　　saber (syphilitic) A50.56 *[M90.80]*
　toe (acquired) M20.60
　　congenital Q66.9
　　hallux valgus M20.10
　　　left M20.12
　　　right M20.11
　　hallux rigidus M20.20
　　　left M20.22
　　　right M20.21
　　hammer toe M20.40
　　　left M20.42
　　　right M20.41
　　left M20.62
　　right M20.61
　　specified hallux NEC M20.30
　　　left M20.32
　　　right M20.31
　　specified NEC M20.50
　　　left M20.52
　　　right M20.51
　tongue (congenital) Q38.3
　　acquired K14.8
　tooth, teeth K00.2
　trachea (rings) (congenital) Q32.1
　　acquired J39.8
　transverse aortic arch (congenital) Q25.4
　tricuspid (leaflets) (valve) I07.8
　　atresia or stenosis Q22.4
　trunk (acquired) M95.8
　　congenital Q89.9
　ulna (acquired) — *see also* Deformity, limb, forearm
　　congenital NEC Q68.8
　urachus, congenital Q64.4
　ureter (opening) (congenital) Q62.8
　　acquired N28.89
　urethra (congenital) Q64.79
　　acquired N36.8
　urinary tract (congenital) Q64.9
　　urachus Q64.4
　uterus (congenital) Q51.9
　　acquired N85.8
　uvula (congenital) Q38.5
　vagina (acquired) N89.8
　　congenital Q52.4
　valgus NEC M21.00
　　ankle M21.079
　　　left M21.072
　　　right M21.071
　　elbow M21.029
　　　left M21.022
　　　right M21.021
　　knee M21.069
　　　left M21.062
　　　right M21.061
　valve, valvular (congenital) (heart) Q24.8
　　acquired — *see* Endocarditis
　varus NEC M21.10
　　ankle M21.179
　　　left M21.172
　　　right M21.171
　　elbow M21.129
　　　left M21.122
　　　right M21.121
　　knee M21.169
　　　left M21.162
　　　right M21.161

Deformity — *continued*
　varus NEC — *continued*
　　tibia — *see* Osteochondrosis, juvenile, tibia
　vas deferens (congenital) Q55.4
　　acquired N50.8
　vein (congenital) Q27.9
　　great Q26.9
　vertebra — *see* Dorsopathy, deforming
　vesicourethral orifice (acquired) N32.8
　　congenital NEC Q64.79
　vessels of optic papilla (congenital) Q14.2
　visual field (contraction) — *see* Defect, visual field
　vitreous body, acquired H43.89
　vulva (congenital) Q52.79
　　acquired N90.8
　wrist (joint) (acquired) — *see also* Deformity, limb, forearm
　　congenital Q68.1
　　contraction — *see* Contraction, joint, wrist

Degeneration, degenerative
　adrenal (capsule) (fatty) (gland) (hyaline) (infectional) E27.8
　amyloid (*see also* Amyloidosis) E85 *[G99.8]*
　anterior cornua, spinal cord G12.29
　aorta, aortic I70.0
　　fatty I77.8
　aortic valve (heart) — *see* Endocarditis, aortic
　arteriovascular — *see* Arteriosclerosis
　artery, arterial (atheromatous) (calcareous) — *see also* Arteriosclerosis
　　cerebral, amyloid E85 *[I68.1]*
　　medial — *see* Arteriosclerosis, extremities
　articular cartilage NEC — *see also* Disorder, cartilage, articular NEC
　　elbow — *see* Derangement, joint, elbow
　　knee — *see* Chondromalacia, patella
　　shoulder — *see* Derangement, joint, shoulder
　atheromatous — *see* Arteriosclerosis
　basal nuclei or ganglia G23.9
　　specified NEC G23.8
　bone NEC — *see* Disorder, bone, specified type NEC
　brachial plexus G54.0
　brain (cortical) (progressive) G31.9
　　alcoholic G31.2
　　arteriosclerotic I67.2
　　childhood G31.9
　　　specified NEC G31.89
　　cystic G31.89
　　　congenital Q04.6
　　in
　　　alcoholism G31.2
　　　beriberi E51.2
　　　cerebrovascular disease I67.9
　　　congenital hydrocephalus Q03.9
　　　　with spina bifida — *see also* Spina bifida
　　　Fabry-Anderson disease E75.21
　　　Gaucher's disease E75.22
　　　Hunter's syndrome E76.1
　　　lipidosis
　　　　cerebral E75.4
　　　　generalized E75.6
　　　mucopolysaccharidosis — *see* Mucopolysaccharidosis
　　　myxedema E03.9 *[G32.8]*
　　　neoplastic disease (*see also* Neoplasm) D49.6 *[G32.8]*
　　　Niemann-Pick disease E75.249 *[G32.8]*
　　　sphingolipidosis E75.3 *[G32.8]*
　　　vitamin B12 deficiency E53.8 *[G32.8]*
　　senile NEC G31.1
　breast N64.8
　Bruch's membrane — *see* Degeneration, choroid
　capillaries (fatty) I78.8
　　amyloid E85 *[I79.8]*
　cardiac — *see also* Degeneration, myocardial
　　valve, valvular — *see* Endocarditis
　cardiorenal — *see* Hypertension, cardiorenal
　cardiovascular — *see also* Disease, cardiovascular
　　renal — *see* Hypertension, cardiorenal
　cerebellar NOS G31.9
　　alcoholic G31.2

Degeneration, degenerative — *continued*
  cerebellar NOS — *continued*
    primary (hereditary) (sporadic) G11.9
  cerebral — *see* Degeneration, brain
  cerebrovascular I67.9
    due to hypertension I67.4
  cervical plexus G54.2
  cervix N88.8
    due to radiation (intended effect) N88.8
      adverse effect or misadventure N99.89
  chamber angle H21.219
    bilateral H21.213
    left H21.212
    right H21.211
  changes, spine or vertebra — *see* Spondylosis
  chorioretinal — *see also* Degeneration, choroid
    hereditary H31.20
  choroid (colloid) (drusen) H31.119
    atrophy — *see* Atrophy, choroidal
    bilateral H31.113
    hereditary — *see* Dystrophy, choroidal,
      hereditary
    left H31.112
    right H31.111
  ciliary body H21.229
    bilateral H21.223
    left H21.222
    right H21.221
  cochlear — *see* category H83.8
  combined (spinal cord) (subacute) E53.8
    [G32.0]
    with anemia (pernicious) D51.0 *[G32.0]*
      due to dietary vitamin B12 deficiency
        D51.3 *[G32.0]*
    in (due to)
      vitamin B12 deficiency E53.8 *[G32.0]*
        anemia D51.9 *[G32.0]*
  conjunctiva H11.10
    concretions — *see* Concretion, conjunctiva
    deposits — *see* Deposit, conjunctiva
    pigmentations — *see* Pigmentation,
      conjunctiva
    pinguecula — *see* Pinguecula
    xerosis — *see* Xerosis, conjunctiva
  cornea H18.40
    calcerous H18.43
      band keratopathy H18.429
        bilateral H18.423
        left H18.422
        right H18.421
    familial, hereditary — *see* Dystrophy, cornea
    hyaline (of old scars) H18.49
    keratomalacia — *see* Keratomalacia
    nodular H18.459
      bilateral H18.453
      left H18.452
      right H18.451
    peripheral H18.469
      bilateral H18.463
      left H18.462
      right H18.461
    senile H18.419
      bilateral H18.413
      left H18.412
      right H18.411
    specified type NEC H18.49
  cortical (cerebellar) (parenchymatous) G31.89
    alcoholic G31.2
    diffuse, due to arteriopathy I67.2
  cutis L98.8
    amyloid E85 *[L99]*
  dental pulp K04.2
  disc disease — *see* Degeneration, intervertebral
    disc NEC
  dorsolateral (spinal cord) — *see* Degeneration,
    combined
  extrapyramidal G25.9
  eye, macular — *see also* Degeneration, macula
    congenital or hereditary — *see* Dystrophy,
      retina
  facet joints — *see* Spondylosis
  fatty
    liver NEC K76.0
      alcoholic K70.0
    placenta — *see* Disorder, placenta,
      malformation
  grey matter (brain) (Alpers') G31.81

Degeneration, degenerative — *continued*
  heart — *see also* Degeneration, myocardial
    amyloid E85 *[I43]*
    atheromatous — *see* Disease, heart,
      ischemic, atherosclerotic
    ischemic — *see* Disease, heart, ischemic
  hepatolenticular (Wilson's) E83.01
  hepatorenal K76.7
  hyaline (diffuse) (generalized)
    localized — *see* Degeneration, by site
  infrapatellar fat pad M79.4
  intervertebral disc NOS
    with
      myelopathy — *see* Disorder, disc, with,
        myelopathy
      radiculitis or radiculopathy — *see*
        Disorder, disc, with, radiculopathy
    cervical, cervicothoracic — *see* Disorder,
      disc, cervical, degeneration
      with
        myelopathy — *see* Disorder, disc,
          cervical, with myelopathy
        neuritis, radiculitis or radiculopathy —
          see Disorder, disc, cervical, with
          neuritis
    lumbar region M51.36
      with
        myelopathy M51.06
        neuritis, radiculitis, radiculopathy or
          sciatica M51.16
    lumbosacral region M51.37
      with
        myelopathy M51.07
        neuritis, radiculitis, radiculopathy or
          sciatica M51.17
    sacrococcygeal region M53.3
    thoracic region M51.34
      with
        myelopathy M51.04
        neuritis, radiculitis, radiculopathy
          M51.14
    thoracolumbar region M51.35
      with
        myelopathy M51.05
        neuritis, radiculitis, radiculopathy
          M51.15
  intestine, amyloid E85 *[K93]*
  iris (pigmentary) H21.239
    bilateral H21.233
    left H21.232
    right H21.231
  ischemic — *see* Ischemia
  joint disease — *see* Osteoarthrosis
  kidney N28.89
    amyloid E85 *[N29]*
    cystic, congenital Q61.9
    fatty N28.89
    polycystic Q61.3
      adult type (autosomal dominant) Q61.2
      infantile type (autosomal recessive)
        Q61.19
        collecting duct dilatation Q61.11
  Kuhnt-Junius — *see* Degeneration, macula
  lens — *see* Cataract
  lenticular (familial) (progressive) (Wilson's) (with
    cirrhosis of liver) E83.01
  liver (diffuse) NEC K76.8
    amyloid E85 *[K77]*
    cystic K76.8
      congenital Q44.6
    fatty NEC K76.0
      alcoholic K70.0
    hypertrophic K76.8
    parenchymatous, acute or subacute K72.00
      with coma K72.01
    pigmentary K76.8
    toxic (acute) K71.9
  lung J98.4
  lymph gland I89.8
    hyaline I89.8
  macula, macular (acquired) (atrophic)
    (exudative) (senile) H35.30
    angioid streaks H35.33
    congenital or hereditary — *see* Dystrophy,
      retina
    cystoid H35.359
      bilateral H35.353

Degeneration, degenerative — *continued*
  macula, macular — *continued*
    cystoid — *continued*
      left H35.352
      right H35.351
    drusen H35.369
      bilateral H35.363
      left H35.362
      right H35.361
    exudative H35.31
    hole H35.349
      bilateral H35.343
      left H35.342
      right H35.341
    nonexudative H35.32
    puckering H35.379
      bilateral H35.373
      left H35.372
      right H35.371
    toxic H35.389
      bilateral H35.383
      left H35.382
      right H35.381
  membranous labyrinth, congenital (causing
    impairment of hearing) Q16.5
  meniscus — *see* Derangement, meniscus
  mitral — *see* Insufficiency, mitral
  Mönckeberg's — *see* Arteriosclerosis,
    extremities
  motor centers, senile G31.1
  multi-system G90.3
  mural — *see* Degeneration, myocardial
  muscle (fatty) (fibrous) (hyaline) (progressive)
    M62.89
    heart — *see* Degeneration, myocardial
  myelin, central nervous system G37.9
  myocardial, myocardium (fatty) (hyaline) (senile)
    I51.5
    with rheumatic fever (conditions in I00)
      I09.0
      active, acute or subacute I01.2
        with chorea I02.0
      inactive or quiescent (with chorea) I09.0
    hypertensive — *see* Hypertension, heart
    rheumatic — *see* Degeneration, myocardial,
      with rheumatic fever
    syphilitic A52.06
  nasal sinus (mucosa) J32.9
    frontal J32.1
    maxillary J32.0
  nerve — *see* Disorder, nerve
  nervous system G31.9
    alcoholic G31.2
    amyloid E85 *[G99.8]*
    autonomic G90.9
    fatty G31.89
    specified NEC G31.89
  nipple N64.8
  olivopontocerebellar (hereditary) (familial)
    G23.8
  osseous labyrinth — *see* category H83.8
  ovary N83.8
    cystic N83.20
    microcystic N83.20
  pallidal pigmentary (progressive) G23.0
  pancreas K86.8
    tuberculous A18.83
  penis N48.89
  pigmentary (diffuse) (general)
    localized — *see* Degeneration, by site
    pallidal (progressive) G23.0
  pineal gland E34.8
  pituitary (gland) E23.6
  placenta O43.899
    first trimester O43.891
    second trimester O43.892
    third trimester O43.893
  popliteal fat pad M79.4
  posterolateral (spinal cord) — *see* Degeneration,
    combined
  pulmonary valve (heart) I37.8
  pulp (tooth) K04.2
  pupillary margin H21.249
    bilateral H21.243
    left H21.242
    right H21.241
  renal — *see* Degeneration, kidney

Degeneration, degenerative — *continued*
retina H35.9
  hereditary (cerebroretinal) (congenital) (juvenile) (macula) (peripheral) (pigmentary) — *see* Dystrophy, retina
  Kuhnt-Junius — *see* Degeneration, macula, hole
  macula (cystic) (exudative) (hole) (nonexudative) (pseudohole) (senile) (toxic) — *see* Degeneration, macula
  peripheral H35.40
    lattice H35.419
      bilateral H35.413
      left H35.412
      right H35.411
    microcystoid H35.429
      bilateral H35.423
      left H35.422
      right H35.421
    paving stone H35.439
      bilateral H35.433
      left H35.432
      right H35.431
  secondary
    pigmentary H35.459
      bilateral H35.453
      left H35.452
      right H35.451
    vitreoretinal H35.469
      bilateral H35.463
      left H35.462
      right H35.461
  senile reticular H35.449
    bilateral H35.443
    left H35.442
    right H35.441
  pigmentary (primary) — *see also* Dystrophy, retina
  secondary — *see* Degeneration, retina, peripheral, secondary
  posterior pole — *see* Degeneration, macula
saccule, congenital (causing impairment of hearing) Q16.5
senile R54
  brain G31.1
  cardiac, heart or myocardium — *see* Degeneration, myocardial
  motor centers G31.1
  vascular — *see* Arteriosclerosis
sinus (cystic) — *see also* Sinusitis
  polypoid J33.1
skin L98.8
  amyloid E85 [L99]
  colloid L98.8
spinal (cord) G31.89
  amyloid E85 [G32.8]
  combined (subacute) — *see* Degeneration, combined
  dorsolateral — *see* Degeneration, combined
  familial NEC G31.89
  fatty G31.89
  funicular — *see* Degeneration, combined
  posterolateral — *see* Degeneration, combined
  subacute combined — *see* Degeneration, combined
  tuberculous A17.81
spleen D73.0
  amyloid E85 [D77]
stomach K31.89
striatonigral G23.2
suprarenal (capsule) (gland) E27.8
synovial membrane (pulpy) — *see* Disorder, synovium, specified type NEC
tapetoretinal — *see* Dystrophy, retina
thymus (gland) E32.8
  fatty E32.8
thyroid (gland) E07.89
tricuspid (heart) (valve) I07.9
tuberculous NEC — *see* Tuberculosis
turbinate J34.8
uterus (cystic) N85.8
vascular (senile) — *see* Arteriosclerosis
  hypertensive — *see* Hypertension
vitreoretinal, secondary — *see* Degeneration, retina, peripheral, secondary, vitreoretinal

Degeneration, degenerative — *continued*
vitreous (body) H43.819
  bilateral H43.813
  left H43.812
  right H43.811
Wallerian — *see* Disorder, nerve
Wilson's hepatolenticular E83.01
Deglutition
paralysis R13.0
  hysterical F44.4
  pneumonia J69.0
Degos' disease I77.8
Dehiscence
cesarean wound O90.0
episiotomy O90.1
operation wound NEC T81.3
perineal wound (postpartum) O90.1
postoperative NEC (abdomen) T81.3
Dehydration E86.0
hypertonic E87.0
hypotonic E87.1
newborn P74.1
Déjérine-Roussy syndrome G93.8
Déjérine-Sottas disease or neuropathy (hypertrophic) G60.0
Déjérine-Thomas atrophy G23.8
Delay, delayed
any plane in pelvis
  complicating delivery O66.9
birth or delivery NOS O63.9
closure, ductus arteriosus (Botalli) P29.3
coagulation — *see* Defect, coagulation
conduction (cardiac) (ventricular) I45.9
delivery, second twin, triplet, etc O63.2
development R62.50
  intellectual (specific) F81.9
  learning F81.9
  physiological R62.50
    specified stage NEC R62.0
  reading F81.0
  sexual E30.0
  speech F80.9
  spelling F81.81
gastric emptying K30
menarche E28.3
menstruation (cause unknown) N91.0
milestone R62.0
passage of meconium (newborn) P76.0
primary respiration P28.9
puberty (constitutional) E30.0
sexual maturation, female E30.0
union, fracture — *see* Fracture, by site
Deletion
autosome Q93.9
chromosome
  with complex rearrangements NEC Q93.7
  part Q93.5
  seen only at prometaphase Q93.8
  short arm
    specified part NEC Q93.5
    4 Q93.3
    5 Q93.4
  specified NEC Q93.8
long arm chromosome 18 or 21 Q93.8
  with complex rearrangements NEC Q93.7
Delhi boil or button B55.1
Delinquency (juvenile) (neurotic) F91.8
group Z72.810
Delirium, delirious (acute or subacute) (not alcoholor drug-induced) (with dementia) R41.0
alcoholic (acute) (tremens) (withdrawal) F10.921
  with intoxication F10.921
    in
      abuse F10.121
      dependence F10.221
due to (secondary to)
  alcohol
    intoxication F10.921
      in
        abuse F10.121
        dependence F10.221
      withdrawal F10.231

Delinquency — *continued*
due to — *continued*
  amphetamine intoxication F15.921
    in
      abuse F15.121
      dependence F15.221
  anxiolytic
    intoxication F13.921
      in
        abuse F13.121
        dependence F13.221
      withdrawal F13.231
  cannabis intoxication (acute) F12.921
    in
      abuse F12.121
      dependence F12.221
  cocaine intoxication (acute) F14.921
    in
      abuse F14.121
      dependence F14.221
  general medical condition F05
  hallucinogen intoxication F16.921
    in
      abuse F16.121
      dependence F16.221
  hypnotic
    intoxication F13.921
      in
        abuse F13.121
        dependence F13.221
      withdrawal F13.231
  inhalant intoxication (acute) F18.921
    in
      abuse F18.121
      dependence F18.221
  multiple etiologies F05
  opioid intoxication (acute) F11.921
    in
      abuse F11.121
      dependence F11.221
  phencyclidine intoxication (acute) F19.921
    in
      abuse F19.121
      dependence F19.221
  psychoactive substance NEC intoxication (acute) F19.921
    in
      abuse F19.121
      dependence F19.221
  sedative
    intoxication F13.921
      abuse F13.121
      dependence F13.221
    withdrawal F13.231
  unknown etiology F05
exhaustion F43.0
hysterical F44.89
puerperal F05
thyroid — *see* Thyrotoxicosis with thyroid storm
traumatic — *see* Injury, intracranial
tremens (alcohol-induced) F10.231
  sedative-induced F13.231
uremic N19
Delivery (single)
cesarean (for)
  abnormal
    cervix — *see* Abnormal, cervix, in pregnancy or childbirth
    pelvis (bony) (deformity) (major) NEC with disproportion (fetopelvic) O33.0
      with obstructed labor O65.0
    presentation or position O32.9
      in multiple gestation O32.5
    uterus, congenital — *see* Abnormal, uterus in pregnancy or childbirth
    vagina — *see* Abnormal, vagina in pregnancy or childbirth
    vulva — *see* Abnormal, vulva in pregnancy and childbirth
  abruptio placentae — *see* Disorder, placenta, abruptio
  acromion presentation O32.2
  anteversion, uterus — *see* Abnormal, uterus in pregnancy or childbirth

Delivery — *continued*
  cesarean — *continued*
    atony, uterus O62.2
    breech presentation O32.1
      incomplete O32.8
    brow presentation O32.3
    cephalopelvic disproportion O33.9
    cerclage –*see* Incompetence, cervix, in pregnancy
    chin presentation O32.3
    cicatrix of cervix — *see* Abnormal, cervix, in pregnancy or childbirth
    contracted pelvis (general)
      inlet O33.2
      outlet O33.3
    cord presentation or prolapse O69.0
    cystocele — *see* category O34.8
    deformity (acquired) (congenital)
      pelvic organs or tissues NEC — *see* category O34.8
      pelvis (bony) NEC O33.0
    displacement, uterus NEC — *see* Abnormal, uterus in pregnancy or childbirth
    disproportion NOS O33.9
    distress
      fetal O77.9
      maternal O75.0
    eclampsia — *see* Eclampsia
    face presentation O32.3
    failed
      forceps O66.5
      trial of labor NOS O66.40
        following previous cesarean section O66.41
      vacuum extraction O66.5
      ventouse O66.5
    fetal-maternal hemorrhage O43.019
      first trimester O43.011
      second trimester O43.012
      third trimester O43.013
    fetus, fetal
      disproportion due to fetal deformity NEC O33.7
      distress O77.9
      prematurity O60.9
        second trimester O60.2
        third trimester O60.3
    hemorrhage (intrapartum) O67.9
      with coagulation defect O67.0
      specified cause NEC O67.8
    high head at term O32.4
    hydrocephalic fetus O33.6
    incarceration of uterus — *see* Abnormal, uterus in pregnancy or childbirth
    incoordinate uterine action O62.4
    increased size, fetus O33.5
    inertia, uterus O62.2
      primary O62.0
      secondary O62.1
    lateroversion, uterus — *see* Abnormal, uterus in pregnancy or childbirth
    mal lie O32.9
    malposition
      fetus O32.9
        in multiple gestation O32.5
      pelvic organs or tissues NEC — *see* category O34.8
      uterus NEC — *see* Abnormal, uterus in pregnancy or childbirth
    malpresentation NOS O32.9
      in multiple gestation O32.5
    maternal
      diabetes mellitus — *see* Diabetes, complicating childbirth
      heart disease NEC — *see* Disease, circulatory system, obstetric
    meconium in liquor O77.0
    oblique presentation O32.2
    oversize fetus O33.5
    pelvic tumor NEC — *see* category O34.8
    placenta previa — *see* Disorder, placenta, previa
    placental insufficiency — *see* category O36.5
    polyp, cervix — *see* Abnormal, cervix, in pregnancy or childbirth
    poor dilatation, cervix O62.0
    pre-eclampsia — *see* Pre-eclampsia

Delivery — *continued*
  cesarean — *continued*
    previous
      cesarean section O34.21
      surgery (to)
        cervix — *see* Abnormal, cervix, in pregnancy or childbirth
        gynecological NEC — *see* category O34.8
        uterus O34.29
        vagina — *see* Abnormal, vagina in pregnancy or childbirth
    prolapse
      arm or hand O32.2
      uterus — *see* Abnormal, uterus in pregnancy or childbirth
    prolonged labor NOS O63.9
    rectocele — *see* category O34.8
    retroversion — *see* Abnormal, uterus in pregnancy or childbirth
      uterus — *see* Abnormal, uterus in pregnancy or childbirth
    rigid
      cervix — *see* Abnormal, cervix, in pregnancy or childbirth
      pelvic floor — *see* category O34.8
      perineum — *see* Abnormal, vulva in pregnancy and childbirth
      vagina — *see* Abnormal, vagina in pregnancy or childbirth
      vulva — *see* Abnormal, vulva in pregnancy and childbirth
    sacculation, pregnant uterus — *see* Abnormal, uterus in pregnancy or childbirth
    scar(s)
      cervix — *see* Abnormal, cervix, in pregnancy or childbirth
      cesarean section O34.21
      uterus O34.29
    Shirodkar suture in situ — *see* Incompetence, cervix, in pregnancy
    shoulder presentation O32.2
    stenosis or stricture, cervix — *see* Abnormal, cervix, in pregnancy or childbirth
    transverse presentation or lie O32.2
    tumor, pelvic organs or tissues NEC — *see* category O34.8
      cervix — *see* Abnormal, cervix, in pregnancy or childbirth
    umbilical cord presentation or prolapse O69.0
  completely normal case O80
  complicated O75.9
    by
      abnormal, abnormality (of)
        forces of labor O62.9
          specified type NEC O62.8
        glucose tolerance test O99.821
        uterine contractions NOS O62.9
      abruptio placentae — *see* Disorder, placenta, abruptio
      abuse (physical) (suspected) O94.330
        confirmed O94.331
        psychological (suspected) O94.530
          confirmed O94.531
        sexual (suspected) O94.430
          confirmed O94.431
      adherent placenta O72.0
        without hemorrhage O73.0
      anesthetic death O74.8
      annular detachment of cervix O71.3
      apoplexy (cerebral) — *see* Disease, circulatory system, obstetric
      atony, uterus O62.2
      Bandl's ring O62.4
      bleeding — *see* Delivery, complicated by, hemorrhage
      blood disorder O99.12
      cerebral hemorrhage — *see* Disease, circulatory system, obstetric
      cervical dystocia (hypotonic) O62.0
      compression of cord (umbilical) NEC O69.2
        affecting fetus P02.5
      contraction, contracted ring O62.4

Delivery — *continued*
  complicated — *continued*
    by — *continued*
      cord (umbilical)
        around neck, tightly or with compression O69.1
        bruising O69.5
        complication O69.9
          specified NEC O69.8
        compression NEC O69.2
        entanglement O69.2
        hematoma O69.5
        presentation O69.0
        prolapse O69.0
        short O69.3
        thrombosis (vessels) O69.5
        vascular lesion O69.5
      Couvelaire uterus — *see* Disorder, placenta, abruptio
      death of fetus, early O02.1
      delay following rupture of membranes (spontaneous) — *see* Rupture, membranes, premature
      diastasis recti (abdominis) O71.89
      dilatation
        bladder O66.8
        cervix incomplete, poor or slow O62.0
      diseased placenta — *see* Disorder, placenta
      disruptio uteri — *see* Delivery, complicated by, rupture, uterus
      distress
        fetal O77.9
          with meconium in amniotic fluid O77.0
        abnormal
          acid-base balance O68
          heart rate or rhythm O76
        due to drugs O77.1
        specified sign NEC O77.8
        maternal O75.0
      dysfunction, uterus NOS O62.9
        hypertonic O62.4
        hypotonic O62.2
          primary O62.0
          secondary O62.1
        incoordinate O62.4
      eclampsia O15.1
      embolism (pulmonary) — *see* Embolism, obstetric
      endocrine or metabolic disease NEC O99.22
      fetal
        death, early O02.1
        deformity O66.3
        distress — *see* Delivery, complicated by, distress, fetal
        hypoxia O77.9
      fever during labor O75.2
      gastrointestinal disease NEC O99.62
      gestational diabetes O24.425
        diet controlled O24.420
        insulin (and diet) controlled O24.424
      hematoma O71.7
        ischial spine O71.7
        pelvic O71.7
        subdural — *see* Disease, circulatory system, obstetric
        vagina O71.7
        vulva or perineum O71.7
      hemorrhage (uterine) O67.9
        accidental — *see* Disorder, placenta, abruptio
        associated with
          afibrinogenemia O67.0
          coagulation defect O67.0
          hyperfibrinolysis O67.0
          hypofibrinogenemia O67.0
        cerebral — *see* Disease, circulatory system, obstetric
        due to
          low-lying placenta — *see* Disorder, placenta, previa
          placenta previa — *see* Disorder, placenta, previa

Delivery — *continued*
  complicated — *continued*
    by — *continued*
      hemorrhage — *continued*
        due to — *continued*
          premature separation of placenta
            (normally implanted) — *see*
            Disorder, placenta, abruptio
          retained placenta O72.0
          trauma (obstetric) O67.8
          uterine leiomyoma O67.8
        placenta NEC O67.8
        postpartum NEC (atonic) (immediate)
          O72.1
          with retained or trapped placenta
            O72.0
          delayed O72.2
          secondary O72.2
          third stage O72.0
      hourglass contraction, uterus O62.4
      hypertension — *see* Hypertension,
        complicating pregnancy
      incomplete dilatation (cervix) O62.0
      incoordinate uterus contractions O62.4
      inertia, uterus O62.2
        affecting fetus P03.6
        primary O62.0
        secondary O62.1
      infantile
        genitalia NEC — *see* category O34.8
        uterus — *see* Abnormal, uterus in
          pregnancy or childbirth
      injury (to mother) O71.9
        nonobstetric O94.22
          caused by abuse — *see* Delivery,
            complicated by, abuse
      intrauterine fetal death, early O02.1
      inversion, uterus O71.2
      laceration (perineal) O70.9
        anus (sphincter) O70.2
          with mucosa O70.3
        bladder (urinary) O71.5
        bowel O71.5
        cervix (uteri) O71.3
        fourchette O70.0
        hymen O70.0
        labia O70.0
        pelvic
          floor O70.1
          organ NEC O71.5
        perineum, perineal O70.9
          first degree O70.0
          fourth degree O70.3
          muscles O70.1
          second degree O70.1
          skin O70.0
          slight O70.0
          third degree O70.2
        peritoneum O71.5
        rectovaginal (septum) (without perineal
          laceration) O71.4
          with perineum O70.2
            with anal or rectal mucosa
              O70.3
        specified NEC O71.89
        sphincter ani O70.2
          with mucosa O70.3
        urethra O71.5
        uterus O71.1
          before labor — *see* Rupture, uterus,
            before labor
          other specified O71.81
        vagina, vaginal (deep) (high) (without
          perineal laceration) O71.4
          with perineum O70.0
          muscles, with perineum O70.1
        vulva O70.0
      malignancy O94.12
      malposition
        placenta (with hemorrhage) — *see*
          Disorder, placenta, previa
        uterus or cervix O65.5
      meconium in liquor — *see* Delivery,
        complicated by, distress, fetal

Delivery — *continued*
  complicated — *continued*
    by — *continued*
      metrorrhexis — *see* Delivery, complicated
        by, rupture, uterus
      obstetric trauma O71.9
        specified NEC O71.89
      obstruction — *see* Labor, obstructed
      pathological retraction ring, uterus O62.4
      penetration, pregnant uterus by
        instrument O71.1
      perforation — *see* Delivery, complicated
        by, laceration
      placenta, placental
        ablatio — *see* Disorder, placenta,
          abruptio
        abnormality — *see* Abnormal, placenta
        abruptio — *see* Disorder, placenta,
          abruptio
        accreta O72.0
          without hemorrhage O73.0
        adherent (with hemorrhage) O72.0
          without hemorrhage O73.0
        detachment (premature) — *see*
          Disorder, placenta, abruptio
        disorder — *see* Disorder, placenta
        hemorrhage NEC O67.8
        increta (with hemorrhage) O72.0
          without hemorrhage O73.0
        low (implantation) — *see* Disorder,
          placenta, previa
        malformation — *see* Abnormal,
          placenta
        malposition — *see* Disorder, placenta,
          previa
        percreta O72.0
          without hemorrhage O73.0
        previa (central) (lateral) (marginal)
          (partial) — *see* Disorder,
          placenta, previa
        retained (with hemorrhage) O72.0
          without hemorrhage O73.0
        separation (premature) — *see*
          Disorder, placenta, abruptio
        vicious insertion — *see* Disorder,
          placenta, previa
      precipitate labor O62.3
        affecting fetus P03.5
      premature rupture, membranes — *see*
        Rupture, membranes, premature
      previous
        cesarean section O34.21
        surgery
          cervix — *see* Abnormal, cervix, in
            pregnancy or childbirth
          gynecological NEC — *see* category
            O34.8
          perineum — *see* Abnormal, vulva in
            pregnancy and childbirth
          uterus NEC O34.29
          vagina — *see* Abnormal, vagina in
            pregnancy or childbirth
          vulva — *see* Abnormal, vulva in
            pregnancy and childbirth
      primipara, elderly or old – code to specific
        condition complicating delivery
      prolapse
        arm or hand O32.8
        cord (umbilical) O69.0
        foot or leg O32.8
        uterus — *see* Abnormal, uterus in
          pregnancy or childbirth
      prolonged labor O63.9
        first stage O63.0
        second stage O63.1
      respiratory disease NEC O99.52
      retained membranes or portions of
        placenta O72.2
        without hemorrhage O73.1
      retarded birth O63.9
      retention of secundines (with
        hemorrhage) O72.0
        without hemorrhage O73.0
        partial O72.2
          without hemorrhage O73.1

Delivery — *continued*
  complicated — *continued*
    by — *continued*
      rupture
        bladder (urinary) O71.5
        cervix O71.3
        pelvic organ NEC O71.5
        perineum (without mention of other
          laceration) — *see* Delivery,
          complicated by, laceration,
          perineum
        urethra O71.5
        uterus (during or after labor) O71.1
          before labor — *see* Rupture, uterus,
            before labor
      sacculation, pregnant uterus — *see*
        Abnormal, uterus in pregnancy or
        childbirth
      scar(s)
        cervix — *see* Abnormal, cervix, in
          pregnancy or childbirth
        cesarean section O34.21
        uterus NEC O34.29
      separation, pubic bone (symphysis pubis)
        O71.6
      shock O75.1
      shoulder presentation O64.4
      skin disorder NEC O99.73
      spasm, cervix O62.4
      specified condition NEC O99.88
      stenosis or stricture, cervix O65.5
      stillbirth, early O02.1
      streptococcus B carrier state O99.831
      stress, fetal — *see* Delivery, complicated
        by, distress, fetal
      tear — *see* Delivery, complicated by,
        laceration
      tetanic uterus O62.4
      trauma (obstetrical) O71.9
        non-obstetric O94.22
      tumor, pelvic organs or tissues NEC
        O65.5
      uterine inertia O62.2
        primary O62.0
        secondary O62.1
      vasa previa O69.4
      velamentous insertion of cord O69.8
  delayed NOS O63.9
    following rupture of membranes
      artificial O75.5
      spontaneous — *see* Rupture, membranes,
        premature
    second twin, triplet, etc. O63.2
  difficult NEC
    previous, affecting management of
      pregnancy — *see* Antenatal, care, high
      risk pregnancy, history of, specified
      obstetric problem NEC
  early onset (spontaneous) O60.9
    second trimester O60.2
    third trimester O60.3
  forceps, low following failed vacuum extraction
    O66.5
  missed (at or near term) O36.4
  normal O80
  precipitate O62.3
  premature or preterm NOS O60.9
    previous, affecting management of
      pregnancy — *see* Antenatal, care, high
      risk pregnancy, history of, specified
      obstetric problem NEC
    second trimester O60.2
    third trimester O60.3
  spontaneous O80
  term pregnancy NOS O80
  threatened premature — *see* False, labor
  uncomplicated O80
  vaginal, following previous cesarean section
    O34.21

Delusions (paranoid) — *see* Disorder, delusional

Dementia (degenerative) (primary) (old age)
  (persisting) F03
  alcoholic F10.97
    with dependence F10.27
  Alzheimer's type — *see* Disease, Alzheimer's
  arteriosclerotic — *see* Dementia, vascular

Dementia — *continued*
atypical, Alzheimer's type — *see* Disease, Alzheimer's, specified NEC
congenital — *see* Retardation, mental
in (due to)
  alcohol F10.97
    with dependence F10.27
  Alzheimer's disease — *see* Disease, Alzheimer's
  arteriosclerotic brain disease— *see* Dementia, vascular
  cerebral lipidoses E75.4 *[F02.80]*
    with behavioral disturbance E75.4 *[F02.81]*
  Creutzfeldt-Jakob disease A81.0 *[F02.80]*
    with behavioral disturbance A81.0 *[F02.81]*
  epilepsy G40.90 *[F02.80]*
    with behavioral disturbance G40.90 *[F02.81]*
  general paralysis of the insane A52.17 *[F02.80]*
    with behavioral disturbance A52.17 *[F02.81]*
  hepatolenticular degeneration E83.01 *[F02.80]*
    with behavioral disturbance E83.01 *[F02.81]*
  human immunodeficiency virus (HIV) disease B20 *[F02.80]*
    with behavioral disturbance B20 *[F02.81]*
  Huntington's disease or chorea G10 *[F02.80]*
    with behavioral disturbance G10 *[F02.81]*
  hypercalcemia E83.52 *[F02.80]*
    with behavioral disturbance E83.52 *[F02.81]*
  hypothyroidism, acquired E03.9 *[F02.80]*
    with behavioral disturbance E03.9 *[F02.81]*
    due to iodine deficiency E01.8 *[F02.80]*
      with behavioral disturbance E01.8 *[F02.81]*
  inhalants F18.97
    with dependence F18.27
  multiple
    etiologies F03
  sclerosis G35 *[F02.80]*
    with behavioral disturbance G35 *[F02.81]*
  neurosyphilis A52.17 *[F02.80]*
    with behavioral disturbance A52/17 *[F02.81]*
    juvenile A50.49 *[F02.80]*
      with behavioral disturbance A50.49 *[F02.81]*
  niacin deficiency E52 *[F02.80]*
    with behavioral disturbance E52 *[F02.81]*
  paralysis agitans G20 *[F02.80]*
    with behavioral disturbance G20 *[F02.81]*
  Parkinson's disease (parkinsonism) G20 *[F02.80]*
    with behavioral disturbance G20 *[F02.81]*
  pellagra E52 *[F02.80]*
    with behavioral disturbance E52 *[F02.81]*
  Pick's G31.0 *[F02.80]*
    with behavioral disturbance G31.0 *[F02.81]*
  polyarteritis nodosa M30.0 *[F02.80]*
    with behavioral disturbance M30.0 *[F02.81]*
  psychoactive drug F19.97
    with dependence F19.27
    inhalants F18.97
      with dependence F18.27
    sedatives, hypnotics or anxiolytics F13.97
      with dependence F13.27
  sedatives, hypnotics or anxiolytics F13.97
    with dependence F13.27
  systemic lupus erythematosus M32.9 *[F02.80]*
    with behavioral disturbance M32.9 *[F02.81]*
  trypanosomiasis
    African B56.9 *[F02.80]*
      with behavioral disturbance B56.9 *[F02.81]*
  unknown etiology F03

Dementia — *continued*
in — *continued*
  vitamin B$_{12}$ deficiency E53.8 *[F02.80]*
    with behavioral disturbance E53.8 *[F02.81]*
  volatile solvents F18.97
    with dependence F18.27
infantile, infantilis F84.3
multi-infarct — *see* Dementia, vascular
paralytica, paralytic (syphilitic) A52.17
  juvenilis A50.45 *[F02.80]*
    with behavioral disturbance A50.45 *[F02.81]*
paretic A52.17
praecox — *see* Schizophrenia
presenile F03
  Alzheimer's type — *see* Disease, Alzheimer's, early onset
primary degenerative F03
progressive, syphilitic A52.17
senile F03
  with acute confusional state F05
  Alzheimer's type — *see* Disease, Alzheimer's, late onset
  depressed or paranoid type F03
uremic N18.8 *[F02.80]*
  with behavioral disturbance N18.8 *[F02.81]*
vascular (acute onset) (mixed) (multi-infarct) (subcortical) F01.50
  with behavioral disturbance F01.51

Demineralization, bone — *see* Osteoporosis
Demodex folliculorum (infestation) B88.0
Demophobia F40.248
Demoralization R45.3
Demyelination, demyelinization
central nervous system G37.9
  specified NEC G37.8
corpus callosum (central) G37.1
disseminated, acute G36.9
  specified NEC G36.8
global G35
in optic neuritis G36.0
Dengue (classical) (fever) A90
hemorrhagic A91
sandfly A93.1
Dennie-Marfan syphilitic syndrome A50.45
Dens evaginatus, in dente or invaginatus K00.2
Density
increased, bone (disseminated) (generalized) (spotted) — *see* Disorder, bone, density and structure, specified type NEC
lung (nodular) J98.4
Dental — *see also* condition
examination Z01.20
  with abnormal findings Z01.21
Dentia praecox K00.6
Denticles (pulp) K04.2
Dentigerous cyst K09.0
Dentin
irregular (in pulp) K04.3
opalescent K00.5
secondary (in pulp) K04.3
sensitive K03.8
Dentinogenesis imperfecta K00.5
Dentinoma (M9271/0) D16.5
upper jaw (bone) D16.4
Dentition (syndrome) K00.7
delayed K00.6
difficult K00.7
precocious K00.6
premature K00.6
retarded K00.6
Dependence (syndrome) F19.20
with remission F19.21
alcohol (ethyl) (methyl) (without remission) F10.20
  with
    amnestic disorder, persisting F10.26
    anxiety disorder F10.280
    dementia, persisting F10.27
    intoxication F10.229
      with delirium F10.221
      uncomplicated F10.220
    mood disorder F10.24

Dependence — *continued*
alcohol — *continued*
  with — *continued*
    psychotic disorder F10.259
      with
        delusions F10.250
        hallucinations F10.251
    remission F10.21
    sexual dysfunction F10.281
    sleep disorder F10.282
    specified disorder NEC F10.288
    withdrawal F10.239
      with
        delirium F10.231
        perceptual disturbance F10.232
      uncomplicated F10.230
  complicating
    childbirth O99.314
    pregnancy O99.313
      first trimester O99.310
      second trimester O99.311
      third trimester O99.312
    puerperium O99.315
  counselling and surveillance Z71.41
  detoxification therapy Z51.89
  rehabilitation measures Z51.89
amobarbital — *see* Dependence, drug, sedative
amphetamine(s) (type) — *see* Dependence, drug, stimulant NEC
amytal (sodium) — *see* Dependence, drug, sedative
analgesic NEC F55.8
anesthetic (agent) (gas) (general) (local) NEC — *see* Dependence, drug, psychoactive NEC
anxiolytic NEC — *see* Dependence, drug, sedative
barbital(s) — *see* Dependence, drug, sedative
barbiturate(s) (compounds) (drugs classifiable to T42.30-T42.33) — *see* Dependence, drug, sedative
benzedrine — *see* Dependence, drug, stimulant NEC
bhang — *see* Dependence, drug, cannabis
bromide(s) NEC — *see* Dependence, drug, sedative
caffeine — *see* Dependence, drug, stimulant NEC
cannabis (sativa) (indica) (resin) (derivatives) (type) — *see* Dependence, drug, cannabis
chloral (betaine) (hydrate) — *see* Dependence, drug, sedative
chlordiazepoxide — *see* Dependence, drug, sedative
coca (leaf) (derivatives) — *see* Dependence, drug, cocaine
cocaine — *see* Dependence, drug, cocaine
codeine — *see* Dependence, drug, opioid
combinations of drugs F19.20
dagga — *see* Dependence, drug, cannabis
demerol — *see* Dependence, drug, opioid
dexamphetamine — *see* Dependence, drug, stimulant NEC
dexedrine — *see* Dependence, drug, stimulant NEC
dextromethorphan — *see* Dependence, drug, opioid
dextromoramide — *see* Dependence, drug, opioid
dextro-nor-pseudo-ephedrine — *see* Dependence, drug, stimulant NEC
dextrorphan — *see* Dependence, drug, opioid
diazepam — *see* Dependence, drug, sedative
dilaudid — *see* Dependence, drug, opioid
D-lysergic acid diethylamide — *see* Dependence, drug, hallucinogen
drug NEC F19.20
  cannabis F12.20
    with
      anxiety disorder F12.280
      intoxication F12.229
        with
          delirium F12.221
          perceptual disturbance F12.222
        uncomplicated F12.220
      other specified disorder F12.288

©2002 Ingenix, Inc.

Dependence — continued
drug NEC — continued
cannabis — continued
with — continued
psychosis F12.259
delusions F12.250
hallucinations F12.251
unspecified disorder F12.29
in remission F12.21
cocaine F14.20
with
anxiety disorder F14.280
intoxication F14.229
with
delirium F14.221
perceptual disturbance F14.222
uncomplicated F14.220
mood disorder F14.24
other specified disorder F14.288
psychosis F14.259
delusions F14.250
hallucinations F14.251
sexual dysfunction F14.281
sleep disorder F14.282
unspecified disorder F14.29
withdrawal F14.23
in remission F14.21
complicating pregnancy, childbirth or the
puerperium — see Dependence, drug,
obstetric
affecting fetus or newborn P04.49
cocaine P04.41
withdrawal symptoms in newborn P96.1
counselling and surveillance Z71.51
detoxification therapy NEC Z51.89
hallucinogen F16.20
with
anxiety disorder F16.280
flashbacks F16.283
intoxication F16.229
with delirium F16.221
uncomplicated F16.220
mood disorder F16.24
other specified disorder F16.288
perception disorder, persisting
F16.283
psychosis F16.259
delusions F16.250
hallucinations F16.251
unspecified disorder F16.29
in remission F16.21
in remission F19.21
inhalant F18.20
with
amnestic disorder F13.26
anxiety disorder F18.280
dementia, persisting F18.27
intoxication F18.229
with delirium F18.221
uncomplicated F18.220
mood disorder F18.24
other specified disorder F18.288
psychosis F18.259
delusions F18.250
hallucinations F18.251
sexual dysfunction F13.281
sleep disorder F13.282
unspecified disorder F18.29
withdrawal F13.239
with
delirium F13.231
perceptual disturbance F13.232
uncomplicated F13.230
in remission F18.21
nicotine F17.200
with disorder F17.209
remission F17.201
specified disorder NEC F17.208
withdrawal F17.203
chewing tobacco F17.220
with disorder F17.229
remission F17.221
specified disorder NEC F17.228
withdrawal F17.223

Dependence — continued
drug NEC — continued
nicotine — continued
cigarettes F17.210
with disorder F17.219
remission F17.211
specified disorder NEC F17.218
withdrawal F17.213
specified product NEC F17.290
with disorder F17.299
remission F17.291
specified disorder NEC F17.298
withdrawal F17.293
obstetric complicating
childbirth O99.324
pregnancy O99.323
first trimester O99.320
second trimester O99.321
third trimester O99.322
puerperium O99.325
opioid F11.20
with
intoxication F11.229
with
delirium F11.221
perceptual disturbance F11.222
uncomplicated F11.220
mood disorder F11.24
other specified disorder F11.288
psychosis F11.259
delusions F11.250
hallucinations F11.251
sexual dysfunction F11.281
sleep disorder F11.282
unspecified disorder F11.29
withdrawal F11.23
in remission F11.21
psychoactive NEC F19.20
with
amnestic disorder F19.26
anxiety disorder F19.280
dementia F19.27
intoxication F19.229
with
delirium F19.221
perceptual disturbance F19.222
uncomplicated F19.220
mood disorder F19.24
other specified disorder F19.288
psychosis F19.259
delusions F19.250
hallucinations F19.251
sexual dysfunction F19.281
sleep disorder F19.282
unspecified disorder F19.29
withdrawal F19.239
with
delirium F19.231
perceptual disturbance F19.232
uncomplicated F19.230
rehabilitation measures Z51.89
sedative, hypnotic or anxiolytic F13.20
with
amnestic disorder F13.26
anxiety disorder F13.280
dementia, persisting F13.27
intoxication F13.229
with delirium F13.221
uncomplicated F13.220
mood disorder F13.24
other specified disorder F13.288
psychosis F13.259
delusions F13.250
hallucinations F13.251
sexual dysfunction F13.281
sleep disorder F13.282
unspecified disorder F13.29
withdrawal F13.239
with
delirium F13.231
perceptual disturbance F13.232
uncomplicated F13.230
in remission F13.21

Dependence — continued
drug NEC — continued
stimulant NEC F15.20
with
anxiety disorder F15.280
intoxication F15.229
with
delirium F15.221
perceptual disturbance F15.222
uncomplicated F15.220
mood disorder F15.24
other specified disorder F15.288
psychosis F15.259
delusions F15.250
hallucinations F15.251
sexual dysfunction F15.281
sleep disorder F15.282
unspecified disorder F15.29
withdrawal F15.23
in remission F15.21
suspected damage to fetus affecting
management of pregnancy O35.5
ethyl
alcohol (without remission) F10.20
with remission F10.21
bromide — see Dependence, drug, sedative
carbamate F19.20
chloride F19.20
morphine — see Dependence, drug, opioid
ganja — see Dependence, drug, cannabis
glue (airplane) (sniffing) — see Dependence,
drug, inhalant
glutethimide — see Dependence, drug, sedative
hallucinogenics — see Dependence, drug,
hallucinogen
hashish — see Dependence, drug, cannabis
hemp — see Dependence, drug, cannabis
heroin (salt) (any) — see Dependence, drug,
opioid
hypnotic NEC — see Dependence, drug,
sedative
Indian hemp — see Dependence, drug,
cannabis
inhalants — see Dependence, drug, inhalant
khat — see Dependence, drug, stimulant NEC
laudanum — see Dependence, drug, opioid
LSD(-25) (derivatives) — see Dependence, drug,
hallucinogen
luminal — see Dependence, drug, sedative
lysergic acid — see Dependence, drug,
hallucinogen
maconha — see Dependence, drug, cannabis
marihuana — see Dependence, drug, cannabis
meprobamate — see Dependence, drug,
sedative
mescaline — see Dependence, drug,
hallucinogen
methadone — see Dependence, drug, opioid
methamphetamine(s) — see Dependence, drug,
stimulant NEC
methaqualone — see Dependence, drug,
sedative
methyl
alcohol (without remission) F10.20
with remission F10.21
bromide — see Dependence, drug, sedative
morphine — see Dependence, drug, opioid
phenidate — see Dependence, drug,
stimulant NEC
sulfonal — see Dependence, drug, sedative
morphine (sulfate) (sulfite) (type) — see
Dependence, drug, opioid
narcotic (drug) NEC — see Dependence, drug,
opioid
nembutal — see Dependence, drug, sedative
neraval — see Dependence, drug, sedative
neravan — see Dependence, drug, sedative
neurobarb — see Dependence, drug, sedative
nicotine — see Dependence, drug, nicotine
nitrous oxide F19.20
nonbarbiturate sedatives and tranquilizers with
similar effect — see Dependence, drug,
sedative
on
aspirator Z99.0
care provider, because (of) Z74.0
impaired mobility Z74.0

Dependence — *continued*
on — *continued*
  care provider, because — *continued*
    need for
      assistance with personal care Z74.1
      continuous supervision Z74.3
    no other household member able to
      render care Z74.2
    specified reason NEC Z74.8
  iron lung Z99.1
  machine Z99.9
    enabling NEC Z99.8
    specified type NEC Z99.8
  renal dialysis Z99.2
  respirator Z99.1
  wheelchair Z99.3
opiate — *see* Dependence, drug, opioid
opioids — *see* Dependence, drug, opioid
opium (alkaloids) (derivatives) (tincture) — *see* Dependence, drug, opioid
paraldehyde — *see* Dependence, drug, sedative
paregoric — *see* Dependence, drug, opioid
PCP (phencyclidine) F19.20
pentobarbital — *see* Dependence, drug, sedative
pentobarbitone (sodium) — *see* Dependence, drug, sedative
pentothal — *see* Dependence, drug, sedative
peyote — *see* Dependence, drug, hallucinogen
phencyclidine (PCP) (and related substances) F19.20
phenmetrazine — *see* Dependence, drug, stimulant NEC
phenobarbital — *see* Dependence, drug, sedative
polysubstance F19.20
psilocibin, psilocin, psilocyn, psilocyline — *see* Dependence, drug, hallucinogen
psychostimulant NEC — *see* Dependence, drug, stimulant NEC
secobarbital — *see* Dependence, drug, sedative
seconal — *see* Dependence, drug, sedative
sedative NEC — *see* Dependence, drug, sedative
specified drug NEC — *see* Dependence, drug
stimulant NEC — *see* Dependence, drug, stimulant NEC
substance NEC — *see* Dependence, drug
tobacco — *see* Dependence, drug, nicotine
  counselling and surveillance Z71.6
tranquilizer NEC — *see* Dependence, drug, sedative
vitamin B6 E53.1
volatile solvents — *see* Dependence, drug, inhalant

Dependency
care-provider Z74.9
passive F60.7
reactions (persistent) F60.7

Depersonalization (in neurotic state) (neurotic) (syndrome) F48.1

Depletion
extracellular fluid E86.1
plasma E86.1
potassium E87.6
  nephropathy N25.8
salt or sodium E87.1
  causing heat exhaustion or prostration T67.4
  nephropathy N28.9
volume NOS E86.9

Depolarization, premature I49.4
atrial I49.1
junctional I49.2
specified NEC I49.4
ventricular I49.3

Deposit
bone in Boeck's sarcoid D86.89
calcareous, calcium — *see* Calcification
cholesterol
  retina H35.89
  vitreous (body) (humor) — *see* Deposit, crystalline
conjunctiva H11.119
  bilateral H11.113
  left H11.112

Deposit — *continued*
conjunctiva — *continued*
  right H11.111
cornea H18.009
  argentous H18.029
    bilateral H18.023
    left H18.022
    right H18.021
  bilateral H18.003
  due to metabolic disorder H18.039
    bilateral H18.033
    left H18.032
    right H18.031
  Kayser-Fleischer ring — *see* Kayser-Fleischer ring
  left H18.002
  pigmentation — *see* Pigmentation, cornea
  right H18.001
crystalline, vitreous (body) (humor) H43.20
  bilateral H43.23
  left H43.22
  right H43.21
hemosiderin in old scars of cornea — *see* Pigmentation, cornea, stromal
metallic in lens — *see* Cataract, specified NEC
skin R23.8
tooth, teeth (betel) (black) (green) (materia alba) (orange) (tobacco) K03.6
urate, kidney — *see* Calculus, kidney

Depraved appetite — *see* Pica

Depression (acute) (mental) F32.9
agitated (single episode) F32.2
anaclitic — *see* Disorder, adjustment
anxiety F41.8
  persistent F34.1
arches — *see also* Deformity, limb, flat foot
  congenital Q66.5
atypical (single episode) F32.8
basal metabolic rate R94.8
bone marrow D75.8
central nervous system R09.2
cerebral R29.81
  newborn P91.4
cerebrovascular I67.9
chest wall M95.4
climacteric (single episode) F32.8
endogenous (without psychotic symptoms) F33.2
  with psychotic symptoms F33.3
functional activity R68.8
hysterical F44.89
involutional (single episode) F32.8
major F32.2
  with psychotic symptoms F32.3
major (recurrent) — *see* Disorder, depressive, recurrent
manic-depressive — *see* Disorder, depressive, recurrent
masked (single episode) F32.8
medullary G93.8
menopausal (single episode) F32.8
metatarsus — *see* Depression, arches
monopolar F33.9
nervous F34.1
neurotic F34.1
nose M95.0
postnatal F53
postpartum F53
post-psychotic of schizophrenia F32.8
post-schizophrenic F32.8
psychogenic (reactive) (single episode) F32.9
psychoneurotic F34.1
psychotic (single episode) F32.3
  recurrent F33.3
reactive (psychogenic) (single episode) F32.9
  psychotic (single episode) F32.3
recurrent — *see* Disorder, depressive, recurrent
respiratory center G93.8
seasonal — *see* Disorder, depressive, recurrent
senile F03
severe, single episode F32.2
skull Q67.4
specified NEC (single episode) F32.8
sternum M95.4
visual field — *see* Defect, visual field
vital (recurrent) (without psychotic symptoms) F33.2

Depression — *continued*
vital — *continued*
  with psychotic symptoms F33.3
  single episode F32.2

Deprivation
cultural Z60.3
effects NOS T73.9
  specified NEC T73.8
emotional NEC Z65.8
  affecting infant or child — *see* Maltreatment, child, psychological
food T73.0
protein — *see* Malnutrition
social Z60.4
  affecting infant or child — *see* Maltreatment, child, psychological
specified NEC T73.8
vitamins — *see* Deficiency, vitamin
water T73.1

Derangement
ankle (internal) — *see* Derangement, joint, ankle
cartilage (articular) NEC — *see also* Disorder, cartilage, articular NEC
  knee, meniscus — *see* Derangement, meniscus
  recurrent — *see* Dislocation, recurrent
cruciate ligament, anterior, current injury — *see* Sprain, knee, cruciate, anterior
elbow (internal) — *see* Derangement, joint, elbow
hip (joint) (internal) (old) — *see* Derangement, joint, hip
joint (internal) M24.9
  ankylosis — *see* Ankylosis, joint
  articular cartilage M24.10
    ankle M24.173
      left M24.172
      right M24.171
    elbow M24.129
      left M24.122
      right M24.121
    foot M24.176
      left M24.175
      right M24.174
    hand M24.149
      left M24.142
      right M24.141
    hip M24.159
      left M24.152
      right M24.151
    knee M24.169
      left M24.162
      right M24.161
    loose body — *see* Loose, body
    shoulder M24.119
      left M24.112
      right M24.111
    vertebra M24.18
    wrist M24.139
      left M24.132
      right M24.131
  contracture — *see* Contraction, joint
  current injury — *see also* Dislocation
    knee, meniscus or cartilage — *see* Tear, meniscus
  dislocation
    pathological — *see* Dislocation, pathological
    recurrent — *see* Dislocation, recurrent
  knee — *see* Derangement, knee
  ligament — *see* Disorder, ligament
  loose body — *see* Loose, body
  recurrent — *see* Dislocation, recurrent
  specified type NEC M24.80
    ankle M24.873
      left M24.872
      right M24.871
    elbow M24.829
      left M24.822
      right M24.821
    foot joint M24.876
      left M24.875
      right M24.874

©2002 Ingenix, Inc.

Derangement — *continued*
  joint — *continued*
    specified type NEC — *continued*
      hand joint M24.849
        left M24.842
        right M24.841
      hip M24.859
        left M24.852
        right M24.851
      knee M24.869
        left M24.862
        right M24.861
      shoulder M24.819
        left M24.812
        right M24.811
      specified joint NEC M24.88
      wrist M24.839
        left M24.832
        right M24.831
    temporomandibular M26.69
  knee (recurrent) M23.90
    left M23.92
    ligament disruption, spontaneous M23.609
      anterior cruciate M23.619
        left M23.612
        right M23.611
      capsular M23.679
        left M23.672
        right M23.671
      instability, chronic M23.50
        left M23.52
        right M23.51
      lateral collateral M23.649
        left M23.642
        right M23.641
      left M23.602
      medial collateral M23.639
        left M23.632
        right M23.631
      posterior cruciate M23.629
        left M23.622
        right M23.621
      right M23.601
    loose body M23.40
      left M23.42
      right M23.41
    meniscus M23.309
      cystic M23.009
        lateral M23.002
          anterior horn M23.049
            left M23.042
            right M23.041
          left M23.001
          posterior horn M23.059
            left M23.052
            right M23.051
        right M23.000
        specified NEC M23.069
          left M23.062
          right M23.061
        left M23.007
        medial M23.005
          anterior horn M23.019
            left M23.012
            right M23.011
          left M23.004
          posterior horn M23.029
            left M23.022
            right M23.021
        right M23.003
        specified NEC M23.039
          left M23.032
          right M23.031
        right M23.006
      degenerate — *see* Derangement, knee,
        meniscus, specified NEC
      detached — *see* Derangement, knee,
        meniscus, specified NEC
      due to old tear or injury M23.209
        lateral M23.202
          anterior horn M23.249
            left M23.242
            right M23.241
          left M23.201
          posterior horn M23.259
            left M23.252

Derangement — *continued*
  knee — *continued*
    meniscus — *continued*
      due to old tear or injury — *continued*
        lateral — *continued*
          posterior horn — *continued*
            right M23.251
          right M23.200
          specified NEC M23.269
            left M23.262
            right M23.261
        left M23.207
        medial M23.205
          anterior horn M23.219
            left M23.212
            right M23.211
          left M23.204
          posterior horn M23.229
            left M23.222
            right M23.221
          right M23.203
          specified NEC M23.239
            left M23.232
            right M23.231
        right M23.206
      retained — *see* Derangement, knee,
        meniscus, specified NEC
      specified NEC M23.309
        lateral M23.302
          anterior horn M23.349
            left M23.342
            right M23.341
          left M23.301
          posterior horn M23.359
            left M23.352
            right M23.351
          right M23.300
          specified NEC M23.369
            left M23.362
            right M23.361
        left M23.307
        medial M23.305
          anterior horn M23.319
            left M23.312
            right M23.311
          left M23.304
          posterior horn M23.329
            left M23.322
            right M23.321
          right M23.303
          specified NEC M23.339
            left M23.332
            right M23.331
        right M23.306
      right M23.91
      specified NEC — *see* category M23.8
    low back NEC — *see* Dorsopathy, specified
      NEC
    meniscus — *see* Derangement, knee, meniscus
    mental — *see* Psychosis
    patella, specified NEC — *see* Disorder, patella,
      derangement NEC
    semilunar cartilage (knee) — *see* Derangement,
      knee, meniscus, specified NEC
    shoulder (internal) — *see* Derangement, joint,
      shoulder

Dercum's disease E88.2

Derealization (neurotic) F48.1

Dermal — *see* condition

Dermaphytid — *see* Dermatophytosis

Dermatitis (eczematous) L30.9
  ab igne L59.0
  acarine B88.0
  actinic (due to sun) L57.8
    other than from sun L59.8
  allergic — *see* Dermatitis, contact, allergic
  ambustionis, due to burn or scald — *see* Burn
  amebic A06.7
  ammonia L22
  arsenical (ingested) L27.8
  artefacta L98.1
    psychogenic F54
  atopic L20.9
    psychogenic F54
    specified NEC L20.89

Dermatitis — *continued*
  berlock, berloque L56.2
  blastomycotic B40.3
  blister beetle L24.8
  bullous, bullosa L13.9
    mucosynechial, atrophic L12.1
    seasonal L30.8
    specified NEC L13.8
  calorica L59.0
    due to burn or scald — *see* Burn
  caterpillar L24.8
  cercarial B65.3
  combustionis L59.0
    due to burn or scald — *see* Burn
  congelationis T69.1
  contact (occupational) L25.9
    allergic L23.9
      due to
        chemical products L23.5
          adhesives L23.1
          cosmetics L23.2
          drugs in contact with skin L23.3
          dyes L23.4
        food in contact with skin L23.6
        metals L23.0
        plants, non-food L23.7
        specified agent NEC L23.8
    due to
      chemical products L25.3
      cosmetics L25.0
      drugs in contact with skin L25.1
      dyes L25.2
      food in contact with skin L25.4
      plants, non-food L25.5
      specified agent NEC L25.8
    irritant L24.9
      due to
        chemical products L24.5
          cosmetics L24.3
          detergents L24.0
          drugs in contact with skin L24.4
          oils and greases L24.1
          solvents L24.2
        food in contact with skin L24.6
        plants, non-food L24.7
        specified agent NEC L24.8
  contusiformis L52
  diabetic — *see* E09-E13 with .63
  diaper L22
  diphtheritica A36.3
  dry skin L85.3
  due to
    acetone (contact) (irritant) L24.2
    acids (contact) (irritant) L24.5
    adhesive(s) (allergic) (contact) (plaster) L23.1
      irritant L24.5
    alcohol (irritant) (skin contact) (substances
      in T51.00-T51.93) L24.2
      taken internally L27.8
    alkalis (contact) (irritant) L24.5
    arsenic (ingested) L27.8
    carbon disulfide (contact) (irritant) L24.2
    caustics (contact) (irritant) L24.5
    cement (contact) L25.3
      allergic L23.5
      irritant L24.5
    cereal (ingested) L27.2
    chemical(s) NEC L25.3
      in contact with skin L25.3
        allergic L23.5
        irritant NEC L24.5
      taken internally L27.8
    chlorocompounds L24.2
    chromium (allergic) (contact) L23.0
      irritant L24.8
    coffee (ingested) L27.2
    cold weather L30.8
    cosmetics (contact) L25.0
      allergic L23.2
      irritant L24.3
    cyclohexanes L24.2
    Demodex species B88.0
    Dermanyssus gallinae B88.0
    detergents (contact) (irritant) L24.0
    dichromate (allergic) L23.0
      irritant L24.5

Dermatitis — *continued*
due to — *continued*
drugs and medicaments (correct substance properly administered) (generalized) (internal use) L27.0
external — *see* Dermatitis, due to, drugs, in contact with skin
wrong substance given or taken (by accident) T49.91
administered with intent to harm by
another person T49.93
self T49.92
circumstances undetermined T49.94
specified substance — *see* Table of Drugs and Chemicals
in contact with skin L25.1
allergic L23.3
irritant L24.4
localized skin eruption L27.1
overdose or wrong substance given or taken (by accident) T50.901
administered with intent to harm by
another person T50.903
self T50.902
circumstances undetermined T50.904
specified substance — *see* Table of Drugs and Chemicals
dyes (contact) L25.2
allergic L23.4
irritant L24.8
epidermophytosis — *see* Dermatophytosis
esters L24.2
external irritant NEC L24.9
fish (ingested) L27.2
flour (ingested) L27.2
food (ingested) L27.2
in contact with skin L25.4
allergic L23.6
irritant L24.6
fruit (ingested) L27.2
furs (allergic) (contact) L23.8
irritant L24.8
glues — *see* Dermatitis, due to, adhesives
glycols L24.2
greases NEC (contact) (irritant) L24.1
hot
objects and materials — *see* Burn
weather or places L59.0
hydrocarbons L24.2
infrared rays L59.8
ingestion, ingested substance L27.9
chemical NEC L27.8
drugs and medicaments (correct substance properly administered)— *see* Dermatitis, due to, drugs
food L27.2
specified NEC L27.8
insecticide in contact with skin L25.3
allergic L23.5
irritant L24.5
internal agent L27.9
drugs and medicaments (generalized) — *see* Dermatitis, due to, drugs
food L27.2
irradiation — *see* Dermatitis, due to, radioactive substance
ketones L24.2
lacquer tree (allergic) (contact) L23.7
light (sun) NEC L57.8
acute L56.8
other L59.8
Liponyssoides sanguineus B88.0
low temperature L30.8
meat (ingested) L27.2
metals, metal salts (allergic) (contact) L23.0
irritant L24.8
milk (ingested) L27.2
nickel (allergic) (contact) L23.0
irritant L24.8
nylon (allergic) (contact) L23.5
irritant L24.5
oils NEC (contact) (irritant) L24.1
paint solvent (contact) (irritant) L24.2

petroleum products (contact) (irritant) (substances in T52.00-T52.93) L24.2
plants NEC (contact) L25.5
allergic L23.7
irritant L24.7
plasters (adhesive) (any) (allergic) (contact) L23.1
irritant L24.5
plastic (allergic) (contact) L23.5
irritant L24.5
preservatives (contact) — *see* Dermatitis, due to, chemical, in contact with skin
primrose (allergic) (contact) L23.7
primula (allergic) (contact) L23.7
radiation L59.8
nonionizing (chronic exposure) L57.8
sun NEC L57.8
acute L56.8
radioactive substance L58.9
acute L58.0
chronic L58.1
radium L58.9
acute L58.0
chronic L58.1
ragweed (allergic) (contact) L23.7
Rhus (allergic) (contact) (diversiloba) (radicans) (toxicodendron) (venenata) (verniciflua) L23.7
rubber (allergic) (contact) L23.5
Senecio jacobaea (allergic) (contact) L23.7
solvents (contact) (irritant) (substances in T52.00-T53.93) L24.2
specified agent NEC (contact) L25.8
allergic L23.8
irritant L24.8
sunshine NEC L57.8
acute L56.8
tetrachlorethylene (contact) (irritant) L24.2
toluene (contact) (irritant) L24.2
turpentine (contact) L25.3
allergic L23.5
irritant L24.2
ultraviolet rays (sun NEC) (chronic exposure) L57.8
acute L56.8
vaccine or vaccination (correct substance properly administered) L27.0
overdose or wrong substance given or taken (by accident) T50.901
administered with intent to harm by
another person T50.903
self T50.902
circumstances undetermined T50.904
varicose veins — *see* Varix, leg, with, inflammation
X-rays L58.9
acute L58.0
chronic L58.1
dyshydrotic L30.1
dysmenorrheica N94.6
escharotica — *see* Burn
exfoliative, exfoliativa (generalized) L26
neonatorum L00
eyelid — *see also* Dermatosis, eyelid
allergic H01.119
left H01.116
lower H01.115
upper H01.114
right H01.113
lower H01.112
upper H01.111
contact — *see* Dermatitis, eyelid, allergic
due to
Demodex species B88.0
herpes (zoster) B02.39
simplex B00.59
eczematous H01.139
left H01.136
lower H01.135
upper H01.134
right H01.133
lower H01.132
upper H01.131
facta, factitia, factitial L98.1
psychogenic F54

flexural NEC L20.82
friction L30.4
fungus B36.9
specified type NEC B36.8
gangrenosa, gangrenous L88
infantum I96
harvest mite B88.0
heat L59.0
herpesviral, vesicular (ear) (lip) B00.1
herpetiformis (bullous) (erythematous) (pustular) (vesicular) L13.0
juvenile L12.2
senile L12.0
hiemalis L30.8
hypostatic, hypostatica — *see* Varix, leg, with, inflammation
infectious eczematoid L30.3
infective L30.3
irritant — *see* Dermatitis, contact, irritant
Jacquet's (diaper dermatitis) L22
Leptus B88.0
lichenified NEC L28.0
medicamentosa (generalized) (internal use) — *see* Dermatitis, due to drugs
mite B88.0
multiformis L13.0
juvenile L12.2
napkin L22
neurotica L13.0
nummular L30.0
papillaris capillitii L73.0
pellagrous E52
perioral L71.0
photocontact L56.2
polymorpha dolorosa L13.0
pruriginosa L13.0
pruritic NEC L30.8
psychogenic F54
purulent L08.0
pustular
contagious B08.0
subcorneal L13.1
pyococcal L08.0
pyogenica L08.0
repens L40.2
Ritter's (exfoliativa) L00
Schamberg's L81.7
schistosome B65.3
seasonal bullous L30.8
seborrheic L21.9
infantile L21.1
specified NEC L21.8
sensitization NOS L23.9
septic L08.0
solare L57.8
specified NEC L30.8
stasis I87.2
with varicose ulcer — *see* Varix, leg, with, ulcer, with inflammation
due to postphlebitic syndrome I87.0
suppurative L08.0
traumatic NEC L30.4
trophoneurotica L13.0
ultraviolet (sun) (chronic exposure) L57.8
acute L56.8
varicose — *see* Varix, leg, with, inflammation
vegetans L10.1
verrucosa B43.0
vesicular, herpesviral B00.1
Dermatoarthritis, lipoid E78.81
Dermatochalasis, eyelid H02.839
left H02.836
lower H02.835
upper H02.834
right H02.833
lower H02.832
upper H02.831
Dermatofibroma (lenticulare) (M8832/0) — *see also* Neoplasm, skin, benign
protuberans (M8832/1) — *see* Neoplasm, skin, uncertain behavior

©2002 Ingenix, Inc.

Dermatofibrosarcoma (M8832/3) — see
    Neoplasm, skin, malignant
    protuberans (M8832/3) — see Neoplasm, skin,
      malignant
      pigmented (M8833/3) — see Neoplasm,
        malignant
Dermatographia L50.3
Dermatolysis (exfoliativa) (congenital) Q82.8
    acquired L57.4
    eyelids — see Blepharochalasis
    palpebrarum — see Blepharochalasis
    senile L57.4
Dermatomegaly NEC Q82.8
Dermatomucosomyositis M33.10
    with
      myopathy M33.12
      respiratory involvement M33.11
      specified organ involvement NEC M33.19
Dermatomycosis B36.9
    furfuracea B36.0
    specified type NEC B36.8
Dermatomyositis (acute) (chronic) — see also
    Dermatopolymyositis
    in (due to) neoplastic disease (see also
      Neoplasm) D49.9 [M36.0]
Dermatoneuritis of children — see Poisoning,
    mercury
Dermatophilosis A48.8
Dermatophytid L30.2
Dermatophytide — see Dermatophytosis
Dermatophytosis (epidermophyton) (infection)
    (Microsporum) (tinea) (Trichophyton) B35.9
    beard B35.0
    body B35.4
    capitis B35.0
    corporis B35.4
    deep-seated B35.8
    disseminated B35.8
    foot B35.3
    granulomatous B35.8
    groin B35.6
    hand B35.2
    nail B35.1
    perianal (area) B35.6
    scalp B35.0
    specified NEC B35.8
Dermatopolymyositis M33.90
    with
      myopathy M33.92
      respiratory involvement M33.91
      specified organ involvement NEC M33.99
    in neoplastic disease (see also Neoplasm) D49.9
      [M36.0]
    juvenile M33.00
      with
        myopathy M33.02
        respiratory involvement M33.01
        specified organ involvement NEC M33.09
    specified NEC M33.10
      myopathy M33.12
      respiratory involvement M33.11
      specified organ involvement NEC M33.19
Dermatopolyneuritis — see Poisoning, mercury
Dermatorrhexis Q79.6
    acquired L57.4
Dermatosclerosis — see also Scleroderma
    localized L94.0
Dermatosis L98.9
    Andrews' L08.89
    Bowen's (M8081/2) — see Neoplasm, skin, in
      situ
    bullous L13.9
      specified NEC L13.8
    exfoliativa L26
    eyelid (noninfectious)
      dermatitis — see Dermatitis, eyelid
      discoid lupus erythematosus — see Lupus,
        erythematosus, eyelid
      xeroderma — see Xeroderma, acquired,
        eyelid
    factitial L98.1
    febrile neutrophilic L98.2
    gonococcal A54.89

Dermatosis — continued
    herpetiformis L13.0
      juvenile L12.2
    menstrual NEC L98.8
    neutrophilic, febrile L98.2
    occupational — see Dermatitis, contact
    papulosa nigra L82.1
    pigmentary L81.9
      progressive L81.7
      Schamberg's L81.7
    psychogenic F54
    purpuric, pigmented L81.7
    pustular, subcorneal L13.1
    transient acantholytic L11.1
Dermographia, dermographism L50.3
Dermoid (cyst) (M9084/0) — see also Neoplasm,
    benign
    with malignant transformation (M9084/3)
      C56.9
      left side C56.1
      right side C56.0
    due to radiation (nonionizing) L57.8
Dermopathy, infiltrative with thyrotoxicosis —
    see Thyrotoxicosis
Dermophytosis — see Dermatophytosis
Descemetocele H18.739
    bilateral H18.733
    left H18.732
    right H18.731
Descemet's membrane — see condition
Descending — see condition
Descensus uteri — see Prolapse, uterus
Desensitization to allergens Z51.89
Desert
    rheumatism B38.0
    sore — see Ulcer, skin
Desertion (newborn) — see Maltreatment,
    abandonment
Desmoid (extra-abdominal) (tumor) (M8821/1) —
    see Neoplasm, connective tissue, uncertain
    behavior
    abdominal (M8822/1) D48.1
Despondency F32.9
Desquamation, skin R23.4
Destruction, destructive — see also Damage
    articular facet — see also Derangement, joint,
      specified type NEC
      vertebra — see Spondylosis
    bone — see also Disorder, bone, specified type
      NEC
      syphilitic A52.77
    joint — see also Derangement, joint, specified
      type NEC
      sacroiliac M53.3
    rectal sphincter K62.8
    septum (nasal) J34.8
    tuberculous NEC — see Tuberculosis
    tympanum, tympanic membrane
      (nontraumatic) — see Disorder, tympanic
      membrane, specified NEC
    vertebral disc — see Degeneration,
      intervertebral disc
Destructiveness — see also Disorder, conduct
    adjustment reaction — see Disorder,
      adjustment
Desultory labor O62.2
Detachment
    cartilage — see Sprain
    cervix, annular N88.8
      complicating delivery O71.3
    choroid (old) (postinfectional) (simple)
      (spontaneous) H31.409
      bilateral H31.403
      hemorrhagic H31.419
        bilateral H31.413
        left H31.412
        right H31.411
      left H31.402
      right H31.401
      serous H31.429
        bilateral H31.423
        left H31.422
        right H31.421
    ligament — see Sprain

Detachment — continued
    meniscus (knee) — see also Derangement,
      knee, meniscus, specified NEC
      current injury — see Tear, meniscus
      due to old tear or injury — see
        Derangement, knee, meniscus, due to
        old tear
    placenta (premature) — see Disorder, placenta,
      abruptio
    retina (without retinal break) (serous) H33.20
      with retinal
        break H33.009
          bilateral H33.003
          giant H33.039
            bilateral H33.033
            left H33.032
            right H33.031
          left H33.002
          multiple H33.029
            bilateral H33.023
            left H33.022
            right H33.021
          right H33.001
          single H33.019
            bilateral H33.013
            left H33.012
            right H33.011
        dialysis H33.049
          bilateral H33.043
          left H33.042
          right H33.041
        bilateral H33.23
        left H33.22
        pigment epithelium — see Degeneration,
          retina, separation of layers, pigment
          epithelium detachment
        rhegmatogenous — see Detachment, retina,
          with retinal, break
        right H33.21
        specified NEC H33.5
        total H33.059
          bilateral H33.053
          left H33.052
          right H33.051
        traction H33.40
          bilateral H33.43
          left H33.42
          right H33.41
    vitreous (body) H43.89
Detergent asthma J69.8
Deterioration
    epileptic F06.8
    general physical R53.81
    heart, cardiac — see Degeneration, myocardial
    mental — see Psychosis
    myocardial, myocardium — see Degeneration,
      myocardial
    senile (simple) R54
Detoxification therapy (alcohol) (drug) Z51.89
Deuteranomaly (anomalous trichromat) H53.53
Deuteranopia (complete) (incomplete) H53.53
Development
    abnormal, bone Q79.9
    arrested R62.50
      bone — see Arrest, development or growth,
        bone
      child R62.50
      due to malnutrition E45
      fetus — see also Slow, fetal growth
        affecting management of pregnancy —
          see category O36.5
    defective, congenital — see also Anomaly, by
      site
      cauda equina Q06.3
      left ventricle Q24.8
        in hypoplastic left heart syndrome Q23.4
      valve Q24.8
        pulmonary Q22.2
    delayed (see also Delay, development) R62.50
      arithmetical skills F81.2
      language (skills) (expressive) F80.1
      learning skill F81.9
      mixed skills F88
      motor coordination F82
      reading F81.0
      specified learning skill NEC F81.89

Development — *continued*
 delayed (*see also* Delay, development) —
   continued
   speech F80.9
   spelling F81.81
   written expression F81.81
 imperfect, congenital — *see also* Anomaly, by
   site
   heart Q24.9
   lungs Q33.6
 incomplete — *see also* Slow, fetal growth
   bronchial tree Q32.8
   organ or site not listed — *see* Hypoplasia, by
     site
   respiratory system Q34.9
 sexual, precocious NEC E30.1
 tardy, mental — *see* Retardation, mental
Developmental — *see* condition
Devergie's disease (pityriasis rubra pilaris) L44.0
Deviation
 conjugate palsy (eye) (spastic) H51.0
 esophagus (acquired) K22.8
 eye, skew H51.8
 midline (jaw) (teeth) (dental arch) M26.2
   specified site NEC — *see* Malposition
 nasal septum J34.2
   congenital Q67.4
 organ or site, congenital NEC — *see*
     Malposition, congenital
 septum (nasal) (acquired) J34.2
   congenital Q67.4
 sexual F65.9
   bestiality F65.89
   egodystonic homosexuality F66
   erotomania F52.8
   exhibitionism F65.2
   fetishism, fetishistic F65.0
     transvestism F65.1
   frotteurism F65.81
   homosexuality, ego-dystonic F66
     pedophilic F65.4
   masochism F65.51
   multiple F65.89
   necrophilia F65.89
   nymphomania F52.8
   pederosis F65.4
   pedophilia F65.4
   sadism, sadomasochism F65.52
   satyriasis F52.8
   specified type NEC F65.89
   transvestism F64.1
   voyeurism F65.3
 teeth, midline M26.2
 trachea J39.8
 ureter, congenital Q62.61
Device
 cerebral ventricle (communicating) in situ
     Z98.2
 contraceptive — *see* Contraceptive, device
 drainage, cerebrospinal fluid, in situ Z98.2
Devic's disease G36.0
Devil's
 grip B33.0
 pinches (purpura simplex) D69.2
Devitalized tooth K04.99
Devonshire colic — *see* Poisoning, lead
Dextraposition, aorta Q20.3
 in tetralogy of Fallot Q21.3
Dextrinosis, limit (debrancher enzyme deficiency)
   E74.03
Dextrocardia (true) Q24.0
 with
   complete transposition of viscera Q89.3
   situs inversus Q89.3
Dextrotransposition, aorta Q20.3
d-glycericacidemia E72.59
Dhat syndrome F48.8
Dhobi itch B35.6
Di George's syndrome D82.1
Di Guglielmo's disease (M9841/3) C94.00
 in remission C94.01

Diabetes, diabetic (mellitus) (familial) (sugar)
   E14.9
 with complication E14.8
   angiopathy E14.51
     with
       gangrene E14.52
       ulcer E14.622
         foot E14.621
   arthropathy E14.618
     neuropathic E14.610
   circulatory complication E14.59
     peripheral angiopathy E14.51
       with gangrene E14.52
   coma (hyperosmolar) (NKHHC) E14.01
     hypoglycemic E14.641
     insulin E14.641
     ketoacidotic E14.11
   dermatitis E14.620
   gangrene E14.52
   hyperglycemia E14.65
   hyperosmolarity E14.00
     with coma E14.01
   hypoglycemia E14.620
     with coma E14.641
   ketoacidosis E14.10
     with coma E14.11
   neurological complication E14.40
     amyotrophy E14.44
     autonomic (poly)neuropathy E14.43
     mononeuropathy E14.41
     myasthenia E14.44
     neuralgia E14.42
     polyneuropathy E14.42
       autonomic E14.43
     specified NEC E14.49
   ophthalmic complication E14.30
     cataract E14.33
     retinopathy (background) E14.31
       proliferative E14.32
     specified NEC E14.39
   oral complication E14.638
     periodontal disease E14.630
   osteomyelitis E14.69
   renal complication E14.29
     Ebstein's disease E14.22
       with renal failure E14.23
     failure E14.23
     nephropathy E14.21
       with renal failure E14.23
     specified NEC E14.29
   skin complication E14.628
     dermatitis E14.620
     ulcer E14.622
       foot E14.621
   specified complication NEC E14.69
 amyotrophy E14.44
   in
     diabetes due to underlying condition
         E08.44
     drug-induced diabetes E09.44
     insulin-dependent (type I) diabetes
         E10.44
     noninsulin-dependent (type II) diabetes
         E11.44
     specified diabetes NEC E13.44
 angiopathy E14.51
   with gangrene E14.52
   in
     diabetes due to underlying condition
         E08.51
       with gangrene E08.52
     drug-induced diabetes E09.51
       with gangrene E09.52
     insulin-dependent (type I) diabetes
         E10.51
       with gangrene E10.52
     noninsulin-dependent (type II) diabetes
         E11.51
       with gangrene E11.52
     specified diabetes NEC E13.51
       with gangrene E13.52
 arising in pregnancy — *see* Diabetes,
   gestational

Diabetes, diabetic — *continued*
 arthropathy E14.618
   in
     diabetes due to underlying condition
         E08.618
       neuropathic E08.610
     drug-induced diabetes E09.618
       neuropathic E09.610
     insulin-dependent (type I) diabetes
         E10.618
       neuropathic E10.610
     noninsulin-dependent (type II) diabetes
         E11.618
       neuropathic E11.610
     specified diabetes NEC E13.618
       neuropathic E13.610
   neuropathic E14.610
     in
       diabetes due to underlying condition
           E08.610
       drug-induced diabetes E09.610
       insulin-dependent (type I) diabetes
           E10.610
       noninsulin-dependent (type II) diabetes
           E11.610
       specified diabetes NEC E13.610
 asymptomatic R73.0
 ataxia E14.49
   in
     diabetes due to underlying condition
         E08.49
     drug-induced diabetes E09.49
     insulin-dependent (type I) diabetes
         E10.49
     noninsulin-dependent (type II) diabetes
         E11.49
     specified diabetes NEC E13.49
 autonomic neuropathy (peripheral) E14.43
   in
     diabetes due to underlying condition
         E08.43
     drug-induced diabetes E09.43
     insulin-dependent (type I) diabetes
         E10.43
     noninsulin-dependent (type II) diabetes
         E11.43
     specified diabetes NEC E13.43
 bone change E14.69
   in
     diabetes due to underlying condition
         E08.69
     drug-induced diabetes E09.69
     insulin-dependent (type I) diabetes
         E10.69
     noninsulin-dependent (type II) diabetes
         E11.69
     specified diabetes NEC E13.69
 brittle — *see* Diabetes, insulin-dependent
 bronze, bronzed E83.11
 cataract E14.33
   in
     diabetes due to underlying condition
         E08.33
     drug-induced diabetes E09.33
     insulin-dependent (type I) diabetes
         E10.33
     noninsulin-dependent (type II) diabetes
         E11.33
     specified diabetes NEC E13.33
 chemical R73.0
 circulatory E14.59
   angiopathy E14.51
     with gangrene E14.52
   in
     diabetes due to underlying condition
         E08.59
       angiopathy E08.51
         with gangrene E08.52
     drug-induced diabetes E09.59
       angiopathy E09.51
         with gangrene E09.52
     insulin-dependent (type I) diabetes
         E10.59
       angiopathy E10.51
         with gangrene E10.52

©2002 Ingenix, Inc.

Diabetes, diabetic — *continued*
circulatory — *continued*
  in — *continued*
    noninsulin-dependent (type II) diabetes E11.59
      angiopathy E11.51
        with gangrene E11.52
    specified diabetes NEC E13.59
      angiopathy E13.51
        with gangrene E13.52
coma (hyperosmolar) (NKHHC) E14.01
  hypoglycemic E14.641
    in
      diabetes due to underlying condition E08.641
      drug-induced diabetes E09.641
      insulin-dependent (type I) diabetes E10.641
      noninsulin-dependent (type II) diabetes E11.641
      specified diabetes NEC E13.641
  in
    diabetes due to underlying condition E08.01
    drug-induced diabetes E09.01
    noninsulin-dependent (type II) diabetes E11.01
    specified diabetes NEC E13.01
  insulin-induced — *see* Diabetes, coma, hypoglycemic
  ketoacidotic E14.11
    in
      diabetes due to underlying condition E08.11
      drug-induced diabetes E09.11
      insulin-dependent (type I) diabetes E10.11
      specified diabetes NEC E13.11
complicating
  childbirth O24.92
    arising during pregnancy — *see* Diabetes, gestational
    specified as pre-existing O24.32
      specified NEC O24.82
      type I — *see* Diabetes, insulin-dependent
      type II — *see* Diabetes, type II
  pregnancy O24.919
    affecting fetus or newborn P70.1
    arising during pregnancy (gestational) — *see* Diabetes, gestational
    first trimester O24.911
    second trimester O24.912
    specified as pre-existing O24.319
      first trimester O24.311
      juvenile onset — *see* Diabetes, insulin-dependent
      second trimester O24.312
      specified NEC O24.819
        first trimester O24.811
        second trimester O24.812
        third trimester O24.813
      third trimester O24.313
      type I — *see* Diabetes, insulin-dependent
      type II — *see* Diabetes, type II
    third trimester O24.913
  puerperium O24.93
    arising during pregnancy — *see* Diabetes, gestational
    specified as pre-existing O24.33
      specified NEC O24.83
      type I — *see* Diabetes, insulin-dependent
      type II — *see* Diabetes, type II
congenital — *see* Diabetes, insulin-dependent
dietary counselling and surveillance Z71.3
dorsal sclerosis E14.49
  in
    diabetes due to underlying condition E08.49
    drug-induced diabetes E09.49
    insulin-dependent (type I) diabetes E10.49
    noninsulin-dependent (type II) diabetes E11.49

Diabetes, diabetic — *continued*
dorsal sclerosis — *continued*
  in — *continued*
    specified diabetes NEC E13.49
due to
  drug or chemical E09.9
    with complication E09.8
      acetonemia E09.10
        with coma E09.11
      acidosis E09.10
        with coma E09.11
      angiopathy E09.51
        with gangrene E09.52
      arthropathy E09.618
        neuropathic E09.610
      circulatory complication E09.59
        peripheral angiopathy E09.51
          with gangrene E09.52
      coma E09.11
        hypoglycemic E09.641
        insulin E09.641
      dermatitis E09.620
      hyperglycemia E09.65
      hypoglycemia E09.640
        with coma E09.641
      ketosis, ketoacidosis E09.10
        with coma E09.11
      neurological complication E09.40
        amyotrophy E09.44
        autonomic (poly)neuropathy E09.43
        mononeuropathy E09.41
        myasthenia E09.44
        neuralgia E09.42
        polyneuropathy E09.42
          autonomic E09.43
        specified NEC E09.49
      ophthalmic complication E09.30
        cataract E09.33
        retinopathy (background) E09.31
          proliferative E09.32
        specified NEC E09.39
      oral complication E09.638
        periodontal disease E09.630
      renal complication E09.29
        Ebstein's disease E09.22
          with renal failure E09.23
        failure E09.23
        Kimmelstiel-Wilson disease E09.21
          with renal failure E09.23
        nephropathy E09.21
          with renal failure E09.23
        specified NEC E09.29
      specified complication NEC E09.69
      skin complication E09.628
        dermatitis E09.620
        ulcer E09.622
          foot E09.621
      ulcer E09.622
        foot E09.621
  underlying condition E08.9
    with complication E08.8
      acetonemia E08.10
        with coma E08.11
      acidosis E08.10
        with coma E08.11
      angiopathy E08.51
        with gangrene E08.52
      arthropathy E08.618
        neuropathic E08.610
      circulatory complication E08.59
        peripheral angiopathy E08.51
          with gangrene E08.52
      coma E08.11
        hypoglycemic E08.641
        insulin E08.641
      dermatitis E08.620
      hyperglycemia E08.65
      hypoglycemia E08.640
        with coma E08.641
      ketosis, ketoacidosis E08.10
        with coma E08.11
      neurological complication E08.40
        amyotrophy E08.44
        autonomic (poly)neuropathy E08.43
        mononeuropathy E08.41
        myasthenia E08.44

Diabetes, diabetic — *continued*
due to — *continued*
  underlying condition — *continued*
    with complication — *continued*
      neurological complication — *continued*
        neuralgia E08.42
        polyneuropathy E08.42
          autonomic E08.43
          specified NEC E08.49
      ophthalmic complication E08.30
        cataract E08.33
        retinopathy (background) E08.31
          proliferative E08.32
        specified NEC E08.39
      oral complication E08.638
        periodontal disease E08.630
      renal complication E08.29
        Ebstein's disease E08.22
          with renal failure E08.23
        failure E08.23
        Kimmelstiel-Wilson disease E08.21
          with renal failure E08.23
        nephropathy E08.21
          with renal failure E08.23
        specified NEC E08.29
      specified complication NEC E08.69
      skin complication E08.628
        dermatitis E08.620
        ulcer E08.622
          foot E08.621
      ulcer E08.622
        foot E08.621
Ebstein's disease E14.22
  with renal failure E14.23
  in
    diabetes due to underlying condition E08.22
      with renal failure E08.23
    drug-induced diabetes E09.22
      with renal failure E09.23
    insulin-dependent (type I) diabetes E10.22
      with renal failure E10.23
    noninsulin-dependent (type II) diabetes E11.22
      with renal failure E11.23
    specified diabetes NEC E13.22
      with renal failure E13.23
gangrene E14.52
  in
    diabetes due to underlying condition E08.52
    drug-induced diabetes E09.52
    insulin-dependent (type I) diabetes E10.52
    noninsulin-dependent (type II) diabetes E11.52
    specified diabetes NEC E13.52
gastroparalysis E14.43
  in
    diabetes due to underlying condition E08.43
    drug-induced diabetes E09.43
    insulin-dependent (type I) diabetes E10.43
    noninsulin-dependent (type II) diabetes E11.43
    specified diabetes NEC E13.43
gastroparesis E14.43
  in
    diabetes due to underlying condition E08.43
    drug-induced diabetes E09.43
    insulin-dependent (type I) diabetes E10.43
    noninsulin-dependent (type II) diabetes E11.43
    specified diabetes NEC E13.43
gestational (in pregnancy) O24.415
  affecting fetus or newborn P70.0
  diet-controlled O24.410
  in childbirth O24.425
    diet-controlled O24.420
    insulin (and diet) controlled O24.424
  insulin (and diet) controlled O24.414

Diabetes, diabetic — *continued*
    gestational — *continued*
        puerperal O24.435
            diet-controlled O24.430
            insulin (and diet) controlled O24.434
    glaucoma E14.39
        in
            diabetes due to underlying condition
                E08.39
            drug-induced diabetes E09.39
            insulin-dependent (type I) diabetes
                E10.39
            noninsulin-dependent (type II) diabetes
                E11.39
            specified diabetes NEC E13.39
    glomerulosclerosis (intercapillary) E14.21
        in
            diabetes due to underlying condition
                E08.21
            drug-induced diabetes E09.21
            insulin-dependent (type I) diabetes
                E10.21
            noninsulin-dependent (type II) diabetes
                E11.21
            specified diabetes NEC E13.21
    glycogenosis, secondary E14.69
        in
            diabetes due to underlying condition
                E08.69
            drug-induced diabetes E09.69
            insulin-dependent (type I) diabetes
                E10.69
            noninsulin-dependent (type II) diabetes
                E11.69
            specified diabetes NEC E13.69
    hemochromatosis E83.11
    hyperosmolar coma E14.01
        in
            diabetes due to underlying condition
                E08.01
            drug-induced diabetes E09.01
            noninsulin-dependent (type II) diabetes
                E11.01
            specified diabetes NEC E13.01
    hyperosmolarity E14.00
        with coma E14.01
        in
            diabetes due to underlying condition
                E08.00
                with coma E08.01
            drug-induced diabetes E09.00
                with coma E09.01
            noninsulin-dependent (type II) diabetes
                E11.00
                with coma E11.01
            specified diabetes NEC E13.00
                with coma E13.01
    hypertension-nephrosis syndrome E14.29
        in
            diabetes due to underlying condition
                E08.29
            drug-induced diabetes E09.29
            insulin-dependent (type I) diabetes
                E10.29
            noninsulin-dependent (type II) diabetes
                E11.29
            specified diabetes NEC E13.29
    hypoglycemia E14.640
        with coma E14.641
        in
            diabetes due to underlying condition
                E08.640
                with coma E08.641
            drug-induced diabetes E09.640
                with coma E09.641
            insulin-dependent (type I) diabetes
                E10.640
                with coma E10.641
            noninsulin-dependent (type II) diabetes
                E11.640
                with coma E11.641
            specified diabetes NEC E13.640
                with coma E13.641
    insipidus E23.2
        nephrogenic N25.1
        pituitary E23.2

Diabetes, diabetic — *continued*
    insipidus — *continued*
        vasopressin resistant N25.1
    insulin-dependent E10.9
        with complication E10.8
            acetonemia E10.10
                with coma E10.11
            acidosis E10.10
                with coma E10.11
            angiopathy E10.51
                with gangrene E10.52
            arthropathy E10.618
                neuropathic E10.610
            circulatory complication E10.59
                peripheral angiopathy E10.51
                    with gangrene E10.52
            coma E10.11
                hypoglycemic E10.641
                insulin E10.641
            dermatitis E10.620
            hyperglycemia E10.65
            hypoglycemia E10.640
                with coma E10.641
            ketosis, ketoacidosis E10.10
                with coma E10.11
            neurological complication E10.40
                amyotrophy E10.44
                autonomic (poly)neuropathy E10.43
                mononeuropathy E10.41
                myasthenia E10.44
                neuralgia E10.42
                polyneuropathy E10.42
                    autonomic E10.43
                specified NEC E10.49
            ophthalmic complication E10.30
                cataract E10.33
                retinopathy (background) E10.31
                    proliferative E10.32
                specified NEC E10.39
            oral complication E10.638
                periodontal disease E10.630
            renal complication E10.29
                Ebstein's disease E10.22
                    with renal failure E10.23
                failure E10.23
                Kimmelstiel-Wilson disease E10.21
                    with renal failure E10.23
                nephropathy E10.21
                    with renal failure E10.23
                specified NEC E10.29
            skin complication E10.628
                dermatitis E10.620
                ulcer E10.622
                    foot E10.621
            specified complication NEC E10.69
            ulcer E10.622
                foot E10.621
        complicating
            childbirth O24.02
            pregnancy O24.019
                first trimester O24.011
                second trimester O24.012
                third trimester O24.013
            puerperium O24.03
    intercapillary glomerulosclerosis E14.21
        in
            diabetes due to underlying condition
                E08.21
            drug-induced diabetes E09.21
            insulin-dependent (type I) diabetes
                E10.21
            noninsulin-dependent (type II) diabetes
                E11.21
            specified diabetes NEC E13.21
    intracapillary glomerulosclerosis E14.21
        in
            diabetes due to underlying condition
                E08.21
            drug-induced diabetes E09.21
            insulin-dependent (type I) diabetes
                E10.21
            noninsulin-dependent (type II) diabetes
                E11.21
            specified diabetes NEC E13.21

Diabetes, diabetic — *continued*
    iritis E14.39
        in
            diabetes due to underlying condition
                E08.39
            drug-induced diabetes E09.39
            insulin-dependent (type I) diabetes
                E10.39
            noninsulin-dependent (type II) diabetes
                E11.39
            specified diabetes NEC E13.39
    juvenile-onset — *see* Diabetes, insulin-
        dependent
    ketosis-prone — *see* Diabetes, insulin-
        dependent
    Kimmelstiel (-Wilson) disease (intercapillary
        glomerulosclerosis) E14.21
        in
            diabetes due to underlying condition
                E08.21
            drug-induced diabetes E09.21
            insulin-dependent (type I) diabetes
                E10.21
            noninsulin-dependent (type II) diabetes
                E11.21
            specified diabetes NEC E13.21
    Lancereaux's (with marked emaciation) E14.69
        in
            diabetes due to underlying condition
                E08.69
            drug-induced diabetes E09.69
            insulin-dependent (type I) diabetes
                E10.69
            noninsulin-dependent (type II) diabetes
                E11.69
            specified diabetes NEC E13.69
    latent R73.0
    lipoidosis E14.69
        in
            diabetes due to underlying condition
                E08.69
            drug-induced diabetes E09.69
            insulin-dependent (type I) diabetes
                E10.69
            noninsulin-dependent (type II) diabetes
                E11.69
            specified diabetes NEC E13.69
    macular edema E14.32
        in
            diabetes due to underlying condition
                E08.32
            drug-induced diabetes E09.32
            insulin-dependent (type I) diabetes
                E10.32
            noninsulin-dependent (type II) diabetes
                E11.32
            specified diabetes NEC E13.32
    malnutrition-related (insulin-or non-insulin-
        dependent) — *see* Diabetes, due to,
        underlying condition
    microaneurysms, retinal E14.31
        in
            diabetes due to underlying condition
                E08.31
            drug-induced diabetes E09.31
            insulin-dependent (type I) diabetes
                E10.31
            noninsulin-dependent (type II) diabetes
                E11.31
            specified diabetes NEC E13.31
    mononeuropathy E14.41
        in
            diabetes due to underlying condition
                E08.41
            drug-induced diabetes E09.41
            insulin-dependent (type I) diabetes
                E10.41
            noninsulin-dependent (type II) diabetes
                E11.41
            specified diabetes NEC E13.41
    neonatal (transient) P70.2
    nephropathy E14.21
        with renal failure E14.23
        in
            diabetes due to underlying condition
                E08.21

©2002 Ingenix, Inc.

Diabetes, diabetic — *continued*
  nephropathy — *continued*
    in — *continued*
      diabetes due to underlying condition — *continued*
        with renal failure E08.23
      drug-induced diabetes E09.21
        with renal failure E09.23
      insulin-dependent (type I) diabetes E10.21
        with renal failure E10.23
      noninsulin-dependent (type II) diabetes E11.21
        with renal failure E11.23
      specified diabetes NEC E13.21
        with renal failure E13.23
  nephrosis (Kimmelstiel-Wilson disease) E14.21
    with renal failure E14.23
    in
      diabetes due to underlying condition E08.21
        with renal failure E08.23
      drug-induced diabetes E09.21
        with renal failure E09.23
      insulin-dependent (type I) diabetes E10.21
        with renal failure E10.23
      noninsulin-dependent (type II) diabetes E11.21
        with renal failure E11.23
      specified diabetes NEC E13.21
        with renal failure E13.23
  neuralgia E14.42
    in
      diabetes due to underlying condition E08.42
      drug-induced diabetes E09.42
      insulin-dependent (type I) diabetes E10.42
      noninsulin-dependent (type II) diabetes E11.42
      specified diabetes NEC E13.42
  neuritis E14.42
    in
      diabetes due to underlying condition E08.42
      drug-induced diabetes E09.42
      insulin-dependent (type I) diabetes E10.42
      noninsulin-dependent (type II) diabetes E11.42
      specified diabetes NEC E13.42
  neuropathic arthropathy E14.610
    in
      diabetes due to underlying condition E08.610
      drug-induced diabetes E09.610
      insulin-dependent (type I) diabetes E10.610
      noninsulin-dependent (type II) diabetes E11.610
      specified diabetes NEC E13.610
  neuropathy E14.40
    in
      diabetes due to underlying condition E08.40
      drug-induced diabetes E09.40
      insulin-dependent (type I) diabetes E10.40
      noninsulin-dependent (type II) diabetes E11.40
      specified diabetes NEC E13.40
  nonclinical R73.0
  oral complication E14.638
    in
      diabetes due to underlying condition E08.638
        periodontal disease E08.630
      drug-induced diabetes E09.638
        periodontal disease E09.630
      insulin-dependent (type I) diabetes E10.638
        periodontal disease E10.630
      noninsulin-dependent (type II) diabetes E11.638
        periodontal disease E11.630

Diabetes, diabetic — *continued*
  oral complication — *continued*
    in — *continued*
      specified diabetes NEC E13.638
        periodontal disease E13.630
    periodontal disease E14.630
  osteomyelitis E14.69
    in
      diabetes due to underlying condition E08.69
      drug-induced diabetes E09.69
      insulin-dependent (type I) diabetes E10.69
      noninsulin-dependent (type II) diabetes E11.69
      specified diabetes NEC E13.69
  peripheral autonomic neuropathy E14.43
    in
      diabetes due to underlying condition E08.43
      drug-induced diabetes E09.43
      insulin-dependent (type I) diabetes E10.43
      noninsulin-dependent (type II) diabetes E11.43
      specified diabetes NEC E13.43
  phosphate E83.39
  polyneuropathy E14.42
    autonomic E14.43
    in
      diabetes due to underlying condition E08.42
        autonomic E08.43
      drug-induced diabetes E09.42
        autonomic E09.43
      insulin-dependent (type I) diabetes E10.42
        autonomic E10.43
      noninsulin-dependent (type II) diabetes E11.42
        autonomic E11.43
      specified diabetes NEC E13.42
        autonomic E13.43
  renal E74.8
  retinal
    edema E14.32
      in
        diabetes due to underlying condition E08.32
        drug-induced diabetes E09.32
        insulin-dependent (type I) diabetes E10.32
        noninsulin-dependent (type II) diabetes E11.32
        specified diabetes NEC E13.32
    hemorrhage E14.31
      in
        diabetes due to underlying condition E08.31
        drug-induced diabetes E09.31
        insulin-dependent (type I) diabetes E10.31
        noninsulin-dependent (type II) diabetes E11.31
        specified diabetes NEC E13.31
    microaneurysms E14.31
      in
        diabetes due to underlying condition E08.31
        drug-induced diabetes E09.31
        insulin-dependent (type I) diabetes E10.31
        noninsulin-dependent (type II) diabetes E11.31
        specified diabetes NEC E13.31
    retinitis E14.31
      in
        diabetes due to underlying condition E08.31
        drug-induced diabetes E09.31
        insulin-dependent (type I) diabetes E10.31
        noninsulin-dependent (type II) diabetes E11.31
        specified diabetes NEC E13.31

Diabetes, diabetic — *continued*
  retinopathy (background) E14.31
    in
      diabetes due to underlying condition E08.31
      drug-induced diabetes E09.31
      insulin-dependent (type I) diabetes E10.31
      noninsulin-dependent (type II) diabetes E11.31
      specified diabetes NEC E13.31
    proliferative E14.32
    in
      diabetes due to underlying condition E08.32
      drug-induced diabetes E09.32
      insulin-dependent (type I) diabetes E10.32
      noninsulin-dependent (type II) diabetes E11.32
      specified diabetes NEC E13.32
  specified NEC E13.9
    with complication E13.8
      acetonemia E13.10
        with coma E13.11
      acidosis E13.10
        with coma E13.11
      angiopathy E13.51
        with gangrene E13.52
      arthropathy E13.618
        neuropathic E13.610
      circulatory complication E13.59
        peripheral angiopathy E13.51
          with gangrene E13.52
      coma (hyperosmolar) (NKHHC) E13.01
        hypoglycemic E13.641
        insulin E13.641
        ketoacidotic E13.11
      dermatitis E13.620
      hyperglycemia E13.65
      hypoglycemia E13.640
        with coma E13.641
      ketosis, ketoacidosis E13.10
        with coma E13.11
      neurological complication E13.40
        amyotrophy E13.44
        autonomic (poly)neuropathy E13.43
        mononeuropathy E13.41
        myasthenia E13.44
        neuralgia E13.42
        polyneuropathy E13.42
          autonomic E13.43
        specified NEC E13.49
      ophthalmic complication E13.30
        cataract E13.33
        retinopathy (background) E13.31
          proliferative E13.32
          specified NEC E13.39
      oral complication E13.638
        periodontal disease E13.630
      renal complication E13.29
        Ebstein's disease E13.22
          with renal failure E13.23
        failure E13.23
        Kimmelstiel-Wilson disease E13.21
          with renal failure E13.23
        nephropathy E13.21
          with renal failure E13.23
        specified NEC E13.29
      skin complication E13.628
        dermatitis E13.620
        ulcer E13.622
          foot E13.621
      specified complication NEC E13.69
      ulcer E13.622
        foot E13.621
  steroid-induced
    correct substance properly administered — *see* Diabetes, due to, drug or chemical
    overdose or wrong substance given or taken — *see* category T38.0
  stress R73.0
  subclinical R73.0
  subliminal R73.0
  type I — *see* Diabetes, insulin-dependent

Diabetes, diabetic — *continued*
  type II E11.9
    with complication E11.8
      angiopathy E11.51
        with gangrene E11.52
      arthropathy E11.618
        neuropathic E11.610
      circulatory complication E11.59
        peripheral angiopathy E11.51
          with gangrene E11.52
      coma E11.01
        hypoglycemic E11.641
        insulin E11.641
      dermatitis E11.620
      hyperglycemia E11.65
      hypoglycemia E11.640
        with coma E11.641
      neurological complication E11.40
        amyotrophy E11.44
        autonomic (poly)neuropathy E11.43
        mononeuropathy E11.41
        myasthenia E11.44
        neuralgia E11.42
        polyneuropathy E11.42
          autonomic E11.43
        specified NEC E11.49
      ophthalmic complication E11.30
        cataract E11.33
        retinopathy (background) E11.31
          proliferative E11.32
        specified NEC E11.39
      oral complication E11.638
        periodontal disease E11.630
      renal complication E11.29
        Ebstein's disease E11.22
          with renal failure E11.23
        failure E11.23
        Kimmelstiel-Wilson disease E11.21
          with renal failure E11.23
        nephropathy E11.21
          with renal failure E11.23
        specified NEC E11.29
      skin complication E11.628
        dermatitis E11.620
        ulcer E11.622
          foot E11.621
      specified complication NEC E11.69
      ulcer E11.622
        foot E11.621
  complicating
    childbirth O24.12
    pregnancy O24.119
      first trimester O24.111
      second trimester O24.112
      third trimester O24.113
    puerperium O24.13
  ulcer E14.622
    foot E14.621
    in
      diabetes due to underlying condition E08.622
        foot E08.621
      drug-induced diabetes E09.622
        foot E09.621
      insulin-dependent (type I) diabetes E10.622
        foot E10.621
      noninsulin-dependent (type II) diabetes E11.622
        foot E11.621
      specified diabetes NEC E13.622
        foot E13.621
  unstable — *see* Diabetes, insulin-dependent
  xanthoma E14.69
    in
      diabetes due to underlying condition E08.69
      drug-induced diabetes E09.69
      insulin-dependent (type I) diabetes E10.69
      noninsulin-dependent (type II) diabetes E11.69
      specified diabetes NEC E13.69

Diacyclothrombopathia D69.1

Diagnosis deferred R69

Dialysis (intermittent) (treatment)
  renal status only Z99.2
  retina, retinal — *see* Detachment, retina, with retinal, dialysis

Diamond-Blackfan anemia (congenital hypoplastic) D61.4

Diamond-Gardener syndrome (autoerythrocyte sensitization) D69.2

Diaper rash L22

Diaphragm — *see* condition

Diaphragmalgia R07.1

Diaphragmatitis, diaphragmitis J98.6

Diaphysial aclasis Q78.6

Diaphysitis — *see* Osteomyelitis, specified type NEC

Diarrhea, diarrheal (disease) (infantile) (inflammatory) R19.7
  achlorhydric K31.83
  allergic K52.2
  amebic (*see also* Amebiasis) A06.0
    with abscess — *see* Abscess, amebic
    acute A06.0
    chronic A06.1
    nondysenteric A06.2
  and vomiting, epidemic A08.1
  bacillary — *see* Dysentery, bacillary
  balantidial A07.0
  cachectic NEC K52.8
  Chilomastix A07.8
  choleriformis A00.1
  chronic (noninfective) K52.9
  coccidial A07.3
  Cochin-China K90.1
    strongyloidiasis B78.0
  Dientamoeba A07.8
  dietetic K52.2
  due to
    bacteria A04.9
      specified NEC A04.8
    Campylobacter A04.5
    Capillaria philippinensis B81.1
    Clostridium perfringens (C) (F) A04.8
    Cryptosporidium A07.2
    Escherichia coli A04.4
      enteroaggregative A04.4
      enterohemorrhagic A04.3
      enteroinvasive A04.2
      enteropathogenic A04.0
      enterotoxigenic A04.1
      specified NEC A04.4
    food hypersensitivity K52.2
    Necator americanus B76.1
    S. japonicum B65.2
    specified organism NEC A08.5
      bacterial A04.8
      viral A08.3
    Staphylococcus A04.8
    Trichuris trichiuria B79
    virus — *see* Enteritis, viral
    Yersinia enterocolitica A04.6
  dysenteric A09
  epidemic A09
  flagellate A07.9
  Flexner's (ulcerative) A03.1
  functional K59.1
    following gastrointestinal surgery K91.89
    psychogenic F45.8
  Giardia lamblia A07.1
  giardial A07.1
  hill K90.1
  infectious A09
  malarial — *see* Malaria
  mite B88.0
  mycotic NEC B49 *[K93]*
  neonatal (noninfective) P78.3
  nervous F45.8
  neurogenic K59.1
  noninfective K52.9
  postgastrectomy K91.89
  postvagotomy K91.89
  presumed noninfectious K52.9
  protozoal A07.9
    specified NEC A07.8
  psychogenic F45.8
  specified
    bacterium NEC A04.8

Diarrhea, diarrheal — *continued*
  specified — *continued*
    virus NEC A08.3
  strongyloidiasis B78.0
  toxic K52.1
  trichomonal A07.8
  tropical K90.1
  tuberculous A18.32
  viral — *see* Enteritis, viral

Diastasis
  cranial bones M84.88
    congenital NEC Q75.8
  joint (traumatic) — *see* Dislocation
  muscle M62.00
    ankle M62.079
      left M62.072
      right M62.071
    congenital Q79.8
    foot M62.079
      left M62.072
      right M62.071
    forearm M62.039
      left M62.032
      right M62.031
    hand M62.049
      left M62.042
      right M62.041
    lower leg M62.069
      left M62.062
      right M62.061
    pelvic region M62.059
      left M62.052
      right M62.051
    shoulder region M62.019
      left M62.012
      right M62.011
    specified site NEC M62.08
    thigh M62.059
      left M62.052
      right M62.051
    upper arm M62.029
      left M62.022
      right M62.021
  recti (abdomen)
    complicating delivery O71.89
    congenital Q79.59

Diastema, tooth, teeth M26.3

Diastematomyelia Q06.2

Diataxia, cerebral, infantile G80.4

Diathesis
  allergic — *see* History, allergy
  bleeding (familial) D69.9
  cystine (familial) E72.00
  gouty — *see* Gout
  hemorrhagic (familial) D69.9
    newborn NEC P53
  spasmophilic R29.0

Diaz's disease or osteochondrosis (juvenile) (talus) — *see* Osteochondrosis, juvenile, tarsus

Dibothriocephalus, dibothriocephaliasis (latus) (infection) (infestation) B70.0
  larval B70.1

Dicephalus, dicephaly Q89.4

Dichotomy, teeth K00.2

Dichromat, dichromatopsia (congenital) — *see* Deficiency, color vision

Dichuchwa A65

Dicroceliasis B66.2

Didelphia, didelphys — *see* Double uterus

Didymytis N45.1
  with orchitis N45.3

Dietary
  inadequacy or deficiency E63.9
  surveillance and counselling Z71.3

Dietl's crisis N13.8

Dieulafoy's disease or ulcer K25.0

Difficult, difficulty (in)
  acculturation Z60.3
  feeding R63.3
    newborn P92.9
      breast P92.5
      specified NEC P92.8

©2002 Ingenix, Inc.

Difficult, difficulty — *continued*
  feeding — *continued*
    nonorganic (infant or child) F98.29
  intubation, in anesthesia T88.4
  mechanical, gastroduodenal stoma K91.89
    causing obstruction K91.3
  reading (developmental) F81.0
    secondary to emotional disorders F93.9
  spelling (specific) F81.81
    with reading disorder F81.89
    due to inadequate teaching Z55.8
  swallowing — *see* Dysphagia
  walking R26.2
  work
    conditions NEC Z56.5
    schedule Z56.3
Diffuse — *see* condition
DiGeorge's syndrome (thymic hypoplasia) D82.1
Digestive — *see* condition
Diktyoma (M9501/3) — *see* Neoplasm, malignant
Dilaceration, tooth K00.4
Dilatation
  anus K59.8
    venule — *see* Hemorrhoids
  aorta (focal) (general) — *see* Aneurysm, aorta
  artery — *see* Aneurysm
  bladder (sphincter) N32.8
    congenital Q64.79
  blood vessel I99.8
  bronchial J47.9
    with
      acute exacerbation J47.1
      lower respiratory infection J47.0
  calyx (due to obstruction) — *see*
    Hydronephrosis
  capillaries I78.8
  cardiac (acute) (chronic) — *see also*
    Hypertrophy, cardiac
    congenital Q24.8
      valve NEC Q24.8
        pulmonary Q22.2
    valve — *see* Endocarditis
  cavum septi pellucidi Q06.8
  cervix (uteri) — *see also* Incompetency, cervix
    incomplete, poor, slow complicating delivery
      O62.0
  colon K59.3
    congenital Q43.1
    psychogenic F45.8
  common duct (acquired) K83.8
    congenital Q44.5
  cystic duct (acquired) K82.8
    congenital Q44.5
  duct, mammary — *see* Ectasia, mammary duct
  duodenum K59.8
  esophagus K22.8
    congenital Q39.5
    due to achalasia K22.0
  eustachian tube, congenital Q17.8
  gallbladder K82.8
  gastric — *see* Dilatation, stomach
  heart (acute) (chronic) — *see also* Hypertrophy,
    cardiac
    congenital Q24.8
    valve — *see* Endocarditis
  ileum K59.8
    psychogenic F45.8
  jejunum K59.8
    psychogenic F45.8
  kidney (calyx) (collecting structures) (cystic)
    (parenchyma) (pelvis) (idiopathic) N28.89
  lacrimal passages or duct — *see* Disorder,
    lacrimal system, changes
  lymphatic vessel I89.0
  mammary duct — *see* Ectasia, mammary duct
  Meckel's diverticulum (congenital) Q43.0
  myocardium (acute) (chronic) — *see*
    Hypertrophy, cardiac
  organ or site, congenital NEC — *see* Distortion
  pancreatic duct K86.8
  pericardium — *see* Pericarditis
  pharynx J39.2
  prostate N42.89
  pulmonary
    artery (idiopathic) I28.8
    valve, congenital Q22.2

Dilatation — *continued*
  pupil H57.04
  rectum K59.3
  saccule, congenital Q16.5
  salivary gland (duct) K11.8
  sphincter ani K62.8
  stomach K31.89
    acute K31.0
    psychogenic F45.8
  submaxillary duct K11.8
  trachea, congenital Q32.1
  ureter (idiopathic) N28.82
    congenital Q62.2
    due to obstruction N13.4
  urethra (acquired) N36.8
  vasomotor I73.9
  vein I86.8
  ventricular, ventricle (acute) (chronic) — *see*
    also Hypertrophy, cardiac
    cerebral, congenital Q04.8
  venule NEC I86.8
  vesical orifice N32.8
Dilated, dilation — *see* Dilatation
Diminished, diminution
  hearing (acuity) — *see* Deafness
  sense or sensation (cold) (heat) (tactile)
    (vibratory) R20.8
  vision NEC H54.7
  vital capacity R94.2
Diminuta taenia B71.0
Dimitri-Sturge-Weber disease Q85.8
Dimple
  parasacral, pilonidal or postanal — *see* Cyst,
    pilonidal
Dioctophyme renalis (infection) (infestation)
    B83.8
Dipetalonemiasis B74.4
Diphallus Q55.69
Diphtheria, diphtheritic (gangrenous)
    (hemorrhagic) A36.9
  carrier (suspected) Z22.2
  cutaneous A36.3
  faucial A36.0
  infection of wound A36.3
  inoculation (not sick) Z23
  laryngeal A36.2
  myocarditis A36.81
  nasal, anterior A36.89
  nasopharyngeal A36.1
  neurological complication A36.89
  pharyngeal A36.0
  specified site NEC A36.89
  tonsillar A36.0
Diphyllobothriasis (intestine) B70.0
  larval B70.1
Diplacusis H93.229
  bilateral H93.223
  left H93.222
  right H93.221
Diplegia (upper limbs) G83.0
  facial G51.0
  infantile or congenital (cerebral) (spastic)
    (spinal) G80.1
  lower limbs G82.20
Diplococcus, diplococcal — *see* condition
Diplopia H53.2
Dipsomania F10.20
  with
    psychosis — *see* Psychosis, alcoholic
    remission F10.21
Dipylidiasis B71.1
Direction, teeth, abnormal M26.3
Dirofilariasis B74.8
Dirt-eating child F98.3
Disability
  heart — *see* Disease, heart
  knowledge acquisition F81.9
  learning F81.9
  limiting activities Z73.6
  spelling, specific F81.81
Disappearance of family member Z63.4

Disarticulation — *see* Amputation
  meaning traumatic amputation — *see*
    Amputation, traumatic
Disaster, cerebrovascular I64
Discharge (from)
  abnormal finding in — *see* Abnormal, specimen
  breast (female) (male) N64.5
  diencephalic autonomic idiopathic — *see*
    Epilepsy, special syndrome
  ear — *see also* Otorrhea
    blood — *see* Otorrhagia
  excessive urine R35.8
  nipple N64.5
  penile R36.9
  postnasal — *see* Sinusitis
  prison, anxiety concerning Z65.2
  urethral R36.9
    without blood R36.0
    hematospermia R36.1
  vaginal N89.8
Discitis, diskitis M46.40
  cervical region M46.42
  cervicothoracic region M46.43
  lumbar region M46.46
  lumbosacral region M46.47
  multiple sites M46.49
  occipito-atlanto-axial region M46.41
  pyogenic — *see* Infection, intervertebral disc,
    pyogenic
  sacrococcygeal region M46.48
  thoracic region M46.44
  thoracolumbar region M46.45
Discoid
  meniscus (congenital) Q68.609
    lateral Q68.669
      anterior horn Q68.649
        left Q68.642
        right Q68.641
      posterior horn Q68.659
        left Q68.652
        right Q68.651
      left Q68.662
      right Q68.661
    left Q68.602
    medial Q68.639
      anterior horn Q68.619
        left Q68.612
        right Q68.611
      posterior horn Q68.629
        left Q68.622
        right Q68.621
      left Q68.632
      right Q68.631
    right Q68.601
  semilunar cartilage (congenital) — *see*
    Derangement, knee, meniscus, specified
    NEC
Discoloration
  nails L60.8
  teeth (posteruptive) K03.7
    during formation K00.8
Discomfort
  chest R07.89
  visual H53.149
    bilateral H53.143
    left H53.142
    right H53.141
Discontinuity, ossicles, ear H74.20
  bilateral H74.23
  left H74.22
  right H74.21
Discord (with)
  boss Z56.4
  classmates Z55.4
  counselor Z64.4
  employer Z56.4
  family Z63.8
  fellow employees Z56.4
  landlord Z59.2
  lodgers Z59.2
  neighbors Z59.2
  parents and in-laws Z63.1
  probation officer Z64.4
  social worker Z64.4
  spouse or partner (perpetrator) Z69.12
    victim Z69.11

Discord — *continued*
  teachers Z55.4
  workmates Z56.4
Discordant connection
  atrioventricular (congenital) Q20.5
  ventriculoarterial Q20.3
Discrepancy, leg length (acquired) (upper) — *see also* Deformity, limb, unequal length
  congenital — *see* Defect, reduction, lower limb
  lower leg — *see* Deformity, limb, unequal length
Discrimination
  ethnic Z60.5
  political Z60.5
  racial Z60.5
  religious Z60.5
  sex Z60.5
Disease, diseased — *see also* Syndrome
  absorbent system I87.8
  acid peptic K30
  Acosta's T70.29
  Adams-Stokes (-Morgagni) (syncope with heart block) I45.9
  Addison's anemia (pernicious) D51.0
  adenoids (and tonsils) J35.9
  adrenal (capsule) (cortex) (gland) (medullary) E27.9
    hyperfunction E27.0
    specified NEC E27.8
  ainhum L94.6
  airway, obstructive, chronic J44.9
    due to
      cotton dust J66.0
      specific organic dusts NEC J66.8
  akamushi (scrub typhus) A75.3
  Albers-Schönberg's (marble bones) Q78.2
  Albert's — *see* Tendinitis, Achilles
  alimentary canal K63.9
  alligator-skin Q80.9
    acquired L85.0
  alpha heavy chain (M9762/3) C88.1
  alpine T70.29
  altitude T70.20
  alveolar ridge
    edentulous K06.9
      specified NEC K06.8
  alveoli, teeth K08.9
  Alzheimer's G30.90
    with behavioral disturbance G30.91
    early onset G30.00
      with behavioral disturbance G30.01
    late onset G30.10
      with behavioral disturbance G30.11
    specified NEC G30.80
      with behavioral disturbance G30.81
  amyloid — *see* Amyloidosis
  Andersen's (glycogenosis IV) E74.09
  Andes T70.29
  Andrews' (bacterid) L08.89
  angiospastic I73.9
    cerebral G45.9
    vein I87.8
  anterior
    chamber H21.9
    horn cell G12.29
  antiglomerular basement membrane (antiGBM) antibody M31.0
    tubulo-interstitial nephritis N12
  antral — *see* Sinusitis, maxillary
  anus K62.9
    specified NEC K62.8
  aorta (nonsyphilitic) I77.9
    syphilitic NEC A52.02
  aortic (heart) (valve) I35.9
    rheumatic I06.9
  Apollo B30.3
  aponeuroses — *see* Enthesopathy
  appendix K38.9
    specified NEC K38.8
  aqueous (chamber) H21.9
  Arnold-Chiari — *see* Arnold-Chiari disease
  arterial I77.9
    occlusive — *see* Occlusion, by site
      due to stricture or stenosis I77.1
  arteriocardiorenal — *see* Hypertension, cardiorenal
  arteriolar (generalized) (obliterative) I77.9

Disease, diseased — *see also* Syndrome — *continued*
  arteriorenal — *see* Hypertension, kidney
  arteriosclerotic — *see also* Arteriosclerosis
    cardiovascular — *see* Disease, heart, ischemic, atherosclerotic
    coronary (artery) — *see* Disease, heart, ischemic, atherosclerotic
    heart — *see* Disease, heart, ischemic, atherosclerotic
  artery I77.9
    cerebral I67.9
    coronary — *see* Disease, heart, ischemic, atherosclerotic
  arthropod-borne NOS (viral) A94
    specified type NEC A93.8
  atticoantral, chronic H66.20
    left H66.22
      with right H66.23
    right H66.21
      with left H66.23
  auditory canal — *see* Disorder, ear, external
  auricle, ear NEC — *see* Disorder, pinna
  Australian X A83.4
  autoimmune (systemic) NOS M35.9
    hemolytic (cold type) (warm type) D59.1
      drug-induced D59.0
    thyroid E06.3
  aviator's — *see* Effect, adverse, high altitude
  Ayala's Q78.5
  Ayerza's (pulmonary artery sclerosis with pulmonary hypertension) I27.0
  Babington's (familial hemorrhagic telangiectasia) I78.0
  bacterial A49.9
    specified NEC A48.8
    zoonotic A28.9
      specified type NEC A28.8
  Baelz's (cheilitis glandularis apostematosa) K13.0
  bagasse J67.1
  balloon — *see* Effect, adverse, high altitude
  Bang's (brucella abortus) A23.1
  Bannister's T78.3
  barometer makers' — *see* Poisoning, mercury
  Barraquer (-Simons') (progressive lipodystrophy) E88.1
  Bartholin's gland N75.9
  basal ganglia G25.9
    degenerative G23.9
      specified NEC G23.8
    specified NEC G25.8
  Basedow's (exophthalmic goiter) — *see* Hyperthyroidism, with, goiter (diffuse)
  Bateman's B08.1
  Batten-Steinert G71.1
  Battey A31.0
  Beard's (neurasthenia) F48.8
  Becker's (idiopathic mural endomyocardial disease) I42.3
  Begbie's (exophthalmic goiter) — *see* Hyperthyroidism, with, goiter (diffuse)
  Beigel's (white piedra) B36.2
  behavioral, organic F07.9
  Benson's — *see* Deposit, crystalline
  Bernard-Soulier (thrombopathy) D69.1
  Bernhardt (-Roth) — *see* Mononeuropathy, lower limb, meralgia paresthetica
  Biermer's (pernicious anemia) D51.0
  bile duct (common) (hepatic) K83.9
    with calculus, stones — *see* Calculus, bile duct
    specified NEC K83.8
  biliary (tract) K83.9
    specified NEC K83.8
  Billroth's — *see* Spina bifida
  bird fancier's J67.2
  black lung J60
  bladder N32.9
    in (due to)
      schistosomiasis (bilharziasis) B65.0 [N33]
    specified NEC N32.8
  bleeder's D66
  blood D75.9
    forming organs D75.9
    vessel I99.9
  Bloodgood's — *see* Mastopathy, cystic

Disease, diseased — *see also* Syndrome — *continued*
  Bodechtel-Guttmann (subacute sclerosing panencephalitis) A81.1
  bone — *see also* Disorder, bone
    aluminum M83.4
    fibrocystic NEC
      jaw M27.49
  bone-marrow D75.9
  Borna A83.9
  Bornholm (epidemic pleurodynia) B33.0
  Bouchard's (myopathic dilatation of the stomach) K31.0
  Bouillaud's (rheumatic heart disease) I01.9
  Bourneville (-Brissaud) (tuberous sclerosis) Q85.1
  Bouveret (-Hoffmann) (paroxysmal tachycardia) I47.9
  bowel K63.9
    functional K59.9
      psychogenic F45.0
  brain G93.9
    arterial, artery I67.9
    arteriosclerotic I67.2
    congenital Q04.9
    degenerative — *see* Degeneration, brain
    inflammatory — *see* Encephalitis
    organic G93.9
      arteriosclerotic I67.2
    parasitic NEC B71.9 [G94]
    Pick's G31.0
      dementia in G31.0 [F02.80]
        with behavioral disturbance G31.0 [F02.81]
    senile NEC G31.1
    specified NEC G93.8
  breast (see also Disorder, breast) N64.9
    cystic (chronic) — *see* Mastopathy, cystic
    fibrocystic — *see* Mastopathy, cystic
    Paget's (M8540/3)
      female, unspecified side C50.00
        left side C50.02
        right side C50.01
      male, unspecified side C50.05
        left side C50.04
        right side C50.03
    specified NEC N64.8
  Breda's — *see* Yaws
  Bretonneau's (diphtheritic malignant angina) A36.0
  Bright's — *see* Nephritis
  Brill's (recrudescent typhus) A75.1
  Brill-Zinsser (recrudescent typhus) A75.1
  Brion-Kayser — *see* Fever, paratyphoid
  broad
    beta E78.2
    ligament (noninflammatory) N83.9
      inflammatory — *see* Disease, pelvis, inflammatory
    specified NEC N83.8
  Brocq-Duhring (dermatitis herpetiformis) L13.0
  Brocq's
    meaning
      dermatitis herpetiformis L13.0
      prurigo L28.2
  bronchopulmonary J98.4
  bronchus NEC J98.0
  bronze Addison's E27.1
    tuberculous A18.7
  budgerigar fancier's J67.2
  bullous L13.9
    chronic of childhood L12.2
    specified NEC L13.8
  Buerger's (thromboangiitis obliterans) I73.1
  Bürger-Grütz (essential familial hyperlipemia) E78.3
  bursa — *see* Bursopathy
  caisson T70.3
  California — *see* Coccidioidomycosis
  capillaries I78.9
    specified NEC I78.8
  Carapata A68.0
  cardiac — *see* Disease, heart
  cardiopulmonary, chronic I27.9
  cardiorenal (hepatic) (hypertensive) (vascular) — *see* Hypertension, cardiorenal

©2002 Ingenix, Inc.

Disease, diseased — *see also* Syndrome — *continued*
cardiovascular I51.6
  atherosclerotic — *see* Disease, heart, ischemic, atherosclerotic
  congenital Q28.9
    fetus or newborn P29.9
      specified NEC P29.8
  hypertensive — *see* Hypertension, heart
  renal (hypertensive) — *see* Hypertension, cardiorenal
  syphilitic (asymptomatic) A52.00
cartilage — *see* Disorder, cartilage
Castellani's A69.8
cat-scratch A28.1
Cavare's (familial periodic paralysis) G72.3
cecum K63.9
celiac (adult) (infantile) K90.0
cellular tissue L98.9
central core G71.2
cerebellar, cerebellum — *see* Disease, brain
cerebral — *see also* Disease, brain
  degenerative — *see* Degeneration, brain
cerebrospinal G96.9
cerebrovascular I67.9
  acute I67.8
    embolic I63.4
      puerperal, postpartum, childbirth — *see* Disease, circulatory system, obstetric
    thrombotic I63.3
  arteriosclerotic I67.2
  embolic I66.9
  occlusive I66.9
    puerperal, postpartum, childbirth — *see* Disease, circulatory system, obstetric
  specified NEC I67.8
  thrombotic I66.9
cervix (uteri) (noninflammatory) N88.9
  inflammatory — *see* Cervicitis
  specified NEC N88.8
Chabert's A22.9
Chandler's (osteochondritis dissecans, hip) — *see* Osteochondritis, dissecans, hip
Charlouis — *see* Yaws
Chédiak-Steinbrinck (-Higashi) (congenital gigantism of peroxidase granules) D72.0
chest J98.9
Chiari's (hepatic vein thrombosis) I82.0
Chicago B40.9
Chignon (white piedra) B36.2
chigo, chigoe B88.1
childhood granulomatous D71
Chinese liver fluke B66.1
chlamydial A74.9
  specified NEC A74.89
cholecystic K82.9
choroid H31.9
  specified NEC H31.8
Christmas D67
chronic bullous of childhood L12.2
chylomicron retention E78.3
ciliary body H21.9
  specified NEC H21.8
circulatory (system) NEC I99.8
  fetus or newborn P29.9
  obstetric complicating
    childbirth O99.42
    pregnancy O99.419
      first trimester O99.411
      second trimester O99.412
      third trimester O99.413
    puerperium O99.43
  syphilitic A52.00
    congenital A50.54 *[I98]*
climacteric (female) N95.1
  male N50.8
coagulation factor deficiency (congenital) — *see* Defect, coagulation
coccidioidal — *see* Coccidioidomycosis
cold
  agglutinin or hemoglobinuria D59.1
    paroxysmal D59.6
  hemagglutinin (chronic) D59.1
collagen NOS (nonvascular) (vascular) M35.9
  specified NEC M35.8

Disease, diseased — *see also* Syndrome — *continued*
colon K63.9
  functional K59.9
    congenital Q43.2
  ischemic K55.0
combined system — *see* Degeneration, combined
compressed air T70.3
Concato's (pericardial polyserositis) I31.1
  pleural — *see* Pleurisy, with effusion
conjunctiva H11.9
  chlamydial A74.0
  specified NEC H11.89
  viral B30.9
    specified NEC B30.8
connective tissue, systemic (diffuse) M35.9
  in (due to)
    hypogammaglobulinemia D80.1 *[M36.8]*
    ochronosis E70.29 *[M36.8]*
  specified NEC M35.8
Conor and Bruch's (boutonneuse fever) A77.1
Cooper's — *see* Mastopathy, cystic
Cori's (glycogenosis III) E74.03
corkhandler's or corkworker's J67.3
cornea H18.9
  specified NEC H18.89
coronary (artery) — *see* Disease, heart, ischemic, atherosclerotic
  congenital Q24.5
  ostial, syphilitic (aortic) (mitral) (pulmonary) A52.03
corpus cavernosum N48.9
  specified NEC N48.89
Cotugno's — *see* Sciatica
coxsackie (virus) NEC B34.1
cranial nerve NOS G52.9
Creutzfeldt-Jakob A81.0
Crocq's (acrocyanosis) I73.8
Crohn's — *see* Enteritis, regional
cystic
  breast (chronic) — *see* Mastopathy, cystic
  kidney, congenital Q61.9
  liver, congenital Q44.6
  lung J98.4
    congenital Q33.0
cytomegalic inclusion (generalized) B25.9
  with pneumonia B25.0
  congenital P35.1
cytomegaloviral B25.9
  specified NEC B25.8
Czerny's (periodic hydrarthrosis of the knee) — *see* Effusion, joint, knee
Daae (-Finsen) (epidemic pleurodynia) B33.0
Darling's — *see* Histoplasmosis capsulati
Débove's (splenomegaly) R16.1
deer fly — *see* Tularemia
Degos' I77.8
demyelinating, demyelinizating (nervous system) G37.9
  multiple sclerosis G35
  specified NEC G37.8
dense deposit (*see also* N00-N07 with fourth character .6) N05.6
deposition, hydroxyapatite — *see* Disease, hydroxyapatite deposition
de Quervain's (tendon sheath) M65.4
  thyroid (subacute granulomatous thyroiditis) E06.1
Devergie's (pityriasis rubra pilaris) L44.0
Devic's G36.0
diaphorase deficiency D74.0
diaphragm J98.6
diarrheal, infectious NEC A09
digestive system K92.9
  specified NEC K92.8
disc, degenerative — *see* Degeneration, intervertebral disc
discogenic — *see also* Displacement, intervertebral disc NEC
  with myelopathy — *see* Disorder, disc, with, myelopathy
diverticular — *see* Diverticula
Dubois (thymus) A50.59
Duchenne-Griesinger G71.0

Disease, diseased — *see also* Syndrome — *continued*
Duchenne's
  muscular dystrophy G71.0
  pseudohypertrophy, muscles G71.0
ductless glands E34.9
Duhring's (dermatitis herpetiformis) L13.0
duodenum K31.9
  specified NEC K31.89
Dupré's (meningism) R29.1
Dupuytren's (muscle contracture) M72.0
Durand-Nicholas-Favre (climatic bubo) A55
Duroziez's (congenital mitral stenosis) Q23.2
ear — *see* Disorder, ear
Eberth's — *see* Fever, typhoid
Ebola (virus) A98.4
Ebstein's
  heart Q22.5
  meaning diabetes — *see* E09-E13 with .22
Echinococcus — *see* Echinococcus
echovirus NEC B34.1
Eddowes' (brittle bones and blue sclera) Q78.0
edentulous (alveolar) ridge K06.9
  specified NEC K06.8
Edsall's T67.2
Eichstedt's (pityriasis versicolor) B36.0
Ellis-van Creveld (chondroectodermal dysplasia) Q77.6
end-stage renal N18.0
endocrine glands or system NEC E34.9
endomyocardial (eosinophilic) I42.3
English (rickets) E55.0
enteroviral, enterovirus NEC B34.1
  central nervous system NEC A88.8
epidemic B99.9
  specified NEC B99.8
epididymis N50.9
Erb-Goldflam G70.0
Erb (-Landouzy) G71.0
esophagus K22.9
  functional K22.4
  psychogenic F45.8
  specified NEC K22.8
Eulenburg's (congenital paramyotonia) G71.1
eustachian tube — *see* Disorder, eustachian tube
external
  auditory canal — *see* Disorder, ear, external
  ear — *see* Disorder, ear, external
extrapyramidal G25.9
  specified NEC G25.8
eye H57.9
  anterior chamber H21.9
  inflammatory NEC H57.8
  muscle (external) — *see* Strabismus
  specified NEC H57.8
  syphilitic — *see* Oculopathy, syphilitic
eyeball H44.9
  specified NEC H44.89
eyelid — *see* Disorder, eyelid
  specified NEC — *see* Disorder, eyelid, specified type NEC
eyeworm of Africa B74.3
facial nerve (seventh) G51.9
  newborn (birth injury) P11.3
fallopian tube (noninflammatory) N83.9
  inflammatory — *see* Salpingo-oophoritis
  specified NEC N83.8
familial periodic paralysis G72.3
Fanconi's (congenital pancytopenia) D61.0
fascia NEC *see also* Disorder, muscle
  inflammatory — *see* Myositis
  specified NEC M62.89
Fauchard's (periodontitis) K05.3
Favre-Durand-Nicolas (climatic bubo) A55
Fede's K14.0
Feer's — *see* Poisoning, mercury
female pelvic inflammatory (*see also* Disease, pelvis, inflammatory) N73.9
  syphilitic (secondary) A51.42
  tuberculous A18.17
Fernels' (aortic aneurysm) I71.9
fetal NEC, known or suspected, affecting management of pregnancy O35.8
fibrocaseous of lung — *see* Tuberculosis, pulmonary
fibrocystic — *see* Fibrocystic disease
Fiedler's (leptospiral jaundice) A27.0

Disease, diseased — *see also* Syndrome — *continued*
  fifth B08.3
  file-cutter's — *see* Poisoning, lead
  fish-skin Q80.9
    acquired L85.0
  Flajani (-Basedow) (exophthalmic goiter) — *see* Hyperthyroidism, with, goiter (diffuse)
  flax-dresser's J66.1
  fluke — *see* Infestation, fluke
  foot and mouth B08.8
  foot process — *see* Nephrosis
  Forbes' (glycogenosis III) E74.03
  Fordyce-Fox (apocrine miliaria) L75.2
  Fordyce's (ectopic sebaceous glands) (mouth) Q38.6
  Fothergill's
    neuralgia — *see* Neuralgia, trigeminal
    scarlatina anginosa A38.9
  Fournier's N49.3
  fourth D00.0
  Fox (-Fordyce) (apocrine miliaria) L75.2
  Francis' — *see* Tularemia
  Frei's (climatic bubo) A55
  Friedreich's
    combined systemic or ataxia G11.1
    myoclonia G25.3
  frontal sinus — *see* Sinusitis, frontal
  fungus NEC B49
  Gaisböck's (polycythemia hypertonica) D75.1
  gallbladder K82.9
    calculus — *see* Calculus, gallbladder
    cholecystitis — *see* Cholecystitis
    cholesterolosis K82.4
    fistula — *see* Fistula, gallbladder
    hydrops K82.1
    obstruction — *see* Obstruction, gallbladder
    perforation K82.2
    specified NEC K82.8
  gamma heavy chain (M9763/3) C88.2
  Gamna's (siderotic splenomegaly) D73.2
  Gamstorp's (adynamia episodica hereditaria) G72.3
  Gandy-Nanta (siderotic splenomegaly) D73.2
  ganister J62.8
  gastric — *see* Disease, stomach
  gastrointestinal (tract) K92.9
    amyloid E85 [K93]
    functional K59.9
      psychogenic F45.8
    specified NEC K92.8
  Gee (-Herter) (-Heubner) (-Thaysen) (nontropical sprue) K90.0
  generalized neoplastic (M8000/6) C80
  genital organs
    female N94.9
    male N50.9
  Gerhardt's (erythromelalgia) I73.8
  Gibert's (pityriasis rosea) L42
  Gierke's (glycogenosis I) E74.01
  Gilles de la Tourette's (motor-verbal tic) F95.2
  gingiva K06.9
    specified NEC K06.8
  gland (lymph) I89.9
  Glanzmann's (hereditary hemorrhagic thrombasthenia) D69.1
  glass-blower's (cataract) — *see* Cataract, specified NEC
  salivary gland hypertrophy K11.1
  Glisson's — *see* Rickets
  globe H44.9
    specified NEC H44.89
  glomerular — *see also* Glomerulonephritis
    with edema — *see* Nephrosis
    acute — *see* Nephritis, acute
    minimal change N04.0
    rapidly progressive N01.9
  glycogen storage E74.00
    Andersen's E74.09
    Cori's E74.03
    Forbes' E74.03
    generalized E74.00
    glucose-6-phosphatase deficiency E74.01
    heart E74.02 [I43]
    hepatorenal E74.09
    Hers' E74.09
    liver and kidney E74.01
    McArdle's E74.04

Disease, diseased — *see also* Syndrome — *continued*
  glycogen storage — *continued*
    muscle phosphofructokinase E74.09
    myocardium E74.02 [I43]
    Pompe's E74.02
    Tauri's E74.09
    type 0 E74.09
    type I E74.01
    type II E74.02
    type III E74.03
    type IV E74.09
    type V E74.04
    type VI-XI E74.09
    Von Gierke's E74.01
  Goldflam-Erb G70.0
  Goldstein's (familial hemorrhagic telangiectasia) I78.0
  gonococcal NOS A54.9
  graft-versus-host (GVH) (bone marrow) T86.01
  grainhandler's J67.0
  granulomatous (childhood) (chronic) D71
  Graves' (exophthalmic goiter) — *see* Hyperthyroidism, with, goiter (diffuse)
  Griesinger's — *see* Ancylostomiasis
  Grisel's M43.6
  Gruby's (tinea tonsurans) B35.0
  Guillain-Barré G61.0
  Guinon's (motor-verbal tic) F95.2
  gum K06.9
  gynecological N94.9
  H (Hartnup's) E72.02
  Haff — *see* Poisoning, arsenic
  Hageman (congenital factor XII deficiency) D68.2
  hair (color) (shaft) L67.9
    follicles L73.9
      specified NEC L73.8
  Hamman's (spontaneous mediastinal emphysema) J98.2
  hand, foot and mouth B08.4
  Hansen's — *see* Leprosy
  Harada's — *see* Vogt-Koyanagi syndrome
  Hartnup (pellagra-cerebellar ataxia-renal aminoaciduria) E72.02
  Hart's (pellagra-cerebellar ataxia-renal aminoaciduria) E72.02
  Hashimoto's (struma lymphomatosa) E06.3
  Hb — *see* Disease, hemoglobin
  heart (organic) I51.9
    with
      acute pulmonary edema — *see* Failure, ventricular, left
      rheumatic fever (conditions in I00)
        active I01.9
          with chorea I02.0
          specified NEC I01.8
        inactive or quiescent (with chorea) I09.9
          specified NEC I09.89
    amyloid E85 [I43]
    aortic (valve) I35.9
    arteriosclerotic or sclerotic (senile) — *see* Disease, heart, ischemic, atherosclerotic
    artery, arterial — *see* Disease, heart, ischemic, atherosclerotic
    beer drinkers' I42.6
    beriberi (wet) E51.12
    black I27.0
    congenital Q24.9
      cyanotic Q24.9
      specified NEC Q24.8
    congestive — *see* Failure, heart, congestive
    coronary — *see* Disease, heart, ischemic
    cryptogenic I51.9
    fibroid — *see* Myocarditis
    functional I51.8
      psychogenic F45.8
    glycogen storage E74.02 [I43]
    gonococcal A54.83
    hypertensive — *see* Hypertension, heart
    hyperthyroid (*see also* Hyperthyroidism) E05.90 [I43]
      with thyroid storm E05.91 [I43]

Disease, diseased — *see also* Syndrome — *continued*
  heart — *continued*
    ischemic (chronic or with a stated duration of over 4 weeks) I25.9
      with
        aneurysm (heart) I25.3
          coronary artery I25.4
        acute or with a stated duration of 4 weeks or less I24.9
          specified NEC I24.8
        without myocardial infarction I24.9
          with coronary (artery) occlusion I24.0
      atherosclerotic (of) I25.10
        with angina pectoris I25.11
          angiospastic (Prinzmetal) I25.13
          specified form NEC I25.19
          unstable I25.12
        coronary artery bypass graft I25.700
          with angina pectoris I25.709
            with documented spasm I25.702
            specified type NEC I25.708
            unstable I25.701
          autologous (vein) I25.710
            with angina pectoris I25.719
              with documented spasm I25.712
              specified type NEC I25.718
              unstable I25.711
          artery I25.720
            with angina pectoris I25.729
              with documented spasm I25.722
              specified type NEC I25.728
              unstable I25.721
          nonautologous biological I25.730
            with angina pectoris I25.739
              with documented spasm I25.732
              specified type NEC I25.738
              unstable I25.731
          specified NEC I25.790
            with angina pectoris I25.799
              with documented spasm I25.792
              specified type NEC I25.798
              unstable I25.791
      asymptomatic I25.6
      cardiomyopathy I25.5
      diagnosed on ECG or other special investigation, but currently presenting no symptoms I25.6
      silent I25.6
      specified form NEC I25.8
    kyphoscoliotic I27.1
    meningococcal A39.50
      endocarditis A39.51
      myocarditis A39.52
      pericarditis A39.53
    mitral I05.9
      specified NEC I05.8
    muscular — *see* Degeneration, myocardial
    psychogenic (functional) F45.8
    pulmonary (chronic) I27.9
      acute I26.0
      in schistosomiasis B65.9 [I52]
      specified NEC I27.8
    rheumatic (chronic) (inactive) (old) (quiescent) (with chorea) I09.9
      active or acute I01.9
        with chorea (acute) (rheumatic) (Sydenham's) I02.0
      specified NEC I09.89
    senile — *see* Myocarditis
    syphilitic A52.06
      aortic A52.03
        aneurysm A52.01
      congenital A50.54 [I52]
    thyrotoxic (*see also* Thyrotoxicosis) E05.90 [I43]
      with thyroid storm E05.91 [I43]
    valve, valvular (obstructive) (regurgitant) — *see also* Endocarditis
      congenital NEC Q24.8
      pulmonary Q22.3

©2002 Ingenix, Inc.

Disease, diseased — *see also* Syndrome — *continued*
heart — *continued*
  vascular — *see* Disease, cardiovascular
heavy chain
  alpha (M9762/3) C88.1
  gamma (M9763/3) C88.2
Hebra's
  pityriasis
    maculata et circinata L42
    rubra pilaris L44.0
  prurigo L28.2
hematopoietic organs D75.9
hemoglobin or Hb
  abnormal (mixed) NEC D58.2
    with thalassemia D56.9
  AS genotype D57.3
  C (Hb-C) D58.2
    with other abnormal hemoglobin NEC D58.2
    elliptocytosis D58.1
    Hb-S D57.2
    sickle-cell D57.2
    thalassemia D56.9
  D (Hb-D) D58.2
  E (Hb-E) D58.2
  elliptocytosis D58.1
  H (Hb-H) (thalassemia) D56.0
    with other abnormal hemoglobin NEC D56.9
  I thalassemia D56.9
  M D74.0
  S or SS — *see* Disease, sickle-cell
  SC D57.2
  SD D57.2
  SE D57.2
  spherocytosis D58.0
  unstable, hemolytic D58.2
hemolytic (fetus) (newborn) P55.9
  autoimmune (cold type) (warm type) D59.1
  drug-induced D59.0
  due to or with
    incompatibility
      ABO (blood group) P55.1
      blood (group) (Duffy) (K(ell)) (Kidd) (Lewis) (M) (S) NEC P55.8
      Rh (blood group) (factor) P55.0
      Rh negative mother P55.0
    specified type NEC P55.8
  unstable hemoglobin D58.2
hemorrhagic D69.9
  newborn P53
Henoch (-Schönlein) (purpura nervosa) D69.0
hepatic — *see* Disease, liver
hepatolenticular E83.01
heredodegenerative NEC
  spinal cord G95.89
herpesviral, disseminated B00.7
Hers' (glycogenosis VI) E74.09
Herter (-Gee) (-Heubner) (nontropical sprue) K90.0
Heubner-Herter (nontropical sprue) K90.0
high fetal gene or hemoglobin thalassemia D56.9
Hildenbrand's — *see* Typhus
hip (joint) M25.9
  congenital Q65.8
  suppurative M00.9
  tuberculous A18.02
Hirschfeld's (acute diabetes mellitus) E14.8
His (-Werner) (trench fever) A79.0
Hodgson's I71.9
  ruptured I71.8
Holla — *see* Spherocytosis
hookworm B76.9
  specified NEC B76.8
host-versus-graft (immune or nonimmune) T86.91
  heart T86.21
  kidney T86.11
  liver T86.41
human immunodeficiency virus (HIV) B20
Huntington's G10
Hutchinson's (cheiropompholyx) L30.1
hyaline (diffuse) (generalized)
  membrane (lung) (newborn) P22.0
    adult J80

Disease, diseased — *see also* Syndrome — *continued*
hydatid — *see* Echinococcus
hydroxyapatite deposition M11.00
  ankle M11.079
    left M11.072
    right M11.071
  elbow M11.029
    left M11.022
    right M11.021
  foot joint M11.079
    left M11.072
    right M11.071
  hand joint M11.049
    left M11.042
    right M11.041
  hip M11.059
    left M11.052
    right M11.051
  knee M11.069
    left M11.062
    right M11.061
  multiple site M11.09
  shoulder M11.019
    left M11.012
    right M11.011
  vertebra M11.08
  wrist M11.039
    left M11.032
    right M11.031
hyperkinetic — *see* Hyperkinesia
hypertensive — *see* Hypertension
hypophysis E23.7
Iceland G93.3
I-cell E77.0
ill-defined R68.8
immune D89.9
immunoproliferative (M9760/3) C88.9
  small intestinal (M9764/3) C88.3
  specified NEC C88.7
inclusion B25.9
  salivary gland B25.9
infectious, infective B99.9
  complicating pregnancy, childbirth or puerperium — *see* Disease, infectious, obstetric
  congenital P37.9
    specified NEC P37.8
  obstetric
    complicating
      childbirth O98.92
      pregnancy O98.919
        first trimester O98.911
        second trimester O98.912
        third trimester O98.913
      puerperium O98.93
    gonorrhea — *see* Gonorrhea, obstetric
    protozoal disease — *see* Disease, protozoal, obstetric
    specified infection NEC complicating
      childbirth O98.82
      pregnancy O98.819
        first trimester O98.811
        second trimester O98.812
        third trimester O98.813
      puerperium O98.83
    STD NEC — *see* Disease, sexually transmitted, obstetric
    streptococcus B — *see* Infection, streptococcus, B genitourinary, obstetric
    syphilis — *see* Syphilis, obstetric
    tuberculosis — *see* Tuberculosis, obstetric
    viral
      hepatitis — *see* Hepatitis, viral, obstetric
      infection NEC — *see* Disease, viral, obstetric
  specified NEC B99.8
inflammatory
  penis N48.29
    abscess N48.21
    cellulitis N48.22
  prepuce N47.7
    balanoposthitis N47.6

Disease, diseased — *see also* Syndrome — *continued*
inflammatory — *continued*
  tubo-ovarian — *see* Salpingo-oophoritis
intervertebral disc — *see also* Disorder, disc
  with myelopathy — *see* Disorder, disc, with, myelopathy
  cervical, cervicothoracic — *see* Disorder, disc, cervical
  with
    myelopathy — *see* Disorder, disc, cervical, with myelopathy
    neuritis, radiculitis or radiculopathy — *see* Disorder, disc, cervical, with neuritis
    specified NEC — *see* Disorder, disc, cervical, specified type NEC
  lumbar (with)
    myelopathy M51.06
    neuritis, radiculitis, radiculopathy or sciatica M51.16
    specified NEC M51.86
  lumbosacral (with)
    myelopathy M51.07
    neuritis, radiculitis, radiculopathy or sciatica M51.17
    specified NEC M51.87
  specified NEC — *see* Disorder, disc, specified NEC
  thoracic (with)
    myelopathy M51.04
    neuritis, radiculitis or radiculopathy M51.14
    specified NEC M51.84
  thoracolumbar (with)
    myelopathy M51.05
    neuritis, radiculitis or radiculopathy M51.15
    specified NEC M51.85
intestine K63.9
  functional K59.9
    psychogenic F45.8
    specified NEC K59.8
  organic K63.9
  protozoal A07.9
  specified NEC K63.8
iris H21.9
  specified NEC H21.8
iron metabolism or storage E83.10
island (scrub typhus) A75.3
itai-itai — *see* Poisoning, cadmium
Jakob-Creutzfeldt A81.0
jaw M27.9
  fibrocystic M27.49
  specified NEC M27.8
jigger B88.1
joint — *see also* Disorder, joint
  Charcôt's — *see* Arthropathy, Charcôt's
  degenerative — *see also* Arthrosis
    multiple M15.9
    spine — *see* Spondylosis
  hypertrophic — *see* Arthrosis
  sacroiliac M53.3
  specified NEC — *see* Disorder, joint, specified type NEC
  spine NEC — *see* Dorsopathy
  suppurative — *see* Arthritis, pyogenic or pyemic
Jourdain's (acute gingivitis) K05.0
Kaschin-Beck (endemic polyarthritis) M12.10
  ankle M12.179
    left M12.172
    right M12.171
  elbow M12.129
    left M12.122
    right M12.121
  foot joint M12.179
    left M12.172
    right M12.171
  hand joint M12.149
    left M12.142
    right M12.141
  hip M12.159
    left M12.152
    right M12.151
  knee M12.169
    left M12.162

Disease, diseased — *see also* Syndrome — *continued*

Kaschin-Beck — *continued*
  knee — *continued*
    right M12.161
  multiple site M12.19
  shoulder M12.119
    left M12.112
    right M12.111
  vertebra M12.18
  wrist M12.139
    left M12.132
    right M12.131
Katayama B65.2
Kedani (scrub typhus) A75.3
Keshan E59
kidney (functional) (pelvis) — *see also* Disease, renal
  cystic (congenital) Q61.9
  fibrocystic (congenital) Q61.8
  in (due to)
    schistosomiasis (bilharziasis) B65.9 *[N29]*
  polycystic Q61.3
    adult type Q61.2
    childhood type Q61.19
      collecting duct dilatation Q61.11
Kimmelstiel (-Wilson) (intercapillary polycystic (congenital) glomerulosclerosis — *see* E09-E13 with .21
Kinnier Wilson's (hepatolenticular degeneration) E83.01
kissing — *see* Mononucleosis, infectious
Kleb's — *see* Nephritis
Klippel-Feil (brevicollis) Q76.1
Köhler-Pellegrini-Stieda (calcification, knee joint) — *see* Bursitis, tibial collateral
König's (osteochondritis dissecans) — *see* Osteochondritis, dissecans
Korsakoff's (nonalcoholic) F04
  alcoholic F10.96
    with dependence F10.26
Kostmann's (infantile genetic agranulocytosis) D70.0
kuru A81.8
Kyasanur Forest A98.2
labyrinth, ear — *see* Disorder, ear, inner
lacrimal system — *see* Disorder, lacrimal system
Lafora's G25.3
Lancereaux-Mathieu (leptospiral jaundice) A27.0
Landry's G61.0
Larrey-Weil (leptospiral jaundice) A27.0
larynx J38.7
legionnaire's A48.1
  nonpneumonic A48.2
Lenegre's I44.2
lens H27.9
  specified NEC H27.8
Lev's (acquired complete heart block) I44.2
Lichtheim's (subacute combined sclerosis with pernicious anemia) D51.0
Lightwood's (renal tubular acidosis) N25.8
Lignac's (cystinosis) E72.04
lip K13.0
lipid-storage E75.6
  specified NEC E75.5
Lipschütz's N76.6
liver (chronic) (organic) K76.9
  alcoholic (chronic) K70.9
    acute — *see* Disease, liver, alcoholic, hepatitis
    cirrhosis K70.30
      with ascites K70.31
    failure K70.40
      with coma K70.41
    fatty liver K70.0
    fibrosis K70.2
    hepatitis K70.10
      with ascites K70.11
    sclerosis K70.2
  cystic, congenital Q44.6
  drug-induced (idiosyncratic) (toxic) (predictable) (unpredictable) — *see* Disease, liver, toxic
  fibrocystic (congenital) Q44.6

Disease, diseased — *see also* Syndrome — *continued*

liver — *continued*
  fluke
    Chinese B66.1
    oriental B66.1
    sheep B66.3
  glycogen storage E74.09 *[K77]*
  in (due to)
    schistosomiasis (bilharziasis) B65.9 *[K77]*
  inflammatory K75.9
    autoimmune hepatitis K75.4
    specified NEC K75.8
  polycystic (congenital) Q44.6
  toxic K71.9
    with
      cholestasis K71.0
      cirrhosis (liver) K71.7
      fibrosis (liver) K71.7
      focal nodular hyperplasia K71.8
      hepatic granuloma K71.8
      hepatic necrosis K71.10
        with coma K71.11
      hepatitis NEC K71.6
        acute K71.2
        chronic
          active K71.50
            with ascites K71.51
          lobular K71.4
          persistent K71.3
        lupoid K71.50
          with ascites K71.51
      peliosis hepatis K71.8
      veno-occlusive disease (VOD) of liver K71.8
  alcoholic — *see* Disease, liver, alcoholic
  veno-occlusive K76.5
Lobo's (keloid blastomycosis) B48.0
Lobstein's (brittle bones and blue sclera) Q78.0
Ludwig's (submaxillary cellulitis) K12.2
luetic — *see* Syphilis
lumbosacral region M53.87
lung J98.4
  black J60
  congenital Q33.9
  cystic J98.4
    congenital Q33.0
  fibroid (chronic) — *see* Fibrosis, lung
  fluke B66.4
    oriental B66.4
  in
    amyloidosis E85 *[J99]*
    sarcoidosis D86.0
    Sjögren's syndrome M35.02
    systemic
      lupus erythematosus M32.13
      sclerosis M34.81
  interstitial J84.9
    acute B59
    specified NEC J84.8
  obstructive (chronic) J44.9
    with
      acute
        exacerbation NEC J44.1
        lower respiratory infection (except influenza) J44.0
      alveolitis, allergic J67.9
      asthma J44.9
      bronchiectasis J47.9
        with
          acute exacerbation J47.1
          lower respiratory infection J47.0
      bronchitis J44.9
      emphysema J44.9
      hypersensitivity pneumonitis J67.9
  polycystic J98.4
    congenital Q33.0
  rheumatoid (diffuse) (interstitial) — *see* Rheumatoid, lung
Lutembacher's (atrial septal defect with mitral stenosis) Q21.1
Lyme A69.20
lymphatic (gland) (system) (channel) (vessel) I89.9

Disease, diseased — *see also* Syndrome — *continued*

lymphoproliferative NEC (M9970/1) D47.7
  T-gamma (M9768/1) D47.7
  X-linked D82.3
Magitot's M27.2
malarial — *see* Malaria
malignant (M8000/3) — *see also* Neoplasm, malignant
Manson's B65.1
maple bark J67.6
maple-syrup-urine E71.0
Marburg (virus) A98.3
Marion's (bladder neck obstruction) N32.0
Marsh's (exophthalmic goiter) — *see* Hyperthyroidism, with, goiter (diffuse)
mastoid (process) — *see* Disorder, ear, middle
Mathieu's (leptospiral jaundice) A27.0
Maxcy's A75.2
McArdle (-Schmid-Pearson) (glycogenosis V) E74.04
mediastinum J98.5
Mediterranean D56.9
medullary center (idiopathic) (respiratory) G93.8
Meige's (chronic hereditary edema) Q82.0
meningeal — *see* Meningitis
meningococcal — *see* Infection, meningococcal
mental F99
  organic F06.9
mesenchymal M35.9
mesenteric embolic K55.0
metabolic, metabolism E88.9
  bilirubin E80.7
metal-polisher's J62.8
metastatic (M8000/6) — *see* Metastasis
middle ear — *see* Disorder, ear, middle
Mikulicz's (dryness of mouth, absent or decreased lacrimation) K11.1
Milroy's (chronic hereditary edema) Q82.0
Minamata — *see* Poisoning, mercury
minicore G71.2
Minor's G95.19
Minot's (hemorrhagic disease, newborn) P53
Minot-von Willebrand-Jürgens (angiohemophilia) D68.0
Mitchell's (erythromelalgia) I73.8
mitral (valve) I05.9
  nonrheumatic I34.9
mixed connective tissue M35.1
Monge's T70.29
Morgagni-Adams-Stokes (syncope with heart block) I45.9
Morgagni's (syndrome) (hyperostosis frontalis interna) M85.2
Morton's (with metatarsalgia) — *see* Lesion, nerve, plantar
Morvan's G95.0
motor neuron (bulbar) (familial) (mixed type) (spinal) G12.20
  amyotrophic lateral sclerosis G12.21
  progressive bulbar palsy G12.22
  specified NEC G12.29
moldy hay J67.0
moyamoya I67.5
multicore G71.2
muscle *see also* Disorder, muscle
  inflammatory — *see* Myositis
  ocular (external) — *see* Strabismus
musculoskeletal system, soft tissue — *see also* Disorder, soft tissue
  specified NEC — *see* Disorder, soft tissue, specified type NEC
mushroom workers' J67.5
mycotic B49
myeloproliferative (chronic) (M9960/1) D47.1
myocardium, myocardial (*see also* Degeneration, myocardial) I51.5
  primary (idiopathic) I42.9
myoneural G70.9
Naegeli's D69.1
nails L60.9
  specified NEC L60.8
Nairobi (sheep virus) A93.8
nasal J34.9
nemaline body G71.2
neoplastic, generalized (M8000/6) C80
nerve — *see* Disorder, nerve

©2002 Ingenix, Inc.

Disease, diseased — *see also* Syndrome — *continued*
  nervous system G98.8
    affecting management of
      childbirth O99.354
      pregnancy O99.353
        first trimester O99.350
        second trimester O99.351
        third trimester O99.352
      puerperium O99.355
    autonomic G90.9
    central G96.9
      specified NEC G96.8
    congenital Q07.9
    parasympathetic G90.9
    specified NEC G98.8
    sympathetic G90.9
    vegetative G90.9
  neuromuscular system G70.9
  Newcastle B30.8
  Nicolas (-Durand) -Favre (climatic bubo) A55
  nipple N64.9
    Paget's (M8540/3)
      female, unspecified side C50.00
        left side C50.02
        right side C50.01
      male, unspecified side C50.05
        left side C50.04
        right side C50.03
  Nishimoto (-Takeuchi) I67.5
  nonarthropod-borne NOS (viral) B34.9
    enterovirus NEC B34.1
  nonautoimmune hemolytic D59.4
    drug-induced D59.2
  Nonne-Milroy-Meige (chronic hereditary edema) Q82.0
  nose J34.9
  nucleus pulposus — *see* Disorder, disc
  nutritional E63.9
  oast-house-urine E72.19
  ocular
    herpesviral B02.30
    zoster B00.50
  obliterative vascular I77.1
  Ohara's — *see* Tularemia
  Opitz's (congestive splenomegaly) D73.2
  Oppenheim-Urbach (necrobiosis lipoidica diabeticorum) — *see* E09-E13 with .63
  optic nerve NEC — *see* Disorder, nerve, optic
  orbit — *see* Disorder, orbit
  Oriental liver fluke B66.1
  Oriental lung fluke B66.4
  Ormond's N13.8
  Oropouche virus A93.0
  Osler-Rendu (familial hemorrhagic telangiectasia) I78.0
  osteofibrocystic E21.0
  Otto's M16.9
  outer ear — *see* Disorder, ear, external
  ovary (noninflammatory) N83.9
    cystic N83.20
    inflammatory — *see* Salpingo-oophoritis
    polycystic E28.2
    specified NEC N83.8
  ovum (complicating pregnancy) O02.0
  Owren's (congenital) — *see* Defect, coagulation
  pancreas K86.9
    cystic K86.2
    fibrocystic E84.9
    specified NEC K86.8
  panvalvular I08.9
    specified NEC I08.8
  parametrium (noninflammatory) N83.9
  parasitic B89
    cerebral NEC B71.9 [G94]
    complicating pregnancy, childbirth or puerperium — *see* Disease, infectious, obstetric
    intestinal NOS B82.9
    mouth B37.0
    skin NOS B88.9
    specified type — *see* Infestation
    tongue B37.0
  parathyroid (gland) E21.5
    specified NEC E21.4
  Parkinson's G20
  parodontal K05.6

Disease, diseased — *see also* Syndrome — *continued*
  Parrot's (syphilitic osteochondritis) A50.02
  Parry's (exophthalmic goiter) — *see* Hyperthyroidism, with, goiter (diffuse)
  Parson's (exophthalmic goiter) — *see* Hyperthyroidism, with, goiter (diffuse)
  Paxton's (white piedra) B36.2
  pearl-worker's — *see* Osteomyelitis, specified type NEC
  Pellegrini-Stieda (calcification, knee joint) — *see* Bursitis, tibial collateral
  pelvis, pelvic
    female NOS N94.9
      specified NEC N94.8
    gonococcal (acute) (chronic) A54.24
    inflammatory (female) N73.9
      acute N73.0
      chronic N73.1
      complicating pregnancy O23.50
        first trimester O23.51
        second trimester O23.52
        third trimester O23.53
      following ectopic or molar pregnancy O08.0
      specified NEC N73.8
      syphilitic (secondary) A51.42
        late A52.76
      tuberculous A18.17
    organ, female N94.9
    peritoneum, female NEC N94.8
  penis N48.9
    inflammatory N48.29
      abscess N48.21
      cellulitis N48.22
    specified NEC N48.89
  periapical tissues NOS K04.90
  periodontal K05.6
    specified NEC K05.5
  periosteum — *see* Disorder, bone, specified type NEC
  peripheral
    arterial I73.9
    autonomic nervous system G90.9
    nerves — *see* Polyneuropathy
    vascular NOS I73.9
  peritoneum K66.9
    pelvic, female NEC N94.8
    specified NEC K66.8
  persistent mucosal (middle ear) H66.20
    left H66.22
      with right H66.23
    right H66.21
      with left H66.23
  Petit's — *see* Hernia, abdomen, specified site NEC
  pharynx J39.2
    specified NEC J39.2
  Phocas' — *see* Mastopathy, cystic
  photochromogenic (acid-fast bacilli) (pulmonary) A31.0
    nonpulmonary A31.9
  Pick's
    brain G31.0
      with dementia G31.0 [F02.80]
        with behavioral disturbance G31.0 [F02.81]
      cerebral atrophy G31.0
        with dementia G31.0 [F02.80]
          with behavioral disturbance G31.0 [F02.81]
    liver (pericardial pseudocirrhosis of liver) I31.1
    pericardium (pericardial pseudocirrhosis of liver) I31.1
    polyserositis (pericardial pseudocirrhosis of liver) I31.1
  pigeon fancier's J67.2
  pineal gland E34.8
  pink — *see* Poisoning, mercury
  Pinkus' (lichen nitidus) L44.1
  pinna (noninfective) — *see* Disorder, pinna
  pinworm B80
  Piry virus A93.8
  pituitary (gland) E23.7
  pituitary-snuff-taker's J67.8

Disease, diseased — *see also* Syndrome — *continued*
  placenta complicating pregnancy or childbirth — *see* Disorder, placenta
  pleura (cavity) J94.9
    specified NEC J94.8
  pneumatic drill (hammer) T75.21
  Pollitzer's (hidradenitis suppurativa) L73.2
  polycystic
    kidney or renal Q61.3
      adult type Q61.2
      childhood type Q61.19
        collecting duct dilatation Q61.11
    liver or hepatic Q44.6
    lung or pulmonary J98.4
      congenital Q33.0
    ovary, ovaries E28.2
    spleen Q89.09
  Pompe's (glycogenosis II) E74.02
  Posada-Wernicke B38.9
  Potain's (pulmonary edema) J18.2
  pregnancy NEC — *see* Pregnancy
  prepuce N47.8
    inflammatory N47.7
      balanoposthitis N47.6
  Pringle's (tuberous sclerosis) Q85.1
  prion A81.9
    specified NEC A81.8
  prostate N42.9
    specified NEC N42.89
  protozoal B64
    acanthamebiasis — *see* Acanthamebiasis
    African trypanosomiasis — *see* African trypanosomiasis
    babesiosis B60.0
    Chagas disease — *see* Chagas disease
    intestine, intestinal A07.9
    leishmaniasis — *see* Leishmaniasis
    malaria — *see* Malaria
    naegleriasis B60.2
    obstetric complicating
      childbirth O98.62
      pregnancy O98.619
        first trimester O98.611
        second trimester O98.612
        third trimester O98.613
      puerperium O98.63
    pneumocystosis B59
    specified organism NEC B60.8
    toxoplasmosis — *see* Toxoplasmosis
  pseudo-Hurler's E77.0
  psychiatric F99
  psychotic — *see* Psychosis
  Puente's (simple glandular cheilitis) K13.0
  puerperal — *see* Puerperal
  pulmonary — *see also* Disease, lung
    artery I28.9
    heart I27.9
      specified NEC I27.8
    hypertensive (vascular) I27.0
    valve I37.9
    rheumatic I09.89
  pulp (dental) NOS K04.90
  pulseless M31.4
  Putnam's (subacute combined sclerosis with pernicious anemia) D51.0
  Pyle (-Cohn) (craniometaphyseal dysplasia) Q78.5
  ragpicker's or ragsorter's A22.1
  Raynaud's –*see* Raynaud's disease
  Reclus' (cystic) — *see* Mastopathy, cystic
  rectum K62.9
    specified NEC K62.8
  Refsum's (heredopathia atactica polyneuritiformis) G60.1
  renal (functional) (pelvis) N28.9
    with
      edema — *see* Nephrosis
      glomerular lesion — *see* Glomerulonephritis
        with edema — *see* Nephrosis
      interstitial nephritis N12
    acute — *see* Nephritis, acute
    chronic — *see* Nephritis, chronic

Disease, diseased — *see also* Syndrome — *continued*
renal — *continued*
　complicating pregnancy O26.839
　　with hypertension
　　　secondary (pre-existing) — *see* Hypertension, complicating pregnancy, pre-existing, secondary
　　first trimester O26.831
　　second trimester O26.832
　　third trimester O26.833
　cystic, congenital Q61.9
　diabetic — *see* E09-E13 with .29
　end-stage (failure) N18.0
　fibrocystic (congenital) Q61.8
　hypertensive — *see* Hypertension, kidney
　lupus M32.14
　phosphate-losing (tubular) N25.0
　polycystic (congenital) Q61.3
　　adult type Q61.2
　　childhood type Q61.19
　　　collecting duct dilatation Q61.11
　rapidly progressive N01.9
　subacute N04.9
Rendu-Osler-Weber (familial hemorrhagic telangiectasia) I78.0
renovascular (arteriosclerotic) — *see* Hypertension, kidney
respiratory (tract) J98.9
　acute or subacute NOS J06.9
　　due to
　　　chemicals, gases, fumes or vapors (inhalation) J68.3
　　　external agent J70.9
　　　　specified NEC J70.8
　　　radiation J70.0
　　noninfectious J39.8
　chronic NOS J98.9
　　due to
　　　chemicals, gases, fumes or vapors J68.4
　　　external agent J70.9
　　　　specified NEC J70.8
　　　radiation J70.1
　fetus or newborn P27.9
　　specified NEC P27.8
　due to
　　chemicals, gases, fumes or vapors J68.9
　　　acute or subacute NEC J68.3
　　　chronic J68.4
　　external agent J70.9
　　　specified NEC J70.8
　newborn P28.9
　　specified type NEC P28.8
　upper J39.9
　　acute or subacute J06.9
　　noninfectious NEC J39.8
　　specified NEC J39.8
　　streptococcal J06.9
retina, retinal H35.9
　Batten's or Batten-Mayou E75.4 [H36]
　specified NEC H35.89
rheumatoid — *see* Arthritis, rheumatoid
rickettsial NOS A79.9
　specified type NEC A79.8
Riga (-Fede) (cachectic aphthae) K14.0
Riggs' (compound periodontitis) K05.3
Ritter's L00
Rivalta's (cervicofacial actinomycosis) A42.2
Robles' (onchocerciasis) B73.1
Roger's (congenital interventricular septal defect) Q21.0
Rosenthal's (factor XI deficiency) D68.1
Rossbach's (hyperchlorhydria) K30
Ross River B33.1
Roth (-Bernhardt) — *see* Mononeuropathy, lower limb, meralgia paresthetica
Runeberg's (progressive pernicious anemia) D51.0
sacroiliac NEC M53.3
salivary gland or duct K11.9
　inclusion B25.9
　specified NEC K11.8
　virus B25.9
sandworm B76.9
Schimmelbusch's — *see* Mastopathy, cystic

Disease, diseased — *see also* Syndrome — *continued*
Schmorl's — *see* Schmorl's disease or nodes
Schönlein (-Henoch) (purpura rheumatica) D69.0
Schottmüller's — *see* Fever, paratyphoid
Schultz's (agranulocytosis) — *see* Agranulocytosis
sclera H15.9
　specified NEC H15.89
scrofulous (tuberculous) A18.2
scrotum N50.9
sebaceous glands L73.9
semilunar cartilage, cystic — *see also* Derangement, knee, meniscus, cystic
seminal vesicle N50.9
serum NEC T80.6
sexually transmitted A64.9
　anogenital
　　herpesviral infection — *see* Herpes, anogenital
　　warts A63.0
　chancroid A57
　chlamydial infection — *see* Chlamydia
　complicating pregnancy, childbirth or the puerperium — *see* Disease, sexually transmitted, obstetric
　gonorrhea — *see* Gonorrhea
　granuloma inguinale A58
　obstetric complicating
　　childbirth O98.32
　　pregnancy O98.319
　　　first trimester O98.311
　　　second trimester O98.312
　　　third trimester O98.313
　　puerperium O98.33
　specified organism NEC A63.8
　syphilis — *see* Syphilis
　trichomoniasis — *see* Trichomoniasis
shimamushi (scrub typhus) A75.3
shipyard B30.0
sickle-cell D57.1
　with
　　crisis D57.0
　elliptocytosis D57.8
　spherocytosis D57.8
　thalassemia D57.4
silo-filler's J68.8
simian B B00.4
Simons' (progressive lipodystrophy) E88.1
sinus — *see* Sinusitis
Sirkari's B55.0
sixth B08.2
skin L98.9
　due to metabolic disorder NEC E88.9 [L99]
　specified NEC L98.8
slim (HIV) B20
small vessel I73.9
Sneddon-Wilkinson (subcorneal pustular dermatosis) L13.1
South African creeping B88.0
spinal (cord) G95.9
　congenital Q06.9
　specified NEC G95.89
spine — *see also* Spondylopathy
　joint — *see* Dorsopathy
　tuberculous A18.01
spinocerebellar (hereditary) G11.9
　specified NEC G11.8
spleen D73.9
　amyloid E85 [D77]
　organic D73.9
　polycystic Q89.09
　postinfectional D73.8
sponge-diver's — *see* Toxicity, venom, marine animal, sea anemone
Steiner's G71.1
Sticker's (erythema infectiosum) B08.3
Stieda's (calcification, knee joint) — *see* Bursitis, tibial collateral
Stokes' (exophthalmic goiter) — *see* Hyperthyroidism, with, goiter (diffuse)
Stokes-Adams (syncope with heart block) I45.9
stomach K31.9
　functional, psychogenic F45.8
　specified NEC K31.89
stonemason's J62.8

Disease, diseased — *see also* Syndrome — *continued*
storage
　glycogen — *see* Disease, glycogen storage
　mucopolysaccharide — *see* Mucopolysaccharidosis
striatopallidal system NEC G25.8
Stuart-Prower (congenital factor X deficiency) D68.2
Stuart's (congenital factor X deficiency) D68.2
subcutaneous tissue — *see* Disease, skin
supporting structures of teeth K08.9
　specified NEC K08.8
suprarenal (capsule) (gland) E27.9
　hyperfunction E27.0
　specified NEC E27.8
sweat glands L74.9
　specified NEC L74.8
Swift (-Feer) — *see* Poisoning, mercury
swimming-pool granuloma A31.1
Sylvest's (epidemic pleurodynia) B33.0
sympathetic nervous system G90.9
synovium — *see* Disorder, synovium
syphilitic — *see* Syphilis
systemic tissue mast cell (M9741/3) C96.2
Tangier E78.6
Tarral-Besnier (pityriasis rubra pilaris) L44.0
Tauri's E74.09
tear duct — *see* Disorder, lacrimal system
tendon, tendinous — *see also* Disorder, tendon
　nodular — *see* Trigger finger
terminal vessel I73.9
testis N50.9
Thaysen-Gee (nontropical sprue) K90.0
Thomsen's G71.1
throat J39.2
　septic J02.0
thromboembolic — *see* Embolism
thymus (gland) E32.9
　specified NEC E32.8
thyroid (gland) E07.9
　heart (*see also* Hyperthyroidism) E05.90 [I43]
　　with thyroid storm E05.91 [I43]
　specified NEC E07.89
Tietze's M94.0
tongue K14.9
　specified NEC K14.8
tonsils, tonsillar (and adenoids) J35.9
tooth, teeth K08.9
　hard tissues K03.9
　　specified NEC K03.8
　pulp NEC K04.99
　specified NEC K08.8
Tourette's F95.2
trachea NEC J39.8
tricuspid I07.9
　nonrheumatic I36.9
triglyceride-storage E75.5
trophoblastic — *see* Mole, hydatidiform
tsutsugamushi A75.3
tube (fallopian) (noninflammatory) N83.9
　inflammatory — *see* Salpingitis
　specified NEC N83.8
tuberculous NEC — *see* Tuberculosis
tubo-ovarian (noninflammatory) N83.9
　inflammatory — *see* Salpingo-oophoritis
　specified NEC N83.8
tubotympanic, chronic — *see* Otitis, media, suppurative, chronic, tubotympanic
tubulo-interstitial N15.9
　specified NEC N15.8
tympanum — *see* Disorder, tympanic membrane
Uhl's Q22.6
Underwood's (sclerema neonatorum) P83.0
Unverricht (-Lundborg) G25.3
Urbach-Oppenheim (necrobiosis lipoidica diabeticorum) — *see* E09-E13 with .63
ureter N28.9
　in (due to)
　　schistosomiasis (bilharziasis) B65.0 [N29]
urethra N36.9
　specified NEC N36.8
urinary (tract) N39.9
　bladder N32.9
　　specified NEC N32.8

©2002 Ingenix, Inc.

Disease, diseased — *see also* Syndrome — *continued*
urinary — *continued*
  specified NEC N39.8
uterus (noninflammatory) N85.9
  infective — *see* Endometritis
  inflammatory — *see* Endometritis
  specified NEC N85.8
uveal tract (anterior) H21.9
  posterior H31.9
vagabond's B85.1
vagina, vaginal (noninflammatory) N89.9
  inflammatory NEC N76.8
  specified NEC N89.8
valve, valvular I38
  multiple I08.9
    specified NEC I08.8
van Creveld-von Gierke (glycogenosis I) E74.01
vas deferens N50.9
vascular I99.9
  arteriosclerotic — *see* Arteriosclerosis
  ciliary body NEC — *see* Disorder, iris, vascular
  hypertensive — *see* Hypertension
  iris NEC — *see* Disorder, iris, vascular
  obliterative I77.1
    peripheral I73.9
  occlusive I99.8
  peripheral (occlusive) I73.9
    in diabetes mellitus — *see* E09-E13 with .51
vasomotor I73.9
vasospastic I73.9
vein I87.9
venereal (*see also* Disease, sexually transmitted) A64.9
  chlamydial NEC A56.8
    anus A56.3
    genitourinary NOS A56.2
    pharynx A56.4
    rectum A56.3
  cystitis A64.0
  female NEC A64.4
  fifth A55
  male NEC A64.2
  penis A64.1
  sixth A55
  specified nature or type NEC A63.8
  urethritis A64.0
  urinary NEC A64.8
  vagina A64.3
vertebra, vertebral — *see also* Spondylopathy
  disc — *see* Disorder, disc
vibration — *see* Vibration, adverse effects
viral, virus (*see also* Disease, by type of virus) B34.9
  arbovirus NOS A94
  arthropod-borne NOS A94
  congenital P35.9
    specified NEC P35.8
  Hantaan A98.5
    pulmonary syndrome B33.4
  human immunodeficiency (HIV) B20
  Kunjin A83.4
  nonarthropod-borne NOS B34.9
  obstetric
    complicating
      childbirth O98.52
      pregnancy O98.519
        first trimester O98.511
        second trimester O98.512
        third trimester O98.513
      puerperium O98.53
  hepatitis — *see* Hepatitis, viral, obstetric
  Powassan A84.8
  Rocio (encephalitis) A83.6
  suspected damage to fetus affecting management of pregnancy O35.3
  Tahyna B33.8
  vesicular stomatitis A93.8
vitreous H43.9
  specified NEC H43.89
vocal cord J38.3
Volkmann's, acquired T79.6
von Eulenburg's (congenital paramyotonia) G71.1
von Gierke's (glycogenosis I) E74.01

Disease, diseased — *see also* Syndrome — *continued*
von Graefe's — *see* Strabismus, paralytic, ophthalmoplegia, progressive
von Willebrand (-Jürgens) (angiohemophilia) D68.0
Vrolik's (osteogenesis imperfecta) Q78.0
vulva (noninflammatory) N90.9
  inflammatory NEC N76.8
  specified NEC N90.8
Wallgren's (obstruction of splenic vein with collateral circulation) I87.8
Wassilieff's (leptospiral jaundice) A27.0
wasting NEC R64
  due to malnutrition E41
Waterhouse-Friderichsen A39.1
Wegner's (syphilitic osteochondritis) A50.02
Weil's (leptospiral jaundice of lung) A27.0
Weir Mitchell's (erythromelalgia) I73.8
Werdnig-Hoffmann G12.0
Wermer's E31.1
Werner-His (trench fever) A79.0
Werner-Schultz (agranulocytosis) — *see* Agranulocytosis
Wernicke-Posadas B38.9
whipworm B79
white blood cells D72.9
  specified NEC D72.8
white-spot, meaning lichen sclerosus et atrophicus L90.0
  penis N48.0
  vulva N90.4
Wilkie's K55.1
Wilkinson-Sneddon (subcorneal pustular dermatosis) L13.1
Willis' — *see* Diabetes
Wilson's (hepatolenticular degeneration) E83.01
winter vomiting (epidemic) A08.1
woolsorter's A22.1
zoonotic, bacterial A28.9
  specified type NEC A28.8

Disfigurement (due to scar) L90.5

Disgerminoma — *see* Dysgerminoma

DISH (diffuse idiopathic skeletal hyperostosis) — *see* Hyperostosis, ankylosing

Disinsertion, retina — *see* Detachment, retina

Disintegration, complete, of the body R68.8

Dislocatable hip, congenital Q65.6

Dislocation (articular)
with fracture — *see* Fracture
acromioclavicular (joint)
  with displacement
    100%-200% S43.129
      left S43.122
      right S43.121
    more than 200% S43.139
      left S43.132
      right S43.131
  inferior S43.149
    left S43.142
    right S43.141
  posterior S43.159
    left S43.152
    right S43.151
ankle S93.06
  left S93.05
  right S93.04
astragalus — *see* Dislocation, ankle
atlantoaxial S13.121
atlantooccipital S13.111
atloidooccipital S13.111
breast bone S23.29
capsule, joint – code by site under Dislocation
carpal (bone) — *see* Dislocation, wrist
carpometacarpal (joint) NEC S63.056
  left S63.055
  right S63.054
  thumb S63.046
    left S63.045
    right S63.044
cartilage (joint) – code by site under Dislocation
cervical spine (vertebra) — *see* Dislocation, vertebra, cervical
chronic — *see* Dislocation, recurrent
clavicle — *see* Dislocation, acromioclavicular joint

Dislocation — *continued*
coccyx S33.2
congenital NEC Q68.8
coracoid — *see* Dislocation, shoulder
costal cartilage S23.29
costochondral S23.29
cricoarytenoid articulation S13.29
cricothyroid articulation S13.29
dorsal vertebra — *see* Dislocation, vertebra, thoracic
ear ossicle — *see* Discontinuity, ossicles, ear
elbow S53.106
  congenital Q68.8
  left S53.105
  pathological — *see* Dislocation, pathological NEC, elbow
  radial head alone — *see* Dislocation, radial head
  recurrent — *see* Dislocation, recurrent, elbow
  right S53.104
  traumatic S53.106
    anterior S53.116
      left S53.115
      right S53.114
    lateral S53.146
      left S53.145
      right S53.144
    left S53.105
    medial S53.136
      left S53.135
      right S53.134
    posterior S53.126
      left S53.125
      right S53.124
    right S53.104
    specified type NEC S53.196
      left S53.195
      right S53.194
eye, nontraumatic — *see* Luxation, globe
eyeball, nontraumatic — *see* Luxation, globe
femur
  distal end — *see* Dislocation, knee
  proximal end — *see* Dislocation, hip
fibula
  distal end — *see* Dislocation, ankle
  proximal end — *see* Dislocation, knee
finger S63.259
  index S63.258
    left S63.251
    right S63.250
  interphalangeal S63.279
    distal S63.299
      index S63.298
        left S63.291
        right S63.290
      little S63.298
        left S63.297
        right S63.296
      middle S63.298
        left S63.293
        right S63.292
      ring S63.298
        left S63.295
        right S63.294
    index S63.278
      left S63.271
      right S63.270
    little S63.278
      left S63.277
      right S63.276
    middle S63.278
      left S63.273
      right S63.272
    proximal S63.289
      index S63.288
        left S63.281
        right S63.280
      little S63.288
        left S63.287
        right S63.286
      middle S63.288
        left S63.283
        right S63.282
      ring S63.288
        left S63.285

Dislocation — *continued*
  pathological NEC — *continued*
    ankle — *continued*
      right M24.371
    elbow M24.329
      left M24.322
      right M24.321
    foot joint M24.376
      left M24.375
      right M24.374
    hand joint M24.349
      left M24.342
      right M24.341
    hip M24.359
      left M24.352
      right M24.351
    knee M24.369
      left M24.362
      right M24.361
    lumbosacral joint — *see* category M53.2
    pelvic region — *see* Dislocation, pathological, hip
    sacroiliac — *see* category M53.2
    shoulder M24.319
      left M24.312
      right M24.311
    specified joint NEC M24.38
    vertebra M24.38
    wrist M24.339
      left M24.332
      right M24.331
  pelvis NEC S33.30
    specified NEC S33.39
  phalanx
    finger or hand — *see* Dislocation, finger
    foot or toe — *see* Dislocation, toe
  prosthesis, internal — *see* Complications, prosthetic device, by site, mechanical
  radial head S53.006
    anterior S53.016
      left S53.015
      right S53.014
    left S53.005
    posterior S53.026
      left S53.025
      right S53.024
    right S53.004
    specified type NEC S53.096
      left S53.095
      right S53.094
  radiocarpal (joint) S63.026
    left S63.025
    right S63.024
  radiohumeral (joint) — *see* Dislocation, radial head
  radioulnar (joint)
    distal S63.016
      left S63.015
      right S63.014
    proximal — *see* Dislocation, elbow
  radius
    distal end — *see* Dislocation, wrist
    proximal end — *see* Dislocation, radial head
  recurrent M24.40
    ankle M24.473
      left M24.472
      right M24.471
    elbow M24.429
      left M24.422
      right M24.421
    finger M24.446
      left M24.445
      right M24.444
    foot joint M24.476
      left M24.475
      right M24.474
    hand joint M24.443
      left M24.442
      right M24.441
    hip M24.459
      left M24.452
      right M24.451
    joint NEC M24.48
    knee M24.469
      left M24.462
      patella — *see* Dislocation, patella, recurrent

Dislocation — *continued*
  recurrent — *continued*
    knee — *continued*
      right M24.461
    patella — *see* Dislocation, patella, recurrent
    sacroiliac — *see* category M53.2
    shoulder M24.419
      left M24.412
      right M24.411
    toe M24.479
      left M24.478
      right M24.477
    vertebra — *see also* category M43.5
      atlantoaxial M43.4
        with myelopathy M43.3
    wrist M24.439
      left M24.432
      right M24.431
  rib (cartilage) S23.29
  sacrococcygeal S33.2
  sacroiliac (joint) (ligament) S33.2
    congenital Q74.2
    recurrent — *see* category M53.2
  sacrum S33.2
  scaphoid (bone) (hand) (wrist) — *see* Dislocation, wrist
    foot — *see* Dislocation, foot
  scapula — *see* Dislocation, shoulder, girdle, scapula
  semilunar cartilage, knee — *see* Tear, meniscus
  septal cartilage (nose) S03.1
  septum (nasal) (old) J34.2
  sesamoid bone – code by site under Dislocation
  shoulder (blade) (ligament) (joint) (traumatic) S43.006
    acromioclavicular — *see* Dislocation, acromioclavicular
    chronic — *see* Dislocation, recurrent, shoulder
    congenital Q68.8
    girdle S43.306
      left S43.305
      right S43.304
      scapula S43.316
        left S43.315
        right S43.314
      specified site NEC S43.396
        left S43.395
        right S43.394
    humerus S43.006
      anterior S43.016
        left S43.015
        right S43.014
      inferior S43.036
        left S43.035
        right S43.034
      posterior S43.026
        left S43.025
        right S43.024
    left S43.005
    pathological — *see* Dislocation, pathological NEC, shoulder
    recurrent — *see* Dislocation, recurrent, shoulder
    right S43.004
    specified type NEC S43.086
      left S43.085
      right S43.084
  spine
    cervical — *see* Dislocation, vertebra, cervical
    congenital Q76.49
    due to birth trauma P11.5
    lumbar — *see* Dislocation, vertebra, lumbar
    thoracic — *see* Dislocation, vertebra, thoracic
  spontaneous — *see* Dislocation, pathological
  sternoclavicular (joint) S43.206
    anterior S43.216
      left S43.215
      right S43.214
    left S43.205
    posterior S43.226
      left S43.225
      right S43.224
    right S43.204
  sternum S23.29

Dislocation — *continued*
  subglenoid — *see* Dislocation, shoulder
  symphysis pubis S33.4
    obstetric (traumatic) O71.6
  talus — *see* Dislocation, ankle
  tarsal (bone(s)) (joint(s)) — *see* Dislocation, foot
  tarsometatarsal (joint(s)) — *see* Dislocation, foot
  temporomandibular (joint) S03.0
  thigh, proximal end — *see* Dislocation, hip
  thorax S23.20
    specified site NEC S23.29
    vertebra — *see* Dislocation, vertebra
  thumb S63.106
    interphalangeal joint — *see* Dislocation, interphalangeal (joint), thumb
    left S63.105
    metacarpophalangeal joint — *see* Dislocation, metacarpophalangeal (joint), thumb
    right S63.104
  thyroid cartilage S13.29
  tibia
    distal end — *see* Dislocation, ankle
    proximal end — *see* Dislocation, knee
  tibiofibular (joint)
    distal — *see* Dislocation, ankle
    superior — *see* Dislocation, knee
  toe(s) S93.106
    great S93.106
      interphalangeal joint S93.113
        left S93.112
        right S93.111
      metatarsophalangeal joint S93.123
        left S93.122
        right S93.121
    interphalangeal joint S93.119
    left S93.105
    lesser S93.106
      interphalangeal joint S93.116
        left S93.115
        right S93.114
      metatarsophalangeal joint S93.126
        left S93.125
        right S93.124
    metatarsophalangeal joint S93.129
    right S93.104
  tooth S03.2
  trachea S23.29
  ulna
    distal end S63.076
      left S63.075
      right S63.074
    proximal end — *see* Dislocation, elbow
  ulnohumeral (joint) — *see* Dislocation, elbow
  vertebra (articular process) (body)
    cervical S13.101
      atlantoaxial joint S13.121
      atlantooccipital joint S13.111
      atloidooccipital joint S13.111
      joint between
        C0 and C1 S13.111
        C1 and C2 S13.121
        C2 and C3 S13.131
        C3 and C4 S13.141
        C4and C5 S13.151
        C5and C6 S13.161
        C6and C7 S13.171
        C7and T1 S13.181
      occipitoatloid joint S13.111
    congenital Q76.49
    lumbar S33.101
      joint between
        L1and L2 S33.111
        L2and L3 S33.121
        L3 and L4 S33.131
        L4and L5 S33.141
    partial — *see* Subluxation, by site
    recurrent NEC — *see* category M43.5
    thoracic S23.101
      joint between
        T1and T2 S23.111
        T2and T3 S23.121
        T3 and T4 S23.123
        T4and T5 S23.131
        T5 and T6 S23.133
        T6 and T7 S23.141
        T7 and T8 S23.143

Dislocation — *continued*
vertebra — *continued*
  thoracic — *continued*
    joint between — *continued*
      T8 and T9 S23.151
      T9 and T10 S23.153
      T10 and T11 S23.161
      T11 and T12 S23.163
      T12 and L1 S23.171
  wrist (carpal bone) S63.006
    carpometacarpal joint — *see* Dislocation,
      carpometacarpal (joint)
    distal radioulnar joint — *see* Dislocation,
      radioulnar (joint), distal
    left S63.005
    metacarpal bone, proximal — *see*
      Dislocation, metacarpal (bone),
      proximal end
    midcarpal — *see* Dislocation, midcarpal
      (joint)
    radiocarpal joint — *see* Dislocation,
      radiocarpal (joint)
    recurrent — *see* Dislocation, recurrent, wrist
    right S63.004
    specified site NEC S63.096
      left S63.095
      right S63.094
    ulna — *see* Dislocation, ulna, distal end
    xiphoid cartilage S23.29

Disorder (of) — *see also* Disease
acantholytic L11.9
  specified NEC L11.8
acute
  psychotic — *see* Psychosis, acute
  stress F43.0
adjustment F43.20
  with
    anxiety F43.22
      with depressed mood F43.23
    conduct disturbance F43.24
      with emotional disturbance F43.25
    depressed mood F43.21
      with anxiety F43.23
    other specified symptom F43.29
adrenal (capsule) (gland) (medullary) E27.9
  specified NEC E27.8
adrenogenital E25.9
  drug-induced E25.8
  iatrogenic E25.8
  idiopathic E25.8
adult personality (and behavior) F69
  specified NEC F68.8
affective (mood) — *see* Disorder, mood
aggressive, unsocialized F91.1
alcohol-related F10.99
  with
    amnestic disorder, persisting F10.96
    anxiety disorder F10.980
    dementia, persisting F10.97
    intoxication F10.929
      with delirium F10.921
      uncomplicated F10.920
    mood disorder F10.94
    other specified F10.988
    psychotic disorder F10.959
      with
        delusions F10.950
        hallucinations F10.951
    sexual dysfunction F10.981
    sleep disorder F10.988
  in
    abuse F10.19
      with
        anxiety disorder F10.180
        intoxication F10.129
          with delirium F10.121
          uncomplicated F10.120
        other specified disorder F10.188
        psychotic disorder F10.159
          with
            delusions F10.150
            hallucinations F10.151
        sexual dysfunction F10.181
        sleep disorder F10.182
        uncomplicated F10.10

Disorder — *see also* Disease — *continued*
alcohol-related — *continued*
  in — *continued*
    dependence F10.29
      with
        amnestic disorder, persisting
          F10.26
        anxiety disorder F10.280
        dementia, persisting F10.27
        intoxication F10.229
          with delirium F10.221
          uncomplicated F10.220
        mood disorder F10.24
        other specified disorder F10.288
        psychotic disorder F10.259
          with
            delusions F10.250
            hallucinations F10.251
        sexual dysfunction F10.281
        sleep disorder F10.282
        withdrawal F10.239
          with
            delirium F10.231
            perceptual disturbance
              F10.232
          uncomplicated F10.230
    in remission F10.21
    uncomplicated F10.20
allergic — *see* Allergy
alveolar NEC J84.0
amino-acid
  cystathioninuria E72.19
  cystinosis E72.04
  cystinuria E72.01
  glycinuria E72.09
  homocystinuria E72.11
  metabolism — *see* Disturbance, metabolism,
    amino-acid
  specified NEC E72.8
  neonatal, transitory P74.8
  renal transport NEC E72.09
  transport NEC E72.09
amnesic, amnestic
  alcohol-induced F10.96
    with dependence F10.26
  due to (secondary to) general medical
    condition F04
  psychoactive NEC-induced F19.96
    with
      abuse F19.16
      dependence F19.26
  sedative, hypnotic or anxiolytic-induced
    F13.96
    with dependence F13.26
anaerobic glycolysis with anemia D55.2
anxiety F41.9
  due to (secondary to)
    alcohol F10.980
    amphetamine F15.980
      in
        abuse F15.180
        dependence F15.280
    anxiolytic F13.980
      in
        abuse F13.180
        dependence F13.280
    caffeine F15.980
      in
        abuse F15.180
        dependence F15.280
    cannabis F12.980
      in
        abuse F12.180
        dependence F12.280
    cocaine F14.980
      in
        abuse F14.180
        dependence F14.180
    general medical condition F06.4
    hallucinogen F16.980
      in
        abuse F16.180
        dependence F16.280

Disorder — *see also* Disease — *continued*
anxiety — *continued*
  due to — *continued*
    hypnotic F13.980
      in
        abuse F13.180
        dependence F13.280
    inhalant F18.980
      in
        abuse F18.180
        dependence F18.280
    phencyclidine F19.980
      in
        abuse F19.180
        dependence F19.280
    psychoactive substance NEC F19.980
      in
        abuse F19.180
        dependence F19.280
    sedative F13.980
      in
        abuse F13.180
        dependence F13.280
    volatile solvents F18.980
      in
        abuse F18.180
        dependence F18.280
  generalized F41.1
  mixed
    with depression (mild) F41.8
    specified NEC F41.3
  organic F06.4
  phobic F40.9
    of childhood F40.8
    specified NEC F41.8
aortic valve — *see* Endocarditis, aortic
aromatic amino-acid metabolism E70.9
  specified NEC E70.8
arteriole NEC I77.8
artery NEC I77.8
articulation — *see* Disorder, joint
attachment (childhood)
  disinhibited F94.2
  reactive F94.1
attention-deficit hyperactivity F90.9
  combined type F90.2
  hyperactive type F90.1
  inattentive type F90.0
  specified type NEC F90.8
autistic F84.0
autonomic nervous system G90.9
  specified NEC G90.8
avoidant, child or adolescent F40.10
balance
  acid-base E87.8
    mixed E87.4
  electrolyte E87.8
  fluid NEC E87.8
behavioral (disruptive) — *see* Disorder, conduct
beta-amino-acid metabolism E72.8
bile acid and cholesterol metabolism E78.70
  Barth syndrome E78.71
  other specified E78.79
  Smith-Lemli-Opitz syndrome E78.72
bilirubin excretion E80.6
binocular
  movement H51.9
    convergence
      excess H51.12
      insufficiency H51.11
    internuclear ophthalmoplegia — *see*
      Ophthalmoplegia, internuclear
    palsy of conjugate gaze H51.0
    specified type NEC H51.8
  vision NEC — *see* Disorder, vision, binocular
bipolar (I) F31.9
  current episode
    depressed F31.9
      with psychotic features F31.5
      without psychotic features F31.30
        mild F31.31
        moderate F31.32
        severe (without psychotic features)
          F31.4
          with psychotic features F31.5
    hypomanic F31.0

Disorder — *see also* Disease — *continued*
  bipolar — *continued*
    current episode — *continued*
      manic F31.9
        with psychotic features F31.2
        without psychotic features F31.10
          mild F31.11
          moderate F31.12
          severe (without psychotic features) F31.13
          with psychotic features F31.2
      mixed F31.60
        mild F31.61
        moderate F31.62
        severe (without psychotic features) F31.63
        with psychotic features F31.64
      severe depression (without psychotic features) F31.4
        with psychotic features F31.5
    in remission (currently) F31.70
      in full remission
        most recent episode
          depressed F31.76
          hypomanic F31.72
          manic F31.74
          mixed F31.78
      in partial remission
        most recent episode
          depressed F31.75
          hypomanic F31.71
          manic F31.73
          mixed F31.77
    specified NEC F31.89
    II F31.81
    organic F06.30
    single manic episode F30.9
      mild F30.11
      moderate F30.12
      severe (without psychotic symptoms) F30.13
      with psychotic symptoms F30.2
  bladder N32.9
    functional NEC N31.9
    in schistosomiasis B65.0 [N33]
    specified NEC N32.8
  blood
    in congenital early syphilis A50.09 [D77]
  body dysmorphic F45.22
  bone M89.9
    continuity M84.9
      specified type NEC M84.80
        ankle M84.879
          left M84.872
          right M84.871
        fibula M84.869
          left M84.864
          right M84.863
        foot M84.879
          left M84.872
          right M84.871
        hand M84.849
          left M84.842
          right M84.841
        humerus M84.829
          left M84.822
          right M84.821
        neck M84.88
        pelvis M84.859
        radius M84.839
          left M84.834
          right M84.833
        rib M84.88
        shoulder M84.819
          left M84.812
          right M84.811
        skull M84.88
        thigh M84.859
          left M84.852
          right M84.851
        tibia M84.869
          left M84.862
          right M84.861
        ulna M84.839
          left M84.832
          right M84.831

Disorder — *see also* Disease — *continued*
  bone — *continued*
    continuity — *continued*
      specified type NEC — *continued*
        vertebra M84.88
    density and structure M85.9
      cyst — *see also* Cyst, bone, specified type NEC
        aneurysmal — *see* Cyst, bone, aneurysmal
        solitary — *see* Cyst, bone, solitary
      diffuse idiopathic skeletal hyperostosis — *see* Hyperostosis, ankylosing
      fibrous dysplasia (monostotic) — *see* Dysplasia, fibrous, bone
      fluorosis — *see* Fluorosis, skeletal
      hyperostosis of skull M85.2
      osteitis condensans — *see* Osteitis, condensans
      specified type NEC M85.80
        ankle M85.879
          left M85.872
          right M85.871
        foot M85.879
          left M85.872
          right M85.871
        forearm M85.839
          left M85.832
          right M85.831
        hand M85.849
          left M85.842
          right M85.841
        lower leg M85.869
          left M85.862
          right M85.861
        multiple sites M85.89
        neck M85.88
        rib M85.88
        shoulder M85.819
          left M85.812
          right M85.811
        skull M85.88
        thigh M85.859
          left M85.852
          right M85.851
        upper arm M85.829
          left M85.822
          right M85.821
        vertebra M85.88
    development and growth NEC M89.20
      carpus M89.249
        left M89.242
        right M89.241
      clavicle M89.219
        left M89.212
        right M89.211
      femur M89.259
        left M89.252
        right M89.251
      fibula M89.269
        left M89.264
        right M89.263
      finger M89.249
        left M89.242
        right M89.241
      humerus M89.229
        left M89.222
        right M89.221
      ilium M89.259
      ischium M89.259
      metacarpus M89.249
        left M89.242
        right M89.241
      metatarsus M89.279
        left M89.272
        right M89.271
      multiple sites M89.29
      neck M89.28
      radius M89.239
        left M89.234
        right M89.233
      rib M89.28
      scapula M89.219
        left M89.212
        right M89.211
      skull M89.28

Disorder — *see also* Disease — *continued*
  bone — *continued*
    development and growth NEC — *continued*
      tarsus M89.279
        left M89.272
        right M89.271
      tibia M89.269
        left M89.262
        right M89.261
      toe M89.279
        left M89.272
        right M89.271
      ulna M89.239
        left M89.232
        right M89.231
      vertebra M89.28
    specified type NEC M89.80
      carpus M89.84
      clavicle M89.81
      femur M89.85
      fibula M89.86
      finger M89.84
      humerus M89.82
      ilium M89.85
      ischium M89.85
      metacarpus M89.84
      metatarsus M89.87
      multiple sites M89.89
      neck M89.88
      radius M89.83
      rib M89.88
      scapula M89.81
      skull M89.88
      tarsus M89.87
      tibia M89.86
      toe M89.87
      ulna M89.83
      vertebra M89.88
  brachial plexus G54.0
  branched-chain amino-acid metabolism E71.2
    specified NEC E71.19
  breast N64.9
    agalactia — *see* Agalactia
    associated with
      lactation O92.92
      pregnancy O92.909
        first trimester O92.901
        second trimester O92.902
        third trimester O92.903
      puerperium O92.91
    cracked nipple — *see* Cracked nipple
    galactorrhea — *see* Galactorrhea
    hypogalactia O92.4
    lactation disorder NEC O92.7
    mastitis — *see* Mastitis
    nipple infection — *see* Infection, nipple
    retracted nipple — *see* Retraction, nipple
    specified type NEC N64.8
      associated with
        pregnancy O92.219
          first trimester O92.211
          second trimester O92.212
          third trimester O92.213
        puerperium O92.22
  Briquet's F45.0
  cannabis use — *see* Disorder, drug-related, cannabis
  carbohydrate
    absorption, intestinal NEC E74.39
    metabolism (congenital) E74.9
      specified NEC E74.8
  cardiac, functional I51.8
  cardiovascular system I51.6
    psychogenic F45.8
  carnitine metabolism E71.329
  cartilage M94.9
    articular NOS — *see* Derangement, joint, articular cartilage
      chondrocalcinosis — *see* Chondrocalcinosis
    specified type NEC M94.80
      ankle M94.87
      articular — *see* Disorder, cartilage, articular
      foot M94.87
      forearm M94.83

Disorder — *see also* Disease — *continued*
  cartilage — *continued*
    specified type NEC — *continued*
      hand M94.84
      lower leg M94.86
      multiple sites M94.89
      pelvic region M94.85
      rib M94.88
      shoulder M94.81
      skull M94.88
      specified site NEC M94.88
      thigh M94.85
      upper arm M94.82
      vertebra M94.88
  catatonic
    due to (secondary to) a general medical condition F06.1
    organic F06.1
  cervical
    region NEC M53.82
    root (nerve) NEC G54.2
  character NEC F68.8
  childhood disintegrative NEC F84.3
  cholesterol and bile acid metabolism E78.70
    Barth syndrome E78.71
    other specified E78.79
    Smith-Lemli-Opitz syndrome E78.72
  choroid H31.9
    atrophy — *see* Atrophy, choroid
    degeneration — *see* Degeneration, choroid
    detachment — *see* Detachment, choroid
    dystrophy — *see* Dystrophy, choroid
    hemorrhage — *see* Hemorrhage, choroid
    rupture — *see* Rupture, choroid
    scar — *see* Scar, chorioretinal
    solar retinopathy — *see* Retinopathy, solar
    specified type NEC H31.8
  ciliary body — *see also* Disorder, iris
    degeneration — *see* Degeneration, ciliary body
  coagulation (factor) (*see also* Defect, coagulation) D68.9
    newborn, transient P61.6
  coccyx NEC M53.3
  cognitive F09
    due to (secondary to) general medical condition F06.9
      mixed F06.8
    mild F06.8
    persisting R41.89
      due to
        alcohol F10.97
          with dependence F10.27
        anxiolytics F13.97
          with dependence F13.27
        hypnotics F13.97
          with dependence F13.27
        sedatives F13.97
          with dependence F13.27
        specified substance NEC F19.97
          with
            abuse F19.17
            dependence F19.27
  conduct (childhood) F91.9
    adjustment reaction — *see* Disorder, adjustment
    adolescent onset type F91.2
    childhood onset type F91.1
    compulsive F63.9
    confined to family context F91.0
    depressive F91.8
    group type F91.2
    hyperkinetic — *see* Disorder, attention-deficit hyperactivity
    oppositional defiance F91.3
    socialized F91.2
    solitary aggressive type F91.1
    specified NEC F91.8
    unsocialized (aggressive) F91.1
  conduction, heart I45.9
  conjunctiva H11.9
    infection — *see* Conjunctivitis
  connective tissue, localized L94.9
    specified NEC L94.8
  conversion — *see* Disorder, dissociative
  convulsive (secondary) — *see* Convulsions

Disorder — *see also* Disease — *continued*
  cornea H18.9
    deformity — *see* Deformity, cornea
    degeneration — *see* Degeneration, cornea
    deposits — *see* Deposit, cornea
    due to contact lens H18.829
      bilateral H18.823
      left H18.822
      right H18.821
      specified as edema — *see* Edema, cornea
    edema — *see* Edema, cornea
    keratitis — *see* Keratitis
    keratoconjunctivitis — *see* Keratoconjunctivitis
    membrane change — *see* Change, corneal membrane
    neovascularization — *see* Neovascularization, cornea
    scar — *see* Opacity, cornea
    specified type NEC H18.89
    ulcer — *see* Ulcer, cornea
  corpus cavernosum N48.9
  cranial nerve — *see* Disorder, nerve, cranial
  cyclothymic F34.0
  defiant oppositional F91.3
  delusional (persistent) (systematized) F22
    induced F24
  depersonalization F48.1
  depressive F32.9
    major
      with psychotic symptoms F32.3
      in remission (full) F32.5
        partial F32.4
      recurrent F33.9
      single episode F32.9
        mild F32.0
        moderate F32.1
        severe (without psychotic symptoms) F32.2
          with psychotic symptoms F32.3
    organic F06.31
    recurrent F33.9
      current episode
        mild F33.0
        moderate F33.1
        severe (without psychotic symptoms) F33.2
          with psychotic symptoms F33.3
      in remission F33.40
        full F33.42
        partial F33.41
      specified NEC F33.8
    single episode — *see* Episode, depressive
  developmental F89
    arithmetical skills F81.2
    coordination (motor) F82
    expressive writing F81.81
    language (receptive type) F80.2
      expressive F80.1
    learning F81.9
      arithmetical F81.2
      reading F81.0
    mixed F88
    motor coordination or function F82
    pervasive F84.9
      specified NEC F84.8
    phonological F80.0
    reading F81.0
    scholastic skills — *see also* Disorder, learning
      mixed F81.89
    specified NEC F88
    speech F80.9
      and language disorder F80.9
      articulation F80.0
    written expression F81.81
  diaphragm J98.6
  digestive (system) K92.9
    fetus or newborn P78.9
      specified NEC P78.89
    postprocedural — *see* Complication, gastrointestinal
    psychogenic F45.8
  disc (intervertebral) M51.9
    with
      myelopathy
        cervical region M50.00

Disorder — *see also* Disease — *continued*
  disc — *continued*
    with — *continued*
      myelopathy — *continued*
        cervicothoracic region M50.03
        lumbar region M51.06
        lumbosacral region M51.07
        occipito-atlanto-axial region M50.01
        sacrococcygeal region M53.3
        thoracic region M51.04
        thoracolumbar region M51.05
      radiculopathy
        cervical region M50.10
        cervicothoracic region M50.13
        lumbar region M51.16
        lumbosacral region M51.17
        occipito-atlanto-axial region M50.11
        sacrococcygeal region M53.3
        thoracic region M51.14
        thoracolumbar region M51.15
    cervical M50.90
      with
        myelopathy M50.00
          cervicothoracic region M50.03
          occipito-atlanto-axial region M50.01
        neuritis, radiculitis or radiculopathy M50.10
          cervicothoracic region M50.13
          occipito-atlanto-axial region M50.11
    cervicothoracic region M50.93
    degeneration M50.30
      cervicothoracic region M50.33
      occipito-atlanto-axial region M50.31
    displacement M50.20
      cervicothoracic region M50.23
      occipito-atlanto-axial region M50.21
    occipito-atlanto-axial region M50.91
    specified type NEC M50.80
      cervicothoracic region M50.83
      occipito-atlanto-axial region M50.81
    specified NEC
      lumbar region M51.86
      lumbosacral region M51.87
      sacrococcygeal region M53.3
      thoracic region M51.84
      thoracolumbar region M51.85
  disinhibited attachment (childhood) F94.2
  disintegrative, childhood NEC F84.3
  disruptive behavior F98.9
  dissocial personality F60.2
  dissociative F44.9
    affecting
      motor function F44.4
        and sensation F44.7
      sensation F44.6
        and motor function F44.7
    brief reactive F43.0
    due to (secondary to) general medical condition F06.8
    mixed F44.7
    organic F06.8
    other specified NEC F44.89
  double heterozygous sickling D57.2
  dream anxiety F51.5
  drug-related F19.99
    with
      amnestic disorder F19.96
      anxiety disorder F19.980
      dementia F19.97
      intoxication F19.929
        with
          delirium F19.921
          perceptual disturbance F19.922
        uncomplicated F19.920
      mood disorder F19.94
      other specified disorder F19.988
      psychotic disorder F19.959
        with
          delusions F19.950
          hallucinations F19.951
      sexual dysfunction F19.981
      sleep disorder F19.982
      withdrawal F19.939
        with
          delirium F19.931

Disorder — see also Disease — continued
  drug-related — continued
    with — continued
      withdrawal — continued
        with — continued
          dependence F19.239
            with
              delirium F19.231
              perceptual disturbance
                F19.232
              uncomplicated F19.230
          perceptual disturbance F19.932
          uncomplicated F19.930
        uncomplicated F19.90
    cannabis F12.99
      with
        anxiety disorder F12.980
        intoxication F12.929
          with
            delirium F12.921
            perceptual disturbance F12.922
          uncomplicated F12.920
        other specified disorder F12.988
        psychotic disorder F12.959
          with
            delusions F12.950
            hallucinations F12.951
      in
        abuse — see Abuse, drug, cannabis
        dependence — see Dependence, drug,
          cannabis
      uncomplicated F12.90
    cocaine F14.99
      with
        anxiety disorder F14.980
        intoxication F14.929
          with
            delirium F14.921
            perceptual disturbance F14.922
          uncomplicated F14.920
        mood disorder F14.94
        other specified disorder F14.988
        psychotic disorder F14.959
          with
            delusions F14.950
            hallucinations F14.951
        sexual dysfunction F14.981
        sleep disorder F14.982
      in
        abuse — see Abuse, drug, cocaine
        dependence — see Dependence, drug,
          cocaine
      uncomplicated F14.90
    hallucinogen F16.99
      with
        anxiety disorder F16.980
        flashbacks F16.983
        intoxication F16.929
          with delirium F16.921
          uncomplicated F16.920
        mood disorder F16.94
        other specified disorder F16.988
        perception disorder, persisting
          F16.983
        psychotic disorder F16.959
          with
            delusions F16.950
            hallucinations F16.951
        uncomplicated F16.90
      in
        abuse — see Abuse, drug,
          hallucinogen
        dependence — see Dependence, drug,
          hallucinogen
    in
      abuse — see Abuse, drug
      dependence — see Dependence, drug
    inhalant F18.99
      with
        anxiety disorder F18.980
        dementia, persisting F18.97
        intoxication F18.929
          with delirium F18.921
          uncomplicated F18.920
        mood disorder F18.94
        other specified disorder F18.988

Disorder — see also Disease — continued
  drug-related — continued
    inhalant — continued
      with — continued
        psychotic disorder F18.959
          with
            delusions F18.950
            hallucinations F18.951
      in
        abuse — see Abuse, drug, inhalant
        dependence — see Dependence, drug,
          inhalant
      uncomplicated F18.90
    nicotine — see Dependence, nicotine
    opioid F11.99
      with
        intoxication F11.929
          with
            delirium F11.921
            perceptual disturbance F11.922
          uncomplicated F11.920
        mood disorder F11.94
        other specified disorder F11.988
        psychotic disorder F11.959
          with
            delusions F11.950
            hallucinations F11.951
        sexual dysfunction F11.981
        sleep disorder F11.982
        withdrawal F11.93
      in
        abuse — see Abuse, drug, opioid
        dependence — see Dependence, drug,
          opioid
      uncomplicated F11.90
    sedative F13.99
      with
        amnestic disorder, persisting F13.96
        anxiety disorder F13.980
        dementia, persisting F13.97
        intoxication F13.929
          with delirium F13.921
          uncomplicated F13.920
        mood disorder F13.94
        other specified disorder F13.988
        psychotic disorder F13.959
          with
            delusions F13.950
            hallucinations F13.951
        sexual dysfunction F13.981
        sleep disorder F13.982
        withdrawal F13.939
          with
            delirium F13.931
            dependence F13.239
              with
                delirium F13.231
                perceptual disturbance
                  F13.232
                uncomplicated F13.230
            perceptual disturbance F13.932
            uncomplicated F13.930
      in
        abuse — see Abuse, drug, sedative
        dependence — see Dependence, drug,
          sedative
      uncomplicated F13.90
    stimulant NEC F15.99
      with
        anxiety disorder F15.980
        intoxication F15.929
          with
            delirium F15.921
            perceptual disturbance F15.922
          uncomplicated F15.920
        mood disorder F15.94
        other specified disorder F15.988
        psychotic disorder F15.959
          with
            delusions F15.950
            hallucinations F15.951
        sexual dysfunction F15.981
        sleep disorder F15.982
        withdrawal F15.93

Disorder — see also Disease — continued
  drug-related — continued
    stimulant NEC — continued
      in
        abuse — see Abuse, drug, stimulant
        dependence — see Dependence, drug,
          stimulant
      uncomplicated F15.90
  dysmorphic body F45.1
  dysthymic F34.1
  ear H93.90
    bilateral H93.93
    bleeding — see Otorrhagia
    deafness — see Deafness
    degenerative H93.009
      bilateral H93.003
      left H93.002
      right H93.001
    discharge — see Otorrhea
    external H61.90
      auditory canal stenosis — see Stenosis,
        external ear canal
      bilateral H61.93
      exostosis — see Exostosis, external ear
        canal
      left H61.92
      impacted cerumen — see Impaction,
        cerumen
      otitis — see Otitis, externa
      perichondritis — see Perichondritis, ear
      pinna — see Disorder, pinna
      right H61.91
      specified type NEC H61.899
        bilateral H61.893
        left H61.892
        right H61.891
    inner H83.90
      bilateral H83.93
      left H83.92
      right H83.91
      vestibular dysfunction — see Disorder,
        vestibular function
    left H93.92
    middle H74.90
      bilateral H74.93
      left H74.92
      ossicle — see Abnormal, ear ossicles
      polyp — see Polyp, ear (middle)
      right H74.91
    postprocedural — see Complications, ear,
      procedure
    right H93.91
  eating (adult) (psychogenic) F50.9
    anorexia — see Anorexia
    bulimia F50.2
    child F98.29
      pica F98.3
      rumination disorder F98.21
    pica F50.8
      childhood F98.3
  electrolyte (balance) NEC E87.8
    with
      abortion — see Abortion by type
        complicated by specified condition
          NEC
      ectopic pregnancy O08.5
      molar pregnancy O08.5
    acidosis (metabolic) (respiratory) E87.2
    alkalosis (metabolic) (respiratory) E87.3
  elimination, transepidermal L87.9
    specified NEC L87.8
  emotional (persistent) F34.9
    of childhood F93.9
      specified NEC F93.8
  endocrine E34.9
    postprocedural E89.9
    specified NEC E89.8
  erythematous — see Erythema
  esophagus K22.9
    functional K22.4
    psychogenic F45.8
  eustachian tube H69.90
    bilateral H69.93
    infection — see Salpingitis, eustachian
    left H69.92

Disorder — *see also* Disease — *continued*
  eustachian tube — *continued*
    obstruction — *see* Obstruction, eustachian
      tube
    patulous — *see* Patulous, eustachian tube
    right H69.91
    specified NEC H69.80
      bilateral H69.83
      left H69.82
      right H69.81
  extrapyramidal G25.9
    specified type NEC G25.8
  eye H57.9
    postprocedural H59.91
      specified NEC H59.89
    specified type NEC H57.8
  eyelid H02.9
    cyst — *see* Cyst, eyelid
    degenerative H02.70
      chloasma — *see* Chloasma, eyelid
      madarosis — *see* Madarosis
      specified type NEC H02.79
      vitiligo — *see* Vitiligo, eyelid
      xanthelasma — *see* Xanthelasma
    dermatochalasis — *see* Dermatochalasis
    edema — *see* Edema, eyelid
    elephantiasis — *see* Elephantiasis, eyelid
    foreign body, retained — *see* Foreign body,
      retained, eyelid
    function H02.59
      abnormal innervation syndrome — *see*
        Syndrome, abnormal innervation
      blepharochalasis — *see* Blepharochalasis
      blepharoclonus — *see* Blepharoclonus
      blepharophimosis — *see*
        Blepharophimosis
      blepharoptosis — *see* Blepharoptosis
      lagophthalmos — *see* Lagophthalmos
      lid retraction — *see* Retraction, lid
      hypertrichosis — *see* Hypertrichosis, eyelid
    specified type NEC H02.89
    vascular H02.879
      left H02.876
        lower H02.875
        upper H02.874
      right H02.873
        lower H02.872
        upper H02.871
  factitious F68.10
    with predominantly
      psychological symptoms F68.11
        with physical symptoms F68.13
      physical symptoms F68.12
        with psychological symptoms F68.13
  factor, coagulation — *see* Defect, coagulation
  fatty acid
    metabolism E71.30
    oxidation
      LCAD E71.310
      MCAD E71.311
      SCAD E71.312
      specified deficiency NEC E71.318
  feeding (infant or child) — *see also* Disorder,
    eating
    mismanagement R63.3
  feigned (with obvious motivation) Z76.5
    without obvious motivation — *see* Disorder,
      factitious
  female
    hypoactive sexual desire F52.0
    orgasmic F52.31
    sexual arousal F52.22
  fetus or newborn P96.9
    specified NEC P96.8
  fibroblastic M72.9
    specified NEC M72.8
  fluid balance E87.8
  follicular (skin) L73.9
    specified NEC L73.8
  fructose metabolism E74.10
    essential fructosuria E74.11
    fructokinase deficiency E74.11
    fructose-1, 6-diphosphatase deficiency
      E74.19
    hereditary fructose intolerance E74.12
    other specified E74.10
  functional polymorphonuclear neutrophils D71

Disorder — *see also* Disease — *continued*
  gamma-glutamyl cycle E72.8
  gastric (functional) K31.9
    motility K30
    psychogenic F45.8
    secretion K30
  gastrointestinal (functional) NOS K92.9
    newborn P78.9
    psychogenic F45.8
  gender-identity or -role F64.9
    childhood F64.2
    effect on relationship F66
    egodystonic F66
    of adolescence or adulthood
      (nontranssexual) F64.1
    specified NEC F64.8
    uncertainty F66
  genitourinary system
    female N94.9
    male N50.9
    psychogenic F45.8
  globe H44.9
    degenerated condition H44.50
      absolute glaucoma H44.519
        bilateral H44.513
        left H44.512
        right H44.511
      atrophy H44.529
        bilateral H44.523
        left H44.522
        right H44.521
      leucocoria H44.539
        bilateral H44.533
        left H44.532
        right H44.531
    degenerative H44.30
      chalcosis H44.319
        bilateral H44.313
        left H44.312
        right H44.311
      myopia H44.20
        bilateral H44.23
        left H44.22
        right H44.21
      siderosis H44.329
        bilateral H44.323
        left H44.322
        right H44.321
      specified type NEC H44.399
        bilateral H44.393
        left H44.392
        right H44.391
    endophthalmitis — *see* Endophthalmitis
    foreign body, retained — *see* Foreign body,
      intraocular, old, retained
    hemophthalmos — *see* Hemophthalmos
    hypotony H44.40
      due to
        ocular fistula H44.429
          bilateral H44.423
          left H44.422
          right H44.421
        specified disorder NEC H44.439
          bilateral H44.433
          left H44.432
          right H44.431
      flat anterior chamber H44.419
        bilateral H44.413
        left H44.412
        right H44.411
      primary H44.449
        bilateral H44.443
        left H44.442
        right H44.441
    luxation — *see* Luxation, globe
    specified type NEC H44.89
  glomerular (in) N05.9
    amyloidosis E85 *[N08]*
    cryoglobulinemia D89.1 *[N08]*
    disseminated intravascular coagulation D65
      [N08]
    Fabry's disease E75.21 *[N08]*
    familial lecithin cholesterol acyltransferase
      deficiency E78.6 *[N08]*
    Goodpasture's syndrome M31.0
    hemolytic-uremic syndrome D59.3

Disorder — *see also* Disease — *continued*
  glomerular — *continued*
    Henoch (-Schönlein) purpura D69.0 *[N08]*
    malariae malaria B52.0
    multiple myeloma (M9732/3) C90.00 *[N08]*
    mumps B26.83
    polyarteritis nodosa M30.0 *[N08]*
    schistosomiasis B65.9 *[N08]*
    septicemia NEC A41.9 *[N08]*
      streptococcal A40.9 *[N08]*
    sickle-cell disorders D57.8 *[N08]*
    strongyloidiasis B78.9 *[N08]*
    subacute bacterial endocarditis I33.0 *[N08]*
    syphilis A52.75
    systemic lupus erythematosus M32.14
    thrombotic thrombocytopenic purpura
      M31.1 *[N08]*
    Waldenström's macroglobulinemia
      (M9761/3) C88.0 *[N08]*
    Wegener's granulomatosis M31.31
  gluconeogenesis E74.4
  glucosaminoglycan metabolism — *see* Disorder,
    metabolism, glucosaminoglycan
  glycine metabolism E72.50
    d-glycericacidemia E72.59
    hyperhydroxyprolinemia E72.59
    hyperoxaluria E72.53
    hyperprolinemia E72.59
    non-ketotic hyperglycinemia E72.51
    oxalosis E72.53
    oxaluria E72.53
    sarcosinemia E72.59
    trimethylaminuria E72.52
  glycoprotein metabolism E77.9
    specified NEC E77.8
  habit (and impulse) F63.9
    involving sexual behavior NEC F65.9
    specified NEC F63.89
  heart action I49.9
  hematological D75.9
    fetus or newborn (transient) P61.9
      specified NEC P61.8
  hematopoietic organs D75.9
  hemorrhagic NEC D69.9
    drug-induced D68.5
    due to circulating intrinsic anticoagulants
      D68.3
    following childbirth O72.3
  hemostasis — *see* Defect, coagulation
  histidine metabolism E70.40
    histidinemia E70.41
    other specified E70.49
  hyperkinetic — *see* Disorder, attention-deficit
    hyperactivity
  hyperleucine-isoleucinemia E71.19
  hypervalinemia E71.19
  hypoactive sexual desire F52.0
  hypochondriacal F45.20
    body dysmorphic F45.22
    neurosis F45.21
    other specified F45.29
  identity
    dissociative F44.81
    of childhood F93.8
  immune mechanism (immunity) D89.9
    specified type NEC D89.8
  impaired renal tubular function N25.9
    specified NEC N25.8
  impulse (control) F63.9
  inflammatory
    penis N48.29
      abscess N48.21
      cellulitis N48.22
  in diseases classified elsewhere – code first
    underlying disease
    biliary tract *[K87]*
    bullous *[L14]*
    cerebral arteritis *[I68.2]*
    erythema *[L54]*
    extrapyramidal *[G26]*
    gallbladder *[K87]*
    keratoderma *[L86]*
    lens NEC *[H28]*
      bilateral *[H28]*
      left *[H28]*
      right *[H28]*

©2002 Ingenix, Inc.

Disorder — *see also* Disease — *continued*
  in diseases classified elsewhere – code first
    underlying disease — *continued*
     mastoid NEC *[H75.80]*
      bilateral *[H75.83]*
      left *[H75.82]*
      right *[H75.81]*
     metabolic *[E90]*
     middle ear NEC *[H75.80]*
      bilateral *[H75.83]*
      left *[H75.82]*
      right *[H75.81]*
     mononeuropathy *[G59]*
     movement *[G26]*
     nutritional *[E90]*
     pancreas *[K87]*
     papulosquamous *[L45]*
     Parkinsonism *[G22]*
     urethra *[N37]*
     vertiginous *[H82.9]*
      bilateral *[H82.3]*
      left *[H82.2]*
      right *[H82.1]*
  inhalant use — *see* Disorder, drug-related,
    inhalant
  integument, fetus or newborn P83.9
    specified NEC P83.8
  intermittent explosive F63.81
  internal secretion pancreas — *see* Increased,
    secretion, pancreas, endocrine
  intestine, intestinal
    carbohydrate absorption NEC E74.39
     postoperative K91.2
    functional NEC K59.9
     postoperative K91.89
    psychogenic F45.8
    vascular K55.9
     chronic K55.1
     specified NEC K55.8
  iris H21.9
    adhesions — *see* Adhesions, iris
    atrophy — *see* Atrophy, iris
    chamber angle recession — *see* Recession,
     chamber angle
    cyst — *see* Cyst, iris
    degeneration — *see* Degeneration, iris
    iridodialysis — *see* Iridodialysis
    iridoschisis — *see* Iridoschisis
    miotic pupillary cyst — *see* Cyst, pupillary
    pupillary
     abnormality — *see* Abnormality, pupillary
     membrane — *see* Membrane, pupillary
    specified type NEC H21.8
    vascular H21.10
     bilateral H21.13
     hyphema H21.00
      bilateral H21.03
      left H21.02
      right H21.01
     left H21.12
     right H21.11
  iron metabolism E83.10
    hemochromatosis E83.11
    other specified E83.19
  isovaleric acidemia E71.110
  jaw, developmental M27.0
    temporomandibular — *see* Anomaly,
     dentofacial, temporomandibular joint
  joint M25.9
    derangement — *see* Derangement, joint
    effusion — *see* Effusion, joint
    fistula — *see* Fistula, joint
    hemarthrosis — *see* Hemarthrosis
    instability — *see* Instability, joint
    osteophyte — *see* Osteophyte
    pain — *see* Pain, joint
    psychogenic F45.8
    specified type NEC M25.80
     ankle M25.879
      left M25.872
      right M25.871
     elbow M25.829
      left M25.822
      right M25.821
     foot joint M25.879
      left M25.872
      right M25.871

Disorder — *see also* Disease — *continued*
  joint — *continued*
    specified type NEC — *continued*
     hand joint M25.849
      left M25.842
      right M25.841
     hip M25.859
      left M25.852
      right M25.851
     knee M25.869
      left M25.862
      right M25.861
     shoulder M25.819
      left M25.812
      right M25.811
     specified joint NEC M25.88
     wrist M25.839
      left M25.832
      right M25.831
    stiffness — *see* Stiffness, joint
  ketone metabolism E71.33
  kidney N28.9
    functional (tubular) N25.9
    in
     schistosomiasis B65.9 *[N29]*
    tubular function N25.9
    specified NEC N25.8
  lacrimal system H04.9
    changes H04.69
     fistula — *see* Fistula, lacrimal
    gland H04.19
     atrophy — *see* Atrophy, lacrimal gland
     cyst — *see* Cyst, lacrimal, gland
     dacryops — *see* Dacryops
     dislocation — *see* Dislocation, lacrimal
      gland
     dry eye syndrome — *see* Syndrome, dry
      eye
     infection — *see* Dacryoadenitis
     granuloma — *see* Granuloma, lacrimal
     inflammation — *see* Inflammation, lacrimal
     obstruction — *see* Obstruction, lacrimal
     specified NEC H04.89
  lactation NEC O92.7
  language (developmental) F80.9
    expressive F80.1
    mixed receptive and expressive F80.2
    receptive F80.2
  late luteal phase dysphoric N94.8
  learning (specific) F81.9
    acalculia R48.8
    alexia R48.0
    mathematics F81.2
    reading F81.0
    specified NEC F81.89
    spelling F81.81
    written expression F81.81
  lens H27.9
    aphakia — *see* Aphakia
    cataract — *see* Cataract
    dislocation — *see* Dislocation, lens
    specified type NEC H27.8
  ligament M24.20
    ankle M24.273
     left M24.272
     right M24.271
    attachment, spine — *see* Enthesopathy,
     spinal
    elbow M24.229
     left M24.222
     right M24.221
    foot joint M24.276
     left M24.275
     right M24.274
    hand joint M24.249
     left M24.242
     right M24.241
    hip M24.259
     left M24.252
     right M24.251
    knee — *see* Derangement, knee, specified
     NEC
    shoulder M24.219
     left M24.212
     right M24.211
    vertebra M24.28

Disorder — *see also* Disease — *continued*
  ligament — *continued*
    wrist M24.239
     left M24.232
     right M24.231
  ligamentous attachments — *see also*
    Enthesopathy
    spine — *see* Enthesopathy, spinal
  lipid
    metabolism, congenital E78.9
    storage E75.6
     specified NEC E75.5
  lipoprotein
    deficiency (familial) E78.6
    metabolism E78.9
     specified NEC E78.89
  liver K76.9
    malarial B54 *[K77]*
  low back — *see also* Dorsopathy, specified NEC
    psychogenic F45.4
  lumbosacral
    plexus G54.1
    root (nerve) NEC G54.4
  lung, interstitial, drug-induced J70.4
    acute J70.2
    chronic J70.3
  lysine and hydroxylysine metabolism E72.3
  male
    erectile — *see* Dysfunction, sexual, male,
     erectile
    hypoactive sexual desire F52.0
    orgasmic F52.32
  manic F30.9
    organic F06.33
  mastoid — *see also* Disorder, ear, middle
    postprocedural — *see* Complications, ear,
     procedure
  membranes or fluid, amniotic O41.90
    first trimester O41.91
    second trimester O41.92
    third trimester O41.93
  meniscus — *see* Derangement, knee, meniscus
  menopausal N95.9
    specified NEC N95.8
  menstrual N92.6
    psychogenic F45.8
    specified NEC N92.5
  mental (or behavioral) (nonpsychotic) F99
    affecting management of
     childbirth O99.344
     pregnancy O99.343
      first trimester O99.340
      second trimester O99.341
      third trimester O99.342
     puerperium O99.345
    due to (secondary to)
     amphetamine — *see* Disorder, drug-
      related, stimulant
     brain disease, damage and dysfunction
      F06.9
     caffeine use — *see* Disorder, drug-related,
      stimulant
     cannabis use — *see* Disorder, drug-
      related, cannabis
     general medical condition F06.9
     sedative or hypnotic use — *see* Disorder,
      drug-related, sedative
     tobacco (nicotine) use — *see* Dependence,
      drug, nicotine
    following organic brain damage F07.9
     frontal lobe syndrome F07.0
     personality change F07.0
     postconcussional syndrome F07.81
     specified NEC F07.89
    infancy, childhood or adolescence F98.9
    neurotic — *see* Neurosis
    organic or symptomatic F06.9
    presenile, psychotic F03
    previous, affecting management of
     pregnancy — *see* Antenatal, care, high
      risk pregnancy, history of, specified
      obstetric problem NEC
    psychoneurotic — *see* Neurosis
    psychotic — *see* Psychosis
    puerperal F53
    senile, psychotic NEC F03

Disorder — *see also* Disease — *continued*
  metabolism NOS E88.9
    amino-acid E72.9
      aromatic E70.9
        albinism — *see* Albinism
        histidine E70.40
          histidinemia E70.41
          other specified E70.49
        hyperphenylalaninemia EE70.1
          classical phenylketonuria E70.0
        other specified E70.8
        tryptophan E70.5
        tyrosine E70.20
          hypertyrosinemia E70.21
          other specified E70.29
      branched chain E71.2
        3-methylglutaconic aciduria E71.111
        hyperleucine-isoleucinemia E71.19
        hypervalinemia E71.19
        isovaleric acidemia E71.110
        maple syrup urine disease E71.0
        methylmalonic acidemia E71.120
        organic aciduria NEC E71.118
        other specified E71.19
        proprionate NEC E71.128
        proprionic acidemia E71.121
      glycine E72.50
        d-glycericacidemia E72.59
        hyperhydroxyprolinemia E72.59
        hyperoxaluria E72.53
        hyperprolinemia E72.59
        non-ketotic hyperglycinemia E72.51
        other specified E72.59
        sarcosinemia E72.59
        trimethylaminuria E72.52
      hydroxylysine E72.3
      lysine E72.3
      ornithine E72.4
      other specified E72.8
        beta-amino acid E72.8
        gamma-glutamyl cycle E72.8
      straight-chain E72.8
      sulfur-bearing E72.10
        homocystinuria E72.11
        methylenetetrahydrofolate reductase
          deficiency E72.12
        other specified E72.19
    bile acid and cholesterol metabolism E78.70
    bilirubin E80.7
      specified NEC E80.6
    calcium E83.50
      hypercalcemia E83.52
      hypocalcemia E83.51
      other specified E83.59
    carbohydrate E74.9
      specified NEC E74.8
    cholesterol and bile acid metabolism E78.70
    congenital E88.9
    copper E83.00
      Wilson's disease E83.01
      specified type NEC E83.09
    cystinuria E72.01
    following
      ectopic pregnancy O08.5
      molar pregnancy O08.5
    fructose E74.10
    galactose E74.20
    glucosaminoglycan E76.9
      mucopolysaccharidosis — *see*
        Mucopolysaccharidosis
      specified NEC E76.8
    glutamine E72.8
    glycine E72.50
    glycogen storage (hepatorenal) E74.01
    glycoprotein E77.9
      specified NEC E77.8
    glycosaminoglycan E76.9
      specified NEC E76.8
    in labor and delivery O75.89
    iron E83.10
    isoleucine E71.19
    leucine E71.19
    lipoid E78.9
    lipoprotein E78.9
      specified NEC E78.89

Disorder — *see also* Disease — *continued*
  metabolism NOS — *continued*
    magnesium E83.40
      hypermagnesemia E83.41
      hypomagnesemia E83.42
      other specified E83.49
    mineral E83.9
      specified NEC E83.8
    mitochondrial E88.30
      MELAS syndrome E88.31
      MERFF syndrome E88.32
      other specified E88.39
    ornithine E72.4
    phosphorus E83.30
      acid phosphatase deficiency E83.39
      hypophosphatasia E83.39
      hypophosphatemia E83.39
        familial E83.31
      other specified E83.39
      pseudovitamin D deficiency E83.32
    plasma protein NEC E88.09
    porphyrin — *see* Porphyria
    postprocedural E89.9
      specified NEC E89.8
    purine E79.9
      specified NEC E79.8
    pyrimidine E79.9
      specified NEC E79.8
    pyruvate E74.4
    serine E72.8
    sodium E87.8
    specified NEC E88.8
    threonine E72.8
    valine E71.19
    zinc E83.2
  methylmalonic acidemia E71.120
  micturition NEC R39.19
    feeling of incomplete emptying R39.14
    hesitancy R39.11
    poor stream R39.12
    psychogenic F45.8
    split stream R39.13
    straining R39.16
    urgency R39.15
  mild cognitive F06.8
  mitochondrial metabolism E88.30
  mitral (valve) — *see* Endocarditis, mitral
  mixed
    anxiety and depressive F41.8
    of scholastic skills (developmental) F81.89
    receptive expressive language F80.2
  mood F39
    bipolar — *see* Disorder, bipolar
    depressive — *see* Disorder, depressive
    due to (secondary to)
      alcohol F10.959
      amphetamine F15.94
        in
          abuse F15.14
          dependence F15.24
      anxiolytic F13.94
        in
          abuse F13.14
          dependence F13.24
      cocaine F14.94
        in
          abuse F14.14
          dependence F14.24
      general medical condition F06.30
      hallucinogen F16.94
        in
          abuse F16.14
          dependence F16.24
      hypnotic F13.94
        in
          abuse F13.14
          dependence F13.24
      inhalant F18.94
        in
          abuse F18.14
          dependence F18.24
      opioid F11.94
        in
          abuse F11.14
          dependence F11.24

Disorder — *see also* Disease — *continued*
  mood — *continued*
    due to — *continued*
      phencyclidine (PCP) F19.94
        in
          abuse F19.14
          dependence F19.24
      physiological condition F06.30
        with
          depressive features F06.31
          major depressive-like episode
            F06.32
          manic features F06.33
          mixed features F06.34
      psychoactive substance NEC F19.94
        in
          abuse F19.14
          dependence F19.24
      sedative F13.94
        in
          abuse F13.14
          dependence F13.24
      volatile solvents F18.94
        in
          abuse F18.14
          dependence F18.24
    manic episode F30.9
      with psychotic symptoms F30.2
      in remission (full) F30.4
        partial F30.3
      specified type NEC F30.8
      without psychotic symptoms F30.10
        mild F30.11
        moderate F30.12
        severe F30.13
    organic F06.30
      right hemisphere F07.89
    persistent F34.9
      cyclothymia F34.0
      dysthymia F34.1
      specified type NEC F34.8
    recurrent F39
    right hemisphere organic F07.89
  movement G25.9
    drug-induced G25.70
      akathisia G25.71
      specified NEC G25.79
    hysterical F44.4
    specified NEC G25.8
    stereotyped F98.4
    treatment-induced G25.9
  multiple personality F44.81
  muscle M62.9
    attachment, spine — *see* Enthesopathy,
      spinal
    in trichinellosis — *see* Trichinellosis, with
      muscle disorder
    psychogenic F45.8
    specified type NEC M62.89
    tone, newborn P94.9
      specified NEC P94.8
  muscular
    attachments — *see also* Enthesopathy
      spine — *see* Enthesopathy, spinal
    urethra N36.44
  musculoskeletal system, soft tissue — *see*
    Disorder, soft tissue
    postprocedural M96.9
    psychogenic F45.8
  myoneural G70.9
    due to lead G70.1
    specified NEC G70.8
    toxic G70.1
  myotonic G71.1
  neck region NEC — *see* Dorsopathy, specified
    NEC
  nerve G58.9
    abducent NEC — *see* Strabismus, paralytic,
      sixth nerve
    accessory G52.8
    acoustic — *see* category H93.3
    auditory — *see* category H93.3
    auriculotemporal G50.8
    axillary G54.0
    cerebral — *see* Disorder, nerve, cranial

©2002 Ingenix, Inc.

Disorder — *see also* Disease — *continued*
  nerve — *continued*
    cranial G52.9
      eighth — *see* category H93.3
      eleventh G52.8
      fifth G50.9
      first G52.0
      fourth NEC — *see* Strabismus, paralytic,
        fourth nerve
      multiple G52.7
      ninth G52.1
      second NEC — *see* Disorder, nerve, optic
      seventh NEC G51.9
      sixth NEC — *see* Strabismus, paralytic,
        sixth nerve
      specified NEC G52.8
      tenth G52.2
      third NEC — *see* Strabismus, paralytic,
        third nerve
      twelfth G52.3
    entrapment — *see* Neuropathy, entrapment
    facial G51.9
      specified NEC G51.8
    femoral — *see* Lesion, nerve, femoral
    glossopharyngeal NEC G52.1
    hypoglossal G52.3
    intercostal G58.0
    lateral
      cutaneous of thigh — *see*
        Mononeuropathy, lower limb,
        meralgia paresthetica
      popliteal — *see* Lesion, nerve, popliteal
    lower limb — *see* Mononeuropathy, lower
      limb
    medial popliteal — *see* Lesion, nerve,
      popliteal, medial
    median NEC — *see* Lesion, nerve, median
    multiple G58.7
    oculomotor NEC — *see* Strabismus,
      paralytic, third nerve
    olfactory G52.0
    optic NEC H47.099
      bilateral H47.093
      hemorrhage into sheath — *see*
        Hemorrhage, optic nerve
      ischemic H47.019
        bilateral H47.013
        left H47.012
        right H47.011
      left H47.092
      right H47.091
    peroneal — *see* Lesion, nerve, popliteal
    phrenic G58.8
    plantar — *see* Lesion, nerve, plantar
    pneumogastric G52.2
    posterior tibial — *see* Syndrome, tarsal
      tunnel
    radial — *see* Lesion, nerve, radial
    recurrent laryngeal G52.2
    root G54.9
      specified NEC G54.8
    sciatic NEC — *see* Lesion, nerve, sciatic
    specified NEC G58.8
      lower limb — *see* Mononeuropathy, lower
        limb, specified NEC
      upper limb — *see* Mononeuropathy,
        upper limb, specified NEC
    sympathetic G90.9
    tibial — *see* Lesion, nerve, popliteal, medial
    trigeminal G50.9
      specified NEC G50.8
    trochlear NEC — *see* Strabismus, paralytic,
      fourth nerve
    ulnar — *see* Lesion, nerve, ulnar
    upper limb — *see* Mononeuropathy, upper
      limb
    vagus G52.2
  nervous system G98.8
    autonomic (peripheral) G90.9
      specified NEC G90.8
    central G96.9
      specified NEC G96.8
    parasympathetic G90.9
    specified NEC G98.8
    sympathetic G90.9
    vegetative G90.9
  neurohypophysis NEC E23.3

Disorder — *see also* Disease — *continued*
  neurological NEC R29.81
  neuromuscular G70.9
    hereditary NEC G71.9
    specified NEC G70.8
    toxic G70.1
  neurotic F48.9
    specified NEC F48.8
  neutrophil, polymorphonuclear D71
  nicotine use — *see* Dependence, drug, nicotine
  nightmare F51.5
  nose J34.9
    specified NEC J34.8
  obsessive-compulsive F42
  odontogenesis NOS K00.9
  oesophagus — *see* Disorder, esophagus
  opioid use — *see* Disorder, drug-related, opioid
  oppositional defiant F91.3
  optic
    chiasm H47.49
      due to
        inflammatory disorder H47.41
        neoplasm H47.42
        vascular disorder H47.43
    disc H47.399
      bilateral H47.393
      coloboma — *see* Coloboma, optic disc
      drusen — *see* Drusen, optic disc
      left H47.392
      pseudopapilledema — *see*
        Pseudopapilledema
      right H47.391
    radiations — *see* Disorder, visual, pathway
    tracts — *see* Disorder, visual, pathway
  orbit H05.9
    cyst — *see* Cyst, orbit
    deformity — *see* Deformity, orbit
    edema — *see* Edema, orbit
    enophthalmos — *see* Enophthalmos
    exophthalmos — *see* Exophthalmos
    hemorrhage — *see* Hemorrhage, orbit
    inflammation — *see* Inflammation, orbit
    myopathy — *see* Myopathy, extraocular
      muscles
    retained foreign body — *see* Foreign body,
      orbit, old
    specified type NEC H05.89
  organic
    anxiety F06.4
    catatonic F06.1
    delusional F06.2
    dissociative F06.8
    emotionally labile (asthenic) F06.8
    mood (affective) F06.30
    schizophrenia-like F06.2
  orgasmic (female) F52.31
    male F52.32
  ornithine metabolism E72.4
  overactive, associated with mental retardation
    and stereotyped movements F84.4
  overanxious F41.1
    of childhood F93.8
  pain
    (secondary) due to a general medical
      condition R52.9
    associated with psychological factors F45.4
  pancreatic internal secretion E16.9
    specified NEC E16.8
  panic F41.0
    with agoraphobia F40.01
  papulosquamous L44.9
    specified NEC L44.8
  paranoid F22
    induced F24
    shared F24
  parathyroid (gland) E21.5
    specified NEC E21.4
  parietoalveolar NEC J84.0
  paroxysmal, mixed R56.8
  patella M22.90
    chondromalacia — *see* Chondromalacia,
      patella
    derangement NEC M22.30
      left M22.32
      right M22.31
    left M22.92

Disorder — *see also* Disease — *continued*
  patella — *continued*
    recurrent
      dislocation — *see* Dislocation, patella,
        recurrent
      subluxation — *see* Dislocation, patella,
        recurrent, incomplete
    right M22.91
    specified NEC M22.80
      left M22.82
      right M22.81
  patellofemoral M22.20
    left M22.22
    right M22.21
  pentose phosphate pathway with anemia D55.1
  perception, due to hallucinogens F16.983
    in
      abuse F16.183
      dependence F16.283
  peripheral nervous system NEC G64
  peroxisomal E71.40
    biogenesis
      neonatal adrenoleukodystrophy E71.411
      specified disorder NEC E71.418
      Zellweger syndrome E71.410
    rhizomelic chondrodysplasia punctata
      E71.440
    specified form NEC E71.448
      group 1 E71.418
      group 2 E71.43
      group 3 E71.442
    X-linked adrenoleukodystrophy
      adolescent E71.421
      adrenomyeloneuropathy E71.422
      childhood E71.420
      specified form NEC E71.428
    Zellweger-like syndrome E71.441
  persistent
    (somatoform) pain F45.4
    affective (mood) F34.9
  personality (*see also* Personality) F60.9
    affective F34.0
    aggressive F60.3
    amoral F60.2
    anankastic F60.5
    antisocial F60.2
    anxious F60.6
    asocial F60.2
    asthenic F60.7
    avoidant F60.6
    borderline F60.3
    change (secondary) due to general medical
      condition F07.0
    compulsive F60.5
    cyclothymic F34.0
    dependent (passive) F60.7
    depressive F34.1
    dissocial F60.2
    emotional instability F60.3
    expansive paranoid F60.0
    explosive F60.3
    following organic brain damage F07.9
    histrionic F60.4
    hyperthymic F34.0
    hypothymic F34.1
    hysterical F60.4
    immature F60.89
    inadequate F60.7
    labile F60.3
    mixed (nonspecific) F60.89
    moral deficiency F60.2
    narcissistic F60.81
    negativistic F60.89
    obsessional F60.5
    obsessive(-compulsive) F60.5
    organic F07.9
    overconscientious F60.5
    paranoid F60.0
    passive(-dependent) F60.7
    passive-aggressive F60.89
    pathological NEC F60.9
    pseudosocial F60.2
    psychopathic F60.2
    schizoid F60.1
    schizotypal F21
    self-defeating F60.7
    specified NEC F60.89

Disorder — *see also* Disease — *continued*
  personality (*see also* Personality) — *continued*
    type A F60.5
    unstable (emotional) F60.3
  pervasive, developmental F84.9
  phobic anxiety, childhood F40.8
  phosphate-losing tubular N25.0
  pigmentation L81.9
    choroid, congenital Q14.3
    diminished melanin formation L81.6
    iron L81.8
    specified NEC L81.8
  pinna (noninfective) H61.109
    bilateral H61.103
    deformity, acquired H61.119
      bilateral H61.113
      left H61.112
      right H61.111
    hematoma H61.129
      bilateral H61.123
      left H61.122
      right H61.121
    left H61.102
    perichondritis — *see* Perichondritis, ear
    right H61.101
    specified type NEC H61.199
      bilateral H61.193
      left H61.192
      right H61.191
  pituitary gland E23.7
    iatrogenic (postprocedural) E89.3
    specified NEC E23.6
  placenta O43.90
    abruptio O45.90
      with coagulation defect O45.009
        afibrinogenemia O45.019
          first trimester O45.011
          second trimester O45.012
          third trimester O45.013
        disseminated intravascular
          coagulation O45.029
          first trimester O45.021
          second trimester O45.022
          third trimester O45.023
        first trimester O45.001
        second trimester O45.002
        specified defect NEC O45.099
          first trimester O45.091
          second trimester O45.092
          third trimester O45.093
        third trimester O45.003
      first trimester O45.91
      second trimester O45.92
      specified type NEC — *see* category O45.8
      third trimester O45.93
    dysfunction O43.819
      first trimester O43.811
      second trimester O43.812
      third trimester O43.813
    fetomaternal transfusion syndrome O43.019
      first trimester O43.011
      second trimester O43.012
      third trimester O43.013
    fetus-to-fetus transfusion syndrome
      O43.029
      first trimester O43.021
      second trimester O43.022
      third trimester O43.023
    first trimester O43.91
    infarction O43.829
      first trimester O43.821
      second trimester O43.822
      third trimester O43.823
    malformation O43.109
      circumvallate O43.119
        first trimester O43.111
        second trimester O43.112
        third trimester O43.113
      first trimester O43.101
      second trimester O43.102
      specified type NEC O43.199
        first trimester O43.191
        second trimester O43.192
        third trimester O43.193
      third trimester O43.103

Disorder — *see also* Disease — *continued*
  placenta — *continued*
    malformation — *continued*
      velamentous cord insertion O43.129
        first trimester O43.121
        second trimester O43.122
        third trimester O43.123
    premature separation — *see* Disorder,
      placenta, abruptio
    previa (with hemorrhage) O44.10
      first trimester O44.11
      second trimester O44.12
      third trimester O44.13
      without hemorrhage O44.00
        first trimester O44.01
        second trimester O44.02
        third trimester O44.03
    second trimester O43.92
    specified type NEC O43.899
      first trimester O43.891
      second trimester O43.892
      third trimester O43.893
    third trimester O43.93
  platelets D69.1
  plexus G54.9
    specified NEC G54.8
  polymorphonuclear neutrophils D71
  porphyrin metabolism — *see* Porphyria
  postconcussional F07.81
  posthallucinogen perception F16.983
    in
      abuse F16.183
      dependence F16.283
  postmenopausal N95.9
    specified NEC N95.8
  post-traumatic stress F43.10
    acute F43.0
    chronic F43.12
  prepuce N47.8
  propionic acidemia E71.121
  prostate N42.9
    specified NEC N42.89
  psychoactive substance use — *see* Disorder,
    drug-related
  psychogenic NOS (*see also* condition) F45.9
    anxiety F41.8
    appetite F50.9
    asthenic F48.8
    cardiovascular (system) F45.8
    compulsive F42
    cutaneous F54
    depressive F32.9
    digestive (system) F45.8
    dysmenorrheic F45.8
    dyspneic F45.8
    endocrine (system) F54
    eye NEC F45.8
    feeding — *see* Disorder, eating
    functional NEC F45.8
    gastric F45.8
    gastrointestinal (system) F45.8
    genitourinary (system) F45.8
    heart (function) (rhythm) F45.8
    hyperventilatory F45.8
    hypochondriacal — *see* Disorder,
      hypochondriacal
    intestinal F45.8
    joint F45.8
    learning F81.9
    limb F45.8
    lymphatic (system) F45.8
    menstrual F45.8
    micturition F45.8
    monoplegic NEC F44.4
    motor F44.4
    muscle F45.8
    musculoskeletal F45.8
    neurocirculatory F45.8
    obsessive F42
    occupational F48.8
    organ or part of body NEC F45.8
    paralytic NEC F44.4
    phobic F40.9
    physical NEC F45.8
    rectal F45.8
    respiratory (system) F45.8
    rheumatic F45.8

Disorder — *see also* Disease — *continued*
  psychogenic NOS (*see also* condition) —
    continued
    sexual (function) F52.9
    skin (allergic) (eczematous) F54
    sleep F51.9
    specified part of body NEC F45.8
    stomach F45.8
  psychological F99
    associated with
      disease classified elsewhere F54
      egodystonic orientation F66
      sexual
        development F66
        relationship F66
      uncertainty about gender identity F66
  psychomotor NEC F44.4
    hysterical F44.4
  psychoneurotic — *see also* Neurosis
    mixed NEC F48.8
  psychophysiologic — *see* Disorder, somatoform
  psychosexual F65.9
    development F66
    identity of childhood F64.2
  psychosomatic NOS — *see* Disorder,
    somatoform
    multiple F45.0
    undifferentiated F45.1
  psychotic (due to) — *see also* Psychosis
    acute F23
    alcohol(-induced), alcoholic F10.959
      in
        abuse F10.159
        dependence F10.259
    amphetamine F15.959
      in
        abuse F15.159
        dependence F15.259
    anxiolytic F13.959
      in
        abuse F13.159
        dependence F13.259
    brief F23
    cannabis F12.959
      in
        abuse F12.159
        dependence F12.259
    cocaine F14.959
      in
        abuse F14.159
        dependence F14.259
    delusional F22
      acute F23
    general medical condition with
      delusions F06.2
      hallucinations F06.0
    hallucinogen F16.959
      in
        abuse F16.159
        dependence F16.259
    hypnotic F13.959
      in
        abuse F13.159
        dependence F13.259
    induced F24
    inhalant F18.959
      in
        abuse F18.159
        dependence F18.259
    opioid F11.959
      in
        abuse F11.159
        dependence F11.259
    phencyclidine (PCP) F19.959
      in
        abuse F19.159
        dependence F19.259
    polymorphic, acute F23
    psychoactive substance NEC F19.959
      in
        abuse F19.159
        dependence F19.259
    residual and late-onset
      alcohol-induced F10.97
        with dependence F10.27

©2002 Ingenix, Inc.

Disorder — *see also* Disease — *continued*
  psychotic — *see also* Psychosis — *continued*
    residual and late-onset — *continued*
      drug-induced — *see* Dementia, in (due to), psychoactive drug
      sedative F13.959
        in
          abuse F13.159
          dependence F13.259
      transient (acute) F23
  puberty E30.9
    specified NEC E30.8
  pulmonary (valve) — *see* Endocarditis, pulmonary
  purine metabolism E79.9
  pyrimidine metabolism E79.9
  pyruvate metabolism E74.4
  reactive attachment (childhood) F94.1
  reading R48.0
    developmental (specific) F81.0
  receptive language F80.2
  receptor, hormonal, peripheral E34.5
  recurrent brief depressive F33.8
  reflex R29.2
  refraction H52.7
    aniseikonia H52.32
    anisometropia H52.31
    astigmatism — *see* Astigmatism
    hypermetropia — *see* Hypermetropia
    myopia — *see* Myopia
    presbyopia H52.4
    specified NEC H52.6
  relationship F68.8
    due to sexual orientation F66
  renal function, impaired (tubular) N25.9
  respiratory function, impaired — *see also* Failure, respiration
    postprocedural — *see* Complication, postoperative, respiratory system
    psychogenic F45.8
  retina H35.9
    angioid streaks H35.33
    changes in vascular appearance H35.019
      bilateral H35.013
      left H35.012
      right H35.011
    degeneration — *see* Degeneration, retina
    dystrophy (hereditary) — *see* Dystrophy, retina
    edema H35.81
    hemorrhage — *see* Hemorrhage, retina
    ischemia H35.82
    macular degeneration — *see* Degeneration, macula
    microaneurysms H35.049
      bilateral H35.043
      left H35.042
      right H35.041
    microvascular abnormality NEC H35.09
    neovascularization — *see* Neovascularization, retina
    retinopathy — *see* Retinopathy
    separation of layers H35.70
      central serous chorioretinopathy H35.719
        bilateral H35.713
        left H35.712
        right H35.711
      pigment epithelium detachment (serous) H35.729
        bilateral H35.723
        hemorrhagic H35.739
          bilateral H35.733
          left H35.732
          right H35.731
        left H35.722
        right H35.721
    specified type NEC H35.89
    telangiectasis — *see* Telangiectasis, retina
    vasculitis — *see* Vasculitis, retina
  right hemisphere organic affective F07.89
  rumination (infant or child) F98.21
  sacrum, sacrococcygeal NEC M53.3
  schizoaffective F25.9
    bipolar type F25.8
    depressive type F25.1
    manic type F25.0
    mixed type F25.8

Disorder — *see also* Disease — *continued*
  schizoaffective — *continued*
    specified NEC F25.8
  schizoid of childhood F84.5
  schizophreniform F20.81
    brief F23
  schizotypal (personality) F21
  secretion, thyrocalcitonin E07.0
  seizure R56.9
  sense of smell R43.1
    psychogenic F45.8
  separation anxiety, of childhood F93.0
  sexual
    arousal, female F52.22
    aversion F52.1
    function, psychogenic F52.9
    maturation F66
    nonorganic F52.9
    orientation (egodystonic) (preference) F66
    preference (*see also* Deviation, sexual) F65.9
      fetishistic transvestism F65.1
    relationship F66
  shyness, of childhood and adolescence F40.10
  sibling rivalry F93.8
  sickle-cell (sickling) (homozygous) D57.1
    with crisis D57.0
    double heterozygous D57.2
    heterozygous D57.3
    specified type NEC D57.8
    trait D57.3
  sinus (nasal) J34.9
    specified NEC J34.8
  skin L98.9
    atrophic L90.9
      specified NEC L90.8
    fetus or newborn P83.9
      specified NEC P83.8
    granulomatous L92.9
      specified NEC L92.8
    hypertrophic L91.9
      specified NEC L91.8
    infiltrative NEC L98.6
    psychogenic (allergic) (eczematous) F54
  sleep G47.9
    breathing-related — *see* Apnea, sleep
    circadian rhythm G47.2
      psychogenic F51.20
        delayed sleep phase type F51.23
        jet-lag type F51.21
        other specified F51.29
        shift work type F51.22
    due to
      alcohol F10.982
      amphetamine F15.982
        in
          abuse F15.182
          dependence F15.282
      anxiolytic F13.982
        in
          abuse F13.182
          dependence F13.282
      caffeine F15.982
        in
          abuse F15.182
          dependence F15.282
      cocaine F14.982
        in
          abuse F14.182
          dependence F14.282
      hypnotic F13.982
        in
          abuse F13.182
          dependence F13.282
      opioid F11.982
        in
          abuse F11.182
          dependence F11.282
      psychoactive substance NEC F19.982
        in
          abuse F19.182
          dependence F19.282
      sedative F13.982
        in
          abuse F13.182
          dependence F13.282
    emotional F51.9

Disorder — *see also* Disease — *continued*
  sleep — *continued*
    excessive somnolence G47.1
      psychogenic F51.1
    hypersomnia type G47.1
      psychogenic F51.1
    initiating or maintaining G47.0
      psychogenic F51.0
    insomnia type G47.0
      psychogenic F51.0
    mixed type G47.8
    nightmares F51.5
    nonorganic F51.9
      specified NEC F51.8
    parasomnia type G47.8
    specified NEC G47.8
    terrors F51.4
    walking F51.3
  sleep-wake pattern or schedule — *see* Disorder, sleep, circadian rhythm
  social
    anxiety of childhood F40.10
    functioning in childhood F94.9
      specified NEC F94.8
  soft tissue M79.9
    ankle M79.9
    due to use, overuse and pressure M70.90
      ankle M70.979
        left M70.972
        right M70.971
      bursitis — *see* Bursitis
      foot M70.979
        left M70.972
        right M70.971
      forearm M70.939
        left M70.932
        right M70.931
      hand M70.949
        left M70.942
        right M70.941
      lower leg M70.969
        left M70.962
        right M70.961
      multiple sites M70.99
      pelvic region M70.959
        left M70.952
        right M70.951
      shoulder region M70.919
        left M70.912
        right M70.911
      specified site NEC M70.98
      specified type NEC M70.80
        ankle M70.879
          left M70.872
          right M70.871
        foot M70.879
          left M70.872
          right M70.871
        forearm M70.839
          left M70.832
          right M70.831
        hand M70.849
          left M70.842
          right M70.841
        lower leg M70.869
          left M70.862
          right M70.861
        multiple sites M70.89
        pelvic region M70.859
          left M70.852
          right M70.851
        shoulder region M70.819
          left M70.812
          right M70.811
        specified site NEC M70.88
        thigh M70.859
          left M70.852
          right M70.851
        upper arm M70.829
          left M70.822
          right M70.821
      thigh M70.959
        left M70.952
        right M70.951
      upper arm M70.929
        left M70.922

Disorder — *see also* Disease — *continued*
  soft tissue — *continued*
    due to use, overuse and pressure —
        continued
      upper arm — *continued*
        right M70.921
    foot M79.9
    forearm M79.9
    hand M79.9
    lower leg M79.9
    multiple sites M79.9
    occupational — *see* Disorder, soft tissue,
        due to use, overuse and pressure
    pelvic region M79.9
    shoulder region M79.9
    specified site NEC M79.9
    specified type NEC M79.8
    thigh M79.9
    upper arm M79.9
  somatization F45.0
  somatoform F45.9
    pain (persistent) F45.4
    somatization (multiple) (long-lasting) F45.0
    specified NEC F45.8
    undifferentiated F45.1
  somnolence, excessive G47.1
  specific
    arithmetical F81.2
    developmental, of motor F82
    reading F81.0
    speech and language F80.9
    spelling F81.81
    written expression F81.81
  speech R47.9
    articulation (functional) (specific) F80.0
    developmental F80.9
    specified NEC R47.89
  spelling (specific) F81.81
  spine — *see also* Dorsopathy
    ligamentous or muscular attachments,
        peripheral — *see* Enthesopathy, spinal
    specified NEC — *see* Dorsopathy, specified
        NEC
  stereotyped, habit or movement F98.4
  stomach (functional) — *see* Disorder, gastric
  stress F43.9
    post-traumatic F43.10
      acute F43.0
      chronic F43.12
  sulfur-bearing amino-acid metabolism E72.10
  sweat gland (eccrine) L74.9
    apocrine L75.9
      specified NEC L75.8
    specified NEC L74.8
  synovium M67.90
    acromioclavicular M67.919
      left M67.912
      right M67.911
    ankle M67.979
      left M67.972
      right M67.971
    elbow M67.929
      left M67.922
      right M67.921
    foot M67.979
      left M67.972
      right M67.971
    forearm M67.939
      left M67.932
      right M67.931
    hand M67.949
      left M67.942
      right M67.941
    hip M67.959
      left M67.952
      right M67.951
    knee M67.969
      left M67.962
      right M67.961
    multiple sites M67.99
    rupture — *see* Rupture, synovium
    shoulder M67.919
      left M67.912
      right M67.911
    specified type NEC M67.80
      acromioclavicular M67.819
        left M67.812

Disorder — *see also* Disease — *continued*
  synovium — *continued*
    specified type NEC — *continued*
      acromioclavicular — *continued*
        right M67.811
      ankle M67.879
        left M67.872
        right M67.871
      elbow M67.829
        left M67.822
        right M67.821
      foot M67.879
        left M67.872
        right M67.871
      hand M67.849
        left M67.842
        right M67.841
      hip M67.859
        left M67.852
        right M67.851
      knee M67.869
        left M67.862
        right M67.861
      multiple sites M67.89
      wrist M67.839
        left M67.832
        right M67.831
    synovitis — *see* Synovitis
    upper arm M67.929
      left M67.922
      right M67.921
    wrist M67.939
      left M67.932
      right M67.931
  temperature regulation, fetus or newborn P81.9
    specified NEC P81.8
  temporomandibular joint — *see* Anomaly,
      dentofacial, temporomandibular joint
  tendon M67.90
    acromioclavicular M67.919
      left M67.912
      right M67.911
    ankle M67.979
      left M67.972
      right M67.971
    contracture — *see* Contracture, tendon
    elbow M67.929
      left M67.922
      right M67.921
    foot M67.979
      left M67.972
      right M67.971
    forearm M67.939
      left M67.932
      right M67.931
    hand M67.949
      left M67.942
      right M67.941
    hip M67.959
      left M67.952
      right M67.951
    knee M67.969
      left M67.962
      right M67.961
    multiple sites M67.99
    rupture — *see* Rupture, tendon
    shoulder M67.919
      left M67.912
      right M67.911
    specified type NEC M67.80
      acromioclavicular M67.819
        left M67.814
        right M67.813
      ankle M67.879
        left M67.874
        right M67.873
      elbow M67.829
        left M67.824
        right M67.823
      foot M67.879
        left M67.874
        right M67.873
      hand M67.849
        left M67.844
        right M67.843

Disorder — *see also* Disease — *continued*
  tendon — *continued*
    specified type NEC — *continued*
      hip M67.859
        left M67.854
        right M67.853
      knee M67.869
        left M67.864
        right M67.863
      multiple sites M67.89
      trunk M67.88
      wrist M67.839
        left M67.834
        right M67.833
    synovitis — *see* Synovitis
    tendinitis — *see* Tendinitis
    tenosynovitis — *see* Tenosynovitis
    upper arm M67.929
      left M67.922
      right M67.921
    trunk M67.98
    wrist M67.939
      left M67.932
      right M67.931
  thoracic root (nerve) NEC G54.3
  thyrocalcitonin hypersecretion E07.0
  thyroid (gland) E07.9
    function NEC, neonatal, transitory P72.2
    iodine-deficiency related E01.8
    specified NEC E07.89
  tic — *see* Tic
  tobacco use — *see* Dependence, drug, nicotine
  tooth K08.9
    development K00.9
      specified NEC K00.8
    eruption K00.6
      with abnormal position M26.3
  Tourette's F95.2
  trance and possession F44.89
  tricuspid (valve) — *see* Endocarditis, tricuspid
  tryptophan metabolism E70.5
  tubular, phosphate-losing N25.0
  tubulo-interstitial (in)
    brucellosis A23.9 *[N16]*
    cystinosis E72.04
    diphtheria A36.84
    glycogen storage disease E74.00 *[N16]*
    leukemia NEC (M9800/3) C95.90 *[N16]*
    lymphoma NEC (M9590/3) C85.90 *[N16]*
    mixed cryoglobulinemia D89.1 *[N16]*
    multiple myeloma (M9732/3) C90.00 *[N16]*
    Salmonella infection A02.25
    sarcoidosis D86.84
    septicemia A41.9 *[N16]*
      streptococcal A40.9 *[N16]*
    systemic lupus erythematosus M32.15
    toxoplasmosis B58.83
    transplant rejection T86.91 *[N16]*
    Wilson's disease E83.01 *[N16]*
  tubulo-renal function, impaired N25.9
    specified NEC N25.8
  tympanic membrane H73.90
    atrophy — *see* Atrophy, tympanic membrane
    bilateral H73.93
    infection — *see* Myringitis
    left H73.92
    perforation — *see* Perforation, tympanum
    right H73.91
    specified NEC H73.899
      bilateral H73.893
      left H73.892
      right H73.891
  unsocialized aggressive F91.1
  urea cycle metabolism E72.20
    argininemia E72.21
    arginosuccinic aciduria E72.22
    citrullinemia E72.23
    ornithine transcarbamylase deficiency
        E72.24
    other specified E72.29
  ureter (in) N28.9
    schistosomiasis B65.0 *[N29]*
    tuberculosis A18.11
  urethra N36.9
    specified NEC N36.8
  urinary system N39.9
    specified NEC N39.8

Disorder — see also Disease — continued
　valve, heart
　　aortic — see Endocarditis, aortic
　　mitral — see Endocarditis, mitral
　　pulmonary — see Endocarditis, pulmonary
　　rheumatic
　　　aortic — see Endocarditis, aortic,
　　　　rheumatic
　　　mitral — see Endocarditis, mitral
　　　pulmonary — see Endocarditis,
　　　　pulmonary, rheumatic
　　　tricuspid — see Endocarditis, tricuspid
　　tricuspid — see Endocarditis, tricuspid
　vestibular function H81.90
　　bilateral H81.93
　　left H81.92
　　right H81.91
　　specified NEC — see category H81.8
　　vertigo — see Vertigo
　vision, binocular H53.30
　　abnormal retinal correspondence H53.31
　　diplopia H53.2
　　fusion with defective stereopsis H53.32
　　simultaneous perception H53.33
　　suppression H53.34
　visual
　　cortex
　　　blindness H47.619
　　　　left brain H47.612
　　　　right brain H47.611
　　　due to
　　　　inflammatory disorder H47.629
　　　　　left brain H47.622
　　　　　right brain H47.621
　　　　neoplasm H47.639
　　　　　left brain H47.632
　　　　　right brain H47.631
　　　　vascular disorder H47.649
　　　　　left brain H47.642
　　　　　right brain H47.641
　　pathway H47.7
　　　due to
　　　　inflammatory disorder H47.519
　　　　　left H47.512
　　　　　right H47.511
　　　　neoplasm H47.529
　　　　　left H47.522
　　　　　right H47.521
　　　　vascular disorder H47.539
　　　　　left H47.532
　　　　　right H47.531
　　optic chiasm — see Disorder, optic,
　　　chiasm
　vitreous body H43.9
　　crystalline deposits — see Deposit,
　　　crystalline
　　degeneration — see Degeneration, vitreous
　　hemorrhage — see Hemorrhage, vitreous
　　opacities — see Opacity, vitreous
　　prolapse — see Prolapse, vitreous
　　specified type NEC H43.89
　voice R49.9
　　specified type NEC R49.8
　volatile solvent use — see Disorder, drug-
　　related, inhalant
　withdrawing, child or adolescent F40.10
Disorientation R41.0
　psychogenic F44.89
Displacement, displaced
　acquired traumatic of bone, cartilage, joint,
　　tendon NEC — see Dislocation
　adrenal gland (congenital) Q89.1
　appendix, retrocecal (congenital) Q43.8
　auricle (congenital) Q17.4
　bladder (acquired) N32.8
　　congenital Q64.19
　brachial plexus (congenital) Q07.8
　brain stem, caudal (congenital) Q04.8
　canaliculus (lacrimalis), congenital Q10.6
　cardia through esophageal hiatus (congenital)
　　Q40.1
　cerebellum, caudal (congenital) Q04.8
　cervix — see Malposition, uterus
　colon (congenital) Q43.3

Displacement, displaced — continued
　device, implant or graft (see also
　　Complications, by site and type,
　　mechanical) T85.9
　　arterial graft NEC — see Complication,
　　　cardiovascular device, mechanical,
　　　vascular
　　breast (implant) T85.42
　　catheter NEC T85.628
　　　dialysis (renal) T82.42
　　　　intraperitoneal T85.621
　　　infusion NEC T82.524
　　　　spinal (epidural) (subdural) T85.620
　　　urinary (indwelling) T83.021
　　　　cystostomy T83.020
　　electronic (electrode) (pulse generator)
　　　(stimulator) — see Complication,
　　　electronic stimulator
　　fixation, internal (orthopedic) NEC — see
　　　Complication, fixation device,
　　　mechanical
　　gastrointestinal — see Complications,
　　　prosthetic device, mechanical,
　　　gastrointestinal device
　　genital NEC T83.428
　　　intrauterine contraceptive device T83.32
　　　penile prosthesis T83.420
　　heart NEC — see Complication,
　　　cardiovascular device, mechanical
　　joint prosthesis — see Complications, joint
　　　prosthesis, mechanical
　　ocular — see Complications, prosthetic
　　　device, mechanical, ocular device
　　orthopedic NEC — see Complication,
　　　orthopedic, device or graft, mechanical
　　specified NEC T85.628
　　urinary NEC — see also Complication,
　　　genitourinary, device, urinary,
　　　mechanical
　　　graft T83.22
　　vascular NEC — see Complication,
　　　cardiovascular device, mechanical
　　ventricular intracranial shunt T85.02
　electronic stimulator
　　bone T84.320
　　cardiac — see Complications, cardiac device,
　　　electronic
　　nervous system — see Complication,
　　　prosthetic device, mechanical,
　　　electronic nervous system stimulator
　　urinary — see Complications, electronic
　　　stimulator, urinary
　epithelium
　　columnar of cervix N87.9
　　cuboidal, beyond limits of external os Q51.8
　esophageal mucosa into cardia of stomach,
　　congenital Q39.8
　esophagus (acquired) K22.8
　　congenital Q39.8
　eyeball (acquired) (lateral) (old) — see
　　Displacement, globe
　　congenital Q15.8
　　current — see Avulsion, eye
　fallopian tube (acquired) N83.4
　　congenital Q50.6
　　opening (congenital) Q50.6
　gallbladder (congenital) Q44.1
　gastric mucosa (congenital) Q40.2
　globe (acquired) (old) (lateral) H05.219
　　bilateral H05.213
　　current — see Avulsion, eye
　　left H05.212
　　right H05.211
　heart (congenital) Q24.8
　　acquired I51.8
　hymen (upward) (congenital) Q52.4
　intervertebral disc NEC
　　with myelopathy — see Disorder, disc, with,
　　　myelopathy
　　cervical, cervicothoracic (with) M50.20
　　　myelopathy — see Disorder, disc,
　　　　cervical, with myelopathy
　　　neuritis, radiculitis or radiculopathy —
　　　　see Disorder, disc, cervical, with
　　　　neuritis
　　due to major trauma — see Dislocation,
　　　vertebra

Displacement, displaced — continued
　intervertebral disc NEC — continued
　　lumbar region M51.26
　　　with
　　　　myelopathy M51.06
　　　　neuritis, radiculitis, radiculopathy or
　　　　　sciatica M51.16
　　lumbosacral region M51.27
　　　with
　　　　myelopathy M51.07
　　　　neuritis, radiculitis, radiculopathy or
　　　　　sciatica M51.17
　　sacrococcygeal region M53.3
　　thoracic region M51.24
　　　with
　　　　myelopathy M51.04
　　　　neuritis, radiculitis, radiculopathy
　　　　　M51.14
　　thoracolumbar region M51.25
　　　with
　　　　myelopathy M51.05
　　　　neuritis, radiculitis, radiculopathy
　　　　　M51.15
　intrauterine device T83.32
　kidney (acquired) N28.83
　　congenital Q63.2
　lachrymal, lacrimal apparatus or duct
　　(congenital) Q10.6
　lens, congenital Q12.1
　macula (congenital) Q14.1
　Meckel's diverticulum Q43.0
　nail (congenital) Q84.6
　　acquired L60.8
　oesophagus (acquired) — see Displacement,
　　esophagus
　opening of Wharton's duct in mouth Q38.4
　organ or site, congenital NEC — see
　　Malposition, congenital
　ovary (acquired) N83.4
　　congenital Q50.39
　　free in peritoneal cavity (congenital) Q50.39
　　into hernial sac N83.4
　oviduct (acquired) N83.4
　　congenital Q50.6
　parathyroid (gland) E21.4
　parotid gland (congenital) Q38.4
　punctum lacrimale (congenital) Q10.6
　sacro-iliac (joint) (congenital) Q74.2
　　current injury S33.2
　　old — see category M53.2
　salivary gland (any) (congenital) Q38.4
　spleen (congenital) Q89.09
　stomach, congenital Q40.2
　sublingual duct Q38.4
　tongue (downward) (congenital) Q38.3
　tooth, teeth M26.3
　trachea (congenital) Q32.1
　ureter or ureteric opening or orifice (congenital)
　　Q62.62
　uterine opening of oviducts or fallopian tubes
　　Q50.6
　uterus, uterine — see Malposition, uterus
　ventricular septum Q21.0
　　with rudimentary ventricle Q20.4
Disproportion (fetopelvic) O33.9
　caused by
　　conjoined twins O33.7
　　contraction pelvis (general) O33.1
　　　causing obstruction O65.1
　　　inlet O33.2
　　　outlet O33.3
　　fetal
　　　ascites O33.7
　　　deformity NEC O33.7
　　　hydrocephalus O33.6
　　　hydrops O33.7
　　　meningomyelocele O33.7
　　　sacral teratoma O33.7
　　　tumor O33.7
　　hydrocephalic fetus O33.6
　　pelvis, pelvic, abnormality (bony) NEC O33.0
　　　causing obstructed labor O65.0
　　unusually large fetus O33.5
　causing obstructed labor O65.4
　cephalopelvic O33.9
　　causing obstructed labor O65.4
　fetal (with normally formed fetus) O33.5

Disproportion — *continued*
fiber-type G71.2
mixed maternal and fetal origin O33.4
specified NEC O33.8

Disruptio uteri — *see* Rupture, uterus

Disruption
ciliary body NEC H21.8
family Z63.8
involving divorce or separation Z63.5
iris NEC H21.8
ligament(s) — *see also* Sprain
knee
current injury — *see* Dislocation, knee
old (chronic) — *see* Derangement, knee, instability
spontaneous NEC — *see* Derangement, knee, disruption ligament
marital (perpetrator) Z69.12
involving divorce Z63.5
victim Z60.11
ossicular chain — *see* Discontinuity, ossicles, ear
pelvic circle (stable) S32.810
unstable S32.811
wound
episiotomy O90.1
operation T81.3
cesarean O90.0
perineal (obstetric) O90.1

Dissatisfaction with
employment Z56.9
school environment Z55.4

Dissecting — *see* condition

Dissection
aorta (ruptured) I71.00
abdominal I71.02
thoracic I71.01
thoracoabdominal I71.03
artery
cerebral (nonruptured) I67.0
ruptured — *see* Hemorrhage, intracranial, subarachnoid
vascular I99.8
wound — *see* Wound, open

Disseminated — *see* condition

Dissocial behavior, without manifest psychiatric disorder Z03.8

Dissociation
auriculoventricular or atrioventricular (AV) (any degree) (isorhythmic) I45.8
with heart block I44.2
interference I45.8

Dissociative reaction, state F44.9

Dissolution, vertebra — *see* Osteoporosis

Distension, distention
abdomen R14.0
bladder N32.8
cecum K63.8
colon K63.8
gallbladder K82.8
intestine K63.8
kidney N28.89
liver K76.8
seminal vesicle N50.8
stomach K31.89
acute K31.0
psychogenic F45.8
ureter — *see* Dilatation, ureter
uterus N85.8

Distoma hepaticum infestation B66.3

Distomiasis B66.9
bile passages B66.3
hemic B65.9
hepatic B66.3
due to Clonorchis sinensis B66.1
intestinal B66.5
liver B66.3
due to Clonorchis sinensis B66.1
lung B66.4
pulmonary B66.4

Distomolar (fourth molar) K00.1
causing crowding M26.3

Disto-occlusion M26.2

Distortion (congenital)
adrenal (gland) Q89.1
arm NEC Q68.8
bile duct or passage Q44.5
bladder Q64.79
brain Q04.9
cervix (uteri) Q51.9
chest (wall) Q67.8
bones Q76.8
clavicle Q74.0
clitoris Q52.6
coccyx Q76.49
common duct Q44.5
coronary Q24.5
cystic duct Q44.5
ear (auricle) (external) Q17.3
inner Q16.5
middle Q16.4
ossicles Q16.3
endocrine NEC Q89.2
eustachian tube Q17.8
eye (adnexa) Q15.8
face bone(s) NEC Q75.8
fallopian tube Q50.6
femur NEC Q68.8
fibula NEC Q68.8
finger(s) Q68.1
foot Q66.9
genitalia, genital organ(s)
female Q52.8
external Q52.79
internal NEC Q52.8
gyri Q04.8
hand bone(s) Q68.1
heart (auricle) (ventricle) Q24.8
valve (cusp) Q24.8
hepatic duct Q44.5
humerus NEC Q68.8
hymen Q52.4
intrafamilial communications Z63.8
jaw NEC M26.8
labium (majus) (minus) Q52.79
leg NEC Q68.8
lens Q12.8
liver Q44.7
lumbar spine Q76.49
with disproportion O33.8
causing obstructed labor O65.0
lumbosacral (joint) (region) Q76.49
kyphosis — *see* Kyphosis, congenital
lordosis — *see* Lordosis, congenital
nerve Q07.8
nose Q30.8
organ
of Corti Q16.5
or site not listed — *see* Anomaly, by site
ossicles, ear Q16.3
oviduct Q50.6
pancreas Q45.3
parathyroid (gland) Q89.2
pituitary (gland) Q89.2
radius NEC Q68.8
sacroiliac joint Q74.2
sacrum Q76.49
scapula Q74.0
shoulder girdle Q74.0
skull bone(s) NEC Q75.8
with
anencephalus Q00.0
encephalocele — *see* Encephalocele
hydrocephalus Q03.9
with spina bifida — *see* Spina bifida, with hydrocephalus
microcephaly Q02
spinal cord Q06.8
spine Q76.49
kyphosis — *see* Kyphosis, congenital
lordosis — *see* Lordosis, congenital
spleen Q89.09
sternum NEC Q76.7
thorax (wall) Q67.8
bony Q76.8
thymus (gland) Q89.2
thyroid (gland) Q89.2
tibia NEC Q68.8
toe(s) Q66.9
tongue Q38.3

Distortion — *continued*
trachea (cartilage) Q32.1
ulna NEC Q68.8
ureter Q62.8
urethra Q64.79
causing obstruction Q64.39
uterus Q51.9
vagina Q52.4
vertebra Q76.49
kyphosis — *see* Kyphosis, congenital
lordosis — *see* Lordosis, congenital
visual — *see* Disturbance, vision
vulva Q52.79
wrist (bones) (joint) Q68.8

Distress
abdomen — *see* Pain, abdominal
epigastric R10.13
fetal (syndrome) P19.9
affecting
labor and delivery — *see* Delivery, complicated by, distress, fetal
management of pregnancy (unrelated to labor or delivery) O36.899
first noted
at birth P19.2
before onset of labor P19.0
during labor and delivery P19.1
manifested by abnormal heart rate (bradycardia) (tachycardia) or rhythm P03.819
first noted
before onset of labor P03.810
during labor and delivery P03.811
gastrointestinal (functional) K30
psychogenic F45.8
intestinal (functional) NOS K59.9
psychogenic F45.8
intrauterine — *see* Distress, fetal
maternal, during labor and delivery O75.0
respiratory R06.00
adult J80
newborn P22.9
specified NEC P22.8
orthopnea R06.01
psychogenic F45.8
shortness of breath R06.02
specified type NEC R06.09
syndrome (idiopathic) (newborn) (type I) P22.0
adult J80
type II P22.1

Distribution vessel, atypical Q27.9
coronary artery Q24.5
precerebral Q28.1

Districhiasis L68.8

Disturbance — *see also* Disease
absorption K90.9
calcium E58
carbohydrate K90.4
fat K90.4
pancreatic K90.3
protein K90.4
starch K90.4
vitamin — *see* Deficiency, vitamin
acid-base equilibrium E87.8
mixed E87.4
activity and attention (with hyperkinesis) — *see* Disorder, attention-deficit hyperactivity
amino acid transport E72.00
assimilation, food K90.9
auditory nerve, except deafness — *see* category H93.3
behavior — *see* Disorder, conduct
blood clotting (mechanism) (*see also* Defect, coagulation) D68.9
cerebral
nerve — *see* Disorder, nerve, cranial
status, newborn P91.9
specified NEC P91.8
circulatory I99.9
conduct (*see also* Disorder, conduct) F91.9
adjustment reaction — *see* Disorder, adjustment
compulsive F63.9
disruptive F91.9

©2002 Ingenix, Inc.

Disturbance — *see also* Disease — *continued*
  conduct (*see also* Disorder, conduct) —
    continued
    hyperkinetic — *see* Disorder, attention-
      deficit hyperactivity
    socialized F91.2
    specified NEC F91.8
    unsocialized F91.1
  coordination R27.8
  cranial nerve — *see* Disorder, nerve, cranial
  deep sensibility — *see* Disturbance, sensation
  digestive K30
    psychogenic F45.8
  electrolyte — *see also* Imbalance, electrolyte
    newborn, transitory P74.4
      hyperammonemia P74.6
      potassium balance P74.3
      sodium balance P74.2
      specified type NEC P74.4
  emotions specific to childhood and adolescence
    F93.9
    with
      anxiety and fearfulness NEC F93.8
      elective mutism F94.0
      oppositional disorder F91.3
      sensitivity (withdrawal) F40.10
      shyness F40.10
      social withdrawal F40.10
    involving relationship problems F93.8
    mixed F93.8
    specified NEC F93.8
  endocrine (gland) E34.9
    neonatal, transitory P72.9
      specified NEC P72.8
  equilibrium R42
  feeding R63.3
    newborn P92.9
    nonorganic origin — *see* Disorder, eating
  fructose metabolism E74.10
  gait — *see* Gait
    hysterical F44.4
    psychogenic F44.4
  gastrointestinal (functional) K30
    psychogenic F45.8
  habit, child F98.9
  hearing, except deafness and tinnitus — *see*
    Abnormal, auditory perception
  heart, functional (conditions in I44-I50)
    due to presence of (cardiac) prosthesis I97.1
    postoperative I97.89
      cardiac surgery I97.1
  hormones E34.9
  innervation uterus (parasympathetic)
    (sympathetic) N85.8
  keratinization NEC
    gingiva K05.1
    lip K13.0
    oral (mucosa) (soft tissue) K13.2
    tongue K13.2
  learning (specific) — *see* Disorder, learning
  memory — *see* Amnesia
    mild, following organic brain damage F06.8
  mental F99
    associated with diseases classified elsewhere
      F54
  metabolism E88.9
    with
      abortion — *see* Abortion, by type with
        other specified complication
      ectopic pregnancy O08.5
      molar pregnancy O08.5
    amino-acid E72.9
      aromatic E70.9
      branched-chain E71.2
      straight-chain E72.8
      sulfur-bearing E72.10
    ammonia E72.20
    arginine E72.21
    arginosuccinic acid E72.22
    carbohydrate E74.9
    cholesterol E78.9
    citrulline E72.23
    cystathionine E72.19
    general E88.9
    glutamine E72.8
    histidine E70.40
    homocystine E72.19

Disturbance — *see also* Disease — *continued*
  metabolism — *continued*
    hydroxylysine E72.3
    in labor or delivery O75.89
    iron E83.10
    lipoid E78.9
    lysine E72.3
    methionine E72.19
    neonatal, transitory P74.9
      calcium and magnesium P71.9
        specified type NEC P71.8
      carbohydrate metabolism P70.9
        specified type NEC P70.8
      specified NEC P74.8
    ornithine E72.4
    phosphate E83.39
    sodium NEC E87.8
    threonine E72.8
    tryptophan E70.5
    tyrosine E70.20
    urea cycle E72.20
  motor R29.2
  nervous, functional R45.0
  neuromuscular mechanism (eye), due to
    syphilis A52.15
  nutritional E63.9
    nail L60.3
  ocular motion H51.9
    psychogenic F45.8
  oculogyric H51.9
    psychogenic F45.8
  oculomotor H51.9
    psychogenic F45.8
  olfactory nerve R43.1
  optic nerve NEC — *see* Disorder, nerve, optic
  oral epithelium, including tongue K13.2
  perceptual due to
    alcohol withdrawal F10.232
    amphetamine intoxication F15.922
      in
        abuse F15.122
        dependence F15.222
    anxiolytic withdrawal F13.232
    cannabis intoxication (acute) F12.922
      in
        abuse F12.122
        dependence F12.222
    cocaine intoxication (acute) F14.922
      in
        abuse F14.122
        dependence F14.222
    hypnotic withdrawal F13.232
    opioid intoxication (acute) F11.922
      in
        abuse F11.122
        dependence F11.222
    phencyclidine intoxication (acute) F19.922
      in
        abuse F19.122
        dependence F19.222
    sedative withdrawal F13.232
  personality (pattern) (trait) (*see also* Disorder,
    personality) F60.9
    following organic brain damage F07.9
  polyglandular E31.9
    specified NEC E31.8
  potassium balance, newborn P74.3
  psychogenic F45.9
  psychomotor F44.4
  pupillary — *see* Anomaly, pupil, function
  reflex R29.2
  rhythm, heart I49.9
  salivary secretion K11.7
  sensation (cold) (heat) (localization) (tactile
    discrimination) (texture) (vibratory) NEC
    R20.9
    hysterical F44.6
    skin R20.9
      anesthesia R20.0
      hyperesthesia R20.3
      hypoesthesia R20.1
      paresthesia R20.2
      specified type NEC R20.8
    smell R43.9
      and taste (mixed) R43.8
      anosmia R43.0
      parosmia R43.1

Disturbance — *see also* Disease — *continued*
  sensation NEC — *continued*
    smell — *continued*
      specified NEC R43.8
    taste R43.9
      and smell (mixed) R43.8
      parageusia R43.2
      specified NEC R43.8
  sensory — *see* Disturbance, sensation
  situational (transient) — *see also* Disorder,
    adjustment
    acute F43.0
  sleep G47.9
    nonorganic origin F51.9
  smell — *see* Disturbance, sensation, smell
  sociopathic F60.2
  sodium balance, newborn P74.2
  speech R47.9
    developmental F80.9
    specified NEC R47.89
  stomach (functional) K31.9
  sympathetic (nerve) G90.9
  taste — *see* Disturbance, sensation, taste
  temperature
    regulation, newborn P81.9
      specified NEC P81.8
    sense R20.8
      hysterical F44.6
  tooth
    eruption K00.6
    formation K00.4
    structure, hereditary NEC K00.5
  touch — *see* Disturbance, sensation
  vascular I99.9
    arteriosclerotic — *see* Arteriosclerosis
  vasomotor I73.9
  vasospastic I73.9
  vision, visual H53.9
    specified NEC H53.8
    subjective H53.10
      day blindness H53.11
      discomfort H53.149
        bilateral H53.143
        left H53.142
        right H53.141
      distortions of shape and size H53.18
      loss
        sudden H53.139
          bilateral H53.133
          left H53.132
          right H53.131
        transient H53.129
          bilateral H53.123
          left H53.122
          right H53.121
      specified type NEC H53.19
  voice R49.9
    psychogenic F44.4
    specified NEC R49.8
Diuresis R35.8
Diver's palsy, paralysis or squeeze T70.3
Diverticulitis (acute) K57.92
  bladder — *see* Cystitis
  ileum — *see* Diverticulitis, intestine, small
  intestine K57.92
    with
      abscess, perforation or peritonitis K57.80
        with bleeding K57.81
      bleeding K57.93
    congenital Q43.8
    large K57.32
      with
        abscess, perforation or peritonitis
          K57.20
          with bleeding K57.21
        bleeding K57.33
        small intestine K57.52
          with
            abscess, perforation or
              peritonitis K57.40
              with bleeding K57.41
            bleeding K57.53

Diverticulitis — continued
  intestine — continued
    small K57.12
      with
        abscess, perforation or peritonitis
          K57.00
          with bleeding K57.01
        bleeding K57.13
        large intestine K57.52
        with
          abscess, perforation or
            peritonitis K57.40
            with bleeding K57.41
          bleeding K57.53
Diverticulosis K57.90
  with bleeding K57.91
  large intestine K57.30
    with
      bleeding K57.31
      small intestine K57.50
        with bleeding K57.51
  small intestine K57.10
    with
      bleeding K57.11
      large intestine K57.50
        with bleeding K57.51
Diverticulum, diverticula (multiple) K57.90
  appendix (noninflammatory) K38.2
  bladder (sphincter) N32.3
    congenital Q64.6
  bronchus (congenital) Q32.8
    acquired J98.0
  calyx, calyceal (kidney) N28.89
  cardia (stomach) K31.4
  cecum — see Diverticulosis, intestine, large
    congenital Q43.8
  colon — see Diverticulosis, intestine, large
    congenital Q43.8
  duodenum — see Diverticulosis, intestine,
    small
    congenital Q43.8
  epiphrenic (esophagus) K22.5
  esophagus (congenital) Q39.6
    acquired (epiphrenic) (pulsion) (traction)
      K22.5
  eustachian tube — see Disorder, eustachian
    tube, specified NEC
  fallopian tube N83.8
  gastric K31.4
  heart (congenital) Q24.8
  ileum — see Diverticulosis, intestine, small)
  jejunum — see Diverticulosis, intestine, small
  kidney (pelvis) (calyces) N28.89
    with calculus — see Calculus, kidney
  Meckel's (displaced) (hypertrophic) Q43.0
  midthoracic K22.5
  organ or site, congenital NEC — see Distortion
  pericardium (congenital) (cyst) Q24.8
    acquired I31.8
  pharyngoesophageal (congenital) Q39.6
    acquired K22.5
  pharynx (congenital) Q38.7
  rectosigmoid — see Diverticulosis, intestine,
    large
    congenital Q43.8
  rectum — see Diverticulosis, intestine, large
  Rokitansky's K22.5
  seminal vesicle N50.8
  sigmoid — see Diverticulosis, intestine, large
    congenital Q43.8
  stomach (acquired) K31.4
    congenital Q40.2
  trachea (acquired) J39.8
  ureter (acquired) N28.89
    congenital Q62.8
  ureterovesical orifice N28.89
  urethra (acquired) N36.1
    congenital Q64.79
  ventricle, left (congenital) Q24.8
  vesical N32.3
    congenital Q64.6
  Zenker's (esophagus) K22.5
Division
  cervix uteri (acquired) N88.8
  external os into two openings by frenum Q51.8
  glans penis Q55.69
  labia minora (congenital) Q52.79

Division — continued
  ligament (partial or complete) (current) — see
    also Sprain
    with open wound — see Wound, open
  muscle (partial or complete) (current) — see
    also Injury, muscle
    with open wound — see Wound, open
  nerve (traumatic) — see Injury, nerve
  spinal cord — see Injury, spinal cord, by region
  vein I87.8
Divorce, causing family disruption Z63.5
Dix-Hallpike neurolabyrinthitis — see
  Neuronitis, vestibular
Dizziness R42
  hysterical F44.89
  psychogenic F45.8
  DMAC (disseminated mycobacterium
    aviumintracellulare complex A31.2
DNR (do not resuscitate) Z66
Doan-Wiseman syndrome (primary splenic
  neutropenia) — see Agranulocytosis
Doehle-Heller aortitis A52.02
Dog bite — see Bite
Dohle body panmyelopathic syndrome D72.0
Dolichocephaly Q67.2
Dolichocolon Q43.8
Dolichostenomelia — see Syndrome, Marfan's
Donohue's syndrome E34.8
Donor (organ or tissue) Z52.9
  blood (whole) Z52.000
    autologous Z52.010
    specified donor NEC Z52.090
    specified component NEC Z52.008
      autologous Z52.018
      specified donor NEC Z52.098
    stem cells Z52.001
      autologous Z52.011
      specified donor NEC Z52.091
  bone Z52.20
    autologous Z52.21
    marrow Z52.3
    specified type NEC Z52.29
  cornea Z52.5
  kidney Z52.4
  lung Z52.8
  lymphocyte Z52.8
  potential, examination of Z00.5
  skin Z52.10
    autologous Z52.11
    specified type NEC Z52.19
  specified organ or tissue NEC Z52.8
Donovanosis A58
Dorsalgia M54.9
  psychogenic F45.4
  specified NEC M54.89
Dorsopathy M53.9
  deforming M43.9
    specified NEC — see category M43.8
  specified NEC M53.80
    cervical region M53.82
    cervicothoracic region M53.83
    lumbar region M53.86
    lumbosacral region M53.87
    occipito-atlanto-axial region M53.81
    sacrococcygeal region M53.88
    thoracic region M53.84
    thoracolumbar region M53.85
Double
  albumin E88.09
  aortic arch Q25.4
  auditory canal Q17.8
  auricle (heart) Q20.8
  bladder Q64.79
  cervix Q51.8
    with doubling of uterus (and vagina) Q51.10
      with obstruction Q51.11
  external os Q51.8
  inlet ventricle Q20.4
  kidney with double pelvis (renal) Q63.0
  meatus urinarius Q64.75
  monster Q89.4
  outlet
    left ventricle Q20.2
    right ventricle Q20.1

Double — continued
  pelvis (renal) with double ureter Q62.5
  tongue Q38.3
  ureter (one or both sides) Q62.5
    with double pelvis (renal) Q62.5
  urethra Q64.74
  urinary meatus Q64.75
  uterus Q51.2
    with
      doubling of cervix (and vagina) Q51.10
        with obstruction Q51.11
    in pregnancy or childbirth — see Anomaly,
      uterus, in pregnancy or childbirth
      causing obstructed labor O65.0
  vagina Q52.1
    with doubling of uterus (and cervix) Q51.10
      with obstruction Q51.11
  vision H53.2
  vulva Q52.79
Douglas' pouch, cul-de-sac — see condition
Down's disease or syndrome — see Trisomy, 21
Dracontiasis B72
Dracunculiasis, dracunculosis B72
Drainage, suprapubic, bladder N32.2
Dream state, hysterical F44.89
Dreschlera (hawaiiensis) (infection) B43.8
Drepanocytic anemia — see Disease, sickle-cell
Dresbach's syndrome (elliptocytosis) D58.1
Dressler's syndrome I24.1
Drift, ulnar — see Deformity, limb, specified type
  NEC, forearm
Drinking (alcohol)
  excessive, to excess NEC (without dependence)
    F10.10
    habitual (continual) (without remission)
      F10.20
      with remission F10.21
Drop
  attack NEC R55
  finger — see Deformity, finger
  foot — see Deformity, limb, foot, drop
  toe — see Deformity, toe, specified NEC
  wrist — see Deformity, limb, wrist drop
Dropped heart beats I45.9
Dropsy, dropsical — see also Hydrops
  abdomen R18
  brain — see Hydrocephalus
  cardiac, heart — see Failure, heart, congestive
  cardiorenal I13.2
  fetus or newborn due to isoimmunization P56.0
  gangrenous — see Gangrene
  heart — see Failure, heart, congestive
  kidney — see Nephrosis
  lung — see Edema, lung
  pericardium — see Pericarditis
Drowned, drowning T75.1
Drowsiness R40.0
Drug
  abuse counseling and surveillance Z71.51
  addiction — see Dependence
  adverse effect NEC, correct substance properly
    administered T88.7
  dependence — see Dependence
  detoxification therapy Z51.89
  habit — see Dependence
  harmful use — see Disorder, drug-related
  overdose — see Table of Drugs and Chemicals
  poisoning — see Table of Drugs and Chemicals
  rehabilitation measures Z51.89
  resistant organism infection Z06
  use NEC
    obstetric complicating
      childbirth O99.324
      pregnancy O99.323
        first trimester O99.320
        second trimester O99.321
        third trimester O99.322
      puerperium O99.325
  wrong substance given or taken in error — see
    Table of Drugs and Chemicals
Drunkenness (without dependence) F10.129
  acute in alcoholism F10.229
  chronic (without remission) F10.20
    with remission F10.21

Drunkenness — *continued*
  pathological (without dependence) F10.129
    with dependence F10.229
  sleep F51.9
Drusen
  macula (degenerative) (retina) — *see*
    Degeneration, macula, drusen
  optic disc H47.329
    bilateral H47.323
    left H47.322
    right H47.321
Dry, dryness — *see also* condition
  larynx J38.7
  mouth R68.2
    due to dehydration E86.0
  nose J34.8
  socket (teeth) M27.3
  throat J39.2
DSAP L56.5
Duane's syndrome
  left H50.812
  right H50.811
Dubin-Johnson disease or syndrome E80.6
Dubois' disease (thymus gland) A50.59 *[E35]*
Dubowitz' syndrome Q87.1
Duchenne-Aran muscular atrophy G12.21
Duchenne-Griesinger disease G71.0
Duchenne's
  disease or syndrome
    motor neuron disease G12.21
    muscular dystrophy G71.0
  locomotor ataxia (syphilitic) A52.11
  paralysis G71.0
    birth injury P14.0
    muscular dystrophy G71.0
Ducrey's chancre A57
Duct, ductus — *see* condition
Duhring's disease (dermatitis herpetiformis) L13.0
Dullness, cardiac (decreased) (increased) R01.2
Dumb ague — *see* Malaria
Dumbness — *see* Aphasia
Dumdum fever B55.0
Dumping syndrome (postgastrectomy) K91.1
Duodenitis (nonspecific) (peptic) K29.80
  with bleeding K29.81
Duodenocholangitis — *see* Cholangitis
Duodenum, duodenal — *see* condition
Duplay's bursitis or periarthritis — *see* Tendinitis, calcific, shoulder
Duplication, duplex — *see also* Accessory
  alimentary tract Q45.8
  anus Q43.4
  appendix (and cecum) Q43.4
  biliary duct (any) Q44.5
  bladder Q64.79
  cecum (and appendix) Q43.4
  chromosome NEC
    with complex rearrangements NEC Q92.5
    seen only at prometaphase Q92.8
  cystic duct Q44.5
  digestive organs Q45.8
  esophagus Q39.8
  frontonasal process Q75.8
  intestine (large) (small) Q43.4
  kidney Q63.0
  liver Q44.7
  oesophagus Q39.8
  pancreas Q45.3
  penis Q55.69
  placenta — *see* Abnormal, placenta, specified type NEC
  respiratory organs NEC Q34.8
  salivary duct Q38.4
  spinal cord (incomplete) Q06.2
  stomach Q40.2
Dupré's disease (meningism) R29.1
Dupuytren's contraction or disease M72.0
Durand-Nicolas-Favre disease A55
Duroziez's disease (congenital mitral stenosis) Q23.2

Dust exposure (inorganic) Z58.1
  occupational Z57.2
  reticulation — *see also* Pneumoconiosis
    organic dusts J66.8
Dutton's relapsing fever (West African) A68.1
Dwarfism E34.3
  achondroplastic Q77.4
  congenital E34.3
  constitutional E34.3
  hypochondroplastic Q77.4
  hypophyseal E23.0
  infantile E34.3
  Laron-type E34.3
  Lorain(-Levi) type E23.0
  metatropic Q77.8
  nephrotic-glycosuric (with hypophosphatemic rickets) E72.09
  nutritional E45
  pancreatic K86.8
  pituitary E23.0
  psychosocial E34.3
  renal N25.0
  thanatophoric Q77.1
Dyke-Young anemia (secondary) (symptomatic) D59.8
Dysacusis — *see* Abnormal, auditory perception
Dysadrenocortism E27.9
  hyperfunction E27.0
Dysarthria R47.1
  following
    cerebrovascular disease I69.928
      cerebral infarction I69.328
      intracerebral hemorrhage I69.128
      nontraumatic intracranial hemorrhage NEC I69.228
      specified disease NEC I69.828
      stroke NOS I69.428
      subarachnoid hemorrhage I69.028
Dysautonomia (familial) G90.1
Dysbarism T70.3
Dysbasia R26.2
  angiosclerotica intermittens I73.9
  hysterical F44.4
  lordotica (progressiva) G24.1
  nonorganic origin F44.4
  psychogenic F44.4
Dysbetalipoproteinemia (familial) E78.2
Dyscalculia R48.8
  developmental F81.2
Dyschezia K59.0
Dyschondroplasia (with hemangiomata) Q78.4
Dyschromia (skin) L81.9
Dyscollagenosis M35.9
Dyscranio-pygo-phalangy Q87.0
Dyscrasia
  blood (with) D75.9
    antepartum hemorrhage — *see* Hemorrhage, antepartum, with coagulation defect
    fetus or newborn P61.9
      specified type NEC P61.8
    intrapartum hemorrhage O67.0
    puerperal, postpartum O72.3
    polyglandular, pluriglandular E31.9
Dysendocrinism E34.9
Dysentery, dysenteric (catarrhal) (diarrhea) (epidemic) (hemorrhagic) (infectious) (sporadic) (tropical) A09
  abscess, liver A06.4
  amebic (*see also* Amebiasis) A06.0
    with abscess — *see* Abscess, amebic
    acute A06.0
    chronic A06.1
  arthritis A09 (*see also* category M01)
    bacillary A03.9 (*see also* category M01)
  bacillary A03.9
    arthritis A03.9 (*see also* category M01)
    Boyd A03.2
    Flexner A03.1
    Schmitz(-Stutzer) A03.0
    Shiga(-Kruse) A03.0
    Shigella A03.9
      boydii A03.2
      dysenteriae A03.0
      flexneri A03.1

Dysentery, dysenteric — *continued*
  bacillary — *continued*
    Shigella — *continued*
      group A A03.0
      group B A03.1
      group C A03.2
      group D A03.3
      sonnei A03.3
      specified type NEC A03.8
    Sonne A03.3
    specified type NEC A03.8
  balantidial A07.0
  Balantidium coli A07.0
  Boyd's A03.2
  candidal B37.82
  Chilomastix A07.8
  Chinese A03.9
  coccidial A07.3
  Dientamoeba (fragilis) A07.8
  Embadomonas A07.8
  Entamoeba, entamebic — *see* Dysentery, amebic
  Flexner-Boyd A03.2
  Flexner's A03.1
  Giardia lamblia A07.1
  Hiss-Russell A03.1
  Lamblia A07.1
  leishmanial B55.0
  malarial — *see* Malaria
  metazoal B82.0
  monilial B37.82
  protozoal A07.9
  Salmonella A02.0
  schistosomal B65.1
  Schmitz(-Stutzer) A03.0
  Shiga(-Kruse) A03.0
  Shigella NOS — *see* Dysentery, bacillary
  Sonne A03.3
  strongyloidiasis B78.0
  trichomonal A07.8
  viral (*see also* Enteritis, viral) A08.4
Dysequilibrium R42
Dysesthesia R20.8
  hysterical F44.6
Dysfibrinogenemia (congenital) D68.2
Dysfunction
  adrenal E27.9
    hyperfunction E27.0
  ambulatory (transient) following surgery Z48.8
  autonomic
    due to alcohol G31.2
    somatoform F45.8
  bladder N31.9
    neurogenic NOS — *see* Dysfunction, bladder, neuromuscular
    neuromuscular NOS N31.9
      atonic (motor) (sensory) N31.2
      autonomous N31.2
      flaccid N31.2
      nonreflex N31.2
      overactive N31.3
      reflex N31.1
      specified NEC N31.8
      uninhibited N31.0
  bleeding, uterus N93.8
  cerebral G93.8
  colon K59.9
    psychogenic F45.8
  colostomy K94.03
  cystic duct K82.8
  cystostomy (stoma) — *see* Complications, cystostomy
  ejaculatory N53.19
    anejaculatory orgasm N53.13
    painful N53.12
    premature F52.4
    retarded N53.11
  endocrine NOS E34.9
  endometrium N85.8
  enterostomy K94.13
  gallbladder K82.8
  gastrostomy (stoma) K94.23
  gland, glandular NOS E34.9
  heart I51.8
  hemoglobin D75.8
  hepatic K76.8

Dysfunction — continued
- hypophysis E23.3
- hypothalamic NEC E23.3
- ileostomy (stoma) K94.13
- jejunostomy (stoma) K94.13
- kidney — see Disease, renal
- labyrinthine — see category H83.2
- liver K76.8
- male—see Dysfunction, sexual, male
- orgasmic (female) F52.31
  - male F52.32
- ovary E28.9
  - specified NEC E28.8
- papillary muscle I51.8
- parathyroid E21.4
- physiological NEC R68.8
  - psychogenic F59
- pineal gland E34.8
- pituitary (gland) E23.3
- placental O43.819
  - first trimester O43.811
  - second trimester O43.812
  - third trimester O43.813
- platelets D69.1
- polyglandular E31.9
  - specified NEC E31.8
- psychophysiologic F59
- psychosexual F52.9
  - with
    - dyspareunia F52.6
    - premature ejaculation F52.4
    - vaginismus F52.5
- pylorus K31.9
- rectum K59.9
  - psychogenic F45.8
- segmental — see Dysfunction, somatic
- senile R54
- sexual (due to) R37
  - alcohol F10.981
  - amphetamine F15.981
    - in
      - abuse F15.181
      - dependence F15.281
  - anxiolytic F13.981
    - in
      - abuse F13.181
      - dependence F13.281
  - cocaine F14.981
    - in
      - abuse F14.181
      - dependence F14.281
  - excessive sexual drive F52.8
  - failure of genital response (male) F52.21
    - female F52.22
  - female N94.9
    - anhedonia F52.0
    - aversion F52.1
    - dyspareunia N94.1
      - psychogenic F52.6
    - frigidity F52.22
    - nymphomania F52.8
    - orgasmic F52.31
    - psychogenic F52.9
      - anhedonia F52.0
      - aversion F52.1
      - dyspareunia F52.6
      - frigidity F52.22
      - nymphomania F52.8
      - orgasmic F52.31
      - vaginismus F52.5
    - vaginismus N94.2
      - psychogenic F52.5
  - hypnotic F13.981
    - in
      - abuse F13.181
      - dependence F13.281
  - inhibited orgasm (female) F52.31
    - male F52.32
  - lack
    - of sexual enjoyment F52.1
    - or loss of sexual desire F52.0
  - male N53.9
    - anejaculatory orgasm N53.13
    - ejaculatory N53.19
      - painful N53.12
      - premature F52.4
      - retarded N53.11

Dysfunction — continued
- sexual — continued
  - male — continued
    - erectile N52.9
      - drug induced N52.2
      - due to
        - disease classified elsewhere N52.1
        - drug N52.2
      - post-operative N52.39
        - following
          - prostatectomy N52.34
            - radical N52.31
          - radical cystectomy N52.32
          - urethral surgery N52.33
      - psychogenic F52.21
      - specified cause NEC N52.8
      - vasculogenic
        - arterial insufficiency N52.01
          - with corporo-venous occlusive N52.03
        - corporo-venous occlusive N52.02
          - with arterial insufficiency N52.03
    - impotence—see Dysfunction, sexual, male, erectile
    - psychogenic F52.9
      - anhedonia F52.0
      - aversion F52.1
      - erectile F52.21
      - orgasmic F52.32
      - premature ejaculation F52.4
      - satyriasis F52.8
      - specified type NEC F52.8
    - specified type NEC N53.8
  - nonorganic F52.9
    - specified NEC F52.8
  - opioid F11.981
    - in
      - abuse F11.181
      - dependence F11.281
  - orgasmic dysfunction (female) F52.31
    - male F52.32
  - premature ejaculation F52.4
  - psychoactive substances NEC F19.981
    - in
      - abuse F19.181
      - dependence F19.281
  - psychogenic F52.9
  - sedative F13.981
    - in
      - abuse F13.181
      - dependence F13.281
  - sexual aversion F52.1
  - vaginismus (nonorganic) (psychogenic) F52.5
- sinoatrial node I49.5
- somatic M99.09
  - abdomen M99.09
  - acromioclavicular M99.07
  - cervical region M99.01
  - cervicothoracic M99.01
  - costochondral M99.08
  - costovertebral M99.08
  - head region M99.00
  - hip M99.05
  - lower extremity M99.06
  - lumbar region M99.03
  - lumbosacral M99.03
  - occipitocervical M99.00
  - pelvic region M99.05
  - pubic M99.05
  - rib cage M99.08
  - sacral region M99.04
  - sacrococcygeal M99.04
  - sacroiliac M99.04
  - specified NEC M99.09
  - sternochondral M99.08
  - sternoclavicular M99.07
  - thoracic region M99.02
  - thoracolumbar M99.02
  - upper extremity M99.07
- somatoform autonomic F45.8
- stomach K31.89
  - psychogenic F45.8
- suprarenal E27.9
  - hyperfunction E27.0
- symbolic R48.9
  - specified type NEC R48.8

Dysfunction — continued
- temporomandibular (joint) (joint-pain syndrome) M26.69
- testicular (endocrine) E29.9
  - specified NEC E29.8
- thymus E32.9
- thyroid E07.9
- ureterostomy (stoma) — see Complications, stoma, urinary tract
- urethrostomy (stoma) — see Complications, stoma, urinary tract
- uterus, complicating delivery O62.9
  - hypertonic O62.4
  - hypotonic O62.2
    - primary O62.0
    - secondary O62.1
- ventricular I51.9
  - with congestive heart failure I50.0

Dysgenesis
- gonadal (due to chromosomal anomaly) Q96.9
  - pure Q56.1
- renal Q60.5
  - bilateral Q60.4
  - unilateral Q60.3
- reticular D72.0

Dysgerminoma (M9060/3)
- specified site — see Neoplasm, malignant
- unspecified site
  - female C56.9
  - male C62.90

Dysgeusia R43.2

Dysgraphia R27.8

Dyshidrosis, dysidrosis L30.1

Dyskaryotic cervical smear R87.6

Dyskeratosis L85.8
- cervix — see Dysplasia, cervix
- congenital Q82.8
- uterus NEC N85.8

Dyskinesia G24.9
- biliary (cystic duct or gallbladder) K82.8
- esophagus K22.4
- hysterical F44.4
- intestinal K59.8
- neuroleptic-induced (tardive) G24.02
- nonorganic origin F44.4
- orofacial (idiopathic) G24.4
- psychogenic F44.4
- tardive (oral) G24.4
  - drug-induced G24.02
- trachea J39.8
- tracheobronchial J98.09

Dyslalia (developmental) F80.0

Dyslexia R48.0
- developmental F81.0

Dysmaturity — see also Light for dates
- pulmonary (newborn) (Wilson-Mikity) P27.0

Dysmenorrhea (essential) (exfoliative) N94.6
- congestive (syndrome) N94.6
- primary N94.4
- psychogenic F45.8
- secondary N94.5

Dysmetria R27.8

Dysmorphism (due to)
- alcohol Q86.0
- exogenous cause NEC Q86.8
- hydantoin Q86.1
- warfarin Q86.2

Dysmorphophobia (nondelusional) F45.22
- delusional F22

Dysnomia R47.01

Dysorexia R63.0
- psychogenic F50.8

Dysostosis
- cleidocranial, cleidocranialis Q74.0
- craniofacial Q75.1
- Fairbank's (idiopathic familial generalized osteophytosis) Q78.9
- mandibulofacial (incomplete) Q75.4
- multiplex E76.01
- oculomandibular Q75.5

Dyspareunia (female) N94.1
- male N53.12
- nonorganic F52.6
- psychogenic F52.6

Dyspareunia — *continued*
secondary N94.1

Dyspepsia (allergic) (atonic) (congenital)
(functional) (gastrointestinal) (occupational)
(reflex) K30
intestinal K59.8
nervous F45.8
neurotic F45.8
psychogenic F45.8

Dysphagia R13.1
following
cerebrovascular disease I69.991
cerebral infarction I69.391
intracerebral hemorrhage I69.191
nontraumatic intracranial hemorrhage
NEC I69.291
specified disease NEC I69.891
stroke NOS I69.491
subarachnoid hemorrhage I69.091
functional (hysterical) F45.8
hysterical F45.8
nervous (hysterical) F45.8
psychogenic F45.8
sideropenic D50.1
spastica K22.4

Dysphagocytosis, congenital D71

Dysphasia R47.02
developmental
expressive type F80.1
receptive type F80.2
following
cerebrovascular disease I69.921
cerebral infarction I69.321
intracerebral hemorrhage I69.121
nontraumatic intracranial hemorrhage
NEC I69.221
specified disease NEC I69.821
stroke NOS I69.421
subarachnoid hemorrhage I69.021

Dysphonia R49.0
functional F44.4
hysterical F44.4
psychogenic F44.4
spastica J38.3

Dysphoria, postpartal O90.6

Dyspituitarism E23.3

Dysplasia — *see also* Anomaly
acetabular, congenital Q65.8
arrhythmogenic right ventricular I42.8
arterial, fibromuscular I77.3
asphyxiating thoracic (congenital) Q77.2
brain Q07.9
bronchopulmonary, perinatal P27.1
cervix (uteri) N87.9
mild N87.0
moderate N87.1
severe NEC N87.2
chondroectodermal Q77.6
craniometaphyseal Q78.5
dentinal K00.5
diaphyseal, progressive Q78.3
dystrophic Q77.5
ectodermal (anhidrotic) (congenital) (hereditary)
Q82.4
hydrotic Q82.8
epithelial, uterine cervix — *see* Dysplasia,
cervix
eye (congenital) Q11.2
fibrous
bone NEC (monostotic) M85.00
ankle M85.079
left M85.072
right M85.071
foot M85.079
left M85.072
right M85.071
forearm M85.039
left M85.032
right M85.031
hand M85.049
left M85.042
right M85.041
lower leg M85.069
left M85.062
right M85.061

Dysplasia — *see also* Anomaly — *continued*
fibrous — *continued*
bone NEC — *continued*
multiple site M85.09
neck M85.08
rib M85.08
shoulder M85.019
left M85.012
right M85.011
skull M85.08
specified site NEC M85.08
thigh M85.059
left M85.052
right M85.051
toe M85.079
left M85.072
right M85.071
upper arm M85.029
left M85.022
right M85.021
vertebra M85.08
diaphyseal, progressive Q78.3
jaw M27.8
polyostotic Q78.1
florid osseous (M9275/0) D16.5
upper jaw (bone) D16.4
hip, congenital Q65.8
joint, congenital Q74.8
kidney Q61.4
leg Q74.2
lung, congenital (not associated with short
gestation) Q33.6
mammary (female) (gland) (benign) N60.90
cyst (solitary) — *see* Cyst, breast
cystic — *see* Mastopathy, cystic
duct ectasia — *see* Ectasia, mammary duct
fibroadenosis — *see* Fibroadenosis, breast
fibrosclerosis — *see* Fibrosclerosis, breast
left N60.92
male N60.95
left N60.94
right N60.93
right N60.91
specified type NEC (female) N60.80
left N60.82
male N60.85
left N60.84
right N60.83
right N60.81
metaphyseal Q78.5
muscle Q79.8
oculodentodigital Q87.0
periapical (cemental) (cemento-osseous)
(M9272/0) D16.5
upper jaw (bone) D16.4
periosteum — *see* Disorder, bone, specified
type NEC
polyostotic fibrous Q78.1
renal Q61.4
retinal, congenital Q14.1
right ventricular, arrhythmogenic I42.8
septo-optic Q04.4
spinal cord Q06.1
spondyloepiphyseal Q77.7
thymic, with immunodeficiency D82.1
vagina N89.3
mild N89.0
moderate N89.1
severe NEC N89.2
vulva N90.3
mild N90.0
moderate N90.1
severe NEC N90.2

Dyspnea (nocturnal) (paroxysmal) R06.00
asthmatic (bronchial) J45.90
with
acute exacerbation J45.91
bronchitis J45.90
with
acute exacerbation J45.91
status asthmaticus J45.92
chronic J44.9
status asthmaticus J45.92
cardiac — *see* Failure, ventricular, left
cardiac — *see* Failure, ventricular, left
functional F45.8
hyperventilation R06.4

Dyspnea — *continued*
hysterical F45.8
newborn
orthopnea R06.01
psychogenic F45.8
shortness of breath R06.02
specified type NEC R06.09
uremic N19

Dyspraxia R27.8
developmental (syndrome) F82

Dysproteinemia E88.09

Dysreflexia, autonomic G90.4

Dysrhythmia
cardiac I49.9
newborn P29.1
occurring before birth P03.819
before onset of labor P03.810
during labor P03.811
postoperative I97.89
long term effect of cardiac surgery I97.1
cerebral or cortical — *see* Epilepsy

Dyssomnia — *see* Disorder, sleep

Dysthymia F34.1

Dysthyroidism E07.9

Dystocia O66.9
cervical (hypotonic) O62.2
primary O62.0
secondary O62.1
contraction ring O62.4
fetal O66.9
abnormality NEC O66.3
conjoined twins O66.3
oversize O66.2
maternal O66.9
positional O64.9
shoulder (girdle) O66.0
causing obstructed labor O66.0
uterine NEC O62.4

Dystonia G24.9
deformans progressive G24.1
drug-induced G24.00
acute G24.01
specified NEC G24.09
tardive dyskinesia G24.02
idiopathic G24.1
familial G24.1
nonfamilial G24.2
orofacial G24.4
lenticularis G24.8
musculorum deformans G24.1
orofacial (idiopathic) G24.4
specified NEC G24.8
torsion (idiopathic) G24.1
symptomatic (nonfamilial) G24.2

Dystonic movements R25.8

Dystrophy, dystrophia
adiposogenital E23.6
Becker's type G71.0
choroid (hereditary) H31.20
central areolar H31.22
choroideremia H31.21
gyrate atrophy H31.23
specified type NEC H31.29
cornea (hereditary) H18.50
endothelial H18.51
epithelial H18.52
granular H18.53
lattice H18.54
macular H18.55
specified type NEC H18.59
Duchenne's type G71.0
due to malnutrition E45
Erb's G71.0
Fuchs' H18.52
Gower's muscular G71.0
hair L67.8
infantile neuraxonal G31.89
Landouzy-Déjérine G71.0
Leyden-Möbius G71.0
muscular G71.0
benign (Becker type) G71.0

Dystrophy, dystrophia — *continued*
  muscular — *continued*
    congenital (hereditary) (progressive) G71.2
      myotonic G71.1
    distal G71.0
    Duchenne type G71.0
    Emery-Dreifuss G71.0
    Erb type G71.0
    facioscapulohumeral G71.0
    Gower's G71.0
    hereditary (progressive) G71.0
    Landouzy-Déjérine type G71.0
    limb-girdle G71.0
    myotonic G71.1
    progressive (hereditary) G71.0
      Charcot-Marie(-Tooth) type G60.0
    pseudohypertrophic (infantile) G71.0
    severe (Duchenne type) G71.0
  myocardium, myocardial — *see* Degeneration,
    myocardial
  myotonic, myotonica G71.1
  nail L60.3
    congenital Q84.6
  nutritional E45
  ocular G71.0
  oculocerebrorenal E72.03
  oculopharyngeal G71.0
  ovarian N83.8
  polyglandular E31.8
  reflex (sympathetic) — *see* Syndrome, pain,
    complex regional I
  retinal (hereditary) H35.50
    in
      lipid storage disorders E75.6 *[H36]*
      systemic lipidoses E75.6 *[H36]*
    involving
      pigment epithelium H35.54
      sensory area H35.53
    pigmentary H35.52
    vitreoretinal H35.51
  Salzmann's nodular — *see* Degeneration,
    cornea, nodular
  scapuloperoneal G71.0
  skin NEC L98.8
  sympathetic (reflex) — *see* Syndrome, pain,
    complex regional I
  tapetoretinal H35.54
  thoracic, asphyxiating Q77.2
  unguium L60.3
    congenital Q84.6
  vitreoretinal H35.51
  vulva N90.4
  yellow (liver) — *see* Failure, hepatic
Dysuria R30.0
  psychogenic F45.8

E

Eales' disease — *see* Vasculitis, retina
Ear — *see also* condition
  piercing Z41.3
  tropical B36.8
  wax (impacted) H61.20
    left H61.22
      with right H61.23
    right H61.21
      with left H61.23
Earache — *see* category H92.0
Eaton-Lambert syndrome C34.90 *[G73.1]*
Eberth's disease (typhoid fever) A01.00
Ebola virus disease A98.4
Ebstein's
  anomaly or syndrome (heart) Q22.5
  disease (renal tubular degeneration in diabetes)
    — *see* Diabetes, Ebstein's disease
Eccentro-osteochondrodysplasia E76.29
Ecchondroma (M9210/0) — *see* Neoplasm, bone,
  benign
Ecchondrosis (M9210/1) D48.0
Ecchymosis R58
  conjunctiva — *see* Hemorrhage, conjunctiva
  eye (traumatic) — *see* Contusion, eyeball
  eyelid (traumatic) — *see* Contusion, eyelid
  fetus or newborn P54.5
  spontaneous R23.3
  traumatic — *see* Contusion

Echinococciasis — *see* Echinococcus
Echinococcosis — *see* Echinococcus
Echinococcus (infection) B67.90
  granulosus B67.4
    bone B67.2
    liver B67.0
    lung B67.1
    multiple sites B67.32
    specified site NEC B67.39
    thyroid B67.31 *[E35]*
  liver NOS B67.8
    granulosus B67.0
    multilocularis B67.5
  lung NEC B67.99
    granulosus B67.1
    multilocularis B67.69
  multilocularis B67.7
    liver B67.5
    multiple sites B67.61
    specified site NEC B67.69
  specified site NEC B67.99
    granulosus B67.39
    multilocularis B67.69
  thyroid NEC B67.99
    granulosus B67.31 *[E35]*
    multilocularis B67.69 *[E35]*
Echinorhynchiasis B83.8
Echinostomiasis B66.8
Echolalia R48.8
**Echovirus, as cause of disease classified
  elsewhere** B97.12
Eclampsia, eclamptic (coma) (convulsions)
  (delirium) (with hypertension) NEC O15.9
  during labor and delivery O15.1
  male R56.9
  not associated with pregnancy or childbirth
    R56.9
  postpartum O15.2
  pregnancy O15.00
    second trimester O15.02
    third trimester O15.03
  puerperal O15.2
  uremic N19
Economic circumstances affecting care Z59.9
Economo's disease A85.8
Ectasia, ectasis
  aorta — *see* Aneurysm, aorta
  breast — *see* Ectasia, mammary duct
  capillary I78.8
  cornea H18.719
    bilateral H18.713
    left H18.712
    right H18.711
  mammary duct N60.40
    left N60.42
    male N60.45
      left N60.44
      right N60.43
    right N60.41
  salivary gland (duct) K11.8
  sclera — *see* Sclerectasia
Ecthyma L08.0
  contagiosum B08.0
  gangrenosum L88
  infectiosum B08.0
Ectocardia Q24.8
Ectodermal dysplasia (anhidrotic) Q82.4
Ectodermosis erosiva pluriorificialis L51.1
Ectopic, ectopia (congenital)
  abdominal viscera Q45.8
    due to defect in anterior abdominal wall
      Q79.59
  ACTH syndrome E24.3
  adrenal gland Q89.1
  anus Q43.5
  atrial beats I49.1
  beats I49.4
    atrial I49.1
    ventricular I49.3
  bladder Q64.10
  bone and cartilage in lung Q33.5
  brain Q04.8
  breast tissue Q83.8
  cardiac Q24.8
  cerebral Q04.8

Ectopic, ectopia — *continued*
  cordis Q24.8
  endometrium — *see* Endometriosis
  gastric mucosa Q40.2
  gestation — *see* Pregnancy, by site
  heart Q24.8
  hormone secretion NEC E34.2
  kidney (crossed) (pelvis) Q63.2
  lens, lentis Q12.1
  mole — *see* Pregnancy, by site
  organ or site NEC — *see* Malposition,
    congenital
  pancreas Q45.3
  pregnancy — *see* Pregnancy, ectopic
  pupil — *see* Abnormality, pupillary
  renal Q63.2
  sebaceous glands of mouth Q38.6
  spleen Q89.09
  testis Q53.00
    bilateral Q53.02
    unilateral Q53.01
  thyroid Q89.2
  tissue in lung Q33.5
  ureter Q62.63
  ventricular beats I49.3
  vesicae Q64.10
Ectromelia Q73.8
  lower limb — *see* Defect, reduction, limb, lower,
    specified type NEC
  upper limb — *see* Defect, reduction, limb,
    upper, specified type NEC
Ectropion H02.109
  cervix N86
    with cervicitis N72
  congenital Q10.1
  eyelid (paralytic) H02.109
    cicatricial H02.119
      left H02.116
        lower H02.115
        upper H02.114
      right H02.113
        lower H02.112
        upper H02.111
    congenital Q10.1
    left H02.106
      lower H02.105
      upper H02.104
    mechanical H02.129
      left H02.126
        lower H02.125
        upper H02.124
      right H02.123
        lower H02.122
        upper H02.121
    right H02.103
      lower H02.102
      upper H02.101
    senile H02.139
      left H02.136
        lower H02.135
        upper H02.134
      right H02.133
        lower H02.132
        upper H02.131
    spastic H02.149
      left H02.146
        lower H02.145
        upper H02.144
      right H02.143
        lower H02.142
        upper H02.141
  iris H21.8
  lip (acquired) K13.0
    congenital Q38.0
  urethra N36.8
  uvea H21.8
Eczema (acute) (chronic) (erythematous) (fissum)
  (rubrum) (squamous) (*see also* Dermatitis)
  L30.9
  contact — *see* Dermatitis, contact
  dyshydrotic L30.1
  external ear — *see* Otitis, externa, acute,
    eczematoid
  flexural L20.82
  herpeticum B00.0
  hypertrophicum L28.0

©2002 Ingenix, Inc.

Eczema (*see also* Dermatitis) — *continued*
hypostatic — *see* Varix, leg, with, inflammation
impetiginous L01.1
infantile (due to any substance) L20.83
   intertriginous L21.1
   seborrheic L21.1
intertriginous NEC L30.4
   infantile L21.1
intrinsic (allergic) L20.84
lichenified NEC L28.0
marginatum (hebrae) B35.6
pustular L30.3
stasis — *see* Varix, leg, with, inflammation
vaccination, vaccinatum T88.1
varicose — *see* Varix, leg, with, inflammation
Eczematid L30.2
Eddowes (-Spurway) syndrome Q78.0
Edema, edematous (infectious) (pitting) (toxic)
R60.9
with nephritis — *see* Nephrosis
allergic T78.3
amputation stump (surgical) (late effect) T87.8
angioneurotic (allergic) (any site) (with urticaria)
   T78.3
   hereditary D84.1
angiospastic I73.9
Berlin's (traumatic) S05.80
   left S05.82
   right S05.81
brain G93.6
   due to birth injury P11.0
   fetus or newborn (anoxia or hypoxia) P52.4
      birth injury P11.0
   traumatic — *see* Injury, intracranial,
      cerebral edema
cardiac — *see* Failure, heart, congestive
cardiovascular — *see* Failure, heart, congestive
cerebral — *see* Edema, brain
cerebrospinal — *see* Edema, brain
cervix (uteri) (acute) N88.8
   puerperal, postpartum O90.8
chronic hereditary Q82.0
circumscribed, acute T78.3
   hereditary D84.1
complicating pregnancy — *see* Edema,
   gestational
conjunctiva H11.429
   bilateral H11.423
   left H11.422
   right H11.421
cornea H18.20
   idiopathic H18.229
      bilateral H18.223
      left H18.222
      right H18.221
   secondary H18.239
      bilateral H18.233
      due to contact lens H18.219
         bilateral H18.213
         left H18.212
         right H18.211
      left H18.232
      right H18.231
due to
   lymphatic obstruction I89.0
   salt retention E87.0
epiglottis — *see* Edema, glottis
essential, acute T78.3
   hereditary D84.1
extremities, lower — *see* Edema, legs
eyelid NEC H02.849
   left H02.846
      lower H02.845
      upper H02.844
   right H02.843
      lower H02.842
      upper H02.841
familial, hereditary Q82.0
famine — *see* Malnutrition, severe
fetus or newborn P83.30
   hydrops fetalis — *see* Hydrops, fetalis
   specified NEC P83.39
generalized R60.1
gestational O12.00
   with proteinuria O12.20
      first trimester O12.21
      second trimester O12.22

Edema, edematous — *continued*
gestational — *continued*
   with proteinuria — *continued*
      third trimester O12.23
   first trimester O12.01
   second trimester O12.02
   third trimester O12.03
glottis, glottic, glottidis (obstructive) (passive)
   J38.4
   allergic T78.3
      hereditary D84.1
heart — *see* Failure, heart, congestive
heat T67.7
hereditary Q82.0
inanition — *see* Malnutrition, severe
intracranial G93.6
iris H21.8
joint — *see* Effusion, joint
larynx — *see* Edema, glottis
legs R60.0
   due to venous obstruction I87.1
   hereditary Q82.0
localized R60.0
   due to venous obstruction I87.1
lower limbs — *see* Edema, legs
lung J81.1
   acute J81.0
      with heart condition or failure — *see*
         Failure, ventricular, left
      due to
         chemicals, fumes or vapors
            (inhalation) J68.1
         external agent J70.9
            specified NEC J70.8
         radiation J70.0
      meaning failure, left ventricle I50.1
   chemical (acute) J68.1
      chronic J68.4
   chronic J81.1
      due to
         chemicals, gases, fumes or vapors
            (inhalation) J68.4
         external agent J70.9
            specified NEC J70.8
         radiation J70.1
   due to
      external agent J70.9
         specified NEC J70.8
      high altitude T70.29
      near drowning T75.1
   following obstetric procedure O75.4
   terminal J81.1
lymphatic I89.0
   due to mastectomy I97.2
macula H35.81
   diabetic — *see* Diabetes, macular edema
malignant — *see* Gangrene, gas
Milroy's Q82.0
nasopharynx J39.2
newborn P83.30
   hydrops fetalis — *see* Hydrops, fetalis
   specified NEC P83.39
nutritional — *see also* Malnutrition, severe
   with dyspigmentation, skin and hair E40
optic disc or nerve — *see* Papilledema
orbit H05.229
   bilateral H05.223
   left H05.222
   right H05.221
pancreas K86.8
papilla, optic — *see* Papilledema
penis N48.89
periodic T78.3
   hereditary D84.1
pharynx J39.2
pulmonary — *see* Edema, lung
Quincke's T78.3
   hereditary D84.1
renal — *see* Nephrosis
retina H35.81
   diabetic — *see* Diabetes, macular edema
salt E87.0
scrotum N50.8
seminal vesicle N50.8
spermatic cord N50.8
spinal (cord) (vascular) (nontraumatic) G95.19
starvation — *see* Malnutrition, severe

Edema, edematous — *continued*
subglottic — *see* Edema, glottis
supraglottic — *see* Edema, glottis
testis N44.8
tunica vaginalis N50.8
vas deferens N50.8
vulva (acute) N90.8
Edsall's disease T67.2
Educational handicap Z55.9
specified NEC Z55.8
Edward's syndrome — *see* Trisomy, 18
Effect, adverse
abnormal gravitational (G) forces or states
   T75.81
abuse — *see* Maltreatment
air pressure T70.9
   specified NEC T70.8
altitude (high) — *see* Effect, adverse, high
   altitude
anesthesia (*see also* Anesthesia) T88.5
   in labor and delivery O74.9
      affecting fetus or newborn P04.0
   in pregnancy — *see* Complications,
      anesthesia, in, pregnancy
   local, toxic
      in labor and delivery O74.4
      postpartum, puerperal O89.3
   postpartum, puerperal O89.9
   specified NEC T88.5
      in labor and delivery O74.8
      postpartum, puerperal O89.8
   spinal and epidural T88.5
      headache T88.5
         in labor and delivery O74.5
         postpartum, puerperal O89.4
      specified NEC
         in labor and delivery O74.6
         postpartum, puerperal O89.5
antitoxin — *see* Complications, vaccination
atmospheric pressure T70.9
   due to explosion T70.8
   high T70.3
   low — *see* Effect, adverse, high altitude
   specified effect NEC T70.8
biological, correct substance properly
   administered — *see* Effect, adverse, drug
blood (derivatives) (serum) (transfusion) — *see*
   Complications, transfusion
chemical substance — *see* Table of Drugs and
   Chemicals
cobalt, radioactive T66
cold (temperature) (weather) T69.9
   chilblains T69.1
   frostbite — *see* Frostbite
   specified effect NEC T69.8
drugs and medicaments NEC T88.7
   correct substance properly administered
      T88.7
   overdose or wrong substance given or taken
      (by accident) T50.901
      administered with intent to harm by
         another person T50.903
         self T50.902
      circumstances undetermined T50.904
      specified drug — *see* Table of Drugs and
         Chemicals
electric current, electricity (shock) T75.4
   burn — *see* Burn
exertion (excessive) T73.3
exposure — *see* Exposure
external cause NEC T75.89
fallout (radioactive) NOS T66
fluoroscopy NOS T66
foodstuffs T78.1
   allergic reaction — *see* Allergy, food
   causing anaphylaxis — *see* Shock,
      anaphylactic, food
   noxious — *see* Poisoning, food, noxious
gases, fumes, or vapors — *see* Table of Drugs
   and Chemicals
glue (airplane) sniffing — *see* Disorder, drug-
   related, inhalant
heat — *see* Heat
high altitude NEC T70.29
   anoxia T70.20

Effect, adverse — *continued*
  high altitude NEC — *continued*
    on
      ears T70.0
      sinuses T70.1
      polycythemia D75.1
  high pressure fluids T70.8
  hot weather — *see* Heat
  hunger T73.0
  immersion, foot — *see* Immersion
  immunization — *see* Complications,
    vaccination
  immunological agents — *see* Complications,
    vaccination
  implantation (removable) of isotope or radium
    NOS T66
  infrared (radiation) (rays) NOS T66
    dermatitis or eczema L59.8
  infusion — *see* Complications, infusion
  ingestion or injection of isotope (therapeutic)
    NOS T66
  irradiation NOS T66
  isotope (radioactive) NOS T66
  lack of care of infants — *see* Maltreatment,
    child
  lightning — *see* Lightning
  medical care T88.9
    specified NEC T88.8
  medicinal substance, correct, properly
    administered — *see* Effect, adverse, drug
  mesothorium NOS T66
  motion T75.3
  noise, on inner ear — *see* category H83.3
  overheated places — *see* Heat
  polonium NOS T66
  psychosocial, of work environment Z56.5
  radiation (diagnostic) (infrared) (natural source)
    (therapeutic) (ultraviolet) (X-ray) NOS T66
    dermatitis or eczema — *see* Dermatitis, due
      to, radiation
    fibrosis of lung J70.1
    pneumonitis J70.0
    pulmonary manifestations
      acute J70.0
      chronic J70.1
    skin L59.9
    suspected damage to fetus affecting
      management of pregnancy O35.6
  radioactive substance NOS T66
    dermatitis or eczema — *see* Radiodermatitis
  radioactivity NOS T66
  radiotherapy NOS T66
    dermatitis or eczema — *see* Radiodermatitis
  radium NOS T66
  reduced temperature T69.9
    immersion foot or hand — *see* Immersion
    specified effect NEC T69.8
  roentgen rays, roentgenography,
    roentgenoscopy NOS T66
  serum (prophylactic) (therapeutic) NEC T80.6
  specified NEC T78.8
    external cause NEC T75.89
  strangulation — *see* Asphyxia, traumatic
  submersion T75.1
  teletherapy NOS T66
  thirst T73.1
  toxic — *see* Toxicity
  transfusion — *see* Complications, transfusion
  ultraviolet (radiation) (rays) NOS T66
    burn (*see* Burn)
    dermatitis or eczema — *see* Dermatitis, due
      to, ultraviolet rays
      acute L56.8
  uranium NOS T66
  vaccine (any) — *see* Complications, vaccination
  vibration — *see* Vibration, adverse effects
  water pressure NEC T70.9
    specified NEC T70.8
  weightlessness T75.82
  whole blood — *see* Complications, transfusion
  work environment Z56.5
  X-rays NOS T66
    dermatitis or eczema — *see* Radiodermatitis
Effect(s) (of) (from) — *see* Effect, adverse NEC
Effects, late — *see* Sequelae

Effluvium
  anagen L65.1
  telogen L65.0
Effort syndrome (psychogenic) F45.8
Effusion
  amniotic fluid — *see* Rupture, membranes,
    premature
  brain (serous) G93.6
  bronchial — *see* Bronchitis
  cerebral G93.6
  cerebrospinal — *see also* Meningitis
    vessel G93.6
  chest — *see* Effusion, pleura
  chylous, chyliform (pleura) J94.0
  intracranial G93.6
  joint M25.40
    ankle M25.473
      left M25.472
      right M25.471
    elbow M25.429
      left M25.422
      right M25.421
    foot joint M25.476
      left M25.475
      right M25.474
    hand joint M25.449
      left M25.442
      right M25.441
    hip M25.459
      left M25.452
      right M25.451
    knee M25.469
      left M25.462
      right M25.461
    shoulder M25.419
      left M25.412
      right M25.411
    specified joint NEC M25.48
    wrist M25.439
      left M25.432
      right M25.431
  meninges — *see* Meningitis
  pericardium, pericardial (noninflammatory)
    I31.3
    acute — *see* Pericarditis, acute
  peritoneal (chronic) R18
  pleura, pleurisy, pleuritic, pleuropericardial
    J90
    chylous, chyliform J94.0
    due to systemic lupus erythematosis M32.13
    fetus or newborn P28.8
    influenzal J10.1
    malignant C78.2
    tuberculous NEC A15.6
      primary (progressive) A15.7
  spinal — *see* Meningitis
  thorax, thoracic — *see* Effusion, pleura
Egg shell nails L60.3
  congenital Q84.6
Egyptian splenomegaly B65.1
Ehrlichiosis A77.40
  due to
    E. chafeensis A77.41
    E. sennetsu A79.2
    specified organism NEC A77.49
Ehlers-Danlos syndrome Q79.6
Eichstedt's disease B36.0
Eisenmenger's defect, complex, or syndrome
  Q21.8
Ejaculation
  premature F52.4
  semen, painful N53.12
    psychogenic F52.6
Ekbom's syndrome (restless legs) G25.8
Ekman's syndrome (brittle bones and blue sclera)
  Q78.0
Elastic skin Q82.8
  acquired L57.4
Elastofibroma (M8820/0) — *see* Neoplasm,
  connective tissue, benign
Elastoma (juvenile) Q82.8
  Miescher's L87.2
Elastomyofibrosis I42.4

Elastosis
  actinic, solar L57.8
  atrophicans (senile) L57.4
  perforans serpiginosa L87.2
  senilis L57.4
Elbow — *see* condition
Electric current, electricity, effects
  (concussion) (fatal) (nonfatal) (shock) T75.4
  burn — *see* Burn
Electric feet syndrome E53.8
Electrocution T75.4
Electrolyte imbalance E87.8
  with
    abortion — *see* Abortion by type complicated
      by specified condition NEC
    ectopic pregnancy O08.5
    molar pregnancy O08.5
Elephantiasis (nonfilarial) I89.0
  arabicum — *see* Infestation, filarial
  bancroftian B74.0
  congenital (any site) (hereditary) Q82.0
  due to
    Brugia (malayi) B74.1
      timori B74.2
    mastectomy I97.2
    Wuchereria (bancrofti) B74.0
  eyelid H02.859
    left H02.856
      lower H02.855
      upper H02.854
    right H02.853
      lower H02.852
      upper H02.851
  filarial, filariensis — *see* Infestation, filarial
  glandular I89.0
  graecorum A30.9
  lymphangiectatic I89.0
  lymphatic vessel I89.0
    due to mastectomy I97.2
  scrotum (nonfilarial) I89.0
  streptococcal I89.0
  surgical I97.89
    postmastectomy I97.2
  telangiectodes I89.0
  vulva (nonfilarial) N90.8
Elevated, elevation
  antibody titer R76.0
  basal metabolic rate R94.8
  blood pressure — *see also* Hypertension
    reading (incidental) (isolated) (nonspecific),
      no diagnosis of hypertension R03.0
  body temperature (of unknown origin) R50.9
  conjugate, eye H51.0
  diaphragm, congenital Q79.1
  erythrocyte sedimentation rate R70.0
  immunoglobulin level R76.89
  indolacetic acid R82.5
  lactic acid dehydrogenase (LDH) level R74.0
  leukocyte count R72.0
  prostate specific antigen (PSA) R76.81
  Rh titer T80.4
  scapula, congenital Q74.0
  sedimentation rate R70.0
  SGOT R74.0
  SGPT R74.0
  transaminase level R74.0
  urine level of
    catecholamine R82.5
    indoleacetic acid R82.5
    l7-ketosteroids R82.5
    steroids R82.5
    vanillylmandelic acid (VMA) R82.5
  venous pressure I87.8
Elliptocytosis (congenital) (hereditary) D58.1
  Hb C (disease) D58.1
  hemoglobin disease D58.1
  sickle-cell (disease) D57.8
    trait D57.3
Ellison-Zollinger syndrome E16.4
Ellis-van Creveld syndrome (chondroectodermal
  dysplasia) Q77.6
Elongated, elongation (congenital) — *see also*
  Distortion
  bone Q79.9

©2002 Ingenix, Inc.

Elongated, elongation — *see also* Distortion —
　　continued
　cervix (uteri) Q51.8
　　acquired N88.4
　　hypertrophic N88.4
　colon Q43.8
　common bile duct Q44.5
　cystic duct Q44.5
　frenulum, penis Q55.69
　labia minora (acquired) N90.6
　ligamentum patellae Q74.1
　petiolus (epiglottidis) Q31.8
　tooth, teeth K00.2
　uvula Q38.6

Eltor cholera A00.1

Emaciation (due to malnutrition) E41

Embadomoniasis A07.8

Embedded tooth, teeth K01.0
　with abnormal position (same or adjacent
　　tooth) M26.3
　root only K08.3

Embolic — *see* condition

Embolism (multiple) (paradoxical) (septic) I74.9
　air (any site) (traumatic) T79.0
　　following
　　　abortion — *see* Abortion by type
　　　　complicated by embolism
　　　ectopic pregnancy O08.2
　　　infusion, therapeutic injection or
　　　　transfusion T80.0
　　　molar pregnancy O08.2
　　　procedure NEC T81.7
　　in pregnancy, childbirth or puerperium —
　　　see Embolism, obstetric
　amniotic fluid (pulmonary) — *see also*
　　Embolism, obstetric
　　following
　　　abortion — *see* Abortion by type
　　　　complicated by embolism
　　　ectopic pregnancy O08.2
　　　molar pregnancy O08.2
　aorta, aortic I74.10
　　abdominal I74.0
　　bifurcation I74.0
　　saddle I74.0
　　thoracic I74.11
　artery I74.9
　　auditory, internal I65.8
　　basilar — *see* Occlusion, artery, basilar
　　carotid (common) (internal) — *see* Occlusion,
　　　artery, carotid
　　cerebellar (anterior inferior) (posterior
　　　inferior) (superior) I66.3
　　cerebral — *see* Occlusion, artery, cerebral
　　choroidal (anterior) I66.8
　　communicating posterior I66.8
　　coronary — *see also* Infarct, myocardium
　　　not resulting in infarction I24.0
　　extremity I74.4
　　　lower I74.3
　　　upper I74.2
　　hypophyseal I66.8
　　iliac I74.5
　　limb I74.4
　　　lower I74.3
　　　upper I74.2
　　mesenteric (with gangrene) K55.0
　　ophthalmic — *see* Occlusion, artery, retina
　　peripheral I74.4
　　pontine I66.8
　　precerebral — *see* Occlusion, artery,
　　　precerebral
　　pulmonary — *see* Embolism, pulmonary
　　renal N28.0
　　retinal — *see* Occlusion, artery, retina
　　specified NEC I74.8
　　vertebral — *see* Occlusion, artery, vertebral
　basilar (artery) I65.1
　birth, mother — *see* Embolism, obstetric
　blood clot
　　following
　　　abortion — *see* Abortion by type
　　　　complicated by embolism
　　　ectopic or molar pregnancy O08.2
　　in pregnancy, childbirth or puerperium —
　　　see Embolism, obstetric

Embolism — *continued*
　brain — *see also* Occlusion, artery, cerebral
　　following
　　　abortion — *see* Abortion by type
　　　　complicated by embolism
　　　ectopic or molar pregnancy O08.2
　　　puerperal, postpartum, childbirth — *see*
　　　　Embolism, obstetric
　capillary I78.8
　cardiac — *see also* Infarct, myocardium
　　not resulting in infarction I24.0
　carotid (artery) (common) (internal) — *see*
　　Occlusion, artery, carotid
　cavernous sinus (venous) — *see* Embolism,
　　intracranial venous sinus
　cerebral — *see* Occlusion, artery, cerebral
　coronary (artery or vein) (systemic) — *see*
　　Occlusion, coronary
　due to device, implant or graft — *see also*
　　Complications, by site and type, specified
　　NEC
　　arterial graft NEC T82.818
　　breast (implant) T85.81
　　catheter NEC T85.81
　　　dialysis (renal) T82.818
　　　　intraperitoneal T85.81
　　　infusion NEC T82.818
　　　　spinal (epidural) (subdural) T85.81
　　　urinary (indwelling) T83.81
　　electronic (electrode) (pulse generator)
　　　(stimulator)
　　　bone T84.81
　　　cardiac T82.817
　　　nervous system (brain) (peripheral nerve)
　　　　(spinal) T85.81
　　　urinary T83.81
　　fixation, internal (orthopedic) NEC T84.81
　　gastrointestinal (bile duct) (esophagus)
　　　T85.81
　　genital NEC T83.81
　　heart (graft) (valve) T82.817
　　joint prosthesis T84.81
　　ocular (corneal graft) (orbital implant)
　　　T85.81
　　orthopedic (bone graft) NEC T86.838
　　specified NEC T85.81
　　urinary (graft) NEC T83.81
　　vascular NEC T82.818
　　ventricular intracranial shunt T85.81
　extremities I74.4
　　lower I80.3
　　　arterial I74.3
　　upper I74.2
　eye H34.9
　fat (cerebral) (pulmonary) (systemic) T79.1
　　following
　　　abortion — *see* Abortion by type
　　　　complicated by embolism
　　　ectopic or molar pregnancy O08.2
　　complicating delivery — *see* Embolism,
　　　obstetric
　femoral (artery) I74.3
　　vein — *see* Phlebitis, leg, femoral vein
　following
　　abortion — *see* Abortion by type complicated
　　　by embolism
　　ectopic or molar pregnancy O08.2
　　infusion, therapeutic injection or transfusion
　　　air T80.0
　　　thrombus T80.1
　heart (fatty) — *see also* Infarct, myocardium
　　not resulting in infarction I24.0
　hepatic (vein) I82.0
　iliac (artery) I74.5
　iliofemoral I74.5
　in pregnancy, childbirth or puerperium — *see*
　　Embolism, obstetric
　intestine (artery) (vein) (with gangrene) K55.0
　intracranial — *see also* Occlusion, artery,
　　cerebral
　　venous sinus (any) G08
　　　nonpyogenic I67.6
　intraspinal venous sinuses or veins G08
　　nonpyogenic G95.19
　kidney (artery) N28.0
　lateral sinus (venous) — *see* Embolism,
　　intracranial, venous sinus

Embolism — *continued*
　leg I80.3
　　arterial I74.3
　longitudinal sinus (venous) — *see* Embolism,
　　intracranial, venous sinus
　lung (massive) — *see* Embolism, pulmonary
　meninges I66.8
　mesenteric (artery) (vein) (with gangrene) K55.0
　obstetric (in) (pulmonary)
　　childbirth O88.82
　　　air O88.02
　　　amniotic fluid O88.12
　　　blood clot O88.22
　　　fat O88.82
　　　pyemic O88.32
　　　septic O88.32
　　　specified type NEC O88.82
　　pregnancy O88.819
　　　air O88.019
　　　　first trimester O88.011
　　　　second trimester O88.012
　　　　third trimester O88.013
　　　amniotic fluid O88.119
　　　　first trimester O88.111
　　　　second trimester O88.112
　　　　third trimester O88.113
　　　blood clot O88.219
　　　　first trimester O88.211
　　　　second trimester O88.212
　　　　third trimester O88.213
　　　fat O88.819
　　　　first trimester O88.811
　　　　second trimester O88.812
　　　　third trimester O88.813
　　　pyemic O88.319
　　　　first trimester O88.311
　　　　second trimester O88.312
　　　　third trimester O88.313
　　　septic O88.319
　　　　first trimester O88.311
　　　　second trimester O88.312
　　　　third trimester O88.313
　　　specified type NEC O88.819
　　　　first trimester O88.811
　　　　second trimester O88.812
　　　　third trimester O88.813
　　puerperal O88.83
　　　air O88.03
　　　blood clot O88.23
　　　fat O88.83
　　　pyemic O88.33
　　　septic O88.33
　　　specified type NEC O88.83
　ophthalmic — *see* Occlusion, artery, retina
　penis N48.81
　peripheral artery NEC I74.8
　pituitary E23.6
　popliteal (artery) I74.3
　portal (vein) I81
　postoperative T81.7
　precerebral artery — *see* Occlusion, artery,
　　precerebral
　puerperal — *see* Embolism, obstetric
　pulmonary (artery) (vein) I26.9
　　with acute cor pulmonale I26.0
　　following
　　　abortion — *see* Abortion by type
　　　　complicated by embolism
　　　ectopic or molar pregnancy O08.2
　　in pregnancy, childbirth or puerperium —
　　　see Embolism, obstetric
　pyemic (multiple) — *see also* Septicemia
　　enterococcal A41.81
　　following
　　　abortion — *see* Abortion by type
　　　　complicated by embolism
　　　ectopic or molar pregnancy O08.2
　　Hemophilus influenzae A41.3
　　pneumococcal A40.3
　　　with pneumonia J13
　　puerperal, postpartum, childbirth (any
　　　organism) — *see* Embolism, obstetric
　　specified organism NEC A41.89
　　staphylococcal A41.2
　　streptococcal A40.9

Embolism — continued
  renal (artery) N28.0
    vein I82.3
  retina, retinal — see Occlusion, artery, retina
  saddle (aorta) I74.0
  septic complicating abortion — see Abortion, by
    type, complicated by, embolism
  septicemic — see Septicemia
  sinus — see Embolism, intracranial, venous
    sinus
  soap complicating abortion — see Abortion, by
    type, complicated by, embolism
  spinal cord G95.19
    pyogenic origin G06.1
  spleen, splenic (artery) I74.8
  thrombus (thromboembolism) following
    infusion, therapeutic injection or
    transfusion T80.1
  upper extremity I74.2
  vein I82.9
    cerebral I67.6
    coronary — see also Infarct, myocardium
      not resulting in infarction I24.0
    hepatic I82.0
    mesenteric (with gangrene) K55.0
    portal I81
    pulmonary — see Embolism, pulmonary
    renal I82.3
    specified NEC I82.8
  vena cava I82.2
  venous sinus G08
  vessels of brain — see Occlusion, artery,
    cerebral

Embolus — see Embolism

Embryoma (M9080/1) — see also Neoplasm,
  uncertain behavior
  benign (M9080/0) — see Neoplasm, benign
  kidney (M8960/3) C64.9
    left C64.1
    right C64.0
  liver (M8970/3) C22.0
  malignant (M9080/3) — see also Neoplasm,
    malignant
    kidney (M8960/3) C64.9
      left C64.1
      right C64.0
    liver (M8970/3) C22.0
    testis (M9070/3) C62.90
      descended (scrotal) C62.10
        left side C62.12
        right side C62.11
      left side C62.92
      right side C62.91
      undescended C62.00
        left side C62.02
        right side C62.01
  testis (M9070/3) C62.90
    descended (scrotal) C62.10
      left side C62.12
      right side C62.11
    left side C62.92
    right side C62.91
    undescended C62.00
      left side C62.02
      right side C62.01

Embryonic
  circulation Q28.9
  heart Q28.9
  vas deferens Q55.4

Embryopathia NOS Q89.9

Embryotoxon Q13.4

Emesis — see Vomiting

Emotionality, pathological F60.3

Emotogenic disease — see Disorder, psychogenic

Emphysema (atrophic) (bullous) (chronic)
  (interlobular) (lung) (obstructive) (pulmonary)
  (senile) (vesicular) J43.9
  cellular tissue (traumatic) T79.7
    surgical T81.82
  centrilobular J43.2
  compensatory J98.3
  congenital (interstitial) P25.0
  conjunctiva H11.89
  connective tissue (traumatic) T79.7
    surgical T81.82

Emphysema — continued
  due to chemicals, gases, fumes or vapors J68.4
  eyelid(s) — see Disorder, eyelid, specified type
    NEC
    surgical T81.82
    traumatic T79.7
  fetus or newborn (interstitial) P25.0
  heart I27.9
  interstitial J98.2
    congenital P25.0
    perinatal period P25.0
  laminated tissue T79.7
    surgical T81.82
  mediastinal J98.2
    fetus or newborn P25.2
  orbit, orbital — see Disorder, orbit, specified
    type NEC
  panacinar J43.1
  panlobular J43.1
  specified NEC J43.8
  subcutaneous (traumatic) T79.7
    nontraumatic J98.2
    postprocedural T81.82
    surgical T81.82
  surgical T81.82
  thymus (gland) (congenital) E32.8
  traumatic (subcutaneous) T79.7
  unilateral J43.0

Empty nest syndrome Z60.0

Empyema (acute) (chest) (double) (pleura)
  (supradiaphragmatic) (thorax) J86.9
  with fistula J86.0
  accessory sinus (chronic) — see Sinusitis
  antrum (chronic) — see Sinusitis, maxillary
  brain (any part) — see Abscess, brain
  ethmoidal (chronic) (sinus) — see Sinusitis,
    ethmoidal
  extradural — see Abscess, extradural
  frontal (chronic) (sinus) — see Sinusitis, frontal
  gallbladder K81.0
  mastoid (process) (acute) — see Mastoiditis,
    acute
  maxilla, maxillary M27.2
    sinus (chronic) — see Sinusitis, maxillary
  nasal sinus (chronic) — see Sinusitis
  sinus (accessory) (chronic) (nasal) — see
    Sinusitis
  sphenoidal (sinus) (chronic) — see Sinusitis,
    sphenoidal
  subarachnoid — see Abscess, extradural
  subdural — see Abscess, subdural
  tuberculous A15.6
  ureter — see Ureteritis
  ventricular — see Abscess, brain

En coup de sabre lesion L94.1

Enamel pearls K00.2

Enameloma K00.2

Enanthema, viral B09

Encephalitis (chronic) (hemorrhagic) (idiopathic)
  (nonepidemic) (spurious) (subacute) G04.9
  acute — see also Encephalitis, viral A86
    disseminated (postimmunization)
      (postinfectious) (postvaccination)
      G04.0
      postimmunization G04.0
    inclusion body A85.8
  arboviral, arbovirus NEC A85.2
  arthropod-borne NEC (viral) A85.2
  Australian A83.4
  California (virus) A83.5
  Central European (tick-borne) A84.1
  Czechoslovakian A84.1
  Dawson's (inclusion body) A81.1
  diffuse sclerosing A81.1
  disseminated, acute G04.0
  due to
    cat scratch disease A28.1
    malaria — see Malaria
    rickettsiosis — see Rickettsiosis
    smallpox inoculation G04.0
    typhus — see Typhus
  Eastern equine A83.2
  endemic (viral) A86
  epidemic NEC (viral) A86
  equine (acute) (infectious) (viral) A83.9
    Eastern A83.2

Encephalitis — continued
  equine — continued
    Venezuelan A92.2
    Western A83.1
  Far Eastern (tick-borne) A84.0
  following vaccination or other immunization
    procedure G04.0
  herpes zoster B02.0
  herpesviral B00.4
  Ilheus (virus) A83.8
  inclusion body A81.1
  in (due to)
    actinomycosis A42.82
    adenovirus A85.1
    African trypanosomiasis B56.9 [G05]
    Chagas' disease (chronic) B57.42
    cytomegalovirus B25.8
    enterovirus A85.0
    herpes (simplex) virus B00.4
    infectious disease NEC B99 [G05]
    influenza J10.89
    listeriosis A32.12
    measles B05.0
    mumps B26.2
    naegleriasis B60.2
    parasitic disease NEC B89 [G05]
    poliovirus A80.9 [G05]
    rubella B06.01
    syphilis
      congenital A50.42
      late A52.14
    systemic lupus erythematosus M32.19
    toxoplasmosis (acquired) B58.2
      congenital P37.1
    tuberculosis A17.82
    zoster B02.0
  infectious (acute) (virus) NEC A86
  Japanese (B type) A83.0
  La Crosse A83.5
  lead — see Poisoning, lead
  lethargica (acute) (infectious) A85.8
  louping ill A84.8
  lupus erythematosus, systemic M32.19
  lymphatica A87.2
  Mengo A85.8
  meningococcal A39.81
  Murray Valley A83.4
  otitic NEC H66.40 [G05]
  parasitic NOS B71.9
  periaxial G37.0
  periaxialis (concentrica) (diffuse) G37.5
  postchickenpox B01.1
  postexanthematous NEC B09
  postimmunization G04.0
  postmeasles B05.0
  postvaccinal G04.0
  postvaricella B01.1
  postviral NEC A86
  Powassan A84.8
  Rio Bravo A85.8
  Russian
    autumnal A83.0
    spring-summer (taiga) A84.0
  saturnine — see Poisoning, lead
  specified NEC G04.8
  St. Louis A83.3
  subacute sclerosing A81.1
  summer A83.0
  suppurative G04.8
  tick-borne A84.9
  Torula, torular (cryptococcal) B45.1
  toxic NEC G92
  trichinosis B75 [G05]
  type
    B A83.0
    C A83.3
  van Bogaert's A81.1
  Venezuelan equine A92.2
  Vienna A85.8
  viral, virus A86
    arthropod-borne NEC A85.2
      mosquito-borne A83.9
        Australian X disease A83.4
        California virus A83.5
        Eastern equine A83.2
        Japanese (B type) A83.0
        Murray Valley A83.4

Encephalitis — continued
  viral, virus — continued
    arthropod-borne NEC — continued
      mosquito-borne — continued
        specified NEC A83.8
        St. Louis A83.3
        type B A83.0
        type C A83.3
        Western equine A83.1
      tick-borne A84.9
        biundulant A84.1
        central European A84.1
        Czechoslovakian A84.1
        diphasic meningoencephalitis A84.1
        Far Eastern A84.0
        Russian spring-summer (taiga) A84.0
        specified NEC A84.8
      specified type NEC A85.8
    Western equine A83.1
Encephalocele Q01.9
  frontal Q01.0
  nasofrontal Q01.1
  occipital Q01.2
  specified NEC Q01.8
Encephalocystocele — see Encephalocele
Encephalomalacia (brain) (cerebellar) (cerebral) —
    see Softening, brain
Encephalomeningitis — see Meningoencephalitis
Encephalomeningocele — see Encephalocele
Encephalomeningomyelitis — see
    Meningoencephalitis
Encephalomyelitis (see also Encephalitis) G04.9
  acute disseminated (postimmunization) G04.0
    postinfectious G04.0
  benign myalgic G93.3
  due to or resulting from vaccination (any)
      G04.0
  equine A83.9
    Eastern A83.2
    Venezuelan A92.2
    Western A83.1
  myalgic, benign G93.3
  postchickenpox B01.1
  postinfectious NEC G04.8
  postmeasles B05.0
  postvaccinal G04.0
  postvaricella B01.1
  rubella B06.01
  specified NEC G04.8
  Venezuelan equine A92.2
Encephalomyelocele — see Encephalocele
Encephalomyelomeningitis — see
    Meningoencephalitis
Encephalomyelopathy G96.9
Encephalomyeloradiculitis (acute) G61.0
Encephalomyeloradiculoneuritis (acute)
    (Guillain-Barr) G61.0
Encephalomyeloradiculopathy G96.9
Encephalopathia hyperbilirubinemica, newborn
    P57.9
  due to isoimmunization (conditions in P55)
      P57.0
Encephalopathy (acute) G93.4
  alcoholic G31.2
  anoxic — see Damage, brain, anoxic
  arteriosclerotic I67.2
  centrolobar progressive (Schilder) G37.0
  congenital Q07.9
  demyelinating callosal G37.1
  hepatic — see Failure, hepatic
  hyperbilirubinemic, newborn P57.9
    due to isoimmunization (conditions in P55)
        P57.0
  hypertensive I67.4
  hypoglycemic E16.2
  hypoxic — see Damage, brain, anoxic
  in (due to)
    birth injury P11.1
    hyperinsulinism E16.1 [G94]
    influenza J10.89
    lack of vitamin (see also Deficiency, vitamin)
        E56.9 [G32.8]
    neoplastic disease (see also Neoplasm)
        D49.9 [G13.1]

Encephalopathy — continued
  in — continued
    serum (nontherapeutic) (therapeutic) T80.6
    syphilis A52.17
    trauma (postconcussional) F07.81
      current injury — see Injury, intracranial
    vaccination G04.0
  lead — see Poisoning, lead
  myoclonic, early, symptomatic — see Epilepsy,
      generalized, specified NEC
  necrotizing, subacute (Leigh) G31.82
  pellagrous E52 [G32.8]
  portosystemic — see Failure, hepatic
  postcontusional F07.81
    current injury — see Injury, intracranial,
        diffuse
  posthypoglycemic (coma) E16.1 [G94]
  postradiation G93.8
  saturnine — see Poisoning, lead
  spongiform, subacute (viral) A81.0
  toxic G92
  traumatic (postconcussional) F07.81
    current injury — see Injury, intracranial
  vitamin B deficiency NEC E53.9 [G32.8]
    vitamin B1 E51.2
  Wernicke's E51.2
Encephalorrhagia — see Hemorrhage,
    intracranial, intracerebral
Encephalosis, posttraumatic F07.81
Enchondroma (M9220/0) — see also Neoplasm,
    bone, benign
Enchondromatosis (cartilaginous) (multiple)
    Q78.4
Encopresis R15
  functional F98.1
  nonorganic origin F98.1
  psychogenic F98.1
Encounter with health service (for) Z76.9
  administrative purpose only Z02.9
    examination for
      adoption Z02.82
      armed forces Z02.3
      disability determination Z02.71
      driving license Z02.4
      employment Z02.1
      insurance Z02.6
      medical certificate NEC Z02.79
      paternity testing Z02.81
      residential institution admission Z02.2
      school admission Z02.0
      sports Z02.5
    specified reason NEC Z02.89
  instruction
    childbirth Z32.1
    child care (postpartal) (prenatal) Z32.2
  radiotherapy Z51.0
  specified NEC Z76.8
  sterilization Z30.2
  therapeutic drug level monitoring Z51.81
Encystment — see Cyst
Endarteritis (bacterial, subacute) (infective)
    (septic) I77.6
  brain I67.7
  cerebral or cerebrospinal I67.7
  deformans — see Arteriosclerosis
  embolic — see Embolism
  obliterans — see also Arteriosclerosis
    pulmonary I28.8
  pulmonary I28.8
  retina — see Vasculitis, retina
  senile — see Arteriosclerosis
  syphilitic A52.09
    brain or cerebral A52.04
    congenital A50.54 [I79.8]
  tuberculous A18.89
Endemic — see condition
Endocarditis (chronic) (nonbacterial thrombotic)
    (valvular) I38
  with rheumatic fever (conditions in I00)
    active — see Endocarditis, acute, rheumatic
    inactive or quiescent (with chorea) I09.1
  acute or subacute I33.9
    infective I33.0
    rheumatic (aortic) (mitral) (pulmonary)
        (tricuspid) I01.1

Endocarditis — continued
  acute or subacute — continued
    rheumatic — continued
      with chorea (acute) (rheumatic)
          (Sydenham's) I02.0
  aortic (heart) (nonrheumatic) (valve) I35.8
    with
      mitral disease I08.0
        with tricuspid (valve) disease I08.3
          active or acute I01.1
            with chorea (acute) (rheumatic)
                (Sydenham's) I02.0
      rheumatic fever (conditions in I00)
        active — see Endocarditis, acute,
            rheumatic
        inactive or quiescent (with chorea)
            I06.9
      tricuspid (valve) disease I08.2
        with mitral (valve) disease I08.3
    acute or subacute I33.9
    arteriosclerotic I35.8
    rheumatic I06.9
      with mitral disease I08.0
        with tricuspid (valve) disease I08.3
          active or acute I01.1
            with chorea (acute) (rheumatic)
                (Sydenham's) I02.0
        active or acute I01.1
          with chorea (acute) (rheumatic)
              (Sydenham's) I02.0
        specified NEC I06.8
    specified cause NEC I35.8
    syphilitic A52.03
  arteriosclerotic I38
  atypical verrucous (Libman-Sacks) M32.11
  bacterial (acute) (any valve) (subacute) I33.0
  candidal B37.6 [I39]
  congenital I42.4
  constrictive I33.0
  Coxiella burnetii A78 [I39]
  Coxsackie B33.21
  due to
    prosthetic cardiac valve T82.6
    Q fever A78 [I39]
    Serratia marcescens I33.0
    typhoid (fever) A01.02
  fetal I42.4
  gonococcal A54.83
  infectious or infective (acute) (any valve)
      (subacute) I33.0
  lenta (acute) (any valve) (subacute) I33.0
  Libman-Sacks M32.11
  listerial A32.82
  Löffler's I42.3
  malignant (acute) (any valve) (subacute) I33.0
  meningococcal A39.51
  mitral (chronic) (double) (fibroid) (heart)
      (inactive) (valve) (with chorea) I05.9
    with
      aortic (valve) disease I08.0
        with tricuspid (valve) disease I08.3
          active or acute I01.1
            with chorea (acute) (rheumatic)
                (Sydenham's) I02.0
      rheumatic fever (conditions in I00)
        active — see Endocarditis, acute,
            rheumatic
        inactive or quiescent (with chorea)
            I05.9
      tricuspid (valve) disease I08.1
        with aortic (valve) disease I08.3
    active or acute I01.1
      with chorea (acute) (rheumatic)
          (Sydenham's) I02.0
    bacterial I33.0
    arteriosclerotic I34.8
    nonrheumatic I34.8
      acute or subacute I33.9
    specified NEC I05.8
  monilial B37.6
  multiple valves I08.9
    specified disorders I08.8
  mycotic (acute) (any valve) (subacute) I33.0
  pneumococcal (acute) (any valve) (subacute)
      I33.0

Endocarditis — continued
  pulmonary (chronic) (heart) (valve) I37.8
    with rheumatic fever (conditions in I00)
      active — see Endocarditis, acute,
        rheumatic
      inactive or quiescent (with chorea) I09.89
        with aortic, mitral or tricuspid disease
          I08.8
    acute or subacute I33.9
      rheumatic I01.1
        with chorea (acute) (rheumatic)
          (Sydenham's) I02.0
    arteriosclerotic I37.8
    congenital Q22.2
    rheumatic (chronic) (inactive) (with chorea)
      I09.89
      active or acute I01.1
        with chorea (acute) (rheumatic)
          (Sydenham's) I02.0
    syphilitic A52.03
  purulent (acute) (any valve) (subacute) I33.0
  Q fever A78 [I39]
  rheumatic (chronic) (inactive) (with chorea)
    I09.1
    active or acute (aortic) (mitral) (pulmonary)
      (tricuspid) I01.1
      with chorea (acute) (rheumatic)
        (Sydenham's) I02.0
  rheumatoid — see Rheumatoid, carditis
  septic (acute) (any valve) (subacute) I33.0
  streptococcal (acute) (any valve) (subacute)
    I33.0
  subacute — see Endocarditis, acute
  suppurative (acute) (any valve) (subacute) I33.0
  syphilitic A52.03
  toxic I33.9
  tricuspid (chronic) (heart) (inactive) (rheumatic)
    (valve) (with chorea) I07.9
    with
      aortic (valve) disease I08.2
        mitral (valve) disease I08.3
      mitral (valve) disease I08.1
        aortic (valve) disease I08.3
      rheumatic fever (conditions in I00)
        active — see Endocarditis, acute,
          rheumatic
        inactive or quiescent (with chorea)
          I07.8
    active or acute I01.1
      with chorea (acute) (rheumatic)
        (Sydenham's) I02.0
    arteriosclerotic I36.8
    nonrheumatic I36.8
      acute or subacute I33.9
    specified cause, except rheumatic I36.8
  tuberculous — see Tuberculosis, endocarditis
  typhoid A01.02
  ulcerative (acute) (any valve) (subacute) I33.0
  vegetative (acute) (any valve) (subacute) I33.0
  verrucous (atypical) (nonbacterial)
    (nonrheumatic) M32.11

Endocardium, endocardial — see also condition
  cushion defect Q21.2
Endocervicitis — see also Cervicitis
  due to intrauterine (contraceptive) device T83.6
  hyperplastic N72
Endocrine — see condition
Endocrinopathy, pluriglandular E31.9
Endodontitis K04.0
Endomastoiditis — see Mastoiditis
Endometrioma N80.9
Endometriosis N80.9
  appendix N80.5
  bladder N80.8
  bowel N80.5
  broad ligament N80.3
  cervix N80.0
  colon N80.5
  cul-de-sac (Douglas') N80.3
  exocervix N80.0
  fallopian tube N80.2
  female genital organ NEC N80.8
  gallbladder N80.8
  in scar of skin N80.6
  internal N80.0

Endometriosis — continued
  intestine N80.5
  lung N80.8
  myometrium N80.0
  ovary N80.1
  parametrium N80.3
  pelvic peritoneum N80.3
  peritoneal (pelvic) N80.3
  rectovaginal septum N80.4
  rectum N80.5
  round ligament N80.3
  skin (scar) N80.6
  specified site NEC N80.8
  stromal (M8931/1) D39.0
  umbilicus N80.8
  uterus (internal) N80.0
  vagina N80.4
  vulva N80.8
Endometritis (decidual) (nonspecific) (purulent)
  (senile (atrophic)) (septic) (suppurative)
  N71.9
  with ectopic pregnancy O08.0
  acute N71.0
  blenorrhagic (gonococcal) (acute) (chronic)
    A54.24
  cervix, cervical (with erosion or ectropion) —
    see also Cervicitis
    hyperplastic N72
  chlamydial A56.11
  chronic N71.1
  complicating pregnancy O23.50
    first trimester O23.51
    second trimester O23.52
    third trimester O23.53
  following
    abortion — see Abortion by type complicated
      by genital infection
    ectopic or molar pregnancy O08.0
  gonococcal, gonorrheal (acute) (chronic) A54.24
  hyperplastic N85.0
    cervix N72
  puerperal, postpartum, childbirth O86.1
  subacute N71.0
  tuberculous A18.17
Endometrium — see condition
Endomyocarditis — see Endocarditis
Endomyocardiopathy, South African I42.3
Endomyofibrosis I42.3
Endomyometritis — see Endometritis
Endopericarditis — see Endocarditis
Endoperineuritis — see Disorder, nerve
Endophlebitis — see Phlebitis
Endophthalmia — see Endophthalmitis, purulent
Endophthalmitis (acute) (infective) (metastatic)
  (subacute) H44.009
  gonorrheal A54.39
  in (due to)
    cysticercosis B69.1
    onchocerciasis B73.01
    toxocariasis B83.0 [H45.1]
  panuveitis — see Panuveitis
  parasitic H44.129
    bilateral H44.123
    left H44.122
    right H44.121
  purulent H44.009
    bilateral H44.003
    left H44.002
    panophthalmitis — see Panophthalmitis
    right H44.001
  vitreous abscess H44.029
    bilateral H44.023
    left H44.022
    right H44.021
  specified NEC H44.19
  sympathetic — see Uveitis, sympathetic
Endosalpingioma (M8932/0) D28.2
Endosteitis — see Osteomyelitis
Endothelioma, bone (M9260/3) — see Neoplasm,
  bone, malignant
Endotheliosis (hemorrhagic infectional) D69.8
Endotrachelitis — see Cervicitis
Engelmann (-Camurati) syndrome Q78.3
English disease — see Rickets

Engman's disease L30.3
Engorgement
  breast N64.5
    newborn P83.4
    puerperal, postpartum O92.7
  lung (passive) — see Edema, lung
  pulmonary (passive) — see Edema, lung
  stomach K31.89
  venous, retina — see Occlusion, retina, vein,
    engorgement
Enlargement, enlarged — see also Hypertrophy
  adenoids J35.2
    with tonsils J35.3
  alveolar ridge K08.8
    congenital — see Anomaly, alveolar
  apertures of diaphragm (congenital) Q79.1
  gingival K06.1
  heart, cardiac — see Hypertrophy, cardiac
  lacrimal gland, chronic H04.039
    bilateral H04.033
    left H04.032
    right H04.031
  liver — see Hypertrophy, liver
  lymph gland or node R59.9
    generalized R59.1
    localized R59.0
  orbit H05.349
    bilateral H05.343
    left H05.342
    right H05.341
  organ or site, congenital NEC — see Anomaly,
    by site
  parathyroid (gland) E21.0
  pituitary fossa R93.0
  prostate, simple — see Hyperplasia, prostate
  sella turcica R93.0
  spleen — see Splenomegaly
  thymus (gland) (congenital) E32.0
  thyroid (gland) — see Goiter
  tongue K14.8
  tonsils J35.1
    with adenoids J35.3
  uterus N85.2
Enophthalmos H05.409
  bilateral H05.403
  due to
    orbital tissue atrophy H05.419
      bilateral H05.413
      left H05.412
      right H05.411
    trauma or surgery H05.429
      bilateral H05.423
      left H05.422
      right H05.421
  left H05.402
  right H05.401
Enostosis M27.8
Entamebic, entamebiasis — see Amebiasis
Entanglement
  umbilical cord(s) O69.2
    with compression O69.2
    around neck (with compression) O69.1
    of twins in monoamniotic sac O69.2
Enteralgia — see Pain, abdominal
Enteric — see condition
Enteritis (acute) (diarrheal) (hemorrhagic)
  (noninfective) (septic) K52.9
  aertrycke infection A02.0
  allergic K52.2
  amebic (acute) A06.0
    with abscess — see Abscess, amebic
    chronic A06.1
      with abscess — see Abscess, amebic
      nondysenteric A06.2
    nondysenteric A06.2
  bacillary NOS A03.9
  bacterial A04.9
    specified NEC A04.8
  candidal B37.82
  Chilomastix A07.8
  choleriformis A00.1
  chronic (noninfective) K52.9
    ulcerative — see Colitis, ulcerative
  cicatrizing (chronic) — see Enteritis, regional,
    small intestine
  Clostridium botulinum A05.1

Enteritis — *continued*
  coccidial A07.3
  dietetic K52.2
  due to
    food hypersensitivity K52.2
    infectious organism (bacterial) (viral) — *see*
        Enteritis, infectious
    Yersinia enterocolitica A04.6
  eltor A00.1
  epidemic (infectious) A09
  fulminant K55.0
  gangrenous — *see* Enteritis, infectious
  giardial A07.1
  infectious NOS A09
    due to
      adenovirus A08.2
      Aerobacter aerogenes A04.8
      Arizona (bacillus) A02.0
      bacteria NOS A04.9
        specified NEC A04.8
      Campylobacter A04.5
      Clostridium perfringens A04.8
      Enterobacter aerogenes A04.8
      enterovirus A08.3
      Escherichia coli A04.4
        enteroaggregative A04.4
        enterohemorrhagic A04.3
        enteroinvasive A04.2
        enteropathogenic A04.0
        enterotoxigenic A04.1
        specified NEC A04.4
      specified
        bacteria NEC A04.8
        virus NEC A08.3
      Staphylococcus A04.8
      virus NEC A08.4
        specified type NEC A08.3
      Yersinia enterocolitica A04.6
    specified organism NEC A08.5
  influenzal J10.81
  ischemic K55.9
    acute K55.0
    chronic K55.1
  microsporidial A07.8
  mucomembranous, myxomembranous — *see*
      Syndrome, irritable bowel
  mucous — *see* Syndrome, irritable bowel
  necroticans A05.2
  necrotizing of fetus or newborn P77
  neurogenic — *see* Syndrome, irritable bowel
  newborn necrotizing P77
  parasitic NEC B82.9
  paratyphoid (fever) — *see* Fever, paratyphoid
  presumed noninfectious K52.9
  protozoal A07.9
    specified NEC A07.8
  regional (of) K50.95
    with
      complication K50.90
        abscess K50.94
        fistula K50.93
        intestinal obstruction K50.92
        rectal bleeding K50.91
        specified complication NEC K50.99
    large intestine (colon) (rectum) K50.15
      with
        complication K50.10
          abscess K50.14
          fistula K50.13
          intestinal obstruction K50.12
          rectal bleeding K50.11
          small intestine involvement K50.85
            with
              complication K50.80
                abscess K50.84
                fistula K50.83
                intestinal obstruction
                    K50.82
                rectal bleeding K50.81
                specified complication NEC
                    K50.89
          specified complication NEC K50.19

Enteritis — *continued*
  regional — *continued*
    small intestine (duodenum) (ileum)
        (jejunum) K50.05
      with
        complication K50.00
          abscess K50.04
          fistula K50.03
          intestinal obstruction K50.02
          large intestine involvement K50.85
            with
              complication K50.80
                abscess K50.84
                fistula K50.83
                intestinal obstruction
                    K50.82
                rectal bleeding K50.81
                specified complication NEC
                    K50.89
          rectal bleeding K50.01
          specified complication NEC K50.09
  rotaviral A08.0
  Salmonella, salmonellosis (arizonae) (cholerae-
      suis) (enteritidis) (typhimurium) A02.0
  segmental — *see* Enteritis, regional
  Shigella — *see* Infection, Shigella
  spasmodic, spastic — *see* Syndrome, irritable
      bowel
  staphylococcal A04.8
    due to food A05.0
  toxic K52.1
  trichomonal A07.8
  tuberculous A18.32
  typhosa A01.00
  ulcerative (chronic) — *see* Colitis, ulcerative
  viral A08.4
    adenovirus A08.2
    enterovirus A08.3
    Rotavirus A08.0
    small round structured A08.1
    virus specified NEC A08.3

Enterobiasis B80

Enterobius vermicularis (infection) (infestation)
    B80

Enterocele — *see also* Hernia, abdomen
  pelvic, pelvis (acquired) (congenital) N81.5
  vagina, vaginal (acquired) (congenital) NEC
      N81.5

Enterocolitis (*see also* Enteritis) K52.9
  due to Clostridium difficile A04.7
  fulminant ischemic K55.0
  granulomatous — *see* Enteritis, regional
  hemorrhagic (acute) K55.0
    chronic K55.1
  ischemic K55.9
  necrotizing
    due to Clostridium difficile A04.7
    fetus or newborn P77
  radiation K52.0
    newborn P77
  ulcerative (chronic) K51.05
    with
      complication K51.00
        abscess K51.04
        fistula K51.03
        obstruction K51.02
        rectal bleeding K51.01
        specified complication NEC K51.09

Enterogastritis — *see* Enteritis
Enterolith, enterolithiasis (impaction) K56.4
Enteropathy K63.9
  gluten-sensitive K90.0
  hemorrhagic, terminal K55.0
  protein-losing K90.4
Enteroperitonitis — *see* Peritonitis
Enteroptosis K63.4
Enterorrhagia K92.2
Enterospasm — *see also* Syndrome, irritable,
    bowel
  psychogenic F45.8
Enterostenosis — *see* Obstruction, intestine
Enterostomy
  complication — *see* Complication, enterostomy
  status Z93.4

**Enterovirus, as cause of disease classified
    elsewhere** B97.10
  coxsackievirus B97.11
  echovirus B97.12
  other specified B97.19

Enthesopathy (peripheral) M77.9
  Achilles tendinitis — *see* Tendinitis, Achilles
  ankle and tarsus M77.9
    specified type NEC — *see* Enthesopathy,
        foot, specified type NEC
  anterior tibial syndrome — *see* Enthesopathy,
      lower limb, lower leg, specified type NEC
  calcaneal spur — *see* Spur, bone, calcaneal
  elbow region M77.8
    lateral epicondylitis — *see* Epicondylitis,
        lateral
    medial epicondylitis — *see* Epicondylitis,
        medial
  foot NEC M77.9
    metatarsalgia — *see* Metatarsalgia
    specified type NEC M77.50
      left M77.52
      right M77.51
  forearm M77.9
  gluteal tendinitis — *see* Tendinitis, gluteal
  hand M77.9
  hip — *see* Enthesopathy, lower limb, thigh,
      specified type NEC
  iliac crest spur — *see* Spur, bone, iliac crest
  iliotibial band syndrome — *see* Syndrome,
      iliotibial band
  knee — *see* Enthesopathy, lower limb, lower
      leg, specified type NEC
  lateral epicondylitis — *see* Epicondylitis, lateral
  lower limb M76.90
    Achilles tendinitis — *see* Tendinitis, Achilles
    ankle M76.979
      left M76.972
      right M76.971
      specified type NEC M76.879
        left M76.872
        right M76.871
    anterior tibial syndrome — *see*
        Enthesopathy, lower limb, lower leg,
        specified type NEC
    gluteal tendinitis — *see* Tendinitis, gluteal
    iliac crest spur — *see* Spur, bone, iliac crest
    iliotibial band syndrome — *see* Syndrome,
        iliotibial band
    lower leg M76.969
      left M76.962
      right M76.961
      specified type NEC M76.869
        left M76.862
        right M76.861
    multiple sites M76.99
    patellar tendinitis — *see* Tendinitis, patellar
    pelvic region — *see* Enthesopathy, lower
        limb, thigh
    peroneal tendinitis — *see* Tendinitis,
        peroneal
    posterior tibial syndrome — *see*
        Enthesopathy, lower limb, lower leg,
        specified type NEC
    psoas tendinitis — *see* Tendinitis, psoas
    shoulder M77.9
    specified type NEC M76.80
      ankle — *see* Enthesopathy, lower limb,
          ankle, specified type NEC
      lower leg — *see* Enthesopathy, lower
          limb, lower leg, specified type NEC
      multiple sites M76.89
      pelvic region — *see* Enthesopathy, lower
          limb, thigh, specified type NEC
      thigh — *see* Enthesopathy, lower limb,
          thigh, specified type NEC
    thigh M76.959
      left M76.952
      right M76.951
      specified type NEC M76.859
        left M76.852
        right M76.851
    tibial collateral bursitis — *see* Bursitis, tibial
        collateral
  medial epicondylitis — *see* Epicondylitis,
      medial
  metatarsalgia — *see* Metatarsalgia

Enthesopathy — *continued*
  multiple sites M77.9
  patellar tendinitis — *see* Tendinitis, patellar
  pelvis M77.9
  periarthritis of wrist — *see* Periarthritis, wrist
  peroneal tendinitis — *see* Tendinitis, peroneal
  posterior tibial syndrome — *see* Enthesopathy, lower limb, lower leg, specified type NEC
  psoas tendinitis — *see* Tendinitis, psoas
  shoulder region — *see* Lesion, shoulder
  specified site NEC M77.9
  specified type NEC M77.8
  spinal M46.00
    cervical region M46.02
    cervicothoracic region M46.03
    lumbar region M46.06
    lumbosacral region M46.07
    multiple sites M46.09
    occipito-atlanto-axial region M46.01
    sacrococcygeal region M46.08
    thoracic region M46.04
    thoracolumbar region M46.05
  tibial collateral bursitis — *see* Bursitis, tibial collateral
  upper arm M77.9
  wrist and carpus NEC M77.8
    calcaneal spur — *see* Spur, bone, calcaneal
    periarthritis of wrist — *see* Periarthritis, wrist

Entomophobia F40.218
Entomophthoromycosis B46.8
Entrance, air into vein — *see* Embolism, air
Entrapment, nerve — *see* Neuropathy, entrapment
Entropion (eyelid) (paralytic) H02.009
  cicatricial H02.019
    left H02.016
      lower H02.015
      upper H02.014
    right H02.013
      lower H02.012
      upper H02.011
  congenital Q10.2
  left H02.006
    lower H02.005
    upper H02.004
  mechanical H02.029
    left H02.026
      lower H02.025
      upper H02.024
    right H02.023
      lower H02.022
      upper H02.021
  right H02.003
    lower H02.002
    upper H02.001
  senile H02.039
    left H02.036
      lower H02.035
      upper H02.034
    right H02.033
      lower H02.032
      upper H02.031
  spastic H02.049
    left H02.046
      lower H02.045
      upper H02.044
    right H02.043
      lower H02.042
      upper H02.041
Enucleated eye (traumatic, current) S05.70
  left S05.72
  right S05.71
Enuresis R32
  functional F98.0
  habit disturbance F98.0
  nocturnal R32
    psychogenic F98.0
  nonorganic origin F98.0
  psychogenic F98.0
Eosinopenia — *see* Agranulocytosis
Eosinophilia (allergic) (hereditary) (idiopathic) (secondary) D72.1
  infiltrative J82
  Löffler's J82

Eosinophilia — *continued*
  pulmonary NEC J82
  tropical (pulmonary) J82
Eosinophilia-myalgia syndrome M35.8
Ependymitis (acute) (cerebral) (chronic) (granular) — *see* Encephalomyelitis
Ependymoblastoma (M9392/3)
  specified site — *see* Neoplasm, malignant
  unspecified site C71.9
Ependymoma (epithelial) (malignant) (M9391/3)
  anaplastic (M9392/3)
    specified site — *see* Neoplasm, malignant
    unspecified site C71.9
  benign (M9391/0)
    specified site — *see* Neoplasm, benign
    unspecified site D33.2
  myxopapillary (M9394/1) D43.2
    specified site — *see* Neoplasm, uncertain behavior
    unspecified site D43.2
  papillary (M9393/1) D43.2
    specified site — *see* Neoplasm, uncertain behavior
    unspecified site D43.2
  specified site — *see* Neoplasm, malignant
  unspecified site C71.9
Ependymopathy G93.8
Ephelis, ephelides L81.2
Epiblepharon (congenital) Q10.3
Epicanthus, epicanthic fold (eyelid) (congenital) Q10.3
Epicondylitis (elbow)
  lateral M77.10
    left M77.12
    right M77.11
  medial M77.00
    left M77.02
    right M77.01
Epicystitis — *see* Cystitis
Epidemic — *see* condition
Epidermidalization, cervix — *see* Dysplasia, cervix
Epidermis, epidermal — *see* condition
Epidermodysplasia verruciformis B07
Epidermolysis
  bullosa (congenital) Q81.9
    acquired L12.30
      drug-induced L12.31
      specified cause NEC L12.35
    dystrophica Q81.2
    letalis Q81.1
    simplex Q81.0
    specified NEC Q81.8
  necroticans combustiformis L51.2
    due to drug
      correct substance properly administered L51.2
      overdose or wrong substance given or taken (by accident) T50.901
      administered with intent to harm by another person T50.903
      self T50.902
      circumstances undetermined T50.904
      specified drug — *see* Table of Drugs and Chemicals
Epidermophytid — *see* Dermatophytosis
Epidermophytosis (infected) — *see* Dermatophytosis
Epididymis — *see* condition
Epididymitis (acute) (nonvenereal) (recurrent) (residual) N45.1
  with orchitis N45.3
  blennorrhagic (gonococcal) A54.23
  caseous (tuberculous) A18.15
  chlamydial A56.19
  filarial B74.9
  gonococcal A54.23
  syphilitic A52.76
  tuberculous A18.15
Epididymo-orchitis (*see also* Epididymitis) N45.3
Epidural — *see* condition
Epigastrium, epigastric — *see* condition
Epigastrocele — *see* Hernia, ventral

Epiglottis — *see* condition
Epiglottitis, epiglottiditis (acute) J05.1
  chronic J37.0
Epignathus Q89.4
Epilepsy, epileptic, epilepsia (attack) (cerebral) (convulsion) (fit) (seizure) G40.90
  with
    complex partial seizures — *see* Epilepsy, focal
    grand mal seizures on awakening — *see* Epilepsy, generalized
    myoclonic absences — *see* Epilepsy, generalized, specified NEC
    myoclonic-astatic seizures — *see* Epilepsy, generalized, specified NEC
    simple partial seizures — *see* Epilepsy, focal
    status epilepticus G40.91
  abdominal — *see* Epilepsy, specified NEC
  akinetic — *see* Epilepsy, generalized
  automatism — *see* Epilepsy, focal, with complex partial seizures
  Bravais-jacksonian — *see* Epilepsy, focal
  childhood (benign) (with)
    absence — *see* Epilepsy, generalized
    centrotemporal EEG spikes — *see* Epilepsy, focal, idiopathic
    occipital EEG paroxysms — *see* Epilepsy, focal, idiopathic
  climacteric — *see* Epilepsy, specified NEC
  clonic — *see* Epilepsy, generalized
  clouded state — *see* Epilepsy, specified NEC
  coma — *see* Epilepsy, specified NEC
  cortical (focal) (motor) — *see* Epilepsy, focal
  cysticercosis B69.0
  deterioration (mental) F06.8
  due to syphilis A52.19
  equivalent — *see* Epilepsy, specified NEC
  focal (symptomatic) (with simple partial seizures) G40.10
    with
      complex partial seizures G40.20
        with status epilepticus G40.21
      status epilepticus G40.11
    idiopathic G40.00
      with status epilepticus G40.01
  generalized (idiopathic) G40.30
    with status epilepticus G40.31
    specified NEC G40.40
      with status epilepticus G40.41
  grand mal NOS (*see also* Epilepsy, generalized) G40.60
    with status epilepticus G40.61
    on awakening — *see* Epilepsy, generalized
  jacksonian (motor) (sensory) — *see* Epilepsy, focal
  juvenile absence — *see* Epilepsy, generalized
  Kojevnikov's (Kozhevnikof's) — *see* Epilepsy, special syndrome
  laryngeal R05
  limbic system — *see* Epilepsy, focal, with complex partial seizures
  localization-related (focal) (partial) — *see* Epilepsy, focal
  major — *see* Epilepsy, generalized
  minor — *see* Epilepsy, generalized
  mixed (type) — *see* Epilepsy, generalized
  motor partial — *see* Epilepsy, focal
  musicogenic — *see* Epilepsy, specified NEC
  myoclonus, myoclonic — *see* Epilepsy, generalized
  parasitic NOS B71.9 *[G94]*
  partial (focalized) — *see* Epilepsy, focal
  partialis continua — *see* Epilepsy, special syndrome
  peripheral — *see* Epilepsy, specified NEC
  petit mal NOS (*see also* Epilepsy, generalized) G40.70
    with status epilepticus G40.71
  procursiva — *see* Epilepsy, focal, with complex partial seizures
  progressive (familial) myoclonic — *see* Epilepsy, generalized
  psychomotor — *see* Epilepsy, focal, with complex partial seizures
  psychosensory — *see* Epilepsy, focal, with complex partial seizures
  reflex — *see* Epilepsy, specified NEC

©2002 Ingenix, Inc.

Epilepsy, epileptic, epilepsia — *continued*
  related to external cause — *see* Epilepsy,
    special syndrome
  senile — *see* Epilepsy, specified NEC
  sleep G47.4
  somatomotor — *see* Epilepsy, focal
  somatosensory — *see* Epilepsy, focal
  special syndrome G40.50
    with status epilepticus G40.51
    specified NEC G40.80
      with status epilepticus G40.81
  syndrome — *see* Epilepsy
  temporal lobe — *see* Epilepsy, focal, with
    complex partial seizures
  tonic(-clonic) — *see* Epilepsy, generalized
  twilight F05
  uncinate (gyrus) — *see* Epilepsy, focal, with
    complex partial seizures
  Unverricht(-Lundborg) (familial myoclonic) —
    see Epilepsy, generalized
  visceral — *see* Epilepsy, specified NEC
  visual — *see* Epilepsy, specified NEC
Epiloia Q85.1
Epimenorrhea N92.0
Epipharyngitis — *see* Nasopharyngitis
Epiphora H04.209
  bilateral H04.203
  due to
    excess lacrimation H04.219
      bilateral H04.213
      left H04.212
      right H04.211
    insufficient drainage H04.229
      bilateral H04.223
      left H04.222
      right H04.221
  left H04.202
  right H04.201
Epiphyseal arrest — *see* Arrest, epiphyseal
Epiphyseolysis, epiphysiolysis — *see*
    Osteochondropathy
Epiphysitis — *see also* Osteochondropathy
  juvenile M92.9
  syphilitic (congenital) A50.02 *[M90.80]*
Epiplocele — *see* Hernia, abdomen
Epiploitis — *see* Peritonitis
Epiplosarcomphalocele — *see* Hernia, umbilicus
Episcleritis (suppurative) H15.109
  bilateral H15.103
  in (due to)
    syphilis A52.71
    tuberculosis A18.51
  left H15.102
  nodular H15.129
    bilateral H15.123
    left H15.122
    right H15.121
  periodica fugax H15.119
    angioneurotic — *see* Edema, angioneurotic
    bilateral H15.113
    left H15.112
    right H15.111
  right H15.101
  syphilitic (late) A52.71
  tuberculous A18.51
Episode
  affective, mixed F39
  brain (apoplectic) I64
  cerebral (apoplectic) I64
  depersonalization (in neurotic state) F48.1
  depressive F32.9
    major F32.9
      mild F32.0
      moderate F32.1
      severe (without psychotic symptoms)
        F32.2
        with psychotic symptoms F32.3
    recurrent F33.9
      brief F33.8
    specified NEC F32.8
  hypomanic F30.8
  manic F30.9
    with
      psychotic symptoms F30.2

Episode — *continued*
  manic — *continued*
    with — *continued*
      remission (full) F30.4
        partial F30.3
      other specified F30.8
      recurrent F31.89
      without psychotic symptoms F30.10
        mild F30.11
        moderate F30.12
        severe (without psychotic symptoms)
          F30.13
          with psychotic symptoms F30.2
  psychotic F23
    organic F06.8
  schizophrenic (acute) NEC, brief F23
Epispadias (female) (male) Q64.0
Episplenitis D73.8
Epistaxis (multiple) R04.0
  hereditary I78.0
  vicarious menstruation N94.8
Epithelioma (malignant) (M8011/3) — *see also*
    Neoplasm, malignant
  adenoides cysticum (M8100/0) — *see*
    Neoplasm, skin, benign
  basal cell (M8090/3) — *see* Neoplasm, skin,
    malignant
  benign (M8011/0) — *see* Neoplasm, benign
  Bowen's (M8081/2) — *see* Neoplasm, skin, in
    situ
  calcifying, of Malherbe (M8110/0) — *see*
    Neoplasm, skin, benign
  external site — *see* Neoplasm, skin, malignant
  intraepidermal, Jadassohn (M8096/0) — *see*
    Neoplasm, skin, benign
  squamous cell (M8070/3) — *see* Neoplasm,
    malignant
Epitheliomatosis pigmented Q82.1
Epitheliopathy, multifocal placoid pigment
    H30.149
  bilateral H30.143
  left H30.142
  right H30.141
Epithelium, epithelial — *see* condition
Epituberculosis (with atelectasis) (allergic) A15.7
Eponychia Q84.6
Epstein's
  nephrosis or syndrome — *see* Nephrosis
  pearl K09.8
Epulis (gingiva) (fibrous) (giant cell) K06.8
Equinia A24.0
Equinovarus (congenital) (talipes) Q66.0
  acquired — *see* Deformity, limb, clubfoot
Equivalent
  convulsive (abdominal) — *see* Epilepsy,
    specified NEC
  epileptic (psychic) — *see* Epilepsy, focal, with
    complex partial seizures
Erb (-Duchenne) paralysis (birth injury)
    (newborn) P14.0
Erb-Goldflam disease or syndrome G70.0
Erb's
  disease G71.0
  palsy, paralysis (brachial) (birth) (newborn)
    P14.0
  spinal (spastic) syphilitic A52.17
  pseudohypertrophic muscular dystrophy G71.0
Erdheim's syndrome (acromegalic
    macrospondylitis) E22.0
Erection, painful (persistent) — *see* Priapism
Ergosterol deficiency (vitamin D) E55.9
  with
    adult osteomalacia M83.8
    rickets — *see* Rickets
Ergotism — *see also* Poisoning, food, noxious,
    plant
  from ergot used as drug (migraine therapy) —
    see Table of Drugs and Chemicals
Erosio interdigitalis blastomycetica B37.2
Erosion
  artery I77.2
    without rupture I77.8

Erosion — *continued*
  bone — *see* Disorder, bone, density and
    structure, specified NEC
  bronchus J98.0
  cartilage (joint) — *see* Disorder, cartilage,
    specified type NEC
  cervix (uteri) (acquired) (chronic) (congenital)
    N86
    with cervicitis N72
  cornea (nontraumatic) — *see* Ulcer, cornea
    recurrent H18.839
      bilateral H18.833
      left H18.832
      right H18.831
    traumatic — *see* Abrasion, cornea
  dental (idiopathic) (occupational) (due to diet,
    drugs or vomiting) K03.2
  duodenum, postpyloric — *see* Ulcer, duodenum
  esophagus K22.1
  gastric — *see* Ulcer, stomach
  gastrojejunal — *see* Ulcer, gastrojejunal
  intestine K63.3
  lymphatic vessel I89.8
  pylorus, pyloric (ulcer) — *see* Ulcer, stomach
  spine, aneurysmal A52.09
  stomach — *see* Ulcer, stomach
  teeth (idiopathic) (occupational) (due to diet,
    drugs or vomiting) K03.2
  urethra N36.8
  uterus N85.8
Erotomania F52.8
Error
  metabolism, inborn — *see* Disorder, metabolism
  refractive — *see* Disorder, refraction
Eructation R14.2
  nervous or psychogenic F45.8
Eruption
  creeping B76.9
  drug (generalized) (taken internally) L27.0
    fixed L27.1
    in contact with skin — *see* Dermatitis, due
      to drugs
    localized L27.1
  Hutchinson, summer L56.4
  Kaposi's varicelliform B00.0
  napkin L22
  polymorphous light (sun) L56.4
  recalcitrant pustular L13.8
  ringed R23.8
  skin (nonspecific) R21
    creeping (meaning hookworm) B76.9
    due to inoculation/vaccination (generalized)
      (*see also* Dermatitis, due to, vaccine)
      L27.0
      localized L27.1
    erysipeloid A26.0
    feigned L98.1
    Kaposi's varicelliform B00.0
    lichenoid L28.0
    meaning dermatitis — *see* Dermatitis
    toxic NEC L53.0
  tooth, teeth, abnormal (incomplete) (late)
    (premature) (sequence) K00.6
  vesicular R23.8
Erysipelas (gangrenous) (infantile) (newborn)
    (phlegmonous) (suppurative) A46
  external ear A46 *[H62.40]*
  puerperal, postpartum O86.8
Erysipeloid A26.9
  cutaneous (Rosenbach's) A26.0
  disseminated A26.8
  septicemia A26.7
  specified NEC A26.8
Erythema, erythematous (infectional)
    (inflammation) L53.9
  ab igne L59.0
  annulare (centrifugum) (rheumaticum) L53.1
  arthriticum epidemicum A25.1
  brucellum — *see* Brucellosis
  chronic figurate L53.3
  chronicum migrans (Borrelia burgdorferi)
    A69.20
  diaper L22
  due to
    chemical NEC L53.0
      in contact with skin L25.3

Erythema, erythematous — *continued*
  drug (internal use)*see* Dermatitis, due to, drugs
  elevatum diutinum L95.1
  endemic E52
  epidemic, arthritic A25.1
  figuratum perstans L53.3
  gluteal L22
  heat – code by site under Burn, first degree
  ichthyosiforme congenitum bullous Q80.3
  induratum (nontuberculous) L52
    tuberculous A18.4
  infectiosum B08.3
  intertrigo L30.4
  iris L51.1 *[H22]*
  marginatum L53.2
    in (due to) acute rheumatic fever I00
  medicamentosum — *see* Dermatitis, due to, drugs
  migrans A26.0
    chronicum A69.20
      tongue K14.1
  multiforme L51.9
    bullous, bullosum L51.1
    conjunctiva L51.1 *[H13]*
    nonbullous L51.0
    pemphigoides L12.0
    specified NEC L51.8
  napkin L22
  neonatorum P83.8
    toxic P83.1
  nodosum L52
    tuberculous A18.4
  palmar L53.8
  pernio T69.1
  rash, newborn P83.8
  scarlatiniform (recurrent) (exfoliative) L53.8
  solare L55.0
  specified NEC L53.8
  toxic, toxicum NEC L53.0
    newborn P83.1
  tuberculous (primary) A18.4
Erythematous, erythematosus — *see* condition
Erythermalgia (primary) I73.8
Erythralgia I73.8
Erythrasma L08.1
Erythredema (polyneuropathy) — *see* Poisoning, mercury
Erythremia (acute) (M9841/3) C94.00
  chronic (M9842/3) C94.10
    in remission C94.11
  in remission C94.01
  secondary D75.1
Erythroblastopenia (*see also* Aplasia, red cell) D60.9
  congenital D61.0
Erythroblastophthisis D61.0
Erythroblastosis (fetalis) (newborn) P55.9
  due to
    ABO (antibodies) (incompatibility) (isoimmunization) P55.1
    Rh (antibodies) (incompatibility) (isoimmunization) P55.0
Erythrocyanosis (crurum) I73.8
Erythrocythemia (M9841/3) — *see* Erythremia
Erythrocytosis (megalosplenic)
  familial D75.0
  oval, hereditary — *see* Elliptocytosis
  secondary D75.1
  stress D75.1
Erythroderma (secondary) (*see also* Erythema) L53.9
  bullous ichthyosiform, congenital Q80.3
  desquamativum L21.1
  ichthyosiform, congenital (bullous) Q80.3
  neonatorum P83.8
  psoriaticum L40.8
Erythrogenesis imperfecta D61.0
Erythroleukemia (M9840/3) C94.00
  in remission C94.01
Erythromelalgia I73.8
Erythrophagocytosis D75.8
Erythrophobia F40.298
Erythroplakia, oral epithelium, and tongue K13.2

Erythroplasia (Queyrat) (M8080/2)
  specified site — *see* Neoplasm, skin, in situ
  unspecified site D07.4
Escherichia (E.) coli, as cause of disease classified elsewhere B96.2
Esophagismus K22.4
Esophagitis (acute) (alkaline) (chemical) (chronic) (infectional) (necrotic) (peptic) (postoperative) K20
  candidal B37.81
  reflux K21.0
  tuberculous A18.83
Esophagocele K22.5
Esophagomalacia K22.8
Esophagospasm K22.4
Esophagostenosis K22.2
Esophagostomiasis B81.8
Esophagotracheal — *see* condition
Esophagus — *see* condition
Esophoria H50.51
  convergence, excess H51.12
  divergence, insufficiency H51.8
Esotropia — *see* Strabismus, convergent concomitant
Espundia B55.2
Essential — *see* condition
Esthesioneuroblastoma (M9522/3) C30.0
Esthesioneurocytoma (M9521/3) C30.0
Esthesioneuroepithelioma (M9523/3) C30.0
Esthiomene A55
Estivo-autumnal malaria (fever) B50.9
Estrangement Z63.5
Estriasis — *see* Myiasis
Ethanolism — *see* Alcoholism
Etherism — *see* Dependence, drug, inhalant
Ethmoid, ethmoidal — *see* condition
Ethmoiditis (chronic) (purulent) (nonpurulent) — *see also* Sinusitis, ethmoidal
  influenzal J10.1
  Woakes' J33.1
Ethylism — *see* Alcoholism
Eulenburg's disease (congenital paramyotonia G71.1
Eumycetoma B47.0
Eunuchoidism E29.1
  hypogonadotropic E23.0
European blastomycosis — *see* Cryptococcosis
Eustachian — *see* condition
Evaluation (for) (of)
  development state
    adolescent Z00.3
    infant or child Z00.10
      with abnormal findings Z00.11
    period of
      delayed growth in childhood Z00.70
        with abnormal findings Z00.71
      rapid growth in childhood Z00.2
    puberty Z00.3
  growth and developmental state (period of rapid growth) Z00.2
    child Z00.10
      with abnormal findings Z00.11
      delayed growth Z00.70
        with abnormal findings Z00.71
  mental health (status) Z00.8
    requested by authority Z04.6
  period of
    delayed growth in childhood Z00.70
      with abnormal findings Z00.71
    rapid growth in childhood Z00.2
  suspected condition — *see* Observation
Evans' syndrome D69.3
Eventration — *see also* Hernia, ventral
  colon into chest — *see* Hernia, diaphragm
  diaphragm (congenital) Q79.1
Eversion
  bladder N32.8
  cervix (uteri) N86
    with cervicitis N72

Eversion — *continued*
  foot NEC — *see also* Deformity, valgus, ankle
    congenital Q66.6
  punctum lacrimale (postinfectional) (senile) H04.529
    bilateral H04.523
    left H04.522
    right H04.521
  ureter (meatus) N28.89
  urethra (meatus) N36.8
  uterus N81.4
Evisceration
  birth injury P15.8
  operative wound T81.3
  traumatic NEC
    eye — *see* Enucleated eye
Evulsion — *see* Avulsion
Ewing's sarcoma or tumor (M9260/3) — *see* Neoplasm, bone, malignant
Examination (general) (routine) (of) (for) Z00.010
  with abnormal findings Z00.011
  adolescent (development state) Z00.3
  allergy Z01.8
  annual (periodic) (physical) Z00.010
    with abnormal findings Z00.011
    gynecological Z01.40
      with abnormal findings Z01.41
  blood pressure Z01.30
    with abnormal findings Z01.31
  cancer staging — *see* Neoplasm, malignant
  cervical Papanicolaou smear Z12.4
    as part of routine gynecological examination Z01.40
  chest X-ray Z00.030
    with abnormal findings Z00.031
    for suspected tuberculosis Z03.8
  child care (routine) Z00.10
    with abnormal findings Z00.11
  clinical research control or normal comparison Z00.6
  contraceptive (drug) maintenance (routine) Z30.8
    device (intrauterine) Z30.44
  dental Z01.20
    with abnormal findings Z01.21
  developmental testing (child) (infant) Z00.10
    with abnormal findings Z00.11
  donor (potential) Z00.5
  ear Z01.10
    with abnormal findings Z01.11
  eye Z01.00
    with abnormal findings Z01.01
  following
    accident NEC Z04.3
      transport Z04.1
      work Z04.2
    assault, alleged
      adult Z04.71
      child Z04.72
    motor vehicle accident Z04.1
    rape, alleged (victim or culprit) Z04.4
    seduction, alleged (victim or culprit) Z04.4
    treatment (for) Z09
      combined NEC Z09
        fracture Z09
          malignant neoplasm Z08
        malignant neoplasm Z08
        mental disorder Z09
        specified condition NEC Z09
  follow-up (routine) (following) Z09
    chemotherapy NEC Z09
      malignant neoplasm Z08
    fracture Z09
    malignant neoplasm Z08
    postpartum Z39.2
    psychotherapy Z09
    radiotherapy NEC Z09
      malignant neoplasm Z08
    surgery NEC Z09
      malignant neoplasm Z08
  gynecological Z01.40
    with abnormal findings Z01.41
    for contraceptive maintenance Z30.8
  health — *see* Examination, medical
  hearing Z01.10
    with abnormal findings Z01.11

                                                                      ©2002 *Ingenix, Inc.*

Examination — *continued*
  infant or child Z00.10
    with abnormal findings Z00.11
  inflicted injury, alleged
    adult Z04.71
    child Z04.72
  laboratory Z00.020
    with abnormal findings Z00.021
  lactating mother Z39.1
  medical (for) (of) Z00.010
    with abnormal findings Z00.011
    administrative purpose only Z02.9
      specified NEC Z02.89
    admission to
      armed forces Z02.3
      old age home Z02.2
      prison Z02.89
      residential institution Z02.2
      school Z02.0
      summer camp Z02.89
    adoption Z02.82
    blood alcohol or drug level Z02.83
    camp (summer) Z02.89
    child, routine Z00.10
      with abnormal findings Z00.11
    clinical research, normal subject Z00.6
    control subject in clinical research Z00.6
    donor (potential) Z00.5
    driving license Z02.4
    general Z00.010
      with abnormal findings Z00.011
    immigration Z02.89
    infant or child Z00.10
      with abnormal findings Z00.11
    insurance purposes Z02.6
    marriage Z02.89
    medicolegal reasons NEC Z04.8
    naturalization Z02.89
    participation in sport Z02.5
    paternity testing Z02.81
    population survey Z00.8
    pre-employment Z02.1
    preschool children
      for admission to school Z02.0
    prisoners
      for entrance into prison Z02.89
    recruitment for armed forces Z02.3
    specified NEC Z00.8
    sport competition Z02.5
  medicolegal reason NEC Z04.8
  pelvic (annual) (periodic) Z01.40
    with abnormal findings Z01.41
  period of rapid growth in childhood Z00.2
  periodic (annual) (routine) Z00.010
    with abnormal findings Z00.011
  postpartum
    immediately after delivery Z39.0
    routine follow-up Z39.2
  prenatal (normal pregnancy) — *see* Antenatal,
    care
  psychiatric NEC Z00.8
    follow-up not needing further care Z09
    requested by authority Z04.6
  radiological NEC Z00.030
    with abnormal findings Z00.031
  rape or seduction, alleged (victim or culprit)
    Z04.4
  sensitization Z01.8
  skin (hypersensitivity) Z01.8
  special (*see also* Examination, by type) Z01.9
    specified type NEC Z01.8
  specified type or reason NEC Z04.8
  teeth Z01.20
    with abnormal findings Z01.21
  vision Z01.00
    with abnormal findings Z01.01
  well baby Z00.10
    with abnormal findings Z00.11
Exanthem, exanthema — *see also* Rash
  with enteroviral vesicular stomatitis B08.4
  Boston A88.0
  epidemic with meningitis A88.0 [G02]
  subitum B08.2
  viral, virus B09
    specified type NEC B08.8

Excess, excessive, excessively
  alcohol level in blood R78.0
  androgen (ovarian) E28.1
  attrition, tooth, teeth K03.0
  carotene, carotin (dietary) E67.1
  cold, effects of T69.9
    specified effect NEC T69.8
  convergence H51.12
  crying in infant R68.11
  development, breast N62
  divergence H51.8
  drinking (alcohol) NEC (without dependence)
    F10.10
    habitual (continual) (without remission)
      F10.20
  eating R63.2
  estrogen E28.0
  fat — *see also* Obesity
    in heart — *see* Degeneration, myocardial
    localized E65
  foreskin N47.8
  gas R14.8
  glucagon E16.3
  heat — *see* Heat
  kalium E87.5
  large
    colon K59.3
      congenital Q43.8
    fetus or infant P08.0
      with obstructed labor O66.2
      affecting management of pregnancy
        O36.60
        first trimester O36.61
        second trimester O36.62
        third trimester O36.63
      causing disproportion O33.5
    organ or site, congenital NEC — *see*
      Anomaly, by site
  long
    organ or site, congenital NEC — *see*
      Anomaly, by site
  menstruation (with regular cycle) N92.0
    with irregular cycle N92.1
  natrium E87.0
  number of teeth K00.1
    causing crowding M26.3
  nutrient (dietary) NEC R63.2
  potassium (K) E87.5
  salivation K11.7
  secretion — *see also* Hypersecretion
    milk O92.6
    sputum R09.3
    sweat R61.9
  sexual drive F52.8
  short
    organ or site, congenital NEC — *see*
      Anomaly, by site
    umbilical cord in labor or delivery O69.3
  skin, eyelid (acquired) — *see* Blepharochalasis
    congenital Q10.3
  sodium (Na) E87.0
  sputum R09.3
  sweating R61.9
  thirst R63.1
    due to deprivation of water T73.1
  vitamin
    A (dietary) E67.0
      administered as drug (chronic) (prolonged
        excessive intake) E67.0
      overdose or wrong substance given or
        taken — *see* category T45.2
    D (dietary) E67.3
      administered as drug (chronic) (prolonged
        excessive intake) E67.3
      overdose or wrong substance given or
        taken — *see* category T45.2
  weight
    gain R63.5
    loss R63.4
Excitability, abnormal, under minor stress
  (personality disorder) F60.3
Excitation
  anomalous atrioventricular I45.6
  psychogenic F30.8
  reactive (from emotional stress, psychological
    trauma) F30.8

Excitement
  hypomanic F30.8
  manic F30.9
  mental, reactive (from emotional stress,
    psychological trauma) F30.8
  state, reactive (from emotional stress,
    psychological trauma) F30.8
Excoriation (traumatic) — *see also* Abrasion
  neurotic L98.1
Exercise Z51.89
Exfoliation, teeth, due to systemic causes
  K08.0
Exfoliative — *see* condition
Exhaustion, exhaustive (physical NEC) R53.82
  battle F43.0
  cardiac — *see* Failure, heart
  complicating pregnancy O26.819
    first trimester O26.811
    second trimester O26.812
    third trimester O26.813
  delirium F43.0
  due to
    cold T69.8
    excessive exertion T73.3
    exposure T73.2
    neurasthenia F48.8
    pregnancy O26.819
      first trimester O26.811
      second trimester O26.812
      third trimester O26.813
  fetus or newborn P96.8
  heart — *see* Failure, heart
  heat (*see also* Heat, exhaustion) T67.5
    due to
      salt depletion T67.4
      water depletion T67.3
  maternal, complicating delivery O75.81
  mental F48.8
  myocardium, myocardial — *see* Failure, heart
  nervous F48.8
  old age R54
  psychogenic F48.8
  psychosis F43.0
  senile R54
  vital NEC Z73.0
Exhibitionism F65.2
Exocervicitis — *see* Cervicitis
Exomphalos Q79.2
  meaning hernia — *see* Hernia, umbilicus
Exophoria H50.52
  convergence, insufficiency H51.11
  divergence, excess H51.8
Exophthalmos H05.20
  congenital Q15.8
  constant NEC H05.249
    bilateral H05.243
    left H05.242
    right H05.241
  displacement, globe — *see* Displacement, globe
  due to thyrotoxicosis (hyperthyroidism) — *see*
    Hyperthyroidism, with, goiter (diffuse)
  dysthyroid — *see* Hyperthyroidism, with, goiter
    (diffuse)
  goiter — *see* Hyperthyroidism, with, goiter
    (diffuse)
  intermittent NEC H05.259
    bilateral H05.253
    left H05.252
    right H05.251
  malignant — *see* Hyperthyroidism, with, goiter
    (diffuse)
  orbital
    edema — *see* Edema, orbit
    hemorrhage — *see* Hemorrhage, orbit
  pulsating NEC H05.269
    bilateral H05.263
    left H05.262
    right H05.261
  thyrotoxic, thyrotropic — *see* Hyperthyroidism,
    with, goiter (diffuse)
Exostosis — *see also* Disorder, bone
  cartilaginous (M9210/0) — *see* Neoplasm,
    bone, benign
  congenital (multiple) Q78.6

Exostosis — see also Disorder, bone — continued
external ear canal H61.819
bilateral H61.813
left H61.812
right H61.811
gonococcal A54.49
jaw (bone) M27.8
multiple, congenital Q78.6
orbit H05.359
bilateral H05.353
left H05.352
right H05.351
osteocartilaginous (M9210/0) — see Neoplasm,
bone, benign
syphilitic A52.77

Exotropia — see Strabismus, divergent
concomitant

Explanation of
investigation finding Z71.2
medication Z71.89

Exposure (to) (see also Contact, with) T75.89
acariasis Z20.7
agricultural toxic agents (gases) (liquids)
(solids) (vapors) Z57.4
nonoccupational Z58.5
AIDS virus Z20.6
air
contaminants NEC Z58.1
occupational NEC Z57.39
dust Z57.2
tobacco smoke Z57.31
pollution NEC Z58.1
occupational NEC Z57.39
dust Z57.2
tobacco smoke Z57.31
asbestos Z58.82
cholera Z20.0
cold, effects of T69.9
specified effect NEC T69.8
communicable disease Z20.9
specified NEC Z20.8
disaster Z65.5
discrimination Z60.5
dust NEC Z58.1
occupational Z57.2
effects of T73.9
exhaustion due to T73.2
extreme temperature (occupational) Z57.6
nonoccupational Z58.5
German measles Z20.4
gonorrhea Z20.2
human immunodeficiency virus (HIV) Z20.6
human T-lymphotropic virus type-1 (HTLV-1)
Z20.8
industrial toxic agents (gases) (liquids) (solids)
(vapors) Z57.5
nonoccupational Z58.5
infestation (parasitic) NEC Z20.7
intestinal infectious disease Z20.0
lead Z58.81
noise Z58.0
occupational Z57.0
occupational risk factor Z57.9
specified NEC Z57.8
parasitic disease NEC Z20.7
pediculosis Z20.7
persecution Z60.5
poliomyelitis Z20.8
pollution NEC Z58.5
air contaminants NEC Z58.1
occupational Z57.39
dust Z57.2
tobacco smoke Z57.31
dust NEC Z58.1
occupational Z57.2
noise NEC Z58.0
occupational Z57.0
occupational Z57.8
soil Z58.3
specified NEC Z58.5
occupational Z57.8
water Z58.2
rabies Z20.3
radiation NEC Z58.4
occupational Z57.1
rubella Z20.4
sexually-transmitted disease Z20.2

Exposure (see also Contact, with) — continued
smallpox (laboratory) Z20.8
soil pollution Z58.3
occupational Z57.8
syphilis Z20.2
terrorism Z65.4
torture Z65.4
toxic agents (gases) (liquids) (solids) (vapors)
agricultural Z57.4
nonoccupational Z58.5
industrial NEC Z57.5
nonoccupational Z58.5
tuberculosis Z20.1
venereal disease Z20.2
vibration Z58.89
occupational Z57.7
viral disease NEC Z20.8
hepatitis Z20.5
war Z65.5
water pollution Z58.2

Exsanguination — see Hemorrhage

Exstrophy
abdominal contents Q45.8
bladder Q64.10
cloacal Q64.12
specified type NEC Q64.19
supravesical fissure Q64.11

Extensive — see condition

Extra — see also Accessory
marker chromosomes (normal individual)
Q92.61
in abnormal individual Q92.62
rib Q76.6
cervical Q76.5

Extrasystoles (ventricular) I49.4
atrial I49.1

Extrauterine gestation or pregnancy — see
Pregnancy, by site

Extravasation
blood R58
chyle into mesentery I89.8
pelvicalyceal N13.8
pyelosinus N13.8
urine (from ureter) R39.0

Extremity — see condition, limb

Extrophy — see Exstrophy

Extroversion
bladder Q64.19
uterus N81.4
complicating delivery O71.2
postpartal (old) N81.4

Extrusion
breast implant (prosthetic) T85.42
eye implant (globe) (ball) T85.328
intervertebral disc — see Displacement,
intervertebral disc
ocular lens implant (prosthetic) — see
Complications, intraocular lens
vitreous — see Prolapse, vitreous

Exudate
pleural — see Effusion, pleura
retina H35.89

Exudative — see condition

Eye, eyeball, eyelid — see condition

Eyestrain — see Disturbance, vision, subjective

Eyeworm disease of Africa B74.3

F

Faber's syndrome (achlorhydric anemia) D50.9

Fabry (-Anderson) disease E75.21

Faciocephalalgia, autonomic (see also
Neuropathy, peripheral, autonomic) G90.0

Factor(s)
psychic, associated with diseases classified
elsewhere F54
psychological
affecting physical conditions F54
or behavioral
affecting general medical condition F54
associated with disorders or diseases
classified elsewhere F54

Failure, failed
abortion — see Abortion, attempted
aortic (valve) I35.8
rheumatic I06.8
attempted abortion — see Abortion, attempted
biventricular I50.9
bone marrow — see Anemia, aplastic
cardiac — see Failure, heart
cardiorenal (chronic) I50.9
hypertensive I13.2
cardiorespiratory (see also Failure, heart) R09.2
specified during or due to a cardiac
procedure T81.89
long term effect of cardiac surgery I97.1
non-cardiac procedure T81.84
cardiovascular (chronic) — see Failure, heart
cerebrovascular I67.9
cervical dilatation in labor O62.0
circulation, circulatory (peripheral) R57.9
compensation — see Disease, heart
compliance with medical treatment or regimen
— see Noncompliance
congestive — see Failure, heart, congestive
descent of head (at term) of pregnancy (mother)
O32.4
engagement of head (term of pregnancy)
(mother) O32.4
erection (penile) F52.21
examination(s), anxiety concerning Z55.2
expansion terminal respiratory units (newborn)
(primary) P28.0
fetal head to enter pelvic brim (mother) O32.4
forceps NOS (with subsequent cesarean
section) O66.5
gain weight R62.51
genital response (male) F52.21
female F52.22
heart (acute) (sudden) I50.9
with
acute pulmonary edema — see Failure,
ventricular, left
decompensation — see Failure, heart,
congestive
dilatation — see Disease, heart
arteriosclerotic I70.90
combined left-right sided I50.0
compensated I50.0
complicating
anesthesia (general) (local) or other
sedation
in labor and delivery O74.2
in pregnancy — see Complications,
anesthesia, in, pregnancy,
cardiac
postpartum, puerperal O89.1
delivery (cesarean) (instrumental) O75.4
surgery T81.89
congestive (compensated) (decompensated)
I50.0
with rheumatic fever (conditions in I00)
active I01.8
inactive or quiescent (with chorea)
I09.81
hypertensive I11.0
with renal disease I13.0
with renal failure I13.2
newborn P29.0
rheumatic (chronic) (inactive) (with
chorea) I09.81
active or acute I01.8
with chorea I02.0
decompensated I50.0
degenerative — see Degeneration,
myocardial
due to presence of cardiac prosthesis I97.1
following cardiac surgery I97.1
high output NOS I50.9
hypertensive I11.0
with renal disease I13.0
with renal failure I13.2
left (ventricular) — see Failure, ventricular,
left
low output (syndrome) NOS I50.9
newborn P29.0
organic — see Disease, heart
postoperative I97.89
cardiac surgery I97.1

Failure, failed — *continued*
  heart — *continued*
    rheumatic (chronic) (inactive) I09.9
    right (ventricular) (secondary to left heart
      failure) — *see* Failure, heart,
      congestive
    senile R54
    specified during or due to a procedure
      T81.89
      long term effect of cardiac surgery I97.1
    thyrotoxic (*see also* Thyrotoxicosis) E05.90
      [I43]
      with thyroid storm E05.91 *[I43]*
    valvular — *see* Endocarditis
  hepatic K72.90
    with coma K72.91
    acute or subacute K72.00
      with coma K72.01
      due to drugs K71.10
        with coma K71.11
    alcoholic (acute) (chronic) (subacute) K70.40
      with coma K70.41
    chronic K72.10
      with coma K72.11
      due to drugs (acute) (subacute) (chronic)
        K71.10
        with coma K71.11
    due to drugs (acute) (subacute) (chronic)
      K71.10
      with coma K71.11
    postoperative K91.81
  hepatorenal K76.7
    postoperative K91.82
  induction (of labor) O61.9
    abortion — *see* Abortion, attempted
    by
      oxytocic drugs O61.0
      prostaglandins O61.0
    instrumental O61.1
    mechanical O61.1
    medical O61.0
    specified NEC O61.8
    surgical O61.1
  intubation during anesthesia T88.4
    in pregnancy — *see* Complications,
      anesthesia, in, pregnancy, failed
      intubation
    labor and delivery O74.7
    postpartum, puerperal O89.6
  involution, thymus (gland) E32.0
  kidney — *see* Failure, renal
  lactation (complete) O92.3
    partial O92.4
  Leydig's cell, adult E29.1
  liver — *see* Failure, hepatic
  menstruation at puberty N91.0
  mitral I05.8
  myocardial, myocardium (*see also* Failure,
    heart) I50.9
    chronic (*see also* Failure, heart, congestive)
      I50.0
    congestive (*see also* Failure, heart,
      congestive) I50.0
  orgasm (female) (psychogenic) F52.31
    male F52.32
  ovarian (primary) E28.3
    iatrogenic E89.4
    postprocedural (postablative)
      (postirradiation) (postsurgical) E89.4
  ovulation causing infertility N97.0
  polyglandular, autoimmune E31.0
  renal N19
    with
      hypertension I12.0
      hypertensive heart disease (conditions in
        I11) I13.1
        with heart failure (congestive) I13.2
      tubular necrosis (acute) N17.0
    acute N17.9
      with
        cortical necrosis N17.1
        medullary necrosis N17.2
        tubular necrosis N17.0
      specified NEC N17.8
    chronic N18.9
      end stage renal disease N18.0

Failure, failed — *continued*
  renal — *continued*
    chronic — *continued*
      hypertensive (*see also* Hypertension,
        kidney) I12.0
    congenital P96.0
    end stage (chronic) N18.0
    following
      abortion — *see* Abortion by type
        complicated by specified condition
        NEC
      crushing T79.5
      ectopic or molar pregnancy O08.4
      labor and delivery (acute) O90.4
    hypertensive (*see also* Hypertension, kidney)
      I12.0
    postprocedural N99.0
  respiration, respiratory J96.9
    acute J96.0
      with chronic J96.2
    center G93.8
    chronic J96.1
      with acute J96.2
    newborn P28.5
    postprocedural J95.82
  rotation
    cecum Q43.3
    colon Q43.3
    intestine Q43.3
    kidney Q63.2
  segmentation — *see also* Fusion
    fingers — *see* Syndactylism, complex, fingers
    toes Q70.2
    vertebra Q76.49
      with scoliosis Q76.3
  seminiferous tubule, adult E29.1
  senile (general) R54
  sexual arousal (male) F52.21
    female F52.22
  testicular endocrine function E29.1
  to thrive (child) R62.51
    adult R62.7
  transplant T86.92
    bone T86.831
      marrow T86.09
        graft vs host disease T86.01
    cornea T86.841
    heart T86.22
      with lung(s) T86.32
    intestine T86.891
    kidney T86.12
    liver T86.42
    lung(s) T86.811
      with heart T86.32
    pancreas T86.891
    skin (allograft) (autograft) T86.821
    specified organ or tissue NEC T86.891
  trial of labor (with subsequent cesarean
    section) O66.40
    following previous cesarean section O66.41
  urinary — *see* Failure, renal
  vacuum extraction NOS (with subsequent
    cesarean section) O66.5
  ventouse NOS (with subsequent cesarean
    section) O66.5
  ventricular (*see also* Failure, heart) I50.9
    left I50.1
      with rheumatic fever (conditions in I00)
        active I01.8
          with chorea I02.0
        inactive or quiescent (with chorea)
          I09.81
      hypertensive (*see also* Hypertension,
        heart) I11.0
      rheumatic (chronic) (inactive) (with
        chorea) I09.81
        active or acute I01.8
          with chorea I02.0
    right (*see also* Failure, heart, congestive)
      I50.0
  vital centers, fetus or newborn P91.8
Fainting (fit) R55
Fallen arches — *see* Deformity, limb, flat foot
Falling, any organ or part — *see* Prolapse

Fallopian
  insufflation Z31.41
  tube — *see* condition
Fallot's
  pentalogy Q21.3
  tetrad or tetralogy Q21.3
  triad or trilogy Q22.2
Fallout, radioactive (adverse effect) NOS T66
False — *see also* condition
  croup J38.5
  joint — *see* Nonunion, fracture
  labor (pains) O47.9
    after 37 completed weeks of gestation O47.1
    before 37 completed weeks of gestation
      O47.00
      second trimester O47.02
      third trimester O47.03
  passage, urethra (prostatic) N36.0
  pregnancy F45.8
Family, familial — *see also* condition
  disruption Z63.8
    involving divorce or separation Z63.5
  planning advice Z30.09
  problem Z63.9
    specified NEC Z63.8
Famine (effects of) T73.0
  edema — *see* Malnutrition, severe
Fanconi (-de Toni) (-Debré) syndrome E72.09
  with cystinosis E72.04
Fanconi's anemia (congenital pancytopenia)
  D61.0
Farber's disease or syndrome E75.29
Farcy A24.0
Farmer's
  lung J67.0
  skin L57.8
Farsightedness — *see* Hypermetropia
Fascia — *see* condition
Fasciculation R25.3
Fasciitis M72.59
  diffuse (eosinophilic) M35.4
  infective M72.52
    necrotizing M72.51
  necrotizing M72.51
  nodular M72.3
  perirenal (with ureteral obstruction) N13.5
    with infection N13.6
  plantar M72.2
  specified NEC M72.59
  traumatic (old) M72.59
  current – code by site under Sprain
Fascioliasis B66.3
Fasciolopsis, fasciolopsiasis (intestinal) B66.5
Fascioscapulohumeral myopathy G71.0
Fast pulse R00.0
Fat
  embolism — *see* Embolism, fat
  excessive — *see also* Obesity
    in heart — *see* Degeneration, myocardial
  in stool R19.5
  localized (pad) E65
    heart — *see* Degeneration, myocardial
    knee M79.4
    retropatellar M79.4
  necrosis
    breast N64.1
    mesentery K65.8
    omentum K65.8
  pad E65
    knee M79.4
Fatigue R53.82
  auditory deafness — *see* Deafness
  combat F43.0
  complicating pregnancy O26.819
    first trimester O26.811
    second trimester O26.812
    third trimester O26.813
  general R53.82
    psychogenic F48.8
  heat (transient) T67.6
  muscle M62.89
  myocardium — *see* Failure, heart
  neoplasm-related R53.0
  nervous, neurosis F48.8

Fatigue — *continued*
  operational F48.8
  psychogenic (general) F48.8
  senile R54
  voice R49.8
Fatness — *see* Obesity
Fatty — *see also* condition
  apron E65
  degeneration — *see* Degeneration, fatty
  heart (enlarged) — *see* Degeneration,
    myocardial
  liver NEC K76.0
    alcoholic K70.0
  necrosis — *see* Degeneration, fatty
Fauces — *see* condition
Fauchard's disease (periodontitis) K05.3
Faucitis J02.9
Favism (anemia) D55.0
Favus — *see* Dermatophytosis
Fazio-Londe disease or syndrome G12.1
Fear complex or reaction F40.9
Fear of — *see* Phobia
Feared complaint unfounded Z71.1
Febricula (continued) (simple) R50.9
Febris, febrile — *see also* Fever
  flava (*see also* Fever, yellow) A95.9
  melitensis A23.0
  pestis — *see* Plague
  puerperalis O85
  recurrens — *see* Fever, relapsing
  rubra A38.9
Fecal — *see* condition
Fecalith (impaction) K56.4
  appendix K38.1
  congenital P76.8
Fede's disease K14.0
Feeble rapid pulse due to shock following injury T79.4
Feeble-minded F70
Feeding
  difficulties and mismanagement R63.3
  faulty R63.3
  formula check (infant) Z00.10
  improper R63.3
  problem R63.3
    newborn P92.9
      specified NEC P92.8
    nonorganic (adult) — *see* Disorder, eating
Feer's disease — *see* Poisoning, mercury
Feet — *see* condition
Feigned illness Z76.5
Feil-Klippel syndrome (brevicollis) Q76.1
Feinmesser's (hidrotic) ectodermal dysplasia Q82.4
Felinophobia F40.218
Felon — *see also* Cellulitis, digit
  with lymphangitis — *see* Lymphangitis, acute, digit
Felty's syndrome M05.00
  ankle M05.079
    left M05.072
    right M05.071
  elbow M05.029
    left M05.022
    right M05.021
  foot joint M05.079
    left M05.072
    right M05.071
  hand joint M05.049
    left M05.042
    right M05.041
  hip M05.059
    left M05.052
    right M05.051
  knee M05.069
    left M05.062
    right M05.061
  multiple site M05.09
  shoulder M05.019
    left M05.012
    right M05.011
  vertebra — *see* Spondylitis, ankylosing

Felty's syndrome — *continued*
  wrist M05.039
    left M05.032
    right M05.031
Femur, femoral — *see* condition
Fenestration, fenestrated — *see also* Imperfect, closure
  aortico-pulmonary Q21.4
  cusps, heart valve NEC Q24.8
    pulmonary Q22.2
  pulmonic cusps Q22.2
Fernell's disease (aortic aneurysm) I71.9
Fertile eunuch syndrome E23.0
Fetal — *see* Fetus
Fetalis uterus Q51.8
Fetid
  breath R19.6
  sweat L75.0
Fetishism F65.0
  transvestic F65.1
Fetus, fetal — *see also* condition
  alcohol syndrome (dysmorphic) Q86.0
  compressus (mother) O31.00
    first trimester O31.01
    second trimester O31.02
    third trimester O31.03
  hydantoin syndrome Q86.1
  lung tissue P28.0
  papyraceous (mother) — *see* Fetus compressus
Fever (inanition) (of unknown origin) R50.9
  with
    chills R50.0
      in malarial regions B54
    rigors R50.0
  abortus A23.1
  Aden (dengue) A90
  African tick-borne A68.1
  American
    mountain (tick) A93.2
    spotted A77.0
  aphthous B08.8
  arbovirus, arboviral A94
    hemorrhagic A94
    specified NEC A93.8
  Argentinian hemorrhagic A96.0
  Assam B55.0
  Australian Q A78
  Bangkok hemorrhagic A91
  Barmah forest A92.8
  Bartonella A44.0
  bilious, hemoglobinuric B50.8
  blackwater B50.8
  blister B00.1
  Bolivian hemorrhagic A96.1
  Bonvale dam T73.3
  boutonneuse A77.1
  brain — *see* Encephalitis
  Brazilian purpuric A48.4
  breakbone A90
  Bullis A77.0
  Bunyamwera A92.8
  Burdwan B55.0
  Bwamba A92.8
  Cameroon — *see* Malaria
  Canton A75.9
  catarrhal (acute) J00
    chronic J31.0
  cat-scratch A28.1
  Central Asian hemorrhagic A98.0
  cerebral — *see* Encephalitis
  cerebrospinal meningococcal A39.0
  Chagres B50.9
  Chandipura A92.8
  Changuinola A93.1
  Charcôt's (biliary) (hepatic) (intermittent) — *see* Calculus, bile duct
  Chikungunya (viral) (hemorrhagic) A92.0
  Chitral A93.1
  Colombo — *see* Fever, paratyphoid
  Colorado tick (virus) A93.2
  congestive (remittent) — *see* Malaria
  Congo virus A98.0
  continued malarial B50.9
  Corsican — *see* Malaria
  Crimean-Congo hemorrhagic A98.0
  Cyprus — *see* Brucellosis

Fever — *continued*
  dandy A90
  deer fly — *see* Tularemia
  dengue (virus) A90
    hemorrhagic A91
    sandfly A93.1
  desert B38.0
  due to heat T67.0
  enteric A01.00
  enteroviral exanthematous (Boston exanthem) A88.0
  ephemeral (of unknown origin) R50.9
  epidemic hemorrhagic A98.5
  erysipelatous — *see* Erysipelas
  estivo-autumnal (malarial) B50.9
  famine A75.0
  five day A79.0
  following delivery O86.4
  Fort Bragg A27.89
  gastroenteric A01.00
  gastromalarial — *see* Malaria
  Gibraltar — *see* Brucellosis
  glandular — *see* Mononucleosis, infectious
  Guama (viral) A92.8
  Haverhill A25.1
  hay (allergic) J30.1
    with asthma (bronchial) J45.00
      with
        acute exacerbation J45.01
        status asthmaticus J45.02
    due to
      allergen other than pollen J30.8
      pollen, any plant or tree J30.1
  heat (effects) T67.0
  hematuric, bilious B50.8
  hemoglobinuric (malarial) (bilious) B50.8
  hemorrhagic (arthropod-borne) NOS A94
    with renal syndrome A98.5
    arenaviral A96.9
      specified NEC A96.8
    Argentinian A96.0
    Bangkok A91
    Bolivian A96.1
    Central Asian A98.0
    Chikungunya A92.0
    Crimean-Congo A98.0
    dengue (virus) A91
    epidemic A98.5
    Junin (virus) A96.0
    Korean A98.5
    Kyasanur forest A98.2
    Machupo (virus) A96.1
    mite-borne A93.8
    mosquito-borne A92.8
    Omsk A98.1
    Philippine A91
    Russian A98.5
    Singapore A91
    Southeast Asia A91
    Thailand A91
    tick-borne NEC A93.8
    viral A99
      specified NEC A98.8
  hepatic — *see* Cholecystitis
  herpetic — *see* Herpes
  icterohemorrhagic A27.0
  Indiana A93.8
  infective B99.9
    specified NEC B99.8
  intermittent (bilious) — *see also* Malaria
    of unknown origin R50.9
    pernicious B50.9
  iodide
    correct substance properly administered R50.9
    overdose or wrong substance given or taken — *see* category T48.4
  Japanese river A75.3
  jungle — *see also* Malaria
    yellow A95.0
  Junin (virus) hemorrhagic A96.0
  Katayama B65.2
  kedani A75.3
  Kenya (tick) A77.1
  Kew Garden A79.1
  Korean hemorrhagic A98.5
  Lassa A96.2

©2002 Ingenix, Inc.

Fever — *continued*
  Lone Star A77.0
  Machupo (virus) hemorrhagic A96.1
  malaria, malarial — *see* Malaria
  Malta A23.9
  Marseilles A77.1
  marsh — *see* Malaria
  Mayaro (viral) A92.8
  Mediterranean — *see* Brucellosis
    familial E85
    tick A77.1
  meningeal — *see* Meningitis
  Meuse A79.0
  Mexican A75.2
  mianeh A68.1
  miasmatic — *see* Malaria
  mosquito-borne (viral) A92.9
    hemorrhagic A92.8
  mountain — *see also* Brucellosis
    meaning Rocky Mountain spotted fever
      A77.0
    tick (American) (Colorado) (viral) A93.2
  Mucambo (viral) A92.8
  mud A27.9
  Neapolitan — *see* Brucellosis
  newborn P81.9
    environmental P81.0
  Nine-Mile A78
  non-exanthematous tick A93.2
  North Asian tick-borne A77.2
  Omsk hemorrhagic A98.1
  O'nyong-nyong (viral) A92.1
  Oropouche (viral) A93.0
  Oroya A44.0
  paludal — *see* Malaria
  Panama (malarial) B50.9
  Pappataci A93.1
  paratyphoid A01.4
    A A01.1
    B A01.2
    C A01.3
  parrot A70
  periodic (Mediterranean) E85
  persistent (of unknown origin) R50.8
  petechial A39.0
  pharyngoconjunctival B30.2
  Philippine hemorrhagic A91
  phlebotomus A93.1
  Piry (virus) A93.8
  Pixuna (viral) A92.8
  Plasmodium ovale B53.0
  polioviral (nonparalytic) A80.4
  Pontiac A48.2
  postoperative (due to infection) T81.4
  pretibial A27.89
  puerperal O85
  putrid — *see* Septicemia
  pyemic — *see* Septicemia
  Q A78
  quadrilateral A78
  quartan (malaria) B52.9
  Queensland (coastal) (tick) A77.3
  quintan A79.0
  rabbit — *see* Tularemia
  rat-bite A25.9
    due to
      Spirillum A25.0
      Streptobacillus moniliformis A25.1
  recurrent — *see* Fever, relapsing
  relapsing (Borrelia) A68.9
    Carter's (Asiatic) A68.1
    Dutton's (West African) A68.1
    Koch's A68.9
    louse-borne A68.0
    Novy's
      louse-borne A68.0
      tick-borne A68.1
    Obermeyer's (European) A68.0
    tick-borne A68.1
  remittent (bilious) (congestive) (gastric) — *see*
    Malaria
  rheumatic (active) (acute) (chronic) (subacute)
    I00
    with central nervous system involvement
      I02.9
    active with heart involvement — *see* category
      I01

Fever — *continued*
  rheumatic — *continued*
    inactive or quiescent with
      cardiac hypertrophy I09.89
      carditis I09.9
      endocarditis I09.1
        aortic (valve) I06.9
          with mitral (valve) disease I08.0
        mitral (valve) I05.9
          with aortic (valve) disease I08.0
        pulmonary (valve) I09.89
        tricuspid (valve) I07.8
      heart disease NEC I09.89
      heart failure (congestive) (conditions in
        I50.0, I50.9) I09.81
      left ventricular failure (conditions in
        I50.1) I09.81
      myocarditis, myocardial degeneration
        (conditions in I51.4) I09.0
      pancarditis I09.9
      pericarditis I09.2
  Rift Valley (viral) A92.4
  Rocky Mountain spotted A77.0
  rose J30.1
  Ross River B33.1
  Russian hemorrhagic A98.5
  San Joaquin (Valley) B38.0
  sandfly A93.1
  Sao Paulo A77.0
  scarlet A38.9
  septic — *see* Septicemia
  seven day (leptospirosis) (autumnal) (Japanese)
    A27.89
    dengue A90
  shin-bone A79.0
  Singapore hemorrhagic A91
  solar A90
  sore B00.1
  South African tick-bite A68.1
  Southeast Asia hemorrhagic A91
  spinal — *see* Meningitis
  spirillary A25.0
  splenic — *see* Anthrax
  spotted A77.9
    American A77.0
    Brazilian A77.0
    cerebrospinal meningitis A39.0
    Colombian A77.0
    due to Rickettsia
      australis A77.3
      conorii A77.1
      rickettsii A77.0
      sibirica A77.2
      specified type NEC A77.8
    Ehrlichiosis A77.40
      due to
        E. chafeensis A77.41
        specified organism NEC A77.49
    Rocky Mountain A77.0
  steroid
    correct substance properly administered
      R50.9
    overdose or wrong substance given or taken
      — *see* category T38.0
  streptobacillary A25.1
  subtertian B50.9
  Sumatran mite A75.3
  sun A90
  swamp A27.9
  swine A02.8
  sylvatic, yellow A95.0
  Tahyna A83.5
  tertian — *see* Malaria, tertian
  Thailand hemorrhagic A91
  thermic T67.0
  three-day A93.1
  tick
    American mountain A93.2
    Colorado A93.2
    Kemerovo A93.8
    Mediterranean A77.1
    mountain A93.2
    nonexanthematous A93.2
    Quaranfil A93.8
  tick-bite NEC A93.8
  tick-borne (hemorrhagic) NEC A93.8
  trench A79.0

Fever — *continued*
  tsutsugamushi A75.3
  typhogastric A01.00
  typhoid (abortive) (hemorrhagic) (intermittent)
    (malignant) A01.00
    complicated by
      arthritis A01.04
      heart involvement A01.02
      meningitis A01.01
      osteomyelitis A01.05
      pneumonia A01.03
      specified NEC A01.09
  typhomalarial — *see* Malaria
  typhus — *see* Typhus (fever)
  undulant — *see* Brucellosis
  unknown origin R50.9
  uremic N19
  uveoparotid D86.89
  valley B38.0
  Venezuelan equine A92.2
  vesicular stomatitis A93.8
  viral hemorrhagic — *see* Fever, hemorrhagic, by
    type of virus
  Volhynian A79.0
  Wesselsbron (viral) A92.8
  West
    African B50.8
    Nile (viral) A92.3
  Whitmore's — *see* Melioidosis
  Wolhynian A79.0
  worm B83.9
  yellow A95.9
    jungle A95.0
    sylvatic A95.0
    urban A95.1
  Zika (viral) A92.8

Fibrillation
  atrial or auricular (established) I48.0
  cardiac I49.8
  heart I49.8
  muscular M62.89
  ventricular I49.01

Fibrin
  ball or bodies, pleural (sac) J94.1
  chamber, anterior (eye) (gelatinous exudate) —
    see Iridocyclitis, acute

Fibrinogenolysis — *see* Fibrinolysis

Fibrinogenopenia D68.89
  acquired D65
  congenital D68.2

Fibrinolysis (hemorrhagic) (acquired) D65
  antepartum hemorrhage — *see* Hemorrhage,
    antepartum, with coagulation defect
  following
    abortion — *see* Abortion by type complicated
      by hemorrhage
    ectopic or molar pregnancy O08.1
  intrapartum O67.0
  newborn, transient P60
  postpartum O72.3

Fibrinopenia (hereditary) D68.2
  acquired D68.4

Fibrinopurulent — *see* condition

Fibrinous — *see* condition

Fibroadenoma (M9010/0)
  cellular intracanalicular (female) (M9020/0)
    D24.00
    left D24.02
    male D24.10
      left D24.12
      right D24.11
    right D24.01
  giant (female) (M9016/0) D24.00
    left D24.02
    male D24.10
      left D24.12
      right D24.11
    right D24.01
  intracanalicular (M9011/0)
    cellular (female) (M9020/0) D24.00
    left D24.02
    male D24.10
      left D24.12
      right D24.11
    right D24.01

Fibroadenoma — continued
  intracanalicular — continued
    giant (female) (M9020/0) D24.00
      left D24.02
      male D24.10
        left D24.12
        right D24.11
      right D24.01
    specified site — see Neoplasm, benign
    unspecified site (female) D24.00
      left D24.02
      male D24.10
        left D24.12
        right D24.11
      right D24.01
  juvenile (female) (M9030/0) D24.00
    left D24.02
    male D24.10
      left D24.12
      right D24.11
    right D24.01
  pericanalicular (M9012/0)
    specified site — see Neoplasm, benign
    unspecified site (female) D24.00
      left D24.02
      male D24.10
        left D24.12
        right D24.11
      right D24.01
  phyllodes (female) (M9020/0) D24.00
    left D24.02
    male D24.10
      left D24.12
      right D24.11
    right D24.01
  prostate — see Hyperplasia, prostate, localized
  specified site NEC — see Neoplasm, benign
  unspecified site (female) D24.00
    left D24.02
    male D24.10
      left D24.12
      right D24.11
    right D24.01

Fibroadenosis, breast (chronic) (cystic) (diffuse) (female) (periodic) (segmental) N60.20
  left N60.22
  male N60.25
    left N60.24
    right N60.23
  right N60.21

Fibroangioma (M9160/0) — see also Neoplasm, benign
  juvenile (M9160/0)
    specified site — see Neoplasm, benign
    unspecified site D10.6

Fibrochondrosarcoma (M9220/3) — see Neoplasm, cartilage, malignant

Fibrocystic
  disease — see also Fibrosis, cystic
    breast — see Mastopathy, cystic
    jaw M27.49
    kidney (congenital) Q61.8
    liver Q44.6
    pancreas E84.9
  kidney (congenital) Q61.8

Fibrodysplasia ossificans progressiva — see Myositis, ossificans, progressiva

Fibroelastosis (cordis) (endocardial) (endomyocardial) I42.4

Fibroid (tumor) (M8890/0) — see also Neoplasm, connective tissue, benign
  disease, lung (chronic) — see Fibrosis, lung
  heart (disease) — see Myocarditis
  in pregnancy or childbirth — see category O34.1
    causing obstructed labor O65.5
  induration, lung (chronic) — see Fibrosis, lung
  lung — see Fibrosis, lung
  pneumonia (chronic) — see Fibrosis, lung
  uterus D25.9

Fibrolipoma (M8851/0) — see Lipoma

Fibroliposarcoma (M8850/3) — see Neoplasm, connective tissue, malignant

Fibroma (M8810/0) — see also Neoplasm, connective tissue, benign
  ameloblastic (M9330/0) D16.5
    upper jaw (bone) D16.4
  bone (nonossifying) — see Disorder, bone, specified type NEC
    ossifying (M9262/0) — see Neoplasm, bone, benign
  cementifying (M9274/0) — see Neoplasm, bone, benign
  chondromyxoid (M9241/0) — see Neoplasm, bone, benign
  desmoplastic (M8823/1) — see Neoplasm, connective tissue, uncertain behavior
  durum (M8810/0) — see Neoplasm, connective tissue, benign
  fascial (M8813/0) — see Neoplasm, connective tissue, benign
  invasive (M8821/1) — see Neoplasm, connective tissue, uncertain behavior
  molle (M8851/0) — see Lipoma
  myxoid (M8811/0) — see Neoplasm, connective tissue, benign
  nasopharynx, nasopharyngeal (juvenile) (M9160/0) D10.6
  nonosteogenic (nonossifying) — see Dysplasia, fibrous
  odontogenic (central) (M9321/0) D16.5
    peripheral (M9322/0) D16.5
      upper jaw (bone) D16.4
    upper jaw (bone) D16.4
  ossifying (M9262/0) — see Neoplasm, bone, benign
  periosteal (M8812/0) — see Neoplasm, bone, benign
  prostate — see Hyperplasia, prostate, localized
  soft (M8851/0) — see Lipoma

Fibromatosis M72.9
  abdominal (M8822/1) — see Neoplasm, connective tissue, uncertain behavior
  aggressive (M8821/1) — see Neoplasm, connective tissue, uncertain behavior
  congenital generalized (M8824/1) — see Neoplasm, connective tissue, uncertain behavior
  Dupuytren's M72.0
  gingival K06.1
  palmar (fascial) M72.0
  plantar (fascial) M72.2
  pseudosarcomatous (proliferative) (subcutaneous) M72.4
  retroperitoneal D48.3
  specified NEC M72.8

Fibromyalgia — see Rheumatism

Fibromyoma (M8890/0) — see also Neoplasm, connective tissue, benign
  uterus (corpus) — see also Leiomyoma, uterus
    in pregnancy or childbirth — see Fibroid, in pregnancy or childbirth
    causing obstructed labor O65.5

Fibromyositis — see Rheumatism

Fibromyxolipoma (M8852/0) D17.9

Fibromyxoma (M8811/0) — see Neoplasm, connective tissue, benign

Fibromyxosarcoma (M8811/3) — see Neoplasm, connective tissue, malignant

Fibro-odontoma, ameloblastic (M9290/0) D16.5
  upper jaw (bone) D16.4

Fibro-osteoma (M9262/0) — see Neoplasm, bone, benign

Fibroplasia, retrolental H35.1

Fibropurulent — see condition

Fibrosarcoma (M8810/3) — see also Neoplasm, connective tissue, malignant
  ameloblastic (M9330/3) C41.1
    upper jaw (bone) C41.0
  congenital (M8814/3) — see Neoplasm, connective tissue, malignant
  fascial (M8813/3) — see Neoplasm, connective tissue, malignant
  infantile (M8814/3) — see Neoplasm, connective tissue, malignant
  odontogenic (M9330/3) C41.1
    upper jaw (bone) C41.0

Fibrosarcoma — see also Neoplasm, connective tissue, malignant — continued
  periosteal (M8812/3) — see Neoplasm, bone, malignant

Fibrosclerosis
  breast N60.30
    left N60.32
    male N60.35
      left N60.34
      right N60.33
    right N60.31
  multifocal M35.5
  penis (corpora cavernosa) N48.6

Fibrosis, fibrotic
  adrenal (gland) E27.8
  amnion — see category O41.8
  anal papillae K62.8
  arteriocapillary — see Arteriosclerosis
  bladder N32.8
    interstitial — see Cystitis, chronic, interstitial
    localized submucosal — see Cystitis, chronic, interstitial
    panmural — see Cystitis, chronic, interstitial
  breast — see Fibrosclerosis, breast
  capillary — see also Arteriosclerosis I70.90
    lung (chronic) — see Fibrosis, lung
  cardiac — see Myocarditis
  cervix N88.8
  chorion — see category O41.8
  corpus cavernosum (sclerosing) N48.6
  cystic (of pancreas) E84.9
    with
      combined manifestations E84.8
      fecal impaction E84.1
      intestinal manifestations E84.1
        due to enzyme replacement therapy E84.20
        distal obstruction syndrome E84.21
        fecal impaction E84.21
        other specified E84.29
      pulmonary manifestations E84.0
    specified NEC E84.8
  due to device, implant or graft (see also Complications, by site and type, specified NEC) T85.82
    arterial graft NEC T82.828
    breast (implant) T85.82
    catheter NEC T85.82
      dialysis (renal) T82.828
        intraperitoneal T85.82
      infusion NEC T82.828
        spinal (epidural) (subdural) T85.82
      urinary (indwelling) T83.82
    electronic (electrode) (pulse generator) (stimulator)
      bone T84.82
      cardiac T82.827
      nervous system (brain) (peripheral nerve) (spinal) T85.82
      urinary T83.82
    fixation, internal (orthopedic) NEC T84.82
    gastrointestinal (bile duct) (esophagus) T85.82
    genital NEC T83.82
    heart NEC T82.827
    joint prosthesis T84.82
    ocular (corneal graft) (orbital implant) NEC T85.82
    orthopedic NEC T84.82
    specified NEC T85.82
    urinary NEC T83.82
    vascular NEC T82.828
    ventricular intracranial shunt T85.82
  ejaculatory duct N50.8
  endocardium — see Endocarditis
  endomyocardial (tropical) I42.3
  epididymis N50.8
  eye muscle — see Strabismus, mechanical
  heart — see Myocarditis
  hepatic — see Fibrosis, liver
  hepatolienal (portal hypertension) K76.6
  hepatosplenic (portal hypertension) K76.6
  infrapatellar fat pad M79.4
  intrascrotal N50.8
  kidney N26.9

©2002 Ingenix, Inc.

Fibrosis, fibrotic — *continued*
  liver K74.0
    with sclerosis K74.2
    alcoholic K70.2
  lung (atrophic) (capillary) (chronic) (confluent)
    (massive) (perialveolar) (peribronchial)
    J84.1
    with
      anthracosilicosis J60
      anthracosis J60
      asbestosis J61
      bagassosis J67.1
      bauxite J63.1
      berylliosis J63.2
      byssinosis J66.0
      calcicosis J62.8
      chalicosis J62.8
      dust reticulation J64
      farmer's lung J67.0
      ganister disease J62.8
      graphite J63.3
      pneumoconiosis NOS J64
      siderosis J63.4
      silicosis J62.8
    congenital P27.8
    diffuse (idiopathic) (interstitial) J84.1
      chemicals, gases, fumes or vapors
        (inhalation) J68.4
      talc J62.0
    following radiation J70.1
    idiopathic J84.1
    postinflammatory J84.1
    silicotic J62.8
    tuberculous — *see* Tuberculosis, pulmonary
  lymphatic gland I89.8
  median bar — *see* Hyperplasia, prostate
  mediastinum (idiopathic) J98.5
  meninges G96.1
  myocardium, myocardial — *see* Myocarditis
  ovary N83.8
  oviduct N83.8
  pancreas K86.8
  penis NEC N48.6
  pericardium I31.0
  perineum, in pregnancy or childbirth — *see*
    Abnormal, vulva in pregnancy and
    childbirth
    causing obstructed labor O65.5
  placenta O43.899
    first trimester O43.891
    second trimester O43.892
    third trimester O43.893
  pleura J94.1
  popliteal fat pad M79.4
  prostate (chronic) — *see* Hyperplasia, prostate
  pulmonary — *see also* Fibrosis, lung
    congenital P27.8
  rectal sphincter K62.8
  retroperitoneal, idiopathic (with ureteral
    obstruction) N13.5
    with infection N13.6
  scrotum N50.8
  seminal vesicle N50.8
  senile R54
  skin L90.5
  spermatic cord N50.8
  spleen D73.8
    in schistosomiasis (bilharziasis) B65.9 *[D77]*
  subepidermal nodular (M8832/0) — *see*
    Neoplasm, skin, benign
  submucous (oral) (tongue) K13.5
  testis N44.8
    chronic, due to syphilis A52.76
  thymus (gland) E32.8
  tongue, submucous K13.5
  tunica vaginalis N50.8
  uterus (non-neoplastic) N85.8
  vagina N89.8
  valve, heart — *see* Endocarditis
  vas deferens N50.8
  vein I87.8

Fibrositis (periarticular) (rheumatoid) — *see*
  Rheumatism
  nodular, chronic (Jaccoud's) (rheumatoid) —
    see Arthropathy, postrheumatic, chronic

Fibrothorax J94.1

Fibrotic — *see* Fibrosis

Fibrous — *see* condition

Fibroxanthoma (M8830/0) — *see also* Neoplasm,
  connective tissue, benign
  atypical (M8830/1) — *see* Neoplasm,
    connective tissue, uncertain behavior
  malignant (M8830/3) — *see* Neoplasm,
    connective tissue, malignant

Fibroxanthosarcoma (M8830/3) — *see* Neoplasm,
  connective tissue, malignant

Fiedler's
  disease (icterohemorrhagic leptospirosis) A27.0
  myocarditis (acute) I40.1

Fifth disease B08.3
  venereal A55

Filaria, filarial, filariasis — *see* Infestation,
  filarial

Filatov's disease — *see* Mononucleosis, infectious

File-cutter's disease — *see* Poisoning, lead

Filling defect
  biliary tract R93.2
  bladder R93.4
  duodenum R93.3
  gallbladder R93.2
  gastrointestinal tract R93.3
  intestine R93.3
  kidney R93.4
  stomach R93.3
  ureter R93.4

Fimbrial cyst Q50.4

Financial problem affecting care NOS Z59.9
  bankruptcy Z59.8
  foreclosure on loan Z59.8

Findings, abnormal, without diagnosis
  17-ketosteroids, elevated R82.5
  acetonuria R82.4
  alcohol in blood R78.0
  anisocytosis R71.8
  bacteriuria N39.0
  bicarbonate E87.8
  bile in urine R82.2
  blood sugar (high) R73.0
    low E16.2
  casts, urine R82.99
  catecholamines R82.5
  cells, urine R82.99
  chloride E87.8
  chyluria R82.0
  cloudy
    dialysis effluent R88.0
    urine R82.90
  crystals, urine R82.99
  echocardiogram R93.1
  electrolyte level, urinary R82.99
  function study NEC R94.8
    bladder R94.8
    endocrine NEC R94.7
      thyroid R94.6
    kidney R94.4
    liver R94.5
    pancreas R94.8
    placenta R94.8
    pulmonary R94.2
    spleen R94.8
  gallbladder, nonvisualization R93.2
  glucose (tolerance test) R73.0
  glycosuria R81
  heart
    shadow R93.1
    sounds R01.2
  hematinuria R82.3
  hematocrit drop (precipitous) R71.0
  hemoglobinuria R82.3
  in blood (of substance not normally found in
    blood) R78.9
    addictive drug NEC R78.4
    alcohol (excessive level) R78.0
    cocaine R78.2
    hallucinogen R78.3
    heavy metals (abnormal level) R78.7
    lithium (abnormal level) R78.89
    opiate drug R78.1
    psychotropic drug R78.5
    specified substance NEC R78.89
    steroid agent R78.6

Findings, abnormal, without diagnosis —
  continued
  indolacetic acid, elevated R82.5
  ketonuria R82.4
  lactic acid dehydrogenase (LDH) R74.0
  mammogram R92.8
    microcalcification R92.0
  mediastinal shift R93.1
  melanin, urine R82.99
  myoglobinuria R82.1
  nonvisualization of gallbladder R93.2
  odor of urine NOS R82.90
  Papanicolaou cervix R87.6
  pneumoencephalogram R93.0
  poikilocytosis R71.8
  potassium (deficiency) E87.6
    excess E87.5
  PPD R76.1
  radiologic (X-ray) R93.8
    abdomen R93.5
    biliary tract R93.2
    breast R92.8
    gastrointestinal tract R93.3
    genitourinary organs R93.4
    head R93.0
    intrathoracic organs NEC R93.1
    placenta R93.8
    retroperitoneum R93.5
    skin R93.8
    skull R93.0
    subcutaneous tissue R93.8
  red blood cell (count) (morphology) (sickling)
    (volume) R71.8
  scan NEC R94.8
    bladder R94.8
    bone R94.8
    kidney R94.4
    liver R94.5
    lung R94.2
    pancreas R94.8
    placental R94.8
    spleen R94.8
    thyroid R94.6
  sedimentation rate, elevated R70.0
  SGOT R74.0
  SGPT R74.0
  sodium (deficiency) E87.1
    excess E87.0
  specified body fluid NEC R88.8
  thyroid (function) (metabolic rate) (scan)
    (uptake) R94.6
  transaminase (level) R74.0
  tuberculin skin test (without active
    tuberculosis) R76.1
  urine R82.90
    acetone R82.4
    bacteria N39.0
    bile R82.2
    casts or cells R82.99
    chyle R82.0
    culture positive R82.7
    glucose R81
    hemoglobin R82.3
    ketone R82.4
    sugar R81
  vanillylmandelic acid (VMA), elevated R82.5
  vectorcardiogram (VCG) R93.1
  ventriculogram R93.0
  white blood cell (count) (differential)
    (morphology) D72.9
  xerography R92.8

Finger — *see* condition

Fire, Saint Anthony's — *see* Erysipelas

Fire-setting
  pathological (compulsive) F63.1
  without manifest psychiatric disorder Z03.8

Fish hook stomach K31.89

Fishmeal-worker's lung J67.8

Fissure, fissured
  anus, anal K60.2
    acute K60.0
    chronic K60.1
    congenital Q43.8
  ear, lobule, congenital Q17.8
  epiglottis (congenital) Q31.8

Fissure, fissured — *continued*
  larynx J38.7
    congenital Q31.8
  lip K13.0
    congenital — *see* Cleft, lip
  nipple N64.0
    associated with
      lactation O92.13
      pregnancy O92.119
        first trimester O92.111
        second trimester O92.112
        third trimester O92.113
      puerperium O92.12
  nose Q30.2
  palate (congenital) — *see* Cleft, palate
  skin R23.4
  spine (congenital) — *see also* Spina bifida
    with hydrocephalus — *see* Spina bifida, by
      site, with hydrocephalus
  tongue (acquired) K14.5
    congenital Q38.3

Fistula (cutaneous) L98.8
  abdomen (wall) K63.2
    bladder N32.2
    intestine NEC K63.2
    ureter N28.89
    uterus N82.5
  abdominorectal K63.2
  abdominosigmoidal K63.2
  abdominothoracic J86.0
  abdominouterine N82.5
    congenital Q51.7
  abdominovesical N32.2
  accessory sinuses — *see* Sinusitis
  actinomycotic — *see* Actinomycosis
  alveolar antrum — *see* Sinusitis, maxillary
  alveolar process K04.6
  anorectal K60.5
  antrobuccal — *see* Sinusitis, maxillary
  antrum — *see* Sinusitis, maxillary
  anus, anal (recurrent) (infectional) K60.3
    congenital Q43.6
      with absence, atresia and stenosis Q42.2
    tuberculous A18.32
  aorta-duodenal I77.2
  appendix, appendicular K38.3
  arteriovenous (acquired) (nonruptured) I77.0
    brain I67.1
      congenital Q28.2
        ruptured I60.8
      ruptured I60.8
    cerebral — *see* Fistula, arteriovenous, brain
    congenital (peripheral) — *see also*
      Malformation, arteriovenous
      brain Q28.2
        ruptured I60.8
      coronary Q24.5
      pulmonary Q25.7
    coronary I25.4
      congenital Q24.5
    pulmonary I28.0
      congenital Q25.7
    surgically created (for dialysis) Z99.2
      complication — *see* Complication,
        arteriovenous, fistula, surgically
        created
      traumatic — *see* Injury, blood vessel
  artery I77.2
  aural (mastoid) — *see* Mastoiditis, chronic
  auricle — *see also* Disorder, pinna, specified
    type NEC
    congenital Q18.1
  Bartholin's gland N82.8
  bile duct (common) (hepatic) K83.3
    with calculus, stones — *see* Calculus, bile
      duct
  biliary (tract) — *see* Fistula, bile duct
  bladder (sphincter) NEC (*see also* Fistula,
    vesico-) N32.2
    into seminal vesicle N32.2
  bone — *see also* Disorder, bone, specified type
    NEC
    with osteomyelitis, chronic — *see*
      Osteomyelitis, chronic, with draining
      sinus

Fistula — *continued*
  brain G93.8
    arteriovenous (acquired) I67.1
      congenital Q28.2
  branchial (cleft) Q18.0
  branchiogenous Q18.0
  breast N61
    puerperal, postpartum or gestational, due to
      mastitis (purulent) — *see* Mastitis,
      obstetric, purulent
  bronchial J86.0
  bronchocutaneous, bronchomediastinal,
    bronchopleural,
    bronchopleuromediastinal (infective)
    J86.0
    tuberculous NEC A15.5
  bronchoesophageal J86.0
    congenital Q39.2
      with atresia of esophagus Q39.1
  bronchovisceral J86.0
  buccal cavity (infective) K12.2
  cecosigmoidal K63.2
  cecum K63.2
  cerebrospinal (fluid) G96.0
  cervical, lateral Q18.1
  cervicoaural Q18.1
  cervicosigmoidal N82.4
  cervicovesical N82.1
  cervix N82.8
  chest (wall) J86.0
  cholecystenteric — *see* Fistula, gallbladder
  cholecystocolic — *see* Fistula, gallbladder
  cholecystocolonic — *see* Fistula, gallbladder
  cholecystoduodenal — *see* Fistula, gallbladder
  cholecystogastric — *see* Fistula, gallbladder
  cholecystointestinal — *see* Fistula, gallbladder
  choledochoduodenal — *see* Fistula, bile duct
  cholocolic K82.3
  coccyx — *see* Sinus, pilonidal
  colon K63.2
  colostomy K94.09
  common duct — *see* Fistula, bile duct
  congenital, site not listed — *see* Anomaly, by
    site
  coronary, arteriovenous I25.4
    congenital Q24.5
  costal region J86.0
  cul-de-sac, Douglas' N82.8
  cystic duct — *see also* Fistula, gallbladder
    congenital Q44.5
  dental K04.6
  diaphragm J86.0
  duodenum K31.6
  ear (external) (canal) — *see* Disorder, ear,
    external, specified type NEC
  enterocolic K63.2
  enterocutaneous K63.2
  enterouterine N82.4
    congenital Q51.7
  enterovaginal N82.4
    congenital Q52.2
    large intestine N82.3
    small intestine N82.2
  enterovesical N32.1
  epididymis N50.8
    tuberculous A18.15
  esophagobronchial J86.0
    congenital Q39.2
      with atresia of esophagus Q39.1
  esophagocutaneous K22.8
  esophagopleural-cutaneous J86.0
  esophagotracheal J86.0
    congenital Q39.2
      with atresia of esophagus Q39.1
  esophagus K22.8
    congenital Q39.2
      with atresia of esophagus Q39.1
  ethmoid — *see* Sinusitis, ethmoidal
  eyeball (cornea) (sclera) — *see* Disorder, globe,
    hypotony
  eyelid H01.8
  fallopian tube, external N82.5
  fecal K63.2
    congenital Q43.6
  from periapical abscess K04.6
  frontal sinus — *see* Sinusitis, frontal

Fistula — *continued*
  gallbladder K82.3
    with calculus, cholelithiasis, stones — *see*
      Calculus, gallbladder
  gastric K31.6
  gastrocolic K31.6
    congenital Q40.2
    tuberculous A18.32
  gastroenterocolic K31.6
  gastroesophageal K31.6
  gastrojejunal K31.6
  gastrojejunocolic K31.6
  genital tract (female) N82.9
    specified NEC N82.8
    to intestine NEC N82.4
    to skin N82.5
  hepatic artery-portal vein, congenital Q26.6
  hepatopleural J86.0
  hepatopulmonary J86.0
  ileorectal or ileosigmoidal K63.2
  ileovaginal N82.2
  ileovesical N32.1
  ileum K63.2
  in ano K60.3
    tuberculous A18.32
  inner ear (labyrinth) — *see* category H83.1
  intestine NEC K63.2
  intestinocolonic (abdominal) K63.2
  intestinoureteral N28.89
  intestinouterine N82.4
  intestinovaginal N82.4
    large intestine N82.3
    small intestine N82.2
  intestinovesical N32.1
  ischiorectal (fossa) K61.3
  jejunum K63.2
  joint M25.10
    ankle M25.173
      left M25.172
      right M25.171
    elbow M25.129
      left M25.122
      right M25.121
    foot joint M25.176
      left M25.175
      right M25.174
    hand joint M25.149
      left M25.142
      right M25.141
    hip M25.159
      left M25.152
      right M25.151
    knee M25.169
      left M25.162
      right M25.161
    shoulder M25.119
      left M25.112
      right M25.111
    specified joint NEC M25.18
    tuberculous — *see* Tuberculosis, joint
    wrist M25.139
      left M25.132
      right M25.131
  kidney N28.89
  labium (majus) (minus) N82.8
  labyrinth — *see* category H83.1
  lacrimal (gland) (sac) H04.619
    bilateral H04.613
    left H04.612
    right H04.611
  lacrimonasal duct — *see* Fistula, lacrimal
  laryngotracheal, congenital Q34.8
  larynx J38.7
  lip K13.0
    congenital Q38.0
  lumbar, tuberculous A18.01
  lung J86.0
  lymphatic I89.8
  mammary (gland) N61
  mastoid (process) (region) — *see* Mastoiditis,
    chronic
  maxillary J32.0
  medial, face and neck Q18.8
  mediastinal J86.0
  mediastinobronchial J86.0
  mediastinocutaneous J86.0
  middle ear — *see* category H74.8

©2002 Ingenix, Inc.

Fistula — continued
  mouth K12.2
  nasal J34.8
    sinus — *see* Sinusitis
  nasopharynx J39.2
  nipple N64.0
  nose J34.8
  oral (cutaneous) K12.2
    maxillary J32.0
    nasal (with cleft palate) — *see* Cleft, palate
  orbit, orbital — *see* Disorder, orbit, specified
    type NEC
  oroantral J32.0
  oviduct, external N82.5
  palate (hard) M27.8
  pancreatic K86.8
  pancreaticoduodenal K86.8
  parotid (gland) K11.4
    region K12.2
  penis N48.89
  perianal K60.3
  pericardium (pleura) (sac) — *see* Pericarditis
  pericecal K63.2
  perineorectal K60.4
  perineosigmoidal K63.2
  perineum, perineal (with urethral involvement)
    NEC N36.0
    tuberculous A18.13
    ureter N28.89
  perirectal K60.4
    tuberculous A18.32
  peritoneum K65.9
  pharyngoesophageal J39.2
  pharynx J39.2
    branchial cleft (congenital) Q18.0
  pilonidal (infected) (rectum) — *see* Sinus,
    pilonidal
  pleura, pleural, pleurocutaneous,
    pleuroperitoneal J86.0
    tuberculous NEC A15.6
  pleuropericardial I31.8
  portal vein-hepatic artery, congenital Q26.6
  postauricular H70.819
    bilateral H70.813
    left H70.812
    right H70.811
  postoperative, persistent T81.83
    specified site — *see* Fistula, by site
  preauricular (congenital) Q18.1
  prostate N42.89
  pulmonary J86.0
    arteriovenous I28.0
      congenital Q25.7
    tuberculous — *see* Tuberculosis, pulmonary
  pulmonoperitoneal J86.0
  rectolabial N82.4
  rectosigmoid (intercommunicating) K63.2
  rectoureteral N28.89
  rectourethral N36.0
    congenital Q64.73
  rectouterine N82.4
    congenital Q51.7
  rectovaginal N82.3
    congenital Q52.2
    tuberculous A18.18
  rectovesical N32.1
    congenital Q64.79
  rectovesicovaginal N82.3
  rectovulval N82.4
    congenital Q52.79
  rectum (to skin) K60.4
    congenital Q43.6
      with absence, atresia and stenosis Q42.0
    tuberculous A18.32
  renal N28.89
  retroauricular — *see* Fistula, postauricular
  salivary duct or gland (any) K11.4
    congenital Q38.4
  scrotum (urinary) N50.8
    tuberculous A18.15
  semicircular canals — *see* category H83.1
  sigmoid K63.2
    to bladder N32.1
  sinus — *see* Sinusitis
  skin L98.8
    to genital tract (female) N82.5
  splenocolic D73.8
  stercoral K63.2

Fistula — continued
  stomach K31.6
  sublingual gland K11.4
  submandibular gland K11.4
  submaxillary (gland) K11.4
    region K12.2
  thoracic J86.0
    duct I89.8
  thoracoabdominal J86.0
  thoracogastric J86.0
  thoracointestinal J86.0
  thorax J86.0
  thyroglossal duct Q89.2
  thyroid E07.89
  trachea, congenital (external) (internal) Q32.1
  tracheoesophageal J86.0
    congenital Q39.2
      with atresia of esophagus Q39.1
    following tracheostomy J95.04
  traumatic arteriovenous — *see* Injury, blood
    vessel, by site
  tuberculous – code by site under Tuberculosis
  typhoid A01.09
  umbilicourinary Q64.8
  urachus, congenital Q64.4
  ureter (persistent) N28.89
  ureteroabdominal N28.89
  ureterorectal N28.89
  ureterosigmoido-abdominal N28.89
  ureterovaginal N82.1
  ureterovesical N32.2
  urethra N36.0
    congenital Q64.79
    tuberculous A18.13
  urethroperineal N36.0
  urethroperineovesical N32.2
  urethrorectal N36.0
    congenital Q64.73
  urethroscrotal N50.8
  urethrovaginal N82.1
  urethrovesical N32.2
  urinary (tract) (persistent) (recurrent) N36.0
  uteroabdominal N82.5
    congenital Q51.7
  uteroenteric, uterointestinal N82.4
    congenital Q51.7
  uterorectal N82.4
    congenital Q51.7
  uteroureteric N82.1
  uterourethral Q51.7
  uterovaginal N82.8
  uterovesical N82.1
    congenital Q51.7
  uterus N82.8
  vagina (postpartal) (wall) N82.8
  vaginocutaneous (postpartal) N82.5
  vaginointestinal NEC N82.4
    large intestine N82.3
    small intestine N82.2
  vaginoperineal N82.5
  vasocutaneous, congenital Q55.7
  vesical NEC N32.2
  vesicoabdominal N32.2
  vesicocervicovaginal N82.1
  vesicocolic N32.1
  vesicocutaneous N32.2
  vesicoenteric N32.1
  vesicointestinal N32.1
  vesicometrorectal N82.4
  vesicoperineal N32.2
  vesicorectal N32.1
    congenital Q64.79
  vesicosigmoidal N32.1
  vesicosigmoidovaginal N82.3
  vesicoureteral N32.2
  vesicoureterovaginal N82.1
  vesicourethral N32.2
  vesicourethrorectal N32.1
  vesicouterine N82.1
    congenital Q51.7
  vesicovaginal N82.0
  vulvorectal N82.4
    congenital Q52.79

Fit R56.9
  apoplectic I64
  epileptic — *see* Epilepsy
  fainting R55

Fit — continued
  hysterical F44.5
  newborn P90
Fitting (of)
  artificial
    arm — *see* Admission, adjustment, artificial,
      arm
    breast Z44.3
    eye Z44.2
    leg — *see* Admission, adjustment, artificial,
      leg
  brain neuropacemaker Z46.2
    implanted Z45.42
  colostomy belt Z46.8
  contact lenses Z46.0
  cystostomy device Z46.6
  dentures Z46.3
  device NOS Z46.9
    abdominal Z46.8
    nervous system Z46.2
      implanted — *see* Admission, adjustment,
        device, implanted, nervous system
    orthodontic Z46.4
    orthoptic Z46.0
    orthotic Z46.8
    prosthetic (external) Z44.9
      breast Z44.3
      dental Z46.3
      eye Z44.2
      specified NEC Z44.8
    specified NEC Z46.8
    substitution
      auditory Z46.2
        implanted — *see* Admission,
          adjustment, device, implanted,
          hearing device
      nervous system Z46.2
        implanted — *see* Admission,
          adjustment, device, implanted,
          nervous system
      visual Z46.2
        implanted Z45.31
      urinary Z46.6
  glasses (reading) Z46.0
  hearing aid Z46.1
  ileostomy device Z46.8
  intestinal appliance NEC Z46.8
  neuropacemaker Z46.2
    implanted Z45.42
  orthodontic device Z46.4
  orthopedic device (brace) (cast) (corset) (shoes)
    Z46.8
  pacemaker (cardiac) Z45.018
    nervous system (brain) (peripheral nerve)
      (spinal cord) Z46.2
      implanted Z45.42
    pulse generator Z45.010
  prosthesis (external) Z44.9
    arm — *see* Admission, adjustment, artificial,
      arm
    breast Z44.3
    dental Z46.3
    eye Z44.2
    leg — *see* Admission, adjustment, artificial,
      leg
    specified NEC Z44.8
  spectacles Z46.0
  wheelchair Z46.8

Fitzhugh-Curtis syndrome (gonococcal) A54.85

Fitz's syndrome (acute hemorrhagic pancreatitis)
  K85.8

Fixation
  joint — *see* Ankylosis
  larynx J38.7
  stapes — *see* Ankylosis, ear ossicles
    deafness — *see* Deafness, conductive
  uterus (acquired) — *see* Malposition, uterus
  vocal cord J38.3

Flabby ridge K06.8

Flaccid — *see also* condition
  palate, congenital Q38.5

Flail
  chest S22.59
    bilateral S22.53
    left S22.52
    newborn (birth injury) P13.8

Flail — continued
  chest — continued
    right S22.51
  joint (paralytic) M25.20
    ankle M25.279
      left M25.272
      right M25.271
    elbow M25.229
      left M25.222
      right M25.221
    foot joint M25.279
      left M25.272
      right M25.271
    hand joint M25.249
      left M25.242
      right M25.241
    hip M25.259
      left M25.252
      right M25.251
    knee M25.269
      left M25.262
      right M25.261
    shoulder M25.219
      left M25.212
      right M25.211
    specified joint NEC M25.28
    wrist M25.239
      left M25.232
      right M25.231

Flajani's disease — see Hyperthyroidism, with, goiter (diffuse)

Flashbacks (residual to hallucinogen use) F16.283

Flap, liver K71.3

Flat
  chamber (eye) — see Disorder, globe, hypotony, flat anterior chamber
  chest, congenital Q67.8
  foot (acquired) (fixed type) (painful) (postural) — see also Deformity, limb, flat foot
    congenital Q66.5
    rachitic (late effect) E64.3
    rocker bottom Q66.5
    rigid Q66.5
    spastic (everted) Q66.5
    vertical talus, congenital Q66.5
  organ or site, congenital NEC — see Anomaly, by site
  pelvis M95.5
    with disproportion (fetopelvic) O33.0
      causing obstructed labor O65.0
    congenital Q74.2

Flatau-Schilder disease G37.0

Flatback syndrome M40.30
  lumbar region M40.36
  lumbosacral region M40.37
  sacrococcygeal region M40.38
  thoracolumbar region M40.35

Flattening
  head, femur M89.85
  hip — see Coxa, plana
  lip (congenital) Q18.8
  nose (congenital) Q67.4
    acquired M95.0

Flatulence R14.3
  psychogenic F45.8

Flatus R14.3
  vaginalis N89.8

Flax-dresser's disease J66.1

Flea bite — see Injury, bite, insect

Flecks, glaucomatous (subcapsular) — see Cataract, complicated

Fleischer (-Kayser) ring (cornea) — see Kayser-Fleischer ring

Fleshy mole O02.0

Flexibilitas cerea — see Catalepsy

Flexion
  cervix — see Malposition, uterus
  contracture, joint — see Contraction, joint
  deformity, joint — see also Deformity, flexion
    hip (congenital) Q65.8
  uterus — see also Malposition, uterus
    lateral   see Lateroversion, uterus

Flexner-Boyd dysentery A03.2

Flexner's dysentery A03.1

Flexure — see Flexion

Flint murmur (aortic insufficiency) I35.1

Floater, vitreous — see Opacity, vitreous

Floating
  cartilage (joint) — see also Loose, body, joint
    knee — see Derangement, knee, loose body
  gallbladder, congenital Q44.1
  kidney N28.89
    congenital Q63.8
  spleen D73.8

Flooding N92.0

Floor — see condition

Floppy baby syndrome (nonspecific) P94.2

Flu — see also Influenza
  intestinal NEC A08.4

Fluctuating blood pressure I99.8

Fluid
  abdomen R18
  chest J94.8
  heart — see Failure, heart, congestive
  joint — see Effusion, joint
  loss (acute) E86.9
    with
      hypernatremia E87.0
      hyponatremia E87.1
  lung — see Edema, lung
  peritoneal cavity R18
  pleural cavity J94.8
  retention E87.7

Flukes NEC — see also Infestation, fluke
  blood NEC — see Schistosomiasis
  liver B66.3

Fluor (vaginalis) N89.8
  trichomonal or due to Trichomonas (vaginalis) A59.00

Fluorosis
  dental K00.3
  skeletal M85.10
    ankle M85.179
      left M85.172
      right M85.171
    foot M85.179
      left M85.172
      right M85.171
    forearm M85.139
      left M85.132
      right M85.131
    hand M85.149
      left M85.142
      right M85.141
    lower leg M85.169
      left M85.162
      right M85.161
    multiple site M85.19
    neck M85.18
    rib M85.18
    shoulder M85.119
      left M85.112
      right M85.111
    skull M85.18
    specified site NEC M85.18
    thigh M85.159
      left M85.152
      right M85.151
    toe M85.179
      left M85.172
      right M85.171
    upper arm M85.129
      left M85.122
      right M85.121
    vertebra M85.18

Flush syndrome E34.0

Flushing R23.2
  menopausal N95.1

Flutter
  atrial or auricular I48.1
  heart I49.02
  ventricular I49.02

Fochier's abscess – code by site under Abscess

Focus, Assmann's — see Tuberculosis, pulmonary

Fogo selvagem L10.3

Foix-Alajouanine syndrome G95.19

Fold, folds (anomalous) — see also Anomaly, by site
  Descemet's membrane — see Change, corneal membrane, Descemet's, fold
  epicanthic Q10.3
  heart Q24.8

Folie à deux F24

Follicle
  cervix (nabothian) (ruptured) N88.8
  graafian, ruptured, with hemorrhage N83.0
  nabothian N88.8

Follicular — see condition

Folliculitis (superficial) L73.9
  abscedens et suffodiens L66.3
  cyst N83.0
  decalvans L66.2
  deep — see Furuncle, by site
  gonococcal (acute) (chronic) A54.01
  keloid, keloidalis L73.0
  pustular L01.02
  ulerythematosa reticulata L66.4

Folliculome lipidique (M8641/0)
  specified site — see Neoplasm, benign
  unspecified site
    female D27.9
    male D29.20

Følling's disease E70.0

Follow-up — see Examination, follow-up

Fong's syndrome (hereditary osteo-onychodysplasia) Q78.5

Food
  allergy L27.2
  asphyxia (from aspiration or inhalation) — see Asphyxia, food
  choked on — see Asphyxia, food
  deprivation T73.0
    specified kind of food NEC E63.8
  intoxication — see Poisoning, food
  lack of T73.0
  poisoning — see Poisoning, food
  rejection NEC — see Disorder, eating
  strangulation or suffocation — see Asphyxia, food
  toxemia — see Poisoning, food

Foot — see condition

Foramen ovale (nonclosure) (patent) (persistent) Q21.1

Forbes' glycogen storage disease E74.03

Fordyce-Fox disease L75.2

Fordyce's disease (mouth) Q38.6

Forearm — see condition

Foreign body
  with
    laceration — see Laceration, with foreign body, by site
    puncture wound — see Puncture, with foreign body, by site
  accidentally left following a procedure T81.509
    aspiration T81.506
      resulting in
        adhesions T81.516
        obstruction T81.526
        perforation T81.536
        specified complication NEC T81.596
    cardiac catheterization T81.505
      resulting in
        acute reaction T81.60
          aseptic peritonitis T81.61
          specified NEC T81.69
        adhesions T81.515
        obstruction T81.525
        perforation T81.535
        specified complication NEC T81.595
    endoscopy T81.504
      resulting in
        adhesions T81.514
        obstruction T81.524
        perforation T81.534
        specified complication NEC T81.594
    immunization T81.503
      resulting in
        adhesions T81.513
        obstruction T81.523

Foreign body — *continued*
  accidentally left following a procedure —
    continued
    immunization — *continued*
      resulting in — *continued*
        perforation T81.533
        specified complication NEC T81.593
    infusion T81.501
      resulting in
        adhesions T81.511
        obstruction T81.521
        perforation T81.531
        specified complication NEC T81.591
    injection T81.503
      resulting in
        adhesions T81.513
        obstruction T81.523
        perforation T81.533
        specified complication NEC T81.593
    kidney dialysis T81.502
      resulting in
        adhesions T81.512
        obstruction T81.522
        perforation T81.532
        specified complication NEC T81.592
    packing removal T81.507
      resulting in
        acute reaction T81.60
          aseptic peritonitis T81.61
          specified NEC T81.69
        adhesions T81.517
        obstruction T81.527
        perforation T81.537
        specified complication NEC T81.597
    puncture T81.506
      resulting in
        adhesions T81.516
        obstruction T81.526
        perforation T81.536
        specified complication NEC T81.596
    specified procedure NEC T81.508
      resulting in
        acute reaction T81.60
          aseptic peritonitis T81.61
          specified NEC T81.69
        adhesions T81.518
        obstruction T81.528
        perforation T81.538
        specified complication NEC T81.598
    surgical operation T81.500
      resulting in
        acute reaction T81.60
          aseptic peritonitis T81.61
          specified NEC T81.69
        adhesions T81.510
        obstruction T81.520
        perforation T81.530
        specified complication NEC T81.590
    transfusion T81.501
      resulting in
        adhesions T81.511
        obstruction T81.521
        perforation T81.531
        specified complication NEC T81.591
    causing
      acute reaction T81.60
        aseptic peritonitis T81.61
        specified complication NEC T81.69
      adhesions T81.519
      aseptic peritonitis T81.61
      obstruction T81.529
      perforation T81.539
      specified complication NEC T81.599
  alimentary tract T18.9
    anus T18.5
    colon T18.4
    esophagus — *see* Foreign body, esophagus
    mouth T18.0
    multiple sites T18.8
    rectosigmoid (junction) T18.5
    rectum T18.5
    small intestine T18.3
    specified site NEC T18.8
    stomach T18.2
  anterior chamber (eye) S05.50
    left S05.52

Foreign body — *continued*
  anterior chamber — *continued*
    right S05.51
  auditory canal — *see* Foreign body, entering
    through orifice, ear
  bronchus T17.508
    causing
      asphyxiation T17.500
        food (bone) (*seed*) T17.520
        gastric contents (vomitus) T17.510
        specified type NEC T17.590
      injury NEC T17.508
        food (bone) (*seed*) T17.528
        gastric contents (vomitus) T17.518
        specified type NEC T17.598
  canthus — *see* Foreign body, conjunctival sac
  ciliary body (eye) S05.50
    left S05.52
    right S05.51
  conjunctival sac T15.10
    left T15.12
    right T15.11
  cornea T15.00
    left T15.02
    right T15.01
  entering through orifice
    accessory sinus T17.0
    alimentary canal T18.9
      multiple parts T18.8
      specified part NEC T18.8
    alveolar process T18.0
    antrum (Highmore's) T17.0
    anus T18.5
    appendix T18.4
    auditory canal — *see* Foreign body, entering
      through orifice, ear
    auricle — *see* Foreign body, entering
      through orifice, ear
    bladder T19.1
    bronchioles — *see* Foreign body, respiratory
      tract, specified site NEC
    bronchus (main) — *see* Foreign body,
      bronchus
    buccal cavity T18.0
    canthus (inner) — *see* Foreign body,
      conjunctival sac
    cecum T18.4
    cervix (canal) (uteri) T19.3
    colon T18.4
    conjunctival sac — *see* Foreign body,
      conjunctival sac
    cornea — *see* Foreign body, cornea
    digestive organ or tract NOS T18.9
      multiple parts T18.8
      specified part NEC T18.8
    duodenum T18.3
    ear (external) T16.9
      left T16.2
      right T16.1
    esophagus — *see* Foreign body, esophagus
    eye (external) NOS T15.90
      conjunctival sac — *see* Foreign body,
        conjunctival sac
      cornea — *see* Foreign body, cornea
      left T15.92
        specified part NEC T15.82
      right T15.91
        specified part NEC T15.81
      specified part NEC T15.80
    eyeball — *see also* Foreign body, entering
      through orifice, eye, specified part NEC
      with penetrating wound — *see* Puncture,
        eyeball
    eyelid — *see also* Foreign body, conjunctival
      sac
      with
        laceration — *see* Laceration, eyelid,
          with foreign body
        puncture — *see* Puncture, eyelid, with
          foreign body
        superficial injury — *see* Foreign body,
          superficial, eyelid
    gastrointestinal tract T18.9
      multiple parts T18.8
      specified part NEC T18.8
    genitourinary tract T19.9
      multiple parts T19.8

Foreign body — *continued*
  entering through orifice — *continued*
    genitourinary tract — *continued*
      specified part NEC T19.8
    globe — *see* Foreign body, entering through
      orifice, eyeball
    gum T18.0
    Highmore's antrum T17.0
    hypopharynx — *see* Foreign body, pharynx
    ileum T18.3
    intestine (small) T18.3
      large T18.4
    lacrimal apparatus (punctum) — *see* Foreign
      body, entering through orifice, eye,
      specified part NEC
    large intestine T18.4
    larynx — *see* Foreign body, larynx
    lung — *see* Foreign body, respiratory tract,
      specified site NEC
    maxillary sinus T17.0
    mouth T18.0
    nasal sinus T17.0
    nasopharynx — *see* Foreign body, pharynx
    nose (passage) T17.1
    nostril T17.1
    oral cavity T18.0
    palate T18.0
    penis T19.8
    pharynx — *see* Foreign body, pharynx
    piriform sinus — *see* Foreign body, pharynx
    rectosigmoid (junction) T18.5
    rectum T18.5
    respiratory tract — *see* Foreign body,
      respiratory tract
    sinus (accessory) (frontal) (maxillary) (nasal)
      T17.0
      piriform — *see* Foreign body, pharynx
    small intestine T18.3
    stomach T18.2
    suffocation by — *see* Asphyxia, food
    tear ducts or glands — *see* Foreign body,
      entering through orifice, eye, specified
      part NEC
    throat — *see* Foreign body, pharynx
    tongue T18.0
    tonsil, tonsillar (fossa) — *see* Foreign body,
      pharynx
    trachea — *see* Foreign body, trachea
    ureter T19.8
    urethra T19.0
    uterus (any part) T19.3
    vagina T19.2
    vulva T19.2
  esophagus T18.108
    causing
      injury NEC T18.108
        food (bone) (*seed*) T18.128
        gastric contents (vomitus) T18.118
        specified type NEC T18.198
      tracheal compression T18.100
        food (bone) (*seed*) T18.120
        gastric contents (vomitus) T18.110
        specified type NEC T18.190
  genitourinary tract T19.9
    bladder T19.1
    multiple parts T19.8
    penis T19.4
    specified site NEC T19.8
    urethra T19.0
    uterus T19.3
      IUD Z97.5
    vagina T19.2
      contraceptive device Z97.5
    vulva T19.2
  granuloma (old) (soft tissue) — *see also*
    Granuloma, foreign body
    skin L92.3
  in
    laceration — *see* Laceration, by site, with
      foreign body
    puncture wound — *see* Puncture, by site,
      with foreign body
    soft tissue (residual) M79.5
  inadvertently left in operation wound — *see*
    Foreign body, accidentally left during a
    procedure
  ingestion, ingested NOS T18.9

Foreign body — *continued*
  superficial, without major open wound —
    continued
    eyelid — *continued*
      right S00.251
    face S00.85
    finger(s) S60.459
      index S60.458
        left S60.451
        right S60.450
      little S60.458
        left S60.457
        right S60.456
      middle S60.458
        left S60.453
        right S60.452
      ring S60.458
        left S60.455
        right S60.454
    flank S30.851
    foot (except toe(s) alone) S90.859
      left S90.852
      right S90.851
      toe — *see* Foreign body, superficial, toe
    forearm S50.859
      elbow only — *see* Foreign body,
        superficial, elbow
      left S50.852
      right S50.851
    forehead S00.85
    genital organs, external
      female S30.856
      male S30.855
    groin S30.851
    gum S00.552
    hand S60.559
      left S60.552
      right S60.551
    head S00.95
      ear — *see* Foreign body, superficial, ear
      eyelid — *see* Foreign body, superficial,
        eyelid
      lip S00.551
      nose S00.35
      oral cavity S00.552
      scalp S00.05
      specified site NEC S00.85
    heel — *see* Foreign body, superficial, foot
    hip S70.259
      left S70.252
      right S70.251
    inguinal region S30.851
    interscapular region S20.459
    jaw S00.85
    knee S80.259
      left S80.252
      right S80.251
    labium (majus) (minus) S30.854
    larynx S10.15
    leg (lower) S80.859
      knee — *see* Foreign body, superficial,
        knee
      left S80.852
      right S80.851
      upper — *see* Foreign body, superficial,
        thigh
    lip S00.551
    lower back S30.850
    lumbar region S30.850
    malar region S00.85
    mammary — *see* Foreign body, superficial,
      breast
    mastoid region S00.85
    mouth S00.552
    nail
      finger — *see* Foreign body, superficial,
        finger
      toe — *see* Foreign body, superficial, toe
    nape S10.85
    nasal S00.35
    neck S10.95
      specified site NEC S10.85
      throat S10.15
    nose S00.35
    occipital region S00.05
    oral cavity S00.552

Foreign body — *continued*
  superficial, without major open wound —
    continued
    orbital region — *see* Foreign body,
      superficial, eyelid
    palate S00.552
    palm — *see* Foreign body, superficial, hand
    parietal region S00.05
    pelvis S30.850
    penis S30.852
    perineum
      female S30.854
      male S30.850
    periocular area — *see* Foreign body,
      superficial, eyelid
    phalanges
      finger — *see* Foreign body, superficial,
        finger
      toe — *see* Foreign body, superficial, toe
    pharynx S10.15
    pinna — *see* Foreign body, superficial, ear
    popliteal space — *see* Foreign body,
      superficial, knee
    prepuce S30.852
    pubic region S30.850
    pudendum
      female S30.856
      male S30.855
    sacral region S30.850
    scalp S00.05
    scapular region — *see* Foreign body,
      superficial, shoulder
    scrotum S30.853
    shin — *see* Foreign body, superficial, leg
    shoulder S40.259
      left S40.252
      right S40.251
    sternal region S20.359
    submaxillary region S00.85
    submental region S00.85
    subungual
      finger(s) — *see* Foreign body, superficial,
        finger
      toe(s) — *see* Foreign body, superficial, toe
    supraclavicular fossa S10.85
    supraorbital S00.85
    temple S00.85
    temporal region S00.85
    testis S30.853
    thigh S70.359
      left S70.352
      right S70.351
    thorax, thoracic (wall) S20.95
      back S20.459
        left S20.452
        right S20.451
      front S20.359
        left S20.352
        right S20.351
    throat S10.15
    thumb S60.359
      left S60.352
      right S60.351
    toe(s) (lesser) S90.456
      great S90.453
        left S90.452
        right S90.451
      left S90.455
      right S90.454
    tongue S00.552
    trachea S10.15
    tunica vaginalis S30.853
    tympanum, tympanic membrane — *see*
      Foreign body, superficial, ear
    uvula S00.552
    vagina S30.854
    vocal cords S10.15
    vulva S30.854
    wrist S60.859
      left S60.852
      right S60.851
  swallowed T18.9
  trachea T17.408
    causing
      asphyxiation T17.400
        food (bone) (seed) T17.420
        gastric contents (vomitus) T17.410

Foreign body — *continued*
  trachea — *continued*
    causing — *continued*
      asphyxiation — *continued*
        specified type NEC T17.490
      injury NEC T17.408
        food (bone) (seed) T17.428
        gastric contents (vomitus) T17.418
        specified type NEC T17.498
  vitreous (humor) S05.50
    left S05.52
    right S05.51

Forestier's disease — *see* Hyperostosis,
  ankylosing
Formation
  hyalin in cornea — *see* Degeneration, cornea
  sequestrum in bone (due to infection) — *see*
    Osteomyelitis, chronic
  valve
    colon, congenital Q43.8
    ureter (congenital) Q62.39
Formication R20.2
Fort Bragg fever A27.89
Fossa — *see also* condition
  pyriform — *see* condition
Fothergill's
  disease (trigeminal neuralgia) — *see also*
    Neuralgia, trigeminal
  scarlatina anginosa A38.9
Foul breath R19.6
Foundling Z76.1
Fournier's disease or gangrene N49.2
Fourth
  cranial nerve — *see* condition
  molar K00.1
Foville's (peduncular) **disease or syndrome**
  G46.3
Fox (-Fordyce) disease (apocrine miliaria) L75.2
Fracture (abduction) (adduction) (separation)
  acetabulum S32.409
    column
      anterior (displaced) (iliopubic) S32.433
        left S32.432
        nondisplaced S32.436
          left S32.435
          right S32.434
        right S32.431
      posterior (displaced) (ilioischial) S32.443
        left S32.442
        nondisplaced S32.446
          left S32.445
          right S32.444
        right S32.441
    dome (displaced) S32.483
      left S32.482
      nondisplaced S32.486
        left S32.485
        right S32.484
      right S32.481
    left S32.402
    right S32.401
    specified NEC S32.499
      left S32.492
      right S32.491
    transverse (displaced) S32.453
      with associated posterior wall fracture
        (displaced) S32.463
        left S32.462
        nondisplaced S32.466
          left S32.465
          right S32.464
        right S32.461
      left S32.452
      nondisplaced S32.456
        left S32.455
        right S32.454
      right S32.451
    wall
      anterior (displaced) S32.413
        left S32.412
        nondisplaced S32.416
          left S32.415
          right S32.414
        right S32.411

Fracture — *continued*
  acetabulum — *continued*
    wall — *continued*
      medial (displaced) S32.473
        left S32.472
        nondisplaced S32.476
          left S32.475
          right S32.474
        right S32.471
      posterior (displaced) S32.423
        with associated transverse fracture
          (displaced) S32.463
          left S32.462
          nondisplaced S32.466
            left S32.465
            right S32.464
          right S32.461
        left S32.422
        nondisplaced S32.426
          left S32.425
          right S32.424
        right S32.421
  acromion — *see* Fracture, scapula, acromial
    process
  alveolus S02.83
    mandible S02.82
    maxilla S02.81
  ankle S82.899
    bimalleolar (displaced) S82.843
      left S82.842
      nondisplaced S82.846
        left S82.845
        right S82.844
      right S82.841
    lateral malleolus only (displaced) S82.63
      left S82.62
      nondisplaced S82.66
        left S82.65
        right S82.64
      right S82.61
    left S82.892
    medial malleolus (displaced) S82.53
      associated with Maisonneuve's fracture —
        see Fracture, Maisonneuve's
      left S82.52
      nondisplaced S82.56
        left S82.55
        right S82.54
      right S82.51
    right S82.891
    talus — *see* Fracture, tarsal, talus
    trimalleolar (displaced) S82.853
      left S82.852
      nondisplaced S82.856
        left S82.855
        right S82.854
      right S82.851
  arm (upper) — *see also* Fracture, humerus,
    shaft
    humerus — *see* Fracture, humerus
    radius — *see* Fracture, radius
    ulna — *see* Fracture, ulna
  astragalus — *see* Fracture, tarsal, talus
  atlas — *see* Fracture, neck, cervical vertebra,
    first
  axis — *see* Fracture, neck, cervical vertebra,
    second
  back — *see* Fracture, vertebra
  Barton's — *see* Barton's fracture
  base of skull — *see* Fracture, skull, base
  Bennett's — *see* Bennett's fracture
  bimalleolar — *see* Fracture, ankle, bimalleolar
  blow-out S02.3
  bone T14.90
    birth injury P13.9
    following insertion of orthopedic implant,
      joint prosthesis or bone plate M96.60
    in (due to) neoplastic disease NEC — *see*
      Fracture, pathological, due to,
      neoplastic disease
    pathological (cause unknown) — *see*
      Fracture, pathological
  breast bone — *see* Fracture, sternum
  bucket handle (semilunar cartilage) — *see* Tear,
    meniscus
  calcaneus — *see* Fracture, tarsal, calcaneus

Fracture — *continued*
  carpal bone(s) S62.109
    capitate (displaced) S62.133
      left S62.132
      nondisplaced S62.136
        left S62.135
        right S62.134
      right S62.131
    cuneiform — *see* Fracture, carpal bone,
      triquetrum
    hamate (body) (displaced) S62.143
      hook process (displaced) S62.153
        left S62.152
        nondisplaced S62.156
          left S62.155
          right S62.154
        right S62.151
      left S62.142
      nondisplaced S62.146
        left S62.145
        right S62.144
      right S62.141
    larger multangular — *see* Fracture, carpal
      bones, trapezium
    left S62.102
    lunate (displaced) S62.123
      left S62.122
      nondisplaced S62.126
        left S62.125
        right S62.124
      right S62.121
    navicular S62.009
      distal pole (displaced) S62.013
        left S62.012
        nondisplaced S62.016
          left S62.015
          right S62.014
        right S62.011
      left S62.002
      middle third (displaced) S62.023
        left S62.022
        nondisplaced S62.026
          left S62.025
          right S62.024
        right S62.021
      proximal third (displaced) S62.033
        left S62.032
        nondisplaced S62.036
          left S62.035
          right S62.034
        right S62.031
      right S62.001
      volar tuberosity — *see* Fracture, carpal
        bones, navicular, distal pole
    os magnum — *see* Fracture, carpal bones,
      capitate
    pisiform (displaced) S62.163
      left S62.162
      nondisplaced S62.166
        left S62.165
        right S62.164
      right S62.161
    right S62.101
    semilunar — *see* Fracture, carpal bones,
      lunate
    smaller multangular — *see* Fracture, carpal
      bones, trapezoid
    trapezium (displaced) S62.173
      left S62.172
      nondisplaced S62.176
        left S62.175
        right S62.174
      right S62.171
    trapezoid (displaced) S62.183
      left S62.182
      nondisplaced S62.186
        left S62.185
        right S62.184
      right S62.181
    triquetrum (displaced) S62.113
      left S62.112
      nondisplaced S62.116
        left S62.115
        right S62.114
      right S62.111

Fracture — *continued*
  carpal bone(s) — *continued*
    unciform — *see* Fracture, carpal bones,
      hamate
  cervical — *see* Fracture, vertebra, cervical
  clavicle S42.009
    acromial end (displaced) S42.033
      left S42.032
      nondisplaced S42.036
        left S42.035
        right S42.034
      right S42.031
    birth injury P13.4
    lateral end — *see* Fracture, clavicle,
      acromial end
    left S42.002
    right S42.001
    shaft (displaced) S42.023
      left S42.022
      nondisplaced S42.026
        left S42.025
        right S42.024
      right S42.021
    sternal end (anterior) (displaced) S42.013
      left S42.012
      nondisplaced S42.019
        left S42.018
        right S42.017
      posterior S42.016
        left S42.015
        right S42.014
      right S42.011
  coccyx S32.2
  collapsed — *see* Collapse, vertebra
  collar bone — *see* Fracture, clavicle
  Colles' — *see* Colles' fracture
  compression, not due to trauma — *see*
    Collapse, vertebra
  coronoid process — *see* Fracture, ulna, upper
    end, coronoid process
  costochondral, costosternal junction — *see*
    Fracture, rib
  cranium — *see* Fracture, skull
  cricoid cartilage S12.8
  cuboid (ankle) — *see* Fracture, tarsal, cuboid
  cuneiform
    foot — *see* Fracture, tarsal, cuneiform
    wrist — *see* Fracture, carpal, triquetrum
  delayed union — *see* Delay, union, fracture
    due to
      birth injury — *see* Birth, injury, fracture
      osteoporosis — *see* Osteoporosis, with
        fracture
  Dupuytren's — *see* Fracture, ankle, lateral
    malleolus
  elbow S42.409
  ethmoid (bone) (sinus) — *see* Fracture, skull,
    base
  face bone S02.92
  fatigue — *see also* Fracture, stress
    vertebra M48.40
      cervical region M48.42
      cervicothoracic region M48.43
      lumbar region M48.46
      lumbosacral region M48.47
      occipito-atlanto-axial region M48.41
      sacrococcygeal region M48.48
      thoracic region M48.44
      thoracolumbar region M48.45
  femur, femoral S72.90
    birth injury P13.2
    condyles, epicondyles — *see* Fracture,
      femur, lower end
    distal end — *see* Fracture, femur, lower end
    epiphysis
      head — *see* Fracture, femur, upper end,
        epiphysis
      lower — *see* Fracture, femur, lower end,
        epiphysis
      upper — *see* Fracture, femur, upper end,
        epiphysis
    following insertion of implant, prosthesis or
      plate M96.669
      left M96.662
      right M96.661
    head — *see* Fracture, femur, upper end,
      head

Fracture — *continued*
  femur, femoral — *continued*
    intertrochanteric — *see* Fracture, femur, trochanteric
    intratrochanteric — *see* Fracture, femur, trochanteric
    left S72.92
    lower end S72.409
      condyle (displaced) S72.413
        left S72.412
        lateral (displaced) S72.423
          left S72.422
          nondisplaced S72.426
            left S72.425
            right S72.424
          right S72.421
        medial (displaced) S72.433
          left S72.432
          nondisplaced S72.436
            left S72.435
            right S72.434
          right S72.431
        nondisplaced S72.416
          left S72.415
          right S72.414
        right S72.411
      epiphysis (displaced) S72.443
        left S72.442
        nondisplaced S72.446
          left S72.445
          right S72.444
        right S72.441
      left S72.402
      physeal S79.109
        left S79.102
        right S79.101
        Salter-Harris
          Type I S79.119
            left S79.112
            right S79.111
          Type II S79.129
            left S79.122
            right S79.121
          Type III S79.139
            left S79.132
            right S79.131
          Type IV S79.149
            left S79.142
            right S79.141
        specified NEC S79.199
          left S79.192
          right S79.191
      right S72.401
      specified NEC S72.499
        left S72.492
        right S72.491
      supracondylar (displaced) S72.453
        with intracondylar extension (displaced) S72.463
          left S72.462
          nondisplaced S72.466
            left S72.465
            right S72.464
          right S72.461
        left S72.452
        nondisplaced S72.456
          left S72.455
          right S72.454
        right S72.451
      torus S72.479
        left S72.472
        right S72.471
    neck — *see* Fracture, femur, upper end, neck
    pertrochanteric — *see* Fracture, femur, trochanteric
    right S72.91
    shaft (lower third) (middle third) (upper third) S72.309
      comminuted (displaced) S72.353
        left S72.352
        nondisplaced S72.356
          left S72.355
          right S72.354
        right S72.351
      left S72.302

Fracture — *continued*
  femur, femoral — *continued*
    shaft — *continued*
      oblique (displaced) S72.333
        left S72.332
        nondisplaced S72.336
          left S72.335
          right S72.334
        right S72.301
      segmental (displaced) S72.363
        left S72.362
        nondisplaced S72.366
          left S72.365
          right S72.364
        right S72.361
      specified NEC S72.399
        left S72.392
        right S72.391
      spiral (displaced) S72.343
        left S72.342
        nondisplaced S72.346
          left S72.345
          right S72.344
        right S72.341
      transverse (displaced) S72.323
        left S72.322
        nondisplaced S72.326
          left S72.325
          right S72.324
        right S72.321
    specified site NEC — *see* category S72.8
    subtrochanteric (region) (section) (displaced) S72.23
      left S72.22
      nondisplaced S72.26
        left S72.25
        right S72.24
      right S72.21
    transcervical — *see* Fracture, femur, upper end, neck
    transtrochanteric — *see* Fracture, femur, trochanteric
    trochanteric S72.109
      apophyseal (displaced) S72.143
        left S72.142
        nondisplaced S72.146
          left S72.145
          right S72.144
        right S72.141
      greater trochanter (displaced) S72.113
        left S72.112
        nondisplaced S72.116
          left S72.115
          right S72.114
        right S72.111
      intertrochanteric (displaced) S72.133
        left S72.132
        nondisplaced S72.136
          left S72.135
          right S72.134
        right S72.131
      left S72.102
      lesser trochanter (displaced) S72.123
        left S72.122
        nondisplaced S72.126
          left S72.125
          right S72.124
        right S72.121
      right S72.101
    upper end S72.009
      apophyseal (displaced) S72.133
        left S72.132
        nondisplaced S72.136
          left S72.135
          right S72.134
        right S72.131
      cervicotrochanteric — *see* Fracture, femur, upper end, neck, base
      epiphysis (displaced) S72.023
        left S72.022
        nondisplaced S72.026
          left S72.025
          right S72.024
        right S72.021

Fracture — *continued*
  femur, femoral — *continued*
    upper end — *continued*
      head S72.059
        articular (displaced) S72.063
          left S72.062
          nondisplaced S72.066
            left S72.065
            right S72.064
          right S72.061
        left S72.052
        right S72.051
        specified NEC S72.099
          left S72.092
          right S72.091
      intertrochanteric (displaced) S72.143
        left S72.142
        nondisplaced S72.146
          left S72.145
          right S72.144
        right S72.141
      intracapsular S72.019
        left S72.012
        right S72.011
      left S72.002
      midcervical (displaced) S72.033
        left S72.032
        nondisplaced S72.036
          left S72.035
          right S72.034
        right S72.031
      neck S72.009
        base (displaced) S72.043
          left S72.042
          nondisplaced S72.046
            left S72.045
            right S72.044
          right S72.041
        left S72.002
        right S72.001
        specified NEC S72.099
          left S72.092
          right S72.091
      pertrochanteric — *see* Fracture, femur, upper end, trochanteric
      physeal S79.009
        left S79.002
        right S79.001
        Salter-Harris type I S79.019
          left S79.012
          right S79.011
        specified NEC S79.099
          left S79.092
          right S79.091
      right S72.001
      subcapital (displaced) — *see* Fracture, femur, upper end, intracapsular
      subtrochanteric (displaced) S72.23
        left S72.22
        nondisplaced S72.26
          left S72.25
          right S72.24
        right S72.21
      transcervical — *see* Fracture, femur, upper end, midcervical
      trochanteric S72.109
        greater (displaced) S72.113
          left S72.112
          nondisplaced S72.116
            left S72.115
            right S72.114
          right S72.111
        lesser (displaced) S72.123
          left S72.122
          nondisplaced S72.126
            left S72.125
            right S72.124
          right S72.121
        left S72.102
        right S72.101
  fetus — *see* Birth, injury, fracture
  fibula (shaft) (styloid) S82.409
    comminuted (displaced) S82.453
      left S82.452
      nondisplaced S82.456
        left S82.455

Fracture — *continued*
  fibula — *continued*
    comminuted — *continued*
      nondisplaced — *continued*
        right S82.454
        right S82.451
    following insertion of implant, prosthesis or
      plate M96.679
      left M96.672
      right M96.671
    involving ankle or malleolus — *see* Fracture,
      fibula, lateral malleolus
    lateral malleolus (displaced) S82.63
      left S82.62
      nondisplaced S82.66
        left S82.65
        right S82.64
      right S82.61
    left S82.402
    lower end
      physeal S89.309
        left S89.302
        right S89.301
        Salter-Harris
          Type I S89.319
            left S89.312
            right S89.311
          Type II S89.329
            left S89.322
            right S89.321
        specified NEC S89.399
          left S89.392
          right S89.391
      specified NEC S82.839
        left S82.832
        right S82.831
      torus S82.829
        left S82.822
        right S82.821
    oblique (displaced) S82.433
      left S82.432
      nondisplaced S82.436
        left S82.435
        right S82.434
      right S82.431
    right S82.401
    segmental (displaced) S82.463
      left S82.462
      nondisplaced S82.466
        left S82.465
        right S82.464
      right S82.461
    specified NEC S82.499
      left S82.492
      right S82.491
    spiral (displaced) S82.443
      left S82.442
      nondisplaced S82.446
        left S82.445
        right S82.444
      right S82.441
    transverse (displaced) S82.423
      left S82.422
      nondisplaced S82.426
        left S82.425
        right S82.424
      right S82.421
    upper end
      physeal S89.209
        left S89.202
        right S89.201
        Salter-Harris
          Type I S89.219
            left S89.212
            right S89.211
          Type II S89.229
            left S89.222
            right S89.221
        specified NEC S89.299
          left S89.292
          right S89.291
      specified NEC S82.839
        left S82.832
        right S82.831

Fracture — *continued*
  fibula — *continued*
    upper end — *continued*
      torus S82.819
        left S82.812
        right S82.811
  finger (except thumb) S62.609
    distal phalanx (displaced) S62.639
      nondisplaced S62.669
    index S62.608
      distal phalanx (displaced) S62.638
        left S62.631
        nondisplaced S62.668
          left S62.661
          right S62.660
        right S62.630
      left S62.601
      medial phalanx (displaced) S62.628
        left S62.621
        nondisplaced S62.658
          left S62.651
          right S62.650
        right S62.620
      proximal phalanx (displaced) S62.618
        left S62.611
        nondisplaced S62.648
          left S62.641
          right S62.640
        right S62.610
      right S62.600
    little S62.608
      distal phalanx (displaced) S62.638
        left S62.637
        nondisplaced S62.668
          left S62.667
          right S62.666
        right S62.636
      left S62.607
      medial phalanx (displaced) S62.628
        left S62.627
        nondisplaced S62.658
          left S62.657
          right S62.656
        right S62.626
      proximal phalanx (displaced) S62.618
        left S62.617
        nondisplaced S62.648
          left S62.647
          right S62.646
        right S62.616
      right S62.606
    medial phalanx (displaced) S62.629
      nondisplaced S62.659
    middle S62.608
      distal phalanx (displaced) S62.638
        left S62.633
        nondisplaced S62.668
          left S62.663
          right S62.662
        right S62.632
      left S62.603
      medial phalanx (displaced) S62.628
        left S62.623
        nondisplaced S62.658
          left S62.653
          right S62.652
        right S62.622
      proximal phalanx (displaced) S62.618
        left S62.613
        nondisplaced S62.648
          left S62.643
          right S62.642
        right S62.612
      right S62.602
    proximal phalanx (displaced) S62.619
      nondisplaced S62.649
    ring S62.608
      distal phalanx (displaced) S62.638
        left S62.635
        nondisplaced S62.668
          left S62.665
          right S62.664
        right S62.634
      left S62.605
      medial phalanx (displaced) S62.628
        left S62.625

Fracture — *continued*
  finger — *continued*
    ring — *continued*
      medial phalanx — *continued*
        nondisplaced S62.658
          left S62.655
          right S62.654
        right S62.624
      proximal phalanx (displaced) S62.618
        left S62.615
        nondisplaced S62.648
          left S62.645
          right S62.644
        right S62.614
      right S62.604
    thumb — *see* Fracture, thumb
  following insertion of orthopedic implant, joint
    prosthesis or bone plate M96.60
    femur M96.669
      left M96.662
      right M96.661
    fibula M96.679
      left M96.672
      right M96.671
    humerus M96.629
      left M96.622
      right M96.621
    pelvis M96.65
    radius M96.639
      left M96.632
      right M96.631
    specified bone NEC M96.69
    tibia M96.679
      left M96.672
      right M96.671
    ulna M96.639
      left M96.632
      right M96.631
  foot S92.909
    astragalus — *see* Fracture, tarsal, talus
    calcaneus — *see* Fracture, tarsal, calcaneus
    cuboid — *see* Fracture, tarsal, cuboid
    cuneiform — *see* Fracture, tarsal, cuneiform
    left S92.902
    metatarsal — *see* Fracture, metatarsal
    navicular — *see* Fracture, tarsal, navicular
    right S92.901
    talus — *see* Fracture, tarsal, talus
    tarsal — *see* Fracture, tarsal
    toe — *see* Fracture, toe
  forearm S52.90
    left S52.92
    radius — *see* Fracture, radius
    right S52.91
    ulna — *see* Fracture, ulna
  fossa (anterior) (middle) (posterior) S02.19
  frontal (bone) (skull) S02.0
    sinus S02.19
  glenoid (cavity) (scapula) — *see* Fracture,
    scapula, glenoid cavity
  greenstick — *see* Fracture, by site
  hallux — *see* Fracture, toe, great
  hand S62.90
    carpal — *see* Fracture, carpal bone
    finger (except thumb) — *see* Fracture, finger
    left S62.92
    metacarpal — *see* Fracture, metacarpal
    navicular (scaphoid) (hand) — *see* Fracture,
      carpal bone, navicular
    right S62.91
    thumb — *see* Fracture, thumb
  healed or old
  with complications – code by Nature of the
    complication
  heel bone — *see* Fracture, tarsal, calcaneus
  hip — *see* Fracture, femur, neck
  humerus S42.309
    anatomical neck– *see* Fracture, humerus,
      upper end
    articular process — *see* Fracture, humerus,
      lower end
    capitellum — *see* Fracture, humerus, lower
      end, condyle, lateral
    distal end — *see* Fracture, humerus, lower
      end

©2002 Ingenix, Inc.

Fracture — *continued*
  humerus — *continued*
    epiphysis
      lower — *see* Fracture, humerus, lower end, physeal
      upper — *see* Fracture, humerus, upper end, physeal
    external condyle — *see* Fracture, humerus, lower end, condyle, lateral
    following insertion of implant, prosthesis or plate M96.629
      left M96.622
      right M96.621
    great tuberosity — *see* Fracture, humerus, upper end, greater tuberosity
    intercondylar — *see* Fracture, humerus, lower end
    internal epicondyle — *see* Fracture, humerus, lower end, epicondyle, medial
    left S42.302
    lesser tuberosity — *see* Fracture, humerus, upper end, specified NEC
    lower end S42.409
      condyle
        lateral (displaced) S42.453
          left S42.452
          nondisplaced S42.456
            left S42.455
            right S42.454
          right S42.451
        medial (displaced) S42.463
          left S42.462
          nondisplaced S42.466
            left S42.465
            right S42.464
          right S42.461
      epicondyle
        lateral (displaced) S42.433
          left S42.432
          nondisplaced S42.436
            left S42.435
            right S42.434
          right S42.431
        medial (displaced) S42.443
          incarcerated S42.449
            left S42.448
            right S42.447
          left S42.442
          nondisplaced S42.446
            left S42.445
            right S42.444
          right S42.441
      left S42.402
      physeal S49.109
        left S49.102
        right S49.101
        Salter-Harris
          Type I S49.119
            left S49.112
            right S49.111
          Type II S49.129
            left S49.122
            right S49.121
          Type III S49.139
            left S49.132
            right S49.131
          Type IV S49.149
            left S49.142
            right S49.141
          specified NEC S49.199
            left S49.192
            right S49.191
      right S42.401
      specified NEC (displaced) S42.493
        left S42.492
        nondisplaced S42.496
          left S42.495
          right S42.494
        right S42.491
      supracondylar (simple) (displaced) S42.413
        comminuted (displaced) S42.423
          left S42.422
          nondisplaced S42.426
            left S42.425

Fracture — *continued*
  humerus — *continued*
    lower end — *continued*
      supracondylar — *continued*
        comminuted — *continued*
          nondisplaced — *continued*
            right S42.424
            right S42.421
          left S42.412
          nondisplaced S42.416
            left S42.415
            right S42.414
          right S42.411
      torus S42.489
        left S42.482
        right S42.481
      transcondylar (displaced) S42.473
        left S42.472
        nondisplaced S42.476
          left S42.475
          right S42.474
        right S42.471
    proximal end — *see* Fracture, humerus, upper end
    right S42.301
    shaft S42.309
      comminuted (displaced) S42.353
        left S42.352
        nondisplaced S42.356
          left S42.355
          right S42.354
        right S42.351
      greenstick S42.319
        left S42.312
        right S42.311
      left S42.302
      oblique (displaced) S42.333
        left S42.332
        nondisplaced S42.336
          left S42.335
          right S42.334
        right S42.331
      right S42.301
      segmental (displaced) S42.363
        left S42.362
        nondisplaced S42.366
          left S42.365
          right S42.364
        right S42.361
      specified NEC S42.399
        left S42.392
        right S42.391
      spiral (displaced) S42.343
        left S42.342
        nondisplaced S42.346
          left S42.345
          right S42.344
        right S42.341
      transverse (displaced) S42.323
        left S42.322
        nondisplaced S42.326
          left S42.325
          right S42.324
        right S42.321
    supracondylar — *see* Fracture, humerus, lower end
    surgical neck — *see* Fracture, humerus, upper end, surgical neck
    trochlea — *see* Fracture, humerus, lower end, condyle, medial
    tuberosity — *see* Fracture, humerus, upper end
    upper end S42.209
      anatomical neck — *see* Fracture, humerus, upper end, specified NEC
      articular head — *see* Fracture, humerus, upper end, specified NEC
      epiphysis — *see* Fracture, humerus, upper end, physeal
      greater tuberosity (displaced) S42.253
        left S42.252
        nondisplaced S42.256
          left S42.255
          right S42.254
        right S42.251
      left S42.202

Fracture — *continued*
  humerus — *continued*
    upper end — *continued*
      lesser tuberosity (displaced) S42.263
        left S42.262
        nondisplaced S42.266
          left S42.265
          right S42.264
        right S42.261
      physeal S49.009
        left S49.002
        right S49.001
        Salter-Harris
          Type I S49.019
            left S49.012
            right S49.011
          Type II S49.029
            left S49.022
            right S49.021
          Type III S49.039
            left S49.032
            right S49.031
          Type IV S49.049
            left S49.042
            right S49.041
          specified NEC S49.099
            left S49.092
            right S49.091
      right S42.201
      specified NEC (displaced) S42.293
        left S42.292
        nondisplaced S42.296
          left S42.295
          right S42.294
        right S42.291
      surgical neck (displaced) S42.213
        four-part S42.249
          left S42.242
          right S42.241
        left S42.212
        nondisplaced S42.216
          left S42.215
          right S42.214
        right S42.211
        three-part S42.239
          left S42.232
          right S42.231
        two-part (displaced) S42.223
          left S42.222
          nondisplaced S42.226
            left S42.225
            right S42.224
          right S42.221
      torus S42.279
        left S42.272
        right S42.271
      transepiphyseal — *see* Fracture, humerus, upper end, physeal
  hyoid bone S12.8
  ilium S32.309
    with disruption of pelvic circle — *see* Disruption, pelvic circle
    avulsion (displaced) S32.313
      left S32.312
      nondisplaced S32.316
        left S32.315
        right S32.314
      right S32.311
    left S32.302
    right S32.301
    specified NEC S32.399
      left S32.392
      right S32.391
  impaction, impacted – code as Fracture, by site
  innominate bone — *see* Fracture, ilium
  instep — *see* Fracture, foot
  ischium S32.609
    with disruption of pelvic circle — *see* Disruption, pelvic circle
    avulsion (displaced) S32.613
      left S32.612
      nondisplaced S32.616
        left S32.615
        right S32.614
      right S32.611

Fracture — *continued*
 ischium — *continued*
  left S32.602
  right S32.601
  specified NEC S32.699
   left S32.692
   right S32.691
 jaw (bone) (lower) — *see* Fracture, mandible
  upper — *see* Fracture, maxilla
 knee cap — *see* Fracture, patella
 larynx S12.8
 late effects — *see* Sequelae, fracture
 leg (lower) S82.90
  ankle — *see* Fracture, ankle
  femur — *see* Fracture, femur
  fibula — *see* Fracture, fibula
  left S82.92
  malleolus — *see* Fracture, ankle
  patella — *see* Fracture, patella
  right S82.91
  specified site NEC S82.899
   left S82.892
   right S82.891
  tibia — *see* Fracture, tibia
 lumbar spine — *see* Fracture, vertebra, lumbar
 lumbosacral spine S32.9
 Maisonneuve's (displaced) S82.863
  left S82.862
  nondisplaced S82.866
   left S82.865
   right S82.864
  right S82.861
 malar bone — *see* Fracture, maxilla
 malleolus — *see* Fracture, ankle
 malunion — *see* Malunion, fracture
 mandible (lower jaw) S02.60
  angle of jaw S02.65
  body, unspecified S02.68
  condylar process S02.61
  coronoid process S02.63
  ramus, unspecified S02.64
  specified site NEC S02.69
  subcondylar S02.62
  symphysis S02.66
 manubrium (sterni) S22.21
  dissociation from sternum S22.23
 march — *see* Fracture, foot
 maxilla, maxillary (bone) sinus) (superior)
   (upper jaw) S02.40
  inferior — *see* Fracture, mandible
  LeFort I S02.41
  LeFort II S02.42
  LeFort III S02.43
 metacarpal S62.309
  base (displaced) S62.319
   nondisplaced S62.349
  fifth S62.308
   base (displaced) S62.318
    left S62.317
    nondisplaced S62.348
     left S62.347
     right S62.346
    right S62.316
   left S62.307
   neck (displaced) S62.338
    left S62.337
    nondisplaced S62.368
     left S62.367
     right S62.366
    right S62.336
   right S62.306
   shaft (displaced) S62.328
    left S62.327
    nondisplaced S62.358
     left S62.357
     right S62.356
    right S62.326
   specified NEC S62.398
    left S62.397
    right S62.396
  first S62.209
   base NEC (displaced) S62.233
    left S62.232
    nondisplaced S62.236
     left S62.235
     right S62.234
    right S62.231

Fracture — *continued*
 metacarpal — *continued*
  first — *continued*
   Bennett's — *see* Bennett's fracture
   left S62.202
   neck (displaced) S62.253
    left S62.252
    nondisplaced S62.256
     left S62.255
     right S62.254
    right S62.251
   right S62.201
   shaft (displaced) S62.243
    left S62.242
    nondisplaced S62.246
     left S62.245
     right S62.244
    right S62.241
   specified NEC S62.299
    left S62.292
    right S62.291
  fourth S62.308
   base (displaced) S62.318
    left S62.315
    nondisplaced S62.348
     left S62.345
     right S62.344
    right S62.314
   left S62.305
   neck (displaced) S62.338
    left S62.335
    nondisplaced S62.368
     left S62.365
     right S62.364
    right S62.334
   right S62.304
   shaft (displaced) S62.328
    left S62.325
    nondisplaced S62.358
     left S62.355
     right S62.354
    right S62.324
   specified NEC S62.398
    left S62.395
    right S62.394
  left S62.302
  neck (displaced) S62.339
   nondisplaced S62.369
  right S62.301
  Rolando's — *see* Rolando's fracture
  second S62.308
   base (displaced) S62.318
    left S62.311
    nondisplaced S62.348
     left S62.341
     right S62.340
    right S62.310
   left S62.301
   neck (displaced) S62.338
    left S62.331
    nondisplaced S62.368
     left S62.361
     right S62.360
    right S62.330
   right S62.300
   shaft (displaced) S62.328
    left S62.321
    nondisplaced S62.358
     left S62.351
     right S62.350
    right S62.320
   specified NEC S62.398
    left S62.391
    right S62.390
  shaft (displaced) S62.329
   nondisplaced S62.359
  third S62.308
   base (displaced) S62.318
    left S62.313
    nondisplaced S62.348
     left S62.343
     right S62.342
    right S62.312
   left S62.303
   neck (displaced) S62.338
    left S62.333

Fracture — *continued*
 metacarpal — *continued*
  third — *continued*
   neck — *continued*
    nondisplaced S62.368
     left S62.363
     right S62.362
    right S62.332
   right S62.302
   shaft (displaced) S62.328
    left S62.323
    nondisplaced S62.358
     left S62.353
     right S62.352
    right S62.322
   specified NEC S62.398
    left S62.393
    right S62.392
  specified NEC S62.399
 metastatic (M8000/6) (*see also* Neoplasm) —
   see Fracture, pathological, due to,
   neoplastic disease
 metatarsal bone S92.309
  fifth (displaced) S92.353
   left S92.352
   nondisplaced S92.356
    left S92.355
    right S92.354
   right S92.351
  first (displaced) S92.313
   left S92.312
   nondisplaced S92.316
    left S92.315
    right S92.314
   right S92.311
  fourth (displaced) S92.343
   left S92.342
   nondisplaced S92.346
    left S92.345
    right S92.344
   right S92.341
  left S92.302
  right S92.301
  second (displaced) S92.323
   left S92.322
   nondisplaced S92.326
    left S92.325
    right S92.324
   right S92.321
  third (displaced) S92.333
   left S92.332
   nondisplaced S92.336
    left S92.335
    right S92.334
   right S92.331
 Monteggia's — *see* Monteggia's fracture
 multiple
  hand (and wrist) NEC — *see* Fracture, by
    site
  ribs — *see* Fracture, rib, multiple
 nasal (bone(s)) S02.2
 navicular (scaphoid) (foot) — *see also* Fracture,
   tarsal, navicular
  hand — *see* Fracture, carpal, navicular
 neck S12.9
  cervical vertebra S12.9
   fifth (displaced) S12.400
    nondisplaced S12.401
    specified type NEC (displaced) S12.490
     nondisplaced S12.491
   first (displaced) S12.000
    burst (stable) S12.01
     unstable S12.02
    lateral mass (displaced) S12.040
     nondisplaced S12.041
    nondisplaced S12.001
    posterior arch (displaced) S12.030
     nondisplaced S12.031
    specified type NEC (displaced) S12.090
     nondisplaced S12.091
   fourth (displaced) S12.300
    nondisplaced S12.301
    specified type NEC (displaced) S12.390
     nondisplaced S12.391
   second (displaced) S12.100
    nondisplaced S12.101

    ©2002 Ingenix, Inc.

Fracture — *continued*
  neck — *continued*
    cervical vertebra — *continued*
      dens (anterior) (displaced) (type II)
          S12.110
        nondisplaced S12.112
        posterior S12.111
        specified type NEC (displaced)
            S12.120
          nondisplaced S12.121
      specified type NEC (displaced) S12.190
        nondisplaced S12.191
      seventh (displaced) S12.600
        nondisplaced S12.601
        specified type NEC (displaced) S12.690
          displaced S12.691
      sixth (displaced) S12.500
        nondisplaced S12.501
        specified type NEC (displaced) S12.590
          displaced S12.591
      third (displaced) S12.200
        nondisplaced S12.201
        specified type NEC (displaced) S12.290
          displaced S12.291
    hyoid bone S12.8
    larynx S12.8
    specified site NEC S12.8
    thyroid cartilage S12.8
    trachea S12.8
  neoplastic NEC — *see* Fracture, pathological,
      due to, neoplastic disease
  neural arch — *see* Fracture, vertebra
  newborn — *see* Birth, injury, fracture
  nontraumatic — *see* Fracture, pathological
  nonunion — *see* Nonunion, fracture
  nose, nasal (bone) (septum) S02.2
  occiput — *see* Fracture, skull, base, occiput
  odontoid process — *see* Fracture, neck, cervical
      vertebra, second
  olecranon (process) (ulna) — *see* Fracture,
      ulna, upper end, olecranon process
  orbit, orbital (bone) (region) S02.89
    floor (blow-out) S02.3
    roof S02.19
  os
    calcis — *see* Fracture, tarsal, calcaneus
    magnum — *see* Fracture, carpal, capitate
    pubis — *see* Fracture, pubis
  palate S02.89
  parietal bone (skull) S02.0
  patella S82.009
    comminuted (displaced) S82.043
      left S82.042
      nondisplaced S82.046
        left S82.045
        right S82.044
      right S82.041
    left S82.002
    longitudinal (displaced) S82.023
      left S82.022
      nondisplaced S82.026
        left S82.025
        right S82.024
      right S82.021
    osteochondral (displaced) S82.013
      left S82.012
      nondisplaced S82.016
        left S82.015
        right S82.014
      right S82.011
    right S82.001
    specified NEC S82.099
      left S82.092
      right S82.091
    transverse (displaced) S82.033
      left S82.032
      nondisplaced S82.036
        left S82.035
        right S82.034
      right S82.031
  pathological M84.40
    ankle M84.473
      left M84.472
      right M84.471
    carpus M84.443
      left M84.442

Fracture — *continued*
  pathological — *continued*
    carpus — *continued*
      right M84.441
    clavicle M84.419
      left M84.412
      right M84.411
    due to
      neoplastic disease NEC (M8000/1) (*see
          also* Neoplasm) M84.50
        ankle M84.573
          left M84.572
          right M84.571
        carpus M84.549
          left M84.542
          right M84.541
        clavicle M84.519
          left M84.512
          right M84.511
        femur M84.553
          left M84.552
          right M84.551
        fibula M84.569
          left M84.564
          right M84.563
        finger M84.549
          left M84.542
          right M84.541
        hip M84.559
        humerus M84.529
          left M84.522
          right M84.521
        ilium M84.550
        ischium M84.550
        metacarpus M84.549
          left M84.542
          right M84.541
        metatarsus M84.576
          left M84.575
          right M84.574
        neck M84.58
        radius M84.539
          left M84.534
          right M84.533
        rib M84.58
        scapula M84.519
          left M84.512
          right M84.511
        skull M84.58
        tarsus M84.576
          left M84.575
          right M84.574
        tibia M84.569
          left M84.562
          right M84.561
        toe M84.576
          left M84.575
          right M84.574
        ulna M84.539
          left M84.532
          right M84.531
        vertebra M84.58
      osteoporosis M80.80
        disuse — *see* Osteoporosis, specified
            type NEC, with pathological
            fracture
        drug-induced — *see* Osteoporosis,
            drug induced, with pathological
            fracture
        idiopathic — *see* Osteoporosis,
            specified type NEC, with
            pathological fracture
        postmenopausal — *see* Osteoporosis,
            postmenopausal, with
            pathological fracture
        postoophorectomy — *see* Osteoporosis,
            postoophorectomy, with
            pathological fracture
        postsurgical malabsorption — *see*
            Osteoporosis, specified type
            NEC, with pathological fracture
        specified cause NEC — *see*
            Osteoporosis, specified type
            NEC, with pathological fracture

Fracture — *continued*
  pathological — *continued*
    due to — *continued*
      specified disease NEC M84.60
        ankle M84.673
          left M84.672
          right M84.671
        carpus M84.649
          left M84.642
          right M84.641
        clavicle M84.619
          left M84.612
          right M84.611
        femur M84.653
          left M84.652
          right M84.651
        fibula M84.669
          left M84.664
          right M84.663
        finger M84.649
          left M84.642
          right M84.641
        hip M84.659
        humerus M84.629
          left M84.622
          right M84.621
        ilium M84.650
        ischium M84.650
        metacarpus M84.649
          left M84.642
          right M84.641
        metatarsus M84.676
          left M84.675
          right M84.674
        neck M84.68
        radius M84.639
          left M84.634
          right M84.633
        rib M84.68
        scapula M84.619
          left M84.612
          right M84.611
        skull M84.68
        tarsus M84.676
          left M84.675
          right M84.674
        tibia M84.669
          left M84.662
          right M84.661
        toe M84.676
          left M84.675
          right M84.674
        ulna M84.639
          left M84.632
          right M84.631
        vertebra M84.68
    femur M84.453
      left M84.452
      right M84.451
    fibula M84.469
      left M84.464
      right M84.463
    finger M84.446
      left M84.445
      right M84.444
    hip M84.459
    humerus M84.429
      left M84.422
      right M84.421
    ilium M84.454
    ischium M84.454
    metacarpus M84.443
      left M84.442
      right M84.441
    metatarsus M84.476
      left M84.475
      right M84.474
    neck M84.48
    pelvis M84.454
    radius M84.439
      left M84.434
      right M84.433
    rib M84.48
    scapula M84.419
      left M84.412
      right M84.411

Fracture — *continued*
pathological — *continued*
  skull M84.48
  tarsus M84.476
    left M84.475
    right M84.474
  tibia M84.469
    left M84.462
    right M84.461
  toe M84.479
    left M84.478
    right M84.477
  ulna M84.439
    left M84.432
    right M84.431
  vertebra M84.48
pedicle (of vertebral arch) — *see* Fracture, vertebra
pelvis, pelvic (bone) S32.9
  acetabulum — *see* Fracture, acetabulum
  following insertion of implant, prosthesis or plate M96.65
  ilium — *see* Fracture, ilium
  ischium — *see* Fracture, ischium
  multiple with disruption of pelvic circle — *see* Disruption, pelvic circle
  pubis — *see* Fracture, pubis
  specified site NEC S32.89
  sacrum — *see* Fracture, sacrum
phalanx
  foot — *see* Fracture, toe
  hand — *see* Fracture, finger
pisiform — *see* Fracture, carpal, pisiform
pond — *see* Fracture, skull
prosthetic device, internal — *see* Complications, prosthetic device, by site, mechanical
pubis S32.50
  with disruption of pelvic circle — *see* Disruption, pelvic circle
  specified site NEC S32.59
  superior rim S32.519
    left S32.512
    right S32.511
radius S52.90
  distal end — *see* Fracture, radius, lower end
  following insertion of implant, prosthesis or plate M96.639
    left M96.632
    right M96.631
  head — *see* Fracture, radius, upper end, head
  lower end S52.509
    Barton's — *see* Barton's fracture
    Colles' — *see* Colles' fracture
    extraarticular NEC S52.559
      left S52.552
      right S52.551
    intraarticular NEC S52.579
      left S52.572
      right S52.571
    left S52.502
    physeal S59.209
      left S59.202
      right S59.201
      Salter-Harris
        Type I S59.219
          left S59.212
          right S59.211
        Type II S59.229
          left S59.222
          right S59.221
        Type III S59.239
          left S59.232
          right S59.231
        Type IV S59.249
          left S59.242
          right S59.241
        specified NEC S59.299
          left S59.292
          right S59.291
    right S52.501
    Smith's — *see* Smith's fracture
    specified NEC S52.599
      left S52.592
      right S52.591

Fracture — *continued*
radius — *continued*
  lower end — *continued*
    styloid process (displaced) S52.513
      left S52.512
      nondisplaced S52.516
        left S52.515
        right S52.514
      right S52.511
    torus S52.529
      left S52.522
      right S52.521
  neck — *see* Fracture, radius, upper end
  proximal end — *see* Fracture, radius, upper end
  shaft S52.309
    bent bone S52.389
      left S52.382
      right S52.381
    comminuted (displaced) S52.353
      left S52.352
      nondisplaced S52.356
        left S52.355
        right S52.354
      right S52.351
    Galeazzi's — *see* Galeazzi's fracture
    greenstick S52.319
      left S52.312
      right S52.311
    left S52.302
    oblique (displaced) S52.333
      left S52.332
      nondisplaced S52.336
        left S52.335
        right S52.334
      right S52.331
    right S52.301
    segmental (displaced) S52.363
      left S52.362
      nondisplaced S52.366
        left S52.365
        right S52.364
      right S52.361
    specified NEC S52.399
      left S52.392
      right S52.391
    spiral (displaced) S52.343
      left S52.342
      nondisplaced S52.346
        left S52.345
        right S52.344
      right S52.341
    transverse (displaced) S52.323
      left S52.322
      nondisplaced S52.326
        left S52.325
        right S52.324
      right S52.321
  upper end S52.109
    head (displaced) S52.123
      left S52.122
      nondisplaced S52.126
        left S52.125
        right S52.124
      right S52.121
    left S52.102
    neck (displaced) S52.133
      left S52.132
      nondisplaced S52.136
        left S52.135
        right S52.134
      right S52.131
    right S52.101
    specified NEC S52.189
      left S52.182
      right S52.181
    physeal S59.109
      left S59.102
      right S59.101
      Salter-Harris
        Type I S59.119
          left S59.112
          right S59.111
        Type II S59.129
          left S59.122
          right S59.121

Fracture — *continued*
radius — *continued*
  upper end — *continued*
    physeal — *continued*
      Salter-Harris — *continued*
        Type III S59.139
          left S59.132
          right S59.131
        Type IV S59.149
          left S59.142
          right S59.141
        specified NEC S59.199
          left S59.192
          right S59.191
    torus S52.119
      left S52.112
      right S52.111
ramus
  inferior or superior, pubis — *see* Fracture, pubis
  mandible — *see* Fracture, mandible
rib S22.39
  with flail chest — *see* Flail, chest
  left S22.32
    multiple S22.42
  multiple S22.49
    with flail chest — *see* Flail, chest
    bilateral S22.43
    left S22.42
    right S22.41
  right S22.31
    multiple S22.41
root, tooth — *see* Fracture, tooth
sacrum S32.10
  specified NEC S32.19
  Type
    1 S32.14
    2 S32.15
    3 S32.16
    4 S32.17
  Zone
    I S32.119
      displaced (minimally) S32.111
      severely S32.112
      nondisplaced S32.110
    II S32.129
      displaced (minimally) S32.121
      severely S32.122
      nondisplaced S32.120
    III S32.139
      displaced (minimally) S32.131
      severely S32.132
      nondisplaced S32.130
scaphoid (hand) — *see also* Fracture, carpal, navicular
  foot — *see* Fracture, tarsal, navicular
scapula S42.109
  acromial process (displaced) S42.123
    left S42.122
    nondisplaced S42.126
      left S42.125
      right S42.124
    right S42.121
  body (displaced) S42.113
    left S42.112
    nondisplaced S42.116
      left S42.115
      right S42.114
    right S42.111
  coracoid process (displaced) S42.133
    left S42.132
    nondisplaced S42.136
      left S42.135
      right S42.134
    right S42.131
  glenoid cavity (displaced) S42.143
    left S42.142
    nondisplaced S42.146
      left S42.145
      right S42.144
    right S42.141
  left S42.102
  neck (displaced) S42.153
    left S42.152
    nondisplaced S42.156
      left S42.155

©2002 Ingenix, Inc.

Fracture — *continued*
  scapula — *continued*
    neck — *continued*
      nondisplaced — *continued*
        right S42.154
      right S42.151
      right S42.101
      specified NEC S42.199
        left S42.192
        right S42.191
  semilunar bone, wrist — *see* Fracture, carpal, lunate
  sequelae — *see* Sequelae, fracture
  sesamoid bone
    hand — *see* Fracture, carpal
    other – code by site under Fracture
  shepherd's — *see* Fracture, tarsal, talus
  shoulder (girdle) S42.90
    blade — *see* Fracture, scapula
    left S42.92
    right S42.91
  sinus (ethmoid) (frontal) S02.19
  skull S02.91
    base S02.10
      occiput S02.119
        condyle S02.113
          type I S02.110
          type II S02.111
          type III S02.112
        specified NEC S02.118
      specified NEC S02.19
    birth injury P13.0
    frontal bone S02.0
    parietal bone S02.0
    specified site NEC S02.89
    temporal bone S02.19
    vault S02.0
  Smith's — *see* Smith's fracture
  specified bone following insertion of implant, prosthesis or plate M96.69
  sphenoid (bone) (sinus) S02.19
  spine — *see* Fracture, vertebra
  spinous process — *see* Fracture, vertebra
  spontaneous (cause unknown) — *see* Fracture, pathological
  stave (of thumb) — *see* Fracture, metacarpal, first
  sternum S22.20
    with flail chest — *see* Flail, chest
    body S22.22
    manubrium S22.21
    xiphoid (process) S22.24
  stress M84.30
    ankle M84.373
      left M84.372
      right M84.371
    carpus M84.343
      left M84.342
      right M84.341
    clavicle M84.319
      left M84.312
      right M84.311
    femur M84.353
      left M84.352
      right M84.351
    fibula M84.369
      left M84.364
      right M84.363
    finger M84.346
      left M84.345
      right M84.344
    hip M84.359
    humerus M84.329
      left M84.322
      right M84.321
    ilium M84.350
    ischium M84.350
    metacarpus M84.343
      left M84.342
      right M84.341
    metatarsus M84.376
      left M84.375
      right M84.374
    neck — *see* Fracture, fatigue, vertebra
    radius M84.339
      left M84.334
      right M84.333

Fracture — *continued*
  stress — *continued*
    rib M84.38
    scapula M84.319
      left M84.312
      right M84.311
    skull M84.38
    tarsus M84.376
      left M84.375
      right M84.374
    tibia M84.369
      left M84.362
      right M84.361
    toe M84.379
      left M84.378
      right M84.377
    ulna M84.339
      left M84.332
      right M84.331
    vertebra — *see* Fracture, fatigue, vertebra
  supracondylar, elbow — *see* Fracture, humerus, lower end, supracondylar
  symphysis pubis — *see* Fracture, pubis
  talus (ankle bone) — *see* Fracture, tarsal, talus
  tarsal bone(s) S92.209
    astragalus — *see* Fracture, tarsal, talus
    calcaneus S92.009
      anterior process (displaced) S92.023
        left S92.022
        nondisplaced S92.026
          left S92.025
          right S92.024
        right S92.021
      body (displaced) S92.013
        left S92.012
        nondisplaced S92.016
          left S92.015
          right S92.014
        right S92.011
      extraarticular NEC (displaced) S92.053
        left S92.052
        nondisplaced S92.056
          left S92.055
          right S92.054
        right S92.051
      intraarticular (displaced) S92.063
        left S92.062
        nondisplaced S92.066
          left S92.065
          right S92.064
        right S92.061
      left S92.002
      right S92.001
      tuberosity (displaced) S92.043
        avulsion (displaced) S92.033
          left S92.032
          nondisplaced S92.036
            left S92.035
            right S92.034
          right S92.031
        left S92.042
        nondisplaced S92.046
          left S92.045
          right S92.044
        right S92.041
    cuboid (displaced) S92.213
      left S92.212
      nondisplaced S92.216
        left S92.215
        right S92.214
      right S92.211
    cuneiform
      intermediate (displaced) S92.233
        left S92.232
        nondisplaced S92.236
          left S92.235
          right S92.234
        right S92.231
      lateral (displaced) S92.223
        left S92.222
        nondisplaced S92.226
          left S92.225
          right S92.224
        right S92.221
      medial (displaced) S92.243
        left S92.242

Fracture — *continued*
  tarsal bone(s) — *continued*
    cuneiform — *continued*
      medial — *continued*
        nondisplaced S92.246
          left S92.245
          right S92.244
        right S92.241
      left S92.202
    navicular (displaced) S92.253
      left S92.252
      nondisplaced S92.256
        left S92.255
        right S92.254
      right S92.251
    right S92.201
    scaphoid — *see* Fracture, tarsal, navicular
    talus S92.109
      avulsion (displaced) S92.153
        left S92.152
        nondisplaced S92.156
          left S92.155
          right S92.154
        right S92.151
      body (displaced) S92.123
        left S92.122
        nondisplaced S92.126
          left S92.125
          right S92.124
        right S92.121
      dome (displaced) S92.143
        left S92.142
        nondisplaced S92.146
          left S92.145
          right S92.144
        right S92.141
      head (displaced) S92.123
        left S92.122
        nondisplaced S92.126
          left S92.125
          right S92.124
        right S92.121
      lateral process (displaced) S92.143
        left S92.142
        nondisplaced S92.146
          left S92.145
          right S92.144
        right S92.141
      left S92.102
      neck (displaced) S92.113
        left S92.112
        nondisplaced S92.116
          left S92.115
          right S92.114
        right S92.111
      posterior process (displaced) S92.133
        left S92.132
        nondisplaced S92.136
          left S92.135
          right S92.134
        right S92.131
      right S92.101
      specified NEC S92.199
        left S92.192
        right S92.191
  temporal bone (styloid) S02.19
  thorax (bony) S22.9
    with flail chest — *see* Flail, chest
    rib S22.39
      left S22.32
        multiple S22.42
      multiple S22.49
        with flail chest — *see* Flail, chest
        bilateral S22.43
        left S22.42
        right S22.41
      right S22.31
        multiple S22.41
    sternum S22.20
      body S22.22
      manubrium S22.21
      xiphoid process S22.24
    vertebra (displaced) S22.009
      burst (stable) S22.001
        unstable S22.002

Fracture — continued
  thorax — continued
    vertebra — continued
      eighth S22.069
        burst (stable) S22.061
          unstable S22.062
        specified type NEC S22.068
        wedge compression S22.060
      eleventh S22.089
        burst (stable) S22.081
          unstable S22.082
        specified type NEC S22.088
        wedge compression S22.080
      fifth S22.059
        burst (stable) S22.051
          unstable S22.052
        specified type NEC S22.058
        wedge compression S22.050
      first S22.019
        burst (stable) S22.011
          unstable S22.012
        specified type NEC S22.018
        wedge compression S22.010
      fourth S22.049
        burst (stable) S22.041
          unstable S22.042
        specified type NEC S22.048
        wedge compression S22.040
      ninth S22.079
        burst (stable) S22.071
          unstable S22.072
        specified type NEC S22.078
        wedge compression S22.070
      nondisplaced S22.001
      second S22.029
        burst (stable) S22.021
          unstable S22.022
        specified type NEC S22.028
        wedge compression S22.020
      seventh S22.069
        burst (stable) S22.061
          unstable S22.062
        specified type NEC S22.068
        wedge compression S22.060
      sixth S22.059
        burst (stable) S22.051
          unstable S22.052
        specified type NEC S22.058
        wedge compression S22.050
      specified type NEC S22.008
      tenth S22.079
        burst (stable) S22.071
          unstable S22.072
        specified type NEC S22.078
        wedge compression S22.070
      third S22.039
        burst (stable) S22.031
          unstable S22.032
        specified type NEC S22.038
        wedge compression S22.030
      twelfth S22.089
        burst (stable) S22.081
          unstable S22.082
        specified type NEC S22.088
        wedge compression S22.080
      wedge compression S22.000
  thumb S62.509
    distal phalanx (displaced) S62.523
      left S62.522
      nondisplaced S62.526
        left S62.525
        right S62.524
      right S62.521
    left S62.502
    proximal phalanx (displaced) S62.513
      left S62.512
      nondisplaced S62.516
        left S62.515
        right S62.514
      right S62.511
    right S62.501
  thyroid cartilage S12.8
  tibia (shaft) S82.209
    comminuted (displaced) S82.253
      left S82.252

Fracture — continued
  tibia — continued
    comminuted — continued
      nondisplaced S82.256
        left S82.255
        right S82.254
      right S82.251
    condyles — see Fracture, tibia, upper end
    distal end — see Fracture, tibia, lower end
    epiphysis
      lower — see Fracture, tibia, lower end
      upper — see Fracture, tibia, upper end
    following insertion of implant, prosthesis or
        plate M96.679
      left M96.672
      right M96.671
    head (involving knee joint) — see Fracture,
        tibia, upper end
    intercondyloid eminence — see Fracture,
        tibia, upper end
    involving ankle or malleolus — see Fracture,
        ankle, medial malleolus
    left S82.202
    lower end S82.309
      left S82.302
      physeal S89.109
        left S89.102
        right S89.101
        Salter-Harris
          Type I S89.119
            left S89.112
            right S89.111
          Type II S89.129
            left S89.122
            right S89.121
          Type III S89.139
            left S89.132
            right S89.131
          Type IV S89.149
            left S89.142
            right S89.141
        specified NEC S89.199
          left S89.192
          right S89.191
      pilon (displaced) S82.873
        left S82.872
        nondisplaced S82.876
          left S82.875
          right S82.874
        right S82.871
      right S82.301
      specified NEC S82.399
        left S82.392
        right S82.391
      torus S82.319
        left S82.312
        right S82.311
    malleolus — see Fracture, ankle, medial
        malleolus
    oblique (displaced) S82.233
      left S82.232
      nondisplaced S82.236
        left S82.235
        right S82.234
      right S82.231
    pilon — see Fracture, tibia, lower end, pilon
    proximal end — see Fracture, tibia, upper
        end
    right S82.201
    segmental (displaced) S82.263
      left S82.262
      nondisplaced S82.266
        left S82.265
        right S82.264
      right S82.261
    specified NEC S82.299
      left S82.292
      right S82.291
    spine — see Fracture, upper end, spine
    spiral (displaced) S82.243
      left S82.242
      nondisplaced S82.246
        left S82.245
        right S82.244
      right S82.241

Fracture — continued
  tibia — continued
    transverse (displaced) S82.223
      left S82.222
      nondisplaced S82.226
        left S82.225
        right S82.224
      right S82.221
    tuberosity — see Fracture, tibia, upper end,
        tuberosity
    upper end S82.109
      bicondylar (displaced) S82.143
        left S82.142
        nondisplaced S82.146
          left S82.145
          right S82.144
        right S82.141
      lateral condyle (displaced) S82.123
        left S82.122
        nondisplaced S82.126
          left S82.125
          right S82.124
        right S82.121
      left S82.102
      medial condyle (displaced) S82.133
        left S82.132
        nondisplaced S82.136
          left S82.135
          right S82.134
        right S82.131
      physeal S89.009
        left S89.002
        right S89.001
        Salter-Harris
          Type I S89.019
            left S89.012
            right S89.011
          Type II S89.029
            left S89.022
            right S89.021
          Type III S89.039
            left S89.032
            right S89.031
          Type IV S89.049
            left S89.042
            right S89.041
        specified NEC S89.099
          left S89.092
          right S89.091
      plateau — see Fracture, tibia, upper end,
          bicondylar
      right S82.101
      spine (displaced) S82.113
        left S82.112
        nondisplaced S82.116
          left S82.115
          right S82.114
        right S82.111
      torus S82.169
        left S82.162
        right S82.161
      specified NEC S82.199
        left S82.192
        right S82.191
      tuberosity (displaced) S82.153
        left S82.152
        nondisplaced S82.156
          left S82.155
          right S82.154
        right S82.151
  toe S92.919
    great (displaced) S92.403
      distal phalanx (displaced) S92.423
        left S92.422
        nondisplaced S92.426
          left S92.425
          right S92.424
        right S92.421
      left S92.402
      nondisplaced S92.406
        left S92.405
        right S92.404
      proximal phalanx (displaced) S92.413
        left S92.412
        nondisplaced S92.416
          left S92.415

©2002 Ingenix, Inc.

Fracture — *continued*
  toe — *continued*
    great — *continued*
      proximal phalanx — *continued*
        nondisplaced — *continued*
          right S92.414
        right S92.411
      right S92.401
      specified NEC S92.499
        left S92.492
        right S92.491
      left S92.912
      lesser (displaced) S92.503
        distal phalanx (displaced) S92.533
          left S92.532
          nondisplaced S92.536
            left S92.535
            right S92.534
          right S92.531
        left S92.502
        medial phalanx (displaced) S92.523
          left S92.522
          nondisplaced S92.526
            left S92.525
            right S92.524
          right S92.521
        nondisplaced S92.506
          left S92.505
          right S92.504
        proximal phalanx (displaced) S92.513
          left S92.512
          nondisplaced S92.516
            left S92.515
            right S92.514
          right S92.511
        right S92.501
        specified NEC S92.599
          left S92.592
          right S92.591
      right S92.911
  tooth (root) S02.5
  trachea (cartilage) S12.8
  transverse process — *see* Fracture, vertebra
  trapezium or trapezoid bone — *see* Fracture, carpal
  trimalleolar — *see* Fracture, ankle, trimalleolar
  triquetrum (cuneiform of carpus) — *see* Fracture, carpal, triquetrum
  trochanter — *see* Fracture, femur, trochanteric
  tuberosity (external) – code by site under Fracture
  ulna (shaft) S52.209
    bent bone S52.283
      left S52.282
      right S52.281
    coronoid process — *see* Fracture, ulna, upper end, coronoid process
    distal end — *see* Fracture, ulna, lower end
    following insertion of implant, prosthesis or plate M96.639
      left M96.632
      right M96.631
    head — *see* Fracture, ulna, upper end
    left S52.202
    lower end S52.609
      left S52.602
      physeal S59.009
        left S59.002
        right S59.001
      Salter-Harris
        Type I S59.019
          left S59.012
          right S59.011
        Type II S59.029
          left S59.022
          right S59.021
        Type III S59.039
          left S59.032
          right S59.031
        Type IV S59.049
          left S59.042
          right S59.041
      specified NEC S59.099
        left S59.092
        right S59.091

Fracture — *continued*
  ulna — *continued*
    lower end — *continued*
      right S52.601
      specified NEC S52.699
        left S52.692
        right S52.691
      styloid process (displaced) S52.613
        left S52.612
        nondisplaced S52.616
          left S52.615
          right S52.614
        right S52.611
      torus S52.629
        left S52.622
        right S52.621
    proximal end — *see* Fracture, ulna, upper end
    right S52.201
    shaft S52.209
      comminuted (displaced) S52.253
        left S52.252
        nondisplaced S52.256
          left S52.255
          right S52.254
        right S52.251
      greenstick S52.219
        left S52.212
        right S52.211
      left S52.202
      Monteggia's — *see* Monteggia's fracture
      oblique (displaced) S52.233
        left S52.232
        nondisplaced S52.236
          left S52.235
          right S52.234
        right S52.231
      right S52.201
      segmental (displaced) S52.263
        left S52.262
        nondisplaced S52.266
          left S52.265
          right S52.264
        right S52.261
      specified NEC S52.299
        left S52.292
        right S52.291
      spiral (displaced) S52.243
        left S52.242
        nondisplaced S52.246
          left S52.245
          right S52.244
        right S52.241
      transverse (displaced) S52.223
        left S52.222
        nondisplaced S52.226
          left S52.225
          right S52.224
        right S52.221
    upper end S52.009
      coronoid process (displaced) S52.043
        left S52.042
        nondisplaced S52.046
          left S52.045
          right S52.044
        right S52.041
      left S52.002
      olecranon process (displaced) S52.023
        with intraarticular extension S52.033
        left S52.022
          with intraarticular extension S52.032
        nondisplaced S52.026
          with intraarticular extension S52.036
          left S52.025
            with intraarticular extension S52.035
          right S52.024
            with intraarticular extension S52.034
        right S52.021
          with intraarticular extension S52.031
      right S52.001

Fracture — *continued*
  ulna — *continued*
    upper end — *continued*
      specified NEC S52.099
        left S52.092
        right S52.091
      torus S52.019
        left S52.012
        right S52.011
  unciform — *see* Fracture, carpal, hamate
  vault of skull S02.0
  vertebra, vertebral (arch) (body) (column) (neural arch) (pedicle) (spinous process) (transverse process)
    atlas — *see* Fracture, neck, cervical vertebra, first
    axis — *see* Fracture, neck, cervical vertebra, second
    cervical (teardrop) S12.9
      axis — *see* Fracture, neck, cervical vertebra, second
      first (atlas) — *see* Fracture, neck, cervical vertebra, first
      second (axis) — *see* Fracture, neck, cervical vertebra, second
    coccyx S32.2
    dorsal — *see* Fracture, thorax, vertebra
    fetus or newborn (birth injury) P11.5
    lumbar S32.009
      burst (stable) S32.001
        unstable S32.002
      fifth S32.059
        burst (stable) S32.051
          unstable S32.052
        specified type NEC S32.058
        wedge compression S32.050
      first S32.019
        burst (stable) S32.011
          unstable S32.012
        specified type NEC S32.018
        wedge compression S32.010
      fourth S32.049
        burst (stable) S32.041
          unstable S32.042
        specified type NEC S32.048
        wedge compression S32.040
      second S32.029
        burst (stable) S32.021
          unstable S32.022
        specified type NEC S32.028
        wedge compression S32.020
      specified type NEC S32.008
      third S32.039
        burst (stable) S32.031
          unstable S32.032
        specified type NEC S32.038
        wedge compression S32.030
      wedge compression S32.000
    metastatic (M8000/6) (*see also* Neoplasm) — *see* Collapse, vertebra, in, specified disease NEC
    sacrum S32.10
      specified NEC S32.19
      Type
        1 S32.14
        2 S32.15
        3 S32.16
        4 S32.17
      Zone
        I S32.119
          displaced (minimally) S32.111
            severely S32.112
          nondisplaced S32.110
        II S32.129
          displaced (minimally) S32.121
            severely S32.122
          nondisplaced S32.120
        III S32.139
          displaced (minimally) S32.131
            severely S32.132
          nondisplaced S32.130
    thoracic — *see* Fracture, thorax, vertebra
  vertex S02.0
  vomer (bone) S02.2
  wrist S62.109
    carpal — *see* Fracture, carpal bone

Fracture — *continued*
  wrist — *continued*
    left S62.102
    navicular (scaphoid) (hand) — *see* Fracture, carpal, navicular
    right S62.101
  xiphisternum, xiphoid (process) S22.24
  zygoma S02.44

Fragile, fragility
  autosomal site Q95.5
  bone, congenital (with blue sclera) Q78.0
  capillary (hereditary) D69.8
  hair L67.8
  nails L60.3
  non-sex chromosome site Q95.5
  X chromosome Q99.2

Fragilitas
  crinium L67.8
  ossium (with blue sclerae) (hereditary) Q78.0
  unguium L60.3
    congenital Q84.6

Frambesia, frambesial (tropica) — *see also* Yaws
  initial lesion or ulcer A66.0
  primary A66.0

Frambeside
  gummatous A66.4
  of early yaws A66.2

Frambesioma A66.1

Franceschetti-Klein (-Wildervanck) disease or syndrome Q75.4

Francis' disease — *see* Tularemia

Franklin's disease (M9763/3) C88.2

Frank's essential thrombocytopenia D69.3

Fraser's syndrome Q87.0

Freckle(s) L81.2
  malignant melanoma in (M8742/3) — *see* Melanoma
  melanotic (Hutchinson's) (M8742/2) — *see* Melanoma, in situ

Frederickson's hyperlipoproteinemia, type
  I and V E78.3
  IIA E78.0
  IIB and III E78.2
  IV E78.1

Freeman Sheldon syndrome Q87.0

Freezing — *see also* Effect, adverse, cold T69.9

Freiberg's disease (infraction of metatarsal head or osteochondrosis) — *see* Osteochondrosis, juvenile, metatarsus

Frei's disease A55

Fremitus, friction, cardiac R01.2

Frenum, frenulum
  external os Q51.8
  tongue (shortening) (congenital) Q38.1

Frequency micturition (nocturnal) R35.0
  psychogenic F45.8

Frey's syndrome (auriculotemporal syndrome) G50.8

Friction
  burn — *see* Burn, by site
  fremitus, cardiac R01.2
  precordial R01.2
  sounds, chest R09.89

Friderichsen-Waterhouse syndrome or disease A39.1

Friedländer's B (bacillus) **NEC** (*see also* condition) A49.8

Friedreich's
  ataxia G11.1
  combined systemic disease G11.1
  facial hemihypertrophy Q67.4
  sclerosis (cerebellum) (spinal cord) G11.1

Frigidity F52.22

Fröhlich's syndrome E23.6

Frontal — *see also* condition
  lobe syndrome F07.0

Frostbite (superficial) T33.90
  with
    partial thickness skin loss — *see* Frostbite (superficial), by site
    tissue necrosis T34.90

Frostbite — *continued*
  abdominal wall T33.3
    with tissue necrosis T34.3
  ankle T33.819
    with tissue necrosis T34.819
      left T34.812
      right T34.811
    left T33.812
    right T33.811
  arm T33.40
    with tissue necrosis T34.40
      left T34.42
      right T34.41
    finger(s) — *see* Frostbite, finger
    hand — *see* Frostbite, hand
    left T33.42
    right T33.41
    wrist — *see* Frostbite, wrist
  ear T33.019
    with tissue necrosis T34.019
      left T34.012
      right T34.011
    left T33.012
    right T33.011
  face T33.09
    with tissue necrosis T34.09
  finger T33.539
    with tissue necrosis T34.539
      left T34.532
      right T34.531
    left T33.532
    right T33.531
  foot T33.829
    with tissue necrosis T34.829
      left T34.822
      right T34.821
    left T33.822
    right T33.821
  hand T33.529
    with tissue necrosis T34.529
      left T34.522
      right T34.521
    left T33.522
    right T33.521
  head T33.09
    with tissue necrosis T34.09
    ear — *see* Frostbite, ear
    nose — *see* Frostbite, nose
  hip (and thigh) T33.60
    with tissue necrosis T34.60
      left T34.62
      right T34.61
    left T33.62
    right T33.61
  knee T33.70
    with tissue necrosis T34.70
      left T34.72
      right T34.71
    left T33.72
    right T33.71
  leg T33.99
    with tissue necrosis T34.99
    ankle — *see* Frostbite, ankle
    foot — *see* Frostbite, foot
    knee — *see* Frostbite, knee
    lower T33.70
      with tissue necrosis T34.70
        left T34.72
        right T34.71
      left T33.72
      right T33.71
    thigh — *see* Frostbite, hip
    toe — *see* Frostbite, toe
  limb
    lower T33.99
      with tissue necrosis T34.99
    upper — *see* Frostbite, arm
  neck T33.1
    with tissue necrosis T34.1
  nose T33.02
    with tissue necrosis T34.02
  pelvis T33.3
    with tissue necrosis T34.3
  specified site NEC T33.99
    with tissue necrosis T34.99
  thigh — *see* Frostbite, hip

Frostbite — *continued*
  thorax T33.2
    with tissue necrosis T34.2
  toes T33.839
    with tissue necrosis T34.839
      left T34.832
      right T34.831
    left T33.832
    right T33.831
  trunk T33.99
    with tissue necrosis T34.99
  wrist T33.519
    with tissue necrosis T34.519
      left T34.512
      right T34.511
    left T33.512
    right T33.511

Frotteurism F65.81

Frozen — *see also* Effect, adverse, cold T69.9
  shoulder — *see* Capsulitis, adhesive

Fructokinase deficiency E74.11

Fructose 1,6 diphosphatase deficiency E74.19

Fructosemia (benign) (essential) E74.19

Fructosuria (benign) (essential) E74.11

Fuchs'
  black spot (myopic) — *see* Disorder, globe, degenerative, myopia
  dystrophy (corneal endothelium) H18.52
  heterochromic cyclitis — *see* Cyclitis, Fuchs' heterochromic

Fucosidosis E77.1

Fugue R68.8
  dissociative F44.1
  hysterical (dissociative) F44.1
  postictal in epilepsy — *see* Epilepsy
  reaction to exceptional stress (transient) F43.0

Fulminant, fulminating — *see* condition

Functional — *see also* condition
  bleeding (uterus) N93.8

Functioning, intellectual, borderline R41.83

Fundus — *see* condition

Fungemia NOS B49

Fungus, fungous
  cerebral G93.8
  disease NOS B49
  infection — *see* Infection, fungus

Funiculitis (acute) (chronic) (endemic) N49.1
  gonococcal (acute) (chronic) A54.23
  tuberculous A18.15

Funnel
  breast (acquired) M95.4
    congenital Q67.6
    late effect of rickets E64.3
  chest (acquired) M95.4
    congenital Q67.6
    late effect of rickets E64.3
  pelvis (acquired) M95.5
    with disproportion (fetopelvic) O33.3
      causing obstructed labor O65.3
    congenital Q74.2

FUO (fever of unknown origin) R50.9

Furfur L21.0
  microsporon B36.0

Furrier's lung J67.8

Furrowed K14.5
  nail(s) (transverse) L60.4
    congenital Q84.6
  tongue K14.5
    congenital Q38.3

Furuncle L02.92
  abdominal wall L02.221
  ankle — *see* Furuncle, lower limb
  anus K61.0
  antecubital space — *see* Furuncle, upper limb
  arm — *see* Furuncle, upper limb
  auditory canal, external — *see* Abscess, ear, external
  auricle (ear) — *see* Abscess, ear, external
  axilla (region) L02.429
    left L02.422
    right L02.421
  back (any part) L02.222
  breast N61

©2002 Ingenix, Inc.

Furuncle — *continued*
buttock L02.32
cheek (external) L02.02
chest wall L02.223
chin L02.02
corpus cavernosum N48.21
ear, external — *see* Abscess, ear, external
external auditory canal — *see* Abscess, ear, external
eyelid — *see* Abscess, eyelid
face L02.02
femoral (region) — *see* Furuncle, lower limb
finger — *see* Furuncle, hand
flank L02.221
foot L02.629
    left L02.622
    right L02.621
forehead L02.02
gluteal (region) L02.32
groin L02.224
hand L02.529
    left L02.522
    right L02.521
head L02.821
    face L02.02
hip — *see* Furuncle, lower limb
kidney — *see* Abscess, kidney
knee — *see* Furuncle, lower limb
labium (majus) (minus) N76.4
lacrimal
    gland — *see* Dacryoadenitis
    passages (duct) (sac) — *see* Inflammation, lacrimal, passages, acute
leg (any part) — *see* Furuncle, lower limb
lower limb L02.429
    left L02.426
    right L02.425
malignant A22.0
mouth K12.2
navel L02.226
neck L02.12
nose J34.0
orbit, orbital — *see* Abscess, orbit
palmar (space) — *see* Furuncle, hand
partes posteriores L02.32
pectoral region L02.223
penis N48.21
perineum L02.225
pinna — *see* Abscess, ear, external
popliteal — *see* Furuncle, lower limb
prepatellar — *see* Furuncle, lower limb
scalp L02.821
seminal vesicle N49.0
shoulder — *see* Furuncle, upper limb
specified site NEC L02.828
submandibular K12.2
temple (region) L02.02
thumb — *see* Furuncle, hand
toe — *see* Furuncle, foot
trunk L02.229
    abdominal wall L02.221
    back L02.222
    chest wall L02.223
    groin L02.224
    perineum L02.225
    umbilicus L02.226
umbilicus L02.226
upper limb L02.429
    left L02.424
    right L02.423
vulva N76.4
Furunculosis — *see* Abscess, by site
Fusion, fused (congenital)
astragaloscaphoid Q74.2
atria Q21.1
auditory canal Q16.1
auricles, heart Q21.1
binocular with defective stereopsis H53.32
bone Q79.8
cervical spine M43.22
choanal Q30.0
commissure, mitral valve Q23.2
cusps, heart valve NEC Q24.8
    mitral Q23.2
    pulmonary Q22.1
    tricuspid Q22.4
ear ossicles Q16.3

Fusion, fused — *continued*
fingers — *see* Syndactyly, complex, fingers
hymen Q52.3
joint (acquired) — *see also* Ankylosis
    congenital Q74.8
kidneys (incomplete) Q63.1
labium (majus) (minus) Q52.5
larynx and trachea Q34.8
limb, congenital Q74.8
    lower Q74.2
    upper Q74.0
lobes, lung Q33.8
lumbosacral (acquired) M43.27
    congenital Q76.49
    surgical Z98.1
nares, nose, nasal, nostril(s) Q30.0
organ or site not listed — *see* Anomaly, by site
ossicles Q79.9
    auditory Q16.3
pulmonic cusps Q22.1
ribs Q76.6
sacroiliac (joint) (acquired) M43.25
    congenital Q74.2
    surgical Z98.1
spine (acquired) NEC M43.20
    arthrodesis status Z98.1
    cervical region M43.22
    cervicothoracic region M43.23
    congenital Q76.49
    lumbar M43.26
    lumbosacral region M43.27
    occipito-atlanto-axial region M43.21
    postoperative status Z98.1
    sacrococcygeal region M43.28
    thoracic region M43.24
    thoracolumbar region M43.25
sublingual duct with submaxillary duct at opening in mouth Q38.4
testes Q55.1
toes Q70.2
tooth, teeth K00.2
trachea and esophagus Q39.8
twins Q89.4
vagina Q52.4
ventricles, heart Q21.0
vertebra (arch) — *see* Fusion, spine
vulva Q52.5
Fusospirillosis (mouth) (tongue) (tonsil) A69.1
Fussy baby R68.12

G

Gain in weight (abnormal) (excessive) — *see also* Weight, gain
pregnancy O26.00
    first trimester O26.01
    second trimester O26.02
    third trimester O26.03
Gaisböck's disease (polycythemia hypertonica) D75.1
Gait abnormality R26.9
ataxic R26.0
falling R26.81
hysterical (ataxic) (staggering) F44.4
paralytic R26.1
spastic R26.1
specified type NEC R26.89
staggering R26.0
unsteadiness R26.82
walking difficulty NEC R26.2
Galactocele (breast) N64.8
puerperal, postpartum O92.7
Galactokinase deficiency E74.29
Galactophoritis N61
gestational, puerperal, postpartum — *see* Mastitis, obstetric, purulent
Galactorrhea O92.6
not associated with childbirth N64.3
Galactosemia (classic) (congenital) E74.21
Galactosuria E74.29
Galacturia R82.0
schistosomiasis (bilharziasis) B65.0
Galeazzi's fracture S52.379
left S52.372
right S52.371
Galen's vein — *see* condition
Galeophobia F40.218
Gall duct — *see* condition
Gallbladder — *see also* condition
acute K81.0
Gallop rhythm R00.8
Gallstone (colic) (cystic duct) (gallbladder) (impacted) (multiple) — *see also* Calculus, gallbladder
with
    cholecystitis — *see* Calculus, gallbladder, with cholecystitis
    bile duct (common) (hepatic) — *see* Calculus, bile duct
causing intestinal obstruction K56.3
specified NEC K80.80
    with obstruction K80.81
Gambling Z72.6
pathological (compulsive) F63.0
Gammopathy
associated with lymphoplasmacytic dyscrasia (M9765/1) D47.2
monoclonal (M9765/1) D47.2
    of undetermined significance D89.2
polyclonal D89.0
Gamna's disease (siderotic splenomegaly) D73.1
Gamophobia F40.298
Gampsodactylia (congenital) Q66.7
Gamstorp's disease (adynamia episodica hereditaria) G72.3
Gandy-Nanta disease (siderotic splenomegaly) D73.1
Gang
activity, without manifest psychiatric disorder Z03.8
membership offenses Z72.810
Gangliocytoma (M9490/0) D36.10
Ganglioglioma (M9505/1) — *see* Neoplasm, uncertain behavior
Ganglion (compound) (diffuse) (joint) (tendon (sheath)) M67.40
ankle M67.479
    left M67.472
    right M67.471
foot M67.479
    left M67.472
    right M67.471

Ganglion — *continued*
  forearm M67.439
    left M67.432
    right M67.431
  hand M67.449
    left M67.442
    right M67.441
  lower leg M67.469
    left M67.462
    right M67.461
  multiple sites M67.49
  of yaws (early) (late) A66.6
  pelvic region M67.459
    left M67.452
    right M67.451
  periosteal — *see* Periostitis
  shoulder region M67.419
    left M67.412
    right M67.411
  specified site NEC M67.48
  thigh region M67.459
    left M67.452
    right M67.451
  tuberculous A18.09
  upper arm M67.429
    left M67.422
    right M67.421
  wrist M67.439
    left M67.432
    right M67.431
Ganglioneuroblastoma (M9490/3) — *see* Neoplasm, nerve, malignant
Ganglioneuroma (M9490/0) D36.10
  malignant (M9490/3) — *see* Neoplasm, nerve, malignant
Ganglioneuromatosis (M9491/0) D36.10
Ganglionitis
  fifth nerve — *see* Neuralgia, trigeminal
  gasserian (postherpetic) (postzoster) B02.21
  geniculate G51.1
    newborn (birth injury) P11.3
    postherpetic, postzoster B02.21
  herpes zoster B02.21
  postherpetic geniculate B02.21
Gangliosidosis E75.10
  GM1 E75.19
  GM2 E75.00
    other specified E75.09
    Sandhoff disease E75.01
    Tay-Sachs disease E75.02
  GM3 E75.19
  mucolipidosis IV E75.11
Gangosa A66.5
Gangrene, gangrenous (connective tissue) (dropsical) (dry) (moist) (skin) (ulcer) I96
  with diabetes (mellitus) — *see* Diabetes, gangrene
  abdomen (wall) I96
  alveolar M27.3
  appendix K35.9
    with perforation, peritonitis, or rupture K35.0
  arteriosclerotic (general) (senile) — *see* Arteriosclerosis, extremities, with, gangrene
  auricle I96
  Bacillus welchii A48.0
  bladder (infectious) — *see* Cystitis, specified type NEC
  bowel, cecum, or colon — *see* Gangrene, intestine
  Clostridium perfringens or welchii A48.0
  cornea H18.89
  corpora cavernosa N48.29
    noninfective N48.89
  cutaneous, spreading I96
  decubital — *see* Decubitus
  diabetic (any site) — *see* Diabetes, gangrene
  epidemic — *see* Poisoning, food, noxious, plant
  epididymis (infectional) N45.1
  erysipelas — *see* Erysipelas
  emphysematous — *see* Gangrene, gas
  extremity (lower) (upper) I96
  Fournier's N49.3
  fusospirochetal A69.0
  gallbladder — *see* Cholecystitis, acute

Gangrene, gangrenous — *continued*
  gas (bacillus) A48.0
    following
      abortion — *see* Abortion by type complicated by infection
      ectopic or molar pregnancy O08.0
  glossitis K14.0
  hernia — *see* Hernia, by site, with gangrene
  intestine, intestinal (hemorrhagic) (massive) K55.0
    with
      mesenteric embolism K55.0
      obstruction — *see* Obstruction, intestine
  laryngitis J04.0
  limb (lower) (upper) I96
  lung J85.0
    spirochetal A69.8
  lymphangitis I89.1
  Meleney's (synergistic) — *see* Ulcer, skin
  mesentery K55.0
    with
      embolism K55.0
      intestinal obstruction — *see* Obstruction, intestine
  mouth A69.0
  ovary — *see* Oophoritis
  pancreas K85.8
  penis N48.29
    noninfective N48.89
  perineum I96
  pharynx — *see also* Pharyngitis
    Vincent's A69.1
  presenile I73.1
  progressive synergistic — *see* Ulcer, skin
  pulmonary J85.0
  pulpal (dental) K04.1
  quinsy J36
  Raynaud's (symmetric gangrene) I73.01
  retropharyngeal J39.2
  scrotum N49.2
    noninfective N50.8
  senile (atherosclerotic) — *see* Arteriosclerosis, extremities, with, gangrene
  spermatic cord N49.1
    noninfective N50.8
  spine I96
  spirochetal NEC A69.8
  spreading cutaneous I96
  stomatitis A69.0
  symmetrical I73.01
  testis (infectional) N45.2
    noninfective N44.8
  throat — *see also* Pharyngitis
    diphtheritic A36.0
    Vincent's A69.1
  thyroid (gland) E07.89
  tooth (pulp) K04.1
  tuberculous NEC — *see* Tuberculosis
  tunica vaginalis N49.1
    noninfective N50.8
  umbilicus I96
  uterus — *see* Endometritis
  uvulitis K12.2
  vas deferens N49.1
    noninfective N50.8
  vulva N76.8
Ganister disease J62.8
Ganser's syndrome (hysterical) F44.89
Gardner-Diamond syndrome (autoerythrocyte sensitization) D69.2
Gargoylism E76.01
Garré's disease, osteitis (sclerosing), osteomyelitis — *see* Osteomyelitis, specified type NEC
Garrod's pad, knuckle M72.1
Gartner's duct
  cyst Q50.5
  persistent Q50.6
Gas
  asphyxiation, inhalation, poisoning, suffocation NEC — *see* Table of Drugs and Chemicals
  excessive R14.8
  gangrene A48.0
    following
      abortion — *see* Abortion by type complicated by infection

Gas — *continued*
  gangrene — *continued*
    following — *continued*
      ectopic or molar pregnancy O08.0
  on stomach R14.8
  pains R14.1
Gastralgia — *see also* Pain, abdominal
  psychogenic F45.4
Gastrectasis K31.0
  psychogenic F45.8
Gastric — *see* condition
Gastrinoma (M8153/1)
  malignant (M8153/3)
    pancreas C25.4
    specified site NEC — *see* Neoplasm, malignant
    unspecified site C25.4
  specified site — *see* Neoplasm, uncertain behavior
  unspecified site D37.7
Gastritis (simple) K29.70
  with bleeding K29.71
  acute (erosive) K29.00
    with bleeding K29.01
  alcoholic K29.20
    with bleeding K29.21
  allergic K29.60
    with bleeding K29.61
  atrophic (chronic) K29.40
    with bleeding K29.41
  chronic (antral) (fundal) K29.50
    with bleeding K29.51
    atrophic K29.40
      with bleeding K29.41
    superficial K29.30
      with bleeding K29.31
  dietary counseling and surveillance Z71.3
  due to diet deficiency E63.9 *[K93]*
  eosinophilic K52.8
  giant hypertrophic K29.60
    with bleeding K29.61
  granulomatous K29.60
    with bleeding K29.61
  hypertrophic (mucosa) K29.60
    with bleeding K29.61
  nervous F54
  spastic K29.60
    with bleeding K29.61
  specified NEC K29.60
    with bleeding K29.61
  superficial chronic K29.30
    with bleeding K29.31
  tuberculous A18.83
Gastrocarcinoma (M8010/3) — *see* Neoplasm, malignant, stomach
Gastrocolic — *see* condition
Gastrodisciasis, gastrodiscoidiasis B66.8
Gastroduodenitis K29.90
  with bleeding K29.91
  virus, viral A08.4
    specified type NEC A08.3
Gastrodynia — *see* Pain, abdominal
Gastroenteritis (acute) (chronic (noninfective)) (septic) (*see also* Enteritis) K52.9
  allergic K52.2
  dietetic K52.2
  due to
    Cryptosporidium A07.2
    food poisoning — *see* Intoxication, foodborne
    radiation K52.0
  eosinophilic K52.8
  epidemic (infectious) A09
  food hypersensitivity K52.2
  infectious — *see* Enteritis, infectious
  nonbacterial of infancy A08.5
  noninfective K52.9
    specified NEC K52.8
  rotaviral A08.0
  Salmonella A02.0
  toxic K52.1
  viral NEC A08.4
    acute infectious A08.3
    epidemic A08.1
      type Norwalk A08.1
    infantile (acute) A08.3

©2002 Ingenix, Inc.

Gastroenteritis (see also Enteritis) — continued
  viral NEC — continued
    Norwalk agent A08.1
    rotaviral A08.0
    severe of infants A08.3
    specified type NEC A08.3
Gastroenteropathy — see also Gastroenteritis
  acute, due to Norwalk agent A08.1
Gastroenteroptosis K63.4
  Gastroesophageal lacerationhemorrhage
    syndrome K22.6
Gastrointestinal — see condition
Gastrojejunal — see condition
Gastrojejunitis, noninfective (presumed) — see
  Enteritis
Gastrojejunocolic — see condition
Gastroliths K31.89
Gastromalacia K31.89
Gastroparalysis K31.89
  diabetic — see Diabetes, gastroparalysis
Gastroparesis K31.89
  diabetic — see Diabetes, gastroparesis
Gastroptosis K31.89
Gastrorrhagia K92.2
  psychogenic F45.8
Gastroschisis (congenital) Q79.3
Gastrospasm (neurogenic) (reflex) K31.89
  neurotic F45.8
  psychogenic F45.8
Gastrostaxis — see Gastritis, with bleeding
Gastrostenosis K31.89
Gastrostomy
  attention to Z43.1
  status Z93.1
Gastrosuccorrhea (continuous) (intermittent)
  K31.89
  neurotic F45.8
  psychogenic F45.8
Gatophobia F40.218
Gaucher's disease or splenomegaly (adult)
  (infantile) E75.22
Gee (-Herter) (-Thaysen) **disease** (nontropical
  sprue) K90.0
Gélineau's syndrome G47.4
Gemination, tooth, teeth K00.2
Gemistocytoma (M9411/3)
  specified site — see Neoplasm, malignant
  unspecified site C71.9
General, generalized — see condition
Genital — see condition
Genito-anorectal syndrome A55
Genitourinary system — see condition
Genu
  congenital Q74.1
  extrorsum (acquired) — see also Deformity,
    varus, knee
    congenital Q74.1
    late effect of rickets E64.3
  introrsum (acquired) — see also Deformity,
    valgus, knee
    congenital Q74.1
    late effect of rickets E64.3
  rachitic (old) E64.3
  recurvatum (acquired) — see also Deformity,
    limb, specified type NEC, lower leg
    congenital Q68.2
    late effect of rickets E64.3
  valgum (acquired) (knock-knee) — see also
    Deformity, valgus, knee
    congenital Q74.1
    late effect of rickets E64.3
  varum (acquired) (bowleg) — see also
    Deformity, varus, knee
    congenital Q74.1
    late effect of rickets E64.3
Geographic tongue K14.1
Geophagia — see Pica
Gerbode defect Q21.0
Geotrichosis B48.3
  stomatitis B48.3 [K93]
Gephyrophobia F40.242

Gerhardt's
  disease (erythromelalgia) I73.8
  syndrome (vocal cord paralysis) J38.00
    bilateral J38.02
    unilateral J38.01
German measles — see also Rubella
  exposure to Z20.4
Germinoblastoma (diffuse) (M9676/3) C83.20
  follicular (M9692/3) C82.10
Germinoma (M9064/3) — see Neoplasm,
  malignant
Gerontoxon — see Degeneration, cornea, senile
Gerstmann's syndrome (developmental) F81.2
Gestation (period) — see also Pregnancy
  ectopic — see Pregnancy, by site
  multiple O30.90
    first trimester O30.91
    second trimester O30.92
    specified NEC — see category O30.8
    third trimester O30.93
Ghon tubercle, primary infection A15.7
Ghost
  teeth K00.4
  vessels (cornea) H16.419
    bilateral H16.413
    left H16.412
    right H16.411
Ghoul hand A66.3
Giannotti-Crosti disease L44.4
Giant
  cell
    epulis K06.8
    peripheral granuloma K06.8
  esophagus, congenital Q39.5
  kidney, congenital Q63.3
  oesophagus, congenital Q39.5
  urticaria T78.3
    hereditary D84.1
Giardiasis A07.1
Gibert's disease or pityriasis L42
Giddiness R42
  hysterical F44.89
  psychogenic F45.8
Gierke's disease (glycogenosis I) E74.01
Gigantism (cerebral) (hypophyseal) (pituitary)
  E22.0
  constitutional E34.4
Gilbert's disease or syndrome E80.4
Gilchrist's disease B40.9
Gilford-Hutchinson disease E34.8
Gilles de la Tourette's disease or syndrome
  (motor-verbal tic) F95.2
Gingivitis K05.1
  acute (catarrhal) K05.0
    necrotizing A69.1
  chronic (desquamative) (hyperplastic) (simple
    marginal) (ulcerative) K05.1
  expulsiva K05.3
  necrotizing ulcerative (acute) A69.1
  pellagrous E52 [K93]
    acute necrotizing A69.1
  Vincent's A69.1
Gingivoglossitis K14.0
Gingivopericementitis K05.3
Gingivosis K05.1
Gingivostomatitis K05.1
  herpesviral B00.2
  necrotizing ulcerative (acute) A69.1
Gland, glandular — see condition
Glanders A24.0
Glanzmann (-Naegeli) **disease or**
  thrombasthenia D69.1
Glass-blower's disease (cataract) — see Cataract,
  specified NEC
Glaucoma H40.9
  with
    increased episcleral venous pressure
      H40.819
      bilateral H40.813
      left H40.812
      right H40.811

Glaucoma — continued
  with — continued
    pseudoexfoliation of lens — see Glaucoma,
      open angle, primary, capsular
  absolute H44.519
    bilateral H44.513
    left H44.512
    right H44.511
  angle-closure (primary) H40.20
    acute H40.219
      bilateral H40.213
      left H40.212
      right H40.211
    chronic H40.229
      bilateral H40.223
      left H40.222
      right H40.221
    intermittent H40.239
      bilateral H40.233
      left H40.232
      right H40.231
    residual stage H40.249
      bilateral H40.243
      left H40.242
      right H40.241
  borderline H40.0
  capsular (with pseudoexfoliation of lens) — see
    Glaucoma, open angle, primary, capsular
  childhood Q15.0
  closed angle — see Glaucoma, angle-closure
  congenital Q15.0
  corticosteroid-induced — see Glaucoma,
    secondary, drugs
  hypersecretion H40.829
    bilateral H40.823
    left H40.822
    right H40.821
  in (due to)
    amyloidosis E85 [H42]
    aniridia Q13.1 [H42]
    concussion of globe — see Glaucoma,
      secondary, trauma
    dislocation of lens — see Glaucoma,
      secondary
    disorder of lens NEC — see Glaucoma,
      secondary
    drugs — see Glaucoma, secondary, drugs
    endocrine disease NOS E34.9 [H42]
    eye
      inflammation — see Glaucoma,
        secondary, inflammation
      trauma — see Glaucoma, secondary,
        trauma
    hypermature cataract — see Glaucoma,
      secondary
    iridocyclitis — see Glaucoma, secondary,
      inflammation
    lens disorder — see Glaucoma, secondary,
    Lowe's syndrome E72.03 [H42]
    metabolic disease NOS E88.9 [H42]
    ocular disorders NEC — see Glaucoma,
      secondary
    onchocerciasis B73.02
    pupillary block — see Glaucoma, secondary
    retinal vein occlusion — see Glaucoma,
      secondary
    Rieger's anomaly Q13.81 [H42]
    rubeosis of iris — see Glaucoma, secondary
    tumor of globe — see Glaucoma, secondary
  infantile Q15.0
  low tension — see Glaucoma, open angle, low-
    tension
  narrow angle — see Glaucoma, angle-closure
  newborn Q15.0
  noncongestive (chronic) — see Glaucoma, open
    angle
  nonobstructive — see Glaucoma, open angle
  obstructive — see also Glaucoma, angle-closure
    due to lens changes — see Glaucoma,
      secondary
  open angle H40.10
    primary H40.11
      capsular (with pseudoexfoliation of lens)
        H40.149
      bilateral H40.143
      left H40.142
      right H40.141

Glaucoma — continued
  open angle — continued
    primary — continued
      low-tension H40.129
        bilateral H40.123
        left H40.122
        right H40.121
      pigmentary H40.139
        bilateral H40.133
        left H40.132
        right H40.131
      residual stage H40.159
        bilateral H40.153
        left H40.152
        right H40.151
  phacolytic — see Glaucoma, secondary
  pigmentary — see Glaucoma, open angle, pigmentary
  postinfectious — see Glaucoma, secondary, inflammation
  secondary (to) H40.50
    bilateral H40.53
    drugs H40.60
      bilateral H40.63
      left H40.62
      right H40.61
    inflammation H40.40
      bilateral H40.43
      left H40.42
      right H40.41
    left H40.52
    right H40.51
    trauma H40.30
      bilateral H40.33
      left H40.32
      right H40.31
  simple (chronic) — see Glaucoma, open angle
  simplex — see Glaucoma, open angle
  specified type NEC H40.89
  suspect H40.0
  syphilitic A52.71
  traumatic — see also Glaucoma, secondary, trauma
    newborn (birth injury) P15.3
  tuberculous A18.59
Glaucomatous flecks (subcapsular) — see Cataract, complicated
Glazed tongue K14.4
Gleet (gonococcal) A54.01
Glénard's disease K63.4
Glioblastoma (multiforme) (M9440/3)
  with sarcomatous component (M9442/3)
    specified site — see Neoplasm, malignant
    unspecified site C71.9
  giant cell (M9441/3)
    specified site — see Neoplasm, malignant
    unspecified site C71.9
  specified site — see Neoplasm, malignant
  unspecified site C71.9
Glioma (malignant) (M9380/3)
  astrocytic (M9400/3)
    specified site — see Neoplasm, malignant
    unspecified site C71.9
  mixed (M9382/3)
    specified site — see Neoplasm, malignant
    unspecified site C71.9
  nose Q30.8
  specified site NEC — see Neoplasm, malignant
  subependymal (M9383/1) D43.2
    specified site — see Neoplasm, uncertain behavior
    unspecified site D43.2
  unspecified site C71.9
Gliomatosis cerebri (M9381/3) C71.0
Glioneuroma (M9505/1) — see Neoplasm, uncertain behavior
Gliosarcoma (M9380/3)
  specified site — see Neoplasm, malignant
  unspecified site C71.9
Gliosis (cerebral) G93.8
  spinal G95.89
Glisson's disease — see Rickets
Globinuria R82.3
Globus (hystericus) F45.8

Glomangioma (M8712/0) D18.00
  intra-abdominal D18.03
  intracranial D18.02
  skin D18.01
  specified site NEC D18.09
Glomangiomyoma (M8713/0) D18.00
  intra-abdominal D18.03
  intracranial D18.02
  skin D18.01
  specified site NEC D18.09
Glomangiosarcoma (M8710/3) — see Neoplasm, connective tissue, malignant
Glomerular
  disease in syphilis A52.75
  nephritis — see Glomerulonephritis
Glomerulitis — see Glomerulonephritis
Glomerulonephritis N05.9
  with edema — see Nephrosis
  acute N00.9
  chronic N03.9
  crescentic (diffuse) NEC (see also N00-N07 with fourth character .7) N05.7
  dense deposit (see also N00-N07 with fourth character .6) N05.6
  diffuse
    crescentic (see also N00-N07 with fourth character .7) N05.7
    endocapillary proliferative (see also N00-N07 with fourth character .4) N05.4
    membranous (see also N00-N07 with fourth character .2) N05.2
    mesangial proliferative (see also N00-N07 with fourth character .3) N05.3
    mesangiocapillary (see also N00-N07 with fourth character .5) N05.5
    sclerosing (see also Failure, renal, chronic) N18.9
  endocapillary proliferative (diffuse) NEC (see also N00-N07 with fourth character .4) N05.4
  extracapillary NEC (see also N00-N07 with fourth character .7) N05.7
  focal (and segmental) (see also N00-N07 with fourth character .1) N05.1
  hypocomplementemic — see Glomerulonephritis, membranoproliferative
  IgA — see Nephropathy, IgA
  immune complex (circulating) NEC N05.8
  in (due to)
    amyloidosis E85 [N08]
    bilharziasis B65.9 [N08]
    cryoglobulinemia D89.1 [N08]
    defibrination syndrome D65 [N08]
    diabetes mellitus — see Diabetes, glomerulosclerosis
    disseminated intravascular coagulation D65 [N08]
    Fabry(-Anderson) disease E75.21 [N08]
    Goodpasture's syndrome M31.0
    hemolytic-uremic syndrome D59.3
    Henoch(-Schönlein) purpura D69.0 [N08]
    lecithin cholesterol acyltransferase deficiency E78.6 [N08]
    multiple myeloma (M9732/3) C90.00 [N08]
    Plasmodium malariae B52.0
    polyarteritis nodosa M30.0 [N08]
    schistosomiasis B65.9 [N08]
    septicemia A41.9 [N08]
    sickle-cell disorders D57.0-D57.8 [N08]
    strongyloidiasis B78.9 [N08]
    subacute bacterial endocarditis I33.0 [N08]
    syphilis (late) congenital A50.59 [N08]
    systemic lupus erythematosus M32.14
    thrombotic thrombocytopenic purpura M31.1 [N08]
    typhoid fever A01.09
    Waldenström's macroglobulinemia (M9761/3) C88.0 [N08]
    Wegener's granulomatosis M31.31
  latent or quiescent N03.9
  lobular, lobulonodular — see Glomerulonephritis, membranoproliferative
  membranoproliferative (diffuse) (type 1 or 3) (see also N00-N07 with fourth character .5) N05.5

Glomerulonephritis — continued
  membranoproliferative (see also N00-N07 with fourth character .5) — continued
    dense deposit (type 2) NEC (see also N00-N07 with fourth character .6) N05.6
  membranous (diffuse) NEC (see also N00-N07 with fourth character .2) N05.2
  mesangial
    IgA/IgG — see Nephropathy, IgA
    proliferative (diffuse) NEC (see also N00-N07 with fourth character .3) N05.3
  mesangiocapillary (diffuse) NEC (see also N00-N07 with fourth character .5) N05.5
  necrotic, necrotizing NEC (see also N00-N07 with fourth character .8) N05.8
  nodular — see Glomerulonephritis, membranoproliferative
  poststreptococcal NEC N05.9
    acute N00.9
    chronic N03.9
    rapidly progressive N01.9
  proliferative NEC (see also N00-N07 with fourth character .8) N05.8
    diffuse (lupus) M32.14
  rapidly progressive N01.9
  sclerosing, diffuse (see also Failure, renal, chronic) N18.9
  specified pathology NEC (see also N00-N07 with fourth character .8) N05.8
  subacute N01.9
Glomerulopathy — see Glomerulonephritis
Glomerulosclerosis — see also Sclerosis, renal
  intercapillary (nodular) (with diabetes) — see Diabetes, glomerulosclerosis
  intracapillary — see Diabetes, glomerulosclerosis
Glossagra K14.6
Glossalgia K14.6
Glossitis (chronic superficial) (gangrenous) (Moeller's) K14.0
  areata exfoliativa K14.1
  atrophic K14.4
  benign migratory K14.1
  cortical superficial, sclerotic K14.0
  Hunter's D51.0
  interstitial, sclerous K14.0
  median rhomboid K14.2
  pellagrous E52 [K93]
  superficial, chronic K14.0
Glossocele K14.8
Glossodynia K14.6
  exfoliativa K14.4
Glossoncus K14.8
Glossopathy K14.9
Glossophytia K14.3
Glossoplegia K14.8
Glossoptosis K14.8
Glossopyrosis K14.6
Glossotrichia K14.3
Glossy skin L90.8
Glottis — see condition
Glottitis — see Glossitis
Glucagonoma (M8152/0)
  malignant (M8152/3)
    pancreas C25.4
    specified site NEC — see Neoplasm, malignant
    unspecified site C25.4
  pancreas D13.7
  specified site NEC — see Neoplasm, benign
  unspecified site D13.7
Glucoglycinuria E72.51
Glucose-galactose malabsorption E74.39
Glue
  ear — see Otitis, media, nonsuppurative, chronic, mucoid
  sniffing (airplane) — see Disorder, drug-related, inhalant
Glutaric aciduria E72.3
Glycinemia E72.51
Glycinuria (renal) (with ketosis) E72.09

Glycogen
infiltration — *see* Disease, glycogen storage
storage disease — *see* Disease, glycogen storage
Glycogenosis (diffuse) (generalized) — *see also*
Disease, glycogen storage
cardiac E74.02 *[I43]*
diabetic, secondary — *see* Diabetes,
glycogenesis, secondary
Glycopenia E16.2
Glycosuria R81
renal E74.8
Gnathostoma spinigerum (infection) (infestation)
gnathostomiasis (wandering swelling) B83.1
Goiter (plunging) (substernal) E04.9
with
hyperthyroidism (recurrent) — *see*
Hyperthyroidism, with, goiter
thyrotoxicosis — *see* Hyperthyroidism, with,
goiter
adenomatous — *see* Goiter, nodular
cancerous (M8000/3) C73
congenital (nontoxic) E03.0
diffuse E03.0
parenchymatous E03.0
transitory, with normal functioning P72.0
cystic E04.2
due to iodine-deficiency E01.1
due to
enzyme defect in synthesis of thyroid
hormone E07.1
iodine-deficiency (endemic) E01.2
dyshormonogenetic (familial) E07.1
endemic (iodine-deficiency) E01.2
diffuse E01.0
multinodular E01.1
exophthalmic — *see* Hyperthyroidism, with,
goiter
iodine-deficiency (endemic) E01.2
diffuse E01.0
multinodular E01.1
nodular E01.1
lingual Q89.2
lymphadenoid E06.3
malignant (M8000/3) C73
multinodular (cystic) (nontoxic) E04.2
toxic or with hyperthyroidism E05.20
with thyroid storm E05.21
neonatal NEC P72.0
nodular (nontoxic) (due to) E04.9
with
hyperthyroidism E05.20
with thyroid storm E05.21
thyrotoxicosis E05.20
with thyroid storm E05.21
endemic E01.1
iodine-deficiency E01.1
sporadic E04.9
toxic E05.20
with thyroid storm E05.21
nontoxic E04.9
diffuse (colloid) E04.0
multinodular E04.2
simple E04.0
specified NEC E04.8
uninodular E04.1
simple E04.0
toxic — *see* Hyperthyroidism, with, goiter
uninodular (nontoxic) E04.1
toxic or with hyperthyroidism E05.10
with thyroid storm E05.11
Goiter-deafness syndrome E07.1
Goldberg-Maxwell syndrome E34.5
Goldblatt's hypertension or kidney I70.1
Goldenhar (-Gorlin) syndrome Q87.0
Goldflam-Erb disease or syndrome G70.0
Goldscheider's disease Q81.8
Goldstein's disease (familial hemorrhagic
telangiectasia) I78.0
Golfer's elbow — *see* Epicondylitis, medial
Gonadoblastoma (M9073/1)
specified site — *see* Neoplasm, uncertain
behavior
unspecified site
female D39.10
male D40.10

Gonarthrosis M17.9
post-traumatic (unilateral) M17.30
bilateral M17.2
left M17.32
right M17.31
primary (unilateral) M17.10
bilateral M17.0
left M17.12
right M17.11
secondary NEC (unilateral) M17.5
bilateral M17.4
Gonecystitis — *see* Vesiculitis
Gongylonemiasis B83.8
Goniosynechiae — *see* Adhesions, iris,
goniosynechiae
Gonococcemia A54.86
Gonococcus, gonococcal (disease) (infection) (*see
also* condition) A54.9
anus A54.6
bursa, bursitis A54.49
complicating pregnancy, childbirth or
puerperium — *see* Gonorrhea, obstetric
conjunctiva, conjunctivitis (neonatorum)
A54.31
endocardium A54.83
eye A54.30
conjunctivitis A54.31
iridocyclitis A54.32
keratitis A54.33
newborn A54.31
other specified A54.39
fallopian tubes (acute) (chronic) A54.24
genitourinary (organ) (system) (tract) (acute)
A54.00
lower A54.00
with abscess (accessory gland)
(periurethral) A54.1
upper (*see also* condition) A54.29
heart A54.83
iridocyclitis A54.32
joint A54.42
lymphatic (gland) (node) A54.89
meninges, meningitis A54.81
musculoskeletal A54.40
arthritis A54.42
osteomyelitis A54.43
other specified A54.49
spondylopathy A54.41
obstetric complicating
childbirth O98.22
pregnancy O98.219
first trimester O98.211
second trimester O98.212
third trimester O98.213
puerperium O98.23
pelviperitonitis A54.24
pelvis (acute) (chronic) A54.24
pharynx A54.5
proctitis A54.6
pyosalpinx (acute) (chronic) A54.24
rectum A54.6
skin A54.89
specified site NEC A54.89
tendon sheath A54.49
throat A54.5
urethra (acute) (chronic) A54.01
with abscess (accessory gland) (periurethral)
A54.1
vulva (acute) (chronic) A54.02
Gonocytoma (M9073/1)
specified site — *see* Neoplasm, uncertain
behavior
unspecified site
female D39.10
male D40.10
Gonorrhea (acute) (chronic) A54.9
Bartholin's gland (acute) (chronic) (purulent)
A54.02
with abscess (accessory gland) (periurethral)
A54.1
bladder A54.01
cervix A54.03
complicating pregnancy, childbirth or
puerperium — *see* Gonorrhea, obstetric
conjunctiva, conjunctivitis (neonatorum)
A54.31
contact Z20.2

Gonorrhea — *continued*
Cowper's gland (with abscess) A54.1
exposure to Z20.2
fallopian tube (acute) (chronic) A54.24
kidney (acute) (chronic) A54.21
lower genitourinary tract A54.00
with abscess (accessory gland) (periurethral)
A54.1
obstetric complicating
childbirth O98.22
pregnancy O98.219
first trimester O98.211
second trimester O98.212
third trimester O98.213
puerperium O98.23
ovary (acute) (chronic) A54.24
pelvis (acute) (chronic) A54.24
female pelvic inflammatory disease A54.24
penis A54.09
prostate (acute) (chronic) A54.22
seminal vesicle (acute) (chronic) A54.23
specified site not listed — *see also* Gonococcus
A54.89
spermatic cord (acute) (chronic) A54.23
urethra A54.01
with abscess (accessory gland) (periurethral)
A54.1
vagina A54.02
vas deferens (acute) (chronic) A54.23
vulva A54.02
Goodall's disease A08.1
Goodpasture's syndrome M31.0
Gopalan's syndrome (burning feet) E53.0
Gorlin-Chaudry-Moss syndrome Q87.0
Gottron's papules L94.4
Gougerot's syndrome (trisymptomatic) L81.7
Gougerot-Blum syndrome (pigmented purpuric
lichenoid dermatitis) L81.7
Gougerot-Carteaud disease or syndrome
(confluent reticulate papillomatosis) L83
Gouley's syndrome (constrictive pericarditis)
I31.1
Goundou A66.6
Gout, gouty M10.9
drug-induced M10.20
ankle M10.279
left M10.272
right M10.271
elbow M10.229
left M10.222
right M10.221
foot joint M10.279
left M10.272
right M10.271
hand joint M10.249
left M10.242
right M10.241
hip M10.259
left M10.252
right M10.251
knee M10.269
left M10.262
right M10.261
multiple site M10.29
shoulder M10.219
left M10.212
right M10.211
specified joint NEC M10.28
wrist M10.239
left M10.232
right M10.231
idiopathic M10.00
ankle M10.079
left M10.072
right M10.071
elbow M10.029
left M10.022
right M10.021
foot joint M10.079
left M10.072
right M10.071
hand joint M10.049
left M10.042
right M10.041

Gout, gouty — *continued*
  idiopathic — *continued*
    hip M10.059
      left M10.052
      right M10.051
    knee M10.069
      left M10.062
      right M10.061
    multiple site M10.09
    shoulder M10.019
      left M10.012
      right M10.011
    specified joint NEC M10.08
    wrist M10.039
      left M10.032
      right M10.031
  in (due to) renal impairment M10.30
    ankle M10.379
      left M10.372
      right M10.371
    elbow M10.329
      left M10.322
      right M10.321
    foot joint M10.379
      left M10.372
      right M10.371
    hand joint M10.349
      left M10.342
      right M10.341
    hip M10.359
      left M10.352
      right M10.351
    knee M10.369
      left M10.362
      right M10.361
    multiple site M10.39
    shoulder M10.319
      left M10.312
      right M10.311
    specified joint NEC M10.38
    wrist M10.339
      left M10.332
      right M10.331
  lead-induced M10.10
    ankle M10.179
      left M10.172
      right M10.171
    elbow M10.129
      left M10.122
      right M10.121
    foot joint M10.179
      left M10.172
      right M10.171
    hand joint M10.149
      left M10.142
      right M10.141
    hip M10.159
      left M10.152
      right M10.151
    knee M10.169
      left M10.162
      right M10.161
    multiple site M10.19
    shoulder M10.119
      left M10.112
      right M10.111
    specified joint NEC M10.18
    wrist M10.139
      left M10.132
      right M10.131
  primary — *see* Gout, idiopathic
  saturnine — *see* Gout, lead-induced
  secondary NEC M10.40
    ankle M10.479
      left M10.472
      right M10.471
    elbow M10.429
      left M10.422
      right M10.421
    foot joint M10.479
      left M10.472
      right M10.471
    hand joint M10.449
      left M10.442
      right M10.441

Gout, gouty — *continued*
  secondary NEC — *continued*
    hip M10.459
      left M10.452
      right M10.451
    knee M10.469
      left M10.462
      right M10.461
    multiple site M10.49
    shoulder M10.419
      left M10.412
      right M10.411
    specified joint NEC M10.48
    wrist M10.439
      left M10.432
      right M10.431
  syphilitic (*see also* category M14.8) A52.77
  tophi NEC — *see* Gout by type
    ear (*see also* category H62.8) M10.08
    heart M10.08 *[I43]*

Gower's
  muscular dystrophy G71.0
  syndrome (vasovagal attack) R55

Gradenigo's syndrome — *see* Otitis, media, suppurative, acute

Graefe's disease — *see* Strabismus, paralytic, ophthalmoplegia, progressive

Graft-versus-host (GVH) **disease** (bone marrow) T86.01

Grainhandler's disease or lung J67.8

Grain mite (itch) B88.0

Grand mal — *see* Epilepsy, grand mal

Grand multipara status only (not pregnant) Z64.1
  pregnant — *see* Pregnancy, complicated by, grand multiparity

Granite worker's lung J62.8

Granular — *see also* condition
  inflammation, pharynx J31.2
  kidney (contracting) — *see* Sclerosis, renal
  liver K74.6

Granulation tissue (abnormal) (excessive) L92.9
  postmastoidectomy cavity — *see* Complications, postmastoidectomy, granulation

Granulocytopenia (primary) (malignant) — *see* Agranulocytosis

Granuloma L92.9
  abdomen K66.8
    from residual foreign body L92.3
    pyogenicum L98.0
  actinic L57.5
  annulare (perforating) L92.0
  apical K04.5
  aural — *see* Otitis, externa, specified NEC
  beryllium (skin) L92.3
  bone (from residual foreign body) — *see also* Osteomyelitis, specified type NEC
    eosinophilic D76.0
  brain (any site) G06.0
    schistosomiasis B65.9 *[G07]*
  canaliculus lacrimalis — *see* Granuloma, lacrimal
  candidal (cutaneous) B37.2
  cerebral (any site) G06.0
  coccidioidal (primary) (progressive) B38.7
    lung B38.1
    meninges B38.4
  colon K63.8
  conjunctiva H11.229
    bilateral H11.223
    left H11.222
    right H11.221
  dental K04.5
  ear, middle — *see* Cholesteatoma
  eosinophilic D76.0
    bone D76.0
    lung D76.0
    oral mucosa K13.4
    skin L92.2
  eyelid H01.8
  facial(e) L92.2
  foreign body (in soft tissue) NEC M60.20
    ankle M60.279
      left M60.272
      right M60.271

Granuloma — *continued*
  foreign body NEC — *continued*
    foot M60.279
      left M60.272
      right M60.271
    forearm M60.239
      left M60.232
      right M60.231
    hand M60.249
      left M60.242
      right M60.241
    in operation wound — *see* Foreign body, accidentally left following a procedure
    lower leg M60.269
      left M60.262
      right M60.261
    pelvic region M60.259
      left M60.252
      right M60.251
    shoulder region M60.219
      left M60.212
      right M60.211
    skin L92.3
    specified site NEC M60.28
    subcutaneous tissue L92.3
    thigh M60.259
      left M60.252
      right M60.251
    upper arm M60.229
      left M60.222
      right M60.221
  gangraenescens M31.2
  genito-inguinale A58
  giant cell (central) (reparative) (jaw) M27.1
    gingiva (peripheral) K06.8
  gland (lymph) I88.8
  hepatic NEC K75.3
    in (due to)
      berylliosis J63.2 *[K77]*
      sarcoidosis D86.89
  Hodgkin's (M9661/3) C81.70
  ileum K63.8
  infectious B99.9
    specified NEC B99.8
  inguinale (Donovan) (venereal) A58
  intestine NEC K63.8
  intracranial (any site) G06.0
  intraspinal (any part) G06.1
  iridocyclitis — *see* Iridocyclitis, chronic
  jaw (bone) (central) M27.1
    reparative giant cell M27.1
  kidney (*see also* Infection, kidney) N15.8
  lacrimal H04.819
    bilateral H04.813
    left H04.812
    right H04.811
  larynx J38.7
  lethal midline (faciale(e)) M31.2
  liver NEC — *see* Granuloma, hepatic
  lung (infectious) — *see also* Fibrosis, lung
    coccidioidal B38.1 *[J99]*
    eosinophilic D76.0
  Majocchi's B35.8
  malignant (facial(e)) M31.2
  mandible (central) M27.1
  midline (lethal) M31.2
  monilial (cutaneous) B37.2
  nasal sinus — *see* Sinusitis
  operation wound T81.89
    foreign body — *see* Foreign body, accidentally left following a procedure
    stitch T81.89
    talc — *see* Foreign body, accidentally left following a procedure
  oral mucosa K13.4
  orbit, orbital H05.119
    bilateral H05.113
    left H05.112
    right H05.111
  paracoccidioidal B41.8
  penis, venereal A58
  periapical K04.5
  peritoneum K66.8
    due to ova of helminths NOS (*see also* Helminthiasis) B83.9 *[K67]*

©2002 Ingenix, Inc.

Granuloma — continued
  postmastoidectomy cavity — see Complications, postmastoidectomy, recurrent cholesteatoma
  prostate N42.89
  pudendi (ulcerating) A58
  pulp, internal (tooth) K03.3
  pyogenic, pyogenicum (of) (skin) L98.0
    gingiva K06.8
    maxillary alveolar ridge K04.5
    oral mucosa K13.4
  rectum K62.8
  reticulohistiocytic D76.3
  rubrum nasi L74.8
  Schistosoma — see Schistosomiasis
  septic (skin) L98.0
  silica (skin) L92.3
  sinus (accessory) (infective) (nasal) — see Sinusitis
  skin L92.9
    from residual foreign body L92.3
    pyogenicum L98.0
  spine
    syphilitic (epidural) A52.19
    tuberculous A18.01
  stitch (postoperative) T81.89
  suppurative (skin) L98.0
  swimming pool A31.1
  talc — see also Granuloma, foreign body
    in operation wound — see Foreign body, accidentally left following a procedure
  telangiectaticum (skin) L98.0
  trichophyticum B35.8
  tropicum A66.4
  umbilicus L92.9
    newborn P38
  urethra N36.8
  uveitis — see Iridocyclitis, chronic
  vagina A58
  venereum A58
  vocal cord J38.3
Granulomatosis L92.9
  lymphoid (M9766/1) D47.7
  miliary (listerial) A32.89
  necrotizing, respiratory M31.30
  progressive septic D71
  specified NEC L92.8
  Wegener's M31.30
    with renal involvement M31.31
Granulomatous tissue (abnormal) (excessive) L92.9
Granulosis rubra nasi L74.8
Graphite fibrosis (of lung) J63.3
Graphospasm F48.8
  organic G25.8
Grating scapula M89.81
Gravel (urinary) — see Calculus, urinary
Graves' disease — see Hyperthyroidism, with, goiter
Gravis — see condition
Grawitz tumor (M8312/3) C64.9
  left C64.1
  right C64.0
Gray syndrome (newborn) P93.0
Grayness, hair (premature) L67.1
  congenital Q84.2
Green sickness D50.8
Greenfield's disease
  meaning
    concentric sclerosis (encephalitis periaxialis concentrica) G37.5
    metachromatic leukodystrophy E75.25
  Greenstick fracture – code as Fracture, by site
Grey syndrome (newborn) P93.0
Griesinger's disease B76.9
Grinder's lung or pneumoconiosis J62.8
Grinding, teeth F45.8
Grip
  Dabney's B33.0
  devil's B33.0
Grippe, grippal — see also Influenza
  Balkan A78
  summer, of Italy A93.1

Grisel's disease M43.6
Groin — see condition
Grooved tongue K14.5
Ground itch B76.9
Grover's disease or syndrome L11.1
Growing pains, children R29.898
Growth (fungoid) (neoplastic) (new) — see also Neoplasm
  adenoid (vegetative) J35.8
  benign (M8000/0) — see Neoplasm, benign
  malignant (M8000/3) — see Neoplasm, malignant
  rapid, childhood Z00.2
  secondary (M8000/6) — see Neoplasm, secondary
Gruby's disease B35.0
Gubler-Millard paralysis or syndrome G46.3
Guerin-Stern syndrome Q74.3
Guillain-Barré disease or syndrome G61.0
  sequelae G65.0
Guinea worms (infection) (infestation) B72
Guinon's disease (motor-verbal tic) F95.2
Gull's disease E03.4
Gum — see condition
Gumboil K04.6
Gumma (syphilitic) A52.79
  artery A52.09
    cerebral A52.04
  bone A52.77
    of yaws (late) A66.6
  brain A52.19
  cauda equina A52.19
  central nervous system A52.3
  ciliary body A52.71
  congenital A50.59
  eyelid A52.71
  heart A52.06
  intracranial A52.19
  iris A52.71
  kidney A52.75
  larynx A52.73
  leptomeninges A52.19
  liver A52.74
  meninges A52.19
  myocardium A52.06
  nasopharynx A52.73
  neurosyphilitic A52.3
  nose A52.73
  orbit A52.71
  palate (soft) A52.79
  penis A52.76
  pericardium A52.06
  pharynx A52.73
  pituitary A52.79
  scrofulous (tuberculous) A18.4
  skin A52.79
  specified site NEC A52.79
  spinal cord A52.19
  tongue A52.79
  tonsil A52.73
  trachea A52.73
  tuberculous A18.4
  ulcerative due to yaws A66.4
  ureter A52.75
  yaws A66.4
    bone A66.6
Gunn's syndrome Q07.8
Gunshot wound — see also Wound, open
  fracture – code as Fracture, by site
  internal organs — see Injury, by site
Gynandrism Q56.0
Gynandroblastoma (M8632/1)
  specified site — see Neoplasm, uncertain behavior
  unspecified site
    female D39.10
    male D40.10
Gynecological examination (periodic) (routine) Z01.40
  with abnormal findings Z01.41
Gynecomastia N62
Gynephobia F40.291
Gyrate scalp Q82.8

H

H (Hartnup's) disease E72.02
Haas' disease or osteochondrosis (juvenile) (head of humerus) — see Osteochondrosis, juvenile, humerus
Habit, habituation
  chorea F95.8
  disturbance, child F98.9
  drug — see Dependence, drug
  laxative F55.2
  spasm — see Tic
  tic — see Tic
Haemophilus (H.) influenzae, as cause of disease classified elsewhere B96.3
Haff disease — see Poisoning, mercury
Hageman's factor defect, deficiency or disease D68.2
Haglund's disease or osteochondrosis (juvenile) (os tibiale externum) — see Osteochondrosis, juvenile, tarsus
Hailey-Hailey disease Q82.8
Hair — see also condition
  plucking F63.3
    in stereotyped movement disorder F98.4
Hairball in stomach T18.2
Hair-pulling, pathological (compulsive) F63.3
Hairy black tongue K14.3
Half vertebra Q76.49
Halitosis R19.6
Hallerman-Streiff syndrome Q87.0
Hallervorden-Spatz disease G23.0
Hallopeau's acrodermatitis or disease L40.2
Hallucination R44.3
  auditory R44.0
  gustatory R44.2
  olfactory R44.2
  specified NEC R44.2
  tactile R44.2
  visual R44.1
Hallucinosis (chronic) F28
  alcoholic (acute) F10.951
    in
      abuse F10.151
      dependence F10.251
  drug-induced F19.951
    cannabis F12.951
    cocaine F14.951
    hallucinogen F16.151
    in
      abuse F19.151
        cannabis F12.151
        cocaine F14.151
        hallucinogen F16.151
        inhalant F18.151
        opioid F11.151
        sedative, anxiolytic or hypnotic F13.151
        stimulant NEC F15.151
      dependence F19.251
        cannabis F12.251
        cocaine F14.251
        hallucinogen F16.251
        inhalant F18.251
        opioid F11.251
        sedative, anxiolytic or hypnotic F13.251
        stimulant NEC F15.251
    inhalant F18.951
    opioid F11.951
    sedative, anxiolytic or hypnotic F13.951
    stimulant NEC F15.951
  organic F06.0
Hallux
  deformity (acquired) NEC — see Deformity, toe, specified hallux NEC
  malleus (acquired) NEC — see Deformity, toe, hammer toe
  rigidus (acquired) — see also Deformity, toe, hallux rigidus
    congenital Q74.2
    late effect of rickets E64.3

Hallux — *continued*
  valgus (acquired) — *see also* Deformity, toe, hallux valgus
    congenital Q66.8
  varus (acquired) — *see also* Deformity, toe, specified hallux NEC
    congenital Q66.3

Halo, visual H53.19

Hamartoma, hamartoblastoma Q85.9
  epithelial (gingival), odontogenic, central or peripheral (M9321/0) D16.5
    upper jaw (bone) D16.4

Hamartosis Q85.9

Hamman-Rich syndrome J84.1

Hammer toe (acquired) **NEC** — *see also* Deformity, toe, hammer toe
  congenital Q66.8
  late effect of rickets E64.3

Hand — *see* condition

Handicap, handicapped
  educational Z55.9
    specified NEC Z55.8

Hand-Schüller-Christian disease or syndrome D76.0

Hanging (asphyxia) (strangulation) (suffocation) — *see* Asphyxia, traumatic, due to mechanical threat

Hangnail — *see also* Cellulitis, digit
  with lymphangitis — *see* Lymphangitis, acute, digit

Hangover (alcohol) F10.129

Hanhart's syndrome Q87.0

Hanot-Chauffard (-Troisier) syndrome E83.19

Hanot's cirrhosis or disease K74.3

Hansen's disease — *see* Leprosy

Hantaan virus disease A98.5
  pulmonary syndrome B33.4

Harada's disease or syndrome — *see* Vogt-Koyanagi syndrome

Hardening
  artery — *see* Arteriosclerosis
  brain G93.8

Harelip (complete) (incomplete) — *see* Cleft, lip

Harlequin (fetus) Q80.4

Harley's disease D59.6

Harmful use (of)
  alcohol F10.10
  anxiolytics — *see* Abuse, drug, sedative
  cannabinoids — *see* Abuse, drug, cannabis
  cocaine — *see* Abuse, drug, cocaine
  drug — *see* Abuse, drug
  hallucinogens — *see* Abuse, drug, hallucinogen
  hypnotics — *see* Abuse, drug, sedative
  opioids — *see* Abuse, drug, opioid
  PCP (phencyclidine) — *see* Abuse, drug NEC
  sedatives — *see* Abuse, drug, sedative
  stimulants NEC — *see* Abuse, drug, stimulant

Harris' lines — *see* Arrest, epiphyseal

Hartnup's disease E72.02

Harvester's lung J67.0

Harvesting ovum for in vitro fertilization Z31.89

Hashimoto's disease or thyroiditis E06.3

Hashitoxicosis (transient) E06.3

Hassal-Henle bodies or warts (cornea) H18.49

Haut mal — *see* Epilepsy, grand mal

Haverhill fever A25.1

Hay fever J30.1

Hayem-Widal syndrome D59.8

Haygarth's nodes M15.8

Haymaker's lung J67.0

Hb (abnormal)
  disease — *see* Disease, hemoglobin
  trait — *see* Trait

Head — *see* condition

Headache R51
  allergic NEC G44.8
  cluster (chronic) (episodic) G44.0
  drug-induced NEC G44.4
  emotional F45.4

Headache — *continued*
  histamine G44.0
  lumbar puncture G97.1
  migraine (type) G43.9
  nonorganic origin F45.4
  postspinal puncture G97.1
  post-traumatic, chronic G44.3
  psychogenic F45.4
  specified syndrome NEC G44.8
  spinal and epidural anesthesia-induced T88.5
    in labor and delivery O74.5
    in pregnancy — *see* Complications, anesthesia, in, pregnancy, spinal, headache
    postpartum, puerperal O89.4
  spinal fluid loss (from puncture) G97.1
  tension (chronic) (episodic) G44.2
  vascular G44.1

Health
  advice Z71.9
  check-up (routine) Z00.010
    with abnormal findings Z00.011
    infant or child Z00.10
      with abnormal findings Z00.11
    occupational Z04.8
  education Z71.9
  instruction Z71.9
  services provided because (of)
    bedfast status Z74.0
    boarding school residence Z59.3
    holiday relief for person providing home care Z75.5
    inadequate
      economic resources NOS Z59.9
      housing Z59.1
    lack of housing Z59.0
    need for
      assistance with personal care Z74.1
      continuous supervision Z74.3
    no care available in home Z74.2
    person living alone Z60.2
    poverty NEC Z59.6
      extreme Z59.5
    residence in institution Z59.3
    specified cause NEC Z59.8

Healthy
  infant
    accompanying sick mother Z76.3
    receiving care Z76.2
  person accompanying sick person Z76.3

Hearing examination Z01.10
  with abnormal findings Z01.11

Heart — *see* condition

Heart beat
  abnormality R00.9
    specified NEC R00.8
  awareness R00.2
  rapid R00.0
  slow R00.1

Heartburn R12
  psychogenic F45.8

Heat (effects) T67.9
  apoplexy T67.0
  burn — *see also* Burn L55.9
  collapse T67.1
  cramps T67.2
  dermatitis or eczema L59.0
  edema T67.7
  erythema – code by site under Burn, first degree
  excessive T67.9
    specified effect NEC T67.8
  exhaustion T67.5
    anhydrotic T67.3
    due to
      salt (and water) depletion T67.4
      water depletion T67.3
        with salt depletion T67.4
  fatigue (transient) T67.6
  fever T67.0
  hyperpyrexia T67.0
  prickly L74.0
  prostration — *see* Heat, exhaustion
  pyrexia T67.0
  rash L74.0
  specified effect NEC T67.8
  stroke T67.0

Heat — *continued*
  sunburn — *see* Sunburn
  syncope T67.1

Heavy-for-dates NEC (fetus or infant) P08.1
  exceptionally (4500g or more) P08.0

Hebephrenia, hebephrenic (schizophrenia) F20.1

Heberden's disease or nodes (with arthropathy) M15.1

Hebra's
  pityriasis L26
  prurigo L28.2

Heel — *see* condition

Heerfordt's disease D86.89

Hegglin's anomaly or syndrome D72.0

Heilmeyer-Schoner disease (M9842/3) C94.10
  in remission C94.11

Heine-Medin disease A80.9

Heinz body anemia, congenital D58.2

Heliophobia F40.228

Heller's disease or syndrome F84.3

Hellp syndrome O14.10

Helminthiasis — *see also* Infestation, helminth
  Ancylostoma B76.0
  intestinal B82.0
    mixed types (types classifiable to more than one of the titles B65.0-B81.3 and B81.8) B81.4
    specified type NEC B81.8
  mixed types (intestinal) (types classifiable to more than one of the titles B65.0-B81.3 and B81.8) B81.4
  Necator (americanus) B76.1
  specified type NEC B83.8

Heloma L84

Hemangioblastoma (M9161/1) — *see also* Neoplasm, connective tissue, uncertain behavior
  malignant (M9161/3) — *see* Neoplasm, connective tissue, malignant

Hemangioendothelioma (M9130/1) — *see also* Neoplasm, uncertain behavior
  benign (M9130/0) D18.00
    intra-abdominal D18.03
    intracranial D18.02
    skin D18.01
    specified site NEC D18.09
  bone (diffuse) (M9130/3) — *see* Neoplasm, bone, malignant
  epithelioid (M9133/1) — *see also* Neoplasm, uncertain behavior
    malignant (M9133/3) — *see* Neoplasm, malignant
  malignant (M9130/3) — *see* Neoplasm, connective tissue, malignant

Hemangiofibroma (M9160/0) — *see* Neoplasm, benign

Hemangiolipoma (M8861/0) — *see* Lipoma

Hemangioma (M9120/0) D18.00
  arteriovenous (M9123/0) D18.00
    intra-abdominal D18.03
    intracranial D18.02
    skin D18.01
    specified site NEC D18.09
  capillary (M9131/0) D18.00
    intra-abdominal D18.03
    intracranial D18.02
    skin D18.01
    specified site NEC D18.09
  cavernous (M9121/0) D18.00
    intra-abdominal D18.03
    intracranial D18.02
    skin D18.01
    specified site NEC D18.09
  epithelioid (M9125/0) D18.00
    intra-abdominal D18.03
    intracranial D18.02
    skin D18.01
    specified site NEC D18.09
  histiocytoid (M9126/0) D18.00
    intra-abdominal D18.03
    intracranial D18.02
    skin D18.01
    specified site NEC D18.09

Hemangioma — *continued*
  infantile (M9131/0) D18.00
    intra-abdominal D18.03
    intracranial D18.02
    skin D18.01
    specified site NEC D18.09
  intra-abdominal D18.03
  intracranial D18.02
  intramuscular (M9132/0) D18.00
    intra-abdominal D18.03
    intracranial D18.02
    skin D18.01
    specified site NEC D18.09
  juvenile (M9131/0) D18.00
  malignant (M9120/3) — *see* Neoplasm,
    connective tissue, malignant
  plexiform (M9131/0) D18.00
    intra-abdominal D18.03
    intracranial D18.02
    skin D18.01
    specified site NEC D18.09
  racemose (M9123/0) D18.00
    intra-abdominal D18.03
    intracranial D18.02
    skin D18.01
    specified site NEC D18.09
  sclerosing (M8832/0) — *see* Neoplasm, skin,
    benign
  simplex (M9131/0) D18.00
    intra-abdominal D18.03
    intracranial D18.02
    skin D18.01
    specified site NEC D18.09
  skin D18.01
  specified site NEC D18.09
  venous (M9122/0) D18.00
    intra-abdominal D18.03
    intracranial D18.02
    skin D18.01
    specified site NEC D18.09
  verrucous keratotic (M9142/0) D18.00
    intra-abdominal D18.03
    intracranial D18.02
    skin D18.01
    specified site NEC D18.09

Hemangiomatosis (systemic) I78.8
  involving single site (M9120/0) — *see*
    Hemangioma

Hemangiopericytoma (M9150/1) — *see also*
  Neoplasm, connective tissue, uncertain
  behavior
  benign (M9150/0) — *see* Neoplasm, connective
    tissue, benign
  malignant (M9150/3) — *see* Neoplasm,
    connective tissue, malignant

Hemangiosarcoma (M9120/3) — *see* Neoplasm,
  connective tissue, malignant

Hemarthrosis (nontraumatic) M25.00
  ankle M25.073
    left M25.072
    right M25.071
  elbow M25.029
    left M25.022
    right M25.021
  foot joint M25.076
    left M25.075
    right M25.074
  hand joint M25.049
    left M25.042
    right M25.041
  hip M25.059
    left M25.052
    right M25.051
  in hemophilic arthropathy — *see* Arthropathy,
    hemophilic
  knee M25.069
    left M25.062
    right M25.061
  shoulder M25.019
    left M25.012
    right M25.011
  specified joint NEC M25.08
  traumatic — *see* Sprain, by site
  wrist M25.039
    left M25.032
    right M25.031

Hematemesis K92.0
  with ulcer – code by site under Ulcer, with
    hemorrhage K27.4
  newborn, neonatal P54.0
    due to swallowed maternal blood P78.2

Hematidrosis L74.8

Hematinuria — *see also* Hemoglobinuria
  malarial B50.8

Hematobilia K83.8

Hematocele
  female NEC N94.8
    with ectopic pregnancy O00.9
    ovary N83.8
  male N50.1

Hematochyluria — *see also* Infestation, filarial
  schistosomiasis (bilharziasis) B65.0

Hematocolpos (with hematometra or
  hematosalpinx) N89.7

Hematocornea — *see* Pigmentation, cornea,
  stromal

Hematogenous — *see* condition

Hematoma (traumatic) (skin surface intact) — *see
  also* Contusion
  with
    injury of internal organs — *see* Injury, by
      site
    open wound — *see* Wound, open
  amputation stump (surgical) (late) T87.8
  aorta, dissecting I71.00
    abdominal I71.02
    thoracic I71.01
    thoracoabdominal I71.03
  arterial (complicating trauma) — *see* Injury,
    blood vessel, by site
  auricle — *see* Contusion, ear
    nontraumatic — *see* Disorder, pinna,
      hematoma
  birth injury NEC P15.8
  brain (traumatic)
    with
      cerebral laceration or contusion (diffuse)
        — *see* Injury, intracranial, diffuse
      focal — *see* Injury, intracranial, focal
    cerebellar, traumatic S06.371
      with loss of consciousness S06.379
        brief (<1 hour) S06.372
        minor (1-6 hours) S06.373
        moderate (6-24 hours) S06.374
        prolonged (>24 hours) S06.375
          without return to consciousness
            S06.376
    fetus or newborn NEC P52.4
      birth injury P10.1
    intracerebral, traumatic — *see* Injury,
      intracranial, intracerebral hemorrhage
    nontraumatic — *see* Hemorrhage,
      intracranial
    subarachnoid, arachnoid, traumatic — *see*
      Injury, intracranial, subarachnoid
      hemorrhage
    subdural, traumatic — *see* Injury,
      intracranial, subdural hemorrhage
  breast (nontraumatic) N64.8
  broad ligament (nontraumatic) N83.7
    traumatic S37.892
  cerebellar, traumatic S06.371
    with loss of consciousness S06.379
      brief (<1 hour) S06.372
      minor (1-6 hours) S06.373
      moderate (6-24 hours) S06.374
      prolonged (>24 hours) S06.375
        without return to consciousness
          S06.376
  cerebral — *see* Hematoma, brain
  cesarean section wound O90.2
  complicating delivery (perineal) (pelvic) (vagina)
    (vulva) O71.7
  corpus cavernosum (nontraumatic) N48.89
  epididymis (nontraumatic) N50.1
  epidural (traumatic) — *see* Injury, intracranial,
    epidural hemorrhage
    spinal — *see* Injury, spinal cord, by region
  episiotomy O90.2
  face, birth injury P15.4

Hematoma — *see also* Contusion — *continued*
  genital organ NEC (nontraumatic)
    female (nonobstetric) N94.8
      traumatic S30.202
    male N50.1
      traumatic S30.201
  internal organs — *see* Injury, by site
  intracerebral, traumatic — *see* Injury,
    intracranial, intracerebral hemorrhage
  intraoperative of
    operative site during
      circulatory system procedure I97.43
        due to accidental laceration I97.51
      digestive system procedure K91.63
        due to accidental laceration K91.71
      ear procedure H95.23
        due to accidental laceration H95.31
      endocrine system procedure E36.03
        due to accidental puncture E36.11
      eye procedure
      genitourinary system procedure N99.63
        due to accidental puncture N99.71
      mastoid procedure H95.23
        due to accidental laceration H95.31
      musculoskeletal system procedure
        M96.813
        due to accidental puncture M96.821
      nervous system procedure G97.33
        due to accidental puncture G97.41
      respiratory system procedure J95.63
        due to accidental puncture J95.71
      skin procedure L76.03
        due to accidental puncture L76.11
      spleen procedure D78.03
        with accidental puncture D78.11
    specified site NEC during
      circulatory system procedure I97.44
        due to accidental laceration I97.52
      digestive system procedure K91.64
        due to accidental laceration K91.72
      ear procedure H95.24
        due to accidental laceration H95.32
      endocrine system procedure E36.04
        due to accidental puncture E36.12
      genitourinary system procedure N99.64
        due to accidental puncture N99.72
      mastoid procedure H95.24
        due to accidental laceration H95.32
      musculoskeletal system procedure
        M96.814
        due to accidental puncture M96.822
      nervous system procedure G97.34
        due to accidental puncture G97.42
      respiratory system procedure J95.64
        due to accidental puncture J95.72
      skin procedure L76.04
        due to accidental puncture L76.12
      spleen procedure D78.04
        with accidental puncture D78.12
  labia (nontraumatic) (nonobstetric) N90.8
  liver (subcapsular) (nontraumatic) K76.8
    birth injury P15.0
  mediastinum — *see* Injury, intrathoracic
  mesosalpinx (nontraumatic) N83.7
    traumatic S37.529
      bilateral S37.522
      unilateral S37.521
  muscle – code by site under Contusion
  obstetrical surgical wound O90.2
  orbit, orbital (nontraumatic) — *see also*
    Hemorrhage, orbit
    traumatic — *see* Contusion, orbit
  pelvis (female) (nontraumatic) (nonobstetric)
    N94.8
    obstetric O71.7
    traumatic — *see* Injury, by site
  penis (nontraumatic) N48.89
    birth injury P15.5
  perineal S30.23
    complicating delivery O71.7
  perirenal — *see* Injury, kidney
  pinna — *see* Contusion, ear
    nontraumatic — *see* Disorder, pinna,
      hematoma
  placenta O43.899
    first trimester O43.891

Hematoma — *see also* Contusion — *continued*
placenta — *continued*
second trimester O43.892
third trimester O43.893
postoperative of
operative site following
circulatory system procedure I97.47
due to accidental laceration I97.51
digestive system procedure K91.67
due to accidental laceration K91.71
ear procedure H95.27
due to accidental laceration H95.31
endocrine system procedure E36.07
due to accidental puncture E36.11
eye procedure
genitourinary system procedure N99.67
due to accidental puncture N99.71
mastoid procedure H95.27
due to accidental laceration H95.31
musculoskeletal system procedure
M96.817
due to accidental laceration M96.821
nervous system procedure G97.37
due to accidental puncture G97.41
respiratory system procedure J95.67
due to accidental puncture J95.72
skin procedure L76.07
due to accidental puncture L76.11
spleen procedure D78.07
with accidental puncture D78.11
specified site NEC following
circulatory system procedure I97.48
due to accidental laceration I97.52
digestive system procedure K91.68
due to accidental laceration K91.72
ear procedure H95.28
due to accidental puncture H95.32
endocrine system procedure E36.08
due to accidental puncture E36.12
genitourinary system procedure N99.68
due to accidental puncture N99.72
mastoid procedure H95.28
due to accidental puncture H95.32
musculoskeletal system procedure
M96.818
due to accidental laceration M96.822
nervous system procedure G97.38
due to accidental puncture G97.42
respiratory system procedure J95.68
due to accidental puncture J95.72
skin procedure L76.08
due to accidental puncture L76.12
spleen procedure D78.08
with accidental puncture D78.12
retroperitoneal (nontraumatic) K66.1
traumatic S36.892
scrotum, superficial S30.22
birth injury P15.5
seminal vesicle (nontraumatic) N50.1
traumatic S37.892
spermatic cord (traumatic) S37.892
nontraumatic N50.1
spinal (cord) (meninges) — *see also* Injury,
spinal cord, by region
fetus or newborn (birth injury) P11.5
spleen D73.5
intraoperative D78.03
with accidental puncture D78.11
postoperative D78.07
with accidental puncture D78.11
sternocleidomastoid, birth injury P15.2
sternomastoid, birth injury P15.2
subarachnoid (traumatic) — *see* Injury,
intracranial, subarachnoid hemorrhage
fetus or newborn (nontraumatic) P52.5
due to birth injury P10.3
nontraumatic — *see* Hemorrhage,
intracranial, subarachnoid
subdural (traumatic) — *see* Injury, intracranial,
subdural hemorrhage
fetus or newborn (localized) P52.8
birth injury P10.0
nontraumatic — *see* Hemorrhage,
intracranial, subdural
superficial, fetus or newborn P54.5

Hematoma — *see also* Contusion — *continued*
testis (nontraumatic) N50.1
birth injury P15.5
tunica vaginalis (nontraumatic) N50.1
umbilical cord, complicating delivery O69.5
uterine ligament (broad) (nontraumatic) N83.7
traumatic S37.62
vagina (ruptured) (nontraumatic) N89.8
complicating delivery O71.7
vas deferens (nontraumatic) N50.1
traumatic S37.892
vitreous — *see* Hemorrhage, vitreous
vulva (nontraumatic) (nonobstetric) N90.8
complicating delivery O71.7
fetus or newborn (birth injury) P15.5
Hematometra N85.7
with hematocolpos N89.7
Hematomyelia (central) G95.19
fetus or newborn (birth injury) P11.5
traumatic T14.90
Hematomyelitis G04.9
Hematoperitoneum — *see* Hemoperitoneum
Hematophobia F40.230
Hematopneumothorax (*see* Hemothorax)
Hematoporphyria — *see* Porphyria
Hematorachis, hematorrhachis G95.19
fetus or newborn (birth injury) P11.5
Hematosalpinx N83.6
with
hematocolpos N89.7
hematometra N85.7
with hematocolpos N89.7
infectional — *see* Salpingitis
Hematospermia R36.1
Hematothorax (*see* Hemothorax)
Hematuria R31.9
benign (familial) (of childhood) — *see also*
Hematuria, idiopathic
essential microscopic R31.1
endemic (*see also* Schistosomiasis) B65.0
gross R31.0
idiopathic N02.9
with glomerular lesion
crescentic (diffuse) glomerulonephritis
N02.7
dense deposit disease N02.6
endocapillary proliferative
glomerulonephritis N02.4
focal and segmental hyalinosis or
sclerosis N02.1
membranoproliferative (diffuse) N02.5
membranous (diffuse) N02.2
mesangial proliferative (diffuse) N02.3
mesangiocapillary (diffuse) N02.5
minor abnormality N02.0
proliferative NEC N02.8
specified pathology NEC N02.8
intermittent — *see* Hematuria, idiopathic
malarial B50.8
microscopic R31.2
benign essential R31.1
paroxysmal — *see also* Hematuria, idiopathic
nocturnal D59.5
persistent — *see* Hematuria, idiopathic
recurrent — *see* Hematuria, idiopathic
sulphonamide, sulfonamide
correct substance properly administered
R31.9
overdose or wrong substance given or taken
— *see* category T37.0
tropical (*see also* Schistosomiasis) B65.0
tuberculous A18.13
Hemeralopia (day blindness) H53.11
vitamin A deficiency E50.5
Hemi-akinesia R41.4
Hemianalgesia R20.0
Hemianencephaly Q00.0
Hemianesthesia R20.0
Hemianopia, hemianopsia (heteronymous)
H53.47
homonymous H53.46
syphilitic A52.71
Hemiathetosis R25.8

Hemiatrophy R68.8
cerebellar G31.9
face, facial, progressive (Romberg) G51.8
tongue K14.8
Hemiballism(us) G25.5
Hemicardia Q24.8
Hemicephalus, hemicephaly Q00.0
Hemichorea G25.5
Hemicrania
congenital malformation Q00.0
meaning migraine G43.9
paroxysmal, chronic G44.0
Hemidystrophy — *see* Hemiatrophy
Hemiectromelia Q73.8
Hemihypalgesia R20.8
Hemihypesthesia R20.1
Hemi-inattention R41.4
Hemimelia Q73.8
lower limb — *see* Defect, reduction, lower limb,
specified type NEC
upper limb — *see* Defect, reduction, upper
limb, specified type NEC
Hemiparalysis — *see* Hemiplegia
Hemiparesis — *see* Hemiplegia
Hemiparesthesia R20.2
Hemiparkinsonism G20
Hemiplegia G81.90
with involvement of
dominant side (right) G81.91
left G81.92
left (nondominant) side G81.94
dominant G81.92
nondominant side (left) G81.94
right G81.93
right (dominant) side G81.91
nondominant G81.93
acute I64
alternans facialis G83.89
apoplectic (current episode) I64
arteriosclerotic I63.8
ascending NEC G81.90
spinal G95.89
attack (current episode) I64
brain (current episode) I64
cerebral (current episode) I64
congenital (cerebral) (spastic) (spinal) G80.2
cortical (current episode) I64
embolic (current episode) I63.4
flaccid G81.00
with involvement of
dominant side (right) G81.01
left G81.02
left (nondominant side) G81.04
dominant G81.02
nondominant side (left) G81.04
right G81.03
right (dominant side) G81.01
nondominant G81.03
following
cerebrovascular disease I69.959
cerebral infarction I69.359
dominant (right) I69.351
left I69.352
left (nondominant) I69.354
dominant I69.352
nondominant (left) I69.354
right I69.353
right (dominant) I69.351
nondominant I69.353
dominant (right) I69.951
left I69.952
intracerebral hemorrhage I69.159
dominant (right) I69.151
left I69.152
left (nondominant) I69.154
dominant I69.152
nondominant (left) I69.154
right I69.153
right (dominant) I69.151
nondominant I69.153
left (nondominant) I69.954
dominant I69.952
nondominant (left) I69.954
right I69.953

©2002 Ingenix, Inc.

Hemiplegia — *continued*
  following — *continued*
    cerebrovascular disease — *continued*
      nontraumatic intracranial hemorrhage
          NEC I69.259
        dominant (right) I69.251
          left I69.252
        left (nondominant) I69.254
          dominant I69.252
        nondominant (left) I69.254
          right I69.253
        right (dominant) I69.251
          nondominant I69.253
      right (dominant) I69.951
        nondominant I69.953
      specified disease NEC I69.859
        dominant (right) I69.851
          left I69.852
        left (nondominant) I69.854
          dominant I69.852
        nondominant (left) I69.854
          right I69.853
        right (dominant) I69.851
          nondominant I69.853
      stroke NOS I69.459
        dominant (right) I69.451
          left I69.452
        left (nondominant) I69.454
          dominant I69.452
        nondominant (left) I69.454
          right I69.453
        right (dominant) I69.451
          nondominant I69.453
      subarachnoid hemorrhage I69.059
        dominant (right) I69.051
          left I69.052
        left (nondominant) I69.054
          dominant I69.052
        nondominant (left) I69.054
          right I69.053
        right (dominant) I69.051
          nondominant I69.053
  hypertensive (current episode) I64
  hysterical F44.4
  infantile (postnatal) G80.2
  newborn NEC P91.8
    birth injury P11.9
  seizure (current episode) I64
  spastic G81.10
    with involvement of
      dominant side (right) G81.11
        left G81.12
      left (nondominant) side G81.14
        dominant G81.12
      nondominant side (left) G81.14
        right G81.13
      right (dominant) side G81.11
        nondominant G81.13
    congenital or infantile G80.2
  thrombotic (current episode) I63.3
Hemisection, spinal cord — *see* Injury, spinal
    cord, by region
Hemispasm (facial) R25.2
Hemisporosis B48.8
Hemitremor R25.1
Hemivertebra Q76.49
  failure of segmentation with scoliosis Q76.3
  fusion with scoliosis Q76.3
Hemochromatosis (diabetic) (hereditary) (liver)
    (myocardium) (primary idiopathic)
    (secondary) E83.11
  with refractory anemia (M9982/1) D46.1
Hemoglobin — *see also* condition
  abnormal (disease) — *see* Disease, hemoglobin
  AS genotype D57.3
  fetal, hereditary persistence (HPFH) D56.4
  low NOS D64.9
  S (Hb S), heterozygous D57.3
Hemoglobinemia D59.9
  due to blood transfusion T80.8
  paroxysmal D59.6
    nocturnal D59.5
Hemoglobinopathy (mixed) D58.2
  with thalassemia D56.9

Hemoglobinopathy — *continued*
  sickle-cell D57.1
    with thalassemia D57.4
Hemoglobinuria R82.3
  with anemia, hemolytic, acquired (chronic) NEC
      D59.6
  cold (agglutinin) (paroxysmal) (with Raynaud's
      syndrome) D59.6
  due to exertion or hemolysis NEC D59.6
  intermittent D59.6
  malarial B50.8
  march D59.6
  nocturnal (paroxysmal) D59.5
  paroxysmal (cold) D59.6
    nocturnal D59.5
Hemolymphangioma (M9175/0) D18.1
Hemolysis
  intravascular
    with
      abortion — *see* Abortion, by type,
          complicated by, hemorrhage
      ectopic or molar pregnancy O08.1
      hemorrhage
        antepartum — *see* Hemorrhage,
            antepartum
        intrapartum — *see also* Hemorrhage,
            complicating, delivery O67.0
      postpartum O72.3
  neonatal (excessive) P58.8
Hemolytic — *see* condition
Hemopericardium I31.2
  following acute myocardial infarction (current
      complication) I23.0
  newborn P54.8
  traumatic — *see* Injury, heart, with
      hemopericardium
Hemoperitoneum K66.1
  infectional K65.9
  traumatic S36.899
    with open wound — *see* Wound, open, with
        penetration into peritoneal cavity
Hemophilia (classical) (familial) (hereditary) D66
  A D66
  B D67
  C D68.1
  calcipriva (*see also* Defect, coagulation) D68.4
  nonfamilial (*see also* Defect, coagulation) D68.4
  vascular D68.0
Hemophthalmos H44.819
  bilateral H44.813
  left H44.812
  right H44.811
Hemopneumothorax — *see also* Hemothorax
  traumatic S27.2
Hemoptysis R04.2
  newborn P26.9
  tuberculous — *see* Tuberculosis, pulmonary
Hemorrhage, hemorrhagic (concealed) R58
  abdomen R58
  accidental antepartum — *see* Hemorrhage,
      antepartum
  adenoid J35.8
  adrenal (capsule) (gland) E27.4
    medulla E27.8
    newborn P54.4
  after delivery — *see* Hemorrhage, postpartum
  alveolar
    lung, newborn P26.8
    process K08.8
  alveolus K08.8
  amputation stump (surgical) M96.815
    secondary, delayed T87.8
  anemia (chronic) D50.0
    acute D62
  antepartum (with) O46.90
    with coagulation defect O46.009
      afibrinogenemia O46.019
        first trimester O46.011
        second trimester O46.012
        third trimester O46.013
      disseminated intravascular coagulation
          O46.029
        first trimester O46.021
        second trimester O46.022
        third trimester O46.023

Hemorrhage, hemorrhagic — *continued*
  antepartum — *continued*
    with coagulation defect — *continued*
      first trimester O46.001
      hypofibrinogenemia — *see* Hemorrhage,
          antepartum, with coagulation
          defect, afibrinogenemia
      second trimester O46.002
      specified defect NEC O46.099
        first trimester O46.091
        second trimester O46.092
        third trimester O46.093
      third trimester O46.003
    before 20 weeks gestation O20.9
      specified type NEC O20.8
      threatened abortion O20.0
    due to
      abruptio placenta — *see* Disorder,
          placenta, abruptio
      leiomyoma, uterus — *see* Hemorrhage,
          antepartum, specified cause NEC
      placenta previa — *see* Disorder, placenta,
          previa
    first trimester O46.91
    previous, affecting management of
        pregnancy — *see* Antenatal, care, high
        risk pregnancy, history of, specified
        obstetric problem NEC
    second trimester O46.92
    specified cause NEC — *see* category O46.8
    third trimester O46.93
  anus (sphincter) K62.5
  apoplexy (stroke) — *see* Hemorrhage,
      intracranial, intracerebral
  arachnoid — *see* Hemorrhage, intracranial,
      subarachnoid
  artery R58
    brain — *see* Hemorrhage, intracranial,
        intracerebral
  basilar (ganglion) I61.0
  bladder N32.8
  bowel K92.2
    newborn P54.3
  brain (miliary) (nontraumatic) — *see*
      Hemorrhage, intracranial, intracerebral
    due to
      birth injury P10.1
      syphilis A52.05
    epidural or extradural (traumatic) — *see*
        Injury, intracranial, epidural
        hemorrhage
    fetus or newborn P52.4
      birth injury P10.1
    puerperal, postpartum, childbirth — *see*
        Disease, circulatory system, obstetric
    subarachnoid — *see* Hemorrhage,
        intracranial, subarachnoid
    subdural — *see* Hemorrhage, intracranial,
        subdural
  brainstem (nontraumatic) I61.3
    traumatic S06.381
      with loss of consciousness S06.389
        brief (<1 hour) S06.382
        minor (1-6 hours) S06.383
        moderate (6-24 hours) S06.384
        prolonged (>24 hours) S06.385
        without return to consciousness
            S06.386
  breast N64.5
  bronchial tube — *see* Hemorrhage, lung
  bronchopulmonary — *see* Hemorrhage, lung
  bronchus — *see* Hemorrhage, lung
  bulbar I61.5
  capillary I78.8
    primary D69.8
  cecum K92.2
  cerebellar, cerebellum (nontraumatic) I61.4
    fetus or newborn P52.6
    traumatic S06.371
      with loss of consciousness S06.379
        brief (<1 hour) S06.372
        minor (1-6 hours) S06.373
        moderate (6-24 hours) S06.374
        prolonged (>24 hours) S06.375
        without return to consciousness
            S06.376

Hemorrhage, hemorrhagic — *continued*
  cerebral, cerebrum — *see also* Hemorrhage, intracranial, intracerebral
    fetus or newborn (anoxic) P52.4
      birth injury P10.1
    lobe I61.1
  cerebromeningeal I61.8
  cerebrospinal — *see* Hemorrhage, intracranial, intracerebral
  cervix (uteri) (stump) NEC N88.8
  chamber, anterior (eye) — *see* Hyphema
  childbirth — *see* Hemorrhage, complicating, delivery
  choroid H31.309
    bilateral H31.303
    expulsive H31.319
      bilateral H31.313
      left H31.312
      right H31.311
    left H31.302
    right H31.301
  ciliary body — *see* Hyphema
  cochlea — *see* category H83.8
  colon K92.2
  complicating
    abortion — *see* Abortion, by type, complicated by, hemorrhage
    delivery O67.9
      associated with coagulation defect (afibrinogenemia) (DIC) (hyperfibrinolysis) O67.0
      specified cause NEC O67.8
      due to
        low-lying placenta — *see* Disorder, placenta, previa
        placenta previa — *see* Disorder, placenta, previa
        premature separation of placenta — *see* Disorder, placenta, abruptio
        retained
          placenta O72.0
          products of conception O72.2
          secundines O72.2
            partial O72.2
        trauma O67.8
        uterine leiomyoma O67.8
    ectopic or molar pregnancy (subsequent episode) O08.1
    surgical procedure — *see* Hemorrhage, intraoperative
  conjunctiva H11.30
    bilateral H11.33
    left H11.32
    newborn P54.8
    right H11.31
  cord, newborn (stump) P51.9
  corpus luteum (ruptured) cyst N83.1
  cortical (brain) I61.1
  cranial — *see* Hemorrhage, intracranial
  cutaneous R23.3
    due to autosensitivity, erythrocyte D69.2
    fetus or newborn P54.5
  delayed
    following ectopic or molar pregnancy O08.1
    postpartum O72.2
  diathesis (familial) D69.9
  disease D69.9
    fetus or newborn P53
    specified type NEC D69.8
  due to or associated with
    afibrinogenemia or other coagulation defect (conditions in category D65D69)
      antepartum — *see* Hemorrhage, antepartum, with coagulation defect
      intrapartum O67.0
    device, implant or graft (*see also* Complications, by site and type, specified NEC) T85.83
      arterial graft NEC T82.838
      breast T85.83
      catheter NEC T85.83
        dialysis (renal) T82.838
          intraperitoneal T85.83
        infusion NEC T82.838
          spinal (epidural) (subdural) T85.83
        urinary (indwelling) T83.83

Hemorrhage, hemorrhagic — *continued*
  due to or associated with — *continued*
    device, implant or graft (*see also* Complications, by site and type, specified NEC) — *continued*
      electronic (electrode) (pulse generator) (stimulator)
        bone T84.83
        cardiac T82.837
        nervous system (brain) (peripheral nerve) (spinal) T85.83
        urinary T83.83
      fixation, internal (orthopedic) NEC T84.83
      gastrointestinal (bile duct) (esophagus) T85.83
      genital NEC T83.83
      heart NEC T82.837
      joint prosthesis T84.83
      ocular (corneal graft) (orbital implant) NEC T85.83
      orthopedic NEC T84.83
        bone graft T86.838
      specified NEC T85.83
      urinary NEC T83.83
      vascular NEC T82.838
      ventricular intracranial shunt T85.83
  duodenum, duodenal K92.2
    ulcer — *see* Ulcer, duodenum, with hemorrhage
  dura mater — *see* Hemorrhage, intracranial, subdural
  endotracheal — *see* Hemorrhage, lung
  epicranial subaponeurotic (massive), birth injury P12.2
  epidural (traumatic) — *see also* Injury, intracranial, epidural hemorrhage
    nontraumatic I62.1
  esophagus K22.8
    varix I85.01
      secondary I85.11
  excessive, following ectopic gestation (subsequent episode) O08.1
  extradural (traumatic) — *see* Injury, intracranial, epidural hemorrhage
    birth injury P10.8
    fetus or newborn (anoxic) (nontraumatic) P52.8
    nontraumatic I62.1
  eye NEC H57.8
    fundus — *see* Hemorrhage, retina
    lid — *see* Disorder, eyelid, specified type NEC
  fallopian tube N83.6
  fetal, fetus P50.9
    from
      cut end of co-twin's cord P50.5
      placenta P50.2
      ruptured cord P50.1
      vasa previa P50.0
    into
      co-twin P50.3
        affecting management of pregnancy or puerperium O43.029
        first trimester O43.021
        second trimester O43.022
        third trimester O43.023
      maternal circulation P50.4
        affecting management of pregnancy or puerperium O43.019
        first trimester O43.011
        second trimester O43.012
        third trimester O43.013
    specified NEC P50.8
  fetal-maternal P50.4
    affecting management of pregnancy or puerperium O43.019
      first trimester O43.011
      second trimester O43.012
      third trimester O43.013
  fibrinogenolysis — *see* Fibrinolysis
  fibrinolytic (acquired) — *see* Fibrinolysis
  from
    ear (nontraumatic) — *see* Otorrhagia
    tracheostomy stoma J95.01
  fundus, eye — *see* Hemorrhage, retina
  funis — *see* Hemorrhage, umbilicus, cord

Hemorrhage, hemorrhagic — *continued*
  gastric — *see* Hemorrhage, stomach
  gastroenteric K92.2
    newborn P54.3
  gastrointestinal (tract) K92.2
    newborn P54.3
  genitourinary (tract) NOS R31.9
  gingiva K06.8
  globe (eye) — *see* Hemophthalmos
  graafian follicle cyst (ruptured) N83.0
  gum K06.8
  heart I51.8
  hypopharyngeal (throat) R58
  intermenstrual (regular) N92.3
    irregular N92.1
  internal (organs) NEC R58
    capsule I61.0
    ear — *see* category H83.8
    newborn P54.8
  intestine K92.2
    newborn P54.3
  intra-abdominal R58
  intra-alveolar (lung), newborn P26.8
  intracerebral (nontraumatic) — *see* Hemorrhage, intracranial, intracerebral
  intracranial (nontraumatic) I62.9
    birth injury P10.9
    complicating pregnancy, childbirth and puerperium — *see* Disease, circulatory system, obstetric
    epidural, nontraumatic I62.1
    extradural, nontraumatic I62.1
    fetus or newborn P52.9
      specified NEC P52.8
    intracerebral (nontraumatic) (in) I61.9
      brain stem I61.3
      cerebellum I61.4
      fetus or newborn P52.4
        birth injury P10.1
      hemisphere I61.2
        cortical (superficial) I61.1
        subcortical (deep) I61.0
      intraventricular I61.5
      multiple localized I61.6
      specified NEC I61.8
      superficial I61.1
      traumatic (diffuse) — *see* Injury, intracranial, diffuse
        focal — *see* Injury, intracranial, focal
    subarachnoid (nontraumatic) (from) I60.9
      fetus or newborn P52.5
        birth injury P10.3
      intracranial (cerebral) artery I60.7
        anterior communicating I60.2
        basilar I60.4
        carotid siphon and bifurcation I60.0
        communicating I60.7
          anterior I60.2
          posterior I60.3
        middle cerebral I60.1
        posterior communicating I60.3
        specified artery NEC I60.6
        vertebral I60.5
      puerperal, childbirth, pregnancy — *see* Disease, circulatory system, obstetric
      specified NEC I60.8
      traumatic S06.61
        with loss of consciousness S06.60
          brief (<1 hour) S06.62
          minor (1-6 hours) S06.63
          moderate (1-24 hours) S06.64
          prolonged (>24 hours) S06.65
            without return to consciousness S06.66
    subdural (nontraumatic) I62.00
      acute I62.01
      birth injury P10.0
      chronic I62.03
      fetus or newborn (anoxic) (hypoxic) P52.8
        birth injury P10.0
      spinal G95.19
      subacute I62.02
      traumatic — *see* Injury, intracranial, subdural hemorrhage

©2002 Ingenix, Inc.

Hemorrhage, hemorrhagic — continued
  intracranial — continued
    traumatic — see Injury, intracranial, focal
      brain injury
  intramedullary NEC G95.19
  intraocular — see Hemophthalmos
  intraoperative of
    operative site during
      circulatory system procedure I97.418
        cardiac
          bypass I97.411
          catheterization I97.410
        due to accidental laceration I97.51
      digestive system procedure K91.61
        due to accidental laceration K91.71
      ear procedure H95.21
        due to accidental laceration H95.31
      endocrine system procedure E36.01
        due to accidental laceration E36.11
      eye procedure H59.31
        due to accidental laceration H59.41
      genitourinary system procedure N99.61
        due to accidental laceration N99.71
      mastoid procedure H95.21
        due to accidental laceration H95.31
      musculoskeletal system procedure
        M96.811
        due to accidental laceration M96.821
      nervous system procedure G97.31
        due to accidental laceration G97.41
      respiratory system procedure J95.61
        due to accidental laceration J95.71
      skin procedure L76.01
        due to accidental laceration L76.11
      spleen procedure D78.01
        with accidental puncture D78.11
    specified site NEC during
      circulatory system procedure I97.42
        due to accidental laceration I97.52
      ear procedure H95.22
        due to accidental laceration H95.32
      endocrine system procedure E36.02
        due to accidental laceration E36.12
      eye procedure H59.32
        due to accidental laceration H59.42
      genitourinary system procedure N99.62
        due to accidental laceration N99.72
      mastoid procedure H95.22
        due to accidental laceration H95.32
      musculoskeletal system procedure
        M96.812
        due to accidental laceration M96.822
      nervous system procedure G97.32
        due to accidental laceration G97.42
      respiratory system procedure J95.62
        due to accidental laceration J95.72
      skin procedure L76.02
        due to accidental laceration L76.12
      spleen procedure D78.02
        due to accidental laceration D78.12
  intrapartum — see Hemorrhage, complicating,
    delivery
  intrapelvic
    female N94.8
    male K66.1
  intraperitoneal K66.1
  intrapontine I61.3
  intrauterine N85.7
    complicating delivery — see also
      Hemorrhage, complicating, delivery
      O67.9
    postpartum — see Hemorrhage, postpartum
  intraventricular I61.5
    fetus or newborn (nontraumatic) P52.3
      due to birth injury P10.2
      grade
        1 P52.0
        2 P52.1
        3 P52.2
  intravesical N32.8
  iris (postinfectional) (postinflammatory) (toxic)
    — see Hyphema
  joint (nontraumatic) — see Hemarthrosis
  kidney N28.89
  knee (joint) (nontraumatic) — see
    Hemarthrosis, knee

Hemorrhage, hemorrhagic — continued
  labyrinth — see category H83.8
  lenticular striate artery I61.0
  ligature, vessel — see Hemorrhage,
    postoperative
  liver K76.8
  lung R04.8
    newborn P26.9
      massive P26.1
      specified NEC P26.8
    tuberculous — see Tuberculosis, pulmonary
  massive umbilical, newborn P51.0
  mediastinum — see Hemorrhage, lung
  medulla I61.3
  membrane (brain) I60.8
    spinal cord — see Hemorrhage, spinal cord
  meninges, meningeal (brain) (middle) I60.8
    spinal cord — see Hemorrhage, spinal cord
  mesentery K66.1
  metritis — see Endometritis
  mouth K13.7
  mucous membrane NEC R58
    newborn P54.8
  muscle M62.89
  nail (subungual) L60.8
  nasal turbinate R04.0
    newborn P54.8
  navel, newborn P51.9
  newborn P54.9
    specified NEC P54.8
  nipple N64.5
  nose R04.0
    newborn P54.8
  omentum K66.1
  optic nerve (sheath) H47.029
    bilateral H47.023
    left H47.022
    right H47.021
  orbit, orbital H05.239
    bilateral H05.233
    left H05.232
    right H05.231
  ovary NEC N83.8
  oviduct N83.6
  pancreas K86.8
  parathyroid (gland) (spontaneous) E21.4
  parturition — see Hemorrhage, complicating,
    delivery
  penis N48.89
  pericardium, pericarditis I31.2
  peritoneum, peritoneal K66.1
  peritonsillar tissue J35.8
    due to infection J36
  petechial R23.3
    due to autosensitivity, erythrocyte D69.2
  pituitary (gland) E23.6
  pleura — see Hemorrhage, lung
  polioencephalitis, superior E51.2
  polymyositis — see Polymyositis
  pons, pontine I61.3
  posterior fossa (nontraumatic) I61.8
    fetus or newborn P52.6
  postmenopausal N95.0
  postnasal R04.0
  postoperative
    operative site following
      circulatory system procedure I97.45
        due to accidental laceration I97.51
      digestive system procedure K91.65
        due to accidental laceration K91.71
      ear procedure H95.25
        due to accidental laceration H95.31
      endocrine system procedure E36.05
        due to accidental laceration E36.11
      eye procedure H59.35
        due to accidental laceration H59.41
      genitourinary system procedure N99.65
        due to accidental laceration N99.71
      mastoid procedure H95.25
        due to accidental laceration H95.31
      musculoskeletal system procedure
        M96.815
        due to accidental laceration M96.821
      nervous system procedure G97.35
        due to accidental laceration G97.41
      respiratory system procedure J95.65
        due to accidental laceration J95.71

Hemorrhage, hemorrhagic — continued
  postoperative — continued
    operative site following — continued
      skin procedure L76.05
        due to accidental laceration L76.11
      spleen procedure D78.05
        with accidental puncture D78.11
    specified site NEC following
      circulatory system procedure I97.46
        due to accidental laceration I97.52
      ear procedure H95.26
        due to accidental laceration H95.32
      endocrine system procedure E36.06
        due to accidental laceration E36.12
      genitourinary system procedure N99.66
        due to accidental laceration N99.72
      mastoid procedure H95.26
        due to accidental laceration H95.32
      musculoskeletal system procedure
        M96.816
        due to accidental laceration M96.822
      nervous system procedure G97.36
        due to accidental laceration G97.42
      respiratory system procedure J95.66
        due to accidental laceration J95.72
      skin procedure L76.06
        due to accidental laceration L76.12
      spleen procedure D78.06
        due to accidental laceration D78.12
  postpartum NEC (following delivery of placenta)
    O72.1
    delayed or secondary O72.2
    retained placenta O72.0
    third stage O72.0
  pregnancy — see Hemorrhage, antepartum
  preretinal — see Hemorrhage, retina
  prostate N42.1
  puerperal — see Hemorrhage, postpartum
    delayed or secondary O72.2
  pulmonary R04.8
    newborn P26.9
      massive P26.1
      specified NEC P26.8
    tuberculous — see Tuberculosis, pulmonary
  purpura (primary) D69.3
  rectum (sphincter) K62.5
    newborn P54.2
  recurring, following initial hemorrhage at time
    of injury T79.2
  renal N28.89
  respiratory passage or tract R04.9
    specified NEC R04.8
  retina, retinal (vessels) H35.60
    bilateral H35.63
    diabetic — see Diabetes, retinal, hemorrhage
    left H35.62
    right H35.61
  retroperitoneal R58
  scalp R58
  scrotum N50.1
  secondary (nontraumatic) R58
    following initial hemorrhage at time of injury
    T79.2
  seminal vesicle N50.1
  skin R23.3
    fetus or newborn P54.5
  slipped umbilical ligature P51.8
  spermatic cord N50.1
  spinal (cord) G95.19
    fetus or newborn (birth injury) P11.5
  spleen D73.5
    intraoperative D78.01
      with accidental puncture D78.11
    postoperative D78.05
      with accidental puncture D78.11
  stomach K92.2
    newborn P54.3
    ulcer — see Ulcer, stomach, with
      hemorrhage
  subarachnoid (nontraumatic) — see
    Hemorrhage, intracranial, subarachnoid
  subconjunctival — see also Hemorrhage,
    conjunctiva
    birth injury P15.3
  subcortical (brain) I61.0
  subcutaneous R23.3
  subdiaphragmatic R58

Hemorrhage, hemorrhagic — *continued*
  subdural (acute) (nontraumatic) — *see*
    Hemorrhage, intracranial, subarachnoid
  subependymal
    fetus or newborn P52.0
      with intraventricular extension P52.1
        and intracerebral extension P52.2
  subhyaloid — *see* Hemorrhage, retina
  subperiosteal — *see* Disorder, bone, specified
    type NEC
  subretinal — *see* Hemorrhage, retina
  subtentorial — *see* Hemorrhage, intracranial,
    subarachnoid
  subungual L60.8
  suprarenal (capsule) (gland) E27.4
    newborn P54.4
  tentorium (traumatic) NEC — *see* Hemorrhage,
    brain
    fetus or newborn (birth injury) P10.4
  testis N50.1
  third stage (postpartum) O72.0
  thorax — *see* Hemorrhage, lung
  throat R04.1
  thymus (gland) E32.8
  thyroid (cyst) (gland) E07.89
  tongue K14.8
  tonsil J35.8
  trachea — *see* Hemorrhage, lung
  tracheobronchial R04.8
    newborn P26.0
  traumatic – code to specific injury
    cerebellar — *see* Hemorrhage, brain
    intracranial — *see* Hemorrhage, brain
    recurring or secondary (following initial
      hemorrhage at time of injury) T79.2
  tuberculous NEC — *see also* Tuberculosis,
    pulmonary A15.0
  tunica vaginalis N50.1
  ulcer – code by site under Ulcer, with
    hemorrhage K27.4
  umbilicus, umbilical
    cord
      after birth, newborn P51.9
      complicating delivery O69.5
        affecting fetus or newborn P51.9
        from ruptured cord P50.1
    newborn P51.9
      massive P51.0
      slipped ligature P51.8
    stump P51.9
  unavoidable (antepartum) (due to placenta
    previa) — *see* Disorder, placenta, previa
  urethra (idiopathic) N36.8
  uterus, uterine (abnormal) N93.9
    climacteric N92.4
    complicating delivery — *see* Hemorrhage,
      complicating, delivery
    dysfunctional or functional N93.8
    intermenstrual (regular) N92.3
      irregular N92.1
    postmenopausal N95.0
    postpartum — *see* Hemorrhage, postpartum
    preclimacteric or premenopausal N92.4
    prepubertal N93.8
    pubertal N92.2
  vagina (abnormal) N93.9
    newborn P54.6
  vas deferens N50.1
  vasa previa O69.4
    affecting fetus or newborn P50.0
  ventricular I61.5
  vesical N32.8
  viscera NEC R58
    newborn P54.8
  vitreous (humor) (intraocular) H43.10
    bilateral H43.13
    left H43.12
    right H43.11
  vulva N90.8
Hemorrhoids I84.20
  bleeding I84.101
  complicating
    pregnancy O22.40
      first trimester O22.41
      second trimester O22.42
      third trimester O22.43
    puerperium O87.2

Hemorrhoids — *continued*
  external I84.22
    with internal I84.23
      bleeding I84.131
      prolapsed I84.132
      strangulated I84.133
      thrombosed I84.03
      ulcerated I84.134
    bleeding I84.121
    prolapsed I84.122
    strangulated I84.123
    thrombosed I84.02
    ulcerated I84.124
  internal I84.21
    with external I84.23
      bleeding I84.131
      prolapsed I84.132
      strangulated I84.133
      thrombosed I84.03
      ulcerated I84.134
    bleeding I84.111
    prolapsed I84.112
    strangulated I84.113
    thrombosed I84.01
    ulcerated I84.114
  prolapsed I84.102
  skin tags, residual I84.6
  strangulated I84.103
  thrombosed I84.00
  ulcerated I84.104
Hemosalpinx N83.6
  with
    hematocolpos N89.7
    hematometra N85.7
      with hematocolpos N89.7
Hemosiderosis (dietary) E83.19
  pulmonary, idiopathic E83.19 *[J99]*
  transfusion T80.8
Hemothorax (bacterial) (nontuberculous) J94.2
  newborn P54.8
  traumatic S27.1
    with pneumothorax S27.2
  tuberculous NEC A15.6
Henoch (-Schönlein) disease or syndrome
  (purpura) D69.0
Henpue, henpuye A66.6
Hepar lobatum (syphilitic) A52.74
Hepatalgia K76.8
Hepatitis K75.9
  acute NEC K72.00
    with coma K72.01
    alcoholic — *see* Hepatitis, alcoholic
    infectious B15.9
      with hepatic coma B15.0
  alcoholic (acute) (chronic) K70.10
    with ascites K70.11
  amebic — *see* Abscess, liver, amebic
  anicteric, acute (viral) — *see* Hepatitis, viral
  antigen-associated (HAA) — *see* Hepatitis, viral,
    type B
  Australia-antigen (positive) — *see* Hepatitis,
    viral, type B
  autoimmune K75.4
  catarrhal (acute) B15.9
    with hepatic coma B15.0
  cholangiolitic K75.8
  cholestatic K75.8
  chronic K73.9
    active NEC K73.2
    lobular NEC K73.1
    persistent NEC K73.0
    specified NEC K73.8
  cytomegaloviral B25.1
  due to ethanol (acute) (chronic) — *see*
    Hepatitis, alcoholic
  epidemic B15.9
    with hepatic coma B15.0
  fetus or newborn P59.29
  from injection (blood) (plasma) (serum) (other
    substance) (*see also* Hepatitis, viral type
    B) B16.9
  fulminant NEC (viral) — *see* Hepatitis, viral
  granulomatous NEC K75.3
  herpesviral B00.81
  homologous serum — *see* Hepatitis, viral, type
    B

Hepatitis — *continued*
  in (due to)
    mumps B26.81
    toxoplasmosis (acquired) B58.1
      congenital (active) P37.1 *[K77]*
  infectious, infective (acute) (chronic) (subacute)
    B15.9
    with hepatic coma B15.0
  inoculation — *see* Hepatitis, viral, type B
  interstitial (chronic) K74.6
  lupoid NEC K73.2
  malignant NEC (with hepatic failure) K72.90
    with coma K72.91
  neonatal (toxic) P59.29
  postimmunization — *see* Hepatitis, viral, type B
  post-transfusion — *see* Hepatitis, viral, type B
  reactive, nonspecific K75.2
  serum — *see* Hepatitis, viral, type B
  specified type NEC
    with hepatic failure — *see* Failure, hepatic
  syphilitic (late) A52.74
    congenital (early) A50.08 *[K77]*
      late A50.59 *[K77]*
    secondary A51.45
  toxic (*see also* Disease, liver, toxic) K71.6
  tuberculous A18.83
  viral, virus (acute) B19.9
    with hepatic coma B19.0
    chronic B18.9
      specified NEC B18.8
    type
      B B18.1
        with delta-agent B18.0
      C B18.2
    complicating pregnancy, childbirth or
      puerperium — *see* Hepatitis, viral,
      obstetric
    congenital P35.3
    coxsackie B33.8 *[K77]*
    cytomegalic inclusion B25.1
    non-A, non-B B17.8
    obstetric complicating
      childbirth O98.42
      pregnancy O98.419
        first trimester O98.411
        second trimester O98.412
        third trimester O98.413
      puerperium O98.43
    specified type NEC (with or without coma)
      B17.8
    type
      A B15.9
        with hepatic coma B15.0
      B B16.9
        with
          delta-agent (coinfection) (without
            hepatic coma) B16.1
            with hepatic coma B16.0
          hepatic coma (without delta-agent
            coinfection) B16.2
      C B17.1
      E B17.2
      non-A, non-B B17.8
Hepatization lung (acute) — *see* Pneumonia,
    lobar
Hepatoblastoma (M8970/3) C22.2
Hepatocarcinoma (M8170/3) C22.0
Hepatocholangiocarcinoma (M8180/3) C22.0
Hepatocholangioma, benign (M8180/0) D13.4
Hepatocholangitis K75.8
Hepatolenticular degeneration E83.01
Hepatoma (malignant) (M8170/3) C22.0
  benign (M8170/0) D13.4
  embryonal (M8970/3) C22.0
Hepatomegaly — *see also* Hypertrophy, liver
  with splenomegaly R16.2
  congenital Q44.7
  in infectious mononucleosis
    (gammaherpesviral) B27.09
Hepatoptosis K76.8
**Hepatorenal syndrome following labor and
    delivery** O90.4
Hepatosis K76.8

©2002 Ingenix, Inc.

Hepatosplenomegaly R16.2
  hyperlipemic (Bürger-Grütz type) E78.3 *[K77]*
Hereditary — *see* condition
Heredodegeneration, macular — *see* Dystrophy, retina
Heredopathia atactica polyneuritiformis G60.1
Heredosyphilis — *see* Syphilis, congenital
Herlitz' syndrome Q81.1
Hermansky-Pudlak syndrome E70.331
Hermaphrodite, hermaphroditism (true) Q56.0
  46,XX with streak gonads Q99.1
  46,XX/46,XY Q99.0
  46,XY with streak gonads Q99.1
  chimera 46,XX/46,XY Q99.0
Hernia, hernial (acquired) (recurrent) K46.9
  with
    gangrene — *see* Hernia, by site, with, gangrene
    incarceration — *see* Hernia, by site, with, obstruction
    irreducible — *see* Hernia, by site, with, obstruction
    obstruction — *see* Hernia, by site, with, obstruction
    strangulation — *see* Hernia, by site, with, obstruction
  abdomen, abdominal K46.9
    with
      gangrene (and obstruction) K46.1
      obstruction K46.0
    femoral — *see* Hernia, femoral
    incisional — *see* Hernia, incisional
    inguinal — *see* Hernia, inguinal
    specified site NEC K45.8
      with
        gangrene (and obstruction) K45.1
        obstruction K45.0
    umbilical — *see* Hernia, umbilical
    wall — *see* Hernia, ventral
  appendix — *see* Hernia, abdomen
  bladder (mucosa) (sphincter)
    congenital (female) (male) Q79.51
    female N81.1
    male N32.8
  brain, congenital — *see* Encephalocele
  cartilage, vertebra — *see* Displacement, intervertebral disc
  cerebral, congenital — *see also* Encephalocele
    endaural Q01.8
  ciliary body (traumatic) S05.20
    left S05.22
    right S05.21
  colon — *see* Hernia, abdomen
  Cooper's — *see* Hernia, abdomen, specified site NEC
  crural — *see* Hernia, femoral
  diaphragm, diaphragmatic K44.9
    with
      gangrene (and obstruction) K44.1
      obstruction K44.0
    congenital Q79.0
  direct (inguinal) — *see* Hernia, inguinal
  diverticulum, intestine — *see* Hernia, abdomen
  double (inguinal) — *see* Hernia, inguinal, bilateral
  epigastric — *see* Hernia, ventral
  esophageal hiatus — *see* Hernia, hiatal
  external (inguinal) — *see* Hernia, inguinal
  fallopian tube N83.4
  fascia M62.89
  femoral K41.9
    with
      gangrene (and obstruction) K41.4
      obstruction K41.3
    bilateral K41.2
      with
        gangrene (and obstruction) K41.1
        obstruction K41.0
    unilateral K41.9
      with
        gangrene (and obstruction) K41.4
        obstruction K41.3
  foramen magnum G93.5
    congenital Q01.8

Hernia, hernial — *continued*
  funicular (umbilical) — *see also* Hernia, umbilicus
    spermatic (cord) — *see* Hernia, inguinal
  gastrointestinal tract — *see* Hernia, abdomen
  Hesselbach's — *see* Hernia, abdomen, specified site NEC
  hiatal (esophageal) (sliding) K44.9
    with
      gangrene (and obstruction) K44.1
      obstruction K44.0
    congenital Q40.1
  incarcerated — *see also* Hernia, by site, with obstruction
    with gangrene — *see* Hernia, by site, with gangrene
  incisional K43.91
    with
      gangrene (and obstruction) K43.11
      obstruction K43.01
  indirect (inguinal) — *see* Hernia, inguinal
  inguinal (direct) (external) (funicular) (indirect) (internal) (oblique) (scrotal) (sliding) K40.9
    with
      gangrene (and obstruction) K40.4
      obstruction K40.3
    bilateral K40.2
      with
        gangrene (and obstruction) K40.1
        obstruction K40.0
    unilateral K40.9
      with
        gangrene (and obstruction) K40.4
        obstruction K40.3
  internal — *see also* Hernia, abdomen
    inguinal — *see* Hernia, inguinal
  interstitial — *see* Hernia, abdomen
  intervertebral cartilage or disc — *see* Displacement, intervertebral disc
  intestine, intestinal — *see* Hernia, by site
  intra-abdominal — *see* Hernia, abdomen
  iris (traumatic) S05.20
    left S05.22
    right S05.21
  irreducible — *see also* Hernia, by site, with obstruction
    with gangrene — *see* Hernia, by site, with gangrene
  ischiatic — *see* Hernia, abdomen, specified site NEC
  ischiorectal — *see* Hernia, abdomen, specified site NEC
  lens (traumatic) S05.20
    left S05.22
    right S05.21
  linea (alba) (semilunaris) — *see* Hernia, ventral
  Littre's — *see* Hernia, abdomen
  lumbar — *see* Hernia, abdomen, specified site NEC
  lung (subcutaneous) J98.4
  mediastinum J98.5
  mesenteric (internal) — *see* Hernia, abdomen
  muscle (sheath) M62.89
  nucleus pulposus — *see* Displacement, intervertebral disc
  oblique (inguinal) — *see* Hernia, inguinal
  obstructive — *see also* Hernia, by site, with obstruction
    with gangrene — *see* Hernia, by site, with gangrene
  obturator — *see* Hernia, abdomen, specified site NEC
  omental — *see* Hernia, abdomen
  ovary N83.4
  oviduct N83.4
  paraesophageal — *see also* Hernia, diaphragm
    congenital Q40.1
  paraumbilical — *see* Hernia, umbilicus
  perineal — *see* Hernia, abdomen, specified site NEC
  Petit's — *see* Hernia, abdomen, specified site NEC
  postoperative — *see* Hernia, incisional
  pregnant uterus — *see* Abnormal, uterus in pregnancy or childbirth
  prevesical N32.8

Hernia, hernial — *continued*
  properitoneal — *see* Hernia, abdomen, specified site NEC
  pudendal — *see* Hernia, abdomen, specified site NEC
  rectovaginal N81.6
  retroperitoneal — *see* Hernia, abdomen, specified site NEC
  Richter's — *see* Hernia, abdomen, with obstruction
  Rieux's, Riex's — *see* Hernia, abdomen, specified site NEC
  sac condition (adhesion) (dropsy) (inflammation) (laceration) (suppuration) – code by site under Hernia
  sciatic — *see* Hernia, abdomen, specified site NEC
  scrotum, scrotal — *see* Hernia, inguinal
  sliding (inguinal) — *see also* Hernia, inguinal
    hiatus — *see* Hernia, hiatal
  spigelian — *see* Hernia, ventral
  spinal — *see* Spina bifida
  strangulated — *see also* Hernia, by site, with obstruction
    with gangrene — *see* Hernia, by site, with gangrene
  supra-umbilicus — *see* Hernia, ventral
  tendon — *see* Disorder, tendon, specified type NEC
  Treitz's (fossa) — *see* Hernia, abdomen, specified site NEC
  tunica vaginalis Q55.29
  umbilicus, umbilical K42.9
    with
      gangrene (and obstruction) K42.1
      obstruction K42.0
  ureter N28.89
  urethra, congenital Q64.79
  urinary meatus, congenital Q64.79
  uterus N81.4
    pregnant — *see* Abnormal, uterus in pregnancy or childbirth
  vaginal (anterior) (wall) N81.1
  Velpeau's — *see* Hernia, femoral
  ventral K43.90
    with
      gangrene (and obstruction) K43.10
      obstruction K43.00
    incisional K43.91
      with
        gangrene (and obstruction) K43.11
        obstruction K43.01
    specified NEC K43.99
      with
        gangrene (and obstruction) K43.19
        obstruction K43.09
  vesical
    congenital (female) (male) Q79.51
    female N81.1
    male N32.8
  vitreous (into wound) S05.20
    into anterior chamber — *see* Prolapse, vitreous
    left S05.22
    right S05.21
Herniation — *see also* Hernia
  brain (stem) G93.5
  cerebral G93.5
  mediastinum J98.5
  nucleus pulposus — *see* Displacement, intervertebral disc
Herpangina B08.5
Herpes, herpetic B00.9
  anogenital A60.9
    perianal skin A60.1
    rectum A60.1
    urogenital tract A60.00
      cervix A60.03
      male genital organ NEC A60.02
      penis A60.01
      specified site NEC A60.09
      vagina A60.04
      vulva A60.04
  blepharitis (zoster) B02.39
    simplex B00.59
  circinatus B35.4
    bullosus L12.0

Herpes, herpetic — continued
  conjunctivitis B02.31
  cornea B02.33
  encephalitis B00.4
  eye (zoster) B02.30
    simplex B00.50
  eyelid (zoster) B02.39
    simplex B00.59
  facialis B00.1
  febrilis B00.1
  geniculate ganglionitis B02.21
  genital, genitalis A60.00
    female A60.09
    male A60.01
  gestational, gestationis O26.40
    first trimester O26.41
    second trimester O26.42
    third trimester O26.43
  gingivostomatitis B00.2
  iridocyclitis (simplex) B00.51
    zoster B02.32
  iris (vesicular erythema multiforme) L51.1
  iritis (simplex) B00.51
  keratitis (simplex) (dendritic) (disciform)
    (interstitial) B00.52
    zoster (interstitial) B02.33
  keratoconjunctivitis (simplex) B00.52
    zoster B02.33
  labialis B00.1
  lip B00.1
  meningitis (simplex) B00.3
    zoster B02.1
  ophthalmicus (zoster) NEC B02.30
    simplex B00.50
  penis A60.01
  perianal skin A60.1
  pharyngitis, pharyngotonsillitis B00.2
  rectum A60.1
  scrotum A60.02
  septicemia B00.7
  simplex B00.9
    complicated NEC B00.89
    congenital P35.2
    external ear B00.1
    eyelid B00.59
    hepatitis B00.81
    keratitis (interstitial) B00.52
    specified complication NEC B00.89
    visceral B00.89
  stomatitis B00.2
  tonsurans B35.0
  visceral B00.89
  vulva A60.04
  whitlow B00.89
  zoster (see also condition) B02.9
    auricularis B02.21
    complicated NEC B02.8
    disseminated B02.7
    encephalitis B02.0
    eye(lid) B02.39
    geniculate ganglionitis B02.21
    keratitis (interstitial) B02.33
    meningitis B02.1
    neuritis, neuralgia B02.29
    ophthalmicus NEC B02.30
    oticus B02.21
    polyneuropathy B02.23
    specified complication NEC B02.8
    trigeminal neuralgia B02.22
Herpetophobia F40.218
Herrick's anemia — see Disease, sickle-cell
Hers' disease E74.09
Herter-Gee syndrome K90.0
Herxheimer's reaction T78.2
Hesitancy of micturition R39.11
Hesselbach's hernia — see Hernia, abdomen, specified site NEC
Heterochromia (congenital) Q13.2
  cataract — see Cataract, complicated
  cyclitis (Fuchs) — see Cyclitis, Fuchs' heterochromic
  hair L67.1
  iritis — see Cyclitis, Fuchs' heterochromic

Heterochromia — continued
  retained metallic foreign body (nonmagnetic) — see Foreign body, intraocular, old, retained
    magnetic — see Foreign body, intraocular, old, retained, magnetic
  uveitis — see Cyclitis, Fuchs' heterochromic
Heterophoria — see Strabismus, heterophoria
Heterophyes, heterophyiasis (small intestine) B66.8
Heterotopia, heterotopic — see also Malposition, congenital
  cerebralis Q04.8
Heterotropia — see Strabismus
Heubner-Herter disease K90.0
Hexadactylism Q69.9
Hibernoma (M8880/0) — see Lipoma
Hiccup, hiccough R06.6
  epidemic B33.0
  psychogenic F45.8
Hidradenitis (axillaris) (suppurative) L73.2
Hidradenoma (nodular) (M8400/0) — see also Neoplasm, skin, benign
  clear cell (M8402/0) — see Neoplasm, skin, benign
  papillary (M8405/0) — see Neoplasm, skin, benign
Hidrocystoma (M8404/0) — see Neoplasm, skin, benign
High
  altitude effects T70.20
    anoxia T70.20
    on
      ears T70.0
      sinuses T70.1
    polycythemia D75.1
  arch
    foot Q66.7
    palate, congenital Q38.5
  arterial tension — see Hypertension
  basal metabolic rate R94.8
  blood pressure — see also Hypertension
    reading (incidental) (isolated) (nonspecific), without diagnosis of hypertension R03.0
  diaphragm (congenital) Q79.1
  expressed emotional level within family Z63.8
  head at term O32.4
  palate, congenital Q38.5
  risk
    environment (physical) NOS Z58.9
      occupational NOS Z57.9
        specified NEC Z57.8
      specified NEC Z58.89
    infant NEC Z76.2
    sexual behavior (heterosexual) Z72.51
      bisexual Z72.53
      homosexual Z72.52
  temperature (of unknown origin) R50.9
  thoracic rib Q76.6
Hildenbrand's disease A75.0
Hilum — see condition
Hip — see condition
Hippel's disease Q85.8
Hippophobia F40.218
Hippus H57.09
Hirschsprung's disease or megacolon Q43.1
Hirsutism, hirsuties L68.0
Hirudiniasis
  external B88.3
  internal B83.4
Hiss-Russell dysentery A03.1
Histidinemia, histidinuria E70.41
Histiocytoma (M8832/0) — see also Neoplasm, skin, benign
  fibrous (M8830/0) — see also Neoplasm, skin, benign
    atypical (M8830/1) — see Neoplasm, connective tissue, uncertain behavior
    malignant (M8830/3) — see Neoplasm, connective tissue, malignant

Histiocytosis D76.3
  acute differentiated progressive (M9722/3) C96.0
  Langerhans' cell NEC D76.0
  lipid, lipoid (essential) D76.0
  malignant (M9720/3) C96.1
  mononuclear phagocytes NEC D76.1
    Langerhans' cells D76.0
  sinus, with massive lymphadenopathy D76.3
  syndrome NEC D76.3
  X D76.0
    acute (progressive) (M9722/3) C96.0
    chronic D76.0
Histoplasmosis B39.9
  with pneumonia NEC B39.2 [J17]
  African B39.5
  American — see Histoplasmosis, capsulati
  capsulati B39.4
    disseminated B39.3
    generalized B39.3
    pulmonary B39.2
      acute B39.0
      chronic B39.1
  Darling's B39.4
  duboisii B39.5
  lung NEC B39.2
History (personal) **of**
  abuse Z91.8
  alcohol dependence F10.21
  allergy to
    analgesic agent NEC Z88.6
    anesthetic Z88.4
    antibiotic agent NEC Z88.1
    anti-infective agent NEC Z88.3
    contrast media Z91.041
    drugs, medicaments and biological substances Z88.9
      specified NEC Z88.8
    food Z91.018
      additives Z91.02
      eggs Z91.012
      milk products Z91.011
      peanuts Z91.010
      seafood Z91.013
      specified food NEC Z91.018
    insect Z91.038
      bee Z91.030
    latex Z91.040
    medicinal agents Z88.9
      specified NEC Z88.8
    narcotic agent NEC Z88.5
    nonmedicinal agents Z91.048
    penicillin Z88.0
    serum Z88.7
    specified NEC Z91.09
    sulfonamides Z88.2
    vaccine Z88.7
  anticoagulant use (long term) Z79.1
    with hemorrhage D68.5
  arthritis Z87.3
  aspirin use (long term) Z79.8
  benign neoplasm Z86.018
    brain Z86.011
    colonic polyps Z86.010
  childhood abuse — see Maltreatment, child, history of, by type
  chromosomal abnormality Z87.89
  congenital malformation Z87.79
    hypospadias Z87.71
  contraception Z92.0
  disease or disorder (of) Z87.89
    blood and blood-forming organs Z86.2
    circulatory system Z86.79
      specified condition NEC Z86.79
      thrombophlebitis Z86.72
      venous thrombosis or embolism Z86.71
    digestive system Z87.19
      colonic polyp Z86.010
      peptic ulcer disease Z87.11
      specified condition NEC Z87.19
    ear Z86.6
    endocrine Z86.39
      diabetic foot ulcer Z86.31
      specified type NEC Z86.39
    eye Z86.6
    genital system Z87.4
    hematological Z86.2

©2002 Ingenix, Inc.

History of — *continued*
  disease or disorder — *continued*
    immune mechanism Z86.2
    infectious Z86.19
      malaria Z86.13
      poliomyelitis Z86.12
      specified NEC Z86.19
      tuberculosis Z86.11
    mental NEC Z87.89
    metabolic Z86.39
      diabetic foot ulcer Z86.31
      specified type NEC Z86.39
    musculoskeletal Z87.3
    nervous system Z86.6
    nutritional Z86.39
    obstetric Z87.5
    parasitic Z86.19
    respiratory system Z87.0
    sense organs Z86.6
    skin Z87.2
    specified site or type NEC Z87.89
    subcutaneous tissue Z87.2
    trophoblastic Z87.5
    urinary system Z87.4
  drug dependence F11 -F19 with .11
  family of
    alcohol abuse Z81.1
    allergy NEC Z84.8
    anemia Z83.2
    arthritis Z82.6
    asthma Z82.5
    blindness Z82.1
    chromosomal anomaly Z82.79
    chronic
      disabling disease NEC Z82.8
      lower respiratory disease Z82.5
    congenital malformations and deformations Z82.79
      polycystic kidney Z82.71
    consanguinity Z84.3
    deafness Z82.2
    diabetes mellitus Z83.3
    disability NEC Z82.8
    disease or disorder (of)
      allergic NEC Z84.8
      behavioral NEC Z81.8
      blood and blood-forming organs Z83.2
      cardiovascular NEC Z82.4
      chronic disabling NEC Z82.8
      digestive Z83.7
      ear NEC Z83.5
      endocrine Z83.4
      eye NEC Z83.5
      genitourinary NEC Z84.2
      hematological Z83.2
      immune mechanism Z83.2
      infectious NEC Z83.1
      ischemic heart Z82.4
      kidney Z84.1
      mental NEC Z81.8
      metabolic Z83.4
      musculoskeletal Z82.6
      neurological NEC Z82.0
      nutritional NEC Z83.4
      parasitic NEC Z83.1
      psychiatric NEC Z81.8
      respiratory NEC Z83.6
      skin and subcutaneous tissue NEC Z84.0
      specified NEC Z84.8
    drug abuse NEC Z81.3
    epilepsy Z82.0
    hearing loss Z82.2
    human immunodeficiency virus (HIV) infection Z83.0
    Huntington's chorea Z82.0
    leukemia Z80.6
    malignant neoplasm (of) NOS Z80.9
      breast Z80.3
      bronchus Z80.1
      digestive organ Z80.0
      gastrointestinal tract Z80.0
      genital organ Z80.49
        ovary Z80.41
        prostate Z80.42
        specified organ NEC Z80.49
        testis Z80.43

History of — *continued*
  family of — *continued*
    malignant neoplasm — *continued*
      hematopoietic NEC Z80.7
      intrathoracic organ NEC Z80.2
      lung Z80.1
      lymphatic NEC Z80.7
      ovary Z80.41
      prostate Z80.42
      respiratory organ NEC Z80.2
      specified site NEC Z80.8
      testis Z80.43
      trachea Z80.1
      urinary organ or tract Z80.59
        kidney Z80.51
    mental
      disorder NEC Z81.8
      retardation Z81.0
    polycystic kidney Z82.71
    psychiatric disorder Z81.8
    psychoactive substance abuse NEC Z81.3
    respiratory condition, chronic NEC Z82.5
    self-harmful behavior Z81.8
    skin condition Z84.0
    specified condition NEC Z84.8
    stroke (cerebrovascular) Z82.3
    substance abuse NEC Z81.4
      alcohol Z81.1
      drug NEC Z81.3
      psychoactive NEC Z81.3
      tobacco Z81.2
    tobacco abuse Z81.2
    violence, violent behavior Z81.8
    visual loss Z82.1
  hyperthermia, malignant Z88.4
  in situ neoplasm Z86.008
    breast Z86.000
  injury NEC Z91.8
  irradiation Z92.3
  malignant neoplasm (of) Z85.9
    bone Z85.822
      secondary Z85.863
    brain Z85.831
      secondary Z85.862
    breast Z85.3
    bronchus Z85.11
    digestive organ Z85.00
      anus Z85.04
      colon Z85.03
      esophagus Z85.01
      large intestine Z85.03
      lip Z85.819
        specified site NEC Z85.818
      liver Z85.05
        secondary Z85.861
      oral cavity Z85.819
        specified site NEC Z85.818
        tongue Z85.810
      rectosigmoid junction Z85.04
      rectum Z85.04
      small intestine Z85.09
      specified site NEC Z85.09
      stomach Z85.02
    endocrine gland Z85.848
      thyroid Z85.840
    eye Z85.830
    gastrointestinal tract — *see* History, malignant neoplasm, digestive organ
    genital organ (female) Z85.40
      male Z85.45
        epididymis Z85.48
        prostate Z85.46
        specified NEC Z85.49
        testis Z85.47
      ovary Z85.43
      specified NEC Z85.44
      uterus Z85.42
        cervix Z85.41
    intrathoracic organ Z85.20
      bronchus Z85.11
      heart Z85.29
      lung Z85.11
        secondary Z85.860
      mediastinum Z85.29
      pleura Z85.29
      thymus Z85.29

History of — *continued*
  malignant neoplasm — *continued*
    intrathoracic organ — *continued*
      trachea Z85.12
    liver Z85.05
      secondary Z85.861
    lung Z85.11
      secondary Z85.860
    nervous system Z85.838
      brain Z85.831
        secondary Z85.862
    oral cavity Z85.819
      specified site NEC Z85.818
      tongue Z85.810
    pharynx Z85.819
      specified site NEC Z85.818
    respiratory organ Z85.20
      bronchus Z85.11
      glottis Z85.21
      larynx Z85.21
      lung Z85.11
        secondary Z85.860
      nasal cavity Z85.22
      sinus Z85.22
      subglottis Z85.21
      supraglottis Z85.21
      trachea Z85.12
      vocal cord Z85.21
    skin Z85.821
      melanoma Z85.820
    soft tissue Z85.828
      skin Z85.821
        melanoma Z85.820
    specified site NEC Z85.85
      secondary Z85.868
    thyroid Z85.840
    trachea Z85.12
    urinary organ or tract Z85.50
      bladder Z85.51
      kidney Z85.52
        pelvis Z85.53
      specified NEC Z85.59
  maltreatment Z91.8
  neglect (in)
    adult Z91.41
    childhood Z61.812
  neoplasm
    benign Z86.018
      brain Z86.011
      colon polyp Z86.010
    in situ Z86.008
      breast Z86.000
    malignant — *see* History of, malignant neoplasm
    uncertain behavior Z86.03
  nicotine dependence Z87.82
  noncompliance with medical treatment or regimen — *see* Noncompliance
  nutritional deficiency Z86.39
  parasuicide (attempt) Z91.5
  perinatal problems Z87.89
  physical trauma NEC Z91.8
    self-harm or suicide attempt Z91.5
  poisoning NEC Z91.8
    self-harm or suicide attempt Z91.5
  poor personal hygiene Z91.8
  psychiatric disorder NEC Z87.89
  psychological trauma NEC Z91.49
  radiation therapy Z92.3
  respiratory condition, chronic, NEC Z87.0
  risk factors NEC Z91.8
  self-harm Z91.5
  self-poisoning attempt Z91.5
  sex reassignment Z87.81
  sleep-wake cycle problem Z91.3
  specified NEC Z87.89
  substance abuse NEC F10-F19 with .11
  suicide attempt Z91.5
  surgery (major) NEC Z92.4
    sex reassignment Z87.81
    transplant — *see* Transplant
  trauma NEC Z91.8
    psychological NEC Z91.49
    self-harm Z91.5
  unhealthy sleep-wake cycle Z91.3
  use of medicaments (long term) — *see* Use, medicaments for a long term

His-Werner disease A79.0
HIV B20
  laboratory evidence (nonconclusive) R75
  positive, seropositive Z21
  nonconclusive test in infants R75
Hives (bold) — *see* Urticaria
Hoarseness R49.0
Hobo Z59.0
Hodgkin's
  disease (M9650/3) C81.90
    lymphocytic
      depletion (M9653/3) C81.30
        diffuse fibrosis (M9654/3) C81.30
        nodes (of)
          arm C81.34
          axilla C81.34
          head, face and neck C81.31
          inguinal C81.35
          intra-abdominal C81.33
          intrapelvic C81.36
          intrathoracic C81.32
          leg C81.35
          multiple sites C81.38
        reticular (M9655/3) C81.30
        spleen C81.37
      predominance (M9657/3) C81.00
        diffuse (M9658/3) C81.00
        nodes (of)
          arm C81.94
          axilla C81.94
          head, face and neck C81.91
          inguinal C81.95
          intra-abdominal C81.93
          intrapelvic C81.96
          intrathoracic C81.92
          leg C81.95
          multiple sites C81.98
        nodular (M9659/3) C81.00
        spleen C81.07
    lymphocytic-histiocytic predominance
      (M9657/3) C81.00
    mixed cellularity (M9652/3) C81.20
      nodes (of)
        arm C81.24
        axilla C81.24
        head, face and neck C81.21
        inguinal C81.25
        intra-abdominal C81.23
        intrapelvic C81.26
        intrathoracic C81.22
        leg C81.25
        multiple sites C81.28
      nodular sclerosis (M9666/3) C81.10
      spleen C81.27
    nodes (of)
      arm C81.94
      axilla C81.94
      head, face and neck C81.91
      inguinal C81.95
      intra-abdominal C81.93
      intrapelvic C81.96
      intrathoracic C81.92
      leg C81.95
      multiple sites C81.98
    nodular sclerosis (M9663/3) C81.10
      cellular phase (M9664/3) C81.10
      lymphocytic
        depletion (M9667/3) C81.10
        predominance (M9665/3) C81.10
      mixed cellularity (M9666/3) C81.10
      nodes (of)
        arm C81.14
        axilla C81.14
        head, face and neck C81.11
        inguinal C81.15
        intra-abdominal C81.13
        intrapelvic C81.16
        intrathoracic C81.12
        leg C81.15
        multiple sites C81.18
      spleen C81.17
      syncytial variant (M9667/3) C81.10
    specified type NEC C81.70
      nodes (of)
        arm C81.74

Hodgkin's — *continued*
  disease — *continued*
    specified type NEC — *continued*
      nodes — *continued*
        axilla C81.74
        head, face and neck C81.71
        inguinal C81.75
        intra-abdominal C81.73
        intrapelvic C81.76
        intrathoracic C81.72
        leg C81.75
        multiple sites C81.78
      spleen C81.77
    spleen C81.97
    granuloma (M9661/3) C81.70
    lymphoma, malignant (M9650/3) C81.90
    paragranuloma (nodular) (M9660/3) C81.70
    sarcoma (M9662/3) C81.70
Hodgson's disease I71.2
  ruptured I71.1
Hoffa-Kastert disease E88.8
Hoffa's disease E88.8
Hoffmann-Bouveret syndrome I47.9
Hoffmann's syndrome E03.9 [G73.7]
Hole (round)
  macula — *see* Degeneration, macula, hole
  retina (without detachment) — *see also* Break,
    retina, round hole
    with detachment — *see* Detachment, retina,
      with retinal, break
Holiday relief care Z75.5
Hollenhorst's plaque — *see* Occlusion, artery,
  retina
Hollow foot (congenital) Q66.7
  acquired — *see* Deformity, limb, foot, specified
    NEC
Holoprosencephaly Q04.2
Holt-Oram syndrome Q87.2
Homelessness Z59.0
Homesickness — *see* Disorder, adjustment
Homocystinemia, homocystinuria E72.11
Homogentisate 1,2-dioxygenase deficiency
  E70.29
Homologous serum hepatitis (prophylactic)
  (therapeutic) — *see* Hepatitis, viral, type B
Honeycomb lung J98.4
  congenital Q33.0
Hooded
  clitoris Q52.6
  penis Q55.69
Hookworm (anemia) (disease) (infection)
  (infestation) B76.9
  specified NEC B76.8
Hordeolum (eyelid) (externum) (recurrent)
  H00.019
  internum H00.029
    left H00.026
      lower H00.025
      upper H00.024
    right H00.023
      lower H00.022
      upper H00.021
  left H00.016
    lower H00.015
    upper H00.014
  right H00.013
    lower H00.012
    upper H00.011
Horn
  cutaneous L85.8
  nail L60.2
  congenital Q84.6
Horner (-Claude Bernard) syndrome G90.2
  traumatic — *see* Injury, nerve, cervical
    sympathetic
Horseshoe kidney (congenital) Q63.1
Horton's headache or neuralgia G44.0
Hospital hopper syndrome — *see* Disorder,
  factitious
Hospitalism in children — *see* Disorder,
  adjustment

Hostility R45.5
  towards child Z62.3
Hourglass (contracture) — *see also* Contraction,
  hourglass
  stomach K31.89
    congenital Q40.2
    stricture K31.2
Household, housing circumstance affecting
  care Z59.9
  specified NEC Z59.8
Housemaid's knee — *see* Bursitis, prepatellar
Hudson (-Stähli) line (cornea) — *see*
  Pigmentation, cornea, anterior
Human
  bite (open wound) — *see also* Bite
    intact skin surface — *see* Bite, superficial
  immunodeficiency virus (HIV) disease (infection)
    B20
    asymptomatic status Z21
    contact Z20.6
    counseling Z71.7
    dementia B20 [F02.80]
    exposure to Z20.6
    laboratory evidence R75
    type-2 (HIV 2) as cause of disease classified
      elsewhere B97.35
  T-cell lymphotropic virus
    type-1 (HTLV-I) infection B33.3
      as cause of disease classified elsewhere
        B97.33
    carrier Z22.6
    type-2 (HTLV-II) as cause of disease
      classified elsewhere B97.34
Humidifier lung or pneumonitis J67.7
Humiliation (experience) **in childhood** Z61.3
Humpback (acquired) — *see* Kyphosis
Hunchback (acquired) — *see* Kyphosis
Hunger T73.0
  air, psychogenic F45.8
Hunner's ulcer — *see* Cystitis, chronic,
  interstitial
Hunter's
  glossitis D51.0
  syndrome E76.1
Huntington's disease or chorea G10
  with dementia G10 [F02.80]
    with behavioral disturbance G10 [F02.81]
Hunt's
  disease or syndrome (herpetic geniculate
    ganglionitis) B02.21
    dyssynergia cerebellaris myoclonica G11.1
  neuralgia B02.21
Hurler (-Scheie) disease or syndrome E76.02
Hurst's disease G36.1
Hurthle cell
  adenocarcinoma (M8290/3) C73
  adenoma (M8290/0) D34
  carcinoma (M8290/3) C73
  tumor (M8290/0) D34
Hutchinson-Boeck disease or syndrome — *see*
  Sarcoidosis
Hutchinson-Gilford disease or syndrome E34.8
Hutchinson's
  disease meaning
    angioma serpiginosum L81.7
    pompholyx L30.1
    prurigo estivalis L56.4
    summer eruption or summer prurigo L56.4
  melanotic freckle (M8742/2) — *see* Melanoma,
    in situ
    malignant melanoma in (M8742/3) — *see*
      Melanoma
  teeth or incisors (congenital syphilis) A50.52
  triad (congenital syphilis) A50.53
Hyalin plaque, sclera, senile H15.89
Hyaline membrane (disease) (lung) (pulmonary)
  (newborn) P22.0
Hyalinosis
  cutis (et mucosae) E78.89
  focal and segmental (glomerular) — *see* N00-
    N07 with fourth character .1

Hyalitis, hyalosis, asteroid — *see also* Deposit,
crystalline
  syphilitic (late) A52.71
Hydatid
  cyst or tumor — *see* Echinococcus
  mole — *see* Hydatidiform mole
  Morgagni's
    female Q52.8
    male Q55.4
Hydatidiform mole (benign) (complicating
pregnancy) (delivered) (undelivered) O01.9
  classical O01.0
  complete O01.0
  incomplete O01.1
  invasive (M9100/1) D39.2
  malignant (M9100/1) D39.2
  partial O01.1
  previous, affecting pregnancy — *see* Antenatal,
care, high risk pregnancy, history of,
molar pregnancy
Hydatidosis — *see* Echinococcus
Hydradenitis (axillaris) (suppurative) L73.2
Hydradenoma (M8400/0) — *see* Hidradenoma
Hydramnios O40.9
  first trimester O40.1
  second trimester O40.2
  third trimester O40.3
Hydrancephaly, hydranencephaly Q04.3
  with spina bifida — *see* Spina bifida, with
hydrocephalus
Hydrargyrism NEC — *see* Poisoning, mercury
Hydrarthrosis — *see also* Effusion, joint
  gonococcal A54.42
  intermittent M12.40
    ankle M12.479
      left M12.472
      right M12.471
    elbow M12.429
      left M12.422
      right M12.421
    foot joint M12.479
      left M12.472
      right M12.471
    hand joint M12.449
      left M12.442
      right M12.441
    hip M12.459
      left M12.452
      right M12.451
    knee M12.469
      left M12.462
      right M12.461
    multiple site M12.49
    shoulder M12.419
      left M12.412
      right M12.411
    specified joint NEC M12.48
    wrist M12.439
      left M12.432
      right M12.431
  of yaws (early) (late) (*see also* category M14.8)
A66.6
  syphilitic (late) A52.77
    congenital A50.55 [M12.80]
Hydremia D64.8
Hydrencephalocele (congenital) — *see*
Encephalocele
Hydrencephalomeningocele (congenital) — *see*
Encephalocele
Hydroa R23.8
  aestivale L56.4
  vacciniforme L56.4
Hydroadenitis (axillaris) (suppurative) L73.2
Hydrocalycosis — *see* Hydronephrosis
Hydrocele (testis) (tunica vaginalis) N43.3
  canal of Nuck N94.8
  congenital P83.5
  encysted N43.0
  female NEC N94.8
  fetus or newborn P83.5
  infected N43.1
  round ligament N94.8
  specified NEC N43.2
  spermatic cord N43.5

Hydrocele — *continued*
  spinalis — *see* Spina bifida
  vulva N90.8
Hydrocephalus (acquired) (external) (internal)
(malignant) (recurrent) G91.9
  aqueduct Sylvius stricture Q03.0
  causing disproportion O33.6
    with obstructed labor O66.3
  communicating G91.0
  congenital (external) (internal) Q03.9
    with spina bifida Q05.4
      cervical Q05.0
      dorsal Q05.1
      lumbar Q05.2
      lumbosacral Q05.2
      sacral Q05.3
      thoracic Q05.1
      thoracolumbar Q05.1
    specified NEC Q03.8
  due to toxoplasmosis (congenital) P37.1
  fetus (suspected), affecting management of
pregnancy O35.0
  foramen Magendie block (acquired) G91.1
    congenital (*see also* Hydrocephalus,
congenital) Q03.1
  in (due to)
    infectious disease NEC G91.4
    neoplastic disease NEC (M8000/1) (*see also*
Neoplasm) G91.4
    parasitic disease G91.4
  newborn Q03.9
    with spina bifida — *see* Spina bifida, with
hydrocephalus
  noncommunicating G91.1
  normal-pressure G91.2
  obstructive G91.1
  post-traumatic NEC G91.3
  secondary G91.4
    post traumatic G91.3
  specified NEC G91.8
  syphilitic, congenital A50.49
Hydrocolpos (congenital) N89.8
Hydrocystoma (M8404/0) — *see* Neoplasm, skin,
benign
Hydroencephalocele (congenital) — *see*
Encephalocele
Hydroencephalomeningocele (congenital) — *see*
Encephalocele
Hydrohematopneumothorax — *see* Hemothorax
Hydromeningitis — *see* Meningitis
Hydromeningocele (spinal) — *see also* Spina
bifida
  cranial — *see* Encephalocele
Hydrometra N85.8
Hydrometrocolpos N89.8
Hydromicrocephaly Q02
Hydromphalos (since birth) Q45.8
Hydromyelia Q06.4
Hydromyelocele — *see* Spina bifida
Hydronephrosis (atrophic) (early) (functionless)
(intermittent) (primary) (secondary) NEC
N13.30
  with
    infection N13.6
    obstruction (by) (of)
      renal calculus N13.2
        with infection N13.6
      ureteral NEC N13.1
        with infection N13.6
        calculus N13.2
          with infection N13.6
      ureteropelvic junction (congenital) Q62.0
        with infection N13.6
      ureteral stricture NEC N13.1
        with infection N13.6
  congenital Q62.0
  specified type NEC N13.39
  tuberculous A18.11
Hydropericarditis — *see* Pericarditis
Hydropericardium — *see* Pericarditis
Hydroperitoneum R18
Hydrophobia — *see* Rabies
Hydrophthalmos Q15.0

Hydropneumohemothorax — *see* Hemothorax
Hydropneumopericarditis — *see* Pericarditis
Hydropneumopericardium — *see* Pericarditis
Hydropneumothorax J94.8
  traumatic — *see* Injury, intrathoracic, lung
  tuberculous NEC A15.6
Hydrops R60.9
  abdominis R18
  amnii (complicating pregnancy) — *see*
Hydramnios
  articulorum intermittens — *see* Hydrarthrosis,
intermittent
  cardiac — *see* Failure, heart, congestive
  causing obstructed labor (mother) O66.3
  endolymphatic — *see* category H81.0
  fetal(is) or newborn (idiopathic) P83.2
    affecting management of pregnancy O36.20
    due to
      ABO isoimmunization P56.0
        affecting management of pregnancy —
see Isoimmunization, affecting
management of pregnancy
      hemolytic disease NEC P56.9
      isoimmunization (ABO) (Rh) P56.0
      Rh incompatibility P56.0
        affecting management of pregnancy —
see Isoimmunization, affecting
management of pregnancy, Rh
    first trimester O36.21
    second trimester O36.22
    third trimester O36.23
  gallbladder K82.1
  joint — *see* Effusion, joint
  labyrinth — *see* category H81.0
  nutritional — *see* Malnutrition, severe
  pericardium — *see* Pericarditis
  pleura — *see* Hydrothorax
  spermatic cord — *see* Hydrocele
Hydropyonephrosis N13.6
Hydrorachis Q06.4
Hydrorrhea (nasal) J34.8
  pregnancy — *see* Rupture, membranes,
premature
Hydrosadenitis (axillaris) (suppurative) L73.2
Hydrosalpinx (fallopian tube) (follicularis) N70.11
Hydrothorax (double) (pleura) J94.8
  chylous (nonfilarial) I89.8
    filarial (*see also* Infestation, filarial) B74.9
[J91]
  traumatic — *see* Injury, intrathoracic
  tuberculous NEC (non primary) A15.6
Hydroureter (*see also* Hydronephrosis) N13.4
  with infection N13.6
  congenital Q62.39
Hydroureteronephrosis — *see* Hydronephrosis
Hydrourethra N36.8
Hydroxykynureninuria E70.8
Hydroxylysinemia E72.3
Hydroxyprolinemia E72.59
Hygroma (congenital) (cystic) (M9173/0) D18.1
  praepatellare, prepatellar — *see* Bursitis,
prepatellar
Hymen — *see* condition
Hymenolepis, hymenolepiasis (diminuta)
(infection) (infestation) (nana) B71.0
Hypalgesia R20.8
Hyperacidity (gastric) K31.89
  psychogenic F45.8
Hyperactive, hyperactivity
  basal cell, uterine cervix — *see* Dysplasia,
cervix
  bowel sounds R19.12
  cervix epithelial (basal) — *see* Dysplasia, cervix
  child F90.9
    attention deficit — *see* Disorder, attention-
deficit hyperactivity
  gastrointestinal K31.89
    psychogenic F45.8
  nasal mucous membrane J34.3
  stomach K31.89
  thyroid (gland) — *see* Hyperthyroidism

Hyperacusis H93.239
  bilateral H93.233
  left H93.232
  right H93.231
Hyperadrenalism E27.5
Hyperadrenocorticism E24.9
  congenital E25.0
  iatrogenic
    correct substance properly administered
      E24.2
    overdose or wrong substance given or taken
      — see category T38.0
  not associated with Cushing's syndrome E27.0
  pituitary-dependent E24.0
Hyperaldosteronism E26.9
  primary (due to (bilateral) adrenal hyperplasia)
    E26.0
  secondary E26.1
Hyperalgesia R20.8
Hyperalimentation R63.2
  carotene, carotin E67.1
  specified NEC E67.8
  vitamin
    A E67.0
    D E67.3
Hyperaminoaciduria
  arginine E72.21
  cystine E72.01
  lysine E72.3
  ornithine E72.4
Hyperammonemia (congenital) E72.20
Hyperazotemia — see Uremia
Hyperbetalipoproteinemia (familial) E78.0
  with prebetalipoproteinemia E78.2
Hyperbilirubinemia
  constitutional E80.6
  familial conjugated E80.6
  neonatal (transient) — see Jaundice, fetus or
    newborn
Hypercalcemia, hypocalciuric, familial E83.52
Hypercalciuria, idiopathic E83.52
Hypercapnia — see also Hyperventilation
  newborn P84
Hypercarotenemia, hypercarotinemia (dietary)
  E67.1
Hypercementosis K03.4
Hyperchloremia E87.8
Hyperchlorhydria K31.89
  neurotic F45.8
  psychogenic F45.8
Hypercholesterinemia — see
  Hypercholesterolemia
Hypercholesterolemia (essential) (familial)
  (hereditary) (primary) (pure) E78.0
  with hyperglyceridemia, endogenous E78.2
  dietary counseling and surveillance Z71.3
Hyperchylia gastrica, psychogenic F45.8
Hyperchylomicronemia (familial) (primary) E78.3
  with hyperbetalipoproteinemia E78.3
Hypercoagulation (state) D68.618
  primary D68.618
    activated protein C resistance D68.610
    factor V Leiden mutation D68.610
    prothrombin gene mutation D68.611
  secondary D68.62
Hypercorticalism, pituitary-dependent E24.0
Hypercorticosolism — see Cushing's syndrome
Hypercorticosteronism
  correct substance properly administered E24.2
  overdose or wrong substance given or taken —
    see category T38.0
Hypercortisonism
  correct substance properly administered E24.2
  overdose or wrong substance given or taken —
    see category T38.0
Hyperelectrolytemia E87.8
Hyperemesis R11.3
  with nausea R11.0
  gravidarum (mild) O21.0
    with
      carbohydrate depletion O21.1
      dehydration O21.1

Hyperemesis — continued
  gravidarum — continued
    with — continued
      electrolyte imbalance O21.1
      metabolic disturbance O21.1
      severe (with metabolic disturbance) O21.1
  projectile R11.2
  psychogenic F45.8
Hyperemia (acute) (passive) R68.8
  anal mucosa K62.8
  bladder N32.8
  cerebral I67.8
  conjunctiva H11.439
    bilateral H11.433
    left H11.432
    right H11.431
  ear internal, acute — see category H83.0
  enteric K59.8
  eye — see Hyperemia, conjunctiva
  eyelid (active) (passive) — see Disorder, eyelid,
    specified type NEC
  intestine K59.8
  iris — see Disorder, iris, vascular
  kidney N28.89
  labyrinth — see category H83.0
  liver (active) K76.8
  lung (passive) — see Edema, lung
  pulmonary (passive) — see Edema, lung
  renal N28.89
  retina H35.89
  stomach K31.89
Hyperesthesia (body surface) R20.3
  larynx (reflex) J38.7
    hysterical F44.89
  pharynx (reflex) J39.2
    hysterical F44.89
Hyperestrogenism (drug-induced) (iatrogenic)
  E28.0
Hyperfibrinolysis — see Fibrinolysis
Hyperfructosemia E74.19
Hyperfunction
  adrenal cortex, not associated with Cushing's
    syndrome E27.0
  medulla E27.5
    adrenomedullary E27.5
    virilism E25.9
      congenital E25.0
  ovarian E28.8
  pancreas K86.8
  parathyroid (gland) E21.3
  pituitary (gland) (anterior) E22.9
    specified NEC E22.8
  polyglandular E31.1
  testicular E29.0
Hypergammaglobulinemia D89.2
  polyclonal D89.0
  Waldenström's D89.0
Hypergastrinemia E16.4
Hyperglobulinemia R77.1
Hyperglycemia, hyperglycemic R73.9
  coma — see Diabetes, coma
  postpancreatectomy E89.1
Hyperglyceridemia (endogenous) (essential)
  (familial) (hereditary) (pure) E78.1
  mixed E78.3
Hyperglycinemia (non-ketotic) E72.51
Hypergonadism
  ovarian E28.8
  testicular (primary) (infantile) E29.0
Hyperheparinemia — see Circulating
  anticoagulants
Hyperhidrosis, hyperidrosis R61.9
  generalized R61.1
  localized R61.0
  psychogenic F45.8
Hyperhistidinemia E70.41
Hyperhydroxyprolinemia E72.59
Hyperinsulinism (functional) E16.1
  with
    coma (hypoglycemic) E15
    encephalopathy E16.1 [G94]
  ectopic E16.1
  therapeutic misadventure (from administration
    of insulin) — see category T38.3

Hyperkalemia E87.5
Hyperkeratosis (see also Keratosis) L85.9
  cervix — see Dysplasia, cervix
  due to yaws (early) (late) (palmar or plantar)
    A66.3
  follicularis Q82.8
    penetrans (in cutem) L87.0
  palmoplantaris climacterica L85.1
  pinta A67.1
  senile (with pruritus) L57.0
  universalis congenita Q80.8
  vocal cord J38.3
  vulva N90.4
Hyperkinesia, hyperkinetic (disease) (reaction)
  (syndrome) (childhood) (adolescence) — see
  also Disorder, attention-deficit hyperactivity
  with mental retardation and stereotyped
    movements F84.4
  heart I51.8
Hyperleucine-isoleucinemia E71.19
Hyperlipemia, hyperlipidemia E78.5
  combined familial E78.4
  group
    A E78.0
    B E78.1
    C E78.2
    D E78.3
  mixed E78.2
  specified NEC E78.4
Hyperlipidosis E75.6
  hereditary NEC E75.5
Hyperlipoproteinemia E78.5
  Fredrickson's type
    I E78.3
    IIa E78.0
    IIb E78.2
    III E78.2
    IV E78.1
    V E78.3
  low-density-lipoprotein-type (LDL) E78.0
  very-low-density-lipoprotein-type (VLDL) E78.1
Hyperlucent lung, unilateral J43.0
Hyperlysinemia E72.3
Hypermagnesemia E83.41
  neonatal P71.8
Hypermaturity (fetus or newborn) P08.2
Hypermenorrhea N92.0
Hypermethioninemia E72.19
Hypermetropia (congenital) H52.00
  bilateral H52.03
  left H52.02
  right H52.01
Hypermobility, hypermotility
  cecum — see Syndrome, irritable bowel
  coccyx — see category M53.2
  colon — see Syndrome, irritable bowel
    psychogenic F45.8
  ileum K58.9
  intestine — see also Syndrome, irritable bowel
    K58.9
    psychogenic F45.8
  meniscus (knee) — see Derangement, knee,
    meniscus
  scapula — see Instability, joint, shoulder
  stomach K31.89
    psychogenic F45.8
  syndrome M35.7
  urethra N36.41
    with intrinsic sphincter deficiency N36.43
Hypernasality R49.21
Hypernatremia E87.0
Hypernephroma (M8312/3) C64.9
  left C64.1
  right C64.0
Hyperopia — see Hypermetropia
Hyperorexia nervosa F50.2
Hyperornithinemia E72.4
Hyperosmia R43.1
Hyperosmolality E87.0

©2002 Ingenix, Inc.

Hyperostosis (monomelic) — *see also* Disorder, bone, density and structure, specified NEC
  ankylosing (spine) M48.10
    cervical region M48.12
    cervicothoracic region M48.13
    lumbar region M48.16
    lumbosacral region M48.17
    multiple sites M48.19
    occipito-atlanto-axial region M48.11
    sacrococcygeal region M48.18
    thoracic region M48.14
    thoracolumbar region M48.15
  cortical (skull) M85.2
    infantile — *see* Disorder, bone, specified type NEC
  frontal, internal of skull M85.2
  interna frontalis M85.2
  skeletal, diffuse idiopathic — *see* Hyperostosis, ankylosing
  skull M85.2
    congenital Q75.8
  vertebral, ankylosing — *see* Hyperostosis, ankylosing
Hyperovarism E28.8
Hyperoxaluria (primary) E72.53
Hyperparathyroidism E21.3
  primary E21.0
  secondary NEC E21.1
    renal N25.8
  specified NEC E21.2
Hyperpathia R20.8
Hyperperistalsis R19.2
  psychogenic F45.8
Hyperpermeability, capillary I78.8
Hyperphagia R63.2
Hyperphenylalaninemia NEC E70.1
Hyperphoria (alternating) H50.53
Hyperphosphatemia E83.39
Hyperpiesis, hyperpiesia — *see* Hypertension
Hyperpigmentation — *see also* Pigmentation
  melanin NEC L81.4
  postinflammatory L81.0
Hyperpinealism E34.8
Hyperpituitarism E22.9
Hyperplasia, hyperplastic
  adenoids J35.2
  adrenal (capsule) (cortex) (gland) E27.8
    with
      sexual precocity (male) E25.9
        congenital E25.0
      virilism, adrenal E25.9
        congenital E25.0
      virilization (female) E25.9
        congenital E25.0
    congenital E25.0
    salt-losing E25.0
  adrenomedullary E27.5
  appendix (lymphoid) K38.0
  artery, fibromuscular I77.3
  bone — *see also* Hypertrophy, bone
    marrow D75.8
  breast — *see* Hypertrophy, breast
  C-cell, thyroid E07.0
  cementation (tooth) (teeth) K03.4
  cervical gland R59.0
  cervix (uteri) (basal cell) (endometrium) (polypoid) — *see also* Dysplasia, cervix
    congenital Q51.8
  clitoris, congenital Q52.6
  denture K06.2
  endocervicitis N72
  endometrium, endometrial (cystic) (glandular) (glandular-cystic) (polypoid) N85.0
    cervix — *see* Dysplasia, cervix
  epithelial L85.9
    focal, oral, including tongue K13.2
    nipple N62
    skin L85.9
    tongue K13.2
    vaginal wall N89.3
  erythroid D75.8
  genital
    female NEC N94.8
    male N50.8

Hyperplasia, hyperplastic — *continued*
  gingiva K06.1
  glandularis cystica uteri (interstitialis) N85.0
  gum K06.1
  hymen, congenital Q52.4
  irritative, edentulous (alveolar) K06.2
  jaw M26.09
    alveolar M26.79
    lower M26.03
      alveolar M26.72
    upper M26.01
      alveolar M26.71
  kidney (congenital) Q63.3
  labia N90.6
    epithelial N90.3
  liver (congenital) Q44.7
    nodular, focal K76.8
  lymph gland or node R59.9
  mandible, mandibular M26.03
    alveolar M26.72
    unilateral condylar M27.8
  maxilla, maxillary M26.01
    alveolar M26.71
  myometrium, myometrial N85.2
  nose
    lymphoid J34.8
    polypoid J33.9
  oral mucosa (irritative) K13.6
  organ or site, congenital NEC — *see* Anomaly, by site
  ovary N83.8
  palate, papillary (irritative) K13.6
  pancreatic islet cells E16.9
    alpha E16.8
      with excess
        gastrin E16.4
        glucagon E16.3
    beta E16.1
  parathyroid (gland) E21.0
  pharynx (lymphoid) J39.2
  prostate (adenofibromatous) (nodular) N40.90
    with
      hematuria N40.92
        with obstruction N40.93
      obstruction N40.91
        with hematuria N40.93
      specified complication NEC N40.99
    hypertrophy (benign) (smooth) (soft) N40.00
      with
        hematuria N40.02
          with obstruction N40.03
        obstruction N40.01
          with hematuria N40.03
        specified complication NEC N40.09
    localized N40.20
      with
        hematuria N40.22
          with obstruction N40.23
        obstruction N40.21
          with hematuria N40.23
        specified complication NEC N40.29
    nodular (multiple) N40.10
      with
        hematuria N40.12
          with obstruction N40.13
        obstruction N40.11
          with hematuria N40.13
        specified complication NEC N40.19
  renal artery I77.8
  reticulo-endothelial (cell) D75.8
  salivary gland (any) K11.1
  Schimmelbusch's — *see* Mastopathy, cystic
  suprarenal capsule (gland) E27.8
  thymus (gland) (persistent) E32.0
  thyroid (gland) — *see* Goiter
  tonsils (faucial) (infective) (lingual) (lymphoid) J35.1
    with adenoids J35.3
    unilateral condylar M27.8
  uterus, uterine N85.2
    endometrium (glandular) N85.0
      adenomatous N85.1
      atypical (adenomatous) N85.1
  vulva N90.6
    epithelial N90.3
Hyperpnea — *see* Hyperventilation

Hyperpotassemia E87.5
Hyperprebetalipoproteinemia (familial) E78.1
Hyperprolactinemia E22.1
Hyperprolinemia (type I) (type II) E72.59
Hyperproteinemia E88.09
Hyperprothrombinemia, causing coagulation factor deficiency D68.4
Hyperpyrexia R50.9
  heat (effects) T67.0
  malignant, due to anesthetic T88.3
  rheumatic — *see* Fever, rheumatic
  unknown origin R50.9
Hyper-reflexia R29.2
Hypersalivation K11.7
Hypersecretion
  ACTH (not associated with Cushing's syndrome) E27.0
    pituitary E24.0
  adrenaline E27.5
  adrenomedullary E27.5
  androgen (testicular) E29.0
    ovarian (drug-induced) (iatrogenic) E28.1
  calcitonin E07.0
  catecholamine E27.5
  corticoadrenal E24.9
  cortisol E24.9
  epinephrine E27.5
  estrogen E28.0
  gastric K31.89
    psychogenic F45.8
  gastrin E16.4
  glucagon E16.3
  hormone(s)
    ACTH (not associated with Cushing's syndrome) E27.0
      pituitary E24.0
    antidiuretic E22.2
    growth E22.0
    intestinal NEC E34.1
    ovarian androgen E28.1
    pituitary E22.9
    testicular E29.0
    thyroid stimulating E05.80
      with thyroid storm E05.81
  insulin — *see* Hyperinsulinism
  lacrimal glands — *see* Epiphora
  medulloadrenal E27.5
  milk O92.6
  ovarian androgens E28.1
  salivary gland (any) K11.7
  thyrocalcitonin E07.0
  upper respiratory J39.8
Hypersegmentation, leukocytic, hereditary D72.0
Hypersensitive, hypersensitiveness, hypersensitivity — *see also* Allergy
  carotid sinus G90.0
  colon — *see* Irritable, colon
  drug — *see* Allergy, drug
  gastrointestinal K52.2
    psychogenic F45.8
  labyrinth — *see* category H83.2
  pain R20.8
  pneumonitis — *see* Pneumonitis, allergic
  reaction T78.4
    upper respiratory tract NEC J39.3
Hypersomnia (organic) G47.1
  nonorganic origin F51.1
  primary F51.1
Hypersplenia, hypersplenism D73.1
Hyperstimulation, ovaries (associated with induced ovulation) N98.1
Hypersusceptibility — *see* Allergy
Hypertelorism (ocular) (orbital) Q75.2
Hypertension, hypertensive (accelerated) (benign) (essential) (idiopathic) (malignant) (systemic) I10
  with
    heart involvement (conditions in I51.4-I51.9 due to hypertension) — *see* Hypertension, heart
    kidney involvement — *see* Hypertension, kidney

Hypertension, hypertensive — *continued*
  with — *continued*
    renal sclerosis (conditions in N26) — *see*
      Hypertension, kidney
  benign, intracranial G93.2
  cardiorenal (disease) I13.9
    with
      heart failure I13.0
        and renal failure I13.2
      renal failure I13.1
        and heart failure (congestive) I13.2
  cardiovascular
    disease (arteriosclerotic) (sclerotic) — *see*
      Hypertension, heart
    renal (disease) (sclerosis) — *see*
      Hypertension, cardiorenal
  complicating
    childbirth O10.92
      with
        heart disease O10.12
          with renal disease O10.32
        renal disease O10.22
          with heart disease O10.32
      essential O10.02
      secondary O10.42
    pregnancy O16.9
      first trimester O16.1
      gestational (transient) (without
        proteinuria) O13.9
        with proteinuria O14.90
          mild pre-eclampsia O14.00
            second trimester O14.02
            third trimester O14.03
          second trimester O14.92
          severe pre-eclampsia O14.10
            second trimester O14.12
            third trimester O14.13
          third trimester O14.93
      first trimester O13.1
      second trimester O13.2
      third trimester O13.3
    pre-existing O10.919
      with
        heart disease O10.119
          with renal disease O10.319
            first trimester O10.311
            second trimester O10.312
            third trimester O10.313
          first trimester O10.111
          second trimester O10.112
          third trimester O10.113
        proteinuria O11.9
          first trimester O11.1
          second trimester O11.2
          third trimester O11.3
        renal disease O10.219
          with heart disease O10.319
            first trimester O10.311
            second trimester O10.312
            third trimester O10.313
          first trimester O10.211
          second trimester O10.212
          third trimester O10.213
      first trimester O10.911
      second trimester O10.912
      third trimester O10.913
      essential O10.019
        first trimester O10.011
        second trimester O10.012
        third trimester O10.013
      first trimester O10.911
      second trimester O10.912
      secondary O10.419
        first trimester O10.411
        second trimester O10.412
        third trimester O10.413
      third trimester O10.913
      second trimester O16.2
      third trimester O16.3
    puerperium O10.93
      with
        heart disease O10.13
          with renal disease O10.33
        renal disease O10.23
          with heart disease O10.33
      essential O10.03

Hypertension, hypertensive — *continued*
  complicating — *continued*
    puerperium — *continued*
      secondary O10.43
  due to
    endocrine disorders I15.2
    pheochromocytoma I15.2
    renal disorders NEC I15.1
      arterial I15.0
    renovascular disorders I15.0
    specified disease NEC I15.8
  encephalopathy I67.4
  gestational (without significant proteinuria)
    (pregnancy-induced) (transient) O13.9
    with significant proteinuria — *see* Pre-
      eclampsia
    first trimester O13.1
    second trimester O13.2
    third trimester O13.3
  Goldblatt's I70.1
  heart (disease) (conditions in I51.4-I51.9 due to
    hypertension) I11.9
    with
      heart failure (congestive) I11.0
      renal disease I13.9
        with
          heart failure I13.0
            with renal failure I13.2
          renal failure I13.1
            with heart failure I13.2
  intracranial (benign) G93.2
  kidney I12.9
    with
      heart disease I13.9
        with
          heart failure I13.0
            with renal failure I13.2
          renal failure I13.1
            with heart failure I13.2
      renal failure I12.0
  lesser circulation I27.0
  maternal (of pregnancy) NEC — *see*
    Hypertension, complicating pregnancy
  newborn P29.2
    pulmonary (persistent) P29.3
  ocular H40.0
  portal (due to chronic liver disease) (idiopathic)
    K76.6
    in (due to) schistosomiasis (bilharziasis)
      B65.9 *[K77]*
  postoperative I97.3
  psychogenic F45.8
  pulmonary (artery) I27.0
    of newborn (persistent) P29.3
  renal — *see* Hypertension, kidney
  renovascular I15.0
  secondary I15.9
    due to
      endocrine disorders I15.2
      pheochromocytoma I15.2
      renal disorders NEC I15.1
        arterial I15.0
      renovascular disorders I15.0
      specified NEC I15.8
  transient of pregnancy — *see* Hypertension,
    complicating pregnancy

Hyperthecosis ovary E28.8

Hyperthermia (of unknown origin) — *see also*
  Hyperpyrexia
  malignant, due to anesthesia T88.3
  newborn, environmental P81.0

Hyperthyroid (recurrent) — *see* Hyperthyroidism

Hyperthyroidism (latent) (pre-adult) (recurrent)
  E05.90
  with
    goiter (diffuse) E05.00
      with thyroid storm E05.01
      nodular (multinodular) E05.20
        with thyroid storm E05.21
      uninodular E05.10
        with thyroid storm E05.11
    storm E05.91
  due to ectopic thyroid tissue E05.30
    with thyroid storm E05.31
  neonatal, transitory P72.1
  specified NEC E05.80
    with thyroid storm E05.81

Hypertony, hypertonia, hypertonicity
  bladder N31.8
  congenital P94.1
  stomach K31.89
    psychogenic F45.8
  uterus, uterine (contractions) (complicating
    delivery) O62.4

Hypertrichosis L68.9
  congenital Q84.2
  eyelid H02.869
    left H02.866
      lower H02.865
      upper H02.864
    right H02.863
      lower H02.862
      upper H02.861
  lanuginosa Q84.2
    acquired L68.1
  localized L68.2
  specified NEC L68.8

Hypertriglyceridemia, essential E78.1

Hypertrophy, hypertrophic
  adenofibromatous, prostate — *see* Hyperplasia,
    prostate
  adenoids (infective) J35.2
    with tonsils J35.3
  adrenal cortex E27.8
  alveolar process or ridge — *see* Anomaly,
    alveolar
  anal papillae K62.8
  artery I77.8
    congenital NEC Q27.8
      digestive system Q27.8
      lower limb Q27.8
      specified site NEC Q27.8
      upper limb Q27.8
  arthritis — *see* Arthrosis
  auricular — *see* Hypertrophy, cardiac
  Bartholin's gland N75.8
  bile duct (common) (hepatic) K83.8
  bladder (sphincter) (trigone) N32.8
  bone M89.30
    carpus M89.349
      left M89.342
      right M89.341
    clavicle M89.319
      left M89.312
      right M89.311
    femur M89.359
      left M89.352
      right M89.351
    fibula M89.369
      left M89.364
      right M89.363
    finger M89.349
      left M89.342
      right M89.341
    humerus M89.329
      left M89.322
      right M89.321
    ilium M89.359
    ischium M89.359
    metacarpus M89.349
      left M89.342
      right M89.341
    metatarsus M89.379
      left M89.372
      right M89.371
    multiple sites M89.39
    neck M89.38
    radius M89.339
      left M89.334
      right M89.333
    rib M89.38
    scapula M89.319
      left M89.312
      right M89.311
    skull M89.38
    tarsus M89.379
      left M89.372
      right M89.371
    tibia M89.369
      left M89.362
      right M89.361
    toe M89.379
      left M89.372

©2002 Ingenix, Inc.

Hypertrophy, hypertrophic — *continued*
bone — *continued*
 toe — *continued*
  right M89.371
 ulna M89.339
  left M89.332
  right M89.331
 vertebra M89.38
brain G93.8
breast N62
 cystic — *see* Mastopathy, cystic
 fetus or newborn P83.4
 pubertal, massive N62
 puerperal, postpartum — *see* Disorder,
  breast, specified type NEC
 senile (parenchymatous) N62
cardiac (chronic) (idiopathic) I51.7
 with rheumatic fever (conditions in I00)
  active I01.8
  inactive or quiescent (with chorea) I09.89
 congenital NEC Q24.8
 fatty — *see* Degeneration, myocardial
 hypertensive — *see* Hypertension, heart
 rheumatic (with chorea) I09.89
  active or acute I01.8
   with chorea I02.0
 valve — *see* Endocarditis
cartilage — *see* Disorder, cartilage, specified
  type NEC
cecum — *see* Megacolon
cervix (uteri) N88.8
 congenital Q51.8
 elongation N88.4
clitoris (cirrhotic) N90.8
 congenital Q52.6
colon — *see also* Megacolon
 congenital Q43.2
conjunctiva, lymphoid H11.89
corpora cavernosa N48.89
cystic duct K82.8
duodenum K31.89
endometrium (glandular) N85.0
 atypical (adenomatous) N85.1
 cervix N88.8
epididymis N50.8
esophageal hiatus (congenital) Q79.1
 with hernia — *see* Hernia, hiatal
eyelid — *see* Disorder, eyelid, specified type
  NEC
fat pad M79.4
foot (congenital) Q74.2
frenulum, frenum (tongue) K14.8
 lip K13.0
gallbladder K82.8
gastric mucosa K29.60
 with bleeding K29.61
gland, glandular R59.9
 generalized R59.1
 localized R59.0
gum (mucous membrane) K06.1
heart (idiopathic) — *see also* Hypertrophy,
  cardiac
 valve — *see also* Endocarditis I38
hemifacial Q67.4
hepatic — *see* Hypertrophy, liver
hiatus (esophageal) Q79.1
hilus gland R59.0
hymen, congenital Q52.4
ileum K63.8
intestine NEC K63.8
jejunum K63.8
kidney (compensatory) N28.81
 congenital Q63.3
labium (majus) (minus) N90.6
ligament — *see* Disorder, ligament
lingual tonsil (infective) J35.1
 with adenoids J35.3
lip K13.0
 congenital Q18.6
liver R16.0
 acute K76.8
 congenital Q44.7
 cirrhotic — *see* Cirrhosis, liver
 fatty — *see* Fatty, liver
lymph, lymphatic gland R59.9
 generalized R59.1
 localized R59.0

Hypertrophy, hypertrophic — *continued*
lymph, lymphatic gland — *continued*
 tuberculous — *see* Tuberculosis, lymph
  gland
mammary gland — *see* Hypertrophy, breast
Meckel's diverticulum (congenital) Q43.0
median bar — *see* Hyperplasia, prostate
meibomian gland — *see* Chalazion
meniscus, knee, congenital Q74.1
metatarsal head — *see* Hypertrophy, bone,
  metatarsus
metatarsus — *see* Hypertrophy, bone,
  metatarsus
mucous membrane
 alveolar ridge K06.2
 gum K06.1
 nose (turbinate) J34.3
muscle M62.89
muscular coat, artery I77.8
myocardium — *see also* Hypertrophy, cardiac
 idiopathic I42.2
myometrium N85.2
nail L60.2
 congenital Q84.5
nasal J34.8
 alae J34.8
 bone J34.8
 cartilage J34.8
 mucous membrane (septum) J34.3
 sinus J34.8
 turbinate J34.3
nasopharynx, lymphoid (infectional) (tissue)
  (wall) J35.2
nipple N62
organ or site, congenital NEC — *see* Anomaly,
  by site
ovary N83.8
palate (hard) M27.8
 soft K13.7
pancreas, congenital Q45.3
parathyroid (gland) E21.0
parotid gland K11.1
penis N48.89
pharyngeal tonsil J35.2
pharynx J39.2
 lymphoid (infectional) (tissue) (wall) J35.2
pituitary (anterior) (fossa) (gland) E23.6
prepuce (congenital) N47.8
 female N90.8
prostate (asymptomatic) (benign) (early)
  (recurrent) — *see also* Hyperplasia,
  prostate, hypertrophy
 adenofibromatous — *see also* Hyperplasia,
  prostate, localized
 congenital Q55.4
pseudomuscular G71.0
pylorus (adult) (muscle) (sphincter) K31.1
 congenital or infantile Q40.0
rectal, rectum (sphincter) K62.8
rhinitis (turbinate) J31.0
salivary gland (any) K11.1
 congenital Q38.4
scaphoid (tarsal) — *see* Hypertrophy, bone,
  tarsus
scar L91.0
scrotum N50.8
seminal vesicle N50.8
sigmoid — *see* Megacolon
spermatic cord N50.8
spleen — *see* Splenomegaly
spondylitis — *see* Spondylosis
stomach K31.89
sublingual gland K11.1
submandibular gland K11.1
suprarenal cortex (gland) E27.8
synovial NEC M67.20
 acromioclavicular M67.219
  left M67.212
  right M67.211
 ankle M67.279
  left M67.272
  right M67.271
 elbow M67.229
  left M67.222
  right M67.221
 foot M67.279
  left M67.272

Hypertrophy, hypertrophic — *continued*
synovial NEC — *continued*
 foot — *continued*
  right M67.271
 hand M67.249
  left M67.242
  right M67.241
 hip M67.259
  left M67.252
  right M67.251
 knee M67.269
  left M67.262
  right M67.261
 multiple sites M67.29
 specified site NEC M67.28
 wrist M67.239
  left M67.232
  right M67.231
tendon — *see* Disorder, tendon, specified type
  NEC
testis N44.8
 congenital Q55.29
thymic, thymus (gland) (congenital) E32.0
thyroid (gland) — *see* Goiter
toe (congenital) Q74.2
 acquired — *see also* Deformity, toe, specified
  NEC
tongue K14.8
 congenital Q38.2
 papillae (foliate) K14.3
tonsils (faucial) (infective) (lingual) (lymphoid)
  J35.1
 with adenoids J35.3
tunica vaginalis N50.8
ureter N28.89
urethra N36.8
uterus N85.2
 neck (with elongation) N88.4
 puerperal O90.8
uvula K13.7
vagina N89.8
vas deferens N50.8
vein I87.8
ventricle, ventricular (heart) — *see also*
  Hypertrophy, cardiac
 congenital Q24.8
 in tetralogy of Fallot Q21.3
verumontanum N36.8
vocal cord J38.3
vulva N90.6
 stasis (nonfilarial) N90.6

Hypertropia
 left H50.212
 right H50.211

Hypertyrosinemia E70.21
Hyperuricemia (asymptomatic) E79.0
Hypervalinemia E71.19
Hyperventilation (tetany) R06.4
 hysterical F45.8
 psychogenic F45.8
 syndrome F45.8
Hypervitaminosis (dietary) NEC E67.8
 A E67.0
  reaction to sudden overdose — *see* category
   T45.2
 B6 E67.2
 D E67.3
  reaction to sudden overdose — *see* category
   T45.2
 from excessive administration or use of vitamin
  preparations (chronic) E67.8
  reaction to sudden overdose — *see* category
   T45.2
 K E67.8
  overdose or wrong substance given or taken
   — *see* category T45.7
Hypervolemia E87.7
Hypesthesia R20.1
 cornea — *see* Anesthesia, cornea
Hyphema H21.00
 bilateral H21.03
 left H21.02
 right H21.01
 traumatic S05.10
  left S05.12
  right S05.11

Hypnotherapy NEC Z51.89
Hypoacidity, gastric K31.89
  psychogenic F45.8
Hypoadrenalism, hypoadrenia E27.4
  primary E27.1
  tuberculous A18.7
Hypoadrenocorticism E27.4
  pituitary E23.0
  primary E27.1
Hypoalbuminemia E88.09
Hypoaldosteronism E27.4
Hypoalphalipoproteinemia E78.6
Hypobarism T70.29
Hypobaropathy T70.29
Hypobetalipoproteinemia (familial) E78.6
Hypocalcemia E83.51
  dietary E58
  neonatal P71.1
    due to cow's milk P71.0
  phosphate-loading (newborn) P71.1
Hypochloremia E87.8
Hypochlorhydria K31.89
  neurotic F45.8
  psychogenic F45.8
Hypochondria, hypochondriac, hypochondriasis (reaction) F45.21
Hypochondrogenesis Q77.0
Hypochondroplasia Q77.4
Hypochromasia, blood cells D50.8
Hypodontia — see Anodontia
Hypoeosinophilia D72.8
Hypoesthesia R20.1
Hypofibrinogenemia D68.89
  acquired D65
  congenital (hereditary) D68.2
Hypofunction
  adrenocortical E27.4
    drug-induced E27.3
    postprocedural E89.6
    primary E27.1
  adrenomedullary, postprocedural E89.6
  cerebral R29.81
  corticoadrenal NEC E27.4
  intestinal K59.8
  labyrinth — see category H83.2
  ovary E28.3
  pituitary (gland) (anterior) E23.0
  testicular E29.1
    postprocedural (postsurgical) (postirradiation) (iatrogenic) E89.5
Hypogalactia O92.4
Hypogammaglobulinemia (see also Agammaglobulinemia) D80.1
  hereditary D80.0
  nonfamilial D80.1
  transient, of infancy D80.7
Hypogenitalism (congenital) — see Hypogonadism
Hypoglossia Q38.3
Hypoglycemia (spontaneous) E16.2
  coma E15
    diabetic — see Diabetes, coma
  dietary counseling and surveillance Z71.3
  drug-induced E16.0
    with coma (nondiabetic) E15
  due to insulin E16.0
    with coma (nondiabetic) E15
    therapeutic misadventure — see category T38.3
  functional, nonhyperinsulinemic E16.1
  iatrogenic E16.0
    with coma (nondiabetic) E15
  in infant of diabetic mother P70.1
    gestational diabetes P70.0
  infantile E16.1
  leucine-induced E71.19
  neonatal (transitory) P70.4
    iatrogenic P70.3
    maternal diabetes P70.1
      gestational P70.0
  reactive (not drug-induced) E16.1
  transitory neonatal P70.4

Hypogonadism
  female E28.3
  hypogonadotropic E23.0
  male E29.1
  ovarian (primary) E28.3
  pituitary E23.0
  testicular (primary) E29.1
Hypohidrosis, hypoidrosis L74.4
Hypoinsulinemia, postprocedural E89.1
Hypokalemia E87.6
Hypoleukocytosis — see Agranulocytosis
Hypolipoproteinemia (alpha) (beta) E78.6
Hypomagnesemia E83.42
  neonatal P71.2
Hypomania, hypomanic reaction F30.8
Hypomenorrhea — see Oligomenorrhea
Hypometabolism R63.8
Hypomotility
  gastrointestinal (tract) K01.00
    psychogenic F45.8
  intestine K59.8
    psychogenic F45.8
  stomach K31.89
    psychogenic F45.8
Hyponasality R49.22
Hyponatremia E87.1
Hypo-osmolality E87.1
Hypo-ovarianism, hypo-ovarism E28.3
Hypoparathyroidism E20.9
  familial E20.8
  idiopathic E20.0
  neonatal, transitory P71.4
  postprocedural E89.2
  specified NEC E20.8
Hypopharyngitis — see Laryngopharyngitis
Hypophoria H50.53
Hypophosphatemia, hypophosphatasia (acquired) (congenital) (renal) E83.39
  familial E83.31
Hypophyseal, hypophysis — see also condition
  dwarfism E23.0
  gigantism E22.0
Hypopiesis — see Hypotension
Hypopinealism E34.8
Hypopituitarism (juvenile) E23.0
  drug-induced E23.1
  due to
    hypophysectomy E89.3
    radiotherapy E89.3
  iatrogenic NEC E23.1
  postirradiation E89.3
  postpartum E23.0
  postprocedural E89.3
Hypoplasia, hypoplastic
  adrenal (gland), congenital Q89.1
  alimentary tract, congenital Q45.8
    upper Q40.8
  anus, anal (canal) Q42.3
    with fistula Q42.2
  aorta, aortic Q25.4
    ascending, in hypoplastic left heart syndrome Q23.4
    valve Q23.1
      in hypoplastic left heart syndrome Q23.4
  areola, congenital Q83.8
  arm (congenital) — see Defect, reduction, upper limb
  artery (peripheral) Q27.8
    brain (congenital) Q28.3
    coronary Q24.5
    digestive system Q27.8
    lower limb Q27.8
    pulmonary Q25.7
      functional, unilateral J43.0
    retinal (congenital) Q14.1
    specified site NEC Q27.8
    umbilical Q27.0
    upper limb Q27.8
  auditory canal Q17.8
    causing impairment of hearing Q16.9
  biliary duct or passage Q44.5
  bone NOS Q79.9
    face Q75.8

Hypoplasia, hypoplastic — continued
  bone NOS — continued
    marrow D61.9
      megakaryocytic D69.4
    skull — see Hypoplasia, skull
  brain Q02
    gyri Q04.3
    part of Q04.3
  breast (areola), congenital Q83.8
  bronchus Q32.8
  cardiac Q24.8
  carpus — see Defect, reduction, upper limb, specified type NEC
  cecum Q42.8
  cementum K00.4
  cephalic Q02
  cerebellum Q04.3
  cervix (uteri), congenital Q51.8
  clavicle (congenital) Q74.0
  coccyx Q76.49
  colon Q42.9
    specified NEC Q42.8
  corpus callosum Q04.0
  cricoid cartilage Q31.2
  digestive organ(s) or tract NEC Q45.8
    upper (congenital) Q40.8
  ear (auricle) (lobe) Q17.2
    middle Q16.4
  enamel of teeth (neonatal) (postnatal) (prenatal) K00.4
  endocrine (gland) NEC Q89.2
  endometrium N85.8
  epididymis (congenital) Q55.4
  epiglottis Q31.2
  erythroid, congenital D61.0
  esophagus (congenital) Q39.8
  eustachian tube Q17.8
  eye Q11.2
  eyelid (congenital) Q10.3
  face Q18.8
    bone(s) Q75.8
  femur (congenital) — see Defect, reduction, lower limb, specified type NEC
  fibula (congenital) — see Defect, reduction, lower limb, specified type NEC
  finger (congenital) — see Defect, reduction, upper limb, specified type NEC
  focal dermal Q82.8
  foot — see Defect, reduction, lower limb, specified type NEC
  gallbladder Q44.0
  genitalia, genital organ(s)
    female, congenital Q52.8
      external Q52.79
      internal NEC Q52.8
    in adiposogenital dystrophy E23.6
  glottis Q31.2
  hair Q84.2
  hand (congenital) — see Defect, reduction, upper limb, specified type NEC
  heart Q24.8
  humerus (congenital) — see Defect, reduction, upper limb, specified type NEC
  intestine (small) Q41.9
    large Q42.9
      specified NEC Q42.8
  jaw M26.09
    alveolar M26.79
    lower M26.04
      alveolar M26.74
    upper M26.02
      alveolar M26.73
  kidney(s) Q60.5
    bilateral Q60.4
    unilateral Q60.3
  labium (majus) (minus), congenital Q52.79
  larynx Q31.2
  left heart syndrome Q23.4
  leg (congenital) — see Defect, reduction, lower limb
  limb Q73.8
    lower (congenital) — see Defect, reduction, lower limb
    upper (congenital) — see Defect, reduction, upper limb
  liver Q44.7

©2002 Ingenix, Inc.

Hypoplasia, hypoplastic — *continued*
lung (lobe) (not associated with short gestation) Q33.6
  associated with short gestation P28.0
mammary (areola), congenital Q83.8
mandible, mandibular M26.04
  alveolar M26.74
  unilateral condylar M27.8
maxillary M26.02
  alveolar M26.73
medullary D61.9
megakaryocytic D69.4
metacarpus — *see* Defect, reduction, upper limb, specified type NEC
metatarsus — *see* Defect, reduction, lower limb, specified type NEC
muscle Q79.8
nail(s) Q84.6
nose, nasal Q30.1
osseous meatus (ear) Q17.8
ovary, congenital Q50.39
pancreas Q45.0
parathyroid (gland) Q89.2
parotid gland Q38.4
patella Q74.1
pelvis, pelvic girdle Q74.2
penis (congenital) Q55.62
peripheral vascular system Q27.8
  digestive system Q27.8
  lower limb Q27.8
  specified site NEC Q27.8
  upper limb Q27.8
pituitary (gland) (congenital) Q89.2
pulmonary (not associated with short gestation) Q33.6
  artery, functional J43.0
  associated with short gestation P28.0
radioulnar — *see* Defect, reduction, upper limb, specified type NEC
radius — *see* Defect, reduction, upper limb
rectum Q42.1
  with fistula Q42.0
respiratory system NEC Q34.8
rib Q76.6
right heart syndrome Q22.6
sacrum Q76.49
scapula Q74.0
scrotum Q55.1
shoulder girdle Q74.0
skin Q82.8
skull (bone) Q75.8
  with
    anencephaly Q00.0
    encephalocele — *see* Encephalocele
    hydrocephalus Q03.9
      with spina bifida — *see* Spina bifida, by site, with hydrocephalus
    microcephaly Q02
spinal (cord) (ventral horn cell) Q06.1
spine Q76.49
sternum Q76.7
tarsus — *see* Defect, reduction, lower limb, specified type NEC
testis Q55.1
thymic, with immunodeficiency D82.1
thymus (gland) Q89.2
  with immunodeficiency D82.1
thyroid (gland) E03.1
  cartilage Q31.2
tibiofibular (congenital) — *see* Defect, reduction, lower limb, specified type NEC
toe — *see* Defect, reduction, lower limb, specified type NEC
tongue Q38.3
Turner's K00.4
ulna (congenital) — *see* Defect, reduction, upper limb
umbilical artery Q27.0
unilateral condylar M27.8
ureter Q62.8
uterus, congenital Q51.8
vagina Q52.4
vascular NEC peripheral Q27.8
  brain Q28.3
  digestive system Q27.8
  lower limb Q27.8
  specified site NEC Q27.8

Hypoplasia, hypoplastic — *continued*
vascular NEC peripheral — *continued*
  upper limb Q27.8
vein(s) (peripheral) Q27.8
  brain Q28.3
  digestive system Q27.8
  great Q26.8
  lower limb Q27.8
  specified site NEC Q27.8
  upper limb Q27.8
vena cava (inferior) (superior) Q26.8
vertebra Q76.49
vulva, congenital Q52.79
zonule (ciliary) Q12.8
Hypopotassemia E87.6
Hypoproconvertinemia, congenital (hereditary) D68.2
Hypoproteinemia E77.8
Hypoprothrombinemia (congenital) (hereditary) (idiopathic) D68.2
  acquired D68.4
  newborn, transient P61.6
Hypoptyalism K11.7
Hypopyon (eye) (anterior chamber) — *see* Iridocyclitis, acute, hypopyon
Hypopyrexia R68.0
Hyporeflexia R29.2
Hyposecretion
  ACTH E23.0
  antidiuretic hormone E23.2
  ovary E28.3
  salivary gland (any) K11.7
  vasopressin E23.2
Hyposegmentation, leukocytic, hereditary D72.0
Hyposiderinemia D50.9
Hyposomnia G47.0
  nonorganic origin F51.0
Hypospadias Q54.9
  balanic Q54.0
  coronal Q54.0
  glandular Q54.0
  penile Q54.1
  penoscrotal Q54.2
  perineal Q54.3
  specified NEC Q54.8
Hypospermatogenesis — *see* Oligospermia
Hyposplenism D73.0
Hypostasis pulmonary, passive — *see* Edema, lung
Hypostatic — *see* condition
Hyposthenuria N28.89
Hypotension (arterial) (constitutional) I95.9
  chronic I95.8
  drug-induced I95.2
  iatrogenic I95.3
    drug-induced I95.2
  idiopathic (permanent) I95.0
  intracranial, following ventricular shunting (ventriculostomy) G97.2
  maternal, syndrome (following labor and delivery) O26.50
    first trimester O26.51
    second trimester O26.52
    third trimester O26.53
  neurogenic, orthostatic G90.3
  orthostatic (chronic) I95.1
    neurogenic G90.3
  postural I95.1
  specified NEC I95.8
Hypothermia (accidental) T68
  anesthetic T88.5
  low environmental temperature T68
  neonatal P80.9
    environmental (mild) NEC P80.8
    mild P80.8
    severe (chronic) (cold injury syndrome) P80.0
    specified NEC P80.8
  not associated with low environmental temperature R68.0
Hypothyroidism (acquired) E03.9
  congenital (without goiter) E03.1
    with goiter (diffuse) E03.0

Hypothyroidism — *continued*
due to
  exogenous substance NEC E03.2
  iodine-deficiency, acquired E01.8
    subclinical E02
  irradiation therapy E89.0
  medicament NEC E03.2
  P-aminosalicylic acid (PAS) E03.2
  phenylbutazone E03.2
  resorcinol E03.2
  sulfonamide E03.2
  surgery E89.0
  thiourea group drugs E03.2
iatrogenic NEC E03.2
iodine-deficiency (acquired) E01.8
  congenital — *see* Syndrome, iodinedeficiency, congenital
  subclinical E02
neonatal, transitory P72.2
postinfectious E03.3
postirradiation E89.0
postprocedural E89.0
postsurgical E89.0
specified NEC E03.8
subclinical, iodine-deficiency related E02
Hypotonia, hypotonicity, hypotony
bladder N31.2
congenital (benign) P94.2
eye — *see* Disorder, globe, hypotony
Hypotrichosis — *see* Alopecia
Hypotropia
left H50.222
right H50.221
Hypoventilation R06.89
Hypovitaminosis — *see* Deficiency, vitamin
Hypovolemia E86.1
surgical shock T81.1
traumatic (shock) T79.4
Hypoxia — *see also* Anoxia
cerebral, during a procedure NEC G97.81
  resulting from a procedure NEC G97.82
fetal, complicating delivery O77.9
intrauterine P19.9
  first noted
    before onset of labor P19.0
    during labor and delivery P19.1
myocardial — *see* Insufficiency, coronary
newborn P84
Hypsarhythmia — *see* Epilepsy, generalized, specified NEC
Hysteralgia, pregnant uterus O26.899
first trimester O26.891
second trimester O26.892
third trimester O26.893
Hysteria, hysterical (conversion) (dissociative state) F44.9
anxiety F41.8
convulsions F44.5
psychosis, acute F44.9
Hysteroepilepsy F44.5

I

Ichthyoparasitism due to Vandellia cirrhosa B88.8
Ichthyosis (congenital) Q80.9
acquired L85.0
fetalis Q80.4
hystrix Q80.8
lamellar Q80.2
lingual K13.2
palmaris and plantaris Q82.8
simplex Q80.0
vera Q80.8
vulgaris Q80.0
X-linked Q80.1
Ichthyotoxism — *see* Poisoning, fish
bacterial — *see* Intoxication, foodborne
Icteroanemia, hemolytic (acquired) D59.9
congenital — *see* Spherocytosis
Icterus — *see also* Jaundice
conjunctiva R17
newborn P59.9
gravis, fetus or newborn P55.0
hematogenous (acquired) D59.9

Icterus — *see also* Jaundice — *continued*
hemolytic (acquired) D59.9
congenital — *see* Spherocytosis
hemorrhagic (acute) (leptospiral) (spirochetal) A27.0
newborn P53
infectious B15.9
with hepatic coma B15.0
leptospiral A27.0
spirochetal A27.0
neonatorum — *see* Jaundice, fetus or newborn
spirochetal A27.0
Ictus solaris, solis T67.0
Identity disorder (child) F64.9
gender role F64.2
psychosexual F64.2
Id reaction (due to bacteria) L30.2
Idioglossia F80.0
Idiopathic — *see* condition
Idiosyncrasy — *see* Allergy
drug, medicament and biological — *see* Allergy, drug
Idiot, idiocy (congenital) F73
amaurotic (Bielschowsky (-Jansky)) (family) (infantile (late)) (juvenile (late)) (Vogt-Spielmeyer) E75.4
microcephalic Q02
IgE asthma J45.00
Ileitis (chronic) — *see also* Enteritis K52.9
regional (ulcerative) — *see* Enteritis, regional, small intestine
segmental — *see* Enteritis, regional
terminal (ulcerative) — *see* Enteritis, regional, small intestine
Ileocolitis (*see also* Enteritis) K52.9
regional — *see* Enteritis, regional
ulcerative (chronic) K51.15
with
complication K51.10
abscess K51.14
fistula K51.13
obstruction K51.12
rectal bleeding K51.11
specified complication NEC K51.19
Ileostomy
attention to Z43.2
malfunctioning K94.13
status Z93.2
with complication — *see* Complications, enterostomy
Ileotyphus — *see* Typhoid
Ileum — *see* condition
Ileus (bowel) (colon) (inhibitory) (intestine) (neurogenic) K56.7
adynamic K56.0
due to gallstone (in intestine) K56.3
duodenal (chronic) K31.5
gallstone K56.3
mechanical NEC K56.6
meconium P75
myxedema K59.8
newborn
due to meconium P75
transitory P76.1
obstructive K56.6
paralytic K56.0
Iliac — *see* condition
Illegitimacy (unwanted pregnancy) Z64.0
supervision of high-risk pregnancy O09.70
first trimester O09.71
second trimester O09.72
third trimester O09.73
Illiteracy Z55.0
Illness — *see also* Disease R69
manic-depressive — *see* Disorder, bipolar
Imbalance R26.82
autonomic G90.8
constituents of food intake E63.1
electrolyte E87.8
with molar pregnancy O08.5
due to hyperemesis gravidarum O21.1
following ectopic or molar pregnancy O08.5
neonatal, transitory NEC P74.4
potassium P74.3

Imbalance — *continued*
electrolyte — *continued*
neonatal, transitory NEC — *continued*
sodium P74.2
endocrine E34.9
eye muscle NOS H50.9
hormone E34.9
hysterical F44.4
labyrinth — *see* category H83.2
posture R29.3
protein-energy — *see* Malnutrition
sympathetic G90.8
Imbecile, imbecility (I.Q. 35-49) F71
Imbedding, intrauterine device T83.39
Imbibition, cholesterol (gallbladder) K82.4
Imbrication, teeth M26.3
Imerslund (-Gräsbeck) syndrome D51.1
Immature — *see also* Immaturity
birth (less than 37 completed weeks) *see* Preterm infant, newborn
extremely (less than 28 completed weeks) — *see* Immaturity, extreme
personality F60.89
Immaturity (less than 37 completed weeks) — *see* Preterm infant, newborn
extreme P07.20
with gestation of:
less than 24 weeks P07.21
24-26 weeks P07.22
27 weeks P07.23
fetus or infant light-for-dates — *see* Light-for-dates
lung, fetus or newborn P28.0
organ or site NEC — *see* Hypoplasia
pulmonary, fetus or newborn P28.0
reaction F60.89
sexual (female) (male), after puberty E30.0
Immersion T75.1
foot or hand T69.00
hand
left T69.02
right T69.01
foot
left T69.04
right T69.03
Immobile, immobility
intestine K59.8
syndrome (paraplegic) M62.3
Immunization — *see also* Vaccination Z23
ABO — *see* Incompatibility, ABO
affecting management of pregnancy — *see* category O36.1
in fetus or newborn P55.1
complication — *see* Complications, vaccination
not done Z28.9
because (of)
contraindication Z28.0
patient's belief Z28.1
previous infection Z28.81
specified reason NEC Z28.89
of patient Z28.29
unspecified patient reason Z28.20
Rh factor — *see* Incompatibility, Rh
affecting management of pregnancy O36.00
first trimester O36.01
second trimester O36.02
third trimester O36.03
from transfusion T80.4
Immunocytoma (M9671/3) — *see* Lymphoma, non-Hodgkin's, diffuse, small cell
Immunodeficiency D84.9
with
adenosine-deaminase deficiency D81.3
antibody defects D80.9
specified type NEC D80.8
hyperimmunoglobulinemia D80.6
increased immunoglobulin M (IgM) D80.5
major defect D82.9
specified type NEC D82.8
partial albinism D82.8
short-limbed stature D82.2
thrombocytopenia and eczema D82.0
antibody with
hyperimmunoglobulinemia D80.6
near-normal immunoglobulins D80.6

Immunodeficiency — *continued*
autosomal recessive, Swiss type D80.0
combined D81.9
biotin-dependent carboxylase D81.819
biotinidase D81.810
holocarboxylase synthetase D81.818
specified type NEC D81.818
severe (SCID) D81.9
with
low or normal B-cell numbers D81.2
low T and B-cell numbers D81.1
reticular dysgenesis D81.0
specified type NEC D81.89
common variable D83.9
with
abnormalities of B-cell numbers and function D83.0
autoantibodies to B or T-cells D83.2
immunoregulatory T-cell disorders D83.1
specified type NEC D83.8
following hereditary defective response to Epstein-Barr virus (EBV) D82.3
selective, immunoglobulin
A (IgA) D80.2
G (IgG) (subclasses) D80.3
M (IgM) D80.4
severe combined (SCID) D81.9
specified type NEC D84.8
to Rh factor, affecting the management of pregnancy, fetus or newborn P55.0
X-linked, with increased IgM D80.5
Immunotherapy, prophylactic Z51.89
Impaction, impacted
bowel, colon, rectum (fecal) K56.4
by gallstone K56.3
calculus — *see* Calculus
cerumen (ear) (external) H61.20
bilateral H61.23
left H61.22
right H61.21
cuspid — *see* Impaction, tooth
dental (same or adjacent tooth) K01.1
fecal, feces K56.4
fracture — *see* Fracture, by site
gallbladder — *see* Calculus, gallbladder
gallstone(s) — *see* Calculus, gallbladder
bile duct (common) (hepatic) — *see* Calculus, bile duct
cystic duct — *see* Calculus, gallbladder
in intestine, with obstruction (any part) K56.3
intestine (calculous) (fecal) NEC K56.4
gallstone, with ileus K56.3
intrauterine device (IUD) T83.39
molar — *see* Impaction, tooth
shoulder, causing obstructed labor O66.0
tooth, teeth K01.1
with abnormal position (same or adjacent tooth) M26.3
turbinate J34.8
Impaired, impairment (function)
auditory discrimination — *see* Abnormal, auditory perception
glucose tolerance R73.0
hearing — *see* Deafness
heart — *see* Disease, heart
kidney — *see also* Failure, renal
disorder resulting from N25.9
specified NEC N25.8
liver K72.90
with coma K72.91
mastication K08.8
mobility
ear ossicles — *see* Ankylosis, ear ossicles
requiring care provider Z74.0
myocardium, myocardial — *see* Insufficiency, myocardial
rectal sphincter R19.8
renal — *see also* Failure, renal
disorder resulting from N25.9
specified NEC N25.8
tolerance, glucose R73.0
vision H54.7
both eyes H54.3
Impediment, speech R47.9
psychogenic (childhood) F98.8
slurring R47.81

Impediment, speech — *continued*
  specified NEC R47.89
Impending
  coronary syndrome I20.0
  delirium tremens F10.239
  myocardial infarction I20.0
Imperception auditory (acquired) — *see also*
  Deafness
  congenital F80.2
Imperfect
  aeration, lung (newborn) NEC — *see* Atelectasis
  closure (congenital)
    alimentary tract NEC Q45.8
      upper Q40.8
    atrioventricular ostium Q21.2
    atrium (secundum) Q21.1
    branchial cleft or sinus Q18.0
    choroid Q14.3
    cricoid cartilage Q31.8
    cusps, heart valve NEC Q24.8
      pulmonary Q22.3
    ductus
      arteriosus Q25.0
      Botalli Q25.0
    ear drum (causing impairment of hearing)
      Q16.4
    esophagus with communication to bronchus
      or trachea Q39.1
    eyelid Q10.3
    foramen
      botalli Q21.1
      ovale Q21.1
    genitalia, genital organ(s) or system
      female Q52.8
        external Q52.79
        internal NEC Q52.8
      male Q55.8
    glottis Q31.8
    interatrial ostium or septum Q21.1
    interauricular ostium or septum Q21.1
    interventricular ostium or septum Q21.0
    larynx Q31.8
    lip — *see* Cleft, lip
    nasal septum Q30.3
    nose Q30.2
    omphalomesenteric duct Q43.0
    optic nerve entry Q14.2
    organ or site not listed — *see* Anomaly, by
      site
    ostium
      interatrial Q21.1
      interauricular Q21.1
      interventricular Q21.0
    palate — *see* Cleft, palate
    preauricular sinus Q18.1
    retina Q14.1
    roof of orbit Q75.8
    sclera Q13.5
    septum
      aorticopulmonary Q21.4
      atrial (secundum) Q21.1
      between aorta and pulmonary artery
        Q21.4
      heart Q21.9
      interatrial (secundum) Q21.1
      interauricular (secundum) Q21.1
      interventricular Q21.0
        in tetralogy of Fallot Q21.3
      nasal Q30.3
      ventricular Q21.0
        with pulmonary stenosis or atresia,
          dextraposition of aorta, and
          hypertrophy of right ventricle
          Q21.3
        in tetralogy of Fallot Q21.3
    skull Q75.0
      with
        anencephaly Q00.0
        encephalocele — *see* Encephalocele
        hydrocephalus Q03.9
          with spina bifida — *see* Spina
            bifida, by site, with
            hydrocephalus
        microcephaly Q02
    spine (with meningocele) — *see* Spina bifida
    trachea Q32.1

Imperfect — *continued*
  closure — *continued*
    tympanic membrane (causing impairment of
      hearing) Q16.4
    uterus Q51.8
    vitelline duct Q43.0
  erection — *see* Dysfunction, sexual, male,
    erectile
  fusion — *see* Imperfect, closure
  inflation, lung (newborn) — *see* Atelectasis
  posture R29.3
  rotation, intestine Q43.3
  septum, ventricular Q21.0
Imperfectly descended testis — *see* Cryptorchid
Imperforate (congenital) — *see also* Atresia
  anus Q42.3
    with fistula Q42.2
  cervix (uteri) Q51.8
  esophagus Q39.0
    with tracheoesophageal fistula Q39.1
  hymen Q52.3
  jejunum Q41.1
  pharynx Q38.8
  rectum Q42.1
    with fistula Q42.0
  urethra Q64.39
  vagina Q52.4
Impervious (congenital) — *see also* Atresia
  anus Q42.3
    with fistula Q42.2
  bile duct Q44.2
  esophagus Q39.0
    with tracheoesophageal fistula Q39.1
  intestine (small) Q41.9
    large Q42.9
      specified NEC Q42.8
  rectum Q42.1
    with fistula Q42.0
  ureter — *see* Atresia, ureter
  urethra Q64.39
Impetiginization of dermatoses L01.1
Impetigo (any organism) (any site) (circinate)
  (contagiosa) (simplex) (vulgaris) L01.00
  Bockhart's L01.02
  bullous, bullosa L01.03
  external ear L01.00 [H62.40]
  follicularis L01.02
  furfuracea L30.5
  herpetiformis L40.1
    nonobstetrical L40.1
  neonatorum L01.03
  nonbullous L01.01
  specified type NEC L01.09
  ulcerative L01.09
Impingement, soft tissue between teeth M26.2
Implant, endometrial N80.9
Implantation
  anomalous — *see* Anomaly, by site
    ureter Q62.63
  cyst
    external area or site (skin) NEC L72.0
    iris — *see* Cyst, iris, implantation
    vagina N89.8
    vulva N90.7
  dermoid (cyst) — *see* Implantation, cyst
  placenta, low or marginal — *see* Placenta,
    previa
Impotence (sexual) (psychogenic) F52.21
  counseling Z70.1
  organic origin NEC — *see* Dysfunction, sexual,
    male, erectile
Impression, basilar Q75.8
Imprisonment, anxiety concerning Z65.1
Improper care (child) (newborn) — *see* Neglect
Improperly tied umbilical cord (causing
  hemorrhage) P51.8
Inability to swallow — *see* Aphagia
Inaccessible, inaccessibility
  health care NEC Z75.3
    due to
      waiting period Z75.2
        for admission to facility elsewhere
          Z75.1
  other helping agencies Z75.4

Inactive — *see* condition
Inadequate, inadequacy
  biologic, constitutional, functional, or social
    F60.7
  development
    child R62.50
    fetus — *see* Slow, fetal growth
      affecting management of pregnancy —
        see category O36.5
    genitalia
      after puberty NEC E30.0
      congenital
        female Q52.8
          external Q52.79
          internal Q52.8
        male Q55.8
    lungs Q33.6
      associated with short gestation P28.0
    organ or site not listed — *see* Anomaly, by
      site
  diet (causing nutritional deficiency) E63.9
  drinking water supply Z58.6
  eating habits Z72.4
  environment, household Z59.1
  family support Z63.2
  food (supply) NEC Z59.4
    hunger effects T73.0
  functional F60.7
  household care, due to
    family member
      handicapped or ill Z74.2
      on vacation Z75.5
      temporarily away from home Z74.2
    technical defects in home Z59.1
    temporary absence from home of person
      rendering care Z74.2
  housing (heating) (space) Z59.1
  income (financial) Z59.6
  intrafamilial communication Z63.8
  material resources Z59.6
  mental — *see* Retardation, mental
  parental supervision or control of child Z62.0
  personality F60.7
  prenatal care affecting management of
    pregnancy O09.30
    first trimester O09.31
    second trimester O09.32
    third trimester O09.33
  pulmonary
    function R06.89
      newborn P28.5
    ventilation, newborn P28.5
  social F60.7
    insurance Z59.7
    skills NEC Z73.4
  supervision of child by parent Z62.0
  teaching affecting education Z55.8
  welfare support Z59.7
Inanition R64
  with edema — *see* Malnutrition, severe
  due to
    deprivation of food T73.0
    malnutrition — *see* Malnutrition
  fever R50.9
Inappropriate
  diet or eating habits Z72.4
  secretion
    antidiuretic hormone (ADH) (excessive)
      E22.2
      deficiency E23.2
    pituitary (posterior) E22.2
Inattention at or after birth — *see* Neglect
Incarceration, incarcerated
  enterocele K46.0
    gangrenous K46.1
  epiplocele K46.0
    gangrenous K46.1
  exophthalmos K42.0
    gangrenous K42.1
  hernia — *see also* Hernia, by site, with
    obstruction
    with gangrene — *see* Hernia, by site, with
      gangrene
  iris, in wound — *see* Injury, eye, laceration,
    with prolapse

Incarceration, incarcerated — continued
  lens, in wound — see Injury, eye, laceration,
      with prolapse
  omphalocele K42.0
  prison, anxiety concerning Z65.1
  rupture — see Hernia, by site
  sarcoepiplocele K46.0
      gangrenous K46.1
  sarcoepiplomphalocele K42.0
      with gangrene K42.1
  uterus N85.8
      gravid — see category O34.5
          causing obstructed labor O65.5

Incident, cerebrovascular I64

Incineration (entire body) (from fire,
      conflagration, electricity or lightning) T29

Incised wound
  external — see Laceration
  internal organs — see Injury, by site

Incision, incisional
  hernia — see Hernia, ventral
  surgical, complication — see Complications,
      surgical procedure
  traumatic
      external — see Laceration
      internal organs — see Injury, by site

Inclusion
  azurophilic leukocytic D72.0
  blennorrhea (neonatal) (newborn) P39.1
  gallbladder in liver (congenital) Q44.1

Incompatibility
  ABO
      affecting management of pregnancy — see
          category O36.1
      fetus or newborn P55.1
      infusion or transfusion reaction T80.3
  blood (group) (Duffy) (K(ell)) (Kidd) (Lewis) (M)
      (S) NEC
      affecting management of pregnancy — see
          category O36.1
      fetus or newborn P55.8
      infusion or transfusion reaction T80.3
  divorce or estrangement Z63.5
  Rh (blood group) (factor) Z31.82
      affecting management of pregnancy O36.00
          first trimester O36.01
          second trimester O36.02
          third trimester O36.03
      fetus or newborn P55.0
      infusion or transfusion reaction T80.4
  rhesus — see Incompatibility, Rh

Incompetency, incompetent, incompetence
  annular
      aortic (valve) — see Insufficiency, aortic
      mitral (valve) I34.0
      pulmonary valve (heart) I37.1
  aortic (valve) — see Insufficiency, aortic
  cardiac valve — see Endocarditis
  cervix, cervical (os) N88.3
      in pregnancy O34.30
          first trimester O34.31
          second trimester O34.32
          third trimester O34.33
  esophagogastric (junction) (sphincter) K22.0
  mitral (valve) — see Insufficiency, mitral
  pelvic fundus N81.8
  pulmonary valve (heart) I37.1
      congenital Q22.3
  tricuspid (annular) (valve) — see Insufficiency,
      tricuspid
  valvular — see Endocarditis
  vein, venous (saphenous) (varicose) — see
      Varix, leg

Incomplete — see also condition
  bladder, emptying R33.9
  expansion lungs (newborn) NEC — see
      Atelectasis
  rotation, intestine Q43.3

Incontinence R32
  anal sphincter R15
  feces R15
      nonorganic origin F98.1
  overflow N39.49
  psychogenic F45.8
  rectal R15
  reflex N39.49

Incontinence — continued
  stress (female) (male) N39.3
  urethral sphincter R32
  urge N39.41
  urine R32
      continuous N39.45
      mixed N39.46
      nocturnal N39.44
      nonorganic origin F98.0
      overflow N39.49
      post dribbling N39.43
      reflex N39.49
      specified NEC N39.49
      stress (female) (male) N39.3
      total N39.49
      unaware N39.42
      urge N39.41

Incontinentia pigmenti Q82.3

Incoordinate, incoordination
  esophageal-pharyngeal (newborn) — see
      Dysphagia
  muscular R27.8
  uterus (action) (contractions) (complicating
      delivery) O62.4

Increase, increased
  abnormal, in development R63.8
  androgens (ovarian) E28.1
  anticoagulants (antithrombin) (anti-VIIIa) (anti-
      IXa) (anti-Xa) (anti-XIa) — see Circulating
      anticoagulants)
  cold sense R20.8
  estrogen E28.0
  function
      adrenal
          cortex — see Cushing's syndrome
          medulla E27.5
      pituitary (gland) (anterior) (lobe) E22.9
          posterior E22.2
  heat sense R20.8
  intracranial pressure (benign) G93.2
  permeability, capillaries I78.8
  pressure, intracranial G93.2
  secretion
      gastrin E16.4
      glucagon E16.3
      pancreas, endocrine E16.9
          growth hormone-releasing hormone
              E16.8
          pancreatic polypeptide E16.8
          somatostatin E16.8
          vasoactive-intestinal polypeptide E16.8
  sphericity, lens Q12.4
  splenic activity D73.1
  venous pressure I87.8
      portal K76.6

Incrustation, cornea, foreign body (lead) (zinc)—
      see Foreign body, cornea

Incyclophoria H50.54

Incyclotropia — see Cyclotropia

Indeterminate sex Q56.4

India rubber skin Q82.8

Indigestion (acid) (bilious) (functional) K30
  catarrhal K31.89
  due to decomposed food NOS A05.9
  nervous F45.8
  psychogenic F45.8

Indirect — see condition

Induratio penis plastica N48.7

Induration, indurated
  brain G93.8
  breast (fibrous) N64.5
      puerperal, postpartum O92.22
  broad ligament N83.8
  chancre
      anus A51.1
      congenital A50.07
      extragenital NEC A51.2
  corpora cavernosa (penis) (plastic) N48.7
  liver (chronic) K76.8
  lung (black) (brown) (chronic) (fibroid) — see
      Fibrosis, lung
  penile (plastic) N48.7
  phlebitic — see Phlebitis
  skin R23.4

Inebriety (without dependence) — see Alcohol,
      intoxication

Inefficiency, kidney — see Failure, renal

Inelasticity, skin R23.4

Inequality, leg (length) (acquired) — see also
      Deformity, limb, unequal length
  congenital — see Defect, reduction, lower limb
  lower leg — see Deformity, limb, unequal
      length

Inertia
  bladder (neurogenic) N31.2
  stomach K31.89
      psychogenic F45.8
  uterus, uterine during labor O62.2
      primary O62.0
      secondary O62.1
  vesical (neurogenic) N31.2

Infancy, infantile, infantilism — see also
      condition
  celiac K90.0
  genitalia, genitals (after puberty) E30.0
      in pregnancy or childbirth NEC — see
          category O34.8
          causing obstructed labor O65.5
  Herter's (nontropical sprue) K90.0
  intestinal K90.0
  Lorain E23.0
  pancreatic K86.8
  pelvis M95.5
      with disproportion (fetopelvic) O33.1
          causing obstructed labor O65.1
  pituitary E23.0
  renal N25.0
  sexual (with obesity) E30.0
  uterus — see Infantile, genitalia

Infant(s) — see also Infancy
  excessive crying R68.11
  irritable child R68.12
  lack of care — see Neglect
  liveborn (singleton) Z38.2
      born in hospital Z38.00
          by cesarean Z38.01
      born outside hospital Z38.1
      multiple NEC Z38.8
          born in hospital Z38.68
              by cesarean Z38.69
          born outside hospital Z38.7
      quadruplet Z38.8
          born in hospital Z38.63
              by cesarean Z38.64
          born outside hospital Z38.7
      quintuplet Z38.8
          born in hospital Z38.65
              by cesarean Z38.66
          born outside hospital Z38.7
      triplet Z38.8
          born in hospital Z38.61
              by cesarean Z38.62
          born outside hospital Z38.7
      twin Z38.5
          born in hospital Z38.30
              by cesarean Z38.31
          born outside hospital Z38.4
  of diabetic mother (syndrome of) P70.1
      gestational diabetes P70.0

Infantile — see also condition
  genitalia, genitals E30.0
  os, uterine E30.0
  penis E30.0
  testis E29.1
  uterus E30.0

Infantilism — see Infancy

Infarct, infarction
  adrenal (capsule) (gland) E27.4
  appendices epiploicae K55.0
  bowel K55.0
  brain (stem) — see Infarct, cerebral
  breast N64.8
  brewer's (kidney) N28.0
  cardiac — see Infarct, myocardium
  cerebellar — see Infarct, cerebral
  cerebral I63.9
      due to
          cerebral venous thrombosis, nonpyogenic
              I63.6

©2002 Ingenix, Inc.

Infarct, infarction — *continued*
  cerebral — *continued*
    due to — *continued*
      embolism
        cerebral arteries I63.4
        precerebral arteries I63.1
      occlusion NEC
        cerebral arteries I63.5
        precerebral arteries I63.2
      stenosis NEC
        cerebral arteries I63.5
        precerebral arteries I63.2
      thrombosis
        cerebral arteries I63.3
        precerebral arteries I63.0
    puerperal, postpartum, childbirth — *see* Disease, circulatory, obstetric
    specified NEC I63.8
  colon (acute) (agnogenic) (embolic) (hemorrhagic) (nonocclusive) (nonthrombotic) (occlusive) (segmental) (thrombotic) (with gangrene) K55.0
  coronary artery — *see* Infarct, myocardium
  embolic — *see* Embolism
  fallopian tube N83.8
  gallbladder K82.8
  heart — *see* Infarct, myocardium
  hepatic K76.3
  hypophysis (anterior lobe) E23.6
  impending (myocardium) I20.0
  intestine (acute) (agnogenic) (embolic) (hemorrhagic) (nonocclusive) (nonthrombotic) (occlusive) (thrombotic) (with gangrene) K55.0
  kidney N28.0
  liver K76.3
  lung (embolic) (thrombotic) — *see* Embolism, pulmonary
  lymph node I89.8
  mesentery, mesenteric (embolic) (thrombotic) (with gangrene) K55.0
  muscle (ischemic) M62.20
    ankle M62.279
      left M62.272
      right M62.271
    foot M62.279
      left M62.272
      right M62.271
    forearm M62.239
      left M62.232
      right M62.231
    hand M62.249
      left M62.242
      right M62.241
    lower leg M62.269
      left M62.262
      right M62.261
    pelvic region M62.259
      left M62.252
      right M62.251
    shoulder region M62.219
      left M62.212
      right M62.211
    specified site NEC M62.28
    thigh M62.259
      left M62.252
      right M62.251
    upper arm M62.229
      left M62.222
      right M62.221
  myocardium, myocardial (acute) (with stated duration of 4 weeks or less) (with hypertension) I21.9
    with symptoms after 4 weeks from date of infarction I25.8
    chronic or with a stated duration of over 4 weeks I25.8
    diagnosed on ECG, but presenting no symptoms I25.2
    healed or old I25.2
    nontransmural I21.4
    past (diagnosed on ECG or other investigation, but currently presenting no symptoms) I25.2
    syphilitic A52.06

Infarct, infarction — *continued*
  myocardium, myocardial — *continued*
    subsequent (recurrent) I22.9
      anterior (anteroapical) (anterolateral) (anteroseptal) (wall) I22.0
      diaphragmatic (wall) I22.1
      inferior (diaphragmatic) (inferolateral) (inferoposterior) (wall) I22.1
      lateral (apical-lateral) (basal-lateral) (high) I22.8
      posterior (posterobasal) (posterolateral) (posteroseptal) (true) I22.8
      septal I22.8
      specified NEC I22.8
      subendocardial I22.3
      transmural I22.2
        anterior (anteroapical) (anterolateral) (anteroseptal) (wall) I22.0
        diaphragmatic (wall) I22.1
        inferior (diaphragmatic) (inferolateral) (inferoposterior) (wall) I22.1
        lateral (apical-lateral) (basal-lateral) (high) I22.8
        posterior (posterobasal) (posterolateral) (posteroseptal) (true) I22.8
        specified NEC I22.8
    syphilitic A52.06
    transmural I21.3
      anterior (wall) (anteroapical) (anterolateral) (anteroseptal) I21.0
      inferior (diaphragmatic) (inferolateral) (inferoposterior) (wall) I21.1
      lateral (apical-lateral) (basal-lateral) (high) I21.2
      posterior (posterobasal) (posterolateral) (posteroseptal) (true) I21.2
      septal I21.2
      specified NEC I21.2
  nontransmural I21.4
  omentum K55.0
  ovary N83.8
  pancreas
  papillary muscle — *see* Infarct, myocardium
  parathyroid gland E21.4
  pituitary (gland) E23.6
  placenta (complicating pregnancy) O43.829
    first trimester O43.821
    second trimester O43.822
    third trimester O43.823
  prostate N42.89
  pulmonary (artery) (vein) (hemorrhagic) — *see* Embolism, pulmonary
  renal (embolic) (thrombotic) N28.0
  retina, retinal (artery) — *see* Occlusion, artery, retina
  spinal (cord) (acute) (embolic) (nonembolic) G95.11
  spleen D73.5
    embolic or thrombotic I74.8
  subchorionic — *see* Infarct, placenta
  subendocardial (acute) (nontransmural) I21.4
  suprarenal (capsule) (gland) E27.4
  testis N50.1
  thrombotic — *see also* Thrombosis
    artery, arterial — *see* Embolism
  thyroid (gland) E07.89
  urge
    healed or old, currently presenting no symptoms I25.2
    impending I20.0
    past (diagnosed on ECG or other investigation, but currently presenting no symptoms) I25.2
    with symptoms NEC I25.8
    previous, currently presenting no symptoms I25.2
  ventricle (heart) — *see* Infarct, myocardium
Infecting — *see* condition
Infection, infected, infective (opportunistic) B99.9
  with
    drug resistant organism (*see also* specific organism) Z06
    lymphangitis — *see* Lymphangitis
  abscess (skin) – code by site under Abscess
  Absidia — *see* Mucormycosis

Infection, infected, infective — *continued*
  Acanthocheilonema (perstans) (streptocerca) B74.4
  accessory sinus (chronic) — *see* Sinusitis
  achorion — *see* Dermatophytosis
  Acremonium falciforme B47.0
  acromioclavicular M00.9
  Actinobacillus (actinomycetem-comitans) A28.8
    mallei A24.0
    muris A25.1
  Actinomadura B47.1
  Actinomyces (israelii) — *see also* Actinomycosis A42.9
  Actinomycetales — *see* Actinomycosis
  actinomycotic NOS — *see* Actinomycosis
  adenoid (and tonsil) J03.90
    chronic J35.02
  adenovirus NEC
    as cause of disease classified elsewhere B97.0
    unspecified nature or site B34.0
  aerogenes capsulatus A48.0
  aertrycke — *see* Infection, salmonella
  alimentary canal NOS — *see* Enteritis, infectious
  Allescheria boydii B48.2
  Alternaria B48.8
  alveolus, alveolar (process) K04.7
  Ameba, amebic (histolytica) — *see* Amebiasis
  amniotic fluid, sac or cavity O41.109
    chorioamnionitis O41.129
      first trimester O41.121
      second trimester O41.122
      third trimester O41.123
    first trimester O41.101
    second trimester O41.102
    third trimester O41.103
    placentitis O41.149
      first trimester O41.141
      second trimester O41.142
      third trimester O41.143
  amputation stump (surgical) — *see* Complication, amputation stump, infection
  Ancylostoma (duodenalis) B76.0
  Anisakiasis, Anisakis larvae B81.0
  anthrax — *see* Anthrax
  antrum (chronic) — *see* Sinusitis, maxillary
  anus, anal (papillae) (sphincter) K62.8
  arbovirus (arbor virus) A94
    specified type NEC A93.8
  artificial insemination N98.0
  Ascaris lumbricoides — *see* Ascariasis
  Ascomycetes B47.0
  Aspergillus (flavus) (fumigatus) (terreus) — *see* Aspergillosis
  atypical
    acid-fast (bacilli) — *see* Mycobacterium, atypical
    mycobacteria — *see* Mycobacterium, atypical
    virus A81.9
      specified type NEC A81.8
  auditory meatus (external) — *see* Otitis, externa, infective
  auricle (ear) — *see* Otitis, externa, infective
  axillary gland (lymph) L04.2
  Bacillus A49.9
    abortus A23.1
    anthracis — *see* Anthrax
    Ducrey's (any location) A57
    Flexner's A03.1
    fragilis, as cause of disease classified elsewhere B96.6
    Friedländer's NEC A49.8
    gas (gangrene) A48.0
    mallei A24.0
    melitensis A23.0
    paratyphoid, paratyphosus A01.4
      A A01.1
      B A01.2
      C A01.3
    Shiga(-Kruse) A03.0
    suipestifer — *see* Infection, salmonella
    swimming pool A31.1
    typhosa A01.00
    welchii — *see* Gangrene, gas

Infection, infected, infective — *continued*
  bacterial NOS A49.9
    agent NEC, as cause of disease classified
      elsewhere B96.89
    specified NEC A48.8
  Bacterium
    paratyphosum A01.4
      A A01.1
      B A01.2
      C A01.3
    typhosum A01.00
  Bacteroides NEC A49.8
  Balantidium coli A07.0
  Bartholin's gland N75.8
  Basidiobolus B46.8
  bile duct (common) (hepatic) — *see* Cholangitis
  bladder — *see* Cystitis
  Blastomyces, blastomycotic — *see also*
    Blastomycosis
    brasiliensis — *see* Paracoccidioidomycosis
    dermatitidis — *see* Blastomycosis
    European — *see* Cryptococcosis
    Loboi B48.0
    North American B40.9
    South American — *see*
      Paracoccidioidomycosis
  blood stream — *see* Septicemia
  bone — *see* Osteomyelitis
  Bordetella — *see* Whooping cough
  Borrelia bergdorfi A69.20
  brain (*see also* Encephalitis) G04.9
    membranes — *see* Meningitis
    septic G06.0
    meninges — *see* Meningitis, bacterial
  branchial cyst Q18.0
  breast — *see* Mastitis
  bronchus — *see* Bronchitis
  Brucella A23.9
    abortus A23.1
    canis A23.3
    melitensis A23.0
    mixed A23.8
    specified NEC A23.8
    suis A23.2
  Brugia (malayi) B74.1
    timori B74.2
  bursa — *see* Bursitis, infective
  buttocks (skin) L08.9
  Campylobacter, intestinal A04.5
    as cause of disease classified elsewhere
      B96.81
  Candida (albicans) (tropicalis) — *see*
    Candidiasis
  candiru B88.8
  Capillaria (intestinal) B81.1
    hepatica B83.8
    philippinensis B81.1
  cartilage — *see* Disorder, cartilage, specified
    type NEC
  cat liver fluke B66.0
  cellulitis – code by site under Cellulitis
  Cephalosporium falciforme B47.0
  cerebrospinal — *see* Meningitis
  cervical gland (lymph) L04.0
  cervix — *see* Cervicitis
  cesarean section wound (puerperal) O86.0
  cestodes — *see* Infestation, cestodes
  Chilomastix (intestinal) A07.8
  Chlamydia, chlamydial A74.9
    anus A56.3
    genitourinary tract A56.2
      lower A56.00
        specified NEC A56.19
    lymphogranuloma A55
    pharynx A56.4
    psittaci A70
    rectum A56.3
    sexually transmitted NEC A56.8
  cholera — *see* Cholera
  Cladosporium
    bantianum (brain abscess) B43.1
    carrionii B43.0
    castellanii B36.1
    trichoides (brain abscess) B43.1
    werneckii B36.1
  Clonorchis (sinensis) (liver) B66.1

Infection, infected, infective — *continued*
  Clostridium NEC
    bifermentans A48.0
    botulinum A05.1
    congenital P39.8
    difficile
      as cause of disease classified elsewhere
        B96.89
      foodborne (disease) A05.8
      gas gangrene A48.0
      necrotizing enterocolitis A05.8
      septicemia A41.4
    gas-forming NEC A48.0
    histolyticum A48.0
    novyi, causing gas gangrene A48.0
    oedematiens A48.0
    perfringens
      as cause of disease classified elsewhere
        B96.7
      due to food A05.2
      foodborne (disease) A05.2
      gas gangrene A48.0
      septicemia A41.4
    septicum, causing gas gangrene A48.0
    sordellii, causing gas gangrene A48.0
    welchii
      as cause of disease classified elsewhere
        B96.7
      foodborne (disease) A05.2
      gas gangrene A48.0
      necrotizing enteritis A05.2
      septicemia A41.4
  Coccidioides (immitis) — *see*
    Coccidioidomycosis
  colon — *see* Enteritis, infectious
  colostomy K94.02
  common duct — *see* Cholangitis
  congenital NOS P39.9
    Candida (albicans) P37.5
    Clostridium, other than Clostridium tetani
      P39.8
    cytomegalovirus P35.1
    Escherichia coli P39.8
      sepsis P36.4
    hepatitis, viral P35.3
    herpes simplex P35.2
    infectious or parasitic disease P37.9
      specified NEC P37.8
    listeriosis (disseminated) P37.2
    malaria NEC P37.4
      falciparum P37.3
    Plasmodium falciparum P37.3
    poliomyelitis P35.8
    rubella P35.0
    Salmonella P39.8
    skin P39.4
    streptococcal NEC P39.8
      sepsis P36.1
        group B P36.0
    toxoplasmosis (acute) (subacute) (chronic)
      P37.1
    tuberculosis P37.0
    urinary (tract) P39.3
    vaccinia P35.8
    virus P35.9
      specified type NEC P35.8
  Conidiobolus B46.8
  coronavirus NEC B34.2
    as cause of disease classified elsewhere
      B97.2
  corpus luteum — *see* Salpingo-oophoritis
  Corynebacterium diphtheriae — *see* Diphtheria
  Coxiella burnetii A78
  coxsackie — *see* Coxsackie
  Cryptococcus neoformans — *see*
    Cryptococcosis
  Cryptosporidium A07.2
  Cunninghamella — *see* Mucormycosis
  cyst — *see* Cyst
  cystic duct (*see also* Cholecystitis) K81.9
  Cysticercus cellulosae — *see* Cysticercosis
  cytomegalovirus, cytomegaloviral B25.9
    congenital P35.1
    maternal, maternal care for (suspected)
      damage to fetus O35.3

Infection, infected, infective — *continued*
  cytomegalovirus, cytomegaloviral — *continued*
    mononucleosis B27.10
      with
        complication NEC B27.19
        meningitis B27.12
        polyneuropathy B27.11
  delta-agent (acute), in hepatitis B carrier B17.0
  dental (pulpal origin) K04.7
  Deuteromycetes B47.0
  Dicrocoelium dendriticum B66.2
  Dipetalonema (perstans) (streptocerca) B74.4
  diphtherial — *see* Diphtheria
  Diphyllobothrium (adult) (latum) (pacificum)
    B70.0
    larval B70.1
  Diplogonoporus (grandis) B71.8
  Dipylidium caninum B71.1
  Dirofilaria B74.8
  Dracunculus medinensis B72
  Drechslera (hawaiiensis) B43.8
  Ducrey Haemophilus (any location) A57
  due to or resulting from
    artificial insemination N98.0
    device, implant or graft (*see also*
      Complications, by site and type,
      infection or inflammation) T85.79
      arterial graft NEC T82.7
      breast (implant) T85.79
      catheter NEC T85.79
      dialysis (renal) T82.7
        intraperitoneal T85.71
      infusion NEC T82.7
        spinal (epidural) (subdural) T85.79
      urinary (indwelling) T83.51
      electronic (electrode) (pulse generator)
      (stimulator)
        bone T84.7
        cardiac T82.7
        nervous system (brain) (peripheral
          nerve) (spinal) T85.79
        urinary T83.59
      fixation, internal (orthopedic) NEC — *see*
        Complication, fixation device,
        infection
      gastrointestinal (bile duct) (esophagus)
        T85.79
      genital NEC T83.6
      heart NEC T82.7
        valve (prosthesis) T82.6
        graft T82.7
      joint prosthesis — *see* Complication, joint
        prosthesis, infection
      ocular (corneal graft) (orbital implant)
        NEC T85.79
      orthopedic NEC T84.7
      specified NEC T85.79
      urinary NEC T83.59
      vascular NEC T82.7
      ventricular intracranial shunt T85.79
    immunization or vaccination T88.0
    infusion, injection or transfusion NEC T80.2
  injury NEC – code by site under Wound, open
  surgery T81.4
  during labor NEC O75.3
  ear (middle) — *see also* Otitis media
    external — *see* Otitis, externa, infective
    inner — *see* category H83.0
  Eberthella typhosa A01.00
  Echinococcus — *see* Echinococcus
  echovirus
    as cause of disease classified elsewhere
      B97.12
    unspecified nature or site B34.1
  endocardium I33.0
  endocervix — *see* Cervicitis
  Entamoeba — *see* Amebiasis
  enteric — *see* Enteritis, infectious
  Enterobius vermicularis B80
  enterostomy K94.12
  enterovirus B34.1
    as cause of disease classified elsewhere
      B97.10
      coxsackievirus B97.11
      echovirus B97.12
      specified NEC B97.19
  Entomophthora B46.8

Infection, infected, infective — *continued*
　Epidermophyton — *see* Dermatophytosis
　epididymis — *see* Epididymitis
　episiotomy (puerperal) O86.0
　Erysipelothrix (insidiosa) (rhusiopathiae) — *see*
　　　Erysipeloid
　erythema infectiosum B08.3
　Escherichia (E.) coli NEC A49.8
　　as cause of disease classified elsewhere
　　　B96.2
　　congenital P39.8
　　　sepsis P36.4
　　generalized A41.51
　　intestinal — *see* Enteritis, infectious, due to,
　　　Escherichia coli
　ethmoidal (chronic) (sinus) — *see* Sinusitis,
　　　ethmoidal
　eustachian tube (ear) — *see* Salpingitis,
　　　eustachian
　external auditory canal (meatus) NEC — *see*
　　　Otitis, externa, infective
　eye (purulent) — *see* Endophthalmitis, purulent
　eyelid — *see* Inflammation, eyelid
　fallopian tube — *see* Salpingo-oophoritis
　Fasciola (gigantica) (hepatica) (indica) B66.3
　Fasciolopsis (buski) B66.5
　fetus P39.9
　　intra-amniotic NEC P39.2
　filarial — *see* Infestation, filarial
　finger (skin) L08.9
　　nail fungus B35.1
　fish tapeworm B70.0
　　larval B70.1
　flagellate, intestinal A07.9
　fluke — *see* Infestation, fluke
　focal
　　teeth (pulpal origin) K04.7
　　tonsils J35.01
　Fonsecaea (compactum) (pedrosoi) B43.0
　food — *see* Intoxication, foodborne
　foot (skin) L08.9
　　dermatophytic fungus B35.3
　Francisella tularensis — *see* Tularemia
　frontal (sinus) (chronic) — *see* Sinusitis, frontal
　fungus NOS B49
　　beard B35.0
　　dermatophytic — *see* Dermatophytosis
　　foot B35.3
　　groin B35.6
　　hand B35.2
　　nail B35.1
　　pathogenic to compromised host only B48.8
　　perianal (area) B35.6
　　scalp B35.0
　　skin B36.9
　　　foot B35.3
　　　hand B35.2
　　　toenails B35.1
　Fusarium B48.8
　gallbladder — *see* Cholecystitis
　gas bacillus — *see* Gangrene, gas
　gastrointestinal — *see* Enteritis, infectious
　generalized NEC — *see* Septicemia
　genital organ or tract
　　complicating pregnancy O23.50
　　　first trimester O23.51
　　　second trimester O23.52
　　　third trimester O23.53
　　female — *see* Disease, pelvis, inflammatory
　　following ectopic or molar pregnancy O08.0
　　male N49.9
　　　multiple sites N49.8
　　　specified NEC N49.8
　　puerperal, postpartum, childbirth NEC
　　　O86.1
　　　major or generalized O85
　　　minor or localized O86.1
　genitourinary tract NEC
　　in pregnancy O23.90
　　　first trimester O23.91
　　　second trimester O23.92
　　　third trimester O23.93
　Ghon tubercle, primary A15.7
　Giardia lamblia A07.1
　gingiva (chronic) K05.1
　　acute K05.0
　glanders A24.0

Infection, infected, infective — *continued*
　glenosporopsis B48.0
　Gnathostoma (spinigerum) B83.1
　Gongylonema B83.8
　gonococcal — *see* Gonococcus
　gram-negative bacilli NOS A49.9
　guinea worm B72
　gum (chronic) K05.1
　　acute K05.0
　Haemophilus — *see* Infection, Hemophilus
　heart — *see* Carditis
　Helicobacter pylori A04.5
　　as cause of disease classified elsewhere
　　　B96.81
　helminths B83.9
　　intestinal B82.0
　　　mixed (types classifiable to more than one
　　　　of the titles B65.0-B81.3 and
　　　　B81.8) B81.4
　　　specified type NEC B81.8
　　specified type NEC B83.8
　Hemophilus
　　aegyptius, systemic A48.4
　　ducrey (any location) A57
　　influenzae NEC A49.2
　　　as cause of disease classified elsewhere
　　　　B96.3
　　　generalized A41.3
　herpes (simplex) — *see also* Herpes
　　congenital P35.2
　　disseminated B00.7
　　zoster B02.9
　herpesvirus, herpesviral — *see* Herpes
　Heterophyes (heterophyes) B66.8
　Histoplasma — *see* Histoplasmosis
　　American B39.4
　　capsulatum B39.4
　hookworm B76.9
　human
　　papilloma virus A63.0
　　T-cell lymphotropic virus type-1 (HTLV-1)
　　　B33.3
　hydrocele N43.0
　Hymenolepis B71.0
　hypopharynx — *see* Pharyngitis
　inguinal (lymph) glands L04.1
　　due to soft chancre A57
　intervertebral disc, pyogenic M46.30
　　cervical region M46.32
　　cervicothoracic region M46.33
　　lumbar region M46.36
　　lumbosacral region M46.37
　　multiple sites M46.39
　　occipito-atlanto-axial region M46.31
　　sacrococcygeal region M46.38
　　thoracic region M46.34
　　thoracolumbar region M46.35
　intestine, intestinal — *see* Enteritis, infectious
　intra-amniotic, fetus P39.2
　intrauterine (complicating pregnancy) — *see
　　also* Endometritis, complicating
　　　pregnancy
　　puerperal (postpartum) (with sepsis) O85
　　specified infection NEC, fetus P39.2
　Isospora belli or hominis A07.3
　Japanese B encephalitis A83.0
　jaw (bone) (lower) (upper) M27.2
　joint — *see* Arthritis, pyogenic or pyemic
　kidney (cortex) (hematogenous) N15.9
　　with calculus N20.0
　　　with hydronephrosis N13.6
　　complicating pregnancy O23.00
　　　with a predominantly sexual mode of
　　　　transmission NEC O98.319
　　　　first trimester O98.311
　　　　second trimester O98.312
　　　　third trimester O98.313
　　　first trimester O23.01
　　　second trimester O23.02
　　　third trimester O23.03
　　following ectopic gestation O08.89
　　pelvis and ureter (cystic) N28.85
　　puerperal (postpartum) O86.21
　　specified NEC N15.8
　Klebsiella (K.) pneumoniae NEC A49.8
　　as cause of disease classified elsewhere
　　　B96.1

Infection, infected, infective — *continued*
　knee (skin) NEC L08.9
　　joint M00.9
　Koch's — *see* Tuberculosis
　labia (majora) (minora) (acute) — *see* Vulvitis
　lacrimal
　　gland — *see* Dacryoadenitis
　　passages (duct) (sac) — *see* Inflammation,
　　　lacrimal, passages
　lancet fluke B66.2
　larynx NEC J38.7
　leg (skin) NOS L08.9
　Legionella pneumophila A48.1
　　nonpneumonic A48.2
　Leishmania — *see also* Leishmaniasis
　　aethiopica B55.1
　　braziliensis B55.2
　　chagasi B55.0
　　donovani B55.0
　　infantum B55.0
　　major B55.1
　　mexicana B55.1
　　tropica B55.1
　lentivirus, as cause of disease classified
　　elsewhere B97.31
　Leptosphaeria senegalensis B47.0
　Leptospira interrogans A27.9
　　autumnalis A27.89
　　canicola A27.89
　　hebdomadis A27.89
　　icterohaemorrhagiae A27.0
　　pomona A27.89
　　specified type NEC A27.89
　　icterohaemorrhagiae A27.0
　leptospirochetal NEC — *see* Leptospirosis
　Listeria monocytogenes — *see also* Listeriosis
　　congenital P37.2
　Loa loa B74.3
　　with conjunctival infestation B74.3
　　eyelid B74.3
　Loboa loboi B48.0
　local, skin (staphylococcal) (streptococcal)
　　L08.9
　　abscess – code by site under Abscess
　　cellulitis – code by site under Cellulitis
　　specified NEC L08.89
　　ulcer — *see* Ulcer, skin
　Loefflerella mallei A24.0
　lung NEC J98.4
　　atypical Mycobacterium A31.0
　　spirochetal A69.8
　　tuberculous — *see* Tuberculosis, pulmonary
　　virus — *see* Pneumonia, viral
　lymph gland — *see also* Lymphadenitis, acute
　　mesenteric I88.0
　lymphoid tissue, base of tongue or posterior
　　pharynx, NEC (chronic) J35.03
　Madurella (grisea) (mycetomii) B47.0
　major
　　following ectopic or molar pregnancy O08.0
　　puerperal, postpartum, childbirth O85
　Malassezia furfur B36.0
　Malleomyces
　　mallei A24.0
　　pseudomallei (whitmori) — *see* Melioidosis
　mammary gland N61
　Mansonella (ozzardi) (perstans) (streptocerca)
　　B74.4
　mastoid — *see* Mastoiditis
　maxilla, maxillary M27.2
　　sinus (chronic) — *see* Sinusitis, maxillary
　mediastinum J98.5
　Medina (worm) B72
　meibomian cyst or gland — *see* Hordeolum
　meninges — *see* Meningitis, bacterial
　meningococcal (*see also* condition) A39.9
　　adrenals A39.1
　　brain A39.81
　　cerebrospinal A39.0
　　conjunctiva A39.89
　　endocardium A39.51
　　heart A39.50
　　　endocardium A39.51
　　　myocardium A39.52
　　　pericardium A39.53
　　joint A39.83
　　meninges A39.0

Infection, infected, infective — *continued*
  meningococcal (*see also* condition) — *continued*
    meningococcemia A39.4
      acute A39.2
      chronic A39.3
    myocardium A39.52
    pericardium A39.53
    retrobulbar neuritis A39.82
    specified site NEC A39.89
  mesenteric lymph nodes or glands NEC I88.0
  Metagonimus B66.8
  metatarsophalangeal M00.9
  Microsporum, microsporic — *see* Dermatophytosis
  mixed flora (bacterial) NEC A49.8
  Monilia — *see* Candidiasis
  Monosporium apiospermum B48.2
  mouth, parasitic B37.0
  Mucor — *see* Mucormycosis
  muscle NEC — *see* Myositis, infective
  mycelium NOS B49
  mycetoma
    actinomycotic NEC B47.1
    mycotic NEC B47.0
  Mycobacterium, mycobacterial — *see* Mycobacterium
  Mycoplasma NEC A49.3
    pneumoniae, as cause of disease classified elsewhere B96.0
  mycotic NOS B49
    pathogenic to compromised host only B48.8
    skin NOS B36.9
  myocardium NEC I40.0
  nail (chronic) — *see also* Cellulitis, digit
    with lymphangitis — *see* Lymphangitis, acute, digit
    finger fungus B35.1
    ingrowing L60.0
    toe fungus B35.1
  nasal sinus (chronic) — *see* Sinusitis
  nasopharynx — *see* Nasopharyngitis
  navel L08.82
    newborn P38
  Necator americanus B76.1
  Neisseria — *see* Gonococcus
  Neotestudina rosatii B47.0
  newborn P39.9
    skin P39.4
    specified type NEC P39.8
  nipple N61
    associated with
      lactation O91.03
      pregnancy O91.019
        first trimester O91.011
        second trimester O91.012
        third trimester O91.013
      puerperium O91.02
  Nocardia — *see* Nocardiosis
  obstetrical surgical wound (puerperal) O86.0
  Oesophagostomum (apiostomum) B81.8
  Oestrus ovis — *see* Myiasis
  Oidium albicans B37.9
  Onchocerca (volvulus) — *see* Onchocerciasis
  oncovirus, as cause of disease classified elsewhere B97.32
  operation wound T81.4
  Opisthorchis (felineus) (viverrini) B66.0
  orbit, orbital — *see* Inflammation, orbit
  orthopoxvirus NEC B08.0
  ovary — *see* Salpingo-oophoritis
  Oxyuris vermicularis B80
  pancreas (acute) K85.8
    abscess K85.0
  papillomavirus, as cause of disease classified elsewhere B97.7
  papovavirus NEC B34.4
  Paracoccidioides brasiliensis — *see* Paracoccidioidomycosis
  Paragonimus (westermani) B66.4
  parainfluenza virus B34.8
  parameningococcus NOS A39.9
  parasitic B89
  Parastrongylus
    cantonensis B83.2
    costaricensis B81.3

Infection, infected, infective — *continued*
  Parastrongylus — *continued*
    parathyroid A01.4
      Type A A01.1
      Type B A01.2
      Type C A01.3
  paraurethral ducts N34.2
  parotid gland — *see* Sialoadenitis
  parvovirus NEC B34.3
    as cause of disease classified elsewhere B97.6
  Pasteurella NEC A28.0
    multocida A28.0
    pestis — *see* Plague
    pseudotuberculosis A28.0
    septica (cat bite) (dog bite) A28.0
    tularensis — *see* Tularemia
  pelvic, female — *see* Disease, pelvis, inflammatory
  Penicillium (marneffei) B48.4
  penis (glans) (retention) NEC N48.29
  periapical K04.5
  peridental, periodontal K05.2
  perinatal period P39.9
    specified type NEC P39.8
  perineal repair (puerperal) O86.0
  periorbital — *see* Inflammation, orbit
  perirectal K62.8
  perirenal — *see* Infection, kidney
  peritoneal — *see* Peritonitis
  periureteral N28.89
  Petriellidium boydii B48.2
  pharynx — *see also* Pharyngitis
    coxsackievirus B08.5
    posterior, lymphoid (chronic) J35.03
  Phialophora
    gougerotii (subcutaneous abscess or cyst) B43.2
    jeanselmei (subcutaneous abscess or cyst) B43.2
    verrucosa (skin) B43.0
  Piedraia hortae B36.3
  pinta A67.9
    intermediate A67.1
    late A67.2
    mixed A67.3
    primary A67.0
  pinworm B80
  pityrosporum furfur B36.0
  pleuro-pneumonia-like organism (PPLO) NEC A49.8
    as cause of disease classified elsewhere B96.0
  pneumococcus, pneumococcal NEC A49.1
    as cause of disease classified elsewhere B95.3
    generalized (purulent) A40.3
      with pneumonia J13
  Pneumocystis carinii (pneumonia) B59
  postoperative wound T81.4
  post-traumatic NEC T79.3
  postvaccinal T88.0
  prepuce NEC N47.7
    with penile inflammation N47.6
  prion — *see* Disease, prion
  prostate (capsule) — *see* Prostatitis
  Proteus (mirabilis) (morganii) (vulgaris) NEC A49.8
    as cause of disease classified elsewhere B96.4
  protozoal B64
    intestinal A07.9
    specified NEC A07.8
  Pseudoallescheria boydii B48.2
  Pseudomonas NEC A49.8
    as cause of disease classified elsewhere B96.5
    mallei A24.0
    pneumonia J15.1
    pseudomallei — *see* Melioidosis
  puerperal O86.4
    genitourinary tract NEC O86.8
    major or generalized O85
    minor O86.4
    specified NEC O86.8
  pulmonary — *see* Infection, lung
  purulent — *see* Abscess

Infection, infected, infective — *continued*
  pyemic — *see* Septicemia
  Pyrenochaeta romeroi B47.0
  Q fever A78
  rectum (sphincter) K62.8
  renal — *see also* Infection, kidney
    pelvis and ureter (cystic) N28.85
  reovirus, as cause of disease classified elsewhere B97.5
  respiratory (tract) NEC J98.8
    acute J22
    chronic J98.8
    influenzal (upper) (acute) J10.1
    lower (acute) J22
      chronic — *see* Bronchitis, chronic
    rhinovirus J00
    syncytial virus, as cause of disease classified elsewhere B97.4
    upper (acute) NOS J06.9
      chronic J39.8
      streptococcal J06.9
    viral NOS J06.9
  resulting from
    presence of internal prosthesis, implant, graft — *see* Complications, by site and type, infection
  retortamoniasis A07.8
  retrovirus B33.3
    as cause of disease classified elsewhere B97.30
    human
      immunodeficiency, type 2 [HIV 2] B97.35
      T-cell lymphotropic
        type I [HTLV-I] B97.33
        type II [HTLV-II] B97.34
    lentivirus B97.31
    oncovirus B97.32
    specified NEC B97.39
  Rhinosporidium (*seeberi*) B48.1
  rhinovirus
    as cause of disease classified elsewhere B97.8
    unspecified nature or site B34.8
  Rhizopus — *see* Mucormycosis
  rickettsial NOS A79.9
  roundworm (large) NOS — *see* Ascariasis
  rubella — *see* Rubella
  Saccharomyces — *see* Candidiasis
  salivary duct or gland (any) — *see* Sialoadenitis
  Salmonella (aertrycke) (arizonae) (callinarum) (choleraesuis) (enteritidis) (suipestifer) (typhimurium) A02.9
    with
      (gastro)enteritis A02.0
      septicemia A02.1
      specified manifestation NEC A02.8
    congenital P39.8
    due to food (poisoning) A02.9
    hirschfeldii A01.3
    localized A02.20
      arthritis A02.23
      meningitis A02.21
      osteomyelitis A02.24
      pneumonia A02.22
      pyelonephritis A02.25
      specified NEC A02.29
    paratyphi A01.4
      A A01.1
      B A01.2
      C A01.3
    schottmuelleri A01.2
    typhi, typhosa — *see* Typhoid
  Sarcocystis A07.8
  scabies B86
  Schistosoma — *see* Infestation, Schistosoma
  scrotum (acute) NEC N49.2
  secondary, burn T79.3
  seminal vesicle — *see* Vesiculitis
  septic
    generalized — *see* Septicemia
    localized, skin — *see* Abscess
  septicemic — *see* Septicemia
  sheep liver fluke B66.3
  Shigella A03.9
    boydii A03.2
    dysenteriae A03.0

©2002 Ingenix, Inc.

Infection, infected, infective — *continued*
　Shigella — *continued*
　　flexneri A03.1
　　group
　　　A A03.0
　　　B A03.1
　　　C A03.2
　　　D A03.3
　　Schmitz (-Stutzer) A03.0
　　schmitzii A03.0
　　shigae A03.0
　　sonnei A03.3
　　specified NEC A03.8
　sinus (accessory) (chronic) (nasal) — *see also*
　　　Sinusitis
　　pilonidal — *see* Sinus, pilonidal
　　skin NEC L08.89
　Skene's duct or gland — *see* Urethritis
　skin (local) (staphylococcal) (streptococcal)
　　　L08.9
　　abscess – code by site under Abscess
　　cellulitis – code by site under Cellulitis
　　due to fungus B36.9
　　　specified type NEC B36.8
　　mycotic B36.9
　　　specified type NEC B36.8
　　newborn P39.4
　　ulcer — *see* Ulcer, skin
　slow virus A81.9
　　specified NEC A81.8
　Sparganum (mansoni) (proliferum) (baxteri)
　　　B70.1
　specific — *see also* Syphilis
　　to perinatal period — *see* Infection,
　　　congenital
　specified NEC B99.8
　spermatic cord NEC N49.1
　sphenoidal (sinus) — *see* Sinusitis, sphenoidal
　spinal cord NOS (*see also* Myelitis) G04.9
　　abscess G06.1
　　meninges — *see* Meningitis
　　streptococcal G04.8
　Spirillum A25.0
　spirochetal NOS A69.9
　　lung A69.8
　　specified NEC A69.8
　Spirometra larvae B70.1
　spleen D73.8
　Sporotrichum, Sporothrix (schenckii) — *see*
　　　Sporotrichosis
　staphylococcal NEC A49.0
　　as cause of disease classified elsewhere
　　　B95.8
　　food poisoning A05.0
　　generalized (purulent) A41.2
　　pneumonia — *see* Pneumonia,
　　　staphylococcal
　Stellantchasmus falcatus B66.8
　streptobacillus moniliformis A25.1
　streptococcal NEC A49.1
　　as cause of disease classified elsewhere
　　　B95.5
　　B genitourinary complicating
　　　childbirth O98.82
　　　pregnancy O98.819
　　　　first trimester O98.811
　　　　second trimester O98.812
　　　　third trimester O98.813
　　　puerperium O98.83
　　congenital P39.8
　　　sepsis P36.1
　　　　group B P36.0
　　generalized (purulent) A40.9
　Streptomyces B47.1
　Strongyloides (stercoralis) — *see*
　　　Strongyloidiasis
　stump (amputation) (surgical) — *see*
　　　Complication, amputation stump,
　　　infection
　subcutaneous tissue, local L08.9
　suipestifer — *see* Infection, salmonella
　swimming pool bacillus A31.1
　systemic — *see* Septicemia
　Taenia — *see* Infestation, Taenia
　Taeniarhynchus saginatus B68.1
　tapeworm — *see* Infestation, tapeworm

Infection, infected, infective — *continued*
　tendon (sheath) — *see* Tenosynovitis, infective
　　　NEC
　Ternidens diminutus B81.8
　testis — *see* Orchitis
　threadworm B80
　throat — *see* Pharyngitis
　thyroglossal duct K14.8
　toe (skin) L08.9
　　cellulitis (with lymphangitis), fungus B35.1
　　nail fungus B35.1
　tongue NEC K14.0
　　parasitic B37.0
　tonsil (and adenoid) (faucial) (lingual)
　　　(pharyngeal) — *see* Tonsillitis
　tooth, teeth K04.7
　　periapical K04.7
　　peridental, periodontal K05.2
　　pulp K04.0
　　socket M27.3
　Torula histolytica — *see* Cryptococcosis
　Toxocara (canis) (cati) (felis) B83.0
　Toxoplasma gondii — *see* Toxoplasma
　trachea, chronic J42
　traumatic NEC T79.3
　trematode NEC — *see* Infestation, fluke
　trench fever A79.0
　Treponema pallidum — *see* Syphilis
　Trichinella (spiralis) B75
　Trichomonas A59.9
　　cervix A59.09
　　intestine A07.8
　　prostate A59.02
　　specified site NEC A59.8
　　urethra A59.03
　　urogenitalis A59.00
　　vagina A59.01
　　vulva A59.01
　Trichophyton, trichophytic — *see*
　　　Dermatophytosis
　Trichosporon (beigelii) cutaneum B36.2
　Trichostrongylus B81.2
　Trichuris (trichiura) B79
　Trombicula (irritans) B88.0
　Trypanosoma
　　brucei
　　　gambiense B56.0
　　　rhodesiense B56.1
　　cruzi — *see* Chagas' disease
　tubal — *see* Salpingo-oophoritis
　tuberculous NEC — *see* Tuberculosis
　tubo-ovarian — *see* Salpingo-oophoritis
　tunica vaginalis N49.1
　tympanic membrane NEC — *see* Myringitis
　typhoid (abortive) (ambulant) (bacillus) — *see*
　　　Typhoid
　typhus A75.9
　　flea-borne A75.2
　　mite-borne A75.3
　　recrudescent A75.1
　　tick-borne A77.9
　　　African A77.1
　　　North Asian A77.2
　umbilicus L08.82
　　newborn P38
　ureter N28.86
　urethra — *see* Urethritis
　urinary (tract) N39.0
　　bladder — *see* Cystitis
　　complicating
　　　abortion — *see* Abortion, by type,
　　　　complicated by infection, urinary
　　　　tract
　　　pregnancy O23.40
　　　　first trimester O23.41
　　　　second trimester O23.42
　　　　specified type NEC O23.30
　　　　　first trimester O23.31
　　　　　second trimester O23.32
　　　　　third trimester O23.33
　　　　third trimester O23.43
　　kidney — *see* Infection, kidney
　　newborn P39.3
　　puerperal (postpartum) O86.20
　　tuberculous A18.13
　　urethra — *see* Urethritis
　uterus, uterine — *see* Endometritis

Infection, infected, infective — *continued*
　vaccination T88.0
　vagina (acute) — *see* Vaginitis
　varicella B01.9
　varicose veins — *see* Varix
　vas deferens NEC N49.1
　vesical — *see* Cystitis
　Vibrio
　　cholerae A00.0
　　　El Tor A00.1
　　parahaemolyticus (food poisoning) A05.3
　Vincent's (gum) (mouth) (tonsil) A69.1
　virus, viral NOS B34.9
　　adenovirus
　　　as cause of disease classified elsewhere
　　　　B97.0
　　　unspecified nature or site B34.0
　　arborvirus, arbovirus arthropod-borne A94
　　as cause of disease classified elsewhere
　　　B97.8
　　　adenovirus B97.0
　　　coronavirus B97.2
　　　coxsackievirus B97.11
　　　echovirus B97.12
　　　enterovirus B97.10
　　　　coxsackievirus B97.11
　　　　echovirus B97.12
　　　　specified NEC B97.19
　　　human
　　　　immunodeficiency, type 2 [HIV 2]
　　　　　B97.35
　　　　T-cell lymphotropic,
　　　　　type I [HTLV-I] B97.33
　　　　　type II [HTLV-II] B97.34
　　　papillomavirus B97.7
　　　parvovirus B97.6
　　　reovirus B97.5
　　　respiratory syncytial B97.4
　　　retrovirus B97.30
　　　　human
　　　　　immunodeficiency, type 2 [HIV 2]
　　　　　　B97.35
　　　　　T-cell lymphotropic,
　　　　　　type I [HTLV-I] B97.33
　　　　　　type II [HTLV-II] B97.34
　　　　lentivirus B97.31
　　　　oncovirus B97.32
　　　　specified NEC B97.39
　　　specified NEC B97.8
　　central nervous system A89
　　　atypical A81.9
　　　　specified NEC A81.8
　　　enterovirus NEC A88.8
　　　　meningitis A87.0
　　　slow virus A81.9
　　　　specified NEC A81.8
　　　specified NEC A88.8
　　chest J98.8
　　coxsackie — *see also* Infection, coxsackie
　　　B34.1
　　　as cause of disease classified elsewhere
　　　　B97.11
　　ECHO
　　　as cause of disease classified elsewhere
　　　　B97.12
　　　unspecified nature or site B34.1
　　encephalitis, tick-borne A84.9
　　enterovirus, as cause of disease classified
　　　elsewhere B97.10
　　　coxsackievirus B97.11
　　　echovirus B97.12
　　　specified NEC B97.19
　　exanthem NOS B09
　　human papilloma as cause of disease
　　　classified elsewhere B97.7
　　intestine — *see* Enteritis, viral
　　respiratory syncytial
　　　as cause of disease classified elsewhere
　　　　B97.4
　　　bronchopneumonia J12.1
　　　common cold syndrome J00
　　　nasopharyngitis (acute) J00
　　rhinovirus
　　　as cause of disease classified elsewhere
　　　　B97.8
　　　unspecified nature or site B34.8

Infection, infected, infective — continued
- virus, viral NOS — continued
  - slow A81.9
    - specified NEC A81.8
  - specified type NEC
    - as cause of disease classified elsewhere B97.8
    - unspecified nature or site B34.8
  - unspecified nature or site B34.9
- vulva (acute) — see Vulvitis
- whipworm B79
- worms B83.9
  - specified type NEC B83.8
- wound (local) (post-traumatic) NEC T79.3
  - with
    - open wound – code as Wound, open
  - postoperative T81.4
  - surgical T81.4
- Wuchereria (bancrofti) B74.0
  - malayi B74.1
- yeast — see Candidiasis
- yellow fever — see Fever, yellow
- Yersinia
  - enterocolitica (intestinal) A04.6
  - pestis — see Plague
  - pseudotuberculosis A28.2
- Zeis' gland — see Hordeolum
- zoonotic bacterial NOS A28.9
- Zopfia senegalensis B47.0

Infective, infectious — see condition

Infertility
- female N97.9
  - associated with
    - anovulation N97.0
    - cervical (mucus) disease or anomaly N97.3
    - congenital anomaly
      - cervix N97.3
      - fallopian tube N97.1
      - uterus N97.2
      - vagina N97.8
    - dysmucorrhea N97.3
    - fallopian tube disease or anomaly N97.1
    - male factors N97.8
    - pituitary-hypothalamic origin E23.0
    - specified origin NEC N97.8
    - Stein-Leventhal syndrome E28.2
    - uterine disease or anomaly N97.2
    - vaginal disease or anomaly N97.8
  - due to
    - cervical anomaly N97.3
    - fallopian tube anomaly N97.1
    - ovarian failure E28.3
    - Stein-Leventhal syndrome E28.2
    - uterine anomaly N97.2
    - vaginal anomaly N97.3
  - nonimplantation N97.2
  - origin
    - cervical N97.3
    - tubal (block) (occlusion) (stenosis) N97.1
    - uterine N97.2
    - vaginal N97.3
  - previous, requiring supervision of pregnancy O09.00
    - first trimester O09.01
    - second trimester O09.02
    - third trimester O09.03
- male N46.9
  - azoospermia N46.01
    - extratesticular cause N46.029
      - drug therapy N46.021
      - efferent duct obstruction N46.023
      - infection N46.022
      - radiation N46.024
      - specified cause NEC N46.029
      - systemic disease N46.025
  - oligospermia N46.11
    - extratesticular cause N46.129
      - drug therapy N46.121
      - efferent duct obstruction N46.123
      - infection N46.122
      - radiation N46.124
      - specified cause NEC N46.129
      - systemic disease N46.125
  - specified type NEC N46.8
- relative N96

Infestation B88.9
- Acanthocheilonema (perstans) (streptocerca) B74.4
- Acariasis B88.0
  - demodex folliculorum B88.0
  - sarcoptes scabiei B86
  - trombiculae B88.0
- Agamofilaria streptocerca B74.4
- Ancylostoma, ankylostoma (braziliense) (caninum) (ceylanicum) (duodenale) B76.0
  - americanum B76.1
  - new world B76.1
- Anisakis larvae, anisakiasis B81.0
- arthropod NEC B88.2
- Ascaris lumbricoides — see Ascariasis
- Balantidium coli A07.0
- beef tapeworm B68.1
- Bothriocephalus (latus) B70.0
  - larval B70.1
- broad tapeworm B70.0
  - larval B70.1
- Brugia (malayi) B74.1
  - timori B74.2
- candiru B88.8
- Capillaria
  - hepatica B83.8
  - philippinensis B81.1
- cat liver fluke B66.0
- cestodes B71.9
  - diphyllobothrium — see Infestation, diphyllobothrium
  - dipylidiasis B71.1
  - hymenolepiasis B71.0
  - specified type NEC B71.8
- chigger B88.0
- chigo, chigoe B88.1
- Clonorchis (sinensis) (liver) B66.1
- coccidial A07.3
- crab-lice B85.3
- Cysticercus cellulosae — see Cysticercosis
- Demodex (folliculorum) B88.0
- Dermanyssus gallinae B88.0
- Dermatobia (hominis) — see Myiasis
- Dibothriocephalus (latus) B70.0
  - larval B70.1
- Dicrocoelium dendriticum B66.2
- Diphyllobothrium (adult) (latum) (intestinal) (pacificum) B70.0
  - larval B70.1
- Diplogonoporus (grandis) B71.8
- Dipylidium caninum B71.1
- Distoma hepaticum B66.3
- dog tapeworm B71.1
- Dracunculus medinensis B72
- dragon worm B72
- dwarf tapeworm B71.0
- Echinococcus — see Echinococcus
- Echinostomum ilocanum B66.8
- Entamoeba (histolytica) — see Infection, Ameba
- Enterobius vermicularis B80
- eyelid
  - in (due to)
    - leishmaniasis B55.1
    - loiasis B74.3
    - onchocerciasis B73.00
    - phthiriasis B85.3
  - parasitic NOS B89
- eyeworm B74.3
- Fasciola (gigantica) (hepatica) (indica) B66.3
- Fasciolopsis (buski) (intestine) B66.5
- filarial B74.9
  - bancroftian B74.0
  - conjunctiva B74.3
  - due to
    - Acanthocheilonema (perstans) (streptocerca) B74.4
    - Brugia (malayi) B74.1
      - timori B74.2
    - Dracunculus medinensis B72
    - guinea worm B72
    - loa loa B74.3
    - Mansonella (ozzardi) (perstans) (streptocerca) B74.4
    - Onchocerca volvulus B73.00
      - eye B73.00
      - eyelid B73.09
    - Wuchereria (bancrofti) B74.0

Infestation — continued
- filarial — continued
  - Malayan B74.1
  - ozzardi B74.4
  - specified type NEC B74.8
- fish tapeworm B70.0
  - larval B70.1
- fluke B66.9
  - blood NOS — see Schistosomiasis
  - cat liver B66.0
  - intestinal B66.5
  - liver (sheep) B66.3
    - cat B66.0
    - Chinese B66.1
    - due to clonorchiasis B66.1
    - oriental B66.1
  - lancet B66.2
  - lung (oriental) B66.4
  - sheep liver B66.3
  - specified type NEC B66.8
- fly larvae — see Myiasis
- Gasterophilus (intestinalis) — see Myiasis
- Gastrodiscoides hominis B66.8
- Giardia lamblia A07.1
- Gnathostoma (spinigerum) B83.1
- Gongylonema B83.8
- guinea worm B72
- helminth B83.9
  - angiostrongyliasis B83.2
    - intestinal B81.3
  - gnathostomiasis B83.1
  - hirudiniasis, internal B83.4
  - intestinal B82.0
    - angiostrongyliasis B81.3
    - anisakiasis B81.0
    - ascariasis — see Ascariasis
    - capillariasis B81.1
    - cysticercosis — see Cysticercosis
    - diphyllobothriasis — see Infestation, diphyllobothriasis
    - dracunculiasis B72
    - echinococcus — see Echinococcosis
    - enterobiasis B80
  - filariasis — see Infestation, filarial
  - fluke — see Infestation, fluke
  - hookworm — see Infestation, hookworm
  - mixed (types classifiable to more than one of the titles B65.0-B81.3 and B81.8) B81.4
  - onchocerciasis — see Onchocerciasis
  - schistosomiasis — see Infestation, schistosoma
  - specified
    - cestode NEC — see Infestation, cestode
    - type NEC B81.8
  - strongyloidiasis — see Strongyloidiasis
  - taenia — see Infestation, taenia
  - trichinellosis B75
  - trichostrongyliasis B81.2
  - trichuriasis B79
  - specified type NEC B83.8
  - syngamiasis B83.3
  - visceral larva migrans B83.0
- Heterophyes (heterophyes) B66.8
- hookworm B76.9
  - ancylostomiasis B76.0
  - necatoriasis B76.1
  - specified type NEC B76.8
- Hymenolepis (diminuta) (nana) B71.0
- intestinal NEC B82.9
- leeches (aquatic) (land) — see Hirudiniasis
- Leishmania — see Leishmaniasis
- lice, louse — see Infestation, Pediculus
- Linguatula B88.8
- Liponyssoides sanguineus B88.0
- Loa loa B74.3
  - conjunctival B74.3
  - eyelid B74.3
- louse — see Infestation, Pediculus
- maggots — see Myiasis
- Mansonella (ozzardi) (perstans) (streptocerca) B74.4
- Medina (worm) B72
- Metagonimus (yokogawai) B66.8
- microfilaria streptocerca B74.4
  - eye B73.00

©2002 Ingenix, Inc.

Infestation — *continued*
  microfilaria streptocerca — *continued*
    eyelid B73.09
  mites B88.9
    scabic B86
  Monilia (albicans) — *see* Candidiasis
  mouth B37.0
  Necator americanus B76.1
  nematode NEC (intestinal) B82.0
    Ancylostoma B76.0
    conjunctiva NEC B83.9
    Enterobius vermicularis B80
    Gnathostoma spinigerum B83.1
    intestinal NEC B81.8
    physaloptera B80
    trichostrongylus B81.2
    trichuris (trichuria) B79
  Oesophagostomum (apiostomum) B81.8
  Oestrus ovis (*see also* Myiasis) B87.9
  Onchocerca (volvulus) — *see* Onchocerciasis
  Opisthorchis (felineus) (viverrini) B66.0
  orbit, parasitic NOS B89
  Oxyuris vermicularis B80
  Paragonimus (westermani) B66.4
  parasite, parasitic B89
    eyelid B89
    intestinal NOS B82.9
    mouth B37.0
    skin B88.9
    tongue B37.0
  Parastrongylus
    cantonensis B83.2
    costaricensis B81.3
  Pediculus B85.2
    body B85.1
    capitis (humanus) (any site) B85.0
    corporis (humanus) (any site) B85.1
    head B85.0
    mixed (classifiable to more than one of the titles B85.0-B85.3) B85.4
    pubis (any site) B85.3
  Pentastoma B88.8
  Phthirus (pubis) (any site) B85.3
    with any infestation classifiable to B85.0-B85.2 B85.4
  pinworm B80
  pork tapeworm (adult) B68.0
  protozoal NEC B88.8
  pubic, louse B85.3
  rat tapeworm B71.0
  red bug B88.0
  roundworm (large) NOS — *see* Ascariasis
  sandflea B88.1
  Sarcoptes scabiei B86
  scabies B86
  Schistosoma B65.9
    bovis B65.8
    cercariae B65.3
    haematobium B65.0
    intercalatum B65.8
    japonicum B65.2
    mansoni B65.1
    mattheei B65.8
    mekongi B65.8
    specified type NEC B65.8
    spindale B65.8
  screw worms — *see* Myiasis
  skin NOS B88.9
  Sparganum (mansoni) (proliferum) (baxteri) B70.1
    larval B70.1
  specified type NEC B88.8
  Spirometra larvae B70.1
  Stellantchasmus falcatus B66.8
  Strongyloides stercoralis — *see* Strongyloidiasis
  Taenia B68.9
    diminuta B71.0
    echinococcus — *see* Echinococcus
    mediocanellata B68.1
    nana B71.0
    saginata B68.1
    solium (intestinal form) B68.0
      larval form — *see* Cysticercosis
  Taeniarhynchus saginatus B68.1
  tapeworm B71.9
    beef B68.1
    broad B70.0
      larval B70.1

Infestation — *continued*
  tapeworm — *continued*
    dog B71.1
    dwarf B71.0
    fish B70.0
      larval B70.1
    pork B68.0
    rat B71.0
  Ternidens diminutus B81.8
  Tetranychus molestissimus B88.0
  threadworm B80
  tongue B37.0
  Toxocara (canis) (cati) (felis) B83.0
  trematode(s) NEC — *see* Infestation, fluke
  Trichinella (spiralis) B75
  Trichocephalus B79
  Trichomonas — *see* Trichomoniasis
  Trichostrongylus B81.2
  Trichuris (trichiura) B79
  Trombicula (irritans) B88.0
  Tunga penetrans B88.1
  Uncinaria americana B76.1
  Vandellia cirrhosa B88.8
  whipworm B79
  worms B83.9
    intestinal B82.0
  Wuchereria (bancrofti) B74.0

Infiltrate, infiltration
  amyloid (generalized) (localized) — *see* Amyloidosis
  calcareous NEC R89.7
    localized — *see* Degeneration, by site
  calcium salt R89.7
  cardiac
    fatty — *see* Degeneration, myocardial
    glycogenic E74.02
  corneal — *see* Edema, cornea
  eyelid — *see* Inflammation, eyelid
  glycogen, glycogenic — *see* Disease, glycogen storage
  heart, cardiac
    fatty — *see* Degeneration, myocardial
    glycogenic E74.02 *[I43]*
  inflammatory in vitreous H43.89
  kidney N28.89
  leukemic (M9800/3) — *see* Leukemia
  liver K76.8
    fatty — *see* Fatty, liver NEC
    glycogen (*see also* Disease, glycogen storage) E74.03 *[K77]*
  lung (eosinophilic) J82
  lymphatic (M9820/3) (*see also* Leukemia, lymphatic) C91.90
    gland I88.9
  muscle, fatty M62.89
  myocardium, myocardial
    fatty — *see* Degeneration, myocardial
    glycogenic E74.02 *[I43]*
  pulmonary J82
    with eosinophilia J82
  thymus (gland) (fatty) E32.8
  urine R39.0
  vitreous body H43.89

Infirmity R68.8
  senile R54

Inflammation, inflamed, inflammatory (with exudation)
  abducent (nerve) — *see* Strabismus, paralytic, sixth nerve
  accessory sinus (chronic) — *see* Sinusitis
  adrenal (gland) E27.8
  alveoli, teeth M27.3
    scorbutic E54 *[K93]*
  anal canal, anus K62.8
  antrum (chronic) — *see* Sinusitis, maxillary
  appendix — *see* Appendicitis
  arachnoid — *see* Meningitis
  areola N61
    puerperal, postpartum or gestational — *see* Infection, nipple
  areolar tissue NOS L08.9
  artery — *see* Arteritis
  auditory meatus (external) — *see* Otitis, externa
  Bartholin's gland N75.8
  bile duct (common) (hepatic) or passage — *see* Cholangitis

Inflammation, inflamed, inflammatory — *continued*
  bladder — *see* Cystitis
  bone — *see* Osteomyelitis
  brain — *see also* Encephalitis
    membrane — *see* Meningitis
  breast N61
    puerperal, postpartum, gestational — *see* Mastitis, obstetric
  broad ligament — *see* Disease, pelvis, inflammatory
  bronchi — *see* Bronchitis
  catarrhal J00
  cecum — *see* Appendicitis
  cerebral — *see also* Encephalitis
    membrane — *see* Meningitis
  cerebrospinal
    meningococcal A39.0
  cervix (uteri) — *see* Cervicitis
  chest J98.8
  chorioretinal H30.90
    bilateral H30.103
    cyclitis — *see* Cyclitis
    disseminated H30.109
      bilateral H30.103
      generalized H30.139
        bilateral H30.133
        left H30.132
        right H30.131
      left H30.102
      peripheral H30.129
        bilateral H30.123
        left H30.122
        right H30.121
      posterior pole H30.119
        bilateral H30.113
        left H30.112
        right H30.111
      right H30.101
    epitheliopathy — *see* Epitheliopathy
    focal H30.009
      bilateral H30.003
      juxtapapillary H30.019
        bilateral H30.013
        left H30.012
        right H30.011
      left H30.002
      macular H30.049
        bilateral H30.043
        left H30.042
        right H30.041
      paramacular — *see* Inflammation, chorioretinal, focal, macular
      peripheral H30.039
        bilateral H30.033
        left H30.032
        right H30.031
      posterior pole H30.029
        bilateral H30.023
        left H30.022
        right H30.021
      right H30.001
    left H30.92
    right H30.91
    specified type NEC H30.80
      bilateral H30.83
      left H30.82
      right H30.81
  choroid — *see* Inflammation, chorioretinal
  chronic, postmastoidectomy cavity — *see* Complications, postmastoidectomy, inflammation
  colon — *see* Enteritis
  connective tissue (diffuse) NEC — *see* Disorder, soft tissue, specified type NEC
  cornea — *see* Keratitis
  corpora cavernosa N48.29
  cranial nerve — *see* Disorder, nerve, cranial
  Douglas' cul-de-sac or pouch (chronic) N73.0
  due to device, implant or graft — *see also* Complications, by site and type, infection or inflammation
    arterial graft T82.7
    breast (implant) T85.79
    catheter T85.79
      dialysis (renal) T82.7
        intraperitoneal T85.71

Inflammation, inflamed, inflammatory —
continued
  due to device, implant or graft — *see also*
    Complications, by site and type, infection
    or inflammation — *continued*
    catheter — *continued*
      infusion T82.7
        spinal (epidural) (subdural) T85.79
        urinary (indwelling) T83.51
      electronic (electrode) (pulse generator)
        (stimulator)
        bone T84.7
        cardiac T82.7
        nervous system (brain) (peripheral nerve)
          (spinal) T85.79
        urinary T83.59
    fixation, internal (orthopedic) NEC — *see*
      Complication, fixation device, infection
    gastrointestinal (bile duct) (esophagus)
      T85.79
    genital NEC T83.6
    heart NEC T82.7
      valve (prosthesis) T82.6
      graft T82.7
    joint prosthesis — *see* Complication, joint
      prosthesis, infection
    ocular (corneal graft) (orbital implant) NEC
      T85.79
    orthopedic NEC T84.7
    specified NEC T85.79
    urinary NEC T83.59
    vascular NEC T82.7
    ventricular intracranial shunt T85.79
  duodenum K29.80
    with bleeding K29.81
  dura mater — *see* Meningitis
  ear (middle) — *see also* Otitis, media
    external — *see* Otitis, externa
    inner — *see* category H83.0
  epididymis — *see* Epididymitis
  esophagus K20
  ethmoidal (sinus) (chronic) — *see* Sinusitis,
    ethmoidal
  eustachian tube (catarrhal) — *see* Salpingitis,
    eustachian
  eyelid H01.9
    abscess — *see* Abscess, eyelid
    blepharitis — *see* Blepharitis
    chalazion — *see* Chalazion
    dermatosis (noninfectious) — *see*
      Dermatosis, eyelid
    hordeolum — *see* Hordeolum
    specified NEC H01.8
  fallopian tube — *see* Salpingo-oophoritis
  fascia — *see* Myositis
  follicular, pharynx J31.2
  frontal (sinus) (chronic) — *see* Sinusitis, frontal
  gallbladder — *see* Cholecystitis
  gastric — *see* Gastritis
  gastrointestinal — *see* Enteritis
  genital organ (internal) (diffuse)
    female — *see* Disease, pelvis, inflammatory
    male N49.9
      multiple sites N49.8
      specified NEC N49.8
  gland (lymph) — *see* Lymphadenitis
  glottis — *see* Laryngitis
  granular, pharynx J31.2
  gum K05.1
  heart — *see* Carditis
  hepatic duct — *see* Cholangitis
  ileum — *see also* Enteritis
    regional or terminal — *see* Enteritis, regional
  intestine (any part) — *see* Enteritis
  jaw (acute) (bone) (chronic) (lower) (suppurative)
    (upper) M27.2
  joint NEC — *see* Arthritis
    sacroiliac M46.1
  kidney — *see* Nephritis
  knee (joint) M13.169
    tuberculous A18.02
  labium (majus) (minus) — *see* Vulvitis
  lacrimal
    gland — *see* Dacryoadenitis
    passages (duct) (sac) — *see also*
      Dacryocystitis
      canaliculitis — *see* Canaliculitis, lacrimal

Inflammation, inflamed, inflammatory —
continued
  larynx — *see* Laryngitis
  leg NOS L08.9
  lip K13.0
  liver (capsule) — *see also* Hepatitis
    chronic K73.9
    suppurative K75.0
  lung (acute) — *see also* Pneumonia
    chronic J98.4
  lymph gland or node — *see* Lymphadenitis
  lymphatic vessel — *see* Lymphangitis
  maxilla, maxillary M27.2
    sinus (chronic) — *see* Sinusitis, maxillary
  membranes of brain or spinal cord — *see*
    Meningitis
  meninges — *see* Meningitis
  mouth K12.1
  muscle — *see* Myositis
  myocardium — *see* Myocarditis
  nasal sinus (chronic) — *see* Sinusitis
  nasopharynx — *see* Nasopharyngitis
  navel L08.82
    newborn P38
  nerve NEC — *see* Neuralgia
  nipple N61
    puerperal, postpartum or gestational — *see*
      Infection, nipple
  nose — *see* Rhinitis
  oculomotor (nerve) — *see* Strabismus,
    paralytic, third nerve
  optic nerve — *see* Neuritis, optic
  orbit (chronic) H05.10
    acute H05.00
      abscess — *see* Abscess, orbit
      cellulitis — *see* Cellulitis, orbit
      osteomyelitis — *see* Osteomyelitis, orbit
      periostitis — *see* Periostitis, orbital
      tenonitis — *see* Tenonitis, eye
    granuloma — *see* Granuloma, orbit
    myositis — *see* Myositis, orbital
  ovary — *see* Salpingo-oophoritis
  oviduct — *see* Salpingo-oophoritis
  pancreas (acute) — *see* Pancreatitis
  parametrium N73.0
  parotid region L08.9
  pelvis, female — *see* Disease, pelvis,
    inflammatory
  penis (corpora cavernosa) N48.29
  perianal K62.8
  pericardium — *see* Pericarditis
  perineum (female) (male) L08.9
  perirectal K62.8
  peritoneum — *see* Peritonitis
  periuterine — *see* Disease, pelvis, inflammatory
  perivesical — *see* Cystitis
  petrous bone (acute) (chronic) — *see* Petrositis
  pharynx (acute) — *see* Pharyngitis
  pia mater — *see* Meningitis
  pleura — *see* Pleurisy
  prostate — *see also* Prostatitis
    specified type NEC N41.8
  rectosigmoid — *see* Rectosigmoiditis
  rectum (*see also* Proctitis) K62.8
  respiratory, upper (*see also* Infection,
    respiratory, upper) J06.9
    acute, due to radiation J70.8
    chronic, due to external agent — *see*
      condition, respiratory, chronic, due to
    due to
      chemicals, gases, fumes or vapors
        (inhalation) J68.2
      radiation J70.1
  retina — *see* Chorioretinitis
  retrocecal — *see* Appendicitis
  retroperitoneal — *see* Peritonitis
  salivary duct or gland (any) (suppurative) — *see*
    Sialoadenitis
  scorbutic, alveoli, teeth E54 *[K93]*
  scrotum N49.2
  seminal vesicle — *see* Vesiculitis
  sigmoid — *see* Enteritis
  sinus — *see* Sinusitis
  Skene's duct or gland — *see* Urethritis
  skin L08.9
  spermatic cord N49.1
  sphenoidal (sinus) — *see* Sinusitis, sphenoidal

Inflammation, inflamed, inflammatory —
continued
  spinal
    cord — *see* Encephalitis
    membrane — *see* Meningitis
    nerve — *see* Disorder, nerve
  spine — *see* Spondylopathy, inflammatory
  spleen (capsule) D73.8
  stomach — *see* Gastritis
  subcutaneous tissue L08.9
  suprarenal (gland) E27.8
  synovial — *see* Tenosynovitis
  tendon (sheath) NEC — *see* Tenosynovitis
  testis — *see* Orchitis
  throat (acute) — *see* Pharyngitis
  thymus (gland) E32.8
  thyroid (gland) — *see* Thyroiditis
  tongue K14.0
  tonsil — *see* Tonsillitis
  trachea — *see* Tracheitis
  trochlear (nerve) — *see* Strabismus, paralytic,
    fourth nerve
  tubal — *see* Salpingo-oophoritis
  tuberculous NEC — *see* Tuberculosis
  tubo-ovarian — *see* Salpingo-oophoritis
  tunica vaginalis N49.1
  tympanic membrane — *see* Tympanitis
  umbilicus, umbilical L08.82
    newborn P38
  uterine ligament — *see* Disease, pelvis,
    inflammatory
  uterus (catarrhal) — *see* Endometritis
  uveal tract (anterior) NOS — *see also*
    Iridocyclitis
    posterior — *see* Chorioretinitis
  vagina — *see* Vaginitis
  vas deferens N49.1
  vein — *see also* Phlebitis
    intracranial or intraspinal (septic) G08
    thrombotic I80.9
      leg — *see* Phlebitis, leg
      lower extremity — *see* Phlebitis, leg
  vocal cord J38.3
  vulva — *see* Vulvitis
  Wharton's duct (suppurative) — *see*
    Sialoadenitis

Inflation, lung, imperfect (newborn) — *see*
  Atelectasis

Influenza, influenzal (bronchial) (epidemic)
  (respiratory (upper)) J10.1
  with
    digestive manifestations J10.81
    enteritis J10.81
    gastroenteritis J10.81
    involvement of
      gastrointestinal tract J10.81
      nervous system NEC J10.89
    laryngitis J10.1
    manifestations NEC J10.89
    meningismus J10.89
    myocarditis J10.89
    pharyngitis J10.1
    pleural effusion NEC J10.1
    respiratory manifestations NEC J10.1
    upper respiratory infection (acute) NEC
      J10.1
  summer, of Italy A93.1

Influenza-like disease — *see* Influenza

Infraction, Freiberg's (metatarsal head) — *see*
  Osteochondrosis, juvenile, metatarsus

**Infusion complication, misadventure, or
  reaction** — *see* Complications, infusion

Ingestion
  chemical — *see* Table of Drugs and Chemicals
  drug or medicament
    correct substance properly administered
      T88.7
    overdose or wrong substance given or taken
      (by accident) T50.901
      administered with intent to harm by
        another person T50.903
        self T50.902
      circumstances undetermined T50.904
      specified drug — *see* Table of Drugs and
        Chemicals

©2002 Ingenix, Inc.

Ingestion — continued
  foreign body — see Foreign body, alimentary tract
  tularemia A21.3

Ingrowing
  hair (beard) L73.1
  nail (finger) (toe) L60.0

Inguinal — see also condition
  testicle Q53.9
    bilateral Q53.21
    unilateral Q53.11

Inhalation
  anthrax A22.1
  carbon monoxide — see Poisoning, carbon monoxide
  flame T27.3
  food or foreign body — see Asphyxia, food
  gases, fumes, or vapors NEC T59.91
    administered with intent to harm by another person T59.93
      self T59.92
    circumstances undetermined T59.94
    specified agent — see Table of Drugs and Chemicals
  liquid or vomitus — see Asphyxia
  meconium (newborn) P24.0
  mucus — see Asphyxia, mucus
  oil or gasoline (causing suffocation) — see Asphyxia, food
  smoke — see Toxicity, vapors
  steam — see Toxicity, vapors
  stomach contents or secretions — see also Asphyxia, food
    due to anesthesia (general) (local) or other sedation T88.5
    in labor and delivery O74.0
    in pregnancy — see Complications, anesthesia, in, pregnancy, pulmonary
    postpartum, puerperal O89.01

Inhibition, orgasm
  female F52.32
  male F52.31

Inhibitor, systemic lupus erythematosus (presence of) D68.81

Iniencephalus, iniencephaly Q00.2

Injection, traumatic jet (air) (industrial) (water) (paint or dye) T70.4

Injury (see also specified injury type) T14.90
  abdomen, abdominal S39.91
    blood vessel — see Injury, blood vessel, abdomen
    cavity — see Injury, intra-abdominal
    contusion S30.1
    internal — see Injury, intra-abdominal
    intra-abdominal organ — see Injury, intra-abdominal
    nerve — see Injury, nerve, abdomen
    open — see Wound, open, abdomen
    specified NEC S39.81
    superficial — see Injury, superficial, abdomen
  Achilles tendon S86.009
    laceration S86.029
      left S86.022
      right S86.021
    left S86.002
    right S86.001
    specified type NEC S86.099
      left S86.092
      right S86.091
    strain S86.019
      left S86.012
      right S86.011
  acoustic, resulting in deafness — see Injury, nerve, acoustic
  adrenal (gland) S37.819
    contusion S37.812
    laceration S37.813
    specified type NEC S37.818
  alveolar (process) S09.93
  ankle S99.919
    contusion — see Contusion, ankle
    dislocation — see Dislocation, ankle
    fracture — see Fracture, ankle
    left S99.912

Injury (see also specified injury type) — continued
  ankle — continued
    nerve — see Injury, nerve, ankle
    open — see Wound, open, ankle
    right S99.911
    specified type NEC S99.819
      left S99.812
      right S99.811
    sprain — see Sprain, ankle
    superficial — see Injury, superficial, ankle
  anterior chamber, eye — see Injury, eye, specified site NEC
  anus — see Injury, abdomen
  aorta (thoracic) S25.00
    abdominal S35.00
      laceration (minor) (superficial) S35.01
        major S35.02
      specified type NEC S35.09
    laceration (minor) (superficial) S25.01
      major S25.02
    specified type NEC S25.09
  arm (upper) S49.90
    blood vessel — see Injury, blood vessel, arm
    contusion — see Contusion, arm, upper
    fracture — see Fracture, humerus
    left S49.92
    lower — see Injury, forearm
    muscle — see Injury, muscle, shoulder
    nerve — see Injury, nerve, arm
    open — see Wound, open, arm
    right S49.91
    specified type NEC S49.80
      left S49.82
      right S49.81
    superficial — see Injury, superficial, arm
  artery (complicating trauma) — see also Injury, blood vessel, by site
    cerebral or meningeal — see Injury, intracranial
  auditory canal (external) (meatus) S09.91
  auricle, auris, ear S09.91
  axilla — see Injury, shoulder
  back — see Injury, back, lower
  bile duct — see Injury, gallbladder
  birth — see also Birth, injury P15.9
  bladder (sphincter) S37.20
    at delivery O71.5
    contusion S37.22
    laceration S37.23
    obstetrical trauma O71.5
    specified type NEC S37.28
  blast (air) (hydraulic) (immersion) (underwater) NEC T14.90
    acoustic nerve trauma — see Injury, nerve, acoustic
    bladder — see Injury, bladder, blast injury
    brain — see Concussion
    colon — see Injury, intestine, large, blast injury
    ear (primary) S09.319
      bilateral S09.313
      left S09.312
      right S09.311
      secondary S09.399
        left S09.392
        right S09.391
    generalized T70.8
    lung — see Injury, intrathoracic, lung, blast injury
    multiple body organs T70.8
    peritoneum S36.81
    rectum S36.61
    retroperitoneum S36.898
    small intestine S36.419
      duodenum S36.410
      specified site NEC S36.418
    specified
      intra-abdominal organ NEC S36.898
      pelvic organ NEC S37.899
  blood vessel NEC T14.90
    abdomen S35.90
      aorta — see Injury, aorta, abdominal
      celiac artery — see Injury, blood vessel, celiac artery
      iliac vessel — see Injury, blood vessel, iliac
      laceration S35.91

Injury (see also specified injury type) — continued
  blood vessel NEC — continued
    abdomen — continued
      mesenteric vessel — see Injury, mesenteric
      portal vein — see Injury, blood vessel, portal vein
      renal vessel — see Injury, blood vessel, renal
      specified
        site NEC — see category S35.8
        type NEC S35.99
      splenic vessel — see Injury, blood vessel, splenic
      vena cava — see Injury, vena cava, inferior
    ankle — see Injury, blood vessel, foot
    aorta (abdominal) (thoracic) — see Injury, aorta
    arm (upper) NEC S45.909
      forearm — see Injury, blood vessel, forearm
      laceration S45.919
        left S45.912
        right S45.911
      left S45.902
      right S45.901
      specified
        site NEC S45.809
          laceration S45.819
            left S45.812
            right S45.811
          left S45.802
          right S45.801
          specified type NEC S45.899
            left S45.892
            right S45.891
        type NEC S45.999
          left S45.992
          right S45.991
      superficial vein S45.309
        laceration S45.319
          left S45.312
          right S45.311
        left S45.302
        right S45.301
        specified type NEC S45.399
          left S45.392
          right S45.391
    axillary
      artery S45.009
        laceration S45.019
          left S45.012
          right S45.011
        left S45.002
        right S45.001
        specified type NEC S45.099
          left S45.092
          right S45.091
      vein S45.209
        laceration S45.219
          left S45.212
          right S45.211
        left S45.202
        right S45.201
        specified type NEC S45.299
          left S45.292
          right S45.291
    azygos vein — see Injury, blood vessel, thoracic, specified site NEC
    brachial
      artery S45.109
        laceration S45.119
          left S45.112
          right S45.111
        left S45.102
        right S45.101
        specified type NEC S45.199
          left S45.192
          right S45.191
      vein S45.209
        laceration S45.219
          left S45.212
          right S45.211
        left S45.202
        right S45.201

Injury (*see also* specified injury type) — *continued*
blood vessel NEC — *continued*
  brachial — *continued*
    vein — *continued*
      specified type NEC S45.299
        left S45.292
        right S45.291
  carotid artery (common) (external) (internal, extracranial) S15.009
    internal, intracranial S06.8
    laceration (minor) (superficial) S15.019
      left S15.012
      major S15.029
        left S15.022
        right S15.021
      right S15.011
    left S15.002
    right S15.001
    specified type NEC S15.099
      left S15.092
      right S15.091
  celiac artery S35.219
    branch S35.299
      laceration (minor) (superficial) S35.291
        major S35.292
      specified NEC S35.298
    laceration (minor) (superficial) S35.211
      major S35.212
    specified type NEC S35.218
  cerebral — *see* Injury, intracranial
  deep plantar — *see* Injury, nerve, medial plantar
  digital (hand) — *see* Injury, blood vessel, finger
  dorsal
    artery (foot) S95.009
      laceration S95.019
        left S95.012
        right S95.011
      left S95.002
      right S95.001
      specified type NEC S95.099
        left S95.092
        right S95.091
    vein (foot) S95.209
      laceration S95.219
        left S95.212
        right S95.211
      left S95.202
      right S95.201
      specified type NEC S95.299
        left S95.292
        right S95.291
  due to accidental laceration during procedure — *see* Laceration, accidental complicating surgery
  extremity — *see* Injury, blood vessel, limb
  femoral
    artery (common) (superficial) S75.009
      laceration (minor) (superficial) S75.019
        left S75.012
        major S75.029
          left S75.022
          right S75.021
        right S75.011
      left S75.002
      right S75.001
      specified type NEC S75.099
        left S75.092
        right S75.091
    vein (hip level) (thigh level) S75.109
      laceration (minor) (superficial) S75.119
        left S75.112
        major S75.129
          left S75.122
          right S75.121
        right S75.111
      left S75.102
      right S75.101
      specified type NEC S75.199
        left S75.192
        right S75.191
  finger S65.509
    index S65.508
      laceration S65.518
        left S65.511

Injury (*see also* specified injury type) — *continued*
blood vessel NEC — *continued*
  finger — *continued*
    index — *continued*
      laceration — *continued*
        right S65.510
      left S65.501
      right S65.500
      specified type NEC S65.598
        left S65.591
        right S65.590
    laceration S65.519
    little S65.508
      laceration S65.518
        left S65.517
        right S65.516
        left S65.507
        right S65.506
      specified type NEC S65.598
        left S65.597
        right S65.596
    middle S65.508
      laceration S65.518
        left S65.513
        right S65.512
        left S65.503
        right S65.502
      specified type NEC S65.598
        left S65.593
        right S65.592
    ring S65.508
      laceration S65.518
        left S65.515
        right S65.514
        left S65.505
        right S65.504
      specified type NEC S65.598
        left S65.595
        right S65.594
    specified type NEC S65.599
    thumb — *see* Injury, blood vessel, thumb
  foot S95.909
    dorsal
      artery — *see* Injury, blood vessel, dorsal, artery
      vein — *see* Injury, blood vessel, dorsal, vein
    laceration S95.919
      left S95.912
      right S95.911
    left S95.902
    plantar artery — *see* Injury, blood vessel, plantar artery
    right S95.901
    specified
      site NEC S95.809
        laceration S95.819
          left S95.812
          right S95.811
        left S95.802
        right S95.801
        specified type NEC S95.899
          left S95.892
          right S95.891
      specified type NEC S95.999
        left S95.992
        right S95.991
  forearm S55.909
    laceration S55.919
      left S55.912
      right S55.911
    left S55.902
    radial artery — *see* Injury, blood vessel, radial artery
    right S55.901
    specified
      site NEC S55.809
        laceration S55.819
          left S55.812
          right S55.811
        left S55.802
        right S55.801
        specified type NEC S55.899
          left S55.892
          right S55.891

Injury (*see also* specified injury type) — *continued*
blood vessel NEC — *continued*
  forearm — *continued*
    specified — *continued*
      type NEC S55.999
        left S55.992
        right S55.991
    ulnar artery — *see* Injury, blood vessel, ulnar artery
    vein S55.209
      laceration S55.219
        left S55.212
        right S55.211
      left S55.202
      right S55.201
      specified type NEC S55.299
        left S55.292
        right S55.291
  gastric
    artery — *see* Injury, mesenteric, artery, branch
    vein — *see* Injury, blood vessel, abdomen
  gastroduodenal artery — *see* Injury, mesenteric, artery, branch
  greater saphenous vein (lower leg level) S85.309
    hip (and thigh) level S75.209
      laceration (minor) (superficial) S75.219
        left S75.212
        major S75.229
          left S75.222
          right S75.221
        right S75.211
      left S75.202
      right S75.201
      specified type NEC S75.299
        left S75.292
        right S75.291
    laceration S85.319
      left S85.312
      right S85.311
    left S85.302
    right S85.301
    specified type NEC S85.399
      left S85.392
      right S85.391
  hand (level) S65.909
    finger — *see* Injury, blood vessel, finger
    laceration S65.919
      left S65.912
      right S65.911
    left S65.902
    palmar arch — *see* Injury, blood vessel, palmar arch
    radial artery — *see* Injury, blood vessel, radial artery, hand
    right S65.901
    specified
      site NEC S65.809
        laceration S65.819
          left S65.812
          right S65.811
        left S65.802
        right S65.801
        specified type NEC S65.899
          left S65.892
          right S65.891
      type NEC S65.999
        left S65.992
        right S65.991
    thumb — *see* Injury, blood vessel, thumb
    ulnar artery — *see* Injury, blood vessel, ulnar artery, hand
  head S09.0
    intracranial — *see* Injury, intracranial
    multiple S09.0
  hepatic
    artery — *see* Injury, mesenteric, artery
    vein — *see* Injury, vena cava, inferior
  hip S75.909
    femoral artery — *see* Injury, blood vessel, femoral, artery
    femoral vein — *see* Injury, blood vessel, femoral, vein

Injury (see also specified injury type) — continued
  blood vessel NEC — continued
    hip — continued
      greater saphenous vein — see Injury,
        blood vessel, greater saphenous,
        hip level
      laceration S75.919
        left S75.912
        right S75.911
      left S75.902
      right S75.901
      specified
        site NEC S75.809
          laceration S75.819
            left S75.812
            right S75.811
          left S75.802
          right S75.801
          specified type NEC S75.899
            left S75.892
            right S75.891
        type NEC S75.999
          left S75.992
          right S75.991
    hypogastric (artery) (vein) — see Injury,
      blood vessel, iliac
    iliac S35.50
      artery S35.513
        left S35.512
        right S35.511
      specified vessel NEC S35.59
      uterine vessel — see Injury, blood vessel,
        uterine
      vein S35.516
        left S35.515
        right S35.514
    innominate — see Injury, blood vessel,
      thoracic, innominate
    intercostal (artery) (vein) — see Injury, blood
      vessel, thoracic, intercostal
    jugular vein (external) S15.209
      internal S15.309
        laceration (minor) (superficial) S15.319
          left S15.312
          major S15.329
            left S15.322
            right S15.321
          right S15.311
        left S15.302
        right S15.301
        specified type NEC S15.399
          left S15.392
          right S15.391
      laceration (minor) (superficial) S15.219
        left S15.212
        major S15.229
          left S15.222
          right S15.221
        right S15.211
      left S15.202
      right S15.201
      specified type NEC S15.299
        left S15.292
        right S15.291
    leg (level) (lower) S85.909
      greater saphenous — see Injury, blood
        vessel, greater saphenous
      laceration S85.919
        left S85.912
        right S85.911
      left S85.902
      lesser saphenous — see Injury, blood
        vessel, lesser saphenous
      peroneal artery — see Injury, blood
        vessel, peroneal artery
      popliteal
        artery — see Injury, blood vessel,
          popliteal, artery
        vein — see Injury, blood vessel,
          popliteal, vein
      right S85.901
      specified
        site NEC S85.809
          laceration S85.819
            left S85.812
            right S85.811

Injury (see also specified injury type) — continued
  blood vessel NEC — continued
    leg — continued
      specified — continued
        site NEC — continued
          left S85.802
          right S85.801
          specified type NEC S85.899
            left S85.892
            right S85.891
        type NEC S85.999
          left S85.992
          right S85.991
      thigh — see Injury, blood vessel, hip
      tibial artery — see Injury, blood vessel,
        tibial artery
    lesser saphenous vein (lower leg level)
      S85.409
      laceration S85.419
        left S85.412
        right S85.411
      left S85.402
      right S85.401
      specified type NEC S85.499
        left S85.492
        right S85.491
    limb
      lower — see Injury, blood vessel, leg
      upper — see Injury, blood vessel, arm
    lower back — see Injury, blood vessel,
      abdomen
      specified NEC — see Injury, blood vessel,
        abdomen, specified, site NEC
    mammary (artery) (vein) — see Injury, blood
      vessel, thoracic, specified site NEC
    mesenteric (inferior) (superior)
      artery — see Injury, mesenteric, artery
      vein — see Injury, blood vessel, portal
        vein
    neck S15.9
      specified site NEC S15.8
    ovarian (artery) (vein) — see category S35.8
    palmar arch (superficial) S65.209
      deep S65.309
        laceration S65.319
          left S65.312
          right S65.311
        left S65.302
        right S65.301
        specified type NEC S65.399
          left S65.392
          right S65.391
      laceration S65.219
        left S65.212
        right S65.211
      left S65.202
      right S65.201
      specified type NEC S65.299
        left S65.292
        right S65.291
    pelvis — see Injury, blood vessel, abdomen
      specified NEC — see Injury, blood vessel,
        abdomen, specified, site NEC
    peroneal artery S85.209
      laceration S85.219
        left S85.212
        right S85.211
      left S85.202
      right S85.201
      specified type NEC S85.299
        left S85.292
        right S85.291
    plantar artery (deep) (foot) S95.109
      laceration S95.119
        left S95.112
        right S95.111
      left S95.102
      right S95.101
      specified type NEC S95.199
        left S95.192
        right S95.191
    popliteal
      artery S85.009
        laceration S85.019
          left S85.012
          right S85.011

Injury (see also specified injury type) — continued
  blood vessel NEC — continued
    popliteal — continued
      artery — continued
        left S85.002
        right S85.001
        specified type NEC S85.099
          left S85.092
          right S85.091
      vein S85.509
        laceration S85.519
          left S85.512
          right S85.511
        left S85.502
        right S85.501
        specified type NEC S85.599
          left S85.592
          right S85.591
    portal vein S35.319
      laceration S35.311
      specified type NEC S35.318
    precerebral — see Injury, blood vessel, neck
    pulmonary (artery) (vein) — see Injury, blood
      vessel, thoracic, pulmonary
    radial artery (forearm level) S55.109
      hand and wrist (level) S65.109
        laceration S65.119
          left S65.112
          right S65.111
        left S65.102
        right S65.101
        specified type NEC S65.199
          left S65.192
          right S65.191
      laceration S55.119
        left S55.112
        right S55.111
      left S55.102
      right S55.101
      specified type NEC S55.199
        left S55.192
        right S55.191
    renal
      artery S35.403
        laceration S35.413
          left S35.412
          right S35.411
        left S35.402
        right S35.401
        specified NEC S35.493
          left S35.492
          right S35.491
      vein S35.406
        laceration S35.416
          left S35.415
          right S35.414
        left S35.405
        right S35.404
        specified NEC S35.496
          left S35.495
          right S35.494
    saphenous vein (greater) (lower leg level) —
      see Injury, blood vessel, greater
      saphenous
      hip and thigh level — see Injury, blood
        vessel, greater saphenous, hip level
      lesser — see Injury, blood vessel, lesser
        saphenous
    shoulder
      specified NEC — see Injury, blood vessel,
        arm, specified site NEC
      superficial vein — see Injury, blood
        vessel, arm, superficial vein
    specified NEC T14.90
    splenic
      artery — see Injury, blood vessel, celiac
        artery, branch
      vein S35.329
        laceration S35.321
        specified NEC S35.328
    subclavian — see Injury, blood vessel,
      thoracic, innominate
    thigh — see Injury, blood vessel, hip

Injury (see also specified injury type) — continued
  blood vessel NEC — continued
    thoracic S25.90
      aorta S25.00
        laceration (minor) (superficial) S25.01
          major S25.02
        specified type NEC S25.09
      azygos vein — see Injury, blood vessel, thoracic, specified, site NEC
      innominate
        artery S25.109
          laceration (minor) (superficial) S25.119
            left S25.112
              major S25.129
            left S25.122
              right S25.121
            right S25.111
          left S25.102
          right S25.101
          specified type NEC S25.199
            left S25.192
            right S25.191
        vein S25.309
          laceration (minor) (superficial) S25.319
            left S25.312
              major S25.329
            left S25.322
              right S25.321
            right S25.311
          left S25.302
          right S25.301
          specified type NEC S25.399
            left S25.392
            right S25.391
      intercostal S25.509
        laceration S25.519
          left S25.512
          right S25.511
        left S25.502
        right S25.501
        specified type NEC S25.599
          left S25.592
          right S25.591
      laceration S25.91
      mammary vessel — see Injury, blood vessel, thoracic, specified, site NEC
      pulmonary S25.409
        laceration (minor) (superficial) S25.419
          left S25.412
            major S25.429
            left S25.422
              right S25.421
          right S25.411
        left S25.402
        right S25.401
        specified type NEC S25.499
          left S25.492
          right S25.491
      specified
        site NEC S25.809
          laceration S25.819
            left S25.812
            right S25.811
          left S25.802
          right S25.801
          specified type NEC S25.899
            left S25.892
            right S25.891
        type NEC S25.99
      subclavian — see Injury, blood vessel, thoracic, innominate
      vena cava (superior) S25.20
        laceration (minor) (superficial) S25.21
          major S25.22
        specified type NEC S25.29
    thumb S65.409
      laceration S65.419
        left S65.412
        right S65.411
      left S65.402
      right S65.401
      specified type NEC S65.499
        left S65.492
        right S65.491

Injury (see also specified injury type) — continued
  blood vessel NEC — continued
    tibial artery S85.109
      anterior S85.139
        laceration S85.149
          left S85.142
          right S85.141
        left S85.132
        right S85.131
        specified injury NEC S85.159
          left S85.152
          right S85.151
      laceration S85.119
        left S85.112
        right S85.111
      left S85.102
      posterior S85.169
        laceration S85.179
          left S85.172
          right S85.171
        left S85.162
        right S85.161
        specified injury NEC S85.189
          left S85.182
          right S85.181
      right S85.101
      specified injury NEC S85.129
        left S85.122
        right S85.121
    ulnar artery (forearm level) S55.009
      hand and wrist (level) S65.009
        laceration S65.019
          left S65.012
          right S65.011
        left S65.002
        right S65.001
        specified type NEC S65.099
          left S65.092
          right S65.091
      laceration S55.019
        left S55.012
        right S55.011
      left S55.002
      right S55.001
      specified type NEC S55.099
        left S55.092
        right S55.091
    upper arm (level) — see Injury, blood vessel, arm
    superficial vein — see Injury, blood vessel, arm, superficial vein
    uterine S35.50
      artery S35.533
        left S35.532
        right S35.531
      vein S35.536
        left S35.535
        right S35.534
    vena cava — see Injury, vena cava
    vertebral artery S15.109
      laceration (minor) (superficial) S15.119
        left S15.112
          major S15.129
          left S15.122
            right S15.121
        right S15.111
      left S15.102
      right S15.101
      specified type NEC S15.199
        left S15.192
        right S15.191
    wrist (level) — see Injury, blood vessel, hand
  brachial plexus S14.3
    newborn P14.3
  brain — see Injury, intracranial
    diffuse — see Injury, intracranial, diffuse
    focal — see Injury, intracranial, focal
  brainstem S06.381
    with loss of consciousness S06.389
      brief (<1 hour) S06.382
      minor (1-6 hours) S06.383
      moderate (6-24 hours) S06.384
      prolonged (>24 hours) S06.385
        without return to consciousness S06.386

Injury (see also specified injury type) — continued
  breast NOS S29.9
  broad ligament — see Injury, pelvic organ, specified site NEC
  bronchus, bronchi — see Injury, intrathoracic, bronchus
  brow S09.90
  buttock S39.92
  canthus, eye S05.90
  cardiac plexus — see Injury, nerve, thorax, sympathetic
  cathode ray T66
  cauda equina S34.3
  cavernous sinus — see Injury, intracranial
  cecum — see Injury, colon
  celiac ganglion or plexus — see Injury, nerve, lumbosacral, sympathetic
  cerebellum — see Injury, intracranial
  cerebral — see Injury, intracranial
  cervix (uteri) — see Injury, uterus
  cheek (wall) S09.93
  chest — see Injury, thorax
  childbirth (fetus or newborn) — see also Birth, injury
    maternal NEC O71.9
  chin S09.93
  choroid (eye) — see Injury, eye, specified site NEC
  clitoris S39.93
  coccyx — see also Injury, back, lower
    complicating delivery O71.6
  colon — see Injury, intestine, large
  common bile duct — see Injury, liver
  conjunctiva (superficial) — see Injury, eye, conjunctiva
  conus medullaris — see Injury, spinal, sacral cord
    spermatic — see Injury, pelvic organ, specified site NEC
    spinal — see Injury, spinal cord, by region
  cornea — see Injury, eye, specified site NEC
    abrasion — see Injury, eye, cornea, abrasion
  cortex (cerebral) — see also Injury, intracranial
    visual — see Injury, nerve, optic
  costal region NEC S29.9
  costochondral NEC S29.9
  cranial
    cavity — see Injury, intracranial
    nerve — see Injury, nerve, cranial
  crushing — see Crush
  cutaneous sensory nerve
  cystic duct — see Injury, liver
  delivery (fetus or newborn) P15.9
    maternal NEC O71.9
  Descemet's membrane — see Injury, eyeball, penetrating
  diaphragm — see Injury, intrathoracic, diaphragm
  duodenum — see Injury, intestine, small, duodenum
  ear (auricle) (external) (canal) S09.91
    abrasion — see Abrasion, ear
    bite — see Bite, ear
    blister — see Blister, ear
    bruise — see Contusion, ear
    contusion — see Contusion, ear
    external constriction — see Constriction, external, ear
    hematoma — see Hematoma, ear
    inner — see Injury, ear, middle
    laceration — see Laceration, ear
    middle S09.309
      blast — see Injury, blast, ear
      left S09.302
      right S09.301
      specified NEC S09.399
        left S09.392
        right S09.391
    puncture — see Puncture, ear
    superficial — see Injury, superficial, ear
  eighth cranial nerve (acoustic or auditory) — see Injury, nerve, acoustic
  elbow S59.909
    contusion — see Contusion, elbow
    dislocation — see Dislocation, elbow
    fracture — see Fracture, ulna, upper end
    left S59.902

©2002 Ingenix, Inc.

Injury (*see also* specified injury type) — *continued*
  elbow — *continued*
    open — *see* Wound, open, elbow
      right S59.901
    specified NEC S59.809
      left S59.802
      right S59.801
    sprain — *see* Sprain, elbow
    superficial — *see* Injury, superficial, elbow
  eleventh cranial nerve (accessory) — *see* Injury,
      nerve, accessory
  epididymis S39.93
  epigastric region S39.91
  epiglottis NEC S19.8
  esophageal plexus — *see* Injury, nerve, thorax,
      sympathetic
  esophagus (thoracic part) — *see also* Injury,
      intrathoracic, esophagus
    cervical NEC S19.8
  eustachian tube S09.91
  eye S05.90
    avulsion S05.70
      left S05.72
      right S05.71
    ball — *see* Injury, eyeball
    conjunctiva S05.00
      left S05.02
      right S05.01
    cornea
      abrasion S05.00
        left S05.02
        right S05.01
    laceration S05.30
      with prolapse S05.20
        left S05.22
        right S05.21
      left S05.32
      right S05.31
    lacrimal apparatus S05.80
      left S05.82
      right S05.81
    left S05.92
    orbit penetration S05.40
      left S05.42
      right S05.41
    right S05.91
    specified site NEC S05.80
      left S05.82
      right S05.81
  eyeball S05.80
    contusion S05.10
      left S05.12
      right S05.11
    left S05.82
    penetrating S05.60
      with
        foreign body S05.50
          left S05.52
          right S05.51
        prolapse or loss of intraocular tissue
            S05.20
          left S05.22
          right S05.21
        left S05.62
        right S05.61
      without prolapse or loss of intraocular
          tissue S05.30
        left S05.32
        right S05.31
    right S05.81
    specified type NEC S05.80
  eyebrow S09.93
  eyelid S09.93
    abrasion — *see* Abrasion, eyelid
    contusion — *see* Contusion, eyelid
    open — *see* Wound, open, eyelid
  face S09.93
  fallopian tube S37.509
    bilateral S37.502
      blast injury S37.512
      contusion S37.522
      laceration S37.532
      specified type NEC S37.592
    blast injury (primary) S37.519
      bilateral S37.512

Injury (*see also* specified injury type) — *continued*
  fallopian tube — *continued*
    blast injury — *continued*
      secondary — *see* Injury, fallopian tube,
          specified type NEC
      unilateral S37.511
    contusion S37.529
      bilateral S37.522
      unilateral S37.521
    laceration S37.539
      bilateral S37.532
      unilateral S37.531
    specified type NEC S37.599
      bilateral S37.592
      unilateral S37.591
    unilateral S37.501
      blast injury S37.511
      contusion S37.521
      laceration S37.531
      specified type NEC S37.591
  fascia — *see* Injury, muscle
  fifth cranial nerve (trigeminal) — *see* Injury,
      nerve, trigeminal
  finger (nail) S69.90
    blood vessel — *see* Injury, blood vessel,
        finger
    contusion — *see* Contusion, finger
    dislocation — *see* Dislocation, finger
    fracture — *see* Fracture, finger
    left S69.92
    muscle — *see* Injury, muscle, finger
    nerve — *see* Injury, nerve, digital, finger
    open — *see* Wound, open, finger
    right S69.91
    specified NEC S69.80
      left S69.82
      right S69.81
    sprain — *see* Sprain, finger
    superficial — *see* Injury, superficial, finger
  first cranial nerve (olfactory) — *see* Injury,
      nerve, olfactory
  flank — *see* Injury, abdomen
  foot S99.929
    blood vessel — *see* Injury, blood vessel, foot
    contusion — *see* Contusion, foot
    dislocation — *see* Dislocation, foot
    fracture — *see* Fracture, foot
    left S99.922
    muscle — *see* Injury, muscle, foot
    open — *see* Wound, open, foot
    right S99.921
    specified type NEC S99.829
      left S99.822
      right S99.821
    sprain — *see* Sprain, foot
    superficial — *see* Injury, superficial, foot
  forceps NOS P15.9
  forearm S59.919
    blood vessel — *see* Injury, blood vessel,
        forearm
    contusion — *see* Contusion, forearm
    fracture — *see* Fracture, forearm
    left S59.912
    muscle — *see* Injury, muscle, forearm
    nerve — *see* Injury, nerve, forearm
    open — *see* Wound, open, forearm
    right S59.911
    specified NEC S59.819
      left S59.812
      right S59.811
    superficial — *see* Injury, superficial, forearm
  forehead S09.90
  fourth cranial nerve (trochlear) — *see* Injury,
      nerve, trochlear
  gallbladder S36.129
    contusion S36.122
    laceration S36.123
    specified NEC S36.128
  ganglion
    celiac, coeliac — *see* Injury, nerve,
        lumbosacral, sympathetic
    gasserian — *see* Injury, nerve, trigeminal
    stellate — *see* Injury, nerve, thorax,
        sympathetic
    thoracic sympathetic — *see* Injury, nerve,
        thorax, sympathetic

Injury (*see also* specified injury type) — *continued*
  gasserian ganglion — *see* Injury, nerve,
      trigeminal
  gastric artery — *see* Injury, blood vessel, celiac
      artery, branch
  gastroduodenal artery — *see* Injury, blood
      vessel, celiac artery, branch
  gastrointestinal tract — *see* Injury, intra-
      abdominal
    with open wound into abdominal cavity —
        see Wound, open, with penetration
        into peritoneal cavity
    colon — *see* Injury, intestine, large
    rectum — *see* Injury, intestine, large,
        rectum
      with open wound into abdominal cavity
          S36.61
    specified site NEC — *see* Injury, intra-
        abdominal, specified, site NEC
    stomach — *see* Injury, stomach
    small intestine — *see* Injury, intestine, small
  genital organ(s)
    with or following ectopic or molar pregnancy
        O08.6
    external S39.93
    internal S37.90
      fallopian tube — *see* Injury, fallopian
          tube
      ovary — *see* Injury, ovary
      prostate — *see* Injury, prostate
      seminal vesicle — *see* Injury, pelvis,
          organ, specified site NEC
      uterus — *see* Injury, uterus
      vas deferens — *see* Injury, pelvis, organ,
          specified site NEC
    obstetrical trauma O71.9
  gland
    lacrimal laceration — *see* Injury, eye,
        specified site NEC
    salivary S09.90
    thyroid NEC S19.8
  globe (eye) S05.90
  groin — *see* Injury, abdomen
  gum S09.90
  hand S69.90
    blood vessel — *see* Injury, blood vessel,
        hand
    contusion — *see* Contusion, hand
    fracture — *see* Fracture, hand
    left S69.92
    muscle — *see* Injury, muscle, hand
    nerve — *see* Injury, nerve, hand
    open — *see* Wound, open, hand
    right S69.91
    specified NEC S69.80
      left S69.82
      right S69.81
    sprain — *see* Sprain, hand
    superficial — *see* Injury, superficial, hand
  head S09.90
    with loss of consciousness S06.00
    specified NEC S09.8
  heart S26.90
    with hemopericardium S26.00
      contusion S26.01
      laceration (mild) S26.020
        moderate S26.021
        major S26.022
      specified type NEC S26.09
    contusion S26.91
    laceration S26.92
    specified type NEC S26.99
    without hemopericardium S26.10
      contusion S26.11
      laceration S26.12
      specified type NEC S26.19
  heel — *see* Injury, foot
  hepatic
    artery — *see* Injury, blood vessel, celiac
        artery, branch
    duct — *see* Injury, liver
    vein — *see* Injury, vena cava, inferior
  hip S79.919
    blood vessel — *see* Injury, blood vessel, hip
    contusion — *see* Contusion, hip
    dislocation — *see* Dislocation, hip
    fracture — *see* Fracture, femur, neck

Injury (*see also* specified injury type) — *continued*
- hip — *continued*
  - left S79.912
  - muscle — *see* Injury, muscle, hip
  - nerve — *see* Injury, nerve, hip
  - open — *see* Wound, open, hip
  - right S79.911
  - sprain — *see* Sprain, hip
  - superficial — *see* Injury, superficial, hip
  - specified NEC S79.819
    - left S79.812
    - right S79.811
- hymen S39.93
- hypogastric
  - blood vessel — *see* Injury, blood vessel, iliac
  - plexus — *see* Injury, nerve, lumbosacral, sympathetic
- ileum — *see* Injury, intestine, small
- iliac region S39.91
- infrared rays NOS T66
- instrumental (during surgery) — *see* Laceration, accidental complicating surgery
  - birth injury — *see* Birth, injury
  - nonsurgical — *see* Injury, by site
  - obstetrical O71.9
    - bladder O71.5
    - cervix O71.3
    - high vaginal O71.4
    - perineal NOS O70.9
    - urethra O71.5
    - uterus O71.5
      - with rupture or perforation O71.1
- internal T14.90
  - aorta — *see* Injury, aorta
  - bladder (sphincter) — *see* Injury, bladder
    - with
      - ectopic or molar pregnancy O08.6
      - following ectopic or molar pregnancy O08.6
      - obstetrical trauma O71.5
  - bronchus, bronchi — *see* Injury, intrathoracic, bronchus
  - cecum — *see* Injury, intestine, large
  - cervix (uteri) — *see also* Injury, uterus
    - with ectopic or molar pregnancy O08.6
    - following ectopic or molar pregnancy O08.6
    - obstetrical trauma O71.3
  - chest — *see* Injury, intrathoracic
  - gastrointestinal tract — *see* Injury, intra-abdominal
  - heart — *see* Injury, heart
  - intestine NEC — *see* Injury, intestine
  - intrauterine — *see* Injury, uterus
  - mesentery — *see* Injury, intra-abdominal, specified, site NEC
  - pelvis, pelvic (organ) S37.90
    - following ectopic or molar pregnancy (subsequent episode) O08.6
    - obstetrical trauma NEC O71.5
      - rupture or perforation O71.1
    - specified NEC S39.83
  - rectum — *see* Injury, intestine, large, rectum
  - stomach — *see* Injury, stomach
  - ureter — *see* Injury, ureter
  - urethra (sphincter) following ectopic or molar pregnancy O08.6
  - uterus — *see* Injury, uterus
- interscapular area — *see* Injury, thorax
- intestine
  - large S36.509
    - ascending (right) S36.500
      - blast injury (primary) S36.510
        - secondary S36.590
      - contusion S36.520
      - laceration S36.530
      - specified type NEC S36.590
    - blast injury (primary) S36.519
      - ascending (right) S36.510
      - descending (left) S36.512
      - rectum S36.61
      - sigmoid S36.513
      - specified site NEC S36.518
      - transverse S36.511

Injury (*see also* specified injury type) — *continued*
- intestine — *continued*
  - large — *continued*
    - contusion S36.529
      - ascending (right) S36.520
      - descending (left) S36.522
      - rectum S36.62
      - sigmoid S36.523
      - specified site NEC S36.528
      - transverse S36.521
    - descending (left) S36.502
      - blast injury (primary) S36.512
        - secondary S36.592
      - contusion S36.522
      - laceration S36.532
      - specified type NEC S36.592
    - laceration S36.539
      - ascending (right) S36.530
      - descending (left) S36.532
      - rectum S36.63
      - sigmoid S36.533
      - specified site NEC S36.538
      - transverse S36.531
    - rectum S36.60
      - blast injury (primary) S36.61
        - secondary S36.69
      - contusion S36.62
      - laceration S36.63
      - specified type NEC S36.69
    - sigmoid S36.503
      - blast injury (primary) S36.513
        - secondary S36.593
      - contusion S36.523
      - laceration S36.533
      - specified type NEC S36.593
    - specified
      - site NEC S36.508
        - blast injury (primary) S36.518
          - secondary S36.598
        - contusion S36.528
        - laceration S36.538
        - specified type NEC S36.598
      - type NEC S36.599
        - ascending (right) S36.590
        - descending (left) S36.592
        - rectum S36.69
        - sigmoid S36.593
        - specified site NEC S36.598
        - transverse S36.591
    - transverse S36.501
      - blast injury (primary) S36.511
        - secondary S36.591
      - contusion S36.521
      - laceration S36.531
      - specified type NEC S36.591
  - small S36.409
    - blast injury (primary) S36.419
      - duodenum S36.410
      - secondary S36.499
        - duodenum S36.490
        - specified site NEC S36.498
      - specified site NEC S36.418
    - contusion S36.429
      - duodenum S36.420
      - specified site NEC S36.428
    - duodenum S36.400
      - blast injury (primary) S36.410
        - secondary S36.490
      - contusion S36.420
      - laceration S36.430
      - specified NEC S36.490
    - laceration S36.439
      - duodenum S36.430
      - specified site NEC S36.438
    - specified
      - type NEC S36.499
        - duodenum S36.490
        - specified site NEC S36.498
      - site NEC S36.408
  - intra-abdominal S36.90
    - adrenal gland — *see* Injury, adrenal gland
    - bladder — *see* Injury, bladder
    - colon — *see* Injury, intestine, large
    - contusion S36.92
    - fallopian tube — *see* Injury, fallopian tube
    - gallbladder — *see* Injury, gallbladder

Injury (*see also* specified injury type) — *continued*
- intra-abdominal — *continued*
  - intestine — *see* Injury, intestine
  - laceration S36.93
  - liver — *see* Injury, liver
  - kidney — *see* Injury, kidney
  - ovary — *see* Injury, ovary
  - pancreas — *see* Injury, pancreas
  - pelvic NOS S37.90
  - peritoneum — *see* Injury, intra-abdominal, specified, site NEC
  - prostate — *see* Injury, prostate
  - rectum — *see* Injury, intestine, large, rectum
  - retroperitoneum — *see* Injury, intra-abdominal, specified, site NEC
  - seminal vesicle — *see* Injury, pelvis, organ, specified site NEC
  - small intestine — *see* Injury, intestine, small
  - specified
    - site NEC S36.899
      - contusion S36.892
      - laceration S36.893
      - specified type NEC S36.898
    - type NEC S36.99
  - pelvic S37.90
    - specified
      - site NEC S37.899
        - specified type NEC S37.898
      - type NEC S37.99
  - spleen — *see* Injury, spleen
  - stomach — *see* Injury, stomach
  - ureter — *see* Injury, ureter
  - urethra — *see* Injury, urethra
  - uterus — *see* Injury, uterus
  - vas deferens — *see* Injury, pelvis, organ, specified site NEC
- intracranial S06.91
  - with
    - loss of consciousness S06.90
      - brief (<1 hour) S06.92
      - minor (1-6 hours) S06.93
      - moderate (6-24 hours) S06.94
      - prolonged (>24 hours) S06.95
        - without return to consciousness S06.96
  - cerebellar hemorrhage, traumatic — *see* Injury, intracranial, focal
  - cerebral edema, traumatic S06.11
    - with loss of consciousness S06.10
      - brief (< 1 hour) S06.12
      - minor (1-6 hours) S06.13
      - moderate (6-24 hours) S06.14
      - prolonged (>24 hours) S06.15
        - without return to consciousness S06.16
    - focal S06.17
  - diffuse (axonal) brain injury S06.20
    - with loss of consciousness S06.20
      - moderate (6-24 hours) S06.24
      - prolonged (>24 hours) S06.25
        - without return to consciousness S06.26
  - epidural hemorrhage (traumatic) S06.41
    - with loss of consciousness S06.40
      - brief (<1 hour) S06.42
      - minor (1-6 hours) S06.43
      - moderate (6-24 hours) S06.44
      - prolonged (>24 hours) S06.45
        - without return to consciousness S06.46
  - focal brain injury S06.301
    - with loss of consciousness S06.309
      - brief (< 1 hour) S06.302
      - minor (1-6 hours) S06.303
      - moderate (6-24 hours) S06.304
      - prolonged (>24 hours) S06.305
        - without return to consciousness S06.306
    - contusion — *see* Contusion, cerebral
    - laceration — *see* Laceration, cerebral
  - intracerebral hemorrhage, traumatic S06.361
    - with loss of consciousness S06.369
      - brief (<1 hour) S06.362
      - minor (1-6 hours) S06.363

©2002 Ingenix, Inc.

Injury (*see also* specified injury type) — *continued*
intracranial — *continued*
  intracerebral hemorrhage, traumatic — *continued*
    with loss of consciousness — *continued*
      moderate (6-24 hours) S06.364
      prolonged (>24 hours) S06.365
        without return to consciousness S06.366
    left side S06.351
      with loss of consciousness S06.359
        brief (<1 hour) S06.352
        minor (1-6 hours) S06.353
        moderate (6-24 hours) S06.354
        prolonged (>24 hours) S06.355
          without return to consciousness S06.356
    right side S06.341
      with loss of consciousness S06.349
        brief (<1 hour) S06.342
        minor (1-6 hours) S06.343
        moderate (6-24 hours) S06.344
        prolonged (>24 hours) S06.345
          without return to consciousness S06.346
  subarachnoid hemorrhage, traumatic S06.61
    with loss of consciousness S06.60
      brief (<1 hour) S06.62
      minor (1-6 hours) S06.63
      moderate (1-24 hours) S06.64
      prolonged (>24 hours) S06.65
        without return to consciousness S06.66
  subdural hemorrhage, traumatic S06.51
    with loss of consciousness S06.50
      brief (<1 hour) S06.52
      minor (1-6 hours) S06.53
      moderate (6-24 hours) S06.54
      prolonged (>24 hours) S06.55
        without return to consciousness S06.56
intraocular — *see* Injury, eyeball, penetrating
intrathoracic S27.9
  bronchus S27.409
    bilateral S27.402
    blast injury (primary) S27.419
      bilateral S27.412
      secondary — *see* Injury, intrathoracic, bronchus, specified type NEC
      unilateral S27.411
    contusion S27.429
      bilateral S27.422
      unilatera.l S27.421
    laceration S27.439
      bilateral S27.432
      unilateral S27.431
    specified type NEC S27.499
      bilateral S27.492
      unilateral S27.491
    unilateral S27.401
  diaphragm S27.809
    contusion S27.802
    laceration S27.803
    specified type NEC S27.808
  esophagus (thoracic) S27.819
    contusion S27.812
    laceration S27.813
    specified type NEC S27.818
  heart — *see* Injury, heart
  hemopneumothorax S27.2
  hemothorax S27.1
  lung S27.309
    bilateral S27.302
    blast injury (primary) S27.319
      bilateral S27.312
      secondary — *see* Injury, intrathoracic, lung, specified type NEC
      unilateral S27.311
    contusion S27.329
      bilateral S27.322
      unilateral S27.321
    laceration S27.339
      bilateral S27.332
      unilateral S27.331

Injury (*see also* specified injury type) — *continued*
intrathoracic — *continued*
  lung — *continued*
    specified type NEC S27.399
      bilateral S27.392
      unilateral S27.391
    unilateral S27.301
  pleura S27.60
    laceration S27.63
    specified type NEC S27.69
  pneumothorax S27.0
  specified organ NEC S27.899
    contusion S27.892
    laceration S27.893
    specified type NEC S27.898
  thoracic duct — *see* Injury, intrathoracic, specified organ NEC
  thymus gland — *see* Injury, intrathoracic, specified organ NEC
  trachea, thoracic S27.50
    blast (primary) S27.51
    contusion S27.52
    laceration S27.53
    specified type NEC S27.59
iris — *see* Injury, eye, specified site NEC
  penetrating — *see* Injury, eyeball, penetrating
jaw S09.93
jejunum — *see* Injury, intestine, small
joint NOS T14.90
  old or residual — *see* Disorder, joint, specified type NEC
kidney S37.009
  contusion (minor) S37.019
    major S37.029
  laceration S37.039
    major (massive) (stellate) S37.069
    minor S37.049
    moderate S37.059
  left S37.002
    contusion (minor) S37.012
      major S37.022
    laceration S37.032
      major (massive) (stellate) S37.062
      minor S37.042
      moderate S37.052
      specified type NEC S37.092
  right S37.001
    contusion (minor) S37.011
      major S37.021
    laceration S37.031
      major (massive) (stellate) S37.061
      minor S37.041
      moderate S37.051
    specified type NEC S37.091
  specified type NEC S37.099
knee S89.90
  contusion — *see* Contusion, knee
  dislocation — *see* Dislocation, knee
  left S89.92
  meniscus (lateral) (medial) — *see* Sprain, knee, specified site NEC
    old injury or tear — *see* Derangement, knee, meniscus, due to old injury
  open — *see* Wound, open, knee
  right S89.91
  specified NEC S89.80
    left S89.82
    right S89.81
  sprain — *see* Sprain, knee
  superficial — *see* Injury, superficial, knee
labium (majus) (minus) S39.93
labyrinth, ear S09.91
lacrimal apparatus, duct, gland, or sac — *see* Injury, eye, specified site NEC
larynx NEC S19.8
  with
leg (lower) S89.90
  blood vessel — *see* Injury, blood vessel, leg
  contusion — *see* Contusion, leg
  fracture — *see* Fracture, leg
  left S89.92
  muscle — *see* Injury, muscle, leg
  nerve — *see* Injury, nerve, leg
  open — *see* Wound, open, leg
  right S89.91

Injury (*see also* specified injury type) — *continued*
leg — *continued*
  specified NEC S89.80
    left S89.82
    right S89.81
  superficial — *see* Injury, superficial, leg
lens, eye — *see* Injury, eye, specified site NEC
  penetrating — *see* Injury, eyeball, penetrating
limb T14.90
lip S09.93
liver S36.119
  contusion S36.112
  laceration S36.113
    major (stellate) S36.116
    minor S36.114
    moderate S36.115
    specified NEC S36.118
lower back S39.92
  specified NEC S39.82
lumbar, lumbosacral (region) S39.92
  plexus — *see* Injury, lumbosacral plexus
lumbosacral plexus S34.4
lung — *see* Injury, intrathoracic, lung
lymphatic thoracic duct — *see* Injury, intrathoracic, specified organ NEC
malar region S09.93
mastoid region S09.90
maxilla S09.93
mediastinum — *see* Injury, intrathoracic, specified organ NEC
membrane, brain — *see* Injury, intracranial
meningeal artery — *see* Injury, intracranial, subdural hemorrhage
meninges (cerebral) — *see* Injury, intracranial
mesenteric
  artery
    branch S35.299
      laceration (minor) (superficial) S35.291
        major S35.292
        specified NEC S35.298
    inferior S35.239
      laceration (minor) (superficial) S35.231
        major S35.232
        specified NEC S35.238
    superior S35.229
      laceration (minor) (superficial) S35.221
        major S35.222
        specified NEC S35.228
  plexus (inferior) (superior) — *see* Injury, nerve, lumbosacral, sympathetic
  vein
    inferior S35.349
      laceration S35.341
      specified NEC S35.348
    superior) S35.339
      laceration S35.331
      specified NEC S35.338
mesentery — *see* Injury, intra-abdominal, specified site NEC
mesosalpinx — *see* Injury, pelvic organ, specified site NEC
middle ear S09.91
midthoracic region NOS S29.9
mouth S09.93
multiple NOS T07
muscle (and fascia) (and tendon)
  abdomen S39.001
    laceration S39.021
    specified type NEC S39.091
    strain S39.011
  abductor
    thumb, forearm level — *see* Injury, muscle, thumb, abductor
  adductor
    thigh S76.209
      laceration S76.229
        left S76.222
        right S76.221
      left S76.202
      right S76.201
      specified type NEC S76.299
        left S76.292
        right S76.291
      strain S76.219
        left S76.212
        right S76.211

©2002 Ingenix, Inc.

Injury (*see also* specified injury type) — *continued*
  muscle — *continued*
    finger — *continued*
      middle — *continued*
        intrinsic — *continued*
          laceration — *continued*
            right S66.522
          left S66.503
          right S66.502
          specified type NEC S66.598
            left S66.593
            right S66.592
          strain S66.518
            left S66.513
            right S66.512
      ring
        extensor (forearm level)
          hand level S66.308
            laceration S66.328
              left S66.325
              right S66.324
            left S66.305
            right S66.304
            specified type NEC S66.398
              left S66.395
              right S66.394
            strain S66.318
              left S66.315
              right S66.314
          laceration
            left S56.426
            right S56.425
          left S56.406
          right S56.405
          specified type NEC
            left S56.496
            right S56.495
          strain
            left S56.416
            right S56.415
        flexor (forearm level)
          hand level S66.108
            laceration S66.128
              left S66.125
              right S66.124
            left S66.105
            right S66.104
            specified type NEC S66.198
              left S66.195
              right S66.194
            strain S66.118
              left S66.115
              right S66.114
          laceration
            left S56.126
            right S56.125
          left S56.106
          right S56.105
          specified type NEC
            left S56.196
            right S56.195
          strain
            left S56.116
            right S56.115
        intrinsic S66.508
          laceration S66.528
            left S66.525
            right S66.524
          left S66.505
          right S66.504
          specified type NEC S66.598
            left S66.595
            right S66.594
          strain S66.518
            left S66.515
            right S66.514
      flexor
        finger(s) (other than thumb) — *see* Injury,
            muscle, finger
        forearm level, specified NEC — *see* Injury,
            muscle, forearm, flexor
        thumb — *see* Injury, muscle, thumb,
            flexor
        toe (long) (ankle level) (foot level) — *see*
            Injury, muscle, toe, flexor

Injury (*see also* specified injury type) — *continued*
  muscle — *continued*
    foot S96.909
      intrinsic S96.209
        laceration S96.229
          left S96.222
          right S96.221
        left S96.202
        right S96.201
        specified type NEC S96.299
          left S96.292
          right S96.291
        strain S96.219
          left S96.212
          right S96.211
      laceration S96.929
        left S96.922
        right S96.921
      left S96.902
      long extensor, toe — *see* Injury, muscle,
          toe, extensor
      long flexor, toe — *see* Injury, muscle, toe,
          flexor
      right S96.901
      specified
        site NEC S96.809
          laceration S96.829
            left S96.822
            right S96.821
          left S96.802
          right S96.801
          specified type NEC S96.899
            left S96.892
            right S96.891
          strain S96.819
            left S96.812
            right S96.811
        type NEC S96.999
          left S96.992
          right S96.991
      strain S96.919
        left S96.912
        right S96.911
    forearm (level) S56.909
      extensor S56.509
        laceration S56.529
          left S56.522
          right S56.521
        left S56.502
        right S56.501
        specified type NEC S56.599
          left S56.592
          right S56.591
        strain S56.519
          left S56.512
          right S56.511
      flexor S56.209
        laceration S56.229
          left S56.222
          right S56.221
        left S56.202
        right S56.201
        specified type NEC S56.299
          left S56.292
          right S56.291
        strain S56.219
          left S56.212
          right S56.211
      laceration S56.929
        left S56.922
        right S56.921
      left S56.902
      right S56.901
      specified
        site NEC S56.809
          laceration S56.829
            left S56.822
            right S56.821
          left S56.802
          right S56.801
          specified type NEC S56.899
            left S56.892
            right S56.891
          strain S56.819
            left S56.812

Injury (*see also* specified injury type) — *continued*
  muscle — *continued*
    forearm — *continued*
      specified — *continued*
        site NEC — *continued*
          strain — *continued*
            right S56.811
        type NEC S56.999
          left S56.992
          right S56.991
      strain S56.919
        left S56.912
        right S56.911
    hand (level) S66.909
      laceration S66.929
        left S66.922
        right S66.921
      left S66.902
      right S66.901
      specified
        site NEC S66.809
          laceration S66.829
            left S66.822
            right S66.821
          left S66.802
          right S66.801
          specified type NEC S66.899
            left S66.892
            right S66.891
          strain S66.819
            left S66.812
            right S66.811
        type NEC S66.999
          left S66.992
          right S66.991
      strain S66.919
        left S66.912
        right S66.911
    head S09.10
      laceration S09.12
      specified type NEC S09.19
      strain S09.11
    hip NEC S76.009
      laceration S76.029
        left S76.022
        right S76.021
      left S76.002
      right S76.001
      specified type NEC S76.099
        left S76.092
        right S76.091
      strain S76.019
        left S76.012
        right S76.011
    intrinsic
      ankle and foot level — *see* Injury, muscle,
          foot, intrinsic
      finger (other than thumb) — *see* Injury,
          muscle, finger by site, intrinsic
      foot (level) — *see* Injury, muscle, foot,
          intrinsic
      thumb — *see* Injury, muscle, thumb,
          intrinsic
    leg (level) (lower) S86.909
      Achilles tendon — *see* Injury, Achilles
          tendon
      anterior muscle group — *see* Injury,
          muscle, anterior muscle group
      laceration S86.929
        left S86.922
        right S86.921
      left S86.902
      peroneal muscle group — *see* Injury,
          muscle, peroneal muscle group
      posterior muscle group — *see* Injury,
          muscle, posterior muscle group, leg
          level
      right S86.901
      specified
        site NEC S86.809
          laceration S86.829
            left S86.822
            right S86.821
          left S86.802
          right S86.801

Injury (*see also* specified injury type) — *continued*
muscle — *continued*
　leg — *continued*
　　specified — *continued*
　　　site NEC — *continued*
　　　　specified type NEC S86.899
　　　　　left S86.892
　　　　　right S86.891
　　　　strain S86.819
　　　　　left S86.812
　　　　　right S86.811
　　　type NEC S86.999
　　　　left S86.992
　　　　right S86.991
　　　strain S86.919
　　　　left S86.912
　　　　right S86.911
　long
　　extensor toe, at ankle and foot level —
　　　see Injury, muscle, toe, extensor
　　flexor, toe, at ankle and foot level — *see*
　　　Injury, muscle, toe, flexor
　　head, biceps — *see* Injury, muscle,
　　　biceps, long head
　lower back S39.002
　　laceration S39.022
　　specified type NEC S39.092
　　strain S39.012
　neck (level) S16.9
　　laceration S16.2
　　specified type NEC S16.8
　　strain S16.1
　pelvis S39.003
　　laceration S39.023
　　specified type NEC S39.093
　　strain S39.013
　peroneal muscle group, at leg level (lower)
　　S86.309
　　laceration S86.329
　　　left S86.322
　　　right S86.321
　　left S86.302
　　right S86.301
　　specified type NEC S86.399
　　　left S86.392
　　　right S86.391
　　strain S86.319
　　　left S86.312
　　　right S86.311
　posterior muscle (group)
　　leg level (lower) S86.109
　　　laceration S86.129
　　　　left S86.122
　　　　right S86.121
　　　left S86.102
　　　right S86.101
　　　specified type NEC S86.199
　　　　left S86.192
　　　　right S86.191
　　　strain S86.119
　　　　left S86.112
　　　　right S86.111
　　thigh level S76.309
　　　laceration S76.329
　　　　left S76.322
　　　　right S76.321
　　　left S76.302
　　　right S76.301
　　　specified type NEC S76.399
　　　　left S76.392
　　　　right S76.391
　　　strain S76.319
　　　　left S76.312
　　　　right S76.311
　quadriceps (thigh) S76.109
　　laceration S76.129
　　　left S76.122
　　　right S76.121
　　left S76.102
　　right S76.101
　　specified type NEC S76.199
　　　left S76.192
　　　right S76.191
　　strain S76.119
　　　left S76.112
　　　right S76.111

Injury (*see also* specified injury type) — *continued*
muscle — *continued*
　shoulder S46.909
　　laceration S46.929
　　　left S46.922
　　　right S46.921
　　left S46.902
　　right S46.901
　　rotator cuff — *see* Injury, rotator cuff
　　specified site NEC S46.809
　　　laceration S46.829
　　　　left S46.822
　　　　right S46.821
　　　left S46.802
　　　right S46.801
　　　strain S46.819
　　　　left S46.812
　　　　right S46.811
　　　specified type NEC S46.899
　　　　left S46.892
　　　　right S46.891
　　strain S46.919
　　　left S46.912
　　　right S46.911
　　specified type NEC S46.999
　　　left S46.992
　　　right S46.991
　thigh NEC (level) S76.909
　　adductor — *see* Injury, muscle, adductor,
　　　thigh
　　laceration S76.929
　　　left S76.922
　　　right S76.921
　　left S76.902
　　posterior muscle (group) — *see* Injury,
　　　muscle, posterior muscle, thigh
　　　level
　　quadriceps — *see* Injury, muscle,
　　　quadriceps
　　right S76.901
　　specified
　　　site NEC S76.809
　　　　laceration S76.829
　　　　　left S76.822
　　　　　right S76.821
　　　　left S76.802
　　　　right S76.801
　　　　specified type NEC S76.899
　　　　　left S76.892
　　　　　right S76.891
　　　　strain S76.819
　　　　　left S76.812
　　　　　right S76.811
　　　type NEC S76.999
　　　　left S76.992
　　　　right S76.991
　　strain S76.919
　　　left S76.912
　　　right S76.911
　thorax (level) S29.009
　　back wall S29.002
　　front wall S29.001
　　laceration S29.029
　　　back wall S29.022
　　　front wall S29.021
　　specified type NEC S29.099
　　　back wall S29.092
　　　front wall S29.091
　　strain S29.019
　　　back wall S29.012
　　　front wall S29.011
　thumb
　　abductor (forearm level) S56.309
　　　laceration S56.329
　　　　left S56.322
　　　　right S56.321
　　　left S56.302
　　　right S56.301
　　　specified type NEC S56.399
　　　　left S56.392
　　　　right S56.391
　　　strain S56.319
　　　　left S56.312
　　　　right S56.311

Injury (*see also* specified injury type) — *continued*
muscle — *continued*
　thumb — *continued*
　　extensor (forearm level) S56.309
　　　hand level S66.209
　　　　laceration S66.229
　　　　　left S66.222
　　　　　right S66.221
　　　　left S66.202
　　　　right S66.201
　　　　specified type NEC S66.299
　　　　　left S66.292
　　　　　right S66.291
　　　　strain S66.219
　　　　　left S66.212
　　　　　right S66.211
　　　laceration S56.329
　　　　left S56.322
　　　　right S56.321
　　　left S56.302
　　　right S56.301
　　　specified type NEC S56.399
　　　　left S56.392
　　　　right S56.391
　　　strain S56.319
　　　　left S56.312
　　　　right S56.311
　　flexor (forearm level) S56.009
　　　hand level S66.009
　　　　laceration S66.029
　　　　　left S66.022
　　　　　right S66.021
　　　　left S66.002
　　　　right S66.001
　　　　specified type NEC S66.099
　　　　　left S66.092
　　　　　right S66.091
　　　　strain S66.019
　　　　　left S66.012
　　　　　right S66.011
　　　laceration S56.029
　　　　left S56.022
　　　　right S56.021
　　　left S56.002
　　　right S56.001
　　　specified type NEC S56.099
　　　　left S56.092
　　　　right S56.091
　　　strain S56.019
　　　　left S56.012
　　　　right S56.011
　　　wrist level — *see* Injury, muscle,
　　　　thumb, flexor, hand level
　　intrinsic S66.409
　　　laceration S66.429
　　　　left S66.422
　　　　right S66.421
　　　left S66.402
　　　right S66.401
　　　specified type NEC S66.499
　　　　left S66.492
　　　　right S66.491
　　　strain S66.419
　　　　left S66.412
　　　　right S66.411
　toe — *see also* Injury, muscle, foot
　　extensor, long S96.109
　　　laceration S96.129
　　　　left S96.122
　　　　right S96.121
　　　left S96.102
　　　right S96.101
　　　specified type NEC S96.199
　　　　left S96.192
　　　　right S96.191
　　　strain S96.119
　　　　left S96.112
　　　　right S96.111
　　flexor, long S96.009
　　　laceration S96.029
　　　　left S96.022
　　　　right S96.021
　　　left S96.002
　　　right S96.001

　　　　　　　　　　　　　　　　　　　　　　　©2002 Ingenix, Inc.

Injury (see also specified injury type) — continued
  muscle — continued
    toe — see also Injury, muscle, foot —
      continued
      flexor, long — continued
        specified type NEC S96.099
          left S96.092
          right S96.091
        strain S96.019
          left S96.012
          right S96.011
    triceps S46.309
      laceration S46.329
        left S46.322
        right S46.321
      left S46.302
      right S46.301
      specified type NEC S46.399
        left S46.392
        right S46.391
      strain S46.319
        left S46.312
        right S46.311
    wrist (and hand) level — see Injury, muscle,
      hand
  musculocutaneous nerve — see Injury, nerve,
    musculocutaneous
  myocardium — see Injury, heart
  nape — see Injury, neck
  nasal (septum) (sinus) S09.92
  nasopharynx S09.92
  neck S19.9
    specified NEC S19.8
  nerve
    abdomen S34.9
      peripheral S34.6
      specified site NEC S34.8
    abducens S04.40
      contusion S04.40
        left S04.42
        right S04.41
      laceration S04.40
        left S04.42
        right S04.41
      left S04.42
      right S04.41
      specified type NEC S04.40
        left S04.42
        right S04.41
    abducent — see Injury, nerve, abducens
    accessory S04.70
      contusion S04.70
        left S04.72
        right S04.71
      laceration S04.70
        left S04.72
        right S04.71
      left S04.72
      right S04.71
      specified type NEC S04.70
        left S04.72
        right S04.71
    acoustic S04.60
      contusion S04.60
        left S04.62
        right S04.61
      laceration S04.60
        left S04.62
        right S04.61
      left S04.62
      right S04.61
      specified type NEC S04.60
        left S04.62
        right S04.61
    ankle S94.90
      cutaneous sensory S94.30
        left S94.32
        right S94.31
      left S94.92
      right S94.91
      specified site NEC — see category S94.8
    anterior crural, femoral — see Injury, nerve,
      femoral
    arm (upper) S44.90
      axillary — see Injury, nerve, axillary

Injury (see also specified injury type) — continued
  nerve — continued
    arm — continued
      cutaneous — see Injury, nerve,
        cutaneous, arm
      left S44.92
      median — see Injury, nerve, median,
        upper arm
      musculocutaneous — see Injury, nerve,
        musculocutaneous
      radial — see Injury, nerve, radial, upper
        arm
      right S44.91
      specified site NEC — see category S44.8
      ulnar — see Injury, nerve, ulnar, arm
    auditory — see Injury, nerve, acoustic
    axillary S44.30
      left S44.32
      right S44.31
    brachial plexus — see Injury, brachial
      plexus
    cervical sympathetic S14.5
    cranial S04.9
      contusion S04.9
        left S04.9
        right S04.9
      eighth (acoustic or auditory) — see
        Injury, nerve, acoustic
      eleventh (accessory) — see Injury, nerve,
        accessory
      fifth (trigeminal) — see Injury, nerve,
        trigeminal
      first (olfactory) — see Injury, nerve,
        olfactory
      fourth (trochlear) — see Injury, nerve,
        trochlear
      laceration S04.9
        left S04.9
        right S04.9
      left S04.9
      ninth (glossopharyngeal) — see Injury,
        nerve, glossopharyngeal
      right S04.9
      second (optic) — see Injury, nerve, optic
      seventh (facial) — see Injury, nerve, facial
      sixth (abducent) — see Injury, nerve,
        abducens
      specified
        nerve NEC S04.899
          contusion S04.899
            left S04.892
            right S04.891
          laceration S04.899
            left S04.892
            right S04.891
          left S04.892
          right S04.891
          specified type NEC S04.899
            left S04.892
            right S04.891
        type NEC S04.9
          left S04.9
          right S04.9
      tenth (pneumogastric or vagus) — see
        Injury, nerve, vagus
      third (oculomotor) — see Injury, nerve,
        oculomotor
      twelfth (hypoglossal) — see Injury, nerve,
        hypoglossal
    cutaneous sensory
      ankle (level) S94.30
        left S94.32
        right S94.31
      arm (upper) (level) S44.50
        left S44.52
        right S44.51
      foot (level) — see Injury, nerve, cutaneous
        sensory, ankle
      forearm (level) S54.30
        left S54.32
        right S54.31
      hip (level) S74.20
        left S74.22
        right S74.21

Injury (see also specified injury type) — continued
  nerve — continued
    cutaneous sensory — continued
      leg (lower level) S84.20
        left S84.22
        right S84.21
      shoulder (level) — see Injury, nerve,
        cutaneous sensory, arm
      thigh (level) — see Injury, nerve,
        cutaneous sensory, hip
    deep peroneal — see Injury, nerve, peroneal,
      foot
    digital
      finger S64.40
        index S64.498
          left S64.491
          right S64.490
        little S64.498
          left S64.497
          right S64.496
        middle S64.498
          left S64.493
          right S64.492
        ring S64.498
          left S64.495
          right S64.494
        thumb S64.30
          left S64.32
          right S64.31
      toe — see Injury, nerve, ankle, specified
        site NEC
    eighth cranial (acoustic or auditory) — see
      Injury, nerve, acoustic
    eleventh cranial (accessory) — see Injury,
      nerve, accessory
    facial S04.50
      contusion S04.50
        left S04.52
        right S04.51
      laceration S04.50
        left S04.52
        right S04.51
      left S04.52
      newborn P11.3
      right S04.51
      specified type NEC S04.50
        left S04.52
        right S04.51
    femoral (hip level) (thigh level) S74.10
      left S74.12
      right S74.11
    fifth cranial (trigeminal) — see Injury, nerve,
      trigeminal
    finger (digital) — see Injury, nerve, digital,
      finger
    first cranial (olfactory) — see Injury, nerve,
      olfactory
    foot S94.90
      cutaneous sensory S94.30
        left S94.32
        right S94.31
      deep peroneal S94.20
        left S94.22
        right S94.21
      lateral plantar S94.00
        left S94.02
        right S94.01
      left S94.92
      medial plantar S94.10
        left S94.12
        right S94.11
      right S94.91
      specified site NEC — see category S94.8
    forearm (level) S54.90
      cutaneous sensory — see Injury, nerve,
        cutaneous sensory, forearm
      left S54.92
      median — see Injury, nerve, median
      radial — see Injury, nerve, radial
      right S54.91
      specified site NEC — see category S54.8
      ulnar — see Injury, nerve, ulnar
    fourth cranial (trochlear) — see Injury,
      nerve, trochlear

©2002 Ingenix, Inc.

Injury (*see also* specified injury type) — *continued*
optic (chiasm) (cortex) (nerve) (pathways) — *see* Injury, nerve, optic
orbit, orbital (region) — *see* Injury, eye
  penetrating (with foreign body) — *see* Injury, eye, orbit, penetrating
  specified NEC — *see* Injury, eye, specified site NEC
ovary, ovarian S37.409
  bilateral S37.402
    contusion S37.422
    laceration S37.432
    specified type NEC S37.492
  blood vessel — *see* Injury, blood vessel, ovarian
  contusion S37.429
    bilateral S37.422
    unilateral S37.421
  laceration S37.439
    bilateral S37.432
    unilateral S37.431
  specified type NEC S37.499
    bilateral S37.492
    unilateral S37.491
  unilateral S37.401
    contusion S37.421
    laceration S37.431
    specified type NEC S37.491
palate (hard) (soft) S09.93
pancreas S36.209
  body S36.201
    contusion S36.221
    laceration S36.231
      major S36.261
      minor S36.241
      moderate S36.251
    specified type NEC S36.291
  contusion S36.229
  head S36.200
    contusion S36.220
    laceration S36.230
      major S36.260
      minor S36.240
      moderate S36.250
    specified type NEC S36.290
  laceration S36.239
    major S36.269
    minor S36.249
    moderate S36.259
  specified type NEC S36.299
  tail S36.202
    contusion S36.222
    laceration S36.232
      major S36.262
      minor S36.242
      moderate S36.252
    specified type NEC S36.292
parietal (region) (scalp) S09.90
  lobe — *see* Injury, intracranial
pelvis, pelvic (floor) S39.93
  complicating delivery O70.1
  joint or ligament, complicating delivery O71.6
  organ S37.90
    with ectopic or molar pregnancy O08.6
    complication of abortion — *see* categories O03-O07 with fourth character .3 or .8
    contusion S37.92
    following ectopic or molar pregnancy O08.6
    laceration S37.93
    obstetrical trauma NEC O71.5
    specified
      site NEC S37.899
        contusion S37.892
        laceration S37.893
        specified type NEC S37.898
      type NEC S37.99
  specified NEC S39.83
penis S39.93
perineum S39.93
peritoneum — *see* Injury, intra-abdominal, specified site NEC
periurethral tissue — *see* Injury, urethra

Injury (*see also* specified injury type) — *continued*
phalanges
  foot — *see* Injury, foot
  hand — *see* Injury, hand
pharynx S09.93
pleura — *see* Injury, intrathoracic, pleura
plexus
  brachial — *see* Injury, brachial plexus
  cardiac — *see* Injury, nerve, thorax, sympathetic
  celiac, coeliac — *see* Injury, nerve, lumbosacral, sympathetic
  esophageal — *see* Injury, nerve, thorax, sympathetic
  hypogastric — *see* Injury, nerve, lumbosacral, sympathetic
  lumbar, lumbosacral — *see* Injury, lumbosacral plexus
  mesenteric — *see* Injury, nerve, lumbosacral, sympathetic
  pulmonary — *see* Injury, nerve, thorax, sympathetic
prepuce S39.93
prostate S37.829
  contusion S37.822
  laceration S37.823
  specified type NEC S37.828
pubic region S39.93
pudendum S39.93
pulmonary plexus — *see* Injury, nerve, thorax, sympathetic
radiation NEC T66
radioactive substance or radium NEC T66
rectovaginal septum NEC S39.83
rectum — *see* Injury, intestine, large, rectum
retina — *see* Injury, eye, specified site NEC
  penetrating — *see* Injury, eyeball, penetrating
retroperitoneal — *see* Injury, intra-abdominal, specified site NEC
roentgen rays NEC T66
rotator cuff S46.009
  laceration S46.029
    left S46.022
    right S46.021
  left S46.002
  right S46.001
  specified type NEC S46.099
    left S46.092
    right S46.091
  strain S46.019
    left S46.012
    right S46.011
round ligament — *see* Injury, pelvic organ, specified site NEC
sacral plexus — *see* Injury, lumbosacral plexus
salivary duct or gland S09.93
scalp S09.90
  fetus or newborn (birth injury) P12.9
    due to monitoring (electrode) (sampling incision) P12.4
    specified NEC P12.89
      caput succedaneum P12.81
scapular region — *see* Injury, shoulder
sclera — *see* Injury, eye, specified site NEC
  penetrating — *see* Injury, eyeball, penetrating
scrotum S39.93
second cranial nerve (optic) — *see* Injury, nerve, optic
seminal vesicle — *see* Injury, pelvic organ, specified site NEC
seventh cranial nerve (facial) — *see* Injury, nerve, facial
shoulder S49.90
  blood vessel — *see* Injury, blood vessel, arm
  contusion — *see* Contusion, shoulder
  dislocation — *see* Dislocation, shoulder
  fracture — *see* Fracture, shoulder
  left S49.92
  muscle — *see* Injury, muscle, shoulder
  nerve — *see* Injury, nerve, shoulder
  open — *see* Wound, open, shoulder
  right S49.91
  specified type NEC S49.80
    left S49.82
    right S49.81

Injury (*see also* specified injury type) — *continued*
shoulder — *continued*
  sprain — *see* Sprain, shoulder girdle
  superficial — *see* Injury, superficial, shoulder
sinus
  cavernous — *see* Injury, intracranial
  nasal S09.92
sixth cranial nerve (abducent) — *see* Injury, nerve, abducens
skeleton, birth injury P13.9
  specified part NEC P13.8
skin NEC T14.90
  surface intact — *see* Injury, superficial
skull NEC S09.90
spermatic cord (scrotal) S39.93
  pelvic region — *see* Injury, pelvic organ, specified site NEC
spinal (cord)
  cervical (neck) S14.109
    anterior cord syndrome S14.139
      C1 level S14.131
      C2 level S14.132
      C3 level S14.133
      C4 level S14.134
      C5 level S14.135
      C6 level S14.136
      C7 level S14.137
    Brown-Séquard syndrome S14.149
      C1 level S14.141
      C2 level S14.142
      C3 level S14.143
      C4 level S14.144
      C5 level S14.145
      C6 level S14.146
      C7 level S14.147
    C1 level S14.101
    C2 level S14.102
    C3 level S14.103
    C4 level S14.104
    C5 level S14.105
    C6 level S14.106
    C7 level S14.107
    central cord syndrome S14.129
      C1 level S14.121
      C2 level S14.122
      C3 level S14.123
      C4 level S14.124
      C5 level S14.125
      C6 level S14.126
      C7 level S14.127
    complete lesion S14.119
      C1 level S14.111
      C2 level S14.112
      C3 level S14.113
      C4 level S14.114
      C5 level S14.115
      C6 level S14.116
      C7 level S14.117
    concussion S14.0
    edema S14.0
    incomplete lesion specified NEC S14.159
      C1 level S14.151
      C2 level S14.152
      C3 level S14.153
      C4 level S14.154
      C5 level S14.155
      C6 level S14.156
      C7 level S14.157
    posterior cord syndrome S14.159
      C1 level S14.151
      C2 level S14.152
      C3 level S14.153
      C4 level S14.154
      C5 level S14.155
      C6 level S14.156
      C7 level S14.157
  dorsal — *see* Injury, spinal, thoracic
  lumbar S34.109
    complete lesion S34.119
      C1 level S34.111
      C2 level S34.112
      C3 level S34.113
      C4 level S34.114
      C5 level S34.115
    concussion S34.01

Injury (see also specified injury type) — continued
  spinal — continued
    lumbar — continued
      edema S34.01
      incomplete lesion S34.129
        C1 level S34.121
        C2 level S34.122
        C3 level S34.123
        C4 level S34.124
        C5 level S34.125
        L1 level S34.101
        L2 level S34.102
        L3 level S34.103
        L4 level S34.104
        L5 level S34.105
    nerve root NEC
      cervical — see Injury, nerve, spinal, root, cervical
      dorsal — see Injury, nerve, spinal, root, dorsal
      lumbar S34.21
      sacral S34.22
      thoracic — see Injury, nerve, spinal, root, dorsal
    plexus
      brachial — see Injury, brachial plexus
      lumbosacral — see Injury, lumbosacral plexus
    sacral S34.139
      complete lesion S34.131
      incomplete lesion S34.132
    thoracic S24.109
      anterior cord syndrome S24.139
        T1 level S24.131
        T2-T6 level S24.132
        T7-T10 level S24.133
        T11-T12 level S24.134
      Brown-Séquard syndrome S24.149
        T1 level S24.141
        T2-T6 level S24.142
        T7-T10 level S24.143
        T11-T12 level S24.144
      complete lesion S24.119
        T1 level S24.111
        T2-T6 level S24.112
        T7-T10 level S24.113
        T11-T12 level S24.114
      concussion S24.0
      edema S24.0
      incomplete lesion specified NEC S24.159
        T1 level S24.151
        T2-T6 level S24.152
        T7-T10 level S24.153
        T11-T12 level S24.154
      posterior cord syndrome S24.159
        T1 level S24.151
        T2-T6 level S24.152
        T7-T10 level S24.153
        T11-T12 level S24.154
      T1 level S24.101
      T2-T6 level S24.102
      T7-T10 level S24.103
      T11-T12 level S24.104
    splanchnic nerve — see Injury, nerve, lumbosacral, sympathetic
  spleen S36.00
    contusion S36.029
      major S36.021
      minor S36.020
    laceration S36.039
      major (massive) (stellate) S36.032
      moderate S36.031
      superficial (capsular) (minor) S36.030
    specified type NEC S36.09
  splenic artery — see Injury, blood vessel, celiac artery, branch
  stellate ganglion — see Injury, nerve, thorax, sympathetic
  sternal region S29.9
  stomach S36.30
    contusion S36.32
    laceration S36.33
    specified type NEC S36.39
  subconjunctival — see Injury, eye, conjunctiva
  subcutaneous NEC T14.90
  submaxillary region S09.93

Injury (see also specified injury type) — continued
  submental region S09.93
  subungual
    fingers — see Injury, hand
    toes — see Injury, foot
  superficial
    abdomen, abdominal (wall) S30.92
      abrasion S30.811
      bite S30.871
        insect S30.861
      contusion S30.1
      external constriction S30.841
      foreign body S30.851
    abrasion — see Abrasion, by site
    adnexa, eye NEC — see Injury, eye, specified site NEC
    alveolar process — see Injury, superficial, oral cavity
    ankle S90.919
      abrasion — see Abrasion, ankle
      blister — see Blister, ankle
      bite — see Bite, ankle
      contusion — see Contusion, ankle
      external constriction — see Constriction, external, ankle
      foreign body — see Foreign body, superficial, ankle
      left S90.912
      right S90.911
    anus S30.98
    arm (upper) S40.929
      abrasion — see Abrasion, arm
      bite — see Bite, superficial, arm
      blister — see Blister, arm (upper)
      contusion — see Contusion, arm
      external constriction — see Constriction, external, arm
      foreign body — see Foreign body, superficial, arm
      left S40.922
      right S40.921
    auditory canal (external) (meatus) — see Injury, superficial, ear
    auricle — see Injury, superficial, ear
    axilla — see Injury, superficial, arm
    back — see also Injury, superficial, thorax, back
      lower S30.91
        abrasion S30.810
        contusion S30.0
        external constriction S30.840
        superficial
          bite NEC S30.870
            insect S30.860
          foreign body S30.850
    bite NEC — see Bite, superficial NEC, by site
    blister — see Blister, by site
    breast S20.109
      abrasion — see Abrasion, breast
      bite — see Bite, superficial, breast
      contusion — see Contusion, breast
      external constriction — see Constriction, external, breast
      foreign body — see Foreign body, superficial, breast
      left S20.102
      right S20.101
    brow — see Injury, superficial, head, specified NEC
    buttock S30.91
    calf — see Injury, superficial, leg
    canthus, eye — see Injury, superficial, periocular area
    cheek (external) — see Injury, superficial, head, specified NEC
      internal — see Injury, superficial, oral cavity
    chest wall — see Injury, superficial, thorax
    chin — see Injury, superficial, head NEC
    clitoris S30.95
    conjunctiva — see Injury, eye, conjunctiva
      with foreign body (in conjunctival sac) — see Foreign body, conjunctival sac
    contusion — see Contusion, by site
    costal region — see Injury, superficial, thorax

Injury (see also specified injury type) — continued
  superficial — continued
    digit(s)
      hand — see Injury, superficial, finger
    ear (auricle) (canal) (external) S00.409
      abrasion — see Abrasion, ear
      bite — see Bite, superficial, ear
      contusion — see Contusion, ear
      external constriction — see Constriction, external, ear
      foreign body — see Foreign body, superficial, ear
      left S00.402
      right S00.401
    elbow S50.909
      abrasion — see Abrasion, elbow
      bite — see Bite, superficial, elbow
      blister — see Blister, elbow
      contusion — see Contusion, elbow
      external constriction — see Constriction, external, elbow
      foreign body — see Foreign body, superficial, elbow
      left S50.902
      right S50.901
    epididymis S30.94
    epigastric region S30.92
    epiglottis — see Injury, superficial, throat
    esophagus
      cervical — see Injury, superficial, throat
    external constriction — see Constriction, external, by site
    extremity T14.90
    eyeball NEC — see Injury, eye, specified site NEC
    eyebrow — see Injury, superficial, periocular area
    eyelid S00.209
      abrasion — see Abrasion, eyelid
      bite — see Bite, superficial, eyelid
      contusion — see Contusion, eyelid
      external constriction — see Constriction, external, eyelid
      foreign body — see Foreign body, superficial, eyelid
      left S00.202
      right S00.201
    face NEC — see Injury, superficial, head, specified NEC
    finger(s) S60.949
      abrasion — see Abrasion, finger
      bite — see Bite, superficial, finger
      blister — see Blister, finger
      contusion — see Contusion, finger
      external constriction — see Constriction, external, finger
      foreign body — see Foreign body, superficial, finger
      insect bite — see Bite, insect, finger
      index S60.949
        left S60.941
        right S60.940
      little S60.948
        left S60.947
        right S60.946
      middle S60.948
        left S60.943
        right S60.942
      ring S60.948
        left S60.945
        right S60.944
    flank S30.92
    foot S90.929
      abrasion — see Abrasion, foot
      bite — see Bite, foot
      blister — see Blister, foot
      contusion — see Contusion, foot
      external constriction — see Constriction, external, foot
      foreign body — see Foreign body, superficial, foot
      left S90.922
      right S90.921
    forearm S50.919
      abrasion — see Abrasion, forearm
      bite — see Bite, forearm, superficial

©2002 Ingenix, Inc.

Injury (see also specified injury type) — continued
  superficial — continued
    forearm — continued
      blister — see Blister, forearm
      contusion — see Contusion, forearm
      elbow only — see Injury, superficial,
        elbow
      external constriction — see Constriction,
        external, forearm
      foreign body — see Foreign body,
        superficial, forearm
      left S50.912
      right S50.911
    forehead — see Injury, superficial, head
      NEC
    foreign body — see Foreign body, superficial
    genital organs, external
      female S30.97
      male S30.96
    globe (eye) — see Injury, eye, specified site
      NEC
    groin S30.92
    gum — see Injury, superficial, oral cavity
    hand S60.929
      abrasion — see Abrasion, hand
      bite — see Bite, superficial, hand
      contusion — see Contusion, hand
      external constriction — see Constriction,
        external, hand
      foreign body — see Foreign body,
        superficial, hand
      left S60.922
      right S60.921
    head S00.90
      ear — see Injury, superficial, ear
      eyelid — see Injury, superficial, eyelid
      nose S00.30
      oral cavity S00.502
      scalp S00.00
      specified site NEC S00.80
    heel — see Injury, superficial, foot
    hip S70.919
      abrasion — see Abrasion, hip
      bite — see Bite, superficial, hip
      blister — see Blister, hip
      contusion — see Contusion, hip
      external constriction — see Constriction,
        external, hip
      foreign body — see Foreign body,
        superficial, hip
      left S70.912
      right S70.911
    iliac region — see Injury, superficial,
      abdomen
    inguinal region — see Injury, superficial,
      abdomen
    insect bite — see Bite, insect, by site
    interscapular region — see Injury,
      superficial, thorax, back
    jaw — see Injury, superficial, head, specified
      NEC
    knee S80.919
      abrasion — see Abrasion, knee
      bite — see Bite, superficial, knee
      blister — see Blister, knee
      contusion — see Contusion, knee
      external constriction — see Constriction,
        external, knee
      foreign body — see Foreign body,
        superficial, knee
      left S80.912
      right S80.911
    labium (majus) (minus) S30.95
    lacrimal (apparatus) (gland) (sac) — see
      Injury, eye, specified site NEC
    larynx — see Injury, superficial, throat
    leg (lower) S80.929
      abrasion — see Abrasion, leg
      bite — see Bite, superficial, leg
      contusion — see Contusion, leg
      external constriction — see Constriction,
        external, leg
      foreign body — see Foreign body,
        superficial, leg
      knee — see Injury, superficial, knee
      left S80.922

Injury (see also specified injury type) — continued
  superficial — continued
    leg — continued
      right S80.921
    limb T14.90
    lip S00.501
    lower back S30.91
    lumbar region S30.91
    malar region — see Injury, superficial, head,
      specified NEC
    mammary — see Injury, superficial, breast
    mastoid region — see Injury, superficial,
      head, specified NEC
    mouth — see Injury, superficial, oral cavity
    muscle T14.90
    nail
      finger — see Injury, superficial, finger
      toe — see Injury, superficial, toe
    nasal (septum) — see Injury, superficial,
      nose
    neck S10.90
      specified site NEC S10.80
    nose (septum) S00.30
    occipital region — see Injury, superficial,
      scalp
    oral cavity S00.502
    orbital region — see Injury, superficial,
      periocular area
    palate — see Injury, superficial, oral cavity
    palm — see Injury, superficial, hand
    parietal region — see Injury, superficial,
      scalp
    pelvis S30.91
      girdle — see Injury, superficial, hip
    penis S30.93
    perineum
      female S30.95
      male S30.91
    periocular area S00.209
      abrasion — see Abrasion, eyelid
      bite — see Bite, superficial, eyelid
      contusion — see Contusion, eyelid
      external constriction — see Constriction,
        external, eyelid
      foreign body — see Foreign body,
        superficial, eyelid
      left S00.202
      right S00.201
    phalanges
      finger — see Injury, superficial, finger
      toe — see Injury, superficial, toe
    pharynx — see Injury, superficial, throat
    pinna — see Injury, superficial, ear
    popliteal space — see Injury, superficial,
      knee
    prepuce S30.93
    pubic region S30.91
    pudendum
      female S30.97
      male S30.96
    sacral region S30.91
    scalp S00.00
    scapular region — see Injury, superficial,
      shoulder
    sclera — see Injury, eye, specified site NEC
    scrotum S30.94
    shin — see Injury, superficial, leg
    shoulder S40.919
      abrasion — see Abrasion, shoulder
      bite — see Bite, superficial, shoulder
      blister — see Blister, shoulder
      contusion — see Contusion, shoulder
      external constriction — see Constriction,
        external, shoulder
      foreign body — see Foreign body,
        superficial, shoulder
      left S40.912
      right S40.911
    skin NEC T14.90
    sternal region — see Injury, superficial,
      thorax, front
    subconjunctival — see Injury, eye, specified
      site NEC
    subcutaneous NEC T14.90
    submaxillary region — see Injury,
      superficial, head, specified NEC

Injury (see also specified injury type) — continued
  superficial — continued
    submental region — see Injury, superficial,
      head, specified NEC
    subungual
      finger(s) — see Injury, superficial, finger
      toe(s) — see Injury, superficial, toe
    supraclavicular fossa — see Injury,
      superficial, neck
    supraorbital — see Injury, superficial, head,
      specified NEC
    temple — see Injury, superficial, head,
      specified NEC
    temporal region — see Injury, superficial,
      head, specified NEC
    testis S30.94
    thigh S70.929
      abrasion — see Abrasion, thigh
      bite — see Bite, superficial, thigh
      blister — see Blister, thigh
      contusion — see Contusion, thigh
      external constriction — see Constriction,
        external, thigh
      foreign body — see Foreign body,
        superficial, thigh
      left S70.922
      right S70.921
    thorax, thoracic (wall) S20.90
      abrasion — see Abrasion, thorax
      back S20.409
        left S20.402
        right S20.401
      bite — see Bite, thorax, superficial
      blister — see Blister, thorax
      contusion — see Contusion, thorax
      external constriction — see Constriction,
        external, thorax
      foreign body — see Foreign body,
        superficial, thorax
      front S20.309
        left S20.302
        right S20.301
    throat S10.10
      abrasion S10.11
      bite S10.17
        insect S10.16
      blister S10.12
      contusion S10.0
      external constriction S10.14
      foreign body S10.15
    thumb S60.939
      abrasion — see Abrasion, thumb
      bite — see Bite, superficial, thumb
      blister — see Blister, thumb
      contusion — see Contusion, thumb
      external constriction — see Constriction,
        external, thumb
      foreign body — see Foreign body,
        superficial, thumb
      insect bite — see Bite, insect, thumb
      left S60.932
        specified type NEC S60.392
      right S60.931
        specified type NEC S60.391
      specified type NEC S60.399
    toe(s) S90.936
      abrasion — see Abrasion, toe
      bite — see Bite, toe
      blister — see Blister, toe
      contusion — see Contusion, toe
      external constriction — see Constriction,
        external, toe
      foreign body — see Foreign body,
        superficial, toe
      great S90.933
        left S90.932
        right S90.931
      left S90.935
      right S90.934
    tongue — see Injury, superficial, oral cavity
    tooth, teeth — see Injury, superficial, oral
      cavity
    trachea S10.10
    tunica vaginalis S30.94
    tympanum, tympanic membrane — see
      Injury, superficial, ear

Injury (*see also* specified injury type) — *continued*
  superficial — *continued*
    uvula — *see* Injury, superficial, oral cavity
    vagina S30.95
    vocal cords — *see* Injury, superficial, throat
    vulva S30.95
    wrist S60.919
      left S60.912
      right S60.911
  supraclavicular region — *see* Injury, neck
  supraorbital S09.93
  suprarenal gland (multiple) — *see* Injury, adrenal
  surgical complication (external or internal site) — *see* Laceration, accidental complicating surgery
  temple S09.90
  temporal region S09.90
  tendon — *see also* Injury, muscle, by site
    abdomen — *see* Injury, muscle, abdomen
    Achilles — *see* Injury, Achilles tendon
    lower back — *see* Injury, muscle, lower back
    pelvic organs — *see* Injury, muscle, pelvis
  tenth cranial nerve (pneumogastric or vagus) — *see* Injury, nerve, vagus
  testis S39.93
  thigh S79.929
    blood vessel — *see* Injury, blood vessel, hip
    contusion — *see* Contusion, thigh
    fracture — *see* Fracture, femur
    left S79.922
    muscle — *see* Injury, muscle, thigh
    nerve — *see* Injury, nerve, thigh
    open — *see* Wound, open, thigh
    right S79.921
    specified NEC S79.829
      left S79.822
      right S79.821
    superficial — *see* Injury, superficial, thigh
  third cranial nerve (oculomotor) — *see* Injury, nerve, oculomotor
  thorax, thoracic S29.9
    blood vessel — *see* Injury, blood vessel, thorax
    cavity — *see* Injury, intrathoracic
    dislocation — *see* Dislocation, thorax
    external (wall) S29.9
      contusion — *see* Contusion, thorax
      nerve — *see* Injury, nerve, thorax
      open — *see* Wound, open, thorax
      specified NEC S29.8
      sprain — *see* Sprain, thorax
      superficial — *see* Injury, superficial, thorax
    fracture — *see* Fracture, thorax
    internal — *see* Injury, intrathoracic
    intrathoracic organ — *see* Injury, intrathoracic
    sympathetic ganglion — *see* Injury, nerve, thorax, sympathetic
  throat — *see* Injury, neck
  thumb S69.90
    blood vessel — *see* Injury, blood vessel, thumb
    contusion — *see* Contusion, thumb
    dislocation — *see* Dislocation, thumb
    fracture — *see* Fracture, thumb
    left S69.92
    muscle — *see* Injury, muscle, thumb
    nerve — *see* Injury, nerve, digital, thumb
    open — *see* Wound, open, thumb
    right S69.91
    specified NEC S69.80
      left S69.82
      right S69.81
    sprain — *see* Sprain, thumb
    superficial — *see* Injury, superficial, thumb
  thymus (gland) — *see* Injury, intrathoracic, specified organ NEC
  thyroid (gland) NEC S19.8
  toe S99.929
    contusion — *see* Contusion, toe
    dislocation — *see* Dislocation, toe
    fracture — *see* Fracture, toe
    left S99.922
    muscle — *see* Injury, muscle, toe
    open — *see* Wound, open, toe

Injury (*see also* specified injury type) — *continued*
  toe — *continued*
    right S99.921
    specified type NEC S99.829
      left S99.822
      right S99.821
    sprain — *see* Sprain, toe
    superficial — *see* Injury, superficial, toe
  tongue S09.93
  tonsil S09.93
  tooth S09.93
  trachea (cervical) NEC S19.8
    thoracic — *see* Injury, intrathoracic, trachea, thoracic
  tunica vaginalis S39.93
  twelfth cranial nerve (hypoglossal) — *see* Injury, nerve, hypoglossal
  ultraviolet rays NEC T66
  ureter S37.10
    contusion S37.12
    laceration S37.13
    specified type NEC S37.19
  urethra (sphincter) S37.30
    at delivery O71.5
    contusion S37.32
    laceration S37.33
    specified type NEC S37.38
  uterus, uterine S37.60
    with ectopic or molar pregnancy O08.6
    blood vessel — *see* Injury, blood vessel, iliac
    contusion S37.62
    laceration S37.63
      cervix at delivery O71.3
    rupture associated with obstetrics — *see* Rupture, uterus
    specified type NEC S37.69
  uvula S09.93
  vagina S39.93
    abrasion S30.814
    bite S31.45
      insect S30.864
      superficial NEC S30.874
    contusion S30.23
    crush S38.03
    during delivery — *see* Laceration, vagina, during delivery
    external constriction S30.844
    insect bite S30.864
    laceration S31.41
      with foreign body S31.42
    open wound S31.40
    puncture S31.43
      with foreign body S31.44
    superficial S30.95
      foreign body S30.854
  vas deferens — *see* Injury, pelvic organ, specified site NEC
  vein — *see* Injury, blood vessel
  vena cava (superior) S25.20
    inferior S35.10
      laceration (minor) (superficial) S35.11
        major S35.12
      specified type NEC S35.19
    laceration (minor) (superficial) S25.21
      major S25.22
    specified type NEC S25.29
  vesical (sphincter) — *see* Injury, bladder
  visual cortex — *see* Injury, nerve, optic
  vitreous (humor) S05.90
  vulva S39.93
    abrasion S30.814
    bite S31.45
      insect S30.864
      superficial NEC S30.874
    contusion S30.23
    crush S38.03
    during delivery — *see* Laceration, perineum, female, during delivery
    external constriction S30.844
    insect bite S30.864
    laceration S31.41
      with foreign body S31.42
    open wound S31.40
    puncture S31.43
      with foreign body S31.44
    superficial S30.95
      foreign body S30.854

Injury (*see also* specified injury type) — *continued*
  whiplash (cervical spine) S13.4
  wrist S69.90
    blood vessel — *see* Injury, blood vessel, hand
    contusion — *see* Contusion, wrist
    dislocation — *see* Dislocation, wrist
    fracture — *see* Fracture, wrist
    left S69.92
    muscle — *see* Injury, muscle, hand
    nerve — *see* Injury, nerve, hand
    open — *see* Wound, open, wrist
    right S69.91
    specified NEC S69.80
      left S69.82
      right S69.81
    sprain — *see* Sprain, wrist
    superficial — *see* Injury, superficial, wrist
  X-ray NEC T66

Inoculation — *see also* Vaccination
  complication or reaction — *see* Complications, vaccination

Insanity, insane — *see also* Psychosis
  adolescent — *see* Schizophrenia
  confusional F28
    acute or subacute F05
  delusional F22
  senile F03

Insect
  bite — *see* Bite, insect, by site
  venomous, poisoning NEC (by) — *see* Venom, arthropod

Insertion
  cord (umbilical) lateral or velamentous O43.129
    first trimester O43.121
    second trimester O43.122
    third trimester O43.123
  placenta, vicious — *see* Placenta, previa

Insolation (sunstroke) T67.0

Insomnia (organic) G47.0
  nonorganic origin F51.0
  primary F51.0

Inspiration
  food or foreign body — *see* Asphyxia, food
  mucus — *see* Asphyxia, mucus

Inspissated bile syndrome (newborn) P59.1

Instability
  emotional (excessive) F60.3
  joint (post-traumatic) M25.30
    ankle M25.373
      left M25.372
      right M25.371
    due to old ligament injury — *see* Disorder, ligament
    elbow M25.329
      left M25.322
      right M25.321
    flail — *see* Flail, joint
    foot M25.376
      left M25.375
      right M25.374
    hand M25.349
      left M25.342
      right M25.341
    hip M25.359
      left M25.352
      right M25.351
    knee M25.369
      left M25.362
      right M25.361
    lumbosacral — *see* category M53.2
    sacroiliac — *see* category M53.2
    secondary to
      old ligament injury — *see* Disorder, ligament
      removal of joint prosthesis M96.89
    shoulder (region) M25.319
      left M25.312
      right M25.311
    specified site NEC M25.38
    spine — *see* category M53.2
    wrist M25.339
      left M25.332
      right M25.331

©2002 Ingenix, Inc.

Instability — *continued*
knee (chronic) M23.50
left M23.52
right M23.51
lumbosacral — *see* category M53.2
nervous F48.8
personality (emotional) F60.3
spine — *see* Instability, joint, spine
vasomotor R55
Institutional syndrome (childhood) F94.2
Institutionalization, affecting child Z62.2
disinhibited attachment F94.2
Insufficiency, insufficient
accommodation, old age H52.4
adrenal (gland) E27.4
primary E27.1
adrenocortical E27.4
drug-induced E27.3
iatrogenic E27.3
primary E27.1
anus K62.8
aortic (valve) I35.1
with
mitral (valve) disease I08.0
with tricuspid (valve) disease I08.3
stenosis I35.2
tricuspid (valve) disease I08.2
with mitral (valve) disease I08.3
congenital Q23.1
rheumatic I06.1
with
mitral (valve) disease I08.0
with tricuspid (valve) disease I08.3
stenosis I06.2
with mitral (valve) disease I08.0
with tricuspid (valve) disease
I08.3
tricuspid (valve) disease I08.2
with mitral (valve) disease I08.3
specified cause NEC I35.1
syphilitic A52.03
arterial I77.1
basilar G45.0
carotid (hemispheric) G45.1
cerebral I67.8
coronary (acute or subacute) I24.9
mesenteric K55.1
peripheral I73.9
precerebral (multiple) (bilateral) G45.2
vertebral G45.0
arteriovenous I99.8
biliary K83.8
cardiac — *see also* Insufficiency, myocardial
complicating surgery T81.89
due to presence of (cardiac) prosthesis I97.1
postoperative I97.89
long term effect of cardiac surgery I97.1
specified during or due to a procedure
T81.89
cardiorenal, hypertensive I13.2
cardiovascular — *see* Disease, cardiovascular
cerebrovascular (acute) I67.8
with transient focal neurological signs and
symptoms G45.8
circulatory NEC I99.8
fetus or newborn P29.8
convergence H51.11
coronary (acute or subacute) I24.8
chronic or with a stated duration of over 4
weeks I25.8
corticoadrenal E27.4
primary E27.1
dietary E63.9
divergence H51.8
food T73.0
gastroesophageal K22.8
gonadal
ovary E28.3
testis E29.1
heart — *see also* Insufficiency, myocardial
newborn P29.0
valve — *see* Endocarditis
hepatic — *see* Failure, hepatic
idiopathic autonomic G90.0
kidney — *see* Failure, renal
lacrimal (secretion) — *see* Syndrome, dry eye
passages — *see* Stenosis, lacrimal

Insufficiency, insufficient — *continued*
liver — *see* Failure, hepatic
lung — *see* Insufficiency, pulmonary
mental (congenital) — *see* Retardation, mental
mesenteric K55.1
mitral (valve) I34.0
with
aortic valve disease I08.0
with tricuspid (valve) disease I08.3
obstruction or stenosis I05.2
with aortic valve disease I08.0
tricuspid (valve) disease I08.1
with aortic valve disease I08.3
congenital Q23.3
rheumatic I05.1
with
aortic valve disease I08.0
with tricuspid (valve) disease I08.3
obstruction or stenosis I05.2
with aortic valve disease I08.0
with tricuspid (valve) disease
I08.3
tricuspid (valve) disease I08.1
tricuspid (valve) disease I08.1
with aortic valve disease I08.3
active or acute I01.1
with chorea, rheumatic (Sydenham's)
I02.0
specified cause, except rheumatic I34.0
muscle — *see also* Disease, muscle
heart — *see* Insufficiency, myocardial
ocular NEC H50.9
myocardial, myocardium (with arteriosclerosis)
I50.9
with
rheumatic fever (conditions in I00) I09.0
active, acute or subacute I01.2
with chorea I02.0
inactive or quiescent (with chorea)
I09.0
congenital Q24.8
hypertensive — *see* Hypertension, heart
newborn P29.0
rheumatic I09.0
active, acute, or subacute I01.2
syphilitic A52.06
nourishment T73.0
organic R68.8
ovary E28.3
postablative E89.4
pancreatic K86.8
parathyroid (gland) E20.9
peripheral vascular (arterial) I73.9
pituitary E23.0
placental (mother) — *see* category O36.5
platelets D69.6
prenatal care affecting management of
pregnancy O09.30
first trimester O09.31
second trimester O09.32
third trimester O09.33
progressive pluriglandular E31.0
pulmonary J98.4
acute, following surgery (nonthoracic) J95.2
thoracic J95.1
chronic, following surgery J95.3
following
shock J80
trauma J80
newborn P28.5
valve I37.1
with stenosis I37.2
congenital Q22.2
rheumatic I09.89
with aortic, mitral or tricuspid (valve)
disease I08.8
pyloric K31.89
renal — *see also* Failure, renal
postprocedural N99.0
respiratory R06.89
newborn P28.5
rotation — *see* Malrotation
social insurance Z59.7
suprarenal E27.4
primary E27.1
tarso-orbital fascia, congenital Q10.3
testis E29.1

Insufficiency, insufficient — *continued*
thyroid (gland) (acquired) E03.9
congenital E03.1
tricuspid (valve) (rheumatic) I07.1
with
aortic (valve) disease I08.2
with mitral (valve) disease I08.3
mitral (valve) disease I08.1
with aortic (valve) disease I08.3
obstruction or stenosis I07.2
with aortic (valve) disease I08.2
with mitral (valve) disease I08.3
congenital Q22.8
nonrheumatic I36.1
with stenosis I36.2
urethral sphincter R32
valve, valvular (heart) — *see* Endocarditis
vascular I99.8
intestine K55.9
mesenteric K55.1
peripheral I73.9
renal — *see* Hypertension, kidney
venous (chronic) (peripheral) I87.2
ventricular — *see* Insufficiency, myocardial
welfare support Z59.7
Insufflation, fallopian Z31.41
Insular — *see* condition
Insulinoma (M8151/0)
malignant (M8151/3)
pancreas C25.4
Insulinoma (M8151/0)
specified site NEC — *see* Neoplasm,
malignant
unspecified site C25.4
pancreas D13.7
specified site NEC — *see* Neoplasm, benign
unspecified site D13.7
Insuloma (M8151/0) — *see* Insulinoma
Insult (acute), brain, cerebrovascular or vascular
I64
Intermenstrual — *see* condition
Intermittent — *see* condition
Internal — *see* condition
Interruption
bundle of His I44.30
phase-shift, sleep cycle
sleep phase-shift, or 24 hour sleep-wake cycle
Interstitial — *see* condition
Intertrigo L30.4
labialis K13.0
Intervertebral disc — *see* condition
Intestine, intestinal — *see* condition
Intolerance
carbohydrate K90.4
disaccharide, hereditary E73.0
fat NEC K90.4
pancreatic K90.3
food K90.4
dietary counseling and surveillance Z71.3
fructose E74.10
hereditary E74.12
glucose(-galactose) E74.39
gluten K90.0
lactose E73.9
specified NEC E73.8
lysine E72.3
milk NEC K90.4
lactose E73.9
protein K90.4
starch NEC K90.4
sucrose(-isomaltose) E74.31
Intoxicated NEC (without dependence) — *see*
Alcohol, intoxication
Intoxication
acid E87.2
alcoholic (acute) (without dependence) — *see*
Alcohol, intoxication
alimentary canal K52.1
amphetamine (without dependence) — *see*
Abuse, drug, stimulant, with intoxication
with dependence — *see* Dependence, drug,
stimulant, with intoxication
anxiolytic (acute) (without dependence) — *see*
Abuse, drug, sedative, with intoxication

Iridocyclitis — continued
  subacute — see Iridocyclitis, acute
  sympathetic — see Uveitis, sympathetic
  syphilitic (secondary) A51.43
  tuberculous (chronic) A18.54
  Vogt-Koyanagi — see Vogt-Koyanagi syndrome
Iridocyclochoroiditis (panuveitis) — see
  Panuveitis
Iridodialysis H21.539
  bilateral H21.533
  left H21.532
  right H21.531
Iridodonesis H21.8
Iridoplegia (complete) (partial) (reflex) H57.09
Iridoschisis H21.259
  bilateral H21.253
  left H21.252
  right H21.251
Iris — see also condition
  bombé — see Membrane, pupillary
Iritis — see also Iridocyclitis
  chronic — see Iridocyclitis, chronic
  diabetic — see E09-E13 with .39
  due to
    herpes simplex B00.51
    leprosy A30.9 [H22]
  gonococcal A54.32
  gouty M10.9 [H22]
  granulomatous — see Iridocyclitis, chronic
  lens induced — see Iridocyclitis, lens-induced
  papulosa (syphilitic) A52.71
  rheumatic — see Iridocyclitis, chronic
  syphilitic (secondary) A51.43
    congenital (early) A50.01 [H22]
    late A52.71
  tuberculous A18.54
Iron — see condition
Iron-miner's lung J63.4
Irradiated enamel (tooth, teeth) K03.8
Irradiation effects, adverse T66
Irreducible, irreducibility — see condition
Irregular, irregularity
  action, heart I49.9
  alveolar process K08.8
  bleeding N92.6
  breathing R06.89
  contour of cornea (acquired) — see Deformity,
    cornea
    congenital Q13.4
  dentin (in pulp) K04.3
  eye movements H55.89
    nystagmus — see Nystagmus
    saccadic H55.81
  labor O62.2
  menstruation (cause unknown) N92.6
  periods N92.6
  prostate N42.9
  pupil — see Abnormality, pupillary
  respiratory R06.89
  septum (nasal) J34.2
  shape, organ or site, congenital NEC — see
    Distortion
  sleep-wake rhythm, nonorganic origin — see
    Disorder, sleep, circadian rhythm,
    psychogenic
Irritable, irritability R45.4
  bladder N32.8
  bowel (syndrome) K58.9
    with diarrhea K58.0
    psychogenic F45.8
  bronchial — see Bronchitis
  cerebral, in newborn P91.3
  colon K58.9
    with diarrhea K58.0
    psychogenic F45.8
  duodenum K59.8
  heart (psychogenic) F45.8
  hip — see Derangement, joint, specified type
    NEC, hip
  ileum K59.8
  infant R68.12
  jejunum K59.8
  rectum K59.8
  stomach K31.89
    psychogenic F45.8

Irritable, irritability — continued
  sympathetic G90.8
  urethra N36.8
Irritation
  anus K62.8
  axillary nerve G54.0
  bladder N32.8
  brachial plexus G54.0
  bronchial — see Bronchitis
  cervical plexus G54.2
  cervix — see Cervicitis
  choroid, sympathetic — see Endophthalmitis
  cranial nerve — see Disorder, nerve, cranial
  gastric K31.89
    psychogenic F45.8
  globe, sympathetic — see Uveitis, sympathetic
  labyrinth — see category H83.2
  lumbosacral plexus G54.1
  meninges (traumatic) — see Injury, intracranial
    nontraumatic — see Meningismus
  nerve — see Disorder, nerve
  nervous R45.0
  penis N48.89
  perineum NEC L29.3
  peripheral autonomic nervous system G90.8
  peritoneum — see Peritonitis
  pharynx J39.2
  plantar nerve — see Lesion, nerve, plantar
  spinal (cord) (traumatic) — see also Injury,
    spinal cord, by region
    nerve G58.9
      root NEC — see Radiculopathy
    nontraumatic — see Myelopathy
  stomach K31.89
    psychogenic F45.8
  sympathetic nerve NEC G90.8
  ulnar nerve — see Lesion, nerve, ulnar
  vagina N89.8
Ischemia, ischemic I99.8
  brain — see Ischemia, cerebral
  bowel (transient)
    acute K55.0
    chronic K55.1
    due to mesenteric artery insufficiency K55.1
  cardiac (see Disease, heart, ischemic)
  cardiomyopathy I25.5
  cerebral (chronic) (generalized) I67.8
    arteriosclerotic I67.2
    intermittent G45.9
    newborn P91.0
    puerperal, postpartum, childbirth — see
      Disease, circulatory, obstetric
    recurrent focal G45.8
    transient G45.9
  colon chronic(due to mesenteric artery
    insufficiency K55.1
  coronary — see Disease, heart, ischemic
  heart (chronic or with a stated duration of over
    4 weeks) I25.9
    acute or with a stated duration of 4 weeks
      or less I24.9
    subacute I24.9
  infarction, muscle — see Infarct, muscle
  intestine (large) (small) (transient) K55.9
    acute K55.0
    chronic K55.1
    due to mesenteric artery insufficiency K55.1
  kidney N28.0
  mesenteric, acute K55.0
  muscle, traumatic T79.6
  myocardium, myocardial (chronic or with a
    stated duration of over 4 weeks) I25.9
    acute, without myocardial infarction I24.0
    silent (asymptomatic) I25.6
    transient of newborn P29.4
  renal N28.0
  retina, retinal — see Occlusion, artery, retina
  small bowel
    acute K55.0
    chronic K55.1
    due to mesenteric artery insufficiency
  spinal cord G95.11
  subendocardial — see Insufficiency, coronary
Ischial spine — see condition
Ischialgia — see Sciatica
Ischiopagus Q89.4

Ischium, ischial — see condition
Ischuria R34
Iselin's disease or osteochondrosis — see
  Osteochondrosis, juvenile, metatarsus
Islands of
  parotid tissue in
    lymph nodes Q38.6
    neck structures Q38.6
  submaxillary glands in
    fascia Q38.6
    lymph nodes Q38.6
    neck muscles Q38.6
Islet cell tumor, pancreas (M8150/0) D13.7
Isoimmunization NEC — see also Incompatibility
  affecting management of pregnancy (ABO) —
    see also category O36.1
    Rh O36.00
      first trimester O36.01
      second trimester O36.02
      third trimester O36.03
  fetus or newborn P55.9
    with
      hydrops fetalis P56.0
      kernicterus P57.0
    ABO (blood groups) P55.1
    Rhesus (Rh) factor P55.0
    specified type NEC P55.8
Isolation, isolated Z51.89
  dwelling Z59.8
  family Z63.7
  social Z60.4
Isoleucinosis E71.19
Isomerism atrial appendages (with asplenia or
  polysplenia) Q20.6
Isosporiasis, isosporosis A07.3
Isovaleric acidemia E71.110
Issue of
  medical certificate (cause of death) Z02.79
    for disability determination Z02.71
  repeat prescription (appliance) (glasses)
    (medicinal substance, medicament,
    medicine) Z76.0
    contraceptive pill Z30.41
    device (intrauterine) Z30.44
Itch, itching — see also Pruritus
  baker's L25.4
    allergic L23.6
    irritant L24.6
  barber's B35.0
  bricklayer's L25.3
    allergic L23.5
    irritant L24.5
  cheese B88.0
  clam digger's B65.3
  coolie B76.9
  copra B88.0
  dew B76.9
  dhobi B35.6
  filarial — see Infestation, filarial
  grain B88.0
  grocer's B88.0
  ground B76.9
  harvest B88.0
  jock B35.6
  Malabar B35.5
    beard B35.0
    foot B35.3
    scalp B35.0
  meaning scabies B86
  Norwegian B86
  perianal L29.0
  poultrymen's B88.0
  sarcoptic B86
  scrub B88.0
  seven year Z63.0
    meaning scabies B86
  straw B88.0
  swimmer's B65.3
  water B76.9
  winter L29.8
Ivemark's syndrome (asplenia with congenital
  heart disease) Q89.01
Ivory bones Q78.2
Ixodiasis NEC B88.8

J

Jaccoud's syndrome — see Arthropathy, postrheumatic, chronic

Jackson's
  membrane Q43.3
  paralysis or syndrome G83.89
  veil Q43.3

Jacquet's dermatitis (diaper dermatitis) L22

Jadassohn-Pellizari's disease or anetoderma L90.2

Jadassohn's
  blue nevus (M8780/0) — see Nevus
  intraepidermal epithelioma (M8096/0) — see Neoplasm, skin, benign

Jaffe-Lichtenstein (-Uehlinger) syndrome — see Dysplasia, fibrous, bone NEC

Jakob-Creutzfeldt disease or syndrome A81.0
  with dementia A81.0 [F02]

Jaksch-Luzet disease D64.8

Jamaican
  neuropathy G92
  paraplegic tropical ataxic-spastic syndrome G92

Janet's disease F48.8

Janiceps Q89.4

Jansky-Bielschowsky amaurotic idiocy E75.4

Japanese
  B-type encephalitis A83.0
  river fever R17

Jaundice (yellow) R17
  acholuric (familial) (splenomegalic) — see also Spherocytosis
    acquired D59.8
  breast-milk (inhibitor) P59.3
  catarrhal (acute) B15.9
    with hepatic coma B15.0
  cholestatic (benign) R17
  due to or associated with
    delivery due to delayed conjugation P59.0
      preterm delivery P59.0
  epidemic (catarrhal)
    with hepatic coma B15.0
    leptospiral A27.0
    spirochetal A27.0
  familial nonhemolytic E80.4
    congenital E80.5
  febrile (acute) B15.9
    with hepatic coma B15.0
    leptospiral A27.0
    spirochetal A27.0
  fetus or newborn (physiological) P59.9
    due to or associated with
      ABO
        antibodies P55.1
        incompatibility, maternal/fetal P55.1
        isoimmunization P55.1
      absence or deficiency of enzyme system for bilirubin conjugation (congenital) P59.8
      bleeding P58.1
      breast milk inhibitors to conjugation P59.3
        associated with preterm delivery P59.0
      bruising P58.0
      Crigler-Najjar syndrome E80.5
      delayed conjugation P59.8
        associated with preterm delivery P59.0
      drugs or toxins
        given to newborn P58.42
        transmitted from mother P58.41
      excessive hemolysis P58.9
        due to
          bleeding P58.1
          bruising P58.0
          drugs or toxins
            given to newborn P58.42
            transmitted from mother P58.41
          infection P58.2
          polycythemia P58.3
          swallowed maternal blood P58.5
        specified type NEC P58.8
      galactosemia E74.21
      Gilbert's syndrome E80.4

Jaundice — continued
  fetus or newborn — continued
    due to or associated with — continued
      hemolytic disease P55.9
        ABO isoimmunization P55.1
        Rh isoimmunization P55.0
        specified NEC P55.8
      hepatocellular damage P59.20
        specified NEC P59.29
      hereditary hemolytic anemia P58.8
      hypothyroidism, congenital E03.1
      incompatibility, maternal/fetal NOS P55.9
      infection P58.2
      inspissated bile syndrome P59.1
      isoimmunization NOS P55.9
      mucoviscidosis E84.9
      polycythemia P58.3
      preterm delivery P59.0
      Rh
        antibodies P55.0
        incompatibility, maternal/fetal P55.0
        isoimmunization P55.0
      specified cause NEC P59.8
      swallowed maternal blood P58.5
    spherocytosis (congenital) D58.0
  hematogenous D59.9
  hemolytic (acquired) D59.9
    congenital — see Spherocytosis
  hemorrhagic (acute) (leptospiral) (spirochetal) A27.0
    newborn P53
  infectious (acute) (subacute) B15.9
    with hepatic coma B15.0
    leptospiral A27.0
    spirochetal A27.0
  leptospiral (hemorrhagic) A27.0
  malignant K72.90
  newborn — see Jaundice, fetus or newborn
  neonatal — see Jaundice, fetus or newborn
  nonhemolytic congenital familial (Gilbert) E80.4
  nuclear, newborn — see Kernicterus of newborn
  obstructive K83.1
  post-immunization — see Hepatitis, viral, type, B
  post-transfusion — see Hepatitis, viral, type, B
  regurgitation K83.1
  serum — see Hepatitis, viral, type, B
  spirochetal (hemorrhagic) A27.0
  symptomatic R17
    newborn P59.9

Jaw — see condition

Jaw-winking phenomenon or syndrome Q07.8

Jealousy
  alcoholic F10.988
  childhood F93.8
  sibling F93.8

Jejunitis — see Enteritis

Jejunostomy status Z93.4

Jejunum, jejunal — see condition

Jensen's disease — see Inflammation, chorioretinal, focal, juxtapapillary

Jerks, myoclonic G25.3

Jeune's disease Q77.2

Jigger disease B88.1

Job's syndrome (chronic granulomatous disease) D71

Joint — see also condition
  mice — see Loose, body, joint
    knee M23.40
      left M23.42
      right M23.41

Jordan's anomaly or syndrome D72.0

Joseph-Diamond-Blackfan anemia (congenital hypoplastic) D61.0

Jungle yellow fever A95.0

Jüngling's disease — see Sarcoidosis

Juvenile — see condition

K

Kahler's disease (M9732/3) C90.00
  in remission C90.01

Kakke E51.11

Kala-azar B55.0

Kallmann's syndrome E23.0

Kanner's syndrome (autism) — see Psychosis, childhood

Kaposi's
  dermatosis (xeroderma pigmentosum) Q82.1
  lichen ruber L44.0
    acuminatus L44.0
  sarcoma (M9140/3)
    colon C46.4
    connective tissue C46.1
    gastrointestinal organ C46.4
    lung C46.50
      left C46.52
      right C46.51
    lymph node (multiple) C46.3
    palate (hard) (soft) C46.2
    rectum C46.4
    skin (multiple sites) C46.0
    specified site NEC C46.7
    stomach C46.4
    unspecified site C46.9
  varicelliform eruption B00.0
  vaccinia T88.1

Kartagener's syndrome or triad (sinusitis, bronchiectasis, situs inversus) Q89.3

Karyotype
  with abnormality except iso (Xq) Q96.2
  45, X Q96.0
  46, X
    iso (Xq) Q96.1
  46, XX Q98.3
    with streak gonads Q50.32
    hermaphrodite (true) Q99.1
    male Q98.3
  46, XY
    with streak gonads Q56.1
    female Q97.3
    hermaphrodite (true) Q99.1
  47, XXX Q97.0
  47, XXY Q98.0
  47, XYY Q98.5

Kaschin-Beck disease — see Disease, Kaschin-Beck

Katayama's disease or fever B65.2

Kawasaki's syndrome M30.3

Kayser-Fleischer ring (cornea) (pseudosclerosis) E83.01 [H18.049]
  bilateral E83.01 [H18.043]
  left E83.01 [H18.042]
  right E83.01 [H18.041]

Kaznelson's syndrome (congenital hypoplastic anemia) D61.4

Kearns-Sayre syndrome H49.819
  bilateral H49.813
  left H49.812
  right H49.811

Kedani fever A75.3

Kelis L91.0

Kelly (-Patterson) syndrome (sideropenic dysphagia) D50.1

Keloid, cheloid L91.0
  acne L73.0
  Addison's L94.0
  cornea see Opacity, cornea
  Hawkin's L91.0
  scar L91.0

Keloma L91.0

Kenya fever A77.1

Keratectasia — see also Ectasia, cornea
  congenital Q13.4

Keratitis (nodular) (nonulcerative) (simple) (zonular) H16.9
  with ulceration (central) (marginal) (perforated) (ring) — see Ulcer, cornea
  actinic — see Photokeratitis
  arborescens (herpes simplex) B00.52
  areolar — see Keratitis, macular
  bullosa H16.8

©2002 Ingenix, Inc.

Keratitis — *continued*
  deep H16.309
    specified type NEC H16.399
  dendritic(a) (herpes simplex) B00.52
  disciform(is) (herpes simplex) B00.52
    varicella B01.81
  filamentary H16.129
    bilateral H16.123
    left H16.122
    right H16.121
  gonococcal (congenital or prenatal) A54.33
  herpes, herpetic (simplex) B00.52
    zoster B02.33
  in (due to)
    acanthamebiasis B60.13
    adenovirus B30.0
    exanthema (*see also* Exanthem) B09
    herpes (simplex) virus B00.52
    measles B05.81
    syphilis A50.31
    tuberculosis A18.52
    zoster B02.33
  interstitial (nonsyphilitic) H16.309
    bilateral H16.303
    diffuse H16.329
      bilateral H16.323
      left H16.322
      right H16.321
    herpes, herpetic (simplex) B00.52
      zoster B02.33
    left H16.302
    right H16.301
    sclerosing H16.339
      bilateral H16.333
      left H16.332
      right H16.331
    specified type NEC H16.399
      bilateral H16.393
      left H16.392
      right H16.391
    syphilitic (congenital) (late) A50.31
    tuberculous A18.52
  macular H16.119
    bilateral H16.113
    left H16.112
    right H16.111
  nummular — *see* Keratitis, macular
  oyster shuckers' H16.8
  parenchymatous — *see* Keratitis, interstitial
  petrificans H16.8
  postmeasles B05.81
  punctata
    leprosa A30.9
    syphilitic (profunda) A50.31
  punctate H16.149
    bilateral H16.143
    left H16.142
    right H16.141
  purulent H16.8
  rosacea L71.8
  sclerosing — *see* Keratitis, interstitial, sclerosing
  specified type NEC H16.8
  superficial (stellate) (striate) H16.109
    with conjunctivitis — *see* Keratoconjunctivitis
    bilateral H16.103
    due to light — *see* Photokeratitis
    filamentary — *see* Keratitis, filamentary
    left H16.102
    macular — *see* Keratitis, macular
    punctate — *see* Keratitis, punctate
    right H16.101
  suppurative H16.8
  syphilitic (congenital) (prenatal) A50.31
  trachomatous A71.1
    sequelae B94.0
  tuberculous A18.52
  vesicular H16.8
  xerotic (*see also* Keratomalacia) H16.8
    vitamin A deficiency E50.4
Keratoacanthoma L85.8
Keratocele — *see* Descemetocele
Keratoconjunctivitis H16.209
  Acanthamoeba B60.13
  adenoviral B30.0
  bilateral H16.203

Keratoconjunctivitis — *continued*
  epidemic B30.0
  exposure H16.219
    bilateral H16.213
    left H16.212
    right H16.211
  herpes, herpetic (simplex) B00.52
    zoster B02.33
  in exanthema (*see also* Exanthem) B09
  infectious B30.0
  lagophthalmic — *see* Keratoconjunctivitis, specified type NEC
  left H16.202
  neurotrophic H16.239
    bilateral H16.233
    left H16.232
    right H16.231
  phlyctenular H16.259
    bilateral H16.253
    left H16.252
    right H16.251
  postmeasles B05.81
  right H16.201
  shipyard B30.0
  sicca (Sjogren's) M35.01
    not Sjogren's H16.229
      bilateral H16.223
      left H16.222
      right H16.221
  specified type NEC H16.299
    bilateral H16.293
    left H16.292
    right H16.291
  tuberculous (phlyctenular) A18.52
  vernal H16.269
    bilateral H16.263
    left H16.262
    right H16.261
Keratoconus H18.609
  bilateral H18.603
  congenital Q13.4
  in Down's syndrome Q90.9 [*H19.8*]
  left H18.602
  right H18.601
  stable H18.619
    bilateral H18.613
    left H18.612
    right H18.611
  unstable H18.629
    bilateral H18.623
    left H18.622
    right H18.621
Keratocyst (dental) (odontogenic) K09.0
Keratoderma, keratodermia (congenital) (palmaris et plantaris) (symmetrical) Q82.8
  acquired L85.1
  climactericum L85.1
  gonococcal A54.89
  gonorrheal A54.89
  punctata L85.2
  Reiter's — *see* Reiter's disease
Keratodermatocele — *see* Descemetocele
Keratoglobus (congenital) Q15.8
  with glaucoma Q15.0
Keratohemia — *see* Pigmentation, cornea, stromal
Keratoiritis — *see also* Iridocyclitis
  syphilitic A50.39
  tuberculous A18.54
Keratoma L57.0
  palmaris and plantaris hereditarium Q82.8
  senile L57.0
Keratomalacia H18.449
  bilateral H18.443
  left H18.442
  right H18.441
  vitamin A deficiency E50.4
Keratomegaly Q13.4
Keratomycosis B49
  nigrans, nigricans (palmaris) B36.1
Keratopathy H18.9
  band H18.429
    bilateral H18.423
    left H18.422
    right H18.421

Keratopathy — *continued*
  bullous H18.10
    bilateral H18.13
    left H18.12
    right H18.11
Keratoscleritis, tuberculous A18.52
Keratosis L57.0
  actinic L57.0
  arsenical L85.8
  congenital, specified NEC Q80.8
  female genital NEC N94.8
  follicularis Q82.8
    acquired L11.0
    congenita Q82.8
    et parafollicularis in cutem penetrans L87.0
    spinulosa (decalvans) Q82.8
    vitamin A deficiency E50.8
  gonococcal A54.89
  male genital (external) N50.8
  nigricans L83
  obturans, external ear (canal) — *see* Cholesteatoma, external ear
  palmaris et plantaris (inherited) (symmetrical) Q82.8
    acquired L85.1
  penile N48.89
  pharynx J39.2
  pilaris, acquired L85.8
  punctata (palmaris et plantaris) L85.2
  scrotal N50.8
  seborrheic L82.1
    inflamed L82.0
  senile L57.0
  solar L57.0
  tonsillaris J35.8
  vagina N89.4
  vegetans Q82.8
  vitamin A deficiency E50.8
  vocal cord J38.3
Kerato-uveitis — *see* Iridocyclitis
Kerunoparalysis T75.09
Kerion (celsi) B35.0
Kernicterus of newborn (not due to isoimmunization) P57.9
  due to isoimmunization (conditions in P55.0-P55.9) P57.0
  specified type NEC P57.8
Keshan disease E59
Ketoacidosis E87.2
  diabetic — *see* Diabetes, by type, with complication, ketosis
Ketonuria R82.4
Ketosis NEC E88.8
  diabetic — *see* Diabetes, by type, with complication, ketosis
Kew Garden fever A79.1
Kidney — *see* condition
Kienböck's disease — *see also* Osteochondrosis, juvenile, hand, carpal lunate
  adult M93.1
Kimmelstiel (-Wilson) disease — *see* Diabetes, Kimmelstiel (-Wilson) disease
Kink, kinking
  artery I77.1
  hair (acquired) L67.8
  ileum or intestine — *see* Obstruction, intestine
  Lane's — *see* Obstruction, intestine
  organ or site, congenital NEC — *see* Anomaly, by site
  ureter (pelvic junction) N13.5
    with
      hydronephrosis N13.1
        with infection N13.6
      pyelonephritis (chronic) N11.1
    congenital Q62.39
  vein(s) I87.8
    caval I87.1
    peripheral I87.1
Kinnier Wilson's disease (hepatolenticular degeneration) E83.01
Kissing spine M48.20
  cervical region M48.22
  cervicothoracic region M48.23
  lumbar region M48.26

Kissing spine — continued
  lumbosacral region M48.27
  occipito-atlanto-axial region M48.21
  sacrococcygeal region M48.28
  thoracic region M48.24
  thoracolumbar region M48.25
Klatskin's tumor (M8162/3) C22.1
Klauder's disease A26.8
Klebs' disease — see Glomerulonephritis
Klebsiella (K.) pneumoniae, as cause of disease classified elsewhere B96.1
Kleine-Levin syndrome G47.8
Kleptomania F63.2
Klinefelter's syndrome Q98.4
  karyotype 47,XXY Q98.0
  male with more than two X chromosomes Q98.1
Klippel-Feil deficiency, disease, or syndrome (brevicollis) Q76.1
Klippel's disease I67.2
Klippel-Trenaunay (-Weber) syndrome Q87.2
Klumpke (-Déjerine) palsy, paralysis (birth) (newborn) P14.1
Knee — see condition
Knock knee (acquired) — see also Deformity, valgus, knee
  congenital Q74.1
Knot(s)
  intestinal, syndrome (volvulus) K56.2
  surfer T14.90
  umbilical cord (true) O69.2
Knotting (of)
  hair L67.8
  intestine K56.2
Knuckle pad (Garrod's) M72.1
Koch's
  infection — see Tuberculosis
  relapsing fever A68.9
Koch-Weeks' conjunctivitis — see Conjunctivitis, acute, mucopurulent
Köebner's syndrome Q81.8
Köenig's disease (osteochondritis dissecans) — see Osteochondritis, dissecans
Köhler-Pellegrini-Steida disease or syndrome (calcification, knee joint) — see Bursitis, tibial collateral
Köhler's disease
  patellar — see Osteochondrosis, juvenile, patella
  tarsal navicular — see Osteochondrosis, juvenile, tarsus
Koilonychia L60.3
  congenital Q84.6
Kojevnikov's, Kozhevnikof's epilepsy G40.50
  with status epilepticus G40.51
Koplik's spots B05.9
Kopp's asthma E32.8
Korsakoff's (Wernicke) disease, psychosis or syndrome (alcoholic) F10.96
  with dependence F10.26
  drug-induced — see Disorder, drug-related, by type, with amnestic disorder
  nonalcoholic F04
Korsakov's disease, psychosis or syndrome — see Korsakoff's disease
Korsakow's disease, psychosis or syndrome — see Korsakoff's disease
Kostmann's disease or syndrome (infantile genetic agranulocytosis) — see Agranulocytosis
Krabbe's
  disease E75.23
  syndrome, congenital muscle hypoplasia Q79.8
Kraepelin-Morel disease — see Schizophrenia
Kraft-Weber-Dimitri disease Q85.8
Kraurosis
  ani K62.8
  penis N48.0
  vagina N89.8
  vulva N90.4
Kreotoxism A05.9

Krukenberg's
  spindle — see Pigmentation, cornea, posterior
  tumor (M8490/6) C79.60
    left C79.62
    right C79.61
Kufs' disease E75.4
Kugelberg-Welander disease G12.1
Kuhnt-Junius degeneration — see Degeneration, macula
Kulchitsky's cell carcinoma (carcinoid tumor of intestine) E34.0
Kümmell's disease or spondylitis — see Spondylopathy, traumatic
Kupffer cell sarcoma (M9124/3) C22.3
Kuru A81.8
Kussmaul's
  disease M30.0
  respiration E87.2
    in diabetic acidosis — see Diabetes, by type with ketoacidosis
Kwashiorkor E40
  marasmic, marasmus type E42
Kyasanur Forest disease A98.2
Kyphoscoliosis, kyphoscoliotic (acquired) — see Scoliosis)
  congenital Q67.5
  heart (disease) I27.1
  sequelae of rickets (see also category M49.8) E64.3
  tuberculous A18.01
Kyphosis, kyphotic (acquired) M40.209
  cervical region M40.202
  cervicothoracic region M40.203
  congenital Q76.419
    cervical region Q76.412
    cervicothoracic region Q76.413
    occipito-atlanto-axial region Q76.411
    thoracic region Q76.414
    thoracolumbar region Q76.415
  Morquio-Brailsford type (spinal) (see also category M49.8) E76.219
  occipito-atlanto-axial region M40.201
  postlaminectomy M96.3
  postradiation therapy M96.2
  postural (adolescent) M40.00
    cervical region M40.02
    cervicothoracic region M40.03
    occipito-atlanto-axial region M40.01
    thoracic region M40.04
    thoracolumbar region M40.05
  secondary NEC M40.10
    cervical region M40.12
    cervicothoracic region M40.13
    occipito-atlanto-axial region M40.11
    thoracic region M40.14
    thoracolumbar region M40.15
  specified type NEC M40.299
    cervical region M40.292
    cervicothoracic region M40.293
    occipito-atlanto-axial region M40.291
    thoracic region M40.294
    thoracolumbar region M40.295
  sequelae of rickets (see also category M49.8) E64.3
  syphilitic, congenital (see also category M49.8) A50.56
  thoracic region M40.204
  thoracolumbar region M40.205
  tuberculous A18.01
Kyrle's disease L87.0

L

Labia, labium — see condition
Labile
  blood pressure R09.89
  vasomotor system I73.9
Labioglossal paralysis G12.29
Labium leporinum — see Cleft, lip
Labor — see also Delivery
  arrested active phase O62.1
  desultory O62.2
  dyscoordinate O62.4

Labor — see also Delivery — continued
  early onset (before 37 completed weeks' gestation) O60.9
    second trimester O60.2
    third trimester O60.3
  false O47.9
    at or after 37 completed weeks of gestation O47.1
    before 37 completed weeks of gestation O47.00
      second trimester O47.02
      third trimester O47.03
  hypertonic O62.4
  hypotonic O62.2
    primary O62.0
    secondary O62.1
  incoordinate O62.4
  irregular O62.2
  long — see Labor, prolonged
  missed O36.4
  obstructed O66.9
    by or due to
      abnormal
        cervix O65.5
        pelvic organs or tissues O65.5
        pelvis (bony) O65.9
          specified NEC O65.8
        presentation or position O64.9
        size, fetus O66.2
        soft parts (of pelvis) O65.5
        uterus O65.5
        vagina O65.5
      acromion presentation O64.4
      anteversion, cervix or uterus O65.5
      bicornis or bicornate uterus O65.5
      breech presentation O64.1
      brow presentation O64.3
      cephalopelvic disproportion (normally formed fetus) O65.4
      chin presentation O64.2
      cicatrix of cervix — see category O34.4
      compound presentation O64.5
      conditions in O32.0-O32.9 O64.9
      congenital uterine malformation O65.5
      contraction, contracted
        pelvis (general) O65.1
          inlet O65.2
          mid-cavity O65.3
          outlet O65.3
      cystocele O65.5
      deep transverse arrest O64.0
      deformity (acquired) (congenital)
        pelvic organs or tissues NEC O65.5
        pelvis (bony) NEC O65.0
      displacement uterus O65.5
      disproportion, fetopelvic NEC O65.4
      double uterus (congenital) O65.5
      face presentation O64.2
        to pubes O64.0
      failure, fetal head to enter pelvic brim O64.8
      fibroid (tumor) (uterus) O65.5
      hydrocephalic fetus O66.3
      impacted shoulders O66.0
      incarceration of uterus O65.5
      lateroversion, uterus or cervix O65.5
      locked twins O66.1
      mal lie O64.9
      malposition
        fetus NOS O64.9
        pelvic organs or tissues NEC O65.5
      malpresentation O64.9
        specified NEC O64.8
      nonengagement of fetal head O64.8
      oblique presentation O64.4
      oversize fetus O66.2
      pelvic tumor NEC O65.5
      persistent occipitoposterior, posterior or transverse O64.0
      prolapse
        arm or hand O64.4
        foot or leg O64.8
        uterus O65.5
      rectocele O65.5
      retroversion, uterus or cervix O65.5

Labor — *see also* Delivery — *continued*
  obstructed — *continued*
    by or due to — *continued*
      rigid
        cervix O65.5
        pelvic floor O65.5
        perineum or vulva O65.5
        vagina O65.5
      shoulder
        distocia or impaction O66.0
        presentation O64.4
      stenosis O65.5
      transverse
        arrest (deep) O64.0
        presentation or lie O64.8
    specified NEC O66.8
  precipitate O62.3
  premature or preterm O60.9
    second trimester O60.2
    third trimester O60.3
  prolonged or protracted O63.9
    first stage O63.0
    second stage O63.1

Labored breathing — *see* Hyperventilation

Labyrinthitis (circumscribed) (destructive) (diffuse) (inner ear) (latent) (purulent) (suppurative) — *see also* category H83.0
  syphilitic A52.79

Laceration
  with abortion — *see* Abortion, by type, complicated by laceration of pelvic organs
  abdomen, abdominal S31.91
    with foreign body S31.92
    wall S31.119
      with
        foreign body S31.129
        penetration into peritoneal cavity S31.619
          with foreign body S31.629
      epigastric region S31.112
        with
          foreign body S31.122
          penetration into peritoneal cavity S31.612
            with foreign body S31.622
      left
        lower quadrant S31.114
          with
            foreign body S31.124
            penetration into peritoneal cavity S31.614
              with foreign body S31.624
        upper quadrant S31.111
          with
            foreign body S31.121
            penetration into peritoneal cavity S31.611
              with foreign body S31.621
      periumbilic region S31.115
        with
          foreign body S31.125
          penetration into peritoneal cavity S31.615
            with foreign body S31.625
      right
        lower quadrant S31.113
          with
            foreign body S31.123
            penetration into peritoneal cavity S31.613
              with foreign body S31.623
        upper quadrant S31.110
          with
            foreign body S31.120
            penetration into peritoneal cavity S31.610
              with foreign body S31.620
  accidental, complicating surgery — *see* Complications, surgical, accidental puncture or laceration
  Achilles tendon S86.029
    left S86.022
    right S86.021
  adrenal gland S37.813
  alveolar (process) — *see* Laceration, oral cavity

Laceration — *continued*
  ankle S91.019
    with
      foreign body S91.029
      fracture S91.069
    left S91.012
      with
        foreign body S91.022
        fracture S91.062
    right S91.011
      with
        foreign body S91.021
        fracture S91.061
  antecubital space — *see* Laceration, elbow
  anus S31.831
    with
      ectopic or molar pregnancy O08.6
      foreign body S31.832
    complicating delivery O70.2
      with laceration of anal or rectal mucosa O70.3
    following ectopic or molar pregnancy O08.6
    nontraumatic, nonpuerperal — *see* Fissure, anus
  arm (upper) S41.119
    with foreign body S41.129
    left S41.112
      with foreign body S41.122
    lower — *see* Laceration, forearm
    right S41.111
      with foreign body S41.121
  auditory canal (external) (meatus) — *see* Laceration, ear
  auricle, ear — *see* Laceration, ear
  axilla — *see* Laceration, arm
  back — *see also* Laceration, thorax, back
    lower S31.010
      with
        foreign body S31.020
          with penetration into retroperitoneal space S31.021
        penetration into retroperitoneal space S31.011
  bile duct S36.13
  bladder S37.23
    with ectopic or molar pregnancy O08.6
    following ectopic or molar pregnancy O08.6
    obstetrical trauma O71.5
  blood vessel — *see* Injury, blood vessel
  bowel — *see also* Laceration, intestine
    with ectopic or molar pregnancy O08.6
    complicating abortion — *see* Abortion, by type, complicated by, specified condition NEC
    following ectopic or molar pregnancy O08.6
    obstetrical trauma O71.5
  brain (any part) (cortex) (diffuse) (membrane) — *see also* Injury, intracranial, diffuse
    during birth P10.8
      with hemorrhage P10.1
    focal — *see* Injury, intracranial, focal brain injury
  brainstem S06.381
    with loss of consciousness S06.389
      brief (<1 hour) S06.382
      minor (1-6 hours) S06.383
      moderate (6-24 hours) S06.384
      prolonged (>24 hours) S06.385
        without return to consciousness S06.386
  breast S21.019
    with foreign body S21.029
    left S21.012
      with foreign body S21.022
    right S21.011
      with foreign body S21.021
  broad ligament S37.893
    with ectopic or molar pregnancy O08.6
    following ectopic or molar pregnancy O08.6
    laceration syndrome N83.8
    obstetrical trauma O71.6
    syndrome (laceration) N83.8
  buttock S31.801
    with foreign body S31.802
    left S31.821
      with foreign body S31.822

Laceration — *continued*
  buttock — *continued*
    right S31.811
      with foreign body S31.812
  calf — *see* Laceration, leg
  canaliculus lacrimalis — *see* Laceration, eyelid
  canthus, eye — *see* Laceration, eyelid
  capsule, joint — *see* Sprain
  causing eversion of cervix uteri (old) N86
  central (perineal), complicating delivery O70.9
  cerebellum, traumatic S06.371
    with loss of consciousness S06.379
      brief (<1 hour) S06.372
      minor (1-6 hours) S06.373
      moderate (6-24 hours) S06.374
      prolonged (>24 hours) S06.375
        without return to consciousness S06.376
  cerebral S06.331
    with loss of consciousness S06.339
      brief (<1 hour) S06.332
      minor (1-6 hours) S06.333
      moderate (6-24 hours) S06.334
      prolonged (>24 hours) S06.335
        without return to consciousness S06.336
    left side S06.321
      with loss of consciousness S06.329
        brief (<1 hour) S06.322
        minor (1-6 hours) S06.323
        moderate (6-24 hours) S06.324
        prolonged (>24 hours) S06.325
          without return to consciousness S06.326
    during birth P10.8
      with hemorrhage P10.1
    right side S06.311
      with loss of consciousness S06.319
        brief (<1 hour) S06.312
        minor (1-6 hours) S06.313
        moderate (6-24 hours) S06.314
        prolonged (>24 hours) S06.315
          without return to consciousness S06.316
  cervix (uteri)
    with ectopic or molar pregnancy O08.6
    following ectopic or molar pregnancy O08.6
    nonpuerperal, nontraumatic N88.1
    obstetrical trauma (current) O71.3
    old (postpartal) N88.1
    traumatic S37.63
  cheek (external) S01.419
    with foreign body S01.429
    left S01.412
      with foreign body S01.422
    right S01.411
      with foreign body S01.421
    internal — *see* Laceration, oral cavity
  chest wall — *see* Laceration, thorax
  chin — *see* Laceration, head, specified site NEC
  chordae tendinae I51.1
    concurrent with acute myocardial infarction — *see* Infarct, myocardium
    following acute myocardial infarction (current complication) I23.4
  clitoris — *see* Laceration, vulva
  colon — *see* Laceration, intestine, large, colon
  common bile duct S36.13
  cortex (cerebral) — *see* Injury, intracranial, diffuse
  costal region — *see* Laceration, thorax
  cystic duct S36.13
  diaphragm S27.803
  digit(s)
    hand — *see* Laceration, finger
    foot — *see* Laceration, toe
  duodenum S36.430
  ear (canal) (external) S01.319
    with foreign body S01.329
    left S01.312
      with foreign body S01.322
    right S01.311
      with foreign body S01.321
    drum S09.20
      left S09.22
      right S09.21

Laceration — *continued*
elbow S51.019
  with
    foreign body S51.029
    fracture S51.069
  left S51.012
    with
      foreign body S51.022
      fracture S51.062
  right S51.011
    with
      foreign body S51.021
      fracture S51.061
epididymis — *see* Laceration, testis
epigastric region — *see* Laceration, abdomen, wall, epigastric region
esophagus K22.8
  traumatic
    cervical S11.21
      with foreign body S11.22
    thoracic S27.813
eye(ball) S05.30
  with prolapse or loss of intraocular tissue S05.20
    left S05.22
    right S05.21
  left S05.32
  penetrating S05.60
    left S05.62
    right S05.61
  right S05.31
eyebrow — *see* Laceration, eyelid
eyelid S01.119
  with foreign body S01.129
  left S01.112
    with foreign body S01.122
  right S01.111
    with foreign body S01.121
face NEC — *see* Laceration, head, specified site NEC
fallopian tube S37.539
  bilateral S37.532
  unilateral S37.531
finger(s) S61.219
  with
    damage to nail S61.319
      with
        foreign body S61.329
        fracture S61.369
    foreign body S61.229
    fracture S61.269
  index S61.218
    with
      damage to nail S61.318
        with
          foreign body S61.328
          fracture S61.368
      foreign body S61.228
      fracture S61.268
    left S61.211
      with
        damage to nail S61.311
          with
            foreign body S61.321
            fracture S61.361
        foreign body S61.221
        fracture S61.261
    right S61.210
      with
        damage to nail S61.310
          with
            foreign body S61.320
            fracture S61.360
        foreign body S61.220
        fracture S61.260
  little S61.218
    with
      damage to nail S61.318
        with
          foreign body S61.328
          fracture S61.368
      foreign body S61.228
      fracture S61.268
    left S61.217
      with
        damage to nail S61.317

Laceration — *continued*
finger(s) — *continued*
  little — *continued*
    left — *continued*
      with — *continued*
        damage to nail — *continued*
          with
            foreign body S61.327
            fracture S61.367
          foreign body S61.227
          fracture S61.267
    right S61.216
      with
        damage to nail S61.316
          with
            foreign body S61.326
            fracture S61.366
          foreign body S61.226
          fracture S61.266
  middle S61.218
    with
      damage to nail S61.318
        with
          foreign body S61.328
          fracture S61.368
      foreign body S61.228
      fracture S61.268
    left S61.213
      with
        damage to nail S61.313
          with
            foreign body S61.323
            fracture S61.363
        foreign body S61.223
        fracture S61.263
    right S61.212
      with
        damage to nail S61.312
          with
            foreign body S61.322
            fracture S61.362
        foreign body S61.222
        fracture S61.262
  ring S61.218
    with
      damage to nail S61.318
        with
          foreign body S61.328
          fracture S61.368
      foreign body S61.228
      fracture S61.268
    left S61.215
      with
        damage to nail S61.315
          with
            foreign body S61.325
            fracture S61.365
        foreign body S61.225
        fracture S61.265
    right S61.214
      with
        damage to nail S61.314
          with
            foreign body S61.324
            fracture S61.364
        foreign body S61.224
        fracture S61.264
flank S31.119
  with foreign body S31.129
foot (except toe(s) alone) S91.319
  with foreign body S91.329
  left S91.312
    with foreign body S91.322
  right S91.311
    with foreign body S91.321
  toe — *see* Laceration, toe
forearm S51.819
  with
    foreign body S51.829
    fracture of radius or ulna S51.869
  elbow only — *see* Laceration, elbow
  left S51.812
    with
      foreign body S51.822
      fracture of radius or ulna S51.862

Laceration — *continued*
forearm — *continued*
  right S51.811
    with
      foreign body S51.821
      fracture of radius or ulna S51.861
forehead — *see* Laceration, head, specified site NEC
fourchette O70.0
  with ectopic or molar pregnancy O08.6
  complicating delivery O70.0
  following ectopic or molar pregnancy O08.6
gallbladder S36.123
genital organs, external
  female S31.512
    with foreign body S31.522
    vagina — *see* Laceration, vagina
    vulva — *see* Laceration, vulva
  male S31.511
    with foreign body S31.521
    penis — *see* Laceration, penis
    scrotum — *see* Laceration, scrotum
    testis — *see* Laceration, testis
groin — *see* Laceration, abdomen, wall
gum — *see* Laceration, oral cavity
hand S61.419
  with
    foreign body S61.429
    fracture S61.469
  finger — *see* Laceration, finger
  left S61.412
    with
      foreign body S61.422
      fracture S61.462
  right S61.411
    with
      foreign body S61.421
      fracture S61.461
  thumb — *see* Laceration, thumb
head S01.91
  with foreign body S01.92
  cheek — *see* Laceration, cheek
  ear — *see* Laceration, ear
  eyelid — *see* Laceration, eyelid
  lip — *see* Laceration, lip
  nose — *see* Laceration, nose
  oral cavity — *see* Laceration, oral cavity
  scalp S01.01
    with foreign body S01.02
  specified site NEC S01.81
    with foreign body S01.82
  temporomandibular area — *see* Laceration, cheek
heart — *see* Injury, heart, laceration
heel — *see* Laceration, foot
hepatic duct S36.13
hip S71.019
  with foreign body S71.029
  left S71.012
    with foreign body S71.022
  right S71.011
    with foreign body S71.021
hymen — *see* Laceration, vagina
hypochondrium — *see* Laceration, abdomen, wall
hypogastric region — *see* Laceration, abdomen, wall
ileum S36.438
inguinal region — *see* Laceration, abdomen, wall
instep — *see* Laceration, foot
internal organ — *see* Injury, by site
interscapular region — *see* Laceration, thorax, back
intestine
  large
    colon S36.539
      ascending S36.530
      descending S36.532
      sigmoid S36.533
      specified site NEC S36.538
    rectum S36.63
    transverse S36.531
  small S36.439
    duodenum S36.430
    specified site NEC S36.438

©2002 Ingenix, Inc.

Laceration — *continued*
  intra-abdominal organ S36.93
    intestine — *see* Laceration, intestine
    liver — *see* Laceration, liver
    pancreas — *see* Laceration, pancreas
    peritoneum S36.81
    specified site NEC S36.893
    spleen — *see* Laceration, spleen
    stomach — *see* Laceration, stomach
  intracranial NEC — *see also* Injury,
      intracranial, diffuse
    birth injury P10.9
  jaw — *see* Laceration, head, specified site NEC
  jejunum S36.438
  joint capsule — *see* Sprain, by site
  kidney S37.039
    left S37.032
    major (massive) (stellate) S37.069
      left S37.062
      right S37.061
    minor S37.049
      left S37.042
      right S37.041
    moderate S37.059
      left S37.052
      right S37.051
    right S37.031
  knee S81.019
    with foreign body S81.029
    left S81.012
      with foreign body S81.022
    right S81.011
      with foreign body S81.021
  labium (majus) (minus) — *see* Laceration, vulva
  lacrimal duct — *see* Laceration, eyelid
  large intestine — *see* Laceration, intestine,
      large
  larynx S11.011
    with foreign body S11.012
  leg (lower) S81.819
    with foreign body S81.829
    foot — *see* Laceration, foot
    knee — *see* Laceration, knee
    left S81.812
      with foreign body S81.822
    right S81.811
      with foreign body S81.821
    upper — *see* Laceration, thigh
  ligament — *see* Sprain
  lip S01.511
    with foreign body S01.521
  liver S36.113
    major (stellate) S36.116
    minor S36.114
    moderate S36.115
  loin — *see* Laceration, abdomen, wall
  lower back — *see* Laceration, back, lower
  lumbar region — *see* Laceration, back, lower
  lung S27.339
    bilateral S27.332
    unilateral S27.331
  malar region — *see* Laceration, head, specified
      site NEC
  mammary — *see* Laceration, breast
  mastoid region — *see* Laceration, head,
      specified site NEC
  meninges — *see* Injury, intracranial, diffuse
  meniscus — *see* Tear, meniscus
  mesentery S36.893
  mesosalpinx S37.539
    bilateral S37.532
    unilateral S37.531
  mouth — *see* Laceration, oral cavity
  muscle — *see* Injury, muscle
  nail
    finger — *see* Laceration, finger, with damage
        to nail
    toe — *see* Laceration, toe, with damage to
        nail
  nasal (septum) (sinus) — *see* Laceration, nose
  nasopharynx — *see* Laceration, head, specified
      site NEC
  neck S11.91
    with foreign body S11.92
    involving
      cervical esophagus S11.21
        with foreign body S11.22

Laceration — *continued*
  neck — *continued*
    larynx — *see* Laceration, larynx
    pharynx — *see* Laceration, pharynx
    thyroid gland — *see* Laceration, thyroid
        gland
    trachea — *see* Laceration, trachea
    specified site NEC S11.81
      with foreign body S11.82
  nerve — *see* Injury, nerve
  nose (septum) (sinus) S01.21
    with foreign body S01.22
  ocular NOS S05.30
    adnexa NOS S01.119
      left S01.112
      right S01.111
    left S05.32
    right S05.31
  oral cavity S01.512
    with foreign body S01.522
  orbit (eye) — *see* Wound, open, ocular, orbit
  ovary S37.439
    bilateral S37.432
    unilateral S37.431
  palate — *see* Laceration, oral cavity
  palm — *see* Laceration, hand
  pancreas S36.239
    body S36.231
      major S36.261
      minor S36.241
      moderate S36.251
    head S36.230
      major S36.260
      minor S36.240
      moderate S36.250
    major S36.269
    minor S36.249
    moderate S36.259
    tail S36.232
      major S36.262
      minor S36.242
      moderate S36.252
  pelvic S31.010
    with
      foreign body S31.020
        penetration into retroperitoneal cavity
            S31.021
      penetration into retroperitoneal cavity
          S31.011
    floor — *see also* Laceration, back, lower
      with ectopic or molar pregnancy O08.6
      complicating delivery O70.1
      following ectopic or molar pregnancy
          O08.6
      old (postpartal) N81.8
    organ S37.93
      with ectopic or molar pregnancy O08.6
      adrenal gland S37.813
      bladder S37.23
      fallopian tube — *see* Laceration, fallopian
          tube
      following ectopic or molar pregnancy
          O08.6
      kidney — *see* Laceration, kidney
      obstetrical trauma O71.5
      ovary — *see* Laceration, ovary
      prostate S37.823
      specified site NEC S37.893
      ureter S37.13
      urethra S37.33
      uterus S37.63
  penis S31.21
    with foreign body S31.22
  perineum
    female S31.41
      with
        ectopic or molar pregnancy O08.6
        foreign body S31.42
      during delivery O70.9
        first degree O70.0
        fourth degree O70.3
        second degree O70.1
        third degree O70.2
      involving
        anus (sphincter) O70.2
        fourchette O70.0

Laceration — *continued*
  perineum — *continued*
    female — *continued*
      involving — *continued*
        hymen O70.0
        labia O70.0
        pelvic floor O70.1
        perineal muscles O70.1
        rectovaginal septum O70.2
          with anal or rectal mucosa O70.3
        skin O70.0
        sphincter (anal) O70.2
          with anal or rectal mucosa O70.3
        vagina O70.0
        vaginal muscles O70.1
        vulva O70.0
      old (postpartal) N81.8
      postpartal N81.8
      secondary (postpartal) O90.1
    male S31.119
      with foreign body S31.129
  periocular area (with or without lacrimal
      passages) — *see* Laceration, eyelid
  peritoneum S36.893
  periumbilic region — *see* Laceration, abdomen,
      wall, periumbilic
  periurethral tissue — *see* Laceration, urethra
  phalanges
    finger — *see* Laceration, finger
    toe — *see* Laceration, toe
  pharynx S11.21
    with foreign body S11.22
  pinna — *see* Laceration, ear
  popliteal space — *see* Laceration, knee
  prepuce — *see* Laceration, penis
  prostate S37.823
  pubic region S31.119
    with foreign body S31.129
  pudendum — *see* Laceration, genital organs,
      external
  rectovaginal septum — *see* Laceration, vagina
  rectum S36.63
  retroperitoneum S36.893
  round ligament S37.893
  sacral region — *see* Laceration, back, lower
  sacroiliac region — *see* Laceration, back, lower
  salivary gland — *see* Laceration, oral cavity
  scalp S01.01
    with foreign body S01.02
  scapular region — *see* Laceration, shoulder
  scrotum S31.31
    with foreign body S31.32
  seminal vesicle S37.893
  shin — *see* Laceration, leg
  shoulder S41.019
    with foreign body S41.029
    left S41.012
      with foreign body S41.022
    right S41.011
      with foreign body S41.021
  small intestine — *see* Laceration, intestine,
      small
  spermatic cord — *see* Laceration, testis
  spinal cord (meninges) — *see also* Injury,
      spinal cord, by region
    due to injury at birth P11.5
    fetus or newborn (birth injury) P11.5
  spleen S36.039
    major (massive) (stellate) S36.032
    moderate S36.031
    superficial (minor) S36.030
  sternal region — *see* Laceration, thorax, front
  stomach S36.33
  submaxillary region — *see* Laceration, head,
      specified site NEC
  submental region — *see* Laceration, head,
      specified site NEC
  subungual
    finger(s) — *see* Laceration, finger, with
        damage to nail
    toe(s) — *see* Laceration, toe, with damage to
        nail
  suprarenal gland — *see* Laceration, adrenal
      gland
  temple, temporal region — *see* Laceration,
      head, specified site NEC

Laceration — *continued*
 temporomandibular area — *see* Laceration, cheek
 tendon — *see also* Injury, muscle or tendon
  Achilles S86.029
   left S86.022
   right S86.021
 tentorium cerebelli — *see* Injury, intracranial, diffuse
 testis S31.31
  with foreign body S31.32
 thigh S71.119
  with foreign body S71.129
  left S71.112
   with foreign body S71.122
  right S71.111
   with foreign body S71.121
 thorax, thoracic (wall) S21.91
  with foreign body S21.92
   back S21.229
   front S21.129
  back S21.219
   with foreign body S21.229
   left S21.212
    with foreign body S21.222
   right S21.211
    with foreign body S21.221
  breast — *see* Laceration, breast
  front S21.119
   with foreign body S21.129
   left S21.112
    with foreign body S21.122
   right S21.111
    with foreign body S21.121
 thumb S61.019
  with
   damage to nail S61.119
    with
     foreign body S61.129
     fracture S61.169
   foreign body S61.029
   fracture S61.069
  left S61.012
   with
    damage to nail S61.112
     with
      foreign body S61.122
      fracture S61.162
    foreign body S61.022
    fracture S61.062
  right S61.011
   with
    damage to nail S61.111
     with
      foreign body S61.121
      fracture S61.161
    foreign body S61.021
    fracture S61.061
 thyroid gland S11.11
  with foreign body S11.12
 toe(s) S91.119
  with
   damage to nail S91.219
    with
     foreign body S91.229
     fracture S91.269
   foreign body S91.129
   fracture S91.169
  great S91.113
   with
    damage to nail S91.213
     with
      foreign body S91.223
      fracture S91.263
    foreign body S91.123
    fracture S91.163
   left S91.112
    with
     damage to nail S91.212
      with
       foreign body S91.222
       fracture S91.262
     foreign body S91.122
     fracture S91.162

Laceration — *continued*
 toe(s) — *continued*
  great — *continued*
   right S91.111
    with
     damage to nail S91.211
      with
       foreign body S91.221
       fracture S91.261
     foreign body S91.121
     fracture S91.161
  lesser S91.116
   with
    damage to nail S91.216
     with
      foreign body S91.226
      fracture S91.266
    foreign body S91.126
    fracture S91.166
   left S91.115
    with
     damage to nail S91.215
      with
       foreign body S91.225
       fracture S91.265
     foreign body S91.125
     fracture S91.165
   right S91.114
    with
     damage to nail S91.214
      with
       foreign body S91.224
       fracture S91.264
     foreign body S91.124
     fracture S91.164
 tongue — *see* Laceration, oral cavity
 trachea S11.021
  with foreign body S11.022
 tunica vaginalis — *see* Laceration, testis
 tympanum, tympanic membrane — *see* Laceration, ear, drum
 umbilical region S31.115
  with foreign body S31.125
 ureter S37.13
 urethra S37.33
  with or following ectopic or molar pregnancy O08.6
  obstetrical trauma O71.5
 uterus S37.63
  with ectopic or molar pregnancy O08.6
  following ectopic or molar pregnancy O08.6
  nonpuerperal, nontraumatic N85.8
  obstetrical trauma NEC O71.1
  old (postpartal) N85.8
 uvula — *see* Laceration, oral cavity
 vagina S31.41
  with
   ectopic or molar pregnancy O08.6
   foreign body S31.42
  during delivery O71.4
   with perineal laceration — *see* Laceration, perineum, female, during delivery
  following ectopic or molar pregnancy O08.6
  nonpuerperal, nontraumatic N89.8
  old (postpartal) N89.8
 vas deferens S37.893
 vesical — *see* Laceration, bladder
 vulva S31.41
  with
   ectopic or molar pregnancy O08.6
   foreign body S31.42
  complicating delivery O70.0
  following ectopic or molar pregnancy O08.6
  nonpuerperal, nontraumatic N90.8
  old (postpartal) N90.8
 wrist S61.519
  with
   foreign body S61.529
   fracture S61.569
  left S61.512
   with
    foreign body S61.522
    fracture S61.562
  right S61.511
   with
    foreign body S61.521
    fracture S61.561

Lack of
 achievement in school Z55.3
 adequate food Z59.4
 appetite — *see* Anorexia
 care
  in home Z74.2
  of infant (at or after birth) T76.02
   confirmed T74.02
 coordination R27.9
  ataxia R27.0
  specified type NEC R27.8
 development (physiological) R62.50
  failure to thrive (child) R62.51
   adult R62.7
  short stature R62.52
  specified type NEC R62.59
 financial resources Z59.6
 food T73.0
 growth R62.50
 heating Z59.1
 housing (permanent) (temporary) Z59.0
  adequate Z59.1
 learning experiences in childhood Z62.8
 leisure time (affecting life-style) Z73.2
 material resources Z59.6
 memory — *see also* Amnesia
  mild, following organic brain damage F06.8
 ovulation N97.0
 parental supervision or control of child Z62.0
 person able to render necessary care Z74.2
 physical exercise Z72.3
 play experience in childhood Z62.8
 prenatal care O09.30
  first trimester O09.31
  second trimester O09.32
  third trimester O09.33
 relaxation (affecting life-style) Z73.2
 sexual
  desire F52.0
  enjoyment F52.1
 shelter Z59.0

Lack of
 supervision of child by parent Z62.0
 water T73.1

Lacrimal — *see* condition

Lacrimation, abnormal — *see* Epiphora

Lacrimonasal duct — *see* condition

Lactation, lactating (breast) (puerperal, postpartum)
 defective O92.4
 disorder NEC O92.7
 excessive O92.6
 failed (complete) O92.3
  partial O92.4
 mastitis NEC — *see* Mastitis, obstetric
 mother (care and/or examination) Z39.1
 nonpuerperal N64.3

Lacticemia, excessive E87.2

Lacunar skull Q75.8

Laennec's cirrhosis K74.6
 alcoholic K70.30
  with ascites K70.31

Lafora's disease G40.30
 with status epilepticus G40.31

Lag, lid (nervous) — *see* Retraction, lid

Lagophthalmos (eyelid) (nervous) H02.209
 cicatricial H02.219
  left H02.216
   lower H02.215
   upper H02.214
  right H02.213
   lower H02.212
   upper H02.211
 keratoconjunctivitis — *see* Keratoconjunctivitis
 left H02.206
  lower H02.205
  upper H02.204
 mechanical H02.229
  left H02.226
   lower H02.225
   upper H02.224
  right H02.223
   lower H02.222
   upper H02.221

©2002 Ingenix, Inc.

Lagophthalmos — *continued*
   paralytic H02.239
      left H02.236
         lower H02.235
         upper H02.234
      right H02.233
         lower H02.232
         upper H02.231
      right H02.203
         lower H02.202
         upper H02.201
Laki-Lorand factor deficiency — *see* Defect,
      coagulation, specified type NEC
Lalling F80.0
Lambert-Eaton syndrome C34.90 *[G73.1]*
Lambliasis, lambliosis A07.1
Landau-Kleffner syndrome F80.3
Landouzy-Déjérine dystrophy or
      facioscapulohumeral atrophy G71.0
Landouzy's disease (icterohemorrhagic
      leptospirosis) A27.0
Landry-Guillain-Barré, syndrome or paralysis
      G61.0
Landry's disease or paralysis G61.0
Lane's
   band Q43.3
   kink — *see* Obstruction, intestine
   syndrome K90.2
Langdon Down's syndrome — *see* Trisomy, 21
Large
   baby (regardless of gestational age) P08.1
   ear, congenital Q17.1
   fetus — *see* Oversize fetus
   physiological cup Q14.2
Large-for-dates NEC (fetus or infant) P08.1
   affecting management of pregnancy — *see*
      Pregnancy, complicated by, fetal, excess
      growth
   exceptionally (4500g or more) P08.0
Larsen-Johansson disease orosteochondrosis —
      see Osteochondrosis, juvenile, patella
Larsen's syndrome (flattened facies and multiple
      congenital dislocations) Q74.8
Larva migrans
   cutaneous B76.9
      Ancylostoma B76.0
   visceral B83.0
Laryngeal — *see* condition
Laryngismus (stridulus) J38.5
   congenital Q31.4
   diphtheritic A36.2
Laryngitis (acute) (edematous) (fibrinous)
      (infective) (infiltrative) (malignant)
      (membranous) (phlegmonous)
      (pneumococcal) (pseudomembranous) (septic)
      (subglottic) (suppurative) (ulcerative) J04.0
   with
      influenza, flu, or grippe J10.1
      tracheitis (acute) — *see* Laryngotracheitis
   atrophic J37.0
   catarrhal J37.0
   chronic J37.0
      with tracheitis (chronic) J37.1
   diphtheritic A36.2
   due to external agent — *see* Inflammation,
      respiratory, upper, due to
   Hemophilus influenzae J04.0
   H. influenzae J04.0
   hypertrophic J37.0
   influenzal J10.1
   obstructive J05.0
   sicca J37.0
   spasmodic J05.0
      acute J04.0
   streptococcal J04.0
   stridulous J05.0
   syphilitic (late) A52.73
      congenital A50.59 *[J99]*
      early A50.03 *[J99]*
   tuberculous A15.5
   Vincent's A69.1
Laryngocele (congenital) (ventricular) Q31.3
Laryngofissure J38.7

Laryngopharyngitis (acute) J06.0
   chronic J37.0
   due to external agent — *see* Inflammation,
      respiratory, upper, due to
Laryngoplegia J38.00
   bilateral J38.02
   unilateral J38.01
Laryngoptosis J38.7
Laryngospasm J38.5
Laryngostenosis J38.6
Laryngotracheitis (acute) (Infectional) (infective)
      (viral) J04.2
   atrophic J37.1
   catarrhal J37.1
   chronic J37.1
   diphtheritic A36.2
   due to external agent — *see* Inflammation,
      respiratory, upper, due to
   Hemophilus influenzae J04.2
   hypertrophic J37.1
   influenzal J10.1
   pachydermic J38.7
   sicca J37.1
   spasmodic J38.5
      acute J05.0
   streptococcal J04.2
   stridulous J38.5
   syphilitic (late) A52.73
      congenital A50.59 *[J99]*
      early A50.03 *[J99]*
   tuberculous A15.5
   Vincent's A69.1
Laryngotracheobronchitis — *see* Bronchitis
Larynx, laryngeal — *see* condition
Lassa fever A96.2
Lassitude — *see* Weakness
Late
   talker R62.0
   walker R62.0
Late effect(s) — *see* Sequelae
Latent — *see* condition
Laterocession — *see* Lateroversion
Lateroflexion — *see* Lateroversion
Lateroversion
   cervix — *see* Lateroversion, uterus
   uterus, uterine (cervix) (postinfectional)
      (postpartal, old) N85.4
      congenital Q51.8
      in pregnancy or childbirth — *see* category
         O34.5
Lathyrism — *see* Poisoning, food, noxious, plant
Launois' syndrome (pituitary gigantism) E22.0
Launois-Bensaude adenolipomatosis E88.8
Laurence-Moon (-Bardet)-Biedl syndrome Q87.89
Lax, laxity — *see also* Relaxation
   ligament(ous) — *see also* Disorder, ligament
      familial M35.7
      knee — *see* Derangement, knee
   skin (acquired) L57.4
      congenital Q82.8
Laxative habit F55.2
Lazy leukocyte syndrome D70.8
Lead miner's lung J63.6
Leak, leakage
   amniotic fluid — *see* Rupture, membranes,
      premature
   blood (microscopic), fetal, into maternal
      circulation affecting management of
      pregnancy — *see* Pregnancy, complicated
      by, placenta, transfusion syndrome
   cerebrospinal fluid G96.0
      from spinal (lumbar) puncture G97.0
   device, implant or graft — *see also*
      Complications, by site and type,
      mechanical
      arterial graft NEC — *see* Complication,
         cardiovascular device, mechanical,
         vascular
      breast (implant) T85.43
      catheter NEC T85.638
         cystostomy T83.030
         dialysis (renal) T82.43
            intraperitoneal T85.631

Leak, leakage — *continued*
   device, implant or graft — *see also*
      Complications, by site and type,
      mechanical — *continued*
      catheter NEC — *continued*
         infusion NEC T82.534
            spinal (epidural) (subdural) T85.630
         urinary (indwelling) T83.031
      gastrointestinal — *see* Complications,
         prosthetic device, mechanical,
         gastrointestinal device
      genital NEC T83.498
         penile prosthesis T83.490
      heart NEC — *see* Complication,
         cardiovascular device, mechanical
      ocular NEC — *see* Complications, prosthetic
         device, mechanical, ocular device
      orthopedic NEC — *see* Complication,
         orthopedic, device, mechanical
      specified NEC T85.638
      urinary NEC — *see also* Complication,
         genitourinary, device, urinary,
         mechanical
         graft T83.23
      vascular NEC — *see* Complication,
         cardiovascular device, mechanical
      ventricular intracranial shunt T85.03
Leaky heart — *see* Endocarditis
Learning defect (specific) F81.9
Leather bottle stomach (M8142/3) C16.9
Leber's
   congenital amaurosis H35.50
   optic atrophy (hereditary) H47.22
Lederer's anemia D59.1
Leeches (external) — *see* Hirudiniasis
Leg — *see* condition
Legg (-Calvé)-Perthes disease, syndrome or
      osteochondrosis M91.10
   left M91.12
   right M91.11
Legionellosis A48.1
   nonpneumonic A48.2
Legionnaire's
   disease A48.1
      nonpneumonic A48.2
   pneumonia A48.1
Leigh's disease G31.82
Leiner's disease L21.1
Leiofibromyoma (M8890/0) — *see* Leiomyoma
Leiomyoblastoma (M8891/0) — *see* Neoplasm,
      connective tissue, benign
Leiomyofibroma (M8890/0) — *see also*
      Neoplasm, connective tissue, benign
   uterus (cervix) (corpus) D25.9
Leiomyoma (M8890/0) — *see also* Neoplasm,
      connective tissue, benign
   bizarre (M8893/0) — *see* Neoplasm, connective
      tissue, benign
   cellular (M8892/0) — *see* Neoplasm, connective
      tissue, benign
   epithelioid (M8891/0) — *see* Neoplasm,
      connective tissue, benign
   uterus (cervix) (corpus) D25.9
      intramural D25.1
      submucous D25.0
      subserosal D25.2
   vascular (M8894/0) — *see* Neoplasm,
      connective tissue, benign
Leiomyoma, leiomyomatosis (intravascular)
      (M8890/1) — *see* Neoplasm, connective
      tissue, uncertain behavior
Leiomyosarcoma (M8890/3) — *see also*
      Neoplasm, connective tissue, malignant
   epithelioid (M8891/3) — *see* Neoplasm,
      connective tissue, malignant
   myxoid (M8896/3) — *see* Neoplasm, connective
      tissue, malignant
Leishmaniasis B55.9
   American (mucocutaneous) B55.2
      cutaneous B55.1
   Asian Desert B55.1
   Brazilian B55.2
   cutaneous (any type) B55.1

Leishmaniasis — continued
  dermal — see also Leishmaniasis, cutaneous
    post-kala-azar B55.0
  eyelid B55.1
  infantile B55.0
  Mediterranean B55.0
  mucocutaneous (American) (New World) B55.2
  naso-oral B55.2
  nasopharyngeal B55.2
  old world B55.1
  tegumentaria diffusa B55.1
  vaccination, prophylactic (against) Z23
  visceral B55.0
Leishmanoid, dermal — see also Leishmaniasis,
    cutaneous
  post-kala-azar B55.0
Lenegre's disease I44.2
Lengthening, leg — see Deformity, limb, unequal
    length
Lennert's lymphoma (M9704/3) — see
    Lymphoma, non-Hodgkin's type,
    lymphoepithelioid
Lennox-Gastaut syndrome G40.40
  with status epilepticus G40.41
Lens — see condition
Lenticonus (anterior) (posterior) (congenital) Q12.8
Lenticular degeneration, progressive E83.01
Lentiglobus (posterior) (congenital) Q12.8
Lentigo (congenital) L81.4
  maligna (M8742/2) — see also Melanoma, in
      situ
    melanoma (M8742/3) — see Melanoma
**Lentivirus, as cause of disease classified
    elsewhere** B97.31
Leontiasis
  ossium M85.2
  syphilitic (late) A52.78
    congenital A50.59
Lepothrix A48.8
Lepra — see Leprosy
Leprechaunism E34.8
Leprosy A30.9
  with muscle disorder A30.9 [M63.80]
    ankle A30.9 [M63.879]
      left A30.9 [M63.872]
      right A30.9 [M63.871]
    foot A30.9 [M63.879]
      left A30.9 [M63.872]
      right A30.9 [M63.871]
    forearm A30.9 [M63.839]
      left A30.9 [M63.832]
      right A30.9 [M63.831]
    hand A30.9 [M63.849]
      left A30.9 [M63.842]
      right A30.9 [M63.841]
    lower leg A30.9 [M63.869]
      left A30.9 [M63.862]
      right A30.9 [M63.861]
    multiple sites A30.9 [M63.89]
    pelvic region A30.9 [M63.859]
      left A30.9 [M63.852]
      right A30.9 [M63.851]
    shoulder region A30.9 [M63.819]
      left A30.9 [M63.812]
      right A30.9 [M63.811]
    specified site NEC A30.9 [M63.88]
    thigh A30.9 [M63.859]
      left A30.9 [M63.852]
      right A30.9 [M63.851]
    upper arm A30.9 [M63.829]
      left A30.9 [M63.822]
      right A30.9 [M63.821]
  anesthetic A30.9
  BB A30.3
  BL A30.4
  borderline (infiltrated) (neuritic) A30.3
    lepromatous A30.4
    tuberculoid A30.2
  BT A30.2
  dimorphous (infiltrated) (neuritic) A30.3
  I A30.0
  indeterminate (macular) (neuritic) A30.0
  lepromatous (diffuse) (infiltrated) (macular)
      (neuritic) (nodular) A30.5

Leprosy — continued
  LL A30.5
  macular (early) (neuritic) (simple) A30.9
  maculoanesthetic A30.9
  mixed A30.3
  neural A30.9
  nodular A30.5
  primary neuritic A30.3
  specified type NEC A30.8
  TT A30.1
  tuberculoid (major) (minor) A30.1
Leptocytosis, hereditary D56.9
Leptomeningitis (chronic) (circumscribed)
    (hemorrhagic) (nonsuppurative) — see
    Meningitis
Leptomeningopathy G96.1
Leptospiral — see condition
Leptospirochetal — see condition
Leptospirosis A27.9
  canicola A27.89
  due to Leptospira interrogans serovar
      icterohaemorrhagiae A27.0
  icterohemorrhagica A27.0
  pomona A27.89
  Weil's disease A27.0
Leptus dermatitis B88.0
Leriche's syndrome (aortic bifurcation occlusion)
    I74.0
Leri's pleonosteosis Q78.8
Leri-Weill syndrome Q77.8
Lermoyez' syndrome — see Vertigo, peripheral
    NEC
Lesbianism, ego-dystonic F66
Lesch-Nyhan syndrome E79.1
Leser-Trélat disease L82.1
  inflamed L82.0
Lesion (nontraumatic)
  abducens nerve — see Strabismus, paralytic,
      sixth nerve
  alveolar process K08.9
  angiocentric immunoproliferative (M9766/1)
      D47.7
  anorectal K62.9
  aortic (valve) I35.9
  auditory nerve — see category H93.3
  basal ganglion G25.9
  bile duct — see Disease, bile duct
  biomechanical M99.9
    specified type NEC M99.89
      abdomen M99.89
      acromioclavicular M99.87
      cervical region M99.81
      cervicothoracic M99.81
      costochondral M99.88
      costovertebral M99.88
      head region M99.80
      hip M99.85
      lower extremity M99.86
      lumbar region M99.83
      lumbosacral M99.83
      occipitocervical M99.80
      pelvic region M99.85
      pubic M99.85
      rib cage M99.88
      sacral region M99.84
      sacrococcygeal M99.84
      sacroiliac M99.84
      specified NEC M99.89
      sternochondral M99.88
      sternoclavicular M99.87
      thoracic region M99.82
      thoracolumbar M99.82
      upper extremity M99.87
  bladder N32.9
  bone — see Disorder, bone
  brachial plexus G54.0
  brain G93.9
    congenital Q04.9
    vascular I67.9
      degenerative I67.9
      hypertensive I67.4
  buccal cavity K13.7
  calcified — see Calcification
  canthus — see Disorder, eyelid

Lesion — continued
  carate — see Pinta, lesions
  cardia K22.9
  cardiac — see also Disease, heart I51.9
    congenital Q24.9
    valvular — see Endocarditis
  cauda equina G83.4
  cecum K63.9
  cerebral — see Lesion, brain
  cerebrovascular I67.9
    degenerative I67.9
    hypertensive I67.4
  cervical (nerve) root NEC G54.2
  chiasmal — see Disorder, optic, chiasm
  chorda tympani G51.8
  coin, lung R91
  colon K63.9
  congenital — see Anomaly, by site
  conjunctiva H11.9
  coronary artery — see Ischemia, heart
  cranial nerve G52.9
    eighth — see Disorder, ear
    eleventh G52.9
    fifth G50.9
    first G52.0
    fourth — see Strabismus, paralytic, fourth
        nerve
    seventh G51.9
    sixth — see Strabismus, paralytic, sixth
        nerve
    tenth G52.2
    twelfth G52.3
  cystic — see Cyst
  degenerative — see Degeneration
  duodenum K31.9
  edentulous (alveolar) ridge, associated with
      trauma, due to traumatic occlusion
      K06.2
  en coup de sabre L94.1
  eyelid — see Disorder, eyelid
  gasserian ganglion G50.8
  gastric K31.9
  gastroduodenal K31.9
  gastrointestinal K63.9
  gingiva, associated with trauma K06.2
  glomerular
    focal and segmental — see N00-N07 with
        fourth character .1
    minimal change — see N00-N07 with fourth
        character .0
  heart (organic) — see Disease, heart
  hyperchromic, due to pinta (carate) A67.1
  hyperkeratotic — see Hyperkeratosis
  hypothalamic E23.7
  ileocecal K63.9
  ileum K63.9
  iliohypogastric nerve G57.80
    left G57.82
    right G57.81
  inflammatory — see Inflammation
  intestine K63.9
  intracerebral — see Lesion, brain
  intrachiasmal (optic) — see Disorder, optic,
      chiasm
  intracranial, space-occupying R90.0
  joint — see Disorder, joint
    sacroiliac (old) M53.3
  keratotic — see Keratosis
  kidney — see Disease, renal
  laryngeal nerve (recurrent) G52.2
  lip K13.0
  liver K76.9
  lumbosacral
    plexus G54.1
    root (nerve) NEC G54.4
  lung (coin) R91
  maxillary sinus J32.0
  mitral I05.9
  motor cortex NEC G93.8
  mouth K13.7
  nerve G58.9
    femoral G57.20
      left G57.22
      right G57.21
    median G56.10
      carpal tunnel syndrome — see Syndrome,
          carpal tunnel

©2002 Ingenix, Inc.

Lesion — *continued*
  nerve — *continued*
    median — *continued*
      left G56.12
      right G56.11
    plantar G57.60
      left G57.62
      right G57.61
    popliteal (lateral) G57.30
      left G57.32
      medial G57.40
        left G57.42
        right G57.41
      right G57.31
    radial G56.30
      left G56.32
      right G56.31
    sciatic G57.00
      left G57.02
      right G57.01
    ulnar G56.20
      left G56.22
      right G56.21
  nervous system, congenital Q07.9
  nonallopathic — *see* Lesion, biomechanical
  nose (internal) J34.8
  obstructive — *see* Obstruction
  obturator nerve G57.80
    left G57.82
    right G57.81
  oral mucosa K13.7
  organ or site NEC — *see* Disease, by site
  osteolytic — *see* Osteolysis
  peptic K27.9
  periodontal, due to traumatic occlusion K05.5
  pharynx J39.2
  pigment, pigmented (skin) L81.9
  pinta — *see* Pinta, lesions
  polypoid — *see* Polyp
  prechiasmal (optic) — *see* Disorder, optic, chiasm
  primary — *see also* Syphilis, primary A51.0
    carate A67.0
    pinta A67.0
    yaws A66.0
  pulmonary J98.4
    valve I37.9
  pylorus K31.9
  radiation T66
  radium T66
  rectosigmoid K63.9
  retina, retinal H35.9
  sacroiliac (joint) (old) M53.3
  salivary gland K11.9
    benign lymphoepithelial K11.8
  saphenous nerve G57.80
    left G57.82
    right G57.81
  sciatic nerve G57.00
    left G57.02
    right G57.01
  secondary — *see* Syphilis, secondary
  shoulder (region) M75.90
    left M75.92
    right M75.91
    specified NEC M75.80
      left M75.82
      right M75.81
  sigmoid K63.9
  sinus (accessory) (nasal) J34.8
  skin L98.9
    suppurative L08.0
  spinal cord G95.9
    congenital Q06.9
  spleen D73.8
  stomach K31.9
  syphilitic — *see* Syphilis
  tertiary — *see* Syphilis, tertiary
  thoracic root (nerve) NEC G54.3
  tonsillar fossa J35.9
  tooth, teeth K08.9
    white spot K02.0
  traumatic — *see* specific type of injury by site
  tricuspid (valve) I07.9
    nonrheumatic I36.9
  trigeminal nerve G50.9
  ulcerated or ulcerative — *see* Ulcer, skin

Lesion — *continued*
  uterus N85.9
  vagus nerve G52.2
  valvular — *see* Endocarditis
  vascular I99.9
    affecting central nervous system I67.9
    following trauma T14.90
    umbilical cord, complicating delivery O69.5
  warty — *see* Verruca
  X-ray (radiation) T66
Lethargic — *see* condition
Lethargy R53.82
Letterer-Siwe's disease (M9722/3) C96.0
  Leuc(o)for any term beginning thus — *see* Leuk(o)
Leukemia, leukemic (congenital) (M9800/3) C95.90
  acute (M9801/3) C95.00
    in remission C95.01
  adult T-cell (M9827/3) C91.50
    in remission C91.51
  aleukemic (M9804/3) C95.70
    in remission C95.71
  basophilic (M9870/3) C92.70
    in remission C92.71
  blast (cell) (M9801/3) C95.00
    in remission C95.01
  blastic (M9801/3) C95.00
    granulocytic (M9861/3) C92.00
      in remission C92.01
    in remission C95.01
  chronic (M9803/3) C95.10
    in remission C95.11
  compound (M9800/3) C94.70
    in remission C94.71
  eosinophilic (M9880/3) C92.70
    in remission C92.71
  granulocytic (M9860/3) C92.90
    acute (M9861/3) C92.00
      in remission C92.01
    aleukemic (M9864/3) C92.70
      in remission C92.71
    blastic (M9861/3) C92.00
      in remission C92.01
    chronic (M9863/3) C92.10
      in remission C92.11
    in remission C92.91
    subacute (M9862/3) C92.20
      in remission C92.21
  hairy cell (M9940/3) C91.40
    in remission C91.41
  histiocytic (M9890/3) C93.90
    in remission C93.91
  in remission C95.91
  lymphatic (M9820/3) C91.90
    acute (M9821/3) C91.00
      in remission C91.01
    aleukemic (M9824/3) C91.70
      in remission C91.71
    chronic (M9823/3) C91.10
      in remission C91.11
    in remission C91.91
    subacute (M9822/3) C91.20
      in remission C91.21
  lymphoblastic (M9821/3) C91.00
    in remission C91.01
  lymphocytic (M9820/3) C91.90
    acute (M9821/3) C91.00
      in remission C91.01
    aleukemic (M9824/3) C91.70
      in remission C91.71
    chronic (M9823/3) C91.10
      in remission C91.11
    in remission C91.91
    subacute (M9822/3) C91.20
      in remission C91.21
  lymphogenous (M9820/3) — *see* Leukemia, lymphoid
  lymphoid (M9820/3) C91.90
    acute (M9821/3) C91.00
      in remission C91.01
    aleukemic (M9824/3) C91.70
      in remission C91.71
    blastic (M9821/3) C91.00
      in remission C91.01

Leukemia, leukemic — *continued*
  lymphoid — *continued*
    chronic (M9823/3) C91.10
      in remission C91.11
      in remission C91.91
    subacute (M9822/3) C91.20
      in remission C91.21
  lymphosarcoma cell (M9850/3) C94.70
    in remission C94.71
  mast cell (M9900/3) C94.30
    in remission C94.31
  megakaryocytic (M9910/3) C94.20
    in remission C94.21
  mixed (cell) (M9800/3) C94.70
    in remission C94.71
  monoblastic (acute) (M9891/3) C93.00
    in remission C93.01
  monocytic (M9890/3) C93.90
    acute (M9891/3) C93.00
      in remission C93.01
    aleukemic (M9894/3) C93.70
      in remission C93.71
    chronic (M9893/3) C93.10
      in remission C93.11
      in remission C93.91
    Naegeli-type (M9863/3) C92.10
      in remission C92.11
    subacute (M9892/3) C93.20
      in remission C93.21
  monocytoid (M9890/3) C93.90
    acute (M9891/3) C93.00
      in remission C93.01
    aleukemic (M9894/3) C93.70
      in remission C93.71
    chronic (M9893/3) C93.10
      in remission C93.11
      in remission C93.91
    myelogenous (M9863/3) C92.10
      in remission C92.11
    subacute (M9892/3) C93.20
      in remission C93.21
  monomyelocytic (M9860/3) — *see* Leukemia, myelomonocytic
  myeloblastic (acute) (M9861/3) C92.00
    in remission C92.01
  myelocytic (M9860/3) C92.90
    acute (M9861/3) C92.00
      in remission C92.01
    in remission C92.91
    chronic (M9863/3) C92.10
      in remission C92.11
  myelogenous (M9860/3) C92.90
    acute (M9861/3) C92.00
      in remission C92.01
    aleukemic (M9864/3) C92.70
      in remission C92.71
    chronic (M9863/3) C92.10
      in remission C92.11
      in remission C92.91
    subacute (M9862/3) C92.20
      in remission C92.21
  myeloid (M9860/3) C92.90
    acute (M9861/3) C92.00
      in remission C92.01
    aleukemic (M9864/3) C92.70
      in remission C92.71
    chronic (M9863/3) C92.10
      in remission C92.11
      in remission C92.91
    subacute (M9862/3) C92.20
      in remission C92.21
  myelomonocytic (M9860/3) C92.90
    acute (M9867/3) C92.50
      in remission C92.51
    chronic (M9868/3) C92.10
      in remission C92.11
      in remission C92.91
  Naegeli-type monocytic (M9863/3) C92.10
    in remission C92.11
  neutrophilic (M9800/3) C92.10
    in remission C92.11
  plasma cell (M9830/3) C90.10
    in remission C90.11
  plasmacytic (M9830/3) C90.10
    in remission C90.11
  prolymphocytic (M9825/3) C91.30
    in remission C91.31

Leukemia, leukemic — *continued*
  promyelocytic, acute (M9866/3) C92.40
    in remission C92.41
  stem cell (M9801/3) C95.00
    in remission C95.01
  subacute (M9802/3) C95.20
    in remission C95.21
  thrombocytic (M9910/3) C94.20
    in remission C94.21
  undifferentiated (M9801/3) C95.00
    in remission C95.01
  x-ray T66
Leukemoid reaction (lymphocytic) (monocytic)
    (myelocytic) D72.8
Leukocoria — *see* Disorder, globe, degenerated
    condition, leucocoria
Leukocytosis D72.8
  eosinophilic D72.1
Leukoderma, leukodermia NEC L81.5
  syphilitic A51.39
    late A52.79
Leukodystrophy E75.29
Leukoedema, oral epithelium K13.2
Leukoencephalitis (postinfectious) G04.8
  acute (subacute) hemorrhagic G36.1
    postimmunization or postvaccinal G04.0
  subacute sclerosing A81.1
  van Bogaert's (sclerosing) A81.1
Leukoencephalopathy — *see also*
    Encephalopathy
  acute necrotizing hemorrhagic (postinfectious)
    B89
    postimmunization or postvaccinal G04.0
  metachromatic E75.25
  multifocal (progressive) A81.2
  postimmunization and postvaccinal G04.0
  progressive multifocal A81.2
  van Bogaert's (sclerosing) A81.1
  vascular, progressive I67.3
Leukoerythroblastosis D64.8
Leukokeratosis — *see also* Leukoplakia
  mouth K13.2
  nicotina palati K13.2
  tongue K13.2
  vocal cord J38.3
Leukokraurosis vulva(e) N90.4
Leukoma (cornea) — *see also* Opacity, cornea
  adherent H17.00
    bilateral H17.03
    left H17.02
    right H17.01
  interfering with central vision — *see* Opacity,
    cornea, central
Leukomalacia, cerebral, newborn P91.2
Leukomelanopathy, hereditary D72.0
Leukonychia (punctata) (striata) L60.8
  congenital Q84.4
Leukopathia unguium L60.8
  congenital Q84.4
Leukopenia (malignant) — *see also*
    Agranulocytosis -chemotherapy (cancer)
    induced D70.1
  congenital D70.0
  cyclic D70.0
  drug induced NEC D70.2
    due to cytoreductive cancer chemotherapy
      D70.1
  familial D70.0
  infantile genetic D70.0
  periodic D70.0
  transitory neonatal P61.5
Leukopenic — *see* condition
Leukoplakia
  anus K62.8
  bladder (postinfectional) N32.8
  buccal K13.2
  cervix (uteri) N88.0
  esophagus K22.8
  gingiva K13.2
  hairy (oral mucosa) (tongue) K13.3
  kidney (pelvis) N28.89
  larynx J38.7
  lip K13.2
  mouth K13.2

Leukoplakia — *continued*
  oral epithelium, including tongue (mucosa)
    K13.2
  palate K13.2
  pelvis (kidney) N28.89
  penis (infectional) N48.0
  rectum K62.8
  syphilitic (late) A52.79
  tongue K13.2
  ureter (postinfectional) N28.89
  urethra (postinfectional) N36.8
  uterus N85.8
  vagina N89.4
  vocal cord J38.3
  vulva N90.4
Leukorrhea N89.8
  due to Trichomonas (vaginalis) A59.00
  trichomonal A59.00
Leukosarcoma (M9850/3) C94.70
  in remission C94.71
Levocardia (isolated) Q24.1
  with situs inversus Q89.3
Levotransposition Q20.5
Lev's disease or syndrome (acquired) (complete
    heart block) I44.2
Levulosuria — *see* Fructosuria
Levurid L30.2
Leyden-Moebius dystrophy G71.0
Leydig cell
  carcinoma (M8650/3)
    specified site — *see* Neoplasm, malignant
    unspecified site
      female C56.9
        left C56.1
        right C56.0
      male C62.90
        left C62.92
        right C62.91
  tumor (M8650/1)
    benign (M8650/0)
      specified site — *see* Neoplasm, benign
      unspecified site
        female D27.9
          left D27.1
          right D27.0
        male D29.20
          left D29.22
          right D29.21
    malignant (M8650/3)
      specified site — *see* Neoplasm, malignant
      unspecified site
        female C56.9
        male C62.90
          left C62.92
          right C62.91
    specified site — *see* Neoplasm, uncertain
      behavior
    unspecified site
      female D39.10
        left D39.12
        right D39.11
      male D40.10
        left D40.12
        right D40.11
Leydig-Sertoli cell tumor (M8631/0)
  specified site — *see* Neoplasm, benign
  unspecified site
    female D27.9
      left D27.1
      right D27.0
    male D29.20
      left D29.22
      right D29.21
Liar, pathologic F60.2
Libman-Sacks disease M32.11
Lice (infestation) B85.2
  body (Pediculus corporis) B85.1
  crab B85.3
  head (Pediculus capitis) B85.0
  mixed (classifiable to more than one of the
    titles B85.0-B85.3) B85.4
  pubic (Phthirus pubis) B85.3

Lichen L28.0
  albus L90.0
    penis N48.0
    vulva N90.4
  amyloidosis E85 [L99]
  atrophicus L90.0
    penis N48.0
    vulva N90.4
  congenital Q82.8
  myxedematosus L98.5
  nitidus L44.1
  pilaris Q82.8
    acquired L85.8
  planopilaris L66.1
  planus (chronicus) L43.9
    annularis L43.8
    bullous L43.1
    follicular L66.1
    hypertrophic L43.0
    moniliformis L44.3
    of Wilson L43.9
    specified NEC L43.8
    subacute (active) L43.3
    tropicus L43.3
  ruber
    acuminatus L44.0
    moniliformis L44.3
    planus L43.9
  sclerosus (et atrophicus) L90.0
    penis N48.0
    vulva N90.4
  scrofulosus (primary) (tuberculous) A18.4
  simplex (chronicus) (circumscriptus) L28.0
  striatus L44.2
  urticatus L28.2
Lichenification L28.0
Lichenoides tuberculosis (primary) A18.4
Lichtheim's disease or syndrome — *see*
    Degeneration, combined
Lie, abnormal (maternal care) — *see* Presentation,
    fetal, abnormal
Lien migrans D73.8
Ligament — *see* condition
Light
  fetus or newborn for gestational age — *see*
    Light for dates
  headedness R42
Light-for-dates (infant) P05.00
  with weight of
    499 grams or less P05.01
    500-749 grams P05.02
    750-999 grams P05.03
    1000-1249 grams P05.04
    1250-1499 grams P05.05
    1500-1749 grams P05.06
    1750-1999 grams P05.07
    2000-2499 grams P05.08
  and small-for-dates — *see* Small for dates
  affecting management of pregnancy — *see*
    category O36.5
Lightning (effects) (stroke) (struck by) T75.00
  burn — *see* Burn
  foot E53.8
  shock T75.01
  specified effect NEC T75.09
Lightwood-Albright syndrome N25.8
Lightwood's disease or syndrome (renal tubular
    acidosis) N25.8
**Lignac (-de Toni) (-Fanconi) (-Debré) disease or
    syndrome** E72.09
  with cystinosis E72.04
Ligneous thyroiditis E06.5
Likoff's syndrome I20.8
Limb — *see* condition
Limbic epilepsy personality syndrome F07.0
Limitation, limited
  activities due to disability Z73.6
  cardiac reserve — *see* Disease, heart
  eye muscle duction, traumatic — *see*
    Strabismus, mechanical
Lindau (-von Hippel) disease Q85.8
Line(s)
  Dcau's L60.4
  Harris' — *see* Arrest, epiphyseal

©2002 Ingenix, Inc.

Line(s) — *continued*
  Hudson's (cornea) — *see* Pigmentation, cornea, anterior
  Stähli's (cornea) — *see* Pigmentation, cornea, anterior

Linea corneae senilis — *see* Change, cornea, senile

Lingua
  geographica K14.1
  nigra (villosa) K14.3
  plicata K14.5
  tylosis K13.2

Lingual — *see* condition

Linguatulosis B88.8

Linitis (gastric) **plastica** (M8142/3) C16.9

Lip — *see* condition

Lipedema — *see* Edema

Lipemia — *see also* Hyperlipidemia
  retina, retinalis E78.3

Lipidosis E75.6
  cerebral (infantile) (juvenile) (late) E75.4
  cerebroretinal E75.4
  cerebroside E75.22
  cholesterol (cerebral) E75.5
  glycolipid E75.21
  hepatosplenomegalic E78.3
  sphingomyelin — *see* Niemann-Pick disease or syndrome
  sulfatide E75.29

Lipoadenoma (M8324/0) — *see* Neoplasm, benign

Lipoblastoma (M8881/0) — *see* Lipoma

Lipoblastomatosis (M8881/0) — *see* Lipoma

Lipochondrodystrophy E76.01

Lipochrome histiocytosis (familial) D71

Lipodystrophia progressiva E88.1

Lipodystrophy (progressive) E88.1
  insulin E88.1
  intestinal K90.81

Lipofibroma (M8851/0) — *see* Lipoma

Lipofuscinosis, neuronal (with ceroidosis) E75.4

Lipogranuloma, sclerosing L92.8

Lipogranulomatosis E78.89

Lipoid — *see also* condition
  histiocytosis D76.0
    essential E75.29
  nephrosis — *see* Nephrosis
  proteinosis of Urbach E78.89

Lipoidemia — *see* Hyperlipidemia

Lipoidosis — *see* Lipidosis

Lipoma (M8850/0) D17.9
  fetal (M8881/0) D17.9
  fat cell (M8880/0) D17.9
  infiltrating (M8856/0) D17.9
  intramuscular (M8856/0) D17.9
  pleomorphic (M8854/0) D17.9
  site classification
    arms (skin) (subcutaneous) D17.20
      left D17.22
      right D17.21
    connective tissue D17.30
      intra-abdominal D17.5
      intrathoracic D17.4
      peritoneum D17.7
      retroperitoneum D17.7
      specified site NEC D17.39
      spermatic cord D17.6
    face (skin) (subcutaneous) D17.0
    head (skin) (subcutaneous) D17.0
    intra-abdominal D17.5
    intrathoracic D17.4
    legs (skin) (subcutaneous) D17.20
      left D17.24
      right D17.23
    neck (skin) (subcutaneous) D17.0
    peritoneum D17.7
    retroperitoneum D17.7
    skin D17.30
      specified site NEC D17.39
    specified site NEC D17.7
    spermatic cord D17.6
    subcutaneous D17.30
      specified site NEC D17.39

Lipoma — *continued*
  site classification — *continued*
    trunk (skin) (subcutaneous) D17.1
    unspecified D17.9
  spindle cell (M8857/0) D17.9

Lipomatosis E88.2
  dolorosa (Dercum) E88.2
  fetal (M8881/0) — *see* Lipoma
  Launois-Bensaude E88.8

Lipomyoma (M8860/0) — *see* Lipoma

Lipomyxoma (M8852/0) — *see* Lipoma

Lipomyxosarcoma (M8852/3) — *see* Neoplasm, connective tissue, malignant

Lipoprotein metabolism disorder E78.9

Lipoproteinemia E78.5
  broad-beta E78.2
  floating-beta E78.2
  hyper-pre-beta E78.1

Liposarcoma (M8850/3) — *see also* Neoplasm, connective tissue, malignant
  dedifferentiated (M8858/3) — *see* Neoplasm, connective tissue, malignant
  differentiated type (M8851/3) — *see* Neoplasm, connective tissue, malignant
  embryonal (M8852/3) — *see* Neoplasm, connective tissue, malignant
  mixed type (M8855/3) — *see* Neoplasm, connective tissue, malignant
  myxoid (M8852/3) — *see* Neoplasm, connective tissue, malignant
  pleomorphic (M8854/3) — *see* Neoplasm, connective tissue, malignant
  round cell (M8853/3) — *see* Neoplasm, connective tissue, malignant
  well differentiated type (M8851/3) — *see* Neoplasm, connective tissue, malignant

Liposynovitis prepatellaris E88.8

Lipping, cervix N86

Lipschütz disease or ulcer N76.6

Lipuria R82.0
  schistosomiasis (bilharziasis) B65.0

Lisping F80.0

Lissauer's paralysis A52.17

Lissencephalia, lissencephaly Q04.3

Listeriosis, listerellosis A32.9
  congenital (disseminated) P37.2
  cutaneous A32.0
  fetal P37.2
  neonatal (disseminated) P37.2
  oculoglandular A32.81
  specified NEC A32.89
  suspected damage to fetus affecting management of pregnancy O35.8

Lithemia E79.0

Lithiasis — *see* Calculus

Lithosis J62.8

Lithuria R82.99

Litigation, anxiety concerning Z65.3

Little leaguer's elbow — *see* Epicondylitis, medial

Little's disease G80.9

Littre's
  gland — *see* condition
  hernia — *see* Hernia, abdomen

Littritis — *see* Urethritis

Livedo (annularis) (racemosa) (reticularis) R23.1

Liver — *see* condition

Living alone (problems with) Z60.2
  with handicapped person Z74.2

Lloyd's syndrome (M8360/1) — *see* Adenomatosis, endocrine

Loa loa, loaiasis, loasis B74.3

Lobar — *see* condition

Lobomycosis B48.0

Lobo's disease B48.0

Lobotomy syndrome F07.0

Lobstein (-Ekman) disease or syndrome Q78.0

Lobster-claw hand Q71.60
  bilateral Q71.63
  left Q71.62
  right Q71.61

Lobulation (congenital) — *see also* Anomaly, by site
  kidney, fetal Q63.1
  liver, abnormal Q44.7
  spleen Q89.09

Lobule, lobular — *see* condition

Local, localized — *see* condition

Locked-in state G83.5

Locked twins causing obstructed labor O66.1

Locking
  joint — *see* Derangement, joint, specified type NEC
  knee — *see* Derangement, knee

Lockjaw — *see* Tetanus

Löffler's
  endocarditis I42.3
  eosinophilia J82
  pneumonia J82
  syndrome (eosinophilic pneumonitis) J82

Loiasis (with conjunctival infestation) (eyelid) B74.3

Lone Star fever A77.0

Long
  labor O63.9
    first stage O63.0
    second stage O63.1
  term use (current) of
    anticoagulants Z79.1
      with hemorrhage D68.5
    aspirin Z79.8
    medicaments NEC Z79.8

Longitudinal stripes or grooves, nails L60.8
  congenital Q84.6

Loop
  intestine — *see* Volvulus
  vascular on papilla (optic) Q14.2

Loose — *see also* condition
  body
    joint M24.00
      ankle M24.073
        left M24.072
        right M24.071
      elbow M24.029
        left M24.022
        right M24.021
      hand M24.049
        left M24.042
        right M24.041
      hip M24.059
        left M24.052
        right M24.051
      knee M23.40
        left M23.42
        right M23.41
      shoulder (region) M24.019
        left M24.012
        right M24.011
      specified site NEC M24.08
      vertebra M24.08
      toe M24.076
        left M24.075
        right M24.074
      wrist M24.039
        left M24.032
        right M24.031
    knee M23.40
      left M23.42
      right M23.41
    sheath, tendon — *see* Disorder, tendon, specified type NEC
  cartilage — *see* Loose, body, joint
  tooth, teeth K08.8

Loosening epiphysis — *see* Osteochondropathy

Looser-Milkman (-Debray) syndrome M83.8

Lop ear (deformity) Q17.3

Lorain (-Levi) short stature syndrome E23.0

Lordosis M40.50
  acquired — *see* Lordosis, specified type NEC
  congenital Q76.429
    lumbar region Q76.426
    lumbosacral region Q76.427
    sacral region Q76.428
    sacrococcygeal region Q76.428

Lordosis — *continued*
  congenital — *continued*
    thoracolumbar region Q76.425
  lumbar region M40.56
  lumbosacral region M40.57
  postsurgical M96.4
  postural — *see* Lordosis, specified type NEC
  rachitic (late effect) (*see also* category M49.8)
    E64.3
  sacrococcygeal region M40.58
  sequelae of rickets (*see also* category M49.8)
    E64.3
  specified type NEC M40.40
    lumbar region M40.46
    lumbosacral region M40.47
    sacrococcygeal region M40.48
    thoracolumbar region M40.45
  thoracolumbar region M40.55
  tuberculous A18.01

Loss (of)
  appetite R63.0
    hysterical F50.8
    nonorganic origin F50.8
    psychogenic F50.8
  blood — *see* Hemorrhage
  control, sphincter, rectum R15
    nonorganic origin F98.1
  consciousness, transient R55
    traumatic — *see* Injury, intracranial
  elasticity, skin R23.4
  family (member) in childhood Z61.0
  fluid (acute) E86.9
    with
      hypernatremia E87.0
      hyponatremia E87.1
    fetus or newborn P74.1
  function of labyrinth — *see* category H83.2
  hair, nonscarring — *see* Alopecia
  hearing — *see* Deafness
  height R29.890
  limb or member, traumatic, current — *see*
    Amputation, traumatic
  love relationship in childhood Z61.0
  memory — *see also* Amnesia
    mild, following organic brain damage F06.8
  mind — *see* Psychosis
  organ or part — *see* Absence, by site, acquired
  ossicles, ear (partial) H74.329
    bilateral H74.323
    left H74.322
    right H74.321
  parent in childhood Z61.0
  self-esteem, in childhood Z61.3
  sense of
    smell — *see* Disturbance, sensation, smell
    taste — *see* Disturbance, sensation, taste
    touch R20.8
  sensory R44.9
    dissociative F44.6
  sexual desire F52.0
  sight (acquired) (complete) (congenital) — *see*
    Blindness
  substance of
    bone — *see* Disorder, bone, density and
      structure, specified NEC
    cartilage — *see* Disorder, cartilage, specified
      type NEC
      auricle (ear) — *see* Disorder, pinna,
        specified type NEC
    vitreous (humor) H15.89
  tooth, teeth due to accident, extraction or local
    periodontal disease K08.1
  vision, visual H54.7
    both eyes H54.3
    one eye H54.60
      left (normal vision on right) H54.62
      right (normal vision on left) H54.61
    specified as blindness — *see* Blindness
    subjective
      sudden H53.139
        bilateral H53.133
        left H53.132
        right H53.131
      transient H53.129
        bilateral H53.123
        left H53.122
        right H53.121

Loss — *continued*
  vitreous — *see* Prolapse, vitreous
  voice — *see* Aphonia
  weight (abnormal) (cause unknown) R63.4

Louis-Bar syndrome (ataxia-telangiectasia) G11.3

Louping ill (encephalitis) A84.8

Louse, lousiness — *see* Lice

Low
  achiever, school Z55.3
  back syndrome M54.5
  basal metabolic rate R94.8
  birthweight (2499 grams or less) P07.10
    with weight of
      1000-1249 grams P07.14
      1250-1499 grams P07.15
      1500-1749 grams P07.16
      1750-1999 grams P07.17
      2000-2499 grams P07.18
    extreme (999 grams or less) P07.00
      with weight of
        499 grams or less P07.01
        500-749 grams P07.02
        750-999 grams P07.03
    for gestational age — *see* Light for dates
  blood pressure — *see also* Hypotension
    reading (incidental) (isolated) (nonspecific)
      R03.1
  cardiac reserve — *see* Disease, heart
  function — *see also* Hypofunction
    kidney — *see* Failure, renal
  hemoglobin D64.9
  implantation, placenta — *see* Placenta, previa
  income Z59.6
  insertion, placenta — *see* Placenta, previa
  level of literacy Z55.0
  lying
    kidney N28.89
    organ or site, congenital — *see* Malposition,
      congenital
    placenta — *see* Placenta, previa
  output syndrome (cardiac) — *see* Failure, heart
  platelets (blood) — *see* Thrombocytopenia
  reserve, kidney N28.89
  salt syndrome E87.1
  self esteem R45.81
  set ears Q17.4
  vision H54.2
    one eye (other eye normal) H54.50
      left (normal vision on right) H54.52
      other eye blind — *see* Blindness
      right (normal vision on left) H54.51

Low-density-lipoprotein-type (LDL)
  hyperlipoproteinemia E78.0

Lowe's syndrome E72.03

Lown-Ganong-Levine syndrome I45.6

LSD reaction (acute) (without dependence) F16.90
  with dependence F16.20

L-shaped kidney Q63.8

Ludwig's angina or disease K12.2

Lues (venerea), luetic — *see* Syphilis

Luetscher's syndrome (dehydration) E86.0

Lumbago, lumbalgia M54.5
  with sciatica M54.4
    due to intervertebral disc disorder M51.17
  due to displacement, intervertebral disc
    M51.27
    with sciatica M51.17

Lumbar — *see* condition

Lumbarization, vertebra, congenital Q76.49

Lumbermen's itch B88.0

Lump — *see* Mass

Lunacy — *see* Psychosis

Lung — *see* condition

Lupoid (miliary) of Boeck D86.3

Lupus
  discoid (local) L93.0
  erythematosus (discoid) (local) L93.0
    disseminated — *see* Lupus, erythematosus,
      systemic
    eyelid H01.129
      left H01.126
        lower H01.125
        upper H01.124

Lupus — *continued*
  erythematosus — *continued*
    eyelid — *continued*
      right H01.123
        lower H01.122
        upper H01.121
    profundus L93.2
    specified NEC L93.2
    subacute cutaneous L93.1
    systemic M32.9
      with
        with organ or system involvement M32.10
          endocarditis M32.11
          lung M32.13
          pericarditis M32.12
          renal (glomerular) M32.14
            tubulo-interstitial M32.15
          specified organ or system NEC M32.19
      drug-induced M32.0
      inhibitor (presence of) D68.81
      specified NEC M32.8
  exedens A18.4
  hydralazine
    correct substance properly administered
      M32.0
    overdose or wrong substance given or taken
      — *see* category T46.5
  nephritis (chronic) M32.14
  nontuberculous, not disseminated L93.0
  panniculitis L93.2
  pernio (Besnier) D86.3
  systemic — *see* Lupus, erythematosus,
    systemic
  tuberculous A18.4
    eyelid A18.4
  vulgaris A18.4
    eyelid A18.4

Luteinoma (M8610/0) D27.9
  left D27.1
  right D27.0

Lutembacher's disease or syndrome (atrial
  septal defect with mitral stenosis) Q21.1

Luteoma (M8610/0) D27.9
  left D27.1
  right D27.0

Lutz (-Splendore-de Almeida) disease — *see*
  Paracoccidioidomycosis

Luxation — *see also* Dislocation
  eyeball (nontraumatic) — *see* Luxation, globe
    birth injury P15.3
  globe, nontraumatic H44.829
    bilateral H44.823
    left H44.822
    right H44.821
  lacrimal gland — *see* Dislocation, lacrimal
    gland
  lens (old) (partial) (spontaneous)
    congenital
      syphilitic A50.39

Lycanthropy F22

Lyell's syndrome L51.2
  due to drug
    correct substance properly administered
      L51.2
    overdose or wrong substance given or taken
      (by accident) T50.901
      administered with intent to harm by
        another person T50.903
        self T50.902
      circumstances undetermined T50.904
      specified drug   *see* Table of Drugs and
        Chemicals

Lyme disease A69.20

Lymph
  gland or node — *see* condition
  scrotum — *see* Infestation, filarial

Lymphadenitis I88.9
  with ectopic or molar pregnancy O08.0
  acute L04.9
    axilla L04.2
    face L04.0
    head L04.0
    hip L04.3

Lymphadenitis — *continued*
  acute — *continued*
    limb
      lower L04.3
      upper L04.2
    neck L04.0
    shoulder L04.2
    specified site NEC L04.8
    trunk L04.1
  anthracosis (occupational) J60
  any site, except mesenteric I88.9
    chronic I88.1
    subacute I88.1
  breast
    gestational — *see* Mastitis, obstetric
    puerperal, postpartum (nonpurulent) O91.22
  chancroidal (congenital) A57
  chronic I88.1
    mesenteric I88.0
  due to
    Brugia (malayi) B74.1
      timori B74.2
    chlamydial lymphogranuloma A55
    diphtheria (toxin) A36.89
    lymphogranuloma venereum A55
    Wuchereria bancrofti B74.0
  following ectopic or molar pregnancy O08.0
  gonorrheal A54.89
  infective — *see* Lymphadenitis, acute
  mesenteric (acute) (chronic) (nonspecific) (subacute) I88.0
    due to Salmonella typhi A01.09
    tuberculous A18.39
  mycobacterial A31.8
  purulent — *see* Lymphadenitis, acute
  pyogenic — *see* Lymphadenitis, acute
  regional, nonbacterial A28.1
  septic — *see* Lymphadenitis, acute
  subacute, unspecified site I88.1
  suppurative — *see* Lymphadenitis, acute
  syphilitic (early) (secondary) A51.49
    late A52.79
  tuberculous — *see* Tuberculosis, lymph gland
  venereal (chlamydial) A55
Lymphadenoid goiter E06.3
Lymphadenopathy (generalized) R59.1
  angioimmunoblastic (M9767/1) D47.7
  due to toxoplasmosis (acquired) B58.89
    congenital (acute) (subacute) (chronic) P37.1
  localized R59.0
  syphilitic (early) (secondary) A51.49
Lymphadenosis R59.1
Lymphangiectasis I89.0
  conjunctiva H11.89
  postinfectional I89.0
  scrotum I89.0
Lymphangiectatic elephantiasis, nonfilarial I89.0
Lymphangioendothelioma (M9170/0) D18.1
  malignant (M9170/3) — *see* Neoplasm, connective tissue, malignant
Lymphangioma (M9170/0) D18.1
  capillary (M9171/0) D18.1
  cavernous (M9172/0) D18.1
  cystic (M9173/0) D18.1
  malignant (M9170/3) — *see* Neoplasm, connective tissue, malignant
Lymphangiomyoma (M9174/0) D18.1
Lymphangiomyomatosis (M9174/1) — *see* Neoplasm, connective tissue, uncertain behavior
Lymphangiosarcoma (M9170/3) — *see* Neoplasm, connective tissue, malignant
Lymphangitis I89.1
  with
    abscess – code by site under Abscess
    cellulitis – code by site under Cellulitis
  ectopic or molar pregnancy O08.0
  acute L03.91
    abdominal wall L03.321
    ankle — *see* Lymphangitis, acute, lower limb
    arm — *see* Lymphangitis, acute, upper limb
    auricle (ear) — *see* Lymphangitis, acute, ear
    axilla L03.129
      left L03.122

Lymphangitis — *continued*
  acute — *continued*
    axilla — *continued*
      right L03.121
    back (any part) L03.322
    buttock L03.327
    cervical (meaning neck) L03.222
    cheek (external) L03.212
    chest wall L03.323
    digit
      finger — *see* Lymphangitis, acute, finger
      toe — *see* Lymphangitis, acute, toe
    ear (external) H60.10
      bilateral H60.13
      left H60.12
      right H60.11
    external auditory canal — *see* Lymphangitis, acute, ear
    eyelid — *see* Abscess, eyelid
    face NEC L03.212
    finger (intrathecal) (periosteal) (subcutaneous) (subcuticular) L03.029
      left L03.022
      right L03.021
    foot — *see* Lymphangitis, acute, lower limb
    gluteal (region) L03.327
    groin L03.324
    hand — *see* Lymphangitis, acute, upper limb
    head NEC L03.891
      face (any part, except ear, eye and nose) L03.212
    heel — *see* Lymphangitis, acute, lower limb
    hip — *see* Lymphangitis, acute, lower limb
    jaw (region) L03.212
    knee — *see* Lymphangitis, acute, lower limb
    leg — *see* Lymphangitis, acute, lower limb
    lower limb L03.129
      left L03.126
      right L03.125
      toe — *see* Lymphangitis, acute, toe
    navel L03.326
    neck (region) L03.222
    orbit, orbital — *see* Cellulitis, orbit
    pectoral (region) L03.323
    perineal, perineum L03.325
    scalp (any part) L03.891
    shoulder — *see* Lymphangitis, acute, upper limb
    specified site NEC L03.898
    thigh — *see* Lymphangitis, acute, lower limb
    thumb (intrathecal) (periosteal) (subcutaneous) (subcuticular) — *see* Lymphangitis, acute, finger
    toe (intrathecal) (periosteal) (subcutaneous) (subcuticular) L03.049
      left L03.042
      right L03.041
    trunk L03.329
      abdominal wall L03.321
      back (any part) L03.322
      buttock L03.327
      chest wall L03.323
      groin L03.324
      perineal, perineum L03.325
      umbilicus L03.326
    umbilicus L03.326
    upper limb L03.129
      axilla — *see* Lymphangitis, acute, axilla
      finger — *see* Lymphangitis, acute, finger
      left L03.124
      right L03.123
      thumb — *see* Lymphangitis, acute, finger
      wrist — *see* Lymphangitis, acute, upper limb
  breast
    gestational — *see* Mastitis, obstetric
  chancroidal A57
  chronic (any site) I89.1
  due to
    Brugia (malayi) B74.1
      timori B74.2
    Wuchereria bancrofti B74.0
  following ectopic or molar pregnancy O08.89
  penis
    acute N48.29
    gonococcal (acute) (chronic) A54.09
  puerperal, postpartum, childbirth O86.8

Lymphangitis — *continued*
  strumous, tuberculous A18.2
  subacute (any site) I89.1
  tuberculous — *see* Tuberculosis, lymph gland
Lymphatic (vessel) — *see* condition
Lymphatism E32.8
Lymphectasia I89.0
Lymphedema (acquired) — *see also* Elephantiasis
  congenital Q82.0
  hereditary (chronic) (idiopathic) Q82.0
  postmastectomy I97.2
  praecox I89.0
  secondary I89.0
  surgical NEC I97.89
    postmastectomy (syndrome) I97.2
Lymphoblastic — *see* condition
Lymphoblastoma (diffuse) (M9685/3) — *see* Lymphoma, non-Hodgkin's type, diffuse, lymphoblastic
  giant follicular (M9685/3) — *see* Lymphoma, non-Hodgkin's type, diffuse, lymphoblastic
  macrofollicular (M9685/3) — *see* Lymphoma, non-Hodgkin's type, diffuse, lymphoblastic
Lymphocele I89.8
Lymphocytic
  chorioencephalitis (acute) (serous) A87.2
  choriomeningitis (acute) (serous) A87.2
  meningoencephalitis A87.2
Lymphocytoma, benign cutis L98.8
Lymphocytosis (symptomatic) D72.8
  infectious (acute) B33.8
Lymphoepithelioma (M8082/3) — *see* Neoplasm, malignant
Lymphogranuloma (malignant) (M9650/3) — *see also* Hodgkin's, disease
  chlamydial A55
  inguinale A55
  venereum (any site) (chlamydial) (with stricture of rectum) A55
Lymphogranulomatosis (malignant) (M9650/3) — *see also* Hodgkin's, disease
  benign (Boeck's sarcoid) (Schaumann's) D86.1
Lymphohistiocytosis, hemophagocytic D76.1
Lymphoid — *see* condition
Lymphoma (malignant) (M9590/3) C85.90
  adult T-cell (M9827/3) C91.50
    in remission C91.51
  angiocentric T-cell (M9713/3) — *see* Lymphoma, non-Hodgkin's type, specified type NEC
  angioimmunoblastic (M9705/3) — *see* Lymphoma, non-Hodgkin's type, T-cell, peripheral
  B-cell NEC (M9590/3) — *see* Lymphoma, non-Hodgkin's type, B-cell unspecified
    monocytoid (M9711/3) — *see* Lymphoma, non-Hodgkin's type, specified type NEC
  B-precursor NEC (M9590/3) — *see* Lymphoma, non-Hodgkin's type, B-cell unspecified
  Burkitt's (small noncleaved, diffuse) (undifferentiated) (M9687/3) — *see* Lymphoma, non-Hodgkin's type, diffuse, Burkitt's
  centroblastic (diffuse) (M9683/3)– *see* Lymphoma, non-Hodgkin's type, diffuse, large cell
    follicular (M9697/3) — *see* Lymphoma, non-Hodgkin's type, follicular, specified type NEC
  centroblastic-centrocytic (diffuse) (M9676/3) — *see* Lymphoma, non-Hodgkin's type, diffuse, mixed small and large cell
    follicular (M9692/3) — *see* Lymphoma, non-Hodgkin's type, follicular, mixed small cleaved cell and large cell
  centrocytic (M9674/3) — *see* Lymphoma, non-Hodgkin's type, diffuse, small cell, cleaved

Lymphoma — *continued*
   cleaved cell (diffuse) (M9672/3) — *see*
      Lymphoma, non-Hodgkin's type, diffuse,
      small cell, cleaved
     with
       large cell, follicular (M9691/3) — *see*
         Lymphoma, non-Hodgkin's type,
         follicular, mixed small cleaved cell
         and large cell
       noncleaved, large cell (M9680/3) — *see*
         Lymphoma, non-Hodgkin's type,
         diffuse, large cell
   follicular (M9695/3) — *see* Lymphoma, non-
      Hodgkin's type, follicular, small
      cleaved cell
   large (diffuse) (M9681/3) — *see* Lymphoma,
      non-Hodgkin's type, diffuse, large cell
     follicular (M9698/3) — *see* Lymphoma,
      non-Hodgkin's type, follicular, large
      cell
   small (diffuse) (M9672/3) — *see* Lymphoma,
      non-Hodgkin's type, diffuse, small cell,
      cleaved
   convoluted cell (M9685/3) — *see* Lymphoma,
      non-Hodgkin's type, diffuse,
      lymphoblastic
   cutaneous (M9709/3) — *see* Lymphoma, non-
      Hodgkin's type, T-cell
   diffuse (M9595/3) — *see* Lymphoma, non-
      Hodgkin's type, diffuse
   histiocytic (M9680/3) — *see* Lymphoma,
      non-Hodgkin's type, diffuse, large cell
   large cell (M9680/3) — *see* Lymphoma, non-
      Hodgkin's type, diffuse, large cell
     noncleaved (M9682/3) — *see* Lymphoma,
      non-Hodgkin's type, diffuse, large
      cell
   lymphocytic (well differentiated) (M9670/3)
      — *see* Lymphoma, non-Hodgkin's type,
      diffuse, small cell
     intermediate differentiation (M9673/3) —
      see Lymphoma, non-Hodgkin's
      type, diffuse, small cell
     poorly differentiated (M9672/3) — *see*
      Lymphoma, non-Hodgkin's type,
      diffuse, small cell, cleaved
   mixed cell type (M9675/3) — *see*
      Lymphoma, non-Hodgkin's type,
      diffuse, mixed small and large cell
   lymphocytic-histiocytic (M9675/3) — *see*
      Lymphoma, non-Hodgkin's type,
      diffuse, mixed small and large cell
   small and large cell (M9675/3) — *see*
      Lymphoma, non-Hodgkin's type,
      diffuse, mixed small and large cell
   noncleaved (large cell) (M9682/3) — *see*
      Lymphoma, non-Hodgkin's type,
      diffuse, large cell
     small cell (M9686/3) — *see* Lymphoma,
      non-Hodgkin's type, diffuse,
      undifferentiated
   reticulum cell sarcoma (M9593/3) — *see*
      Lymphoma, non-Hodgkin's type,
      diffuse, large cell
   small cell (lymphocytic) (M9670/3) — *see*
      Lymphoma, non-Hodgkin's type,
      diffuse, small cell
     cleaved (M9672/3) — *see* Lymphoma,
      non-Hodgkin's type, diffuse, small
      cell, cleaved
     noncleaved, Burkitt's (M9687/3) — *see*
      Lymphoma, non-Hodgkin's type,
      diffuse, Burkitt's
   follicular (nodular) (with or without diffuse
      areas) (M9690/3) — *see* Lymphoma, non-
      Hodgkin's type, follicular
   centroblastic (M9697/3) — *see* Lymphoma,
      non-Hodgkin's type, follicular,
      specified type NEC
   centrocytic (M9692/3) — *see* Lymphoma,
      non-Hodgkin's type, follicular,
      mixed small cleaved cell and large
      cell
   histiocytic (M9698/3) — *see* Lymphoma,
      non-Hodgkin's type, follicular, large
      cell

Lymphoma — *continued*
   follicular — *continued*
     large cell (cleaved) (noncleaved) (M9698/3)
      — *see* Lymphoma, non-Hodgkin's type,
      follicular, large cell
     mixed cell type (M9691/3) — *see*
      Lymphoma, non-Hodgkin's type,
      follicular, mixed small cleaved cell and
      large cell
     noncleaved (large cell) (M9698/3) — *see*
      Lymphoma, non-Hodgkin's type,
      follicular, large cell
     small cleaved cell (M9695/3) — *see*
      Lymphoma, non-Hodgkin's type,
      follicular, small cleaved cell
      and large cell (M9691/3) — *see*
        Lymphoma, non-Hodgkin's type,
        follicular, mixed small cleaved cell
        and large cell
   histiocytic (M9698/3) — *see* Lymphoma, non-
      Hodgkin's type, follicular, large cell
    true (M9723/3) C96.3
   Hodgkin's (M9650/3) — *see* Hodgkin's, disease
   immunoblastic (large type) (diffuse) (M9684/3)
      — *see* Lymphoma, non-Hodgkin's type,
      diffuse, immunoblastic
   large cell (diffuse) (M9680/3) — *see* Lymphoma,
      non-Hodgkin's type, diffuse, large cell
     with
      small cell, mixed diffuse (M9675/3) — *see*
        Lymphoma, non-Hodgkin's type,
        diffuse, mixed small and large cell
      small cleaved, mixed, follicular (M9691/3)
        — *see* Lymphoma, non-Hodgkin's
        type, follicular, mixed small cleaved
        cell and large cell
     Ki-1+ (M9714/3) — *see* Lymphoma, non-
      Hodgkin's type, specified type NEC
     noncleaved and cleaved (M9680/3) — *see*
      Lymphoma, non-Hodgkin's type,
      diffuse, large cell
   Lennert's (M9704/3) — *see* Lymphoma, non-
      Hodgkin's type, lymphoepithelioid
   leukemia, adult T-cell (M9827/3) C91.50
     in remission C91.51
   lymphoblastic (diffuse) (M9685/3) — *see*
      Lymphoma, non-Hodgkin's type, diffuse,
      lymphoblastic
   lymphocytic (diffuse) (small) (M9670/3) — *see*
      Lymphoma, non-Hodgkin's type, diffuse,
      small cell
     nodular (M9690/3) — *see* Lymphoma, non-
      Hodgkin's type, follicular, small
      cleaved cell
     intermediate differentiation (M9694/3) —
      see Lymphoma, non-Hodgkin's
      type, follicular, small cleaved cell
     poorly differentiated (M9696/3) — *see*
      Lymphoma, non-Hodgkin's type,
      follicular, small cleaved cell
     well differentiated (M9693/3) — *see*
      Lymphoma, non-Hodgkin's type,
      follicular, small cleaved cell
   lymphoepithelioid (M9704/3) — *see*
      Lymphoma, non-Hodgkin's type,
      lymphoepithelioid
   lymphoplasmacytoid (M9671/3) — *see*
      Lymphoma, non-Hodgkin's type, diffuse,
      small cell
   lymphoplasmatic (M9671/3) — *see* Lymphoma,
      non-Hodgkin's type, diffuse, small cell
   mantle zone (M9673/3) — *see* Lymphoma, non-
      Hodgkin's type, diffuse, small cell
   Mediterranean (M9764/3) C88.3
   mixed cell type
     diffuse (M9675/3) — *see* Lymphoma, non-
      Hodgkin's type, diffuse, mixed small
      and large cell
     follicular (M9691/3) — *see* Lymphoma, non-
      Hodgkin's type, follicular, mixed small
      cleaved cell and large cell

Lymphoma — *continued*
   mixed cell type — *continued*
     lymphocytic-histiocytic (diffuse) (M9675/3)
      — *see* Lymphoma, non-Hodgkin's type,
      diffuse, mixed small and large cell
     nodular (M9691/3) — *see* Lymphoma,
      non-Hodgkin's type, follicular,
      mixed small cleaved cell and large
      cell
     small and large cell (diffuse) (M9675/3) —
      see Lymphoma, non-Hodgkin's type,
      diffuse, mixed small and large cell
     small cleaved and large cell, follicular
      (M9691/3) — *see* Lymphoma, non-
      Hodgkin's type, follicular, mixed small
      cleaved cell and large cell
   monocytoid B-cell (M9711/3) — *see*
      Lymphoma, non-Hodgkin's type, specified
      type NEC
   nodular (with or without diffuse areas)
      (M9690/3) — *see* Lymphoma, non-
      Hodgkin's type, follicular
     histiocytic (M9698/3) — *see* Lymphoma,
      non-Hodgkin's type, follicular, large
      cell
     lymphocytic (M9690/3) — *see* Lymphoma,
      non-Hodgkin's type, follicular, small
      cleaved cell
      intermediate differentiation (M9693/3) —
        see Lymphoma, non-Hodgkin's
        type, follicular, small cleaved cell
      poorly differentiated (M9696/3) — *see*
        Lymphoma, non-Hodgkin's type,
        follicular, small cleaved cell
      well differentiated (M9693/3) — *see*
        Lymphoma, non-Hodgkin's type,
        follicular, small cleaved cell
     mixed (cell type) (M9691/3) — *see*
      Lymphoma, non-Hodgkin's type,
      follicular, mixed small cleaved cell and
      large cell
     mixed lymphocytic-histiocytic (M9691/3) —
      see Lymphoma, non-Hodgkin's type,
      follicular, mixed small cleaved cell and
      large cell
   non-Burkitt's, undifferentiated cell (M9686/3)
      — *see* Lymphoma, non-Hodgkin's type,
      diffuse, undifferentiated
   noncleaved (diffuse) (M9682/3) — *see*
      Lymphoma, non-Hodgkin's type, diffuse,
      large cell
     follicular (M9698/3) — *see* Lymphoma, non-
      Hodgkin's type, follicular, large cell
     large cell (diffuse) (M9682/3) — *see*
      Lymphoma, non-Hodgkin's type,
      diffuse, large cell
     follicular (M9698/3) — *see* Lymphoma,
      non-Hodgkin's type, follicular, large
      cell
     small cell (diffuse) (M9686/3) — *see*
      Lymphoma, non-Hodgkin's type,
      diffuse, undifferentiated
   non-Hodgkin's type (M9591/3) C85.90
     axilla nodes C85.94
     B-cell unspecified C85.10
      axilla nodes C85.14
      extranodal site C85.19
      head, face and neck nodes C85.11
      inguinal nodes C85.15
      intra-abdominal nodes C85.13
      intrapelvic nodes C85.16
      intrathoracic nodes C85.12
      lower limb nodes C85.15
      multiple sites C85.18
      spleen C85.17
      upper limb nodes C85.14
     diffuse C83.90
      axilla nodes C83.94
      Burkitt's C83.70
       axilla nodes C83.74
       extranodal site C83.79
       head, face and neck nodes C83.71
       inguinal nodes C83.75
       intra-abdominal nodes C83.73
       intrapelvic nodes C83.76
       intrathoracic nodes C83.72
       lower limb nodes C83.75

Lymphoma — *continued*
  non-Hodgkin's type — *continued*
    diffuse — *continued*
      Burkitt's — *continued*
        multiple sites C83.78
        spleen C83.77
        upper limb nodes C83.74
      extranodal site C83.99
      head, face and neck nodes C83.91
      immunoblastic C83.40
        axilla nodes C83.44
        extranodal site C83.49
        head, face and neck nodes C83.41
        inguinal nodes C83.45
        intra-abdominal nodes C83.43
        intrapelvic nodes C83.46
        intrathoracic nodes C83.42
        lower limb nodes C83.45
        multiple sites C83.48
        spleen C83.47
        upper limb nodes C83.44
      inguinal nodes C83.95
      intra-abdominal nodes C83.93
      intrapelvic nodes C83.96
      intrathoracic nodes C83.92
      large cell C83.30
        axilla nodes C83.34
        extranodal site C83.39
        head, face and neck nodes C83.31
        inguinal nodes C83.35
        intra-abdominal nodes C83.33
        intrapelvic nodes C83.36
        intrathoracic nodes C83.32
        lower limb nodes C83.35
        multiple sites C83.38
        spleen C83.37
        upper limb nodes C83.34
      lower limb nodes C83.95
      lymphoblastic C83.50
        axilla nodes C83.54
        extranodal site C83.59
        head, face and neck nodes C83.51
        inguinal nodes C83.55
        intra-abdominal nodes C83.53
        intrapelvic nodes C83.56
        intrathoracic nodes C83.52
        lower limb nodes C83.55
        multiple sites C83.58
        spleen C83.57
        upper limb nodes C83.54
      mixed small and large cell C83.20
        axilla nodes C83.24
        extranodal site C83.29
        head, face and neck nodes C83.21
        inguinal nodes C83.25
        intra-abdominal nodes C83.23
        intrapelvic nodes C83.26
        intrathoracic nodes C83.22
        lower limb nodes C83.25
        multiple sites C83.28
        spleen C83.27
        upper limb nodes C83.24
      multiple sites C83.98
      small cell C83.00
        axilla nodes C83.04
        cleaved C83.10
          axilla nodes C83.14
          extranodal site C83.19
          head, face and neck nodes C83.11
          inguinal nodes C83.15
          intra-abdominal nodes C83.13
          intrapelvic nodes C83.16
          intrathoracic nodes C83.12
          lower limb nodes C83.15
          multiple sites C83.18
          spleen C83.17
          upper limb nodes C83.14
        extranodal site C83.09
        head, face and neck nodes C83.01
        inguinal nodes C83.05
        intra-abdominal nodes C83.03
        intrapelvic nodes C83.06

Lymphoma — *continued*
  non-Hodgkin's type — *continued*
    diffuse — *continued*
      small cell — *continued*
        intrathoracic nodes C83.02
        lower limb nodes C83.05
        multiple sites C83.08
        spleen C83.07
        upper limb nodes C83.04
      specified type NEC C83.80
        axilla nodes C83.84
        extranodal site C83.89
        head, face and neck nodes C83.81
        inguinal nodes C83.85
        intra-abdominal nodes C83.83
        intrapelvic nodes C83.86
        intrathoracic nodes C83.82
        lower limb nodes C83.85
        multiple sites C83.88
        spleen C83.87
        upper limb nodes C83.84
      spleen C83.97
      undifferentiated C83.60
        axilla nodes C83.64
        extranodal site C83.69
        head, face and neck nodes C83.61
        inguinal nodes C83.65
        intra-abdominal nodes C83.63
        intrapelvic nodes C83.66
        intrathoracic nodes C83.62
        lower limb nodes C83.65
        multiple sites C83.68
        spleen C83.67
        upper limb nodes C83.64
      upper limb nodes C83.94
    extranodal site C85.99
    follicular C82.90
      axilla nodes C82.94
      extranodal site C82.99
      head, face and neck nodes C82.91
      inguinal nodes C82.95
      intra-abdominal nodes C82.93
      intrapelvic nodes C82.96
      intrathoracic nodes C82.92
      large cell C82.20
        axilla nodes C82.24
        extranodal site C82.29
        head, face and neck nodes C82.21
        inguinal nodes C82.25
        intra-abdominal nodes C82.23
        intrapelvic nodes C82.26
        intrathoracic nodes C82.22
        lower limb nodes C82.25
        multiple sites C82.28
        spleen C82.27
        upper limb nodes C82.24
      lower limb nodes C82.95
      mixed small cleaved cell and large cell C82.10
        axilla nodes C82.14
        extranodal site C82.19
        head, face and neck nodes C82.11
        inguinal nodes C82.15
        intra-abdominal nodes C82.13
        intrapelvic nodes C82.16
        intrathoracic nodes C82.12
        lower limb nodes C82.15
        multiple sites C82.18
        spleen C82.17
        upper limb nodes C82.14
      multiple sites C82.98
      small cleaved cell C82.00
        axilla nodes C82.04
        extranodal site C82.09
        head, face and neck nodes C82.01
        inguinal nodes C82.05
        intra-abdominal nodes C82.03
        intrapelvic nodes C82.06
        intrathoracic nodes C82.02
        lower limb nodes C82.05
        multiple sites C82.08
        spleen C82.07
        upper limb nodes C82.04
      specified type NEC C82.70
        axilla nodes C82.74
        extranodal site C82.79

Lymphoma — *continued*
  non-Hodgkin's type — *continued*
    follicular — *continued*
      specified type NEC — *continued*
        head, face and neck nodes C82.71
        inguinal nodes C82.75
        intra-abdominal nodes C82.73
        intrapelvic nodes C82.76
        intrathoracic nodes C82.72
        lower limb nodes C82.75
        multiple sites C82.78
        spleen C82.77
        upper limb nodes C82.74
      spleen C82.97
      upper limb nodes C85.94
    head, face and neck nodes C85.91
    inguinal nodes C85.95
    intra-abdominal nodes C85.93
    intrapelvic nodes C85.96
    intrathoracic nodes C85.92
    lower limb nodes C85.95
    lymphoepithelioid C84.30
      axilla nodes C84.34
      extranodal site C84.39
      head, face and neck nodes C84.31
      inguinal nodes C84.35
      intra-abdominal nodes C84.33
      intrapelvic nodes C84.36
      intrathoracic nodes C84.32
      lower limb nodes C84.35
      multiple sites C84.38
      spleen C84.37
      upper limb nodes C84.34
    lymphosarcoma C85.00
      axilla nodes C85.04
      extranodal site C85.09
      head, face and neck nodes C85.01
      inguinal nodes C85.05
      intra-abdominal nodes C85.03
      intrapelvic nodes C85.06
      intrathoracic nodes C85.02
      lower limb nodes C85.05
      multiple sites C85.08
      spleen C85.07
      upper limb nodes C85.04
    multiple sites C85.98
    mycosis fungoides C84.00
      axilla nodes C84.04
      extranodal site C84.09
      head, face and neck nodes C84.01
      inguinal nodes C84.05
      intra-abdominal nodes C84.03
      intrapelvic nodes C84.06
      intrathoracic nodes C84.02
      lower limb nodes C84.05
      multiple sites C84.08
      spleen C84.07
      upper limb nodes C84.04
    Sèzary's disease C84.10
      axilla nodes C84.14
      extranodal site C84.19
      head, face and neck nodes C84.11
      inguinal nodes C84.15
      intra-abdominal nodes C84.13
      intrapelvic nodes C84.16
      intrathoracic nodes C84.12
      lower limb nodes C84.15
      multiple sites C84.18
      spleen C84.17
      upper limb nodes C84.14
    specified type NEC C85.70
      axilla nodes C85.74
      extranodal site C85.79
      head, face and neck nodes C85.71
      inguinal nodes C85.75
      intra-abdominal nodes C85.73
      intrapelvic nodes C85.76
      intrathoracic nodes C85.72
      lower limb nodes C85.75
      multiple sites C85.78
      spleen C85.77
      upper limb nodes C85.74
    spleen C85.97
    T-cell C84.50
      axilla nodes C84.54
      extranodal site C84.59

Lymphoma — *continued*
  non-Hodgkin's type — *continued*
    T-cell — *continued*
      head, face and neck nodes C84.51
      inguinal nodes C84.55
      intra-abdominal nodes C84.53
      intrapelvic nodes C84.56
      intrathoracic nodes C84.52
      lower limb nodes C84.55
      multiple sites C84.58
      peripheral C84.40
        axilla nodes C84.44
        extranodal site C84.49
        head, face and neck nodes C84.41
        inguinal nodes C84.45
        intra-abdominal nodes C84.43
        intrapelvic nodes C84.46
        intrathoracic nodes C84.42
        lower limb nodes C84.45
        multiple sites C84.48
        spleen C84.47
        upper limb nodes C84.44
      spleen C84.57
      upper limb nodes C84.54
      T-zone C84.20
        axilla nodes C84.24
        extranodal site C84.29
        head, face and neck nodes C84.21
        inguinal nodes C84.25
        intra-abdominal nodes C84.23
        intrapelvic nodes C84.26
        intrathoracic nodes C84.22
        lower limb nodes C84.25
        multiple sites C84.28
        spleen C84.27
        upper limb nodes C84.24
      upper limb nodes C85.94
    peripheral T-cell (M9702/3) — *see* Lymphoma, non-Hodgkin's type, T-cell, peripheral
    AILD (M9705/3) — *see* Lymphoma, non-Hodgkin's type, T-cell, peripheral
    angioimmunoblastic lymphadenopathy with dysproteinemia (M9705/3) — *see* Lymphoma, non-Hodgkin's type, T-cell, peripheral
    pleomorphic
      medium and large cell (M9707/3) — *see* Lymphoma, non-Hodgkin's type, T-cell, peripheral
      small cell (M9706/3) — *see* Lymphoma, non-Hodgkin's type, T-cell, peripheral
    plasmacytic (M9671/3) — *see* Lymphoma, non-Hodgkin's type, diffuse, small cell
    plasmacytoid (M9671/3) — *see* Lymphoma, non-Hodgkin's type, diffuse, small cell
    small cell (diffuse) (M9670/3) — *see* Lymphoma, non-Hodgkin's type, diffuse, small cell
      with large cell, mixed (diffuse) (M9675/3) — *see* Lymphoma, non-Hodgkin's type, diffuse, mixed small and large cell
      cleaved (diffuse) (M9672/3) — *see* Lymphoma, non-Hodgkin's type, diffuse, small cell, cleaved
      and large cell, mixed, follicular (M9691/3) — *see* Lymphoma, non-Hodgkin's type, follicular, mixed small cleaved cell and large cell
      follicular (M9695/3) — *see* Lymphoma, non-Hodgkin's type, follicular, small cleaved cell
    lymphocytic (diffuse) (M9670/3) — *see* Lymphoma, non-Hodgkin's type, diffuse, small cell
    noncleaved (diffuse) (M9686/3) — *see* Lymphoma, non-Hodgkin's type, diffuse, undifferentiated
      Burkitt's (M9687/3) — *see* Lymphoma, non-Hodgkin's type, diffuse, Burkitt's
    T-cell NEC (M9590/3) — *see* Lymphoma, non-Hodgkin's type, T-cell
  adult (M9827/3) C91.50
    in remission C91.51

Lymphoma — *continued*
  T-cell NEC — *see* Lymphoma, non-Hodgkin's type, T-cell — *continued*
    angiocentric (M9713/3) — *see* Lymphoma, non-Hodgkin's type, specified type NEC
    peripheral (M9702/3) — *see* Lymphoma, non-Hodgkin's type, T-cell, peripheral
    AILD (M9705/3) — *see* Lymphoma, non-Hodgkin's type, T-cell, peripheral
    angioimmunoblastic lymphadenopathy with dysproteinemia (M9705/3) — *see* Lymphoma, non-Hodgkin's type, T-cell, peripheral
    pleomorphic
      medium and large cell (M9707/3) — *see* Lymphoma, non-Hodgkin's type, T-cell, peripheral
      small cell (M9706/3) — *see* Lymphoma, non-Hodgkin's type, T-cell, peripheral
    true histiocytic (M9723/3) C96.3
    T-zone (M9703/3) — *see* Lymphoma, non-Hodgkin's type, T-zone
    undifferentiated cell (M9686/3) — *see* Lymphoma, non-Hodgkin's type, diffuse, undifferentiated
      Burkitt's type (M9687/3) — *see* Lymphoma, non-Hodgkin's type, diffuse, Burkitt's
      non-Burkitt's (M9686/3) — *see* Lymphoma, non-Hodgkin's type, diffuse, undifferentiated

Lymphomatosis (M9590/3) — *see* Lymphoma
Lymphopathia venereum, veneris A55
Lymphopenia D72.8
Lymphoproliferation, X-linked disease D82.3
Lymphoreticulosis, benign (of inoculation) A28.1
Lymphorrhea I89.8
Lymphosarcoma (diffuse) (M9592/3) — *see* Lymphoma, non-Hodgkin's type, lymphosarcoma
  cell leukemia (M9850/3) C94.70
    in remission C94.71
  diffuse (M9610/3) — *see* Lymphoma, non-Hodgkin's type, diffuse, lymphoblastic
    with plasmacytoid differentiation (M9611/3) — *see* Lymphoma, non-Hodgkin's type
    lymphoplasmacytic (M9611/3) — *see* Lymphoma, non-Hodgkin's type
  follicular (giant) (M9690/3) — *see* Lymphoma, non-Hodgkin's type, follicular
    lymphoblastic (M9696/3) — *see* Lymphoma, non-Hodgkin's type, follicular
    lymphocytic, intermediate differentiation (M9694/3) — *see* Lymphoma, non-Hodgkin's type, follicular
    mixed cell type (M9691/3) — *see* Lymphoma, non-Hodgkin's type, follicular
  giant follicular (M9690/3) — *see* Lymphoma, non-Hodgkin's type, follicular
  Hodgkin's (M9650/3) — *see* Hodgkin's, disease
  immunoblastic (M9612/3) — *see* Lymphoma, non-Hodgkin's type
  lymphoblastic (diffuse) (M9630/3) — *see* Lymphoma, non-Hodgkin's type, diffuse, lymphoblastic
    follicular (M9696/3) — *see* Lymphoma, non-Hodgkin's type, follicular
    nodular (M9696/3) — *see* Lymphoma, non-Hodgkin's type, follicular
  lymphocytic (diffuse) (M9620/3) — *see* Lymphoma, non-Hodgkin's type, diffuse, lymphoblastic
    intermediate differentiation (diffuse) (M9621/3) — *see* Lymphoma, non-Hodgkin's type, diffuse, lymphoblastic
    follicular (M9694/3) — *see* Lymphoma, non-Hodgkin's type, follicular
    nodular (M9694/3) — *see* Lymphoma, non-Hodgkin's type, follicular
  mixed cell type (diffuse) (M9613/3) — *see* Lymphoma, non-Hodgkin's type
    follicular (M9691/3) — *see* Lymphoma, non-Hodgkin's type, follicular

Lymphosarcoma — *see* Lymphoma, non-Hodgkin's type, lymphosarcoma — *continued*
  mixed cell type — *see* Lymphoma, non-Hodgkin's type — *continued*
    nodular (M9691/3) — *see* Lymphoma, non-Hodgkin's type, follicular
  nodular (M9690/3) — *see* Lymphoma, non-Hodgkin's type, follicular
    lymphoblastic (M9696/3) — *see* Lymphoma, non-Hodgkin's type, follicular
    lymphocytic, intermediate differentiation (M9694/3) — *see* Lymphoma, non-Hodgkin's type, follicular
    mixed cell type (M9691/3) — *see* Lymphoma, non-Hodgkin's type, follicular
  prolymphocytic (M9631/3) — *see* Lymphoma, non-Hodgkin's type, diffuse, lymphoblastic
  reticulum cell (M9640/3) — *see* Lymphoma, non-Hodgkin's type, diffuse, mixed small and large cell
Lymphostasis I89.8
Lypemania — *see* Melancholia
Lysine and hydroxylysine metabolism disorder E72.3
Lyssa — *see* Rabies

M

Macacus ear Q17.3
Maceration, wet feet, tropical (syndrome)
  left T69.04
  right T69.03
MacLeod's syndrome J43.0
Macrocephalia, macrocephaly Q75.3
Macrocheilia, macrochilia (congenital) Q18.6
Macrocolon (see also Megacolon) Q43.1
Macrocornea Q15.8
  with glaucoma Q15.0
Macrocytic — *see* condition
Macrocytosis D75.8
Macrodactylia, macrodactylism (fingers) (thumbs) Q74.0
  toes Q74.2
Macrodontia K00.2
Macrogenia M26.05
Macrogenitosomia (adrenal) (male) (praecox) E25.9
  congenital E25.0
Macroglobulinemia (idiopathic) (primary) C88.0
  Waldenström's (M9761/3) C88.0
Macroglossia (congenital) Q38.2
  acquired K14.8
Macrognathia, macrognathism (congenital) (mandibular) (maxillary) M26.09
Macrogyria (congenital) Q04.8
Macrohydrocephalus — *see* Hydrocephalus
Macromastia — *see* Hypertrophy, breast
Macrophthalmos Q11.3
  in congenital glaucoma Q15.0
Macropsia H53.18
Macrosigmoid K59.3
  congenital Q43.2
Macrospondylitis, acromegalic E22.0
Macrostomia (congenital) Q18.4
Macrotia (external ear) (congenital) Q17.1
Macula
  cornea, corneal — *see* Opacity, cornea
  degeneration (atrophic) (exudative) (senile) — *see also* Degeneration, macula
  hereditary — *see* Dystrophy, retina
  Maculae ceruleae -B85.1
Maculopathy, toxic — *see* Degeneration, macula, toxic
Madarosis (eyelid) H02.729
  left H02.726
    lower H02.725
    upper H02.724
  right H02.723
    lower H02.722

©2002 Ingenix, Inc.

Madarosis — *continued*
  right — *continued*
    upper H02.721
Madelung's
  deformity (radius) Q74.0
  disease
    radial deformity Q74.0
    symmetrical lipomas, neck E88.8
Madness — *see* Psychosis
Madura
  foot B47.9
    actinomycotic B47.1
    mycotic B47.0
Maduromycosis B47.0
Maffucci's syndrome Q78.4
Magnesium metabolism disorder — *see*
  Disorder, metabolism, magnesium
Main en griffe (acquired) — *see also* Deformity,
  limb, clawhand
  congenital Q74.0
Maintenance
  chemotherapy NEC Z51.81
    neoplasm Z51.1
  radiotherapy Z51.0
Majocchi's
  disease L81.7
  granuloma B35.8
Major — *see* condition
Malabar itch (any site) B35.5
Malabsorption K90.9
  calcium K90.89
  carbohydrate K90.4
  disaccharide E73.9
  fat K90.4
  galactose E74.20
  glucose(-galactose) E74.39
  intestinal K90.9
    specified NEC K90.89
  isomaltose E74.31
  lactose E73.9
  methionine E72.19
  monosaccharide E74.39
  postgastrectomy K91.2
  postsurgical K91.2
  protein K90.4
  starch K90.4
  sucrose E74.39
  syndrome K90.9
    postsurgical K91.2
Malacia, bone (adult) M83.9
  juvenile — *see* Rickets
Malacoplakia
  bladder N32.8
  pelvis (kidney) N28.89
  ureter N28.89
  urethra N36.8
Malacosteon, juvenile — *see* Rickets
Maladaptation — *see* Maladjustment
Maladie de Roger Q21.0
Maladjustment
  conjugal Z63.0
    involving divorce or estrangement Z63.5
  educational Z55.4
  family Z63.9
  marital Z63.0
    involving divorce or estrangement Z63.5
  occupational NEC Z56.89
  simple, adult — *see* Disorder, adjustment
  situational — *see* Disorder, adjustment
  social Z60.9
    due to
      acculturation difficulty Z60.3
      discrimination and persecution
        (perceived) Z60.5
      exclusion and isolation Z60.4
      life-cycle (phase of life) transition Z60.0
      rejection Z60.4
      specified reason NEC Z60.8
Malaise R53.81
Malakoplakia — *see* Malacoplakia

Malaria, malarial (fever) B54
  with
    blackwater fever B50.8
      hemoglobinuric (bilious) B50.8
      hemoglobinuria B50.8
  accidentally induced (therapeutically) – code by
    type under Malaria
  algid B50.9
  cerebral B50.0 *[G94]*
  clinically diagnosed (without parasitological
    confirmation) B54
  complicating pregnancy, childbirth or
    puerperium — *see* Disease, protozoal,
    obstetric
  congenital NEC P37.4
    falciparum P37.3
  congestion, congestive B54
  continued (fever) B50.9
  estivo-autumnal B50.9
  falciparum B50.9
    with complications NEC B50.8
      cerebral B50.0 *[G94]*
      severe B50.8
  hemorrhagic B54
  malariae B52.9
    with
      complications NEC B52.8
      glomerular disorder B52.0
  malignant (tertian) — *see* Malaria, falciparum
  mixed infections – code to first listed type in
    B50-B53
  ovale B53.0
  parasitologically confirmed NEC B53.8
  pernicious, acute — *see* Malaria, falciparum
  Plasmodium (P.)
    falciparum NEC — *see* Malaria, falciparum
    malariae NEC B52.9
      with Plasmodium
        falciparum (and or vivax) — *see*
          Malaria, falciparum
        vivax — *see also* Malaria, vivax
          and falciparum — *see* Malaria,
            falciparum
    ovale B53.0
      with Plasmodium malariae — *see also*
        Malaria, malariae
      and vivax — *see also* Malaria, vivax
        and falciparum — *see* Malaria,
          falciparum
    simian B53.1
      with Plasmodium malariae — *see also*
        Malaria, malariae
      and vivax — *see also* Malaria, vivax
        and falciparum — *see* Malaria,
          falciparum
    vivax NEC B51.9
      with Plasmodium falciparum — *see*
        Malaria, falciparum
  quartan — *see* Malaria, malariae
  quotidian — *see* Malaria, falciparum
  recurrent B54
  remittent B54
  specified type NEC (parasitologically confirmed)
    B53.8
  spleen B54
  subtertian (fever) — *see* Malaria, falciparum
  tertian (benign) — *see also* Malaria, vivax
    malignant B50.9
  tropical B50.9
  typhoid B54
  vivax B51.9
    with
      complications NEC B51.8
      ruptured spleen B51.0
Malassimilation K90.9
Malassez's disease (cystic) N50.8
Mal de los pintos — *see* Pinta
Mal de mer T75.3
Maldescent, testis Q53.9
  bilateral Q53.20
    abdominal Q53.21
    perineal Q53.22
  unilateral Q53.10
    abdominal Q53.11
    perineal Q53.12

Maldevelopment — *see also* Anomaly
  brain Q07.9
  colon Q43.9
  hip Q74.2
    congenital dislocation Q65.2
      bilateral Q65.1
      unilateral Q65.00
        left Q65.02
        right Q65.01
  mastoid process Q75.8
  middle ear Q16.4
    except ossicles Q16.4
    ossicles Q16.3
  ossicles Q16.3
  spine Q76.49
  toe Q74.2
Male type pelvis Q74.2
  with disproportion (fetopelvic) O33.3
    causing obstructed labor O65.3
Malformation (congenital) — *see also* Anomaly
  adrenal gland Q89.1
  affecting multiple systems with skeletal
    changes NEC Q87.5
  alimentary tract Q45.9
    specified type NEC Q45.8
    upper Q40.9
      specified type NEC Q40.8
  aorta Q25.9
    atresia Q25.2
    coarctation (preductal) (postductal) Q25.1
    patent ductus arteriosus Q25.0
    specified type NEC Q25.4
    stenosis (supravalvular) Q25.3
  aortic valve Q23.9
    specified NEC Q23.8
  arteriovenous, aneurysmatic (congenital)
    Q27.30
    brain Q28.2
    cerebral Q28.2
    peripheral Q27.30
      digestive system Q27.33
      lower limb Q27.32
      other specified site Q27.39
      renal vessel Q27.34
      upper limb Q27.31
    precerebral vessels (nonruptured) Q28.0
  auricle
    ear (congenital) Q17.3
      acquired H61.119
        left H61.112
          with right H61.113
        right H61.111
          with left H61.113
  bile duct Q44.5
  bladder Q64.79
    aplasia Q64.5
    diverticulum Q64.6
    exstrophy — *see* Exstrophy, bladder
    neck obstruction Q64.31
  bone Q79.9
    face Q75.9
      specified type NEC Q75.8
    skull Q75.9
      specified type NEC Q75.8
  brain (multiple) Q04.9
    arteriovenous Q28.2
    specified type NEC Q04.8
  branchial cleft Q18.2
  breast Q83.9
    specified type NEC Q83.8
  broad ligament Q50.6
  bronchus Q32.8
  bursa Q79.9
  cardiac
    chambers Q20.9
      specified type NEC Q20.8
    septum Q21.9
      specified type NEC Q21.8
  cerebral Q04.9
    vessels Q28.3
  cervix uteri Q51.9
    specified type NEC Q51.8
  Chiari
    Type I G93.5
    Type II Q07.01
  choroid (congenital) Q14.3
    plexus Q07.8

Mallet finger (acquired) — *see* Deformity, finger, mallet finger
  congenital Q74.0
  sequelae of rickets E64.3
Malleus A24.0
Mal lie — *see* Presentation, fetal
Mallory's bodies R89.7
Mallory-Weiss syndrome K22.6
Malnutrition E46
  degree
    first E44.1
    mild E44.1
    moderate E44.0
    second E44.0
    severe (protein-energy) E43
      intermediate form E42
        with
          kwashiorkor (and marasmus) E42
          marasmus E41
    third E43
  following gastrointestinal surgery K91.2
  in
    childbirth O25.2
    pregnancy O25.10
      first trimester O25.11
      second trimester O25.12
      third trimester O25.13
    puerperium O25.3
  intrauterine or fetal P05.2
    light-for-dates — *see* Light for dates
    small-for-dates — *see* Small for dates
  lack of care, or neglect (child) (infant) T76.02
    confirmed T74.02
  malignant E40
  protein E46
    calorie
      mild E44.1
      moderate E44.0
      severe E43
        intermediate form E42
          with
            kwashiorkor (and marasmus) E42
            marasmus E41
    energy E46
      mild E44.1
      moderate E44.0
      severe E43
        intermediate form E42
          with
            kwashiorkor (and marasmus) E42
            marasmus E41
    severe (protein-energy) E43
      with
        kwashiorkor (and marasmus) E42
        marasmus E41
Malocclusion (teeth) M26.4
  due to
    abnormal swallowing M26.5
    accessory teeth (causing crowding) M26.3
    dentofacial abnormality NEC M26.8
    displaced or missing teeth M26.3
    impacted teeth M26.3
    mouth breathing M26.5
    supernumerary teeth M26.3
    thumb sucking M26.3
    tongue, lip or finger habits M26.5
    temporomandibular (joint) M26.69
Mal perforant — *see* Ulcer, lower limb
Malposition
  cervix — *see* Malposition, uterus
  congenital
    adrenal (gland) Q89.1
    alimentary tract Q45.8
      lower Q43.8
      upper Q40.8
    aorta Q25.4
    appendix Q43.8
    arterial trunk Q25.4
    artery (peripheral) Q27.8
      coronary Q24.5
      digestive system Q27.8
      lower limb Q27.8
      pulmonary Q25.7

Malposition — *continued*
  congenital — *continued*
    artery — *continued*
      specified site NEC Q27.8
      upper limb Q27.8
    auditory canal Q17.8
      causing impairment of hearing Q16.9
    auricle (ear) Q17.4
      causing impairment of hearing Q16.9
      cervical Q18.2
    biliary duct or passage Q44.5
    bladder (mucosa) — *see* Exstrophy, bladder
    brachial plexus Q07.8
    brain tissue Q04.8
    breast Q83.8
    bronchus Q32.8
    cecum Q43.8
    clavicle Q74.0
    colon Q43.8
    digestive organ or tract NEC Q45.8
      lower Q43.8
      upper Q40.8
    ear (auricle) (external) Q17.4
      ossicles Q16.3
    endocrine (gland) NEC Q89.2
    epiglottis Q31.8
    eustachian tube Q17.8
    eye Q15.8
    facial features Q18.8
    fallopian tube Q50.6
    finger(s) Q68.1
      supernumerary Q69.0
    foot Q66.9
    gallbladder Q44.1
    gastrointestinal tract Q45.8
    genitalia, genital organ(s) or tract
      female Q52.8
        external Q52.79
        internal NEC Q52.8
      male Q55.8
    glottis Q31.8
    hand Q68.1
    heart Q24.8
      dextrocardia Q24.0
        with complete transposition of viscera Q89.3
    hepatic duct Q44.5
    hip (joint) Q65.8
    intestine (large) (small) Q43.8
      with anomalous adhesions, fixation or malrotation Q43.3
    joint NEC Q68.8
    kidney Q63.2
    larynx Q31.8
    limb Q68.8
      lower Q68.8
      upper Q68.8
    liver Q44.7
    lung (lobe) Q33.8
    nail(s) Q84.6
    nerve Q07.8
    nervous system NEC Q07.8
    nose, nasal (septum) Q30.8
    organ or site not listed — *see* Anomaly, by site
    ovary Q50.39
    pancreas Q45.3
    parathyroid (gland) Q89.2
    patella Q74.1
    peripheral vascular system Q27.8
    pituitary (gland) Q89.2
    respiratory organ or system NEC Q34.8
    rib (cage) Q76.6
      supernumerary in cervical region Q76.5
    scapula Q74.0
    shoulder Q74.0
    spinal cord Q06.8
    spleen Q89.09
    sternum NEC Q76.7
    stomach Q40.2
    symphysis pubis Q74.2
    thymus (gland) Q89.2
    thyroid (gland) (tissue) Q89.2
      cartilage Q31.8
    toe(s) Q66.9
      supernumerary Q69.2
    tongue Q38.3

Malposition — *continued*
  congenital — *continued*
    trachea Q32.1
    ureter Q62.60
      deviation Q62.61
      displacement Q62.62
      ectopia Q62.63
      specified type NEC Q62.69
    uterus Q51.8
    vein(s) (peripheral) Q27.8
      great Q26.8
    vena cava (inferior) (superior) Q26.8
  device, implant or graft (*see also* Complications, by site and type, mechanical) T85.628
    arterial graft NEC — *see* Complication, cardiovascular device, mechanical, vascular
    breast (implant) T85.42
    catheter NEC T85.628
      cystostomy T83.020
      dialysis (renal) T82.42
        intraperitoneal T85.621
      infusion NEC T82.524
        spinal (epidural) (subdural) T85.620
      urinary (indwelling) T83.021
    electronic (electrode) (pulse generator) (stimulator)
      bone T84.320
      cardiac T82.129
        electrode T82.120
        pulse generator T82.121
        specified type NEC T82.128
      nervous system — *see* Complication, prosthetic device, mechanical, electronic nervous system stimulator
      urinary — *see* Complication, genitourinary, device, urinary, mechanical
    fixation, internal (orthopedic) NEC — *see* Complication, fixation device, mechanical
    gastrointestinal — *see* Complications, prosthetic device, mechanical, gastrointestinal device
    genital NEC T83.428
      intrauterine contraceptive device T83.32
      penile prosthesis T83.420
    heart NEC — *see* Complication, cardiovascular device, mechanical
    joint prosthesis — *see* Complication, joint prosthesis, mechanical
    ocular NEC — *see* Complications, prosthetic device, mechanical, ocular device
    orthopedic NEC — *see* Complication, orthopedic, device, mechanical
    specified NEC T85.628
    urinary NEC — *see also* Complication, genitourinary, device, urinary, mechanical
      graft T83.22
    vascular NEC — *see* Complication, cardiovascular device, mechanical
    ventricular intracranial shunt T85.02
  fetus NEC — *see also* Presentation, fetal
    causing obstructed labor O64.9
    in multiple gestation (of one fetus or more) O32.5
      causing obstructed labor O64.8
  gallbladder K82.8
  gastrointestinal tract, congenital Q45.8
  heart, congenital NEC Q24.8
  pelvic organs or tissues NEC
    in pregnancy or childbirth — *see* category O34.8
      causing obstructed labor O65.5
  placenta — *see* Placenta, previa
  stomach K31.89
    congenital Q40.2
  tooth, teeth (with impaction) M26.3
  uterus (acute) (acquired) (adherent) (asymptomatic) (postinfectional) (postpartal, old) N85.4
    anteflexion or anteversion N85.4
      congenital Q51.8

Malposition — *continued*
  uterus — *continued*
    anteflexion or anteversion — *continued*
      in pregnancy or childbirth — *see*
        Abnormal, uterus in pregnancy or
        childbirth
        causing obstructed labor O65.5
    flexion N85.4
      lateral — *see* Lateroversion, uterus
    in pregnancy or childbirth — *see* category
      O34.5
      causing obstructed labor O65.5
    inversion N85.5
    lateral (flexion) (version) — *see*
      Lateroversion, uterus
    retroflexion or retroversion — *see*
      Retroversion, uterus

Malposture R29.3

Malpresentation, fetus — *see* Presentation, fetal

Malrotation
  cecum Q43.3
  colon Q43.3
  intestine Q43.3
  kidney Q63.2

Maltreatment (suspected) (syndrome) (of)
  adult T76.91
    abandonment T76.01
      confirmed T74.01
    confirmed T74.91
    history of Z91.41
    neglect T76.01
      confirmed T74.01
    physical abuse T76.11
      confirmed T74.11
    psychological abuse T76.31
      confirmed T74.31
      history of Z91.49
    sexual abuse T76.21
      confirmed T74.21
  child T76.92
    abandonment T76.02
      confirmed T74.02
    confirmed T74.92
    history of Z61.819
    neglect T76.02
      confirmed T74.02
      history of Z61.812
    physical abuse T76.12
      confirmed T74.12
      history of Z61.810
    psychological abuse T76.32
      confirmed T74.32
      history of Z61.811
    sexual abuse T76.22
      confirmed T74.22
      history of Z61.810
  personal history of Z91.8

Malta fever — *see* Brucellosis

Maltworker's lung J67.4

Malunion, fracture — *see* Fracture, by site

Mammillitis N61
  puerperal, postpartum O91.02

Mammitis — *see* Mastitis

Mammogram (examination) Z12.39
  routine Z12.31

Mammoplasia N62

Management (of)
  bone conduction hearing device (implanted)
    Z45.320
  cardiac pacemaker NEC Z45.018
  cerebrospinal fluid drainage device Z45.41
  cochlear device (implanted) Z45.321
  contraceptive Z30.9
    specified NEC Z30.8
  implanted device Z45.9
    specified NEC Z45.8
  infusion pump Z45.1
  procreative Z31.9
    male factor infertility in female Z31.81
    specified NEC Z31.89
  prosthesis (external) (*see also* Fitting) Z44.9
    implanted Z45.9
      specified NEC Z45.8
  renal dialysis catheter Z45.2
  vascular access device Z45.2

Mangled — *see* specified injury by site

Mania (monopolar) — *see also* Disorder, mood, manic episode
  with psychotic symptoms F30.2
  without psychotic symptoms F30.10
    mild F30.11
    moderate F30.12
    severe F30.13
  Bell's F30.8
  chronic (recurrent) F31.89
  hysterical F44.89
  puerperal F30.8
  recurrent F31.89

Manic-depressive insanity, psychosis, or syndrome — *see* Disorder, bipolar

Mannosidosis E77.1

Mansonelliasis, mansonellosis B74.4

Manson's
  disease B65.1
  schistosomiasis B65.1

Manual — *see* condition

Maple-bark-stripper's lung (disease) J67.6

Maple-syrup-urine disease E71.0

Marable's syndrome (celiac artery compression) I77.4

Marasmus E41
  due to malnutrition E41
  intestinal E41
  nutritional E41
  senile R54
  tuberculous NEC — *see* Tuberculosis

Marble
  bones Q78.2
  skin R23.8

Marburg virus disease A98.3

March
  fracture — *see* Fracture, metatarsal
  hemoglobinuria D59.6

Marchesani (-Weill) syndrome Q87.0

Marchiafava (-Bignami) syndrome or disease G37.1

Marchiafava-Micheli syndrome D59.5

Marcus Gunn's syndrome Q07.8

Marfan's syndrome — *see* Syndrome, Marfan's

Marginal implantation, placenta — *see* Placenta, previa

Marie-Bamberger disease — *see* Osteoarthropathy, hypertrophic, specified NEC

Marie-Charcot-Tooth neuropathic muscular atrophy G60.0

Marie's
  cerebellar ataxia (late-onset) G11.2
  disease or syndrome (acromegaly) E22.0

Marie-Strümpell arthritis, disease or spondylitis — *see* Spondylitis, ankylosing

Marion's disease (bladder neck obstruction) N32.0

Marital conflict Z63.0

Mark
  port wine Q82.5
  raspberry Q82.5
  strawberry Q82.5
  stretch L90.6
  tattoo L81.8

Marker heterochromatin — *see* Extra, marker chromosomes

Maroteaux-Lamy syndrome (mild) (severe) E76.29

Marrow (bone)
  arrest D61.9
  poor function D75.8

Marseilles fever A77.1

Marsh fever — *see* Malaria

Marshall's (hidrotic) **ectodermal dysplasia** Q82.4

Marsh's disease (exophthalmic goiter) E05.00
  with storm E05.01

Masculinization (female) **with adrenal hyperplasia** E25.9
  congenital E25.0

Masculinovoblastoma (M8670/0) D27.9
  left D27.1
  right D27.0

Masochism (sexual) F65.51

Mason's lung J62.8

Mass
  abdominal R19.00
    epigastric R19.06
    generalized R19.07
    left lower quadrant R19.04
    left upper quadrant R19.02
    periumbilic R19.05
    right lower quadrant R19.03
    right upper quadrant R19.01
    specified site NEC R19.09
  breast N63
  chest R22.2
  cystic — *see* Cyst
  ear — *see* category H93.8
  head R22.0
  intra-abdominal (diffuse) (generalized) — *see* Mass, abdominal
  kidney N28.89
  liver R16.0
  localized (skin) R22.9
    chest R22.2
    head R22.0
    limb
      lower R22.40
        bilateral R22.43
        left R22.42
        right R22.41
      upper R22.30
        bilateral R22.33
        left R22.32
        right R22.31
    neck R22.1
    trunk R22.2
  lung R90.8
  malignant (M8000/3) — *see* Neoplasm, malignant
  neck R22.1
  pelvic (diffuse) (generalized) — *see* Mass, abdominal
  specified organ NEC — *see* Disease, by site
  splenic R16.1
  substernal thyroid — *see* Goiter
  superficial (localized) R22.9
  umbilical (diffuse) (generalized) R19.09

Massive — *see* condition

Mast cell
  disease, systemic tissue (M9741/3) C96.2
  leukemia (M9900/3) C94.30
    in remission C94.31
  sarcoma (M9740/3) C96.2
  tumor (M9740/1) D47.0
    malignant (M9740/3) C96.2

Mastalgia N64.4
  psychogenic F45.4

Masters-Allen syndrome N83.8

Mastitis (acute) (diffuse) (nonpuerperal) (subacute) N61
  chronic (cystic) — *see* Mastopathy, cystic
  cystic (Schimmelbusch's type) — *see* Mastopathy, cystic
  fibrocystic — *see* Mastopathy, cystic
  infective N61
    newborn P39.0
  interstitial, gestational or puerperal — *see* Mastitis, obstetric
  neonatal (noninfective) P83.4
    infective P39.0
  obstetric (interstitial) (nonpurulent)
    associated with
      lactation O91.23
      pregnancy O91.219
        first trimester O91.211
        second trimester O91.212
        third trimester O91.213
      puerperium O91.22
    purulent
      associated with
        lactation O91.13
        pregnancy O91.119
          first trimester O91.111
          second trimester O91.112

Mastitis — *continued*
  obstetric — *continued*
    purulent — *continued*
      associated with — *continued*
        pregnancy — *continued*
          third trimester O91.113
        puerperium O91.12
    periductal — *see* Ectasia, mammary duct
    phlegmonous — *see* Mastopathy, cystic
    plasma cell — *see* Ectasia, mammary duct
Mastocytoma (M9740/1) D47.0
  malignant (M9740/3) C96.2
Mastocytosis Q82.2
  malignant (M9741/3) C96.2
Mastodynia N64.4
  psychogenic F45.4
Mastoid — *see* condition
Mastoidalgia — *see* category H92.0
Mastoiditis (coalescent) (hemorrhagic)
  (suppurative) H70.90
  acute, subacute H70.009
    bilateral H70.003
    complicated NEC H70.099
      bilateral H70.093
      left H70.092
      right H70.091
    subperiosteal H70.019
      bilateral H70.013
      left H70.012
      right H70.011
    left H70.002
    right H70.001
  bilateral H70.93
  chronic (necrotic) (recurrent) H70.10
    bilateral H70.13
    left H70.12
    right H70.11
  in (due to)
    infectious disease NEC B99 [H75.00]
      bilateral B99 [H75.03]
      left B99 [H75.02]
      right B99 [H75.01]
    parasitic disease NEC B89 [H75.00]
      bilateral B89 [H75.03]
      left B89 [H75.02]
      right B89 [H75.01]
    tuberculosis A18.03
  left H70.92
  petrositis — *see* Petrositis
  postauricular fistula — *see* Fistula,
    postauricular
  right H70.91
  specified NEC H70.899
    bilateral H70.893
    left H70.892
    right H70.891
  tuberculous A18.03
Mastopathy, mastopathia N64.9
  chronica cystica — *see* Mastopathy, cystic
  cystic (chronic) (diffuse) (female) N60.10
    with epithelial proliferation N60.30
      left N60.32
      male N60.35
        left N60.34
        right N60.33
      right N60.31
    left N60.12
    male N60.15
      left N60.14
      right N60.13
    right N60.11
  diffuse cystic — *see* Mastopathy, cystic
  estrogenic, oestrogenica N64.8
  ovarian origin N64.8
Mastoplasia, mastoplastia N62
Masturbation (excessive) F98.8
Maternal
  care (for) (known) (suspected)
    abnormality (*see also* condition)
      cervix uteri NEC (polyp) (stenosis)
        (stricture) (surgery) (tumor) — *see*
        category O34.4
        incompetence O34.30
          affecting fetus P01.0
          first trimester O34.31

Maternal — *continued*
  care — *continued*
    abnormality (*see also* condition) — *continued*
      cervix uteri NEC — *see* category O34.4 —
        continued
        incompetence — *continued*
          second trimester O34.32
          third trimester O34.33
      gravid uterus NEC (incarceration)
        (prolapse) (retroversion) — *see*
        category O34.5
      pelvic organs O34.90
        first trimester O34.91
        second trimester O34.92
        specified NEC — *see* category O34.8
        third trimester O34.93
      vagina (septate) (stenosis) (stricture)
        (surgery) (tumor) — *see* category
        O34.6
      vulva and perineum (fibrosis) (surgery)
        (tumor) — *see* category O34.7
    breech presentation O32.1
      affecting fetus P01.7
    central nervous system malformation, fetus
      O35.0
    cervical
      cerclage — *see* Maternal, care for,
        cervical, incompetence
      incompetence O34.30
        affecting fetus P01.0
        first trimester O34.31
        second trimester O34.32
        third trimester O34.33
    chromosomal abnormality, fetus O35.1
    compound presentation O32.6
      affecting fetus P01.7
    congenital malformation, uterus — *see*
      category O34.0
    damage to fetus from
      alcohol O35.4
      drugs O35.5
      maternal
        alcohol addiction O35.4
        cytomegalovirus infection O35.3
        drug addiction O35.5
        listeriosis O35.8
        rubella O35.3
        toxoplasmosis O35.8
        viral disease O35.3
      medical procedure NEC O35.7
      radiation O35.6
    disproportion (fetopelvic), due to O33.9
      deformity of maternal pelvic bones O33.0
      fetal deformity NEC O33.7
      generally contracted maternal pelvis
        O33.1
      hydrocephalic fetus O33.6
      inlet contraction, maternal pelvis O33.2
      mixed maternal and fetal origin O33.4
      origin NEC O33.8
      outlet contraction, maternal pelvis O33.3
      unusually large fetus O33.5
    excessive fetal growth O36.60
      first trimester O36.61
      second trimester O36.62
      third trimester O36.63
    face, brow and chin presentation O32.3
      affecting fetus P01.7
    fetal
      abnormality O35.9
        specified NEC O35.8
      anencephaly O35.0
      damage O35.9
        specified NEC O35.8
      problem O36.90
        first trimester O36.91
        second trimester O36.92
        specified NEC O36.899
          first trimester O36.891
          second trimester O36.892
          third trimester O36.893
        third trimester O36.93
      spina bifida O35.0
    habitual aborter (during pregnancy) O26.20
      first trimester O26.21

Maternal — *continued*
  care — *continued*
    habitual aborter — *continued*
      second trimester O26.22
      third trimester O26.23
    hereditary disease, fetus O35.2
    high head at term (pregnancy) O32.4
    hydrops fetalis NEC (not due to
      isoimmunization) O36.20
      first trimester O36.21
      second trimester O36.22
      third trimester O36.23
    incompatibility — *see* Maternal, care,
      isoimmunization
    intrauterine death (late) O36.4
    isoimmunization (ABO) — *see also* category
      O36.1
      Rh (rhesus) (anti-D) O36.00
        first trimester O36.01
        second trimester O36.02
        third trimester O36.03
    malpresentation (fetus) O32.9
      affecting fetus P01.7
      specified NEC O32.8
    multiple gestation with malpresentation of
      one fetus or more O32.5
      affecting fetus P01.5
    placental insufficiency — *see also* category
      O36.5
      affecting fetus P02.29
    poor fetal growth — *see* category O36.5
    Shirodkar suture — *see* Maternal, care for,
      cervical, incompetence
    transverse and oblique lie O32.2
      affecting fetus P01.7
    tumor, corpus uteri — *see* category O34.1
    unstable lie O32.0
      affecting fetus P01.7
    uterine scar from previous surgery O34.29
      previous cesarean section O34.21
    viable fetus in abdominal pregnancy O36.70
      affecting fetus P01.4
      first trimester O36.71
      second trimester O36.72
      third trimester O36.73
  condition, affecting fetus or newborn P00.9
    abdominal pregnancy P01.4
    abnormal
      membranes P02.9
        chorioamnionitis P02.7
        specified NEC P02.8
      placenta (functional) (morphological)
        P02.20
        specified NEC P02.29
      uterine contractions P03.6
    abruptio placenta P02.1
    amnionitis P02.7
    anesthesia or analgesia P04.0
    antepartum hemorrhage P02.1
    breech
      delivery and extraction P03.0
      presentation P01.7
    cesarean delivery P03.4
    chorioamnionitis P02.7
    circulatory disease NEC P00.3
      hypertensive disorder P00.0
    compression cord P02.5
      due to prolapse P02.4
    death P01.6
    diabetes mellitus (conditions in E09-E13)
      P70.1
      manifesting diabetes in infant P70.2
    ectopic pregnancy P01.4
    face presentation P01.7
      at delivery P03.1
    forceps delivery P03.2
    hydramnios P01.3
    hypertensive disorder P00.0
    hypertonic labor P03.6
    incompetent cervix P01.0
    infectious disease P00.2
    influenza
      manifest influenza in the infant P35.8
    injury P00.5

Maternal — *continued*
  condition, affecting fetus or newborn —
    continued
    malaria P00.2
      manifest malaria NEC in infant or fetus
        P37.4
        falciparum P37.3
    malnutrition P00.4
    malpresentation P01.7
      during delivery P03.1
    medical procedure NEC P00.7
    membranitis P02.7
    multiple pregnancy P01.5
    noxious substance transmitted via breast
      milk or placenta P04.9
    nutritional disorder P00.4
    oligohydramnios P01.2
      due to premature rupture of membranes
        P01.1
    parasitic disease P00.2
    persistent occipitoposterior presentation
      P03.1
    placenta previa P02.0
    placental
      separation NEC P02.1
        placenta previa P02.0
      transfusion syndrome P02.3
    placentitis P02.7
    polyhydramnios P01.3
    precipitate delivery P03.5
    pre-existing condition NEC P00.8
    pregnancy complication P01.9
      specified NEC P01.8
    premature rupture of membranes P01.1
    prolapsed cord P02.4
    rapid second stage P03.5
    renal disease P00.1
    respiratory disease NEC P00.3
      infectious P00.2
    rubella (conditions in B06)
      manifest rubella in the infant or fetus
        P35.0
    surgical procedure P00.6
    syphilis (conditions in A50-A53)
      manifest syphilis in the infant or fetus —
        see Syphilis, congenital, early,
        symptomatic
    toxoplasmosis (conditions in B58)
      manifest toxoplasmosis (acute) (subacute)
        (chronic) in the infant or fetus
        P37.1
    transmission of chemical substance through
      the placenta P04.9
    transverse lie P01.7
      at delivery P03.1
    triplet pregnancy P01.5
    twin pregnancy P01.5
    tumor, vagina — *see* category O34.6
    umbilical cord complication P02.60
      compression P02.5
        due to prolapse P02.4
      specified NEC P02.69
    unstable lie P01.7
      at delivery P03.1
    urinary tract disease P00.1
    uterine inertia P03.6
    vasa previa P02.69
    ventouse delivery P03.3
Maternity — *see* Delivery
Matheiu's disease (leptospiral jaundice) A27.0
Mauclaire's disease or osteochondrosis — *see*
  Osteochondrosis, juvenile, hand, metacarpal
Maxcy's disease A75.2
Maxilla, maxillary — *see* condition
May (-Hegglin) anomaly or syndrome D72.0
McArdle (-Schmid) (-Pearson) disease (glycogen
  storage) E74.04
McCune-Albright syndrome Q78.1
McQuarrie's syndrome (idiopathic familial
  hypoglycemia) E16.2
Meadow's syndrome Q86.1
Measles (black) (hemorrhagic) (suppressed) B05.9
  with
    complications NEC B05.89
    encephalitis B05.0

Measles — *continued*
  with — *continued*
    intestinal complications B05.4
    keratitis (keratoconjunctivitis) B05.81
    meningitis B05.1
    otitis media B05.3
    pneumonia B05.2
  French — *see* Rubella
  German — *see* Rubella
  Liberty — *see* Rubella
  vaccination, prophylactic (against) Z23
Meatitis, urethral — *see* Urethritis
Meatus, meatal — *see* condition
Meat-wrappers' asthma J68.9
Meckel-Gruber syndrome Q61.9
Meckel's diverticulitis, diverticulum (displaced)
  (hypertrophic) Q43.0
Meconium
  ileus, fetus or newborn P75
  in liquor — *see* Distress, fetal
    complicating labor and delivery O68
  obstruction, fetus or newborn P76.0
    in mucoviscidosis E84.1
  passage of — *see* Distress, fetal
  peritonitis P78.0
  plug syndrome (newborn) NEC P76.0
Median — *see also* condition
  arcuate ligament syndrome I77.4
  bar (prostate) (vesical orifice) — *see*
    Hyperplasia, prostate
  rhomboid glossitis K14.2
Mediastinal shift R93.1
Mediastinitis (acute) (chronic) J98.5
  syphilitic A52.73
  tuberculous A15.8
Mediastinopericarditis — *see also* Pericarditis
  acute I30.9
  adhesive I31.0
  chronic I31.8
  rheumatic I09.2
Mediastinum, mediastinal — *see* condition
Medical services provided for — *see* Health,
  services provided because (of)
Medicine poisoning (by accident) (by overdose)
  (wrong substance given or taken in error)
  T50.901
  administered with intent to harm by
    another person T50.903
    self T50.902
  circumstances undetermined T50.904
  specified drug or substance — *see* Table of
    Drugs and Chemicals
Mediterranean
  disease or syndrome (hemipathic) D56.9
  fever A23.9
    familial E85
  kala-azar B55.0
  leishmaniasis B55.0
  tick fever A77.1
Medulla — *see* condition
Medullary cystic kidney Q61.5
Medullated fibers
  optic (nerve) Q14.8
  retina Q14.1
Medulloblastoma (M9470/3)
  desmoplastic (M9471/3) C71.6
  specified site — *see* Neoplasm, malignant
  unspecified site C71.6
Medulloepithelioma (M9501/3) — *see also*
  Neoplasm, malignant
  teratoid (M9502/3) — *see* Neoplasm, malignant
Medullomyoblastoma (M9472/3)
  specified site — *see* Neoplasm, malignant
  unspecified site C71.6
Meekeren-Ehlers-Danlos syndrome Q79.6
Megacolon (acquired) (functional) (not
  Hirschsprung's disease) (in) K59.3
  Chagas' disease B57.32
  congenital, congenitum (aganglionic) Q43.1
  Hirschsprung's (disease) Q43.1
  toxic K59.3

Megaesophagus (functional) K22.0
  congenital Q39.5
  in (due to) Chagas' disease B57.31
Megalencephaly Q04.5
Megalerythema (epidemic) B08.3
Megaloappendix Q43.8
Megalocephalus, megalocephaly NEC Q75.3
Megalocornea Q15.8
  with glaucoma Q15.0
Megalocytic anemia D53.9
Megalodactylia (fingers) (thumbs) (congenital)
  Q74.0
  toes Q74.2
Megaloduodenum Q43.8
Megaloesophagus (functional) K22.0
  congenital Q39.5
Megalogastria (acquired) K31.89
  congenital Q40.2
Megalophthalmos Q11.3
Megalopsia H53.18
Megalosplenia — *see* Splenomegaly
Megaloureter N28.82
  congenital Q62.2
Megarectum K62.8
Megasigmoid K59.3
  congenital Q43.2
Megaureter N28.82
  congenital Q62.2
Megavitamin-B6 syndrome E67.2
Megrim — *see* Migraine
Meibomian
  cyst, infected — *see* Hordeolum
  gland — *see* condition
  sty, stye — *see* Hordeolum
Meibomitis — *see* Hordeolum
Meige-Milroy disease (chronic hereditary edema)
  Q82.0
Meige's syndrome Q82.0
Melalgia, nutritional E53.8
Melancholia F32.9
  climacteric (single episode) F32.8
    recurrent episode F33.9
  hypochondriac F45.29
  intermittent (single episode) F32.8
    recurrent episode F33.9
  involutional (single episode) E32.8
    recurrent episode F33.9
  menopausal (single episode) F32.8
    recurrent episode F33.9
  puerperal F32.8
  reactive (emotional stress or trauma) F32.3
  recurrent F33.9
  senile F03
  stuporous (single episode) F32.8
    recurrent episode F33.9
Melanemia R79.89
Melanoameloblastoma (M9363/0) — *see*
  Neoplasm, bone, benign
Melanoblastoma (M8720/3) — *see* Melanoma
Melanocarcinoma (M8720/3) — *see* Melanoma
Melanocytoma, eyeball (M8726/0) D31.40
  left D31.42
  right D31.41
Melanoderma, melanodermia L81.4
Melanodontia, infantile K02.4
Melanodontoclasia K02.4
Melanoepithelioma (M8720/3) — *see* Melanoma
Melanoma (malignant) (M8720/3) C43.9
  acral lentiginous, malignant (M8744/3)
  amelanotic (M8730/3)
  balloon cell (M8722/3)
  benign (M8720/0) — *see* Nevus
  desmoplastic, malignant (M8745/3)
  epithelioid cell (M8771/3)
    with spindle cell, mixed (M8770/3)
  in
    giant pigmented nevus (M8761/3)
    Hutchinson's melanotic freckle (M8742/3)
    junctional nevus (M8740/3)
    precancerous melanosis (M8741/3)

Melanoma — *continued*
 in situ (M8720/2) D03.9
  abdominal wall D03.5
  ala nasi D03.39
  ankle D03.70
   left D03.72
   right D03.71
  anus, anal (margin) (skin) D03.5
  arm D03.60
   left D03.62
   right D03.61
  auditory canal D03.20
   left D03.22
   right D03.21
  auricle (ear) D03.20
   left D03.22
   right D03.21
  auricular canal (external) D03.20
   left D03.22
   right D03.21
  axilla, axillary fold D03.5
  back D03.5
  breast D03.5
  brow D03.39
  buttock D03.5
  canthus (eye) D03.10
   left D03.12
   right D03.11
  cheek (external) D03.39
  chest wall D03.5
  chin D03.39
  choroid D03.8
  conjunctiva D03.8
  ear (external) D03.20
   left D03.22
   right D03.21
  external meatus (ear) D03.20
   left D03.22
   right D03.21
  eye D03.8
  eyebrow D03.39
  eyelid (lower) (upper) D03.10
   left D03.12
   right D03.11
  face D03.30
   specified NEC D03.39
  female genital organ (external) NEC D03.8
  finger D03.60
   left D03.62
   right D03.61
  flank D03.5
  foot D03.70
   left D03.72
   right D03.71
  forearm D03.60
   left D03.62
   right D03.61
  forehead D03.39
  foreskin D03.8
  gluteal region D03.5
  groin D03.5
  hand D03.60
   left D03.62
   right D03.61
  heel D03.70
   left D03.72
   right D03.71
  helix D03.20
   left D03.22
   right D03.21
  hip D03.70
   left D03.72
   right D03.71
  interscapular region D03.5
  iris D03.8
  jaw D03.39
  knee D03.70
   left D03.72
   right D03.71
  labium (majus) (minus) D03.8
  lacrimal gland D03.8
  leg D03.70
   left D03.72
   right D03.71
  lip (lower) (upper) D03.0
  lower limb NEC D03.70
   left D03.72

Melanoma — *continued*
 in situ — *continued*
  lower limb NEC — *continued*
   right D03.71
  male genital organ (external) NEC D03.8
  nail D03.9
   finger D03.60
    left D03.62
    right D03.61
   toe D03.70
    left D03.72
    right D03.71
  neck D03.4
  nose (external) D03.39
  orbit D03.8
  penis D03.8
  perianal skin D03.5
  perineum D03.5
  pinna D03.20
   left D03.22
   right D03.21
  popliteal fossa or space D03.70
   left D03.72
   right D03.71
  prepuce D03.8
  pubes D03.5
  pudendum D03.8
  retina D03.8
  retrobulbar D03.8
  scalp D03.4
  scrotum D03.8
  shoulder D03.60
   left D03.62
   right D03.61
  specified site NEC D03.8
  submammary fold D03.5
  temple D03.39
  thigh D03.70
   left D03.72
   right D03.71
  toe D03.70
   left D03.72
   right D03.71
  trunk NEC D03.5
  umbilicus D03.5
  upper limb NEC D03.60
   left D03.62
   right D03.61
  vulva D03.8
 juvenile (M8770/0) — *see* Nevus
 malignant, of soft parts except skin (M9044/3)
   — *see* Neoplasm, connective tissue,
   malignant
 metastatic
  breast C79.81
  genital organ C79.82
  specified site NEC (M8720/6) C79.89
  unspecified site (M8720/6) C80
 neurotropic, malignant (M8745/3)
 nodular (M8721/3)
 regressing, malignant (M8723/3)
 skin C43.9
  abdominal wall C43.5
  ala nasi C43.39
  ankle C43.70
   left C43.72
   right C43.71
  anus, anal C21.0
   margin (skin) C43.5
  arm C43.60
   left C43.62
   right C43.61
  auditory canal (external) C43.20
   left C43.22
   right C43.21
  auricle (ear) C43.20
   left C43.22
   right C43.21
  auricular canal (external) C43.20
   left C43.22
   right C43.21
  axilla, axillary fold C43.5
  back C43.5
  breast (female) (male) C43.5
  brow C43.39
  buttock C43.5

Melanoma — *continued*
 skin — *continued*
  canthus (eye) C43.10
   left C43.12
   right C43.11
  cheek (external) C43.39
  chest wall C43.5
  chin C43.39
  choroid C69.30
   left C69.32
   right C69.31
  conjunctiva C69.00
   left C69.02
   right C69.01
  ear (external) C43.20
   left C43.22
   right C43.21
  elbow C43.60
   left C43.62
   right C43.61
  external meatus (ear) C43.20
   left C43.22
   right C43.21
  eye C69.90
   left C69.92
   right C69.91
  eyebrow C43.39
  eyelid (lower) (upper) C43.10
   left C43.12
   right C43.11
  face C43.30
   specified NEC C43.39
  female genital organ (external) NEC C51.9
  finger C43.60
   left C43.62
   right C43.61
  flank C43.5
  foot C43.70
   left C43.72
   right C43.71
  forearm C43.60
   left C43.62
   right C43.61
  forehead C43.39
  foreskin C60.0
  glabella C43.39
  gluteal region C43.5
  groin C43.5
  hand C43.60
   left C43.62
   right C43.61
  heel C43.70
   left C43.72
   right C43.71
  helix C43.20
   left C43.22
   right C43.21
  hip C43.70
   left C43.72
   right C43.71
  interscapular region C43.5
  iris C69.40
   left C69.42
   right C69.41
  jaw (external) C43.39
  knee C43.70
   left C43.72
   right C43.71
  labium C51.9
   majus C51.0
   minus C51.1
  lacrimal gland C69.50
   left C69.52
   right C69.51
  leg C43.70
   left C43.72
   right C43.71
  lip (lower) (upper) C43.0
  liver (primary) C22.9
  lower limb NEC C43.70
   left C43.72
   right C43.71
  male genital organ (external) NEC C63.9
  nail C43.9
   finger C43.60
    left C43.62

Melanoma — *continued*
 skin — *continued*
  nail — *continued*
   finger — *continued*
    right C43.61
   toe C43.70
    left C43.72
    right C43.71
  nasolabial groove C43.39
  nates C43.5
  neck C43.4
  nose (external) C43.39
  orbit C69.60
   left C69.62
   right C69.61
  palpebra C43.10
   left C43.12
   right C43.11
  penis C60.9
  perianal skin C43.5
  perineum C43.5
  pinna C43.20
   left C43.22
   right C43.21
  popliteal fossa or space C43.70
   left C43.72
   right C43.71
  prepuce C60.0
  pubes C43.5
  pudendum C51.9
  retina C69.20
   left C69.22
   right C69.21
  retrobulbar C69.60
   left C69.62
   right C69.61
  scalp C43.4
  scrotum C63.2
  shoulder C43.60
   left C43.62
   right C43.61
  skin NEC C43.9
  specified site NEC — *see* Neoplasm,
    malignant
  submammary fold C43.5
  temple C43.39
  thigh C43.70
   left C43.72
   right C43.71
  toe C43.70
   left C43.72
   right C43.71
  trunk NEC C43.5
  umbilicus C43.5
  upper limb NEC C43.60
   left C43.62
   right C43.61
  vulva C51.9
 spindle cell (M8772/3)
  with epithelioid, mixed (M8770/3)
  type A (M8773/3) C69.40
   left C69.42
   right C69.41
  type B (M8774/3) C69.40
   left C69.42
   right C69.41
 superficial spreading (M8743/3)
Melanosarcoma (M8720/3) — *see also* Melanoma
 epithelioid cell (M8771/3) — *see* Melanoma
Melanosis L81.4
 addisonian E27.1
  tuberculous A18.7
 adrenal E27.1
 colon K63.8
 conjunctiva — *see* Pigmentation, conjunctiva
  congenital Q13.89
 cornea (presenile) (senile) — *see also*
    Pigmentation, cornea
  congenital Q13.4
 eye NEC H57.8
  congenital Q15.8
 lenticularis progressiva Q82.1
 liver K76.8

Melanosis — *continued*
 precancerous (M8741/2) — *see also* Melanoma,
    in situ
  malignant melanoma in (M8741/3) — *see*
    Melanoma
 Riehl's L81.4
 sclera H15.89
  congenital Q13.89
 suprarenal E27.1
 tar L81.4
 toxic L81.4
Melanuria R82.91
MELAS syndrome E88.31
Melasma L81.1
 adrenal (gland) E27.1
 suprarenal (gland) E27.1
Melena K92.1
 with ulcer – code by site under Ulcer, with
    hemorrhage K27.4
 due to swallowed maternal blood P78.2
 newborn, neonatal P54.1
  due to swallowed maternal blood P78.2
Meleney's
 gangrene (cutaneous) — *see* Ulcer, skin
 ulcer (chronic undermining) — *see* Ulcer, skin
Melioidosis A24.4
 acute A24.1
 chronic A24.2
 fulminating A24.1
 pneumonia A24.1
 pulmonary (chronic) A24.2
  acute A24.1
  subacute A24.2
 septicemia A24.1
 specified NEC A24.3
 subacute A24.2
Melitensis, febris A23.0
Melkersson (-Rosenthal) syndrome G51.2
Mellitus, diabetes — *see* Diabetes
Melorheostosis (bone) — *see* Disorder, bone,
    density and structure, specified NEC
Meloschisis Q18.4
Melotia Q17.4
Membrana
 capsularis lentis posterior Q13.89
 epipapillaris Q14.2
Membranacea placenta — *see* Malformation,
    placenta, specified type NEC
Membranaceous uterus N85.8
Membrane(s), membranous — *see also* condition
 cyclitic — *see* Membrane, pupillary
 folds, congenital — *see* Web
 Jackson's Q43.3
 over face (causing asphyxia), fetus or newborn
    P28.9
 premature rupture — *see* Rupture,
    membranes, premature
 pupillary H21.40
  bilateral H21.43
  left H21.42
  persistent Q13.89
  right H21.41
 retained (with hemorrhage) (complicating
    delivery) O72.2
  without hemorrhage O73.1
 secondary cataract — *see* Cataract, secondary
 unruptured (causing asphyxia) — *see* Asphyxia,
    newborn
 vitreous — *see* Opacity, vitreous, membranes
    and strands
Membranitis — *see* Chorioamnionitis
Memory disturbance, lack or loss — *see also*
    Amnesia
 mild, following organic brain damage F06.8
Menadione deficiency E56.1
Menarche
 delayed E30.0
 precocious E30.1
Mendacity, pathologic F60.2
Mendelson's syndrome (due to anesthesia) J95.4
 in labor and delivery O74.0
 in pregnancy — *see* Complications, anesthesia,
    in, pregnancy, pulmonary

Mendelson's syndrome — *continued*
 obstetric O74.0
 postpartum, puerperal O89.01
Ménétrier's disease or syndrome K29.60
 with bleeding K29.61
Ménière's disease, syndrome or vertigo — *see*
    category H81.0
Meninges, meningeal — *see* condition
Meningioma (M9530/0) — *see also* Neoplasm,
    meninges, benign
 angioblastic (M9535/0) — *see* Neoplasm,
    meninges, benign
 angiomatous (M9534/0) — *see* Neoplasm,
    meninges, benign
 endotheliomatous (M9531/0) — *see* Neoplasm,
    meninges, benign
 fibroblastic (M9532/0) — *see* Neoplasm,
    meninges, benign
 fibrous (M9532/0) — *see* Neoplasm, meninges,
    benign
 hemangioblastic (M9535/0) — *see* Neoplasm,
    meninges, benign
 hemangiopericytic (M9536/0) — *see* Neoplasm,
    meninges, benign
 malignant (M9530/3) — *see* Neoplasm,
    meninges, malignant
 meningiothelial (M9531/0) — *see* Neoplasm,
    meninges, benign
 meningotheliomatous (M9531/0) — *see*
    Neoplasm, meninges, benign
 mixed (M9537/0) — *see* Neoplasm, meninges,
    benign
 multiple (M9530/1) — *see* Neoplasm,
    meninges, uncertain behavior
 papillary (M9538/1) — *see* Neoplasm,
    meninges, uncertain behavior
 psammomatous (M9533/0) — *see* Neoplasm,
    meninges, benign
 syncytial (M9531/0) — *see* Neoplasm,
    meninges, benign
 transitional (M9537/0) — *see* Neoplasm,
    meninges, benign
Meningiomatosis (diffuse) (M9530/1) — *see*
    Neoplasm, meninges, uncertain behavior
Meningism — *see* Meningismus
Meningismus (infectional) (pneumococcal) R29.1
 due to serum or vaccine R29.1
 influenzal J10.89
Meningitis (basal) (basic) (brain) (cerebral)
    (cervical) (congestive) (diffuse) (hemorrhagic)
    (infantile) (membranous) (metastatic)
    (nonspecific) (pontine) (progressive) (simple)
    (spinal) (subacute) (sympathetic) (toxic)
    G03.9
 abacterial G03.0
 actinomycotic A42.81
 adenoviral A87.1
 arbovirus A87.8
 aseptic (acute) G03.0
 bacterial G00.9
  Escherichia coli (E. coli) G00.8
  Friedländer (bacillus) G00.8
  gram-negative G00.9
  H. influenzae G00.0
  Klebsiella G00.8
  pneumococcal G00.1
  specified organism NEC G00.8
  staphylococcal G00.3
  streptococcal (acute) G00.2
 benign recurrent (Mollaret) G03.2
 candidal B37.5
 caseous (tuberculous) A17.0
 cerebrospinal A39.0
 chronic NEC G03.1
 clear cerebrospinal fluid NEC G03.0
 coxsackievirus A87.0
 cryptococcal B45.1
 diplococcal (gram positive) A39.0
 echovirus A87.0
 enteroviral A87.0
 eosinophilic B83.2
 epidemic NEC A39.0
 Escherichia coli (E. coli) G00.8
 fibrinopurulent G00.9
  specified organism NEC G00.8
 Friedländer (bacillus) G00.8

Meningitis — *continued*
- gonococcal A54.81
- gram-negative cocci G00.9
- gram-positive cocci G00.9
- Haemophilus (influenzae) G00.0
- H. influenzae G00.0
- in (due to)
  - adenovirus A87.1
  - African trypanosomiasis B56.9
  - anthrax A22.8
  - bacterial disease NEC A48.8 *[G01]*
  - Chagas' disease (chronic) B57.41
  - chickenpox B01.0
  - coccidioidomycosis B38.4
  - Diplococcus pneumoniae G00.1
  - enterovirus A87.0
  - herpes (simplex) virus B00.3
    - zoster B02.1
  - infectious mononucleosis B27.92
  - leptospirosis A27.81
  - Listeria monocytogenes A32.11
  - Lyme disease A69.21
  - measles B05.1
  - mumps (virus) B26.1
  - neurosyphilis (late) A52.13
  - parasitic disease NEC B89 *[G02]*
  - poliovirus A80.9 *[G02]*
  - preventive immunization, inoculation or vaccination G03.8
  - rubella B06.02
  - Salmonella infection A02.21
  - specified cause NEC G03.8
  - typhoid fever A01.01
  - varicella B01.0
  - viral disease NEC A87.8
  - whooping cough A37.90
  - zoster B02.1
- infectious G00.9
- influenzal (H. influenzae) G00.0
- Klebsiella G00.8
- leptospiral (aseptic) A27.81
- lymphocytic (acute) (benign) (serous) A87.2
- meningococcal A39.0
- Mima polymorpha G00.8
- Mollaret (benign recurrent) G03.2
- monilial B37.5
- mycotic NEC B49 *[G02]*
- Neisseria A39.0
- nonbacterial G03.0
- nonpyogenic NEC G03.0
- ossificans G96.1
- pneumococcal G00.1
- poliovirus A80.9 *[G02]*
- postmeasles B05.1
- purulent G00.9
  - specified organism NEC G00.8
- pyogenic G00.9
  - specified organism NEC G00.8
- Salmonella (arizonae) (Cholerae-Suis) (enteritidis) (typhimurium) A02.21
- septic G00.9
  - specified organism NEC G00.8
- serosa circumscripta NEC G03.0
- serous NEC G93.2
- specified organism NEC G00.8
- sporotrichosis B42.81
- staphylococcal G00.3
- sterile G03.9
- streptococcal (acute) G00.2
- suppurative G00.9
  - specified organism NEC G00.8
- syphilitic (late) (tertiary) A52.13
  - acute A51.41
  - congenital A50.41
  - secondary A51.41
- Torula histolytica (cryptococcal) B45.1
- traumatic (complication of injury) T79.8
- tuberculous A17.0
- typhoid A01.01
- viral NEC A87.9
- Yersinia pestis A20.3

Meningocele (spinal) — *see also* Spina bifida
- with hydrocephalus — *see* Spina bifida, by site, with hydrocephalus
- acquired (traumatic) G96.1
- cerebral — *see* Encephalocele

Meningocerebritis — *see* Meningoencephalitis

Meningococcemia A39.4
- acute A39.2
- chronic A39.3

Meningococcus, meningococcal (*see also* condition) A39.9
- adrenalitis, hemorrhagic A39.1
- carrier (suspected) of Z22.31
- meningitis (cerebrospinal) A39.0

Meningoencephalitis (*see also* Encephalitis) G04.9
- acute NEC (*see also* Encephalitis, viral) A86
- bacterial NEC G04.2
- California A83.5
- diphasic A84.1
- eosinophilic B83.2
- epidemic A39.81
- herpesviral, herpetic B00.4
- in (due to)
  - blastomycosis NEC B40.81
  - free-living amebae B60.2
  - Hemophilus influenzae (H .influenzae) G04.2
  - herpes B00.4
  - H. influenzae G00.0
  - Lyme disease A69.22
  - mercury — *see* category T56.1
  - mumps B26.2
  - Naegleria (amebae) (organisms) (fowleri) B60.2
  - Parastrongylus cantonensis B83.2
  - toxoplasmosis (acquired) B58.2
    - congenital P37.1
- infectious (acute) (viral) A86
- influenzal (H. influenzae) G04.2
- Listeria monocytogenes A32.12
- lymphocytic (serous) A87.2
- mumps B26.2
- parasitic NEC B71.9 *[G05]*
- pneumococcal G00.1
- primary amebic B60.2
- specific (syphilitic) A52.14
- specified organism NEC G04.8
- staphylococcal G04.2
- streptococcal G04.2
- syphilitic A52.14
- toxic NEC G92
  - due to mercury — *see* category T56.1
- tuberculous A17.82
- virus NEC A86

Meningoencephalocele — *see also* Encephalocele
- syphilitic A52.19
- congenital A50.49

Meningoencephalomyelitis — *see* Meningoencephalitis
- acute NEC (viral) A86
  - disseminated (postimmunization or postvaccination) (postinfectious) G04.0
- due to
  - actinomycosis A42.82
  - Torula B45.1
  - Toxoplasma or toxoplasmosis (acquired) B58.2
    - congenital P37.1
- postimmunization or postvaccination G04.0

Meningoencephalomyelopathy G96.9

Meningoencephalopathy G96.9

Meningomyelitis — *see also* Meningoencephalitis
- bacterial NEC G04.2
- blastomycotic NEC B40.81
- cryptococcal B45.1
- meningococcal A39.81
- syphilitic A52.14
- tuberculous A17.82

Meningomyelocele — *see also* Spina bifida
- fetal, causing obstructed labor (mother) O66.3
- syphilitic A52.19

Meningomyeloneuritis — *see* Meningoencephalitis

Meningoradiculitis — *see* Meningitis

Meningovascular — *see* condition

Menkes' disease or syndrome E83.09
- meaning maple-syrup-urine disease E71.0

Menometrorrhagia N92.1

Menopause, menopausal (symptoms) (syndrome) N95.1
- arthritis (any site) NEC — *see* Arthritis, specified form NEC
- artificial N95.3
- bleeding N92.4
- crisis N95.1
- depression (single episode) F32.8
  - agitated (single episode) F32.2
    - recurrent episode F33.9
  - psychotic (single episode) F32.8
    - recurrent episode F33.9
- melancholia (single episode) F32.8
  - recurrent episode F33.9
- paranoid state F22
- postsurgical N95.3
- premature E28.3
  - postirradiation E89.4
  - postsurgical E89.4
- psychoneurosis N95.1
- psychosis NEC F28
- surgical N95.3
- toxic polyarthritis NEC — *see* Arthritis, specified form NEC

Menorrhagia (primary) N92.0
- climacteric N92.4
  - menopausal N92.4
- menopausal N92.4
- postclimacteric N95.0
- postmenopausal N95.0
- preclimacteric or premenopausal N92.4
- pubertal (menses retained) N92.2

Menostaxis N92.0

Menses, retention N94.8

Menstrual — *see* Menstruation

Menstruation
- absent — *see* Amenorrhea
- anovulatory N97.0
- cycle, irregular N92.6
- delayed N91.0
- disorder N93.9
  - psychogenic F45.8
- during pregnancy O20.8
- excessive (with regular cycle) N92.0
  - with irregular cycle N92.1
  - at puberty N92.2
- frequent N92.0
- infrequent — *see* Oligomenorrhea
- irregular N92.6
  - specified NEC N92.5
- latent N92.5
- membranous N92.5
- painful (primary) (secondary) — *see* Dysmenorrhea
- passage of clots N92.0
- period, normal Z71.1
- precocious E30.1
- protracted N92.5
- rare — *see* Oligomenorrhea
- retained N94.8
- retrograde N92.5
- scanty — *see* Oligomenorrhea
- suppression N94.8
- vicarious (nasal) N94.8

Mental — *see also* condition
- deficiency — *see* Retardation, mental
- deterioration — *see* Psychosis
- disorder — *see* Disorder, mental
- exhaustion F48.8
- insufficiency (congenital) — *see* Retardation, mental
- observation without need for further medical care Z03.8
- retardation — *see* Retardation, mental
- subnormality — *see* Retardation, mental
- upset — *see* Disorder, mental

Meralgia paresthetica G57.10
- left G57.12
- right G57.11

Mercurial — *see* condition

Mercurialism — *see* category T56.1

MERFF syndrome E88.32

Merkel cell tumor (M8247/3) — *see* Neoplasm, skin, malignant

Merocele — *see* Hernia, femoral
Meromelia
  lower limb — *see* Defect, reduction, lower limb
    intercalary
      femur — *see* Defect, reduction, lower
        limb, specified type NEC
      tibiofibular (complete) (incomplete) —
        see Defect, reduction, lower limb
  upper limb — *see* Defect, reduction, upper limb
    intercalary, humeral, radioulnar — *see*
      Agenesis, arm, with hand present
Merzbacher-Pelizaeus disease E75.29
Mesaortitis — *see* Aortitis
Mesarteritis — *see* Arteritis
Mesencephalitis — *see* Encephalitis
Mesenchymoma (M8990/1) — *see also*
  Neoplasm, connective tissue, uncertain
  behavior
  benign (M8990/0) — *see* Neoplasm, connective
    tissue, benign
  malignant (M8990/3) — *see* Neoplasm,
    connective tissue, malignant
Mesentery, mesenteric — *see* condition
Mesiodens, mesiodentes K00.1
  causing crowding M26.3
Mesio-occlusion M26.2
Mesocolon — *see* condition
Mesonephroma (malignant) (M9110/3) — *see*
  Neoplasm, malignant
  benign (M9110/0) — *see* Neoplasm, benign
Mesophlebitis — *see* Phlebitis
Mesostromal dysgenesia Q13.89
Mesothelioma (malignant) (M9050/3) C45.9
  benign (M9050/0)
    mesentery D19.1
    mesocolon D19.1
    omentum D19.1
    peritoneum D19.1
    pleura D19.0
    specified site NEC D19.7
    unspecified site D19.9
  biphasic (M9053/3) C45.9
    benign (M9053/0)
      mesentery D19.1
      mesocolon D19.1
      omentum D19.1
      peritoneum D19.1
      pleura D19.0
      specified site NEC D19.7
      unspecified site D19.9
  cystic (M9055/1) D48.4
  epithelioid (M9052/3) C45.9
    benign (M9052/0)
      mesentery D19.1
      mesocolon D19.1
      omentum D19.1
      peritoneum D19.1
      pleura D19.0
      specified site NEC D19.7
      unspecified site D19.9
  fibrous (M9051/3) C45.9
    benign (M9051/0)
      mesentery D19.1
      mesocolon D19.1
      omentum D19.1
      peritoneum D19.1
      pleura D19.0
      specified site NEC D19.7
      unspecified site D19.9
  site classification
    liver C45.7
    lung C45.7
    mediastinum C45.7
    mesentery C45.1
    mesocolon C45.1
    omentum C45.1
    pericardium C45.2
    peritoneum C45.1
    pleura C45.0
      parietal C45.0
    retroperitoneum C45.7
    specified site NEC C45.7
    unspecified C45.9
Metagonimiasis B66.8

Metagonimus infestation (intestine) B66.8
Metal
  pigmentation L81.8
  polisher's disease J62.8
Metamorphopsia H53.18
Metaplasia
  apocrine (breast) — *see* Dysplasia, mammary,
    specified type NEC
  cervix (squamous) — *see* Dysplasia, cervix
  endometrium (squamous) (uterus) N85.8
  kidney (pelvis) (squamous) N28.89
  myelogenous D73.1
  myeloid (agnogenic) (megakaryocytic) D73.1
  spleen D73.1
  squamous cell, bladder N32.8
Metastasis, metastatic
  abscess — *see* Abscess
  calcification E83.59
  cancer, neoplasm or disease (M8000/6) C80
    from specified site (M8000/3) — *see*
      Neoplasm, malignant, by site
    to specified site (M8000/6) — *see* Neoplasm,
      secondary, by site
  deposits (in) (M8000/6) — *see* Neoplasm,
    secondary, by site
  pneumonia A41.89
  spread (to) (M8000/6) — *see* Neoplasm,
    secondary, by site
Metastrongyliasis B83.8
Metatarsalgia M77.40
  anterior G57.60
    left G57.62
    right G57.61
  left M77.42
  Morton's G57.60
    left G57.62
    right G57.61
  right M77.41
Metatarsus, metatarsal — *see also* condition
  valgus (adductus), congenital Q66.6
  varus (adductus) (congenital) Q66.2
Methemoglobinemia D74.9
  acquired (with sulfhemoglobinemia) D74.8
  congenital D74.0
  enzymatic (congenital) D74.0
  Hb M disease D74.0
  hereditary D74.0
  toxic D74.8
Methemoglobinuria — *see* Hemoglobinuria
Methioninemia E72.19
Methylmalonic acidemia E71.120
Metritis (catarrhal) (hemorrhagic) (septic)
  (suppurative) — *see also* Endometritis
  cervical — *see* Cervicitis
Metropathia hemorrhagica N93.8
Metroperitonitis — *see* Peritonitis, pelvic, female
Metrorrhagia N92.1
  climacteric N92.4
  menopausal N92.4
  postpartum NEC (atonic) (following delivery of
    placenta) O72.1
    delayed or secondary O72.2
  preclimacteric or premenopausal N92.4
  psychogenic F45.8
Metrorrhexis — *see* Rupture, uterus
Metrosalpingitis N70.91
Metrostaxis N93.8
Metrovaginitis — *see* Endometritis
Meyer-Schwickerath and Weyers syndrome
  Q87.0
Meynert's amentia (nonalcoholic) F04
  alcoholic F10.96
    with dependence F10.26
Mibelli's disease (porokeratosis) Q82.8
Mice, joint — *see* Loose, body, joint
  knee M23.40
    left M23.42
    right M23.41
Micrencephalon, micrencephaly Q02
Microaneurysm, retinal — *see also* Disorder,
  retina, microaneurysms
  diabetic — *see* E09-E13 with .31

Microangiopathy (peripheral) I73.9
  thrombotic M31.1
Microcephalus, microcephalic, microcephaly
  Q02
  due to toxoplasmosis (congenital) P37.1
Microcheilia Q18.7
Microcolon (congenital) Q43.8
Microcornea (congenital) Q13.4
Microcytic — *see* condition
Microdontia K00.2
Microdrepanocytosis D56.8
Microembolism, retinal — *see* Occlusion, artery,
  retina
Microencephalon Q02
Microfilaria streptocerca infestation B73.1
Microgastria (congenital) Q40.2
Microgenia M26.06
Microgenitalia, congenital
  female Q52.8
  male Q55.8
Microglioma (M9594/3) — *see* Lymphoma, non-
  Hodgkin's type, specified type NEC
Microglossia (congenital) Q38.3
Micrognathia, micrognathism (congenital)
  (mandibular) (maxillary) M26.09
Microgyria (congenital) Q04.3
Microinfarct of heart — *see* Insufficiency,
  coronary
Microlentia (congenital) Q12.8
Microlithiasis, alveolar, pulmonary J84.0
Micromyelia (congenital) Q06.8
Micropenis Q55.62
Microphakia (congenital) Q12.8
Microphthalmos, microphthalmia (congenital)
  Q11.2
  due to toxoplasmosis P37.1
Micropsia H53.18
Microsporidiosis B60.8
  intestinal A07.8
Microsporon furfur infestation B36.0
Microsporosis — *see also* Dermatophytosis
  nigra B36.1
Microstomia (congenital) Q18.5
Microtia (congenital) (external ear) Q17.2
Microtropia H50.40
Micturition
  disorder NEC R39.19
    psychogenic F45.8
  frequency R35.0
    psychogenic F45.8
  hesitancy R39.11
  incomplete emptying R39.14
  nocturnal R35.1
  painful R30.9
    dysuria R30.0
    psychogenic F45.8
    tenesmus R30.1
  poor stream R39.12
  split stream R39.13
  straining R39.16
  urgency R39.15
Mid plane — *see* condition
Middle
  ear — *see* condition
  lobe (right) syndrome J98.19
Miescher's elastoma L87.2
Mietens' syndrome Q87.2
Migraine (idiopathic) G43.9
  with aura (acute-onset) (prolonged) (typical)
    G43.10
    with status migrainosus G43.11
  without aura G43.00
    with status migrainosus G43.01
  abdominal (syndrome) G43.10
    with status migrainosus G43.11
  allergic (histamine) G43.8
  atypical G43.00
  basilar G43.10
    with status migrainosus G43.11

©2002 Ingenix, Inc.

Migraine — *continued*
classical G43.10
with status migrainosus G43.11
common G43.00
with status migrainosus G43.01
complicated G43.3
equivalent(s) G43.10
with status migrainosus G43.11
hemiplegic (familial) G43.10
with status migrainosus G43.11
menstrual N94.3
ophthalmic G43.8
ophthalmoplegic G43.8
retinal G43.8
specified NEC G43.8
variant G43.8
Migrant, social Z59.0
Migration, anxiety concerning Z60.3
Migratory, migrating — *see also* condition
person Z59.0
testis Q55.29
Mikity-Wilson disease or syndrome P27.0
Mikulicz' disease or syndrome K11.8
Miliaria L74.3
alba L74.1
apocrine L75.2
crystallina L74.1
profunda L74.2
rubra L74.0
tropicalis L74.2
Miliary — *see* condition
Milium L72.0
colloid L57.8
Milk
crust L21.0
excessive secretion O92.6
poisoning — *see* Poisoning, food, noxious
retention O92.7
sickness — *see* Poisoning, food, noxious
spots I31.0
Milk-alkali disease or syndrome E83.59
Milk-leg (deep vessels) (nonpuerperal) — *see also*
Phlebitis, leg, femoral vein
complicating pregnancy O22.30
first trimester O22.31
second trimester O22.32
third trimester O22.33
puerperal, postpartum, childbirth O87.1
Milkman's disease or syndrome M83.8
Milky urine — *see* Chyluria
Millard-Gubler (-Foville) paralysis or syndrome
G46.3
Millar's asthma J38.5
Miller-Fisher's syndrome G61.0
Mills' disease — *see* Hemiplegia
Millstone maker's pneumoconiosis J62.8
Milroy's disease (chronic hereditary edema)
Q82.0
Minamata disease T26.10
left T26.12
right T26.11
Minkowski-Chauffard syndrome — *see*
Spherocytosis
Miners' asthma or lung J60
Minkowski-Chauffard syndrome — *see*
Spherocytosis
Minor — *see* condition
Minor's disease (hematomyelia) G95.19
Minot's disease (hemorrhagic disease), newborn
P53
Minot-von Willebrand-Jurgens disease or
syndrome (angiohemophilia) D68.0
Minus (and plus) **hand** (intrinsic) —
Deformity, limb, specified type NEC, forearm
Miosis (pupil) H57.03
Mirizzi's syndrome (hepatic duct stenosis) K83.1
Mirror writing F81.0
Misadventure (prophylactic) (therapeutic) (*see*
also Complications) T88.9
administration of insulin (by accident) — *see*
category T38.3

Misadventure (*see also* Complications) —
continued
infusion — *see* Complications, infusion
local applications (of fomentations, plasters,
etc.) T88.9
burn or scald — *see* Burn
specified NEC T88.8
medical care (early) (late) T88.9
adverse effect of drugs or chemicals — *see*
Table of Drugs and Chemicals
burn or scald — *see* Burn
specified NEC T88.8
radiation NEC T66
radiotherapy NEC T66
specified NEC T88.8
surgical procedure (early) (late) — *see*
Complications, surgical procedure
transfusion — *see* Complications, transfusion
vaccination or other immunological procedure
— *see* Complications, vaccination
Miscarriage O03.9
Mismanagement of feeding R63.3
Misplaced, misplacement
ear Q17.4
kidney (acquired) N28.89
congenital Q63.2
organ or site, congenital NEC — *see*
Malposition, congenital
Missed
abortion O02.1
delivery O36.4
Missing — *see* Absence
Misuse of drugs F19.99
Mitchell's disease (erythromelalgia) I73.8
Mite(s) (infestation) B88.9
diarrhea B88.0
grain (itch) B88.0
hair follicle (itch) B88.0
in sputum B88.0
Mitral — *see* condition
Mittelschmerz N94.0
Mixed — *see* condition
Mobile, mobility
cecum Q43.3
excessive — *see* Hypermobility
gallbladder, congenital Q44.1
kidney N28.89
organ or site, congenital NEC — *see*
Malposition, congenital
Mobitz heart block (atrioventricular) I44.30
Moebius, Möbius
disease (ophthalmoplegic migraine) G43.8
syndrome Q87.0
congenital oculofacial paralysis (with other
anomalies) Q87.0
ophthalmoplegic migraine G43.8
Moeller's glossitis (vitamin B deficiency) E53.9
[K93]
Mohr's syndrome (Types I and II) Q87.0
Mola destruens (M9100/1) D39.2
Molar pregnancy O01.9
Molarization of premolars K00.2
Molding, head (during birth) P13.1
Mole (pigmented) (M8720/0) — *see also* Nevus
blood O02.0
Breus' O02.0
cancerous (M8720/3) — *see* Melanoma
carneous O02.0
destructive (M9100/1) D39.2
fleshy O02.0
hydatid, hydatidiform (benign) (complicating
pregnancy) (delivered) (undelivered) O01.9
classical O01.0
complete O01.0
incomplete O01.1
invasive (M9100/1) D39.2
malignant (M9100/1) D39.2
partial O01.1
previous, affecting management of
pregnancy O09.10
first trimester O09.11
second trimester O09.12

Mole — *see also* Nevus — *continued*
hydatid, hydatidiform — *continued*
previous, affecting management of
pregnancy — *continued*
third trimester O09.13
intrauterine O02.0
invasive (hydatidiform) (M9100/1) D39.2
malignant
meaning
malignant hydatidiform mole (M9100/1)
D39.2
melanoma (M8720/3) — *see* Melanoma
nonhydatidiform O02.0
nonpigmented (M8730/0) — *see* Nevus
pregnancy NEC O02.0
skin (M8720/0) — *see* Nevus
tubal O00.1
vesicular — *see* Mole, hydatidiform
Molimen, molimina (menstrual) N94.3
Molluscum contagiosum (epitheliale) B08.1
Mönckeberg's arteriosclerosis, disease, or
sclerosis — *see* Arteriosclerosis, extremities
Mondini's malformation (cochlea) Q16.5
Mondor's disease I80.8
Monge's disease T70.29
Monilethrix (congenital) Q84.1
Moniliasis — *see also* Candidiasis B37.9
neonatal P37.5
Monkey malaria B53.1
Monkeypox B04
Monoarthritis M13.10
ankle M13.179
left M13.172
right M13.171
elbow M13.129
left M13.122
right M13.121
foot joint M13.179
left M13.172
right M13.171
hand joint M13.149
left M13.142
right M13.141
hip M13.159
left M13.152
right M13.151
knee M13.169
left M13.162
right M13.161
shoulder M13.119
left M13.112
right M13.111
wrist M13.139
left M13.132
right M13.131
Monoblastic — *see* condition
Monochromat(ism), monochromatopsia
(acquired) (congenital) H53.51
Monocytic — *see* condition
Monocytosis (symptomatic) D72.8
Monomania — *see* Psychosis
Mononeuritis G58.9
cranial nerve — *see* Disorder, nerve, cranial
femoral nerve G57.20
left G57.22
right G57.21
lateral
cutaneous nerve of thigh G57.10
left G57.12
right G57.11
popliteal nerve G57.30
left G57.32
right G57.31
lower limb G57.90
left G57.92
right G57.91
specified nerve NEC G57.80
left G57.82
right G57.81
medial popliteal nerve G57.40
left G57.42
right G57.41
median nerve G56.10
left G56.12

Mononeuritis — *continued*
  median nerve — *continued*
    right G56.11
  multiplex G58.7
  plantar nerve G57.60
    left G57.62
    right G57.61
  posterior tibial nerve G57.50
    left G57.52
    right G57.51
  radial nerve G56.30
    left G56.32
    right G56.31
  sciatic nerve G57.00
    left G57.02
    right G57.01
  specified NEC G58.8
  tibial nerve G57.40
    left G57.42
    right G57.41
  ulnar nerve G56.20
    left G56.22
    right G56.21
  upper limb G56.90
    left G56.92
    right G56.91
    specified nerve NEC G56.80
      left G56.82
      right G56.81
  vestibular — *see* category H93.3
Mononeuropathy G58.9
  carpal tunnel syndrome — *see* Syndrome, carpal tunnel
  diabetic NEC — *see* E09-E13 with .41
  femoral nerve — *see* Lesion, nerve, femoral
  ilioinguinal nerve G57.80
    left G57.82
    right G57.81
  intercostal G58.0
  lower limb G57.90
    causalgia — *see* Causalgia, lower limb
    femoral nerve — *see* Lesion, nerve, femoral
    left G57.92
    meralgia paresthetica G57.10
      left G57.12
      right G57.11
    plantar nerve — *see* Lesion, nerve, plantar
    popliteal nerve — *see* Lesion, nerve, popliteal
    right G57.91
    sciatic nerve — *see* Lesion, nerve, sciatic
    specified NEC G57.80
      left G57.82
      right G57.81
    tarsal tunnel syndrome — *see* Syndrome, tarsal tunnel
  median nerve — *see* Lesion, nerve, median
  multiplex G58.7
  obturator nerve G57.80
    left G57.82
    right G57.81
  popliteal nerve — *see* Lesion, nerve, popliteal
  radial nerve — *see* Lesion, nerve, radial
  saphenous nerve G57.80
    left G57.82
    right G57.81
  specified NEC G58.8
  tarsal tunnel syndrome — *see* Syndrome, tarsal tunnel
  tuberculous A17.83
  ulnar nerve — *see* Lesion, nerve, ulnar
  upper limb G56.90
    carpal tunnel syndrome — *see* Syndrome, carpal tunnel
    causalgia — *see* Causalgia
    left G56.92
    median nerve — *see* Lesion, nerve, median
    radial nerve — *see* Lesion, nerve, radial
    right G56.91
    specified site NEC G56.80
      left G56.82
      right G56.81
    ulnar nerve — *see* Lesion, nerve, ulnar
Mononucleosis, infectious B27.90
  with
    complication NEC B27.99
    meningitis B27.92
    polyneuropathy B27.91

Mononucleosis, infectious — *continued*
  cytomegaloviral B27.10
    with
      complication NEC B27.19
      meningitis B27.12
      polyneuropathy B27.11
  Epstein-Barr (virus) B27.00
    with
      complication NEC B27.09
      meningitis B27.02
      polyneuropathy B27.01
  gammaherpesviral B27.00
    with
      complication NEC B27.09
      meningitis B27.02
      polyneuropathy B27.01
  specified NEC B27.80
    with
      complication NEC B27.89
      meningitis B27.82
      polyneuropathy B27.81

Monoplegia G83.30
  with involvement of
    dominant (right) side G83.31
      left G83.32
    left (nondominant) side G83.34
      dominant G83.32
    nondominant (left) side G83.34
      right G83.33
    right (dominant) side G83.31
      nondominant G83.33
  congenital or infantile (cerebral) (spinal) G80.8
  embolic (current episode) I63.4
  following
    cerebrovascular disease
      cerebral infarction
        lower limb I69.349
          dominant (right) I69.341
            left I69.342
          left (nondominant) I69.344
            dominant I69.342
          nondominant (left) I69.344
            right I69.343
          right (dominant) I69.341
            nondominant I69.343
        upper limb I69.339
          dominant (right) I69.331
            left I69.332
          left (nondominant) I69.334
            dominant I69.332
          nondominant (left) I69.334
            right I69.333
          right (dominant) I69.331
            nondominant I69.333
      intracerebral hemorrhage
        lower limb I69.149
          dominant (right) I69.141
            left I69.142
          left (nondominant) I69.144
            dominant I69.142
          nondominant (left) I69.144
            right I69.143
          right (dominant) I69.141
            nondominant I69.143
        upper limb I69.139
          dominant (right) I69.131
            left I69.132
          left (nondominant) I69.134
            dominant I69.132
          nondominant (left) I69.134
            right I69.133
          right (dominant) I69.131
            nondominant I69.133
      lower limb I69.949
        dominant (right) I69.941
          left I69.942
        left (nondominant) I69.944
          dominant I69.942
        nondominant (left) I69.944
          right I69.943
        right (dominant) I69.941
          nondominant I69.943

Monoplegia — *continued*
  following — *continued*
    cerebrovascular disease — *continued*
      nontraumatic intracranial hemorrhage NEC
        lower limb I69.249
          dominant (right) I69.241
            left I69.242
          left (nondominant) I69.244
            dominant I69.242
          nondominant (left) I69.244
            right I69.243
          right (dominant) I69.241
            nondominant I69.243
        upper limb I69.239
          dominant (right) I69.231
            left I69.232
          left (nondominant) I69.234
            dominant I69.232
          nondominant (left) I69.234
            right I69.233
          right (dominant) I69.231
            nondominant I69.233
    specified disease NEC
      lower limb I69.849
        dominant (right) I69.841
          left I69.842
        left (nondominant) I69.844
          dominant I69.842
        nondominant (left) I69.844
          right I69.843
        right (dominant) I69.841
          nondominant I69.843
      upper limb I69.839
        dominant (right) I69.831
          left I69.832
        left (nondominant) I69.834
          dominant I69.832
        nondominant (left) I69.834
          right I69.833
        right (dominant) I69.831
          nondominant I69.833
    stroke NOS
      lower limb I69.449
        dominant (right) I69.441
          left I69.442
        left (nondominant) I69.444
          dominant I69.442
        nondominant (left) I69.444
          right I69.443
        right (dominant) I69.441
          nondominant I69.443
      upper limb I69.439
        dominant (right) I69.431
          left I69.432
        left (nondominant) I69.434
          dominant I69.432
        nondominant (left) I69.434
          right I69.433
        right (dominant) I69.431
          nondominant I69.433
    subarachnoid hemorrhage
      lower limb I69.049
        dominant (right) I69.041
          left I69.042
        left (nondominant) I69.044
          dominant I69.042
        nondominant (left) I69.044
          right I69.043
        right (dominant) I69.041
          nondominant I69.043
      upper limb I69.039
        dominant (right) I69.031
          left I69.032
        left (nondominant) I69.034
          dominant I69.032
        nondominant (left) I69.034
          right I69.033
        right (dominant) I69.031
          nondominant I69.033
    upper limb I69.939
      dominant (right) I69.931
        left I69.932
      left (nondominant) I69.934
        dominant I69.932

Monoplegia — continued
  following — continued
    cerebrovascular disease — continued
      upper limb — continued
        nondominant (left) I69.934
        right I69.933
        right (dominant) I69.931
          nondominant I69.933
  hysterical (transient) F44.4
  infantile (cerebral) (spinal) G80.8
  lower limb G83.10
    with involvement of
      dominant (right) side G83.11
        left G83.12
      left (nondominant) side G83.14
        dominant G83.12
      nondominant (left) side G83.14
        right G83.13
      right (dominant) side G83.11
        nondominant G83.13
  psychogenic (conversion reaction) F44.4
  thrombotic (current episode) I63.3
  transient R29.81
  upper limb G83.20
    with involvement of
      dominant (right) side G83.21
        left G83.22
      left (nondominant) side G83.24
        dominant G83.22
      nondominant (left) side G83.24
        right G83.23
      right (dominant) side G83.21
        nondominant G83.23

Monorchism, monorchidism Q55.0
Monosomy — see also Deletion, chromosome
  Q93.9
  specified NEC Q93.8
  whole chromosome
    meiotic nondisjunction Q93.0
    mitotic nondisjunction Q93.1
    mosaicism Q93.1
  X Q96.9
Monster, monstrosity (single) Q89.7
  acephalic Q00.0
  twin Q89.4
Monteggia's fracture (-dislocation) S52.279
  left S52.272
  right S52.271
Mooren's ulcer (cornea) — see Ulcer, cornea,
  Mooren's
Moore's syndrome G40.80
  with status epilepticus G40.81
Mooser-Neill reaction A75.2
Mooser's bodies A75.2
Morbidity not stated or unknown R69
Morbilli — see Measles
Morbus (see also Disease)
  angelicus, anglorum E55.0
  Beigel B36.2
  caducus — see Epilepsy
  celiacus K90.0
  comitialis — see Epilepsy
  cordis — see also Disease, heart I51.9
    valvulorum — see Endocarditis
  coxae senilis M16.9
    tuberculous A18.02
  hemorrhagicus neonatorum P53
  maculosus neonatorum P54.5
  senilis — see Osteoarthrosis
Morel (-Stewart) (-Morgagni) syndrome M85.2
Morel-Kraepelin disease — see Schizophrenia
Morel-Moore syndrome M85.2
Morgagni's
  cyst, organ, hydatid, or appendage
    female Q52.8
    male Q55.4
  syndrome M85.2
Morgagni-Stokes-Adams syndrome I45.9
Morgagni-Stewart-Morel syndrome M85.2
Morgagni-Turner (-Albright) syndrome Q96.9
Moria F07.0
Moron (I.Q. 50-69) F70
Morphea L94.0

Morphinism (without remission) F11.20
  with remission F11.21
Morphinomania (without remission) F11.20
  with remission F11.21
Morquio (-Ullrich) (-Brailsford) disease or
  syndrome — see Mucopolysaccharidosis
Mortification (dry) (moist) — see Gangrene
Morton's metatarsalgia (neuralgia) (neuroma)
  (syndrome) G57.60
  left G57.62
  right G57.61
Morvan's disease or syndrome G60.8
Mosaicism, mosaic (autosomal) (chromosomal)
  45,X/other cell lines NEC with abnormal sex
    chromosome Q96.4
  45,X/46,XX Q96.3
  sex chromosome
    female Q97.8
    lines with various numbers of X
      chromosomes Q97.2
    male Q98.7
  XY Q96.3
Moschowitz' disease M31.1
Mother yaw A66.0
Motion sickness (from travel, any vehicle) (from
  roundabouts or swings) T75.3
Mottled, mottling, teeth (enamel) (endemic)
  (nonendemic) K00.3
Mounier-Kuhn syndrome J47.9
  with
    acute exacerbation J47.1
    lower respiratory infection J47.0
Mountain
  sickness T70.29
    with polycythemia , acquired (acute) D75.1
  tick fever A93.2
Mouse, joint — see Loose, body, joint
  knee M23.40
    left M23.42
    right M23.41
Mouth — see condition
Movable
  coccyx — see category M53.2
  kidney N28.89
    congenital Q63.8
  spleen D73.8
Movements, dystonic R25.8
Moyamoya disease I67.5
Mucha-Habermann disease L41.0
Mucinosis (cutaneous) (focal) (papular) (skin)
  L98.5
  oral K13.7
Mucocele
  appendix K38.8
  buccal cavity K13.7
  gallbladder K82.1
  lacrimal sac, chronic H04.439
    bilateral H04.433
    left H04.432
    right H04.431
  nasal sinus J34.1
  salivary gland (any) K11.6
  sinus (accessory) (nasal) J34.1
  turbinate (bone) (middle) (nasal) J34.1
  uterus N85.8
Mucolipidosis
  I E77.1
  II, III E77.0
  IV E75.11
Mucopolysaccharidosis E76.3
  ß-gluduronidase deficiency E76.29
  cardiopathy E76.3 [I52]
  Hunter's syndrome E76.1
  Hurler's syndrome E76.01
  Hurler-Scheie syndrome E76.02
  Maroteaux-Lamy syndrome E76.29
  Morquio syndrome E76.219
    A E76.210
    B E76.211
    classic E76.210
  Sanfilippo syndrome E76.22
  Scheie's syndrome E76.03
  specified NEC E76.29

Mucopolysaccharidosis — continued
  type
    I
      Hurler's syndrome E76.01
      Hurler-Scheie syndrome E76.02
      Scheie's syndrome E76.03
    II E76.1
    III E76.22
    IV E76.219
    IVA E76.210
    IVB E76.211
    VI E76.29
    VII E76.29
Mucormycosis B46.5
  cutaneous B46.3
  disseminated B46.4
  gastrointestinal B46.2
  generalized B46.4
  pulmonary B46.0
  rhinocerebral B46.1
  skin B46.3
  subcutaneous B46.3
Mucositis necroticans agranulocytica — see
  Agranulocytosis
Mucous — see also condition
  patches (syphilitic) A51.39
    congenital A50.07
Mucoviscidosis E84.9
  with meconium obstruction E84.1
Mucus
  asphyxia or suffocation — see Asphyxia, mucus
  in stool R19.5
  plug — see Asphyxia, mucus
Muguet B37.0
Mulberry molars (congenital syphilis) A50.52
Mullerian mixed tumor (M8950/3)
  specified site — see Neoplasm, malignant
  unspecified site C54.9
Multicystic kidney Q61.8
Multiparity (grand) Z64.1
  affecting management of pregnancy, labor and
    delivery (supervision only) O09.40
    first trimester O09.41
    second trimester O09.42
    third trimester O09.43
  requiring contraceptive management — see
    Contraception
Multipartita placenta — see Malformation,
  placenta, specified type NEC
Multiple, multiplex — see also condition
  digits (congenital) Q69.9
  personality F44.81
Mumps B26.9
  arthritis B26.85
  complication NEC B26.89
  encephalitis B26.2
  hepatitis B26.81
  meningitis (aseptic) B26.1
  meningoencephalitis B26.2
  myocarditis B26.82
  oophoritis B26.89
  orchitis B26.0
  pancreatitis B26.3
  polyneuropathy B26.84
Mumu (see also Infestation, filarial) B74.9 [N51]
Münchhausen's syndrome — see Disorder,
  factitious
Münchmeyer's syndrome — see Myositis,
  ossificans, progressiva
Mural — see condition
Murmur (cardiac) (heart) (organic) R01.1
  abdominal R19.15
  aortic (valve) — see Endocarditis, aortic
  benign R01.0
  diastolic — see Endocarditis
  Flint I35.1
  functional R01.0
  Graham Steell I37.1
  innocent R01.0
  mitral (valve) — see Insufficiency, mitral
  nonorganic R01.0
  presystolic, mitral — see Insufficiency, mitral
  pulmonic (valve) I37.8
  systolic (valvular) — see Endocarditis

Murmur — *continued*
  tricuspid (valve) I07.9
  valvular — *see* Endocarditis
Murri's disease (intermittent hemoglobinuria)
  D59.6
Muscle, muscular — *see also* condition
  carnitine (palmityltransferase) deficiency
    E71.328
Musculoneuralgia — *see* Neuralgia
Mushroom-workers' (pickers') **disease or lung**
  J67.5
Mushrooming hip — *see* Derangement, joint,
  specified NEC, hip
Mutation
  factor V Leiden D68.610
  prothrombin gene D68.611
Mutism — *see also* Aphasia
  deaf (acquired) (congenital) NEC H91.3
  elective (adjustment reaction) (childhood) F94.0
  hysterical F44.4
  selective (childhood) F94.0
Myalgia M79.1
  epidemic (cervical) B33.0
  psychogenic F45.4
  traumatic NEC T14.90
Myasthenia, myasthenic G70.9
  congenital G70.2
  cordis — *see* Failure, heart
  developmental G70.2
  gravis G70.0
    neonatal, transient P94.0
    pseudoparalytica G70.0
  stomach, psychogenic F45.8
  syndrome
    in
      botulism A05.1
      diabetes mellitus — *see* E09-E13 with .44
      malignant neoplasm NEC (M8000/3) (*see*
        also Neoplasm, malignant) C80
        [G73.3]
      pernicious anemia D51.0 *[G73.3]*
      thyrotoxicosis E05.90 *[G73.3]*
        with thyroid storm E05.91 *[G73.3]*
Mycelium infection B49
Mycetismus — *see* Poisoning, food, noxious,
  mushroom
Mycetoma B47.9
  actinomycotic B47.1
  bone (mycotic) B47.9 *[M90.80]*
  eumycotic B47.0
  foot B47.9
    actinomycotic B47.1
    mycotic B47.0
  madurae NEC B47.9
    mycotic B47.0
  maduromycotic B47.0
  mycotic B47.0
  nocardial B47.1
Mycobacteriosis — *see* Mycobacterium
Mycobacterium, mycobacterial (infection) A31.9
  anonymous A31.9
  atypical A31.9
    cutaneous A31.1
    pulmonary A31.0
      tuberculous — *see* Tuberculosis,
        pulmonary
    specified site NEC A31.8
  avium (intracellulare complex) A31.0
  balnei A31.1
  Battey A31.0
  chelonei A31.8
  cutaneous A31.1
  extrapulmonary systemic A31.8
  fortuitum A31.8
  intracellulare (Battey bacillus) A31.0
  kansasii (yellow bacillus) A31.0
  kakaferifu A31.8
  kasongo A31.8
  leprae (*see also* Leprosy) A30.9
  luciflavum A31.1
  marinum (M. balnei) A31.1
  nonspecific — *see* Mycobacterium, atypical
  pulmonary (atypical) A31.0
    tuberculous — *see* Tuberculosis, pulmonary
  scrofulaceum A31.8

Mycobacterium, mycobacterial — *continued*
  simiae A31.8
  systemic, extrapulmonary A31.8
  szulgai A31.8
  terrae A31.8
  triviale A31.8
  tuberculosis (human, bovine) — *see*
    Tuberculosis
  ulcerans A31.1
  xenopi A31.8
Mycoplasma (M.) pneumoniae, as cause of
  disease classified elsewhere B96.0
Mycosis, mycotic B49
  cutaneous NEC B36.9
  ear B36.8
  fungoides (M9700/3) (extranodal) (solid organ)
    C84.00
    lymph nodes (of)
      axilla C84.04
      face C84.01
      head C84.01
      inguinal region C84.05
      intra-abdominal C84.03
      intrapelvic C84.06
      intrathoracic C84.02
      lower limb C84.05
      neck C84.01
      upper limb C84.04
    multiple sites C84.08
    spleen C84.07
  mouth B37.0
  opportunistic B48.8
  skin NEC B36.9
  specified NEC B48.8
  stomatitis B37.0
  vagina, vaginitis (candidal) B37.3
Mydriasis (pupil) H57.04
Myelatelia Q06.1
Myelinoclasis, perivascular, acute
  (postinfectious) B89
  postimmunization or postvaccinal G04.0
Myelinolysis, pontine, central G37.2
Myelitis (acute) (ascending) (childhood) (chronic)
  (descending) (diffuse) (disseminated)
  (pressure) (progressive) (spinal cord)
  (subacute) G04.9
  necrotizing, subacute G37.4
  optic neuritis in G36.0
  postimmunization G04.0
  postinfectious NEC G04.8
  postvaccinal G04.0
  specified NEC G04.8
  syphilitic (transverse) A52.14
  transverse, acute (in demyelinating diseases of
    central nervous system) G37.3
  tuberculous A17.82
Myeloblastic — *see* condition
Myeloblastoma
  granular cell (M9580/0) — *see also* Neoplasm,
    connective tissue
    malignant (M9580/3) — *see* Neoplasm,
      connective tissue, malignant
    tongue (M9580/0) D10.1
Myelocele — *see* Spina bifida
Myelocystocele — *see* Spina bifida
Myelocytic — *see* condition
Myelodysplasia (M9989/1) D46.9
  specified NEC D46.7
  spinal cord (congenital) Q06.1
Myeloencephalitis — *see* Encephalitis
Myelofibrosis (with myeloid metaplasia)
  (M9961/1) D47.1
  acute (M9932/3) C94.50
    in remission C94.51
Myelogenous — *see* condition
Myeloid — *see* condition
Myelokathexis D70.9
Myeloleukodystrophy E75.29
Myelolipoma (M8870/0) — *see* Lipoma
Myeloma (multiple) (M9732/3) C90.00
  in remission C90.01
  monostotic (M9731/3) C90.20
    in remission C90.21

Myeloma — *continued*
  monostotic — *continued*
    plasma cell (M9732/3) C90.00
      in remission C90.01
    solitary (M9731/3) C90.20
      in remission C90.21
Myelomalacia G95.89
Myelomata, multiple (M9732/3) C90.00
  in remission C90.01
Myelomatosis (M9732/3) C90.00
  in remission C90.01
Myelomeningitis — *see* Meningoencephalitis
Myelomeningocele (spinal cord) — *see* Spina
  bifida
Myelo-osteo-musculodysplasia hereditaria
  Q79.8
Myelopathic — *see* condition
Myelopathy (spinal cord) G95.9
  drug-induced G95.89
  in (due to)
    degeneration or displacement, intervertebral
      disc NEC — *see* Disorder, disc, with,
      myelopathy
    infection — *see* Encephalitis
    intervertebral disc disorder — *see also*
      Disorder, disc, with, myelopathy
    mercury — *see* category T56.1
    neoplastic disease (*see also* Neoplasm)
      D49.9 *[G99.2]*
    pernicious anemia D51.0 *[G99.2]*
    spondylosis — *see* Spondylosis, with
      myelopathy NEC
  necrotic (subacute) (vascular) G95.19
  radiation-induced G95.89
  spondylogenic NEC — *see* Spondylosis, with
    myelopathy NEC
  toxic G95.89
  transverse, acute G37.3
  vascular G95.19
  vitamin B12 E53.8 *[G32.0]*
Myeloradiculitis G04.9
Myeloradiculodysplasia (spinal) Q06.1
Myelosarcoma (M9930/3) C92.30
  in remission C92.31
Myelosclerosis D75.8
  with myeloid metaplasia (M9961/1) D47.1
  disseminated, of nervous system G35
  megakaryocytic (with myeloid metaplasia)
    (M9961/1) D47.1
Myelosis
  acute (M9861/3) C92.00
    in remission C92.01
  aleukemic (M9864/3) C92.70
    in remission C92.71
  chronic (M9863/3) C92.10
    in remission C92.11
  erythremic (M9840/3) C94.00
    in remission C94.01
    acute (M9841/3) C94.00
      in remission C94.01
  megakaryocytic (M9910/3) C94.20
    in remission C94.21
Myelosis
  subacute (M9862/3) C92.20
    in remission C92.21
Myiasis (cavernous) B87.9
  aural B87.4
  creeping B87.0
  cutaneous B87.0
  dermal B87.0
  ear (external) (middle) B87.4
  eye B87.2
  genitourinary B87.81
  intestinal B87.82
  laryngeal B87.3
  nasopharyngeal B87.3
  ocular B87.2
  orbit B87.2
  skin B87.0
  specified site NEC B87.89
  traumatic B87.1
  wound B87.1
Myoadenoma, prostate — *see* Hyperplasia,
  prostate

©2002 Ingenix, Inc.

Myoblastoma
  granular cell (M9580/0) — *see also* Neoplasm,
    connective tissue, benign
    malignant (M9580/3) — *see* Neoplasm,
      connective tissue, malignant
  tongue (M9580/0) D10.1
Myocardial — *see* condition
Myocardiopathy (congestive) (constrictive)
  (familial) (hypertrophic nonobstructive)
  (idiopathic) (infiltrative) (obstructive)
  (primary) (restrictive) (sporadic) (*see also*
  Cardiomyopathy) I42.9
  alcoholic I42.6
  cobalt-beer I42.6
  glycogen storage E74.02 [I43]
  hypertrophic obstructive I42.1
  in (due to)
    beriberi E51.12 [I43]
    cardiac glycogenosis E74.02 [I43]
    Friedreich's ataxia G11.1 [I43]
    myotonia atrophica G71.1 [I43]
    progressive muscular dystrophy G71.0 [I43]
  obscure (African) I42.8
  secondary I42.7
  thyrotoxic E05.90 [I43]
    with storm E05.91 [I43]
  toxic NEC I42.7
Myocarditis (with arteriosclerosis) (chronic)
  (fibroid) (interstitial) (old) (progressive)
  (senile) I51.4
  with
    rheumatic fever (conditions in I00) I09.0
      active — *see* Myocarditis, acute,
        rheumatic
      inactive or quiescent (with chorea) I09.0
  active I40.9
    rheumatic I01.2
      with chorea (acute) (rheumatic)
        (Sydenham's) I02.0
  acute or subacute (interstitial) I40.9
    due to
      streptococcus (beta-hemolytic) I01.2
    idiopathic I40.1
    rheumatic I01.2
      with chorea (acute) (rheumatic)
        (Sydenham's) I02.0
    specified NEC I40.8
  aseptic of newborn B33.22
  bacterial (acute) I40.0
  Coxsackie (virus) B33.22
  diphtheritic A36.81
  eosinophilic I40.1
  epidemic of newborn (Coxsackie) B33.22
  Fiedler's (acute) (isolated) I40.1
  giant cell (acute) (subacute) I40.1
  gonococcal A54.83
  granulomatous (idiopathic) (isolated)
    (nonspecific) I40.1
  hypertensive — *see* Hypertension, heart
  idiopathic (granulomatous) I40.1
  in (due to)
    diphtheria A36.81
    epidemic louse-borne typhus A75.0 [I41]
    Lyme disease A69.29
    sarcoidosis D86.85
    scarlet fever A38.1
    toxoplasmosis (acquired) B58.81
    typhoid A01.02
    typhus NEC A75.9 [I41]
  infective I40.0
  influenzal J10.89
  isolated (acute) I40.1
  meningococcal A39.52
  mumps B26.82
  nonrheumatic, active I40.9
  parenchymatous I40.9
  pneumococcal I40.0
  rheumatic (chronic) (inactive) (with chorea)
    I09.0
    active or acute I01.2
      with chorea (acute) (rheumatic)
        (Sydenham's) I02.0
  rheumatoid — *see* Rheumatoid, carditis
  septic I40.0
  staphylococcal I40.0
  suppurative I40.0
  syphilitic (chronic) A52.06

Myocarditis — *continued*
  toxic I40.8
    rheumatic — *see* Myocarditis, acute,
      rheumatic
  tuberculous A18.84
  typhoid A01.02
  valvular — *see* Endocarditis
  virus, viral I40.0
    of newborn (Coxsackie) B33.22
Myocardium, myocardial — *see* condition
Myocardosis — *see* Cardiomyopathy
Myoclonus, myoclonic, myoclonia (familial)
  (essential) (multifocal) (simplex) G25.3
  drug-induced G25.3
  epilepsy, familial (progressive) G25.3
  epileptica G40.30
    with status epilepticus G40.31
  facial G51.3
  familial progressive G25.3
  Friedreich's G25.3
  jerks G25.3
  massive G25.3
  pharyngeal J39.2
Myodiastasis — *see* Diastasis, muscle
Myoendocarditis — *see* Endocarditis
Myoepithelioma (M8982/0) — *see* Neoplasm,
  benign
Myofasciitis (acute) — *see* Myositis
Myofibroma (M8890/0) — *see also* Neoplasm,
  connective tissue, benign
  uterus (cervix) (corpus) — *see* Leiomyoma
Myofibromatosis (M8824/1) D48.1
Myofibrosis M62.89
  heart — *see* Myocarditis
  scapulohumeral — *see* Lesion, shoulder,
    specified NEC
Myofibrositis — *see also* Rheumatism
  scapulohumeral — *see* Lesion, shoulder,
    specified NEC
Myoglobulinuria, myoglobinuria (primary) R82.1
Myokymia, facial G51.4
Myolipoma (M8860/0) — *see also* Lipoma
  unspecified site D30.00
Myoma (M8895/0) — *see also* Neoplasm,
  connective tissue, benign
  malignant (M8895/3) — *see* Neoplasm,
    connective tissue, malignant
  prostate — *see* Hyperplasia, prostate, localized
  uterus (cervix) (corpus) — *see* Leiomyoma
Myomalacia M62.89
Myometritis — *see* Endometritis
Myometrium — *see* condition
Myonecrosis, clostridial A48.0
Myopathy G72.9
  alcoholic G72.1
  benign congenital G70.9
  central core G70.9
  centronuclear G71.2
  congenital (benign) G71.2
  distal G71.0
  drug-induced G72.0
  endocrine NEC E34.9 [G73.7]
  extraocular muscles H05.829
    bilateral H05.823
    left H05.822
    right H05.821
  facioscapulohumeral G71.0
  hereditary G71.9
    specified NEC G71.8
  in (due to)
    Addison's disease E27.1 [G73.7]
    alcohol G72.1
    amyloidosis E85 [G73.7]
    cretinism E00.9 [G73.7]
    Cushing's syndrome E24.9 [G73.7]
    drugs G72.0
    endocrine disease NEC E34.9 [G73.7]
    giant cell arteritis M31.6 [G73.7]
    glycogen storage disease E74.00 [G73.7]
    hyperadrenocorticism E24.9 [G73.7]
    hyperparathyroidism NEC E21.3 [G73.7]
    hypoparathyroidism E20.9 [G73.7]
    hypopituitarism E23.0 [G73.7]
    hypothyroidism E03.9 [G73.7]

Myopathy — *continued*
  in — *continued*
    infectious disease NEC B99 [G73.7]
    lipid storage disease E75.6 [G73.7]
    malignant neoplasm NEC (M8000/3) (*see*
      also Neoplasm, malignant) C80 [M63]
    metabolic disease NEC E88.9 [G73.7]
    myxedema E03.9 [G73.7]
    parasitic disease NEC B89 [G73.7]
    polyarteritis nodosa M30.0 [G73.7]
    rheumatoid arthritis — *see* Rheumatoid,
      myopathy
    sarcoidosis D86.87
    scleroderma M34.82
    sicca syndrome M35.03
    Sjögren's syndrome M35.03
    systemic lupus erythematosus M32.19
    thyrotoxicosis (hyperthyroidism) E05.90
      [G73.7]
      with thyroid storm E05.91 [G73.7]
    toxic agent NEC G72.2
  inflammatory NEC G72.4
  limb-girdle G71.0
  mitochondrial NEC G71.3
  myotubular G71.2
  nemaline G71.2
  ocular G71.0
  oculopharyngeal G71.0
  primary G71.9
    specified NEC G71.8
  progressive NEC G72.8
  rod G71.2
  scapulohumeral G71.0
  specified NEC G72.8
  toxic G72.2
Myopericarditis — *see also* Pericarditis
  chronic rheumatic I09.2
Myopia (axial) (congenital) (progressive) H52.10
  bilateral H52.13
  degenerative (malignant) — *see* Disorder, globe,
    degenerative, myopia
  left H52.12
  malignant — *see* Disorder, globe, degenerative,
    myopia
  pernicious — *see* Disorder, globe, degenerative,
    myopia
  progressive high (degenerative) — *see* Disorder,
    globe, degenerative, myopia
  right H52.11
Myosarcoma (M8895/3) — *see* Neoplasm,
  connective tissue, malignant
Myosis (pupil) H57.03
  stromal (endolymphatic) (M8931/1) D39.0
Myositis M60.9
  clostridial A48.0
  due to posture — *see* Myositis, specified type
    NEC
  epidemic B33.0
  fibrosa or fibrous (chronic), Volkmann's T79.6
  foreign body granuloma — *see* Granuloma,
    foreign body
  in (due to)
    bilharziasis B65.9 [M63]
    cysticercosis B69.81
    leprosy A30.9 [M63]
    mycosis B49 [M63]
    sarcoidosis D86.87
    schistosomiasis B65.9 [M63]
    syphilis
      late A52.78
      secondary A51.49
    toxoplasmosis (acquired) B58.82
    trichinellosis B75 [M63]
    tuberculosis A18.09
  infective M60.009
    lower limb M60.005
      ankle M60.072
        left M60.071
        right M60.070
      foot M60.075
        left M60.074
        right M60.073
      left M60.004
      lower leg M60.069
        left M60.062
        right M60.061

Myositis — *continued*
  infective — *continued*
    lower limb — *continued*
      right M60.003
      thigh M60.059
        left M60.052
        right M60.051
      toe M60.078
        left M60.077
        right M60.076
    multiple sites M60.09
    specified site NEC M60.08
    upper limb M60.002
      finger M60.046
        left M60.045
        right M60.044
      forearm M60.039
        left M60.032
        right M60.031
      hand M60.043
        left M60.042
        right M60.041
      left M60.001
      right M60.000
      shoulder region M60.019
        left M60.012
        right M60.011
      upper arm M60.029
        left M60.022
        right M60.021
  interstitial M60.10
    ankle M60.179
      left M60.172
      right M60.171
    foot M60.179
      left M60.172
      right M60.171
    forearm M60.139
      left M60.132
      right M60.131
    hand M60.149
      left M60.142
      right M60.141
    lower leg M60.169
      left M60.162
      right M60.161
    multiple sites M60.19
    shoulder region M60.119
      left M60.112
      right M60.111
    specified site NEC M60.18
    thigh M60.159
      left M60.152
      right M60.151
    upper arm M60.129
      left M60.122
      right M60.121
  mycotic B49 [M63]
  orbital, chronic H05.129
    bilateral H05.123
    left H05.122
    right H05.121
  ossificans or ossifying (circumscripta) — *see also* Ossification, muscle, specified NEC
    in (due to)
      burns M61.30
        ankle M61.379
          left M61.372
          right M61.371
        foot M61.379
          left M61.372
          right M61.371
        forearm M61.339
          left M61.332
          right M61.331
        hand M61.349
          left M61.342
          right M61.341
        lower leg M61.369
          left M61.362
          right M61.361
        multiple sites M61.39
        pelvic region M61.359
          left M61.352
          right M61.351

Myositis — *continued*
  ossificans or ossifying — *see also* Ossification, muscle, specified NEC — *continued*
  in — *continued*
    burns — *continued*
      shoulder region M61.319
        left M61.312
        right M61.311
      specified site NEC M61.38
      thigh M61.359
        left M61.352
        right M61.351
      upper arm M61.329
        left M61.322
        right M61.321
      quadriplegia or paraplegia M61.20
        ankle M61.279
          left M61.272
          right M61.271
        foot M61.279
          left M61.272
          right M61.271
        forearm M61.239
          left M61.232
          right M61.231
        hand M61.249
          left M61.242
          right M61.241
        lower leg M61.269
          left M61.262
          right M61.261
        multiple sites M61.29
        pelvic region M61.259
          left M61.252
          right M61.251
        shoulder region M61.219
          left M61.212
          right M61.211
        specified site NEC M61.28
        thigh M61.259
          left M61.252
          right M61.251
        upper arm M61.229
          left M61.222
          right M61.221
  progressiva M61.10
    ankle M61.173
      left M61.172
      right M61.171
    finger M61.146
      left M61.145
      right M61.144
    foot M61.176
      left M61.175
      right M61.174
    forearm M61.139
      left M61.132
      right M61.131
    hand M61.143
      left M61.142
      right M61.141
    lower leg M61.169
      left M61.162
      right M61.161
    multiple sites M61.19
    pelvic region M61.159
      left M61.152
      right M61.151
    shoulder region M61.119
      left M61.112
      right M61.111
    specified site NEC M61.18
    thigh M61.159
      left M61.152
      right M61.151
    toe M61.179
      left M61.178
      right M61.177
    upper arm M61.129
      left M61.122
      right M61.121
  traumatica M61.00
    ankle M61.079
      left M61.072
      right M61.071

Myositis — *continued*
  ossificans or ossifying — *see also* Ossification, muscle, specified NEC — *continued*
  traumatica — *continued*
    foot M61.079
      left M61.072
      right M61.071
    forearm M61.039
      left M61.032
      right M61.031
    hand M61.049
      left M61.042
      right M61.041
    lower leg M61.069
      left M61.062
      right M61.061
    multiple sites M61.09
    pelvic region M61.059
      left M61.052
      right M61.051
    shoulder region M61.019
      left M61.012
      right M61.011
    specified site NEC M61.08
    thigh M61.059
      left M61.052
      right M61.051
    upper arm M61.029
      left M61.022
      right M61.021
  purulent — *see* Myositis, infective
  specified type NEC M60.80
    ankle M60.879
      left M60.872
      right M60.871
    foot M60.879
      left M60.872
      right M60.871
    forearm M60.839
      left M60.832
      right M60.831
    hand M60.849
      left M60.842
      right M60.841
    lower leg M60.869
      left M60.862
      right M60.861
    multiple sites M60.89
    pelvic region M60.859
      left M60.852
      right M60.851
    shoulder region M60.819
      left M60.812
      right M60.811
    specified site NEC M60.88
    thigh M60.859
      left M60.852
      right M60.851
    upper arm M60.829
      left M60.822
      right M60.821
  suppurative — *see* Myositis, infective
  traumatic (old) — *see* Myositis, specified type NEC

Myospasia impulsiva F95.2

Myotonia (acquisita) (intermittens) M62.89
  atrophica G71.1
  chondrodystrophic G71.1
  congenita G71.1
  drug-induced G71.1
  dystrophica G71.1
  symptomatic G71.1

Myotonic pupil — *see* Anomaly, pupil, function, tonic pupil

Myriapodiasis B88.2

Myringitis H73.20
  with otitis media — *see* Otitis, media
  acute H73.009
    bilateral H73.003
    bullous H73.019
      bilateral H73.013
      left H73.012
      right H73.011
    left H73.002
    right H73.001

©2002 Ingenix, Inc.

Myringitis — continued
  acute — continued
    specified NEC H73.099
      bilateral H73.093
      left H73.092
      right H73.091
    bilateral H73.23
    bullous — see Myringitis, acute, bullous
  chronic H73.10
    bilateral H73.13
    left H73.12
    right H73.11
    left H73.22
    right H73.21
Mysophobia F40.228
Mytilotoxism — see Poisoning, fish
Myxadenitis labialis K13.0
Myxedema (adult) (idiocy) (infantile) (juvenile) (see
  also Hypothyroidism) E03.9
  circumscribed E05.90
    with storm E05.91
  coma E03.5
  congenital E00.1
  cutis L98.5
  localized (pretibial) E05.90
    with storm E05.91
  papular L98.5
Myxochondrosarcoma (M9220/3) — see
  Neoplasm, cartilage, malignant
Myxofibroma (M8811/0) — see Neoplasm,
  connective tissue, benign
  odontogenic (M9320/0) D16.5
    upper jaw (bone) D16.4
Myxofibrosarcoma (M8811/3) — see Neoplasm,
  connective tissue, malignant
Myxolipoma (M8852/0) D17.9
Myxoliposarcoma (M8852/3) — see Neoplasm,
  connective tissue, malignant
Myxoma (M8840/0) — see also Neoplasm,
  connective tissue, benign
  nerve sheath (M9562/0) — see Neoplasm,
    nerve, benign
  odontogenic (M9320/0) D16.5
    upper jaw (bone) D16.4
Myxosarcoma (M8840/3) — see Neoplasm,
  connective tissue, malignant

N

Naegeli's
  disease Q82.8
  leukemia, monocytic (M9863/3) C92.10
    in remission C92.11
Naegleriasis (with meningoencephalitis) B60.2
Naffziger's syndrome G54.0
Naga sore — see Ulcer, skin
Nägele's pelvis M95.5
  with disproportion (fetopelvic) O33.0
    causing obstructed labor O65.0
Nail — see also condition
  biting F98.8
  patella syndrome Q87.2
Nanism, nanosomia — see Dwarfism
Nanophyetiasis B66.8
Nanukayami A27.89
Napkin rash L22
Narcolepsy G47.4
Narcosis
  carbon dioxide (respiratory) R06.89
  due to drug
    correct substance properly administered
      R41.89
    overdose or wrong substance given or taken
      (by accident) T40.601
      administered with intent to harm by
        another person T40.603
        self T40.602
      circumstances undetermined T40.604
      specified drug — see Table of Drugs and
        Chemicals
Narcotism — see Dependence

Narrow
  anterior chamber angle H40.0
  pelvis — see Contraction, pelvis
Narrowing
  artery I77.1
    auditory, internal I65.8
    basilar — see Occlusion, artery, basilar
    carotid — see Occlusion, artery, carotid
    cerebellar — see Occlusion, artery,
      cerebellar
    cerebral — see Occlusion artery, cerebral
    choroidal — see Occlusion, artery, cerebral,
      specified NEC
    communicating posterior — see Occlusion,
      artery, cerebral, specified NEC
    coronary — see also Disease, heart,
      ischemic, atherosclerotic
      congenital Q24.5
      syphilitic A50.54 [I52]
      due to syphilis NEC A52.06
    hypophyseal — see Occlusion, artery,
      cerebral, specified NEC
    pontine — see Occlusion, artery, cerebral,
      specified NEC
    precerebral — see Occlusion, artery,
      precerebral
    vertebral — see Occlusion, artery, vertebral
  auditory canal (external) — see Stenosis,
    external ear canal
  eustachian tube — see Obstruction, eustachian
    tube
  eyelid — see Disorder, eyelid function
  larynx J38.6
  mesenteric artery K55.0
  palate M26.8
  palpebral fissure — see Disorder, eyelid
    function
  ureter N13.5
    with infection N13.6
  urethra — see Stricture, urethra
Narrowness, abnormal, eyelid Q10.3
Nasal — see condition
Nasolachrymal, nasolacrimal — see condition
Nasopharyngeal — see also condition
  pituitary gland Q89.2
  torticollis M43.6
Nasopharyngitis (acute) (infective) (septic)
  (streptococcal) (subacute) J00
  chronic (suppurative) (ulcerative) J31.1
Nasopharynx, nasopharyngeal — see condition
Natal tooth, teeth K00.6
Nausea R11.1
  with vomiting R11.0
  epidemic A08.1
  gravidarum — see Hyperemesis, gravidarum
  marina T75.3
  navalis T75.3
Navel — see condition
Neapolitan fever — see Brucellosis
Nearsightedness — see Myopia
Near-syncope R55
Nebula, cornea — see Opacity, cornea
Necator americanus infestation B76.1
Necatoriasis B76.1
Neck — see condition
Necrobiosis R68.8
  lipoidica NEC L92.1
    with diabetes — see E09-E13 with .63
Necrolysis, toxic epidermal L51.2
  due to drug
    correct substance properly administered
      L51.2
    overdose or wrong substance given or taken
      (by accident) T50.901
      administered with intent to harm by
        another person T50.903
        self T50.902
      circumstances undetermined T50.904
      specified drug — see Table of Drugs and
        Chemicals
Necrophilia F65.89

Necrosis, necrotic (ischemic) — see also
  Gangrene
  adrenal (capsule) (gland) E27.4
  amputation stump (surgical) (late) T87.50
  arm
    left T87.52
    right T87.51
  leg
    left T87.54
    right T87.53
  antrum J32.0
  aorta (hyaline) — see also Aneurysm, aorta
    cystic medial — see Dissection, aorta
  artery I77.5
  bladder (aseptic) (sphincter) N32.8
  bone — see also Osteomyelitis
    aseptic or avascular — see also
      Osteonecrosis
    idiopathic M87.00
      carpus — see Osteonecrosis,
        idiopathic, carpus
      clavicle — see Osteonecrosis,
        idiopathic, clavicle
      femur — see Osteonecrosis, idiopathic,
        femur
      fibula — see Osteonecrosis, idiopathic,
        fibula
      finger — see Osteonecrosis, idiopathic,
        finger
      humerus — see Osteonecrosis,
        idiopathic, humerus
      ilium M87.050
      ischium M87.050
      metacarpus — see Osteonecrosis,
        idiopathic, metacarpus
      metatarsus — see Osteonecrosis,
        idiopathic, metatarsus
      neck M87.08
      radius — see Osteonecrosis,
        idiopathic, radius
      rib M87.08
      scapula — see Osteonecrosis,
        idiopathic, scapula
      skull M87.08
      tarsus — see Osteonecrosis,
        idiopathic, tarsus
      tibia — see Osteonecrosis, idiopathic,
        tibia
      toe — see Osteonecrosis, idiopathic,
        toe
      ulna — see Osteonecrosis, idiopathic,
        ulna
      vertebra M87.08
    ethmoid J32.2
    jaw M27.2
    specified NEC — see Osteonecrosis, specified
      type NEC
    tuberculous — see Tuberculosis, bone
  brain I67.8
  breast (aseptic) (fat) (segmental) N64.1
  bronchus J98.0
  central nervous system NEC I67.8
  cerebellar I67.8
  cerebral I67.8
  cornea H18.40
  cortical (acute) (renal) N17.1
  cystic medial (aorta) — see Dissection, aorta
  dental pulp K04.1
  esophagus K22.8
  ethmoid (bone) J32.2
  eyelid — see Disorder, eyelid, degenerative
  fat, fatty (generalized) — see also Disorder, soft
    tissue, specified type NEC
    breast (aseptic) (segmental) N64.1
    localized — see Degeneration, by site, fatty
    mesentery K65.8
    omentum K65.8
    pancreas K86.8
    peritoneum K65.8
    skin (subcutaneous), newborn P83.0
    subcutaneous, due to birth injury P15.6
  gallbladder — see Cholecystitis, acute
  heart — see Infarct, myocardium
  hip, aseptic or avascular — see Osteonecrosis,
    by type, femur
  intestine (acute) (hemorrhagic) (massive) K55.0
  jaw M27.2

Necrosis, necrotic — *see also* Gangrene —
  continued
  kidney (bilateral) N28.0
    acute N17.9
    cortical (acute) (bilateral) N17.1
      with ectopic or molar pregnancy O08.4
    medullary (bilateral) (in acute renal failure)
      (papillary) — *see* Pyelitis
    papillary (bilateral) (in acute renal failure) —
      see Pyelitis
    tubular N17.0
      with ectopic or molar pregnancy O08.4
      complicating
        abortion — *see* Abortion, by type,
          complicated by, tubular necrosis
        ectopic or molar pregnancy O08.4
        pregnancy — *see* Pregnancy,
          complicated by, diseases of,
          specified type or system NEC
      following ectopic or molar pregnancy
        O08.4
      traumatic T79.5
  larynx J38.7
  liver (with hepatic failure) (cell) *see* Failure,
    hepatic
    complicating
      childbirth O26.62
      pregnancy O26.619
        first trimester O26.611
        second trimester O26.612
        third trimester O26.613
      puerperium O26.63
    hemorrhagic, central K76.2
  lung J85.0
  lymphatic gland — *see* Lymphadenitis, acute
  mammary gland (fat) (segmental) N64.1
  mastoid (chronic) — *see* Mastoiditis, chronic
  medullary (acute) (renal) N17.2
  mesentery K55.0
    fat K65.8
  mitral valve — *see* Insufficiency, mitral
  myocardium, myocardial — *see* Infarct,
    myocardium
  nose J34.0
  omentum (with mesenteric infarction) K55.0
    fat K65.8
  orbit, orbital — *see* Osteomyelitis, orbit
  ossicles, ear — *see* Abnormal, ear ossicles
  ovary N70.92
  pancreas (aseptic) (duct) (fat) K86.8
    acute (infective) K85.8
    infective K85.8
  papillary (acute) (renal) N17.2
  peritoneum (with mesenteric infarction) K55.0
    fat K65.8
  pharynx J02.9
    in granulocytopenia — *see* Neutropenia
    Vincent's A69.1
  phosphorus — *see* category T54.2
  pituitary (gland) (postpartum) (Sheehan) E23.0
  placenta O43.829
    first trimester O43.821
    second trimester O43.822
    third trimester O43.823
  pressure — *see* Decubitus
  pulmonary J85.0
  pulp (dental) K04.1
  radiation — *see* Necrosis, by site
  radium — *see* Necrosis, by site
  renal — *see* Necrosis, kidney
  sclera H15.89
  scrotum N50.8
  skin or subcutaneous tissue NEC I96
  spine, spinal (column) — *see also*
    Osteonecrosis, by type, vertebra
    cord G95.19
  spleen D73.5
  stomach K31.89
  stomatitis (ulcerative) A69.0
  subcutaneous fat, fetus or newborn P83.8
  subendocardial (acute) I21.4
    chronic I25.8
  suprarenal (capsule) (gland) E27.4
  testis N50.8
  thymus (gland) E32.8
  tonsil J35.8
  trachea J39.8

Necrosis, necrotic — *see also* Gangrene —
  continued
  tuberculous NEC — *see* Tuberculosis
  tubular (acute) (anoxic) (renal) (toxic) N17.0
    postprocedural N99.0
  vagina N89.8
  vertebra — *see also* Osteonecrosis, by type,
    vertebra
    tuberculous A18.01
  X-ray — *see* Necrosis, by site

Necrospermia — *see* Infertility, male

Need (for)
  care provider because (of)
    assistance with personal care Z74.1
    continuous supervision required Z74.3
    impaired mobility Z74.0
    no other household member able to render
      care Z74.2
    specified reason NEC Z74.8
  immunization — *see* Vaccination
  vaccination — *see* Vaccination

Neglect (newborn) T76.02
  adult T76.01
    confirmed T74.01
    history of Z91.41
  confirmed T74.02
  emotional, in childhood Z62.8
  hemispatial R41.4
  left-sided R41.4
  sensory R41.4
  visuospatial R41.4

Neisserian infection NEC — *see* Gonococcus

Nelaton's syndrome G60.8

Nelson's syndrome E24.1

Nematodiasis (intestinal) B82.0
  Ancylostoma B76.0

Neonatal — *see also* condition
  tooth, teeth K00.6

Neonatorum — *see* condition

Neoplasia
  endocrine, multiple (MEN) (M8360/1) — *see
    also* Adenomatosis, endocrine D44.8
  intraepithelial
    cervix (uteri) (CIN) N87.9
      grade I N87.0
      grade II N87.1
      grade III (severe dysplasia) (M8077/2)
        D06.9
    vagina (VAIN) N89.3
      grade I N89.0
      grade II N89.1
      grade III (severe dysplasia) (M8077/2)
        D07.2
    vulva (VIN) N90.3
      grade I N90.0
      grade II N90.1
      grade III (severe dysplasia) (M8077/2)
        D07.1

Neovascularization
  ciliary body — *see* Disorder, iris, vascular
  cornea H16.409
    bilateral H16.403
    deep H16.449
      bilateral H16.443
      left H16.442
      right H16.441
    ghost vessels — *see* Ghost, vessels
    left H16.402
    localized H16.439
      bilateral H16.433
      left H16.432
      right H16.431
    pannus — *see* Pannus
    right H16.401
  iris — *see* Disorder, iris, vascular
  retina H35.059
    bilateral H35.053
    left H35.052
    right H35.051

Nephralgia N23

Nephritis, nephritic (albuminuric) (azotemic)
  (congenital) (disseminated) (epithelial)
  (familial) (focal) granulomatous)
  (hemorrhagic) (infantile) (nonsuppurative)
  excretory) (uremic) N05.9
  with
    dense deposit disease N05.6
    diffuse
      crescentic glomerulonephritis N05.7
      endocapillary proliferative
        glomerulonephritis N05.4
      membranous glomerulonephritis N05.2
      mesangial proliferative glomerulonephritis
        N05.3
      mesangiocapillary glomerulonephritis
        N05.5
    edema — *see* Nephrosis
    focal and segmental glomerular lesions
      N05.1
    foot process disease N04.9
    glomerular lesion
      diffuse sclerosing (*see also* Failure, renal,
        chronic) N18.9
    hypocomplementemic — *see* Nephritis,
      membranoproliferative
    IgA — *see* Nephropathy, IgA
    lobular, lobulonodular — *see* Nephritis,
      membranoproliferative
    nodular — *see* Nephritis,
      membranoproliferative
  lesion of
    glomerulonephritis, proliferative N04.4
    renal necrosis N05.9
  minor glomerular abnormality N05.0
  specified morphological changes NEC N05.8
  acute N00.9
    with
      dense deposit disease N00.6
      diffuse
        crescentic glomerulonephritis N00.7
        endocapillary proliferative
          glomerulonephritis N00.4
        membranous glomerulonephritis
          N00.2
        mesangial proliferative
          glomerulonephritis N00.3
        mesangiocapillary glomerulonephritis
          N00.5
      focal and segmental glomerular lesions
        N00.1
      minor glomerular abnormality N00.0
      specified morphological changes NEC
        N00.8
  amyloid E85 [N08]
  antiglomerular basement membrane (anti-
    GBM) antibody NEC
    in Goodpasture's syndrome M31.0
  antitubular basement membrane (tubulo-
    interstitial) NEC N12
    toxic — *see* Nephropathy, toxic
  arteriolar — *see* Hypertension, kidney
  arteriosclerotic — *see* Hypertension, kidney
  ascending — *see* Nephritis, tubulo-interstitial
  atrophic N03.9
  Balkan (endemic) N15.0
  calculous, calculus — *see* Calculus, kidney
  cardiac — *see* Hypertension, kidney
  cardiovascular — *see* Hypertension, kidney
  chronic N03.9
    with
      dense deposit disease N03.6
      diffuse
        crescentic glomerulonephritis N03.7
        endocapillary proliferative
          glomerulonephritis N03.4
        membranous glomerulonephritis
          N03.2
        mesangial proliferative
          glomerulonephritis N03.3
        mesangiocapillary glomerulonephritis
          N03.5
      focal and segmental glomerular lesions
        N03.1
      minor glomerular abnormality N03.0
      specified morphological changes NEC
        N03.8

©2002 Ingenix, Inc.

Nephritis, nephritic — *continued*
  chronic — *continued*
    arteriosclerotic — *see* Hypertension, kidney
  cirrhotic N26.9
  croupous N00.9
  degenerative — *see* Nephrosis
  diffuse sclerosing — *see* Failure, renal, chronic
  due to
    diabetes mellitus — *see* E09-E13 with .21
    subacute bacterial endocarditis I33.0
    systemic lupus erythematosus (chronic) M32.14
    typhoid fever A01.09
  gonococcal (acute) (chronic) A54.21
  hypocomplementemic — *see* Nephritis, membranoproliferative
  IgA — *see* Nephropathy, IgA
  immune complex (circulating) NEC N05.8
  infective — *see* Nephritis, tubulo-interstitial
  interstitial — *see* Nephritis, tubulo-interstitial
  lead N14.3
  membranoproliferative (diffuse) (type 1 or 3) (*see also* N00-N07 with fourth character .5) N05.5
    type 2 (*see also* N00-N07 with fourth character .6) N05.6
  minimal change N04.0
  necrotic, necrotizing NEC (*see also* N00-N07 with fourth character .8) N05.8
  nephrotic — *see* Nephrosis
  nodular — *see* Nephritis, membranoproliferative
  polycystic Q61.3
    adult type Q61.2
    autosomal
      dominant Q61.2
      recessive Q61.19
    childhood type Q61.19
    infantile type Q61.19
  poststreptococcal N05.9
    acute N00.9
    chronic N03.0
    rapidly progressive N01.9
  proliferative NEC (*see also* N00-N07 with fourth character .8) N05.8
  puerperal (postpartum) O90.8
  purulent — *see* Nephritis, tubulo-interstitial
  rapidly progressive N01.9
    with
      dense deposit disease N01.6
      diffuse
        crescentic glomerulonephritis N01.7
        endocapillary proliferative glomerulonephritis N01.4
        membranous glomerulonephritis N01.2
        mesangial proliferative glomerulonephritis N01.3
        mesangiocapillary glomerulonephritis N01.5
      focal and segmental glomerular lesions N01.1
      minor glomerular abnormality N01.0
      specified morphological changes NEC N01.8
  salt losing or wasting NEC N28.89
  saturnine N14.3
  sclerosing, diffuse — *see* Failure, renal, chronic
  septic — *see* Nephritis, tubulo-interstitial
  specified pathology NEC (*see also* N00-N07 with fourth character .8) N05.8
  subacute N01.9
  suppurative — *see* Nephritis, tubulo-interstitial
  syphilitic (late) A52.75
    congenital A50.59 [N08]
    early (secondary) A51.44
  toxic — *see* Nephropathy, toxic
  tubal, tubular — *see* Nephritis, tubulo-interstitial
  tuberculous A18.11
  tubulo-interstitial (in) N12
    acute (infectious) N10
    chronic (infectious) N11.9
      nonobstructive N11.8
        reflux-associated N11.0
      obstructive N11.1
      specified NEC N11.8

Nephritis, nephritic — *continued*
  tubulo-interstitial — *continued*
    due to
      brucellosis A23.9 [N16]
      cryoglobulinemia D89.1 [N16]
      glycogen storage disease E74.00 [N16]
      Sjögren's syndrome M35.04
    vascular — *see* Hypertension, kidney
    war N00.9

Nephroblastoma (epithelial) (mesenchymal) (M8960/3) C64.9
  left C64.1
  right C64.0

Nephrocalcinosis E83.59 [N29]

Nephrocystitis, pustular — *see* Nephritis, tubulo-interstitial

Nephrolithiasis (congenital) (pelvis) (recurrent) — *see also* Calculus, kidney
  gouty M10.08
  uric acid M10.08

Nephroma (M8960/3) C64.9
  left C64.1
  mesoblastic (M8960/1) D41.00
    left D41.02
    right D41.01
  right C64.0

Nephronephritis — *see* Nephrosis

Nephronophthisis Q61.5

Nephropathia epidemica A98.5

Nephropathy (*see also* Nephritis) N28.9
  with
    edema — *see* Nephrosis
    glomerular lesion — *see* Glomerulonephritis
  amyloid, hereditary E85
  analgesic N14.0
    with medullary necrosis, acute N17.2
  Balkan (endemic) N15.0
  chemical — *see* Nephropathy, toxic
  diabetic — *see* E09-E13 with .21
  drug-induced N14.2
    specified NEC N14.1
  heavy metal-induced N14.3
  hereditary NEC N07.9
    with
      dense deposit disease N07.6
      diffuse
        crescentic glomerulonephritis N07.7
        endocapillary proliferative glomerulonephritis N07.4
        membranous glomerulonephritis N07.2
        mesangial proliferative glomerulonephritis N07.3
        mesangiocapillary glomerulonephritis N07.5
      focal and segmental glomerular lesions N07.1
      minor glomerular abnormality N07.0
      specified morphological changes NEC N07.8
  hypercalcemic N25.8
  hypertensive — *see* Hypertension, kidney
  hypokalemic (vacuolar) N25.8
  IgA N02.8
    with glomerular lesion N02.9
      focal and segmental hyalinosis or sclerosis N02.1
      membranoproliferative (diffuse) N02.5
      membranous (diffuse) N02.2
      mesangial proliferative (diffuse) N02.3
      mesangiocapillary (diffuse) N02.5
      proliferative NEC N02.8
      specified pathology NEC N02.8
  lead N14.3
  mesangial (IgA/IgG) — *see* Nephropathy, IgA
  obstructive N13.8
  phenacetin N17.2
  phosphate-losing N25.0
  potassium depletion N25.8
  pregnancy-related O26.839
    first trimester O26.831
    second trimester O26.832
    third trimester O26.833
  proliferative NEC (*see also* N00-N07 with fourth character .8) N05.8

Nephropathy (*see also* Nephritis) — *continued*
  protein-losing N25.8
  saturnine N14.3
  sickle-cell (*see also* Disease, sickle-cell) D57.1 [N08]
  toxic NEC N14.4
    due to
      drugs N14.2
        analgesic N14.0
        specified NEC N14.1
      heavy metals N14.3
  vasomotor N17.0
  water-losing N25.8

Nephroptosis N28.83

Nephropyosis — *see* Abscess, kidney

Nephrorrhagia N28.89

Nephrosclerosis (arteriolar) (arteriosclerotic) (chronic) (hyaline) — *see also* Hypertension, kidney
  hyperplastic — *see* Hypertension, kidney
  senile N26.9

Nephrosis, nephrotic (Epstein's) (syndrome) (congenital) N04.9
  with glomerular lesion N04.1
    foot process disease N04.9
    hypocomplementemic N04.5
  acute N04.9
  anoxic — *see* Nephrosis, tubular
  chemical — *see* Nephrosis, tubular
  cholemic K76.7
  complicating pregnancy O26.839
    first trimester O26.831
    second trimester O26.832
    third trimester O26.833
  diabetic — *see* E09-E13 with .21
  hemoglobin N10
  hemoglobinuric — *see* Nephrosis, tubular
  in
    amyloidosis E85 [N08]
    diabetes mellitus — *see* E09-E13 with .21
    epidemic hemorrhagic fever A98.5
    malaria (malariae) B52.0
  ischemic — *see* Nephrosis, tubular
  lipoid N04.9
  lower nephron — *see* Nephrosis, tubular
  malarial (malariae) B52.0
  minimal change N04.0
  myoglobin N10
  necrotizing — *see* Nephrosis, tubular
  osmotic (sucrose) N25.8
  radiation N04.9
  syphilitic (late) A52.75
  toxic — *see* Nephrosis, tubular
  tubular (acute) N17.0
    postprocedural N99.0
    radiation N04.9

Nephrosonephritis, hemorrhagic (endemic) A98.5

Nephrostomy
  attention to Z43.6
  status Z93.6

Nerve — *see also* condition
  injury — *see* Injury, nerve, by body site

Nerves R45.0

Nervous (*see also* condition) R45.0
  heart F45.8
  stomach F45.8
  tension R45.0

Nervousness R45.0

Nesidioblastoma (M8150/0)
  pancreas D13.7
  specified site NEC — *see* Neoplasm, benign
  unspecified site D13.7

Nettleship's syndrome Q82.2

Neumann's disease or syndrome L10.1

Neuralgia, neuralgic (acute) M79.2
  accessory (nerve) G52.8
  acoustic (nerve) — *see* category H93.3
  auditory (nerve) — *see* category H93.3
  ciliary G44.0
  cranial
    nerve — *see also* Disorder, nerve, cranial
      fifth or trigeminal — *see* Neuralgia, trigeminal

Neuralgia, neuralgic — *continued*
 cranial — *continued*
  postherpetic, postzoster B02.29
 ear — *see* category H92.0
 facialis vera G51.1
 Fothergill's — *see* Neuralgia, trigeminal
 glossopharyngeal (nerve) G52.1
 Horton's G43.8
 Hunt's B02.21
 hypoglossal (nerve) G52.3
 infraorbital — *see* Neuralgia, trigeminal
 malarial — *see* Malaria
 migrainous G44.0
 Morton's G57.60
  left G57.62
  right G57.61
 nerve, cranial — *see* Disorder, nerve, cranial
 nose G52.0
 occipital M54.81
 olfactory G52.0
 penis N48.9
 perineum R10.2
 postherpetic NEC B02.29
  trigeminal B02.22
 pubic region R10.2
 scrotum R10.2
 Sluder's G90.0
 specified nerve NEC G58.8
 spermatic cord R10.2
 sphenopalatine (ganglion) G44.8
 trifacial — *see* Neuralgia, trigeminal
 trigeminal G50.0
  postherpetic, postzoster B02.22
 vagus (nerve) G52.2
 writer's F48.8
  organic G25.8
Neurapraxia — *see* Injury, nerve
Neurasthenia F48.8
 cardiac F45.8
 gastric F45.8
 heart F45.8
Neurilemmoma (M9560/0) — *see also* Neoplasm,
  nerve, benign
 acoustic (nerve) D33.3
 malignant (M9560/3) — *see also* Neoplasm,
  nerve, malignant
  acoustic (nerve) C72.40
   left C72.42
   right C72.41
Neurilemmosarcoma (M9560/3) — *see* Neoplasm,
  nerve, malignant
Neurinoma (M9560/0) — *see* Neoplasm, nerve,
  benign
Neurinomatosis (M9560/1) — *see* Neoplasm,
  nerve, uncertain behavior
Neuritis (rheumatoid) — *see also* Neuralgia
 abducens (nerve) — *see* Strabismus, paralytic,
  sixth nerve
 accessory (nerve) G52.8
 acoustic (nerve) — *see also* category H93.3
  in (due to)
   infectious disease NEC B99 *[H94.00]*
    bilateral B99 *[H94.03]*
    left B99 *[H94.02]*
    right B99 *[H94.01]*
   parasitic disease NEC B89 *[H94.00]*
    bilateral B99 *[H94.03]*
    left B99 *[H94.02]*
    right B99 *[H94.01]*
  syphilitic A52.15
 alcoholic G62.1
  with psychosis — *see* Psychosis, alcoholic
 amyloid, any site E85 *[G63]*
 arising during pregnancy O26.829
  first trimester O26.821
  second trimester O26.822
  third trimester O26.823
 auditory (nerve) — *see* category H93.3
 brachial — *see* Radiculopathy
  due to displacement, intervertebral disc —
   see Disorder, disc, cervical, with
   neuritis
 cranial nerve
  due to Lyme disease A69.22
  eighth or acoustic or auditory — *see*
   category H93.3

Neuritis — *see also* Neuralgia — *continued*
 cranial nerve — *continued*
  eleventh or accessory g52.8
  fifth or trigeminal G51.1
  first or olfactory G52.0
  fourth or trochlear — *see* Strabismus,
   paralytic, fourth nerve
  second or optic — *see* Neuritis, optic
  seventh or facial G51.8
   newborn (birth injury) P11.3
  sixth or abducent — *see* Strabismus,
   paralytic, sixth nerve
  tenth or vagus G52.2
  third or oculomotor — *see* Strabismus,
   paralytic, third nerve
  twelfth or hypoglossal G52.3
 Déjérine-Sottas G60.0
 diabetic (mononeuropathy) — *see* E09-E13 with
   .41
  polyneuropathy — *see* E09-E13 with .42
 due to
  beriberi E51.11 *[G63]*
  displacement, prolapse or rupture,
   intervertebral disc — *see* Disorder,
   disc, with, radiculopathy
  herniation, nucleus pulposus M51.9 *[G55]*
 endemic E51.11 *[G63]*
 facial G51.8
  newborn (birth injury) P11.3
 general — *see* Polyneuropathy
 geniculate ganglion G51.1
  due to herpes (zoster) B02.21
 gouty M10.00 *[G63]*
 hypoglossal (nerve) G52.3
 ilioinguinal (nerve) G57.90
  left G57.92
  right G57.91
 infectious (multiple) NEC G61.0
 interstitial hypertrophic progressive G60.0
 lumbar M54.16
 lumbosacral M54.17
 multiple — *see also* Polyneuropathy
  endemic E51.11
  infective, acute G61.0
 multiplex endemica E51.11
 nerve root — *see* Radiculopathy
 oculomotor (nerve) — *see* Strabismus,
  paralytic, third nerve
 olfactory nerve G52.0
 optic (nerve) (hereditary) (sympathetic) H46.9
  with demyelination G36.0
  in myelitis G36.0
  nutritional H46.2
  papillitis — *see* Papillitis, optic
  retrobulbar H46.10
   left H46.12
   right H46.11
  specified type NEC H46.8
  toxic H46.3
 peripheral (nerve) G62.9
  complicating pregnancy or puerperium
   O26.829
   first trimester O26.821
   second trimester O26.822
   third trimester O26.823
  multiple — *see* Polyneuropathy
  single — *see* Mononeuritis
 pneumogastric (nerve) G52.2
 postherpetic, postzoster B02.29
 pregnancy-related O26.829
  first trimester O26.821
  second trimester O26.822
  third trimester O26.823
 progressive hypertrophic interstitial G60.0
 puerperal, postpartum O90.8
 retrobulbar — *see also* Neuritis, optic,
  retrobulbar
  in (due to)
   late syphilis A52.15
   meningococcal infection A39.82
  meningococcal A39.82
  syphilitic A52.15
 sciatic (nerve) — *see also* Sciatica
  due to displacement of intervertebral disc —
   see Disorder, disc, with, radiculopathy
 serum T80.6
 shoulder-girdle G54.5

Neuritis — *see also* Neuralgia — *continued*
 specified nerve NEC G58.8
 spinal (nerve) root — *see* Radiculopathy
 syphilitic A52.79
 thenar (median) G56.10
  left G56.12
  right G56.11
 thoracic M54.14
 toxic NEC G62.2
 trochlear (nerve) — *see* Strabismus, paralytic,
  fourth nerve
 vagus (nerve) G52.2
Neuroastrocytoma (M9505/1) — *see* Neoplasm,
  uncertain behavior
Neuroavitaminosis E56.9 *[G99.8]*
Neuroblastoma (M9500/3)
 olfactory (M9522/3) C30.0
 specified site — *see* Neoplasm, malignant
 unspecified site C74.90
Neurochorioretinitis — *see* Chorioretinitis
Neurocirculatory asthenia F45.8
Neurocysticercosis B69.0
Neurocytoma (M9506/0) — *see* Neoplasm, benign
Neurodermatitis (circumscribed) (circumscripta)
  (local) L28.0
 atopic L20.81
 diffuse (Brocq) L20.81
 disseminated L20.81
Neuroencephalomyelopathy, optic G36.0
Neuroepithelioma (M9503/3) — *see also*
  Neoplasm, malignant
 olfactory (M9523/3) C30.0
Neurofibroma (M9540/0) — *see also* Neoplasm,
  nerve, benign
 melanotic (M9541/0) — *see* Neoplasm, nerve,
  benign
 multiple — *see* Neurofibromatosis
 plexiform (M9550/0) — *see* Neoplasm, nerve,
  benign
Neurofibromatosis (multiple) (nonmalignant)
  Q85.0
 malignant (M9540/3) — *see* Neoplasm, nerve,
  malignant
Neurofibrosarcoma (M9540/3) — *see* Neoplasm,
  nerve, malignant
Neurogenic — *see also* condition
 bladder — *see also* Dysfunction, bladder,
  neuromuscular N31.9
  cauda equina syndrome G83.4
 bowel NEC K59.2
 heart F45.8
Neuroglioma (M9505/1) — *see* Neoplasm,
  uncertain behavior
Neurolabyrinthitis (of Dix and Hallpike) — *see*
  Neuronitis, vestibular
Neurolathyrism — *see* Poisoning, food, noxious,
  plant
Neuroleprosy A30.9
Neuroma (M9570/0) — *see also* Neoplasm, nerve,
  benign
 acoustic (nerve) (M9560/0) D33.3
 amputation (stump) (traumatic) (surgical
  complication) (late) T87.30
  arm
   left T87.32
   right T87.31
  leg
   left T87.34
   right T87.33
 digital (toe) G57.60
  left G57.62
  right G57.61
 interdigital (toe) G58.8
  lower limb G57.80
   left G57.82
   right G57.81
  upper limb G56.80
   left G56.82
   right G56.81
 intermetatarsal G57.80
  left G57.82
  right G57.81

©2002 Ingenix, Inc.

Neuroma — *see also* Neoplasm, nerve, benign — *continued*
- Morton's G57.60
  - left G57.62
  - right G57.61
- nonneoplastic
  - arm G56.90
    - left G56.92
    - right G56.91
  - leg G57.90
    - left G57.92
    - right G57.91
  - lower extremity G57.90
    - left G57.92
    - right G57.91
  - upper extremity G56.90
    - left G56.92
    - right G56.91
- optic (nerve) D33.3
- plantar G57.60
  - left G57.62
  - right G57.61
- plexiform (M9550/0) — *see* Neoplasm, nerve, benign
- surgical (nonneoplastic)
  - arm G56.90
    - left G56.92
    - right G56.91
  - leg G57.90
    - left G57.92
    - right G57.91
  - lower extremity G57.90
    - left G57.92
    - right G57.91
  - upper extremity G56.90
    - left G56.92
    - right G56.91

Neuromyalgia — *see* Neuralgia
Neuromyasthenia (epidemic) (postinfectious) G93.3
Neuromyelitis G36.9
- ascending G61.0
- optica G36.0
Neuromyopathy G70.9
- paraneoplastic D49.9 *[G13.0]*
Neuromyotonia (Isaacs) G71.1
Neuronevus (M8725/0) — *see* Nevus
Neuronitis G58.9
- ascending (acute) G57.20
  - left G57.22
  - right G57.21
- vestibular H81.23
  - left H81.21
    - with right H81.22
  - right H81.20
    - with left H81.22
Neuroparalytic — *see* condition
Neuropathy, neuropathic G62.9
- alcoholic G62.1
  - with psychosis — *see* Psychosis, alcoholic
- arm G56.90
  - left G56.92
  - right G56.91
- autonomic, peripheral — *see* Neuropathy, peripheral, autonomic
- axillary G56.90
  - left G56.92
  - right G56.91
- bladder N31.9
  - atonic (motor) (sensory) N31.2
  - autonomous N31.2
  - flaccid N31.2
  - nonreflex N31.2
  - overactive N31.3
  - reflex N31.1
  - uninhibited N31.0
- brachial plexus G54.0
- carcinomatous C80 *[G13.0]*
- cervical plexus G54.2
- chronic
  - progressive segmentally demyelinating G62.8
  - relapsing demyelinating G62.8
  - Déjérine-Sottas G60.0

Neuropathy, neuropathic — *continued*
- diabetic — *see* E09-E13 with .40
  - mononeuropathy — *see* E09-E13 with .41
  - polyneuropathy — *see* E09-E13 with .42
- entrapment G58.9
  - iliohypogastric nerve G57.80
    - left G57.82
    - right G57.81
  - ilioinguinal nerve G57.80
    - left G57.82
    - right G57.81
  - lateral cutaneous nerve of thigh G57.10
    - left G57.12
    - right G57.11
  - median nerve G56.00
    - left G56.02
    - right G56.01
  - obturator nerve G57.80
    - left G57.82
    - right G57.81
  - peroneal nerve G57.30
    - left G57.32
    - right G57.31
  - posterior tibial nerve G57.50
    - left G57.52
    - right G57.51
  - saphenous nerve G57.80
    - left G57.82
    - right G57.81
  - ulnar nerve G56.20
    - left G56.22
    - right G56.21
- facial nerve G51.9
- hereditary G60.9
  - motor and sensory (types I-IV) G60.0
  - sensory G60.8
  - specified NEC G60.8
- hypertrophic G60.0
  - Charcot-Marie-Tooth G60.0
  - Déjérine-Sottas G60.0
  - interstitial progressive G60.0
  - of infancy G60.0
  - Refsum G60.1
- idiopathic G60.9
  - progressive G60.3
  - specified NEC G60.8
- in association with hereditary ataxia G60.2
- intercostal G58.0
- ischemic — *see* Disorder, nerve
- Jamaica (ginger) G62.2
- leg NEC G57.90
  - left G57.92
  - right G57.91
- lower extremity G57.90
  - left G57.92
  - right G57.91
- lumbar plexus G54.1
- median nerve G56.10
  - left G56.12
  - right G56.11
- motor and sensory — *see also* Polyneuropathy
  - hereditary (types I-IV) G60.0
- multiple (acute) (chronic) — *see* Polyneuropathy
- optic (nerve) — *see also* Neuritis, optic
  - ischemic — *see* Disorder, nerve, optic, ischemic
- paraneoplastic (sensorial) (Denny Brown) D49.9 *[G13.0]*
- peripheral (nerve) (*see also* Polyneuropathy) G62.9
  - autonomic G90.9
    - idiopathic G90.0
    - in (due to)
      - amyloidosis E85 *[G99.0]*
      - diabetes mellitus — *see* E09-E13 with .43
      - endocrine disease NEC E34.9 *[G99.0]*
      - gout M10.00 *[G99.0]*
      - hyperthyroidism E05.90 *[G99.0]*
        - with thyroid storm E05.91 *[G99.0]*
      - metabolic disease NEC E88.9 *[G99.0]*
    - idiopathic G60.9
      - progressive G60.3
    - in (due to)
      - antitetanus serum G62.0
      - arsenic G62.2
      - drugs NEC G62.0

Neuropathy, neuropathic — *continued*
- peripheral (*see also* Polyneuropathy) — *continued*
  - in — *continued*
    - lead G62.2
    - organophosphate compounds G62.2
    - toxic agent NEC G62.2
  - plantar nerves G57.60
    - left G57.62
    - right G57.61
  - progressive hypertrophic interstitial G60.9
  - radicular NEC — *see* Radiculopathy
  - sacral plexus G54.1
  - sciatic G57.00
    - left G57.02
    - right G57.01
  - serum G61.1
  - toxic NEC G62.2
  - trigeminal sensory G50.8
  - ulnar nerve G56.20
    - left G56.22
    - right G56.21
  - uremic N18.8 *[G63]*
  - vitamin B12 E53.8 *[G63]*
    - with anemia (pernicious) D51.0 *[G63]*
    - due to dietary deficiency D51.3 *[G63]*
Neurophthisis — *see also* Disorder, nerve
- peripheral, diabetic — *see* E09-E13 with .42
Neuroretinitis — *see* Chorioretinitis
Neuroretinopathy, hereditary optic H47.22
Neurosarcoma (M9540/3) — *see* Neoplasm, nerve, malignant
Neurosclerosis — *see* Disorder, nerve
Neurosis, neurotic F48.9
- anankastic F42
- anxiety (state) F41.1
  - panic type F41.0
- asthenic F48.8
- bladder F45.8
- cardiac (reflex) F45.8
- cardiovascular F45.8
- character F60.9
- climacteric N95.1
- colon F45.8
- compensation F68.8
- compulsive, compulsion F42
- conversion F44.9
- craft F48.8
- cutaneous F45.8
- depersonalization F48.1
- depressive (reaction) (type) F34.1
- environmental F48.8
- excoriation L98.1
- fatigue F48.8
- functional — *see* Disorder, somatoform
- gastric F45.8
- gastrointestinal F45.8
- heart F45.8
- hypochondriacal F45.21
- hysterical F44.9
- incoordination F45.8
  - larynx F45.8
  - vocal cord F45.8
- intestine F45.8
- larynx (sensory) F45.8
  - hysterical F44.4
- menopause N95.1
- mixed NEC F48.8
- musculoskeletal F45.8
- obsessional F42
- obsessive-compulsive F42
- occupational F48.8
- ocular NEC F45.8
- organ — *see* Disorder, somatoform
- pharynx F45.8
- phobic F40.9
- posttraumatic (acute) (situational) F43.9
- psychasthenic (type) F48.8
- railroad F48.8
- rectum F45.8
- respiratory F45.8
- rumination F45.8
- sexual F65.9
- situational F48.8
- social F40.10
  - generalized F40.11

Neurosis, neurotic — *continued*
  specified type NEC F48.8
  state F48.9
    with depersonalization episode F48.1
  stomach F45.8
  traumatic F43.10
    acute F43.11
    chronic F43.12
  vasomotor F45.8
  visceral F45.8
  war F48.8
Neurospongioblastosis diffusa Q85.1
Neurosyphilis (arrested) (early) (gumma) (late)
      (latent) (recurrent) (relapse) A52.3
  with ataxia (cerebellar) (locomotor) (spastic)
      (spinal) A52.19
  aneurysm (cerebral) A52.05
  arachnoid (adhesive) A52.13
  arteritis (any artery) (cerebral) A52.04
  asymptomatic A52.2
  congenital A50.40
  dura (mater) A52.13
  general paresis A52.17
  hemorrhagic A52.05
  juvenile (asymptomatic) (meningeal) A50.40
  leptomeninges (aseptic) A52.13
  meningeal, meninges (adhesive) A52.13
  meningitis A52.12
  meningovascular (diffuse) A52.13
  optic atrophy A52.15
  parenchymatous (degenerative) A52.19
  paresis, paretic A52.17
    juvenile A50.45
  remission in (sustained) A52.3
  serological (without symptoms) A52.2
  specified nature or site NEC A52.19
  tabes, tabetic (dorsalis) A52.11
    juvenile A50.45
  taboparesis A52.17
    juvenile A50.45
  thrombosis (cerebral) A52.05
  vascular (cerebral) NEC A52.05
Neurothekeoma (M9562/0) — *see* Neoplasm,
      nerve, benign
Neurotic — *see* Neurosis
Neurotoxemia — *see* Toxemia
Neutroclusion M26.2
Neutropenia, neutropenic (chronic) (genetic)
      (idiopathic) (immune) (infantile) (malignant)
      (pernicious) (splenic) (splenomegaly) D70.9
  congenital (primary) D70.0
  cyclic D70.4
  cytoreductive cancer chemotherapy sequela
      D70.1
  drug-induced (toxic) D70.2
    due to cytoreductive cancer chemotherapy
      D70.1
  neonatal, transitory (isoimmune) (maternal
      transfer) P61.5
  periodic D70.4
  secondary (cyclic) (periodic) (splenic) D70.3
    drug-induced D70.2
      due to cytoreductive cancer
        chemotherapy D70.1
Neutrophilia, hereditary giant D72.0
Nevocarcinoma (M8720/3) — *see* Melanoma
Nevus (M8720/0) D22.9
  achromic (M8730/0)
  amelanotic (M8730/0)
  angiomatous (M9120/0) D18.00
    intra-abdominal D18.03
    intracranial D18.02
    skin D18.01
    specified site NEC D18.09
  araneus I78.1
  balloon cell (M8722/0)
  bathing trunk (M8761/1) D48.5
  blue (M8780/0)
    cellular (M8790/0)
    giant (M8790/0)
    Jadassohn's (M8780/0)
    malignant (M8780/3) — *see* Melanoma
  capillary (M9131/0) D18.00
    intra-abdominal D18.03
    intracranial D18.02
    skin D18.01

Nevus — *continued*
  capillary — *continued*
    specified site NEC D18.09
  cavernous (M9121/0) D18.00
    intra-abdominal D18.03
    intracranial D18.02
    skin D18.01
    specified site NEC D18.09
  cellular (M8720/0)
    blue (M8790/0)
  choroid D31.30
    left D31.32
    right D31.31
  comedonicus Q82.5
  compound (M8760/0)
  conjunctiva (M8720/0) D31.00
    left D31.02
    right D31.01
  dermal (M8750/0)
    with epidermal nevus (M8760/0)
  dysplastic (M8727/0)
  epitheloid cell (M8771/0)
    with spindle cell (M8770/0)
  eye D31.90
    left D31.92
    right D31.91
  flammeus Q82.5
  hairy (M8720/0)
  halo (M8723/0)
  hemangiomatous (M9120/0) D18.00
    intra-abdominal D18.03
    intracranial D18.02
    skin D18.01
    specified site NEC D18.09
  intradermal (M8750/0)
  intraepidermal (M8740/0)
  involuting (M8724/0)
  iris D31.40
    left D31.42
    right D31.41
  Jadassohn's blue (M8780/0)
  junction, junctional (M8740/0)
    malignant melanoma in (M8740/3) C43.9
  juvenile (M8770/0)
  lacrimal gland D31.50
    left D31.52
    right D31.51
  lymphatic (M9170/0) D18.1
  magnocellular (M8726/0)
    specified site — *see* Neoplasm, benign
    unspecified site D31.40
  malignant (M8720/3) — *see* Melanoma
  meaning hemangioma (M9120/0) D18.00
    intra-abdominal D18.03
    intracranial D18.02
    skin D18.01
    specified site NEC D18.09
  melanotic (pigmented) (M8720/0)
  mouth (mucosa) D10.30
    specified site NEC D10.39
    white sponge Q38.6
  multiplex Q85.1
  non-neoplastic I78.1
  nonpigmented (M8730/0)
  nonvascular (M8720/0)
  oral mucosa D10.30
    specified site NEC D10.39
    white sponge Q38.6
  orbit D31.60
    left D31.62
    right D31.61
  papillaris (M8720/0)
  papillomatosus (M8720/0)
  pigmented (M8720/0)
    giant (M8761/1) — *see also* Neoplasm, skin,
      uncertain behavior D48.5
      malignant melanoma in (M8761/3) — *see*
        Melanoma
  pilosus (M8720/0)
  portwine Q82.5
  regressing (M8723/0)
  retina D31.20
    left D31.22
    right D31.21
  retrobulbar D31.60
    left D31.62
    right D31.61
  sanguineous Q82.5

Nevus — *continued*
  senile I78.1
  skin D22.9
    abdominal wall D22.5
    ala nasi D22.39
    ankle D22.70
      left D22.72
      right D22.71
    anus, anal D22.5
    arm D22.60
      left D22.62
      right D22.61
    auditory canal (external) D22.20
      left D22.22
      right D22.21
    auricle (ear) D22.20
      left D22.22
      right D22.21
    auricular canal (external) D22.20
      left D22.22
      right D22.21
    axilla, axillary fold D22.5
    back D22.5
    breast D22.5
    brow D22.39
    buttock D22.5
    canthus (eye) D22.10
      left D22.12
      right D22.11
    cheek (external) D22.39
    chest wall D22.5
    chin D22.39
    ear (external) D22.20
      left D22.22
      right D22.21
    external meatus (ear) D22.20
      left D22.22
      right D22.21
    eyebrow D22.39
    eyelid (lower) (upper) D22.10
      left D22.12
      right D22.11
    face D22.30
      specified NEC D22.39
    female genital organ (external) NEC D28.0
    finger D22.60
      left D22.62
      right D22.61
    flank D22.5
    foot D22.70
      left D22.72
      right D22.71
    forearm D22.60
      left D22.62
      right D22.61
    forehead D22.39
    foreskin D29.0
    genital organ (external) NEC
      female D28.0
      male D29.9
    gluteal region D22.5
    groin D22.5
    hand D22.60
      left D22.62
      right D22.61
    heel D22.70
      left D22.72
      right D22.71
    helix D22.20
      left D22.22
      right D22.21
    hip D22.70
      left D22.72
      right D22.71
    interscapular region D22.5
    jaw D22.39
    knee D22.70
      left D22.72
      right D22.71
    labium (majus) (minus) D28.0
    leg D22.70
      left D22.72
      right D22.71
    lip (lower) (upper) D22.0
    lower limb D22.70
      left D22.72
      right D22.71

Nevus — *continued*
  skin — *continued*
    male genital organ (external) D29.9
    nail D22.9
      finger D22.60
        left D22.62
        right D22.61
      toe D22.70
        left D22.72
        right D22.71
    nasolabial groove D22.39
    nates D22.5
    neck D22.4
    nose (external) D22.39
    palpebra D22.10
      left D22.12
      right D22.11
    penis D29.0
    perianal skin D22.5
    perineum D22.5
    pinna D22.20
      left D22.22
      right D22.21
    popliteal fossa or space D22.70
      left D22.72
      right D22.71
    prepuce D29.0
    pubes D22.5
    pudendum D28.0
    scalp D22.4
    scrotum D29.4
    shoulder D22.60
      left D22.62
      right D22.61
    skin D22.9
    specified site NEC — *see* Neoplasm, benign
    submammary fold D22.5
    temple D22.39
    thigh D22.70
      left D22.72
      right D22.71
    toe D22.70
      left D22.72
      right D22.71
    trunk NEC D22.5
    umbilicus D22.5
    upper limb D22.60
      left D22.62
      right D22.61
    vulva D28.0
  spider I78.1
  spindle cell (M8772/0)
    with epithelioid cell (M8770/0)
  stellar I78.1
  strawberry Q82.5
  Sutton's (M8723/0)
  unius lateris Q82.5
  Unna's Q82.5
  vascular Q82.5
  verrucous Q82.5
Newborn (infant) (liveborn) (singleton) Z38.2
  born in hospital Z38.00
    by cesarean Z38.01
  born outside hospital Z38.1
  multiple born NEC Z38.8
    born in hospital Z38.68
      by cesarean Z38.69
    born outside hospital Z38.7
  quadruplet Z38.8
    born in hospital Z38.63
      by cesarean Z38.64
    born outside hospital Z38.7
  quintuplet Z38.8
    born in hospital Z38.65
      by cesarean Z38.66
    born outside hospital Z38.7
  triplet Z38.8
    born in hospital Z38.61
      by cesarean Z38.62
    born outside hospital Z38.7
  twin Z38.5
    born in hospital Z38.30
      by cesarean Z38.31
    born outside hospital Z38.4
Newcastle conjunctivitis or disease B30.8
Nezelof's syndrome (pure alymphocytosis) D81.4

Niacin (amide) deficiency E52
Nicolas (-Durand) -Favre disease A55
Nicotine — *see* Tobacco
Nicotinic acid deficiency E52
Niemann-Pick disease or syndrome E75.249
  specified NEC E75.248
  type
    A E75.240
    B E75.241
    C E75.242
    D E75.243
Night
  blindness — *see* Blindness, night
  sweats R61.9
  terrors (child) F51.4
Nightmares (REM sleep type) F51.5
Nipple — *see* condition
Nisbet's chancre A57
Nishimoto (-Takeuchi) disease I67.5
Nitritoid crisis or reaction — *see* Crisis, nitritoid
Nitrosohemoglobinemia D74.8
Njovera A65
No
  diagnosis (feared complaint unfounded) Z71.1
  disease (found) Z04.9
Nocardiosis, nocardiasis A43.9
  cutaneous A43.1
  lung A43.0
  pneumonia A43.0
  pulmonary A43.0
  specified site NEC A43.8
Nocturia R35.1
  psychogenic F45.8
Nocturnal — *see* condition
Nodal rhythm I49.8
Node(s) — *see also* Nodule
  Bouchard's (with arthropathy) M15.2
  Haygarth's M15.8
  Heberden's (with arthropathy) M15.1
  larynx J38.7
  lymph — *see* condition
  milker's B08.0
  Osler's I33.0
  Schmorl's — *see* Schmorl's disease
  singer's J38.2
  teacher's J38.2
  tuberculous — *see* Tuberculosis, lymph gland
  vocal cord J38.2
Nodule(s), nodular
  actinomycotic — *see* Actinomycosis
  breast NEC N63
  colloid (cystic), thyroid E04.9
  cutaneous — *see* Swelling, localized
  endometrial (stromal) (M8930/0) D26.1
  Haygarth's M15.8
  inflammatory — *see* Inflammation
  juxta-articular
    syphilitic A52.77
    yaws A66.7
  larynx J38.7
  milker's B08.0
  prostate — *see* Hyperplasia, prostate
  rheumatoid M06.30
    ankle M06.379
      left M06.372
      right M06.371
    elbow M06.329
      left M06.322
      right M06.321
    foot joint M06.379
      left M06.372
      right M06.371
    hand joint M06.349
      left M06.342
      right M06.341
    hip M06.359
      left M06.352
      right M06.351
    knee M06.369
      left M06.362
      right M06.361
    multiple site M06.39
    shoulder M06.319
      left M06.312

Nodule(s), nodular — *continued*
  rheumatoid — *continued*
    shoulder — *continued*
      right M06.311
    vertebra M06.38
    wrist M06.339
      left M06.332
      right M06.331
  scrotum (inflammatory) N49.2
  singer's J38.2
  solitary, lung J98.4
  subcutaneous — *see* Swelling, localized
  teacher's J38.2
  thyroid (gland) (nontoxic) E04.1
    with thyrotoxicosis E05.20
      with thyroid storm E05.21
    toxic or with hyperthyroidism E05.20
      with thyroid storm E05.21
  vocal cord J38.2
Noise exposure Z58.0
  occupational Z57.0
Noma (gangrenous) (hospital) (infective) A69.0
  auricle I96
  mouth A69.0
  pudendi N76.8
  vulvae N76.8
Nomad, nomadism Z59.0
Nonautoimmune hemolytic anemia D59.4
  drug-induced D59.2
Nonclosure — *see also* Imperfect, closure
  ductus arteriosus (Botallo's) Q25.0
  foramen
    botalli Q21.1
    ovale Q21.1
Noncompliance Z91.19
  with
    dietary regimen Z91.13
    medication regimen Z91.12
      dosage reduction causing withdrawal Z91.11
Nondescent (congenital) — *see also* Malposition, congenital
  cecum Q43.3
  colon Q43.3
  testicle Q53.9
    bilateral Q53.20
      abdominal Q53.21
      perineal Q53.22
    unilateral Q53.10
      abdominal Q53.11
      perineal Q53.12
Nondevelopment
  brain Q02
    part of Q04.3
  heart Q24.8
  organ or site, congenital NEC — *see* Hypoplasia
Nonengagement
  head NEC O32.4
    in labor, causing obstructed labor O64.8
Nonexanthematous tick fever A93.2
Nonexpansion, lung (newborn) P28.0
Nonfunctioning
  cystic duct (*see also* Disease, gallbladder) K82.8
  gallbladder (*see also* Disease, gallbladder) K82.8
  kidney — *see* Failure, renal
  labyrinth — *see* category H83.2
Non-Hodgkin's lymphoma NEC (M9591/3) — *see* Lymphoma, non-Hodgkin's type
Nonimplantation, ovum N97.2
Noninsufflation, fallopian tube N97.1
Non-ketotic hyperglycinemia E72.51
Nonne-Milroy syndrome Q82.0
Nonovulation N97.0
Nonpatent fallopian tube N97.1
Nonpneumatization, lung NEC P28.0
Nonretention food R11.3
  with nausea R11.0
  projectile R11.2
Nonrotation — *see* Malrotation
Nonsecretion, urine — *see* Anuria

Nonunion
> fracture — *see* Fracture, by site
> organ or site, congenital NEC — *see* Imperfect, closure
> symphysis pubis, congenital Q74.2

Nonvisualization, gallbladder R93.2

Nonvital, nonvitalized tooth K04.99

Noonan's syndrome Q87.1

Normal
> delivery O80
> menses Z71.1
> state (feared complaint unfounded) Z71.1

Normocytic anemia (infectional) **due to blood loss** (chronic) D50.0
> acute D62

Norrie's disease (congenital) Q15.8

North American blastomycosis B40.9

Norwegian itch B86

Nose, nasal — *see* condition

Nosebleed R04.0

Nose-picking F98.8

Nosomania F45.21

Nosophobia F45.22

Nostalgia F43.20

Notch of iris Q13.2

Notching nose, congenital (tip) Q30.2

Nothnagel's
> syndrome — *see* Strabismus, paralytic, third nerve
> vasomotor acroparesthesia I73.8

Novy's relapsing fever A68.9
> louse-borne A68.0
> tick-borne A68.1

Noxious
> foodstuffs, poisoning by — *see* Poisoning, food, noxious, plant
> substances transmitted through placenta or breast milk P04.9
> > obstetric anesthetic or analgesic P04.0

Nucleus pulposus — *see* condition

Numbness R20.0

Nuns' knee — *see* Bursitis, prepatellar

Nutcracker esophagus K22.4

Nutmeg liver K76.1

Nutrient element deficiency E61.9
> specified NEC E61.8

Nutrition deficient or insufficient — *see also* Malnutrition E46
> due to
> > insufficient food T73.0
> > lack of
> > > care (child) T76.02
> > > > adult T76.01
> > > food T73.0

Nutritional stunting E45

Nyctalopia (night blindness) — *see* Blindness, night

Nycturia R35.1
> psychogenic F45.8

Nymphomania F52.8

Nystagmus H55.00
> benign paroxysmal — *see* Vertigo, benign paroxysmal
> central positional — *see* category H81.4
> congenital H55.01
> dissociated H55.04
> latent H55.02
> miners' H55
> positional
> > benign paroxysmal — *see* category H81.4
> > central — *see* category H81.4
> specified form NEC H55.09
> visual deprivation H55.03

O

Obermeyer's relapsing fever (European) A68.0

Obesity (simple) E66.9
> with alveolar hyperventilation E66.2
> adrenal E27.8
> constitutional E66.8
> dietary counseling and surveillance Z71.3
> drug-induced E66.1
> due to
> > drug E66.1
> > excess calories E66.09
> > > morbid E66.01
> endocrine E66.8
> endogenous E66.8
> familial E66.8
> glandular E66.8
> hypothyroid — *see* Hypothyroidism
> nutritional E66.09
> pituitary E23.6
> specified type NEC E66.8

Oblique — *see* condition

Obliteration
> appendix (lumen) K38.8
> artery I77.1
> bile duct (noncalculous) K83.1
> common duct (noncalculous) K83.1
> cystic duct — *see* Obstruction, gallbladder
> disease, arteriolar I77.1
> endometrium N85.8
> eye, anterior chamber — *see* Disorder, globe, hypotony
> fallopian tube N97.1
> lymphatic vessel I89.0
> > due to mastectomy I97.2
> organ or site, congenital NEC — *see* Atresia, by site
> placental blood vessels O43.829
> > first trimester O43.821
> > second trimester O43.822
> > third trimester O43.823
> ureter N13.5
> > with infection N13.6
> urethra — *see* Stricture, urethra
> vein I87.8
> vestibule (oral) K08.8

Observation (for) (without need for further medical care) Z04.9
> accident NEC Z04.3
> > at work Z04.2
> > transport Z04.1
> adverse effect of drug Z03.6
> cardiovascular disease Z03.8
> alleged rape or seduction Z04.4
> criminal assault Z04.8
> development state
> > adolescent Z00.3
> > infant or child Z00.10
> > > with abnormal findings Z00.11
> > period of rapid growth in childhood Z00.2
> > puberty Z00.3
> disease
> > cardiovascular NEC Z03.8
> > heart NEC Z03.8
> > mental Z03.8
> > myocardial infarction Z03.8
> > nervous system Z03.8
> > specified NEC Z03.8
> dissocial behavior, without manifest psychiatric disorder Z03.8
> fire-setting (behavior), without manifest psychiatric disorder Z03.8
> following work accident Z04.2
> gang activity (behavior), without manifest psychiatric disorder Z03.8
> growth and development state — *see* Observation, development state
> injuries (accidental) NEC — *see also* Observation, accident
> > inflicted NEC Z04.8
> > > during alleged rape or seduction Z04.4
> malignant neoplasm, suspected Z03.8
> myocardial infarction Z03.8
> postpartum
> > immediately after delivery Z39.0
> > routine follow-up Z39.2

Observation — *continued*
> pregnancy (normal) (without complication) Z34.90
> > first trimester Z34.91
> > high risk O09.90
> > > first trimester O09.91
> > > second trimester O09.92
> > > third trimester O09.93
> > second trimester Z34.92
> > third trimester Z34.93
> rape or seduction (alleged) Z04.4
> shoplifting (behavior), without manifest psychiatric disorder Z03.8
> suicide attempt, alleged NEC Z03.8
> > self-poisoning Z03.6
> suspected (undiagnosed) (unproven)
> > accident at work Z04.2
> > adult battering victim Z04.71
> > behavioral disorder Z03.8
> > cardiovascular disease NEC Z03.8
> > child battering victim Z04.72
> > condition NEC Z03.8
> > drug poisoning or adverse effect Z03.6
> > infectious disease not requiring isolation Z03.8
> > inflicted injury NEC Z04.8
> > malignant neoplasm Z03.8
> > mental disorder Z03.8
> > myocardial infarction Z03.8
> > neoplasm Z03.8
> > nervous system disorder Z03.8
> > suicide attempt, alleged Z03.8
> > > self-poisoning Z03.6
> > toxic effects from ingested substance (drug) (poison) Z03.6
> > tuberculosis Z03.8
> toxic effects from ingested substance (drug) (poison) Z03.6
> tuberculosis, suspected Z03.8

Obsession, obsessional state F42

Obsessive-compulsive neurosis or reaction F42

Obstetric embolism, septic — *see* Embolism, obstetric, septic

Obstetrical trauma (complicating delivery) O71.9
> with or following ectopic or molar pregnancy O08.6
> specified type NEC O71.89

Obstipation — *see* Constipation

Obstruction, obstructed, obstructive
> airway J98.8
> > with
> > > allergic alveolitis J67.9
> > > asthma J45.90
> > > > with
> > > > > acute exacerbation J45.91
> > > > > status asthmaticus J45.92
> > > bronchiectasis J47.9
> > > > with
> > > > > acute exacerbation J47.1
> > > > > lower respiratory infection J47.0
> > > bronchitis (chronic) J44.9
> > > emphysema J43.9
> > chronic J44.9
> > > with
> > > > allergic alveolitis — *see* Pneumonitis, hypersensitivity
> > > > bronchiectasis J47.9
> > > > > with
> > > > > > acute exacerbation J47.1
> > > > > > lower respiratory infection J47.0
> > due to
> > > foreign body — *see* Foreign body, by site, causing asphyxia
> > > inhalation of fumes or vapors J68.9
> > > laryngospasm J38.5
> ampulla of Vater K83.1
> aortic (heart) (valve) — *see* Stenosis, aortic
> aortoiliac I74.0
> aqueduct of Sylvius G91.1
> > congenital Q03.0
> > > with spina bifida — *see* Spina bifida, by site, with hydrocephalus
> Arnold-Chiari — *see* Arnold-Chiari disease
> artery (see also Embolism, artery) I74.9
> > basilar (complete) (partial) — *see* Occlusion, artery, basilar

Obstruction, obstructed, obstructive —
  continued
    artery (*see also* Embolism, artery) — *continued*
      carotid (complete) (partial) — *see* Occlusion, artery, carotid
      cerebellar — *see* Occlusion, artery, cerebellar
      cerebral (anterior) (middle) (posterior) — *see* Occlusion, artery, cerebral
      precerebral — *see* Occlusion, artery, precerebral
      renal N28.0
      retinal NEC — *see* Occlusion, artery, retina
      vertebral (complete) (partial) — *see* Occlusion, artery, vertebral
    band (intestinal) K56.6
    bile duct or passage (common) (hepatic) (noncalculous) K83.1
      with calculus K80.51
      congenital (causing jaundice) Q44.3
    biliary (duct) (tract) K83.1
      gallbladder K82.0
    bladder-neck (acquired) N32.0
      congenital Q64.31
    bowel — *see* Obstruction, intestine
    bronchus J98.0
    canal, ear — *see* Stenosis, external ear canal
    cardia K22.2
    caval veins (inferior) (superior) I87.1
    cecum — *see* Obstruction, intestine
    circulatory I99.8
    colon — *see* Obstruction, intestine
    common duct (noncalculous) K83.1
    coronary (artery) — *see* Occlusion, coronary
    cystic duct — *see also* Obstruction, gallbladder
      with calculus K80.21
    device, implant or graft (*see also* Complications, by site and type, mechanical) T85.628
      arterial graft NEC — *see* Complication, cardiovascular device, mechanical, vascular
      catheter NEC T85.628
        cystostomy T83.090
        dialysis (renal) T82.49
          intraperitoneal T85.691
        infusion NEC T82.594
          spinal (epidural) (subdural) T85.690
        urinary (indwelling) T83.091
      due to infection T85.79
      gastrointestinal — *see* Complications, prosthetic device, mechanical, gastrointestinal device
      genital NEC T83.498
        intrauterine contraceptive device T83.39
        penile prosthesis T83.490
      heart NEC — *see* Complication, cardiovascular device, mechanical
      joint prosthesis — *see* Complication, joint prosthesis, mechanical
      orthopedic NEC — *see* Complication, orthopedic, device, mechanical
      specified NEC T85.628
      urinary NEC — *see also* Complication, genitourinary, device, urinary, mechanical
        graft T83.29
      vascular NEC — *see* Complication, cardiovascular device, mechanical
      ventricular intracranial shunt T85.09
    due to foreign body accidentally left in operative wound T81.529
    duodenum K31.5
    ejaculatory duct N50.8
    esophagus K22.2
    eustachian tube (complete) (partial) H68.109
      bilateral H68.103
      cartilagenous (extrinsic) H68.139
        bilateral H68.133
        intrinsic H68.129
          bilateral H68.123
          left H68.122
          right H68.121
        left H68.132
        right H68.131
      left H68.102

Obstruction, obstructed, obstructive —
  continued
    eustachian tube — *continued*
      osseous H68.119
        bilateral H68.113
        left H68.112
        right H68.111
      right H68.101
    fallopian tube (bilateral) N97.1
    fecal K56.4
      with hernia — *see* Hernia, by site, with obstruction
    foramen of Monro (congenital) Q03.8
      with spina bifida — *see* Spina bifida, by site, with hydrocephalus
    foreign body — *see* Foreign body
    gallbladder K82.0
      with calculus, stones K80.21
      congenital Q44.1
    gastric outlet K31.1
    gastrointestinal — *see* Obstruction, intestine
    hepatic K76.8
      duct (noncalculous) K83.1
    ileum — *see* Obstruction, intestine
    iliofemoral (artery) I74.5
    intestine (mechanical) (neurogenic) (paroxysmal) (postinfective) (reflex) K56.6
      with
        adhesions (intestinal) (peritoneal) K56.5
      adynamic K56.0
      by gallstone K56.3
      congenital (small) Q41.9
        large Q42.9
          specified part NEC Q42.8
      newborn P76.9
        due to
          fecaliths P76.8
          inspissated milk P76.2
          meconium (plug) P76.0
            in mucoviscidosis E84.1
        specified NEC P76.8
      postoperative K91.3
      volvulus K56.2
    intracardiac ball valve prosthesis T82.09
    jejunum — *see* Obstruction, intestine
    labor — *see also* Labor, obstructed
      due to
        bony pelvis (conditions in O33.0-O33.9) O65.0
        pelvic deformity O65.0
        fetopelvic disproportion O65.4
        impacted shoulder O66.0
        malposition (fetus) O64.9
        maternal pelvic abnormality O65.9
          specified NEC O65.8
        persistent occipitoposterior or transverse position O64.0
        soft tissues and organs of pelvis (conditions in O34.00-O34.93) O65.5
      specified NEC O66.8
    lacrimal (passages) (duct)
      by
        dacryolith — *see* Dacryolith
        stenosis — *see* Stenosis, lacrimal
      congenital Q10.5
      neonatal H04.539
        bilateral H04.533
        left H04.532
        right H04.531
    lacrimonasal duct — *see* Obstruction, lacrimal
    lacteal, with steatorrhea K90.2
    laryngitis — *see* Laryngitis
    larynx NEC J38.6
      congenital Q31.8
    lung J98.4
      disease, chronic J44.9
    lymphatic I89.0
    meconium (plug)
      fetus or newborn P76.0
        due to fecaliths P76.0
        in mucoviscidosis E84.1
    mitral — *see* Stenosis, mitral
    nasal J34.8
    nasolacrimal duct — *see also* Obstruction, lacrimal
      congenital Q10.5

Obstruction, obstructed, obstructive —
  continued
    nasopharynx J39.2
    nose J34.8
    organ or site, congenital NEC — *see* Atresia, by site
    pancreatic duct K86.8
    parotid duct or gland K11.8
    pelviureteral junction N13.5
      congenital Q62.11
    pharynx J39.2
    portal (circulation) (vein) I81
    prostate — *see also* Hyperplasia, prostate, with obstruction
      valve (urinary) N32.0
    pulmonary valve (heart) I37.0
    pyelonephritis (chronic) N11.1
    pylorus
      adult K31.1
      congenital or infantile Q40.0
    rectosigmoid — *see* Obstruction, intestine
    rectum K62.4
    renal
      outflow N13.8
      pelvis, congenital Q62.39
    respiratory J98.8
      chronic J44.9
    retinal (vessels) H34.9
    salivary duct (any) K11.8
      with calculus K11.5
    sigmoid — *see* Obstruction, intestine
    sinus (accessory) (nasal) J34.8
    Stensen's duct K11.8
    stomach NEC K31.89
      acute K31.0
      congenital Q40.2
      due to pylorospasm K31.3
    submandibular duct K11.8
    submaxillary gland K11.8
      with calculus K11.5
    thoracic duct I89.0
    thrombotic — *see* Thrombosis
    trachea J39.8
    tracheostomy airway J95.03
    tricuspid (valve) — *see* Stenosis, tricuspid
    upper respiratory, congenital Q34.8
    ureter (functional) (pelvic junction) NEC N13.5
      with
        hydronephrosis N13.1
          with infection N13.6
        pyelonephritis (chronic) N11.1
      congenital Q62.39
      due to calculus — *see* Calculus, ureter
    urethra NEC N36.8
      congenital Q64.39
    urinary (moderate) N13.9
      organ or tract (lower) N13.9
      prostatic valve N32.0
    uropathy N13.9
    uterus N85.8
    vagina N89.5
    valvular — *see* Endocarditis
    vein, venous I87.1
      caval (inferior) (superior) I87.1
      thrombotic — *see* Thrombosis
    vena cava (inferior) (superior) I87.1
    vesical NEC N32.0
    vesicourethral orifice N32.0
      congenital Q64.31
    vessel NEC I99.8

Obturator — *see* condition

Occlusal wear, teeth K03.0

Occlusio pupillae — *see* Membrane, pupillary

Occlusion, occluded
  anus K62.4
    congenital Q42.3
      with fistula Q42.2
  aortoiliac (chronic) I74.0
  aqueduct of Sylvius G91.1
    congenital Q03.0
      with spina bifida — *see* Spina bifida, by site, with hydrocephalus

Occlusion, occluded — *continued*
  artery (*see also* Embolism, artery) I74.9
    auditory, internal I65.8
    basilar I65.1
      with
        infarction I63.2
          due to
            embolism I63.1
            thrombosis I63.0
        other precerebral artery I65.3
      bilateral I65.3
    brain or cerebral I66.9
      with infarction (due to) I63.5
        embolism I63.4
        thrombosis I63.3
    carotid I65.2
      with
        infarction I63.2
          due to
            embolism I63.1
            thrombosis I63.0
        other precerebral artery I65.3
      bilateral I65.3
    cerebellar (anterior inferior) (posterior
      inferior) (superior) I66.3
      with infarction I63.5
        due to
          embolism I63.4
          thrombosis I63.3
    cerebral I66.9
      with infarction I63.5
        due to
          embolism I63.4
          thrombosis I63.3
      anterior I66.1
        with infarction I63.5
          due to
            embolism I63.4
            thrombosis I63.3
      bilateral I66.4
      middle I66.0
        with infarction I63.5
          due to
            embolism I63.4
            thrombosis I63.3
      multiple or bilateral I66.4
        with infarction I63.5
          due to
            embolism I63.4
            thrombosis I63.3
      posterior I66.2
        with infarction I63.5
          due to
            embolism I63.4
            thrombosis I63.3
      specified NEC I66.8
        with infarction I63.5
          due to
            embolism I63.4
            thrombosis I63.3
    choroidal (anterior) — *see* Occlusion, artery,
      cerebral, specified NEC
    communicating posterior — *see* Occlusion,
      artery, cerebral, specified NEC
    coronary (acute) (thrombotic) (without
      myocardial infarction) I24.0
      with myocardial infarction — *see*
        Infarction, myocardium
      healed or old I25.2
    hypophyseal — *see* Occlusion, artery,
      precerebral, specified NEC
    iliac I74.5
    lower extremities due to stenosis or stricture
      I77.1
    mesenteric (embolic) (thrombotic) K55.0
    perforating — *see* Occlusion, artery,
      cerebral, specified NEC
    peripheral I77.9
      thrombotic or embolic I74.4
    pontine — *see* Occlusion, artery, cerebral,
      specified NEC
    precerebral I65.9
      with infarction I63.2
        due to
          embolism I63.1
          thrombosis I63.0

Occlusion, occluded — *continued*
  artery (*see also* Embolism, artery) — *continued*
    precerebral — *continued*
      basilar — *see* Occlusion, artery, basilar
      carotid — *see* Occlusion, artery, carotid
      complicating
        childbirth O88.22
        pregnancy O88.219
          first trimester O88.211
          second trimester O88.212
          third trimester O88.213
      multiple or bilateral I65.3
        with infarction I63.2
          due to
            embolism I63.1
            thrombosis I63.0
      puerperal O88.23
      specified NEC I65.8
        with infarction I63.2
          due to
            embolism I00.1
            thrombosis I63.0
      vertebral — *see* Occlusion, artery,
        vertebral
    renal N28.0
    retinal
      central H34.10
        bilateral H34.13
        left H34.12
        right H34.11
      partial H34.219
        bilateral H34.213
        left H34.212
        right H34.211
      branch H34.239
        bilateral H34.233
        left H34.232
        right H34.231
      transient H34.00
        left H34.02
        right H34.01
    spinal — *see* Occlusion, artery, precerebral,
      vertebral
    vertebral I65.0
      with
        infarction I63.2
          due to
            embolism I63.1
            thrombosis I63.0
        other precerebral artery I65.3
      bilateral I65.3
  basilar artery — *see* Occlusion, artery, basilar
  bile duct (common) (hepatic) (noncalculous)
    K83.1
  bowel — *see* Obstruction, intestine
  carotid (artery) (common) (internal) — *see*
    Occlusion, artery, carotid
  cerebellar (artery) — *see* Occlusion, artery,
    cerebellar
  cerebral (artery) — *see* Occlusion, artery,
    cerebral
  cerebrovascular — *see also* Occlusion, artery,
    cerebral
    with infarction I63.5
    diffuse (without infarction) I66.9
  cervical canal — *see* Stricture, cervix
  cervix (uteri) — *see* Stricture, cervix
  choanal Q30.0
  choroidal (artery) I65.8
  colon — *see* Obstruction, intestine
  communicating posterior artery — *see*
    Occlusion, artery, precerebral, specified
    NEC
  coronary (artery) (vein) (thrombotic) — *see also*
    Infarct, myocardium
    healed or old I25.2
    not resulting in infarction I24.0
  cystic duct — *see* Obstruction, gallbladder
  embolic — *see* Embolism
  fallopian tube N97.1
    congenital Q50.6
  gallbladder — *see also* Obstruction, gallbladder
    congenital (causing jaundice) Q44.1
  gingiva, traumatic K06.2
  hymen N89.6
    congenital Q52.3

Occlusion, occluded — *continued*
  hypophyseal (artery) — *see* Occlusion, artery,
    precerebral, specified NEC
  iliac artery I74.5
  intestine — *see* Obstruction, intestine
  lacrimal passages — *see* Obstruction, lacrimal
  lung J98.4
  lymph or lymphatic channel I89.0
  mammary duct N64.8
  mesenteric artery (embolic) (thrombotic) K55.0
  nose J34.8
    congenital Q30.0
  organ or site, congenital NEC — *see* Atresia, by
    site
  oviduct N97.1
    congenital Q50.6
  peripheral arteries
    due to stricture or stenosis I77.1
    upper extremity I74.3
  pontine (artery) — *see* Occlusion, artery,
    precerebral, specified NEC
  posterior lingual, of mandibular teeth M26.2
  precerebral artery — *see* Occlusion, artery,
    precerebral
  punctum lacrimale — *see* Obstruction, lacrimal
  pupil — *see* Membrane, pupillary
  pylorus, adult (*see also* Stricture, pylorus)
    K31.1
  renal artery N28.0
  retina, retinal
    artery — *see* Occlusion, artery, retinal
    vein (central) H34.819
      bilateral H34.813
      engorgement H34.829
        bilateral H34.823
        left H34.822
        right H34.821
      left H34.812
      right H34.811
      tributary H34.839
        bilateral H34.833
        left H34.832
        right H34.831
    vessels H34.9
  spinal artery — *see* Occlusion, artery,
    precerebral, vertebral
  teeth (mandibular) (posterior lingual) M26.2
  thoracic duct I89.0
  thrombotic — *see* Thrombosis, artery
  traumatic
    edentulous (alveolar) ridge K06.2
    gingiva K06.2
    periodontal K05.5
  tubal N97.1
  ureter (complete) (partial) N13.5
    congenital Q62.10
  ureteropelvic junction N13.5
    congenital Q62.11
  ureterovesical orifice N13.5
    congenital Q62.12
  urethra — *see* Stricture, urethra
  uterus N85.8
  vagina N89.5
  vascular NEC I99.8
  vein — *see* Thrombosis
    retinal — *see* Occlusion, retinal, vein
  vena cava (inferior) (superior) I82.2
  ventricle (brain) NEC G91.1
  vertebral (artery) — *see* Occlusion, artery,
    vertebral
  vessel (blood) I99.8
  vulva N90.5

Occupational
  problems NEC Z56.89
  therapy Z51.89

Ochlophobia — *see* Agoraphobia

Ochronosis (endogenous) E70.29

Ocular muscle — *see* condition

Oculogyric crisis or disturbance H51.8
  psychogenic F45.8

Oculomotor syndrome H51.9

Oculopathy
  syphilitic NEC A52.71
    congenital
      early A50.01 *[H58]*
      late A50.30

©2002 Ingenix, Inc.

Oculopathy — *continued*
  syphilitic NEC — *continued*
    early (secondary) A51.43
    late A52.71
Oddi's sphincter spasm K83.4
Odontalgia K08.8
Odontoameloblastoma (M9311/0) D16.5
  upper jaw (bone) D16.4
Odontoclasia K02.4
Odontodysplasia, regional K00.4
Odontogenesis imperfecta K00.5
Odontoma (M9280/0) D16.5
  ameloblastic (M9311/0) D16.5
    upper jaw (bone) D16.4
  complex (M9282/0) D16.5
    upper jaw (bone) D16.4
  compound (M9281/0) D16.5
    upper jaw (bone) D16.4
  fibroameloblastic (M9290/0) D16.5
    upper jaw (bone) D16.4
  upper jaw (bone) (M9280/0) D16.4
Odontomyelitis (closed) (open) K04.0
Odontorrhagia K08.8
Odontosarcoma, ameloblastic (M9290/3) C41.1
  upper jaw (bone) C41.0
Oedema, oedematous — *see* Edema
Oesophag(o)— *see* Esophag(o)-
Oestriasis — *see* Myiasis
Oguchi's disease H53.63
Ohara's disease — *see* Tularemia
Oidiomycosis — *see* Candidiasis
Oidium albicans infection — *see* Candidiasis
Old age (without mention of debility) R54
  dementia F03
Olfactory — *see* condition
Oligemia — *see* Anemia
Oligoastrocytoma, mixed (M9382/3)
  specified site — *see* Neoplasm, malignant
  unspecified site C71.9
Oligocythemia D64.9
Oligodendroblastoma (M9460/3)
  specified site — *see* Neoplasm, malignant
  unspecified site C71.9
Oligodendroglioma (M9450/3)
  anaplastic type (M9451/3)
    specified site — *see* Neoplasm, malignant
    unspecified site C71.9
  specified site — *see* Neoplasm, malignant
  unspecified site C71.9
Oligodontia — *see* Anodontia
Oligoencephalon Q02
Oligohidrosis L74.4
Oligohydramnios O41.00
  first trimester O41.01
  second trimester O41.02
  third trimester O41.03
Oligohydrosis L74.4
Oligomenorrhea N91.5
  primary N91.3
  secondary N91.4
Oligophrenia — *see also* Retardation, mental
  phenylpyruvic E70.0
Oligospermia N46.11
  due to
    drug therapy N46.121
    efferent duct obstruction N46.123
    infection N46.122
    radiation N46.124
    specified cause NEC N46.129
    systemic disease N46.125
Oligotrichia — *see* Alopecia
Oliguria R34
  with, complicating or following ectopic or molar
    pregnancy O08.4
  postprocedural N99.0
Ollier's disease Q78.4
Omentitis — *see* Peritonitis
Omenotocele — *see* Hernia, abdomen, specified
  site NEC
Omentum, omental — *see* condition

Omphalitis (congenital) (newborn) (with mild
  hemorrhage) P38
  not of newborn L08.82
  tetanus A33
Omphalocele Q79.2
Omphalomesenteric duct, persistent Q43.0
Omphalorrhagia, newborn P51.9
Omsk hemorrhagic fever A98.1
Onanism (excessive) F98.8
Onchocerciasis, onchocercosis B73.1
  with
    eye disease B73.00
      endophthalmitis B73.01
      eyelid B73.09
      glaucoma B73.02
      specified NEC B73.09
  eye NEC B73.00
  eyelid B73.09
Oncocytoma (M8290/0) — *see* Neoplasm, benign
Oncovirus, as cause of disease classified
  elsewhere B97.32
Ondine's curse — *see* Apnea, sleep
Oneirophrenia F23
Onychauxis L60.2
  congenital Q84.5
Onychia — *see also* Cellulitis, digit
  with lymphangitis — *see* Lymphangitis, acute,
    digit
  candidal B37.2
  dermatophytic B35.1
Onychitis — *see also* Cellulitis, digit
  with lymphangitis — *see* Lymphangitis, acute,
    digit
Onychocryptosis L60.0
Onychodystrophy L60.3
  congenital Q84.6
Onychogryphosis, onychogryposis L60.2
Onycholysis L60.1
Onychomadesis L60.8
Onychomalacia L60.3
Onychomycosis (finger) (toe) B35.1
Onycho-osteodysplasia Q79.8
Onychophagia F98.8
Onychophosis L60.8
Onychoptosis L60.8
Onychorrhexis L60.3
  congenital Q84.6
Onychoschizia L60.3
Onyxis (finger) (toe) L60.0
Onyxitis — *see also* Cellulitis, digit
  with lymphangitis — *see* Lymphangitis, acute,
    digit
Oophoritis (cystic) (infectional) (interstitial)
  N70.92
  with salpingitis N70.93
  acute N70.02
    with salpingitis N70.03
  chronic N70.12
    with salpingitis N70.13
  complicating abortion — *see* Abortion, by type,
    complicated by, oophoritis
Oophorocele N83.4
Opacity, opacities
  cornea H17.9
    central H17.10
      bilateral H17.13
      left H17.12
      right H17.11
    congenital Q13.3
    degenerative — *see* Degeneration, cornea
    hereditary — *see* Dystrophy, cornea
    inflammatory — *see* Keratitis
    minor H17.819
      bilateral H17.813
      left H17.812
      right H17.811
    peripheral H17.829
      bilateral H17.823
      left H17.822
      right H17.821
    sequelae of trachoma (healed) B94.0

Opacity, opacities — *continued*
  cornea — *continued*
    specified NEC H17.89
  enamel (teeth) (fluoride) (nonfluoride) K00.3
  lens — *see* Cataract
  snowball — *see* Deposit, crystalline
  vitreous (humor) NEC H43.399
    bilateral H43.393
    congenital Q14.0
    left H43.392
    membranes and strands H43.319
      bilateral H43.313
      left H43.312
      right H43.311
    right H43.391
Opalescent dentin (hereditary) K00.5
Open, opening
  abnormal, organ or site, congenital — *see*
    Imperfect, closure
  angle with
    borderline intraocular pressure H40.0
    cupping of discs H40.0
    glaucoma (primary) — *see* Glaucoma, open
      angle
  bite (anterior) (posterior) M26.2
  false — *see* Imperfect, closure
  wound — *see* Wound, open
Operation R69
Operational fatigue F48.8
Operative — *see* condition
Operculitis (chronic) K05.3
  acute K05.2
Operculum — *see* Break, retina
Ophiasis L63.2
Ophthalmia (*see also* Conjunctivitis) H10.9
  actinic rays — *see* Photokeratitis
  allergic (acute) — *see* Conjunctivitis, acute,
    atopic
  blennorrhagic (gonococcal) (neonatorum)
    A54.31
  diphtheritic A36.86
  Egyptian A71.1
  electrica — *see* Photokeratitis
  gonococcal (neonatorum) A54.31
  metastatic — *see* Endophthalmitis, purulent
  migraine G43.8
  neonatorum, newborn P39.1
    gonococcal A54.31
  nodosa H16.249
    bilateral H16.243
    left H16.242
    right H16.241
  purulent — *see* Conjunctivitis, acute,
    mucopurulent
  spring — *see* Conjunctivitis, acute, atopic
  sympathetic — *see* Uveitis, sympathetic
Ophthalmitis — *see* Ophthalmia
Ophthalmocele (congenital) Q15.8
Ophthalmoneuromyelitis G36.0
Ophthalmoplegia — *see also* Strabismus,
  paralytic
  anterior internuclear — *see* Ophthalmoplegia,
    internuclear
  ataxia-areflexia G61.0
  diabetic — *see* E09-E13 with .39
  exophthalmic E05.00
    with thyroid storm E05.01
  external H49.889
    bilateral H49.883
    left H49.882
    progressive H49.40
      with pigmentary retinopathy — *see*
        Kearns-Sayre syndrome
      bilateral H49.43
      left H49.42
      right H49.41
    right H49.881
    total H49.30
      bilateral H49.33
      left H49.32
      right H49.31
  internal (complete) (total) H52.519
    bilateral H52.513
    left H52.512
    right H52.511

Ophthalmoplegia — *see also* Strabismus,
  paralytic — *continued*
  internuclear H51.20
    bilateral H51.23
    left H51.22
    right H51.21
  migraine G43.8
  Parinaud's H49.889
    bilateral H49.883
    left H49.882
    right H49.881
  progressive external — *see* Ophthalmoplegia,
    external, progressive
  supranuclear, progressive G23.1
  total (external) — *see* Ophthalmoplegia,
    external, total
Opioid(s) — *see* Disorder, drug-related, opioid
Opisthognathism M26.09
Opisthorchiasis (felineus) (viverrini) B66.0
Opitz' disease D73.2
Opiumism — *see* Dependence, drug, opioid
Oppenheim's disease G70.2
Oppenheim-Urbach disease E88.8
Optic nerve — *see* condition
Orbit — *see* condition
Orchioblastoma (M9071/3) C62.90
  left C62.92
  right C62.91
Orchitis (gangrenous) (nonspecific) (septic)
  (suppurative) N45.2
  blennorrhagic (gonococcal) (acute) (chronic)
    A54.23
  chlamydial A56.19
  filarial B74.9
  gonococcal (acute) (chronic) A54.23
  mumps B26.0
  syphilitic A52.76
  tuberculous A18.15
Orf (virus disease) B08.0
Organ of Morgagni (persistence of)
  female Q52.8
  male Q55.4
Organic — *see also* condition
  heart — *see* Disease, heart
  insufficiency R68.8
Oriental
  bilharziasis B65.2
  schistosomiasis B65.2
Orientation, sexual, egodystonic (bisexual,
  heterosexual, homosexual, prepubertal) F66
Orifice — *see* condition
**Origin of both great vessels from right
  ventricle** Q20.1
Ormond's disease (with ureteral obstruction)
  N13.5
  with infection N13.6
Ornithine metabolism disorder E72.4
Ornithinemia (Type I) (Type II) E72.4
Ornithosis A70
  with pneumonia A70
Orotaciduria, oroticaciduria (congenital)
  (hereditary) (pyrimidine deficiency) D53.0
Orotic aciduria (congenital) (hereditary)
  (pyrimidine deficiency) E79.8
  anemia D53.0
Orthodontics Z51.89
  adjustment Z46.4
  fitting Z46.4
Orthopnea R06.01
Orthoptic training Z51.89
Os, uterus — *see* condition
Osgood-Schlatter disease or osteochondrosis —
  see Osteochondrosis, juvenile, tibia
Osler (-Weber) -Rendu disease I78.0
Osler's nodes I33.0
Osmidrosis L75.0
Osseous — *see* condition
Ossification
  artery — *see* Arteriosclerosis
  auricle (ear) — *see* Disorder, pinna, specified
    type NEC

Ossification — *continued*
  bronchial J98.0
  cardiac — *see* Degeneration, myocardial
  cartilage (senile) — *see* Disorder, cartilage,
    specified type NEC
  coronary (artery) — *see* Disease, heart,
    ischemic, atherosclerotic
  diaphragm J98.6
  ear, middle — *see* Otosclerosis
  falx cerebri G96.1
  fontanel, premature Q75.0
  heart — *see also* Degeneration, myocardial
    valve — *see* Endocarditis
  larynx J38.7
  ligament — *see* Disorder, tendon, specified type
    NEC
    posterior longitudinal — *see* Spondylopathy,
      specified NEC
  meninges (cerebral) (spinal) G96.1
  multiple, eccentric centers — *see* Disorder,
    bone, development or growth
  muscle — *see also* Calcification, muscle
    due to burns — *see* Myositis, ossificans, in,
      burns
    paralytic — *see* Myositis, ossificans, in,
      quadriplegia
    progressive — *see* Myositis, ossificans,
      progressiva
    specified NEC M61.50
      ankle M61.579
        left M61.572
        right M61.571
      foot M61.579
        left M61.572
        right M61.571
      forearm M61.539
        left M61.532
        right M61.531
      hand M61.549
        left M61.542
        right M61.541
      lower leg M61.569
        left M61.562
        right M61.561
      multiple sites M61.59
      pelvic region M61.559
        left M61.552
        right M61.551
      shoulder region M61.519
        left M61.512
        right M61.511
      specified site NEC M61.58
      thigh M61.559
        left M61.552
        right M61.551
      upper arm M61.529
        left M61.522
        right M61.521
    traumatic — *see* Myositis, ossificans,
      traumatica
  myocardium, myocardial — *see* Degeneration,
    myocardial
  penis N48.89
  periarticular — *see* Disorder, joint, specified
    type NEC
  pinna — *see* Disorder, pinna, specified type
    NEC
  rider's bone — *see* Ossification, muscle,
    specified NEC
  sclera H15.89
  subperiosteal, post-traumatic — *see* Disorder,
    bone, specified type NEC
  tendon — *see* Disorder, tendon, specified type
    NEC
  trachea J39.8
  tympanic membrane — *see* Disorder, tympanic
    membrane, specified NEC
  vitreous (humor) — *see* Deposit, crystalline
Osteitis — *see also* Osteomyelitis
  alveolar M27.3
  condensans M85.30
    ankle M85.379
      left M85.372
      right M85.371

Osteitis — *see also* Osteomyelitis — *continued*
  condensans — *continued*
    foot M85.379
      left M85.372
      right M85.371
    forearm M85.339
      left M85.332
      right M85.331
    hand M85.349
      left M85.342
      right M85.341
    lower leg M85.369
      left M85.362
      right M85.361
    multiple site M85.39
    neck M85.38
    rib M85.38
    shoulder M85.319
      left M85.312
      right M85.311
    skull M85.38
    specified site NEC M85.38
    thigh M85.359
      left M85.352
      right M85.351
    toe M85.379
      left M85.372
      right M85.371
    upper arm M85.329
      left M85.322
      right M85.321
    vertebra M85.38
  deformans M88.9
  in (due to)
    malignant neoplasm of bone (M8000/3)
      C41.9 *[M90.60]*
    neoplastic disease (*see also* Neoplasm)
      D49.9 *[M90.60]*
      carpus D49.9 *[M90.649]*
        left D49.9 *[M90.642]*
        right D49.9 *[M90.641]*
      clavicle D49.9 *[M90.619]*
        left D49.9 *[M90.612]*
        right D49.9 *[M90.611]*
      femur D49.9 *[M90.659]*
        left D49.9 *[M90.652]*
        right D49.9 *[M90.651]*
      fibula D49.9 *[M90.669]*
        left D49.9 *[M90.662]*
        right D49.9 *[M90.661]*
      finger D49.9 *[M90.649]*
        left D49.9 *[M90.642]*
        right D49.9 *[M90.641]*
      humerus D49.9 *[M90.629]*
        left D49.9 *[M90.622]*
        right D49.9 *[M90.621]*
      ilium D49.9 *[M90.659]*
      ischium D49.9 *[M90.659]*
      metacarpus D49.9 *[M90.649]*
        left D49.9 *[M90.642]*
        right D49.9 *[M90.641]*
      metatarsus D49.9 *[M90.679]*
        left D49.9 *[M90.672]*
        right D49.9 *[M90.671]*
      multiple sites D49.9 *[M90.69]*
      neck D49.9 *[M90.68]*
      radius D49.9 *[M90.639]*
        left D49.9 *[M90.632]*
        right D49.9 *[M90.631]*
      rib D49.9 *[M90.68]*
      scapula D49.9 *[M90.619]*
        left D49.9 *[M90.612]*
        right D49.9 *[M90.611]*
      skull D49.9 *[M90.68]*
      tarsus D49.9 *[M90.679]*
        left D49.9 *[M90.672]*
        right D49.9 *[M90.671]*
      tibia D49.9 *[M90.669]*
        left D49.9 *[M90.662]*
        right D49.9 *[M90.661]*
      toe D49.9 *[M90.679]*
        left D49.9 *[M90.672]*
        right D49.9 *[M90.671]*

©2002 Ingenix, Inc.

Osteitis — *see also* Osteomyelitis — *continued*
deformans — *continued*
  in — *continued*
    neoplastic disease — *continued*
      ulna D49.9 [M90.639]
        left D49.9 [M90.632]
        right D49.9 [M90.631]
      vertebra D49.9 [M90.68]
    skull M88.0
    specified NEC — *see* Paget's disease, bone,
      by site
    vertebra M88.1
  due to yaws A66.6
  fibrosa NEC — *see* Cyst, bone, by site
    circumscripta — *see* Dysplasia, fibrous,
      bone NEC
    cystica (generalisata) E21.0
    disseminata Q78.1
    osteoplastica E21.0
  fragilitans Q78.0
  Garr,'s (sclerosing) — *see* Osteomyelitis,
    specified type NEC
  jaw (acute) (chronic) (lower) (suppurative)
    (upper) M27.2
  parathyroid E21.0
  petrous bone (acute) (chronic) — *see* Petrositis
  sclerotic, nonsuppurative — *see* Osteomyelitis,
    specified type NEC
  tuberculosa A18.09
    cystica D86.89
    multiplex cystoides D86.89
Osteoarthritis — *see also* Arthrosis
  post-traumatic NEC M19.92
    ankle M19.179
      left M19.172
      right M19.171
    elbow M19.129
      left M19.122
      right M19.121
    foot joint M19.179
      left M19.172
      right M19.171
    hand joint M19.149
      first carpometacarpal joint M18.30
        bilateral M18.2
        left M18.32
        right M18.31
      left M19.142
      right M19.141
    hip M16.50
      bilateral M16.4
      left M16.52
      right M16.51
    knee M17.30
      bilateral M17.2
      left M17.32
      right M17.31
    shoulder M19.119
      left M19.112
      right M19.111
    wrist M19.139
      left M19.132
      right M19.131
  primary M19.91
    ankle M19.079
      left M19.072
      right M19.071
    elbow M19.029
      left M19.022
      right M19.021
    foot joint M19.079
      left M19.072
      right M19.071
    hand joint M19.049
      first carpometacarpal joint M18.10
        bilateral M18.0
        left M18.12
        right M18.11
      left M19.042
      right M19.041
    hip M16.10
      bilateral M16.0
      left M16.12
      right M16.11

Osteoarthritis — *continued*
  primary — *continued*
    knee M17.10
      bilateral M17.0
      left M17.12
      right M17.11
    shoulder M19.019
      left M19.012
      right M19.011
    spine — *see* Spondylosis
    wrist M19.039
      left M19.032
      right M19.031
  secondary M19.93
    ankle M19.279
      left M19.272
      right M19.271
    elbow M19.229
      left M19.222
      right M19.221
    foot joint M19.279
      left M19.272
      right M19.271
    hand joint M19.249
      first carpometacarpal joint M18.50
        bilateral M18.4
        left M18.52
        right M18.51
      left M19.242
      right M19.241
    hip M16.7
      bilateral M16.6
    knee M17.5
      bilateral M17.4
    multiple M15.3
    shoulder M19.219
      left M19.212
      right M19.211
    spine — *see* Spondylosis
    wrist M19.239
      left M19.232
      right M19.231
Osteoarthropathy (hypertrophic) (*see also*
  Osteoarthrosis) M19.90
  ankle — *see* Osteoarthritis, primary, ankle
  elbow — *see* Osteoarthritis, primary, elbow
  foot joint — *see* Osteoarthritis, primary, foot
  hand joint — *see* Osteoarthritis, primary, hand
    joint
  multiple site — *see* Osteoarthritis, primary,
    multiple joint
  pulmonary — *see also* Osteoarthropathy,
    specified type NEC
    hypertrophic — *see* Osteoarthropathy,
      hypertrophic, specified type NEC
  secondary hypertrophic — *see*
    Osteoarthropathy, specified type NEC
  shoulder — *see* Osteoarthritis, primary,
    shoulder
  specified joint NEC — *see* Osteoarthritis,
    primary, specified joint NEC
  specified type NEC M89.40
    carpus M89.449
      left M89.442
      right M89.441
    clavicle M89.419
      left M89.412
      right M89.411
    femur M89.459
      left M89.452
      right M89.451
    fibula M89.469
      left M89.462
      right M89.461
    finger M89.449
      left M89.442
      right M89.441
    humerus M89.429
      left M89.422
      right M89.421
    ilium M89.459
    ischium M89.459
    metacarpus M89.449
      left M89.442
      right M89.441

Osteoarthropathy (*see also* Osteoarthrosis) —
  continued
  specified type NEC — *continued*
    metatarsus M89.479
      left M89.472
      right M89.471
    multiple sites M89.49
    neck M89.48
    radius M89.439
      left M89.432
      right M89.431
    rib M89.48
    scapula M89.419
      left M89.412
      right M89.411
    skull M89.48
    tarsus M89.479
      left M89.472
      right M89.471
    tibia M89.469
      left M89.462
      right M89.461
    toe M89.479
      left M89.472
      right M89.471
    ulna M89.439
      left M89.432
      right M89.431
    vertebra M89.48
  secondary — *see* Osteoarthropathy, specified
    type NEC
  spine — *see* Spondylosis
  wrist — *see* Osteoarthritis, primary, wrist
Osteoarthrosis (degenerative) (hypertrophic)
  (joint) — *see also* Arthrosis
  deformans alkaptonurica E70.29 [M36.8]
  erosive M15.4
  generalized M15.9
    primary M15.0
  polyarticular M15.9
  primary — *see* Arthrosis, primary NEC
  secondary NEC — *see* Arthrosis, secondary
    NEC
  spine — *see* Spondylosis
Osteoblastoma (M9200/0) — *see* Neoplasm,
  bone, benign
  aggressive (M9200/1) — *see* Neoplasm, bone,
    uncertain behavior
Osteochondroarthrosis deformans endemica —
  see Disease, Kaschin-Beck
Osteochondritis — *see also* Osteochondropathy,
  by site
  Brailsford's — *see* Osteochondrosis, juvenile,
    radius
  dissecans M93.20
    ankle M93.279
      left M93.272
      right M93.271
    elbow M93.229
      left M93.222
      right M93.221
    foot M93.279
      left M93.272
      right M93.271
    hand M93.249
      left M93.242
      right M93.241
    hip M93.259
      left M93.252
      right M93.251
    knee M93.269
      left M93.262
      right M93.261
    multiple sites M93.29
    shoulder joint M93.219
      left M93.212
      right M93.211
    specified site NEC M93.28
    wrist M93.239
      left M93.232
      right M93.231
  juvenile M92.9
    patellar — *see* Osteochondrosis, juvenile,
      patella

Osteochondritis — *see also* Osteochondropathy,
  by site — *continued*
   syphilitic (congenital) (early) A50.02 *[M90.80]*
     ankle A50.02 *[M90.879]*
      left A50.02 *[M90.872]*
      right A50.02 *[M90.871]*
     elbow A50.02 *[M90.829]*
      left A50.02 *[M90.822]*
      right A50.02 *[M90.821]*
     foot A50.02 *[M90.879]*
      left A50.02 *[M90.872]*
      right A50.02 *[M90.871]*
     forearm A50.02 *[M90.839]*
      left A50.02 *[M90.832]*
      right A50.02 *[M90.831]*
     hand A50.02 *[M90.849]*
      left A50.02 *[M90.842]*
      right A50.02 *[M90.841]*
     hip A50.02 *[M90.859]*
      left A50.02 *[M90.852]*
      right A50.02 *[M90.851]*
     knee A50.02 *[M90.869]*
      left A50.02 *[M90.862]*
      right A50.02 *[M90.861]*
     multiple sites A50.02 *[M90.89]*
     shoulder joint A50.02 *[M90.819]*
      left A50.02 *[M90.812]*
      right A50.02 *[M90.811]*
     specified site NEC A50.02 *[M90.88]*
Osteochondrodysplasia Q78.9
  with defects of growth of tubular bones and
    spine Q77.9
   specified NEC Q77.8
  specified NEC Q78.8
Osteochondrodystrophy E78.9
Osteochondrolysis — *see* Osteochondritis,
  dissecans
Osteochondroma (M9210/0) — *see* Neoplasm,
  bone, benign
Osteochondromatosis (M9210/1) D48.0
  syndrome Q78.4
Osteochondromyxosarcoma (M9180/3) — *see*
  Neoplasm, bone, malignant
Osteochondropathy M93.90
  ankle M93.979
   left M93.972
   right M93.971
  elbow M93.929
   left M93.922
   right M93.921
  foot M93.979
   left M93.972
   right M93.971
  hand M93.949
   left M93.942
   right M93.941
  hip M93.959
   left M93.952
   right M93.951
  Kienböck's disease of adults M93.1
  knee M93.969
   left M93.962
   right M93.961
  multiple joints M93.99
  osteochondritis dissecans — *see*
    Osteochondritis, dissecans
  osteochondrosis — *see* Osteochondrosis
  shoulder region M93.919
   left M93.912
   right M93.911
  slipped upper femoral epiphysis — *see* Slipped,
    epiphysis, upper femoral
  specified joint NEC M93.98
  specified type NEC M93.80
   ankle M93.879
    left M93.872
    right M93.871
   elbow M93.829
    left M93.822
    right M93.821
   foot M93.879
    left M93.872
    right M93.871
   hand M93.849
    left M93.842
    right M93.841

Osteochondropathy — *continued*
  specified type NEC — *continued*
   hip M93.859
    left M93.852
    right M93.851
   knee M93.869
    left M93.862
    right M93.861
   multiple joints M93.89
   shoulder region M93.819
    left M93.812
    right M93.811
   specified joint NEC M93.88
   wrist M93.839
    left M93.832
    right M93.831
  syphilitic, congenital
   early A50.02 *[M90.80]*
   late A50.56 *[M90.80]*
  wrist M93.939
   left M93.932
   right M93.931
Osteochondrosarcoma (M9180/3) — *see*
  Neoplasm, bone, malignant
Osteochondrosis — *see also* Osteochondropathy,
  by site
  acetabulum (juvenile) M91.0
  adult — *see* Osteochondropathy, specified type
    NEC, by site
  astragalus (juvenile) — *see* Osteochondrosis,
    juvenile, tarsus
  Blount's — *see* Osteochondrosis, juvenile, tibia
  Buchanan's M91.0
  Burns' — *see* Osteochondrosis, juvenile, ulna
  calcaneus (juvenile) — *see* Osteochondrosis,
    juvenile, tarsus
  capitular epiphysis (femur) (juvenile) — *see*
    Legg-Calve-Perthes disease
  carpal (juvenile) (lunate) (scaphoid) — *see*
    Osteochondrosis, juvenile, hand, carpal
    lunate
   adult M93.1
  coxae juvenilis — *see* Legg-Calve-Perthes
    disease
  deformans juvenilis, coxae — *see* Legg-Calve-
    Perthes disease
  Diaz's — *see* Osteochondrosis, juvenile, tarsus
  dissecans (knee) (shoulder) — *see*
    Osteochondritis, dissecans
  femoral capital epiphysis (juvenile) — *see* Legg-
    Calve-Perthes disease
  femur (head), juvenile — *see* Legg-Calve-
    Perthes disease
  fibula (juvenile) — *see* Osteochondrosis,
    juvenile, fibula
  foot NEC (juvenile) M92.8
  Freiberg's — *see* Osteochondrosis, juvenile,
    metatarsus
  Haas' (juvenile) — *see* Osteochondrosis,
    juvenile, humerus
  Haglund's — *see* Osteochondrosis, juvenile,
    tarsus
  hip (juvenile) — *see* Legg-Calve-Perthes disease
  humerus (capitulum) (head) (juvenile) — *see*
    Osteochondrosis, juvenile, humerus
  ilium, iliac crest (juvenile) M91.0
  ischiopubic synchondrosis M91.0
  Iselin's — *see* Osteochondrosis, juvenile,
    metatarsus
  juvenile, juvenilis M92.9
   after congenital dislocation of hip reduction
      — *see* Osteochondrosis, juvenile, hip,
      specified NEC
   arm — *see* Osteochondrosis, juvenile, upper
     limb NEC
   capitular epiphysis (femur) — *see* Legg-
     Calve-Perthes disease
   clavicle, sternal epiphysis — *see*
     Osteochondrosis, juvenile, upper limb
     NEC
   coxae — *see* Legg-Calve-Perthes disease
   deformans M92.9
   fibula M92.50
    left M92.52
    right M92.51
   foot NEC M92.8

Osteochondrosis — *see also* Osteochondropathy,
  by site — *continued*
  juvenile, juvenilis — *continued*
   hand M92.209
    carpal lunate M92.219
     left M92.212
     right M92.211
    left M92.202
    metacarpal head M92.229
     left M92.222
     right M92.221
    right M92.201
    specified site NEC M92.299
     left M92.292
     right M92.291
   head of femur — *see* Legg-Calve-Perthes
    disease
   hip and pelvis M91.90
    coxa plana — *see* Coxa, plana
    femoral head — *see* Legg-Calve-Perthes
     disease
    left M91.92
    pelvis M91.0
    pseudocoxalgia — *see* Pseudocoxalgia
    right M91.91
    specified NEC M91.80
     left M91.82
     right M91.81
   humerus M92.00
    left M92.02
    right M92.01
   limb
    lower NEC M92.8
    upper NEC — *see* Osteochondrosis,
     juvenile, upper limb NEC
   medial cuneiform bone — *see*
    Osteochondrosis, juvenile, tarsus
   metatarsus M92.70
    left M92.72
    right M92.71
   patella M92.40
    left M92.42
    right M92.41
   radius M92.10
    left M92.12
    right M92.11
   specified site NEC M92.8
   spine M42.00
    cervical region M42.02
    cervicothoracic region M42.03
    lumbar region M42.06
    lumbosacral region M42.07
    multiple sites M42.09
    occipito-atlanto-axial region M42.01
    sacrococcygeal region M42.08
    thoracic region M42.04
    thoracolumbar region M42.05
   tarsus M92.60
    left M92.62
    right M92.61
   tibia M92.50
    left M92.52
    right M92.51
   ulna M92.10
    left M92.12
    right M92.11
   upper limb NEC M92.30
    left M92.32
    right M92.31
   vertebra (body) (epiphyseal plates) (Calvés)
    (Scheuermann's) — *see*
    Osteochondrosis, juvenile, spine
  Kienböck's — *see* Osteochondrosis, juvenile,
    hand, carpal lunate
  Köhler's
   patellar — *see* Osteochondrosis, juvenile,
    patella
   tarsal navicular — *see* Osteochondrosis,
    juvenile, tarsus
  Legg-Perthes (-Calvé) (-Waldenström) — *see*
    Legg-Calve-Perthes disease
  limb
   lower NEC (juvenile) M92.8
   upper NEC (juvenile) — *see*
    Osteochondrosis, juvenile, upper limb
    NEC

©2002 Ingenix, Inc.

Osteochondrosis — *see also* Osteochondropathy, by site — *continued*
  lunate bone (carpal) (juvenile) — *see also* Osteochondrosis, juvenile, hand, carpal lunate
    adult M93.1
  Mauclaire's — *see* Osteochondrosis, juvenile, hand, metacarpal
  metacarpal (head) (juvenile) — *see* Osteochondrosis, juvenile, hand, metacarpal
  metatarsus (fifth) (head) (juvenile) (second) — *see* Osteochondrosis, juvenile, metatarsus
  navicular (juvenile) — *see* Osteochondrosis, juvenile, tarsus
  os
    calcis (juvenile) — *see* Osteochondrosis, juvenile, tarsus
    tibiale externum (juvenile) — *see* Osteochondrosis, juvenile, tarsus
  Osgood-Schlatter — *see* Osteochondrosis, juvenile, tibia
  Panner's — *see* Osteochondrosis, juvenile, humerus
  patellar center (juvenile) (primary) (secondary) — *see* Osteochondrosis, juvenile, patella
  pelvis (juvenile) M91.0
  Pierson's M91.0
  radius (head) (juvenile) — *see* Osteochondrosis, juvenile, radius
  Scheuermann's — *see* Osteochondrosis, juvenile, spine
  Sever's — *see* Osteochondrosis, juvenile, tarsus
  Sinding-Larsen — *see* Osteochondrosis, juvenile, patella
  spine M42.9
    adult M42.10
      cervical region M42.12
      cervicothoracic region M42.13
      lumbar region M42.16
      lumbosacral region M42.17
      multiple sites M42.19
      occipito-atlanto-axial region M42.11
      sacrococcygeal region M42.18
      thoracic region M42.14
      thoracolumbar region M42.15
    juvenile — *see* Osteochondrosis, juvenile, spine
  symphysis pubis (juvenile) M91.0
  syphilitic (congenital) A50.02
  talus (juvenile) — *see* Osteochondrosis, juvenile, tarsus
  tarsus (navicular) (juvenile) — *see* Osteochondrosis, juvenile, tarsus
  tibia (proximal) (tubercle) (juvenile) — *see* Osteochondrosis, juvenile, tibia
  tuberculous — *see* Tuberculosis, bone
  ulna (lower) (juvenile) — *see* Osteochondrosis, juvenile, ulna
  van Neck's M91.0
  vertebral — *see* Osteochondrosis, spine
Osteoclastoma (M9250/1) D48.0
  malignant (M9250/3) — *see* Neoplasm, bone, malignant
Osteodynia — *see* Disorder, bone, specified type NEC
Osteodystrophy Q78.9
  azotemic N25.0
  congenital Q78.9
  parathyroid, secondary E21.1
  renal N25.0
Osteofibroma (M9262/0) — *see* Neoplasm, bone, benign
Osteofibrosarcoma (M9182/3) — *see* Neoplasm, bone, malignant
Osteogenesis imperfecta Q78.0
Osteogenic — *see* condition
Osteolysis M89.50
  carpus M89.549
    left M89.542
    right M89.541
  clavicle M89.519
    left M89.512
    right M89.511

Osteolysis — *continued*
  femur M89.559
    left M89.552
    right M89.551
  fibula M89.569
    left M89.562
    right M89.561
  finger M89.549
    left M89.542
    right M89.541
  humerus M89.529
    left M89.522
    right M89.521
  ilium M89.559
  ischium M89.559
  metacarpus M89.549
    left M89.542
    right M89.541
  metatarsus M89.579
    left M89.572
    right M89.571
  multiple sites M89.59
  neck M89.58
  radius M89.539
    left M89.532
    right M89.531
  rib M89.58
  scapula M89.519
    left M89.512
    right M89.511
  skull M89.58
  tarsus M89.579
    left M89.572
    right M89.571
  tibia M89.569
    left M89.562
    right M89.561
  toe M89.579
    left M89.572
    right M89.571
  ulna M89.539
    left M89.532
    right M89.531
  vertebra M89.58
Osteoma (M9180/0) — *see also* Neoplasm, bone, benign
  osteoid (M9191/0) — *see also* Neoplasm, bone, benign
    giant (M9200/0) — *see* Neoplasm, bone, benign
Osteomalacia M83.9
  adult M83.9
    drug-induced NEC M83.5
    due to
      malabsorption (postsurgical) M83.2
      malnutrition M83.3
    specified NEC M83.8
  aluminium-induced M83.4
  infantile — *see* Rickets
  juvenile — *see* Rickets
  pelvis M83.8
  puerperal M83.0
  senile M83.1
  vitamin-D-resistant in adults E83.31 *[M90.80]*
    carpus E83.31 *[M90.849]*
      left E83.31 *[M90.842]*
      right E83.31 *[M90.841]*
    clavicle E83.31 *[M90.819]*
      left E83.31 *[M90.812]*
      right E83.31 *[M90.811]*
    femur E83.31 *[M90.859]*
      left E83.31 *[M90.852]*
      right E83.31 *[M90.851]*
    fibula E83.31 *[M90.869]*
      left E83.31 *[M90.862]*
      right E83.31 *[M90.861]*
    finger E83.31 *[M90.849]*
      left E83.31 *[M90.842]*
      right E83.31 *[M90.841]*
    humerus E83.31 *[M90.829]*
      left E83.31 *[M90.822]*
      right E83.31 *[M90.821]*
    ilium E83.31 *[M90.859]*
    ischium E83.31 *[M90.859]*
    metacarpus E83.31 *[M90.849]*
      left E83.31 *[M90.842]*
      right E83.31 *[M90.841]*

Osteomalacia — *continued*
  vitamin-D-resistant in adults — *continued*
    metatarsus E83.31 *[M90.879]*
      left E83.31 *[M90.872]*
      right E83.31 *[M90.871]*
      multiple sites E83.31 *[M90.89]*
    neck E83.31 *[M90.88]*
    radius E83.31 *[M90.839]*
      left E83.31 *[M90.832]*
      right E83.31 *[M90.831]*
    rib E83.31 *[M90.88]*
    scapula E83.31 *[M90.819]*
      left E83.31 *[M90.812]*
      right E83.31 *[M90.811]*
    skull E83.31 *[M90.88]*
    tarsus E83.31 *[M90.879]*
      left E83.31 *[M90.872]*
      right E83.31 *[M90.871]*
    tibia E83.31 *[M90.869]*
      left E83.31 *[M90.862]*
      right E83.31 *[M90.861]*
    toe E83.31 *[M90.879]*
      left E83.31 *[M90.872]*
      right E83.31 *[M90.871]*
    ulna E83.31 *[M90.839]*
      left E83.31 *[M90.832]*
      right E83.31 *[M90.831]*
    vertebra E83.31 *[M90.88]*
Osteomyelitis (general) (infective) (localized) (neonatal) (purulent) (septic) (staphylococcal) (streptococcal) (suppurative) (with periostitis) M86.9
  acute M86.10
    carpus M86.149
      left M86.142
      right M86.141
    clavicle M86.119
      left M86.112
      right M86.111
    femur M86.159
      left M86.152
      right M86.151
    fibula M86.169
      left M86.162
      right M86.161
    finger M86.149
      left M86.142
      right M86.141
    hematogenous M86.00
      carpus M86.049
        left M86.042
        right M86.041
      clavicle M86.019
        left M86.012
        right M86.011
      femur M86.059
        left M86.052
        right M86.051
      fibula M86.069
        left M86.062
        right M86.061
      finger M86.049
        left M86.042
        right M86.041
      humerus M86.029
        left M86.022
        right M86.021
      ilium M86.059
      ischium M86.059
      mandible M27.2
      metacarpus M86.049
        left M86.042
        right M86.041
      metatarsus M86.079
        left M86.072
        right M86.071
      multiple sites M86.09
      neck M86.08
      orbit H05.029
        bilateral H05.023
        left H05.022
        right H05.021
      petrous bone — *see* Petrositis
      radius M86.039
        left M86.032
        right M86.031

Osteomyelitis — *continued*
  acute — *continued*
    hematogenous — *continued*
      rib M86.08
      scapula M86.019
        left M86.012
        right M86.011
      skull M86.08
      tarsus M86.079
        left M86.072
        right M86.071
      tibia M86.069
        left M86.062
        right M86.061
      toe M86.079
        left M86.072
        right M86.071
      ulna M86.039
        left M86.032
        right M86.031
      vertebra — *see* Osteomyelitis, vertebra
    humerus M86.129
      left M86.122
      right M86.121
    ilium M86.159
    ischium M86.159
    mandible M27.2
    metacarpus M86.149
      left M86.142
      right M86.141
    metatarsus M86.179
      left M86.172
      right M86.171
    multiple sites M86.19
    neck M86.18
    orbit H05.029
      bilateral H05.023
      left H05.022
      right H05.021
    petrous bone — *see* Petrositis
    radius M86.139
      left M86.132
      right M86.131
    rib M86.18
    scapula M86.119
      left M86.112
      right M86.111
    skull M86.18
    tarsus M86.179
      left M86.172
      right M86.171
    tibia M86.169
      left M86.162
      right M86.161
    toe M86.179
      left M86.172
      right M86.171
    ulna M86.139
      left M86.132
      right M86.131
    vertebra — *see* Osteomyelitis, vertebra
  chronic (or old) M86.60
    with draining sinus M86.40
      carpus M86.449
        left M86.442
        right M86.441
      clavicle M86.419
        left M86.412
        right M86.411
      femur M86.459
        left M86.452
        right M86.451
      fibula M86.469
        left M86.462
        right M86.461
      finger M86.449
        left M86.442
        right M86.441
      humerus M86.429
        left M86.422
        right M86.421
      ilium M86.459
      ischium M86.459
      mandible M27.2

Osteomyelitis — *continued*
  chronic — *continued*
    with draining sinus — *continued*
      metacarpus M86.449
        left M86.442
        right M86.441
      metatarsus M86.479
        left M86.472
        right M86.471
      multiple sites M86.49
      neck M86.48
      orbit H05.029
        bilateral H05.023
        left H05.022
        right H05.021
      petrous bone — *see* Petrositis
      radius M86.439
        left M86.432
        right M86.431
      rib M86.48
      scapula M86.419
        left M86.412
        right M86.411
      skull M86.48
      tarsus M86.479
        left M86.472
        right M86.471
      tibia M86.469
        left M86.462
        right M86.461
      toe M86.479
        left M86.472
        right M86.471
      ulna M86.439
        left M86.432
        right M86.431
      vertebra — *see* Osteomyelitis, vertebra
    carpus M86.649
      left M86.642
      right M86.641
    clavicle M86.619
      left M86.612
      right M86.611
    femur M86.659
      left M86.652
      right M86.651
    fibula M86.669
      left M86.662
      right M86.661
    finger M86.649
      left M86.642
      right M86.641
    hematogenous NEC M86.50
      carpus M86.549
        left M86.542
        right M86.541
      clavicle M86.519
        left M86.512
        right M86.511
      femur M86.559
        left M86.552
        right M86.551
      fibula M86.569
        left M86.562
        right M86.561
      finger M86.549
        left M86.542
        right M86.541
      humerus M86.529
        left M86.522
        right M86.521
      ilium M86.559
      ischium M86.559
      mandible M27.2
      metacarpus M86.549
        left M86.542
        right M86.541
      metatarsus M86.579
        left M86.572
        right M86.571
      multifocal M86.30
        carpus M86.349
          left M86.342
          right M86.341

Osteomyelitis — *continued*
  chronic — *continued*
    hematogenous NEC — *continued*
      multifocal — *continued*
        clavicle M86.319
          left M86.312
          right M86.311
        femur M86.359
          left M86.352
          right M86.351
        fibula M86.369
          left M86.362
          right M86.361
        finger M86.349
          left M86.342
          right M86.341
        humerus M86.329
          left M86.322
          right M86.321
        ilium M86.359
        ischium M86.359
        metacarpus M86.349
          left M86.342
          right M86.341
        metatarsus M86.379
          left M86.372
          right M86.371
        multiple sites M86.39
        neck M86.38
        radius M86.339
          left M86.332
          right M86.331
        rib M86.38
        scapula M86.319
          left M86.312
          right M86.311
        skull M86.38
        tarsus M86.379
          left M86.372
          right M86.371
        tibia M86.369
          left M86.362
          right M86.361
        toe M86.379
          left M86.372
          right M86.371
        ulna M86.339
          left M86.332
          right M86.331
        vertebra — *see* Osteomyelitis, vertebra
      multiple sites M86.59
      neck M86.58
      orbit H05.029
        bilateral H05.023
        left H05.022
        right H05.021
      petrous bone — *see* Petrositis
      radius M86.539
        left M86.532
        right M86.531
      rib M86.58
      scapula M86.519
        left M86.512
        right M86.511
      skull M86.58
      tarsus M86.579
        left M86.572
        right M86.571
      tibia M86.569
        left M86.562
        right M86.561
      toe M86.579
        left M86.572
        right M86.571
      ulna M86.539
        left M86.532
        right M86.531
      vertebra — *see* Osteomyelitis, vertebra
    humerus M86.629
      left M86.622
      right M86.621
    ilium M86.659
    ischium M86.659
    mandible M27.2

Osteomyelitis — *continued*
  chronic — *continued*
    metacarpus M86.649
      left M86.642
      right M86.641
    metatarsus M86.679
      left M86.672
      right M86.671
    multifocal — *see* Osteomyelitis, chronic,
      hematogenous, multifocal
    multiple sites M86.69
    neck M86.68
    orbit H05.029
      bilateral H05.023
      left H05.022
      right H05.021
    petrous bone — *see* Petrositis
    radius M86.639
      left M86.632
      right M86.631
    rib M86.68
    scapula M86.619
      left M86.612
      right M86.611
    skull M86.68
    tarsus M86.679
      left M86.672
      right M86.671
    tibia M86.669
      left M86.662
      right M86.661
    toe M86.679
      left M86.672
      right M86.671
    ulna M86.639
      left M86.632
      right M86.631
    vertebra — *see* Osteomyelitis, vertebra
  echinococcal B67.2
  Garr,'s — *see* Osteomyelitis, specified type NEC
  jaw (acute) (chronic) (lower) (neonatal)
    (suppurative) (upper) M27.2
  nonsuppurating — *see* Osteomyelitis, specified
    type NEC
  orbit H05.029
    bilateral H05.023
    left H05.022
    right H05.021
  petrous bone — *see* Petrositis
  Salmonella (arizonae) (cholerae-suis)
    (enteritidis) (typhimurium) A02.24
  sclerosing, nonsuppurative — *see*
    Osteomyelitis, specified type NEC
  specified type NEC — *see also* category M86.8
    mandible M27.2
    orbit H05.029
      bilateral H05.023
      left H05.022
      right H05.021
    petrous bone — *see* Petrositis
    vertebra — *see* Osteomyelitis, vertebra
  subacute M86.20
    carpus M86.249
      left M86.242
      right M86.241
    clavicle M86.219
      left M86.212
      right M86.211
    femur M86.259
      left M86.252
      right M86.251
    fibula M86.269
      left M86.262
      right M86.261
    finger M86.249
      left M86.242
      right M86.241
    humerus M86.229
      left M86.222
      right M86.221
    mandible M27.2
    metacarpus M86.249
      left M86.242
      right M86.241
    metatarsus M86.279
      left M86.272
      right M86.271

Osteomyelitis — *continued*
  subacute — *continued*
    multiple sites M86.29
    neck M86.28
    orbit H05.029
      bilateral H05.023
      left H05.022
      right H05.021
    petrous bone — *see* Petrositis
    radius M86.239
      left M86.232
      right M86.231
    rib M86.28
    scapula M86.219
      left M86.212
      right M86.211
    skull M86.28
    tarsus M86.279
      left M86.272
      right M86.271
    tibia M86.269
      left M86.262
      right M86.261
    toe M86.279
      left M86.272
      right M86.271
    ulna M86.239
      left M86.232
      right M86.231
    vertebra — *see* Osteomyelitis, vertebra
  syphilitic A52.77
    congenital (early) A50.02 *[M90.80]*
  tuberculous — *see* Tuberculosis, bone
  typhoid A01.05
  vertebra M46.20
    cervical region M46.22
    cervicothoracic region M46.23
    lumbar region M46.26
    lumbosacral region M46.27
    occipito-atlanto-axial region M46.21
    sacrococcygeal region M46.28
    thoracic region M46.24
    thoracolumbar region M46.25

Osteomyelofibrosis D75.8

Osteomyelosclerosis D75.8

Osteonecrosis M87.9
  due to
    drugs — *see* Osteonecrosis, secondary, due
      to, drugs
    trauma — *see* Osteonecrosis, secondary, due
      to, trauma
  idiopathic aseptic M87.00
    ankle M87.073
      left M87.072
      right M87.071
    carpus M87.039
      left M87.037
      right M87.038
    clavicle M87.019
      left M87.012
      right M87.011
    femur M87.059
      left M87.052
      right M87.051
    fibula M87.066
      left M87.065
      right M87.064
    finger M87.046
      left M87.045
      right M87.044
    humerus M87.029
      left M87.022
      right M87.021
    ilium M87.050
    ischium M87.050
    metacarpus M87.043
      left M87.042
      right M87.041
    metatarsus M87.076
      left M87.075
      right M87.074
    neck M87.08
    pelvis M87.050
    radius M87.033
      left M87.032
      right M87.031

Osteonecrosis — *continued*
  idiopathic aseptic — *continued*
    rib M87.08
    scapula M87.019
      left M87.012
      right M87.011
    skull M87.08
    tarsus M87.076
      left M87.075
      right M87.074
    tibia M87.063
      left M87.062
      right M87.061
    toe M87.079
      left M87.078
      right M87.077
    ulna M87.036
      left M87.035
      right M87.034
    vertebra M87.08
  secondary NEC M87.30
    carpus M87.349
      left M87.342
      right M87.341
    clavicle M87.319
      left M87.312
      right M87.311
    due to
      drugs M87.10
        carpus M87.149
          left M87.142
          right M87.141
        clavicle M87.119
          left M87.112
          right M87.111
        femur M87.159
          left M87.152
          right M87.151
        fibula M87.169
          left M87.162
          right M87.161
        finger M87.149
          left M87.142
          right M87.141
        humerus M87.129
          left M87.122
          right M87.121
        ilium M87.159
        ischium M87.159
        metacarpus M87.149
          left M87.142
          right M87.141
        metatarsus M87.179
          left M87.172
          right M87.171
        multiple sites M87.19
        neck M87.18
        radius M87.139
          left M87.132
          right M87.131
        rib M87.18
        scapula M87.119
          left M87.112
          right M87.111
        skull M87.18
        tarsus M87.179
          left M87.172
          right M87.171
        tibia M87.169
          left M87.162
          right M87.161
        toe M87.179
          left M87.172
          right M87.171
        ulna M87.139
          left M87.132
          right M87.131
        vertebra M87.18
      hemoglobinopathy NEC D58.2 *[M90.50]*
        carpus D58.2 *[M90.549]*
          left D58.2 *[M90.542]*
          right D58.2 *[M90.541]*
        clavicle D58.2 *[M90.519]*
          left D58.2 *[M90.512]*
          right D58.2 *[M90.511]*

Osteonecrosis — *continued*
  secondary NEC — *continued*
    due to — *continued*
      hemoglobinopathy NEC — *continued*
        femur D58.2 *[M90.559]*
          left D58.2 *[M90.552]*
          right D58.2 *[M90.551]*
        fibula D58.2 *[M90.569]*
          left D58.2 *[M90.562]*
          right D58.2 *[M90.561]*
        finger D58.2 *[M90.549]*
          left D58.2 *[M90.542]*
          right D58.2 *[M90.541]*
        humerus D58.2 *[M90.529]*
          left D58.2 *[M90.522]*
          right D58.2 *[M90.521]*
        ilium D58.2 *[M90.559]*
        ischium D58.2 *[M90.559]*
        metacarpus D58.2 *[M90.549]*
          left D58.2 *[M90.542]*
          right D58.2 *[M90.541]*
        metatarsus D58.2 *[M90.579]*
          left D58.2 *[M90.572]*
          right D58.2 *[M90.571]*
        multiple sites D58.2 *[M90.59]*
        neck D58.2 *[M90.58]*
        radius D58.2 *[M90.539]*
          left D58.2 *[M90.532]*
          right D58.2 *[M90.531]*
        rib D58.2 *[M90.58]*
        scapula D58.2 *[M90.519]*
          left D58.2 *[M90.512]*
          right D58.2 *[M90.511]*
        skull D58.2 *[M90.58]*
        tarsus D58.2 *[M90.579]*
          left D58.2 *[M90.572]*
          right D58.2 *[M90.571]*
        tibia D58.2 *[M90.569]*
          left D58.2 *[M90.562]*
          right D58.2 *[M90.561]*
        toe D58.2 *[M90.579]*
          left D58.2 *[M90.572]*
          right D58.2 *[M90.571]*
        ulna D58.2 *[M90.539]*
          left D58.2 *[M90.532]*
          right D58.2 *[M90.531]*
        vertebra D58.2 *[M90.58]*
      trauma (previous) M87.20
        carpus M87.249
          left M87.242
          right M87.241
        clavicle M87.219
          left M87.212
          right M87.211
        femur M87.259
          left M87.252
          right M87.251
        fibula M87.269
          left M87.262
          right M87.261
        finger M87.249
          left M87.242
          right M87.241
        humerus M87.229
          left M87.222
          right M87.221
        ilium M87.259
        ischium M87.259
        metacarpus M87.249
          left M87.242
          right M87.241
        metatarsus M87.279
          left M87.272
          right M87.271
        multiple sites M87.29
        neck M87.28
        radius M87.239
          left M87.232
          right M87.231
        rib M87.28
        scapula M87.219
          left M87.212
          right M87.211
        skull M87.28

Osteonecrosis — *continued*
  secondary NEC — *continued*
    due to — *continued*
      trauma — *continued*
        tarsus M87.279
          left M87.272
          right M87.271
        tibia M87.269
          left M87.262
          right M87.261
        toe M87.279
          left M87.272
          right M87.271
        ulna M87.239
          left M87.232
          right M87.231
        vertebra M87.28
      femur M87.359
        left M87.352
        right M87.351
      fibula M87.369
        left M87.362
        right M87.361
      finger M87.349
        left M87.342
        right M87.341
      humerus M87.329
        left M87.322
        right M87.321
      ilium M87.359
      in
        caisson disease T70.3 *[M90.50]*
          carpus T70.3 *[M90.549]*
            left T70.3 *[M90.542]*
            right T70.3 *[M90.541]*
          clavicle T70.3 *[M90.519]*
            left T70.3 *[M90.512]*
            right T70.3 *[M90.511]*
          femur T70.3 *[M90.559]*
            left T70.3 *[M90.552]*
            right T70.3 *[M90.551]*
          fibula T70.3 *[M90.569]*
            left T70.3 *[M90.562]*
            right T70.3 *[M90.561]*
          finger T70.3 *[M90.549]*
            left T70.3 *[M90.542]*
            right T70.3 *[M90.541]*
          humerus T70.3 *[M90.529]*
            left T70.3 *[M90.522]*
            right T70.3 *[M90.521]*
          ilium T70.3 *[M90.559]*
          ischium T70.3 *[M90.559]*
          metacarpus T70.3 *[M90.549]*
            left T70.3 *[M90.542]*
            right T70.3 *[M90.541]*
          metatarsus T70.3 *[M90.579]*
            left T70.3 *[M90.572]*
            right T70.3 *[M90.571]*
          multiple sites T70.3 *[M90.59]*
          neck T70.3 *[M90.58]*
          radius T70.3 *[M90.539]*
            left T70.3 *[M90.532]*
            right T70.3 *[M90.531]*
          rib T70.3 *[M90.58]*
          scapula T70.3 *[M90.519]*
            left T70.3 *[M90.512]*
            right T70.3 *[M90.511]*
          skull T70.3 *[M90.58]*
          tarsus T70.3 *[M90.579]*
            left T70.3 *[M90.572]*
            right T70.3 *[M90.571]*
          tibia T70.3 *[M90.569]*
            left T70.3 *[M90.562]*
            right T70.3 *[M90.561]*
          toe T70.3 *[M90.579]*
            left T70.3 *[M90.572]*
            right T70.3 *[M90.571]*
          ulna T70.3 *[M90.539]*
            left T70.3 *[M90.532]*
            right T70.3 *[M90.531]*
          vertebra T70.3 *[M90.58]*
      ischium M87.359
      metacarpus M87.349
        left M87.342
        right M87.341

Osteonecrosis — *continued*
  secondary NEC — *continued*
    metatarsus M87.379
      left M87.372
      right M87.371
    multiple site M87.39
    neck M87.38
    radius M87.339
      left M87.332
      right M87.331
    rib M87.38
    scapula M87.319
      left M87.312
      right M87.311
    skull M87.38
    tarsus M87.379
      left M87.372
      right M87.371
    tibia M87.369
      left M87.362
      right M87.361
    toe M87.379
      left M87.372
      right M87.371
    ulna M87.339
      left M87.332
      right M87.331
    vertebra M87.38
    specified type NEC M87.80
      carpus M87.84
      clavicle M87.81
      femur M87.85
      fibula M87.86
      finger M87.84
      humerus M87.82
      ilium M87.85
      ischium M87.85
      metacarpus M87.84
      metatarsus M87.87
      multiple sites M87.89
      neck M87.88
      radius M87.83
      rib M87.88
      scapula M87.81
      skull M87.88
      tarsus M87.87
      tibia M87.86
      toe M87.87
      ulna M87.83
      vertebra M87.88

Osteo-onycho-arthro-dysplasia Q79.8
Osteo-onychodysplasia, hereditary Q79.8
Osteopathia condensans disseminata Q78.8
Osteopathy — *see also* Osteomyelitis, Osteonecrosis, Osteoporosis
  after poliomyelitis M89.60
    carpus M89.649
      left M89.642
      right M89.641
    clavicle M89.619
      left M89.612
      right M89.611
    femur M89.659
      left M89.652
      right M89.651
    fibula M89.669
      left M89.662
      right M89.661
    finger M89.649
      left M89.642
      right M89.641
    humerus M89.629
      left M89.622
      right M89.621
    ilium M89.659
    ischium M89.659
    metacarpus M89.649
      left M89.642
      right M89.641
    metatarsus M89.679
      left M89.672
      right M89.671
    multiple sites M89.69
    neck M89.68

©2002 Ingenix, Inc.

Osteopathy — *see also* Osteomyelitis,
    Osteonecrosis, Osteoporosis — *continued*
    after poliomyelitis — *continued*
      radius M89.639
        left M89.632
        right M89.631
      rib M89.68
      scapula M89.619
        left M89.612
        right M89.611
      skull M89.68
      tarsus M89.679
        left M89.672
        right M89.671
      tibia M89.669
        left M89.662
        right M89.661
      toe M89.679
        left M89.672
        right M89.671
      ulna M89.639
        left M89.632
        right M89.631
      vertebra M89.68
    in (due to)
      renal osteodystrophy N25.0
      specified diseases classified elsewhere — *see*
        category M90.8

Osteoperiostitis — *see* Osteomyelitis, specified
    type NEC

Osteopetrosis (familial) Q78.2

Osteophyte M25.70
    ankle M25.773
      left M25.772
      right M25.771
    elbow M25.729
      left M25.722
      right M25.721
    foot joint M25.776
      left M25.775
      right M25.774
    hand joint M25.749
      left M25.742
      right M25.741
    hip M25.759
      left M25.752
      right M25.751
    knee M25.769
      left M25.762
      right M25.761
    shoulder M25.719
      left M25.712
      right M25.711
    specified joint NEC M25.78
    wrist M25.739
      left M25.732
      right M25.731

Osteopoikilosis Q78.8

Osteoporosis
    with pathological fracture M80.80
    disuse M81.8
      with pathological fracture — *see*
        Osteoporosis, specified type NEC, with
        pathological fracture
    drug-induced — *see* Osteoporosis, specified
      type NEC
    idiopathic — *see* Osteoporosis, specified type
      NEC
      with patholgical fracture — *see*
        Osteoporosis, specified type NEC, with
        pathological fracture
    localized M81.60
      carpus M81.649
        left M81.642
        right M81.641
      clavicle M81.619
        left M81.612
        right M81.611
      fibula M81.669
        left M81.662
        right M81.661
      finger M81.649
        left M81.642
        right M81.641

Osteoporosis — *continued*
    localized — *continued*
      humerus M81.629
        left M81.622
        right M81.621
      ilium M81.659
        left M81.652
        right M81.651
      ischium M81.659
        left M81.652
        right M81.651
      metacarpus M81.649
        left M81.642
        right M81.641
      metatarsus M81.679
        left M81.672
        right M81.671
      pelvis M81.659
        left M81.652
        right M81.651
      radius M81.639
        left M81.632
        right M81.631
      scapula M81.619
        left M81.612
        right M81.611
      tarsus M81.679
        left M81.672
        right M81.671
      tibia M81.669
        left M81.662
        right M81.661
      toe M81.679
        left M81.672
        right M81.671
      ulna M81.639
        left M81.632
        right M81.631
      vertebra M81.68
    postmenopausal M81.0
      with pathological fracture M80.00
        carpus M80.049
          left M80.042
          right M80.041
        clavicle M80.019
          left M80.012
          right M80.011
        fibula M80.069
          left M80.062
          right M80.061
        finger M80.049
          left M80.042
          right M80.041
        humerus M80.029
          left M80.022
          right M80.021
        ilium M80.059
          left M80.052
          right M80.051
        ischium M80.059
          left M80.052
          right M80.051
        metacarpus M80.049
          left M80.042
          right M80.041
        metatarsus M80.079
          left M80.072
          right M80.071
        pelvis M80.059
          left M80.052
          right M80.051
        radius M80.039
          left M80.032
          right M80.031
        scapula M80.019
          left M80.012
          right M80.011
        tarsus M80.079
          left M80.072
          right M80.071
        tibia M80.069
          left M80.062
          right M80.061
        toe M80.079
          left M80.072
          right M80.071

Osteoporosis — *continued*
    postmenopausal — *continued*
      with pathological fracture — *continued*
        ulna M80.039
          left M80.032
          right M80.031
        vertebra M80.08
    postoophorectomy — *see* Osteoporosis,
      specified type NEC
    postsurgical malabsorption M81.8
      with pathological fracture — *see*
        Osteoporosis, specified type NEC, with
        pathological fracture
    post-traumatic — *see* Osteoporosis, specified
      type NEC
    senile — *see also* Osteoporosis, specified type
      NEC
      with pathological fracture — *see*
        Osteoporosis, specified type NEC, with
        pathological fracture
    specified type NEC M81.8
      with pathological fracture M80.80
        carpus M80.849
          left M80.842
          right M80.841
        clavicle M80.819
          left M80.812
          right M80.811
        fibula M80.869
          left M80.862
          right M80.861
        finger M80.849
          left M80.842
          right M80.841
        humerus M80.829
          left M80.822
          right M80.821
        ilium M80.859
          left M80.852
          right M80.851
        ischium M80.859
          left M80.852
          right M80.851
        metacarpus M80.849
          left M80.842
          right M80.841
        metatarsus M80.879
          left M80.872
          right M80.871
        pelvis M80.859
          left M80.852
          right M80.851
        radius M80.839
          left M80.832
          right M80.831
        scapula M80.819
          left M80.812
          right M80.811
        tarsus M80.879
          left M80.872
          right M80.871
        tibia M80.869
          left M80.862
          right M80.861
        toe M80.879
          left M80.872
          right M80.871
        ulna M80.839
          left M80.832
          right M80.831
        vertebra M80.88

Osteopsathyrosis (idiopathica) Q78.0

Osteoradionecrosis, jaw (acute) (chronic) (lower)
    (suppurative) (upper) M27.2

Osteosarcoma (M9180/3) — *see also* Neoplasm,
    bone, malignant
    chondroblastic (M9181/3) — *see* Neoplasm,
      bone, malignant
    fibroblastic (M9182/3) — *see* Neoplasm, bone,
      malignant
    in Paget's disease of bone (M9184/3) — *see*
      Neoplasm, bone, malignant
    juxtacortical (M9190/3) — *see* Neoplasm, bone,
      malignant
    parosteal (M9190/3) — *see* Neoplasm, bone,
      malignant

Osteosarcoma — *see also* Neoplasm, bone, malignant — *continued*
  small cell (M9185/3) — *see* Neoplasm, bone, malignant
  telangiectatic (M9183/3) — *see* Neoplasm, bone, malignant

Osteosclerosis (fragilitas) (generalisata) Q78.2
  myelofibrosis D75.8

Osteosclerotic anemia D64.8

Osteosis
  cutis L94.2
  renal fibrocystic N25.0

Österreicher-Turner syndrome Q87.2

Ostium
  atrioventriculare commune Q21.2
  primum (arteriosum) (defect) (persistent) Q21.2
  secundum (arteriosum) (defect) (patent) (persistent) Q21.1

Ostrum-Furst syndrome Q75.8

Otalgia — *see* category H92.0

Otitis (acute) H66.90
  with effusion — *see also* Otitis, media, nonsuppurative
    purulent — *see* Otitis, media, suppurative
  adhesive — *see* category H74.1
  chronic — *see also* Otitis, media, chronic
    with effusion — *see also* Otitis, media, nonsuppurative, chronic
  externa H60.90
    abscess — *see* Abscess, ear, external
    acute (noninfective) H60.509
      actinic H60.519
        bilateral H60.513
        left H60.512
        right H60.511
      bilateral H60.503
      chemical H60.529
        bilateral H60.523
        left H60.522
        right H60.521
      contact H60.539
        bilateral H60.533
        left H60.532
        right H60.531
      eczematoid H60.549
        bilateral H60.543
        left H60.542
        right H60.541
      infective — *see* Otitis, externa, infective
      left H60.502
      reactive H60.559
        bilateral H60.553
        left H60.552
        right H60.551
      right H60.501
      specified NEC H60.599
        bilateral H60.593
        left H60.592
        right H60.591
    bilateral H60.93
    cellulitis — *see* Cellulitis, ear
    chronic H60.63
      bilateral H60.62
      left H60.61
      right H60.60
    diffuse — *see* Otitis, externa, infective, diffuse
    hemorrhagic — *see* Otitis, externa, infective, hemorrhagic
    in (due to)
      aspergillosis B44.89
      candidiasis B37.84
      erysipelas A46 [H62.40]
      herpes (simplex) virus infection B00.1
        zoster B02.8
      impetigo L01.00 [H62.40]
      infectious disease NEC B99 [H62.40]
        bilateral B99 [H62.43]
        left B99 [H62.42]
        right B99 [H62.41]
      mycosis NEC B36.9 [H62.40]
      parasitic disease NEC B89 [H62.40]
      viral disease NEC B34.9 [H62.40]
      zoster B02.8

Otitis — *continued*
  externa — *continued*
    infective NEC H60.399
      abscess — *see* Abscess, ear, external
      bilateral H60.393
      cellulitis — *see* Cellulitis, ear
      diffuse H60.319
        bilateral H60.313
        left H60.312
        right H60.311
      hemorrhagic H60.329
        bilateral H60.323
        left H60.322
        right H60.321
      left H60.392
      right H60.391
      swimmer's ear — *see* Swimmer's, ear
    left H60.92
    malignant H60.20
      bilateral H60.23
      left H60.22
      right H60.21
    mycotic B36.9 [H62.40]
    necrotizing — *see* Otitis, externa, malignant
    Pseudomonas aeruginosa — *see* Otitis, externa, malignant
    reactive — *see* Otitis, externa, acute, reactive
    right H60.91
    specified NEC — *see* category H60.8
    tropical B36.8
  insidiosa — *see* Otosclerosis
  interna — *see* category H83.0
  media (hemorrhagic) (staphylococcal) (streptococcal) H66.90
    with effusion (nonpurulent) — *see* Otitis, media, nonsuppurative
    acute, subacute H66.90
      allergic — *see* Otitis, media, nonsuppurative, acute, allergic
      bilateral H66.93
      exudative — *see* Otitis, media, nonsuppurative, acute
      mucoid — *see* Otitis, media, nonsuppurative, acute
      necrotizing — *see also* Otitis, media, suppurative, acute
        in
          measles B05.3
          scarlet fever A38.0
      nonsuppurative NEC — *see* Otitis, media, nonsuppurative, acute
      purulent — *see* Otitis, media, suppurative, acute
      sanguinous — *see* Otitis, media, nonsuppurative, acute
      secretory — *see* Otitis, media, nonsuppurative, acute, serous
      seromucinous — *see* Otitis, media, nonsuppurative, acute
      serous — *see* Otitis, media, nonsuppurative, acute, serous
      suppurative — *see* Otitis, media, suppurative, acute
    allergic — *see* Otitis, media, nonsuppurative
    bilateral H66.93
    catarrhal — *see* Otitis, media, nonsuppurative
    chronic H66.90
      with effusion (nonpurulent) — *see* Otitis, media, nonsuppurative, chronic
      allergic — *see* Otitis, media, nonsuppurative, chronic, allergic
      benign suppurative — *see* Otitis, media, suppurative, chronic, tubotympanic
      catarrhal — *see* Otitis, media, nonsuppurative, chronic, serous
      exudative — *see* Otitis, media, nonsuppurative, chronic
      mucinous — *see* Otitis, media, nonsuppurative, chronic, mucoid
      mucoid — *see* Otitis, media, nonsuppurative, chronic, mucoid
      nonsuppurative NEC — *see* Otitis, media, nonsuppurative, chronic

Otitis — *continued*
  media — *continued*
    chronic — *continued*
      purulent — *see* Otitis, media, suppurative, chronic
      secretory — *see* Otitis, media, nonsuppurative, chronic, mucoid
      seromucinous — *see* Otitis, media, nonsuppurative, chronic
      serous — *see* Otitis, media, nonsuppurative, chronic, serous
      suppurative — *see* Otitis, media, suppurative, chronic
      transudative — *see* Otitis, media, nonsuppurative, chronic, mucoid
    exudative — *see* Otitis, media, nonsuppurative
    in (due to)
      influenza J10.89
      measles B05.3
      scarlet fever A38.0
      tuberculosis A18.6
      viral disease NEC B34.9 [H67.0]
        bilateral B34.9 [H67.3]
        left B34.9 [H67.2]
        right B34.9 [H67.1]
    left H66.92
    mucoid — *see* Otitis, media, nonsuppurative
    nonsuppurative H65.90
      acute or subacute NEC H65.199
        allergic H65.119
          bilateral H65.113
          left H65.112
          right H65.111
          recurrent H65.117
            bilateral H65.116
            left H65.115
            right H65.114
        bilateral H65.193
        left H65.192
        right H65.191
        recurrent H65.197
          bilateral H65.196
          left H65.195
          right H65.194
        secretory — *see* Otitis, media, nonsuppurative, serous
        serous H65.00
          bilateral H65.03
          left H65.02
          right H65.01
          recurrent H65.07
            bilateral H65.06
            left H65.05
            right H65.04
      bilateral H65.93
      chronic H65.499
        allergic H65.419
          bilateral H65.413
          left H65.412
          right H65.411
        bilateral H65.493
        left H65.492
        right H65.491
        mucoid H65.30
          bilateral H65.33
          left H65.32
          right H65.31
        serous H65.20
          bilateral H65.23
          left H65.22
          right H65.21
      left H65.92
      right H65.91
    postmeasles B05.3
    purulent — *see* Otitis, media, suppurative
    right H66.91
    secretory — *see* Otitis, media, nonsuppurative
    seromucinous — *see* Otitis, media, nonsuppurative
    serous — *see* Otitis, media, nonsuppurative

Otitis — *continued*
  media — *continued*
    suppurative H66.40
      acute H66.009
        with rupture of ear drum H66.019
          bilateral H66.013
          left H66.012
          right H66.011
        bilateral H66.003
        left H66.002
        recurrent H66.007
          with rupture of ear drum H66.017
            bilateral H66.016
            left H66.015
            right H66.014
          bilateral H66.006
          left H66.005
          right H66.004
        right H66.001
      bilateral H66.43
      chronic — *see also* category H66.3
        atticoantral H66.20
          bilateral H66.23
          left H66.22
          right H66.21
        benign — *see* Otitis, media,
          suppurative, chronic,
          tubotympanic
        tubotympanic H66.10
          bilateral H66.13
          left H66.12
          right H66.11
      left H66.42
      right H66.41
      transudative — *see* Otitis, media,
        nonsuppurative
      tuberculous A18.6
Otocephaly Q18.2
Otolith syndrome — *see* category H81.8
Otomycosis (diffuse) NEC B36.9 *[H62.40]*
  in
    aspergillosis B44.89
    candidiasis B37.84
    moniliasis B37.84
Otoporosis — *see* Otosclerosis
Otorrhagia (nontraumatic) H92.20
  bilateral H92.23
  left H92.22
  right H92.21
  traumatic – code by Type of injury
Otorrhea H92.10
  bilateral H92.13
  cerebrospinal G96.0
  left H92.12
  right H92.11
Otosclerosis (general) H80.90
  bilateral H80.93
  cochlear (endosteal) H80.20
    bilateral H80.23
    left H80.22
    right H80.21
  involving
    otic capsule — *see* Otosclerosis, cochlear
    oval window
      nonobliterative H80.00
        bilateral H80.03
        left H80.02
        right H80.01
      obliterative H80.10
        bilateral H80.13
        left H80.12
        right H80.11
    round window — *see* Otosclerosis, cochlear
  left H80.92
  nonobliterative — *see* Otosclerosis, involving,
    oval window, nonobliterative
  obliterative — *see* Otosclerosis, involving, oval
    window, obliterative
  right H80.91
  specified NEC H80.80
    bilateral H80.83
    left H80.82
    right H80.81
Otospongiosis — *see* Otosclerosis

Otto's disease or pelvis M24.7
Outcome of delivery Z37.9
  multiple births Z37.9
    all liveborn Z37.50
      quadruplets Z37.52
      quintuplets Z37.53
      sextuplets Z37.54
      specified number NEC Z37.59
      triplets Z37.51
    all stillborn Z37.7
    some liveborn Z37.60
      quadruplets Z37.62
      quintuplets Z37.63
      sextuplets Z37.64
      specified number NEC Z37.69
      triplets Z37.61
  single NEC Z37.9
    liveborn Z37.0
    stillborn Z37.1
  twins NEC Z37.9
    both liveborn Z37.2
    both stillborn Z37.4
    one liveborn, one stillborn Z37.3
Outlet — *see* condition
Outstanding ears (bilateral) Q17.5
Ovalocytosis (congenital) (hereditary) — *see*
  Elliptocytosis
Ovarian — *see* Condition
Ovariocele N83.4
Ovaritis (cystic) — *see* Oophoritis
Ovary, ovarian — *see also* condition
  resistant syndrome E28.3
  vein syndrome N13.8
Overactive — *see also* Hyperfunction
  adrenal cortex NEC E27.0
  bladder N31.3
  disorder, associated with mental retardation
    and stereotyped movements F84.4
  hypothalamus E23.3
  thyroid — *see* Hyperthyroidism
Overactivity R46.3
  child — *see* Disorder, attention-deficit
    hyperactivity
Overbite (deep) (excessive) (horizontal) (vertical)
  M26.2
Overbreathing — *see* Hyperventilation
Overconscientious personality F60.5
Overdevelopment — *see* Hypertrophy
Overdistension — *see* Distension
Overdose, overdosage (by accident) (drug)
  T50.901
  administered with intent to harm by
    another person T50.903
      self T50.902
  circumstances undetermined T50.904
  specified drug or substance — *see* Table of
    Drugs and Chemicals
Overeating R63.2
  nonorganic origin F50.8
  psychogenic F50.8
Overexertion (effects) (exhaustion) T73.3
Overexposure (effects) T73.9
  exhaustion T73.2
Overfeeding — *see* Overeating
  newborn P92.4
Overgrowth, bone — *see* Hypertrophy, bone
Overheated (places) (effects) — *see* Heat
Overjet M26.2
Overlaid, overlying (suffocation) — *see* Asphyxia,
  traumatic, due to mechanical threat
Overlapping toe (acquired) — *see also* Deformity,
  toe, specified NEC
  congenital (fifth toe) Q66.8
Overload
  fluid E87.7
  potassium (K) E87.5
  sodium (Na) E87.0
Overnutrition — *see* Hyperalimentation
Overproduction — *see also* Hypersecretion
  ACTH E27.0
  catecholamine E27.5
  growth hormone E22.0

Overprotection, child by parent Z62.1
Overriding
  aorta Q25.4
  finger (acquired) — *see* Deformity, finger
    congenital Q68.1
  toe (acquired) — *see also* Deformity, toe,
    specified NEC
    congenital Q66.8
Oversize fetus P08.1
  affecting management of pregnancy O36.60
    first trimester O36.61
    second trimester O36.62
    third trimester O36.63
  causing disproportion O33.5
    with obstructed labor O66.2
  exceptionally large (more than 4500g.) P08.0
Overstrained R53.82
  heart — *see* Hypertrophy, cardiac
Overweight — *see* Obesity
Overwork R53.82
Oviduct — *see* condition
Ovotestis Q56.0
Ovulation (cycle)
  failure or lack of N97.0
  pain N94.0
Ovum — *see* condition
Owren's disease or syndrome (parahemophilia)
  D68.2
Ox heart — *see* Hypertrophy, cardiac
Oxalosis E72.53
Oxaluria E72.53
Oxycephaly, oxycephalic Q75.0
  syphilitic, congenital A50.02
Oxyuriasis B80
Oxyuris vermicularis (infestation) B80
Ozena J31.0

O

Pachyderma, pachydermia L85.9
  larynx (verrucosa) J38.7
Pachydermatocele (congenital) Q82.8
Pachydermoperiostosis — *see also*
  Osteoarthropathy, hypertrophic, specified
  type NEC
  clubbed nail M89.40 *[L62]*
Pachygyria Q04.3
Pachymeningitis (adhesive) (basal) (brain) (cervical)
  (chronic) (circumscribed) (external) (fibrous)
  (hemorrhagic) (hypertrophic) (internal) (purulent)
  (spinal) (suppurative) — *see* Meningitis
Pachyonychia (congenital) Q84.5
Pacinian tumor (M9507/0) — *see* Neoplasm,
  skin, benign
Pad, knuckle or Garrod's M72.1
Paget-Schroetter syndrome I82.8
Paget's disease
  with infiltrating duct carcinoma (M8541/3) —
    see Neoplasm, breast, malignant
  bone M88.9
    carpus M88.849
      left M88.842
      right M88.841
    clavicle M88.819
      left M88.812
      right M88.811
    femur M88.859
      left M88.852
      right M88.851
    fibula M88.869
      left M88.862
      right M88.861
    finger M88.849
      left M88.842
      right M88.841
    humerus M88.829
      left M88.822
      right M88.821
    ilium M88.859
    in neoplastic disease — *see* Osteitis,
      deformans, in neoplastic disease
    ischium M88.859

Paget's disease — continued
- bone — continued
  - metacarpus M88.849
    - left M88.842
    - right M88.841
  - metatarsus M88.879
    - left M88.872
    - right M88.871
  - multiple sites M88.89
  - neck M88.88
  - radius M88.839
    - left M88.832
    - right M88.831
  - rib M88.88
  - scapula M88.819
    - left M88.812
    - right M88.811
  - skull M88.0
  - tarsus M88.879
    - left M88.872
    - right M88.871
  - tibia M88.869
    - left M88.862
    - right M88.861
  - toe M88.879
    - left M88.872
    - right M88.871
  - ulna M88.839
    - left M88.832
    - right M88.831
  - vertebra M88.88
- breast (M8540/3) (female) C50.00
  - left C50.02
  - male C50.05
    - left C50.04
    - right C50.03
  - right C50.01
- extramammary (M8542/3) — see also Neoplasm, skin, malignant
  - anus (M8542/3) C21.0
    - margin (M8542/3) C44.5
    - skin (M8542/3) C44.5
- intraductal carcinoma (M8543/3) — see Neoplasm, breast, malignant
- malignant (M8540/3)
  - breast (female) C50.00
    - left C50.02
    - male C50.05
      - left C50.04
      - right C50.03
    - right C50.01
  - specified site NEC (M8542/3) — see Neoplasm, skin, malignant
  - unspecified site (female) C50.00
    - male C50.05
- mammary — see Paget's disease, breast
- nipple — see Paget's disease, breast
- osteitis deformans — see Paget's disease, bone

Pain(s) R52.9
- abdominal R10.9
  - colic R10.83
  - generalized R10.84
    - with acute abdomen R10.0
  - lower R10.30
    - left quadrant R10.32
    - pelvic or perineal R10.2
    - periumbilical R10.33
    - right quadrant R10.31
  - rebound — see Tenderness, abdominal, rebound
  - severe with abdominal rigidity R10.0
  - tenderness — see Tenderness, abdominal
  - upper R10.10
    - epigastric R10.13
    - left quadrant R10.12
    - right quadrant R10.11
- acute — see Pain, specified site NEC, acute
- adnexa (uteri) R10.2
- anginoid — see Pain, precordial
- anus K62.8
- arm — see Pain, limb, upper
- back (postural) — see Dorsalgia
- bladder R39.8
  - associated with micturition — see Micturition, painful
- bone — see Disorder, bone, specified type NEC

Pain(s) — continued
- breast N64.4
  - psychogenic F45.4
- broad ligament R10.2
- cecum — see Pain, abdominal
- cervicobrachial M53.1
- chest (central) R07.9
  - anterior wall R07.89
  - ischemic I20.9
  - on breathing R07.1
  - pleurodynia R07.81
  - precordial R07.2
  - wall (anterior) R07.89
- chronic — see Pain, specified site NEC, chronic
- coccyx M53.3
- colon — see Pain, abdominal
- coronary — see Angina
- costochondral R07.1
- diaphragm R07.1
- due to device, implant or graft (see also Complications, by site and type, specified NEC) T85.84
  - arterial graft NEC T82.848
  - breast (implant) T85.84
  - catheter NEC T85.84
    - dialysis (renal) T82.848
      - intraperitoneal T85.84
    - infusion NEC T82.848
      - spinal (epidural) (subdural) T85.84
    - urinary (indwelling) T83.84
  - electronic (electrode) (pulse generator) (stimulator)
    - bone T84.84
    - cardiac T82.847
    - nervous system (brain) (peripheral nerve) (spinal) T85.84
    - urinary T83.84
  - fixation, internal (orthopedic) NEC T84.84
  - gastrointestinal (bile duct) (esophagus) T85.84
  - genital NEC T83.84
  - heart NEC T82.847
  - infusion NEC T85.84
  - joint prosthesis T84.84
  - ocular (corneal graft) (orbital implant) NEC T85.84
  - orthopedic NEC T84.84
  - specified NEC T85.84
  - urinary NEC T83.84
  - vascular NEC T82.848
  - ventricular intracranial shunt T85.84
- ear — see category H92.0
- epigastric, epigastrium R10.13
- eye — see Pain, ocular
- face, facial R51
  - atypical G50.1
- false (labor) — see Labor, false
- female genital organs NEC N94.8
- finger — see Pain, limb, upper
- flank — see Pain, abdominal
- foot — see Pain, limb, lower
- gallbladder K82.9
- gas (intestinal) R14.1
- gastric — see Pain, abdominal
- generalized R52.9
- genital organ
  - female N94.8
  - male N50.8
  - psychogenic F45.4
- groin — see Pain, abdominal, lower
- hand — see Pain, limb, upper
- head — see Headache
- heart — see Pain, precordial
- infra-orbital — see Neuralgia, trigeminal
- intermenstrual N94.0
- jaw M27.8
- joint M25.50
  - ankle M25.579
    - left M25.572
    - right M25.571
  - elbow M25.529
    - left M25.522
    - right M25.521
  - finger M79.646
    - left M79.645
    - right M79.644

Pain(s) — continued
- joint — continued
  - foot M79.673
    - left M79.672
    - right M79.671
  - hand M79.643
    - left M79.642
    - right M79.641
  - hip M25.559
    - left M25.552
    - right M25.551
  - knee M25.569
    - left M25.562
    - right M25.561
  - psychogenic F45.4
  - shoulder M25.519
    - left M25.512
    - right M25.511
  - toe M79.676
    - left M79.675
    - right M79.674
  - wrist M25.539
    - left M25.532
    - right M25.531
- kidney N23
- labor, false or spurious — see Labor, false
- laryngeal R07.0
- leg — see Pain, limb, lower
- limb M79.609
  - lower M79.606
    - foot M79.673
      - left M79.672
      - right M79.671
    - left M79.605
    - lower leg M79.669
      - left M79.662
      - right M79.661
    - right M79.604
    - thigh M79.659
      - left M79.652
      - right M79.651
    - toe M79.676
      - left M79.675
      - right M79.674
  - upper M79.603
    - finger M79.646
      - left M79.645
      - right M79.644
    - forearm M79.639
      - left M79.632
      - right M79.631
    - hand M79.643
      - left M79.642
      - right M79.641
    - left M79.602
    - right M79.601
    - upper arm M79.629
      - left M79.622
      - right M79.621
- loin M54.5
- low back M54.5
- lumbar region M54.5
- mastoid — see category H92.0
- maxilla M27.8
- metacarpophalangeal (joint) — see Pain, joint, hand
- metatarsophalangeal (joint) — see Pain, joint, foot
- mouth K13.7
- muscle — see Myalgia
- nasal J34.8
- nasopharynx J39.2
- neck NEC M54.2
  - psychogenic F45.4
- nerve NEC — see Neuralgia
- neuromuscular — see Neuralgia
- nose J34.8
- ocular H57.10
  - bilateral H57.13
  - left H57.12
  - right H57.11
- ophthalmic — see Pain, ocular
- orbital region — see Pain, ocular
- ovary N94.8
- over heart — see Pain, precordial
- ovulation N94.0
- pelvic (female) R10.2

©2002 Ingenix, Inc.

Pain(s) — continued
  penis N48.89
    psychogenic F45.4
  pericardial — see Pain, precordial
  perineal, perineum R10.2
  pharynx J39.2
  pleura, pleural, pleuritic R07.89
  precordial (region) R07.2
    psychogenic F45.4
  psychogenic (persistent) (any site) F45.4
  radicular (spinal) — see Radiculopathy
  rectum K62.8
  respiration R07.1
  retrosternal R07.2
  rheumatoid, muscular — see Myalgia
  rib R07.81
  root (spinal) — see Radiculopathy
  round ligament (stretch) R10.2
  sciatic — see Sciatica
  scrotum N50.8
    psychogenic F45.4
  seminal vesicle N50.8
  shoulder — see Lesion, shoulder, specified NEC
  specified site NEC R52.9
    acute R52.00
      due to neoplasm R52.02
      postoperative R52.01
      specified cause NEC R52.09
    chronic R52.20
      due to neoplasm R52.22
      intractable R52.10
        due to neoplasm R52.12
        postoperative R52.11
        specified cause NEC R52.19
      postoperative R52.21
      specified cause NEC R52.29
  spermatic cord N50.8
  spinal root — see Radiculopathy
  spine M54.9
    cervical M54.2
    low back M54.5
      with sciatica M54.4
    thoracic M54.6
  stomach — see Pain, abdominal
    psychogenic F45.4
  substernal R07.2
  temporomandibular (joint) M26.62
  testis N50.8
    psychogenic F45.4
  thoracic spine M54.6
    with radicular and visceral pain M54.14
  throat R07.0
  tibia — see Pain, limb, lower
  toe — see Pain, limb, lower
  tongue K14.6
  tooth K08.8
  trigeminal — see Neuralgia, trigeminal
  ureter N23
  urinary (organ) (system) N23
  uterus NEC N94.8
    psychogenic F45.4
  vagina R10.2
  vertebrogenic (syndrome) — see Dorsalgia,
      specified NEC
  vesical R39.8
    associated with micturition — see
        Micturition, painful
  vulva R10.2
Painful — see also Pain
  coitus
    female N94.1
    male N53.12
    psychogenic F52.6
  ejaculation (semen) N53.12
    psychogenic F52.6
  erection — see Priapism
  feet syndrome E53.8
  menstruation — see Dysmenorrhea
    psychogenic F45.8
  micturition — see Micturition, painful
  respiration R07.1
  scar NEC L90.5
  wire sutures T81.89
Painter's colic — see category T56.0
Palate — see condition
Palatoplegia K13.7

Palatoschisis — see Cleft, palate
Palilalia R48.8
Palliative care Z51.5
Pallor R23.1
  optic disc, temporal — see Atrophy, optic
Palmar — see also condition
  fascia — see condition
Palpable
  cecum K63.8
  kidney N28.89
  ovary N83.8
  prostate N42.9
  spleen — see Splenomegaly
Palpitations (heart) R00.2
  psychogenic F45.8
Palsy — see also Paralysis
  atrophic diffuse (progressive) G12.22
  Bell's — see also Palsy, facial
    newborn P11.3
  brachial plexus NEC G54.0
    fetus or newborn (birth injury) P14.3
  brain — see Palsy, cerebral
  bulbar (progressive) (chronic) G12.22
    of childhood (Fazio-Londe) G12.1
    pseudo NEC G12.29
    supranuclear NEC G12.22
  cerebral (congenital) (infantile) G80.9
    ataxic G80.4
    athetoid G80.3
    diplegic (spastic) G80.1
    dyskinetic G80.3
    hemiplegic G80.2
    mixed G80.8
    monoplegic NEC G80.8
    not congenital or infantile, acute I64
    paraplegic NEC G80.8
      spastic G80.1
    quadriplegic G80.8
    spastic G80.0
      not congenital or infantile G83.89
    specified NEC G80.8
    syphilitic A52.12
      congenital A50.49
    tetraplegic G80.8
  cranial nerve — see also Disorder, nerve,
      cranial
    multiple G52.7
      in
        infectious disease B99 [G53]
        neoplastic disease (see also Neoplasm)
            D49.9 [G53]
        parasitic disease B89 [G53]
        sarcoidosis D86.82
  creeping G12.22
  diver's T70.3
  Erb's P14.0
  facial G51.0
    newborn (birth injury) P11.3
  glossopharyngeal G52.1
  Klumpke(-Déjérine) P14.1
  lead — see category T56.0
  median nerve (tardy) G56.10
    left G56.12
    right G56.11
  nerve G58.9
    specified NEC G58.8
  peroneal nerve (acute) (tardy G57.30
    left G57.32
    right G57.31
  pseudobulbar NEC G12.29
  radial nerve (acute) G56.30
    left G56.32
    right G56.31
  seventh nerve — see also Palsy, facial
    newborn P11.3
  shaking — see Parkinsonism
  spastic (cerebral) (spinal) G80.9
  ulnar nerve (tardy) G56.20
    left G56.22
    right G56.21
  wasting G12.29
Paludism — see Malaria
Panangiitis M30.0

Panaris, panaritium — see also Cellulitis, digit
  with lymphangitis — see Lymphangitis, acute,
      digit
Panarteritis nodosa M30.0
  brain or cerebral I67.7
Pancake heart R93.1
  with cor pulmonale (chronic) I27.9
Pancarditis (acute) (chronic) I51.8
  rheumatic I09.89
    active or acute I01.8
Pancoast's syndrome or tumor (M8010/3)
    C34.10
  left C34.12
  right C34.11
Pancreas, pancreatic — see condition
Pancreatitis (acute (recurrent)) (annular)
    (apoplectic) (calcareous) (edematous)
    (hemorrhagic) (malignant) (subacute)
    (suppurative) K85.8
  chronic (infectious) K86.1
    alcohol-induced K86.0
    recurrent K86.1
    relapsing K86.1
  cystic (chronic) K86.1
  cytomegaloviral B25.2
  fibrous (chronic) K86.1
  gangrenous K85.8
  interstitial (chronic) K86.1
    acute K85.8
  mumps B26.3
  recurrent (chronic) K86.1
  relapsing, chronic K86.1
  syphilitic A52.74
Pancreatoblastoma (M8971/3) — see Neoplasm,
    pancreas, malignant
Pancreolithiasis K86.8
Pancytolysis D75.8
Pancytopenia (acquired) D61.9
  with malformations D61.0
  congenital D61.0
Panencephalitis, subacute, sclerosing A81.1
Panhematopenia D61.9
  congenital D61.0
  constitutional D61.0
  splenic, primary D73.1
Panhemocytopenia D61.9
  congenital D61.0
  constitutional D61.0
Panhypogonadism E29.1
Panhypopituitarism E23.0
  prepubertal E23.0
Panic (attack) (state) F41.0
  reaction to exceptional stress (transient) F43.0
Panmyelopathy, familial, constitutional D61.0
Panmyelophthisis D61.9
  congenital D61.0
Panmyelosis (acute) (M9931/1) C94.40
  in remission C94.41
Panner's disease — see Osteochondrosis,
    juvenile, humerus
Panneuritis endemica E51.11
Panniculitis (nodular) (nonsuppurative) M79.3
  back M54.00
    cervical region M54.02
    cervicothoracic region M54.03
    lumbar region M54.06
    lumbosacral region M54.07
    multiple sites M54.09
    occipito-atlanto-axial region M54.01
    sacrococcygeal region M54.08
    thoracic region M54.04
    thoracolumbar region M54.05
  lupus L93.2
  neck M54.02
    cervicothoracic region M54.03
    occipito-atlanto-axial region M54.01
  relapsing M35.6
Panniculus adiposus (abdominal) E65

Pannus (allergic) (cornea) (degenerativus) (keratic)
H16.429
  bilateral H16.423
  left H16.422
  right H16.421
  trachomatosus, trachomatous (active) A71.1
Panophthalmitis H44.019
  bilateral H44.013
  left H44.012
  right H44.011
Pansinusitis (chronic) (hyperplastic) (nonpurulent)
(purulent) J32.4
  acute J01.40
    recurrent J01.41
  tuberculous A15.8
Panuveitis (sympathetic) H44.119
  bilateral H44.113
  left H44.112
  right H44.111
Panvalvular disease I08.9
  specified NEC I08.8
Papanicolaou smear, cervix Z12.4
  as part of routine gynecological examination
Z01.40
  for suspected neoplasm Z12.4
    no disease found Z03.8
  nonspecific abnormal finding R87.6
  routine Z01.40
Papilledema (choked disc) H47.10
  associated with
    decreased ocular pressure H47.12
    increased intracranial pressure H47.11
    retinal disorder H47.13
  Foster Kennedy syndrome H47.149
    bilateral H47.143
    left H47.142
    right H47.141
Papillitis H46.00
  anus K62.8
  chronic lingual K14.4
  necrotizing, kidney N17.2
  optic H46.00
    left H46.02
    right H46.01
  rectum K62.8
  renal, necrotizing N17.2
  tongue K14.0
Papilloma (M8050/0) — *see also* Neoplasm,
benign
  acuminatum (female) (male) (anogenital) A63.0
  benign pinta (primary) A67.0
  bladder (urinary) (transitional cell) (M8120/1)
D41.4
    benign (M8120/0) D30.3
  choroid plexus (lateral ventricle) (third
ventricle) (M9390/0) D33.0
    anaplastic (M9390/3) C71.5
    fourth ventricle D33.1
    malignant (M9390/3) C71.5
  ductal (M8503/0)
  dyskeratotic (M8052/0)
  epidermoid (M8052/0)
  hyperkeratotic (M8052/0)
  intracystic (M8504/0)
  intraductal (M8503/0)
  inverted (M8053/0)
  keratotic (M8052/0)
  parakeratotic (M8052/0)
  renal pelvis (transitional cell) (M8120/1)
D41.10
    benign (M8120/0) D30.10
      left D30.12
      right D30.11
    left D41.12
    right D41.11
  Schneiderian (M8121/0)
    specified site — *see* Neoplasm, benign
    unspecified site D14.0
  serous surface (M8461/0)
    borderline malignancy (M8461/1)
      specified site — *see* Neoplasm, uncertain
behavior
      unspecified site D39.10
    specified site — *see* Neoplasm, benign
    unspecified site D27.0

Papilloma — *see also* Neoplasm, benign —
continued
  squamous (cell) (M8052/0)
  transitional (cell) (M8120/0)
    bladder (urinary) (M8120/1) D41.4
    inverted type (M8121/1) — *see* Neoplasm,
uncertain behavior
    renal pelvis (M8120/1) D41.10
      left D41.12
      right D41.11
    ureter (M8120/1) D41.20
      left D41.22
      right D41.21
  ureter (transitional cell) (M8120/1) D41.20
    benign (M8120/0) D30.20
      left D30.22
      right D30.21
    left D41.22
    right D41.21
  urothelial (M8120/1) — *see* Neoplasm,
uncertain behavior
  verrucous (M8051/0)
  villous (M8261/1) — *see* Neoplasm, uncertain
behavior
    adenocarcinoma in (M8261/3) — *see*
Neoplasm, malignant
      in situ (M8261/2) — *see* Neoplasm, in
situ
  yaws, plantar or palmar A66.1
Papillomata, multiple, of yaws A66.1
Papillomatosis (M8060/0) — *see also* Neoplasm,
benign
  confluent and reticulated L83
  cystic, breast — *see* Mastopathy, cystic
  ductal, breast — *see* Mastopathy, cystic
  intraductal (diffuse) (M8505/0) — *see*
Neoplasm, benign
  subareolar duct (M8506/0) (female) D24.00
    left D24.02
    male D24.10
      left D24.12
      right D24.11
    right D24.01
**Papillomavirus, as cause of disease classified
elsewhere** B97.7
Papillon-Léage and Psaume syndrome Q87.0
Papule(s) R23.8
  carate (primary) A67.0
  fibrous, of nose (M8724/0) D22.39
  Gottron's L94.4
  pinta (primary) A67.0
Papulosis
  lymphomatoid L41.2
  malignant I77.8
Papyraceous fetus, complicating pregnancy
O31.00
  first trimester O31.01
  second trimester O31.02
  third trimester O31.03
Para-albuminemia E88.09
Paracephalus Q89.7
Parachute mitral valve Q23.2
Paracoccidioidomycosis B41.9
  disseminated B41.7
  generalized B41.7
  mucocutaneous-lymphangitic B41.8
  pulmonary B41.0
  specified NEC B41.8
  visceral B41.8
Paradentosis K05.4
Paraffinoma T88.8
Paraganglioma (M8680/1)
  adrenal (M8700/0) D35.00
    left D35.02
    right D35.01
    malignant (M8700/3) C74.10
      left C74.12
      right C74.11
  aortic body (M8691/1) D44.7
    malignant (M8691/3) C75.5
  carotid body (M8692/1) D44.6
    malignant (M8692/3) C75.4

Paraganglioma — *continued*
  chromaffin (M8700/0) — *see also* Neoplasm,
benign
    malignant (M8700/3) — *see* Neoplasm,
malignant
  extra-adrenal (M8693/1)
    malignant (M8693/3)
      specified site — *see* Neoplasm, malignant
      unspecified site C75.5
    specified site — *see* Neoplasm, uncertain
behavior
    unspecified site D44.7
  gangliocytic (M8683/0)
    specified site — *see* Neoplasm, benign
    unspecified site D13.2
  glomus jugulare (M8690/1) D44.7
    malignant (M8690/3) C75.5
  jugular (M8690/1) D44.7
  malignant (M8680/3)
    specified site — *see* Neoplasm, malignant
    unspecified site C75.5
  nonchromaffin (M8693/1)
    malignant (M8693/3)
      specified site — *see* Neoplasm, malignant
      unspecified site C75.5
    specified site — *see* Neoplasm, uncertain
behavior
    unspecified site D44.7
  parasympathetic (M8682/1)
    specified site — *see* Neoplasm, uncertain
behavior
    unspecified site D44.7
  specified site — *see* Neoplasm, uncertain
behavior
  sympathetic (M8681/1)
    specified site — *see* Neoplasm, uncertain
behavior
    unspecified site D44.7
  unspecified site D44.7
Parageusia R43.2
  psychogenic F45.8
Paragonimiasis B66.4
Paragranuloma, Hodgkin's (M9660/3) — *see*
Hodgkin's, disease, specified type NEC
Parahemophilia (*see also* Defect, coagulation)
D68.2
Parakeratosis R23.4
  variegata L41.0
Paralysis, paralytic (complete) (incomplete) G83.9
  with
    syphilis A52.17
  abducens, abducent (nerve) — *see* Strabismus,
paralytic, sixth nerve
  abductor, lower extremity G57.90
    left G57.92
    right G57.91
  accessory nerve G52.8
  accommodation — *see also* Paresis, of
accommodation
    hysterical F44.89
  acoustic nerve (except Deafness) — *see*
category H93.3
  agitans — *see also* Parkinsonism
    arteriosclerotic G21.8
  alternating (oculomotor) G83.89
  amyotrophic G12.21
  ankle G57.90
    left G57.92
    right G57.91
  anus (sphincter) K62.8
  apoplectic (current episode) I64
  arm — *see* Monoplegia, upper limb
  arteriosclerotic (current episode) I63.8
  ascending (spinal), acute G61.0
  association G12.29
  asthenic bulbar G70.0
  ataxic (hereditary) G11.9
    general (syphilitic) A52.17
  atrophic G58.9
    infantile, acute — *see* Poliomyelitis, paralytic
    progressive G12.22
    spinal (acute) — *see* Poliomyelitis, paralytic
  attack I64
  axillary G54.0
  Babinski-Nageotte's G83.89

©2002 Ingenix, Inc.

Paralysis, paralytic — *continued*
- Bell's G51.0
  - newborn P11.3
- Benedikt's G46.3
- birth injury P14.9
  - spinal cord P11.5
- bladder (neurogenic) (sphincter) N31.2
  - puerperal, postpartum O90.8
- bowel, colon or intestine K56.0
- brachial plexus G54.0
  - birth injury P14.3
  - newborn (birth injury) P14.3
- brain G83.9
  - diplegia G83.0
  - triplegia G83.89
- bronchial J98.0
- Brown-Séquard G83.81
- bulbar (chronic) (progressive) G12.22
  - infantile — *see* Poliomyelitis, paralytic
  - poliomyelitic — *see* Poliomyelitis, paralytic
  - pseudo G12.29
  - supranuclear G12.22
- bulbospinal G70.0
- cardiac — *see also* Failure, heart I50.9
- cerebrocerebellar, diplegic infantile G80.1
- cervical
  - plexus G54.2
  - sympathetic G90.2
- Cestan-Chenais G46.3
- Charcot-Marie-Tooth type G60.0
- Clark's G80.9
- colon K56.0
- compressed air T70.3
- compression
  - arm G56.90
    - left G56.92
    - right G56.91
  - leg G57.90
    - left G57.92
    - right G57.91
  - lower extremity G57.90
    - left G57.92
    - right G57.91
  - upper extremity G56.90
    - left G56.92
    - right G56.91
- congenital (cerebral) (spinal) G80.9
  - spastic G80.0
- conjugate movement (gaze) (of eye) H51.0
  - cortical (nuclear) (supranuclear) H51.0
- cordis — *see* Failure, heart
- cranial or cerebral nerve G52.9
- creeping G12.22
- crossed leg G83.89
- crutch — *see* Injury, brachial plexus
- deglutition R13.0
  - hysterical F44.4
- dementia A52.17
- descending (spinal) NEC G12.29
- diaphragm (flaccid) J98.6
  - due to accidental section of phrenic nerve during procedure — *see* Puncture, accidental complicating surgery
- digestive organs NEC K59.8
- diplegic — *see* Diplegia
- divergence (nuclear) H51.8
- diver's T70.3
- Duchenne's G12.21
  - birth injury P14.0
- due to intracranial or spinal birth injury — *see* Palsy, cerebral
- embolic (current episode) I63.4
- Erb (-Duchenne) (birth) (newborn) P14.0
- Erb's syphilitic spastic spinal A52.17
- esophagus K22.8
- eye muscle (extrinsic) H49.9
  - intrinsic — *see also* Paresis, of accommodation
- facial (nerve) G51.0
  - birth injury P11.3
  - congenital P11.3
  - following operation NEC — *see* Puncture, accidental complicating surgery
  - newborn (birth injury) P11.3
- familial (recurrent) (periodic) G72.3
  - spastic G11.4
- fauces J39.2

Paralysis, paralytic — *continued*
- finger G56.90
  - left G56.92
  - right G56.91
- gait R26.1
- gastric nerve G52.2
- gaze, conjugate H51.0
- general (progressive) (syphilitic) A52.17
  - juvenile A50.45
- glottis J38.00
  - bilateral J38.02
  - unilateral J38.01
- gluteal G54.1
- Gubler(-Millard) G46.3
- hand — *see* Monoplegia, upper limb
- heart — *see* Arrest, cardiac
- hemiplegic — *see* Hemiplegia
- hyperkalemic periodic (familial) G72.3
- hypertensive (current episode) I64
- hypoglossal (nerve) G52.3
- hypokalemic periodic G72.3
- hysterical F44.4
- ileus K56.0
- infantile — *see also* Poliomyelitis, paralytic
  - bulbar — *see* Poliomyelitis, paralytic
  - cerebral — *see* Palsy, cerebral
  - spastic G80.0
- infective — *see* Poliomyelitis, paralytic
- inferior nuclear G83.9
- internuclear — *see* Ophthalmoplegia, internuclear
- intestine K56.0
- iris H57.09
  - due to diphtheria (toxin) A36.89
- ischemic, Volkmann's (complicating trauma) T79.6
- Jackson's G83.89
- jake — *see* Poisoning, food, noxious, plant
- Jamaica ginger (jake) G62.2
- juvenile general A50.45
- Klumpke (-Déjérine) (birth) (newborn) P14.1
- labioglossal (laryngeal) (pharyngeal) G12.29
- Landry's G61.0
- laryngeal nerve (bilateral) (recurrent) (superior) (unilateral) J38.00
  - bilateral J38.02
  - unilateral J38.01
- larynx J38.00
  - bilateral J38.02
  - due to diphtheria (toxin) A36.2
  - unilateral J38.01
- lateral G12.21
- lead — *see* category T56.0
- left side — *see* Hemiplegia
- leg G83.10
  - with involvement of
    - dominant side G83.11
    - nondominant side G83.12
  - both — *see* Paraplegia
  - crossed G83.89
  - hysterical F44.4
  - psychogenic F44.4
  - transient or transitory R29.81
    - traumatic NEC — *see* Injury, nerve, leg
- levator palpebrae superioris — *see* Blepharoptosis, paralytic
- limb — *see* Monoplegia
- lip K13.0
- Lissauer's A52.17
- lower limb — *see* Monoplegia, lower limb
  - both — *see* Paraplegia
- lung J98.4
- median nerve G56.10
  - left G56.12
  - right G56.11
- medullary (tegmental) G83.89
- mesencephalic NEC G83.89
  - tegmental G83.89
- middle alternating G83.89
- monoplegic — *see* Monoplegia
- motor G83.9

Paralysis, paralytic — *continued*
- muscle, muscular NEC G72.8
  - due to nerve lesion G58.9
  - eye (extrinsic) H49.9
    - intrinsic — *see* Paresis, of accommodation
    - oblique — *see* Strabismus, paralytic, fourth nerve
  - iris sphincter H21.9
  - ischemic (Volkmann's) (complicating trauma) T79.6
  - progressive G12.21
  - pseudohypertrophic G71.0
- musculocutaneous nerve G56.90
  - left G56.92
  - right G56.91
- musculospiral G56.90
  - left G56.92
  - right G56.91
- nerve — *see also* Disorder, nerve
  - abducent — *see* Strabismus, paralytic, sixth nerve
  - accessory G52.8
  - auditory (except Deafness) — *see* category H93.3
  - birth injury P14.9
  - cranial or cerebral G52.9
  - facial G51.0
    - birth injury P11.3
    - newborn (birth injury) P11.3
  - fourth or trochlear — *see* Strabismus, paralytic, fourth nerve
  - newborn (birth injury) P14.9
  - oculomotor — *see* Strabismus, paralytic, third nerve
  - phrenic (birth injury) P14.2
  - radial — *see* Lesion, nerve, radial
  - seventh or facial G51.0
    - newborn (birth injury) P11.3
  - sixth or abducent — *see* Strabismus, paralytic, sixth nerve
  - syphilitic A52.15
  - third or oculomotor — *see* Strabismus, paralytic, third nerve
  - trigeminal G50.9
  - trochlear — *see* Strabismus, paralytic, fourth nerve
  - ulnar G56.20
    - left G56.22
    - right G56.21
- normokalemic periodic G72.3
- ocular H49.9
  - alternating G83.89
- oculofacial, congenital (Moebius) Q87.0
- oculomotor (external bilateral) (nerve) — *see* Strabismus, paralytic, third nerve
- palate (soft) K13.7
- paratrigeminal G50.9
- periodic (familial) (hyperkalemic) (hypokalemic) (myotonic) (normokalemic) (secondary) G72.3
- peripheral autonomic nervous system — *see* Neuropathy, peripheral, autonomic
- peroneal (nerve) G57.30
  - left G57.32
  - right G57.31
- pharynx J39.2
- phrenic nerve G56.80
  - left G56.82
  - right G56.81
- plantar nerve(s) G57.60
  - left G57.62
  - right G57.61
- pneumogastric nerve G52.2
- poliomyelitis (current) — *see* Poliomyelitis, paralytic
- popliteal nerve G57.30
  - left G57.32
  - right G57.31
- postepileptic transitory G83.84
- progressive (atrophic) (bulbar) (spinal) G12.22
  - general A52.17
  - infantile acute — *see* Poliomyelitis, paralytic
- pseudobulbar G12.29
- pseudohypertrophic (muscle) G71.0
- psychogenic F44.4

Paralysis, paralytic — *continued*
  quadriceps G57.90
    left G57.92
    right G57.91
  quadriplegic — *see* Tetraplegia
  radial nerve — *see* Lesion, nerve, radial
  rectus muscle (eye) H49.9
  respiratory (muscle) (system) (tract) R06.81
    center NEC G93.8
    congenital P28.8
    newborn P28.8
  right side — *see* Hemiplegia
  Saturday night G56.30
    left G56.32
    right G56.31
  saturnine — *see* category T56.0
  sciatic nerve G57.00
    left G57.02
    right G57.01
  seizure (current episode) I64
  senile G83.9
  shaking — *see* Parkinsonism
  shock I64
  shoulder G56.90
    left G56.92
    right G56.91
  spastic G83.9
    cerebral infantile G80.0
    congenital (cerebral) (spinal) G80.0
    familial G11.4
    hereditary G11.4
    infantile G80.0
    not infantile or congenital (cerebral) G83.9
    syphilitic (spinal) A52.17
  sphincter, bladder — *see* Paralysis, bladder
  spinal (cord) G83.9
    accessory nerve G52.8
    acute — *see* Poliomyelitis, paralytic
    ascending acute G61.0
    atrophic (acute) — *see also* Poliomyelitis, paralytic
      spastic, syphilitic A52.17
    congenital G80.9
    infantile — *see* Poliomyelitis, paralytic
    hereditary G95.89
    progressive G12.21
    sequelae NEC G83.89
    spastic NEC G80.0
  sternomastoid G52.8
  stomach K31.89
    nerve G52.2
  stroke (current episode) I64
  subcapsularis G56.80
    left G56.82
    right G56.81
  supranuclear G12.29
  sympathetic G90.8
    cervical G90.2
    nervous system — *see* Neuropathy, peripheral, autonomic
  syndrome G83.9
    specified NEC G83.89
  syphilitic spastic spinal (Erb's) A52.17
  thigh G57.90
    left G57.92
    right G57.91
  throat J39.2
    diphtheritic A36.0
    muscle J39.2
  thrombotic (current episode) I63.3
  thumb G56.90
    left G56.92
    right G56.91
  tick — *see* Toxicity, venom, arthropod, specified NEC
  Todd's (postepileptic transitory paralysis) G83.84
  toe G57.60
    left G57.62
    right G57.61
  tongue K14.8
  transient R29.5
    arm or leg NEC R29.81
    traumatic NEC — *see* Injury, nerve
  trapezius G52.8
  traumatic, transient NEC — *see* Injury, nerve

Paralysis, paralytic — *continued*
  trembling — *see* Parkinsonism
  triceps brachii G56.90
    left G56.92
    right G56.91
  trigeminal nerve G50.9
  trochlear (nerve) — *see* Strabismus, paralytic, fourth nerve
  ulnar nerve G56.20
    left G56.22
    right G56.21
  upper limb — *see* Monoplegia, upper limb
  uremic N18.8 *[G99.8]*
  uveoparotitic D86.89
  uvula K13.7
    postdiphtheritic A36.0
  vagus nerve G52.2
  vasomotor NEC G90.8
  velum palati K13.7
  vesical — *see* Paralysis, bladder
  vestibular nerve (except Vertigo) — *see* category H93.3
  vocal cords J38.00
    bilateral J38.02
    unilateral J38.01
  Volkmann's (complicating trauma) T79.6
  wasting G12.29
  Weber's G46.3
  wrist G56.90
    left G56.92
    right G56.91

Paramedial urethrovesical orifice Q64.79

Paramenia N92.6

Parametritis (*see also* Disease, pelvis, inflammatory) N73.2
  acute N73.0
  complicating abortion — *see* Abortion, by type, complicated by, parametritis

Parametrium, parametric — *see* condition

Paramnesia — *see* Amnesia

Paramolar K00.1
  causing crowding M26.3

Paramyloidosis E85

Paramyoclonus multiplex G25.3

Paramyotonia (congenita) G71.1

Parangi — *see* Yaws

Paranoia (querulans) F22
  senile F03

Paranoid
  dementia (senile) F03
    praecox — *see* Schizophrenia
  personality F60.0
  psychosis (climacteric) (involutional) (menopausal) F22
    psychogenic (acute) F23
    senile F03
  reaction (acute) F23
    chronic F22
  schizophrenia F20.0
  state (climacteric) (involutional) (menopausal) (simple) F22
    senile F03
  tendencies F60.0
  traits F60.0
  trends F60.0
  type, psychopathic personality F60.0

Paraparesis — *see* Paraplegia

Paraphasia R47.02

Paraphilia F65.9

Paraphimosis (congenital) N47.2
  chancroidal A57

Paraphrenia, paraphrenic (late) F22
  schizophrenia F20.0

Paraplegia (lower) G82.20
  ataxic — *see* Degeneration, combined, spinal cord
  complete G82.21
  congenital or infantile (cerebral) (spinal) G80.8
    spastic G80.1
  familial spastic G11.4
  functional (hysterical) F44.4
  hereditary, spastic G11.4
  hysterical F44.4
  incomplete G82.22

Paraplegia — *continued*
  infantile G80.4
  Pott's A18.01
  psychogenic F44.4
  spastic
    Erb's spinal, syphilitic A52.17
    hereditary G11.4
    tropical G04.1
  syphilitic (spastic) A52.17
  tropical spastic G04.1

Paraproteinemia D89.2
  benign (familial) D89.2
  monoclonal (M9765/1) D47.2
  secondary to malignant disease (M9765/1) D47.2

Parapsoriasis L41.9
  en plaques L41.4
  guttata L41.1
  large plaque L41.4
  retiform, retiformis L41.5
  small plaque L41.3
  specified NEC L41.8
  varioliformis (acuta) L41.0

Parasitic — *see also* condition
  disease NEC B89
  stomatitis B37.0
  sycosis (beard) (scalp) B35.0
  twin Q89.4

Parasitism B89
  intestinal B82.9
  skin B88.9
  specified — *see* Infestation

Parasitophobia F40.218

Parasomnia G47.8
  nonorganic origin F51.9

Paraspadias Q54.9

Paraspasmus facialis G51.8

Parasuicide (attempt)
  history of (personal) Z91.5
    in family Z81.8
  observation following alleged attempt Z03.8

Parathyroid gland — *see* condition

Parathyroid tetany E20.9

Paratrachoma A74.0

Paratyphilitis — *see* Appendicitis

Paratyphoid (fever) — *see* Fever, paratyphoid

Paratyphus — *see* Fever, paratyphoid

Paraurethral duct Q64.79
  nonorganic origin F51.5

Paraurethritis — *see also* Urethritis
  gonococcal (acute) (chronic) (with abscess) A54.1

Paravaccinia NEC B08.0

Paravaginitis — *see* Vaginitis

Parencephalitis — *see also* Encephalitis
  sequelae G09

Paresis — *see also* Paralysis
  accommodation — *see* Paresis, of accommodation
  Bernhardt's G57.10
    left G57.12
    right G57.11
  bladder (sphincter) — *see also* Paralysis, bladder
    tabetic A52.17
  bowel, colon or intestine K56.0
  extrinsic muscle, eye H49.9
  general (progressive) (syphilitic) A52.17
    juvenile A50.45
  heart — *see* Failure, heart
  insane (syphilitic) A52.17
  juvenile (general) A50.45
  of accommodation H52.529
    bilateral H52.523
    left H52.522
    right H52.521
  peripheral progressive (idiopathic) G60.3
  pseudohypertrophic G71.0
  senile G83.9
  syphilitic (general) A52.17
    congenital A50.45
  vesical NEC N31.2

©2002 Ingenix, Inc.

Paresthesia — see also Disturbance, sensation
  Bernhardt G57.10
    left G57.12
    right G57.11
Paretic — see condition
Parinaud's
  conjunctivitis H10.8
  oculoglandular syndrome H10.8
  ophthalmoplegia H49.889
    bilateral H49.883
    left H49.882
    right H49.881
Parkinsonism (idiopathic) (primary) G20
  associated with orthostatic hypotension
    (idiopathic) (symptomatic) G90.3
  due to
    drugs NEC G21.1
      neuroleptic G21.0
    postencephalitic G21.3
  secondary G21.9
    due to
      arteriosclerosis G21.8
      drugs NEC G21.1
        neuroleptic G21.0
      encephalitis G21.3
      external agents NEC G21.2
      syphilis A52.19
      specified NEC G21.8
    syphilitic A52.19
    treatment-induced NEC G21.1
Parkinson's disease, syndrome or tremor — see Parkinsonism
Parodontitis — see Periodontitis
Parodontosis K05.4
Paronychia — see also Cellulitis, digit
  with lymphangitis — see Lymphangitis, acute, digit
  candidal (chronic) B37.2
  tuberculous (primary) A18.4
Parorexia (psychogenic) F50.8
Parosmia R43.1
  psychogenic F45.8
Parotid gland — see condition
Parotitis, parotiditis (allergic) (nonspecific toxic) (purulent) (septic) (suppurative) see also Sialoadenitis
  epidemic — see Mumps
  infectious — see Mumps
  postoperative K91.89
  surgical K91.89
Parrot fever A70
Parrot's disease (early congenital syphilitic pseudoparalysis) A50.02
Parry-Romberg syndrome G51.8
Parry's disease or syndrome E05.00
  with thyroid storm E05.01
Pars planitis — see Cyclitis
Parsonage (-Aldren) -Turner syndrome G54.5
Parson's disease (exophthalmic goiter) E05.00
  with thyroid storm E05.01
Particolored infant Q82.8
Parturition — see Delivery
Parulis K04.6
Parvovirus, as cause of disease classified elsewhere B97.6
Pasini and Pierini's atrophoderma L90.3
Passage
  false, urethra N36.0
  of sounds or bougies — see Attention to, artificial, opening
Passive — see condition
Pasteurella septica A28.0
Pasteurellosis — see Infection, Pasteurella
PAT (paroxysmal atrial tachycardia) I47.1
Patau's syndrome — see Trisomy, 13
Patches
  mucous (syphilitic) A51.39
    congenital A50.07
  smokers' (mouth) K13.2
Patellar — see condition

Patent — see also Imperfect, closure
  canal of Nuck Q52.4
  cervix N88.3
    complicating pregnancy — see Pregnancy, complicated by, incompetent cervix
  ductus arteriosus or Botallo's Q25.0
  foramen
    botalli Q21.1
    ovale Q21.1
  interauricular septum Q21.1
  interventricular septum Q21.1
  omphalomesenteric duct Q43.0
  os (uteri) — see Patent, cervix
  ostium secundum Q21.1
  urachus Q64.4
  vitelline duct Q43.0
Paterson (-Brown) (-Kelly) syndrome or web D50.1
Pathologic, pathological — see also condition
  asphyxia R09.0
  fire-setting F63.1
  gambling F63.0
  ovum O02.0
  resorption, tooth K03.3
  stealing F63.2
Pathology (of) — see Disease
Pattern, sleep-wake, irregular G47.2
Patulous
  eustachian tube H69.00
    bilateral H69.03
    left H69.02
    right H69.01
Pause, sinoatrial I49.5
Paxton's disease B36.8
Pearl(s)
  enamel K00.2
  Epstein's K09.8
Pearl-worker's disease — see Osteomyelitis, specified type NEC
Pectenosis K62.4
Pectoral — see condition
Pectus
  carinatum (congenital) Q67.7
    acquired M95.4
    rachitic (late effect) E64.3
  excavatum (congenital) Q67.6
    acquired M95.4
    rachitic (late effect) E64.3
  recurvatum (congenital) Q67.6
Pedatrophia E41
Pederosis F65.4
Pediculosis (infestation) B85.2
  capitis (head-louse) (any site) B85.0
  corporis (body-louse) (any site) B85.1
  eyelid B85.0
  mixed (classifiable to more than one of the titles B85.0-B85.3) B85.4
  pubis (pubic louse) (any site) B85.3
  vestimenti B85.1
  vulvae B85.3
Pediculus (infestation) — see Pediculosis
Pedophilia F65.4
Peg-shaped teeth K00.2
Pelade — see Alopecia, areata
Pelger-Huët anomaly or syndrome D72.0
Peliosis (rheumatica) D69.0
  hepatis K76.4
    with toxic liver disease K71.8
Pelizaeus-Merzbacher disease E75.29
Pellagra (alcoholic) (with polyneuropathy) E52
Pellagra-cerebellar-ataxia-renal aminoaciduria syndrome E72.02
Pellegrini (-Stieda) disease or syndrome — see Bursitis, tibial collateral
Pellizzi's syndrome E34.8
Pel's crisis A52.17
Pelvic — see also condition
  examination (periodic) (routine) Z01.40
    with abnormal findings Z01.41
  kidney, congenital Q63.2
Pelviolithiasis — see Calculus, kidney

Pelviperitonitis — see also Peritonitis, pelvic
  gonococcal A54.24
  puerperal O85
Pelvis — see condition or type
Pemphigoid L12.9
  benign, mucous membrane L12.1
  bullous L12.0
  cicatricial L12.1
  juvenile L12.2
  ocular L12.1
  specified NEC L12.8
Pemphigus L10.9
  benign familial (chronic) Q82.8
  Brazilian L10.3
  circinatus L13.0
  conjunctiva L12.1
  drug-induced L10.5
  erythematosus L10.4
  foliaceous L10.2
  gangrenous — see Gangrene
  neonatorum L01.03
  ocular L12.1
  paraneoplastic L10.81
  specified NEC L10.89
  syphilitic (congenital) A50.06
  vegetans L10.1
  vulgaris L10.0
  wildfire L10.3
Pendred's syndrome E07.1
Pendulous
  abdomen, in pregnancy — see Pregnancy, complicated by, abnormal, pelvic organs or tissues NEC
  breast N64.8
Penetrating wound — see also Puncture
  with internal injury — see Injury, by site
  eyeball — see Puncture, eyeball
  orbit (with or without foreign body) — see Puncture, orbit
  uterus by instrument with or following ectopic or molar pregnancy O08.6
Penicillosis B48.4
Penis — see condition
Penitis N48.29
Pentalogy of Fallot Q21.8
Pentasomy X syndrome Q97.1
Pentosuria (essential) E74.8
Peregrinating patient — see Disorder, factitious
Perforation, perforated (nontraumatic)
  accidental during procedure (blood vessel) (nerve) (organ) — see Puncture, accidental complicating surgery
  antrum — see Sinusitis, maxillary
  appendix K35.0
    with peritoneal abscess K35.1
  atrial septum, multiple Q21.1
  attic, ear — see Perforation, tympanum, attic
  bile duct (common) (hepatic) K83.2
    cystic K82.2
  bladder (urinary)
    with or following ectopic or molar pregnancy O08.6
    obstetrical trauma O71.5
    traumatic S37.28
      at delivery O71.5
  bowel K63.1
    with or following ectopic or molar pregnancy O08.6
    fetus or newborn P78.0
    obstetrical trauma O71.5
    traumatic — see Laceration, intestine
  broad ligament N83.8
    with or following ectopic or molar pregnancy O08.6
    obstetrical trauma O71.6
  by
    device, implant or graft (see also Complications, by site and type, mechanical) T85.628
      arterial graft NEC — see Complication, cardiovascular device, mechanical, vascular
      breast (implant) T85.49

Perforation, perforated — *see* Puncture,
accidental complicating surgery — *continued*
by — *continued*
device, implant or graft (*see also*
Complications, by site and type,
mechanical) — *continued*
catheter NEC T85.628
cystostomy T83.090
dialysis (renal) T82.49
intraperitoneal T85.691
infusion NEC T82.594
spinal (epidural) (subdural) T85.690
urinary (indwelling) T83.091
electronic (electrode) (pulse generator)
(stimulator)
bone T84.390
cardiac T82.199
electrode T82.190
pulse generator T82.191
specified type NEC T82.198
nervous system — *see* Complication,
prosthetic device, mechanical,
electronic nervous system
stimulator
urinary — *see* Complication,
genitourinary, device, urinary,
mechanical
fixation, internal (orthopedic) NEC — *see*
Complication, fixation device,
mechanical
gastrointestinal — *see* Complications,
prosthetic device, mechanical,
gastrointestinal device
genital NEC T83.498
intrauterine contraceptive device
T83.39
penile prosthesis T83.490
heart NEC — *see* Complication,
cardiovascular device, mechanical
joint prosthesis — *see* Complication, joint
prosthesis, mechanical
ocular NEC — *see* Complications,
prosthetic device, mechanical,
ocular device
orthopedic NEC — *see* Complication,
orthopedic, device, mechanical
specified NEC T85.628
urinary NEC — *see also* Complication,
genitourinary, device, urinary,
mechanical
graft T83.29
vascular NEC — *see* Complication,
cardiovascular device, mechanical
ventricular intracranial shunt T85.09
foreign body left accidentally in operative
wound T81.539
instrument (any) during a procedure,
accidental — *see* Puncture, accidental
complicating surgery
cecum K35.0
with peritoneal abscess K35.1
cervix (uteri) N88.8
with or following ectopic or molar pregnancy
O08.6
obstetrical trauma O71.3
colon K63.1
fetus or newborn P78.0
obstetrical trauma O71.5
traumatic — *see* Laceration, intestine, large
common duct (bile) K83.2
cornea (due to ulceration) — *see* Ulcer, cornea,
perforated
cystic duct K82.2
diverticulum (intestine) K57.80
with bleeding K57.81
large intestine K57.20
with
bleeding K57.21
small intestine K57.40
with bleeding K57.41
small intestine K57.00
with
bleeding K57.01
large intestine K57.40
with bleeding K57.41
ear drum — *see* Perforation, tympanum

Perforation, perforated — *see* Puncture,
accidental complicating surgery — *continued*
esophagus K22.3
ethmoidal sinus — *see* Sinusitis, ethmoidal
frontal sinus — *see* Sinusitis, frontal
gallbladder K82.2
heart valve — *see* Endocarditis
ileum K63.1
fetus or newborn P78.0
obstetrical trauma O71.5
traumatic — *see* Laceration, intestine, small
instrumental, surgical (accidental) (blood
vessel) (nerve) (organ) — *see* Puncture,
accidental complicating surgery
intestine NEC K63.1
with ectopic or molar pregnancy O08.6
fetus or newborn P78.0
obstetrical trauma O71.5
traumatic — *see* Laceration, intestine
ulcerative NEC K63.1
fetus or newborn P78.0
jejunum, jejunal K63.1
obstetrical trauma O71.5
traumatic — *see* Laceration, intestine, small
ulcer — *see* Ulcer, gastrojejunal, with
perforation
mastoid (antrum) (cell) — *see* Disorder,
mastoid, specified NEC
maxillary sinus — *see* Sinusitis, maxillary
membrana tympani — *see* Perforation,
tympanum
nasal
septum J34.8
congenital Q30.3
syphilitic A52.73
sinus J34.8
congenital Q30.8
due to sinusitis — *see* Sinusitis
palate — *see also* Cleft, palate
syphilitic A52.79
palatine vault — *see also* Cleft, palate, hard
syphilitic A52.79
congenital A50.59
pars flaccida (ear drum) — *see* Perforation,
tympanum, attic
pelvic
floor S31.030
with
ectopic or molar pregnancy O08.6
penetration into retroperitoneal space
S31.031
retained foreign body S31.040
with penetration into
retroperitoneal space S31.041
following ectopic or molar pregnancy
O08.6
obstetrical trauma O70.1
organ S37.99
adrenal gland S37.818
bladder — *see* Perforation, bladder
fallopian tube S37.599
bilateral S37.592
unilateral S37.591
kidney S37.099
left S37.092
right S37.091
obstetrical trauma O71.5
ovary S37.499
bilateral S37.492
unilateral S37.491
prostate S37.828
specified organ NEC S37.898
ureter — *see* Perforation, ureter
urethra — *see* Perforation, urethra
uterus — *see* Perforation, uterus
perineum — *see* Laceration, perineum
pharynx J39.2
rectum K62.8
fetus or newborn P78.0
obstetrical trauma O71.5
traumatic S36.63
sigmoid K63.1
fetus or newborn P78.0
obstetrical trauma O71.5
traumatic S36.533
sinus (accessory) (chronic) (nasal) J34.8
sphenoidal sinus — *see* Sinusitis, sphenoidal

Perforation, perforated — *see* Puncture,
accidental complicating surgery — *continued*
surgical (accidental) (by instrument) (blood
vessel) (nerve) (organ) — *see* Puncture,
accidental complicating surgery
traumatic
external — *see* Puncture
eye — *see* Puncture, eyeball
internal organ — *see* Injury, by site
tympanum (membrane) (persistent post-
traumatic) (postinflammatory) H72.90
with otitis media — *see* Otitis, media
attic H72.10
bilateral H72.13
left H72.12
multiple — *see* Perforation, tympanum,
multiple
right H72.11
total — *see* Perforation, tympanum, total
bilateral H72.93
central H72.00
bilateral H72.03
left H72.02
multiple — *see* Perforation, tympanum,
multiple
right H72.01
total — *see* Perforation, tympanum, total
left H72.92
marginal NEC — *see* category H72.2
multiple H72.819
bilateral H72.813
left H72.812
right H72.811
pars flaccida — *see* Perforation, tympanum,
attic
right H72.91
total H72.829
bilateral H72.823
left H72.822
right H72.821
traumatic, current episode S09.20
left S09.22
right S09.21
typhoid, gastrointestinal — *see* Typhoid
ulcer — *see* Ulcer, by site, with perforation
ureter N28.89
traumatic S37.19
urethra N36.8
with ectopic or molar pregnancy O08.6
following ectopic or molar pregnancy O08.6
obstetrical trauma O71.5
traumatic S37.38
at delivery O71.5
uterus
with ectopic or molar pregnancy O08.6
by intrauterine contraceptive device T83.39
following ectopic or molar pregnancy O08.6
obstetrical trauma O71.1
traumatic S37.69
obstetric O71.1
uvula K13.7
syphilitic A52.79
vagina — *see also* Puncture, vagina O71.4
Periadenitis mucosa necrotica recurrens K12.0
Periappendicitis (acute) — *see* Appendicitis
Periarteritis nodosa (disseminated) (infectious)
(necrotizing) M30.0
Periarthritis (joint) — *see also* Enthesopathy
Duplay's — *see* Capsulitis, adhesive
gonococcal A54.42
humeroscapularis — *see* Capsulitis, adhesive
scapulohumeral — *see* Capsulitis, adhesive
shoulder — *see* Capsulitis, adhesive
wrist M77.20
left M77.22
right M77.21
Periarthrosis (angioneural) — *see* Enthesopathy
Pericapsulitis, adhesive (shoulder) — *see*
Capsulitis, adhesive
Pericarditis (with decompensation) (with effusion)
I31.9
with rheumatic fever (conditions in I00)
active — *see* Pericarditis, rheumatic
inactive or quiescent I09.2

©2002 Ingenix, Inc.

Pericarditis — continued
acute (hemorrhagic) (infective) (nonrheumatic) (Sicca) I30.9
with chorea (acute) (rheumatic) (Sydenham's) I02.0
benign I30.8
nonspecific I30.0
rheumatic I01.0
with chorea (acute) (Sydenham's) I02.0
adhesive or adherent (chronic) (external) (internal) I31.0
acute — see Pericarditis, acute
rheumatic I09.2
bacterial (acute) (subacute) (with serous or seropurulent effusion) I30.1
calcareous I31.1
cholesterol (chronic) I31.8
acute I30.9
chronic (nonrheumatic) I31.9
rheumatic I09.2
constrictive (chronic) I31.1
coxsackie B33.23
fibrinocaseous (tuberculous) A18.84
fibrinopurulent I30.1
fibrinous I30.8
fibrous I31.0
gonococcal A54.83
idiopathic I30.0
in systemic lupus erythematosus M32.12
infective I30.1
meningococcal A39.53
neoplastic (chronic) I31.8
acute I30.9
obliterans, obliterating I31.0
plastic I31.0
pneumococcal I30.1
postinfarction I24.1
purulent I30.1
rheumatic (active) (acute) (with effusion) (with pneumonia) I01.0
with chorea (acute) (rheumatic) (Sydenham's) I02.0
chronic or inactive (with chorea) I09.2
rheumatoid — see Rheumatoid, carditis
septic I30.1
serofibrinous I30.8
staphylococcal I30.1
streptococcal I30.1
suppurative I30.1
syphilitic A52.06
tuberculous A18.84
uremic N18.8 [I32]
viral I30.1
Pericardium, pericardial — see condition
Pericellulitis — see Cellulitis
Pericementitis (chronic) (suppurative) — see also Periodontitis
acute K05.2
Perichondritis
auricle — see Perichondritis, ear
bronchus J98.0
ear (external) H61.009
acute H61.019
bilateral H61.013
left H61.012
right H61.011
bilateral H61.003
chronic H61.029
bilateral H61.023
left H61.022
right H61.021
left H61.002
right H61.001
external auditory canal — see Perichondritis, ear
larynx J38.7
syphilitic A52.73
typhoid A01.09
nose J34.8
pinna — see Perichondritis, ear
trachea J39.8
Periclasia K05.4
Pericoronitis (chronic) K05.3
acute K05.2
Pericystitis N30.90
with hematuria N30.91

Peridiverticulitis (intestine) K57.92
cecum — see Diverticulitis, intestine, large
colon — see Diverticulitis, intestine, large
duodenum — see Diverticulitis, intestine, small
intestine — see Diverticulitis, intestine
jejunum — see Diverticulitis, intestine, small
rectosigmoid — see Diverticulitis, intestine, large
rectum — see Diverticulitis, intestine, large
sigmoid — see Diverticulitis, intestine, large
Periendocarditis — see Endocarditis
Periepididymitis N45.1
Perifolliculitis L01.02
abscedens, caput, scalp L66.3
capitis, abscedens (et suffodiens) L66.3
superficial pustular L01.02
Perihepatitis K65.8
Perilabyrinthitis (acute) — see category H83.0
Perimeningitis — see Meningitis
Perimetritis — see Endometritis
Perimetrosalpingitis — see Salpingo-oophoritis
Perinephric, perinephritic — see condition
Perinephritis — see also Infection, kidney
purulent — see Abscess, kidney
Perineum, perineal — see condition
Perineuritis NEC — see Neuralgia
Periodic — see condition
Periodontitis (chronic) (complex) (compound) (local) (simplex) K05.3
acute K05.2
apical K04.5
acute (pulpal origin) K04.4
Periodontoclasia K05.4
Periodontosis (juvenile) K05.4
Periods — see also Menstruation
heavy N92.0
irregular N92.6
shortened intervals (irregular) N92.1
Perionychia — see also Cellulitis, digit
with lymphangitis — see Lymphangitis, acute, digit
Periophoritis — see Salpingo-oophoritis
Periorchitis N45.2
Periosteum, periosteal — see condition
Periostitis (albuminosa) (circumscribed) (diffuse) (infective) (monomelic) — see also Osteomyelitis
alveolar M27.3
alveolodental M27.3
dental M27.3
gonorrheal A54.43
jaw (lower) (upper) M27.2
orbit H05.039
bilateral H05.033
left H05.032
right H05.031
syphilitic A52.77
congenital (early) A50.02 [M90.80]
secondary A51.46
tuberculous — see Tuberculosis, bone
yaws (hypertrophic) (early) (late) A66.6 [M90.80]
Periostosis (hyperplastic) — see also Disorder, bone, specified type NEC
with osteomyelitis — see Osteomyelitis, specified type NEC
Periphlebitis — see Phlebitis
Periproctitis K62.8
Periprostatitis — see Prostatitis
Perirectal — see condition
Perirenal — see condition
Perisalpingitis — see Salpingo-oophoritis
Perisplenitis (infectional) D73.8
Peristalsis, visible or reversed R19.2
Peritendinitis — see Enthesopathy
Peritoneum, peritoneal — see condition

Peritonitis (adhesive) (fibrinous) (hemorrhagic) (idiopathic) (localized) (perforative) (primary) (with adhesions) (with effusion) K65.9
with or following
abscess K65.0
appendicitis K35.0
with peritoneal abscess K35.1
diverticular disease (intestine) K57.80
with bleeding K57.81
large intestine K57.20
with
bleeding K57.21
small intestine K57.40
with bleeding K57.41
small intestine K57.00
with
bleeding K57.01
large intestine K57.40
with bleeding K57.41
ectopic or molar pregnancy O08.0
acute K65.0
aseptic T81.61
bile, biliary K65.8
chemical T81.61
chlamydial A74.81
complicating abortion — see Abortion, by type, complicated by, pelvic peritonitis
congenital P78.1
chronic proliferative K65.8
diaphragmatic K65.0
diffuse K65.0
diphtheritic A36.89
disseminated K65.0
due to
bile K65.8
foreign
body or object accidentally left following a procedure (instrument) (sponge) (swab) T81.599
substance accidentally left during a procedure (chemical) (powder) (talc) T81.61
talc T81.61
urine K65.8
fibrocaseous (tuberculous) A18.31
fibropurulent K65.0
following ectopic or molar pregnancy O08.0
general(ized) K65.0
gonococcal A54.85
meconium (newborn) P78.0
neonatal P78.1
meconium P78.0
pancreatic K65.0
paroxysmal, familial E85
benign E85
pelvic
female N73.5
acute N73.3
chronic N73.4
with adhesions N73.6
male K65.0
periodic, familial E85
proliferative, chronic K65.8
puerperal, postpartum, childbirth O85
purulent K65.0
septic K65.0
subdiaphragmatic K65.0
subphrenic K65.0
suppurative K65.0
syphilitic A52.74
congenital (early) A50.08 [K67]
talc T81.61
tuberculous A18.31
urine K65.8
Peritonsillar — see condition
Peritonsillitis J36
Perityphlitis K37
Periureteritis N28.89
Periurethral — see condition
Periurethritis (gangrenous) — see Urethritis
Periuterine — see condition
Perivaginitis — see Vaginitis
Perivasculitis, retinal — see Vasculitis, retina
Perivasitis (chronic) N49.1
Perivesiculitis (seminal) — see Vesiculitis

Perlèche NEC K13.0
  due to
    candidiasis B37.83
    moniliasis B37.83
    riboflavin deficiency E53.0
    vitamin B2 (riboflavin) deficiency E53.0
      [K93]
Pernicious — see condition
Pernio, perniosis T69.1
Persecution
  delusion F22
  social Z60.5
Perseveration (tonic) R48.8
Persistence, persistent (congenital)
  anal membrane Q42.3
    with fistula Q42.2
  arteria stapedia Q16.3
  atrioventricular canal Q21.2
  branchial cleft Q18.0
  bulbus cordis in left ventricle Q21.8
  canal of Cloquet Q14.0
  capsule (opaque) Q12.8
  cilioretinal artery or vein Q14.8
  cloaca Q43.7
  communication — see Fistula, congenital
  convolutions
    aortic arch Q25.4
    fallopian tube Q50.6
    oviduct Q50.6
    uterine tube Q50.6
  double aortic arch Q25.4
  ductus arteriosus (Botalli) Q25.0
  fetal
    circulation P29.3
    form of cervix (uteri) Q51.8
    hemoglobin, hereditary (HPFH) D56.4
  foramen
    Botalli Q21.1
    ovale Q21.1
  Gartner's duct Q50.6
  hemoglobin, fetal (hereditary) (HPFH) D56.4
  hyaloid
    artery (generally incomplete) Q14.8
    system Q14.8
  hymen, in pregnancy or childbirth — see
      Pregnancy, complicated by, abnormal,
      vulva
  lanugo Q84.2
  left
    posterior cardinal vein Q26.8
    root with right arch of aorta Q25.4
    superior vena cava Q26.1
  Meckel's diverticulum Q43.0
  mucosal disease (middle ear) — see Otitis,
      media, suppurative, chronic,
      tubotympanic
  nail(s), anomalous Q84.6
  occipitoposterior or transverse O64.0
  omphalomesenteric duct Q43.0
  organ or site not listed — see Anomaly, by site
  ostium
    atrioventriculare commune Q21.2
    primum Q21.2
    secundum Q21.1
  ovarian rests in fallopian tube Q50.6
  pancreatic tissue in intestinal tract Q43.8
  primary (deciduous)
    teeth K00.6
    vitreous hyperplasia Q14.0
  pupillary membrane Q13.89
  right aortic arch Q25.4
  rhesus (Rh) titer T80.4
  sinus
    urogenitalis
      female Q52.8
      male Q55.8
    venosus with imperfect incorporation in
        right auricle Q26.8
  thymus (gland) (hyperplasia) E32.0
  thyroglossal duct Q89.2
  thyrolingual duct Q89.2
  truncus arteriosus or communis Q20.0
  tunica vasculosa lentis Q12.2
  umbilical sinus Q64.4
  urachus Q64.4
  vitelline duct Q43.0

Person (with)
  admitted for clinical research, as a control
      subject Z00.6
  awaiting admission to adequate facility
      elsewhere Z75.1
  concern (normal) about sick person in family
      Z63.6
  consulting on behalf of another Z71.0
  feared
    complaint in whom no diagnosis was made
        Z71.1
    condition not demonstrated Z71.1
  feigning illness Z76.5
  living (in)
    alone Z60.2
    boarding school Z59.3
    residential institution Z59.3
    without
      adequate housing (heating) (space) Z59.1
      housing (permanent) (temporary) Z59.0
      person able to render necessary care Z74.2
      shelter Z59.0
  on waiting list Z75.1
  sick or handicapped in family Z63.6
  "worried well" Z71.1
Personality (disorder) F60.9
  accentuation of traits (type A pattern) Z73.1
  affective F34.0
  aggressive F60.3
  amoral F60.2
  anacastic, anankastic F60.5
  antisocial F60.2
  anxious F60.6
  asocial F60.2
  asthenic F60.7
  avoidant F60.6
  borderline F60.3
  change due to organic condition (enduring)
      F07.0
  compulsive F60.5
  cycloid F34.0
  cyclothymic F34.0
  dependent F60.7
  depressive F34.1
  dissocial F60.2
  dual F44.81
  eccentric F60.89
  emotionally unstable F60.3
  expansive paranoid F60.0
  explosive F60.3
  fanatic F60.0
  haltose type F60.89
  histrionic F60.4
  hyperthymic F34.0
  hypothymic F34.1
  hysterical F60.4
  immature F60.89
  inadequate F60.7
  labile (emotional) F60.3
  mixed (nonspecific) F60.81
  morally defective F60.2
  multiple F44.81
  narcissistic F60.81
  obsessional F60.5
  obsessive(-compulsive) F60.5
  organic F07.0
  overconscientious F60.5
  paranoid F60.0
  passive(-dependent) F60.7
  passive-aggressive F60.89
  pathologic F60.9
  pattern defect or disturbance F60.9
  pseudopsychopathic (organic) F07.0
  pseudoretarded (organic) F07.0
  psychoinfantile F60.4
  psychoneurotic NEC F60.89
  psychopathic F60.2
  querulant F60.0
  sadistic F60.89
  schizoid F60.1
  self-defeating F60.7
  sensitive paranoid F60.0
  sociopathic (amoral) (antisocial) (asocial)
      (dissocial) F60.2
  specified NEC F60.89
  type A Z73.1
  unstable (emotional) F60.3

Perthes' disease — see Legg-Calve-Perthes
    disease
Pertussis — see also Whooping cough
  vaccination, prophylactic (against) Z23
Perversion, perverted
  appetite F50.8
    psychogenic F50.8
  function
    pituitary gland E23.2
      posterior lobe E22.2
  sense of smell and taste R43.8
    psychogenic F45.8
  sexual — see Deviation, sexual
Pervious, congenital — see also Imperfect,
    closure
  ductus arteriosus Q25.0
Pes (congenital) — see also Talipes
  acquired — see also Deformity, limb, foot,
      specified NEC
    planus   see Deformity, limb, flat foot
  adductus Q66.8
  cavus Q66.7
  deformity NEC, acquired — see Deformity,
      limb, foot, specified NEC
  planus (acquired) (any degree) — see also
      Deformity, limb, flat foot
    congenital Q66.5
    rachitic (late effect) E64.3
  valgus Q66.6
Pest, pestis — see Plague
Petechia, petechiae R23.3
  fetus or newborn P54.5
Petechial typhus A75.9
Peter's anomaly Q13.4
Petit mal G40.70
  with
    grand mal seizures G40.60
      with status epilepticus G40.61
    status epilepticus G40.71
  epilepsy (idiopathic) (juvenile) (childhood)
      G40.30
    with status epilepticus G40.31
  impulsive G40.30
    with status epilepticus G40.31
Petit's hernia — see Hernia, abdomen, specified
    site NEC
Petrellidosis B48.2
Petrositis H70.209
  acute H70.219
    bilateral H70.213
    left H70.212
    right H70.211
  bilateral H70.203
  chronic H70.229
    bilateral H70.223
    left H70.222
    right H70.221
  left H70.202
  right H70.201
Peutz-Jeghers disease or syndrome Q85.8
Peyronie's disease N48.6
Pfeiffer's disease — see Mononucleosis,
    infectious
Phagedena (dry) (moist) (sloughing) — see also
    Gangrene
  geometric L88
  penis N48.29
  tropical — see Ulcer, skin
  vulva N76.6
Phagedenic — see condition
Phakoma H35.89
Phakomatosis (see also specific eponymous
    syndromes) Q85.9
  Bourneville's Q85.1
  specified NEC Q85.8
Phantom limb syndrome (without pain) G54.7
  with pain G54.6
Pharyngeal pouch syndrome D82.1

©2002 Ingenix, Inc.

Pharyngitis (acute) (catarrhal) (gangrenous) (infective) (malignant) (membranous) (phlegmonous) (pseudomembranous) (simple) (subacute) (suppurative) (ulcerative) (viral) J02.9
  with influenza, flu, or grippe J10.1
  aphthous B08.5
  atrophic J31.2
  chlamydial A56.4
  chronic (atrophic) (granular) (hypertrophic) J31.2
  coxsackievirus B08.5
  diphtheritic A36.0
  enteroviral vesicular B08.5
  follicular (chronic) J31.2
  fusospirochetal A69.1
  gonococcal A54.5
  granular (chronic) J31.2
  herpesviral B00.2
  hypertrophic J31.2
  infectional, chronic J31.2
  influenzal J10.1
  lymphonodular, acute (enteroviral) B08.8
  pneumococcal J02.8
  purulent J02.9
  putrid J02.9
  septic J02.0
  sicca J31.2
  specified organism NEC J02.8
  staphylococcal J02.8
  streptococcal J02.0
  syphilitic, congenital (early) A50.03
  tuberculous A15.8
  vesicular, enteroviral B08.5
  viral NEC J02.8
Pharyngoconjunctivitis, viral B30.2
Pharyngolaryngitis (acute) J06.0
  chronic J37.0
Pharyngoplegia J39.2
Pharyngotonsillitis, herpesviral B00.2
Pharyngotracheitis, chronic J42
Pharynx, pharyngeal — see condition
Phenomenon
  Arthus' — see Arthus' phenomenon
  jaw-winking Q07.8
  lupus erythematosus (LE) cell M32.9
  Raynaud's (secondary) I73.00
    with gangrene I73.01
  vasomotor R55
  vasospastic I73.9
  vasovagal R55
  Wenckebach's I44.1
Phenylketonuria E70.1
  classical E70.0
  maternal E70.1
Pheochromoblastoma (M8700/3)
  specified site — see Neoplasm, malignant
  unspecified site C74.10
Pheochromocytoma (M8700/0)
  malignant (M8700/3)
    specified site — see Neoplasm, malignant
    unspecified site C74.10
  specified site — see Neoplasm, benign
  unspecified site D35.00
Pheohyphomycosis — see Chromomycosis
Pheomycosis — see Chromomycosis
Phimosis (congenital) (due to infection) N47.1
  chancroidal A57
Phlebectasia — see also Varix
  congenital Q27.4
Phlebitis (infective) (pyemic) (septic) (suppurative) I80.9
  blue — see Phlebitis, leg, deep
  breast, superficial I80.8
  cavernous (venous) sinus — see Phlebitis, intracranial (venous) sinus
  cerebral (venous) sinus — see Phlebitis, intracranial (venous) sinus
  chest wall, superficial I80.8
  complicating pregnancy — see Thrombophlebitis, antepartum
  cranial (venous) sinus — see Phlebitis, intracranial (venous) sinus
  deep (vessels) — see Phlebitis, leg, deep

Phlebitis — continued
  due to implanted device — see Complications, by site and type, specified NEC
  during or resulting from a procedure T81.7
  femoral vein I80.10
    bilateral I80.13
    left I80.12
    right I80.11
  following infusion, therapeutic injection or transfusion T80.1
  gestational — see Phlebopathy, gestational
  hepatic veins I80.8
  iliofemoral — see Phlebitis, femoral vein
  intracranial (venous) sinus (any) G08
    antepartum O22.50
      first trimester O22.51
      second trimester O22.52
      third trimester O22.53
    nonpyogenic I67.6
  intraspinal venous sinuses and veins G08
    nonpyogenic G95.19
  lateral (venous) sinus — see Phlebitis, intracranial (venous) sinus
  leg I80.3
    antepartum — see Thrombophlebitis, antepartum
    deep (vessels) NEC I80.209
      bilateral I80.203
      left I80.202
      popliteal vein I80.219
        bilateral I80.213
        left I80.212
        right I80.211
      right I80.201
      specified vessel NEC I80.299
        bilateral I80.293
        left I80.292
        right I80.291
      tibial vein I80.229
        bilateral I80.223
        left I80.222
        right I80.221
    femoral vein I80.10
      bilateral I80.13
      left I80.12
      right I80.11
    superficial (vessels) I80.00
      bilateral I80.03
      left I80.02
      right I80.01
  longitudinal sinus — see Phlebitis, intracranial (venous) sinus
  lower limb — see Phlebitis, leg
  migrans, migrating (superficial) I82.1
  pelvic
    with ectopic or molar pregnancy O08.0
    following ectopic or molar pregnancy O08.0
    puerperal, postpartum O87.1
  popliteal vein — see Phlebitis, leg, deep, popliteal
  portal (vein) K75.1
  postoperative T81.7
  pregnancy — see Thrombophlebitis, antepartum
  puerperal, postpartum, childbirth O87.9
    deep O87.1
    pelvic O87.1
    superficial O87.0
  retina — see Vasculitis, retina
  saphenous (accessory) (great) (long) (small) — see Phlebitis, leg, superficial
  sinus (meninges) — see Phlebitis, intracranial (venous) sinus
  specified site NEC I80.8
  syphilitic A52.09
  tibial vein — see Phlebitis, leg, deep, tibial
  ulcerative I80.9
    leg — see Phlebitis, leg
  umbilicus I80.8
  uterus (septic) — see Endometritis
  varicose (leg) (lower limb) — see Varix, leg, with, inflammation
Phlebofibrosis I87.8
Pholeboliths I87.8

Phlebopathy
  gestational O22.90
    first trimester O22.91
    second trimester O22.92
    third trimester O22.93
  puerperal O87.9
Phlebosclerosis I87.8
Phlebothrombosis — see also Thrombosis
  antepartum — see Thrombophlebitis, antepartum
  pregnancy — see Thrombophlebitis, antepartum
  puerperal — see Thrombophlebitis, puerperal
Phlebotomus fever A93.1
Phlegmasia
  alba dolens O87.1
    nonpuerperal — see Phlebitis, femoral vein
  cerulea dolens — see Phlebitis, leg, deep
Phlegmon — see Abscess
Phlegmonous — see condition
Phlyctenulosis (allergic) (keratoconjunctivitis) (nontuberculous) — see also Keratoconjunctivitis
  cornea — see Keratoconjunctivitis
  tuberculous A18.52
Phobia, phobic F40.9
  animal F40.218
    spiders F40.210
  examination F40.298
  reaction F40.9
  simple F40.298
  social F40.10
    generalized F40.11
  specific (isolated) F40.298
    animal F40.218
      spiders F40.210
    blood F40.230
    injection F40.231
    injury F40.233
    men F40.290
    natural environment F40.228
      thunderstorms F40.220
    situational F40.248
      bridges F40.242
      closed in spaces F40.240
      flying F40.243
      heights F40.241
    specified focus NEC F40.298
    transfusion F40.231
    women F40.291
  specified NEC F40.8
    medical care NEC F40.232
  state F40.9
Phocas' disease — see Mastopathy, cystic
Phocomelia Q73.1
  lower limb — see Agenesis, leg, with foot present
  upper limb — see Agenesis, arm, with hand present
Phoria H50.50
Phosphate-losing tubular disorder N25.0
Phosphatemia E83.39
Phosphaturia E83.39
Photodermatitis (sun) L56.8
  chronic L57.8
  due to drug L56.8
  light other than sun L59.8
Photokeratitis H16.139
  bilateral H16.133
  left H16.132
  right H16.131
Photophobia H53.19
Photophthalmia — see Photokeratitis
Photopsia H53.19
Photoretinitis — see Retinopathy, solar
Photosensitivity, photosensitization (sun) **skin** L56.8
  light other than sun L59.8
Phrenitis — see Encephalitis
Phrynoderma (vitamin A deficiency) E50.8
Phthiriasis (pubis) B85.3
  with any infestation classifiable to B85.0-B85.2 B85.4

Phthirus infestation — see Phthiriasis
Phthisis — see also Tuberculosis
  bulbi (infectional) — see Disorder, globe, degenerated condition, atrophy
  eyeball (due to infection) — see Disorder, globe, degenerated condition, atrophy
Phycomycosis — see Zygomycosis
Physalopteriasis B81.8
Physical therapy NEC Z51.89
Phytobezoar T18.9
  intestine T18.3
  stomach T18.2
Pian — see Yaws
Pianoma A66.1
Pica F50.8
  in adults F50.8
  infant or child F98.3
Picking, nose F98.8
Pick-Niemann disease — see Niemann-Pick disease or syndrome
Pick's
  cerebral atrophy G31.0
  disease or syndrome (brain) G31.0
    dementia in G31.0 [F02]
    liver I31.1
    pericardium I31.1
    polyserositis I31.1
    tubular adenoma (M8640/0)
      specified site — see Neoplasm, benign
      unspecified site
        female D27.9
        male D29.20
          left D29.22
          right D29.21
Pickwickian syndrome E66.2
Piebaldism E70.39
Piedra (beard) (scalp) B36.8
  black B36.3
  white B36.2
Pierre Robin deformity or syndrome Q87.0
Pierson's disease or osteochondrosis M91.0
Pig-bel A05.2
Pigeon
  breast or chest (acquired) M95.4
    congenital Q67.7
    rachitic (late effect) E64.3
  breeder's disease or lung J67.2
  fancier's disease or lung J67.2
  toe — see Deformity, toe, specified NEC
Pigmentation (abnormal) (anomaly) L81.9
  conjunctiva H11.139
    bilateral H11.133
    left H11.132
    right H11.131
  cornea (anterior) H18.019
    bilateral H18.013
    left H18.012
    posterior H18.059
      bilateral H18.053
      left H18.052
      right H18.051
    right H18.011
    stromal H18.069
      bilateral H18.063
      left H18.062
      right H18.061
  diminished melanin formation NEC L81.6
  iron L81.8
  lids, congenital Q82.8
  limbus corneae — see Pigmentation, cornea
  metals L81.8
  optic papilla, congenital Q14.2
  retina, congenital (grouped) (nevoid) Q14.1
  scrotum, congenital Q82.8
  tattoo L81.8
Piles — see Hemorrhoids
Pili
  annulati or torti (congenital) Q84.1
  incarnati L73.1
Pill roller hand (intrinsic) — see Parkinsonism

Pilomatrixoma (M8110/0) — see Neoplasm, skin, benign
  malignant (M8110/3) — see Neoplasm, skin, malignant
Pilonidal — see condition
Pimple R23.8
Pinched nerve — see Neuropathy, entrapment
Pindborg tumor (M9340/0) D16.5
  upper jaw (bone) (M9340/0) D16.4
Pineal body or gland — see condition
Pinealoblastoma (M9362/3) C75.3
Pinealoma (M9360/1) D44.5
  malignant (M9360/3) C75.3
Pineoblastoma (M9362/3) C75.3
Pineocytoma (M9361/1) D44.5
Pinguecula H11.159
  bilateral H11.153
  left H11.152
  right H11.151
Pinhole meatus (see also Stricture, urethra) N35.9
Pink
  disease — see category T56.1
  eye — see Conjunctivitis, acute, mucopurulent
Pinkus' disease (lichen nitidus) L44.1
Pinpoint
  meatus — see Stricture, urethra
  os (uteri) — see Stricture, cervix
Pins and needles R20.2
Pinta A67.9
  cardiovascular lesions A67.2
  chancre (primary) A67.0
  erythematous plaques A67.1
  hyperchromic lesions A67.1
  hyperkeratosis A67.1
  lesions A67.9
    cardiovascular A67.2
    hyperchromic A67.1
    intermediate A67.1
    late A67.2
    mixed A67.3
    primary A67.0
    skin (achromic) (cicatricial) (dyschromic) A67.2
      hyperchromic A67.1
      mixed (achromic and hyperchromic) A67.3
  papule (primary) A67.0
  skin lesions (achromic) (cicatricial) (dyschromic) A67.2
    hyperchromic A67.1
    mixed (achromic and hyperchromic) A67.3
  vitiligo A67.2
Pintids A67.1
Pinworm (disease) (infection) (infestation) B80
Piroplasmosis B60.0
Pistol wound — see Gunshot wound
Pitchers' elbow — see Derangement, joint, specified type NEC, elbow
Pithecoid pelvis Q74.2
  with disproportion (fetopelvic) O33.0
    causing obstructed labor O65.0
Pithiatism F48.8
Pitted — see Pitting
Pitting — see also Edema R60.9
  lip R60.0
  nail L60.8
  teeth K00.4
Pituitary gland — see condition
Pituitary-snuff-taker's disease J67.8
Pityriasis (capitis) L21.0
  alba L30.5
  circinata (et maculata) L42
  furfuracea L21.0
  Hebra's L26
  lichenoides L41.0
    chronica L41.1
    et varioliformis (acuta) L41.0
  maculata (et circinata) L30.5
  nigra B36.1
  pilaris, Hebra's L44.0
  rosea L42

Pityriasis — continued
  rotunda L44.8
  rubra (Hebra) pilaris L44.0
  simplex L30.5
  specified type NEC L30.5
  streptogenes L30.5
  versicolor (scrotal) B36.0
Placenta, placental (see also condition)
  ablatio — see Disorder, placenta, abruptio
  abnormal, abnormality — see Disorder, placenta, malformation
  abruptio — see Disorder, placenta, abruptio
  accreta (with hemorrhage) O72.0
    without hemorrhage O73.0
  adherent (with postpartum hemorrhage) O72.0
    without hemorrhage O73.0
  battledore — see Disorder, placenta, malformation, specified type NEC
  bipartita — see Disorder, placenta, malformation, specified type NEC
  circumvallata — see Disorder, placenta, malformation, circumvallate
  cyst (amniotic) — see Disorder, placenta, malformation, specified type NEC
  deficiency — see Pregnancy, management affected by, fetal, poor growth
  detachment (partial) (premature) (with hemorrhage) — see Disorder, placenta, abruptio
  dimidiata — see Disorder, placenta, malformation, specified type NEC
  disease — see Disorder, placenta
  duplex — see Disorder, placenta, malformation, specified type NEC
  dysfunction — see Disorder, placenta
  fenestrata — see Disorder, placenta, malformation, specified type NEC
  fibrosis — see Disorder, placenta, specified type NEC
  hematoma — see Disorder, placenta, specified type NEC
  hemorrhage — see also Hemorrhage, antepartum
    abruptio placentae — see Disorder, placenta, abruptio
    placenta previa — see Disorder, placenta, previa
  hyperplasia — see Disorder, placenta, specified type NEC
  increta (with postpartum hemorrhage) O72.0
    without hemorrhage O73.0
  infarction — see Disorder, placenta, infarction
  insertion, vicious — see Disorder, placenta, previa
  insufficiency, affecting management of pregnancy — see Pregnancy, management affected by, fetal, poor growth
  lateral — see Disorder, placenta, previa
  low implantation or insertion (with hemorrhage) — see Disorder, placenta, previa
  low-lying — see Disorder, placenta, previa
  malformation — see Disorder, placenta, malformation
  malposition — see Disorder, placenta, previa
  marginal sinus (hemorrhage) (rupture) O44.10
  membranacea — see Disorder, placenta, malformation, specified type NEC
  multilobed — see Disorder, placenta, malformation, specified type NEC
  multipartita — see Disorder, placenta, malformation, specified type NEC
  necrosis — see Disorder, placenta, specified type NEC
  percreta (with postpartum hemorrhage) O72.0
    without hemorrhage O73.0
  polyp O90.8
  previa (central) (complete) (marginal) (partial) (total) (with hemorrhage) O44.10
    first trimester O44.11
    second trimester O44.12
    third trimester O44.13
    without hemorrhage O44.00
      first trimester O44.01
      second trimester O44.02
      third trimester O44.03

©2002 Ingenix, Inc.

Placenta, placental (*see also* condition) — continued
  retention (with postpartum hemorrhage) O72.0
    without hemorrhage O73.0
    fragments, complicating puerperium (delayed hemorrhage) O72.2
      without hemorrhage O73.1
  separation (normally implanted) (partial) (premature) (with hemorrhage) — *see* Disorder, placenta, abruptio
  septuplex — *see* Disorder, placenta, malformation, specified type NEC
  small — *see* Pregnancy, management affected by, fetal, poor growth
  softening (premature) — *see* Disorder, placenta, specified type NEC
  spuria — *see* Disorder, placenta, malformation, specified type NEC
  succenturiata — *see* Disorder, placenta, malformation, specified type NEC
  syphilitic A52.76
  transmission of chemical substance — *see* Absorption, chemical, through placenta
  trapped (with postpartum hemorrhage) O72.0
    without hemorrhage O73.0
  tripartita, triplex — *see* Disorder, placenta, malformation, specified type NEC
  varicose vessels — *see* Disorder, placenta, specified type NEC
  Placentitis complicating pregnancy — *see* Pregnancy, complicated by, placentitis

Plagiocephaly Q67.3
Plague A20.9
  abortive A20.8
  ambulatory A20.8
  asymptomatic A20.8
  bubonic A20.0
  cellulocutaneous A20.1
  cutaneobubonic A20.1
  lymphatic gland A20.0
  meningitis A20.3
  pharyngeal A20.8
  pneumonic (primary) (secondary) A20.2
  pulmonary, pulmonic A20.2
  septicemic A20.7
  tonsillar A20.8
    septicemic A20.7
  vaccination, prophylactic (against) Z23

Planning, family
  contraception Z30.9
  procreation Z31.6

Plaque(s)
  artery, arterial — *see* Arteriosclerosis
  calcareous — *see* Calcification
  epicardial I31.8
  erythematous, of pinta A67.1
  Hollenhorst's — *see* Occlusion, artery, retina
  pleural (without asbestos) J92.9
    with asbestos J92.0
  tongue K13.2

Plasmacytoma (extramedullary) (solitary) (M9731/3) C90.20
  in remission C90.21
Plasmacytosis D72.8
Plaster ulcer — *see* Decubitus
Platybasia Q75.8
Platyonychia (congenital) Q84.6
  acquired L60.8
Platypelloid pelvis M95.5
  with disproportion (fetopelvic) O33.0
    causing obstructed labor O65.0
  congenital Q74.2
Platyspondylisis Q76.49
Plaut (-Vincent) disease — *see also* Vincent's A69.1
Plethora R23.2
  newborn P61.1
Pleura, pleural — *see* condition
Pleuralgia R07.89

Pleurisy (acute) (adhesive) (chronic) (costal) (diaphragmatic) (double) (dry) (fibrinous) (fibrous) (interlobar) (latent) (plastic) (primary) (residual) (sicca) (sterile) (subacute) (unresolved) R09.1
  with
    adherent pleura J86.0
    effusion J90
      chylous, chyliform J94.0
      influenzal J10.1
      tuberculous (non primary) A15.6
        primary (progressive) A15.7
    influenza, flu, or grippe J10.1
    tuberculosis — *see* Pleurisy, tuberculous (non primary)
  encysted — *see* Pleurisy, with effusion
  exudative — *see* Pleurisy, with effusion
  fibrinopurulent, fibropurulent — *see* Pyothorax
  hemorrhagic — *see* Hemothorax
  influenzal J10.1
  pneumococcal J90
  purulent — *see* Pyothorax
  septic — *see* Pyothorax
  serofibrinous — *see* Pleurisy, with effusion
  seropurulent — *see* Pyothorax
  serous — *see* Pleurisy, with effusion
  staphylococcal J86.9
  streptococcal J90
  suppurative — *see* Pyothorax
  traumatic (post) (current) — *see* Injury, intrathoracic, pleura
  tuberculous (with effusion) (non primary) A15.6
    primary (progressive) A15.7
Pleuritis sicca — *see* Pleurisy
Pleurobronchopneumonia — *see* Pneumonia, broncho-
Pleurodynia R07.81
  epidemic B33.0
  viral B33.0
Pleuropericarditis — *see also* Pericarditis
  acute I30.9
Pleuropneumonia (acute) (bilateral) (double) (septic) (*see also* Pneumonia) J18.8
  chronic — *see* Fibrosis, lung
Pleuro-pneumonia-like-organism (PPLO), **as cause of disease classified elsewhere** B96.0
Pleurorrhea — *see* Pleurisy, with effusion
Plexitis, brachial G54.0
Plica
  polonica B85.0
  syndrome, knee M67.50
    left M67.52
    right M67.51
  tonsil J35.8
Plicated tongue K14.5
Plug
  bronchus NEC J98.0
  meconium (newborn) NEC syndrome P76.0
  mucus — *see* Asphyxia, mucus
Plumbism — *see* category T56.0
Plummer's disease E05.20
  with thyroid storm E05.21
Plummer-Vinson syndrome D50.1
Pluricarential syndrome of infancy E40
Plus (and minus) hand (intrinsic) — *see* Deformity, limb, specified type NEC, forearm
Pneumathemia — *see* Air, embolism
Pneumatic hammer (drill) **syndrome** T75.21
Pneumatocele (lung) J98.4
  intracranial G93.8
  tension J44.9
Pneumatosis
  cystoides intestinalis K63.8
  intestinalis K63.8
  peritonei K66.8
Pneumaturia R39.8
Pneumoblastoma (M8972/3) — *see* Neoplasm, lung, malignant
Pneumocephalus G93.8
Pneumococcemia A40.3
Pneumococcus, pneumococcal — *see* condition

Pneumoconiosis (due to) (inhalation of) J64
  with tuberculosis (any type in A15-A16) J65
  aluminum J63.0
  asbestos J61
  bagasse, bagassosis J67.1
  bauxite J63.1
  beryllium J63.2
  coal miners' (simple) J60
  coalworkers' (simple) J60
  collier's J60
  cotton dust J66.0
  diatomite (diatomaceous earth) J62.8
  dust
    inorganic NEC J63.6
    lime J62.8
    marble J62.8
    organic NEC J66.8
  fumes or vapors (from silo) J68.9
  graphite J63.3
  grinder's J62.8
  kaolin J62.8
  mica J62.8
  millstone maker's J62.8
  mineral fibers NEC J61
  miner's J60
  moldy hay J67.0
  potter's J62.8
  rheumatoid — *see* Rheumatoid, lung
  sandblaster's J62.8
  silica, silicate NEC J62.8
    with carbon J60
  stonemason's J62.8
  talc (dust) J62.0
Pneumocystis carinii pneumonia B59
Pneumocystosis (with pneumonia) B59
Pneumohemopericardium I31.2
Pneumohemothorax J94.2
  traumatic S27.2
Pneumohydropericardium — *see* Pericarditis
Pneumohydrothorax — *see* Hydrothorax
Pneumomediastinum J98.2
  congenital or perinatal P25.2
Pneumomycosis B49 [*J99*]
Pneumonia (acute) (Alpenstich) (benign) (bilateral) (brain) (cerebral) (circumscribed) (congestive) (creeping) (delayed resolution) (double) (epidemic) (fever) (flash) (fulminant) (fungoid) (granulomatous) (hemorrhagic) (incipient) (infantile) (infectious) (infiltration) (insular) (intermittent) (latent) (migratory) (organized) (overwhelming) (primary (atypical)) (progressive) (pseudolobar) (purulent) (resolved) (secondary) (senile) (septic) (suppurative) (terminal) (true) (unresolved) (vesicular) J18.9
  with
    lung abscess J85.1
      due to specified organism — *see* Pneumonia, in (due to)
  adenoviral J12.0
  adynamic J18.2
  alba A50.04
  allergic (eosinophilic) J82
  alveolar — *see* Pneumonia, lobar
  anaerobes J15.8
  anthrax A22.1
  apex, apical — *see* Pneumonia, lobar
  Ascaris B77.81
  aspiration J69.0
    due to
      aspiration of microorganisms
        bacterial J15.9
        viral J12.9
      food (regurgitated) J69.0
      gastric secretions J69.0
      milk (regurgitated) J69.0
      oils, essences J69.1
      solids, liquids NEC J69.8
      vomitus J69.0
    newborn P24.9
      meconium P24.0
  atypical J18.9
  bacillus J15.9
    specified NEC J15.8

Pneumonia — *continued*
- bacterial J15.9
  - specified NEC J15.8
- Bacteroides (fragilis) (oralis) (melaninogenicus) J15.8
- basal, basic, basilar — *see* Pneumonia, lobar
- broncho-, bronchial (confluent) (croupous) (diffuse) (disseminated) (hemorrhagic) (involving lobes) (lobar) (terminal) J18.0
  - allergic (eosinophilic) J82
  - aspiration — *see* Pneumonia, aspiration
  - bacterial J15.9
    - specified NEC J15.8
  - chronic — *see* Fibrosis, lung
  - diplococcal J13
  - Eaton's agent J15.7
  - Escherichia coli (E. coli) J15.5
  - Friedländer's bacillus J15.0
  - Hemophilus influenzae J14
  - hypostatic J18.2
  - inhalation (*see also* Pneumonia, aspiration due to fumes or vapors (chemical) J68.0
    - of oils or essences J69.1
  - Klebsiella (pneumoniae) J15.0
  - lipid, lipoid J69.1
    - endogenous J84.8
  - Mycoplasma (pneumoniae) J15.7
  - pleuro-pneumonia-like-organisms (PPLO) J15.7
  - pneumococcal J13
  - Proteus J15.6
  - Pseudomonas J15.1
  - Serratia marcescens J15.6
  - specified organism NEC J16.8
  - staphylococcal — *see* Pneumonia, staphylococcal
  - streptococcal NEC J15.4
    - group B J15.3
    - pneumoniae J13
  - viral, virus — *see* Pneumonia, viral
- Butyrivibrio (fibriosolvens) J15.8
- Candida B37.1
- caseous — *see* Tuberculosis, pulmonary
- catarrhal — *see* Pneumonia, broncho
- chlamydial J16.0
  - congenital P23.1
- cholesterol J84.8
- cirrhotic (chronic) — *see* Fibrosis, lung
- Clostridium (haemolyticum) (novyi) J15.8
- confluent — *see* Pneumonia, broncho
- congenital (infective) P23.9
  - aspiration P24.9
  - due to
    - bacterium NEC P23.6
    - Chlamydia P23.1
    - Escherichia coli P23.4
    - Haemophilus influenzae P23.6
    - infective organism NEC P23.8
    - Klebsiella pneumoniae P23.6
    - Mycoplasma P23.6
    - Pseudomonas P23.5
    - Staphylococcus P23.2
    - Streptococcus (except group B) P23.6
      - group B P23.3
    - viral agent P23.0
  - specified NEC P23.8
- croupous — *see* Pneumonia, lobar
- cytomegalic inclusion B25.0
- cytomegaloviral B25.0
- deglutition — *see* Pneumonia, aspiration
- desquamative interstitial J84.8
- diffuse — *see* Pneumonia, broncho
- diplococcal, diplococcus (broncho-) (lobar) J13
- disseminated (focal) — *see* Pneumonia, broncho
- Eaton's agent J15.7
- embolic, embolism — *see* Embolism, pulmonary
- Enterobacter J15.6
- eosinophilic J82
- Escherichia coli (E. coli) J15.5
- Eubacterium J15.8
- fibrinous — *see* Pneumonia, lobar
- fibroid, fibrous (chronic) — *see* Fibrosis, lung
- Friedländer's bacillus J15.0
- Fusobacterium (nucleatum) J15.8
- gangrenous J85.0
- giant cell (measles) B05.2

Pneumonia — *continued*
- gonococcal A54.84
- gram-negative bacteria NEC J15.6
  - anaerobic J15.8
- Hemophilus influenzae ((broncho) (lobar) J14
- hypostatic (broncho) (lobar) J18.2
- in (due to)
  - actinomycosis A42.0
  - adenovirus J12.0
  - anthrax A22.1
  - ascariasis B77.81
  - aspergillosis B44.9
  - Bacillus anthracis A22.1
  - Bacterium anitratum J15.6
  - candidiasis B37.1
  - chickenpox B01.2
  - Chlamydia J16.0
    - neonatal P23.1
  - coccidioidomycosis B38.2
    - acute B38.0
    - chronic B38.1
  - cytomegalovirus disease B25.0
  - Diplococcus (pneumoniae) J13
  - Eaton's agent J15.7
  - Enterobacter J15.6
  - Escherichia coli (E. coli) J15.5
  - Friedländer's bacillus J15.0
  - fumes and vapors (chemical) (inhalation) J68.0
  - gonorrhea A54.84
  - Hemophilus influenzae (H. influenzae) J14
  - Herellea J15.6
  - histoplasmosis B39.2 *[J17]*
    - acute B39.0 *[J17]*
    - chronic B39.1 *[J17]*
  - Klebsiella (pneumoniae) J15.0
  - measles B05.2
  - Mycoplasma (pneumoniae) J15.7
  - nocardiosis, nocardiasis A43.0
  - ornithosis A70
  - parainfluenza virus J12.2
  - pleuro-pneumonia-like-organism (PPLO) J15.7
  - pneumococcus J13
  - pneumocystosis (Pneumocystis carinii) B59
  - Proteus J15.6
  - Pseudomonas NEC J15.1
    - pseudomallei A24.1
  - psittacosis A70
  - Q fever A78
  - respiratory syncytial virus J12.1
  - rheumatic fever I00 *[J17]*
  - rubella B06.81
  - Salmonella (infection) A02.22
    - typhi A01.03
  - schistosomiasis B65.9 *[J17]*
  - septicemia A41.9 *[J17.0]*
  - Serratia marcescens J15.6
  - specified
    - bacterium NEC J15.8
    - organism NEC J16.8
  - spirochetal NEC A69.8
  - Staphylococcus J15.20
    - aureus J15.21
    - specified NEC J15.29
  - Streptococcus J15.4
    - group B J15.3
    - pneumoniae J13
    - specified NEC J15.4
  - toxoplasmosis B58.3
  - tularemia A21.2
  - typhoid (fever) A01.03
  - varicella B01.2
  - virus — *see* Pneumonia, viral
  - whooping cough A37.91
    - due to
      - Bordetella parapertussis A37.11
      - Bordetella pertussis A37.01
      - specified NEC A37.81
  - Yersinia pestis A20.2
- inhalation of food or vomit — *see* Pneumonia, aspiration
- interstitial J84.9
  - chronic J84.1
  - lymphoid J84.2
  - plasma cell B59
  - pseudomonas J15.1

Pneumonia — *continued*
- Klebsiella (pneumoniae) J15.0
- lipid, lipoid (exogenous) J69.1
  - endogenous J84.2
- lobar (disseminated) (double) (interstitial) J18.1
  - bacterial J15.9
    - specified NEC J15.8
  - chronic — *see* Fibrosis, lung
  - Escherichia coli (E. coli) J15.5
  - Friedländer's bacillus J15.0
  - Hemophilus influenzae J14
  - hypostatic J18.2
  - Klebsiella (pneumoniae) J15.0
  - pneumococcal J13
  - Proteus J15.6
  - Pseudomonas J15.1
  - specified organism NEC J16.8
  - staphylococcal — *see* Pneumonia, staphylococcal
  - streptococcal NEC J15.4
  - Streptococcus pneumoniae J13
  - viral, virus — *see* Pneumonia, viral
- lobular — *see* Pneumonia, broncho
- Löffler's J82
- lymphoid interstitial J84.2
- massive — *see* Pneumonia, lobar
- meconium P24.0
- Mycoplasma (pneumoniae) J15.7
- necrotic J85.0
- neonatal P23.9
  - aspiration P24.9
- nitrogen dioxide J68.9
- orthostatic J18.2
- parainfluenza virus J12.2
- parenchymatous — *see* Fibrosis, lung
- passive J18.2
- patchy — *see* Pneumonia, broncho
- Peptococcus J15.8
- Peptostreptococcus J15.8
- plasma cell (of infants) B59
- pleurolobar — *see* Pneumonia, lobar
- pleuro-pneumonia-like organism (PPLO) J15.7
- pneumococcal (broncho) (lobar) J13
- Pneumocystis (carinii) B59
- postinfectional NEC B99 *[J17]*
- postmeasles B05.2
- Proteus J15.6
- Pseudomonas J15.1
- psittacosis A70
- radiation J70.0
- respiratory syncytial virus J12.1
- resulting from a procedure J95.89
- rheumatic I00 *[J17]*
- Salmonella (arizonae) (cholerae-suis) (enteritidis) (typhimurium) A02.22
  - typhi A01.03
  - typhoid fever A01.03
- segmented, segmental — *see* Pneumonia, broncho
- Serratia marcescens J15.6
- specified NEC J18.8
  - bacterium NEC J15.8
  - organism NEC J16.8
  - virus NEC J12.8
- spirochetal NEC A69.8
- staphylococcal (broncho) (lobar) J15.20
  - aureus J15.21
  - specified NEC J15.29
- static, stasis J18.2
- streptococcal NEC (broncho) (lobar) J15.4
  - group
    - A J15.4
    - B J15.3
    - specified NEC J15.4
- Streptococcus pneumoniae J13
- syphilitic, congenital (early) A50.04
- traumatic (complication) (early) (secondary) T79.8
- tuberculous (any) — *see* Tuberculosis, pulmonary
- tularemic A21.2
- varicella B01.2
- Veillonella J15.8

©2002 Ingenix, Inc.

Pneumonia — *continued*
  viral, virus (broncho) (interstitial) (lobar) J12.9
    adenoviral J12.0
    congenital P23.0
    parainfluenza J12.2
    respiratory syncytial J12.1
    specified NEC J12.8
  white (congenital) A50.04
Pneumonic — *see* condition
Pneumonitis (acute) (primary) — *see also*
  Pneumonia
  air-conditioner J67.7
  allergic (due to) J67.9
    organic dust NEC J67.8
    red cedar dust J67.8
    sequoiosis J67.8
    wood dust J67.8
  aspiration J69.0
    due to
      anesthesia J95.4
        during
          labor and delivery O74.0
          pregnancy — *see* Complications,
            anesthesia, in, pregnancy,
            pulmonary
          puerperium O89.01
      fumes or gases J68.0
      obstetric O74.0
  chemical (due to gases, fumes or vapors)
    (inhalation) J68.0
  cholesterol J84.8
  chronic — *see* Fibrosis, lung
  congenital rubella P35.0
  due to
    beryllium J68.0
    cadmium J68.0
    detergent J69.8
    fluorocarbon-polymer J68.0
    food, vomit (aspiration) J69.0
    fumes or vapors J68.0
    gases, fumes or vapors (inhalation) J68.0
    inhalation
      blood J69.8
      essences J69.1
      food (regurgitated), milk, vomit J69.0
      oils, essences J69.1
      saliva J69.0
      solids, liquids NEC J69.8
    manganese J68.0
    nitrogen dioxide J68.0
    oils, essences J69.1
    solids, liquids NEC J69.8
    toxoplasmosis (acquired) B58.3
      congenital P37.1
    vanadium J68.0
  eosinophilic J82
  hypersensitivity J67.9
    air conditioner lung J67.7
    bagassosis J67.1
    bird fancier's lung J67.2
    farmer's lung J67.0
    maltworker's lung J67.4
    maple bark-stripper's lung J67.6
    mushroom worker's lung J67.5
    specified organic dust NEC J67.8
    suberosis J67.3
  interstitial (chronic) J84.1
    lymphoid J84.2
  lymphoid, interstitial J84.2
  meconium P24.0
  neonatal aspiration P24.9
  postanesthetic
    correct substance properly administered
      J95.4
    in labor and delivery O74.0
    in pregnancy — *see* Complications,
      anesthesia, in, pregnancy, pulmonary
    obstetric O74.0
    overdose or wrong substance given or taken
      (by accident) T41.201
      administered with intent to harm by
        another person T41.203
        self T41.202
      circumstances undetermined T41.204
      specified anesthetic — *see* Table of Drugs
        and Chemicals
  postpartum, puerperal O89.01

Pneumonitis — *see also* Pneumonia — *continued*
  postoperative J95.4
    obstetric O74.0
  radiation J70.0
  rubella, congenital P35.0
  ventilation (air-conditioning) J67.7
  wood-dust J67.8
Pneumonoconiosis — *see* Pneumoconiosis
Pneumoparotid K11.8
Pneumopathy NEC J98.4
  alveolar J84.0
  due to organic dust NEC J66.8
  parietoalveolar J84.0
Pneumopericarditis — *see also* Pericarditis
  acute I30.9
Pneumopericardium — *see also* Pericarditis
  congenital P25.3
  fetus or newborn P25.3
  traumatic (post) — *see* Injury, heart
Pneumophagia (psychogenic) F45.8
Pneumopleurisy, pneumopleuritis (*see also*
  Pneumonia) J18.8
Pneumopyopericardium I30.1
Pneumopyothorax — *see* Pyopneumothorax
  with fistula J86.0
Pneumorrhagia — *see also* Hemorrhage, lung
  tuberculous — *see* Tuberculosis, pulmonary
Pneumothorax J93.9
  acute J93.8
  chronic J93.8
  congenital P25.1
  perinatal period P25.1
  postprocedural J95.81
  specified NEC J93.8
  spontaneous NEC J93.1
    fetus or newborn P25.1
    tension J93.0
  tense valvular, infectional J93.0
  tension (spontaneous) J93.0
  traumatic S27.0
    with hemothorax S27.2
  tuberculous — *see* Tuberculosis, pulmonary
Podagra M10.9
Podencephalus Q01.9
Poikilocytosis R71.8
Poikiloderma L81.6
  Civatte's L57.3
  congenital Q82.8
  vasculare atrophicans L94.5
Poikilodermatomyositis M33.10
  with
    myopathy M33.12
    respiratory involvement M33.11
    specified organ involvement NEC M33.19
Pointed ear (congenital) Q17.3
Poison ivy, oak, sumac or other plant
dermatitis (allergic) (contact) L23.7
Poisoning (acute) — *see also* Table of Drugs and
  Chemicals T65.91
  administered with intent to harm by
    another person T65.93
    self T65.92
  Bacillus B (aertrycke) (cholerae (suis))
    (paratyphosus) (suipestifer) A02.9
    botulinus A05.1
  bacterial toxins A05.9
  berries, noxious — *see* Poisoning, food,
    noxious, berries
  botulism A05.1
  ciguatera fish T61.01
    administered with intent to harm by
      another person T61.03
      self T61.02
    circumstances undetermined T61.04
  circumstances undetermined T65.94
  Clostridium botulinum A05.1
  death-cap (Amanita phalloides) (Amanita verna)
    — *see* Poisoning, food, noxious,
    mushrooms
  drug — *see* Table of Drugs and Chemicals
  epidemic, fish (noxious) — *see* Poisoning,
    seafood
    bacterial A05.9
  fava bean D55.0

Poisoning — *see also* Table of Drugs and
  Chemicals — *continued*
  fish (noxious) T61.91
    administered with intent to harm by
      another person T61.93
      self T61.92
    bacterial — *see* Intoxication, foodborne, by
      agent
    ciguatera fish — *see* Poisoning, ciguatera
      fish
    circumstances undetermined T61.94
    scombroid fish — *see* Poisoning, scombroid
      fish
    specified type NEC T61.771
      administered with intent to harm by
        another person T61.773
        self T61.772
  food (acute) (diseased) (infected) (noxious) NEC
    T62.91
    bacterial — *see* Intoxication, foodborne, by
      agent
    due to
      Bacillus (aertrycke) (choleraesuis)
        (paratyphosus) (suipestifer) A02.9
      botulinus A05.1
      Clostridium (perfringens) Welchii) A05.2
      salmonella (aertrycke) (callinarum)
        (choleraesuis) (enteritidis)
        (paratyphi) (suipestifer) A02.9
        with
          gastroenteritis A02.0
          septicemia A02.1
      staphylococcus A05.0
      Vibrio
        parahaemolyticus A05.3
        vulnificus A05.5
    noxious or naturally toxic T62.91
      administered with intent to harm by
        another person T62.93
        self T62.92
      berries — *see* category T62.1
      circumstances undetermined T62.94
      fish — *see* Poisoning, seafood
      mushrooms — *see* category T62.0
      plants NEC — *see* category T62.2
      seafood — *see* Poisoning, seafood
      specified NEC — *see* category T62.8
  ichthyotoxism — *see* Poisoning, seafood
  kreotoxism, food A05.9
  latex T65.811
    administered with intent to harm by
      another person T65.813
      self T65.812
    circumstances undetermined T65.814
  mushroom — *see* Poisoning, food, noxious,
    mushroom
  mussels — *see also* Poisoning, shellfish
    bacterial — *see* Intoxication, foodborne, by
      agent
  noxious foodstuffs — *see* Poisoning, food,
    noxious
  plants, noxious — *see* Poisoning, food, noxious,
    plants NEC
  ptomaine — *see* Poisoning, food
  radiation J70.0
  Salmonella (arizonae) (cholerae-suis)
    (enteritidis) (typhimurium) A02.9
  scombroid fish T61.11
    administered with intent to harm by
      another person T61.13
      self T61.12
    circumstances undetermined T61.14
  seafood (noxious) T61.91
    administered with intent to harm by
      another person T61.93
      self T61.92
    bacterial — *see* Intoxication, foodborne, by
      agent
    circumstances undetermined T61.94
    fish — *see* Poisoning, fish
    shellfish — *see* Poisoning, shellfish
    specified NEC — *see* category T61.8
  shellfish (noxious) T61.781
    administered with intent to harm by
      another person T61.783
      self T61.782

Poisoning — *see also* Table of Drugs and Chemicals — *continued*
  shellfish — *continued*
    bacterial — *see* Intoxication, foodborne, by agent
    ciguatera mollusk — *see* Poisoning, ciguatera fish
    specified substance NEC T65.891
      administered with intent to harm by another person T65.893
        self T65.892
      circumstances undetermined T65.894
    Staphylococcus, food A05.0
Poker spine — *see* Spondylitis, ankylosing
Poland's syndrome Q79.8
Polioencephalitis (acute) (bulbar) A80.9
  inferior G12.22
  influenzal J10.89
  superior hemorrhagic (acute) (Wernicke's) E51.2
  Wernicke's E51.2
Polioencephalomyelitis (acute) (anterior) A80.9
  with beriberi E51.2
Polioencephalopathy, superior hemorrhagic E51.8
  with
    beriberi E51.11
    pellagra E52
Poliomeningoencephalitis — *see* Meningoencephalitis
Poliomyelitis (acute) (anterior) (epidemic) A80.9
  with paralysis (bulbar) — *see* Poliomyelitis, paralytic
  abortive A80.4
  ascending (progressive) — *see* Poliomyelitis, paralytic
  bulbar (paralytic) — *see* Poliomyelitis, paralytic
  congenital P35.8
  nonepidemic A80.9
  nonparalytic A80.4
  paralytic A80.30
    specified NEC A80.39
    vaccine-associated A80.0
    wild virus
      imported A80.1
      indigenous A80.2
  spinal, acute A80.9
  vaccination, prophylactic (against) Z23
Poliosis (eyebrow) (eyelashes) L67.1
  circumscripta, acquired L67.1
Pollakiuria R35.0
  psychogenic F45.8
Pollinosis J30.1
Pollitzer's disease L73.2
Polyadenitis — *see also* Lymphadenitis
  malignant A20.0
Polyangiitis M30.0
  overlap syndrome M30.8
Polyarteritis nodosa M30.0
  with lung involvement M30.1
  juvenile M30.2
  related condition NEC M30.8
Polyarthralgia — *see* Pain, joint
  psychogenic F45.4
Polyarthritis, polyarthropathy (*see also* Arthritis) M13.0
  due to or associated with other specified conditions — *see* Arthritis
  epidemic (Australian) (with exanthema) B33.1
  infective — *see* Arthritis, pyogenic or pyemic
  inflammatory M06.4
  juvenile (chronic) (seronegative) M08.3
  migratory — *see* Fever, rheumatic
  rheumatic, acute — *see* Fever, rheumatic
Polyarthrosis M15.9
  post-traumatic M15.3
  primary M15.0
  specified NEC M15.8
Polycarential syndrome of infancy E40

Polychondritis (atrophic) (chronic) — *see also* Disorder, cartilage, specified type NEC
  relapsing M94.10
    acromioclavicular joint M94.119
      left M94.112
      right M94.111
    ankle M94.179
      left M94.172
      right M94.171
    elbow M94.129
      left M94.122
      right M94.121
    foot joint M94.179
      left M94.172
      right M94.171
    glenohumeral joint M94.119
      left M94.112
      right M94.111
    hand joint M94.149
      left M94.142
      right M94.141
    hip M94.159
      left M94.152
      right M94.151
    knee M94.169
      left M94.162
      right M94.161
    multiple sites M94.19
    rib M94.18
    sacroiliac joint M94.159
    shoulder M94.119
      left M94.112
      right M94.111
    sternoclavicular joint M94.119
      left M94.112
      right M94.111
    vertebral joint M94.18
    wrist M94.139
      left M94.132
      right M94.131
Polycoria Q13.2
Polycystic (disease)
  degeneration, kidney Q61.3
    adult type Q61.2
    infantile type Q61.19
  kidney Q61.3
    autosomal
      dominant Q61.2
      recessive Q61.19
    adult type Q61.2
    childhood type Q61.19
    infantile type Q61.19
  liver Q44.6
  lung J98.4
    congenital Q33.0
  ovary, ovaries E28.2
  spleen Q89.09
Polycythemia (primary) (rubra) (vera) (M9950/1) D45
  acquired D75.1
  benign (familial) D75.0
  due to
    donor twin P61.1
    erythropoietin D75.1
    fall in plasma volume D75.1
    high altitude D75.1
    maternal-fetal transfusion P61.1
    stress D75.1
  emotional D75.1
  erythropoietin D75.1
  familial (benign) D75.0
  Gaisböck's (hypertonica) D75.1
  high altitude D75.1
  hypertonica D75.1
  hypoxemic D75.1
  neonatorum P61.1
  nephrogenous D75.1
  relative D75.1
  secondary D75.1
  spurious D75.1
  stress D75.1
Polycytosis cryptogenica D75.1
Polydactylism, polydactyly Q69.9
  toes Q69.2
Polydipsia R63.1
Polydystrophy, pseudo-Hurler E77.0

Polyembryoma (M9072/3) — *see* Neoplasm, malignant
Polyglandular
  deficiency E31.0
  dyscrasia E31.9
  dysfunction E31.9
  syndrome E31.8
Polyhydramnios O40.9
  first trimester O40.1
  second trimester O40.2
  third trimester O40.3
Polymastia Q83.1
Polymenorrhea N92.0
Polymyalgia M35.3
  arteritica, giant cell M31.5
  rheumatica M35.3
    with giant cell arteritis M31.5
Polymyositis (acute) (chronic) (hemorrhagic) M33.20
  with
    myopathy M33.22
    respiratory involvement M33.21
    skin involvement — *see* Dermatopolymyositis
    specified organ involvement NEC M33.29
  ossificans (generalisata) (progressiva) — *see* Myositis, ossificans, progressiva
Polyneuritis, polyneuritic — *see also* Polyneuropathy
  acute (post-)infective G61.0
  alcoholic G62.1
  cranialis G52.7
  demyelinating, chronic inflammatory G61.8
  diabetic — *see* Diabetes, polyneuropathy
  diphtheritic A36.83
  due to lack of vitamin NEC E56.9 [G63]
  endemic E51.11
  erythredema — *see* category T56.1
  febrile, acute G61.0
  hereditary ataxic G60.1
  idiopathic, acute G61.0
  infective (acute) G61.0
  inflammatory, chronic demyelinating G61.8
  nutritional E63.9 [G63]
  postinfective (acute) G61.0
  specified NEC G62.8
Polyneuropathy (peripheral) G62.9
  alcoholic G62.1
  amyloid (Portuguese) E85 [G63]
  arsenical G62.2
  diabetic — *see* Diabetes, polyneuropathy
  drug-induced G62.0
  hereditary G60.9
    specified NEC G60.8
  idiopathic G60.9
    progressive G60.3
  in (due to)
    alcohol G62.1
      sequelae G65.2
    amyloidosis, familial (Portuguese) E85 [G63]
    antitetanus serum G61.1
    arsenic G62.2
      sequelae G65.2
    avitaminosis NEC E56.9 [G63]
    beriberi E51.11
    collagen vascular disease NEC M35.9 [G63]
    deficiency (of)
      B(-complex) vitamins E53.9 [G63]
      vitamin B6 E53.1 [G63]
    diabetes — *see* Diabetes, polyneuropathy
    diphtheria A36.83
    drug or medicament G62.0
      correct substance, properly administered G62.0
      overdose or wrong substance given or taken (by accident) T50.901
        administered with intent to harm by another person T50.903
          self T50.902
        circumstances undetermined T50.904
        specified drug — *see* Table of Drugs and Chemicals
      sequelae G65.2
    endocrine disease NEC E34.9 [G63]
    herpes zoster B02.23

©2002 Ingenix, Inc.

Polyneuropathy — *continued*
  in (due to) — *continued*
    hypoglycemia E16.2 *[G63]*
    infectious
      disease NEC B99 *[G63]*
      mononucleosis B27.91
    lack of vitamin NEC E56.9 *[G63]*
    lead G62.2
      sequelae G65.2
    leprosy A30.9
    Lyme disease A69.22
    malignant neoplasm NEC (M8000/3) (*see also* Neoplasm, malignant) C80 *[G63]*
    metabolic disease NEC E88.9 *[G63]*
    mumps B26.84
    neoplastic disease (*see also* Neoplasm) D49.9 *[G63]*
    nutritional deficiency NEC E63.9 *[G63]*
    organophosphate compounds G62.2
      sequelae G65.2
    parasitic disease NEC B89 *[G63]*
    pellagra E52 *[G63]*
    polyarteritis nodosa M30.0
    porphyria E80.20 *[G63]*
    radiation G62.8
    rheumatoid arthritis — *see* Rheumatoid, polyneuropathy
    sarcoidosis D86.9
    serum G61.1
    syphilis (late) A52.15
      congenital A50.43
    systemic
      connective tissue disorder M35.9 *[G63]*
      lupus erythematosus M32.19
    toxic agent NEC G62.2
      sequelae G65.2
    triorthocresyl phosphate G62.2
      sequelae G65.2
    tuberculosis A17.89
    uremia N18.8 *[G63]*
    vitamin B12 deficiency E53.8 *[G63]*
      with anemia (pernicious) D51.0 *[G63]*
        due to dietary deficiency D51.3 *[G63]*
    zoster B02.23
  inflammatory G61.9
    sequelae G65.1
    specified NEC G61.8
  lead G62.2
    sequelae G65.2
  nutritional NEC E63.9 *[G63]*
  postherpetic (zoster) B02.23
  progressive G60.3
  radiation-induced G62.8
  sensory (hereditary) (idiopathic) G60.8
  specified NEC G62.8
  syphilitic (late) A52.15
    congenital A50.43
Polyopia H53.8
Polyorchism, polyorchidism Q55.21
Polyostotic fibrous dysplasia Q78.1
Polyotia Q17.0
Polyp, polypus
  accessory sinus J33.8
  adenocarcinoma in (M8210/3) — *see* Neoplasm, malignant
  adenocarcinoma in situ in (M8210/2) — *see* Neoplasm, in situ
  adenoid tissue J33.0
  adenomatous (M8210/0) — *see also* Neoplasm, benign
    adenocarcinoma in (M8210/3) — *see* Neoplasm, malignant
    adenocarcinoma in situ in (M8210/2) — *see* Neoplasm, in situ
    carcinoma in (M8210/3) — *see* Neoplasm, malignant
    carcinoma in situ in (M8210/2) — *see* Neoplasm, in situ
    multiple (M8221/0) — *see* Neoplasm, benign
      adenocarcinoma in (M8221/3) — *see* Neoplasm, malignant
      adenocarcinoma in situ in (M8221/2) — *see* Neoplasm, in situ
  antrum J33.8
  anus, anal (canal) K62.0
  Bartholin's gland N84.3

Polyp, polypus — *continued*
  bladder (M8120/1) D41.4
  carcinoma in (M8210/3) — *see* Neoplasm, malignant
  carcinoma in situ in (M8210/2) — *see* Neoplasm, in situ
  cervix (uteri) N84.1
    in pregnancy or childbirth — *see* Pregnancy, complicated by, abnormal, cervix
    mucous N84.1
    nonneoplastic N84.1
  choanal J33.0
  cholesterol K82.4
  clitoris N84.3
  colon K63.5
    adenomatous D12.6
  corpus uteri N84.0
  dental K04.0
  duodenum K31.7
  ear (middle) H74.40
    bilateral H74.43
    left H74.42
    right H74.41
  endometrium N84.0
  ethmoidal (sinus) J33.8
  fallopian tube N84.8
  female genital tract N84.9
    specified NEC N84.8
  frontal (sinus) J33.8
  gallbladder K82.4
  gingiva, gum K06.8
  labia, labium (majus) (minus) N84.3
  larynx (mucous) J38.1
  malignant (M8000/3) — *see* Neoplasm, malignant
  maxillary (sinus) J33.8
  middle ear — *see* Polyp, ear (middle)
  myometrium N84.0
  nares
    anterior J33.9
    posterior J33.0
  nasal (mucous) J33.9
    cavity J33.9
    septum J33.9
  nasopharyngeal J33.0
  nose (mucous) J33.9
  oviduct N84.8
  pharynx J39.2
  placenta O90.8
  prostate — *see* Hyperplasia, prostate, localized
  pudenda, pudendum N84.8
  pulpal (dental) K04.0
  rectum (nonadenomatous) K62.1
    adenomatous — *see* Polyp, adenomatous
  septum (nasal) J33.0
  sinus (accessory) (ethmoidal) (frontal) (maxillary) (sphenoidal) J33.8
  sphenoidal (sinus) J33.8
  stomach K31.7
    adenomatous (M8210/0) D13.1
  tube, fallopian N84.8
  turbinate, mucous membrane J33.8
  umbilical, newborn P83.6
  ureter N28.89
  urethra N36.2
  uterus (body) (corpus) (mucous) N84.0
    cervix N84.1
    in pregnancy or childbirth — *see* Pregnancy, complicated by, tumor, uterus
  vagina N84.2
  vocal cord (mucous) J38.1
  vulva N84.3
Polyphagia R63.2
Polyploidy Q92.7
Polypoid — *see* condition
Polyposis — *see also* Polyp
  coli (adenomatous) (M8220/0) D12.6
    adenocarcinoma in (M8220/3) C18.9
    adenocarcinoma in situ in (M8220/2) — *see* Neoplasm, in situ
    carcinoma in (M8220/3) C18.9
  familial (M8220/0) D12.6
    adenocarcinoma in situ in (M8220/2) — *see* Neoplasm, in situ

Polyposis — *see also* Polyp — *continued*
  intestinal (adenomatous) (M8220/0) D12.6
  lymphomatous, malignant (M9677/3) — *see* Lymphoma, non-Hodgkin's, diffuse, specified type NEC
  multiple, adenomatous (M8221/0) — *see also* Neoplasm, benign D36.9
Polyradiculitis — *see* Polyneuropathy
Polyradiculoneuropathy (acute) (postinfective) (segmentally demyelinating) G61.0
Polyserositis
  due to pericarditis I31.1
  pericardial I31.1
  periodic, familial E85
  tuberculous A19.9
    acute A19.1
    chronic A19.8
Polysplenia syndrome Q89.09
Polysyndactyly Q70.4
Polytrichia L68.3
Polyunguia Q84.6
Polyuria R35.8
  nocturnal R35.1
  psychogenic F45.8
Pompe's disease (glycogen storage) E74.02
Pompholyx L30.1
Poncet's disease (tuberculous rheumatism) A18.09
Pond fracture — *see* Fracture, skull
Ponos B55.0
Pons, pontine — *see* condition
Poor
  contractions, labor O62.2
  fetal growth NEC — *see* Slow, fetal growth
    affecting management of pregnancy — *see* Pregnancy, management affected by, fetal, poor growth
  personal hygiene R46.0
  prenatal care, affecting management of pregnancy — *see* Pregnancy, complicated by, insufficient, prenatal care
  sucking reflex (newborn) R29.2
  urinary stream R39.12
  vision NEC H54.7
Poradenitis, nostras inguinalis or venerea A55
Porencephaly (congenital) (developmental) (true) Q04.6
  acquired G93.0
  nondevelopmental G93.0
  traumatic (post) F07.89
Porocephaliasis B88.8
Porokeratosis Q82.8
Poroma, eccrine (M8402/0) — *see* Neoplasm, skin, benign
Porphyria (South African) E80.20
  acquired E80.20
  acute intermittent (hepatic) (Swedish) E80.21
  cutanea tarda (hereditary) (symptomatic) E80.1
  due to drugs
    correct substance properly administered E80.20
    overdose or wrong substance given or taken (by accident) T50.901
      administered with intent to harm by another person T50.903
        self T50.902
      circumstances undetermined T50.904
      specified drug — *see* Table of Drugs and Chemicals
  erythropoietic (congenital) (hereditary) E80.0
  hepatocutaneous type E80.1
  secondary E80.20
  toxic NEC E80.20
  variegata E80.20
Porphyrinuria — *see* Porphyria
Porphyruria — *see* Porphyria
Portal — *see* condition
Port wine nevus, mark, or stain Q82.5
Posada-Wernicke disease B38.7
Position
  fetus, abnormal — *see* Presentation, fetal
  teeth, faulty M26.3

Positive
  culture (nonspecific)
    bronchial washings R84.5
    cerebrospinal fluid R83.5
    cervix uteri R87.5
    nasal secretions R84.5
    nipple discharge R89.5
    nose R84.5
    peritoneal fluid R85.5
    pleural fluid R84.5
    prostatic secretions R86.5
    saliva R85.5
    seminal fluid R86.5
    sputum R84.5
    synovial fluid R89.5
    throat scrapings R84.5
    urine R82.7
    vagina R87.5
    vulva R87.5
    wound secretions R89.5
  PPD (skin test) R76.1
  serology, syphilis A53.0
  with signs or symptoms – code as Syphilis, by site and stage
  skin test, tuberculin (without active tuberculosis) R76.1
  test, human immunodeficiency virus (HIV) R75
  VDRL A53.0
  with signs or symptoms – code by site and stage under Syphilis A53.9
  Wassermann reaction A53.0

Postcardiotomy syndrome I97.0

Postcaval ureter Q62.62

Postcholecystectomy syndrome K91.5

Postclimacteric bleeding N95.0

Postcommissurotomy syndrome I97.0

Postconcussional syndrome F07.81

Postcontusional syndrome F07.81

Postcricoid region — see condition

Post-dates (40-42 weeks) (pregnancy) (mother) O48.0
  more than 42 weeks gestation O48.1

Postencephalitic syndrome F07.89

Posterior — see condition

Posterolateral sclerosis (spinal cord) — see Degeneration, combined

Postexanthematous — see condition

Postfebrile — see condition

Postgastrectomy dumping syndrome K91.1

Posthemiplegic chorea — see Monoplegia

Posthemorrhagic anemia (chronic) D50.0
  acute (D62
  newborn P61.3

Postherpetic neuralgia (zoster) B02.29
  trigeminal B02.22

Posthitis N47.7

Postimmunization complication or reaction — see Complications, vaccination

Postinfectious — see condition

Postlaminectomy syndrome NEC M96.1

Postleukotomy syndrome F07.0

Postmastectomy lymphedema (syndrome) I97.2

Postmaturity, postmature (fetus or newborn) (syndrome) P08.2
  affecting management of pregnancy (40 to 42 weeks) O48.0
  more than 42 weeks gestation O48.1

Postmeasles complication NEC (see also condition) B05.89

Postmenopausal endometrium (atrophic) N95.8
  suppurative — see Endometritis

Postnatal — see condition

Postoperative — see Complication, postoperative
  pneumothorax, therapeutic Z98.3
  state NEC Z98.8

Postpancreatectomy hyperglycemia E89.1

Postpartum — see condition

Postpoliomyelitic — see also condition
  osteopathy — see Osteopathy, after poliomyelitis

Postschizophrenic depression F32.8

Postsurgery status — see also Status (post)
  pneumothorax, therapeutic Z98.3

Post-term (40-42 weeks) (pregnancy) (mother) O48.0
  infant P08.2

Post-traumatic brain syndrome, nonpsychotic F07.81

Post-typhoid abscess A01.09

Postures, hysterical F44.2

Postvaccinal reaction or complication — see Complications, vaccination

Postvalvulotomy syndrome I97.0

Potain's
  disease (pulmonary edema) — see Edema, lung
  syndrome (gastrectasis with dyspepsia) K31.0

Potter's
  asthma J62.8
  facies Q60.6
  lung J62.8
  syndrome (with renal agenesis) Q60.6

Pott's
  curvature (spinal) A18.01
  disease or paraplegia A18.01
  spinal curvature A18.01
  tumor, puffy — see Osteomyelitis, specified type NEC

Pouch
  bronchus Q32.8
  Douglas' — see condition
  esophagus, esophageal, congenital Q39.6
    acquired K22.5
  gastric K31.4
  Hartmann's K82.8
  pharynx, pharyngeal (congenital) Q38.7

Poultrymen's itch B88.0

Poverty NEC Z59.6
  extreme Z59.5

Prader-Willi syndrome Q87.1

Preauricular appendage or tag Q17.0

Prebetalipoproteinemia (acquired) (essential) (familial) (hereditary) (primary) (secondary) E78.1
  with chylomicronemia E78.3

Precipitate labor or delivery O62.3

Preclimacteric bleeding (menorrhagia) N92.4

Precocious
  adrenarche E30.1
  menarche E30.1
  menstruation E30.1
  pubarche E30.1
  puberty E30.1
    central E22.8
  sexual development NEC E30.1
  thelarche E30.8

Precocity, sexual (constitutional) (cryptogenic) (female) (idiopathic) (male) E30.1
  with adrenal hyperplasia (congenital) E25.0

Precordial pain R07.2
  psychogenic F45.4

Predeciduous teeth K00.2

Prediabetes, prediabetic R73.0
  complicating
    childbirth O99.88
    pregnancy — see Pregnancy, complicated by, diseases of, specified type or system NEC
    puerperium O99.89

Predislocation status of hip at birth Q65.6

Pre-eclampsia O14.90
  with pre-existing hypertension –see Hypertension, complicating pregnancy, pre-existing, with, proteinuria
  mild O14.00
    second trimester O14.02
    third trimester O14.03
  second trimester O14.92
  severe O14.10
    second trimester O14.12
    third trimester O14.13
  third trimester O14.93

Pre-eruptive color change, teeth, tooth K00.8

Pre-excitation atrioventricular conduction I45.6

Pregnancy (single) (uterine) O00.0
  abdominal (ectopic) O00.0
    affecting fetus P01.4
    viable fetus O36.70
      first trimester O36.71
      second trimester O36.72
      third trimester O36.73
  ampullar O00.1
  broad ligament O00.8
  cervical O00.8
  complicated by — see also Pregnancy, management, affected by
  abnormal, abnormality
    cervix — see category O34.4
      causing obstructed labor O65.5
      incompetence — see Pregnancy, complicated by, incompetent cervix
    cord (umbilical) O69.9
    glucose tolerance NEC O99.820
    pelvic organs or tissues NEC — see category O34.8
      affecting fetus P03.89
      causing obstructed labor O65.5
    pelvis (bony) (major) NEC O33.0
    perineum or vulva — see Pregnancy, complicated by, abnormal, vulva
    placenta, placental (vessel) — see Disorder, placenta, malformation
    position
      placenta — see Disorder, placenta, previa
      uterus — see Pregnancy, complicated by, abnormal, uterus
    uterus — see also category O34.5
      causing obstructed labor O65.5
      cervix — see category O34.4
        incompetence — see Pregnancy, complicated by, incompetent cervix
      congenital — see category O34.0
      polyp — see Pregnancy, complicated by, tumor, uterus
      scar O34.29
        previous cesarean section O34.21
      tumor — see Pregnancy, complicated by, tumor, uterus
    vagina — see category O34.6
      causing obstructed labor O65.5
    vulva — see category O34.7
      causing obstructed labor O65.5
  abortion of one fetus or more in multiple gestation O31.30
    first trimester O31.31
    second trimester O31.32
    spontaneous abortion O31.10
      first trimester O31.11
      second trimester O31.12
      third trimester O31.13
    third trimester O31.33
  abscess or cellulitis
    bladder — see Cystitis, complicating pregnancy
    genital organ or tract — see Pregnancy, complicated by, genital infection
  abuse (physical) (suspected) O94.319
    confirmed O94.329
      first trimester O94.321
      second trimester O94.322
      third trimester O94.323
    first trimester O94.311
    psychological (suspected) O94.519
      confirmed O94.529
        first trimester O94.521
        second trimester O94.522
        third trimester O94.523
      first trimester O94.511
      second trimester O94.512
      third trimester O94.513
    second trimester O94.312

©2002 Ingenix, Inc.

Pregnancy — *continued*
  complicated by — *see also* Pregnancy,
    management, affected by — *continued*
    abuse — *continued*
      sexual (suspected) O94.419
        confirmed O94.429
          first trimester O94.421
          second trimester O94.422
          third trimester O94.423
        first trimester O94.411
        second trimester O94.412
        third trimester O94.413
    adverse effect anesthesia — *see*
      Complications, anesthesia, in,
      pregnancy
    albuminuria — *see* Proteinuria, gestational
    alcohol dependence O99.313
      affecting fetus P04.3
      first trimester O99.310
      second trimester O99.311
      third trimester O99.312
    amnionitis O41.129
      affecting fetus P02.7
      first trimester O41.121
      second trimester O41.122
      third trimester O41.123
    anemia (conditions in D50-D64) O99.019
      first trimester O99.011
      second trimester O99.012
      third trimester O99.013
    atrophy (yellow) (acute) liver (subacute) —
      see Pregnancy, complicated by,
      disorders of liver
    bicornis or bicornuate uterus — *see*
      Pregnancy, complicated by, abnormal,
      uterus
    bone and joint disorders of back, pelvis and
      lower limbs — *see* Pregnancy,
      complicated by, diseases of, specified
      type or system NEC
    breech presentation O32.1
      affecting fetus P01.7
    cardiovascular diseases (conditions in I00-
      I09, I20-I52, I70-I99) — *see*
      Pregnancy, complicated by, diseases
      of, circulatory system
    cerebrovascular disorders (conditions in I60-
      I69) — *see* Pregnancy, complicated by,
      diseases of, circulatory system
    cervicitis — *see* Pregnancy, complicated by,
      genital infection
    chloasma (gravidarum) — *see* Pregnancy,
      complicated by, specified pregnancy-
      related condition NEC
    chorioamnionitis O41.129
      affecting fetus P02.7
      first trimester O41.121
      second trimester O41.122
      third trimester O41.123
    compound presentation O32.6
      affecting fetus P01.7
    conditions in
      A15-A19 — *see* Tuberculosis, obstetric
        complicating, pregnancy
      A50-A53 — *see* Syphilis, obstetric
        complicating, pregnancy
      A54.0 — *see* Gonorrhea, obstetric
        complicating, pregnancy
      A55-A64 — *see* Disease, sexually
        transmitted, obstetric complicating,
        pregnancy
      A80-B09, B25-B34 — *see* Disease, viral,
        obstetric complicating, pregnancy
      B15-B19 — *see* Hepatitis, viral, obstetric
        complicating, pregnancy
      B50-B64 — *see* Disease, protozoal,
        obstetric complicating, pregnancy
      C00-C97 — *see* Pregnancy, complicated
        by, tumor, malignant
      D50-D64 — *see* Pregnancy, complicated
        by, anemia
      D65-D89 — *see* Pregnancy, complicated
        by, diseases of, blood NEC
      E40-E46 — *see* Pregnancy, complicated
        by, malnutrition

Pregnancy — *continued*
  complicated by — *see also* Pregnancy,
    management, affected by — *continued*
    conditions in — *continued*
      F00-F99 — *see* Pregnancy, complicated
        by, mental disorder
      G00-G99 — *see* Pregnancy, complicated
        by, diseases of, nervous system
      H00-H95 — *see* Pregnancy, complicated
        by, diseases of, specified type or
        system NEC
      I00-I09, I20-I99 — *see* Pregnancy,
        complicated by, diseases of,
        circulatory system
      I10, pre-existing — *see* Hypertension,
        complicating, pregnancy, pre-
        existing
      I11.0, I11.9, pre-existing — *see*
        Hypertension, complicating,
        pregnancy, pre-existing, with, heart
        disease
      I12.0, I12.9, pre-existing — *see*
        Hypertension, complicating,
        pregnancy, pre-existing, with, renal
        disease
      I13.0 I13.9, pre-existing — *see*
        Hypertension, complicating,
        pregnancy, pre-existing, with, heart
        disease, with renal disease
      I15.0 -I15.9, pre-existing — *see*
        Hypertension, complicating,
        pregnancy, pre-existing, secondary
      J00-J99 — *see* Pregnancy, complicated
        by, diseases of, respiratory system
      K00-K93 — *see* Pregnancy, complicated
        by, diseases of, digestive system
      K70-K77 — *see* Pregnancy, complicated
        by, disorders of liver
      L00-L99 — *see* Pregnancy, complicated
        by, diseases of, skin and
        subcutaneous tissue
      N00-N07 — *see* Pregnancy, complicated
        by, glomerular diseases
      N10-N99 — *see* Pregnancy, complicated
        by, diseases of, specified type or
        system NEC
      N10-N12, N13.6, N15.1 — *see* Infection,
        kidney, complicating pregnancy
      Q00-Q99 NEC — *see* Pregnancy,
        complicated by, diseases of,
        specified type or system NEC
      R73.0 — *see* Pregnancy, complicated by,
        diseases of, specified type or system
        NEC
      S00-T88 — *see* Pregnancy, complicated
        by, injury or poisoning
    congenital malformations, deformations and
      chromosomal abnormalities NEC —
      see Pregnancy, complicated by,
      diseases of, specified type or system
      NEC
    contracted pelvis (general) O33.1
      inlet O33.2
      outlet O33.3
    convulsions (eclamptic) (uremic) — *see*
      Eclampsia
    cystitis — *see* Cystitis, complicating
      pregnancy
    cystocele — *see* Pregnancy, complicated by,
      abnormal, pelvic organs or tissues
      NEC
    death of fetus (near term) O36.4
      early pregnancy O02.1
      of one fetus or more in multiple gestation
        O31.20
        first trimester O31.21
        second trimester O31.22
        third trimester O31.23
    deciduitis O41.149
      first trimester O41.141
      second trimester O41.142
      third trimester O41.143
    diabetes (mellitus) — *see* Diabetes,
      complicating, pregnancy

Pregnancy — *continued*
  complicated by — *see also* Pregnancy,
    management, affected by — *continued*
    diseases of
      blood NEC (conditions in D65-D77)
        O99.119
        anemia — *see* Pregnancy, complicated
          by, anemia
        first trimester O99.111
        second trimester O99.112
        third trimester O99.113
      circulatory system (conditions in I00-I09,
        I20-I99) O99.419
        affecting fetus P00.3
        first trimester O99.411
        second trimester O99.412
        third trimester O99.413
      digestive system NEC (conditions in K00-
        K93) O99.619
        first trimester O99.611
        second trimester O99.612
        third trimester O99.613
      ear and mastoid process (conditions in
        H60-H95) — *see* Pregnancy,
        complicated by, diseases of,
        specified type or system NEC
      eye and adnexa (conditions in H00-H59)
        — *see* Pregnancy, complicated by,
        diseases of, specified type or system
        NEC
      genitourinary system NEC (conditions in
        N00-N99) — *see* Pregnancy,
        complicated by, diseases of,
        specified type or system NEC
      musculoskeletal system and connective
        tissue (conditions in M00-M99) —
        see Pregnancy, complicated by,
        diseases of, specified type or system
        NEC
      nervous system (conditions in G00-G99)
        O99.353
        first trimester O99.350
        second trimester O99.351
        third trimester O99.352
      respiratory system (conditions in J00-
        J99) O99.519
        affecting fetus P00.3
        first trimester O99.511
        second trimester O99.512
        third trimester O99.513
      skin and subcutaneous tissue (conditions
        in L00-L99) O99.729
        first trimester O99.721
        PUPPP (pruritic urticarial papules and
          plaques of pregnancy) O99.719
          first trimester O99.711
          second trimester O99.712
          third trimester O99.713
        second trimester O99.722
        third trimester O99.723
      specified type or system NEC O26.849
        first trimester O26.841
        second trimester O26.842
        third trimester O26.843
    disorders of liver O26.619
      first trimester O26.611
      second trimester O26.612
      third trimester O26.613
    displacement, uterus NEC — *see* Pregnancy,
      complicated by, abnormal, uterus
    disproportion — *see* Disproportion
    double uterus — *see* Pregnancy, complicated
      by, abnormal, ;uterus
    drug dependence (conditions in F11-F19,
      fourth character .1) O99.323
      affecting fetus P04.49
      first trimester O99.320
      second trimester O99.321
      third trimester O99.322
    early delivery (spontaneous) O60.9
      second trimester O60.2
      third trimester O60.3
    eclampsia, eclamptic (coma) (convulsions)
      (delirium) (nephritis) (uremia) — *see*
      Eclampsia
    edema — *see* Edema, gestational

Pregnancy — *continued*
 complicated by — *see also* Pregnancy,
  management, affected by — *continued*
 effusion, amniotic fluid — *see* category
  O41.8
 elderly
  multigravida O09.529
   first trimester O09.521
   second trimester O09.522
   third trimester O09.523
  primigravida O09.519
   first trimester O09.511
   second trimester O09.512
   third trimester O09.513
 embolism — *see* Embolism, obstetric,
  pregnancy
 endocrine diseases NEC O99.219
  first trimester O99.211
  second trimester O99.212
  third trimester O99.213
 endometritis — *see* Pregnancy, complicated
  by, genital infection
 excessive weight gain O26.00
  first trimester O26.01
  second trimester O26.02
  third trimester O26.03
 exhaustion O26.819
  first trimester O26.811
  second trimester O26.812
  third trimester O26.813
 face presentation O32.3
  affecting fetus P01.7
 failure, fetal head to enter pelvic brim O32.4
 false labor (pains) — *see* Labor, false
 fatigue — *see* Pregnancy, complicated by,
  exhaustion
 fatty metamorphosis of liver — *see*
  Pregnancy, complicated by, disorders
  of liver
 fetal
  abnormality or damage O35.9
   acid-base balance O68
   heart rate or rhythm O76
   specified type NEC O35.8
  acidemia O68
  acidosis O68
  alkalosis O68
  anencephaly O35.0
  bradycardia O76
  central nervous system malformation
   O35.0
  chromosomal abnormality (conditions in
   Q90-Q99) O35.1
  damage from
   amniocentesis O35.7
   biopsy procedures O35.7
   drug addiction O35.5
   hematological investigation O35.7
   intrauterine contraceptive device
    O35.7
   intrauterine surgery O35.7
   maternal
    alcohol addiction O35.4
    cytomegalovirus infection O35.3
    disease NEC O35.8
    drug addiction O35.5
    listeriosis O35.8
    rubella O35.3
    toxoplasmosis O35.8
    viral infection O35.3
   medical procedure NEC O35.7
   radiation O35.6
  death (near term) O36.4
   early pregnancy O02.1
  decreased movement O36.819
   second trimester O36.812
   third trimester O36.813
  disproportion due to deformity (fetal)
   O33.7
  distress O77.9
  excessive growth O36.60
   first trimester O36.61
   second trimester O36.62
   third trimester O36.63

Pregnancy — *continued*
 complicated by — *see also* Pregnancy,
  management, affected by — *continued*
 fetal — *continued*
  growth retardation — *see* Pregnancy,
   management affected by, fetal, poor
   growth
  heart rate irregularity (bradycardia)
   (decelerations) (tachycardia) O76
  hereditary disease O35.2
  hydrocephalus O35.0
  intrauterine death O36.4
  poor growth — *see* category O36.5
  problem O36.90
   first trimester O36.91
   second trimester O36.92
   specified type NEC O36.899
    first trimester O36.891
    second trimester O36.892
    third trimester O36.893
   third trimester O36.93
  spina bifida O35.0
 fibroid (tumor) (uterus) — *see* Pregnancy,
  complicated by, tumor, uterus
 genital infection O23.50
  affecting fetus P00.8
  first trimester O23.51
  second trimester O23.52
  third trimester O23.53
 glomerular diseases (conditions in N00-N07)
  O26.839
  with hypertension, pre-existing — *see*
   Hypertension, complicating,
   pregnancy, pre-existing, with, renal
   disease
  affecting fetus P00.1
  first trimester O26.831
  second trimester O26.832
  third trimester O26.833
 gonococcal infection — *see* Gonorrhea,
  obstetric complicating, pregnancy
 grand multiparity O09.40
  first trimester O09.41
  second trimester O09.42
  third trimester O09.43
 hemorrhage
  antepartum — *see* Hemorrhage,
   antepartum
  before 22 completed weeks' gestation
   O20.9
   specified NEC O20.8
  due to premature separation, placenta —
   see Disorder, placenta, abruptio
  early O20.9
   specified NEC O20.8
  threatened abortion O20.0
 hemorrhoids — *see* Hemorrhoids,
  complicating, pregnancy
 herniation of uterus — *see* Pregnancy,
  complicated by, abnormal, uterus
 high
  head at term O32.4
  risk O09.90
   with
    grand multiparity — *see* Pregnancy,
     complicated by, grand
     multiparity
   history of
    ectopic pregnancy — *see*
     Pregnancy, complicated by,
     previous, trophoblastic
     disease
    infertility — *see* Pregnancy,
     complicated by, infertility,
     previous
    insufficient antenatal care — *see*
     Pregnancy, complicated by,
     insufficient, prenatal care
    molar pregnancy — *see*
     Pregnancy, complicated by,
     previous, trophoblastic
     disease
    neonatal death — *see* Pregnancy,
     complicated by, poor
     obstetric history

Pregnancy — *continued*
 complicated by — *see also* Pregnancy,
  management, affected by — *continued*
 high — *continued*
  risk — *continued*
   with — *continued*
    history of — *continued*
     reproductive problem NEC — *see*
      Pregnancy, complicated by,
      poor obstetric history
     stillbirth — *see* Pregnancy,
      complicated by, poor
      obstetric history
     social problem NEC — *see*
      Pregnancy, complicated by,
      social problem
   elderly
    multigravida — *see* Pregnancy,
     complicated by, elderly,
     multigravida
    primigravida — *see* Pregnancy,
     complicated by, elderly,
     primigravida
   first trimester O09.91
   second trimester O09.92
   specified problem NEC O09.899
    first trimester O09.891
    second trimester O09.892
    third trimester O09.893
   third trimester O09.93
   very young
    multigravida — *see* Pregnancy,
     complicated by, very young,
     multigravida
    primigravida — *see* Pregnancy,
     complicated by, very young,
     primigravida
 hydatidiform mole — *see* Mole, hydatidiform
 hydramnios — *see* Polyhydramnios
 hydrocephalic fetus (disproportion) O33.6
 hydrops
  amnii — *see* Polyhydramnios
  fetalis O36.20
   associated with isoimmunization —
    see Pregnancy, management
    affected by, isoimmunization
   first trimester O36.21
   second trimester O36.22
   third trimester O36.23
 hydrorrhea — *see* Rupture, membranes,
  premature
 hyperemesis (gravidarum) — *see*
  Hyperemesis, gravidarum
 hypertension — *see* Hypertension,
  complicating pregnancy
 hypertensive
  heart and renal disease, pre-existing —
   see Hypertension, complicating,
   pregnancy, pre-existing, with, heart
   disease, with renal disease
  heart disease, pre-existing — *see*
   Hypertension, complicating,
   pregnancy, pre-existing, with, heart
   disease
  renal disease, pre-existing — *see*
   Hypertension, complicating,
   pregnancy, pre-existing, with, renal
   disease
 immune disorders NEC (conditions in D80-
  D89) — *see* Pregnancy, complicated
  by, diseases of, blood NEC
 incarceration, uterus — *see* Pregnancy,
  complicated by, abnormal, uterus
 incompetent cervix O34.30
  affecting fetus P01.0
  first trimester O34.31
  second trimester O34.32
  third trimester O34.33
 infection(s) — *see also* Pregnancy,
  complicated by, infectious or parasitic
  disease
  amniotic fluid or sac O41.109
   affecting fetus P02.7
   first trimester O41.101
   second trimester O41.102
   third trimester O41.103

©2002 Ingenix, Inc.

Pregnancy — *continued*
  complicated by — *see also* Pregnancy,
    management, affected by — *continued*
    infection(s) — *see also* Pregnancy,
      complicated by, infectious or parasitic
      disease — *continued*
      bladder — *see* Cystitis, complicating
       pregnancy
      genital organ or tract — *see* Pregnancy,
       complicated by, genital infection
      genitourinary tract O23.90
       affecting fetus P00.8
       first trimester O23.91
       second trimester O23.92
       streptococcus B O98.819
        first trimester O98.811
        second trimester O98.812
        third trimester O98.813
       third trimester O23.93
      kidney — *see* Infection, kidney,
       complicating pregnancy
      specified NEC — *see* Disease, infectious,
       obstetric, specified infection NEC
       complicating, pregnancy
      urethra — *see* Urethritis, complicating
       pregnancy
      urinary (tract) — *see* Infection, urinary,
       complicating pregnancy
    infectious or parasitic disease O98.919
     affecting fetus P00.2
     first trimester O98.911
     gonorrhea — *see* Gonorrhea, obstetric
      complicating, pregnancy
     protozoal disease — *see* Disease,
      protozoal, obstetric complicating,
      pregnancy
     second trimester O98.912
     sexually transmitted disease NEC — *see*
      Disease, sexually transmitted,
      obstetric complicating, pregnancy
     specified type NEC O98.819
      first trimester O98.811
      second trimester O98.812
      third trimester O98.813
     streptococcus B genitourinary infection —
      see Pregnancy, complicated by,
      infection, genitourinary tract,
      streptococcus B
     syphilis — *see* Syphilis, obstetric
      complicating, pregnancy
     third trimester O98.913
     tuberculosis — *see* Tuberculosis,
      obstetric, complicating, pregnancy
     viral disease — *see also* Disease, viral,
      obstetric complicating, pregnancy
      hepatitis — *see* Hepatitis, viral,
       obstetric complicating,
       pregnancy
    infertility, previous O09.00
     first trimester O09.01
     second trimester O09.02
     third trimester O09.03
    injury or poisoning (conditions in S00-T88)
     O94.219
     affecting fetus P00.5
     due to abuse — *see* Pregnancy,
      complicated by, abuse
     first trimester O94.211
     second trimester O94.212
     third trimester O94.213
    insufficient
     prenatal care O09.30
      first trimester O09.31
      second trimester O09.32
      third trimester O09.33
     weight gain O26.10
      first trimester O26.11
      second trimester O26.12
      third trimester O26.13
    intrauterine fetal death (near term) O36.4
     early pregnancy O02.1
     multiple gestation (one fetus or more)
      O31.20
      first trimester O31.21
      second trimester O31.22
      third trimester O31.23

Pregnancy — *continued*
  complicated by — *see also* Pregnancy,
   management, affected by — *continued*
   malaria — *see* Disease, protozoal, obstetric
    complicating, pregnancy
   malformation
    placenta, placental (vessel) — *see*
     Disorder, placenta, malformation
    uterus (congenital) — *see* Pregnancy,
     complicated by, abnormal, uterus
   malnutrition (conditions in E40-E46) O25.10
    affecting fetus P00.4
    first trimester O25.11
    second trimester O25.12
    third trimester O25.13
   malposition
    fetus — *see* Presentation, fetal
    uterus — *see* Pregnancy, complicated by,
     abnormal, uterus
   malpresentation of fetus — *see also*
    Presentation, fetal
    in multiple gestation O32.5
    specified NEC O32.8
   mental disorders (conditions in F01-F09,
    F20-F99) O99.343
    alcohol use — *see* Alcohol, use,
     uncomplicated, complicating,
     pregnancy
    drug use — *see* Drug, use, obstetric
     complicating, pregnancy
    first trimester O99.340
    second trimester O99.341
    smoking — *see* Tobacco, use,
     complicating, pregnancy
    third trimester O99.342
   mentum presentation O32.3
   metabolic disorders O99.219
    first trimester O99.211
    second trimester O99.212
    third trimester O99.213
   missed
    abortion O02.1
    delivery O36.4
   necrosis, liver (conditions in K72) — *see*
    Pregnancy, complicated by, disorders
    of liver
   neoplasms NEC — *see* Pregnancy,
    complicated by, tumor
   nephropathy NEC — *see* Pregnancy,
    complicated by, renal disease or failure
   nutritional diseases NEC O99.219
    affecting fetus P00.4
    first trimester O99.211
    second trimester O99.212
    third trimester O99.213
   oblique lie or presentation O32.2
    affecting fetus P01.7
   oligohydramnios O41.00
    with premature rupture of membranes —
     see Rupture, membranes,
     premature
    affecting fetus P01.2
    first trimester O41.01
    second trimester O41.02
    third trimester O41.03
   onset of contractions before 37 weeks'
    gestation — *see* Labor, premature or
    preterm
   oophoritis — *see* Pregnancy, complicated by,
    genital infection
   overdose, drug — *see* Pregnancy,
    complicated by, injury or poisoning
   oversize fetus O33.5
   papyraceous fetus — *see* Papyraceous fetus,
    complicating pregnancy
   peripheral neuritis O26.829
    first trimester O26.821
    second trimester O26.822
    third trimester O26.823
   phlebothrombosis — *see* Thrombophlebitis,
    antepartum
   placenta, placental
    abnormality — *see* Disorder, placenta,
     malformation

Pregnancy — *continued*
  complicated by — *see also* Pregnancy,
   management, affected by — *continued*
   placenta, placental — *continued*
    abruptio or ablatio — *see* Disorder,
     placenta, abruptio
    detachment — *see* Disorder, placenta,
     abruptio
    disease — *see* Disorder, placenta
    dysfunction — *see* Disorder, placenta,
     dysfunction
    infarction — *see* Disorder, placenta,
     infarction
    low implantation (with hemorrhage) —
     see Disorder, placenta, previa
    malformation — *see* Disorder, placenta,
     malformation
    malposition (with hemorrhage) — *see*
     Disorder, placenta, previa
    previa (with hemorrhage) — *see* Disorder,
     placenta, previa
    separation, premature — *see* Disorder,
     placenta, abruptio
    transfusion syndrome (fetomaternal)
     O43.019
     affecting fetus P02.3
     fetus-to-fetus O43.029
      first trimester O43.021
      second trimester O43.022
      third trimester O43.023
     first trimester O43.011
     second trimester O43.012
     third trimester O43.013
   placentitis O41.149
    affecting fetus P02.7
    first trimester O41.141
    second trimester O41.142
    third trimester O41.143
   poisoning — *see* Pregnancy, complicated by,
    injury or poisoning
   polyhydramnios — *see* Polyhydramnios
   poor obstetric history — *see* category O09.2
   postmaturity (40 to 42 weeks) O48.0
    more than 42 weeks gestation O48.1
   pre-eclampsia — *see* Pre-eclampsia
   premature rupture of membranes — *see*
    Rupture, membranes, premature
   previous
    infertility — *see* Pregnancy, complicated
     by, infertility, previous
    nonobstetric condition — *see* Pregnancy,
     complicated by, high, risk, specified
     problem NEC
    poor obstetric history — *see* Pregnancy,
     complicated by, poor obstetric
     history
    premature delivery — *see* Pregnancy,
     complicated by, poor obstetric
     history
    trophoblastic disease or ectopic
     pregnancy (conditions in O00 and
     O01) O09.10
     first trimester O09.11
     second trimester O09.12
     third trimester O09.13
   primigravida
    elderly (supervision only) — *see*
     Pregnancy, complicated by, elderly,
     primigravida
    very young (supervision only) — *see*
     Pregnancy, complicated by, very
     young, primigravida
   prolapse, uterus — *see* Pregnancy,
    complicated by, abnormal, uterus
   proteinuria — *see* Proteinuria, gestational
   protozoal diseases — *see* Disease, protozoal,
    obstetric complicating, pregnancy
   pruritus (neurogenic) — *see* Pregnancy,
    complicated by, specified pregnancy-
    related condition NEC
   psychosis or psychoneurosis — *see*
    Pregnancy, complicated by, mental
    disorder
   ptyalism — *see* Pregnancy, complicated by,
    specified pregnancy-related condition
    NEC

Pregnancy — *continued*
  complicated by — *see also* Pregnancy,
    management, affected by — *continued*
    pyelitis — *see* Infection, kidney,
      complicating pregnancy
    renal disease or failure NEC O26.839
      with secondary hypertension, pre-existing
        — *see* Hypertension, complicating,
        pregnancy, pre-existing, secondary
      affecting fetus P00.1
      first trimester O26.831
      hypertensive, pre-existing — *see*
        Hypertension, complicating,
        pregnancy, pre-existing, with, renal
        disease
      second trimester O26.832
      third trimester O26.833
    retention, retained
      dead ovum O02.0
      intrauterine contraceptive device O26.30
        first trimester O26.31
        second trimester O26.32
        third trimester O26.33
    retroversion, uterus — *see* Pregnancy,
      complicated by, abnormal, uterus
    Rh immunization, incompatibility or
      sensitization — *see* Pregnancy,
      management affected by,
      isoimmunization, Rhesus
  rupture
    amnion (premature) — *see* Rupture,
      membranes, premature
    membranes (premature) — *see* Rupture,
      membranes, premature
    uterus (during labor) — *see* Rupture,
      uterus
  salivation (excessive) — *see* Pregnancy,
    complicated by, specified pregnancy-
    related condition NEC
  salpingitis — *see* Pregnancy, complicated by,
    genital infection
  salpingo-oophoritis — *see* Pregnancy,
    complicated by, genital infection
  septicemia (conditions in A40, A41) — *see*
    Disease, infectious, obstetric, specified
    infection NEC complicating, pregnancy
  specified pregnancy-related condition NEC
    O26.899
    affecting fetus P03.89
    first trimester O26.891
    second trimester O26.892
    third trimester O26.893
  signs of fetal hypoxia (unrelated to labor or
    delivery) O36.899
    first trimester O36.891
    second trimester O36.892
    third trimester O36.893
  social problem O09.70
    first trimester O09.71
    second trimester O09.72
    third trimester O09.73
  specified condition NEC O26.899
    first trimester O26.891
    second trimester O26.892
    third trimester O26.893
  spurious labor pains — *see* Labor, false
  streptococcus B carrier state O99.830
  superfecundation — *see* category O30.8
    complicated by obstructed labor O66.6
  superfetation — *see* category O30.8
  syphilis (conditions in A50-A53) — *see*
    Syphilis, obstetric complicating,
    pregnancy
  threatened
    abortion O20.0
    delivery O47.9
      at or after 37 completed weeks of
        gestation O47.1
      before 37 completed weeks of gestation
        O47.00
        second trimester O47.02
        third trimester O47.03
  thrombophlebitis — *see* Thrombophlebitis,
    antepartum
  thrombosis — *see* Thrombophlebitis,
    antepartum

Pregnancy — *continued*
  complicated by — *see also* Pregnancy,
    management, affected by — *continued*
    torsion of uterus — *see* Pregnancy,
      complicated by, abnormal, uterus
    toxemia — *see* Pre-eclampsia
    transverse lie or presentation O32.2
      affecting fetus P01.7
    tuberculosis (conditions in A15-A19) — *see*
      Tuberculosis, obstetric complicating,
      pregnancy
    tumor (benign) — *see also* Pregnancy,
      complicated by, diseases of, specified
      type or system NEC
      malignant O94.119
        first trimester O94.111
        second trimester O94.112
        third trimester O94.113
      ovary — *see* Pregnancy, complicated by,
        tumor, pelvic organs or tissues NEC
      pelvic organs or tissues NEC — *see*
        category O34.8
        causing obstructed labor O65.5
      uterus (body) — *see* category O34.1
        causing obstructed labor O65.5
      cervix — *see* category O34.4
        causing obstructed labor O65.5
      vagina — *see* category O34.6
        causing obstructed labor O65.5
      vulva — *see* category O34.7
        causing obstructed labor O65.5
    unstable lie O32.0
      affecting fetus P01.7
    urethritis — *see* Urethritis, complicating
      pregnancy
    uterus bicornis — *see* Pregnancy,
      complicated by, abnormal, uterus
    vaginitis or vulvitis — *see* Pregnancy,
      complicated by, genital infection
    varicose
      placental vessels — *see* Disorder,
        placenta, specified type NEC
      veins — *see* Varix, complicating,
        pregnancy
    venereal disease NEC (conditions in A64) —
      see Disease, sexually transmitted,
      obstetric complicating, pregnancy
    venous disorders O22.90
      cerebral venous thrombosis — *see*
        Phlebitis, intracranial, antepartum
      first trimester O22.91
      hemorrhoids — *see* Hemorrhoids,
        complicating, pregnancy
      second trimester O22.92
      specified type NEC — *see* category O22.8
      third trimester O22.93
      thrombophlebitis — *see*
        Thrombophlebitis, antepartum
      varicose veins — *see* Varix, complicating,
        pregnancy
    viral diseases (conditions in A80-B09, B25-
      B34) — *see* Disease, viral, obstetric
      complicating, pregnancy
    very young
      multigravida O09.629
        first trimester O09.621
        second trimester O09.622
        third trimester O09.623
      primigravida O09.619
        first trimester O09.611
        second trimester O09.612
        third trimester O09.613
    vomiting O21.9
      due to diseases classified elsewhere
        O21.8
      hyperemesis gravidarum — *see*
        Hyperemesis, gravidarum
      late (occurring after the 20th week of
        gestation) O21.2
  complications NOS O26.90
    first trimester O26.91
    second trimester O26.92
    third trimester O26.93
  concealed — *see* Pregnancy, complicated by,
    insufficient, prenatal care

Pregnancy — *continued*
  continuing after
    abortion of one fetus or more O31.30
      first trimester O31.31
      second trimester O31.32
      spontaneous abortion O31.10
        first trimester O31.11
        second trimester O31.12
        third trimester O31.13
      third trimester O31.33
    intrauterine death of one fetus or more
      O31.20
      first trimester O31.21
      second trimester O31.22
      third trimester O31.23
  cornual O00.8
  ectopic (ruptured) O00.9
    abdominal O00.0
      with viable fetus O36.70
        first trimester O36.71
        second trimester O36.72
        third trimester O36.73
    affecting fetus P01.4
    cervical O00.8
    cornual O00.8
    intraligamentous O00.8
    mural O00.8
    ovarian O00.2
    specified site NEC O00.8
    tubal (ruptured) O00.1
  examination, pregnancy not confirmed Z32.0
  extrauterine — *see* Pregnancy, ectopic
  fallopian O00.1
  false F45.8
  hidden — *see* Pregnancy, complicated by,
    insufficient, prenatal care
  illegitimate (unwanted) Z64.0
    supervision of high-risk pregnancy — *see*
      Pregnancy, complicated by, social
      problem
  in double uterus — *see* Pregnancy, complicated
    by, abnormal, uterus
  incidental finding Z33.1
  interstitial O00.8
  intraligamentous O00.8
  intramural O00.8
  intraperitoneal O00.0
  isthmian O00.1
  management affected by — *see also* Pregnancy,
    complicated by
    abnormal, abnormality
      fetus (suspected) O35.9
        specified NEC O35.8
      placenta — *see* Disorder, placenta,
        malformation
    antibodies (maternal)
      anti-D — *see* Pregnancy, management
        affected by, isoimmunization, Rh
      blood group — *see* Pregnancy,
        management affected by,
        isoimmunization
    death, fetal (near term) O36.4
    early pregnancy O02.1
    diseases of the nervous system (conditions
      in G00-G99) O99.353
      first trimester O99.350
      second trimester O99.351
      third trimester O99.352
    elderly primigravida (supervision only) — *see*
      Pregnancy, complicated by, elderly,
      primigravida
    fetal (suspected)
      abnormality or damage O35.9
        acid-base balance O68
        heart rate or rhythm O76
        specified NEC O35.8
      acidemia O68
      anencephaly O35.0
      bradycardia O76
      central nervous system malformation
        O35.0
      chromosomal abnormality (conditions in
        Q90-Q99) O35.1

©2002 Ingenix, Inc.

Pregnancy — *continued*
management affected by — *see also* Pregnancy, complicated by — *continued*
fetal — *continued*
damage from
amniocentesis O35.7
biopsy procedures O35.7
drug addiction O35.5
hematological investigation O35.7
intrauterine contraceptive device O35.7
intrauterine surgery O35.7
maternal
alcohol addiction O35.4
cytomegalovirus infection O35.3
disease NEC O35.8
drug addiction O35.5
listeriosis O35.8
rubella O35.3
toxoplasmosis O35.8
viral infection O35.3
medical procedure NEC O35.7
radiation O35.6
death (near term) O36.4
early pregnancy O02.1
distress O77.9
excessive growth O36.60
first trimester O36.61
second trimester O36.62
third trimester O36.63
growth retardation — *see* Pregnancy, management affected by, fetal, poor growth
hereditary disease O35.2
hydrocephalus O35.0
intrauterine death O36.4
poor growth — *see* category O36.5
spina bifida O35.0
fetomaternal hemorrhage — *see* Pregnancy, complicated by, placenta, transfusion syndrome
hereditary disease in family, (possibly) affecting fetus O35.2
high-risk pregnancy NEC — *see* Pregnancy, complicated by, high risk
incompatibility, blood groups — *see* Pregnancy, management affected by, isoimmunization
insufficient prenatal care (supervision only) — *see* Pregnancy, complicated by, insufficient, prenatal care
intrauterine death (late) O36.4
isoimmunization (ABO) — *see also* category O36.1
Rh(esus) O36.00
first trimester O36.01
second trimester O36.02
third trimester O36.03
large-for-dates fetus — *see* Pregnancy, management affected by, fetal, excessive growth
light-for-dates fetus — *see* Pregnancy, management affected by, fetal, poor growth
mental disorder (conditions in F00-F99) — *see* Pregnancy, complicated by, mental disorder
multiparity (grand) (supervision only) — *see* Pregnancy, complicated by, grand multiparity
poor obstetric history (conditions classified to O10-O92) — *see* Pregnancy, complicated by, poor obstetric history
postmaturity (40 to 42 weeks) O48.0
more than 42 weeks gestation O48.1
previous
abortion — *see* Pregnancy, complicated by, poor obstetric history
habitual O26.2
first trimester O26.21
second trimester O26.22
third trimester O26.23
cesarean section O34.21

Pregnancy — *continued*
management affected by — *see also* Pregnancy, complicated by — *continued*
previous — *continued*
difficult delivery — *see* Pregnancy, complicated by, poor obstetric history
forceps delivery — *see* Pregnancy, complicated by, poor obstetric history
hemorrhage, antepartum or postpartum — *see* Pregnancy, complicated by, poor obstetric history
hydatidiform mole — *see* Pregnancy, complicated by, previous, trophoblastic disease
infertility — *see* Pregnancy, complicated by, infertility, previous
malignancy NEC — *see* Pregnancy, complicated by, high, risk, specified problem NEC
nonobstetrical condition — *see* Pregnancy, complicated by, high, risk, specified problem NEC
premature delivery — *see* Pregnancy, complicated by, poor obstetric history
trophoblastic disease (conditions in O01) — *see* Pregnancy, complicated by, previous, trophoblastic disease
vesicular mole — *see* Pregnancy, complicated by, previous, trophoblastic disease
prolonged pregnancy (more than 42 weeks gestation) O48.1
small-for-dates fetus — *see* Pregnancy, management affected by, fetal, poor growth
social problem — *see* Pregnancy, complicated by, social problem
very young primigravida (supervision only) — *see* Pregnancy, complicated by, very young, primigravida
mesometric (mural) O00.8
molar NEC O02.0
hydatiform — *see* Mole, hydatidiform
multiple O30.90
affecting fetus P01.5
complicated NEC — *see* category O31.8
first trimester O30.91
quadruplet — *see* Pregnancy, quadruplet
quintuplet — *see* Pregnancy, quintuplet
second trimester O30.92
sextuplet — *see* Pregnancy, sextuplet
specified number NEC — *see* category O30.8
third trimester O30.92
triplet — *see* Pregnancy, triplet
twin — *see* Pregnancy, twin
mural O00.8
normal (supervision of) Z34.90
first Z34.00
first trimester Z34.01
second trimester Z34.02
third trimester Z34.03
first trimester Z34.91
second trimester Z34.92
subsequent Z34.80
first trimester Z34.81
second trimester Z34.82
third trimester Z34.83
third trimester Z34.93
observation NEC — *see* Pregnancy, normal
ovarian O00.2
postmature (40 to 42 weeks) O48.0
more than 42 weeks gestation O48.1
post-term (40 to 42 weeks) O48.0
more than 42 weeks gestation O48.1
prenatal care only –*see also* Pregnancy, normal
high risk — *see* Pregnancy, complicated by, high, risk
prolonged (more than 42 weeks gestation) O48.1
quadruplet O30.20
first trimester O30.21
second trimester O30.22
third trimester O30.23
quintuplet — *see* category O30.8

Pregnancy — *continued*
sextuplet — *see* category O30.8
spurious F45.8
supervision (of) (for) — *see also* Pregnancy, management affected by
high-risk — *see* Pregnancy, complicated by, high, risk
normal — *see* Pregnancy, normal
triplet O30.10
first trimester O30.11
second trimester O30.12
third trimester O30.13
tubal (with abortion) (with rupture) O00.1
twin O30.009
first trimester O30.001
monoamniotic/monochorionic O30.019
first trimester O30.011
second trimester O30.012
third trimester O30.013
second trimester O30.002
specified NEC O30.099
first trimester O30.091
second trimester O30.092
third trimester O30.093
third trimester O30.003
unconfirmed Z32.0
undelivered (no other diagnosis) Z33.1
unwanted Z64.0

Preiser's disease — *see* Osteonecrosis, secondary, due to, trauma, metacarpus

Pre-kwashiorkor — *see* Malnutrition, severe

Preleukemia (syndrome) (M9989/1) D46.9

Preluxation, hip, congenital Q65.6

Premature — *see also* condition
adrenarche E27.0
aging E34.8
beats I49.4
atrial I49.1
auricular I49.1
supraventricular I49.1
birth NEC — *see* Preterm infant, newborn
closure, foramen ovale Q21.8
contraction
atrial I49.1
atrioventricular I49.2
auricular I49.1
auriculoventricular I49.2
heart (extrasystole) I49.4
junctional I49.2
ventricular I49.3
delivery O60.9
second trimester O60.2
third trimester O60.3
ejaculation F52.4
infant NEC — *see* Preterm infant, newborn
light-for-dates — *see* Light for dates
lungs P28.0
menopause E28.3
newborn — *see* Prematurity
puberty E30.1
rupture membranes or amnion — *see* Rupture, membranes, premature
senility E34.8
separation, placenta (partial) — *see* Disorder, placenta, abruptio
thelarche E30.8
ventricular systole I49.3

Prematurity NEC (less than 37 completed weeks) — *see* Preterm infant, newborn
extreme (less than 28 completed weeks) — *see* Immaturity, extreme

Premenstrual tension (syndrome) N94.3

Premolarization, cuspids K00.2

Prenatal
care, normal pregnancy — *see* Pregnancy, normal
screening Z36

Preparatory care for subsequent treatment NEC Z51.89
for dialysis Z49.01
peritoneal Z49.02

Prepartum — *see* condition

Preponderance, left or right ventricular I51.7

Prepuce — *see* condition

Presbycardia R54
Presbycusis, presbyacusia H91.10
    bilateral H91.13
    left H91.12
    right H91.11
Presbyesophagus K22.8
Presbyophrenia F03
Presbyopia H52.4
Prescription of contraceptives (initial) Z30.019
    implantable subdermal Z30.012
    injectable Z30.013
    intrauterine contraceptive device Z30.014
    pills Z30.011
    repeat Z30.40
       implantable subdermal Z30.42
       injectable Z30.43
       intrauterine contraceptive device Z30.44
       pills Z30.41
       specified type NEC Z30.49
    specified type NEC Z30.018
Presence (of)
    ankle-joint implant (functional) (prosthesis) Z96.669
       left Z96.662
       right Z96.661
    aortocoronary (bypass) graft Z95.1
    arterial-venous shunt (dialysis) Z99.2
    artificial
       eye (globe) Z97.0
       heart (mechanical) Z95.89
          valve Z95.2
       larynx Z96.3
       lens (intraocular) Z96.1
       limb (complete) (partial) Z97.10
          arm
             bilateral Z97.15
             left Z97.12
             right Z97.11
          leg
             bilateral Z97.16
             left Z97.14
             right Z97.13
    audiological implant (functional) Z96.29
    bladder implant (functional) Z96.0
    bone
       conduction hearing device Z96.29
       implant (functional) NEC Z96.7
       joint (prosthesis) — see Presence, joint implant
    cardiac
       defibrillator (functional) Z95.81
       implant or graft Z95.9
          specified type NEC Z95.89
       pacemaker Z95.0
    cerebrospinal fluid drainage device Z98.2
    cochlear implant (functional) Z96.21
    contact lens(es) Z97.3
    coronary artery graft or prosthesis Z95.51
    CSF shunt Z98.2
    dental prosthesis device Z97.2
    device (external) NEC Z97.8
       implanted (functional) Z96.9
          specified NEC Z96.89
       prosthetic Z97.8
    ear implant Z96.20
       cochlear implant Z96.21
       myringotomy tube Z96.22
       specified type NEC Z96.29
    elbow-joint implant (functional) (prosthesis) Z96.629
       left Z96.622
       right Z96.621
    endocrine implant (functional) Z96.4
    eustachian tube stent or device (functional) Z96.29
    external hearing-aid or device Z97.4
    finger-joint implant (functional) (prosthetic)
       bilateral Z96.693
       left Z96.692
       right Z96.691
    functional implant Z96.9
       specified NEC Z96.89
    hearing-aid or device (external) Z97.4
       implant (bone) (cochlear) (functional) Z96.21

Presence — continued
    heart valve implant (functional) NEC Z95.4
       prosthetic Z95.2
       specified type NEC Z95.4
       xenogenic Z95.3
    hip-joint implant (functional) (prosthesis) Z96.649
       bilateral Z96.643
       left Z96.642
       right Z96.641
    implanted device (artificial) (functional) (prosthetic) Z96.9
       automatic cardiac defibrillator Z95.81
       cardiac pacemaker Z95.0
       cochlear Z96.21
       dental Z96.5
       heart valve Z95.4
          prosthetic Z95.2
          xenogenic Z95.3
       insulin pump Z96.4
       intraocular lens Z96.1
       joint Z96.60
          ankle Z96.669
             left Z96.662
             right Z96.661
          elbow Z96.629
             left Z96.622
             right Z96.621
          finger Z96.698
             bilateral Z96.693
             left Z96.692
             right Z96.691
          hip Z96.649
             bilateral Z96.643
             left Z96.642
             right Z96.641
          knee Z96.659
             bilateral Z96.653
             left Z96.652
             right Z96.651
          shoulder Z96.619
             left Z96.612
             right Z96.611
          specified NEC Z96.698
          wrist Z96.639
             left Z96.632
             right Z96.631
       larynx Z96.3
       myringotomy tube Z96.22
       otological Z96.20
          cochlear Z96.21
          eustachian stent Z96.29
          myringotomy Z96.22
          specified NEC Z96.29
          stapes Z96.29
       skin Z96.81
       skull plate Z96.7
       specified NEC Z96.89
       urogenital Z96.0
    insulin pump (functional) Z96.4
    intestinal bypass or anastomosis Z98.0
    intraocular lens (functional) Z96.1
    intrauterine contraceptive device (IUD) Z97.5
    intravascular implant (functional) (prosthetic) NEC Z95.9
       coronary artery Z95.51
       defibrillator Z95.81
       peripheral vessel Z95.89
          with angioplasty Z95.83
    joint implant (prosthetic) (any) Z96.60
       ankle — see Presence, ankle joint implant
       elbow — see Presence, elbow joint implant
       finger — see Presence, finger joint implant
       hip — see Presence, hip joint implant
       knee — see Presence, knee joint implant
       shoulder — see Presence, shoulder joint implant
       specified joint NEC Z96.698
       wrist — see Presence, wrist joint implant
    knee-joint implant (functional) (prosthesis) Z96.659
       bilateral Z96.653
       left Z96.652
       right Z96.651

Presence — continued
    laryngeal implant (functional) Z96.3
    mandibular implant (dental) Z96.5
    myringotomy tube(s) Z96.22
    orthopedic-joint implant (prosthetic) (any) — see Presence, joint implant
    otological implant (functional) Z96.29
    shoulder-joint implant (functional) (prosthesis) Z96.619
       left Z96.612
       right Z96.611
    skull-plate implant Z96.7
    spectacles Z97.3
    stapes implant (functional) Z96.29
    tendon implant (functional) (graft) Z96.7
    tooth root(s) implant Z96.5
    ureteral stent Z96.0
    urethral stent Z96.0
    urogenital implant (functional) Z96.0
    vascular implant or device Z95.9
       access port device Z95.89
       specified type NEC Z95.89
    wrist-joint implant (functional) (prosthesis) Z96.639
       left Z96.632
       right Z96.631
Presenile — see also condition
    dementia F03
    premature aging E34.8
Presentation, fetal
    abnormal O32.9
       causing obstructed labor O64.9
          specified NEC O64.8
       in multiple gestation (one or more) O32.5
       specified NEC O32.8
    arm O32.2
       causing obstructed labor O64.4
    breech (mother) O32.1
       causing obstructed labor O64.1
       footling O32.8
          causing obstructed labor O64.8
       incomplete O32.8
          causing obstructed labor O64.8
    brow (mother) O32.3
       causing obstructed labor O64.3
    chin (mother) O32.3
       causing obstructed labor O64.2
    compound O32.6
       causing obstructed labor O64.5
    cord O69.0
    extended head (mother) O32.3
       causing obstructed labor O64.3
    face (mother) O32.3
       causing obstructed labor O64.2
       to pubes O32.3
          causing obstructed labor O64.0
    footling O32.8
       causing obstructed labor O64.8
    hand O32.2
       causing obstructed labor O64.4
    leg or foot, NEC O32.1
       causing obstructed labor O64.1
    mentum (mother) O32.3
       causing obstructed labor O64.2
    oblique (mother) O32.2
       causing obstructed labor O64.4
    shoulder O32.2
       causing obstructed labor O64.4
    transverse (mother) O32.2
       causing obstructed labor O64.8
    unstable O32.0
Prespondylolisthesis (congenital) Q76.2
Pressure
    area, skin ulcer — see Decubitus
    birth, fetus or newborn P15.9
    brachial plexus G54.0
    brain G93.5
       injury at birth NEC P11.1
    cerebral — see Pressure, brain
    chest R07.89
    cone, tentorial G93.5
    hyposystolic — see also Hypotension
       incidental reading, without diagnosis of hypotension R03.1

Pressure — *continued*
 increased
  intracranial (benign) G93.2
   injury at birth P11.0
  intraocular H40.0
 lumbosacral plexus G54.1
 mediastinum J98.5
 necrosis (chronic) — *see* Decubitus
 sore (chronic) — *see* Decubitus
 spinal cord G95.2
 ulcer (chronic) — *see* Decubitus
 venous, increased I87.8

Pre-syncope R55

Preterm-infant, newborn P07.30
 with gestation of:
  28-31 weeks P07.31
  32-36 weeks P07.32

Previa
 placenta (with hemorrhage) — *see* Disorder, placenta, previa
 vasa O69.4

Priapism N48.30
 due to
  disease classified elsewhere N48.32
  drug N48.33
  specified cause NEC N48.39
  trauma N48.31

Prickling sensation (skin) R20.2

Prickly heat L74.0

Primary — *see* condition

Primigravida
 elderly, affecting management of pregnancy, labor and delivery (supervision only) — *see* Pregnancy, complicated by, elderly, primigravida
 very young, affecting management of pregnancy, labor and delivery (supervision only) — *see* Pregnancy, complicated by, very young, primigravida

Primipara
 elderly, affecting management of pregnancy, labor and delivery (supervision only) — *see* Pregnancy, complicated by, elderly, primigravida
 very young, affecting management of pregnancy, labor and delivery (supervision only) — *see* Pregnancy, complicated by, very young, primigravida

Primus varus (bilateral) Q66.3

P.R.I.N.D I64

Pringle's disease (tuberous sclerosis) Q85.1

Prinzmetal angina I20.1

Prizefighter ear — *see* Cauliflower ear

Problem (with) (related to)
 academic Z55.8
 acculturation Z60.3
 adjustment (to)
  change of job Z56.1
  life-cycle transition Z60.0
  pension Z60.0
  retirement Z60.0
 adopted child Z63.8
 aged
  in-law Z63.1
  parent Z63.1
  person NEC Z63.8
 alcoholism in family Z63.7
 atypical parenting situation Z60.1
 bankruptcy Z59.8
 behavioral (adult) F69
 birth of sibling affecting child Z61.2
 care (of)
  provider dependency Z74.9
   specified NEC Z74.8
  sick or handicapped person in family or household Z63.6
 career choice Z56.89
 child
  abuse (affecting the child) — *see* Maltreatment, child
  custody or support proceedings Z65.3
 child-rearing Z62.9
  specified NEC Z62.8

Problem — *continued*
 communication (developmental) F80.9
 conflict or discord (with)
  boss Z56.4
  classmates Z55.4
  counselor Z64.4
  employer Z56.4
  family Z63.9
   specified NEC Z63.8
  probation officer Z64.4
  social worker Z64.4
  teachers Z55.4
  workmates Z56.4
 conviction in legal proceedings Z65.0
  with imprisonment Z65.1
 counselor Z64.4
 creditors Z59.8
 digestive K92.9
 ear — *see* Disorder, ear
 economic Z59.9
  affecting care Z59.9
  specified NEC Z59.8
 education Z55.9
  specified NEC Z55.8
 employment Z56.9
  change of job Z56.1
  discord Z56.4
  environment Z56.5
  sexual harassment Z56.81
  specified NEC Z56.89
  stress NEC Z56.6
  stressful schedule Z56.3
  threat of job loss Z56.2
  unemployment Z56.0
 enuresis, child F98.0
 eye H57.9
 failed examinations (school) Z55.2
 family Z63.9
  specified NEC Z63.8
 feeding (elderly) (infant) R63.3
  newborn P92.9
   breast P92.5
   overfeeding P92.4
   slow P92.2
   specified NEC P92.8
   underfeeding P92.3
  nonorganic F50.8
 fetal, affecting management of pregnancy — *see* Pregnancy, complicated by, fetal, problem
 finance Z59.9
  specified NEC Z59.8
 foreclosure on loan Z59.8
 foster child Z63.8
 frightening experience(s) in childhood Z61.7
 genital NEC
  female N94.9
  male N50.9
 health care Z75.9
  specified NEC Z75.89
 hearing — *see* Deafness
 homelessness Z59.0
 housing Z59.9
  inadequate Z59.1
  isolated Z59.8
  specified NEC Z59.8
 identity (of childhood) F93.8
 illegitimate pregnancy (unwanted) Z64.0
 illiteracy Z55.0
 impaired mobility Z74.0
 imprisonment or incarceration Z65.1
 inadequate teaching affecting education Z55.8
 inappropriate parental pressure Z62.6
 influencing health status NEC Z91.8
 in-law Z63.1
 institutionalization, affecting child Z62.2
 intrafamilial communication Z63.8
 jealousy, child F93.8
 landlord Z59.2
 language (developmental) F80.9
 learning (developmental) F81.9
 legal Z65.3
  conviction without imprisonment Z65.0
  imprisonment Z65.1
  release from prison Z65.2
 life-management Z73.9
  specified NEC Z73.8

Problem — *continued*
 life-style Z72.9
  gambling Z72.6
  high-risk sexual behavior (heterosexual) Z72.51
   bisexual Z72.53
   homosexual Z72.52
  inappropriate eating habits Z72.4
  self-damaging behavior NEC Z72.89
  specified NEC Z72.89
  tobacco use Z72.0
 literacy Z55.9
  low level Z55.0
  specified NEC Z55.8
 living alone Z60.2
 lodgers Z59.2
 loss of love relationship in childhood Z61.0
 marital Z63.0
  involving
   divorce Z63.5
   estrangement Z63.5
   gender identity F66
 mastication K08.8
 medical
  care, within family Z63.6
  facilities Z75.9
   specified NEC Z75.89
 mental F48.9
 multiparity Z64.1
 negative life events in childhood Z61.9
  altered pattern of family relationships Z61.2
  frightening experience Z61.7
  loss of
   love relationship Z61.0
   self-esteem Z61.3
  physical abuse (alleged) — *see* Maltreatment, child
  removal from home Z61.1
  sexual abuse Z61.810
  specified event NEC Z61.88
 neighbor Z59.2
 neurological NEC R29.81
 new step-parent affecting child Z61.2
 none (feared complaint unfounded) Z71.1
 occupational NEC Z56.89
 parent Z63.1
 parent-child Z61.9
 personal hygiene Z91.8
 personality F60.81
 phase-of-life transition, adjustment Z60.0
 physical environment Z58.9
  exposure to
   asbestos Z58.82
   lead Z58.81
   noise Z58.0
   pollution Z58.5
    air Z58.1
    soil Z58.3
    water Z58.2
   radiation Z58.4
  occupational Z57.9
   exposure to
    air contaminants Z57.39
     dust Z57.2
     tobacco smoke Z57.31
    industrial toxins Z57.5
     agricultural Z57.4
    noise Z57.0
    radiation Z57.1
    temperature extremes Z57.6
    vibration Z57.7
   specified problem NEC Z57.8
  specified problem NEC Z58.89
 presence of sick or handicapped person in family or household Z63.7
  needing care Z63.6
 primary support group (family) Z63.9
  specified NEC Z63.8
 probation officer Z64.4
 psychiatric F99
 psychosexual (development) F66
 psychosocial Z65.9
  specified NEC Z65.8
 relationship Z63.9
  childhood F93.8
 release from prison Z65.2
 removal from home affecting child Z61.1

Problem — *continued*
  seeking and accepting known hazardous and harmful
    behavioral or psychological interventions Z65.8
    chemical, nutritional or physical interventions Z65.8
  sexual function (nonorganic) F52.9
  sight H54.7
  sleep disorder, child F51.9
  smell — *see* Disturbance, sensation, smell
  social
    environment Z60.9
      specified NEC Z60.8
    exclusion and rejection Z60.4
    worker Z64.4
  speech R47.9
    developmental F80.9
    specified NEC R47.89
  swallowing — *see* Dysphagia
  taste — *see* Disturbance, sensation, taste
  tic, child F95.0
  underachievement in school Z55.3
  unemployment Z56.0
    threatened Z56.2
  unwanted pregnancy Z64.0
  upbringing Z62.9
    specified NEC Z62.8
  urinary N39.9
  voice production R47.89
  work schedule (stressful) Z56.3
Procedure (surgical)
  elective — *see* Surgery, elective
    ear piercing Z41.3
    specified NEC Z41.8
  for purpose other than remedying health state Z41.9
    specified NEC Z41.8
  not done Z53.9
    because of
      administrative reasons Z53.8
      contraindication Z53.09
        smoking Z53.01
      patient's decision Z53.20
        for reasons of belief or group pressure Z53.1
        left AMA Z53.21
        specified reason NEC Z53.29
      specified reason NEC Z53.8
Procidentia (uteri) N81.3
Proctalgia K62.8
  fugax K59.4
  spasmodic K59.4
    psychogenic F45.4
Proctitis K62.8
  amebic (acute) A06.0
  chlamydial A56.3
  gonococcal A54.6
  granulomatous — *see* Enteritis, regional, large intestine
  herpetic A60.1
  radiation K62.7
  tuberculous A18.32
  ulcerative (chronic) K51.25
    with
      complication K51.20
        abscess K51.24
        fistula K51.23
        obstruction K51.22
        rectal bleeding K51.21
        specified complication NEC K51.29
Proctocele
  female (without uterine prolapse) N81.6
    with uterine prolapse N81.2
      complete N81.3
  male K62.3
Proctocolitis, mucosal K51.55
  with
    complication K51.50
      abscess K51.54
      fistula K51.53
      obstruction K51.52
      rectal bleeding K51.51
      specified complication NEC K51.59
Proctoptosis K62.3

Proctorrhagia K62.5
Proctosigmoiditis K63.8
  ulcerative (chronic) — *see* Rectosigmoiditis, ulcerative
Proctospasm K59.4
  psychogenic F45.8
Profichet's disease — *see* Disorder, soft tissue, specified type NEC
Progeria E34.8
Prognathism (mandibular) (maxillary) M26.19
Progonoma (melanotic) (M9363/0) — *see* Neoplasm, benign
Progressive — *see* condition
Prolactinoma (M8271/0)
  specified site — *see* Neoplasm, benign
  unspecified site D35.2
Prolapse, prolapsed
  anus, anal (canal) (sphincter) K62.2
  arm or hand O32.2
    causing obstructed labor O64.4
  bladder (mucosa) (sphincter) (acquired)
    congenital Q79.4
    female N81.1
    male N32.8
  breast implant (prosthetic) T85.49
  cecostomy K94.19
  cecum K63.4
  cervix, cervical (stump) (hypertrophied) N81.2
    anterior lip, obstructing labor O65.5
    congenital Q51.8
    postpartal, old N81.2
  ciliary body (traumatic) — *see* Laceration, eye(ball), with prolapse or loss of interocular tissue
  colon (pedunculated) K63.4
  colostomy K94.09
  disc (intervertebral) — *see* Displacement, intervertebral disc
  eye implant (orbital) T85.398
    lens (ocular) — *see* Complications, intraocular lens
  fallopian tube N83.4
  fetal limb NEC O32.8
  gastric (mucosa) K31.89
  genital, female N81.9
    specified NEC N81.8
  globe, nontraumatic — *see* Luxation, globe
  ileostomy bud K94.19
  intervertebral disc — *see* Displacement, intervertebral disc
  intestine (small) K63.4
  iris (traumatic) — *see* Laceration, eye(ball), with prolapse or loss of interocular tissue
    nontraumatic H21.8
  kidney N28.83
    congenital Q63.2
  laryngeal muscles or ventricle J38.7
  liver K76.8
  meatus urinarius N36.8
  mitral (valve) I34.1
  ocular lens implant — *see* Complications, intraocular lens
  organ or site, congenital NEC — *see* Malposition, congenital
  ovary N83.4
  pelvic floor, female N81.8
  perineum, female N81.8
  rectum (mucosa) (sphincter) K62.3
    due to trichuris trichuria B79
  spleen D73.8
  stomach K31.89
  umbilical cord
    complicating delivery O69.0
  urachus, congenital Q64.4
  ureter N28.89
    with obstruction N13.5
      with infection N13.6
  ureterovesical orifice N28.89
  urethra (acquired) (infected) (mucosa) N36.8
    congenital Q64.71
  urinary meatus N36.8
    congenital Q64.72
  uterovaginal N81.4
    complete N81.3
    incomplete N81.2

Prolapse, prolapsed — *continued*
  uterus (with prolapse of vagina) N81.4
    complete N81.3
    congenital Q51.8
    first degree N81.2
    in pregnancy or childbirth — *see* Pregnancy, complicated by, abnormal, uterus
    incomplete N81.2
    postpartal (old) N81.4
    second degree N81.2
    third degree N81.3
  uveal (traumatic) — *see* Laceration, eye(ball), with prolapse or loss of interocular tissue
  vagina (anterior) (wall) N81.1
    with prolapse of uterus N81.4
      complete N81.3
      incomplete N81.2
    posterior wall N81.6
    posthysterectomy N99.3
  vitreous (humor) H43.00
    bilateral H43.03
    in wound — *see* Laceration, eye(ball), with prolapse or loss of interocular tissue
    left H43.02
    right H43.01
  womb — *see* Prolapse, uterus
Prolapsus, female N81.9
  specified NEC N81.8
Proliferative — *see* condition
Prolonged, prolongation (of)
  bleeding (time) (idiopathic) — *see* Defect, coagulation
  coagulation (time) — *see* Defect, coagulation
  gestation syndrome P08.2
  interval I44.0
  labor O63.9
    first stage O63.0
    second stage O63.1
  pregnancy (more than 42 weeks gestation) O48.1
  prothrombin time — *see* Defect, coagulation
  uterine contractions in labor O62.4
Prominence, prominent
  auricle (congenital) (ear) Q17.5
  ischial spine or sacral promontory
    with disproportion (fetopelvic) O33.0
      causing obstructed labor O65.0
  nose (congenital) acquired M95.0
Promiscuity — *see* High, risk, sexual behavior
Pronation
  ankle — *see* Deformity, limb, foot, specified NEC
  foot — *see also* Deformity, limb, foot, specified NEC
    congenital Q74.2
Prophylactic
  administration of
    antibiotics Z51.89
    antitoxin, any Z51.89
    antivenin Z51.89
    diphtheria antitoxin Z51.89
    gamma globulin Z51.89
    immune sera (gamma globulin) Z51.89
    RhoGAM Z51.89
    tetanus antitoxin Z51.89
  chemotherapy Z51.89
  immunotherapy Z51.89
  measure Z51.89
    specified NEC Z51.89
  organ removal (for neoplasia management) Z40.00
    breast Z40.01
    ovary Z40.02
    specified site NEC Z40.09
  surgery Z40.9
    for risk factors related to malignant neoplasm — *see* Prophylactic, organ removal
    specified NEC Z40.8
Propionic acidemia E71.121
Proptosis (ocular) — *see also* Exophthalmos
  thyroid — *see* Hyperthyroidism, with goiter
Prosecution, anxiety concerning Z65.3
Prostadynia N42.81
Prostate, prostatic — *see* condition

©2002 Ingenix, Inc.

Prostatism — see Hyperplasia, prostate
Prostatitis (congestive) (suppurative) (with
　　　cystitis) N41.9
　　acute N41.00
　　　with hematuria N41.01
　　cavitary N41.8
　　chronic N41.10
　　　with hematuria N41.11
　　diverticular N41.8
　　due to Trichomonas (vaginalis) A59.02
　　fibrous N41.10
　　　with hematuria N41.11
　　gonococcal (acute) (chronic) A54.22
　　granulomatous N41.4
　　hypertrophic N41.10
　　　with hematuria N41.11
　　subacute N41.10
　　　with hematuria N41.11
　　trichomonal A59.02
　　tuberculous A18.14
Prostatocystitis N41.3
Prostatorrhea N42.89
Prostatosis N42.82
Prostration R53.82
　　heat — see also Heat, exhaustion
　　　anhydrotic T67.3
　　　due to
　　　　salt (and water) depletion T67.4
　　　　water depletion T67.3
　　nervous F48.8
　　senile R54
Protanomaly (anomalous trichromat) H53.54
Protanopia (complete) (incomplete) H53.54
Protein
　　deficiency NEC — see Malnutrition
　　malnutrition — see Malnutrition
　　sickness (prophylactic) (therapeutic) T80.6
Proteinemia R77.9
Proteinosis
　　alveolar (pulmonary) J84.0
　　lipid or lipoid (of Urbach) E78.89
Proteinuria R80.9
　　Bence Jones R80.3
　　complicating pregnancy — see Proteinuria,
　　　gestational
　　superimposed on pre-existing hypertensive
　　　disorder — see Hypertension,
　　　complicating, pregnancy, preexisting,
　　　with, proteinuria
　　gestational O12.10
　　　with edema O12.20
　　　　first trimester O12.21
　　　　second trimester O12.22
　　　　third trimester O12.23
　　　first trimester O12.11
　　　second trimester O12.12
　　　superimposed on pre-existing hypertensive
　　　　disorder — see Hypertension,
　　　　complicating, pregnancy, preexisting,
　　　　with, proteinuria
　　　third trimester O12.13
　　idiopathic R80.0
　　isolated R80.0
　　　with glomerular lesion N06.9
　　　　dense deposit disease N06.6
　　　　diffuse
　　　　　crescentic glomerulonephritis N06.7
　　　　　endocapillary proliferative
　　　　　　glomerulonephritis N06.4
　　　　　mesangiocapillary glomerulonephritis
　　　　　　N06.5
　　　　focal and segmental hyalinosis or
　　　　　sclerosis N06.1
　　　　membranous (diffuse) N06.2
　　　　mesangial proliferative (diffuse) N06.3
　　　　minimal change N06.0
　　　　specified pathology NEC N06.8
　　orthostatic R80.2
　　　with glomerular lesion — see Proteinuria,
　　　　isolated, with glomerular lesion
　　persistent R80.1
　　　with glomerular lesion — see Proteinuria,
　　　　isolated, with glomerular lesion

Proteinuria — continued
　　postural R80.2
　　　with glomerular lesion — see Proteinuria,
　　　　isolated, with glomerular lesion
　　pre-eclamptic — see Pre-eclampsia
　　specified type NEC R80.8
Proteolysis, pathologic D65
Proteus (mirabilis) (morganii), as cause of
　　disease classified elsewhere B96.4
Protoporphyria, erythropoietic E80.0
Protozoal — see also condition
　　disease B64
　　　specified NEC B60.8
Protrusion, protrusio
　　acetabuli M24.7
　　acetabulum (into pelvis) M24.7
　　device, implant or graft (see also
　　　Complications, by site and type,
　　　mechanical) T85.628
　　　arterial graft NEC — see Complication,
　　　　cardiovascular device, mechanical,
　　　　vascular
　　　breast (implant) T85.49
　　　catheter NEC T85.628
　　　　cystostomy T83.090
　　　　dialysis (renal) T82.49
　　　　　intraperitoneal T85.691
　　　　infusion NEC T82.594
　　　　　spinal (epidural) (subdural) T85.690
　　　　urinary (indwelling) T83.091
　　　electronic (electrode) (pulse generator)
　　　　(stimulator)
　　　　bone T84.390
　　　　nervous system — see Complication,
　　　　　prosthetic device, mechanical,
　　　　　electronic nervous system
　　　　　stimulator
　　　fixation, internal (orthopedic) NEC — see
　　　　Complication, fixation device,
　　　　mechanical
　　　gastrointestinal — see Complications,
　　　　prosthetic device, mechanical,
　　　　gastrointestinal device
　　　genital NEC T83.498
　　　　intrauterine contraceptive device T83.39
　　　　penile prosthesis T83.490
　　　heart NEC — see Complication,
　　　　cardiovascular device, mechanical
　　　joint prosthesis — see Complication, joint
　　　　prosthesis, mechanical
　　　ocular NEC — see Complications, prosthetic
　　　　device, mechanical, ocular device
　　　orthopedic NEC — see Complication,
　　　　orthopedic, device, mechanical
　　　specified NEC T85.628
　　　urinary NEC — see also Complication,
　　　　genitourinary, device, urinary,
　　　　mechanical
　　　　graft T83.29
　　　vascular NEC — see Complication,
　　　　cardiovascular device, mechanical
　　　ventricular intracranial shunt T85.09
　　intervertebral disc — see Displacement,
　　　intervertebral disc
　　nucleus pulposus — see Displacement,
　　　intervertebral disc
Prune belly (syndrome) Q79.4
Prurigo (ferox) (gravis) (Hebrae) (Hebra's) (mitis)
　　(simplex) L28.2
　　Besnier's L20.0
　　estivalis L56.4
　　nodularis L28.1
　　psychogenic F45.8
Pruritus, pruritic (essential) L29.9
　　ani, anus L29.0
　　　psychogenic F45.8
　　anogenital L29.3
　　　psychogenic F45.8
　　due to onchocerca volvulus B73.1
　　gravidarum — see Pregnancy, complicated by,
　　　specified pregnancy-related condition
　　　NEC
　　hiemalis L29.8
　　neurogenic (any site) F45.8
　　perianal L29.0
　　psychogenic (any site) F45.8

Pruritus, pruritic — continued
　　scroti, scrotum L29.1
　　　psychogenic F45.8
　　senile, senilis L29.8
　　specified NEC L29.8
　　　psychogenic F45.8
　　Trichomonas A59.9
　　vulva, vulvae L29.2
　　　psychogenic F45.8
Pseudarthrosis, pseudoarthrosis (bone) — see
　　Nonunion, fracture
　　clavicle, congenital Q74.0
　　joint, following fusion or arthrodesis M96.0
Pseudoaneurysm — see Aneurysm
Pseudoangioma I81
Pseudoangina (pectoris) — see Angina
Pseudoarteriosus Q28.8
Pseudoarthrosis — see Pseudarthrosis
Pseudochromhidrosis L67.8
Pseudocirrhosis, liver, pericardial I31.1
Pseudocowpox B08.0
Pseudocoxalgia M91.30
　　left M91.32
　　right M91.31
Pseudocroup J38.5
Pseudo-Cushing's syndrome, alcohol-induced
　　E24.4
Pseudocyesis F45.8
Pseudocyst
　　lung J98.4
　　pancreas K86.3
　　retina — see Cyst, retina
Pseudoelephantiasis neuroarthritica Q82.0
Pseudoexfoliation, capsule (lens) — see Cataract,
　　specified NEC
Pseudofolliculitis barbae L73.1
Pseudoglioma H44.89
Pseudohemophilia (Bernuth's) (hereditary) (type
　　B) D68.0
　　Type A D69.8
　　vascular D69.8
Pseudohermaphroditism Q56.3
　　adrenal E25.8
　　female Q56.2
　　　with adrenocortical disorder E25.8
　　　without adrenocortical disorder Q56.2
　　　adrenal, congenital E25.0
　　male Q56.1
　　　with
　　　　adrenocortical disorder E25.8
　　　　androgen resistance E34.5
　　　　cleft scrotum Q56.1
　　　　feminizing testis E34.5
　　　　5-alpha-reductase deficiency E29.1
　　　without gonadal disorder Q56.1
　　　adrenal E25.8
Pseudo-Hurler's polydystrophy E77.0
Pseudohydrocephalus G93.2
Pseudohypertrophic muscular dystrophy (Erb's)
　　G71.0
Pseudohypertrophy, muscle G71.0
Pseudohypoparathyroidism E20.1
Pseudoleukemia, infantile D64.8
Pseudomembranous — see condition
Pseudomenses (newborn) P54.6
Pseudomenstruation (newborn) P54.6
Pseudomeningocele (cerebral) (infective) (spinal)
　　(surgical) G96.1
Pseudomonas
　　aeruginosa, as cause of disease classified
　　　elsewhere B96.5
　　mallei infection A24.0
　　　as cause of disease classified elsewhere
　　　　B96.5
　　pseudomallei, as cause of disease classified
　　　elsewhere B96.5
Pseudomyotonia G71.1
Pseudomyxoma peritonei (M8480/6) C78.6
Pseudoneuritis, optic (nerve) (disc) (papilla),
　　congenital Q14.2

Pseudo-obstruction intestine (chronic) (idiopathic) (intermittent secondary) (primary) K59.8
Pseudopapilledema H47.339
   bilateral H47.333
   congenital Q14.2
   left H47.332
   right H47.331
Pseudoparalysis
   arm or leg R29.81
   atonic, congenital P94.2
Pseudopelade L66.0
Pseudophakia Z96.1
Pseudopolycythemia D75.1
Pseudopolyposis of colon K51.45
   with
      complication K51.40
         abscess K51.44
         fistula K51.43
         obstruction K51.42
         rectal bleeding K51.41
         specified complication NEC K51.49
Pseudopseudohypoparathyroidism E20.1
Pseudopterygium H11.819
   bilateral H11.813
   left H11.812
   right H11.811
Pseudoptosis (eyelid) — see Blepharochalasis
Pseudopuberty, precocious
   female heterosexual E25.8
   male isosexual E25.8
Pseudorickets (renal) N25.0
Pseudorubella B08.2
Pseudoscierema, newborn P83.8
Pseudosclerosis (brain)
   of Westphal (Strümpell) E83.01
   Jakob's A81.0
   spastic A81.0
      with dementia A81.0 [F02]
Pseudotetanus — see Convulsions
Pseudotetany R29.0
   hysterical F44.5
Pseudotruncus arteriosus Q25.4
Pseudotuberculosis A28.2
   enterocolitis A04.8
   pasteurella (infection) A28.0
Pseudotumor
   cerebri G93.2
   orbital — see Inflammation, orbit
Pseudoxanthoma elasticum Q82.8
Psilosis (sprue) (tropical) K90.1
   nontropical K90.0
Psittacosis A70
Psoitis M60.88
Psoriasis L40.9
   arthropathic L40.50
      arthritis mutilans L40.52
      distal interphalangeal L40.51
      juvenile L40.54
      other specified L40.59
      spondylitis L40.53
   buccal K13.2
   flexural L40.8
   guttate L40.4
   mouth K13.2
   nummular L40.0
   plaque L40.0
   psychogenic F54
   pustular (generalized) L40.1
      palmaris et plantaris L40.3
   specified NEC L40.8
   vulgaris L40.0
Psychalgia F45.4
Psychasthenia F48.8
Psychiatric disorder or problem F99
Psychoanalysis (therapy) Z51.89
Psychogenic — see also condition
   factors associated with physical conditions F54
Psychological and behavioral factors affecting medical condition F59

Psychoneurosis, psychoneurotic — see also Neurosis
   anxiety (state) F41.1
   climacteric N95.1
   depersonalization F48.1
   hypochondriacal F45.21
   hysteria F44.9
   neurasthenic F48.8
   personality NEC F60.89
Psychopathy, psychopathic
   affectionless F94.2
   autistic F84.5
   constitution, post-traumatic F07.81
   personality — see Disorder, personality
   sexual — see Deviation, sexual
   state F60.2
Psychosexual identity disorder of childhood F64.2
Psychosis, psychotic F29
   acute (transient) F23
      hysterical F44.9
   affecting management of
      pregnancy — see Pregnancy, complicated by, mental disorders
      puerperium F53
   affective — see Disorder, mood
   alcoholic F10.959
      with
         abuse F10.159
         anxiety disorder F10.980
            with
               abuse F10.180
               dependence F10.280
         delirium tremens F10.231
         delusions F10.950
            with
               abuse F10.150
               dependence F10.250
         dementia F10.97
            with dependence F10.27
         dependence F10.259
         hallucinosis F10.951
            with
               abuse F10.151
               dependence F10.251
         mood disorder F10.94
            with
               abuse F10.14
               dependence F10.24
         paranoia F10.950
            with
               abuse F10.150
               dependence F10.250
         persisting amnesia F10.96
            with dependence F10.26
        amnestic confabulatory F10.96
         with dependence F10.26
        delirium tremens F10.231
        Korsakoff's, Korsakov's, Korsakow's F10.26
        paranoid type F10.950
         with
            abuse F10.150
            dependence F10.250
   anergastic — see Psychosis, organic
   arteriosclerotic (simple type) (uncomplicated) F01.50
      with behavioral disturbance F01.51
   childhood F84.0
      atypical F84.8
   climacteric — see Psychosis, involutional
   confusional F29
      acute or subacute F05
      reactive F23
   cycloid F23
   depressive — see Disorder, depressive
   disintegrative (childhood) F84.3
   drug-induced — see F11-F19 with .959
      paranoid and hallucinatory states — see F11-F19 with .950 or .951
   due to or associated with
      addiction, drug — see F11 F19 with .159
      dependence
         alcohol F10.259
         drug — see F11-F19 with .259
      epilepsy F06.8
      Huntington's chorea F06.8

Psychosis, psychotic — continued
   due to or associated with — continued
      ischemia, cerebrovascular (generalized) F06.8
      multiple sclerosis F06.8
      physical disease F06.8
      presenile dementia F03
      senile dementia F03
      vascular disease (arteriosclerotic) (cerebral) F01.50
         with behavioral disturbance F01.51
   epileptic F06.8
   episode F23
      due to or associated with physical condition F06.8
   exhaustive F43.0
   hallucinatory, chronic F28
   hypomanic F30.8
   hysterical (acute) F44.9
   induced F24
   infantile F84.0
      atypical F84.8
   infective (acute) (subacute) F05
   involutional F28
      depressive — see Disorder, depressive
      melancholic — see Disorder, depressive
      paranoid (state) F22
   Korsakoff's, Korsakov's, Korsakow's (nonalcoholic) F04
      alcoholic F10.96
         in dependence F10.26
      induced by other psychoactive substance — see F11-F19 with .96
   mania, manic (single episode) F30.2
      recurrent type F31.89
   manic-depressive — see Disorder, mood
   menopausal — see Psychosis, involutional
   mixed schizophrenic and affective F25.8
   multi-infarct (cerebrovascular) F01.50
      with behavioral disturbance F01.51
   nonorganic F29
      specified NEC F28
   organic F09
      due to or associated with
         arteriosclerosis (cerebral) — see Psychosis, arteriosclerotic
         cerebrovascular disease, arteriosclerotic — see Psychosis, arteriosclerotic
         childbirth — see Psychosis, puerperal
         Creutzfeldt-Jakob disease or syndrome A81.0 [F02]
         dependence, alcohol F10.259
         disease
            alcoholic liver F10.259
            brain, arteriosclerotic — see Psychosis, arteriosclerotic
            cerebrovascular F01.50
               with behavioral disturbance F01.51
            Creutzfeldt-Jakob A81.0 [F02]
            endocrine or metabolic F06.8
               acute or subacute F05
            liver, alcoholic F10.259
         epilepsy transient (acute) F05
         infection
            brain (intracranial) F06.8
               acute or subacute F05
         intoxication
            alcoholic (acute) F10.259
      drug F11 F19 with .259
         ischemia, cerebrovascular (generalized) — see Psychosis, arteriosclerotic
         puerperium — see Psychosis, puerperal
         trauma, brain (birth) (from electric current) (surgical) F06.8
            acute or subacute F05
      infective F06.8
         acute or subacute F05
      post-traumatic F06.8
         acute or subacute F05
   paranoiac F22
   paranoid (climacteric) (involutional) (menopausal) F22
   psychogenic (acute) F23
   schizophrenic F20.0
   senile F03

Psychosis, psychotic — *continued*
  postpartum F53
  presbyophrenic (type) F03
  presenile F03
  psychogenic (paranoid) F23
    depressive F32.3
  puerperal F53
    specified type — *see* Psychosis, by type
  reactive (brief) (transient) (emotional stress)
      (psychological trauma) F23
    depressive F32.3
      recurrent F33.3
    excitative type F30.8
  schizoaffective F25.9
    depressive type F25.1
    manic type F25.0
  schizophrenia, schizophrenic — *see*
      Schizophrenia
  schizophrenia-like, in epilepsy F06.2
  schizophreniform F20.81
    affective type F25.9
    brief F23
    confusional type F23
    depressive type F25.1
    manic type F25.0
    mixed type F25.8
  senile NEC F03
    depressed or paranoid type F03
    simple deterioration F03
  specified type – code to condition
  shared F24
  situational (reactive) F23
  symbiotic (childhood) F84.3
  symptomatic F09
Psychosomatic — *see* Disorder, psychosomatic
Psychosyndrome, organic F07.9
Psychotherapy Z51.89
Psychotic episode due to or associated with
    physical condition F06.9
Pterygium (eye) H11.009
  amyloid H11.019
    bilateral H11.013
    left H11.012
    right H11.011
  bilateral H11.003
  central H11.029
    bilateral H11.023
    left H11.022
    right H11.021
  colli Q18.3
  double H11.039
    bilateral H11.033
    left H11.032
    right H11.031
  left H11.002
  peripheral
    progressive H11.059
      bilateral H11.053
      left H11.052
      right H11.051
    stationary H11.049
      bilateral H11.043
      left H11.042
      right H11.041
  recurrent H11.069
    bilateral H11.063
    left H11.062
    right H11.061
  right H11.001
Ptilosis (eyelid) — *see* Madarosis
Ptomaine (poisoning) — *see* Poisoning, food
Ptosis — *see also* Blepharoptosis
  adiposa (false) — *see* Blepharoptosis
  cecum K63.4
  colon K63.4
  congenital (eyelid) Q10.0
    specified site NEC — *see* Anomaly, by site
  eyelid — *see* Blepharoptosis
    congenital Q10.0
  gastric K31.89
  intestine K63.4
  kidney N28.83
  liver K76.8
  renal N28.83
  splanchnic K63.4

Ptosis — *see also* Blepharoptosis — *continued*
  spleen D73.8
  stomach K31.89
  viscera K63.4
Ptyalism (periodic) K11.7
  hysterical F45.8
  pregnancy — *see* Pregnancy, complicated by,
      specified pregnancy-related condition
      NEC
  psychogenic F45.8
Ptyalolithiasis K11.5
Pubarche, precocious E30.1
Pubertas praecox E30.1
Puberty (development state) Z00.3
  bleeding (excessive) N92.2
  delayed E30.0
  precocious (constitutional) (cryptogenic)
      (idiopathic) E30.1
    central E22.8
    due to
      ovarian hyperfunction E28.1
        estrogen E28.0
      testicular hyperfunction E29.0
  premature E30.1
    due to
      adrenal cortical hyperfunction E25.8
      pineal tumor E34.8
      pituitary (anterior) hyperfunction E22.8
Puckering, macula — *see* Degeneration, macula,
    puckering
Pudenda, pudendum — *see* condition
Puente's disease (simple glandular cheilitis)
    K13.0
Puerperal, puerperium
  abnormal glucose tolerance test O99.822
  abscess
    areola O91.02
      associated with lactation O91.03
    Bartholin's gland O86.1
    breast O91.12
      associated with lactation O91.13
    cervix (uteri) O86.1
    genital organ O86.1
    kidney O86.21
    mammary O91.12
      associated with lactation O91.13
    nipple O91.02
      associated with lactation O91.03
    peritoneum O85
    subareolar O91.12
      associated with lactation O91.13
    urinary tract — *see* Puerperal, infection,
        urinary
    uterus O86.1
    vagina (wall) O86.1
    vaginorectal O86.1
    vulvovaginal gland O86.1
  adnexitis O86.1
  afibrinogenemia, or other coagulation defect
      O72.3
  albuminuria (acute) (subacute) — *see*
      Proteinuria, gestational
  anemia O99.03
    other blood disorder O99.13
  anesthetic death O89.8
  apoplexy O99.43
  blood dyscrasia O72.3
  cardiomyopathy O90.3
  cerebrovascular disorder (conditions in I60-I69)
      O99.43
  cervicitis O86.1
  coagulopathy (any) O72.3
  complications O90.9
    specified NEC O90.8
  convulsions — *see* Eclampsia
  cystitis O86.22
  cystopyelitis O86.29
  delirium NEC F05
  disease O90.9
    breast NEC O92.22
    cerebrovascular (acute) O99.43
    nonobstetric NEC O99.89
    renal NEC O90.8
    tubo-ovarian O86.1
    Valsuani's O99.03

Puerperal, puerperium — *continued*
  disorder O90.9
    lactation O92.7
    nonobstetric NEC O99.89
  disruption
    cesarean wound O90.0
    episiotomy wound O90.1
    perineal laceration wound O90.1
  eclampsia (with pre-existing hypertension)
      O15.2
  embolism (pulmonary) (blood clot) — *see*
      Embolism, obstetric, puerperal
  endocrine or metabolic disease NEC O99.23
  endophlebitis — *see* Puerperal, phlebitis
  endotrachelitis O86.1
  failure
    lactation (complete) O92.3
      partial O92.4
    renal, acute O90.4
  fever (sepsis) O85
    pyrexia (of unknown origin) O86.4
  fissure, nipple O92.12
    associated with lactation O92.13
  fistula
    breast (due to mastitis) O91.12
      associated with lactation O91.13
    nipple O91.02
      associated with lactation O91.03
  galactophoritis O91.22
    associated with lactation O91.23
  galactorrhea O92.6
  gastrointestinal disease NEC O99.63
  gestational diabetes O24.435
    diet controlled O24.430
    insulin (and diet) controlled O24.434
  glomerular diseases (conditions in N00-N07)
      O90.8
    with hypertension, pre-existing — *see*
        Hypertension, complicating,
        pregnancy, pre-existing, with, renal
        disease
  hematoma, subdural O99.43
  hemiplegia, cerebral O99.43
  hemorrhage O72.1
    brain O99.43
    bulbar O99.43
    cerebellar O99.43
    cerebral O99.43
    cortical O99.43
    delayed or secondary O72.2
    extradural O99.43
    internal capsule O99.43
    intracranial O99.43
    intrapontine O99.43
    meningeal O99.43
    pontine O99.43
    retained placenta O72.0
    subarachnoid O99.43
    subcortical O99.43
    subdural O99.43
    third stage O72.0
    uterine, delayed O72.2
    ventricular O99.43
  hemorrhoids O87.2
  hepatorenal syndrome O90.4
  hypertrophy, breast O92.22
  induration breast (fibrous) O92.22
  infection O86.4
    cervix O86.1
    generalized O85
    genital tract NEC O86.1
      minor or localized NEC O86.1
      obstetric surgical wound O86.0
    kidney (bacillus coli) O86.21
    nipple O91.02
      associated with lactation O91.03
    peritoneum O85
    renal O86.21
    specified NEC O86.8
    urinary (asymptomatic) (tract) NEC O86.20
      bladder O86.22
      kidney O86.21
      specified site NEC O86.29
      urethra O86.22
    vagina O86.1
    vein — *see* Puerperal, phlebitis
  ischemia, cerebral O99.43

Puerperal, puerperium — *continued*
- lymphangitis O86.8
  - breast O91.22
    - associated with lactation O91.23
- malignancy O94.13
- mammillitis O91.02
  - associated with lactation O91.03
- mammitis O91.22
  - associated with lactation O91.23
- mania F30.8
- mastitis O91.22
  - associated with lactation O91.23
  - purulent O91.12
    - associated with lactation O91.13
- melancholia — *see* Disorder, depressive
- metroperitonitis O85
- metrorrhagia — *see* Hemorrhage, postpartum
- metrosalpingitis O86.1
- metrovaginitis O86.1
- milk leg O87.1
- monoplegia, cerebral O99.43
- mood disturbance O90.6
- necrosis, liver (acute) (subacute) (conditions in category K72.0) O26.63
  - with renal failure O90.4
- occlusion, precerebral artery O99.43
- paralysis
  - bladder (sphincter) O90.8
  - cerebral O99.43
- paralytic stroke O99.43
- parametritis O85
- paravaginitis O86.1
- pelviperitonitis O85
- perimetritis O86.1
- perimetrosalpingitis O85
- perinephritis O86.21
- periphlebitis — *see* Puerperal phlebitis
- peritoneal infection O85
- peritonitis (pelvic) O85
- perivaginitis O86.1
- phlebitis O87.9
  - deep O87.1
  - pelvic O87.1
  - superficial O87.0
- phlebothrombosis, deep O87.1
- phlegmasia alba dolens O87.1
- placental polyp O90.8
- pneumonia, embolic — *see* Embolism, obstetric, puerperal
- pre-eclampsia — *see* Pre-eclampsia
- psychosis F53
- pyelitis O86.21
- pyelocystitis O86.29
- pyelonephritis O86.21
- pyelonephrosis O86.21
- pyemia O85
- pyocystitis O86.29
- pyohemia O85
- pyometra O86.1
- pyonephritis O86.21
- pyosalpingitis O86.1
- pyrexia (of unknown origin) O86.4
- renal
  - disease NEC O90.8
  - failure O90.4
- respiratory disease NEC O99.53
- retention
  - decidua — *see* Retention, decidua
  - placenta — *see* Retention, placenta
  - secundines — *see* Retention, secundines
- salpingo-ovaritis O86.1
- salpingoperitonitis O85
- secondary perineal tear O90.1
- sepsis (pelvic) O85
- septicemia O85
- skin disorder NEC O99.74
- specified condition NEC O99.89
- streptococcus B carrier state O99.832
- stroke O99.43
- subinvolution (uterus) O90.8
- suppuration — *see* Puerperal, abscess
- tetanus A34
- thelitis O91.02
  - associated with lactation O91.03
- thrombocytopenia O72.3
- thrombophlebitis (superficial) O87.0
  - deep O87.1
  - pelvic O87.1

Puerperal, puerperium — *continued*
- thrombosis (venous) — *see* Thrombosis, puerperal
- thyroiditis O90.5
- toxemia (eclamptic) (pre-eclamptic) (with convulsions) O15.2
- trauma, non-obstetric O94.23
  - caused by abuse (physical) (suspected) O94.340
    - confirmed O94.341
  - psychological (suspected) O94.540
    - confirmed O94.541
  - sexual (suspected) O94.440
    - confirmed O94.441
- uremia (due to renal failure) O90.4
- urethritis O86.22
- vaginitis O86.1
- varicose veins (legs) O87.4
  - vulva or perineum O87.8
- vulvitis O86.1
- vulvovaginitis O86.1
- white leg O87.1

Pulmolithiasis J98.4
Pulmonary — *see* condition
Pulpitis (acute) (anachoretic) (chronic) (hyperplastic) (putrescent) (suppurative) (ulcerative) K04.0
Pulpless tooth K04.99
Pulse
- alternating R00.8
- bigeminal R00.8
- fast R00.0
- feeble, rapid due to shock following injury T79.4
- rapid R00.0
- weak R09.89

Pulsus alternans or trigeminus R00.8
Punch drunk F07.81
Punctum lacrimale occlusion — *see* Obstruction, lacrimal
Puncture
- abdomen, abdominal S31.93
  - with foreign body S31.94
  - wall S31.139
    - with
      - foreign body S31.149
      - penetration into peritoneal cavity S31.639
        - with foreign body S31.649
    - epigastric region S31.132
      - with
        - foreign body S31.142
        - penetration into peritoneal cavity S31.632
          - with foreign body S31.642
    - left
      - lower quadrant S31.134
        - with
          - foreign body S31.144
          - penetration into peritoneal cavity S31.634
            - with foreign body S31.644
      - upper quadrant S31.131
        - with
          - foreign body S31.141
          - penetration into peritoneal cavity S31.631
            - with foreign body S31.641
    - periumbilic region S31.135
      - with
        - foreign body S31.145
        - penetration into peritoneal cavity S31.635
          - with foreign body S31.645
    - right
      - lower quadrant S31.133
        - with
          - foreign body S31.143
          - penetration into peritoneal cavity S31.633
            - with foreign body S31.643

Puncture — *continued*
- abdomen, abdominal — *continued*
  - wall — *continued*
    - right — *continued*
      - upper quadrant S31.130
        - with
          - foreign body S31.140
          - penetration into peritoneal cavity S31.630
            - with foreign body S31.640
- accidental, complicating surgery — *see* Complication, surgical, accidental puncture or laceration
- alveolar (process) — *see* Puncture, oral cavity
- ankle S91.039
  - with
    - foreign body S91.049
    - fracture S91.069
  - left S91.032
    - with
      - foreign body S91.042
      - fracture S91.062
  - right S91.031
    - with
      - foreign body S91.041
      - fracture S91.061
- anus S31.833
  - with foreign body S31.834
- arm (upper) S41.139
  - with foreign body S41.149
  - left S41.132
    - with foreign body S41.142
  - lower — *see* Puncture, forearm
  - right S41.131
    - with foreign body S41.141
- auditory canal (external) (meatus) — *see* Puncture, ear
- auricle, ear — *see* Puncture, ear
- axilla — *see* Puncture, arm
- back — *see also* Puncture, thorax, back
  - lower S31.030
    - with
      - foreign body S31.040
        - with penetration into retroperitoneal space S31.041
      - penetration into retroperitoneal space S31.031
- bladder (traumatic) S37.28
  - nontraumatic N32.8
- breast S21.039
  - with foreign body S21.049
  - left S21.032
    - with foreign body S21.042
  - right S21.031
    - with foreign body S21.041
- buttock S31.803
  - with foreign body S31.804
  - left S31.823
    - with foreign body S31.824
  - right S31.813
    - with foreign body S31.814
- by
  - device, implant or graft — *see* Complications, by site and type, mechanical
  - foreign body left accidentally in operative wound T81.539
  - instrument (any) during a procedure, accidental — *see* Puncture, accidental complicating surgery
- calf — *see* Puncture, leg
- canaliculus lacrimalis — *see* Puncture, eyelid
- canthus, eye — *see* Puncture, eyelid
- cervical esophagus S11.23
  - with foreign body S11.24
- cheek (external) S01.439
  - with foreign body S01.449
  - left S01.432
    - with foreign body S01.442
  - right S01.431
    - with foreign body S01.441
  - internal — *see* Puncture, oral cavity
- chest wall — *see* Puncture, thorax
- chin — *see* Puncture, head, specified site NEC
- clitoris — *see* Puncture, vulva
- costal region — *see* Puncture, thorax

©2002 Ingenix, Inc.

Puncture — continued
- digit(s)
  - hand — see Puncture, finger
  - foot — see Puncture, toe
- ear (canal) (external) S01.339
  - with foreign body S01.349
  - left S01.332
    - with foreign body S01.342
  - right S01.331
    - with foreign body S01.341
  - drum S09.20
    - left S09.22
    - right S09.21
- elbow S51.039
  - with
    - foreign body S51.049
    - fracture S51.069
  - left S51.032
    - with
      - foreign body S51.042
      - fracture S51.062
  - right S51.031
    - with
      - foreign body S51.041
      - fracture S51.061
- epididymis — see Puncture, testis
- epigastric region — see Puncture, abdomen, wall, epigastric
- epiglottis S11.83
  - with foreign body S11.84
- esophagus
  - cervical S11.23
    - with foreign body S11.24
  - thoracic S27.818
- eyeball S05.60
  - with foreign body S05.50
    - left S05.52
    - right S05.51
  - left S05.62
  - right S05.61
- eyebrow — see Puncture, eyelid
- eyelid S01.139
  - with foreign body S01.149
  - left S01.132
    - with foreign body S01.142
  - right S01.131
    - with foreign body S01.141
- face NEC — see Puncture, head, specified site NEC
- finger(s) S61.239
  - with
    - damage to nail S61.339
      - with
        - foreign body S61.349
        - fracture S61.369
    - foreign body S61.249
    - fracture S61.269
  - index S61.238
    - with
      - damage to nail S61.338
        - with
          - foreign body S61.348
          - fracture S61.368
      - foreign body S61.248
      - fracture S61.268
    - left S61.231
      - with
        - damage to nail S61.331
          - with
            - foreign body S61.341
            - fracture S61.361
        - foreign body S61.241
        - fracture S61.261
    - right S61.230
      - with
        - damage to nail S61.330
          - with
            - foreign body S61.340
            - fracture S61.360
        - foreign body S61.240
        - fracture S61.260

Puncture — continued
- finger(s) — continued
  - little S61.238
    - with
      - damage to nail S61.338
        - with
          - foreign body S61.348
          - fracture S61.368
      - foreign body S61.248
      - fracture S61.268
    - left S61.237
      - with
        - damage to nail S61.337
          - with
            - foreign body S61.347
            - fracture S61.367
        - foreign body S61.247
        - fracture S61.267
    - right S61.236
      - with
        - damage to nail S61.336
          - with
            - foreign body S61.346
            - fracture S61.366
        - foreign body S61.246
        - fracture S61.266
  - middle S61.238
    - with
      - damage to nail S61.338
        - with
          - foreign body S61.348
          - fracture S61.368
      - foreign body S61.248
      - fracture S61.268
    - left S61.233
      - with
        - damage to nail S61.333
          - with
            - foreign body S61.343
            - fracture S61.363
        - foreign body S61.243
        - fracture S61.263
    - right S61.232
      - with
        - damage to nail S61.332
          - with
            - foreign body S61.342
            - fracture S61.362
        - foreign body S61.242
        - fracture S61.262
  - ring S61.238
    - with
      - damage to nail S61.338
        - with
          - foreign body S61.348
          - fracture S61.368
      - foreign body S61.248
      - fracture S61.268
    - left S61.235
      - with
        - damage to nail S61.335
          - with
            - foreign body S61.345
            - fracture S61.365
        - foreign body S61.245
        - fracture S61.265
    - right S61.234
      - with
        - damage to nail S61.334
          - with
            - foreign body S61.344
            - fracture S61.364
        - foreign body S61.244
        - fracture S61.264
- flank S31.139
  - with foreign body S31.149
- foot (except toe(s) alone) S91.339
  - with foreign body S91.349
  - left S91.332
    - with foreign body S91.342
  - right S91.331
    - with foreign body S91.341
  - toe — see Puncture, toe

Puncture — continued
- forearm S51.839
  - with
    - foreign body S51.849
    - fracture of radius or ulna S51.869
  - elbow only — see Puncture, elbow
  - left S51.832
    - with
      - foreign body S51.842
      - fracture of radius or ulna S51.862
  - right S51.831
    - with
      - foreign body S51.841
      - fracture of radius or ulna S51.861
- forehead — see Puncture, head, specified site NEC
- genital organs, external
  - female S31.532
    - with foreign body S31.542
    - vagina — see Puncture, vagina
    - vulva — see Puncture, vulva
  - male S31.531
    - with foreign body S31.541
    - penis — see Puncture, penis
    - scrotum — see Puncture, scrotum
    - testis — see Puncture, testis
- groin — see Puncture, abdomen, wall
- gum — see Puncture, oral cavity
- hand S61.439
  - with
    - foreign body S61.449
    - fracture S61.469
  - finger — see Puncture, finger
  - left S61.432
    - with
      - foreign body S61.442
      - fracture S61.462
  - right S61.431
    - with
      - foreign body S61.441
      - fracture S61.461
  - thumb — see Puncture, thumb
- head S01.93
  - with foreign body S01.94
  - cheek — see Puncture, cheek
  - ear — see Puncture, ear
  - eyelid — see Puncture, eyelid
  - lip — see Puncture, oral cavity
  - nose — see Puncture, nose
  - oral cavity — see Puncture, oral cavity
  - scalp S01.03
    - with foreign body S01.04
  - specified site NEC S01.83
    - with foreign body S01.84
  - temporomandibular area — see Puncture, cheek
- heart S26.99
  - with hemopericardium S26.09
  - without hemopericardium S26.19
- heel — see Puncture, foot
- hip S71.039
  - with foreign body S71.049
  - left S71.032
    - with foreign body S71.042
  - right S71.031
    - with foreign body S71.041
- hymen — see Puncture, vagina
- hypochondrium — see Puncture, abdomen, wall
- hypogastric region — see Puncture, abdomen, wall
- inguinal region — see Puncture, abdomen, wall
- instep — see Puncture, foot
- internal organs — see Injury, by site
- interscapular region — see Puncture, thorax, back
- intestine
  - large
    - colon S36.599
      - ascending S36.590
      - descending S36.592
      - sigmoid S36.593
      - specified site NEC S36.598
      - transverse S36.591
    - rectum S36.69

Puncture — *continued*
  intestine — *continued*
    small S36.499
      duodenum S36.490
      specified site NEC S36.498
  intra-abdominal organ S36.99
    gallbladder S36.128
    intestine — *see* Puncture, intestine
    liver S36.118
    pancreas — *see* Puncture, pancreas
    peritoneum S36.81
    specified site NEC S36.898
    spleen S36.09
    stomach S36.39
  jaw — *see* Puncture, head, specified site NEC
  knee S81.039
    with foreign body S81.049
    left S81.032
      with foreign body S81.042
    right S81.031
      with foreign body S81.041
  labium (majus) (minus) — *see* Puncture, vulva
  lacrimal duct — *see* Puncture, eyelid
  larynx S11.013
    with foreign body S11.014
  leg (lower) S81.839
    with foreign body S81.849
    foot — *see* Puncture, foot
    knee — *see* Puncture, knee
    left S81.832
      with foreign body S81.842
    right S81.831
      with foreign body S81.841
    upper — *see* Puncture, thigh
  lip S01.531
    with foreign body S01.541
  loin — *see* Puncture, abdomen, wall
  lower back — *see* Puncture, back, lower
  lumbar region — *see* Puncture, back, lower
  malar region — *see* Puncture, head, specified site NEC
  mammary — *see* Puncture, breast
  mastoid region — *see* Puncture, head, specified site NEC
  mouth — *see* Puncture, oral cavity
  nail
    finger — *see* Puncture, finger, with damage to nail
    toe — *see* Puncture, toe, with damage to nail
  nasal (septum) (sinus) — *see* Puncture, nose
  nasopharynx — *see* Puncture, head, specified site NEC
  neck S11.93
    with foreign body S11.94
    involving
      cervical esophagus — *see* Puncture, cervical esophagus
      larynx — *see* Puncture, larynx
      pharynx — *see* Puncture, pharynx
      thyroid gland — *see* Puncture, thyroid gland
      trachea — *see* Puncture, trachea
    specified site NEC S11.83
      with foreign body S11.84
  nose (septum) (sinus) S01.23
    with foreign body S01.24
  ocular — *see* Puncture, eyeball
  oral cavity S01.532
    with foreign body S01.542
  orbit S05.40
    left S05.42
    right S05.41
  palate — *see* Puncture, oral cavity
  palm — *see* Puncture, hand
  pancreas S36.299
    body S36.291
    head S36.290
    tail S36.292
  pelvis — *see* Puncture, back, lower
  penis S31.23
    with foreign body S31.24
  perineum
    female S31.43
      with foreign body S31.44
    male S31.139
      with foreign body S31.149

Puncture — *continued*
  periocular area (with or without lacrimal passages) — *see* Puncture, eyelid
  phalanges
    finger — *see* Puncture, finger
    toe — *see* Puncture, toe
  pharynx S11.23
    with foreign body S11.24
  pinna — *see* Puncture, ear
  popliteal space — *see* Puncture, knee
  prepuce — *see* Puncture, penis
  pubic region S31.139
    with foreign body S31.149
  pudendum — *see* Puncture, genital organs, external
  rectovaginal septum — *see* Puncture, vagina
  sacral region — *see* Puncture, back, lower
  sacroiliac region — *see* Puncture, back, lower
  salivary gland — *see* Puncture, oral cavity
  scalp S01.03
    with foreign body S01.04
  scapular region — *see* Puncture, shoulder
  scrotum S31.33
    with foreign body S31.34
  shin — *see* Puncture, leg
  shoulder S41.039
    with foreign body S41.049
    left S41.032
      with foreign body S41.042
    right S41.031
      with foreign body S41.041
  spermatic cord — *see* Puncture, testis
  sternal region — *see* Puncture, thorax, front
  submaxillary region — *see* Puncture, head, specified site NEC
  submental region — *see* Puncture, head, specified site NEC
  subungual
    finger(s) — *see* Puncture, finger, with damage to nail
    toe — *see* Puncture, toe, with damage to nail
  supraclavicular fossa — *see* Puncture, neck, specified site NEC
  temple, temporal region — *see* Puncture, head, specified site NEC
  temporomandibular area — *see* Puncture, cheek
  testis S31.33
    with foreign body S31.34
  thigh S71.139
    with foreign body S71.149
    left S71.132
      with foreign body S71.142
    right S71.131
      with foreign body S71.141
  thorax, thoracic (wall) S21.93
    with foreign body S21.94
    back S21.239
      with foreign body S21.249
      left S21.232
        with foreign body S21.242
      right S21.231
        with foreign body S21.241
    breast — *see* Puncture, breast
    front S21.139
      with foreign body S21.149
      left S21.132
        with foreign body S21.142
      right S21.131
        with foreign body S21.141
  throat — *see* Puncture, neck
  thumb S61.039
    with
      damage to nail S61.139
        with
          foreign body S61.149
          fracture S61.169
      foreign body S61.049
      fracture S61.069
    left S61.032
      with
        damage to nail S61.132
          with
            foreign body S61.142
            fracture S61.162
        foreign body S61.042
        fracture S61.062

Puncture — *continued*
  thumb — *continued*
    right S61.031
      with
        damage to nail S61.131
          with
            foreign body S61.141
            fracture S61.161
        foreign body S61.041
        fracture S61.061
  thyroid gland S11.13
    with foreign body S11.14
  toe(s) S91.139
    with
      damage to nail S91.239
        with
          foreign body S91.249
          fracture S91.269
      foreign body S91.149
      fracture S91.169
    great S91.133
      with
        damage to nail S91.233
          with
            foreign body S91.243
            fracture S91.263
        foreign body S91.143
        fracture S91.163
      left S91.132
        with
          damage to nail S91.232
            with
              foreign body S91.242
              fracture S91.262
          foreign body S91.142
          fracture S91.162
      right S91.131
        with
          damage to nail S91.231
            with
              foreign body S91.241
              fracture S91.261
          foreign body S91.141
          fracture S91.161
    lesser S91.136
      with
        damage to nail S91.236
          with
            foreign body S91.246
            fracture S91.266
        foreign body S91.146
        fracture S91.166
      left S91.135
        with
          damage to nail S91.235
            with
              foreign body S91.245
              fracture S91.265
          foreign body S91.145
          fracture S91.165
      right S91.134
        with
          damage to nail S91.234
            with
              foreign body S91.244
              fracture S91.264
          foreign body S91.144
          fracture S91.164
  tongue — *see* Puncture, oral cavity
  trachea S11.023
    with foreign body S11.024
  tunica vaginalis — *see* Puncture, testis
  tympanum, tympanic membrane S09.20
    left S09.22
    right S09.21
  umbilical region S31.135
    with foreign body S31.145
  uvula — *see* Puncture, oral cavity
  vagina S31.43
    with foreign body S31.44
  vocal cords S11.83
    with foreign body S11.84
  vulva S31.43
    with foreign body S31.44

©2002 Ingenix, Inc.

Puncture — *continued*
  wrist S61.539
    with
      foreign body S61.549
      fracture S61.569
    left S61.532
      with
        foreign body S61.542
        fracture S61.562
    right S61.531
      with
        foreign body S61.541
        fracture S61.561
PUO (pyrexia of unknown origin) R50.9
Pupillary membrane (persistent) Q13.89
Pupillotonia — *see* Anomaly, pupil, function, tonic pupil
Purpura D69.2
  abdominal D69.0
  allergic D69.0
  anaphylactoid D69.0
  annularis telangiectodes L81.7
  arthritic D69.0
  autoerythrocyte sensitization D69.2
  autoimmune D69.0
  bacterial D69.0
  Bateman's (senile) D69.2
  capillary fragility (hereditary) (idiopathic)D69.8
  cryoglobulinemic D89.1
  Devil's pinches D69.2
  fibrinolytic — *see* Fibrinolysis
  fulminans, fulminous D65
  gangrenous D65
  hemorrhagic, hemorrhagica D69.3
    not due to thrombocytopenia D69.0
  Henoch(-Schönlein) (allergic) D69.0
  hypergammaglobulinemic (benign)
    (Waldenström's) D89.0
  idiopathic (thrombocytopenic) D69.3
    nonthrombocytopenic D69.0
  infectious D69.0
  malignant D69.0
  neonatorum P54.5
  nervosa D69.0
  newborn P54.5
  nonthrombocytopenic D69.2
    hemorrhagic D69.0
    idiopathic D69.0
  nonthrombopenic D69.2
  peliosis rheumatica D69.0
  post-transfusion D69.5
  primary D69.0
  primitive D69.0
  red cell membrane sensitivity D69.2
  rheumatica D69.0
  Schönlein(-Henoch) (allergic) D69.0
  scorbutic E54 [D77]
  senile D69.2
  simplex D69.2
  symptomatica D69.0
  telangiectasia annularis L81.7
  thrombocytopenic (congenital) (hereditary)
    D69.4
    idiopathic D69.3
    neonatal, transitory P61.0
    thrombotic M31.1
  thrombohemolytic — *see* Fibrinolysis
  thrombolytic — *see* Fibrinolysis
  thrombopenic (congenital) (hereditary) D69.4
  thrombotic, thrombocytopenic M31.1
  toxic D69.0
  vascular D69.0
  visceral symptoms D69.0
Purpuric spots R23.3
Purulent — *see* condition
Pus
  in
    stool R19.5
    urine N39.0
  tube (rupture) — *see* Salpingo-oophoritis
Pustular rash L08.0
Pustule (nonmalignant) L08.9
  malignant A22.0
Pustulosis palmaris et plantaris L40.3

Putnam (-Dana) disease or syndrome — *see* Degeneration, combined
Putrescent pulp (dental) K04.1
Pyarthritis, pyarthrosis — *see* Arthritis, pyogenic or pyemic
  tuberculous — *see* Tuberculosis, joint
Pyelectasis — *see* Hydronephrosis
Pyelitis (congenital) (uremic) — *see also* Pyelonephritis)
  with
    calculus N20.9
      with hydronephrosis N13.2
    contracted kidney N11.9
  acute N10
  chronic N11.9
    with calculus N20.9
      with hydronephrosis N13.2
  complicating pregnancy — *see* Infection, kidney, complicating pregnancy
  cystica N28.84
  puerperal (postpartum) O86.21
  tuberculous A18.11
Pyelocystitis — *see* Pyelonephritis
Pyelonephritis — *see also* Nephritis, tubulo-interstitial
  with
    calculus N20.9
      with hydronephrosis N13.2
    contracted kidney N11.9
  acute N10
  calculous N20.9
    with hydronephrosis N13.2
  chronic N11.9
    with calculus N20.9
      with hydronephrosis N13.2
    associated with ureteral obstruction or stricture N11.1
    nonobstructive N11.8
      with reflux (vesicoureteral) N11.0
    obstructive N11.1
    specified NEC N11.8
  complicating pregnancy — *see* Infection, kidney, complicating pregnancy
  in (due to)
    brucellosis A23.9 [N16]
    cryoglobulinemia (mixed) D89.1 [N16]
    cystinosis E72.04
    diphtheria A36.84
    glycogen storage disease E74.09 [N16]
    leukemia NEC (M9800/3) C95.90 [N16]
    lymphoma NEC (M9590/3) C85.90 [N16]
    multiple myeloma (M9732/3) C90.00 [N16]
    obstruction N11.1
    Salmonella infection A02.25
    sarcoidosis D86.84
    septicemia A41.9 [N16]
    Sjögren's disease M35.04
    toxoplasmosis B58.83
    transplant rejection T86.91 [N16]
    Wilson's disease E83.01 [N16]
  nonobstructive N12
    with reflux (vesicoureteral) N11.0
    chronic N11.8
  syphilitic A52.75
Pyelonephrosis (obstructive) N11.1
  chronic N11.9
Pyelophlebitis I80.8
Pyeloureteritis cystica N28.85
Pyemia, pyemic (fever) (infection) (purulent) — *see also* Septicemia
  joint — *see* Arthritis, pyogenic or pyemic
  liver K75.1
  pneumococcal A40.3
  portal K75.1
  postvaccinal T88.0
  specified organism NEC A41.89
  tuberculous — *see* Tuberculosis, miliary
Pygopagus Q89.4
Pyknoepilepsy, pyknolepsy (idiopathic) G40.30
  with status epilepticus G40.31
Pylephlebitis K75.1
Pyle's syndrome Q78.5
Pylethrombophlebitis K75.1
Pylethrombosis K75.1

Pyloritis K29.90
  with bleeding K29.91
Pylorospasm (reflex) **NEC** K31.3
  congenital or infantile Q40.0
  newborn Q40.0
  neurotic F45.8
  psychogenic F45.8
Pylorus, pyloric — *see* condition
Pyoarthrosis — *see* Arthritis, pyogenic or pyemic
Pyocele
  mastoid — *see* Mastoiditis, acute
  sinus (accessory) — *see* Sinusitis
  turbinate (bone) J32.9
  urethra (*see also* Urethritis) N34.0
Pyocolpos — *see* Vaginitis
Pyocystitis N30.80
  with hematuria N30.81
Pyoderma, pyodermia L08.0
  gangrenosum L88
  newborn P39.4
  phagedenic L88
  vegetans L08.81
Pyodermatitis L08.0
  vegetans L08.81
Pyogenic — *see* condition
Pyohydronephrosis N13.6
Pyometra, pyometrium, pyometritis — *see* Endometritis
Pyomyositis (tropical) — *see* Myositis, infective
Pyonephritis N12
Pyonephrosis N13.6
  tuberculous A18.11
Pyo-oophoritis — *see* Salpingo-oophoritis
Pyo-ovarium — *see* Salpingo-oophoritis
Pyopericarditis, pyopericardium I30.1
Pyophlebitis — *see* Phlebitis
Pyopneumopericardium I30.1
Pyopneumothorax (infective) J86.9
  with fistula J86.0
  tuberculous NEC A15.6
Pyorrhea (alveolar) (alveolaris) K05.3
  degenerative K05.4
Pyosalpinx, pyosalpingitis — *see also* Salpingo-oophoritis
Pyosepticemia — *see* Septicemia
Pyothorax J86.9
  with fistula J86.0
  tuberculous NEC A15.8
Pyoureter N28.89
  tuberculous A18.11
Pyramidopallidonigral syndrome G20
Pyrexia (of unknown origin) R50.9
  atmospheric T67.0
  during labor NEC O75.2
  heat T67.0
  newborn, environmentally-induced P81.0
  persistent R50.8
  puerperal O86.4
Pyroglobulinemia NEC E88.09
Pyromania F63.1
Pyrosis R12
Pyuria (bacterial) N39.0

Q

Q fever A78
  with pneumonia A78
Quadricuspid aortic valve Q23.8
Quadrilateral fever A78
Quadriplegia — *see also* Tetraplegia
  functional R53.2
Quadruplet, pregnancy — *see* Pregnancy, quadruplet
Quarrelsomeness F60.3
Queensland fever A77.3
Quervain's disease M65.4
  thyroid E06.1

Queyrat's erythroplasia (M8080/2)
  penis D07.4
  specified site — *see* Neoplasm, skin, in situ
  unspecified site D07.4
Quincke's disease or edema T78.3
  hereditary D84.1
Quinsy (gangrenous) J36
Quintan fever A79.0
Quintuplet, pregnancy — *see* Pregnancy, quintuplet

R

Rabbit fever — *see* Tularemia
Rabies A82.9
  contact Z20.3
  exposure to Z20.3
  inoculation reaction — *see* Complications, vaccination
  sylvatic A82.0
  urban A82.1
  vaccination, prophylactic (against) Z23
Rachischisis — *see* Spina bifida
Rachitic — *see also* condition
  deformities of spine (late effect) (*see also* category M49.8) E64.3
  pelvis (late effect) E64.3
    with disproportion (fetopelvic) O33.0
     causing obstructed labor O65.0
Rachitis, rachitism (acute) (tarda) — *see also* Rickets
  renalis N25.0
  sequelae E64.3
Radial nerve — *see* condition
Radiation
  burn — *see* Burn
  effects NOS T66
  exposure Z58.4
    occupational Z57.1
  sickness NOS T66
Radiculitis (pressure) (vertebrogenic) — *see* Radiculopathy
Radiculomyelitis — *see also* Encephalitis
  toxic, due to
    Clostridium tetani A35
    Corynebacterium diphtheriae A36.82
Radiculopathy M54.10
  cervical region M54.12
  cervicothoracic region M54.13
  due to displacement of intervertebral disc *see* Disorder, disc, with, radiculopathy
  lumbar region M54.16
  lumbosacral region M54.17
  occipito-atlanto-axial region M54.11
  postherpetic B02.29
  sacrococcygeal region M54.18
  syphilitic A52.11
  thoracic region (with visceral pain) M54.14
  thoracolumbar region M54.15
Radioactive substances, adverse effect T66
Radiodermal burns (acute, chronic, or occupational) — *see* Burn
Radiodermatitis L58.9
  acute L58.0
  chronic L58.1
Radionecrosis T66
Radiotherapy session Z51.0
Radium, adverse effect T66
Rage, meaning rabies — *see* Rabies
Rag sorters' disease A22.1
Raillietiniasis B71.8
Railroad neurosis F48.8
Railway spine F48.8
Raised — *see also* Elevated
  antibody titer R76.0
Rake teeth, tooth M26.3
Rales R09.89
Ramifying renal pelvis Q63.8
Ramsay-Hunt disease or syndrome — *see also* Hunt's disease B02.21
  meaning dyssynergia cerebellaris myoclonica G11.1

Ranula K11.6
  congenital Q38.6
Rape
  adult T76.21
  alleged, observation or examination
    adult Z04.71
    child Z04.72
  child T76.22
  confirmed
    adult T74.21
    child T74.22
Rapid
  feeble pulse, due to shock, following injury T79.4
  heart (beat) R00.0
    psychogenic F45.8
  second stage (delivery) O62.3
  time-zone change syndrome — *see* Disorder, sleep, circadian rhythm, psychogenic
Rarefaction, bone — *see* Disorder, bone, density and structure, specified NEC
Rash (toxic) R21
  canker A38.9
  diaper L22
  drug (internal use) L27.0
    contact — *see also* Dermatitis, due to, drugs, external L25.1
  following immunization T88.1
  food — *see* Dermatitis, due to, food
  heat L74.0
  napkin (psoriasiform) L22
  nettle — *see* Urticaria
  pustular L08.0
  rose R21
    epidemic B06.9
  scarlet A38.9
  serum (prophylactic) (therapeutic) T80.6
  wandering tongue K14.1
Rasmussen's aneurysm — *see* Tuberculosis, pulmonary
Rat-bite fever A25.9
  due to Streptobacillus moniliformis A25.1
  spirochetal (morsus muris) A25.0
Rathke's pouch tumor (M9350/1) D44.3
Raymond (-Cestan) syndrome I65.8
Raynaud's disease, phenomenon or syndrome (secondary) I73.00
  with gangrene (symmetric) I73.01
RDS (newborn) (type I) P22.0
  type II P22.1
Reaction — *see also* Disorder
  adaptation — *see* Disorder, adjustment
  adjustment (anxiety) (conduct disorder) (depressiveness) (distress) — *see* Disorder, adjustment
    with
      mutism, elective (child) (adolescent) F94.0
  affective — *see* Disorder, mood
  allergic — *see* Allergy
  anaphylactic — *see* Shock, anaphylactic
  anesthesia — *see* Anesthesia, complication
  antitoxin (prophylactic) (therapeutic) — *see* Complications, vaccination
  anxiety F41.1
  Arthus — *see* Arthus' phenomenon
  asthenic F48.8
  compulsive F42
  conversion F44.9
  crisis, acute F43.0
  deoxyribonuclease (DNA) (DNase) hypersensitivity D69.2
  depressive (single episode) F32.9
    affective (single episode) F31.4
      recurrent episode F33.9
    neurotic F34.1
    psychoneurotic F34.1
    psychotic F32.3
    recurrent — *see* Disorder, depressive, recurrent
  dissociative F44.9
  drug NEC T88.7
    addictive — *see* Dependence, drug
      transmitted via placenta or breast milk — *see* Absorption, drug, addictive, through placenta

Reaction — *see also* Disorder — *continued*
  drug NEC — *continued*
    allergic — *see* Allergy, drug
    correct substance properly administered T88.7
    lichenoid L43.2
    newborn P93.8
      gray baby syndrome P93.0
    obstetric anesthetic or analgesic O74.9
      affecting fetus or newborn P93.8
        gray baby syndrome P93.0
    overdose or poisoning (by accident) T50.901
      administered with intent to harm by another person T50.903
      self T50.902
      circumstances undetermined T50.904
      specified drug — *see* Table of Drugs and Chemicals
    photoallergic L56.1
    phototoxic L56.0
    withdrawal — *see* Dependence, by drug, with, withdrawal
      infant of dependent mother P96.1
      newborn P96.1
    wrong substance given or taken (by accident) T50.901
      administered with intent to harm by another person T50.903
      self T50.902
      circumstances undetermined T50.904
      specified drug — *see* Table of Drugs and Chemicals
  fear F40.9
    child (abnormal) F93.8
  fluid loss, cerebrospinal G97.1
  foreign
    body NEC — *see* Granuloma, foreign body
      in operative wound (inadvertently left) — *see* Foreign body, accidentally left following a procedure
    substance accidentally left during a procedure (chemical) (powder) (talc) T81.60
      aseptic peritonitis T81.61
      body or object (instrument) (sponge) (swab) — *see* Foreign body, accidentally left following a procedure
      specified reaction NEC T81.69
  grief — *see* Disorder, adjustment
  Herxheimer's T78.2
  hyperkinetic — *see* Hyperkinesia
  hypochondriacal F45.20
  hypoglycemic, due to insulin E16.0
    with coma (diabetic) — *see* Diabetes, coma
      nondiabetic E15
    therapeutic misadventure — *see* category T38.3
  hypomanic F30.8
  hysterical F44.9
  immunization — *see* Complications, vaccination
  incompatibility
    blood group (ABO) (infusion) (transfusion) T80.3
    Rh (factor) (infusion) (transfusion) T80.4
  inflammatory — *see* Infection
  infusion — *see* Complications, infusion
  inoculation (immune serum) — *see* Complications, vaccination
  insulin T78.4
  involutional psychotic — *see* Disorder, depressive
  leukemoid (lymphocytic) (monocytic) (myelocytic) D72.8
  LSD (acute) — *see* Disorder, drug-related, hallucinogen
  lumbar puncture G97.1
  manic-depressive — *see* Disorder, bipolar
  neurasthenic F48.8
  neurogenic — *see* Neurosis
  neurotic F48.9
  neurotic-depressive F34.1
  nitritoid — *see* Crisis, nitritoid
  obsessive-compulsive F42
  organic, acute or subacute *see* Delirium

©2002 Ingenix, Inc.

Reaction — *see also* Disorder — *continued*
  paranoid (acute) F23
    chronic F22
    senile F03
  passive dependency F60.7
  phobic F40.9
  postradiation T66
  post-traumatic stress, uncomplicated Z73.3
  psychogenic F99
  psychoneurotic — *see also* Neurosis
    compulsive F42
    depersonalization F48.1
    depressive F34.1
    hypochondriacal F45.20
    neurasthenic F48.8
    obsessive F42
  psychophysiologic — *see* Disorder, somatoform
  psychosomatic — *see* Disorder, somatoform
  psychotic — *see* Psychosis
  radiation T66
  scarlet fever toxin — *see* Complications, vaccination
  schizophrenic F23
    acute (brief) (undifferentiated) F23
    latent F21
    undifferentiated (acute) (brief) F23
  serological for syphilis — *see* Serology for syphilis
  serum (prophylactic) (therapeutic) T80.6
    immediate T80.5
  situational — *see* Disorder, adjustment
  somatization — *see* Disorder, somatoform
  spinal puncture G97.1
  stress (severe) F43.9
    acute (agitation) ("daze") (disorientation) (disturbance of consciousness) (flight reaction) (fugue) F43.0
    specified NEC F43.8
  surgical procedure — *see* Complications, surgical procedure
  tetanus antitoxin — *see* Complications, vaccination
  toxic, to local anesthesia T81.89
    in labor and delivery O74.4
    in pregnancy — *see* Complications, anesthesia, in, pregnancy, toxic reaction to local
    postpartum, puerperal O89.3
  toxin-antitoxin — *see* Complications, vaccination
  transfusion (blood) (bone marrow) (lymphocytes) (allergic) — *see* Complications, transfusion
  tuberculin skin test, abnormal R76.1
  ultraviolet T66
  vaccination (any) — *see* Complications, vaccination
  withdrawing, child or adolescent F93.8
  X-ray T66
Reactive depression — *see* Reaction, depressive
Rearrangement
  chromosomal
    balanced (in) Q95.9
      abnormal individual (autosomal) Q95.2
      non-sex (autosomal) chromosomes Q95.2
      sex/non-sex chromosomes Q95.3
      specified NEC Q95.8
Recalcitrant patient — *see* Noncompliance
Recanalization, thrombus — *see* Thrombosis
Recession, receding
  chamber angle (eye) H21.559
    bilateral H21.553
    left H21.552
    right H21.551
  chin M26.09
  gingival (generalized) (localized) (postinfective) (postoperative) K06.0
Recklinghausen's disease (M9540/1) Q85.0
  bones E21.0
Reclus' disease (cystic) — *see* Mastopathy, cystic
Recrudescent typhus (fever) A75.1
Recruitment, auditory H93.219
  bilateral H93.213
  left H93.212
  right H93.211

Rectalgia K62.8
Rectitis K62.8
Rectocele
  female (without uterine prolapse) N81.6
    with uterine prolapse N81.4
      incomplete N81.2
  in pregnancy — *see* Pregnancy, complicated by, abnormal, pelvic organs or tissues NEC
  male K62.3
Rectosigmoid junction — *see* condition
Rectosigmoiditis K63.8
  ulcerative (chronic) K51.35
    with
      complication K51.30
        abscess K51.34
        fistula K51.33
        obstruction K51.32
        rectal bleeding K51.31
        specified complication NEC K51.39
Rectourethral — *see* condition
Rectovaginal — *see* condition
Rectovesical — *see* condition
Rectum, rectal — *see* condition
Recurrent — *see* condition
Red bugs B88.0
Red-cedar lung or pneumonitis J67.8
Reduced ventilatory or vital capacity R94.2
Redundant, redundancy
  anus (congenital) Q43.8
  clitoris N90.8
  colon (congenital) Q43.8
  foreskin (congenital) N47.8
  intestine (congenital) Q43.8
  labia N90.6
  organ or site, congenital NEC — *see* Accessory
  panniculus (abdominal) E65
  prepuce (congenital) N47.8
  pylorus K31.89
  rectum (congenital) Q43.8
  scrotum N50.8
  sigmoid (congenital) Q43.8
  skin (of face) L57.4
    eyelids — *see* Blepharochalasis
  stomach K31.89
Reduplication — *see* Duplication
Reflex R29.2
  hyperactive gag J39.2
  pupillary, abnormal — *see* Anomaly, pupil, function
  vasoconstriction I73.9
  vasovagal R55
Reflux
  esophageal K21.9
    with esophagitis K21.0
  gastroesophageal K21.9
    with esophagitis K21.0
  mitral — *see* Insufficiency, mitral
  ureteral — *see* Reflux, vesicoureteral
  vesicoureteral (with scarring) N13.70
    with
      nephropathy N13.729
        with hydroureter N13.739
          bilateral N13.732
          unilateral N13.731
        bilateral N13.722
        unilateral N13.721
        without hydroureter N13.729
          bilateral N13.722
          unilateral N13.721
      pyelonephritis (chronic) N11.1
    congenital Q62.7
    without nephropathy N13.71
Reforming, artificial openings — *see* Attention to, artificial, opening
Refractive error — *see* Disorder, refraction
Refsum's disease or syndrome G60.1
Refusal of
  food, psychogenic F50.8
  treatment (because of) Z53.20
    left AMA Z53.21
    patient's decision NEC Z53.29
    reasons of belief or group pressure Z53.1
Regional — *see* condition

Regulation, feeding (elderly) (infant) R63.3
Regurgitation
  aortic (valve) — *see* Insufficiency, aortic
  food — *see also* Vomiting
    with reswallowing — *see* Rumination
    newborn P92.1
  gastric contents — *see* Vomiting
  heart — *see* Endocarditis
  mitral (valve) — *see* Insufficiency, mitral
    congenital Q23.3
  myocardial — *see* Endocarditis
  pulmonary (valve) (heart) I37.1
    congenital Q22.2
    syphilitic A52.03
  tricuspid — *see* Insufficiency, tricuspid
  valve, valvular — *see* Endocarditis
  vesicoureteral — *see* Reflux, vesicoureteral
Rehabilitation (alcohol) (cardiac) (drug) (occupational) (smoking) (speech) (vocational) Z51.89
Reifenstein's syndrome E34.5
Reinsertion, contraceptive device Z30.44
Reiter's disease, syndrome, or urethritis M02.30
  ankle M02.379
    left M02.372
    right M02.371
  elbow M02.329
    left M02.322
    right M02.321
  foot joint M02.379
    left M02.372
    right M02.371
  hand joint M02.349
    left M02.342
    right M02.341
  hip M02.359
    left M02.352
    right M02.351
  knee M02.369
    left M02.362
    right M02.361
  multiple site M02.39
  shoulder M02.319
    left M02.312
    right M02.311
  vertebra M02.38
  wrist M02.339
    left M02.332
    right M02.331
Rejchmann's disease or syndrome K31.89
Rejection
  food, psychogenic F50.8
  transplant T86.91
    bone T86.830
      marrow T86.09
    cornea T86.840
    heart T86.21
      with lung(s) T86.31
    intestine T86.890
    kidney T86.11
    liver T86.41
    lung(s) T86.810
      with heart T86.31
    organ (immune or nonimmune cause) T86.91
    pancreas T86.890
    skin (allograft) (autograft) T86.820
    specified NEC T86.890
Relapsing fever A68.9
  Carter's (Asiatic) A68.0
  Dutton's (West African) A68.1
  Koch's A68.9
  louse-borne (epidemic) A68.0
  Novy's (American) A68.1
  Obermeyers' (European) A68.0
  Spirillum A68.9
  tick-borne (endemic) A68.1
Relaxation
  anus (sphincter) K62.8
    psychogenic F45.8
  arch (foot) — *see also* Deformity, limb, flat foot
    congenital Q66.5
  back ligaments — *see* Instability, joint, spine
  bladder (sphincter) N31.2
  cardioesophageal K21.9

Relaxation — continued
  cervix — see Incompetency, cervix
  diaphragm J98.6
  joint (capsule) (ligament) (paralytic) — see Flail, joint
    congenital NEC Q74.8
  lumbosacral (joint) — see category M53.2
  pelvic floor N81.8
  perineum N81.8
  posture R29.3
  rectum (sphincter) K62.8
  sacroiliac (joint) — see category M53.2
  scrotum N50.8
  urethra (sphincter) N36.44
  vesical N31.2
Release from prison, anxiety concerning Z65.2
Remains
  canal of Cloquet Q14.0
  capsule (opaque) Q14.8
Remission in
  bipolar affective disorder — see Disorder, bipolar, in remission
  recurrent depressive disorder — see Disorder, depressive, recurrent, in remission
Remittent fever (malarial) B54
Remnant
  canal of Cloquet Q14.0
  capsule (opaque) Q14.8
  cervix, cervical stump (acquired) (postoperative) N88.8
  cystic duct, postcholecystectomy K91.5
  fingernail L60.8
    congenital Q84.6
  meniscus, knee — see Derangement, knee, meniscus, specified NEC
  thyroglossal duct Q89.2
  tonsil J35.8
    infected (chronic) J35.01
  urachus Q64.4
Removal (from) (of)
  cardiac pulse generator (battery) (end-of-life) Z45.010
  catheter (urinary) (indwelling) Z46.6
    from artificial opening — see Attention to, artificial, opening
    vascular NEC Z45.2
  device
    contraceptive Z30.44
  dressing Z48.0
  home in childhood (to foster home or institution) Z61.1
  ileostomy Z43.2
  myringotomy device (stent) (tube) Z45.8
  organ, prophylactic (for neoplasia management) — see Prophylactic, organ removal
  suture Z48.0
  vascular access device or catheter Z45.2
Ren
  arcuatus Q63.1
  mobile, mobilis N28.89
    congenital Q63.8
  unguliformis Q63.1
Renal — see condition
Rendu-Osler-Weber disease or syndrome I78.0
Reninoma (M8361/1) D41.00
  left D41.02
  right D41.01
Renon-Delille syndrome E23.3
Reovirus, as cause of disease classified elsewhere B97.5
Repair
  pelvic floor, previous, in pregnancy — see Pregnancy, complicated by, abnormal, pelvic organs or tissues NEC
  scarred tissue Z48.8
    breast Z48.8
    head and neck Z48.8
    lower extremity Z48.8
    specified NEC Z48.8
    trunk Z48.8
    upper extremity Z48.8
Replaced chromosome by dicentric ring Q93.2

Replacement by artificial or mechanical device or prosthesis of
  bladder Z96.0
  blood vessel NEC Z95.89
  bone NEC Z96.7
  cochlea Z96.21
  coronary artery Z95.51
  eustachian tube Z96.29
  eye globe Z97.0
  heart Z95.89
    valve NEC Z95.4
  intestine Z96.89
  joint Z96.60
    hip — see Presence, hip joint implant
    knee — see Presence, knee joint implant
    specified site NEC Z96.698
  larynx Z96.3
  lens Z96.1
  limb(s) — see Presence, artificial, limb
  mandible NEC (for tooth root implant(s) Z96.5
  organ NEC Z96.89
  peripheral vessel NEC Z95.89
  stapes Z96.29
  teeth Z97.2
  tendon Z96.7
  tissue NEC Z96.89
  tooth root(s) Z96.5
  vessel NEC Z95.89
    coronary (artery) Z95.51
Request for expert evidence Z04.8
Reserve, decreased or low
  cardiac — see Disease, heart
  kidney N28.89
Residual — see also condition
  ovary syndrome N99.81
  state, schizophrenic F20.5
  urine R39.19
Resorption
  dental (roots) K03.3
    alveoli M26.79
  teeth (external) (internal) (pathological) (roots) K03.3
Respiration
  Cheyne-Stokes R06.3
  decreased due to shock, following injury T79.4
  disorder of, psychogenic F45.8
  insufficient, or poor R06.89
    newborn P28.5
  painful R07.1
  sighing, psychogenic F45.8
Respiratory — see also condition
  distress syndrome (newborn) (type I) P22.0
    type II P22.1
  syncytial virus, as cause of disease classified elsewhere B97.4
Respite care Z75.5
Response (drug)
  photoallergic L56.1
  phototoxic L56.0
Restless legs (syndrome) G25.8
Restlessness R45.1
Restriction of housing space Z59.1
Restoration of organ continuity from previous sterilization (tuboplasty) (vasoplasty) Z31.0
  aftercare Z31.42
Rests, ovarian, in fallopian tube Q50.6
Restzustand (schizophrenic) F20.5
Retained — see Retention
Retardation
  development, developmental, specific — see Disorder, developmental
  endochondral bone growth — see Disorder, bone, development or growth
  growth R62.50
    due to malnutrition E45
    fetus — see also Slow, fetal growth
      affecting management of pregnancy — see Pregnancy, complicated by, fetal, poor growth
    intrauterine growth — see also Slow, fetal growth
      affecting management of pregnancy — see Pregnancy, complicated by, fetal, poor growth

Retardation — continued
  mental F79
    with
      autistic features F84.9
      overactivity and stereotyped movements F84.4
    mild (I.Q. 50-69) F70
    moderate (I.Q. 35-49) F71
    profound (I.Q. under 20) F73
    severe (I.Q. 20-34) F72
    specified level NEC F78
  motor function, specific F82
  physical (child) R62.50
    due to malnutrition E45
    fetus — see Slow, fetal growth
  reading (specific) F81.0
  spelling (specific) (without reading disorder) F81.81
Retching — see Vomiting
Retention, retained
  bladder — see Retention, urine
  carbon dioxide E87.2
  cyst — see Cyst
  dead
    fetus (at or near term) (mother) O36.4
      early fetal death O02.1
    ovum O02.0
  decidua (fragments) (following delivery) (with hemorrhage) O72.2
    with abortion — see Abortion, by type
    without hemorrhage O73.1
  deciduous tooth K00.6
  dental root K08.3
  fecal — see Constipation
  fetus
    dead O36.4
      early O02.1
  fluid R60.9
  foreign body — see also Foreign body, retained
    current trauma - code as Foreign body, by site or type
  gastric K31.89
  intrauterine contraceptive device, in pregnancy — see Pregnancy, complicated by, retention, intrauterine device
  membranes (complicating delivery) (with hemorrhage) O72.2
    with abortion — see Abortion, by type
    without hemorrhage O73.1
  meniscus — see Derangement, meniscus
  menses N94.8
  milk (puerperal, postpartum) O92.7
  nitrogen, extrarenal R39.2
  ovary syndrome N99.81
  placenta (total) (with hemorrhage) O72.0
    without hemorrhage O73.0
    portions or fragments (with hemorrhage) O72.2
      without hemorrhage O73.1
  products of conception
    early pregnancy (dead fetus) O02.1
    following
      abortion — see Abortion, by type
      delivery (with hemorrhage) O72.2
        without hemorrhage O73.1
    secundines (following delivery) (with hemorrhage) O72.2
      with abortion — see Abortion, by type
      without hemorrhage O73.0
      complicating puerperium (delayed hemorrhage) O72.2
      partial O72.2
        without hemorrhage O73.1
  smegma, clitoris N90.8
  urine R33.9
    drug-induced R33.0
    organic R33.8
      drug-induced R33.0
    psychogenic F45.8
  water (in tissues) — see Edema
Reticulation, dust — see Pneumoconiosis
Reticulocytosis R70.1
Reticuloendotheliosis
  acute infantile (M9722/3) C96.0
  leukemic (M9941/3) C91.40
    in remission C91.41

Reticuloendotheliosis — *continued*
  malignant (M9720/3) — *see* Lymphoma, non-
    Hodgkin's, specified type NEC
  nonlipid (M9722/3) C96.0
Reticulohistiocytoma (giant-cell) D76.3
Reticuloid, actinic L57.1
Reticulolymphosarcoma (diffuse) (M9675/3) —
  see Lymphoma, non-Hodgkin's, diffuse,
  mixed small and large cell
  follicular (M9691/3) — *see* Lymphoma, non-
    Hodgkin's, follicular, mixed small cleaved
    cell and large cell
  nodular (M9691/3) — *see* Lymphoma, non-
    Hodgkin's, follicular, mixed small cleaved
    cell and large cell
Reticulosarcoma (M9593/3) — *see* Lymphoma,
  non-Hodgkin's, diffuse, large cell
  diffuse — *see* Lymphoma, non-Hodgkin's,
    diffuse, large cell
  nodular (M9593/3) — *see* Lymphoma, non-
    Hodgkin's, follicular, large cell
  pleomorphic cell type (M9593/3) — *see*
    Lymphoma, non-Hodgkin's, diffuse, large
    cell
Reticulosis (skin)
  acute of infancy (M9722/3) C96.0
  hemophagocytic, familial D76.1
  histiocytic medullary (M9720/3) C96.1
  lipomelanotic I89.8
  malignant (midline) (M9713/3) — *see*
    Lymphoma, non-Hodgkin's, specified type
    NEC
  nonlipid (M9722/3) C96.0
  polymorphic (9713/3) — *see* Lymphoma, non-
    Hodgkin's, specified type NEC
  Sézary's (M9701/3) — *see* Lymphoma, non-
    Hodgkin's, Sézary's disease
Retina, retinal — *see* condition
Retinitis — *see also* Inflammation, chorioretinal
  albuminurica N18.8 *[H32]*
  diabetic — *see* Diabetes, retinitis
  disciformis — *see* Degeneration, macula
  focal — *see* Inflammation, chorioretinal, focal
  gravidarum — *see* Pregnancy, complicated by,
    specified pregnancy-related condition
    NEC
  juxtapapillaris — *see* Inflammation,
    chorioretinal, focal, juxtapapillary
  luetic — *see* Retinitis, syphilitic
  pigmentosa H35.52
  proliferans — *see* Disorder, globe, degenerative,
    specified type NEC
  proliferating — *see* Disorder, globe,
    degenerative, specified type NEC
  renal N18.8 *[H32]*
  syphilitic (early) (secondary) A51.43
    central, recurrent A52.71
    congenital (early) A50.01 *[H32]*
    late A52.71
  tuberculous A18.53
Retinoblastoma (M9510/3) C69.20
  differentiated (M9511/3) C69.20
    left C69.22
    right C69.21
  left C69.22
  right C69.21
  undifferentiated (M9512/3) C69.20
    left C69.22
    right C69.21
Retinochoroiditis — *see also* Inflammation,
  chorioretinal
  disseminated — *see* Inflammation,
    chorioretinal, disseminated
    syphilitic A52.71
  focal — *see* Inflammation, chorioretinal
  juxtapapillaris — *see* Inflammation,
    chorioretinal, focal, juxtapapillary
Retinopathy (background) (Coats') H35.9
  arteriosclerotic I70.90 *[H36]*
  atherosclerotic I70.90 *[H36]*
  central serous — *see* Chorioretinopathy, central
    serous
  diabetic — *see* Diabetes, retinopathy

Retinopathy — *continued*
  exudative H35.029
    bilateral H35.023
    left H35.022
    right H35.021
  hypertensive H35.039
    bilateral H35.033
    left H35.032
    right H35.031
  in (due to)
    diabetes — *see* Diabetes, retinopathy
    sickle-cell disorders D57.1 *[H36]*
  of prematurity H35.1
  pigmentary, congenital — *see* Dystrophy, retina
  proliferative NEC H35.20
    bilateral H35.23
    diabetic — *see* Diabetes, retinopathy,
      proliferative
    left H35.22
    right H35.21
    sickle-cell D57.1 *[H36]*
  solar H31.029
    bilateral H31.023
    left H31.022
    right H31.021
Retinoschisis H33.109
  bilateral H33.103
  congenital Q14.1
  left H33.102
  right H33.101
  specified type NEC H33.199
    bilateral H33.193
    left H33.192
    right H33.191
Retortamoniasis A07.8
Retractile testis Q55.22
Retraction
  cervix — *see* Retroversion, uterus
  drum (membrane) — *see* Disorder, tympanic
    membrane, specified NEC
  finger — *see* Deformity, finger
  lid H02.539
    left H02.536
      lower H02.535
      upper H02.534
    right H02.533
      lower H02.532
      upper H02.531
  lung J98.4
  mediastinum J98.5
  nipple N64.5
    associated with
      lactation O92.03
      pregnancy O92.019
        first trimester O92.011
        second trimester O92.012
        third trimester O92.013
      puerperium O92.02
    congenital Q83.8
  palmar fascia M72.0
  pleura — *see* Pleurisy
  ring, uterus (Bandl's) (pathological) O62.4
  sternum (congenital) Q76.7
    acquired M95.4
  uterus — *see* Retroversion, uterus
  valve (heart) — *see* Endocarditis
Retraining
  activities of daily living NEC Z51.89
  cardiac Z51.89
Retrobulbar — *see* condition
Retrocecal — *see* condition
Retrocession — *see* Retroversion
Retrodisplacement — *see* Retroversion
Retroflection, retroflexion — *see* Retroversion
Retrognathia, retrognathism (mandibular)
  (maxillary) M26.19
Retrograde menstruation N92.5
Retroperineal — *see* condition
Retroperitoneal — *see* condition
Retroperitonitis — *see* Peritonitis
Retropharyngeal — *see* condition
Retroplacental — *see* condition
Retroposition — *see* Retroversion

Retrosternal thyroid (congenital) Q89.2
Retroversion, retroverted
  cervix — *see* Retroversion, uterus
  female NEC — *see* Retroversion, uterus
  iris H21.8
  testis (congenital) Q55.29
  uterus (acquired) (acute) (any degree)
    (asymptomatic) (cervix) (postinfectional)
    (postpartal, old) N85.4
    congenital Q51.8
    in pregnancy — *see* Pregnancy, complicated
      by, abnormal, uterus
Retrovirus, as cause of disease classified
  elsewhere B97.30
  human
    immunodeficiency, type 2 [HIV 2] B97.35
    T-cell lymphotropic
      type I [HTLV-I] B97.33
      type II [HTLV-II] B97.34
  lentivirus B97.31
  oncovirus B97.32
  specified NEC B97.39
Retrusion, premaxilla (developmental) M26.09
Rett's disease or syndrome F84.2
Reverse peristalsis R19.2
Reye's syndrome G93.7
Rh (factor)
  hemolytic disease (fetus or newborn) P55.0
  incompatibility, immunization or sensitization
    affecting management of pregnancy — *see*
      Pregnancy, management affected by,
      isoimmunization, Rh
    fetus or newborn P55.0
    transfusion reaction T80.4
  negative mother affecting fetus or newborn
    P55.0
  titer elevated T80.4
  transfusion reaction T80.4
Rhabdomyoma (M8900/0) — *see also* Neoplasm,
  connective tissue, benign
  adult (M8904/0) — *see* Neoplasm, connective
    tissue, benign
  fetal (M8903/0) — *see* Neoplasm, connective
    tissue, benign
  glycogenic (M8904/0) — *see* Neoplasm,
    connective tissue, benign
Rhabdomyosarcoma (M8900/3) — *see also*
  Neoplasm, connective tissue, malignant
  alveolar (M8920/3) — *see* Neoplasm,
    connective tissue, malignant
  embryonal (M8910/3) — *see* Neoplasm,
    connective tissue, malignant
  mixed type (M8902/3) — *see* Neoplasm,
    connective tissue, malignant
  pleomorphic (M8901/3) — *see* Neoplasm,
    connective tissue, malignant
Rhabdosarcoma (M8900/3) — *see*
  Rhabdomyosarcoma
Rhesus (factor) **incompatibility** — *see* Rh,
  incompatibility
Rheumatic (acute) (subacute) (chronic)
  adherent pericardium I09.2
  coronary arteritis I01.9
  degeneration, myocardium I09.0
  fever (acute) — *see* Fever, rheumatic
  heart — *see* Disease, heart, rheumatic
  myocardial degeneration — *see* Degeneration,
    myocardium
  myocarditis (chronic) (inactive) (with chorea)
    I09.0
    active or acute I01.2
    with chorea (acute) (rheumatic)
      (Sydenham's) I02.0
  pancarditis, acute I01/8
    with chorea (acute (rheumatic) Sydenham's)
      i02/0
  pericarditis (active) (acute) (with effusion) (with
    pneumonia) I01.0
    with chorea (acute) (rheumatic)
      (Sydenham's) I02.0
    chronic or inactive I09.2
  pneumonia I00 *[J17]*
  torticollis M43.6
  typhoid fever A01.09

Rheumatism (articular) (neuralgic) (nonarticular) M79.0
  intercostal, meaning Tietze's disease M94.0
  palindromic (any site) M12.30
    ankle M12.379
      left M12.372
      right M12.371
    elbow M12.329
      left M12.322
      right M12.321
    foot joint M12.379
      left M12.372
      right M12.371
    hand joint M12.349
      left M12.342
      right M12.341
    hip M12.359
      left M12.352
      right M12.351
    knee M12.369
      left M12.362
      right M12.361
    multiple site M12.39
    shoulder M12.319
      left M12.312
      right M12.311
    specified joint NEC M12.38
    wrist M12.339
      left M12.332
      right M12.331
  sciatic M54.4
Rheumatoid — see also condition
  arthritis — see also Arthritis, rheumatoid
    with involvement of organs NEC M05.60
      ankle M05.679
        left M05.672
        right M05.671
      elbow M05.629
        left M05.622
        right M05.621
      foot joint M05.679
        left M05.672
        right M05.671
      hand joint M05.649
        left M05.642
        right M05.641
      hip M05.659
        left M05.652
        right M05.651
      knee M05.669
        left M05.662
        right M05.661
      multiple site M05.69
      shoulder M05.619
        left M05.612
        right M05.611
      vertebra — see Spondylitis, ankylosing
      wrist M05.639
        left M05.632
        right M05.631
    seronegative — see Arthritis, rheumatoid, seronegative
    seropositive — see Arthritis, rheumatoid, seropositive
  carditis M05.30
    ankle M05.379
      left M05.372
      right M05.371
    elbow M05.329
      left M05.322
      right M05.321
    foot joint M05.379
      left M05.372
      right M05.371
    hand joint M05.349
      left M05.342
      right M05.341
    hip M05.359
      left M05.352
      right M05.351
    knee M05.369
      left M05.362
      right M05.361
    multiple site M05.39

Rheumatoid — see also condition — continued
  carditis — continued
    shoulder M05.319
      left M05.312
      right M05.311
    vertebra — see Spondylitis, ankylosing
    wrist M05.339
      left M05.332
      right M05.331
  endocarditis — see Rheumatoid, carditis
  lung (disease) M05.10
    ankle M05.179
      left M05.172
      right M05.171
    elbow M05.129
      left M05.122
      right M05.121
    foot joint M05.179
      left M05.172
      right M05.171
    hand joint M05.149
      left M05.142
      right M05.141
    hip M05.159
      left M05.152
      right M05.151
    knee M05.169
      left M05.162
      right M05.161
    multiple site M05.19
    shoulder M05.119
      left M05.112
      right M05.111
    vertebra — see Spondylitis, ankylosing
    wrist M05.139
      left M05.132
      right M05.131
  myocarditis — see Rheumatoid, carditis
  myopathy M05.40
    ankle M05.479
      left M05.472
      right M05.471
    elbow M05.429
      left M05.422
      right M05.421
    foot joint M05.479
      left M05.472
      right M05.471
    hand joint M05.449
      left M05.442
      right M05.441
    hip M05.459
      left M05.452
      right M05.451
    knee M05.469
      left M05.462
      right M05.461
    multiple site M05.49
    shoulder M05.419
      left M05.412
      right M05.411
    vertebra — see Spondylitis, ankylosing
    wrist M05.439
      left M05.432
      right M05.431
  pericarditis — see Rheumatoid, carditis
  polyarthritis — see Arthritis, rheumatoid
  polyneuropathy M05.50
    ankle M05.579
      left M05.572
      right M05.571
    elbow M05.529
      left M05.522
      right M05.521
    foot joint M05.579
      left M05.572
      right M05.571
    hand joint M05.549
      left M05.542
      right M05.541
    hip M05.559
      left M05.552
      right M05.551
    knee M05.569
      left M05.562
      right M05.561

Rheumatoid — see also condition — continued
  polyneuropathy — continued
    multiple site M05.59
    shoulder M05.519
      left M05.512
      right M05.511
    vertebra — see Spondylitis, ankylosing
    wrist M05.539
      left M05.532
      right M05.531
  vasculitis M05.20
    ankle M05.279
      left M05.272
      right M05.271
    elbow M05.229
      left M05.222
      right M05.221
    foot joint M05.279
      left M05.272
      right M05.271
    hand joint M05.249
      left M05.242
      right M05.241
    hip M05.259
      left M05.252
      right M05.251
    knee M05.269
      left M05.262
      right M05.261
    multiple site M05.29
    shoulder M05.219
      left M05.212
      right M05.211
    vertebra — see Spondylitis, ankylosing
    wrist M05.239
      left M05.232
      right M05.231
Rhinitis (atrophic) (catarrhal) (chronic) (croupous) (fibrinous) (granulomatous) (hyperplastic) (hypertrophic) (membranous) (obstructive) (purulent) (suppurative) (ulcerative) J31.0
  with
    hay fever J45.00
    sore throat — see Nasopharyngitis
  acute J00
  allergic J30.9
    with asthma J45.00
      with
        acute exacerbation J45.01
        status asthmaticus J45.02
    due to
      food J30.5
      pollen J30.1
    nonseasonal J30.8
    perennial J30.8
    seasonal NEC J30.2
    specified NEC J30.8
  infective J00
  pneumococcal J00
  syphilitic A52.73
    congenital A50.05 [J99]
  tuberculous A15.8
  vasomotor J30.0
Rhinoantritis (chronic) — see Sinusitis, maxillary
Rhinodacryolith — see Dacryolith
Rhinolith (nasal sinus) J34.8
Rhinomegaly J34.8
Rhinopharyngitis (acute) (subacute) — see also Nasopharyngitis
  chronic J31.1
  destructive ulcerating A66.5
  mutilans A66.5
Rhinophyma L71.1
Rhinorrhea J34.8
  cerebrospinal (fluid) G96.0
  paroxysmal — see Rhinitis, allergic
  spasmodic — see Rhinitis, allergic
Rhinosalpingitis — see Salpingitis, eustachian
Rhinoscleroma A48.8
Rhinosporidiosis B48.1
Rhinovirus infection NEC B34.8

©2002 Ingenix, Inc.

Rhythm
atrioventricular nodal I49.8
disorder I49.9
coronary sinus I49.8
ectopic I49.8
nodal I49.8
escape I49.9
heart, abnormal I49.9
idioventricular I44.2
nodal I49.8
sleep, inversion G47.2
nonorganic origin — see Disorder, sleep, circadian rhythm, psychogenic

Rhytidosis facialis L98.8

Rib — see also condition
cervical Q76.5

Riboflavin deficiency E53.0

Rice bodies — see also Loose, body, joint
knee M23.40
left M23.42
right M23.41

Richter's hernia — see Hernia, abdomen, with obstruction

Ricinism — see Poisoning, food, noxious, plant

Rickets (active) (acute) (adolescent) (chest wall) (congenital) (current) (infantile) (intestinal) E55.0
adult — see Osteomalacia
celiac K90.0
hypophosphatemic with nephrotic-glycosuric dwarfism E72.09
inactive E64.3
kidney N25.0
renal N25.0
sequelae, any E64.3
vitamin-D-resistant E83.31 [M90.80]

Rickettsial disease A79.9
specified type NEC A79.8

Rickettsialpox (Rickettsia akari) A79.1

Rickettsiosis A79.9
due to
Ehrlichia sennetsu A79.2
Rickettsia akari (rickettsialpox) A79.1
specified type NEC A79.8
tick-borne A77.9
vesicular A79.1

Rider's bone — see Ossification, muscle, specified NEC

Ridge, alveolus — see also condition
flabby K06.8

Ridged ear, congenital Q17.3

Riedel's
lobe, liver Q44.7
struma, thyroiditis or disease E06.5

Rieger's anomaly or syndrome Q13.81

Riehl's melanosis L81.4

Rietti-Greppi-Micheli anemia D56.9

Rieux's hernia — see Hernia, abdomen, specified site NEC

Riga (-Fede) disease K14.0

Riggs' disease K05.3

Right middle lobe syndrome J98.11

Rigid, rigidity — see also condition
abdominal R19.30
with severe abdominal pain R10.0
epigastric R19.36
generalized R19.37
left lower quadrant R19.34
left upper quadrant R19.32
periumbilic R19.35
right lower quadrant R19.33
right upper quadrant R19.31
articular, multiple, congenital Q68.8
cervix (uteri) in pregnancy — see Pregnancy, complicated by, abnormal, cervix
hymen (acquired) (congenital) N89.6
nuchal R29.1
pelvic floor in pregnancy — see Pregnancy, complicated by, abnormal, pelvic organs or tissues NEC
perineum or vulva in pregnancy — see Pregnancy, complicated by, abnormal, vulva

Rigid, rigidity — see also condition — continued
spine — see Dorsopathy, specified NEC
vagina in pregnancy — see Pregnancy, complicated by, abnormal, vagina

Rigors R68.8
with fever R50.0

Riley-Day syndrome G90.1

Ring(s)
aorta (vascular) Q25.4
Bandl's O62.4
contraction, complicating delivery O62.4
esophageal, lower (muscular) K22.2
Fleischer's (cornea) E83.01 [H18.049]
hymenal, tight (acquired) (congenital) N89.6
Kayser-Fleischer (cornea) — see Kayser-Fleischer ring
retraction, uterus, pathological O62.4
Schatzki's (esophagus) (lower) K22.4
congenital Q39.8
Soemmerring's — see Cataract, secondary
vascular (congenital) Q25.8
aorta Q25.4

Ringed hair (congenital) Q84.1

Ringworm B35.9
beard B35.0
black dot B35.0
body B35.4
Burmese B35.5
corporeal B35.4
foot B35.3
groin B35.6
hand B35.2
honeycomb B35.0
nails B35.1
perianal (area) B35.6
scalp B35.0
specified NEC B35.8
Tokelau B35.5

Rise, venous pressure I87.8

Risk, suicidal Z91.5

Ritter's disease L00

Rivalry, sibling F93.8

Rivalta's disease A42.2

River blindness B73.01

Robert's pelvis Q74.2
with disproportion (fetopelvic) O33.0
causing obstructed labor O65.0

Robin (-Pierre) syndrome Q87.0

Robinow-Silvermann-Smith syndrome Q87.1

Robinson's (hidrotic) **ectodermal dysplasia or syndrome** Q82.4

Robles' disease — see Onchocerciasis

Rocky Mountain (spotted) **fever** A77.0

Roentgen ray, adverse effect T66

Roetheln — see Rubella

Roger's disease Q21.0

Rokitansky-Aschoff sinuses (gallbladder) K82.8

Rolando's fracture (displaced) S62.223
left S62.222
nondisplaced S62.226
left S62.225
right S62.224
right S62.221

Romberg's disease or syndrome G51.8

Roof, mouth — see condition

Rosacea L71.9
acne L71.9
keratitis L71.8
specified NEC L71.8

Rosary, rachitic E55.0

Rose
cold J30.1
fever J30.1
rash R21
epidemic B06.9

Rosenbach's erysipeloid A26.0

Rosenthal's disease or syndrome D68.1

Roseola B09
infantum B08.2

Rossbach's disease K31.89
psychogenic F45.8

Ross River disease or fever B33.1

Rostan's asthma (cardiac) — see Failure, ventricular, left

Rotation
anomalous, incomplete or insufficient, intestine Q43.3
cecum (congenital) Q43.3
colon (congenital) Q43.3
spine, incomplete or insufficient — see Dorsopathy, deforming, specified NEC
tooth, teeth M26.3
vertebra, incomplete or insufficient — see Dorsopathy, deforming, specified NEC

Roth (-Bernhardt) disease or syndrome — see Meralgia paraesthetica

Rothmund (-Thomson) syndrome Q82.8

Rotor's disease or syndrome E80.6

Round
back (with wedging of vertebrae) — see Kyphosis
sequelae of rickets (see also category M49.8) E64.3
worms (large) (infestation) — see Ascariasis

Roussy-Lévy syndrome G60.0

Rubella (German measles) B06.9
complicating pregnancy, childbirth or the puerperium — see Disease, viral, obstetric
complication NEC B06.09
neurological B06.00
congenital P35.0
contact Z20.4
exposure to Z20.4
maternal
manifest rubella in infant P35.0
care for (suspected) damage to fetus O35.3
suspected damage to fetus affecting management of pregnancy O35.3
specified complications NEC B06.89
vaccination, prophylactic (against) Z23

Rubeola (meaning measles) — see Measles
meaning rubella — see Rubella

Rubeosis, iris — see Disorder, iris, vascular

Rubinstein-Taybi syndrome Q87.2

Rudimentary (congenital) — see also Agenesis
arm — see Defect, reduction, upper limb
bone Q79.9
cervix uteri Q51.8
eye Q11.2
lobule of ear Q17.3
patella Q74.1
respiratory organs in thoracopagus Q89.4
tracheal bronchus Q32.8
uterus Q51.8
in male Q56.1
vagina Q52.0

Ruled out condition — see Observation, suspected

Rumination R11.3
with nausea R11.0
disorder of infancy F98.21
neurotic F42
newborn P92.1
obsessional F42
psychogenic F42

Runeberg's disease D51.0

Runge's syndrome (postmaturity) P08.2

Rupia (syphilitic) A51.39
congenital A50.06
tertiary A52.79

Rupture, ruptured
abscess (spontaneous) – code by site under Abscess
aneurysm — see Aneurysm
anus (sphincter) — see Laceration, anus
aorta, aortic I71.8
abdominal I71.3
arch I71.1
ascending I71.1
descending I71.8
abdominal I71.3
thoracic I71.1
syphilitic A52.01
thoracoabdominal I71.5

Rupture, ruptured — *continued*
  aorta, aortic — *continued*
    thorax, thoracic I71.1
    transverse I71.1
    traumatic — *see* Injury, aorta, laceration,
      major
    valve or cusp (*see also* Endocarditis, aortic)
      I35.8
  appendix (with peritonitis) K35.0
    with peritoneal abscess K35.1
  arteriovenous fistula, brain I60.8
  artery I77.2
    brain — *see* Hemorrhage, intracranial,
      intracerebral
    coronary — *see* Infarct, myocardium
    heart — *see* Infarct, myocardium
    pulmonary I28.8
    traumatic (complication) — *see* Injury, blood
      vessel
  bile duct (common) (hepatic) K83.2
    cystic K82.2
  bladder (sphincter) (nontraumatic)
      (spontaneous) N32.8
    following ectopic or molar pregnancy O08.6
    obstetrical trauma O71.5
    traumatic S37.28
  blood vessel — *see also* Hemorrhage
    brain — *see* Hemorrhage, intracranial,
      intracerebral
    heart — *see* Infarct, myocardium
    traumatic (complication) — *see* Injury, blood
      vessel, laceration, major, by site
  bone — *see* Fracture
  bowel (nontraumatic) K63.1
  brain
    aneurysm (congenital) — *see also*
      Hemorrhage, intracranial,
      subarachnoid
      syphilitic A52.05
    hemorrhagic — *see* Hemorrhage,
      intracranial, intracerebral
  capillaries I78.8
  cardiac (auricle) (ventricle) (wall) I21.9
    concurrent with acute myocardial infarction
      — *see* Infarct, myocardium
    following acute myocardial infarction
      (current complication) I23.3
      with hemopericardium I23.0
    infectional I40.9
    traumatic — *see* Injury, heart
  cartilage (articular) (current) — *see also* Sprain
    knee S83.30
      left S83.32
      right S83.31
    semilunar — *see* Tear, meniscus
  cecum (with peritonitis) K65.0
    with peritoneal abscess K35.1
    traumatic S36.598
  celiac artery, traumatic — *see* Injury, blood
      vessel, celiac artery, laceration, major
  cerebral aneurysm (congenital) (*see*
      Hemorrhage, intracranial, subarachnoid)
  cervix (uteri)
    with ectopic or molar pregnancy O08.6
    following ectopic or molar pregnancy O08.6
    obstetrical trauma O71.3
    traumatic S37.69
  chordae tendineae NEC I51.1
    concurrent with acute myocardial infarction
      — *see* Infarct, myocardium
    following acute myocardial infarction
      (current complication) I23.4
  choroid (direct) (indirect) (traumatic) H31.329
    bilateral H31.323
    left H31.322
    right H31.321
  circle of Willis I60.6
  colon (nontraumatic) K63.1
    traumatic — *see* Injury, intestine, large
  cornea (traumatic) — *see* Injury, eye, laceration
  coronary (artery) (thrombotic) — *see* Infarct,
      myocardium
  corpus luteum (infected) (ovary) N83.1
  cyst — *see* Cyst
  cystic duct K82.2

Rupture, ruptured — *continued*
  Descemet's membrane — *see* Change, corneal
      membrane, Descemet's, rupture
    traumatic — *see* Injury, eye, laceration
  diaphragm, traumatic — *see* Injury,
      intrathoracic, diaphragm
  disc — *see* Rupture, intervertebral disc
  diverticulum (intestine) K57.80
    with bleeding K57.81
    bladder N32.3
    large intestine K57.20
      with
        bleeding K57.21
        small intestine K57.40
          with bleeding K57.41
    small intestine K57.00
      with
        bleeding K57.01
        large intestine K57.40
          with bleeding K57.41
  duodenal stump K31.89
  ear drum (nontraumatic) — *see also*
      Perforation, tympanum
    traumatic S09.20
      due to blast injury — *see* Injury, blast,
        ear
      left S09.22
      right S09.21
  esophagus K22.3
  eye (without prolapse or loss of intraocular
      tissue) — *see* Injury, eye, laceration
  fallopian tube NEC (nonobstetric)
      (nontraumatic) N83.8
    due to pregnancy O00.1
  fontanel P13.1
  gallbladder K82.2
    traumatic S36.128
  gastric — *see also* Rupture, stomach
    vessel K92.2
  globe (eye) (traumatic) — *see* Injury, eye,
      laceration
  graafian follicle (hematoma) N83.0
  heart — *see* Rupture, cardiac
  hymen (nontraumatic) (nonintentional) N89.8
  internal organ, traumatic — *see* Injury, by site
  intervertebral disc — *see* Displacement,
      intervertebral disc
    traumatic-*see* Rupture, traumatic,
      intervertebral disc
  intestine NEC (nontraumatic) K63.1
    traumatic — *see* Injury, intestine
  iris — *see also* Abnormality, pupillary
    traumatic — *see* Injury, eye, laceration
  joint capsule, traumatic — *see* Sprain
  kidney (traumatic) S37.069
    birth injury P15.8
    left S37.062
    nontraumatic N28.89
    right S37.061
  lacrimal duct (traumatic) — *see* Injury, eye,
      specified site NEC
  lens (cataract) (traumatic) — *see* Cataract,
      traumatic
  ligament, traumatic — *see* Rupture, traumatic,
      ligament, by site
  liver S36.116
    birth injury P15.0
  lymphatic vessel I89.8
  marginal sinus (placental) (with hemorrhage) —
      see Hemorrhage, antepartum, specified
      cause NEC
  membrana tympani (nontraumatic) — *see*
      Perforation, tympanum
  membranes (spontaneous)
    artificial
      delayed delivery following O75.5
    delayed delivery following — *see* Rupture,
      membranes, premature

Rupture, ruptured — *continued*
  membranes — *continued*
    premature O42.90
      with onset of labor
        within 24 hours O42.00
          after 37 weeks gestation O42.02
          before 38 weeks gestation O42.019
            first trimester O42.011
            second trimester O42.012
            third trimester O42.013
        after 24 hours O42.10
          after 37 weeks gestation O42.12
          before 38 weeks gestation O42.119
            first trimester O42.111
            second trimester O42.112
            third trimester O42.113
      after 37 weeks gestation O42.92
      before 38 weeks gestation O42.919
        first trimester O42.911
        second trimester O42.912
        third trimester O42.913
  meningeal artery I60.8
  meniscus (knee) — *see also* Tear, meniscus
    old — *see* Derangement, meniscus
    site other than knee – code as Sprain
  mesenteric artery, traumatic — *see* Injury,
      mesenteric, artery, laceration, major
  mesentery (nontraumatic) K66.8
    traumatic — *see* Injury, intra-abdominal,
      specified, site NEC
  mitral (valve) I34.8
  muscle (traumatic) — *see also* Injury, muscle
    diastasis — *see* Diastasis, muscle
    nontraumatic M62.10
      ankle M62.179
        left M62.172
        right M62.171
      foot M62.179
        left M62.172
        right M62.171
      forearm M62.139
        left M62.132
        right M62.131
      hand M62.149
        left M62.142
        right M62.141
      lower leg M62.169
        left M62.162
        right M62.161
      pelvic region M62.159
        left M62.152
        right M62.151
      shoulder region M62.119
        left M62.112
        right M62.111
      specified site NEC M62.18
      thigh M62.159
        left M62.152
        right M62.151
      upper arm M62.129
        left M62.122
        right M62.121
  musculotendinous junction NEC, nontraumatic
      — *see* Rupture, tendon, spontaneous
  mycotic aneurysm causing cerebral
      hemorrhage — *see* Hemorrhage,
      intracranial, subarachnoid
  myocardium, myocardial — *see* Infarct,
      myocardium
    traumatic — *see* Injury, heart
  nontraumatic, meaning hernia — *see* Hernia
  obstructed — *see* Hernia, by site, obstructed
  operation wound T81.3
  ovary, ovarian N83.8
    corpus luteum cyst N83.1
    follicle (graafian) N83.0
  oviduct (nonobstetric) (nontraumatic) N83.8
    due to pregnancy O00.1
  pancreas (nontraumatic) K86.8
    traumatic S36.299
  papillary muscle NEC I51.2
    following acute myocardial infarction
      (current complication) I23.5

©2002 Ingenix, Inc.

Rupture, ruptured — *continued*
  pelvic
    floor, complicating delivery O70.1
    organ NEC, obstetrical trauma O71.5
  perineum (nonobstetric) (nontraumatic) N90.8
    complicating delivery O70.9
      first degree O70.0
      fourth degree O70.3
      second degree O70.1
      third degree O70.2
  postoperative wound T81.3
  prostate (traumatic) S37.828
  pulmonary
    artery I28.8
    valve (heart) I37.8
    vein I28.8
    vessel I28.8
  pus tube — *see* Salpingitis
  pyosalpinx — *see* Salpingitis
  rectum (nontraumatic) K63.1
    traumatic S36.69
  retina, retinal (traumatic) (without detachment)
      — *see also* Break, retina
    with detachment — *see* Detachment, retina,
      with retinal, break
  rotator cuff (complete) (incomplete)
      (nontraumatic) — *see* Syndrome, rotator
      cuff
  sclera — *see* Injury, eye, laceration
  sigmoid (nontraumatic) K63.1
    traumatic S36.593
  spinal cord — *see also* Injury, spinal cord, by
      region
    due to injury at birth P11.5
    fetus or newborn (birth injury) P11.5
  spleen (traumatic) S36.09
    birth injury P15.1
    congenital (birth injury) P15.1
    due to P. vivax malaria B51.0
    nontraumatic D73.5
    spontaneous D73.5
  splenic vein R58
    traumatic — *see* Injury, blood vessel, portal
      vein
  stomach (nontraumatic) (spontaneous) K31.89
    traumatic S36.39
  supraspinatus (complete) (incomplete)
      (nontraumatic) — *see* Syndrome, rotator
      cuff
  symphysis pubis
    obstetric O71.6
    traumatic S33.4
  synovium (cyst) M66.10
    ankle M66.173
      left M66.172
      right M66.171
    elbow M66.129
      left M66.122
      right M66.121
    finger M66.146
      left M66.145
      right M66.144
    foot M66.176
      left M66.175
      right M66.174
    forearm M66.139
      left M66.132
      right M66.131
    hand M66.143
      left M66.142
      right M66.141
    pelvic region M66.159
      left M66.152
      right M66.151
    shoulder region M66.119
      left M66.112
      right M66.111
    specified site NEC M66.18
    thigh M66.159
      left M66.152
      right M66.151
    toe M66.179
      left M66.178
      right M66.177

Rupture, ruptured — *continued*
  synovium — *continued*
    upper arm M66.129
      left M66.122
      right M66.121
    wrist M66.139
      left M66.132
      right M66.131
  tendon (traumatic) — *see also* Injury, muscle
    nontraumatic — *see* Rupture, tendon,
      spontaneous
    spontaneous M66.9
      ankle M66.879
        left M66.872
        right M66.871
      extensor M66.20
        ankle M66.279
          left M66.272
          right M66.271
        foot M66.279
          left M66.272
          right M66.271
        forearm M66.239
          left M66.232
          right M66.231
        hand M66.249
          left M66.242
          right M66.241
        lower leg M66.269
          left M66.262
          right M66.261
        multiple sites M66.29
        pelvic region M66.259
          left M66.252
          right M66.251
        shoulder region M66.219
          left M66.212
          right M66.211
        specified site NEC M66.28
        thigh M66.259
          left M66.252
          right M66.251
        upper arm M66.229
          left M66.222
          right M66.221
      flexor M66.30
        ankle M66.379
          left M66.372
          right M66.371
        foot M66.379
          left M66.372
          right M66.371
        forearm M66.339
          left M66.332
          right M66.331
        hand M66.349
          left M66.342
          right M66.341
        lower leg M66.369
          left M66.362
          right M66.361
        multiple sites M66.39
        pelvic region M66.359
          left M66.352
          right M66.351
        shoulder region M66.319
          left M66.312
          right M66.311
        specified site NEC M66.38
        thigh M66.359
          left M66.352
          right M66.351
        upper arm M66.329
          left M66.322
          right M66.321
      foot M66.879
        left M66.872
        right M66.871
      forearm M66.839
        left M66.832
        right M66.831
      hand M66.849
        left M66.842
        right M66.841

Rupture, ruptured — *continued*
  tendon — *see also* Injury, muscle — *continued*
    spontaneous — *continued*
      lower leg M66.869
        left M66.862
        right M66.861
      multiple sites M66.89
      pelvic region M66.859
        left M66.852
        right M66.851
      shoulder region M66.819
        left M66.812
        right M66.811
      specified
        site NEC M66.88
        tendon M66.80
      thigh M66.859
        left M66.852
        right M66.851
      upper arm M66.829
        left M66.822
        right M66.821
  thoracic duct I89.8
  tonsil J35.8
  traumatic
    aorta — *see* Injury, aorta, laceration, major
    diaphragm — *see* Injury, intrathoracic,
      diaphragm
    external site — *see* Wound, open, by site
    eye — *see* Injury, eye, laceration
    internal organ — *see* Injury, by site
    intervertebral disc
      cervical S13.0
      lumbar S33.0
      thoracic S23.0
    kidney S37.069
      left S37.062
      right S37.061
    ligament — *see also* Sprain
      ankle — *see* Sprain, ankle
      carpus — *see* Rupture, traumatic,
        ligament, wrist
      collateral (hand) — *see* Rupture,
        traumatic, ligament, finger,
        collateral
      finger (metacarpophalangeal)
          (interphalangeal) S63.409
        collateral S63.419
          index S63.418
            left S63.411
            right S63.410
          little S63.418
            left S63.417
            right S63.416
          middle S63.418
            left S63.413
            right S63.412
          ring S63.418
            left S63.415
            right S63.414
        index S63.408
          left S63.401
          right S63.400
        little S63.408
          left S63.407
          right S63.406
        middle S63.408
          left S63.403
          right S63.402
        palmar S63.429
          index S63.428
            left S63.421
            right S63.420
          little S63.428
            left S63.427
            right S63.426
          middle S63.428
            left S63.423
            right S63.422
          ring S63.428
            left S63.425
            right S63.424
        ring S63.408
          left S63.405
          right S63.404

Rupture, ruptured — *continued*
  traumatic — *continued*
    ligament — *see also* Sprain — *continued*
      finger — *continued*
        specified site NEC S63.499
          index S63.498
            left S63.491
            right S63.490
          little S63.498
            left S63.497
            right S63.496
          middle S63.498
            left S63.493
            right S63.492
          ring S63.498
            left S63.495
            right S63.494
        volar plate S63.439
          index S63.438
            left S63.431
            right S63.430
          little S63.438
            left S63.437
            right S63.436
          middle S63.438
            left S63.433
            right S63.432
          ring S63.438
            left S63.435
            right S63.434
    foot — *see* Sprain, foot
    radial collateral S53.20
      left S53.22
      right S53.21
    radiocarpal — *see* Rupture, traumatic,
      ligament, wrist, radiocarpal
    ulnar collateral S53.30
      left S53.32
      right S53.31
    ulnocarpal — *see* Rupture, traumatic,
      ligament, wrist, ulnocarpal
    wrist S63.309
      collateral S63.319
        left S63.312
        right S63.311
      left S63.302
      radiocarpal S63.329
        left S63.322
        right S63.321
      right S63.301
      specified site NEC S63.399
        left S63.392
        right S63.391
      ulnocarpal (palmar) S63.339
        left S63.332
        right S63.331
   liver S36.116
   membrana tympani — *see* Rupture, ear
      drum, traumatic
   muscle or tendon — *see* Injury, muscle
   myocardium — *see* Injury, heart
   pancreas S36.299
   rectum S36.69
   sigmoid S36.593
   spleen S36.09
   stomach S36.39
   symphysis pubis S33.4
   tympanum, tympanic (membrane) — *see*
      Rupture, ear drum, traumatic
   ureter S37.19
   uterus S37.69
   vagina — *see* Injury, vagina
   vena cava — *see* Injury, vena cava,
      laceration, major
  tricuspid (heart) (valve) I07.8
  tube, tubal (nonobstetric) (nontraumatic) N83.8
   abscess — *see* Salpingitis
   due to pregnancy O00.1
  tympanum, tympanic (membrane)
      (nontraumatic) — *see also* Perforation,
      tympanum
   with otitis media — *see* Otitis media
   traumatic — *see* Rupture, ear drum,
      traumatic
  umbilical cord, complicating delivery O69.8
   affecting fetus or newborn P50.1

Rupture, ruptured — *continued*
  ureter (traumatic) S37.19
   nontraumatic N28.89
  urethra (nontraumatic) N36.8
   with ectopic or molar pregnancy O08.6
   following ectopic or molar pregnancy O08.6
   obstetrical trauma O71.5
   traumatic S37.38
  uterosacral ligament (nonobstetric)
      (nontraumatic) N83.8
  uterus (traumatic) S37.69
   before labor O71.00
    second trimester O71.02
    third trimester O71.03
   during or after labor O71.1
    affecting fetus or newborn P03.89
   nonpuerperal, nontraumatic N85.8
   pregnant (during labor) O71.1
    before labor O71.00
     second trimester O71.02
     third trimester O71.03
  vagina — *see* Injury, vagina
  valve, valvular (heart) — *see* Endocarditis
  varicose vein — *see* Varix
  varix — *see* Varix
  vena cava R58
   traumatic — *see* Injury, vena cava,
      laceration, major
  vesical (urinary) N32.8
  vessel (blood) R58
   pulmonary I28.8
   traumatic — *see* Injury, blood vessel
  viscus R19.8
  vulva complicating delivery O70.0
Russell-Silver syndrome Q87.1
Russian spring-summer type encephalitis A84.0
Rust's disease (tuberculous cervical spondylitis)
  A18.01
Rytand-Lipsitch syndrome I44.2

S

Saber, sabre shin or tibia (syphilitic) A50.56
  [M90.80]
Sac lacrimal — *see* condition
Saccharomyces infection B37.9
Saccharopinuria E72.3
Saccular — *see* condition
Sacculation
  aorta (nonsyphilitic) — *see* Aneurysm, aorta
  bladder N32.3
  intralaryngeal (congenital) (ventricular) Q31.3
  larynx (congenital) (ventricular) Q31.3
  organ or site, congenital — *see* Distortion
  pregnant uterus — *see* Pregnancy, complicated
    by, abnormal, uterus
  ureter N28.89
  urethra N36.1
  vesical N32.3
Sachs' amaurotic familial idiocy or disease
  E75.02
Sachs-Tay disease E75.02
Sacks-Libman disease M32.11
Sacralgia M53.3
Sacralization M43.27
Sacrodynia M53.3
Sacroiliac joint — *see* condition
Sacroiliitis NEC M46.1
Sacrum — *see* condition
Saddle
  back — *see* Lordosis
  embolus, aorta I74.0
  nose M95.0
   due to syphilis A50.57
Sadism (sexual) F65.52
Sadness, postpartal O90.6
Sadomasochism F65.50
Saemisch's ulcer (cornea) — *see* Ulcer, cornea,
  central
Sahib disease B55.0
Sailors' skin L57.8
Saint
  Anthony's fire — *see* Erysipelas
  triad — *see* Hernia, diaphragm
  Vitus' dance — *see* Chorea, Sydenham's
Salaam
  attack(s) G40.40
  tic R25.8
Salicylism
  abuse F55.8
  overdose or wrong substance given or taken —
    see category T39.0
Salivary duct or gland — *see* condition
Salivation, excessive K11.7
Salmonella — *see* Infection, Salmonella
Salmonellosis A02.0
Salpingitis (catarrhal) (fallopian tube) (nodular)
  (pseudofollicular) (purulent) (septic) N70.91
  with oophoritis N70.93
  acute N70.01
   with oophoritis N70.03
  chlamydial A56.11
  chronic N70.11
   with oophoritis N70.13
  complicating abortion — *see* Abortion, by type,
    complicated by, salpingitis
  ear — *see* Salpingitis, eustachian
  eustachian (tube) H68.009
   acute H68.019
    bilateral H68.013
    left H68.012
    right H68.011
   bilateral H68.003
   chronic H68.029
    bilateral H68.023
    left H68.022
    right H68.021
   left H68.002
   right H68.001
  follicularis N70.11
   with oophoritis N70.13
  gonococcal (acute) (chronic) A54.24

©2002 Ingenix, Inc.

Salpingitis — *continued*
  interstitial, chronic N70.11
    with oophoritis N70.13
  isthmica nodosa N70.11
    with oophoritis N70.13
  specific (gonococcal) (acute) (chronic) A54.24
  tuberculous (acute) (chronic) A18.17
  venereal (gonococcal) (acute) (chronic) A54.24
Salpingocele N83.4
Salpingo-oophoritis (catarrhal) (purulent)
  (ruptured) (septic) (suppurative) N70.93
  acute N70.03
    with ectopic or molar pregnancy O08.0
    following ectopic or molar pregnancy O08.0
    gonococcal A54.24
  chronic N70.13
  complicating pregnancy — *see* Pregnancy,
    complicated by, genital infection
  following ectopic or molar pregnancy O08.0
  gonococcal (acute) (chronic) A54.24
  puerperal O86.1
  specific (gonococcal) (acute) (chronic) A54.24
  subacute N70.03
  tuberculous (acute) (chronic) A18.17
  venereal (gonococcal) (acute) (chronic) A54.24
Salpingo-ovaritis — *see* Salpingo-oophoritis
Salpingoperitonitis — *see* Salpingo-oophoritis
Salzmann's nodular dystrophy — *see*
  Degeneration, cornea, nodular
Sampson's cyst or tumor N80.1
San Joaquin (Valley) **fever** B38.0
Sandblaster's asthma, lung or pneumoconiosis
  J62.8
Sander's disease (paranoia) F22
Sandfly fever A93.1
Sandhoff's disease E75.01
Sanfilippo (Type B) (Type C) (Type D) **syndrome**
  E76.22
Sanger-Brown ataxia G11.2
Sao Paulo fever or typhus A77.0
Saponification, mesenteric K65.8
Sarcocele (benign)
  syphilitic A52.76
    congenital A50.59
Sarcocystosis A07.8
Sarcoepiplocele — *see* Hernia
Sarcoepiplomphalocele Q79.2
Sarcoid — *see also* Sarcoidosis
  arthropathy D86.86
  Boeck's D86.9
  Darier-Roussy D86.3
  iridocyclitis D86.83
  meningitis D86.81
  myocarditis D86.85
  myositis D86.87
  pyelonephritis D86.84
  Spiegler-Fendt L08.89
Sarcoidosis D86.9
  with
    cranial nerve palsies D86.82
    hepatic granuloma D86.89
    polyarthritis D86.86
    tubulo-interstitial nephropathy D86.84
  combined sites NEC D86.89
  lung D86.0
    and lymph nodes D86.2
  lymph nodes D86.1
    and lung D86.2
  meninges D86.81
  skin D86.3
  specified type NEC D86.89
Sarcoma (M8800/3) — *see also* Neoplasm,
  connective tissue, malignant
  alveolar soft part (M9581/3) — *see* Neoplasm,
    connective tissue, malignant
  ameloblastic (M9330/3) C41.1
    upper jaw (bone) C41.0
  botryoid (M8910/3) — *see* Neoplasm,
    connective tissue, malignant
  botryoides (M8910/3) — *see* Neoplasm,
    connective tissue, malignant
  cerebellar (M9480/3) C71.6
    circumscribed (arachnoidal) (M9471/3) C71.6

Sarcoma — *see also* Neoplasm, connective tissue,
  malignant — *continued*
  circumscribed (arachnoidal) cerebellar
    (M9471/3) C71.6
  clear cell (M9044/3) — *see also* Neoplasm,
    connective tissue, malignant
    kidney (M8964/3) C64.9
      left C64.1
      right C64.0
  embryonal (M8991/3) — *see* Neoplasm,
    connective tissue, malignant
  endometrial (stromal) (M8930/3) C54.1
    isthmus C54.0
  epithelioid (cell) (M8804/3) — *see* Neoplasm,
    connective tissue, malignant
  Ewing's (M9260/3) — *see* Neoplasm, bone,
    malignant
  germinoblastic (diffuse) (M9683/3) — *see*
    Lymphoma, non-Hodgkin's type, diffuse,
    large cell
    follicular (M9697/3) — *see* Lymphoma, non-
      Hodgkin's type, follicular, specified
      type NEC
  giant cell (except of bone) (M8802/3) — *see*
    also Neoplasm, connective tissue,
    malignant
    bone (M9250/3) — *see* Neoplasm, bone,
      malignant
  glomoid (M8710/3) — *see* Neoplasm,
    connective tissue, malignant
  granulocytic (M9930/3) C92.30
    in remission C92.31
  hemangioendothelial (M9130/3) — *see*
    Neoplasm, connective tissue, malignant
  hemorrhagic, multiple (M9140/3) — *see*
    Sarcoma, Kaposi's
  Hodgkin's (M9662/3) — *see* Hodgkin's, disease,
    specified type NEC
  immunoblastic (diffuse) (M9684/3) — *see*
    Lymphoma, non-Hodgkin's type, diffuse,
    immunoblastic
  Kaposi's (M9140/3)
    colon C46.4
    connective tissue C46.1
    gastrointestinal organ C46.4
    lung C46.50
      left C46.52
      right C46.51
    lymph node(s) C46.3
    palate (hard) (soft) C46.2
    rectum C46.4
    skin C46.0
    specified site NEC C46.7
    stomach C46.4
    unspecified site C46.9
  Kupffer cell (M9124/3) C22.3
  leptomeningeal (M9530/3) — *see* Neoplasm,
    meninges, malignant
  liver NEC C22.4
  lymphangioendothelial (M9170/3) — *see*
    Neoplasm, connective tissue, malignant
  lymphoblastic (M9685/3) — *see* Lymphoma,
    non-Hodgkin's type, diffuse,
    lymphoblastic
  lymphocytic (M9670/3) — *see* Lymphoma, non-
    Hodgkin's type, diffuse, small cell
  mast cell (M9740/3) C96.2
  melanotic (M8720/3) — *see* Melanoma
  meningeal (M9530/3) — *see* Neoplasm,
    meninges, malignant
  meningothelial (M9530/3) — *see* Neoplasm,
    meninges, malignant
  mesenchymal (M8800/3) — *see also* Neoplasm,
    connective tissue, malignant
    mixed (M8990/3) — *see* Neoplasm,
      connective tissue, malignant
  mesothelial (M9050/3) — *see* Mesothelioma
  monstrocellular (M9481/3)
    specified site — *see* Neoplasm, malignant
    unspecified site C71.9
  myeloid (M9930/3) C92.30
    in remission C92.31
  neurogenic (M9540/3) — *see* Neoplasm, nerve,
    malignant
  odontogenic (M9270/3) C41.1
    upper jaw (bone) C41.0

Sarcoma — *see also* Neoplasm, connective tissue,
  malignant — *continued*
  osteoblastic (M9180/3) — *see* Neoplasm, bone,
    malignant
  osteogenic (M9180/3) — *see also* Neoplasm,
    bone, malignant
    juxtacortical (M9190/3) — *see* Neoplasm,
      bone, malignant
    periosteal (M9190/3) — *see* Neoplasm, bone,
      malignant
  periosteal (M8812/3) — *see also* Neoplasm,
    bone, malignant
    osteogenic (M9190/3) — *see* Neoplasm,
      bone, malignant
  plasma cell (M9731/3) C90.20
    in remission C90.21
  pleomorphic cell (M8802/3) — *see* Neoplasm,
    connective tissue, malignant
  reticulum cell (diffuse) (M9593/3) — *see*
    Lymphoma, non-Hodgkin's type, diffuse,
    large cell
    nodular (M9698/3) — *see* Lymphoma, non-
      Hodgkin's type, follicular, large cell
    pleomorphic cell type (M9680/3) — *see*
      Lymphoma, non-Hodgkin's type,
      diffuse, large cell
  rhabdoid (M8963/3) — *see* Neoplasm,
    malignant
  round cell (M8803/3) — *see* Neoplasm,
    connective tissue, malignant
  small cell (M8803/3) — *see* Neoplasm,
    connective tissue, malignant
  soft tissue (M8800/3) — *see* Neoplasm,
    connective tissue, malignant
  spindle cell (M8801/3) — *see* Neoplasm,
    connective tissue, malignant
  stromal (endometrial) (M8930/3) C54.1
    isthmus (M8930/3) C54.0
  synovial (M9040/3) — *see also* Neoplasm,
    connective tissue, malignant
    biphasic (M9043/3) — *see* Neoplasm,
      connective tissue, malignant
    epithelioid cell (M9042/3) — *see* Neoplasm,
      connective tissue, malignant
    spindle cell (M9041/3) — *see* Neoplasm,
      connective tissue, malignant
Sarcomatosis
  meningeal (M9539/3) — *see* Neoplasm,
    meninges, malignant
  specified site NEC (M8800/3) — *see* Neoplasm,
    connective tissue, malignant
  unspecified site (M8800/6) C80
Sarcosinemia E72.59
Sarcosporidiosis (intestinal) A07.8
Saturnine — *see* condition
Saturnism
  overdose or wrong substance given or taken —
    see category T56.0
Satyriasis F52.8
Sauriasis — *see* Ichthyosis
SBE (subacute bacterial endocarditis) I28.8
Scabs R23.4
Scabies (any site) B86
Scaglietti-Dagnini syndrome E22.0
Scald — *see* Burn
Scalenus anticus (anterior) **syndrome** G54.0
Scales R23.4
Scaling, skin R23.4
Scalp — *see* condition
Scapegoating affecting child Z62.3
Scaphocephaly Q75.0
Scapulalgia M89.81
Scapulohumeral myopathy G71.0
Scar, scarring (*see also* Cicatrix) L90.5
  adherent L90.5
  atrophic L90.5
  cervix
    in pregnancy or childbirth — *see* Pregnancy,
      complicated by, abnormal cervix
  cheloid L91.0
  chorioretinal H31.009
    bilateral H31.003
    left H31.002

Scar, scarring (*see also* Cicatrix) — *continued*
  chorioretinal — *continued*
    posterior pole macula H31.019
      bilateral H31.013
      left H31.012
      right H31.011
    postsurgical — *see* Complication, eye,
      postoperative, retinal detachment
      surgery, chorioretinal scar
    right H31.001
    solar retinopathy H31.029
      bilateral H31.023
      left H31.022
      right H31.021
    specified type NEC H31.099
      bilateral H31.093
      left H31.092
      right H31.091
  choroid — *see* Scar, chorioretinal
  conjunctiva H11.249
    bilateral H11.243
    left H11.242
    right H11.241
  cornea H17.9
    xerophthalmic — *see also* Opacity, cornea
      vitamin A deficiency E50.6
  due to
    previous cesarean section, complicating
      pregnancy or childbirth O34.21
  duodenum, obstructive K31.5
  hypertrophic L91.0
  keloid L91.0
  labia N90.8
  lung (base) J98.4
  macula — *see* Scar, chorioretinal, posterior
    pole
  muscle M62.89
  myocardium, myocardial I25.2
  painful L90.5
  posterior pole (eye) — *see* Scar, chorioretinal,
    posterior pole
  psychic Z91.49
  retina — *see* Scar, chorioretinal
  trachea J39.8
  uterus N85.8
    in pregnancy O34.29
  vagina N89.8
    postoperative N99.2
  vulva N90.8

Scarabiasis B88.2

Scarlatina (anginosa) (maligna) (ulcerosa) A38.9
  myocarditis (acute) A38.1
    old — *see* Myocarditis
  otitis media A38.0

Scarlet fever (albuminuria) (angina) A38.9

Schamberg's disease (progressive pigmentary
  dermatosis) L81.7

Schatzki's ring (acquired) (esophagus) (lower)
  K22.2
  congenital Q39.8

Schaufenster krankheit I20.8

Schaumann's
  benign lymphogranulomatosis D86.1
  disease or syndrome — *see* Sarcoidosis

Scheie's syndrome E76.03

Schenck's disease B42.1

Scheuermann's disease or osteochondrosis —
  see Osteochondrosis, juvenile, spine

Schilder (-Flatau) disease G37.0

Schilling-type monocytic leukemia (M9890/3)
  C93.90
  in remission C93.91

**Schimmelbusch's disease, cystic mastitis, or
  hyperplasia** — *see* Mastopathy, cystic

Schistosoma infestation — *see* Infestation,
  Schistosoma

Schistosomiasis B65.9
  with muscle disorder B65.9 [*M63.80*]
    ankle B65.9 [*M63.879*]
      left B65.9 [*M63.872*]
      right B65.9 [*M63.871*]
    foot B65.9 [*M63.879*]
      left B65.9 [*M63.872*]
      right B65.9 [*M63.871*]

Schistosomiasis — *continued*
  with muscle disorder — *continued*
    forearm B65.9 [*M63.839*]
      left B65.9 [*M63.832*]
      right B65.9 [*M63.831*]
    hand B65.9 [*M63.849*]
      left B65.9 [*M63.842*]
      right B65.9 [*M63.841*]
    lower leg B65.9 [*M63.869*]
      left B65.9 [*M63.862*]
      right B65.9 [*M63.861*]
    multiple sites B65.9 [*M63.89*]
    pelvic region B65.9 [*M63.859*]
      left B65.9 [*M63.852*]
      right B65.9 [*M63.851*]
    shoulder region B65.9 [*M63.819*]
      left B65.9 [*M63.812*]
      right B65.9 [*M63.811*]
    specified site NEC B65.9 [*M63.88*]
    thigh B65.9 [*M63.859*]
      left B65.9 [*M63.852*]
      right B65.9 [*M63.851*]
    upper arm B65.9 [*M63.829*]
      left B65.9 [*M63.822*]
      right B65.9 [*M63.821*]
  Asiatic B65.2
  bladder B65.0
  chestermani B65.8
  colon B65.1
  cutaneous B65.3
  due to
    S. haematobium B65.0
    S. japonicum B65.2
    S. mansoni B65.1
    S. mattheii B65.8
  Eastern B65.2
  genitourinary tract B65.0
  intestinal B65.1
  lung NEC B65.9 [*J99*]
    pneumonia B65.9 [*J17*]
  Manson's (intestinal) B65.1
  oriental B65.2
  pulmonary NEC B65.9 [*J99*]
    pneumonia B65.9
  Schistosoma
    haematobium B65.0
    japonicum B65.2
    mansoni B65.1
  specified type NEC B65.8
  urinary B65.0
  vesical B65.0

Schizencephaly Q04.6

Schizoaffective psychosis F25.9

Schizodontia K00.2

Schizoid personality F60.1

Schizophrenia, schizophrenic F20.9
  acute (brief) (undifferentiated) F23
  atypical (form) F20.3
  borderline F21
  catalepsy F20.2
  catatonic (type) (excited) (withdrawn) F20.2
  cenesthopathic, cenesthesiopathic F20.89
  childhood type F84.5
  chronic undifferentiated F20.5
  cyclic F25.0
  disorganized (type) F20.1
  flexibilitas cerea F20.2
  hebephrenic (type) F20.1
  incipient F21
  latent F21
  negative type F20.5
  paranoid (type) F20.0
  paraphrenic F20.0
  post-psychotic depression F32.8
  prepsychotic F21
  prodromal F21
  pseudoneurotic F21
  pseudopsychopathic F21
  reaction F23
  residual (state) (type) F20.5
  restzustand F20.5
  schizoaffective (type) — *see* Psychosis,
    schizoaffective
  simple (type) F20.89
  simplex F20.89
  specified type NEC F20.89

Schizophrenia, schizophrenic — *continued*
  stupor F20.2
  syndrome of childhood F84.5
  undifferentiated (type) F20.3
    chronic F20.5

Schizothymia (persistent) F60.1

Schlatter-Osgood disease or osteochondrosis —
  see Osteochondrosis, juvenile, tibia

Schlatter's tibia — *see* Osteochondrosis, juvenile,
  tibia

Schmidt's syndrome (polyglandular,
  autoimmune) E31.0

Schmincke's carcinoma or tumor (M8082/3) —
  see Neoplasm, nasopharynx, malignant

Schmitz (-Stutzer) dysentery A03.0

Schmorl's disease or nodes
  lumbar region M51.46
  lumbosacral region M51.47
  sacrococcygeal region M53.3
  thoracic region M51.44
  thoracolumbar region M51.45

Schneiderian
  carcinoma (M8121/3)
    specified site — *see* Neoplasm, malignant
    unspecified site C30.0
  papilloma (M8121/0)
    specified site — *see* Neoplasm, benign
    unspecified site D14.0

Scholte's syndrome (malignant carcinoid) E34.0

**Scholz (-Bielchowsky-Henneberg) disease or
  syndrome** E75.25

Schönlein (-Henoch) disease or purpura
  (primary) (rheumatic) D69.0

Schottmuller's disease A01.4

Schroeder's syndrome (endocrine hypertensive)
  E27.0

Schüller-Christian disease or syndrome D76.0

Schultze type acroparesthesia, simple I73.8

Schultz's disease or syndrome — *see*
  Agranulocytosis

Schwalbe-Ziehen-Oppenheim disease G24.1

Schwannoma (M9560/0) — *see also* Neoplasm,
  nerve, benign
  malignant (M9560/3) — *see also* Neoplasm,
    nerve, malignant
    with rhabdomyoblastic differentiation
      (M9561/3) — *see* Neoplasm, nerve,
      malignant
  melanocytic (9560/0) — *see* Neoplasm, nerve,
    benign
  pigmented (M9560/0) — *see* Neoplasm, nerve,
    benign

Schwartz (-Jampel) syndrome Q78.8

Schwartz-Bartter syndrome E22.2

Schweniger-Buzzi anetoderma L90.1

Sciatic — *see* condition

Sciatica (infective) M54.30
  with lumbago M54.4
  due to intervertebral disc disorder — *see*
    Disorder, disc, with, radiculopathy
  due to displacement of intervertebral disc (with
    lumbago) — *see* Disorder, disc, with,
    radiculopathy
  left M54.32
  right M54.31

Scimitar syndrome Q26.8

Sclera — *see* condition

Sclerectasia H15.849
  bilateral H15.843
  left H15.842
  right H15.841

Scleredema
  adultorum — *see* Sclerosis, systemic
  Buschke's — *see* Sclerosis, systemic
  newborn P83.0

Sclerema (adiposum) (edematosum) (neonatorum)
  (newborn) P83.0
  adultorum *see* Sclerosis, systemic

Scleriasis — *see* Scleroderma

©2002 Ingenix, Inc.

Scleritis H15.009
  with corneal involvement H15.049
    bilateral H15.043
    left H15.042
    right H15.041
  anterior H15.019
    bilateral H15.013
    left H15.012
    right H15.011
  bilateral H15.003
  brawny H15.029
    bilateral H15.023
    left H15.022
    right H15.021
  in (due to) zoster B02.34
  left H15.002
  posterior H15.039
    bilateral H15.033
    left H15.032
    right H15.031
  right H15.001
  specified type NEC H15.099
    bilateral H15.093
    left H15.092
    right H15.091
  syphilitic A52.71
  tuberculous (nodular) A18.51
Sclerochoroiditis H31.8
Scleroconjunctivitis — see Scleritis
Sclerocystic ovary syndrome E28.2
Sclerodactyly, sclerodactylia L94.3
Scleroderma, sclerodermia (acrosclerotic)
  (diffuse) (generalized) (progressive)
  (pulmonary) — see also Sclerosis, systemic
  circumscribed L94.0
  linear L94.1
  localized L94.0
  newborn P83.8
Sclerokeratitis H16.8
  tuberculous A18.52
Scleroma nasi A48.8
Scleromalacia (perforans) H15.059
  bilateral H15.053
  left H15.052
  right H15.051
Scleromyxedema L98.5
Sclérose en plaques G35
Sclerosis, sclerotic
  adrenal (gland) E27.8
  Alzheimer's — see Disease, Alzheimer's
  amyotrophic (lateral) G12.21
  aorta, aortic I70.0
    valve — see Endocarditis, aortic
  artery, arterial, arteriolar, arteriovascular —
    see Arteriosclerosis
  ascending multiple G35
  brain (generalized) (lobular) G37.9
    artery, arterial I67.2
    atrophic lobar G31.0
      dementia in G31.0 [F02]
    diffuse G37.0
    disseminated G35
    insular G35
    Krabbe's E75.23
    miliary G35
    multiple G35
    presenile (Alzheimer's) — see Disease,
      Alzheimer's, early onset
    senile (arteriosclerotic) I67.2
    stem, multiple G35
    tuberous Q85.1
  bulbar, multiple G35
  bundle of His I44.39
  cardiac — see Disease, heart, ischemic,
    atherosclerotic
  cardiorenal — see Hypertension, cardiorenal
  cardiovascular — see also Disease,
    cardiovascular
    renal — see Hypertension, cardiorenal
  cerebellar — see Sclerosis, brain
  cerebral — see Sclerosis, brain
  cerebrospinal (disseminated) (multiple) G35
  cerebrovascular I67.2
  choroid — see Degeneration, choroid

Sclerosis, sclerotic — continued
  combined (spinal cord) — see also
    Degeneration, combined
    multiple G35
  concentric (Balo) G37.5
  cornea — see Opacity, cornea
  coronary (artery) — see Disease, heart,
    ischemic, atherosclerotic
  corpus cavernosum
    female N90.8
    male N48.6
  diffuse (brain) (spinal cord) G37.0
  disseminated G35
  dorsal G35
  dorsolateral (spinal cord) — see Degeneration,
    combined
  endometrium N85.5
  extrapyramidal G25.9
  eye, nuclear (senile) — see Cataract, senile,
    nuclear
  focal and segmental (glomerular) (see also N00-
    N07 with fourth character .1) N05.1
  Friedreich's (spinal cord) G11.1
  funicular (spermatic cord) N50.8
  general (vascular) — see Arteriosclerosis
  gland (lymphatic) I89.8
  hepatic K74.1
  hereditary
    cerebellar G11.9
    spinal (Friedreich's ataxia) G11.1
  insular G35
  kidney — see Sclerosis, renal
  larynx J38.7
  lateral (amyotrophic) (descending) (primary)
    (spinal) G12.21
  lens, senile nuclear — see Cataract, senile,
    nuclear
  liver K74.1
    with fibrosis K74.2
    alcoholic K70.2
    cardiac K76.1
  lobar, atrophic (of brain) G31.0
    dementia in G31.0 [F02]
  lung — see Fibrosis, lung
  mastoid — see Mastoiditis, chronic
  mitral I05.8
  Mönckeberg's (medial) — see Arteriosclerosis,
    extremities
  multiple (brain stem) (cerebral) (generalized)
    (spinal cord) G35
  myocardium, myocardial — see Disease, heart,
    ischemic, atherosclerotic
  nuclear (senile), eye — see Cataract, senile,
    nuclear
  ovary N83.8
  pancreas K86.8
  penis N48.6
  peripheral arteries — see Arteriosclerosis,
    extremities
  plaques G35
  pluriglandular E31.8
  polyglandular E31.8
  posterolateral (spinal cord) — see Degeneration,
    combined
  presenile (Alzheimer's) — see Disease,
    Alzheimer's, early onset
  primary, lateral G12.29
  progressive, systemic M34.0
  pulmonary — see Fibrosis, lung
    artery I27.0
    valve (heart) — see Endocarditis, pulmonary
  renal N26.9
    with
      cystine storage disease E72.09
      hypertension — see Hypertension, kidney
      hypertensive heart disease (conditions in
        I11) — see Hypertension, cardiorenal
      arteriolar (hyaline) (hyperplastic) — see
        Hypertension, kidney
  retina (senile) (vascular) H35.00
  senile (vascular) — see Arteriosclerosis
  spinal (cord) (progressive) G95.89
    ascending G61.0
    combined — see also Degeneration, combined
      multiple G35
      syphilitic A52.11
    disseminated G35

Sclerosis, sclerotic — continued
  spinal — continued
    dorsolateral — see Degeneration, combined
    hereditary (Friedreich's) (mixed form) G11.1
    lateral (amyotrophic) G12.21
    multiple G35
    posterior (syphilitic) A52.11
  stomach K31.89
  subendocardial, congenital I42.4
  systemic M34.9
    with
      lung involvement M34.81
      myopathy M34.82
      polyneuropathy M34.83
    drug-induced M34.2
    due to chemicals NEC M34.2
    progressive M34.0
    specified NEC M34.89
  tricuspid (heart) (valve) I07.8
  tuberous (brain) Q85.1
  tympanic membrane — see Disorder, tympanic
    membrane, specified NEC
  valve, valvular (heart) — see Endocarditis
  vascular — see Arteriosclerosis
  vein I87.8
Scoliosis (acquired) (postural) M41.9
  adolescent (idiopathic) — see Scoliosis,
    idiopathic, juvenile
  congenital Q67.5
    due to bony malformation Q76.3
    failure of segmentation (hemivertebra) Q76.3
    hemivertebra fusion Q76.3
    postural Q67.5
  idiopathic M41.20
    adolescent M41.129
      cervical region M41.122
      cervicothoracic region M41.123
      lumbar region M41.126
      lumbosacral region M41.127
      multiple sites M41.129
      occipito-atlanto-axial region M41.121
      sacrococcygeal region M41.128
      thoracic region M41.124
      thoracolumbar region M41.125
    cervical region M41.22
    cervicothoracic region M41.23
    infantile M41.00
      cervical region M41.02
      cervicothoracic region M41.03
      lumbar region M41.06
      lumbosacral region M41.07
      occipito-atlanto-axial region M41.01
      sacrococcygeal region M41.08
      thoracic region M41.04
      thoracolumbar region M41.05
    juvenile M41.119
      cervical region M41.112
      cervicothoracic region M41.113
      lumbar region M41.116
      lumbosacral region M41.117
      multiple sites M41.119
      occipito-atlanto-axial region M41.111
      sacrococcygeal region M41.118
      thoracic region M41.114
      thoracolumbar region M41.115
    lumbar region M41.26
    lumbosacral region M41.27
    occipito-atlanto-axial region M41.21
    sacrococcygeal region M41.28
    thoracic region M41.24
    thoracolumbar region M41.25
  neuromuscular M41.40
    cervical region M41.42
    cervicothoracic region M41.43
    lumbar region M41.46
    lumbosacral region M41.47
    occipito-atlanto-axial region M41.41
    sacrococcygeal region M41.48
    thoracic region M41.44
    thoracolumbar region M41.45
  paralytic — see Scoliosis, neuromuscular
  postradiation therapy M96.5
  rachitic (late effect or sequelae) E64.3 [M49.80]
    cervical region E64.3 [M49.82]
    cervicothoracic region E64.3 [M49.83]
    lumbar region E64.3 [M49.86]
    lumbosacral region E64.3 [M49.87]

Scoliosis — continued
  rachitic — continued
    multiple sites E64.3 *[M49.89]*
    occipito-atlanto-axial region E64.3 *[M49.81]*
    sacrococcygeal region E64.3 *[M49.88]*
    thoracic region E64.3 *[M49.84]*
    thoracolumbar region E64.3 *[M49.85]*
  sciatic M54.4
  secondary (to) NEC M41.50
    cerebral palsy, Friedreich's ataxia, poliomyelitis, neuromuscular disorders — *see* Scoliosis, neuromuscular
    cervical region M41.52
    cervicothoracic region M41.53
    lumbar region M41.56
    lumbosacral region M41.57
    occipito-atlanto-axial region M41.51
    sacrococcygeal region M41.58
    thoracic region M41.54
    thoracolumbar region M41.55
  specified form NEC M41.80
    cervical region M41.82
    cervicothoracic region M41.83
    lumbar region M41.86
    lumbosacral region M41.87
    occipito-atlanto-axial region M41.81
    sacrococcygeal region M41.88
    thoracic region M41.84
    thoracolumbar region M41.85
  thoracogenic M41.30
    thoracic region M41.34
    thoracolumbar region M41.35
  tuberculous A18.01

Scoliotic pelvis
  with disproportion (fetopelvic) O33.0
    causing obstructed labor O65.0

Scorbutus, scorbutic — *see also* Scurvy
  anemia D53.2

Scotoma (arcuate) (Bjerrum) (central) (ring) — *see also* Defect, visual field, localized, scotoma
  scintillating H53.19

Scratch — *see* Abrasion

Screening (for) Z13.9
  alcoholism Z13.89
  anemia Z13.0
  anomaly, congenital Z13.89
  antenatal Z36
  arterial hypertension Z13.6
  arthropod-borne viral disease NEC Z11.5
  bacteriuria, asymptomatic Z13.89
  behavioral disorder Z13.89
  bronchitis, chronic Z13.83
  brucellosis Z11.2
  cardiovascular disorder Z13.6
  cataract Z13.5
  chlamydial diseases Z11.8
  cholera Z11.0
  chromosomal abnormalities Z13.89
    by amniocentesis Z36
    postnatal Z13.89
  congenital
    dislocation of hip Z13.89
    eye disorder Z13.5
    malformation or deformation Z13.89
  contamination NEC Z13.88
  cystic fibrosis Z13.228
  dengue fever Z11.5
  dental disorder Z13.84
  depression Z13.89
  developmental handicap Z13.4
    in early childhood Z13.4
  diabetes mellitus Z13.1
  diphtheria Z11.2
  disease or disorder Z13.9
    bacterial NEC Z11.2
      intestinal infectious Z11.0
      respiratory tuberculosis Z11.1
    blood or blood-forming organ Z13.0
    cardiovascular Z13.6
    Chagas' Z11.6
    chlamydial Z11.8
    dental Z13.89
    developmental Z13.4
    digestive tract NEC Z13.818
      lower GI Z13.811
      upper GI Z13.810

Screening — continued
  disease or disorder — continued
    ear Z13.5
    endocrine Z13.29
    eye Z13.5
    genitourinary Z13.89
    heart Z13.6
    human immunodeficiency virus (HIV) infection Z11.4
    immunity Z13.0
    infection
      intestinal Z11.0
        specified NEC Z11.6
    infectious Z11.9
    mental Z13.89
    metabolic Z13.228
    neurological Z13.89
    nutritional Z13.21
      metabolic Z13.228
        lipoid disorders Z13.220
    protozoal Z11.6
      intestinal Z11.0
    respiratory Z13.83
    rheumatic Z13.828
    rickettsial Z11.8
    sexually-transmitted NEC Z11.3
      human immunodeficiency virus (HIV) Z11.4
    sickle-cell (trait) Z13.0
    skin Z13.89
    specified NEC Z13.89
    spirochetal Z11.8
    thyroid Z13.29
    vascular Z13.6
    venereal Z11.3
    viral NEC Z11.5
      human immunodeficiency virus (HIV) Z11.4
      intestinal Z11.0
  emphysema Z13.83
  encephalitis, viral (mosquitoor tick-borne) Z11.5
  exposure to contaminants (toxic) Z13.88
  fever
    dengue Z11.5
    hemorrhagic Z11.5
    yellow Z11.5
  filariasis Z11.6
  galactosemia Z13.228
  gastrointestinal condition Z13.818
  genitourinary condition Z13.89
  glaucoma Z13.5
  gonorrhea Z11.3
  gout Z13.89
  helminthiasis (intestinal) Z11.6
  hematopoietic malignancy Z12.89
  hemoglobinopathies NEC Z13.0
    antenatal Z36
  hemorrhagic fever Z11.5
  Hodgkin's disease Z12.89
  human immunodeficiency virus (HIV) Z11.4
  hypertension Z13.6
  immunity disorders Z13.0
  infection
    mycotic Z11.8
    parasitic Z11.8
  ingestion of radioactive substance Z13.88
  intestinal
    helminthiasis Z11.6
    infectious disease Z11.0
  leishmaniasis Z11.6
  leprosy Z11.2
  leptospirosis Z11.8
  leukemia Z12.89
  lymphoma Z12.89
  malaria Z11.6
  malnutrition Z13.29
    metabolic Z13.228
    nutritional Z13.21
  measles Z11.5
  mental
    disorder Z13.89
    retardation Z13.4
  metabolic errors, inborn Z13.228
  multiphasic Z13.89
  musculoskeletal disorder Z13.828
    osteoporosis Z13.820

Screening — continued
  mycoses Z11.8
  myocardial infarction (acute) Z13.6
  neoplasm (malignant) (of) Z12.9
    bladder Z12.6
    blood Z12.89
    breast Z12.39
      routine mammogram Z12.31
    cervix Z12.4
    colon Z12.11
    genitourinary organs NEC Z12.79
      bladder Z12.6
      cervix Z12.4
      ovary Z12.73
      prostate Z12.5
      testis Z12.71
      vagina Z12.72
    hematopoietic system Z12.89
    intestinal tract Z12.10
      colon Z12.11
      rectum Z12.12
      small intestine Z12.13
    lung Z12.2
    lymph (glands) Z12.89
    nervous system Z12.82
    oral cavity Z12.81
    prostate Z12.5
    rectum Z12.12
    respiratory organs Z12.2
    small intestine Z12.13
    specified site NEC Z12.89
    stomach Z12.0
  nephropathy Z13.89
  neurological condition Z13.89
  obesity Z13.89
  osteoporosis Z13.820
  parasitic infestation Z11.9
    specified NEC Z11.8
  phenylketonuria Z13.228
  plague Z11.2
  poisoning (chemical) (heavy metal) Z13.88
  poliomyelitis Z11.5
  postnatal, chromosomal abnormalities Z13.89
  prenatal Z36
  protozoal disease Z11.6
    intestinal Z11.0
  pulmonary tuberculosis Z11.1
  radiation exposure Z13.88
  respiratory condition Z13.83
  respiratory tuberculosis Z11.1
  rheumatoid arthritis Z13.828
  rubella Z11.5
  schistosomiasis Z11.6
  sexually-transmitted disease NEC Z11.3
    human immunodeficiency virus (HIV) Z11.4
  sickle-cell disease or trait Z13.0
  skin condition Z13.89
  sleeping sickness Z11.6
  special Z13.9
    specified NEC Z13.89
  syphilis Z11.3
  tetanus Z11.2
  trachoma Z11.8
  trypanosomiasis Z11.6
  tuberculosis, respiratory Z11.1
  venereal disease Z11.3
  viral encephalitis (mosquitoor tick-borne) Z11.5
  whooping cough Z11.2
  worms, intestinal Z11.6
  yaws Z11.8
  yellow fever Z11.5

Scrofula, scrofulosis (tuberculosis of cervical lymph glands) A18.2

Scrofulide (primary) (tuberculous) A18.4

Scrofuloderma, scrofulodermia (any site) (primary) A18.4

Scrofulosus lichen (primary) (tuberculous) A18.4

Scrofulous — *see* condition

Scrotal tongue K14.5

Scrotum — *see* condition

Scurvy, scorbutic E54
  anemia D53.2
  gum E54 *[K93]*
  infantile E54
  rickets E55.9 *[M90.80]*

©2002 Ingenix, Inc.

Seasickness T75.3

Seatworm (infection) (infestation) B80

Sebaceous — *see also* condition
 cyst — *see* Cyst, sebaceous

Seborrhea, seborrheic R23.8
 capillitii R23.8
 capitis L21.0
 dermatitis L21.9
  infantile L21.1
 eczema L21.9
  infantile L21.1
 sicca L21.0

Seckel's syndrome Q87.1

Seclusion, pupil — *see* Membrane, pupillary

Secondary
 dentin (in pulp) K04.3
 neoplasm, secondaries (M8000/6) — *see* Table
  of neoplasms, secondary

Secretion
 antidiuretic hormone, inappropriate E22.2
 catecholamine, by pheochromocytoma E27.5
 hormone
  antidiuretic, inappropriate (syndrome) E22.2
  by
   carcinoid tumor E34.0
   pheochromocytoma E27.5
  ectopic NEC E34.2
 urinary
  excessive R35.8
  suppression R34

Section
 cesarean, previous, in pregnancy or childbirth
  O34.21
 nerve, traumatic — *see* Injury, nerve

Segmentation, incomplete (congenital) — *see
 also* Fusion
 bone NEC Q78.8
 lumbosacral (joint) (vertebra) Q76.49

Seitelberger's syndrome (infantile neuraxonal
 dystrophy) G31.89

Seizure(s) (*see also* Convulsions) R56.9
 akinetic — *see* Epilepsy, generalized
 apoplexy, apoplectic I64
 atonic — *see* Epilepsy, generalized
 autonomic (hysterical) F44.5
 brain or cerebral I64
 convulsive — *see* Convulsions
 cortical (focal) (motor) — *see* Epilepsy, focal
 epileptic — *see* Epilepsy
 epileptiform, epileptoid R56.8
  focal — *see* Epilepsy, focal
 febrile R56.0
 heart — *see* Disease, heart
 hysterical F44.5
 Jacksonian (focal) (motor type) (sensory type) —
  see Epilepsy, focal
 newborn P90
 paralysis I64
 uncinate G40.20
  with status epilepticus G40.21

Selenium deficiency, dietary E59

Self-damaging behavior (life-style) Z72.89

Self-harm (attempted)
 history (personal) Z91.5
  in family Z81.8
 observation following (alleged) attempt Z03.8

Self-mutilation (history) Z91.5

Self-poisoning
 history (personal) Z91.5
  in family Z81.8
 observation following (alleged) attempt Z03.6

Semicoma R40.1

Seminal vesiculitis N49.0

Seminoma (M9061/3) C62.90
 anaplastic (M9062/3)
  specified site — *see* Neoplasm, malignant
  unspecified site C62.90
   left C62.92
   right C62.91
 left C62.92
 right C62.91
 specified site — *see* Neoplasm, malignant

Seminoma — *continued*
 spermatocytic (M9063/3)
  specified site — *see* Neoplasm, malignant
  unspecified site C62.90
   left C62.92
   right C62.91

Senear-Usher disease or syndrome L10.4

Senectus R54

Senescence (without mention of psychosis) R54

Senile, senility (*see also* condition) R54
 with
  acute confusional state F05
  mental changes NOS F03
  psychosis NEC — *see* Psychosis, senile
 asthenia R54
 cervix (atrophic) N88.8
 debility R54
 endometrium (atrophic) N85.8
 fallopian tube (atrophic) — *see* Atrophy,
  fallopian tube
 heart (failure) R54
 ovary (atrophic) — *see* Atrophy, ovary
 premature E34.8
 vagina, vaginitis (atrophic) N95.2
 wart L82.1

Sensation
 burning (skin) R20.8
  tongue K14.6
 loss of R20.8
 prickling (skin) R20.2
 tingling (skin) R20.2

Sense loss
 smell — *see* Disturbance, sensation, smell
 taste — *see* Disturbance, sensation, taste
 touch R20.8

Sensibility disturbance (cortical) (deep)
 (vibratory) R20.9

Sensitive, sensitivity — *see also* Allergy
 carotid sinus G90.0
 child (excessive) F93.8
 cold, autoimmune D59.1
 dentin K03.8
 methemoglobin D74.8
 tuberculin, without clinical or radiological
  symptoms R76.1
 visual
  glare H53.71
  impaired contrast H53.72

Sensitiver Beziehungswahn F22

Sensitization, auto-erythrocytic D69.2

Separation
 anxiety, abnormal (of childhood) F93.0
 apophysis, traumatic – code as Fracture, by
  site
 choroid — *see* Detachment, choroid
 epiphysis, epiphyseal
  nontraumatic — *see also*
   Osteochondropathy, specified type
   NEC
  upper femoral — *see* Slipped, epiphysis,
   upper femoral
 traumatic – code as Fracture, by site
 fracture — *see* Fracture
 infundibulum cardiac from right ventricle by a
  partition Q24.3
 joint (traumatic) (current) – code by site under
  Dislocation
 placenta (normally implanted) (premature) —
  see Disorder, placenta, abruptio
 pubic bone, obstetrical trauma O71.6
 retina, retinal — *see* Detachment, retina
 symphysis pubis, obstetrical trauma O71.6
 tracheal ring, incomplete, congenital Q32.1

Sepsis (generalized) — *see also* Septicemia
 with ectopic or molar pregnancy O08.82
 bacterial, newborn P36.9
  due to
   anaerobes NEC P36.5
   Escherichia coli P36.4
   Staphylococcus NEC P36.3
    aureus P36.2
   Streptococcus NEC P36.1
    group B P36.0
  specified type NEC P36.8
 buccal K12.2

Sepsis — *see also* Septicemia — *continued*
 dental (pulpal origin) K04.0
 due to device, implant or graft T85.79
  arterial graft NEC T82.7
  breast (implant) T85.79
  catheter NEC T85.79
   dialysis (renal) T82.7
    intraperitoneal T85.71
   infusion NEC T82.7
    spinal (epidural) (subdural) T85.79
   urinary (indwelling) T83.51
  electronic (electrode) (pulse generator)
   (stimulator)
   bone T84.7
   cardiac T82.7
   nervous system (brain) (peripheral nerve)
    (spinal) T85.79
   urinary T83.59
  fixation, internal (orthopedic) — *see*
   Complication, fixation device, infection
  gastrointestinal (bile duct) (esophagus)
   T85.79
  genital T83.6
  heart NEC T82.7
   valve (prosthesis) T82.6
   graft T82.7
  joint prosthesis — *see* Complication, joint
   prosthesis, infection
  ocular (corneal graft) (orbital implant)
   T85.79
  orthopedic NEC T84.7
   fixation device, internal — *see*
    Complication, fixation device,
    infection
  specified NEC T85.79
  urinary T83.59
  vascular T82.7
  ventricular intracranial shunt T85.79
 following ectopic or molar pregnancy O08.82
  immunization T88.0
  infusion, therapeutic injection or transfusion
   T80.2
 intraocular — *see* Endophthalmitis, purulent
 localized
  in operation wound T81.4
  skin — *see* Abscess
 malleus A24.0
 newborn P36.9
  due to
   anaerobes NEC P36.5
   Escherichia coli P36.4
   Staphylococcus NEC P36.3
    aureus P36.2
   Streptococcus NEC P36.1
    group B P36.0
  specified NEC P36.8
 oral K12.2
 pelvic, puerperal, postpartum, childbirth O85
 puerperal, postpartum, childbirth (pelvic) O85
 skin, localized — *see* Abscess
 tracheostomy stoma J95.02
 umbilical (newborn) (organism unspecified) P38
  tetanus A33
 urinary N39.0

Septate — *see* Septum

Septic — *see also* condition
 arm — *see also* Cellulitis, upper limb
  with lymphangitis — *see* Lymphangitis,
   acute, upper limb
 embolus — *see* Embolism
 finger — *see also* Cellulitis, digit
  with lymphangitis — *see* Lymphangitis,
   acute, digit
 foot — *see also* Cellulitis, lower limb
  with lymphangitis — *see* Lymphangitis,
   acute, lower limb
 gallbladder (acute) K81.0
 hand — *see also* Cellulitis, upper limb
  with lymphangitis — *see* Lymphangitis,
   acute, upper limb
 joint — *see* Arthritis, pyogenic or pyemic
 leg — *see also* Cellulitis, lower limb
  with lymphangitis — *see* Lymphangitis,
   acute, lower limb
 mouth K12.2

Septic — see also condition — continued
  nail — see also Cellulitis, digit
    with lymphangitis — see Lymphangitis, acute, digit
  sore — see also Abscess
    throat J02.0
      streptococcal J02.0
  spleen (acute) D73.8
  teeth, tooth (pulpal origin) K04.4
  throat — see Pharyngitis
  thrombus — see Thrombosis
  toe — see also Cellulitis, digit
    with lymphangitis — see Lymphangitis, acute, digit
  tonsils, chronic J35.01
    with adenoiditis J35.03
  umbilical cord P38
  uterus — see Endometritis
Septicemia, septicemic (generalized) (suppurative) A41.9
  with ectopic or molar pregnancy O08.82
  actinomycotic A42.7
  adrenal hemorrhage syndrome (meningococcal) A39.1
  anaerobic A41.4
  anthrax A22.7
  Bacillus anthracis A22.7
  Bacteroides A41.4
  Brucella — see Brucellosis
  candidal B37.89
  Clostridium A41.4
  cryptogenic A41.9
  due to infusion, therapeutic injection or transfusion T80.2
  during labor O75.3
  enterococcal A41.81
  Erysipelothrix (rhusiopathiae) (erysipeloid) A26.7
  Escherichia coli A41.51
  extraintestinal yersiniosis A28.2
  following
    abortion O06.5
      failed attempted O07.5
        by physician O07.0
      induced O06.5
        by
          non-physician O05.5
          physician O04.5
      spontaneous O03.5
        incomplete O03.0
    ectopic or molar pregnancy O08.82
    immunization T88.0
    infusion, therapeutic injection or transfusion T80.2
    surgical procedure T81.4
  gangrenous A41.9
  gonococcal A54.86
  gram-negative (organism) A41.50
    anaerobic A41.4
    Escherichia coli A41.51
    Pseudomonas aeruginosa A41.52
    Serratia A41.53
    specified NEC A41.59
  Hemophilus influenzae A41.3
  herpesviral B00.7
  herpetic B00.7
  Listeria monocytogenes A32.7
  melioidosis A24.1
  meningeal — see Meningitis
  meningococcal A39.4
    acute A39.2
    chronic A39.3
  newborn NEC — see Sepsis, newborn
  Pasteurella multocida A28.0
  plague A20.7
  pneumococcal A40.3
  postabortal O08.0
  postoperative T81.4
  postprocedural T81.4
  puerperal, postpartum O85
  Salmonella (arizonae) (Cholerae-Suis) (enteritidis) (typhimurium) A02.1
  Shigella — see Dysentery, bacillary
  specified organism NEC A41.89
  Staphylococcus, staphylococcal A41.2
    aureus A41.0
    coagulase-negative A41.1
    specified NEC A41.1

Septicemia, septicemic — continued
  Streptococcus, streptococcal A40.9
    agalactiae A40.1
    group
      A A40.0
      B A40.1
      D A41.81
    neonatal P36.1
    pneumoniae A40.3
    pyogenes A40.0
    specified NEC A40.8
  suipestifer A02.1
  tularemic A21.7
  Yersinia pestis A20.7
Septum, septate (congenital) — see also Anomaly, by site
  anal Q42.3
    with fistula Q42.2
  aqueduct of Sylvius Q03.0
    with spina bifida — see Spina bifida, by site, with hydrocephalus
  uterus — see Double, uterus
  vagina Q52.1
    in pregnancy — see Pregnancy, complicated by, abnormal vagina
    causing obstructed labor O65.5
Sequelae (of) — see also condition
  abscess, intracranial or intraspinal (conditions in G06) G09
  amputation – code to injury with terminal extension of p
  burn and corrosion – code to injury with terminal extension of p
  calcium deficiency E64.8
  cerebrovascular disease NEC — see Sequelae, disease, cerebrovascular, specified type NEC
  childbirth O93
  contusion – code to injury with terminal extension of p
  corrosion — see Sequelae, burn and corrosion
  crushing injury – code to injury with terminal extension of p
  disease
    cerebrovascular I69.90
      hemorrhage
        intracerebral — see Sequelae, hemorrhage, intracerebral
        intracranial, nontraumatic NEC — see Sequelae, hemorrhage, intracranial, nontraumatic
        subarachnoid — see Sequelae, hemorrhage, subarachnoid
      manifested by
        aphasia I69.920
        apraxia I69.990
        cognitive defects I69.91
        dysarthria I69.928
        dysphagia I69.991
        dysphasia I69.921
        hemiplegia I69.959
          dominant (right) I69.951
            left I69.952
          left (nondominant) I69.954
            dominant I69.952
          nondominant (left) I69.954
            right I69.953
          right (dominant) I69.951
            nondominant I69.953
        language deficit NEC I69.928
        monoplegia
          lower limb I69.949
            dominant (right) I69.941
              left I69.942
            left (nondominant) I69.944
              dominant I69.942
            nondominant (left) I69.944
              right I69.943
            right (dominant) I69.941
              nondominant I69.943
          upper limb I69.939
            dominant (right) I69.931
              left I69.932
            left (nondominant) I69.934
              dominant I69.932

Sequelae — see also condition — continued
  disease — continued
    cerebrovascular — continued
      manifested by — continued
        monoplegia — continued
          upper limb — continued
            nondominant (left) I69.934
              right I69.933
            right (dominant) I69.931
              nondominant I69.933
        paralytic syndrome I69.969
          bilateral I69.965
          dominant (right) I69.961
            left I69.962
          left I69.964
            dominant I69.962
          nondominant (left) I69.964
            right I69.963
          right (dominant) I69.961
            nondominant I69.963
        specified effect NEC I69.998
        speech deficit I69.928
      specified type NEC I69.80
        aphasia I69.820
        apraxia I69.890
        cognitive defects I69.81
        dysarthria I69.828
        dysphagia I69.891
        dysphasia I69.821
        hemiplegia I69.859
          dominant (right) I69.851
            left I69.852
          left (nondominant) I69.854
            dominant I69.852
          nondominant (left) I69.854
            right I69.853
          right (dominant) I69.851
            nondominant I69.853
        language deficit I69.828
        monoplegia
          lower limb I69.849
            dominant (right) I69.841
              left I69.842
            left (nondominant) I69.844
              dominant I69.842
            nondominant (left) I69.844
              right I69.843
            right (dominant) I69.841
              nondominant I69.843
          upper limb I69.839
            dominant (right) I69.831
              left I69.832
            left (nondominant) I69.834
              dominant I69.832
            nondominant (left) I69.834
              right I69.833
            right (dominant) I69.831
              nondominant I69.833
        paralytic syndrome I69.869
          bilateral I69.865
          dominant (right) I69.861
            left I69.862
          left (nondominant) I69.864
            dominant I69.862
          nondominant (left) I69.864
            right I69.863
          right (dominant) I69.861
            nondominant I69.863
        specified effect NEC I69.898
        speech deficit I69.828
      stroke NOS — see Sequelae, stroke NOS
  dislocation – code to injury with terminal extension of p
  encephalitis or encephalomyelitis (conditions in G04) G09
    in infectious disease NEC B94.8
    viral B94.1
  external cause – code to injury with terminal extension of p
  foreign body entering natural orifice – code to injury with terminal extension of p
  fracture – code to injury with terminal extension of p
  frostbite – code to injury with terminal extension of p
  Hansen's disease B92

©2002 Ingenix, Inc.

Sequelae — *see also* condition — *continued*
  hemorrhage
    intracerebral I69.10
      aphasia I69.120
      apraxia I69.190
      cognitive defects I69.11
      dysarthria I69.128
      dysphagia I69.191
      dysphasia I69.121
      hemiplegia I69.159
        dominant (right) I69.151
          left I69.152
        left (nondominant) I69.154
          dominant I69.152
        nondominant (left) I69.154
          right I69.153
        right (dominant) I69.151
        nondominant I69.153
      language deficit NEC I69.128
      monoplegia
        lower limb I69.149
          dominant (right) I69.141
            left I69.142
          left (nondominant) I69.144
            dominant I69.142
          nondominant (left) I69.144
            right I69.143
          right (dominant) I69.141
            nondominant I69.143
        upper limb I69.139
          dominant (right) I69.131
            left I69.132
          left (nondominant) I69.134
            dominant I69.132
          nondominant (left) I69.134
            right I69.133
          right (dominant) I69.131
            nondominant I69.133
      paralytic syndrome I69.169
        bilateral I69.165
        dominant (right) I69.161
          left I69.162
        left (nondominant) I69.164
          dominant I69.162
        nondominant (left) I69.164
          right I69.163
        right (dominant) I69.161
          nondominant I69.163
      specified effect NEC I69.198
      speech deficit NEC I69.128
    intracranial, nontraumatic I69.20
      aphasia I69.220
      apraxia I69.290
      cognitive defects I69.21
      dysarthria I69.228
      dysphagia I69.291
      dysphasia I69.221
      hemiplegia I69.259
        dominant (right) I69.251
          left I69.252
        left (nondominant) I69.254
          dominant I69.252
        nondominant (left) I69.254
          right I69.253
        right (dominant) I69.251
          nondominant I69.253
      language deficit NEC I69.228
      monoplegia
        lower limb I69.249
          dominant (right) I69.241
            left I69.242
          left (nondominant) I69.244
            dominant I69.242
          nondominant (left) I69.244
            right I69.243
          right (dominant) I69.241
            nondominant I69.243
        upper limb I69.239
          dominant (right) I69.231
            left I69.232
          left (nondominant) I69.234
            dominant I69.232
          nondominant (left) I69.234
            right I69.233

Sequelae — *see also* condition — *continued*
  hemorrhage — *continued*
    intracranial, nontraumatic — *continued*
      monoplegia — *continued*
        upper limb — *continued*
          right (dominant) I69.231
            nondominant I69.233
      paralytic syndrome I69.269
        bilateral I69.265
        dominant (right) I69.261
          left I69.262
        left (nondominant) I69.264
          dominant I69.262
        nondominant (left) I69.264
          right I69.263
        right (dominant) I69.261
          nondominant I69.263
      specified effect NEC I69.298
      speech deficit NEC I69.228
    subarachnoid I69.00
      aphasia I69.020
      apraxia I69.090
      cognitive defects I69.01
      dysarthria I69.028
      dysphagia I69.091
      dysphasia I69.021
      hemiplegia I69.059
        dominant (right) I69.051
          left I69.052
        left (nondominant) I69.054
          dominant I69.052
        nondominant (left) I69.054
          right I69.053
        right (dominant) I69.051
          nondominant I69.053
      language deficit NEC I69.028
      monoplegia
        lower limb I69.049
          dominant (right) I69.041
            left I69.042
          left (nondominant) I69.044
            dominant I69.042
          nondominant (left) I69.044
            right I69.043
          right (dominant) I69.041
            nondominant I69.043
        upper limb I69.039
          dominant (right) I69.031
            left I69.032
          left (nondominant) I69.034
            dominant I69.032
          nondominant (left) I69.034
            right I69.033
          right (dominant) I69.031
            nondominant I69.033
      paralytic syndrome I69.069
        bilateral I69.065
        dominant (right) I69.061
          left I69.062
        left (nondominant) I69.064
          dominant I69.062
        nondominant (left) I69.064
          right I69.063
        right (dominant) I69.061
          nondominant I69.063
      specified effect NEC I69.098
      speech deficit NEC I69.028
  hepatitis, viral B94.2
  hyperalimentation E68
  infarction
    cerebral I69.30
      aphasia I69.320
      apraxia I69.390
      cognitive defects I69.31
      dysarthria I69.328
      dysphagia I69.391
      dysphasia I69.321
      hemiplegia I69.359
        dominant (right) I69.351
          left I69.352
        left (nondominant) I69.354
          dominant I69.352
        nondominant (left) I69.354
          right I69.353
        right (dominant) I69.351
          nondominant I69.353

Sequelae — *see also* condition — *continued*
  infarction — *continued*
    cerebral — *continued*
      language deficit NEC I69.328
      monoplegia
        lower limb I69.349
          dominant (right) I69.341
            left I69.342
          left (nondominant) I69.344
            dominant I69.342
          nondominant (left) I69.344
            right I69.343
          right (dominant) I69.341
            nondominant I69.343
        upper limb I69.339
          dominant (right) I69.331
            left I69.332
          left (nondominant) I69.334
            dominant I69.332
          nondominant (left) I69.334
            right I69.333
          right (dominant) I69.331
            nondominant I69.333
      paralytic syndrome I69.369
        bilateral I69.365
        dominant (right) I69.361
          left I69.362
        left (nondominant) I69.364
          dominant I69.362
        nondominant (left) I69.364
          right I69.363
        right (dominant) I69.361
          nondominant I69.363
      specified effect NEC I69.398
      speech deficit NEC I69.328
  infection, pyogenic, intracranial or intraspinal G09
  infectious disease B94.9
    specified NEC B94.8
  injury – code to injury with terminal extension of p
  leprosy B92
  meningitis
    bacterial (conditions in G00) G09
    other or unspecified cause (conditions in G03) G09
  muscle (and tendon) injury – code to injury with terminal extension of p
  myelitis — *see* Sequelae, encephalitis
  niacin deficiency E64.8
  nutritional deficiency E64.9
    specified NEC E64.8
  obstetrical condition O93
  parasitic disease B94.9
  phlebitis or thrombophlebitis of intracranial or intraspinal venous sinuses and veins (conditions in G08) G09
  poisoning – code to poisoning with terminal extension of p
    nonmedicinal substance — *see* Sequelae, toxic effect, nonmedicinal substance
  poliomyelitis (acute) B91
  pregnancy O93
  protein-energy malnutrition E64.0
  puerperium O93
  radiation T66
  rickets E64.3
  selenium deficiency E64.8
  sprain and strain – code to injury with terminal extension of p
  stroke NOS I69.40
    aphasia I69.420
    apraxia I69.490
    cognitive defects I69.41
    dysarthria I69.428
    dysphagia I69.491
    dysphasia I69.421
    hemiplegia I69.459
      dominant (right) I69.451
        left I69.452
      left (nondominant) I69.454
        dominant I69.452
      nondominant (left) I69.454
        right I69.453
      right (dominant) I69.451
        nondominant I69.453
    language deficit NEC I69.428

Sequelae — *see also* condition — *continued*
  stroke — *continued*
    monoplegia
      lower limb I69.449
        dominant (right) I69.441
          left I69.442
        left (nondominant) I69.444
          dominant I69.442
        nondominant (left) I69.444
          right I69.443
        right (dominant) I69.441
          nondominant I69.443
      upper limb I69.439
        dominant (right) I69.431
          left I69.432
        left (nondominant) I69.434
          dominant I69.432
        nondominant (left) I69.434
          right I69.433
        right (dominant) I69.431
          nondominant I69.433
    paralytic syndrome I69.469
      bilateral I69.465
      dominant (right) I69.461
        left I69.462
      left (nondominant) I69.464
        dominant I69.462
      nondominant (left) I69.464
        right I69.463
      right (dominant) I69.461
        nondominant I69.463
    specified effect NEC I69.498
    speech deficit NEC I69.428
  tendon and muscle injury – code to injury with
      terminal extension of p
  thiamine deficiency E64.8
  trachoma B94.0
  tuberculosis B90.9
    bones and joints B90.2
    central nervous system B90.0
    genitourinary B90.1
    pulmonary (respiratory) B90.9
    specified organs NEC B90.8
  viral
    encephalitis B94.1
    hepatitis B94.2
  vitamin deficiency NEC E64.8
    A E64.1
    B E64.8
    C E64.2
  wound, open – code to injury with terminal
      extension of p
Sequestration — *see also* Sequestrum
  lung, congenital Q33.2
Sequestrum
  bone — *see* Osteomyelitis, chronic
  dental M27.2
  jaw bone M27.2
  orbit — *see* Osteomyelitis, orbit
  sinus (accessory) (nasal) — *see* Sinusitis
Sequoiosis lung or pneumonitis J67.8
Serology for syphilis
  doubtful
    with signs or symptoms – code by site and
        stage under Syphilis
    follow-up of latent syphilis — *see* Syphilis,
        latent
  negative, with signs or symptoms – code by site
      and stage under Syphilis
  positive A53.0
    with signs or symptoms – code by site and
        stage under Syphilis
  reactivated A53.0
Seroma — *see* Hematoma
Seropurulent — *see* condition
Serositis, multiple K65.8
  pericardial I31.1
  peritoneal K65.8
Serous — *see* condition
Sertoli cell
  adenoma (M8640/0)
    specified site — *see* Neoplasm, benign
    unspecified site
      female D27.9
      male D29.20

Sertoli cell — *continued*
  carcinoma (M8640/3)
    specified site — *see* Neoplasm, malignant
    unspecified site (male) C62.90
      female C56.9
      left C62.92
      right C62.91
  tumor (M8640/0)
    with lipid storage (M8641/0)
      specified site — *see* Neoplasm, benign
      unspecified site
        female D27.9
        male D29.20
    specified site — *see* Neoplasm, benign
    unspecified site
      female D27.9
      male D29.20
Sertoli-Leydig cell tumor (M8631/0)
  specified site — *see* Neoplasm, benign
  unspecified site
    female D27.9
    male D29.20
Serum
  allergy, allergic reaction T80.6
    shock T80.5
  arthritis T80.6
  complication or reaction NEC T80.6
  disease NEC T80.6
  hepatitis — *see also* Hepatitis, viral, type B
    carrier (suspected) of Z22.51
  intoxication T80.6
  neuritis T80.6
  neuropathy G61.1
  poisoning NEC T80.6
  rash NEC T80.6
  reaction NEC T80.6
  sickness NEC T80.6
  urticaria T80.6
Sesamoiditis — *see* Osteomyelitis, specified type
    NEC
Sever's disease or osteochondrosis — *see*
    Osteochondrosis, juvenile, tarsus
Sex
  chromosome mosaics Q97.8
    lines with various numbers of X
        chromosomes Q97.2
  education Z70.8
Sextuplet pregnancy — *see* Pregnancy, sextuplet
Sexual
  function, disorder of (psychogenic) F52.9
  immaturity (female) (male) E30.0
  impotence (psychogenic) organic origin NEC —
      see Dysfunction, sexual, male
  precocity (constitutional) (cryptogenic) (female)
      (idiopathic) (male) E30.1
Sexuality, pathologic — *see* Deviation, sexual
Sézary's disease or syndrome (M9701/3) — *see*
    Lymphoma, non-Hodgkin's type, Sézary's
    disease
Shadow, lung R91
Shaking palsy or paralysis — *see* Parkinsonism
Shallowness, acetabulum — *see* Derangement,
    joint, specified type NEC, hip
Shaver's disease J63.1
Sheath (tendon) — *see* condition
Sheathing, retinal vessels H35.00
Shedding
  nail L60.8
  premature, primary (deciduous) teeth K00.6
Sheehan's disease or syndrome E23.0
Shelf, rectal K62.8
Shell teeth K00.5
Shellshock (current) F43.0
  lasting state — *see* Disorder, post-traumatic
    stress
Shield kidney Q63.1
Shift
  auditory threshold (temporary) H93.249
    bilateral H93.243
    left H93.242
    right H93.241
  mediastinal R93.8

Shifting sleep-work schedule (affecting sleep)
    F51.22
Shiga (-Kruse) dysentery A03.0
Shiga's bacillus A03.0
Shigella (dysentery) — *see* Dysentery, bacillary
Shigellosis A03.9
  Group A A03.0
  Group B A03.1
  Group C A03.2
  Group D A03.3
Shin splints T79.6
Shingles — *see* Herpes, zoster
Shipyard disease or eye B30.0
Shirodkar suture, in pregnancy — *see*
    Pregnancy, complicated by, incompetent
    cervix
Shock R57.9
  with ectopic or molar pregnancy O08.3
  adrenal (cortical) (Addisonian) E27.2
  adverse food reaction (anaphylactic) — *see*
      Shock, anaphylactic, food
  allergic — *see* Shock, anaphylactic
  anaphylactic T78.2
    chemical — *see* Table of Drugs and
        Chemicals
    drug or medicinal substance
      correct substance properly administered
          T88.6
      overdose or wrong substance given or
          taken (by accident) T50.901
        administered with intent to harm by
            another person T50.903
          self T50.902
        circumstances undetermined T50.904
        specified drug — *see* Table of Drugs
            and Chemicals
    following sting(s) — *see* Venom
    food T78.00
      additives T78.06
      dairy products T78.07
      eggs T78.08
      fish T78.03
        shellfish T78.02
      fruit T78.04
      milk T78.07
      nuts T78.05
        peanuts T78.01
      peanuts T78.01
      seeds T78.05
      specified type NEC T78.09
      vegetable T78.04
    immunization T80.5
    serum T80.5
  anaphylactoid — *see* Shock, anaphylactic
  anesthetic
    correct substance properly administered
        T88.2
    overdose or wrong substance given or taken
        — *see* category T41.1
    specified anesthetic — *see* Table of Drugs
        and Chemicals
  birth, fetus or newborn NEC P96.8
  cardiogenic R57.0
  chemical substance — *see* Table of Drugs and
      Chemicals
  complicating ectopic or molar pregnancy O08.3
  culture — *see* Disorder, adjustment
  drug T78.2
    correct substance properly administered
        T88.6
    overdose or wrong substance given or taken
        (by accident) T50.901
      administered with intent to harm by
          another person T50.903
        self T50.902
      circumstances undetermined T50.904
      specified drug — *see* Table of Drugs and
          Chemicals
  during or after labor and delivery O75.1
  electric T75.4
  endotoxic R57.8
    due to surgical procedure T81.1
    during or following procedure T81.1

Shock — *continued*
  following
    ectopic or molar pregnancy O08.3
    injury (immediate) (delayed) T79.4
    labor and delivery O75.1
  food (anaphylactic) — *see* Shock, anaphylactic,
    food
  hematologic R57.8
  hemorrhagic
    surgery (intraoperative) (postoperative) T81.1
    trauma T79.4
  hypovolemic R57.1
    surgical T81.1
    traumatic T79.4
  insulin E15
    therapeutic misadventure — *see* category
      T38.3
  kidney N17.0
    traumatic (following crushing) T79.5
  lightning T75.01
  lung J80
  obstetric O75.1
    with ectopic or molar pregnancy O08.3
    following ectopic or molar pregnancy O08.3
  paralysis, paralytic I64
    due to trauma T79.4
  pleural (surgical) T81.1
    due to trauma T79.4
  postoperative T81.1
    with ectopic or molar pregnancy O08.3
    following ectopic or molar pregnancy O08.3
  psychic F43.0
  septic A41.9
    with ectopic or molar pregnancy O08.82
    due to
      infusion, therapeutic injection or
        transfusion T80.2
      surgical procedure T81.1
    following ectopic or molar pregnancy O08.82
  specified NEC R57.8
  surgical T81.1
  therapeutic misadventure NEC T81.1
  thyroxin
    overdose or wrong substance given or taken
      — *see* category T38.1
  toxic, syndrome A48.3
  transfusion — *see* Complications, transfusion
  traumatic (immediate) (delayed) T79.4

Shoemaker's chest M95.4

Short, shortening, shortness
  arm (acquired) — *see also* Deformity, limb,
    unequal length
    congenital — *see* Defect, reduction, upper
      limb, specified type NEC
    forearm — *see* Deformity, limb, unequal
      length
  bowel syndrome K91.2
  breath R06.02
  common bile duct, congenital Q44.5
  cord (umbilical), complicating delivery O69.3
  cystic duct, congenital Q44.5
  esophagus (congenital) Q39.8
  femur (acquired) — *see* Deformity, limb,
    unequal length, femur
    congenital — *see* Defect, reduction, lower
      limb, longitudinal, femur
  frenum, frenulum, linguae (congenital) Q38.1
  hip (acquired) — *see also* Deformity, limb,
    unequal length
    congenital Q65.8
  leg (acquired) — *see also* Deformity, limb,
    unequal length
    congenital — *see* Defect, reduction, lower
      limb, specified type NEC
    lower leg — *see also* Deformity, limb,
      unequal length
  limbed stature, with immunodeficiency D82.2
  lower limb (acquired) — *see also* Deformity,
    limb, unequal length
    congenital — *see* Defect, reduction, lower
      limb, specified type NEC
  organ or site, congenital NEC — *see* Distortion
  palate, congenital Q38.5
  radius (acquired) — *see also* Deformity, limb,
    unequal length
    congenital — *see* Defect, reduction, upper
      limb, longitudinal, radius

Short, shortening, shortness — *continued*
  rib syndrome Q77.2
  stature NEC — *see* Dwarfism
  tendon — *see also* Contraction, tendon
    with contracture of joint — *see* Contraction,
      joint
    Achilles (acquired) M67.00
      congenital Q66.8
      left M67.02
      right M67.01
    congenital Q79.8
  thigh (acquired) — *see also* Deformity, limb,
    unequal length, femur
    congenital — *see* Defect, reduction, lower
      limb, longitudinal, femur
  tibialis anterior (tendon) — *see* Contraction,
    tendon
  umbilical cord
    complicating delivery O69.3
  upper limb, congenital — *see* Defect, reduction,
    upper limb, specified type NEC
  urethra N36.8
  uvula, congenital Q38.5
  vagina (congenital) Q52.4

Shortsightedness — *see* Myopia

Shoshin (acute fulminating beriberi) E51.11

Shoulder — *see* condition

Shovel-shaped incisors K00.2

Shower, thromboembolic — *see* Embolism

Shunt
  arterial-venous (dialysis) Z99.2
  arteriovenous, pulmonary (acquired) I28.0
    congenital Q25.7
  cerebral ventricle (communicating) in situ
    Z98.2
  surgical, prosthetic, with complications — *see*
    Complications, cardiovascular, device or
    implant

Shutdown, renal — *see* Failure, renal

Shy-Drager syndrome G90.3

Sialadenitis, sialadenosis (any gland) (chronic)
  (periodic) (suppurative) — *see* Sialoadenitis

Sialectasia K11.8

Sialidosis E77.1

Sialitis, silitis (any gland) (chronic) (suppurative)
  — *see* Sialoadenitis

Sialoadenitis (any gland) (periodic) (suppurative)
  K11.20
  acute K11.21
    recurrent K11.22
  chronic K11.23

Sialoadenopathy K11.9

Sialoangitis — *see* Sialoadenitis

Sialodochitis (fibrinosa) — *see* Sialoadenitis

Sialodocholithiasis K11.5

Sialolithiasis K11.5

Sialometaplasia, necrotizing K11.8

Sialorrhea — *see also* Ptyalism
  periodic — *see* Sialoadenitis

Sialosis K11.7

Siamese twin Q89.4

Sibling rivalry Z63.8
  affecting child Z61.2

Sicard's syndrome G52.7

Sicca syndrome M35.00
  with
    keratoconjunctivitis M35.01
    lung involvement M35.02
    myopathy M35.03
    renal tubulo-interstitial disorders M35.04
  specified organ involvement NEC M35.09

Sick R69
  or handicapped person in family Z63.7
    needing care at home Z63.6
  sinus (syndrome) I49.5

Sick-euthyroid syndrome E07.81

Sickle-cell
  anemia — *see* Disease, sickle-cell
  trait D57.3

Sicklemia — *see also* Disease, sickle-cell
  trait D57.3

Sickness
  air (travel) T75.3
  airplane T75.3
  alpine T70.29
  altitude T70.20
  Andes T70.29
  aviator's T70.29
  balloon T70.29
  car T75.3
  compressed air T70.3
  decompression T70.3
  green D50.9
  milk — *see* Poisoning, food, noxious
  motion T75.3
  mountain T70.20
    acute D75.1
  protein T80.6
  radiation T66
  roundabout (motion) T75.3
  sea T75.3
  serum NEC T80.6
  sleeping (African) B56.9
    by Trypanosoma B56.9
      brucei
        gambiense B56.0
        rhodesiense B56.1
      East African B56.1
      Gambian B56.0
      Rhodesian B56.1
      West African B56.0
  swing (motion) T75.3
  train (railway) (travel) T75.3
  travel (any vehicle) T75.3

Sideropenia — *see* Anemia, iron deficiency

Siderosilicosis J62.8

Siderosis (lung) J63.4
  eye (globe) — *see* Disorder, globe, degenerative,
    siderosis

Siemens' syndrome (ectodermal dysplasia) Q82.8

Sighing R06.89
  psychogenic F45.8

Sigmoid — *see also* condition
  flexure — *see* condition
  kidney Q63.1

Sigmoiditis — *see also* Enteritis
  infectious A09
  noninfectious K52.9

Silfverskiöld's syndrome Q78.9

Silicosiderosis J62.8

Silicosis, silicotic (simple) (complicated) J62.8
  with tuberculosis J65

Silicotuberculosis J65

Silo-fillers' disease J68.8

Silver's syndrome Q87.1

Simian malaria B53.1

Simmonds' cachexia or disease E23.0

Simons' disease or syndrome (progressive
  lipodystrophy) E88.1

Simple, simplex — *see* condition

Simulation, conscious (of illness) Z76.5

Sinding-Larsen disease or osteochondrosis —
  see Osteochondrosis, juvenile, patella

Singapore hemorrhagic fever A91

Singer's node or nodule J38.2

Single
  atrium Q21.2
  coronary artery Q24.5
  umbilical artery Q27.0
  ventricle Q20.4

Singultus R06.6
  epidemicus B33.0

Sinus — *see also* Fistula
  abdominal K63.8
  arrest I45.5
  arrhythmia I49.8
  bradycardia I49.8
    chronic I49.5
  branchial cleft (internal) (external) Q18.0
  coccygeal — *see* Sinus, pilonidal
  dental K04.6
  dermal (congenital) Q06.8
    with abscess Q06.8
    coccygeal, pilonidal — *see* Sinus, coccygeal

©2002 Ingenix, Inc.

Softening — *continued*
  brain (necrotic) (progressive) — *continued*
    hemorrhagic — *see* Hemorrhage,
      intracranial, intracerebral
    occlusive I63.5
    thrombotic I63.3
    cartilage — *see* Disorder, cartilage, specified
      type NEC
    cerebellar — *see* Softening, brain
    cerebral — *see* Softening, brain
    cerebrospinal — *see* Softening, brain
    myocardial, heart — *see* Degeneration,
      myocardial
    spinal cord G95.89
    stomach K31.89
Soldier's
  heart F45.8
  patches I31.0
Solitary
  cyst, kidney N28.1
  kidney, congenital Q60.0
Solvent abuse — *see* Disorder, drug-related,
  inhalant
Somatization reaction, somatic reaction — *see*
  Disorder, somatoform
Somnambulism F51.3
  hysterical F44.89
Somnolence R40.0
  nonorganic origin F51.1
  periodic G47.8
Sonne dysentery A03.3
Soor B37.0
Sore
  chiclero B55.1
  Delhi B55.1
  desert — *see* Ulcer, skin
  eye — *see* Pain, ocular
  Lahore B55.1
  mouth K13.7
    canker K12.0
  muscle — *see* Myalgia
  Naga — *see* Ulcer, skin
  of skin — *see* Ulcer, skin
  oriental B55.1
  pressure — *see* Decubitus
  skin L98.9
  soft A57
  throat (acute) — *see also* Pharyngitis
    with influenza, flu, or grippe J10.1
    chronic J31.2
    coxsackie (virus) B08.5
    diphtheritic A36.0
    herpesviral B00.2
    influenzal J10.1
    septic J02.0
    streptococcal (ulcerative) J02.0
    viral NEC J02.8
      coxsackie B08.5
  tropical — *see* Ulcer, skin
  veldt — *see* Ulcer, skin
Soto's syndrome (cerebral gigantism) Q87.3
South African cardiomyopathy syndrome I42.8
Southeast Asian hemorrhagic fever A91
Spacing, abnormal, tooth, teeth M26.3
Spade-like hand (congenital) Q68.1
Spading nail L60.8
  congenital Q84.6
Spanish collar N47.1
Sparganosis B70.1
Spasm(s), spastic, spasticity (*see also* condition)
  R25.2
  accommodation — *see* Spasm, of
    accommodation
  ampulla of Vater K83.4
  anus, ani (sphincter) (reflex) K59.4
    psychogenic F45.8
  artery I73.9
    cerebral G45.9
  Bell's G51.3
  bladder (sphincter, external or internal) N32.8
    psychogenic F45.8
  bronchus, bronchiole J98.0
  cardia K22.0
  cardiac I20.1

Spasm(s), spastic, spasticity (*see also* condition)
  — *continued*
  carpopedal — *see* Tetany
  cerebral (arteries) (vascular) G45.9
  cervix, complicating delivery O62.4
  ciliary body (of accommodation) — *see* Spasm,
    of accommodation
  colon K58.9
    with diarrhea K58.0
    psychogenic F45.8
  common duct K83.8
  compulsive — *see* Tic
  conjugate H51.8
  coronary (artery) I20.1
  diaphragm (reflex) R06.6
    epidemic B33.0
    psychogenic F45.8
  duodenum K59.8
  epidemic diaphragmatic (transient) B33.0
  esophagus (diffuse) K22.4
    psychogenic F45.8
  facial G51.3
  fallopian tube N83.8
  gastrointestinal (tract) K31.89
    psychogenic F45.8
  glottis J38.5
    hysterical F44.4
    psychogenic F45.8
      conversion reaction F44.4
    reflex through recurrent laryngeal nerve
      J38.5
  habit — *see* Tic
  heart I20.1
  hemifacial (clonic) G51.3
  hourglass — *see* Contraction, hourglass
  hysterical F44.4
  infantile G40.40
    with status epilepticus G40.41
  inferior oblique, eye H51.8
  intestinal — *see also* Syndrome, irritable bowel
    K58.9
    psychogenic F45.8
  larynx, laryngeal J38.5
    hysterical F44.4
    psychogenic F45.8
      conversion reaction F44.4
  levator palpebrae superioris — *see* Disorder,
    eyelid function
  lightning G40.40
    with status epilepticus G40.41
  nerve, trigeminal g51.0
  nervous F45.8
  nodding F98.4
  occupational F48.8
  oculogyric H51.8
    psychogenic F45.8
  of accommodation H52.539
    bilateral H52.533
    left H52.532
    right H52.531
  ophthalmic artery — *see* Occlusion, artery,
    retina
  perineal, female N94.8
  peroneo-extensor — *see also* Deformity, limb,
    flat foot
  pharynx (reflex) J39.2
    hysterical F45.8
    psychogenic F45.8
  psychogenic F45.8
  pylorus NEC K31.3
    adult hypertrophic K31.89
    congenital or infantile Q40.0
    psychogenic F45.8
  rectum (sphincter) K59.4
    psychogenic F45.8
  retinal (artery) — *see* Occlusion, artery, retina
  sigmoid — *see also* Syndrome, irritable bowel
    K58.9
    psychogenic F45.8
  sphincter of Oddi K83.4
  stomach K31.89
    neurotic F45.8
  throat J39.2
    hysterical F45.8
    psychogenic F45.8
  tic F95.9
    chronic F95.1
    transient of childhood F95.0

Spasm(s), spastic, spasticity (*see also* condition)
  — *continued*
  tongue K14.8
  torsion (progressive) G24.1
  trigeminal nerve — *see* Neuralgia, trigeminal
  ureter N13.5
  urethra (sphincter) N35.9
  uterus N85.8
    complicating labor O62.4
  vagina N94.2
    psychogenic F52.5
  vascular I73.9
  vasomotor I73.9
  vein NEC I87.8
  viscera — *see* Pain, abdominal
Spasmodic — *see* condition
Spasmophilia — *see* Tetany
Spasmus nutans F98.4
Spastic, spasticity — *see also* Spasm
  child (congenital) (cerebral) (paralysis) G80.0
  cerebral, child G80.0
Speaker's throat R49.8
Specific, specified — *see* condition
Speech
  defect, disorder, disturbance, impediment
    R47.9
    psychogenic, in childhood and adolescence
      F98.8
    slurring R47.81
    specified NEC R47.89
Spencer's disease A08.1
Spens' syndrome (syncope with heart block)
  I45.9
Sperm counts (fertility testing) Z31.41
  postvasectomy Z30.8
  reversal Z31.42
Spermatic cord — *see* condition
Spermatocele N43.40
  congenital Q55.4
  multiple N43.42
  single N43.41
Spermatocystitis N49.0
Spermatocytoma (M9063/3) C62.90
  left C62.92
  right C62.91
  specified site — *see* Neoplasm, malignant
Spermatorrhea N50.8
Sphacelus — *see* Gangrene
Sphenoidal — *see* condition
Sphenoiditis (chronic) — *see* Sinusitis,
  sphenoidal
Sphenopalatine ganglion neuralgia G90.0
Sphericity, increased, lens (congenital) Q12.4
Spherocytosis (congenital) (familial) (hereditary)
  D58.0
  hemoglobin disease D58.0
  sickle-cell (disease) D57.8
Spherophakia Q12.4
Sphincter — *see* condition
Sphincteritis, sphincter of Oddi — *see*
  Cholangitis
Sphingolipidosis E75.3
  specified NEC E75.29
Sphingomyelinosis E75.3
Spicule tooth K00.2
Spider
  fingers — *see* Syndrome, Marfan's
  nevus I78.1
  toes — *see* Syndrome, Marfan's
  vascular I78.1
Spiegler-Fendt
  benign lymphocytoma L98.8
  sarcoid L08.0
Spielmeyer-Vogt disease E75.4
Spina bifida (aperta) Q05.9
  with hydrocephalus Q05.4
  cervical Q05.5
    with hydrocephalus Q05.0
  dorsal Q05.6
    with hydrocephalus Q05.1

Spina bifida (aperta) — *continued*
  fetus (suspected), affecting management of
    pregnancy O35.0
  lumbar Q05.7
    with hydrocephalus Q05.2
  lumbosacral Q05.7
    with hydrocephalus Q05.2
  occulta Q76.0
  sacral Q05.8
    with hydrocephalus Q05.3
  thoracic Q05.6
    with hydrocephalus Q05.1
  thoracolumbar Q05.6
    with hydrocephalus Q05.1
Spindle, Krukenberg's — *see* Pigmentation,
  cornea, posterior
Spine, spinal — *see* condition
Spiradenoma (eccrine) (M8403/0) — *see*
  Neoplasm, skin, benign
Spirillosis A25.0
Spirillum
  minus A25.0
  obermeieri infection A68.0
Spirochetal — *see* condition
Spirochetosis A69.9
  arthritic, arthritica A69.9
  bronchopulmonary A69.8
  icterohemorrhagic A27.0
  lung A69.8
Spirometrosis B70.1
Spitting blood — *see* Hemoptysis
Splanchnoptosis K63.4
Spleen, splenic — *see* condition
Splenectasis — *see* Splenomegaly
Splenitis (interstitial) (malignant) (nonspecific)
  D73.8
  malarial B54
  tuberculous A18.85
Splenocele D73.8
Splenomegaly, splenomegalia (Bengal)
  (cryptogenic) (idiopathic) (tropical) R16.1
  with hepatomegaly R16.2
  cirrhotic D73.2
  congenital Q89.09
  congestive, chronic D73.2
  Egyptian B65.1
  Gaucher's E75.22
  malarial (*see also* Malaria) B54 *[D77]*
  neutropenic — *see* Agranulocytosis
  Niemann-Pick — *see* Niemann-Pick disease or
    syndrome
  siderotic D73.2
  syphilitic A52.79
    congenital (early) A50.08 *[D77]*
Splenopathy D73.9
Splenoptosis D73.8
Splinter — *see* Foreign body, superficial, by site
Split, splitting
  foot Q72.70
    bilateral Q72.73
    left Q72.72
    right Q72.71
  heart sounds R01.2
  lip, congenital — *see* Cleft, lip
  nails L60.3
  urinary stream R39.13
Spondylarthrosis — *see* Spondylosis
Spondylitis (chronic) — *see also* Spondylopathy,
  inflammatory
  ankylopoietica — *see* Spondylitis, ankylosing
  ankylosing (chronic) M45.9
    with lung involvement M45.9 *[J99]*
    cervical region M45.2
    cervicothoracic region M45.3
    juvenile M08.1
    lumbar region M45.6
    lumbosacral region M45.7
    multiple sites M45.0
    occipito-atlanto-axial region M45.1
    sacrococcygeal region M45.8
    thoracic region M45.4
    thoracolumbar region M45.5

Spondylitis (chronic) — *see also* Spondylopathy,
  inflammatory — *continued*
  atrophic (ligamentous) — *see* Spondylitis,
    ankylosing
  deformans (chronic) — *see* Spondylosis
  gonococcal A54.41
  gouty M10.08
  in (due to)
    brucellosis A23.9 *[M49.80]*
      cervical region A23.9 *[M49.82]*
      cervicothoracic region A23.9 *[M49.83]*
      lumbar region A23.9 *[M49.86]*
      lumbosacral region A23.9 *[M49.87]*
      multiple sites A23.9 *[M49.89]*
      occipito-atlanto-axial region A23.9
        [M49.81]
      sacrococcygeal region A23.9 *[M49.88]*
      thoracic region A23.9 *[M49.84]*
      thoracolumbar region A23.9 *[M49.85]*
    enterobacteria (*see also* category M49.8)
      A04.9
    tuberculosis A18.01
  infectious NEC — *see* Spondylopathy, infective
  juvenile ankylosing (chronic) M08.1
  Kümmell's — *see* Spondylopathy, traumatic
  Marie-Strümpell — *see* Spondylitis, ankylosing
  muscularis — *see* Spondylopathy, specified
    NEC
  psoriatic L40.53
  rheumatoid — *see* Spondylitis, ankylosing
  rhizomelica — *see* Spondylitis, ankylosing
  sacroiliac NEC M46.1
  senescent, senile — *see* Spondylosis
  traumatic (chronic) or post-traumatic — *see*
    Spondylopathy, traumatic
  tuberculous A18.01
  typhosa A01.05
Spondylarthrosis — *see* Spondylosis
Spondylolisthesis (acquired) (degenerative)
  M43.10
  with disproportion (fetopelvic) O33.0
    causing obstructed labor O65.0
  cervical region M43.12
  cervicothoracic region M43.13
  congenital Q76.2
  lumbar region M43.16
  lumbosacral region M43.17
  multiple sites M43.19
  occipito-atlanto-axial region M43.11
  sacrococcygeal region M43.18
  thoracic region M43.14
  thoracolumbar region M43.15
  traumatic (old) M43.10
    acute
      fifth cervical (displaced) S12.430
        nondisplaced S12.431
        specified type NEC (displaced) S12.450
          nondisplaced S12.451
        type III S12.44
      fourth cervical (displaced) S12.330
        nondisplaced S12.331
        specified type NEC (displaced) S12.350
          nondisplaced S12.351
        type III S12.34
      second cervical (displaced) S12.130
        nondisplaced S12.131
        specified type NEC (displaced) S12.150
          nondisplaced S12.151
        type III S12.14
      seventh cervical (displaced) S12.630
        nondisplaced S12.631
        specified type NEC (displaced) S12.650
          nondisplaced S12.651
        type III S12.64
      sixth cervical (displaced) S12.530
        nondisplaced S12.531
        specified type NEC (displaced) S12.550
          nondisplaced S12.551
        type III S12.54
      third cervical (displaced) S12.230
        nondisplaced S12.231
        specified type NEC (displaced) S12.250
          nondisplaced S12.251
        type III S12.24

Spondylolysis (acquired) M43.00
  cervical region M43.02
  cervicothoracic region M43.03
  congenital Q76.2
  lumbar region M43.06
  lumbosacral region M43.07
    with disproportion (fetopelvic) O33.0
      causing obstructed labor O65.8
  multiple sites M43.09
  occipito-atlanto-axial region M43.01
  sacrococcygeal region M43.08
  thoracic region M43.04
  thoracolumbar region M43.05
Spondylopathy M48.9
  infective NEC M46.50
    cervical region M46.52
    cervicothoracic region M46.53
    lumbar region M46.56
    lumbosacral region M46.57
    multiple sites M46.59
    occipito-atlanto-axial region M46.51
    sacrococcygeal region M46.58
    thoracic region M46.54
    thoracolumbar region M46.55
  inflammatory M46.90
    cervical region M46.92
    cervicothoracic region M46.93
    lumbar region M46.96
    lumbosacral region M46.97
    multiple sites M46.99
    occipito-atlanto-axial region M46.91
    sacrococcygeal region M46.98
    specified type NEC M46.80
      cervical region M46.82
      cervicothoracic region M46.83
      lumbar region M46.86
      lumbosacral region M46.87
      multiple sites M46.89
      occipito-atlanto-axial region M46.81
      sacrococcygeal region M46.88
      thoracic region M46.84
      thoracolumbar region M46.85
    thoracic region M46.94
    thoracolumbar region M46.95
  neuropathic, in
    syringomyelia and syringobulbia G95.0
    tabes dorsalis A52.11
  specified NEC — *see* category M48.8
  traumatic M48.30
    cervical region M48.32
    cervicothoracic region M48.33
    lumbar region M48.36
    lumbosacral region M48.37
    occipito-atlanto-axial region M48.31
    sacrococcygeal region M48.38
    thoracic region M48.34
    thoracolumbar region M48.35
Spondylosis M47.9
  with
    disproportion (fetopelvic) O33.0
      causing obstructed labor O65.0
    myelopathy NEC M47.10
      cervical region M47.12
      cervicothoracic region M47.13
      lumbar region M47.16
      lumbosacral region M47.17
      occipito-atlanto-axial region M47.11
      sacrococcygeal region M47.18
      thoracic region M47.14
      thoracolumbar region M47.15
    radiculopathy M47.20
      cervical region M47.22
      cervicothoracic region M47.23
      lumbar region M47.26
      lumbosacral region M47.27
      occipito-atlanto-axial region M47.21
      sacrococcygeal region M47.28
      thoracic region M47.24
      thoracolumbar region M47.25
  traumatic — *see* Spondylopathy, traumatic
  without myelopathy or radiculopathy M47.819
    cervical region M47.812
    cervicothoracic region M47.813
    lumbar region M47.816
    lumbosacral region M47.817
    occipito-atlanto-axial region M47.811
    sacrococcygeal region M47.818

Spondylosis — *continued*
  without myelopathy or radiculopathy — *continued*
    thoracic region M47.814
    thoracolumbar region M47.815

Sponge
  inadvertently left in operation wound — *see* Foreign body, accidentally left following a procedure
  kidney (medullary) Q61.5

Sponge-diver's disease — *see* Toxicity, venom, marine animal, sea anemone

Spongioblastoma (M9422/3)
  multiforme (M9440/3)
    specified site — *see* Neoplasm, malignant
    unspecified site C71.9
  polare (M9423/3)
    specified site — *see* Neoplasm, malignant
    unspecified site C71.9
  primitive polar (M9443/3)
    specified site — *see* Neoplasm, malignant
    unspecified site C71.9
  specified site — *see* Neoplasm, malignant
  unspecified site C71.9

Spongioneuroblastoma (M9504/3) — *see* Neoplasm, malignant

Spontaneous — *see also* condition
  fracture (cause unknown) — *see* Fracture, pathological

Spoon nail L60.3
  congenital Q84.6

Sporadic — *see* condition

Sporothrix schenckii infection — *see* Sporotrichosis

Sporotrichosis B42.9
  arthritis B42.82
  disseminated B42.7
  generalized B42.7
  lymphocutaneous (fixed) (progressive) B42.1
  pulmonary B42.0
  specified NEC B42.89

Spots, spotting
  Bitot's — *see also* Pigmentation, conjunctiva
    in the young child E50.1
    vitamin A deficiency E50.1
  café, au lait L81.3
  Cayenne pepper I78.1
  cotton wool, retina — *see* Occlusion, artery, retina
  de Morgan's (senile angiomas) I78.1
  Fuchs' black (myopic) — *see* Disorder, globe, degenerative, myopia
  intermenstrual (regular) N92.0
    irregular N92.1
  Koplik's B05.9
  liver L81.4
  purpuric R23.3
  ruby I78.1

Spotted fever — *see* Fever, spotted N92.3

Sprain, strain (joint) (ligament) (muscle) (tendon)
  Achilles tendon S86.019
    left S86.012
    right S86.011
  acromioclavicular joint or ligament S43.50
    left S43.52
    right S43.51
  ankle S93.409
    calcaneofibular ligament S93.419
      left S93.412
      right S93.411
    deltoid ligament S93.429
      left S93.422
      right S93.421
    internal collateral ligament — *see* Sprain, ankle, specified ligament NEC
    left S93.402
    right S93.401
    specified ligament NEC S93.499
      left S93.492
      right S93.491
    talofibular ligament — *see* Sprain, ankle, specified ligament NEC
    tibiofibular ligament S93.439
      left S93.432
      right S93.431

Sprain, strain — *continued*
  anterior longitudinal, cervical S13.4
  atlas, atlanto-axial, atlanto-occipital S13.4
  breast bone — *see* Sprain, sternum
  calcaneofibular — *see* Sprain, ankle
  carpal — *see* Sprain, wrist
  carpometacarpal — *see* Sprain, hand, specified site NEC
  cartilage
    costal S23.41
    semilunar (knee) — *see* Sprain, knee, specified site NEC
      with current tear — *see* Tear, meniscus
    thyroid region S13.5
    xiphoid — *see* Sprain, sternum
  cervical, cervicodorsal, cervicothoracic S13.4
  chondrosternal S23.421
  coracoclavicular S43.80
    left S43.82
    right S43.81
  coracohumeral S43.419
    left S43.412
    right S43.411
  coronary, knee — *see* Sprain, knee, specified site NEC
  costal cartilage S23.41
  cricoarytenoid articulation or ligament S13.5
  cricothyroid articulation S13.5
  cruciate, knee — *see* Sprain, knee, cruciate
  deltoid, ankle — *see* Sprain, ankle
  dorsal (spine) S23.3
  elbow S53.409
    left S53.402
    right S53.401
    radial collateral ligament S53.439
      left S53.432
      right S53.431
    radiohumeral S53.419
      left S53.412
      right S53.411
    rupture
      radial collateral ligament — *see* Rupture, traumatic, ligament, radial collateral
      ulnar collateral ligament — *see* Rupture, traumatic, ligament, ulnar collateral
    specified type NEC S53.499
      left S53.492
      right S53.491
    ulnar collateral ligament S53.449
      left S53.442
      right S53.441
    ulnohumeral S53.429
      left S53.422
      right S53.421
  femur, head — *see* Sprain, hip
  fibular collateral, knee — *see* Sprain, knee, collateral
  fibulocalcaneal — *see* Sprain, ankle
  finger(s) S63.619
    index S63.618
      left S63.611
      right S63.610
    interphalangeal (joint) S63.639
      index S63.638
        left S63.631
        right S63.630
      little S63.638
        left S63.637
        right S63.636
      middle S63.638
        left S63.633
        right S63.632
      ring S63.638
        left S63.635
        right S63.634
    little S63.618
      left S63.617
      right S63.616
    metacarpophalangeal (joint) S63.659
      index S63.658
        left S63.651
        right S63.650
      little S63.658
        left S63.657
        right S63.656

Sprain, strain — *continued*
  finger(s) — *continued*
    metacarpophalangeal — *continued*
      middle S63.658
        left S63.653
        right S63.652
      ring S63.658
        left S63.655
        right S63.654
    middle S63.618
      left S63.613
      right S63.612
    ring S63.618
      left S63.615
      right S63.614
    specified site NEC S63.699
      index S63.698
        left S63.691
        right S63.690
      little S63.698
        left S63.697
        right S63.696
      middle S63.698
        left S63.693
        right S63.692
      ring S63.698
        left S63.695
        right S63.694
  foot S93.609
    left S93.602
    right S93.601
    specified ligament NEC S93.699
      left S93.692
      right S93.691
    tarsal ligament S93.619
      left S93.612
      right S93.611
    tarsometatarsal ligament S93.629
      left S93.622
      right S93.621
    toe — *see* Sprain, toe
  hand S63.90
    finger — *see* Sprain, finger
    left S63.92
    right S63.91
    specified site NEC — *see* category S63.8
    thumb — *see* Sprain, thumb
  head S03.9
  hip S73.109
    iliofemoral ligament S73.119
      left S73.112
      right S73.111
    ischiocapsular (ligament) S73.129
      left S73.122
      right S73.121
    left S73.102
    right S73.101
    specified NEC S73.199
      left S73.192
      right S73.191
  iliofemoral — *see* Sprain, hip
  innominate
    acetabulum — *see* Sprain, hip
    sacral junction S33.6
  internal
    collateral, ankle — *see* Sprain, ankle
    semilunar cartilage — *see* Sprain, knee, specified site NEC
  interphalangeal
    finger — *see* Sprain, finger, interphalangeal (joint)
    toe — *see* Sprain, toe, interphalangeal joint
  ischiocapsular — *see* Sprain, hip
  ischiofemoral — *see* Sprain, hip
  jaw (articular disc) (cartilage) (meniscus) S03.4
    old M26.69
  knee S83.90
    collateral ligament S83.409
      lateral (fibular) S83.429
        left S83.422
        right S83.421
      left S83.402
      medial (tibial) S83.419
        left S83.412
        right S83.411
      right S83.401

Sprain, strain — continued
knee — continued
  cruciate ligament S83.509
    anterior S83.519
      left S83.512
      right S83.511
    left S83.502
    posterior S83.529
      left S83.522
      right S83.521
    right S83.501
  lateral (fibular) collateral ligament S83.429
    left S83.422
    right S83.421
  left S83.92
  medial (tibial) collateral ligament S83.419
    left S83.412
    right S83.411
  patellar ligament S83.819
    left S83.812
    right S83.811
  right S83.91
  specified site NEC S83.899
    left S83.892
    right S83.891
  superior tibiofibular joint (ligament) S83.60
    left S83.62
    right S83.61
lateral collateral, knee — see Sprain, knee, collateral
lumbar (spine) S33.5
lumbosacral S33.9
mandible (articular disc) S03.4
  old M26.69
medial collateral, knee — see Sprain, knee, collateral
meniscus
  jaw S03.4
    old M26.69
  knee — see Sprain, knee, specified site NEC
    with current tear — see Tear, meniscus
      old — see Derangement, knee, meniscus, due to old tear
  mandible S03.4
    old M26.69
metacarpal (distal) (proximal) — see Sprain, hand, specified site NEC
metacarpophalangeal — see Sprain, finger, metacarpophalangeal (joint)
metatarsophalangeal — see Sprain, toe, metatarsophalangeal joint
midcarpal — see Sprain, hand, specified site NEC
midtarsal — see Sprain, foot, specified site NEC
neck S13.9
  anterior longitudinal cervical ligament S13.4
  atlanto-axial joint S13.4
  atlanto-occipital joint S13.4
  cervical spine S13.4
  cricoarytenoid ligament S13.5
  cricothyroid ligament S13.5
  specified site NEC S13.8
  thyroid region (cartilage) S13.5
nose S03.8
orbicular, hip — see Sprain, hip
patella — see Sprain, knee, specified site NEC
pelvis NEC S33.8
phalanx
  finger — see Sprain, finger
  toe — see Sprain, toe
pubofemoral — see Sprain, hip
radiocarpal — see Sprain, wrist
radiohumeral — see Sprain, elbow
radius, collateral — see Rupture, traumatic, ligament, radial collateral
rib (cage) S23.41
rotator cuff (capsule) S43.429
  left S43.422
  right S43.421
sacroiliac (region)
  chronic or old — see category M53.2
  joint S33.6
scaphoid (hand) — see Sprain, hand, specified site NEC
scapula(r) — see Sprain, shoulder girdle, specified site NEC

Sprain, strain — continued
semilunar cartilage (knee) — see Sprain, knee, specified site NEC
  with current tear — see Tear, meniscus
    old — see Derangement, knee, meniscus, due to old tear
shoulder joint S43.409
  acromioclavicular joint (ligament) — see Sprain, acromioclavicular joint
  blade — see Sprain, shoulder, girdle, specified site NEC
  coracoclavicular joint (ligament) — see Sprain, coracoclavicular joint
  coracohumeral ligament — see Sprain, coracohumeral joint
  girdle S43.90
    left S43.92
    right S43.91
    specified site NEC S43.80
      left S43.82
      right S43.81
  left S43.402
  right S43.401
  rotator cuff — see Sprain, rotator cuff
  specified site NEC S43.499
    left S43.492
    right S43.491
  sternoclavicular joint (ligament) — see Sprain, sternoclavicular joint
spine
  cervical S13.4
  lumbar S33.5
  thoracic S23.3
sternoclavicular joint S43.60
  left S43.62
  right S43.61
sternum S23.429
  chondrosternal joint S23.421
  specified site NEC S23.428
  sternoclavicular (joint) (ligament) S23.420
symphysis
  jaw S03.4
    old M26.69
  mandibular S03.4
    old M26.69
talofibular — see Sprain, ankle
tarsal — see Sprain, foot, specified site NEC
tarsometatarsal — see Sprain, foot, specified site NEC
temporomandibular S03.4
  old M26.69
thorax S23.9
  specified site NEC S23.8
  spine S23.3
thorax S23.9
  ribs S23.41
  specified site NEC S23.8
  spine S23.3
  sternum — see Sprain, sternum
thumb S63.609
  interphalangeal (joint) S63.629
    left S63.622
    right S63.621
  left S63.602
  metacarpophalangeal (joint) S63.649
    left S63.642
    right S63.641
  right S63.601
  specified site NEC S63.689
    left S63.682
    right S63.681
thyroid cartilage or region S13.5
tibia (proximal end) — see Sprain, knee, specified site NEC
tibial collateral, knee — see Sprain, knee, collateral
tibiofibular
  distal — see Sprain, ankle
  superior — see Sprain, knee, specified site NEC
toe(s) S93.509
  great S93.503
    left S93.502
    right S93.501

Sprain, strain — continued
toe(s) — continued
  interphalangeal joint S93.519
    great S93.513
      left S93.512
      right S93.511
    lesser S93.516
      left S93.515
      right S93.514
  lesser S93.506
    left S93.505
    right S93.504
  metatarsophalangeal joint S93.529
    great S93.523
      left S93.522
      right S93.521
    lesser S93.526
      left S93.525
      right S93.524
ulna, collateral — see Rupture, traumatic, ligament, ulnar collateral
ulnohumeral — see Sprain, elbow
wrist S63.509
  carpal S63.519
    left S63.512
    right S63.511
  left S63.502
  radiocarpal S63.529
    left S63.522
    right S63.521
  right S63.501
  specified site NEC S63.599
    left S63.592
    right S63.591
  xiphoid cartilage — see Sprain, sternum
Sprengel's deformity (congenital) Q74.0
Sprue (tropical) K90.1
  celiac K90.0
  idiopathic K90.0
  meaning thrush B37.0
  nontropical K90.0
Spur, bone — see also Enthesopathy
  calcaneal M77.30
    left M77.32
    right M77.31
  iliac crest M76.20
    left M76.22
    right M76.21
  nose (septum) J34.8
Spurway's syndrome Q78.0
Sputum
  abnormal (amount) (color) (odor) (purulent) R09.3
  blood-stained R04.2
  excessive (cause unknown) R09.3
Squamous — see also condition
  epithelium in
    cervical canal (congenital) Q51.8
    uterine mucosa (congenital) Q51.8
Squashed nose M95.0
  congenital Q67.4
Squeeze, divers' T70.3
Squint — see also Strabismus
  accommodative — see Strabismus, convergent concomitant
St. Hubert's disease A82.9
Stab — see also Laceration
  internal organs — see Injury, by site
Stafne's cyst or cavity M27.0
Staggering gait R26.0
  hysterical F44.4
Staghorn calculus — see Calculus, kidney
Stähli's line (cornea) (pigment) — see Pigmentation, cornea, anterior
Stain, staining
  port wine Q82.5
  tooth, teeth (hard tissues) (extrinsic) K03.6
    due to
      accretions K03.6
      deposits (betel) (black) (green) (materia alba) (orange) (soft) (tobacco) K03.6
      metals (copper) (silver) K03.7
      nicotine K03.6
      pulpal bleeding K03.7
      tobacco K03.6

©2002 Ingenix, Inc.

Stain, staining — *continued*
  tooth, teeth — *continued*
    intrinsic K00.8
Stammering F98.5
Standstill
  auricular I45.5
  cardiac — *see* Arrest, cardiac
  sinoatrial I45.5
  ventricular — *see* Arrest, cardiac
Stannosis J63.5
Stanton's disease — *see* Melioidosis
Staphylitis (acute) (catarrhal) (chronic)
  (gangrenous) (membranous) (suppurative)
  (ulcerative) K12.2
Staphylococcal scalded skin syndrome L00
Staphylococcemia A41.2
Staphylococcus, staphylococcal — *see also*
  condition
  as cause of disease classified elsewhere B95.8
  aureus, as cause of disease classified elsewhere
    B95.6
  specified NEC, as cause of disease classified
    elsewhere B95.7
Staphyloma (sclera)
  cornea H18.729
    bilateral H18.723
    left H18.722
    right H18.721
  equatorial H15.819
    bilateral H15.813
    left H15.812
    right H15.811
  localized (anterior) H15.829
    bilateral H15.823
    left H15.822
    right H15.821
  posticum H15.839
    bilateral H15.833
    left H15.832
    right H15.831
  ring H15.859
    bilateral H15.853
    left H15.852
    right H15.851
Stargardt's disease — *see* Dystrophy, retina
Starvation (inanition) (due to lack of food)T73.0
  edema — *see* Malnutrition, severe
Stasis
  bile (noncalculous) K83.1
  bronchus J98.0
    with infection — *see* Bronchitis
  cardiac — *see* Failure, heart, congestive
  cecum K59.8
  colon K59.8
  dermatitis — *see* Varix, leg, with, inflammation
  duodenal K31.5
  eczema — *see* Varix, leg, with, inflammation
  foot T69.00
    left T69.04
    right T69.03
  ileocecal coil K59.8
  ileum K59.8
  intestinal K59.8
  jejunum K59.8
  kidney N19
  liver (cirrhotic) K76.1
  lymphatic I89.8
  pneumonia J18.2
  pulmonary — *see* Edema, lung
  rectal K59.8
  renal N19
    tubular N17.0
  ulcer — *see* Varix, leg, with, ulcer
  urine — *see* Retention, urine
  venous I87.8
State (of)
  affective and paranoid, mixed, organic
    psychotic F06.8
  agitated R45.1
    acute reaction to stress F43.0
  anxiety (neurotic) F41.1
  apprehension F41.1
  burn-out Z73.0
  climacteric, female N95.1
    following induced menopause N95.3

State — *continued*
  clouded epileptic or paroxysmal G40.80
    with status epilepticus G40.81
  compulsive F42
    mixed with obsessional thoughts F42
  confusional (psychogenic) F44.89
    acute — *see also* Delirium
      with
        arteriosclerotic dementia F01.50
          with behavioral disturbance F01.51
        senility or dementia F05
      alcoholic F10.231
    epileptic F05
    reactive (from emotional stress,
      psychological trauma) F44.89
    subacute — *see* Delirium
  convulsive — *see* Convulsions
  crisis F43.0
  depressive F32.9
    neurotic F34.1
  dissociative F44.9
  emotional shock (stress) R45.7
  hypercoagulation — *see* Hypercoagulation
  locked-in G83.5
  menopausal N95.1
    artificial N95.3
    following induced menopause N95.3
  neurotic F48.9
    with depersonalization F48.1
  obsessional F42
  oneiroid (schizophrenia-like) F23
  organic
    hallucinatory (nonalcoholic) F06.0
    paranoid (-hallucinatory) F06.2
  panic F41.0
  paranoid F22
    climacteric F22
    involutional F22
    menopausal F22
    organic F06.2
    senile F03
    simple F22
  persistent vegetative R40.3
  phobic F40.9
  postleukotomy F07.0
  pregnant — *see* Pregnancy
  psychogenic, twilight F44.89
  psychopathic (constitutional) F60.2
  psychotic, organic — *see also* Psychosis, organic
    mixed paranoid and affective F06.8
    senile or presenile F03
    transient NEC F06.8
      with
        hallucinations F06.0
        depression F06.31
  residual schizophrenic F20.5
  restlessness R45.1
  stress (emotional) R45.7
  tension (mental) F48.9
    specified NEC F48.8
  transient organic psychotic NEC F06.8
    depressive type F06.31
    hallucinatory type F06.30
  twilight
    epileptic F05
    psychogenic F44.89
  vegetative, persistent R40.3
  vital exhaustion Z73.0
  withdrawal, see Withdrawal, state
Status (post)
  absence, epileptic — *see* Epilepsy, by type, with
    status epilepticus
  adrenalectomy (unilateral) (bilateral) E89.6
  anastomosis Z98.0
  angioplasty (peripheral) Z95.82
    with implant Z95.83
    coronary artery Z95.50
      with implant Z95.51
      specified type NEC Z95.59
  anginosus I20.9
  aortocoronary bypass Z95.1
  arthrodesis Z98.1
  artificial opening (of) Z93.9
    gastrointestinal tract Z93.4
    specified NEC Z93.8
    urinary tract Z93.6
    vagina Z93.8

Status — *continued*
  asthmaticus — *see* Asthma, by type, with
    status asthmaticus
  cholecystectomy Z90.4
  colectomy (complete) (partial) Z90.4
  colostomy Z93.3
  convulsivus idiopathicus — *see* Epilepsy, by
    type, with status epilepticus
  coronary artery angioplasty — *see* Status,
    angioplasty, coronary artery
  cystectomy (urinary bladder) Z90.6
  cystostomy Z93.50
    appendico-vesicostomy Z93.52
    cutaneous Z93.51
    specified NEC Z93.59
  dialysis Z99.2
  donor — *see* Donor
  enterostomy Z93.4
  epileptic, epilepticus — *see* Epilepsy, by type,
    with status epilepticus
  gastrectomy (complete) (partial) Z90.3
  gastrostomy Z93.1
  grand mal G40.61
  human immunodeficiency virus (HIV) infection,
    asymptomatic Z21
  hysterectomy (complete) (partial) Z90.71
  ileostomy Z93.2
  immaturity Z91.729
    less than 28 weeks Z91.720
    28-37 weeks Z91.721
  intestinal bypass Z98.0
  jejunostomy Z93.4
  laryngectomy Z90.02
  low birth weight Z91.719
    less than 500 grams Z91.710
    500-999 grams Z91.711
    1000-1499 grams Z91.712
    1500-1999 grams Z91.713
    2000-2500 grams Z91.714
  lymphaticus E32.8
  marmoratus G80.3
  mastectomy (unilateral) (bilateral) Z90.1
  medicament regimen for a long term (current)
    NEC Z79.8
    antibiotics Z79.2
    anticoagulants Z79.1
      with hemorrhage D68.5
    aspirin Z79.8
    hormone, post-menopausal Z79.3
    multiple Z79.4
  nephrectomy (unilateral) (bilateral) Z90.5
  nephrostomy Z93.6
  oophorectomy (unilateral) (bilateral) Z90.79
  organ replacement
    by artificial or mechanical device or
      prosthesis of
      artery Z95.89
      bladder Z96.0
      blood vessel Z95.89
      breast Z97.8
      eye globe Z97.0
      heart Z95.89
        valve Z95.2
      intestine Z97.8
      joint Z96.60
        hip — *see* Presence, hip joint implant
        knee — *see* Presence, knee joint
          implant
        specified site NEC Z96.698
      kidney Z97.8
      larynx Z96.3
      lens Z96.1
      limbs — *see* Presence, artificial, limb
      liver Z97.8
      lung Z97.8
      pancreas Z97.8
    by organ transplant (heterologous)
      (homologous) — *see* Transplant
  pacemaker
    brain Z96.89
    cardiac Z95.0
    specified NEC Z96.89
  pancreatectomy Z90.4
  petit mal G40.71
  pneumonectomy (complete) (partial) Z90.2
  pneumothorax, therapeutic Z98.3

Status — *continued*
postcommotio cerebri F07.81
postoperative NEC Z98.8
  pneumothorax, therapeutic Z98.3
postpartum (routine follow-up) Z39.2
  care immediately after delivery Z39.0
postsurgical NEC Z98.8
  pneumothorax, therapeutic Z98.3
prosthesis coronary angioplasty Z95.51
pseudophakia Z96.1
renal dialysis Z99.2
reversed jejunal transposition (for bypass) Z98.0
salpingo-oophorectomy (unilateral) (bilateral) Z90.79
shunt
  arteriovenous (for dialysis) Z99.2
  cerebrospinal fluid Z98.2
  ventricular (communicating) (for drainage) Z98.2
splenectomy D73.0
thymicolymphaticus E32.8
thymicus E32.8
thymolymphaticus E32.8
thyroidectomy (hypothyroidism) E89.0
tracheostomy Z93.0
transplant — *see* Transplant
tubal ligation Z98.51
ureterostomy Z93.6
urethrostomy Z93.6
vagina, artificial Z93.8
vasectomy Z98.52

Stealing
child problem F91.8
  in company with others Z72.810
pathological (compulsive) F63.2

Steam burn — *see* Burn

Steatocystoma multiplex L72.2

Steatoma L72.1
eyelid (cystic) — *see* Dermatosis, eyelid
infected — *see* Hordeolum

Steatorrhea (chronic) K90.4
with lacteal obstruction K90.2
idiopathic (adult) (infantile) K90.0
pancreatic K90.3
primary K90.0
tropical K90.1

Steatosis E88.8
heart — *see* Degeneration, myocardial
kidney N28.89
liver NEC K76.0

Steele-Richardson-Olszewski disease or syndrome G23.1

Steinbrocker's syndrome G90.8

Steinert's disease G71.1

Stein-Leventhal syndrome E28.2

Stein's syndrome E28.2

Stenocardia I20.8

Stenocephaly Q75.8

Stenosis, stenotic (cicatricial) — *see also* Stricture
ampulla of Vater K83.1
anus, anal (canal) (sphincter) K62.4
  and rectum K62.4
  congenital Q42.3
    with fistula Q42.2
aorta (ascending) (supraventricular) (congenital) Q25.3
  arteriosclerotic I70.0
  calcified I70.0
aortic (valve) I35.0
  with insufficiency I35.2
  congenital Q23.0
  rheumatic I06.0
    with
      incompetency, insufficiency or regurgitation I06.2
        with mitral (valve) disease I08.0
          with tricuspid (valve) disease I08.3
      mitral (valve) disease I08.0
        with tricuspid (valve) disease I08.3
      tricuspid (valve) disease I08.2
        with mitral (valve) disease I08.3
  specified cause NEC I35.0
  syphilitic A52.03

Stenosis, stenotic — *see also* Stricture — *continued*
aqueduct of Sylvius (congenital) Q03.0
  with spina bifida — *see* Spina bifida, by site, with hydrocephalus
  acquired G91.1
artery I77.1
  celiac I77.4
  cerebral — *see* Occlusion, artery, cerebral
  pulmonary (congenital) Q25.6
    acquired I28.8
  renal I70.1
bile duct (common) (hepatic) K83.1
  congenital Q44.3
bladder-neck (acquired) N32.0
  congenital Q64.31
brain G93.8
bronchus J98.0
  congenital Q32.3
  syphilitic A52.72
cardia (stomach) K22.2
  congenital Q40.2
cardiovascular — *see* Disease, cardiovascular
caudal M48.08
cervix, cervical (canal) N88.2
  congenital Q51.8
  in pregnancy or childbirth — *see* Pregnancy, complicated by, abnormal cervix
colon — *see also* Obstruction, intestine
  congenital Q42.9
    specified NEC Q42.8
colostomy K94.03
common (bile) duct K83.1
  congenital Q44.3
coronary (artery) — *see* Disease, heart, ischemic, atherosclerotic
cystic duct — *see* Obstruction, gallbladder
due to presence of device, implant or graft (*see also* Complications, by site and type, specified NEC) T85.85
  arterial graft NEC T82.858
  breast (implant) T85.85
  catheter T83.85
    dialysis (renal) T82.858
      intraperitoneal T85.85
    infusion NEC T82.858
      spinal (epidural) (subdural) T85.85
    urinary (indwelling) T83.85
  fixation, internal (orthopedic) NEC T84.85
  gastrointestinal (bile duct) (esophagus) T85.85
  genital NEC T83.85
  heart NEC T82.857
  joint prosthesis T84.85
  ocular (corneal graft) (orbital implant) NEC T85.85
  orthopedic NEC T84.85
  specified NEC T85.85
  urinary NEC T83.85
  vascular NEC T82.858
  ventricular intracranial shunt T85.85
duodenum K31.5
  congenital Q41.0
ejaculatory duct NEC N50.8
endocervical os — *see* Stenosis, cervix
enterostomy K94.13
esophagus K22.2
  congenital Q39.3
  syphilitic A52.79
    congenital A50.59 *[K23]*
eustachian tube — *see* Obstruction, eustachian tube
external ear canal (acquired) H61.309
  bilateral H61.303
  congenital Q16.1
  due to
    inflammation H61.329
      bilateral H61.323
      left H61.322
      right H61.321
    trauma H61.319
      bilateral H61.313
      left H61.312
      right H61.311
  left H61.302
  right H61.301

Stenosis, stenotic — *see also* Stricture — *continued*
external ear canal — *continued*
  specified cause NEC H61.399
    bilateral H61.393
    left H61.392
    right H61.391
gallbladder — *see* Obstruction, gallbladder
glottis J38.6
heart valve (congenital)
  aortic Q23.0
  mitral Q23.2
  pulmonary Q22.1
  tricuspid Q22.4
hepatic duct K83.1
hymen N89.6
hypertrophic subaortic (idiopathic) I42.1
ileum K56.6
  congenital Q41.2
infundibulum cardia Q24.3
intervertebral foramina — *see also* Lesion, biomechanical, specified NEC
  connective tissue M99.79
    abdomen M99.79
    cervical region M99.71
    cervicothoracic M99.71
    head region M99.70
    lumbar region M99.73
    lumbosacral M99.73
    occipitocervical M99.70
    sacral region M99.74
    sacrococcygeal M99.74
    sacroiliac M99.74
    specified NEC M99.79
    thoracic region M99.72
    thoracolumbar M99.72
  disc M99.79
    abdomen M99.79
    cervical region M99.71
    cervicothoracic M99.71
    head region M99.70
    lower extremity M99.76
    lumbar region M99.73
    lumbosacral M99.73
    occipitocervical M99.70
    pelvic M99.75
    rib cage M99.78
    sacral region M99.74
    sacrococcygeal M99.74
    sacroiliac M99.74
    specified NEC M99.79
    thoracic region M99.72
    thoracolumbar M99.72
    upper extremity M99.77
  osseous M99.69
    abdomen M99.69
    cervical region M99.61
    cervicothoracic M99.61
    head region M99.60
    lower extremity M99.66
    lumbar region M99.63
    lumbosacral M99.63
    occipitocervical M99.60
    pelvic M99.65
    rib cage M99.68
    sacral region M99.64
    sacrococcygeal M99.64
    sacroiliac M99.64
    specified NEC M99.69
    thoracic region M99.62
    thoracolumbar M99.62
    upper extremity M99.67
  subluxation — *see* Stenosis, intervertebral foramina, osseous
intestine — *see also* Obstruction, intestine
  congenital (small) Q41.9
    large Q42.9
      specified NEC Q42.8
    specified NEC Q41.8
jejunum K56.6
  congenital Q41.1
lacrimal (passage)
  canaliculi H04.549
    bilateral H04.543
    left H04.542
    right H04.541

©2002 Ingenix, Inc.

Stenosis, stenotic — *see also* Stricture — *continued*
  lacrimal — *continued*
    congenital Q10.5
    duct H04.559
      bilateral H04.553
      left H04.552
      right H04.551
    punctum H04.569
      bilateral H04.563
      left H04.562
      right H04.561
    sac H04.579
      bilateral H04.573
      left H04.572
      right H04.571
  lacrimonasal duct — *see* Stenosis, lacrimal, duct
    congenital Q10.5
  larynx J38.6
    congenital NEC Q31.8
      subglottic Q31.1
    syphilitic A52.73
      congenital A50.59 *[J99]*
  mitral (chronic) (inactive) (valve) I05.0
    with
      aortic valve disease I08.0
      incompetency, insufficiency or regurgitation I05.2
    active or acute I01.1
      with rheumatic or Sydenham's chorea I02.0
    congenital Q23.2
    specified cause, except rheumatic I34.2
    syphilitic A52.03
  myocardium, myocardial — *see also* Degeneration, myocardial
    hypertrophic subaortic (idiopathic) I42.1
  nares (anterior) (posterior) J34.8
    congenital Q30.0
  nasal duct — *see also* Stenosis, lacrimal, duct
    congenital Q10.5
  nasolacrimal duct — *see also* Stenosis, lacrimal, duct
    congenital Q10.5
  neural canal — *see also* Lesion, biomechanical, specified NEC
    connective tissue M99.49
      abdomen M99.49
      cervical region M99.41
      cervicothoracic M99.41
      head region M99.40
      lower extremity M99.46
      lumbar region M99.43
      lumbosacral M99.43
      occipitocervical M99.40
      pelvic M99.45
      rib cage M99.48
      sacral region M99.44
      sacrococcygeal M99.44
      sacroiliac M99.44
      specified NEC M99.49
      thoracic region M99.42
      thoracolumbar M99.42
      upper extremity M99.47
    intervertebral disc M99.59
      abdomen M99.59
      cervical region M99.51
      cervicothoracic M99.51
      head region M99.50
      lower extremity M99.56
      lumbar region M99.53
      lumbosacral M99.53
      occipitocervical M99.50
      pelvic M99.55
      rib cage M99.58
      sacral region M99.54
      sacrococcygeal M99.54
      sacroiliac M99.54
      specified NEC M99.59
      thoracic region M99.52
      thoracolumbar M99.52
      upper extremity M99.57
    osseous M99.39
      abdomen M99.39
      cervical region M99.31

Stenosis, stenotic — *see also* Stricture — *continued*
  neural canal — *continued*
    osseous — *continued*
      cervicothoracic M99.31
      head region M99.30
      lower extremity M99.36
      lumbar region M99.33
      lumbosacral M99.33
      pelvic M99.35
      rib cage M99.38
      occipitocervical M99.30
      sacral region M99.34
      sacrococcygeal M99.34
      sacroiliac M99.34
      specified NEC M99.39
      thoracic region M99.32
      thoracolumbar M99.32
      upper extremity M99.37
    subluxation M99.29
      cervical region M99.21
      cervicothoracic M99.21
      head region M99.20
      lower extremity M99.26
      lumbar region M99.23
      lumbosacral M99.23
      occipitocervical M99.20
      pelvic M99.25
      rib cage M99.28
      sacral region M99.24
      sacrococcygeal M99.24
      sacroiliac M99.24
      specified NEC M99.29
      thoracic region M99.22
      thoracolumbar M99.22
      upper extremity M99.27
  oesophagus — *see* Stenosis, esophagus
  organ or site, congenital NEC — *see* Atresia, by site
  papilla of Vater K83.1
  pulmonary (artery) (congenital) Q25.6
    with ventricular septal defect, transposition of aorta, and hypertrophy of right ventricle Q21.3
    acquired I28.8
    in tetralogy of Fallot Q21.3
    infundibular Q24.3
    valve I37.0
      with insufficiency I37.2
      congenital Q22.1
      rheumatic I09.89
        with aortic, mitral or tricuspid (valve) disease I08.8
    subvalvular Q24.3
    vein, acquired I28.8
    vessel NEC I28.8
  pulmonic (congenital) Q22.1
    infundibular Q24.3
    subvalvular Q24.3
  pylorus (hypertrophic) (acquired) K31.1
    adult K31.1
    congenital Q40.0
    infantile Q40.0
  rectum (sphincter) — *see* Stricture, rectum
  renal artery I70.1
    congenital Q27.1
  salivary duct (any) K11.8
  sphincter of Oddi K83.1
  spinal M48.00
    cervical region M48.02
    cervicothoracic region M48.03
    lumbar region M48.06
    lumbosacral region M48.07
    occipito-atlanto-axial region M48.01
    sacrococcygeal region M48.08
    thoracic region M48.04
    thoracolumbar region M48.05
  stomach, hourglass K31.2
  subaortic (congenital) Q24.4
    hypertrophic (idiopathic) I42.1
  subglottic
    congenital Q31.1
    postprocedural J95.5
  trachea J39.8
    congenital Q32.1
    syphilitic A52.73
    tuberculous NEC A15.5

Stenosis, stenotic — *see also* Stricture — *continued*
  tracheostomy J95.03
  tricuspid (valve) I07.0
    with
      aortic (valve) disease I08.2
      incompetency, insufficiency or regurgitation I07.2
        with aortic (valve) disease I08.2
          with mitral (valve) disease I08.3
      mitral (valve) disease I08.1
        with aortic (valve) disease I08.3
    congenital Q22.4
    nonrheumatic I36.0
      with insufficiency I36.2
  tubal N97.1
  ureter — *see* Atresia, ureter
  ureteropelvic junction, congenital Q62.11
  ureterovesical orifice, congenital Q62.12
  urethra (valve) — *see also* Stricture, urethra
    congenital Q64.32
  urinary meatus, congenital Q64.33
  vagina N89.5
    congenital Q52.4
    in pregnancy — *see* Pregnancy, complicated by, abnormal vagina
    causing obstructed labor O65.5
  valve (cardiac) (heart) — *see also* Endocarditis
    congenital
      aortic Q23.0
      mitral Q23.2
      pulmonary Q22.1
      tricuspid Q22.4
  vena cava (inferior) (superior) I87.1
    congenital Q26.0
  vesicourethral orifice Q64.31
  vulva N90.5

Stercolith (impaction) K56.4
  appendix K38.1

Stercoraceous, stercoral ulcer K63.3
  anus or rectum K62.6

Stereotypies NEC F98.4

Sterility — *see* Infertility

Sternalgia — *see* Angina

Sternopagus Q89.4

Sternum bifidum Q76.7

Steroid
  effects (adverse) (adrenocortical) (iatrogenic) cushingoid
    overdose or wrong substance given or taken — *see* category T38.0
    diabetes
      correct substance properly administered — *see* Diabetes, specified NEC
      overdose or wrong substance given or taken — *see* category T38.0
    due to
      correct substance properly administered E27.3
      overdose or wrong substance given or taken — *see* category T38.0
    fever
      correct substance properly administered R50.9
      overdose or wrong substance given or taken — *see* category T38.0
    withdrawal
      correct substance properly administered E27.3
      overdose or wrong substance given or taken — *see* category T38.0

Stevens-Johnson disease or syndrome L51.1

Stewart-Morel syndrome M85.2

Sticker's disease B08.3

Sticky eye — *see* Conjunctivitis, acute, mucopurulent

Stieda's disease — *see* Bursitis, tibial collateral

Stiff neck — *see* Torticollis

Stiff-man syndrome G25.8

Stiffness, joint NEC M25.60
  ankle M25.673
    left M25.672
    right M25.671
  ankylosis — *see* Ankylosis, joint

Stiffness, joint NEC — continued
- contracture — see Contraction, joint
- elbow M25.629
  - left M25.622
  - right M25.621
- foot M25.676
  - left M25.675
  - right M25.674
- hand M25.649
  - left M25.642
  - right M25.641
- hip M25.659
  - left M25.652
  - right M25.651
- knee M25.669
  - left M25.662
  - right M25.661
- shoulder M25.619
  - left M25.612
  - right M25.611
- wrist M25.639
  - left M25.632
  - right M25.631

Stigmata congenital syphilis A50.59

Stillbirth P95

Still-Felty syndrome — see Felty's syndrome

Still's disease or syndrome (juvenile) M08.20
- adult-onset M06.1
- ankle M08.279
  - left M08.272
  - right M08.271
- elbow M08.229
  - left M08.222
  - right M08.221
- foot joint M08.279
  - left M08.272
  - right M08.271
- hand joint M08.249
  - left M08.242
  - right M08.241
- hip M08.259
  - left M08.252
  - right M08.251
- knee M08.269
  - left M08.262
  - right M08.261
- multiple site M08.29
- shoulder M08.219
  - left M08.212
  - right M08.211
- vertebra M08.28
- wrist M08.239
  - left M08.232
  - right M08.231

Stimulation, ovary E28.1

Sting (venomous) (with allergic or anaphylactic shock) — see Toxicity, venom

Stippled epiphyses Q78.8

Stitch
- abscess T81.4
- burst (in operation wound) T81.3

Stokes-Adams disease or syndrome I45.9

Stokes' disease E05.00
- with thyroid storm E05.01

Stokvis (-Talma) disease D74.8

Stoma malfunction
- colostomy K94.03
- enterostomy K94.13
- gastrostomy K94.23
- ileostomy K94.13
- tracheostomy J95.03

Stomach — see condition

Stomatitis (denture) (ulcerative) K12.1
- angular K13.0
  - due to dietary or vitamin deficiency E53.0
- aphthous K12.0
- candidal B37.0
- catarrhal K12.1
- diphtheritic A36.89
- due to
  - dietary deficiency E53.0
  - thrush B37.0
  - vitamin deficiency
    - B group NEC E53.9 *[K93]*
    - B2 (riboflavin) E53.0 *[K93]*

Stomatitis — continued
- epidemic B08.8
- epizootic B08.8
- follicular K12.1
- gangrenous A69.0
- Geotrichum B48.3
- herpesviral, herpetic B00.2
- herpetiformis K12.0
- malignant K12.1
- membranous acute K12.1
- monilial B37.0
- mycotic B37.0
- necrotizing ulcerative A69.0
- parasitic B37.0
- septic K12.1
- spirochetal A69.1
- suppurative (acute) K12.2
- ulceromembranous A69.1
- vesicular K12.1
  - with exanthem (enteroviral) B08.4
  - virus disease A93.8
- Vincent's A69.1

Stomatocytosis D58.8

Stomatomycosis B37.0

Stomatorrhagia K13.7

Stone(s) — see also Calculus
- bladder (diverticulum) N21.0
- cystine E72.09
- heart syndrome I50.1
- kidney N20.0
- prostate N42.0
- pulpal (dental) K04.2
- renal N20.0
- salivary gland or duct (any) K11.5
- urethra (impacted) N21.1
- urinary (duct) (impacted) (passage) N20.9
  - bladder (diverticulum) N21.0
  - lower tract N21.9
  - specified NEC N21.8
- xanthine E79.8 *[N22]*

Stonecutter's lung J62.8

Stonemason's asthma, disease, lung or pneumoconiosis J62.8

Stoppage
- heart — see Arrest, cardiac
- urine — see Retention, urine

Storm, thyroid — see Thyrotoxicosis

Strabismus (congenital) (nonparalytic) H50.9
- concomitant H50.40
  - convergent — see Strabismus, convergent concomitant
  - divergent — see Strabismus, divergent concomitant
- convergent concomitant H50.00
  - accommodative component H50.45
  - alternating H50.05
    - with
      - A pattern H50.06
      - specified nonconcomitances NEC H50.08
      - V pattern H50.07
    - monocular
      - with
        - A pattern
          - left H50.022
          - right H50.021
        - specified nonconcomitances NEC
          - left H50.042
          - right H50.041
        - V pattern
          - left H50.032
          - right H50.031
    - intermittent
      - alternating H50.32
        - left H50.312
        - right H50.311
      - left H50.012
      - right H50.011
  - cyclotropia
    - left H50.432
    - right H50.431

Strabismus — continued
- divergent concomitant H50.10
  - alternating H50.15
    - with
      - A pattern H50.16
      - specified noncomitances NEC H50.18
      - V pattern H50.17
  - monocular
    - with
      - A pattern
        - left H50.122
        - right H50.121
      - specified noncomitances NEC
        - left H50.142
        - right H50.141
      - V pattern
        - left H50.132
        - right H50.131
  - intermittent
    - alternating H50.34
    - left H50.332
    - right H50.331
  - left H50.112
  - right H50.111
- Duane's syndrome
  - left H50.812
  - right H50.811
- due to adhesions, scars H50.60
- heterophoria H50.50
  - alternating H50.55
  - cyclophoria H50.54
  - esophoria H50.51
  - exophoria H50.52
  - vertical H50.53
- heterotropia H50.40
  - intermittent H50.30
- hypertropia
  - left H50.212
  - right H50.211
- hypotropia
  - left H50.222
  - right H50.221
- latent H50.50
- mechanical H50.60
  - Brown's sheath syndrome
    - left H50.612
    - right H50.611
  - specified type NEC H50.69
- monofixation syndrome H50.44
- paralytic H49.9
  - abducens nerve H49.20
    - bilateral H49.23
    - left H49.22
    - right H49.21
  - fourth nerve H49.10
    - bilateral H49.13
    - left H49.12
    - right H49.11
  - Kearns-Sayre syndrome H49.819
    - bilateral H49.813
    - left H49.812
    - right H49.811
  - ophthalmoplegia (external)
    - progressive H49.40
      - with pigmentary retinopathy H49.819
        - bilateral H49.813
        - left H49.812
        - right H49.811
      - bilateral H49.43
      - left H49.42
      - right H49.41
    - total H49.30
      - bilateral H49.33
      - left H49.32
      - right H49.31
  - sixth nerve H49.20
    - bilateral H49.23
    - left H49.22
    - right H49.21
  - specified type NEC H49.889
    - bilateral H49.883
    - left H49.882
    - right H49.881
  - third nerve H49.00
    - bilateral H10.03
    - left H49.02

©2002 Ingenix, Inc.

Strabismus — *continued*
　paralytic — *continued*
　　third nerve — *continued*
　　　right H49.01
　　trochlear nerve H49.10
　　　bilateral H49.13
　　　left H49.12
　　　right H49.11
　　specified type NEC H50.89
　　vertical H50.2
Strain — *see also* Sprain
　eye NEC — *see* Disturbance, vision, subjective
　heart — *see* Disease, heart
　low back M54.5
　mental NOS Z73.3
　　work-related Z56.6
　muscle M62.89
　　traumatic — *see* Sprain
　postural — *see also* Disorder, soft tissue, due
　　to use
　physical NOS Z73.3
　　work-related Z56.6
　psychological NEC Z73.3
Strand, vitreous — *see* Opacity, vitreous,
　membranes and strands
Strangulation, strangulated — *see also*
　Asphyxia, traumatic
　appendix K38.8
　bladder-neck N32.0
　bowel or colon K56.2
　food or foreign body — *see* Asphyxia, food
　hemorrhoids — *see* Hemorrhoids, with
　　complication
　hernia — *see also* Hernia, by site, with
　　obstruction
　　with gangrene — *see* Hernia, by site, with
　　　gangrene
　intestine (large) (small) K56.2
　　with hernia — *see also* Hernia, by site, with
　　　obstruction
　　　with gangrene — *see* Hernia, by site, with
　　　　gangrene
　mesentery K56.2
　mucus — *see* Asphyxia, mucus
　omentum K56.2
　organ or site, congenital NEC — *see* Atresia, by
　　site
　ovary — *see* Torsion, ovary
　penis N48.89
　　foreign body T19.8
　rupture — *see* Hernia, by site, with obstruction
　stomach due to hernia — *see also* Hernia, by
　　site, with obstruction
　　with gangrene — *see* Hernia, by site, with
　　　gangrene
　vesicourethral orifice N32.0
Strangury R30.0
Straw itch B88.0
Strawberry
　gallbladder K82.4
　mark Q82.5
　tongue (red) (white) K14.3
Streak(s)
　macula, angioid H35.33
　ovarian Q50.32
Strephosymbolia F81.0
　secondary to organic lesion R48.8
Streptobacillary fever A25.1
Streptobacillosis A25.1
Streptobacillus moniliformis A25.1
Streptococcemia — *see* Septicemia, streptococcal
Streptococcus, streptococcal — *see also*
　　condition
　as cause of disease classified elsewhere B95.5
　group
　　A, as cause of disease classified elsewhere
　　　B95.0
　　B, as cause of disease classified elsewhere
　　　B95.1
　　D, as cause of disease classified elsewhere
　　　B95.2
　pneumoniae, as cause of disease classified
　　elsewhere B95.3
　specified NEC, as cause of disease classified
　　elsewhere B95.4

Streptomycosis B47.1
Streptotrichosis A48.8
Stress
　fetal — *see* Distress, fetal
　mental NEC Z73.3
　　work-related Z56.6
　physical NEC Z73.3
　　work-related Z56.6
　polycythemia D75.1
　reaction — *see* Reaction, stress
　work schedule Z56.3
Stretching, nerve — *see* Injury, nerve
Striae albicantes, atrophicae or distensae
　(cutis) L90.6
Stricture R68.8
　ampulla of Vater K83.1
　anus (sphincter) K62.4
　　congenital Q42.3
　　　with fistula Q42.2
　　infantile Q42.3
　　　with fistula Q42.2
　aorta (ascending) (congenital) Q25.3
　　arteriosclerotic I70.0
　　calcified I70.0
　　supravalvular, congenital Q25.3
　aortic (valve) — *see* Stenosis, aortic
　aqueduct of Sylvius (congenital) Q03.0
　　with spina bifida — *see* Spina bifida, by site,
　　　with hydrocephalus
　　acquired G91.1
　artery I77.1
　　basilar — *see* Occlusion, artery, basilar
　　carotid — *see* Occlusion, artery, carotid
　　celiac I77.4
　　congenital (peripheral) Q27.8
　　　cerebral Q28.3
　　　coronary Q24.5
　　　digestive system Q27.8
　　　lower limb Q27.8
　　　retinal Q14.1
　　　specified site NEC Q27.8
　　　umbilical Q27.0
　　　upper limb Q27.8
　　coronary — *see* Disease, heart, ischemic,
　　　atherosclerotic
　　　congenital Q24.5
　　precerebral — *see* Occlusion, artery,
　　　precerebral
　　pulmonary (congenital) Q25.6
　　　acquired I28.8
　　renal I70.1
　　vertebral — *see* Occlusion, artery, vertebral
　auditory canal (external) (congenital)
　　acquired — *see* Stenosis, external ear canal
　bile duct (common) (hepatic) K83.1
　　congenital Q44.3
　　postoperative K91.89
　bladder N32.8
　　neck N32.0
　bowel — *see* Obstruction, intestine
　brain G93.8
　bronchus J98.0
　　congenital Q32.3
　　syphilitic A52.72
　cardia (stomach) K22.2
　　congenital Q40.2
　cardiac — *see also* Disease, heart
　　orifice (stomach) K22.2
　cecum — *see* Obstruction, intestine
　cervix, cervical (canal) N88.2
　　congenital Q51.8
　　in pregnancy — *see* Pregnancy, complicated
　　　by, abnormal cervix
　　　causing obstructed labor O65.5
　colon — *see also* Obstruction, intestine
　　congenital Q42.9
　　　specified NEC Q42.8
　colostomy K94.03
　common (bile) duct K83.1
　coronary (artery) — *see* Disease, heart,
　　ischemic, atherosclerotic
　cystic duct — *see* Obstruction, gallbladder
　digestive organs NEC, congenital Q45.8
　duodenum K31.5
　　congenital Q41.0

Stricture — *continued*
　ear canal (external) (congenital) Q16.1
　　acquired — *see* Stricture, auditory canal,
　　　acquired
　ejaculatory duct N50.8
　enterostomy K94.13
　esophagus K22.2
　　congenital Q39.3
　　syphilitic A52.79
　　　congenital A50.59 *[K23]*
　eustachian tube — *see also* Obstruction,
　　eustachian tube
　　congenital Q17.8
　fallopian tube N97.1
　　gonococcal A54.24
　　tuberculous A18.17
　gallbladder — *see* Obstruction, gallbladder
　glottis J38.6
　heart — *see also* Disease, heart
　　valve (*see also* Endocarditis) I38
　　　aortic Q23.0
　　　mitral Q23.4
　　　pulmonary Q22.1
　　　tricuspid Q22.4
　hepatic duct K83.1
　hourglass, of stomach K31.2
　hymen N89.6
　hypopharynx J39.2
　ileum K56.6
　　congenital Q41.2
　intestine — *see also* Obstruction, intestine
　　congenital (small) Q41.9
　　　large Q42.9
　　　　specified NEC Q42.8
　　　specified NEC Q41.8
　　ischemic K55.1
　jejunum K56.6
　　congenital Q41.1
　lacrimal passages — *see also* Stenosis, lacrimal
　　congenital Q10.5
　larynx J38.6
　　congenital NEC Q31.8
　　　subglottic Q31.1
　　syphilitic A52.73
　　　congenital A50.59 *[J99]*
　meatus
　　ear (congenital) Q16.1
　　　acquired — *see* Stricture, auditory canal,
　　　　acquired
　　osseous (ear) (congenital) Q16.1
　　　acquired — *see* Stricture, auditory canal,
　　　　acquired
　　urinarius — *see also* Stricture, urethra
　　　congenital Q64.33
　mitral (valve) — *see* Stenosis, mitral
　myocardium, myocardial I51.5
　　hypertrophic subaortic (idiopathic) I42.1
　nares (anterior) (posterior) J34.8
　　congenital Q30.0
　nasal duct — *see also* Stenosis, lacrimal, duct
　　congenital Q10.5
　nasolacrimal duct — *see also* Stenosis,
　　lacrimal, duct
　　congenital Q10.5
　nasopharynx J39.2
　　syphilitic A52.73
　nose J34.8
　　congenital Q30.0
　nostril (anterior) (posterior) J34.8
　　congenital Q30.0
　　syphilitic A52.73
　　　congenital A50.59 *[J99]*
　oesophagus — *see* Stricture, esophagus
　organ or site, congenital NEC — *see* Atresia, by
　　site
　os uteri — *see* Stricture, cervix
　osseous meatus (ear) (congenital) Q16.1
　　acquired — *see* Stricture, auditory canal,
　　　acquired
　oviduct — *see* Stricture, fallopian tube
　pelviureteric junction (congenital) Q62.0
　penis, by foreign body T19.8
　pharynx J39.2
　prostate N42.89
　pulmonary, pulmonic
　　artery (congenital) Q25.6
　　　acquired I28.8

Stricture — *continued*
  pulmonary, pulmonic — *continued*
    artery (congenital) — *continued*
      noncongenital I28.8
    infundibulum (congenital) Q24.3
    valve I37.0
      congenital Q22.1
    vein, acquired I28.8
    vessel NEC I28.8
  punctum lacrimale — *see also* Stenosis,
    lacrimal, punctum
    congenital Q10.5
  pylorus (hypertrophic) K31.1
    adult K31.1
    congenital Q40.0
    infantile Q40.0
  rectosigmoid K56.6
  rectum (sphincter) K62.4
    congenital Q42.1
      with fistula Q42.0
    due to
      chlamydial lymphogranuloma A55
      irradiation K91.89
      lymphogranuloma venereum A55
    gonococcal A54.6
    inflammatory (chlamydial) A55
    syphilitic A52.74
    tuberculous A18.32
  renal artery I70.1
    congenital Q27.1
  salivary duct or gland (any) K11.8
  sigmoid (flexure) — *see* Obstruction, intestine
  spermatic cord N50.8
  stoma (following) (of)
    colostomy K94.03
    enterostomy K94.13
    gastrostomy K94.23
    ileostomy K94.13
    tracheostomy J95.03
  stomach K31.89
    congenital Q40.2
    hourglass K31.2
  subaortic Q24.4
    hypertrophic (acquired) (idiopathic) I42.1
  subglottic J38.6
  syphilitic NEC A52.79
  trachea J39.8
    congenital Q32.1
    syphilitic A52.73
    tuberculous NEC A15.5
  tracheostomy J95.03
  tricuspid (valve) — *see* Stenosis, tricuspid
  tunica vaginalis N50.8
  ureter (postoperative) N13.5
    with
      hydronephrosis N13.1
        with infection N13.6
      pyelonephritis (chronic) N11.1
    congenital — *see* Atresia, ureter
    tuberculous A18.11
  ureteropelvic junction (congenital) Q62.0
  ureterovesical orifice N13.5
    with infection N13.6
  urethra (organic) (spasmodic) N35.9
    associated with schistosomiasis B65.0 *[N29]*
    congenital Q64.39
      valvular (posterior) Q64.2
    due to
      infection — *see* Stricture, urethra,
        postinfective
      trauma — *see* Stricture, urethra, post-
        traumatic
    gonococcal, gonorrheal A54.01
    infective NEC — *see* Stricture, urethra,
      postinfective
    late effect of injury — *see* Stricture, urethra,
      post-traumatic
    postcatheterization — *see* Stricture, urethra,
      postprocedural
    postinfective NEC
      female N35.12
      male N35.119
        anterior urethra N35.114
        bulbous urethra N35.112
        meatal N35.111
        membranous urethra N35.113
    postobstetric N35.021

Stricture — *continued*
  urethra — *continued*
    postoperative — *see* Stricture, urethra,
      postprocedural
    postprocedural
      female N99.12
      male N99.114
        anterior urethra N99.113
        bulbous urethra N99.111
        meatal N99.110
        membranous urethra N99.112
    post-traumatic
      female N35.028
        due to childbirth N35.021
      male N35.014
        anterior urethra N35.013
        bulbous urethra N35.011
        meatal N35.010
        membranous urethra N35.012
    sequela of
      childbirth N35.021
      injury — *see* Stricture, urethra, post-
        traumatic
    specified cause NEC N35.8
    syphilitic A52.76
    traumatic — *see* Stricture, urethra, post-
      traumatic
    valvular (posterior), congenital Q64.2
  urinary meatus — *see* Stricture, urethra
  uterus, uterine (synechiae) N85.6
    os (external) (internal) — *see* Stricture,
      cervix
  vagina (outlet) — *see* Stenosis, vagina
  valve (cardiac) (heart) — *see also* Endocarditis
    congenital
      aortic Q23.0
      mitral Q23.2
      pulmonary Q22.1
      tricuspid Q22.4
  vas deferens N50.8
    congenital Q55.4
  vein I87.1
  vena cava (inferior) (superior) NEC I87.1
    congenital Q26.0
  vesicourethral orifice N32.0
    congenital Q64.31
  vulva (acquired) N90.5
Stridor R06.1
  congenital (larynx) Q31.4
Stridulous — *see* condition
Stroke (apoplectic) (brain) (paralytic) I64
  epileptic — *see* Epilepsy
  heart — *see* Disease, heart
  heat T67.0
  lightning — *see* Lightning
Stromatosis, endometrial (M8931/1) D39.0
Strongyloidiasis, strongyloidosis B78.9
  cutaneous B78.1
  disseminated B78.7
  intestinal B78.0
Strophulus pruriginosus L28.2
Struck by lightning — *see* Lightning
Struma — *see also* Goiter
  Hashimoto E06.3
  lymphomatosa E06.3
  nodosa (simplex) E04.9
    endemic E01.2
      multinodular E01.1
    multinodular E04.2
      iodine-deficiency related E01.1
    toxic or with hyperthyroidism E05.20
      with thyroid storm E05.21
      multinodular E05.20
        with thyroid storm E05.21
      uninodular E05.10
        with thyroid storm E05.11
    toxicosa E05.20
      with thyroid storm E05.21
      multinodular E05.20
        with thyroid storm E05.21
      uninodular E05.10
        with thyroid storm E05.11
    uninodular E04.1
  ovarii (M9090/0) D27.9
    with carcinoid (M9091/1) D39.10

Struma — *see also* Goiter — *continued*
  ovarii — *continued*
    with carcinoid — *continued*
      left D39.12
      right D39.11
    left D27.1
    malignant (M9090/3) C56.9
      left C56.1
      right C56.0
    right D27.0
  Riedel's E06.5
Strumipriva cachexia E03.4
Strümpell-Marie spine — *see* Spondylitis,
  ankylosing
Strümpell-Westphal pseudosclerosis E83.01
Stuart deficiency disease (factor X) D68.2
Stuart-Prower factor deficiency (factor X) D68.2
Student's elbow — *see* Bursitis, elbow, olecranon
Stump — *see* Amputation
Stunting, nutritional E45
Stupor (catatonic) R40.1
  depressive F32.8
  dissociative F44.2
  manic F30.2
  manic-depressive F31.89
  psychogenic (anergic) F44.2
  reaction to exceptional stress (transient) F43.0
Sturge (-Weber) (-Dimitri) (-Kalischer) disease or
  syndrome Q85.8
Stuttering F98.5
Sty, stye (external) (internal) (meibomian)
  (zeisian) — *see* Hordeolum
Subacidity, gastric K31.89
  psychogenic F45.8
Subacute — *see* condition
Subarachnoid — *see* condition
Subcortical — *see* condition
Subcostal syndrome, nerve compression — *see*
  Mononeuropathy, upper limb, specified site
  NEC
Subcutaneous, subcuticular — *see* condition
Subdural — *see* condition
Subendocardium — *see* condition
Subependymoma (M9383/1)
  specified site — *see* Neoplasm, uncertain
    behavior
  unspecified site D43.2
Suberosis J67.3
Subglossitis — *see* Glossitis
Subhemophilia D66
Subinvolution
  breast (postlactational) (postpuerperal) N64.8
  puerperal O90.8
  uterus (chronic) (nonpuerperal) N85.3
    puerperal O90.8
Sublingual — *see* condition
Sublinguitis — *see* Sialoadenitis
Subluxatable hip Q65.6
Subluxation — *see also* Dislocation
  acromioclavicular S43.119
    left S43.112
    right S43.111
  ankle S93.03
    left S93.02
    right S93.01
  atlantoaxial, recurrent M43.4
    with myelopathy M43.3
  carpometacarpal (joint) NEC S63.053
    left S63.052
    right S63.051
    thumb S63.043
      left S63.042
      right S63.041
  complex, vertebral — *see* Complex, subluxation
  congenital — *see also* Malposition, congenital
    hip — *see* Dislocation, hip, congenital,
      partial
    joint (excluding hip)
      lower limb Q68.8
      shoulder Q68.8
      upper limb Q68.8

         ©2002 Ingenix, Inc.

Subluxation — *see also* Dislocation — *continued*
elbow (traumatic) S53.103
  anterior S53.113
    left S53.112
    right S53.111
  lateral S53.143
    left S53.142
    right S53.141
  left S53.102
  medial S53.133
    left S53.132
    right S53.131
  posterior S53.123
    left S53.122
    right S53.121
  right S53.101
  specified type NEC S53.193
    left S53.192
    right S53.191
finger S63.209
  index S63.208
    left S63.201
    right S63.200
  interphalangeal S63.229
    distal S63.249
      index S63.248
        left S63.241
        right S63.240
      little S63.248
        left S63.247
        right S63.246
      middle S63.248
        left S63.243
        right S63.242
      ring S63.248
        left S63.245
        right S63.244
    index S63.228
      left S63.221
      right S63.220
    little S63.228
      left S63.227
      right S63.226
    middle S63.228
      left S63.223
      right S63.222
    proximal S63.239
      index S63.238
        left S63.231
        right S63.230
      little S63.238
        left S63.237
        right S63.236
      middle S63.238
        left S63.233
        right S63.232
      ring S63.238
        left S63.235
        right S63.234
    ring S63.228
      left S63.225
      right S63.224
  little S63.208
    left S63.207
    right S63.206
  metacarpophalangeal S63.219
    index S63.218
      left S63.211
      right S63.210
    little S63.218
      left S63.217
      right S63.216
    middle S63.218
      left S63.213
      right S63.212
    ring S63.218
      left S63.215
      right S63.214
  middle S63.208
    left S63.203
    right S63.202
  ring S63.208
    left S63.205
    right S63.204

Subluxation — *see also* Dislocation — *continued*
foot S93.303
  left S93.302
  right S93.301
  specified site NEC S93.333
    left S93.332
    right S93.331
  tarsal joint S93.313
    left S93.312
    right S93.311
  tarsometatarsal joint S93.323
    left S93.322
    right S93.321
  toe — *see* Subluxation, toe
hip S73.003
  anterior S73.033
    left S73.032
    obturator S73.023
      left S73.022
      right S73.021
    right S73.031
  central S73.043
    left S73.042
    right S73.041
  left S73.002
  posterior S73.013
    left S73.012
    right S73.011
  right S73.001
interphalangeal (joint)
  finger S63.229
    distal joint S63.249
      index S63.248
        left S63.241
        right S63.240
      little S63.248
        left S63.247
        right S63.246
      middle S63.248
        left S63.243
        right S63.242
      ring S63.248
        left S63.245
        right S63.244
    index S63.228
      left S63.221
      right S63.220
    little S63.228
      left S63.227
      right S63.226
    middle S63.228
      left S63.223
      right S63.222
    proximal joint S63.239
      index S63.238
        left S63.231
        right S63.230
      little S63.238
        left S63.237
        right S63.236
      middle S63.238
        left S63.233
        right S63.232
      ring S63.238
        left S63.235
        right S63.234
    ring S63.228
      left S63.225
      right S63.224
  thumb S63.123
    distal joint S63.143
      left S63.142
      right S63.141
    left S63.122
    proximal joint S63.133
      left S63.132
      right S63.131
    right S63.121
  toe S93.139
    great S93.133
      left S93.132
      right S93.131
    lesser S93.136
      left S93.135
      right S93.134

Subluxation — *see also* Dislocation — *continued*
knee S83.103
  cap — *see* Subluxation, patella
  left S83.102
  patella — *see* Subluxation, patella
  proximal tibia
    anteriorly S83.113
      left S83.112
      right S83.111
    laterally S83.143
      left S83.142
      right S83.141
    medially S83.133
      left S83.132
      right S83.131
    posteriorly S83.123
      left S83.122
      right S83.121
  right S83.101
  specified type NEC S83.193
    left S83.192
    right S83.191
lens — *see* Dislocation, lens, partial
ligament, traumatic — *see* Sprain, by site
metacarpal (bone)
  proximal end S63.063
    left S63.062
    right S63.061
metacarpophalangeal (joint)
  finger S63.219
    index S63.218
      left S63.211
      right S63.210
    little S63.218
      left S63.217
      right S63.216
    middle S63.218
      left S63.213
      right S63.212
    ring S63.218
      left S63.215
      right S63.214
  thumb S63.113
    left S63.112
    right S63.111
metatarsophalangeal joint S93.149
  great toe S93.143
    left S93.142
    right S93.141
  lesser toe S93.146
    left S93.145
    right S93.144
midcarpal (joint) S63.033
  left S63.032
  right S63.031
patella S83.003
  lateral S83.013
    left S83.012
    right S83.011
  left S83.002
  recurrent (nontraumatic) — *see* Dislocation,
    patella, recurrent, incomplete
  right S83.001
  specified type NEC S83.093
    left S83.092
    right S83.091
pathological — *see* Dislocation, pathological
radial head S53.003
  anterior S53.013
    left S53.012
    right S53.011
  left S53.002
  posterior S53.023
    left S53.022
    right S53.021
  right S53.001
  specified type NEC S53.093
    left S53.092
    right S53.091
radiocarpal (joint) S63.023
  left S63.022
  right S63.021
radioulnar (joint)
  distal S63.013
    left S63.012
    right S63.011

Subluxation — *see also* Dislocation — *continued*
  radioulnar — *continued*
    proximal — *see* Subluxation, elbow
  shoulder
    congenital Q68.8
    girdle S43.303
      left S43.302
      right S43.301
      scapula S43.313
        left S43.312
        right S43.311
      specified site NEC S43.393
        left S43.392
        right S43.391
    traumatic S43.003
      anterior S43.013
        left S43.012
        right S43.011
      inferior S43.033
        left S43.032
        right S43.031
      left S43.002
      posterior S43.023
        left S43.022
        right S43.021
      right S43.001
      specified type NEC S43.083
        left S43.082
        right S43.081
  sternoclavicular (joint) S43.203
    anterior S43.213
      left S43.212
      right S43.211
    left S43.202
    posterior S43.223
      left S43.222
      right S43.221
    right S43.201
  symphysis (pubis)
    complicating
      childbirth O26.72
      pregnancy O26.719
        first trimester O26.711
        second trimester O26.712
        third trimester O26.713
      puerperium O26.73
  thumb S63.103
    interphalangeal joint — *see* Subluxation, interphalangeal (joint), thumb
    left S63.102
    metacarpophalangeal joint — *see* Subluxation, metacarpophalangeal (joint), thumb
    right S63.101
  toe(s) S93.103
    great S93.103
      interphalangeal joint S93.133
        left S93.132
        right S93.131
      metatarsophalangeal joint S93.143
        left S93.142
        right S93.141
    interphalangeal joint S93.139
    left S93.102
    lesser S93.103
      interphalangeal joint S93.136
        left S93.135
        right S93.134
      metatarsophalangeal joint S93.146
        left S93.145
        right S93.144
    metatarsophalangeal joint S93.149
    right S93.101
  ulnohumeral joint — *see* Subluxation, elbow
  vertebral
    recurrent NEC — *see* category M43.5
    traumatic
      cervical S13.100
        atlantoaxial joint S13.120
        atlantooccipital joint S13.110
        atloidooccipital joint S13.110
        joint between
          C0 and C1 S13.110
          C1 and C2 S13.120
          C2 and C3 S13.130
          C3 and C4 S13.140

Subluxation — *see also* Dislocation — *continued*
  vertebral — *continued*
    traumatic — *continued*
      cervical — *continued*
        joint between — *continued*
          C4 and C5 S13.150
          C5 and C6 S13.160
          C6 and C7 S13.170
          C7 and T1 S13.180
        occipitoatloid joint S13.110
      lumbar S33.100
        joint between
          L1 and L2 S33.110
          L2 and L3 S33.120
          L3 and L4 S33.130
          L4 and L5 S33.140
      thoracic S23.100
        joint between
          T1 and T2 S23.110
          T2 and T3 S23.120
          T3 and T4 S23.122
          T4 and T5 S23.130
          T5 and T6 S23.132
          T6 and T7 S23.140
          T7 and T8 S23.142
          T8 and T9 S23.150
          T9 and T10 S23.152
          T10 and T11 S23.160
          T11 and T12 S23.162
          T12 and L1 S23.170
  ulna
    distal end S63.073
      left S63.072
      right S63.071
    proximal end — *see* Subluxation, elbow
  wrist (carpal bone) S63.003
    carpometacarpal joint — *see* Subluxation, carpometacarpal (joint)
    distal radioulnar joint — *see* Subluxation, radioulnar (joint), distal
    left S63.002
    metacarpal bone, proximal — *see* Subluxation, metacarpal (bone), proximal end
    midcarpal — *see* Subluxation, midcarpal (joint)
    radiocarpal joint — *see* Subluxation, radiocarpal (joint)
    recurrent — *see* Dislocation, recurrent, wrist
    right S63.001
    specified site NEC S63.093
      left S63.092
      right S63.091
    ulna — *see* Subluxation, ulna, distal end

Submaxillary — *see* condition

Submersion (fatal) (nonfatal) T75.1

Submucous — *see* condition

Subnormal, subnormality
  accommodation (old age) H52.4
  mental F79
    mild F70
    moderate F71
    profound F73
    severe F72
  temperature (accidental) T68

Subphrenic — *see* condition

Subscapular nerve — *see* condition

Subseptus uterus Q51.8

Subsiding appendicitis K36

Substernal thyroid E04.9
  congenital Q89.2

Substitution disorder F44.9

Subtentorial — *see* condition

Subthyroidism (acquired) — *see also* Hypothyroidism
  congenital E03.1

Succenturiate placenta — *see* Disorder, placenta, malformation, specified type NEC

Sucking thumb, child (excessive) F98.8

Sudamen, sudamina L74.1

Sudanese kala-azar B55.0

Sudden
  death, cause unknown, infant P96.6
  heart failure — *see* Failure, heart

Sudden — *continued*
  hearing loss — *see* Deafness, sudden

Sudeck's atrophy, disease, or syndrome — *see* Algoneurodystrophy

Suffocation — *see* Asphyxia, traumatic

Sugar
  blood
    high R73.9
    low E16.2
  in urine R81

Suicide, suicidal (attempted) T14.91
  by poisoning — *see* Table of Drugs and Chemicals
  history of (personal) Z91.5
    in family Z81.8
  observation following alleged attempt Z03.8
  risk Z91.5
  tendencies Z91.5
  trauma — *see* nature of injury by site

Suipestifer infection — *see* Infection, salmonella

Sulfhemoglobinemia, sulphemoglobinemia (acquired) (with methemoglobinemia) D74.8

Sumatran mite fever A75.3

Summer — *see* condition

Sunburn L55.9
  first degree L55.0
  second degree L55.1
  third degree L55.2

Sunken acetabulum — *see* Derangement, joint, specified type NEC, hip

Sunstroke T67.0

Superfecundation — *see* Pregnancy, multiple

Superfetation — *see* Pregnancy, multiple

Superinvolution (uterus) N85.8

Supernumerary (congenital)
  aortic cusps Q23.8
  auditory ossicles Q16.3
  bone Q79.8
  breast Q83.1
  carpal bones Q74.0
  cusps, heart valve NEC Q24.8
    aortic Q23.8
    mitral Q23.2
    pulmonary Q22.3
  digit(s) Q69.9
  ear (lobule) Q17.0
  fallopian tube Q50.6
  finger Q69.0
  hymen Q52.4
  kidney Q63.0
  lacrimonasal duct Q10.6
  lobule (ear) Q17.0
  mitral cusps Q23.2
  muscle Q79.8
  nipple(s) Q83.3
  organ or site not listed — *see* Accessory
  ossicles, auditory Q16.3
  ovary Q50.31
  oviduct Q50.6
  pulmonary, pulmonic cusps Q22.3
  rib Q76.6
    cervical or first (syndrome) Q76.5
  roots (of teeth) K00.2
  spleen Q89.09
  tarsal bones Q74.2
  teeth K00.1
    causing crowding M26.3
  testis Q55.29
  thumb Q69.1
  toe Q69.2
  uterus Q51.2
  vagina Q52.1
  vertebra Q76.49

Supervision (of)
  contraceptive — *see* Prescription, contraceptives
  dietary (for) Z71.3
    allergy (food) Z71.3
    colitis Z71.3
    diabetes mellitus Z71.3
    food allergy or intolerance Z71.3
    gastritis Z71.3
    hypercholesterolemia Z71.3
    hypoglycemia Z71.3
    intolerance (food) Z71.3

©2002 Ingenix, Inc.

Supervision (of) — *continued*
  obesity Z71.3
    specified NEC Z71.3
  healthy infant or child Z76.2
    foundling Z76.1
  high-risk pregnancy — *see* Pregnancy,
    complicated by, high, risk
  lactation Z39.1
  pregnancy — *see* Pregnancy, supervision of
Supplemental teeth K00.1
  causing crowding M26.3
Suppression
  binocular vision H53.34
  lactation O92.5
  menstruation N94.8
  ovarian secretion E28.3
  renal — *see* Failure, renal
  urine, urinary secretion R34
Suppuration, suppurative — *see also* condition
  accessory sinus (chronic) — *see* Sinusitis
  adrenal gland
  antrum (chronic) — *see* Sinusitis, maxillary
  bladder — *see* Cystitis
  brain G06.0
    sequelae G09
  breast N61
    puerperal, postpartum or gestational — *see*
      Mastitis, obstetric, purulent
  dental periosteum M27.3
  ear (middle) — *see also* Otitis, media
    external NEC — *see* Otitis, externa, infective
    internal — *see* category H83.0
  ethmoidal (chronic) (sinus) — *see* Sinusitis,
    ethmoidal
  fallopian tube — *see* Salpingo-oophoritis
  frontal (chronic) (sinus) — *see* Sinusitis, frontal
  gallbladder (acute) K81.0
  gum K05.2
  intracranial G06.0
  joint — *see* Arthritis, pyogenic or pyemic
  labyrinthine — *see* category H83.0
  lung — *see* Abscess, lung
  mammary gland N61
    puerperal, postpartum O91.12
      associated with lactation O91.13
  maxilla, maxillary M27.2
    sinus (chronic) — *see* Sinusitis, maxillary
  muscle — *see* Myositis, infective
  nasal sinus (chronic) — *see* Sinusitis
  pancreas, acute K85.8
  parotid gland — *see* Sialoadenitis
  pelvis, pelvic
    female — *see* Disease, pelvis, inflammatory
    male K65.0
  pericranial — *see* Osteomyelitis
  salivary duct or gland (any) — *see* Sialoadenitis
  sinus (accessory) (chronic) (nasal) — *see*
    Sinusitis
  sphenoidal sinus (chronic) — *see* Sinusitis,
    sphenoidal
  thymus (gland) E32.1
  thyroid (gland) E06.0
  tonsil — *see* Tonsillitis
  uterus — *see* Endometritis
Suprarenal (gland) — *see* condition
Suprascapular nerve — *see* condition
Suprasellar — *see* condition
Surfer's knots or nodules T14.90
Surgery
  cosmetic Z41.1
    hair transplant Z41.1
  elective Z41.9
    breast augmentation or reduction (cosmetic)
      Z41.1
    circumcision, ritual or routine (in absence of
      medical indication) Z41.2
    cosmetic NEC Z41.1
    ear piercing Z41.3
    face lift (cosmetic) Z41.1
    specified type NEC Z41.8
  not done — *see* Procedure, surgical, not done
  plastic
    breast augmentation or reduction Z41.1
    corrective, restorative — *see* Surgery,
      reconstructive

Surgery — *continued*
  plastic — *continued*
    cosmetic Z41.1
      breast augmentation or reduction Z41.1
      face lift Z41.1
    face lift Z41.1
    following healed injury or operation — *see*
      Surgery, reconstructive
    for unacceptable cosmetic appearance Z41.1
    specified type NEC Z41.8
  previous, in pregnancy or childbirth
    cervix — *see* Pregnancy, complicated by,
      abnormal cervix
    pelvic soft tissues NEC — *see* Pregnancy,
      complicated by, abnormal pelvic
      organs or tissues NEC
    perineum or vulva — *see* Pregnancy,
      complicated by, abnormal vulva
    uterus O34.29
      causing obstructed labor O65.5
    vagina — *see* Pregnancy, complicated by,
      abnormal vagina
  prophylactic — *see* Prophylactic, organ removal
Surgical
  emphysema T81.82
  operation R69
  procedures, complication or misadventure —
    see Complications, surgical procedures
  shock T81.1
Surveillance (of) (for) — *see also* Observation
  alcohol abuse Z71.41
  contraceptive — *see* Prescription,
    contraceptives
  dietary Z71.3
  drug abuse Z71.51
Suspected condition, ruled out — *see*
  Observation, suspected
Suspended uterus
  in pregnancy or childbirth — *see* Pregnancy,
    complicated by, abnormal uterus
Sutton's nevus (M8723/0) D22.9
Suture
  burst (in operation wound) T81.3
  inadvertently left in operation wound — *see*
    Foreign body, accidentally left following a
    procedure
  removal Z48.0
Swab inadvertently left in operation wound —
  see Foreign body, accidentally left following
  a procedure
Swallowed, swallowing
  difficulty — *see* Dysphagia
  foreign body — *see* Foreign body, alimentary
    tract
Swan-neck deformity (finger) — *see* Deformity,
  finger, swan-neck
Swearing, compulsive F42
  in Gilles de la Tourette's syndrome F95.2
Sweat, sweats
  fetid L75.0
  night R61.9
Sweating, excessive R61.9
Sweet's disease or dermatosis L98.2
Swelling (of)
  abdomen, abdominal (not referable to any
    particular organ) — *see* Mass, abdominal
  adrenal gland, cloudy E27.3
  ankle — *see* Effusion, joint, ankle
  arm M79.8
    forearm M79.8
  breast N63
  Calabar B74.3
  cervical gland R59.0
  chest, localized R22.2
  ear — *see* category H93.8
  extremity (lower) (upper) — *see* Disorder, soft
    tissue, specified type NEC
  finger M79.8
  foot M79.8
  glands R59.9
    generalized R59.1
    localized R59.0
  hand M79.8
  head (localized) R22.0
  inflammatory — *see* Inflammation

Swelling — *continued*
  intra-abdominal — *see* Mass, abdominal
  joint — *see* Effusion, joint
  leg M79.8
    lower M79.8
  limb — *see* Disorder, soft tissue, specified type
    NEC
  localized (skin) R22.9
    chest R22.2
    head R22.0
    limb
      lower — *see* Mass, localized, limb, lower
      upper — *see* Mass, localized, limb, upper
    neck R22.1
    trunk R22.2
  neck (localized) R22.1
  pelvic — *see* Mass, abdominal
  scrotum N50.8
  splenic — *see* Splenomegaly
  testis N50.8
  toe M79.8
  umbilical R19.09
  wandering, due to Gnathostoma (spinigerum)
    B83.1
  white — *see* Tuberculosis, arthritis
Swift (-Feer) disease
  overdose or wrong substance given or taken —
    see category T56.1
Swimmer's
  cramp T75.1
  ear H60.339
    bilateral H60.333
    left H60.332
    right H60.331
  itch B65.3
Swimming in the head R42
Swollen — *see* Swelling
Sycosis L73.8
  barbae (not parasitic) L73.8
  contagiosa (mycotic) B35.0
  lupoides L73.8
  mycotic B35.0
  parasitic B35.0
  vulgaris L73.8
Sydenham's chorea — *see* Chorea, Sydenham's
Sylvatic yellow fever A95.0
Sylvest's disease B33.0
Symblepharon H11.239
  bilateral H11.233
  congenital Q10.3
  left H11.232
  right H11.231
Symond's syndrome G93.2
Sympathetic — *see* condition
Sympatheticotonia G90.8
Sympathicoblastoma (M9500/3)
  specified site — *see* Neoplasm, malignant
  unspecified site C74.90
Sympathicogonioma (M9500/3) — *see*
  Sympathicoblastoma
Sympathoblastoma (M9500/3) — *see*
  Sympathicoblastoma
Sympathogonioma (M9500/3) — *see*
  Sympathicoblastoma
Symphalangy (fingers) (toes) Q70.9
Symptoms NEC R68.8
  breast NEC N64.5
  development NEC R63.8
  factitious, self-induced — *see* Disorder,
    factitious
  genital organs, female R10.2
  involving
    abdomen NEC R19.8
    appearance NEC R46.89
    awareness R41.9
      altered mental status R41.82
      amnesia — *see* Amnesia
      borderline intellectual functioning R41.83
      coma — *see* Coma
      disorientation R41.0
      neurologic neglect syndrome R41.4
      senile cognitive decline R41.81
      specified symptom NEC R41.89
    behavior NEC R46.89

Symptoms NEC — *continued*
  involving — *continued*
    cardiovascular system NEC R09.89
    chest NEC R09.89
    circulatory system NEC R09.89
    cognitive functions R41.9
      altered mental status R41.82
      amnesia — *see* Amnesia
      borderline intellectual functioning R41.83
      coma — *see* Coma
      disorientation R41.0
      neurologic neglect syndrome R41.4
      senile cognitive decline R41.81
      specified symptom NEC R41.89
    development NEC R62.50
    digestive system NEC R19.8
    emotional state NEC R45.89
    food and fluid intake R63.8
    general perceptions and sensations R44.9
      specified NEC R44.8
    musculoskeletal system R29.91
    nervous system R29.90
    pelvis NEC R19.8
    respiratory system NEC R09.89
    skin and integument R23.9
    urinary system R39.9
  menopausal N95.1
  metabolism NEC R63.8
  neurotic F48.8
  of infancy R68.19
  pelvis NEC, female R10.2
  skin and integument NEC R23.8
  subcutaneous tissue NEC R23.8

Sympus Q74.2

Syncephalus Q89.4

Synchondrosis
  abnormal (congenital) Q78.8
  ischiopubic M91.0

Synchysis (scintillans) (senile) (vitreous body) H43.89

Syncope (near) (pre-) R55
  anginosa I20.8
  bradycardia R00.1
  cardiac R55
  carotid sinus G90.0
  due to spinal (lumbar) puncture G97.1
  heart R55
  heat T67.1
  laryngeal R05
  psychogenic F48.8
  tussive R05
  vasoconstriction R55
  vasodepressor R55
  vasomotor R55
  vasovagal R55

Syndactylism, syndactyly Q70.9
  complex (with synostosis) Q70.9
    fingers Q70.00
      bilateral Q70.03
      left Q70.02
      right Q70.01
    toes Q70.2
  fingers Q70.10
    bilateral Q70.13
    left Q70.12
    right Q70.11
  simple (without synostosis) Q70.9
    fingers Q70.10
      bilateral Q70.13
      left Q70.12
      right Q70.11
    toes Q70.3
  toes Q70.3

Syndrome — *see also* Disease
  48, XXXX Q97.1
  49, XXXXX Q97.1
  abdominal
    acute R10.0
    migraine G43.10
      with status migrainosus G43.11
    muscle deficiency Q79.4
  abnormal innervation H02.519
    left H02.516
      lower H02.515
      upper H02.514

Syndrome — *see also* Disease — *continued*
  abnormal innervation — *continued*
    right H02.513
      lower H02.512
      upper H02.511
  acid pulmonary aspiration, obstetric O74.0
  acquired immunodeficiency — *see* Human, immunodeficiency virus (HIV) disease
  acute abdominal R10.0
  Adair-Dighton Q78.0
  Adams-Stokes (-Morgagni) I45.9
  adiposogenital E23.6
  adrenal
    hemorrhage (meningococcal) A39.1
    meningococcic A39.1
  adrenocortical — *see* Cushing's syndrome
  adrenogenital E25.9
    congenital, associated with enzyme deficiency E25.0
  afferent loop NEC K91.89
  alcohol withdrawal (without convulsions) — *see* Dependence, alcohol, with, withdrawal
  Alder's D72.0
  Aldrich (-Wiskott) D82.0
  Alport's Q87.810
    with chronic renal failure Q87.811
  alveolar hypoventilation E66.2
  alveolocapillary block J84.1
  amnesic, amnestic (confabulatory) (due to) — *see* Disorder, amnesic
  amyostatic (Wilson's disease) E83.01
  androgen resistance E34.5
  anginal — *see* Angina
  ankyloglossia superior Q38.1
  anterior
    chest wall R07.89
    cord G83.82
    spinal artery G95.19
      compression M47.00
        cervical region M47.02
        cervicothoracic region M47.03
        lumbar region M47.06
        lumbosacral region M47.07
        occipito-atlanto-axial region M47.01
        sacrococcygeal region M47.08
        thoracic region M47.04
        thoracolumbar region M47.05
  antibody deficiency D80.9
    agammaglobulinemic D80.1
      hereditary D80.0
    congenital D80.0
    hypogammaglobulinemic D80.1
      hereditary D80.0
  anticardiolipin D68.89
  antiphospholipid (-antibody) D68.89
  aortic
    arch M31.4
    bifurcation I74.0
  aortomesenteric duodenum occlusion K31.5
  arcuate ligament I77.4
  argentaffin, argintaffinoma E34.0
  Arnold-Chiari — *see* Arnold-Chiari disease
  Arrillaga-Ayerza I27.0
  Asherman's N85.6
  aspiration, of newborn (massive) P24.9
    meconium P24.0
  ataxia-telangiectasia G11.3
  auriculotemporal G50.8
  autoerythrocyte sensitization (Gardner-Diamond) D69.2
  autoimmune polyglandular E31.0
  autosomal — *see* Abnormal, autosomes
  Avellis' G83.89
  Ayerza (-Arrillaga) I27.0
  Babinski-Nageotte G83.89
  Bakwin-Krida Q79.8
  Ballantyne (-Runge) (postmaturity) P08.2
  bare lymphocyte D81.6
  Barré-Guillain G61.0
  Barré-Liéou M53.0
  Barrett's K22.1
  Barsony-Polgar K22.4
  Barsony-Teschendorf K22.4
  Bartter's E26.8
  Basedow's E05.00
    with thyroid storm E05.01
  basilar artery G45.0

Syndrome — *see also* Disease — *continued*
  Batten-Steinert G71.1
  battered
    baby or child — *see* Maltreatment, child, physical abuse
    spouse — *see* Maltreatment, adult, physical abuse
  Beau's I51.5
  Beck's I65.8
  Benedikt's G83.89
  Béquez César (-Steinbrinck-Chédiak-Higashi) D72.0
  Bernhardt-Roth — *see* Meralgia paresthetica
  Bernheim's I50.0
  big spleen D73.1
  bilateral polycystic ovarian E28.2
  Bing-Horton's G43.8
  Björck (-Thorsen) E34.0
  black
    lung J60
    widow spider bite — *see* Toxicity, venom, spider, black widow
  Blackfan-Diamond D61.4
  blind loop K90.2
    congenital Q43.8
    postsurgical K91.2
  blue sclera Q78.0
  Boder-Sedgewick G11.3
  Boerhaave's K22.3
  Bouillaud's I01.9
  Bourneville (-Pringle) Q85.1
  Bouveret (-Hoffman) I47.9
  brachial plexus G54.0
  bradycardia-tachycardia I49.5
  brain (nonpsychotic) F06.9
    with psychosis, psychotic reaction F09
    acute or subacute — *see* Delirium
    congenital — *see* Retardation, mental
    organic F06.9
      post-traumatic (nonpsychotic) F07.81
        psychotic F06.8
    personality change F07.0
    postcontusional F07.81
    post-traumatic, nonpsychotic F07.81
    psycho-organic F06.9
    psychotic F06.8
  brain stem stroke G46.3
  Brandt's L08.0
  broad ligament laceration N83.8
  Brock's J98.11
  bronze baby P83.8
  Brown-Sequard G83.81
  bubbly lung P27.0
  Buchem's M85.2
  Budd-Chiari I82.0
  bulbar (progressive) G12.22
  Bürger-Grütz E78.3
  Burke's K86.8
  burning feet E53.9
  Bywaters' T79.5
  carcinogenic thrombophlebitis I82.1
  carcinoid E34.0
  cardiac asthma I50.1
  cardiacos negros I27.0
  cardiopulmonary-obesity E66.2
  cardiorenal — *see* Hypertension, cardiorenal
  cardiorespiratory distress (idiopathic), newborn P22.0
  cardiovascular renal — *see* Hypertension, cardiorenal
  carotid
    artery (hemispheric) (internal) G45.1
    body G90.0
    sinus G90.0
  carpal tunnel G56.00
    left G56.02
    right G56.01
  Cassidy (-Scholte) M34.0
  cat-cry Q93.4
  cauda equina G83.4
  causalgia — *see* Causalgia
  celiac K90.0
    artery compression I77.4
    axis I77.4
  cerebellar
    hereditary G11.9
    stroke G46.4

©2002 Ingenix, Inc.

Syndrome — see also Disease — continued
- cerebellomedullary malformation — see Spina bifida
- cerebral
  - artery
    - anterior G46.1
    - middle G46.0
    - posterior G46.2
  - gigantism E22.0
- cervical (root) M53.1
  - disc — see Disorder, disc, cervical, with neuritis
  - fusion Q76.1
  - posterior, sympathicus M53.0
  - rib Q76.5
  - sympathetic paralysis G90.2
- cervicobrachial (diffuse) M53.1
- cervicocranial M53.0
- cervicodorsal outlet G54.2
- cervicothoracic outlet G54.0
- Céstan (-Raymond) I65.8
- Charcot's (angina cruris) (intermittent claudication) I73.9
- Charcot-Weiss-Baker G90.0
- Chédiak-Higashi (-Steinbrinck) D72.0
- chest wall R07.1
- Chiari's (hepatic vein thrombosis) I82.0
- Chilaiditi's Q43.3
- child maltreatment — see Maltreatment, child
- chondrocostal junction M94.0
- chondroectodermal dysplasia Q77.6
- chromosome 4 short arm deletion Q93.3
- chromosome 5 short arm deletion Q93.4
- chronic
  - pain personality F68.8
- Clarke-Hadfield K86.8
- Clerambault's automatism G93.8
- Clifford's (postmaturity) P08.2
- climacteric N95.1
- Clouston's (hidrotic ectodermal dysplasia) Q82.4
- clumsiness, clumsy child F82
- cluster headache G44.0
- cold injury (newborn) P80.0
- combined immunity deficiency D81.9
- compartment (deep) (posterior) T79.6
- compression T79.5
  - anterior spinal and vertebral artery — see Syndrome, anterior, spinal artery, compression
  - cauda equina G83.4
  - celiac artery I77.4
- concussion F07.81
- congenital
  - affecting multiple systems NEC Q87.89
  - facial diplegia Q87.0
  - muscular hypertrophy-cerebral Q87.89
  - oculo-auriculovertebral Q87.0
  - oculofacial diplegia (Moebius) Q87.0
  - rubella (manifest) P35.0
- congestion-fibrosis (pelvic), female N94.8
- congestive dysmenorrhea N94.6
- connective tissue M35.9
  - overlap NEC M35.1
- conus medullaris G95.81
- cor pulmonale I27.9
- cord
  - anterior G83.82
  - posterior G83.83
- coronary, insufficiency or intermediate I20.0
- Costen's (complex) M26.62
- costochondral junction M94.0
- costoclavicular G54.0
- costovertebral E22.0
- craniovertebral M53.0
- Creutzfeldt-Jakob A81.0
- cri-du-chat Q93.4
- crib death R99
- cricopharyngeal — see Dysphagia
- croup J05.0
- CRPS I — see Syndrome, pain, complex regional I
- crush T79.5
- cubital tunnel — see Lesion, nerve, ulnar
- Curschmann (-Batten) (-Steinert) G71.1
- Cushing's E24.9
  - alcohol-induced E24.4
  - due to
    - alcohol
      - drugs E24.2

Syndrome — see also Disease — continued
- Cushing's — continued
  - due to — continued
    - ectopic ACTH E24.3
    - overproduction of pituitary ACTH E24.0
  - drug-induced E24.2
  - overdose or wrong substance given or taken — see Steroid, effects, cushingoid
  - pituitary-dependent E24.0
  - specified type NEC E24.8
- cryptophthalmos Q87.0
- cystic duct stump K91.5
- Dana-Putnam D51.0
- Danbolt (-Closs) L08.0
- Dandy-Walker Q03.0
  - with spina bifida Q07.01
- Danlos' Q79.8
- defibrination — see also Fibrinolysis
  - with
    - antepartum hemorrhage — see Hemorrhage, antepartum
    - intrapartum hemorrhage — see Hemorrhage, complicating, delivery
    - premature separation of placenta — see Disorder, placenta, abruptio
  - fetus or newborn P60
  - postpartum O72.3
- Degos' I77.8
- Déjérine-Roussy G93.8
- delayed sleep phase G47.2
- demyelinating G37.9
- dependence — see F10-F19 with fourth character .1
- depersonalization (-derealization) F48.1
- de Toni-Fanconi (-Debré) E72.09
  - with cystinosis E72.04
- diabetes mellitus-hypertension-nephrosis — see Diabetes, nephrosis
- diabetes mellitus in newborn infant P70.2
- diabetes-nephrosis — see Diabetes, nephrosis
- diabetic amyotrophy — see Diabetes, amyotrophy
- Diamond-Blackfan D61.4
- Diamond-Gardener D69.2
- DIC (diffuse or disseminated intravascular coagulopathy) D65
- di George's D82.1
- Dighton's Q78.0
- disequilibrium E87.8
- Döhle body-panmyelopathic D72.0
- dorsolateral medullary G46.4
- Dresbach's (elliptocytosis) D58.1
- Dressler's (postmyocardial infarction) I24.1
- drug withdrawal, infant of dependent mother P96.1
- dry eye H04.129
  - bilateral H04.123
  - left H04.122
  - right H04.121
- due to abnormality
  - chromosomal Q99.9
    - sex
      - female phenotype Q97.9
      - male phenotype Q98.9
    - specified NEC Q99.8
- dumping (postgastrectomy) K91.1
  - nonsurgical K31.89
- Dupré's (meningism) R29.1
- dyspraxia, developmental F82
- Eagle-Barrett Q79.4
- Ebstein's Q22.5
- ectopic ACTH E24.3
- eczema-thrombocytopenia D82.0
- Eddowes' Q78.0
- effort (psychogenic) F45.8
- Eisenmenger's Q21.8
- Ehlers-Danlos Q79.6
- Ekman's Q78.0
- electric feet E53.8
- Ellis-van Creveld Q77.6
- empty nest Z60.0
- endocrine-hypertensive E27.0
- entrapment — see Neuropathy, entrapment
- eosinophilia-myalgia M35.8
- epidemic vomiting A08.1
- epileptic — see Epilepsy
- Erb (-Oppenheim) -Goldflam G70.0

Syndrome — see also Disease — continued
- Erdheim's E22.0
- erythrocyte fragmentation D59.4
- exhaustion F48.8
- extrapyramidal G25.9
  - specified NEC G25.8
- eye retraction — see Strabismus
- eyelid-malar-mandible Q87.0
- Faber's D50.9
- facial pain, paroxysmal G50.0
- Fallot's Q21.3
- familial eczema-thrombocytopenia (Wiskott-Aldrich) D82.0
- Fanconi (-de Toni) (-Debré) E72.09
  - with cystinosis E72.04
- Fanconi's (anemia) (congenital pancytopenia) D61.0
- fatigue F48.8
  - postviral G93.3
- faulty bowel habit K59.3
- Feil-Klippel (brevicollis) Q76.1
- Felty's — see Felty's syndrome
- fertile eunuch E23.0
- fetal
  - alcohol (dysmorphic) Q86.0
  - hydantoin Q86.1
- Fiedler's I40.1
- first arch Q87.0
- Fisher's G61.0
- Fitz's K85.8
- Flajani (-Basedow) E05.00
  - with thyroid storm E05.01
- flatback — see Flatback syndrome
- floppy
  - baby P94.2
  - mitral valve I34.1
- flush E34.0
- Foix-Alajouanine G95.19
- Fong's Q79.8
- foramen magnum G93.5
- Foville's (peduncular) G83.89
- fragile X Q99.2
- Frey's (auriculotemporal) G50.8
- Friderichsen-Waterhouse A39.1
- Froin's G95.89
- frontal lobe F07.0
- functional
  - bowel K59.9
  - prepubertal castrate E29.1
- Gaisböck's D75.1
- ganglion (basal ganglia brain) G25.9
  - geniculi G51.1
- Gardner-Diamond D69.2
- gastroesophageal
  - junction K22.0
  - laceration-hemorrhage K22.6
- gastrojejunal loop obstruction K91.89
- Gee-Herter-Heubner K90.0
- Gelineau's G47.4
- genito-anorectal A55
- giant platelet (Bernard-Soulier) D69.1
- Gilles de la Tourette's F95.2
- goiter-deafness E07.1
- Goldfam-Erb G70.0
- Gopalan' (burning feet) E53.8
- Gougerot-Blum L81.7
- Gouley's I31.1
- Gower's R55
- gray or grey (newborn) P93.0
  - platelet D69.1
- Gubler-Millard G83.89
- Guillain-Barré (-Strohl) G61.0
- gustatory sweating G50.8
- Hadfield-Clarke K86.8
- Hamman's J98.19
- hand-shoulder G90.8
- Harada — see Vogt-Koyanagi syndrome
- Hayem-Faber D50.9
- headache NEC G44.8
- Heberden's I20.8
- Hedinger's E34.0
- Hegglin's D72.0
- hemolytic-uremic D59.3
- hemophagocytic, infection-associated D76.2
- Henoch-Schönlein D69.0
- hepatic flexure K59.8
- hepatorenal K76.7
  - following delivery O90.4

Syndrome — *see also* Disease — *continued*
  hepatorenal — *continued*
    postoperative or postprocedural K91.82
    postpartum, puerperal O90.4
  hepatourologic K76.7
  Herter (-Gee) (nontropical sprue) K90.0
  Heubner-Herter K90.0
  Heyd's K76.7
  Hilger's G90.0
  histamine-like (fish poisoning) — *see* Poisoning, fish
  histiocytosis NEC D76.3
  HIV infection, acute B20
  Hoffmann-Werdnig G12.0
  Hollander-Simons E88.1
  Hoppe-Goldflam G70.0
  hunterian glossitis K14.4
  Hutchinson's triad A50.53
  hyperabduction G54.0
  hypereosinophilic (idiopathic) D72.1
  hyperimmunoglobulin E (IgE) D82.4
  hyperkalemic E87.5
  hyperkinetic — *see* Hyperkinesia
  hypermobility M35.7
  hypernatremia E87.0
  hyperosmolarity E87.0
  hypersomnia-bulimia G47.8
  hypersplenic D73.1
  hypertransfusion, newborn P61.1
  hyperventilation F45.8
  hyperviscosity (-of serum)
    polycythemic D75.1
    sclerothymic D58.8
  hypoglycemic (familial) (neonatal) E16.2
  hypokalemic E87.6
  hyponatremic E87.1
  hypopituitarism E23.0
  hypoplastic left-heart Q23.4
  hypopotassemia E87.6
  hyposmolality E87.1
  hypotension, maternal O26.50
    first trimester O26.51
    second trimester O26.52
    third trimester O26.53
  ICF (intravascular coagulation-fibrinolysis) D65
  idiopathic
    cardiorespiratory distress, newborn P22.0
    nephrotic (infantile) N04.9
  iliotibial band M76.30
    left M76.32
    right M76.31
  immobility, immobilization (paraplegic) M62.3
  immunity deficiency, combined D81.9
  immunodeficiency
    acquired — *see* Human, immunodeficiency virus (HIV) disease
    combined D81.9
  impending coronary I20.0
  impingement, shoulder M75.40
    left M75.42
    right M75.41
  inappropriate secretion of antidiuretic hormone E22.2
  infant
    death, sudden (SIDS) P96.6
    of diabetic mother P70.1
    gestational diabetes P70.0
  infantilism (pituitary) E23.0
  inferior vena cava I87.1
  inspissated bile (newborn) P59.1
  institutional (childhood) F94.2
  intermediate coronary (artery) I20.0
  internal carotid artery I65.2
  interspinous ligament — *see* Spondylopathy, specified NEC
  intestinal
    carcinoid E34.0
    knot K56.2
  intravascular coagulation-fibrinolysis (ICF) D65
  iodine-deficiency, congenital E00.9
    type
      mixed E00.2
      myxedematous E00.1
      neurological E00.0
  IRDS (idiopathic respiratory distress, newborn) P22.0

Syndrome — *see also* Disease — *continued*
  irritable
    bowel K58.9
      with diarrhea K58.0
      psychogenic F45.8
    heart (psychogenic) F45.8
    weakness F48.8
  ischemic bowel (transient) K55.9
    chronic K55.1
    due to mesenteric artery insufficiency K55.1
  IVC (intravascular coagulopathy) D65
  Ivemark's Q89.01
  Jaccoud's — *see* Arthropathy, postrheumatic, chronic
  Jackson's G83.89
  Jakob-Creutzfeldt A81.0
  jaw-winking Q07.8
  jet lag F51.21
  Job's D71
  Joseph-Diamond-Blackfan D61.4
  jugular foramen G52.7
  Kanner's (autism) F84.0
  Kartagener's Q89.3
  Kelly's D50.1
  Kimmelstiel-Wilson — *see* Diabetes, nephrosis
  Klippel-Feil (brevicollis) Q76.1
  Köhler-Pellegrini-Steida — *see* Bursitis, tibial collateral
  König's K59.8
  Korsakoff (-Wernicke) (nonalcoholic) F04
    alcoholic F10.26
  Kostmann's D70.0
  Krabbe's congenital muscle hypoplasia Q79.8
  labyrinthine — *see* category H83.2
  lacunar NEC G46.7
  Larsen's Q74.8
  lateral
    cutaneous nerve of thigh — *see* Meralgia paresthetica
    medullary G46.4
  Launois' E22.0
  lazy
    leukocyte D70.9
    posture M62.3
  lenticular, progressive E83.01
  Leopold-Levi's E05.90
  Lev's I44.2
  Lichtheim's D51.0
  Lightwood's N25.8
  Lignac (de Toni) (-Fanconi) (-Debré) E72.09
    with cystinosis E72.04
  Likoff's I20.8
  limbic epilepsy personality F07.0
  liver-kidney K76.7
  lobotomy F07.0
  Löffler's J82
  long arm 18 or 21 deletion Q93.8
  Louis-Barré G11.3
  low
    atmospheric pressure T70.20
    back M54.5
      psychogenic F45.4
    output (cardiac) I50.9
  lower radicular, newborn (birth injury) P14.8
  Luetscher's (dehydration) E86.0
  Lutembacher's Q21.1
  malabsorption K90.9
    postsurgical K91.2
  magnesium-deficiency R29.0
  malabsorption K90.9
    postsurgical K91.2
  malformation, congenital, due to
    alcohol Q86.0
    exogenous cause NEC Q86.8
    hydantoin Q86.1
    warfarin Q86.2
  malignant
    carcinoid E34.0
    neuroleptic G21.0
  Mallory-Weiss K22.6
  mandibulofacial dysostosis Q75.4
  manic-depressive — *see* Disorder, bipolar, affective
  maple-syrup-urine E71.0
  Marable's I77.4

Syndrome — *see also* Disease — *continued*
  Marfan's Q87.40
    with
      cardiovascular manifestations Q87.418
        aortic dilation Q87.410
      ocular manifestations Q87.42
      skeletal manifestations Q87.43
  Marie's (acromegaly) E22.0
  maternal hypotension — *see* Syndrome, hypotension, maternal
  maternofetal placental transfusion — *see* Disorder, placenta, fetomaternal transfusion syndrome
  May (-Hegglin) D72.0
  McArdle (-Schmidt) (-Pearson) E74.04
  McQuarrie's E16.2
  meconium plug (newborn) P76.0
  median arcuate ligament I77.4
  Meekeren-Ehlers-Danlos Q79.6
  megavitamin-B6 E67.2
  Meige G24.4
  MELAS E88.31
  Mendelson's O74.0
  menopause N95.1
    postartificial N95.3
  menstruation N94.3
  MERFF E88.32
  mesenteric
    artery (superior) K55.1
    vascular insufficiency K55.1
  metastatic carcinoid E34.0
  micrognathia-glossoptosis Q87.0
  midbrain NEC G93.8
  middle lobe (lung) J98.19
  middle radicular G54.0
  migraine G43.9
  Mikulicz's K11.1
  milk-alkali E83.52
  Millard-Gubler G83.89
  Miller-Fisher G61.0
  Minkowski-Chauffard D58.0
  Mirizzi's K83.1
  Möbius, ophthalmoplegic migraine G43.8
  monofixation H50.44
  Morel-Moore M85.2
  Morel-Morgagni M85.2
  Morgagni (-Morel) (-Stewart) M85.2
  Morgagni-Adams-Stokes I45.9
  mucocutaneous lymph node (acute febrile) (MCLS) M30.3
  multiple operations — *see* Disorder, factitious
  myasthenic G70.9
    in
      diabetes mellitus — *see* Diabetes, amyotrophy
      endocrine disease NEC E34.9 *[G73.3]*
      neoplastic disease (*see also* Neoplasm) D49.9 *[G73.3]*
      thyrotoxicosis (hyperthyroidism) E05.90 *[G73.3]*
        with thyroid storm E05.91 *[G73.3]*
  myelodysplastic (M9989/1) D46.9
    specified NEC D46.7
  myeloproliferative (chronic) (M9960/1) D47.1
  Naffziger's G54.0
  nail patella Q87.2
  nephritic — *see also* Nephritis
    with edema — *see* Nephrosis
    acute N00.9
    chronic N03.9
    rapidly progressive N01.9
  nephrotic (congenital) — *see also* Nephrosis
    with
      dense deposit disease N04.6
      diffuse
        crescentic glomerulonephritis N04.7
        endocapillary proliferative glomerulonephritis N04.4
        membranous glomerulonephritis N04.2
        mesangial proliferative glomerulonephritis N04.3
        mesangiocapillary glomerulonephritis N04.5
      focal and segmental glomerular lesions N04.1
      minor glomerular abnormality N04.0

Syndrome — *see also* Disease — *continued*
nephrotic — *see also* Nephrosis — *continued*
  with — *continued*
    specified morphological changes NEC
      N04.8
    diabetic — *see* Diabetes, nephrosis
neurologic neglect R41.4
Nezelof's D81.4
Nonne-Milroy-Meige Q82.0
Nothnagel's vasomotor acroparesthesia I73.8
oculomotor H51.9
ophthalmoplegia-cerebellar ataxia — *see*
  Strabismus, paralytic, third nerve
oral-facial-digital Q87.0
organic
  affective F06.30
amnesic (not alcoholor drug-induced) F04
  depressive F06.31
  hallucinosis F06.0
  personality F07.0
Ormond's N13.8
oro-facial-digital Q87.0
Osler-Weber-Rendu I78.0
osteoporosis-osteomalacia M83.8
Osterreicher-Turner Q79.8
otolith — *see* category H81.8
oto-palatal-digital Q87.0
outlet (thoracic) G54.0
ovarian vein N13.8
ovary
  polycystic E28.2
  resistant E28.3
  sclerocystic E28.2
Owren's D68.2
Paget-Schroetter I82.8
pain — *see also* Pain
  complex regional I G90.50
    lower limb G90.529
      bilateral G90.523
      left G90.522
      right G90.521
    specified site NEC G90.59
    upper limb G90.519
      bilateral G90.513
      left G90.512
      right G90.511
  complex regional II — *see* Causalgia
painful
  bruising D69.2
  feet E53.8
  prostate N42.81
paralysis agitans — *see* Parkinsonism
paralytic G83.9
  specified NEC G83.89
Parinaud's H51.0
parkinsonian — *see* Parkinsonism
Parkinson's — *see* Parkinsonism
paroxysmal facial pain G50.0
Parry's E05.00
  with thyroid storm E05.01
Parsonage (-Aldren) -Turner G54.5
Paterson (-Brown) (-Kelly) D50.1
pectoral girdle I77.8
pectoralis minor I77.8
Pelger-Huet D72.0
pellagra-cerebellar ataxia-renal aminoaciduria
  E72.02
pellagroid E52
Pellegrini-Stieda — *see* Bursitis, tibial collateral
pelvic congestion-fibrosis, female N94.8
penta X Q97.1
peptic ulcer — *see* Ulcer, peptic
perabduction I77.8
periurethral fibrosis N13.8
phantom limb (without pain) G54.7
  with pain G54.6
pharyngeal pouch D82.1
Pick's (heart) (liver) I31.1
Pickwickian E66.2
PIE (pulmonary infiltration with eosinophilia)
  J82
pigmentary pallidal degeneration progressive)
  G23.0
pineal E34.8
pituitary E22.0

Syndrome — *see also* Disease — *continued*
placental
  dysfunction — *see* Disorder, placenta,
    dysfunction
  insufficiency — *see* Disorder, placenta,
    dysfunction
  transfusion (mother) — *see* Pregnancy,
    complicated by, placenta, transfusion
    syndrome
plantar fascia M72.2
Plummer-Vinson D50.1
pluricarential of infancy E40
plurideficiency E40
pluriglandular (compensatory) (M8360/1)
  D44.8
  autoimmune E31.0
pneumatic hammer T75.21
polyangiitis overlap M30.8
polycarential of infancy E40
polyglandular (M8360/1) D44.8
  autoimmune E31.0
polysplenia Q89.09
pontine NEC G93.8
popliteal
  artery entrapment I77.8
  web Q87.89
postartificial menopause N95.3
postcardiotomy I97.0
postcholecystectomy K91.5
postcommissurotomy I97.0
postconcussional F07.81
postcontusional F07.81
postencephalitic F07.89
posterior
  cervical sympathetic M53.0
  cord G83.83
  fossa compression G93.5
  inferior cerebellar artery I64
postgastrectomy (dumping) K91.1
postgastric surgery K91.1
postinfarction I24.1
postirradiation T66
postlaminectomy NEC M96.1
postleukotomy F07.0
postmastectomy lymphedema I97.2
postmature (of newborn) P08.2
postmyocardial infarction I24.1
postoperative NEC T81.9
  blind loop K90.2
postpartum panhypopituitary (Sheehan) E23.0
postphlebitic I87.0
postvagotomy K91.1
postvalvulotomy I97.0
postviral NEC R53.82
  fatigue G93.3
Potain's K31.0
potassium intoxication E87.5
precerebral artery (multiple) (bilateral) G45.2
preinfarction I20.0
preleukemic (M9989/1) D46.9
premature senility E34.8
premenstrual tension N94.3
Prinzmetal-Massumi R07.1
prolonged gestation P08.2
prune belly Q79.4
pseudocarpal tunnel (sublimis) — *see*
  Syndrome, carpal tunnel
pseudoparalytica G70.0
pseudo-Turner's Q87.1
psycho-organic (nonpsychotic severity) F07.9
  acute or subacute F05
  depressive type F06.31
  hallucinatory type F06.0
  nonpsychotic severity F07.0
  specified NEC F07.89
pulmonary
  arteriosclerosis I27.0
  dysmaturity (Wilson-Mikity) P27.0
  hypoperfusion (idiopathic) P22.0
  renal (hemorrhagic) (Goodpasture's) M31.0
pure
  motor lacunar G46.5
  sensory lacunar G46.6
Putnam-Dana D51.0
pyramidopallidonigral G20
pyriformis — *see* Lesion, nerve, sciatic
radicular NEC — *see* Radiculopathy
  upper limbs, newborn (birth injury) P14.3

Syndrome — *see also* Disease — *continued*
rapid time-zone change F51.21
Raymond (-Céstan) I65.8
Raynaud's I73.00
  with gangrene I73.01
RDS (respiratory distress syndrome, newborn)
  P22.0
reactive airways dysfunction J68.3
Refsum's G60.1
Reifenstein's E34.5
renal glomerulohyalinosis-diabetic — *see*
  Diabetes, nephrosis
Rendu-Osler-Weber I78.0
residual ovary N99.81
resistant ovary E28.3
respiratory distress (idiopathic) (newborn)
  (type I) P22.0
  adult J80
  type II P22.1
restless legs G25.8
retroperitoneal fibrosis N13.8
Reye's G93.7
Ridley's I50.1
right
  heart, hypoplastic Q22.6
  ventricular obstruction — *see* Failure, heart,
    congestive
rotator cuff, shoulder M75.10
  left M75.12
  right M75.11
Roth — *see* Meralgia paresthetica
rubella (congenital) P35.0
Runge's (postmaturity) P08.2
Ruvalcaba-Myhre-Smith E71.321
Rytand-Lipsitch I44.2
salt
  depletion E87.1
    due to heat NEC T67.8
      causing heat exhaustion or prostration
        T67.4
  low E87.1
salt-losing N28.89
Scaglietti-Dagnini E22.0
scalenus anticus (anterior) G54.0
scapulocostal — *see* Mononeuropathy, upper
  limb, specified site NEC
scapuloperoneal G71.0
schizophrenic, of childhood NEC F84.5
Scholte's E34.0
Schroeder's E27.0
Schwartz (-Jampel) Q79.8
Schwartz-Bartter E22.2
scimitar Q26.8
sclerocystic ovary E28.2
Seitelberger's G31.89
septicemic adrenal hemorrhage A39.1
serous meningitis G93.2
shaken infant T74.4
shock (traumatic) T79.4
  kidney N17.0
    following crush injury T79.5
  toxic A48.3
shock-lung J80
short
  bowel K91.2
  rib Q77.2
shoulder-hand — *see* Algoneurodystrophy
sicca — *see* Sicca syndrome
sick
  cell E87.1
  sinus I49.5
sick-euthyroid E07.81
sideropenic D50.1
Siemens' ectodermal dysplasia Q82.4
Silfverskold's Q78.9
Simon's E88.1
sinus tarsi — *see* Syndrome, tarsal tunnel
sinusitis-bronchiectasis-situs inversus Q89.3
sirenomelia Q87.2
Slocumb's E27.0
Sluder's
Sneddon-Wilkinson L13.1
Sotos' E22.0
South African cardiomyopathy I42.8
spasmodic
  upward movement, eyes H51.8
  winking F95.8

Syndrome — *see also* Disease — *continued*
Spen's I45.9
splenic
  agenesis Q89.01
  flexure K59.8
  neutropenia D70.8
Spurway's Q78.0
staphylococcal scalded skin L00
Stein-Leventhal E28.2
Stein's E28.2
Stewart-Morel M85.2
stiff man G25.8
Still-Felty — *see* Felty's syndrome
Stokes (-Adams) I45.9
stone heart I50.1
straight back, congenital Q76.49
stroke I64
subclavian steal G45.8
subcoracoid-pectoralis minor G54.0
subcostal nerve compression I77.8
subphrenic interposition Q43.3
sudden infant death (SIDS) P96.6
superior
  cerebellar artery I63.8
  mesenteric artery K55.1
  vena cava I87.1
supine hypotensive (maternal) — *see*
  Syndrome, hypotension, maternal
suprarenal cortical E27.0
supraspinatus — *see* Syndrome, rotator cuff
swallowed blood P78.2
sweat retention L74.0
Symond's G93.2
sympathetic
  cervical paralysis G90.2
  pelvic, female N94.8
tachycardia-bradycardia I49.5
TAR (thrombocytopenia with absent radius)
  Q87.2
tarsal tunnel G57.50
  left G57.52
  right G57.51
teething K00.7
tegmental G93.8
telangiectasic-pigmentation-cataract Q82.8
temporal pyramidal apex — *see* Otitis, media,
  suppurative, acute
temporomandibular joint-pain-dysfunction
  M26.62
Terry's — *see* Disorder, globe, degenerative,
  myopia
testicular feminization E34.5
thalamic G93.8
thoracic outlet (compression) G54.0
Thorson-Björck E34.0
thrombocytopenia with absent radius (TAR)
  Q87.2
thyroid-adrenocortical insufficiency E31.0
tibial (anterior) (posterior) — *see* Enthesopathy,
  lower limb, lower leg, specified type NEC
Tietze's M94.0
time-zone (rapid) F51.21
Toni-Fanconi E72.09
  with cystinosis E72.04
Touraine's Q79.8
toxic shock A48.3
traumatic vasospastic T75.22
triple X, female Q97.0
trisomy Q92.9
  13 Q91.7
    meiotic nondisjunction Q91.4
    mitotic nondisjunction Q91.5
    mosaicism Q91.5
    translocation Q91.6
  18 Q91.3
    meiotic nondisjunction Q91.0
    mitotic nondisjunction Q91.1
    mosaicism Q91.1
    translocation Q91.2
  20 Q92.8
  21 Q90.9
    meiotic nondisjunction Q90.0
    mitotic nondisjunction Q90.1
    mosaicism Q90.1
    translocation Q90.2
  22 Q92.8

Syndrome — *see also* Disease — *continued*
tropical wet feet T69.00
  left T69.04
  right T69.03
Trousseau's I82.1
tumor lysis N17.8
twin (to twin) transfusion
  mother — *see* Pregnancy, complicated by,
    placenta, transfusion syndrome
  recipient twin P61.1
Unverricht (-Lundborg) G25.3
upward gaze H51.8
uremia, chronic — *see* Failure, renal, chronic
urethral N34.3
urethro-oculo-articular — *see* Reiter's disease
urohepatic K76.7
vago-hypoglossal G52.7
vascular NEC in cerebrovascular disease G46.8
vasomotor I73.9
vasospastic (traumatic) T75.22
vasovagal R55
van Buchem's M85.2
van der Hoeve's Q78.0
VATER Q87.2
vena cava (inferior) (superior) (obstruction) I87.1
vertebral
  artery G45.0
    compression — *see* Syndrome, anterior,
     spinal artery, compression
  steal G45.0
vertebro-basilar artery G45.0
vertebrogenic (pain) — *see* Dorsalgia, specified
  NEC
vertiginous — *see* Disorder, vestibular function
Vinson-Plummer D50.1
virus B34.9
visceral larva migrans B83.0
visual disorientation H53.8
vitamin B6 deficiency E53.1
vitreous (touch) — *see* Complication, eye,
  postoperative, cataract surgery, vitreous
  touch
Volkmann's T79.6
von Schroetter's I82.8
von Willebrand (-Jürgen) D68.0
Waldenström-Kjellberg D50.1
Wallenberg's I64
water retention E87.7
Waterhouse (-Friderichsen) A39.1
Weber-Gubler G83.89
Weber-Leyden G83.89
Weber's G83.89
Weingarten's (tropical eosinophilia) J82
Weiss-Baker G90.0
Werdnig-Hoffman G12.0
Wermer's E31.1
Wernicke-Korsakoff (nonalcoholic) F04
  alcoholic F10.26
Westphal-Strümpell E83.01
wet
  feet (maceration) (tropical) T69.00
    left T69.04
    right T69.03
  lung, newborn P22.1
whiplash S13.4
whistling face Q87.0
Wilkie's K55.1
Wilkinson-Sneddon L13/1
Willebrand (-Jürgens) D68.0
Wilson's (hepatolenticular degeneration) D83.0
Wiskott-Aldrich D82.0
withdrawal — *see* Withdrawal, state
  drug
    infant of dependent mother P96.1
    therapeutic use, newborn P96.2
Woakes' (ethmoiditis) J33.1
Wright's (hyperabduction) I77.8
X I20.9
XXXX Q97.1
XXXXX Q97.1
XXXXY Q98.1
XXY Q98.0
yellow nail L60.5
Zahorsky's B08.5

Synechia (anterior) (iris) (posterior) (pupil) — *see
also* Adhesions, iris
  intra-uterine (traumatic) N85.6

Synesthesia R20.8
Syngamiasis, syngamosis B83.3
Synodontia K00.2
Synorchidism, synorchism Q55.1
Synostosis (congenital) Q78.8
  astragalo-scaphoid Q74.2
  radioulnar Q74.0
Synovial sarcoma (M9040/3) — *see* Neoplasm,
  connective tissue, malignant
Synovioma (malignant) (M9040/3) — *see also*
  Neoplasm, connective tissue, malignant
  benign (M9040/0) — *see* Neoplasm, connective
    tissue, benign
Synoviosarcoma (M9040/3) — *see* Neoplasm,
  connective tissue, malignant
Synovitis — *see also* Tenosynovitis
  crepitant
    hand M70.049
      left M70.042
      right M70.041
    wrist M70.039
      left M70.032
      right M70.031
  gonococcal A54.49
  gouty — *see* Gout, idiopathic
  in (due to)
    crystals — *see* Arthritis, in, crystals
    gonorrhea A54.49
    syphilis (late) A52.78
    use, overuse, pressure — *see* Disorder, soft
      tissue, due to use
  infective NEC — *see* Tenosynovitis, infective
    NEC
  specified NEC — *see* Tenosynovitis, specified
    type NEC
  syphilitic A52.78
    congenital (early) A50.02
  toxic — *see* Synovitis, transient
  transient M67.30
    ankle M67.379
      left M67.372
      right M67.371
    elbow M67.329
      left M67.322
      right M67.321
    foot joint M67.379
      left M67.372
      right M67.371
    hand joint M67.349
      left M67.342
      right M67.341
    hip M67.359
      left M67.352
      right M67.351
    knee M67.369
      left M67.362
      right M67.361
    multiple site M67.39
    pelvic region M67.359
      left M67.352
      right M67.351
    shoulder M67.319
      left M67.312
      right M67.311
    specified joint NEC M67.38
    wrist M67.339
      left M67.332
      right M67.331
  traumatic, current — *see* Sprain
  tuberculous — *see* Tuberculosis, synovitis
  villonodular (pigmented) M12.20
    ankle M12.279
      left M12.272
      right M12.271
    elbow M12.229
      left M12.222
      right M12.221
    foot joint M12.279
      left M12.272
      right M12.271
    hand joint M12.249
      left M12.242
      right M12.241
    hip M12.259
      left M12.252

©2002 Ingenix, Inc.

Synovitis — *see also* Tenosynovitis — *continued*
  villonodular — *continued*
    hip — *continued*
      right M12.251
    knee M12.269
      left M12.262
      right M12.261
    multiple site M12.29
    pelvic region M12.259
      left M12.252
      right M12.251
    shoulder M12.219
      left M12.212
      right M12.211
    specified joint NEC M12.28
    wrist M12.239
      left M12.232
      right M12.231
Syphilid A51.39
  congenital A50.06
  newborn A50.06
  tubercular (late) A52.79
Syphilis, syphilitic (acquired) A53.9
  abdomen (late) A52.79
  acoustic nerve A52.15
  adenopathy (secondary) A51.49
  adrenal (gland) (with cortical hypofunction) A52.79
  age under 2 years NOS — *see also* Syphilis, congenital, early
    acquired A51.9
  alopecia (secondary) A51.32
  anemia (late) A52.79 *[D63.8]*
  aneurysm (aorta) (ruptured) A52.01
    central nervous system A52.05
    congenital A50.54 *[I79.0]*
  anus (late) A52.74
    primary A51.1
    secondary A51.39
  aorta (arch) (abdominal) (thoracic) A52.02
    aneurysm A52.01
  aortic (insufficiency) (regurgitation) (stenosis) A52.03
    aneurysm A52.01
  arachnoid (adhesive) (cerebral) (spinal) A52.13
  asymptomatic — *see* Syphilis, latent
  ataxia (locomotor) A52.11
  atrophoderma maculatum A51.39
  auricular fibrillation A52.06
  bladder (late) A52.76
  bone A52.77
    secondary A51.46
  brain A52.17
  breast (late) A52.79
  bronchus (late) A52.72
  bubo (primary) A51.0
  bulbar palsy A52.19
  bursa (late) A52.78
  cardiac decompensation A52.06
  cardiovascular A52.00
  causing death under 2 years of age — *see also* Syphilis, congenital, early
    stated to be acquired A51.9
  central nervous system (late) (recurrent) (relapse) (tertiary) A52.3
    with
      ataxia A52.11
      general paralysis A52.17
        juvenile A50.45
      paresis (general) A52.17
        juvenile A50.45
      tabes (dorsalis) A52.11
        juvenile A50.45
      taboparesis A52.11
        juvenile A50.45
    aneurysm A52.05
    congenital A50.40
    juvenile A50.40
    remission in (sustained) A52.3
    serology doubtful, negative, or positive A52.3
    specified nature or site NEC A52.19
    vascular A52.05
  cerebral A52.17
    meningovascular A52.13
    nerves (multiple palsies) A52.15
    sclerosis A52.17
    thrombosis A52.05

Syphilis, syphilitic — *continued*
  cerebrospinal (tabetic type) A52.12
  cerebrovascular A52.05
  cervix (late) A52.76
  chancre (multiple) A51.0
    extragenital A51.2
    Rollet's A51.0
  Charcot's joint A52.16
  chorioretinitis A51.43
    congenital A50.01
    late A52.71
    prenatal A50.01
  choroiditis — *see* Syphilitic chorioretinitis
  choroidoretinitis — *see* Syphilitic chorioretinitis
  ciliary body (secondary) A51.43
    late A52.71
  colon (late) A52.74
  combined spinal sclerosis A52.11
  complicating pregnancy, childbirth or puerperium — *see* Syphilis, obstetric
  condyloma (latum) A51.31
  congenital A50.9
    with
      paresis (general) A50.45
      tabes (dorsalis) A50.45
      taboparesis A50.45
    chorioretinitis, choroiditis A50.01 *[H32]*
    early, or less than 2 years after birth NEC A50.2
      with manifestations — *see* Syphilis, congenital, early, symptomatic
      latent (without manifestations) A50.1
        negative spinal fluid test A50.1
        serology positive A50.1
      symptomatic A50.09
        cutaneous A50.06
        mucocutaneous A50.07
        oculopathy A50.01
        osteochondropathy A50.02
        pharyngitis A50.03
        pneumonia A50.04
        rhinitis A50.05
        visceral A50.08
      interstitial keratitis A50.31
      juvenile neurosyphilis A50.45
    late, or 2 years or more after birth NEC A50.7
      chorioretinitis, choroiditis A50.32
      interstitial keratitis A50.31
      juvenile neurosyphilis A50.45
      latent (without manifestations) A50.6
        negative spinal fluid test A50.6
        serology positive A50.6
      symptomatic or with manifestations NEC A50.59
        arthropathy A50.55
        cardiovascular A50.54
        Clutton's joints A50.51
        Hutchinson's teeth A50.52
        Hutchinson's triad A50.53
        osteochondropathy A50.56
        saddle nose A50.57
  conjugal A53.9
    tabes A52.11
  conjunctiva (late) A52.71
  contact Z20.2
  cord bladder A52.19
  cornea, late A52.71
  coronary (artery) (sclerosis) A52.06
  coryza, congenital A50.05
  cranial nerve A52.15
    multiple palsies A52.15
  cutaneous — *see* Syphilis, skin
  dacryocystitis (late) A52.71
  degeneration, spinal cord A52.12
  dementia paralytica A52.17
    juvenilis A50.45
  destruction of bone A52.77
  dilatation, aorta A52.01
  due to blood transfusion A53.9
  dura mater A52.13
  ear A52.79
    inner A52.79
      nerve (eighth) A52.15
      neurorecurrence A52.15
  early A51.9
    cardiovascular A52.00

Syphilis, syphilitic — *continued*
  early — *continued*
    central nervous system A52.3
    latent (without manifestations) (less than 2 years after infection) A51.5
      negative spinal fluid test A51.5
      serological relapse after treatment A51.5
      serology positive A51.5
    relapse (treated, untreated) A51.9
    skin A51.39
    symptomatic A51.9
      extragenital chancre A51.2
      primary, except extragenital chancre A51.0
      secondary (*see also* Syphilis, secondary) A51.39
        relapse (treated, untreated) A51.49
    ulcer A51.39
  eighth nerve (neuritis) A52.15
  endemic A65
  endocarditis A52.03
    aortic A52.03
    pulmonary A52.03
  epididymis (late) A52.76
  epiglottis (late) A52.73
  epiphysitis (congenital) (early) A50.02 *[M90.80]*
  episcleritis (late) A52.71
  esophagus A52.79
  eustachian tube A52.73
  exposure to Z20.2
  eye A52.71
  eyelid (late) (with gumma) A52.71
  fallopian tube (late) A52.76
  fracture A52.77
  gallbladder (late) A52.74
  gastric (polyposis) (late) A52.74
  general A53.9
    paralysis A52.17
      juvenile A50.45
  genital (primary) A51.0
  glaucoma A52.71
  gumma NEC A52.79
    cardiovascular system A52.00
    central nervous system A52.3
    congenital A50.59
  heart (block) (decompensation) (disease) (failure) A52.06 *[I52]*
    valve NEC A52.03
  hemianesthesia A52.19
  hemianopsia A52.71
  hemiparesis A52.17
  hemiplegia A52.17
  hepatic artery A52.09
  hepatis A52.74
  hepatomegaly, congenital A50.08
  hereditaria tarda — *see* Syphilis, congenital, late
  hereditary — *see* Syphilis, congenital
  Hutchinson's teeth A50.52
  hyalitis A52.71
  inactive — *see* Syphilis, latent
  infantum — *see* Syphilis, congenital
  inherited — *see* Syphilis, congenital
  internal ear A52.79
  intestine (late) A52.74
  iris, iritis (secondary) A51.43
    late A52.71
  joint (late) A52.77
  keratitis (congenital) (interstitial) (late) A50.31
  kidney (late) A52.75
  lacrimal passages (late) A52.71
  larynx (late) A52.73
  late A52.9
    cardiovascular A52.00
    central nervous system A52.3
    kidney A52.75
    latent or 2 years or more after infection (without manifestations) A52.8
      negative spinal fluid test A52.8
      serology positive A52.8
    paresis A52.17
    specified site NEC A52.79
    symptomatic or with manifestations A52.79
    tabes A52.11
  latent A53.0
    with signs or symptoms – code by site and stage under Syphilis

Syphilis, syphilitic — *continued*
  latent — *continued*
    central nervous system A52.2
    date of infection unspecified A53.0
    early, or less than 2 years after infection A51.5
      follow-up of latent syphilis A53.0
        date of infection unspecified A53.0
        late, or 2 years or more after infection A52.8
    late, or 2 years or more after infection A52.8
    positive serology (only finding) A53.0
      date of infection unspecified A53.0
      early, or less than 2 years after infection A51.5
      late, or 2 years or more after infection A52.8
  lens (late) A52.71
  leukoderma A51.39
    late A52.79
  lienitis A52.79
  lip A51.39
    chancre (primary) A51.2
    late A52.79
  Lissauer's paralysis A52.17
  liver A52.74
  locomotor ataxia A52.11
  lung A52.72
  lymph gland (early) (secondary) A51.49
    late A52.79
  lymphadenitis (secondary) A51.49
  macular atrophy of skin A51.39
    striated A52.79
  maternal, affecting fetus or newborn
    manifest syphilis in infant — *see* category A50
  mediastinum (late) A52.73
  meninges (adhesive) (brain) (spinal cord) A52.13
  meningitis A52.13
    acute (secondary) A51.41
    congenital A50.41
  meningoencephalitis A52.14
  meningovascular A52.13
    congenital A50.41
  mesarteritis A52.09
    brain A52.04
  middle ear A52.77
  mitral stenosis A52.03
  monoplegia A52.17
  mouth (secondary) A51.39
    late A52.79
  mucocutaneous (secondary) A51.39
    late A52.79
  mucous
    membrane (secondary) A51.39
      late A52.79
    patches A51.39
      congenital A50.07
  mulberry molars A50.52
  muscle A52.78
  myocardium A52.06
  nasal sinus (late) A52.73
  neonatorum — *see* Syphilis, congenital
  nephrotic syndrome (secondary) A51.44
  nerve palsy (any cranial nerve) A52.15
    multiple A52.15
  nervous system, central A52.3
  neuritis A52.15
    acoustic A52.15
  neurorecidive of retina A52.19
  neuroretinitis A52.19
  newborn — *see* Syphilis, congenital
  nodular superficial (late) A52.79
  nonvenereal A65
  nose (late) A52.73
    saddle back deformity A50.57
  obstetric complicating
    childbirth O98.12
    pregnancy O98.119
      first trimester O98.111
      second trimester O98.112
      third trimester O98.113
    puerperium O98.13
  occlusive arterial disease A52.09
  oculopathy A52.71

Syphilis, syphilitic — *continued*
  oesophagus (late) A52.79
  ophthalmic (late) A52.71
  optic nerve (atrophy) (neuritis) (papilla) A52.15
  orbit (late) A52.71
  organic A53.9
  osseous (late) A52.77
  osteochondritis (congenital) (early) A50.02 [M90.80]
  osteoporosis A52.77
  ovary (late) A52.76
  oviduct (late) A52.76
  palate (late) A52.79
  pancreas (late) A52.74
  paralysis A52.17
    general A52.17
      juvenile A50.45
  paresis (general) A52.17
    juvenile A50.45
  paresthesia A52.19
  Parkinson's disease or syndrome A52.19
  paroxysmal tachycardia A52.06
  pemphigus (congenital) A50.06
  penis (chancre) A51.0
    late A52.76
  pericardium A52.06
  perichondritis, larynx (late) A52.73
  periosteum (late) A52.77
    congenital (early) A50.02 [M90.80]
    early (secondary) A51.46
  peripheral nerve A52.79
  petrous bone (late) A52.77
  pharynx (late) A52.73
    secondary A51.39
  pituitary (gland) A52.79
  placenta — *see* Syphilis, obstetric
  pleura (late) A52.73
  pneumonia, white A50.04
  pontine lesion A52.17
  portal vein A52.09
  primary A51.0
    anal A51.1
    and secondary — *see* Syphilis, secondary
    central nervous system A52.3
    extragenital chancre NEC A51.2
    fingers A51.2
    genital A51.0
    lip A51.2
    specified site NEC A51.2
    tonsils A51.2
  prostate (late) A52.76
  ptosis (eyelid) A52.71
  pulmonary (late) A52.72
    artery A52.09
  pyelonephritis (late) A52.75
  recently acquired, symptomatic A51.9
  rectum (late) A52.74
  respiratory tract (late) A52.73
  retina
    late A52.71
  retrobulbar neuritis A52.15
  salpingitis A52.76
  sclera (late) A52.71
  sclerosis
    cerebral A52.17
    coronary A52.06
    multiple A52.11
  scotoma (central) A52.71
  scrotum (late) A52.76
  secondary (and primary) A51.49
    adenopathy A51.49
    anus A51.39
    bone A51.46
    chorioretinitis, choroiditis A51.43
    hepatitis A51.45
    liver A51.45
    lymphadenitis A51.49
    meningitis (acute) A51.41
    mouth A51.39
    mucous membranes A51.39
    periosteum, periostitis A51.46
    pharynx A51.39
    relapse (treated, untreated) A51.49
    skin A51.39
    specified form NEC A51.49
    tonsil A51.39
    ulcer A51.39
    viscera NEC A51.49

Syphilis, syphilitic — *continued*
  secondary — *continued*
    vulva A51.39
  seminal vesicle (late) A52.76
  seronegative with signs or symptoms – code by site and stage under Syphilis
  seropositive
    with signs or symptoms – code by site and stage under Syphilis
    follow-up of latent syphilis — *see* Syphilis, latent
    only finding — *see* Syphilis, latent
  seventh nerve (paralysis) A52.15
  sinus, sinusitis (late) A52.73
  skeletal system A52.77
  skin (with ulceration) (early) (secondary) A51.39
    late or tertiary A52.79
  small intestine A52.74
  spastic spinal paralysis A52.17
  spermatic cord (late) A52.76
  spinal (cord) A52.12
  spleen A52.79
  splenomegaly A52.79
  spondylitis A52.77
  staphyloma A52.71
  stigmata (congenital) A50.59
  stomach A52.74
  synovium A52.78
  tabes dorsalis (late) A52.11
    juvenile A50.45
  tabetic type A52.11
    juvenile A50.45
  taboparesis A52.11
    juvenile A50.45
  tachycardia A52.06
  tendon (late) A52.78
  tertiary A52.9
    with symptoms NEC A52.79
    cardiovascular A52.00
    central nervous system A52.3
    multiple NEC A52.79
    specified site NEC A52.79
  testis A52.76
  thorax A52.73
  throat A52.73
  thymus (gland) (late) A52.79
  thyroid (late) A52.79
  tongue (late) A52.79
  tonsil (lingual) (late) A52.73
    primary A51.2
    secondary A51.39
  trachea (late) A52.73
  tunica vaginalis (late) A52.76
  ulcer (any site) (early) (secondary) A51.39
    late A52.79
    perforating A52.79
      foot A52.11
  urethra (late) A52.76
  urogenital (late) A52.76
  uterus (late) A52.76
  uveal tract (secondary) A51.43
    late A52.71
  uveitis (secondary) A51.43
    late A52.71
  uvula (late) (perforated) A52.79
  vagina A51.0
    late A52.76
  valvulitis NEC A52.03
  vascular A52.00
    brain (cerebral) A52.05
  ventriculi A52.74
  vesicae urinariae (late) A52.76
  viscera (abdominal) (late) A52.74
    secondary A51.49
  vitreous (opacities) (late) A52.71
    hemorrhage A52.71
  vulva A51.0
    late A52.76
    secondary A51.39
Syphiloma A52.79
  cardiovascular system A52.00
  central nervous system A52.3
  circulatory system A52.00
  congenital A50.59
Syphilophobia F45.29
Syringadenoma (M8400/0) — *see also* Neoplasm, skin, benign

Syringadenoma — see also Neoplasm, skin, benign — continued
  papillary (M8406/0) — see Neoplasm, skin, benign
Syringobulbia G95.0
Syringocystadenoma (M8400/0) — see Neoplasm, skin, benign
  papillary (M8406/0) — see Neoplasm, skin, benign
Syringoma (M8407/0) — see also Neoplasm, skin, benign
  chondroid (M8940/0) — see Neoplasm, skin, benign
Syringomyelia G95.0
Syringomyelitis — see Encephalitis
Syringomyelocele — see Spina bifida
Syringopontia G95.0
System, systemic — see also condition
  disease, combined — see Degeneration, combined
  lupus erythematosus M32.9
    inhibitor present D68.81

T

Tabacism, tabacosis, tabagism
  meaning dependence (without remission) F17.200
  with
    disorder F17.209
      remission F17.201
      specified disorder NEC F17.208
      withdrawal F17.203
Tabardillo A75.9
  flea-borne A75.2
  louse-borne A75.0
Tabes, tabetic A52.10
  with
    central nervous system syphilis A52.10
    Charcot's joint A52.16
    cord bladder A52.19
    crisis, viscera (any) A52.19
    paralysis, general A52.17
    paresis (general) A52.17
    perforating ulcer (foot) A52.19
  arthropathy (Charcot) A52.16
  bladder A52.19
  bone A52.11
  cerebrospinal A52.12
  congenital A50.45
  conjugal A52.10
  dorsalis A52.11
    juvenile A50.49
  juvenile A50.49
  latent A52.19
  mesenterica A18.39
  paralysis, insane, general A52.17
  spasmodic A52.17
  syphilis (cerebrospinal) A52.12
Taboparalysis A52.17
Taboparesis (remission) A52.17
  juvenile A50.45
Tachyalimentation K91.2
Tachyarrhythmia, tachyrhythmia — see Tachycardia
Tachycardia R00.0
  atrial I47.1
  auricular I47.1
  fetal — see Distress, fetal
  nodal I47.1
  non-paroxysmal AV nodal I45.8
  paroxysmal I47.9
    with sinus bradycardia I49.5
    atrial (PAT) I47.1
    atrioventricular (AV) I47.1
      psychogenic F54
    junctional I47.1
    nodal I47.1
    psychogenic (atrial) (supraventricular) (ventricular) F54
    supraventricular I47.1
      psychogenic F54
    ventricular I47.2
      psychogenic F54
  psychogenic F45.8

Tachycardia — continued
  sick sinus I49.5
  sinoauricular I47.1
  sinus I47.1
  supraventricular I47.1
  ventricular (paroxysmal) I47.2
    psychogenic F54
Tachypnea R06.82
  hysterical F45.8
  newborn (idiopathic) (transitory) P22.1
  psychogenic F45.8
  transitory, of newborn P22.1
Taenia (infection) (infestation) B68.9
  diminuta B71.0
  echinococcal infestation B67.90
  mediocanellata B68.1
  nana B71.0
  saginata B68.1
  solium (intestinal form) B68.0
    larval form — see Cysticercosis
Taeniasis (intestine) — see Taenia
Tag (hypertrophied skin) (infected) L91.8
  adenoid J35.8
  anus I84.6
  hemorrhoidal I84.6
  hymen N89.8
  perineal N90.8
  preauricular Q17.0
  rectum I84.6
  sentinel I84.6
  skin L91.8
    accessory (congenital) Q82.8
    anus I84.6
    congenital Q82.8
    preauricular Q17.0
    rectum I84.6
  tonsil J35.8
  urethra, urethral N36.8
  vulva N90.8
Tahyna fever B33.8
Takahara's disease E80.3
Takayasu's disease or syndrome M31.4
Talcosis (pulmonary) J62.0
Talipes (congenital) Q66.8
  acquired, planus — see Deformity, limb, flat foot
  asymmetric Q66.8
  calcaneovalgus Q66.4
  calcaneovarus Q66.1
  calcaneus Q66.8
  cavus Q66.7
  equinovalgus Q66.6
  equinovarus Q66.0
  equinus Q66.8
  percavus Q66.7
  planovalgus Q66.6
  planus (acquired) (any degree) — see also Deformity, limb, flat foot
    congenital Q66.5
    due to rickets (sequelae) E64.3
  valgus Q66.6
  varus Q66.3
Tall stature, constitutional E34.4
Talma's disease M62.89
Tamponade, heart — see Pericarditis
Tanapox (virus disease) B08.8
Tangier disease E78.6
Tantrum, child problem F91.8
Tapeworm (infection) (infestation) — see Infestation, tapeworm
Tapia's syndrome G52.7
TAR (thrombocytopenia with absent radius) **syndrome** Q87.2
Tarral-Besnier disease L44.0
Tarsal tunnel syndrome — see Syndrome, tarsal tunnel
Tarsalgia — see Pain, limb, lower
Tarsitis (eyelid) H01.8
  syphilitic A52.71
  tuberculous A18.4
Tartar (teeth) (dental calculus) K03.6
Tattoo (mark) L81.8
Tauri's disease E74.09

Taurodontism K00.2
Taussig-Bing syndrome Q20.1
Taybi's syndrome Q87.2
Tay-Sachs amaurotic familial idiocy or disease E75.02
Teacher's node or nodule J38.2
Tear, torn (traumatic) — see also Laceration
  with abortion — see Abortion
  anus, anal (sphincter) S31.831
    complicating delivery O70.2
      with mucosa O70.3
    nontraumatic, nonpuerperal — see Fissure, anus
  articular cartilage, old — see Disorder, cartilage, articular NEC
  bladder
    with ectopic or molar pregnancy O08.6
    following ectopic or molar pregnancy O08.6
    obstetrical O71.5
    traumatic — see Injury, bladder
  bowel
    with ectopic or molar pregnancy O08.6
    following ectopic or molar pregnancy O08.6
    obstetrical trauma O71.5
  broad ligament
    with ectopic or molar pregnancy O08.6
    following ectopic or molar pregnancy O08.6
    obstetrical trauma O71.6
  bucket handle (knee) (meniscus) — see Tear, meniscus
  capsule, joint — see Sprain
  cartilage — see also Sprain
    articular, old — see Disorder, cartilage, articular NEC
  cervix
    with ectopic or molar pregnancy O08.6
    following ectopic or molar pregnancy O08.6
    obstetrical trauma (current) O71.3
    old N88.1
    traumatic — see Injury, uterus
  internal organ — see Injury, by site
  knee cartilage
    articular (current) S83.30
    left S83.32
    old — see Derangement, knee, meniscus, due to old tear
    right S83.31
  ligament — see Sprain
  meniscus (knee) (current injury) S83.209
    bucket-handle S83.202
      left S83.201
      right S83.200
    lateral
      bucket-handle S83.259
        left S83.252
        right S83.251
      complex S83.279
        left S83.272
        right S83.271
      peripheral S83.269
        left S83.262
        right S83.261
      specified type NEC S83.289
        left S83.282
        right S83.281
    left S83.207
    medial
      bucket-handle S83.219
        left S83.212
        right S83.211
      complex S83.239
        left S83.232
        right S83.231
      peripheral S83.229
        left S83.222
        right S83.221
      specified type NEC S83.249
        left S83.242
        right S83.241
    old — see Derangement, knee, meniscus, due to old tear
    right S83.206
    site other than knee – code as Sprain
    specified type NEC S83.205
      left S83.204
      right S83.203

Tear, torn — *see also* Laceration — *continued*
  muscle — *see* Injury, muscle
  pelvic
    floor, complicating delivery O70.1
    organ NEC, obstetrical trauma O71.5
      with ectopic or molar pregnancy O08.6
      following ectopic or molar pregnancy
        O08.6
  perineal, secondary O90.1
  periurethral tissue, obstetrical trauma O71.5
    with ectopic or molar pregnancy O08.6
    following ectopic or molar pregnancy O08.6
  rectovaginal septum — *see* Laceration, vagina
  retina, retinal (without detachment) (horseshoe)
    — *see also* Break, retina, horseshoe
    with detachment — *see* Detachment, retina,
      with retinal, break
  rotator cuff (complete) (incomplete)
    (nontraumatic) — *see* Syndrome, rotator
    cuff
  semilunar cartilage, knee — *see* Tear, meniscus
  supraspinatus (complete) (incomplete)
    (nontraumatic) — *see* Syndrome, rotator
    cuff
  tendon — *see* Injury, muscle
  tentorial, at birth P10.4
  umbilical cord
    affecting fetus or newborn P50.1
    complicating delivery O69.8
  urethra
    with ectopic or molar pregnancy O08.6
    following ectopic or molar pregnancy O08.6
    obstetrical trauma O71.5
  uterus — *see* Injury, uterus
  vagina — *see* Laceration, vagina
  vessel, from catheter — *see* Puncture,
    accidental complicating surgery
  vulva, complicating delivery O70.0

Tear-stone — *see* Dacryolith

Teeth — *see also* condition
  grinding F45.8

Teething (syndrome) K00.7

Telangiectasia, telangiectasis (verrucous) I78.1
  ataxic (cerebellar) (Louis-Bar) G11.3
  familial I78.0
  hemorrhagic, hereditary (congenital) (senile)
    I78.0
  hereditary, hemorrhagic (congenital) (senile)
    I78.0
  retina H35.079
    bilateral H35.073
    left H35.072
    right H35.071
  spider I78.1

Telephone scatologia F65.89

Telescoped bowel or intestine K56.1
  congenital Q43.8

Teletherapy, adverse effect T66

Temperature
  body, high (of unknown origin) R50.9
  cold, trauma from T69.9
    newborn P80.0
    specified effect NEC T69.8

Temple — *see* condition

Temporal — *see* condition

Temporomandibular joint pain-dysfunction
  syndrome M26.62

Temporosphenoidal — *see* condition

Tendency
  bleeding — *see* Defect, coagulation
  suicide Z91.5

Tenderness, abdominal R10.819
  epigastric R10.816
  generalized R10.817
  left lower quadrant R10.814
  left upper quadrant R10.812
  periumbilic R10.815
  right lower quadrant R10.813
  right upper quadrant R10.811
  rebound R10.829
    epigastric R10.826
    generalized R10.827
    left lower quadrant R10.824
    left upper quadrant R10.822
    periumbilic R10.825

Tenderness, abdominal — *continued*
  rebound — *continued*
    right lower quadrant R10.823
    right upper quadrant R10.821

Tendinitis, tendonitis — *see also* Enthesopathy
  Achilles M76.60
    left M76.62
    right M76.61

Tendinitis, tendonitis — *see also* Enthesopathy
  — *continued*
  adhesive — *see* Tenosynovitis, specified type NEC
    shoulder — *see* Capsulitis, adhesive
  bicipital M75.20
    left M75.22
    right M75.21
  calcific M65.20
    ankle M65.279
      left M65.272
      right M65.271
    foot M65.279
      left M65.272
      right M65.271
    forearm M65.239
      left M65.232
      right M65.231
    hand M65.249
      left M65.242
      right M65.241
    lower leg M65.269
      left M65.262
      right M65.261
    multiple sites M65.29
    pelvic region M65.259
      left M65.252
      right M65.251
    shoulder M75.30
      left M75.32
      right M75.31
    specified site NEC M65.28
    thigh M65.259
      left M65.252
      right M65.251
    upper arm M65.229
      left M65.222
      right M65.221
  due to use, overuse, pressure — *see also*
    Disorder, soft tissue, due to use
    specified NEC — *see* Disorder, soft tissue,
      due to use, specified NEC
  gluteal M76.00
    left M76.02
    right M76.01
  patellar M76.50
    left M76.52
    right M76.51
  peroneal M76.70
    left M76.72
    right M76.71
  psoas M76.10
    left M76.12
    right M76.11
  tibialis (anterior) (posterior) — *see*
    Enthesopathy, lower limb, lower leg,
    specified type NEC
  trochanteric — *see* Bursitis, hip, trochanteric

Tendon — *see* condition

Tendosynovitis — *see* Tenosynovitis

Tenesmus (rectal) R19.8
  vesical R30.1

Tennis elbow — *see* Epicondylitis, lateral

Tenonitis — *see also* Tenosynovitis
  eye (capsule) H05.049
    bilateral H05.043
    left H05.042
    right H05.041

Tenontosynovitis — *see* Tenosynovitis

Tenontothecitis — *see* Tenosynovitis

Tenophyte — *see* Disorder, synovium, specified
  type NEC

Tenosynovitis M65.9
  adhesive — *see* Tenosynovitis, specified type
    NEC
    shoulder — *see* Capsulitis, adhesive
  bicipital (calcifying) — *see* Tendinitis, bicipital
  gonococcal A54.49

Tenosynovitis — *continued*
  in (due to)
    crystals — *see* Arthritis, in, crystals
    gonorrhea A54.49
    syphilis (late) A52.78
    use, overuse, pressure — *see also* Disorder,
      soft tissue, due to use
      specified NEC — *see* Disorder, soft tissue,
        due to use, specified NEC
  infective NEC M65.10
    ankle M65.179
      left M65.172
      right M65.171
    foot M65.179
      left M65.172
      right M65.171
    forearm M65.139
      left M65.132
      right M65.131
    hand M65.149
      left M65.142
      right M65.141
    lower leg M65.169
      left M65.162
      right M65.161
    multiple sites M65.19
    pelvic region M65.159
      left M65.152
      right M65.151
    shoulder region M65.119
      left M65.112
      right M65.111
    specified site NEC M65.18
    thigh M65.159
      left M65.152
      right M65.151
    upper arm M65.129
      left M65.122
      right M65.121
  radial styloid M65.4
  shoulder region M65.9
    adhesive — *see* Capsulitis, adhesive
  specified type NEC M65.80
    ankle M65.879
      left M65.872
      right M65.871
    foot M65.879
      left M65.872
      right M65.871
    forearm M65.839
      left M65.832
      right M65.831
    hand M65.849
      left M65.842
      right M65.841
    lower leg M65.869
      left M65.862
      right M65.861
    multiple sites M65.89
    pelvic region M65.859
      left M65.852
      right M65.851
    shoulder region M65.819
      left M65.812
      right M65.811
    specified site NEC M65.88
    thigh M65.859
      left M65.852
      right M65.851
    upper arm M65.829
      left M65.822
      right M65.821
  tuberculous — *see* Tuberculosis, tenosynovitis

Tenovaginitis — *see* Tenosynovitis

Tension
  arterial, high — *see also* Hypertension
    without diagnosis of hypertension R03.0
  headache G44.2
  nervous R45.0
  pneumothorax J93.0
  premenstrual N94.3
  state (mental) F48.9

Tentorium — *see* condition

Teratencephalus Q89.8

Teratism Q89.7

Teratoblastoma (malignant) (M9080/3) — *see* Neoplasm, malignant

Teratocarcinoma (M9081/3) — *see also* Neoplasm, malignant
  liver C22.7

Teratoma (solid) (M9080/1) — *see also* Neoplasm, uncertain behavior
  with embryonal carcinoma, mixed (M9081/3) — *see* Neoplasm, malignant
  with malignant transformation (M9084/3) — *see* Neoplasm, malignant
  adult (cystic) (M9080/0) — *see* Neoplasm, benign
  benign (M9080/0) — *see* Neoplasm, benign
  combined with choriocarcinoma (M9101/3) — *see* Neoplasm, malignant
  cystic (adult) (M9080/0) — *see* Neoplasm, benign
  differentiated (M9080/0) — *see* Neoplasm, benign
  embryonal (M9080/3) — *see also* Neoplasm, malignant
    liver C22.7
  immature (M9080/3) — *see* Neoplasm, malignant
  liver (M9080/3) C22.7
    adult, benign, cystic, differentiated type or mature (M9080/0) D13.4
  malignant (M9080/3) — *see also* Neoplasm, malignant
    anaplastic (M9082/3) — *see* Neoplasm, malignant
    intermediate (M9083/3) — *see* Neoplasm, malignant
    trophoblastic (M9102/3)
      specified site — *see* Neoplasm, malignant
      unspecified site C62.90
    undifferentiated (M9082/3) — *see* Neoplasm, malignant
  mature (M9080/1) — *see* Neoplasm, uncertain behavior
  ovary (M9080/0) D27.9
    embryonal, immature or malignant (M9080/3) C56.9
      left C56.1
      right C56.0
    left D27.1
    right D27.0
  sacral, fetal, causing obstructed labor (mother) O66.3
  solid (M9080/1) — *see* Neoplasm, uncertain behavior
  testis (M9080/3) C62.90
    adult, benign, cystic, differentiated type or mature (M9080/0) D29.20
      left D29.22
      right D29.21
    left C62.92
    right C62.91
    scrotal C62.10
      left C62.12
      right C62.11
    undescended C62.00
      left C62.02
      right C62.01

Termination
  anomalous — *see also* Malposition, congenital
    right pulmonary vein Q26.3
  pregnancy — *see* Abortion

Ternidens diminutus infestation B81.8

Ternidensiasis B81.8

Terror(s) night (child) F51.4

Terrorism, victim of Z65.4

Terry's syndrome — *see* Disorder, globe, degenerative, myopia

Tertiary — *see* condition

Test(s)
  adequacy (for dialysis)
    hemodialysis Z49.31
    peritoneal Z49.32
  AIDS virus Z01.8
  allergens Z01.8
  basal metabolic rate Z01.8
  blood pressure Z01.30
    abnormal reading — *see* Blood, pressure

Test(s) — *continued*
  blood-alcohol Z04.8
    positive — *see* Findings, abnormal, in blood
  blood-drug Z04.8
    positive — *see* Findings, abnormal, in blood
  cardiac pulse generator (battery) Z45.010
  developmental, infant or child Z00.10
    with abnormal findings Z00.11
  fertility Z31.41
  hearing Z01.10
    with abnormal findings Z01.11
  HIV (human immunodeficiency virus)
    nonconclusive in infants R75
    positive Z21
    seropositive Z21
  intelligence NEC Z01.8
    infant or child Z00.10
      with abnormal findings Z00.11
  laboratory Z00.020
    with abnormal finding Z00.021
    for medicolegal reason NEC Z04.8
  Mantoux (for tuberculosis) Z11.1
    abnormal result R76.1
  pregnancy, positive first pregnancy — *see* Pregnancy, normal, first
  procreative Z31.49
    fertility Z31.41
  skin, diagnostic
    allergy Z01.8
    bacterial disease Z01.8
      special screening examination — *see* Screening, by name of disease
    hypersensitivity Z01.8
    Mantoux Z11.1
    tuberculin Z11.1
  specified NEC Z01.8
  tuberculin Z11.1
    abnormal result R76.1
  vision Z01.00
    with abnormal findings Z01.01
  Wassermann Z11.3
    positive — *see* Serology for syphilis, positive

Testicle, testicular, testis — *see also* condition
  feminization syndrome E34.5
  migrans Q55.29

Tetanus, tetanic (cephalic) (convulsions) A35
  with
    abortion A34
    ectopic or molar pregnancy O08.0
  following ectopic or molar pregnancy O08.0
  inoculation Z23
    reaction (due to serum) — *see* Complications, vaccination
  neonatorum A33
  obstetrical A34
  puerperal, postpartum, childbirth A34

Tetany (due to) R29.0
  alkalosis E87.3
  associated with rickets E55.0
  convulsions R29.0
    hysterical F44.5
  functional (hysterical) F44.5
  hyperkinetic R29.0
    hysterical F44.5
  hyperpnea R06.89
    hysterical F44.5
    psychogenic F45.8
  hyperventilation — *see* Hyperventilation
  hysterical F44.5
  neonatal (without calcium or magnesium deficiency) P71.3
  parathyroid (gland) E20.9
  parathyroprival E89.2
  post-(para)thyroidectomy E89.2
  postoperative E89.2
  pseudotetany R29.0
  psychogenic (conversion reaction) F44.5

Tetralogy of Fallot Q21.3

Tetraplegia G82.50
  complete
    C1-C4 level G82.51
    C5-C7 level G82.53
  congenital or infantile (cerebral) (spinal) G80.8
  embolic (current episode) I63.4
  incomplete
    C1-C4 level G82.52
    C5-C7 level G82.54

Tetraplegia — *continued*
  functional R53.2
  newborn P11.9
  thrombotic (current episode) I63.3
  traumatic — — *code* to injury with terminal extension of p
    current episode — *see* Injury, spinal (cord), cervical

Thailand hemorrhagic fever A91

Thalassanemia — *see* Thalassemia

Thalassemia (anemia) (disease) D56.9
  with other hemoglobinopathy NEC D56.9
  alpha (major) (severe) (triple gene defect) D56.0
    minor D56.3
  beta (severe) (sickle-cell) D56.1
    minor D56.3
  delta-beta (homozygous) D56.2
    minor D56.3
  intermedia D56.1
  major D56.1
  minor D56.3
  mixed (with other hemoglobinopathy) D56.9
  specified type NEC D56.8
  trait D56.3
  variants D56.8

Thanatophoric dwarfism or short stature Q77.1

Thaysen-Gee disease (nontropical sprue) K90.0

Thaysen's disease K90.0

Thecoma (M8600/0) D27.9
  left D27.1
  luteinized (M8601/0) D27.9
    left D27.1
    right D27.0
  malignant (M8600/3) C56.9
    left C56.1
    right C56.0
  right D27.0

Thelarche, premature E30.8

Thelaziasis B83.8

Thelitis N61
  puerperal, postpartum or gestational — *see* Infection, nipple

Therapeutic — *see* condition

Therapy Z51.9
  aversive (behavior) NEC Z51.89
    alcohol Z51.89
    drug Z51.89
  blood transfusion, without reported diagnosis Z51.89
  breathing Z51.89
  detoxification
    alcohol Z51.89
    drug Z51.89
  intravenous (IV) without reported diagnosis Z51.89
    following surgery Z48.8
  occupational Z51.89
  orthoptic Z51.89
  physical NEC Z51.89
  psychodynamic NEC Z51.89
  radiation Z51.0
  speech Z51.89
  vocational Z51.89

Thermic — *see* condition

Thermography (abnormal) R93.8
  breast R92.8

Thermoplegia T67.0

Thesaurismosis, glycogen — *see* Disease, glycogen storage

Thiamin deficiency E51.9
  specified NEC E51.8

Thiaminic deficiency with beriberi E51.11

Thibierge-Weissenbach syndrome — *see* Sclerosis, systemic

Thickening
  bone — *see* Hypertrophy, bone
  breast N64.5
  epidermal L85.9
    specified NEC L85.8
  hymen N89.6
  larynx J38.7
  nail L60.2
    congenital Q84.5
  periosteal — *see* Hypertrophy, bone

Thickening — continued
  pleura J92.9
    with asbestos J92.0
  skin R23.4
  subepiglottic J38.7
  tongue K14.8
  valve, heart — see Endocarditis
Thigh — see condition
Thinning vertebra — see Spondylopathy,
  specified NEC
Thirst, excessive R63.1
  due to deprivation of water T73.1
Thomsen's disease G71.1
Thoracic — see also condition
  kidney Q63.2
  outlet syndrome G54.0
Thoracogastroschisis (congenital) Q79.8
Thoracopagus Q89.4
Thorax — see condition
Thorn's syndrome N28.89
Thorson-Björck syndrome E34.0
Threadworm (infection) (infestation) B80
Threatened
  abortion O20.0
    with subsequent abortion O03.9
  job loss, anxiety concerning Z56.2
  labor — see Labor, false
  loss of job, anxiety concerning Z56.2
  miscarriage O20.0
  unemployment, anxiety concerning Z56.2
Three-day fever A93.1
Threshers' lung J67.0
Thrix annulata (congenital) Q84.1
Throat — see condition
Thrombasthenia (Glanzmann) (hemorrhagic)
  (hereditary) D69.1
Thromboangiitis I73.1
  obliterans (general) I73.1
    cerebral I67.8
    vessels
      brain I67.8
      spinal cord I67.8
Thromboarteritis — see Arteritis
Thromboasthenia (Glanzmann) (hemorrhagic)
  (hereditary) D69.1
Thrombocytasthenia (Glanzmann) D69.1
Thrombocythemia (essential) (hemorrhagic)
  (idiopathic) (primary) (M9962/1) D47.3
Thrombocytopathy (dystrophic) (granulopenic)
  D69.1
Thrombocytopenia, thrombocytopenic D69.6
  with absent radius (TAR) Q87.2
  congenital D69.4
  dilutional D69.5
  due to
    drugs D69.5
    extracorporeal circulation of blood D69.5
    massive blood transfusion D69.5
    platelet alloimmunization D69.5
  essential D69.3
  hereditary D69.4
  idiopathic D69.3
  neonatal, transitory P61.0
    due to
      exchange transfusion P61.0
      idiopathic maternal thrombocytopenia
        P61.0
      isoimmunization P61.0
  primary NEC D69.4
    idiopathic D69.3
  puerperal, postpartum O72.3
  secondary D69.5
  transient neonatal P61.0
Thrombocytosis, essential D75.2
Thromboembolism — see Embolism
Thrombopathy (Bernard-Soulier) D69.1
  constitutional D68.0
  Willebrand-Jurgens D68.0
Thrombopenia — see Thrombocytopenia

Thrombophlebitis I80.9
  antepartum O22.90
    deep O22.30
      first trimester O22.31
      second trimester O22.32
      third trimester O22.33
    first trimester O22.91
    second trimester O22.92
    superficial O22.20
      first trimester O22.21
      second trimester O22.22
      third trimester O22.23
    third trimester O22.93
  cavernous (venous) sinus G08
    complicating pregnancy O22.50
      first trimester O22.51
      second trimester O22.52
      third trimester O22.53
    nonpyogenic I67.6
  cerebral (sinus) (vein) G08
    nonpyogenic I67.6
    sequelae G09
  due to implanted device — see Complications,
    by site and type, specified NEC
  during or resulting from a procedure NEC
    T81.7
  femoral — see Phlebitis, leg, femoral vein
  following infusion, perfusion, therapeutic
    injection or transfusion T80.1
  hepatic (vein) I80.8
  idiopathic, recurrent I82.1
  iliofemoral — see Phlebitis, leg, femoral vein
  intracranial venous sinus (any) G08
    nonpyogenic I67.6
    sequelae G09
  intraspinal venous sinuses and veins G08
    nonpyogenic G95.19
  lateral (venous) sinus G08
    nonpyogenic I67.6
  leg — see Phlebitis, leg
  longitudinal (venous) sinus G08
    nonpyogenic I67.6
  lower extremity — see Phlebitis, leg
  migrans, migrating I82.1
  pelvic
    with ectopic or molar pregnancy O08.0
    following ectopic or molar pregnancy O08.0
    puerperal O87.1
  popliteal vein — see Phlebitis, leg, deep,
    popliteal
  portal (vein) K75.1
  postoperative T81.7
  pregnancy — see Thrombophlebitis,
    antepartum
  puerperal, postpartum, childbirth O87.9
    deep O87.1
    pelvic O87.1
    superficial O87.0
  saphenous (greater) (lesser) — see Phlebitis,
    leg, superficial
  sinus (intracranial) G08
    nonpyogenic I67.6
  specified site NEC I80.8
  tibial vein — see Phlebitis, leg, deep, tibial
Thrombosis, thrombotic (bland) (multiple)
  (progressive) (septic) (silent) (vein) (vessel)
  I82.9
  antepartum — see Thrombophlebitis,
    antepartum
  aorta, aortic I74.10
    abdominal I74.0
    bifurcation I74.0
    saddle I74.0
    specified site NEC I74.19
    terminal I74.0
    thoracic I74.11
    valve — see Endocarditis, aortic
  apoplexy I63.3
  appendix, septic K35.9
  artery, arteries (postinfectional) I74.9
    auditory, internal — see Occlusion, artery,
      precerebral, specified NEC
    basilar — see Occlusion, artery, basilar
    carotid (common) (internal) — see Occlusion,
      artery, carotid

Thrombosis, thrombotic — continued
  artery, arteries — continued
    cerebellar (anterior inferior) (posterior
      inferior) (superior) — see Occlusion,
      artery, cerebellar
    cerebral — see Occlusion, artery, cerebral
    choroidal (anterior) — see Occlusion, artery,
      cerebral, specified NEC
    communicating, posterior — see Occlusion,
      artery, cerebral, specified NEC
    coronary — see also Infarct, myocardium
      not resulting in infarction I24.0
    hepatic I74.8
    hypophyseal — see Occlusion, artery,
      cerebral, specified NEC
    iliac I74.5
    limb I74.4
      lower I74.3
      upper I74.2
    meningeal, anterior or posterior — see
      Occlusion, artery, cerebral, specified
      NEC
    mesenteric (with gangrene) K55.0
    ophthalmic — see Occlusion, artery, retina
    pontine — see Occlusion, artery, cerebral,
      specified NEC
    precerebral — see Occlusion, artery,
      precerebral
    pulmonary (iatrogenic) — see Embolism,
      pulmonary
    renal N28.0
    retinal — see Occlusion, artery, retina
    spinal, anterior or posterior G95.11
    traumatic T14.90
    vertebral — see Occlusion, artery, vertebral
  atrium, auricular — see also Infarct,
    myocardium
    following acute myocardial infarction
      (current complication) I23.6
    not resulting in infarction I24.0
  axillary (vein) I82.8
  basilar (artery) — see Occlusion, artery, basilar
  brain (artery) (stem) — see also Occlusion,
    artery, cerebral
    due to syphilis A52.05
    puerperal O99.43
    sinus — see Thrombosis, intracranial
      venous sinus
  capillary I78.8
  cardiac — see also Infarct, myocardium
    not resulting in infarction I24.0
    valve — see Endocarditis
  carotid (artery) (common) (internal) — see
    Occlusion, artery, carotid
  cavernous (venous) sinus — see Thrombosis,
    intracranial venous sinus
  cerebellar artery (anterior inferior) (posterior
    inferior) (superior) I65.8
  cerebral (artery) — see Occlusion, artery,
    cerebral
  cerebrovenous sinus — see also Thrombosis,
    intracranial venous sinus
    pregnancy — see Thrombophlebitis,
      cavernous sinus, complicating
      pregnancy
    puerperium O87.3
  coronary (artery) (vein) — see also Infarct,
    myocardium
    not resulting in infarction I24.0
  corpus cavernosum N48.89
  cortical I66.9
  deep — see Phlebitis, leg, deep
  due to device, implant or graft (see also
    Complications, by site and type, specified
    NEC) T85.86
    arterial graft NEC T82.868
    breast (implant) T85.86
    catheter NEC T85.86
      dialysis (renal) T82.868
        intraperitoneal T85.86
      infusion NEC T82.868
        spinal (epidural) (subdural) T85.86
      urinary (indwelling) T83.86
    electronic (electrode) (pulse generator)
      (stimulator)
      bone T84.86
      cardiac I82.867

©2002 Ingenix, Inc.

Thrombosis, thrombotic — *continued*
due to device, implant or graft (*see also*
Complications, by site and type, specified
NEC) — *continued*
electronic — *continued*
nervous system (brain) (peripheral nerve)
(spinal) T85.86
urinary T83.86
fixation, internal (orthopedic) NEC T84.86
gastrointestinal (bile duct) (esophagus)
T85.86
due to device, implant or graft (*see also*
Complications, by site and type, specified
NEC) — *continued*
genital NEC T83.86
heart T82.867
joint prosthesis T84.86
ocular (corneal graft) (orbital implant) NEC
T85.86
orthopedic NEC T84.86
specified NEC T85.86
urinary NEC T83.86
vascular NEC T82.868
ventricular intracranial shunt T85.86
during the puerperium — *see* Thrombosis,
puerperal
effort I82.8
endocardial — *see also* Infarct, myocardium
not resulting in infarction I24.0
eye — *see* Occlusion, retina
femoral (vein) — *see also* Phlebitis, leg, femoral
vein
artery I74.3
genital organ
female NEC N94.8
pregnancy — *see* Thrombophlebitis,
antepartum
male N50.1
gestational — *see* Phlebopathy, gestational
heart (chamber) — *see also* Infarct,
myocardium
not resulting in infarction I24.0
hepatic (vein) I82.0
artery I74.8
iliac (vein) — *see also* Phlebitis, leg, deep
(vessel) NEC, specified vessel NEC
artery I74.5
iliofemoral — *see* Phlebitis, leg, femoral vein
intestine (with gangrene) K55.0
intracardiac NEC (apical) (atrial) (auricular)
(ventricular) (old) I51.3
intracranial (arterial) I66.9
venous sinus (any) G08
nonpyogenic origin I67.6
pregnancy — *see* Thrombophlebitis,
cavernous sinus, complicating
pregnancy
puerperium O87.3
intramural — *see also* Infarct, myocardium
not resulting in infarction I24.0
intraspinal venous sinuses and veins G08
nonpyogenic G95.19
jugular (bulb) I82.8
kidney (artery) N28.0
lateral (venous) sinus — *see* Thrombosis,
intracranial venous sinus
leg — *see also* Phlebitis, leg
arterial I74.3
liver (venous) I82.0
artery I74.8
portal vein I81
longitudinal (venous) sinus — *see* Thrombosis,
intracranial venous sinus
lower limb — *see* Thrombosis, leg
lung (iatrogenic) (postoperative) — *see*
Embolism, pulmonary
meninges (brain) (arterial) I66.8
mesenteric (artery) (with gangrene) K55.0
vein (inferior) (superior) I81
mitral I34.8
mural — *see also* Infarct, myocardium
not resulting in infarction I24.0
omentum (with gangrene) K55.0
ophthalmic — *see* Occlusion, retina
pampiniform plexus (male) N50.1
parietal — *see also* Infarct, myocardium
not resulting in infarction I24.0

Thrombosis, thrombotic — *continued*
penis, superficial vein N48.81
peripheral arteries I74.4
upper I74.3
portal I81
due to syphilis A52.09
precerebral artery — *see* Occlusion, artery,
precerebral
pregnancy — *see also* Thrombophlebitis,
antepartum
cerebral venous (sinus) — *see*
Thrombophlebitis, cavernous sinus,
complicating pregnancy
deep-vein — *see* Thrombophlebitis,
antepartum, deep
following ectopic or molar pregnancy O08.7
puerperal, postpartum O87.9
brain (artery) O99.43
venous (sinus) O87.3
cardiac O99.43
cerebral (artery) O99.43
venous (sinus) O87.3
superficial O87.0
pulmonary (artery) (iatrogenic) (postoperative)
(vein) — *see* Embolism, pulmonary
renal (artery) N28.0
vein I82.3
resulting from presence of device, implant or
graft — *see* Complications, by site and
type, specified NEC
retina, retinal — *see* Occlusion, retina
scrotum N50.1
seminal vesicle N50.1
sigmoid (venous) sinus — *see* Thrombosis,
intracranial venous sinus
sinus, intracranial (any) — *see* Thrombosis,
intracranial venous sinus
specified site NEC I82.8
spermatic cord N50.1
spinal cord (arterial) G95.11
due to syphilis A52.09
pyogenic origin G06.1
spleen, splenic D73.5
artery I74.8
testis N50.1
traumatic T14.90
tricuspid I07.8
tunica vaginalis N50.1
umbilical cord (vessels), complicating delivery
O69.5
vas deferens N50.1
vena cava (inferior) (superior) I82.2
ventricle — *see also* Infarct, myocardium
following acute myocardial infarction
(current complication) I23.6
not resulting in infarction I24.0
Thrombus — *see* Thrombosis
Thrush — *see also* Candidiasis
oral B37.0
newborn P37.5
vaginal B37.3
Thumb — *see also* condition
sucking (child problem) F98.8
Thymitis E32.8
Thymoma (benign) (M8580/0) D15.0
malignant (M8580/3) C37
Thymus, thymic (gland) — *see* condition
Thyrocele — *see* Goiter
Thyroglossal — *see also* condition
cyst Q89.2
duct, persistent Q89.2
Thyroid (gland) (body) — *see also* condition
lingual Q89.2
nodule (cystic) (nontoxic) (single) E04.1
Thyroiditis E06.9
acute (nonsuppurative) (pyogenic) (suppurative)
E06.0
autoimmune E06.3
chronic (nonspecific) (sclerosing) E06.5
with thyrotoxicosis, transient E06.2
fibrous E06.5
lymphadenoid E06.3
lymphocytic E06.3
lymphoid E06.3
de Quervain's E06.1
drug-induced E06.4

Thyroiditis — *continued*
fibrous (chronic) E06.5
giant-cell (follicular) E06.1
granulomatous (de Quervain) (subacute) E06.1
Hashimoto's (struma lymphomatosa) E06.3
iatrogenic E06.4
ligneous E06.5
lymphocytic (chronic) E06.3
lymphoid E06.3
lymphomatous E06.3
nonsuppurative E06.1
postpartum, puerperal O90.5
pseudotuberculous E06.1
pyogenic E06.0
radiation E06.4
Riedel's E06.5
subacute (granulomatous) E06.1
suppurative E06.0
tuberculous A18.81
viral E06.1
woody E06.5
Thyrolingual duct, persistent Q89.2
Thyromegaly E01.0
Thyrotoxic
crisis — *see* Thyrotoxicosis
heart disease or failure (*see also*
Thyrotoxicosis) E05.90 [I43]
with thyroid storm E05.91 [I43]
storm — *see* Thyrotoxicosis
Thyrotoxicosis (recurrent) E05.90
with
goiter (diffuse) E05.00
with thyroid storm E05.01
adenomatous uninodular E05.10
with thyroid storm E05.11
multinodular E05.20
with thyroid storm E05.21
nodular E05.20
with thyroid storm E05.21
uninodular E05.10
with thyroid storm E05.11
thyroid storm E05.91
infiltrative
dermopathy E05.00
with thyroid storm E05.01
ophthalmopathy E05.00
with thyroid storm E05.01
single thyroid nodule E05.10
with thyroid storm E05.11
thyroid storm E05.91
due to
ectopic thyroid nodule or tissue E05.30
with thyroid storm E05.31
ingestion of (excessive) thyroid material
E05.40
with thyroid storm E05.41
overproduction of thyroid-stimulating
hormone E05.80
with thyroid storm E05.81
specified cause NEC E05.80
with thyroid storm E05.81
factitia E05.40
with thyroid storm E05.41
heart E05.90 [I43]
with thyroid storm E05.91 [I43]
failure E05.90 [I43]
neonatal (transient) P72.1
transient with chronic thyroiditis E06.2
Tibia vara — *see* Osteochondrosis, juvenile, tibia
Tic (disorder) F95.9
breathing F95.8
child problem F95.0
compulsive F95.1
de la Tourette F95.2
degenerative (generalized) (localized) G25.6
facial G25.6
disorder
chronic
motor F95.1
vocal F95.1
combined vocal and multiple motor F95.2
transient F95.0
douloureux G50.0
atypical G50.1
postherpetic, postzoster B02.22
drug-induced G25.6

Tic — *continued*
eyelid F95.8
habit F95.9
chronic F95.1
transient of childhood F95.0
lid, transient of childhood F95.0
motor-verbal F95.2
occupational F48.8
orbicularis F95.8
transient of childhood F95.0
organic origin G25.6
postchoreic G25.6
psychogenic, compulsive F95.1
salaam R25.8
spasm (motor or vocal) F95.9
chronic F95.1
transient of childhood F95.0
specified NEC F95.8
Tick-borne — *see* condition
Tietze's disease or syndrome M94.0
Tight, tightness
anus K62.8
chest R07.89
fascia (lata) M62.89
foreskin (congenital) N47.1
hymen, hymenal ring N89.6
introitus (acquired) (congenital) N89.6
rectal sphincter K62.8
tendon — *see* Short, tendon
urethral sphincter N35.9
Tilting vertebra — *see* Dorsopathy, deforming,
specified NEC
Timidity, child F93.8
Tin-miner's lung J63.5
Tinea (intersecta) (tarsi) B35.9
amiantacea L44.8
asbestina B35.0
barbae B35.0
beard B35.0
black dot B35.0
blanca B36.2
capitis B35.0
corporis B35.4
cruris B35.6
flava B36.0
foot B35.3
furfuracea B36.0
imbricata (Tokelau) B35.5
kerion B35.0
manuum B35.2
microsporic — *see* Dermatophytosis
nigra B36.1
nodosa — *see* Piedra
pedis B35.3
scalp B35.0
specified site NEC B35.8
sycosis B35.0
tonsurans B35.0
trichophytic — *see* Dermatophytosis
unguium B35.1
versicolor B36.0
Tingling sensation (skin) R20.2
Tinnitus (audible) (aurium) (subjective) — *see*
category H93.1
Tipping pelvis M95.5
with disproportion (fetopelvic) O33.0
causing obstructed labor O65.0
Tiredness R53.82
Tissue — *see* condition
Tobacco (nicotine)
dependence — *see* Dependence, drug, nicotine
harmful use Z72.0
heart — *see* Tobacco, toxic effect
maternal use, affecting fetus or newborn P04.2
toxic effect T65.291
administered with intent to harm by
another person T65.293
self T65.292
chewing tobacco T65.211
administered with intent to harm by
another person T65.213
self T65.212
circumstances undetermined T65.214

Tobacco — *continued*
toxic effect — *continued*
cigarettes T65.221
administered with intent to harm by
another person T65.223
self T65.222
circumstances undetermined T65.224
circumstances undetermined T65.294
use Z72.0
complicating
childbirth O99.334
pregnancy O99.333
first trimester O99.330
second trimester O99.331
third trimester O99.332
puerperium O99.335
counseling and surveillance Z71.6
withdrawal state — *see* Dependence, drug,
nicotine
Tocopherol deficiency E56.0
Todd's
cirrhosis K74.3
paralysis (postepileptic) (transitory) G83.84
Toe — *see* condition
Toilet, artificial opening — *see* Attention to,
artificial, opening
Tokelau (ringworm) B35.5
Tollwut — *see* Rabies
Tommaselli's disease
correct substance properly administered R31.9
overdose or wrong substance given or taken —
see category T37.2
Tongue — *see also* condition
tie Q38.1
Tonic pupil — *see* Anomaly, pupil, function, tonic
pupil
Toni-Fanconi syndrome (cystinosis) E72.09
with cystinosis E72.04
Tonsil — *see* condition
Tonsillitis (acute) (catarrhal) (croupous)
(follicular) (gangrenous) (infective) (lacunar)
(lingual) (malignant) (membranous)
(parenchymatous) (phlegmonous)
(pseudomembranous) (purulent) (septic)
(subacute) (suppurative) (toxic) (ulcerative)
(vesicular) (viral) J03.90
chronic J35.01
with adenoiditis J35.03
diphtheritic A36.0
hypertrophic J35.01
with adenoiditis J35.03
recurrent J03.91
specified organism NEC J03.80
recurrent J03.81
staphylococcal J03.80
recurrent J03.81
streptococcal J03.00
recurrent J03.01
tuberculous A15.8
Vincent's A69.1
Tooth, teeth — *see* condition
Toothache K08.8
Topagnosis R20.8
Tophi — *see also* Gout, tophi M10.9
heart M10.08 *[143]*
Torn — *see* Tear
Tornwaldt's cyst or disease J39.2
Torsion
accessory tube — *see* Torsion, fallopian tube
adnexa (female) — *see* Torsion, fallopian tube
aorta, acquired I77.1
appendix epididymis N44.01
bile duct (common) (hepatic) K83.8
congenital Q44.5
bowel, colon or intestine K56.2
cervix — *see* Malposition, uterus
cystic duct K82.8
dystonia — *see* Dystonia, torsion
epididymis (appendix) N44.01
fallopian tube N83.52
with ovary N83.53
gallbladder K82.8
congenital Q44.1

Torsion — *continued*
hydatid of Morgagni (female) — *see* Torsion,
fallopian tube
kidney (pedicle) (leading to infarction) N28.0
Meckel's diverticulum (congenital) Q43.0
mesentery K56.2
omentum K56.2
organ or site, congenital NEC — *see* Anomaly,
by site
ovary (pedicle) N83.51
with fallopian tube N83.53
congenital Q50.2
oviduct — *see* Torsion, fallopian tube
penis N48.89
congenital Q55.69
spasm — *see* Dystonia, torsion
spermatic cord
extravaginal N44.02
intravaginal N44.03
spleen D73.5
testis, testicle N44.00
appendix N44.04
tibia — *see* Deformity, limb, specified type
NEC, lower leg
uterus — *see* Malposition, uterus
Torticollis (intermittent) (spastic) M43.6
congenital (sternomastoid) Q68.0
due to birth injury P15.2
hysterical F44.4
psychogenic F45.8
conversion reaction F44.4
rheumatoid M06.88
spasmodic G24.3
traumatic, current S13.4
Tortipelvis G24.1
Tortuous
artery I77.1
organ or site, congenital NEC — *see* Distortion
retinal vessel, congenital Q14.1
ureter N13.8
urethra N36.8
vein — *see* Varix
Torture, victim of Z65.4
Torula, torular (histolytica) (infection) — *see*
Cryptococcosis
Torulosis — *see* Cryptococcosis
Torus (mandibularis) (palatinus) M27.0
Touraine's syndrome Q79.8
Tourette's syndrome F95.2
Tower skull Q75.0
with exophthalmos Q87.0
Toxemia R68.8
bacterial — *see* Septicemia
burn — *see* Burn
eclamptic (with pre-existing hypertension) —
see Eclampsia
erysipelatous — *see* Erysipelas
fatigue R68.8
food — *see* Poisoning, food
gastrointestinal K52.1
intestinal K52.1
kidney — *see* Uremia
malarial — *see* Malaria
myocardial — *see* Myocarditis, toxic
of pregnancy — *see* Pre-eclampsia
pre-eclamptic — *see* Pre-eclampsia
septic — *see* Septicemia
small intestine K52.1
staphylococcal, due to food A05.0
stasis R68.8
uremic — *see* Uremia
urinary — *see* Uremia
Toxemica cerebropathia psychica (nonalcoholic)
F04
alcoholic — *see* Alcohol, amnestic disorder
Toxic (poisoning) — *see also* condition T65.91
from drug or nonmedicinal substance — *see*
Table of Drugs and Chemicals
shock syndrome A48.3
thyroid (gland) — *see* Thyrotoxicosis
Toxicemia — *see* Toxemia
Toxicity T65.91
fava bean D55.0
food, noxious — *see* Poisoning, food

Toxicity — *continued*
  from drug or nonmedicinal substance — *see*
      Table of Drugs and Chemicals
  mycotoxin food contaminant T64.81
      administered with intent to harm by
          another person T64.83
          self T64.82
      aflatoxin T64.01
          administered with intent to harm by
              another person T64.03
              self T64.02
          circumstances undetermined T64.04
      circumstances undetermined T64.84
  vapors
      accidental T59.91
      assault T59.93
      carbon
          monoxide — *see* Poisoning, carbon
              monoxide
          dioxide — *see* category T59.7
      chlorine gas — *see* category T59.4
      circumstances undetermined T59.94
      fluorine gas — *see* category T59.5
      formaldehyde — *see* category T59.2
      hydrogen
          fluoride — *see* Toxicity, vapors, fluorine
              gas
          sulfide — *see* category T59.6
      lacrimogenic gas — *see* category T59.3
      nitrogen oxide — *see* category T59.0
      self inflicted T59.92
      specified type NEC
          accidental T59.891
          assault T59.893
          circumstances undetermined T59.894
          self inflicted T59.892
      sulfur dioxide — *see* category T59.1
  venom T63.91
      administered with intent to harm by
          another person T63.93
          self T63.92
      amphibian T63.831
          administered with intent to harm by
              another person T63.833
              self T63.832
          circumstances undetermined T63.834
          frog T63.811
              administered with intent to harm by
                  another person T63.813
                  self T63.812
              circumstances undetermined T63.814
          toad T63.821
              administered with intent to harm by
                  another person T63.823
                  self T63.822
              circumstances undetermined T63.824
      arthropod T63.481
          administered with intent to harm by
              another person T63.483
              self T63.482
          ant T63.421
              administered with intent to harm by
                  another person T63.423
                  self T63.422
              circumstances undetermined T63.424
          bee T63.441
              administered with intent to harm by
                  another person T63.443
                  self T63.442
          caterpillar T63.431
              administered with intent to harm by
                  another person T63.433
                  self T63.432
              circumstances undetermined T63.434
          centipede T63.411
              administered with intent to harm by
                  another person T63.413
                  self T63.412
              circumstances undetermined T63.414
          circumstances undetermined T63.484
          hornet T63.451
              administered with intent to harm by
                  another person T63.453
                  self T63.452
              circumstances undetermined T63.454

Toxicity — *continued*
  venom — *continued*
      arthropod — *continued*
          millipede T63.411
              administered with intent to harm by
                  another person T63.413
                  self T63.412
              circumstances undetermined T63.414
          spider — *see* Toxicity, venom, spider
          wasp T63.461
              administered with intent to harm by
                  another person T63.463
                  self T63.462
              circumstances undetermined T63.464
      circumstances undetermined T63.94
      marine animal T63.691
          administered with intent to harm by
              another person T63.693
              self T63.692
          circumstances undetermined T63.694
          fish T63.591
              administered with intent to harm by
                  another person T63.593
                  self T63.592
              circumstances undetermined T63.594
          jellyfish T63.621
              administered with intent to harm by
                  another person T63.623
                  self T63.622
              circumstances undetermined T63.624
              Portuguese man-o-war T63.611
                  administered with intent to harm by
                      another person T63.613
                      self T63.612
                  circumstances undetermined
                      T63.614
          sea anemone T63.631
              administered with intent to harm by
                  another person T63.633
                  self T63.632
              circumstances undetermined T63.634
          shellfish T63.691
              administered with intent to harm by
                  another person T63.693
                  self T63.692
              circumstances undetermined T63.694
          starfish T63.691
              administered with intent to harm by
                  another person T63.693
                  self T63.692
              circumstances undetermined T63.694
          stingray T63.511
              administered with intent to harm by
                  another person T63.513
                  self T63.512
              circumstances undetermined T63.514
      plant T63.791
          administered with intent to harm by
              another person T63.793
              self T63.792
          circumstances undetermined T63.794
          marine T63.711
              administered with intent to harm by
                  another person T63.713
                  self T63.712
              circumstances undetermined T63.714
      reptile T63.191
          administered with intent to harm by
              another person T63.193
              self T63.192
          circumstances undetermined T63.194
          gila monster T63.111
              administered with intent to harm by
                  another person T63.113
                  self T63.112
              circumstances undetermined T63.114
          lizard NEC T63.121
              administered with intent to harm by
                  another person T63.123
                  self T63.122
              circumstances undetermined T63.124
          snake — *see* Toxicity, venom, snake
      scorpion — *see* category T63.2
      snake T63.001
          administered with intent to harm by
              another person T63.003

Toxicity — *continued*
  venom — *continued*
      snake — *continued*
          administered with intent to harm by —
              continued
              self T63.002
          African snake NEC T63.081
              administered with intent to harm by
                  another person T63.083
                  self T63.082
              circumstances undetermined T63.084
          American snake NEC T63.061
              administered with intent to harm by
                  another person T63.063
                  self T63.062
              circumstances undetermined T63.064
          Asian snake NEC T63.081
              administered with intent to harm by
                  another person T63.083
                  self T63.082
              circumstances undetermined T63.084
          Australian snake NEC T63.071
              administered with intent to harm by
                  another person T63.073
                  self T63.072
              circumstances undetermined T63.074
          circumstances undetermined T63.004
          cobra T63.041
              administered with intent to harm by
                  another person T63.043
                  self T63.042
              circumstances undetermined T63.044
          coral snake T63.021
              administered with intent to harm by
                  another person T63.023
                  self T63.022
              circumstances undetermined T63.024
          North American snake NEC T63.061
              administered with intent to harm by
                  another person T63.063
                  self T63.062
              circumstances undetermined T63.064
          rattlesnake T63.011
              administered with intent to harm by
                  another person T63.013
                  self T63.012
              circumstances undetermined T63.014
          sea snake T63.031
              administered with intent to harm by
                  another person T63.033
                  self T63.032
              circumstances undetermined T63.034
          South American snake NEC T63.061
              administered with intent to harm by
                  another person T63.063
                  self T63.062
              circumstances undetermined T63.064
          specified snake NEC T63.091
              administered with intent to harm by
                  another person T63.093
                  self T63.092
              circumstances undetermined T63.094
          taipan T63.031
              administered with intent to harm by
                  another person T63.033
                  self T63.032
              circumstances undetermined T63.034
      specified animal NEC T63.891
          administered with intent to harm by
              another person T63.893
              self T63.892
          circumstances undetermined T63.894
      spider T63.301
          administered with intent to harm by
              another person T63.303
              self T63.302
          black widow T63.311
              administered with intent to harm by
                  another person T63.313
                  self T63.312
              circumstances undetermined T63.314
          brown recluse T63.331
              administered with intent to harm by
                  another person T63.333
                  self T63.332
              circumstances undetermined T63.334

Toxicity — *continued*
  venom — *continued*
    spider — *continued*
      circumstances undetermined T63.304
      specified NEC T63.391
        administered with intent to harm by
          another person T63.393
          self T63.392
        circumstances undetermined T63.394
      tarantula T63.321
        administered with intent to harm by
          another person T63.323
          self T63.322
        circumstances undetermined T63.324

Toxicosis — *see also* Toxemia
  capillary, hemorrhagic D69.0

Toxinfection, gastrointestinal K52.1

Toxocariasis B83.0

Toxoplasma, toxoplasmosis (acquired) B58.9
  with
    hepatitis B58.1
    meningoencephalitis B58.2
    ocular involvement B58.00
    other organ involvement B58.89
    pneumonia, pneumonitis B58.3
  congenital (acute) (subacute) (chronic) P37.1
  maternal, manifest toxoplasmosis in infant or
    fetus (acute) (subacute) (chronic) P37.1
  suspected damage to fetus affecting
    management of pregnancy O35.8

Trabeculation, bladder N32.8

Trachea — *see* condition

Tracheitis (acute) (catarrhal) (infantile)
  (membranous) (plastic) (pneumococcal)
  (septal) (suppurative) (viral) J04.1
  with
    bronchitis (15 years of age and above) J40
      acute or subacute — *see* Bronchitis,
        acute
      chronic J42
      tuberculous NEC A15.5
      under 15 years of age J20.9
    laryngitis (acute) J04.2
      chronic J37.1
      tuberculous NEC A15.5
  chronic J42
    with
      bronchitis (chronic) J42
      laryngitis (chronic) J37.1
  diphtheritic (membranous) A36.89
  due to external agent — *see* Inflammation,
    respiratory, upper, due to
  streptococcal J04.1
  syphilitic A52.73
  tuberculous A15.5

Trachelitis (nonvenereal) — *see* Cervicitis

Tracheobronchial — *see* condition

Tracheobronchitis (15 years of age and above) —
  see also Bronchitis
  due to
    Bordetella bronchiseptica A37.80
      with pneumonia A37.81
    Francisella tularensis A21.8

Tracheobronchopneumonitis — *see* Pneumonia,
  broncho-

Tracheocele (external) (internal) J39.8
  congenital Q32.1

Tracheomalacia J39.8
  congenital Q32.0

Tracheopharyngitis
  chronic J42
  due to external agent — *see* Inflammation,
    respiratory, upper, due to

Tracheostenosis J39.8

Tracheostomy
  complication — *see* Complication, tracheostomy
  status Z93.0
    attention to Z43.0
    malfunctioning J95.03

Trachoma, trachomatous A71.9
  active (stage) A71.1
  contraction of conjunctiva A71.1
  dubium A71.0
  initial (stage) A71.0

Trachoma, trachomatous — *continued*
  healed or sequelae B94.0
  pannus A71.1
  Türck's J37.0

Train sickness T75.3

Training (in)
  activities of daily living Z51.89
  orthoptic Z51.89

Trait(s) D57.3
  Hb-S D57.3
  hemoglobin
    abnormal NEC D58.2
      with thalassemia D56.3
    C — *see* Disease, hemoglobin C
    S (Hb-S) D57.3
  Lepore D56.3
  personality, accentuated Z73.1
  sickle-cell D57.3
    with elliptocytosis or spherocytosis D57.3
  type A personality Z73.1

Tramp Z59.0

Trance R41.89
  hysterical F44.89

Transection
  abdomen (partial) S38.3
  aorta (incomplete) — *see also* Injury, aorta
    complete — *see* Injury, aorta, laceration,
      major
  carotid artery (incomplete) — *see also* Injury,
    blood vessel, carotid, laceration
    complete — *see* Injury, blood vessel, carotid,
      laceration, major
  celiac artery (incomplete) S35.211
    branch (incomplete) S35.291
      complete S35.292
    complete S35.212
  innominate
    artery (incomplete) — *see also* Injury, blood
      vessel, thoracic, innominate, artery,
      laceration
      complete — *see* Injury, blood vessel,
        thoracic, innominate, artery,
        laceration, major
    vein (incomplete) — *see also* Injury, blood
      vessel, thoracic, innominate, vein,
      laceration
      complete — *see* Injury, blood vessel,
        thoracic, innominate, vein,
        laceration, major
  jugular vein (external) (incomplete) — *see also*
    Injury, blood vessel, jugular vein,
    laceration
    complete — *see* Injury, blood vessel, jugular
      vein, laceration, major
    internal (incomplete) — *see also* Injury,
      blood vessel, jugular vein, internal,
      laceration
      complete — *see* Injury, blood vessel,
        jugular vein, internal, laceration,
        major
  mesenteric artery (incomplete) — *see also*
    Injury, mesenteric, artery, laceration
    complete — *see* Injury, mesenteric artery,
      laceration, major
  pulmonary vessel (incomplete) — *see also*
    Injury, blood vessel, thoracic, pulmonary,
    laceration
    complete — *see* Injury, blood vessel,
      thoracic, pulmonary, laceration, major
  subclavian — *see* Transection, innominate
  vena cava (incomplete) — *see also* Injury, vena
    cava
    complete — *see* Injury, vena cava,
      laceration, major
  vertebral artery (incomplete) — *see also* Injury,
    blood vessel, vertebral, laceration
    complete — *see* Injury, blood vessel,
      vertebral, laceration, major

Transaminasemia R74.0

Transfusion
  blood
    without reported diagnosis Z51.89
    incompatible T80.3
    reaction or complication — *see*
      Complications, transfusion

Transfusion — *continued*
  fetomaternal (mother) — *see* Pregnancy,
    complicated by, placenta, transfusion
    syndrome
  maternofetal (mother) — *see* Pregnancy,
    complicated by, placenta, transfusion
    syndrome
  placental (syndrome) (mother) — *see*
    Pregnancy, complicated by, placenta,
    transfusion syndrome
  reaction (adverse) — *see* Complications,
    transfusion
  twin-to-twin — *see* Pregnancy, complicated by,
    placenta, transfusion syndrome, fetus to
    fetus

Transient (meaning homeless) (*see also* condition)
  Z59.0

Translocation
  balanced autosomal Q95.9
    in normal individual Q95.0
  chromosomes NEC Q99.8
    balanced and insertion in normal individual
      Q95.0
  Down's syndrome Q90.2
  trisomy
    13 Q91.6
    18 Q91.2
    21 Q90.2

Translucency, iris — *see* Degeneration, iris

**Transmission of chemical substances through
the placenta** — *see* Absorption, chemical,
through placenta

Transparency, lung, unilateral J43.0

Transplant(ed) (status) Z94.9
  bone Z94.6
    marrow Z94.81
  candidate Z75.81
  complication — *see* Complication, transplant
  cornea Z94.7
  heart Z94.1
    and lung(s) Z94.3
    valve Z95.4
      prosthetic Z95.2
      xenogenic Z95.3
  intestine Z94.82
  kidney Z94.0
  liver Z94.4
  lung(s) Z94.2
    and heart Z94.3
  organ (failure) (infection) (rejection)Z94.9
  pancreas Z94.83
  skin Z94.5
  social Z60.3
  specified organ or tissue NEC Z94.89
  stem cells Z94.84
  tissue Z94.9

Transplants, ovarian, endometrial N80.1

Transposed — *see* Transposition

Transposition (congenital) — *see also*
  Malposition, congenital
  abdominal viscera Q89.3
  aorta (dextra) Q20.3
  appendix Q43.8
  colon Q43.8
  corrected Q20.5
  great vessels (complete) (partial) Q20.3
  heart Q24.0
    with complete transposition of viscera Q89.3
  intestine (large) (small) Q43.8
  reversed jejunal (for bypass) (status) Z98.0
  stomach Q40.2
    with general transposition of viscera Q89.3
  tooth, teeth M26.3
  vessels, great (complete) (partial) Q20.3
  viscera (abdominal) (thoracic) Q89.3

Transsexualism F64.1

Transverse — *see also* condition
  arrest (deep), in labor O64.0
  lie (mother) O32.2
    causing obstructed labor O64.8

Transvestism, transvestitism (dual-role) F64.1
  fetishistic F65.1

Trapped placenta (with hemorrhage) O72.0
  without hemorrhage O73.0

Trauma, traumatism — *see also* Injury
  acoustic — *see* category H83.3
  birth — *see* Birth, injury
  complicating ectopic or molar pregnancy O08.6
  during delivery O71.9
  following ectopic or molar pregnancy O08.6
  obstetric O71.9
    specified NEC O71.89
  previous major, affecting management of
    pregnancy — *see* Pregnancy, complicated
    by, high, risk, specified problem NEC
Traumatic — *see* condition
Treacher Collins syndrome Q75.4
Treitz's hernia — *see* Hernia, abdomen, specified
  site NEC
Trematode infestation — *see* Infestation, fluke
Trematodiasis — *see* Infestation, fluke
Trembling paralysis — *see* Parkinsonism
Tremor R25.1
  drug-induced G25.1
  essential (benign) G25.0
  familial G25.0
  hereditary G25.0
  hysterical F44.4
  intention G25.2
  mercurial — *see* category T56.1
  Parkinson's — *see* Parkinsonism
  psychogenic (conversion reaction) F44.4
  senilis R54
  specified type NEC G25.2
Trench
  fever A79.0
  foot — *see* Immersion, foot
  mouth A69.1
Treponema pallidum infection — *see* Syphilis
Treponematosis
  due to
    T. pallidum — *see* Syphilis
    T. pertenue — *see* Yaws
Triad
  Hutchinson's (congenital syphilis) A50.53
  Kartagener's Q89.3
  Saint's — *see* Hernia, diaphragm
Trichiasis (eyelid) H02.059
  with entropion — *see* Entropion
  left H02.056
    lower H02.055
    upper H02.054
  right H02.053
    lower H02.052
    upper H02.051
Trichinella spiralis (infection) (infestation) B75
**Trichinellosis, trichiniasis, trichinelliasis,
  trichinosis** B75
  with muscle disorder B75 *[M63.80]*
    ankle B75 *[M63.879]*
      left B75 *[M63.872]*
      right B75 *[M63.871]*
    foot B75 *[M63.879]*
      left B75 *[M63.872]*
      right B75 *[M63.871]*
    forearm B75 *[M63.839]*
      left B75 *[M63.832]*
      right B75 *[M63.831]*
    hand B75 *[M63.849]*
      left B75 *[M63.842]*
      right B75 *[M63.841]*
    lower leg B75 *[M63.869]*
      left B75 *[M63.862]*
      right B75 *[M63.861]*
    multiple sites B75 *[M63.89]*
    pelvic region B75 *[M63.859]*
      left B75 *[M63.852]*
      right B75 *[M63.851]*
    shoulder region B75 *[M63.819]*
      left B75 *[M63.812]*
      right B75 *[M63.811]*
    specified site NEC B75 *[M63.88]*
    thigh B75 *[M63.859]*
      left B75 *[M63.852]*
      right B75 *[M63.851]*
    upper arm B75 *[M63.829]*
      left B75 *[M63.822]*
      right B75 *[M63.821]*

Trichobezoar T18.9
  intestine T18.3
  stomach T18.2
Trichocephaliasis, trichocephalosis B79
Trichocephalus infestation B79
Trichoclasis L67.8
Trichoepithelioma (M8100/0) — *see also*
  Neoplasm, skin, benign
  malignant (M8100/3) — *see* Neoplasm, skin,
    malignant
Trichofolliculoma (M8101/0) — *see* Neoplasm,
  skin, benign
Tricholemmoma (M8102/0) — *see* Neoplasm,
  skin, benign
Trichomoniasis A59.9
  bladder A59.03
  cervix A59.09
  intestinal A07.8
  prostate A59.02
  seminal vesicles A59.09
  specified site NEC A59.8
  urethra A59.03
  urogenitalis A59.00
  vagina A59.01
  vulva A59.01
Trichomycosis
  axillaris A48.8
  nodosa, nodularis B36.8
Trichonodosis L67.8
Trichophytid, trichophyton infection — *see*
  Dermatophytosis
Trichophytobezoar T18.9
  intestine T18.3
  stomach T18.2
Trichophytosis — *see* Dermatophytosis
Trichoptilosis L67.8
Trichorrhexis (nodosa) (invaginata) L67.0
Trichosis axillaris A48.8
Trichosporosis nodosa B36.2
Trichostasis spinulosa (congenital) Q84.1
Trichostrongyliasis, trichostrongylosis (small
  intestine) B81.2
Trichostrongylus infection B81.2
Trichotillomania F63.3
Trichromat, trichromatopsia, anomalous
  (congenital) H53.55
Trichuriasis B79
Trichuris trichiura (infection) (infestation) (any
  site) B79
Tricuspid (valve) — *see* condition
Trifid — *see also* Accessory
  kidney (pelvis) Q63.8
  tongue Q38.3
Trigeminal neuralgia — *see* Neuralgia, trigeminal
Trigeminy R00.8
Trigger finger (acquired) M65.30
  congenital Q74.0
  index finger M65.329
    left M65.322
    right M65.321
  little finger M65.359
    left M65.352
    right M65.351
  middle finger M65.339
    left M65.332
    right M65.331
  ring finger M65.349
    left M65.342
    right M65.341
  thumb M65.319
    left M65.312
    right M65.311
Trigonitis (bladder) (chronic)
  (pseudomembranous) N30.30
  with hematuria N30.31
Trigonocephaly Q75.0
Trilocular heart — *see* Cor triloculare
Trimethylaminuria E88.8
Tripartite placenta — *see* Malformation,
  placenta, specified type NEC
Triphalangeal thumb Q74.0

Triple — *see also* Accessory
  kidneys Q63.0
  uteri Q51.8
  X, female Q97.0
Triplegia G83.89
  congenital or infantile G80.8
Triplet (fetus or newborn) — *see also* Newborn,
  triplet
  complicating pregnancy — *see* Pregnancy,
    triplet
Triplication — *see* Accessory
Triploidy Q92.7
Trismus R25.2
  neonatorum A33
  newborn A33
Trisomy (syndrome) Q92.9
  autosomes Q92.9
  chromosome specified NEC Q92.8
    partial Q92.2
      due to unbalanced translocation Q92.5
    whole (nonsex chromosome)
      meiotic nondisjunction Q92.0
      mitotic nondisjunction Q92.1
      mosaicism Q92.1
      specified NEC Q92.8
  due to
    dicentrics — *see* Extra, marker
      chromosomes
    extra rings — *see* Extra, marker
      chromosomes
    isochromosomes — *see* Extra, marker
      chromosomes
  specified NEC Q92.8
  whole chromosome Q92.9
    meiotic nondisjunction Q92.0
    mitotic nondisjunction Q92.1
    mosaicism Q92.1
    partial Q92.9
    specified NEC Q92.8
  13 (partial) Q91.7
    meiotic nondisjunction Q91.4
    mitotic nondisjunction Q91.5
    mosaicism Q91.5
    translocation Q91.6
  18 (partial) Q91.3
    meiotic nondisjunction Q91.0
    mitotic nondisjunction Q91.1
    mosaicism Q91.1
    translocation Q91.2
  20 Q92.8
  21 (partial) Q90.9
    meiotic nondisjunction Q90.0
    mitotic nondisjunction Q90.1
    mosaicism Q90.1
    translocation Q90.2
  22 Q92.8
Tritanomaly, tritanopia H53.55
Trombiculosis, trombiculiasis, trombidiosis
  B88.0
Trophedema (congenital) (hereditary) Q82.0
Trophoblastic disease — *see also* Mole,
  hydatidiform
  previous, affecting management of pregnancy
    — *see* Pregnancy, complicated by,
    previous, trophoblastic disease
Tropholymphedema Q82.0
Trophoneurosis NEC G96.8
  disseminated M34.9
Tropical — *see* condition
Trouble — *see also* Disease
  heart — *see* Disease, heart
  kidney — *see* Disease, renal
  nervous R45.0
  sinus — *see* Sinusitis
Trousseau's syndrome (thrombophlebitis
  migrans) I82.1
Truancy, childhood
  socialized F91.2
  unsocialized F91.1
Truncus
  arteriosus (persistent) Q20.0
  communis Q20.0
Trunk — *see* condition

Trypanosomiasis
African B56.9
by Trypanosoma brucei
gambiense B56.0
rhodesiense B56.1
American — *see* Chagas' disease
Brazilian — *see* Chagas' disease
by Trypanosoma
brucei gambiense B56.0
brucei rhodesiense B56.1
cruzi — *see* Chagas' disease
gambiensis, Gambian B56.0
rhodesiensis, Rhodesian B56.1
South American — *see* Chagas' disease
where
African trypanosomiasis is prevalent B56.9
Chagas' disease is prevalent B57.2

T-shaped incisors K00.2

Tsutsugamushi (disease) (fever) A75.3

Tube, tubal, tubular — *see* condition

Tubercle — *see also* Tuberculosis
brain, solitary A17.81
Darwin's Q17.8
Ghon, primary infection A15.7

Tuberculid, tuberculide (indurating, subcutaneous) (lichenoid) (miliary) (papulonecrotic) (primary) (skin) A18.4

Tuberculoma — *see also* Tuberculosis
brain A17.81
meninges (cerebral) (spinal) A17.1
spinal cord A17.81

Tuberculosis, tubercular, tuberculous
(calcification) (calcified) (caseous) (chromogenic acid-fast bacilli) (degeneration) (fibrocaseous) (fistula) (interstitial) (isolated circumscribed lesions) (necrosis) (parenchymatous) (ulcerative) A15.9
with pneumoconiosis (any condition in J60-J64) J65
abdomen (lymph gland) A18.39
abscess (respiratory) A15.9
bone A18.03
hip A18.02
knee A18.02
sacrum A18.01
specified site NEC A18.03
spinal A18.01
vertebra A18.01
brain A17.81
breast A18.89
Cowper's gland A18.15
dura (mater) (cerebral) (spinal) A17.81
epidural (cerebral) (spinal) A17.81
female pelvis A18.17
frontal sinus A15.8
genital organs NEC A18.10
genitourinary A18.10
gland (lymphatic) — *see* Tuberculosis, lymph gland
hip A18.02
intestine A18.32
ischiorectal A18.32
joint NEC A18.02
hip A18.02
knee A18.02
specified NEC A18.02
vertebral A18.01
kidney A18.11
knee A18.02
lumbar (spine) A18.01
lung — *see* Tuberculosis, pulmonary
meninges (cerebral) (spinal) A17.0
muscle A18.09
perianal (fistula) A18.32
perinephritic A18.11
perirectal A18.32
rectum A18.32
retropharyngeal A15.8
sacrum A18.01
scrofulous A18.2
scrotum A18.15
skin (primary) A18.4
spinal cord A17.81
spine or vertebra (column) A18.01
subdiaphragmatic A18.31
testis A18.15

Tuberculosis, tubercular, tuberculous — *continued*
abscess — *continued*
urinary A18.13
uterus A18.17
accessory sinus — *see* Tuberculosis, sinus
Addison's disease A18.7
adenitis — *see* Tuberculosis, lymph gland
adenoids A15.8
adenopathy — *see* Tuberculosis, lymph gland
adherent pericardium A18.84
adnexa (uteri) A18.17
adrenal (capsule) (gland) A18.7
alimentary canal A18.32
anemia A18.89
ankle (joint) (bone) A18.02
anus A18.32
apex, apical — *see* Tuberculosis, pulmonary
appendicitis, appendix A18.32
arachnoid A17.0
artery, arteritis A18.89
cerebral A18.89
arthritis (chronic) (synovial) A18.02
spine or vertebra (column) A18.01
articular — *see* Tuberculosis, joint
ascites A18.31
asthma — *see* Tuberculosis, pulmonary
axilla, axillary (gland) A18.2
bilateral — *see* Tuberculosis, pulmonary
bladder A18.12
bone A18.03
hip A18.02
knee A18.02
limb NEC A18.03
sacrum A18.01
spine or vertebral column A18.01
bowel (miliary) A18.32
brain A17.81
breast A18.89
broad ligament A18.17
bronchi, bronchial, bronchus A15.5
ectasia, ectasis (bronchiectasis) — *see* Tuberculosis, pulmonary
fistula A15.5
primary (progressive) A15.7
gland or node A15.4
primary (progressive) A15.7
lymph gland or node A15.4
primary (progressive) A15.7
bronchiectasis — *see* Tuberculosis, pulmonary
bronchitis A15.5
bronchopleural A15.6
bronchopneumonia, bronchopneumonic — *see* Tuberculosis, pulmonary
bronchorrhagia A15.5
bronchotracheal A15.5
bronze disease A18.7
buccal cavity A18.83
bulbourethral gland A18.15
bursa A18.09
cachexia A15.9
cardiomyopathy A18.84
caries — *see* Tuberculosis, bone
cartilage A18.02
intervertebral A18.01
catarrhal — *see* Tuberculosis, respiratory
cecum A18.32
cellulitis (primary) A18.4
cerebellum A17.81
cerebral, cerebrum A17.81
cerebrospinal A17.81
meninges A17.0
cervical (lymph gland or node) A18.2
cervicitis, cervix (uteri) A18.16
chest — *see* Tuberculosis, respiratory
chorioretinitis A18.53
choroid, choroiditis A18.53
ciliary body A18.54
colitis A18.32
collier's J65
colliquativa (primary) A18.4
colon A18.32
complex, primary A15.7
complicating pregnancy, childbirth or puerperium — *see* Tuberculosis, obstetric
congenital P37.0
conjunctiva A18.59
connective tissue (systemic) A18.89

Tuberculosis, tubercular, tuberculous — *continued*
contact Z20.1
cornea (ulcer) A18.52
Cowper's gland A18.15
coxae A18.02
coxalgia A18.02
cul-de-sac of Douglas A18.17
curvature, spine A18.01
cutis (colliquativa) (primary) A18.4
cyst, ovary A18.18
cystitis A18.12
dactylitis A18.03
diarrhea A18.32
diffuse — *see* Tuberculosis, miliary
digestive tract A18.32
disseminated — *see* Tuberculosis, miliary
duodenum A18.32
dura (mater) (cerebral) (spinal) A17.0
abscess (cerebral) (spinal) A17.81
dysentery A18.32
ear (external) (inner) (middle) A18.6
bone A18.03
external (primary) A18.4
skin (primary) A18.4
elbow A18.02
emphysema — *see* Tuberculosis, pulmonary
empyema A15.6
encephalitis A17.82
endarteritis A18.89
endocarditis A18.84
aortic A18.84
mitral A18.84
pulmonary A18.84
tricuspid A18.84
endocrine glands NEC A18.82
endometrium A18.17
enteric, enterica, enteritis A18.32
enterocolitis A18.32
epididymis, epididymitis A18.15
epidural abscess (cerebral) (spinal) A17.81
epiglottis A15.5
episcleritis A18.51
erythema (induratum) (nodosum) (primary) A18.4
esophagus A18.83
eustachian tube A18.6
exposure (to) Z20.1
exudative — *see* Tuberculosis, pulmonary
eye A18.50
glaucoma A18.59
eyelid (primary) (lupus) A18.4
fallopian tube (acute) (chronic) A18.17
fascia A18.09
fauces A15.8
female pelvic inflammatory disease A18.17
finger A18.03
first infection A15.7
gallbladder A18.83
ganglion A18.09
gastritis A18.83
gastrocolic fistula A18.32
gastroenteritis A18.32
gastrointestinal tract A18.32
general, generalized — *see* Tuberculosis, miliary
genital organs A18.10
genitourinary A18.10
genu A18.02
glandula suprarenalis A18.7
glandular, general A18.2
glottis A15.5
grinder's J65
gum A18.83
hand A18.03
heart A18.84
hematogenous — *see* Tuberculosis, miliary
hemoptysis — *see* Tuberculosis, pulmonary
hemorrhage NEC — *see* Tuberculosis, pulmonary
hemothorax A15.6
hepatitis A18.83
hilar lymph nodes A15.4
primary (progressive) A15.7
hip (joint) (disease) (bone) A18.02
hydropneumothorax A15.6
hydrothorax A15.6
hypoadrenalism A18.7

Tuberculosis, tubercular, tuberculous —
continued
hypopharynx A15.8
ileocecal (hyperplastic) A18.32
ileocolitis A18.32
ileum A18.32
iliac spine (superior) A18.03
immunological findings only A15.7
indurativa (primary) A18.4
infantile A15.7
infection A15.9
  without clinical manifestations A15.7
infraclavicular gland A18.2
inguinal gland A18.2
inguinalis A18.2
intestine (any part) A18.32
iridocyclitis A18.54
iris, iritis A18.54
ischiorectal A18.32
jaw A18.03
jejunum A18.32
joint A18.02
  vertebral A18.01
keratitis (interstitial) A18.52
keratoconjunctivitis A18.52
kidney A18.11
knee (joint) A18.02
kyphosis, kyphoscoliosis A18.01
laryngitis A15.5
larynx A15.5
leptomeninges, leptomeningitis (cerebral)
  (spinal) A17.0
lichenoides (primary) A18.4
linguae A18.83
lip A18.83
liver A18.83
lordosis A18.01
lung — *see* Tuberculosis, pulmonary
lupus vulgaris A18.4
lymph gland or node (peripheral) A18.2
  abdomen A18.39
  bronchial A15.4
    primary (progressive) A15.7
  cervical A18.2
  hilar A15.4
    primary (progressive) A15.7
  intrathoracic A15.4
    primary (progressive) A15.7
  mediastinal A15.4
    primary (progressive) A15.7
  mesenteric A18.39
  retroperitoneal A18.39
  tracheobronchial A15.4
    primary (progressive) A15.7
lymphadenitis — *see* Tuberculosis, lymph
  gland
lymphangitis — *see* Tuberculosis, lymph gland
lymphatic (gland) (vessel) — *see* Tuberculosis,
  lymph gland
mammary gland A18.89
marasmus A15.9
mastoiditis A18.03
mediastinal lymph gland or node A15.4
  primary (progressive) A15.7
mediastinitis A15.8
  primary (progressive) A15.7
mediastinum A15.8
  primary (progressive) A15.7
medulla A17.81
melanosis, Addisonian A18.7
meninges, meningitis (basilar) (cerebral)
  (cerebrospinal) (spinal) A17.0
meningoencephalitis A17.82
mesentery, mesenteric (gland or node) A18.39
miliary A19.9
  acute A19.2
    multiple sites A19.1
    single specified site A19.0
  chronic A19.8
  specified NEC A19.8
millstone makers' J65
miner's J65
molder's J65
mouth A18.83
multiple A19.9
  acute A19.1
  chronic A19.8

Tuberculosis, tubercular, tuberculous —
continued
muscle A18.09
myelitis A17.82
myocardium, myocarditis A18.84
nasal (passage) (sinus) A15.8
nasopharynx A15.8
neck gland A18.2
nephritis A18.11
nerve (mononeuropathy) A17.83
nervous system A17.9
nose (septum) A15.8
obstetric complicating
  childbirth O98.02
  pregnancy O98.019
    first trimester O98.011
    second trimester O98.012
    third trimester O98.013
  puerperium O98.03
ocular A18.50
omentum A18.31
oophoritis (acute) (chronic) A18.17
optic (nerve trunk) (papilla) A18.59
orbit A18.59
orchitis A18.15
organ, specified NEC A18.89
osseous — *see* Tuberculosis, bone
osteitis — *see* Tuberculosis, bone
osteomyelitis — *see* Tuberculosis, bone
otitis media A18.6
ovary, ovaritis (acute) (chronic) A18.17
oviduct (acute) (chronic) A18.17
pachymeningitis A17.0
palate (soft) A18.83
pancreas A18.83
papulonecrotic(a) (primary) A18.4
parathyroid glands A18.82
paronychia (primary) A18.4
parotid gland or region A18.83
pelvis (bony) A18.03
penis A18.15
peribronchitis A15.5
pericardium, pericarditis A18.84
perichondritis, larynx A15.5
periostitis — *see* Tuberculosis, bone
perirectal fistula A18.32
peritoneum NEC A18.31
peritonitis A18.31
pharynx, pharyngitis A15.8
phlyctenulosis (keratoconjunctivitis) A18.52
phthisis NEC — *see* Tuberculosis, pulmonary
pituitary gland A18.82
placenta — *see* Tuberculosis, obstetric
pleura, pleural, pleurisy, pleuritis (fibrinous)
  (obliterative) (purulent) (simple plastic)
  (with effusion) A15.6
  primary (progressive) A15.7
pneumonia, pneumonic — *see* Tuberculosis,
  pulmonary
pneumothorax (spontaneous) (tense valvular) —
  see Tuberculosis, pulmonary
polyneuropathy A17.89
polyserositis A19.9
  acute A19.1
  chronic A19.8
potter's J65
prepuce A18.15
primary (complex) A15.7
proctitis A18.32
prostate, prostatitis A18.14
pulmonalis — *see* Tuberculosis, pulmonary
pulmonary (cavitated) (fibrotic) (infiltrative)
  (nodular) A15.0
  childhood type or first infection A15.7
  primary (complex) A15.7
pyelitis A18.11
pyelonephritis A18.11
pyemia — *see* Tuberculosis, miliary
pyonephrosis A18.11
pyopneumothorax A15.6
pyothorax A15.6
rectum (fistula) (with abscess) A18.32
reinfection stage — *see* Tuberculosis, pulmonary
renal A18.11
renis A18.11
respiratory A15.9
  primary A15.7
  specified site NEC A15.8

Tuberculosis, tubercular, tuberculous —
continued
retina, retinitis A18.53
retroperitoneal (lymph gland or node) A18.39
rheumatism NEC A18.09
rhinitis A15.8
sacroiliac (joint) A18.01
sacrum A18.01
salivary gland A18.83
salpingitis (acute) (chronic) A18.17
sandblaster's J65
sclera A18.51
scoliosis A18.01
scrofulous A18.2
scrotum A18.15
seminal tract or vesicle A18.15
senile A15.9
septic — *see* Tuberculosis, miliary
shoulder (joint) A18.02
  blade A18.03
sigmoid A18.32
sinus (any nasal) A15.8
  bone A18.03
  epididymis A18.15
skeletal NEC A18.03
skin (any site) (primary) A18.4
small intestine A18.32
soft palate A18.83
spermatic cord A18.15
spine, spinal (column) A18.01
  cord A17.81
  medulla A17.81
  membrane A17.0
  meninges A17.0
spleen, splenitis A18.85
spondylitis A18.01
sternoclavicular joint A18.02
stomach A18.83
stonemason's J65
subcutaneous tissue (cellular) (primary) A18.4
subcutis (primary) A18.4
subdeltoid bursa A18.83
submaxillary (region) A18.83
supraclavicular gland A18.2
suprarenal (capsule) (gland) A18.7
swelling, joint (*see also* Tuberculosis, joint)
  A18.02 (*see also* category M01)
symphysis pubis A18.02
synovitis A18.09
  articular A18.02
  spine or vertebra A18.01
systemic — *see* Tuberculosis, miliary
tarsitis A18.4
tendon (sheath) — *see* Tuberculosis, tenosynovitis
tenosynovitis A18.09
  spine or vertebra A18.01
testis A18.15
throat A15.8
thymus gland A18.82
thyroid gland A18.81
tongue A18.83
tonsil, tonsillitis A15.8
trachea, tracheal A15.5
  lymph gland or node A15.4
    primary (progressive) A15.7
tracheobronchial A15.5
  lymph gland or node A15.4
    primary (progressive) A15.7
tubal (acute) (chronic) A18.17
tunica vaginalis A18.15
ulcer (skin) (primary) A18.4
  bowel or intestine A18.32
specified NEC – code under Tuberculosis, by
  site
unspecified site A15.9
ureter A18.11
urethra, urethral (gland) A18.13
urinary organ or tract A18.13
uterus A18.17
uveal tract A18.54
uvula A18.83
vaccination, prophylactic (against) Z23
vagina A18.18
vas deferens A18.15
verruca, verrucosa (cutis) (primary) A18.4
vertebra (column) A18.01
vesiculitis A18.15
vulva A18.18

Tuberculosis, tubercular, tuberculous —
  continued
  wrist (joint) A18.02
Tuberculum
  Carabelli — *see* Note at K00.2
  occlusal — *see* Note at K00.2
  paramolare K00.2
Tuberous sclerosis (brain) Q85.1
Tubo-ovarian — *see* condition
Tuboplasty, after previous sterilization Z31.0
  aftercare Z31.42
Tubotympanitis, catarrhal (chronic) — *see* Otitis,
    media, nonsuppurative, chronic, serous
Tularemia A21.9
  with
    conjunctivitis A21.1
    pneumonia A21.2
  abdominal A21.3
  bronchopneumonic A21.2
  conjunctivitis A21.1
  cryptogenic A21.3
  enteric A21.3
  gastrointestinal A21.3
  generalized A21.7
  ingestion A21.3
  intestinal A21.3
  oculoglandular A21.1
  ophthalmic A21.1
  pneumonia (any), pneumonic A21.2
  pulmonary A21.2
  septicemia A21.7
  specified NEC A21.8
  typhoidal A21.7
  ulceroglandular A21.0
  vaccination, prophylactic (against) Z23
Tularensis conjunctivitis A21.1
Tumefaction — *see also* Swelling
  liver — *see* Hypertrophy, liver
Tumor — *see also* Neoplasm, unspecified behavior
  acinar cell (M8550/1) — *see* Neoplasm,
    uncertain behavior
  acinic cell (M8550/1) — *see* Neoplasm,
    uncertain behavior
  adenocarcinoid (M8245/3) — *see* Neoplasm,
    malignant
  adenomatoid (M9054/0) — *see also* Neoplasm,
    benign
    odontogenic (M9300/0) D16.5
    upper jaw (bone) D16.4
  adnexal (skin) (M8390/0) — *see* Neoplasm,
    skin, benign
  adrenal
    cortical (benign) (M8370/0) D35.00
      left D35.02
      malignant (M8370/3) C74.00
        left C74.02
        right C74.01
      right D35.01
    rest (M8671/0) — *see* Neoplasm, benign
  alpha-cell (M8152/0)
    malignant (M8152/3)
      pancreas C25.4
      specified site NEC — *see* Neoplasm,
        malignant
      unspecified site C25.4
    pancreas D13.7
    specified site NEC — *see* Neoplasm, benign
    unspecified site D13.7
  aneurysmal — *see* Aneurysm
  aortic body (M8691/1) D44.7
    malignant (M8691/3) C75.5
  Askin's (M8803/3) — *see* Neoplasm, connective
    tissue, malignant
  basal cell (M8090/1) — *see also* Neoplasm,
    skin, uncertain behavior D48.5
  Bednar (M8833/3) — *see* Neoplasm, malignant
  benign (unclassified) (M8000/0) — *see*
    Neoplasm, benign
  beta-cell (M8151/0)
    malignant (M8151/3)
      pancreas C25.4
      specified site NEC — *see* Neoplasm,
        malignant
      unspecified site C25.4
    pancreas D13.7

Tumor — *see also* Neoplasm, unspecified behavior
  — *continued*
  beta-cell — *continued*
    specified site NEC — *see* Neoplasm, benign
    unspecified site D13.7
  Brenner (M9000/0) D27.9
    borderline malignancy (M9000/1) D39.10
      left D39.12
      right D39.11
    left D27.1
    malignant (M9000/3) C56.9
      left C56.1
      right C56.0
    proliferating (M9000/1) D39.10
      left D39.12
      right D39.11
    right D27.0
  bronchial alveolar, intravascular (M9134/1)
    D38.1
  Brooke's (M8100/0) — *see* Neoplasm, skin,
    benign
  brown fat (M8880/0) — *see* Lipoma
  Burkitt's (M9687/3) — *see* Burkitt's lymphoma
  calcifying epithelial odontogenic (M9340/0)
    D16.5
    upper jaw (bone) D16.4
  carcinoid (M8240/3) — *see* Carcinoid
  carotid body (M8692/1) D44.6
    malignant (M8692/3) C75.4
  cells — *see also* Neoplasm, unspecified
    behavior
    benign (M8001/0) — *see* Neoplasm, benign
    malignant (M8001/3) — *see* Neoplasm,
      malignant
    uncertain whether benign or malignant
      (M8001/1) — *see* Neoplasm, uncertain
      behavior
  cervix, in pregnancy or childbirth — *see*
    Pregnancy, complicated by, tumor,
    uterus, cervix
  chondromatous giant cell (M9230/0) — *see*
    Neoplasm, bone, benign
  chromaffin (M8700/0) — *see also* Neoplasm,
    benign
    malignant (M8700/3) — *see* Neoplasm,
      malignant
  Cock's peculiar L72.1
  Codman's (M9230/0) — *see* Neoplasm, bone,
    benign
  dentigerous, mixed (M9282/0) D16.5
    upper jaw (bone) D16.4
  dermoid (M9084/0) — *see* Neoplasm, benign
    with malignant transformation (M9084/3)
      C56.9
      left C56.1
      right C56.0
  desmoid (extra-abdominal) (M8821/1) — *see*
    also Neoplasm, connective tissue,
    uncertain behavior
    abdominal (M8822/1) — *see* Neoplasm,
      connective tissue, uncertain behavior
  embolus (M8000/6) — *see* Neoplasm,
    secondary
  embryonal (mixed) (M9080/1) — *see also*
    Neoplasm, uncertain behavior
    liver (M9080/3) C22.7
  endodermal sinus (M9071/3)
    specified site — *see* Neoplasm, malignant
    unspecified site
      female C56.9
        left C56.1
        right C56.0
      male C62.90
  endometrioid of low malignant potential
    (M8380/1) — *see* Neoplasm, uncertain
    behavior
  epithelial
    benign (M8010/0) — *see* Neoplasm, benign
    malignant (M8010/3) — *see* Neoplasm,
      malignant
  Ewing's (M9260/3) — *see* Neoplasm, bone,
    malignant
  fatty (M8850/0) — *see* Lipoma
  fetal, causing obstructed labor (mother) O66.3
  fibroid (M8890/0) — *see* Leiomyoma
  G cell (M8153/1)
    malignant (M8153/3)

Tumor — *see also* Neoplasm, unspecified behavior
  — *continued*
  G cell — *continued*
    malignant — *continued*
      pancreas C25.4
      specified site NEC — *see* Neoplasm,
        malignant
      unspecified site C25.4
    specified site — *see* Neoplasm, uncertain
      behavior
    unspecified site D37.7
  germ cell (M9064/3) — *see also* Neoplasm,
    malignant
    mixed (M9085/3) — *see* Neoplasm,
      malignant
  ghost cell, odontogenic (M9302/0) D16.5
    upper jaw (bone) D16.4
  giant cell ((M8003/1) — *see also* Neoplasm,
    uncertain behavior
    bone (M9250/1) D48.0
      malignant (M9250/3) — *see* Neoplasm,
        bone, malignant
    chondromatous (M9230/0) — *see* Neoplasm,
      bone, benign
    malignant (M8003/3) — *see* Neoplasm,
      malignant
    soft parts (M9251/1) — *see* Neoplasm,
      connective tissue, uncertain behavior
      malignant (M9251/3) — *see* Neoplasm,
        connective tissue, malignant
  glomus (M8711/0) D18.00
    intra-abdominal D18.03
    intracranial D18.02
    jugulare (M8690/1) D44.7
      malignant (M8690/3) C75.5
    skin D18.01
    specified site NEC D18.09
  gonadal stromal (M8590/1) — *see* Neoplasm,
    uncertain behavior
  granular cell (M9580/0) — *see also* Neoplasm,
    connective tissue, benign
    malignant (M9580/3) — *see* Neoplasm,
      connective tissue, malignant
  granulosa cell (M8620/1) D39.10
    juvenile (M8622/1) D39.10
    left D39.12
    malignant (M8620/3) C56.9
      left C56.1
      right C56.0
    right D39.11
  granulosa cell-theca cell (M8621/1) D39.10
    left D39.12
    malignant (M8621/3) C56.9
      left C56.1
      right C56.0
    right D39.11
  Grawitz's (M8312/3) C64.9
    left C64.1
    right C64.0
  hemorrhoidal — *see* Hemorrhoids
  hilar cell (M8660/0) D27.9
    left D27.1
    right D27.0
  hilus cell (M8660/0) D27.9
    left D27.1
    right D27.0
  Hurthle cell (benign) (M8290/0) D34
    malignant (M8290/3) C73
  hydatid — *see* Echinococcus
  hypernephroid (M8311/1) — *see also*
    Neoplasm, uncertain behavior
  interstitial cell (M8650/1) — *see also*
    Neoplasm, uncertain behavior
    benign (M8650/0) — *see* Neoplasm, benign
    malignant (M8650/3) — *see* Neoplasm,
      malignant
  intravascular bronchial alveolar D49.1
  islet cell (M8150/1)
    malignant (M8150/3)
      pancreas C25.4
      specified site NEC — *see* Neoplasm,
        malignant
      unspecified site C25.4
    pancreas D13.7
    specified site NEC — *see* Neoplasm, benign
    unspecified site D13.7

Tumor — *see also* Neoplasm, unspecified behavior — *continued*

juxtaglomerular (M8361/1) D41.00
  left D41.02
  right D41.01
Klatskin's (M8162/3) C22.1
Krukenberg's (M8490/6) C79.60
  left C79.62
  right C79.61
Leydig cell (M8650/1)
  benign (M8650/0)
    specified site — *see* Neoplasm, benign
    unspecified site
      female D27.9
      male D29.20
  malignant (M8650/3)
    specified site — *see* Neoplasm, malignant
    unspecified site
      female C56.9
      male C62.90
  specified site — *see* Neoplasm, uncertain behavior
  unspecified site
    female D39.10
    male D40.10
lipid cell, ovary (M8670/0) D27.9
  left D27.1
  right D27.0
lipoid cell, ovary (M8670/0) D27.9
  left D27.1
  right D27.0
malignant (M8000/3) — *see also* Neoplasm, malignant
  fusiform cell (type) (M8004/3) — *see* Neoplasm, malignant
  giant cell (type) (M8003/3) — *see* Neoplasm, malignant
  mixed NEC (M8940/3) — *see* Neoplasm, malignant
  small cell (type) (M8002/3) — *see* Neoplasm, malignant
  spindle cell (type) (M8004/3) — *see* Neoplasm, malignant
  unclassified (M8000/3) — *see* Neoplasm, malignant
mast cell (M9740/1) D47.0
  malignant (M9740/3) C96.2
melanotic, neuroectodermal (M9363/0) — *see* Neoplasm, benign
Merkel cell (M8247/3) — *see* Neoplasm, skin, malignant
mesenchymal
  malignant (M8800/3) — *see* Neoplasm, connective tissue, malignant
  mixed (M8990/1) — *see* Neoplasm, connective tissue, uncertain behavior
mesodermal, mixed (M8951/3) — *see also* Neoplasm, malignant
  liver C22.4
mesonephric (M9110/1) — *see also* Neoplasm, uncertain behavior
  malignant (M9110/3) — *see* Neoplasm, malignant
metastatic
  from specified site (M8000/3) — *see* Neoplasm, malignant, by site
  of specified site — *see* Neoplasm, malignant, by site
  to specified site (M8000/6) — *see* Neoplasm, secondary, by site
mixed NEC (M8940/0) — *see also* Neoplasm, benign
  malignant (M8940/3) — *see* Neoplasm, malignant
mucinous of low malignant potential (M8472/3)
  specified site — *see* Neoplasm, malignant
  unspecified site C56.9
mucocarcinoid (M8243/3)
  specified site — *see* Neoplasm, malignant
  unspecified site C18.1
mucoepidermoid (M8430/1) — *see* Neoplasm, uncertain behavior
Mullerian, mixed (M8950/3)
  specified site — *see* Neoplasm, malignant
  unspecified site C54.9
myoepithelial (M8982/0) — *see* Neoplasm, benign

Tumor — *see also* Neoplasm, unspecified behavior — *continued*

neuroectodermal (peripheral) (M9364/3) — *see* Neoplasm, malignant
  primitive (M9473/3)
    specified site — *see* Neoplasm, malignant
    unspecified site C71.9
neurogenic olfactory (M9520/3) C30.0
nonencapsulated sclerosing (M8350/3) C73
odontogenic (M9270/1) D48.0
  adenomatoid (M9300/0) D16.5
    upper jaw (bone) D16.4
  benign (M9270/0) D16.5
    upper jaw (bone) D16.4
  calcifying epithelial (M9340/0) D16.5
    upper jaw (bone) D16.4
  malignant (M9270/3) C41.1
    upper jaw (bone) C41.0
  squamous (M9312/0) D16.5
    upper jaw (bone) D16.4
ovarian stromal (M8590/1) D39.10
  left D39.12
  right D39.11
ovary, in pregnancy — *see* Pregnancy, complicated by, abnormal, pelvic organs or tissues NEC
pacinian (M9507/0) — *see* Neoplasm, skin, benign
Pancoast's (M8010/3) — *see* Pancoast's syndrome
papillary (M8050/0) — *see also* Papilloma
  cystic (M8452/1) D37.7
  mucinous of low malignant potential (M8473/3) C56.9
    left C56.1
    right C56.0
    specified site — *see* Neoplasm, malignant
    unspecified site C56.9
  serous of low malignant potential (M8462/3)
    specified site — *see* Neoplasm, malignant
    unspecified site C56.9
pelvic, in pregnancy or childbirth — *see* Pregnancy, complicated by, abnormal, pelvic organs or tissues NEC
phantom F45.8
phyllodes (M9020/1)
  female D48.60
    left D48.62
    right D48.61
  male D48.65
    left D48.64
    right D48.63
  benign (M9020/0) D24.00
    left D24.02
    male D24.10
      left D24.12
      right D24.11
    right D24.01
  malignant (M9020/3) — *see* Neoplasm, breast, malignant
Pindborg (M9340/0) D16.5
  upper jaw (bone) D16.4
placental site trophoblastic (M9104/1) D39.2
plasma cell (malignant) (M9731/3) C90.20
  in remission C90.21
polyvesicular vitelline (M9071/3)
  specified site — *see* Neoplasm, malignant
  unspecified site
    female C56.9
    male C62.90
Pott's puffy -*see* Osteomyelitis, specified NEC
Rathke's pouch (M9350/1) D44.3
retinal anlage (M9363/0) — *see* Neoplasm, benign
salivary gland type, mixed (M8940/0) — *see* Neoplasm, salivary gland, benign
  malignant (M8940/3) — *see* Neoplasm, salivary gland, malignant
Sampson's N80.1
Schmincke's (M8082/3) — *see* Neoplasm, nasopharynx, malignant
sclerosing stromal (M8602/2) D27.9
  left D27.1
  right D27.0
sebaceous — *see* Cyst, sebaceous
secondary (M8000/6) — *see* Neoplasm, secondary

Tumor — *see also* Neoplasm, unspecified behavior — *continued*

serous of low malignant potential (M8442/3)
  specified site — *see* Neoplasm, malignant
  unspecified site C56.9
Sertoli cell (M8640/0)
  with lipid storage (M8641/0)
    specified site — *see* Neoplasm, benign
    unspecified site
      female D27.9
      male D29.20
  specified site — *see* Neoplasm, benign
  unspecified site
    female D27.9
    male D29.20
Sertoli-Leydig cell (M8631/0)
  specified site — *see* Neoplasm, benign
  unspecified site
    female D27.9
    male D29.20
sex cord(-stromal) (M8590/1) — *see* Neoplasm, uncertain behavior
  with annular tubules (M8623/1) D39.10
    left D39.12
    right D39.11
skin appendage (M8390/0) — *see* Neoplasm, skin, benign
smooth muscle (M8897/1) — *see* Neoplasm, connective tissue, uncertain behavior
soft tissue
  benign (M8800/0) — *see* Neoplasm, connective tissue, benign
  malignant (M8800/3) — *see* Neoplasm, connective tissue, malignant
sternomastoid (congenital) Q68.0
sweat gland (M8400/1) — *see also* Neoplasm, skin, uncertain behavior
  benign (M8400/0) — *see* Neoplasm, skin, benign
  malignant (M8400/3) — *see* Neoplasm, skin, malignant
syphilitic, brain A52.17
testicular stromal (M8590/1) D40.10
  left D40.12
  right D40.11
theca cell (M8600/0) D27.9
  left D27.1
  right D27.0
theca cell-granulosa cell (M8621/1) D39.10
  left D39.12
  right D39.11
Triton, malignant (M9561/3) — *see* Neoplasm, nerve, malignant
trophoblastic, placental site (M9104/1) D39.2
turban (M8200/0) D23.4
uterus (body), in pregnancy or childbirth — *see* Pregnancy, complicated by, tumor, uterus
vagina, in pregnancy or childbirth — *see* Pregnancy, complicated by, abnormal, vagina
varicose — *see* Varix
von Recklinghausen's — *see* Neurofibromatosis
vulva or perineum, in pregnancy or childbirth — *see* Pregnancy, complicated by, abnormal, vulva
  causing obstructed labor O65.5
Warthin's (M8561/0) — *see* Neoplasm, salivary gland, benign
Wilms' (M8960/3) C64.9
  left C64.1
  right C64.0
yolk sac (M9071/3)
  specified site — *see* Neoplasm, malignant
  unspecified site
    female C56.9
    male C62.90

Tumorlet (M8040/1) — *see* Neoplasm, uncertain behavior

Tungiasis B88.1

Tunica vasculosa lentis Q12.2

Turban tumor (M8200/0) D23.4

Türck's trachoma J37.0

Turner-Kieser syndrome Q79.8

Turner-like syndrome Q87.1

Turner's
  hypoplasia (tooth) K00.4

Turner's — *continued*
  syndrome Q96.9
    specified NEC Q96.8
  tooth K00.4
Turner-Ullrich syndrome Q96.9
Tussis convulsiva — *see* Whooping cough
Twilight state
  epileptic F05
  psychogenic F44.89
Twin (fetus or newborn) — *see also* Newborn, twin
  complicating pregnancy — *see* Pregnancy, twin
  conjoined Q89.4
Twinning, teeth K00.2
Twist, twisted
  bowel, colon or intestine K56.2
  hair (congenital) Q84.1
  mesentery K56.2
  omentum K56.2
  organ or site, congenital NEC — *see* Anomaly, by site
  ovarian pedicle — *see* Torsion, ovary
Twitching R25.3
Tylosis (acquired) L84
  buccalis K13.2
  linguae K13.2
  palmaris et plantaris (congenital) (inherited) Q82.8
    acquired L85.1
Tympanism R14.0
Tympanites (abdominal) (intestinal) R14.0
Tympanitis — *see* Myringitis
Tympanosclerosis — *see* category H74.0
Tympanum — *see* condition
Tympany
  abdomen R14.0
  chest R09.89
Type A behavior pattern Z73.1
Typhlitis — *see* Appendicitis
Typhoenteritis — *see* Typhoid
Typhoid (abortive) (ambulant) (any site) (clinical) (fever) (hemorrhagic) (infection) (intermittent) (malignant) (rheumatic) (Widal negative) A01.00
  with pneumonia A01.03
  abdominal A01.09
  arthritis A01.04
  carrier (suspected) of Z22.0
  cholecystitis (current) A01.09
  endocarditis A01.02
  heart involvement A01.02
  inoculation reaction — *see* Complications, vaccination
  meningitis A01.01
  mesenteric lymph nodes A01.09
  myocarditis A01.02
  osteomyelitis A01.05
  perichondritis, larynx A01.09
  pneumonia A01.03
  spine A01.05
  specified NEC A01.09
  ulcer (perforating) A01.09
  vaccination, prophylactic (against) Z23
Typhomalaria (fever) — *see* Malaria
Typhomania A01.00
Typhoperitonitis A01.09
Typhus (fever) A75.9
  abdominal, abdominalis — *see* Typhoid
  African tick A77.1
  amarillic A95.9
  brain A75.9 *[G94]*
  cerebral A75.9 *[G94]*
  classical A75.0
  due to Rickettsia
    prowazekii A75.0
      recrudescent A75.1
    tsutsugamushi A75.3
    typhi A75.2
  endemic (flea-borne) A75.2
  epidemic (louse-borne) A75.0
  exanthematic NEC A75.0
  exanthematicus SAI A75.0
    brillii SAI A75.1
    mexicanus SAI A75.2

Typhus — *continued*
  exanthematicus SAI — *continued*
    typhus murinus A75.2
  flea-borne A75.2
  India tick A77.1
  Kenya (tick) A77.1
  louse-borne A75.0
  Mexican A75.2
  mite-borne A75.3
  murine A75.2
  North Asian tick-borne A77.2
  petechial A75.9
  Queensland tick A77.3
  rat A75.2
  recrudescent A75.1
  recurrens — *see* Fever, relapsing
  Sao Paulo A77.0
  scrub (China) (India) (Malaysia) (New Guinea) A75.3
  shop (of Malaysia) A75.2
  Siberian tick A77.2
  tick-borne A77.9
  tropical (mite-borne) A75.3
Tyrosinemia E70.21
  newborn, transitory P74.5
Tyrosinosis E70.21
Tyrosinuria E70.29

U

Uhl's anomaly or disease Q24.8
Ulcer, ulcerated, ulcerating, ulceration, ulcerative L98.499
  alveolar process M27.3
  amebic (intestine) A06.1
    skin A06.7
  anastomotic — *see* Ulcer, gastrojejunal
  anorectal K62.6
  antral — *see* Ulcer, stomach
  anus (sphincter) (solitary) K62.6
    varicose — *see* Varicose, ulcer, anus
  aphthous (oral) (recurrent) K12.0
    genital organ(s)
      female N76.6
      male N50.8
  artery I77.2
  atrophic — *see* Ulcer, skin
  back L98.429
    with
      bone necrosis L98.424
      exposed fat layer L98.422
      muscle necrosis L98.423
      skin breakdown only L98.421
    decubitus — *see* Ulcer, decubitus, by site
  Barrett's (chronic of esophagus) K22.1
  bile duct (common) (hepatic) K83.8
  bladder (solitary) (sphincter) NEC N32.8
    bilharzial B65.9 *[N33]*
    in schistosomiasis (bilharzial) B65.9 *[N33]*
    submucosal — *see* Cystitis, interstitial
    tuberculous A18.12
  bleeding K27.4
  bone — *see* Osteomyelitis, specified type NEC
  bowel — *see* Ulcer, intestine
  breast N61
  bronchus J98.0
  buccal (cavity) (traumatic) K12.1
  Buruli A31.1
  buttock L98.419
    with
      bone necrosis L98.414
      exposed fat layer L98.412
      muscle necrosis L98.413
      skin breakdown only L98.411
    decubitus — *see* Ulcer, decubitus, buttock
  cancerous (M8000/3) — *see* Neoplasm, malignant
  cardia K22.1
  cardioesophageal (peptic) K22.1
  cecum — *see* Ulcer, intestine
  cervix (uteri) (decubitus) (trophic) N86
    with cervicitis N72
  chancroidal A57
  chiclero B55.1
  chronic (cause unknown) — *see* Ulcer, skin
  Cochin-China B55.1
  colon — *see* Ulcer, intestine

Ulcer, ulcerated, ulcerating, ulceration, ulcerative — *continued*
  conjunctiva H10.8
  cornea H16.009
    with hypopyon H16.039
      bilateral H16.033
      left H16.032
      right H16.031
    bilateral H16.003
    central H16.019
      bilateral H16.013
      left H16.012
      right H16.011
    dendritic (herpes simplex) B00.52
    left H16.002
    marginal H16.049
      bilateral H16.043
      left H16.042
      right H16.041
    Mooren's H16.059
      bilateral H16.053
      left H16.052
      right H16.051
    mycotic H16.069
      bilateral H16.063
      left H16.062
      right H16.061
    perforated H16.079
      bilateral H16.073
      left H16.072
      right H16.071
    right H16.001
    ring H16.029
      bilateral H16.023
      left H16.022
      right H16.021
    tuberculous (phlyctenular) A18.52
  corpus cavernosum (chronic) N48.5
  crural — *see* Ulcer, lower limb
  Curling's — *see* Ulcer, peptic, acute
  Cushing's — *see* Ulcer, peptic, acute
  cystic duct K82.8
  cystitis (interstitial) — *see* Cystitis, interstitial
  decubitus L89.90
    with
      bone necrosis L89.94
      exposed fat layer L89.92
      muscle necrosis L89.93
      skin breakdown only L89.91
    back L89.009
      with
        bone necrosis L89.004
        contiguous site of buttock L89.20
          with
            bone necrosis L89.24
            exposed fat layer L89.22
            muscle necrosis L89.23
            skin breakdown only L89.21
        exposed fat layer L89.002
        muscle necrosis L89.003
        skin breakdown only L89.001
      lower
        left L89.049
          with
            bone necrosis L89.044
            exposed fat layer L89.042
            muscle necrosis L89.043
            skin breakdown only L89.041
        right L89.039
          with
            bone necrosis L89.034
            exposed fat layer L89.032
            muscle necrosis L89.033
            skin breakdown only L89.031
      upper
        left L89.029
          with
            bone necrosis L89.024
            exposed fat layer L89.022
            muscle necrosis L89.023
            skin breakdown only L89.021
        right L89.019
          with
            bone necrosis L89.014
            exposed fat layer L89.012
            muscle necrosis L89.013

©2002 Ingenix, Inc.

Ulcer, ulcerated, ulcerating, ulceration,
    ulcerative — continued
  decubitus — continued
    back — continued
      upper — continued
        right — continued
          with — continued
            skin breakdown only L89.011
    buttock L89.109
      with
        bone necrosis L89.104
        contiguous site of back L89.20
          with
            bone necrosis L89.24
            exposed fat layer L89.22
            muscle necrosis L89.23
            skin breakdown only L89.21
        exposed fat layer L89.102
        muscle necrosis L89.103
        skin breakdown only L89.101
    left L89.129
      with
        bone necrosis L89.124
        exposed fat layer L89.122
        muscle necrosis L89.123
        skin breakdown only L89.121
    right L89.119
      with
        bone necrosis L89.114
        exposed fat layer L89.112
        muscle necrosis L89.113
        skin breakdown only L89.111
    sacral region L89.059
      with
        bone necrosis L89.054
        exposed fat layer L89.052
        muscle necrosis L89.053
        skin breakdown only L89.051
    specified site NEC L89.80
      with
        bone necrosis L89.84
        exposed fat layer L89.82
        muscle necrosis L89.83
        skin breakdown only L89.81
  dendritic, cornea (herpes simplex) B00.52
  diabetes, diabetic — see Diabetes, ulcer
  Dieulafoy's K25.0
  due to
    infection NEC — see Ulcer, skin
    radiation NEC L59.8
    trophic disturbance (any region) — see
      Ulcer, skin
    X-ray L58.1
  duodenum, duodenal (eroded) (peptic) K26.9
    with
      hemorrhage K26.4
        and perforation K26.6
      perforation K26.5
    acute K26.3
      with
        hemorrhage K26.0
          and perforation K26.2
        perforation K26.1
    chronic K26.7
      with
        hemorrhage K26.4
          and perforation K26.6
        perforation K26.5
  dysenteric A09
  elusive — see Cystitis, interstitial
  endocarditis (acute) (chronic) (subacute) I28.8
  epiglottis J38.7
  esophagus (peptic) K22.1
    due to
      aspirin K22.1
      ingestion of chemical or medicament
        K22.1
    fungal K22.1
    infective K22.1
    varicose — see Varix, esophagus
  eyelid (region) H01.8
  fauces J39.2
  Fenwick (-Hunner) (solitary) — see Cystitis,
    interstitial
  fistulous — see Ulcer, skin
  foot (indolent) (trophic) — see Ulcer, lower limb

Ulcer, ulcerated, ulcerating, ulceration,
    ulcerative — continued
  frambesial, initial A66.0
  frenum (tongue) K14.0
  gallbladder or duct K82.8
  gangrenous — see Gangrene
  gastric — see Ulcer, stomach
  gastrocolic — see Ulcer, gastrojejunal
  gastroduodenal — see Ulcer, peptic
  gastroesophageal — see Ulcer, stomach
  gastrointestinal — see Ulcer, gastrojejunal
  gastrojejunal (peptic) K28.9
    with
      hemorrhage K28.4
        and perforation K28.6
      perforation K28.5
    acute K28.3
      with
        hemorrhage K28.0
          and perforation K28.2
        perforation K28.1
    chronic K28.7
      with
        hemorrhage K28.4
          and perforation K28.6
        perforation K28.5
  gastrojejunocolic — see Ulcer, gastrojejunal
  gingiva K06.8
  gingivitis K05.1
  glottis J38.7
  granuloma of pudenda A58
  gum K06.8
  gumma, due to yaws A66.4
  heel — see Ulcer, lower limb
  hemorrhoids — see Hemorrhoids
  Hunner's — see Cystitis, interstitial
  hypopharynx J39.2
  hypopyon (chronic) (subacute) — see Ulcer,
    cornea, with hypopyon
  hypostaticum — see Ulcer, varicose
  ileum — see Ulcer, intestine
  intestine, intestinal K63.3
    with perforation K63.1
    amebic A06.1
    duodenal — see Ulcer, duodenum
    granulocytopenic (with hemorrhage) — see
      Neutropenia
    marginal — see Ulcer, gastrojejunal
    perforating K63.1
    primary, small intestine K63.3
    rectum K62.6
    stercoraceous, stercoral K63.3
    tuberculous A18.32
    typhoid (fever) — see Typhoid
    varicose I86.8
  jejunum, jejunal — see Ulcer, gastrojejunal
  keratitis — see Ulcer, cornea
  knee — see Ulcer, lower limb
  labium (majus) (minus) N76.6
  laryngitis — see Laryngitis
  larynx (aphthous) (contact) J38.7
    diphtheritic A36.2
  leg — see Ulcer, lower limb
  lip K13.0
  Lipschütz's N76.6
  lower limb (atrophic) (chronic) (neurogenic)
      (perforating) (pyogenic) (trophic) (tropical)
      L97.909
    with
      bone necrosis L97.904
      exposed fat layer L97.902
      muscle necrosis L97.903
      skin breakdown only L97.901
    ankle L97.309
      with
        bone necrosis L97.304
        exposed fat layer L97.302
        muscle necrosis L97.303
        skin breakdown only L97.301
      left L97.329
        with
          bone necrosis L97.324
          exposed fat layer L97.322
          muscle necrosis L97.323
          skin breakdown only L97.321

Ulcer, ulcerated, ulcerating, ulceration,
    ulcerative — continued
  lower limb — continued
    ankle — continued
      right L97.319
        with
          bone necrosis L97.314
          exposed fat layer L97.312
          muscle necrosis L97.313
          skin breakdown only L97.311
    calf L97.209
      with
        bone necrosis L97.204
        exposed fat layer L97.202
        muscle necrosis L97.203
        skin breakdown only L97.201
      left L97.229
        with
          bone necrosis L97.224
          exposed fat layer L97.222
          muscle necrosis L97.223
          skin breakdown only L97.221
      right L97.219
        with
          bone necrosis L97.214
          exposed fat layer L97.212
          muscle necrosis L97.213
          skin breakdown only L97.211
    decubitus — see Ulcer, decubitus, by site
    foot specified NEC L97.509
      with
        bone necrosis L97.504
        exposed fat layer L97.502
        muscle necrosis L97.503
        skin breakdown only L97.501
      left L97.529
        with
          bone necrosis L97.524
          exposed fat layer L97.522
          muscle necrosis L97.523
          skin breakdown only L97.521
      right L97.519
        with
          bone necrosis L97.514
          exposed fat layer L97.512
          muscle necrosis L97.513
          skin breakdown only L97.511
    heel L97.409
      with
        bone necrosis L97.404
        exposed fat layer L97.402
        muscle necrosis L97.403
        skin breakdown only L97.401
      left L97.429
        with
          bone necrosis L97.424
          exposed fat layer L97.422
          muscle necrosis L97.423
          skin breakdown only L97.421
      right L97.419
        with
          bone necrosis L97.414
          exposed fat layer L97.412
          muscle necrosis L97.413
          skin breakdown only L97.411
    left L97.929
      with
        bone necrosis L97.924
        exposed fat layer L97.922
        muscle necrosis L97.923
        skin breakdown only L97.921
    lower leg NOS L97.909
      with
        bone necrosis L97.904
        exposed fat layer L97.902
        muscle necrosis L97.903
        skin breakdown only L97.901
      left L97.929
        with
          bone necrosis L97.924
          exposed fat layer L97.922
          muscle necrosis L97.923
          skin breakdown only L97.921
      right L97.919
        with
          bone necrosis L97.914

Ulcer, ulcerated, ulcerating, ulceration, ulcerative — *continued*
- lower limb — *continued*
  - lower leg NOS — *continued*
    - right — *continued*
      - with — *continued*
        - exposed fat layer L97.912
        - muscle necrosis L97.913
        - skin breakdown only L97.911
    - specified site NEC L97.809
      - with
        - bone necrosis L97.804
        - exposed fat layer L97.802
        - muscle necrosis L97.803
        - skin breakdown only L97.801
      - left L97.829
        - with
          - bone necrosis L97.824
          - exposed fat layer L97.822
          - muscle necrosis L97.823
          - skin breakdown only L97.821
      - right L97.819
        - with
          - bone necrosis L97.814
          - exposed fat layer L97.812
          - muscle necrosis L97.813
          - skin breakdown only L97.811
    - midfoot L97.409
      - with
        - bone necrosis L97.404
        - exposed fat layer L97.402
        - muscle necrosis L97.403
        - skin breakdown only L97.401
      - left L97.429
        - with
          - bone necrosis L97.424
          - exposed fat layer L97.422
          - muscle necrosis L97.423
          - skin breakdown only L97.421
      - right L97.419
        - with
          - bone necrosis L97.414
          - exposed fat layer L97.412
          - muscle necrosis L97.413
          - skin breakdown only L97.411
    - right L97.919
      - with
        - bone necrosis L97.914
        - exposed fat layer L97.912
        - muscle necrosis L97.913
        - skin breakdown only L97.911
    - thigh L97.109
      - with
        - bone necrosis L97.104
        - exposed fat layer L97.102
        - muscle necrosis L97.103
        - skin breakdown only L97.101
      - left L97.129
        - with
          - bone necrosis L97.124
          - exposed fat layer L97.122
          - muscle necrosis L97.123
          - skin breakdown only L97.121
      - right L97.119
        - with
          - bone necrosis L97.114
          - exposed fat layer L97.112
          - muscle necrosis L97.113
          - skin breakdown only L97.111
    - toe L97.509
      - with
        - bone necrosis L97.504
        - exposed fat layer L97.502
        - muscle necrosis L97.503
        - skin breakdown only L97.501
      - left L97.529
        - with
          - bone necrosis L97.524
          - exposed fat layer L97.522
          - muscle necrosis L97.523
          - skin breakdown only L97.521
      - right L97.519
        - with
          - bone necrosis L97.514
          - exposed fat layer L97.512

Ulcer, ulcerated, ulcerating, ulceration, ulcerative — *continued*
- lower limb — *continued*
  - toe — *continued*
    - right — *continued*
      - with — *continued*
        - muscle necrosis L97.513
        - skin breakdown only L97.511
  - leprous A30.1
  - syphilitic A52.19
  - varicose — *see* Varix, leg, with, ulcer
- luetic — *see* Ulcer, syphilitic
- lung J98.4
  - tuberculous — *see* Tuberculosis, pulmonary
- malignant (M8000/3) — *see* Neoplasm, malignant
- marginal NEC — *see* Ulcer, gastrojejunal
- meatus (urinarius) N34.2
- Meckel's diverticulum Q43.0
- Meleney's (chronic undermining) — *see* Ulcer, skin
- Mooren's (cornea) — *see* Ulcer, cornea, Mooren's
- mycobacterial (skin) A31.1
- nasopharynx J39.2
- navel cord (newborn) P38
- neck, uterus N86
- neurogenic NEC — *see* Ulcer, skin
- nose, nasal (passage) (infective) (septum) J34.0
  - skin — *see* Ulcer, skin
  - spirochetal A69.8
  - varicose (bleeding) I86.8
- oral mucosa (traumatic) K12.1
- palate (soft) K12.1
- penis (chronic) N48.5
- peptic (site unspecified) K27.9
  - with
    - hemorrhage K27.4
      - and perforation K27.6
    - perforation K27.5
  - acute K27.3
    - with
      - hemorrhage K27.0
        - and perforation K27.2
      - perforation K27.1
  - chronic K27.7
    - with
      - hemorrhage K27.4
        - and perforation K27.6
      - perforation K27.5
  - newborn P78.82
  - perforating K27.5
- skin — *see* Ulcer, skin
- peritonsillar J35.8
- phagedenic (tropical) — *see* Ulcer, skin
- pharynx J39.2
- phlebitis — *see* Phlebitis
- plaster — *see* Decubitus
- popliteal space — *see* Ulcer, lower limb
- postpyloric — *see* Ulcer, duodenum
- prepuce N47.7
- prepyloric — *see* Ulcer, stomach
- pressure — *see* Decubitus
- primary of intestine K63.3
  - with perforation K63.1
- prostate N41.9
- pyloric — *see* Ulcer, stomach
- rectosigmoid K63.3
  - with perforation K63.1
- rectum (sphincter) (solitary) K62.6
  - stercoraceous, stercoral K62.6
  - varicose — *see* Varicose, ulcer, anus
- retina — *see* Inflammation, chorioretinal
- rodent (M8090/3) — *see also* Neoplasm, skin, malignant
- sclera — *see* Scleritis
- scrofulous (tuberculous) A18.2
- scrotum N50.8
  - tuberculous A18.15
  - varicose I86.1
- seminal vesicle N50.8
- sigmoid — *see* Ulcer, intestine
- skin (atrophic) (chronic) (neurogenic) (non-healing) (perforating) (pyogenic) (trophic) (tropical) L98.499
  - with gangrene — *see* Gangrene
  - amebic A06.7
  - back — *see* Ulcer, back

Ulcer, ulcerated, ulcerating, ulceration, ulcerative — *continued*
- skin — *continued*
  - buttock — *see* Ulcer, buttock
  - decubitus — *see* Ulcer, decubitus
  - lower limb — *see* Ulcer, lower limb
  - mycobacterial A31.1
  - specified site NEC L98.499
    - with
      - bone necrosis L98.494
      - exposed fat layer L98.492
      - muscle necrosis L98.493
      - skin breakdown only L98.491
  - tuberculous (primary) A18.4
  - varicose — *see* Ulcer, varicose
- sloughing — *see* Ulcer, skin
- solitary, anus or rectum (sphincter) K62.6
- sore throat J02.9
  - streptococcal J02.0
- spermatic cord N50.8
- spine (tuberculous) A18.01
- stasis (venous) — *see* Varix, leg, with, ulcer
- stercoraceous, stercoral K63.3
  - with perforation K63.1
  - anus or rectum K62.6
- stoma, stomal — *see* Ulcer, gastrojejunal
- stomach (eroded) (peptic) (round) K25.9
  - with
    - hemorrhage K25.4
      - and perforation K25.6
    - perforation K25.5
  - acute K25.3
    - with
      - hemorrhage K25.0
        - and perforation K25.2
      - perforation K25.1
  - chronic K25.7
    - with
      - hemorrhage K25.4
        - and perforation K25.6
      - perforation K25.5
- stomal — *see* Ulcer, gastrojejunal
- stomatitis K12.1
- stress — *see* Ulcer, peptic
- strumous (tuberculous) A18.2
- submucosal, bladder — *see* Cystitis, interstitial
- syphilitic (any site) (early) (secondary) A51.39
  - late A52.79
  - perforating A52.79
    - foot A52.11
- testis N50.8
- thigh — *see* Ulcer, lower limb
- throat J39.2
  - diphtheritic A36.0
- toe — *see* Ulcer, lower limb
- tongue (traumatic) K14.0
- tonsil J35.8
  - diphtheritic A36.0
- trachea J39.8
- trophic — *see* Ulcer, skin
- tropical — *see* Ulcer, skin
- tuberculous — *see* Tuberculosis, ulcer
- tunica vaginalis N50.8
- turbinate J34.8
- typhoid (perforating) — *see* Typhoid
- umbilicus (newborn) P38
- unspecified site — *see* Ulcer, skin
- urethra (meatus) — *see* Urethritis
- uterus N85.8
  - cervix N86
    - with cervicitis N72
  - neck N86
    - with cervicitis N72
- vagina N76.5
  - in Behçet's disease M35.2 [N77.0]
  - pessary N89.8
- valve, heart I33.0
- varicose (lower limb, any part) — *see also* Varix, leg, with, ulcer
  - anus — *see* Varicose, ulcer, anus
  - broad ligament I86.2
  - esophagus — *see* Varix, esophagus
  - inflamed or infected — *see* Varix, leg, with, ulcer, with inflammation
  - nasal septum I86.8
  - perineum I86.3
  - rectum — *see* Varicose, ulcer, anus

Ulcer, ulcerated, ulcerating, ulceration, ulcerative — *continued*
  skin — *continued*
    scrotum I86.1
    specified site NEC I86.8
    sublingual I86.0
    vulva I86.3
  vas deferens N50.8
  vulva (acute) (infectional) N76.6
    in (due to)
      Behçet's disease M35.2 *[N77.0]*
      herpesviral (herpes simplex) infection
        A60.04
      tuberculosis A18.18
  vulvobuccal, recurring N76.6
  X-ray L58.1
  yaws A66.4
Ulcerosa scarlatina A38.8
Ulcus — *see also* Ulcer
  cutis tuberculosum A18.4
  duodeni — *see* Ulcer, duodenum
  durum (syphilitic) A51.0
    extragenital A51.2
  gastrojejunale — *see* Ulcer, gastrojejunal
  hypostaticum — *see* Ulcer, varicose
  molle (cutis) (skin) A57
  serpens corneae — *see* Ulcer, cornea, central
  ventriculi — *see* Ulcer, stomach
Ulegyria Q04.8
Ulerythema
  ophryogenes, congenital Q84.2
  sycosiforme L73.8
Ullrich (-Bonnevie) (-Turner) syndrome Q87.1
Ullrich-Feichtiger syndrome Q87.0
Ulnar — *see* condition
Ulorrhagia, ulorrhea K06.8
Umbilicus, umbilical — *see* condition
Unavailability (of)
  bed at medical facility Z75.1
  health service-related agencies Z75.4
  medical facilities (at) Z75.3
    due to
      investigation by social service agency Z75.2
      lack of services at home Z75.0
      remoteness from facility Z75.3
      waiting list Z75.1
    home Z75.0
    outpatient clinic Z75.3
  schooling Z55.1
  social service agencies Z75.4
Uncinaria americana infestation B76.9
Uncinariasis B76.9
Uncongenial work Z56.5
Unconscious(ness) — *see* Coma
Under observation — *see* Observation
Underachievement in school Z55.3
Underdevelopment — *see also* Undeveloped
  nose Q30.1
  sexual E30.0
Underfeeding, newborn P92.3
Undernourishment — *see* Malnutrition
Undernutrition — *see* Malnutrition
Underweight R63.6
  for gestational age — *see* Light for dates
Underwood's disease P83.0
Undescended — *see also* Malposition, congenital
  cecum Q43.3
  colon Q43.3
  testicle — *see* Cryptorchid
Undetermined cause R69
Undeveloped, undevelopment — *see also*
    Hypoplasia
  brain (congenital) Q02
  cerebral (congenital) Q02
  heart Q24.8
  lung Q33.6
  testis E29.1
  uterus E30.0
Undiagnosed (disease) R69
Undulant fever — *see* Brucellosis
Unemployment, anxiety concerning Z56.0
  threatened Z56.2

Unequal length (acquired) (limb) — *see also*
    Deformity, limb, unequal length
  leg — *see also* Deformity, limb, unequal length
    congenital Q72.90
      bilateral Q72.93
      left Q72.92
      right Q72.91
Unextracted dental root K08.3
Unguis incarnatus L60.0
Unhappiness R45.2
Unicornate uterus Q51.4
Unilateral — *see also* condition
  development, breast N64.8
  organ or site, congenital NEC — *see* Agenesis,
    by site
Unilocular heart Q20.8
Union, abnormal — *see also* Fusion
  larynx and trachea Q34.8
Universal mesentery Q43.3
Unknown cause, morbidity R69
Unsatisfactory
  surroundings Z59.1
    physical environment Z58.9
      specified NEC Z58.89
    work Z56.5
Unsoundness of mind — *see* Psychosis
Unspecified cause, morbidity R69
Unstable
  back NEC — *see* Instability, joint, spine
  hip (congenital) Q65.6
    acquired — *see* Derangement, joint,
      specified type NEC, hip
  joint — *see* Instability, joint
    secondary to removal of joint prosthesis
      M96.89
  lie (mother) O32.0
  lumbosacral joint (congenital)
    acquired — *see* category M53.2
    sacroiliac — *see* category M53.2
  spine NEC — *see* Instability, joint, spine
Unsteadiness on feet R26.82
Untruthfulness, child problem F91.8
Unverricht (-Lundborg) disease or epilepsy
  G40.30
  with status epilepticus G40.31
Unwanted pregnancy Z64.0
Upbringing, institutional Z62.2
Upper respiratory — *see* condition
Upset
  gastric K30
  gastrointestinal K30
    psychogenic F45.8
  intestinal (large) (small) K59.9
    psychogenic F45.8
  menstruation N93.9
  mental F48.9
  stomach K30
    psychogenic F45.8
Urachus — *see also* condition
  patent or persistent Q64.4
Urbach-Oppenheim disease E88.8
Urbach's lipoid proteinosis E78.89
Urbach-Wiethe disease E78.89
Urban yellow fever A95.1
Urea
  blood, high — *see* Uremia
  cycle metabolism disorder — *see* Disorder, urea
    cycle metabolism
Uremia, uremic (coma) N19
  with
    ectopic or molar pregnancy O08.4
    polyneuropathy N19 *[G63]*
  chronic — *see* Failure, renal, chronic
  complicating
    ectopic or molar pregnancy O08.4
    hypertension I12.0
  congenital P96.0
  extrarenal R39.2
  following ectopic or molar pregnancy O08.4
  hypertensive I12.0
  newborn P96.0
  prerenal R39.2

Ureter, ureteral — *see* condition
Ureteralgia N23
Ureterectasis — *see* Hydroureter
Ureteritis N28.89
  cystica N28.86
  due to calculus N20.1
    with calculus, kidney N20.2
      with hydronephrosis N13.2
  gonococcal (acute) (chronic) A54.21
  nonspecific N28.89
Ureterocele N28.89
  congenital (orthotopic) Q62.31
    ectopic Q62.32
Ureterolith, ureterolithiasis — *see* Calculus,
  ureter
Ureterostomy
  attention to Z43.6
  status Z93.6
Urethra, urethral — *see* condition
Urethralgia R39.8
Urethritis (anterior) (posterior) N34.2
  calculous N21.1
  candidal B37.41
  chlamydial A56.01
  complicating pregnancy O23.20
    first trimester O23.21
    second trimester O23.22
    third trimester O23.23
  diplococcal (gonococcal) A54.01
    with abscess (accessory gland) (periurethral)
      A54.1
  gonococcal A54.01
    with abscess (accessory gland) (periurethral)
      A54.1
  nongonococcal N34.1
    Reiter's — *see* Reiter's disease
  nonspecific N34.1
  nonvenereal N34.1
  postmenopausal N34.2
  puerperal O86.29
  Reiter's — *see* Reiter's disease
  specified NEC N34.2
  trichomonal or due to Trichomonas (vaginalis)
    A59.03
  venereal NEC (nongonococcal) A64.0
Urethrocele N81.0
  with
    cystocele N81.1
    prolapse of uterus — *see* Prolapse, uterus
Urethrolithiasis (with colic or infection) N21.1
Urethrorectal — *see* condition
Urethrorrhagia N36.8
Urethrorrhea R36.9
Urethrostomy
  attention to Z43.6
  status Z93.6
Urethrotrigonitis — *see* Trigonitis
Urethrovaginal — *see* condition
Urhidrosis, uridrosis L74.8
Uric acid in blood (increased) E79.0
Uricacidemia (asymptomatic) E79.0
Uricemia (asymptomatic) E79.0
Uricosuria R82.99
Urinary — *see* condition
Urination
  frequent R35.0
  painful R30.9
Urine
  blood in — *see* Hematuria
  discharge, excessive R35.8
  enuresis, nonorganic origin F98.0
  extravasation R39.0
  frequency R35.0
  incontinence R32
    nonorganic origin F98.0
  intermittent stream R39.19
  pus in N39.0
  retention or stasis R33.9
    organic R33.8
      drug-induced R33.0
    psychogenic F45.8

Urine — continued
  secretion
    deficient R34
    excessive R35.8
    frequency R35.0
  stream
    intermittent R39.19
    slowing R39.19
    splitting R39.13
    weak R39.12
Urinemia — see Uremia
Urinoma, urethra N36.8
Uroarthritis, infectious (Reiter's) — see Reiter's disease
Urodialysis R34
Urolithiasis — see Calculus, urinary
Uronephrosis — see Hydronephrosis
Uropathy N39.9
  obstructive N13.9
    specified NEC N13.8
  reflux N13.9
    specified NEC N13.8
  vesicoureteral reflux-associated — see Reflux, vesicoureteral
Urosepsis N39.0
Urticaria L50.9
  with angioneurotic edema T78.3
    hereditary D84.1
  allergic L50.0
  cholinergic L50.5
  chronic L50.8
  cold, familial L50.2
  contact L50.6
  dermatographic L50.3
  due to
    cold or heat L50.2
    drugs L50.0
    food L50.0
    inhalants L50.0
    plants L50.6
    serum T80.6
  factitial L50.3
  giant T78.3
    hereditary D84.1
  gigantea T78.3
  idiopathic L50.1
  larynx T78.3
    hereditary D84.1
  neonatorum P83.8
  nonallergic L50.1
  papulosa (Hebra) L28.2
  pigmentosa Q82.2
  recurrent periodic L50.8
  serum T80.6
  solar L56.3
  specified type NEC L50.8
  thermal (cold) (heat) L50.2
  vibratory L50.4
  xanthelasmoidea Q82.2
Use (of)
  anticoagulant for a long term (current) Z79.1
    with hemorrhage D68.5
  aspirin for a long term (current) Z79.8
  harmful
    alcohol — see Abuse, alcohol
    drugs — see Abuse, drug, by type
    inhalants — see Abuse, drug, inhalant
    nonprescribed drugs, non-dependence producing — see Abuse, non-psychoactive substance
    patent medicines — see Abuse, non-psychoactive substance
      maternal, affecting fetus or newborn P04.2
    volatile solvents — see Abuse, drug, inhalant
  medicaments for a long term (current) NEC Z79.8
    antibiotics Z79.2
    anticoagulants Z79.1
      with hemorrhage D68.5
    hormones, postmenopausal Z79.3
    insulin Z79.4
    multiple prescribed Z79.7
    specified NEC Z79.8
  tobacco Z72.0

Usher-Senear disease or syndrome L10.4
Uta B55.1
Uteromegaly N85.2
Uterovaginal — see condition
Uterovesical — see condition
Uveal — see condition
Uveitis (anterior) — see also Iridocyclitis
  acute — see Iridocyclitis, acute
  chronic — see Iridocyclitis, chronic
  due to toxoplasmosis B58.09
    congenital P37.1 [H22]
  granulomatous — see Iridocyclitis, chronic
  heterochromic — see Cyclitis, Fuchs' heterochromic
  lens-induced — see Iridocyclitis, lens-induced
  posterior — see Chorioretinitis
  sympathetic H44.139
    bilateral H44.133
    left H44.132
    right H44.131
  syphilitic (secondary) A51.43
    congenital (early) A50.01 [H22]
    late A52.71
  tuberculous A18.54
Uveoencephalitis — see Inflammation, chorioretinal
Uveokeratitis — see Iridocyclitis
Uveoparotitis D86.89
Uvula — see condition
Uvulitis (acute) (catarrhal) (chronic) (membranous) (suppurative) (ulcerative) K12.2

Vaccination (prophylactic) Z23
  complication or reaction — see Complications, vaccination
Vaccinia (generalized) (localized) T88.1
  congenital P35.8
  without vaccination B08.0
Vacuum, in sinus (accessory) (nasal) J34.8
Vagabond, vagabondage Z59.0
Vagabond's disease B85.1
Vagina, vaginal — see condition
Vaginalitis (tunica) (testis) N49.1
Vaginismus (reflex) N94.2
  functional F52.5
  nonorganic F52.5
  psychogenic F52.5
  secondary N94.2
Vaginitis (acute) (circumscribed) (diffuse) (emphysematous) (nonvenereal) (ulcerative) N76.0
  with ectopic or molar pregnancy O08.0
  amebic A06.82
  atrophic, postmenopausal N95.2
  blennorrhagic (gonococcal) A54.02
  candidal B37.3
  chlamydial A56.02
  chronic N76.1
  complicating pregnancy — see Infection, genital organ or tract, complicating pregnancy
  due to Trichomonas (vaginalis) A59.01
  following ectopic or molar pregnancy O08.0
  gonococcal A54.02
    with abscess (accessory gland) (periurethral) A54.1
  granuloma A58
  in (due to)
    candidiasis B37.3
    herpesviral (herpes simplex) infection A60.04
    pinworm infection B80 [N77.1]
  monilial B37.3
  mycotic (candidal) B37.3
  postmenopausal atrophic N95.2
  puerperal (postpartum) O86.1
  senile (atrophic) N95.2
  subacute or chronic N76.1
  syphilitic (early) A51.0
    late A52.76
  trichomonal A59.01
  tuberculous A18.18
  venereal NOS A64.3
Vagotonia G52.2
Vagrancy Z59.0
VAIN — see Neoplasia, intraepithelial, vagina
Vallecula — see condition
Valley fever B38.0
Valsuani's disease — see Anemia, obstetric
Valve, valvular (formation) — see also condition
  cerebral ventricle (communicating) in situ Z98.2
  cervix, internal os Q51.8
  congenital NEC — see Atresia, by site
  ureter (pelvic junction) (vesical orifice) Q62.39
  urethra (congenital) (posterior) Q64.2
Valvulitis (chronic) — see Endocarditis
Valvulopathy — see Endocarditis
Van Bogaert's leukoencephalopathy (sclerosing) (subacute) A81.1
Van Bogaert-Scherer-Epstein disease or syndrome E75.5
Van Buchem's syndrome M85.2
Van Creveld-von Gierke disease E74.01
Van der Hoeve (-de Kleyn) syndrome Q78.0
Van der Woude's syndrome Q38.0
Van Neck's disease or osteochondrosis M91.0
Vanillism L23.6
Vanishing lung J44.9
Vapor asphyxia or suffocation T65.91
  specified agent — see Table of Drugs and Chemicals
Variance, lethal ball, prosthetic heart valve T82.09

Variants, thalassemic D56.8
Variations in hair color L67.1
Varicella B01.9
  with
    complications NEC B01.89
    encephalitis B01.1
    meningitis B01.0
    pneumonia B01.2
  congenital P35.8
Varices — *see* Varix
Varicocele (scrotum) (thrombosed) I86.1
  ovary I86.2
  perineum I86.3
  spermatic cord (ulcerated) I86.1
Varicose
  aneurysm (ruptured) I77.0
  dermatitis — *see* Varix, leg, with, inflammation
  eczema — *see* Varix, leg, with, inflammation
  phlebitis — *see* Varix, with, inflammation
  placental vessel — *see* Disorder, placenta,
    specified type NEC
  tumor — *see* Varix
  ulcer (lower limb, any part) — *see also* Varix,
    leg, with, ulcer
    anus — *see* Hemorrhoids, with complication
    esophagus — *see* Varix, esophagus
    inflamed or infected — *see* Varix, leg, with,
      ulcer, with inflammation
    nasal septum I86.8
    perineum I86.3
    rectum — *see* Varicose, ulcer, anus
    scrotum I86.1
    specified site NEC I86.8
  vein — *see* Varix
  vessel — *see* Varix, leg
    placenta — *see* Disorder, placenta, specified
      type NEC
Varicosis, varicosities, varicosity — *see* Varix
Variola (major) (minor) B03
Varioloid B03
Varix (lower limb) (ruptured) I83.90
  with
    inflammation or infection I83.10
      with ulcer I83.209
    stasis dermatitis I83.10
      with ulcer I83.209
    ulcer I83.009
      with inflammation or infection I83.209
  aneurysmal I77.0
  anus — *see* Hemorrhoids
  bladder I86.2
  broad ligament I86.2
  complicating
    childbirth (lower extremity) O87.4
      anus or rectum O87.2
      genital (vagina, vulva or perineum) O87.8
    pregnancy (lower extremity) O22.00
      anus or rectum O22.40
        first trimester O22.41
        second trimester O22.42
        third trimester O22.43
      first trimester O22.01
      genital (vagina, vulva or perineum) O22.10
        first trimester O22.11
        second trimester O22.12
        third trimester O22.13
      second trimester O22.02
      third trimester O22.03
    puerperium (lower extremity) O87.4
      anus or rectum O87.2
      genital (vagina, vulva, perineum) O87.8
  congenital (any site) Q27.8
  esophagus (idiopathic) (primary) (ulcerated)
    I85.00
    bleeding I85.01
    congenital Q27.8
    in (due to)
      alcoholic liver disease I85.10
        bleeding I85.11
      cirrhosis of liver I85.10
        bleeding I85.11
      portal hypertension I85.10
        bleeding I85.11
      schistosomiasis I85.10
        bleeding I85.11

Varix — *continued*
  esophagus — *continued*
    in — *continued*
      toxic liver disease I85.10
        bleeding I85.11
    secondary I85.10
      bleeding I85.11
  gastric I86.4
  inflamed or infected I83.10
    ulcerated I83.209
  labia (majora) I86.3
  leg I83.90
    with
      inflammation I83.10
        with ulcer — *see* Varix, leg, with,
          ulcer, with inflammation by site
      ulcer I83.009
        with inflammation I83.209
        ankle I83.003
          with inflammation I83.203
        calf I83.002
          with inflammation I83.202
        foot NEC I83.005
          with inflammation I83.205
        heel I83.004
          with inflammation I83.204
        lower leg NEC I83.008
          with inflammation I83.208
        midfoot I83.004
          with inflammation I83.204
        thigh I83.001
          with inflammation I83.201
    bilateral I83.93
      with
        ulcer I83.009
          with inflammation I83.209
    left I83.92
      with
        inflammation I83.12
          with ulcer — *see* Varix, leg, with,
            ulcer, with inflammation by
            site
        ulcer I83.029
          with inflammation I83.229
          ankle I83.023
            with inflammation I83.223
          calf I83.022
            with inflammation I83.222
          foot NEC I83.025
            with inflammation I83.225
          heel I83.024
            with inflammation I83.224
          lower leg NEC I83.028
            with inflammation I83.228
          midfoot I83.024
            with inflammation I83.224
          thigh I83.021
            with inflammation I83.221
    right I83.91
      with
        inflammation I83.11
          with ulcer — *see* Varix, leg, with,
            ulcer, with inflammation by
            site
        ulcer I83.019
          with inflammation I83.219
          ankle I83.013
            with inflammation I83.213
          calf I83.012
            with inflammation I83.212
          foot NEC I83.015
            with inflammation I83.215
          heel I83.014
            with inflammation I83.214
          lower leg NEC I83.018
            with inflammation I83.218
          midfoot I83.014
            with inflammation I83.214
          thigh I83.011
            with inflammation I83.211
  nasal septum I86.8
  orbit I86.8
    congenital Q27.8
  ovary I86.2
  papillary I78.1
  pelvis I86.2

Varix — *continued*
  perineum I86.3
    complicating
      pregnancy O22.10
        first trimester O22.11
        second trimester O22.12
        third trimester O22.13
      puerperium O87.8
  pharynx I86.8
  placenta — *see* Disorder, placenta, specified
    type NEC
  rectum — *see* Hemorrhoids, internal
  renal papilla I86.8
  retina H35.09
  scrotum (ulcerated) I86.1
  sigmoid colon I86.8
  specified site NEC I86.8
  spinal (cord) (vessels) I86.8
  spleen, splenic (vein) (with phlebolith) I86.8
  stomach I86.4
  sublingual I86.0
  ulcerated I83.009
    inflamed or infected I83.209
  uterine ligament I86.2
  vagina I86.8
    complicating
      pregnancy O22.10
        first trimester O22.11
        second trimester O22.12
        third trimester O22.13
      puerperium O87.8
  vocal cord I86.8
  vulva I86.3
    complicating
      pregnancy O22.10
        first trimester O22.11
        second trimester O22.12
        third trimester O22.13
      puerperium O87.8
Vas deferens — *see* condition
Vas deferentitis N49.1
Vasa previa O69.4
  hemorrhage from, affecting fetus or newborn
    P50.0
Vascular — *see also* condition
  loop on optic papilla Q14.2
  spasm I73.9
  spider I78.1
Vascularization, cornea — *see*
  Neovascularization, cornea
Vasculitis I77.6
  allergic D69.0
  cryoglobulinemic D89.1
  disseminated I77.6
  hypocomplementemic M31.8
  kidney I77.8
  livedoid L95.0
  nodular L95.8
  retina H35.069
    bilateral H35.063
    left H35.062
    right H35.061
  rheumatic — *see* Fever, rheumatic
  rheumatoid — *see* Rheumatoid, vasculitis
  skin (limited to) L95.9
    specified NEC L95.8
Vasculopathy, necrotizing M31.9
  specified NEC M31.8
Vasitis (nodosa) N49.1
  tuberculous A18.15
Vasodilation I73.9
Vasomotor — *see* condition
Vasoplasty, after previous sterilization Z31.0
  aftercare Z31.42
Vasospasm I73.9
  cerebral (artery) G45.9
  nerve
    arm — *see* Mononeuropathy, upper limb
    brachial plexus G54.0
    cervical plexus G54.2
    leg — *see* Mononeuropathy, lower limb
  peripheral NOS I73.9
  retina (artery) — *see* Occlusion, artery, retina

Vasospastic — *see* condition
Vasovagal attack (paroxysmal) R55
  psychogenic F45.8
VATER syndrome Q87.2
Vater's ampulla — *see* condition
Vegetation, vegetative
  adenoid (nasal fossa) J35.8
  endocarditis (acute) (any valve) (subacute) I33.0
  heart (mycotic) (valve) I33.0
Veil
  Jackson's Q43.3
  over face (causing asphyxia) P28.9
Vein, venous — *see* condition
Veldt sore — *see* Ulcer, skin
Velpeau's hernia — *see* Hernia, femoral
Venereal
  bubo A55
  disease A64.9
  granuloma inguinale A58
  lymphogranuloma (Durand-Nicolas-Favre) A55
Venofibrosis I87.8
Venom, venomous — *see also* Toxicity, venom
  bite or sting (animal or insect) (with allergic or anaphylactic shock) T63.91
    administered with intent to harm by another person T63.93
      self T63.92
    amphibian — *see* Toxicity, venom, amphibian
    arthropod NEC — *see* Toxicity, venom, arthropod
    circumstances undetermined T63.94
    fish — *see* Toxicity, venom, fish
    frog — *see* Toxicity, venom, frog
    insect — *see* Toxicity, venom, arthropod
    jellyfish — *see* Toxicity, venom, marine animal
    lizard — *see* Toxicity, venom, reptile
    marine animal NEC — *see* Toxicity, venom, marine animal
    reptile NEC — *see* Toxicity, venom, reptile
    sea anemone — *see* Toxicity, venom, marine animal, sea anemone
    shellfish — *see* Toxicity, venom, marine animal, shellfish
    snake T63.001
      administered with intent to harm by another person T63.003
        self T63.002
      American snake NEC T63.061
        administered with intent to harm by another person T63.063
          self T63.062
        circumstances undetermined T63.064
      Asian snake NEC T63.081
        administered with intent to harm by another person T63.083
          self T63.082
        circumstances undetermined T63.084
      Australian snake NEC T63.071
        administered with intent to harm by another person T63.073
          self T63.072
        circumstances undetermined T63.074
      circumstances undetermined T63.004
      cobra T63.041
        administered with intent to harm by another person T63.043
          self T63.042
        circumstances undetermined T63.044
      coral snake T63.021
        administered with intent to harm by another person T63.023
          self T63.022
        circumstances undetermined T63.024
      rattlesnake T63.011
        administered with intent to harm by another person T63.013
          self T63.012
        circumstances undetermined T63.014
      sea snake T63.031
        administered with intent to harm by another person T63.033
          self T63.032
        circumstances undetermined T63.034

Venom, venomous — *see also* Toxicity, venom — *continued*
  bite — *continued*
    snake — *continued*
      specified snake NEC T63.091
        administered with intent to harm by another person T63.093
          self T63.092
        circumstances undetermined T63.094
    spider — *see* Toxicity, venom, spider
  poisoning — *see* Venom, bite or sting
Venous — *see* condition
Ventilator lung, newborn P27.8
Ventral — *see* condition
Ventricle, ventricular — *see also* condition
  escape I49.3
  inversion Q20.5
Ventriculitis (cerebral) G04.9
Ventriculostomy status Z98.2
Vernet's syndrome G52.7
Verneuil's disease (syphilitic bursitis) A52.78
Verruca (filiformis) (plana) (plana juvenilis) (plantaris) (simplex) (viral) (vulgaris) B07
  acuminata A63.0
  necrogenica (primary) (tuberculosa) A18.4
  seborrheica L82.1
    inflamed L82.0
  senile (seborrheic) L82.1
    inflamed L82.0
  tuberculosa (primary) A18.4
  venereal A63.0
Verrucosities — *see* Verruca
Verruga peruana, peruviana A44.1
Version
  with extraction
  cervix — *see* Malposition, uterus
  uterus (postinfectional) (postpartal, old) — *see* Malposition, uterus
Vertebra, vertebral — *see* condition
Vertical talus Q66.8
Vertigo R42
  auditory — *see* Vertigo, aural
  aural H81.319
    bilateral H81.313
    left H81.312
    right H81.311
  benign paroxysmal (positional) H81.13
    bilateral H81.12
    left H81.11
    right H81.10
  central (origin) — *see* category H81.4
  cerebral — *see* category H81.4
  Dix and Hallpike (epidemic) — *see* Neuronitis, vestibular
  due to infrasound T75.23
  epidemic A88.1
    Dix and Hallpike — *see* Neuronitis, vestibular
    Pedersen's — *see* Neuronitis, vestibular
    vestibular neuronitis — *see* Neuronitis, vestibular
  epileptic G40.80
    with status epilepticus G40.81
  hysterical F44.89
  infrasound T75.23
  labyrinthine — *see* category H81.0
  laryngeal R05
  malignant positional — *see* category H81.4
  Ménière's — *see* category H81.0
  menopausal N95.1
  otogenic — *see* Vertigo, aural
  paroxysmal positional, benign — *see* Vertigo, benign paroxysmal
  Pedersen's (epidemic) — *see* Neuronitis, vestibular
  peripheral NEC H81.399
    bilateral H81.393
    left H81.392
    right H81.391
  positional
    benign paroxysmal — *see* Vertigo, benign paroxysmal
    malignant — *see* category H81.4

Very-low-density-lipoprotein-type (VLDL) **hyperlipoproteinemia** E78.1
Vesania — *see* Psychosis
Vesical — *see* condition
Vesicle
  cutaneous R23.8
  seminal — *see* condition
  skin R23.8
Vesicocolic — *see* condition
Vesicoperineal — *see* condition
Vesicorectal — *see* condition
Vesicourethrorectal — *see* condition
Vesicovaginal — *see* condition
Vesicular — *see* condition
Vesiculitis (seminal) N49.0
  amebic A06.82
  gonorrheal (acute) (chronic) A54.23
  trichomonal A59.09
  tuberculous A18.15
Vestibulitis (ear) — *see also* category H83.0
  nose (external) J34.8
Vestibulopathy, acute peripheral (recurrent) — *see* Neuronitis, vestibular
Vestige, vestigial — *see also* Persistence
  branchial Q18.0
  structures in vitreous Q14.0
Vibration
  adverse effects T75.20
    pneumatic hammer syndrome T75.21
    specified effect NEC T75.29
    vasospastic syndrome T75.22
    vertigo from infrasound T75.23
  exposure (occupational) Z57.7
  vertigo T75.23
Vibriosis A28.9
Victim (of)
  crime Z65.4
  disaster Z65.5
  terrorism Z65.4
  torture Z65.4
  war Z65.5
Vidal's disease L28.0
Villaret's syndrome G52.7
Villous — *see* condition
VIN — *see* Neoplasia, intraepithelial, vulva
Vincent's infection (angina) (gingivitis) A69.1
  stomatitis A69.0
Vinson-Plummer syndrome D50.1
Violence, physical R45.6
Viosterol deficiency — *see* Deficiency, calciferol
Vipoma (M8155/3) — *see* Neoplasm, malignant
Viremia B34.9
Virilism (adrenal) E25.0
Virilization (female) (suprarenal) E25.0
  isosexual E28.2
Virulent bubo A57
Virus, viral — *see also* condition
  as cause of disease classified elsewhere B97.8
  cytomegalovirus B25.9
  human immunodeficiency (HIV) — *see* Human, immunodeficiency virus (HIV) disease
  infection — *see* Infection, virus
  specified NEC B34.8
Viscera, visceral — *see* condition
Visceroptosis K63.4
Visible peristalsis R19.2
Vision, visual
  binocular, suppression H53.34
  blurred, blurring H53.8
    hysterical F44.6
  defect, defective NEC H54.7
  disorientation (syndrome) H53.8
  disturbance H53.9
    hysterical F44.6
  double H53.2
  examination Z01.00
    with abnormal findings Z01.01
  field, limitation (defect) — *see* Defect, visual field
  hallucinations R44.1
  halos H53.19

Vision, visual — *continued*
loss — *see* Loss, vision
  sudden — *see* Disturbance, vision,
    subjective, loss, sudden
low (both eyes) — *see* Low, vision
perception, simultaneous without fusion
  H53.33
Vitality, lack or want of R53.82
newborn P96.8
Vitamin deficiency — *see* Deficiency, vitamin
Vitelline duct, persistent Q43.0
Vitiligo L80
eyelid H02.739
  left H02.736
    lower H02.735
    upper H02.734
  right H02.733
    lower H02.732
    upper H02.731
pinta A67.2
vulva N90.8
Vitreoretinopathy, proliferative — *see also*
  Retinopathy, proliferative
with retinal detachment — *see* Detachment,
  retina, traction
Vitreous — *see also* condition
touch syndrome — *see* Complication, eye,
  postoperative, cataract surgery, vitreous
  touch
Vocal cord — *see* condition
Vocational rehabilitation Z51.89
Vogt-Koyanagi syndrome H20.829
bilateral H20.823
left H20.822
right H20.821
Vogt's disease or syndrome G80.3
Vogt-Spielmeyer amaurotic idiocy or disease
  E75.4
Voice
change R49.9
  specified NEC R49.8
loss — *see* Aphonia
Volhynian fever A79.0
Volkmann's ischemic contracture or paralysis
  (complicating trauma) T79.6
Volvulus (bowel) (colon) (duodenum) (intestine)
  K56.2
with perforation K56.2
congenital Q43.8
fallopian tube — *see* Torsion, fallopian tube
oviduct — *see* Torsion, fallopian tube
stomach (due to absence of gastrocolic
  ligament) K31.89
Vomiting (fecal matter) (stercoral) R11.3
with nausea R11.0
asphyxia — *see* Foreign body, by site, causing
  asphyxia, gastric contents
bilious (cause unknown) R11.3
  with nausea R11.0
  following gastro-intestinal surgery K91.0
blood — *see* Hematemesis
causing asphyxia, choking, or suffocation —
  see Asphyxia, food
cyclical R11.3
  with nausea R11.0
  psychogenic F50.8
epidemic A08.1
following gastrointestinal surgery K91.0
  psychogenic F50.8
functional K31.89
hysterical F50.8
nervous F50.8
neurotic F50.8
newborn P92.0
of or complicating pregnancy O21.9
  due to
    diseases classified elsewhere O21.8
    specific cause NEC O21.8
  early (before the end of the 22nd week of
    gestation) (mild) O21.0
    with metabolic disturbance O21.1
  late (after 22 completed weeks gestation)
    O21.2

Vomiting — *continued*
periodic R11.3
  with nausea R11.0
  psychogenic F50.8
projectile R11.2
psychogenic F50.8
uremic — *see* Uremia
winter (epidemic) A08.1
Vomito negro — *see* Fever, yellow
Von Bezold's abscess — *see* Mastoiditis, acute
Von Economo-Cruchet disease A85.8
Von Eulenburg's disease G71.1
Von Gierke's disease E74.01
Von Hippel (-Lindau) disease or syndrome
  Q85.8
Von Jaksch's anemia or disease D64.8
Von Recklinghausen's
disease (neurofibromatosis) Q85.0
bones E21.0
Von Schroetter's syndrome I82.8
Von Willebrand (-Jurgens) (-Minot) disease or
  syndrome D68.0
Von Zumbusch's disease L40.1
Voyeurism F65.3
Vrolik's disease Q78.0
Vulva — *see* condition
Vulvismus N94.2
Vulvitis (acute) (allergic) (aphthous) (atrophic)
  (hypertrophic) (intertriginous) (senile) N76.2
with ectopic or molar pregnancy O08.0
adhesive, congenital Q52.79
blennorrhagic (gonococcal) A54.02
candidal B37.3
Vulvitis (acute) (allergic) (aphthous) (atrophic)
  (hypertrophic) (intertriginous) (senile) N76.2
chlamydial A56.02
complicating pregnancy — *see* Infection, genital
  organ or tract, complicating pregnancy
due to Haemophilus ducreyi A57
following ectopic or molar pregnancy O08.0
gonococcal A54.02
  with abscess (accessory gland) (periurethral)
    A54.1
herpesviral A60.04
leukoplakic N90.4
monilial B37.3
puerperal (postpartum) O86.1
subacute or chronic N76.3
syphilitic (early) A51.0
  late A52.76
trichomonal A59.01
tuberculous A18.18
Vulvodynia R10.2
Vulvorectal — *see* condition
Vulvovaginitis (acute) — *see* Vaginitis

W

Waiting list, person on Z75.1
for transplant Z75.81
undergoing social agency investigation Z75.2
Waldenström-Kjellberg syndrome D50.1
Waldenström's
hypergammaglobulinemia D89.0
syndrome or macroglobulinemia (M9761/3)
  C88.0
Walking
difficulty R26.2
  psychogenic F44.4
sleep F51.3
  hysterical F44.89
Wall, abdominal — *see* condition
Wallenberg's disease or syndrome G46.3
Wallgren's disease I87.8
Wandering
gallbladder, congenital Q44.1
kidney, congenital Q63.8
organ or site, congenital NEC — *see*
  Malposition, congenital, by site
pacemaker (heart) I49.8
spleen D73.8
War neurosis F48.8

Wart (common) (digitate) (filiform) (infectious)
  (juvenile) (plantar) (viral) B07
anogenital region (venereal) A63.0
external genital organs (venereal) A63.0
Hassal-Henle's (of cornea) H18.49
Peruvian A44.1
prosector (tuberculous) A18.4
seborrheic L82.1
  inflamed L82.0
senile (seborrheic) L82.1
  inflamed L82.0
tuberculous A18.4
venereal A63.0
Warthin's tumor (M8561/0) — *see* Neoplasm,
  salivary gland, benign
Wassilieff's disease A27.0
Wasting
disease R64
  due to malnutrition E41
extreme (due to malnutrition) E41
muscle NEC — *see* Atrophy, muscle
Water
clefts (senile cataract) — *see* Cataract, senile,
  incipient
deprivation of T73.1
intoxication E87.7
itch B76.9
lack of T73.1
loading E87.7
on
  brain — *see* Hydrocephalus
  chest J94.8
poisoning E87.7
pollution (exposure to) Z58.2
Waterbrash R12
Waterhouse (-Friderichsen) syndrome or
  disease (meningococcal) A39.1
Water-losing nephritis N25.8
Watsoniasis B66.8
Wax in ear — *see* Impaction, cerumen
Weak, weakness (generalized) R53.1
arches (acquired) — *see also* Deformity, limb,
  flat foot
  congenital Q66.5
bladder (sphincter) R32
foot (double) — *see* Weak, arches
heart, cardiac — *see* Failure, heart
mind F70
muscle M62.81
myocardium — *see* Failure, heart
newborn P96.8
pelvic fundus N81.8
senile R54
valvular — *see* Endocarditis
Weaning from ventilator or respirator
  (mechanical) Z51.89
Wear, worn, tooth, teeth (approximal) (hard
  tissues) (interproximal) (occlusal) K03.0
Weather, weathered
effects of
  cold T69.9
    specified effect NEC T69.8
  hot — *see* Heat
skin L57.8
Weaver's syndrome Q87.3
Web, webbed (congenital)
esophagus Q39.4
fingers — *see* Syndactylism, simple
larynx (glottic) (subglottic) Q31.0
neck (pterygium colli) Q18.3
Paterson-Kelly D50.1
popliteal syndrome Q87.89
toes Q70.3
Weber-Christian disease M35.6
Weber-Cockayne syndrome (epidermolysis
  bullosa) Q81.8
Weber-Gubler syndrome G46.3
Weber-Leyden syndrome G46.3
Weber-Osler syndrome I78.0
Weber's paralysis or syndrome G46.3
Wedge-shaped or wedging vertebra — *see*
  Collapse, vertebra NEC

Wound, open — *continued*
 auditory canal (external) (meatus) — *see*
  Wound, open, ear
 auricle, ear — *see* Wound, open, ear
 axilla — *see* Wound, open, arm
 back — *see also* Wound, open, thorax, back
  lower S31.000
   with penetration into retroperitoneal
    space S31.001
   bite — *see* Bite, back, lower
   laceration — *see* Laceration, back, lower
   puncture — *see* Puncture, back, lower
 bite — *see* Bite
 blood vessel — *see* Injury, blood vessel
 breast S21.009
  with amputation — *see* Amputation,
   traumatic, breast
  bite — *see* Bite, breast
  laceration — *see* Laceration, breast
  left S21.002
  puncture — *see* Puncture, breast
  right S21.001
 buttock S31.809
  bite — *see* Bite, buttock
  laceration — *see* Laceration, buttock
  left S31.829
  puncture — *see* Puncture, buttock
  right S31.819
 calf — *see* Wound, open, leg
 canaliculus lacrimalis — *see* Wound, open,
  eyelid
 canthus, eye — *see* Wound, open, eyelid
 cervical esophagus S11.20
  bite S11.25
  laceration — *see* Laceration, esophagus,
   traumatic, cervical
  puncture — *see* Puncture, cervical
   esophagus
 cheek (external) S01.409
  bite — *see* Bite, cheek
  laceration — *see* Laceration, cheek
  left S01.402
  puncture — *see* Puncture, cheek
  right S01.401
  internal — *see* Wound, open, oral cavity
 chest wall — *see* Wound, open, thorax
 chin — *see* Wound, open, head, specified site
  NEC
 choroid — *see* Wound, open, ocular
 ciliary body (eye) — *see* Wound, open, ocular
 clitoris S31.40
  with amputation — *see* Amputation,
   traumatic, clitoris
  bite S31.45
  laceration — *see* Laceration, vulva
  puncture — *see* Puncture, vulva
 conjunctiva — *see* Wound, open, ocular
 cornea — *see* Wound, open, ocular
 costal region — *see* Wound, open, thorax
 Descemet's membrane — *see* Wound, open,
  ocular
 digit(s)
  foot — *see* Wound, open, toe
  hand — *see* Wound, open, finger
 ear (canal) (external) S01.309
  with amputation — *see* Amputation,
   traumatic, ear
  bite — *see* Bite, ear
  laceration — *see* Laceration, ear
  left S01.302
  puncture — *see* Puncture, ear
  right S01.301
  drum S09.20
   left S09.22
   right S09.21
 elbow S51.009
  with fracture of elbow S51.069
   left S51.062
   right S51.061
  bite — *see* Bite, elbow
  laceration — *see* Laceration, elbow
  left S51.002
  puncture — *see* Puncture, elbow
  right S51.001
 epididymis — *see* Wound, open, testis

Wound, open — *continued*
 epigastric region S31.102
  with penetration into peritoneal cavity
   S31.602
  bite — *see* Bite, abdomen, wall, epigastric
   region
  laceration — *see* Laceration, abdomen, wall,
   epigastric region
  puncture — *see* Puncture, abdomen, wall,
   epigastric region
 epiglottis — *see* Wound, open, neck, specified
  site NEC
 esophagus (thoracic) S27.819
  cervical — *see* Wound, open, cervical
   esophagus
  laceration S27.813
  specified type NEC S27.818
 eye — *see* Wound, open, ocular
 eyeball — *see* Wound, open, ocular
 eyebrow — *see* Wound, open, eyelid
 eyelid S01.109
  bite — *see* Bite, eyelid
  laceration — *see* Laceration, eyelid
  left S01.102
  puncture — *see* Puncture, eyelid
  right S01.101
 face NEC — *see* Wound, open, head, specified
  site NEC
 finger(s) S61.209
  with
   amputation — *see* Amputation,
    traumatic, finger
   damage to nail S61.309
    with fracture S61.369
   fracture S61.269
  bite — *see* Bite, finger
  index S61.208
   with
    damage to nail S61.308
     with fracture S61.368
    fracture S61.268
   left S61.201
    with
     damage to nail S61.301
      with fracture S61.361
     fracture S61.261
   right S61.200
    with
     damage to nail S61.300
      with fracture S61.360
     fracture S61.260
  laceration — *see* Laceration, finger
  little S61.208
   with
    damage to nail S61.308
     with fracture S61.368
    fracture S61.268
   left S61.207
    with damage to nail S61.307
   right S61.206
    with damage to nail S61.306
  middle S61.208
   with
    damage to nail S61.308
     with fracture S61.368
    fracture S61.268
   left S61.203
    with damage to nail S61.303
   right S61.202
    with damage to nail S61.302
  puncture — *see* Puncture, finger
  ring S61.208
   with
    damage to nail S61.308
     with fracture S61.368
    fracture S61.268
   left S61.205
    with damage to nail S61.305
   right S61.204
    with damage to nail S61.304
 flank — *see* Wound, open, abdomen, wall
 foot (except toe(s) alone) S91.309
  with amputation — *see* Amputation,
   traumatic, foot
  bite — *see* Bite, foot
  laceration — *see* Laceration, foot

Wound, open — *continued*
 foot — *continued*
  left S91.302
  puncture — *see* Puncture, foot
  right S91.301
  toe — *see* Wound, open, toe
 forearm S51.809
  with
   amputation — *see* Amputation,
    traumatic, forearm
   fracture of radius and ulna S51.869
    left S51.862
    right S51.861
  bite — *see* Bite, forearm
  elbow only — *see* Wound, open, elbow
  laceration — *see* Laceration, forearm
  left S51.802
  puncture — *see* Puncture, forearm
  right S51.801
 forehead — *see* Wound, open, head, specified
  site NEC
 genital organs, external
  with amputation — *see* Amputation,
   traumatic, genital organs
  bite — *see* Bite, genital organ
  female S31.502
   vagina S31.40
   vulva S31.40
  laceration — *see* Laceration, genital organ
  male S31.501
   penis S31.20
   scrotum S31.30
   testes S31.30
  puncture — *see* Puncture, genital organ
 globe (eye) — *see* Wound, open, ocular
 groin — *see* Wound, open, abdomen, wall
 gum — *see* Wound, open, oral cavity
 hand S61.409
  with
   amputation — *see* Amputation,
    traumatic, hand
   fracture S61.469
    left S61.462
    right S61.461
  bite — *see* Bite, hand
  finger(s) — *see* Wound, open, finger
  laceration — *see* Laceration, hand
  left S61.402
  puncture — *see* Puncture, hand
  right S61.401
  thumb — *see* Wound, open, thumb
 head S01.90
  bite — *see* Bite, head
  cheek — *see* Wound, open, cheek
  ear — *see* Wound, open, ear
  eyelid — *see* Wound, open, eyelid
  laceration — *see* Laceration, head
  lip — *see* Wound, open, lip
  nose S01.20
  oral cavity — *see* Wound, open, oral cavity
  puncture — *see* Puncture, head
  scalp — *see* Wound, open, scalp
  specified site NEC S01.80
  temporomandibular area — *see* Wound,
   open, cheek
 heel — *see* Wound, open, foot
 hip S71.009
  with amputation — *see* Amputation,
   traumatic, hip
  bite — *see* Bite, hip
  laceration — *see* Laceration, hip
  left S71.002
  puncture — *see* Puncture, hip
  right S71.001
 hymen S31.40
  bite — *see* Bite, vulva
  laceration — *see* Laceration, vagina
  puncture — *see* Puncture, vagina
 hypochondrium S31.109
  bite — *see* Bite, hypochondrium
  laceration — *see* Laceration, hypochondrium
  puncture — *see* Puncture, hypochondrium
 hypogastric region S31.109
  bite — *see* Bite, hypogastric region
  laceration — *see* Laceration, hypogastric
   region

Wound, open — *continued*
  hypogastric region — *continued*
    puncture — *see* Puncture, hypogastric
      region
  iliac (region) — *see* Wound, open, inguinal
    region
  inguinal region S31.109
    bite — *see* Bite, abdomen, wall, lower
      quadrant
    laceration — *see* Laceration, inguinal region
    puncture — *see* Puncture, inguinal region
  instep — *see* Wound, open, foot
  interscapular region — *see* Wound, open,
    thorax, back
  intraocular — *see* Wound, open, ocular
  iris — *see* Wound, open, ocular
  jaw — *see* Wound, open, head, specified site
    NEC
  knee S81.009
    bite — *see* Bite, knee
    laceration — *see* Laceration, knee
    left S81.002
    puncture — *see* Puncture, knee
    right S81.001
  labium (majus) (minus) — *see* Wound, open,
    vulva
  laceration — *see* Laceration, by site
  lacrimal duct — *see* Wound, open, eyelid
  larynx S11.019
    bite — *see* Bite, larynx
    laceration — *see* Laceration, larynx
    puncture — *see* Puncture, larynx
  left
    lower quadrant S31.104
      with penetration into peritoneal cavity
        S31.604
      bite — *see* Bite, abdomen, wall, left, lower
        quadrant
      laceration — *see* Laceration, abdomen,
        wall, left, lower quadrant
      puncture — *see* Puncture, abdomen,
        wall, left, lower quadrant
    upper quadrant S31.101
      with penetration into peritoneal cavity
        S31.601
      bite — *see* Bite, abdomen, wall, left,
        upper quadrant
      laceration — *see* Laceration, abdomen,
        wall, left, upper quadrant
      puncture — *see* Puncture, abdomen,
        wall, left, upper quadrant
  leg (lower) S81.809
    with amputation — *see* Amputation,
      traumatic, leg
    ankle — *see* Wound, open, ankle
    bite — *see* Bite, leg
    foot — *see* Wound, open, foot
    knee — *see* Wound, open, knee
    laceration — *see* Laceration, leg
    left S81.802
    puncture — *see* Puncture, leg
    right S81.801
    toe — *see* Wound, open, toe
    upper — *see* Wound, open, thigh
  lip S01.501
    bite — *see* Bite, lip
    laceration — *see* Laceration, lip
    puncture — *see* Puncture, lip
  loin S31.109
    bite — *see* Bite, abdomen, wall
    laceration — *see* Laceration, loin
    puncture — *see* Puncture, loin
  lower back — *see* Wound, open, back, lower
  lumbar region — *see* Wound, open, back, lower
  malar region — *see* Wound, open, head,
    specified site NEC
  mammary — *see* Wound, open, breast
  mastoid region — *see* Wound, open, head,
    specified site NEC
  mouth — *see* Wound, open, oral cavity
  nail
    finger — *see* Wound, open, finger, with
      damage to nail
    toe — *see* Wound, open, toe, with damage to
      nail
  nape (neck) — *see* Wound, open, neck

Wound, open — *continued*
  nasal (septum) (sinus) — *see* Wound, open,
    nose
  nasopharynx — *see* Wound, open, head,
    specified site NEC
  neck S11.90
    bite — *see* Bite, neck
    involving
      cervical esophagus S11.20
      larynx — *see* Wound, open, larynx
      pharynx S11.20
      thyroid S11.10
      trachea (cervical) S11.029
        bite — *see* Bite, trachea
        laceration S11.021
          with foreign body S11.022
        puncture S11.023
          with foreign body S11.024
    laceration — *see* Laceration, neck
    puncture — *see* Puncture, neck
    specified site NEC S11.80
      specified type NEC S11.89
  nose (septum) (sinus) S01.20
    with amputation — *see* Amputation,
      traumatic, nose
    bite — *see* Bite, nose
    laceration — *see* Laceration, nose
    puncture — *see* Puncture, nose
  ocular S05.90
    avulsion (traumatic enucleation) S05.70
      left S05.72
      right S05.71
    eyeball S05.60
      with foreign body S05.50
        left S05.52
        right S05.51
      left S05.62
      right S05.61
    eyelid — *see* Wound, open, eyelid
    laceration and rupture S05.30
      with prolapse or loss of intraocular tissue
        S05.20
        left S05.22
        right S05.21
      left S05.32
      right S05.31
    left S05.92
    orbit (penetrating) (with or without foreign
      body) S05.40
      left S05.42
      right S05.41
    periocular area — *see* Wound, open, eyelid
    right S05.91
    specified NEC S05.80
      left S05.82
      right S05.81
  oral cavity S01.502
    bite S01.552
    laceration — *see* Laceration, oral cavity
    puncture — *see* Puncture, oral cavity
  orbit — *see* Wound, open, ocular, orbit
  palate — *see* Wound, open, oral cavity
  palm — *see* Wound, open, hand
  pelvis, pelvic — *see also* Wound, open, back,
    lower
    girdle — *see* Wound, open, hip
  penetrating — *see* Puncture, by site
  penis S31.20
    with amputation — *see* Amputation,
      traumatic, penis
    bite S31.25
    laceration — *see* Laceration, penis
    puncture — *see* Puncture, penis
  perineum
    bite — *see* Bite, perineum
    female S31.502
    laceration — *see* Laceration, perineum
    male S31.501
    puncture — *see* Puncture, perineum
  periocular area (with or without lacrimal
    passages) — *see* Wound, open, eyelid
  periumbilic region S31.105
    with penetration into peritoneal cavity
      S31.605
    bite — *see* Bite, abdomen, wall, periumbilic
      region

Wound, open — *continued*
  periumbilic region — *continued*
    laceration — *see* Laceration, abdomen, wall,
      periumbilic region
    puncture — *see* Puncture, abdomen, wall,
      periumbilic region
  phalanges
    finger — *see* Wound, open, finger
    toe — *see* Wound, open, toe
  pharynx S11.20
  pinna — *see* Wound, open, ear
  popliteal space — *see* Wound, open, knee
  prepuce — *see* Wound, open, penis
  pubic region — *see* Wound, open, back, lower
  pudendum — *see* Wound, open, genital organs,
    external
  puncture wound — *see* Puncture
  rectovaginal septum — *see* Wound, open,
    vagina
  right
    lower quadrant S31.103
      with penetration into peritoneal cavity
        S31.603
      bite — *see* Bite, abdomen, wall, right,
        lower quadrant
      laceration — *see* Laceration, abdomen,
        wall, right, lower quadrant
      puncture — *see* Puncture, abdomen,
        wall, right, lower quadrant
    upper quadrant S31.100
      with penetration into peritoneal cavity
        S31.600
      bite — *see* Bite, abdomen, wall, right,
        upper quadrant
      laceration — *see* Laceration, abdomen,
        wall, right, upper quadrant
      puncture — *see* Puncture, abdomen,
        wall, right, upper quadrant
  sacral region — *see* Wound, open, back, lower
  sacroiliac region — *see* Wound, open, back,
    lower
  salivary gland — *see* Wound, open, oral cavity
  scalp S01.00
    bite S01.05
    laceration — *see* Laceration, scalp
    puncture — *see* Puncture, scalp
  scalpel, fetus or newborn (birth injury) P15.8
  scapular region — *see* Wound, open, shoulder
  sclera — *see* Wound, open, ocular
  scrotum S31.30
    with amputation — *see* Amputation,
      traumatic, scrotum
    bite S31.35
    laceration — *see* Laceration, scrotum
    puncture — *see* Puncture, scrotum
  shin — *see* Wound, open, leg
  shoulder S41.009
    with amputation — *see* Amputation,
      traumatic, arm
    bite — *see* Bite, shoulder
    laceration — *see* Laceration, shoulder
    left S41.002
    puncture — *see* Puncture, shoulder
    right S41.001
  skin NOS T14.90
  spermatic cord — *see* Wound, open, testis
  sternal region — *see* Wound, open, thorax,
    front wall
  submaxillary region — *see* Wound, open, head,
    specified site NEC
  submental region — *see* Wound, open, head,
    specified site NEC
  subungual
    finger(s) — *see* Wound, open, finger
    toe(s) — *see* Wound, open, toe
  supraclavicular region — *see* Wound, open,
    neck, specified site NEC
  temple, temporal region — *see* Wound, open,
    head, specified site NEC
  temporomandibular area — *see* Wound, open,
    cheek
  testis S31.30
    with amputation — *see* Amputation,
      traumatic, testes
    bite S31.35
    laceration — *see* Laceration, testis
    puncture — *see* Puncture, testis

©2002 Ingenix, Inc.

Wound, open — *continued*
  thigh S71.109
    with amputation — *see* Amputation,
      traumatic, hip
    bite — *see* Bite, thigh
    laceration — *see* Laceration, thigh
    left S71.102
    puncture — *see* Puncture, thigh
    right S71.101
  thorax, thoracic (wall) S21.90
    back S21.209
      left S21.202
      right S21.201
    bite — *see* Bite, thorax
    breast — *see* Wound, open, breast
    front S21.109
      left S21.102
      right S21.101
    laceration — *see* Laceration, thorax
    puncture — *see* Puncture, thorax
  throat — *see* Wound, open, neck
  thumb S61.009
    with
      amputation — *see* Amputation,
        traumatic, thumb
      damage to nail S61.109
        with fracture S61.169
      fracture S61.069
    bite — *see* Bite, thumb
    laceration — *see* Laceration, thumb
    left S61.002
      with
        damage to nail S61.102
          with fracture S61.162
        fracture S61.062
    puncture — *see* Puncture, thumb
    right S61.001
      with
        damage to nail S61.101
          with fracture S61.161
        fracture S61.061
  thyroid (gland) — *see* Wound, open, neck,
    thyroid
  toe(s) S91.109
    with
      amputation — *see* Amputation,
        traumatic, toe
      damage to nail S91.209
        with fracture S91.269
      fracture S91.169
    bite — *see* Bite, toe
    great S91.103
      with
        damage to nail S91.203
          with fracture S91.263
        fracture S91.163
      left S91.102
        with
          damage to nail S91.202
            with fracture S91.262
          fracture S91.162
      right S91.101
        with
          damage to nail S91.201
            with fracture S91.261
          fracture S91.161
    laceration — *see* Laceration, toe
    lesser S91.106
      with
        damage to nail S91.206
          with fracture S91.266
        fracture S91.166
      left S91.105
        with
          damage to nail S91.205
            with fracture S91.265
          fracture S91.165
      right S91.104
        with
          damage to nail S91.204
            with fracture S91.264
          fracture S91.164
    puncture — *see* Puncture, toe
  tongue — *see* Wound, open, oral cavity
  trachea (cervical region) — *see* Wound, open,
    neck, trachea

Wound, open — *continued*
  tunica vaginalis — *see* Wound, open, testis
  tympanum, tympanic membrane S09.20
    laceration — *see* Laceration, ear, drum
    left S09.22
    puncture — *see* Puncture, tympanum
    right S09.21
  umbilical region — *see* Wound, open, abdomen,
    wall, periumbilic region
  uvula — *see* Wound, open, oral cavity
  vagina S31.40
    bite S31.45
    laceration — *see* Laceration, vagina
    puncture — *see* Puncture, vagina
  vocal cord S11.039
    bite — *see* Bite, vocal cord
    laceration S11.031
      with foreign body S11.032
    puncture S11.033
      with foreign body S11.034
  vitreous (humor) — *see* Wound, open, ocular
  vulva S31.40
    with amputation — *see* Amputation,
      traumatic, vulva
    bite S31.45
    laceration — *see* Laceration, vulva
    puncture — *see* Puncture, vulva
  wrist S61.509
    with fracture S61.569
    bite — *see* Bite, wrist
    laceration — *see* Laceration, wrist
    left S61.502
      with fracture S61.562
    puncture — *see* Puncture, wrist
    right S61.501
      with fracture S61.561

Wright's syndrome G54.0

Wrist — *see* condition

Wrong drug (by accident) (given in error) T50.901
  administered with intent to harm by
    another person T50.903
    self T50.902
  circumstances undetermined T50.904
  specified drug or substance — *see* Table of
    Drugs and Chemicals

Wry neck — *see* Torticollis

Wuchereria (bancrofti) **infestation** B74.0

Wuchereriasis B74.0

Wuchernde Struma Langhans (M8332/3) C73

X

Xanthelasma (eyelid) (palpebrarum) H02.60
  left H02.66
    lower H02.65
    upper H02.64
  right H02.63
    lower H02.62
    upper H02.61

Xanthelasmatosis (essential) E78.2

Xanthinuria, hereditary E79.8

Xanthoastrocytoma, pleomorphic (M9424/3)
  specified site — *see* Neoplasm, malignant
  unspecified site C71.9

Xanthofibroma (M8830/0) — *see* Neoplasm,
  connective tissue, benign

Xanthogranuloma D76.3

Xanthoma(s), xanthomatosis (primary) (familial)
  (hereditary) E75.5
  with
    hyperlipoproteinemia
      Type I E78.3
      Type III E78.2
      Type IV E78.1
      Type V E78.3
  bone (generalisata) D76.0
  cerebrotendinous E75.5
  cutaneotendinous E75.5
  disseminatum (skin) E78.2
  eruptive E78.2
  hypercholesterinemic E78.0
  hypercholesterolemic E78.0
  hyperlipidemic E78.5
  joint E75.5
  multiple (skin) E78.2

Xanthoma(s), xanthomatosis — *continued*
  tendon (sheath) E75.5
  tubo-eruptive E78.2
  tuberosum E78.2
  tuberous E78.2
  verrucous, oral mucosa K13.4

Xanthosis R23.8

Xenophobia F40.10

Xeroderma — *see also* Ichthyosis
  acquired L85.0
  eyelid H01.149
    left H01.146
      lower H01.145
      upper H01.144
    right H01.143
      lower H01.142
      upper H01.141
  pigmentosum Q82.1
  vitamin A deficiency E50.8

Xerophthalmia (vitamin A deficiency) E50.7
  unrelated to vitamin A deficiency — *see*
    Keratoconjunctivitis

Xerosis
  conjunctiva H11.149
    with Bitot's spots — *see also* Pigmentation,
      conjunctiva
        vitamin A deficiency E50.1
    bilateral H11.143
    left H11.142
    right H11.141
    vitamin A deficiency E50.0
  cornea H18.89
    with ulceration — *see* Ulcer, cornea
      vitamin A deficiency E50.3
    vitamin A deficiency E50.2
  cutis L85.3
  skin L85.3

Xerostomia K11.7

Xiphopagus Q89.4

XO syndrome Q96.9

X-ray (of)
  abnormal findings — *see* Abnormal, diagnostic
    imaging
  breast (mammogram) (routine) Z12.31
  chest
    for suspected tuberculosis Z03.8
    routine Z00.030
      with abnormal findings Z00.031
  effects, adverse T66
  routine NEC Z00.030
    with abnormal findings Z00.031

XXXXY syndrome Q98.1

XXY syndrome Q98.0

Y

Yaba pox virus disease B08.8

Yawning R06.89
  psychogenic F45.8

Yaws A66.9
  bone lesions A66.6
  butter A66.1
  chancre A66.0
  cutaneous, less than five years after infection
    A66.2
  early (cutaneous) (macular) (maculopapular)
    (micropapular) (papular) A66.2
    frambeside A66.2
    skin lesions NEC A66.2
  eyelid A66.2
  ganglion A66.6
  gangosis, gangosa A66.5
  gumma, gummata A66.4
    bone A66.6
  gummatous
    frambeside A66.4
    osteitis A66.6
    periostitis A66.6
  hydrarthrosis (*see also* category M14.8) A66.6
  hyperkeratosis (early) (late) A66.3
  initial lesions A66.0
  joint lesions (*see also* category M14.8) A66.6
  juxta-articular nodules A66.7
  late nodular (ulcerated) A66.4

Yaws — *continued*
  latent (without clinical manifestations) (with
      positive serology) A66.8
  mother A66.0
  mucosal A66.7
  multiple papillomata A66.1
  nodular, late (ulcerated) A66.4
  osteitis A66.6
  papilloma, plantar or palmar A66.1
  periostitis (hypertrophic) A66.6
  specified NEC A66.7
  ulcers A66.4
  wet crab A66.1
Yeast infection — *see* Candidiasis
Yellow
  atrophy (liver) — *see* Failure, hepatic
  fever — *see* Fever, yellow
  jack — *see* Fever, yellow
  jaundice — *see* Jaundice
  nail syndrome L60.5
Yersiniosis — *see also* Infection, Yersinia
  extraintestinal A28.2
  intestinal A04.6

Z

Zahorsky's syndrome (herpangina) B08.5
Zellweger's syndrome Q87.89
Zenker's diverticulum (esophagus) K22.5
Ziehen-Oppenheim disease G24.1
Zieve's syndrome K70.0
Zinc
  deficiency, dietary E60
  metabolism disorder E83.2
Zollinger-Ellison syndrome E16.4
Zona — *see* Herpes, zoster
Zoophobia F40.218
Zoster (herpes) — *see* Herpes, zoster
Zygomycosis B46.9
  specified NEC B46.8
Zymotic — *see* condition

©2002 Ingenix, Inc.

	Malignant					
	Primary	**Secondary**	**Ca in situ**	**Benign**	**Uncertain Behavior**	**Unspecified**
Neoplasm, neoplastic	C76.9	C79.9	D09.9	D36.9	D48.9	D49.9

Notes — 1. The list below gives the code numbers for neoplasms by anatomical site. For each site there are six possible code numbers according to whether the neoplasm in question is malignant, benign, in situ, of uncertain behavior, or of unspecified nature. The description of the neoplasm will often indicate which of the six columns is appropriate; e.g., malignant melanoma of skin, benign fibroadenoma of breast, carcinoma in situ of cervix uteri.

Where such descriptors are not present, the remainder of the Index should be consulted where guidance is given to the appropriate column for each morphological (histological) variety listed; e.g., Mesonephroma — see Neoplasm, malignant; Embryoma — see also Neoplasm, uncertain behavior; Disease, Bowen's — see Neoplasm, skin, in situ. However, the guidance in the Index can be overridden if one of the descriptors mentioned above is present; e.g., malignant adenoma of colon is coded to C18.9 and not to D12.6 as the adjective "malignant" overrides the Index entry "Adenoma — see also Neoplasm, benign."

*2. Sites marked with the sign * (e.g., face NEC*) should be classified to malignant neoplasm of skin of these sites if the variety of neoplasm is a squamous cell carcinoma or an epidermoid carcinoma and to benign neoplasm of skin of these sites if the variety of neoplasm is a papilloma (any type).*

	Primary	Secondary	Ca in situ	Benign	Uncertain Behavior	Unspecified
abdomen, abdominal	C76.2	C79.89	D09.7	D36.7	D48.7	D49.8
cavity	C76.2	C79.89	D09.7	D36.7	D48.7	D49.8
organ	C76.2	C79.89	D09.7	D36.7	D48.7	D49.8
viscera	C76.2	C79.89	D09.7	D36.7	D48.7	D49.8
wall	C44.5	C79.2	D04.5	D23.5	D48.5	D49.2
connective tissue	C49.4	C79.89	—	D21.4	D48.1	D49.2
abdominopelvic	C76.7	C79.89	D09.7	D36.7	D48.7	D49.8
accessory sinus — see Neoplasm, sinus						
acoustic nerve (unspecified side)	C72.40	C79.49	—	D33.3	D43.3	D49.7
left side	C72.42	C79.49	—	D33.3	D43.3	D49.7
right side	C72.41	C79.49	—	D33.3	D43.3	D49.7
acromion (process)						
left side	C40.02	C79.51	—	D16.02	D48.0	D49.2
marrow NEC	C96.9	C79.52	—	—	—	D47.9
right side	C40.01	C79.51	—	D16.01	D48.0	D49.2
marrow NEC	C96.9	C79.52	—	—	—	D47.9
unspecified side	C40.00	C79.51	—	D16.00	D48.0	D49.2
marrow NEC	C96.9	C79.52	—	—	—	D47.9
adenoid (pharynx) (tissue)	C11.1	C79.89	D00.08	D10.6	D37.05	D49.0
adipose tissue (see also Neoplasm, connective tissue)	C49.9	C79.89	—	D21.9	D48.1	D49.2
adnexa (uterine)	C57.4	C79.89	D07.39	D28.7	D39.7	D49.5
adrenal						
capsule (unspecified side)	C74.90	C79.70	D09.3	D35.00	D44.10	D49.7
left side	C74.92	C79.72	D09.3	D35.02	D44.12	D49.7
right side	C74.91	C79.71	D09.3	D35.01	D44.11	D49.7
cortex (unspecified side)	C74.00	C79.70	D09.3	D35.00	D44.10	D49.7
left side	C74.02	C79.72	D09.3	D35.02	D44.12	D49.7
right side	C74.01	C79.71	D09.3	D35.01	D44.11	D49.7
gland (unspecified side)	C74.90	C79.70	D09.3	D35.00	D44.10	D49.7
left side	C74.92	C79.72	D09.3	D35.02	D44.12	D49.7
right side	C74.91	C79.71	D09.3	D35.01	D44.11	D49.7
medulla (unspecified side)	C74.10	C79.70	D09.3	D35.00	D44.10	D49.7
left side	C74.12	C79.72	D09.3	D35.02	D44.12	D49.7
right side	C74.11	C79.71	D09.3	D35.01	D44.11	D49.7
unspecified site (unspecified side)	C74.90	C79.70	D09.3	D35.00	D44.10	D49.7
left side	C74.92	C79.72	D09.3	D35.02	D44.12	D49.7
right side	C74.91	C79.71	D09.3	D35.01	D44.11	D49.7
ala nasi (external)	C44.3	C79.2	D04.39	D23.39	D48.5	D49.2
alimentary canal or tract NEC	C26.9	C78.80	D01.9	D13.9	D37.9	D49.0
alveolar	C03.9	C79.89	D00.03	D10.39	D37.09	D49.0
mucosa	C03.9	C79.89	D00.03	D10.39	D37.09	D49.0
lower	C03.1	C79.89	D00.03	D10.39	D37.09	D49.0
upper	C03.0	C79.89	D00.03	D10.39	D37.09	D49.0
ridge or process	C41.1	C79.51	—	D16.5	D48.0	D49.2
carcinoma	C03.9	—	—	—	—	—
lower	C03.1	—	—	—	—	—
upper	C03.0	—	—	—	—	—
lower	C41.1	C79.51	—	D16.5	D48.0	D49.2
marrow NEC	C96.9	C79.52	—	—	—	D47.9
marrow NEC	C96.9	C79.52	—	—	—	D47.9
mucosa	C03.9	C79.89	D00.03	D10.39	D37.09	D49.0
lower	C03.1	C79.89	D00.03	D10.39	D37.09	D49.0
upper	C03.0	C79.89	D00.03	D10.39	D37.09	D49.0
upper	C41.0	C79.51	—	D16.4	D48.0	D49.2
marrow NEC	C96.9	C79.52	—	—	—	D47.9
sulcus	C06.1	C79.89	D00.02	D10.39	D37.09	D49.0

	Malignant			Benign	Uncertain Behavior	Unspecified
	Primary	**Secondary**	**Ca in situ**	**Benign**	**Uncertain Behavior**	**Unspecified**
Neoplasm, neoplastic — *continued*						
alveolus	C03.9	C79.89	D00.03	D10.39	D37.09	D49.0
lower	C03.1	C79.89	D00.03	D10.39	D37.09	D49.0
upper	C03.0	C79.89	D00.03	D10.39	D37.09	D49.0
ampulla of Vater	C24.1	C78.89	D01.5	D13.5	D37.6	D49.0
ankle (unspecified side) NEC*	C76.50	C79.89	D04.70	D36.7	D48.7	D49.8
left side	C76.52	C79.89	D04.72	D36.7	D48.7	D49.8
right side	C76.51	C79.89	D04.71	D36.7	D48.7	D49.8
anorectum, anorectal (junction)	C21.8	C78.5	D01.3	D12.9	D37.7	D49.0
antecubital fossa or space (unspecified side)*	C76.40	C79.89	D04.60	D36.7	D48.7	D49.8
left side	C76.42	C79.89	D04.62	D36.7	D48.7	D49.8
right side	C76.41	C79.89	D04.61	D36.7	D48.7	D49.8
antrum (Highmore) (maxillary)	C31.0	C78.39	D02.3	D14.0	D38.5	D49.1
pyloric	C16.3	C78.89	D00.2	D13.1	D37.1	D49.0
tympanicum	C30.1	C78.39	D02.3	D14.0	D38.5	D49.1
anus, anal	C21.0	C78.5	D01.3	D12.9	D37.7	D49.0
canal	C21.1	C78.5	D01.3	D12.9	D37.7	D49.0
cloacogenic zone	C21.2	C78.5	D01.3	D12.9	D37.7	D49.0
margin	C44.5	C79.2	D04.5	D23.5	D48.5	D49.2
overlapping lesion with rectosigmoid junction or rectum	C21.8	—	—	—	—	—
skin	C44.5	C79.2	D04.5	D23.5	D48.5	D49.2
sphincter	C21.1	C78.5	D01.3	D12.9	D37.7	D49.0
aorta (thoracic)	C49.3	C79.89	—	D21.3	D48.1	D49.2
abdominal	C49.4	C79.89	—	D21.4	D48.1	D49.2
aortic body	C75.5	C79.89	—	D35.6	D44.7	D49.7
aponeurosis	C49.9	C79.89	—	D21.9	D48.1	D49.2
palmar (unspecified side)	C49.10	C79.89	—	D21.10	D48.1	D49.2
left side	C49.12	C79.89	—	D21.12	D48.1	D49.2
right side	C49.11	C79.89	—	D21.11	D48.1	D49.2
plantar (unspecified side)	C49.20	C79.89	—	D21.20	D48.1	D49.2
left side	C49.22	C79.89	—	D21.22	D48.1	D49.2
right side	C49.21	C79.89	—	D21.21	D48.1	D49.2
appendix	C18.1	C78.5	D01.0	D12.1	D37.3	D49.0
arachnoid	C70.9	C79.49	—	D32.9	D42.9	D49.7
cerebral	C70.0	C79.32	—	D32.0	D42.0	D49.7
spinal	C70.1	C79.49	—	D32.1	D42.1	D49.7
areola						
female (unspecified side)	C50.00	C79.81	D05.90	D24.00	D48.60	D49.3
left side	C50.02	C79.81	D05.92	D24.02	D48.62	D49.3
right side	C50.01	C79.81	D05.91	D24.01	D48.61	D49.3
male (unspecified side)	C50.05	C79.81	D05.95	D24.10	D48.65	D49.3
left side	C50.04	C79.81	D05.94	D24.12	D48.64	D49.3
right side	C50.03	C79.81	D05.93	D24.11	D48.63	D49.3
arm (unspecified side) NEC*	C76.40	C79.89	D04.60	D36.7	D48.7	D49.8
left side	C76.42	C79.89	D04.61	D36.7	D48.7	D49.8
right side	C76.41	C79.89	D04.62	D36.7	D48.7	D49.8
artery — see Neoplasm, connective tissue						
aryepiglottic fold	C13.1	C79.89	D00.08	D10.7	D37.05	D49.0
hypopharyngeal aspect	C13.1	C79.89	D00.08	D10.7	D37.05	D49.0
laryngeal aspect	C32.1	C78.39	D02.0	D14.1	D38.0	D49.1
marginal zone	C13.1	C79.89	D00.08	D10.7	D37.05	D49.0
arytenoid (cartilage)	C32.3	C78.39	D02.0	D14.1	D38.0	D49.1
fold — see Neoplasm, aryepiglottic						
atlas	C41.2	C79.51	—	D16.6	D48.0	D49.2
marrow NEC	C96.9	C79.52	—	—	—	D47.9
atrium, cardiac	C38.0	C79.89	—	D15.1	D48.7	D49.8
auditory						
canal (external) (skin) (unspecified side)	C44.20	C79.2	D04.20	D23.20	D48.5	D49.2
left side	C44.22	C79.2	D04.22	D23.22	D48.5	D49.2
right side	C44.21	C79.2	D04.21	D23.21	D48.5	D49.2
internal	C30.1	C78.39	D02.3	D14.0	D38.5	D49.1
nerve (unspecified side)	C72.40	C79.49	—	D33.3	D43.3	D49.7
left side	C72.42	C79.49	—	D33.3	D43.3	D49.7
right side	C72.41	C79.49	—	D33.3	D43.3	D49.7
tube	C30.1	C78.39	D02.3	D14.0	D38.5	D49.1
opening	C11.2	C79.89	D00.08	D10.6	D37.05	D49.0

©2002 Ingenix, Inc.

	Malignant			Benign	Uncertain Behavior	Unspecified
	Primary	Secondary	Ca in situ			
Neoplasm, neoplastic — *continued*						
auricle, ear						
left side	C44.22	C79.2	D04.22	D23.22	D48.5	D49.2
cartilage	C49.0	C79.89	—	D21.0	D48.1	D49.2
right side	C44.21	C79.2	D04.21	D23.21	D48.5	D49.2
cartilage	C49.0	C79.89	—	D21.0	D48.1	D49.2
unspecified side	C44.20	C79.2	D04.20	D23.20	D48.5	D49.2
cartilage	C49.0	C79.89	—	D21.0	D48.1	D49.2
auricular canal (external)						
left side	C44.22	C79.2	D04.22	D23.22	D48.5	D49.2
internal	C30.1	C78.39	D02.3	D14.0	D38.5	D49.2
right side	C44.21	C79.2	D04.21	D23.21	D48.5	D49.2
internal	C30.1	C78.39	D02.3	D14.0	D38.5	D49.2
unspecified side	C44.20	C79.2	D04.20	D23.20	D48.5	D49.2
internal	C30.1	C78.39	D02.3	D14.0	D38.5	D49.2
autonomic nerve or nervous system NEC						
(see also Neoplasm, nerve, peripheral)	C47.9	C79.89	—	D36.10	D48.2	D49.2
axilla, axillary	C76.1	C79.89	D09.7	D36.7	D48.7	D49.8
fold	C44.5	C79.2	D04.5	D23.5	D48.5	D49.2
back NEC*	C76.7	C79.89	D04.5	D36.7	D48.7	D49.8
Bartholin's gland	C51.0	C79.82	D07.1	D28.0	D39.7	D49.5
basal ganglia	C71.0	C79.31	—	D33.0	D43.0	D49.6
basis pedunculi	C71.7	C79.31	—	D33.1	D43.1	D49.6
bile or biliary (tract)	C24.9	C78.89	D01.5	D13.5	D37.6	D49.0
canaliculi (biliferi) (intrahepatic)	C22.1	C78.89	D01.5	D13.4	D37.6	D49.0
canals, interlobular	C22.1	C78.89	D01.5	D13.4	D37.6	D49.0
overlapping lesion	C24.8	—	—	—	—	—
duct or passage (common) (cystic) (extrahepatic)	C24.0	C78.89	D01.5	D13.5	D37.6	D49.0
interlobular	C22.1	C78.89	D01.5	D13.4	D37.6	D49.0
intrahepatic	C22.1	C78.89	D01.5	D13.4	D37.6	D49.0
and extrahepatic	C24.8	C78.89	D01.5	D13.5	D37.6	D49.0
overlapping lesion with gallbladder	C24.8	—	—	—	—	—
bladder (urinary)	C67.9	C79.11	D09.0	D30.3	D41.4	D49.4
dome	C67.1	C79.11	D09.0	D30.3	D41.4	D49.4
neck	C67.5	C79.11	D09.0	D30.3	D41.4	D49.4
orifice	C67.9	C79.11	D09.0	D30.3	D41.4	D49.4
ureteric	C67.6	C79.11	D09.0	D30.3	D41.4	D49.4
urethral	C67.5	C79.11	D09.0	D30.3	D41.4	D49.4
overlapping lesion	C67.8	—	—	—	—	—
sphincter	C67.8	C79.11	D09.0	D30.3	D41.4	D49.4
trigone	C67.0	C79.11	D09.0	D30.3	D41.4	D49.4
urachus	C67.7	—	D09.0	D30.3	D41.4	D49.4
wall	C67.9	C79.11	D09.0	D30.3	D41.4	D49.4
anterior	C67.3	C79.11	D09.0	D30.3	D41.4	D49.4
lateral	C67.2	C79.11	D09.0	D30.3	D41.4	D49.4
posterior	C67.4	C79.11	D09.0	D30.3	D41.4	D49.4
blood vessel — see Neoplasm, connective tissue						
bone (periosteum)	C41.9	C79.51	—	D16.9	D48.0	D49.2

Note: Carcinomas and adenocarcinomas, of any type other than intraosseous or odontogenic, of the sites listed under "Neoplasm, bone" should be considered as constituting metastatic spread from an unspecified primary site and coded to C79.51 for morbidity coding and to C80.1 for underlying cause a death coding.

	Malignant			Benign	Uncertain Behavior	Unspecified
	Primary	Secondary	Ca in situ			
acetabulum	C41.4	C79.51	—	D16.8	D48.0	D49.2
marrow NEC	C96.9	C79.52	—	—	—	D47.9
acromion (process)						
left side	C40.02	C79.51	—	D16.02	D48.0	D49.2
marrow NEC	C96.9	C79.52	—	—	—	D47.9
right side	C40.01	C79.51	—	D16.01	D48.0	D49.2
marrow NEC	C96.9	C79.52	—	—	—	D47.9
unspecified side	C40.00	C79.51	—	D16.00	D48.0	D49.2
marrow NEC	C96.9	C79.52	—	—	—	D47.9
ankle						
left side	C40.32	C79.51	—	D16.32	D48.0	D49.2
marrow NEC	C96.9	C79.52	—	—	—	D47.9
right side	C40.31	C79.51	—	D16.31	D48.0	D49.2
marrow NEC	C96.9	C79.52	—	—	—	D47.9
unspecified side	C40.30	C79.51	—	D16.30	D48.0	D49.2
marrow NEC	C96.9	C79.52	—	—	—	D47.9

		Malignant					
		Primary	Secondary	Ca in situ	Benign	Uncertain Behavior	Unspecified
Neoplasm, neoplastic — *continued*							
bone — *continued*							
arm NEC							
left side		C40.02	C79.51	—	D16.02	D48.0	D49.2
marrow NEC		C96.9	C79.52	—	—	—	D47.9
right side		C40.01	C79.51	—	D16.01	D48.0	D49.2
marrow NEC		C96.9	C79.52	—	—	—	D47.9
unspecified side		C40.00	C79.51	—	D16.00	D48.0	D49.2
marrow NEC		C96.9	C79.52	—	—	—	D47.9
astragalus							
left side		C40.32	C79.51	—	D16.32	D48.0	D49.2
marrow NEC		C96.9	C79.52	—	—	—	D47.9
right side		C40.31	C79.51	—	D16.31	D48.0	D49.2
marrow NEC		C96.9	C79.52	—	—	—	D47.9
unspecified side		C40.30	C79.51	—	D16.30	D48.0	D49.2
marrow NEC		C96.9	C79.52	—	—	—	D47.9
atlas		C41.2	C79.51	—	D16.6	D48.0	D49.2
marrow NEC		C96.9	C79.52	—	—	—	D47.9
axis		C41.2	C79.51	—	D16.6	D48.0	D49.2
marrow NEC		C96.9	C79.52	—	—	—	D47.9
back NEC		C41.2	C79.51	—	D16.6	D48.0	D49.2
marrow NEC		C96.9	C79.52	—	—	—	D47.9
calcaneus							
left side		C40.32	C79.51	—	D16.32	D48.0	D49.2
marrow NEC		C96.9	C79.52	—	—	—	D47.9
right side		C40.31	C79.51	—	D16.31	D48.0	D49.2
marrow NEC		C96.9	C79.52	—	—	—	D47.9
unspecified side		C40.30	C79.51	—	D16.30	D48.0	D49.2
marrow NEC		C96.9	C79.52	—	—	—	D47.9
calvarium		C41.0	C79.51	—	D16.4	D48.0	D49.2
marrow NEC		C96.9	C79.52	—	—	—	D47.9
carpus (any)							
left side		C40.12	C79.51	—	D16.12	D48.0	D49.2
marrow NEC		C96.9	C79.52	—	—	—	D47.9
right side		C40.11	C79.51	—	D16.11	D48.0	D49.2
marrow NEC		C96.9	C79.52	—	—	—	D47.9
unspecified side		C40.10	C79.51	—	D16.10	D48.0	D49.2
marrow NEC		C96.9	C79.52	—	—	—	D47.9
cartilage NEC		C41.9	C79.51	—	D16.9	D48.0	D49.2
clavicle		C41.3	C79.51	—	D16.7	D48.0	D49.2
marrow NEC		C96.9	C79.52	—	—	—	D47.9
clivus		C41.0	C79.51	—	D16.4	D48.0	D49.2
marrow NEC		C96.9	C79.52	—	—	—	D47.9
coccygeal vertebra		C41.4	C79.51	—	D16.8	D48.0	D49.2
marrow NEC		C96.9	C79.52	—	—	—	D47.9
coccyx		C41.4	C79.51	—	D16.8	D48.0	D49.2
marrow NEC		C96.9	C79.52	—	—	—	D47.9
costal cartilage		C41.3	C79.51	—	D16.7	D48.0	D49.2
costovertebral joint		C41.3	C79.51	—	D16.7	D48.0	D49.2
marrow NEC		C96.9	C79.52	—	—	—	D47.9
cranial		C41.0	C79.51	—	D16.4	D48.0	D49.2
marrow NEC		C96.9	C79.52	—	—	—	D47.9
cuboid							
left side		C40.32	C79.51	—	D16.32	D48.0	D49.2
marrow NEC		C96.9	C79.52	—	—	—	D47.9
right side		C40.31	C79.51	—	D16.31	D48.0	D49.2
marrow NEC		C96.9	C79.52	—	—	—	D47.9
unspecified side		C40.30	C79.51	—	D16.30	D48.0	D49.2
marrow NEC		C96.9	C79.52	—	—	—	D47.9
cuneiform		C41.9	C79.51	—	D16.9	D48.0	D49.2
ankle							
left side		C40.32	C79.51	—	D16.32	D48.0	D49.2
marrow NEC		C96.9	C79.52	—	—	—	D47.9
right side		C40.31	C79.51	—	D16.31	D48.0	D49.2
marrow NEC		C96.9	C79.52	—	—	—	D47.9
unspecified side		C40.30	C79.51	—	D16.30	D48.0	D49.2
marrow NEC		C96.9	C79.52	—	—	—	D47.9

©2002 Ingenix, Inc.

	Malignant					
	Primary	**Secondary**	**Ca in situ**	**Benign**	**Uncertain Behavior**	**Unspecified**
Neoplasm, neoplastic — *continued*						
bone — *continued*						
cuneiform — *continued*						
wrist						
left side	C40.12	C79.51	—	D16.12	D48.0	D49.2
marrow NEC	C96.9	C79.52	—	—	—	D47.9
right side	C40.11	C79.51	—	D16.11	D48.0	D49.2
marrow NEC	C96.9	C79.52	—	—	—	D47.9
unspecified side	C40.10	C79.51	—	D16.10	D48.0	D49.2
marrow NEC	C96.9	C79.52	—	—	—	D47.9
digital						
finger						
left side	C40.12	C79.51	—	D16.12	D48.0	D49.2
marrow NEC	C96.9	C79.52	—	—	—	D47.9
right side	C40.11	C79.51	—	D16.11	D48.0	D49.2
marrow NEC	C96.9	C79.52	—	—	—	D47.9
unspecified side	C40.10	C79.51	—	D16.10	D48.0	D49.2
marrow NEC	C96.9	C79.52	—	—	—	D47.9
toe						
left side	C40.32	C79.51	—	D16.32	D48.0	D49.2
marrow NEC	C96.9	C79.52	—	—	—	D47.9
right side	C40.31	C79.51	—	D16.31	D48.0	D49.2
marrow NEC	C96.9	C79.52	—	—	—	D47.9
unspecified side	C40.30	C79.51	—	D16.30	D48.0	D49.2
marrow NEC	C96.9	C79.52	—	—	—	D47.9
unspecified site						
left side	C40.92	C79.51	—	D16.9	D48.0	D49.2
marrow NEC	C96.9	C79.52	—	—	—	D47.9
right side	C40.91	C79.51	—	D16.9	D48.0	D49.2
marrow NEC	C96.9	C79.52	—	—	—	D47.9
unspecified side	C40.90	C79.51	—	D16.9	D48.0	D49.2
marrow NEC	C96.9	C79.52	—	—	—	D47.9
elbow						
left side	C40.02	C79.51	—	D16.02	D48.0	D49.2
marrow NEC	C96.9	C79.52	—	—	—	D47.9
right side	C40.01	C79.51	—	D16.01	D48.0	D49.2
marrow NEC	C96.9	C79.52	—	—	—	D47.9
unspecified side	C40.00	C79.51	—	D16.00	D48.0	D49.2
marrow NEC	C96.9	C79.52	—	—	—	D47.9
ethmoid (labyrinth)	C41.0	C79.51	—	D16.4	D48.0	D49.2
marrow NEC	C96.9	C79.52	—	—	—	D47.9
face	C41.0	C79.51	—	D16.4	D48.0	D49.2
lower jaw	C41.1	C79.51	—	D16.5	D48.0	D49.2
marrow NEC	C96.9	C79.52	—	—	—	D47.9
marrow NEC	C96.9	C79.52	—	—	—	D47.9
femur (any part)						
left side	C40.22	C79.51	—	D16.22	D48.0	D49.2
marrow NEC	C96.9	C79.52	—	—	—	D47.9
right side	C40.21	C79.51	—	D16.21	D48.0	D49.2
marrow NEC	C96.9	C79.52	—	—	—	D47.9
unspecified side	C40.20	C79.51	—	D16.20	D48.0	D49.2
marrow NEC	C96.9	C79.52	—	—	—	D47.9
fibula (any part)						
left side	C40.22	C79.51	—	D16.22	D48.0	D49.2
marrow NEC	C96.9	C79.52	—	—	—	D47.9
right side	C40.21	C79.51	—	D16.21	D48.0	D49.2
marrow NEC	C96.9	C79.52	—	—	—	D47.9
unspecified side	C40.20	C79.51	—	D16.20	D48.0	D49.2
marrow NEC	C96.9	C79.52	—	—	—	D47.9
finger (any)						
left side	C40.12	C79.51	—	D16.12	D48.0	D49.2
marrow NEC	C96.9	C79.52	—	—	—	D47.9
right side	C40.11	C79.51	—	D16.11	D48.0	D49.2
marrow NEC	C96.9	C79.52	—	—	—	D47.9
unspecified side	C40.10	C79.51	—	D16.10	D48.0	D49.2
marrow NEC	C96.9	C79.52	—	—	—	D47.9

	Malignant			Benign	Uncertain Behavior	Unspecified
	Primary	Secondary	Ca in situ			
Neoplasm, neoplastic — *continued*						
bone — *continued*						
foot						
left side	C40.32	C79.51	—	D16.32	D48.0	D49.2
marrow NEC	C96.9	C79.52	—	—	—	D47.9
right side	C40.31	C79.51	—	D16.31	D48.0	D49.2
marrow NEC	C96.9	C79.52	—	—	—	D47.9
unspecified side	C40.30	C79.51	—	D16.30	D48.0	D49.2
marrow NEC	C96.9	C79.52	—	—	—	D47.9
forearm						
left side	C40.02	C79.51	—	D16.02	D48.0	D49.2
marrow NEC	C96.9	C79.52	—	—	—	D47.9
right side	C40.01	C79.51	—	D16.01	D48.0	D49.2
marrow NEC	C96.9	C79.52	—	—	—	D47.9
unspecified side	C40.00	C79.51	—	D16.00	D48.0	D49.2
marrow NEC	C96.9	C79.52	—	—	—	D47.9
frontal	C41.0	C79.51	—	D16.4	D48.0	D49.2
marrow NEC	C96.9	C79.52	—	—	—	D47.9
hand						
left side	C40.12	C79.51	—	D16.12	D48.0	D49.2
marrow NEC	C96.9	C79.52	—	—	—	D47.9
right side	C40.11	C79.51	—	D16.11	D48.0	D49.2
marrow NEC	C96.9	C79.52	—	—	—	D47.9
unspecified side	C40.10	C79.51	—	D16.10	D48.0	D49.2
marrow NEC	C96.9	C79.52	—	—	—	D47.9
heel						
left side	C40.32	C79.51	—	D16.32	D48.0	D49.2
marrow NEC	C96.9	C79.52	—	—	—	D47.9
right side	C40.31	C79.51	—	D16.31	D48.0	D49.2
marrow NEC	C96.9	C79.52	—	—	—	D47.9
unspecified side	C40.30	C79.51	—	D16.30	D48.0	D49.2
marrow NEC	C96.9	C79.52	—	—	—	D47.9
hip	C41.4	C79.51	—	D16.8	D48.0	D49.2
marrow NEC	C96.9	C79.52	—	—	—	D47.9
humerus (any part)						
left side	C40.02	C79.51	—	D16.02	D48.0	D49.2
marrow NEC	C96.9	C79.52	—	—	—	D47.9
right side	C40.01	C79.51	—	D16.01	D48.0	D49.2
marrow NEC	C96.9	C79.52	—	—	—	D47.9
unspecified side	C40.00	C79.51	—	D16.00	D48.0	D49.2
marrow NEC	C96.9	C79.52	—	—	—	D47.9
hyoid	C41.0	C79.51	—	D16.4	D48.0	D49.2
marrow NEC	C96.9	C79.52	—	—	—	D47.9
ilium	C41.4	C79.51	—	D16.8	D48.0	D49.2
marrow NEC	C96.9	C79.52	—	—	—	D47.9
innominate	C41.4	C79.51	—	D16.8	D48.0	D49.2
marrow NEC	C96.9	C79.52	—	—	—	D47.9
intervertebral cartilage or disc	C41.2	C79.51	—	D16.6	D48.0	D49.2
marrow NEC	C96.9	C79.52	—	—	—	D47.9
ischium	C41.4	C79.51	—	D16.8	D48.0	D49.2
marrow NEC	C96.9	C79.52	—	—	—	D47.9
jaw (lower)	C41.1	C79.51	—	D16.5	D48.0	D49.2
marrow NEC	C96.9	C79.52	—	—	—	D47.9
upper	C41.0	C79.51	—	D16.4	D48.0	D49.2
marrow NEC	C96.9	C79.52	—	—	—	D47.9
knee						
left side	C40.22	C79.51	—	D16.22	D48.0	D49.2
marrow NEC	C96.9	C79.52	—	—	—	D47.9
right side	C40.21	C79.51	—	D16.21	D48.0	D49.2
marrow NEC	C96.9	C79.52	—	—	—	D47.9
unspecified side	C40.20	C79.51	—	D16.20	D48.0	D49.2
marrow NEC	C96.9	C79.52	—	—	—	D47.9
leg NEC						
left side	C40.22	C79.51	—	D16.22	D48.0	D49.2
marrow NEC	C96.9	C79.52	—	—	—	D47.9
right side	C40.21	C79.51	—	D16.21	D48.0	D49.2
marrow NEC	C96.9	C79.52	—	—	—	D47.9

©2002 Ingenix, Inc.

	Malignant			Benign	Uncertain Behavior	Unspecified
	Primary	Secondary	Ca in situ	Benign	Uncertain Behavior	Unspecified
Neoplasm, neoplastic — *continued*						
bone — *continued*						
leg NEC — *continued*						
unspecified side	C40.20	C79.51	—	D16.20	D48.0	D49.2
marrow NEC	C96.9	C79.52	—	—	—	D47.9
limb NEC						
lower						
long bones						
left side	C40.20	C79.51	—	D16.21	D48.0	D49.2
marrow NEC	C96.9	C79.52	—	—	—	D47.9
right side	C40.22	C79.51	—	D16.22	D48.0	D49.2
marrow NEC	C96.9	C79.52	—	—	—	D47.9
unspecified side	C40.21	C79.51	—	D16.20	D48.0	D49.2
marrow NEC	C96.9	C79.52	—	—	—	D47.9
short bones						
left side	C40.32	C79.51	—	D16.32	D48.0	D49.2
marrow NEC	C96.9	C79.52	—	—	—	D47.9
right side	C40.31	C79.51	—	D16.31	D48.0	D49.2
marrow NEC	C96.9	C79.52	—	—	—	D47.9
unspecified side	C40.30	C79.51	—	D16.30	D48.0	D49.2
marrow NEC	C96.9	C79.52	—	—	—	D47.9
unspecified site						
left side	C40.22	C79.51	—	D16.22	D48.0	D49.2
marrow NEC	C96.9	C79.52	—	—	—	D47.9
right side	C40.21	C79.51	—	D16.21	D48.0	D49.2
marrow NEC	C96.9	C79.52	—	—	—	D47.9
unspecified side	C40.20	C79.51	—	D16.20	D48.0	D49.2
marrow NEC	C96.9	C79.52	—	—	—	D47.9
unspecified site						
left side	C40.92	C79.51	—	D16.9	D48.0	D49.2
marrow NEC	C96.9	C79.52	—	—	—	D47.9
right side	C40.91	C79.51	—	D16.9	D48.0	D49.2
marrow NEC	C96.9	C79.52	—	—	—	D47.9
unspecified side	C40.90	C79.51	—	D16.9	D48.0	D49.2
marrow NEC	C96.9	C79.52	—	—	—	D47.9
upper						
long bones						
left side	C40.02	C79.51	—	D16.02	D48.0	D49.2
marrow NEC	C96.9	C79.52	—	—	—	D47.9
right side	C40.01	C79.51	—	D16.01	D48.0	D49.2
marrow NEC	C96.9	C79.52	—	—	—	D47.9
unspecified side	C40.00	C79.51	—	D16.00	D48.0	D49.2
marrow NEC	C96.9	C79.52	—	—	—	D47.9
short bones						
left side	C40.12	C79.51	—	D16.12	D48.0	D49.2
marrow NEC	C96.9	C79.52	—	—	—	D47.9
right side	C40.11	C79.51	—	D16.11	D48.0	D49.2
marrow NEC	C96.9	C79.52	—	—	—	D47.9
unspecified side	C40.10	C79.51	—	D16.10	D48.0	D49.2
marrow NEC	C96.9	C79.52	—	—	—	D47.9
unspecified site						
left side	C40.02	C79.51	—	D16.02	D48.0	D49.2
marrow NEC	C96.9	C79.52	—	—	—	D47.9
right side	C40.01	C79.51	—	D16.01	D48.0	D49.2
marrow NEC	C96.9	C79.52	—	—	—	D47.9
unspecified side	C40.00	C79.51	—	D16.00	D48.0	D49.2
marrow NEC	C96.9	C79.52	—	—	—	D47.9
long						
lower limbs NEC						
left side	C40.22	C79.51	—	D16.22	D48.0	D49.2
marrow NEC	C96.9	C79.52	—	—	—	D47.9
right side	C40.21	C79.51	—	D16.21	D48.0	D49.2
marrow NEC	C96.9	C79.52	—	—	—	D47.9
unspecified side	C40.20	C79.51	—	D16.20	D48.0	D49.2
marrow NEC	C96.9	C79.52	—	—	—	D47.9

			Malignant					
			Primary	**Secondary**	**Ca in situ**	**Benign**	**Uncertain Behavior**	**Unspecified**
Neoplasm, neoplastic — *continued*								
bone — *continued*								
long — *continued*								
unspecified site								
left side			C40.92	C79.51	—	D16.9	D48.0	D49.2
marrow NEC			C96.9	C79.52	—	—	—	D47.9
right side			C40.91	C79.51	—	D16.9	D48.0	D49.2
marrow NEC			C96.9	C79.52	—	—	—	D47.9
unspecified side			C40.90	C79.51	—	D16.9	D48.0	D49.2
marrow NEC			C96.9	C79.52	—	—	—	D47.9
upper limbs NEC								
left side			C40.02	C79.51	—	D16.02	D48.0	D49.2
marrow NEC			C96.9	C79.52	—	—	—	D47.9
right side			C40.01	C79.51	—	D16.01	D48.0	D49.2
marrow NEC			C96.9	C79.52	—	—	—	D47.9
unspecified side			C40.00	C79.51	—	D16.00	D48.0	D49.2
marrow NEC			C96.9	C79.52	—	—	—	D47.9
malar			C41.0	C79.51	—	D16.4	D48.0	D49.2
marrow NEC			C96.9	C79.52	—	—	—	D47.9
mandible			C41.1	C79.51	—	D16.5	D48.0	D49.2
marrow NEC			C96.9	C79.52	—	—	—	D47.9
marrow NEC			C96.9	C79.52	—	—	—	D47.9
mastoid			C41.0	C79.51	—	D16.4	D48.0	D49.2
marrow NEC			C96.9	C79.52	—	—	—	D47.9
maxilla, maxillary (superior)			C41.0	C79.51	—	D16.4	D48.0	D49.2
marrow NEC			C96.9	C79.52	—	—	—	D47.9
inferior			C41.1	C79.51	—	D16.5	D48.0	D49.2
marrow NEC			C96.9	C79.52	—	—	—	D47.9
metacarpus (any)								
left side			C40.12	C79.51	—	D16.12	D48.0	D49.2
marrow NEC			C96.9	C79.52	—	—	—	D47.9
right side			C40.11	C79.51	—	D16.11	D48.0	D49.2
marrow NEC			C96.9	C79.52	—	—	—	D47.9
unspecified side			C40.10	C79.51	—	D16.10	D48.0	D49.2
marrow NEC			C96.9	C79.52	—	—	—	D47.9
metatarsus (any)								
left side			C40.32	C79.51	—	D16.32	D48.0	D49.2
marrow NEC			C96.9	C79.52	—	—	—	D47.9
right side			C40.31	C79.51	—	D16.31	D48.0	D49.2
marrow NEC			C96.9	C79.52	—	—	—	D47.9
unspecified side			C40.30	C79.51	—	D16.30	D48.0	D49.2
marrow NEC			C96.9	C79.52	—	—	—	D47.9
navicular								
ankle								
left side			C40.32	C79.51	—	D16.32	D48.0	D49.2
marrow NEC			C96.9	C79.52	—	—	—	D47.9
right side			C40.31	C79.51	—	D16.31	D48.0	D49.2
marrow NEC			C96.9	C79.52	—	—	—	D47.9
unspecified side			C40.30	C79.51	—	D16.30	D48.0	D49.2
marrow NEC			C96.9	C79.52	—	—	—	D47.9
hand								
left side			C40.12	C79.51	—	D16.12	D48.0	D49.2
marrow NEC			C96.9	C79.52	—	—	—	D47.9
right side			C40.11	C79.51	—	D16.11	D48.0	D49.2
marrow NEC			C96.9	C79.52	—	—	—	D47.9
unspecified side			C40.10	C79.51	—	D16.10	D48.0	D49.2
marrow NEC			C96.9	C79.52	—	—	—	D47.9
unspecified site								
left side			C40.32	C79.51	—	D16.32	D48.0	D49.2
marrow NEC			C96.9	C79.52	—	—	—	D47.9
right side			C40.31	C79.51	—	D16.31	D48.0	D49.2
marrow NEC			C96.9	C79.52	—	—	—	D47.9
unspecified side			C40.30	C79.51	—	D16.30	D48.0	D49.2
marrow NEC			C96.9	C79.52	—	—	—	D47.9
nose, nasal			C41.0	C79.51	—	D16.4	D48.0	D49.2
marrow NEC			C96.9	C79.52	—	—	—	D47.9

©2002 Ingenix, Inc.

	Malignant			Benign	Uncertain Behavior	Unspecified
	Primary	Secondary	Ca in situ			
Neoplasm, neoplastic — *continued*						
bone — *continued*						
occipital	C41.0	C79.51	—	D16.4	D48.0	D49.2
marrow NEC	C96.9	C79.52	—	—	—	D47.9
orbit	C41.0	C79.51	—	D16.4	D48.0	D49.2
marrow NEC	C96.9	C79.52	—	—	—	D47.9
parietal	C41.0	C79.51	—	D16.4	D48.0	D49.2
marrow NEC	C96.9	C79.52	—	—	—	D47.9
patella						
left side	C40.32	C79.51	—	D16.32	D48.0	D49.2
marrow NEC	C96.9	C79.52	—	—	—	D47.9
right side	C40.31	C79.51	—	D16.31	D48.0	D49.2
marrow NEC	C96.9	C79.52	—	—	—	D47.9
unspecified side	C40.30	C79.51	—	D16.30	D48.0	D49.2
marrow NEC	C96.9	C79.52	—	—	—	D47.9
pelvic	C41.4	C79.51	—	D16.8	D48.0	D49.2
marrow NEC	C96.9	C79.52	—	—	—	D47.9
phalanges						
foot						
left side	C40.32	C79.51	—	D16.32	D48.0	D49.2
marrow NEC	C96.9	C79.52	—	—	—	D47.9
right side	C40.31	C79.51	—	D16.31	D48.0	D49.2
marrow NEC	C96.9	C79.52	—	—	—	D47.9
unspecified side	C40.30	C79.51	—	D16.30	D48.0	D49.2
marrow NEC	C96.9	C79.52	—	—	—	D47.9
hand						
left side	C40.12	C79.51	—	D16.12	D48.0	D49.2
marrow NEC	C96.9	C79.52	—	—	—	D47.9
right side	C40.11	C79.51	—	D16.11	D48.0	D49.2
marrow NEC	C96.9	C79.52	—	—	—	D47.9
unspecified side	C40.10	C79.51	—	D16.10	D48.0	D49.2
marrow NEC	C96.9	C79.52	—	—	—	D47.9
unspecified site						
left side	C40.92	C79.51	—	D16.9	D48.0	D49.2
marrow NEC	C96.9	C79.52	—	—	—	D47.9
right side	C40.91	C79.51	—	D16.9	D48.0	D49.2
marrow NEC	C96.9	C79.52	—	—	—	D47.9
unspecified side	C40.90	C79.51	—	D16.9	D48.0	D49.2
marrow NEC	C96.9	C79.52	—	—	—	D47.9
pubic	C41.4	C79.51	—	D16.8	D48.0	D49.2
marrow NEC	C96.9	C79.52	—	—	—	D47.9
radius (any part)						
left side	C40.02	C79.51	—	D16.02	D48.0	D49.2
marrow NEC	C96.9	C79.52	—	—	—	D47.9
right side	C40.01	C79.51	—	D16.01	D48.0	D49.2
marrow NEC	C96.9	C79.52	—	—	—	D47.9
unspecified side	C40.00	C79.51	—	D16.00	D48.0	D49.2
marrow NEC	C96.9	C79.52	—	—	—	D47.9
rib	C41.3	C79.51	—	D16.7	D48.0	D49.2
marrow NEC	C96.9	C79.52	—	—	—	D47.9
sacral vertebra	C41.4	C79.51	—	D16.8	D48.0	D49.2
marrow NEC	C96.9	C79.52	—	—	—	D47.9
sacrum	C41.4	C79.51	—	D16.8	D48.0	D49.2
marrow NEC	C96.9	C79.52	—	—	—	D47.9
scaphoid						
of ankle						
left side	C40.32	C79.51	—	D16.32	D48.0	D49.2
marrow NEC	C96.9	C79.52	—	—	—	D47.9
right side	C40.31	C79.51	—	D16.31	D48.0	D49.2
marrow NEC	C96.9	C79.52	—	—	—	D47.9
unspecified side	C40.30	C79.51	—	D16.30	D48.0	D49.2
marrow NEC	C96.9	C79.52	—	—	—	D47.9
of hand						
left side	C40.12	C79.51	—	D16.12	D48.0	D49.2
marrow NEC	C96.9	C79.52	—	—	—	D47.9
right side	C40.11	C79.51	—	D16.11	D48.0	D49.2
marrow NEC	C96.9	C79.52	—	—	—	D47.9

| | Malignant | | | | | |
	Primary	Secondary	Ca in situ	Benign	Uncertain Behavior	Unspecified
Neoplasm, neoplastic — *continued*						
bone — *continued*						
scaphoid — *continued*						
of hand — *continued*						
unspecified side	C40.10	C79.51	—	D16.10	D48.0	D49.2
marrow NEC	C96.9	C79.52	—	—	—	D47.9
unspecified site						
left side	C40.12	C79.51	—	D16.12	D48.0	D49.2
marrow NEC	C96.9	C79.52	—	—	—	D47.9
right side	C40.11	C79.51	—	D16.11	D48.0	D49.2
marrow NEC	C96.9	C79.52	—	—	—	D47.9
unspecified side	C40.10	C79.51	—	D16.10	D48.0	D49.2
marrow NEC	C96.9	C79.52	—	—	—	D47.9
scapula (any part)						
left side	C40.02	C79.51	—	D16.02	D48.0	D49.2
marrow NEC	C96.9	C79.52	—	—	—	D47.9
right side	C40.01	C79.51	—	D16.01	D48.0	D49.2
marrow NEC	C96.9	C79.52	—	—	—	D47.9
unspecified side	C40.00	C79.51	—	D16.00	D48.0	D49.2
marrow NEC	C96.9	C79.52	—	—	—	D47.9
sella turcica	C41.0	C79.51	—	D16.4	D48.0	D49.2
marrow NEC	C96.9	C79.52	—	—	—	D47.9
short						
lower limb						
left side	C40.32	C79.51	—	D16.32	D48.0	D49.2
marrow NEC	C96.9	C79.52	—	—	—	D47.9
right side	C40.31	C79.51	—	D16.31	D48.0	D49.2
marrow NEC	C96.9	C79.52	—	—	—	D47.9
unspecified side	C40.30	C79.51	—	D16.30	D48.0	D49.2
marrow NEC	C96.9	C79.52	—	—	—	D47.9
unspecified site						
left side	C40.92	C79.51	—	D16.9	D48.0	D49.2
marrow NEC	C96.9	C79.52	—	—	—	D47.9
right side	C40.91	C79.51	—	D16.9	D48.0	D49.2
marrow NEC	C96.9	C79.52	—	—	—	D47.9
unspecified side	C40.90	C79.51	—	D16.9	D48.0	D49.2
marrow NEC	C96.9	C79.52	—	—	—	D47.9
upper limb						
left side	C40.12	C79.51	—	D16.12	D48.0	D49.2
marrow NEC	C96.9	C79.52	—	—	—	D47.9
right side	C40.11	C79.51	—	D16.11	D48.0	D49.2
marrow NEC	C96.9	C79.52	—	—	—	D47.9
unspecified side	C40.10	C79.51	—	D16.10	D48.0	D49.2
marrow NEC	C96.9	C79.52	—	—	—	D47.9
shoulder						
left side	C40.02	C79.51	—	D16.02	D48.0	D49.2
marrow NEC	C96.9	C79.52	—	—	—	D47.9
right side	C40.01	C79.51	—	D16.01	D48.0	D49.2
marrow NEC	C96.9	C79.52	—	—	—	D47.9
unspecified side	C40.00	C79.51	—	D16.00	D48.0	D49.2
marrow NEC	C96.9	C79.52	—	—	—	D47.9
skeleton, skeletal NEC	C41.9	C79.51	—	D16.9	D48.0	D49.2
marrow NEC	C96.9	C79.52	—	—	—	D47.9
skull	C41.0	C79.51	—	D16.4	D48.0	D49.2
marrow NEC	C96.9	C79.52	—	—	—	D47.9
sphenoid	C41.0	C79.51	—	D16.4	D48.0	D49.2
marrow NEC	C96.9	C79.52	—	—	—	D47.9
spine, spinal (column)	C41.2	C79.51	—	D16.6	D48.0	D49.2
coccyx	C41.4	C79.51	—	D16.8	D48.0	D49.2
marrow NEC	C96.9	C79.52	—	—	—	D47.9
marrow NEC	C96.9	C79.52	—	—	—	D47.9
sacrum	C41.4	C79.51	—	D16.8	D48.0	D49.2
marrow NEC	C96.9	C79.52	—	—	—	D47.9
sternum	C41.3	C79.51	—	D16.7	D48.0	D49.2
marrow NEC	C96.9	C79.52	—	—	—	D47.9

©2002 Ingenix, Inc.

	Malignant			Benign	Uncertain Behavior	Unspecified
	Primary	Secondary	Ca in situ			
Neoplasm, neoplastic — *continued*						
bone — *continued*						
tarsus (any)						
left side	C40.32	C79.51	—	D16.32	D48.0	D49.2
marrow NEC	C96.9	C79.52	—	—	—	D47.9
right side	C40.31	C79.51	—	D16.31	D48.0	D49.2
marrow NEC	C96.9	C79.52	—	—	—	D47.9
unspecified side	C40.30	C79.51	—	D16.30	D48.0	D49.2
marrow NEC	C96.9	C79.52	—	—	—	D47.9
temporal	C41.0	C79.51	—	D16.4	D48.0	D49.2
marrow NEC	C96.9	C79.52	—	—	—	D47.9
thumb						
left side	C40.12	C79.51	—	D16.12	D48.0	D49.2
marrow NEC	C96.9	C79.52	—	—	—	D47.9
right side	C40.11	C79.51	—	D16.11	D48.0	D49.2
marrow NEC	C96.9	C79.52	—	—	—	D47.9
unspecified side	C40.10	C79.51	—	D16.10	D48.0	D49.2
marrow NEC	C96.9	C79.52	—	—	—	D47.9
tibia (any part)						
left side	C40.22	C79.51	—	D16.22	D48.0	D49.2
marrow NEC	C96.9	C79.52	—	—	—	D47.9
right side	C40.21	C79.51	—	D16.21	D48.0	D49.2
marrow NEC	C96.9	C79.52	—	—	—	D47.9
unspecified side	C40.20	C79.51	—	D16.20	D48.0	D49.2
marrow NEC	C96.9	C79.52	—	—	—	D47.9
toe (any)						
left side	C40.32	C79.51	—	D16.32	D48.0	D49.2
marrow NEC	C96.9	C79.52	—	—	—	D47.9
right side	C40.31	C79.51	—	D16.31	D48.0	D49.2
marrow NEC	C96.9	C79.52	—	—	—	D47.9
unspecified side	C40.30	C79.51	—	D16.30	D48.0	D49.2
marrow NEC	C96.9	C79.52	—	—	—	D47.9
trapezium						
left side	C40.12	C79.51	—	D16.12	D48.0	D49.2
marrow NEC	C96.9	C79.52	—	—	—	D47.9
right side	C40.11	C79.51	—	D16.11	D48.0	D49.2
marrow NEC	C96.9	C79.52	—	—	—	D47.9
unspecified side	C40.10	C79.51	—	D16.10	D48.0	D49.2
marrow NEC	C96.9	C79.52	—	—	—	D47.9
trapezoid						
left side	C40.12	C79.51	—	D16.12	D48.0	D49.2
marrow NEC	C96.9	C79.52	—	—	—	D47.9
right side	C40.11	C79.51	—	D16.11	D48.0	D49.2
marrow NEC	C96.9	C79.52	—	—	—	D47.9
unspecified side	C40.10	C79.51	—	D16.10	D48.0	D49.2
marrow NEC	C96.9	C79.52	—	—	—	D47.9
turbinate	C41.0	C79.51	—	D16.4	D48.0	D49.2
marrow NEC	C96.9	C79.52	—	—	—	D47.9
ulna (any part)						
left side	C40.02	C79.51	—	D16.02	D48.0	D49.2
marrow NEC	C96.9	C79.52	—	—	—	D47.9
right side	C40.01	C79.51	—	D16.01	D48.0	D49.2
marrow NEC	C96.9	C79.52	—	—	—	D47.9
unspecified side	C40.00	C79.51	—	D16.00	D48.0	D49.2
marrow NEC	C96.9	C79.52	—	—	—	D47.9
unciform						
left side	C40.12	C79.51	—	D16.12	D48.0	D49.2
marrow NEC	C96.9	C79.52	—	—	—	D47.9
right side	C40.11	C79.51	—	D16.11	D48.0	D49.2
marrow NEC	C96.9	C79.52	—	—	—	D47.9
unspecified side	C40.10	C79.51	—	D16.10	D48.0	D49.2
marrow NEC	C96.9	C79.52	—	—	—	D47.9
vertebra (column)	C41.2	C79.51	—	D16.6	D48.0	D49.2
coccyx	C41.4	C79.51	—	D16.8	D48.0	D49.2
marrow NEC	C96.9	C79.52	—	—	—	D47.9
marrow NEC	C96.9	C79.52	—	—	—	D47.9

©2002 Ingenix, Inc.

	Malignant					
	Primary	Secondary	Ca in situ	Benign	Uncertain Behavior	Unspecified
Neoplasm, neoplastic — *continued*						
bone — *continued*						
vertebra — *continued*						
sacrum	C41.4	C79.51	—	D16.8	D48.0	D49.2
marrow NEC	C96.9	C79.52	—	—	—	D47.9
vomer	C41.0	C79.51	—	D16.4	D48.0	D49.2
marrow NEC	C96.9	C79.52	—	—	—	D47.9
wrist						
left side	C40.12	C79.51	—	D16.12	D48.0	D49.2
marrow NEC	C96.9	C79.52	—	—	—	D47.9
right side	C40.11	C79.51	—	D16.11	D48.0	D49.2
marrow NEC	C96.9	C79.52	—	—	—	D47.9
unspecified side	C40.10	C79.51	—	D16.10	D48.0	D49.2
marrow NEC	C96.9	C79.52	—	—	—	D47.9
xiphoid process	C41.3	C79.51	—	D16.7	D48.0	D49.2
marrow NEC	C96.9	C79.52	—	—	—	D47.9
zygomatic	C41.0	C79.51	—	D16.4	D48.0	D49.2
marrow NEC	C96.9	C79.52	—	—	—	D47.9
book-leaf (mouth)	C06.89	C79.89	D00.00	D10.39	D37.09	D49.0
bowel — see Neoplasm, intestine						
brachial plexus (unspecified side)	C47.10	C79.89	—	D36.12	D48.2	D49.2
left side	C47.12	C79.89	—	D36.12	D48.2	D49.2
right side	C47.11	C79.89	—	D36.12	D48.2	D49.2
brain NEC	C71.9	C79.31	—	D33.2	D43.2	D49.6
basal ganglia	C71.0	C79.31	—	D33.0	D43.0	D49.6
cerebellopontine angle	C71.6	C79.31	—	D33.1	D43.1	D49.6
cerebellum NOS	C71.6	C79.31	—	D33.1	D43.1	D49.6
cerebrum	C71.0	C79.31	—	D33.0	D43.0	D49.6
choroid plexus	C71.7	C79.31	—	D33.1	D43.1	D49.6
corpus callosum	C71.8	C79.31	—	D33.2	D43.2	D49.6
corpus striatum	C71.0	C79.31	—	D33.0	D43.0	D49.6
cortex (cerebral)	C71.0	C79.31	—	D33.0	D43.0	D49.6
frontal lobe	C71.1	C79.31	—	D33.0	D43.0	D49.6
globus pallidus	C71.0	C79.31	—	D33.0	D43.0	D49.6
hippocampus	C71.2	C79.31	—	D33.0	D43.0	D49.6
hypothalamus	C71.0	C79.31	—	D33.0	D43.0	D49.6
internal capsule	C71.0	C79.31	—	D33.0	D43.0	D49.6
medulla oblongata	C71.7	C79.31	—	D33.1	D43.1	D49.6
meninges	C70.0	C79.32	—	D32.0	D42.0	D49.7
midbrain	C71.7	C79.31	—	D33.1	D43.1	D49.6
occipital lobe	C71.4	C79.31	—	D33.0	D43.0	D49.6
overlapping lesion	C71.8	C79.31	—	—	—	—
parietal lobe	C71.3	C79.31	—	D33.0	D43.0	D49.6
peduncle	C71.7	C79.31	—	D33.1	D43.1	D49.6
pons	C71.7	C79.31	—	D33.1	D43.1	D49.6
stem	C71.7	C79.31	—	D33.1	D43.1	D49.6
tapetum	C71.8	C79.31	—	D33.2	D43.2	D49.6
temporal lobe	C71.2	C79.31	—	D33.0	D43.0	D49.6
thalamus	C71.0	C79.31	—	D33.0	D43.0	D49.6
uncus	C71.2	C79.31	—	D33.0	D43.0	D49.6
ventricle (floor)	C71.5	C79.31	—	D33.0	D43.0	D49.6
fourth	C71.7	C79.31	—	D33.1	D43.1	D49.6
branchial (cleft) (cyst) (vestiges)	C10.4	C79.89	D00.08	D10.5	D37.05	D49.0
breast (connective tissue) (glandular tissue) (soft parts)						
female						
areola (unspecified side)	C50.00	C79.81	D05.90	D24.00	D48.60	D49.3
left side	C50.02	C79.81	D05.92	D24.02	D48.62	D49.3
right side	C50.01	C79.81	D05.91	D24.01	D48.61	D49.3
axillary tail (unspecified side)	C50.60	C79.81	D05.90	D24.00	D48.60	D49.3
left side	C50.62	C79.81	D05.92	D24.02	D48.62	D49.3
right side	C50.61	C79.81	D05.91	D24.01	D48.61	D49.3
central portion (unspecified side)	C50.10	C79.81	D05.90	D24.00	D48.60	D49.3
left side	C50.12	C79.81	D05.92	D24.02	D48.62	D49.3
right side	C50.11	C79.81	D05.91	D24.01	D48.61	D49.3
ectopic sites (unspecified side)	C50.80	C79.81	D05.90	D24.00	D48.60	D49.3
left side	C50.82	C79.81	D05.92	D24.02	D48.62	D49.3
right side	C50.81	C79.81	D05.91	D24.01	D48.61	D49.3

©2002 Ingenix, Inc.

	Malignant					
	Primary	Secondary	Ca in situ	Benign	Uncertain Behavior	Unspecified
Neoplasm, neoplastic — *continued*						
breast — *continued*						
female — *continued*						
inner (unspecified side)	C50.80	C79.81	D05.90	D24.00	D48.60	D49.3
left side	C50.82	C79.81	D05.92	D24.02	D48.62	D49.3
right side	C50.81	C79.81	D05.91	D24.01	D48.61	D49.3
lower (unspecified side)	C50.80	C79.81	D05.90	D24.00	D48.60	D49.3
left side	C50.82	C79.81	D05.92	D24.02	D48.62	D49.3
right side	C50.81	C79.81	D05.91	D24.01	D48.61	D49.3
lower-inner quadrant (unspecified side)	C50.30	C79.81	D05.90	D24.00	D48.60	D49.3
left side	C50.32	C79.81	D05.92	D24.02	D48.62	D49.3
right side	C50.31	C79.81	D05.91	D24.01	D48.61	D49.3
lower-outer quadrant (unspecified side)	C50.50	C79.81	D05.90	D24.00	D48.60	D49.3
left side	C50.52	C79.81	D05.92	D24.02	D48.62	D49.3
right side	C50.51	C79.81	D05.91	D24.01	D48.61	D49.3
mastectomy site (skin)	C44.5	C79.2	—	—	—	—
specified as breast tissue (unspecified side)	C50.80	C79.81	—	—	—	—
left side	C50.82	C79.81	—	—	—	—
right side	C50.81	C79.81	—	—	—	—
midline (unspecified side)	C50.80	C79.81	D05.90	D24.00	D48.60	D49.3
left side	C50.82	C79.81	D05.92	D24.02	D48.62	D49.3
right side	C50.81	C79.81	D05.91	D24.01	D48.61	D49.3
nipple (unspecified side)	C50.00	C79.81	D05.90	D24.00	D48.60	D49.3
left side	C50.02	C79.81	D05.92	D24.02	D48.62	D49.3
right side	C50.01	C79.81	D05.91	D24.01	D48.61	D49.3
outer (unspecified side)	C50.80	C79.81	D05.90	D24.00	D48.60	D49.3
left side	C50.82	C79.81	D05.92	D24.02	D48.62	D49.3
right side	C50.81	C79.81	D05.91	D24.01	D48.61	D49.3
overlapping lesion (unspecified side)	C50.80	—	—	—	—	—
left side	C50.82	—	—	—	—	—
right side	C50.8	—	—	—	—	—
skin	C44.5	C79.2	D04.5	D23.5	D48.5	D49.2
tail (axillary) (unspecified side)	C50.60	C79.81	D05.90	D24.00	D48.60	D49.3
left side	C50.62	C79.81	D05.92	D24.02	D48.62	D49.3
right side	C50.61	C79.81	D05.91	D24.01	D48.61	D49.3
unspecified site (unspecified side)	C50.90	C79.81	D05.90	D24.00	D48.60	D49.3
left side	C50.92	C79.81	D05.92	D24.02	D48.62	D49.3
right side	C50.91	C79.81	D05.91	D24.01	D48.61	D49.3
upper (unspecified side)	C50.80	C79.81	D05.90	D24.00	D48.60	D49.3
left side	C50.82	C79.81	D05.92	D24.02	D48.62	D49.3
right side	C50.81	C79.81	D05.91	D24.01	D48.61	D49.3
upper-inner quadrant (unspecified side)	C50.20	C79.81	D05.90	D24.00	D48.60	D49.3
left side	C50.22	C79.81	D05.92	D24.02	D48.62	D49.3
right side	C50.21	C79.81	D05.91	D24.01	D48.61	D49.3
upper-outer quadrant (unspecified side)	C50.40	C79.81	D05.90	D24.00	D48.60	D49.3
left side	C50.42	C79.81	D05.92	D24.02	D48.62	D49.3
right side	C50.41	C79.81	D05.91	D24.01	D48.61	D49.3
male						
areola (unspecified side)	C50.05	C79.81	D05.95	D24.10	D48.65	D49.3
left side	C50.04	C79.81	D05.94	D24.12	D48.64	D49.3
right side	C50.03	C79.81	D05.93	D24.11	D48.63	D49.3
axillary tail (unspecified side)	C50.65	C79.81	D05.95	D24.10	D48.65	D49.3
left side	C50.64	C79.81	D05.94	D24.12	D48.64	D49.3
right side	C50.63	C79.81	D05.93	D24.11	D48.63	D49.3
central portion (unspecified side)	C50.15	C79.81	D05.95	D24.10	D48.65	D49.3
left side	C50.14	C79.81	D05.94	D24.12	D48.64	D49.3
right side	C50.13	C79.81	D05.93	D24.11	D48.63	D49.3
ectopic sites (unspecified side)	C50.85	C79.81	D05.95	D24.10	D48.65	D49.3
left side	C50.84	C79.81	D05.94	D24.12	D48.64	D49.3
right side	C50.83	C79.81	D05.93	D24.11	D48.63	D49.3
inner (unspecified side)	C50.85	C79.81	D05.95	D24.10	D48.65	D49.3
left side	C50.84	C79.81	D05.94	D24.12	D48.64	D49.3
right side	C50.83	C79.81	D05.93	D24.11	D48.63	D49.3
lower (unspecified side)	C50.85	C79.81	D05.95	D24.10	D48.65	D49.3
left side	C50.84	C79.81	D05.94	D24.12	D48.64	D49.3
right side	C50.83	C79.81	D05.93	D24.11	D48.63	D49.3

	Malignant					
	Primary	**Secondary**	**Ca in situ**	**Benign**	**Uncertain Behavior**	**Unspecified**
Neoplasm, neoplastic — *continued*						
breast — *continued*						
lower-inner quadrant (unspecified side)	C50.35	C79.81	D05.95	D24.10	D48.65	D49.3
left side	C50.34	C79.81	D05.94	D24.12	D48.64	D49.3
right side	C50.33	C79.81	D05.93	D24.11	D48.63	D49.3
lower-outer quadrant (unspecified side)	C50.55	C79.81	D05.95	D24.10	D48.65	D49.3
left side	C50.54	C79.81	D05.94	D24.12	D48.64	D49.3
right side	C50.53	C79.81	D05.93	D24.11	D48.63	D49.3
mastectomy site (skin)	C44.5	C79.2	—	—	—	—
specified as breast tissue (unspecified side)	C50.85	C79.81	—	—	—	—
left side	C50.84	C79.81	—	—	—	—
right side	C50.83	C79.81	—	—	—	—
midline (unspecified side)	C50.85	C79.81	D05.95	D24.10	D48.65	D49.3
left side	C50.84	C79.81	D05.94	D24.12	D48.64	D49.3
right side	C50.83	C79.81	D05.93	D24.11	D48.63	D49.3
nipple (unspecified side)	C50.05	C79.81	D05.95	D24.10	D48.65	D49.3
left side	C50.04	C79.81	D05.94	D24.12	D48.64	D49.3
right side	C50.03	C79.81	D05.93	D24.11	D48.63	D49.3
outer (unspecified side)	C50.85	C79.81	D05.95	D24.10	D48.65	D49.3
left side	C50.84	C79.81	D05.94	D24.12	D48.64	D49.3
right side	C50.83	C79.81	D05.93	D24.11	D48.63	D49.3
overlapping lesion (unspecified side)	C50.85	—	—	—	—	—
left side	C50.84	—	—	—	—	—
right side	C50.83	—	—	—	—	—
skin	C44.5	C79.2	D04.5	D23.5	D48.5	D49.2
tail (axillary) (unspecified side)	C50.65	C79.81	D05.95	D24.10	D48.65	D49.3
left side	C50.64	C79.81	D05.94	D24.12	D48.64	D49.3
right side	C50.63	C79.81	D05.93	D24.11	D48.63	D49.3
unspecified site (unspecified side)	C50.95	C79.81	D05.95	D24.10	D48.65	D49.3
left side	C50.94	C79.81	D05.94	D24.12	D48.64	D49.3
right side	C50.93	C79.81	D05.93	D24.11	D48.63	D49.3
upper (unspecified side)	C50.85	C79.81	D05.95	D24.10	D48.65	D49.3
left side	C50.84	C79.81	D05.94	D24.12	D48.64	D49.3
right side	C50.83	C79.81	D05.93	D24.11	D48.63	D49.3
upper-inner quadrant (unspecified side)	C50.25	C79.81	D05.95	D24.10	D48.65	D49.3
left side	C50.24	C79.81	D05.94	D24.12	D48.64	D49.3
right side	C50.23	C79.81	D05.93	D24.11	D48.63	D49.3
upper-outer quadrant (unspecified side)	C50.45	C79.81	D05.95	D24.10	D48.65	D49.3
left side	C50.44	C79.81	D05.94	D24.12	D48.64	D49.3
right side	C50.43	C79.81	D05.93	D24.11	D48.63	D49.3
mastectomy site (skin)	C44.5	C79.2	—	—	—	—
specified as breast tissue						
female (unspecified side)	C50.80	C79.81	—	—	—	—
left side	C50.82	C79.81	—	—	—	—
right side	C50.81	C79.81	—	—	—	—
male (unspecified side)	C50.85	C79.81	—	—	—	—
left side	C50.84	C79.81	—	—	—	—
right side	C50.83	C79.81	—	—	—	—
skin	C44.5	C79.2	D04.5	D23.5	D48.5	D49.2
broad ligament	C57.1	C79.82	D07.39	D28.2	D39.7	D49.5
bronchiogenic, bronchogenic (lung) (unspecified side)	C34.90	C78.00	D02.20	D14.30	D38.1	D49.1
left side	C34.92	C78.02	D02.22	D14.32	D38.1	D49.1
right side	C34.91	C78.01	D02.21	D14.31	D38.1	D49.1
bronchiole (unspecified side)	C34.90	C78.00	D02.20	D14.30	D38.1	D49.1
left side	C34.92	C78.02	D02.22	D14.32	D38.1	D49.1
right side	C34.91	C78.01	D02.21	D14.31	D38.1	D49.1
bronchus						
carina (unspecified side)	C34.00	C78.00	D02.20	D14.30	D38.1	D49.1
left side	C34.02	C78.02	D02.22	D14.32	D38.1	D49.1
right side	C34.01	C78.01	D02.21	D14.31	D38.1	D49.1
lower lobe of lung (unspecified side)	C34.30	C78.00	D02.20	D14.30	D38.1	D49.1
left side	C34.32	C78.02	D02.22	D14.32	D38.1	D49.1
right side	C34.31	C78.01	D02.21	D14.31	D38.1	D49.1
main (unspecified side)	C34.00	C78.00	D02.20	D14.30	D38.1	D49.1
left side	C34.02	C78.02	D02.22	D14.32	D38.1	D49.1
right side	C34.01	C78.01	D02.21	D14.31	D38.1	D49.1
middle lobe of lung	C34.2	C78.01	D02.21	D14.31	D38.1	D49.1

©2002 *Ingenix, Inc.*

	Malignant					
	Primary	Secondary	Ca in situ	Benign	Uncertain Behavior	Unspecified
Neoplasm, neoplastic — *continued*						
bronchus — *continued*						
overlapping lesion (unspecified side)	C34.80	—	—	—	—	—
left side	C34.82	—	—	—	—	—
right side	C34.81	—	—	—	—	—
unspecified site (unspecified side)	C34.90	C78.00	D02.20	D14.30	D38.1	D49.1
left side	C34.92	C78.02	D02.22	D14.32	D38.1	D49.1
right side	C34.91	C78.01	D02.21	D14.31	D38.1	D49.1
upper lobe of lung (unspecified side)	C34.10	C78.00	D02.20	D14.30	D38.1	D49.1
left side	C34.12	C78.02	D02.22	D14.32	D38.1	D49.1
right side	C34.11	C78.01	D02.21	D14.31	D38.1	D49.1
brow	C44.31	C79.2	D04.39	D23.39	D48.5	D49.2
buccal (cavity)	C06.9	C79.89	D00.00	D10.30	D37.09	D49.0
commissure	C06.0	C79.89	D00.02	D10.39	D37.09	D49.0
groove (lower) (upper)	C06.1	C79.89	D00.02	D10.39	D37.09	D49.0
mucosa	C06.0	C79.89	D00.02	D10.39	D37.09	D49.0
sulcus (lower) (upper)	C06.1	C79.89	D00.02	D10.39	D37.09	D49.0
bulbourethral gland	C68.0	C79.19	D09.19	D30.4	D41.3	D49.5
bursa — *see* Neoplasm, connective tissue						
buttock NEC*	C76.3	C79.89	D04.5	D36.7	D48.7	D49.8
caecum — *see* Neoplasm, cecum						
calf (unspecified side)*	C76.50	C79.89	D04.70	D36.7	D48.7	D49.8
left side	C76.52	C79.89	D04.72	D36.7	D48.7	D49.8
right side	C76.51	C79.89	D04.71	D36.7	D48.7	D49.8
calvarium	C41.0	C79.51	—	D16.4	D48.0	D49.2
marrow NEC	C96.9	C79.52	—	—	—	D47.9
calyx, renal (unspecified side)	C65.9	C79.00	D09.19	D30.10	D41.10	D49.5
left side	C65.1	C79.02	D09.19	D30.12	D41.12	D49.5
right side	C65.0	C79.01	D09.19	D30.11	D41.11	D49.5
canal						
anal	C21.1	C78.5	D01.3	D12.9	D37.7	D49.0
auditory (external) (unspecified side)	C44.20	C79.2	D04.20	D23.20	D48.5	D49.2
left side	C44.22	C79.2	D04.22	D23.22	D48.5	D49.2
right side	C44.21	C79.2	D04.21	D23.21	D48.5	D49.2
auricular (external) (unspecified side)	C44.20	C79.2	D04.20	D23.20	D48.5	D49.2
left side	C44.22	C79.2	D04.22	D23.22	D48.5	D49.2
right side	C44.21	C79.2	D04.21	D23.21	D48.5	D49.2
canaliculi, biliary (biliferi) (intrahepatic)	C22.1	C78.89	D01.5	D13.4	D37.6	D49.0
canthus (eye) (inner) (outer) (unspecified side)	C44.10	C79.2	D04.10	D23.10	D48.5	D49.2
left side	C44.12	C79.2	D04.12	D23.12	D48.5	D49.2
right side	C44.11	C79.2	D04.11	D23.11	D48.5	D49.2
capillary — *see* Neoplasm, connective tissue						
caput coli	C18.0	C78.5	D01.0	D12.0	D37.4	D49.0
cardia (gastric)	C16.0	C78.89	D00.2	D13.1	D37.1	D49.0
cardiac orifice (stomach)	C16.0	C78.89	D00.2	D13.1	D37.1	D49.0
cardio-esophageal junction	C16.0	C78.89	D00.2	D13.1	D37.1	D49.0
cardio-esophagus	C16.0	C78.89	D00.2	D13.1	D37.1	D49.0
carina (bronchus) (unspecified side)	C34.00	C78.00	D02.20	D14.30	D38.1	D49.1
left side	C34.02	C78.02	D02.22	D14.32	D38.1	D49.1
right side	C34.01	C78.01	D02.21	D14.31	D38.1	D49.1
carotid (artery)	C49.0	C79.89	—	D21.0	D48.1	D49.2
body	C75.4	C79.89	—	D35.5	D44.6	D49.7
carpus (any bone)						
left side	C40.12	C79.51	—	D16.12	D48.0	D49.2
marrow NEC	C96.9	C79.52	—	—	—	D47.9
right side	C40.11	C79.51	—	D16.11	D48.0	D49.2
marrow NEC	C96.9	C79.52	—	—	—	D47.9
unspecified side	C40.10	C79.51	—	D16.10	D48.0	D49.2
marrow NEC	C96.9	C79.52	—	—	—	D47.9
cartilage (articular) (joint) NEC (*see also* Neoplasm, bone)	C41.9	C79.51	—	D16.9	D48.0	D49.2
arytenoid	C32.3	C78.39	D02.0	D14.1	D38.0	D49.1
auricular	C49.0	C79.89	—	D21.0	D48.1	D49.2
bronchi (unspecified side)	C34.00	C78.39	—	D14.30	D38.1	D49.1
left side	C34.02	C78.39	—	D14.32	D38.1	D49.1
right side	C34.01	C78.39	—	D14.31	D38.1	D49.1
connective tissue — *see* Neoplasm, connective tissue						
costal	C41.3	C79.51	—	D16.7	D48.0	D49.2

| | Malignant | | | | | |
	Primary	Secondary	Ca in situ	Benign	Uncertain Behavior	Unspecified
Neoplasm, neoplastic — *continued*						
cartilage NEC (see also Neoplasm, bone) — *continued*						
cricoid	C32.3	C78.39	D02.0	D14.1	D38.0	D49.1
cuneiform	C32.3	C78.39	D02.0	D14.1	D38.0	D49.1
ear (external)	C49.0	C79.89	—	D21.0	D48.1	D49.2
ensiform	C41.3	C79.51	—	D16.7	D48.0	D49.2
epiglottis	C32.1	C78.39	D02.0	D14.1	D38.0	D49.1
anterior surface	C10.1	C79.89	D00.08	D10.5	D37.05	D49.0
eyelid	C49.0	C79.89	—	D21.0	D48.1	D49.2
intervertebral	C41.2	C79.51	—	D16.6	D48.0	D49.2
larynx, laryngeal	C32.3	C78.39	D02.0	D14.1	D38.0	D49.1
nose, nasal	C30.0	C78.39	D02.3	D14.0	D38.5	D49.1
pinna	C49.0	C79.89	—	D21.0	D48.1	D49.2
rib	C41.3	C79.51	—	D16.7	D48.0	D49.2
semilunar (knee) (unspecified side)	C40.20	C79.51	—	D16.20	D48.0	D49.2
left side	C40.22	C79.51	—	D16.22	D48.0	D49.2
right side	C40.21	C79.51	—	D16.21	D48.0	D49.2
thyroid	C32.3	C78.39	D02.0	D14.1	D38.0	D49.1
trachea	C33	C78.39	D02.1	D14.2	D38.1	D49.1
cauda equina	C72.1	C79.49	—	D33.4	D43.4	D49.7
cavity						
buccal	C06.9	C79.89	D00.00	D10.30	D37.09	D49.0
nasal	C30.0	C78.39	D02.3	D14.0	D38.5	D49.1
oral	C06.9	C79.89	D00.00	D10.30	D37.09	D49.0
peritoneal	C48.2	C78.6	—	D20.1	D48.4	D49.0
tympanic	C30.1	C78.39	D02.3	D14.0	D38.5	D49.1
cecum	C18.0	C78.5	D01.0	D12.0	D37.4	D49.0
central nervous system — see also Neoplasm, nervous system						
white matter	C71.0	C79.31	—	D33.0	D43.0	D49.6
cerebellopontine (angle)	C71.6	C79.31	—	D33.1	D43.1	D49.6
cerebellum, cerebellar	C71.6	C79.31	—	D33.1	D43.1	D49.6
cerebrum, cerebral (cortex) (hemisphere) (white matter)	C71.0	C79.31	—	D33.0	D43.0	D49.6
meninges	C70.0	C79.32	—	D32.0	D42.0	D49.7
peduncle	C71.7	C79.31	—	D33.1	D43.1	D49.6
ventricle	C71.5	C79.31	—	D33.0	D43.0	D49.6
fourth	C71.7	C79.31	—	D33.1	D43.1	D49.6
cervical region	C76.0	C79.89	D09.7	D36.7	D48.7	D49.8
cervix (cervical) (uteri) (uterus)	C53.9	C79.82	D06.9	D26.0	D39.0	D49.5
canal	C53.0	C79.82	D06.0	D26.0	D39.0	D49.5
endocervix (canal) (gland)	C53.0	C79.82	D06.0	D26.0	D39.0	D49.5
exocervix	C53.1	C79.82	D06.1	D26.0	D39.0	D49.5
external os	C53.1	C79.82	D06.1	D26.0	D39.0	D49.5
internal os	C53.0	C79.82	D06.0	D26.0	D39.0	D49.5
nabothian gland	C53.0	C79.82	D06.0	D26.0	D39.0	D49.5
overlapping lesion	C53.8	—	—	—	—	—
squamocolumnar junction	C53.8	C79.82	D06.7	D26.0	D39.0	D49.5
stump	C53.8	C79.82	D06.7	D26.0	D39.0	D49.5
cheek	C76.0	C79.89	D09.7	D36.7	D48.7	D49.8
external	C44.31	C79.2	D04.39	D23.39	D48.5	D49.2
inner aspect	C06.0	C79.89	D00.02	D10.39	D37.09	D49.0
internal	C06.0	C79.89	D00.02	D10.39	D37.09	D49.0
mucosa	C06.0	C79.89	D00.02	D10.39	D37.09	D49.0
chest (wall) NEC	C76.1	C79.89	D09.7	D36.7	D48.7	D49.8
chiasma opticum (unspecified side)	C72.30	C79.49	—	D33.3	D43.3	D49.7
left side	C72.32	C79.49	—	D33.3	D43.3	D49.7
right side	C72.31	C79.49	—	D33.3	D43.3	D49.7
chin	C44.31	C79.2	D04.39	D23.39	D48.5	D49.2
choana	C11.3	C79.89	D00.08	D10.6	D37.05	D49.0
cholangiole	C22.1	C78.89	D01.5	D13.4	D37.6	D49.0
choledochal duct	C24.0	C78.89	D01.5	D13.5	D37.6	D49.0
choroid						
left side	C69.32	C79.49	D09.22	D31.32	D48.7	D49.8
plexus	C71.5	C79.31	—	D33.0	D43.0	D49.6
right side	C69.31	C79.49	D09.21	D31.31	D48.7	D49.8
plexus	C71.5	C79.31	—	D33.0	D43.0	D49.6
unspecified side	C69.30	C79.49	D09.20	D31.30	D48.7	D49.8
plexus	C71.5	C79.31	—	D33.0	D43.0	D49.6

©2002 Ingenix, Inc.

| | Malignant | | | | | |
	Primary	Secondary	Ca in situ	Benign	Uncertain Behavior	Unspecified
Neoplasm, neoplastic — *continued*						
ciliary body (unspecified side)	C69.40	C79.49	D09.20	D31.40	D48.7	D49.8
left side	C69.42	C79.49	D09.22	D31.42	D48.7	D49.8
right side	C69.41	C79.49	D09.21	D31.41	D48.7	D49.8
clavicle	C41.3	C79.51	—	D16.7	D48.0	D49.2
marrow NEC	C96.9	C79.52	—	—	—	D47.9
clitoris	C51.2	C79.82	D07.1	D28.0	D39.7	D49.5
clivus	C41.0	C79.51	—	D16.4	D48.0	D49.2
marrow NEC	C96.9	C79.52	—	—	—	D47.9
cloacogenic zone	C21.2	C78.5	D01.3	D12.9	D37.7	D49.0
coccygeal						
body or glomus	C75.5	C79.89	—	D35.6	D44.7	D49.7
vertebra	C41.4	C79.51	—	D16.8	D48.0	D49.2
marrow NEC	C96.9	C79.52	—	—	—	D47.9
coccyx	C41.4	C79.51	—	D16.8	D48.0	D49.2
marrow NEC	C96.9	C79.52	—	—	—	D47.9
colon — see also Neoplasm, intestine, large						
and rectum	C19	C78.5	D01.1	D12.7	D37.5	D49.0
column, spinal — see Neoplasm, spine						
columnella	C44.31	C79.2	D04.39	D23.39	D48.5	D49.2
commissure						
labial, lip	C00.6	C79.89	D00.01	D10.39	D37.01	D49.0
laryngeal	C32.0	C78.39	D02.0	D14.1	D38.0	D49.1
common (bile) duct	C24.0	C78.89	D01.5	D13.5	D37.6	D49.0
concha						
left side	C44.22	C79.2	D04.22	D23.22	D48.5	D49.2
nose	C30.0	C78.39	D02.3	D14.0	D38.5	D49.1
right side	C44.21	C79.2	D04.21	D23.21	D48.5	D49.2
nose	C30.0	C78.39	D02.3	D14.0	D38.5	D49.1
unspecified side	C44.20	C79.2	D04.20	D23.20	D48.5	D49.2
nose	C30.0	C78.39	D02.3	D14.0	D38.5	D49.1
conjunctiva (unspecified side)	C69.00	C79.49	D09.20	D31.00	D48.7	D49.8
left side	C69.02	C79.49	D09.22	D31.02	D48.7	D49.8
right side	C69.01	C79.49	D09.21	D31.01	D48.7	D49.8
connective tissue NEC	C49.9	C79.89		D21.9	D48.1	D49.2

Note — For neoplasms of connective tissue (blood vessel, bursa, fascia, ligament, muscle, synovia, tendon, etc.) or of morphological types that indicate connective tissue, code according to the list under "Neoplasm, connective tissue;" for sites that do not appear in this list, code to neoplasm of that site; e.g., liposarcoma, shoulder C49.10, leiomyosarcoma, stomach C16.9 *Morphological types that indicate connective tissue appear in their proper place in the alphabetic index with the instruction "see Neoplasm, connective tissue ...."*

abdomen	C49.4	C79.89	—	D21.4	D48.1	D49.2
abdominal wall	C49.4	C79.89	—	D21.4	D48.1	D49.2
ankle (unspecified side)	C49.20	C79.89	—	D21.20	D48.1	D49.2
left side	C49.22	C79.89	—	D21.22	D48.1	D49.2
right side	C49.21	C79.89	—	D21.21	D48.1	D49.2
antecubital fossa or space (unspecified side)	C49.10	C79.89	—	D21.20	D48.1	D49.2
left side	C49.12	C79.89	—	D21.22	D48.1	D49.2
right side	C49.11	C79.89	—	D21.21	D48.1	D49.2
arm (unspecified side)	C49.10	C79.89	—	D21.10	D48.1	D49.2
left side	C49.12	C79.89	—	D21.12	D48.1	D49.2
right side	C49.11	C79.89	—	D21.11	D48.1	D49.2
auricle (ear)	C49.0	C79.89	—	D21.0	D48.1	D49.2
axilla	C49.3	C79.89	—	D21.3	D48.1	D49.2
back	C49.6	C79.89	—	D21.6	D48.1	D49.2
breast — see Neoplasm, breast						
buttock	C49.5	C79.89	—	D21.5	D48.1	D49.2
calf (unspecified side)	C49.20	C79.89	—	D21.20	D48.1	D49.2
left side	C49.22	C79.89	—	D21.22	D48.1	D49.2
right side	C49.21	C79.89	—	D21.21	D48.1	D49.2
cervical region	C49.0	C79.89	—	D21.0	D48.1	D49.2
cheek	C49.0	C79.89	—	D21.0	D48.1	D49.2
chest (wall)	C49.3	C79.89	—	D21.3	D48.1	D49.2
chin	C49.0	C79.89	—	D21.0	D48.1	D49.2
diaphragm	C49.3	C79.89	—	D21.3	D48.1	D49.2
ear (external)	C49.0	C79.89	—	D21.0	D48.1	D49.2

	Malignant					
	Primary	Secondary	Ca in situ	Benign	Uncertain Behavior	Unspecified
Neoplasm, neoplastic — *continued*						
connective tissue NEC — *continued*						
elbow (unspecified side)	C49.10	C79.89	—	D21.10	D48.1	D49.2
left side	C49.12	C79.89	—	D21.12	D48.1	D49.2
right side	C49.11	C79.89	—	D21.11	D48.1	D49.2
extrarectal	C49.5	C79.89	—	D21.5	D48.1	D49.2
extremity	C49.9	C79.89	—	D21.9	D48.1	D49.2
lower (unspecified side)	C49.20	C79.89	—	D21.20	D48.1	D49.2
left side	C49.22	C79.89	—	D21.22	D48.1	D49.2
right side	C49.21	C79.89	—	D21.21	D48.1	D49.2
upper (unspecified side)	C49.10	C79.89	—	D21.10	D48.1	D49.2
left side	C49.12	C79.89	—	D21.12	D48.1	D49.2
right side	C49.11	C79.89	—	D21.11	D48.1	D49.2
eyelid	C49.0	C79.89	—	D21.0	D48.1	D49.2
face	C49.0	C79.89	—	D21.0	D48.1	D49.2
finger (unspecified side)	C49.10	C79.89	—	D21.10	D48.1	D49.2
left side	C49.12	C79.89	—	D21.12	D48.1	D49.2
right side	C49.11	C79.89	—	D21.11	D48.1	D49.2
flank	C49.6	C79.89	—	D21.6	D48.1	D49.2
foot (unspecified side)	C49.20	C79.89	—	D21.20	D48.1	D49.2
left side	C49.22	C79.89	—	D21.22	D48.1	D49.2
right side	C49.21	C79.89	—	D21.21	D48.1	D49.2
forearm (unspecified side)	C49.10	C79.89	—	D21.10	D48.1	D49.2
left side	C49.12	C79.89	—	D21.12	D48.1	D49.2
right side	C49.11	C79.89	—	D21.11	D48.1	D49.2
forehead	C49.0	C79.89	—	D21.0	D48.1	D49.2
gluteal region	C49.5	C79.89	—	D21.5	D48.1	D49.2
great vessels NEC	C49.3	C79.89	—	D21.3	D48.1	D49.2
groin	C49.5	C79.89	—	D21.5	D48.1	D49.2
hand (unspecified side)	C49.10	C79.89	—	D21.10	D48.1	D49.2
left side	C49.12	C79.89	—	D21.12	D48.1	D49.2
right side	C49.11	C79.89	—	D21.11	D48.1	D49.2
head	C49.0	C79.89	—	D21.0	D48.1	D49.2
heel (unspecified side)	C49.20	C79.89	—	D21.20	D48.1	D49.2
left side	C49.22	C79.89	—	D21.22	D48.1	D49.2
right side	C49.21	C79.89	—	D21.21	D48.1	D49.2
hip (unspecified side)	C49.20	C79.89	—	D21.20	D48.1	D49.2
left side	C49.22	C79.89	—	D21.22	D48.1	D49.2
right side	C49.21	C79.89	—	D21.21	D48.1	D49.2
hypochondrium	C49.4	C79.89	—	D21.4	D48.1	D49.2
iliopsoas muscle	C49.5	C79.89	—	D21.5	D48.1	D49.2
infraclavicular region	C49.3	C79.89	—	D21.3	D48.1	D49.2
inguinal (canal) (region)	C49.5	C79.89	—	D21.5	D48.1	D49.2
intrathoracic	C49.3	C79.89	—	D21.3	D48.1	D49.2
ischiorectal fossa	C49.5	C79.89	—	D21.5	D48.1	D49.2
jaw	C03.9	C79.89	D00.03	D10.39	D48.1	D49.0
knee (unspecified side)	C49.20	C79.89	—	D21.20	D48.1	D49.2
left side	C49.22	C79.89	—	D21.22	D48.1	D49.2
right side	C49.21	C79.89	—	D21.21	D48.1	D49.2
leg (unspecified side)	C49.20	C79.89	—	D21.20	D48.1	D49.2
left side	C49.22	C79.89	—	D21.22	D48.1	D49.2
right side	C49.21	C79.89	—	D21.21	D48.1	D49.2
limb NEC	C49.9	C79.89	—	D21.9	D48.1	D49.2
lower (unspecified side)	C49.20	C79.89	—	D21.20	D48.1	D49.2
left side	C49.22	C79.89	—	D21.22	D48.1	D49.2
right side	C49.21	C79.89	—	D21.21	D48.1	D49.2
upper (unspecified side)	C49.10	C79.89	—	D21.10	D48.1	D49.2
left side	C49.12	C79.89	—	D21.12	D48.1	D49.2
right side	C49.11	C79.89	—	D21.11	D48.1	D49.2
nates	C49.5	C79.89	—	D21.5	D48.1	D49.2
neck	C49.0	C79.89	—	D21.0	D48.1	D49.2
orbit (unspecified side)	C69.60	C79.49	D09.20	D31.60	D48.7	D49.8
left side	C69.62	C79.49	D09.22	D31.62	D48.7	D49.8
right side	C69.61	C79.49	D09.21	D61.61	D48.7	D49.8
overlapping lesion	C49.8	—	—	—	—	—
pararectal	C49.5	C79.89	—	D21.5	D48.1	D49.2

©2002 Ingenix, Inc.

	Malignant					
	Primary	**Secondary**	**Ca in situ**	**Benign**	**Uncertain Behavior**	**Unspecified**
Neoplasm, neoplastic — *continued*						
connective tissue NEC — *continued*						
para-urethral	C49.5	C79.89	—	D21.5	D48.1	D49.2
paravaginal	C49.5	C79.89	—	D21.5	D48.1	D49.2
pelvis (floor)	C49.5	C79.89	—	D21.5	D48.1	D49.2
pelvo-abdominal	C49.8	C79.89	—	D21.6	D48.1	D49.2
perineum	C49.5	C79.89	—	D21.5	D48.1	D49.2
perirectal (tissue)	C49.5	C79.89	—	D21.5	D48.1	D49.2
periurethral (tissue)	C49.5	C79.89	—	D21.5	D48.1	D49.2
popliteal fossa or space (unspecified side)	C49.20	C79.89	—	D21.20	D48.1	D49.2
left side	C49.22	C79.89	—	D21.22	D48.1	D49.2
right side	C49.21	C79.89	—	D21.21	D48.1	D49.2
presacral	C49.5	C79.89	—	D21.5	D48.1	D49.2
psoas muscle	C49.4	C79.89	—	D21.4	D48.1	D49.2
pterygoid fossa	C49.0	C79.89	—	D21.0	D48.1	D49.2
rectovaginal septum or wall	C49.5	C79.89	—	D21.5	D48.1	D49.2
rectovesical	C49.5	C79.89	—	D21.5	D48.1	D49.2
retroperitoneum	C48.0	C78.6	—	D20.0	D48.3	D49.0
sacrococcygeal region	C49.5	C79.89	—	D21.5	D48.1	D49.2
scalp	C49.0	C79.89	—	D21.0	D48.1	D49.2
scapular region	C49.3	C79.89	—	D21.3	D48.1	D49.2
shoulder (unspecified side)	C49.10	C79.89	—	D21.10	D48.1	D49.2
left side	C49.12	C79.89	—	D21.12	D48.1	D49.2
right side	C49.11	C79.89	—	D21.11	D48.1	D49.2
skin (dermis) NEC	C44.9	C79.2	D04.9	D23.9	D48.5	D49.2
submental	C49.0	C79.89	—	D21.0	D48.1	D49.2
supraclavicular region	C49.0	C79.89	—	D21.0	D48.1	D49.2
temple	C49.0	C79.89	—	D21.0	D48.1	D49.2
temporal region	C49.0	C79.89	—	D21.0	D48.1	D49.2
thigh (unspecified side)	C49.20	C79.89	—	D21.20	D48.1	D49.2
left side	C49.22	C79.89	—	D21.22	D48.1	D49.2
right side	C49.21	C79.89	—	D21.21	D48.1	D49.2
thoracic (duct) (wall)	C49.3	C79.89	—	D21.3	D48.1	D49.2
thorax	C49.3	C79.89	—	D21.3	D48.1	D49.2
thumb (unspecified side)	C49.10	C79.89	—	D21.10	D48.1	D49.2
left side	C49.12	C79.89	—	D21.12	D48.1	D49.2
right side	C49.11	C79.89	—	D21.11	D48.1	D49.2
toe (unspecified side)	C49.20	C79.89	—	D21.20	D48.1	D49.2
left side	C49.22	C79.89	—	D21.22	D48.1	D49.2
right side	C49.21	C79.89	—	D21.21	D48.1	D49.2
trunk	C49.6	C79.89	—	D21.6	D48.1	D49.2
umbilicus	C49.4	C79.89	—	D21.4	D48.1	D49.2
vesicorectal	C49.5	C79.89	—	D21.5	D48.1	D49.2
wrist (unspecified side)	C49.10	C79.89	—	D21.10	D48.1	D49.2
left side	C49.12	C79.89	—	D21.12	D48.1	D49.2
right side	C49.11	C79.89	—	D21.11	D48.1	D49.2
conus medullaris	C72.0	C79.49	—	D33.4	D43.4	D49.7
cord (true) (vocal)	C32.0	C78.39	D02.0	D14.1	D38.0	D49.1
false	C32.1	C78.39	D02.0	D14.1	D38.0	D49.1
spermatic (unspecified side)	C63.10	C79.82	D07.69	D29.7	D40.7	D49.5
left side	C63.12	C79.82	D07.69	D29.7	D40.7	D49.5
right side	C63.11	C79.82	D07.69	D29.7	D40.7	D49.5
spinal (cervical) (lumbar) (thoracic)	C72.0	C79.49	—	D33.4	D43.4	D49.7
cornea (limbus) (unspecified side)	C69.10	C79.49	D09.20	D31.10	D48.7	D49.8
left side	C69.12	C79.49	D09.22	D31.12	D48.7	D49.8
right side	C69.11	C79.49	D09.21	D31.11	D48.7	D49.8
corpus						
albicans (unspecified side)	C56.9	C79.60	D07.39	D27.9	D39.10	D49.5
left side	C56.1	C79.62	D07.39	D27.1	D39.12	D49.5
right side	C56.0	C79.61	D07.39	D27.0	D39.11	D49.5
callosum, brain	C71.0	C79.31	—	D33.2	D43.2	D49.6
cavernosum	C60.2	C79.82	D07.4	D29.0	D40.7	D49.5
gastric	C16.2	C78.89	D00.2	D13.1	D37.1	D49.0
penis	C60.2	C79.82	D07.4	D29.0	D40.7	D49.5
striatum, cerebrum	C71.0	C79.31	—	D33.0	D43.0	D49.6

	Malignant					
	Primary	**Secondary**	**Ca in situ**	**Benign**	**Uncertain Behavior**	**Unspecified**
Neoplasm, neoplastic — *continued*						
corpus — *continued*						
uteri	C54.9	C79.82	D07.0	D26.1	D39.0	D49.5
isthmus	C54.0	C79.82	D07.0	D26.1	D39.0	D49.5
cortex						
adrenal (unspecified side)	C74.00	C79.70	D09.3	D35.00	D44.10	D49.7
left side	C74.02	C79.72	D09.3	D35.02	D44.12	D49.7
right side	C74.01	C79.71	D09.3	D35.01	D44.11	D49.7
cerebral	C71.0	C79.31	—	D33.0	D43.0	D49.6
costal cartilage	C41.3	C79.51	—	D16.7	D48.0	D49.2
costovertebral joint	C41.3	C79.51	—	D16.7	D48.0	D49.2
marrow NEC	C96.9	C79.52	—	—	—	D47.9
Cowper's gland	C68.0	C79.19	D09.19	D30.4	D41.3	D49.5
cranial (fossa, any)	C71.9	C79.31	—	D33.2	D43.2	D49.6
meninges	C70.0	C79.32	—	D32.0	D42.0	D49.7
nerve	C72.50	C79.49	—	D33.3	D43.3	D49.7
specified NEC	C72.59	C79.49	—	D33.3	D43.3	D49.7
craniobuccal pouch	C75.2	C79.89	D09.3	D35.2	D44.3	D49.7
craniopharyngeal (duct) (pouch)	C75.2	C79.89	D09.3	D35.3	D44.4	D49.7
cricoid	C13.0	C79.89	D00.08	D10.7	D37.05	D49.0
cartilage	C32.3	C79.39	D02.0	D14.1	D38.0	D49.1
cricopharynx	C13.0	C79.89	D00.08	D10.7	D37.05	D49.0
crypt of Morgagni	C21.8	C78.5	D01.3	D12.9	D37.7	D49.0
crystalline lens (unspecified side)	C69.40	C79.49	D09.20	D31.40	D48.7	D49.8
left side	C69.42	C79.49	D09.22	D31.42	D48.7	D49.8
right side	C69.41	C79.49	D09.21	D31.41	D48.7	D49.8
cul-de-sac (Douglas')	C48.1	C78.6	—	D20.1	D48.4	D49.0
cuneiform cartilage	C32.3	C78.39	D02.0	D14.1	D38.0	D49.1
cutaneous — *see* Neoplasm, skin						
cutis — *see* Neoplasm, skin						
cystic (bile) duct (common)	C24.0	C78.89	D01.5	D13.5	D37.6	D49.0
dermis — *see* Neoplasm, skin						
diaphragm	C49.3	C79.89	—	D21.3	D48.1	D49.2
digestive organs, system, tube, or tract NEC	C26.9	C78.89	D01.9	D13.9	D37.9	D49.0
disc, intervertebral	C41.2	C79.51	—	D16.6	D48.0	D49.2
marrow NEC	C96.9	C79.52	—	—	—	D47.9
disease, generalized	C80.0	C80.0	D09.9	D36.9	D48.9	C80.0
disseminated	C80.0	C80.0	D09.9	D36.9	D48.9	C80.0
Douglas' cul-de-sac or pouch	C48.1	C78.6	—	D20.1	D48.4	D49.0
duodenojejunal junction	C17.8	C78.4	D01.49	D13.39	D37.2	D49.0
duodenum	C17.0	C78.4	D01.41	D14.2	D37.2	D49.0
dura (cranial) (mater)	C70.9	C79.49	—	D32.9	D42.9	D49.7
cerebral	C70.0	C79.32	—	D32.0	D42.0	D49.7
spinal	C70.1	C79.49	—	D32.1	D42.1	D49.7
ear (external)						
left side	C44.22	C79.2	D04.22	D23.22	D48.5	D49.2
auricle or auris	C44.22	C79.2	D04.22	D23.22	D48.5	D49.2
canal, external	C44.22	C79.2	D04.22	D23.22	D48.5	D49.2
cartilage	C49.0	C79.89	—	D21.0	D48.1	D49.2
external meatus	C44.22	C79.2	D04.22	D23.22	D48.5	D49.2
inner	C30.1	C78.39	D02.3	D14.0	D38.5	D49.1
lobule	C44.22	C79.2	D04.22	D23.22	D48.5	D49.2
middle	C30.1	C78.39	D02.3	D14.0	D38.5	D49.1
overlapping lesion with accessory sinuses	C31.8	—	—	—	—	—
skin	C44.22	C79.2	D04.22	D23.22	D48.5	D49.2
right side	C44.21	C79.2	D04.21	D23.21	D48.5	D49.2
auricle or auris	C44.21	C79.2	D04.21	D23.21	D48.5	D49.2
canal, external	C44.21	C79.2	D04.21	D23.21	D48.5	D49.2
cartilage	C49.0	C79.89	—	D21.0	D48.1	D49.2
external meatus	C44.21	C79.2	D04.21	D23.21	D48.5	D49.2
inner	C30.1	C78.39	D02.3	D14.0	D38.5	D49.1
lobule	C44.21	C79.2	D04.21	D23.21	D48.5	D49.2
middle	C30.1	C78.39	D02.3	D14.0	D38.5	D49.1
overlapping lesion with accessory sinuses	C31.8	—	—	—	—	—
skin	C44.21	C79.2	D04.21	D23.21	D48.5	D49.2
unspecified side	C44.20	C79.2	D04.20	D23.20	D48.5	D49.2
auricle or auris	C44.20	C79.2	D04.20	D23.20	D48.5	D49.2

©2002 Ingenix, Inc.

	Malignant					
	Primary	**Secondary**	**Ca in situ**	**Benign**	**Uncertain Behavior**	**Unspecified**
Neoplasm, neoplastic — *continued*						
ear — *continued*						
unspecified side — *continued*						
canal, external	C44.20	C79.2	D04.20	D23.20	D48.5	D49.2
cartilage	C49.0	C79.89	—	D21.0	D48.1	D49.2
external meatus	C44.20	C79.2	D04.20	D23.20	D48.5	D49.2
inner	C30.1	C78.39	D02.3	D14.0	D38.5	D49.1
lobule	C44.20	C79.2	D04.20	D23.20	D48.5	D49.2
middle	C30.1	C78.39	D02.3	D14.0	D38.5	D49.1
overlapping lesion with accessory sinuses	C31.8	—	—	—	—	—
skin	C44.20	C79.2	D04.20	D23.20	D48.5	D49.2
earlobe (unspecified side)	C44.20	C79.2	D04.20	D23.20	D48.5	D49.2
left side	C44.22	C79.2	D04.22	D23.22	D48.5	D49.2
right side	C44.21	C79.2	D04.21	D23.21	D48.5	D49.2
ejaculatory duct	C63.7	C79.82	D07.69	D29.7	D40.7	D49.5
elbow (unspecified side) NEC*	C76.40	C79.89	D04.60	D36.7	D48.7	D49.8
left side	C76.42	C79.89	D04.62	D36.7	D48.7	D49.8
right side	C76.41	C79.89	D04.61	D36.7	D48.7	D49.8
endocardium	C38.0	C79.89	—	D15.1	D48.7	D49.8
endocervix (canal) (gland)	C53.0	C79.82	D06.0	D26.0	D39.0	D49.5
endocrine gland NEC	C75.9	C79.89	D09.3	D35.9	D44.9	D49.7
pluriglandular NEC	C75.8	C79.89	D09.3	D35.8	D44.8	D49.7
endometrium (gland) (stroma)	C54.1	C79.82	D07.0	D26.1	D39.0	D49.5
ensiform cartilage	C41.3	C79.51	—	D16.7	D48.0	D49.2
enteric — see Neoplasm, intestine						
ependyma (brain)	C71.5	C79.31	—	D33.0	D43.0	D49.6
fourth ventricle	C71.7	C79.31	—	D33.1	D43.1	D49.6
epicardium	C38.0	C79.89	—	D15.1	D48.7	D49.8
epididymis (unspecified side)	C63.00	C79.82	D07.69	D29.30	D40.7	D49.5
left side	C63.02	C79.82	D07.69	D29.32	D40.7	D49.5
right side	C63.01	C79.82	D07.69	D29.31	D40.7	D49.5
epidural	C72.9	C79.49	—	D33.9	D43.9	D49.7
epiglottis	C32.1	C78.39	D02.0	D14.1	D38.0	D49.1
anterior aspect or surface	C10.1	C79.89	D00.08	D10.5	D37.05	D49.0
cartilage	C32.3	C78.39	D02.0	D14.1	D38.0	D49.1
free border (margin)	C10.1	C79.89	D00.08	D10.5	D37.05	D49.0
junctional region	C10.8	C79.89	D00.08	D10.5	D37.05	D49.0
posterior (laryngeal) surface	C32.1	C78.39	D02.0	D14.1	D38.0	D49.1
suprahyoid portion	C32.1	C78.39	D02.0	D14.1	D38.0	D49.1
esophagogastric junction	C16.0	C78.89	D00.2	D13.1	D37.1	D49.0
esophagus	C15.9	C78.89	D00.1	D13.0	D37.7	D49.0
abdominal	C15.5	C78.89	D00.1	D13.0	D37.7	D49.0
cervical	C15.3	C78.89	D00.1	D13.0	D37.7	D49.0
distal (third)	C15.5	C78.89	D00.1	D13.0	D37.7	D49.0
lower (third)	C15.5	C78.89	D00.1	D13.0	D37.7	D49.0
middle (third)	C15.4	C78.89	D00.1	D13.0	D37.7	D49.0
overlapping lesion	C15.8	—	—	—	—	—
proximal (third)	C15.3	C78.89	D00.1	D13.0	D37.7	D49.0
thoracic	C15.4	C78.89	D00.1	D13.0	D37.7	D49.0
upper (third)	C15.3	C78.89	D00.1	D13.0	D37.7	D49.0
ethmoid (sinus)	C31.1	C78.39	D02.3	D14.0	D38.5	D49.1
bone or labyrinth	C41.0	C79.51	—	D16.4	D48.0	D49.2
marrow NEC	C96.9	C79.52	—	—	—	D47.9
Eustachian tube	C30.1	C78.39	D02.3	D14.0	D38.5	D49.1
exocervix	C53.1	C79.82	D06.1	D26.0	D39.0	D49.5
external						
meatus (ear) (unspecified side)	C44.20	C79.2	D04.20	D23.20	D48.5	D49.2
left side	C44.22	C79.2	D04.22	D23.22	D48.5	D49.2
right side	C44.21	C79.2	D04.21	D23.21	D48.5	D49.2
os, cervix uteri	C53.1	C79.82	D06.1	D26.0	D39.0	D49.5
extradural	C72.9	C79.49	—	D33.9	D43.9	D49.7
extrahepatic (bile) duct	C24.0	C78.89	D01.5	D13.5	D37.6	D49.0
overlapping lesion with gallbladder	C24.8	—	—	—	—	—
extraocular muscle (unspecified side)	C69.60	C79.49	D09.20	D31.60	D48.7	D49.8
left side	C69.62	C79.49	D09.22	D31.62	D48.7	D49.8
right side	C69.61	C79.49	D09.21	D31.61	D48.7	D49.8
extrarectal	C76.3	C79.89	D09.7	D36.7	D48.7	D49.8

	Malignant					
	Primary	Secondary	Ca in situ	Benign	Uncertain Behavior	Unspecified
Neoplasm, neoplastic — *continued*						
extremity*	C76.7	C79.89	D04.8	D36.7	D48.7	D49.8
lower (unspecified side)*	C76.50	C79.89	D04.70	D36.7	D48.7	D49.8
left side	C76.52	C79.89	D04.72	D36.7	D48.7	D49.8
right side	C76.51	C79.89	D04.71	D36.7	D48.7	D49.8
upper (unspecified side)*	C76.40	C79.89	D04.60	D36.7	D48.7	D49.8
left side	C76.42	C79.89	D04.62	D36.7	D48.7	D49.8
right side	C76.41	C79.89	D04.61	D36.7	D48.7	D49.8
eye NEC						
left side	C69.92	C79.49	D09.22	D31.92	D48.7	D49.8
overlapping lesion	C69.82	—	—	—	—	—
right side	C69.91	C79.49	D09.21	D31.91	D48.7	D49.8
overlapping lesion	C69.81	—	—	—	—	—
unspecified side	C69.90	C79.49	D09.20	D31.90	D48.7	D49.8
overlapping lesion	C69.80	—	—	—	—	—
eyeball (unspecified side)	C69.40	C79.49	D09.20	D31.40	D48.7	D49.8
left side	C69.42	C79.49	D09.22	D31.42	D48.7	D49.8
right side	C69.41	C79.49	D09.21	D31.41	D48.7	D49.8
eyebrow	C44.31	C79.2	D04.39	D23.39	D48.5	D49.2
eyelid (lower) (skin) (upper)						
left side	C44.12	C79.2	D04.12	D23.12	D48.5	D49.2
cartilage	C49.0	C79.89	—	D21.0	D48.1	D49.2
right side	C44.11	C79.2	D04.11	D23.11	D48.5	D49.2
cartilage	C49.0	C79.89	—	D21.0	D48.1	D49.2
unspecified side	C44.10	C79.2	D04.10	D23.10	D48.5	D49.2
cartilage	C49.0	C79.89	—	D21.0	D48.1	D49.2
face NEC*	C76.0	C79.89	D04.39	D36.7	D48.7	D49.8
fallopian tube (accessory) (unspecified side)	C57.00	C79.82	D07.39	D28.2	D39.7	D49.5
left side	C57.02	C79.82	D07.39	D28.2	D39.7	D49.5
right side	C57.01	C79.82	D07.39	D28.2	D39.7	D49.5
falx (cerebella) (cerebri)	C70.0	C79.32	—	D32.0	D42.0	D49.7
fascia — see also Neoplasm, connective tissue						
palmar (unspecified side)	C49.10	C79.89	—	D21.10	D48.1	D49.2
left side	C49.12	C79.89	—	D21.12	D48.1	D49.2
right side	C49.11	C79.89	—	D21.11	D48.1	D49.2
plantar (unspecified side)	C49.20	C79.89	—	D21.20	D48.1	D49.2
left side	C49.22	C79.89	—	D21.22	D48.1	D49.2
right side	C49.21	C79.89	—	D21.21	D48.1	D49.2
fatty tissue — see Neoplasm, connective tissue						
fauces, faucial NEC	C10.9	C79.89	D00.00	D10.5	D37.05	D49.0
pillars	C09.1	C79.89	D00.08	D10.5	D37.05	D49.0
tonsil	C09.9	C79.89	D00.08	D10.4	D37.05	D49.0
femur (any part)						
left side	C40.22	C79.51	—	D16.22	D48.0	D49.2
marrow NEC	C96.9	C79.52	—	—	—	D47.9
right side	C40.21	C79.51	—	D16.21	D48.0	D49.2
marrow NEC	C96.9	C79.52	—	—	—	D47.9
unspecified side	C40.20	C79.51	—	D16.20	D48.0	D49.2
marrow NEC	C96.9	C79.52	—	—	—	D47.9
fetal membrane	C58	C79.82	D07.0	D26.7	D39.2	D49.5
fibrous tissue — see Neoplasm, connective tissue						
fibula (any part)						
left side	C40.22	C79.51	—	D16.22	D48.0	D49.2
marrow NEC	C96.9	C79.52	—	—	—	D47.9
right side	C40.21	C79.51	—	D16.21	D48.0	D49.2
marrow NEC	C96.9	C79.52	—	—	—	D47.9
unspecified side	C40.20	C79.51	—	D16.20	D48.0	D49.2
marrow NEC	C96.9	C79.52	—	—	—	D47.9
filum terminale	C72.0	C79.49	—	D33.4	D43.4	D49.7
finger (unspecified side) NEC*	C76.40	C79.89	D04.60	D36.7	D48.7	D49.8
left side	C76.42	C79.89	D04.62	D36.7	D48.7	D49.8
right side	C76.41	C79.89	D04.61	D36.7	D48.7	D49.8
flank NEC*	C76.7	C79.89	D04.5	D36.7	D48.7	D49.8
follicle, nabothian	C53.0	C79.82	D06.0	D26.0	D39.0	D49.5
foot (unspecified side) NEC*	C76.50	C79.89	D04.70	D36.7	D48.7	D49.8
left side	C76.52	C79.89	D04.72	D36.7	D48.7	D49.8
right side	C76.51	C79.89	D04.71	D36.7	D48.7	D49.8

©2002 Ingenix, Inc.

	Malignant					
	Primary	Secondary	Ca in situ	Benign	Uncertain Behavior	Unspecified
Neoplasm, neoplastic — *continued*						
forearm (unspecified side) NEC*	C76.40	C79.89	D04.60	D36.7	D48.7	D49.8
left side	C76.42	C79.89	D04.62	D36.7	D48.7	D49.8
right side	C76.41	C79.89	D04.61	D36.7	D48.7	D49.8
forehead (skin)	C44.31	C79.2	D04.39	D23.39	D48.5	D49.2
foreskin	C60.0	C79.82	D07.4	D29.0	D40.7	D49.5
fornix						
pharyngeal	C11.3	C79.89	D00.08	D10.6	D37.05	D49.0
vagina	C52	C79.82	D07.2	D28.1	D39.7	D49.5
fossa (of)						
anterior (cranial)	C71.9	C79.31	—	D33.2	D43.2	D49.6
cranial	C71.9	C79.31	—	D33.2	D43.2	D49.6
ischiorectal	C76.3	C79.89	D09.7	D36.7	D48.7	D49.8
middle (cranial)	C71.9	C79.31	—	D33.2	D43.2	D49.6
piriform	C12	C79.89	D00.08	D10.7	D37.05	D49.0
pituitary	C75.1	C79.89	D09.3	D35.2	D44.3	D49.7
posterior (cranial)	C71.9	C79.31	—	D33.2	D43.2	D49.6
pterygoid	C49.0	C79.89	—	D21.0	D48.1	D49.2
pyriform	C12	C79.89	D00.08	D10.7	D37.05	D49.0
Rosenmüller	C11.2	C79.89	D00.08	D10.6	D37.05	D49.0
tonsillar	C09.0	C79.89	D00.08	D10.5	D37.05	D49.0
fourchette	C51.9	C79.82	D07.1	D28.0	D39.7	D49.5
frenulum						
labii — see Neoplasm, lip, internal						
linguae	C02.2	C79.89	D00.07	D10.1	D37.02	D49.0
frontal						
bone	C41.0	C79.51	—	D16.4	D48.0	D49.2
marrow NEC	C96.9	C79.52	—	—	—	D47.9
lobe, brain	C71.1	C79.31	—	D33.0	D43.0	D49.6
meninges	C70.0	C79.32	—	D32.0	D42.0	D49.7
pole	C71.1	C79.31	—	D33.0	D43.0	D49.6
sinus	C31.2	C78.39	D02.3	D14.0	D38.5	D49.1
fundus						
stomach	C16.1	C78.89	D00.2	D13.1	D37.1	D49.0
uterus	C54.3	C79.82	D07.0	D26.1	D39.0	D49.5
gall duct (extrahepatic)	C24.0	C78.89	D01.5	D13.5	D37.6	D49.0
intrahepatic	C22.1	C78.89	D01.5	D13.4	D37.6	D49.0
gallbladder	C23	C78.89	D01.5	D13.5	D37.6	D49.0
overlapping lesion with extrahepatic bile ducts	C24.8	—	—	—	—	—
ganglia (see also Neoplasm, nerve, peripheral)	C47.9	C79.89	—	D36.10	D48.2	D49.2
basal	C71.0	C79.31	—	D33.0	D43.0	D49.6
cranial nerve	C72.50	C79.49	—	D33.3	D43.3	D49.7
Gartner's duct	C52	C79.82	D07.2	D28.1	D39.7	D49.5
gastric — see Neoplasm, stomach						
gastrocolic	C26.8	C78.89	D01.9	D13.9	D37.9	D49.0
gastroesophageal junction	C16.0	C78.89	D00.2	D13.1	D37.1	D49.0
gastrointestinal (tract) NEC	C26.9	C78.89	D01.9	D13.9	D37.9	D49.0
generalized	C80.0	C80.0	D09.9	D36.9	D48.9	C80.0
genital organ or tract						
female NEC	C57.9	C79.82	D07.30	D28.9	D39.9	D49.5
overlapping lesion	C57.8	—	—	—	—	—
specified site NEC	C57.7	C79.82	D07.39	D28.7	D39.7	D49.5
male NEC	C63.9	C79.82	D07.60	D29.9	D40.9	D49.5
overlapping lesion	C63.8	—	—	—	—	—
specified site NEC	C63.7	C79.82	D07.69	D29.7	D40.7	D49.5
genitourinary tract						
female	C57.9	C79.82	D07.30	D28.9	D39.9	D49.5
male	C63.9	C79.82	D07.60	D29.9	D40.9	D49.5
gingiva (alveolar) (marginal)	C03.9	C79.89	D00.03	D10.39	D37.09	D49.0
lower	C03.1	C79.89	D00.03	D10.39	D37.09	D49.0
mandibular	C03.1	C79.89	D00.03	D10.39	D37.09	D49.0
maxillary	C03.0	C79.89	D00.03	D10.39	D37.09	D49.0
upper	C03.0	C79.89	D00.03	D10.39	D37.09	D49.0
gland, glandular (lymphatic) (system) — see also Neoplasm, lymph gland						
endocrine NEC	C75.9	C79.89	D09.3	D35.9	D44.9	D49.7
salivary — see Neoplasm, salivary gland						
glans penis	C60.1	C79.82	D07.4	D29.0	D40.7	D49.5

	Malignant			Benign	Uncertain Behavior	Unspecified
	Primary	Secondary	Ca in situ			
Neoplasm, neoplastic — *continued*						
globus pallidus	C71.0	C79.31	—	D33.0	D43.0	D49.6
glomus						
coccygeal	C75.5	C79.89	—	D35.6	D44.7	D49.7
jugularis	C75.5	C79.89	—	D35.6	D44.7	D49.7
glosso-epiglottic fold(s)	C10.1	C79.89	D00.08	D10.5	D37.05	D49.0
glossopalatine fold	C09.1	C79.89	D00.08	D10.5	D37.05	D49.0
glossopharyngeal sulcus	C09.0	C79.89	D00.08	D10.5	D37.05	D49.0
glottis	C32.0	C78.39	D02.0	D14.1	D38.0	D49.1
gluteal region*	C76.3	C79.89	D04.5	D36.7	D48.7	D49.8
great vessels NEC	C49.3	C79.89	—	D21.3	D48.1	D49.2
groin NEC	C76.3	C79.89	D04.5	D36.7	D48.7	D49.8
gum	C03.9	C79.89	D00.03	D10.39	D37.09	D49.0
lower	C03.1	C79.89	D00.03	D10.39	D37.09	D49.0
upper	C03.0	C79.89	D00.03	D10.39	D37.09	D49.0
hand (unspecified side) NEC*	C76.40	C79.89	D04.60	D36.7	D48.7	D49.8
left side	C76.42	C79.89	D04.62	D36.7	D48.7	D49.8
right side	C76.41	C79.89	D04.61	D36.7	D48.7	D49.8
head NEC*	C76.0	C79.89	D04.4	D36.7	D48.7	D49.8
heart	C38.0	C79.89	—	D15.1	D48.7	D49.8
overlapping lesion with mediastinum or pleura	C38.8	—	—	—	—	—
heel (unspecified side) NEC*	C76.50	C79.89	D04.70	D36.7	D48.7	D49.8
left side	C76.52	C79.89	D04.72	D36.7	D48.7	D49.8
right side	C76.51	C79.89	D04.71	D36.7	D48.7	D49.8
helix (unspecified side)	C44.20	C79.2	D04.20	D23.20	D48.5	D49.2
left side	C44.22	C79.2	D04.22	D23.22	D48.5	D49.2
right side	C44.21	C79.2	D04.21	D23.21	D48.5	D49.2
hematopoietic, hemopoietic tissue NEC	C96.9	C79.89	—	—	—	D47.9
hemisphere, cerebral	C71.0	C79.31	—	D33.0	D43.0	D49.6
hemorrhoidal zone	C21.1	C78.5	D01.3	D12.9	D37.7	D49.0
hepatic	C22.9	C78.7	D01.5	D13.4	D37.6	D49.0
duct (bile)	C24.0	C78.89	D01.5	D13.5	D37.6	D49.0
flexure (colon)	C18.3	C78.5	D01.0	D12.3	D37.4	D49.0
primary	C22.8	—	—	—	—	—
hilus of lung (unspecified side)	C34.00	C78.00	D02.20	D14.30	D38.1	D49.1
left side	C34.02	C78.02	D02.22	D14.32	D38.1	D49.1
right side	C34.01	C78.01	D02.21	D14.31	D38.1	D49.1
hip (unspecified side) NEC*	C76.50	C79.89	D04.70	D36.7	D48.7	D49.8
left side	C76.52	C79.89	D04.72	D36.7	D48.7	D49.8
right side	C76.51	C79.89	D04.71	D36.7	D48.7	D49.8
hippocampus, brain	C71.2	C79.31	—	D33.0	D43.0	D49.6
humerus (any part)						
left side	C40.02	C79.51	—	D16.02	D48.0	D49.2
marrow NEC	C96.9	C79.52	—	—	—	D47.9
right side	C40.01	C79.51	—	D16.01	D48.0	D49.2
marrow NEC	C96.9	C79.52	—	—	—	D47.9
unspecified side	C40.00	C79.51	—	D16.00	D48.0	D49.2
marrow NEC	C96.9	C79.52	—	—	—	D47.9
hymen	C52	C79.82	D07.2	D28.1	D39.7	D49.5
hypopharynx, hypopharyngeal NEC	C13.9	C79.89	D00.08	D10.7	D37.05	D49.0
overlapping lesion	C13.8	—	—	—	—	—
postcricoid region	C13.0	C79.89	D00.08	D10.7	D37.05	D49.0
posterior wall	C13.2	C79.89	D00.08	D10.7	D37.05	D49.0
pyriform fossa (sinus)	C12	C79.89	D00.08	D10.7	D37.05	D49.0
wall	C13.9	C79.89	D00.08	D10.7	D37.05	D49.0
posterior	C13.2	C79.89	D00.08	D10.7	D37.05	D49.0
hypophysis	C75.1	C79.89	D09.3	D35.2	D44.3	D49.7
hypothalamus	C71.0	C79.31	—	D33.0	D43.0	D49.6
ileocecum, ileocecal (coil) (junction) (valve)	C18.0	C78.5	D01.0	D12.0	D37.4	D49.0
ileum	C17.2	C78.4	D01.49	D13.39	D37.2	D49.0
ilium	C41.4	C79.51	—	D16.8	D48.0	D49.2
marrow NEC	C96.9	C79.52	—	—	—	D47.9
immunoproliferative NEC	C88.9	—	—	—	—	—
infraclavicular (region)*	C76.1	C79.89	D04.5	D36.7	D48.7	D49.8
inguinal (region)*	C76.3	C79.89	D04.5	D36.7	D48.7	D49.8
insula	C71.0	C79.31	—	D33.0	D43.0	D49.6

	Malignant			Benign	Uncertain Behavior	Unspecified
	Primary	Secondary	Ca in situ			
Neoplasm, neoplastic — *continued*						
insular tissue (pancreas)	C25.4	C78.89	D01.7	D13.7	D37.7	D49.0
brain	C71.0	C79.31	—	D33.0	D43.0	D49.6
interarytenoid fold	C13.1	C79.89	D00.08	D10.7	D37.05	D49.0
hypopharyngeal aspect	C13.1	C79.89	D00.08	D10.7	D37.05	D49.0
laryngeal aspect	C32.1	C79.39	D02.0	D14.1	D38.0	D49.1
marginal zone	C13.1	C79.89	D00.08	D10.7	D37.05	D49.0
interdental papillae	C03.9	C79.89	D00.03	D10.39	D37.09	D49.0
lower	C03.1	C79.89	D00.03	D10.39	D37.09	D49.0
upper	C03.0	C79.89	D00.03	D10.39	D37.09	D49.0
internal						
capsule	C71.0	C79.31	—	D33.0	D43.0	D49.6
os (cervix)	C53.0	C79.82	D06.0	D26.0	D39.0	D49.5
intervertebral cartilage or disc	C41.2	C79.51	—	D16.6	D48.0	D49.2
marrow NEC	C96.9	C79.52		—	—	D47.9
intestine, intestinal	C26.0	C78.80	D01.40	D13.9	D37.7	D49.0
large	C18.9	C78.5	D01.0	D12.6	D37.4	D49.0
appendix	C18.1	C78.5	D01.0	D12.1	D37.3	D49.0
caput coli	C18.0	C78.5	D01.0	D12.0	D37.4	D49.0
cecum	C18.0	C78.5	D01.0	D12.0	D37.4	D49.0
colon	C18.9	C78.5	D01.0	D12.6	D37.4	D49.0
and rectum	C19	C78.5	D01.1	D12.7	D37.5	D49.0
ascending	C18.2	C78.5	D01.0	D12.2	D37.4	D49.0
caput	C18.0	C78.5	D01.0	D12.0	D37.4	D49.0
descending	C18.6	C78.5	D01.0	D12.4	D37.4	D49.0
distal	C18.6	C78.5	D01.0	D12.4	D37.4	D49.0
left	C18.6	C78.5	D01.0	D12.4	D37.4	D49.0
overlapping lesion	C18.8	—	—	—	—	—
pelvic	C18.7	C78.5	D01.0	D12.5	D37.4	D49.0
right	C18.2	C78.5	D01.0	D12.2	D37.4	D49.0
sigmoid (flexure)	C18.7	C78.5	D01.0	D12.5	D37.4	D49.0
transverse	C18.4	C78.5	D01.0	D12.3	D37.4	D49.0
hepatic flexure	C18.3	C78.5	D01.0	D12.3	D37.4	D49.0
ileocecum, ileocecal (coil) (valve)	C18.0	C78.5	D01.0	D12.0	D37.4	D49.0
overlapping lesion	C18.8	—	—	—	—	—
sigmoid flexure (lower) (upper)	C18.7	C78.5	D01.0	D12.5	D37.4	D49.0
splenic flexure	C18.5	C78.5	D01.0	D12.3	D37.4	D49.0
small	C17.9	C78.4	D01.40	D13.30	D37.2	D49.0
duodenum	C17.0	C78.4	D01.49	D13.2	D37.2	D49.0
ileum	C17.2	C78.4	D01.49	D13.39	D37.2	D49.0
jejunum	C17.1	C78.4	D01.49	D13.39	D37.2	D49.0
overlapping lesion	C17.8	—	—	—	—	—
tract NEC	C26.0	C78.89	D01.40	D13.9	D37.7	D49.0
intra-abdominal	C76.2	C79.89	D09.7	D36.7	D48.7	D49.8
intracranial NEC	C71.9	C79.31	—	D33.2	D43.2	D49.6
intrahepatic (bile) duct	C22.1	C78.89	D01.5	D13.4	D37.6	D49.0
intraocular (unspecified side)	C69.40	C79.49	D09.20	D31.40	D48.7	D49.8
left side	C69.42	C79.49	D09.22	D31.42	D48.7	D49.8
right side	C69.41	C79.49	D09.21	D31.41	D48.7	D49.8
intraorbital (unspecified side)	C69.60	C79.49	D09.20	D31.60	D48.7	D49.8
left side	C69.62	C79.49	D09.22	D31.62	D48.7	D49.8
right side	C69.61	C79.49	D09.21	D31.61	D48.7	D49.8
intrasellar	C75.1	C79.89	D09.3	D35.2	D44.3	D49.7
intrathoracic (cavity) (organs NEC)	C76.1	C79.89	D09.7	D36.7	D48.7	D49.8
overlapping lesion with respiratory organs	C39.8	—	—	—	—	—
iris (unspecified side)	C69.40	C79.49	D09.20	D31.40	D48.7	D49.8
left side	C69.42	C79.49	D09.22	D31.42	D48.7	D49.8
right side	C69.41	C79.49	D09.21	D31.41	D48.7	D49.8
ischiorectal (fossa)	C76.3	C79.89	D09.7	D36.7	D48.7	D49.8
ischium	C41.4	C79.51	—	D16.8	D48.0	D49.2
marrow NEC	C96.9	C79.52	—	—	—	D47.9
island of Reil	C71.0	C79.31	—	D33.0	D43.0	D49.6
islands or islets of Langerhans	C25.4	C78.89	D01.7	D13.7	D37.7	D49.0
isthmus uteri	C54.0	C79.82	D07.0	D26.1	D39.0	D49.5

| | Malignant | | | | | |
	Primary	Secondary	Ca in situ	Benign	Uncertain Behavior	Unspecified
Neoplasm, neoplastic — *continued*						
jaw	C76.0	C79.89	D09.7	D36.7	D48.7	D49.8
bone	C41.1	C79.51	—	D16.5	D48.0	D49.2
carcinoma	C03.9	—	—	—	—	—
lower	C03.1	—	—	—	—	—
upper	C03.0	—	—	—	—	—
lower	C41.1	C79.51	—	D16.5	D48.0	D49.2
marrow NEC	C96.9	C79.52	—	—	—	D47.9
marrow NEC	C96.9	C79.52	—	—	—	D47.9
upper	C41.0	C79.51	—	D16.4	D48.0	D49.2
marrow NEC	C96.9	C79.52	—	—	—	D47.9
carcinoma (any type) (lower) (upper)	C76.0	—	—	—	—	—
skin	C44.31	C79.2	D04.39	D23.39	D48.5	D49.2
soft tissues	C03.9	C79.89	D00.03	D10.39	D37.09	D49.0
lower	C03.1	C79.89	D00.03	D10.39	D37.09	D49.0
upper	C03.0	C79.89	D00.03	D10.39	D37.09	D49.0
jejunum	C17.1	C79.89	D01.49	D13.39	D37.2	D49.0
joint NEC (see also Neoplasm, bone)	C41.9	C79.51	—	D16.9	D48.0	D49.2
acromioclavicular (unspecified side)	C40.00	C79.51	—	D16.00	D48.0	D49.2
left side	C40.02	C79.51	—	D16.02	D48.0	D49.2
right side	C40.01	C79.51	—	D16.01	D48.0	D49.2
bursa or synovial membrane — see Neoplasm, connective tissue						
costovertebral	C41.3	C79.51	—	D16.7	D48.0	D49.2
sternocostal	C41.3	C79.51	—	D16.7	D48.0	D49.2
temporomandibular	C41.1	C79.51	—	D16.5	D48.0	D49.2
junction						
anorectal	C21.8	C78.5	D01.3	D12.9	D37.7	D49.0
cardioesophageal	C16.0	C78.89	D00.2	D13.1	D37.1	D49.0
esophagogastric	C16.0	C78.89	D00.2	D13.1	D37.1	D49.0
gastroesophageal	C16.0	C78.89	D00.2	D13.1	D37.1	D49.0
hard and soft palate	C05.9	C79.89	D00.00	D10.39	D37.09	D49.0
ileocecal	C18.0	C78.5	D01.0	D12.0	D37.4	D49.0
pelvirectal	C19	C78.5	D01.1	D12.7	D37.5	D49.0
pelviureteric (unspecified side)	C65.9	C79.00	D09.19	D30.10	D41.10	D49.5
left side	C65.1	C79.02	D09.19	D30.12	D41.12	D49.5
right side	C65.0	C79.01	D09.19	D30.11	D41.11	D49.5
rectosigmoid	C19	C78.5	D01.1	D12.7	D37.5	D49.0
squamocolumnar, of cervix	C53.8	C79.82	D06.7	D26.0	D39.0	D49.5
kidney (parenchymal)						
calyx (unspecified side)	C65.9	C79.00	D09.19	D30.10	D41.10	D49.5
left side	C65.1	C79.02	D09.19	D30.12	D41.12	D49.5
right side	C65.0	C79.01	D09.19	D30.11	D41.11	D49.5
hilus (unspecified side)	C65.9	C79.00	D09.19	D30.10	D41.10	D49.5
left side	C65.1	C79.02	D09.19	D30.12	D41.12	D49.5
right side	C65.0	C79.01	D09.19	D30.11	D41.11	D49.5
pelvis (unspecified side)	C65.9	C79.00	D09.19	D30.10	D41.10	D49.5
left side	C65.1	C79.02	D09.19	D30.12	D41.12	D49.5
right side	C65.0	C79.01	D09.19	D30.11	D41.11	D49.5
unspecified site (unspecified side)	C64.9	C79.00	D09.19	D30.00	D41.00	D49.5
left side	C64.1	C79.02	D09.19	D30.02	D41.02	D49.5
right side	C64.0	C79.01	D09.19	D30.01	D41.01	D49.5
knee (unspecified side) NEC*	C76.50	C79.89	D04.70	D36.7	D48.7	D49.8
left side	C76.52	C79.89	D04.72	D36.7	D48.7	D49.8
right side	C76.51	C79.89	D04.71	D36.7	D48.7	D49.8
labia (skin)	C51.9	C79.82	D07.0	D28.0	D39.7	D49.5
majora	C51.0	C79.82	D07.0	D28.0	D39.7	D49.5
minora	C51.1	C79.82	D07.0	D28.0	D39.7	D49.5
labial — see also Neoplasm, lip						
sulcus (lower) (upper)	C06.1	C79.89	D00.02	D10.39	D37.09	D49.0
labium (skin)	C51.9	C79.82	D07.1	D28.0	D39.7	D49.5
majus	C51.0	C79.82	D07.1	D28.0	D39.7	D49.5
minus	C51.1	C79.82	D07.1	D28.0	D39.7	D49.5
lacrimal						
canaliculi (unspecified side)	C69.50	C79.49	D09.20	D31.50	D48.7	D49.8
left side	C69.52	C79.49	D09.22	D31.52	D48.7	D49.8
right side	C69.51	C79.49	D09.21	D31.51	D48.7	D40.8

©2002 Ingenix, Inc.

	Malignant					
	Primary	Secondary	Ca in situ	Benign	Uncertain Behavior	Unspecified
Neoplasm, neoplastic — *continued*						
lacrimal — *continued*						
duct (nasal) (unspecified side)	C69.50	C79.49	D09.20	D31.50	D48.7	D49.8
left side	C69.52	C79.49	D09.22	D31.52	D48.7	D49.8
right side	C69.51	C79.49	D09.21	D31.51	D48.7	D49.8
gland (unspecified side)	C69.50	C79.49	D09.20	D31.50	D48.7	D49.8
left side	C69.52	C79.49	D09.22	D31.52	D48.7	D49.8
right side	C69.51	C79.49	D09.21	D31.51	D48.7	D49.8
punctum (unspecified side)	C69.50	C79.49	D09.20	D31.50	D48.7	D49.8
left side	C69.52	C79.49	D09.22	D31.52	D48.7	D49.8
right side	C69.51	C79.49	D09.21	D31.51	D48.7	D49.8
sac (unspecified side)	C69.50	C79.49	D09.20	D31.50	D48.7	D49.8
left side	C69.52	C79.49	D09.22	D31.52	D48.7	D49.8
right side	C69.51	C79.49	D09.21	D31.51	D48.7	D49.8
Langerhans, islands or islets	C25.4	C78.89	D01.7	D13.7	D37.7	D49.0
laryngopharynx	C14.1	C79.89	D00.08	D10.7	D37.05	D49.0
larynx, laryngeal NEC	C32.9	C78.39	D02.0	D14.1	D38.0	D49.1
aryepiglottic fold	C32.1	C78.39	D02.0	D14.1	D38.0	D49.1
cartilage (arytenoid) (cricoid) (cuneiform) (thyroid)	C32.3	C78.39	D02.0	D14.1	D38.0	D49.1
commissure (anterior) (posterior)	C32.0	C78.39	D02.0	D14.1	D38.0	D49.1
extrinsic NEC	C32.1	C78.39	D02.0	D14.1	D38.0	D49.1
meaning hypopharynx	C13.9	C79.89	D00.08	D10.7	D37.05	D49.0
interarytenoid fold	C32.1	C78.39	D02.0	D14.1	D38.0	D49.1
intrinsic	C32.0	C78.39	D02.0	D14.1	D38.0	D49.1
overlapping lesion	C32.8	—	—	—	—	—
ventricular band	C32.1	C78.39	D02.0	D14.1	D38.0	D49.1
leg (unspecified side) NEC*	C76.50	C79.89	D04.70	D36.7	D48.7	D49.8
left side	C76.52	C79.89	D04.72	D36.7	D48.7	D49.8
right side	C76.51	C79.89	D04.71	D36.7	D48.7	D49.8
lens, crystalline (unspecified side)	C69.40	C79.49	D09.20	D31.40	D48.7	D49.8
left side	C69.42	C79.49	D09.22	D31.42	D48.7	D49.8
right side	C69.41	C79.49	D09.21	D31.41	D48.7	D49.8
lid (lower) (upper) (unspecified side)	C44.10	C79.2	D04.10	D23.10	D48.5	D49.2
left side	C44.12	C79.2	D04.12	D23.12	D48.5	D49.2
right side	C44.11	C79.2	D04.11	D23.11	D48.5	D49.2
ligament — see also Neoplasm, connective tissue						
broad	C57.1	C79.82	D07.39	D28.2	D39.7	D49.5
Mackenrodt's	C57.7	C79.82	D07.39	D28.7	D39.7	D49.5
non-uterine — see Neoplasm, connective tissue						
round	C57.2	C79.82	—	D28.2	D39.7	D49.5
sacro-uterine	C57.3	C79.82	—	D28.2	D39.7	D49.5
uterine	C57.3	C79.82	—	D28.2	D39.7	D49.5
utero-ovarian	C57.7	C79.82	D07.39	D28.2	D39.7	D49.5
uterosacral	C57.3	C79.82	—	D28.2	D39.7	D49.5
limb*	C76.7	C79.89	D04.8	D36.7	D48.7	D49.8
lower (unspecified side)*	C76.50	C79.89	D04.70	D36.7	D48.7	D49.8
left side	C76.52	C79.89	D04.72	D36.7	D48.7	D49.8
right side	C76.51	C79.89	D04.71	D36.7	D48.7	D49.8
upper (unspecified side)*	C76.40	C79.89	D04.60	D36.7	D48.7	D49.8
left side	C76.42	C79.89	D04.62	D36.7	D48.7	D49.8
right side	C76.41	C79.89	D04.61	D36.7	D48.7	D49.8
limbus of cornea (unspecified side)	C69.10	C79.49	D09.20	D31.10	D48.7	D49.8
left side	C69.12	C79.49	D09.22	D31.12	D48.7	D49.8
right side	C69.11	C79.49	D09.21	D31.11	D48.7	D49.8
lingual NEC (see also Neoplasm, tongue)	C02.9	C79.89	D00.07	D10.1	D37.02	D49.0
lingula, lung (unspecified side)	C34.10	C78.00	D02.20	D14.30	D38.1	D49.1
left side	C34.12	C78.02	D02.22	D14.32	D38.1	D49.1
right side	C34.11	C78.01	D02.21	D14.31	D38.1	D49.1
lip	C00.9	C79.89	D00.01	D10.0	D37.01	D49.0
buccal aspect — see Neoplasm, lip, internal						
commissure	C00.6	C79.89	D00.01	D10.0	D37.01	D49.0
external	C00.2	C79.89	D00.01	D10.0	D37.01	D49.0
lower	C00.1	C79.89	D00.01	D10.0	D37.01	D49.0
upper	C00.0	C79.89	D00.01	D10.0	D37.01	D49.0
frenulum — see Neoplasm, lip, internal						
inner aspect — see Neoplasm, lip, internal						

| | Malignant | | | | | |
	Primary	Secondary	Ca in situ	Benign	Uncertain Behavior	Unspecified
Neoplasm, neoplastic — *continued*						
lip — *continued*						
internal	C00.5	C79.89	D00.01	D10.0	D37.01	D49.0
lower	C00.4	C79.89	D00.01	D10.0	D37.01	D49.0
upper	C00.3	C79.89	D00.01	D10.0	D37.01	D49.0
lipstick area	C00.2	C79.89	D00.01	D10.0	D37.01	D49.0
lower	C00.1	C79.89	D00.01	D10.0	D37.01	D49.0
upper	C00.0	C79.89	D00.01	D10.0	D37.01	D49.0
lower	C00.1	C79.89	D00.01	D10.0	D37.01	D49.0
internal	C00.4	C79.89	D00.01	D10.0	D37.01	D49.0
mucosa — see Neoplasm, lip, internal						
oral aspect — see Neoplasm, lip, internal						
overlaping lesion	C00.8	—	—	—	—	—
with oral cavity or pharynx	C14.8	—				
skin (commissure) (lower) (upper)	C44.0	C79.2	D04.0	D23.0	D48.5	D49.2
upper	C00.0	C79.89	D00.01	D10.0	D37.01	D49.0
internal	C00.3	C79.89	D00.01	D10.0	D37.01	D49.0
vermilion border	C00.2	C79.89	D00.01	D10.0	D37.01	D49.0
lower	C00.1	C79.89	D00.01	D10.0	D37.01	D49.0
upper	C00.0	C79.89	D00.01	D10.0	D37.01	D49.0
liver	C22.9	C78.7	D01.5	D13.4	D37.6	D49.0
primary	C22.8	—	—	—	—	—
lobe						
azygos (unspecified side)	C34.10	C78.00	D02.20	D14.30	D38.1	D49.1
left side	C34.12	C78.02	D02.22	D14.32	D38.1	D49.1
right side	C34.11	C78.01	D02.21	D14.31	D38.1	D49.1
frontal	C71.1	C79.31	—	D33.0	D43.0	D49.6
lower (unspecified side)	C34.30	C78.00	D02.20	D14.30	D38.1	D49.1
left side	C34.32	C78.02	D02.22	D14.32	D38.1	D49.1
right side	C34.31	C78.01	D02.21	D14.31	D38.1	D49.1
middle	C34.2	C78.01	D02.21	D14.31	D38.1	D49.1
occipital	C71.4	C79.31	—	D33.0	D43.0	D49.6
parietal	C71.3	C79.31	—	D33.0	D43.0	D49.6
temporal	C71.2	C79.31	—	D33.0	D43.0	D49.6
upper (unspecified side)	C34.10	C78.00	D02.20	D14.30	D38.1	D49.1
left side	C34.12	C78.02	D02.22	D14.32	D38.1	D49.1
right side	C34.11	C78.01	D02.21	D14.31	D38.1	D49.1
lumbosacral plexus	C47.5	C79.49	—	D36.16	D48.2	D49.2
lung						
azygos lobe (unspecified side)	C34.10	C78.00	D02.20	D14.30	D38.1	D49.1
left side	C34.12	C78.02	D02.22	D14.32	D38.1	D49.1
right side	C34.11	C78.01	D02.21	D14.31	D38.1	D49.1
carina (unspecified side)	C34.00	C78.00	D02.20	D14.30	D38.1	D49.1
left side	C34.02	C78.02	D02.22	D14.32	D38.1	D49.1
right side	C34.01	C78.01	D02.21	D14.31	D38.1	D49.1
hilus (unspecified side)	C34.00	C78.00	D02.20	D14.30	D38.1	D49.1
left side	C34.02	C78.02	D02.22	D14.32	D38.1	D49.1
right side	C34.01	C78.01	D02.21	D14.31	D38.1	D49.1
linqula (unspecified side)	C34.10	C78.00	D02.20	D14.30	D38.1	D49.1
left side	C34.12	C78.02	D02.22	D14.32	D38.1	D49.1
right side	C34.11	C78.01	D02.21	D14.31	D38.1	D49.1
lobe (unspecified side) NEC	C34.90	C78.00	D02.20	D14.30	D38.1	D49.1
left side	C34.92	C78.02	D02.22	D14.32	D38.1	D49.1
right side	C34.91	C78.01	D02.21	D14.31	D38.1	D49.1
lower lobe (unspecified side)	C34.30	C78.00	D02.20	D14.30	D38.1	D49.1
left side	C34.32	C78.02	D02.22	D14.32	D38.1	D49.1
right side	C34.31	C78.01	D02.21	D14.31	D38.1	D49.1
main bronchus (unspecified side)	C34.00	C78.00	D02.20	D14.30	D38.1	D49.1
left side	C34.02	C78.02	D02.22	D14.32	D38.1	D49.1
right side	C34.01	C78.01	D02.21	D14.31	D38.1	D49.1
middle lobe	C34.2	C78.01	D02.21	D14.31	D38.1	D49.1
overlapping lesion (unspecified side)	C34.80	—	—	—	—	—
left side	C34.82	—	—	—	—	—
right side	C34.81	—	—	—	—	—
unspecified site (unspecified side)	C34.90	C78.00	D02.20	D14.30	D38.1	D49.1
left side	C34.92	C78.02	D02.22	D14.32	D38.1	D49.1
right side	C34.91	C78.01	D02.21	D14.31	D38.1	D49.1

©2002 Ingenix, Inc.

	Malignant				Uncertain Behavior	Unspecified
	Primary	Secondary	Ca in situ	Benign		
Neoplasm, neoplastic — *continued*						
lung — *continued*						
upper lobe (unspecified side)	C34.10	C78.00	D02.20	D14.30	D38.1	D49.1
left side	C34.12	C78.02	D02.22	D14.32	D38.1	D49.1
right side	C34.11	C78.01	D02.21	D14.31	D38.1	D49.1
lymph, lymphatic channel NEC (see also Neoplasm, connective tissue)	C49.9	C79.89	—	D21.9	D48.1	D49.2
gland (secondary)	—	C77.9	—	D36.0	D48.7	D49.8
abdominal	—	C77.2	—	D36.0	D48.7	D49.8
aortic	—	C77.2	—	D36.0	D48.7	D49.8
arm	—	C77.3	—	D36.0	D48.7	D49.8
auricular (anterior) (posterior)	—	C77.0	—	D36.0	D48.7	D49.8
axilla, axillary	—	C77.3	—	D36.0	D48.7	D49.8
brachial	—	C77.3	—	D36.0	D48.7	D49.8
bronchial	—	C77.1	—	D36.0	D48.7	D49.8
bronchopulmonary	—	C77.1	—	D36.0	D48.7	D49.8
celiac	—	C77.2	—	D36.0	D48.7	D49.8
cervical	—	C77.0	—	D36.0	D48.7	D49.8
cervicofacial	—	C77.0	—	D36.0	D48.7	D49.8
Cloquet	—	C77.4	—	D36.0	D48.7	D49.8
colic	—	C77.2	—	D36.0	D48.7	D49.8
common duct	—	C77.2	—	D36.0	D48.7	D49.8
cubital	—	C77.3	—	D36.0	D48.7	D49.8
diaphragmatic	—	C77.1	—	D36.0	D48.7	D49.8
epigastric, inferior	—	C77.1	—	D36.0	D48.7	D49.8
epitrochlear	—	C77.3	—	D36.0	D48.7	D49.8
esophageal	—	C77.1	—	D36.0	D48.7	D49.8
face	—	C77.0	—	D36.0	D48.7	D49.8
femoral	—	C77.4	—	D36.0	D48.7	D49.8
gastric	—	C77.2	—	D36.0	D48.7	D49.8
groin	—	C77.4	—	D36.0	D48.7	D49.8
head	—	C77.0	—	D36.0	D48.7	D49.8
hepatic	—	C77.2	—	D36.0	D48.7	D49.8
hilar (pulmonary)	—	C77.1	—	D36.0	D48.7	D49.8
splenic	—	C77.2	—	D36.0	D48.7	D49.8
hypogastric	—	C77.5	—	D36.0	D48.7	D49.8
ileocolic	—	C77.2	—	D36.0	D48.7	D49.8
iliac	—	C77.5	—	D36.0	D48.7	D49.8
infraclavicular	—	C77.3	—	D36.0	D48.7	D49.8
inguina, inguinal	—	C77.4	—	D36.0	D48.7	D49.8
innominate	—	C77.1	—	D36.0	D48.7	D49.8
intercostal	—	C77.1	—	D36.0	D48.7	D49.8
intestinal	—	C77.2	—	D36.0	D48.7	D49.8
intrabdominal	—	C77.2	—	D36.0	D48.7	D49.8
intrapelvic	—	C77.5	—	D36.0	D48.7	D49.8
intrathoracic	—	C77.1	—	D36.0	D48.7	D49.8
jugular	—	C77.0	—	D36.0	D48.7	D49.8
leg	—	C77.4	—	D36.0	D48.7	D49.8
limb						
lower	—	C77.4	—	D36.0	D48.7	D49.8
upper	—	C77.3	—	D36.0	D48.7	D49.8
lower limb	—	C77.4	—	D36.0	D48.7	D49.8
lumbar	—	C77.2	—	D36.0	D48.7	D49.8
mandibular	—	C77.0	—	D36.0	D48.7	D49.8
mediastinal	—	C77.1	—	D36.0	D48.7	D49.8
mesenteric (inferior) (superior)	—	C77.2	—	D36.0	D48.7	D49.8
midcolic	—	C77.2	—	D36.0	D48.7	D49.8
multiple sites in categories C77.0–C77.5	—	C77.8	—	D36.0	D48.7	D49.8
neck	—	C77.0	—	D36.0	D48.7	D49.8
obturator	—	C77.5	—	D36.0	D48.7	D49.8
occipital	—	C77.0	—	D36.0	D48.7	D49.8
pancreatic	—	C77.2	—	D36.0	D48.7	D49.8
para-aortic	—	C77.2	—	D36.0	D48.7	D49.8
paracervical	—	C77.5	—	D36.0	D48.7	D49.8
parametrial	—	C77.5	—	D36.0	D48.7	D49.8
parasternal	—	C77.1	—	D36.0	D48.7	D49.8
parotid	—	C77.0	—	D36.0	D48.7	D49.8
pectoral	—	C77.3	—	D36.0	D48.7	D49.8

	Malignant			Benign	Uncertain Behavior	Unspecified
	Primary	Secondary	Ca in situ			
Neoplasm, neoplastic — *continued*						
lymph, lymphatic channel NEC (see also Neoplasm, connective tissue) — *continued*						
gland — *continued*						
pelvic	—	C77.5	—	D36.0	D48.7	D49.8
peri-aortic	—	C77.2	—	D36.0	D48.7	D49.8
peripancreatic	—	C77.2	—	D36.0	D48.7	D49.8
popliteal	—	C77.4	—	D36.0	D48.7	D49.8
porta hepatis	—	C77.2	—	D36.0	D48.7	D49.8
portal	—	C77.2	—	D36.0	D48.7	D49.8
preauricular	—	C77.0	—	D36.0	D48.7	D49.8
prelaryngeal	—	C77.0	—	D36.0	D48.7	D49.8
presymphysial	—	C77.5	—	D36.0	D48.7	D49.8
pretracheal	—	C77.0	—	D36.0	D48.7	D49.8
primary (any site) NEC	C96.9	—	—	—	—	—
pulmonary (hiler)	—	C77.1	—	D36.0	D48.7	D49.8
pyloric	—	C77.2	—	D36.0	D48.7	D49.8
retroperitoneal	—	C77.2	—	D36.0	D48.7	D49.8
retropharyngeal	—	C77.0	—	D36.0	D48.7	D49.8
Rosenmüller's	—	C77.4	—	D36.0	D48.7	D49.8
sacral	—	C77.5	—	D36.0	D48.7	D49.8
scalene	—	C77.0	—	D36.0	D48.7	D49.8
site NEC	—	C77.9	—	D36.0	D48.7	D49.8
splenic (hilar)	—	C77.2	—	D36.0	D48.7	D49.8
subclavicular	—	C77.3	—	D36.0	D48.7	D49.8
subinguinal	—	C77.4	—	D36.0	D48.7	D49.8
sublingual	—	C77.0	—	D36.0	D48.7	D49.8
submandibular	—	C77.0	—	D36.0	D48.7	D49.8
submaxillary	—	C77.0	—	D36.0	D48.7	D49.8
submental	—	C77.0	—	D36.0	D48.7	D49.8
subscapular	—	C77.3	—	D36.0	D48.7	D49.8
supraclavicular	—	C77.0	—	D36.0	D48.7	D49.8
thoracic	—	C77.1	—	D36.0	D48.7	D49.8
tibial —	C77.4	—	D36.0	D48.7	D49.8	
tracheal	—	C77.1	—	D36.0	D48.7	D49.8
tracheobronchial	—	C77.1	—	D36.0	D48.7	D49.8
upper limb	—	C77.3	—	D36.0	D48.7	D49.8
Virchow's	—	C77.0	—	D36.0	D48.7	D49.8
node — see also Neoplasm, lymph gland						
primary NEC	C96.9	—	—	—	—	—
vessel (see also Neoplasm, connective tissue)	C49.9	C79.89	—	D21.9	D48.1	D49.2
Mackenrodt's ligament	C57.7	C79.82	D07.39	D28.7	D39.7	D49.5
malar	C41.0	C79.51	—	D16.4	D48.0	D49.2
marrow NEC	C96.9	C79.52	—	—	—	D47.9
region — see Neoplasm, cheek						
mammary gland — see Neoplasm, breast						
mandible	C41.1	C79.51	—	D16.5	D48.0	D49.2
alveolar						
mucosa	C03.1	C79.89	D00.03	D10.39	D37.09	D49.0
ridge or process	C41.1	C79.51	—	D16.5	D48.0	D49.2
carcinoma	C03.1	—	—	—	—	—
marrow NEC	C96.9	C79.52	—	—	—	D47.9
carcinoma	C03.1	—	—	—	—	—
marrow NEC	C96.9	C79.52	—	—	—	D47.9
marrow (bone) NEC	C96.9	C79.52	—	—	—	D47.9
mastectomy site (skin)	C44.5	C79.2	—	—	—	—
specified as breast tissue						
female (unspecified side)	C50.80	C79.81	—	—	—	—
left side	C50.82	C79.81	—	—	—	—
right side	C50.81	C79.81	—	—	—	—
male (unspecified side)	C50.85	C79.81	—	—	—	—
left side	C50.84	C79.81	—	—	—	—
right side	C50.83	C79.81	—	—	—	—
mastoid (air cells) (antrum) (cavity)	C30.1	C78.39	D02.3	D14.0	D38.5	D49.1
bone or process	C41.0	C79.51	—	D16.4	D48.0	D49.2
marrow NEC	C96.9	C79.52	—	—	—	D47.9

©2002 Ingenix, Inc.

| | Malignant | | | | | |
	Primary	Secondary	Ca in situ	Benign	Uncertain Behavior	Unspecified
Neoplasm, neoplastic — *continued*						
maxilla, maxillary (superior)	C41.0	C79.51	—	D16.4	D48.0	D49.2
alveolar						
mucosa	C03.0	C79.89	D00.03	D10.39	D37.09	D49.0
ridge or process	C41.0	C79.51	—	D16.4	D48.0	D49.2
carcinoma	C03.0	—	—	—	—	—
marrow NEC	C96.9	C79.52	—	—	—	D47.9
antrum	C31.0	C78.39	D02.3	D14.0	D38.5	D49.1
carcinoma	C03.0	—	—	—	—	—
inferior — *see* Neoplasm, mandible						
marrow NEC	C96.9	C79.52	—	—	—	D47.9
sinus	C31.0	C78.39	D02.3	D14.0	D38.5	D49.1
meatus						
external (ear) (unspecified side)	C44.20	C79.2	D04.20	D23.20	D48.5	D49.2
left side	C44.22	C79.2	D04.22	D23.22	D48.5	D49.2
right side	C44.21	C79.2	D04.21	D23.21	D48.5	D49.2
Meckel's diverticulum	C17.3	C78.4	D01.49	D13.39	D37.2	D49.0
mediastinum, mediastinal	C38.3	C78.1	—	D15.2	D38.3	D49.8
anterior	C38.1	C78.1	—	D15.2	D38.3	D49.8
overlapping lesion with heart or pleura	C38.8	—	—	—	—	—
posterior	C38.2	C78.1	—	D15.2	D38.3	D49.8
medulla						
adrenal (unspecified side)	C74.10	C79.70	D09.3	D35.00	D44.10	D49.7
left side	C74.12	C79.72	D09.3	D35.02	D44.12	D49.7
right side	C74.11	C79.71	D09.3	D35.01	D44.11	D49.7
oblongata	C71.7	C79.31	—	D33.1	D43.1	D49.6
meibomian gland (unspecified side)	C44.10	C79.2	D04.10	D23.10	D48.5	D49.2
left side	C44.12	C79.2	D04.12	D23.12	D48.5	D49.2
right side	C44.11	C79.2	D04.11	D23.11	D48.5	D49.2
melanoma — *see* Melanoma						
meninges	C70.9	C79.49	—	D32.9	D42.9	D49.7
brain	C70.0	C79.32	—	D32.0	D42.0	D49.7
cerebral	C70.0	C79.32	—	D32.0	D42.0	D49.7
crainial	C70.0	C79.32	—	D32.0	D42.0	D49.7
intracranial	C70.0	C79.32	—	D32.0	D42.0	D49.7
spinal (cord)	C70.1	C79.49	—	D32.1	D42.1	D49.7
meniscus, knee joint (lateral) (medial) (unspecified side)	C40.20	C79.51	—	D16.20	D48.0	D49.2
left side	C40.22	C79.51	—	D16.22	D48.0	D49.2
right side	C40.21	C79.51	—	D16.21	D48.0	D49.2
mesentery, mesenteric	C48.1	C78.6	—	D20.1	D48.4	D49.0
mesoappendix	C48.1	C78.6	—	D20.1	D48.4	D49.0
mesocolon	C48.1	C78.6	—	D20.1	D48.4	D49.0
mesopharynx — *see* Neoplasm, oropharynx						
mesosalpinx	C57.1	C79.82	D07.39	D28.2	D39.7	D49.5
mesovarium	C57.1	C79.82	D07.39	D28.2	D39.7	D49.5
metacarpus (any bone)						
left side	C40.12	C79.51	—	D16.12	D48.0	D49.2
marrow NEC	C96.9	C79.52	—	—	—	D47.9
right side	C40.11	C79.51	—	D16.11	D48.0	D49.2
marrow NEC	C96.9	C79.52	—	—	—	D47.9
unspecified side	C40.10	C79.51	—	D16.10	D48.0	D49.2
marrow NEC	C96.9	C79.52	—	—	—	D47.9
metastatic NEC — *see also* Neoplasm, by site, secondary	—	C79.9	—	—	—	—
metatarsus (any bone)						
left side	C40.32	C79.51	—	D16.32	D48.0	D49.2
marrow NEC	C96.9	C79.52	—	—	—	D47.9
right side	C40.31	C79.51	—	D16.31	D48.0	D49.2
marrow NEC	C96.9	C79.52	—	—	—	D47.9
unspecified side	C40.30	C79.51	—	D16.30	D48.0	D49.2
marrow NEC	C96.9	C79.52	—	—	—	D47.9
midbrain	C71.7	C79.31	—	D33.1	D43.1	D49.6
milk duct — *see* Neoplasm, breast						
mons						
pubis	C51.9	C79.82	D07.1	D28.0	D39.7	D49.5
veneris	C51.9	C79.82	D07.1	D28.0	D39.7	D49.5
motor tract	C72.9	C79.49	—	D33.9	D43.9	D49.7
brain	C71.9	C79.31	—	D33.2	D43.2	D49.6

	Malignant			Benign	Uncertain Behavior	Unspecified
	Primary	Secondary	Ca in situ			
Neoplasm, neoplastic — *continued*						
motor tract — *continued*						
cauda equina	C72.1	C79.49	—	D33.4	D43.4	D49.7
spinal	C72.0	C79.49	—	D33.4	D43.4	D49.7
mouth	C06.9	C79.89	D00.00	D10.30	D37.09	D49.0
floor	C04.9	C79.89	D00.06	D10.2	D37.09	D49.0
anterior portion	C04.0	C79.89	D00.06	D10.2	D37.09	D49.0
lateral portion	C04.1	C79.89	D00.06	D10.2	D37.09	D49.0
overlapping lesion	C04.8	—	—	—	—	—
overlapping lesion of						
other parts of mouth	C06.89	—	—	—	—	—
unspecified parts of mouth	C06.80	—	—	—	—	—
roof	C05.9	C79.89	D00.00	D10.39	D37.09	D49.0
specified part NEC	C06.89	C79.89	D00.00	D10.39	D37.09	D49.0
vestibule	C06.1	C79.89	D00.00	D10.39	D37.09	D49.0
mucosa						
alveolar (ridge or process)	C03.9	C79.89	D00.03	D10.39	D37.09	D49.0
lower	C03.1	C79.89	D00.03	D10.39	D37.09	D49.0
upper	C03.0	C79.89	D00.03	D10.39	D37.09	D49.0
buccal	C06.0	C79.89	D00.02	D10.39	D37.09	D49.0
cheek	C06.0	C79.89	D00.02	D10.39	D37.09	D49.0
lip — see Neoplasm, lip, internal						
nasal	C30.0	C78.39	D02.3	D14.0	D38.5	D49.1
oral	C06.0	C79.89	D00.02	D10.39	D37.09	D49.0
Müllerian duct						
female	C57.7	C79.82	D07.39	D28.7	D39.7	D49.5
male	C63.7	C79.82	D07.69	D29.7	D40.7	D49.5
multiple sites NEC	C80.0	C80.0	D09.9	D36.9	D48.9	C80.0
muscle — see also Neoplasm, connective tissue						
extraocular (unspecified side)	C69.60	C79.49	D09.20	D31.60	D48.7	D49.8
left side	C69.62	C79.49	D09.22	D31.62	D48.7	D49.8
right side	C69.61	C79.49	D09.21	D31.61	D48.7	D49.8
myocardium	C38.0	C79.89	—	D15.1	D48.7	D49.8
myometrium	C54.2	C79.82	D07.0	D26.1	D39.0	D49.5
myopericardium	C38.0	C79.89	—	D15.1	D48.7	D49.8
nabothian gland (follicle)	C53.0	C79.82	D06.0	D26.0	D39.0	D49.5
nail C44.9	C79.2	D04.9	D23.9	D48.5	D49.2	
finger (unspecified side)	C44.60	C79.2	D04.60	D23.60	D48.5	D49.2
left side	C44.62	C79.2	D04.62	D23.62	D48.5	D49.2
right side	C44.61	C79.2	D04.61	D23.61	D48.5	D49.2
toe (unspecified side)	C44.70	C79.2	D04.70	D23.70	D48.5	D49.2
left side	C44.72	C79.2	D04.72	D23.72	D48.5	D49.2
right side	C44.71	C79.2	D04.71	D23.71	D48.5	D49.2
nares, naris (anterior) (posterior)	C30.0	C78.39	D02.3	D14.0	D38.5	D49.1
nasal — see Neoplasm, nose						
nasolabial groove	C44.31	C79.2	D04.39	D23.39	D48.5	D49.2
nasolacrimal duct (unspecified side)	C69.50	C79.49	D09.20	D31.50	D48.7	D49.8
left side	C69.52	C79.49	D09.22	D31.52	D48.7	D49.8
right side	C69.51	C79.49	D09.21	D31.51	D48.7	D49.8
nasopharynx, nasopharyngeal	C11.9	C79.89	D00.08	D10.6	D37.05	D49.0
floor	C11.3	C79.89	D00.08	D10.6	D37.05	D49.0
overlapping lesion	C11.8	—	—	—	—	—
roof	C11.0	C79.89	D00.08	D10.6	D37.05	D49.0
wall	C11.9	C79.89	D00.08	D10.6	D37.05	D49.0
anterior	C11.3	C79.89	D00.08	D10.6	D37.05	D49.0
lateral	C11.2	C79.89	D00.08	D10.6	D37.05	D49.0
posterior	C11.1	C79.89	D00.08	D10.6	D37.05	D49.0
superior	C11.0	C79.89	D00.08	D10.6	D37.05	D49.0
nates	C44.5	C79.2	D04.5	D23.5	D48.5	D49.2
neck NEC*	C76.0	C79.89	D09.7	D36.7	D48.7	D49.8
nerve (ganglion)	C47.9	C79.89	—	D36.10	D48.2	D49.2
abducens	C72.59	C79.49	—	D33.3	D43.3	D49.7
accessory (spinal)	C72.59	C79.49	—	D33.3	D43.3	D49.7
acoustic (unspecified side)	C72.40	C79.49	—	D33.3	D43.3	D49.7
left side	C72.42	C79.49	—	D33.3	D43.3	D49.7
right side	C72.41	C79.49	—	D33.3	D43.3	D49.7

©2002 Ingenix, Inc.

| | Malignant | | | | | |
	Primary	Secondary	Ca in situ	Benign	Uncertain Behavior	Unspecified
Neoplasm, neoplastic — *continued*						
nerve — *continued*						
auditory (unspecified side)	C72.40	C79.49	—	D33.3	D43.3	D49.7
left side	C72.42	C79.49	—	D33.3	D43.3	D49.7
right side	C72.41	C79.49	—	D33.3	D43.3	D49.7
autonomic NEC (see also Neoplasm, nerve, peripheral)	C47.9	C79.89	—	D36.10	D48.2	D49.2
brachial (unspecified side)	C47.10	C79.89	—	D36.12	D48.2	D49.2
left side	C47.12	C79.89	—	D36.12	D48.2	D49.2
right side	C47.11	C79.89	—	D36.12	D48.2	D49.2
cranial	C72.50	C79.49	—	D33.3	D43.3	D49.7
specified NEC	C72.59	C79.49	—	D33.3	D43.3	D49.7
facial	C72.59	C79.49	—	D33.3	D43.3	D49.7
femoral (unspecified side)	C47.20	C79.89	—	D36.13	D48.2	D49.2
left side	C47.22	C79.89	—	D36.13	D48.2	D49.2
right side	C47.21	C79.89	—	D36.13	D48.2	D49.2
ganglion NEC (see also Neoplasm, nerve, peripheral)	C47.9	C79.89	—	D36.10	D48.2	D49.2
glossopharyngeal	C72.59	C79.49	—	D33.3	D43.3	D49.7
hypoglossal	C72.59	C79.49	—	D33.3	D43.3	D49.7
intercostal	C47.3	C79.89	—	D36.14	D48.2	D49.2
lumbar	C47.6	C79.89	—	D36.17	D48.2	D49.2
median (unspecified side)	C47.10	C79.89	—	D36.12	D48.2	D49.2
left side	C47.12	C79.89	—	D36.12	D48.2	D49.2
right side	C47.11	C79.89	—	D36.12	D48.2	D49.2
obturator (unspecified side)	C47.20	C79.89	—	D36.13	D48.2	D49.2
left side	C47.22	C79.89	—	D36.13	D48.2	D49.2
right side	C47.21	C79.89	—	D36.13	D48.2	D49.2
oculomotor	C72.59	C79.49	—	D33.3	D43.3	D49.7
olfactory (unspecified side)	C47.20	C79.49	—	D33.3	D43.3	D49.7
left side	C47.22	C79.49	—	D33.3	D43.3	D49.7
right side	C47.21	C79.49	—	D33.3	D43.3	D49.7
optic (unspecified side)	C72.30	C79.49	—	D33.3	D43.3	D49.7
left side	C72.32	C79.49	—	D33.3	D43.3	D49.7
right side	C72.31	C79.49	—	D33.3	D43.3	D49.7
parasympathetic NEC — (see also Neoplasm, nerve, peripheral)	C47.9	C79.89	—	D36.10	D48.2	D49.2
peripheral NEC	C47.9	C79.89	—	D36.10	D48.2	D49.2
abdomen	C47.4	C79.89	—	D36.15	D48.2	D49.2
abdominal wall	C47.4	C79.89	—	D36.15	D48.2	D49.2
ankle (unspecified side)	C47.20	C79.89	—	D36.13	D48.2	D49.2
left side	C47.22	C79.89	—	D36.13	D48.2	D49.2
right side	C47.21	C79.89	—	D36.13	D48.2	D49.2
antecubital fossa or space (unspecified side)	C47.10	C79.89	—	D36.12	D48.2	D49.2
left side	C47.12	C79.89	—	D36.12	D48.2	D49.2
right side	C47.11	C79.89	—	D36.12	D48.2	D49.2
arm (unspecified side)	C47.10	C79.89	—	D36.12	D48.2	D49.2
left side	C47.12	C79.89	—	D36.12	D48.2	D49.2
right side	C47.11	C79.89	—	D36.12	D48.2	D49.2
auricle (ear)	C47.0	C79.89	—	D36.11	D48.2	D49.2
axilla	C47.3	C79.89	—	D36.12	D48.2	D49.2
back	C47.6	C79.89	—	D36.17	D48.2	D49.2
buttock	C47.5	C79.89	—	D36.16	D48.2	D49.2
calf (unspecified side)	C47.20	C79.89	—	D36.13	D48.2	D49.2
left side	C47.22	C79.89	—	D36.13	D48.2	D49.2
right side	C47.21	C79.89	—	D36.13	D48.2	D49.2
cervical region	C47.0	C79.89	—	D36.11	D48.2	D49.2
cheek	C47.0	C79.89	—	D36.11	D48.2	D49.2
chest (wall)	C47.3	C79.89	—	D36.14	D48.2	D49.2
chin	C47.0	C79.89	—	D36.11	D48.2	D49.2
ear (external)	C47.0	C79.89	—	D36.11	D48.2	D49.2
elbow (unspecified side)	C47.10	C79.89	—	D36.12	D48.2	D49.2
left side	C47.12	C79.89	—	D36.12	D48.2	D49.2
right side	C47.11	C79.89	—	D36.12	D48.2	D49.2
extrarectal	C47.5	C79.89	—	D36.16	D48.2	D49.2
extremity	C47.9	C79.89	—	D36.10	D48.2	D49.2
lower (unspecified side)	C47.20	C79.89	—	D36.13	D48.2	D49.2
left side	C47.22	C79.89	—	D36.13	D48.2	D49.2
right side	C47.21	C79.89	—	D36.13	D48.2	D49.2

| | Malignant | | | | | |
	Primary	Secondary	Ca in situ	Benign	Uncertain Behavior	Unspecified
Neoplasm, neoplastic — *continued*						
nerve — *continued*						
peripheral NEC — *continued*						
extremity — *continued*						
upper (unspecified side)	C47.10	C79.89	—	D36.12	D48.2	D49.2
left side	C47.12	C79.89	—	D36.12	D48.2	D49.2
right side	C47.11	C79.89	—	D36.12	D48.2	D49.2
eyelid	C47.0	C79.89	—	D36.11	D48.2	D49.2
face	C47.0	C79.89	—	D36.11	D48.2	D49.2
finger (unspecified side)	C47.10	C79.89	—	D36.12	D48.2	D49.2
left side	C47.12	C79.89	—	D36.12	D48.2	D49.2
right side	C47.11	C79.89	—	D36.12	D48.2	D49.2
flank	C47.6	C79.89	—	D36.17	D48.2	D49.2
foot (unspecified side)	C47.20	C79.89	—	D36.13	D48.2	D49.2
left side	C47.22	C79.89	—	D36.13	D48.2	D49.2
right side	C47.21	C79.89	—	D36.13	D48.2	D49.2
forearm (unspecified side)	C47.10	C79.89	—	D36.12	D48.2	D49.2
left side	C47.12	C79.89	—	D36.12	D48.2	D49.2
right side	C47.11	C79.89	—	D36.12	D48.2	D49.2
forehead	C47.0	C79.89	—	D36.11	D48.2	D49.2
gluteal region	C47.5	C79.89	—	D36.16	D48.2	D49.2
groin	C47.5	C79.89	—	D36.16	D48.2	D49.2
hand (unspecified side)	C47.10	C79.89	—	D36.12	D48.2	D49.2
left side	C47.12	C79.89	—	D36.12	D48.2	D49.2
right side	C47.11	C79.89	—	D36.12	D48.2	D49.2
head	C47.0	C79.89	—	D36.11	D48.2	D49.2
heel (unspecified side)	C47.20	C79.89	—	D36.13	D48.2	D49.2
left side	C47.22	C79.89	—	D36.13	D48.2	D49.2
right side	C47.21	C79.89	—	D36.13	D48.2	D49.2
hip (unspecified side)	C47.20	C79.89	—	D36.13	D48.2	D49.2
left side	C47.22	C79.89	—	D36.13	D48.2	D49.2
right side	C47.21	C79.89	—	D36.13	D48.2	D49.2
infraclavicular region	C47.3	C79.89	—	D36.14	D48.2	D49.2
inguinal (canal) (region)	C47.5	C79.89	—	D36.16	D48.2	D49.2
intrathoracic	C47.3	C79.89	—	D36.14	D48.2	D49.2
ischiorectal fossa	C47.5	C79.89	—	D36.16	D48.2	D49.2
knee (unspecified side)	C47.20	C79.89	—	D36.13	D48.2	D49.2
left side	C47.22	C79.89	—	D36.13	D48.2	D49.2
right side	C47.21	C79.89	—	D36.13	D48.2	D49.2
leg (unspecified side)	C47.20	C79.89	—	D36.13	D48.2	D49.2
left side	C47.22	C79.89	—	D36.13	D48.2	D49.2
right side	C47.21	C79.89	—	D36.13	D48.2	D49.2
limb NEC	C47.9	C79.89	—	D36.10	D48.2	D49.2
lower (unspecified side)	C47.20	C79.89	—	D36.13	D48.2	D49.2
left side	C47.22	C79.89	—	D36.13	D48.2	D49.2
right side	C47.21	C79.89	—	D36.13	D48.2	D49.2
upper (unspecified side)	C47.10	C79.89	—	D36.12	D48.2	D49.2
left side	C47.12	C79.89	—	D36.12	D48.2	D49.2
right side	C47.11	C79.89	—	D36.12	D48.2	D49.2
nates	C47.5	C79.89	—	D36.16	D48.2	D49.2
neck	C47.0	C79.89	—	D36.11	D48.2	D49.2
orbit (unspecified side)	C69.60	C79.49	—	D31.60	D48.7	D49.2
left side	C69.62	C79.49	—	D31.62	D48.7	D49.2
right side	C69.61	C79.49	—	D31.61	D48.7	D49.2
pararectal	C47.5	C79.89	—	D36.16	D48.2	D49.2
paraurethral	C47.5	C79.89	—	D36.16	D48.2	D49.2
paravaginal	C47.5	C79.89	—	D36.16	D48.2	D49.2
pelvis (floor)	C47.5	C79.89	—	D36.16	D48.2	D49.2
pelvoabdominal	C47.8	C79.89	—	D36.17	D48.2	D49.2
perineum	C47.5	C79.89	—	D36.16	D48.2	D49.2
perirectal (tissue)	C47.5	C79.89	—	D36.16	D48.2	D49.2
periurethral (tissue)	C47.5	C79.89	—	D36.16	D48.2	D49.2
popliteal fossa or space (unspecified side)	C47.20	C79.89	—	D36.13	D48.2	D49.2
left side	C47.22	C79.89	—	D36.13	D48.2	D49.2
right side	C47.21	C79.89	—	D36.13	D48.2	D49.2
presacral	C47.5	C79.89	—	D36.16	D48.2	D49.2
pterygoid fossa	C47.0	C79.89	—	D36.11	D48.2	D49.2

©2002 Ingenix, Inc.

		Malignant				
	Primary	**Secondary**	**Ca in situ**	**Benign**	**Uncertain Behavior**	**Unspecified**
Neoplasm, neoplastic — *continued*						
nerve — *continued*						
peripheral NEC — *continued*						
rectovaginal septum or wall	C47.5	C79.89	—	D36.16	D48.2	D49.2
rectovesical	C47.5	C79.89	—	D36.16	D48.2	D49.2
sacrococcygeal region	C47.5	C79.89	—	D36.16	D48.2	D49.2
scalp	C47.0	C79.89	—	D36.11	D48.2	D49.2
scapular region	C47.3	C79.89	—	D36.14	D48.2	D49.2
shoulder (unspecified side)	C47.10	C79.89	—	D36.12	D48.2	D49.2
left side	C47.12	C79.89	—	D36.12	D48.2	D49.2
right side	C47.11	C79.89	—	D36.12	D48.2	D49.2
submental	C47.0	C79.89	—	D36.11	D48.2	D49.2
supraclavicular region	C47.0	C79.89	—	D36.11	D48.2	D49.2
temple	C47.0	C79.89	—	D36.11	D48.2	D49.2
temporal region	C47.0	C79.89	—	D36.11	D48.2	D49.2
thigh (unspecified side)	C47.20	C79.89	—	D36.13	D48.2	D49.2
left side	C47.22	C79.89	—	D36.13	D48.2	D49.2
right side	C47.21	C79.89	—	D36.13	D48.2	D49.2
thoracic (duct) (wall)	C47.3	C79.89	—	D36.14	D48.2	D49.2
thorax	C47.3	C79.89	—	D36.14	D48.2	D49.2
thumb (unspecified side)	C47.10	C79.89	—	D36.12	D48.2	D49.2
left side	C47.12	C79.89	—	D36.12	D48.2	D49.2
right side	C47.11	C79.89	—	D36.12	D48.2	D49.2
toe (unspecified side)	C47.20	C79.89	—	D36.13	D48.2	D49.2
left side	C47.22	C79.89	—	D36.13	D48.2	D49.2
right side	C47.21	C79.89	—	D36.13	D48.2	D49.2
trunk	C47.6	C79.89	—	D36.17	D48.2	D49.2
umbilicus	C47.4	C79.89	—	D36.15	D48.2	D49.2
vesicorectal	C47.5	C79.89	—	D36.16	D48.2	D49.2
wrist (unspecified side)	C47.10	C79.89	—	D36.12	D48.2	D49.2
left side	C47.12	C79.89	—	D36.12	D48.2	D49.2
right side	C47.11	C79.89	—	D36.12	D48.2	D49.2
radial (unspecified side)	C47.10	C79.89	—	D36.12	D48.2	D49.2
left side	C47.12	C79.89	—	D36.12	D48.2	D49.2
right side	C47.11	C79.89	—	D36.12	D48.2	D49.2
sacral	C47.5	C79.89	—	D36.16	D48.2	D49.2
sciatic (unspecified side)	C47.20	C79.89	—	D36.13	D48.2	D49.2
left side	C47.22	C79.89	—	D36.13	D48.2	D49.2
right side	C47.21	C79.89	—	D36.13	D48.2	D49.2
spinal NEC	C47.9	C79.89	—	D36.10	D48.2	D49.2
accessory	C72.59	C79.49	—	D33.3	D43.3	D49.7
sympathetic NEC (see also Neoplasm, nerve, peripheral)	C47.9	C79.89	—	D36.10	D48.2	D49.2
trigeminal	C72.59	C79.49	—	D33.3	D43.3	D49.7
trochlear	C72.59	C79.49	—	D33.3	D43.3	D49.7
ulnar (unspecified side)	C47.10	C79.89	—	D36.12	D48.2	D49.2
left side	C47.12	C79.89	—	D36.12	D48.2	D49.2
right side	C47.11	C79.89	—	D36.12	D48.2	D49.2
vagus	C72.59	C79.49	—	D33.3	D43.3	D49.7
nervous system (central) NEC	C72.9	C79.40	—	D33.9	D43.9	D49.7
autonomic NEC (see also Neoplasm, nerve, peripheral)	C47.9	C79.89	—	D36.10	D48.2	D49.2
brain — see also Neoplasm, brain						
membrane or meninges	C70.0	C79.32	—	D32.0	D42.0	D49.7
overlapping lesion	C72.8	—	—	—	—	—
parasympathetic NEC (see also Neoplasm, nerve, peripheral)	C47.9	C79.89	—	D36.10	D48.2	D49.2
sympathetic NEC (see also Neoplasm, nerve, peripheral)	C47.9	C79.89	—	D36.10	D48.2	D49.2
nipple						
female (unspecified side)	C50.00	C79.81	D05.90	D24.00	D48.60	D49.3
left side	C50.02	C79.81	D05.92	D24.02	D48.62	D49.3
right side	C50.01	C79.81	D05.91	D24.01	D48.61	D49.3
male (unspecified side)	C50.05	C79.81	D05.95	D24.10	D48.65	D49.3
left side	C50.04	C79.81	D05.94	D24.12	D48.64	D49.3
right side	C50.03	C79.81	D05.93	D24.11	D48.63	D49.3
nose, nasal	C76.0	C79.89	D09.7	D36.7	D48.7	D49.8
ala (external) (nasi)	C44.31	C79.2	D04.39	D23.39	D48.5	D49.2
bone	C41.0	C79.51	—	D16.4	D48.0	D49.2
marrow NEC	C96.9	C79.52	—	—	—	D47.9

	Malignant					
	Primary	Secondary	Ca in situ	Benign	Uncertain Behavior	Unspecified
Neoplasm, neoplastic — *continued*						
nose, nasal — *continued*						
cartilage	C30.0	C78.39	D02.3	D14.0	D38.5	D49.1
cavity	C30.0	C78.39	D02.3	D14.0	D38.5	D49.1
overlapping lesion with accessory sinuses	C31.8	—	—	—	—	—
choana	C11.3	C79.89	D00.08	D10.6	D37.05	D49.0
external (skin)	C44.31	C79.2	D04.39	D23.39	D48.5	D49.2
fossa	C30.0	C78.39	D02.3	D14.0	D38.5	D49.1
internal	C30.0	C78.39	D02.3	D14.0	D38.5	D49.1
mucosa	C30.0	C78.39	D02.3	D14.0	D38.5	D49.1
septum	C30.0	C78.39	D02.3	D14.0	D38.5	D49.1
posterior margin	C11.3	C79.89	D00.08	D10.6	D37.05	D49.0
sinus — *see* Neoplasm, sinus						
skin	C44.31	C79.2	D04.39	D23.39	D48.5	D49.2
turbinate (mucosa)	C30.0	C78.39	D02.3	D14.0	D38.5	D49.1
bone	C41.0	C79.51	—	D16.4	D48.0	D49.2
marrow NEC	C96.9	C79.52	—	—	—	D47.9
vestibule	C30.0	C78.39	D02.3	D14.0	D38.5	D49.1
nostril	C30.0	C78.39	D02.3	D14.0	D38.5	D49.1
nucleus pulposus	C41.2	C79.51	—	D16.6	D48.0	D49.2
marrow NEC	C96.9	C79.52	—	—	—	D47.9
occipital						
bone	C41.0	C79.51	—	D16.4	D48.0	D49.2
marrow NEC	C96.9	C79.52	—	—	—	D47.9
lobe or pole, brain	C71.4	C79.31	—	D33.0	D43.0	D49.6
odontogenic — *see* Neoplasm, jaw bone						
oesophagus — *see* Neoplasm, esophagus						
olfactory nerve or bulb (unspecified side)	C72.20	C79.49	—	D33.3	D43.3	D49.7
left side	C72.22	C79.49	—	D33.3	D43.3	D49.7
right side	C72.21	C79.49	—	D33.3	D43.3	D49.7
olive (brain)	C71.7	C79.31	—	D33.1	D43.1	D49.6
omentum	C48.1	C78.6	—	D20.1	D48.4	D49.0
overlaping lesion with retroperitoneum	C48.8	—	—	—	—	—
operculum (brain)	C71.0	C79.31	—	D33.0	D43.0	D49.6
optic nerve, chiasm, or tract (unspecified side)	C72.30	C79.49	—	D33.3	D43.3	D49.7
left side	C72.32	C79.49	—	D33.3	D43.3	D49.7
right side	C72.31	C79.49	—	D33.3	D43.3	D49.7
oral (cavity)	C06.9	C79.89	D00.00	D10.30	D37.09	D49.0
ill-defined	C14.8	C79.89	D00.00	D10.30	D37.09	D49.0
mucosa	C06.9	C79.89	D00.02	D10.39	D37.09	D49.0
overlapping lesion with lip or pharynx	C14.8	—	—	—	—	—
orbit						
autonomic nerve (unspecified side)	C69.60	C79.49	—	D31.60	D48.7	D49.2
left side	C69.62	C79.49	—	D31.62	D48.7	D49.2
right side	C69.61	C79.49	—	D31.61	D48.7	D49.2
bone	C41.0	C79.51	—	D16.4	D48.0	D49.2
marrow NEC	C96.9	C79.52	—	—	—	D47.9
eye (unspecified side)	C69.60	C79.49	D09.20	D31.60	D48.7	D49.8
left side	C69.62	C79.49	D09.22	D31.62	D48.7	D49.8
right side	C69.61	C79.49	D09.21	D31.61	D48.7	D49.8
peripheral nerves (unspecified side)	C69.60	C79.49	—	D31.60	D48.7	D49.2
left side	C69.62	C79.49	—	D31.62	D48.7	D49.2
right side	C69.61	C79.49	—	D31.61	D48.7	D49.2
soft parts (unspecified side)	C69.60	C79.49	D09.20	D31.60	D48.7	D49.8
left side	C69.62	C79.49	D09.22	D31.62	D48.7	D49.8
right side	C69.61	C79.49	D09.21	D31.61	D48.7	D49.8
unspecified site (unspecified side)	C69.60	C79.49	D09.20	D31.60	D48.7	D49.8
left side	C69.62	C79.49	D09.22	D31.62	D48.7	D49.8
right side	C69.61	C79.49	D09.21	D31.61	D48.7	D49.8
organ of Zuckerkandl	C75.5	C79.89	—	D35.6	D44.7	D49.7
oropharynx	C10.9	C79.89	D00.08	D10.5	D37.05	D49.0
branchial cleft (vestige)	C10.4	C79.89	D00.08	D10.5	D37.05	D49.0
junctional region	C10.8	C79.89	D00.08	D10.5	D37.05	D49.0
lateral wall	C10.2	C79.89	D00.08	D10.5	D37.05	D49.0
overlapping lesion	C10.8	—	—	—	—	—
pillars or fauces	C09.1	C79.89	D00.08	D10.5	D37.05	D49.0
posterior wall	C10.3	C79.89	D00.08	D10.5	D37.05	D49.0

©2002 Ingenix, Inc.

	Malignant					
	Primary	**Secondary**	**Ca in situ**	**Benign**	**Uncertain Behavior**	**Unspecified**
Neoplasm, neoplastic — *continued*						
oropharynx — *continued*						
vallecula	C10.0	C79.89	D00.08	D10.5	D37.05	D49.0
os						
external	C53.1	C79.82	D06.1	D26.0	D39.0	D49.5
internal	C53.0	C79.82	D06.0	D26.0	D39.0	D49.5
ovary (unspecified side)	C56.9	C79.60	D07.39	D27.9	D39.10	D49.5
left side	C56.1	C79.62	D07.39	D27.1	D39.12	D49.5
right side	C56.0	C79.61	D07.39	D27.0	D39.11	D49.5
oviduct (unspecified side)	C57.00	C79.82	D07.39	D28.2	D39.7	D49.5
left side	C57.02	C79.82	D07.39	D28.2	D39.7	D49.5
right side	C57.01	C79.82	D07.39	D28.2	D39.7	D49.5
palate	C05.9	C79.89	D00.00	D10.39	D37.09	D49.0
hard	C05.0	C79.89	D00.05	D10.39	D37.09	D49.0
junction of hard and soft palate	C05.9	C79.89	D00.00	D10.39	D37.09	D49.0
overlapping lesions	C05.8	—	—	—	—	—
soft	C05.1	C79.89	D00.04	D10.39	D37.09	D49.0
nasopharyngeal surface	C11.3	C79.89	D00.08	D10.6	D37.05	D49.0
posterior surface	C11.3	C79.89	D00.08	D10.6	D37.05	D49.0
superior surface	C11.3	C79.89	D00.08	D10.6	D37.05	D49.0
palatoglossal arch	C09.1	C79.89	D00.00	D10.5	D37.09	D49.0
palatopharyngeal arch	C09.1	C79.89	D00.00	D10.5	D37.09	D49.0
pallium	C71.0	C79.31	—	D33.0	D43.0	D49.6
palpebra (unspecified side)	C44.10	C79.2	D04.10	D23.10	D48.5	D49.2
left side	C44.12	C79.2	D04.12	D23.12	D48.5	D49.2
right side	C44.11	C79.2	D04.11	D23.11	D48.5	D49.2
pancreas	C25.9	C78.89	D01.7	D13.6	D37.7	D49.0
body	C25.1	C78.89	D01.7	D13.6	D37.7	D49.0
duct (of Santorini) (of Wirsung)	C25.3	C78.89	D01.7	D13.6	D37.7	D49.0
ectopic tissue	C25.7	C78.89	—	D13.6	D37.7	D49.0
head	C25.0	C78.89	D01.7	D13.6	D37.7	D49.0
islet cells	C25.4	C78.89	D01.7	D13.7	D37.7	D49.0
neck	C25.7	C78.89	D01.7	D13.6	D37.7	D49.0
overlapping lesion	C25.8	—	—	—	—	—
tail	C25.2	C78.89	D01.7	D13.6	D37.7	D49.0
para-aortic body	C75.5	C79.89	—	D35.6	D44.7	D49.7
paraganglion NEC	C75.5	C79.89	—	D35.6	D44.7	D49.7
parametrium	C57.3	C79.82	—	D28.2	D39.7	D49.5
paranephric	C48.0	C78.6	—	D20.0	D48.3	D49.0
pararectal	C76.3	C79.89	—	D36.7	D48.7	D49.8
parasagittal (region)	C76.0	C79.89	D09.7	D36.7	D48.7	D49.8
parasellar	C72.9	C79.49	—	D33.9	D43.7	D49.7
parathyroid (gland)	C75.0	C79.89	D09.3	D35.1	D44.2	D49.7
paraurethral	C76.3	C79.89	—	D36.7	D48.7	D49.8
gland	C68.1	C79.19	D09.19	D30.7	D41.7	D49.5
paravaginal	C76.3	C79.89	—	D36.7	D48.7	D49.8
parenchyma, kidney (unspecified side)	C64.9	C79.00	D09.19	D30.00	D41.00	D49.5
left side	C64.1	C79.02	D09.19	D30.02	D41.02	D49.5
right side	C64.0	C79.01	D09.19	D30.01	D41.01	D49.5
parietal						
bone	C41.0	C79.51	—	D16.4	D48.0	D49.2
marrow NEC	C96.9	C79.52	—	—	—	D47.9
lobe, brain	C71.3	C79.31	—	D33.0	D43.0	D49.6
paroophoron	C57.1	C79.82	D07.39	D28.2	D39.7	D49.5
parotid (duct) (gland)	C07	C79.89	D00.00	D11.0	D37.030	D49.0
parovarium	C57.1	C79.82	D07.39	D28.2	D39.7	D49.5
patella						
left side	C40.32	C79.51	—	D16.32	D48.0	D49.2
marrow NEC	C96.9	C79.52	—	—	—	D47.9
right side	C40.31	C79.51	—	D16.31	D48.0	D49.2
marrow NEC	C96.9	C79.52	—	—	—	D47.9
unspecified side	C40.30	C79.51	—	D16.30	D48.0	D49.2
marrow NEC	C96.9	C79.52	—	—	—	D47.9
peduncle, cerebral	C71.7	C79.31	—	D33.1	D43.1	D49.6
pelvirectal junction	C19	C78.5	D01.1	D12.7	D37.5	D49.0
pelvis, pelvic	C76.3	C79.89	D09.7	D36.7	D48.7	D49.8
bone	C41.4	C79.51	—	D16.8	D48.0	D49.2

| | Malignant | | | | | |
	Primary	Secondary	Ca in situ	Benign	Uncertain Behavior	Unspecified
Neoplasm, neoplastic — *continued*						
pelvis, pelvic — *continued*						
marrow NEC	C96.9	C79.52	—	—	—	D47.9
floor	C76.3	C79.89	D09.7	D36.7	D48.7	D49.8
renal (unspecified side)	C65.9	C79.00	D09.19	D30.10	D41.10	D49.5
left side	C65.1	C79.02	D09.19	D30.12	D41.12	D49.5
right side	C65.0	C79.01	D09.19	D30.11	D41.11	D49.5
viscera	C76.3	C79.89	D09.7	D36.7	D48.7	D49.8
wall	C76.3	C79.89	D09.7	D36.7	D48.7	D49.8
pelvo-abdominal	C76.8	C79.89	D09.7	D36.7	D48.7	D49.8
penis	C60.9	C79.82	D07.4	D29.0	D40.7	D49.5
body	C60.2	C79.82	D07.4	D29.0	D40.7	D49.5
corpus (cavernosum)	C60.2	C79.82	D07.4	D29.0	D40.7	D49.5
glans	C60.1	C79.82	D07.4	D29.0	D40.7	D49.5
skin NEC	C60.9	C79.82	D07.4	D29.0	D40.7	D49.5
periadrenal (tissue)	C48.0	C78.6	—	D20.0	D48.3	D49.0
perianal (skin)	C44.5	C79.2	D04.5	D23.5	D48.5	D49.2
pericardium	C38.0	C79.89	—	D15.1	D48.7	D49.8
perinephric	C48.0	C78.6	—	D20.0	D48.3	D49.0
perineum	C76.3	C79.89	D09.7	D36.7	D48.7	D49.8
periodontal tissue NEC	C03.9	C79.89	D00.03	D10.39	D37.09	D49.0
periosteum — *see Neoplasm, bone*						
peripancreatic	C48.0	C78.6	—	D20.0	D48.3	D49.0
peripheral nerve NEC	C47.9	C79.89	—	D36.10	D48.2	D49.2
perirectal (tissue)	C76.3	C79.89	—	D36.7	D48.7	D49.8
perirenal (tissue)	C48.0	C78.6	—	D20.0	D48.3	D49.0
peritoneum, peritoneal (cavity)	C48.2	C78.6	—	D20.1	D48.4	D49.0
overlapping lesion	C48.8	—	—	—	—	—
with digestive organs	C26.8	—	—	—	—	—
parietal	C48.1	C78.6	—	D20.1	D48.4	D49.0
pelvic	C48.1	C78.6	—	D20.1	D48.4	D49.0
specified part NEC	C48.1	C78.6	—	D20.1	D48.4	D49.0
peritonsillar (tissue)	C76.0	C79.89	D09.7	D36.7	D48.7	D49.8
periurethral tissue	C76.3	C79.89	—	D36.7	D48.7	D49.8
phalanges						
foot						
left side	C40.32	C79.51	—	D16.32	D48.0	D49.2
marrow NEC	C96.9	C79.52	—	—	—	D47.9
right side	C40.31	C79.51	—	D16.31	D48.0	D49.2
marrow NEC	C96.9	C79.52	—	—	—	D47.9
unspecified side	C40.30	C79.51	—	D16.30	D48.0	D49.2
marrow NEC	C96.9	C79.52	—	—	—	D47.9
hand						
left side	C40.12	C79.51	—	D16.12	D48.0	D49.2
marrow NEC	C96.9	C79.52	—	—	—	D47.9
right side	C40.11	C79.51	—	D16.11	D48.0	D49.2
marrow NEC	C96.9	C79.52	—	—	—	D47.9
unspecified side	C40.10	C79.51	—	D16.10	D48.0	D49.2
marrow NEC	C96.9	C79.52	—	—	—	D47.9
unspecified site						
left side	C40.92	C79.51	—	D16.9	D48.0	D49.2
marrow NEC	C96.9	C79.52	—	—	—	D47.9
right side	C40.91	C79.51	—	D16.9	D48.0	D49.2
marrow NEC	C96.9	C79.52	—	—	—	D47.9
unspecified side	C40.90	C79.51	—	D16.9	D48.0	D49.2
marrow NEC	C96.9	C79.52	—	—	—	D47.9
pharynx, pharyngeal	C14.0	C79.89	D00.08	D10.9	D37.05	D49.0
bursa	C11.1	C79.89	D00.08	D10.6	D37.05	D49.0
fornix	C11.3	C79.89	D00.08	D10.6	D37.05	D49.0
recess	C11.2	C79.89	D00.08	D10.6	D37.05	D49.0
region	C14.0	C79.89	D00.08	D10.9	D37.05	D49.0
tonsil	C11.1	C79.89	D00.08	D10.6	D37.05	D49.0
wall (lateral) (posterior)	C14.0	C79.89	D00.08	D10.9	D37.05	D49.0
pia mater	C70.9	C79.40	—	D32.9	D42.9	D49.7
cerebral	C70.0	C79.32	—	D32.0	D42.0	D49.7
cranial	C70.0	C79.32	—	D32.0	D42.0	D49.7
spinal	C70.1	C79.49	—	D32.1	D42.1	D49.7

©2002 Ingenix, Inc.

| | Malignant | | | | | |
	Primary	Secondary	Ca in situ	Benign	Uncertain Behavior	Unspecified
Neoplasm, neoplastic — *continued*						
pillars of fauces	C09.1	C79.89	D00.08	D10.5	D37.05	D49.0
pineal (body) (gland)	C75.3	C79.89	D09.3	D35.4	D44.5	D49.7
pinna (ear) NEC						
left side	C44.22	C79.2	D04.22	D23.22	D48.5	D49.2
cartilage	C49.0	C79.89	—	D21.0	D48.1	D49.2
right side	C44.21	C79.2	D04.21	D23.21	D48.5	D49.2
cartilage	C49.0	C79.89	—	D21.0	D48.1	D49.2
unspecified side	C44.20	C79.2	D04.20	D23.20	D48.5	D49.2
cartilage	C49.0	C79.89	—	D21.0	D48.1	D49.2
piriform fossa or sinus	C12	C79.89	D00.08	D10.7	D37.05	D49.0
pituitary (body) (fossa) (gland) (lobe)	C75.1	C79.89	D09.3	D35.2	D44.3	D49.7
placenta	C58	C79.82	D07.0	D26.7	D39.2	D49.5
pleura, pleural (cavity)	C38.4	C78.2	—	D19.0	D38.2	D49.1
overlapping lesion with heart or mediastinum	C38.8	—	—	—	—	—
parietal	C38.4	C78.2	—	D19.0	D38.2	D49.1
visceral	C38.4	C78.2	—	D19.0	D38.2	D49.1
plexus						
brachial	C47.10	C79.89	—	D36.12	D48.2	D49.2
left side	C47.12	C79.89	—	D36.12	D48.2	D49.2
right side	C47.11	C79.89	—	D36.12	D48.2	D49.2
cervical	C47.0	C79.89	—	D36.11	D48.2	D49.2
choroid	C71.5	C79.31	—	D33.0	D43.0	D49.6
lumbosacral	C47.5	C79.89	—	D36.16	D48.2	D49.2
sacral	C47.5	C79.89	—	D36.16	D48.2	D49.2
pluri-endocrine	C75.8	C79.89	D09.3	D35.8	D44.8	D49.7
pole						
frontal	C71.1	C79.31	—	D33.0	D43.0	D49.6
occipital	C71.4	C79.31	—	D33.0	D43.0	D49.6
pons (varolii)	C71.7	C79.31	—	D33.1	D43.1	D49.6
popliteal fossa or space (unspecified side)*	C76.50	C79.89	D04.70	D36.7	D48.7	D49.8
left side	C76.52	C79.89	D04.72	D36.7	D48.7	D49.8
right side	C76.51	C79.89	D04.71	D36.7	D48.7	D49.8
postcricoid (region)	C13.0	C79.89	D00.08	D10.7	D37.05	D49.0
posterior fossa (cranial)	C71.9	C79.31	—	D33.2	D43.2	D49.6
postnasal space	C11.9	C79.89	D00.08	D10.6	D37.05	D49.0
prepuce	C60.0	C79.82	D07.4	D29.0	D40.7	D49.5
prepylorus	C16.4	C78.89	D00.2	D13.1	D37.1	D49.0
presacral (region)	C76.3	C79.89	—	D36.7	D48.7	D49.8
prostate (gland)	C61	C79.82	D07.5	D29.1	D40.0	D49.5
utricle	C68.0	C79.19	D09.19	D30.4	D41.3	D49.5
pterygoid fossa	C49.0	C79.89	—	D21.0	D48.1	D49.2
pubic bone	C41.4	C79.51	—	D16.8	D48.0	D49.2
marrow NEC	C96.9	C79.52	—	—	—	D47.9
pudenda, pudendum (female)	C51.9	C79.82	D07.1	D28.0	D39.7	D49.5
pulmonary (unspecified side) (see also Neoplasm, lung)	C34.90	C78.00	D02.20	D14.30	D38.1	D49.1
left side	C34.92	C78.02	D02.22	D14.32	D38.1	D49.1
right side	C34.91	C78.01	D02.21	D14.31	D38.1	D49.1
putamen	C71.0	C79.31	—	D33.0	D43.0	D49.6
pyloric						
antrum	C16.3	C78.89	D00.2	D13.1	D37.1	D49.0
canal	C16.4	C78.89	D00.2	D13.1	D37.1	D49.0
pylorus	C16.4	C78.89	D00.2	D13.1	D37.1	D49.0
pyramid (brain)	C71.7	C79.31	—	D33.1	D43.1	D49.6
pyriform fossa or sinus	C12	C79.89	D00.08	D10.7	D37.05	D49.0
radius (any part)						
left side	C40.02	C79.51	—	D16.02	D48.0	D49.2
marrow NEC	C96.9	C79.52	—	—	—	D47.9
right side	C40.01	C79.51	—	D16.01	D48.0	D49.2
marrow NEC	C96.9	C79.52	—	—	—	D47.9
unspecified side	C40.00	C79.51	—	D16.00	D48.0	D49.2
marrow NEC	C96.9	C79.52	—	—	—	D47.9
Rathke's pouch	C75.1	C79.89	D09.3	D35.2	D44.3	D49.7
rectosigmoid (junction)	C19	C78.5	D01.1	D12.7	D37.5	D49.0
overlapping lesion with anus or rectum	C21.8	—	—	—	—	—
rectouterine pouch	C48.1	C78.6	—	D20.1	D48.4	D49.0
rectovaginal septum or wall	C76.3	C79.89	D09.7	D36.7	D48.7	D49.8

	Malignant			Benign	Uncertain Behavior	Unspecified
	Primary	Secondary	Ca in situ			
Neoplasm, neoplastic — *continued*						
rectovesical septum	C76.3	C79.89	D09.7	D36.7	D48.7	D49.8
rectum (ampulla)	C20	C78.5	D01.2	D12.8	D37.5	D49.0
and colon	C19	C78.5	D01.1	D12.7	D37.5	D49.0
overlapping lesion with anus or rectosigmoid junction	C21.8	—	—	—	—	—
renal						
calyx (unspecified side)	C65.9	C79.00	D09.19	D30.10	D41.10	D49.5
left side	C65.1	C79.02	D09.19	D30.12	D41.12	D49.5
right side	C65.0	C79.01	D09.19	D30.11	D41.11	D49.5
hilus (unspecified side)	C65.9	C79.00	D09.19	D30.10	D41.10	D49.5
left side	C65.1	C79.02	D09.19	D30.12	D41.12	D49.5
right side	C65.0	C79.01	D09.19	D30.11	D41.11	D49.5
parenchyma (unspecified side)	C64.9	C79.00	D09.19	D30.00	D41.00	D49.5
left side	C64.1	C79.02	D09.19	D30.02	D41.02	D49.5
right side	C64.0	C79.01	D09.19	D30.01	D41.01	D49.5
pelvis (unspecified side)	C65.9	C79.00	D09.19	D30.10	D41.10	D49.5
left side	C65.1	C79.02	D09.19	D30.12	D41.12	D49.5
right side	C65.0	C79.01	D09.19	D30.11	D41.11	D49.5
unspecified site (unspecified side)	C64.9	C79.00	D09.19	D30.00	D41.00	D49.5
left side	C64.1	C79.02	D09.19	D30.02	D41.02	D49.5
right side	C64.0	C79.01	D09.19	D30.01	D41.01	D49.5
respiratory						
organs or system NEC	C39.9	C78.30	D02.4	D14.4	D38.6	D49.1
overlapping lesion with intrathoracic organs	C39.8	—	—	—	—	—
specified sites NEC	C39.8	C78.39	D02.3	D15.7	D38.5	D49.1
tract NEC	C39.9	C78.30	D02.4	D14.4	D38.5	D49.1
upper	C39.0	C78.30	D02.4	D14.4	D38.5	D49.1
retina (unspecified side)	C69.20	C79.49	D09.20	D31.20	D48.7	D49.8
left side	C69.22	C79.49	D09.22	D31.22	D48.7	D49.8
right side	C69.21	C79.49	D09.21	D31.21	D48.7	D49.8
retrobulbar (unspecified side)	C69.60	C79.49	—	D31.60	D48.7	D49.8
left side	C69.62	C79.49	—	D31.62	D48.7	D49.8
right side	C69.61	C79.49	—	D31.61	D48.7	D49.8
retrocecal	C48.0	C78.6		D20.0	D48.3	D49.0
retromolar (area) (triangle) (trigone)	C06.2	C79.89	D00.00	D10.39	D37.09	D49.0
retro-orbital	C76.0	C79.89	D09.7	D36.7	D48.7	D49.8
retroperitoneal (space) (tissue)	C48.0	C78.6	—	D20.0	D48.3	D49.0
overlapping lesion	C48.8	—	—	—	—	—
retroperitoneum	C48.0	C78.6	—	D20.0	D48.3	D49.0
overlapping lesion	C48.8	—	—	—	—	—
retropharyngeal	C14.0	C79.89	D00.08	D10.9	D37.05	D49.0
retrovesical (septum)	C76.3	C79.89	D09.7	D36.7	D48.7	D49.8
rhinencephalon	C71.0	C79.31	—	D33.0	D43.0	D49.6
rib	C41.3	C79.51	—	D16.7	D48.0	D49.2
marrow NEC	C96.9	C79.52	—	—	—	D47.9
Rosenmüller's fossa	C11.2	C79.89	D00.08	D10.6	D37.05	D49.0
round ligament	C57.2	C79.82	—	D28.2	D39.7	D49.5
sacrococcyx, sacrococcygeal	C41.4	C79.51	—	D16.8	D48.0	D49.2
marrow NEC	C96.9	C79.52	—	—	—	D47.9
region	C76.3	C79.89	D09.7	D36.7	D48.7	D49.8
sacrouterine ligament	C57.3	C79.82	—	D28.2	D39.7	D49.5
sacrum, sacral (vertebra)	C41.4	C79.51	—	D16.8	D48.0	D49.2
marrow NEC	C96.9	C79.52	—	—	—	D47.9
salivary gland or duct (major)	C08.9	C79.89	D00.00	D11.9	D37.039	D49.0
minor NEC	C06.9	C79.89	D00.00	D10.39	D37.04	D49.0
overlapping lesion	C08.8	—	—	—	—	—
parotid	C07	C79.89	D00.00	D11.0	D37.030	D49.0
pluriglandular	C08.8	C79.89	D00.00	D11.9	D37.039	D49.0
sublingual	C08.1	C79.89	D00.00	D11.7	D37.031	D49.0
submandibular	C08.0	C79.89	D00.00	D11.7	D37.032	D49.0
submaxillary	C08.0	C79.89	D00.00	D11.7	D37.032	D49.0
salpinx (uterine) (unspecified side)	C57.00	C79.82	D07.39	D28.2	D39.7	D49.5
left side	C57.02	C79.82	D07.39	D28.2	D39.7	D49.5
right side	C57.01	C79.82	D07.39	D28.2	D39.7	D49.5
Santorini's duct	C25.3	C78.89	D01.7	D13.6	D37.7	D49.0
scalp	C44.4	C79.2	D04.4	D23.4	D48.5	D49.2

©2002 Ingenix, Inc.

	Malignant					
	Primary	**Secondary**	**Ca in situ**	**Benign**	**Uncertain Behavior**	**Unspecified**
Neoplasm, neoplastic — *continued*						
scapula (any part)						
left side	C40.02	C79.51	—	D16.02	D48.0	D49.2
marrow NEC	C96.9	C79.52	—	—	—	D47.9
right side	C40.01	C79.51	—	D16.01	D48.0	D49.2
marrow NEC	C96.9	C79.52	—	—	—	D47.9
unspecified side	C40.00	C79.51	—	D16.00	D48.0	D49.2
marrow NEC	C96.9	C79.52	—	—	—	D47.9
scapular region	C76.1	C79.89	D09.7	D36.7	D48.7	D49.8
scar NEC (see also Neoplasm, skin)	C44.9	C79.2	D04.9	D23.9	D48.5	D49.2
sciatic nerve (unspecified side)	C47.20	C79.89	—	D36.13	D48.2	D49.2
left side	C47.22	C79.89	—	D36.13	D48.2	D49.2
right side	C47.21	C79.89	—	D36.13	D48.2	D49.2
sclera (unspecified side)	C69.40	C79.49	D09.20	D31.40	D48.7	D49.8
left side	C69.42	C79.49	D09.22	D31.42	D48.7	D49.8
right side	C69.41	C79.49	D09.21	D31.41	D48.7	D49.8
scrotum (skin)	C63.2	C79.82	D07.61	D29.4	D40.7	D49.5
sebaceous gland — see Neoplasm, skin						
sella turcica	C75.1	C79.89	D09.3	D35.2	D44.3	D49.7
bone	C41.0	C79.51	—	D16.4	D48.0	D49.2
marrow NEC	C96.9	C79.52	—	—	—	D47.9
semilunar cartilage (knee) (unspecified side)	C40.20	C79.51	—	D16.20	D48.0	D49.2
left side	C40.22	C79.51	—	D16.22	D48.0	D49.2
right side	C40.21	C79.51	—	D16.21	D48.0	D49.2
seminal vesicle	C63.7	C79.82	D07.69	D29.7	D40.7	D49.5
septum						
nasal	C30.0	C78.39	D02.3	D14.0	D38.5	D49.1
posterior margin	C11.3	C79.89	D00.08	D10.6	D37.05	D49.0
rectovaginal	C76.3	C79.89	D09.7	D36.7	D48.7	D49.8
rectovesical	C76.3	C79.89	D09.7	D36.7	D48.7	D49.8
urethrovaginal	C57.9	C79.82	D07.30	D28.9	D39.9	D49.5
vesicovaginal	C57.9	C79.82	D07.30	D28.9	D39.9	D49.5
shoulder NEC* (unspecified side)	C76.40	C79.89	D04.60	D36.7	D48.7	D49.8
left side	C76.42	C79.89	D04.62	D36.7	D48.7	D49.8
right side	C76.41	C79.89	D04.61	D36.7	D48.7	D49.8
sigmoid flexure (lower) (upper)	C18.7	C78.5	D01.0	D12.5	D37.4	D49.0
sinus (accessory)	C31.9	C78.39	D02.3	D14.0	D38.5	D49.1
bone (any)	C41.0	C79.51	—	D16.4	D48.0	D49.2
marrow NEC	C96.9	C79.52	—	—	—	D47.9
ethmoidal	C31.1	C78.39	D02.3	D14.0	D38.5	D49.1
frontal	C31.2	C78.39	D02.3	D14.0	D38.5	D49.1
maxillary	C31.0	C78.39	D02.3	D14.0	D38.5	D49.1
nasal, paranasal NEC	C31.9	C78.39	D02.3	D14.0	D38.5	D49.1
overlapping lesion	C31.8	—	—	—	—	—
pyriform	C12	C79.89	D00.08	D10.7	D37.05	D49.0
sphenoid	C31.3	C78.39	D02.3	D14.0	D38.5	D49.1
skeleton, skeletal NEC	C41.9	C79.51	—	D16.9	D48.0	D49.2
marrow NEC	C96.9	C79.52	—	—	—	D47.9
Skene's gland	C68.1	C79.19	D09.19	D30.7	D41.7	D49.5
skin NEC	C44.9	C79.2	D04.9	D23.9	D48.5	D49.2
abdominal wall	C44.5	C79.2	D04.5	D23.5	D48.5	D49.2
ala nasi	C44.31	C79.2	D04.39	D23.39	D48.5	D49.2
ankle (unspecified side)	C44.70	C79.2	D04.70	D23.70	D48.5	D49.2
left side	C44.72	C79.2	D04.72	D23.72	D48.5	D49.2
right side	C44.71	C79.2	D04.71	D23.71	D48.5	D49.2
antecubital space (unspecified side)	C44.60	C79.2	D04.60	D23.60	D48.5	D49.2
left side	C44.62	C79.2	D04.62	D23.62	D48.5	D49.2
right side	C44.61	C79.2	D04.61	D23.61	D48.5	D49.2
anus	C44.5	C79.2	D04.5	D23.5	D48.5	D49.2
arm (unspecified side)	C44.60	C79.2	D04.60	D23.60	D48.5	D49.2
left side	C44.62	C79.2	D04.62	D23.62	D48.5	D49.2
right side	C44.61	C79.2	D04.61	D23.61	D48.5	D49.2
auditory canal (external) (unspecified side)	C44.20	C79.2	D04.20	D23.20	D48.5	D49.2
left side	C44.22	C79.2	D04.22	D23.22	D48.5	D49.2
right side	C44.21	C79.2	D04.21	D23.21	D48.5	D49.2
auricle (ear) (unspecified side)	C44.20	C79.2	D04.20	D23.20	D48.5	D49.2
left side	C44.22	C79.2	D04.22	D23.22	D48.5	D49.2

| | Malignant | | | | | |
	Primary	Secondary	Ca in situ	Benign	Uncertain Behavior	Unspecified
Neoplasm, neoplastic — *continued*						
skin NEC — *continued*						
auricle — *continued*						
right side	C44.21	C79.2	D04.21	D23.21	D48.5	D49.2
auricular canal (external) (unspecified side)	C44.20	C79.2	D04.20	D23.20	D48.5	D49.2
left side	C44.22	C79.2	D04.22	D23.22	D48.5	D49.2
right side	C44.21	C79.2	D04.21	D23.21	D48.5	D49.2
axilla, axillary fold	C44.5	C79.2	D04.5	D23.5	D48.5	D49.2
back	C44.5	C79.2	D04.5	D23.5	D48.5	D49.2
breast	C44.5	C79.2	D04.5	D23.5	D48.5	D49.2
brow	C44.31	C79.2	D04.39	D23.39	D48.5	D49.2
buttock	C44.5	C79.2	D04.5	D23.5	D48.5	D49.2
calf (unspecified side)	C44.70	C79.2	D04.70	D23.70	D48.5	D49.2
left side	C44.72	C79.2	D04.72	D23.72	D48.5	D49.2
right side	C44.71	C79.2	D04.71	D23.71	D48.5	D49.2
canthus (eye) (inner) (outer) (unspecified side)	C44.10	C79.2	D04.10	D23.10	D48.5	D49.2
left side	C44.12	C79.2	D04.12	D23.12	D48.5	D49.2
right side	C44.11	C79.2	D04.11	D23.11	D48.5	D49.2
cervical region	C44.4	C79.2	D04.4	D23.4	D48.5	D49.2
cheek (external)	C44.31	C79.2	D04.39	D23.39	D48.5	D49.2
chest (wall)	C44.5	C79.2	D04.5	D23.5	D48.5	D49.2
chin	C44.31	C79.2	D04.39	D23.39	D48.5	D49.2
clavicular area	C44.5	C79.2	D04.5	D23.5	D48.5	D49.2
clitoris	C51.2	C79.82	D07.1	D28.0	D39.7	D49.5
columnella	C44.31	C79.2	D04.39	D23.39	D48.5	D49.2
concha (unspecified side)	C44.20	C79.2	D04.20	D23.20	D48.5	D49.2
left side	C44.22	C79.2	D04.22	D23.22	D48.5	D49.2
right side	C44.21	C79.2	D04.21	D23.21	D48.5	D49.2
ear (external) (unspecified side)	C44.20	C79.2	D04.20	D23.20	D48.5	D49.2
left side	C44.22	C79.2	D04.22	D23.22	D48.5	D49.2
right side	C44.21	C79.2	D04.21	D23.21	D48.5	D49.2
elbow (unspecified side)	C44.60	C79.2	D04.60	D23.60	D48.5	D49.2
left side	C44.62	C79.2	D04.62	D23.62	D48.5	D49.2
right side	C44.61	C79.2	D04.61	D23.61	D48.5	D49.2
eyebrow	C44.31	C79.2	D04.39	D23.39	D48.5	D49.2
eyelid (unspecified side)	C44.10	C79.2	D04.10	D23.10	D48.5	D49.2
left side	C44.12	C79.2	D04.12	D23.12	D48.5	D49.2
right side	C44.11	C79.2	D04.11	D23.11	D48.5	D49.2
face NEC	C44.30	C79.2	D04.30	D23.30	D48.5	D49.2
female genital organs (external)	C51.9	C79.82	D07.1	D28.0	D39.7	D49.5
clitoris	C51.2	C79.82	D07.1	D28.0	D39.7	D49.5
labium NEC	C51.9	C79.82	D07.1	D28.0	D39.7	D49.5
majus	C51.0	C79.82	D07.1	D28.0	D39.7	D49.5
minus	C51.1	C79.82	D07.1	D28.0	D39.7	D49.5
pudendum	C51.9	C79.82	D07.1	D28.0	D39.7	D49.5
vulva	C51.9	C79.82	D07.1	D28.0	D39.7	D49.5
finger (unspecified side)	C44.60	C79.2	D04.60	D23.60	D48.5	D49.2
left side	C44.62	C79.2	D04.62	D23.62	D48.5	D49.2
right side	C44.61	C79.2	D04.61	D23.61	D48.5	D49.2
flank	C44.5	C79.2	D04.5	D23.5	D48.5	D49.2
foot (unspecified side)	C44.70	C79.2	D04.70	D23.70	D48.5	D49.2
left side	C44.72	C79.2	D04.72	D23.72	D48.5	D49.2
right side	C44.71	C79.2	D04.71	D23.71	D48.5	D49.2
forearm (unspecified side)	C44.60	C79.2	D04.60	D23.60	D48.5	D49.2
left side	C44.62	C79.2	D04.62	D23.62	D48.5	D49.2
right side	C44.61	C79.2	D04.61	D23.61	D48.5	D49.2
forehead	C44.31	C79.2	D04.39	D23.39	D48.5	D49.2
glabella	C44.31	C79.2	D04.39	D23.39	D48.5	D49.2
gluteal region	C44.5	C79.2	D04.5	D23.5	D48.5	D49.2
groin	C44.5	C79.2	D04.5	D23.5	D48.5	D49.2
hand (unspecified side)	C44.60	C79.2	D04.60	D23.60	D48.5	D49.2
left side	C44.62	C79.2	D04.62	D23.62	D48.5	D49.2
right side	C44.61	C79.2	D04.61	D23.61	D48.5	D49.2
head NEC	C44.4	C79.2	D04.4	D23.4	D48.5	D49.2
heel (unspecified side)	C44.70	C79.2	D04.70	D23.70	D48.5	D49.2
left side	C44.72	C79.2	D04.72	D23.72	D48.5	D49.2
right side	C44.71	C79.2	D04.71	D23.71	D48.5	D49.2

©2002 Ingenix, Inc.

	Malignant					
	Primary	Secondary	Ca in situ	Benign	Uncertain Behavior	Unspecified
Neoplasm, neoplastic — *continued*						
skin NEC — *continued*						
helix (unspecified side)	C44.20	C79.2	D04.20	D23.20	D48.5	D49.2
left side	C44.22	C79.2	D04.22	D23.22	D48.5	D49.2
right side	C44.21	C79.2	D04.21	D23.21	D48.5	D49.2
hip (unspecified side)	C44.70	C79.2	D04.70	D23.70	D48.5	D49.2
left side	C44.72	C79.2	D04.72	D23.72	D48.5	D49.2
right side	C44.71	C79.2	D04.71	D23.71	D48.5	D49.2
infraclavicular region	C44.5	C79.2	D04.5	D23.5	D48.5	D49.2
inguinal region	C44.5	C79.2	D04.5	D23.5	D48.5	D49.2
jaw	C44.31	C79.2	D04.39	D23.39	D48.5	D49.2
knee (unspecified side)	C44.70	C79.2	D04.70	D23.70	D48.5	D49.2
left side	C44.72	C79.2	D04.72	D23.72	D48.5	D49.2
right side	C44.71	C79.2	D04.71	D23.71	D48.5	D49.2
labia						
majora	C51.0	C79.82	D07.1	D28.0	D39.7	D49.5
minora	C51.1	C79.82	D07.1	D28.0	D39.7	D49.5
leg (unspecified side)	C44.70	C79.2	D04.70	D23.70	D48.5	D49.2
left side	C44.72	C79.2	D04.72	D23.72	D48.5	D49.2
right side	C44.71	C79.2	D04.71	D23.71	D48.5	D49.2
lid (lower) (upper) (unspecified side)	C44.10	C79.2	D04.10	D23.10	D48.5	D49.2
left side	C44.12	C79.2	D04.12	D23.12	D48.5	D49.2
right side	C44.11	C79.2	D04.11	D23.11	D48.5	D49.2
limb NEC	C44.9	C79.2	D04.9	D23.9	D48.5	D49.2
lower (unspecified side)	C44.70	C79.2	D04.70	D23.70	D48.5	D49.2
left side	C44.72	C79.2	D04.72	D23.72	D48.5	D49.2
right side	C44.71	C79.2	D04.71	D23.71	D48.5	D49.2
upper (unspecified side)	C44.60	C79.2	D04.60	D23.60	D48.5	D49.2
left side	C44.62	C79.2	D04.62	D23.62	D48.5	D49.2
right side	C44.61	C79.2	D04.61	D23.61	D48.5	D49.2
lip (lower) (upper)	C44.0	C79.2	D04.0	D23.0	D48.5	D49.2
male genital organs	C63.9	C79.82	D07.60	D29.9	D40.7	D49.5
penis	C60.9	C79.82	D07.4	D29.0	D40.7	D49.5
prepuce	C60.0	C79.82	D07.4	D29.0	D40.7	D49.5
scrotum	C63.2	C79.82	D07.61	D29.4	D40.7	D49.5
mastectomy site (skin)	C44.5	C79.2	—	—	—	—
specified as breast tissue						
female (unspecified side)	C50.80	C79.81	—	—	—	—
left side	C50.82	C79.81	—	—	—	—
right side	C50.81	C79.81	—	—	—	—
male (unspecified side)	C50.85	C79.81	—	—	—	—
left side	C50.84	C79.81	—	—	—	—
right side	C50.83	C79.81	—	—	—	—
meatus, acoustic (external) (unspecified side)	C44.20	C79.2	D04.20	D23.20	D48.5	D49.2
left side	C44.22	C79.2	D04.22	D23.22	D48.5	D49.2
right side	C44.21	C79.2	D04.21	D23.21	D48.5	D49.2
melanotic — *see* Melanoma						
nates	C44.5	C79.2	D04.5	D23.5	D48.5	D49.2
neck	C44.4	C79.2	D04.4	D23.4	D48.5	D49.2
nose (external)	C44.31	C79.2	D04.39	D23.39	D48.5	D49.2
overlapping lesion	C44.8	—	—	—	—	—
palm (unspecified side)	C44.60	C79.2	D04.60	D23.60	D48.5	D49.2
left side	C44.62	C79.2	D04.62	D23.62	D48.5	D49.2
right side	C44.61	C79.2	D04.61	D23.61	D48.5	D49.2
palpebra (unspecified side)	C44.10	C79.2	D04.10	D23.10	D48.5	D49.2
left side	C44.12	C79.2	D04.12	D23.12	D48.5	D49.2
right side	C44.11	C79.2	D04.11	D23.11	D48.5	D49.2
penis NEC	C60.9	C79.82	D07.4	D29.0	D40.7	D49.5
perianal	C44.5	C79.2	D04.5	D23.5	D48.5	D49.2
perineum	C44.5	C79.2	D04.5	D23.5	D48.5	D49.2
pinna (unspecified side)	C44.20	C79.2	D04.20	D23.20	D48.5	D49.2
left side	C44.22	C79.2	D04.22	D23.22	D48.5	D49.2
right side	C44.21	C79.2	D04.21	D23.21	D48.5	D49.2
plantar (unspecified side)	C44.70	C79.2	D04.70	D23.70	D48.5	D49.2
left side	C44.72	C79.2	D04.72	D23.72	D48.5	D49.2
right side	C44.71	C79.2	D04.71	D23.71	D48.5	D49.2

	Malignant			Benign	Uncertain Behavior	Unspecified
	Primary	Secondary	Ca in situ			
Neoplasm, neoplastic — *continued*						
skin NEC — *continued*						
popliteal fossa or space (unspecified side)	C44.70	C79.2	D04.70	D23.70	D48.5	D49.2
left side	C44.72	C79.2	D04.72	D23.72	D48.5	D49.2
right side	C44.71	C79.2	D04.71	D23.71	D48.5	D49.2
prepuce	C60.0	C79.82	D07.4	D29.0	D40.7	D49.5
pubes	C44.5	C79.2	D04.5	D23.5	D48.5	D49.2
sacrococcygeal region	C44.5	C79.2	D04.5	D23.5	D48.5	D49.2
scalp	C44.4	C79.2	D04.4	D23.4	D48.5	D49.2
scapular region	C44.5	C79.2	D04.5	D23.5	D48.5	D49.2
scrotum	C63.2	C79.82	D07.61	D29.4	D40.7	D49.5
shoulder (unspecified side)	C44.60	C79.2	D04.60	D23.60	D48.5	D49.2
left side	C44.62	C79.2	D04.62	D23.62	D48.5	D49.2
right side	C44.61	C79.2	D04.61	D23.61	D48.5	D49.2
sole (foot) (unspecified side)	C44.70	C79.2	D04.70	D23.70	D48.5	D49.2
left side	C44.72	C79.2	D04.72	D23.72	D48.5	D49.2
right side	C44.71	C79.2	D04.71	D23.71	D48.5	D49.2
specified sites NEC	C44.8	C79.2	D04.8	D23.9	D48.5	D49.2
submammary fold	C44.5	C79.2	D04.5	D23.5	D48.5	D49.2
supraclavicular region	C44.4	C79.2	D04.4	D23.4	D48.5	D49.2
temple	C44.31	C79.2	D04.39	D23.39	D48.5	D49.2
thigh (unspecified side)	C44.70	C79.2	D04.70	D23.70	D48.5	D49.2
left side	C44.72	C79.2	D04.72	D23.72	D48.5	D49.2
right side	C44.71	C79.2	D04.71	D23.71	D48.5	D49.2
thoracic wall	C44.5	C79.2	D04.5	D23.5	D48.5	D49.2
thumb (unspecified side)	C44.60	C79.2	D04.60	D23.60	D48.5	D49.2
left side	C44.62	C79.2	D04.62	D23.62	D48.5	D49.2
right side	C44.61	C79.2	D04.61	D23.61	D48.5	D49.2
toe (unspecified side)	C44.70	C79.2	D04.70	D23.70	D48.5	D49.2
left side	C44.72	C79.2	D04.72	D23.72	D48.5	D49.2
right side	C44.71	C79.2	D04.71	D23.71	D48.5	D49.2
tragus (unspecified side)	C44.20	C79.2	D04.20	D23.20	D48.5	D49.2
left side	C44.22	C79.2	D04.22	D23.22	D48.5	D49.2
right side	C44.21	C79.2	D04.21	D23.21	D48.5	D49.2
trunk	C44.5	C79.2	D04.5	D23.5	D48.5	D49.2
umbilicus	C44.5	C79.2	D04.5	D23.5	D48.5	D49.2
vulva	C51.9	C79.82	D07.1	D28.0	D39.7	D49.5
wrist (unspecified side)	C44.60	C79.2	D04.60	D23.60	D48.5	D49.2
left side	C44.62	C79.2	D04.62	D23.62	D48.5	D49.2
right side	C44.61	C79.2	D04.61	D23.61	D48.5	D49.2
skull	C41.0	C79.51	—	D16.4	D48.0	D49.2
marrow NEC	C96.9	C79.52	—	—	—	D47.9
soft parts or tissues — *see* Neoplasm, connective tissue						
specified site NEC	C76.7	C79.89	D09.7	D36.7	D48.7	D49.8
spermatic cord (unspecified side)	C63.10	C79.82	D07.69	D29.7	D40.7	D49.5
left side	C63.12	C79.82	D07.69	D29.7	D40.7	D49.5
right side	C63.11	C79.82	D07.69	D29.7	D40.7	D49.5
sphenoid	C31.3	C78.39	D02.3	D14.0	D38.5	D49.1
bone	C41.0	C79.51	—	D16.4	D48.0	D49.2
marrow NEC	C96.9	C79.52	—	—	—	D47.9
sinus	C31.3	C78.39	D02.3	D14.0	D38.5	D49.1
sphincter						
anal	C21.1	C78.5	D01.3	D12.9	D37.7	D49.0
of Oddi	C24.0	C78.89	D01.5	D13.5	D37.6	D49.0
spine, spinal (column)	C41.2	C79.51	—	D16.6	D48.0	D49.2
bulb	C71.7	C79.31	—	D33.1	D43.1	D49.6
coccyx	C41.4	C79.51	—	D16.8	D48.0	D49.2
marrow NEC	C96.9	C79.52	—	—	—	D47.9
cord (cervical) (lumbar) (sacral) (thoracic)	C72.0	C79.49	—	D33.4	D43.4	D49.7
dura mater	C70.1	C79.49	—	D32.1	D42.1	D49.7
lumbosacral	C41.2	C79.51	—	D16.6	D48.0	D49.2
marrow NEC	C96.9	C79.52	—	—	—	D47.9
marrow NEC	C96.9	C79.52	—	—	—	D47.9
membrane	C70.1	C79.49	—	D32.1	D42.1	D49.7
meninges	C70.1	C79.49	—	D32.1	D42.1	D49.7
nerve (root)	C47.9	C79.89	—	D36.10	D48.2	D49.2
pia mater	C70.1	C79.49	—	D32.1	D42.1	D49.7

©2002 Ingenix, Inc.

| | Malignant | | | | | |
	Primary	Secondary	Ca in situ	Benign	Uncertain Behavior	Unspecified
Neoplasm, neoplastic — *continued*						
spine, spinal — *continued*						
root	C47.9	C79.89	—	D36.10	D48.2	D49.2
sacrum	C41.4	C79.51	—	D16.8	D48.0	D49.2
marrow NEC	C96.9	C79.52	—	—	—	D47.9
spleen, splenic NEC	C26.1	C78.89	D01.7	D13.9	D37.7	D49.0
flexure (colon)	C18.5	C78.5	D01.0	D12.3	D37.4	D49.0
stem, brain	C71.7	C79.31	—	D33.1	D43.1	D49.6
Stensen's duct	C07	C79.89	D00.00	D11.0	D37.030	D49.0
sternum	C41.3	C79.51	—	D16.7	D48.0	D49.2
marrow NEC	C96.9	C79.52	—	—	—	D47.9
stomach	C16.9	C78.89	D00.2	D13.1	D37.1	D49.0
antrum (pyloric)	C16.3	C78.89	D00.2	D13.1	D37.1	D49.0
body	C16.2	C78.89	D00.2	D13.1	D37.1	D49.0
cardia	C16.0	C78.89	D00.2	D13.1	D37.1	D49.0
cardiac orifice	C16.0	C78.89	D00.2	D13.1	D37.1	D49.0
corpus	C16.2	C78.89	D00.2	D13.1	D37.1	D49.0
fundus	C16.1	C78.89	D00.2	D13.1	D37.1	D49.0
greater curvature NEC	C16.6	C78.89	D00.2	D13.1	D37.1	D49.0
lesser curvature NEC	C16.5	C78.89	D00.2	D13.1	D37.1	D49.0
overlapping lesion	C16.8	—	—	—	—	—
prepylorus	C16.4	C78.89	D00.2	D13.1	D37.1	D49.0
pylorus	C16.4	C78.89	D00.2	D13.1	D37.1	D49.0
wall NEC	C16.9	C78.89	D00.2	D13.1	D37.1	D49.0
anterior NEC	C16.8	C78.89	D00.2	D13.1	D37.1	D49.0
posterior NEC	C16.8	C78.89	D00.2	D13.1	D37.1	D49.0
stroma, endometrial	C54.1	C79.82	D07.0	D26.1	D39.0	D49.5
stump, cervical	C53.8	C79.82	D06.7	D26.0	D39.0	D49.5
subcutaneous (nodule) (tissue) NEC — *see Neoplasm, connective tissue*						
subdural	C70.9	C79.32	—	D32.9	D42.9	D49.7
subglottis, subglottic	C32.2	C78.39	D02.0	D14.1	D38.0	D49.1
sublingual	C04.9	C79.89	D00.06	D10.2	D37.09	D49.0
gland or duct	C08.1	C79.89	D00.00	D11.7	D37.031	D49.0
submandibular gland	C08.0	C79.89	D00.00	D11.7	D37.032	D49.0
submaxillary gland or duct	C08.0	C79.89	D00.00	D11.7	D37.032	D49.0
submental	C76.0	C79.89	D09.7	D36.7	D48.7	D49.8
subpleural (unspecified side)	C34.90	C78.00	—	D14.30	D38.1	D49.1
left side	C34.92	C78.02	—	D14.32	D38.1	D49.1
right side	C34.91	C78.01	—	D14.31	D38.1	D49.1
substernal	C38.1	C78.1	—	D15.2	D38.3	D49.8
sudoriferous, sudoriparous gland, site unspecified	C44.9	C79.2	D04.9	D23.9	D48.5	D49.2
specified site — *see Neoplasm, skin*						
supraclavicular region	C76.0	C79.89	D09.7	D36.7	D48.7	D49.8
supraglottis	C32.1	C78.39	D02.0	D14.1	D38.0	D49.1
suprarenal						
capsule (unspecified side)	C74.90	C79.70	D09.3	D35.00	D44.10	D49.7
left side	C74.92	C79.72	D09.3	D35.02	D44.12	D49.7
right side	C74.91	C79.71	D09.3	D35.01	D44.11	D49.7
cortex (unspecified side)	C74.00	C79.70	D09.3	D35.00	D44.10	D49.7
left side	C74.02	C79.72	D09.3	D35.02	D44.12	D49.7
right side	C74.01	C79.71	D09.3	D35.01	D44.11	D49.7
gland (unspecified side)	C74.90	C79.70	D09.3	D35.00	D44.10	D49.7
left side	C74.92	C79.72	D09.3	D35.02	D44.12	D49.7
right side	C74.91	C79.71	D09.3	D35.01	D44.11	D49.7
medulla (unspecified side)	C74.10	C79.70	D09.3	D35.00	D44.10	D49.7
left side	C74.12	C79.72	D09.3	D35.02	D44.12	D49.7
right side	C74.11	C79.71	D09.3	D35.01	D44.11	D49.7
unspecified site (unspecified side)	C74.90	C79.70	D09.3	D35.00	D44.10	D49.7
left side	C74.92	C79.72	D09.3	D35.02	D44.12	D49.7
right side	C74.91	C79.71	D09.3	D35.01	D44.11	D49.7
suprasellar (region)	C71.9	C79.31	—	D33.2	D43.2	D49.6
supratentorial (brain) NEC	C71.0	C79.31	—	D33.0	D43.0	D49.6
sweat gland (apocrine) (eccrine), site unspecified	C44.9	C79.2	D04.9	D23.9	D48.5	D49.2
specified site — *see Neoplasm, skin*						
sympathetic nerve or nervous system NEC	C47.9	C79.89	—	D36.10	D48.2	D49.2
symphysis pubis	C41.4	C79.51	—	D16.8	D48.0	D49.2
marrow NEC	C96.9	C79.52	—	—	—	D47.9

| | Malignant | | | | | |
	Primary	Secondary	Ca in situ	Benign	Uncertain Behavior	Unspecified
Neoplasm, neoplastic — *continued*						
synovial membrane — see Neoplasm, connective tissue						
tapetum, brain	C71.8	C79.31	—	D33.2	D43.2	D49.6
tarsus (any bone)						
left side	C40.32	C79.51	—	D16.32	D48.0	D49.2
marrow NEC	C96.9	C79.52	—	—	—	D47.9
right side	C40.31	C79.51	—	D16.31	D48.0	D49.2
marrow NEC	C96.9	C79.52	—	—	—	D47.9
unspecified side	C40.30	C79.51	—	D16.30	D48.0	D49.2
marrow NEC	C96.9	C79.52	—	—	—	D47.9
temple (skin)	C44.31	C79.2	D04.39	D23.39	D48.5	D49.2
temporal						
bone	C41.0	C79.51	—	D16.4	D48.0	D49.2
marrow NEC	C96.9	C79.52	—	—	—	D47.9
lobe or pole	C71.2	C79.31	—	D33.0	D43.0	D49.6
region	C76.0	C79.89	D09.7	D36.7	D48.7	D49.8
skin	C44.31	C79.2	D04.39	D23.39	D48.5	D49.2
tendon (sheath) — see Neoplasm, connective tissue						
tentorium (cerebelli)	C70.0	C79.32	—	D32.0	D42.0	D49.7
testis, testes						
descended (unspecified side)	C62.10	C79.82	D07.69	D29.20	D40.10	D49.5
left side	C62.12	C79.82	D07.69	D29.22	D40.12	D49.5
right side	C62.11	C79.82	D07.69	D29.21	D40.11	D49.5
ectopic (unspecified side)	C62.00	C79.82	D07.69	D29.20	D40.10	D49.5
left side	C62.02	C79.82	D07.69	D29.22	D40.12	D49.5
right side	C62.01	C79.82	D07.69	D29.21	D40.11	D49.5
retained (unspecified side)	C62.00	C79.82	D07.69	D29.20	D40.10	D49.5
left side	C62.02	C79.82	D07.69	D29.22	D40.12	D49.5
right side	C62.01	C79.82	D07.69	D29.21	D40.11	D49.5
scrotal (unspecified side)	C62.10	C79.82	D07.69	D29.20	D40.10	D49.5
left side	C62.12	C79.82	D07.69	D29.22	D40.12	D49.5
right side	C62.11	C79.82	D07.69	D29.21	D40.11	D49.5
undescended (unspecified side)	C62.00	C79.82	D07.69	D29.20	D40.10	D49.5
left side	C62.02	C79.82	D07.69	D29.22	D40.12	D49.5
right side	C62.01	C79.82	D07.69	D29.21	D40.11	D49.5
unspecified site (unspecified side)	C62.90	C79.82	D07.69	D29.20	D40.10	D49.5
left side	C62.92	C79.82	D07.69	D29.22	D40.12	D49.5
right side	C62.91	C79.82	D07.69	D29.21	D40.11	D49.5
thalamus	C71.0	C79.31	—	D33.0	D43.0	D49.6
thigh (unspecified side) NEC*	C76.50	C79.89	D04.70	D36.7	D48.7	D49.8
left side	C76.52	C79.89	D04.72	D36.7	D48.7	D49.8
right side	C76.51	C79.89	D04.71	D36.7	D48.7	D49.8
thorax, thoracic (cavity) (organs NEC)	C76.1	C79.89	D09.7	D36.7	D48.7	D49.8
duct	C49.3	C79.89	—	D21.3	D48.1	D49.2
wall NEC	C76.1	C79.89	D09.7	D36.7	D48.7	D49.8
throat	C14.0	C79.89	D00.08	D10.9	D37.05	D49.0
thumb (unspecified side) NEC*	C76.40	C79.89	D04.60	D36.7	D48.7	D49.8
left side	C76.42	C79.89	D04.62	D36.7	D48.7	D49.8
right side	C76.41	C79.89	D04.61	D36.7	D48.7	D49.8
thymus (gland)	C37	C79.89	—	D15.0	D38.4	D49.8
overlapping lesion with heart or mediastinum	C38.8	—	—	—	—	—
thyroglossal duct	C73	C79.89	D09.3	D34	D44.0	D49.7
thyroid (gland)	C73	C79.89	D09.3	D34	D44.0	D49.7
cartilage	C32.3	C78.39	D02.0	D14.1	D38.0	D49.1
tibia (any part)						
left side	C40.22	C79.51	—	D16.22	D48.0	D49.2
marrow NEC	C96.9	C79.52	—	—	—	D47.9
right side	C40.21	C79.51	—	D16.21	D48.0	D49.2
marrow NEC	C96.9	C79.52	—	—	—	D47.9
unspecified side	C40.20	C79.51	—	D16.20	D48.0	D49.2
marrow NEC	C96.9	C79.52	—	—	—	D47.9
toe (unspecified side) NEC*	C76.50	C79.89	D04.70	D36.7	D47.7	D49.8
left side	C76.52	C79.89	D04.72	D36.7	D47.7	D49.8
right side	C76.51	C79.89	D04.71	D36.7	D47.7	D49.8
tongue	C02.9	C79.89	D00.07	D10.1	D37.02	D49.0
anterior (two-thirds) NEC	C02.3	C79.89	D00.07	D10.1	D37.02	D49.0
dorsal surface	C02.0	C79.89	D00.07	D10.1	D37.02	D49.0

©2002 Ingenix, Inc.

	Malignant					
	Primary	Secondary	Ca in situ	Benign	Uncertain Behavior	Unspecified
Neoplasm, neoplastic — *continued*						
tongue — *continued*						
anterior NEC — *continued*						
ventral surface	C02.2	C79.89	D00.07	D10.1	D37.02	D49.0
base (dorsal surface)	C01	C79.89	D00.07	D10.1	D37.02	D49.0
border (lateral)	C02.1	C79.89	D00.07	D10.1	D37.02	D49.0
dorsal surface NEC	C02.0	C79.89	D00.07	D10.1	D37.02	D49.0
fixed part NEC	C01	C79.89	D00.07	D10.1	D37.02	D49.0
foreamen cecum	C02.0	C79.89	D00.07	D10.1	D37.02	D49.0
frenulum linguae	C02.2	C79.89	D00.07	D10.1	D37.02	D49.0
junctional zone	C02.8	C79.89	D00.07	D10.1	D37.02	D49.0
margin (lateral)	C02.1	C79.89	D00.07	D10.1	D37.02	D49.0
midline NEC	C02.0	C79.89	D00.07	D10.1	D37.02	D49.0
mobile part NEC	C02.3	C79.89	D00.07	D10.1	D37.02	D49.0
overlapping lesion	C02.8	—	—	—	—	—
posterior (third)	C01	C79.89	D00.07	D10.1	D37.02	D49.0
root	C01	C79.89	D00.07	D10.1	D37.02	D49.0
surface (dorsal)	C02.0	C79.89	D00.07	D10.1	D37.02	D49.0
base	C01	C79.89	D00.07	D10.1	D37.02	D49.0
ventral	C02.2	C79.89	D00.07	D10.1	D37.02	D49.0
tip	C02.1	C79.89	D00.07	D10.1	D37.02	D49.0
tonsil	C02.4	C79.89	D00.07	D10.1	D37.02	D49.0
tonsil	C09.9	C79.89	D00.08	D10.4	D37.05	D49.0
fauces, faucial	C09.9	C79.89	D00.08	D10.4	D37.05	D49.0
lingual	C02.4	C79.89	D00.07	D10.1	D37.02	D49.0
palatine	C09.9	C79.89	D00.08	D10.4	D37.05	D49.0
pharyngeal	C11.1	C79.89	D00.08	D10.6	D37.05	D49.0
pillar (anterior) (posterior)	C09.1	C79.89	D00.08	D10.5	D37.05	D49.0
tonsillar fossa	C09.0	C79.89	D00.08	D10.5	D37.05	D49.0
tooth socket NEC	C03.9	C79.89	D00.03	D10.39	D37.09	D49.0
trachea (cartilage) (mucosa)	C33	C78.39	D02.1	D14.2	D38.1	D49.1
overlapping lesion with bronchus or lung (unspecified side)	C34.80	—	—	—	—	—
left side	C34.82	—	—	—	—	—
right side	C34.81	—	—	—	—	—
tracheobronchial						
overlapping lesion with lung (unspecified side)	C34.80	—	—	—	—	—
left side	C34.82	—	—	—	—	—
right side	C34.81	—	—	—	—	—
unspecified site (unspecified side)	C34.80	C78.39	D02.1	D14.2	D38.1	D49.1
left side	C34.82	C78.39	D02.1	D14.2	D38.1	D49.1
right side	C34.81	C78.39	D02.1	D14.2	D38.1	D49.1
tragus (unspecified side)	C44.20	C79.2	D04.20	D23.20	D48.5	D49.2
left side	C44.22	C79.2	D04.22	D23.22	D48.5	D49.2
right side	C44.21	C79.2	D04.21	D23.21	D48.5	D49.2
trunk NEC*	C76.7	C79.89	D04.5	D36.7	D48.7	D49.8
tubo-ovarian	C57.8	C79.82	D07.39	D28.7	D39.7	D49.5
tunica vaginalis	C63.7	C79.82	D07.69	D29.7	D40.7	D49.5
turbinate (bone)	C41.0	C79.51	—	D16.4	D48.0	D49.2
marrow NEC	C96.9	C79.52	—	—	—	D47.9
nasal	C30.0	C78.39	D02.3	D14.0	D38.5	D49.1
tympanic cavity	C30.1	C78.39	D02.3	D14.0	D38.5	D49.1
ulna (any part)						
left side	C40.02	C79.51	—	D16.01	D48.0	D49.2
marrow NEC	C96.9	C79.52	—	—	—	D47.9
right side	C40.01	C79.51	—	D16.02	D48.0	D49.2
marrow NEC	C96.9	C79.52	—	—	—	D47.9
unspecified side	C40.00	C79.51	—	D16.00	D48.0	D49.2
marrow NEC	C96.9	C79.52	—	—	—	D47.9
umbilicus, umbilical	C44.5	C79.2	D04.5	D23.5	D48.5	D49.2
uncus, brain	C71.2	C79.31	—	D33.0	D43.0	D49.6
unknown site or unspecified	C76.9	C79.9	D09.9	D36.9	D48.9	D49.9
urachus	C67.7	C79.11	D09.0	D30.3	D41.4	D49.4
ureter, ureteral						
orifice (bladder)	C67.6	C79.11	D09.0	D30.3	D41.4	D49.4
unspecified site (unspecified side)	C66.9	C79.19	D09.19	D30.20	D41.20	D49.5
left side	C66.1	C79.19	D09.19	D30.22	D41.22	D49.5
right side	C66.0	C79.19	D09.19	D30.21	D41.21	D49.5

| | Malignant | | | | | |
	Primary	Secondary	Ca in situ	Benign	Uncertain Behavior	Unspecified
Neoplasm, neoplastic — *continued*						
ureter-bladder (junction)	C67.6	C79.11	D09.0	D30.3	D41.4	D49.4
urethra, urethral (gland)	C68.0	C79.19	D09.19	D30.4	D41.3	D49.5
orifice, internal	C67.5	C79.11	D09.0	D30.3	D41.4	D49.4
urethrovaginal (septum)	C57.9	C79.82	D07.39	D28.9	D39.7	D49.5
urinary organ or system NEC	C68.9	C79.10	D09.10	D30.9	D41.9	D49.5
bladder — see Neoplasm, bladder						
overlapping lesion	C68.8	—	—	—	—	—
specified sites NEC	C68.8	C79.19	D09.19	D30.7	D41.7	D49.5
utero-ovarian	C57.8	C79.82	D07.39	D28.7	D39.7	D49.5
ligament	C57.1	C79.82	D07.39	D28.2	D39.7	D49.5
uterosacral ligament	C57.3	C79.82	—	D28.2	D39.7	D49.5
uterus, uteri, uterine	C55	C79.82	D07.0	D26.9	D39.0	D49.5
adnexa NEC	C57.4	C79.82	D07.39	D28.7	D39.7	D49.5
overlapping lesion	C57.8	—	—	—	—	—
body	C54.9	C79.82	D07.0	D26.1	D39.0	D49.5
overlapping lesion	C54.8	—	—	—	—	—
cervix	C53.9	C79.82	D06.9	D26.0	D39.0	D49.5
cornu	C54.9	C79.82	D07.0	D26.1	D39.0	D49.5
corpus	C54.9	C79.82	D07.0	D26.1	D39.0	D49.5
endocervix (canal) (gland)	C53.0	C79.82	D06.0	D26.0	D39.0	D49.5
endometrium	C54.1	C79.82	D07.0	D26.1	D39.0	D49.5
exocervix	C53.1	C79.82	D06.1	D26.0	D39.0	D49.5
external os	C53.1	C79.82	D06.1	D26.0	D39.0	D49.5
fundus	C54.3	C79.82	D07.0	D26.1	D39.0	D49.5
internal os	C53.0	C79.82	D06.0	D26.0	D39.0	D49.5
isthmus	C54.0	C79.82	D07.0	D26.1	D39.0	D49.5
ligament	C57.3	C79.82	—	D28.2	D39.7	D49.5
broad	C57.1	C79.82	D07.39	D28.2	D39.7	D49.5
round	C57.2	C79.82	—	D28.2	D39.7	D49.5
lower segment	C54.0	C79.82	D07.0	D26.1	D39.0	D49.5
myometrium	C54.2	C79.82	D07.0	D26.1	D39.0	D49.5
squamocolumnar junction	C53.8	C79.82	D06.7	D26.0	D39.0	D49.5
tube (unspecified side)	C57.00	C79.82	D07.39	D28.2	D39.7	D49.5
left side	C57.02	C79.82	D07.39	D28.2	D39.7	D49.5
right side	C57.01	C79.82	D07.39	D28.2	D39.7	D49.5
utricle, prostatic	C68.0	C79.19	D09.19	D30.4	D41.3	D49.5
uveal tract (unspecified side)	C69.40	C79.49	D09.20	D31.40	D48.7	D49.8
left side	C69.42	C79.49	D09.22	D31.42	D48.7	D49.8
right side	C69.41	C79.49	D09.21	D31.41	D48.7	D49.8
uvula	C05.2	C79.89	D00.04	D10.39	D37.09	D49.0
vagina, vaginal (fornix) (vault) (wall)	C52	C79.82	D07.2	D28.1	D39.7	D49.5
vaginovesical	C57.9	C79.82	D07.30	D28.9	D39.9	D49.5
septum	C57.9	C79.82	D07.30	D28.9	D39.9	D49.5
vallecula (epiglottis)	C10.0	C79.89	D00.08	D10.5	D37.05	D49.0
vascular — see Neoplasm, connective tissue						
vas deferens (unspecified side)	C63.10	C79.82	D07.69	D29.7	D40.7	D49.5
left side	C63.12	C79.82	D07.69	D29.7	D40.7	D49.5
right side	C63.11	C79.82	D07.69	D29.7	D40.7	D49.5
Vater's ampulla	C24.1	C78.89	D01.5	D13.5	D37.6	D49.0
vein, venous — see Neoplasm, connective tissue						
vena cava (abdominal) (inferior)	C49.4	C79.89	—	D21.4	D48.1	D49.2
superior	C49.3	C79.89	—	D21.3	D48.1	D49.2
ventricle (cerebral) (floor) (lateral) (third)	C71.5	C79.31	—	D33.0	D43.0	D49.6
cardiac (left) (right)	C38.0	C79.89	—	D15.1	D48.7	D49.8
fourth	C71.7	C79.31	—	D33.1	D43.1	D49.6
ventricular band of larynx	C32.1	C78.39	D02.0	D14.1	D38.0	D49.1
ventriculus — see Neoplasm, stomach						
vermillion border — see Neoplasm, lip						
vermis, cerebellum	C71.6	C79.31	—	D33.1	D43.1	D49.6
vertebra (column)	C41.2	C79.51	—	D16.6	D48.0	D49.2
coccyx	C41.4	C79.51	—	D16.8	D48.0	D49.2
marrow NEC	C96.9	C79.52	—	—	—	D47.9
marrow NEC	C96.9	C79.52	—	—	—	D47.9
sacrum	C41.4	C79.51	—	D16.8	D48.0	D49.2
marrow NEC	C96.9	C79.52	—	—	—	D47.9

©2002 Ingenix, Inc.

	Malignant					
	Primary	**Secondary**	**Ca in situ**	**Benign**	**Uncertain Behavior**	**Unspecified**
Neoplasm, neoplastic — *continued*						
vesical — see Neoplasm, bladder						
vesicle, seminal	C63.7	C79.82	D07.69	D29.7	D40.7	D49.5
vesicocervical tissue	C57.9	C79.82	D07.30	D28.9	D39.9	D49.5
vesicorectal	C76.3	C79.82	D09.7	D36.7	D48.7	D49.8
vesicovaginal	C57.9	C79.82	D07.30	D28.9	D39.9	D49.5
septum	C57.9	C79.82	D07.39	D28.9	D39.7	D49.5
vessel (blood) — see Neoplasm, connective tissue						
vestibular gland, greater	C51.0	C79.82	D07.1	D28.0	D39.7	D49.5
vestibule						
mouth	C06.1	C79.89	D00.00	D10.30	D37.09	D49.0
nose	C30.0	C78.39	D02.3	D14.0	D38.5	D49.1
Virchow's gland	—	C77.0	—	D36.0	D48.7	D49.8
viscera NEC	C76.7	C79.89	D09.7	D36.7	D48.7	D49.8
vocal cords (true)	C32.0	C78.39	D02.0	D14.1	D38.0	D49.1
false	C32.1	C78.39	D02.0	D14.1	D38.0	D49.1
vomer	C41.0	C79.51	—	D16.4	D48.0	D49.2
marrow NEC	C96.9	C79.52	—	—	—	D47.9
vulva	C51.9	C79.82	D07.1	D28.0	D39.7	D49.5
vulvovaginal gland	C51.9	C79.82	D07.1	D28.0	D39.7	D49.5
Waldeyer's ring	C14.2	C79.89	D00.08	D10.9	D37.05	D49.0
Wharton's duct	C08.0	C79.89	D00.00	D11.7	D37.032	D49.0
white matter (central) (cerebral)	C71.0	C79.31	—	D33.0	D43.0	D49.6
windpipe	C33	C78.39	D02.1	D14.2	D38.1	D49.1
Wirsung's duct	C25.3	C78.89	D01.7	D13.6	D37.7	D49.0
wolffian (body) (duct)						
female	C57.7	C79.82	D07.39	D28.7	D39.7	D49.5
male	C63.7	C79.82	D07.69	D29.7	D40.7	D49.5
womb — see Neoplasm, uterus						
wrist (unspecified side) NEC*	C76.40	C79.89	D04.60	D36.7	D48.7	D49.8
left side	C76.42	C79.89	D04.62	D36.7	D48.7	D49.8
right side	C76.41	C79.89	D04.61	D36.7	D48.7	D49.8
xiphoid process	C41.3	C79.51	—	D16.7	D48.0	D49.2
Zuckerkandl's organ	C75.5	C79.89	—	D35.6	D44.7	D49.7

Abandonment (causing exposure to weather conditions) (with intent to injure or kill) NEC — *see* Maltreatment

Abuse (adult) (child) (mental) (physical) (sexual) — *see* Maltreatment

Accident (to) X58.8
- aircraft (in transit) (powered) — *see also* Accident, transport, aircraft
  - due to, caused by cataclysm — *see* Forces of nature, by type
- animal-rider — *see* Accident, transport, animal-rider
- animal-drawn vehicle — *see* Accident, transport, animal-drawn vehicle occupant
- automobile — *see* Accident, transport, car occupant
- bare foot water skiier V94.4
- boat, boating — *see also* Accident, watercraft
  - striking swimmer
    - powered V94.11
    - unpowered V94.12
- bus — *see* Accident, transport, bus occupant
- cable car, not on rails V98.0
  - on rails — *see* Accident, transport, streetcar occupant
- car — *see* Accident, transport, car occupant
- caused by, due to
  - animal NEC W64
  - chain hoist W24.0
  - cold (excessive) — *see* Exposure, cold
  - corrosive liquid, substance — *see* Table of Drugs and Chemicals
  - cutting or piercing instrument — *see* Contact, with, by type of instrument
  - drive belt W24.0
  - electric
    - current — *see* Exposure, electric current
    - motor (*see also* Contact, with, by type of machine) W31.3
    - current (of) W86.8
  - environmental factor NEC X58.8
  - explosive material — *see* Explosion
  - fire, flames — *see* Exposure, fire
  - firearm missile — *see* Discharge, firearm by type
  - heat (excessive) — *see* Heat
  - hot — *see* Contact, with, hot
  - ignition — *see* Ignition
  - lifting device W24.0
  - lightning X33
    - causing fire — *see* Exposure, fire
  - machine, machinery — *see* Contact, with, by type of machine
  - natural factor NEC X58.8
  - pulley (block) W24.0
  - radiation — *see* Radiation
  - steam X13.1
    - inhalation X13.0
    - pipe X16
  - thunderbolt X33
    - causing fire — *see* Exposure, fire
  - transmission device W24.1
- coach — *see* Accident, transport, bus occupant
- coal car — *see* Accident, transport, industrial vehicle occupant
- diving — *see also* Fall, into, water
  - with
    - drowning or submersion — *see* Drowning
- forklift — *see* Accident, transport, industrial vehicle occupant
- heavy transport vehicle NOS — *see* Accident, transport, truck occupant
- ice yacht V98.2
- in
  - medical, surgical procedure
    - as, or due to misadventure — *see* Misadventure
    - causing an abnormal reaction or later complication without mention of misadventure (*see also* Complication of or following, by type of procedure) Y84.9
- land yacht V98.1
- late effect of — *see* W00-X58 with q as terminal character
- logging car — *see* Accident, transport, industrial vehicle occupant

Accident — *continued*
- machine, machinery — *see also* Contact, with, by type of machine
  - on board watercraft V93.69
    - explosion — *see* Explosion, in, watercraft
    - fire — *see* Burn, on board watercraft
    - powered craft V93.63
      - ferry boat V93.61
      - fishing boat V93.62
      - jetskis V93.63
      - liner V93.61
      - merchant ship V93.60
      - passenger ship V93.61
      - sailboat V93.64
- mine tram — *see* Accident, transport, industrial vehicle occupant
- motor scooter — *see* Accident, transport, motorcyclist
- motor vehicle NOS (traffic) (*see also* Accident, transport) V89.2
  - nontraffic V89.0
  - three-wheeled NOS — *see* Accident, transport, three wheeled motor vehicle occupant
- motorcycle NOS — *see* Accident, transport, motorcyclist
- nonmotor vehicle NOS (nontraffic) (*see also* Accident, transport) V89.1
  - traffic NOS V89.3
- nontraffic (victim's mode of transport NOS) V88.9
  - collision (between) V88.7
    - bus and truck V88.5
    - car and:
      - bus V88.3
      - pickup V88.2
      - three-wheeled motor vehicle V88.0
      - train V88.6
      - truck V88.4
      - two-wheeled motor vehicle V88.0
      - van V88.2
    - specified vehicle NEC and:
      - three-wheeled motor vehicle V88.1
      - two-wheeled motor vehicle V88.1
    - known mode of transport — *see* Accident, transport, by type of vehicle
  - noncollision V88.8
- on board watercraft V93.89
  - powered craft V93.83
    - ferry boat V93.81
    - fishing boat V93.82
    - jetskis V93.83
    - liner V93.81
    - merchant ship V93.80
    - passenger ship V93.81
  - unpowered craft V93.88
    - canoe V93.85
    - inflatable V93.86
      - in tow
        - recreational V94.31
        - specified NEC V94.32
    - kayak V93.85
    - sailboat V93.84
    - surf-board V93.88
    - water skis V93.87
    - windsurfer V93.88
- parachutist V97.29
  - entangled in object V97.21
  - injured on landing V97.22
- pedal cycle — *see* Accident, transport, pedal cyclist
- pedestrian (on foot)
  - with
    - another pedestrian W51
      - with fall W03
        - due to ice or snow W00.0
    - on pedestrian conveyance NEC 09
    - roller skater (in-line) V00.01
    - skate boarder V00.02
    - transport vehicle — *see* Accident, transport
  - on pedestrian conveyance — *see* Accident, transport, pedestrian, conveyance
- pick-up truck or van — *see* Accident, transport, pickup truck occupant

Accident — *continued*
- quarry truck — *see* Accident, transport, industrial vehicle occupant
- railway vehicle (any) (in motion) — *see* Accident, transport, railway vehicle occupant
  - due to cataclysm — *see* Forces of nature, by type
- scooter (non-motorized) — *see* Accident, transport, pedestrian, conveyance, scooter
- sequelae of — *see* W00-X58 with q as terminal character
- skateboard — *see* Accident, transport, pedestrian, conveyance, skateboard
- ski(ing) — *see* Accident, transport, pedestrian, conveyance
  - lift V98.3
- specified cause NEC X58.8
- streetcar — *see* Accident, transport, streetcar occupant
- traffic (victim's mode of transport NOS) V87.9
  - collision (between) V87.7
    - bus and truck V87.5
    - car and:
      - bus V87.3
      - pickup V87.2
      - three-wheeled motor vehicle V87.0
      - train V87.6
      - truck V87.4
      - two-wheeled motor vehicle V87.0
      - van V87.2
    - specified vehicle NEC and:
      - three-wheeled motor vehicle V87.1
      - two-wheeled motor vehicle V87.1
    - known mode of transport — *see* Accident, transport, by type of vehicle
  - noncollision V87.8
- transport (involving injury to) V99
  - 18 wheeler — *see* Accident, transport, truck occupant
  - agricultural vehicle occupant (nontraffic) V84.9
    - driver V84.5
    - hanger-on V84.7
    - passenger V84.6
    - traffic V84.3
      - driver V84.0
      - hanger-on V84.2
      - passenger V84.1
    - while boarding or alighting V84.4
  - aircraft
    - occupant injured (in)
      - nonpowered craft accident V96.9
        - balloon V96.00
          - collision V96.03
          - crash V96.01
          - explosion V96.05
          - fire V96.04
          - forced landing V96.02
          - specified type NEC V96.09
        - glider V96.20
          - collision V96.23
          - crash V96.21
          - explosion V96.25
          - fire V96.24
          - forced landing V96.22
          - specified type NEC V96.29
        - hang glider V96.10
          - collision V96.13
          - crash V96.11
          - explosion V96.15
          - fire V96.14
          - forced landing V96.12
          - specified type NEC V96.19
        - specified craft NEC V96.8
      - powered craft accident V95.9
        - fixed wing NEC
          - commercial V95.30
            - collision V95.33
            - crash V95.31
            - explosion V95.35
            - fire V95.34
            - forced landing V95.32
            - specified type NEC V95.39

Accident — *continued*
  transport — *continued*
    aircraft — *continued*
      occupant injured — *continued*
        powered craft accident — *continued*
          fixed wing NEC — *continued*
            private V95.20
              collision V95.23
              crash V95.21
              explosion V95.25
              fire V95.24
              forced landing V95.22
              specified type NEC V95.29
          glider V95.10
            collision V95.13
            crash V95.11
            explosion V95.15
            fire V95.14
            forced landing V95.12
            specified type NEC V95.19
          helicopter V95.00
            collision V95.03
            crash V95.01
            explosion V95.05
            fire V95.04
            forced landing V95.02
            specified type NEC V95.09
          spacecraft V95.40
            collision V95.43
            crash V95.41
            explosion V95.45
            fire V95.44
            forced landing V95.42
            specified type NEC V95.49
          specified craft NEC V95.8
          ultralight V95.10
            collision V95.13
            crash V95.11
            explosion V95.15
            fire V95.14
            forced landing V95.12
            specified type NEC V95.19
        specified accident NEC V97.0
        while boarding or alighting V97.1
      person (injured by)
        falling from, in or on aircraft V97.0
        machinery on aircraft V97.8
        on ground with aircraft involvement V97.39
        rotating propeller V97.32
        struck by object falling from aircraft V97.31
        sucked into aircraft jet V97.33
        while boarding or alighting aircraft V97.1
    airport (battery powered) passenger vehicle — *see* Accident, transport, industrial vehicle occupant
    all-terrain vehicle occupant (nontraffic) V86.99
      driver V86.59
      dune buggy — *see* Accident, transport, dune buggy occupant
      hanger-on V86.79
      passenger V86.69
      snowmobile — *see* Accident, transport, snowmobile occupant
      traffic V86.39
        driver V86.09
        hanger-on V86.29
        passenger V86.19
      while boarding or alighting V86.49
    ambulance occupant (traffic) V86.31
      driver V86.01
      hanger-on V86.21
      nontraffic V86.91
        driver V86.51
        hanger-on V86.71
        passenger V86.61
      passenger V86.11
      while boarding or alighting V86.41
    animal-drawn vehicle occupant (in) V80.929
      collision (with)
        animal V80.12
          being ridden V80.711
        animal-drawn vehicle V80.721

Accident — *continued*
  transport — *continued*
    animal-drawn vehicle occupant — *continued*
      collision — *continued*
        bus V80.42
        car V80.42
        fixed or stationary object V80.82
        military vehicle V80.920
        nonmotor vehicle V80.791
        pedal cycle V80.22
        pedestrian V80.12
        pickup V80.42
        railway train or vehicle V80.62
        specified motor vehicle NEC V80.52
        streetcar V80.731
        truck V80.42
        two- or three-wheeled motor vehicle V80.32
        van V80.42
      noncollision V80.02
      specified circumstance NEC V80.928
    animal-rider V80.919
      collision (with)
        animal V80.11
          being ridden V80.710
        animal-drawn vehicle V80.720
        bus V80.41
        car V80.41
        fixed or stationary object V80.81
        military vehicle V80.910
        nonmotor vehicle V80.790
        pedal cycle V80.21
        pedestrian V80.11
        pickup V80.41
        railway train or vehicle V80.61
        specified motor vehicle NEC V80.51
        streetcar V80.730
        truck V80.41
        two- or three-wheeled motor vehicle V80.31
        van V80.41
      noncollision V80.018
        specified as horse rider V80.010
      specified circumstance NEC V80.918
    armored car — *see* Accident, transport, truck occupant
    battery-powered truck (baggage) (mail) — *see* Accident, transport, industrial vehicle occupant
    bus occupant V79.9
      collision (with)
        animal (traffic) V70.9
          being ridden (traffic) V76.9
            nontraffic V76.3
            while boarding or alighting V76.4
          nontraffic V70.3
            while boarding or alighting V70.4
        animal-drawn vehicle (traffic) V76.9
          nontraffic V76.3
          while boarding or alighting V76.4
        bus (traffic) V74.9
          nontraffic V74.3
          while boarding or alighting V74.4
        car (traffic) V73.9
          nontraffic V73.3
          while boarding or alighting V73.4
        motor vehicle NOS (traffic) V79.60
          nontraffic V79.20
          specified type NEC (traffic) V79.69
            nontraffic V79.29
        pedal cycle (traffic) V71.9
          nontraffic V71.3
          while boarding or alighting V71.4
        pickup truck (traffic) V73.9
          nontraffic V73.3
          while boarding or alighting V73.4
        railway vehicle (traffic) V75.9
          nontraffic V75.3
          while boarding or alighting V75.4
        specified vehicle NEC (traffic) V76.9
          nontraffic V76.3
          while boarding or alighting V76.4
        stationary object (traffic) V77.9
          nontraffic V77.3
          while boarding or alighting V77.4

Accident — *continued*
  transport — *continued*
    bus occupant — *continued*
      collision — *continued*
        streetcar (traffic) V76.9
          nontraffic V76.3
          while boarding or alighting V76.4
        three-wheeled motor vehicle (traffic) V72.9
          nontraffic V72.3
          while boarding or alighting V72.4
        truck (traffic) V74.9
          nontraffic V74.3
          while boarding or alighting V74.4
        two-wheeled motor vehicle (traffic) V72.9
          nontraffic V72.3
          while boarding or alighting V72.4
        van (traffic) V73.9
          nontraffic V73.3
          while boarding or alighting V73.4
      driver
        collision (with)
          animal (traffic) V70.5
            being ridden (traffic) V76.5
              nontraffic V76.0
            nontraffic V70.0
          animal-drawn vehicle (traffic) V76.5
            nontraffic V76.0
          bus (traffic) V74.5
            nontraffic V74.0
          car (traffic) V73.5
            nontraffic V73.0
          motor vehicle NOS (traffic) V79.40
            nontraffic V79.00
            specified type NEC (traffic) V79.49
              nontraffic V79.09
          pedal cycle (traffic) V71.5
            nontraffic V71.0
          pickup truck (traffic) V73.5
            nontraffic V73.0
          railway vehicle (traffic) V75.5
            nontraffic V75.0
          specified vehicle NEC (traffic) V76.5
            nontraffic V76.0
          stationary object (traffic) V77.5
            nontraffic V77.0
          streetcar (traffic) V76.5
            nontraffic V76.0
          three-wheeled motor vehicle (traffic) V72.5
            nontraffic V72.0
          truck (traffic) V74.5
            nontraffic V74.0
          two-wheeled motor vehicle (traffic) V72.5
            nontraffic V72.0
          van (traffic) V73.5
            nontraffic V73.0
        noncollision accident (traffic) V78.5
          nontraffic V78.0
      noncollision accident (traffic) V78.9
        nontraffic V78.3
        while boarding or alighting V78.4
      nontraffic V79.3
      hanger-on
        collision (with)
          animal (traffic) V70.7
            being ridden (traffic) V76.7
              nontraffic V76.2
            nontraffic V70.2
          animal-drawn vehicle (traffic) V76.7
            nontraffic V76.2
          bus (traffic) V74.7
            nontraffic V74.2
          car (traffic) V73.7
            nontraffic V73.2
          pedal cycle (traffic) V71.7
            nontraffic V71.2
          pickup truck (traffic) V73.7
            nontraffic V73.2
          railway vehicle (traffic) V75.7
            nontraffic V75.2

©2002 Ingenix, Inc.

©2002 Ingenix, Inc.

Accident — *continued*
  transport — *continued*
    occupant — *continued*
      animal-drawn vehicle — *see* Accident, transport, animal-drawn vehicle occupant
      automobile — *see* Accident, transport, car occupant
      balloon V96.00
      battery-powered vehicle — *see* Accident, transport, industrial vehicle occupant
      bicycle — *see* Accident, transport, pedal cyclist
        motorized — *see* Accident, transport, motorcycle rider
      boat NEC — *see* Accident, watercraft
      bulldozer — *see* Accident, transport, construction vehicle occupant
      bus — *see* Accident, transport, bus occupant
      cable car (on rails) — *see also* Accident, transport, streetcar occupant
        not on rails V98.0
      car — *see also* Accident, transport, car occupant
        cable (on rails) — *see also* Accident, transport, streetcar occupant
        not on rails V98.0
      coach — *see* Accident, transport, bus occupant
      coal-car — *see* Accident, transport, industrial vehicle occupant
      digger — *see* Accident, transport, construction vehicle occupant
      dump truck — *see* Accident, transport, construction vehicle occupant
      earth-leveler — *see* Accident, transport, construction vehicle occupant
      farm machinery (self-propelled) — *see* Accident, transport, agricultural vehicle occupant
      forklift — *see* Accident, transport, industrial vehicle occupant
      glider (unpowered) V96.20
        hang V96.10
        powered (microlight) (ultralight) — *see* Accident, transport, aircraft, occupant, powered, glider
      glider (unpowered) NEC V96.20
      hang-glider V96.10
      harvester — *see* Accident, transport, agricultural vehicle occupant
      heavy (transport) vehicle — *see* Accident, transport, truck occupant
      helicopter — *see* Accident, transport, aircraft, occupant, helicopter
      ice-yacht V98.2
      kite (carrying person) V96.8
      land-yacht V98.1
      logging car — *see* Accident, transport, industrial vehicle occupant
      mechanical shovel — *see* Accident, transport, construction vehicle occupant
      microlight — *see* Accident, transport, aircraft, occupant, powered, glider
      minibus — *see* Accident, transport, car occupant
      minivan — *see* Accident, transport, car occupant
      moped — *see* Accident, transport, motorcycle
      motor scooter — *see* Accident, transport, motorcycle
      motorcycle (with sidecar) — *see* Accident, transport, motorcycle
      pedal cycle — *see also* Accident, transport, pedal cyclist
      pick-up (truck) — *see* Accident, transport, pickup truck occupant
      railway (train) (vehicle) (subterranean) (elevated) — *see* Accident, transport, railway vehicle occupant

Accident — *continued*
  transport — *continued*
    occupant — *continued*
      rickshaw — *see* Accident, transport, pedal cycle
        motorized — *see* Accident, transport, three-wheeled motor vehicle)
        pedal driven — *see* Accident, transport, pedal cyclist
      road-roller — *see* Accident, transport, construction vehicle occupant
      ship NOS V94.9
      ski-lift (chair) (gondola) V98.3
      snowmobile — *see* Accident, transport, snowmobile occupant
      spacecraft, spaceship — *see* Accident, transport, aircraft, occupant, spacecraft
      sport utility vehicle — *see* Accident, transport, car occupant
      streetcar (interurban) (operating on public street or highway) — *see* Accident, transport, streetcar occupant
      SUV — *see* Accident, transport, car occupant
      téléférique V98.0
      three-wheeled vehicle (motorized) — *see also* Accident, transport, three-wheeled motor vehicle occupant
        nonmotorized — *see* Accident, transport, pedal cycle
      tractor (farm) (and trailer) — *see* Accident, transport, agricultural vehicle occupant
      train — *see* Accident, transport, railway vehicle occupant
      tram — *see* Accident, transport, streetcar occupant
        in mine or quarry — *see* Accident, transport, industrial vehicle occupant
      tricycle — *see* Accident, transport, pedal cycle
        motorized — *see* Accident, transport, three-wheeled motor vehicle
      trolley — *see* Accident, transport, streetcar occupant
        in mine or quarry — *see* Accident, transport, industrial vehicle occupant
      tub, in mine or quarry — *see* Accident, transport, industrial vehicle occupant
      ultralight — *see* Accident, transport, aircraft, occupant, powered, glider
      van — *see* Accident, transport, van occupant
      vehicle NEC V89.9
        heavy transport — *see* Accident, transport, truck occupant
        motor (traffic) NEC V89.2
        nontraffic NEC V89.0
      watercraft NOS V94.9
        causing drowning — *see* Drowning, resulting from accident to boat
  parachutist V97.29
    after accident to aircraft — *see* Accident, transport, aircraft
    entangled in object V97.21
    injured on landing V97.22
  pedal cyclist V19.9
    collision (with)
      animal (traffic) 10.9
        being ridden (traffic) V16.9
          nontraffic 16.2
            while boarding or alighting V16.3
        nontraffic V10.2
          while boarding or alighting V10.3
      animal-drawn vehicle (traffic) V16.9
        nontraffic V16.2
          while boarding or alighting V16.3
      bus (traffic) V14.9
        nontraffic V14.2
          while boarding or alighting V14.3
      car (traffic) V13.9
        nontraffic V13.2

Accident — *continued*
  transport — *continued*
    pedal cyclist — *continued*
      collision — *continued*
        car — *continued*
          while boarding or alighting V13.3
        motor vehicle NOS (traffic) V19.60
          nontraffic V19.20
          specified type NEC (traffic) V19.69
            nontraffic V19.29
        pedal cycle (traffic) V11.9
          nontraffic V11.2
          while boarding or alighting V11.3
        pickup truck (traffic) V13.9
          nontraffic V13.2
          while boarding or alighting V13.3
        railway vehicle (traffic) V15.9
          nontraffic V15.2
          while boarding or alighting V15.3
        specified vehicle NEC (traffic) V16.9
          nontraffic V16.2
          while boarding or alighting V16.3
        stationary object (traffic) V17.9
          nontraffic V17.2
          while boarding or alighting V17.3
        streetcar (traffic) V16.9
          nontraffic V16.2
          while boarding or alighting V16.3
        three-wheeled motor vehicle (traffic) V12.9
          nontraffic V12.2
          while boarding or alighting V12.3
        truck (traffic) V14.9
          nontraffic V14.2
          while boarding or alighting V14.3
        two-wheeled motor vehicle (traffic) V12.9
          nontraffic V12.2
          while boarding or alighting V12.3
        van (traffic) V13.9
          nontraffic V13.2
          while boarding or alighting V13.3
      driver
        collision (with)
          animal (traffic) V10.4
            being ridden (traffic) V16.4
              nontraffic V16.0
            nontraffic V10.0
          animal-drawn vehicle (traffic) V16.4
            nontraffic V16.0
          bus (traffic) V14.4
            nontraffic V14.0
          car (traffic) V13.4
            nontraffic V13.0
          motor vehicle NOS (traffic) V19.40
            nontraffic V19.00
            specified type NEC (traffic) V19.49
              nontraffic V19.09
          pedal cycle (traffic) V11.4
            nontraffic V11.0
          pickup truck (traffic) V13.4
            nontraffic V13.0
          railway vehicle (traffic) V15.4
            nontraffic V15.0
          specified vehicle NEC (traffic) V16.4
            nontraffic V16.0
          stationary object (traffic) V17.4
            nontraffic V17.0
          streetcar (traffic) V16.4
            nontraffic V16.0
          three-wheeled motor vehicle (traffic) V12.4
            nontraffic V12.0
          truck (traffic) V14.4
            nontraffic V14.0
          two-wheeled motor vehicle (traffic) V12.4
            nontraffic V12.0
          van (traffic) V13.4
            nontraffic V13.0
        noncollision accident (traffic) V18.4
          nontraffic V18.0

Accident — *continued*
  transport — *continued*
    pedal cyclist — *continued*
      noncollision accident (traffic) V18.9
        nontraffic V18.2
        while boarding or alighting V18.3
      nontraffic V19.3
      passenger
        collision (with)
          animal (traffic) V10.5
            being ridden (traffic) V16.5
              nontraffic V16.1
            nontraffic V10.1
          animal-drawn vehicle (traffic) V16.5
            nontraffic V16.1
          bus (traffic) V14.5
            nontraffic V14.1
          car (traffic) V13.5
            nontraffic V13.1
          motor vehicle NOS (traffic) V19.50
            nontraffic V19.10
            specified type NEC (traffic) V19.59
              nontraffic V19.19
          pedal cycle (traffic) V11.5
            nontraffic V11.1
          pickup truck (traffic) V13.5
            nontraffic V13.1
          railway vehicle (traffic) V15.5
            nontraffic V15.1
          specified vehicle NEC (traffic) V16.5
            nontraffic V16.1
          stationary object (traffic) V17.5
            nontraffic V17.1
          streetcar (traffic) V16.5
            nontraffic V16.1
          three-wheeled motor vehicle (traffic) V12.5
            nontraffic V12.1
          truck (traffic) V14.5
            nontraffic V14.1
          two-wheeled motor vehicle (traffic) V12.5
            nontraffic V12.1
          van (traffic) V13.5
            nontraffic V13.1
        noncollision accident (traffic) V18.5
          nontraffic V18.1
        specified type NEC V19.88
        military vehicle V19.81
    pedestrian
      conveyance occupant V09.9
        babystroller V00.828
          collision (with) V09.9
            animal being ridden or animal drawn vehicle V06.99
              nontraffic V06.09
              traffic V06.19
            bus or heavy transport V04.99
              nontraffic V04.09
              traffic V04.19
            car V03.99
              nontraffic V03.09
              traffic V03.19
            pedal cycle V01.99
              nontraffic V01.09
              traffic V01.19
            pick-up truck or van V03.99
              nontraffic V03.09
              traffic V03.19
            railway (train) (vehicle) V05.99
              nontraffic V05.09
              traffic V05.19
            streetcar V06.99
              nontraffic V06.09
              traffic V06.19
            stationary object V00.822
            two- or three-wheeled motor vehicle V02.99
              nontraffic V02.09
              traffic V02.19
            vehicle V09.9
              animal-drawn V06.99
                nontraffic V06.09
                traffic V06.19

Accident — *continued*
  transport — *continued*
    pedestrian — *continued*
      conveyance occupant — *continued*
        babystroller — *continued*
          collision — *continued*
            vehicle — *continued*
              motor
                nontraffic V09.00
                traffic V09.20
          fall V00.821
          nontraffic V09.1
            involving motor vehicle NEC V09.00
          traffic V09.3
            involving motor vehicle NEC V09.20
        flat-bottomed NEC V00.388
          collision (with) V09.9
            animal being ridden or animal drawn vehicle V06.99
              nontraffic V06.09
              traffic V06.19
            bus or heavy transport V04.99
              nontraffic V04.09
              traffic V04.19
            car V03.99
              nontraffic V03.09
              traffic V03.19
            pedal cycle V01.99
              nontraffic V01.09
              traffic V01.19
            pick-up truck or van V03.99
              nontraffic V03.09
              traffic V03.19
            railway (train) (vehicle) V05.99
              nontraffic V05.09
              traffic V05.19
            stationary object V00.382
            streetcar V06.99
              nontraffic V06.09
              traffic V06.19
            two- or three-wheeled motor vehicle V02.99
              nontraffic V02.09
              traffic V02.19
            vehicle V09.9
              animal-drawn V06.99
                nontraffic V06.09
                traffic V06.19
              motor
                nontraffic V09.00
                traffic V09.20
        fall V00.381
        nontraffic V09.1
          involving motor vehicle NEC V09.00
        snow
          board — *see* Accident, transport, pedestrian, conveyance, snow board
          ski — *see* Accident, transport, pedestrian, conveyance, skis (snow)
        traffic V09.3
          involving motor vehicle NEC V09.20
        gliding type NEC V00.288
          collision (with) V09.9
            animal being ridden or animal drawn vehicle V06.99
              nontraffic V06.09
              traffic V06.19
            bus or heavy transport V04.99
              nontraffic V04.09
              traffic V04.19
            car V03.99
              nontraffic V03.09
              traffic V03.19
            pedal cycle V01.99
              nontraffic V01.09
              traffic V01.19
            pick-up truck or van V03.99
              nontraffic V03.09
              traffic V03.19

Accident — *continued*
  transport — *continued*
    pedestrian — *continued*
      conveyance occupant — *continued*
        gliding type NEC — *continued*
          collision — *continued*
            railway (train) (vehicle) V05.99
              nontraffic V05.09
              traffic V05.19
            stationary object V00.282
            streetcar V06.99
              nontraffic V06.09
              traffic V06.19
            two- or three-wheeled motor vehicle V02.99
              nontraffic V02.09
              traffic V02.19
            vehicle V09.9
              animal-drawn V06.99
                nontraffic V06.09
                traffic V06.19
              motor
                nontraffic V09.00
                traffic V09.20
          fall V00.281
          ice skate — *see* Accident, transport, pedestrian, conveyance, ice skate
          nontraffic V09.1
            involving motor vehicle NEC V09.00
          sled — *see* Accident, transport, pedestrian, conveyance, sled
          traffic V09.3
            involving motor vehicle NEC V09.20
         ice skates V00.218
          collision (with) V09.9
            animal being ridden or animal drawn vehicle V06.99
              nontraffic V06.09
              traffic V06.19
            bus or heavy transport V04.99
              nontraffic V04.09
              traffic V04.19
            car V03.99
              nontraffic V03.09
              traffic V03.19
            pedal cycle V01.99
              nontraffic V01.09
              traffic V01.19
            pick-up truck or van V03.99
              nontraffic V03.09
              traffic V03.19
            railway (train) (vehicle) V05.99
              nontraffic V05.09
              traffic V05.19
            streetcar V06.99
              nontraffic V06.09
              traffic V06.19
            stationary object V00.212
            two- or three-wheeled motor vehicle V02.99
              nontraffic V02.09
              traffic V02.19
            vehicle V09.9
              animal-drawn V06.99
                nontraffic V06.09
                traffic V06.19
              motor
                nontraffic V09.00
                traffic V09.20
          fall V00.211
          nontraffic V09.1
            involving motor vehicle NEC V09.00
          traffic V09.3
            involving motor vehicle NEC V09.20
         nontraffic V09.1
          involving motor vehicle V09.00
            military V09.01
            specified type NEC V09.09

Accident — *continued*
 transport — *continued*
  pedestrian — *continued*
   conveyance occupant — *continued*
    roller skates (non in-line) V00.128
     collision (with) V09.9
      animal being ridden or animal
       drawn vehicle V06.91
        nontraffic V06.01
        traffic V06.11
      bus or heavy transport V04.91
       nontraffic V04.01
       traffic V04.11
      car V03.91
       nontraffic V03.01
       traffic V03.11
      pedal cycle V01.91
       nontraffic V01.01
       traffic V01.11
      pick-up truck or van V03.91
       nontraffic V03.01
       traffic V03.11
      railway (train) (vehicle) V05.91
       nontraffic V05.01
       traffic V05.11
      streetcar V06.91
       nontraffic V06.01
       traffic V06.11
      stationary object V00.122
      two- or three-wheeled motor
       vehicle V02.91
        nontraffic V02.01
        traffic V02.11
      vehicle V09.9
       animal-drawn V06.91
        nontraffic V06.01
        traffic V06.11
       motor
        nontraffic V09.00
        traffic V09.20
     fall V00.121
    in-line V00.118
     collision — *see also* Accident,
      transport, pedestrian,
      conveyance occupant, roller
      skates, collision
      with stationary object V00.112
     fall V00.111
     nontraffic V09.1
      involving motor vehicle NEC
       V09.00
     traffic V09.3
      involving motor vehicle NEC
       V09.20
    rolling type NEC V00.188
     collision (with) V09.9
      animal being ridden or animal
       drawn vehicle V06.99
        nontraffic V06.09
        traffic V06.19
      bus or heavy transport V04.99
       nontraffic V04.09
       traffic V04.19
      car V03.99
       nontraffic V03.09
       traffic V03.19
      pedal cycle V01.99
       nontraffic V01.09
       traffic V01.19
      pick-up truck or van V03.99
       nontraffic V03.09
       traffic V03.19
      railway (train) (vehicle) V05.99
       nontraffic V05.09
       traffic V05.19
      stationary object V00.182
      streetcar V06.99
       nontraffic V06.09
       traffic V06.19
      two- or three-wheeled motor
       vehicle V02.99
        nontraffic V02.09
        traffic V02.19

Accident — *continued*
 transport — *continued*
  pedestrian — *continued*
   conveyance occupant — *continued*
    rolling type NEC — *continued*
     collision — *continued*
      vehicle V09.9
       animal-drawn V06.99
        nontraffic V06.09
        traffic V06.19
       motor
        nontraffic V09.00
        traffic V09.20
    fall V00.181
    in-line roller skate — *see* Accident,
     transport, pedestrian,
     conveyance, roller skate, in-
     line
    nontraffic V09.1
     involving motor vehicle NEC
      V09.00
    roller skate — *see* Accident,
     transport, pedestrian,
     conveyance, roller skate
    scooter (non-motorized) — *see*
     Accident, transport,
     pedestrian, conveyance,
     scooter
    skateboard — *see* Accident,
     transport, pedestrian,
     conveyance, skateboard
    traffic V09.3
     involving motor vehicle NEC
      V09.20
    scooter (non-motorized) V00.148
     collision (with) V09.9
      animal being ridden or animal
       drawn vehicle V06.99
        nontraffic V06.09
        traffic V06.19
      bus or heavy transport V04.99
       nontraffic V04.09
       traffic V04.19
      car V03.99
       nontraffic V03.09
       traffic V03.19
      pedal cycle V01.99
       nontraffic V01.09
       traffic V01.19
      pick-up truck or van V03.99
       nontraffic V03.09
       traffic V03.19
      railway (train) (vehicle) V05.99
       nontraffic V05.09
       traffic V05.19
      streetcar V06.99
       nontraffic V06.09
       traffic V06.19
      stationary object V00.142
      two- or three-wheeled motor
       vehicle V02.99
        nontraffic V02.09
        traffic V02.19
      vehicle V09.9
       animal-drawn V06.99
        nontraffic V06.09
        traffic V06.19
       motor
        nontraffic V09.00
        traffic V09.20
    fall V00.141
    nontraffic V09.1
     involving motor vehicle NEC
      V09.00
    traffic V09.3
     involving motor vehicle NEC
      V09.20
    skate board V00.138
     collision (with) V09.9
      animal being ridden or animal
       drawn vehicle V06.92
        nontraffic V06.02
        traffic V06.12
      bus or heavy transport V04.92
       nontraffic V04.02
       traffic V04.12

Accident — *continued*
 transport — *continued*
  pedestrian — *continued*
   conveyance occupant — *continued*
    skate board — *continued*
     collision — *continued*
      car V03.92
       nontraffic V03.02
       traffic V03.12
      pedal cycle V01.92
       nontraffic V01.02
       traffic V01.12
      pick-up truck or van V03.92
       nontraffic V03.02
       traffic V03.12
      railway (train) (vehicle) V05.92
       nontraffic V05.02
       traffic V05.12
      streetcar V06.92
       nontraffic V06.02
       traffic V06.12
      stationary object V00.132
      two- or three-wheeled motor
       vehicle V02.92
        nontraffic V02.02
        traffic V02.12
      vehicle V09.9
       animal-drawn V06.92
        nontraffic V06.02
        traffic V06.12
       motor
        nontraffic V09.00
        traffic V09.20
    fall V00.131
    nontraffic V09.1
     involving motor vehicle NEC
      V09.00
    traffic V09.3
     involving motor vehicle NEC
      V09.20
    sled V00.228
     collision (with) V09.9
      animal being ridden or animal
       drawn vehicle V06.99
        nontraffic V06.09
        traffic V06.19
      bus or heavy transport V04.99
       nontraffic V04.09
       traffic V04.19
      car V03.99
       nontraffic V03.09
       traffic V03.19
      pedal cycle V01.99
       nontraffic V01.09
       traffic V01.19
      pick-up truck or van V03.99
       nontraffic V03.09
       traffic V03.19
      railway (train) (vehicle) V05.99
       nontraffic V05.09
       traffic V05.19
      streetcar V06.99
       nontraffic V06.09
       traffic V06.19
      stationary object V00.222
      two- or three-wheeled motor
       vehicle V02.99
        nontraffic V02.09
        traffic V02.19
      vehicle V09.9
       animal-drawn V06.99
        nontraffic V06.09
        traffic V06.19
       motor
        nontraffic V09.00
        traffic V09.20
    fall V00.221
    nontraffic V09.1
     involving motor vehicle NEC
      V09.00
    traffic V09.3
     involving motor vehicle NEC
      V09.20

Accident — *continued*
  transport — *continued*
    pedestrian — *continued*
      conveyance occupant — *continued*
        skis (snow) V00.328
          collision (with) V09.9
            animal being ridden or animal
              drawn vehicle V06.99
              nontraffic V06.09
              traffic V06.19
            bus or heavy transport V04.99
              nontraffic V04.09
              traffic V04.19
            car V03.99
              nontraffic V03.09
              traffic V03.19
            pedal cycle V01.99
              nontraffic V01.09
              traffic V01.19
            pick-up truck or van V03.99
              nontraffic V03.09
              traffic V03.19
            railway (train) (vehicle) V05.99
              nontraffic V05.09
              traffic V05.19
            streetcar V06.99
              nontraffic V06.09
              traffic V06.19
            stationary object V00.322
            two- or three-wheeled motor
              vehicle V02.99
              nontraffic V02.09
              traffic V02.19
            vehicle V09.9
              animal-drawn V06.99
                nontraffic V06.09
                traffic V06.19
              motor
                nontraffic V09.00
                traffic V09.20
        fall V00.321
        nontraffic V09.1
          involving motor vehicle NEC
            V09.00
        traffic V09.3
          involving motor vehicle NEC
            V09.20
        snow board V00.318
          collision (with) V09.9
            animal being ridden or animal
              drawn vehicle V06.99
              nontraffic V06.09
              traffic V06.19
            bus or heavy transport V04.99
              nontraffic V04.09
              traffic V04.19
            car V03.99
              nontraffic V03.09
              traffic V03.19
            pedal cycle V01.99
              nontraffic V01.09
              traffic V01.19
            pick-up truck or van V03.99
              nontraffic V03.09
              traffic V03.19
            railway (train) (vehicle) V05.99
              nontraffic V05.09
              traffic V05.19
            streetcar V06.99
              nontraffic V06.09
              traffic V06.19
            stationary object V00.312
            two- or three-wheeled motor
              vehicle V02.99
              nontraffic V02.09
              traffic V02.19
            vehicle V09.9
             animal-drawn V06.99
              nontraffic V06.09
              traffic V06.19
             motor
              nontraffic V09.00
              traffic V09.20
        fall V00.311

Accident — *continued*
  transport — *continued*
    pedestrian — *continued*
      conveyance occupant — *continued*
        snow board — *continued*
          nontraffic V09.1
            involving motor vehicle NEC
              V09.00
          traffic V09.3
            involving motor vehicle NEC
              V09.20
        specified type NEC V00.898
          collision (with) V09.9
            animal being ridden or animal
              drawn vehicle V06.99
              nontraffic V06.09
              traffic V06.19
            bus or heavy transport V04.99
              nontraffic V04.09
              traffic V04.19
            car V03.99
              nontraffic V03.09
              traffic V03.19
            pedal cycle V01.99
              nontraffic V01.09
              traffic V01.19
            pick-up truck or van V03.99
              nontraffic V03.09
              traffic V03.19
            railway (train) (vehicle) V05.99
              nontraffic V05.09
              traffic V05.19
            streetcar V06.99
              nontraffic V06.09
              traffic V06.19
            stationary object V00.892
            two- or three-wheeled motor
              vehicle V02.99
              nontraffic V02.09
              traffic V02.19
            vehicle V09.9
             animal-drawn V06.99
              nontraffic V06.09
              traffic V06.19
             motor
              nontraffic V09.00
              traffic V09.20
        fall V00.891
        nontraffic V09.1
          involving motor vehicle NEC
            V09.00
        traffic V09.3
          involving motor vehicle NEC
            V09.20
      traffic V09.3
        involving motor vehicle V09.20
          military V09.21
          specified type NEC V09.29
      wheelchair (powered) V00.818
        collision (with) V09.9
          animal being ridden or animal
            drawn vehicle V06.99
            nontraffic V06.09
            traffic V06.19
          bus or heavy transport V04.99
            nontraffic V04.09
            traffic V04.19
          car V03.99
            nontraffic V03.09
            traffic V03.19
          pedal cycle V01.99
            nontraffic V01.09
            traffic V01.19
          pick-up truck or van V03.99
            nontraffic V03.09
            traffic V03.19
          railway (train) (vehicle) V05.99
            nontraffic V05.09
            traffic V05.19
          streetcar V06.99
            nontraffic V06.09
            traffic V06.19
          stationary object V00.812

Accident — *continued*
  transport — *continued*
    pedestrian — *continued*
      conveyance occupant — *continued*
        wheelchair — *continued*
          collision — *continued*
            two- or three-wheeled motor
              vehicle V02.99
              nontraffic V02.09
              traffic V02.19
            vehicle V09.9
             animal-drawn V06.99
              nontraffic V06.09
              traffic V06.19
             motor
              nontraffic V09.00
              traffic V09.20
        fall V00.811
        nontraffic V09.1
          involving motor vehicle NEC
            V09.00
        traffic V09.3
          involving motor vehicle NEC
            V09.20
      on foot — *see also* Accident, pedestrian
        collision (with)
          animal being ridden or animal drawn
            vehicle V06.90
            nontraffic V06.00
            traffic V06.10
          bus or heavy transport V04.90
            nontraffic V04.00
            traffic V04.10
          car V03.90
            nontraffic V03.00
            traffic V03.10
          pedal cycle V01.90
            nontraffic V01.00
            traffic V01.10
          pick-up truck or van V03.90
            nontraffic V03.00
            traffic V03.10
          railway (train) (vehicle) V05.90
            nontraffic V05.00
            traffic V05.10
          streetcar V06.90
            nontraffic V06.00
            traffic V06.10
          two- or three-wheeled motor vehicle
            V02.90
            nontraffic V02.00
            traffic V02.10
          vehicle V09.9
            animal-drawn V06.90
             nontraffic V06.00
             traffic V06.10
            motor
             nontraffic V09.00
             traffic V09.20
        nontraffic V09.1
          involving motor vehicle V09.00
           military V09.01
           specified type NEC V09.09
        traffic V09.3
          involving motor vehicle V09.20
           military V09.21
           specified type NEC V09.29
      person NEC (unknown way or transportation)
        V99
      collision (between)
        bus (with)
          heavy transport vehicle (traffic)
            V87.5
          nontraffic V88.5
        car (with)
          nontraffic V88.5
          bus (traffic) V87.3
           nontraffic V88.3
          heavy transport vehicle (traffic)
            V87.4
           nontraffic V88.4
          pick-up truck or van (traffic) V87.2
           nontraffic V88.2
          train or railway vehicle (traffic) V87.6
           nontraffic V88.6

Accident — *continued*
  transport — *continued*
    person NEC — *continued*
      collision — *continued*
        car — *continued*
          two- or three-wheeled motor vehicle (traffic) V87.0
            nontraffic V88.0
          motor vehicle (traffic) NEC V87.7
            nontraffic V88.7
          two- or three-wheeled vehicle (with) (traffic)
            motor vehicle NEC V87.1
            nontraffic V88.1
          nonmotor vehicle (collision) (noncollision) (traffic) V87.9
            nontraffic V88.9
    pickup truck occupant V59.9
      collision (with)
        animal (traffic) V50.9
          being ridden (traffic) V56.9
            nontraffic V56.3
            while boarding or alighting V56.4
          nontraffic V50.3
          while boarding or alighting V50.4
        animal-drawn vehicle (traffic) V56.9
          nontraffic V56.3
          while boarding or alighting V56.4
        bus (traffic) V54.9
          nontraffic V54.3
          while boarding or alighting V54.4
        car (traffic) V53.9
          nontraffic V53.3
          while boarding or alighting V53.4
        motor vehicle NOS (traffic) V59.60
          nontraffic V59.20
          specified type NEC (traffic) V59.69
            nontraffic V59.29
        pedal cycle (traffic) V51.9
          nontraffic V51.3
          while boarding or alighting V51.4
        pickup truck (traffic) V53.9
          nontraffic V53.3
          while boarding or alighting V53.4
        railway vehicle (traffic) V55.9
          nontraffic V55.3
          while boarding or alighting V55.4
        specified vehicle NEC (traffic) V56.9
          nontraffic V56.3
          while boarding or alighting V56.4
        stationary object (traffic) V57.9
          nontraffic V57.3
          while boarding or alighting V57.4
        streetcar (traffic) V56.9
          nontraffic V56.3
          while boarding or alighting V56.4
        three-wheeled motor vehicle (traffic) V52.9
          nontraffic V52.3
          while boarding or alighting V52.4
        truck (traffic) V54.9
          nontraffic V54.3
          while boarding or alighting V54.4
        two-wheeled motor vehicle (traffic) V52.9
          nontraffic V52.3
          while boarding or alighting V52.4
        van (traffic) V53.9
          nontraffic V53.3
          while boarding or alighting V53.4
      driver
        collision (with)
          animal (traffic) V50.5
            being ridden (traffic) V56.5
              nontraffic V56.0
            nontraffic V50.0
          animal-drawn vehicle (traffic) V56.5
            nontraffic V56.0
          bus (traffic) V54.5
            nontraffic V54.0
          car (traffic) V53.5
            nontraffic V53.0
          motor vehicle NOS (traffic) V59.40
            nontraffic V59.00

Accident — *continued*
  transport — *continued*
    pickup truck occupant — *continued*
      driver — *continued*
        collision — *continued*
          motor vehicle NOS — *continued*
            specified type NEC (traffic) V59.49
              nontraffic V59.09
          pedal cycle (traffic) V51.5
            nontraffic V51.0
          pickup truck (traffic) V53.5
            nontraffic V53.0
          railway vehicle (traffic) V55.5
            nontraffic V55.0
          specified vehicle NEC (traffic) V56.5
            nontraffic V56.0
          stationary object (traffic) V57.5
            nontraffic V57.0
          streetcar (traffic) V56.5
            nontraffic V56.0
          three-wheeled motor vehicle (traffic) V52.5
            nontraffic V52.0
          truck (traffic) V54.5
            nontraffic V54.0
          two-wheeled motor vehicle (traffic) V52.5
            nontraffic V52.0
          van (traffic) V53.5
            nontraffic V53.0
        noncollision accident (traffic) V58.5
          nontraffic V58.0
      noncollision accident (traffic) V58.9
        nontraffic V58.3
        while boarding or alighting V58.4
      nontraffic V59.3
      hanger-on
        collision (with)
          animal (traffic) V50.7
            being ridden (traffic) V56.7
              nontraffic V56.2
            nontraffic V50.2
          animal-drawn vehicle (traffic) V56.7
            nontraffic V56.2
          bus (traffic) V54.7
            nontraffic V54.2
          car (traffic) V53.7
            nontraffic V53.2
          pedal cycle (traffic) V51.7
            nontraffic V51.2
          pickup truck (traffic) V53.7
            nontraffic V53.2
          railway vehicle (traffic) V55.7
            nontraffic V55.2
          specified vehicle NEC (traffic) V56.7
            nontraffic V56.2
          stationary object (traffic) V57.7
            nontraffic V57.2
          streetcar (traffic) V56.7
            nontraffic V56.2
          three-wheeled motor vehicle (traffic) V52.7
            nontraffic V52.2
          truck (traffic) V54.7
            nontraffic V54.2
          two-wheeled motor vehicle (traffic) V52.7
            nontraffic V52.2
          van (traffic) V53.7
            nontraffic V53.2
        noncollision accident (traffic) V58.7
          nontraffic V58.2
      passenger
        collision (with)
          animal (traffic) V50.6
            being ridden (traffic) V56.6
              nontraffic V56.1
            nontraffic V50.1
          animal-drawn vehicle (traffic) V56.6
            nontraffic V56.1
          bus (traffic) V54.6
            nontraffic V54.1
          car (traffic) V53.6
            nontraffic V53.1

Accident — *continued*
  transport — *continued*
    pickup truck occupant — *continued*
      passenger — *continued*
        collision — *continued*
          motor vehicle NOS (traffic) V59.50
            nontraffic V59.10
            specified type NEC (traffic) V59.59
              nontraffic V59.19
          pedal cycle (traffic) V51.6
            nontraffic V51.1
          pickup truck (traffic) V53.6
            nontraffic V53.1
          railway vehicle (traffic) V55.6
            nontraffic V55.1
          specified vehicle NEC (traffic) V56.6
            nontraffic V56.1
          stationary object (traffic) V57.6
            nontraffic V57.1
          streetcar (traffic) V56.6
            nontraffic V56.1
          three-wheeled motor vehicle (traffic) V52.6
            nontraffic V52.1
          truck (traffic) V54.6
            nontraffic V54.1
          two-wheeled motor vehicle (traffic) V52.6
            nontraffic V52.1
          van (traffic) V53.6
            nontraffic V53.1
        noncollision accident (traffic) V58.6
          nontraffic V58.1
      specified type NEC V59.88
      military vehicle V59.81
    quarry truck — *see* Accident, transport, industrial vehicle occupant
    race car — *see* Accident, transport, motor vehicle NEC occupant
    railway vehicle occupant V81.9
      collision (with) V81.3
        motor vehicle (non-military) (traffic) V81.1
          military V81.83
          nontraffic V81.0
        rolling stock V81.2
        specified object NEC V81.3
      during derailment V81.7
        with antecedent collision — *see* Accident, transport, railway vehicle occupant, collision
      explosion V81.81
      fall (in railway vehicle) V81.5
        during derailment V81.7
          with antecedent collision — *see* Accident, transport, railway vehicle occupant, collision
        from railway vehicle V81.6
          during derailment V81.7
            with antecedent collision — *see* Accident, transport, railway vehicle occupant, collision
        while boarding or alighting V81.4
      fire V81.81
      object falling onto train V81.82
      specified type NEC V81.89
      while boarding or alighting V81.4
    ski lift V98.3
    snowmobile occupant (nontraffic) V86.92
      driver V86.52
      hanger-on V86.72
      passenger V86.62
      traffic V86.32
        driver V86.02
        hanger-on V86.22
        passenger V86.12
      while boarding or alighting V86.42
    specified NEC V98.8
    sport utility vehicle occupant — *see also* Accident, transport, car occupant
      collision (with)
        stationary object (traffic) V47.91
          nontraffic V47.31

Accident — *continued*
  transport — *continued*
    sport utility vehicle occupant — *continued*
      driver
        collision (with)
          stationary object (traffic) V47.51
            nontraffic V47.01
      passenger
        collision (with)
          stationary object (traffic) V47.61
            nontraffic V47.11
    streetcar occupant V82.9
      collision (with) V82.3
        motor vehicle (traffic) V82.1
        nontraffic V82.0
        rolling stock V82.2
      during derailment V82.7
        with antecedent collision — *see*
            Accident, transport, streetcar
            occupant, collision
      fall (in streetcar) V82.5
        during derailment V82.7
          with antecedent collision — *see*
            Accident, transport, streetcar
            occupant, collision
        from streetcar V82.6
          during derailment V82.7
            with antecedent collision — *see*
              Accident, transport,
              streetcar occupant, collision
          while boarding or alighting V82.4
      while boarding or alighting V82.4
      specified type NEC V82.8
      while boarding or alighting V82.4
    three-wheeled motor vehicle occupant V39.9
      collision (with)
        animal (traffic) V30.9
          being ridden (traffic) V36.9
            nontraffic V36.3
            while boarding or alighting V36.4
          nontraffic V30.3
          while boarding or alighting V30.4
        animal-drawn vehicle (traffic) V36.9
          nontraffic V36.3
          while boarding or alighting V36.4
        bus (traffic) V34.9
          nontraffic V34.3
          while boarding or alighting V34.4
        car (traffic) V33.9
          nontraffic V33.3
          while boarding or alighting V33.4
        motor vehicle NOS (traffic) V39.60
          nontraffic V39.20
          specified type NEC (traffic) V39.69
            nontraffic V39.29
        pedal cycle (traffic) V31.9
          nontraffic V31.3
          while boarding or alighting V31.4
        pickup truck (traffic) V33.9
          nontraffic V33.3
          while boarding or alighting V33.4
        railway vehicle (traffic) V35.9
          nontraffic V35.3
          while boarding or alighting V35.4
        specified vehicle NEC (traffic) V36.9
          nontraffic V36.3
          while boarding or alighting V36.4
        stationary object (traffic) V37.9
          nontraffic V37.3
          while boarding or alighting V37.4
        streetcar (traffic) V36.9
          nontraffic V36.3
          while boarding or alighting V36.4
        three-wheeled motor vehicle (traffic)
          V32.9
          nontraffic V32.3
          while boarding or alighting V32.4
        truck (traffic) V34.9
          nontraffic V34.3
          while boarding or alighting V34.4
        two-wheeled motor vehicle (traffic)
          V32.9
          nontraffic V32.3
          while boarding or alighting V32.4

Accident — *continued*
  transport — *continued*
    three-wheeled motor vehicle occupant —
      continued
      collision — *continued*
        van (traffic) V33.9
          nontraffic V33.3
          while boarding or alighting V33.4
      driver
        collision (with)
          animal (traffic) V30.5
            being ridden (traffic) V36.5
              nontraffic V36.0
            nontraffic V30.0
          animal-drawn vehicle (traffic) V36.5
            nontraffic V36.0
          bus (traffic) V34.5
            nontraffic V34.0
          car (traffic) V33.5
            nontraffic V33.0
          motor vehicle NOS (traffic) V39.40
            nontraffic V39.00
          specified type NEC (traffic) V39.49
            nontraffic V39.09
          pedal cycle (traffic) V31.5
            nontraffic V31.0
          pickup truck (traffic) V33.5
            nontraffic V33.0
          railway vehicle (traffic) V35.5
            nontraffic V35.0
          specified vehicle NEC (traffic) V36.5
            nontraffic V36.0
          stationary object (traffic) V37.5
            nontraffic V37.0
          streetcar (traffic) V36.5
            nontraffic V36.0
          three-wheeled motor vehicle (traffic)
            V32.5
            nontraffic V32.0
          truck (traffic) V34.5
            nontraffic V34.0
          two-wheeled motor vehicle (traffic)
            V32.5
            nontraffic V32.0
          van (traffic) V33.5
            nontraffic V33.0
        noncollision accident (traffic) V38.5
          nontraffic V38.0
      noncollision accident (traffic) V38.9
        nontraffic V38.3
        while boarding or alighting V38.4
      nontraffic V39.3
      hanger-on
        collision (with)
          animal (traffic) V30.7
            being ridden (traffic) V36.7
              nontraffic V36.2
            nontraffic V30.2
          animal-drawn vehicle (traffic) V36.7
            nontraffic V36.2
          bus (traffic) V34.7
            nontraffic V34.2
          car (traffic) V33.7
            nontraffic V33.2
          pedal cycle (traffic) V31.7
            nontraffic V31.2
          pickup truck (traffic) V33.7
            nontraffic V33.2
          railway vehicle (traffic) V35.7
            nontraffic V35.2
          specified vehicle NEC (traffic) V36.7
            nontraffic V36.2
          stationary object (traffic) V37.7
            nontraffic V37.2
          streetcar (traffic) V36.7
            nontraffic V36.2
          three-wheeled motor vehicle (traffic)
            V32.7
            nontraffic V32.2
          truck (traffic) V34.7
            nontraffic V34.2
          two-wheeled motor vehicle (traffic)
            V32.7
            nontraffic V32.2

Accident — *continued*
  transport — *continued*
    three-wheeled motor vehicle occupant —
      continued
      hanger-on — *continued*
        collision — *continued*
          van (traffic) V33.7
            nontraffic V33.2
        noncollision accident (traffic) V38.7
          nontraffic V38.2
      passenger
        collision (with)
          animal (traffic) V30.6
            being ridden (traffic) V36.6
              nontraffic V36.1
            nontraffic V30.1
          animal-drawn vehicle (traffic) V36.6
            nontraffic V36.1
          bus (traffic) V34.6
            nontraffic V34.1
          car (traffic) V33.6
            nontraffic V33.1
          motor vehicle NOS (traffic) V39.50
            nontraffic V39.10
          specified type NEC (traffic) V39.59
            nontraffic V39.19
          pedal cycle (traffic) V31.6
            nontraffic V31.1
          pickup truck (traffic) V33.6
            nontraffic V33.1
          railway vehicle (traffic) V35.6
            nontraffic V35.1
          specified vehicle NEC (traffic) V36.6
            nontraffic V36.1
          stationary object (traffic) V37.6
            nontraffic V37.1
          streetcar (traffic) V36.6
            nontraffic V36.1
          three-wheeled motor vehicle (traffic)
            V32.6
            nontraffic V32.1
          truck (traffic) V34.6
            nontraffic V34.1
          two-wheeled motor vehicle (traffic)
            V32.6
            nontraffic V32.1
          van (traffic) V33.6
            nontraffic V33.1
        noncollision accident (traffic) V38.6
          nontraffic V38.1
      specified type NEC V39.89
      military vehicle V39.81
    tractor (farm) (and trailer) — *see* Accident,
      transport, agricultural vehicle occupant
    tram — *see* Accident, transport, streetcar
      in mine or quarry — *see* Accident,
        transport, industrial vehicle
        occupant
    trolley — *see* Accident, transport, streetcar
      in mine or quarry — *see* Accident,
        transport, industrial vehicle
        occupant
    truck (heavy) occupant V69.9
      collision (with)
        animal (traffic) V60.9
          being ridden (traffic) V66.9
            nontraffic V66.3
            while boarding or alighting V66.4
          nontraffic V60.3
          while boarding or alighting V60.4
        animal-drawn vehicle (traffic) V66.9
          nontraffic V66.3
          while boarding or alighting V66.4
        bus (traffic) V64.9
          nontraffic V64.3
          while boarding or alighting V64.4
        car (traffic) V63.9
          nontraffic V63.3
          while boarding or alighting V63.4
        motor vehicle NOS (traffic) V69.60
          nontraffic V69.20
          specified type NEC (traffic) V69.69
            nontraffic V69.29

©2002 Ingenix, Inc.

Accident — *continued*
  transport — *continued*
    truck occupant — *continued*
      collision — *continued*
        pedal cycle (traffic) V61.9
          nontraffic V61.3
          while boarding or alighting V61.4
        pickup truck (traffic) V63.9
          nontraffic V63.3
          while boarding or alighting V63.4
        railway vehicle (traffic) V65.9
          nontraffic V65.3
          while boarding or alighting V65.4
        specified vehicle NEC (traffic) V66.9
          nontraffic V66.3
          while boarding or alighting V66.4
        stationary object (traffic) V67.9
          nontraffic V67.3
          while boarding or alighting V67.4
        streetcar (traffic) V66.9
          nontraffic V66.3
          while boarding or alighting V66.4
        three-wheeled motor vehicle (traffic) V62.9
          nontraffic V62.3
          while boarding or alighting V62.4
        truck (traffic) V64.9
          nontraffic V64.3
          while boarding or alighting V64.4
        two-wheeled motor vehicle (traffic) V62.9
          nontraffic V62.3
          while boarding or alighting V62.4
        van (traffic) V63.9
          nontraffic V63.3
          while boarding or alighting V63.4
    driver
      collision (with)
        animal (traffic) V60.5
          being ridden (traffic) V66.5
            nontraffic V66.0
          nontraffic V60.0
        animal-drawn vehicle (traffic) V66.5
          nontraffic V66.0
        bus (traffic) V64.5
          nontraffic V64.0
        car (traffic) V63.5
          nontraffic V63.0
        motor vehicle NOS (traffic) V69.40
          nontraffic V69.00
          specified type NEC (traffic) V69.49
            nontraffic V69.09
        pedal cycle (traffic) V61.5
          nontraffic V61.0
        pickup truck (traffic) V63.5
          nontraffic V63.0
        railway vehicle (traffic) V65.5
          nontraffic V65.0
        specified vehicle NEC (traffic) V66.5
          nontraffic V66.0
        stationary object (traffic) V67.5
          nontraffic V67.0
        streetcar (traffic) V66.5
          nontraffic V66.0
        three-wheeled motor vehicle (traffic) V62.5
          nontraffic V62.0
        truck (traffic) V64.5
          nontraffic V64.0
        two-wheeled motor vehicle (traffic) V62.5
          nontraffic V62.0
        van (traffic) V63.5
          nontraffic V63.0
      noncollision accident (traffic) V68.5
        nontraffic V68.0
    dump — *see* Accident, transport, construction vehicle occupant
    hanger-on
      collision (with)
        animal (traffic) V60.7
          being ridden (traffic) V66.7
            nontraffic V66.2
          nontraffic V60.2

Accident — *continued*
  transport — *continued*
    truck occupant — *continued*
      hanger-on — *continued*
        collision — *continued*
          animal-drawn vehicle (traffic) V66.7
            nontraffic V66.2
          bus (traffic) V64.7
            nontraffic V64.2
          car (traffic) V63.7
            nontraffic V63.2
          pedal cycle (traffic) V61.7
            nontraffic V61.2
          pickup truck (traffic) V63.7
            nontraffic V63.2
          railway vehicle (traffic) V65.7
            nontraffic V65.2
          specified vehicle NEC (traffic) V66.7
            nontraffic V66.2
          stationary object (traffic) V67.7
            nontraffic V67.2
          streetcar (traffic) V66.7
            nontraffic V66.2
          three-wheeled motor vehicle (traffic) V62.7
            nontraffic V62.2
          truck (traffic) V64.7
            nontraffic V64.2
          two-wheeled motor vehicle (traffic) V62.7
            nontraffic V62.2
          van (traffic) V63.7
            nontraffic V63.2
        noncollision accident (traffic) V68.7
          nontraffic V68.2
      noncollision accident (traffic) V68.9
        nontraffic V68.3
        while boarding or alighting V68.4
      nontraffic V69.3
    passenger
      collision (with)
        animal (traffic) V60.6
          being ridden (traffic) V66.6
            nontraffic V66.1
          nontraffic V60.1
        animal-drawn vehicle (traffic) V66.6
          nontraffic V66.1
        bus (traffic) V64.6
          nontraffic V64.1
        car (traffic) V63.6
          nontraffic V63.1
        motor vehicle NOS (traffic) V69.50
          nontraffic V69.10
          specified type NEC (traffic) V69.59
            nontraffic V69.19
        pedal cycle (traffic) V61.6
          nontraffic V61.1
        pickup truck (traffic) V63.6
          nontraffic V63.1
        railway vehicle (traffic) V65.6
          nontraffic V65.1
        specified vehicle NEC (traffic) V66.6
          nontraffic V66.1
        stationary object (traffic) V67.6
          nontraffic V67.1
        streetcar (traffic) V66.6
          nontraffic V66.1
        three-wheeled motor vehicle (traffic) V62.6
          nontraffic V62.1
        truck (traffic) V64.6
          nontraffic V64.1
        two-wheeled motor vehicle (traffic) V62.6
          nontraffic V62.1
        van (traffic) V63.6
          nontraffic V63.1
      noncollision accident (traffic) V68.6
        nontraffic V68.1
    pickup — *see* Accident, transport, pickup truck occupant
    specified type NEC V69.88
      military vehicle V69.81

Accident — *continued*
  transport — *continued*
    van occupant V59.9
      collision (with)
        animal (traffic) V50.9
          being ridden (traffic) V56.9
            nontraffic V56.3
            while boarding or alighting V56.4
          nontraffic V50.3
          while boarding or alighting V50.4
        animal-drawn vehicle (traffic) V56.9
          nontraffic V56.3
          while boarding or alighting V56.4
        bus (traffic) V54.9
          nontraffic V54.3
          while boarding or alighting V54.4
        car (traffic) V53.9
          nontraffic V53.3
          while boarding or alighting V53.4
        motor vehicle NOS (traffic) V59.60
          nontraffic V59.20
          specified type NEC (traffic) V59.69
            nontraffic V59.29
        pedal cycle (traffic) V51.9
          nontraffic V51.3
          while boarding or alighting V51.4
        pickup truck (traffic) V53.9
          nontraffic V53.3
          while boarding or alighting V53.4
        railway vehicle (traffic) V55.9
          nontraffic V55.3
          while boarding or alighting V55.4
        specified vehicle NEC (traffic) V56.9
          nontraffic V56.3
          while boarding or alighting V56.4
        stationary object (traffic) V57.9
          nontraffic V57.3
          while boarding or alighting V57.4
        streetcar (traffic) V56.9
          nontraffic V56.3
          while boarding or alighting V56.4
        three-wheeled motor vehicle (traffic) V52.9
          nontraffic V52.3
          while boarding or alighting V52.4
        truck (traffic) V54.9
          nontraffic V54.3
          while boarding or alighting V54.4
        two-wheeled motor vehicle (traffic) V52.9
          nontraffic V52.3
          while boarding or alighting V52.4
        van (traffic) V53.9
          nontraffic V53.3
          while boarding or alighting V53.4
      driver
        collision (with)
          animal (traffic) V50.5
            being ridden (traffic) V56.5
              nontraffic V56.0
            nontraffic V50.0
          animal-drawn vehicle (traffic) V56.5
            nontraffic V56.0
          bus (traffic) V54.5
            nontraffic V54.0
          car (traffic) V53.5
            nontraffic V53.0
          motor vehicle NOS (traffic) V59.40
            nontraffic V59.00
            specified type NEC (traffic) V59.49
              nontraffic V59.09
          pedal cycle (traffic) V51.5
            nontraffic V51.0
          pickup truck (traffic) V53.5
            nontraffic V53.0
          railway vehicle (traffic) V55.5
            nontraffic V55.0
          specified vehicle NEC (traffic) V56.5
            nontraffic V56.0
          stationary object (traffic) V57.5
            nontraffic V57.0
          streetcar (traffic) V56.5
            nontraffic V56.0

Accident — *continued*
  transport — *continued*
    van occupant — *continued*
      driver — *continued*
        collision — *continued*
          three-wheeled motor vehicle (traffic) V52.5
            nontraffic V52.0
          truck (traffic) V54.5
            nontraffic V54.0
          two-wheeled motor vehicle (traffic) V52.5
            nontraffic V52.0
          van (traffic) V53.5
            nontraffic V53.0
        noncollision accident (traffic) V58.5
          nontraffic V58.0
        noncollision accident (traffic) V58.9
          nontraffic V58.3
        while boarding or alighting V58.4
      nontraffic V59.3
      hanger-on
        collision (with)
          animal (traffic) V50.7
            being ridden (traffic) V56.7
              nontraffic V56.2
            nontraffic V50.2
          animal-drawn vehicle (traffic) V56.7
            nontraffic V56.2
          bus (traffic) V54.7
            nontraffic V54.2
          car (traffic) V53.7
            nontraffic V53.2
          pedal cycle (traffic) V51.7
            nontraffic V51.2
          pickup truck (traffic) V53.7
            nontraffic V53.2
          railway vehicle (traffic) V55.7
            nontraffic V55.2
          specified vehicle NEC (traffic) V56.7
            nontraffic V56.2
          stationary object (traffic) V57.7
            nontraffic V57.2
          streetcar (traffic) V56.7
            nontraffic V56.2
          three-wheeled motor vehicle (traffic) V52.7
            nontraffic V52.2
          truck (traffic) V54.7
            nontraffic V54.2
          two-wheeled motor vehicle (traffic) V52.7
            nontraffic V52.2
          van (traffic) V53.7
            nontraffic V53.2
        noncollision accident (traffic) V58.7
          nontraffic V58.2
      passenger
        collision (with)
          animal (traffic) V50.6
            being ridden (traffic) V56.6
              nontraffic V56.1
            nontraffic V50.1
          animal-drawn vehicle (traffic) V56.6
            nontraffic V56.1
          bus (traffic) V54.6
            nontraffic V54.1
          car (traffic) V53.6
            nontraffic V53.1
          motor vehicle NOS (traffic) V59.50
            nontraffic V59.10
            specified type NEC (traffic) V59.59
              nontraffic V59.19
          pedal cycle (traffic) V51.6
            nontraffic V51.1
          pickup truck (traffic) V53.6
            nontraffic V53.1
          railway vehicle (traffic) V55.6
            nontraffic V55.1
          specified vehicle NEC (traffic) V56.6
            nontraffic V56.1
          stationary object (traffic) V57.6
            nontraffic V57.1

Accident — *continued*
  transport — *continued*
    van occupant — *continued*
      passenger — *continued*
        collision — *continued*
          streetcar (traffic) V56.6
            nontraffic V56.1
          three-wheeled motor vehicle (traffic) V52.6
            nontraffic V52.1
          truck (traffic) V54.6
            nontraffic V54.1
          two-wheeled motor vehicle (traffic) V52.6
            nontraffic V52.1
          van (traffic) V53.6
            nontraffic V53.1
        noncollision accident (traffic) V58.6
          nontraffic V58.1
      specified type NEC V59.88
        military vehicle V59.81
    watercraft occupant — *see* Accident, watercraft
    vehicle NEC V89.9
    animal-drawn NEC — *see* Accident, transport, animal-drawn vehicle occupant
    special
      agricultural — *see* Accident, transport, agricultural vehicle occupant
      construction — *see* Accident, transport, construction vehicle occupant
      industrial — *see* Accident, transport, industrial vehicle occupant
      three-wheeled NEC (motorized) — *see* Accident, transport, three-wheeled motor vehicle occupant
  watercraft V94.9
    causing
      drowning — *see* Drowning, due to, accident to, watercraft
      injury NEC V91.89
        crushed between craft and object V91.19
          powered craft V91.13
            ferry boat V91.11
            fishing boat V91.12
            jetskis V91.13
            liner V91.11
            merchant ship V91.10
            passenger ship V91.11
          unpowered craft V91.18
            canoe V91.15
            inflatable V91.16
            kayak V91.15
            sailboat V91.14
            surf-board V91.18
            windsurfer V91.18
        fall on board V91.29
          powered craft V91.23
            ferry boat V91.21
            fishing boat V91.22
            jetskis V91.23
            liner V91.21
            merchant ship V91.20
            passenger ship V91.21
          unpowered craft
            canoe V91.25
            inflatable V91.26
            kayak V91.25
            sailboat V91.24
        fire on board causing burn V91.09
          powered craft V91.03
            ferry boat V91.01
            fishing boat V91.02
            jetskis V91.03
            liner V91.01
            merchant ship V91.00
            passenger ship V91.01
          unpowered craft V91.08
            canoe V91.05
            inflatable V91.06
            kayak V91.05
            sailboat V91.04
            surf-board V91.08

Accident — *continued*
  watercraft — *continued*
    causing — *continued*
      injury — *continued*
        fire on board causing burn — *continued*
          unpowered craft — *continued*
            water skis V91.07
            windsurfer V91.08
        hit by falling object V91.39
          powered craft V91.33
            ferry boat V91.31
            fishing boat V91.32
            jetskis V91.33
            liner V91.31
            merchant ship V91.30
            passenger ship V91.31
          unpowered craft V91.38
            canoe V91.35
            inflatable V91.36
            kayak V91.35
            sailboat V91.34
            surf-board V91.38
            water skis V91.37
            windsurfer V91.38
        specified type NEC V91.89
          powered craft V91.83
            ferry boat V91.81
            fishing boat V91.82
            jetskis V91.83
            liner V91.81
            merchant ship V91.80
            passenger ship V91.81
          unpowered craft V91.88
            canoe V91.85
            inflatable V91.86
            kayak V91.85
            sailboat V91.84
            surf-board V91.88
            water skis V91.87
            windsurfer V91.88
      due to, caused by cataclysm — *see* Forces of nature, by type
      nonpowered, struck by
        nonpowered vessel V94.22
        powered vessel V94.21
      specified type NEC V94.8
      striking swimmer
        powered V94.11
        unpowered V94.12

Acid throwing (assault) Y08.89

Activity of victim at time of event Y93.8
  activities of daily living NEC Y93.21
  bowling Y93.016
  butchering Y93.13
  caregiving activities Y93.3
  computer keyboarding Y93.11
  crafts Y93.19
    knitting Y93.14
    sewing Y93.15
    specified NEC Y93.19
  do it yourself project Y93.8
  electronic equipment Y93.59
    cellular telephone Y93.51
    headphone Y93.52
  gardening Y93.49
  golf Y93.015
  hiking Y93.011
  household activities Y93.22
  jogging Y93.012
  leisure (hobbies) (entertainment) (volunteer activity) Y93.8
  meat cutting Y93.13
  personal hygiene Y93.21
  riding Y93.013
  skating Y93.018
  skiing Y93.018
  snow shoveling Y93.41
  specified activity NEC Y93.8
  sports Y93.018
    group
      baseball Y93.022
      football Y93.020
      lacrosse Y93.023
      soccer Y93.024
      softball Y93.021

©2002 Ingenix, Inc.

Bite, bitten by — continued
- mammal NEC W55.89
  - marine W56.89
- marine animal (nonvenomous) W56.89
- millipede W57
- mammal NEC W55.81
- moray eel W56.51
- mouse W53.01
- person(s) (accidentally) W50.3
  - with intent to injure or kill Y04.1
  - as, or caused by, a crowd or human stampede (with fall) W52
  - assault Y04.1
  - homicide (attempt) Y04.1
  - in
    - fight Y04.1
- pig W55.41
- raccoon W55.51
- rat W53.11
- reptile W59.81
  - lizard W59.01
  - snake W59.11
  - turtle W59.21
    - terrestrial W59.81
- rodent W53.81
  - mouse W53.01
  - rat W53.11
  - specified NEC W53.81
  - squirrel W53.21
- shark W56.41
- sheep W55.31
- snake (nonvenomous) W59.11
- spider (nonvenomous) X57
- squirrel W53.21

Blast (air) **in war operations** Y36.2
- from nuclear explosion — see War operations, nuclear weapons
- underwater Y36.0

Blizzard X37.2

Blood alcohol level Y90.9
- less than 20mg/100ml Y90.0
- presence in blood, level not specified Y90.9
- 20-39mg/100ml Y90.1
- 40-59mg/100ml Y90.2
- 60-79mg/100ml Y90.3
- 80-99mg/100ml Y90.4
- 100-119mg/100ml Y90.5
- 120-199mg/100ml Y90.6
- 200-239mg/100ml Y90.7
- 240mg/100ml or more Y90.8

Blow X58.8
- by law enforcing agent, police (on duty) — see Legal, intervention, manhandling
  - blunt object — see Legal, intervention, blunt object

Blowing up — see Explosion

Brawl (hand) (fists) (foot) Y04.0

Breakage (accidental) (part of)
- ladder (causing fall) W11
- scaffolding (causing fall) W12

Broken
- glass, contact with — see Contact, with, glass
- power line (causing electric shock) W85

Bumping against, into (accidentally)
- object NEC W22.8
  - with fall — see Fall, due to, bumping against, object
  - caused by crowd or human stampede (with fall) W52
  - sports equipment W21.9
- person(s) W51
  - with fall W03
    - due to ice or snow W00.0
  - assault Y04.2
  - caused by, a crowd or human stampede (with fall) W52
  - homicide (attempt) Y04.2
- sports equipment W21.9

Burn, burned, burning (accidental) (by) (from) (on)
- acid NEC — see Table of Drugs and Chemicals
- bed linen — see Exposure, fire, uncontrolled, in building, bed
- blowtorch X08.8
  - with ignition of clothing NEC X06.2
    - nightwear X05

Burn, burned, burning — continued
- bonfire, campfire (controlled) — see also Exposure, fire, controlled, not in building
  - uncontrolled — see Exposure, fire, uncontrolled, not in building
- candle X08.8
  - with ignition of clothing NEC X06.2
    - nightwear X05
- caustic liquid, substance (external) (internal) NEC — see Table of Drugs and Chemicals
- chemical (external) (internal) — see also Table of Drugs and Chemicals
  - in war operations (chemical weapons) Y36.7
- cigar(s) or cigarette(s) X08.8
  - with ignition of clothing NEC X06.2
    - nightwear X05
- clothes, clothing NEC (from controlled fire) X06.2
  - with conflagration — see Exposure, fire, uncontrolled, building
    - not in building or structure — see Exposure, fire, uncontrolled, not in building
- cooker (hot) X15.8
  - stated as undetermined whether accidental or intentional Y27.3
  - suicide (attempt) X77.3
- electric blanket X16
- engine (hot) X17
- fire, flames — see Exposure, fire
- flare, Very pistol — see Discharge, firearm NEC
- heat
  - from appliance (electrical) (household) X15.8
    - cooker X15.8
    - hotplate X15.2
    - kettle X15.8
    - light bulb X15.8
    - saucepan X15.3
    - skillet X15.3
    - stove X15.0
    - stated as undetermined whether accidental or intentional Y27.3
    - suicide (attempt) X77.3
    - toaster X15.1
  - in local application or packing during medical or surgical procedure Y63.5
- heating
  - appliance, radiator or pipe X16
- homicide (attempt) — see Assault, burning
- hot
  - air X14.1
  - cooker X15.8
  - drink X10.0
  - engine X17
  - fat X10.2
  - fluid NEC X12
  - food X10.1
  - gases X14.1
  - heating appliance X16
  - household appliance NEC X15.8
  - kettle X15.8
  - liquid NEC X12
  - machinery X17
  - metal (molten) (liquid) NEC X18
  - object (not producing fire or flames) NEC X19
  - oil (cooking) X10.2
  - pipe(s) X16
  - radiator X16
  - saucepan (glass) (metal) X15.3
  - stove (kitchen) X15.0
  - substance NEC X19
    - caustic or corrosive NEC — see Table of Drugs and Chemicals
  - toaster X15.1
  - tool X17
  - vapor X13.1
  - water (tap) — see Contact, with, hot, tap water
- hotplate X15.2
  - suicide (attempt) X77.3
- ignition — see Ignition
- in war operations — see also War operations, fire
  - nuclear explosion — see War operations, nuclear weapons
  - petrol bomb Y36.31

Burn, burned, burning — continued
- inflicted by other person X97
  - by hot objects, hot vapor, and steam — see Assault, burning, hot object
- internal, from swallowed caustic, corrosive liquid, substance — see Table of Drugs and Chemicals
- iron (hot) X15.8
  - stated as undetermined whether accidental or intentional Y27.3
  - suicide (attempt) X77.3
- kettle (hot) X15.8
  - stated as undetermined whether accidental or intentional Y27.3
  - suicide (attempt) X77.3
- lamp (flame) X08.8
  - with ignition of clothing NEC X06.2
    - nightwear X05
- lighter (cigar) (cigarette) X08.8
  - with ignition of clothing NEC X06.2
    - nightwear X05
- lightning X33
  - causing fire — see Exposure, fire
- liquid (boiling) (hot) NEC X12
  - stated as undetermined whether accidental or intentional Y27.2
  - suicide (attempt) X77.2
- local application of externally applied substance in medical or surgical care Y63.5
- on board watercraft
  - due to
    - accident to watercraft V91.09
      - powered craft V91.03
        - ferry boat V91.01
        - fishing boat V91.02
        - jetskis V91.03
        - liner V91.01
        - merchant ship V91.00
        - passenger ship V91.01
      - unpowered craft V91.08
        - canoe V91.05
        - inflatable V91.06
        - kayak V91.05
        - sailboat V91.04
        - surf-board V91.08
        - water skis V91.07
        - windsurfer V91.08
    - fire on board V93.09
      - ferry boat V93.01
      - fishing boat V93.02
      - jetskis V93.03
      - liner V93.01
      - merchant ship V93.00
      - passenger ship V93.01
      - powered craft NEC V93.03
      - sailboat V93.04
    - specified heat source NEC on board V93.19
      - ferry boat V93.11
      - fishing boat V93.12
      - jetskis V93.13
      - liner V93.11
      - merchant ship V93.10
      - passenger ship V93.11
      - powered craft NEC V93.13
      - sailboat V93.14
- machinery (hot) X17
- matches X08.8
  - with ignition of clothing NEC X06.2
    - nightwear X05
- mattress — see Exposure, fire, uncontrolled, building, bed
- medicament, externally applied Y63.5
- metal (hot) (liquid) (molten) NEC X18
- nightwear (nightclothes, nightdress, gown, pajamas, robe) X05
- object (hot) NEC X19
- pipe (hot) X16
  - smoking X08.8
    - with ignition of clothing NEC X06.2
      - nightwear X05
- radiator (hot) X16
- saucepan (hot) (glass) (metal) X15.3
  - stated as undetermined whether accidental or intentional Y27.3
  - suicide (attempt) X77.3

©2002 Ingenix, Inc.

Burn, burned, burning — *continued*
 self-inflicted X76
  stated as undetermined whether accidental or intentional Y26
 steam X13.1
  pipe X16
   stated as undetermined whether accidental or intentional Y27.8
  stated as undetermined whether accidental or intentional Y27.0
  suicide (attempt) X77.0
 stove (hot) (kitchen) X15.0
  stated as undetermined whether accidental or intentional Y27.3
  suicide (attempt) X77.3
 substance (hot) NEC X19
  boiling X12
   stated as undetermined whether accidental or intentional Y27.2
   suicide (attempt) X77.2
  molten (metal) X18
 suicide (attempt) NEC X76
  hot
   household appliance X77.3
   object X77.9
 stated as undetermined whether accidental or intentional Y27.0
 therapeutic misadventure
  heat in local application or packing during medical or surgical procedure Y63.5
  overdose of radiation Y63.2
 toaster (hot) X15.1
  stated as undetermined whether accidental or intentional Y27.3
  suicide (attempt) X77.3
 tool (hot) X17
 torch, welding X08.8
  with ignition of clothing NEC X06.2
   nightwear X05
 trash fire (controlled) — *see* Exposure, fire, controlled, not in building
  uncontrolled — *see* Exposure, fire, uncontrolled, not in building
 vapor (hot) X13.1
  stated as undetermined whether accidental or intentional Y27.0
  suicide (attempt) X77.0
 Very pistol — *see* Discharge, firearm NEC
Butted by animal W55.89
 bull W55.22
 cow W55.22
 goat W55.32
 horse W55.12
 pig W55.42
 sheep W55.32

C

Caisson disease — *see* Air, pressure, change
Campfire (exposure to) (controlled) — *see also* Exposure, fire, controlled, not in building
 uncontrolled — *see* Exposure, fire, uncontrolled, not in building
Capital punishment (any means) X35.91
Car sickness X51.2
Casualty (not due to war) NEC X58.8
 war — *see* War operations
Cat
 bite W55.01
 scratch W55.03
Cataclysm, cataclysmic (any injury) NEC — *see* Forces of nature
Catching fire — *see* Exposure, fire
Caught
 between
  folding object W23.0
  objects (moving) (stationary and moving) W23.0
   and machinery — *see* Contact, with, by type of machine
   stationary W23.1
  sliding door and door frame W23.0
 by, in
  machinery (moving parts of) — *see* Contact, with, by type of machine
  object NEC W23.2

Caught — *continued*
 by, in — *continued*
  washing machine wringer W23.0
  under packing crate (due to losing grip) W23.1
Cave in caused by cataclysmic earth surface movement or eruption — *see* Landslide
Change(s) in air pressure — *see* Air, pressure, change
Choked, choking (on) (any object except food or vomitus)
 food (bone) (seed) W79
 vomitus W78
Civil insurrection — *see* War operations
Cloudburst (any injury) X37.8
Cold, exposure to (accidental) (excessive) (extreme) (natural) (place) **NEC** — *see* Exposure, cold
Collapse
 building W20.1
  burning (uncontrolled fire) X00.2
 dam or man — made structure (causing earth movement) X36.0
 machinery — *see* Contact, with, by type of machine
 structure W20.1
  burning (uncontrolled fire) X00.2
Collision (accidental) **NEC** (*see also* Accident, transport) V89.9
 pedestrian W51
  with fall W03
   due to ice or snow W00.0
   involving pedestrian conveyance — *see* Accident, transport, pedestrian, conveyance
  and
   crowd or human stampede (with fall) W52
   object W22.8
    with fall — *see* Fall, due to, bumping against, object
  person(s) — *see* Collision, pedestrian
 transport vehicle NEC V89.9
  and
   avalanche, fallen or not moving — *see* Accident, transport
    falling or moving — *see* Landslide
   landslide, fallen or not moving — *see* Accident, transport
    falling or moving — *see* Landslide
   due to cataclysm — *see* Forces of nature, by type
   intentional, purposeful suicide (attempt) — *see* Suicide, collision
Combustion, spontaneous — *see* Ignition
Complication (delayed) **of or following** (medical or surgical procedure) Y84.9
 with misadventure — *see* Misadventure
 amputation of limb(s) Y83.5
 anastomosis (arteriovenous) (blood vessel) (gastrojejunal) (tendon) (natural or artificial material) Y83.2
 aspiration (of fluid) Y84.4
  tissue Y84.8
 biopsy Y84.8
 blood
  sampling Y84.7
  transfusion
   procedure Y84.8
 bypass Y83.2
 catheterization (urinary) Y84.6
  cardiac Y84.0
 colostomy Y83.3
 cystostomy Y83.3
 dialysis (kidney) Y84.1
 drug — *see* Table of Drugs and Chemicals
 due to misadventure — *see* Misadventure
 duodenostomy Y83.3
 electroshock therapy Y84.3
 external stoma, creation of Y83.3
 formation of external stoma Y83.3
 gastrostomy Y83.3
 graft Y83.2
 hypothermia (medically induced) Y84.8

Complication of or following — *continued*
 implant, implantation (of)
  artificial
   internal device (cardiac pacemaker) (electrodes in brain) (heart valve prosthesis) (orthopedic) Y83.1
   material or tissue (for anastomosis or bypass) Y83.2
    with creation of external stoma Y83.3
   natural tissues (for anastomosis or bypass) Y83.2
    with creation of external stoma Y83.3
 infusion
  procedure Y84.8
 injection — *see* Table of Drugs and Chemicals
  procedure Y84.8
 insertion of gastric or duodenal sound Y84.5
 insulin-shock therapy Y84.3
 paracentesis (abdominal) (thoracic) (aspirative) Y84.4
 procedures other than surgical operation — *see* Complication of or following, by type of procedure
 radiological procedure or therapy Y84.2
 removal of organ (partial) (total) NEC Y83.6
 sampling
  blood Y84.7
  fluid NEC Y84.4
  tissue Y84.8
 shock therapy Y84.3
 surgical operation NEC (*see also* Complication of or following, by type of operation) Y83.9
  reconstructive NEC Y83.4
   with
    anastomosis, bypass or graft Y83.2
    formation of external stoma Y83.3
  specified NEC Y83.8
 transfusion — *see also* Table of Drugs and Chemicals
  procedure Y84.8
 transplant, transplantation (heart) (kidney) (liver) (whole organ, any) Y83.0
  partial organ Y83.4
 ureterostomy Y83.3
 vaccination — *see also* Table of Drugs and Chemicals
  procedure Y84.8
Compression
 divers' squeeze — *see* Air, pressure, change
 trachea by
  food (lodged in esophagus) W79
  vomitus (lodged in esophagus) W78
Conflagration — *see* Exposure, fire, uncontrolled
Contact (accidental)
 with
  abrasive wheel (metalworking) W31.1
  alligator
   bite W58.01
   crushing W58.03
   strike W58.02
  amphibian W62.9
   frog W62.0
   toad W62.1
  animal (nonvenomous) NEC W64
   marine W56.89
    bite W56.81
    dolphin — *see* Contact, with, dolphin
    fish NEC — *see* Contact, with, fish
    mammal — *see* Contact, with, mammal, marine
    orca — *see* Contact, with, orca
    sea lion — *see* Contact, with, sea lion
    shark — *see* Contact, with, shark
    strike W56.82
  animate mechanical force NEC W64
  arrow W21.89
   not thrown, projected or falling W45.8
  arthropods (nonvenomous) W57
  axe W27.0
  band-saw (industrial) W31.2
  bayonet — *see* Bayonet wound
  bee(s) X58.8
  bench-saw (industrial) W31.2
  bird W61.99
   bite W61.91

Contact — *continued*
- with — *continued*
  - bird — *continued*
    - chicken — *see* Contact, with, chicken
    - duck — *see* Contact, with, duck
    - goose — *see* Contact, with, goose
    - macaw — *see* Contact, with, macaw
    - parrot — *see* Contact, with, parrot
    - psittacine — *see* Contact, with, psittacine
    - strike W61.92
    - turkey — *see* Contact, with, turkey
  - blender W29.0
  - boiling water X12
    - stated as undetermined whether accidental or intentional Y27.2
    - suicide (attempt) X77.2
  - bore, earth-drilling or mining (land) (seabed) W31.0
  - buffalo — *see* Contact, with, hoof stock NEC
  - bull W55.29
    - bite W55.21
    - strike W55.22
  - bumper cars W31.81
  - camel — *see* Contact, with, hoof stock NEC
  - can
    - lid W45.2
    - opener W27.5
      - powered W29.0
  - cat W55.09
    - bite W55.01
    - scratch W55.03
  - caterpillar (venomous) X58.8
  - centipede (venomous) X58.8
  - chain
    - hoist W24.0
      - agricultural operations W30.89
    - saw W29.3
  - chicken W61.39
    - peck W61.33
    - strike W61.32
  - chisel W27.0
  - circular saw W31.2
  - cobra X58.8
  - combine (harvester) W30.0
  - conveyer belt W24.1
  - cooker (hot) X15.8
    - stated as undetermined whether accidental or intentional Y27.3
    - suicide (attempt) X77.3
  - coral X58.8
  - cotton gin W31.82
  - cow W55.29
    - bite W55.21
    - strike W55.22
  - crane W24.0
    - agricultural operations W30.89
  - crocodile
    - bite W58.11
    - crushing W58.13
    - strike W58.12
  - dagger W26.1
    - stated as undetermined whether accidental or intentional Y28.2
    - suicide (attempt) X78.2
  - dairy equipment W31.82
  - dart W21.89
    - not thrown, projected or falling W45.8
  - deer — *see* Contact, with, hoof stock NEC
  - derrick W24.0
    - agricultural operations W30.89
      - hay W30.2
  - dog W54.8
    - bite W54.0
    - strike W54.1
  - dolphin W56.09
    - bite W56.01
    - strike W56.02
  - donkey — *see* Contact, with, hoof stock NEC
  - drill (powered) W29.8
    - earth (land) (seabed) W31.0
    - nonpowered W27.8
  - drive belt W24.0
    - agricultural operations W30.89
  - dry ice — *see* Exposure, cold, man-made
  - dryer (spin) (clothes) (powered) W29.2

Contact — *continued*
- with — *continued*
  - duck W61.69
    - bite W61.61
    - strike W61.62
  - earth(-)
    - drilling machine (industrial) W31.0
    - scraping machine in stationary use W31.83
  - edge of stiff paper W45.1
  - electric
    - beater W29.0
    - blanket X16
    - fan W29.2
      - commercial W31.82
    - knife W29.1
    - mixer W29.0
  - elevator (building) W24.0
    - agricultural operations W30.89
      - grain W30.3
  - engine(s), hot NEC X17
  - excavating machine W31.0
  - farm machine W30.9
  - feces — *see* Contact, with, by type of animal
  - fer de lance X58.8
  - fish W56.59
    - bite W56.51
    - shark — *see* Contact, with, shark
    - strike W56.52
  - flying horses W31.81
  - forging (metalworking) machine W31.1
  - fork W27.5
  - forklift (truck) W24.0
    - agricultural operations W30.89
  - frog W62.0
  - garden
    - cultivator (powered) W29.3
      - riding W30.89
    - fork W27.1
  - gas turbine W31.3
  - Gila monster X58.8
  - giraffe — *see* Contact, with, hoof stock NEC
  - glass (sharp) (broken) W25
    - with subsequent fall W18.02
    - assault X99.0
    - due to fall — *see* Fall, by type
    - stated as undetermined whether accidental or intentional Y28.0
    - suicide (attempt) X78.0
  - goat W55.39
    - bite W55.31
    - strike W55.32
  - goose W61.59
    - bite W61.51
    - strike W61.52
  - hand
    - saw W27.0
    - tool (not powered) NEC W27.8
      - powered W29.8
  - harvester W30.0
  - hay-derrick W30.2
  - heat NEC X19
    - from appliance (electrical) (household) — *see* Contact, with, hot, household appliance
    - heating appliance X16
  - heating
    - appliance (hot) X16
    - pad (electric) X16
  - hedge-trimmer (powered) W29.3
  - hoe W27.1
  - hoist (chain) (shaft) NEC W24.0
    - agricultural W30.89
  - hoof stock NEC W55.39
    - bite W55.31
    - strike W55.32
  - hornet(s) X58.8
  - horse W55.19
    - bite W55.11
    - strike W55.12
  - hot
    - air X14.1
      - inhalation X14.0
    - cooker X15.8
    - drinks X10.0
    - engine X17

Contact — *continued*
- with — *continued*
  - hot — *continued*
    - fats X10.2
    - fluids NEC X12
      - assault X98.2
      - suicide (attempt) X77.2
      - undetermined whether accidental or intentional Y27.2
    - food X10.1
    - gases X14.1
      - inhalation X14.0
    - heating appliance X16
    - household appliance X15.8
      - assault X98.3
      - cooker X15.8
      - hotplate X15.2
      - kettle X15.8
      - light bulb X15.8
      - object NEC X19
        - assault X98.8
        - stated as undetermined whether accidental or intentional Y27.9
        - suicide (attempt) X77.8
      - saucepan X15.3
      - skillet X15.3
      - stove X15.0
      - stated as undetermined whether accidental or intentional Y27.3
      - suicide (attempt) X77.3
      - toaster X15.1
    - kettle X15.8
    - light bulb X15.8
    - liquid NEC (*see also* Burning) X12
      - drinks X10.0
      - stated as undetermined whether accidental or intentional Y27.2
      - suicide (attempt) X77.2
      - tap water X11.8
        - stated as undetermined whether accidental or intentional Y27.1
        - suicide (attempt) X77.1
    - machinery X17
    - metal (molten) (liquid) NEC X18
    - object (not producing fire or flames) NEC X19
    - oil (cooking) X10.2
    - pipe X16
    - plate X15.2
    - radiator X16
    - saucepan (glass) (metal) X15.3
    - skillet X15.3
    - stove (kitchen) X15.0
    - substance NEC X19
    - tap-water X11.8
      - assault X98.1
      - heated on stove X12
        - stated as undetermined whether accidental or intentional Y27.2
        - suicide (attempt) X77.2
      - in bathtub X11.0
      - running X11.1
      - stated as undetermined whether accidental or intentional Y27.1
      - suicide (attempt) X77.1
    - toaster X15.1
    - tool X17
    - vapors X13.1
      - inhalation X13.0
    - water (tap) X11.8
      - boiling X12
        - stated as undetermined whether accidental or intentional Y27.2
        - suicide (attempt) X77.2
      - heated on stove X12
        - stated as undetermined whether accidental or intentional Y27.2
        - suicide (attempt) X77.2
      - in bathtub X11.0
      - running X11.1

                                          ©2002 Ingenix, Inc.

Contact — *continued*
  with — *continued*
    hot — *continued*
      water — *continued*
        stated as undetermined whether
          accidental or intentional Y27.1
        suicide (attempt) X77.1
      hotplate X15.2
      ice-pick W27.5
      insect (nonvenomous) NEC W57
      kettle (hot) X15.8
      knife W26.0
        assault X99.1
        electric W29.1
        stated as undetermined whether
          accidental or intentional Y28.1
        suicide (attempt) X78.1
      lathe (metalworking) W31.1
        turnings W45.8
        woodworking W31.2
      lawnmower (powered) (ridden) W28
        causing electrocution W86.8
          suicide (attempt) X83.1
        unpowered W27.1
      lift, lifting (devices) W24.0
        agricultural operations W30.89
        shaft W24.0
      liquefied gas — *see* Exposure, cold, man-
        made
      liquid air, hydrogen, nitrogen — *see*
        Exposure, cold, man-made
      lizard (nonvenomous) W59.09
        bite W59.01
        strike W59.02
      llama — *see* Contact, with, hoof stock NEC
      macaw W61.19
        bite W61.11
        strike W61.12
      machine, machinery W31.9
        abrasive wheel W31.1
        agricultural including animal-powered
          W30.9
          combine harvester W30.0
          grain storage elevator W30.3
          hay derrick W30.2
          power take-off device W30.1
          reaper W30.0
          specified NEC W30.89
          thresher W30.0
          transport vehicle, stationary W30.81
        band saw W31.2
        bench saw W31.2
        circular saw W31.2
        commercial NEC W31.82
        drilling, metal (industrial) W31.1
        earth-drilling W31.0
        earthmoving or scraping W31.89
        excavating W31.89
        forging machine W31.1
        gas turbine W31.3
        hot X17
        internal combustion engine W31.3
        land drill W31.0
        lathe W31.1
        lifting (devices) W24.0
        metal drill W31.1
        metalworking (industrial) W31.1
        milling, metal W31.1
        mining W31.0
        molding W31.2
        overhead plane W31.2
        power press, metal W31.1
        prime mover W31.3
        printing W31.89
        radial saw W31.2
        recreational W31.81
        roller-coaster W31.81
        rolling mill, metal W31.1
        sander W31.2
        seabed drill W31.0
        shaft
          hoist W31.0
          lift W31.0
        specified NEC W31.89
        spinning W31.89
        steam engine W31.3

Contact — *continued*
  with — *continued*
    machine, machinery — *continued*
      transmission W24.1
      undercutter W31.0
      water driven turbine W31.3
      weaving W31.89
      woodworking or forming (industrial) W31.2
    mammal (feces) (urine) W55.89
      bull — *see* Contact, with, bull
      cat — *see* Contact, with, cat
      cow — *see* Contact, with, cow
      goat — *see* Contact, with, goat
      hoof stock — *see* Contact, with, hoof stock
      horse — *see* Contact, with, horse
      marine W56.39
        dolphin — *see* Contact, with, dolphin
        orca — *see* Contact, with, orca
        sea lion — *see* Contact, with, sea lion
        specified NEC W56.39
          bite W56.31
          strike W56.32
      pig — *see* Contact, with, pig
      raccoon — *see* Contact, with, raccoon
      rodent — *see* Contact, with, rodent
      sheep — *see* Contact, with, sheep
      specified NEC W55.89
        bite W55.81
        strike W55.82
    marine
      animal W56.89
        bite W56.81
        dolphin — *see* Contact, with, dolphin
        fish NEC — *see* Contact, with, fish
        mammal — *see* Contact, with,
          mammal, marine
        orca — *see* Contact, with, orca
        sea lion — *see* Contact, with, sea lion
        shark — *see* Contact, with, shark
        strike W56.82
    meat
      grinder (domestic) W29.0
        industrial W31.82
        nonpowered W27.5
      slicer (domestic) W29.0
        industrial W31.82
    merry go round W31.81
    metal (hot) (liquid) (molten) NEC X18
    millipede W57
    nail W45.0
      gun W29.4
    needle (sewing) W27.4
      hypodermic (contaminated) W27.3
    object (blunt) NEC
      hot NEC X19
      legal intervention — *see* Legal,
        intervention, blunt object
      sharp NEC W45.8
        inflicted by other person NEC W45.8
          stated as
            intentional homicide (attempt) —
              see Assault, cutting or
              piercing instrument
        legal intervention — *see* Legal,
          intervention, sharp object
        self-inflicted X78.9
    orca W56.29
      bite W56.21
      strike W56.22
    overhead plane W31.2
    paper (as sharp object) W45.1
    paper-cutter W27.6
    parrot W61.09
      bite W61.01
      strike W61.02
    pig W55.49
      bite W55.41
      strike W55.42
    pipe, hot X16
    pitchfork W27.1
    plane (metal) (wood) W27.0
      overhead W31.2
    plant thorns, spines, sharp leaves or other
      mechanisms W60

Contact — *continued*
  with — *continued*
    powered
      garden cultivator W29.3
      household appliance, implement, or
        machine W29.8
      saw (industrial) W31.2
        hand W29.8
    printing machine W31.89
    psittacine bird W61.29
      bite W61.21
      macaw — *see* Contact, with, macaw
      parrot — *see* Contact, with, parrot
      strike W61.22
    pulley (block) (transmission) W24.0
      agricultural operations W30.89
    raccoon W55.59
      bite W55.51
      strike W55.52
    radial-saw (industrial) W31.2
    radiator (hot) X16
    rake W27.1
    rattlesnake X58.8
    reaper W30.0
    reptile W59.89
      lizard — *see* Contact, with, lizard
      snake — *see* Contact, with, snake
      specified NEC W59.89
        bite W59.81
        crushing W59.83
        strike W59.82
      turtle — *see* Contact, with, turtle
    rivet gun (powered) W29.4
    road scraper — *see* Accident, transport,
      construction vehicle
    rodent (feces) (urine) W53.89
      bite W53.81
      mouse W53.09
        bite W53.01
      rat W53.19
        bite W53.11
      specified NEC W53.89
        bite W53.81
      squirrel W53.29
        bite W53.21
    roller coaster W31.81
    rope NEC W24.0
      agricultural operations W30.89
    saliva — *see* Contact, with, by type of animal
    sander W29.8
      industrial W31.2
    saucepan (hot) (glass) (metal) X15.3
    saw W27.0
      band (industrial) W31.2
      bench (industrial) W31.2
      chain W29.3
      hand W27.0
    sawing machine, metal W31.1
    scissors W27.2
    scorpion X58.8
    screwdriver W27.0
      powered W29.8
    sea
      anemone, cucumber or urchin (spine)
        X58.8
      lion W56.19
        bite W56.11
        strike W56.12
    serpent — *see* Contact, with, snake, by type
    sewing-machine (electric) (powered) W29.2
      not powered W27.8
    shaft (hoist) (lift) (transmission) NEC W24.0
      agricultural W30.89
    shark W56.49
      bite W56.41
      strike W56.42
    shears (hand) W27.2
      powered (industrial) W31.1
        domestic W29.2
    sheep W55.39
      bite W55.31
      strike W55.32
    shovel W27.8
      steam — *see* Accident, transport,
        construction vehicle

Contact — *continued*
  with — *continued*
    snake (nonvenomous) W59.19
      bite W59.11
      crushing W59.13
      strike W59.12
    spade W27.1
    spider (venomous) X58.8
    spin-drier W29.2
    spinning machine W31.89
    splinter W45.8
    sports equipment W21.9
    staple gun (powered) W29.8
    steam X13.1
      engine W31.3
      inhalation X13.0
      pipe X16
      shovel W31.89
    stove (hot) (kitchen) X15.0
    substance, hot NEC X19
      molten (metal) X18
    sword W26.1
      assault X99.2
      stated as undetermined whether
          accidental or intentional Y28.2
      suicide (attempt) X78.2
    tarantula X58.8
    thresher W30.0
    tin can lid W45.2
    toad W62.1
    toaster (hot) X15.1
    tool W27.8
      hand (not powered) W27.8
        auger W27.0
        axe W27.0
        can opener W27.5
        chisel W27.0
        fork W27.5
        garden W27.1
        handsaw W27.0
        hoe W27.1
        ice-pick W27.5
        kitchen utensil W27.5
        manual
          lawn mower W27.1
          sewing machine W27.1
        meat grinder W27.5
        needle (sewing) W27.4
          hypodermic (contaminated) W27.3
        paper cutter W27.6
        pitchfork W27.1
        rake W27.1
        scissors W27.2
        screwdriver W27.0
        specified NEC W27.8
        workbench W27.0
      hot X17
      powered W29.8
        blender W29.0
          commercial W31.82
        can opener W29.0
          commercial W31.82
        chainsaw W29.3
        clothes dryer W29.2
          commercial W31.82
        dishwasher W29.2
          commercial W31.82
        edger W29.3
        electric fan W29.2
          commercial W31.82
        electric knife W29.1
        food processor W29.0
          commercial W31.82
        garbage disposal W29.0
          commercial W31.82
        garden tool W29.3
        hedge trimmer W29.3
        ice maker W29.0
          commercial W31.82
        kitchen appliance W29.0
          commercial W31.82
        lawn mower W28
        meat grinder W29.0
          commercial W31.82
        mixer W29.0
          commercial W31.82

Contact — *continued*
  with — *continued*
    tool — *continued*
      powered — *continued*
        rototiller W29.3
        sewing machine W29.2
          commercial W31.82
        washing machine W29.2
          commercial W31.82
      transmission device (belt, cable, chain, gear,
        pinion, shaft) W24.1
        agricultural operations W30.89
      turbine (gas) (water-driven) W31.3
      turkey W61.49
        peck W61.43
        strike W61.42
      turtle (nonvenomous) W59.29
        bite W59.21
        strike W59.22
        terrestrial W59.89
          bite W59.81
          crushing W59.83
          strike W59.82
      under-cutter W31.0
      urine — *see* Contact, with, by type of animal
    vehicle
      agricultural use (transport) — *see*
        Accident, transport, agricultural
        vehicle
        not on public highway W30.81
      industrial use (transport) — *see* Accident,
        transport, industrial vehicle
        not on public highway W31.83
      off-road use (transport) — *see* Accident,
        transport, all-terrain or off-road
        vehicle
        not on public highway W31.83
      special construction use (transport) — *see*
        Accident, transport, construction
        vehicle
        not on public highway W31.83
    venomous
      animal X58.8
      arthropods X58.8
      lizard X58.8
      marine animal NEC X58.8
      marine plant NEC X58.8
      millipedes (tropical) X58.8
      plant(s) X58.8
      snake X58.8
      spider X58.8
      viper X58.8
      washing-machine (powered) W29.2
      wasp X58.8
      weaving-machine W31.89
      winch W24.0
        agricultural operations W30.89
      wire NEC W24.0
        agricultural operations W30.89
      wood slivers W45.8
      yellow jacket X58.8
      zebra — *see* Contact, with, hoof stock NEC

Coup de soleil X32

Crash
  aircraft (in transit) (powered) V95.9
    balloon V96.01
    fixed wing NEC (private) V95.21
      commercial V95.31
    glider V96.21
      hang V96.11
      powered V95.11
    helicopter V95.01
    in war operations — *see* War operations,
      aircraft
    microlight V95.11
    nonpowered V96.9
      specified NEC V96.8
    powered NEC V95.8
    stated as
      homicide (attempt) Y08.81
      suicide (attempt) X83.0
    ultralight V95.11
  spacecraft V95.41
  transport vehicle NEC (*see also* Accident,
    transport) V89.9

Crash — *continued*
  transport vehicle NEC (*see also* Accident,
    transport) — *continued*
    homicide (attempt) Y03.8
    motor NEC (traffic) V89.2
      homicide (attempt) Y03.8
      suicide (attempt) — *see* Suicide, collision

Cruelty (mental) (physical) (sexual) — *see*
  Maltreatment

Crushed (accidentally) X58.8
  between objects (moving) (stationary and
    moving) W23.0
    stationary W23.1
  by
    alligator W58.03
    avalanche NEC — *see* Landslide
    cave-in W20.0
      caused by cataclysmic earth surface
        movement — *see* Landslide
    crocodile W58.13
    crowd or human stampede W52
    falling
      aircraft V97.39
        in war operations — *see* War
          operations, aircraft
      earth, material W20.0
        caused by cataclysmic earth surface
          movement — *see* Landslide
      object NEC W20.8
    landslide NEC — *see* Landslide
    lizard (nonvenomous) W59.09
    machinery — *see* Contact, with, by type of
      machine
    reptile NEC W59.89
    snake (nonvenomous) W59.13
  in
    machinery — *see* Contact, with, by type of
      machine
    object W23.2

Cut, cutting (any part of body) (accidental) — *see*
  also Contact, with, by object or machine
  during medical or surgical treatment as
    misadventure — *see* Misadventure, cut, by
    type of procedure
  homicide (attempt) — *see* Assault, cutting or
    piercing instrument
  inflicted by other person — *see* Assault, cutting
    or piercing instrument
  legal
    execution Y35.91
    intervention — *see* Legal, intervention, sharp
      object
  machine NEC (*see also* Contact, with, by type of
    machine) W31.9
  self-inflicted — *see* Suicide, cutting or piercing
    instrument
  suicide (attempt) — *see* Suicide, cutting or
    piercing instrument
  war operations Y36.4

Cyclone (any injury) X37.1

<hr>

D

**Death due to injury occurring one year or more
  previously** — *see* Sequelae

Decapitation (accidental circumstances) NEC
  X58.8
  homicide X99.9
  legal execution (by guillotine) Y35.91

Dehydration from lack of water X58.8

Deprivation X58.8
  homicidal intent — *see* Maltreatment

Derailment (accidental)
  railway (rolling stock) (train) (vehicle) (without
    antecedent collision) V81.7
    with antecedent collision — *see* Accident,
      transport, railway vehicle occupant
  streetcar (without antecedent collision) V82.7
    with antecedent collision — *see* Accident,
      transport, streetcar occupant

Descent
  parachute (voluntary) (without accident to
    aircraft) V97.29
    due to accident to aircraft — *see* Accident,
      transport, aircraft

©2002 Ingenix, Inc.

Desertion (with intent to injure or kill) — *see* Maltreatment

Destitution X58.8

Disability, late effect or sequela of injury — *see* Sequelae

Discharge (accidental)
  airgun W34.01
    assault X95.01
    homicide (attempt) X95.01
    stated as undetermined whether accidental or intentional Y24.0
    suicide (attempt) X74.01
  BB gun — *see* Discharge, airgun
  firearm (accidental) W34.9
    assault X95.9
    handgun (pistol) (revolver) W32
      assault X93
      homicide (attempt) X93
      legal intervention — *see* Legal, intervention, firearm, handgun
      stated as undetermined whether accidental or intentional Y22
      suicide (attempt) X72
    homicide (attempt) X95.9
    hunting rifle W33.1
      assault X94.1
      homicide (attempt) X94.1
      legal intervention Y35.034
        injuring
          bystander Y35.033
          law enforcement personnel Y35.032
          suspect Y35.031
      stated as undetermined whether accidental or intentional Y23.1
      suicide (attempt) X73.1
    larger W33.9
      assault X94.9
      homicide (attempt) X94.9
      hunting rifle — *see* Discharge, firearm, hunting rifle
      legal intervention — *see* Legal, intervention, firearm by type of firearm
      machine gun — *see* Discharge, firearm, machine gun
      shotgun — *see* Discharge, firearm, shotgun
    specified NEC W33.8
      assault X94.8
      homicide (attempt) X94.8
      legal intervention Y35.094
        injuring
          bystander Y35.093
          law enforcement personnel Y35.092
          suspect Y35.091
      stated as undetermined whether accidental or intentional Y23.8
      suicide (attempt) X73.8
    stated as undetermined whether accidental or intentional Y23.9
    suicide (attempt) X73.9
    legal intervention Y35.004
      injuring
        bystander Y35.003
        law enforcement personnel Y35.002
        suspect Y35.001
      using rubber bullet Y35.044
        injuring
          bystander Y35.043
          law enforcement personnel Y35.042
          suspect Y35.041
    machine gun W33.2
      assault X94.2
      homicide (attempt) X94.2
      legal intervention — *see* Legal, intervention, firearm, machine gun
      stated as undetermined whether accidental or intentional Y23.3
      suicide (attempt) X73.2
    pellet gun — *see* Discharge, airgun
    shotgun W33.0
      assault X94.0
      homicide (attempt) X94.0

Discharge — *continued*
  firearm — *continued*
    shotgun — *continued*
      legal intervention — *see* Legal, intervention, firearm, specified NEC
      stated as undetermined whether accidental or intentional Y23.0
      suicide (attempt) X73.0
    specified NEC W34.8
      assault X95.8
      homicide (attempt) X95.8
      legal intervention — *see* Legal, intervention, firearm, specified NEC
      stated as undetermined whether accidental or intentional Y24.8
      suicide (attempt) X74.8
    stated as undetermined whether accidental or intentional Y24.9
    suicide (attempt) X74.9
    Very pistol W34.8
      assault X95.8
      homicide (attempt) X95.8
      stated as undetermined whether accidental or intentional Y24.8
      suicide (attempt) X74.8
  firework(s) W39
    stated as undetermined whether accidental or intentional Y25
  gas-operated gun NEC W34.09
    airgun — *see* Discharge, airgun
    assault X95.09
    homicide (attempt) X95.09
    paintball gun — *see* Discharge, paintball gun
    stated as undetermined whether accidental or intentional Y24.8
    suicide (attempt) X74.09
  gun NEC — *see also* Discharge, firearm NEC
    air — *see* Discharge, airgun
    BB — *see* Discharge, airgun
    for single hand use — *see* Discharge, firearm, handgun
    hand — *see* Discharge, firearm, handgun
    machine — *see* Discharge, firearm, machine gun
    other specified — *see* Discharge, firearm NEC
    paintball — *see* Discharge, paintball gun
    pellet — *see* Discharge, airgun
  handgun — *see* Discharge, firearm, handgun
  machine gun — *see* Discharge, firearm, machine gun
  paintball gun W34.02
    assault X95.02
    homicide (attempt) X95.02
    stated as undetermined whether accidental or intentional Y24.8
    suicide (attempt) X74.02
  pistol — *see* Discharge, firearm, handgun
    flare — *see* Discharge, firearm, Very pistol
    pellet — *see* Discharge, airgun
    Very — *see* Discharge, firearm, Very pistol
  revolver — *see* Discharge, firearm, handgun
  rifle (hunting) — *see* Discharge, firearm, hunting rifle
  shotgun — *see* Discharge, firearm, shotgun
  spring-operated gun NEC W34.09
    assault X95.09
    homicide (attempt) X95.09
    stated as undetermined whether accidental or intentional Y24.8
    suicide (attempt) X74.09

Disease
  Andes W94.11
  aviator's — *see* Air, pressure
  range W94.11

Diver's disease, palsy, paralysis, squeeze — *see* Air, pressure

Diving (into water) — *see* Accident, diving

Dog bite W54.0

Dragged by transport vehicle NEC (*see also* Accident, transport) V09.9

Drinking poison (accidental) — *see* Table of Drugs and Chemicals

Dropped (accidentally) **while being carried or supported by other person** W04

Drowning (accidental) W74
  assault X92.9
  due to
    accident (to)
      machinery — *see* Contact, with, by type of machine
      watercraft V90.89
        burning V90.29
          powered V90.23
            merchant ship V90.20
            passenger ship V90.21
            fishing boat V90.22
            jetskis V90.23
          unpowered V90.28
            canoe V90.25
            inflatable V90.26
            kayak V90.25
            sailboat V90.24
            water skis V90.27
        crushed V90.39
          powered V90.33
            merchant ship V90.30
            passenger ship V90.31
            fishing boat V90.32
            jetskis V90.33
          unpowered V90.38
            canoe V90.35
            inflatable V90.36
            kayak V90.35
            sailboat V90.34
            water skis V90.37
        overturning V90.09
          powered V90.03
            merchant ship V90.00
            passenger ship V90.01
            fishing boat V90.02
            jetskis V90.03
          unpowered V90.08
            canoe V90.05
            inflatable V90.06
            kayak V90.05
            sailboat V90.04
        sinking V90.19
          powered V90.13
            merchant ship V90.10
            passenger ship V90.11
            fishing boat V90.12
            jetskis V90.13
          unpowered V90.18
            canoe V90.15
            inflatable V90.16
            kayak V90.15
            sailboat V90.14
        specified type NEC V90.89
          powered V90.83
            merchant ship V90.80
            passenger ship V90.81
            fishing boat V90.82
            jetskis V90.83
          unpowered V90.88
            canoe V90.85
            inflatable V90.86
            kayak V90.85
            sailboat V90.84
            water skis V90.87
  avalanche — *see* Landslide
  cataclysmic
    earth surface movement NEC — *see* Forces of nature, earth movement
    storm — *see* Forces of nature, cataclysmic storm
  cloudburst X37.8
  cyclone X37.1
  fall overboard (from) V92.09
    powered craft V92.03
      ferry boat V92.01
      liner V92.01
      merchant ship V92.00
      passenger ship V92.01
      fishing boat V92.02
      jetskis V92.03
    unpowered craft V92.08
      canoe V92.05
      inflatable V92.06
      kayak V92.05
      sailboat V92.04

©2002 Ingenix, Inc.

Explosion — *continued*
blasting (cap) (materials) W40.0
boiler (machinery), not on transport vehicle W35
    on watercraft — *see* Explosion, in, watercraft
butane W40.1
caused by other person X96.9
coal gas W40.1
detonator W40.0
dump (munitions) W40.8
dynamite W40.0
    in
        assault X96.8
        homicide (attempt) X96.8
        legal intervention Y35.114
            injuring
                bystander Y35.113
                law enforcement personnel Y35.112
                suspect Y35.111
        suicide (attempt) X75
explosive (material) W40.9
    gas W40.1
    in blasting operation W40.0
    specified NEC W40.8
        in
            assault X96.8
            homicide (attempt) X96.8
            legal intervention Y35.194
                injuring
                    bystander Y35.193
                    law enforcement personnel Y35.192
                    suspect Y35.191
            suicide (attempt) X75
factory (munitions) W40.8
fertilizer bomb W40.8
    assault X96.3
    homicide (attempt) X96.3
    suicide (attempt) X75
firedamp W40.1
fireworks W39
gas (coal) (explosive) W40.1
    cylinder W36.9
        aerosol can W36.1
        air tank W36.2
        pressurized W36.3
        specified NEC W36.8
gasoline (fumes) (tank) not in moving motor
    vehicle W40.1
    bomb W40.8
        assault X96.1
        homicide (attempt) X96.1
        suicide (attempt) X75
    in motor vehicle — *see* Accident, transport,
        by type of vehicle
grain store W40.8
grenade W40.8
    in
        assault X96.8
        homicide (attempt) X96.8
        legal intervention Y35.194
            injuring
                bystander Y35.193
                law enforcement personnel Y35.192
                suspect Y35.191
        suicide (attempt) X75
homicide (attempt) X96.9
    antipersonnel bomb — *see* Explosion,
        antipersonnel bomb
    fertilizer bomb — *see* Explosion, fertilizer
        bomb
    gasoline bomb — *see* Explosion, gasoline
        bomb
    letter bomb — *see* Explosion, letter bomb
    pipe bomb — *see* Explosion, pipe bomb
    specified NEC X96.8
hose, pressurized W37.8
hot water heater, tank (in machinery) W35
    on watercraft — *see* Explosion, in, watercraft
in, on
    dump W40.8
    factory W40.8
    mine (of explosive gases) NEC W40.1

Explosion — *continued*
in, on — *continued*
    watercraft V93.59
        powered craft V93.53
            ferry boat V93.51
            fishing boat V93.52
            jetskis V93.53
            liner V93.51
            merchant ship V93.50
            passenger ship V93.51
            sailboat V93.54
letter bomb W40.8
    assault X96.2
    homicide (attempt) X96.2
    suicide (attempt) X75
machinery — *see also* Contact, with, by type of
    machine
    on board watercraft — *see* Explosion, in,
        watercraft
    pressure vessel — *see* Explosion, by type of
        vessel
methane W40.1
mine W40.1
missile NEC W40.8
mortar bomb W40.8
    in
        assault X96.8
        homicide (attempt) X96.8
        legal intervention Y35.194
            injuring
                bystander Y35.193
                law enforcement personnel Y35.192
                suspect Y35.191
        suicide (attempt) X75
munitions (dump) (factory) W40.8
pipe, pressurized W37.8
    bomb W40.8
        assault X96.4
        homicide (attempt) X96.4
        suicide (attempt) X75
pressure, pressurized
    cooker W38
    gas tank (in machinery) W36.3
    hose W37.8
    pipe W37.8
    specified device NEC W38
    tire W37.8
        bicycle W37.0
    vessel (in machinery) W38
propane W40.1
self-inflicted X75
shell (artillery) NEC W40.8
    during military operations Y37.2
    in
        legal intervention Y35.124
            injuring
                bystander Y35.123
                law enforcement personnel Y35.122
                suspect Y35.121
    war Y36.2
spacecraft V95.45
steam or water lines (in machinery) W37.8
stove W40.9
stated as undetermined whether accidental or
    intentional Y25
suicide (attempt) X75
tire, pressurized W37.8
    bicycle W37.0
undetermined whether accidental or intentional
    Y25
vehicle tire NEC W37.8
    bicycle W37.0
war operations — *see* War operations, explosion

Exposure (to) X58.8
air pressure change — *see* Air, pressure
cold (accidental) (excessive) (extreme) (natural)
    (place) X31
    assault Y08.89
    due to
        man-made conditions W93.8
            dry ice (contact) W93.01
                inhalation W93.02
            liquid air (contact) (hydrogen) (nitrogen)
                W93.11
                inhalation W93.12
            refrigeration unit (deep freeze) W93.2

Exposure — *continued*
cold — *continued*
    due to — *continued*
        man-made conditions — *continued*
            suicide (attempt) X83.2
        weather (conditions) X31
    homicide (attempt) Y08.89
    self-inflicted X83.2
due to abandonment or neglect — *see*
    Maltreatment
electric current W86.8
    appliance (faulty) W86.8
        domestic W86.0
    caused by other person Y08.89
    conductor (faulty) W86.1
    control apparatus (faulty) W86.1
    electric power generating plant, distribution
        station W86.1
    high-voltage cable W85
    homicide (attempt) Y08.89
    legal execution Y35.91
    lightning X33
    live rail W86.8
    misadventure in medical or surgical
        procedure in electroshock therapy
        Y63.4
    motor (electric) (faulty) W86.8
        domestic W86.0
        self-inflicted X83.1
    specified NEC W86.8
        domestic W86.0
    suicide (attempt) X83.1
    third rail W86.8
    transformer (faulty) W86.1
    transmission lines W85
environmental tobacco smoke X58.1
excessive
    cold — *see* Exposure, cold
    heat (natural) NEC X30
        man-made W92
factor(s) NOS X58.8
    environmental NEC X58.8
        man-made NEC W99
        natural NEC — *see* Forces of nature
    specified NEC X58.8
fire, flames (accidental) X08.8
    assault X97
    campfire — *see* Exposure, fire, controlled,
        not in building
    controlled (in)
        with ignition (of) clothing (*see also*
            Ignition, clothes) X06.2
            nightwear X05
        bonfire — *see* Exposure, fire, controlled,
            not in building
        brazier (in building or structure) — *see*
            also Exposure, fire, controlled,
            building
            not in building or structure — *see*
                Exposure, fire, controlled, not in
                building
        building or structure X02.0
            with
                fall from building X02.3
                injury due to building collapse X02.2
                from building X02.5
                smoke inhalation X02.1
            hit by object from building X02.4
            specified mode of injury NEC X02.8
        fireplace, furnace or stove — *see*
            Exposure, fire, controlled, building
        not in building or structure X03.0
            with
                fall X03.3
                smoke inhalation X03.1
            hit by object X03.4
            specified mode of injury NEC X03.8
        trash — *see* Exposure, fire, controlled, not
            in building
    fireplace — *see* Exposure, fire, controlled,
        building
    fittings or furniture (in building or structure)
        (uncontrolled) — *see* Exposure, fire,
        uncontrolled, building
    forest (uncontrolled) — *see* Exposure, fire,
        uncontrolled, not in building

Exposure — *continued*
  fire, flames — *continued*
    grass (uncontrolled) — *see* Exposure, fire, uncontrolled, not in building
    hay (uncontrolled) — *see* Exposure, fire, uncontrolled, not in building
    homicide (attempt) X97
    ignition of highly flammable material X04
    in, of, on, starting in
      machinery — *see* Contact, with, by type of machine
      motor vehicle (in motion) (*see also* Accident, transport, occupant by type of vehicle) V87.8
        with collision — *see* Collision
      railway rolling stock, train, vehicle V81.81
        with collision — *see* Accident, transport, railway vehicle occupant
      street car (in motion) V82.8
        with collision — *see* Accident, transport, streetcar occupant
      transport vehicle NEC — *see also* Accident, transport
        with collision — *see* Collision
      war operations (by fire-producing device or conventional weapon) — *see also* War operations, fire
      from nuclear explosion — *see* War operation, nuclear weapons
      watercraft (in transit) (not in transit) V91.09
        localized — *see* Burn, on board watercraft, due to, fire on board
        powered craft V91.03
          ferry boat V91.01
          fishing boat V91.02
          jet skis V91.03
          liner V91.01
          merchant ship V91.00
          passenger ship V91.01
        unpowered craft V91.08
          canoe V91.05
          inflatable V91.06
          kayak V91.05
          sailboat V91.04
          surf-board V91.08
          waterskis V91.07
          windsurfer V91.08
    lumber (uncontrolled) — *see* Exposure, fire, uncontrolled, not in building
    mine (uncontrolled) — *see* Exposure, fire, uncontrolled, not in building
    prairie (uncontrolled) — *see* Exposure, fire, uncontrolled, not in building
    resulting from
      explosion — *see* Explosion
      lightning X08.8
    self-inflicted X76
    specified NEC X08.8
    started by other person X97
    stove — *see* Exposure, fire, controlled, building
    stated as undetermined whether accidental or intentional Y26
    suicide (attempt) X76
    tunnel (uncontrolled) — *see* Exposure, fire, uncontrolled, not in building
    uncontrolled
      in building or structure X00.0
        with
          fall from building X00.3
          injury due to building collapse X00.2
          jump from building X00.5
          smoke inhalation X00.1
        bed X08.00
          due to
            cigarette X08.01
            specified material NEC X08.09
        furniture NEC X08.20
          due to
            cigarette X08.21
            specified material NEC X08.29
        hit by object from building X00.4

Exposure — *continued*
  fire, flames — *continued*
    uncontrolled — *continued*
      in building or structure — *continued*
        sofa X08.10
          due to
            cigarette X08.11
            specified material NEC X08.19
        specified mode of injury NEC X00.8
      not in building or structure (any) X01.0
        with
          fall X01.3
          smoke inhalation X01.1
        hit by object X01.4
        specified mode of injury NEC X01.8
      undetermined whether accidental or intentional Y26
  forces of nature NEC — *see* Forces of nature
  G-forces (abnormal) W49
  gravitational forces (abnormal) W49
  heat (natural) NEC — *see* Heat
  high-pressure jet (hydraulic) (pneumatic) W49
  hydraulic jet W49
  inanimate mechanical force W49
  jet, high-pressure (hydraulic) (pneumatic) W49
  lightning X33
    causing fire — *see* Exposure, fire
  mechanical forces NEC W49
    animate NEC W64
    inanimate NEC W49
  noise W42.9
    supersonic W42.0
  noxious substance — *see* Table of Drugs and Chemicals
  pneumatic jet W49
  prolonged in deep-freeze unit or refrigerator W93.2
  radiation — *see* Radiation
  smoke — *see also* Exposure, fire
    tobacco, second hand X58.1
  specified factors NEC X58.8
  sunlight X32
    man-made (sun lamp) W89.8
      tanning bed W89.1
  supersonic waves W42.0
  transmission line(s), electric W85
  vibration W49
  waves
    infrasound W49
    sound W42.9
    supersonic W42.0
  weather NEC — *see* Forces of nature
    with homicidal intent — *see* Maltreatment

F

Factors, supplemental
  alcohol
    blood level
      less than 20mg/100ml Y90.0
      presence in blood, level not specified Y90.9
      20-39mg/100ml Y90.1
      40-59mg/100ml Y90.2
      60-79mg/100ml Y90.3
      80-99mg/100ml Y90.4
      100-119mg/100ml Y90.5
      120-199mg/100ml Y90.6
      200-239mg/100ml Y90.7
      240mg/100ml or more Y90.8
    presence in blood, but level not specified Y90.9
  environmental-pollution-related condition Y97
  nosocomial condition Y95
  work-related condition Y96
Failure
  in suture or ligature during surgical procedure Y65.2
  mechanical, of instrument or apparatus (any) (during any medical or surgical procedure) Y65.8
  sterile precautions (during medical and surgical care) — *see* Misadventure, failure, sterile precautions, by type of procedure

Failure — *continued*
  to
    introduce tube or instrument Y65.4
      endotracheal tube during anesthesia Y65.3
    make curve (transport vehicle) NEC — *see* Accident, transport
    remove tube or instrument Y65.4
Fall, falling (accidental) W19
  building W20.1
    burning (uncontrolled fire) X00.3
  down
    embankment W17.8
    escalator W10.0
    hill W17.8
    ladder W11
    ramp W10.3
    stairs, steps W10.9
  due to
    bumping against
      object W18.00
        sharp glass W18.02
        specified NEC W18.09
        sports equipment W18.01
      person W03
        due to ice or snow W00.0
        on pedestrian conveyance — *see* Accident, transport, pedestrian, conveyance
    collision with another person W03
      due to ice or snow W00.0
      involving pedestrian conveyance — *see* Accident, transport, pedestrian, conveyance
    ice or snow W00.9
      from one level to another W00.2
      on stairs or steps W00.1
      involving pedestrian conveyance — *see* Accident, transport, pedestrian, conveyance
      on same level W00.0
    slipping (on moving sidewalk) W01.0
      with subsequent striking against object W01.10
        furniture W01.190
        sharp object W01.119
          glass W01.110
          power tool or machine W01.111
          specified NEC W01.118
        specified NEC W01.198
    striking against
      object W18.00
        sharp glass W18.02
        specified NEC W18.09
        sports equipment W18.01
      person W03
        due to ice or snow W00.0
        on pedestrian conveyance — *see* Accident, transport, pedestrian, conveyance
  earth (with asphyxia or suffocation (by pressure)) — *see* Earth, falling
  from, off
    aircraft NEC (with accident to aircraft NEC) V97.0
      while boarding or alighting V97.1
    balcony W13.0
    bed W06
    boat, ship, watercraft NEC (with drowning or submersion) — *see* Drowning, due to, fall overboard
      with hitting bottom or object V94.0
    bridge W13.1
    building W13.9
      burning (uncontrolled fire) X00.3
    cavity W17.2
    chair W07
    cliff W15
    dock W17.4
    embankment W17.8
    escalator W10.0
    flagpole W13.8
    furniture NEC W08
    haystack W17.8

Fall, falling — *continued*
  from, off — *continued*
    high place NEC W17.8
      stated as undetermined whether
        accidental or intentional Y30
    hole W17.2
    incline W10.3
    ladder W11
    machine, machinery — *see also* Contact,
      with, by type of machine
      not in operation W17.8
    manhole W17.1
    one level to another NEC W17.8
      intentional, purposeful, suicide (attempt)
        X80
      stated as undetermined whether
        accidental or intentional Y30
    pit W17.2
    playground equipment W09.8
      jungle gym W09.2
      slide W09.0
      swing W09.1
    quarry W17.8
    railing W13.9
    ramp W10.3
    roof W13.2
    scaffolding W12
    stairs, steps W10.9
      curb W10.1
      due to ice or snow W00.1
      escalator W10.0
      incline W10.3
      ramp W10.3
      sidewalk curb W10.1
      specified NEC W10.8
    stepladder W11
    storm drain W17.1
    streetcar NEC V82.6
      with antecedent collision — *see* Accident,
        transport, streetcar occupant
      while boarding or alighting V82.4
    structure NEC W13.8
      burning (uncontrolled fire) X00.3
    table W08
    toilet W18.11
      with subsequent striking against object
        W18.12
    train NEC V81.6
      during derailment (without antecedent
        collision) V81.7
      with antecedent collision — *see*
        Accident, transport, railway
        vehicle occupant
      while boarding or alighting V81.4
    transport vehicle after collision — *see*
      Accident, transport, by type of vehicle,
      collision
    tree W14
    vehicle (in motion) NEC (*see also* Accident,
      transport) V89.9
      motor NEC (*see also* Accident, transport,
        occupant, by type of vehicle) V87.8
      stationary W17.8
        while boarding or alighting — *see*
          Accident, transport, by type of
          vehicle, while boarding or
          alighting
    viaduct W13.8
    wall W13.8
    watercraft — *see also* Drowning, due to, fall
      overboard
      with hitting bottom or object V94.0
    well W17.0
    wheelchair W05
      powered — *see* Accident, transport,
        pedestrian, conveyance occupant,
        specified type NEC
    window W13.4
  in, on
    aircraft NEC V97.0
      with accident to aircraft V97.0
      while boarding or alighting V97.1
    bathtub (empty) W18.2
      filled W16.212
        causing drowning W16.211
    escalator W10.0

Fall, falling — *continued*
  in, on — *continued*
    incline W10.3
    ladder W11
    machine, machinery — *see* Contact, with, by
      type of machine
    object, edged, pointed or sharp (with cut) —
      see Fall, by type
    playground equipment W09.8
      jungle gym W09.2
      slide W09.0
      swing W09.1
    ramp W10.3
    scaffolding W12
    shower W18.2
      causing drowning W16.211
    staircase, stairs, steps W10.9
      curb W10.1
      due to ice or snow W00.1
      escalator W10.0
      incline W10.3
      specified NEC W10.8
    streetcar (without antecedent collision) V82.5
      with antecedent collision — *see* Accident,
        transport, streetcar occupant
      while boarding or alighting V82.4
    train (without antecedent collision) V81.5
      with antecedent collision — *see* Accident,
        transport, railway vehicle occupant
      during derailment (without antecedent
        collision) V81.7
        with antecedent collision — *see*
          Accident, transport, railway
          vehicle occupant
      while boarding or alighting V81.4
    transport vehicle after collision — *see*
      Accident, transport, by type of vehicle,
      collision
    watercraft V93.39
    due to
      accident to craft V91.29
        powered craft V91.23
          ferry boat V91.21
          fishing boat V91.22
          jetskis V91.23
          liner V91.21
          merchant ship V91.20
          passenger ship V91.21
        unpowered craft
          canoe V91.25
          inflatable V91.26
          kayak V91.25
          sailboat V91.24
      powered craft V93.33
        ferry boat V93.31
        fishing boat V93.32
        jetskis V93.33
        liner V93.31
        merchant ship V93.30
        passenger ship V93.31
      unpowered craft V93.38
        canoe V93.35
        inflatable V93.36
        kayak V93.35
        sailboat V93.34
        surf-board V93.38
        windsurfer V93.38
  into
    cavity W17.2
    dock W17.4
    fire — *see* Exposure, fire, by type
    haystack W17.8
    hole W17.2
    lake — *see* Fall, into, water
    manhole W17.1
    moving part of machinery — *see* Contact,
      with, by type of machine
    ocean — *see* Fall, into, water
    opening in surface NEC W17.8
    pit W17.2
    pond — *see* Fall, into, water
    quarry W17.8
    lake — *see* Fall, into, water
    river — *see* Fall, into, water
    shaft W17.8

Fall, falling — *continued*
  into — *continued*
    storm drain W17.1
    stream — *see* Fall, into, water
    swimming pool — *see also* Fall, into, water,
      in, swimming pool
      empty W17.3
    tank W17.8
    water W16.42
      causing drowning W16.41
      from watercraft — *see* Drowning, due to,
        fall overboard
      hitting diving board W21.4
      in
        bathtub W16.212
          causing drowning W16.211
        bucket W16.222
          causing drowning W16.221
        natural body of water W16.112
          causing drowning W16.111
          striking
            bottom W16.122
              causing drowning W16.121
            side W16.132
              causing drowning W16.131
        specified water NEC W16.312
          causing drowning W16.311
          striking
            bottom W16.322
              causing drowning W16.321
            wall W16.332
              causing drowning W16.331
        swimming pool W16.012
          causing drowning W16.011
          striking
            bottom W16.022
              causing drowning W16.021
            wall W16.032
              causing drowning W16.031
        utility bucket W16.222
          causing drowning W16.221
    well W17.0
  involving
    bed W06
    chair W07
    furniture NEC W08
    glass — *see* Fall, by type
    playground equipment W09.8
      jungle gym W09.2
      slide W09.0
      swing W09.1
    roller blades — *see* Accident, transport,
      pedestrian, conveyance
    skateboard(s) — *see* Accident, transport,
      pedestrian, conveyance
    skates (ice) (in line) (roller) — *see* Accident,
      transport, pedestrian, conveyance
    skis — *see* Accident, transport, pedestrian,
      conveyance
    table W08
    wheelchair W05
      powered — *see* Accident, transport,
        pedestrian, conveyance, specified
        type NEC
  object — *see* Struck by, object, falling
  off
    toilet W18.11
      with subsequent striking against object
        W18.12
  out of
    bed W06
    building NEC W13.8
    chair W07
    furniture NEC W08
    wheelchair W05
      powered — *see* Accident, transport,
        pedestrian, conveyance, specified
        type NEC
    window W13.4
  over
    animal W01.0
    cliff W15
    embankment W17.8
    small object W01.0
  rock W20.8

Fall, falling — *continued*
  same level W18.9
    from
      being crushed, pushed, or stepped on by a
        crowd or human stampede W52
      collision, pushing, shoving, by or with
        other person W03
      slipping, stumbling, tripping W01.0
        involving ice or snow W00.0
          involving skates (ice) (roller), skateboard,
            skis — *see* Accident, transport,
            pedestrian, conveyance
  snowslide (avalanche) — *see* Landslide
  stone W20.8
  structure W20.1
    burning (uncontrolled fire) X00.3
  through
    bridge W13.1
    floor W13.3
    roof W13.2
    wall W13.8
    window W13.4
  timber W20.8
  tree (caused by lightning) W20.8
  while being carried or supported by other
    person(s) W04
Fallen on by
  animal (not being ridden) NEC W55.89
    being ridden (*see also* Accident, transport)
      V06
Felo-de-se — *see* Suicide
Fight (hand) (fists) (foot) — *see* Assault, fight
Fire (accidental) — *see* Exposure, fire
Firearm discharge — *see* Discharge, firearm
Fireball effects from nuclear explosion in war
  operations — *see* War operation, nuclear
  weapons
Fireworks (explosion) W39
Flash burns from explosion — *see* Explosion
Flood (any injury) (caused by) X38
  collapse of man-made structure causing earth
    movement X36.0
  tidal wave — *see* Forces of nature, tidal wave
Food (any type) **in**
  air passages (with asphyxia, obstruction, or
    suffocation) W79
  alimentary tract causing asphyxia (due to
    compression of trachea) W79
Forces of nature X39.8
  avalanche X36.1
    causing transport accident — *see* Accident,
      transport, by type of vehicle
  blizzard X37.2
  cataclysmic storm X37.9
    with flood X38
    blizzard X37.2
    cloudburst X37.8
    cyclone X37.1
    dust storm X37.3
    hurricane X37.0
    specified storm NEC X37.8
    storm surge X37.0
    tornado X37.1
    twister X37.1
    typhoon X37.0
  cloudburst X37.8
  cold (natural) X31
  cyclone X37.1
  dam collapse causing earth movement X36.0
  dust storm X37.3
  earth movement X36.1
    earthquake X34
    caused by dam or structure collapse X36.0
  earthquake X34
  flood (caused by) X38
    dam collapse X36.0
    tidal wave — *see* Forces of nature, tidal wave
  heat (natural) X30
  hurricane X37.0
  landslide X36.1
    causing transport accident — *see* Accident,
      transport, by type of vehicle
  lightning X33
    causing fire — *see* Exposure, fire

Forces of nature — *continued*
  mudslide X36.1
    causing transport accident — *see* Accident,
      transport, by type of vehicle
  radiation (natural) X39.08
    radon X39.01
  radon X39.01
  specified force NEC X39.8
  storm surge X37.0
  structure collapse causing earth movement
    X36.0
  sunlight X32
  tidal wave X37.41
    due to
      earthquake or volcanic eruption X37.41
      storm X37.42
  tornado X37.1
  tsunami X37.41
  twister X37.1
  typhoon X37.0
  volcanic eruption X35
Foreign body entering through skin W45.8
  can lid W45.2
  nail W45.0
  paper W45.1
  specified NEC W45.8
  splinter W45.8
Forest fire (exposure to) — *see* Exposure, fire,
  uncontrolled, not in building
Found dead, injured X58.8
  from exposure (to) — *see* Exposure
  on
    highway, road(way), street V89.9
    railway right of way V81.9
Fracture (circumstances unknown or unspecified)
  X58.8
  due to specified cause NEC X58.8
Freezing — *see* Exposure, cold
Frostbite X31
  due to man-made conditions — *see* Exposure,
    cold, man-made
Frozen — *see* Exposure, cold

G

Gored by bull W55.29
Gunshot wound — *see* Discharge, firearm, by type

H

Hailstones, injured by X39.8
Hanged herself or himself — *see* Hanging, self
  inflicted
Hanging (accidental) W76
  caused by other person
    in accidental circumstances W76
  in bed or cradle W75
  legal execution Y35.91
  self-inflicted
    in accidental circumstances W76
Heat (effects of) (excessive) X30
  due to
    man-made conditions W92
      on board watercraft V93.29
        fishing boat V93.22
        merchant ship V93.20
        passenger ship V93.21
        sailboat V93.24
        specified powered craft NEC V93.23
      weather (conditions) X30
  from
    electric heating apparatus causing burning
      X16
    nuclear explosion in war operations — *see*
      War operation, nuclear weapons
  inappropriate in local application or packing in
    medical or surgical procedure Y63.5
Hemorrhage
  delayed following medical or surgical treatment
    without mention of misadventure — *see*
    Complication of or following, by type of
    procedure
  during medical or surgical treatment as
    misadventure — *see* Misadventure, cut, by
    type of procedure

High
  altitude (effects) — *see* Air, pressure, low
  level of radioactivity, effects — *see* Radiation
  pressure (effects) — *see* Air, pressure, high
  temperature, effects *see* Heat
Hit, hitting (accidental) by — *see* Struck by
Hitting against — *see* Striking against
Homicide (attempt) (justifiable) — *see* Assault
Hot
  place, effects — *see also* Heat
  weather, effects X30
House fire (uncontrolled) — *see* Exposure, fire,
  uncontrolled, building
Humidity, causing problem X39.8
Hunger X58.8
  resulting from abandonment or neglect — *see*
    Maltreatment
Hurricane (any injury) X37.0
Hypobarism, hypobaropathy — *see* Air, pressure,
  low

I

Ictus
  caloris — *see also* Heat
  solaris X30
Ignition (accidental) (*see also* Exposure, fire) X08.8
  anesthetic gas in operating room W40.1
  apparel X06.2
    from highly flammable material X04
    nightwear X05
  bed linen (sheets) (spreads) (pillows) (mattress)
    — *see* Exposure, fire, uncontrolled,
    building, bed
  benzine X04
  clothes, clothing NEC (from controlled fire)
    X06.2
    from
      highly flammable material X04
  ether X04
    in operating room W40.1
  explosive material — *see* Explosion
  gasoline X04
  jewelry (plastic) (any) X06.0
  kerosene X04
  material
    explosive — *see* Explosion
    highly flammable with secondary explosion
      X04
  nightwear X05
  paraffin X04
  petrol X04
Immersion (accidental) — *see also* Drowning
  hand or foot due to cold (excessive) X31
Implantation of quills of porcupine W55.89
Inanition (from) (hunger) X58.8
  resulting from homicidal intent — *see*
    Maltreatment
  thirst X58.8
Inappropriate operation performed Y65.5
Inattention after, at birth (homicidal intent)
  (infanticidal intent) — *see* Maltreatment
Incident, adverse
  device
    anesthesiology Y70.8
      accessory Y70.2
      diagnostic Y70.0
      miscellaneous Y70.8
      monitoring Y70.0
      prosthetic Y70.2
      rehabilitative Y70.1
      surgical Y70.3
      therapeutic Y70.1
    cardiovascular Y71.8
      accessory Y71.2
      diagnostic Y71.0
      miscellaneous Y71.8
      monitoring Y71.0
      prosthetic Y71.2
      rehabilitative Y71.1
      surgical Y71.3
      therapeutic Y71.1

©2002 Ingenix, Inc.

Incident, adverse — *continued*
  device — *continued*
    gastroenterology Y73.8
      accessory Y73.2
      diagnostic Y73.0
      miscellaneous Y73.8
      monitoring Y73.0
      prosthetic Y73.2
      rehabilitative Y73.1
      surgical Y73.3
      therapeutic Y73.1
    general
      hospital Y74.8
        accessory Y74.2
        diagnostic Y74.0
        miscellaneous Y74.8
        monitoring Y74.0
        prosthetic Y74.2
        rehabilitative Y74.1
        surgical Y74.3
        therapeutic Y74.1
      surgical Y81.8
        accessory Y81.2
        diagnostic Y81.0
        miscellaneous Y81.8
        monitoring Y81.0
        prosthetic Y81.2
        rehabilitative Y81.1
        surgical Y81.3
        therapeutic Y81.1
    gynecological Y76.8
      accessory Y76.2
      diagnostic Y76.0
      miscellaneous Y76.8
      monitoring Y76.0
      prosthetic Y76.2
      rehabilitative Y76.1
      surgical Y76.3
      therapeutic Y76.1
    medical Y82.9
      specified type NEC Y82.0
    neurological Y75.8
      accessory Y75.2
      diagnostic Y75.0
      miscellaneous Y75.8
      monitoring Y75.0
      prosthetic Y75.2
      rehabilitative Y75.1
      surgical Y75.3
      therapeutic Y75.1
    obstetrical Y76.8
      accessory Y76.2
      diagnostic Y76.0
      miscellaneous Y76.8
      monitoring Y76.0
      prosthetic Y76.2
      rehabilitative Y76.1
      surgical Y76.3
      therapeutic Y76.1
    ophthalmic Y77.8
      accessory Y77.2
      diagnostic Y77.0
      miscellaneous Y77.8
      monitoring Y77.0
      prosthetic Y77.2
      rehabilitative Y77.1
      surgical Y77.3
      therapeutic Y77.1
    orthopedic Y79.8
      accessory Y79.2
      diagnostic Y79.0
      miscellaneous Y79.8
      monitoring Y79.0
      prosthetic Y79.2
      rehabilitative Y79.1
      surgical Y79.3
      therapeutic Y79.1
    otorhinolaryngological Y72.8
      accessory Y72.2
      diagnostic Y72.0
      miscellaneous Y72.8
      monitoring Y72.0
      prosthetic Y72.2
      rehabilitative Y72.1
      surgical Y72.3
      therapeutic Y72.1

Incident, adverse — *continued*
  device — *continued*
    personal use Y74.8
      accessory Y74.2
      diagnostic Y74.0
      miscellaneous Y74.8
      monitoring Y74.0
      prosthetic Y74.2
      rehabilitative Y74.1
      surgical Y74.3
      therapeutic Y74.1
    physical medicine Y80.8
      accessory Y80.2
      diagnostic Y80.0
      miscellaneous Y80.8
      monitoring Y80.0
      prosthetic Y80.2
      rehabilitative Y80.1
      surgical Y80.3
      therapeutic Y80.1
    plastic surgical Y81.8
      accessory Y81.2
      diagnostic Y81.0
      miscellaneous Y81.8
      monitoring Y81.0
      prosthetic Y81.2
      rehabilitative Y81.1
      surgical Y81.3
      therapeutic Y81.1
    radiological Y78.8
      accessory Y78.2
      diagnostic Y78.0
      miscellaneous Y78.8
      monitoring Y78.0
      prosthetic Y78.2
      rehabilitative Y78.1
      surgical Y78.3
      therapeutic Y78.1
    urology Y73.8
      accessory Y73.2
      diagnostic Y73.0
      miscellaneous Y73.8
      monitoring Y73.0
      prosthetic Y73.2
      rehabilitative Y73.1
      surgical Y73.3
      therapeutic Y73.1

Incineration (accidental) — *see* Exposure, fire
Infanticide — *see* Assault
Infrasound waves (causing injury) W49
Ingestion
  foreign body (causing injury) (with obstruction)
    — *see* Foreign body, alimentary canal
  poisonous
    plant(s) X58.8
    substance NEC — *see* Table of Drugs and
      Chemicals
Inhalation
  excessively cold substance, man-made — *see*
    Exposure, cold, man-made
  food (any type) (into respiratory tract) (with
    asphyxia, obstruction respiratory tract,
    suffocation) W79
  foreign body — *see* Foreign body, aspiration
  gastric contents (with asphyxia, obstruction
    respiratory passage, suffocation) W78
  hot air or gases X14.0
  liquid air, hydrogen, nitrogen W93.12
    suicide (attempt) X83.2
  steam X13.0
    assault X98.0
    stated as undetermined whether accidental
      or intentional Y27.0
    suicide (attempt) X77.0
  toxic gas — *see* Table of Drugs and Chemicals
  vomitus (with asphyxia, obstruction respiratory
    passage, suffocation) W78
Injury, injured (accidental(ly)) **NOS** X58.8
  by, caused by, from
    assault — *see* Assault
    law-enforcing agent, police, in course of legal
      intervention — *see* Legal intervention
    suicide (attempt) X83.8
  due to, in
    civil insurrection — *see* War operations

Injury, injured NOS — *continued*
  due to, in — *continued*
    fight (*see also* Assault, fight) Y04.0
    war operations — *see* War operations
  homicide (*see also* Assault) Y09
  inflicted (by)
    in course of arrest (attempted), suppression
      of disturbance, maintenance of order,
      by law-enforcing agents — *see* Legal
      intervention
    other person
      stated as
        accidental X58.8
        intentional, homicide (attempt) —
          Assault
        undetermined whether accidental or
          intentional Y33
  purposely (inflicted) by other person(s) — *see*
    Assault
  self-inflicted X83.8
    stated as accidental X58.8
  specified cause NEC X58.8
  undetermined whether accidental or intentional
    Y33
Insolation, effects X30
Insufficient nourishment X58.8
  homicidal intent — *see* Maltreatment
Interruption of respiration (by)
  food (lodged in esophagus) W79
  vomitus (lodged in esophagus) W78
Intervention, legal — *see* Legal intervention
Intoxication
  drug — *see* Table of Drugs and Chemicals
  poison — *see* Table of Drugs and Chemicals

J

Jammed (accidentally)
  between objects (moving) (stationary and
    moving) W23.0
    stationary W23.1
  in object NEC W23.2
Jogging, excessive X50.01
Jumped, jumping
  before moving object X81
    motor vehicle X82.3
    undetermined whether accidental or
      intentional Y31
  from
    boat (into water) voluntarily, without accident
      (to or on boat) W16.712
      with
        accident to or on boat — *see* Accident,
          watercraft
        drowning or submersion W16.711
          suicide (attempt) X71.3
        striking bottom W16.722
          causing drowning W16.721
    building (*see also* Jumped, from, high place)
      W13.9
      burning (uncontrolled fire) X00.5
    high place NEC W17.8
      suicide (attempt) X80
      undetermined whether accidental or
        intentional Y30
    structure (*see also* Jumped, from, high place)
      W13.9
      burning (uncontrolled fire) X00.5
  into water W16.92
    causing drowning W16.91
    from, off watercraft — *see* Jumped, from,
      boat
    in
      natural body W16.612
        causing drowning W16.611
        striking bottom W16.622
          causing drowning W16.621
      specified place NEC W16.812
        causing drowning W16.811
        striking
          bottom W16.822
            causing drowning W16.821
          wall W16.832
            causing drowning W16.831

Jumped, jumping — *continued*
  into water — *continued*
    in — *continued*
      swimming pool W16.512
        causing drowning W16.511
        striking
          bottom W16.522
            causing drowning W16.521
          wall W16.532
            causing drowning W16.531
    suicide (attempt) X71.3

K

Kicked by
  animal NEC W55.89
  person(s) (accidentally) W50.1
    with intent to injure or kill Y04.0
    as, or caused by, a crowd or human
      stampede (with fall) W52
    assault Y04.0
    homicide (attempt) Y04.0
    in
      fight Y04.0
      legal intervention Y35.814
        injuring
          bystander Y35.813
          law enforcement personnel Y35.812
          suspect Y35.811

Kicking against
  object W22.8
    sports equipment W21.9
    stationary W22.09
      sports equipment W21.89
  person — *see* Striking against, person
  sports equipment W21.9

Killed, killing (accidentally) **NOS** (*see also* Injury)
  X58.8
  in
    action — *see* War operations
    brawl, fight (hand) (fists) (foot) Y04.0
      by weapon — *see also* Assault
        cutting, piercing — *see* Assault, cutting
          or piercing instrument
        firearm — *see* Discharge, firearm, by
          type, homicide
  self
    stated as
      accident NOS X58.8
      suicide — *see* Suicide
      undetermined whether accidental or
        intentional Y33

Knocked down (accidentally) (by) **NOS** X58.8
  animal (not being ridden) NEC — *see also*
    Struck by, by type of animal
    being ridden V06
  crowd or human stampede W52
  person W51
    in brawl, fight Y04.0
  transport vehicle NEC (*see also* Accident,
    transport) V09.9

L

Laceration NEC — *see* Injury

Lack of
  care (helpless person) (infant) (newborn) — *see*
    Maltreatment
  food except as result of abandonment or neglect
    X58.8
    due to abandonment or neglect — *see*
      Maltreatment
  water except as result of transport accident
    X58.8
    due to transport accident — *see* Accident,
      transport, by type
    helpless person, infant, newborn — *see*
      Maltreatment

Landslide (falling on transport vehicle) X36.1
  caused by collapse of man-made structure
    X36.0

Late effect — *see* Sequelae

Legal
  execution Y35.91
  intervention (by) Y35.99
    baton — *see* Legal, intervention, blunt object,
      baton
    bayonet — *see* Legal, intervention, sharp
      object, bayonet
    blow — *see* Legal, intervention, manhandling
    blunt object Y35.304
      baton Y35.314
        injuring
          bystander Y35.313
          law enforcement personnel Y35.312
          suspect Y35.311
      injuring
        bystander Y35.303
        law enforcement personnel Y35.302
        suspect Y35.301
      specified NEC Y35.394
        injuring
          bystander Y35.393
          law enforcement personnel Y35.392
          suspect Y35.391
      stave Y35.394
        injuring
          bystander Y35.393
          law enforcement personnel Y35.392
          suspect Y35.391
    bomb — *see* Legal, intervention, explosive
    cutting or piercing instrument — *see* Legal,
      intervention, sharp object
    dynamite — *see* Legal, intervention,
      explosive, dynamite
    execution, any method Y35.91
    explosive(s) Y35.104
      dynamite Y35.114
        injuring
          bystander Y35.113
          law enforcement personnel Y35.112
          suspect Y35.111
      grenade Y35.194
        injuring
          bystander Y35.193
          law enforcement personnel Y35.192
          suspect Y35.191
      injuring
        bystander Y35.103
        law enforcement personnel Y35.102
        suspect Y35.101
      mortar bomb Y35.194
        injuring
          bystander Y35.193
          law enforcement personnel Y35.192
          suspect Y35.191
      shell Y35.124
        injuring
          bystander Y35.123
          law enforcement personnel Y35.122
          suspect Y35.121
      specified NEC Y35.194
        injuring
          bystander Y35.193
          law enforcement personnel Y35.192
          suspect Y35.191
    firearm(s) (discharge) Y35.004
      handgun Y35.024
        injuring
          bystander Y35.023
          law enforcement personnel Y35.022
          suspect Y35.021
      injuring
        bystander Y35.003
        law enforcement personnel Y35.002
        suspect Y35.001
      machine gun Y35.014
        injuring
          bystander Y35.013
          law enforcement personnel Y35.012
          suspect Y35.011
      rifle pellet Y35.034
        injuring
          bystander Y35.033
          law enforcement personnel Y35.032
          suspect Y35.031

Legal — *continued*
  intervention — *continued*
    firearm(s — *continued*
      rubber bullet Y35.044
        injuring
          bystander Y35.043
          law enforcement personnel Y35.042
          suspect Y35.041
      shotgun — *see* Legal, intervention,
        firearm, specified NEC
      specified NEC Y35.094
        injuring
          bystander Y35.093
          law enforcement personnel Y35.092
          suspect Y35.091
    gas (asphyxiation) (poisoning) Y35.204
      injuring
        bystander Y35.203
        law enforcement personnel Y35.202
        suspect Y35.201
      specified NEC Y35.294
        injuring
          bystander Y35.293
          law enforcement personnel Y35.292
          suspect Y35.291
      tear gas Y35.214
        injuring
          bystander Y35.213
          law enforcement personnel Y35.212
          suspect Y35.211
    grenade — *see* Legal, intervention, explosive,
      grenade
    injuring
      bystander Y35.93
      law enforcement personnel Y35.92
      suspect Y35.91
    late effect (of) — *see* Y35 with q as terminal
      character
    manhandling Y35.814
      injuring
        bystander Y35.813
        law enforcement personnel Y35.812
        suspect Y35.811
    sequelae (of) — *see* Y35 with q as terminal
      character
    sharp objects Y35.404
      bayonet Y35.414
        injuring
          bystander Y35.413
          law enforcement personnel Y35.412
          suspect Y35.411
      injuring
        bystander Y35.403
        law enforcement personnel Y35.402
        suspect Y35.401
      specified NEC Y35.494
        injuring
          bystander Y35.493
          law enforcement personnel Y35.492
          suspect Y35.491
    specified means NEC Y35.894
      injuring
        bystander Y35.892
        law enforcement personnel Y35.891
        suspect Y35.890
    stabbing — *see* Legal, intervention, sharp
      object
    stave — *see* Legal, intervention, blunt object,
      stave
    tear gas — *see* Legal, intervention, gas, tear
      gas
    truncheon — *see* Legal, intervention, blunt
      object, stave

Lifting (heavy objects), **excessive** X50.09
  weights X50.01

Lightning (shock) (stroke) (struck by) X33
  causing fire — *see* Exposure, fire

Loss of control (transport vehicle) **NEC** — *see*
  Accident, transport

Lost at sea NOS — *see* Drowning, due to, fall
  overboard

Low
  pressure (effects) — *see* Air, pressure, low
  temperature (effects) — *see* Exposure, cold

Lying before train, vehicle or other moving object X81
  undetermined whether accidental or intentional Y31

Lynching — *see* Assault

M

Maltreatment (syndrome) **NOS** Y07.50
  by
    boy friend Y07.432
    brother Y07.410
      stepbrother Y07.435
    coach Y07.53
    cousin
      female Y07.491
      male Y07.490
    daycare provider Y07.519
      at-home
        adult care Y07.512
        childcare Y07.510
      care center
        adult care Y07.513
        childcare Y07.511
    family member NEC Y07.499
    father Y07.11
      adoptive Y07.13
      foster Y07.420
      stepfather Y07.430
    girl friend Y07.434
    healthcare provider Y07.529
      mental health Y07.521
      specified NEC Y07.528
    husband Y07.01
    instructor Y07.53
    mother Y07.12
      adoptive Y07.14
      foster Y07.421
      stepmother Y07.433
    nonfamily member NEC Y07.59
    nurse Y07.528
    occupational therapist Y07.528
    partner of parent
      female Y07.04
      male Y07.03
    physical therapist Y07.528
    sister Y07.411
    speech therapist Y07.528
    stepbrother Y07.435
    stepfather Y07.430
    stepmother Y07.433
    stepsister Y07.436
    teacher Y07.53
    wife Y07.02

Mangled (accidentally) **NOS** X58.8

Manhandling (in brawl, fight) Y04.0
  legal intervention — *see* Legal, intervention, manhandling

Manslaughter (nonaccidental) — *see* Assault

Mauled by animal NEC W55.89

Medical procedure, complication of (delayed or as an abnormal reaction without mention of misadventure) — *see* Complication of or following, by specified type of procedure
  due to or as a result of misadventure — *see* Misadventure

Melting (due to fire) (*see also* Exposure, fire)
  apparel NEC X06.3
  clothes, clothing NEC X06.3
    nightwear X05
  fittings or furniture (burning building) (uncontrolled fire) X00.8
  nightwear X05
  plastic jewelry X06.1

Mental cruelty — *see* Maltreatment

Military operations (on military property) (to military personnel) (injury) (by) (in) Y37.9
  air blast Y37.2
  aircraft Y37.1
  asphyxia from
    chemical (weapons) Y37.7
    fire, conflagration Y37.3
      from nuclear explosion Y37.5
    gas or fumes Y37.7
  battle wound NEC Y37.9
  bayonet Y37.4

Military operations — *continued*
  biological warfare agents Y37.6
  blast (air) (effects) Y37.2
    from nuclear explosion Y37.5
    underwater Y37.0
  bomb (antipersonnel) (mortar) (explosion) (fragments) Y37.2
  bullet(s) (from carbine, machine gun, pistol, rifle, shotgun) Y37.4
  burn from
    chemical Y37.7
    fire, conflagration Y37.3
      from nuclear explosion Y37.5
    gas Y37.7
  burning aircraft Y37.1
  chemical Y37.7
  conventional warfare, specified form NEC Y37.4
  crushing by falling aircraft Y37.1
  depth-charge Y37.0
  destruction of aircraft Y37.1
  disability as sequela one year or more after
    injury — *see* Y37 with terminal digit of 7 or 8
  drowning Y37.4
  effect (direct) (secondary) nuclear weapon Y37.5
  explosion Y37.2
    after cessation of hostilities Y37.8
    aircraft Y37.1
    antipersonnel bomb Y37.2
    artillery shell Y37.2
      sea-based Y37.0
    bomb (antipersonnel) (mortar) Y37.2
      atom Y37.5
      hydrogen Y37.5
      nuclear Y37.5
    depth-charge Y37.0
    grenade Y37.2
    guided missile Y37.2
    injury by fragments from Y37.2
    land-mine Y37.2
    marine weapon Y37.0
    mine (land) Y37.2
      at sea or in harbor Y37.0
      marine Y37.0
    missile (explosive) NEC Y37.2
    mortar bomb Y37.2
    munitions (accidental) (being used in war) (dump) (factory) Y37.2
    nuclear (weapon) Y37.5
    own weapons (accidental) Y37.2
    rocket Y37.2
    sea-based artillery shell Y37.0
    torpedo Y37.0
  exposure to ionizing radiation from nuclear explosion Y37.5
  falling aircraft Y37.1
  fire Y37.3
  firearm discharge Y37.4
    stated as undetermined whether accidental or intentional Y23.4
  fireball effects from nuclear explosion Y37.5
  fragments from shell, bomb, grenade, guided missile, mine, rocket, shrapnel Y37.2
  gas or fumes Y37.7
  grenade (explosion) (fragments) Y37.2
  guided missile (explosion) (fragments) Y37.2
    nuclear Y37.5
  heat Y37.3
    due to
      nuclear explosion Y37.5
  land-mine (explosion) (fragments) Y37.2
  laser(s) Y37.7
  late effect of — *see* Y37 with terminal digit of 7 or 8
  lewisite Y37.7
  lung irritant (chemical) (fumes) (gas) Y37.7
  marine mine Y37.0
  mine Y37.2
    at sea Y37.0
    in harbor Y37.0
    land (explosion) (fragments) Y37.2
    marine Y37.0
  missile (guided) (explosion) (fragments) Y37.2
    marine Y37.0
    nuclear Y37.5
  mortar bomb (explosion) (fragments) Y37.2
  mustard gas Y37.7

Military operations — *continued*
  nerve gas Y37.7
  nuclear weapons Y37.5
  phosgene Y37.7
  poisoning (chemical) (fumes) (gas) Y37.7
  radiation, ionizing from nuclear explosion Y37.5
  rocket (explosion) (fragments) Y37.2
  saber, sabre Y37.4
  screening smoke Y37.7
  shell (aircraft) (artillery) (cannon) (land-based) (explosion) (fragments) Y37.2
    sea-based Y37.0
  shooting Y37.4
    bullet(s) Y37.4
    pellet(s) (rifle) (shotgun) Y37.4
  shrapnel Y37.2
  specified NEC Y37.8
  submersion Y37.4
  torpedo Y37.0
  unconventional warfare NEC Y37.7
    biological (warfare) Y37.6
    gas, fumes, chemicals Y37.7
    laser(s) Y37.7
    nuclear weapon Y37.5
    specified NEC Y37.7
  underwater blast Y37.0
  vesicant (chemical) (fumes) (gas) Y37.7
  weapon burst Y37.2

Misadventure(s) to patient(s) during surgical or medical care Y69
  contaminated medical or biological substance (blood, drug, fluid) Y64.9
    administered (by) NEC Y64.9
      immunization Y64.1
      infusion Y64.0
      injection Y64.1
      specified means NEC Y64.8
      transfusion Y64.0
      vaccination Y64.1
  excessive amount of blood or other fluid during transfusion or infusion Y63.0
  failure
    in dosage Y63.9
      electroshock therapy Y63.4
      inappropriate temperature (too hot or too cold) in local application and packing Y63.5
      infusion
        excessive amount of fluid Y63.0
        incorrect dilution of fluid Y63.1
      insulin-shock therapy Y63.4
      nonadministration of necessary drug or biological substance Y63.6
      overdose — *see* Table of Drugs and Chemicals
      radiation, in therapy Y63.2
      radiation
        overdose Y63.2
      specified procedure NEC Y63.8
      transfusion
        excessive amount of blood Y63.0
    mechanical, of instrument or apparatus (any) (during any procedure) Y65.8
    sterile precautions (during procedure) Y62.9
      aspiration of fluid or tissue (by puncture or catheterization, except heart) Y62.6
      biopsy (except needle aspiration) Y62.8
        needle (aspirating) Y62.6
      blood sampling Y62.6
      catheterization Y62.6
        heart Y62.5
      dialysis (kidney) Y62.2
      endoscopic examination Y62.4
      enema Y62.8
      immunization Y62.3
      infusion Y62.1
      injection Y62.3
      needle biopsy Y62.6
      paracentesis (abdominal) (thoracic) Y62.6
      perfusion Y62.2
      puncture (lumbar) Y62.6
      removal of catheter or packing Y62.8
      specified procedure NEC Y62.8
      surgical operation Y62.0

Misadventure(s) to patient(s) during surgical or medical care — continued
failure — continued
  sterile precautions — continued
    transfusion Y62.1
    vaccination Y62.3
  suture or ligature during surgical procedure Y65.2
  to introduce or to remove tube or instrument — see Failure, to
hemorrhage — see Misadventure, cut, by type of procedure
inadvertent exposure of patient to radiation Y63.3
inappropriate
  operation performed Y65.5
  temperature (too hot or too cold) in local application or packing Y63.5
infusion (see also Misadventure, by type, infusion) Y69
  excessive amount of fluid Y63.0
  incorrect dilution of fluid Y63.1
  wrong fluid Y65.1
mismatched blood in transfusion Y65.0
nonadministration of necessary drug or biological substance Y63.6
overdose — see Table of Drugs and Chemicals
  radiation (in therapy) Y63.2
perforation — see Misadventure, cut, by type of procedure
performance of inappropriate operation Y65.5
puncture — see Misadventure, cut, by type of procedure
specified type NEC Y65.8
  failure
    suture or ligature during surgical operation Y65.2
    to introduce or to remove tube or instrument — see Failure, to
  infusion of wrong fluid Y65.1
  performance of inappropriate operation Y65.5
  transfusion of mismatched blood Y65.0
  wrong
    fluid in infusion Y65.1
    placement of endotracheal tube during anesthetic procedure Y65.3
transfusion — see Misadventure, by type, transfusion
  excessive amount of blood Y63.0
  mismatched blood Y65.0
wrong
  drug given in error — see Table of Drugs and Chemicals
  fluid in infusion Y65.1
  placement of endotracheal tube during anesthetic procedure Y65.3

Mismatched blood in transfusion Y65.0
Motion (effects) (sickness) X51.8
accident — see Accident, transport, by type of vehicle
airplane X51.0
boat X51.4
bus X51.3
car X51.2
specified vehicle NEC X51.8
train X51.1
Mountain sickness W94.11
Mudslide (of cataclysmic nature) — see Landslide
Murder (attempt) — see Assault

N
Nail, contact with W45.0
gun W29.4
Neglect (criminal) (homicidal intent) — see Maltreatment
Noise (causing injury) (pollution) W42.9
supersonic W42.0
Nonadministration (of)
drug or biological substance (necessary) Y63.6
surgical and medical care Y66
Nosocomial condition Y95

O
Object
falling
  from, in, on, hitting
    machinery — see Contact, with, by type of machine
set in motion by
  accidental explosion or rupture of pressure vessel W38
  firearm — see Discharge, firearm, by type
  machine(ry) — see Contact, with, by type of machine
Overdose (drug) — see Table of Drugs and Chemicals
radiation Y63.2
Overexertion (lifting) (pulling) (pushing) X50.00
hobby related X50.02
specified activity NEC X50.09
sports related X50.01
Overexposure (accidental) (to)
cold (see also Exposure, cold) X31
  due to man-made conditions — see Exposure, cold, man-made
heat (see also Heat) X30
radiation — see Radiation
radioactivity W88.0
sun (sunburn) X32
weather NEC — see Forces of nature
wind NEC — see Forces of nature
Overheated — see Heat
Overlaid W75
Overturning (accidental)
machinery — see Contact, with, by type of machine
transport vehicle NEC (see also Accident, transport) V89.9
watercraft (causing drowning, submersion) — see also Drowning, due to, accident to, watercraft, overturning
  causing injury except drowning or submersion — see Accident, watercraft, causing, injury NEC

P
Parachute descent (voluntary) (without accident to aircraft) V97.29
due to accident to aircraft — see Accident, transport, aircraft
Pecked by bird W64
Perforation during medical or surgical treatment as misadventure — see Misadventure, cut, by type of procedure
Piercing — see Contact, with, by type of object or machine
Pinched
between objects (moving) (stationary and moving) W23.0
  stationary W23.1
in object W23.2
Pinned under machine(ry) — see Contact, with, by type of machine
Place of occurrence Y92.89
abandoned house Y92.89
airplane Y92.813
airport Y92.520
amusement park Y92.831
apartment (co-op) — see Place of occurrence, residence, apartment
assembly hall Y92.29
bank Y92.510
barn Y92.71
baseball field Y92.320
basketball court Y92.310
beach Y92.832
boarding house — see Place of occurrence, residence, boarding house
boat Y92.814
bowling alley Y92.39
bridge Y92.89
building under construction Y92.61
bus Y92.811
  station Y92.521
cafe Y92.511
campsite Y92.833

Place of occurrence — continued
campus — see Place of occurrence, school
canal Y92.89
car Y92.810
casino Y92.59
children's home — see Place of occurrence, residence, institutional, orphanage
church Y92.22
cinema Y92.26
clubhouse Y92.29
coal pit Y92.64
college (community) Y92.214
condominium — see Place of occurrence, residence, apartment
construction area — see Place of occurrence, industrial and construction area
convalescent home — see Place of occurrence, residence, institutional, nursing home
court-house Y92.240
cricket ground Y92.328
cultural building Y92.258
  art gallery Y92.250
  museum Y92.251
  music hall Y92.252
  opera house Y92.253
  specified NEC Y92.258
  theater Y92.254
dancehall Y92.252
day nursery Y92.210
derelict house Y92.89
desert Y92.820
dock NOS Y92.89
dockyard Y92.62
dormitory — see Place of occurrence, residence, institutional, school dormitory
dry dock Y92.62
factory (building) (premises) Y92.63
farm (land under cultivation) (outbuildings) Y92.79
  barn Y92.71
  chicken coop Y92.72
  field Y92.73
  hen house Y92.72
  house — see Place of occurrence, residence, house
  orchard Y92.74
  specified NEC Y92.79
football field Y92.321
forest Y92.821
freeway Y92.411
gallery Y92.250
garage (commercial) Y92.59
  boarding house Y92.044
  military base Y92.135
  mobile home Y92.025
  nursing home Y92.124
  orphanage Y92.114
  private house Y92.015
  reform school Y92.155
gas station Y92.524
gasworks Y92.69
golf course Y92.39
gravel pit Y92.64
grocery Y92.512
gymnasium Y92.39
handball court Y92.318
harbor Y92.89
harness racing course Y92.39
highway (interstate) Y92.411
hill Y92.828
hockey rink Y92.330
home — see Place of occurrence, residence
hospice — see Place of occurrence, residence, institutional, nursing home
hospital Y92.239
  cafeteria Y92.233
  corridor Y92.232
  operating room Y92.234
  patient
    bathroom Y92.231
    room Y92.230
  specified NEC Y92.238
hotel Y92.59
house — see also Place of occurrence, residence
  abandoned Y92.89
  under construction Y92.61

Place of occurrence — *continued*
sports area — *continued*
skating rink (roller) Y92.331
ice Y92.330
stadium Y92.39
swimming pool Y92.34
squash court Y92.311
stadium Y92.39
steeplechasing course Y92.39
store Y92.512
stream Y92.828
street and highway Y92.410
bike path Y92.482
freeway Y92.411
highway ramp Y92.415
interstate highway Y92.411
local residential or business street Y92.414
motorway Y92.411
parkway Y92.412
parking lot Y92.481
sidewalk Y92.480
specified NEC Y92.488
state road Y92.413
subway car Y92.816
supermarket Y92.512
swamp Y92.828
swimming pool (public) Y92.34
private (at) Y92.095
boarding house Y92.045
military base Y92.136
mobile home Y92.026
nursing home Y92.125
orphanage Y92.115
prison Y92.146
reform school Y92.156
single family residence Y92.016
synagogue Y92.22
television station Y92.59
tennis court Y92.312
theater Y92.254
trade area Y92.59
bank Y92.510
cafe Y92.511
casino Y92.59
garage Y92.59
hotel Y92.59
market Y92.512
office building Y92.59
radio station Y92.59
restaurant Y92.511
shop Y92.513
shopping mall Y92.59
store Y92.512
supermarket Y92.512
television station Y92.59
warehouse Y92.59
trailer park, residential — *see* Place of occurrence, residence, mobile home
trailer site NOS Y92.89
train Y92.815
station Y92.522
truck Y92.812
tunnel under construction Y92.69
university Y92.214
vehicle (transport) Y92.818
airplane Y92.813
boat Y92.814
bus Y92.811
car Y92.810
specified NEC Y92.818
subway car Y92.816
train Y92.815
truck Y92.812
warehouse Y92.59
water reservoir Y92.89
wilderness area Y92.828
desert Y92.820
forest Y92.821
marsh Y92.828
mountain Y92.828
prairie Y92.828
specified NEC Y92.828
swamp Y92.828
workshop Y92.69
yard, private Y92.096
boarding house Y92.046
single family house Y92.017

Place of occurrence — *continued*
yard, private — *continued*
mobile home Y92.027
youth center Y92.29
zoo Y92.89
Plumbism — *see* Table of Drugs and Chemicals, lead
Poisoning (accidental) (by) — *see also* Table of Drugs and Chemicals
by plant, thorns, spines, sharp leaves or other mechanisms NEC X58.8
carbon monoxide
generated by
motor vehicle — *see* Accident, transport
watercraft (in transit) (not in transit) V93.89
ferry boat V93.81
fishing boat V93.82
jet skis V93.83
liner V93.81
merchant ship V93.80
passenger ship V93.81
powered craft NEC V93.83
caused by injection of poisons into skin by plant thorns, spines, sharp leaves X58.8
marine or sea plants (venomous) X58.8
exhaust gas
generated by
motor vehicle — *see* Accident, transport
watercraft (in transit) (not in transit) V93.89
ferry boat V93.81
fishing boat V93.82
jet skis V93.83
liner V93.81
merchant ship V93.80
passenger ship V93.81
powered craft NEC V93.83
fumes or smoke due to
explosion (*see also* Explosion) W40.9
fire — *see* Exposure, fire
ignition — *see* Ignition
gas
in legal intervention — *see* Legal, intervention, gas
legal execution Y35.91
in war operations (chemical weapons) Y36.7
legal
execution Y35.91
intervention by gas — *see* Legal, intervention, gas
Premature cessation (of) **surgical and medical care** Y66
Privation (food) (water) X58.8
due to abandonment or neglect — *see* Maltreatment
Prolonged
sitting in transport vehicle — *see* Travel, by type of vehicle
stay in
high altitude as cause of anoxia, barodontalgia, barotitis or hypoxia W94.11
weightless environment X52
Pulling, excessive — *see* Overexertion
Puncture, puncturing — *see also* Contact, with, by type of object or machine
by
plant thorns, spines, sharp leaves or other mechanisms NEC W60
during medical or surgical treatment as misadventure — *see* Misadventure, cut, by type of procedure
Pushed, pushing (accidental) (injury in) (overexertion) — *see also* Overexertion
by other person(s) (accidental) W51
with fall W03
due to ice or snow W00.0
as, or caused by, a crowd or human stampede (with fall) W52
before moving object Y02
motor vehicle Y03.1
from
high place NEC
in accidental circumstances W17.8

Pushed, pushing — *continued*
by other person(s) — *continued*
from — *continued*
high place NEC — *continued*
stated as
intentional, homicide (attempt) Y01
undetermined whether accidental or intentional Y30
transport vehicle NEC (*see also* Accident, transport) V89.9
stated as
intentional, homicide (attempt) Y08.89

R

Radiation (exposure to)
arc lamps W89.0
atomic power plant (malfunction) NEC W88.1
complication of or abnormal reaction to medical radiotherapy Y84.2
electromagnetic, ionizing W88.0
gamma rays W88.1
in
war operations (from or following nuclear explosion) — *see also* War operation, nuclear weapons
laser(s) Y36.7
inadvertent exposure of patient (receiving test or therapy) Y63.3
infrared (heaters and lamps) W90.1
excessive heat from W92
ionized, ionizing (particles, artificially accelerated)
radioisotopes W88.1
x-rays W88.0
isotopes, radioactive — *see* Radiation, radioactive isotopes
laser(s) W90.2
in war operations Y36.7
misadventure in medical care Y63.2
light sources (man-made visible and ultraviolet) W89.9
natural X32
specified NEC W89.8
tanning bed W89.1
welding light W89.0
man-made visible light W89.9
specified NEC W89.8
tanning bed W89.1
welding light W89.0
microwave W90.8
misadventure in medical or surgical procedure Y63.2
natural NEC X39.08
radon X39.01
overdose (in medical or surgical procedure) Y63.2
radar W90.0
radioactive isotopes (any) W88.1
atomic power plant malfunction W88.1
misadventure in medical or surgical treatment Y63.2
radiofrequency W90.0
radium NEC W88.1
sun X32
ultraviolet (light) (man-made) W89.9
natural X32
specified NEC W89.8
tanning bed W89.1
welding light W89.0
welding arc, torch, or light W89.0
excessive heat from W92
x-rays (hard) (soft) W88.0
Range disease W94.11
Rape (attempted) Y05
Rat bite W53.11
Reaction, abnormal to medical procedure (*see also* Complication of or following, by type of procedure) Y84.9
with misadventure — *see* Misadventure
biologicals — *see* Table of Drugs and Chemicals
drugs — *see* Table of Drugs and Chemicals
vaccine — *see* Table of Drugs and Chemicals

©2002 Ingenix, Inc.

Reduction in
  atmospheric pressure — *see* Air, pressure, change
Repetitive movements X50.10
  hobby related X50.12
  specified activity NEC X50.19
  sports related X50.11
Rock falling on or hitting (accidentally) (person) W20.8
  in cave-in W20.0
Rowing, excessive X50.01
Run over (accidentally) (by)
  animal (not being ridden) NEC W55.89
    being ridden V06
  machinery — *see* Contact, with, by specified type of machine
  transport vehicle NEC (*see also* Accident, transport) V09.9
    intentional homicide (attempt) Y03.0
    motor NEC V09.20
      intentional homicide (attempt) Y03.0
Running
  before moving object X81
    motor vehicle X82.3
  excessive X50.01
Running off, away
  animal (being ridden) (*see also* Accident, transport) V80.918
    not being ridden W55.89
  animal-drawn vehicle NEC (*see also* Accident, transport) V80.928
  highway, road(way), street
    transport vehicle NEC (*see also* Accident, transport) V89.9
Rupture pressurized devices — *see* Explosion, by type of device

S

Saturnism — *see* Table of Drugs and Chemicals, lead
Scald, scalding (accidental) (by) (from) (in) X19
  air (hot) X14.1
  gases (hot) X14.1
  homicide (attempt) — *see* Assault, burning, hot object
  inflicted by other person
    stated as intentional, homicide (attempt) — *see* Assault, burning, hot object
  liquid (boiling) (hot) NEC X12
    stated as undetermined whether accidental or intentional Y27.2
    suicide (attempt) X77.2
  local application of externally applied substance in medical or surgical care Y63.5
  metal (molten) (liquid) (hot) NEC X18
  self-inflicted X77.9
  stated as undetermined whether accidental or intentional Y27.8
  steam X13.1
    assault X98.0
    stated as undetermined whether accidental or intentional Y27.0
    suicide (attempt) X77.0
  suicide (attempt) X77.9
  vapor (hot) X13.1
    assault X98.0
    stated as undetermined whether accidental or intentional Y27.0
    suicide (attempt) X77.0
Scratched by
  cat W55.03
  person(s) (accidentally) W50.4
    with intent to injure or kill Y04.0
    as, or caused by, a crowd or human stampede (with fall) W52
    assault Y04.0
    homicide (attempt) Y04.0
    in
      fight Y04.0
      legal intervention Y35.894
        injuring
          bystander Y35.892
          law enforcement personnel Y35.891
          suspect Y35.890

Seasickness X51.4
Self-harm NEC — *see also* External cause by type, undetermined whether accidental or intentional
  intentional — *see* Suicide
  poisoning NEC — *see* Table of drugs and biologicals, accident
Self-inflicted (injury) **NEC** — *see also* External cause by type, undetermined whether accidental or intentional
  intentional — *see* Suicide
  poisoning NEC — *see* Table of drugs and biologicals, accident
Sequelae (of)
  accident NEC — *see* W00-X58 with q as terminal character
  assault (homicidal) (any means) — *see* X92-Y08 with q as terminal character
  homicide, attempt (any means) — *see* X92-Y08 with q as terminal character
  injury undetermined whether accidentally or purposely inflicted — *see* Y21-Y33 with q as terminal character
  intentional self-harm (classifiable to X71-X83) — *see* X71-X83 with q as terminal character
  legal intervention — *see* Y35 with q as terminal character
  motor vehicle accident — *see* V00-V99 with q as terminal character
  suicide, attempt (any means) — *see* X71-X83 with q as terminal character
  transport accident — *see* V00-V99 with q as terminal character
  war operations — *see* Y36 with terminal digit of 7 or 8
Shock
  electric — *see* Exposure, electric current
  from electric appliance (any) (faulty) W86.8
    domestic W86.0
    suicide (attempt) X83.1
Shooting, shot (accidental(ly)) — *see also* Discharge, firearm, by type
  herself or himself — *see* Discharge, firearm by type, self-inflicted
  homicide (attempt) — *see* Discharge, firearm by type, homicide
  in war operations Y36.4
  inflicted by other person — *see* Discharge, firearm by type, homicide
    accidental — *see* Discharge, firearm, by type of firearm
    legal
    execution Y35.91
    intervention — *see* Legal, intervention, firearm
  self-inflicted — *see* Discharge, firearm by type, suicide
    accidental — *see* Discharge, firearm, by type of firearm
  suicide (attempt) — *see* Discharge, firearm by type, suicide
Shoving (accidentally) **by other person** — *see* Pushing, by other person
Sickness
  air X51.0
  alpine W94.11
  car X51.2
  motion — *see* Motion
  mountain W94.11
  sea X51.4
  travel — *see* Travel
Sinking (accidental)
  watercraft (causing drowning, submersion) — *see also* Drowning, due to, accident to, watercraft, sinking
    causing injury except drowning or submersion — *see* Accident, watercraft, causing, injury NEC
Siriasis X32
Slashed wrists — *see* Cut, selfinflicted

Slipping (accidental) (on same level) (with fall) W01.0
  on
    ice W00.0
      with skates — *see* Accident, transport, pedestrian, conveyance
    mud W01.0
    oil W01.0
    snow W00.0
      with skis — *see* Accident, transport, pedestrian, conveyance
    surface (slippery) (wet) NEC W01.0
Sliver, wood, contact with W45.8
Smoldering (due to fire) — *see* Exposure, fire
Sodomy (attempted) **by force** Y05
Sound waves (causing injury) W42.9
  supersonic W42.0
Splinter, contact with W45.8
Stab, stabbing — *see* Cut
Starvation X58.8
  due to abandonment or neglect — *see* Maltreatment
Stepped on
  by
    animal (not being ridden) NEC W55.89
      being ridden V06
    crowd or human stampede W52
    person W50.0
Stepping on
  object W22.8
    with fall W18.9
    sports equipment W21.9
    stationary W22.09
      sports equipment W21.89
  person W51
    by crowd or human stampede W52
  sports equipment W21.9
Sting
  arthropod, nonvenomous W57
  insect, nonvenomous W57
Storm (cataclysmic) — *see* Forces of nature, cataclysmic storm
Straining, excessive — *see* Overexertion
Strangling — *see* Strangulation
Strangulation (accidental) W76
  by, due to, in
    baby carriage W75
    bed, bed linen W75
    bib W76
    blanket W75
    cot, cradle W75
    other person NEC W76
      in bed W75
    perambulator W75
    pillow W75
    sheet (plastic) W75
    specified cause NEC W76
  self-inflicted
    accidental W76
Strenuous movements — *see* Repetitive movements
Striking against
  airbag (automobile) W22.10
    driver side W22.11
    front passenger side W22.12
    specified NEC W22.19
  bottom when
    diving or jumping into water (in) W16.822
      causing drowning W16.821
      from boat W16.722
        causing drowning W16.721
      natural body W16.622
        causing drowning W16.821
      swimming pool W16.522
        causing drowning W16.521
    falling into water (in) W16.322
      causing drowning W16.321
    fountain — *see* Striking against, bottom when, falling into water, specified NEC
    natural body W16.122
      causing drowning W16.121

Striking against — *continued*
  bottom when — *continued*
    reservoir — *see* Striking against, bottom
      when, falling into water, specified
      NEC
    specified NEC W16.322
      causing drowning W16.321
    swimming pool W16.022
      causing drowning W16.021
  diving board (swimming pool) W21.4
  object W22.8
    with
      drowning or submersion — *see* Drowning
      fall — *see* Fall, due to, bumping against,
        object
      caused by crowd or human stampede (with
        fall) W52
    furniture W22.03
    lamppost W22.02
    sports equipment W21.9
    stationary W22.09
      sports equipment W21.89
    wall W22.01
  person(s) W51
    with fall W03
      due to ice or snow W00.0
    as, or caused by, a crowd or human
      stampede (with fall) W52
    assault Y04.2
    homicide (attempt) Y04.2
  sports equipment W21.9
  wall (when) W22.01
    diving or jumping into water (in) W16.832
      causing drowning W16.831
      swimming pool W16.532
        causing drowning W16.531
    falling into water (in) W16.332
      causing drowning W16.331
      fountain — *see* Striking against, wall
        when, falling into water, specified
        NEC
      natural body W16.132
        causing drowning W16.131
      reservoir — *see* Striking against, wall
        when, falling into water, specified
        NEC
      specified NEC W16.332
        causing drowning W16.331
      swimming pool W16.032
        causing drowning W16.031
    swimming pool (when) W22.042
      causing drowning W22.041
      diving or jumping into water W16.532
        causing drowning W16.531
      falling into water W16.032
        causing drowning W16.031

Struck (accidentally) by
  airbag (automobile) W22.10
    driver side W22.11
    front passenger side W22.12
    specified NEC W22.19
  alligator W58.02
  animal (not being ridden) NEC W55.89
    being ridden V06
  avalanche — *see* Landslide
  ball (hit) (thrown) W21.00
    assault Y08.09
    baseball W21.03
    basketball W21.05
    golf ball W21.04
    football W21.01
    soccer W21.02
    softball W21.07
    specified NEC W21.09
    volleyball W21.06
  bat or racquet
    baseball bat W21.11
      assault Y08.02
    golf club W21.13
      assault Y08.09
    specified NEC W21.19
      assault Y08.09
    tennis racquet W21.12
      assault Y08.09
  bullet — *see also* Discharge, firearm by type
    in war operations Y36.4

Struck by — *continued*
  crocodile W58.12
  dog W54.1
  flare, Very pistol — *see* Discharge, firearm NEC
  hailstones X39.8
  hockey (ice)
    field
      puck W21.221
      stick W21.211
    puck W21.220
    stick W21.210
      assault Y08.01
  landslide — *see* Landslide
  law-enforcement agent (on duty) — *see* Legal,
    intervention, manhandling
    with blunt object — *see* Legal, intervention,
      blunt object
  lightning X33
    causing fire — *see* Exposure, fire
  machine — *see* Contact, with, by type of
    machine
  mammal NEC W55.89
    marine W56.89
  marine animal W56.89
  missile
    firearm — *see* Discharge, firearm by type
    in war operations — *see* War operations,
      missile
  object W22.8
    blunt W22.8
      assault Y00
      suicide (attempt) X79
      undetermined whether accidental or
        intentional Y29
    falling W20.8
      from, in, on
        building W20.1
          burning (uncontrolled fire) X00.4
        cataclysmic
          earth surface movement NEC — *see*
            Landslide
          storm — *see* Forces of nature,
            cataclysmic storm
        cave-in W20.0
        earthquake X34
        machine (in operation) — *see* Contact,
          with, by type of machine
        structure W20.1
          burning X00.4
        transport vehicle (in motion) — *see*
          Accident, transport, by type of
          vehicle
    watercraft V93.49
      due to
        accident to craft V91.39
          powered craft V91.33
            ferry boat V91.31
            fishing boat V91.32
            jetskis V91.33
            liner V91.31
            merchant ship V91.30
            passenger ship V91.31
          unpowered craft V91.38
            canoe V91.35
            inflatable V91.36
            kayak V91.35
            sailboat V91.34
            surf-board V91.38
            windsurfer V91.38
        powered craft V93.43
          ferry boat V93.41
          fishing boat V93.42
          jetskis V93.43
          liner V93.41
          merchant ship V93.40
          passenger ship V93.41
        unpowered craft V93.48
          sailboat V93.44
          surf-board V93.48
          windsurfer V93.48
    moving NEC W20.8
    projected W20.8
      assault Y00
      in sports W21.9
        assault Y08.09

Struck by — *continued*
  object — *continued*
    projected — *continued*
      in sports — *continued*
        ball W21.00
          baseball W21.03
          basketball W21.05
          football W21.01
          golf ball W21.04
          soccer W21.02
          softball W21.07
          specified NEC W21.09
          volleyball W21.06
        bat or racquet
          baseball bat W21.11
            assault Y08.02
          golf club W21.13
            assault Y08.09
          specified NEC W21.19
            assault Y08.09
          tennis racquet W21.12
            assault Y08.09
        hockey (ice)
          field
            puck W21.221
            stick W21.211
          puck W21.220
          stick W21.210
            assault Y08.01
        specified NEC W21.89
    set in motion by explosion — *see* Explosion
    thrown W20.8
      assault Y00
      in sports W21.9
        assault Y08.09
      ball W21.00
        baseball W21.03
        basketball W21.05
        football W21.01
        golf ball W21.04
        soccer W21.02
        soft ball W21.07
        specified NEC W21.09
        volleyball W21.06
      bat or racquet
        baseball bat W21.11
          assault Y08.02
        golf club W21.13
          assault Y08.09
        specified NEC W21.19
          assault Y08.09
        tennis racquet W21.12
          assault Y08.09
      hockey (ice)
        field
          puck W21.221
          stick W21.211
        puck W21.220
        stick W21.210
          assault Y08.01
      specified NEC W21.89
  other person(s) W50.0
    with
      blunt object W22.8
        intentional, homicide (attempt) Y00
        sports equipment W21.9
        undetermined whether accidental or
          intentional Y29
      fall W03
        due to ice or snow W00.0
    as, or caused by, a crowd or human
      stampede (with fall) W52
    assault Y04.2
    homicide (attempt) Y04.2
    in legal intervention Y35.814
      injuring
        bystander Y35.813
        law enforcement personnel Y35.812
        suspect Y35.811
    sports equipment W21.9
  police (on duty) — *see* Legal, intervention,
    manhandling
    with blunt object — *see* Legal, intervention,
      blunt object

©2002 Ingenix, Inc.

Struck by — *continued*
 sports equipment W21.9
  assault Y08.09
  ball W21.00
   baseball W21.03
   basketball W21.05
   football W21.01
   golf ball W21.04
   soccer W21.02
   soft ball W21.07
   specified NEC W21.09
   volleyball W21.06
  bat or racquet
   baseball bat W21.11
    assault Y08.02
   golf club W21.13
    assault Y08.09
   specified NEC W21.19
   tennis racquet W21.12
    assault Y08.09
  cleats (shoe) W21.31
  foot wear NEC W21.39
  football helmet W21.81
  hockey (ice)
   field
    puck W21.221
    stick W21.211
   puck W21.220
   stick W21.210
    assault Y08.01
  skate blades W21.32
  specified NEC W21.89
   assault Y08.09
 thunderbolt X33
  causing fire — *see* Exposure, fire
 transport vehicle NEC (*see also* Accident, transport) V09.9
  intentional, homicide (attempt) Y03.0
  motor NEC (*see also* Accident, transport) V09.20
   homicide Y03.0
 vehicle (transport) NEC — *see* Accident, transport, by type of vehicle
  stationary (falling from jack, hydraulic lift, ramp) W20.8
Stumbling
 over
  animal NEC W64
   with fall W18.09
  carpet, rug or (small) object W22.8
   with fall W18.09
  person W51
   with fall W03
    due to ice or snow W00.0
Submersion (accidental) — *see* Drowning
Suffocation (accidental) (by external means) (by pressure) (mechanical)
 due to, by
  another person in bed W75
  avalanche — *see* Landslide
  bed, bed linen W75
  bib W76
  blanket W75
  cave-in W77
   caused by cataclysmic earth surface movement — *see* Landslide
  explosion — *see* Explosion
  falling earth, other substance W77
  fire — *see* Exposure, fire
  food, any type (aspiration) (ingestion) (inhalation) W79
  ignition — *see* Ignition
  landslide — *see* Landslide
  machine(ry) — *see* Contact, with, by type of machine
  pillow W75
  sheet (plastic) W75
  vomitus (aspiration) (inhalation) W78
 in
  baby carriage W75
  bed W75
  burning building X00.8
  cot, cradle W75
  perambulator W75
 infant while asleep W75

Suicide, suicidal (attempted) (by) X83.8
 blunt object X79
 burning, burns X76
  hot object X77.9
   fluid NEC X77.2
   household appliance X77.3
   specified NEC X77.8
   steam X77.0
   tap water X77.1
   vapors X77.0
 caustic substance — *see* Table of Drugs and Chemicals
 cold, extreme X83.2
 collision of motor vehicle with
  motor vehicle X82.0
  specified NEC X82.8
  train X82.1
  tree X82.2
 crashing of aircraft X83.0
 cut (any part of body) X78.9
 cutting or piercing instrument X78.9
  dagger X78.2
  glass X78.0
  knife X78.1
  specified NEC X78.8
  sword X78.2
 drowning (in) X71.9
  bathtub X71.0
  natural water X71.3
  specified NEC X71.8
  swimming pool X71.1
   following fall X71.2
 electrocution X83.1
 explosive(s) (material) X75
 fire, flames X76
 firearm X74.9
  airgun X74.01
  handgun X72
  hunting rifle X73.1
  larger X73.9
   specified NEC X73.8
  machine gun X73.2
  shotgun X73.0
  specified NEC X74.8
 hanging X83.8
 hot object — *see* Suicide, burning, hot object
 jumping
  before moving object X81
   motor vehicle X82.3
  from high place X80
 late effect of attempt — *see* X71-X83 with q as terminal character
 lying before moving object, train, vehicle X81
 poisoning — *see* Table of Drugs and Chemicals
 puncture (any part of body) — *see* Suicide, cutting or piercing instrument
 scald — *see* Suicide, burning, hot object
 sequelae of attempt — *see* X71-X83 with q as terminal character
 sharp object (any) — *see* Suicide, cutting or piercing instrument
 shooting — *see* Suicide, firearm
 specified means NEC X83.8
 stab (any part of body) — *see* Suicide, cutting or piercing instrument
 steam, hot vapors X77.0
 strangulation X83.8
 submersion — *see* Suicide, drowning
 suffocation X83.8
 wound NEC X83.8
Sunstroke X32
Supersonic waves (causing injury) W42.0
Surgical procedure, complication of (delayed or as an abnormal reaction without mention of misadventure) — *see also* Complication of or following, by type of procedure
 due to or as a result of misadventure — *see* Misadventure
Swallowed, swallowing
 foreign body — *see* Foreign body, alimentary canal
 poison — *see* Table of Drugs and Chemicals
 substance
  caustic or corrosive — *see* Table of Drugs and Chemicals
  poisonous — *see* Table of Drugs and Chemicals

Syndrome
 battered — *see* Maltreatment
 maltreatment — *see* Maltreatment

T

Terrorism (involving) Y38.9
 biological weapons Y38.6
 chemical weapons Y38.7
 conflagration Y38.3
 explosion Y38.2
  destruction of aircraft Y38.1
  marine weapons Y38.0
 fire Y38.3
 firearms Y38.4
 hot substances Y38.3
 nuclear weapons Y38.5
 specified method NEC Y38.8
Tackle in sport W03
Thirst X58.8
Threat to breathing
 aspiration — *see* Aspiration
 due to cave-in, falling earth or substance NEC W77
Thrown (accidentally)
 against part (any) of or object in transport vehicle (in motion) NEC (*see also* Accident, transport)
 from
  high place, homicide (attempt) Y01
  machinery — *see* Contact, with, by type of machine
  transport vehicle NEC (*see also* Accident, transport) V89.9
 off — *see* Thrown, from
Thunderbolt X33
 causing fire — *see* Exposure, fire
Tidal wave (any injury) NEC — *see* Forces of nature, tidal wave
Took
 overdose (drug) — *see* Table of Drugs and Chemicals
 poison — *see* Table of Drugs and Chemicals
Tornado (any injury) X37.1
Torrential rain (any injury) X37.8
Torture — *see* Maltreatment
Trampled by animal NEC W55.89
 being ridden V06
Trapped (accidentally)
 between objects (moving) (stationary and moving) — *see* Caught
 by part (any) of
  motorcycle V29.88
  pedal cycle V19.88
  transport vehicle NEC (*see also* Accident, transport) V89.9
Travel (effects) (sickness) X51.8
 accident — *see* Accident, transport, by type of vehicle
 airplane X51.0
 boat X51.4
 bus X51.3
 car X51.2
 specified vehicle NEC X51.8
 train X51.1
Tree falling on or hitting (accidentally) (person) W20.8
Tripping
 over
  animal W64
   with fall W01.0
  carpet, rug or (small) object W22.8
   with fall W18.09
  person W51
   with fall W03
    due to ice or snow W00.0
Twisted by person(s) (accidentally) W50.2
 with intent to injure or kill Y04.0
 as, or caused by, a crowd or human stampede (with fall) W52
 assault Y04.0
 homicide (attempt) Y04.0

Twisted by person(s) — continued
  in
    fight Y04.0
    legal intervention — *see* Legal, intervention,
      manhandling
Twisting, excessive — *see* Overexertion

U

Undetermined intent (contact) (exposure)
  automobile collision Y32
  blunt object Y29
  drowning (submersion) (in) Y21.9
    bathtub Y21.0
      after fall Y21.1
    natural water (lake) (ocean) (pond) (river)
      (stream) Y21.4
    specified place NEC Y21.8
    swimming pool Y21.2
      after fall Y21.3
  explosive material Y25
  fall, jump or push from high place Y30
  falling, lying or running before moving object
    Y31
  fire Y26
  firearm discharge Y24.9
    airgun (BB) (pellet) Y24.0
    handgun (pistol) (revolver) Y22
    hunting rifle Y23.1
    larger Y23.9
      hunting rifle Y23.1
      machine gun Y23.3
      military Y23.2
      shotgun Y23.0
      specified type NEC Y23.8
    machine gun Y23.3
    military Y23.2
    shotgun Y23.0
    specified type NEC Y24.8
    Very pistol Y24.8
  hot object Y27.9
    fluid NEC Y27.2
    household appliance Y27.3
    specified object NEC Y27.8
    steam Y27.0
    tap water Y27.1
    vapor Y27.0
  jump, fall or push from high place Y30
  lying, falling or running before moving object
    Y31
  motor vehicle crash Y32
  push, fall or jump from high place Y30
  running, falling or lying before moving object
    Y31
  sharp object Y28.9
    dagger Y28.2
    glass Y28.0
    knife Y28.1
    specified object NEC Y28.8
    sword Y28.2
  smoke Y26
  specified event NEC Y33

V

Vibration (causing injury) W49
Victim (of)
  avalanche — *see* Landslide
  earth movements NEC — *see* Forces of nature,
    earth movement
  earthquake X34
  flood — *see* Flood
  landslide — *see* Landslide
  lightning X33
    causing fire — *see* Exposure, fire
  storm (cataclysmic) NEC — *see* Forces of nature,
    cataclysmic storm
  volcanic eruption X35
Volcanic eruption (any injury) X35
Vomitus, gastric contents in air passages (with
  asphyxia, obstruction or suffocation) W78

W

Walked into stationary object (any) W22.09
  furniture W22.03
  lamppost W22.02
  wall W22.01

War operations (during hostilities) (injury) (by) (in)
  Y36.9
  air blast Y36.2
  aircraft
    fixed wing powered
      destruction Y36.128
        shot down Y36.123
      explosion on board Y36.122
      falling and crushing personnel on ground
        Y36.120
      fire on board Y36.121
    helicopter
      destruction Y36.118
        shot down Y36.113
      explosion on board Y36.112
      falling and crushing personnel on ground
        Y36.110
      fire on board Y36.111
    micro-light
      destruction Y36.138
        shot down Y36.133
      explosion on board Y36.132
      falling and crushing personnel on ground
        Y36.130
      fire on board Y36.131
    specified NEC
      destruction Y36.198
        shot down Y36.193
      explosion on board Y36.192
      falling and crushing personnel on ground
        Y36.190
      fire on board Y36.191
    ultra-light
      destruction Y36.138
        shot down Y36.133
      explosion on board Y36.132
      falling and crushing personnel on ground
        Y36.130
      fire on board Y36.131
  asphyxia from
    chemical (weapons) Y36.7
    fire, conflagration — *see also* War operations,
      fire
      from nuclear explosion — *see* War
        operations, nuclear weapons
    gas or fumes Y36.7
  battle wound NEC Y36.9
  bayonet Y36.4
  biological warfare agents Y36.6
  blast (air) (effects) Y36.2
    from nuclear explosion — *see* War
      operations, nuclear weapons
    underwater Y36.0
  bomb (antipersonnel) (mortar) (explosion)
    (fragments) Y36.2
  bullet(s) (from carbine, machine gun, pistol,
    rifle, shotgun) Y36.4
  burn from
    chemical Y36.7
    fire, conflagration — *see also* War operations,
      fire
      from nuclear explosion — *see* War
        operations, nuclear weapons
    gas Y36.7
  burning aircraft — *see* War operations, aircraft
  chemical Y36.7
  conventional warfare, specified form NEC Y36.4
  crushing by falling aircraft Y36.190
    fixed wing powered Y36.120
    helicopter Y36.110
    micro-light or ultra-light Y36.130
    specified NEC Y36.190
  depth-charge Y36.0
  destruction of aircraft — *see* War operations,
    aircraft
  disability as sequela one year or more after
    injury — *see* Y36 with terminal digit of 7
    or 8
  drowning Y36.4
  effect (direct) (secondary) nuclear weapon — *see*
    War operations, nuclear weapons
  explosion Y36.2
    aircraft Y36.192
      fixed wing powered Y36.122
      helicopter Y36.112
      micro-light or ultra-light Y36.132
      specified NEC Y36.192

War operations — continued
  explosion — continued
    antipersonnel bomb Y36.2
    artillery shell Y36.2
      sea-based Y36.0
    bomb (antipersonnel) (mortar) Y36.2
      atom — *see* War operations, nuclear
        weapons
      hydrogen — *see* War operations, nuclear
        weapons
      nuclear — *see* War operations, nuclear
        weapons
    depth-charge Y36.0
    grenade Y36.2
    guided missile Y36.2
    injury by fragments from Y36.2
    land-mine Y36.2
    marine weapon Y36.0
    mine (land) Y36.2
      at sea or in harbor Y36.0
      marine Y36.0
    missile (explosive) NEC — *see* War
      operations, missile
    mortar bomb Y36.2
    munitions (accidental) (being used in war)
      (dump) (factory) Y36.2
    nuclear (weapon) — *see* War operations,
      nuclear weapons
    own weapons (accidental) Y36.2
    rocket Y36.2
    sea-based artillery shell Y36.0
    torpedo Y36.0
  exposure to ionizing radiation from nuclear
    explosion — *see* War operations, nuclear
    weapons
  falling aircraft Y36.190
    fixed wing powered Y36.120
    helicopter Y36.110
    micro-light or ultra-light Y36.130
    specified NEC Y36.190
  fire Y36.35
    due to
      conventional weapon Y36.31
      fire-producing device Y36.32
  firearm discharge Y36.4
  fireball effects from nuclear explosion — *see*
    War operations, nuclear weapons
  fragments from shell, bomb, grenade, guided
    missile, mine, rocket, shrapnel — *see* War
    operations, explosion
  gas or fumes Y36.7
  grenade (explosion) (fragments) Y36.2
  guided missile (explosion) (fragments) Y36.2
    nuclear — *see* War operations, nuclear
      weapons
  heat Y36.35
    due to
      conventional weapon Y36.33
      fire-producing device Y36.34
      nuclear explosion — *see* War operations,
        nuclear weapons
  land-mine (explosion) (fragments) Y36.2
  laser(s) Y36.7
  late effect of — *see* Y36 with terminal digit of 7
    or 8
  lewisite Y36.7
  lung irritant (chemical) (fumes) (gas) Y36.7
  marine mine Y36.0
  mine Y36.2
    at sea Y36.0
    in harbor Y36.0
    land (explosion) (fragments) Y36.2
    marine Y36.0
  missile (guided) (explosion) (fragments) Y36.2
    marine Y36.0
    nuclear — *see* War operations, nuclear
      weapons
  mortar bomb (explosion) (fragments) Y36.2
  mustard gas Y36.7
  nerve gas Y36.7
  nuclear weapons Y36.528
    direct effect Y36.518
      blast effect Y36.510
      fireball effect Y36.512
      heat Y36.513
      radiation exposure Y36.511
      specified NEC Y36.518

War operations — *continued*
  nuclear weapons — *continued*
    secondary effect Y36.528
      blast wave Y36.520
      fire Y36.521
      specified NEC Y36.528
    sequelae Y36.538
      residual radiation exposure Y36.530
      ingestion of radioactivity Y36.531
      inhalation of radioactivity Y36.532
      specified NEC Y36.538
  phosgene Y36.7
  poisoning (chemical) (fumes) (gas) Y36.7
  radiation, ionizing from nuclear explosion — *see*
    War operations, nuclear weapons
  rocket (explosion) (fragments) Y36.2
  saber, sabre Y36.4
  screening smoke Y36.7
  shell (aircraft) (artillery) (cannon) (land-based)
    (explosion) (fragments) Y36.2
    sea-based Y36.0
  shooting Y36.4
    bullet(s) Y36.4
    pellet(s) (rifle) (shotgun) Y36.4
  shrapnel Y36.2
  submersion Y36.4
  torpedo Y36.0
  unconventional warfare NEC Y36.7
    biological (warfare) Y36.6
    gas, fumes, chemicals Y36.7
    laser(s) Y36.7
    nuclear weapon — *see* War operations,
      nuclear weapons
    specified NEC Y36.7
  underwater blast Y36.0
  vesicant (chemical) (fumes) (gas) Y36.7
  weapon burst Y36.2
Washed
  away by flood — *see* Flood
  off road by storm (transport vehicle) — *see*
    Forces of nature, cataclysmic storm
Weather exposure NEC — *see* Forces of nature
Weightlessness (causing injury) (effects of) (in
  spacecraft, real or simulated) X52
Work related condition Y96
Wound (accidental) **NEC** (*see also* Injury) X58.8
  battle (*see also* War operations) Y36.9
  gunshot — *see* Discharge, firearm by type
Wreck transport vehicle NEC (*see also* Accident,
  transport) V89.9
Wrong fluid in infusion Y65.1

CHAPTER I — CERTAIN INFECTIOUS AND PARASITIC DISEASES (A00–B99)

Includes: diseases generally recognized as communicable or transmissible

Use additional code for any associated drug resistance (Z06)

Excludes1:   carrier or suspected carrier of infectious disease (Z22.-)
certain localized infections—see body system-related chapters
infectious and parasitic diseases complicating pregnancy, childbirth and the puerperium (O98.-)
infectious and parasitic diseases specific to the perinatal period (P35-P39)
influenza and other acute respiratory infections (J00-J22)

This chapter contains the following blocks:

A00-A09	Intestinal infectious diseases
A15-A19	Tuberculosis
A20-A28	Certain zoonotic bacterial diseases
A30-A49	Other bacterial diseases
A50-A64	Infections with a predominantly sexual mode of transmission
A65-A69	Other spirochetal diseases
A70-A74	Other diseases caused by chlamydiae
A75-A79	Rickettsioses
A80-A89	Viral infections of the central nervous system
A90-A99	Arthropod-borne viral fevers and viral hemorrhagic fevers
B00-B09	Viral infections characterized by skin and mucous membrane lesions
B15-B19	Viral hepatitis
B20	Human immunodeficiency virus [HIV] disease
B25-B34	Other viral diseases
B35-B49	Mycoses
B50-B64	Protozoal diseases
B65-B83	Helminthiases
B85-B89	Pediculosis, acariasis and other infestations
B90-B94	Sequelae of infectious and parasitic diseases
B95-B97	Bacterial, viral and other infectious agents
B99	Other infectious diseases

INTESTINAL INFECTIOUS DISEASES (A00–A09)

A00 Cholera

A00.0 Cholera due to Vibrio cholerae 01, biovar cholerae
Classical cholera

A00.1 Cholera due to Vibrio cholerae 01, biovar eltor
Cholera eltor

A00.9 Cholera, unspecified

A01 Typhoid and paratyphoid fevers

A01.0 Typhoid fever
Infection due to Salmonella typhi

  A01.00 Typhoid fever, unspecified

  A01.01 Typhoid meningitis

  A01.02 Typhoid fever with heart involvement
    Typhoid endocarditis
    Typhoid myocarditis

  A01.03 Typhoid pneumonia

  A01.04 Typhoid arthritis

  A01.05 Typhoid osteomyelitis

  A01.09 Typhoid fever with other complications

A01.1 Paratyphoid fever A

A01.2 Paratyphoid fever B

A01.3 Paratyphoid fever C

A01.4 Paratyphoid fever, unspecified
Infection due to Salmonella paratyphi NOS

A02 Other salmonella infections
Includes: infection or foodborne intoxication due to any Salmonella species other than S. typhi and S. paratyphi

A02.0 Salmonella enteritis
Salmonellosis

A02.1 Salmonella septicemia

A02.2 Localized salmonella infections

  A02.20 Localized salmonella infection, unspecified

  A02.21 Salmonella meningitis

  A02.22 Salmonella pneumonia

  A02.23 Salmonella arthritis

  A02.24 Salmonella osteomyelitis

  A02.25 Salmonella pyelonephritis
    Salmonella tubulo-interstitial nephropathy

  A02.29 Salmonella with other localized infection

A02.8 Other specified salmonella infections

A02.9 Salmonella infection, unspecified

A03 Shigellosis

A03.0 Shigellosis due to Shigella dysenteriae
Group A shigellosis [Shiga-Kruse dysentery]

A03.1 Shigellosis due to Shigella flexneri
Group B shigellosis

A03.2 Shigellosis due to Shigella boydii
Group C shigellosis

A03.3 Shigellosis due to Shigella sonnei
Group D shigellosis

A03.8 Other shigellosis

A03.9 Shigellosis, unspecified
Bacillary dysentery NOS

A04 Other bacterial intestinal infections
Excludes1:   foodborne intoxications, bacterial (A05.-)
tuberculous enteritis (A18.32)

A04.0 Enteropathogenic Escherichia coli infection

A04.1 Enterotoxigenic Escherichia coli infection

A04.2 Enteroinvasive Escherichia coli infection

A04.3 Enterohemorrhagic Escherichia coli infection

A04.4 Other intestinal Escherichia coli infections
Escherichia coli enteritis NOS

A04.5 Campylobacter enteritis

A04.6 Enteritis due to Yersinia enterocolitica
Excludes1:   extraintestinal yersiniosis (A28.2)

A04.7 Enterocolitis due to Clostridium difficile

A04.8 Other specified bacterial intestinal infections

A04.9 Bacterial intestinal infection, unspecified
Bacterial enteritis NOS

A05 Other bacterial foodborne intoxications
Excludes1:   Escherichia coli infection (A04.0-A04.4)
listeriosis (A32.-)
salmonella foodborne intoxication and infection (A02.-)
toxic effect of noxious foodstuffs (T61-T62)

A05.0 Foodborne staphylococcal intoxication

A05.1 Botulism
Classical foodborne intoxication due to Clostridium botulinum

A05.2 Foodborne Clostridium perfringens [Clostridium welchii] intoxication
Enteritis necroticans
Pig-bel

A05.3 Foodborne Vibrio parahaemolyticus intoxication

A05.4 Foodborne Bacillus cereus intoxication

A05.5 Foodborne Vibrio vulnificus intoxication

A05.8 Other specified bacterial foodborne intoxications

A05.9 Bacterial foodborne intoxication, unspecified

A06 Amebiasis
Includes: infection due to Entamoeba histolytica
Excludes1:   other protozoal intestinal diseases (A07.-)

A06.0 Acute amebic dysentery
Acute amebiasis
Intestinal amebiasis NOS

A06.1 Chronic intestinal amebiasis

A06.2 Amebic nondysenteric colitis

A06.3   **Ameboma of intestine**
     Ameboma NOS

A06.4   **Amebic liver abscess**
     Hepatic amebiasis

A06.5   **Amebic lung abscess**
     Amebic abscess of lung (and liver)

A06.6   **Amebic brain abscess**
     Amebic abscess of brain (and liver) (and lung)

A06.7   **Cutaneous amebiasis**

A06.8   **Amebic infection of other sites**

     A06.81   **Amebic cystitis**

     A06.82   **Other amebic genitourinary infections**
         Amebic balanitis
         Amebic vesiculitis
         Amebic vulvovaginitis

     A06.89   **Other amebic infections**
         Amebic appendicitis
         Amebic splenic abscess

A06.9   **Amebiasis, unspecified**

A07   Other protozoal intestinal diseases

A07.0   **Balantidiasis**
     Balantidial dysentery

A07.1   **Giardiasis [lambliasis]**

A07.2   **Cryptosporidiosis**

A07.3   **Isosporiasis**
     Infection due to Isospora belli and Isospora hominis
     Intestinal coccidiosis
     Isosporosis

A07.4   **Cyclosporiasis**

A07.8   **Other specified protozoal intestinal diseases**
     Intestinal trichomoniasis
     Sarcocystosis
     Sarcosporidiosis

A07.9   **Protozoal intestinal disease, unspecified**
     Flagellate diarrhea
     Protozoal colitis
     Protozoal diarrhea
     Protozoal dysentery

A08   Viral and other specified intestinal infections

     Excludes1:   influenza with involvement of gastrointestinal tract (J10.81)

A08.0   **Rotaviral enteritis**

A08.1   **Acute gastroenteropathy due to Norwalk agent**
     Small round structured virus enteritis

A08.2   **Adenoviral enteritis**

A08.3   **Other viral enteritis**

A08.4   **Viral intestinal infection, unspecified**
     Viral enteritis NOS
     Viral gastroenteritis NOS
     Viral gastroenteropathy NOS

A08.5   **Other specified intestinal infections**

A09   Infectious gastroenteritis and colitis, unspecified

     Includes: infectious colitis NOS
             infectious enteritis NOS
             infectious gastroenteritis NOS

     Excludes1:   colitis NOS (K52.9)
             diarrhea NOS (R19.7)
             enteritis NOS (K52.9)
             gastroenteritis NOS (K52.9)
             noninfective gastroenteritis and colitis, unspecified (K52.9)

TUBERCULOSIS (A15–A19)

     Includes: infections due to Mycobacterium tuberculosis and Mycobacterium bovis

     Excludes1:   congenital tuberculosis (P37.0)
             pneumoconiosis associated with tuberculosis (J65)
             sequelae of tuberculosis (B90.-)
             silicotuberculosis (J65)

A15   Respiratory tuberculosis

A15.0   **Tuberculosis of lung**
     Tuberculous bronchiectasis
     Tuberculous fibrosis of lung
     Tuberculous pneumonia
     Tuberculous pneumothorax

A15.4   **Tuberculosis of intrathoracic lymph nodes**
     Tuberculosis of hilar lymph nodes
     Tuberculosis of mediastinal lymph nodes
     Tuberculosis of tracheobronchial lymph nodes
     Excludes1:   tuberculosis specified as primary (A15.7)

A15.5   **Tuberculosis of larynx, trachea and bronchus**
     Tuberculosis of bronchus
     Tuberculosis of glottis
     Tuberculosis of larynx
     Tuberculosis of trachea

A15.6   **Tuberculous pleurisy**
     Tuberculosis of pleura
     Tuberculous empyema
     Excludes1:   primary respiratory tuberculosis (A15.7)

A15.7   **Primary respiratory tuberculosis**

A15.8   **Other respiratory tuberculosis**
     Mediastinal tuberculosis
     Nasopharyngeal tuberculosis
     Tuberculosis of nose
     Tuberculosis of sinus [any nasal]

A15.9   **Respiratory tuberculosis unspecified**

A17   Tuberculosis of nervous system

A17.0   **Tuberculous meningitis**
     Tuberculosis of meninges (cerebral) (spinal)
     Tuberculous leptomeningitis
     Excludes1:   tuberculous meningoencephalitis (A17.82)

A17.1   **Meningeal tuberculoma**
     Tuberculoma of meninges (cerebral) (spinal)
     Excludes2:   tuberculoma of brain and spinal cord (A17.81)

A17.8   **Other tuberculosis of nervous system**

     A17.81   **Tuberculoma of brain and spinal cord**
         Tuberculous abscess of brain and spinal cord

     A17.82   **Tuberculous meningoencephalitis**
         Tuberculous myelitis

     A17.83   **Tuberculous neuritis**
         Tuberculous mononeuropathy

     A17.89   **Other tuberculosis of nervous system**
         Tuberculous polyneuropathy

A17.9   **Tuberculosis of nervous system, unspecified**

A18   Tuberculosis of other organs

A18.0   **Tuberculosis of bones and joints**

     A18.01   **Tuberculosis of spine**
         Pott's disease or curvature of spine
         Tuberculous arthritis
         Tuberculous osteomyelitis of spine
         Tuberculous spondylitis

     A18.02   **Tuberculous arthritis of other joints**
         Tuberculosis of hip (joint)
         Tuberculosis of knee (joint)

     A18.03   **Tuberculosis of other bones**
         Tuberculous mastoiditis
         Tuberculous osteomyelitis

     A18.09   **Other musculoskeletal tuberculosis**
         Tuberculous myositis
         Tuberculous synovitis
         Tuberculous tenosynovitis

A18.1   **Tuberculosis of genitourinary system**

     A18.10   **Tuberculosis of genitourinary system, unspecified**

     A18.11   **Tuberculosis of kidney and ureter**

     A18.12   **Tuberculosis of bladder**

     A18.13   **Tuberculosis of other urinary organs**
         Tuberculosis urethritis

     A18.14   **Tuberculosis of prostate**

     A18.15   **Tuberculosis of other male genital organs**

     A18.16   **Tuberculosis of cervix**

A18.17 Tuberculous female pelvic inflammatory disease
Tuberculous endometritis
Tuberculous oophoritis and salpingitis
A18.18 Tuberculosis of other female genital organs
Tuberculous ulceration of vulva
A18.2 Tuberculous peripheral lymphadenopathy
Tuberculous adenitis
Excludes2:   tuberculosis of bronchial and mediastinal lymph nodes (A15.4)
tuberculosis of mesenteric and retroperitoneal lymph nodes (A18.39)
tuberculous tracheobronchial adenopathy (A15.4)
A18.3 Tuberculosis of intestines, peritoneum and mesenteric glands
A18.31 Tuberculous peritonitis
Tuberculous ascites
A18.32 Tuberculous enteritis
Tuberculosis of anus and rectum
Tuberculosis of intestine (large) (small)
A18.39 Retroperitoneal tuberculosis
Tuberculosis of mesenteric glands
Tuberculosis of retroperitoneal (lymph glands)
A18.4 Tuberculosis of skin and subcutaneous tissue
Erythema induratum, tuberculous
Lupus excedens
Lupus vulgaris NOS
Lupus vulgaris of eyelid
Scrofuloderma
Excludes2:   lupus erythematosus (L93.-)
lupus NOS (M32.9)
systemic (M32.-)
A18.5 Tuberculosis of eye
Excludes3:   lupus vulgaris of eyelid (A18.4)
A18.50 Tuberculosis of eye, unspecified
A18.51 Tuberculous episcleritis
A18.52 Tuberculous keratitis
Tuberculous interstitial keratitis
Tuberculous keratoconjunctivitis (interstitial) (phlyctenular)
A18.53 Tuberculous chorioretinitis
A18.54 Tuberculous iridocyclitis
A18.59 Other tuberculosis of eye
Tuberculous conjunctivitis
A18.6 Tuberculosis of ear
Tuberculous otitis media
Excludes2:   tuberculous mastoiditis (A18.03)
A18.7 Tuberculosis of adrenal glands
Tuberculous Addison's disease
A18.8 Tuberculosis of other specified organs
A18.81 Tuberculosis of thyroid gland
A18.82 Tuberculosis of other endocrine glands
Tuberculosis of pituitary gland
Tuberculosis of thymus gland
A18.83 Tuberculosis of digestive tract organs, not elsewhere classified
Excludes1:   tuberculosis of intestine (A18.32)
A18.84 Tuberculosis of heart
Tuberculous cardiomyopathy
Tuberculous endocarditis
Tuberculous myocarditis
Tuberculous pericarditis
A18.85 Tuberculosis of spleen
A18.89 Tuberculosis of other sites
Tuberculosis of muscle
Tuberculous cerebral arteritis
A19 Miliary tuberculosis
Includes: disseminated tuberculosis
generalized tuberculosis
tuberculous polyserositis
A19.0 Acute miliary tuberculosis of a single specified site
A19.1 Acute miliary tuberculosis of multiple sites
A19.2 Acute miliary tuberculosis, unspecified
A19.8 Other miliary tuberculosis

A19.9 Miliary tuberculosis, unspecified

CERTAIN ZOONOTIC BACTERIAL DISEASES (A20–A28)

A20 Plague
Includes: infection due to Yersinia pestis
A20.0 Bubonic plague
A20.1 Cellulocutaneous plague
A20.2 Pneumonic plague
A20.3 Plague meningitis
A20.7 Septicemic plague
A20.8 Other forms of plague
Abortive plague
Asymptomatic plague
Pestis minor
A20.9 Plague, unspecified
A21 Tularemia
Includes: deer-fly fever
infection due to Francisella tularensis
rabbit fever
A21.0 Ulceroglandular tularemia
A21.1 Oculoglandular tularemia
Ophthalmic tularemia
A21.2 Pulmonary tularemia
A21.3 Gastrointestinal tularemia
Abdominal tularemia
A21.7 Generalized tularemia
A21.8 Other forms of tularemia
A21.9 Tularemia, unspecified
A22 Anthrax
Includes: infection due to Bacillus anthracis
A22.0 Cutaneous anthrax
Malignant carbuncle
Malignant pustule
A22.1 Pulmonary anthrax
Inhalation anthrax
Ragpicker's disease
Woolsorter's disease
A22.2 Gastrointestinal anthrax
A22.7 Anthrax septicemia
A22.8 Other forms of anthrax
Anthrax meningitis
A22.9 Anthrax, unspecified
A23 Brucellosis
Includes: malta fever
mediterranean fever
undulant fever
A23.0 Brucellosis due to Brucella melitensis
A23.1 Brucellosis due to Brucella abortus
A23.2 Brucellosis due to Brucella suis
A23.3 Brucellosis due to Brucella canis
A23.8 Other brucellosis
A23.9 Brucellosis, unspecified
A24 Glanders and melioidosis
A24.0 Glanders
Infection due to Pseudomonas mallei
Malleus
A24.1 Acute and fulminating melioidosis
Melioidosis pneumonia
Melioidosis septicemia
A24.2 Subacute and chronic melioidosis
A24.3 Other melioidosis
A24.4 Melioidosis, unspecified
Infection due to Pseudomonas pseudomallei NOS
Whitmore's disease
A25 Rat-bite fevers
A25.0 Spirillosis
Sodoku

A25.1 Streptobacillosis
Epidemic arthritic erythema
Haverhill fever
Streptobacillary rat-bite fever

A25.9 Rat-bite fever, unspecified

A26 Erysipeloid

A26.0 Cutaneous erysipeloid
Erythema migrans

A26.7 Erysipelothrix septicemia

A26.8 Other forms of erysipeloid

A26.9 Erysipeloid, unspecified

A27 Leptospirosis

A27.0 Leptospirosis icterohemorrhagica
Leptospiral or spirochetal jaundice (hemorrhagic)
Weil's disease

A27.8 Other forms of leptospirosis

> **A27.81 Aseptic meningitis in leptospirosis**
>
> **A27.89 Other forms of leptospirosis**

A27.9 Leptospirosis, unspecified

A28 Other zoonotic bacterial diseases, not elsewhere classified

A28.0 Pasteurellosis

A28.1 Cat-scratch disease
Cat-scratch fever

A28.2 Extraintestinal yersiniosis
Excludes1:   enteritis due to Yersinia enterocolitica (A04.6)
plague (A20.-)

A28.8 Other specified zoonotic bacterial diseases, not elsewhere classified

A28.9 Zoonotic bacterial disease, unspecified

OTHER BACTERIAL DISEASES (A30–A49)

A30 Leprosy [Hansen's disease]
Includes: infection due to Mycobacterium leprae
Excludes1:   sequelae of leprosy (B92)

A30.0 Indeterminate leprosy
I leprosy

A30.1 Tuberculoid leprosy
TT leprosy

A30.2 Borderline tuberculoid leprosy
BT leprosy

A30.3 Borderline leprosy
BB leprosy

A30.4 Borderline lepromatous leprosy
BL leprosy

A30.5 Lepromatous leprosy
LL leprosy

A30.8 Other forms of leprosy

A30.9 Leprosy, unspecified

A31 Infection due to other mycobacteria
Excludes3:   leprosy (A30.-)
tuberculosis (A15-A19)

A31.0 Pulmonary mycobacterial infection
Infection due to Mycobacterium avium
Infection due to Mycobacterium intracellulare [Battey bacillus]
Infection due to Mycobacterium kansasii

A31.1 Cutaneous mycobacterial infection
Buruli ulcer
Infection due to Mycobacterium marinum
Infection due to Mycobacterium ulcerans

A31.2 Disseminated mycobacterium avium-intracellulare complex (DMAC)
MAC septicemia

A31.8 Other mycobacterial infections

A31.9 Mycobacterial infection, unspecified
Atypical mycobacterial infection NOS
Mycobacteriosis NOS

A32 Listeriosis
Includes: listerial foodborne infection
Excludes1:   neonatal (disseminated) listeriosis (P37.2)

A32.0 Cutaneous listeriosis

A32.1 Listerial meningitis and meningoencephalitis

> **A32.11 Listerial meningitis**
>
> **A32.12 Listerial meningoencephalitis**

A32.7 Listerial septicemia

A32.8 Other forms of listeriosis

> **A32.81 Oculoglandular listeriosis**
>
> **A32.82 Listerial endocarditis**
>
> **A32.89 Other forms of listeriosis**
> Listerial cerebral arteritis

A32.9 Listeriosis, unspecified

A33 Tetanus neonatorum

A34 Obstetrical tetanus

A35 Other tetanus
Tetanus NOS
Excludes1:   tetanus neonatorum (A33)
obstetrical tetanus (A34)

A36 Diphtheria

A36.0 Pharyngeal diphtheria
Diphtheritic membranous angina
Tonsillar diphtheria

A36.1 Nasopharyngeal diphtheria

A36.2 Laryngeal diphtheria
Diphtheritic laryngotracheitis

A36.3 Cutaneous diphtheria
Excludes3:   erythrasma (L08.1)

A36.8 Other diphtheria

> **A36.81 Diphtheritic cardiomyopathy**
> Diphtheritic myocarditis
>
> **A36.82 Diphtheritic radiculomyelitis**
>
> **A36.83 Diphtheritic polyneuritis**
>
> **A36.84 Diphtheritic tubulo-interstitial nephropathy**
>
> **A36.85 Diphtheritic cystitis**
>
> **A36.86 Diphtheritic conjunctivitis**
>
> **A36.89 Other diphtheritic complications**
> Diphtheritic peritonitis

A36.9 Diphtheria, unspecified

A37 Whooping cough

A37.0 Whooping cough due to Bordetella pertussis

> **A37.00 Whooping cough due to Bordetella pertussis without pneumonia**
>
> **A37.01 Whooping cough due to Bordetella pertussis with pneumonia**

A37.1 Whooping cough due to Bordetella parapertussis

> **A37.10 Whooping cough due to Bordetella parapertussis without pneumonia**
>
> **A37.11 Whooping cough due to Bordetella parapertussis with pneumonia**

A37.8 Whooping cough due to other Bordetella species

> **A37.80 Whooping cough due to other Bordetella species without pneumonia**
>
> **A37.81 Whooping cough due to other Bordetella species with pneumonia**

A37.9 Whooping cough, unspecified species

> **A37.90 Whooping cough, unspecified species without pneumonia**
>
> **A37.91 Whooping cough, unspecified species with pneumonia**

A38 Scarlet fever
Includes: scarlatina
Excludes2:   streptococcal sore throat (J02.0)

A38.0 Scarlet fever with otitis media

A38.1 Scarlet fever with myocarditis

A38.8 Scarlet fever with other complications

A38.9   **Scarlet fever, uncomplicated**
    Scarlet fever, NOS

A39   Meningococcal infection

A39.0   **Meningococcal meningitis**

A39.1   **Waterhouse-Friderichsen syndrome**
    Meningococcal hemorrhagic adrenalitis
    Meningococcic adrenal syndrome

A39.2   **Acute meningococcemia**

A39.3   **Chronic meningococcemia**

A39.4   **Meningococcemia, unspecified**

A39.5   **Meningococcal heart disease**

    A39.50   **Meningococcal carditis, unspecified**

    A39.51   **Meningococcal endocarditis**

    A39.52   **Meningococcal myocarditis**

    A39.53   **Meningococcal pericarditis**

A39.8   **Other meningococcal infections**

    A39.81   **Meningococcal encephalitis**

    A39.82   **Meningococcal retrobulbar neuritis**

    A39.83   **Meningococcal arthritis**

    A39.84   **Postmeningococcal arthritis**

    A39.89   **Other meningococcal infections**
      Meningococcal conjunctivitis

A39.9   **Meningococcal infection, unspecified**
    Meningococcal disease NOS

A40   Streptococcal septicemia

    Code first: postprocedural streptococcal septicemia (T81.4)
      streptococcal septicemia during labor (O75.3)
      streptococcal septicemia following abortion or ectopic
       or molar pregnancy (O03-O07, O08.0)
      streptococcal septicemia following immunization (T88.0)
      streptococcal septicemia following infusion, transfusion
       or therapeutic injection (T80.2)
    Excludes1:   neonatal (P36.0-P36.1)
      puerperal sepsis (O85)
      septicemia due to Streptococcus, group D (A41.81)

A40.0   **Septicemia due to streptococcus, group A**

A40.1   **Septicemia due to streptococcus, group B**

A40.3   **Septicemia due to Streptococcus pneumoniae**
    Pneumococcal septicemia

A40.8   **Other streptococcal septicemia**

A40.9   **Streptococcal septicemia, unspecified**

A41   Other septicemia

    Code first: postprocedural septicemia (T81.4)
      septicemia during labor (O75.3)
      septicemia following abortion, ectopic or molar
       pregnancy (O03-O07, O08.0)
      septicemia following immunization (T88.0)
      septicemia following infusion, transfusion or
       therapeutic injection (T80.2)
    Excludes1:   bacteremia NOS (R78.81)
      neonatal (P36.-)
      puerperal septicemia (O85)
      streptococcal septicemia (A40.-)
    Excludes3:   septicemia (due to) (in):
       actinomycotic (A42.7)
       anthrax (A22.7)
       candidal (B37.7)
       Erysipelothrix (A26.7)
       extraintestinal yersiniosis (A28.2)
       gonococcal (A54.86)
       herpesviral (B00.7)
       listerial (A32.7)
       meningococcal (A39.2-A39.4)
       tularemia (A21.7)
      septicemic:
       melioidosis (A24.1)
       plague (A20.7)
      toxic shock syndrome (A48.3)

A41.0   **Septicemia due to Staphylococcus aureus**

A41.1   **Septicemia due to other specified staphylococcus**
    Septicemia due to coagulase-negative staphylococcus

A41.2   **Septicemia due to unspecified staphylococcus**

A41.3   **Septicemia due to Hemophilus influenzae**

A41.4   **Septicemia due to anaerobes**
    Excludes1:   gas gangrene (A48.0)

A41.5   **Septicemia due to other Gram-negative organisms**

    A41.50   **Gram-negative septicemia, unspecified**
      Gram-negative septicemia NOS

    A41.51   **Septicemia due to Escherichia coli [E. coli]**

    A41.52   **Septicemia due to Pseudomonas**
      Pseudomonas aeroginosa

    A41.53   **Septicemia due to Serratia**

    A41.59   **Other Gram-negative septicemia**

A41.8   **Other specified septicemia**

    A41.81   **Septicemia due to Enterococcus**

    A41.89   **Other specified septicemia**

A41.9   **Septicemia, unspecified**
    Septic shock

A42   Actinomycosis

    Excludes1:   actinomycetoma (B47.1)

A42.0   **Pulmonary actinomycosis**

A42.1   **Abdominal actinomycosis**

A42.2   **Cervicofacial actinomycosis**

A42.7   **Actinomycotic septicemia**

A42.8   **Other forms of actinomycosis**

    A42.81   **Actinomycotic meningitis**

    A42.82   **Actinomycotic encephalitis**

    A42.89   **Other forms of actinomycosis**

A42.9   **Actinomycosis, unspecified**

A43   Nocardiosis

A43.0   **Pulmonary nocardiosis**

A43.1   **Cutaneous nocardiosis**

A43.8   **Other forms of nocardiosis**

A43.9   **Nocardiosis, unspecified**

A44   Bartonellosis

A44.0   **Systemic bartonellosis**
    Oroya fever

A44.1   **Cutaneous and mucocutaneous bartonellosis**
    Verruga peruana

A44.8   **Other forms of bartonellosis**

A44.9   **Bartonellosis, unspecified**

A46   Erysipelas

    Excludes1:   postpartum or puerperal erysipelas (O86.8)

A48   Other bacterial diseases, not elsewhere classified

    Excludes1:   actinomycetoma (B47.1)

A48.0   **Gas gangrene**
    Clostridial cellulitis
    Clostridial myonecrosis

A48.1   **Legionnaires' disease**

A48.2   **Nonpneumonic Legionnaires' disease [Pontiac fever]**

A48.3   **Toxic shock syndrome**
    Excludes1:   endotoxic shock NOS (R57.8)
      septicemia NOS (A41.9)

A48.4   **Brazilian purpuric fever**
    Systemic Hemophilus aegyptius infection

A48.8   **Other specified bacterial diseases**

A49   Bacterial infection of unspecified site

    Excludes1:   bacterial agents as the cause of diseases classified to
       other chapters (B95-B96)
      chlamydial infection NOS (A74.9)
      meningococcal infection NOS (A39.9)
      rickettsial infection NOS (A79.9)
      spirochetal infection NOS (A69.9)

A49.0   **Staphylococcal infection, unspecified**

A49.1   **Streptococcal infection, unspecified**

A49.2   **Hemophilus influenzae infection, unspecified**

A49.3   **Mycoplasma infection, unspecified**

A49.8   **Other bacterial infections of unspecified site**

A49.9   **Bacterial infection, unspecified**
> Excludes1:   bacteremia NOS (R78.81)

INFECTIONS WITH A PREDOMINANTLY SEXUAL MODE OF TRANSMISSION (A50–A64)

> Excludes1:   human immunodeficiency virus [HIV] disease (B20)
> nonspecific and nongonococcal urethritis (N34.1)
> Reiter's disease (M02.3-)

A50   Congenital syphilis

A50.0   **Early congenital syphilis, symptomatic**
> Any congenital syphilitic condition specified as early or manifest less than two years after birth.

   A50.01   **Early congenital syphilitic oculopathy**

   A50.02   **Early congenital syphilitic osteochondropathy**

   A50.03   **Early congenital syphilitic pharyngitis**
> Early congenital syphilitic laryngitis

   A50.04   **Early congenital syphilitic pneumonia**

   A50.05   **Early congenital syphilitic rhinitis**

   A50.06   **Early cutaneous congenital syphilis**

   A50.07   **Early mucocutaneous congenital syphilis**

   A50.08   **Early visceral congenital syphilis**

   A50.09   **Other early congenital syphilis, symptomatic**

A50.1   **Early congenital syphilis, latent**
> Congenital syphilis without clinical manifestations, with positive serological reaction and negative spinal fluid test, less than two years after birth.

A50.2   **Early congenital syphilis, unspecified**
> Congenital syphilis NOS less than two years after birth.

A50.3   **Late congenital syphilitic oculopathy**
> Excludes1:   Hutchinson's triad (A50.53)

   A50.30   **Late congenital syphilitic oculopathy, unspecified**

   A50.31   **Late congenital syphilitic interstitial keratitis**

   A50.32   **Late congenital syphilitic chorioretinitis**

   A50.39   **Other late congenital syphilitic oculopathy**

A50.4   **Late congenital neurosyphilis [juvenile neurosyphilis]**
> Use additional code to identify any associated mental disorder.
> Excludes1:   Hutchinson's triad (A50.53)

   A50.40   **Late congenital neurosyphilis, unspecified**
> Juvenile neurosyphilis NOS

   A50.41   **Late congenital syphilitic meningitis**

   A50.42   **Late congenital syphilitic encephalitis**

   A50.43   **Late congenital syphilitic polyneuropathy**

   A50.44   **Late congenital syphilitic optic nerve atrophy**

   A50.45   **Juvenile general paresis**
> Dementia paralytica juvenilis
> Juvenile tabetoparetic neurosyphilis

   A50.49   **Other late congenital neurosyphilis**
> Juvenile tabes dorsalis

A50.5   **Other late congenital syphilis, symptomatic**
> Any congenital syphilitic condition specified as late or manifest two years or more after birth.

   A50.51   **Clutton's joints**

   A50.52   **Hutchinson's teeth**

   A50.53   **Hutchinson's triad**

   A50.54   **Late congenital cardiovascular syphilis**

   A50.55   **Late congenital syphilitic arthropathy**

   A50.56   **Late congenital syphilitic osteochondropathy**

   A50.57   **Syphilitic saddle nose**

   A50.59   **Other late congenital syphilis, symptomatic**

A50.6   **Late congenital syphilis, latent**
> Congenital syphilis without clinical manifestations, with positive serological reaction and negative spinal fluid test, two years or more after birth.

A50.7   **Late congenital syphilis, unspecified**
> Congenital syphilis NOS two years or more after birth.

A50.9   **Congenital syphilis, unspecified**

A51   Early syphilis

A51.0   **Primary genital syphilis**
> Syphilitic chancre NOS

A51.1   **Primary anal syphilis**

A51.2   **Primary syphilis of other sites**

A51.3   **Secondary syphilis of skin and mucous membranes**

   A51.31   **Condyloma latum**

   A51.32   **Syphilitic alopecia**

   A51.39   **Other secondary syphilis of skin**
> Syphilitic leukoderma
> Syphilitic mucous patch
> Excludes1:   late syphilitic leukoderma (A52.79)

A51.4   **Other secondary syphilis**

   A51.41   **Secondary syphilitic meningitis**

   A51.42   **Secondary syphilitic female pelvic disease**

   A51.43   **Secondary syphilitic oculopathy**
> Secondary syphilitic chorioretinitis
> Secondary syphilitic iridocyclitis, iritis
> Secondary syphilitic uveitis

   A51.44   **Secondary syphilitic nephritis**

   A51.45   **Secondary syphilitic hepatitis**

   A51.46   **Secondary syphilitic osteopathy**

   A51.49   **Other secondary syphilitic conditions**
> Secondary syphilitic lymphadenopathy
> Secondary syphilitic myositis

A51.5   **Early syphilis, latent**
> Syphilis (acquired) without clinical manifestations, with positive serological reaction and negative spinal fluid test, less than two years after infection.

A51.9   **Early syphilis, unspecified**

A52   Late syphilis

A52.0   **Cardiovascular and cerebrovascular syphilis**

   A52.00   **Cardiovascular syphilis, unspecified**

   A52.01   **Syphilitic aneurysm of aorta**

   A52.02   **Syphilitic aortitis**

   A52.03   **Syphilitic endocarditis**
> Syphilitic aortic valve incompetence or stenosis
> Syphilitic mitral valve stenosis
> Syphilitic pulmonary valve regurgitation

   A52.04   **Syphilitic cerebral arteritis**

   A52.05   **Other cerebrovascular syphilis**
> Syphilitic cerebral aneurysm (ruptured) (non-ruptured)
> Syphilitic cerebral thrombosis

   A52.06   **Other syphilitic heart involvement**
> Syphilitic coronary artery disease
> Syphilitic myocarditis
> Syphilitic pericarditis

   A52.09   **Other cardiovascular syphilis**

A52.1   **Symptomatic neurosyphilis**

   A52.10   **Symptomatic neurosyphilis, unspecified**

   A52.11   **Tabes dorsalis**
> Locomotor ataxia (progressive)
> Tabetic neurosyphilis

   A52.12   **Other cerebrospinal syphilis**

   A52.13   **Late syphilitic meningitis**

   A52.14   **Late syphilitic encephalitis**

   A52.15   **Late syphilitic neuropathy**
> Late syphilitic acoustic neuritis
> Late syphilitic optic (nerve) atrophy
> Late syphilitic polyneuropathy
> Late syphilitic retrobulbar neuritis

   A52.16   **Charcot's arthropathy (tabetic)**

   A52.17   **General paresis**
> Dementia paralytica

   A52.19   **Other symptomatic neurosyphilis**
> Syphilitic parkinsonism

A52.2   **Asymptomatic neurosyphilis**

A52.3   **Neurosyphilis, unspecified**
> Gumma (syphilitic)
> Syphilis (late)
> Syphiloma

A52.7 **Other symptomatic late syphilis**

  A52.71 **Late syphilitic oculopathy**
Late syphilitic chorioretinitis
Late syphilitic episcleritis

  A52.72 **Syphilis of lung and bronchus**

  A52.73 **Symptomatic late syphilis of other respiratory organs**

  A52.74 **Syphilis of liver and other viscera**
Late syphilitic peritonitis

  A52.75 **Syphilis of kidney and ureter**
Syphilitic glomerular disease

  A52.76 **Other genitourinary symptomatic late syphilis**
Late syphilitic female pelvic inflammatory disease

  A52.77 **Syphilis of bone and joint**

  A52.78 **Syphilis of other musculoskeletal tissue**
Late syphilitic bursitis
Syphilis [stage unspecified] of bursa
Syphilis [stage unspecified] of muscle
Syphilis [stage unspecified] of synovium
Syphilis [stage unspecified] of tendon

  A52.79 **Other symptomatic late syphilis**
Late syphilitic leukoderma
Syphilis of adrenal gland
Syphilis of pituitary gland
Syphilis of thyroid gland
Syphilitic splenomegaly
Excludes1: syphilitic leukoderma (secondary) (A51.39)

A52.8 **Late syphilis, latent**
Syphilis (acquired) without clinical manifestations, with positive serological reaction and negative spinal fluid test, two years or more after infection

A52.9 **Late syphilis, unspecified**

A53 **Other and unspecified syphilis**

A53.0 **Latent syphilis, unspecified as early or late**
Latent syphilis NOS
Positive serological reaction for syphilis

A53.9 **Syphilis, unspecified**
Infection due to Treponema pallidum NOS
Syphilis (acquired) NOS
Excludes1: syphilis NOS under two years of age (A50.2)

A54 **Gonococcal infection**

A54.0 **Gonococcal infection of lower genitourinary tract without periurethral or accessory gland abscess**
Excludes1: gonococcal infection with genitourinary gland abscess (A54.1)
gonococcal infection with periurethral abscess (A54.1)

  A54.00 **Gonococcal infection of lower genitourinary tract, unspecified**

  A54.01 **Gonococcal cystitis and urethritis, unspecified**

  A54.02 **Gonococcal vulvovaginitis, unspecified**

  A54.03 **Gonococcal cervicitis, unspecified**

  A54.09 **Other gonococcal infection of lower genitourinary tract**

A54.1 **Gonococcal infection of lower genitourinary tract with periurethral and accessory gland abscess**
Gonococcal Bartholin's gland abscess

A54.2 **Gonococcal pelviperitonitis and other gonococcal genitourinary infection**

  A54.21 **Gonococcal infection of kidney and ureter**

  A54.22 **Gonococcal prostatitis**

  A54.23 **Gonococcal infection of other male genital organs**
Gonococcal epididymitis
Gonococcal orchitis

  A54.24 **Gonococcal female pelvic inflammatory disease**
Gonococcal pelviperitonitis
Excludes1: gonococcal peritonitis (A54.85)

  A54.29 **Other gonococcal genitourinary infections**

A54.3 **Gonococcal infection of eye**

  A54.30 **Gonococcal infection of eye, unspecified**

  A54.31 **Gonococcal conjunctivitis**
Ophthalmia neonatorum due to gonococcus

  A54.32 **Gonococcal iridocyclitis**

  A54.33 **Gonococcal keratitis**

  A54.39 **Other gonococcal eye infection**
Gonococcal endophthalmia

A54.4 **Gonococcal infection of musculoskeletal system**

  A54.40 **Gonococcal infection of musculoskeletal system, unspecified**

  A54.41 **Gonococcal spondylopathy**

  A54.42 **Gonococcal arthritis**
Excludes2: gonococcal infection of spine (A54.41)

  A54.43 **Gonococcal osteomyelitis**
Excludes2: gonococcal infection of spine (A54.41)

  A54.49 **Gonococcal infection of other musculoskeletal tissue**
Gonococcal bursitis
Gonococcal myositis
Gonococcal synovitis
Gonococcal tenosynovitis

A54.5 **Gonococcal pharyngitis**

A54.6 **Gonococcal infection of anus and rectum**

A54.8 **Other gonococcal infections**

  A54.81 **Gonococcal meningitis**

  A54.82 **Gonococcal brain abscess**

  A54.83 **Gonococcal heart infection**
Gonococcal endocarditis
Gonococcal myocarditis
Gonococcal pericarditis

  A54.84 **Gonococcal pneumonia**

  A54.85 **Gonococcal peritonitis**
Excludes1: gonococcal pelviperitonitis (A54.24)

  A54.86 **Gonococcal septicemia**

  A54.89 **Other gonococcal infections**
Gonococcal keratoderma
Gonococcal lymphadenitis

A54.9 **Gonococcal infection, unspecified**

A55 **Chlamydial lymphogranuloma (venereum)**
Includes: climatic or tropical bubo
Durand-Nicolas-Favre disease
Esthiomene
lymphogranuloma inguinale

A56 **Other sexually transmitted chlamydial diseases**
Includes: sexually transmitted diseases due to Chlamydia trachomatis
Excludes1: neonatal chlamydial conjunctivitis (P39.1)
neonatal chlamydial pneumonia (P23.1)
Excludes2: chlamydial lymphogranuloma (A55)
conditions classified to A74.-

A56.0 **Chlamydial infection of lower genitourinary tract**

  A56.00 **Chlamydial infection of lower genitourinary tract, unspecified**

  A56.01 **Chlamydial cystitis and urethritis**

  A56.02 **Chlamydial vulvovaginitis**

  A56.09 **Other chlamydial infection of lower genitourinary tract**
Chlamydial cervicitis

A56.1 **Chlamydial infection of pelviperitoneum and other genitourinary organs**

  A56.11 **Chlamydial female pelvic inflammatory disease**

  A56.19 **Other chlamydial genitourinary infection**
Chlamydial epididymitis
Chlamydial orchitis

A56.2 **Chlamydial infection of genitourinary tract, unspecified**

A56.3 **Chlamydial infection of anus and rectum**

A56.4 **Chlamydial infection of pharynx**

A56.8 **Sexually transmitted chlamydial infection of other sites**

A57 Chancroid
Ulcus molle

A58 Granuloma inguinale
Donovanosis

A59 Trichomoniasis
Excludes2:   intestinal trichomoniasis (A07.8)

A59.0 Urogenital trichomoniasis

A59.00 Urogenital trichomoniasis, unspecified
Fluor (vaginalis) due to Trichomonas
Leukorrhea (vaginalis) due to Trichomonas

A59.01 Trichomonal vulvovaginitis

A59.02 Trichomonal prostatitis

A59.03 Trichomonal cystitis and urethritis

A59.09 Other urogenital trichomoniasis
Trichomonas cervicitis

A59.8 Trichomoniasis of other sites

A59.9 Trichomoniasis, unspecified

A60 Anogenital herpesviral [herpes simplex] infections

A60.0 Herpesviral infection of genitalia and urogenital tract

A60.00 Herpesviral infection of urogenital system, unspecified

A60.01 Herpesviral infection of penis

A60.02 Herpesviral infection of other male genital organs

A60.03 Herpesviral cervicitis

A60.04 Herpesviral vulvovaginitis
Herpesviral [herpes simplex] ulceration
Herpesviral [herpes simplex] vaginitis
Herpesviral [herpes simplex] vulvitis

A60.09 Herpesviral infection of other urogenital tract

A60.1 Herpesviral infection of perianal skin and rectum

A60.9 Anogenital herpesviral infection, unspecified

A63 Other predominantly sexually transmitted diseases, not elsewhere classified
Excludes2:   molluscum contagiosum (B08.1)
papilloma of cervix (D26.0)

A63.0 Anogenital (venereal) warts
Condyloma acuminatum
Infection due to (human) papillomavirus [HPV]

A63.8 Other specified predominantly sexually transmitted diseases

A64 Unspecified sexually transmitted disease

A64.0 Venereal cystitis and urethritis

A64.1 Venereal infection of penis

A64.2 Venereal disease of other male genital organs

A64.3 Venereal disease of vagina

A64.4 Venereal disease of other female genital organs

A64.8 Venereal disease of other urinary organs

A64.9 Venereal disease, unspecified

OTHER SPIROCHETAL DISEASES (A65–A69)

Excludes3:   leptospirosis (A27.-)
syphilis (A50-A53)

A65 Nonvenereal syphilis
Bejel
Endemic syphilis
Njovera

A66 Yaws
Includes: bouba
frambesia (tropica)
pian

A66.0 Initial lesions of yaws
Chancre of yaws
Frambesia, initial or primary
Initial frambesial ulcer
Mother yaw

A66.1 Multiple papillomata and wet crab yaws
Frambesioma
Pianoma
Plantar or palmar papilloma of yaws

A66.2 Other early skin lesions of yaws
Cutaneous yaws, less than five years after infection
Early yaws (cutaneous) (macular) (maculopapular)
(micropapular) (papular)
Frambeside of early yaws

A66.3 Hyperkeratosis of yaws
Ghoul hand
Hyperkeratosis, palmar or plantar (early) (late) due to yaws
Worm-eaten soles

A66.4 Gummata and ulcers of yaws
Gummatous frambeside
Nodular late yaws (ulcerated)

A66.5 Gangosa
Rhinopharyngitis mutilans

A66.6 Bone and joint lesions of yaws
Yaws ganglion
Yaws goundou
Yaws gumma, bone
Yaws gummatous osteitis or periostitis
Yaws hydrarthrosis
Yaws osteitis
Yaws periostitis (hypertrophic)

A66.7 Other manifestations of yaws
Juxta-articular nodules of yaws
Mucosal yaws

A66.8 Latent yaws
Yaws without clinical manifestations, with positive serology

A66.9 Yaws, unspecified

A67 Pinta [carate]

A67.0 Primary lesions of pinta
Chancre (primary) of pinta
Papule (primary) of pinta

A67.1 Intermediate lesions of pinta
Erythematous plaques of pinta
Hyperchromic lesions of pinta
Hyperkeratosis of pinta
Pintids

A67.2 Late lesions of pinta
Achromic skin lesions of pinta
Cicatricial skin lesions of pinta
Dyschromic skin lesions of pinta

A67.3 Mixed lesions of pinta
Achromic with hyperchromic skin lesions of pinta [carate]

A67.9 Pinta, unspecified

A68 Relapsing fevers
Includes: recurrent fever
Excludes3:   Lyme disease (A69.2-)

A68.0 Louse-borne relapsing fever
Relapsing fever due to Borrelia recurrentis

A68.1 Tick-borne relapsing fever
Relapsing fever due to any Borrelia species other than Borrelia
recurrentis

A68.9 Relapsing fever, unspecified

A69 Other spirochetal infections

A69.0 Necrotizing ulcerative stomatitis
Cancrum oris
Fusospirochetal gangrene
Noma
Stomatitis gangrenosa

A69.1 Other Vincent's infections
Fusospirochetal pharyngitis
Necrotizing ulcerative (acute) gingivitis
Necrotizing ulcerative (acute) gingivostomatitis
Spirochetal stomatitis
Trench mouth
Vincent's angina
Vincent's gingivitis

A69.2 Lyme disease
Erythema chronicum migrans due to Borrelia burgdorferi

A69.20 Lyme disease, unspecified

A69.21 Meningitis due to Lyme disease

A69.22   **Other neurologic disorders in Lyme disease**
Cranial neuritis
Meningoencephalitis
Polyneuropathy

A69.23   **Arthritis due to Lyme disease**

A69.29   **Other conditions associated with Lyme disease**
Myopericarditis due to Lyme disease

A69.8   **Other specified spirochetal infections**

A69.9   **Spirochetal infection, unspecified**

OTHER DISEASES CAUSED BY CHLAMYDIAE (A70–A74)

Excludes1:   sexually transmitted chlamydial diseases (A55-A56)

A70   **Chlamydia psittaci infections**
Ornithosis
Parrot fever
Psittacosis

A71   **Trachoma**

Excludes1:   sequelae of trachoma (B94.0)

A71.0   **Initial stage of trachoma**
Trachoma dubium

A71.1   **Active stage of trachoma**
Granular conjunctivitis (trachomatous)
Trachomatous follicular conjunctivitis
Trachomatous pannus

A71.9   **Trachoma, unspecified**

A74   **Other diseases caused by chlamydiae**

Excludes1:   neonatal chalmydial conjunctivitis (P39.1)
neonatal chlamydial pneumonia (P23.1)
Reiter's disease (M02.3-)
sexually transmitted chlamydial diseases (A55-A56)

Excludes2:   chlamydial pneumonia (J16.0)

A74.0   **Chlamydial conjunctivitis**
Paratrachoma

A74.8   **Other chlamydial diseases**

A74.81   **Chlamydial peritonitis**

A74.89   **Other chlamydial diseases**

A74.9   **Chlamydial infection, unspecified**
Chlamydiosis NOS

RICKETTSIOSES (A75–A79)

A75   **Typhus fever**

Excludes1:   rickettsiosis due to Ehrlichia sennetsu (A79.2)

A75.0   **Epidemic louse-borne typhus fever due to Rickettsia prowazekii**
Classical typhus (fever)
Epidemic (louse-borne) typhus

A75.1   **Recrudescent typhus [Brill's disease]**
Brill-Zinsser disease

A75.2   **Typhus fever due to Rickettsia typhi**
Murine (flea-borne) typhus

A75.3   **Typhus fever due to Rickettsia tsutsugamushi**
Scrub (mite-borne) typhus
Tsutsugamushi fever

A75.9   **Typhus fever, unspecified**
Typhus (fever) NOS

A77   **Spotted fever [tick-borne rickettsioses]**

A77.0   **Spotted fever due to Rickettsia rickettsii**
Rocky Mountain spotted fever
Sao Paulo fever

A77.1   **Spotted fever due to Rickettsia conorii**
African tick typhus
Boutonneuse fever
India tick typhus
Kenya tick typhus
Marseilles fever
Mediterranean tick fever

A77.2   **Spotted fever due to Rickettsia siberica**
North Asian tick fever
Siberian tick typhus

A77.3   **Spotted fever due to Rickettsia australis**
Queensland tick typhus

A77.4   **Ehrlichiosis**

A77.40   **Ehrlichiosis, unspecified**

A77.41   **Ehrlichiosis chafeensis [E. chafeensis]**

A77.49   **Other ehrlichiosis**

A77.8   **Other spotted fevers**

A77.9   **Spotted fever, unspecified**
Tick-borne typhus NOS

A78   **Q fever**
Infection due to Coxiella burnetii
Nine Mile fever
Quadrilateral fever

A79   **Other rickettsioses**

A79.0   **Trench fever**
Quintan fever
Wolhynian fever

A79.1   **Rickettsialpox due to Rickettsia akari**
Kew Garden fever
Vesicular rickettsiosis

A79.2   **Rickettsiosis due to Ehrlichia sennetsu**

A79.8   **Other specified rickettsioses**

A79.9   **Rickettsiosis, unspecified**
Rickettsial infection NOS

VIRAL INFECTIONS OF THE CENTRAL NERVOUS SYSTEM (A80–A89)

Excludes1:   sequelae of poliomyelitis (B91)
sequelae of viral encephalitis (B94.1)

A80   **Acute poliomyelitis**

A80.0   **Acute paralytic poliomyelitis, vaccine-associated**

A80.1   **Acute paralytic poliomyelitis, wild virus, imported**

A80.2   **Acute paralytic poliomyelitis, wild virus, indigenous**

A80.3   **Acute paralytic poliomyelitis, other and unspecified**

A80.30   **Acute paralytic poliomyelitis, unspecified**

A80.39   **Other acute paralytic poliomyelitis**

A80.4   **Acute nonparalytic poliomyelitis**

A80.9   **Acute poliomyelitis, unspecified**

A81   **Atypical virus infections of central nervous system**
Includes: diseases of the central nervous system caused by prions

A81.0   **Creutzfeldt-Jakob disease**
Subacute spongiform encephalopathy (with dementia)

A81.1   **Subacute sclerosing panencephalitis**
Dawson's inclusion body encephalitis
Van Bogaert's sclerosing leukoencephalopathy

A81.2   **Progressive multifocal leukoencephalopathy**
Multifocal leukoencephalopathy NOS

A81.8   **Other slow virus infections of central nervous system**
Kuru

A81.9   **Slow virus infection of central nervous system, unspecified**
Slow virus infection NOS

A82   **Rabies**

A82.0   **Sylvatic rabies**

A82.1   **Urban rabies**

A82.9   **Rabies, unspecified**

A83   **Mosquito-borne viral encephalitis**
Includes: mosquito-borne viral meningoencephalitis
Excludes3:   Venezuelan equine encephalitis (A92.2)
West Nile fever (A92.3-)

A83.0   **Japanese encephalitis**

A83.1   **Western equine encephalitis**

A83.2   **Eastern equine encephalitis**

A83.3   **St Louis encephalitis**

A83.4   **Australian encephalitis**
Kunjin virus disease

A83.5 California encephalitis
California meningoencephalitis
La Crosse encephalitis

A83.6 Rocio virus disease

A83.8 Other mosquito-borne viral encephalitis

A83.9 Mosquito-borne viral encephalitis, unspecified

A84 Tick-borne viral encephalitis
Includes: tick-borne viral meningoencephalitis

A84.0 Far Eastern tick-borne encephalitis [Russian spring-summer encephalitis]

A84.1 Central European tick-borne encephalitis

A84.8 Other tick-borne viral encephalitis
Louping ill
Powassan virus disease

A84.9 Tick-borne viral encephalitis, unspecified

A85 Other viral encephalitis, not elsewhere classified
Includes: specified viral encephalomyelitis NEC
specified viral meningoencephalitis NEC
Excludes1:   benign myalgic encephalomyelitis (G93.3)
encephalitis due to:
cytomegalovirus (B25.8)
herpesvirus [herpes simplex] (B00.4)
measles virus (B05.0)
mumps virus (B26.2)
poliomyelitis virus (A80.-)
zoster (B02.0)
lymphocytic choriomeningitis (A87.2)

A85.0 Enteroviral encephalitis
Enteroviral encephalomyelitis

A85.1 Adenoviral encephalitis
Adenoviral meningoencephalitis

A85.2 Arthropod-borne viral encephalitis, unspecified
Excludes1:   West Nile virus with encephalitis (A92.31)

A85.8 Other specified viral encephalitis
Encephalitis lethargica
Von Economo-Cruchet disease

A86 Unspecified viral encephalitis
Includes: viral encephalomyelitis NOS
viral meningoencephalitis NOS

A87 Viral meningitis
Excludes1:   meningitis due to:
herpesvirus [herpes simplex] (B00.3)
measles virus (B05.1)
mumps virus (B26.1)
poliomyelitis virus (A80.-)
zoster (B02.1)

A87.0 Enteroviral meningitis
Coxsackievirus meningitis
Echovirus meningitis

A87.1 Adenoviral meningitis

A87.2 Lymphocytic choriomeningitis
Lymphocytic meningoencephalitis

A87.8 Other viral meningitis

A87.9 Viral meningitis, unspecified

A88 Other viral infections of central nervous system, not elsewhere classified
Excludes1:   viral encephalitis NOS (A86)
viral meningitis NOS (A87.9)

A88.0 Enteroviral exanthematous fever [Boston exanthem]

A88.1 Epidemic vertigo

A88.8 Other specified viral infections of central nervous system

A89 Unspecified viral infection of central nervous system

ARTHROPOD-BORNE VIRAL FEVERS AND VIRAL HEMORRHAGIC FEVERS (A90–A99)

A90 Dengue fever [classical dengue]
Excludes1:   dengue hemorrhagic fever (A91)

A91 Dengue hemorrhagic fever

A92 Other mosquito-borne viral fevers
Excludes1:   Ross River disease (B33.1)

A92.0 Chikungunya virus disease
Chikungunya (hemorrhagic) fever

A92.1 O'nyong-nyong fever

A92.2 Venezuelan equine fever
Venezuelan equine encephalitis
Venezuelan equine encephalomyelitis virus disease

A92.3 West Nile fever
West Nile virus

     A92.30 West Nile fever without encephalitis
West Nile fever NOS

     A92.31 West Nile fever with encephalitis

A92.4 Rift Valley fever

A92.8 Other specified mosquito-borne viral fevers

A92.9 Mosquito-borne viral fever, unspecified

A93 Other arthropod-borne viral fevers, not elsewhere classified

A93.0 Oropouche virus disease
Oropouche fever

A93.1 Sandfly fever
Pappataci fever
Phlebotomus fever

A93.2 Colorado tick fever

A93.8 Other specified arthropod-borne viral fevers
Piry virus disease
Vesicular stomatitis virus disease [Indiana fever]

A94 Unspecified arthropod-borne viral fever
Includes: arboviral fever NOS
arbovirus infection NOS

A95 Yellow fever

A95.0 Sylvatic yellow fever
Jungle yellow fever

A95.1 Urban yellow fever

A95.9 Yellow fever, unspecified

A96 Arenaviral hemorrhagic fever

A96.0 Junin hemorrhagic fever
Argentinian hemorrhagic fever

A96.1 Machupo hemorrhagic fever
Bolivian hemorrhagic fever

A96.2 Lassa fever

A96.8 Other arenaviral hemorrhagic fevers

A96.9 Arenaviral hemorrhagic fever, unspecified

A98 Other viral hemorrhagic fevers, not elsewhere classified
Excludes1:   chikungunya hemorrhagic fever (A92.0)
dengue hemorrhagic fever (A91)

A98.0 Crimean-Congo hemorrhagic fever
Central Asian hemorrhagic fever

A98.1 Omsk hemorrhagic fever

A98.2 Kyasanur Forest disease

A98.3 Marburg virus disease

A98.4 Ebola virus disease

A98.5 Hemorrhagic fever with renal syndrome
Epidemic hemorrhagic fever
Korean hemorrhagic fever
Russian hemorrhagic fever
Hantaan virus disease
Nephropathia epidemica

A98.8 Other specified viral hemorrhagic fevers

A99 Unspecified viral hemorrhagic fever

VIRAL INFECTIONS CHARACTERIZED BY SKIN AND MUCOUS MEMBRANE LESIONS (B00–B09)

B00 Herpesviral [herpes simplex] infections
>   Excludes1:   congenital herpesviral infections (P35.2)
>   Excludes2:   anogenital herpesviral infection (A60.-)
>   gammaherpesviral mononucleosis (B27.0-)
>   herpangina (B08.5)

B00.0 Eczema herpeticum
>   Kaposi's varicelliform eruption

B00.1 Herpesviral vesicular dermatitis
>   Herpes simplex facialis
>   Herpes simplex labialis
>   Herpes simplex otitis externa
>   Vesicular dermatitis of ear
>   Vesicular dermatitis of lip

B00.2 Herpesviral gingivostomatitis and pharyngotonsillitis
>   Herpesviral pharyngitis

B00.3 Herpesviral meningitis

B00.4 Herpesviral encephalitis
>   Herpesviral meningoencephalitis
>   Simian B disease

B00.5 Herpesviral ocular disease
>   **B00.50   Herpesviral ocular disease, unspecified**
>   **B00.51   Herpesviral iridocyclitis**
>   Herpesviral iritis
>   Herpesviral uveitis, anterior
>   **B00.52   Herpesviral keratitis**
>   Herpesviral keratoconjunctivitis
>   **B00.53   Herpesviral conjunctivitis**
>   **B00.59   Other herpesviral disease of eye**
>   Herpesviral dermatitis of eyelid

B00.7 Disseminated herpesviral disease
>   Herpesviral septicemia

B00.8 Other forms of herpesviral infections
>   **B00.81   Herpesviral hepatitis**
>   **B00.89   Other herpesviral infection**
>   Herpesviral whitlow

B00.9 Herpesviral infection, unspecified
>   Herpes simplex infection NOS

B01 Varicella [chickenpox]
B01.0 Varicella meningitis
B01.1 Varicella encephalitis
>   Postchickenpox encephalitis
>   Varicella encephalomyelitis

B01.2 Varicella pneumonia
B01.8 Varicella with other complications
>   **B01.81   Varicella keratitis**
>   **B01.89   Other varicella complications**

B01.9 Varicella without complication
>   Varicella NOS

B02 Zoster [herpes zoster]
>   Includes: shingles
>   zona

B02.0 Zoster encephalitis
>   Zoster meningoencephalitis

B02.1 Zoster meningitis
B02.2 Zoster with other nervous system involvement
>   **B02.21   Postherpetic geniculate ganglionitis**
>   **B02.22   Postherpetic trigeminal neuralgia**
>   **B02.23   Postherpetic polyneuropathy**
>   **B02.29   Other postherpetic nervous system involvement**
>   Postherpetic radiculopathy

B02.3 Zoster ocular disease
>   **B02.30   Zoster ocular disease, unspecified**
>   **B02.31   Zoster conjunctivitis**
>   **B02.32   Zoster iridocyclitis**
>   **B02.33   Zoster keratitis**
>   Herpes zoster keratoconjunctivitis
>   **B02.34   Zoster scleritis**

>   **B02.39   Other herpes zoster eye disease**
>   Zoster blepharitis

B02.7 Disseminated zoster
B02.8 Zoster with other complications
>   Herpes zoster otitis externa

B02.9 Zoster without complications
>   Zoster NOS

B03 Smallpox
>   In 1980 the 33rd World Health Assembly declared that smallpox had been eradicated. The classification is maintained for surveillance purposes.

B04 Monkeypox

B05 Measles
>   Includes: morbilli
>   Excludes1:   subacute sclerosing panencephalitis (A81.1)

B05.0 Measles complicated by encephalitis
>   Postmeasles encephalitis

B05.1 Measles complicated by meningitis
>   Postmeasles meningitis

B05.2 Measles complicated by pneumonia
>   Postmeasles pneumonia

B05.3 Measles complicated by otitis media
>   Postmeasles otitis media

B05.4 Measles with intestinal complications
B05.8 Measles with other complications
>   **B05.81   Measles keratitis and keratoconjunctivitis**
>   **B05.89   Other measles complications**

B05.9 Measles without complication
>   Measles NOS

B06 Rubella [German measles]
>   Excludes1:   congenital rubella (P35.0)

B06.0 Rubella with neurological complications
>   **B06.00   Rubella with neurological complication, unspecified**
>   **B06.01   Rubella encephalitis**
>   Rubella meningoencephalitis
>   **B06.02   Rubella meningitis**
>   **B06.09   Other neurological complications of rubella**

B06.8 Rubella with other complications
>   **B06.81   Rubella pneumonia**
>   **B06.82   Rubella arthritis**
>   **B06.89   Other rubella complications**

B06.9 Rubella without complication
>   Rubella NOS

B07 Viral warts
>   Includes: verruca simplex
>   verruca vulgaris
>   viral warts due to Human papillomavirus
>   Excludes2:   anogenital (venereal) warts (A63.0)
>   papilloma of bladder (D30.3)
>   papilloma of cervix (D26.0)
>   papilloma larynx (D14.1)

B08 Other viral infections characterized by skin and mucous membrane lesions, not elsewhere classified
>   Excludes1:   vesicular stomatitis virus disease (A93.8)

B08.0 Other orthopoxvirus infections
>   Cowpox
>   Orf virus disease
>   Pseudocowpox [milker's node]
>   Vaccinia
>   Excludes1:   monkeypox (B04)

B08.1 Molluscum contagiosum
B08.2 Exanthema subitum [sixth disease]
B08.3 Erythema infectiosum [fifth disease]
B08.4 Enteroviral vesicular stomatitis with exanthem
>   Hand, foot and mouth disease

B08.5 Enteroviral vesicular pharyngitis
>   Herpangina

B08.8 Other specified viral infections characterized by skin and mucous membrane lesions
Enteroviral lymphonodular pharyngitis
Foot-and-mouth disease
Tanapox virus disease
Yaba pox virus disease

B09 Unspecified viral infection characterized by skin and mucous membrane lesions
Includes: viral enanthema NOS
viral exanthema NOS

VIRAL HEPATITIS (B15–B19)
Excludes1:   sequelae of viral hepatitis (B94.2)
Excludes2:   cytomegaloviral hepatitis (B25.1)
herpesviral [herpes simplex] hepatitis (B00.81)

B15 Acute hepatitis A
B15.0 Hepatitis A with hepatic coma
B15.9 Hepatitis A without hepatic coma
Hepatitis A (acute) (viral) NOS

B16 Acute hepatitis B
B16.0 Acute hepatitis B with delta-agent with hepatic coma
B16.1 Acute hepatitis B with delta-agent without hepatic coma
B16.2 Acute hepatitis B without delta-agent with hepatic coma
B16.9 Acute hepatitis B without delta-agent and without hepatic coma
Hepatitis B (acute) (viral) NOS

B17 Other acute viral hepatitis
B17.0 Acute delta-(super) infection of hepatitis B carrier
B17.1 Acute hepatitis C
B17.2 Acute hepatitis E
B17.8 Other specified acute viral hepatitis
Hepatitis non-A non-B (acute) (viral) NEC

B18 Chronic viral hepatitis
B18.0 Chronic viral hepatitis B with delta-agent
B18.1 Chronic viral hepatitis B without delta-agent
Chronic (viral) hepatitis B
B18.2 Chronic viral hepatitis C
B18.8 Other chronic viral hepatitis
B18.9 Chronic viral hepatitis, unspecified

B19 Unspecified viral hepatitis
B19.0 Unspecified viral hepatitis with coma
B19.9 Unspecified viral hepatitis without coma
Viral hepatitis NOS

HUMAN IMMUNODEFICIENCY VIRUS [HIV] DISEASE (B20)
B20 Human immunodeficiency virus [HIV] disease
Includes: acquired immune deficiency syndrome [AIDS]
AIDS-related complex [ARC]
HIV infection, symptomatic
Use additional code(s) to identify all manifestations of HIV infection.
Excludes1:   asymptomatic human immunodeficiency virus [HIV] infection status (Z21)
exposure to HIV virus (Z20.6)
inconclusive serologic evidence of HIV (R75)

OTHER VIRAL DISEASES (B25–B34)
B25 Cytomegaloviral disease
Excludes1:   congenital cytomegalovirus infection (P35.1)
cytomegaloviral mononucleosis (B27.1-)
B25.0 Cytomegaloviral pneumonitis
B25.1 Cytomegaloviral hepatitis
B25.2 Cytomegaloviral pancreatitis
B25.8 Other cytomegaloviral diseases
Cytomegaloviral encephalitis
B25.9 Cytomegaloviral disease, unspecified

B26 Mumps
Includes: epidemic parotitis
infectious parotitis
B26.0 Mumps orchitis
B26.1 Mumps meningitis
B26.2 Mumps encephalitis
B26.3 Mumps pancreatitis
B26.8 Mumps with other complications
B26.81 Mumps hepatitis
B26.82 Mumps myocarditis
B26.83 Mumps nephritis
B26.84 Mumps polyneuropathy
B26.85 Mumps arthritis
B26.89 Other mumps complications
B26.9 Mumps without complication
Mumps NOS
Mumps parotitis NOS

B27 Infectious mononucleosis
Includes: glandular fever
monocytic angina
Pfeiffer's disease
B27.0 Gammaherpesviral mononucleosis
Mononucleosis due to Epstein-Barr virus
B27.00 Gammaherpesviral mononucleosis without complication
B27.01 Gammaherpesviral mononucleosis with polyneuropathy
B27.02 Gammaherpesviral mononucleosis with meningitis
B27.09 Gammaherpesviral mononucleosis with other complications
Hepatomegaly in gammaherpesviral mononucleosis
B27.1 Cytomegaloviral mononucleosis
B27.10 Cytomegaloviral mononucleosis without complications
B27.11 Cytomegaloviral mononucleosis with polyneuropathy
B27.12 Cytomegaloviral mononucleosis with meningitis
B27.19 Cytomegaloviral mononucleosis with other complication
Hepatomegaly in cytomegaloviral mononucleosis
B27.8 Other infectious mononucleosis
B27.80 Other infectious mononucleosis without complication
B27.81 Other infectious mononucleosis with polyneuropathy
B27.82 Other infectious mononucleosis with meningitis
B27.89 Other infectious mononucleosis with other complication
Hepatomegaly in other infectious mononucleosis
B27.9 Infectious mononucleosis, unspecified
B27.90 Infectious mononucleosis, unspecified without complication
B27.91 Infectious mononucleosis, unspecified with polyneuropathy
B27.92 Infectious mononucleosis, unspecified with meningitis
B27.99 Infectious mononucleosis, unspecified with other complication
Hepatomegaly in unspecified infectious mononucleosis

B30 Viral conjunctivitis
Excludes1:   herpesviral [herpes simplex] ocular disease (B00.5)
ocular zoster (B02.3)
B30.0 Keratoconjunctivitis due to adenovirus
Epidemic keratoconjunctivitis
Shipyard eye
B30.1 Conjunctivitis due to adenovirus
Acute adenoviral follicular conjunctivitis
Swimming-pool conjunctivitis
B30.2 Viral pharyngoconjunctivitis
B30.3 Acute epidemic hemorrhagic conjunctivitis (enteroviral)
Conjunctivitis due to coxsackievirus 24
Conjunctivitis due to enterovirus 70
Hemorrhagic conjunctivitis (acute) (epidemic)

B30.8   Other viral conjunctivitis
Newcastle conjunctivitis

B30.9   Viral conjunctivitis, unspecified

B33   Other viral diseases, not elsewhere classified

B33.0   Epidemic myalgia
Bornholm disease

B33.1   Ross River disease
Epidemic polyarthritis and exanthema
Ross River fever

B33.2   Viral carditis
Coxsackie (virus) carditis

 B33.20   Viral carditis, unspecified

 B33.21   Viral endocarditis

 B33.22   Viral myocarditis

 B33.23   Viral pericarditis

 B33.24   Viral cardiomyopathy

B33.3   Retrovirus infections, not elsewhere classified
Retrovirus infection NOS

B33.4   Hantavirus pulmonary syndrome
Sin nombre virus

B33.8   Other specified viral diseases
Excludes1:   human papillomavirus infection (A63.0)

B34   Viral infection of unspecified site
Excludes1:   cytomegaloviral disease NOS (B25.9)
herpesvirus [herpes simplex] infection NOS (B00.9)
human papillomavirus infection (A63.0)
retrovirus infection NOS (B33.3)
viral agents as the cause of diseases classified to other chapters (B97.-)

B34.0   Adenovirus infection, unspecified

B34.1   Enterovirus infection, unspecified
Coxsackievirus infection NOS
Echovirus infection NOS

B34.2   Coronavirus infection, unspecified

B34.3   Parvovirus infection, unspecified

B34.4   Papovavirus infection, unspecified

B34.8   Other viral infections of unspecified site

B34.9   Viral infection, unspecified
Viremia NOS

MYCOSES (B35–B49)
Excludes2:   hypersensitivity pneumonitis due to organic dust (J67.-)
mycosis fungoides (C84.0-)

B35   Dermatophytosis
Includes: favus
infections due to species of Epidermophyton, Microsporum and Trichophyton
tinea, any type except those in B36.-

B35.0   Tinea barbae and tinea capitis
Beard ringworm
Kerion
Scalp ringworm
Sycosis, mycotic

B35.1   Tinea unguium
Dermatophytic onychia
Dermatophytosis of nail
Onychomycosis
Ringworm of nails

B35.2   Tinea manuum
Dermatophytosis of hand
Hand ringworm

B35.3   Tinea pedis
Athlete's foot
Dermatophytosis of foot
Foot ringworm

B35.4   Tinea corporis
Ringworm of the body

B35.5   Tinea imbricata
Tokelau

B35.6   Tinea cruris
Dhobi itch
Groin ringworm
Jock itch

B35.8   Other dermatophytoses
Disseminated dermatophytosis
Granulomatous dermatophytosis

B35.9   Dermatophytosis, unspecified
Ringworm NOS

B36   Other superficial mycoses

B36.0   Pityriasis versicolor
Tinea flava
Tinea versicolor

B36.1   Tinea nigra
Keratomycosis nigricans palmaris
Microsporosis nigra
Pityriasis nigra

B36.2   White piedra
Tinea blanca

B36.3   Black piedra

B36.8   Other specified superficial mycoses

B36.9   Superficial mycosis, unspecified

B37   Candidiasis
Includes: candidosis
moniliasis
Excludes1:   neonatal candidiasis (P37.5)

B37.0   Candidal stomatitis
Oral thrush

B37.1   Pulmonary candidiasis
Candidal bronchitis
Candidal pneumonia

B37.2   Candidiasis of skin and nail
Candidal onychia
Candidal paronychia
Excludes2:   diaper dermatitis (L22)

B37.3   Candidiasis of vulva and vagina
Candidal vulvovaginitis
Monilial vulvovaginitis
Vaginal thrush

B37.4   Candidiasis of other urogenital sites

 B37.41   Candidal cystitis and urethritis

 B37.42   Candidal balanitis

 B37.49   Other urogenital candidiasis
 Candidal pyelonephritis

B37.5   Candidal meningitis

B37.6   Candidal endocarditis

B37.7   Candidal septicemia
Disseminated candidiasis
Systemic candidiasis

B37.8   Candidiasis of other sites

 B37.81   Candidal esophagitis

 B37.82   Candidal enteritis
 Candidal proctitis

 B37.83   Candidal cheilitis

 B37.84   Candidal otitis externa

 B37.89   Other sites of candidiasis
 Candidal osteomyelitis

B37.9   Candidiasis, unspecified
Thrush NOS

B38   Coccidioidomycosis

B38.0   Acute pulmonary coccidioidomycosis

B38.1   Chronic pulmonary coccidioidomycosis

B38.2   Pulmonary coccidioidomycosis, unspecified

B38.3   Cutaneous coccidioidomycosis

B38.4   Coccidioidomycosis meningitis

B38.7   Disseminated coccidioidomycosis
Generalized coccidioidomycosis

B38.8   Other forms of coccidioidomycosis

 B38.81   Prostatic coccidioidomycosis

 B38.89   Other forms of coccidioidomycosis

B38.9   Coccidioidomycosis, unspecified

B39   Histoplasmosis

Code first associated AIDS (B20)

Use additional code for any associated manifestations, such as:
endocarditis (I39)
meningitis (G02)
pericarditis (I32)
retinitis (H32)

B39.0   Acute pulmonary histoplasmosis capsulati

B39.1   Chronic pulmonary histoplasmosis capsulati

B39.2   Pulmonary histoplasmosis capsulati, unspecified

B39.3   Disseminated histoplasmosis capsulati
Generalized histoplasmosis capsulati

B39.4   Histoplasmosis capsulati, unspecified
American histoplasmosis

B39.5   Histoplasmosis duboisii
African histoplasmosis

B39.9   Histoplasmosis, unspecified

B40   Blastomycosis

Excludes1:   Brazilian blastomycosis (B41.-)
keloidal blastomycosis (B48.0)

B40.0   Acute pulmonary blastomycosis

B40.1   Chronic pulmonary blastomycosis

B40.2   Pulmonary blastomycosis, unspecified

B40.3   Cutaneous blastomycosis

B40.7   Disseminated blastomycosis
Generalized blastomycosis

B40.8   Other forms of blastomycosis

B40.81   Blastomycotic meningoencephalitis
Meningomyelitis due to blastomycosis

B40.89   Other forms of blastomycosis

B40.9   Blastomycosis, unspecified

B41   Paracoccidioidomycosis

Includes: Brazilian blastomycosis
Lutz' disease

B41.0   Pulmonary paracoccidioidomycosis

B41.7   Disseminated paracoccidioidomycosis
Generalized paracoccidioidomycosis

B41.8   Other forms of paracoccidioidomycosis

B41.9   Paracoccidioidomycosis, unspecified

B42   Sporotrichosis

B42.0   Pulmonary sporotrichosis

B42.1   Lymphocutaneous sporotrichosis

B42.7   Disseminated sporotrichosis
Generalized sporotrichosis

B42.8   Other forms of sporotrichosis

B42.81   Cerebral sporotrichosis
Meningitis due to sporotrichosis

B42.82   Sporotrichosis arthritis

B42.89   Other forms of sporotrichosis

B42.9   Sporotrichosis, unspecified

B43   Chromomycosis and pheomycotic abscess

B43.0   Cutaneous chromomycosis
Dermatitis verrucosa

B43.1   Pheomycotic brain abscess
Cerebral chromomycosis

B43.2   Subcutaneous pheomycotic abscess and cyst

B43.8   Other forms of chromomycosis

B43.9   Chromomycosis, unspecified

B44   Aspergillosis

Includes: aspergilloma

B44.0   Invasive pulmonary aspergillosis

B44.1   Other pulmonary aspergillosis

B44.2   Tonsillar aspergillosis

B44.7   Disseminated aspergillosis
Generalized aspergillosis

B44.8   Other forms of aspergillosis

B44.81   Allergic bronchopulmonary aspergillosis

B44.89   Other forms of aspergillosis

B44.9   Aspergillosis, unspecified

B45   Cryptococcosis

B45.0   Pulmonary cryptococcosis

B45.1   Cerebral cryptococcosis
Cryptococcal meningitis
Cryptococcosis meningocerebralis

B45.2   Cutaneous cryptococcosis

B45.3   Osseous cryptococcosis

B45.7   Disseminated cryptococcosis
Generalized cryptococcosis

B45.8   Other forms of cryptococcosis

B45.9   Cryptococcosis, unspecified

B46   Zygomycosis

B46.0   Pulmonary mucormycosis

B46.1   Rhinocerebral mucormycosis

B46.2   Gastrointestinal mucormycosis

B46.3   Cutaneous mucormycosis
Subcutaneous mucormycosis

B46.4   Disseminated mucormycosis
Generalized mucormycosis

B46.5   Mucormycosis, unspecified

B46.8   Other zygomycoses
Entomophthoromycosis

B46.9   Zygomycosis, unspecified
Phycomycosis NOS

B47   Mycetoma

B47.0   Eumycetoma
Madura foot, mycotic
Maduromycosis

B47.1   Actinomycetoma

B47.9   Mycetoma, unspecified
Madura foot NOS

B48   Other mycoses, not elsewhere classified

B48.0   Lobomycosis
Keloidal blastomycosis
Lobo's disease

B48.1   Rhinosporidiosis

B48.2   Allescheriasis
Infection due to Pseudallescheria boydii
Excludes1:   eumycetoma (B47.0)

B48.3   Geotrichosis
Geotrichum stomatitis

B48.4   Penicillosis

B48.8   Other specified mycoses
Adiaspiromycosis
Infection of tissue and organs by alternaria
Infection of tissue and organs by dreschlera
Infection of tissue and organs by fusarium
Infection of tissue and organs by saprophytic fungi NEC

B49   Unspecified mycosis
Fungemia NOS

PROTOZOAL DISEASES (B50–B64)

Excludes1:   amebiasis (A06.-)
other protozoal intestinal diseases (A07.-)

B50   Plasmodium falciparum malaria

Includes: mixed infections of Plasmodium falciparum with any
other Plasmodium species

B50.0   Plasmodium falciparum malaria with cerebral complications
Cerebral malaria NOS

B50.8   Other severe and complicated Plasmodium falciparum malaria
Severe or complicated Plasmodium falciparum malaria NOS

B50.9   Plasmodium falciparum malaria, unspecified

B51 Plasmodium vivax malaria

Includes: mixed infections of Plasmodium vivax with other Plasmodium species, except Plasmodium falciparum

Excludes1:   plasmodium vivav with Plasmodium falciparum (B50.-)

B51.0 Plasmodium vivax malaria with rupture of spleen

B51.8 Plasmodium vivax malaria with other complications

B51.9 Plasmodium vivax malaria without complication
Plasmodium vivax malaria NOS

B52 Plasmodium malariae malaria

Includes: mixed infections of Plasmodium malariae with other Plasmodium species, except Plasmodium falciparum and Plasmodium vivax

Excludes1:   Plasmodium falciparum (B50.-)
Plasmodium vivax (B51.-)

B52.0 Plasmodium malariae malaria with nephropathy

B52.8 Plasmodium malariae malaria with other complications

B52.9 Plasmodium malariae malaria without complication
Plasmodium malariae malaria NOS

B53 Other specified malaria

B53.0 Plasmodium ovale malaria

Excludes1:   Plasmodium ovale with Plasmodium falciparum (B50.-)
Plasmodium ovale with Plasmodium malariae (B52.-)
Plasmodium ovale with Plasmodium vivax (B51.-)

B53.1 Malaria due to simian plasmodia

Excludes1:   Malaria due to simian plasmodia with Plasmodium falciparum (B50.-)
Malaria due to simian plasmodia with Plasmodium malariae (B52.-)
Malaria due to simian plasmodia with Plasmodium ovale (B53.0)
Malaria due to simian plasmodia with Plasmodium vivax (B51.-)

B53.8 Other malaria, not elsewhere classified

B54 Unspecified malaria

B55 Leishmaniasis

B55.0 Visceral leishmaniasis
Kala-azar
Post-kala-azar dermal leishmaniasis

B55.1 Cutaneous leishmaniasis

B55.2 Mucocutaneous leishmaniasis

B55.9 Leishmaniasis, unspecified

B56 African trypanosomiasis

B56.0 Gambiense trypanosomiasis
Infection due to Trypanosoma brucei gambiense
West African sleeping sickness

B56.1 Rhodesiense trypanosomiasis
East African sleeping sickness
Infection due to Trypanosoma brucei rhodesiense

B56.9 African trypanosomiasis, unspecified
Sleeping sickness NOS

B57 Chagas' disease

Includes: American trypanosomiasis
infection due to Trypanosoma cruzi

B57.0 Acute Chagas' disease with heart involvement
Acute Chagas' disease with myocarditis

B57.1 Acute Chagas' disease without heart involvement
Acute Chagas' disease NOS

B57.2 Chagas' disease (chronic) with heart involvement
American trypanosomiasis NOS
Chagas' disease (chronic) NOS
Chagas' disease (chronic) with myocarditis
Trypanosomiasis NOS

B57.3 Chagas' disease (chronic) with digestive system involvement

B57.30 Chagas' disease with digestive system involvement, unspecified

B57.31 Megaesophagus in Chagas' disease

B57.32 Megacolon in Chagas' disease

B57.39 Other digestive system involvement in Chagas' disease

B57.4 Chagas' disease (chronic) with nervous system involvement

B57.40 Chagas' disease with nervous system involvement, unspecified

B57.41 Meningitis in Chagas' disease

B57.42 Meningoencephalitis in Chagas' disease

B57.49 Other nervous system involvement in Chagas' disease

B57.5 Chagas' disease (chronic) with other organ involvement

B58 Toxoplasmosis

Includes: infection due to Toxoplasma gondii

Excludes1:   congenital toxoplasmosis (P37.1)

B58.0 Toxoplasma oculopathy

B58.00 Toxoplasma oculopathy, unspecified

B58.01 Toxoplasma chorioretinitis

B58.09 Other toxoplasma oculopathy
Toxoplasma uveitis

B58.1 Toxoplasma hepatitis

B58.2 Toxoplasma meningoencephalitis

B58.3 Pulmonary toxoplasmosis

B58.8 Toxoplasmosis with other organ involvement

B58.81 Toxoplasma myocarditis

B58.82 Toxoplasma myositis

B58.83 Toxoplasma tubulo-interstitial nephropathy
Toxoplasma pyelonephritis

B58.89 Toxoplasmosis with other organ involvement

B58.9 Toxoplasmosis, unspecified

B59 Pneumocystosis
Pneumonia due to Pneumocystis carinii

B60 Other protozoal diseases, not elsewhere classified

Excludes1:   cryptosporidiosis (A07.2)
isosporiasis (A07.3)

B60.0 Babesiosis
Piroplasmosis

B60.1 Acanthamebiasis

B60.10 Acanthamebiasis, unspecified

B60.11 Meningoencephalitis due to Acanthamoeba (culbertsoni)

B60.12 Conjunctivitis due to Acanthamoeba

B60.13 Keratoconjunctivitis due to Acanthamoeba

B60.19 Other acanthamebic disease

B60.2 Naegleriasis
Primary amebic meningoencephalitis

B60.8 Other specified protozoal diseases
Microsporidiosis

B64 Unspecified protozoal disease

HELMINTHIASES (B65–B83)

B65 Schistosomiasis [bilharziasis]

Includes: snail fever

B65.0 Schistosomiasis due to Schistosoma haematobium [urinary schistosomiasis]

B65.1 Schistosomiasis due to Schistosoma mansoni [intestinal schistosomiasis]

B65.2 Schistosomiasis due to Schistosoma japonicum
Asiatic schistosomiasis

B65.3 Cercarial dermatitis
Swimmer's itch

B65.8 Other schistosomiasis
Infection due to Schistosoma intercalatum
Infection due to Schistosoma mattheei
Infection due to Schistosoma mekongi

B65.9 Schistosomiasis, unspecified

B66 Other fluke infections

B66.0 Opisthorchiasis
Infection due to cat liver fluke
Infection due to Opisthorchis (felineus) (viverrini)

B66.1 Clonorchiasis
Chinese liver fluke disease
Infection due to Clonorchis sinensis
Oriental liver fluke disease

B66.2 Dicroceliasis
Infection due to Dicrocoelium dendriticum
Lancet fluke infection

B66.3 Fascioliasis
Infection due to Fasciola gigantica
Infection due to Fasciola hepatica
Infection due to Fasciola indica
Sheep liver fluke disease

B66.4 Paragonimiasis
Infection due to Paragonimus species
Lung fluke disease
Pulmonary distomiasis

B66.5 Fasciolopsiasis
Infection due to Fasciolopsis buski
Intestinal distomiasis

B66.8 Other specified fluke infections
Echinostomiasis
Heterophyiasis
Metagonimiasis
Nanophyetiasis
Watsoniasis

B66.9 Fluke infection, unspecified

B67 Echinococcosis

Includes: hydatidosis

B67.0 Echinococcus granulosus infection of liver
B67.1 Echinococcus granulosus infection of lung
B67.2 Echinococcus granulosus infection of bone
B67.3 Echinococcus granulosus infection, other and multiple sites
B67.31 Echinococcus granulosus infection, thyroid gland
B67.32 Echinococcus granulosus infection, multiple sites
B67.39 Echinococcus granulosus infection, other sites
B67.4 Echinococcus granulosus infection, unspecified
B67.5 Echinococcus multilocularis infection of liver
B67.6 Echinococcus multilocularis infection, other and multiple sites
B67.61 Echinococcus multilocularis infection, multiple sites
B67.69 Echinococcus multilocularis infection, other sites
B67.7 Echinococcus multilocularis infection, unspecified
B67.8 Echinococcosis, unspecified, of liver
B67.9 Echinococcosis, other and unspecified
B67.90 Echinococcosis, unspecified
Echinococcosis NOS
B67.99 Other echinococcosis

B68 Taeniasis

Excludes1:   cysticercosis (B69.-)

B68.0 Taenia solium taeniasis
Pork tapeworm (infection)

B68.1 Taenia saginata taeniasis
Beef tapeworm (infection)
Infection due to adult tapeworm
Taenia saginata

B68.9 Taeniasis, unspecified

B69 Cysticercosis

Includes: cysticerciasis infection due to larval form of Taenia solium

B69.0 Cysticercosis of central nervous system
B69.1 Cysticercosis of eye
B69.8 Cysticercosis of other sites
B69.81 Myositis in cysticercosis
B69.89 Cysticercosis of other sites
B69.9 Cysticercosis, unspecified

B70 Diphyllobothriasis and sparganosis

B70.0 Diphyllobothriasis
Diphyllobothrium (adult) (latum) (pacificum) infection
Fish tapeworm (infection)
Excludes2:   larval diphyllobothriasis (B70.1)

B70.1 Sparganosis
Infection due to Sparganum (mansoni) (proliferum)
Infection due to Spirometra larva
Larval diphyllobothriasis
Spirometrosis

B71 Other cestode infections

B71.0 Hymenolepiasis
Dwarf tapeworm infection
Rat tapeworm (infection)

B71.1 Dipylidiasis
Dog tapeworm (infection)

B71.8 Other specified cestode infections
Coenurosis

B71.9 Cestode infection, unspecified
Tapeworm (infection) NOS

B72 Dracunculiasis

Includes: guinea worm
infection infection due to Dracunculus medinensis

B73 Onchocerciasis

Includes: onchocerca volvulus infection
onchocercosis
river blindness

B73.0 Onchocerciasis with eye disease
B73.00 Onchocerciasis with eye involvement, unspecified
B73.01 Onchocerciasis with endophthalmitis
B73.02 Onchocerciasis with glaucoma
B73.09 Onchocerciasis with other eye involvement
Infestation of eyelid due to onchocerciasis
B73.1 Onchocerciasis without eye disease

B74 Filariasis

Excludes3:   onchocerciasis (B73)
tropical (pulmonary) eosinophilia NOS (J82)

B74.0 Filariasis due to Wuchereria bancrofti
Bancroftian elephantiasis
Bancroftian filariasis

B74.1 Filariasis due to Brugia malayi
B74.2 Filariasis due to Brugia timori
B74.3 Loiasis
Calabar swelling
Eyeworm disease of Africa
Loa loa infection

B74.4 Mansonelliasis
Infection due to Mansonella ozzardi
Infection due to Mansonella perstans
Infection due to Mansonella streptocerca

B74.8 Other filariases
Dirofilariasis

B74.9 Filariasis, unspecified

B75 Trichinellosis

Includes: infection due to Trichinella species
trichiniasis

B76 Hookworm diseases

Includes: uncinariasis

B76.0 Ancylostomiasis
Infection due to Ancylostoma species

B76.1 Necatoriasis
Infection due to Necator americanus

B76.8 Other hookworm diseases
B76.9 Hookworm disease, unspecified
Cutaneous larva migrans NOS

B77 Ascariasis

Includes: ascaridiasis
roundworm infection

B77.0   Ascariasis with intestinal complications
B77.8   Ascariasis with other complications
    B77.81   Ascariasis pneumonia
    B77.89   Ascariasis with other complications
B77.9   Ascariasis, unspecified

B78   Strongyloidiasis
    Excludes1:   trichostrongyliasis (B81.2)
B78.0   Intestinal strongyloidiasis
B78.1   Cutaneous strongyloidiasis
B78.7   Disseminated strongyloidiasis
B78.9   Strongyloidiasis, unspecified

B79   Trichuriasis
    Includes: trichocephaliasis
              whipworm (disease) (infection)

B80   Enterobiasis
    Includes: oxyuriasis
              pinworm infection
              threadworm infection

B81   Other intestinal helminthiases, not elsewhere classified
    Excludes1:   angiostrongyliasis due to Parastrongylus cantonensis
              (B83.2)
B81.0   Anisakiasis
    Infection due to Anisakis larva
B81.1   Intestinal capillariasis
    Capillariasis NOS
    Infection due to Capillaria philippinensis
    Excludes2:   hepatic capillariasis (B83.8)
B81.2   Trichostrongyliasis
B81.3   Intestinal angiostrongyliasis
    Angiostrongyliasis due to Parastrongylus costaricensis
B81.4   Mixed intestinal helminthiases
    Infection due to intestinal helminths classified to more than one
       of the categories B65.0-B81.3 and B81.8
    Mixed helminthiasis NOS
B81.8   Other specified intestinal helminthiases
    Infection due to Oesophagostomum species [esophagostomiasis]
    Infection due to Ternidens diminutus [ternidensiasis]

B82   Unspecified intestinal parasitism
B82.0   Intestinal helminthiasis, unspecified
B82.9   Intestinal parasitism, unspecified

B83   Other helminthiases
    Excludes1:   capillariasis NOS (B81.1)
    Excludes2:   intestinal capillariasis (B81.1)
B83.0   Visceral larva migrans
    Toxocariasis
B83.1   Gnathostomiasis
    Wandering swelling
B83.2   Angiostrongyliasis due to Parastrongylus cantonensis
    Eosinophilic meningoencephalitis due to Parastrongylus
       cantonensis
    Excludes2:   intestinal angiostrongyliasis (B81.3)
B83.3   Syngamiasis
    Syngamosis
B83.4   Internal hirudiniasis
    Excludes2:   external hirudiniasis (B88.3)
B83.8   Other specified helminthiases
    Acanthocephaliasis
    Gongylonemiasis
    Hepatic capillariasis
    Metastrongyliasis
    Thelaziasis
B83.9   Helminthiasis, unspecified
    Worms NOS
    Excludes1:   intestinal helminthiasis NOS (B82.0)

PEDICULOSIS, ACARIASIS AND OTHER INFESTATIONS
(B85–B89)

B85   Pediculosis and phthiriasis
B85.0   Pediculosis due to Pediculus humanus capitis
    Head-louse infestation
B85.1   Pediculosis due to Pediculus humanus corporis
    Body-louse infestation
B85.2   Pediculosis, unspecified
B85.3   Phthiriasis
    Infestation by crab-louse
    Infestation by Phthirus pubis
B85.4   Mixed pediculosis and phthiriasis
    Infestation classifiable to more than one of the categories
       B85.0-B85.3

B86   Scabies
    Includes: sarcoptic itch

B87   Myiasis
    Includes: infestation by larva of flies
B87.0   Cutaneous myiasis
    Creeping myiasis
B87.1   Wound myiasis
    Traumatic myiasis
B87.2   Ocular myiasis
B87.3   Nasopharyngeal myiasis
    Laryngeal myiasis
B87.4   Aural myiasis
B87.8   Myiasis of other sites
    B87.81   Genitourinary myiasis
    B87.82   Intestinal myiasis
    B87.89   Myiasis of other sites
B87.9   Myiasis, unspecified

B88   Other infestations
B88.0   Other acariasis
    Acarine dermatitis
    Dermatitis due to Demodex species
    Dermatitis due to Dermanyssus gallinae
    Dermatitis due to Liponyssoides sanguineus
    Trombiculosis
    Excludes2:   scabies (B86)
B88.1   Tungiasis [sandflea infestation]
B88.2   Other arthropod infestations
    Scarabiasis
B88.3   External hirudiniasis
    Leech infestation NOS
    Excludes2:   internal hirudiniasis (B83.4)
B88.8   Other specified infestations
    Ichthyoparasitism due to Vandellia cirrhosa
    Linguatulosis
    Porocephaliasis
B88.9   Infestation, unspecified
    Infestation (skin) NOS
    Infestation by mites NOS
    Skin parasites NOS

B89   Unspecified parasitic disease

SEQUELAE OF INFECTIOUS AND PARASITIC DISEASES
(B90–B94)
Note: These categories are to be used to indicate conditions in categories A00-B89 as the cause of sequelae, which are themselves classified elsewhere. The "sequelae" include conditions specified as such; they also include residuals of diseases classifiable to the above categories if there is evidence that the disease itself is no longer present.
Use additional code to identify sequelae

B90   Sequelae of tuberculosis
B90.0   Sequelae of central nervous system tuberculosis
B90.1   Sequelae of genitourinary tuberculosis
B90.2   Sequelae of tuberculosis of bones and joints

B90.8 Sequelae of tuberculosis of other organs
    Excludes2:   sequelae of respiratory tuberculosis (B90.9)

B90.9 Sequelae of respiratory and unspecified tuberculosis
    Sequelae of tuberculosis NOS

B91 Sequelae of poliomyelitis

B92 Sequelae of leprosy

B94 Sequelae of other and unspecified infectious and parasitic diseases

B94.0 Sequelae of trachoma

B94.1 Sequelae of viral encephalitis

B94.2 Sequelae of viral hepatitis

B94.8 Sequelae of other specified infectious and parasitic diseases

B94.9 Sequelae of unspecified infectious and parasitic disease

BACTERIAL, VIRAL AND OTHER INFECTIOUS AGENTS
(B95–B97)

Note: These categories are provided for use as supplementary or additional codes to identify the infectious agent(s) in diseases classified elsewhere.

B95 Streptococcus, Staphylococcus, and Enterococcus as the cause of diseases classified to other chapters

B95.0 Streptococcus, group A, as the cause of diseases classified to other chapters

B95.1 Streptococcus, group B, as the cause of diseases classified to other chapters

B95.2 Enterococcus as the cause of diseases classified elsewhere

B95.3 Streptococcus pneumoniae as the cause of diseases classified to other chapters

B95.4 Other streptococcus as the cause of diseases classified to other chapters

B95.5 Unspecified streptococcus as the cause of diseases classified to other chapters

B95.6 Staphylococcus aureus as the cause of diseases classified to other chapters

B95.7 Other staphylococcus as the cause of diseases classified to other chapters

B95.8 Unspecified staphylococcus as the cause of diseases classified to other chapters

B96 Other bacterial agents as the cause of diseases classified to other chapters

B96.0 Mycoplasma pneumoniae [M. pneumoniae] as the cause of diseases classified to other chapters
    Pleuro-pneumonia-like-organism [PPLO]

B96.1 Klebsiella pneumoniae [K. pneumoniae] as the cause of diseases classified to other chapters

B96.2 Escherichia coli [E. coli] as the cause of diseases classified to other chapters

B96.3 Hemophilus influenzae [H. influenzae] as the cause of diseases classified to other chapters

B96.4 Proteus (mirabilis) (morganii) as the cause of diseases classified to other chapters

B96.5 Pseudomonas (aeruginosa) (mallei) (pseudomallei) as the cause of diseases classified to other chapters

B96.6 Bacillus fragilis [B. fragilis] as the cause of diseases classified to other chapters

B96.7 Clostridium perfringens [C. perfringens] as the cause of diseases classified to other chapters

B96.8 Other specified bacterial agents as the cause of diseases classified to other chapters

    B96.81   Helicobacter pylori [H. pylori] as the cause of diseases classified to other chapters

    B96.89   Other specified bacterial agents as the cause of diseases classified to other chapters

B97 Viral agents as the cause of diseases classified to other chapters

B97.0 Adenovirus as the cause of diseases classified to other chapters

B97.1 Enterovirus as the cause of diseases classified to other chapters

B97.10 Unspecified enterovirus as the cause of diseases classified to other chapters

B97.11 Coxsackievirus as the cause of diseases classified to other chapters

B97.12 Echovirus as the cause of diseases classified to other chapters

B97.19 Other enterovirus as the cause of diseases classified to other chapters

B97.2 Coronavirus as the cause of diseases classified to other chapters

B97.3 Retrovirus as the cause of diseases classified to other chapters
    Excludes1:   Human immunodeficiency virus [HIV] disease (B20)

B97.30 Unspecified retrovirus as the cause of diseases classified to other chapters

B97.31 Lentivirus as the cause of diseases classified to other chapters

B97.32 Oncovirus as the cause of diseases classified to other chapters

B97.33 Human T-cell lymphotrophic virus, type I [HTLV-1] as the cause of diseases classified to other chapters

B97.34 Human T-cell lymphotrophic virus, type II [HTLV-II] as the cause of diseases classified to other chapters

B97.35 Human immunodeficiency virus, type 2 [HIV 2] as the cause of diseases classified to other chapters

B97.39 Other retrovirus as the cause of diseases classified to other chapters

B97.4 Respiratory syncytial virus as the cause of diseases classified to other chapters

B97.5 Reovirus as the cause of diseases classified to other chapters

B97.6 Parvovirus as the cause of diseases classified to other chapters

B97.7 Papillomavirus as the cause of diseases classified to other chapters

B97.8 Other viral agents as the cause of diseases classified to other chapters

OTHER INFECTIOUS DISEASES (B99)

B99 Other and unspecified infectious diseases

B99.8 Other infectious disease

B99.9 Unspecified infectious disease

CHAPTER II — NEOPLASMS (C00–D49)

This chapter contains the following broad groups of neoplasms:

C00-C75	Malignant neoplasms, stated or presumed to be primary, of specified sites, except of lymphoid, hematopoietic and related tissue
C00-C14	Lip, oral cavity and pharynx
C15-C26	Digestive organs
C30-C39	Respiratory and intrathoracic organs
C40-C41	Bone and articular cartilage
C43-C44	Skin
C45-C49	Mesothelial and soft tissue
C50	Breast
C51-C58	Female genital organs
C60-C63	Male genital organs
C64-C68	Urinary tract
C69-C72	Eye, brain and other parts of central nervous system
C73-C75	Thyroid and other endocrine glands
C76-C80	Malignant neoplasms of ill-defined, secondary and unspecified sites
C81-C96	Malignant neoplasms, stated or presumed to be primary, of lymphoid, hematopoietic and related tissue
D00-D09	In situ neoplasms
D10-D36	Benign neoplasms
D37-D48	Neoplasms of uncertain behavior
D49	Neoplasms of unspecified behavior

MALIGNANT NEOPLASMS (C00–C96)

MALIGNANT NEOPLASM OF LIP, ORAL CAVITY AND PHARYNX (C00–C14)

C00 Malignant neoplasm of lip

Excludes1: malignant neoplasm of skin of lip (C43.0, C44.0)
Use additional code to identify:
  alcohol abuse and dependence (F10.-)
  alcohol dependence in remission (F10.21)
  history of tobacco use (Z87.82)
  tobacco dependence (F17.-)
  tobacco use (Z72.0)

C00.0 Malignant neoplasm of external upper lip
  Malignant neoplasm of lipstick area of upper lip
  Malignant neoplasm of upper lip NOS
  Malignant neoplasm of vermilion border of upper lip

C00.1 Malignant neoplasm of external lower lip
  Malignant neoplasm of lower lip NOS
  Malignant neoplasm of lipstick area of lower lip
  Malignant neoplasm of vermilion border of lower lip

C00.2 Malignant neoplasm of external lip, unspecified
  Malignant neoplasm of vermilion border of lip NOS

C00.3 Malignant neoplasm of upper lip, inner aspect
  Malignant neoplasm of buccal aspect of upper lip
  Malignant neoplasm of frenulum of upper lip
  Malignant neoplasm of mucosa of upper lip
  Malignant neoplasm of oral aspect of upper lip

C00.4 Malignant neoplasm of lower lip, inner aspect
  Malignant neoplasm of buccal aspect of lower lip
  Malignant neoplasm of frenulum of lower lip
  Malignant neoplasm of mucosa of lower lip
  Malignant neoplasm of oral aspect of lower lip

C00.5 Malignant neoplasm of lip, unspecified, inner aspect
  Malignant neoplasm of buccal aspect of lip, unspecified
  Malignant neoplasm of frenulum of lip, unspecified
  Malignant neoplasm of mucosa of lip, unspecified
  Malignant neoplasm of oral aspect of lip, unspecified

C00.6 Malignant neoplasm of commissure of lip, unspecified

C00.8 Malignant neoplasm of overlapping sites of lip

C00.9 Malignant neoplasm of lip, unspecified

C01 Malignant neoplasm of base of tongue

Includes: malignant neoplasm of dorsal surface of base of tongue
  malignant neoplasm of fixed part of tongue NOS
  malignant neoplasm of posterior third of tongue
Use additional code to identify:
  alcohol abuse and dependence (F10.-)
  alcohol dependence in remission (F10.21)
  history of tobacco use (Z87.82)
  tobacco dependence (F17.-)
  tobacco use (Z72.0)

C02 Malignant neoplasm of other and unspecified parts of tongue

Use additional code to identify:
  alcohol abuse and dependence (F10.-)
  alcohol dependence in remission (F10.21)
  history of tobacco use (Z87.82)
  tobacco dependence (F17.-)
  tobacco use (Z72.0)

C02.0 Malignant neoplasm of dorsal surface of tongue
  Malignant neoplasm of anterior two-thirds of tongue, dorsal surface
  Excludes2: malignant neoplasm of dorsal surface of base of tongue (C01)

C02.1 Malignant neoplasm of border of tongue
  Malignant neoplasm of tip of tongue

C02.2 Malignant neoplasm of ventral surface of tongue
  Malignant neoplasm of anterior two-thirds of tongue, ventral surface
  Malignant neoplasm of frenulum linguae

C02.3 Malignant neoplasm of anterior two-thirds of tongue, part unspecified
  Malignant neoplasm of middle third of tongue NOS
  Malignant neoplasm of mobile part of tongue NOS

C02.4 Malignant neoplasm of lingual tonsil
  Excludes2: malignant neoplasm of tonsil NOS (C09.9)

C02.8 Malignant neoplasm of overlapping sites of tongue
  Malignant neoplasm of tongue whose point of origin cannot be classified to any one of the categories C01-C02.4

C02.9 Malignant neoplasm of tongue, unspecified

C03 Malignant neoplasm of gum

Includes: malignant neoplasm of alveolar (ridge) mucosa
  malignant neoplasm of gingiva
Excludes2: malignant odontogenic neoplasms (C41.0-C41.1)
Use additional code to identify:
  alcohol abuse and dependence (F10.-)
  alcohol dependence in remission (F10.21)
  history of tobacco use (Z87.82)
  tobacco dependence (F17.-)
  tobacco use (Z72.0)

C03.0 Malignant neoplasm of upper gum

C03.1 Malignant neoplasm of lower gum

C03.9 Malignant neoplasm of gum, unspecified

C04 Malignant neoplasm of floor of mouth

Use additional code to identify:
  alcohol abuse and dependence (F10.-)
  alcohol dependence in remission (F10.21)
  history of tobacco use (Z87.82)
  tobacco dependence (F17.-)
  tobacco use (Z72.0)

C04.0 Malignant neoplasm of anterior floor of mouth
  Malignant neoplasm of anterior to the premolar-canine junction

C04.1 Malignant neoplasm of lateral floor of mouth

C04.8 Malignant neoplasm of overlapping sites of floor of mouth

C04.9 Malignant neoplasm of floor of mouth, unspecified

C05 Malignant neoplasm of palate

Excludes1: Kaposi's sarcoma of palate (C46.2)
Use additional code to identify:
  alcohol abuse and dependence (F10.-)
  alcohol dependence in remission (F10.21)
  history of tobacco use (Z87.82)
  tobacco dependence (F17.-)
  tobacco use (Z72.0)

C05.0 Malignant neoplasm of hard palate

C05.1 Malignant neoplasm of soft palate

> Excludes2: malignant neoplasm of nasopharyngeal surface of
> soft palate (C11.3)

C05.2 Malignant neoplasm of uvula

C05.8 Malignant neoplasm of overlapping sites of palate

C05.9 Malignant neoplasm of palate, unspecified

> Malignant neoplasm of roof of mouth

C06 Malignant neoplasm of other and unspecified parts of mouth

> Use additional code to identify:
> alcohol abuse and dependence (F10.-)
> alcohol dependence in remission (F10.21)
> history of tobacco use (Z87.82)
> tobacco dependence (F17.-)
> tobacco use (Z72.0)

C06.0 Malignant neoplasm of cheek mucosa

> Malignant neoplasm of buccal mucosa NOS
> Malignant neoplasm of internal cheek

C06.1 Malignant neoplasm of vestibule of mouth

> Malignant neoplasm of buccal sulcus (upper) (lower)
> Malignant neoplasm of labial sulcus (upper) (lower)

C06.2 Malignant neoplasm of retromolar area

C06.8 Malignant neoplasm of overlapping sites of other and unspecified parts of mouth

> **C06.80 Malignant neoplasm of overlapping sites of unspecified parts of mouth**
>
> **C06.89 Malignant neoplasm of overlapping sites of other parts of mouth**

C06.9 Malignant neoplasm of mouth, unspecified

> Malignant neoplasm of minor salivary gland, unspecified side
> Malignant neoplasm of oral cavity NOS

C07 Malignant neoplasm of parotid gland

> Use additional code to identify:
> alcohol abuse and dependence (F10.-)
> alcohol dependence, in remission (F10.21)
> exposure to environmental tobacco smoke (X58.1)
> exposure to tobacco smoke in the perinatal period (P96.6)
> history of tobacco use (Z87.82)
> occupational exposure to environmental tobacco smoke (Z57.31)
> tobacco dependence (F17.-)
> tobacco use (Z72.0)

C08 Malignant neoplasm of other and unspecified major salivary glands

> Includes: malignant neoplasm of salivary ducts
> Excludes1: malignant neoplasms of specified minor salivary glands which are classified according to their anatomical location
> Excludes2: malignant neoplasms of minor salivary glands NOS (C06.9)
> malignant neoplasm of parotid gland (C07)
> Use additional code to identify:
> alcohol abuse and dependence (F10.-)
> alcohol dependence, in remission (F10.21)
> exposure to environmental tobacco smoke (X58.1)
> exposure to tobacco smoke in the perinatal period (P96.6)
> history of tobacco use (Z87.82)
> occupational exposure to environmental tobacco smoke (Z57.31)
> tobacco dependence (F17.-)
> tobacco use (Z72.0)

C08.0 Malignant neoplasm of submandibular gland

> Malignant neoplasm of submaxillary gland

C08.1 Malignant neoplasm of sublingual gland

C08.8 Malignant neoplasm of overlapping sites of major salivary glands

> Malignant neoplasm of major salivary glands whose point of origin cannot be classified to any one of the categories C07-C08.1

C08.9 Malignant neoplasm of major salivary gland, unspecified

> Malignant neoplasm of salivary gland (major) NOS

C09 Malignant neoplasm of tonsil

> Excludes2: malignant neoplasm of lingual tonsil (C02.4)
> malignant neoplasm of pharyngeal tonsil (C11.1)
> Use additional code to identify:
> alcohol abuse and dependence (F10.-)
> alcohol dependence, in remission (F10.21)
> exposure to environmental tobacco smoke (X58.1)
> exposure to tobacco smoke in the perinatal period (P96.6)
> history of tobacco use (Z87.82)
> occupational exposure to environmental tobacco smoke (Z57.31)
> tobacco dependence (F17.-)
> tobacco use (Z72.0)

C09.0 Malignant neoplasm of tonsillar fossa

C09.1 Malignant neoplasm of tonsillar pillar (anterior) (posterior)

C09.8 Malignant neoplasm of overlapping sites of tonsil

C09.9 Malignant neoplasm of tonsil, unspecified

> Malignant neoplasm of tonsil NOS
> Malignant neoplasm of faucial tonsils
> Malignant neoplasm of palatine tonsils

C10 Malignant neoplasm of oropharynx

> Excludes2: malignant neoplasm of tonsil (C09.-)
> Use additional code to identify:
> alcohol abuse and dependence (F10.-)
> alcohol dependence, in remission (F10.21)
> exposure to environmental tobacco smoke (X58.1)
> exposure to tobacco smoke in the perinatal period (P96.6)
> history of tobacco use (Z87.82)
> occupational exposure to environmental tobacco smoke (Z57.31)
> tobacco dependence (F17.-)
> tobacco use (Z72.0)

C10.0 Malignant neoplasm of vallecula

C10.1 Malignant neoplasm of anterior surface of epiglottis

> Malignant neoplasm of epiglottis, free border [margin]
> Malignant neoplasm of glossoepiglottic fold(s)
> Excludes2: malignant neoplasm of epiglottis (suprahyoid portion) NOS (C32.1)

C10.2 Malignant neoplasm of lateral wall of oropharynx

C10.3 Malignant neoplasm of posterior wall of oropharynx

C10.4 Malignant neoplasm of branchial cleft

> Malignant neoplasm of branchial cyst [site of neoplasm]

C10.8 Malignant neoplasm of overlapping sites of oropharynx

> Malignant neoplasm of junctional region of oropharynx

C10.9 Malignant neoplasm of oropharynx, unspecified

C11 Malignant neoplasm of nasopharynx

> Use additional code to identify:
> exposure to environmental tobacco smoke (X58.1)
> exposure to tobacco smoke in the perinatal period (P96.6)
> history of tobacco use (Z87.82)
> occupational exposure to environmental tobacco smoke (Z57.31)
> tobacco dependence (F17.-)
> tobacco use (Z72.0)

C11.0 Malignant neoplasm of superior wall of nasopharynx

> Malignant neoplasm of roof of nasopharynx

C11.1 Malignant neoplasm of posterior wall of nasopharynx

> Malignant neoplasm of adenoid
> Malignant neoplasm of pharyngeal tonsil

C11.2 Malignant neoplasm of lateral wall of nasopharynx

> Malignant neoplasm of fossa of Rosenmüller
> Malignant neoplasm of opening of auditory tube
> Malignant neoplasm of pharyngeal recess

C11.3 Malignant neoplasm of anterior wall of nasopharynx

> Malignant neoplasm of floor of nasopharynx
> Malignant neoplasm of nasopharyngeal (anterior) (posterior) surface of soft palate
> Malignant neoplasm of posterior margin of nasal choana
> Malignant neoplasm of posterior margin of nasal septum

C11.8 Malignant neoplasm of overlapping sites of nasopharynx

C11.9 Malignant neoplasm of nasopharynx, unspecified

> Malignant neoplasm of nasopharyngeal wall NOS

C12　Malignant neoplasm of pyriform sinus

Includes:　malignant neoplasm of pyriform fossa
Use additional code to identify:
exposure to environmental tobacco smoke (X58.1)
exposure to tobacco smoke in the perinatal period (P96.6)
history of tobacco use (Z87.82)
occupational exposure to environmental tobacco smoke (Z57.31)
tobacco dependence (F17.-)
tobacco use (Z72.0)

C13　Malignant neoplasm of hypopharynx

Excludes2:　malignant neoplasm of pyriform sinus (C12)
Use additional code to identify:
exposure to environmental tobacco smoke (X58.1)
exposure to tobacco smoke in the perinatal period (P96.6)
history of tobacco use (Z87.82)
occupational exposure to environmental tobacco smoke (Z57.31)
tobacco dependence (F17.-)
tobacco use (Z72.0)

C13.0　Malignant neoplasm of postcricoid region

C13.1　Malignant neoplasm of aryepiglottic fold, hypopharyngeal aspect

Malignant neoplasm of aryepiglottic fold NOS
Malignant neoplasm of interarytenoid fold NOS
Malignant neoplasm of aryepiglottic fold marginal zone
Malignant neoplasm of interarytenoid fold marginal zone

Excludes2:　malignant neoplasm of aryepiglottic fold or interarytenoid fold, laryngeal aspect (C32.1)

C13.2　Malignant neoplasm of posterior wall of hypopharynx

C13.8　Malignant neoplasm of overlapping sites of hypopharynx

C13.9　Malignant neoplasm of hypopharynx, unspecified

Malignant neoplasm of hypopharyngeal wall NOS

C14　Malignant neoplasm of other and ill-defined sites in the lip, oral cavity and pharynx

Excludes1:　malignant neoplasm of oral cavity NOS (C06.9)
Use additional code to identify:
alcohol abuse and dependence (F10.-)
alcohol dependence, in remission (F10.21)
exposure to environmental tobacco smoke (X58.1)
exposure to tobacco smoke in the perinatal period (P96.6)
history of tobacco use (Z87.82)
occupational exposure to environmental tobacco smoke (Z57.31)
tobacco dependence (F17.-)
tobacco use (Z72.0)

C14.0　Malignant neoplasm of pharynx, unspecified

C14.1　Malignant neoplasm of laryngopharynx

C14.2　Malignant neoplasm of Waldeyer's ring

C14.8　Malignant neoplasm of overlapping sites of lip, oral cavity and pharynx

Malignant neoplasm of lip, oral cavity and pharynx whose point of origin cannot be classified to any one of the categories C00-C14.2

Excludes1:　"book leaf" neoplasm [ventral surface of tongue and floor of mouth] (C06.8)

MALIGNANT NEOPLASM OF DIGESTIVE ORGANS (C15–C26)

Excludes1:　Kaposi's sarcoma of gastrointestinal sites (C46.4)

C15　Malignant neoplasm of esophagus

Use additional code to identify:
alcohol abuse and dependence (F10.-)
alcohol dependence, in remission (F10.21)

C15.3　Malignant neoplasm of upper third of esophagus

C15.4　Malignant neoplasm of middle third of esophagus

C15.5　Malignant neoplasm of lower third of esophagus

Excludes1:　malignant neoplasm of cardio-esophageal junction (C16.0)

C15.8　Malignant neoplasm of overlapping sites of esophagus

C15.9　Malignant neoplasm of esophagus, unspecified

C16　Malignant neoplasm of stomach

Use additional code to identify:
alcohol abuse and dependence (F10.-)
alcohol dependence, in remission (F10.21)

C16.0　Malignant neoplasm of cardia

Malignant neoplasm of cardiac orifice
Malignant neoplasm of cardio-esophageal junction
Malignant neoplasm of esophagus and stomach
Malignant neoplasm of gastro-esophageal junction

C16.1　Malignant neoplasm of fundus of stomach

C16.2　Malignant neoplasm of body of stomach

C16.3　Malignant neoplasm of pyloric antrum

Malignant neoplasm of gastric antrum

C16.4　Malignant neoplasm of pylorus

Malignant neoplasm of prepylorus
Malignant neoplasm of pyloric canal

C16.5　Malignant neoplasm of lesser curvature of stomach, unspecified

Malignant neoplasm of lesser curvature of stomach, not classifiable to C16.1-C16.4

C16.6　Malignant neoplasm of greater curvature of stomach, unspecified

Malignant neoplasm of greater curvature of stomach, not classifiable to C16.0-C16.4

C16.8　Malignant neoplasm of overlapping sites of stomach

C16.9　Malignant neoplasm of stomach, unspecified

Gastric cancer NOS

C17　Malignant neoplasm of small intestine

C17.0　Malignant neoplasm of duodenum

C17.1　Malignant neoplasm of jejunum

C17.2　Malignant neoplasm of ileum

Excludes1:　malignant neoplasm of ileocecal valve (C18.0)

C17.3　Meckel's diverticulum

C17.8　Malignant neoplasm of overlapping sites of small intestine

C17.9　Malignant neoplasm of small intestine, unspecified

C18　Malignant neoplasm of colon

C18.0　Malignant neoplasm of cecum

Malignant neoplasm of ileocecal valve

C18.1　Malignant neoplasm of appendix

C18.2　Malignant neoplasm of ascending colon

C18.3　Malignant neoplasm of hepatic flexure

C18.4　Malignant neoplasm of transverse colon

C18.5　Malignant neoplasm of splenic flexure

C18.6　Malignant neoplasm of descending colon

C18.7　Malignant neoplasm of sigmoid colon

Malignant neoplasm of sigmoid (flexure)

Excludes1:　malignant neoplasm of rectosigmoid junction (C19)

C18.8　Malignant neoplasm of overlapping sites of colon

C18.9　Malignant neoplasm of colon, unspecified

Malignant neoplasm of large intestine NOS

C19　Malignant neoplasm of rectosigmoid junction

Includes:　malignant neoplasm of colon with rectum
malignant neoplasm of rectosigmoid (colon)

C20　Malignant neoplasm of rectum

Includes:　malignant neoplasm of rectal ampulla

C21　Malignant neoplasm of anus and anal canal

Excludes3:　malignant melanoma of anal margin (C43.5)
malignant melanoma of anal skin (C43.5)
malignant melanoma of perianal skin (C43.5)
malignant neoplasm of anal margin (C44.5)
malignant neoplasm of anal skin (C44.5)
malignant neoplasm of perianal skin (C44.5)

C21.0　Malignant neoplasm of anus, unspecified

C21.1　Malignant neoplasm of anal canal

Malignant neoplasm of anal sphincter

C21.2　Malignant neoplasm of cloacogenic zone

C21.8 Malignant neoplasm of overlapping sites of rectum, anus and anal canal
  Malignant neoplasm of anorectal junction
  Malignant neoplasm of anorectum
  Malignant neoplasm of rectum, anus and anal canal whose point of origin cannot be classified to any one of the categories C20-C21.1

C22 Malignant neoplasm of liver and intrahepatic bile ducts
  Excludes1: malignant neoplasm of biliary tract NOS (C24.9)
     secondary malignant neoplasm of liver (C78.7)
  Use additional code to identify:
    alcohol abuse and dependence (F10.-)
    alcohol dependence, in remission (F10.21)
    hepatitis B (B16.-, B18.0-B18.1)
    hepatitis C (B17.1, B18.2)

C22.0 Liver cell carcinoma
  Hepatocellular carcinoma
  Hepatoma

C22.1 Intrahepatic bile duct carcinoma
  Cholangiocarcinoma
  Excludes1: malignant neoplasm of hepatic duct (C24.0)

C22.2 Hepatoblastoma
C22.3 Angiosarcoma of liver
  Kupffer cell sarcoma
C22.4 Other sarcomas of liver
C22.7 Other specified carcinomas of liver
C22.8 Malignant neoplasm of liver, primary, unspecified as to type
C22.9 Malignant neoplasm of liver, not specified as primary or secondary

C23 Malignant neoplasm of gallbladder

C24 Malignant neoplasm of other and unspecified parts of biliary tract
  Excludes1: malignant neoplasm of intrahepatic bile duct (C22.1)

C24.0 Malignant neoplasm of extrahepatic bile duct
  Malignant neoplasm of biliary duct or passage NOS
  Malignant neoplasm of common bile duct
  Malignant neoplasm of cystic duct
  Malignant neoplasm of hepatic duct

C24.1 Malignant neoplasm of ampulla of Vater
C24.8 Malignant neoplasm of overlapping sites of biliary tract
  Malignant neoplasm involving both intrahepatic and extrahepatic bile ducts
  Malignant neoplasm of biliary tract whose point of origin cannot be classified to any one of the categories C22.0-C24.1

C24.9 Malignant neoplasm of biliary tract, unspecified

C25 Malignant neoplasm of pancreas
  Use additional code to identify:
    alcohol abuse and dependence (F10.-)
    alcohol dependence, in remission (F10.21)

C25.0 Malignant neoplasm of head of pancreas
C25.1 Malignant neoplasm of body of pancreas
C25.2 Malignant neoplasm of tail of pancreas
C25.3 Malignant neoplasm of pancreatic duct
C25.4 Malignant neoplasm of endocrine pancreas
  Malignant neoplasm of islets of Langerhans
  Use additional code to identify any functional activity.
C25.7 Malignant neoplasm of other parts of pancreas
  Malignant neoplasm of neck of pancreas
C25.8 Malignant neoplasm of overlapping sites of pancreas
C25.9 Malignant neoplasm of pancreas, unspecified

C26 Malignant neoplasm of other and ill-defined digestive organs
  Excludes1: malignant neoplasm of peritoneum and retroperitoneum (C48.-)
C26.0 Malignant neoplasm of intestinal tract, part unspecified
  Malignant neoplasm of intestine NOS
C26.1 Malignant neoplasm of spleen
  Excludes1: Hodgkin's disease (C81.-)
    non-Hodgkin's lymphoma (C82-C85)

C26.8 Malignant neoplasm of overlapping sites of digestive system
  Malignant neoplasm of digestive organs whose point of origin cannot be classified to any one of the categories C15-C26.1
  Excludes1: malignant neoplasm of anus and rectum (C21.8)
    malignant neoplasm of cardio-oesophageal junction (C16.0)
    malignant neoplasm of colon and rectum (C19)

C26.9 Malignant neoplasm of ill-defined sites within the digestive system
  Malignant neoplasm of alimentary canal or tract NOS
  Malignant neoplasm of gastrointestinal tract NOS
  Excludes1: malignant neoplasm of abdominal NOS (C76.2)
    malignant neoplasm of intra-abdominal NOS (C76.2)

MALIGNANT NEOPLASM OF RESPIRATORY AND INTRATHORACIC ORGANS (C30–C39)
  Includes: malignant neoplasm of middle ear
  Excludes1: mesothelioma (C45.-)

C30 Malignant neoplasm of nasal cavity and middle ear
C30.0 Malignant neoplasm of nasal cavity
  Malignant neoplasm of cartilage of nose
  Malignant neoplasm of nasal concha
  Malignant neoplasm of internal nose
  Malignant neoplasm of septum of nose
  Malignant neoplasm of vestibule of nose
  Excludes1: malignant neoplasm of nasal bone (C41.0)
    malignant neoplasm of nose NOS (C76.0)
    malignant neoplasm of olfactory bulb (C72.2-)
    malignant neoplasm of posterior margin of nasal septum and choana (C11.3)
    malignant neoplasm of skin of nose (C43.39, C44.39)
    malignant neoplasm of turbinates (C41.0)

C30.1 Malignant neoplasm of middle ear
  Malignant neoplasm of antrum tympanicum
  Malignant neoplasm of auditory tube
  Malignant neoplasm of eustachian tube
  Malignant neoplasm of inner ear
  Malignant neoplasm of mastoid air cells
  Malignant neoplasm of tympanic cavity
  Excludes1: malignant neoplasm of auricular canal (external) (C43.2-, C44.2-)
    malignant neoplasm of bone of ear (meatus) (C41.0)
    malignant neoplasm of cartilage of ear (C49.0)
    malignant neoplasm of skin of (external) ear (C43.2-, C44.2-)

C31 Malignant neoplasm of accessory sinuses
C31.0 Malignant neoplasm of maxillary sinus
  Malignant neoplasm of antrum (Highmore) (maxillary)
C31.1 Malignant neoplasm of ethmoidal sinus
C31.2 Malignant neoplasm of frontal sinus
C31.3 Malignant neoplasm of sphenoid sinus
C31.8 Malignant neoplasm of overlapping sites of accessory sinuses
C31.9 Malignant neoplasm of accessory sinus, unspecified

C32 Malignant neoplasm of larynx
  Use additional code to identify:
    alcohol abuse and dependence (F10.-)
    alcohol dependence, in remission (F10.21)
    exposure to environmental tobacco smoke (X58.1)
    exposure to tobacco smoke in the perinatal period (P96.6)
    history of tobacco use (Z87.82)
    occupational exposure to environmental tobacco smoke (Z57.31)
    tobacco dependence (F17.-)
    tobacco use (Z72.0)
C32.0 Malignant neoplasm of glottis
  Malignant neoplasm of intrinsic larynx
  Malignant neoplasm of laryngeal commissure (anterior) (posterior)
  Malignant neoplasm of vocal cord (true) NOS

C32.1 **Malignant neoplasm of supraglottis**

    Malignant neoplasm of aryepiglottic fold or interarytenoid fold, laryngeal aspect

    Malignant neoplasm of epiglottis (suprahyoid portion) NOS

    Malignant neoplasm of extrinsic larynx

    Malignant neoplasm of false vocal cord

    Malignant neoplasm of posterior (laryngeal) surface of epiglottis

    Malignant neoplasm of ventricular bands

    Excludes1:   malignant neoplasm of anterior surface of epiglottis (C10.1)

                 malignant neoplasm of aryepiglottic fold or interarytenoid fold:

                    NOS (C13.1)

                    hypopharyngeal aspect (C13.1)

                    marginal zone (C13.1)

C32.2 **Malignant neoplasm of subglottis**

C32.3 **Malignant neoplasm of laryngeal cartilage**

C32.8 **Malignant neoplasm of overlapping sites of larynx**

C32.9 **Malignant neoplasm of larynx, unspecified**

C33 **Malignant neoplasm of trachea**

    Use additional code to identify:

    exposure to environmental tobacco smoke (X58.1)

    exposure to tobacco smoke in the perinatal period (P96.6)

    history of tobacco use (Z87.82)

    occupational exposure to environmental tobacco smoke (Z57.31)

    tobacco dependence (F17.-)

    tobacco use (Z72.0)

C34 **Malignant neoplasm of bronchus and lung**

    Excludes1:   Kaposi's sarcoma of lung (C46.5-)

    Use additional code to identify:

    exposure to environmental tobacco smoke (X58.1)

    exposure to tobacco smoke in the perinatal period (P96.6)

    history of tobacco use (Z87.82)

    occupational exposure to environmental tobacco smoke (Z57.31)

    tobacco dependence (F17.-)

    tobacco use (Z72.0)

C34.0 **Malignant neoplasm of main bronchus**

    Malignant neoplasm of carina

    Malignant neoplasm of hilus (of lung)

    C34.00 **Malignant neoplasm of main bronchus, unspecified side**

    C34.01 **Malignant neoplasm of right main bronchus**

    C34.02 **Malignant neoplasm of left main bronchus**

C34.1 **Malignant neoplasm of upper lobe, bronchus or lung**

    C34.10 **Malignant neoplasm of upper lobe, bronchus or lung, unspecified side**

    C34.11 **Malignant neoplasm of upper lobe, right bronchus or lung**

    C34.12 **Malignant neoplasm of upper lobe, left bronchus or lung**

C34.2 **Malignant neoplasm of middle lobe, right bronchus or lung**

C34.3 **Malignant neoplasm of lower lobe, bronchus or lung**

    C34.30 **Malignant neoplasm of lower lobe, bronchus or lung, unspecified side**

    C34.31 **Malignant neoplasm of lower lobe, right bronchus or lung**

    C34.32 **Malignant neoplasm of lower lobe, left bronchus or lung**

C34.8 **Malignant neoplasm of overlapping sites of bronchus and lung**

    C34.80 **Malignant neoplasm of overlapping sites of bronchus and lung, unspecified side**

    C34.81 **Malignant neoplasm of overlapping sites of right bronchus and lung**

    C34.82 **Malignant neoplasm of overlapping sites of left bronchus and lung**

C34.9 **Malignant neoplasm of bronchus or lung, unspecified**

    C34.90 **Malignant neoplasm of bronchus or lung, unspecified, unspecified side**

    C34.91 **Malignant neoplasm of right bronchus or lung, unspecified**

    C34.92 **Malignant neoplasm of left bronchus or lung, unspecified**

C37 **Malignant neoplasm of thymus**

C38 **Malignant neoplasm of heart, mediastinum and pleura**

    Excludes1:   mesothelioma (C45.-)

C38.0 **Malignant neoplasm of heart**

    Malignant neoplasm of pericardium

    Excludes1:   malignant neoplasm of great vessels (C49.3)

C38.1 **Malignant neoplasm of anterior mediastinum**

C38.2 **Malignant neoplasm of posterior mediastinum**

C38.3 **Malignant neoplasm of mediastinum, part unspecified**

C38.4 **Malignant neoplasm of pleura**

C38.8 **Malignant neoplasm of overlapping sites of heart, mediastinum and pleura**

C39 **Malignant neoplasm of other and ill-defined sites in the respiratory system and intrathoracic organs**

    Excludes1:   intrathoracic malignant neoplasm NOS (C76.1)

                 thoracic malignant neoplasm NOS (C76.1)

    Use additional code to identify:

    exposure to environmental tobacco smoke (X58.1)

    exposure to tobacco smoke in the perinatal period (P96.6)

    history of tobacco use (Z87.82)

    occupational exposure to environmental tobacco smoke (Z57.31)

    tobacco dependence (F17.-)

    tobacco use (Z72.0)

C39.0 **Malignant neoplasm of upper respiratory tract, part unspecified**

C39.8 **Malignant neoplasm of overlapping sites of respiratory and intrathoracic organ**

    Malignant neoplasm of respiratory and intrathoracic organs whose point of origin cannot be classified to any one of the categories C30-C39.0

C39.9 **Malignant neoplasm of lower respiratory tract, part unspecified**

    Malignant neoplasm of respiratory tract NOS

MALIGNANT NEOPLASM OF BONE AND ARTICULAR CARTILAGE (C40–C41)

    Includes: malignant neoplasm of cartilage (articular) (joint)

                 malignant neoplasm of periosteum

    Excludes1:   malignant neoplasm of bone marrow NOS (C96.7)

                 malignant neoplasm of synovia (C49.-)

C40 **Malignant neoplasm of bone and articular cartilage of limbs**

C40.0 **Malignant neoplasm of scapula and long bones of upper limb**

    C40.00 **Malignant neoplasm of scapula and long bones of upper limb, unspecified side**

    C40.01 **Malignant neoplasm of scapula and long bones of right upper limb**

    C40.02 **Malignant neoplasm of scapula and long bones of left upper limb**

C40.1 **Malignant neoplasm of short bones of upper limb**

    C40.10 **Malignant neoplasm of short bones of upper limb, unspecified side**

    C40.11 **Malignant neoplasm of short bones of right upper limb**

    C40.12 **Malignant neoplasm of short bones of left upper limb**

C40.2 **Malignant neoplasm of long bones of lower limb**

    C40.20 **Malignant neoplasm of long bones of lower limb, unspecified side**

    C40.21 **Malignant neoplasm of long bones of right lower limb**

    C40.22 **Malignant neoplasm of long bones of left lower limb**

C40.3 **Malignant neoplasm of short bones of lower limb**

    C40.30 **Malignant neoplasm of short bones of lower limb, unspecified side**

    C40.31 **Malignant neoplasm of short bones of right lower limb**

    C40.32 **Malignant neoplasm of short bones of left lower limb**

C40.8 **Malignant neoplasm of overlapping sites of bone and articular cartilage of limb**

    C40.80 **Malignant neoplasm of overlapping sites of bone and articular cartilage of limb, unspecified side**

    C40.81 **Malignant neoplasm of overlapping sites of bone and articular cartilage of right limb**

C40.82   Malignant neoplasm of overlapping sites of bone and articular cartilage of left limb

C40.9   Malignant neoplasm of bones and articular cartilage of limb, unspecified

C40.90   Malignant neoplasm of bones and articular cartilage of limb, unspecified, unspecified side

C40.91   Malignant neoplasm of bones and articular cartilage of right limb, unspecified

C40.92   Malignant neoplasm of bones and articular cartilage of left limb, unspecified

C41   Malignant neoplasm of bone and articular cartilage of other and unspecified sites

Excludes1:   malignant neoplasm of bones of limbs (C40.-)
malignant neoplasm of cartilage of:
ear (C49.0)
eyelid (C49.0)
larynx (C32.3)
limbs (C40.-)
nose (C30.0)

C41.0   Malignant neoplasm of bones of skull and face

Malignant neoplasm of maxilla (superior)
Malignant neoplasm of orbital bone

Excludes2:   carcinoma, any type except intraosseous or odontogenic of:
maxillary sinus (C31.0)
upper jaw (C03.0)
malignant neoplasm of jaw bone (lower) (C41.1)

C41.1   Malignant neoplasm of mandible

Malignant neoplasm of inferior maxilla
Malignant neoplasm of lower jaw bone

Excludes2:   carcinoma, any type except intraosseous or odontogenic of:
jaw NOS (C03.9)
lower (C03.1)
malignant neoplasm of upper jaw bone (C41.0)

C41.2   Malignant neoplasm of vertebral column

Excludes1:   malignant neoplasm of sacrum and coccyx (C41.4)

C41.3   Malignant neoplasm of ribs, sternum and clavicle

C41.4   Malignant neoplasm of pelvic bones, sacrum and coccyx

C41.8   Malignant neoplasm of overlapping sites of bone and articular cartilage

Malignant neoplasm of bone and articular cartilage whose point of origin cannot be classified to any one of the categories C40-C41.4

C41.9   Malignant neoplasm of bone and articular cartilage, unspecified

MELANOMA AND OTHER MALIGNANT NEOPLASMS OF SKIN
(C43–C44)

Excludes1:   melanoma in situ (D03.-)

C43   Malignant melanoma of skin

Use additional morphology codes M8720-M8790 with behavior code /3

Excludes2:   malignant melanoma of skin of genital organs (C51-C52, C60.-, C63.-)
sites other than skin-code to malignant neoplasm of the site

C43.0   Malignant melanoma of lip

Excludes1:   malignant neoplasm of vermilion border of lip (C00.0-C00.2)

C43.1   Malignant melanoma of eyelid, including canthus

C43.10   Malignant melanoma of eyelid, including canthus, unspecified side

C43.11   Malignant melanoma of right eyelid, including canthus

C43.12   Malignant melanoma of left eyelid, including canthus

C43.2   Malignant melanoma of ear and external auricular canal

C43.20   Malignant melanoma of ear and external auricular canal, unspecified side

C43.21   Malignant melanoma of right ear and external auricular canal

C43.22   Malignant melanoma of left ear and external auricular canal

C43.3   Malignant melanoma of other and unspecified parts of face

C43.30   Malignant melanoma of unspecified part of face

C43.39   Malignant melanoma of other parts of face

C43.4   Malignant melanoma of scalp and neck

C43.5   Malignant melanoma of trunk

Malignant melanoma of anal margin
Malignant melanoma of anal skin
Malignant melanoma of perianal skin
Malignant melanoma of skin of breast

Excludes1:   malignant neoplasm of anus NOS (C21.0)
malignant neoplasm of scrotum (C63.2)

C43.6   Malignant melanoma of upper limb, including shoulder

C43.60   Malignant melanoma of upper limb, including shoulder, unspecified side

C43.61   Malignant melanoma of right upper limb, including shoulder

C43.62   Malignant melanoma of left upper limb, including shoulder

C43.7   Malignant melanoma of lower limb, including hip

C43.70   Malignant melanoma of lower limb, including hip, unspecified side

C43.71   Malignant melanoma of right lower limb, including hip

C43.72   Malignant melanoma of left lower limb, including hip

C43.8   Overlapping malignant melanoma of skin

C43.9   Malignant melanoma of skin, unspecified

Melanoma (malignant) NOS

C44   Other malignant neoplasm of skin

Includes: malignant neoplasm of sebaceous glands
malignant neoplasm of sweat glands

Excludes1:   Kaposi's sarcoma of skin (C46.0)
malignant melanoma of skin (C43.-)
malignant neoplasm of skin of genital organs (C51-C52, C60.-, C63.2)

C44.0   Malignant neoplasm of skin of lip

Malignant neoplasm of basal cell carcinoma of lip

Excludes1:   malignant neoplasm of lip (C00.-)

C44.1   Malignant neoplasm of skin of eyelid, including canthus

Excludes1:   connective tissue of eyelid (C49.0)

C44.10   Malignant neoplasm of skin of eyelid, including canthus, unspecified side

C44.11   Malignant neoplasm of skin of right eyelid, including canthus

C44.12   Malignant neoplasm of skin of left eyelid, including canthus

C44.2   Malignant neoplasm of skin of ear and external auricular canal

Excludes1:   connective tissue of ear (C49.0)

C44.20   Malignant neoplasm of skin of ear and external auricular canal, unspecified side

C44.21   Malignant neoplasm of skin of right ear and external auricular canal

C44.22   Malignant neoplasm of skin of left ear and external auricular canal

C44.3   Malignant neoplasm of skin of other and unspecified parts of face

C44.30   Malignant neoplasm of skin of unspecified part of face

C44.39   Malignant neoplasm of skin of other parts of face

C44.4   Malignant neoplasm of skin of scalp and neck

C44.5   Malignant neoplasm of skin of trunk

Malignant neoplasm of anal margin
Malignant neoplasm of anal skin
Malignant neoplasm of perianal skin
Malignant neoplasm of skin of breast

Excludes1:   anus NOS (C21.0)
scrotum (C63.2)

C44.6   Malignant neoplasm of skin of upper limb, including shoulder

C44.60   Malignant neoplasm of skin of upper limb, including shoulder, unspecified side

C44.61   Malignant neoplasm of skin of right upper limb, including shoulder

C44.62   Malignant neoplasm of skin of left upper limb, including shoulder

C44.7 Malignant neoplasm of skin of lower limb, including hip

C44.70   Malignant neoplasm of skin of lower limb, including hip, unspecified side

C44.71   Malignant neoplasm of skin of right lower limb, including hip

C44.72   Malignant neoplasm of skin of left lower limb, including hip

C44.8 Malignant neoplasm of overlapping sites of skin

C44.9 Malignant neoplasm of skin, unspecified

MALIGNANT NEOPLASMS OF MESOTHELIAL AND SOFT TISSUE
(C45–C49)

C45 Mesothelioma

Use additional morphology code M9050 with behavior code /3

C45.0 Mesothelioma of pleura

Excludes1:   other malignant neoplasm of pleura (C38.4)

C45.1 Mesothelioma of peritoneum

Mesothelioma of cul-de-sac
Mesothelioma of mesentery
Mesothelioma of mesocolon
Mesothelioma of omentum
Mesothelioma of peritoneum (parietal) (pelvic)

Excludes1:   other malignant neoplasm of soft tissue of peritoneum (C48.-)

C45.2 Mesothelioma of pericardium

Excludes1:   other malignant neoplasm of pericardium (C38.0)

C45.7 Mesothelioma of other sites

C45.9 Mesothelioma, unspecified

C46 Kaposi's sarcoma

Use additional morphology code M9140 with behavior code /3
Code first any human immunodeficiency virus [HIV] disease (B20)

C46.0 Kaposi's sarcoma of skin

C46.1 Kaposi's sarcoma of soft tissue

Kaposi's sarcoma of blood vessel
Kaposi's sarcoma of connective tissue
Kaposi's sarcoma of fascia
Kaposi's sarcoma of ligament
Kaposi's sarcoma of lymphatic(s) NEC
Kaposi's sarcoma of muscle

Excludes2:   Kaposi's sarcoma of lymph glands and nodes (C46.3)

C46.2 Kaposi's sarcoma of palate

C46.3 Kaposi's sarcoma of lymph nodes

C46.4 Kaposi's sarcoma of gastrointestinal sites

C46.5 Kaposi's sarcoma of lung

C46.50   Kaposi's sarcoma of lung, unspecified side

C46.51   Kaposi's sarcoma of right lung

C46.52   Kaposi's sarcoma of left lung

C46.7 Kaposi's sarcoma of other sites

C46.9 Kaposi's sarcoma, unspecified

C47 Malignant neoplasm of peripheral nerves and autonomic nervous system

Includes: malignant neoplasm of sympathetic and parasympathetic nerves and ganglia

Excludes1:   Kaposi's sarcoma of soft tissue (C46.1)

C47.0 Malignant neoplasm of peripheral nerves of head, face and neck

Excludes1:   malignant neoplasm of peripheral nerves of orbit (C69.6-)

C47.1 Malignant neoplasm of peripheral nerves of upper limb, including shoulder

C47.10   Malignant neoplasm of peripheral nerves of upper limb, including shoulder, unspecified side

C47.11   Malignant neoplasm of peripheral nerves of right upper limb, including shoulder

C47.12   Malignant neoplasm of peripheral nerves of left upper limb, including shoulder

C47.2 Malignant neoplasm of peripheral nerves of lower limb, including hip

C47.20   Malignant neoplasm of peripheral nerves of lower limb, including hip, unspecified side

C47.21   Malignant neoplasm of peripheral nerves of right lower limb, including hip

C47.22   Malignant neoplasm of peripheral nerves of left lower limb, including hip

C47.3 Malignant neoplasm of peripheral nerves of thorax

C47.4 Malignant neoplasm of peripheral nerves of abdomen

C47.5 Malignant neoplasm of peripheral nerves of pelvis

C47.6 Malignant neoplasm of peripheral nerves of trunk, unspecified

C47.8 Malignant neoplasm of overlapping sites of peripheral nerves and autonomic nervous system

C47.9 Malignant neoplasm of peripheral nerves and autonomic nervous system, unspecified

C48 Malignant neoplasm of retroperitoneum and peritoneum

Excludes1:   Kaposi's sarcoma of connective tissue (C46.1)
mesothelioma (C45.-)

C48.0 Malignant neoplasm of retroperitoneum

C48.1 Malignant neoplasm of specified parts of peritoneum

Malignant neoplasm of cul-de-sac
Malignant neoplasm of mesentery
Malignant neoplasm of mesocolon
Malignant neoplasm of omentum
Malignant neoplasm of parietal peritoneum
Malignant neoplasm of pelvic peritoneum

C48.2 Malignant neoplasm of peritoneum, unspecified

C48.8 Malignant neoplasm of overlapping sites of retroperitoneum and peritoneum

C49 Malignant neoplasm of other connective and soft tissue

Includes: malignant neoplasm of blood vessel
malignant neoplasm of bursa
malignant neoplasm of cartilage
malignant neoplasm of fascia
malignant neoplasm of fat
malignant neoplasm of ligament, except uterine
malignant neoplasm of lymphatic vessel
malignant neoplasm of muscle
malignant neoplasm of synovia
malignant neoplasm of tendon (sheath)

Excludes1:   malignant neoplasm of cartilage (of):
articular (C40-C41)
larynx (C32.3)
nose (C30.0)
malignant neoplasm of connective tissue of:
breast (C50.-)
malignant neoplasm of internal organs-code to malignant neoplasm of the site

Excludes2:   Kaposi's sarcoma of soft tissue (C46.1)
malignant neoplasm of heart (C38.0)
malignant neoplasm of peripheral nerves and autonomic nervous system (C47.-)
malignant neoplasm of peritoneum (C48.2)
malignant neoplasm of retroperitoneum (C48.0)
malignant neoplasm of uterine ligament (C57.3)
mesothelioma (C45.-)

C49.0 Malignant neoplasm of connective and soft tissue of head, face and neck

Malignant neoplasm of connective tissue of ear
Malignant neoplasm of connective tissue of eyelid

Excludes1:   connective tissue of orbit (C69.6-)

C49.1 Malignant neoplasm of connective and soft tissue of upper limb, including shoulder

C49.10   Malignant neoplasm of connective and soft tissue of upper limb, including shoulder, unspecified side

C49.11   Malignant neoplasm of connective and soft tissue of right upper limb, including shoulder

C49.12   Malignant neoplasm of connective and soft tissue of left upper limb, including shoulder

C49.2 Malignant neoplasm of connective and soft tissue of lower limb, including hip

C49.20   Malignant neoplasm of connective and soft tissue of lower limb, including hip, unspecified side

C49.21   Malignant neoplasm of connective and soft tissue of right lower limb, including hip

C49.22   Malignant neoplasm of connective and soft tissue of left lower limb, including hip

C49.3   Malignant neoplasm of connective and soft tissue of thorax
    Malignant neoplasm of axilla
    Malignant neoplasm of diaphragm
    Malignant neoplasm of great vessels
    Excludes1:   malignant neoplasm of breast (C50.-)
                malignant neoplasm of heart (C38.0)
                malignant neoplasm of mediastinum (C38.1-C38.3)
                malignant neoplasm of thymus (C37)

C49.4   Malignant neoplasm of connective and soft tissue of abdomen
    Malignant neoplasm of abdominal wall
    Malignant neoplasm of hypochondrium

C49.5   Malignant neoplasm of connective and soft tissue of pelvis
    Malignant neoplasm of buttock
    Malignant neoplasm of groin
    Malignant neoplasm of perineum

C49.6   Malignant neoplasm of connective and soft tissue of trunk, unspecified
    Malignant neoplasm of back NOS

C49.8   Malignant neoplasm of overlapping sites of connective and soft tissue
    Malignant neoplasm of connective and soft tissue whose point of origin cannot be classified to any one of the categories C47-C49.6

C49.9   Malignant neoplasm of connective and soft tissue, unspecified

MALIGNANT NEOPLASM OF BREAST (C50)

C50   Malignant neoplasm of breast
    Includes: connective tissue of breast
              Paget's disease of breast
              Paget's disease of nipple
    Excludes1: skin of breast (C43.5, C44.5)

C50.0   Malignant neoplasm of nipple and areola

C50.00   Malignant neoplasm of female nipple and areola, unspecified side

C50.01   Malignant neoplasm of right female nipple and areola

C50.02   Malignant neoplasm of left female nipple and areola

C50.03   Malignant neoplasm of right male nipple and areola

C50.04   Malignant neoplasm of left male nipple and areola

C50.05   Malignant neoplasm of male nipple and areola, unspecified side

C50.1   Malignant neoplasm of central portion of breast

C50.10   Malignant neoplasm of central portion of female breast, unspecified side

C50.11   Malignant neoplasm of central portion of right female breast

C50.12   Malignant neoplasm of central portion of left female breast

C50.13   Malignant neoplasm of central portion of right male breast

C50.14   Malignant neoplasm of central portion of left male breast

C50.15   Malignant neoplasm of central portion of male breast, unspecified side

C50.2   Malignant neoplasm of upper-inner quadrant of breast

C50.20   Malignant neoplasm of upper-inner quadrant of female breast, unspecified side

C50.21   Malignant neoplasm of upper-inner quadrant of right female breast

C50.22   Malignant neoplasm of upper-inner quadrant of left female breast

C50.23   Malignant neoplasm of upper-inner quadrant of right male breast

C50.24   Malignant neoplasm of upper-inner quadrant of left male breast

C50.25   Malignant neoplasm of upper-inner quadrant of male breast, unspecified side

C50.3   Malignant neoplasm of lower-inner quadrant of breast

C50.30   Malignant neoplasm of lower-inner quadrant of female breast, unspecified side

C50.31   Malignant neoplasm of lower-inner quadrant of right female breast

C50.32   Malignant neoplasm of lower-inner quadrant of left female breast

C50.33   Malignant neoplasm of lower-inner quadrant of right male breast

C50.34   Malignant neoplasm of lower-inner quadrant of left male breast

C50.35   Malignant neoplasm of lower-inner quadrant of male breast, of unspecified side

C50.4   Malignant neoplasm of upper-outer quadrant of breast

C50.40   Malignant neoplasm of upper-outer quadrant of female breast, unspecified side

C50.41   Malignant neoplasm of upper-outer quadrant of right female breast

C50.42   Malignant neoplasm of upper-outer quadrant of left female breast

C50.43   Malignant neoplasm of upper-outer quadrant of right male breast

C50.44   Malignant neoplasm of upper-outer quadrant of left male breast

C50.45   Malignant neoplasm of upper-outer quadrant of male breast, unspecified side

C50.5   Malignant neoplasm of lower-outer quadrant of breast

C50.50   Malignant neoplasm of lower-outer quadrant of female breast, unspecified side

C50.51   Malignant neoplasm of lower-outer quadrant of right female breast

C50.52   Malignant neoplasm of lower-outer quadrant of left female breast

C50.53   Malignant neoplasm of lower-outer quadrant of right male breast

C50.54   Malignant neoplasm of lower-outer quadrant of left male breast

C50.55   Malignant neoplasm of lower-outer quadrant of male breast, unspecified side

C50.6   Malignant neoplasm of axillary tail of breast

C50.60   Malignant neoplasm of axillary tail of female breast, unspecified side

C50.61   Malignant neoplasm of axillary tail of right female breast

C50.62   Malignant neoplasm of axillary tail of left female breast

C50.63   Malignant neoplasm of axillary tail of right male breast

C50.64   Malignant neoplasm of axillary tail of left male breast

C50.65   Malignant neoplasm of axillary tail of male breast, unspecified side

C50.8   Malignant neoplasm of overlapping sites of breast

C50.80   Malignant neoplasm of overlapping sites of female breast, unspecified side

C50.81   Malignant neoplasm of overlapping sites of right female breast

C50.82   Malignant neoplasm of overlapping sites of left female breast

C50.83   Malignant neoplasm of overlapping sites of right male breast

C50.84   Malignant neoplasm of overlapping sites of left male breast

C50.85   Malignant neoplasm of overlapping sites of male breast, unspecified side

C50.9   Malignant neoplasm of breast, unspecified

C50.90   Malignant neoplasm of female breast, unspecified, unspecified side

C50.91   Malignant neoplasm of right female breast, unspecified

C50.92   Malignant neoplasm of left female breast, unspecified

C50.93   Malignant neoplasm of right male breast, unspecified

C50.94   Malignant neoplasm of left male breast, unspecified

C50.95   Malignant neoplasm of male breast, unspecified side

MALIGNANT NEOPLASM OF FEMALE GENITAL ORGANS

(C51–C58)

Includes: malignant neoplasm of skin of female genital organs

C51 Malignant neoplasm of vulva

Excludes1:   carcinoma in situ of vulva (D07.1)

C51.0   Malignant neoplasm of labium majus

Malignant neoplasm of Bartholin's [greater vestibular] gland

C51.1   Malignant neoplasm of labium minus

C51.2   Malignant neoplasm of clitoris

C51.8   Malignant neoplasm of overlapping sites of vulva

C51.9   Malignant neoplasm of vulva, unspecified

Malignant neoplasm of external female genitalia NOS

Malignant neoplasm of pudendum

C52 Malignant neoplasm of vagina

Excludes1:   carcinoma in situ of vagina (D07.2)

C53 Malignant neoplasm of cervix uteri

Excludes1:   carcinoma in situ of cervix uteri (D06.-)

C53.0   Malignant neoplasm of endocervix

C53.1   Malignant neoplasm of exocervix

C53.8   Malignant neoplasm of overlapping sites of cervix uteri

C53.9   Malignant neoplasm of cervix uteri, unspecified

C54 Malignant neoplasm of corpus uteri

C54.0   Malignant neoplasm of isthmus uteri

Malignant neoplasm of lower uterine segment

C54.1   Malignant neoplasm of endometrium

C54.2   Malignant neoplasm of myometrium

C54.3   Malignant neoplasm of fundus uteri

C54.8   Malignant neoplasm of overlapping sites of corpus uteri

C54.9   Malignant neoplasm of corpus uteri, unspecified

C55 Malignant neoplasm of uterus, part unspecified

C56 Malignant neoplasm of ovary

Use additional code to identify any functional activity

C56.0   Malignant neoplasm of right ovary

C56.1   Malignant neoplasm of left ovary

C56.9   Malignant neoplasm of ovary, unspecified side

C57 Malignant neoplasm of other and unspecified female genital organs

C57.0   Malignant neoplasm of fallopian tube

Malignant neoplasm of oviduct

Malignant neoplasm of uterine tube

C57.00   Malignant neoplasm of fallopian tube, unspecified side

C57.01   Malignant neoplasm of right fallopian tube

C57.02   Malignant neoplasm of left fallopian tube

C57.1   Malignant neoplasm of broad ligament

C57.10   Malignant neoplasm of broad ligament, unspecified side

C57.11   Malignant neoplasm of right broad ligament

C57.12   Malignant neoplasm of left broad ligament

C57.2   Malignant neoplasm of round ligament

C57.20   Malignant neoplasm of round ligament, unspecified side

C57.21   Malignant neoplasm of right round ligament

C57.22   Malignant neoplasm of left round ligament

C57.3   Malignant neoplasm of parametrium

Malignant neoplasm of uterine ligament NOS

C57.4   Malignant neoplasm of uterine adnexa, unspecified

C57.7   Malignant neoplasm of other specified female genital organs

Malignant neoplasm of wolffian body or duct

C57.8   Malignant neoplasm of overlapping sites of female genital organs

Malignant neoplasm of female genital organs whose point of origin cannot be classified to any one of the categories C51-C57.7, C58

Tubo-ovarian malignant neoplasm

Utero-ovarian malignant neoplasm

C57.9   Malignant neoplasm of female genital organ, unspecified

Malignant neoplasm of female genitourinary tract NOS

C58 Malignant neoplasm of placenta

Includes: choriocarcinoma NOS

chorionepithelioma NOS

Excludes1:   chorioadenoma (destruens) (D39.2)

hydatidiform mole NOS (O01.9)

invasive hydatidiform mole (D39.2)

male choriocarcinoma NOS (C62.9-)

malignant hydatidiform mole (D39.2)

MALIGNANT NEOPLASMS OF MALE GENITAL ORGANS

(C60–C63)

Includes: malignant neoplasm of skin of male genital organs

C60 Malignant neoplasm of penis

C60.0   Malignant neoplasm of prepuce

Malignant neoplasm of foreskin

C60.1   Malignant neoplasm of glans penis

C60.2   Malignant neoplasm of body of penis

Malignant neoplasm of corpus cavernosum

C60.8   Malignant neoplasm of overlapping sites of penis

C60.9   Malignant neoplasm of penis, unspecified

Malignant neoplasm of skin of penis NOS

C61 Malignant neoplasm of prostate

Excludes1:   malignant neoplasm of seminal vesicle (C63.7)

C62 Malignant neoplasm of testis

Use additional code to identify any functional activity.

C62.0   Malignant neoplasm of undescended testis

Malignant neoplasm of ectopic testis

Malignant neoplasm of retained testis

C62.00   Malignant neoplasm of undescended testis, unspecified side

C62.01   Malignant neoplasm of undescended right testis

C62.02   Malignant neoplasm of undescended left testis

C62.1   Malignant neoplasm of descended testis

Malignant neoplasm of scrotal testis

C62.10   Malignant neoplasm of descended testis, unspecified side

C62.11   Malignant neoplasm of descended right testis

C62.12   Malignant neoplasm of descended left testis

C62.9   Malignant neoplasm of testis, unspecified

C62.90   Malignant neoplasm of testis, unspecified, unspecified side

C62.91   Malignant neoplasm of right testis, unspecified

C62.92   Malignant neoplasm of left testis, unspecified

C63 Malignant neoplasm of other and unspecified male genital organs

C63.0   Malignant neoplasm of epididymis

C63.00   Malignant neoplasm of epididymis, unspecified side

C63.01   Malignant neoplasm of right epididymis

C63.02   Malignant neoplasm of left epididymis

C63.1   Malignant neoplasm of spermatic cord

C63.10   Malignant neoplasm of spermatic cord, unspecified side

C63.11   Malignant neoplasm of right spermatic cord

C63.12   Malignant neoplasm of left spermatic cord

C63.2   Malignant neoplasm of scrotum

Malignant neoplasm of skin of scrotum

C63.7   Malignant neoplasm of other specified male genital organs

Malignant neoplasm of seminal vesicle

Malignant neoplasm of tunica vaginalis

C63.8 Malignant neoplasm of overlapping sites of male genital organs
Malignant neoplasm of male genital organs whose point of origin cannot be classified to any one of the categories C60-C63.7

C63.9 Malignant neoplasm of male genital organ, unspecified
Malignant neoplasm of male genitourinary tract NOS

MALIGNANT NEOPLASM OF URINARY TRACT (C64–C68)

C64 Malignant neoplasm of kidney, except renal pelvis
Excludes1: malignant neoplasm of renal calyces (C65.-)
malignant neoplasm of renal pelvis (C65.-)

C64.0 Malignant neoplasm of right kidney, except renal pelvis
C64.1 Malignant neoplasm of left kidney, except renal pelvis
C64.9 Malignant neoplasm of kidney, except renal pelvis, unspecified side

C65 Malignant neoplasm of renal pelvis
Includes: malignant neoplasm of pelviureteric junction
malignant neoplasm of renal calyces

C65.0 Malignant neoplasm of right renal pelvis
C65.1 Malignant neoplasm of left renal pelvis
C65.9 Malignant neoplasm of renal pelvis, unspecified side

C66 Malignant neoplasm of ureter
Excludes1: malignant neoplasm of ureteric orifice of bladder (C67.6)

C66.0 Malignant neoplasm of right ureter
C66.1 Malignant neoplasm of left ureter
C66.9 Malignant neoplasm of ureter, unspecified side

C67 Malignant neoplasm of bladder
C67.0 Malignant neoplasm of trigone of bladder
C67.1 Malignant neoplasm of dome of bladder
C67.2 Malignant neoplasm of lateral wall of bladder
C67.3 Malignant neoplasm of anterior wall of bladder
C67.4 Malignant neoplasm of posterior wall of bladder
C67.5 Malignant neoplasm of bladder neck
Malignant neoplasm of internal urethral orifice
C67.6 Malignant neoplasm of ureteric orifice
C67.7 Malignant neoplasm of urachus
C67.8 Malignant neoplasm of overlapping sites of bladder
C67.9 Malignant neoplasm of bladder, unspecified

C68 Malignant neoplasm of other and unspecified urinary organs
Excludes1: malignant neoplasm of female genitourinary tract NOS (C57.9)
malignant neoplasm of male genitourinary tract NOS (C63.9)

C68.0 Malignant neoplasm of urethra
Excludes1: malignant neoplasm of urethral orifice of bladder (C67.5)
C68.1 Malignant neoplasm of paraurethral glands
C68.8 Malignant neoplasm of overlapping sites of urinary organs
Malignant neoplasm of urinary organs whose point of origin cannot be classified to any one of the categories C64-C68.1
C68.9 Malignant neoplasm of urinary organ, unspecified
Malignant neoplasm of urinary system NOS

MALIGNANT NEOPLASMS OF EYE, BRAIN AND OTHER PARTS OF CENTRAL NERVOUS SYSTEM (C69–C72)

C69 Malignant neoplasm of eye and adnexa
Excludes1: malignant neoplasm of connective tissue of eyelid (C49.0)
malignant neoplasm of eyelid (skin) (C43.1-, C44.1-)
malignant neoplasm of optic nerve (C72.3-)
C69.0 Malignant neoplasm of conjunctiva
C69.00 Malignant neoplasm of conjunctiva, unspecified side
C69.01 Malignant neoplasm of right conjunctiva
C69.02 Malignant neoplasm of left conjunctiva

C69.1 Malignant neoplasm of cornea
C69.10 Malignant neoplasm of cornea, unspecified side
C69.11 Malignant neoplasm of right cornea
C69.12 Malignant neoplasm of left cornea
C69.2 Malignant neoplasm of retina
C69.20 Malignant neoplasm of retina, unspecified side
C69.21 Malignant neoplasm of right retina
C69.22 Malignant neoplasm of left retina
C69.3 Malignant neoplasm of choroid
C69.30 Malignant neoplasm of choroid, unspecified side
C69.31 Malignant neoplasm of right choroid
C69.32 Malignant neoplasm of left choroid
C69.4 Malignant neoplasm of ciliary body
Malignant neoplasm of eyeball
C69.40 Malignant neoplasm of ciliary body, unspecified side
C69.41 Malignant neoplasm of right ciliary body
C69.42 Malignant neoplasm of left ciliary body
C69.5 Malignant neoplasm of lacrimal gland and duct
Malignant neoplasm of lacrimal sac
Malignant neoplasm of nasolacrimal duct
C69.50 Malignant neoplasm of lacrimal gland and duct, unspecified side
C69.51 Malignant neoplasm of right lacrimal gland and duct
C69.52 Malignant neoplasm of left lacrimal gland and duct
C69.6 Malignant neoplasm of orbit
Malignant neoplasm of connective tissue of orbit
Malignant neoplasm of extraocular muscle
Malignant neoplasm of peripheral nerves of orbit
Malignant neoplasm of retrobulbar tissue
Malignant neoplasm of retro-ocular tissue
Excludes1: malignant neoplasm of orbital bone (C41.0)
C69.60 Malignant neoplasm of orbit, unspecified side
C69.61 Malignant neoplasm of right orbit
C69.62 Malignant neoplasm of left orbit
C69.8 Malignant neoplasm of overlapping sites of eye and adnexa
C69.80 Malignant neoplasm of overlapping sites of eye and adnexa, unspecified side
C69.81 Malignant neoplasm of overlapping sites of right eye and adnexa
C69.82 Malignant neoplasm of overlapping sites of left eye and adnexa
C69.9 Malignant neoplasm of eye, unspecified
C69.90 Malignant neoplasm of eye, unspecified, unspecified side
C69.91 Malignant neoplasm of right eye, unspecified
C69.92 Malignant neoplasm of left eye, unspecified

C70 Malignant neoplasm of meninges
C70.0 Malignant neoplasm of cerebral meninges
C70.1 Malignant neoplasm of spinal meninges
C70.9 Malignant neoplasm of meninges, unspecified

C71 Malignant neoplasm of brain
Excludes1: malignant neoplasm of cranial nerves (C72.2-C72.5)
retrobulbar malignant neoplasm (C69.6-)
C71.0 Malignant neoplasm of cerebrum, except lobes and ventricles
Malignant neoplasm of corpus callosum
Malignant neoplasm of supratentorial NOS
C71.1 Malignant neoplasm of frontal lobe
C71.2 Malignant neoplasm of temporal lobe
C71.3 Malignant neoplasm of parietal lobe
C71.4 Malignant neoplasm of occipital lobe
C71.5 Malignant neoplasm of cerebral ventricle
Excludes1: malignant neoplasm of fourth cerebral ventricle (C71.7)
C71.6 Malignant neoplasm of cerebellum
C71.7 Malignant neoplasm of brain stem
Malignant neoplasm of fourth cerebral ventricle
Infratentorial malignant neoplasm NOS
C71.8 Malignant neoplasm of overlapping sites of brain
C71.9 Malignant neoplasm of brain, unspecified

C72 **Malignant neoplasm of spinal cord, cranial nerves and other parts of central nervous system**

Excludes1:   malignant neoplasm of meninges (C70.-)
malignant neoplasm of peripheral nerves and autonomic nervous system (C47.-)

C72.0 **Malignant neoplasm of spinal cord**

C72.1 **Malignant neoplasm of cauda equina**

C72.2 **Malignant neoplasm of olfactory nerve**
Malignant neoplasm of olfactory bulb

C72.20 **Malignant neoplasm of olfactory nerve, unspecified side**

C72.21 **Malignant neoplasm of right olfactory nerve**

C72.22 **Malignant neoplasm of left olfactory nerve**

C72.3 **Malignant neoplasm of optic nerve**

C72.30 **Malignant neoplasm of optic nerve, unspecified side**

C72.31 **Malignant neoplasm of right optic nerve**

C72.32 **Malignant neoplasm of left optic nerve**

C72.4 **Malignant neoplasm of acoustic nerve**

C72.40 **Malignant neoplasm of acoustic nerve, unspecified side**

C72.41 **Malignant neoplasm of right acoustic nerve**

C72.42 **Malignant neoplasm of left acoustic nerve**

C72.5 **Malignant neoplasm of other and unspecified cranial nerves**

C72.50 **Malignant neoplasm of unspecified cranial nerve**
Malignant neoplasm of cranial nerve NOS

C72.59 **Malignant neoplasm of other cranial nerves**

C72.8 **Malignant neoplasm of overlapping sites of brain and other parts of central nervous system**
Malignant neoplasm of brain and other parts of central nervous system whose point of origin cannot be classified to any one of the categories C70-C72.5

C72.9 **Malignant neoplasm of central nervous system, unspecified**
Malignant neoplasm of nervous system NOS

MALIGNANT NEOPLASM OF THYROID AND OTHER ENDOCRINE GLANDS (C73–C75)

C73 **Malignant neoplasm of thyroid gland**
Use additional code to identify any functional activity.

C74 **Malignant neoplasm of adrenal gland**

C74.0 **Malignant neoplasm of cortex of adrenal gland**

C74.00 **Malignant neoplasm of cortex of adrenal gland, unspecified side**

C74.01 **Malignant neoplasm of cortex of right adrenal gland**

C74.02 **Malignant neoplasm of cortex of left adrenal gland**

C74.1 **Malignant neoplasm of medulla of adrenal gland**

C74.10 **Malignant neoplasm of medulla of adrenal gland, unspecified side**

C74.11 **Malignant neoplasm of medulla of right adrenal gland**

C74.12 **Malignant neoplasm of medulla of left adrenal gland**

C74.9 **Malignant neoplasm of adrenal gland, unspecified**

C74.90 **Malignant neoplasm of adrenal gland, unspecified, unspecified side**

C74.91 **Malignant neoplasm of right adrenal gland, unspecified**

C74.92 **Malignant neoplasm of left adrenal gland, unspecified**

C75 **Malignant neoplasm of other endocrine glands and related structures**

Excludes1:   malignant neoplasm of adrenal gland (C74.-)
malignant neoplasm of endocrine pancreas (C25.4)
malignant neoplasm of islets of Langerhans (C25.4)
malignant neoplasm of ovary (C56-)
malignant neoplasm of testis (C62.-)
malignant neoplasm of thymus (C37)
malignant neoplasm of thyroid gland (C73)

C75.0 **Malignant neoplasm of parathyroid gland**

C75.1 **Malignant neoplasm of pituitary gland**

C75.2 **Malignant neoplasm of craniopharyngeal duct**

C75.3 **Malignant neoplasm of pineal gland**

C75.4 **Malignant neoplasm of carotid body**

C75.5 **Malignant neoplasm of aortic body and other paraganglia**

C75.8 **Malignant neoplasm with pluriglandular involvement, unspecified**

C75.9 **Malignant neoplasm of endocrine gland, unspecified**

MALIGNANT NEOPLASMS OF ILL–DEFINED, SECONDARY AND UNSPECIFIED SITES (C76–C80)

C76 **Malignant neoplasm of other and ill-defined sites**

Excludes1:   malignant neoplasm of female genitourinary tract NOS (C57.9)
malignant neoplasm of male genitourinary tract NOS (C63.9)
malignant neoplasm of lymphoid, hematopoietic and related tissue (C81-C96)
malignant neoplasm of unspecified site NOS (C80.1)

C76.0 **Malignant neoplasm of head, face and neck**
Malignant neoplasm of cheek NOS
Malignant neoplasm of nose NOS

C76.1 **Malignant neoplasm of thorax**
Intrathoracic malignant neoplasm NOS
Malignant neoplasm of axilla NOS
Thoracic malignant neoplasm NOS

C76.2 **Malignant neoplasm of abdomen**

C76.3 **Malignant neoplasm of pelvis**
Malignant neoplasm of groin NOS
Malignant neoplasm of sites overlapping systems within the pelvis
Rectovaginal (septum) malignant neoplasm
Rectovesical (septum) malignant neoplasm

C76.4 **Malignant neoplasm of upper limb**

C76.40 **Malignant neoplasm of upper limb, unspecified side**

C76.41 **Malignant neoplasm of right upper limb**

C76.42 **Malignant neoplasm of left upper limb**

C76.5 **Malignant neoplasm of lower limb**

C76.50 **Malignant neoplasm of lower limb, unspecified side**

C76.51 **Malignant neoplasm of right lower limb**

C76.52 **Malignant neoplasm of left lower limb**

C76.7 **Malignant neoplasm of other ill-defined sites**

C76.8 **Malignant neoplasm of overlapping sites of other and ill-defined sites**

C77 **Secondary and unspecified malignant neoplasm of lymph nodes**

Excludes1:   malignant neoplasm of lymph nodes, specified as primary (C81-C88, C96.-)

C77.0 **Secondary and unspecified malignant neoplasm of lymph nodes of head, face and neck**
Secondary and unspecified malignant neoplasm of supraclavicular lymph nodes

C77.1 **Secondary and unspecified malignant neoplasm of intrathoracic lymph nodes**

C77.2 **Secondary and unspecified malignant neoplasm of intra-abdominal lymph nodes**

C77.3 **Secondary and unspecified malignant neoplasm of axilla and upper limb lymph nodes**
Secondary and unspecified malignant neoplasm of pectoral lymph nodes

C77.4 **Secondary and unspecified malignant neoplasm of inguinal and lower limb lymph nodes**

C77.5 **Secondary and unspecified malignant neoplasm of intrapelvic lymph nodes**

C77.8 **Secondary and unspecified malignant neoplasm of lymph nodes of multiple regions**

C77.9 **Secondary and unspecified malignant neoplasm of lymph node, unspecified**

C78 **Secondary malignant neoplasm of respiratory and digestive organs**

Excludes1:   lymph node metastases (C77.0)

C78.0 **Secondary malignant neoplasm of lung**

C78.00 **Secondary malignant neoplasm of lung , unspecified side**

C78.01 **Secondary malignant neoplasm of right lung**

C78.02 **Secondary malignant neoplasm of left lung**

C78.1   **Secondary malignant neoplasm of mediastinum**

C78.2   **Secondary malignant neoplasm of pleura**

C78.3   **Secondary malignant neoplasm of other and unspecified respiratory organs**

     C78.30   **Secondary malignant neoplasm of unspecified respiratory organ**

     C78.39   **Secondary malignant neoplasm of other respiratory organs**

C78.4   **Secondary malignant neoplasm of small intestine**

C78.5   **Secondary malignant neoplasm of large intestine and rectum**

C78.6   **Secondary malignant neoplasm of retroperitoneum and peritoneum**
       Malignant ascites NOS

C78.7   **Secondary malignant neoplasm of liver**

C78.8   **Secondary malignant neoplasm of other and unspecified digestive organs**

     C78.80   **Secondary malignant neoplasm of unspecified digestive organ**

     C78.89   **Secondary malignant neoplasm of other digestive organs**

C79   **Secondary malignant neoplasm of other sites**
     Excludes1:   lymph node metastases (C77.0)

C79.0   **Secondary malignant neoplasm of kidney and renal pelvis**

     C79.00   **Secondary malignant neoplasm of kidney and renal pelvis, unspecified side**

     C79.01   **Secondary malignant neoplasm of right kidney and renal pelvis**

     C79.02   **Secondary malignant neoplasm of left kidney and renal pelvis**

C79.1   **Secondary malignant neoplasm of bladder and other and unspecified urinary organs**

     C79.10   **Secondary malignant neoplasm of unspecified urinary organs**

     C79.11   **Secondary malignant neoplasm of bladder**

     C79.19   **Secondary malignant neoplasm of other urinary organs**

C79.2   **Secondary malignant neoplasm of skin**

C79.3   **Secondary malignant neoplasm of brain and cerebral meninges**

     C79.31   **Secondary malignant neoplasm of brain**

     C79.32   **Secondary malignant neoplasm of cerebral meninges**

C79.4   **Secondary malignant neoplasm of other and unspecified parts of nervous system**

     C79.40   **Secondary malignant neoplasm of unspecified part of nervous system**

     C79.49   **Secondary malignant neoplasm of other parts of nervous system**

C79.5   **Secondary malignant neoplasm of bone and bone marrow**

     C79.51   **Secondary malignant neoplasm of bone**

     C79.52   **Secondary malignant neoplasm of bone marrow**

C79.6   **Secondary malignant neoplasm of ovary**

     C79.60   **Secondary malignant neoplasm of ovary, unspecified side**

     C79.61   **Secondary malignant neoplasm of right ovary**

     C79.62   **Secondary malignant neoplasm of left ovary**

C79.7   **Secondary malignant neoplasm of adrenal gland**

     C79.70   **Secondary malignant neoplasm of adrenal gland, unspecified side**

     C79.71   **Secondary malignant neoplasm of right adrenal gland**

     C79.72   **Secondary malignant neoplasm of left adrenal gland**

C79.8   **Secondary malignant neoplasm of other specified sites**

     C79.81   **Secondary malignant neoplasm of breast**

     C79.82   **Secondary malignant neoplasm of genital organs**

     C79.89   **Secondary malignant neoplasm of other specified sites**

C80   **Malignant neoplasm without specification of site**
     Includes: Cancer unspecified site (primary) (secondary)
                   Carcinoma unspecified site (primary) (secondary)
                   Carcinomatosis unspecified site (primary) (secondary)
                   Generalized cancer unspecified site (primary) (secondary)
                   Generalized malignancy unspecified site (primary) (secondary)
                   Malignancy unspecified site (primary) (secondary)
                   Malignant cachexia
                   Multiple cancer unspecified site (primary) (secondary)
                   Primary site unknown

MALIGNANT NEOPLASMS OF LYMPHOID, HEMATOPOIETIC AND RELATED TISSUE (C81–C96)

Use additional morphology codes M959-M994 with behavior code /3

Excludes2:   Kaposi's sarcoma of lymph nodes (C46.3)
            secondary and unspecified neoplasm of lymph nodes (C77.-)
            secondary neoplasm of bone marrow (C79.52)
            secondary neoplasm of spleen (C78.89)

C81   **Hodgkin's disease**
     Use additional morphology codes M9650-M9662 with behavior code /3

C81.0   **Lymphocytic predominance Hodgkin's disease**
     Lymphocytic-histiocytic predominance Hodgkin's disease

     C81.00   **Lymphocytic predominance Hodgkin's disease, unspecified site**

     C81.01   **Lymphocytic predominance Hodgkin's disease, lymph nodes of head, face, and neck**

     C81.02   **Lymphocytic predominance Hodgkin's disease, intrathoracic lymph nodes**

     C81.03   **Lymphocytic predominance Hodgkin's disease, intra-abdominal lymph nodes**

     C81.04   **Lymphocytic predominance Hodgkin's disease, lymph nodes of axilla and upper limb**

     C81.05   **Lymphocytic predominance Hodgkin's disease, lymph nodes of inguinal region and lower limb**

     C81.06   **Lymphocytic predominance Hodgkin's disease, intrapelvic lymph nodes**

     C81.07   **Lymphocytic predominance Hodgkin's disease, spleen**

     C81.08   **Lymphocytic predominance Hodgkin's disease, lymph nodes of multiple sites**

     C81.09   **Lymphocytic predominance Hodgkin's disease, extranodal and solid organ sites**

C81.1   **Nodular sclerosis Hodgkin's disease**

     C81.10   **Nodular sclerosis Hodgkin's disease, unspecified site**

     C81.11   **Nodular sclerosis Hodgkin's disease, lymph nodes of head, face, and neck**

     C81.12   **Nodular sclerosis Hodgkin's disease, intrathoracic lymph nodes**

     C81.13   **Nodular sclerosis Hodgkin's disease, intra-abdominal lymph nodes**

     C81.14   **Nodular sclerosis Hodgkin's disease, lymph nodes of axilla and upper limb**

     C81.15   **Nodular sclerosis Hodgkin's disease, lymph nodes of inguinal region and lower limb**

     C81.16   **Nodular sclerosis Hodgkin's disease, intrapelvic lymph nodes**

     C81.17   **Nodular sclerosis Hodgkin's disease, spleen**

     C81.18   **Nodular sclerosis Hodgkin's disease, lymph nodes of multiple sites**

     C81.19   **Nodular sclerosis Hodgkin's disease, extranodal and solid organ sites**

C81.2   **Mixed cellularity Hodgkin's disease**

     C81.20   **Mixed cellularity Hodgkin's disease, unspecified site**

     C81.21   **Mixed cellularity Hodgkin's disease, lymph nodes of head, face, and neck**

     C81.22   **Mixed cellularity Hodgkin's disease, intrathoracic lymph nodes**

C81.23   Mixed cellularity Hodgkin's disease, intra-abdominal lymph nodes

C81.24   Mixed cellularity Hodgkin's disease, lymph nodes of axilla and upper limb

C81.25   Mixed cellularity Hodgkin's disease, lymph nodes of inguinal region and lower limb

C81.26   Mixed cellularity Hodgkin's disease, intrapelvic lymph nodes

C81.27   Mixed cellularity Hodgkin's disease, spleen

C81.28   Mixed cellularity Hodgkin's disease, lymph nodes of multiple sites

C81.29   Mixed cellularity Hodgkin's disease, extranodal and solid organ sites

C81.3   Lymphocytic depletion Hodgkin's disease

C81.30   Lymphocytic depletion Hodgkin's disease, unspecified site

C81.31   Lymphocytic depletion Hodgkin's disease, lymph nodes of head, face, and neck

C81.32   Lymphocytic depletion Hodgkin's disease, intrathoracic lymph nodes

C81.33   Lymphocytic depletion Hodgkin's disease, intra-abdominal lymph nodes

C81.34   Lymphocytic depletion Hodgkin's disease, lymph nodes of axilla and upper limb

C81.35   Lymphocytic depletion Hodgkin's disease, lymph nodes of inguinal region and lower limb

C81.36   Lymphocytic depletion Hodgkin's disease, intrapelvic lymph nodes

C81.37   Lymphocytic depletion Hodgkin's disease, spleen

C81.38   Lymphocytic depletion Hodgkin's disease, lymph nodes of multiple sites

C81.39   Lymphocytic depletion Hodgkin's disease, extranodal and solid organ sites

C81.7   Other Hodgkin's disease

C81.70   Other Hodgkin's disease, unspecified site

C81.71   Other Hodgkin's disease, lymph nodes of head, face, and neck

C81.72   Other Hodgkin's disease, intrathoracic lymph nodes

C81.73   Other Hodgkin's disease, intra-abdominal lymph nodes

C81.74   Other Hodgkin's disease, lymph nodes of axilla and upper limb

C81.75   Other Hodgkin's disease, lymph nodes of inguinal region and lower limb

C81.76   Other Hodgkin's disease, intrapelvic lymph nodes

C81.77   Other Hodgkin's disease, spleen

C81.78   Other Hodgkin's disease, lymph nodes of multiple sites

C81.79   Other Hodgkin's disease, extranodal and solid organ sites

C81.9   Unspecified Hodgkin's disease

C81.90   Unspecified Hodgkin's disease, unspecified site

C81.91   Unspecified Hodgkin's disease, lymph nodes of head, face, and neck

C81.92   Unspecified Hodgkin's disease, intrathoracic lymph nodes

C81.93   Unspecified Hodgkin's disease, intra-abdominal lymph nodes

C81.94   Unspecified Hodgkin's disease, lymph nodes of axilla and upper limb

C81.95   Unspecified Hodgkin's disease, lymph nodes of inguinal region and lower limb

C81.96   Unspecified Hodgkin's disease, intrapelvic lymph nodes

C81.97   Unspecified Hodgkin's disease, spleen

C81.98   Unspecified Hodgkin's disease, lymph nodes of multiple sites

C81.99   Unspecified Hodgkin's disease, extranodal and solid organ sites

C82   Follicular [nodular] non-Hodgkin's lymphoma

     Includes: follicular non-Hodgkin's lymphoma with or without diffuse areas

     Use additional morphology code M9690 with behavior code /3

C82.0   Small cleaved cell, follicular non-Hodgkin's lymphoma

C82.00   Small cleaved cell, follicular non-Hodgkin's lymphoma, unspecified site

C82.01   Small cleaved cell, follicular non-Hodgkin's lymphoma, lymph nodes of head, face, and neck

C82.02   Small cleaved cell, follicular non-Hodgkin's lymphoma, intrathoracic lymph nodes

C82.03   Small cleaved cell, follicular non-Hodgkin's lymphoma, intra-abdominal lymph nodes

C82.04   Small cleaved cell, follicular non-Hodgkin's lymphoma, lymph nodes of axilla and upper limb

C82.05   Small cleaved cell, follicular non-Hodgkin's lymphoma, lymph nodes of inguinal region and lower limb

C82.06   Small cleaved cell, follicular non-Hodgkin's lymphoma, intrapelvic lymph nodes

C82.07   Small cleaved cell, follicular non-Hodgkin's lymphoma, spleen

C82.08   Small cleaved cell, follicular non-Hodgkin's lymphoma, lymph nodes of multiple sites

C82.09   Small cleaved cell, follicular non-Hodgkin's lymphoma, extranodal and solid organ sites

C82.1   Mixed small cleaved and large cell, follicular non-Hodgkin's lymphoma

C82.10   Mixed small cleaved and large cell, follicular non-Hodgkin's lymphoma, unspecified site

C82.11   Mixed small cleaved and large cell, follicular non-Hodgkin's lymphoma, lymph nodes of head, face, and neck

C82.12   Mixed small cleaved and large cell, follicular non-Hodgkin's lymphoma, intrathoracic lymph nodes

C82.13   Mixed small cleaved and large cell, follicular non-Hodgkin's lymphoma, intra-abdominal lymph nodes

C82.14   Mixed small cleaved and large cell, follicular non-Hodgkin's lymphoma, lymph nodes of axilla and upper limb

C82.15   Mixed small cleaved and large cell, follicular non-Hodgkin's lymphoma, lymph nodes of inguinal region and lower limb

C82.16   Mixed small cleaved and large cell, follicular non-Hodgkin's lymphoma, intrapelvic lymph nodes

C82.17   Mixed small cleaved and large cell, follicular non-Hodgkin's lymphoma, spleen

C82.18   Mixed small cleaved and large cell, follicular non-Hodgkin's lymphoma, lymph nodes of multiple sites

C82.19   Mixed small cleaved and large cell, follicular non-Hodgkin's lymphoma, extranodal and solid organ sites

C82.2   Large cell, follicular non-Hodgkin's lymphoma

C82.20   Large cell, follicular non-Hodgkin's lymphoma, unspecified site

C82.21   Large cell, follicular non-Hodgkin's lymphoma, lymph nodes of head, face, and neck

C82.22   Large cell, follicular non-Hodgkin's lymphoma, intrathoracic lymph nodes

C82.23   Large cell, follicular non-Hodgkin's lymphoma, intra-abdominal lymph nodes

C82.24   Large cell, follicular non-Hodgkin's lymphoma, lymph nodes of axilla and upper limb

C82.25   Large cell, follicular non-Hodgkin's lymphoma, lymph nodes of inguinal region and lower limb

C82.26   Large cell, follicular non-Hodgkin's lymphoma, intrapelvic lymph nodes

C82.27   Large cell, follicular non-Hodgkin's lymphoma, spleen

C82.28   Large cell, follicular non-Hodgkin's lymphoma, lymph nodes of multiple sites

C82.29   Large cell, follicular non-Hodgkin's lymphoma, extranodal and solid organ sites

C82.7   Other types of follicular non-Hodgkin's lymphoma

C82.70   Other types of follicular non-Hodgkin's lymphoma, unspecified site

C82.71   Other types of follicular non-Hodgkin's lymphoma, lymph nodes of head, face, and neck

C82.72   Other types of follicular non-Hodgkin's lymphoma, intrathoracic lymph nodes

C82.73   Other types of follicular non-Hodgkin's lymphoma, intra-abdominal lymph nodes

C82.74   Other types of follicular non-Hodgkin's lymphoma, lymph nodes of axilla and upper limb

C82.75   Other types of follicular non-Hodgkin's lymphoma, lymph nodes of inguinal region and lower limb

C82.76   Other types of follicular non-Hodgkin's lymphoma, intrapelvic lymph nodes

C82.77   Other types of follicular non-Hodgkin's lymphoma, spleen

C82.78   Other types of follicular non-Hodgkin's lymphoma, lymph nodes of multiple sites

C82.79   Other types of follicular non-Hodgkin's lymphoma, extranodal and solid organ sites

C82.9   Follicular non-Hodgkin's lymphoma, unspecified
Nodular non-Hodgkin's lymphoma NOS

C82.90   Unspecified follicular non-Hodgkin's lymphoma, unspecified site

C82.91   Unspecified follicular non-Hodgkin's lymphoma, lymph nodes of head, face, and neck

C82.92   Unspecified follicular non-Hodgkin's lymphoma, intrathoracic lymph nodes

C82.93   Unspecified follicular non-Hodgkin's lymphoma, unspecified, intra-abdominal lymph nodes

C82.94   Unspecified follicular non-Hodgkin's lymphoma, lymph nodes of axilla and upper limb

C82.95   Unspecified follicular non-Hodgkin's lymphoma, lymph nodes of inguinal region and lower limb

C82.96   Unspecified follicular non-Hodgkin's lymphoma, intrapelvic lymph nodes

C82.97   Unspecified follicular non-Hodgkin's lymphoma, spleen

C82.98   Unspecified follicular non-Hodgkin's lymphoma, lymph nodes of multiple sites

C82.99   Unspecified follicular non-Hodgkin's lymphoma, extranodal and solid organ sites

C83   Diffuse non-Hodgkin's lymphoma
Use additional morphology codes M9593, M9595, M967-M968 with behavior code /3

C83.0   Small cell (diffuse) non-Hodgkin's lymphoma

C83.00   Small cell (diffuse) non-Hodgkin's lymphoma, unspecified site

C83.01   Small cell (diffuse) non-Hodgkin's lymphoma, lymph nodes of head, face, and neck

C83.02   Small cell (diffuse) non-Hodgkin's lymphoma, intrathoracic lymph nodes

C83.03   Small cell (diffuse) non-Hodgkin's lymphoma, intra-abdominal lymph nodes

C83.04   Small cell (diffuse) non-Hodgkin's lymphoma, lymph nodes of axilla and upper limb

C83.05   Small cell (diffuse) non-Hodgkin's lymphoma, lymph nodes of inguinal region and lower limb

C83.06   Small cell (diffuse) non-Hodgkin's lymphoma, intrapelvic lymph nodes

C83.07   Small cell (diffuse) non-Hodgkin's lymphoma, spleen

C83.08   Small cell (diffuse) non-Hodgkin's lymphoma, lymph nodes of multiple sites

C83.09   Small cell (diffuse) non-Hodgkin's lymphoma, extranodal and solid organ sites

C83.1   Small cleaved cell (diffuse) non-Hodgkin's lymphoma

C83.10   Small cleaved cell (diffuse) non-Hodgkin's lymphoma, unspecified site

C83.11   Small cleaved cell (diffuse) non-Hodgkin's lymphoma, lymph nodes of head, face, and neck

C83.12   Small cleaved cell (diffuse) non-Hodgkin's lymphoma, intrathoracic lymph nodes

C83.13   Small cleaved cell (diffuse) non-Hodgkin's lymphoma, intra-abdominal lymph nodes

C83.14   Small cleaved cell (diffuse) non-Hodgkin's lymphoma, lymph nodes of axilla and upper limb

C83.15   Small cleaved cell (diffuse) non-Hodgkin's lymphoma, lymph nodes of inguinal region and lower limb

C83.16   Small cleaved cell (diffuse) non-Hodgkin's lymphoma, intrapelvic lymph nodes

C83.17   Small cleaved cell (diffuse) non-Hodgkin's lymphoma, spleen

C83.18   Small cleaved cell (diffuse) non-Hodgkin's lymphoma, lymph nodes of multiple sites

C83.19   Small cleaved cell (diffuse) non-Hodgkin's lymphoma, extranodal and solid organ sites

C83.2   Mixed small and large cell (diffuse) non-Hodgkin's lymphoma

C83.20   Mixed small and large cell (diffuse) non-Hodgkin's lymphoma, unspecified site

C83.21   Mixed small and large cell (diffuse) non-Hodgkin's lymphoma, lymph nodes of head, face, and neck

C83.22   Mixed small and large cell (diffuse) non-Hodgkin's lymphoma, intrathoracic lymph nodes

C83.23   Mixed small and large cell (diffuse) non-Hodgkin's lymphoma, intra-abdominal lymph nodes

C83.24   Mixed small and large cell (diffuse) non-Hodgkin's lymphoma, lymph nodes of axilla and upper limb

C83.25   Mixed small and large cell (diffuse) non-Hodgkin's lymphoma, lymph nodes of inguinal region and lower limb

C83.26   Mixed small and large cell (diffuse) non-Hodgkin's lymphoma, intrapelvic lymph nodes

C83.27   Mixed small and large cell (diffuse) non-Hodgkin's lymphoma, spleen

C83.28   Mixed small and large cell (diffuse) non-Hodgkin's lymphoma, lymph nodes of multiple sites

C83.29   Mixed small and large cell (diffuse) non-Hodgkin's lymphoma, extranodal and solid organ sites

C83.3   Large cell (diffuse) non-Hodgkin's lymphoma
Reticulum cell sarcoma

C83.30   Large cell (diffuse) non-Hodgkin's lymphoma, unspecified site

C83.31   Large cell (diffuse) non-Hodgkin's lymphoma, lymph nodes of head, face, and neck

C83.32   Large cell (diffuse) non-Hodgkin's lymphoma, intrathoracic lymph nodes

C83.33   Large cell (diffuse) non-Hodgkin's lymphoma, intra-abdominal lymph nodes

C83.34   Large cell (diffuse) non-Hodgkin's lymphoma, lymph nodes of axilla and upper limb

C83.35   Large cell (diffuse) non-Hodgkin's lymphoma, lymph nodes of inguinal region and lower limb

C83.36   Large cell (diffuse) non-Hodgkin's lymphoma, intrapelvic lymph nodes

C83.37   Large cell (diffuse) non-Hodgkin's lymphoma, spleen

C83.38   Large cell (diffuse) non-Hodgkin's lymphoma, lymph nodes of multiple sites

C83.39   Large cell (diffuse) non-Hodgkin's lymphoma, extranodal and solid organ sites

C83.4   Immunoblastic (diffuse) non-Hodgkin's lymphoma

C83.40   Immunoblastic (diffuse) non-Hodgkin's lymphoma, unspecified site

C83.41   Immunoblastic (diffuse) non-Hodgkin's lymphoma, lymph nodes of head, face, and neck

C83.42   Immunoblastic (diffuse) non-Hodgkin's lymphoma, intrathoracic lymph nodes

C83.43   Immunoblastic (diffuse) non-Hodgkin's lymphoma, intra-abdominal lymph nodes

C83.44   Immunoblastic (diffuse) non-Hodgkin's lymphoma, lymph nodes of axilla and upper limb

C83.45   Immunoblastic (diffuse) non-Hodgkin's lymphoma, lymph nodes of inguinal region and lower limb

C83.46   Immunoblastic (diffuse) non-Hodgkin's lymphoma, intrapelvic lymph nodes

C83.47   Immunoblastic (diffuse) non-Hodgkin's lymphoma,
          spleen
C83.48   Immunoblastic (diffuse) non-Hodgkin's lymphoma,
          lymph nodes of multiple sites
C83.49   Immunoblastic (diffuse) non-Hodgkin's lymphoma,
          extranodal and solid organ sites
C83.5 Lymphoblastic (diffuse) non-Hodgkin's lymphoma
    C83.50   Lymphoblastic (diffuse) non-Hodgkin's lymphoma,
              unspecified site
    C83.51   Lymphoblastic (diffuse) non-Hodgkin's lymphoma,
              lymph nodes of head, face, and neck
    C83.52   Lymphoblastic (diffuse) non-Hodgkin's lymphoma,
              intrathoracic lymph nodes
    C83.53   Lymphoblastic (diffuse) non-Hodgkin's lymphoma,
              intra-abdominal lymph nodes
    C83.54   Lymphoblastic (diffuse) non-Hodgkin's lymphoma,
              lymph nodes of axilla and upper limb
    C83.55   Lymphoblastic (diffuse) non-Hodgkin's lymphoma,
              lymph nodes of inguinal region and lower limb
    C83.56   Lymphoblastic (diffuse) non-Hodgkin's lymphoma,
              intrapelvic lymph nodes
    C83.57   Lymphoblastic (diffuse) non-Hodgkin's lymphoma,
              spleen
    C83.58   Lymphoblastic (diffuse) non-Hodgkin's lymphoma,
              lymph nodes of multiple sites
    C83.59   Lymphoblastic (diffuse) non-Hodgkin's lymphoma,
              extranodal and solid organ sites
C83.6 Undifferentiated (diffuse) non-Hodgkin's lymphoma
    C83.60   Undifferentiated (diffuse) non-Hodgkin's lymphoma,
              unspecified site
    C83.61   Undifferentiated (diffuse) non-Hodgkin's lymphoma,
              lymph nodes of head, face, and neck
    C83.62   Undifferentiated (diffuse) non-Hodgkin's lymphoma,
              intrathoracic lymph nodes
    C83.63   Undifferentiated (diffuse) non-Hodgkin's lymphoma,
              intra-abdominal lymph nodes
    C83.64   Undifferentiated (diffuse) non-Hodgkin's lymphoma,
              lymph nodes of axilla and upper limb
    C83.65   Undifferentiated (diffuse) non-Hodgkin's lymphoma,
              lymph nodes of inguinal region and lower limb
    C83.66   Undifferentiated (diffuse) non-Hodgkin's lymphoma,
              intrapelvic lymph nodes
    C83.67   Undifferentiated (diffuse) non-Hodgkin's lymphoma,
              spleen
    C83.68   Undifferentiated (diffuse) non-Hodgkin's lymphoma,
              lymph nodes of multiple sites
    C83.69   Undifferentiated (diffuse) non-Hodgkin's lymphoma,
              extranodal and solid organ sites
C83.7 Burkitt's tumor
    C83.70   Burkitt's tumor, unspecified site
    C83.71   Burkitt's tumor, lymph nodes of head, face, and neck
    C83.72   Burkitt's tumor, intrathoracic lymph nodes
    C83.73   Burkitt's tumor, intra-abdominal lymph nodes
    C83.74   Burkitt's tumor, lymph nodes of axilla and upper limb
    C83.75   Burkitt's tumor, lymph nodes of inguinal region and
              lower limb
    C83.76   Burkitt's tumor, intrapelvic lymph nodes
    C83.77   Burkitt's tumor, spleen
    C83.78   Burkitt's tumor, lymph nodes of multiple sites
    C83.79   Burkitt's tumor, extranodal and solid organ sites
C83.8 Other types of diffuse non-Hodgkin's lymphoma
    C83.80   Other types of diffuse non-Hodgkin's lymphoma,
              unspecified site
    C83.81   Other types of diffuse non-Hodgkin's lymphoma,
              lymph nodes of head, face, and neck
    C83.82   Other types of diffuse non-Hodgkin's lymphoma,
              intrathoracic lymph nodes
    C83.83   Other types of diffuse non-Hodgkin's lymphoma, intra-
              abdominal lymph nodes
    C83.84   Other types of diffuse non-Hodgkin's lymphoma,
              lymph nodes of axilla and upper limb

C83.85   Other types of diffuse non-Hodgkin's lymphoma,
          lymph nodes of inguinal region and lower limb
C83.86   Other types of diffuse non-Hodgkin's lymphoma,
          intrapelvic lymph nodes
C83.87   Other types of diffuse non-Hodgkin's lymphoma of
          spleen
C83.88   Other types of diffuse non-Hodgkin's lymphoma,
          lymph nodes of multiple sites
C83.89   Other types of diffuse non-Hodgkin's lymphoma,
          extranodal and solid organ sites
C83.9 Unspecified diffuse non-Hodgkin's lymphoma
    C83.90   Unspecified diffuse non-Hodgkin's lymphoma,
              unspecified site
    C83.91   Unspecified diffuse non-Hodgkin's lymphoma, lymph
              nodes of head, face, and neck
    C83.92   Unspecified diffuse non-Hodgkin's lymphoma,
              intrathoracic lymph nodes
    C83.93   Unspecified diffuse non-Hodgkin's lymphoma, intra-
              abdominal lymph nodes
    C83.94   Unspecified diffuse non-Hodgkin's lymphoma, lymph
              nodes of axilla and upper limb
    C83.95   Unspecified diffuse non-Hodgkin's lymphoma, lymph
              nodes of inguinal region and lower limb
    C83.96   Unspecified diffuse non-Hodgkin's lymphoma,
              intrapelvic lymph nodes
    C83.97   Unspecified diffuse non-Hodgkin's lymphoma, spleen
    C83.98   Unspecified diffuse non-Hodgkin's lymphoma, lymph
              nodes of multiple sites
    C83.99   Unspecified diffuse non-Hodgkin's lymphoma,
              extranodal and solid organ sites

C84 Peripheral and cutaneous T-cell lymphomas
     Use additional morphology code M970 with behavior code /3
C84.0 Mycosis fungoides
    C84.00   Mycosis fungoides, unspecified site
    C84.01   Mycosis fungoides, lymph nodes of head, face, and
              neck
    C84.02   Mycosis fungoides, intrathoracic lymph nodes
    C84.03   Mycosis fungoides, intra-abdominal lymph nodes
    C84.04   Mycosis fungoides, lymph nodes of axilla and upper
              limb
    C84.05   Mycosis fungoides, lymph nodes of inguinal region and
              lower limb
    C84.06   Mycosis fungoides, intrapelvic lymph nodes
    C84.07   Mycosis fungoides, spleen
    C84.08   Mycosis fungoides, lymph nodes of multiple sites
    C84.09   Mycosis fungoides, extranodal and solid organ sites
C84.1 Sézary's disease
    C84.10   Sézary's disease, unspecified site
    C84.11   Sézary's disease, lymph nodes of head, face, and neck
    C84.12   Sézary's disease, intrathoracic lymph nodes
    C84.13   Sézary's disease, intra-abdominal lymph nodes
    C84.14   Sézary's disease, lymph nodes of axilla and upper limb
    C84.15   Sézary's disease, lymph nodes of inguinal region and
              lower limb
    C84.16   Sézary's disease, intrapelvic lymph nodes
    C84.17   Sézary's disease, spleen
    C84.18   Sézary's disease, lymph nodes of multiple site
    C84.19   Sézary's disease, extranodal and solid organ sites
C84.2 T-zone lymphoma
    C84.20   T-zone lymphoma, unspecified site
    C84.21   T-zone lymphoma, lymph nodes of head, face, and
              neck
    C84.22   T-zone lymphoma, intrathoracic lymph nodes
    C84.23   T-zone lymphoma, intra-abdominal lymph nodes
    C84.24   T-zone lymphoma, lymph nodes of axilla and upper
              limb
    C84.25   T-zone lymphoma, lymph nodes of inguinal region and
              lower limb
    C84.26   T-zone lymphoma, intrapelvic lymph nodes
    C84.27   T-zone lymphoma, spleen

C84.28   T-zone lymphoma, lymph nodes of multiple sites

C84.29   T-zone lymphoma, extranodal and solid organ sites

C84.3   Lymphoepithelioid lymphoma

Lennert's lymphoma

C84.30   Lymphoepithelioid lymphoma, unspecified site

C84.31   Lymphoepithelioid lymphoma, lymph nodes of head, face, and neck

C84.32   Lymphoepithelioid lymphoma, intrathoracic lymph nodes

C84.33   Lymphoepithelioid lymphoma, intra-abdominal lymph nodes

C84.34   Lymphoepithelioid lymphoma, lymph nodes of axilla and upper limb

C84.35   Lymphoepithelioid lymphoma, lymph nodes of inguinal region and lower limb

C84.36   Lymphoepithelioid lymphoma, intrapelvic lymph nodes

C84.37   Lymphoepithelioid lymphoma, spleen

C84.38   Lymphoepithelioid lymphoma, lymph nodes of multiple sites

C84.39   Lymphoepithelioid lymphoma, extranodal and solid organ sites

C84.4   Peripheral T-cell lymphoma

C84.40   Peripheral T-cell lymphoma, unspecified site

C84.41   Peripheral T-cell lymphoma, lymph nodes of head, face, and neck

C84.42   Peripheral T-cell lymphoma, intrathoracic lymph nodes

C84.43   Peripheral T-cell lymphoma, intra-abdominal lymph nodes

C84.44   Peripheral T-cell lymphoma, lymph nodes of axilla and upper limb

C84.45   Peripheral T-cell lymphoma, lymph nodes of inguinal region and lower limb

C84.46   Peripheral T-cell lymphoma, intrapelvic lymph nodes

C84.47   Peripheral T-cell lymphoma, spleen

C84.48   Peripheral T-cell lymphoma, lymph nodes of multiple sites

C84.49   Peripheral T-cell lymphoma, extranodal and solid organ sites

C84.5   Other and unspecified T-cell lymphomas

Note: If T-cell lineage or involvement is mentioned in conjunction with a specific lymphoma, code to the more specific description.

C84.50   Other and unspecified T-cell lymphomas, unspecified site

C84.51   Other and unspecified T-cell lymphomas, lymph nodes of head, face, and neck

C84.52   Other and unspecified T-cell lymphomas, intrathoracic lymph nodes

C84.53   Other and unspecified T-cell lymphomas, intra-abdominal lymph nodes

C84.54   Other and unspecified T-cell lymphomas, lymph nodes of axilla and upper limb

C84.55   Other and unspecified T-cell lymphomas, lymph nodes of inguinal region and lower limb

C84.56   Other and unspecified T-cell lymphomas, intrapelvic lymph nodes

C84.57   Other and unspecified T-cell lymphomas, spleen

C84.58   Other and unspecified T-cell lymphomas, lymph nodes of multiple sites

C84.59   Other and unspecified T-cell lymphomas, extranodal and solid organ sites

C85   Other and unspecified types of non-Hodgkin's lymphoma

Use additional morphology codes M9590-M9592, M9594, M9710 with behavior code /3

C85.0   Lymphosarcoma

C85.00   Lymphosarcoma, unspecified site

C85.01   Lymphosarcoma, lymph nodes of head, face, and neck

C85.02   Lymphosarcoma, intrathoracic lymph nodes

C85.03   Lymphosarcoma, intra-abdominal lymph nodes

C85.04   Lymphosarcoma, lymph nodes of axilla and upper limb

C85.05   Lymphosarcoma, lymph nodes of inguinal region and lower limb

C85.06   Lymphosarcoma, intrapelvic lymph nodes

C85.07   Lymphosarcoma, spleen

C85.08   Lymphosarcoma, lymph nodes of multiple sites

C85.09   Lymphosarcoma, extranodal and solid organ sites

C85.1   Unspecified B-cell lymphoma

Note: If B-cell lineage or involvement is mentioned in conjunction with a specific lymphoma, code to the more specific description.

C85.10   Unspecified B-cell lymphoma, unspecified site

C85.11   Unspecified B-cell lymphoma, lymph nodes of head, face, and neck

C85.12   Unspecified B-cell lymphoma, intrathoracic lymph nodes

C85.13   Unspecified B-cell lymphoma, intra-abdominal lymph nodes

C85.14   Unspecified B-cell lymphoma, lymph nodes of axilla and upper limb

C85.15   Unspecified B-cell lymphoma, lymph nodes of inguinal region and lower limb

C85.16   Unspecified B-cell lymphoma, intrapelvic lymph nodes

C85.17   Unspecified B-cell lymphoma, spleen

C85.18   Unspecified B-cell lymphoma, lymph nodes of multiple sites

C85.19   Unspecified B-cell lymphoma, extranodal and solid organ sites

C85.7   Other specified types of non-Hodgkin's lymphoma

Malignant reticuloendotheliosis

Malignant reticulosis

Microglioma

C85.70   Other specified types of non-Hodgkin's lymphoma, unspecified site

C85.71   Other specified types of non-Hodgkin's lymphoma, lymph nodes of head, face, and neck

C85.72   Other specified types of non-Hodgkin's lymphoma, intrathoracic lymph nodes

C85.73   Other specified types of non-Hodgkin's lymphoma, intra-abdominal lymph nodes

C85.74   Other specified types of non-Hodgkin's lymphoma, lymph nodes of axilla and upper limb

C85.75   Other specified types of non-Hodgkin's lymphoma, lymph nodes of inguinal region and lower limb

C85.76   Other specified types of non-Hodgkin's lymphoma, intrapelvic

C85.77   Other specified types of non-Hodgkin's lymphoma, spleen

C85.78   Other specified types of non-Hodgkin's lymphoma, lymph nodes of multiple sites

C85.79   Other specified types of non-Hodgkin's lymphoma, extranodal and solid organ sites

C85.9   Unspecified type non-Hodgkin's lymphoma

Lymphoma NOS

Malignant lymphoma NOS

Non-Hodgkin's lymphoma NOS

C85.90   Unspecified type non-Hodgkin's lymphoma, unspecified site

C85.91   Unspecified type non-Hodgkin's lymphoma, lymph nodes of head, face, and neck

C85.92   Unspecified type non-Hodgkin's lymphoma, intrathoracic lymph nodes

C85.93   Unspecified type non-Hodgkin's lymphoma, intra-abdominal lymph nodes

C85.94   Unspecified type non-Hodgkin's lymphoma, lymph nodes of axilla and upper limb

C85.95   Unspecified type non-Hodgkin's lymphoma, lymph nodes of inguinal region and lower limb

C85.96   Unspecified type non-Hodgkin's lymphoma, intrapelvic lymph nodes

C85.97   Unspecified type non-Hodgkin's lymphoma, spleen

C85.98 Unspecified type non-Hodgkin's lymphoma, lymph nodes of multiple sites

C85.99 Unspecified type non-Hodgkin's lymphoma, extranodal and solid organ sites

C88 Malignant immunoproliferative diseases
Use additional morphology code M976 with behavior code /3

C88.0 Waldenström's macroglobulinemia

C88.1 Alpha heavy chain disease

C88.2 Gamma heavy chain disease
Franklin's disease

C88.3 Immunoproliferative small intestinal disease
Mediterranean disease

C88.7 Other malignant immunoproliferative diseases

C88.9 Malignant immunoproliferative disease, unspecified
Immunoproliferative disease NOS

C90 Multiple myeloma and malignant plasma cell neoplasms
Use additional morphology codes M973, M9830 with behavior code /3

C90.0 Multiple myeloma
Kahler's disease
Myelomatosis
Excludes1:   solitary myeloma (C90.2-)

C90.00 Multiple myeloma not in remission
Multiple myeloma NOS

C90.01 Multiple myeloma in remission

C90.1 Plasma cell leukemia

C90.10 Plasma cell leukemia not in remission
Plasma cell leukemia NOS

C90.11 Plasma cell leukemia in remission

C90.2 Plasmacytoma, extramedullary
Malignant plasma cell tumor NOS
Plasmacytoma NOS
Solitary myeloma

C90.20 Plasmacytoma, extramedullary not in remission
Plasmacytoma, extramedullary NOS

C90.21 Plasmacytoma, extramedullary in remission

C91 Lymphoid leukemia
Use additional morphology codes M9820, M9940-M9941 with behavior code /3

C91.0 Acute lymphoblastic leukemia
Excludes1:   acute exacerbation of chronic lymphocytic leukemia (C91.10)

C91.00 Acute lymphoblastic leukemia, not in remission
Acute lymphoblastic leukemia NOS

C91.01 Acute lymphoblastic leukemia, in remission

C91.1 Chronic lymphocytic leukemia

C91.10 Chronic lymphocytic leukemia, not in remission
Chronic lymphocytic leukemia NOS

C91.11 Chronic lymphocytic leukemia, in remission

C91.2 Subacute lymphocytic leukemia

C91.20 Subacute lymphocytic leukemia, not in remission
Subacute lymphocytic leukemia NOS

C91.21 Subacute lymphocytic leukemia, in remission

C91.3 Prolymphocytic leukemia

C91.30 Prolymphocytic leukemia, not in remission
Prolymphocytic leukemia NOS

C91.31 Prolymphocytic leukemia, in remission

C91.4 Hairy-cell leukemia
Leukemic reticuloendotheliosis

C91.40 Hairy-cell leukemia, not in remission
Hairy-cell leukemia NOS

C91.41 Hairy-cell leukemia, in remission

C91.5 Adult T-cell leukemia

C91.50 Adult T-cell leukemia, not in remission
Adult T-cell leukemia NOS

C91.51 Adult T-cell leukemia, in remission

C91.7 Other lymphoid leukemia

C91.70 Other lymphoid leukemia, not in remission
Other lymphoid leukemia NOS

C91.71 Other lymphoid leukemia, in remission

C91.9 Lymphoid leukemia, unspecified

C91.90 Lymphoid leukemia, unspecified, not in remission
Lymphoid leukemia, unspecified NOS

C91.91 Lymphoid leukemia, unspecified, in remission

C92 Myeloid leukemia
Includes: leukemia granulocytic
leukemia myelogenous
Use additional morphology codes M986-M988, M9930 with behavior code /3

C92.0 Acute myeloid leukemia
Excludes1:   acute exacerbation of chronic myeloid leukemia (C92.10)

C92.00 Acute myeloid leukemia, not in remission
Acute myeloid leukemia NOS

C92.01 Acute myeloid leukemia, in remission

C92.1 Chronic myeloid leukemia

C92.10 Chronic myeloid leukemia, not in remission
Chronic myeloid leukemia NOS

C92.11 Chronic myeloid leukemia, in remission

C92.2 Subacute myeloid leukemia

C92.20 Subacute myeloid leukemia, not in remission
Subacute myeloid leukemia NOS

C92.21 Subacute myeloid leukemia, in remission

C92.3 Myeloid sarcoma
Chloroma
Granulocytic sarcoma

C92.30 Myeloid sarcoma, not in remission
Myeloid sarcoma NOS

C92.31 Myeloid sarcoma, in remission

C92.4 Acute promyelocytic leukemia

C92.40 Acute promyelocytic leukemia, not in remission
Acute promyelocytic leukemia NOS

C92.41 Acute promyelocytic leukemia, in remission

C92.5 Acute myelomonocytic leukemia

C92.50 Acute myelomonocytic leukemia, not in remission
Acute myelomonocytic leukemia NOS

C92.51 Acute myelomonocytic leukemia, in remission

C92.7 Other myeloid leukemia

C92.70 Other myeloid leukemia, not in remission
Other myeloid leukemia NOS

C92.71 Other myeloid leukemia, in remission

C92.9 Myeloid leukemia, unspecified

C92.90 Myeloid leukemia, unspecified, not in remission
Myeloid leukemia, unspecified NOS

C92.91 Myeloid leukemia, unspecified in remission

C93 Monocytic leukemia
Includes: monocytoid leukemia
Use additional morphology code M989 with behavior code /3

C93.0 Acute monocytic leukemia
Excludes1:   acute exacerbation of chronic monocytic leukemia (C93.10)

C93.00 Acute monocytic leukemia, not in remission
Acute monocytic leukemia NOS

C93.01 Acute monocytic leukemia, in remission

C93.1 Chronic monocytic leukemia

C93.10 Chronic monocytic leukemia, not in remission
Chronic monocytic leukemia NOS

C93.11 Chronic monocytic leukemia, in remission

C93.2 Subacute monocytic leukemia

C93.20 Subacute monocytic leukemia, not in remission
Subacute monocytic leukemia NOS

C93.21 Subacute monocytic leukemia, in remission

C93.7 Other monocytic leukemia

C93.70 Other monocytic leukemia, not in remission
Other monocytic leukemia NOS

C93.71 Other monocytic leukemia, in remission

C93.9   **Monocytic leukemia, unspecified**

    C93.90   **Monocytic leukemia, unspecified, not in remission**
         Monocytic leukemia, unspecified NOS

    C93.91   **Monocytic leukemia, unspecified in remission**

C94   **Other leukemias of specified cell type**
     Use additional morphology codes M984, M9850, M9900, M9910,
     M9931-M9932 with behavior code /3

     Excludes1:   leukemic reticuloendotheliosis (C91.4-)
                 plasma cell leukemia (C90.1-)

C94.0   **Acute erythremia and erythroleukemia**
     Acute erythremic myelosis
     Di Guglielmo's disease

    C94.00   **Acute erythremia and erythroleukemia, not in remission**
         Acute erythremia and erythroleukemia NOS

    C94.01   **Acute erythremia and erythroleukemia, in remission**

C94.1   **Chronic erythremia**
     Heilmeyer-Schöner disease

    C94.10   **Chronic erythremia, not in remission**
         Chronic erythremia NOS

    C94.11   **Chronic erythremia, in remission**

C94.2   **Acute megakaryoblastic leukemia**
     Megakaryoblastic (acute) leukemia
     Megakaryocytic (acute) leukemia

    C94.20   **Acute megakaryoblastic leukemia, not in remission**
         Acute megakaryoblastic leukemia NOS

    C94.21   **Acute megakaryoblastic leukemia, in remission**

C94.3   **Mast cell leukemia**

    C94.30   **Mast cell leukemia, not in remission**
         Mast cell leukemia NOS

    C94.31   **Mast cell leukemia, in remission**

C94.4   **Acute panmyelosis**

    C94.40   **Acute panmyelosis, not in remission**
         Acute panmyelosis NOS

    C94.41   **Acute panmyelosis, in remission**

C94.5   **Acute myelofibrosis**

    C94.50   **Acute myelofibrosis, not in remission**
         Acute myelofibrosis NOS

    C94.51   **Acute myelofibrosis, in remission**

C94.7   **Other specified leukemias**
     Lymphosarcoma cell leukemia

    C94.70   **Other specified leukemias, not in remission**
         Other specified leukemias NOS

    C94.71   **Other specified leukemias, in remission**

C95   **Leukemia of unspecified cell type**
     Use additional morphology code M980 with behavior code /3

C95.0   **Acute leukemia of unspecified cell type**
     Blast cell leukemia
     Stem cell leukemia

     Excludes1:   acute exacerbation of unspecified chronic
                 leukemia (C95.10)

    C95.00   **Acute leukemia of unspecified cell type, not in remission**

    C95.01   **Acute leukemia of unspecified cell type, in remission**

C95.1   **Chronic leukemia of unspecified cell type**

    C95.10   **Chronic leukemia of unspecified cell type, not in remission**
         Chronic leukemia of unspecified cell type NOS

    C95.11   **Chronic leukemia of unspecified cell type, in remission**

C95.2   **Subacute leukemia of unspecified cell type**

    C95.20   **Subacute leukemia of unspecified cell type, not in remission**
         Subacute leukemia of unspecified cell type NOS

    C95.21   **Subacute leukemia of unspecified cell type, in remission**

C95.7   **Other leukemia of unspecified cell type**

    C95.70   **Other leukemia of unspecified cell type, not in remission**
         Other leukemia of unspecified cell type NOS

    C95.71   **Other leukemia of unspecified cell type, in remission**

C95.9   **Leukemia, unspecified**

    C95.90   **Leukemia, unspecified, not in remission**
         Leukemia, unspecified NOS

    C95.91   **Leukemia, unspecified, in remission**

C96   **Other and unspecified malignant neoplasms of lymphoid, hematopoietic and related tissue**
     Use additional morphology codes M972, M974 with behavior code /3

C96.0   **Letterer-Siwe disease**
     Nonlipid reticuloendotheliosis
     Nonlipid reticulosis

C96.1   **Malignant histiocytosis**
     Histiocytic medullary reticulosis

C96.2   **Malignant mast cell tumor**
     Malignant mastocytoma
     Malignant mastocytosis
     Mast cell sarcoma

     Excludes1:   mast cell leukemia (C94.30)
                 mastocytosis (cutaneous) (Q82.2)

C96.3   **True histiocytic lymphoma**

C96.7   **Other specified malignant neoplasms of lymphoid, hematopoietic and related tissue**

C96.9   **Malignant neoplasm of lymphoid, hematopoietic and related tissue, unspecified**

IN SITU NEOPLASMS (D00–D09)

Includes: Bowen's disease
               erythroplasia
               grade III intraepithelial neoplasia
               Queyrat's erythroplasia

Use additional morphology codes with behavior code /2

D00   **Carcinoma in situ of oral cavity, esophagus and stomach**
     Excludes1:   melanoma in situ (D03.-)

D00.0   **Carcinoma in situ of lip, oral cavity and pharynx**

     Excludes1:   carcinoma in situ of aryepiglottic fold or
                 interarytenoid fold, laryngeal aspect (D02.0)
                 carcinoma in situ of epiglottis:
                     NOS (D02.0)
                     suprahyoid portion (D02.0)
                 carcinoma in situ of skin of lip (D03.0, D04.0)

     Use additional code to identify:
         exposure to environmental tobacco smoke (X58.1)
         exposure to tobacco smoke in the perinatal period (P96.6)
         history of tobacco use (Z87.82)
         occupational exposure to environmental tobacco smoke
            (Z57.31)
         tobacco dependence (F17.-)
         tobacco use (Z72.0)

    D00.00   **Carcinoma in situ of oral cavity, unspecified site**

    D00.01   **Carcinoma in situ of labial mucosa and vermilion border**

    D00.02   **Carcinoma in situ of buccal mucosa**

    D00.03   **Carcinoma in situ of gingiva and edentulous alveolar ridge**

    D00.04   **Carcinoma in situ of soft palate**

    D00.05   **Carcinoma in situ of hard palate**

    D00.06   **Carcinoma in situ of floor of mouth**

    D00.07   **Carcinoma in situ of tongue**

    D00.08   **Carcinoma in situ of pharynx**
         Carcinoma in situ of aryepiglottic fold NOS
         Carcinoma in situ of hypopharyngeal aspect of
            aryepiglottic fold
         Carcinoma in situ of marginal zone of aryepiglottic fold

D00.1   **Carcinoma in situ of esophagus**

D00.2   **Carcinoma in situ of stomach**

D01   **Carcinoma in situ of other and unspecified digestive organs**
     Excludes1:   melanoma in situ (D03.-)

D01.0   **Carcinoma in situ of colon**

     Excludes1:   carcinoma in situ of rectosigmoid junction
                 (D01.1)

D01.1   **Carcinoma in situ of rectosigmoid junction**

D01.2 Carcinoma in situ of rectum

D01.3 Carcinoma in situ of anus and anal canal
  Excludes1: carcinoma in situ of anal margin (D04.5)
        carcinoma in situ of anal skin (D04.5)
        carcinoma in situ of perianal skin (D04.5)

D01.4 Carcinoma in situ of other and unspecified parts of intestine
  Excludes1: carcinoma in situ of ampulla of Vater (D01.5)

  D01.40 Carcinoma in situ of unspecified part of intestine

  D01.49 Carcinoma in situ of other parts of intestine

D01.5 Carcinoma in situ of liver, gallbladder and bile ducts
  Carcinoma in situ of ampulla of Vater

D01.7 Carcinoma in situ of other specified digestive organs
  Carcinoma in situ of pancreas

D01.9 Carcinoma in situ of digestive organ, unspecified

D02 Carcinoma in situ of middle ear and respiratory system
  Excludes1: melanoma in situ (D03.-)
  Use additional code to identify:
    exposure to environmental tobacco smoke (X58.1)
    exposure to tobacco smoke in the perinatal period (P96.6)
    history of tobacco use (Z87.82)
    occupational exposure to environmental tobacco smoke (Z57.31)
    tobacco dependence (F17.-)
    tobacco use (Z72.0)

D02.0 Carcinoma in situ of larynx
  Carcinoma in situ of aryepiglottic fold or interarytenoid fold, laryngeal aspect
  Carcinoma in situ of epiglottis (suprahyoid portion)
  Excludes1: carcinoma in situ of aryepiglottic fold or interarytenoid fold NOS (D00.08)
        carcinoma in situ of hypopharyngeal aspect (D00.08)
        carcinoma in situ of marginal zone (D00.08)

D02.1 Carcinoma in situ of trachea

D02.2 Carcinoma in situ of bronchus and lung
  D02.20 Carcinoma in situ of bronchus and lung, unspecified side
  D02.21 Carcinoma in situ of right bronchus and lung
  D02.22 Carcinoma in situ of left bronchus and lung

D02.3 Carcinoma in situ of other parts of respiratory system
  Carcinoma in situ of accessory sinuses
  Carcinoma in situ of middle ear
  Carcinoma in situ of nasal cavities
  Excludes1: carcinoma in situ of ear (external) (skin) (D04.2-)
        carcinoma in situ of nose NOS (D09.7)
        carcinoma in situ of skin of nose (D04.3)

D02.4 Carcinoma in situ of respiratory system, unspecified

D03 Melanoma in situ
  Use additional morphology codes M8720-M8790 with behavior code /2

D03.0 Melanoma in situ of lip

D03.1 Melanoma in situ of eyelid, including canthus
  D03.10 Melanoma in situ of eyelid, including canthus, unspecified side
  D03.11 Melanoma in situ of right eyelid, including canthus
  D03.12 Melanoma in situ of left eyelid, including canthus

D03.2 Melanoma in situ of ear and external auricular canal
  D03.20 Melanoma in situ of ear and external auricular canal, unspecified side
  D03.21 Melanoma in situ of right ear and external auricular canal
  D03.22 Melanoma in situ of left ear and external auricular canal

D03.3 Melanoma in situ of other and unspecified parts of face
  D03.30 Melanoma in situ of unspecified part of face
  D03.39 Melanoma in situ of other parts of face

D03.4 Melanoma in situ of scalp and neck

D03.5 Melanoma in situ of trunk
  Melanoma in situ of anal margin
  Melanoma in situ of anal skin
  Melanoma in situ of breast (skin) (soft tissue)
  Melanoma in situ of perianal skin

D03.6 Melanoma in situ of upper limb, including shoulder
  D03.60 Melanoma in situ of upper limb, including shoulder, unspecified side
  D03.61 Melanoma in situ of right upper limb, including shoulder
  D03.62 Melanoma in situ of left upper limb, including shoulder

D03.7 Melanoma in situ of lower limb, including hip
  D03.70 Melanoma in situ of lower limb, including hip, unspecified side
  D03.71 Melanoma in situ of right lower limb, including hip
  D03.72 Melanoma in situ of left lower limb, including hip

D03.8 Melanoma in situ of other sites
  Melanoma in situ of scrotum
  Excludes1: carcinoma in situ of scrotum (D07.61)

D03.9 Melanoma in situ, unspecified

D04 Carcinoma in situ of skin
  Excludes1: erythroplasia of Queyrat (penis) NOS (D07.4)
        melanoma in situ (D03.-)

D04.0 Carcinoma in situ of skin of lip
  Excludes1: carcinoma in situ of vermilion border of lip (D00.01)

D04.1 Carcinoma in situ of skin of eyelid, including canthus
  D04.10 Carcinoma in situ of skin of eyelid, including canthus, unspecified side
  D04.11 Carcinoma in situ of skin of right eyelid, including canthus
  D04.12 Carcinoma in situ of skin of left eyelid, including canthus

D04.2 Carcinoma in situ of skin of ear and external auricular canal
  D04.20 Carcinoma in situ of skin of ear and external auricular canal, unspecfied side
  D04.21 Carcinoma in situ of skin of right ear and external auricular canal
  D04.22 Carcinoma in situ of skin of left ear and external auricular canal

D04.3 Carcinoma in situ of skin of other and unspecified parts of face
  D04.30 Carcinoma in situ of skin of unspecified part of face
  D04.39 Carcinoma in situ of skin of other parts of face

D04.4 Carcinoma in situ of skin of scalp and neck

D04.5 Carcinoma in situ of skin of trunk
  Carcinoma in situ of anal margin
  Carcinoma in situ of anal skin
  Carcinoma in situ of perianal skin
  Carcinoma in situ of skin of breast
  Excludes1: carcinoma in situ of anus NOS (D01.3)
        carcinoma in situ of scrotum (D07.61)
        carcinoma in situ of skin of genital organs (D07.-)

D04.6 Carcinoma in situ of skin of upper limb, including shoulder
  D04.60 Carcinoma in situ of skin of upper limb, including shoulder, unspecified side
  D04.61 Carcinoma in situ of skin of right upper limb, including shoulder
  D04.62 Carcinoma in situ of skin of left upper limb, including shoulder

D04.7 Carcinoma in situ of skin of lower limb, including hip
  D04.70 Carcinoma in situ of skin of lower limb, including hip, unspecified side
  D04.71 Carcinoma in situ of skin of right lower limb, including hip
  D04.72 Carcinoma in situ of skin of left lower limb, including hip

D04.8 Carcinoma in situ of skin of other sites

D04.9 Carcinoma in situ of skin, unspecified

D05 Carcinoma in situ of breast
  Excludes1: carcinoma in situ of skin of breast (D04.5)
        melanoma in situ of breast (skin) (D03.5)
        Paget's disease of breast or nipple (C50.-)

D05.0 Lobular carcinoma in situ of breast

D05.00 Lobular carcinoma in situ of female breast, unspecified side
D05.01 Lobular carcinoma in situ of right female breast
D05.02 Lobular carcinoma in situ of left female breast
D05.03 Lobular carcinoma in situ of right male breast
D05.04 Lobular carcinoma in situ of left male breast
D05.05 Lobular carcinoma in situ of male breast, unspecified side
D05.1 Intraductal carcinoma in situ of breast
D05.10 Intraductal carcinoma in situ of female breast, unspecified side
D05.11 Intraductal carcinoma in situ of right female breast
D05.12 Intraductal carcinoma in situ of left female breast
D05.13 Intraductal carcinoma in situ of right male breast
D05.14 Intraductal carcinoma in situ of left male breast
D05.15 Intraductal carcinoma in situ of male breast, unspecified side
D05.7 Other carcinoma in situ of breast
D05.70 Other carcinoma in situ of female breast, unspecified side
D05.71 Other carcinoma in situ of right female breast
D05.72 Other carcinoma in situ of left female breast
D05.73 Other carcinoma in situ of right male breast
D05.74 Other carcinoma in situ of left male breast
D05.75 Other carcinoma in situ of male breast, unspecified side
D05.9 Unspecified carcinoma in situ of breast
D05.90 Unspecified carcinoma in situ of female breast, unspecified side
D05.91 Unspecified carcinoma in situ of right female breast
D05.92 Unspecified carcinoma in situ of left female breast
D05.93 Unspecified carcinoma in situ of right male breast
D05.94 Unspecified carcinoma in situ of left male breast
D05.95 Unspecified carcinoma in situ of male breast unspecified side

D06 Carcinoma in situ of cervix uteri
Includes: cervical intraepithelial neoplasia [CIN], grade III, with or without severe dysplasia
Excludes1: melanoma in situ of cervix (D03.5)
severe dysplasia of cervix NOS (N87.2)
D06.0 Carcinoma in situ of endocervix
D06.1 Carcinoma in situ of exocervix
D06.7 Carcinoma in situ of other parts of cervix
D06.9 Carcinoma in situ of cervix, unspecified

D07 Carcinoma in situ of other and unspecified genital organs
Excludes1: melanoma in situ of trunk (D03.5)
D07.0 Carcinoma in situ of endometrium
D07.1 Carcinoma in situ of vulva
Vulvar intraepithelial neoplasia [VIN], grade III, with or without severe dysplasia
Excludes1: severe dysplasia of vulva NOS (N90.2)
D07.2 Carcinoma in situ of vagina
Vaginal intraepithelial neoplasia [VIN], grade III, with or without severe dysplasia
Excludes1: severe dysplasia of vagina NOS (N89.2)
D07.3 Carcinoma in situ of other and unspecified female genital organs
D07.30 Carcinoma in situ of unspecified female genital organs
D07.39 Carcinoma in situ of other female genital organs
D07.4 Carcinoma in situ of penis
Erythroplasia of Queyrat NOS
D07.5 Carcinoma in situ of prostate
D07.6 Carcinoma in situ of other and unspecified male genital organs
D07.60 Carcinoma in situ of unspecified male genital organs
D07.61 Carcinoma in situ of scrotum
D07.69 Carcinoma in situ of other male genital organs

D09 Carcinoma in situ of other and unspecified sites
Excludes1: melanoma in situ (D03.-)
D09.0 Carcinoma in situ of bladder
D09.1 Carcinoma in situ of other and unspecified urinary organs
D09.10 Carcinoma in situ of unspecified urinary organ
D09.19 Carcinoma in situ of other urinary organs
D09.2 Carcinoma in situ of eye
Excludes1: carcinoma in situ of skin of eyelid (D04.1-)
D09.20 Carcinoma in situ of eye, unspecified side
D09.21 Carcinoma in situ of right eye
D09.22 Carcinoma in situ of left eye
D09.3 Carcinoma in situ of thyroid and other endocrine glands
Excludes1: carcinoma in situ of endocrine pancreas (D01.7)
carcinoma in situ of ovary (D07.39)
carcinoma in situ of testis (D07.69)
D09.7 Carcinoma in situ of other specified sites
D09.9 Carcinoma in situ, unspecified

BENIGN NEOPLASMS (D10–D36)
Use additional morphology codes with behavior code /0

D10 Benign neoplasm of mouth and pharynx
D10.0 Benign neoplasm of lip
Benign neoplasm of lip (frenulum) (inner aspect) (mucosa) (vermilion border)
Excludes1: benign neoplasm of skin of lip (D22.0, D23.0)
D10.1 Benign neoplasm of tongue
Benign neoplasm of lingual tonsil
D10.2 Benign neoplasm of floor of mouth
D10.3 Other and unspecified parts of mouth
D10.30 Benign neoplasm of unspecified part of mouth
D10.39 Benign neoplasm of other parts of mouth
Benign neoplasm of minor salivary gland NOS
Excludes1: benign odontogenic neoplasms (D16.4-D16.5)
benign neoplasm of mucosa of lip (D10.0)
benign neoplasm of nasopharyngeal surface of soft palate (D10.6)
D10.4 Benign neoplasm of tonsil
Benign neoplasm of tonsil (faucial) (palatine)
Excludes1: benign neoplasm of lingual tonsil (D10.1)
benign neoplasm of pharyngeal tonsil (D10.6)
benign neoplasm of tonsillar fossa (D10.5)
benign neoplasm of tonsillar pillars (D10.5)
D10.5 Benign neoplasm of other parts of oropharynx
Benign neoplasm of epiglottis, anterior aspect
Benign neoplasm of tonsillar fossa
Benign neoplasm of tonsillar pillars
Benign neoplasm of vallecula
Excludes1: benign neoplasm of epiglottis NOS (D14.1)
benign neoplasm of epiglottis, suprahyoid portion (D14.1)
D10.6 Benign neoplasm of nasopharynx
Benign neoplasm of pharyngeal tonsil
Benign neoplasm of posterior margin of septum and choanae
D10.7 Benign neoplasm of hypopharynx
D10.9 Benign neoplasm of pharynx, unspecified

D11 Benign neoplasm of major salivary glands
Excludes1: benign neoplasms of specified minor salivary glands which are classified according to their anatomical location
benign neoplasms of minor salivary glands NOS (D10.39)
D11.0 Benign neoplasm of parotid gland
D11.7 Benign neoplasm of other major salivary glands
Benign neoplasm of sublingual salivary gland
Benign neoplasm of submandibular salivary gland
D11.9 Benign neoplasm of major salivary gland, unspecified

D12 Benign neoplasm of colon, rectum, anus and anal canal
D12.0 Benign neoplasm of cecum
Benign neoplasm of ieocecal valve

D12.1　Benign neoplasm of appendix

D12.2　Benign neoplasm of ascending colon

D12.3　Benign neoplasm of transverse colon
　　　　Benign neoplasm of hepatic flexure
　　　　Benign neoplasm of splenic flexure

D12.4　Benign neoplasm of descending colon

D12.5　Benign neoplasm of sigmoid colon

D12.6　Benign neoplasm of colon, unspecified
　　　　Adenomatosis of colon
　　　　Benign neoplasm of large intestine NOS
　　　　Polyposis (hereditary) of colon

D12.7　Benign neoplasm of rectosigmoid junction

D12.8　Benign neoplasm of rectum

D12.9　Benign neoplasm of anus and anal canal
　　　　Excludes1:　benign neoplasm of anal margin (D22.5, D23.5)
　　　　　　　　　　benign neoplasm of anal skin (D22.5, D23.5)
　　　　　　　　　　benign neoplasm of perianal skin (D22.5, D23.5)

D13　Benign neoplasm of other and ill-defined parts of digestive system

D13.0　Benign neoplasm of esophagus

D13.1　Benign neoplasm of stomach

D13.2　Benign neoplasm of duodenum

D13.3　Benign neoplasm of other and unspecified parts of small intestine
　　　　Excludes1:　benign neoplasm of ileocecal valve (D12.0)

　　D13.30　Benign neoplasm of unspecified part of small intestine

　　D13.39　Benign neoplasm of other parts of small intestine

D13.4　Benign neoplasm of liver
　　　　Benign neoplasm of intrahepatic bile ducts

D13.5　Benign neoplasm of extrahepatic bile ducts

D13.6　Benign neoplasm of pancreas
　　　　Excludes1:　benign neoplasm of endocrine pancreas (D13.7)

D13.7　Benign neoplasm of endocrine pancreas
　　　　Islet cell tumor
　　　　Benign neoplasm of islets of Langerhans
　　　　Use additional code to identify any functional activity.

D13.9　Benign neoplasm of ill-defined sites within the digestive system
　　　　Benign neoplasm of digestive system NOS
　　　　Benign neoplasm of intestine NOS
　　　　Benign neoplasm of spleen

D14　Benign neoplasm of middle ear and respiratory system

D14.0　Benign neoplasm of middle ear, nasal cavity and accessory sinuses
　　　　Benign neoplasm of cartilage of nose
　　　　Excludes1:　benign neoplasm of auricular canal (external) (D22.2-, D23.2-)
　　　　　　　　　　benign neoplasm of bone of ear (D16.4)
　　　　　　　　　　benign neoplasm of bone of nose (D16.4)
　　　　　　　　　　benign neoplasm of cartilage of ear (D21.0)
　　　　　　　　　　benign neoplasm of ear (external) (skin) (D22.2-, D23.2-)
　　　　　　　　　　benign neoplasm of nose NOS (D36.7)
　　　　　　　　　　benign neoplasm of skin of nose (D22.39, D23.39)
　　　　　　　　　　benign neoplasm of olfactory bulb (D33.3)
　　　　　　　　　　benign neoplasm of posterior margin of septum and choanae (D10.6)
　　　　　　　　　　polyp of accessory sinus (J33.8)
　　　　　　　　　　polyp of ear (middle) (H74.4)
　　　　　　　　　　polyp of nasal (cavity) (J33.-)

D14.1　Benign neoplasm of larynx
　　　　Benign neoplasm of epiglottis (suprahyoid portion)
　　　　Excludes1:　benign neoplasm of epiglottis, anterior aspect (D10.5)
　　　　　　　　　　polyp of vocal cord or larynx (J38.1)

D14.2　Benign neoplasm of trachea

D14.3　Benign neoplasm of bronchus and lung

　　D14.30　Benign neoplasm of bronchus and lung, unspecified side

　　D14.31　Benign neoplasm of right bronchus and lung

　　D14.32　Benign neoplasm of left bronchus and lung

D14.4　Benign neoplasm of respiratory system, unspecified

D15　Benign neoplasm of other and unspecified intrathoracic organs
　　　　Excludes1:　benign neoplasm of mesothelial tissue (D19.-)

D15.0　Benign neoplasm of thymus

D15.1　Benign neoplasm of heart
　　　　Excludes1:　benign neoplasm of great vessels (D21.3)

D15.2　Benign neoplasm of mediastinum

D15.7　Benign neoplasm of other specified intrathoracic organs

D15.9　Benign neoplasm of intrathoracic organ, unspecified

D16　Benign neoplasm of bone and articular cartilage
　　　　Excludes1:　benign neoplasm of connective tissue of ear (D21.0)
　　　　　　　　　　benign neoplasm of connective tissue of eyelid (D21.0)
　　　　　　　　　　benign neoplasm of connective tissue of larynx (D14.1)
　　　　　　　　　　benign neoplasm of connective tissue of nose (D14.0)
　　　　　　　　　　benign neoplasm of synovia (D21.-)

D16.0　Benign neoplasm of scapula and long bones of upper limb

　　D16.00　Benign neoplasm of scapula and long bones of upper limb, unspecified side

　　D16.01　Benign neoplasm of scapula and long bones of right upper limb

　　D16.02　Benign neoplasm of scapula and long bones of left upper limb

D16.1　Benign neoplasm of short bones of upper limb

　　D16.10　Benign neoplasm of short bones of upper limb, unspecified side

　　D16.11　Benign neoplasm of short bones of right upper limb

　　D16.12　Benign neoplasm of short bones of left upper limb

D16.2　Benign neoplasm of long bones of lower limb

　　D16.20　Benign neoplasm of long bones of lower limb, unspecified side

　　D16.21　Benign neoplasm of long bones of right lower limb

　　D16.22　Benign neoplasm of long bones of left lower limb

D16.3　Benign neoplasm of short bones of lower limb

　　D16.30　Benign neoplasm of short bones of lower limb, unspecified side

　　D16.31　Benign neoplasm of short bones of right lower limb

　　D16.32　Benign neoplasm of short bones of left lower limb

D16.4　Benign neoplasm of bones of skull and face
　　　　Benign neoplasm of maxilla (superior)
　　　　Benign neoplasm of orbital bone
　　　　Excludes1:　benign neoplasm of lower jaw bone (D16.5)

D16.5　Benign neoplasm of lower jaw bone

D16.6　Benign neoplasm of vertebral column
　　　　Excludes1:　benign neoplasm of sacrum and coccyx (D16.8)

D16.7　Benign neoplasm of ribs, sternum and clavicle

D16.8　Benign neoplasm of pelvic bones, sacrum and coccyx

D16.9　Benign neoplasm of bone and articular cartilage, unspecified

D17　Benign lipomatous neoplasm
　　　　Use additional morphology codes M8850-M8881 with behavior code /0

D17.0　Benign lipomatous neoplasm of skin and subcutaneous tissue of head, face and neck

D17.1　Benign lipomatous neoplasm of skin and subcutaneous tissue of trunk

D17.2　Benign lipomatous neoplasm of skin and subcutaneous tissue of limb

　　D17.20　Benign lipomatous neoplasm of skin and subcutaneous tissue of unspecified limb

　　D17.21　Benign lipomatous neoplasm of skin and subcutaneous tissue of right arm

　　D17.22　Benign lipomatous neoplasm of skin and subcutaneous tissue of left arm

　　D17.23　Benign lipomatous neoplasm of skin and subcutaneous tissue of right leg

　　D17.24　Benign lipomatous neoplasm of skin and subcutaneous tissue of left leg

D17.3　Benign lipomatous neoplasm of skin and subcutaneous tissue of other and unspecified sites

　　D17.30　Benign lipomatous neoplasm of skin and subcutaneous tissue of unspecified sites

D17.39   Benign lipomatous neoplasm of skin and subcutaneous tissue of other sites

D17.4   **Benign lipomatous neoplasm of intrathoracic organs**

D17.5   **Benign lipomatous neoplasm of intra-abdominal organs**

    Excludes1:   benign lipomatous neoplasm of peritoneum and retroperitoneum (D17.7)

D17.6   **Benign lipomatous neoplasm of spermatic cord**

D17.7   **Benign lipomatous neoplasm of other sites**

    Benign lipomatous neoplasm of peritoneum
    Benign lipomatous neoplasm of retroperitoneum

D17.9   **Benign lipomatous neoplasm, unspecified**

    Lipoma NOS

D18 Hemangioma and lymphangioma, any site

    Use additional morphology codes M9120-M9175 with behavior code /0

    Excludes1:   benign neoplasm of glomus jugulare (D35.6)
        blue or pigmented nevus (D22.-)
        nevus NOS (D22.-)
        vascular nevus (Q82.5)

D18.0   **Hemangioma**

    Angioma NOS
    Cavernous nevus

D18.00   **Hemangioma unspecified site**

D18.01   **Hemangioma of skin and subcutaneous tissue**

D18.02   **Hemangioma of intracranial structures**

D18.03   **Hemangioma of intra-abdominal structures**

D18.09   **Hemangioma of other sites**

D18.1   **Lymphangioma, any site**

D19 Benign neoplasm of mesothelial tissue

    Use additional morphology code M905 with behavior code /0

D19.0   **Benign neoplasm of mesothelial tissue of pleura**

D19.1   **Benign neoplasm of mesothelial tissue of peritoneum**

D19.7   **Benign neoplasm of mesothelial tissue of other sites**

D19.9   **Benign neoplasm of mesothelial tissue, unspecified**

    Benign mesothelioma NOS

D20 Benign neoplasm of soft tissue of retroperitoneum and peritoneum

    Excludes1:   benign lipomatous neoplasm of peritoneum and retroperitoneum (D17.7)
        benign neoplasm of mesothelial tissue (D19.-)

D20.0   **Benign neoplasm of soft tissue of retroperitoneum**

D20.1   **Benign neoplasm of soft tissue of peritoneum**

D21 Other benign neoplasms of connective and other soft tissue

    Includes: benign neoplasm of blood vessel
        benign neoplasm of bursa
        benign neoplasm of cartilage
        benign neoplasm of fascia
        benign neoplasm of fat
        benign neoplasm of ligament, except uterine
        benign neoplasm of lymphatic channel
        benign neoplasm of muscle
        benign neoplasm of synovia
        benign neoplasm of tendon (sheath)

    Excludes1:   benign neoplasm of articular cartilage (D16.-)
        benign neoplasm of cartilage of larynx (D14.1)
        benign neoplasm of cartilage of nose (D14.0)
        benign neoplasm of connective tissue of breast (D24.-)
        benign neoplasm of peripheral nerves and autonomic nervous system (D36.1-)
        benign neoplasm of peritoneum (D20.1)
        benign neoplasm of retroperitoneum (D20.0)
        benign neoplasm of uterine ligament, any (D28.2)
        benign neoplasm of vascular tissue (D18.-)
        hemangioma (D18.0-)
        lipomatous neoplasm (D17.-)
        lymphangioma (D18.1)
        uterine leiomyoma (D25.-)

D21.0   **Benign neoplasm of connective and other soft tissue of head, face and neck**

    Benign neoplasm of connective tissue of ear
    Benign neoplasm of connective tissue of eyelid

    Excludes1:   benign neoplasm of connective tissue of orbit (D31.6-)

D21.1   **Benign neoplasm of connective and other soft tissue of upper limb, including shoulder**

D21.10   **Benign neoplasm of connective and other soft tissue of upper limb, including shoulder, unspecified side**

D21.11   **Benign neoplasm of connective and other soft tissue of right upper limb, including shoulder**

D21.12   **Benign neoplasm of connective and other soft tissue of left upper limb, including shoulder**

D21.2   **Benign neoplasm of connective and other soft tissue of lower limb, including hip**

D21.20   **Benign neoplasm of connective and other soft tissue of lower limb, including hip, unspecified side**

D21.21   **Benign neoplasm of connective and other soft tissue of right lower limb, including hip**

D21.22   **Benign neoplasm of connective and other soft tissue of left lower limb, including hip**

D21.3   **Benign neoplasm of connective and other soft tissue of thorax**

    Benign neoplasm of axilla
    Benign neoplasm of diaphragm
    Benign neoplasm of great vessels

    Excludes1:   benign neoplasm of heart (D15.1)
        benign neoplasm of mediastinum (D15.2)
        benign neoplasm of thymus (D15.0)

D21.4   **Benign neoplasm of connective and other soft tissue of abdomen**

D21.5   **Benign neoplasm of connective and other soft tissue of pelvis**

    Excludes1:   benign neoplasm of uterine ligament, any (D28.2)
        uterine leiomyoma (D25.-)

D21.6   **Benign neoplasm of connective and other soft tissue of trunk, unspecified**

    Benign neoplasm of back NOS

D21.9   **Benign neoplasm of connective and other soft tissue, unspecified**

D22 Melanocytic nevi

    Includes: atypical nevus
        blue hairy pigmented nevus
        nevus NOS

    Use additional morphology codes M8720-M8790 with behavior code /0

D22.0   **Melanocytic nevi of lip**

D22.1   **Melanocytic nevi of eyelid, including canthus**

D22.10   **Melanocytic nevi of eyelid, including canthus, unspecified side**

D22.11   **Melanocytic nevi of right eyelid, including canthus**

D22.12   **Melanocytic nevi of left eyelid, including canthus**

D22.2   **Melanocytic nevi of ear and external auricular canal**

D22.20   **Melanocytic nevi of ear and external auricular canal, unspecified side**

D22.21   **Melanocytic nevi of right ear and external auricular canal**

D22.22   **Melanocytic nevi of left ear and external auricular canal**

D22.3   **Melanocytic nevi of other and unspecified parts of face**

D22.30   **Melanocytic nevi of unspecified part of face**

D22.39   **Melanocytic nevi of other parts of face**

D22.4   **Melanocytic nevi of scalp and neck**

D22.5   **Melanocytic nevi of trunk**

    Melanocytic nevi of anal margin
    Melanocytic nevi of anal skin
    Melanocytic nevi of perianal skin
    Melanocytic nevi of skin of breast

D22.6   **Melanocytic nevi of upper limb, including shoulder**

D22.60   **Melanocytic nevi of upper limb, including shoulder, unspecified side**

D22.61   **Melanocytic nevi of right upper limb, including shoulder**

D22.62   Melanocytic nevi of left upper limb, including shoulder
D22.7 Melanocytic nevi of lower limb, including hip
    D22.70   Melanocytic nevi of lower limb, including hip, unspecified side
    D22.71   Melanocytic nevi of right lower limb, including hip
    D22.72   Melanocytic nevi of left lower limb, including hip
D22.9 Melanocytic nevi, unspecified

D23 Other benign neoplasms of skin
    Includes: benign neoplasm of hair follicles
                     benign neoplasm of sebaceous glands
                     benign neoplasm of sweat glands
    Excludes1:   benign lipomatous neoplasms of skin (D17.0-D17.3)
                     melanocytic nevi (D22.-)
D23.0   Other benign neoplasm of skin of lip
        Excludes1:   benign neoplasm of vermilion border of lip (D10.0)
D23.1   Other benign neoplasm of skin of eyelid, including canthus
    D23.10   Other benign neoplasm of skin of eyelid, including canthus, unspecified side
    D23.11   Other benign neoplasm of skin of right eyelid, including canthus
    D23.12   Other benign neoplasm of skin of left eyelid, including canthus
D23.2   Other benign neoplasm of skin of ear and external auricular canal
    D23.20   Other benign neoplasm of skin of ear and external auricular canal, unspecified side
    D23.21   Other benign neoplasm of skin of right ear and external auricular canal
    D23.22   Other benign neoplasm of skin of left ear and external auricular canal
D23.3   Other benign neoplasm of skin of other and unspecified parts of face
    D23.30   Other benign neoplasm of skin of unspecified part of face
    D23.39   Other benign neoplasm of skin of other parts of face
D23.4   Other benign neoplasm of skin of scalp and neck
D23.5   Other benign neoplasm of skin of trunk
        Other benign neoplasm of anal margin
        Other benign neoplasm of anal skin
        Other benign neoplasm of perianal skin
        Other benign neoplasm of skin of breast
        Excludes1:   benign neoplasm of anus NOS (D12.9)
D23.6   Other benign neoplasm of skin of upper limb, including shoulder
    D23.60   Other benign neoplasm of skin of upper limb, including shoulder, unspecified side
    D23.61   Other benign neoplasm of skin of right upper limb, including shoulder
    D23.62   Other benign neoplasm of skin of left upper limb, including shoulder
D23.7 Other benign neoplasm of skin of lower limb, including hip
    D23.70   Other benign neoplasm of skin of lower limb, including hip, unspecified side
    D23.71   Other benign neoplasm of skin of right lower limb, including hip
    D23.72   Other benign neoplasm of skin of left lower limb, including hip
D23.9 Other benign neoplasm of skin, unspecified

D24 Benign neoplasm of breast
    Includes: benign neoplasm of connective tissue of breast
                     benign neoplasm of soft parts of breast
                     fibroadenoma of breast
    Excludes2:   adenofibrosis of breast (N60.2)
                     benign cyst of breast (N60.-)
                     benign mammary dysplasia (N60.-)
                     benign neoplasm of skin of breast (D22.5, D23.5)
                     fibrocystic disease of breast (N60.-)
D24.0 Benign neoplasm of female breast
    D24.00   Benign neoplasm of female breast, unspecified side
    D24.01   Benign neoplasm of right female breast

    D24.02   Benign neoplasm of left female breast
D24.1 Benign neoplasm of male breast
    D24.10   Benign neoplasm of male breast, unspecified side
    D24.11   Benign neoplasm of right male breast
    D24.12   Benign neoplasm of left male breast

D25 Leiomyoma of uterus
    Includes: uterine fibroid
                     uterine fibromyoma
                     uterine myoma
    Use additional morphology code M8890 and behavior code /0
D25.0   Submucous leiomyoma of uterus
D25.1   Intramural leiomyoma of uterus
        Interstitial leiomyoma of uterus
D25.2   Subserosal leiomyoma of uterus
        Subperitoneal leiomyoma of uterus
D25.9   Leiomyoma of uterus, unspecified

D26 Other benign neoplasms of uterus
D26.0   Other benign neoplasm of cervix uteri
D26.1   Other benign neoplasm of corpus uteri
D26.7   Other benign neoplasm of other parts of uterus
D26.9   Other benign neoplasm of uterus, unspecified

D27 Benign neoplasm of ovary
    Use additional code to identify any functional activity.
        Excludes2:   corpus albicans cyst (N83.2)
                      corpus luteum cyst (N83.1)
                      endometrial cyst (N80.1)
                      follicular (atretic) cyst (N83.0)
                      graafian follicle cyst (N83.0)
                      ovarian cyst NEC (N83.2)
                      ovarian retention cyst (N83.2)
D27.0   Benign neoplasm of right ovary
D27.1   Benign neoplasm of left ovary
D27.9   Benign neoplasm of ovary, unspecified side

D28 Benign neoplasm of other and unspecified female genital organs
    Includes: adenomatous polyp
                     benign neoplasm of skin of female genital organs
                     benign teratoma
    Excludes1:   epoophoron cyst (Q50.5)
                     fimbrial cyst (Q50.4)
                     Gartner's duct cyst (Q50.5)
                     parovarian cyst (Q50.5)
D28.0   Benign neoplasm of vulva
D28.1   Benign neoplasm of vagina
D28.2   Benign neoplasm of uterine tubes and ligaments
        Benign neoplasm of fallopian tube
        Benign neoplasm of uterine ligament (broad) (round)
D28.7   Benign neoplasm of other specified female genital organs
D28.9   Benign neoplasm of female genital organ, unspecified

D29 Benign neoplasm of male genital organs
    Includes: benign neoplasm of skin of male genital organs
D29.0   Benign neoplasm of penis
D29.1   Benign neoplasm of prostate
        Excludes1:   hyperplasia of prostate (adenomatous) (N40.2-)
                      prostatic adenoma (N40.2-)
                      prostatic enlargement (N40.0-)
                      prostatic hypertrophy (N40.0-)
D29.2   Benign neoplasm of testis
        Use additional code to identify any functional activity.
    D29.20   Benign neoplasm of testis, unspecified side
    D29.21   Benign neoplasm of right testis
    D29.22   Benign neoplasm of left testis
D29.3   Benign neoplasm of epididymis
    D29.30   Benign neoplasm of epididymis, unspecified side
    D29.31   Benign neoplasm of right epididymis
    D29.32   Benign neoplasm of left epididymis
D29.4   Benign neoplasm of scrotum
        Benign neoplasm of skin of scrotum

D29.7   Benign neoplasm of other male genital organs
Benign neoplasm of seminal vesicle
Benign neoplasm of spermatic cord
Benign neoplasm of tunica vaginalis

D29.9   Benign neoplasm of male genital organ, unspecified

D30   Benign neoplasm of urinary organs

D30.0   Benign neoplasm of kidney
Excludes1:   benign neoplasm of renal calyces (D30.1-)
benign neoplasm of renal pelvis (D30.1-)

D30.00   Benign neoplasm of kidney, unspecified side

D30.01   Benign neoplasm of right kidney

D30.02   Benign neoplasm of left kidney

D30.1   Benign neoplasm of renal pelvis

D30.10   Benign neoplasm of renal pelvis, unspecified side

D30.11   Benign neoplasm of right renal pelvis

D30.12   Benign neoplasm of left renal pelvis

D30.2   Benign neoplasm of ureter
Excludes1:   benign neoplasm of ureteric orifice of bladder (D30.3)

D30.20   Benign neoplasm of ureter, unspecified side

D30.21   Benign neoplasm of right ureter

D30.22   Benign neoplasm of left ureter

D30.3   Benign neoplasm of bladder
Benign neoplasm of ureteric orifice of bladder
Benign neoplasm of urethral orifice of bladder

D30.4   Benign neoplasm of urethra
Excludes1:   benign neoplasm of urethral orifice of bladder (D30.3)

D30.7   Benign neoplasm of other urinary organs
Benign neoplasm of paraurethral glands

D30.9   Benign neoplasm of urinary organ, unspecified
Benign neoplasm of urinary system NOS

D31   Benign neoplasm of eye and adnexa
Excludes1:   benign neoplasm of connective tissue of eyelid (D21.0)
benign neoplasm of optic nerve (D33.3)
benign neoplasm of skin of eyelid (D22.1-, D23.1-)

D31.0   Benign neoplasm of conjunctiva

D31.00   Benign neoplasm of conjunctiva, unspecified side

D31.01   Benign neoplasm of right conjunctiva

D31.02   Benign neoplasm of left conjunctiva

D31.1   Benign neoplasm of cornea

D31.10   Benign neoplasm of cornea, unspecified side

D31.11   Benign neoplasm of right cornea

D31.12   Benign neoplasm of left cornea

D31.2   Benign neoplasm of retina
Excludes1:   hemangioma of retina (D18.09)

D31.20   Benign neoplasm of retina, unspecified side

D31.21   Benign neoplasm of right retina

D31.22   Benign neoplasm of left retina

D31.3   Benign neoplasm of choroid

D31.30   Benign neoplasm of choroid, unspecified side

D31.31   Benign neoplasm of right choroid

D31.32   Benign neoplasm of left choroid

D31.4   Benign neoplasm of ciliary body

D31.40   Benign neoplasm of ciliary body, unspecified side

D31.41   Benign neoplasm of right ciliary body

D31.42   Benign neoplasm of left ciliary body

D31.5   Benign neoplasm of lacrimal gland and duct
Benign neoplasm of lacrimal sac
Benign neoplasm of nasolacrimal duct

D31.50   Benign neoplasm of lacrimal gland and duct, unspecified side

D31.51   Benign neoplasm of right lacrimal gland and duct

D31.52   Benign neoplasm of left lacrimal gland and duct

D31.6   Benign neoplasm of orbit, unspecified
Benign neoplasm of connective tissue of orbit
Benign neoplasm of extraocular muscle
Benign neoplasm of peripheral nerves of orbit
Benign neoplasm of retrobulbar tissue
Benign neoplasm of retro-ocular tissue
Excludes1:   benign neoplasm of orbital bone (D16.4)

D31.60   Benign neoplasm of orbit, unspecified, unspecified side

D31.61   Benign neoplasm of right orbit, unspecified

D31.62   Benign neoplasm of left orbit, unspecified

D31.9   Benign neoplasm of eye, unspecified

D31.90   Benign neoplasm of eye, unspecified, unspecified side

D31.91   Benign neoplasm of right eye, unspecified

D31.92   Benign neoplasm of left eye, unspecified

D32   Benign neoplasm of meninges

D32.0   Benign neoplasm of cerebral meninges

D32.1   Benign neoplasm of spinal meninges

D32.9   Benign neoplasm of meninges, unspecified
Meningioma NOS

D33   Benign neoplasm of brain and other parts of central nervous system
Excludes1:   angioma (D18.0-)
benign neoplasm of meninges (D32.-)
benign neoplasm of peripheral nerves and autonomic nervous system (D36.1-)
hemangioma (D18.0-)
neurofibromatosis (Q85.0)
retro-ocular benign neoplasm (D31.6-)

D33.0   Benign neoplasm of brain, supratentorial
Benign neoplasm of cerebral ventricle
Benign neoplasm of cerebrum
Benign neoplasm of frontal lobe
Benign neoplasm of occipital lobe
Benign neoplasm of parietal lobe
Benign neoplasm of temporal lobe
Excludes1:   benign neoplasm of fourth ventricle (D33.1)

D33.1   Benign neoplasm of brain, infratentorial
Benign neoplasm of brain stem
Benign neoplasm of cerebellum
Benign neoplasm of fourth ventricle

D33.2   Benign neoplasm of brain, unspecified

D33.3   Benign neoplasm of cranial nerves
Benign neoplasm of olfactory bulb

D33.4   Benign neoplasm of spinal cord

D33.7   Benign neoplasm of other specified parts of central nervous system

D33.9   Benign neoplasm of central nervous system, unspecified
Benign neoplasm of nervous system (central) NOS

D34   Benign neoplasm of thyroid gland
Use additional code to identify any functional activity.

D35   Benign neoplasm of other and unspecified endocrine glands
Use additional code to identify any functional activity.
Excludes1:   benign neoplasm of endocrine pancreas (D13.7)
benign neoplasm of ovary (D27.-)
benign neoplasm of testis (D29.2.-)
benign neoplasm of thymus (D15.0)

D35.0   Benign neoplasm of adrenal gland

D35.00   Benign neoplasm of adrenal gland, unspecified side

D35.01   Benign neoplasm of right adrenal gland

D35.02   Benign neoplasm of left adrenal gland

D35.1   Benign neoplasm of parathyroid gland

D35.2   Benign neoplasm of pituitary gland

D35.3   Benign neoplasm of craniopharyngeal duct

D35.4   Benign neoplasm of pineal gland

D35.5   Benign neoplasm of carotid body

D35.6   Benign neoplasm of aortic body and other paraganglia
Benign tumor of glomus jugulare

D35.7   Benign neoplasm of other specified endocrine glands

D35.8   Benign neoplasm with pluriglandular involvement

D35.9   Benign neoplasm of endocrine gland, unspecified

D36 Benign neoplasm of other and unspecified sites

D36.0   Benign neoplasm of lymph nodes

Excludes1:   lymphangioma (D18.1)

D36.1   Benign neoplasm of peripheral nerves and autonomic nervous system

Excludes1:   benign neoplasm of peripheral nerves of orbit (D31.6-)

neurofibromatosis (Q85.0)

D36.10   Benign neoplasm of peripheral nerves and autonomic nervous system, unspecified

D36.11   Benign neoplasm of peripheral nerves and autonomic nervous system of face, head, and neck

D36.12   Benign neoplasm of peripheral nerves and autonomic nervous system, upper limb, including shoulder

D36.13   Benign neoplasm of peripheral nerves and autonomic nervous system of lower limb, including hip

D36.14   Benign neoplasm of peripheral nerves and autonomic nervous system of thorax

D36.15   Benign neoplasm of peripheral nerves and autonomic nervous system of abdomen

D36.16   Benign neoplasm of peripheral nerves and autonomic nervous system of pelvis

D36.17   Benign neoplasm of peripheral nerves and autonomic nervous system of trunk, unspecified

D36.7 Benign neoplasm of other specified sites

Benign neoplasm of nose NOS

D36.9 Benign neoplasm, unspecified site

NEOPLASMS OF UNCERTAIN BEHAVIOR (D37–D48)

Note: Categories D37-D48 classify by site neoplasms of uncertain behavior, i.e., histologic confirmation whether the neoplasm is malignant or benign cannot be made. Such neoplasms are assigned behavior code /1 in the classification of the morphology of neoplasms.

Excludes1:   neoplasms of unspecified behavior (D49-)

D37 Neoplasm of uncertain behavior of oral cavity and digestive organs

D37.0   Neoplasm of uncertain behavior of lip, oral cavity and pharynx

Excludes1:   neoplasm of uncertain behavior of aryepiglottic fold or interarytenoid fold, laryngeal aspect (D38.0)

neoplasm of uncertain behavior of epiglottis NOS (D38.0):

neoplasm of uncertain behavior of skin of lip (D48.5)

neoplasm of uncertain behavior of suprahyoid portion of epiglottis (D38.0)

D37.01   Neoplasm of uncertain behavior of lip

Neoplasm of uncertain behavior of vermilon border of lip

D37.02   Neoplasm of uncertain behavior of tongue

D37.03   Neoplasm of uncertain behavior of the major salivary glands

D37.030   Neoplasm of uncertain behavior of the parotid salivary glands

D37.031   Neoplasm of uncertain behavior of the sublingual salivary glands

D37.032   Neoplasm of uncertain behavior of the submandibular salivary glands

D37.039   Neoplasm of uncertain behavior of the major salivary glands, unspecified

D37.04   Neoplasm of uncertain behavior of the minor salivary glands

Neoplasm of uncertain behavior of submucosal salivary glands of lip

Neoplasm of uncertain behavior of submucosal salivary glands of cheek

Neoplasm of uncertain behavior of submucosal salivary glands of hard palate

Neoplasm of uncertain behavior of submucosal salivary glands of soft palate

D37.05   Neoplasm of uncertain behavior of pharynx

Neoplasm of uncertain behavior of aryepiglottic fold of pharynx NOS

Neoplasm of uncertain behavior of hypopharyngeal aspect of aryepiglottic fold of pharynx

Neoplasm of uncertain behavior of marginal zone of aryepiglottic fold of pharynx

D37.09   Neoplasm of uncertain behavior of other specified sites of the oral cavity

D37.1   Neoplasm of uncertain behavior of stomach

D37.2   Neoplasm of uncertain behavior of small intestine

D37.3   Neoplasm of uncertain behavior of appendix

D37.4   Neoplasm of uncertain behavior of colon

D37.5   Neoplasm of uncertain behavior of rectum

Neoplasm of uncertain behavior of rectosigmoid junction

D37.6   Neoplasm of uncertain behavior of liver, gallbladder and bile ducts

Neoplasm of uncertain behavior of ampulla of Vater

D37.7   Neoplasm of uncertain behavior of other digestive organs

Neoplasm of uncertain behavior of anal canal

Neoplasm of uncertain behavior of anal sphincter

Neoplasm of uncertain behavior of anus NOS

Neoplasm of uncertain behavior of esophagus

Neoplasm of uncertain behavior of intestine NOS

Neoplasm of uncertain behavior of pancreas

Excludes1:   neoplasm of uncertain behavior of anal margin (D48.5)

neoplasm of uncertain behavior of anal skin (D48.5)

neoplasm of uncertain behavior of perianal skin (D48.5)

D37.9   Neoplasm of uncertain behavior of digestive organ, unspecified

D38 Neoplasm of uncertain behavior of middle ear and respiratory and intrathoracic organs

Excludes1:   neoplasm of uncertain behavior of heart (D48.7)

D38.0   Neoplasm of uncertain behavior of larynx

Neoplasm of uncertain behavior of aryepiglottic fold or interarytenoid fold, laryngeal aspect

Neoplasm of uncertain behavior of epiglottis (suprahyoid portion)

Excludes1:   neoplasm of uncertain behavior of aryepiglottic fold or interarytenoid fold NOS (D37.05)

neoplasm of uncertain behavior of hypopharyngeal aspect of aryepiglottic fold (D37.05)

neoplasm of uncertain behavior of marginal zone of aryepiglottic fold (D37.05)

D38.1   Neoplasm of uncertain behavior of trachea, bronchus and lung

D38.2   Neoplasm of uncertain behavior of pleura

D38.3   Neoplasm of uncertain behavior of mediastinum

D38.4   Neoplasm of uncertain behavior of thymus

D38.5   Neoplasm of uncertain behavior of other respiratory organs

Neoplasm of uncertain behavior of accessory sinuses

Neoplasm of uncertain behavior of cartilage of nose

Neoplasm of uncertain behavior of middle ear

Neoplasm of uncertain behavior of nasal cavities

Excludes1:   neoplasm of uncertain behavior of ear (external) (skin) (D48.5)

neoplasm of uncertain behavior of nose NOS (D48.7)

neoplasm of uncertain behavior of skin of nose (D48.5)

D38.6   Neoplasm of uncertain behavior of respiratory organ, unspecified

D39 Neoplasm of uncertain behavior of female genital organs

D39.0   Neoplasm of uncertain behavior of uterus

D39.1   Neoplasm of uncertain behavior of ovary

Use additional code to identify any functional activity.

D39.10   Neoplasm of uncertain behavior of ovary, unspecified side

D39.11   Neoplasm of uncertain behavior of right ovary

D39.12   Neoplasm of uncertain behavior of left ovary

D39.2 Neoplasm of uncertain behavior of placenta
Chorioadenoma destruens
Invasive hydatidiform mole
Malignant hydatidiform mole
Excludes1: hydatidiform mole NOS (O01.9)

D39.7 Neoplasm of uncertain behavior of other female genital organs
Neoplasm of uncertain behavior of skin of female genital organs

D39.9 Neoplasm of uncertain behavior of female genital organ, unspecified

D40 Neoplasm of uncertain behavior of male genital organs
D40.0 Neoplasm of uncertain behavior of prostate
D40.1 Neoplasm of uncertain behavior of testis
  D40.10 Neoplasm of uncertain behavior of testis, unspecified side
  D40.11 Neoplasm of uncertain behavior of right testis
  D40.12 Neoplasm of uncertain behavior of left testis
D40.7 Neoplasm of uncertain behavior of other male genital organs
Neoplasm of uncertain behavior of skin of male genital organs
D40.9 Neoplasm of uncertain behavior of male genital organ, unspecified

D41 Neoplasm of uncertain behavior of urinary organs
D41.0 Neoplasm of uncertain behavior of kidney
Excludes1: neoplasm of uncertain behavior of renal pelvis (D41.1-)
  D41.00 Neoplasm of uncertain behavior of kidney, unspecified side
  D41.01 Neoplasm of uncertain behavior of right kidney
  D41.02 Neoplasm of uncertain behavior of left kidney
D41.1 Neoplasm of uncertain behavior of renal pelvis
  D41.10 Neoplasm of uncertain behavior of renal pelvis, unspecified side
  D41.11 Neoplasm of uncertain behavior of right renal pelvis
  D41.12 Neoplasm of uncertain behavior of left renal pelvis
D41.2 Neoplasm of uncertain behavior of ureter
  D41.20 Neoplasm of uncertain behavior of ureter, unspecified side
  D41.21 Neoplasm of uncertain behavior of right ureter
  D41.22 Neoplasm of uncertain behavior of left ureter
D41.3 Neoplasm of uncertain behavior of urethra
D41.4 Neoplasm of uncertain behavior of bladder
D41.7 Neoplasm of uncertain behavior of other urinary organs
D41.9 Neoplasm of uncertain behavior of urinary organ, unspecified

D42 Neoplasm of uncertain behavior of meninges
D42.0 Neoplasm of uncertain behavior of cerebral meninges
D42.1 Neoplasm of uncertain behavior of spinal meninges
D42.9 Neoplasm of uncertain behavior of meninges, unspecified

D43 Neoplasm of uncertain behavior of brain and central nervous system
Excludes1: neoplasm of uncertain behavior of peripheral nerves and autonomic nervous system (D48.2)
D43.0 Neoplasm of uncertain behavior of brain, supratentorial
Neoplasm of uncertain behavior of cerebral ventricle
Neoplasm of uncertain behavior of cerebrum
Neoplasm of uncertain behavior of frontal lobe
Neoplasm of uncertain behavior of occipital lobe
Neoplasm of uncertain behavior of parietal lobe
Neoplasm of uncertain behavior of temporal lobe
Excludes1: neoplasm of uncertain behavior of fourth ventricle (D43.1)
D43.1 Neoplasm of uncertain behavior of brain, infratentorial
Neoplasm of uncertain behavior of brain stem
Neoplasm of uncertain behavior of cerebellum
Neoplasm of uncertain behavior of fourth ventricle
D43.2 Neoplasm of uncertain behavior of brain, unspecified
D43.3 Neoplasm of uncertain behavior of cranial nerves
D43.4 Neoplasm of uncertain behavior of spinal cord
D43.7 Neoplasm of uncertain behavior of other parts of central nervous system

D43.9 Neoplasm of uncertain behavior of central nervous system, unspecified
Neoplasm of uncertain behavior of nervous system (central) NOS

D44 Neoplasm of uncertain behavior of endocrine glands
Excludes1: neoplasm of uncertain behavior of endocrine pancreas (D37.7)
neoplasm of uncertain behavior of ovary (D39.1-)
neoplasm of uncertain behavior of testis (D40.1-)
neoplasm of uncertain behavior of thymus (D38.4)
D44.0 Neoplasm of uncertain behavior of thyroid gland
D44.1 Neoplasm of uncertain behavior of adrenal gland
Use additional code to identify any functional activity.
  D44.10 Neoplasm of uncertain behavior of adrenal gland, unspecified side
  D44.11 Neoplasm of uncertain behavior of right adrenal gland
  D44.12 Neoplasm of uncertain behavior of left adrenal gland
D44.2 Neoplasm of uncertain behavior of parathyroid gland
D44.3 Neoplasm of uncertain behavior of pituitary gland
Use additional code to identify any functional activity.
D44.4 Neoplasm of uncertain behavior of craniopharyngeal duct
D44.5 Neoplasm of uncertain behavior of pineal gland
D44.6 Neoplasm of uncertain behavior of carotid body
D44.7 Neoplasm of uncertain behavior of aortic body and other paraganglia
D44.8 Neoplasm of uncertain behavior with pluriglandular involvement
Multiple endocrine adenomatosis
D44.9 Neoplasm of uncertain behavior of endocrine gland, unspecified

D45 Polycythemia vera
Use additional morphology code M9950 with behavior code /1.
Excludes1: familial polycythemia (D75.0)
secondary polycythemia (D75.1)

D46 Myelodysplastic syndromes
Use additional morphology code M998 with behavior code /1.
D46.0 Refractory anemia without sideroblasts, so stated
D46.1 Refractory anemia with sideroblasts
D46.2 Refractory anemia with excess of blasts
D46.3 Refractory anemia with excess of blasts with transformation
D46.4 Refractory anemia, unspecified
D46.7 Other myelodysplastic syndromes
D46.9 Myelodysplastic syndrome, unspecified
Myelodysplasia NOS
Preleukemia (syndrome) NOS

D47 Other neoplasms of uncertain behavior of lymphoid, hematopoietic and related tissue
Use additional morphology codes M974, M976, M996-M997 with behavior code /1.
D47.0 Histiocytic and mast cell tumors of uncertain behavior
Mast cell tumor NOS
Mastocytoma NOS
Excludes1: mastocytosis (cutaneous) (Q82.2)
D47.1 Chronic myeloproliferative disease
Myelofibrosis (with myeloid metaplasia)
Myeloproliferative disease, unspecified
Myelosclerosis (megakaryocytic) with myeloid metaplasia
D47.2 Monoclonal gammopathy
D47.3 Essential (hemorrhagic) thrombocythemia
Idiopathic hemorrhagic thrombocythemia
D47.7 Other specified neoplasms of uncertain behavior of lymphoid, hematopoietic and related tissue
D47.9 Neoplasm of uncertain behavior of lymphoid, hematopoietic and related tissue, unspecified
Lymphoproliferative disease NOS

D48 Neoplasm of uncertain behavior of other and unspecified sites

    Excludes1:   neurofibromatosis (nonmalignant) (Q85.0)

D48.0 Neoplasm of uncertain behavior of bone and articular cartilage

    Excludes1:   neoplasm of uncertain behavior of cartilage of ear (D48.1)

               neoplasm of uncertain behavior of cartilage of larynx (D38.0)

               neoplasm of uncertain behavior of cartilage of nose (D38.5)

               neoplasm of uncertain behavior of connective tissue of eyelid (D48.1)

               neoplasm of uncertain behavior of synovia (D48.1)

D48.1 Neoplasm of uncertain behavior of connective and other soft tissue

    Neoplasm of uncertain behavior of connective tissue of ear

    Neoplasm of uncertain behavior of connective tissue of eyelid

    Excludes1:   neoplasm of uncertain behavior of articular cartilage (D48.0)

               neoplasm of uncertain behavior of cartilage of larynx (D38.0)

               neoplasm of uncertain behavior of cartilage of nose (D38.5)

               neoplasm of uncertain behavior of connective tissue of breast (D48.6-)

D48.2 Neoplasm of uncertain behavior of peripheral nerves and autonomic nervous system

    Excludes1:   neoplasm of uncertain behavior of peripheral nerves of orbit (D48.7)

D48.3 Neoplasm of uncertain behavior of retroperitoneum

D48.4 Neoplasm of uncertain behavior of peritoneum

D48.5 Neoplasm of uncertain behavior of skin

    Neoplasm of uncertain behavior of anal margin

    Neoplasm of uncertain behavior of anal skin

    Neoplasm of uncertain behavior of perianal skin

    Neoplasm of uncertain behavior of skin of breast

    Excludes1:   neoplasm of uncertain behavior of anus NOS (D37.7)

               neoplasm of uncertain behavior of skin of genital organs (D39.7, D40.7)

               neoplasm of uncertain behavior of vermilion border of lip (D37.0)

D48.6 Neoplasm of uncertain behavior of breast

    Neoplasm of uncertain behavior of connective tissue of breast

    Cystosarcoma phyllodes

    Excludes1:   neoplasm of uncertain behavior of skin of breast (D48.5)

    D48.60 Neoplasm of uncertain behavior of female breast, unspecified side

    D48.61 Neoplasm of uncertain behavior of right female breast

    D48.62 Neoplasm of uncertain behavior of left female breast

    D48.63 Neoplasm of uncertain behavior of right male breast

    D48.64 Neoplasm of uncertain behavior of left male breast

    D48.65 Neoplasm of uncertain behavior of male breast, unspecified side

D48.7 Neoplasm of uncertain behavior of other specified sites

    Neoplasm of uncertain behavior of eye

    Neoplasm of uncertain behavior of heart

    Neoplasm of uncertain behavior of peripheral nerves of orbit

    Excludes1:   neoplasm of uncertain behavior of connective tissue (D48.1)

               neoplasm of uncertain behavior of skin of eyelid (D48.5)

D48.9 Neoplasm of uncertain behavior, unspecified

D49 Neoplasms of unspecified behavior

    Note: Category D49 classifies by site neoplasms of unspecified morphology and behavior. The term "mass", unless otherwise stated, is not to be regarded as a neoplastic growth.

    Includes: "growth" NOS

               neoplasm NOS

               new growth NOS

               tumor NOS

    Excludes1:   neoplasms of uncertain behavior (D37-D48)

D49.0 Neoplasm of unspecified behavior of digestive system

    Excludes1:   neoplasm of unspecified behavior of margin of anus (D49.2)

               neoplasm of unspecified behavior of perianal skin (D49.2)

               neoplasm of unspecified behavior of skin of anus (D49.2)

D49.1 Neoplasm of unspecified behavior of respiratory system

D49.2 Neoplasm of unspecified behavior of bone, soft tissue, and skin

    Excludes1:   neoplasm of unspecified behavior of anal canal (D49.0)

               neoplasm of unspecified behavior of anus NOS (D49.0)

               neoplasm of unspecified behavior of bone marrow (D49.9)

               neoplasm of unspecified behavior of cartilage of larynx (D49.1)

               neoplasm of unspecified behavior of cartilage of nose (D49.1)

               neoplasm of unspecified behavior of connective tissue of breast (D49.3)

               neoplasm of unspecified behavior of skin of genital organs (D49.5)

               neoplasm of unspecified behavior of vermilion border of lip (D49.0)

D49.3 Neoplasm of unspecified behavior of breast

    Excludes1:   neoplasm of unspecified behavior of skin of breast (D49.2)

D49.4 Neoplasm of unspecified behavior of bladder

D49.5 Neoplasm of unspecified behavior of other genitourinary organs

D49.6 Neoplasm of unspecified behavior of brain

    Excludes1:   neoplasm of unspecified behavior of cerebral meninges (D49.7)

               neoplasm of unspecified behavior of cranial nerves (D49.7)

D49.7 Neoplasm of unspecified behavior of endocrine glands and other parts of nervous system

    Excludes1:   neoplasm of unspecified behavior of peripheral, sympathetic, and parasympathetic nerves and ganglia (D49.2)

D49.8 Neoplasm of unspecified behavior of other specified sites

    Excludes1:   neoplasm of unspecified behavior of eyelid (skin) (D49.2)

               neoplasm of unspecified behavior of eyelid cartilage (D49.2)

               neoplasm of unspecified behavior of great vessels (D49.2)

               neoplasm of unspecified behavior of optic nerve (D49.7)

D49.9 Neoplasm of unspecified behavior of unspecified site

CHAPTER III — DISEASES OF THE BLOOD AND BLOOD–FORMING ORGANS AND CERTAIN DISORDERS INVOLVING THE IMMUNE MECHANISM (D50–D89)

Excludes2:   autoimmune disease (systemic) NOS (M35.9)
certain conditions originating in the perinatal period (P00-P96)
complications of pregnancy, childbirth and the puerperium (O00-O99)
congenital malformations, deformations and chromosomal abnormalities (Q00-Q99)
endocrine, nutritional and metabolic diseases (E00-E90)
human immunodeficiency virus [HIV] disease (B20)
injury, poisoning and certain other consequences of external causes (S00-T98)
neoplasms (C00-D49)
symptoms, signs and abnormal clinical and laboratory findings, not elsewhere classified (R00-R94)

This chapter contains the following blocks:

D50-D53   Nutritional anemias
D55-D59   Hemolytic anemias
D60-D64   Aplastic and other anemias
D65-D69   Coagulation defects, purpura and other hemorrhagic conditions
D70-D78   Other diseases of blood and blood-forming organs
D80-D89   Certain disorders involving the immune mechanism

NUTRITIONAL ANEMIAS (D50–D53)

D50   Iron deficiency anemia

Includes: asiderotic anemia
hypochromic anemia

D50.0   Iron deficiency anemia secondary to blood loss (chronic)
Posthemorrhagic anemia (chronic)
Excludes1:   acute posthemorrhagic anemia (D62)
congenital anemia from fetal blood loss (P61.3)

D50.1   Sideropenic dysphagia
Kelly-Paterson syndrome
Plummer-Vinson syndrome

D50.8   Other iron deficiency anemias
Iron deficiency anemia due to inadequate dietary iron intake

D50.9   Iron deficiency anemia, unspecified

D51   Vitamin B_{12} deficiency anemia

Excludes1:   vitamin B_{12} deficiency (E53.8)

D51.0   Vitamin B_{12} deficiency anemia due to intrinsic factor deficiency
Addison anemia
Biermer anemia
Congenital intrinsic factor deficiency
Pernicious (congenital) anemia

D51.1   Vitamin B_{12} deficiency anemia due to selective vitamin B_{12} malabsorption with proteinuria
Imerslund (-Gräsbeck) syndrome
Megaloblastic hereditary anemia

D51.2   Transcobalamin II deficiency

D51.3   Other dietary vitamin B_{12} deficiency anemia
Vegan anemia

D51.8   Other vitamin B_{12} deficiency anemias

D51.9   Vitamin B_{12} deficiency anemia, unspecified

D52   Folate deficiency anemia

Excludes1:   folate deficiency without anemia (E53.8)

D52.0   Dietary folate deficiency anemia
Nutritional megaloblastic anemia

D52.1   Drug-induced folate deficiency anemia
Use additional external cause code (Chapter XIX) to identify drug.

D52.8   Other folate deficiency anemias

D52.9   Folate deficiency anemia, unspecified
Folic acid deficiency anemia NOS

D53   Other nutritional anemias

Includes: megaloblastic anemia unresponsive to vitamin B_{12} or folate therapy

D53.0   Protein deficiency anemia
Amino-acid deficiency anemia
Orotaciduric anemia
Excludes1:   Lesch-Nyhan syndrome (E79.1)

D53.1   Other megaloblastic anemias, not elsewhere classified
Megaloblastic anemia NOS
Excludes1:   Di Guglielmo's disease (C94.0)

D53.2   Scorbutic anemia
Excludes1:   scurvy (E54)

D53.8   Other specified nutritional anemias
Anemia associated with deficiency of copper
Anemia associated with deficiency of molybdenum
Anemia associated with deficiency of zinc
Excludes1:   nutritional deficiencies without mention of anemia, such as:
copper deficiency NOS (E61.0)
molybdenum deficiency NOS (E61.5)
zinc deficiency NOS (E60)

D53.9   Nutritional anemia, unspecified
Simple chronic anemia
Excludes1:   anemia NOS (D64.9)

HEMOLYTIC ANEMIAS (D55–D59)

D55   Anemia due to enzyme disorders

Excludes1:   drug-induced enzyme deficiency anemia (D59.2)

D55.0   Anemia due to glucose-6-phosphate dehydrogenase [G6PD] deficiency
Favism
G6PD deficiency anemia

D55.1   Anemia due to other disorders of glutathione metabolism
Anemia (due to) enzyme deficiencies, except G6PD, related to the hexose monophosphate [HMP] shunt pathway
Anemia (due to) hemolytic nonspherocytic (hereditary), type I

D55.2   Anemia due to disorders of glycolytic enzymes
Hemolytic nonspherocytic (hereditary) anemia, type II
Hexokinase deficiency anemia
Pyruvate kinase [PK] deficiency anemia
Triose-phosphate isomerase deficiency anemia
Excludes1:   disorders of glycolysis not associated with anemia (E74.8)

D55.3   Anemia due to disorders of nucleotide metabolism

D55.8   Other anemias due to enzyme disorders

D55.9   Anemia due to enzyme disorder, unspecified

D56   Thalassemia

Excludes1:   sickle-cell thalassemia (D57.4)

D56.0   Alpha thalassemia
Alpha thalassemia major
Hemoglobin H disease
Severe alpha thalassemia
Triple gene defect alpha thalassemia
Excludes1:   alpha thalassemia minor (D56.3)
asymptomatic alpha thalassemia (D56.3)
hydrops fetalis due to hemolytic disease (P56.-)

D56.1   Beta thalassemia
Beta thalassemia major
Cooley's anemia
Homozygous beta thalassemia
Severe beta thalassemia
Thalassemia intermedia
Excludes1:   beta thalassemia minor (D56.3)
delta-beta thalassemia (D56.2)

D56.2   Delta-beta thalassemia
Homozygous delta-beta thalassemia
Excludes1:   delta-beta thalassemia minor (D56.3)

D56.3   Thalassemia minor
   Alpha thalassemia minor
   Alpha thalassemia trait
   Beta thalassemia minor
   Delta-beta thalassemia minor
   Excludes1:   alpha thalassemia (D56.0)
                beta thalassemia (D56.1)
                delta-beta thalassemia (D56.2)
D56.4   Hereditary persistence of fetal hemoglobin [HPFH]
D56.8   Other thalassemias
   Excludes1:   sickle cell anemia (D57.-)
                sickle-cell thalassemia (D57.4)
D56.9   Thalassemia, unspecified
   Mediterranean anemia (with other hemoglobinopathy)
   Thalassemia (minor) (mixed) (with other hemoglobinopathy)

D57   Sickle-cell disorders
   Excludes1:   other hemoglobinopathies (D58.-)
D57.0   Sickle-cell anemia with crisis
   Hb-SS disease with crisis
D57.1   Sickle-cell anemia without crisis
   Sickle-cell anemia NOS
   Sickle-cell disease NOS
   Sickle-cell disorder NOS
D57.2   Double heterozygous sickling disorders
   Hb-SC disease
   Hb-SD disease
   Hb-SE disease
D57.3   Sickle-cell trait
   Hb-S trait
   Heterozygous hemoglobin S
D57.4   Sickle-cell thalassemia
   Sickle-cell beta thalassemia
   Thalassemia Hb-S disease
D57.8   Other sickle-cell disorders

D58   Other hereditary hemolytic anemias
   Excludes1:   hemolytic anemia of the newborn (P55.-)
D58.0   Hereditary spherocytosis
   Acholuric (familial) jaundice
   Congenital (spherocytic) hemolytic icterus
   Minkowski-Chauffard syndrome
D58.1   Hereditary elliptocytosis
   Elliptocytosis (congenital)
   Ovalocytosis (congenital) (hereditary)
D58.2   Other hemoglobinopathies
   Abnormal hemoglobin NOS
   Congenital Heinz body anemia
   Hb-C disease
   Hb-D disease
   Hb-E disease
   Hemoglobinopathy NOS
   Unstable hemoglobin hemolytic disease
   Excludes1:   familial polycythemia (D75.0)
                Hb-M disease (D74.0)
                hereditary persistence of fetal hemoglobin [HPFH]
                   (D56.4)
                high-altitude polycythemia (D75.1)
                methemoglobinemia (D74.-)
D58.8   Other specified hereditary hemolytic anemias
   Stomatocytosis
D58.9   Hereditary hemolytic anemia, unspecified

D59   Acquired hemolytic anemia
D59.0   Drug-induced autoimmune hemolytic anemia
   Use additional external cause code (Chapter XIX) to identify
      drug.

D59.1   Other autoimmune hemolytic anemias
   Autoimmune hemolytic disease (cold type) (warm type)
   Chronic cold hemagglutinin disease
   Cold agglutinin disease
   Cold agglutinin hemoglobinuria
   Cold type (secondary) (symptomatic) hemolytic anemia
   Warm type (secondary) (symptomatic) hemolytic anemia
   Excludes1:   Evans' syndrome (D69.3)
                hemolytic disease of fetus and newborn (P55.-)
                paroxysmal cold hemoglobinuria (D59.6)
D59.2   Drug-induced nonautoimmune hemolytic anemia
   Drug-induced enzyme deficiency anemia
   Use additional external cause code (Chapter XIX) to identify
      drug.
D59.3   Hemolytic-uremic syndrome
D59.4   Other nonautoimmune hemolytic anemias
   Mechanical hemolytic anemia
   Microangiopathic hemolytic anemia
   Toxic hemolytic anemia
   Use additional external cause code (Chapter XIX) to identify
      cause.
D59.5   Paroxysmal nocturnal hemoglobinuria [Marchiafava-Micheli]
   Excludes1:   hemoglobinuria NOS (R82.3)
D59.6   Hemoglobinuria due to hemolysis from other external causes
   Hemoglobinuria from exertion
   March hemoglobinuria
   Paroxysmal cold hemoglobinuria
   Use additional external cause code (Chapter XIX) to identify
      cause.
   Excludes1:   hemoglobinuria NOS (R82.3)
D59.8   Other acquired hemolytic anemias
D59.9   Acquired hemolytic anemia, unspecified
   Idiopathic hemolytic anemia, chronic

APLASTIC AND OTHER ANEMIAS (D60–D64)

D60   Acquired pure red cell aplasia [erythroblastopenia]
   Includes: red cell aplasia (acquired) (adult) (with thymoma)
D60.0   Chronic acquired pure red cell aplasia
D60.1   Transient acquired pure red cell aplasia
D60.8   Other acquired pure red cell aplasias
D60.9   Acquired pure red cell aplasia, unspecified

D61   Other aplastic anemias
   Excludes1:   neutropenia (D70.-)
D61.0   Constitutional aplastic anemia
   Fanconi's anemia
   Pancytopenia with malformations
   Excludes1:   congenital red cell aplasia (D61.4)
D61.1   Drug-induced aplastic anemia
   Use additional external cause code (Chapter XIX) to identify
      drug.
D61.2   Aplastic anemia due to other external agents
   Use additional external cause code (Chapter XIX) to identify
      cause.
D61.3   Idiopathic aplastic anemia
D61.4   Congenital red cell aplasia
   Blackfan-Diamond syndrome
   Congenital (pure) red cell aplasia
   Familial hypoplastic anemia
   Primary (pure) red cell aplasia
   Red cell (pure) aplasia of infants
   Excludes1:   acquired pure red cell aplasia (D60.-)
                constitutional aplastic anemia (D61.0)
D61.8   Other specified aplastic anemias
D61.9   Aplastic anemia, unspecified
   Hypoplastic anemia NOS
   Medullary hypoplasia
   Panmyelophthisis

D62   Acute posthemorrhagic anemia
   Excludes1:   anemia due to chronic blood loss (D50.0)
                blood loss anemia NOS (D50.0)
                congenital anemia from fetal blood loss (P61.3)

D63 Anemia in chronic diseases classified elsewhere

D63.0 Anemia in neoplastic disease
Code first neoplasm (C00-D49)

D63.1 Anemia in chronic renal failure
Anemia in end-stage renal disease
Code first underlying renal disease

D63.8 Anemia in other chronic diseases classified elsewhere
Code first underlying disease, such as:
diphyllobothriasis (B70.0)
hookworm disease (B76.0-B76.9)
hypothyroidism (E00.0-E03.9)
malaria (B50.0-B54)
symptomatic late syphilis (A52.79)\
tuberculosis (A18.89)

D64 Other anemias
Excludes1:   refractory anemia (D46.-)

D64.0 Hereditary sideroblastic anemia
Sex-linked hypochromic sideroblastic anemia

D64.1 Secondary sideroblastic anemia due to disease
Code first underlying disease

D64.2 Secondary sideroblastic anemia due to drugs and toxins
Use additional external cause code (Chapter XIX) to identify
drug or toxin

D64.3 Other sideroblastic anemias
Sideroblastic anemia NOS
Pyridoxine-responsive sideroblastic anemia NEC

D64.4 Congenital dyserythropoietic anemia
Dyshematopoietic anemia (congenital)
Excludes1:   Blackfan-Diamond syndrome (D61.4)
Di Guglielmo's disease (C94.0)

D64.8 Other specified anemias
Infantile pseudoleukemia
Leukoerythroblastic anemia

D64.9 Anemia, unspecified

COAGULATION DEFECTS, PURPURA AND OTHER HEMORRHAGIC CONDITIONS (D65–D69)

D65 Disseminated intravascular coagulation [defibrination syndrome]
Includes: afibrinogenemia, acquired
consumption coagulopathy
diffuse or disseminated intravascular coagulation [DIC]
fibrinolytic hemorrhage, acquired
fibrinolytic purpura
purpura fulminans
Excludes1:   disseminated intravascular coagulation (complicating):
abortion or ectopic or molar pregnancy (O00-O07,
O08.1)
in newborn (P60)
pregnancy, childbirth and the puerperium (O45.0,
O46.0, O67.0, O72.3)

D66 Hereditary factor VIII deficiency
Includes: classical hemophilia
deficiency factor VIII (with functional defect)
hemophilia NOS
hemophilia A
Excludes1:   factor VIII deficiency with vascular defect (D68.0)

D67 Hereditary factor IX deficiency
Includes: christmas disease
factor IX deficiency (with functional defect)
hemophilia B
plasma thromboplastin component [PTC] deficiency

D68 Other coagulation defects
Excludes1:   abnormal coagulation profile (R79.2)
coagulation defects complicating:
abortion or ectopic or molar pregnancy (O00-O07,
O08.1)
pregnancy, childbirth and the puerperium (O45.0,
O46.0, O67.0, O72.3)

D68.0 Von Willebrand's disease
Angiohemophilia
Factor VIII deficiency with vascular defect
Vascular hemophilia
Excludes1:   capillary fragility (hereditary) (D69.8)
factor VIII deficiency NOS (D66)
factor VIII deficiency with functional defect (D66)

D68.1 Hereditary factor XI deficiency
Hemophilia C
Plasma thromboplastin antecedent [PTA] deficiency
Rosenthal's disease

D68.2 Hereditary deficiency of other clotting factors
AC globulin deficiency
Congenital afibrinogenemia
Deficiency of factor I [fibrinogen]
Deficiency of factor II [prothrombin]
Deficiency of factor V [labile]
Deficiency of factor VII [stable]
Deficiency of factor X [Stuart-Prower]
Deficiency of factor XII [Hageman]
Deficiency of factor XIII [fibrin stabilizing]
Dysfibrinogenemia (congenital)
Hypoproconvertinemia
Owren's disease
Proaccelerin deficiency

D68.3 Hemorrhagic disorder due to intrinsic circulating anticoagulants
Hemorrhagic disorder due to intrinsic increase in antithrombin
Hemorrhagic disorder due to intrinsic increase in anti-VIIIa
Hemorrhagic disorder due to intrinsic increase in anti-IXa
Hemorrhagic disorder due to intrinsic increase in anti-Xa
Hemorrhagic disorder due to intrinsic increase in anti-XIa
Hyperheparinemia
Excludes1:   drug induced hemorrhagic disorder (D68.5)

D68.4 Acquired coagulation factor deficiency
Deficiency of coagulation factor due to liver disease
Deficiency of coagulation factor due to vitamin K deficiency
Excludes1:   vitamin K deficiency of newborn (P53)

D68.5 Drug-induced hemorrhagic disorder
Use additional external cause code (Chapter XIX) to identify any
administered anticoagulant.
Excludes1:   hemorrhagic disorder due to intrinsic circulating
anticoagulants (D68.3)

D68.6 Hypercoagulation states
Excludes1:   lupus anticoagulant (D68.81)
thrombotic thrombocytopenic purpura (M31.1)

D68.61   Primary hypercoagulation states
Hypercoagulation states NOS

D68.610   Activated protein C resistance
Factor V Leiden mutation

D68.611   Prothrombin gene mutation

D68.618   Other primary hypercoagulation states

D68.62   Secondary hypercoagulation states

D68.8 Other specified coagulation defects
Excludes1:   hemorrhagic disease of newborn (P53)

D68.81   Lupus anticoagulant syndrome
Lupus anticoagulant
Presence of systemic lupus erythematosus [SLE]
inhibitor

D68.89   Other specified coagulation defects

D68.9 Coagulation defect, unspecified

D69 Purpura and other hemorrhagic conditions
Excludes1:   benign hypergammaglobulinemic purpura (D89.0)
cryoglobulinemic purpura (D89.1)
essential (hemorrhagic) thrombocythemia (D47.3)
hemorrhagic thrombocythemia (D47.3)
purpura fulminans (D65)
thrombotic thrombocytopenic purpura (M31.1)
Waldenström's hypergammaglobulinemic purpura
(D89.0)

D69.0 Allergic purpura
Allergic vasculitis
Nonthrombocytopenic hemorrhagic purpura
Nonthrombocytopenic idiopathic purpura
Purpura anaphylactoid
Purpura Henoch (-Schönlein)
Purpura rheumatica
Vascular purpura

D69.1 Qualitative platelet defects
Bernard-Soulier [giant platelet] syndrome
Glanzmann's disease
Grey platelet syndrome
Thromboasthenia (hemorrhagic) (hereditary)
Thrombocytopathy
Excludes1:   von Willebrand's disease (D68.0)

D69.2 Other nonthrombocytopenic purpura
Purpura NOS
Purpura simplex
Senile purpura

D69.3 Idiopathic thrombocytopenic purpura
Evans' syndrome

D69.4 Other primary thrombocytopenia
Excludes1:   thrombocytopenia with absent radius (Q87.2)
transient neonatal thrombocytopenia (P61.0)
Wiskott-Aldrich syndrome (D82.0)

D69.5 Secondary thrombocytopenia
Use additional external cause code (Chapter XIX) to identify cause.
Excludes1:   transient thrombocytopenia of newborn (P61.0)

D69.6 Thrombocytopenia, unspecified

D69.8 Other specified hemorrhagic conditions
Capillary fragility (hereditary)
Vascular pseudohemophilia

D69.9 Hemorrhagic condition, unspecified

OTHER DISEASES OF BLOOD AND BLOOD–FORMING ORGANS
(D70–D78)

D70 Neutropenia
Includes: agranulocytosis
Excludes1:   transient neonatal neutropenia (P61.5)

D70.0 Congenital agranulocytosis
Congenital neutropenia
Infantile genetic agranulocytosis
Kostmann's disease

D70.1 Agranulocytosis secondary to cancer chemotherapy
Code first underlying neoplasm
Use additional external cause code (Chapter XIX) to identify drug.

D70.2 Other drug-induced agranulocytosis
Use additional external cause code (Chapter XIX) to identify drug.

D70.3 Other agranulocytosis

D70.4 Cyclic neutropenia
Periodic neutropenia

D70.8 Other neutropenia

D70.9 Neutropenia, unspecified

D71 Functional disorders of polymorphonuclear neutrophils
Includes: cell membrane receptor complex [CR3] defect
chronic (childhood) granulomatous disease
congenital dysphagocytosis
progressive septic granulomatosis

D72 Other disorders of white blood cells
Excludes1:   basophilia (D75.8)
immunity disorders (D80-D89)
neutropenia (D70)
preleukemia (syndrome) (D46.9)

D72.0 Genetic anomalies of leukocytes
Alder (granulation) (granulocyte) anomaly
Alder syndrome
May-Hegglin (granulation) (granulocyte) anomaly
May-Hegglin syndrome
Pelger-Huët (granulation) (granulocyte) anomaly
Pelger-Huët syndrome
Hereditary leukocytic hypersegmentation
Hereditary leukocytic hyposegmentation
Hereditary leukomelanopathy
Excludes1:   Chediak (-Steinbrinck)-Higashi syndrome (E70.330)

D72.1 Eosinophilia
Allergic eosinophilia
Hereditary eosinophilia
Excludes1:   Löffler's syndrome (J82)
pulmonary eosinophilia (J82)

D72.8 Other specified disorders of white blood cells
Lymphocytic leukemoid reaction
Monocytic leukemoid reaction
Myelocytic leukemoid reaction
Excludes1:   leukemia (C91-C95)
leukocytosis (R72.0)
lymphocytosis (symptomatic) (R72.0)
lymphopenia (R72.1)
monocytosis (symptomatic) (R72.0)
plasmacytosis (R72.0)

D72.9 Disorder of white blood cells, unspecified

D73 Diseases of spleen

D73.0 Hyposplenism
Atrophy of spleen
Excludes1:   asplenia (congenital) (Q89.01)
postsurgical absence of spleen (Z90.81)

D73.1 Hypersplenism
Excludes1:   splenitis, splenomegaly in late syphilis (A52.79)
splenitis, splenomegaly in tuberculosis (A18.85)
splenomegaly NOS (R16.1)
splenomegaly congenital (Q89.0)

D73.2 Chronic congestive splenomegaly

D73.3 Abscess of spleen

D73.4 Cyst of spleen

D73.5 Infarction of spleen
Splenic rupture, nontraumatic
Torsion of spleen
Excludes1:   rupture of spleen due to Plasmodium vivax malaria (B51.0)
traumatic rupture of spleen (S36.03-)

D73.8 Other diseases of spleen
Fibrosis of spleen NOS
Perisplenitis
Splenitis NOS

D73.9 Disease of spleen, unspecified

D74 Methemoglobinemia

D74.0 Congenital methemoglobinemia
Congenital NADH-methemoglobin reductase deficiency
Hemoglobin-M [Hb-M] disease
Methemoglobinemia, hereditary

D74.8 Other methemoglobinemias
Acquired methemoglobinemia (with sulfhemoglobinemia)
Toxic methemoglobinemia
Use additional external cause code (Chapter XIX) to identify cause.

D74.9 Methemoglobinemia, unspecified

D75 Other diseases of blood and blood-forming organs
Excludes2:   acute lymphadenitis (L04.-)
chronic lymphadenitis (I88.1)
enlarged lymph nodes (R59.-)
hypergammaglobulinemia NOS (D89.2)
lymphadenitis NOS (I88.9)
mesenteric lymphadenitis (acute) (chronic) (I88.0)

D75.0   Familial erythrocytosis
Benign polycythemia
Familial polycythemia
Excludes1:   hereditary ovalocytosis (D58.1)

D75.1   Secondary polycythemia
Acquired polycythemia
Emotional polycythemia
Hypoxemic polycythemia
Nephrogenous polycythemia
Polycythemia due to erythropoietin
Polycythemia due to fall in plasma volume
Polycythemia due to high altitude
Polycythemia due to stress
Relative polycythemia
Excludes1:   polycythemia neonatorum (P61.1)
polycythemia vera (D45)

D75.2   Essential thrombocytosis
Excludes1:   essential (hemorrhagic) thrombocythemia (D47.3)

D75.8   Other specified diseases of blood and blood-forming organs
Basophilia

D75.9   Disease of blood and blood-forming organs, unspecified

D76   Certain diseases involving lymphoreticular tissue and reticulohistiocytic system
Excludes1:   Letterer-Siwe disease (C96.0)
malignant histiocytosis (C96.1)
histiocytic medullary reticuloendotheliosis or reticulosis (C96.1)
leukemic reticuloendotheliosis or reticulosis (C91.4-)
lipomelanotic reticuloendotheliosis or reticulosis (I89.8)
malignant reticuloendotheliosis or reticulosis (C85.7-)
nonlipid reticuloendotheliosis or reticulosis (C96.0)

D76.0   Langerhans' cell histiocytosis, not elsewhere classified
Eosinophilic granuloma
Hand-Schüller-Christian disease
Histiocytosis X (chronic)

D76.1   Hemophagocytic lymphohistiocytosis
Familial hemophagocytic reticulosis
Histiocytoses of mononuclear phagocytes other than Langerhans' cells NOS

D76.2   Hemophagocytic syndrome, infection-associated
Use additional code to identify infectious agent or disease.

D76.3   Other histiocytosis syndromes
Reticulohistiocytoma (giant-cell)
Sinus histiocytosis with massive lymphadenopathy
Xanthogranuloma

D77   Other disorders of blood and blood-forming organs in diseases classified elsewhere
Code first underlying disease, such as:
amyloidosis (E85)
congenital early syphilis (A50.0)
echinococcosis (B67.0-B67.9)
malaria (B50.0-B54)
schistosomiasis [bilharziasis] (B65.0-B65.9)
vitamin C deficiency (E54)
Excludes1:   rupture of spleen due to Plasmodium vivax malaria (B51.0)
splenitis, splenomegaly in:
late syphilis (A52.79)
tuberculosis (A18.85)

D78   Intraoperative and postprocedural complications of procedures on the spleen

D78.0   Intraoperative and postprocedural hemorrhage or hematoma complicating procedures on the spleen
Excludes1:   intraoperative hemorrhage or hematoma due to accidental puncture or laceration during a procedure on the spleen (D78.1-)

D78.01   Intraoperative hemorrhage of the spleen during a procedure on the spleen

D78.02   Intraoperative hemorrhage of other organ or structure during a procedure on the spleen

D78.03   Intraoperative hematoma of the spleen during a procedure on the spleen

D78.04   Intraoperative hematoma of other organ or structure during a procedure on the spleen

D78.05   Postprocedural hemorrhage of the spleen following a procedure on the spleen

D78.06   Postprocedural hemorrhage of other organ or structure following a procedure on the spleen

D78.07   Postprocedural hematoma of the spleen following a procedure on the spleen

D78.08   Postprocedural hematoma of other organ or structure following a procedure on the spleen

D78.1   Accidental puncture or laceration during a procedure on the spleen

D78.11   Accidental puncture or laceration of the spleen during a procedure on the spleen

D78.12   Accidental puncture or laceration of other organ or structure during a procedure on the spleen

D78.8   Other intraoperative and postprocedural complications of procedures on the spleen

D78.81   Other intraoperative complications of procedures on the spleen

D78.89   Other postprocedural complications of procedures on the spleen

CERTAIN DISORDERS INVOLVING THE IMMUNE MECHANISM (D80–D89)

Includes: defects in the complement system
immunodeficiency disorders, except human immunodeficiency virus [HIV] disease
sarcoidosis
Excludes1:   autoimmune disease (systemic) NOS (M35.9)
functional disorders of polymorphonuclear neutrophils (D71)
human immunodeficiency virus [HIV] disease (B20)

D80   Immunodeficiency with predominantly antibody defects

D80.0   Hereditary hypogammaglobulinemia
Autosomal recessive agammaglobulinemia (Swiss type)
X-linked agammaglobulinemia [Bruton] (with growth hormone deficiency)

D80.1   Nonfamilial hypogammaglobulinemia
Agammaglobulinemia with immunoglobulin-bearing B-lymphocytes
Common variable agammaglobulinemia [CVAgamma]
Hypogammaglobulinemia NOS

D80.2   Selective deficiency of immunoglobulin A [IgA]

D80.3   Selective deficiency of immunoglobulin G [IgG] subclasses

D80.4   Selective deficiency of immunoglobulin M [IgM]

D80.5   Immunodeficiency with increased immunoglobulin M [IgM]

D80.6   Antibody deficiency with near-normal immunoglobulins or with hyperimmunoglobulinemia

D80.7   Transient hypogammaglobulinemia of infancy

D80.8   Other immunodeficiencies with predominantly antibody defects
Kappa light chain deficiency

D80.9   Immunodeficiency with predominantly antibody defects, unspecified

D81   Combined immunodeficiencies
Excludes1:   autosomal recessive agammaglobulinemia (Swiss type) (D80.0)

D81.0   Severe combined immunodeficiency [SCID] with reticular dysgenesis

D81.1   Severe combined immunodeficiency [SCID] with low T-and B-cell numbers

D81.2   Severe combined immunodeficiency [SCID] with low or normal B-cell numbers

D81.3   Adenosine deaminase [ADA] deficiency

D81.4   Nezelof's syndrome

D81.5   Purine nucleoside phosphorylase [PNP] deficiency

D81.6   Major histocompatibility complex class I deficiency
Bare lymphocyte syndrome

D81.7   Major histocompatibility complex class II deficiency

D81.8   Other combined immunodeficiencies

D81.81 **Biotin-dependent carboxylase deficiency**
Multiple carboxylase deficiency
Excludes1: biotin-dependent carboxylase deficiency
due to dietary deficiency of biotin
(E53.8)

D81.810 **Biotinidase deficiency**
D81.818 **Other biotin-dependent carboxylase deficiency**
Other multiple carboxylase deficiency
Holocarboxylase synthetase deficiency
D81.819 **Biotin-dependent carboxylase deficiency, unspecified**
Multiple carboxylase deficiency, unspecified

D81.89 **Other combined immunodeficiencies**
D81.9 **Combined immunodeficiency, unspecified**
Severe combined immunodeficiency disorder [SCID] NOS

D82 Immunodeficiency associated with other major defects
Excludes1: ataxia telangiectasia [Louis-Bar] (G11.3)

D82.0 **Wiskott-Aldrich syndrome**
Immunodeficiency with thrombocytopenia and eczema
D82.1 **Di George's syndrome**
Pharyngeal pouch syndrome
Thymic alymphoplasia
Thymic aplasia or hypoplasia with immunodeficiency
D82.2 **Immunodeficiency with short-limbed stature**
D82.3 **Immunodeficiency following hereditary defective response to Epstein-Barr virus**
X-linked lymphoproliferative disease
D82.4 **Hyperimmunoglobulin E [IgE] syndrome**
D82.8 **Immunodeficiency associated with other specified major defects**
D82.9 **Immunodeficiency associated with major defect, unspecified**

D83 Common variable immunodeficiency
D83.0 **Common variable immunodeficiency with predominant abnormalities of B-cell numbers and function**
D83.1 **Common variable immunodeficiency with predominant immunoregulatory T-cell disorders**
D83.2 **Common variable immunodeficiency with autoantibodies to B- or T-cells**
D83.8 **Other common variable immunodeficiencies**
D83.9 **Common variable immunodeficiency, unspecified**

D84 Other immunodeficiencies
D84.1 **Lymphocyte function antigen-1 [LFA-1] defect**
D84.1 **Defects in the complement system**
C1 esterase inhibitor [C1-INH] deficiency
D84.8 **Other specified immunodeficiencies**
D84.9 **Immunodeficiency, unspecified**

D86 Sarcoidosis
D86.0 **Sarcoidosis of lung**
D86.1 **Sarcoidosis of lymph nodes**
D86.2 **Sarcoidosis of lung with sarcoidosis of lymph nodes**
D86.3 **Sarcoidosis of skin**
D86.8 **Sarcoidosis of other sites**
D86.81 **Sarcoid meningitis**
D86.82 **Multiple cranial nerve palsies in sarcoidosis**
D86.83 **Sarcoid iridocyclitis**
D86.84 **Sarcoid pyelonephritis**
Tubulo-interstitial nephropathy in sarcoidosis
D86.85 **Sarcoid myocarditis**
D86.86 **Sarcoid arthropathy**
Polyarthritis in sarcoidosis
D86.87 **Sarcoid myositis**
D86.89 **Sarcoidosis of other sites**
Hepatic granuloma
Uveoparotid fever [Heerfordt]
D86.9 **Sarcoidosis, unspecified**

D89 Other disorders involving the immune mechanism, not elsewhere classified
Excludes1: hyperglobulinemia NOS (R77.1)
monoclonal gammopathy (D47.2)
Excludes2: transplant failure and rejection (T86.-)

D89.0 **Polyclonal hypergammaglobulinemia**
Benign hypergammaglobulinemic purpura
Polyclonal gammopathy NOS
Waldenström's hypergammaglobulinemic purpura
D89.1 **Cryoglobulinemia**
Cryoglobulinemic purpura
Cryoglobulinemic vasculitis
Essential cryoglobulinemia
Idiopathic cryoglobulinemia
Mixed cryoglobulinemia
Primary cryoglobulinemia
Secondary cryoglobulinemia
D89.2 **Hypergammaglobulinemia, unspecified**
D89.8 **Other specified disorders involving the immune mechanism, not elsewhere classified**
Excludes1: human immunodeficiency virus disease (B20)
D89.9 **Disorder involving the immune mechanism, unspecified**
Immune disease NOS

CHAPTER IV — ENDOCRINE, NUTRITIONAL AND METABOLIC DISEASES (E00–E90)

Note: All neoplasms, whether functionally active or not, are classified in Chapter II. Appropriate codes in this chapter (i.e., E05.8, E07.0, E16-E31, E34.-) may be used as additional codes to indicate either functional activity by neoplasms and ectopic endocrine tissue or hyperfunction and hypofunction of endocrine glands associated with neoplasms and other conditions classified elsewhere.

Excludes1:   transitory endocrine and metabolic disorders specific to fetus and newborn (P70-P74)

This chapter contains the following blocks:

E00-E07	Disorders of thyroid gland
E08-E13	Diabetes mellitus
E15-E16	Other disorders of glucose regulation and pancreatic internal secretion
E20-E36	Disorders of other endocrine glands
E40-E46	Malnutrition
E50-E64	Other nutritional deficiencies
E65-E68	Obesity and other hyperalimentation
E70-E90	Metabolic disorders

DISORDERS OF THYROID GLAND (E00–E07)

E00 Congenital iodine-deficiency syndrome

Use additional code (F70-F79) to identify associated mental retardation.

Excludes1:   subclinical iodine-deficiency hypothyroidism (E02)

E00.0 Congenital iodine-deficiency syndrome, neurological type
Endemic cretinism, neurological type

E00.1 Congenital iodine-deficiency syndrome, myxedematous type
Endemic hypothyroid cretinism
Endemic cretinism, myxedematous type

E00.2 Congenital iodine-deficiency syndrome, mixed type
Endemic cretinism, mixed type

E00.9 Congenital iodine-deficiency syndrome, unspecified
Congenital iodine-deficiency hypothyroidism NOS
Endemic cretinism NOS

E01 Iodine-deficiency related thyroid disorders and allied conditions

Excludes1:   congenital iodine-deficiency syndrome (E00.-)
subclinical iodine-deficiency hypothyroidism (E02)

E01.0 Iodine-deficiency related diffuse (endemic) goiter

E01.1 Iodine-deficiency related multinodular (endemic) goiter
Iodine-deficiency related nodular goiter

E01.2 Iodine-deficiency related (endemic) goiter, unspecified
Endemic goiter NOS

E01.8 Other iodine-deficiency related thyroid disorders and allied conditions
Acquired iodine-deficiency hypothyroidism NOS

E02 Subclinical iodine-deficiency hypothyroidism

E03 Other hypothyroidism

Excludes1:   iodine-deficiency related hypothyroidism (E00-E02)
postprocedural hypothyroidism (E89.0)

E03.0 Congenital hypothyroidism with diffuse goiter
Congenital parenchymatous goiter (nontoxic)
Congenital goiter (nontoxic) NOS
Excludes1:   transitory congenital goiter with normal function (P72.0)

E03.1 Congenital hypothyroidism without goiter
Aplasia of thyroid (with myxedema)
Congenital atrophy of thyroid
Congenital hypothyroidism NOS

E03.2 Hypothyroidism due to medicaments and other exogenous substances
Use additional external cause code (Chapter XIX) to identify cause

E03.3 Postinfectious hypothyroidism

E03.4 Atrophy of thyroid (acquired)
Excludes1:   congenital atrophy of thyroid (E03.1)

E03.5 Myxedema coma

E03.8 Other specified hypothyroidism

E03.9 Hypothyroidism, unspecified
Myxedema NOS

E04 Other nontoxic goiter

Excludes1:   congenital goiter (NOS) (diffuse) (parenchymatous) (E03.0)
iodine-deficiency related goiter (E00-E02)

E04.0 Nontoxic diffuse goiter
Diffuse (colloid) nontoxic goiter
Simple nontoxic goiter

E04.1 Nontoxic single thyroid nodule
Colloid nodule (cystic) (thyroid)
Nontoxic uninodular goiter
Thyroid (cystic) nodule NOS

E04.2 Nontoxic multinodular goiter
Cystic goiter NOS
Multinodular (cystic) goiter NOS

E04.8 Other specified nontoxic goiter

E04.9 Nontoxic goiter, unspecified
Goiter NOS
Nodular goiter (nontoxic) NOS

E05 Thyrotoxicosis [hyperthyroidism]

Excludes1:   chronic thyroiditis with transient thyrotoxicosis (E06.2)
neonatal thyrotoxicosis (P72.1)

E05.0 Thyrotoxicosis with diffuse goiter
Exophthalmic or toxic goiter NOS
Graves' disease
Toxic diffuse goiter

E05.00 Thyrotoxicosis with diffuse goiter without thyrotoxic crisis or storm

E05.01 Thyrotoxicosis with diffuse goiter with thyrotoxic crisis or storm

E05.1 Thyrotoxicosis with toxic single thyroid nodule
Thyrotoxicosis with toxic uninodular goiter

E05.10 Thyrotoxicosis with toxic single thyroid nodule without thyrotoxic crisis or storm

E05.11 Thyrotoxicosis with toxic single thyroid nodule with thyrotoxic crisis or storm

E05.2 Thyrotoxicosis with toxic multinodular goiter
Toxic nodular goiter NOS

E05.20 Thyrotoxicosis with toxic multinodular goiter without thyrotoxic crisis or storm

E05.21 Thyrotoxicosis with toxic multinodular goiter with thyrotoxic crisis or storm

E05.3 Thyrotoxicosis from ectopic thyroid tissue

E05.30 Thyrotoxicosis from ectopic thyroid tissue without thyrotoxic crisis or storm

E05.31 Thyrotoxicosis from ectopic thyroid tissue with thyrotoxic crisis or storm

E05.4 Thyrotoxicosis factitia

E05.40 Thyrotoxicosis factitia without thyrotoxic crisis or storm

E05.41 Thyrotoxicosis factitia with thyrotoxic crisis or storm

E05.8 Other thyrotoxicosis
Overproduction of thyroid-stimulating hormone
Use additional external cause code (Chapter XIX) to identify cause.

E05.80 Other thyrotoxicosis without thyrotoxic crisis or storm

E05.81 Other thyrotoxicosis with thyrotoxic crisis or storm

E05.9 Thyrotoxicosis, unspecified
Hyperthyroidism NOS

E05.90 Thyrotoxicosis, unspecified without thyrotoxic crisis or storm

E05.91 Thyrotoxicosis, unspecified with thyrotoxic crisis or storm

E06 Thyroiditis

Excludes1: postpartum thyroiditis (O90.5)

E06.0 Acute thyroiditis
Abscess of thyroid
Pyogenic thyroiditis
Suppurative thyroiditis
Use additional code (B95-B97) to identify infectious agent.

E06.1 Subacute thyroiditis
de Quervain thyroiditis
Giant-cell thyroiditis
Granulomatous thyroiditis
Nonsuppurative thyroiditis
Viral thyroiditis
Excludes1: autoimmune thyroiditis (E06.3)

E06.2 Chronic thyroiditis with transient thyrotoxicosis
Excludes1: autoimmune thyroiditis (E06.3)

E06.3 Autoimmune thyroiditis
Hashimoto's thyroiditis
Hashitoxicosis (transient)
Lymphadenoid goiter
Lymphocytic thyroiditis
Struma lymphomatosa

E06.4 Drug-induced thyroiditis
Use additional external cause code (Chapter XIX) to identify drug

E06.5 Other chronic thyroiditis
Chronic fibrous thyroiditis
Chronic thyroiditis NOS
Ligneous thyroiditis
Riedel thyroiditis

E06.9 Thyroiditis, unspecified

E07 Other disorders of thyroid

E07.0 Hypersecretion of calcitonin
C-cell hyperplasia of thyroid
Hypersecretion of thyrocalcitonin

E07.1 Dyshormogenetic goiter
Familial dyshormogenetic goiter
Pendred's syndrome
Excludes1: transitory congenital goiter with normal function (P72.0)

E07.8 Other specified disorders of thyroid

E07.81 Sick-euthyroid syndrome
Euthyroid sick-syndrome

E07.89 Other specified disorders of thyroid
Abnormality of thyroid-binding globulin
Hemorrhage of thyroid
Infarction of thyroid

E07.9 Disorder of thyroid, unspecified

DIABETES MELLITUS (E08–E13)

E08 Diabetes mellitus due to underlying condition
Code first the underlying condition, such as:
Congenital rubella (P35.0)
Cushing's syndrome (E24.-)
Cystic fibrosis (E84.-)
Malignant neoplasm (C00-C96)
Malnutrition (E40-E46)
Pancreatitis and other diseases of the pancreas (K85-K86.-)
Use additional code to identify any insulin use (Z79.7)
Excludes1: drug or chemical induced diabetes mellitus (E09.-)
gestational diabetes (O24.4-)
type 1 diabetes mellitus (E10.-)
type 2 diabetes mellitus (E11.-)
unspecified diabetes mellitus (E14.-)

E08.0 Diabetes mellitus due to underlying condition with hyperosmolarity

E08.00 Diabetes mellitus due to underlying condition with hyperosmolarity without nonketotic hyperglycemic-hyperosmolar coma (NKHHC)

E08.01 Diabetes mellitus due to underlying condition with hyperosmolarity with coma

E08.1 Diabetes mellitus due to underlying condition with ketoacidosis

E08.10 Diabetes mellitus due to underlying condition with ketoacidosis without coma

E08.11 Diabetes mellitus due to underlying condition with ketoacidosis with coma

E08.2 Diabetes mellitus due to underlying condition with renal complications

E08.21 Diabetes mellitus due to underlying condition with diabetic nephropathy
Diabetes mellitus due to underlying condition with intercapillary glomerulosclerosis
Diabetes mellitus due to underlying condition with intracapillary glomerulonephrosis
Diabetes mellitus due to underlying condition with Kimmelstiel-Wilson disease

E08.22 Diabetes mellitus due to underlying condition with Ebstein's disease
Renal tubular degeneration in diabetes mellitus due to underlying condition

E08.23 Diabetes mellitus due to underlying condition with diabetic renal failure
Diabetes mellitus due to underlying condition with renal failure in conditions classified to .21 and .22

E08.29 Diabetes mellitus due to underlying condition with other diabetic renal complication

E08.3 Diabetes mellitus due to underlying condition with ophthalmic complications

E08.30 Diabetes mellitus due to underlying condition with diabetic ophthalmic complication, unspecified

E08.31 Diabetes mellitus due to underlying condition with diabetic background retinopathy
Diabetes mellitus due to underlying condition with diabetic retinopathy NOS

E08.32 Diabetes mellitus due to underlying condition with diabetic proliferative retinopathy

E08.33 Diabetes mellitus due to underlying condition with diabetic cataract

E08.39 Diabetes mellitus due to underlying condition with other diabetic ophthalmic complication

E08.4 Diabetes mellitus due to underlying condition with neurological complications

E08.40 Diabetes mellitus due to underlying condition with diabetic neuropathy, unspecified

E08.41 Diabetes mellitus due to underlying condition with diabetic mononeuropathy

E08.42 Diabetes mellitus due to underlying condition with diabetic polyneuropathy
Diabetes mellitus due to underlying condition with diabetic neuralgia

E08.43 Diabetes mellitus due to underlying condition with diabetic autonomic (poly)neuropathy
Diabetes mellitus due to underlying condition with diabetic gastroparesis

E08.44 Diabetes mellitus due to underlying condition with diabetic amyotrophy
Diabetes mellitus due to underlying condition with diabetic myasthenia

E08.49 Diabetes mellitus due to underlying condition with other diabetic neurological complication

E08.5 Diabetes mellitus due to underlying condition with circulatory complications

E08.51 Diabetes mellitus due to underlying condition with diabetic peripheral angiopathy without gangrene

E08.52 Diabetes mellitus due to underlying condition with diabetic peripheral angiopathy with gangrene
Diabetes mellitus due to underlying condition with diabetic gangrene

E08.59 Diabetes mellitus due to underlying condition with other circulatory complications

E08.6 Diabetes mellitus due to underlying condition with other specified complications

E08.61   Diabetes mellitus due to underlying condition with diabetic arthropathy

 E08.610   Diabetes mellitus due to underlying condition with diabetic neuropathic arthropathy
  Diabetes mellitus due to underlying condition with Charcot's joints

 E08.618   Diabetes mellitus due to underlying condition with other diabetic arthropathy

E08.62   Diabetes mellitus due to underlying condition with skin complications

 E08.620   Diabetes mellitus due to underlying condition with diabetic dermatitis
  Diabetes mellitus due to underlying condition with diabetic necrobiosis lipoidica

 E08.621   Diabetes mellitus due to underlying condition with foot ulcer
  Use additional code to identify site of ulcer (L97.4-, L97.5-)

 E08.622   Diabetes mellitus due to underlying condition with other skin ulcer
  Use additional code to identify site of ulcer (L97.1-L97.9, L98.41-L98.49)

 E08.628   Diabetes mellitus due to underlying condition with other skin complications

E08.63   Diabetes mellitus due to underlying condition with oral complications

 E08.630   Diabetes mellitus due to underlying condition with periodontal disease

 E08.638   Diabetes mellitus due to underlying condition with other oral complications

E08.64   Diabetes mellitus due to underlying condition with hypoglycemia

 E08.640   Diabetes mellitus due to underlying condition with hypoglycemia without coma

 E08.641   Diabetes mellitus due to underlying condition with hypoglycemia with coma

E08.65   Diabetes mellitus due to underlying condition with hyperglycemia

E08.69   Diabetes mellitus due to underlying condition with other specified complication
 Use additional code to identify complication

E08.8   Diabetes mellitus due to underlying condition with unspecified complications

E08.9   Diabetes mellitus due to underlying condition without complications

E09 Drug or chemical induced diabetes mellitus
Use additional code to identify any insulin use (Z79.7)
Use adverse effect external cause code (Chapter XIX) to identify drug or chemical
Excludes1: diabetes mellitus due to underlying condition (E08.-)
  gestational diabetes (O24.4-)
  type 1 diabetes mellitus (E10.-)
  type 2 diabetes mellitus (E11.-)
  unspecified diabetes mellitus (E14.-)

E09.0   Drug or chemical induced diabetes mellitus with hyperosmolarity

 E09.00   Drug or chemical induced diabetes mellitus with hyperosmolarity without nonketotic hyperglycemic-hyperosmolar coma (NKHHC)

 E09.01   Drug or chemical induced diabetes mellitus with hyperosmolarity with coma

E09.1   Drug or chemical induced diabetes mellitus with ketoacidosis

 E09.10   Drug or chemical induced diabetes mellitus with ketoacidosis without coma

 E09.11   Drug or chemical induced diabetes mellitus with ketoacidosis with coma

E09.2   Drug or chemical induced diabetes mellitus with renal complications

 E09.21   Drug or chemical induced diabetes mellitus with diabetic nephropathy
  Drug or chemical induced diabetes mellitus with intercapillary glomerulosclerosis
  Drug or chemical induced diabetes mellitus with intracapillary glomerulonephrosis
  Drug or chemical induced diabetes mellitus with Kimmelstiel-Wilson disease

 E09.22   Drug or chemical induced diabetes mellitus with Ebstein's disease
  Drug or chemical induced diabetes mellitus with renal tubular degeneration

 E09.23   Drug or chemical induced diabetes mellitus with diabetic renal failure
  Drug or chemical induced diabetes mellitus with renal failure in conditions classified to .21 and .22

 E09.29   Drug or chemical induced diabetes mellitus with other diabetic renal complication

E09.3   Drug or chemical induced diabetes mellitus with ophthalmic complications

 E09.30   Drug or chemical induced diabetes mellitus with diabetic ophthalmic complication, unspecified

 E09.31   Drug or chemical induced diabetes mellitus with diabetic background retinopathy
  Drug or chemical induced diabetes mellitus with diabetic retinopathy NOS

 E09.32   Drug or chemical induced diabetes mellitus with diabetic proliferative retinopathy

 E09.33   Drug or chemical induced diabetes mellitus with diabetic cataract

 E09.39   Drug or chemical induced diabetes mellitus with other diabetic ophthalmic complication

E09.4   Drug or chemical induced diabetes mellitus with neurological complications

 E09.40   Drug or chemical induced diabetes mellitus with neurological complications with diabetic neuropathy, unspecified

 E09.41   Drug or chemical induced diabetes mellitus with neurological complications with diabetic mononeuropathy

 E09.42   Drug or chemical induced diabetes mellitus with neurological complications with diabetic polyneuropathy
  Drug or chemical induced diabetes mellitus with diabetic neuralgia

 E09.43   Drug or chemical induced diabetes mellitus with neurological complications with diabetic autonomic (poly)neuropathy
  Drug or chemical induced diabetes mellitus with diabetic gastroparesis

 E09.44   Drug or chemical induced diabetes mellitus with neurological complications with diabetic amyotrophy
  Drug or chemical induced diabetes mellitus with diabetic myasthenia

 E09.49   Drug or chemical induced diabetes mellitus with neurological complications with other diabetic neurological complication

E09.5   Drug or chemical induced diabetes mellitus with circulatory complications

 E09.51   Drug or chemical induced diabetes mellitus with diabetic peripheral angiopathy without gangrene

 E09.52   Drug or chemical induced diabetes mellitus with diabetic peripheral angiopathy with gangrene
  Drug or chemical induced diabetes mellitus with diabetic gangrene

 E09.59   Drug or chemical induced diabetes mellitus with other circulatory complications

E09.6   Drug or chemical induced diabetes mellitus with other specified complications

 E09.61   Drug or chemical induced diabetes mellitus with diabetic arthropathy

E09.610   **Drug or chemical induced diabetes mellitus with diabetic neuropathic arthropathy**
Drug or chemical induced diabetes mellitus with Charcot's joints

E09.618   **Drug or chemical induced diabetes mellitus with other diabetic arthropathy**

E09.62   **Drug or chemical induced diabetes mellitus with skin complications**

E09.620   **Drug or chemical induced diabetes mellitus with diabetic dermatitis**
Drug or chemical induced diabetes mellitus with diabetic necrobiosis lipoidica

E09.621   **Drug or chemical induced diabetes mellitus with foot ulcer**
Use additional code to identify site of ulcer (L97.4-, L97.5-)

E09.622   **Drug or chemical induced diabetes mellitus with other skin ulcer**
Use additional code to identify site of ulcer (L97.1-L97.9, L98.41-L98.49)

E09.628   **Drug or chemical induced diabetes mellitus with other skin complications**

E09.63   **Drug or chemical induced diabetes mellitus with oral complications**

E09.630   **Drug or chemical induced diabetes mellitus with periodontal disease**

E09.638   **Drug or chemical induced diabetes mellitus with other oral complications**

E09.64   **Drug or chemical induced diabetes mellitus with hypoglycemia**

E09.640   **Drug or chemical induced diabetes mellitus with hypoglycemia without coma**

E09.641   **Drug or chemical induced diabetes mellitus with hypoglycemia with coma**

E09.65   **Drug or chemical induced diabetes mellitus with hyperglycemia**

E09.69   **Drug or chemical induced diabetes mellitus with other specified complication**
Use additional code to identify complication

E09.8   **Drug or chemical induced diabetes mellitus with unspecified complications**

E09.9   **Drug or chemical induced diabetes mellitus without complications**

E10   **Type 1 diabetes mellitus**

Includes: brittle diabetes (mellitus)
diabetes (mellitus) due to autoimmune process
diabetes (mellitus) due to immune mediated pancreatic islet β-cell destruction
idiopathic diabetes (mellitus)
juvenile onset diabetes (mellitus)
ketosis-prone diabetes (mellitus)

Excludes1:   diabetes mellitus due to underlying condition (E08.-)
drug or chemical induced diabetes mellitus (E09.-)
gestational diabetes (O24.4-)
type 2 diabetes mellitus (E11.-)
unspecified diabetes mellitus (E14.-)

E10.1   **Type 1 diabetes mellitus with ketoacidosis**

E10.10   **Type 1 diabetes mellitus with ketoacidosis without coma**

E10.11   **Type 1 diabetes mellitus with ketoacidosis with coma**

E10.2   **Type 1 diabetes mellitus with renal complications**

E10.21   **Type 1 diabetes mellitus with diabetic nephropathy**
Type 1 diabetes mellitus with intercapillary glomerulosclerosis
Type 1 diabetes mellitus with intracapillary glomerulonephrosis
Type 1 diabetes mellitus with Kimmelstiel-Wilson disease

E10.22   **Type 1 diabetes mellitus with Ebstein's disease**
Type 1 diabetes mellitus with renal tubular degeneration

E10.23   **Type 1 diabetes mellitus with diabetic renal failure**
Type 1 diabetes mellitus with renal failure in conditions classified to .21 and .22

E10.29   **Type 1 diabetes mellitus with other diabetic renal complication**

E10.3   **Type 1 diabetes mellitus with ophthalmic complications**

E10.30   **Type 1 diabetes mellitus with diabetic ophthalmic complication, unspecified**

E10.31   **Type 1 diabetes mellitus with diabetic background retinopathy**
Type 1 diabetes mellitus with diabetic retinopathy NOS

E10.32   **Type 1 diabetes mellitus with diabetic proliferative retinopathy**

E10.33   **Type 1 diabetes mellitus with diabetic cataract**

E10.39   **Type 1 diabetes mellitus with other diabetic ophthalmic complication**

E10.4   **Type 1 diabetes mellitus with neurological complications**

E10.40   **Type 1 diabetes mellitus with diabetic neuropathy, unspecified**

E10.41   **Type 1 diabetes mellitus with diabetic mononeuropathy**

E10.42   **Type 1 diabetes mellitus with diabetic polyneuropathy**
Type 1 diabetes mellitus with diabetic neuralgia

E10.43   **Type 1 diabetes mellitus with diabetic autonomic (poly)neuropathy**
Type 1 diabetes mellitus with diabetic gastroparesis

E10.44   **Type 1 diabetes mellitus with diabetic amyotrophy**
Type 1 diabetes mellitus with diabetic myasthenia

E10.49   **Type 1 diabetes mellitus with other diabetic neurological complication**

E10.5   **Type 1 diabetes mellitus with circulatory complications**

E10.51   **Type 1 diabetes mellitus with diabetic peripheral angiopathy without gangrene**

E10.52   **Type 1 diabetes mellitus with diabetic peripheral angiopathy with gangrene**
Type 1 diabetes mellitus with diabetic gangrene

E10.59   **Type 1 diabetes mellitus with other circulatory complications**

E10.6   **Type 1 diabetes mellitus with other specified complications**

E10.61   **Type 1 diabetes mellitus with diabetic arthropathy**

E10.610   **Type 1 diabetes mellitus with diabetic neuropathic arthropathy**
Type 1 diabetes mellitus with Charcot's joints

E10.618   **Type 1 diabetes mellitus with other diabetic arthropathy**

E10.62   **Type 1 diabetes mellitus with skin complications**

E10.620   **Type 1 diabetes mellitus with diabetic dermatitis**
Type 1 diabetes mellitus with diabetic necrobiosis lipoidica

E10.621   **Type 1 diabetes mellitus with foot ulcer**
Use additional code to identify site of ulcer (L97.4-, L97.5-)

E10.622   **Type 1 diabetes mellitus with other skin ulcer**
Use additional code to identify site of ulcer (L97.1-L97.9, L98.41-L98.49)

E10.628   **Type 1 diabetes mellitus with other skin complications**

E10.63   **Type 1 diabetes mellitus with oral complications**

E10.630   **Type 1 diabetes mellitus with periodontal disease**

E10.638   **Type 1 diabetes mellitus with other oral complications**

E10.64   **Type 1 diabetes mellitus with hypoglycemia**

E10.640   **Type 1 diabetes mellitus with hypoglycemia without coma**

E10.641   **Type 1 diabetes mellitus with hypoglycemia with coma**

E10.65   **Type 1 diabetes mellitus with hyperglycemia**

E10.69   **Type 1 diabetes mellitus with other specified complication**
Use additional code to identify complication

E10.8   Type 1 diabetes mellitus with unspecified complications

E10.9   Type 1 diabetes mellitus without complications

E11 Type 2 diabetes mellitus

Includes: diabetes (mellitus) due to insulin secretory defect
            insulin resistant diabetes (mellitus)

Use additional code to identify any insulin use (Z79.7)

Excludes1:   diabetes mellitus due to underlying condition (E08.-)
            drug or chemical induced diabetes mellitus (E09.-)
            gestational diabetes (O24.4-)
            type 1 diabetes mellitus (E10.-)
            unspecified diabetes mellitus (E14.-)

E11.0   Type 2 diabetes mellitus with hyperosmolarity

   E11.00   Type 2 diabetes mellitus with hyperosmolarity without nonketotic hyperglycemic-hyperosmolar coma (NKHHC)

   E11.01   Type 2 diabetes mellitus with hyperosmolarity with coma

E11.2   Type 2 diabetes mellitus with renal complications

   E11.21   Type 2 diabetes mellitus with diabetic nephropathy
      Type 2 diabetes mellitus with intercapillary glomerulosclerosis
      Type 2 diabetes mellitus with intracapillary glomerulonephrosis
      Type 2 diabetes mellitus with Kimmelstiel-Wilson disease

   E11.22   Type 2 diabetes mellitus with Ebstein's disease
      Type 2 diabetes mellitus with renal tubular degeneration

   E11.23   Type 2 diabetes mellitus with diabetic renal failure
      Type 2 diabetes mellitus with renal failure in conditions classified to .21 and .22

   E11.29   Type 2 diabetes mellitus with other diabetic renal complication

E11.3   Type 2 diabetes mellitus with ophthalmic complications

   E11.30   Type 2 diabetes mellitus with diabetic ophthalmic complication, unspecified

   E11.31   Type 2 diabetes mellitus with diabetic background retinopathy
      Type 2 diabetes mellitus with diabetic retinopathy NOS

   E11.32   Type 2 diabetes mellitus with diabetic proliferative retinopathy

   E11.33   Type 2 diabetes mellitus with diabetic cataract

   E11.39   Type 2 diabetes mellitus with other diabetic ophthalmic complication

E11.4   Type 2 diabetes mellitus with neurological complications

   E11.40   Type 2 diabetes mellitus with diabetic neuropathy, unspecified

   E11.41   Type 2 diabetes mellitus with diabetic mononeuropathy

   E11.42   Type 2 diabetes mellitus with diabetic polyneuropathy
      Type 2 diabetes mellitus with diabetic neuralgia

   E11.43   Type 2 diabetes mellitus with diabetic autonomic (poly)neuropathy
      Type 2 diabetes mellitus with diabetic gastroparesis

   E11.44   Type 2 diabetes mellitus with diabetic amyotrophy
      Type 2 diabetes mellitus with diabetic myasthenia

   E11.49   Type 2 diabetes mellitus with other diabetic neurological complication

E11.5   Type 2 diabetes mellitus with circulatory complications

   E11.51   Type 2 diabetes mellitus with diabetic peripheral angiopathy without gangrene

   E11.52   Type 2 diabetes mellitus with diabetic peripheral angiopathy with gangrene
      Type 2 diabetes mellitus with diabetic gangrene

   E11.59   Type 2 diabetes mellitus with other circulatory complications

E11.6   Type 2 diabetes mellitus with other specified complications

   E11.61   Type 2 diabetes mellitus with diabetic arthropathy

      E11.610   Type 2 diabetes mellitus with diabetic neuropathic arthropathy
         Type 2 diabetes mellitus with Charcot's joints

      E11.618   Type 2 diabetes mellitus with other diabetic arthropathy

   E11.62   Type 2 diabetes mellitus with skin complications

      E11.620   Type 2 diabetes mellitus with diabetic dermatitis
         Type 2 diabetes mellitus with diabetic necrobiosis lipoidica

      E11.621   Type 2 diabetes mellitus with foot ulcer
         Use additional code to identify site of ulcer (L97.4-, L97.5-)

      E11.622   Type 2 diabetes mellitus with other skin ulcer
         Use additional code to identify site of ulcer (L97.1-L97.9, L98.41-L98.49)

      E11.628   Type 2 diabetes mellitus with other skin complications

   E11.63   Type 2 diabetes mellitus with oral complications

      E11.630   Type 2 diabetes mellitus with periodontal disease

      E11.638   Type 2 diabetes mellitus with other oral complications

   E11.64   Type 2 diabetes mellitus with hypoglycemia

      E11.640   Type 2 diabetes mellitus with hypoglycemia without coma

      E11.641   Type 2 diabetes mellitus with hypoglycemia with coma

   E11.65   Type 2 diabetes mellitus with hyperglycemia

   E11.69   Type 2 diabetes mellitus with other specified complication
      Use additional code to identify complication

E11.8   Type 2 diabetes mellitus with unspecified complications

E11.9   Type 2 diabetes mellitus without complications

E13 Other specified diabetes mellitus

Includes: diabetes mellitus due to genetic defects of β-cell function
            diabetes mellitus due to genetic defects in insulin action

Use additional code to identify any insulin use (Z79.7)

Excludes1:   diabetes (mellitus) due to autoimmune process (E10.-)
            diabetes (mellitus) due to immune mediated pancreatic islet β-cell destruction (E10.-)
            diabetes mellitus due to underlying condition (E08.-)
            drug or chemical induced diabetes mellitus (E09.-)
            gestational diabetes (O24.44)
            type 2 diabetes mellitus (E11.-)
            unspecified diabetes mellitus (E14.-)

E13.0   Other specified diabetes mellitus with hyperosmolarity

   E13.00   Other specified diabetes mellitus with hyperosmolarity without nonketotic hyperglycemic-hyperosmolar coma (NKHHC)

   E13.01   Other specified diabetes mellitus with hyperosmolarity with coma

E13.1   Other specified diabetes mellitus with ketoacidosis

   E13.10   Other specified diabetes mellitus with ketoacidosis without coma

   E13.11   Other specified diabetes mellitus with ketoacidosis with coma

E13.2   Other specified diabetes mellitus with renal complications

   E13.21   Other specified diabetes mellitus with diabetic nephropathy
      Other specified diabetes mellitus with intercapillary glomerulosclerosis
      Other specified diabetes mellitus with intracapillary glomerulonephrosis
      Other specified diabetes mellitus with Kimmelstiel-Wilson disease

   E13.22   Other specified diabetes mellitus with Ebstein's disease
      Other specified diabetes mellitus with renal tubular degeneration

   E13.23   Other specified diabetes mellitus with diabetic renal failure
      Other specified diabetes mellitus with renal failure in conditions classified to .21 and .22

E13.29 Other specified diabetes mellitus with other diabetic renal complication

E13.3 Other specified diabetes mellitus with ophthalmic complications

E13.30 Other specified diabetes mellitus with diabetic ophthalmic complication, unspecified

E13.31 Other specified diabetes mellitus with diabetic background retinopathy
Other specified diabetes mellitus with diabetic retinopathy NOS

E13.32 Other specified diabetes mellitus with diabetic proliferative retinopathy

E13.33 Other specified diabetes mellitus with diabetic cataract

E13.39 Other specified diabetes mellitus with other diabetic ophthalmic complication

E13.4 Other specified diabetes mellitus with neurological complications

E13.40 Other specified diabetes mellitus with diabetic neuropathy, unspecified

E13.41 Other specified diabetes mellitus with diabetic mononeuropathy

E13.42 Other specified diabetes mellitus with diabetic polyneuropathy
Other specified diabetes mellitus with diabetic neuralgia

E13.43 Other specified diabetes mellitus with diabetic autonomic (poly)neuropathy
Other specified diabetes mellitus with diabetic gastroparesis

E13.44 Other specified diabetes mellitus with diabetic amyotrophy
Other specified diabetes mellitus with diabetic myasthenia

E13.49 Other specified diabetes mellitus with other diabetic neurological complication

E13.5 Other specified diabetes mellitus with circulatory complications

E13.51 Other specified diabetes mellitus with diabetic peripheral angiopathy without gangrene

E13.52 Other specified diabetes mellitus with diabetic peripheral angiopathy with gangrene
Other specified diabetes mellitus with diabetic gangrene

E13.59 Other specified diabetes mellitus with other circulatory complications

E13.6 Other specified diabetes mellitus with other specified complications

E13.61 Other specified diabetes mellitus with diabetic arthropathy

E13.610 Other specified diabetes mellitus with diabetic neuropathic arthropathy
Other specified diabetes mellitus with Charcot's joints

E13.618 Other specified diabetes mellitus with other diabetic arthropathy

E13.62 Other specified diabetes mellitus with skin complications

E13.620 Other specified diabetes mellitus with diabetic dermatitis
Other specified diabetes mellitus with diabetic necrobiosis lipoidica

E13.621 Other specified diabetes mellitus with foot ulcer
Use additional code to identify site of ulcer (L97.4-, L97.5-)

E13.622 Other specified diabetes mellitus with other skin ulcer
Use additional code to identify site of ulcer (L97.1-L97.9, L98.41-L98.49)

E13.628 Other specified diabetes mellitus with other skin complications

E13.63 Other specified diabetes mellitus with oral complications

E13.630 Other specified diabetes mellitus with periodontal disease

E13.638 Other specified diabetes mellitus with other oral complications

E13.64 Other specified diabetes mellitus with hypoglycemia

E13.640 Other specified diabetes mellitus with hypoglycemia without coma

E13.641 Other specified diabetes mellitus with hypoglycemia with coma

E13.65 Other specified diabetes mellitus with hyperglycemia

E13.69 Other specified diabetes mellitus with other specified complication
Use additional code to identify complication

E13.8 Other specified diabetes mellitus with unspecified complications

E13.9 Other specified diabetes mellitus without complications

E14 Unspecified diabetes mellitus
Includes:　diabetes (mellitus) NOS
Use additional code to identify any insulin use (Z79.7)
Excludes1:　diabetes mellitus due to underlying condition (E08.-)
drug or chemical induced diabetes mellitus (E09.-)
gestational diabetes (O24.4-)
type 1 diabetes mellitus (E10.-)
type 2 diabetes mellitus (E11.-)

E14.0 Unspecified diabetes mellitus with hyperosmolarity

E14.00 Unspecified diabetes mellitus with hyperosmolarity without nonketotic hyperglycemic-hyperosmolar coma (NKHHC)

E14.01 Unspecified diabetes mellitus with hyperosmolarity with nonketotic hyperglycemic-hyperosmolar (NKHHC) coma

E14.1 Unspecified diabetes mellitus with ketoacidosis

E14.10 Unspecified diabetes mellitus with ketoacidosis without coma

E14.11 Unspecified diabetes mellitus with ketoacidosis with coma

E14.2 Unspecified diabetes mellitus with renal complications

E14.21 Unspecified diabetes mellitus with diabetic nephropathy
Unspecified diabetes mellitus with intercapillary glomerulosclerosis
Unspecified diabetes mellitus with intracapillary glomerulonephrosis
Unspecified diabetes mellitus with Kimmelstiel-Wilson disease

E14.22 Unspecified diabetes mellitus with Ebstein's disease
Unspecified diabetes mellitus with renal tubular degeneration

E14.23 Unspecified diabetes mellitus with diabetic renal failure
Unspecified diabetes mellitus with renal failure in conditions classified to .21 and .22

E14.29 Unspecified diabetes mellitus with other diabetic renal complication

E14.3 Unspecified diabetes mellitus with ophthalmic complications

E14.30 Unspecified diabetes mellitus with diabetic ophthalmic complication, unspecified

E14.31 Unspecified diabetes mellitus with diabetic background retinopathy
Unspecified diabetes mellitus with diabetic retinopathy NOS

E14.32 Unspecified diabetes mellitus with diabetic proliferative retinopathy

E14.33 Unspecified diabetes mellitus with diabetic cataract

E14.39 Unspecified diabetes mellitus with other diabetic ophthalmic complication

E14.4 Unspecified diabetes mellitus with neurological complications

E14.40 Unspecified diabetes mellitus with diabetic neuropathy, unspecified

E14.41 Unspecified diabetes mellitus with diabetic mononeuropathy

E14.42   **Unspecified diabetes mellitus with diabetic polyneuropathy**
  Unspecified diabetes mellitus with diabetic neuralgia

E14.43   **Unspecified diabetes mellitus with diabetic autonomic (poly)neuropathy**
  Unspecified diabetes mellitus with diabetic gastroparesis

E14.44   **Unspecified diabetes mellitus with diabetic amyotrophy**
  Unspecified diabetes mellitus with diabetic myasthenia

E14.49   **Unspecified diabetes mellitus with other diabetic neurological complication**

E14.5   **Unspecified diabetes mellitus with circulatory complications**

E14.51   **Unspecified diabetes mellitus with diabetic peripheral angiopathy without gangrene**

E14.52   **Unspecified diabetes mellitus with diabetic peripheral angiopathy with gangrene**
  Unspecified diabetes mellitus with diabetic gangrene

E14.59   **Unspecified diabetes mellitus with other circulatory complications**

E14.6   **Unspecified diabetes mellitus with other specified complications**

E14.61   **Unspecified diabetes mellitus with diabetic arthropathy**

 E14.610   **Unspecified diabetes mellitus with diabetic neuropathic arthropathy**
   Unspecified diabetes mellitus with Charcot's joints

 E14.618   **Unspecified diabetes mellitus with other diabetic arthropathy**

E14.62   **Unspecified diabetes mellitus with skin complications**

 E14.620   **Unspecified diabetes mellitus with diabetic dermatitis**
   Unspecified diabetes mellitus with diabetic necrobiosis lipoidica

 E14.621   **Unspecified diabetes mellitus with foot ulcer**
   Use additional code to identify site of ulcer (L97.4-, L97.5-)

 E14.622   **Unspecified diabetes mellitus with other skin ulcer**
   Use additional code to identify site of ulcer (L97.1-L97.9, L98.41-L98.49)

 E14.628   **Unspecified diabetes mellitus with other skin complications**

E14.63   **Unspecified diabetes mellitus with oral complications**

 E14.630   **Unspecified diabetes mellitus with periodontal disease**

 E14.638   **Unspecified diabetes mellitus with other oral complications**

E14.64   **Unspecified diabetes mellitus with hypoglycemia**

 E14.640   **Unspecified diabetes mellitus with hypoglycemia without coma**

 E14.641   **Unspecified diabetes mellitus with hypoglycemia with coma**

E14.65   **Unspecified diabetes mellitus with hyperglycemia**

E14.69   **Unspecified diabetes mellitus with other specified complication**
  Use additional code to identify complication

E14.8   **Unspecified diabetes mellitus with unspecified complications**

E14.9   **Unspecified diabetes mellitus without complications**

OTHER DISORDERS OF GLUCOSE REGULATION AND PANCREATIC INTERNAL SECRETION (E15–E16)

E15 Nondiabetic hypoglycemic coma
 Includes: drug-induced insulin coma in nondiabetic
    hyperinsulinism with hypoglycemic coma
    hypoglycemic coma NOS
 Use additional external cause code (Chapter XIX) to identify drug, if drug-induced.

E16 Other disorders of pancreatic internal secretion

E16.0   **Drug-induced hypoglycemia without coma**
  Use additional external cause code (Chapter XIX) to identify drug.

E16.1   **Other hypoglycemia**
  Functional hyperinsulinism
  Functional nonhyperinsulinemic hypoglycemia
  Hyperinsulinism NOS
  Hyperplasia of pancreatic islet beta cells NOS
  Excludes1: hypoglycemia in infant of diabetic mother (P70.1)
     neonatal hypoglycemia (P70.4)

E16.2   **Hypoglycemia, unspecified**

E16.3   **Increased secretion of glucagon**
  Hyperplasia of pancreatic endocrine cells with glucagon excess

E16.4   **Increased secretion of gastrin**
  Hypergastrinemia
  Hyperplasia of pancreatic endocrine cells with gastrin excess
  Zollinger-Ellison syndrome

E16.8   **Other specified disorders of pancreatic internal secretion**
  Increased secretion from endocrine pancreas of growth hormone-releasing hormone
  Increased secretion from endocrine pancreas of pancreatic polypeptide
  Increased secretion from endocrine pancreas of somatostatin
  Increased secretion from endocrine pancreas of vasoactive-intestinal polypeptide

E16.9   **Disorder of pancreatic internal secretion, unspecified**
  Islet-cell hyperplasia NOS
  Pancreatic endocrine cell hyperplasia NOS

DISORDERS OF OTHER ENDOCRINE GLANDS (E20–E35)
 Excludes1: galactorrhea (N64.3)
     gynecomastia (N62)

E20 Hypoparathyroidism
 Excludes1: Di George's syndrome (D82.1)
     postprocedural hypoparathyroidism (E89.2)
     tetany NOS (R29.0)
     transitory neonatal hypoparathyroidism (P71.4)

E20.0   **Idiopathic hypoparathyroidism**

E20.1   **Pseudohypoparathyroidism**

E20.8   **Other hypoparathyroidism**

E20.9   **Hypoparathyroidism, unspecified**
  Parathyroid tetany

E21 Hyperparathyroidism and other disorders of parathyroid gland
 Excludes1: adult osteomalacia (M83.-)
     ectopic hyperparathyroidism (E34.2)
     familial hypocalciuric hypercalcemia (E83.52)
     infantile and juvenile osteomalacia (E55.0)

E21.0   **Primary hyperparathyroidism**
  Hyperplasia of parathyroid
  Osteitis fibrosa cystica generalisata [von Recklinghausen's disease of bone]

E21.1   **Secondary hyperparathyroidism, not elsewhere classified**
  Excludes1: secondary hyperparathyroidism of renal origin (N25.8)

E21.2   **Other hyperparathyroidism**
  Excludes1: familial hypocalciuric hypercalcaemia (E83.52)

E21.3   **Hyperparathyroidism, unspecified**

E21.4   **Other specified disorders of parathyroid gland**

E21.5   **Disorder of parathyroid gland, unspecified**

E22 Hyperfunction of pituitary gland
 Excludes1: Cushing's syndrome (E24.-)
     Nelson's syndrome (E24.1)
     overproduction of ACTH not associated with Cushing's disease (E27.0)
     overproduction of pituitary ACTH (E24.0)
     overproduction of thyroid-stimulating hormone (E05.8-)

E22.0   **Acromegaly and pituitary gigantism**
  Overproduction of growth hormone
  Excludes1: constitutional gigantism (E34.4)
     constitutional tall stature (E34.4)
     increased secretion from endocrine pancreas of growth hormone-releasing hormone (E16.8)

E22.1   Hyperprolactinemia
Use additional external cause code (Chapter XIX) to identify drug, if drug-induced.

E22.2   Syndrome of inappropriate secretion of antidiuretic hormone

E22.8   Other hyperfunction of pituitary gland
Central precocious puberty

E22.9   Hyperfunction of pituitary gland, unspecified

E23   Hypofunction and other disorders of the pituitary gland
Includes: the listed conditions whether the disorder is in the pituitary or the hypothalamus
Excludes1:   postprocedural hypopituitarism (E89.3)

E23.0   Hypopituitarism
Fertile eunuch syndrome
Hypogonadotropic hypogonadism
Idiopathic growth hormone deficiency
Isolated deficiency of gonadotropin
Isolated deficiency of growth hormone
Isolated deficiency of pituitary hormone
Kallmann's syndrome
Lorain-Levi short stature
Necrosis of pituitary gland (postpartum)
Panhypopituitarism
Pituitary cachexia
Pituitary insufficiency NOS
Pituitary short stature
Sheehan's syndrome
Simmonds' disease

E23.1   Drug-induced hypopituitarism
Use additional external cause code (Chapter XIX) to identify drug.

E23.2   Diabetes insipidus
Excludes1:   nephrogenic diabetes insipidus (N25.1)

E23.3   Hypothalamic dysfunction, not elsewhere classified
Excludes1:   Prader-Willi syndrome (Q87.1)
Russell-Silver syndrome (Q87.1)

E23.6   Other disorders of pituitary gland
Abscess of pituitary
Adiposogenital dystrophy

E23.7   Disorder of pituitary gland, unspecified

E24   Cushing's syndrome
Excludes1:   congenital adrenal hyperplasia (E25.0)

E24.0   Pituitary-dependent Cushing's disease
Overproduction of pituitary ACTH
Pituitary-dependent hypercorticalism

E24.1   Nelson's syndrome

E24.2   Drug-induced Cushing's syndrome
Use additional external cause code (Chapter XIX) to identify drug

E24.3   Ectopic ACTH syndrome

E24.4   Alcohol-induced pseudo-Cushing's syndrome

E24.8   Other Cushing's syndrome

E24.9   Cushing's syndrome, unspecified

E25   Adrenogenital disorders
Includes: adrenogenital syndromes, virilizing or feminizing, whether acquired or due to adrenal hyperplasia consequent on inborn enzyme defects in hormone synthesis
female:
adrenal pseudohermaphroditism
heterosexual precocious pseudopuberty
male:
isosexual precocious pseudopuberty
macrogenitosomia praecox
sexual precocity with adrenal hyperplasia
virilization (female)

E25.0   Congenital adrenogenital disorders associated with enzyme deficiency
Congenital adrenal hyperplasia
21-Hydroxylase deficiency
Salt-losing congenital adrenal hyperplasia

E25.8   Other adrenogenital disorders
Idiopathic adrenogenital disorder
Use additional external cause code (Chapter XIX) to identify drug, if drug-induced.

E25.9   Adrenogenital disorder, unspecified
Adrenogenital syndrome NOS

E26   Hyperaldosteronism

E26.0   Primary hyperaldosteronism
Conn's syndrome
Primary aldosteronism due to adrenal hyperplasia (bilateral)

E26.1   Secondary hyperaldosteronism

E26.8   Other hyperaldosteronism
Bartter's syndrome

E26.9   Hyperaldosteronism, unspecified

E27   Other disorders of adrenal gland

E27.0   Other adrenocortical overactivity
Overproduction of ACTH, not associated with Cushing's disease
Premature adrenarche
Excludes1:   Cushing's syndrome (E24.-)

E27.1   Primary adrenocortical insufficiency
Addison's disease
Adrenocortical insufficiency NOS
Autoimmune adrenalitis
Excludes1:   Addison only phenotype adrenoleukodystrophy (E71.428)
amyloidosis (E85)
tuberculous Addison's disease (A18.7)
Waterhouse-Friderichsen syndrome (A39.1)

E27.2   Addisonian crisis
Adrenal crisis
Adrenocortical crisis

E27.3   Drug-induced adrenocortical insufficiency
Use additional external cause code (Chapter XIX) to identify drug.

E27.4   Other and unspecified adrenocortical insufficiency
Adrenal hemorrhage
Adrenal infarction
Adrenocortical insufficiency NOS
Hypoaldosteronism
Excludes1:   adrenoleukodystrophy [Addison-Schilder] (E71.3-)
Waterhouse-Friderichsen syndrome (A39.1)

E27.5   Adrenomedullary hyperfunction
Adrenomedullary hyperplasia
Catecholamine hypersecretion

E27.8   Other specified disorders of adrenal gland
Abnormality of cortisol-binding globulin

E27.9   Disorder of adrenal gland, unspecified

E28   Ovarian dysfunction
Excludes1:   isolated gonadotropin deficiency (E23.0)
postprocedural ovarian failure (E89.4)

E28.0   Estrogen excess
Use additional external cause code (Chapter XIX) to identify drug, if drug-induced.

E28.1   Androgen excess
Hypersecretion of ovarian androgens
Use additional external cause code (Chapter XIX) to identify drug, if drug-induced.

E28.2   Polycystic ovarian syndrome
Sclerocystic ovary syndrome
Stein-Leventhal syndrome

E28.3   Primary ovarian failure
Excludes1:   pure gonadal dysgenesis (Q56.0)
Turner's syndrome (Q96.-)

E28.31   Premature menopause

E28.39   Other primary ovarian failure
Decreased estrogen
Resistant ovary syndrome

E28.8   Other ovarian dysfunction
Ovarian hyperfunction NOS
Excludes1:   postprocedural ovarian failure (E89.4)

E28.9   Ovarian dysfunction, unspecified

E29 Testicular dysfunction
Excludes1:   androgen resistance syndrome (E34.5)
          azoospermia or oligospermia NOS (N46.0-N46.1)
          isolated gonadotropin deficiency (E23.0)
          Klinefelter's syndrome (Q98.0-Q98.2, Q98.4)
          testicular feminization (syndrome) (E34.5)

E29.0 Testicular hyperfunction
Hypersecretion of testicular hormones

E29.1 Testicular hypofunction
Defective biosynthesis of testicular androgen NOS
5-α-reductase deficiency (with male pseudohermaphroditism)
Testicular hypogonadism NOS
Use additional external cause code (Chapter XIX) to identify drug, if drug-induced.
Excludes1:   postprocedural testicular hypofunction (E89.5)

E29.8 Other testicular dysfunction

E29.9 Testicular dysfunction, unspecified

E30 Disorders of puberty, not elsewhere classified

E30.0 Delayed puberty
Constitutional delay of puberty
Delayed sexual development

E30.1 Precocious puberty
Precocious menstruation
Excludes1:   Albright (-McCune) (-Sternberg) syndrome (Q78.1)
          central precocious puberty (E22.8)
          congenital adrenal hyperplasia (E25.0)
          female heterosexual precocious pseudopuberty (E25.-)
          male isosexual precocious pseudopuberty (E25.-)

E30.8 Other disorders of puberty
Premature thelarche

E30.9 Disorder of puberty, unspecified

E31 Polyglandular dysfunction
Excludes1:   ataxia telangiectasia [Louis-Bar] (G11.3)
          dystrophia myotonica [Steinert] (G71.1)
          pseudohypoparathyroidism (E20.1)

E31.0 Autoimmune polyglandular failure
Schmidt's syndrome

E31.1 Polyglandular hyperfunction
Excludes1:   multiple endocrine adenomatosis (D44.8)

E31.8 Other polyglandular dysfunction

E31.9 Polyglandular dysfunction, unspecified

E32 Diseases of thymus
Excludes1:   aplasia or hypoplasia of thymus with immunodeficiency (D82.1)
          myasthenia gravis (G70.0)

E32.0 Persistent hyperplasia of thymus
Hypertrophy of thymus

E32.1 Abscess of thymus

E32.8 Other diseases of thymus
Excludes1:   aplasia or hypoplasia with immunodeficiency (D82.1)
          thymoma (D15.0)

E32.9 Disease of thymus, unspecified

E34 Other endocrine disorders
Excludes1:   pseudohypoparathyroidism (E20.1)

E34.0 Carcinoid syndrome
Note: May be used as an additional code to identify functional activity associated with a carcinoid tumor.

E34.1 Other hypersecretion of intestinal hormones

E34.2 Ectopic hormone secretion, not elsewhere classified
Excludes1:   ectopic ACTH syndrome (E24.3)

E34.3 Short stature, not elsewhere classified
Constitutional short stature
Laron-type short stature
Psychosocial short stature
Short stature NOS
Excludes1:   progeria (E34.8)
          Russell-Silver syndrome (Q87.1)
          short-limbed stature with immunodeficiency (D82.2)
          short stature:
            achondroplastic (Q77.4)
            hypochondroplastic (Q77.4)
            in specific dysmorphic syndromes - code to syndrome - see Alphabetical Index
            nutritional (E45)
            pituitary (E23.0)
            renal (N25.0)

E34.4 Constitutional tall stature
Constitutional gigantism

E34.5 Androgen resistance syndrome
Male pseudohermaphroditism with androgen resistance
Peripheral hormonal receptor disorder
Reifenstein's syndrome
Testicular feminization syndrome

E34.8 Other specified endocrine disorders
Pineal gland dysfunction
Progeria
Excludes2:   pseudohypoparathyroidism (E20.1)

E34.9 Endocrine disorder, unspecified
Endocrine disturbance NOS
Hormone disturbance NOS

E35 Disorders of endocrine glands in diseases classified elsewhere
Code first underlying disease, such as:
late congenital syphilis of thymus gland [Dubois disease] (A50.5)
tuberculous calcification of adrenal gland (B90.8)
Excludes1:   Echinococcus granulosus infection of thyroid gland (B67.3)
          meningococcal hemorrhagic adrenalitis (A39.1)
          syphilis of endocrine gland (A52.79)
          tuberculosis of:
            adrenal gland, except calcification (A18.7)
            endocrine gland NEC (A18.82)
            thyroid gland (A18.81)
          Waterhouse-Friderichsen syndrome (A39.1)

E36 Intraoperative and postprocedural complications of endocrine procedures
Excludes1:   postprocedural endocrine and metabolic disorders, not elsewhere classified (E89.-)

E36.0 Intraoperative and postprocedural hemorrhage or hematoma complicating an endocrine procedure
Excludes1:   intraoperative hemorrhage or hematoma due to accidental puncture or laceration during an endocrine procedure (E36.1-)

E36.01 Intraoperative hemorrhage of an endocrine organ during an endocrine procedure

E36.02 Intraoperative hemorrhage of other organ during an endocrine procedure

E36.03 Intraoperative hematoma of an endocrine organ during an endocrine procedure

E36.04 Intraoperative hematoma of other organ during an endocrine procedure

E36.05 Postprocedural hemorrhage of an endocrine organ following an endocrine procedure

E36.06 Postprocedural hemorrhage of other organ following an endocrine procedure

E36.07 Postprocedural hematoma of an endocrine organ following an endocrine procedure

E36.08 Postprocedural hematoma of other organ following an endocrine procedure

E36.1 Accidental puncture or laceration of an endocrine organ during an endocrine procedure

E36.11 Accidental puncture or laceration of an endocrine organ during an endocrine procedure

E36.12   Accidental puncture or laceration of other organs during an endocrine procedure

E36.8   Other intraoperative and postprocedural complications of endocrine procedures

E36.81   Other intraoperative complications of endocrine procedures

E36.89   Other postprocedural complications of endocrine procedures

MALNUTRITION (E40–E46)

Excludes1:   intestinal malabsorption (K90.-)
             sequelae of protein-calorie malnutrition (E64.0)

Excludes2:   nutritional anemias (D50-D53)
             starvation (T73.0)

E40   Kwashiorkor

Includes: severe malnutrition with nutritional edema with dyspigmentation of skin and hair

Excludes1:   marasmic kwashiorkor (E42)

E41   Nutritional marasmus

Includes: severe malnutrition with marasmus

Excludes1:   marasmic kwashiorkor (E42)

E42   Marasmic kwashiorkor

Includes: severe protein-calorie malnutrition with signs of both kwashiorkor and marasmus
             intermediate form severe protein-calorie malnutrition

E43   Unspecified severe protein-calorie malnutrition

Includes: starvation edema

E44   Protein-calorie malnutrition of moderate and mild degree

E44.0   Moderate protein-calorie malnutrition

E44.1   Mild protein-calorie malnutrition

E45   Retarded development following protein-calorie malnutrition

Includes   nutritional short stature
             nutritional stunting
             physical retardation due to malnutrition

E46   Unspecified protein- calorie malnutrition NOS

Includes: malnutrition
             protein-calorie imbalance NOS

Excludes1:   nutritional deficiency NOS (E63.9)

OTHER NUTRITIONAL DEFICIENCIES (E50–E64)

Excludes2:   nutritional anemias (D50-D53)

E50   Vitamin A deficiency

Excludes1:   sequelae of vitamin A deficiency (E64.1)

E50.0   Vitamin A deficiency with conjunctival xerosis

E50.1   Vitamin A deficiency with Bitot's spot and conjunctival xerosis
             Bitot's spot in the young child

E50.2   Vitamin A deficiency with corneal xerosis

E50.3   Vitamin A deficiency with corneal ulceration and xerosis

E50.4   Vitamin A deficiency with keratomalacia

E50.5   Vitamin A deficiency with night blindness

E50.6   Vitamin A deficiency with xerophthalmic scars of cornea

E50.7   Other ocular manifestations of vitamin A deficiency
             Xerophthalmia NOS

E50.8   Other manifestations of vitamin A deficiency
             Follicular keratosis
             Xeroderma

E50.9   Vitamin A deficiency, unspecified
             Hypovitaminosis A NOS

E51   Thiamine deficiency

Excludes1:   sequelae of thiamine deficiency (E64.8)

E51.1   Beriberi

E51.11   Dry beriberi
             Beriberi NOS
             Beriberi with polyneuropathy

E51.12   Wet beriberi
             Beriberi with cardiovascular manifestations
             Cardiovascular beriberi
             Shoshin disease

E51.2   Wernicke's encephalopathy

E51.8   Other manifestations of thiamine deficiency

E51.9   Thiamine deficiency, unspecified

E52   Niacin deficiency [pellagra]

Includes: niacin (-tryptophan) deficiency
             nicotinamide deficiency
             pellagra (alcoholic)

Excludes1:   sequelae of niacin deficiency (E64.8)

E53   Deficiency of other B group vitamins

Excludes1:   sequelae of vitamin B deficiency (E64.8)

E53.0   Riboflavin deficiency
             Ariboflavinosis
             Vitamin B_2 deficiency

E53.1   Pyridoxine deficiency
             Vitamin B_6 deficiency

Excludes1:   pyridoxine-responsive sideroblastic anemia (D64.3)

E53.8   Deficiency of other specified B group vitamins
             Biotin deficiency
             Cyanocobalamin deficiency
             Folate deficiency
             Folic acid deficiency
             Pantothenic acid deficiency
             Vitamin B_{12} deficiency

Excludes1:   folate deficiency anemia (D52.-)
             vitamin B_{12} deficiency anemia (D51.-)

E53.9   Vitamin B deficiency, unspecified

E54   Ascorbic acid deficiency

Includes: deficiency of vitamin C
             scurvy

Excludes1:   scorbutic anemia (D53.2)
             sequelae of vitamin C deficiency (E64.2)

E55   Vitamin D deficiency

Excludes1:   adult osteomalacia (M83.-)
             osteoporosis (M80-)
             sequelae of rickets (E64.3)

E55.0   Rickets, active
             Infantile osteomalacia
             Juvenile osteomalacia

Excludes1:   celiac rickets (K90.0)
             Crohn's rickets (K50.-)
             hereditary vitamin D-dependent rickets (E83.32)
             inactive rickets (E64.3)
             renal rickets (N25.0)
             sequelae of rickets (E64.3)
             vitamin D-resistant rickets (E83.31)

E55.9   Vitamin D deficiency, unspecified
             Avitaminosis D

E56   Other vitamin deficiencies

Excludes1:   sequelae of other vitamin deficiencies (E64.8)

E56.0   Deficiency of vitamin E

E56.1   Deficiency of vitamin K

Excludes1:   deficiency of coagulation factor due to vitamin K deficiency (D68.4)
             vitamin K deficiency of newborn (P53)

E56.8   Deficiency of other vitamins

E56.9 Vitamin deficiency, unspecified

E58   Dietary calcium deficiency

Excludes1:   disorders of calcium metabolism (E83.5)
             sequelae of calcium deficiency (E64.8)

E59   Dietary selenium deficiency

Includes: Keshan disease

Excludes1:   sequelae of selenium deficiency (E64.8)

E60 Dietary zinc deficiency

E61 Deficiency of other nutrient elements
Use additional external cause code (Chapter XIX) to identify drug, if drug-induced.
Excludes1: disorders of mineral metabolism (E83.-)
iodine deficiency related thyroid disorders (E00-E02)
sequelae of malnutrition and other nutritional deficiencies (E64.-)

E61.0 Copper deficiency
E61.1 Iron deficiency
Excludes1: iron deficiency anemia (D50.-)
E61.2 Magnesium deficiency
E61.3 Manganese deficiency
E61.4 Chromium deficiency
E61.5 Molybdenum deficiency
E61.6 Vanadium deficiency
E61.7 Deficiency of multiple nutrient elements
E61.8 Deficiency of other specified nutrient elements
E61.9 Deficiency of nutrient element, unspecified

E63 Other nutritional deficiencies
Excludes1: dehydration (E86.0)
failure to thrive, adult (R62.7)
failure to thrive, child (R62.51)
feeding problems in newborn (P92.-)
sequelae of malnutrition and other nutritional deficiencies (E64.-)
E63.0 Essential fatty acid [EFA] deficiency
E63.1 Imbalance of constituents of food intake
E63.8 Other specified nutritional deficiencies
E63.9 Nutritional deficiency, unspecified

E64 Sequelae of malnutrition and other nutritional deficiencies
This category is to be used to indicate conditions in categories E43, E44, E46, E50-E63 as the cause of sequelae, which are themselves classified elsewhere. The "sequelae" include conditions specified as such; they also include the late effects of diseases classifiable to the above categories if the disease itself is no longer present
Code first the condition
E64.0 Sequelae of protein-calorie malnutrition
Excludes2: retarded development following protein-calorie malnutrition (E45)
E64.1 Sequelae of vitamin A deficiency
E64.2 Sequelae of vitamin C deficiency
E64.3 Sequelae of rickets
E64.8 Sequelae of other nutritional deficiencies
E64.9 Sequelae of unspecified nutritional deficiency

OBESITY AND OTHER HYPERALIMENTATION (E65–E68)

E65 Localized adiposity
Includes: fat pad

E66 Obesity
Excludes1: adiposogenital dystrophy (E23.6)
lipomatosis NOS (E88.2)
lipomatosis dolorosa [Dercum] (E88.2)
Prader-Willi syndrome (Q87.1)
E66.0 Obesity due to excess calories
E66.01 Morbid obesity due to excess calories
Excludes1: morbid obesity with alveolar hypoventilation (E66.2)
E66.09 Other obesity due to excess calories
E66.1 Drug-induced obesity
Use additional external cause code (Chapter XIX) to identify drug.
E66.2 Extreme obesity with alveolar hypoventilation
Pickwickian syndrome
E66.8 Other obesity
E66.9 Obesity, unspecified
Simple obesity NOS

E67 Other hyperalimentation
Excludes1: hyperalimentation NOS (R63.2)
sequelae of hyperalimentation (E68)
E67.0 Hypervitaminosis A
E67.1 Hypercarotinemia
E67.2 Megavitamin-B$_6$ syndrome
E67.3 Hypervitaminosis D
E67.8 Other specified hyperalimentation

E68 Sequelae of hyperalimentation

METABOLIC DISORDERS (E70–E90)
Excludes1: androgen resistance syndrome (E34.5)
congenital adrenal hyperplasia (E25.0)
Ehlers-Danlos syndrome (Q79.6)
hemolytic anemias attributable to enzyme disorders (D55.-)
Marfan's syndrome (Q87.4)
5-α-reductase deficiency (E29.1)

E70 Disorders of aromatic amino-acid metabolism
E70.0 Classical phenylketonuria
E70.1 Other hyperphenylalaninemias
E70.2 Disorders of tyrosine metabolism
Excludes1: transitory tyrosinemia of newborn (P74.5)
E70.20 Disorder of tyrosine metabolism, unspecified
E70.21 Tyrosinemia
Hypertyrosinemia
E70.29 Other disorders of tyrosine metabolism
Alkaptonuria
Ochronosis
E70.3 Albinism
E70.30 Albinism, unspecified
E70.31 Ocular albinism
E70.310 X-linked ocular albinism
E70.311 Autosomal recessive ocular albinism
E70.318 Other ocular albinism
E70.319 Ocular albinism, unspecified
E70.32 Oculocutaneous albinism
Excludes1: Chediak-Higashi syndrome (E70.330)
Hermansky-Pudlak syndrome (E70.331)
E70.320 Tyrosinase negative oculocutaneous albinism
Albinism I
Oculocutaneous albinism ty-neg
E70.321 Tyrosinase positive oculocutaneous albinism
Albinsim II
Oculocutaneous albinism ty-pos
E70.328 Other oculocutaneous albinism
Cross syndrome
E70.329 Oculocutaneous albinism, unspecified
E70.33 Albinism with hematologic abnormality
E70.330 Chediak-Higashi syndrome
E70.331 Hermansky-Pudlak syndrome
E70.338 Other albinism with hematologic abnormality
E70.339 Albinism with hematologic abnormality, unspecified
E70.39 Other specified albinsim
Piebaldism
E70.4 Disorders of histidine metabolism
E70.40 Disorders of histidine metabolism, unspecified
E70.41 Histidinemia
E70.49 Other disorders of histidine metabolism
E70.5 Disorders of tryptophan metabolism
E70.8 Other disorders of aromatic amino-acid metabolism
E70.9 Disorder of aromatic amino-acid metabolism, unspecified

E71 Disorders of branched-chain amino-acid metabolism and fatty-acid metabolism
E71.0 Maple-syrup-urine disease
E71.1 Other disorders of branched-chain amino-acid metabolism
E71.11 Branched-chain organic acidurias

E71.110   Isovaleric acidemia
E71.111   3-methylglutaconic aciduria
E71.118   Other branched-chain organic acidurias
E71.12   Disorders of propionate metabolism
E71.120   Methylmalonic acidemia
E71.121   Propionic acidemia
E71.128   Other disorders of propionate metabolism
E71.19   Other disorders of branched-chain amino-acid metabolism
    Hyperleucine-isoleucinemia
    Hypervalinemia
E71.2   Disorder of branched-chain amino-acid metabolism, unspecified
E71.3   Disorders of fatty-acid metabolism
    Excludes1:   peroxisomal disorders (E71.4)
            Refsum's disease (G60.1)
            Schilder's disease (G37.0)
E71.30   Disorder of fatty-acid metabolism, unspecified
E71.31   Disorders of fatty-acid oxidation
E71.310   Long chain/very long chain acyl CoA dehydrogenase deficiency
    LCAD
    VLCAD
E71.311   Medium chain acyl CoA dehydrogenase deficiency
    MCAD
E71.312   Short chain acyl CoA dehydrogenase deficiency
    SCAD
E71.313   Glutaric aciduria type II
    Glutaric aciduria type II A
    Glutaric aciduria type II B
    Glutaric aciduria type II C
    Excludes1:   glutaric aciduria (type 1) NOS (E72.3)
E71.318   Other disorders of fatty-acid oxidation
E71.32   Disorders of carnitine metabolism
E71.320   Carnitine insufficiency
E71.321   Ruvalcaba-Myhre-Smith syndrome
E71.322   Secondary carnitine deficiency
E71.328   Other disorders of carnitine metabolism
    Muscle carnitine palmityltransferase deficiency
E71.329   Disorder of carnitine metabolism, unspecified
E71.33   Disorders of ketone metabolism
E71.39   Other disorders of fatty-acid metabolism
    Excludes1:   peroxisomal disorders (E71.4)
E71.4   Peroxisomal disorders
    Excludes1:   Schilder's disease (G37.0)
E71.40   Peroxisomal disorder, unspecified
E71.41   Disorders of peroxisome biogenesis
    Group 1 peroxisomal disorders
    Excludes1:   Refsum's disease (G60.1)
E71.410   Zellweger syndrome
E71.411   Neonatal adrenoleukodystrophy
    Excludes1:   X-linked adrenoleukodystrophy (E71.42-)
E71.418   Other disorders of peroxisome biogenesis
E71.42   X-linked adrenoleukodystrophy
E71.420   Childhood cerebral X-linked adrenoleukodystrophy
E71.421   Adolescent X-linked adrenoleukodystrophy
E71.422   Adrenomyeloneuropathy
E71.428   Other X-linked adrenoleukodystrophy
    Addison only phenotype adrenoleukodystrophy
    Addison-Schilder adrenoleukodystrophy
E71.429   X-linked adrenoleukodystrophy, unspecified
E71.43   Other group 2 peroxisomal disorders
E71.44   Other peroxisomal disorders
E71.440   Rhizomelic chondrodysplasia punctata
    Excludes1:   chondrodysplasia punctata NOS (Q77.3)

E71.441   Zellweger-like syndrome
E71.442   Other group 3 peroxisomal disorders
E71.448   Other peroxisomal disorders

E72   Other disorders of amino-acid metabolism
    Excludes1:   disorders of:
            aromatic amino-acid metabolism (E70.-)
            branched-chain amino-acid metabolism (E71.0-E71.2)
            fatty-acid metabolism (E71.3)
            purine and pyrimidine metabolism (E79.-)
            gout (M10.-)
E72.0   Disorders of amino-acid transport
    Excludes1:   disorders of tryptophan metabolism (E70.5)
E72.00   Disorders of amino-acid transport, unspecified
E72.01   Cystinuria
E72.02   Hartnup's disease
E72.03   Lowe's syndrome
    Use additional code for associated glaucoma (H42)
E72.04   Cystinosis
    Fanconi (-de Toni) (-Debré) syndrome with cystinosis
    Excludes1:   Fanconi (-de Toni) (-Debré) syndrome without cystinosis (E72.09)
E72.09   Other disorders of amino-acid transport
    Fanconi (-de Toni) (-Debré) syndrome, unspecified
E72.1   Disorders of sulphur-bearing amino-acid metabolism
    Excludes1:   cystinosis (E72.04)
            cystinuria (E72.01)
            transcobalamin II deficiency (D51.2)
E72.10   Disorders of sulphur-bearing amino-acid metabolism, unspecified
E72.11   Homocystinuria
    Cystathionine synthase deficiency
E72.12   Methylenetetrahydrofolate reductase deficiency
E72.19   Other disorders of sulphur-bearing amino-acid metabolism
    Cystathioninuria
    Methioninemia
    Sulfite oxidase deficiency
E72.2   Disorders of urea cycle metabolism
    Excludes1:   disorders of ornithine metabolism (E72.4)
E72.20   Disorder of urea cycle metabolism, unspecified
    Hyperammonemia
    Excludes1:   transient hyperammonemia of newborn (P74.6)
E72.21   Argininemia
E72.22   Arginosuccinic aciduria
E72.23   Citrullinemia
E72.24   Ornithine transcarbamylase deficiency
E72.29   Other disorders of urea cycle metabolism
E72.3   Disorders of lysine and hydroxylysine metabolism
    Glutaric aciduria NOS
    Glutaric aciduria (type I)
    Hydroxylysinemia
    Hyperlysinemia
    Excludes1:   glutaric aciduria type II (E71.313)
E72.4   Disorders of ornithine metabolism
    Ornithinemia (types I, II)
    Excludes1:   hereditary choroidal dystrophy (H31.2-)
            ornithine transcarbamylase deficiency (E72.24)
E72.5   Disorders of glycine metabolism
E72.50   Disorder of glycine metabolism, unspecified
E72.51   Non-ketotic hyperglycinemia
E72.52   Trimethylaminuria
E72.53   Hyperoxaluria
    Oxalosis
    Oxaluria
E72.59   Other disorders of glycine metabolism
    D-glycericacidemia
    Hyperhydroxyprolincmia
    Hyperprolinemia (types I, II)
    Sarcosinemia

E72.8   **Other specified disorders of amino-acid metabolism**
Disorders of β-amino-acid metabolism
Disorders of γ-glutamyl cycle
E72.9   **Disorder of amino-acid metabolism, unspecified**

E73   Lactose intolerance
E73.0   **Congenital lactase deficiency**
E73.1   **Secondary lactase deficiency**
E73.8   **Other lactose intolerance**
E73.9   **Lactose intolerance, unspecified**

E74   Other disorders of carbohydrate metabolism
Excludes1:   diabetes mellitus (E09-E13)
hypoglycemia NOS (E16.2)
increased secretion of glucagon (E16.3)
mucopolysaccharidosis (E76.0-E76.3)
E74.0   **Glycogen storage disease**
E74.00   **Glycogen storage disease, unspecified**
E74.01   **Von Gierke's disease**
Type I glycogen storage disease
E74.02   **Pompe's disease**
Cardiac glycogenosis
Type II glycogen storage disease
E74.03   **Cori's disease**
Forbes' disease
Type III glycogen storage disease
E74.04   **McArdle's disease**
Type V glycogen storage disease
E74.09   **Other glycogen storage disease**
Andersen's disease
Hers' disease
Tauri's disease
Glycogen storage disease, types 0, IV, VI-XI
Liver phosphorylase deficiency
Muscle phosphofructokinase deficiency
E74.1   **Disorders of fructose metabolism**
Excludes1:   muscle phosphofructokinase deficiency (E74.09)
E74.10   **Disorder of fructose metabolism, unspecified**
E74.11   **Essential fructosuria**
Fructokinase deficiency
E74.12   **Hereditary fructose intolerance**
Fructosemia
E74.19   **Other disorders of fructose metabolism**
Fructose-1, 6-diphosphatase deficiency
E74.2   **Disorders of galactose metabolism**
E74.20   **Disorders of galactose metabolism, unspecified**
E74.21   **Galactosemia**
E74.29   **Other disorders of galactose metabolism**
Galactokinase deficiency
E74.3   **Other disorders of intestinal carbohydrate absorption**
Excludes2:   lactose intolerance (E73.-)
E74.31   **Sucrase-isomaltase deficiency**
E74.39   **Other disorders of intestinal carbohydrate absorption**
Disorder of intestinal carbohydrate absorption NOS
Glucose-galactose malabsorption
Sucrase deficiency
E74.4   **Disorders of pyruvate metabolism and gluconeogenesis**
Deficiency of phosphoenolpyruvate carboxykinase
Deficiency of pyruvate carboxylase
Deficiency of pyruvate dehydrogenase
Excludes1:   disorders of pyruvate metabolism and gluconeogenesis with anemia (D55.-)
Leigh's syndrome (G31.82)
E74.8   **Other specified disorders of carbohydrate metabolism**
Essential pentosuria
Renal glycosuria
E74.9   **Disorder of carbohydrate metabolism, unspecified**

E75   Disorders of sphingolipid metabolism and other lipid storage disorders
Excludes1:   mucolipidosis, types I-III (E77.0-E77.1)
Refsum's disease (G60.1)

E75.0   **GM$_2$ gangliosidosis**
E75.00   **GM$_2$ gangliosidosis, unspecified**
E75.01   **Sandhoff disease**
E75.02   **Tay-Sachs disease**
E75.09   **Other GM$_2$ gangliosidosis**
Adult GM$_2$ gangliosidosis
Juvenile GM$_2$ gangliosidosis
E75.1   **Other and unspecified gangliosidosis**
E75.10   **Unspecified gangliosidosis**
Gangliosidosis NOS
E75.11   **Mucolipidosis IV**
E75.19   **Other gangliosidosis**
GM$_1$ gangliosidosis
GM$_3$ gangliosidosis
E75.2   **Other sphingolipidosis**
Excludes1:   adrenoleukodystrophy [Addison-Schilder] (E71.30)
E75.21   **Fabry (-Anderson) disease**
E75.22   **Gaucher disease**
E75.23   **Krabbe disease**
E75.24   **Niemann-Pick disease**
E75.240   **Niemann-Pick disease type A**
E75.241   **Niemann-Pick disease type B**
E75.242   **Niemann-Pick disease type C**
E75.243   **Niemann-Pick disease type D**
E75.248   **Other Niemann-Pick disease**
E75.249   **Niemann-Pick disease, unspecified**
E75.25   **Metachromatic leukodystrophy**
E75.29   **Other sphingolipidosis**
Farber's syndrome
Sulfatase deficiency
Sulfatide lipidosis
E75.3   **Sphingolipidosis, unspecified**
E75.4   **Neuronal ceroid lipofuscinosis**
Batten disease
Bielschowsky-Jansky disease
Kufs disease
Spielmeyer-Vogt disease
E75.5   **Other lipid storage disorders**
Cerebrotendinous cholesterosis [van Bogaert-Scherer-Epstein]
Wolman's disease
E75.6   **Lipid storage disorder, unspecified**

E76   Disorders of glycosaminoglycan metabolism
E76.0   **Mucopolysaccharidosis, type I**
E76.01   **Hurler's syndrome**
E76.02   **Hurler-Scheie syndrome**
E76.03   **Scheie's syndrome**
E76.1   **Mucopolysaccharidosis, type II**
Hunter's syndrome
E76.2   **Other mucopolysaccharidoses**
E76.21   **Morquio mucopolysaccharidoses**
E76.210   **Morquio A mucopolysaccharidoses**
Classic Morquio syndrome
Morquio syndrome A
Mucopolysaccharidosis, type IVA
E76.211   **Morquio B mucopolysaccharidoses**
Morquio-like mucopolysaccharidoses
Morquio-like syndrome
Morquio syndrome B
Mucopolysaccharidosis, type IVB
E76.219   **Morquio mucopolysaccharidoses, unspecified**
Morquio syndrome
Mucopolysaccharidosis, type IV
E76.22   **Sanfilippo mucopolysaccharidoses**
Mucopolysaccharidosis, type III (A) (B) (C) (D)
Sanfilippo A syndrome
Sanfilippo B syndrome
Sanfilippo C syndrome
Sanfilippo D syndrome

E76.29　　Other mucopolysaccharidoses
　　　　　　β-Glucuronidase deficiency
　　　　　　Maroteaux-Lamy (mild) (severe) syndrome
　　　　　　Mucopolysaccharidosis, types VI, VII
E76.3　Mucopolysaccharidosis, unspecified
E76.8　Other disorders of glucosaminoglycan metabolism
E76.9　Glucosaminoglycan metabolism disorder, unspecified

E77　Disorders of glycoprotein metabolism
E77.0　Defects in post-translational modification of lysosomal enzymes
　　　　　Mucolipidosis II [I-cell disease]
　　　　　Mucolipidosis III [pseudo-Hurler polydystrophy]
E77.1　Defects in glycoprotein degradation
　　　　　Aspartylglucosaminuria
　　　　　Fucosidosis
　　　　　Mannosidosis
　　　　　Sialidosis [mucolipidosis I]
E77.8　Other disorders of glycoprotein metabolism
E77.9　Disorder of glycoprotein metabolism, unspecified

E78　Disorders of lipoprotein metabolism and other lipidemias
　　　　　Excludes1:　sphingolipidosis (E75.0-E75.3)
E78.0　Pure hypercholesterolemia
　　　　　Familial hypercholesterolemia
　　　　　Fredrickson's hyperlipoproteinemia, type IIa
　　　　　Hyperbetalipoproteinemia
　　　　　Hyperlipidemia, Group A
　　　　　Low-density-lipoprotein-type [LDL] hyperlipoproteinemia
E78.1　Pure hyperglyceridemia
　　　　　Endogenous hyperglyceridemia
　　　　　Fredrickson's hyperlipoproteinemia, type IV
　　　　　Hyperlipidemia, group B
　　　　　Hyperprebetalipoproteinemia
　　　　　Very-low-density-lipoprotein-type [VLDL] hyperlipoproteinemia
E78.2　Mixed hyperlipidemia
　　　　　Broad- or floating-betalipoproteinemia
　　　　　Fredrickson's hyperlipoproteinemia, type IIb or III
　　　　　Hyperbetalipoproteinemia with prebetalipoproteinemia
　　　　　Hypercholesteroemia with endogenous hyperglyceridemia
　　　　　Hyperlipidemia, group C
　　　　　Tubo-eruptive xanthoma
　　　　　Xanthoma tuberosum
　　　　　Excludes1:　cerebrotendinous cholesterosis [van Bogaert-Scherer-Epstein] (E75.5)
E78.3　Hyperchylomicronemia
　　　　　Chylomicron retention disease
　　　　　Fredrickson's hyperlipoproteinemia, type I or V
　　　　　Hyperlipidemia, group D
　　　　　Mixed hyperglyceridemia
E78.4　Other hyperlipidemia
　　　　　Familial combined hyperlipidaemia
E78.5　Hyperlipidemia, unspecified
E78.6　Lipoprotein deficiency
　　　　　Abetalipoproteinemia
　　　　　High-density lipoprotein deficiency
　　　　　Hypoalphalipoproteinemia
　　　　　Hypobetalipoproteinemia (familial)
　　　　　Lecithin cholesterol acyltransferase deficiency
　　　　　Tangier disease
E78.7　Disorders of bile acid and cholesterol metabolism
　　　　　Excludes1:　Niemann-Pick disease type C (E75.242)
E78.70　Disorder of bile acid and cholesterol metabolism, unspecified
E78.71　Barth syndrome
E78.72　Smith-Lemli-Opitz syndrome
E78.79　Other disorders of bile acid and cholesterol metabolism
E78.8　Other disorders of lipoprotein metabolism
E78.81　Lipoid dermatoarthritis
E78.89　Other lipoprotein metabolism disorders
E78.9　Disorder of lipoprotein metabolism, unspecified

E79　Disorders of purine and pyrimidine metabolism
　　　　　Excludes1:　ataxia-telangiectasia (Q87.1)
　　　　　　　　　　　Bloom's syndrome (Q82.8)
　　　　　　　　　　　Cockayne's syndrome (Q87.1)
　　　　　　　　　　　calculus of kidney (N20.0)
　　　　　　　　　　　combined immunodeficiency disorders (D81.-)
　　　　　　　　　　　Fanconi's anemia (D61.0)
　　　　　　　　　　　gout (M10.-)
　　　　　　　　　　　orotaciduric anemia (D53.0)
　　　　　　　　　　　progeria (E34.8)
　　　　　　　　　　　Werner's syndrome (E34.8)
　　　　　　　　　　　xeroderma pigmentosum (Q82.1)
E79.0　Hyperuricemia without signs of inflammatory arthritis and tophaceous disease
　　　　　Asymptomatic hyperuricemia
E79.1　Lesch-Nyhan syndrome
　　　　　HGPRT deficiency
E79.2　Myoadenylate deaminase deficiency
E79.8　Other disorders of purine and pyrimidine metabolism
　　　　　Hereditary xanthinuria
E79.9　Disorder of purine and pyrimidine metabolism, unspecified

E80　Disorders of porphyrin and bilirubin metabolism
　　　　　Includes:　defects of catalase and peroxidase
E80.0　Hereditary erythropoietic porphyria
　　　　　Congenital erythropoietic porphyria
　　　　　Erythropoietic protoporphyria
E80.1　Porphyria cutanea tarda
E80.2　Other and unspecified porphyria
　　　　　Use additional external cause code (Chapter XIX) to identify cause
E80.20　Unspecified porphyria
　　　　　Porphyria NOS
E80.21　Acute intermittent (hepatic) porphyria
E80.29　Other porphyria
　　　　　Hereditary coproporphyria
E80.3　Defects of catalase and peroxidase
　　　　　Acatalasia [Takahara]
E80.4　Gilbert's syndrome
E80.5　Crigler-Najjar syndrome
E80.6　Other disorders of bilirubin metabolism
　　　　　Dubin-Johnson syndrome
　　　　　Rotor's syndrome
E80.7　Disorder of bilirubin metabolism, unspecified

E83　Disorders of mineral metabolism
　　　　　Excludes1:　dietary mineral deficiency (E58-E61)
　　　　　　　　　　　parathyroid disorders (E20-E21)
　　　　　　　　　　　vitamin D deficiency (E55.-)
E83.0　Disorders of copper metabolism
E83.00　Disorder of copper metabolism, unspecified
E83.01　Wilson's disease
E83.09　Other disorders of copper metabolism
　　　　　Menkes' (kinky hair) (steely hair) disease
E83.1　Disorders of iron metabolism
　　　　　Excludes1:　iron deficiency anemia (D50.-)
　　　　　　　　　　　sideroblastic anemia (D64.0-D64.3)
E83.10　Disorder of iron metabolism, unspecified
E83.11　Hemochromatosis
E83.19　Other disorders of iron metabolism
E83.2　Disorders of zinc metabolism
　　　　　Acrodermatitis enteropathica
E83.3　Disorders of phosphorus metabolism
　　　　　Excludes1:　adult osteomalacia (M83.-)
　　　　　　　　　　　osteoporosis (M80)
E83.30　Disorder of phosphorus metabolism, unspecified
E83.31　Familial hypophosphatemia
　　　　　Vitamin D-resistant osteomalacia
　　　　　Vitamin D-resistant rickets
　　　　　Excludes1:　vitamin D-deficiency rickets (E55.0)

E83.32   **Hereditary vitamin D-dependent rickets (type 1)**
          (type 2)
              25-hydroxyvitamin D 1-α-hydroxylase deficiency
              Pseudovitamin D deficiency
              Vitamin D receptor defect
E83.39   **Other disorders of phosphorus metabolism**
              Acid phosphatase deficiency
              Hypophosphatasia
E83.4   **Disorders of magnesium metabolism**
E83.40   **Disorders of magnesium metabolism, unspecified**
E83.41   **Hypermagnesemia**
E83.42   **Hypomagnesemia**
E83.49   **Other disorders of magnesium metabolism**
E83.5   **Disorders of calcium metabolism**
          Excludes1:   chondrocalcinosis (M11.1-M11.2)
                       hyperparathyroidism (E21.0-E21.3)
E83.50   **Unspecified disorder of calcium metabolism**
E83.51   **Hypocalcemia**
E83.52   **Hypercalcemia**
              Familial hypocalciuric hypercalcemia
E83.59   **Other disorders of calcium metabolism**
              Idiopathic hypercalciuria
E83.8   **Other disorders of mineral metabolism**
E83.9   **Disorder of mineral metabolism, unspecified**

E84 **Cystic fibrosis**
        Includes: mucoviscidosis
E84.0   **Cystic fibrosis with pulmonary manifestations**
              Use additional code to identify any infectious organism present,
                 such as:
              Pseudomonas (B96.5)
E84.1   **Meconium ileus in cystic fibrosis**
          Excludes1:   meconium ileus not due to cystic fibrosis (P75)
E84.2   **Cystic fibrosis with gastrointestinal manifestations**
          Excludes1:   meconium ileus in cystic fibrosis (E84.1)
E84.8   **Cystic fibrosis with other manifestations**
E84.9   **Cystic fibrosis, unspecified**

E85 **Amyloidosis**
        Includes: amyloid polyneuropathy (Portuguese)
                     familial Mediterranean fever
                     hemodialysis-associated amyloidosis
                     hereditary amyloid nephropathy
                     heredofamilial (neuropathic) (non-neuropathic)
                        amyloidosis
                     localized amyloidosis
                     organ-limited amyloidosis
                     secondary systemic amyloidosis
        Excludes1:   Alzheimer's disease (G30.0-)

E86 **Volume depletion**
        Excludes1:   dehydration of newborn (P74.1)
                     hypovolemic shock NOS (R57.1)
                     postoperative hypovolemic shock (T81.1)
                     traumatic hypovolemic shock (T79.4)
E86.0   **Dehydration**
E86.1   **Hypovolemia**
              Depletion of volume of plasma or extracellular fluid
E86.9   **Volume depletion, unspecified**

E87 **Other disorders of fluid, electrolyte and acid-base balance**
        Excludes1:   diabetes insipidus (E23.2)
                     electrolyte imbalance associated with hyperemesis
                        gravidarum (O21.1)
                     electrolyte imbalance following ectopic or molar
                        pregnancy (O08.5)
                     familial periodic paralysis (G72.3)
E87.0   **Hyperosmolality and hypernatremia**
              Sodium [Na] excess
              Sodium [Na] overload
E87.1   **Hypo-osmolality and hyponatremia**
              Sodium [Na] deficiency
          Excludes1:   syndrome of inappropriate secretion of
                       antidiuretic hormone (E22.2)

E87.2   **Acidosis**
              Acidosis NOS
              Lactic acidosis
              Metabolic acidosis
              Respiratory acidosis
          Excludes1:   diabetic acidosis (E10.1)
E87.3   **Alkalosis**
              Alkalosis NOS
              Metabolic alkalosis
              Respiratory alkalosis
E87.4   **Mixed disorder of acid-base balance**
E87.5   **Hyperkalemia**
              Potassium [K] excess
              Potassium [K] overload
E87.6   **Hypokalemia**
              Potassium [K] deficiency
E87.7   **Fluid overload**
          Excludes1:   edema NOS (R60.-)
E87.8   **Other disorders of electrolyte and fluid balance, not elsewhere**
        classified
              Electrolyte imbalance NOS
              Hyperchloremia
              Hypochloremia

E88 **Other and unspecified metabolic disorders**
        Use additional external cause code (Chapter XIX) to identify drug, if
           drug-induced.
        Excludes1:   histiocytosis X (chronic) (D76.0)
E88.0   **Disorders of plasma-protein metabolism, not elsewhere**
        classified
          Excludes1:   disorder of lipoprotein metabolism (E78.-)
                       monoclonal gammopathy (D47.2)
                       polyclonal hypergammaglobulinemia (D89.0)
                       Waldenström's macroglobulinemia (C88.0)
E88.01   **α-1-Antitrypsin deficiency**
E88.09   **Other disorders of plasma-protein metabolism, not**
          elsewhere classified
              Bisalbuminemia
E88.1   **Lipodystrophy, not elsewhere classified**
              Lipodystrophy NOS
          Excludes1:   Whipple's disease (K90.81)
E88.2   **Lipomatosis, not elsewhere classified**
              Lipomatosis NOS
              Lipomatosis dolorosa [Dercum]
E88.3   **Mitochondrial metabolism disorders**
          Excludes1:   disorders of pyruvate metabolism (E74.4)
                       Kearns-Sayre syndrome (H49.81)
                       Leber's disease (H47.22)
                       Leigh's encephalopathy (G31.82)
                       Mitochondrial myopathy, NEC (G71.3)
                       Reye's syndrome (G93.7)
E88.30   **Mitochondrial metabolism disorder, unspecified**
E88.31   **MELAS syndrome**
              Mitochondrial myopathy, encephalopathy, lactic
                 acidosis, strokelike episodes
E88.32   **MERRF syndrome**
              Myoclonic epilepsy and ragged-red fibers
E88.39   **Other mitochondrial metabolism disorders**
E88.4   **Dysmetabolic syndrome X**
E88.8   **Other specified metabolic disorders**
              Launois-Bensaude adenolipomatosis
              Trimethylaminuria
E88.9   **Metabolic disorder, unspecified**

E89 **Postprocedural endocrine and metabolic disorders, not elsewhere**
     classified
        Excludes2:   intraoperative and postprocedural complications of
                     endocrine procedures (E36.-)
E89.0   **Postprocedural hypothyroidism**
              Postirradiation hypothyroidism
              Postsurgical hypothyroidism
E89.1   **Postprocedural hypoinsulinemia**
              Postpancreatectomy hyperglycemia
              Postsurgical hypoinsulinemia

E89.2   **Postprocedural hypoparathyroidism**
        Parathyroprival tetany

E89.3   **Postprocedural hypopituitarism**
        Postirradiation hypopituitarism

E89.4   **Postprocedural ovarian failure**

E89.5   **Postprocedural testicular hypofunction**

E89.6   **Postprocedural adrenocortical (-medullary) hypofunction**

E89.8   **Other postprocedural endocrine and metabolic disorders**

E89.9   **Postprocedural endocrine and metabolic disorder, unspecified**

E90 Nutritional and metabolic disorders in diseases classified elsewhere

CHAPTER V — MENTAL AND BEHAVIORAL DISORDERS (F01–F99)

Includes: disorders of psychological development
Excludes2:   symptoms, signs and abnormal clinical laboratory findings, not elsewhere classified (R00-R99)

Note: For definitions of the psychiatric terms and conditions used in this chapter reference the Diagnostic and Statistical Manual of Mental Disorders, fourth edition (DSM-IV) published by the American Psychiatric Association

This chapter contains the following blocks:

F01-F09   Mental disorders due to known physiological conditions
F10-F19   Mental and behavioral disorders due to psychoactive substance use
F20-F29   Schizophrenia, schizotypal and delusional, and other non-mood psychotic disorders
F30-F39   Mood [affective] disorders
F40-F48   Anxiety, dissociative, stress-related, somatoform and other nonpsychotic mental disorders
F50-F59   Behavioral syndromes associated with physiological disturbances and physical factors
F60-F69   Disorders of adult personality and behavior
F70-F79   Mental retardation
F80-F89   Pervasive and specific developmental disorders
F90-F98   Behavioral and emotional disorders with onset usually occurring in childhood and adolescence
F99   Unspecified mental disorder

MENTAL DISORDERS DUE TO KNOWN PHYSIOLOGICAL CONDITIONS (F01–F09)

This block comprises a range of mental disorders grouped together on the basis of their having in common a demonstrable etiology in cerebral disease, brain injury, or other insult leading to cerebral dysfunction. The dysfunction may be primary, as in diseases, injuries, and insults that affect the brain directly and selectively; or secondary, as in systemic diseases and disorders that attack the brain only as one of the multiple organs or systems of the body that are involved.

Code first the underlying physiological condition

F01 Vascular dementia
Vascular dementia as a result of infarction of the brain due to vascular disease, including hypertensive cerebrovascular disease.
Includes: arteriosclerotic dementia
Code first the underlying physiological condition or sequelae of cerebrovascular disease.

F01.5 Vascular dementia
F01.50   Vascular dementia without behavioral disturbance
F01.51   Vascular dementia with behavioral disturbance

F02 Dementia in other diseases classified elsewhere
Code first the underlying physiological condition, such as:
   cerebral lipidosis (E75.-)
   epilepsy (G40.-)
   hepatolenticular degeneration (E83.0)
   human immunodeficiency virus [HIV] disease (B20)
   hypercalcemia (E83.52)
   hypothyroidism, acquired (E00-E03.-)
   intoxications (T36-T65)
   multiple sclerosis (G35)
   niacin deficiency [pellagra] (E52)
   Parkinson's disease (G20)
   polyarteritis nodosa (M30.0)
   systemic lupus erythematosus (M32.-)
   trypanosomiasis (B56.-, B57.-)
   vitamin B deficiency (E53.8)
Excludes2:   dementia in alcohol and psychoactive substance disorders (F10-F19, with .17, .27, .97)
             dementia in Alzheimer's disease (G30.-)
             dementia in neurosyphilis (A52.17)

F02.8 Dementia in other diseases classified elsewhere
F02.80   Dementia in other diseases classified elsewhere, without behavioral disturbance
F02.81   Dementia in other diseases classified elsewhere, with behavioral disturbance

F03 Unspecified dementia
Includes: presenile dementia NOS
               presenile psychosis NOS
               primary degenerative dementia NOS
               senile dementia NOS
               senile dementia depressed or paranoid type
               senile psychosis NOS
Excludes1:   senility NOS (R54)
Excludes2:   senile dementia with delirium or acute confusional state (F05)

F04 Amnestic disorder due to known physiological condition
Includes: Korsakov's psychosis or syndrome, nonalcoholic
Code first the underlying physiological condition
Excludes1:   amnesia NOS (R41.3)
             anterograde amnesia (R41.1)
             dissociative amnesia (F44.0)
             retrograde amnesia (R41.2)
Excludes2:   alcohol-induced or unspecified Korsakov's syndrome (F10.26, F10.96)
             Korsakov's syndrome induced by other psychoactive substances (F13.26, F13.96, F19.16, F19.26, F19.96)

F05 Delirium due to known physiological condition
Includes: acute or subacute brain syndrome
               acute or subacute confusional state (nonalcoholic)
               acute or subacute infective psychosis
               acute or subacute organic reaction
               acute or subacute psycho-organic syndrome
               delirium of mixed etiology
               delirium superimposed on dementia
               sundowning
Code first the underlying physiological condition
Excludes1:   delirium NOS (R41.0)
Excludes2:   delirium tremens alcohol-induced or unspecified (F10.231, F10.931)

F06 Other mental disorders due to known physiological condition
Includes: mental disorders due to endocrine disorder
               mental disorders due to exogenous hormone
               mental disorders due to exogenous toxic substance
               mental disorders due to primary cerebral disease
               mental disorders due to somatic illness
               mental disorders due to systemic disease affecting the brain
Code first the underlying physiological condition
Excludes1:   unspecified dementia (F03)
Excludes2:   dementia as classified in F01-F02
             delirium due to known physiological condition (F05)
             other mental disorders associated with alcohol and other psychoactive substances (F10-F19)

F06.0 Psychotic disorder with hallucinations due to known physiological condition
Organic hallucinatory state (nonalcoholic)
Excludes2:   hallucinations and perceptual disturbance induced by alcohol and other psychoactive substances (F10-F19 with .151, .251, .951)
             schizophrenia (F20.-)

F06.1 Catatonic disorder due to known physiological condition
Excludes1:   catatonic stupor (R40.1)
             stupor NOS (R40.1)
Excludes2:   catatonic schizophrenia (F20.2)
             dissociative stupor (F44.2)

F06.2   Psychotic disorder with delusions due to known physiological condition
Paranoid and paranoid-hallucinatory organic states
Schizophrenia-like psychosis in epilepsy
Excludes2:   alcohol and drug-induced psychotic disorder (F10-F19 with .150, .250, .950)
brief psychotic disorder (F23)
delusional disorder (F22)
schizophrenia (F20.-)

F06.3   Mood disorder due to known physiological condition
Excludes2:   mood disorders due to alcohol and other psychoactive substances (F10-F19 with .14, .24, .94)
mood disorders, not due to known physiological condition or unspecified (F30-F39)
F06.30   Mood disorder due to known physiological condition, unspecified
F06.31   Mood disorder due to known physiological condition with depressive features
F06.32   Mood disorder due to known physiological condition with major depressive-like episode
F06.33   Mood disorder due to known physiological condition with manic features
F06.34   Mood disorder due to known physiological condition with mixed features

F06.4   Anxiety disorder due to known physiological condition
Excludes2:   anxiety disorders due to alcohol and other psychoactive substances (F10-F19 with .180, .280, .980)
anxiety disorders, not due to known physiological condition or unspecified (F40.-, F41.-)

F06.8   Other specified mental disorders due to known physiological condition
Epileptic psychosis NOS
Mild cognitive disorder
Organic dissociative disorder
Organic emotionally labile [asthenic] disorder

F06.9   Unspecified mental disorder due to known physiological condition
Mental disorder NOS due to known physiological condition

F07   Personality and behavioral disorders due to known physiological condition
Code first the underlying physiological condition
F07.0   Personality change due to known physiological condition
Frontal lobe syndrome
Limbic epilepsy personality syndrome
Lobotomy syndrome
Organic personality disorder
Organic pseudopsychopathic personality
Organic pseudoretarded personality
Postleucotomy syndrome
Code first underlying physiological condition
Excludes1:   postconcussional syndrome (F07.8)
postencephalitic syndrome (F07.8)
Excludes2:   specific personality disorder (F60.-)
F07.8   Other personality and behavioral disorders due to known physiological condition
F07.81   Postconcussional syndrome
F07.89   Other personality and behavioral disorders due to known physiological condition
Postencephalitic syndrome
Right hemispheric organic affective disorder
F07.9   Unspecified personality and behavioral disorder due to known physiological condition
Organic psychosyndrome

F09   Unspecified mental disorder due to known physiological condition
Includes: organic brain syndrome NOS
organic mental disorder NOS
organic psychosis NOS
symptomatic psychosis NOS
Code first the underlying physiological condition
Excludes1:   psychosis NOS (F29)

MENTAL AND BEHAVIORAL DISORDERS DUE TO PSYCHOACTIVE SUBSTANCE USE (F10–F19)

F10   Alcohol-related disorders
Use additional code for blood alcohol level, if applicable (Y90.-)
Excludes1:   alcohol use, uncomplicated (Z72.1)
social alcohol use (Z72.1)
F10.1   Alcohol abuse
Excludes1:   alcohol dependence (F10.2-)
alcohol use, unspecified (F10.9-)
F10.10   Alcohol abuse, uncomplicated
F10.12   Alcohol abuse with intoxication
F10.120   Alcohol abuse with intoxication, uncomplicated
F10.121   Alcohol abuse with intoxication delirium
F10.129   Alcohol abuse with intoxication, unspecified
F10.14   Alcohol abuse with alcohol-induced mood disorder
F10.15   Alcohol abuse with alcohol-induced psychotic disorder
F10.150   Alcohol abuse with alcohol-induced psychotic disorder with delusions
F10.151   Alcohol abuse with alcohol-induced psychotic disorder with hallucinations
F10.159   Alcohol abuse with alcohol-induced psychotic disorder, unspecified
F10.18   Alcohol abuse with other alcohol-induced disorders
F10.180   Alcohol abuse with alcohol-induced anxiety disorder
F10.181   Alcohol abuse with alcohol-induced sexual dysfunction
F10.182   Alcohol abuse with alcohol-induced sleep disorder
F10.188   Alcohol abuse with other alcohol-induced disorder
F10.19   Alcohol abuse with unspecified alcohol-induced disorder
F10.2   Alcohol dependence
Excludes1:   alcohol abuse (F10.1-)
alcohol use, unspecified (F10.9-)
Excludes2:   toxic effect of alcohol (T51.0-)
F10.20   Alcohol dependence, uncomplicated
F10.21   Alcohol dependence, in remission
F10.22   Alcohol dependence with intoxication
Excludes1:   alcohol dependence with withdrawal (F10.23-)
F10.220   Alcohol dependence with intoxication, uncomplicated
F10.221   Alcohol dependence with intoxication delirium
F10.229   Alcohol dependence with intoxication, unspecified
F10.23   Alcohol dependence with withdrawal
Excludes1:   alcohol dependence with intoxication (F10.22-)
F10.230   Alcohol dependence with withdrawal, uncomplicated
F10.231   Alcohol dependence with withdrawal delirium
F10.232   Alcohol dependence with withdrawal with perceptual disturbance
F10.239   Alcohol dependence with withdrawal, unspecified
F10.24   Alcohol dependence with alcohol-induced mood disorder
F10.25   Alcohol dependence with alcohol-induced psychotic disorder
F10.250   Alcohol dependence with alcohol-induced psychotic disorder with delusions
F10.251   Alcohol dependence with alcohol-induced psychotic disorder with hallucinations
F10.259   Alcohol dependence with alcohol-induced psychotic disorder, unspecified

F10.26　Alcohol dependence with alcohol-induced persisting amnestic disorder

F10.27　Alcohol dependence with alcohol-induced persisting dementia

F10.28　Alcohol dependence with other alcohol-induced disorders

　　F10.280　Alcohol dependence with alcohol-induced anxiety disorder

　　F10.281　Alcohol dependence with alcohol-induced sexual dysfunction

　　F10.282　Alcohol dependence with alcohol-induced sleep disorder

　　F10.288　Alcohol dependence with other alcohol-induced disorder

F10.29　Alcohol dependence with unspecified alcohol-induced disorder

F10.9　Alcohol use, unspecified

　　Excludes1:　alcohol abuse (F10.1)
　　　　　　　alcohol dependence (F10.2-)
　　　　　　　alcohol use, uncomplicated (Z72.1)
　　　　　　　social alcohol use (Z72.1)

F10.92　Alcohol use, unspecified with intoxication

　　F10.920　Alcohol use, unspecified with intoxication, uncomplicated

　　F10.921　Alcohol use, unspecified with intoxication delirium

　　F10.929　Alcohol use, unspecified with intoxication, unspecified

F10.94　Alcohol use, unspecified with alcohol-induced mood disorder

F10.95　Alcohol use, unspecified with alcohol-induced psychotic disorder

　　F10.950　Alcohol use, unspecified with alcohol-induced psychotic disorder with delusions

　　F10.951　Alcohol use, unspecified with alcohol-induced psychotic disorder with hallucinations

　　F10.959　Alcohol use, unspecified with alcohol-induced psychotic disorder, unspecified

F10.96　Alcohol use, unspecified with alcohol-induced persisting amnestic disorder

F10.97　Alcohol use, unspecified with alcohol-induced persisting dementia

F10.98　Alcohol use, unspecified with other alcohol-induced disorders

　　F10.980　Alcohol use, unspecified with alcohol-induced anxiety disorder

　　F10.981　Alcohol use, unspecified with alcohol-induced sexual dysfunction

　　F10.982　Alcohol use, unspecified with alcohol-induced sleep disorder

　　F10.988　Alcohol use, unspecified with other alcohol-induced disorder

F10.99　Alcohol use, unspecified with unspecified alcohol-induced disorder

F11　Opioid-related disorders

F11.1　Opioid abuse

　　Excludes1:　opioid dependence (F11.2-)
　　　　　　　opioid use, unspecified (F11.9-)

F11.10　Opioid abuse, uncomplicated

F11.12　Opioid abuse with intoxication

　　F11.120　Opioid abuse with intoxication, uncomplicated

　　F11.121　Opioid abuse with intoxication delirium

　　F11.122　Opioid abuse with intoxication with perceptual disturbance

　　F11.129　Opioid abuse with intoxication, unspecified

F11.14　Opioid abuse with opioid-induced mood disorder

F11.15　Opioid abuse with opioid-induced psychotic disorder

　　F11.150　Opioid abuse with opioid-induced psychotic disorder with delusions

　　F11.151　Opioid abuse with opioid-induced psychotic disorder with hallucinations

　　F11.159　Opioid abuse with opioid-induced psychotic disorder, unspecified

F11.18　Opioid abuse with other opioid-induced disorder

　　F11.181　Opioid abuse with opioid-induced sexual dysfunction

　　F11.182　Opioid abuse with opioid-induced sleep disorder

　　F11.188　Opioid abuse with other opioid-induced disorder

F11.19　Opioid abuse with unspecified opioid-induced disorder

F11.2　Opioid dependence

　　Excludes1:　opioid abuse (F11.1-)
　　　　　　　opioid use, unspecified (F11.9-)
　　Excludes2:　opioid poisoning (T40.0-T40.2-)

F11.20　Opioid dependence, uncomplicated

F11.21　Opioid dependence, in remission

F11.22　Opioid dependence with intoxication

　　Excludes1:　opioid dependence with withdrawal (F11.23)

　　F11.220　Opioid dependence with intoxication, uncomplicated

　　F11.221　Opioid dependence with intoxication delirium

　　F11.222　Opioid dependence with intoxication with perceptual disturbance

　　F11.229　Opioid dependence with intoxication, unspecified

F11.23　Opioid dependence with withdrawal

　　Excludes1:　opioid dependence with intoxication (F11.22-)

F11.24　Opioid dependence with opioid-induced mood disorder

F11.25　Opioid dependence with opioid-induced psychotic disorder

　　F11.250　Opioid dependence with opioid-induced psychotic disorder with delusions

　　F11.251　Opioid dependence with opioid-induced psychotic disorder with hallucinations

　　F11.259　Opioid dependence with opioid-induced psychotic disorder, unspecified

F11.28　Opioid dependence with other opioid-induced disorder

　　F11.281　Opioid dependence with opioid-induced sexual dysfunction

　　F11.282　Opioid dependence with opioid-induced sleep disorder

　　F11.288　Opioid dependence with other opioid-induced disorder

F11.29　Opioid dependence with unspecified opioid-induced disorder

F11.9　Opioid use, unspecified

　　Excludes1:　opioid abuse (F11.1-)
　　　　　　　opioid dependence (F11.2-)

F11.90　Opioid use, unspecified, uncomplicated

F11.92　Opioid use, unspecified with intoxication

　　Excludes1:　opioid use, unspecified with withdrawal (F11.93)

　　F11.920　Opioid use, unspecified with intoxication, uncomplicated

　　F11.921　Opioid use, unspecified with intoxication delirium

　　F11.922　Opioid use, unspecified with intoxication with perceptual disturbance

　　F11.929　Opioid use, unspecified with intoxication, unspecified

F11.93　Opioid use, unspecified with withdrawal

　　Excludes1:　opioid use, unspecified with intoxication (F11.92-)

F11.94　Opioid use, unspecified with opioid-induced mood disorder

F11.95　Opioid use, unspecified with opioid-induced psychotic disorder

F11.950   Opioid use, unspecified with opioid-induced psychotic disorder with delusions
F11.951   Opioid use, unspecified with opioid-induced psychotic disorder with hallucinations
F11.959   Opioid use, unspecified with opioid-induced psychotic disorder, unspecified
F11.98   Opioid use, unspecified with other specified opioid-induced disorder
F11.981   Opioid use, unspecified with opioid-induced sexual dysfunction
F11.982   Opioid use, unspecified with opioid-induced sleep disorder
F11.988   Opioid use, unspecified with other opioid-induced disorder
F11.99   Opioid use, unspecified with unspecified opioid-induced disorder

F12 Cannabis-related disorders
   Includes: marijuana
   F12.1   Cannabis abuse
      Excludes1:   cannabis dependence (F12.2-)
                    cannabis use, unspecified (F12.9-)
   F12.10   Cannabis abuse, uncomplicated
   F12.12   Cannabis abuse with intoxication
      F12.120   Cannabis abuse with intoxication, uncomplicated
      F12.121   Cannabis abuse with intoxication delirium
      F12.122   Cannabis abuse with intoxication with perceptual disturbance
      F12.129   Cannabis abuse with intoxication, unspecified
   F12.15   Cannabis abuse with psychotic disorder
      F12.150   Cannabis abuse with psychotic disorder with delusions
      F12.151   Cannabis abuse with psychotic disorder with hallucinations
      F12.159   Cannabis abuse with psychotic disorder, unspecified
   F12.18   Cannabis abuse with other cannabis-induced disorder
      F12.180   Cannabis abuse with cannabis-induced anxiety disorder
      F12.188   Cannabis abuse with other cannabis-induced disorder
   F12.19   Cannabis abuse with unspecified cannabis-induced disorder
   F12.2   Cannabis dependence
      Excludes1:   cannabis abuse (F12.1-)
                    cannabis use, unspecified (F12.9-)
      Excludes2:   cannabis poisoning (T40.7-)
   F12.20   Cannabis dependence, uncomplicated
   F12.21   Cannabis dependence, in remission
   F12.22   Cannabis dependence with intoxication
      F12.220   Cannabis dependence with intoxication, uncomplicated
      F12.221   Cannabis dependence with intoxication delirium
      F12.222   Cannabis dependence with intoxication with perceptual disturbance
      F12.229   Cannabis dependence with intoxication, unspecified
   F12.25   Cannabis dependence with psychotic disorder
      F12.250   Cannabis dependence with psychotic disorder with delusions
      F12.251   Cannabis dependence with psychotic disorder with hallucinations
      F12.259   Cannabis dependence with psychotic disorder, unspecified
   F12.28   Cannabis dependence with other cannabis-induced disorder
      F12.280   Cannabis dependence with cannabis-induced anxiety disorder
      F12.288   Cannabis dependence with other cannabis-induced disorder

   F12.29   Cannabis dependence with unspecified cannabis-induced disorder
   F12.9   Cannabis use, unspecified
      Excludes1:   cannabis abuse (F12.1-)
                    cannabis dependence (F12.2-)
   F12.90   Cannabis use, unspecified, uncomplicated
   F12.92   Cannabis use, unspecified with intoxication
      F12.920   Cannabis use, unspecified with intoxication, uncomplicated
      F12.921   Cannabis use, unspecified with intoxication delirium
      F12.922   Cannabis use, unspecified with intoxication with perceptual disturbance
      F12.929   Cannabis use, unspecified with intoxication, unspecified
   F12.95   Cannabis use, unspecified with psychotic disorder
      F12.950   Cannabis use, unspecified with psychotic disorder with delusions
      F12.951   Cannabis use, unspecified with psychotic disorder with hallucinations
      F12.959   Cannabis use, unspecified with psychotic disorder, unspecified
   F12.98   Cannabis use, unspecified with other cannabis-induced disorder
      F12.980   Cannabis use, unspecified with anxiety disorder
      F12.988   Cannabis use, unspecified with other cannabis-induced disorder
   F12.99   Cannabis use, unspecified with unspecified cannabis-induced disorder

F13 Sedative, hypnotic, or anxiolytic-related disorders
   F13.1   Sedative, hypnotic or anxiolytic-related abuse
      Excludes1:   sedative, hypnotic or anxiolytic-related dependence (F13.2-)
                    sedative, hypnotic, or anxiolytic use, unspecified (F13.9-)
   F13.10   Sedative, hypnotic or anxiolytic abuse, uncomplicated
   F13.12   Sedative, hypnotic or anxiolytic abuse with intoxication
      F13.120   Sedative, hypnotic or anxiolytic abuse with intoxication, uncomplicated
      F13.121   Sedative, hypnotic or anxiolytic abuse with intoxication delirium
      F13.129   Sedative, hypnotic or anxiolytic abuse with intoxication, unspecified
   F13.14   Sedative, hypnotic or anxiolytic abuse with sedative, hypnotic or anxiolytic-induced mood disorder
   F13.15   Sedative, hypnotic or anxiolytic abuse with sedative, hypnotic or anxiolytic-induced psychotic disorder
      F13.150   Sedative, hypnotic or anxiolytic abuse with sedative, hypnotic or anxiolytic-induced psychotic disorder with delusions
      F13.151   Sedative, hypnotic or anxiolytic abuse with sedative, hypnotic or anxiolytic-induced psychotic disorder with hallucinations
      F13.159   Sedative, hypnotic or anxiolytic abuse with sedative, hypnotic or anxiolytic-induced psychotic disorder, unspecified
   F13.18   Sedative, hypnotic or anxiolytic abuse with other sedative, hypnotic or anxiolytic-induced disorders
      F13.180   Sedative, hypnotic or anxiolytic abuse with sedative, hypnotic or anxiolytic-induced anxiety disorder
      F13.181   Sedative, hypnotic or anxiolytic abuse with sedative, hypnotic or anxiolytic-induced sexual dysfunction
      F13.182   Sedative, hypnotic or anxiolytic abuse with sedative, hypnotic or anxiolytic-induced sleep disorder
      F13.188   Sedative, hypnotic or anxiolytic abuse with other sedative, hypnotic or anxiolytic-induced disorder

F13.19   Sedative, hypnotic or anxiolytic abuse with unspecified sedative, hypnotic or anxiolytic-induced disorder

F13.2   Sedative, hypnotic or anxiolytic-related dependence

Excludes1:   sedative, hypnotic or anxiolytic-related abuse (F13.1-)

sedative, hypnotic, or anxiolytic use, unspecified (F13.9-)

Excludes2:   sedative, hypnotic, or anxiolytic poisoning (T42.-)

F13.20   Sedative, hypnotic or anxiolytic dependence, uncomplicated

F13.21   Sedative, hypnotic or anxiolytic dependence, in remission

F13.22   Sedative, hypnotic or anxiolytic dependence with intoxication

Excludes1:   sedative, hypnotic or anxiolytic dependence with withdrawal (F13.23-)

F13.220   Sedative, hypnotic or anxiolytic dependence with intoxication, uncomplicated

F13.221   Sedative, hypnotic or anxiolytic dependence with intoxication delirium

F13.229   Sedative, hypnotic or anxiolytic dependence with intoxication, unspecified

F13.23   Sedative, hypnotic or anxiolytic dependence with withdrawal

Excludes1:   sedative, hypnotic or anxiolytic dependence with intoxication (F13.22-)

F13.230   Sedative, hypnotic or anxiolytic dependence with withdrawal, uncomplicated

F13.231   Sedative, hypnotic or anxiolytic dependence with withdrawal delirium

F13.232   Sedative, hypnotic or anxiolytic dependence with withdrawal with perceptual disturbance

F13.239   Sedative, hypnotic or anxiolytic dependence with withdrawal, unspecified

F13.24   Sedative, hypnotic or anxiolytic dependence with sedative, hypnotic or anxiolytic-induced mood disorder

F13.25   Sedative, hypnotic or anxiolytic dependence with sedative, hypnotic or anxiolytic-induced psychotic disorder

F13.250   Sedative, hypnotic or anxiolytic dependence with sedative, hypnotic or anxiolytic-induced psychotic disorder with delusions

F13.251   Sedative, hypnotic or anxiolytic dependence with sedative, hypnotic or anxiolytic-induced psychotic disorder with hallucinations

F13.259   Sedative, hypnotic or anxiolytic dependence with sedative, hypnotic or anxiolytic-induced psychotic disorder, unspecified

F13.26   Sedative, hypnotic or anxiolytic dependence with sedative, hypnotic or anxiolytic-induced persisting amnestic disorder

F13.27   Sedative, hypnotic or anxiolytic dependence with sedative, hypnotic or anxiolytic-induced persisting dementia

F13.28   Sedative, hypnotic or anxiolytic dependence with other sedative, hypnotic or anxiolytic-induced disorders

F13.280   Sedative, hypnotic or anxiolytic dependence with sedative, hypnotic or anxiolytic-induced anxiety disorder

F13.281   Sedative, hypnotic or anxiolytic dependence with sedative, hypnotic or anxiolytic-induced sexual dysfunction

F13.282   Sedative, hypnotic or anxiolytic dependence with sedative, hypnotic or anxiolytic-induced sleep disorder

F13.288   Sedative, hypnotic or anxiolytic dependence with other sedative, hypnotic or anxiolytic-induced disorder

F13.29   Sedative, hypnotic or anxiolytic dependence with unspecified sedative, hypnotic or anxiolytic-induced disorder

F13.9   Sedative, hypnotic or anxiolytic-related use, unspecified

Excludes1:   sedative, hypnotic or anxiolytic-related abuse (F13.1-)

sedative, hypnotic or anxiolytic-related dependence (F13.2-)

F13.90   Sedative, hypnotic, or anxiolytic use, unspecified, uncomplicated

F13.92   Sedative, hypnotic or anxiolytic use, unspecified with intoxication

Excludes1:   sedative, hypnotic or anxiolytic use, unspecified with withdrawal (F13.93-)

F13.920   Sedative, hypnotic or anxiolytic use, unspecified with intoxication, uncomplicated

F13.921   Sedative, hypnotic or anxiolytic use, unspecified with intoxication delirium

F13.929   Sedative, hypnotic or anxiolytic use, unspecified with intoxication, unspecified

F13.93   Sedative, hypnotic or anxiolytic use, unspecified with withdrawal

Excludes1:   sedative, hypnotic or anxiolytic use, unspecified with intoxication (F13.92-)

F13.930   Sedative, hypnotic or anxiolytic use, unspecified with withdrawal, uncomplicated

F13.931   Sedative, hypnotic or anxiolytic use, unspecified with withdrawal delirium

F13.932   Sedative, hypnotic or anxiolytic use, unspecified with withdrawal with perceptual disturbances

F13.939   Sedative, hypnotic or anxiolytic use, unspecified with withdrawal, unspecified

F13.94   Sedative, hypnotic or anxiolytic use, unspecified with sedative, hypnotic or anxiolytic-induced mood disorder

F13.95   Sedative, hypnotic or anxiolytic use, unspecified with sedative, hypnotic or anxiolytic-induced psychotic disorder

F13.950   Sedative, hypnotic or anxiolytic use, unspecified with sedative, hypnotic or anxiolytic-induced psychotic disorder with delusions

F13.951   Sedative, hypnotic or anxiolytic use, unspecified with sedative, hypnotic or anxiolytic-induced psychotic disorder with hallucinations

F13.959   Sedative, hypnotic or anxiolytic use, unspecified with sedative, hypnotic or anxiolytic-induced psychotic disorder, unspecified

F13.96   Sedative, hypnotic or anxiolytic use, unspecified with sedative, hypnotic or anxiolytic-induced persisting amnestic disorder

F13.97   Sedative, hypnotic or anxiolytic use, unspecified with sedative, hypnotic or anxiolytic-induced persisting dementia

F13.98   Sedative, hypnotic or anxiolytic use, unspecified with other sedative, hypnotic or anxiolytic-induced disorders

F13.980   Sedative, hypnotic or anxiolytic use, unspecified with sedative, hypnotic or anxiolytic-induced anxiety disorder

F13.981   Sedative, hypnotic or anxiolytic use, unspecified with sedative, hypnotic or anxiolytic-induced sexual dysfunction

F13.982   Sedative, hypnotic or anxiolytic use, unspecified with sedative, hypnotic or anxiolytic-induced sleep disorder

F13.988   Sedative, hypnotic or anxiolytic use, unspecified with other sedative, hypnotic or anxiolytic-induced disorder

F13.99 Sedative, hypnotic or anxiolytic use, unspecified with unspecified sedative, hypnotic or anxiolytic-induced disorder

F14 Cocaine-related disorders
Excludes2: other stimulant-related disorders (F15.-)

F14.1 Cocaine abuse
Excludes1: cocaine dependence (F14.2-)
cocaine use, unspecified (F14.9-)

F14.10 Cocaine abuse, uncomplicated

F14.12 Cocaine abuse with intoxication

    F14.120 Cocaine abuse with intoxication, uncomplicated

    F14.121 Cocaine abuse with intoxication with delirium

    F14.122 Cocaine abuse with intoxication with perceptual disturbance

    F14.129 Cocaine abuse with intoxication, unspecified

F14.14 Cocaine abuse with cocaine-induced mood disorder

F14.15 Cocaine abuse with cocaine-induced psychotic disorder

    F14.150 Cocaine abuse with cocaine-induced psychotic disorder with delusions

    F14.151 Cocaine abuse with cocaine-induced psychotic disorder with hallucinations

    F14.159 Cocaine abuse with cocaine-induced psychotic disorder, unspecified

F14.18 Cocaine abuse with other cocaine-induced disorder

    F14.180 Cocaine abuse with cocaine-induced anxiety disorder

    F14.181 Cocaine abuse with cocaine-induced sexual dysfunction

    F14.182 Cocaine abuse with cocaine-induced sleep disorder

    F14.188 Cocaine abuse with other cocaine-induced disorder

F14.19 Cocaine abuse with unspecified cocaine-induced disorder

F14.2 Cocaine dependence
Excludes1: cocaine abuse (F14.1-)
cocaine use, unspecified (F14.9-)
Excludes2: cocaine poisoning (T40.5-)

F14.20 Cocaine dependence, uncomplicated

F14.21 Cocaine dependence, in remission

F14.22 Cocaine dependence with intoxication
Excludes1: cocaine dependence with withdrawal (F14.23)

    F14.220 Cocaine dependence with intoxication, uncomplicated

    F14.221 Cocaine dependence with intoxication delirium

    F14.222 Cocaine dependence with intoxication with perceptual disturbance

    F14.229 Cocaine dependence with intoxication, unspecified

F14.23 Cocaine dependence with withdrawal
Excludes1: cocaine dependence with intoxication (F14.22-)

F14.24 Cocaine dependence with cocaine-induced mood disorder

F14.25 Cocaine dependence with cocaine-induced psychotic disorder

    F14.250 Cocaine dependence with cocaine-induced psychotic disorder with delusions

    F14.251 Cocaine dependence with cocaine-induced psychotic disorder with hallucinations

    F14.259 Cocaine dependence with cocaine-induced psychotic disorder, unspecified

F14.28 Cocaine dependence with other cocaine-induced disorder

    F14.280 Cocaine dependence with cocaine-induced anxiety disorder

    F14.281 Cocaine dependence with cocaine-induced sexual dysfunction

    F14.282 Cocaine dependence with cocaine-induced sleep disorder

    F14.288 Cocaine dependence with other cocaine-induced disorder

F14.29 Cocaine dependence with unspecified cocaine-induced disorder

F14.9 Cocaine use, unspecified
Excludes1: cocaine abuse (F14.1-)
cocaine dependence (F14.2-)

F14.90 Cocaine use, unspecified, uncomplicated

F14.92 Cocaine use, unspecified with intoxication

    F14.920 Cocaine use, unspecified with intoxication, uncomplicated

    F14.921 Cocaine use, unspecified with intoxication delirium

    F14.922 Cocaine use, unspecified with intoxication with perceptual disturbance

    F14.929 Cocaine use, unspecified with intoxication, unspecified

F14.94 Cocaine use, unspecified with cocaine-induced mood disorder

F14.95 Cocaine use, unspecified with cocaine-induced psychotic disorder

    F14.950 Cocaine use, unspecified with cocaine-induced psychotic disorder with delusions

    F14.951 Cocaine use, unspecified with cocaine-induced psychotic disorder with hallucinations

    F14.959 Cocaine use, unspecified with cocaine-induced psychotic disorder, unspecified

F14.98 Cocaine use, unspecified with other specified cocaine-induced disorder

    F14.980 Cocaine use, unspecified with cocaine-induced anxiety disorder

    F14.981 Cocaine use, unspecified with cocaine-induced sexual dysfunction

    F14.982 Cocaine use, unspecified with cocaine-induced sleep disorder

    F14.988 Cocaine use, unspecified with other cocaine-induced disorder

F14.99 Cocaine use, unspecified with unspecified cocaine-induced disorder

F15 Other stimulant-related disorders amphetamine-related disorders
Includes: amphetamine-related disorders
caffeine
Excludes2: cocaine-related disorders (F14.-)

F15.1 Other stimulant abuse
Excludes1: other stimulant dependence (F15.2-)
other stimulant use, unspecified (F15.9-)

F15.10 Other stimulant abuse, uncomplicated

F15.12 Other stimulant abuse with intoxication

    F15.120 Other stimulant abuse with intoxication, uncomplicated

    F15.121 Other stimulant abuse with intoxication delirium

    F15.122 Other stimulant abuse with intoxication with perceptual disturbance

    F15.129 Other stimulant abuse with intoxication, unspecified

F15.14 Other stimulant abuse with stimulant-induced mood disorder

F15.15 Other stimulant abuse with stimulant-induced psychotic disorder

    F15.150 Other stimulant abuse with stimulant-induced psychotic disorder with delusions

    F15.151 Other stimulant abuse with stimulant-induced psychotic disorder with hallucinations

    F15.159 Other stimulant abuse with stimulant-induced psychotic disorder, unspecified

F15.18   Other stimulant abuse with other stimulant-induced disorder

    F15.180   Other stimulant abuse with stimulant-induced anxiety disorder

    F15.181   Other stimulant abuse with stimulant-induced sexual dysfunction

    F15.182   Other stimulant abuse with stimulant-induced sleep disorder

    F15.188   Other stimulant abuse with other stimulant-induced disorder

F15.19   Other stimulant abuse with unspecified stimulant-induced disorder

F15.2   Other stimulant dependence

    Excludes1:   other stimulant abuse (F15.1-)
                   other stimulant use, unspecified (F15.9-)

F15.20   Other stimulant dependence, uncomplicated

F15.21   Other stimulant dependence, in remission

F15.22   Other stimulant dependence with intoxication

    Excludes1:   other stimulant dependence with withdrawal (F15.23)

    F15.220   Other stimulant dependence with intoxication, uncomplicated

    F15.221   Other stimulant dependence with intoxication delirium

    F15.222   Other stimulant dependence with intoxication with perceptual disturbance

    F15.229   Other stimulant dependence with intoxication, unspecified

F15.23   Other stimulant dependence with withdrawal

    Excludes1:   other stimulant dependence with intoxication (F15.22-)

F15.24   Other stimulant dependence with stimulant-induced mood disorder

F15.25   Other stimulant dependence with stimulant-induced psychotic disorder

    F15.250   Other stimulant dependence with stimulant-induced psychotic disorder with delusions

    F15.251   Other stimulant dependence with stimulant-induced psychotic disorder with hallucinations

    F15.259   Other stimulant dependence with stimulant-induced psychotic disorder, unspecified

F15.28   Other stimulant dependence with other stimulant-induced disorder

    F15.280   Other stimulant dependence with stimulant-induced anxiety disorder

    F15.281   Other stimulant dependence with stimulant-induced sexual dysfunction

    F15.282   Other stimulant dependence with stimulant-induced sleep disorder

    F15.288   Other stimulant dependence with other stimulant-induced disorder

F15.29   Other stimulant dependence with unspecified stimulant-induced disorder

F15.9   Other stimulant use, unspecified

    Excludes1:   other stimulant abuse (F15.1-)
                   other stimulant dependence (F15.2-)

F15.90   Other stimulant use, unspecified, uncomplicated

F15.92   Other stimulant use, unspecified with intoxication

    Excludes1:   other stimulant use, unspecified with withdrawal (F15.93)

    F15.920   Other stimulant use, unspecified with intoxication, uncomplicated

    F15.921   Other stimulant use, unspecified with intoxication delirium

    F15.922   Other stimulant use, unspecified with intoxication with perceptual disturbance

    F15.929   Other stimulant use, unspecified with intoxication, unspecified

F15.93   Other stimulant use, unspecifed with withdrawal

    Excludes1:   other stimulant use, unspecified with intoxication (F15.92-)

F15.94   Other stimulant use, unspecified with stimulant-induced mood disorder

F15.95   Other stimulant use, unspecified with stimulant-induced psychotic disorder

    F15.950   Other stimulant use, unspecified with stimulant-induced psychotic disorder with delusions

    F15.951   Other stimulant use, unspecified with stimulant-induced psychotic disorder with hallucinations

    F15.959   Other stimulant use, unspecified with stimulant-induced psychotic disorder, unspecified

F15.98   Other stimulant use, unspecified with other stimulant-induced disorder

    F15.980   Other stimulant use, unspecified with stimulant-induced anxiety disorder

    F15.981   Other stimulant use, unspecified with stimulant-induced sexual dysfunction

    F15.982   Other stimulant use, unspecified with stimulant-induced sleep disorder

    F15.988   Other stimulant use, unspecified with other stimulant-induced disorder

F15.99   Other stimulant use, unspecified with unspecified stimulant-induced disorder

F16   Hallucinogen-related disorders

    Includes: extasy
               PCP
               phencyclidine

F16.1   Hallucinogen abuse

    Excludes1:   hallucinogen dependence (F16.2-)
                   hallucinogen use, unspecified (F16.9-)

F16.10   Hallucinogen abuse, uncomplicated

F16.12   Hallucinogen abuse with intoxication

    F16.120   Hallucinogen abuse with intoxication, uncomplicated

    F16.121   Hallucinogen abuse with intoxication with delirium

    F16.122   Hallucinogen abuse with intoxication with perceptual disturbance

    F16.129   Hallucinogen abuse with intoxication, unspecified

F16.14   Hallucinogen abuse with hallucinogen-induced mood disorder

F16.15   Hallucinogen abuse with hallucinogen-induced psychotic disorder

    F16.150   Hallucinogen abuse with hallucinogen-induced psychotic disorder with delusions

    F16.151   Hallucinogen abuse with hallucinogen-induced psychotic disorder with hallucinations

    F16.159   Hallucinogen abuse with hallucinogen-induced psychotic disorder, unspecified

F16.18   Hallucinogen abuse with other hallucinogen-induced disorder

    F16.180   Hallucinogen abuse with hallucinogen-induced anxiety disorder

    F16.183   Hallucinogen abuse with hallucinogen persisting perception disorder (flashbacks)

    F16.188   Hallucinogen abuse with other hallucinogen-induced disorder

F16.19   Hallucinogen abuse with unspecified hallucinogen-induced disorder

F16.2   Hallucinogen dependence

    Excludes1:   hallucinogen abuse (F16.1-)
                   hallucinogen use, unspecified (F16.9-)

F16.20   Hallucinogen dependence, uncomplicated

F16.21   Hallucinogen dependence, in remission

F16.22   Hallucinogen dependence with intoxication

    F16.220   Hallucinogen dependence with intoxication, uncomplicated

    F16.221   Hallucinogen dependence with intoxication with delirium

F16.229   Hallucinogen dependence with intoxication, unspecified

F16.24   Hallucinogen dependence with hallucinogen-induced mood disorder

F16.25   Hallucinogen dependence with hallucinogen-induced psychotic disorder

F16.250   Hallucinogen dependence with hallucinogen-induced psychotic disorder with delusions

F16.251   Hallucinogen dependence with hallucinogen-induced psychotic disorder with hallucinations

F16.259   Hallucinogen dependence with hallucinogen-induced psychotic disorder, unspecified

F16.28   Hallucinogen dependence with other hallucinogen-induced disorder

F16.280   Hallucinogen dependence with hallucinogen-induced anxiety disorder

F16.283   Hallucinogen dependence with hallucinogen persisting perception disorder (flashbacks)

F16.288   Hallucinogen dependence with other hallucinogen-induced disorder

F16.29   Hallucinogen dependence with unspecified hallucinogen-induced disorder

F16.9   Hallucinogen use, unspecified

Excludes1:   hallucinogen abuse (F16.1-)
hallucinogen dependence (F16.2-)

F16.90   Hallucinogen use, unspecified, uncomplicated

F16.92   Hallucinogen use, unspecified with intoxication

F16.920   Hallucinogen use, unspecified with intoxication, uncomplicated

F16.921   Hallucinogen use, unspecified with intoxication with delirium

F16.929   Hallucinogen use, unspecified with intoxication, unspecified

F16.94   Hallucinogen use, unspecified with hallucinogen-induced mood disorder

F16.95   Hallucinogen use, unspecified with hallucinogen-induced psychotic disorder

F16.950   Hallucinogen use, unspecified with hallucinogen-induced psychotic disorder with delusions

F16.951   Hallucinogen use, unspecified with hallucinogen-induced psychotic disorder with hallucinations

F16.959   Hallucinogen use, unspecified with hallucinogen-induced psychotic disorder, unspecified

F16.98   Hallucinogen use, unspecified with other specified hallucinogen-induced disorder

F16.980   Hallucinogen use, unspecified with hallucinogen-induced anxiety disorder

F16.983   Hallucinogen use, unspecified with hallucinogen persisting perception disorder (flashbacks)

F16.988   Hallucinogen use, unspecified with other hallucinogen-induced disorder

F16.99   Hallucinogen use, unspecified with unspecified hallucinogen-induced disorder

F17   Nicotine dependence

Excludes1:   history of tobacco dependence (Z87.82)
tobacco use NOS (Z72.0)

Excludes2:   tobacco use during pregnancy, childbirth and the puerperium (O99.33-)
toxic effect of nicotine (T65.2-)

F17.2   Nicotine dependence

F17.20   Nicotine dependence, unspecified

F17.200   Nicotine dependence, unspecified, uncomplicated

F17.201   Nicotine dependence, unspecified, in remission

F17.203   Nicotine dependence unspecified, with withdrawal

F17.208   Nicotine dependence, unspecified, with other nicotine-induced disorders

F17.209   Nicotine dependence, unspecified, with unspecified nicotine-induced disorders

F17.21   Nicotine dependence, cigarettes

F17.210   Nicotine dependence, cigarettes, uncomplicated

F17.211   Nicotine dependence, cigarettes, in remission

F17.213   Nicotine dependence, cigarettes, with withdrawal

F17.218   Nicotine dependence, cigarettes, with other nicotine-induced disorders

F17.219   Nicotine dependence, cigarettes, with unspecified nicotine-induced disorders

F17.22   Nicotine dependence, chewing tobacco

F17.220   Nicotine dependence, chewing tobacco, uncomplicated

F17.221   Nicotine dependence, chewing tobacco, in remission

F17.223   Nicotine dependence, chewing tobacco, with withdrawal

F17.228   Nicotine dependence, chewing tobacco, with other nicotine-induced disorders

F17.229   Nicotine dependence, chewing tobacco, with unspecified nicotine-induced disorders

F17.29   Nicotine dependence, other tobacco product

F17.290   Nicotine dependence, other tobacco product, uncomplicated

F17.291   Nicotine dependence, other tobacco product, in remission

F17.292   Nicotine dependence, other tobacco product, with withdrawal

F17.298   Nicotine dependence, other tobacco product, with other nicotine-induced disorders

F17.299   Nicotine dependence, other tobacco product, with unspecified nicotine-induced disorders

F18   Inhalant-related disorders

Includes: volatile solvents

F18.1   Inhalant abuse

Excludes1:   inhalant dependence (F18.2-)
inhalant use, unspecified (F18.9-)

F18.10   Inhalant abuse, uncomplicated

F18.12   Inhalant abuse with intoxication

F18.120   Inhalant abuse with intoxication, uncomplicated

F18.121   Inhalant abuse with intoxication delirium

F18.129   Inhalant abuse with intoxication, unspecified

F18.14   Inhalant abuse with inhalant-induced mood disorder

F18.15   Inhalant abuse with inhalant-induced psychotic disorder

F18.150   Inhalant abuse with inhalant-induced psychotic disorder with delusions

F18.151   Inhalant abuse with inhalant-induced psychotic disorder with hallucinations

F18.159   Inhalant abuse with inhalant-induced psychotic disorder, unspecified

F18.17   Inhalant abuse with inhalant-induced dementia

F18.18   Inhalant abuse with other inhalant-induced disorders

F18.180   Inhalant abuse with inhalant-induced anxiety disorder

F18.188   Inhalant abuse with other inhalant-induced disorder

F18.19   Inhalant abuse with unspecified inhalant-induced disorder

F18.2   Inhalant dependence

Excludes1:   inhalant abuse (F18.1-)
inhalant use, unspecified (F18.9-)

F18.20   Inhalant dependence, uncomplicated

F18.21   Inhalant dependence, in remission

F18.22   Inhalant dependence with intoxication

F18.220 Inhalant dependence with intoxication, uncomplicated

F18.221 Inhalant dependence with intoxication delirium

F18.229 Inhalant dependence with intoxication, unspecified

F18.24 Inhalant dependence with inhalant-induced mood disorder

F18.25 Inhalant dependence with inhalant-induced psychotic disorder

F18.250 Inhalant dependence with inhalant-induced psychotic disorder with delusions

F18.251 Inhalant dependence with inhalant-induced psychotic disorder with hallucinations

F18.259 Inhalant dependence with inhalant-induced psychotic disorder, unspecified

F18.27 Inhalant dependence with inhalant-induced dementia

F18.28 Inhalant dependence with other inhalant-induced disorders

F18.280 Inhalant dependence with inhalant-induced anxiety disorder

F18.288 Inhalant dependence with other inhalant-induced disorder

F18.29 Inhalant dependence with unspecified inhalant-induced disorder

F18.9 Inhalant use, unspecified

Excludes1:   inhalant abuse (F18.1-)
             inhalant dependence (F18.2-)

F18.90 Inhalent use, unspecified, uncomplicated

F18.92 Inhalant use, unspecified with intoxication

F18.920 Inhalant use, unspecified with intoxication, uncomplicated

F18.921 Inhalant use, unspecified with intoxication with delirium

F18.929 Inhalant use, unspecified with intoxication, unspecified

F18.94 Inhalant use, unspecified with inhalant-induced mood disorder

F18.95 Inhalant use, unspecified with inhalant-induced psychotic disorder

F18.950 Inhalant use, unspecified with inhalant-induced psychotic disorder with delusions

F18.951 Inhalant use, unspecified with inhalant-induced psychotic disorder with hallucinations

F18.959 Inhalant use, unspecified with inhalant-induced psychotic disorder, unspecified

F18.97 Inhalant use, unspecified with inhalant-induced persisting dementia

F18.98 Inhalant use, unspecified with other inhalant-induced disorders

F18.980 Inhalant use, unspecified with inhalant-induced anxiety disorder

F18.988 Inhalant use, unspecified with other inhalant-induced disorder

F18.99 Inhalant use, unspecified with unspecified inhalant-induced disorder

F19 Other psychoactive substance-related disorders

Includes: polysubstance drug use (indiscriminate drug use)

F19.1 Other psychoactive substance abuse

Excludes1:   other psychoactive substance dependence (F19.2-)
             other psychoactive substance use, unspecified (F19.9-)

F19.10 Other psychoactive substance abuse, uncomplicated

F19.12 Other psychoactive substance abuse with intoxication

F19.120 Other psychoactive substance abuse with intoxication, uncomplicated

F19.121 Other psychoactive substance abuse with intoxication delirium

F19.122 Other psychoactive substance abuse with intoxication with perceptual disturbances

F19.129 Other psychoactive substance abuse with intoxication, unspecified

F19.14 Other psychoactive substance abuse with psychoactive substance-induced mood disorder

F19.15 Other psychoactive substance abuse with psychoactive substance-induced psychotic disorder

F19.150 Other psychoactive substance abuse with psychoactive substance-induced psychotic disorder with delusions

F19.151 Other psychoactive substance abuse with psychoactive substance-induced psychotic disorder with hallucinations

F19.159 Other psychoactive substance abuse with psychoactive substance-induced psychotic disorder, unspecified

F19.16 Other psychoactive substance abuse with psychoactive substance-induced persisting amnestic disorder

F19.17 Other psychoactive substance abuse with psychoactive substance-induced persisting dementia

F19.18 Other psychoactive substance abuse with other psychoactive substance-induced disorders

F19.180 Other psychoactive substance abuse with psychoactive substance-induced anxiety disorder

F19.181 Other psychoactive substance abuse with psychoactive substance-induced sexual dysfunction

F19.182 Other psychoactive substance abuse with psychoactive substance-induced sleep disorder

F19.188 Other psychoactive substance abuse with other psychoactive substance-induced disorder

F19.19 Other psychoactive substance abuse with unspecified psychoactive substance-induced disorder

F19.2 Other psychoactive substance dependence

Excludes1:   other psychoactive substance abuse (F19.1-)
             other psychoactive substance use, unspecified (F19.9-)

F19.20 Other psychoactive substance dependence, uncomplicated

F19.21 Other psychoactive substance dependence, in remission

F19.22 Other psychoactive substance dependence with intoxication

Excludes1:   other psychoactive substance dependence with withdrawal (F19.23-)

F19.220 Other psychoactive substance dependence with intoxication, uncomplicated

F19.221 Other psychoactive substance dependence with intoxication delirium

F19.222 Other psychoactive substance dependence with intoxication with perceptual disturbance

F19.229 Other psychoactive substance dependence with intoxication, unspecified

F19.23 Other psychoactive substance dependence with withdrawal

Excludes1:   other psychoactive substance dependence with intoxication (F19.22-)

F19.230 Other psychoactive substance dependence with withdrawal, uncomplicated

F19.231 Other psychoactive substance dependence with withdrawal delirium

F19.232 Other psychoactive substance dependence with withdrawal with perceptual disturbance

F19.239 Other psychoactive substance dependence with withdrawal, unspecified

F19.24 Other psychoactive substance dependence with psychoactive substance-induced mood disorder

F19.25 Other psychoactive substance dependence with psychoactive substance-induced psychotic disorder

    F19.250 Other psychoactive substance dependence with psychoactive substance-induced psychotic disorder with delusions

    F19.251 Other psychoactive substance dependence with psychoactive substance-induced psychotic disorder with hallucinations

    F19.259 Other psychoactive substance dependence with psychoactive substance-induced psychotic disorder, unspecified

F19.26 Other psychoactive substance dependence with psychoactive substance-induced persisting amnestic disorder

F19.27 Other psychoactive substance dependence with psychoactive substance-induced persisting dementia

F19.28 Other psychoactive substance dependence with other psychoactive substance-induced disorders

    F19.280 Other psychoactive substance dependence with psychoactive substance-induced anxiety disorder

    F19.281 Other psychoactive substance dependence with psychoactive substance-induced sexual dysfunction

    F19.282 Other psychoactive substance dependence with psychoactive substance-induced sleep disorder

    F19.288 Other psychoactive substance dependence with other psychoactive substance-induced disorder

F19.29 Other psychoactive substance dependence with unspecified psychoactive substance-induced disorder

F19.9 Other psychoactive substance use, unspecified

    Excludes1:   other psychoactive substance abuse (F19.1-)
                other psychoactive substance dependence (F19.2-)

F19.90 Other psychoactive substance use, unspecified, uncomplicated

F19.92 Other psychoactive substance use, unspecified with intoxication

    Excludes1:   other psychoactive substance use, unspecified with withdrawal (F19.93)

    F19.920 Other psychoactive substance use, unspecified with intoxication, uncomplicated

    F19.921 Other psychoactive substance use, unspecified with intoxication with delirium

    F19.922 Other psychoactive substance use, unspecified with intoxication with perceptual disturbance

    F19.929 Other psychoactive substance use, unspecified with intoxication, unspecified

F19.93 Other psychoactive substance use, unspecified with withdrawal

    Excludes1:   other psychoactive substance use, unspecified with intoxication (F19.92-)

    F19.930 Other psychoactive substance use, unspecified with withdrawal, uncomplicated

    F19.931 Other psychoactive substance use, unspecified with withdrawal delirium

    F19.932 Other psychoactive substance use, unspecified with withdrawal with perceptual disturbance

    F19.939 Other psychoactive substance use, unspecified with withdrawal, unspecified

F19.94 Other psychoactive substance use, unspecified with psychoactive substance-induced mood disorder

F19.95 Other psychoactive substance use, unspecified with psychoactive substance-induced psychotic disorder

    F19.950 Other psychoactive substance use, unspecified with psychoactive substance-induced psychotic disorder with delusions

    F19.951 Other psychoactive substance use, unspecified with psychoactive substance-induced psychotic disorder with hallucinations

    F19.959 Other psychoactive substance use, unspecified with psychoactive substance-induced psychotic disorder, unspecified

F19.96 Other psychoactive substance use, unspecified with psychoactive substance-induced persisting amnestic disorder

F19.97 Other psychoactive substance use, unspecified with psychoactive substance-induced persisting dementia

F19.98 Other psychoactive substance use, unspecified with other psychoactive substance-induced disorders

    F19.980 Other psychoactive substance use, unspecified with psychoactive substance-induced anxiety disorder

    F19.981 Other psychoactive substance use, unspecified with psychoactive substance-induced sexual dysfunction

    F19.982 Other psychoactive substance use, unspecified with psychoactive substance-induced sleep disorder

    F19.988 Other psychoactive substance use, unspecified with other psychoactive substance-induced disorder

F19.99 Other psychoactive substance use, unspecified with unspecified psychoactive substance-induced disorder

SCHIZOPHRENIA, SCHIZOTYPAL, DELUSIONAL, AND OTHER NON–MOOD PSYCHOTIC DISORDERS (F20–F29)

F20 **Schizophrenia**

    Excludes1:   brief psychotic disorder (F23)
                cyclic schizophrenia (F25.0)
                mood [affective] disorders with psychotic symptoms (F30.2, F31.2, F31.5, F31.64, F32.3, F33.3)
                schizoaffective disorder (F25.-)
                schizophrenic reaction NOS (F23)

    Excludes2:   schizophrenic reaction in:
                alcoholism (F10.15-, F10.25-, F10.95-)
                brain disease (F06.2)
                epilepsy (F06.2)
                psychoactive drug use (F11-F19 with .15, .25, .95)
                schizotypal disorder (F21)

F20.0 **Paranoid schizophrenia**
    Paraphrenic schizophrenia
    Excludes1:   involutional paranoid state (F22)
                paranoia (F22)

F20.1 **Disorganized schizophrenia**
    Hebephrenic schizophrenia
    Hebephrenia

F20.2 **Catatonic schizophrenia**
    Schizophrenic catalepsy
    Schizophrenic catatonia
    Schizophrenic flexibilitas cerea
    Excludes1:   catatonic stupor (R40.1)

F20.3 **Undifferentiated schizophrenia**
    Atypical schizophrenia
    Excludes1:   acute schizophrenia-like psychotic disorder (F23)
    Excludes2:   post-schizophrenic depression (F32.8)

F20.5 **Residual schizophrenia**
    Restzustand (schizophrenic)
    Schizophrenic residual state

F20.8 **Other schizophrenia**

F20.81 **Schizophreniform disorder**
    Schizophreniform psychosis NOS

F20.89 **Other schizophrenia**
    Cenesthopathic schizophrenia
    Simple schizophrenia

F20.9 **Schizophrenia, unspecified**

F21 Schizotypal disorder

Includes:
borderline schizophrenia
latent schizophrenia
latent schizophrenic reaction
prepsychotic schizophrenia
prodromal schizophrenia
pseudoneurotic schizophrenia
pseudopsychopathic schizophrenia
schizotypal personality disorder

Excludes2:
Asperger's syndrome (F84.5)
schizoid personality disorder (F60.1)

F22 Delusional disorders

Includes:
delusional dysmorphophobia
involutional paranoid state
paranoia
paranoia querulans
paranoid psychosis
paranoid state
paraphrenia (late)
Sensitiver Beziehungswahn

Excludes1:
mood [affective] disorders with psychotic symptoms (F30.2, F31.2, F31.5, F31.64, F32.3, F33.3)
paranoid schizophrenia (F20.0)

Excludes2:
paranoid personality disorder (F60.0)
paranoid psychosis, psychogenic (F23)
paranoid reaction (F23)

F23 Brief psychotic disorder

Includes:
paranoid reaction
psychogenic paranoid psychosis

Excludes2:
mood [affective] disorders with psychotic symptoms (F30.2, F31.2, F31.5, F31.64, F32.3, F33.3)

F24 Shared psychotic disorder

Includes:
folie à deux
induced paranoid disorder
induced psychotic disorder

F25 Schizoaffective disorders

Excludes1:
mood [affective] disorders with psychotic symptoms (F30.2, F31.2, F31.5, F31.64, F32.3, F33.3)
schizophrenia (F20.-)

F25.0 Schizoaffective disorder, bipolar type
Cyclic schizophrenia
Schizoaffective disorder, manic type
Schizoaffective disorder, mixed type
Schizoaffective psychosis, bipolar type
Schizophreniform psychosis, manic type

F25.1 Schizoaffective disorder, depressive type
Schizoaffective psychosis, depressive type
Schizophreniform psychosis, depressive type

F25.8 Other schizoaffective disorders

F25.9 Schizoaffective disorder, unspecified
Schizoaffective psychosis NOS

F28 Other psychotic disorder not due to a substance or known physiological condition
Includes: chronic hallucinatory psychosis

F29 Unspecified psychosis not due to a substance or known physiological condition
Includes: psychosis NOS
Excludes1: mental disorder NOS (F99)
unspecified mental disorder due to known physiological condition (F09)

MOOD [AFFECTIVE] DISORDERS (F30–F39)

F30 Manic episode

Includes:
bipolar disorder, single manic episode
mixed affective episode

Excludes1:
bipolar disorder (F31.-)
major depressive disorder, single episode (F32.-)
major depressive disorder, recurrent (F33.-)

F30.1 Manic episode without psychotic symptoms

F30.10 Manic episode without psychotic symptoms, unspecified
F30.11 Manic episode without psychotic symptoms, mild
F30.12 Manic episode without psychotic symptoms, moderate
F30.13 Manic episode, severe, without psychotic symptoms

F30.2 Manic episode, severe with psychotic symptoms
Manic stupor
Mania with mood-congruent psychotic symptoms
Mania with mood-incongruent psychotic symptoms

F30.3 Manic episode in partial remission

F30.4 Manic episode in full remission

F30.8 Other manic episodes
Hypomania

F30.9 Manic episode, unspecified
Mania NOS

F31 Bipolar disorder

Includes:
manic-depressive illness
manic-depressive psychosis
manic-depressive reaction

Excludes1:
bipolar disorder, single manic episode (F30.-)
major depressive disorder, single episode (F32.-)
major depressive disorder, recurrent (F33.-)

Excludes2: cyclothymia (F34.0)

F31.0 Bipolar disorder, current episode hypomanic

F31.1 Bipolar disorder, current episode manic without psychotic features

F31.10 Bipolar disorder, current episode manic without psychotic features, unspecified
F31.11 Bipolar disorder, current episode manic without psychotic features, mild
F31.12 Bipolar disorder, current episode manic without psychotic features, moderate
F31.13 Bipolar disorder, current episode manic without psychotic features, severe

F31.2 Bipolar disorder, current episode manic severe with psychotic features
Bipolar disorder, current episode manic with mood-congruent psychotic symptoms
Bipolar disorder, current episode manic with mood-incongruent psychotic symptoms

F31.3 Bipolar disorder, current episode depressed, mild or moderate severity

F31.30 Bipolar disorder, current episode depressed, mild or moderate severity, unspecified
F31.31 Bipolar disorder, current episode depressed, mild
F31.32 Bipolar disorder, current episode depressed, moderate

F31.4 Bipolar disorder, current episode depressed, severe, without psychotic features

F31.5 Bipolar disorder, current episode depressed, severe, with psychotic features
Bipolar disorder, current episode depressed with mood-incongruent psychotic symptoms
Bipolar disorder, current episode depressed with mood-congruent psychotic symptoms

F31.6 Bipolar disorder, current episode mixed

F31.60 Bipolar disorder, current episode mixed, unspecified
F31.61 Bipolar disorder, current episode mixed, mild
F31.62 Bipolar disorder, current episode mixed, moderate
F31.63 Bipolar disorder, current episode mixed, severe, without psychotic features
F31.64 Bipolar disorder, current episode mixed, severe, with psychotic features
Bipolar disorder, current episode mixed with mood-congruent psychotic symptoms
Bipolar disorder, current episode mixed with mood-incongruent psychotic symptoms

F31.7 Bipolar disorder, currently in remission

F31.70 Bipolar disorder, currently in remission, most recent episode unspecified
F31.71 Bipolar disorder, in partial remission, most recent episode hypomanic

F31.72 Bipolar disorder, in full remission, most recent episode hypomanic

F31.73 Bipolar disorder, in partial remission, most recent episode manic

F31.74 Bipolar disorder, in full remission, most recent episode manic

F31.75 Bipolar disorder, in partial remission, most recent episode depressed

F31.76 Bipolar disorder, in full remission, most recent episode depressed

F31.77 Bipolar disorder, in partial remission, most recent episode mixed

F31.78 Bipolar disorder, in full remission, most recent episode mixed

F31.8 Other bipolar disorders

F31.81 Bipolar II disorder

F31.89 Other bipolar disorder
Recurrent manic episodes

F31.9 Bipolar disorder, unspecified

F32 Major depressive disorder, single episode

Includes: single episode of agitated depression
single episode of depressive reaction
single episode of major depression
single episode of psychogenic depression
single episode of reactive depression
single episode of vital depression

Excludes1: bipolar disorder (F31-)
manic episode (F30-)
recurrent depressive disorder (F33.-)

Excludes2: adjustment disorder (F43.2)

F32.0 Major depressive disorder, single episode, mild

F32.1 Major depressive disorder, single episode, moderate

F32.2 Major depressive disorder, single episode, severe without psychotic features

F32.3 Major depressive disorder, single episode, severe with psychotic features
Single episode of major depression with mood-congruent psychotic symptoms
Single episode of major depression with mood-incongruent psychotic symptoms
Single episode of major depression with psychotic symptoms
Single episode of psychogenic depressive psychosis
Single episode of psychotic depression
Single episode of reactive depressive psychosis

F32.4 Major depressive disorder, single episode, in partial remission

F32.5 Major depressive disorder, single episode, in full remission

F32.8 Other depressive episodes
Atypical depression
Post-schizophrenic depression
Single episode of "masked" depression NOS

F32.9 Major depressive disorder, single episode, unspecified
Depression NOS
Depressive disorder NOS

F33 Major depressive disorder, recurrent

Includes: recurrent episodes of:
depressive reaction
endogenous depression
major depression
psychogenic depression
reactive depression
seasonal depressive disorder
vital depression

Excludes1: bipolar disorder (F31.-)
manic episode (F30.-)

F33.0 Major depressive disorder, recurrent, mild

F33.1 Major depressive disorder, recurrent, moderate

F33.2 Major depressive disorder, recurrent severe without psychotic features

F33.3 Major depressive disorder, recurrent, severe with psychotic symptoms
Endogenous depression with psychotic symptoms
Recurrent severe episodes of major depression with mood-congruent psychotic symptoms
Recurrent severe episodes of major depression with mood-incongruent psychotic symptoms
Recurrent severe episodes of major depression with psychotic symptoms
Recurrent severe episodes of psychogenic depressive psychosis
Recurrent severe episodes of psychotic depression
Recurrent severe episodes of reactive depressive psychosis

F33.4 Major depressive disorder, recurrent, in remission

F33.40 Major depressive disorder, recurrent, in remission, unspecified

F33.41 Major depressive disorder, recurrent, in partial remission

F33.42 Major depressive disorder, recurrent, in full remission

F33.8 Other recurrent depressive disorders
Recurrent brief depressive episodes

F33.9 Major depressive disorder, recurrent, unspecified
Monopolar depression NOS

F34 Persistent mood [affective] disorders

F34.0 Cyclothymic disorder
Affective personality disorder
Cycloid personality
Cyclothymia
Cyclothymic personality

F34.1 Dysthymic disorder
Depressive neurosis
Depressive personality disorder
Dysthymia
Neurotic depression
Persistent anxiety depression
Excludes2: anxiety depression (mild or not persistent) (F41.8)

F34.8 Other persistent mood [affective] disorders

F34.9 Persistent mood [affective] disorder, unspecified

F39 Unspecified mood [affective] disorder
Includes: affective psychosis NOS

ANXIETY, DISSOCIATIVE, STRESS–RELATED, SOMATOFORM AND OTHER NONPSYCHOTIC MENTAL DISORDERS (F40–F48)

F40 Phobic anxiety disorders

F40.0 Agoraphobia

F40.00 Agoraphobia, unspecified

F40.01 Agoraphobia with panic disorder
Panic disorder with agoraphobia
Excludes1: panic disorder without agoraphobia (F41.0)

F40.02 Agoraphobia without panic disorder

F40.1 Social phobias
Anthropophobia
Social anxiety disorder of childhood
Social neurosis

F40.10 Social phobia, unspecified

F40.11 Social phobia, generalized

F40.2 Specific (isolated) phobias
Excludes2: dysmorphophobia (nondelusional) (F45.22)
nosophobia (F45.22)

F40.21 Animal type phobia

F40.210 Arachnophobia
Fear of spiders

F40.218 Other animal type phobia

F40.22 Natural environment type phobia

F40.220 Fear of thunderstorms

F40.228 Other natural environment type phobia

F40.23 Blood, injection, injury type phobia

F40.230 Fear of blood

F40.231 Fear of injections and transfusions

F40.232 Fear of other medical care

F40.233   Fear of injury
F40.24   Situational type phobia
F40.240   Claustrophobia
F40.241   Acrophobia
F40.242   Fear of bridges
F40.243   Fear of flying
F40.248   Other situational type phobia
F40.29   Other specified phobia
F40.290   Androphobia
Fear of men
F40.291   Gynephobia
Fear of women
F40.298   Other specified phobia
F40.8   Other phobic anxiety disorders
Phobic anxiety disorder of childhood
F40.9   Phobic anxiety disorder, unspecified
Phobia NOS
Phobic state NOS

F41   Other anxiety disorders
Excludes2   anxiety in:
acute stress reaction (F43.0)
transient adjustment reaction (F43.2)
neurasthenia (F48.8)
psychophysiologic disorders (F45.-)
separation anxiety (F93.0)
F41.0   Panic disorder [episodic paroxysmal anxiety] without agoraphobia
Panic attack
Panic state
Excludes1   panic disorder with agoraphobia (F40.01)
F41.1   Generalized anxiety disorder
Anxiety neurosis
Anxiety reaction
Anxiety state
Overanxious disorder
Excludes2:   neurasthenia (F48.8)
F41.3   Other mixed anxiety disorders
F41.8   Other specified anxiety disorders
Anxiety depression (mild or not persistent)
Anxiety hysteria
Mixed anxiety and depressive disorder
F41.9   Anxiety disorder, unspecified
Anxiety NOS

F42   Obsessive-compulsive disorder
Includes: anankastic neurosis
obsessive-compulsive neurosis
Excludes2:   obsessive-compulsive personality (disorder) (F60.5)
obsessive-compulsive symptoms occurring in:
depression (F32-F33)
schizophrenia (F20.-)

F43   Reaction to severe stress, and adjustment disorders
F43.0   Acute stress reaction
Acute crisis reaction
Acute reaction to stress
Combat fatigue
Crisis state
Psychic shock
F43.1   Post-traumatic stress disorder
Traumatic neurosis
F43.10   Post-traumatic stress disorder, unspecified
F43.11   Post-traumatic stress disorder, acute
F43.12   Post-traumatic stress disorder, chronic
F43.2   Adjustment disorders
Culture shock
Grief reaction
Hospitalism in children
Excludes2:   separation anxiety disorder of childhood (F93.0)
F43.20   Adjustment disorder, unspecified
F43.21   Adjustment disorder with depressed mood
F43.22   Adjustment disorder with anxiety

F43.23   Adjustment disorder with mixed anxiety and depressed mood
F43.24   Adjustment disorder with disturbance of conduct
F43.25   Adjustment disorder with mixed disturbance of emotions and conduct
F43.29   Adjustment disorder with other symptoms
F43.8   Other reactions to severe stress
F43.9   Reaction to severe stress, unspecified

F44   Dissociative and conversion disorders
Includes: conversion hysteria
conversion reaction
hysteria
hysterical psychosis
Excludes2:   malingering [conscious simulation] (Z76.5)
F44.0   Dissociative amnesia
Excludes1:   amnesia NOS (R41.3)
anterograde amnesia (R41.1)
retrograde amnesia (R41.2)
Excludes2:   alcohol-or other psychoactive substance-induced amnestic disorder (F10, F13, F19 with .26, .96)
amnestic disorder due to known physiological condition (F04)
postictal amnesia in epilepsy (G40.-)
F44.1   Dissociative fugue
Excludes2:   postictal fugue in epilepsy (G40.-)
F44.2   Dissociative stupor
Excludes1:   catatonic stupor (R40.1)
stupor NOS (R40.1)
Excludes2:   catatonic disorder due to known physiological condition (F06.1)
depressive stupor (F32, F33)
manic stupor (F30, F31)
F44.4   Conversion disorder with motor symptom or deficit
Dissociative motor disorders
Psychogenic aphonia
Psychogenic dysphonia
F44.5   Conversion disorder with seizures or convulsions
Dissociative convulsions
F44.6   Conversion disorder with sensory symptom or deficit
Dissociative anesthesia and sensory loss
Psychogenic deafness
F44.7   Conversion disorder with mixed symptom presentation
F44.8   Other dissociative and conversion disorders
F44.81   Dissociative identity disorder
Multiple personality disorder
F44.89   Other dissociative and conversion disorders
Ganser's syndrome
Psychogenic confusion
Psychogenic twilight state
Trance and possession disorders
F44.9   Dissociative and conversion disorder, unspecified
Dissociative disorder NOS

F45   Somatoform disorders
Excludes2:   dissociative and conversion disorders (F44.-)
factitious disorders (F68.1-)
hair-plucking (F63.3)
lalling (F80.0)
lisping (F80.0)
malingering [conscious simulation] (Z76.5)
nail-biting (F98.8)
psychological or behavioral factors associated with disorders or diseases classified elsewhere (F54)
sexual dysfunction, not due to a substance or known physiological condition (F52.-)
thumb-sucking (F98.8)
tic disorders (in childhood and adolescence) (F95.-)
Tourette's syndrome (F95.2)
trichotillomania (F63.3)
F45.0   Somatization disorder
Multiple psychosomatic disorder

F45.1 Undifferentiated somatoform disorder
Undifferentiated psychosomatic disorder

F45.2 Hypochondriacal disorders

Excludes2:   delusional dysmorphophobia (F22)
fixed delusions about bodily functions or shape (F22)

F45.20   Hypochondriacal disorder, unspecified

F45.21   Hypochondriasis
Hypochondriacal neurosis

F45.22   Body dysmorphic disorder
Dysmorphophobia (nondelusional)
Nosophobia

F45.29   Other hypochondriacal disorders

F45.4 Pain disorder
Psychalgia
Psychogenic backache
Psychogenic headache
Somatoform pain disorder (persistent)

Excludes2:   acute pain (R52.0)
backache NOS (M54.9-)
chronic pain (R52.2)
intractable pain (R52.1)
pain NOS (R52.9)
tension headache (G44.2)

F45.8 Other somatoform disorders
Psychogenic dysmenorrhea
Psychogenic dysphagia, including "globus hystericus"
Psychogenic pruritus
Psychogenic torticollis
Somatoform autonomic dysfunction
Teeth-grinding

F45.9 Somatoform disorder, unspecified
Psychosomatic disorder NOS

F48 Other nonpsychotic mental disorders

F48.1 Depersonalization-derealization syndrome

F48.8 Other specified nonpsychotic mental disorders
Briquet's disorder
Dhat syndrome
Neurasthenia
Occupational neurosis, including writer's cramp
Psychasthenia
Psychasthenic neurosis
Psychogenic syncope

F48.9 Nonpsychotic mental disorder, unspecified
Neurosis NOS

BEHAVIORAL SYNDROMES ASSOCIATED WITH PHYSIOLOGICAL DISTURBANCES AND PHYSICAL FACTORS (F50–F59)

F50 Eating disorders

Excludes1:   anorexia NOS (R63.0)
feeding difficulties and mismanagement (R63.3)
polyphagia (R63.2)

Excludes2:   feeding disorder in infancy or childhood (F98.2-)

F50.0 Anorexia nervosa

Excludes1:   loss of appetite (R63.0)
psychogenic loss of appetitie (F50.8)

F50.00   Anorexia nervosa, unspecified

F50.01   Anorexia nervosa, restricting type

F50.02   Anorexia nervosa, binge eating/purging type
Excludes1:   bulimia nervosa (F50.2)

F50.2 Bulimia nervosa
Bulimia NOS
Hyperorexia nervosa

Excludes1:   anorexia nervosa, binge eating/purging type (F50.02)

F50.8 Other eating disorders
Pica in adults
Psychogenic loss of appetite

Excludes2:   pica of infancy and childhood (F98.3)

F50.9 Eating disorder, unspecified
Atypical anorexia nervosa
Atypical bulimia nervosa

F51 Sleep disorders not due to a substance or known physiological condition

Excludes2:   sleep disorders (organic) (G47.-)

F51.0 Insomnia not due to a substance or known physiological condition
Primary insomnia

Excludes2:   insomnia (due to known physiological condition) (G47.0)

F51.1 Hypersomnia not due to a substance or known physiological condition

Excludes2:   hypersomnia (due to known physiological condition) (G47.1)
narcolepsy (G47.4)

F51.2 Circadian rhythm sleep disorder not due to a substance or known physiological condition
Psychogenic inversion of nyctohemeral rhythm
Psychogenic inversion of sleep rhythm

Excludes2:   disorders of the sleep-wake schedule (due to a known physiological condition) (G47.2)

F51.20   Circadian rhythm sleep disorder not due to a substance or known physiological condition, unspecified type

F51.21   Circadian rhythm sleep disorder not due to a substance or known physiological condition, jet-lag type

F51.22   Circadian rhythm sleep disorder not due to a substance or known physiological condition, shift-work type

F51.23   Circadian rhythm sleep disorder not due to a substance or known physiological condition, delayed sleep phase type

F51.29   Other sleep disorder of circadian rhythm not due to a substance or known physiological condition

F51.3 Sleepwalking [somnambulism]

F51.4 Sleep terrors [night terrors]

F51.5 Nightmare disorder
Dream anxiety disorder

F51.8 Other sleep disorders not due to a substance or known physiological condition

F51.9 Sleep disorder not due to a substance or known physiological condition, unspecified
Emotional sleep disorder NOS

F52 Sexual dysfunction not due to a substance or known physiological condition

Excludes2:   Dhat syndrome (F48.8)

F52.0 Hypoactive sexual desire disorder
Anhedonia (sexual)
Lack or loss of sexual desire

F52.1 Sexual aversion disorder
Sexual aversion and lack of sexual enjoyment

F52.2 Sexual arousal disorders
Failure of genital response

F52.21   Male erectile disorder
Psychogenic impotence
Excludes1:   impotence of organic origin (N52.-)

F52.22   Female sexual arousal disorder
Frigidity

F52.3 Orgasmic disorder
Inhibited orgasm
Psychogenic anorgasmy

F52.31   Female orgasmic disorder

F52.32   Male orgasmic disorder

F52.4 Premature ejaculation

F52.5 Vaginismus not due to a substance or known physiological condition
Psychogenic vaginismus

Excludes2:   vaginismus (due to a known physiological condition) (N94.2)

F52.6 **Dyspareunia not due to a substance or known physiological condition**
Psychogenic dyspareunia
Excludes2: dyspareunia (due to a known physiological condition) (N94.1)

F52.8 **Other sexual dysfunction not due to a substance or known physiological condition**
Excessive sexual drive
Nymphomania
Satyriasis

F52.9 **Unspecified sexual dysfunction not due to a substance or known physiological condition**
Sexual dysfunction NOS

F53 **Puerperal psychosis**
Excludes1: mood disorders with psychotic features (F30.2, F31.2, F31.5, F31.64, F32.3, F33.3)
postpartum dysphoria (O90.6)
psychosis in schizophrenia, schizotypal, delusional, and other psychotic disorders (F20-F29)

F54 **Psychological and behavioral factors associated with disorders or diseases classified elsewhere**
Psychological factors affecting physical conditions
Code first the associated physical disorder, such as:
asthma (J45.-)
dermatitis (L23-L25)
gastric ulcer (K25.-)
mucous colitis (K58.-)
ulcerative colitis (K51.-)
urticaria (L50.-)
Excludes2: tension-type headache (G44.2)

F55 **Abuse of non-psychoactive substances**
Excludes2: abuse of psychoactive substances (F10-F19)
F55.0 **Abuse of antacids**
F55.1 **Abuse of herbal or folk remedies**
F55.2 **Abuse of laxatives**
F55.3 **Abuse of steroids or hormones**
F55.4 **Abuse of vitamins**
F55.8 **Abuse of other non-psychoactive substances**

F59 **Unspecified behavioral syndromes associated with physiological disturbances and physical factors**
Includes: psychogenic physiological dysfunction NOS

DISORDERS OF ADULT PERSONALITY AND BEHAVIOR (F60–F69)

F60 **Specific personality disorders**
F60.0 **Paranoid personality disorder**
Expansive paranoid personality (disorder)
Fanatic personality (disorder)
Querulant personality (disorder)
Paranoid personality (disorder)
Sensitive paranoid personality (disorder)
Excludes2: paranoia (F22)
paranoia querulans (F22)
paranoid psychosis (F22)
paranoid schizophrenia (F20.0)
paranoid state (F22)

F60.1 **Schizoid personality disorder**
Excludes2: Asperger's syndrome (F84.5)
delusional disorder (F22)
schizoid disorder of childhood (F84.5)
schizophrenia (F20.-)
schizotypal disorder (F21)

F60.2 **Antisocial personality disorder**
Amoral personality (disorder)
Asocial personality (disorder)
Dissocial personality disorder
Psychopathic personality (disorder)
Sociopathic personality (disorder)
Excludes1: conduct disorders (F91.-)
Excludes2: borderline personality disorder (F60.3)

F60.3 **Borderline personality disorder**
Aggressive personality (disorder)
Emotionally unstable personality disorder
Explosive personality (disorder)
Excludes2: antisocial personality disorder (F60.2)

F60.4 **Histrionic personality disorder**
Hysterical personality (disorder)
Psychoinfantile personality (disorder)

F60.5 **Obsessive-compulsive personality disorder**
Anankastic personality (disorder)
Compulsive personality (disorder)
Obsessional personality (disorder)
Excludes2: obsessive-compulsive disorder (F42)

F60.6 **Avoidant personality disorder**
Anxious personality disorder

F60.7 **Dependent personality disorder**
Asthenic personality (disorder)
Inadequate personality (disorder)
Passive personality (disorder)

F60.8 **Other specific personality disorders**
F60.81 **Narcissistic personality disorder**
F60.89 **Other specific personality disorders**
Eccentric personality disorder
"Haltlose" type personality disorder
Immature personality disorder
Passive-aggressive personality disorder
Psychoneurotic personality disorder
Self-defeating personality disorder

F60.9 **Personality disorder, unspecified**
Character disorder NOS
Character neurosis NOS
Pathological personality NOS

F63 **Impulse disorders**
Excludes2: habitual excessive use of alcohol or psychoactive substances (F10-F19)
impulse disorders involving sexual behavior (F65.-)

F63.0 **Pathological gambling**
Compulsive gambling
Excludes1: gambling and betting NOS (Z72.6)
Excludes2: excessive gambling by manic patients (F30, F31)
gambling in antisocial personality disorder (F60.2)

F63.1 **Pyromania**
Pathological fire-setting
Excludes2: fire-setting (by) (in):
adult with antisocial personality disorder (F60.2)
alcohol or psychoactive substance intoxication (F10-F19)
conduct disorders (F91.-)
mental disorders due to known physiological condition (F01-F09)
schizophrenia (F20.-)

F63.2 **Kleptomania**
Pathological stealing
Excludes1: shoplifting as the reason for observation for suspected mental disorder (Z03.8)
Excludes2: depressive disorder with stealing (F31-F33)
stealing due to underlying mental condition-code to mental condition
stealing in mental disorders due to known physiological condition (F01-F09)

F63.3 **Trichotillomania**
Hair plucking
Excludes2: other stereotyped movement disorder (F98.4)

F63.8   Other impulse disorders
- **F63.81   Intermittent explosive disorder**
- **F63.89   Other impulse disorders**

F63.9   Impulse disorder, unspecified
Impulse control disorder NOS

F64   Gender identity disorders

F64.1   Gender identity disorder in adolescence and adulthood
Dual role transvestism
Transsexualism
Use additional code to identify sex reassignment status (Z87.81)
Excludes1:   gender identity disorder in childhood (F64.2)
Excludes2:   fetishistic transvestism (F65.1)

F64.2   Gender identity disorder of childhood
Excludes1:   gender identity disorder in adolescence and adulthood (F64.1)
Excludes2:   egodystonic sexual orientation (F66)
sexual maturation disorder (F66)

F64.8   Other gender identity disorders

F64.9   Gender identity disorder, unspecified
Gender-role disorder NOS

F65   Paraphilias

F65.0   Fetishism

F65.1   Transvestic fetishism
Fetishistic transvestism

F65.2   Exhibitionism

F65.3   Voyeurism

F65.4   Pedophilia

F65.5   Sadomasochism
- **F65.50   Sadomasochism, unspecified**
- **F65.51   Sexual masochism**
- **F65.52   Sexual sadism**

F65.8   Other paraphilias
- **F65.81   Frotteurism**
- **F65.89   Other paraphilias**
  Necrophilia

F65.9   Paraphilia, unspecified
Sexual deviation NOS

F66   Other sexual disorders
Includes: egodystonic sexual orientation
sexual maturation disorder
sexual relationship disorder

F68   Other disorders of adult personality and behavior

F68.1   Factitious disorder
Compensation neurosis
Elaboration of physical symptoms for psychological reasons
Hospital hopper syndrome
Münchhausen's syndrome
Peregrinating patient
Excludes2:   factitial dermatitis (L98.1)
person feigning illness (with obvious motivation) (Z76.5)
- **F68.10   Factitious disorder, unspecified**
- **F68.11   Factitious disorder with predominantly psychological signs and symptoms**
- **F68.12   Factitious disorder with predominantly physical signs and symptoms**
- **F68.13   Factitious disorder with combined psychological and physical signs and symptoms**

F68.8   Other specified disorders of adult personality and behavior

F69   Unspecified disorder of adult personality and behavior

MENTAL RETARDATION (F70–F79)

Code first any associated physical or developmental disorders
Excludes1:   borderline intellectual functioning, IQ above 70 to 84 (R41.83)

F70   Mild mental retardation
Includes: IQ level 50-55 to approximately 70
mild mental subnormality

F71   Moderate mental retardation
Includes: IQ level 35-40 to 50-55
moderate mental subnormality

F72   Severe mental retardation
Includes: IQ 20-25 to 35-40
severe mental subnormality

F73   Profound mental retardation
Includes: IQ level below 20-25
profound mental subnormality

F78   Other mental retardation

F79   Unspecified mental retardation
Includes: mental deficiency NOS
mental subnormality NOS

PERVASIVE AND SPECIFIC DEVELOPMENTAL DISORDERS (F80–F89)

F80   Specific developmental disorders of speech and language

F80.0   Phonological disorder
Dyslalia
Functional speech articulation disorder
Lalling
Lisping
Phonological developmental disorder
Speech articulation developmental disorder
Excludes1:   speech articulation impairment due to aphasia NOS (R47.0)
speech articulation impairment due to apraxia (R48.2)
Excludes2:   speech articulation impairment due to hearing loss (H90-H91)
speech articulation impairment due to mental retardation (F70-F79)
speech articulation impairment with expressive language developmental disorder (F80.1)
speech articulation impairment with mixed receptive expressive language developmental disorder (F80.2)

F80.1   Expressive language disorder
Developmental dysphasia or aphasia, expressive type
Excludes1:   mixed receptive-expressive language disorder (F80.2)
dysphasia and aphasia NOS (R47.0)
Excludes2:   acquired aphasia with epilepsy [Landau-Kleffner] (F80.3)
selective mutism (F94.0)
mental retardation (F70-F79)
pervasive developmental disorders (F84.-)

F80.2   Mixed receptive-expressive language disorder
Congenital auditory imperception
Developmental dysphasia or aphasia, receptive type
Developmental Wernicke's aphasia
Word deafness
Excludes1:   dysphasia or aphasia NOS (R47.0)
expressive language disorder (F80.1)
expressive type dysphasia or aphasia (F80.1)
Excludes2:   acquired aphasia with epilepsy [Landau-Kleffner] (F80.3)
pervasive developmental disorders (F84.-)
selective mutism (F94.0)
language delay due to deafness (H90-H91)
mental retardation (F70-F79)

F80.3 Acquired aphasia with epilepsy [Landau-Kleffner]
> Excludes1:   aphasia NOS (R47.0)
> Excludes2:   pervasive developmental disorders (F84.-)

F80.8 Other developmental disorders of speech or language

F80.9 Developmental disorder of speech or language, unspecified
> Communication disorder NOS
> Language disorder NOS

F81 Specific developmental disorders of scholastic skills

F81.0 Specific reading disorder
> "Backward reading"
> Developmental dyslexia
> Specific reading retardation
> Excludes1:   alexia NOS (R48.0)
>   dyslexia NOS (R48.0)

F81.2 Mathematics disorder
> Developmental acalculia
> Developmental arithmetical disorder
> Developmental Gerstmann's syndrome
> Excludes1:   acalculia NOS (R48.8)
> Excludes2:   arithmetical difficulties associated with a reading
>   disorder (F81.0)
>   arithmetical difficulties associated with a spelling
>   disorder (F81.81)
>   arithmetical difficulties due to inadequate
>   teaching (Z55.8)

F81.8 Other developmental disorders of scholastic skills

F81.81 Disorder of written expression
> Specific spelling disorder

F81.89 Other developmental disorders of scholastic skills

F81.9 Developmental disorder of scholastic skills, unspecified
> Knowledge acquisition disability NOS
> Learning disability NOS
> Learning disorder NOS

F82 Specific developmental disorder of motor function
> Includes: clumsy child syndrome
>   developmental coordination disorder
>   developmental dyspraxia
> Excludes1:   abnormalities of gait and mobility (F84.2 R26.-)
>   lack of coordination (R27.-)
> Excludes2:   lack of coordination secondary to mental retardation
>   (F70-F79)

F84 Pervasive developmental disorders
> Use additional code to identify any associated medical condition and
>   mental retardation.

F84.0 Autistic disorder
> Infantile autism
> Infantile psychosis
> Kanner's syndrome
> Excludes1:   Asperger's syndrome (F84.5)

F84.2 Rett's syndrome
> Excludes1:   Asperger's syndrome (F84.5)
>   autistic disorder (F84.0)
>   other childhood disintegrative disorder (F84.3)

F84.3 Other childhood disintegrative disorder
> Dementia infantilis
> Disintegrative psychosis
> Heller's syndrome
> Symbiotic psychosis
> Use additional code to identify any associated neurological
>   condition.
> Excludes1:   Asperger's syndrome (F84.5)
>   autistic disorder (F84.0)
>   Rett's syndrome (F84.2)

F84.5 Asperger's syndrome
> Asperger's disorder
> Autistic psychopathy
> Schizoid disorder of childhood

F84.8 Other pervasive developmental disorders
> Overactive disorder associated with mental retardation and
>   stereotyped movements

F84.9 Pervasive developmental disorder, unspecified
> Atypical autism

F88 Other disorders of psychological development
> Includes: developmental agnosia

F89 Unspecified disorder of psychological development
> Includes: developmental disorder NOS

BEHAVIORAL AND EMOTIONAL DISORDERS WITH ONSET USUALLY OCCURRING IN CHILDHOOD AND ADOLESCENCE (F90–F98)

> Note: Codes within categories F90-F98 may be used regardless of the
> age of a patient. These disorders generally have onset within the
> childhood or adolescent years, but may continue throughout life or
> not be diagnosed until adulthood

F90 Attention-deficit hyperactivity disorders
> Includes: attention deficit disorder with hyperactivity
>   attention deficit syndrome with hyperactivity
> Excludes2:   anxiety disorders (F40.-, F41.-)
>   mood [affective] disorders (F30-F39)
>   pervasive developmental disorders (F84.-)
>   schizophrenia (F20.-)

F90.0 Attention-deficit hyperactivity disorder, predominantly inattentive type

F90.1 Attention-deficit hyperactivity disorder, predominantly hyperactive type

F90.2 Attention-deficit hyperactivity disorder, combined type

F90.8 Attention-deficit hyperactivity disorder, other type

F90.9 Attention-deficit hyperactivity disorder, unspecified type
> Attention-deficit hyperactivity disorder of childhood or
>   adolescence NOS
> Attention-deficit hyperactivity disorder NOS

F91 Conduct disorders
> Excludes1:   antisocial behavior (Z72.81-)
>   antisocial personality disorder (F60.2)
> Excludes2:   conduct problems associated with attention-deficit
>   hyperactivity disorder (F90.-)
>   mood [affective] disorders (F30-F39)
>   pervasive developmental disorders (F84.-)
>   schizophrenia (F20.-)

F91.0 Conduct disorder confined to family context

F91.1 Conduct disorder, childhood-onset type
> Conduct disorder, solitary aggressive type
> Unsocialized aggressive disorder
> Unsocialized conduct disorder

F91.2 Conduct disorder, adolescent-onset type
> Conduct disorder, group type
> Socialized conduct disorder

F91.3 Oppositional defiant disorder

F91.8 Other conduct disorders

F91.9 Conduct disorder, unspecified
> Behavioral disorder NOS
> Conduct disorder NOS
> Disruptive behavior disorder NOS

F93 Emotional disorders with onset specific to childhood

F93.0 Separation anxiety disorder of childhood
> Excludes2:   mood [affective] disorders (F30-F39)
>   nonpsychotic mental disorders (F40-F48)
>   phobic anxiety disorder of childhood (F40.8)
>   social phobia (F40.1)

F93.8 Other childhood emotional disorders
> Identity disorder
> Excludes2:   gender identity disorder of childhood (F64.2)

F93.9 Childhood emotional disorder, unspecified

F94 Disorders of social functioning with onset specific to childhood and adolescence

F94.0 Selective mutism
Elective mutism
Excludes2: pervasive developmental disorders (F84.-)
schizophrenia (F20.-)
specific developmental disorders of speech and language (F80.-)
transient mutism as part of separation anxiety in young children (F93.0)

F94.1 Reactive attachment disorder of childhood
Use additional code to identify any associated failure to thrive or growth retardation
Excludes1: disinhibited attachment disorder of childhood (F94.2)
normal variation in pattern of selective attachment
Excludes2: Asperger's syndrome (F84.5)
maltreatment syndromes (T74.-)
sexual or physical abuse in childhood, resulting in psychosocial problems (Z61.4-Z61.6)

F94.2 Disinhibited attachment disorder of childhood
Affectionless psychopathy
Institutional syndrome
Excludes1: reactive attachment disorder of childhood (F94.l)
Excludes2: Asperger's syndrome (F84.5)
attention-deficit hyperactivity disorders (F90.-)
hospitalism in children (F43.2-)

F94.8 Other childhood disorders of social functioning

F94.9 Childhood disorder of social functioning, unspecified

F95 Tic disorder

F95.0 Transient tic disorder

F95.1 Chronic motor or vocal tic disorder

F95.2 Tourette's disorder
Combined vocal and multiple motor tic disorder [de la Tourette]
Tourette's syndrome

F95.8 Other tic disorders

F95.9 Tic disorder, unspecified
Tic NOS

F98 Other behavioral and emotional disorders with onset usually occurring in childhood and adolescence
Excludes2: breath-holding spells (R06.8)
gender identity disorder of childhood (F64.2)
Kleine-Levin syndrome (G47.8)
obsessive-compulsive disorder (F42)
sleep disorders not due to a substance or known physiological condition (F51.-)

F98.0 Enuresis not due to a substance or known physiological condition
Enuresis (primary) (secondary) of nonorganic origin
Functional enuresis
Psychogenic enuresis
Urinary incontinence of nonorganic origin
Excludes1: enuresis NOS (R32)

F98.1 Encopresis not due to a substance or known physiological condition
Functional encopresis
Incontinence of feces of nonorganic origin
Psychogenic encopresis
Use additional code to identify the cause of any coexisting constipation.
Excludes1: encopresis NOS (R15)

F98.2 Other feeding disorders of infancy and childhood
Excludes1: feeding difficulties and mismanagement (R63.3)
Excludes2: anorexia nervosa and other eating disorders (F50.-)
feeding problems of newborn (P92.-)
pica of infancy or childhood (F98.3)

F98.21 Rumination disorder of infancy

F98.29 Other feeding disorders of infancy mental early childhood

F98.3 Pica of infancy and childhood

F98.4 Stereotyped movement disorders
Stereotype/habit disorder
Excludes1: abnormal involuntary movements (R25.-)
Excludes2: compulsions in obsessive-compulsive disorder (F42)
hair plucking (F63.3)
movement disorders of organic origin (G20-G25)
nail-biting (F98.8)
nose-picking (F98.8)
stereotypies that are part of a broader psychiatric condition (F01-F95)
thumb-sucking (F98.8)
tic disorders (F95.-)
trichotillomania (F63.3)

F98.5 Stuttering [stammering]
Excludes2: cluttering (F98.8)
tic disorders (F95.-)

F98.8 Other specified behavioral and emotional disorders with onset usually occurring in childhood and adolescence
Cluttering
Excessive masturbation
Nail-biting
Nose-picking
Thumb-sucking

F98.9 Unspecified behavioral and emotional disorders with onset usually occurring in childhood and adolescence

UNSPECIFIED MENTAL DISORDER (F99)

F99 Mental disorder, not otherwise specified
Includes: mental illness NOS
Excludes1: unspecified mental disorder due to known physiological condition (F06.9)

CHAPTER VI — DISEASES OF THE NERVOUS SYSTEM (G00–G99)

Excludes2:   certain conditions originating in the perinatal period (P04-P96)
certain infectious and parasitic diseases (A00-B99)
complications of pregnancy, childbirth and the puerperium (O00-O99)
congenital malformations, deformations, and chromosomal abnormalities (Q00-Q99)
endocrine, nutritional and metabolic diseases (E00-E90)
injury, poisoning and certain other consequences of external causes (S00-T98)
neoplasms (C00-D48)
symptoms, signs and abnormal clinical and laboratory findings, not elsewhere classified (R00-R94)

This chapter contains the following blocks:

G00-G09	Inflammatory diseases of the central nervous system
G10-G13	Systemic atrophies primarily affecting the central nervous system
G20-G26	Extrapyramidal and movement disorders
G30-G32	Other degenerative diseases of the nervous system
G35-G37	Demyelinating diseases of the central nervous system
G40-G47	Episodic and paroxysmal disorders
G50-G59	Nerve, nerve root and plexus disorders
G60-G64	Polyneuropathies and other disorders of the peripheral nervous system
G70-G73	Diseases of myoneural junction and muscle
G80-G83	Cerebral palsy and other paralytic syndromes
G90-G99	Other disorders of the nervous system

INFLAMMATORY DISEASES OF THE CENTRAL NERVOUS SYSTEM (G00–G09)

G00 Bacterial meningitis, not elsewhere classified
Includes: bacterial arachnoiditis
bacterial leptomeningitis
bacterial meningitis
bacterial pachymeningitis
Excludes1:   bacterial:
meningoencephalitis (G04.2)
meningomyelitis (G04.2)

G00.0 Hemophilus meningitis
Meningitis due to Hemophilus influenzae

G00.1 Pneumococcal meningitis

G00.2 Streptococcal meningitis
Use additional code to further identify organism (B95.0-B95.5)

G00.3 Staphylococcal meningitis
Use additional code to further identify organism (B95.6-B95.8)

G00.8 Other bacterial meningitis
Meningitis due to Escherichia coli
Meningitis due to Friedländer bacillus
Meningitis due to Klebsiella
Use additional code to further identify organism (B96.-)

G00.9 Bacterial meningitis, unspecified
Meningitis due to gram-negative bacteria, unspecified
Purulent meningitis NOS
Pyogenic meningitis NOS
Suppurative meningitis NOS

G01 Meningitis in bacterial diseases classified elsewhere
Code first underlying disease
Excludes1:   meningitis (in):
gonococcal (A54.81)
leptospirosis (A27.81)
listeriosis (A32.11)
Lyme disease (A69.21)
meningococcal (A39.0)
neurosyphilis (A52.13)
tuberculosis (A17.0)
meningoencephalitis and meningomyelitis in bacterial diseases classified elsewhere (G05)

G02 Meningitis in other infectious and parasitic diseases classified elsewhere
Code first underlying disease, such as:
poliovirus infection (A80.-)
Excludes1:   meningitis (due to):
candidal (B37.5)
coccidioidomycosis (B38.4)
cryptococcal meningitis (B45.1)
herpesviral [herpes simplex] (B00.3)
infectious mononucleosis (B27.-2)
measles (B05.1)
mumps (B26.1)
rubella (B06.02)
varicella [chickenpox] (B01.0)
zoster (B02.1)
meningoencephalitis and meningomyelitis in other infectious and parasitic diseases classified elsewhere (G05)

G03 Meningitis due to other and unspecified causes
Includes: arachnoiditis NOS
leptomeningitis NOS
meningitis NOS
pachymeningitis NOS
Excludes1:   meningoencephalitis (G04.-)
meningomyelitis (G04.-)

G03.0 Nonpyogenic meningitis
Aseptic meningitis
Nonbacterial meningitis

G03.1 Chronic meningitis

G03.2 Benign recurrent meningitis [Mollaret]

G03.8 Meningitis due to other specified causes

G03.9 Meningitis, unspecified
Arachnoiditis (spinal) NOS

G04 Encephalitis, myelitis and encephalomyelitis
Includes: acute ascending myelitis
meningoencephalitis
meningomyelitis
Excludes1:   encephalopathy NOS (G93.4)
Excludes2:   acute transverse myelitis (G37.3)
alcoholic encephalopathy (G31.2)
benign myalgic encephalomyelitis (G93.3)
multiple sclerosis (G35)
subacute necrotizing myelitis (G37.4)
toxic encephalopathy (G92)

G04.0 Acute disseminated encephalitis
Encephalitis, postimmunization
Encephalomyelitis, postimmunization
Use additional external cause code (Chapter XIX) to identify vaccine.

G04.1 Tropical spastic paraplegia

G04.2 Bacterial meningoencephalitis and meningomyelitis, not elsewhere classified

G04.8 Other encephalitis, myelitis and encephalomyelitis

G04.9 Encephalitis, myelitis and encephalomyelitis, unspecified
Ventriculitis (cerebral) NOS

G05 Encephalitis, myelitis and encephalomyelitis in diseases classified elsewhere

    Includes: meningoencephalitis and meningomyelitis in diseases classified elsewhere

    Code first underlying disease, such as:
      poliovirus (A80.-)
      suppurative otitis media (H66.01-H66.4)
      trichinellosis (B75)

    Excludes1:   encephalitis, myelitis and encephalomyelitis (in):
        adenoviral (A85.1)
        cytomegaloviral (B25.8)
        enteroviral (A85.0)
        herpesviral [herpes simplex] (B00.4)
        listerial (A32.12)
        measles (B05.0)
        meningococcal (A39.81)
        mumps (B26.2)
        postchickenpox (B01.1)
        rubella (B06.01)
        systemic lupus erythematosus (M32.19)
        toxoplasmosis (B58.2)
          congenital (P37.1)
        zoster (B02.0)
      eosinophilic meningoencephalitis (B83.2)

G06 Intracranial and intraspinal abscess and granuloma

    Use additional code (B95-B97) to identify infectious agent.

G06.0 Intracranial abscess and granuloma
    Brain [any part] abscess (embolic)
    Cerebellar abscess (embolic)
    Cerebral abscess (embolic)
    Intracranial epidural abscess or granuloma
    Intracranial extradural abscess or granuloma
    Intracranial subdural abscess or granuloma
    Otogenic abscess (embolic)
    Excludes1:   tuberculous intracranial abscess and granuloma (A17.81)

G06.1 Intraspinal abscess and granuloma
    Abscess (embolic) of spinal cord [any part]
    Intraspinal epidural abscess or granuloma
    Intraspinal extradural abscess or granuloma
    Intraspinal subdural abscess or granuloma
    Excludes1:   tuberculous intraspinal abscess and granuloma (A17.81)

G06.2 Extradural and subdural abscess, unspecified

G07 Intracranial and intraspinal abscess and granuloma in diseases classified elsewhere

    Code first, underlying disease, such as:
      schistosomiasis granuloma of brain (B65.-)

    Excludes1:   abscess of brain:
        amebic (A06.6)
        chromomycotic (B43.1)
        gonococcal (A54.82)
        tuberculous (A17.81)
      tuberculoma of meninges (A17.1)

G08 Intracranial and intraspinal phlebitis and thrombophlebitis

    Includes: septic embolism of intracranial or intraspinal venous sinuses and veins
      septic endophlebitis of intracranial or intraspinal venous sinuses and veins
      septic phlebitis of intracranial or intraspinal venous sinuses and veins
      septic thrombophlebitis of intracranial or intraspinal venous sinuses and veins
      septic thrombosis of intracranial or intraspinal venous sinuses and veins

    Excludes1:   intracranial phlebitis and thrombophlebitis complicating:
      abortion, ectopic or molar pregnancy (O00-O07, O08.7)
      pregnancy, childbirth and the puerperium (O22.5, O87.3)
      nonpyogenic intracranial phlebitis and thrombophlebitis (I67.6)
      nonpyogenic intraspinal phlebitis and thrombophlebitis (G95.1)

G09 Sequelae of inflammatory diseases of central nervous system

    Note: This category is to be used to indicate conditions whose primary classification is to G00-G08 as the cause of sequelae, themselves classifiable elsewhere. The "sequelae" include conditions specified as residuals.

SYSTEMIC ATROPHIES PRIMARILY AFFECTING THE CENTRAL NERVOUS SYSTEM (G10–G13)

G10 Huntington's disease

    Includes: Huntington's chorea
      Huntington's dementia

G11 Hereditary ataxia

    Excludes2:   hereditary and idiopathic neuropathy (G60.-)
      infantile cerebral palsy (G80.-)
      metabolic disorders (E70-E90)

G11.0 Congenital nonprogressive ataxia

G11.1 Early-onset cerebellar ataxia
    Early-onset cerebellar ataxia with essential tremor
    Early-onset cerebellar ataxia with myoclonus [Hunt's ataxia]
    Early-onset cerebellar ataxia with retained tendon reflexes
    Friedreich's ataxia (autosomal recessive)
    X-linked recessive spinocerebellar ataxia

G11.2 Late-onset cerebellar ataxia

G11.3 Cerebellar ataxia with defective DNA repair
    Ataxia telangiectasia [Louis-Bar]
    Excludes2:   Cockayne's syndrome (Q87.1)
      other disorders of purine and pyrimidine metabolism (E79.-)
      xeroderma pigmentosum (Q82.1)

G11.4 Hereditary spastic paraplegia

G11.8 Other hereditary ataxias

G11.9 Hereditary ataxia, unspecified
    Hereditary cerebellar ataxia NOS
    Hereditary cerebellar degeneration
    Hereditary cerebellar disease
    Hereditary cerebellar syndrome

G12 Spinal muscular atrophy and related syndromes

G12.0 Infantile spinal muscular atrophy, type I [Werdnig-Hoffman]

G12.1 Other inherited spinal muscular atrophy
    Adult form spinal muscular atrophy
    Childhood form, type II spinal muscular atrophy
    Distal spinal muscular atrophy
    Juvenile form, type III spinal muscular atrophy [Kugelberg-Welander]
    Progressive bulbar palsy of childhood [Fazio-Londe]
    Scapuloperoneal form spinal muscular atrophy

G12.2 Motor neuron disease

G12.20 Motor neuron disease, unspecified

G12.21 Amyotrophic lateral sclerosis
    Progressive spinal muscle atrophy

G12.22　Progressive bulbar palsy
G12.29　Other motor neuron disease
　　　　　Familial motor neuron disease
　　　　　Primary lateral sclerosis
G12.8　Other spinal muscular atrophies and related syndromes
G12.9　Spinal muscular atrophy, unspecified

G13　Systemic atrophies primarily affecting central nervous system in diseases classified elsewhere
G13.0　Paraneoplastic neuromyopathy and neuropathy
　　　　Carcinomatous neuromyopathy
　　　　Sensorial paraneoplastic neuropathy [Denny Brown]
　　　　Code first underlying neoplasm (C00-D48)
G13.1　Other systemic atrophy primarily affecting central nervous system in neoplastic disease
　　　　Paraneoplastic limbic encephalopathy
　　　　Code first underlying neoplasm (C00-D48)
G13.8　Systemic atrophy primarily affecting central nervous system in other diseases classified elsewhere
　　　　Code first underlying disease, such as:
　　　　　cerebellar ataxia (in):
　　　　　　hypothyroidism (E03.-)
　　　　　　myxedematous congenital iodine deficiency (E00.1)

EXTRAPYRAMIDAL AND MOVEMENT DISORDERS (G20–G26)

G20　Parkinson's disease
　　　Includes:　hemiparkinsonism
　　　　　　　　idiopathic Parkinsonism or Parkinson's disease
　　　　　　　　paralysis agitans
　　　　　　　　Parkinsonism or Parkinson's disease NOS
　　　　　　　　primary Parkinsonism or Parkinson's disease

G21　Secondary Parkinsonism
G21.0　Malignant neuroleptic syndrome
　　　　Use additional external cause code (Chapter XIX) to identify drug.
G21.1　Other drug-induced secondary Parkinsonism
　　　　Use additional external cause code (Chapter XIX) to identify drug.
G21.2　Secondary Parkinsonism due to other external agents
　　　　Use additional external cause code (Chapter XIX) to identify external agent.
G21.3　Postencephalitic Parkinsonism
G21.8　Other secondary Parkinsonism
G21.9　Secondary Parkinsonism, unspecified

G22　Parkinsonism in diseases classified elsewhere
　　　Code first underlying disease
　　　Excludes1:　Parkinsonism in:
　　　　　　　　　Huntington's disease (G10)
　　　　　　　　　Shy-Drager syndrome (G90.3)
　　　　　　　　　syphilis (A52.19)

G23　Other degenerative diseases of basal ganglia
　　　Excludes2:　multi-system degeneration of the autonomic nervous system (G90.3)
G23.0　Hallervorden-Spatz disease
　　　　Pigmentary pallidal degeneration
G23.1　Progressive supranuclear ophthalmoplegia [Steele-Richardson-Olszewski]
G23.2　Striatonigral degeneration
G23.8　Other specified degenerative diseases of basal ganglia
　　　　Calcification of basal ganglia
G23.9　Degenerative disease of basal ganglia, unspecified

G24　Dystonia
　　　Includes:　dyskinesia
　　　Excludes2:　athetoid cerebral palsy (G80.3)
G24.0　Drug-induced dystonia
　　　　Use additional external cause code (Chapter XIX) to identify drug
　　　G24.00　Drug-induced dystonia, unspecified
　　　G24.01　Drug-induced acute dystonia
　　　G24.02　Drug-induced tardive dyskinesia

G24.09　Other drug-induced dystonia
G24.1　Idiopathic familial dystonia
　　　　Idiopathic dystonia NOS
G24.2　Idiopathic nonfamilial dystonia
G24.3　Spasmodic torticollis
　　　　Excludes1:　congenital torticollis (Q68.0)
　　　　　　　　　　hysterical torticollis (F44.4)
　　　　　　　　　　psychogenic torticollis (F45.8)
　　　　　　　　　　torticollis NOS (M43.6)
　　　　　　　　　　traumatic recurrent torticollis (S13.4)
G24.4　Idiopathic orofacial dystonia
　　　　Orofacial dyskinesia
G24.5　Blepharospasm
G24.8　Other dystonia
G24.9　Dystonia, unspecified
　　　　Dyskinesia NOS

G25　Other extrapyramidal and movement disorders
G25.0　Essential tremor
　　　　Familial tremor
　　　　Excludes1:　tremor NOS (R25.1)
G25.1　Drug-induced tremor
　　　　Use additional external cause code (Chapter XIX) to identify drug.
G25.2　Other specified forms of tremor
　　　　Intention tremor
G25.3　Myoclonus
　　　　Drug-induced myoclonus
　　　　Use additional external cause code (Chapter XIX) to identify drug, if drug-induced.
　　　　Excludes1:　facial myokymia (G51.4)
　　　　　　　　　　myoclonic epilepsy (G40.-)
G25.4　Drug-induced chorea
　　　　Use additional external cause code (Chapter XIX) to identify drug.
G25.5　Other chorea
　　　　Chorea NOS
　　　　Excludes1:　chorea NOS with heart involvement (I02.0)
　　　　　　　　　　Huntington's chorea (G10)
　　　　　　　　　　rheumatic chorea (I02.-)
　　　　　　　　　　Sydenham's chorea (I02.-)
G25.6　Drug-induced tics and other tics of organic origin
　　　　Use additional external cause code (Chapter XIX) to identify drug, if drug induced
　　　　Excludes1:　habit spasm (F95.9)
　　　　　　　　　　tic NOS (F95.9)
　　　　　　　　　　Tourette's syndrome (F95.2)
G25.7　Other and unspecified drug-induced movement disorders
　　　G25.70　Drug-induced movement disorder, unspecified
　　　G25.71　Drug-induced akathisia
　　　G25.79　Other drug-induced movement disorders
G25.8　Other specified extrapyramidal and movement disorders
　　　　Restless legs syndrome
　　　　Stiff-man syndrome
G25.9　Extrapyramidal and movement disorder, unspecified

G26　Extrapyramidal and movement disorders in diseases classified elsewhere
　　　Code first underlying disease

OTHER DEGENERATIVE DISEASES OF THE NERVOUS SYSTEM (G30–G32)

G30　Alzheimer's disease
　　　Includes:　Alzheimer's dementia senile and presenile forms
　　　Excludes1:　senile degeneration of brain NEC (G31.1)
　　　　　　　　　senile dementia NOS (F03)
　　　　　　　　　senility NOS (R54)
　　　Use additional code for any associated delirium (F05)
G30.0　Alzheimer's disease with early onset
　　　G30.00　Alzheimer's disease with early onset without behavioral disturbance
　　　　　　　　Alzheimer's disease with early onset, NOS

G30.01   Alzheimer's disease with early onset with behavioral disturbance

G30.1 Alzheimer's disease with late onset

G30.10   Alzheimer's disease with late onset without behavioral disturbance
Alzheimer's disease with late onset, NOS

G30.11   Alzheimer's disease with late onset with behavioral disturbance

G30.8 Other Alzheimer's disease

G30.80   Other Alzheimer's disease without behavioral disturbance
Other Alzheimer's disease, NOS

G30.81   Other Alzheimer's disease with behavioral disturbance

G30.9 Alzheimer's disease, unspecified

G30.90   Alzheimer's disease, unspecified without behavioral disturbance
Alzheimer's disease, unspecified

G30.91   Alzheimer's disease, unspecified with behavioral disturbance

G31 Other degenerative diseases of nervous system, not elsewhere classified
Excludes2:   Reye's syndrome (G93.7)

G31.0 Circumscribed brain atrophy
Pick's disease (with dementia)
Progressive isolated aphasia

G31.1 Senile degeneration of brain, not elsewhere classified
Excludes1:   Alzheimer's disease (G30.-)
senility NOS (R54)

G31.2 Degeneration of nervous system due to alcohol
Alcoholic cerebellar ataxia
Alcoholic cerebellar degeneration
Alcoholic cerebral degeneration
Alcoholic encephalopathy
Dysfunction of the autonomic nervous system due to alcohol

G31.8 Other specified degenerative diseases of nervous system

G31.81   Alpers' disease
Grey-matter degeneration

G31.82   Leigh's disease
Subacute necrotizing encephalopathy

G31.89   Other specified degenerative diseases of nervous system

G31.9 Degenerative disease of nervous system, unspecified

G32 Other degenerative disorders of nervous system in diseases classified elsewhere

G32.0 Subacute combined degeneration of spinal cord in diseases classified elsewhere
Dana-Putnam syndrome
Sclerosis of spinal cord (combined) (dorsolateral) (posterolateral)
Code first underlying disease, such as:
vitamin B$_{12}$ deficiency (E53.8)
anemia (D51.9)
dietary (D51.3)
pernicious (D51.0)
Excludes1:   syphilitic combined degeneration of spinal cord (A52.11)

G32.8 Other specified degenerative disorders of nervous system in diseases classified elsewhere
Cerebral degeneration
Degenerative encephalopathy
Code first underlying disease, such as:
cerebral degeneration (due to):
amyloid (E85)
hypothyroidism (E00.-, E03.-)
neoplasm (C00-D48)
vitamin B deficiency, except thiamine (E52-E53.-)
Excludes1:   superior hemorrhagic polioencephalitis [Wernicke's encephalopathy] (E51.2)

DEMYELINATING DISEASES OF THE CENTRAL NERVOUS SYSTEM (G35–G37)

G35 Multiple sclerosis
Includes: disseminated multiple sclerosis
generalized multiple sclerosis
multiple sclerosis NOS
multiple sclerosis of brain stem
multiple sclerosis of cord

G36 Other acute disseminated demyelination
Excludes1:   postinfectious encephalitis and encephalomyelitis NOS (G04.8)

G36.0 Neuromyelitis optica [Devic]
Demyelination in optic neuritis
Excludes1:   optic neuritis NOS (H46)

G36.1 Acute and subacute hemorrhagic leukoencephalitis [Hurst]

G36.8 Other specified acute disseminated demyelination

G36.9 Acute disseminated demyelination, unspecified

G37 Other demyelinating diseases of central nervous system

G37.0 Diffuse sclerosis of central nervous system
Periaxial encephalitis
Schilder's disease
Excludes1:   X linked adrenoleukodystrophy (E71.42-)

G37.1 Central demyelination of corpus callosum

G37.2 Central pontine myelinolysis

G37.3 Acute transverse myelitis in demyelinating disease of central nervous system
Acute transverse myelitis NOS
Excludes1:   multiple sclerosis (G35)
neuromyelitis optica [Devic] (G36.0)

G37.4 Subacute necrotizing myelitis of central nervous system

G37.5 Concentric sclerosis [Baló] of central nervous system

G37.8 Other specified demyelinating diseases of central nervous system

G37.9 Demyelinating disease of central nervous system, unspecified

EPISODIC AND PAROXYSMAL DISORDERS (G40–G47)

G40 Epilepsy
Excludes1:   Landau-Kleffner syndrome (F80.3)
seizure (convulsive) NOS (R56.8)
Todd's paralysis (G83.8)

G40.0 Localization-related (focal) (partial) idiopathic epilepsy and epileptic syndromes with seizures of localized onset
Benign childhood epilepsy with centrotemporal EEG spikes
Childhood epilepsy with occipital EEG paroxysms
Excludes1:   adult onset localization-related epilepsy (G40.1-, G40.2-)

G40.00   Localization-related (focal) (partial) idiopathic epilepsy and epileptic syndromes with seizures of localized onset without status epilepticus

G40.01   Localization-related (focal) (partial) idiopathic epilepsy and epileptic syndromes with seizures of localized onset with status epilepticus

G40.1 Localization-related (focal) (partial) symptomatic epilepsy and epileptic syndromes with simple partial seizures
Attacks without alteration of consciousness
Simple partial seizures developing into secondarily generalized seizures

G40.10   Localization-related (focal) (partial) symptomatic epilepsy and epileptic syndromes with simple partial seizures without status epilepticus

G40.11   Localization-related (focal) (partial) symptomatic epilepsy and epileptic syndromes with simple partial seizures with status epilepticus

G40.2 Localization-related (focal) (partial) symptomatic epilepsy and epileptic syndromes with complex partial seizures
Attacks with alteration of consciousness, often with automatisms
Complex partial seizures developing into secondarily generalized seizures

G40.20   Localization-related (focal) (partial) symptomatic epilepsy and epileptic syndromes with complex partial seizures without status epilepticus

G40.21   Localization-related (focal) (partial) symptomatic epilepsy and epileptic syndromes with complex partial seizures with status epilepticus

G40.3   Generalized idiopathic epilepsy and epileptic syndromes
- Benign myoclonic epilepsy in infancy
- Benign neonatal convulsions (familial)
- Childhood absence epilepsy [pyknolepsy]
- Epilepsy with grand mal seizures on awakening
- Juvenile absence epilepsy
- Juvenile myoclonic epilepsy [impulsive petit mal]
- Nonspecific atonic epileptic seizures
- Nonspecific clonic epileptic seizures
- Nonspecific myoclonic epileptic seizures
- Nonspecific tonic-clonic epileptic seizures
- Nonspecific tonic epileptic seizures

G40.30   Generalized idiopathic epilepsy and epileptic syndromes without status epilepticus

G40.31   Generalized idiopathic epilepsy and epileptic syndromes with status epilepticus

G40.4   Other generalized epilepsy and epileptic syndromes
- Epilepsy with myoclonic absences
- Epilepsy with myoclonic-astatic seizures
- Infantile spasms
- Lennox-Gastaut syndrome
- Salaam attacks
- Symptomatic early myoclonic encephalopathy
- West's syndrome

G40.40   Other generalized epilepsy and epileptic syndromes without status epilepticus

G40.41   Other generalized epilepsy and epileptic syndromes with status epilepticus

G40.5   Special epileptic syndromes
- Epilepsia partialis continua [Kozhevnikof]
- Epileptic seizures related to alcohol
- Epileptic seizures related to drugs
- Epileptic seizures related to hormonal changes
- Epileptic seizures related to sleep deprivation
- Epileptic seizures related to stress

Use additional external cause code (Chapter XIX) to identify drug, if drug-induced.

G40.50   Special epileptic syndromes without status epilepticus

G40.51   Special epileptic syndromes with status epilepticus

G40.6   Grand mal seizures, unspecified

G40.60   Grand mal seizures, unspecified without status epilepticus

G40.61   Grand mal seizures, unspecified with status epilepticus

G40.7   Petit mal, unspecified, without grand mal seizures

G40.70   Petit mal, unspecified, without grand mal seizures without status epilepticus

G40.71   Petit mal, unspecified, without grand mal seizures with status epilepticus

G40.8   Other epilepsy
- Epilepsies and epileptic syndromes undetermined as to whether they are focal or generalized

G40.80   Other epilepsy without status epilepticus

G40.81   Other epilepsy with status epilepticus

G40.9   Epilepsy, unspecified
- Epileptic convulsions NOS
- Epileptic fits NOS
- Epileptic seizures NOS

G40.90   Epilepsy, unspecified without status epilepticus

G40.91   Epilepsy, unspecified with status epilepticus

G43   Migraine
Use additional external cause code (Chapter XIX) to identify drug, if drug-induced.

Excludes1:   headache NOS (R51)

G43.0   Migraine without aura [common migraine]

G43.00   Migraine without aura, without status migrainosus
- Migraine without aura NOS

G43.01   Migraine without aura, with status migrainosus

G43.1   Migraine with aura [classical migraine]
- Basilar migraine
- Familial hemiplegic migraine
- Migraine equivalents
- Migraine with acute-onset aura
- Migraine with aura without headache
- Migraine with prolonged aura
- Migraine with typical aura

G43.10   Migraine with aura, without status migrainosus
- Migraine with aura NOS

G43.11   Migraine with aura, with status migrainosus

G43.3   Complicated migraine

G43.8   Other migraine
- Ophthalmoplegic migraine
- Retinal migraine

G43.9   Migraine, unspecified

G44   Other headache syndromes
Excludes1:   headache NOS (R51)
Excludes2:   atypical facial pain (G50.1)
           trigeminal neuralgia (G50.0)

G44.0   Cluster headache syndrome
- Chronic cluster headache
- Chronic paroxysmal hemicrania
- Episodic cluster headache

G44.1   Vascular headache, not elsewhere classified
- Vascular headache NOS

G44.2   Tension-type headache
- Chronic tension-type headache
- Episodic tension headache
- Tension headache NOS

G44.3   Chronic post-traumatic headache

G44.4   Drug-induced headache, not elsewhere classified
- Use additional external cause code (Chapter XIX) to identify drug.

G44.8   Other specified headache syndromes

G45   Transient cerebral ischemic attacks and related syndromes
Excludes1:   neonatal cerebral ischemia (P91.0)
           transient retinal artery occlusion (H34.0-)

G45.0   Vertebro-basilar artery syndrome

G45.1   Carotid artery syndrome (hemispheric)

G45.2   Multiple and bilateral precerebral artery syndromes

G45.3   Amaurosis fugax

G45.4   Transient global amnesia
Excludes1:   amnesia NOS (R41.3)

G45.8   Other transient cerebral ischemic attacks and related syndromes

G45.9   Transient cerebral ischemic attack, unspecified
- Spasm of cerebral artery
- Transient cerebral ischemia NOS

G46   Vascular syndromes of brain in cerebrovascular diseases
Code first underlying cerebrovascular disease (I60-I69)

G46.0   Middle cerebral artery syndrome

G46.1   Anterior cerebral artery syndrome

G46.2   Posterior cerebral artery syndrome

G46.3   Brain stem stroke syndrome
- Benedikt syndrome
- Claude syndrome
- Foville syndrome
- Millard-Gubler syndrome
- Wallenberg syndrome
- Weber syndrome

G46.4   Cerebellar stroke syndrome

G46.5   Pure motor lacunar syndrome

G46.6   Pure sensory lacunar syndrome

G46.7   Other lacunar syndromes

G46.8   Other vascular syndromes of brain in cerebrovascular diseases

G47 Organic sleep disorders

Excludes2: nightmares (F51.5)
nonorganic sleep disorders (F51.-)
sleep terrors (F51.4)
sleepwalking (F51.3)

G47.0 Organic disorders of initiating and maintaining sleep [organic insomnias]

Insomnia NOS

Excludes2: insomnia not due to a substance or known physiological condition (F51.0)
sleep apnea (G47.3-)

G47.1 Organic disorders of excessive somnolence [organic hypersomnias]

Hypersomnia NOS

Excludes2: hypersomnia not due to a substance or known physiological condition (F51.1)
sleep apnea (G47.3-)

G47.2 Organic disorders of the sleep-wake schedule

Organic delayed sleep phase syndrome
Organic irregular sleep-wake pattern
Sleep-wake schedule disorder NOS

Excludes1: circadian rhythm sleep disorder not due to a substance or known physiological condition (F51.2-)

G47.3 Sleep apnea

Code also any associated underlying condition

Excludes1: pickwickian syndrome (E66.2)
sleep apnea of newborn (P28.3)

G47.30 Sleep apnea, unspecified
Sleep apnea NOS

G47.31 Central sleep apnea

G47.32 Obstructive sleep apnea

G47.33 Mixed sleep apnea

G47.4 Narcolepsy and cataplexy

G47.8 Other organic sleep disorders
Kleine-Levin syndrome

G47.9 Organic sleep disorder, unspecified
Sleep disorder NOS

NERVE, NERVE ROOT AND PLEXUS DISORDERS (G50–G59)

Excludes1: current traumatic nerve, nerve root and plexus disorders —see nerve injury by body region
neuralgia NOS (M79.2)
neuritis NOS (M79.2)
peripheral neuritis in pregnancy (O26.82-)
radiculitis NOS (M54.1-)

G50 Disorders of trigeminal nerve

Includes: disorders of 5th cranial nerve

G50.0 Trigeminal neuralgia
Syndrome of paroxysmal facial pain
Tic douloureux

G50.1 Atypical facial pain

G50.8 Other disorders of trigeminal nerve

G50.9 Disorder of trigeminal nerve, unspecified

G51 Facial nerve disorders

Includes: disorders of 7th cranial nerve

G51.0 Bell's palsy
Facial palsy

G51.1 Geniculate ganglionitis

Excludes1: postherpetic geniculate ganglionitis (B02.21)

G51.2 Melkersson's syndrome
Melkersson-Rosenthal syndrome

G51.3 Clonic hemifacial spasm

G51.4 Facial myokymia

G51.8 Other disorders of facial nerve

G51.9 Disorder of facial nerve, unspecified

G52 Disorders of other cranial nerves

Excludes2: disorders of acoustic [8th] nerve (H93.3)
disorders of optic [2nd] nerve (H46, H47.0)
paralytic strabismus due to nerve palsy (H49.0-H49.2)

G52.0 Disorders of olfactory nerve
Disorders of 1st cranial nerve

G52.1 Disorders of glossopharyngeal nerve
Disorder of 9th cranial nerve
Glossopharyngeal neuralgia

G52.2 Disorders of vagus nerve
Disorders of pneumogastric [10th] nerve

G52.3 Disorders of hypoglossal nerve
Disorders of 12th cranial nerve

G52.7 Disorders of multiple cranial nerves
Polyneuritis cranialis

G52.8 Disorders of other specified cranial nerves

G52.9 Cranial nerve disorder, unspecified

G53 Cranial nerve disorders in diseases classified elsewhere

Code first underlying disease, such as:
neoplasm (C00-D48)

Excludes1: multiple cranial nerve palsy in sarcoidosis (D86.82)
multiple cranial nerve palsy in syphilis (A52.15)
postherpetic geniculate ganglionitis (B02.21)
postherpetic trigeminal neuralgia (B02.22)

G54 Nerve root and plexus disorders

Excludes1: current traumatic nerve root and plexus disorders—see nerve injury by body region
intervertebral disc disorders (M50-M51)
neuralgia or neuritis NOS (M79.2)
neuritis or radiculitis:
brachial NOS (M54.13)
lumbar NOS (M54.16)
lumbosacral NOS (M54.17)
thoracic NOS (M54.14)
radiculitis NOS (M54.10)
radiculopathy NOS (M54.10)
spondylosis (M47.-)

G54.0 Brachial plexus disorders
Thoracic outlet syndrome

G54.1 Lumbosacral plexus disorders

G54.2 Cervical root disorders, not elsewhere classified

G54.3 Thoracic root disorders, not elsewhere classified

G54.4 Lumbosacral root disorders, not elsewhere classified

G54.5 Neuralgic amyotrophy
Parsonage-Aldren-Turner syndrome
Shoulder-girdle neuritis

G54.6 Phantom limb syndrome with pain

G54.7 Phantom limb syndrome without pain
Phantom limb syndrome NOS

G54.8 Other nerve root and plexus disorders

G54.9 Nerve root and plexus disorder, unspecified

G55 Nerve root and plexus compressions in diseases classified elsewhere

Code first underlying disease, such as:
neoplasm (C00-D48)

Excludes1: nerve root compression (due to) (in):
ankylosing spondylitis (M45.-)
dorsopathies (M53.-, M54.-)
intervertebral disc disorders (M50.1.-, M51.1.-)
spondylopathies (M46.-, M48.-)
spondylosis (M47.0-M47.2.-)

G56 Mononeuropathies of upper limb

Excludes1: current traumatic nerve disorder—see nerve injury by body region

G56.0 Carpal tunnel syndrome

G56.00 Carpal tunnel syndrome, unspecified side

G56.01 Carpal tunnel syndrome, right side

G56.02 Carpal tunnel syndrome, left side

G56.1 Other lesions of median nerve

G56.10 Other lesions of median nerve, unspecified side

G56.11 Other lesions of median nerve, right side

G56.12 Other lesions of median nerve, left side

G56.2 Lesion of ulnar nerve
Tardy ulnar nerve palsy

G56.20   Lesion of ulnar nerve, unspecified side
G56.21   Lesion of ulnar nerve, right side
G56.22   Lesion of ulnar nerve, left side
G56.3 Lesion of radial nerve
G56.30   Lesion of radial nerve, unspecified side
G56.31   Lesion of radial nerve, right side
G56.32   Lesion of radial nerve, left side
G56.4 Causalgia of upper limb
Complex regional pain syndrome II of upper limb
Excludes1:   complex regional pain syndrome I (G90.51-)
reflex sympathetic dystrophy (G90.51-)
G56.40   Causalgia of upper limb, unspecified side
G56.41   Causalgia of upper limb, right side
G56.42   Causalgia of upper limb, left side
G56.8 Other mononeuropathies of upper limb
Interdigital neuroma of upper limb
G56.80   Other mononeuropathies of upper limb, unspecified side
G56.81   Other mononeuropathies of upper limb, right side
G56.82   Other mononeuropathies of upper limb, left side
G56.9 Mononeuropathy of upper limb, unspecified
G56.90   Mononeuropathy of upper limb, unspecified, unspecified side
G56.91   Mononeuropathy of upper limb, unspecified, right side
G56.92   Mononeuropathy of upper limb, unspecified, left side

G57 Mononeuropathies of lower limb
Excludes1:   current traumatic nerve disorder—see nerve injury by body region
G57.0 Lesion of sciatic nerve
Excludes1:   sciatica NOS (M54.3-)
Excludes2:   sciatica attributed to intervertebral disc disorder (M51.1.-)
G57.00   Lesion of sciatic nerve, unspecified side
G57.01   Lesion of sciatic nerve, right side
G57.02   Lesion of sciatic nerve, left side
G57.1 Meralgia paresthetica
Lateral cutaneous nerve of thigh syndrome
G57.10   Meralgia paresthetica, unspecified side
G57.11   Meralgia paresthetica, right side
G57.12   Meralgia paresthetica, left side
G57.2 Lesion of femoral nerve
G57.20   Lesion of femoral nerve, unspecified side
G57.21   Lesion of femoral nerve, right side
G57.22   Lesion of femoral nerve, left side
G57.3 Lesion of lateral popliteal nerve
Peroneal nerve palsy
G57.30   Lesion of lateral popliteal nerve, unspecified side
G57.31   Lesion of lateral popliteal nerve, right side
G57.32   Lesion of lateral popliteal nerve, left side
G57.4 Lesion of medial popliteal nerve
G57.40   Lesion of medial popliteal nerve, unspecified side
G57.41   Lesion of medial popliteal nerve, right side
G57.42   Lesion of medial popliteal nerve, left side
G57.5 Tarsal tunnel syndrome
G57.50   Tarsal tunnel syndrome, unspecified side
G57.51   Tarsal tunnel syndrome, right side
G57.52   Tarsal tunnel syndrome, left side
G57.6 Lesion of plantar nerve
Morton's metatarsalgia
G57.60   Lesion of plantar nerve, unspecified side
G57.61   Lesion of plantar nerve, right side
G57.62   Lesion of plantar nerve, left side
G57.7 Causalgia of lower limb
Complex regional pain syndrome II of lower limb
Excludes1:   complex regional pain syndrome I (G90.52-)
reflex sympathetic dystrophy (G90.52-)
G57.70   Causalgia of lower limb, unspecified side
G57.71   Causalgia of lower limb, right side

G57.72   Causalgia of lower limb, left side
G57.8 Other mononeuropathies of lower limb
Interdigital neuroma of lower limb
G57.80   Other mononeuropathies of lower limb, unspecified side
G57.81   Other mononeuropathies of lower limb, right side
G57.82   Other mononeuropathies of lower limb, left side
G57.9 Mononeuropathy of lower limb, unspecified
G57.90   Mononeuropathy of lower limb, unspecified, unspecified side
G57.91   Mononeuropathy of lower limb, unspecified, right side
G57.92   Mononeuropathy of lower limb, unspecified, left side

G58 Other mononeuropathies
G58.0   Intercostal neuropathy
G58.7   Mononeuritis multiplex
G58.8   Other specified mononeuropathies
G58.9   Mononeuropathy, unspecified

G59 Mononeuropathy in diseases classified elsewhere
Code first underlying disease
Excludes1:   diabetic mononeuropathy (E09-E14 with .41)
syphilitic nerve paralysis (A52.19)
syphilitic neuritis (A52.15)
tuberculous mononeuropathy (A17.83)

POLYNEUROPATHIES AND OTHER DISORDERS OF THE PERIPHERAL NERVOUS SYSTEM (G60–G64)

Excludes1:   neuralgia NOS (M79.2)
neuritis NOS (M79.2)
peripheral neuritis in pregnancy (O26.82-)
radiculitis NOS (M54.10)

G60 Hereditary and idiopathic neuropathy
G60.0   Hereditary motor and sensory neuropathy
Charcot-Marie-Tooth disease
Déjérine-Sottas disease
Hereditary motor and sensory neuropathy, types I-IV
Hypertrophic neuropathy of infancy
Peroneal muscular atrophy (axonal type) (hypertrophic type)
Roussy-Lévy syndrome
G60.1   Refsum's disease
Infantile Refsum disease
G60.2   Neuropathy in association with hereditary ataxia
G60.3   Idiopathic progressive neuropathy
G60.8   Other hereditary and idiopathic neuropathies
Dominantly inherited sensory neuropathy
Morvan's disease
Nélaton's syndrome
Recessively inherited sensory neuropathy
G60.9   Hereditary and idiopathic neuropathy, unspecified

G61 Inflammatory polyneuropathy
G61.0   Guillain-Barré syndrome
Acute (post-)infective polyneuritis
G61.1   Serum neuropathy
Use additional external cause code (Chapter XIX) to identify cause.
G61.8   Other inflammatory polyneuropathies
G61.81   Chronic inflammatory demyelinating polyneuritis
G61.89   Other inflammatory polyneuropathies
G61.9   Inflammatory polyneuropathy, unspecified

G62 Other and unspecified polyneuropathies
G62.0   Drug-induced polyneuropathy
Use additional external cause code (Chapter XIX) to identify drug.
G62.1   Alcoholic polyneuropathy
G62.2   Polyneuropathy due to other toxic agents
Use additional external cause code (Chapter XIX) to identify toxic agent.

G62.8   Other specified polyneuropathies

   G62.81   Critical illness polyneuropathy

     Acute motor neuropathy

   G62.82   Radiation-induced polyneuropathy

     Use additional external cause code (Chapter XIX) to identify cause

   G62.89   Other specified polyneuropathies

G62.9   Polyneuropathy, unspecified

   Neuropathy NOS

G63   Polyneuropathy in diseases classified elsewhere

   Code first underlying disease, such as:

     amyloidosis (E85)

     endocrine disease, except diabetes (E00-E07, E15-E16, E20-E34)

     metabolic diseases (E70-E89)

     neoplasm (C00-D48)

     nutritional deficiency (E40-E64)

     uremia (N19)

   Excludes1:   polyneuropathy (in):

     diabetes mellitus (E09-E14 with .42)

     diphtheria (A36.83)

     infectious mononucleosis (B27.0-B27.9 with 1)

     Lyme disease (A69.22)

     mumps (B26.84)

     postherpetic (B02.23)

     rheumatoid arthritis (M05.33)

     scleroderma (M34.83)

     systemic lupus erythematosus (M32.19)

G64   Other disorders of peripheral nervous system

   Disorder of peripheral nervous system NOS

G65   Sequelae of inflammatory and toxic polyneuropathies

G65.0   Sequelae of Guillain-Barré syndrome

G65.1   Sequelae of other inflammatory polyneuropathy

G65.2   Sequelae of toxic polyneuropathy

DISEASES OF MYONEURAL JUNCTION AND MUSCLE (G70–G73)

G70   Myasthenia gravis and other myoneural disorders

   Excludes1:   botulism (A05.1)

     transient neonatal myasthenia gravis (P94.0)

G70.0   Myasthenia gravis

   Use additional external cause code (Chapter XIX) to identify drug, if drug-induced.

G70.1   Toxic myoneural disorders

   Use additional external cause code (Chapter XIX) to identify toxic agent.

G70.2   Congenital and developmental myasthenia

G70.8   Other specified myoneural disorders

G70.9   Myoneural disorder, unspecified

G71   Primary disorders of muscles

   Excludes2:   arthrogryposis multiplex congenita (Q74.3)

     metabolic disorders (E70-E90)

     myositis (M60.-)

G71.0   Muscular dystrophy

   Autosomal recessive, childhood type, muscular dystrophy resembling Duchenne or Becker muscular dystrophy

   Benign [Becker] muscular dystrophy

   Benign scapuloperoneal muscular dystrophy with early contractures [Emery-Dreifuss]

   Distal muscular dystrophy

   Facioscapulohumeral muscular dystrophy

   Limb-girdle muscular dystrophy

   Ocular muscular dystrophy

   Oculopharyngeal muscular dystrophy

   Scapuloperoneal muscular dystrophy

   Severe [Duchenne] muscular dystrophy

   Excludes1:   congenital muscular dystrophy NOS (G71.2)

     congenital muscular dystrophy with specific morphological abnormalities of the muscle fiber (G71.2)

G71.1   Myotonic disorders

   Chondrodystrophic myotonia

   Dominant myotonia congenita [Thomsen]

   Drug-induced myotonia

   Dystrophia myotonica [Steinert]

   Myotonia congenita NOS

   Neuromyotonia [Isaacs]

   Paramyotonia congenita

   Pseudomyotonia

   Recessive myotonia congenita [Becker]

   Symptomatic myotonia

   Use additional external cause code (Chapter XIX) to identify drug, if drug-induced

G71.2   Congenital myopathies

   Central core disease

   Congenital muscular dystrophy NOS

   Congenital muscular dystrophy with specific morphological abnormalities of the muscle fiber

   Fiber-type disproportion

   Minicore disease

   Multicore disease

   Myotubular (centronuclear) myopathy

   Nemaline myopathy

   Excludes1:   arthrogryposis multiplex congenita (Q74.3)

G71.3   Mitochondrial myopathy, not elsewhere classified

   Excludes1:   Kearns-Sayre syndrome (H49.81)

     Leber's disease (H47.21)

     Leigh's encephalopathy (G31.82)

     mitochondrial metabolism disorders (E88.3.-)

     Reye's syndrome (G93.7)

G71.8   Other primary disorders of muscles

G71.9   Primary disorder of muscle, unspecified

   Hereditary myopathy NOS

G72   Other and unspecified myopathies

   Excludes1:   arthrogryposis multiplex congenita (Q74.3)

     dermatopolymyositis (M33.-)

     ischemic infarction of muscle (M62.2.-)

     myositis (M60.-)

     polymyositis (M33.2.-)

G72.0   Drug-induced myopathy

   Use additional external cause code (Chapter XIX) to identify drug.

G72.1   Alcoholic myopathy

   Use additional code to identify:

     alcoholism (F10.-)

     history of alcoholism (F10.11)

G72.2   Myopathy due to other toxic agents

   Use additional external cause code (Chapter XIX) to identify toxic agent.

G72.3   Periodic paralysis

   Hyperkalemic periodic paralysis (familial)

   Hypokalemic periodic paralysis (familial)

   Myotonic periodic paralysis (familial)

   Normokalemic paralysis (familial)

G72.4   Inflammatory myopathy, not elsewhere classified

G72.8   Other specified myopathies

   G72.81   Critical illness myopathy

     Acute necrotizing myopathy

     Acute quadriplegic myopathy

     Intensive care (ICU) myopathy

     Myopathy of critical illness

   G72.89   Other specified myopathies

G72.9   Myopathy, unspecified

G73   Disorders of myoneural junction and muscle in diseases classified elsewhere

G73.1   Eaton-Lambert syndrome

   Code first underlying disease, such as:

     malignant neoplasm of lung (C34.-)

     other neoplastic disease (C00-D48)

G73.3 Other myasthenic syndromes in diseases classified elsewhere
Code first underlying disease, such as:
neoplasm (C00-D498)
thyrotoxicosis (E05.-)
Excludes1:   myasthenic syndromes in diabetes mellitus (E09-E13 with .44)

G73.7 Myopathy in diseases classified elsewhere
Code first underlying disease, such as:
hyperparathyroidism (E21.0, E21.3)
hypoparathyroidism (E20.-)
glycogen storage disease (E74.0)
lipid storage disorders (E75.-)
Excludes1:   myopathy in:
rheumatoid arthritis (M05.32)
sarcoidosis (D86.87)
scleroderma (M34.82)
sicca syndrome [Sjögren] (M35.03)
systemic lupus erythematosus (M32.19)

CEREBRAL PALSY AND OTHER PARALYTIC SYNDROMES
(G80–G83)

G80 Infantile cerebral palsy
Includes: Little's disease
Excludes1:   hereditary spastic paraplegia (G11.4)

G80.0 Spastic cerebral palsy
Congenital spastic paralysis (cerebral)

G80.1 Spastic diplegia

G80.2 Infantile hemiplegia

G80.3 Dyskinetic cerebral palsy
Athetoid cerebral palsy

G80.4 Ataxic cerebral palsy

G80.8 Other infantile cerebral palsy
Congenital quadriplegia
Mixed cerebral palsy syndromes

G80.9 Infantile cerebral palsy, unspecified
Cerebral palsy NOS

G81 Hemiplegia and hemiparesis
Note: This category is to be used only when hemiplegia (complete) (incomplete) is reported without further specification, or is stated to be old or longstanding but of unspecified cause. The category is also for use in multiple coding to identify these types of hemiplegia resulting from any noncongenital neurologic cause.
Excludes1:   congenital and infantile cerebral palsy (G80.-)
hemiplegia and hemiparesis due to sequela of cerebrovascular disease (I69.05-, I69.15-, I69.25-, I69.35-, I69.45-, I69.85-, I69.95-)

G81.0 Flaccid hemiplegia
G81.00   Flaccid hemiplegia affecting unspecified side
G81.01   Flaccid hemiplegia affecting right dominant side
G81.02   Flaccid hemiplegia affecting left dominant side
G81.03   Flaccid hemiplegia affecting right nondominant side
G81.04   Flaccid hemiplegia affecting left nondominant side

G81.1 Spastic hemiplegia
G81.10   Spastic hemiplegia affecting unspecified side
G81.11   Spastic hemiplegia affecting right dominant side
G81.12   Spastic hemiplegia affecting left dominant side
G81.13   Spastic hemiplegia affecting right nondominant side
G81.14   Spastic hemiplegia affecting left nondominant side

G81.9 Hemiplegia, unspecified
G81.90   Hemiplegia, unspecified affecting unspecified side
G81.91   Hemiplegia, unspecified affecting right dominant side
G81.92   Hemiplegia, unspecified affecting left dominant side
G81.93   Hemiplegia, unspecified affecting right nondominant side
G81.94   Hemiplegia, unspecified affecting left nondominant side

G82 Paraplegia (paraparesis) and quadriplegia (quadriparesis)
Note: This category is to be used only when the listed conditions are reported without further specification, or are stated to be old or longstanding but of unspecified cause. The category is also for use in multiple coding to identify these conditions resulting from any noncongenital neurologic cause.
Excludes1:   congenital and infantile cerebral palsy (G80.-)
functional quadriplegia (R26.3)
hysterical paralysis (F44.4)

G82.2 Paraplegia
Paralysis of both lower limbs NOS
Paraparesis (lower) NOS
Paraplegia (lower) NOS
G82.20   Paraplegia, unspecified
G82.21   Paraplegia, complete
G82.22   Paraplegia, incomplete

G82.5 Quadriplegia
G82.50   Quadriplegia, unspecified
G82.51   Quadriplegia, C1-C4 complete
G82.52   Quadriplegia, C1-C4 incomplete
G82.53   Quadriplegia, C5-C7 complete
G82.54   Quadriplegia, C5-C7 incomplete

G83 Other paralytic syndromes
Note: This category is to be used only when the listed conditions are reported without further specification, or are stated to be old or longstanding but of unspecified cause. The category is also for use in multiple coding to identify these conditions resulting from any cause.
Includes: paralysis (complete) (incomplete), except as in G80-G82

G83.0 Diplegia of upper limbs
Diplegia (upper)
Paralysis of both upper limbs

G83.1 Monoplegia of lower limb
Paralysis of lower limb
Excludes1:   monoplegia of lower limbs due to sequela of cerebrovascular disease (I69.04-, I69.14-, I69.24-, I69.34-, I69.44-, I69.84-, I69.94-)
G83.10   Monoplegia of lower limb affecting unspecified side
G83.11   Monoplegia of lower limb affecting right dominant side
G83.12   Monoplegia of lower limb affecting left dominant side
G83.13   Monoplegia of lower limb affecting right nondominant side
G83.14   Monoplegia of lower limb affecting left nondominant side

G83.2 Monoplegia of upper limb
Paralysis of upper limb
Excludes1:   monoplegia of upper limbs due to sequela of cerebrovascular disease (I69.03-, I69.13-, I69.23-, I69.33-, I69.43-, I69.83-, I69.93-)
G83.20   Monoplegia of upper limb affecting unspecified side
G83.21   Monoplegia of upper limb affecting right dominant side
G83.22   Monoplegia of upper limb affecting left dominant side
G83.23   Monoplegia of upper limb affecting right nondominant side
G83.24   Monoplegia of upper limb affecting left nondominant side

G83.3 Monoplegia, unspecified
G83.30   Monoplegia, unspecified affecting unspecified side
G83.31   Monoplegia, unspecified affecting right dominant side
G83.32   Monoplegia, unspecified affecting left dominant side
G83.33   Monoplegia, unspecified affecting right nondominant side
G83.34   Monoplegia, unspecified affecting left nondominant side

G83.4 Cauda equina syndrome
Neurogenic bladder due to cauda equina syndrome
Excludes1:   cord bladder NOS (G95.8)
neurogenic bladder NOS (N31.9)

G83.5 Locked-in state

G83.8 Other specified paralytic syndromes
> Excludes1: paralytic syndromes due to spinal cord injury-
> code to spinal cord injury (S14, S24, S34)

    G83.81 Brown-Sequard syndrome
    G83.82 Anterior cord syndrome
    G83.83 Posterior cord syndrome
    G83.84 Todd's paralysis (postepileptic)
    G83.89 Other specified paralytic syndromes

G83.9 Paralytic syndrome, unspecified

OTHER DISORDERS OF THE NERVOUS SYSTEM (G90–G99)

G90 Disorders of autonomic nervous system
> Excludes1: dysfunction of the autonomic nervous system due to alcohol (G31.2)

G90.0 Idiopathic peripheral autonomic neuropathy
> Carotid sinus syncope

G90.1 Familial dysautonomia [Riley-Day]

G90.2 Horner's syndrome
> Bernard(-Horner) syndrome

G90.3 Multi-system degeneration of the autonomic nervous system
> Neurogenic orthostatic hypotension [Shy-Drager]
> Excludes1: orthostatic hypotension NOS (I95.1)

G90.4 Autonomic dysreflexia
> Code also the underlying cause, such as:
> decubitus ulcer (L89.-)
> fecal impaction (K56.4)
> urinary tract infection (N39.0)

G90.5 Complex regional pain syndrome I (CRPS I)
> Reflex sympathetic dystrophy
> Excludes1: causalgia of lower limb (G57.7-)
> causalgia of upper limb (G56.4-)
> complex regional pain syndrome II of lower limb (G57.7-)
> complex regional pain syndrome II of upper limb (G56.4-)

    G90.50 Complex regional pain syndrome, unspecified
    G90.51 Complex regional pain syndrome of upper limb
      G90.511 Complex regional pain syndrome of right upper limb
      G90.512 Complex regional pain syndrome of left upper limb
      G90.513 Complex regional pain syndrome of upper limb, bilateral
      G90.519 Complex regional pain syndrome of unspecified upper limb
    G90.52 Complex regional pain syndrome of lower limb
      G90.521 Complex regional pain syndrome of right lower limb
      G90.522 Complex regional pain syndrome of left lower limb
      G90.523 Complex regional pain syndrome of lower limb, bilateral
      G90.529 Complex regional pain syndrome of unspecified lower limb
    G90.59 Complex regional pain syndrome of other specified site

G90.8 Other disorders of autonomic nervous system
G90.9 Disorder of the autonomic nervous system, unspecified

G91 Hydrocephalus
> Includes: acquired hydrocephalus
> Excludes1: congenital hydrocephalus (Q03.-)

G91.0 Communicating hydrocephalus
G91.1 Obstructive hydrocephalus
G91.2 Normal-pressure hydrocephalus
G91.3 Post-traumatic hydrocephalus, unspecified

G91.4 Hydrocephalus in diseases classified elsewhere
> Code first underlying condition, such as:
> congenital syphilis (A50.4-)
> neoplasm (C00-D48)
> Excludes1: hydrocephalus due to congenital toxoplasmosis (P37.1)

G91.8 Other hydrocephalus
G91.9 Hydrocephalus, unspecified

G92 Toxic encephalopathy
> Use additional external cause code (Chapter XIX) to identify toxic agent.

G93 Other disorders of brain
G93.0 Cerebral cysts
> Arachnoid cyst
> Porencephalic cyst, acquired
> Excludes1: acquired periventricular cysts of newborn (P91.1)
> congenital cerebral cysts (Q04.6)

G93.1 Anoxic brain damage, not elsewhere classified
> Excludes1: cerebral anoxia due to anesthesia during labor and delivery (O74.3)
> cerebral anoxia due to anesthesia during the puerperium (O89.2)
> neonatal anoxia (P28.9)

G93.2 Benign intracranial hypertension
> Excludes1: hypertensive encephalopathy (I67.4)

G93.3 Postviral fatigue syndrome
> Benign myalgic encephalomyelitis

G93.4 Encephalopathy, unspecified
> Excludes1: alcoholic encephalopathy (G31.2)
> toxic encephalopathy (G92)

G93.5 Compression of brain
> Arnold-Chiari type 1 compression of brain
> Compression of brain (stem)
> Herniation of brain (stem)
> Excludes1: diffuse traumatic compression of brain (S06.2-)
> focal traumatic compression of brain (S06.3-)

G93.6 Cerebral edema
> Excludes1: cerebral edema due to birth injury (P11.0)
> traumatic cerebral edema (S06.1-)

G93.7 Reye's syndrome
> Use additional external cause code (Chapters XIX-XX) to identify cause.

G93.8 Other specified disorders of brain
> Postradiation encephalopathy
> Use additional external cause code (Chapter XX) to identify cause.

G93.9 Disorder of brain, unspecified

G94 Other disorders of brain in diseases classified elsewhere
> Code first underlying disease
> Excludes1: encephalopathy in influenza (J10.89)
> encephalopathy in congenital syphilis (A50.49)
> encephalopathy in syphilis (A52.19)
> hydrocephalus in diseases classified elsewhere (G91.4)

G95 Other diseases of spinal cord
> Excludes2: myelitis (G04.-)

G95.0 Syringomyelia and syringobulbia
G95.1 Vascular myelopathies
> Excludes2: intraspinal phlebitis and thrombophlebitis, except non-pyogenic (G08)

    G95.11 Acute infarction of spinal cord (embolic) (nonembolic)
> Anoxia of spinal cord
> Arterial thrombosis of spinal cord
    G95.19 Other vascular myelopathies
> Edema of spinal cord
> Hematomyelia
> Nonpyogenic intraspinal phlebitis and thrombophlebitis
> Subacute necrotic myelopathy

G95.2 Cord compression, unspecified

G95.8 Other specified diseases of spinal cord

Excludes1:   neurogenic bladder NOS (N31.9)
neurogenic bladder due to cauda equina
syndrome (G83.4)
neuromuscular dysfunction of bladder without
mention of spinal cord lesion (N31.-)

G95.81   Conus medullaris syndrome

G95.89   Other specified diseases of spinal cord
Cord bladder NOS
Drug-induced myelopathy
Radiation-induced myelopathy
Use additional external cause code (Chapters XIX-XX)
to identify external agent.

G95.9 Disease of spinal cord, unspecified
Myelopathy NOS

G96 Other disorders of central nervous system

G96.0 Cerebrospinal fluid leak

Excludes1:   cerebrospinal fluid leak from spinal puncture
(G97.0)

G96.1 Disorders of meninges, not elsewhere classified
Meningeal adhesions (cerebral) (spinal)

G96.8 Other specified disorders of central nervous system

G96.9 Disorder of central nervous system, unspecified

G97 Intraoperative and postprocedural complications and disorders of nervous system, not elsewhere classified

G97.0 Cerebrospinal fluid leak from spinal puncture

G97.1 Other reaction to spinal and lumbar puncture

G97.2 Intracranial hypotension following ventricular shunting

G97.3 Intraoperative and postprocedural hemorrhage or hematoma complicating a nervous system procedure

Excludes1:   intraoperative hemorrhage or hematoma due to
accidental puncture or laceration during a
nervous system procedure (G97.4-)

G97.31   Intraoperative hemorrhage of a nervous system organ during a nervous system procedure

G97.32   Intraoperative hemorrhage of other organ during a nervous system procedure

G97.33   Intraoperative hematoma of a nervous system organ during a nervous system procedure

G97.34   Intraoperative hematoma of other organ during a nervous system procedure

G97.35   Postprocedural hemorrhage of a nervous system organ following a nervous system procedure

G97.36   Postprocedural hemorrhage of other organ following a nervous system procedure

G97.37   Postprocedural hematoma of a nervous system organ following a nervous system procedure

G97.38   Postprocedural hematoma of other organ following a nervous system procedure

G97.4 Accidental puncture or laceration during a nervous system procedure

G97.41   Accidental puncture or laceration of a nervous system structure during a nervous system procedure

G97.42   Accidental puncture or laceration of other organs or structure during a nervous system procedure

G97.8 Other intraoperative and postprocedural complications and disorders of nervous system

G97.81   Other intraoperative complications of nervous system procedure

G97.82   Other postprocedural complications and disorders of nervous system procedure

G97.9 Intraoperative and postprocedural complication and disorder of the nervous system, unspecified

G98 Other disorders of nervous system not elsewhere classified
Includes: nervous system disorder NOS

G98.0 Neurogenic arthritis, not elsewhere classified
Nonsyphilitic neurogenic arthropathy NEC
Nonsyphilitic neurogenic spondylopathy NEC
Excludes1:   spondylopathy (in):
syringomyelia and syringobulbia (G95.0)
tabes dorsalis (A52.11)

G98.8 Other disorders of nervous system
Nervous system disorder NOS

G99 Other disorders of nervous system in diseases classified elsewhere

G99.0 Autonomic neuropathy in diseases classified elsewhere
Code first underlying disease, such as:
amyloidosis (E85)
gout (M10.-)
hyperthyroidism (E05.-)
Excludes1:   diabetic autonomic neuropathy (E09-14 with .43)

G99.2 Myelopathy in diseases classified elsewhere
Code first underlying disease, such as:
neoplasm (C00-D48)
Excludes1:   myelopathy in:
intervertebral disease (M50.0-, M51.0-)
spondylosis (M47.0-, M47.1-)

G99.8 Other specified disorders of nervous system in diseases classified elsewhere
Code first underlying disorder, such as:
amyloidosis (E85)
avitaminosis (E56.9)
uremia (N19)
Excludes1:   nervous system involvement in:
cysticercosis (B69.0)
rubella (B06.0-)
syphilis (A52.1-)

CHAPTER VII — DISEASES OF THE EYE AND ADNEXA (H00-H59)

Excludes2: certain conditions originating in the perinatal period (P04-P96)
certain infectious and parasitic diseases (A00-B99)
complications of pregnancy, childbirth and the puerperium (O00-O99)
congenital malformations, deformations, and chromosomal abnormalities(Q00-Q99)
diabetes mellitus related eye conditions (E09.3-, E10.3-, E11.3-, E13.3-, E14.3)
endocrine, nutritional and metabolic diseases (E00-E90)
injury (trauma) of eye and orbit (S05.-)
injury, poisoning and certain other consequences of external causes (S00-T98)
neoplasms (C00-D48)
symptoms, signs and abnormal clinical and laboratory findings, not elsewhere classified (R00-R94)
syphilis related eye disorders (A50.01, A50.3-, A51.43, A52.71)

This chapter contains the following blocks:

H00-H05	Disorders of eyelid, lacrimal system and orbit
H10-H13	Disorders of conjunctiva
H15-H21	Disorders of sclera, cornea, iris and ciliary body
H25-H28	Disorders of lens
H30-H36	Disorders of choroid and retina
H40-H42	Glaucoma
H43-H45	Disorders of vitreous body and globe
H46-H47	Disorders of optic nerve and visual pathways
H49-H52	Disorders of ocular muscles, binocular movement, accommodation and refraction
H53-H54	Visual disturbances and blindness
H55-H59	Other disorders of eye and adnexa

DISORDERS OF EYELID, LACRIMAL SYSTEM AND ORBIT (H00–H05)

Excludes2: open wound of eyelid (S01.1-)
superficial injury of eyelid (S00.1-, S00.2-)

H00 Hordeolum and chalazion

H00.0 Hordeolum (externum) (internum) of eyelid

H00.01   Hordeolum externum
Hordeolum NOS
Stye

H00.011 Hordeolum externum right upper eyelid

H00.012 Hordeolum externum right lower eyelid

H00.013 Hordeolum externum right eye, unspecified eyelid

H00.014 Hordeolum externum left upper eyelid

H00.015 Hordeolum externum left lower eyelid

H00.016 Hordeolum externum left eye, unspecified eyelid

H00.019 Hordeolum externum unspecified eye, unspecified eyelid

H00.02   Hordeolum internum
Infection of meibomian gland

H00.021 Hordeolum internum right upper eyelid

H00.022 Hordeolum internum right lower eyelid

H00.023 Hordeolum internum right eye, unspecified eyelid

H00.024 Hordeolum internum left upper eyelid

H00.025 Hordeolum internum left lower eyelid

H00.026 Hordeolum internum left eye, unspecified eyelid

H00.029 Hordeolum internum unspecified eye, unspecified eyelid

H00.03   Abscess of eyelid
Furuncle of eyelid

H00.031 Abscess of right upper eyelid

H00.032 Abscess of right lower eyelid

H00.033 Abscess of eyelid right eye, unspecified eyelid

H00.034 Abscess of left upper eyelid

H00.035 Abscess of left lower eyelid

H00.036 Abscess of eyelid left eye, unspecified eyelid

H00.039 Abscess of eyelid unspecified eye, unspecified eyelid

H00.1 Chalazion
Meibomian (gland) cyst
Excludes2: infected meibomian gland (H00.02-)

H00.11   Chalazion right upper eyelid

H00.12   Chalazion right lower eyelid

H00.13   Chalazion right eye, unspecified eyelid

H00.14   Chalazion left upper eyelid

H00.15   Chalazion left lower eyelid

H00.16   Chalazion left eye, unspecified eyelid

H00.19   Chalazion unspecified eye, unspecified eyelid

H01 Other inflammation of eyelid

H01.0 Blepharitis
Excludes1: blepharoconjunctivitis (H10.5-)

H01.00   Unspecified blepharitis

H01.001 Unspecified blepharitis right upper eyelid

H01.002 Unspecified blepharitis right lower eyelid

H01.003 Unspecified blepharitis right eye, unspecified eyelid

H01.004 Unspecified blepharitis left upper eyelid

H01.005 Unspecified blepharitis left lower eyelid

H01.006 Unspecified blepharitis left eye, unspecified eyelid

H01.009 Unspecified blepharitis unspecified eye, unspecified eyelid

H01.01   Ulcerative blepharitis

H01.011 Ulcerative blepharitis right upper eyelid

H01.012 Ulcerative blepharitis right lower eyelid

H01.013 Ulcerative blepharitis right eye, unspecified eyelid

H01.014 Ulcerative blepharitis left upper eyelid

H01.015 Ulcerative blepharitis left lower eyelid

H01.016 Ulcerative blepharitis left eye, unspecified eyelid

H01.019 Ulcerative blepharitis unspecified eye, unspecified eyelid

H01.02   Squamous blepharitis

H01.021 Squamous blepharitis right upper eyelid

H01.022 Squamous blepharitis right lower eyelid

H01.023 Squamous blepharitis right eye, unspecified eyelid

H01.024 Squamous blepharitis left upper eyelid

H01.025 Squamous blepharitis left lower eyelid

H01.026 Squamous blepharitis left eye, unspecified eyelid

H01.029 Squamous blepharitis unspecified eye, unspecified eyelid

H01.1 Noninfectious dermatoses of eyelid

H01.11   Allergic dermatitis of eyelid
Contact dermatitis of eyelid

H01.111 Allergic dermatitis of right upper eyelid

H01.112 Allergic dermatitis of right lower eyelid

H01.113 Allergic dermatitis of right eye, unspecified eyelid

H01.114 Allergic dermatitis of left upper eyelid

H01.115 Allergic dermatitis of left lower eyelid

H01.116 Allergic dermatitis of left eye, unspecified eyelid

H01.119 Allergic dermatitis of unspecified eye, unspecified eyelid

H01.12   Discoid lupus erythematosus of eyelid

H01.121 Discoid lupus erythematosus of right upper eyelid

H01.122 Discoid lupus erythematosus of right lower eyelid

H01.123 Discoid lupus erythematosus of right eye, unspecified eyelid

H01.124 Discoid lupus erythematosus of left upper eyelid

H01.125 Discoid lupus erythematosus of left lower eyelid

H01.126 Discoid lupus erythematosus of left eye, unspecified eyelid

H01.129 Discoid lupus erythematosus of unspecified eye, unspecified eyelid

H01.13 Eczematous dermatitis of eyelid

H01.131 Eczematous dermatitis of right upper eyelid

H01.132 Eczematous dermatitis of right lower eyelid

H01.133 Eczematous dermatitis of right eye, unspecified eyelid

H01.134 Eczematous dermatitis of left upper eyelid

H01.135 Eczematous dermatitis of left lower eyelid

H01.136 Eczematous dermatitis of left eye, unspecified eyelid

H01.139 Eczematous dermatitis of unspecified eye, unspecified eyelid

H01.14 Xeroderma of eyelid

H01.141 Xeroderma of right upper eyelid

H01.142 Xeroderma of right lower eyelid

H01.143 Xeroderma of right eye, unspecified eyelid

H01.144 Xeroderma of left upper eyelid

H01.145 Xeroderma of left lower eyelid

H01.146 Xeroderma of left eye, unspecified eyelid

H01.149 Xeroderma of unspecified eye, unspecified eyelid

H01.8 Other specified inflammations of eyelid

H01.9 Unspecified inflammation of eyelid
Inflammation of eyelid NOS

H02 Other disorders of eyelid

Excludes1: congenital malformations of eyelid (Q10.0-Q10.3)

H02.0 Entropion and trichiasis of eyelid

H02.00 Unspecified entropion of eyelid

H02.001 Unspecified entropion of right upper eyelid

H02.002 Unspecified entropion of right lower eyelid

H02.003 Unspecified entropion of right eye, unspecified eyelid

H02.004 Unspecified entropion of left upper eyelid

H02.005 Unspecified entropion of left lower eyelid

H02.006 Unspecified entropion of left eye, unspecified eyelid

H02.009 Unspecified entropion of unspecified eye, unspecified eyelid

H02.01 Cicatricial entropion of eyelid

H02.011 Cicatricial entropion of right upper eyelid

H02.012 Cicatricial entropion of right lower eyelid

H02.013 Cicatricial entropion of right eye, unspecified eyelid

H02.014 Cicatricial entropion of left upper eyelid

H02.015 Cicatricial entropion of left lower eyelid

H02.016 Cicatricial entropion of left eye, unspecified eyelid

H02.019 Cicatricial entropion of unspecified eye, unspecified eyelid

H02.02 Mechanical entropion of eyelid

H02.021 Mechanical entropion of right upper eyelid

H02.022 Mechanical entropion of right lower eyelid

H02.023 Mechanical entropion of right eye, unspecified eyelid

H02.024 Mechanical entropion of left upper eyelid

H02.025 Mechanical entropion of left lower eyelid

H02.026 Mechanical entropion of left eye, unspecified eyelid

H02.029 Mechanical entropion of unspecified eye, unspecified eyelid

H02.03 Senile entropion of eyelid

H02.031 Senile entropion of right upper eyelid

H02.032 Senile entropion of right lower eyelid

H02.033 Senile entropion of right eye, unspecified eyelid

H02.034 Senile entropion of left upper eyelid

H02.035 Senile entropion of left lower eyelid

H02.036 Senile entropion of left eye, unspecified eyelid

H02.039 Senile entropion of unspecified eye, unspecified eyelid

H02.04 Spastic entropion of eyelid

H02.041 Spastic entropion of right upper eyelid

H02.042 Spastic entropion of right lower eyelid

H02.043 Spastic entropion of right eye, unspecified eyelid

H02.044 Spastic entropion of left upper eyelid

H02.045 Spastic entropion of left lower eyelid

H02.046 Spastic entropion of left eye, unspecified eyelid

H02.049 Spastic entropion of unspecified eye, unspecified eyelid

H02.05 Trichiasis without entropian

H02.051 Trichiasis without entropian right upper eyelid

H02.052 Trichiasis without entropian right lower eyelid

H02.053 Trichiasis without entropian right eye, unspecified eyelid

H02.054 Trichiasis without entropian left upper eyelid

H02.055 Trichiasis without entropian left lower eyelid

H02.056 Trichiasis without entropian left eye, unspecified eyelid

H02.059 Trichiasis without entropian unspecified eye, unspecified eyelid

H02.1 Ectropion of eyelid

H02.10 Unspecified ectropion of eyelid

H02.101 Unspecified ectropion of right upper eyelid

H02.102 Unspecified ectropion of right lower eyelid

H02.103 Unspecified ectropion of right eye, unspecified eyelid

H02.104 Unspecified ectropion of left upper eyelid

H02.105 Unspecified ectropion of left lower eyelid

H02.106 Unspecified ectropion of left eye, unspecified eyelid

H02.109 Unspecified ectropion of unspecified eye, unspecified eyelid

H02.11 Cicatricial ectropion of eyelid

H02.111 Cicatricial ectropion of right upper eyelid

H02.112 Cicatricial ectropion of right lower eyelid

H02.113 Cicatricial ectropion of right eye, unspecified eyelid

H02.114 Cicatricial ectropion of left upper eyelid

H02.115 Cicatricial ectropion of left lower eyelid

H02.116 Cicatricial ectropion of left eye, unspecified eyelid

H02.119 Cicatricial ectropion of unspecified eye, unspecified eyelid

H02.12 Mechanical ectropion of eyelid

H02.121 Mechanical ectropion of right upper eyelid

H02.122 Mechanical ectropion of right lower eyelid

H02.123 Mechanical ectropion of right eye, unspecified eyelid

H02.124 Mechanical ectropion of left upper eyelid

H02.125 Mechanical ectropion of left lower eyelid

H02.126 Mechanical ectropion of left eye, unspecified eyelid

H02.129 Mechanical ectropion of unspecified eye, unspecified eyelid

H02.13 Senile ectropion of eyelid

H02.131   Senile ectropion of right upper eyelid
H02.132   Senile ectropion of right lower eyelid
H02.133   Senile ectropion of right eye, unspecified eyelid
H02.134   Senile ectropion of left upper eyelid
H02.135   Senile ectropion of left lower eyelid
H02.136   Senile ectropion of left eye, unspecified eyelid
H02.139   Senile ectropion of unspecified eye, unspecified eyelid

H02.14   Spastic ectropion of eyelid
H02.141   Spastic ectropion of right upper eyelid
H02.142   Spastic ectropion of right lower eyelid
H02.143   Spastic ectropion of right eye, unspecified eyelid
H02.144   Spastic ectropion of left upper eyelid
H02.145   Spastic ectropion of left lower eyelid
H02.146   Spastic ectropion of left eye, unspecified eyelid
H02.149   Spastic ectropion of unspecified eye, unspecified eyelid

H02.2 Lagophthalmos
H02.20   Unspecified lagophthalmos
H02.201   Unspecified lagophthalmos right upper eyelid
H02.202   Unspecified lagophthalmos right lower eyelid
H02.203   Unspecified lagophthalmos right eye, unspecified eyelid
H02.204   Unspecified lagophthalmos left upper eyelid
H02.205   Unspecified lagophthalmos left lower eyelid
H02.206   Unspecified lagophthalmos left eye, unspecified eyelid
H02.209   Unspecified lagophthalmos unspecified eye, unspecified eyelid

H02.21   Cicatricial lagophthalmos
H02.211   Cicatricial lagophthalmos right upper eyelid
H02.212   Cicatricial lagophthalmos right lower eyelid
H02.213   Cicatricial lagophthalmos right eye, unspecified eyelid
H02.214   Cicatricial lagophthalmos left upper eyelid
H02.215   Cicatricial lagophthalmos left lower eyelid
H02.216   Cicatricial lagophthalmos left eye, unspecified eyelid
H02.219   Cicatricial lagophthalmos unspecifed eye, unspecified eyelid

H02.22   Mechanical lagophthalmos
H02.221   Mechanical lagophthalmos right upper eyelid
H02.222   Mechanical lagophthalmos right lower eyelid
H02.223   Mechanical lagophthalmos right eye, unspecified eyelid
H02.224   Mechanical lagophthalmos left upper eyelid
H02.225   Mechanical lagophthalmos left lower eyelid
H02.226   Mechanical lagophthalmos left eye, unspecified eyelid
H02.229   Mechanical lagophthalmos unspecifed eye, unspecified eyelid

H02.23   Paralytic lagophthalmos
H02.231   Paralytic lagophthalmos right upper eyelid
H02.232   Paralytic lagophthalmos right lower eyelid
H02.233   Paralytic lagophthalmos right eye, unspecified eyelid
H02.234   Paralytic lagophthalmos left upper eyelid
H02.235   Paralytic lagophthalmos left lower eyelid
H02.236   Paralytic lagophthalmos left eye, unspecified eyelid
H02.239   Paralytic lagophthalmos unspecified eye, unspecified eyelid

H02.3 Blepharochalasis
   Pseudoptosis
H02.30   Blepharochalasis unspecified eye, unspecified eyelid
H02.31   Blepharochalasis right upper eyelid
H02.32   Blepharochalasis right lower eyelid

H02.33   Blepharochalasis right eye, unspecified eyelid
H02.34   Blepharochalasis left upper eyelid
H02.35   Blepharochalasis left lower eyelid
H02.36   Blepharochalasis left eye, unspecified eyelid

H02.4 Ptosis of eyelid
H02.40   Unspecified ptosis of eyelid
H02.401   Unspecified ptosis of right eyelid
H02.402   Unspecified ptosis of left eyelid
H02.403   Unspecified ptosis of bilateral eyelids
H02.409   Unspecified ptosis of unspecified eyelid

H02.41   Mechanical ptosis of eyelid
H02.411   Mechanical ptosis of right eyelid
H02.412   Mechanical ptosis of left eyelid
H02.413   Mechanical ptosis of bilateral eyelids
H02.419   Mechanical ptosis of unspecified eyelid

H02.42   Myogenic ptosis of eyelid
H02.421   Myogenic ptosis of right eyelid
H02.422   Myogenic ptosis of left eyelid
H02.423   Myogenic ptosis of bilateral eyelids
H02.429   Myogenic ptosis of unspecified eyelid

H02.43   Paralytic ptosis of eyelid
   Neurogenic ptosis of eyelid
H02.431   Paralytic ptosis of right eyelid
H02.432   Paralytic ptosis of left eyelid
H02.433   Paralytic ptosis of bilateral eyelids
H02.439   Paralytic ptosis unspecified eyelid

H02.5 Other disorders affecting eyelid function
   Excludes2:   blepharospasm (G24.5)
              organic tic (G25.6)
              psychogenic tic (F95.-)

H02.51   Abnormal innervation syndrome
H02.511   Abnormal innervation syndrome right upper eyelid
H02.512   Abnormal innervation syndrome right lower eyelid
H02.513   Abnormal innervation syndrome right eye, unspecified eyelid
H02.514   Abnormal innervation syndrome left upper eyelid
H02.515   Abnormal innervation syndrome left lower eyelid
H02.516   Abnormal innervation syndrome left eye, unspecified eyelid
H02.519   Abnormal innervation syndrome unspecified eye, unspecified eyelid

H02.52   Blepharophimosis
   Ankyloblepharon
H02.521   Blepharophimosis right upper eyelid
H02.522   Blepharophimosis right lower eyelid
H02.523   Blepharophimosis right eye, unspecified eyelid
H02.524   Blepharophimosis left upper eyelid
H02.525   Blepharophimosis left lower eyelid
H02.526   Blepharophimosis left eye, unspecified eyelid
H02.529   Blepharophimosis unspecified eye, unspecified lid

H02.53   Eyelid retraction
   Eyelid lag
H02.531   Eyelid retraction right upper eyelid
H02.532   Eyelid retraction right lower eyelid
H02.533   Eyelid retraction right eye, unspecified eyelid
H02.534   Eyelid retraction left upper eyelid
H02.535   Eyelid retraction left lower eyelid
H02.536   Eyelid retraction left eye, unspecified eyelid
H02.539   Eyelid retraction unspecified eye, unspecified lid

H02.59   Other disorders affecting eyelid function
   Deficient blink reflex
   Sensory disorders

H02.6   **Xanthelasma of eyelid**
- H02.60   Xanthelasma of unspecified eye, unspecified eyelid
- H02.61   Xanthelasma of right upper eyelid
- H02.62   Xanthelasma of right lower eyelid
- H02.63   Xanthelasma of right eye, unspecified eyelid
- H02.64   Xanthelasma of left upper eyelid
- H02.65   Xanthelasma of left lower eyelid
- H02.66   Xanthelasma of left eye, unspecified eyelid

H02.7   **Other and unspecified degenerative disorders of eyelid and periocular area**
- H02.70   Unspecified degenerative disorders of eyelid and periocular area
- H02.71   Chloasma of eyelid and periocular area
  Dyspigmentation of eyelid
  Hyperpigmentation of eyelid
  - H02.711   Chloasma of right upper eyelid and periocular area
  - H02.712   Chloasma of right lower eyelid and periocular area
  - H02.713   Chloasma of right eye, unspecified eyelid and periocular area
  - H02.714   Chloasma of left upper eyelid and periocular area
  - H02.715   Chloasma of left lower eyelid and periocular area
  - H02.716   Chloasma of left eye, uspecified eyelid and periocular area
  - H02.719   Chloasma of unspecified eye, unspecified eyelid and periocular area
- H02.72   Madarosis of eyelid and periocular area
  Hypotrichosis of eyelid
  - H02.721   Madarosis of right upper eyelid and periocular area
  - H02.722   Madarosis of right lower eyelid and periocular area
  - H02.723   Madarosis of right eye, unspecified eyelid and periocular area
  - H02.724   Madarosis of left upper eyelid and periocular area
  - H02.725   Madarosis of left lower eyelid and periocular area
  - H02.726   Madarosis of left eye, uspecified eyelid and periocular area
  - H02.729   Madarosis of unspecified eye, unspecified eyelid and periocular area
- H02.73   Vitiligo of eyelid and periocular area
  Hypopigmentation of eyelid
  - H02.731   Vitiligo of right upper eyelid and periocular area
  - H02.732   Vitiligo of right lower eyelid and periocular area
  - H02.733   Vitiligo of right eye, unspecified eyelid and periocular area
  - H02.734   Vitiligo of left upper eyelid and periocular area
  - H02.735   Vitiligo of left lower eyelid and periocular area
  - H02.736   Vitiligo of left eye, uspecified eyelid and periocular area
  - H02.739   Vitiligo of unspecified eye, unspecified eyelid and periocular area
- H02.79   Other degenerative disorders of eyelid and periocular area

H02.8   **Other specified disorders of eyelid**
- H02.81   Retained foreign body in eyelid
  Excludes1:   laceration of eyelid with foreign body (S01.12-)
  retained intraocular foreign body (H44.6-, H44.7-)
  superficial foreign body of eyelid and periocular area (S00.25-)
  - H02.811   Retained foreign body in right upper eyelid
  - H02.812   Retained foreign body in right lower eyelid
  - H02.813   Retained foreign body in right eye, unspecified eyelid
  - H02.814   Retained foreign body in left upper eyelid

- H02.815   Retained foreign body in left lower eyelid
- H02.816   Retained foreign body in left eye, unspecified eyelid
- H02.819   Retained foreign body in unspecified eye, unspecified eyelid

- H02.82   Cysts of eyelid
  Sebacous cyst of eyelid
  - H02.821   Cysts of right upper eyelid
  - H02.822   Cysts of right lower eyelid
  - H02.823   Cysts of right eye, unspecified eyelid
  - H02.824   Cysts of left upper eyelid
  - H02.825   Cysts of left lower eyelid
  - H02.826   Cysts of left eye, unspecified eyelid
  - H02.829   Cysts of unspecified eye, unspecified eyelid
- H02.83   Dermatochalasis of eyelid
  - H02.831   Dermatochalasis of right upper eyelid
  - H02.832   Dermatochalasis of right lower eyelid
  - H02.833   Dermatochalasis of right eye, unspecified eyelid
  - H02.834   Dermatochalasis of left upper eyelid
  - H02.835   Dermatochalasis of left lower eyelid
  - H02.836   Dermatochalasis of left eye, unspecified eyelid
  - H02.839   Dermatochalasis of unspecified eye, unspecified eyelid
- H02.84   Edema of eyelid
  Hyperemia of eyelid
  - H02.841   Edema of right upper eyelid
  - H02.842   Edema of right lower eyelid
  - H02.843   Edema of right eye, unspecified eyelid
  - H02.844   Edema of left upper eyelid
  - H02.845   Edema of left lower eyelid
  - H02.846   Edema of left eye, unspecified eyelid
  - H02.849   Edema of unspecified eye, unspecified eyelid
- H02.85   Elephantiasis of eyelid
  - H02.851   Elephantiasis of right upper eyelid
  - H02.852   Elephantiasis of right lower eyelid
  - H02.853   Elephantiasis of right eye, unspecified eyelid
  - H02.854   Elephantiasis of left upper eyelid
  - H02.855   Elephantiasis of left lower eyelid
  - H02.856   Elephantiasis of left eye, unspecified eyelid
  - H02.859   Elephantiasis of unspecified eye, unspecified eyelid
- H02.86   Hypertrichosis of eyelid
  - H02.861   Hypertrichosis of right upper eyelid
  - H02.862   Hypertrichosis of right lower eyelid
  - H02.863   Hypertrichosis of right eye, unspecified eyelid
  - H02.864   Hypertrichosis of left upper eyelid
  - H02.865   Hypertrichosis of left lower eyelid
  - H02.866   Hypertrichosis of left eye, unspecified eyelid
  - H02.869   Hypertrichosis of unspecified eye, unspecified eyelid
- H02.87   Vascular anomalies of eyelid
  - H02.871   Vascular anomalies of right upper eyelid
  - H02.872   Vascular anomalies of right lower eyelid
  - H02.873   Vascular anomalies of right eye, unspecified eyelid
  - H02.874   Vascular anomalies of left upper eyelid
  - H02.875   Vascular anomalies of left lower eyelid
  - H02.876   Vascular anomalies of left eye, unspecified eyelid
  - H02.879   Vascular anomalies of unspecified eye, unspecified eyelid
- H02.89   Other specified disorders of eyelid
  Hemorrhage of eyelid

H02.9   **Unspecified disorder of eyelid**
  Disorder of eyelid NOS

H04   **Disorders of lacrimal system**
  Excludes1:   congenital malformations of lacrimal system (Q10.4-Q10.6)

H04.0   Dacryoadenitis
   H04.00   Unspecified dacryoadenitis
      H04.001   Unspecified dacryoadenitis, right lacrimal gland
      H04.002   Unspecified dacryoadenitis, left lacrimal gland
      H04.003   Unspecified dacryoadenitis, bilateral lacrimal glands
      H04.009   Unspecified dacryoadenitis, unspecified lacrimal gland
   H04.01   Acute dacryoadenitis
      H04.011   Acute dacryoadenitis, right lacrimal gland
      H04.012   Acute dacryoadenitis, left lacrimal gland
      H04.013   Acute dacryoadenitis, bilateral lacrimal glands
      H04.019   Acute dacryoadenitis, unspecified lacrimal gland
   H04.02   Chronic dacryoadenitis
      H04.021   Chronic dacryoadenitis, right lacrimal gland
      H04.022   Chronic dacryoadenitis, left lacrimal gland
      H04.023   Chronic dacryoadenitis, bilateral lacrimal gland
      H04.029   Chronic dacryoadenitis, unspecified lacrimal gland
   H04.03   Chronic enlargement of lacrimal gland
      H04.031   Chronic enlargement of right lacrimal gland
      H04.032   Chronic enlargement of left lacrimal gland
      H04.033   Chronic enlargement of bilateral lacrimal glands
      H04.039   Chronic enlargement of unspecified lacrimal gland
H04.1   Other disorders of lacrimal gland
   H04.11   Dacryops
      H04.111   Dacryops of right lacrimal gland
      H04.112   Dacryops of left lacrimal gland
      H04.113   Dacryops of bilateral lacrimal glands
      H04.119   Dacryops of unspecified lacrimal gland
   H04.12   Dry eye syndrome
         Tear film insufficiency, NOS
      H04.121   Dry eye syndrome of right lacrimal gland
      H04.122   Dry eye syndrome of left lacrimal gland
      H04.123   Dry eye syndrome of bilateral lacrimal glands
      H04.129   Dry eye syndrome of unspecified lacrimal gland
   H04.13   Lacrimal cyst
         Lacrimal cystic degeneration
      H04.131   Lacrimal cyst right lacrimal gland
      H04.132   Lacrimal cyst left lacrimal gland
      H04.133   Lacrimal cyst bilateral lacrimal glands
      H04.139   Lacrimal cyst unspecified lacrimal gland
   H04.14   Primary lacrimal gland atrophy
      H04.141   Right primary lacrimal gland atrophy
      H04.142   Left primary lacrimal gland atrophy
      H04.143   Bilateral primary lacrimal gland atrophy
      H04.149   Unspecified primary lacrimal gland atrophy
   H04.15   Secondary lacrimal gland atrophy
      H04.151   Right secondary lacrimal gland atrophy
      H04.152   Left secondary lacrimal gland atrophy
      H04.153   Bilateral secondary lacrimal gland atrophy
      H04.159   Unspecified secondary lacrimal gland atrophy
   H04.16   Lacrimal gland dislocation
      H04.161   Right lacrimal gland dislocation
      H04.162   Left lacrimal gland dislocation
      H04.163   Bilateral lacrimal gland dislocation
      H04.169   Unspecified lacrimal gland dislocation
   H04.19   Other disorders of lacrimal gland
H04.2   Epiphora
   H04.20   Unspecified epiphora
      H04.201   Epiphora, right side
      H04.202   Epiphora, left side
      H04.203   Epiphora, bilateral

      H04.209   Epiphora, unspecified side
   H04.21   Epiphora due to excess lacrimation
      H04.211   Epiphora due to excess lacrimation, right side
      H04.212   Epiphora due to excess lacrimation, left side
      H04.213   Epiphora due to excess lacrimation, bilateral
      H04.219   Epiphora due to excess lacrimation, unspecified side
   H04.22   Epiphora due to insufficient drainage
      H04.221   Epiphora due to insufficient drainage, right side
      H04.222   Epiphora due to insufficient drainage, left side
      H04.223   Epiphora due to insufficient drainage, bilateral
      H04.229   Epiphora due to insufficient drainage, unspecified side
H04.3   Acute and unspecified inflammation of lacrimal passages
      Excludes1:   neonatal dacryocystitis (P39.1)
   H04.30   Unspecified dacryocystitis
      H04.301   Unspecified dacryocystitis of right lacrimal passage
      H04.302   Unspecified dacryocystitis of left lacrimal passage
      H04.303   Unspecified dacryocystitis of bilateral lacrimal passages
      H04.309   Unspecified dacryocystitis of unspecified lacrimal passage
   H04.31   Phlegmonous dacryocystitis
      H04.311   Phlegmonous dacryocystitis of right lacrimal passage
      H04.312   Phlegmonous dacryocystitis of left lacrimal passage
      H04.313   Phlegmonous dacryocystitis of bilateral lacrimal passages
      H04.319   Phlegmonous dacryocystitis of unspecified lacrimal passage
   H04.32   Acute dacryocystitis
         Acute dacryopericystitis
      H04.321   Acute dacryocystitis of right lacrimal passage
      H04.322   Acute dacryocystitis of left lacrimal passage
      H04.323   Acute dacryocystitis of bilateral lacrimal passages
      H04.329   Acute dacryocystitis of unspecified lacrimal passage
   H04.33   Acute lacrimal canaliculitis
      H04.331   Acute lacrimal canaliculitis of right lacrimal passage
      H04.332   Acute lacrimal canaliculitis of left lacrimal passage
      H04.333   Acute lacrimal canaliculitis of bilateral lacrimal passages
      H04.339   Acute lacrimal canaliculitis of unspecified lacrimal passage
H04.4   Chronic inflammation of lacrimal passages
   H04.41   Chronic dacryocystitis
      H04.411   Chronic dacryocystitis of right lacrimal passage
      H04.412   Chronic dacryocystitis of left lacrimal passage
      H04.413   Chronic dacryocystitis of bilateral lacrimal passages
      H04.419   Chronic dacryocystitis of unspecified lacrimal passage
   H04.42   Chronic lacrimal canaliculitis
      H04.421   Chronic lacrimal canaliculitis of right lacrimal passage
      H04.422   Chronic lacrimal canaliculitis of left lacrimal passage
      H04.423   Chronic lacrimal canaliculitis of bilateral lacrimal passages
      H04.429   Chronic lacrimal canaliculitis of unspecified lacrimal passage

H04.43   **Chronic lacrimal mucocele**
    H04.431   **Chronic lacrimal mucocele of right lacrimal passage**
    H04.432   **Chronic lacrimal mucocele of left lacrimal passage**
    H04.433   **Chronic lacrimal mucocele of bilateral lacrimal passages**
    H04.439   **Chronic lacrimal mucocele of unspecified lacrimal passage**
H04.5   **Stenosis and insufficiency of lacrimal passages**
  H04.51   **Dacryolith**
    H04.511   **Dacryolith of right lacrimal passage**
    H04.512   **Dacryolith of left lacrimal passage**
    H04.513   **Dacryolith of bilateral lacrimal passages**
    H04.519   **Dacryolith of unspecified lacrimal passage**
  H04.52   **Eversion of lacrimal punctum**
    H04.521   **Eversion of right lacrimal punctum**
    H04.522   **Eversion of left lacrimal punctum**
    H04.523   **Eversion of bilateral lacrimal punctum**
    H04.529   **Eversion of unspecified lacrimal punctum**
  H04.53   **Neonatal obstruction of nasolacrimal duct**
    Excludes1:   congenital stenosis and stricture of lacrimal duct (Q10.5)
    H04.531   **Neonatal obstruction of right nasolacrimal duct**
    H04.532   **Neonatal obstruction of left nsaolacrimal duct**
    H04.533   **Neonatal obstruction of bilateral nasolacrimal duct**
    H04.539   **Neonatal obstruction of unspecified nasolacrimal duct**
  H04.54   **Stenosis of lacrimal canaliculi**
    H04.541   **Stenosis of right lacrimal canaliculi**
    H04.542   **Stenosis of left lacrimal canaliculi**
    H04.543   **Stenosis of bilateral lacrimal canaliculi**
    H04.549   **Stenosis of unspecified lacrimal canaliculi**
  H04.55   **Acquired stenosis of nasolacrimal duct**
    H04.551   **Acquired stenosis of right nasolacrimal duct**
    H04.552   **Acquired stenosis of left nasolacrimal duct**
    H04.553   **Acquired stenosis of bilateral nasolacrimal duct**
    H04.559   **Acquired stenosis of unspecified nasolacrimal duct**
  H04.56   **Stenosis of lacrimal punctum**
    H04.561   **Stenosis of right lacrimal punctum**
    H04.562   **Stenosis of left lacrimal punctum**
    H04.563   **Stenosis of bilateral lacrimal punctum**
    H04.569   **Stenosis of unspecified lacrimal punctum**
  H04.57   **Stenosis of lacrimal sac**
    H04.571   **Stenosis of right lacrimal sac**
    H04.572   **Stenosis of left lacrimal sac**
    H04.573   **Stenosis of bilateral lacrimal sac**
    H04.579   **Stenosis of unspecified lacrimal sac**
H04.6   **Other changes of lacrimal passages**
  H04.61   **Lacrimal fistula**
    H04.611   **Lacrimal fistula right lacrimal passage**
    H04.612   **Lacrimal fistula left lacrimal passage**
    H04.613   **Lacrimal fistula bilateral lacrimal passages**
    H04.619   **Lacrimal fistula unspecified lacrimal passage**
  H04.69   **Other changes of lacrimal passages**
H04.8   **Other disorders of lacrimal system**
  H04.81   **Granuloma of lacrimal passages**
    H04.811   **Granuloma of right lacrimal passage**
    H04.812   **Granuloma of left lacrimal passage**
    H04.813   **Granuloma of bilateral lacrimal passages**
    H04.819   **Granuloma of unspecified lacrimal passage**
  H04.89   **Other disorders of lacrimal system**
H04.9   **Disorder of lacrimal system, unspecified**

H05   **Disorders of orbit**
    Excludes1:   congenital malformation of orbit (Q10.7)
H05.0   **Acute inflammation of orbit**
  H05.00   **Unspecified acute inflammation of orbit**
  H05.01   **Cellulitis of orbit**
    Abscess of orbit
    H05.011   **Cellulitis of right orbit**
    H05.012   **Cellulitis of left orbit**
    H05.013   **Cellulitis of bilateral orbits**
    H05.019   **Cellulitis of unspecified orbit**
  H05.02   **Osteomyelitis of orbit**
    H05.021   **Osteomyelitis of right orbit**
    H05.022   **Osteomyelitis of left orbit**
    H05.023   **Osteomyelitis of bilateral orbits**
    H05.029   **Osteomyelitis of unspecified orbit**
  H05.03   **Periostitis of orbit**
    H05.031   **Periostitis of right orbit**
    H05.032   **Periostitis of left orbit**
    H05.033   **Periostitis of bilateral orbits**
    H05.039   **Periostitis of unspecified orbit**
  H05.04   **Tenonitis of orbit**
    H05.041   **Tenonitis of right orbit**
    H05.042   **Tenonitis of left orbit**
    H05.043   **Tenonitis of bilateral orbits**
    H05.049   **Tenonitis of unspecified orbit**
H05.1   **Chronic inflammatory disorders of orbit**
  H05.10   **Unspecified chronic inflammatory disorders of orbit**
  H05.11   **Granuloma of orbit**
    Pseudotumor (inflammatory) of orbit
    H05.111   **Granuloma of right orbit**
    H05.112   **Granuloma of left orbit**
    H05.113   **Granuloma of bilateral orbits**
    H05.119   **Granuloma of unspecified orbit**
  H05.12   **Orbital myositis**
    H05.121   **Orbital myositis, right orbit**
    H05.122   **Orbital myositis, left orbit**
    H05.123   **Orbital myositis, bilateral**
    H05.129   **Orbital myositis, unspecified orbit**
H05.2   **Exophthalmic conditions**
  H05.20   **Unspecified exophthalmos**
  H05.21   **Displacement (lateral) of globe**
    H05.211   **Displacement (lateral) of globe, right eye**
    H05.212   **Displacement (lateral) of globe, left eye**
    H05.213   **Displacement (lateral) of globe, bilateral**
    H05.219   **Displacement (lateral) of globe, unspecified eye**
  H05.22   **Edema of orbit**
    Orbital congestion
    H05.221   **Edema of right orbit**
    H05.222   **Edema of left orbit**
    H05.223   **Edema of bilateral orbit**
    H05.229   **Edema of unspecified orbit**
  H05.23   **Hemorrhage of orbit**
    H05.231   **Hemorrhage of right orbit**
    H05.232   **Hemorrhage of left orbit**
    H05.233   **Hemorrhage of bilateral orbit**
    H05.239   **Hemorrhage of unspecified orbit**
  H05.24   **Constant exophthalmos**
    H05.241   **Constant exophthalmos, right eye**
    H05.242   **Constant exophthalmos, left eye**
    H05.243   **Constant exophthalmos, bilateral**
    H05.249   **Constant exophthalmos, unspecified eye**
  H05.25   **Intermittent exophthalmos**
    H05.251   **Intermittent exophthalmos, right eye**
    H05.252   **Intermittent exophthalmos, left eye**
    H05.253   **Intermittent exophthalmos, bilateral**
    H05.259   **Intermittent exophthalmos, unspecified eye**

H05.26   Pulsating exophthalmos
   H05.261   Pulsating exophthalmos, right eye
   H05.262   Pulsating exophthalmos, left eye
   H05.263   Pulsating exophthalmos, bilateral
   H05.269   Pulsating exophthalmos, unspecified eye
H05.3   Deformity of orbit
  Excludes1:   congenital deformity of orbit (Q10.7)
            hypertelorism (Q75.2)
  H05.30   Unspecified deformity of orbit
  H05.31   Atrophy of orbit
   H05.311   Atrophy of right orbit
   H05.312   Atrophy of left orbit
   H05.313   Atrophy of bilateral orbit
   H05.319   Atrophy of unspecified orbit
  H05.32   Deformity of orbit due to bone disease
    Code also associated bone disease
   H05.321   Deformity of right orbit due to bone disease
   H05.322   Deformity of left orbit due to bone disease
   H05.323   Deformity of bilateral orbits due to bone disease
   H05.329   Deformity of unspecified orbit due to bone disease
  H05.33   Deformity of orbit due to trauma or surgery
   H05.331   Deformity of right orbit due to trauma or surgery
   H05.332   Deformity of left orbit due to trauma or surgery
   H05.333   Deformity of bilateral orbits due to trauma or surgery
   H05.339   Deformity of unspecified orbit due to trauma or surgery
  H05.34   Enlargement of orbit
   H05.341   Enlargement of right orbit
   H05.342   Enlargement of left orbit
   H05.343   Enlargement of bilateral orbits
   H05.349   Enlargement of unspecified orbit
  H05.35   Exostosis of orbit
   H05.351   Exostosis of right orbit
   H05.352   Exostosis of left orbit
   H05.353   Exostosis of bilateral orbits
   H05.359   Exostosis of unspecified orbit
H05.4   Enophthalmos
  H05.40   Unspecified enophthalmos
   H05.401   Unspecified enophthalmos, right eye
   H05.402   Unspecified enophthalmos, left eye
   H05.403   Unspecified enophthalmos, bilateral
   H05.409   Unspecified enophthalmos, unspecified eye
  H05.41   Enophthalmos due to atrophy of orbital tissue
   H05.411   Enophthalmos due to atrophy of orbital tissue, right eye
   H05.412   Enophthalmos due to atrophy of orbital tissue, left eye
   H05.413   Enophthalmos due to atrophy of orbital tissue, bilateral
   H05.419   Enophthalmos due to atrophy of orbital tissue, unspecified eye
  H05.42   Enophthalmos due to trauma or surgery
   H05.421   Enophthalmos due to trauma or surgery, right eye
   H05.422   Enophthalmos due to trauma or surgery, left eye
   H05.423   Enophthalmos due to trauma or surgery, bilateral
   H05.429   Enophthalmos due to trauma or surgery, unspecified eye

H05.5   Retained (old) foreign body following penetrating wound of orbit
    Retrobulbar foreign body
  Excludes1:   current penetrating wound of orbit (S05.4-)
  Excludes2:   retained foreign body of eyelid (H02.81-)
           retained intraocular foreign body (H44.6-, H44.7-)
  H05.50   Retained (old) foreign body following penetrating wound of unspecified orbit
  H05.51   Retained (old) foreign body following penetrating wound of right orbit
  H05.52   Retained (old) foreign body following penetrating wound of left orbit
  H05.53   Retained (old) foreign body following penetrating wound of bilateral orbits
H05.8   Other disorders of orbit
  H05.81   Cyst of orbit
    Encephalocele of orbit
   H05.811   Cyst of right orbit
   H05.812   Cyst of left orbit
   H05.813   Cyst of bilateral orbits
   H05.819   Cyst of unspecified orbit
  H05.82   Myopathy of extraocular muscles
   H05.821   Myopathy of extraocular muscles, right orbit
   H05.822   Myopathy of extraocular muscles, left orbit
   H05.823   Myopathy of extraocular muscles, bilateral
   H05.829   Myopathy of extraocular muscles, unspecified orbit
  H05.89   Other disorders of orbit
H05.9   Unspecified disorder of orbit

DISORDERS OF CONJUNCTIVA (H10-H13)

H10 Conjunctivitis
  Excludes1:   keratoconjunctivitis (H16.2-)
  H10.0   Mucopurulent conjunctivitis
   H10.01   Acute follicular conjunctivitis
    H10.011   Acute follicular conjunctivitis, right eye
    H10.012   Acute follicular conjunctivitis, left eye
    H10.013   Acute follicular conjunctivitis, bilateral
    H10.019   Acute follicular conjunctivitis, unspecified eye
   H10.02   Other mucopurulent conjunctivitis
    H10.021   Other mucopurulent conjunctivitis, right eye
    H10.022   Other mucopurulent conjunctivitis, left eye
    H10.023   Other mucopurulent conjunctivitis, bilateral
    H10.029   Other mucopurulent conjunctivitis, unspecified eye
  H10.1   Acute atopic conjunctivitis
    Acute papillary conjunctivitis
   H10.10   Acute atopic conjunctivitis, unspecified eye
   H10.11   Acute atopic conjunctivitis, right eye
   H10.12   Acute atopic conjunctivitis, left eye
   H10.13   Acute atopic conjunctivitis, bilateral
  H10.2   Other acute conjunctivitis
   H10.21   Acute toxic conjunctivitis
    H10.211   Acute toxic conjunctivitis, right eye
    H10.212   Acute toxic conjunctivitis, left eye
    H10.213   Acute toxic conjunctivitis, bilateral
    H10.219   Acute toxic conjunctivitis, unspecified eye
   H10.22   Pseudomembranous conjunctivitis
    H10.221   Pseudomembranous conjunctivitis, right eye
    H10.222   Pseudomembranous conjunctivitis, left eye
    H10.223   Pseudomembranous conjunctivitis, bilateral
    H10.229   Pseudomembranous conjunctivitis, unspecified eye
   H10.23   Serous conjunctivitis, except viral
    Excludes1:   viral conjunctivitis (B30.-)
    H10.231   Serous conjunctivitis, except viral, right eye
    H10.232   Serous conjunctivitis, except viral, left eye
    H10.233   Serous conjunctivitis, except viral, bilateral

H10.239   Serous conjunctivitis, except viral, unspecified eye

H10.3   Unspecified acute conjunctivitis

     Excludes1:   ophthalmia neonatorum NOS (P39.1)

H10.30   Unspecified acute conjunctivitis, unspecified eye

H10.31   Unspecified acute conjunctivitis, right eye

H10.32   Unspecified acute conjunctivitis, left eye

H10.33   Unspecified acute conjunctivitis, bilateral

H10.4   Chronic conjunctivitis

H10.40   Unspecified chronic conjunctivitis

     H10.401   Unspecified chronic conjunctivitis, right eye

     H10.402   Unspecified chronic conjunctivitis, left eye

     H10.403   Unspecified chronic conjunctivitis, bilateral

     H10.409   Unspecified chronic conjunctivitis, unspecified eye

H10.41   Chronic giant papillary conjunctivitis

     H10.411   Chronic giant papillary conjunctivitis, right eye

     H10.412   Chronic giant papillary conjunctivitis, left eye

     H10.413   Chronic giant papillary conjunctivitis, bilateral

     H10.419   Chronic giant papillary conjunctivitis, unspecified eye

H10.42   Simple chronic conjunctivitis

     H10.421   Simple chronic conjunctivitis, right eye

     H10.422   Simple chronic conjunctivitis, left eye

     H10.423   Simple chronic conjunctivitis, bilateral

     H10.429   Simple chronic conjunctivitis, unspecified eye

H10.43   Chronic follicular conjunctivitis

     H10.431   Chronic follicular conjunctivitis, right eye

     H10.432   Chronic follicular conjunctivitis, left eye

     H10.433   Chronic follicular conjunctivitis, bilateral

     H10.439   Chronic follicular conjunctivitis, unspecified eye

H10.44   Vernal conjunctivitis

     Excludes1:   vernal keratoconjunctivitis with limbar and corneal involvement (H16.26-)

H10.45   Other chronic allergic conjunctivitis

H10.5   Blepharoconjunctivitis

H10.50   Unspecified blepharoconjunctivitis

     H10.501   Unspecified blepharoconjunctivitis, right eye

     H10.502   Unspecified blepharoconjunctivitis, left eye

     H10.503   Unspecified blepharoconjunctivitis, bilateral

     H10.509   Unspecified blepharoconjunctivitis, unspecified eye

H10.51   Ligneous conjunctivitis

     H10.511   Ligneous conjunctivitis, right eye

     H10.512   Ligneous conjunctivitis, left eye

     H10.513   Ligneous conjunctivitis, bilateral

     H10.519   Ligneous conjunctivitis, unspecified eye

H10.52   Angular blepharoconjunctivitis

     H10.521   Angular blepharoconjunctivitis, right eye

     H10.522   Angular blepharoconjunctivitis, left eye

     H10.523   Angular blepharoconjunctivitis, bilateral

     H10.529   Angular blepharoconjunctivitis, unspecified eye

H10.53   Contact blepharoconjunctivitis

     H10.531   Contact blepharoconjunctivitis, right eye

     H10.532   Contact blepharoconjunctivitis, left eye

     H10.533   Contact blepharoconjunctivitis, bilateral

     H10.539   Contact blepharoconjunctivitis, unspecified eye

H10.8   Other conjunctivitis

H10.9   Unspecified conjunctivitis

H11   Other disorders of conjunctiva

     Excludes1:   keratoconjunctivitis (H16.2-)

H11.0   Pterygium of eye

     Excludes1:   pseudopterygium (H11.81-)

H11.00   Unspecified pterygium of eye

     H11.001   Unspecified pterygium of right eye

     H11.002   Unspecified pterygium of left eye

     H11.003   Unspecified pterygium of eye, bilateral

     H11.009   Unspecified pterygium of unspecified eye

H11.01   Amyloid pterygium

     H11.011   Amyloid pterygium of right eye

     H11.012   Amyloid pterygium of left eye

     H11.013   Amyloid pterygium of eye, bilateral

     H11.019   Amyloid pterygium of unspecified eye

H11.02   Central pterygium of eye

     H11.021   Central pterygium of right eye

     H11.022   Central pterygium of left eye

     H11.023   Central pterygium of eye, bilateral

     H11.029   Central pterygium of unspecified eye

H11.03   Double pterygium of eye

     H11.031   Double pterygium of right eye

     H11.032   Double pterygium of left eye

     H11.033   Double pterygium of eye, bilateral

     H11.039   Double pterygium of unspecified eye

H11.04   Peripheral pterygium of eye, stationary

     H11.041   Peripheral pterygium, stationary, right eye

     H11.042   Peripheral pterygium, stationary, left eye

     H11.043   Peripheral pterygium, stationary, bilateral

     H11.049   Peripheral pterygium, stationary, unspecified eye

H11.05   Peripheral pterygium of eye, progressive

     H11.051   Peripheral pterygium, progressive, right eye

     H11.052   Peripheral pterygium, progressive, left eye

     H11.053   Peripheral pterygium, progressive, bilateral

     H11.059   Peripheral pterygium, progressive, unspecified eye

H11.06   Recurrent pterygium of eye

     H11.061   Recurrent pterygium of right eye

     H11.062   Recurrent pterygium of left eye

     H11.063   Recurrent pterygium of eye, bilateral

     H11.069   Recurrent pterygium of unspecified eye

H11.1   Conjunctival degenerations and deposits

     Excludes2:   pseudopterygium (H11.81)

H11.10   Unspecified conjunctival degenerations

H11.11   Conjunctival deposits

     H11.111   Conjunctival deposits, right eye

     H11.112   Conjunctival deposits, left eye

     H11.113   Conjunctival deposits, bilateral

     H11.119   Conjunctival deposits, unspecified eye

H11.12   Conjunctival concretions

     H11.121   Conjunctival concretions, right eye

     H11.122   Conjunctival concretions, left eye

     H11.123   Conjunctival concretions, bilateral

     H11.129   Conjunctival concretions, unspecified eye

H11.13   Conjunctival pigmentations

     Conjunctival argyrosis [argyria]

     H11.131   Conjunctival pigmentations, right eye

     H11.132   Conjunctival pigmentations, left eye

     H11.133   Conjunctival pigmentations, bilateral

     H11.139   Conjunctival pigmentations, unspecified eye

H11.14   Conjunctival xerosis NOS

     Excludes1:   xerosis of conjunctiva due to vitamin A deficiency (E50.0, E50.1)

     H11.141   Conjunctival xerosis NOS, right eye

     H11.142   Conjunctival xerosis NOS, left eye

     H11.143   Conjunctival xerosis NOS, bilateral

     H11.149   Conjunctival xerosis NOS, unspecified eye

H11.15   Pinguecula

     H11.151   Pinguecula, right eye

     H11.152   Pinguecula, left eye

     H11.153   Pinguecula, bilateral

     H11.159   Pinguecula, unspecified eye

H11.2　Conjunctival scars
　H11.21　　Conjunctival adhesions and strands (localized)
　　H11.211　Conjunctival adhesions and strands (localized), right eye
　　H11.212　Conjunctival adhesions and strands (localized), left eye
　　H11.213　Conjunctival adhesions and strands (localized), bilateral
　　H11.219　Conjunctival adhesions and strands (localized), unspecified eye
　H11.22　　Conjunctival granuloma
　　H11.221　Conjunctival granuloma, right eye
　　H11.222　Conjunctival granuloma, left eye
　　H11.223　Conjunctival granuloma, bilateral
　　H11.229　Conjunctival granuloma, unspecified
　H11.23　　Symblepharon
　　H11.231　Symblepharon, right eye
　　H11.232　Symblepharon, left eye
　　H11.233　Symblepharon, bilateral
　　H11.239　Symblepharon, unspecified eye
　H11.24　　Scarring of conjunctiva
　　H11.241　Scarring of conjunctiva, right eye
　　H11.242　Scarring of conjunctiva, left eye
　　H11.243　Scarring of conjunctiva, bilateral
　　H11.249　Scarring of conjunctiva, unspecified eye
H11.3　Conjunctival hemorrhage
　Subconjunctival hemorrhage
　H11.30　　Conjunctival hemorrhage, unspecified eye
　H11.31　　Conjunctival hemorrhage, right eye
　H11.32　　Conjunctival hemorrhage, left eye
　H11.33　　Conjunctival hemorrhage, bilateral
H11.4　Other conjunctival vascular disorders and cysts
　H11.41　　Vascular abnormalities of conjunctiva
　　Conjunctival aneurysm
　　H11.411　Vascular abnormalities of conjunctiva, right eye
　　H11.412　Vascular abnormalities of conjunctiva, left eye
　　H11.413　Vascular abnormalities of conjunctiva, bilateral
　　H11.419　Vascular abnormalities of conjunctiva, unspecified eye
　H11.42　　Conjunctival edema
　　H11.421　Conjunctival edema, right eye
　　H11.422　Conjunctival edema, left eye
　　H11.423　Conjunctival edema, bilateral
　　H11.429　Conjunctival edema, unspecified eye
　H11.43　　Conjunctival hyperemia
　　H11.431　Conjunctival hyperemia, right eye
　　H11.432　Conjunctival hyperemia, left eye
　　H11.433　Conjunctival hyperemia, bilateral
　　H11.439　Conjunctival hyperemia, unspecified eye
　H11.44　　Conjunctival cysts
　　H11.441　Conjunctival cysts, right eye
　　H11.442　Conjunctival cysts, left eye
　　H11.443　Conjunctival cysts, bilateral
　　H11.449　Conjunctival cysts, unspecified eye
H11.8　Other specified disorders of conjunctiva
　H11.81　　Pseudopterygium of conjunctiva
　　H11.811　Pseudopterygium of conjunctiva, right eye
　　H11.812　Pseudopterygium of conjunctiva, left eye
　　H11.813　Pseudopterygium of conjunctiva, bilateral
　　H11.819　Pseudopterygium of conjunctiva, unspecified eye
　H11.82　　Conjunctivochalasis
　　H11.821　Conjunctivochalasis, right eye
　　H11.822　Conjunctivochalasis, left eye
　　H11.823　Conjunctivochalasis, bilateral
　　H11.829　Conjunctivochalasis, unspecified eye
　H11.89　　Other specified disorders of conjunctiva

H11.9　Unspecified disorder of conjunctiva

DISORDERS OF SCLERA, CORNEA, IRIS AND CILIARY BODY (H15-H21)

H15　Disorders of sclera
H15.0　Scleritis
　H15.00　　Unspecified scleritis
　　H15.001　Unspecified scleritis, right eye
　　H15.002　Unspecified scleritis, left eye
　　H15.003　Unspecified scleritis, bilateral
　　H15.009　Unspecified scleritis, unspecified eye
　H15.01　　Anterior scleritis
　　H15.011　Anterior scleritis, right eye
　　H15.012　Anterior scleritis, left eye
　　H15.013　Anterior scleritis, bilateral
　　H15.019　Anterior scleritis, unspecified eye
　H15.02　　Brawny scleritis
　　H15.021　Brawny scleritis, right eye
　　H15.022　Brawny scleritis, left eye
　　H15.023　Brawny scleritis, bilateral
　　H15.029　Brawny scleritis, unspecified eye
　H15.03　　Posterior scleritis
　　Sclerotenonitis
　　H15.031　Posterior scleritis, right eye
　　H15.032　Posterior scleritis, left eye
　　H15.033　Posterior scleritis, bilateral
　　H15.039　Posterior scleritis, unspecified eye
　H15.04　　Scleritis with corneal involvement
　　H15.041　Scleritis with corneal involvement, right eye
　　H15.042　Scleritis with corneal involvement, left eye
　　H15.043　Scleritis with corneal involvement, bilateral
　　H15.049　Scleritis with corneal involvement, unspecified eye
　H15.05　　Scleromalacia perforans
　　H15.051　Scleromalacia perforans, right eye
　　H15.052　Scleromalacia perforans, left eye
　　H15.053　Scleromalacia perforans, bilateral
　　H15.059　Scleromalacia perforans, unspecified eye
　H15.09　　Other scleritis
　　Scleral abscess
　　H15.091　Other scleritis, right eye
　　H15.092　Other scleritis, left eye
　　H15.093　Other scleritis, bilateral
　　H15.099　Other scleritis, unspecified eye
H15.1　Episcleritis
　H15.10　　Unspecified episcleritis
　　H15.101　Unspecified episcleritis, right eye
　　H15.102　Unspecified episcleritis, left eye
　　H15.103　Unspecified episcleritis, bilateral
　　H15.109　Unspecified episcleritis, unspecified eye
　H15.11　　Episcleritis periodica fugax
　　H15.111　Episcleritis periodica fugax, right eye
　　H15.112　Episcleritis periodica fugax, left eye
　　H15.113　Episcleritis periodica fugax, bilateral
　　H15.119　Episcleritis periodica fugax, unspecified eye
　H15.12　　Nodular episcleritis
　　H15.121　Nodular episcleritis, right eye
　　H15.122　Nodular episcleritis, left eye
　　H15.123　Nodular episcleritis, bilateral
　　H15.129　Nodular episcleritis, unspecified eye
H15.8　Other disorders of sclera
　Excludes2:　blue sclera (Q13.5)
　　　　　　　degenerative myopia (H44.2-)
　H15.81　　Equatorial staphyloma
　　H15.811　Equatorial staphyloma, right eye
　　H15.812　Equatorial staphyloma, left eye
　　H15.813　Equatorial staphyloma, bilateral

H15.819   Equatorial staphyloma, unspecified eye
H15.82   Localized anterior staphyloma
    H15.821   Localized anterior staphyloma, right eye
    H15.822   Localized anterior staphyloma, left eye
    H15.823   Localized anterior staphyloma, bilateral
    H15.829   Localized anterior staphyloma, unspecified eye
H15.83   Staphyloma posticum
    H15.831   Staphyloma posticum, right eye
    H15.832   Staphyloma posticum, left eye
    H15.833   Staphyloma posticum, bilateral
    H15.839   Staphyloma posticum, unspecified eye
H15.84   Scleral ectasia
    H15.841   Scleral ectasia, right eye
    H15.842   Scleral ectasia, left eye
    H15.843   Scleral ectasia, bilateral
    H15.849   Scleral ectasia, unspecified eye
H15.85   Ring staphyloma
    H15.851   Ring staphyloma, right eye
    H15.852   Ring staphyloma, left eye
    H15.853   Ring staphyloma, bilateral
    H15.859   Ring staphyloma, unspecified eye
H15.89   Other disorders of sclera
H15.9   Unspecified disorder of sclera

H16 Keratitis
H16.0   Corneal ulcer
H16.00   Unspecified corneal ulcer
    H16.001   Unspecified corneal ulcer, right eye
    H16.002   Unspecified corneal ulcer, left eye
    H16.003   Unspecified corneal ulcer, bilateral
    H16.009   Unspecified corneal ulcer, unspecified eye
H16.01   Central corneal ulcer
    H16.011   Central corneal ulcer, right eye
    H16.012   Central corneal ulcer, left eye
    H16.013   Central corneal ulcer, bilateral
    H16.019   Central corneal ulcer, unspecified eye
H16.02   Ring corneal ulcer
    H16.021   Ring corneal ulcer, right eye
    H16.022   Ring corneal ulcer, left eye
    H16.023   Ring corneal ulcer, bilateral
    H16.029   Ring corneal ulcer, unspecified eye
H16.03   Corneal ulcer with hypopyon
    H16.031   Corneal ulcer with hypopyon, right eye
    H16.032   Corneal ulcer with hypopyon, left eye
    H16.033   Corneal ulcer with hypopyon, bilateral
    H16.039   Corneal ulcer with hypopyon, unspecified eye
H16.04   Marginal corneal ulcer
    H16.041   Marginal corneal ulcer, right eye
    H16.042   Marginal corneal ulcer, left eye
    H16.043   Marginal corneal ulcer, bilateral
    H16.049   Marginal corneal ulcer, unspecified eye
H16.05   Mooren's corneal ulcer
    H16.051   Mooren's corneal ulcer, right eye
    H16.052   Mooren's corneal ulcer, left eye
    H16.053   Mooren's corneal ulcer, bilateral
    H16.059   Mooren's corneal ulcer, unspecified eye
H16.06   Mycotic corneal ulcer
    H16.061   Mycotic corneal ulcer, right eye
    H16.062   Mycotic corneal ulcer, left eye
    H16.063   Mycotic corneal ulcer, bilateral
    H16.069   Mycotic corneal ulcer, unspecified eye
H16.07   Perforated corneal ulcer
    H16.071   Perforated corneal ulcer, right eye
    H16.072   Perforated corneal ulcer, left eye
    H16.073   Perforated corneal ulcer, bilateral
    H16.079   Perforated corneal ulcer, unspecified eye

H16.1   Other and unspecified superficial keratitis without conjunctivitis
H16.10   Unspecified superficial keratitis
    H16.101   Unspecified superficial keratitis, right eye
    H16.102   Unspecified superficial keratitis, left eye
    H16.103   Unspecified superficial keratitis, bilateral
    H16.109   Unspecified superficial keratitis, unspecified eye
H16.11   Macular keratitis
    Areolar keratitis
    Nummular keratitis
    Stellate keratitis
    Striate keratitis
    H16.111   Macular keratitis, right eye
    H16.112   Macular keratitis, left eye
    H16.113   Macular keratitis, bilateral
    H16.119   Macular keratitis, unspecified eye
H16.12   Filamentary keratitis
    H16.121   Filamentary keratitis, right eye
    H16.122   Filamentary keratitis, left eye
    H16.123   Filamentary keratitis, bilateral
    H16.129   Filamentary keratitis, unspecified eye
H16.13   Photokeratitis
    Snow blindness
    Welders' keratitis
    H16.131   Photokeratitis, right eye
    H16.132   Photokeratitis, left eye
    H16.133   Photokeratitis, bilateral
    H16.139   Photokeratitis, unspecified eye
H16.14   Punctate keratitis
    H16.141   Punctate keratitis, right eye
    H16.142   Punctate keratitis, left eye
    H16.143   Punctate keratitis, bilateral
    H16.149   Punctate keratitis, unspecified eye
H16.2   Keratoconjunctivitis
H16.20   Unspecified keratoconjunctivitis
    Superficial keratitis with conjunctivitis NOS
    H16.201   Unspecified keratoconjunctivitis, right eye
    H16.202   Unspecified keratoconjunctivitis, left eye
    H16.203   Unspecified keratoconjunctivitis, bilateral
    H16.209   Unspecified keratoconjunctivitis, unspecified eye
H16.21   Exposure keratoconjunctivitis
    H16.211   Exposure keratoconjunctivitis, right eye
    H16.212   Exposure keratoconjunctivitis, left eye
    H16.213   Exposure keratoconjunctivitis, bilateral
    H16.219   Exposure keratoconjunctivitis, unspecified eye
H16.22   Keratoconjunctivitis sicca, not specified as Sjögren's
    Excludes1:   Sjögren's syndrome (M35.01)
    H16.221   Keratoconjunctivitis sicca, not specified as Sjögren's, right eye
    H16.222   Keratoconjunctivitis sicca, not specified as Sjögren's, left eye
    H16.223   Keratoconjunctivitis sicca, not specified as Sjögren's, bilateral
    H16.229   Keratoconjunctivitis sicca, not specified as Sjögren's, unspecified eye
H16.23   Neurotrophic keratoconjunctivitis
    H16.231   Neurotrophic keratoconjunctivitis, right eye
    H16.232   Neurotrophic keratoconjunctivitis, left eye
    H16.233   Neurotrophic keratoconjunctivitis, bilateral
    H16.239   Neurotrophic keratoconjunctivitis, unspecified eye
H16.24   Ophthalmia nodosa
    H16.241   Ophthalmia nodosa, right eye
    H16.242   Ophthalmia nodosa, left eye
    H16.243   Ophthalmia nodosa, bilateral
    H16.249   Ophthalmia nodosa, unspecified eye
H16.25   Phlyctenular keratoconjunctivitis

H16.251   Phlyctenular keratoconjunctivitis, right eye

H16.252   Phlyctenular keratoconjunctivitis, left eye

H16.253   Phlyctenular keratoconjunctivitis, bilateral

H16.259   Phlyctenular keratoconjunctivitis, unspecified eye

H16.26   Vernal keratoconjunctivitis, with limbar and corneal involvement

> Excludes1:   vernal conjunctivitis without limbar and corneal involvement (H10.44)

H16.261   Vernal keratoconjunctivitis, with limbar and corneal involvement, right eye

H16.262   Vernal keratoconjunctivitis, with limbar and corneal involvement, left eye

H16.263   Vernal keratoconjunctivitis, with limbar and corneal involvement, bilateral

H16.269   Vernal keratoconjunctivitis, with limbar and corneal involvement, unspecified eye

H16.29   Other keratoconjunctivitis

H16.291   Other keratoconjunctivitis, right eye

H16.292   Other keratoconjunctivitis, left eye

H16.293   Other keratoconjunctivitis, bilateral

H16.299   Other keratoconjunctivitis, unspecified eye

H16.3   Interstitial and deep keratitis

H16.30   Unspecified interstitial keratitis

H16.301   Unspecified interstitial keratitis, right eye

H16.302   Unspecified interstitial keratitis, left eye

H16.303   Unspecified interstitial keratitis, bilateral

H16.309   Unspecified interstitial keratitis, unspecified eye

H16.31   Corneal abscess

H16.311   Corneal abscess, right eye

H16.312   Corneal abscess, left eye

H16.313   Corneal abscess, bilateral

H16.319   Corneal abscess, unspecified eye

H16.32   Diffuse interstitial keratitis

> Cogan's syndrome

H16.321   Diffuse interstitial keratitis, right eye

H16.322   Diffuse interstitial keratitis, left eye

H16.323   Diffuse interstitial keratitis, bilateral

H16.329   Diffuse interstitial keratitis, unspecified eye

H16.33   Sclerosing keratitis

H16.331   Sclerosing keratitis, right eye

H16.332   Sclerosing keratitis, left eye

H16.333   Sclerosing keratitis, bilateral

H16.339   Sclerosing keratitis, unspecified eye

H16.39   Other interstitial and deep keratitis

H16.391   Other interstitial and deep keratitis, right eye

H16.392   Other interstitial and deep keratitis, left eye

H16.393   Other interstitial and deep keratitis, bilateral

H16.399   Other interstitial and deep keratitis, unspecified eye

H16.4   Corneal neovascularization

H16.40   Unspecified corneal neovascularization

H16.401   Unspecified corneal neovascularization, right eye

H16.402   Unspecified corneal neovascularization, left eye

H16.403   Unspecified corneal neovascularization, bilateral

H16.409   Unspecified corneal neovascularization, unspecified eye

H16.41   Ghost vessels (corneal)

H16.411   Ghost vessels (corneal), right eye

H16.412   Ghost vessels (corneal), left eye

H16.413   Ghost vessels (corneal), bilateral

H16.419   Ghost vessels (corneal), unspecified eye

H16.42   Pannus (corneal)

H16.421   Pannus (corneal), right eye

H16.422   Pannus (corneal), left eye

H16.423   Pannus (corneal), bilateral

H16.429   Pannus (corneal), unspecified eye

H16.43   Localized vascularization of cornea

H16.431   Localized vascularization of cornea, right eye

H16.432   Localized vascularization of cornea, left eye

H16.433   Localized vascularization of cornea, bilateral

H16.439   Localized vascularization of cornea, unspecified eye

H16.44   Deep vascularization of cornea

H16.441   Deep vascularization of cornea, right eye

H16.442   Deep vascularization of cornea, left eye

H16.443   Deep vascularization of cornea, bilateral

H16.449   Deep vascularization of cornea, unspecified eye

H16.8   Other keratitis

H16.9   Unspecified keratitis

H17   Corneal scars and opacities

H17.0   Adherent leukoma

H17.00   Adherent leukoma, unspecifed eye

H17.01   Adherent leukoma, right eye

H17.02   Adherent leukoma, left eye

H17.03   Adherent leukoma, bilateral

H17.1   Central corneal opacity

H17.10   Central corneal opacity, unspecified eye

H17.11   Central corneal opacity, right eye

H17.12   Central corneal opacity, left eye

H17.13   Central corneal opacity, bilateral

H17.8   Other corneal scars and opacities

H17.81   Minor opacity of cornea

> Corneal nebula

H17.811   Minor opacity of cornea, right eye

H17.812   Minor opacity of cornea, left eye

H17.813   Minor opacity of cornea, bilateral

H17.819   Minor opacity of cornea, unspecified eye

H17.82   Peripheral opacity of cornea

H17.821   Peripheral opacity of cornea, right eye

H17.822   Peripheral opacity of cornea, left eye

H17.823   Peripheral opacity of cornea, bilateral

H17.829   Peripheral opacity of cornea, unspecified eye

H17.89   Other corneal scars and opacities

H17.9   Unspecified corneal scar and opacity

H18   Other disorders of cornea

H18.0   Corneal pigmentations and deposits

> Use additional external cause code (Chapter XIX), to identify drug, if drug-induced.

H18.00   Unspecified corneal deposit

H18.001   Unspecified corneal deposit, right eye

H18.002   Unspecified corneal deposit, left eye

H18.003   Unspecified corneal deposit, bilateral

H18.009   Unspecified corneal deposit, unspecified eye

H18.01   Anterior corneal pigmentations

> Staehli's line

H18.011   Anterior corneal pigmentations, right eye

H18.012   Anterior corneal pigmentations, left eye

H18.013   Anterior corneal pigmentations, bilateral

H18.019   Anterior corneal pigmentations, unspecified eye

H18.02   Argentous corneal deposits

H18.021   Argentous corneal deposits, right eye

H18.022   Argentous corneal deposits, left eye

H18.023   Argentous corneal deposits, bilateral

H18.029   Argentous corneal deposits, unspecified eye

H18.03   Corneal deposits in metabolic disorders

> Code also associated metabolic disorder

H18.031   Corneal deposits in metabolic disorders, right eye

H18.032   Corneal deposits in metabolic disorders, left eye

H18.033   Corneal deposits in metabolic disorders, bilateral
H18.039   Corneal deposits in metabolic disorders, unspecified eye

H18.04   Kayser-Fleischer ring
H18.041   Kayser-Fleischer ring, right eye
H18.042   Kayser-Fleischer ring, left eye
H18.043   Kayser-Fleischer ring, bilateral
H18.049   Kayser-Fleischer ring, unspecified eye

H18.05   Posterior corneal pigmentations
Krukenberg's spindle
H18.051   Posterior corneal pigmentations, right eye
H18.052   Posterior corneal pigmentations, left eye
H18.053   Posterior corneal pigmentations, bilateral
H18.059   Posterior corneal pigmentations, unspecified eye

H18.06   Stromal corneal pigmentations
Hematocornea
H18.061   Stromal corneal pigmentations, right eye
H18.062   Stromal corneal pigmentations, left eye
H18.063   Stromal corneal pigmentations, bilateral
H18.069   Stromal corneal pigmentations, unspecified eye

H18.1   Bullous keratopathy
H18.10   Bullous keratopathy, unspecified eye
H18.11   Bullous keratopathy, right eye
H18.12   Bullous keratopathy, left eye
H18.13   Bullous keratopathy, bilateral

H18.2   Other and unspecified corneal edema
H18.20   Unspecified corneal edema
H18.21   Corneal edema secondary to contact lens
Excludes2:   other corneal disorders due to contact lens (H18.82-)
H18.211   Corneal edema secondary to contact lens, right eye
H18.212   Corneal edema secondary to contact lens, left eye
H18.213   Corneal edema secondary to contact lens, bilateral
H18.219   Corneal edema secondary to contact lens, unspecified eye
H18.22   Idiopathic corneal edema
H18.221   Idiopathic corneal edema, right eye
H18.222   Idiopathic corneal edema, left eye
H18.223   Idiopathic corneal edema, bilateral
H18.229   Idiopathic corneal edema, unspecified eye
H18.23   Secondary corneal edema
H18.231   Secondary corneal edema, right eye
H18.232   Secondary corneal edema, left eye
H18.233   Secondary corneal edema, bilateral
H18.239   Secondary corneal edema, unspecified eye

H18.3   Changes of corneal membranes
H18.30   Unspecified corneal membrane change
H18.31   Folds and rupture in Bowman's membrane
H18.311   Folds and rupture in Bowman's membrane, right eye
H18.312   Folds and rupture in Bowman's membrane, left eye
H18.313   Folds and rupture in Bowman's membrane, bilateral
H18.319   Folds and rupture in Bowman's membrane, unspecified eye
H18.32   Folds in Descemet's membrane
H18.321   Folds in Descemet's membrane, right eye
H18.322   Folds in Descemet's membrane, left eye
H18.323   Folds in Descemet's membrane, bilateral
H18.329   Folds in Descemet's membrane, unspecified eye
H18.33   Rupture in Descemet's membrane
H18.331   Rupture in Descemet's membrane, right eye

H18.332   Rupture in Descemet's membrane, left eye
H18.333   Rupture in Descemet's membrane, bilateral
H18.339   Rupture in Descemet's membrane, unspecified eye

H18.4   Corneal degeneration
Excludes1:   Mooren's ulcer (H16.0-)
recurrent erosion of cornea (H18.83-)
H18.40   Unspecified corneal degeneration
H18.41   Arcus senilis
Senile corneal changes
H18.411   Arcus senilis, right eye
H18.412   Arcus senilis, left eye
H18.413   Arcus senilis, bilateral
H18.419   Arcus senilis, unspecified eye
H18.42   Band keratopathy
H18.421   Band keratopathy, right eye
H18.422   Band keratopathy, left eye
H18.423   Band keratopathy, bilateral
H18.429   Band keratopathy, unspecified eye
H18.43   Other calcerous corneal degeneration
H18.44   Keratomalacia
Excludes1:   keratomalacia due to vitamin A deficiency (E50.4)
H18.441   Keratomalacia, right eye
H18.442   Keratomalacia, left eye
H18.443   Keratomalacia, bilateral
H18.449   Keratomalacia, unspecified eye
H18.45   Nodular corneal degeneration
H18.451   Nodular corneal degeneration, right eye
H18.452   Nodular corneal degeneration, left eye
H18.453   Nodular corneal degeneration, bilateral
H18.459   Nodular corneal degeneration, unspecified eye
H18.46   Peripheral corneal degeneration
H18.461   Peripheral corneal degeneration, right eye
H18.462   Peripheral corneal degeneration, left eye
H18.463   Peripheral corneal degeneration, bilateral
H18.469   Peripheral corneal degeneration, unspecified eye
H18.49   Other corneal degeneration

H18.5   Hereditary corneal dystrophies
H18.50   Unspecified hereditary corneal dystrophies
H18.51   Endothelial corneal dystrophy
Fuchs' dystrophy
H18.52   Epithelial (juvenile) corneal dystrophy
H18.53   Granular corneal dystrophy
H18.54   Lattice corneal dystrophy
H18.55   Macular corneal dystrophy
H18.59   Other hereditary corneal dystrophies

H18.6   Keratoconus
H18.60   Keratoconus, unspecified
H18.601   Keratoconus, unspecified, right eye
H18.602   Keratoconus, unspecified, left eye
H18.603   Keratoconus, unspecified, bilateral
H18.609   Keratoconus, unspecified, unspecified eye
H18.61   Keratoconus, stable
H18.611   Keratoconus, stable, right eye
H18.612   Keratoconus, stable, left eye
H18.613   Keratoconus, stable, bilateral
H18.619   Keratoconus, stable, unspecified eye
H18.62   Keratoconus, unstable
Acute hydrops
H18.621   Keratoconus, unstable, right eye
H18.622   Keratoconus, unstable, left eye
H18.623   Keratoconus, unstable, bilateral
H18.629   Keratoconus, unstable, unspecified eye

H18.7   Other and unspecified corneal deformities
Excludes1:   congenital malformations of cornea (Q13.3-Q13.4)
H18.70   Unspecified corneal deformity

H18.71   Corneal ectasia
    H18.711   Corneal ectasia, right eye
    H18.712   Corneal ectasia, left eye
    H18.713   Corneal ectasia, bilateral
    H18.719   Corneal ectasia, unspecified eye
H18.72   Corneal staphyloma
    H18.721   Corneal staphyloma, right eye
    H18.722   Corneal staphyloma, left eye
    H18.723   Corneal staphyloma, bilateral
    H18.729   Corneal staphyloma, unspecified eye
H18.73   Descemetocele
    H18.731   Descemetocele, right eye
    H18.732   Descemetocele, left eye
    H18.733   Descemetocele, bilateral
    H18.739   Descemetocele, unspecified eye
H18.8 Other specified disorders of cornea
H18.81   Anesthesia and hypoesthesia of cornea
    H18.811   Anesthesia and hypoesthesia of cornea, right eye
    H18.812   Anesthesia and hypoesthesia of cornea, left eye
    H18.813   Anesthesia and hypoesthesia of cornea, bilateral
    H18.819   Anesthesia and hypoesthesia of cornea, unspecified eye
H18.82   Corneal disorder due to contact lens
    Excludes2:   corneal edema due to contact lens (H18.21-)
    H18.821   Corneal disorder due to contact lens, right eye
    H18.822   Corneal disorder due to contact lens, left eye
    H18.823   Corneal disorder due to contact lens, bilateral
    H18.829   Corneal disorder due to contact lens, unspecified eye
H18.83   Recurrent erosion of cornea
    H18.831   Recurrent erosion of cornea, right eye
    H18.832   Recurrent erosion of cornea, left eye
    H18.833   Recurrent erosion of cornea, bilateral
    H18.839   Recurrent erosion of cornea, unspecified eye
H18.89   Other specified disorders of cornea
H18.9 Unspecified disorder of cornea

H20 Iridocyclitis
H20.0 Acute and subacute iridocyclitis
    Acute anterior uveitis
    Acute cyclitis
    Acute iritis
    Subacute anterior uveitis
    Subacute cyclitis
    Subacute iritis
    Excludes1:   iridocyclitis, iritis, uveitis (due to) (in):
        diabetes mellitus (E08-E14 with .39)
        diphtheria (A36.89)
        gonococcal (A54.32)
        herpes (simplex) (B00.51)
        herpes zoster (B02.32)
        late congenital syphilis (A50.39)
        late syphilis (A52.71)
        sarcoidosis (D86.83)
        syphilis (A51.43)
        toxoplasmosis (B58.09)
        tuberculosis (A18.54)
H20.00   Unspecified acute and subacute iridocyclitis
H20.01   Primary iridocyclitis
    H20.011   Primary iridocyclitis, right eye
    H20.012   Primary iridocyclitis, left eye
    H20.013   Primary iridocyclitis, bilateral
    H20.019   Primary iridocyclitis, unspecified eye
H20.02   Recurrent acute iridocyclitis
    H20.021   Recurrent acute iridocyclitits, right eye
    H20.022   Recurrent acute iridocyclitits, left eye
    H20.023   Recurrent acute iridocyclitits, bilateral

    H20.029   Recurrent acute iridocyclitits, unspecified eye
H20.03   Secondary infectious iridocyclitis
    H20.031   Secondary infectious iridocyclitis, right eye
    H20.032   Secondary infectious iridocyclitis, left eye
    H20.033   Secondary infectious iridocyclitis, bilateral
    H20.039   Secondary infectious iridocyclitis, unspecified eye
H20.04   Secondary noninfectious iridocyclitis
    H20.041   Secondary noninfectious iridocyclitis, right eye
    H20.042   Secondary noninfectious iridocyclitis, left eye
    H20.043   Secondary noninfectious iridocyclitis, bilateral
    H20.049   Secondary noninfectious iridocyclitis, unspecified eye
H20.05   Hypopyon
    H20.051   Hypopyon, right eye
    H20.052   Hypopyon, left eye
    H20.053   Hypopyon, bilateral
    H20.059   Hypopyon, unspecified eye
H20.1 Chronic iridocyclitis
    Use additional code for any associated cataract (H26.21-)
    Excludes2:   posterior cyclitis (H30.2-)
H20.10   Chronic iridocyclitis, unspecified eye
H20.11   Chronic iridocyclitis, right eye
H20.12   Chronic iridocyclitis, left eye
H20.13   Chronic iridocyclitis, bilateral
H20.2 Lens-induced iridocyclitis
H20.20   Lens-induced iridocyclitis, unspecified eye
H20.21   Lens-induced iridocyclitis, right eye
H20.22   Lens-induced iridocyclitis, left eye
H20.23   Lens-induced iridocyclitis, bilateral
H20.8 Other iridocyclitis
    Excludes2:   glaucomatocyclitis crises (H40.4-)
        posterior cyclitis (H30.2-)
        sympathetic uveitis (H44.13-)
H20.81   Fuchs' heterochromic cyclitis
    H20.811   Fuchs' heterochromic cyclitis, right eye
    H20.812   Fuchs' heterochromic cyclitis, left eye
    H20.813   Fuchs' heterochromic cyclitis, bilateral
    H20.819   Fuchs' heterochromic cyclitis, unspecified eye
H20.82   Vogt-Koyanagi syndrome
    H20.821   Vogt-Koyanagi syndrome, right eye
    H20.822   Vogt-Koyanagi syndrome, left eye
    H20.823   Vogt-Koyanagi syndrome, bilateral
    H20.829   Vogt-Koyanagi syndrome, unspecified eye
H20.9 Unspecified iridocyclitis
    Uveitis NOS

H21 Other disorders of iris and ciliary body
    Excludes2:   sympathetic uveitis (H44.1-)
H21.0 Hyphema
    Excludes1:   traumatic hyphema (S05.1-)
H21.00   Hyphema, unspecified eye
H21.01   Hyphema, right eye
H21.02   Hyphema, left eye
H21.03   Hyphema, bilateral
H21.1 Other vascular disorders of iris and ciliary body
    Neovascularization of iris or ciliary body
    Rubeosis iridis
    Rubeosis of iris
H21.10   Other vascular disorders of iris and ciliary body, unspecified eye
H21.11   Other vascular disorders of iris and ciliary body, right eye
H21.12   Other vascular disorders of iris and ciliary body, left eye
H21.13   Other vascular disorders of iris and ciliary body, bilateral
H21.2 Degeneration of iris and ciliary body
H21.21   Degeneration of chamber angle

H21.211   Degeneration of chamber angle, right eye
H21.212   Degeneration of chamber angle, left eye
H21.213   Degeneration of chamber angle, bilateral
H21.219   Degeneration of chamber angle, unspecified eye

H21.22   **Degeneration of ciliary body**
H21.221   Degeneration of ciliary body, right eye
H21.222   Degeneration of ciliary body, left eye
H21.223   Degeneration of ciliary body, bilateral
H21.229   Degeneration of ciliary body, unspecified eye

H21.23   **Degeneration of iris (pigmentary)**
Translucency of iris
H21.231   Degeneration of iris (pigmentary), right eye
H21.232   Degeneration of iris (pigmentary), left eye
H21.233   Degeneration of iris (pigmentary), bilateral
H21.239   Degeneration of iris (pigmentary), unspecified eye

H21.24   **Degeneration of pupillary margin**
H21.241   Degeneration of pupillary margin, right eye
H21.242   Degeneration of pupillary margin, left eye
H21.243   Degeneration of pupillary margin, bilateral
H21.249   Degeneration of pupillary margin, unspecified eye

H21.25   **Iridoschisis**
H21.251   Iridoschisis, right eye
H21.252   Iridoschisis, left eye
H21.253   Iridoschisis, bilateral
H21.259   Iridoschisis, unspecified eye

H21.26   **Iris atrophy (essential) (progressive)**
H21.261   Iris atrophy (essential) (progressive), right eye
H21.262   Iris atrophy (essential) (progressive), left eye
H21.263   Iris atrophy (essential) (progressive), bilateral
H21.269   Iris atrophy (essential) (progressive), unspecified eye

H21.27   **Miotic pupillary cyst**
H21.271   Miotic pupillary cyst, right eye
H21.272   Miotic pupillary cyst, left eye
H21.273   Miotic pupillary cyst, bilateral
H21.279   Miotic pupillary cyst, unspecified eye

H21.29   **Other iris atrophy**

H21.3   **Cyst of iris, ciliary body and anterior chamber**
Excludes2:   miotic pupillary cyst (H21.27-)

H21.30   **Idiopathic cysts of iris, ciliary body or anterior chamber**
Cyst of iris, ciliary body or anterior chamber NOS
H21.301   Idiopathic cysts of iris, ciliary body or anterior chamber, right eye
H21.302   Idiopathic cysts of iris, ciliary body or anterior chamber, left eye
H21.303   Idiopathic cysts of iris, ciliary body or anterior chamber, bilateral
H21.309   Idiopathic cysts of iris, ciliary body or anterior chamber, unspecified eye

H21.31   **Exudative cysts of iris or anterior chamber**
H21.311   Exudative cysts of iris or anterior chamber, right eye
H21.312   Exudative cysts of iris or anterior chamber, left eye
H21.313   Exudative cysts of iris or anterior chamber, bilateral
H21.319   Exudative cysts of iris or anterior chamber, unspecified eye

H21.32   **Implantation cysts of iris, ciliary body or anterior chamber**
H21.321   Implantation cysts of iris, ciliary body or anterior chamber, right eye
H21.322   Implantation cysts of iris, ciliary body or anterior chamber, left eye
H21.323   Implantation cysts of iris, ciliary body or anterior chamber, bilateral

H21.329   Implantation cysts of iris, ciliary body or anterior chamber, unspecified eye

H21.33   **Parasitic cyst of iris, ciliary body or anterior chamber**
H21.331   Parasitic cyst of iris, ciliary body or anterior chamber, right eye
H21.332   Parasitic cyst of iris, ciliary body or anterior chamber, left eye
H21.333   Parasitic cyst of iris, ciliary body or anterior chamber, bilateral
H21.339   Parasitic cyst of iris, ciliary body or anterior chamber, unspecified eye

H21.34   **Primary cyst of pars plana**
H21.341   Primary cyst of pars plana, right eye
H21.342   Primary cyst of pars plana, left eye
H21.343   Primary cyst of pars plana, bilateral
H21.349   Primary cyst of pars plana, unspecified eye

H21.35   **Exudative cyst of pars plana**
H21.351   Exudative cyst of pars plana, right eye
H21.352   Exudative cyst of pars plana, left eye
H21.353   Exudative cyst of pars plana, bilateral
H21.359   Exudative cyst of pars plana, unspecified eye

H21.4   **Pupillary membranes**
Iris bombé
Pupillary occlusion
Pupillary seclusion
Excludes1:   congenital pupillary membranes (Q13.8)

H21.40   **Pupillary membranes, unspecified eye**
H21.41   **Pupillary membranes, right eye**
H21.42   **Pupillary membranes, left eye**
H21.43   **Pupillary membranes, bilateral**

H21.5   **Other and unspecified adhesions and disruptions of iris and ciliary body**
Excludes1:   corectopia (Q13.2)

H21.50   **Unspecified adhesions of iris**
Synechia (iris) NOS
H21.501   Unspecified adhesions of iris , right eye
H21.502   Unspecified adhesions of iris, left eye
H21.503   Unspecified adhesions of iris, bilateral
H21.509   Unspecified adhesions of iris and ciliary body, unspecified eye

H21.51   **Interior synechiae (iris)**
H21.511   Anterior synechiae (iris), right eye
H21.512   Anterior synechiae (iris), left eye
H21.513   Anterior synechiae (iris), bilateral
H21.519   Anterior synechiae (iris), unspecified eye

H21.52   **Goniosynechiae**
H21.521   Goniosynechiae, right eye
H21.522   Goniosynechiae, left eye
H21.523   Goniosynechiae, bilateral
H21.529   Goniosynechiae, unspecified eye

H21.53   **Iridodialysis**
H21.531   Iridodialysis, right eye
H21.532   Iridodialysis, left eye
H21.533   Iridodialysis, bilateral
H21.539   Iridodialysis, unspecified eye

H21.54   **Posterior synechiae (iris)**
H21.541   Posterior synechiae (iris), right eye
H21.542   Posterior synechiae (iris), left eye
H21.543   Posterior synechiae (iris), bilateral
H21.549   Posterior synechiae (iris), unspecified eye

H21.55   **Recession of chamber angle**
H21.551   Recession of chamber angle, right eye
H21.552   Recession of chamber angle, left eye
H21.553   Recession of chamber angle, bilateral
H21.559   Recession of chamber angle, unspecified eye

H21.56   **Pupillary abnormalities**
Deformed pupil
Ectopic pupil
Rupture of sphincter, pupil
Excludes1:   congenital deformity of pupil (Q13.2-)
H21.561   Pupillary abnormality, right eye
H21.562   Pupillary abnormality, left eye
H21.563   Pupillary abnormality, bilateral
H21.569   Pupillary abnormality, unspecified eye
H21.8   **Other specified disorders of iris and ciliary body**
H21.9   **Unspecified disorder of iris and ciliary body**

DISORDERS OF LENS (H25-H28)

H25   Age-related cataract
Senile cataract
Excludes2:   capsular glaucoma with pseudoexfoliation of lens (H40.1-)
H25.0   **Age-related incipient cataract**
H25.01   **Cortical age-related cataract**
H25.011   Cortical age-related cataract, right eye
H25.012   Cortical age-related cataract, left eye
H25.013   Cortical age-related cataract, bilateral
H25.019   Cortical age-related cataract, unspecified eye
H25.03   **Anterior subcapsular polar age-related cataract**
H25.031   Anterior subcapsular polar age-related cataract, right eye
H25.032   Anterior subcapsular polar age-related cataract, left eye
H25.033   Anterior subcapsular polar age-related cataract, bilateral
H25.039   Anterior subcapsular polar age-related cataract, unspecified eye
H25.04   **Posterior subcapsular polar age-related cataract**
H25.041   Posterior subcapsular polar age-related cataract, right eye
H25.042   Posterior subcapsular polar age-related cataract, left eye
H25.043   Posterior subcapsular polar age-related cataract, bilateral
H25.049   Posterior subcapsular polar age-related cataract, unspecified eye
H25.09   **Other age-related incipient cataract**
Coronary age-related cataract
Punctate age-related cataract
Water clefts
H25.091   Other age-related incipient cataract, right eye
H25.092   Other age-related incipient cataract, left eye
H25.093   Other age-related incipient cataract, bilateral
H25.099   Other age-related incipient cataract, unspecified eye
H25.1   **Age-related nuclear cataract**
Cataracta brunescens
Nuclear sclerosis cataract
H25.10   **Age-related nuclear cataract, unspecified eye**
H25.11   **Age-related nuclear cataract, right eye**
H25.12   **Age-related nuclear cataract, left eye**
H25.13   **Age-related nuclear cataract, bilateral**
H25.2   **Age-related cataract, morgagnian type**
Age-related hypermature cataract
H25.20   **Age-related cataract, morgagnian type, unspecified eye**
H25.21   **Age-related cataract, morgagnian type, right eye**
H25.22   **Age-related cataract, morgagnian type, left eye**
H25.23   **Age-related cataract, morgagnian type, bilateral**
H25.8   **Other age-related cataract**
H25.81   **Combined forms of age-related cataract**
H25.811   Combined forms of age-related cataract, right eye
H25.812   Combined forms of age-related cataract, left eye

H25.813   Combined forms of age-related cataract, bilateral
H25.819   Combined forms of age-related cataract, unspecified eye
H25.89   **Other age-related cataract**
H25.9   **Unspecified age-related cataract**

H26   Other cataract
Excludes1:   congenital cataract (Q12.0)
H26.0   **Infantile and juvenile cataract**
H26.00   **Unspecified infantile and juvenile cataract**
H26.001   Unspecified infantile and juvenile cataract, right eye
H26.002   Unspecified infantile and juvenile cataract, left eye
H26.003   Unspecified infantile and juvenile cataract, bilateral
H26.009   Unspecified infantile and juvenile cataract, unspecified eye
H26.01   **Infantile and juvenile cortical, lamellar, or zonular cataract**
H26.011   Infantile and juvenile cortical, lamellar, or zonular cataract, right eye
H26.012   Infantile and juvenile cortical, lamellar, or zonular cataract, left eye
H26.013   Infantile and juvenile cortical, lamellar, or zonular cataract, bilateral
H26.019   Infantile and juvenile cortical, lamellar, or zonular cataract, unspecified eye
H26.03   **Infantile and juvenile nuclear cataract**
H26.031   Infantile and juvenile nuclear cataract, right eye
H26.032   Infantile and juvenile nuclear cataract, left eye
H26.033   Infantile and juvenile nuclear cataract, bilateral
H26.039   Infantile and juvenile nuclear cataract, unspecified eye
H26.04   **Anterior subcapsular polar infantile and juvenile cataract**
H26.041   Anterior subcapsular polar infantile and juvenile cataract, right eye
H26.042   Anterior subcapsular polar infantile and juvenile cataract, left eye
H26.043   Anterior subcapsular polar infantile and juvenile cataract, bilateral
H26.049   Anterior subcapsular polar infantile and juvenile cataract, unspecified eye
H26.05   **Posterior subcapsular polar infantile and juvenile cataract**
H26.051   Posterior subcapsular polar infantile and juvenile cataract, right eye
H26.052   Posterior subcapsular polar infantile and juvenile cataract, left eye
H26.053   Posterior subcapsular polar infantile and juvenile cataract, bilateral
H26.059   Posterior subcapsular polar infantile and juvenile cataract, unspecified eye
H26.06   **Combined forms of infantile and juvenile cataract**
H26.061   Combined forms of infantile and juvenile cataract, right eye
H26.062   Combined forms of infantile and juvenile cataract, left eye
H26.063   Combined forms of infantile and juvenile cataract cataract, bilateral
H26.069   Combined forms of infantile and juvenile cataract cataract, unspecified eye
H26.09   **Other infantile and juvenile cataract**
H26.1   **Traumatic cataract**
Use additional external cause code (Chapter XX) to identify cause.
H26.10   **Unspecified traumatic cataract**

H26.101   Unspecified traumatic cataract, right eye
H26.102   Unspecified traumatic cataract, left eye
H26.103   Unspecified traumatic cataract, bilateral
H26.109   Unspecified traumatic cataract, unspecified eye
H26.11   **Localized traumatic opacities**
H26.111   Localized traumatic opacities, right eye
H26.112   Localized traumatic opacities, left eye
H26.113   Localized traumatic opacities, bilateral
H26.119   Localized traumatic opacities, unspecified eye
H26.12   **Partially resolved traumatic cataract**
H26.121   Partially resolved traumatic cataract, right eye
H26.122   Partially resolved traumatic cataract, left eye
H26.123   Partially resolved traumatic cataract, bilateral
H26.129   Partially resolved traumatic cataract, unspecified eye
H26.13   **Total traumatic cataract**
H26.131   Total traumatic cataract, right eye
H26.132   Total traumatic cataract, left eye
H26.133   Total traumatic cataract, bilateral
H26.139   Total traumatic cataract, unspecified eye

H26.2   **Complicated cataract**
H26.20   **Unspecified complicated cataract**
Cataracta complicata NOS
H26.21   **Cataract with neovascularization**
Code also associated condition, such as:
chronic iridocyclitis (H20.1-)
H26.211   Cataract with neovascularization, right eye
H26.212   Cataract with neovascularization, left eye
H26.213   Cataract with neovascularization, bilateral
H26.219   Cataract with neovascularization, unspecified eye
H26.22   **Cataract secondary to ocular disorders (degenerative) (inflammatory)**
Code also associated ocular disorder
H26.221   Cataract secondary to ocular disorders (degenerative) (inflammatory), right eye
H26.222   Cataract secondary to ocular disorders (degenerative) (inflammatory), left eye
H26.223   Cataract secondary to ocular disorders (degenerative) (inflammatory), bilateral
H26.229   Cataract secondary to ocular disorders (degenerative) (inflammatory), unspecified eye
H26.23   **Glaucomatous flecks (subcapsular)**
Code first underlying glaucoma (H40-H42)
H26.231   Glaucomatous flecks (subcapsular), right eye
H26.232   Glaucomatous flecks (subcapsular), left eye
H26.233   Glaucomatous flecks (subcapsular), bilateral
H26.239   Glaucomatous flecks (subcapsular), unspecified eye
H26.3   **Drug-induced cataract**
Toxic cataract
Use additional external cause code (Chapter XIX), to identify drug
H26.30   Drug-induced cataract, unspecified eye
H26.31   Drug-induced cataract, right eye
H26.32   Drug-induced cataract, left eye
H26.33   Drug-induced cataract, bilateral
H26.4   **Secondary cataract**
H26.40   Unspecified secondary cataract
H26.41   Soemmering's ring
H26.411   Soemmering's ring, right eye
H26.412   Soemmering's ring, left eye
H26.413   Soemmering's ring, bilateral
H26.419   Soemmering's ring, unspecified eye
H26.49   Other secondary cataract
H26.491   Other secondary cataract, right eye
H26.492   Other secondary cataract, left eye
H26.493   Other secondary cataract, bilateral
H26.499   Other secondary cataract, unspecified eye

H26.8   **Other specified cataract**
H26.9   **Unspecified cataract**

H27   Other disorders of lens
Excludes1: congenital lens malformations (Q12.-)
mechanical complications of intraocular lens implant (T85.2)
pseudophakia (Z96.1)
H27.0   **Aphakia**
Acquired absence of lens
Acquired aphakia
Aphakia due to trauma
Excludes1: cataract extraction status (Z98.4-)
congenital absence of lens (Q12.3)
congenital aphakia (Q12.3)
H27.00   Aphakia, unspecified eye
H27.01   Aphakia, right eye
H27.02   Aphakia, left eye
H27.03   Aphakia, bilateral
H27.1   **Dislocation of lens**
H27.10   Unspecified dislocation of lens
H27.11   Subluxation of lens
H27.111   Subluxation of lens, right eye
H27.112   Subluxation of lens, left eye
H27.113   Subluxation of lens, bilateral
H27.119   Subluxation of lens, unspecified eye
H27.12   Anterior dislocation of lens
H27.121   Anterior dislocation of lens, right eye
H27.122   Anterior dislocation of lens, left eye
H27.123   Anterior dislocation of lens, bilateral
H27.129   Anterior dislocation of lens, unspecified eye
H27.13   Posterior dislocation of lens
H27.131   Posterior dislocation of lens, right eye
H27.132   Posterior dislocation of lens, left eye
H27.133   Posterior dislocation of lens, bilateral
H27.139   Posterior dislocation of lens, unspecified eye
H27.8   **Other specified disorders of lens**
H27.9   **Unspecified disorder of lens**

H28   Cataract in diseases classified elsewhere
Code first underlying disease, such as:
hypoparathyroidism (E20.-)
myotonia (G71.1)
myxedema (E03.-)
protein-calorie malnutrition (E40-E46)
Excludes1: cataract in diabetes mellitus (E08.33, E09.33, E10.33, E11.33, 13.33, E14.33)

DISORDERS OF CHOROID AND RETINA (H30-H36)

H30   Chorioretinal inflammation
H30.0   **Focal chorioretinal inflammation**
Focal chorioretinitis
Focal choroiditis
Focal retinitis
Focal retinochoroiditis
H30.00   Unspecified focal chorioretinal inflammation
Focal chorioretinitis NOS
Focal choroiditis NOS
Focal retinitis NOS
Focal retinochoroiditis NOS
H30.001   Unspecified focal chorioretinal inflammation, right eye
H30.002   Unspecified focal chorioretinal inflammation, left eye
H30.003   Unspecified focal chorioretinal inflammation, bilateral
H30.009   Unspecified focal chorioretinal inflammation, unspecified eye
H30.01   Focal chorioretinal inflammation, juxtapapillary
H30.011   Focal chorioretinal inflammation, juxtapapillary, right eye

H30.012   Focal chorioretinal inflammation, juxtapapillary, left eye

H30.013   Focal chorioretinal inflammation, juxtapapillary, bilateral

H30.019   Focal chorioretinal inflammation, juxtapapillary, unspecified eye

H30.02   Focal chorioretinal inflammation of posterior pole

H30.021   Focal chorioretinal inflammation of posterior pole, right eye

H30.022   Focal chorioretinal inflammation of posterior pole, left eye

H30.023   Focal chorioretinal inflammation of posterior pole, bilateral

H30.029   Focal chorioretinal inflammation of posterior pole, unspecified eye

H30.03   Focal chorioretinal inflammation, peripheral

H30.031   Focal chorioretinal inflammation, peripheral, right eye

H30.032   Focal chorioretinal inflammation, peripheral, left eye

H30.033   Focal chorioretinal inflammation, peripheral, bilateral

H30.039   Focal chorioretinal inflammation, peripheral, unspecified eye

H30.04   Focal chorioretinal inflammation, macular or paramacular

H30.041   Focal chorioretinal inflammataion, macular or paramacular, right eye

H30.042   Focal chorioretinal inflammataion, macular or paramacular, left eye

H30.043   Focal chorioretinal inflammataion, macular or paramacular, bilateral

H30.049   Focal chorioretinal inflammataion, macular or paramacular, unspecified eye

H30.1   Disseminated chorioretinal inflammation
Disseminated chorioretinitis
Disseminated choroiditis
Disseminated retinitis
Disseminated retinochorioditis
Excludes2:   exudative retinopathy (H35.02-)

H30.10   Unspecified disseminated chorioretinal inflammation
Disseminated chorioretinitis NOS
Disseminated choroiditis NOS
Disseminated retinitis NOS
Disseminated retinochorioditis NOS

H30.101   Unspecified disseminated chorioretinal inflammation, right eye

H30.102   Unspecified disseminated chorioretinal inflammation, left eye

H30.103   Unspecified disseminated chorioretinal inflammation, bilateral

H30.109   Unspecified disseminated chorioretinal inflammation, unspecified eye

H30.11   Disseminated chorioretinal inflammation of posterior pole

H30.111   Disseminated chorioretinal inflammation of posterior pole, right eye

H30.112   Disseminated chorioretinal inflammation of posterior pole, left eye

H30.113   Disseminated chorioretinal inflammation of posterior pole, bilateral

H30.119   Disseminated chorioretinal inflammation of posterior pole, unspecified eye

H30.12   Disseminated chorioretinal inflammation, peripheral

H30.121   Disseminated chorioretinal inflammation, peripheral, right eye

H30.122   Disseminated chorioretinal inflammation, peripheral, left eye

H30.123   Disseminated chorioretinal inflammation, peripheral, bilateral

H30.129   Disseminated chorioretinal inflammation, peripheral, unspecified eye

H30.13   Disseminated chorioretinal inflammation, generalized

H30.131   Disseminated chorioretinal inflammation, generalized, right eye

H30.132   Disseminated chorioretinal inflammation, generalized, left eye

H30.133   Disseminated chorioretinal inflammation, generalized, bilateral

H30.139   Disseminated chorioretinal inflammation, generalized, unspecified eye

H30.14   Acute posterior multifocal placoid pigment epitheliopathy

H30.141   Acute posterior multifocal placoid pigment epitheliopathy, right eye

H30.142   Acute posterior multifocal placoid pigment epitheliopathy, left eye

H30.143   Acute posterior multifocal placoid pigment epitheliopathy, bilateral

H30.149   Acute posterior multifocal placoid pigment epitheliopathy, unspecified eye

H30.2   Posterior cyclitis
Pars planitis

H30.20   Posterior cyclitis, unspecified eye

H30.21   Posterior cyclitis, right eye

H30.22   Posterior cyclitis, left eye

H30.23   Posterior cyclitis, bilateral

H30.8   Other chorioretinal inflammations
Harada's disease

H30.80   Other chorioretinal inflammations, unspecified eye

H30.81   Other chorioretinal inflammations, right eye

H30.82   Other chorioretinal inflammations, left eye

H30.83   Other chorioretinal inflammations, bilateral

H30.9   Unspecified chorioretinal inflammation
Chorioretinitis NOS
Choroiditis NOS
Neuroretinitis NOS
Retinitis NOS
Retinochoroiditis NOS

H30.90   Unspecified chorioretinal inflammation, unspecified eye

H30.91   Unspecified chorioretinal inflammation, unspecified, right eye

H30.92   Unspecified chorioretinal inflammation, unspecified, left eye

H30.93   Unspecified chorioretinal inflammation, unspecified, bilateral

H31   Other disorders of choroid

H31.0   Chorioretinal scars

H31.00   Unspecified chorioretinal scars

H31.001   Unspecified chorioretinal scars, right eye

H31.002   Unspecified chorioretinal scars, left eye

H31.003   Unspecified chorioretinal scars, bilateral

H31.009   Unspecified chorioretinal scars, unspecified eye

H31.01   Macula scars of posterior pole (postinflammatory) (post-traumatic)
Excludes1:   postprocedural choriorentinal scar (H59.81-)

H31.011   Macula scars of posterior pole (postinflammatory) (post-traumatic), right eye

H31.012   Macula scars of posterior pole (postinflammatory) (post-traumatic), left eye

H31.013   Macula scars of posterior pole (postinflammatory) (post-traumatic), bilateral

H31.019   Macula scars of posterior pole (postinflammatory) (post-traumatic), unspecified eye

H31.02   Solar retinopathy

H31.021   Solar retinopathy, right eye

H31.022   Solar retinopathy, left eye

H31.023   Solar retinopathy, bilateral

H31.029   Solar retinopathy, unspecified eye

H31.09   Other chorioretinal scars
     H31.091   Other chorioretinal scars, right eye
     H31.092   Other chorioretinal scars, left eye
     H31.093   Other chorioretinal scars, bilateral
     H31.099   Other chorioretinal scars, unspecified eye

H31.1   Choroidal degeneration
     Excludes2:   angioid streaks of macula (H35.33)

H31.10   Unspecified choroidal degeneration
     Choroidal sclerosis NOS
     H31.101   Choroidal degeneration, unspecified, right eye
     H31.102   Choroidal degeneration, unspecified, left eye
     H31.103   Choroidal degeneration, unspecified, bilateral
     H31.109   Choroidal degeneration, unspecified, unspecified eye

H31.11   Age-related choroidal atrophy
     H31.111   Age-related choroidal atrophy, right eye
     H31.112   Age-related choroidal atrophy, left eye
     H31.113   Age-related choroidal atrophy, bilateral
     H31.119   Age-related choroidal atrophy, unspecified eye

H31.12   Diffuse secondary atrophy of choroid
     H31.121   Diffuse secondary atrophy of choroid, right eye
     H31.122   Diffuse secondary atrophy of choroid, left eye
     H31.123   Diffuse secondary atrophy of choroid, bilateral
     H31.129   Diffuse secondary atrophy of choroid, unspecified eye

H31.2   Hereditary choroidal dystrophy
     Excludes2:   hyperornithinemia (E72.4)
                ornithinemia (E72.4)

H31.20   Hereditary choroidal dystrophy, unspecified
H31.21   Choroideremia
H31.22   Choroidal dystrophy (central areolar) (generalized) (peripapillary)
H31.23   Gyrate atrophy, choroid
H31.29   Other hereditary choroidal dystrophy

H31.3   Choroidal hemorrhage and rupture
H31.30   Unspecified choroidal hemorrhage
     H31.301   Unspecified choroidal hemorrhage, right eye
     H31.302   Unspecified choroidal hemorrhage, left eye
     H31.303   Unspecified choroidal hemorrhage, bilateral
     H31.309   Unspecified choroidal hemorrhage, unspecified eye

H31.31   Expulsive choroidal hemorrhage
     H31.311   Expulsive choroidal hemorrhage, right eye
     H31.312   Expulsive choroidal hemorrhage, left eye
     H31.313   Expulsive choroidal hemorrhage, bilateral
     H31.319   Expulsive choroidal hemorrhage, unspecified eye

H31.32   Choroidal rupture
     H31.321   Choroidal rupture, right eye
     H31.322   Choroidal rupture, left eye
     H31.323   Choroidal rupture, bilateral
     H31.329   Choroidal rupture, unspecified eye

H31.4   Choroidal detachment
H31.40   Unspecified choroidal detachment
     H31.401   Unspecified choroidal detachment, right eye
     H31.402   Unspecified choroidal detachment, left eye
     H31.403   Unspecified choroidal detachment, bilateral
     H31.409   Unspecified choroidal detachment, unspecified eye

H31.41   Hemorrhagic choroidal detachment
     H31.411   Hemorrhagic choroidal detachment, right eye
     H31.412   Hemorrhagic choroidal detachment, left eye
     H31.413   Hemorrhagic choroidal detachment, bilateral
     H31.419   Hemorrhagic choroidal detachment, unspecified eye

H31.42   Serous choroidal detachment
     H31.421   Serous choroidal detachment, right eye
     H31.422   Serous choroidal detachment, left eye
     H31.423   Serous choroidal detachment, bilateral
     H31.429   Serous choroidal detachment, unspecified eye

H31.8   Other specified disorders of choroid
H31.9   Unspecified disorder of choroid

H32   Chorioretinal disorders in diseases classified elsewhere
     Code first underlying disease, such as:
     congenital toxoplasmosis (P37.1)
     histoplasmosis (B39.-)
     leprosy (A30.-)
     Excludes1:   chorioretinitis (in):
                toxoplasmosis (acquired) (B58.01)
                tuberculosis (A18.53)

H33   Retinal detachments and breaks
     Excludes1:   detachment of retinal pigment epithelium (H35.72-, H35.73-)

H33.0   Retinal detachment with retinal break
     Rhegmatogenous retinal detachment
     Excludes1:   serous retinal detachment (without retinal break) (H33.2-)

H33.00   Unspecified retinal detachment with retinal break
     H33.001   Unspecified retinal detachment with retinal break, right eye
     H33.002   Unspecified retinal detachment with retinal break, left eye
     H33.003   Unspecified retinal detachment with retinal break, bilateral
     H33.009   Unspecified retinal detachment with retinal break, unspecified eye

H33.01   Retinal detachment with single break
     H33.011   Retinal detachment with single break, right eye
     H33.012   Retinal detachment with single break, left eye
     H33.013   Retinal detachment with single break, bilateral
     H33.019   Retinal detachment with single break, unspecified eye

H33.02   Retinal detachment with multiple breaks
     H33.021   Retinal detachment with multiple breaks, right eye
     H33.022   Retinal detachment with multiple breaks, left eye
     H33.023   Retinal detachment with multiple breaks, bilateral
     H33.029   Retinal detachment with multiple breaks, unspecified eye

H33.03   Retinal detachment with giant retinal tear
     H33.031   Retinal detachment with giant retinal tear, right eye
     H33.032   Retinal detachment with giant retinal tear, left eye
     H33.033   Retinal detachment with giant retinal tear, bilateral
     H33.039   Retinal detachment with giant retinal tear, unspecified eye

H33.04   Retinal detachment with retinal dialysis
     H33.041   Retinal detachment with retinal dialysis, right eye
     H33.042   Retinal detachment with retinal dialysis, left eye
     H33.043   Retinal detachment with retinal dialysis, bilateral
     H33.049   Retinal detachment with retinal dialysis, unspecified eye

H33.05   Total retinal detachment
     H33.051   Total retinal detachment, right eye
     H33.052   Total retinal detachment, left eye
     H33.053   Total retinal detachment, bilateral
     H33.059   Total retinal detachment, unspecified eye

H33.1 Retinoschisis and retinal cysts
> Excludes1:   congenital retinoschisis (Q14.1)
> microcystoid degeneration of retina (H35.42-)

H33.10 Unspecified retinoschisis
- H33.101 Unspecified retinoschisis, right eye
- H33.102 Unspecified retinoschisis, left eye
- H33.103 Unspecified retinoschisis, bilateral
- H33.109 Unspecified retinoschisis, unspecified eye

H33.11 Cyst of ora serrata
- H33.111 Cyst of ora serrata, right eye
- H33.112 Cyst of ora serrata, left eye
- H33.113 Cyst of ora serrata, bilateral
- H33.119 Cyst of ora serrata, unspecified eye

H33.12 Parasitic cyst of retina
- H33.121 Parasitic cyst of retina, right eye
- H33.122 Parasitic cyst of retina, left eye
- H33.123 Parasitic cyst of retina, bilateral
- H33.129 Parasitic cyst of retina, unspecified eye

H33.19 Other retinoschisis and retinal cysts
> Pseudocyst of retina
- H33.191 Other retinoschisis and retinal cysts, right eye
- H33.192 Other retinoschisis and retinal cysts, left eye
- H33.193 Other retinoschisis and retinal cysts, bilateral
- H33.199 Other retinoschisis and retinal cysts, unspecified eye

H33.2 Serous retinal detachment
> Retinal detachment NOS
> Retinal detachment without retinal break
> Excludes1:   central serous chorioretinopathy (H35.71-)

- **H33.20 Serous retinal detachment, unspecified eye**
- **H33.21 Serous retinal detachment, right eye**
- **H33.22 Serous retinal detachment, left eye**
- **H33.23 Serous retinal detachment, bilateral**

H33.3 Retinal breaks without detachment
> Excludes1:   chorioretinal scars after surgery for detachment (H59.81-)
> peripheral retinal degeneration without break (H35.4-)

H33.30 Unspecified retinal break
- H33.301 Unspecified retinal break, right eye
- H33.302 Unspecified retinal break, left eye
- H33.303 Unspecified retinal break, bilateral
- H33.309 Unspecified retinal break, unspecified eye

H33.31 Horseshoe tear of retina without detachment
> Operculum of retina without detachment
- H33.311 Horseshoe tear of retina without detachment, right eye
- H33.312 Horseshoe tear of retina without detachment, left eye
- H33.313 Horseshoe tear of retina without detachment, bilateral
- H33.319 Horseshoe tear of retina without detachment, unspecified eye

H33.32 Round hole of retina without detachment
- H33.321 Round hole, right eye
- H33.322 Round hole, left eye
- H33.323 Round hole, bilateral
- H33.329 Round hole, unspecified eye

H33.33 Multiple defects of retina without detachment
- H33.331 Multiple defects of retina without detachment, right eye
- H33.332 Multiple defects of retina without detachment, left eye
- H33.333 Multiple defects of retina without detachment, bilateral
- H33.339 Multiple defects of retina without detachment, unspecified eye

H33.4 Traction detachment of retina
> Proliferative vitreo-retinopathy with retinal detachment

- H33.40 Traction detachment of retina, unspecified eye
- H33.41 Traction detachment of retina, right eye
- H33.42 Traction detachment of retina, left eye
- H33.43 Traction detachment of retina, bilateral

H33.5 Other retinal detachments

H34 Retinal vascular occlusions
> Excludes1:   amaurosis fugax (G45.3)

H34.0 Transient retinal artery occlusion
- H34.00 Transient retinal artery occlusion, unspecified eye
- H34.01 Transient retinal artery occlusion, right eye
- H34.02 Transient retinal artery occlusion, left eye

H34.1 Central retinal artery occlusion
- H34.10 Central retinal artery occlusion, unspecified eye
- H34.11 Central retinal artery occlusion, right eye
- H34.12 Central retinal artery occlusion, left eye
- H34.13 Central retinal artery occlusion, bilateral

H34.2 Other retinal artery occlusions
H34.21 Partial retinal artery occlusion
> Hollenhorst's plaque
> Retinal microembolism
- H34.211 Partial retinal artery occlusion, right eye
- H34.212 Partial retinal artery occlusion, left eye
- H34.213 Partial retinal artery occlusion, bilateral
- H34.219 Partial retinal artery occlusion, unspecified eye

H34.23 Retinal artery branch occlusion
- H34.231 Retinal artery branch occlusion, right eye
- H34.232 Retinal artery branch occlusion, left eye
- H34.233 Retinal artery branch occlusion, bilateral
- H34.239 Retinal artery branch occlusion, unspecified eye

H34.8 Other retinal vascular occlusions
H34.81 Central retinal vein occlusion
- H34.811 Central retinal vein occlusion, right eye
- H34.812 Central retinal vein occlusion, left eye
- H34.813 Central retinal vein occlusion, bilateral
- H34.819 Central retinal vein occlusion, unspecified eye

H34.82 Venous engorgement
> Incipient retinal vein occlusion
> Partial retinal vein occlusion
- H34.821 Venous engorgement, right eye
- H34.822 Venous engorgement, left eye
- H34.823 Venous engorgement, bilateral
- H34.829 Venous engorgement, unspecified eye

H34.83 Tributary (branch) retinal vein occlusion
- H34.831 Tributary (branch) retinal vein occlusion, right eye
- H34.832 Tributary (branch) retinal vein occlusion, left eye
- H34.833 Tributary (branch) retinal vein occlusion, bilateral
- H34.839 Tributary (branch) retinal vein occlusion, unspecified eye

H34.9 Unspecified retinal vascular occlusion

H35 Other retinal disorders
> Excludes1:   diabetic retinal disorders (E08.31, E08.32, E09.31, E09.32, E10.31, E10.32, E11.31, E11.32, E13.31, E13.32, E14.31, E14.32)

H35.0 Background retinopathy and retinal vascular changes
> Use additional code to identify any associated hypertension (I10)

H35.00 Unspecified background retinopathy
H35.01 Changes in retinal vascular appearance
> Retinal vascular sheathing
- H35.011 Changes in retinal vascular appearance, right eye
- H35.012 Changes in retinal vascular appearance, left eye

     H35.013   **Changes in retinal vascular appearance, bilateral**

     H35.019   **Changes in retinal vascular appearance, unspecified eye**

   H35.02   **Exudative retinopathy**
     Coats retinopathy

     H35.021   **Exudative retinopathy, right eye**

     H35.022   **Exudative retinopathy, left eye**

     H35.023   **Exudative retinopathy, bilateral**

     H35.029   **Exudative retinopathy, unspecified eye**

   H35.03   **Hypertensive retinopathy**

     H35.031   **Hypertensive retinopathy, right eye**

     H35.032   **Hypertensive retinopathy, left eye**

     H35.033   **Hypertensive retinopathy, bilateral**

     H35.039   **Hypertensive retinopathy, unspecified eye**

   H35.04   **Retinal micro-aneurysms NOS**

     H35.041   **Retinal micro-aneurysms NOS, right eye**

     H35.042   **Retinal micro-aneurysms NOS, left eye**

     H35.043   **Retinal micro-aneurysms NOS, bilateral**

     H35.049   **Retinal micro-aneurysms NOS, unspecified eye**

   H35.05   **Retinal neovascularization NOS**

     H35.051   **Retinal neovascularization NOS, right eye**

     H35.052   **Retinal neovascularization NOS, left eye**

     H35.053   **Retinal neovascularization NOS, bilateral**

     H35.059   **Retinal neovascularization NOS, unspecified eye**

   H35.06   **Retinal vasculitis**
     Eales disease
     Retinal perivasculitis

     H35.061   **Retinal vasculitis, right eye**

     H35.062   **Retinal vasculitis, left eye**

     H35.063   **Retinal vasculitis, bilateral**

     H35.069   **Retinal vasculitis, unspecified eye**

   H35.07   **Retinal telangiectasis**

     H35.071   **Retinal telangiectasis, right eye**

     H35.072   **Retinal telangiectasis, left eye**

     H35.073   **Retinal telangiectasis, bilateral**

     H35.079   **Retinal telangiectasis, unspecified eye**

   H35.09   **Other intraretinal microvascular abnormalities**
     Retinal varices

H35.1   Retinopathy of prematurity
   Retrolental fibroplasia

H35.2   Other non-diabetic proliferative retinopathy
   Proliferative vitreo-retinopathy

   Excludes1:   proliferative vitreo-retinopathy with retinal detachment (H33.4-)

   H35.20   **Other non-diabetic proliferative retinopathy, unspecified eye**

   H35.21   **Other non-diabetic proliferative retinopathy, right eye**

   H35.22   **Other non-diabetic proliferative retinopathy, left eye**

   H35.23   **Other non-diabetic proliferative retinopathy, bilateral**

H35.3   Degeneration of macula and posterior pole

   H35.30   **Unspecified macular degeneration (age-related)**

   H35.31   **Nonexudative age-related macular degeneration**
     Atrophic age-related macular degeneration

   H35.32   **Exudative age-related macular degeneration**

   H35.33   **Angioid streaks of macula**

   H35.34   **Macular cyst, hole, or pseudohole**

     H35.341   **Macular cyst, hole, or pseudohole, right eye**

     H35.342   **Macular cyst, hole, or pseudohole, left eye**

     H35.343   **Macular cyst, hole, or pseudohole, bilateral**

     H35.349   **Macular cyst, hole, or pseudohole, unspecified eye**

   H35.35   **Cystoid macular degeneration**

     H35.351   **Cystoid macular degeneration, right eye**

     H35.352   **Cystoid macular degeneration, left eye**

     H35.353   **Cystoid macular degeneration, bilateral**

     H35.359   **Cystoid macular degeneration, unspecified eye**

   H35.36   **Drusen (degenerative) of macula**

     H35.361   **Drusen (degenerative) of macula, right eye**

     H35.362   **Drusen (degenerative) of macula, left eye**

     H35.363   **Drusen (degenerative) of macula, bilateral**

     H35.369   **Drusen (degenerative) of macula, unspecified eye**

   H35.37   **Puckering of macula**

     H35.371   **Puckering of macula, right eye**

     H35.372   **Puckering of macula, left eye**

     H35.373   **Puckering of macula, bilateral**

     H35.379   **Puckering of macula, unspecified eye**

   H35.38   **Toxic maculopathy**
     Use additional external cause code (Chapter XIX) to identify drug, if drug-induced.

     H35.381   **Toxic maculopathy, right eye**

     H35.382   **Toxic maculopathy, left eye**

     H35.383   **Toxic maculopathy, bilateral**

     H35.389   **Toxic maculopathy, unspecified eye**

H35.4   Peripheral retinal degeneration

   Excludes1:   hereditary retinal degeneration (dystrophy) (H35.5-)
     peripheral retinal degeneration with retinal break (H33.3-)

   H35.40   **Unspecified peripheral retinal degeneration**

   H35.41   **Lattice degeneration of retina**
     Palisade degeneration of retina

     H35.411   **Lattice degeneration of retina, right eye**

     H35.412   **Lattice degeneration of retina, left eye**

     H35.413   **Lattice degeneration of retina, bilateral**

     H35.419   **Lattice degeneration of retina, unspecified eye**

   H35.42   **Microcystoid degeneration of retina**

     H35.421   **Microcystoid degeneration of retina, right eye**

     H35.422   **Microcystoid degeneration of retina, left eye**

     H35.423   **Microcystoid degeneration of retina, bilateral**

     H35.429   **Microcystoid degeneration of retina, unspecified eye**

   H35.43   **Paving stone degeneration of retina**

     H35.431   **Paving stone degeneration of retina, right eye**

     H35.432   **Paving stone degeneration of retina, left eye**

     H35.433   **Paving stone degeneration of retina, bilateral**

     H35.439   **Paving stone degeneration of retina, unspecified eye**

   H35.44   **Age-related reticular degeneration of retina**

     H35.441   **Age-related reticular degeneration of retina, right eye**

     H35.442   **Age-related reticular degeneration of retina, left eye**

     H35.443   **Age-related reticular degeneration of retina, bilateral**

     H35.449   **Age-related reticular degeneration of retina, unspecified eye**

   H35.45   **Secondary pigmentary degeneration**

     H35.451   **Secondary pigmentary degeneration, right eye**

     H35.452   **Secondary pigmentary degeneration, left eye**

     H35.453   **Secondary pigmentary degeneration, bilateral**

     H35.459   **Secondary pigmentary degeneration, unspecified eye**

   H35.46   **Secondary vitreoretinal degeneration**

     H35.461   **Secondary vitreoretinal degeneration, right eye**

     H35.462   **Secondary vitreoretinal degeneration, left eye**

     H35.463   **Secondary vitreoretinal degeneration, bilateral**

     H35.469   **Secondary vitreoretinal degeneration, unspecified eye**

H35.5   Hereditary retinal dystrophy

   Excludes1:   dystrophies primarily involving Bruch's membrane (H31.1-)

   H35.50   **Unspecified hereditary retinal dystrophy**

   H35.51   **Vitreoretinal dystrophy**

H35.52 Pigmentary retinal dystrophy
Albipunctate retinal dystrophy
Retinitis pigmentosa
Tapetoretinal dystrophy

H35.53 Other dystrophies primarily involving the sensory retina
Stargardt's disease

H35.54 Dystrophies primarily involving the retinal pigment epithelium
Vitelliform retinal dystrophy

H35.6 Retinal hemorrhage
H35.60 Retinal hemorrhage, unspecified eye
H35.61 Retinal hemorrhage, right eye
H35.62 Retinal hemorrhage, left eye
H35.63 Retinal hemorrhage, bilateral

H35.7 Separation of retinal layers
Excludes1: retinal detachment (serous) (H33.2-)
rhegmatogenous retinal detachment (H33.0-)

H35.70 Unspecified separation of retinal layers
H35.71 Central serous chorioretinopathy
H35.711 Central serous chorioretinopathy, right eye
H35.712 Central serous chorioretinopathy, left eye
H35.713 Central serous chorioretinopathy, bilateral
H35.719 Central serous chorioretinopathy, unspecified eye

H35.72 Serous detachment of retinal pigment epithelium
H35.721 Serous detachment of retinal pigment epithelium, right eye
H35.722 Serous detachment of retinal pigment epithelium, left eye
H35.723 Serous detachment of retinal pigment epithelium, bilateral
H35.729 Serous detachment of retinal pigment epithelium, unspecified eye

H35.73 Hemorrhagic detachment of retinal pigment epithelium
H35.731 Hemorrhagic detachment of retinal pigment epithelium, right eye
H35.732 Hemorrhagic detachment of retinal pigment epithelium, left eye
H35.733 Hemorrhagic detachment of retinal pigment epithelium, bilateral
H35.739 Hemorrhagic detachment of retinal pigment epithelium, unspecified eye

H35.8 Other specified retinal disorders
Excludes2: retinal hemorrhage (H35.6-)
H35.81 Retinal edema
Retinal cotton wool spots
H35.82 Retinal ischemia
H35.89 Other specified retinal disorders

H35.9 Unspecified retinal disorder

H36 Retinal disorders in diseases classified elsewhere
Code first underlying disease, such as:
lipid storage disorders (E75.-)
sickle-cell disorders (D57.-)
Excludes1: arteriosclerotic retinopathy (H35.0-)
diabetic (background) retinopathy (E08.31, E09.31, E10.31, E11.31, E13.31, E14.31)
diabetic proliferative retinopathy (E08.32, E09.32, E10.32, E11.32, E13.32, E14.32)

GLAUCOMA (H40-H42)

H40 Glaucoma
Excludes1: absolute glaucoma (H44.51-)
congenital glaucoma (Q15.0)
traumatic glaucoma due to birth injury (P15.3)

H40.0 Glaucoma suspect
Ocular hypertension

H40.1 Open-angle glaucoma
H40.10 Unspecified open-angle glaucoma

H40.11 Primary open-angle glaucoma
Chronic simple glaucoma
H40.12 Low-tension glaucoma
H40.121 Low-tension glaucoma, right eye
H40.122 Low-tension glaucoma, left eye
H40.123 Low-tension glaucoma, bilateral
H40.129 Low-tension glaucoma, unspecified eye

H40.13 Pigmentary glaucoma
H40.131 Pigmentary glaucoma, right eye
H40.132 Pigmentary glaucoma, left eye
H40.133 Pigmentary glaucoma, bilateral
H40.139 Pigmentary glaucoma, unspecified eye

H40.14 Capsular glaucoma with pseudoexfoliation of lens
H40.141 Capsular glaucoma with pseudoexfoliation of lens, right eye
H40.142 Capsular glaucoma with pseudoexfoliation of lens, left eye
H40.143 Capsular glaucoma with pseudoexfoliation of lens, bilateral
H40.149 Capsular glaucoma with pseudoexfoliation of lens, unspecified eye

H40.15 Residual stage of open-angle glaucoma
H40.151 Residual stage of open-angle glaucoma, right eye
H40.152 Residual stage of open-angle glaucoma, left eye
H40.153 Residual stage of open-angle glaucoma, bilateral
H40.159 Residual stage of open-angle glaucoma, unspecified eye

H40.2 Primary angle-closure glaucoma
Excludes1: aqueous misdirection (H40.83-)
malignant glaucoma (H40.83-)

H40.20 Unspecified primary angle-closure glaucoma
H40.21 Acute angle-closure glaucoma
H40.211 Acute angle-closure glaucoma, right eye
H40.212 Acute angle-closure glaucoma, left eye
H40.213 Acute angle-closure glaucoma, bilateral
H40.219 Acute angle-closure glaucoma, unspecified eye

H40.22 Chronic angle-closure glaucoma
H40.221 Chronic angle-closure glaucoma, right eye
H40.222 Chronic angle-closure glaucoma, left eye
H40.223 Chronic angle-closure glaucoma, bilateral
H40.229 Chronic angle-closure glaucoma, unspecified eye

H40.23 Intermittent angle-closure glaucoma
H40.231 Intermittent angle-closure glaucoma, right eye
H40.232 Intermittent angle-closure glaucoma, left eye
H40.233 Intermittent angle-closure glaucoma, bilateral
H40.239 Intermittent angle-closure glaucoma, unspecified eye

H40.24 Residual stage of angle-closure glaucoma
H40.241 Residual stage of angle-closure glaucoma, right eye
H40.242 Residual stage of angle-closure glaucoma, let eye
H40.243 Residual stage of angle-closure glaucoma, bilateral
H40.249 Residual stage of angle-closure glaucoma, unspecified eye

H40.3 Glaucoma secondary to eye trauma
Code also underlying condition
H40.30 Glaucoma secondary to eye trauma, unspecified eye
H40.31 Glaucoma secondary to eye trauma, right eye
H40.32 Glaucoma secondary to eye trauma, left eye
H40.33 Glaucoma secondary to eye trauma, bilateral

H40.4 Glaucoma secondary to eye inflammation
Code also underlying condition
H40.40 Glaucoma secondary to eye inflammation, unspecified eye

H40.41   Glaucoma secondary to eye inflammation, right eye

H40.42   Glaucoma secondary to eye inflammation, left eye

H40.43   Glaucoma secondary to eye inflammation, bilateral

H40.5   Glaucoma secondary to other eye disorders
> Code also underlying condition

H40.50   Glaucoma secondary to other eye disorders, unspecified eye

H40.51   Glaucoma secondary to other eye disorders, right eye

H40.52   Glaucoma secondary to other eye disorders, left eye

H40.53   Glaucoma secondary to other eye disorders, bilateral

H40.6   Glaucoma secondary to drugs
> Use additional external cause code (Chapter XIX) to identify drug

H40.60   Glaucoma secondary to drugs, unspecified eye

H40.61   Glaucoma secondary to drugs, right eye

H40.62   Glaucoma secondary to drugs, left eye

H40.63   Glaucoma secondary to drugs, bilateral

H40.8   Other glaucoma

H40.81   Glaucoma with increased episcleral venous pressure

      H40.811   Glaucoma with increased episcleral venous pressure, right eye

      H40.812   Glaucoma with increased episcleral venous pressure, left eye

      H40.813   Glaucoma with increased episcleral venous pressure, bilateral

      H40.819   Glaucoma with increased episcleral venous pressure, unspecified eye

H40.82   Hypersecretion glaucoma

      H40.821   Hypersecretion glaucoma, right eye

      H40.822   Hypersecretion glaucoma, left eye

      H40.823   Hypersecretion glaucoma, bilateral

      H40.829   Hypersecretion glaucoma, unspecified eye

H40.83   Aqueous misdirection
> Malignant glaucoma

      H40.831   Aqueous misdirection, right eye

      H40.832   Aqueous misdirection, left eye

      H40.833   Aqueous misdirection, bilateral

      H40.839   Aqueous misdirection, unspecified eye

H40.89   Other specified glaucoma

H40.9   Unspecified glaucoma

H42   Glaucoma in diseases classified elsewhere
> Code first underlying condition, such as:
>   amyloidosis (E85)
>   aniridia (Q13.1)
>   Lowe's syndrome (E72.03)
>   Reiger's anomaly (Q13.81)
>   specified metabolic disorder (E70-E90)
> Excludes1:   glaucoma (in):
>   diabetes mellitus (E08.39, E09.39, E10.39, E11.39, E13.39, E14.39)
>   onchocerciasis (B73.02)
>   syphilis (A52.71)
>   tuberculous (A18.59)

DISORDERS OF VITREOUS BODY AND GLOBE (H43-H45)

H43   Disorders of vitreous body

H43.0   Vitreous prolapse
> Excludes1:   traumatic vitreous prolapse (S05.2-)
>   vitreous syndrome following cataract surgery (H59.0-)

H43.00   Vitreous prolapse, unspecified eye

H43.01   Vitreous prolapse, right eye

H43.02   Vitreous prolapse, left eye

H43.03   Vitreous prolapse, bilateral

H43.1   Vitreous hemorrhage

H43.10   Vitreous hemorrhage, unspecified eye

H43.11   Vitreous hemorrhage, right cyc

H43.12   Vitreous hemorrhage, left eye

H43.13   Vitreous hemorrhage, bilateral

H43.2   Crystalline deposits in vitreous body

H43.20   Crystalline deposits in vitreous body, unspecified eye

H43.21   Crystalline deposits in vitreous body, right eye

H43.22   Crystalline deposits in vitreous body, left eye

H43.23   Crystalline deposits in vitreous body, bilateral

H43.3   Other vitreous opacities

H43.31   Vitreous membranes and strands

      H43.311   Vitreous membranes and strands, right eye

      H43.312   Vitreous membranes and strands, left eye

      H43.313   Vitreous membranes and strands, bilateral

      H43.319   Vitreous membranes and strands, unspecified eye

H43.39   Other vitreous opacities
> Vitreous floaters

      H43.391   Other vitreous opacities, right eye

      H43.392   Other vitreous opacities, left eye

      H43.393   Other vitreous opacities, bilateral

      H43.399   Other vitreous opacities, unspecified eye

H43.8   Other disorders of vitreous body
> Excludes1:   proliferative vitreo-retinopathy with retinal detachment (H33.4-)
> Excludes2:   vitreous abscess (H44.02-)

H43.81   Vitreous degeneration
> Vitreous detachment

      H43.811   Vitreous degeneration, right eye

      H43.812   Vitreous degeneration, left eye

      H43.813   Vitreous degeneration, bilateral

      H43.819   Vitreous degeneration, unspecified eye

H43.89   Other disorders of vitreous body

H43.9   Unspecified disorder of vitreous body

H44   Disorders of globe
> Includes: disorders affecting multiple structures of eye

H44.0   Purulent endophthalmitis
> Use additional code to identify organism

H44.00   Unspecified purulent endophthalmitis

      H44.001   Unspecified purulent endophthalmitis, right eye

      H44.002   Unspecified purulent endophthalmitis, left eye

      H44.003   Unspecified purulent endophthalmitis, bilateral

      H44.009   Unspecified purulent endophthalmitis, unspecified eye

H44.01   Panophthalmitis (acute)

      H44.011   Panophthalmitis (acute), right eye

      H44.012   Panophthalmitis (acute), left eye

      H44.013   Panophthalmitis (acute), bilateral

      H44.019   Panophthalmitis (acute), unspecified eye

H44.02   Vitreous abscess (chronic)

      H44.021   Vitreous abscess (chronic), right eye

      H44.022   Vitreous abscess (chronic), left eye

      H44.023   Vitreous abscess (chronic), bilateral

      H44.029   Vitreous abscess (chronic), unspecified eye

H44.1   Other endophthalmitis
> Excludes2:   ophthalmia nodosa (H16.2-)

H44.11   Panuveitis

      H44.111   Panuveitis, right eye

      H44.112   Panuveitis, left eye

      H44.113   Panuveitis, bilateral

      H44.119   Panuveitis, unspecified eye

H44.12   Parasitic endophthalmitis NOS

      H44.121   Parasitic endophthalmitis NOS, right eye

      H44.122   Parasitic endophthalmitis NOS, left eye

      H44.123   Parasitic endophthalmitis NOS, bilateral

      H44.129   Parasitic endophthalmitis NOS, unspecified eye

H44.13   Sympathetic uveitis

      H44.131   Sympathetic uveitis, right eye

      H44.132   Sympathetic uveitis, left eye

H44.133　Sympathetic uveitis, bilateral
H44.139　Sympathetic uveitis, unspecified eye
H44.19　Other endophthalmitis
H44.2　Degenerative myopia
　　Malignant myopia
H44.20　Degenerative myopia, unspecified eye
H44.21　Degenerative myopia, right eye
H44.22　Degenerative myopia, left eye
H44.23　Degenerative myopia, bilateral
H44.3　Other and unspecified degenerative disorders of globe
H44.30　Unspecified degenerative disorder of globe
H44.31　Chalcosis
H44.311　Chalcosis, right eye
H44.312　Chalcosis, left eye
H44.313　Chalcosis, bilateral
H44.319　Chalcosis, unspecified eye
H44.32　Siderosis of eye
H44.321　Siderosis of eye, right eye
H44.322　Siderosis of eye, left eye
H44.323　Siderosis of eye, bilateral
H44.329　Siderosis of eye, unspecified eye
H44.39　Other degenerative disorders of globe
H44.391　Other degenerative disorders of globe, right eye
H44.392　Other degenerative disorders of globe, left eye
H44.393　Other degenerative disorders of globe, bilateral
H44.399　Other degenerative disorders of globe, unspecified eye
H44.4　Hypotony of eye
H44.40　Unspecified hypotony of eye
H44.41　Flat anterior chamber hypotony of eye
H44.411　Flat anterior chamber hypotony of right eye
H44.412　Flat anterior chamber hypotony of left eye
H44.413　Flat anterior chamber hypotony of eye, bilateral
H44.419　Flat anterior chamber hypotony of unspecified eye
H44.42　Hypotony of eye due to ocular fistula
H44.421　Hypotony of right eye due to ocular fistula
H44.422　Hypotony of left eye due to ocular fistula
H44.423　Hypotony of eye due to ocular fistula, bilateral
H44.429　Hypotony of unspecified eye due to ocular fistula
H44.43　Hypotony of eye due to other ocular disorders
H44.431　Hypotony of eye due to other ocular disorders, right eye
H44.432　Hypotony of eye due to other ocular disorders, left eye
H44.433　Hypotony of eye due to other ocular disorders, bilateral
H44.439　Hypotony of eye due to other ocular disorders,unspecified eye
H44.44　Primary hypotony of eye
H44.441　Primary hypotony of right eye
H44.442　Primary hypotony of left eye
H44.443　Primary hypotony of eye, bilateral
H44.449　Primary hypotony of unspecified eye
H44.5　Degenerated conditions of globe
H44.50　Unspecified degenerated conditions of globe
H44.51　Absolute glaucoma
H44.511　Absolute glaucoma, right eye
H44.512　Absolute glaucoma, left eye
H44.513　Absolute glaucoma, bilateral
H44.519　Absolute glaucoma, unspecified eye
H44.52　Atrophy of globe
　　Phthisis bulb
H44.521　Atrophy of globe, right eye
H44.522　Atrophy of globe, left eye
H44.523　Atrophy of globe, bilateral

H44.529　Atrophy of globe, unspecified eye
H44.53　Leucocoria
H44.531　Leucocoria, right eye
H44.532　Leucocoria, left eye
H44.533　Leucocoria, bilateral
H44.539　Leucocoria, unspecified eye
H44.6　Retained (old) intraocular foreign body, magnetic
Excludes1:　current intraocular foreign body (S05.-)
Excludes2:　retained foreign body in eyelid (H02.81-)
　retained (old) foreign body following penetrating wound of orbit (H05.5-)
H44.60　Unspecified retained (old) intraocular foreign body, magnetic
H44.601　Unspecified retained (old) intraocular foreign body, magnetic, right eye
H44.602　Unspecified retained (old) intraocular foreign body, magnetic, left eye
H44.603　Unspecified retained (old) intraocular foreign body, magnetic, bilateral
H44.609　Unspecified retained (old) intraocular foreign body, magnetic, unspecified eye
H44.61　Retained (old) magnetic foreign body in anterior chamber
H44.611　Retained (old) magnetic foreign body in anterior chamber, right eye
H44.612　Retained (old) magnetic foreign body in anterior chamber, left eye
H44.613　Retained (old) magnetic foreign body in anterior chamber, bilateral
H44.619　Retained (old) magnetic foreign body in anterior chamber, unspecified eye
H44.62　Retained (old) magnetic foreign body in iris or ciliary body
H44.621　Retained (old) magnetic foreign body in iris or ciliary body, right eye
H44.622　Retained (old) magnetic foreign body in iris or ciliary body, left eye
H44.623　Retained (old) magnetic foreign body in iris or ciliary body, bilateral
H44.629　Retained (old) magnetic foreign body in iris or ciliary body, unspecified eye
H44.63　Retained (old) magnetic foreign body in lens
H44.631　Retained (old) magnetic foreign body in lens, right eye
H44.632　Retained (old) magnetic foreign body in lens, left eye
H44.633　Retained (old) magnetic foreign body in lens, bilateral
H44.639　Retained (old) magnetic foreign body in lens, unspecified eye
H44.64　Retained (old) magnetic foreign body in posterior wall of globe
H44.641　Retained (old) magnetic foreign body in posterior wall of globe, right eye
H44.642　Retained (old) magnetic foreign body in posterior wall of globe, left eye
H44.643　Retained (old) magnetic foreign body in posterior wall of globe, bilateral
H44.649　Retained (old) magnetic foreign body in posterior wall of globe, unspecified eye
H44.65　Retained (old) magnetic foreign body in vitreous body
H44.651　Retained (old) magnetic foreign body in vitreous body, right eye
H44.652　Retained (old) magnetic foreign body in vitreous body, left eye
H44.653　Retained (old) magnetic foreign body in vitreous body, bilateral
H44.659　Retained (old) magnetic foreign body in vitreous body, unspecified eye
H44.69　Retained (old) intraocular foreign body, magnetic, in other or multiple sites

    H44.691   Retained (old) intraocular foreign body, magnetic, in other or multiple sites, right eye

    H44.692   Retained (old) intraocular foreign body, magnetic, in other or multiple sites, left eye

    H44.693   Retained (old) intraocular foreign body, magnetic, in other or multiple sites, bilateral

    H44.699   Retained (old) intraocular foreign body, magnetic, in other or multiple sites, unspecified eye

H44.7   Retained (old) intraocular foreign body, nonmagnetic

   Excludes1:   current intraocular foreign body (S05.-)

   Excludes2:   retained foreign body in eyelid (H02.81-)
                 retained (old) foreign body following penetrating wound of orbit (H05.5-)

  H44.70   Unspecified retained (old) intraocular foreign body, nonmagnetic

    H44.701   Unspecified retained (old) intraocular foreign body, nonmagnetic, right eye

    H44.702   Unspecified retained (old) intraocular foreign body, nonmagnetic, left eye

    H44.703   Unspecified retained (old) intraocular foreign body, nonmagnetic, bilateral

    H44.709   Unspecified retained (old) intraocular foreign body, nonmagnetic, unspecified eye
           Retained (old) intraocular foreign body NOS

  H44.71   Retained (nonmagnetic) (old) foreign body in anterior chamber

    H44.711   Retained (nonmagnetic) (old) foreign body in anterior chamber, right eye

    H44.712   Retained (nonmagnetic) (old) foreign body in anterior chamber, left eye

    H44.713   Retained (nonmagnetic) (old) foreign body in anterior chamber, bilateral

    H44.719   Retained (nonmagnetic) (old) foreign body in anterior chamber, unspecified eye

  H44.72   Retained (nonmagnetic) (old) foreign body in iris or ciliary body

    H44.721   Retained (nonmagnetic) (old) foreign body in iris or ciliary body, right eye

    H44.722   Retained (nonmagnetic) (old) foreign body in iris or ciliary body, left eye

    H44.723   Retained (nonmagnetic) (old) foreign body in iris or ciliary body, bilateral

    H44.729   Retained (nonmagnetic) (old) foreign body in iris or ciliary body, unspecified eye

  H44.73   Retained (nonmagnetic) (old) foreign body in lens

    H44.731   Retained (nonmagnetic) (old) foreign body in lens, right eye

    H44.732   Retained (nonmagnetic) (old) foreign body in lens, left eye

    H44.733   Retained (nonmagnetic) (old) foreign body in lens, bilateral

    H44.739   Retained (nonmagnetic) (old) foreign body in lens, unspecified eye

  H44.74   Retained (nonmagnetic) (old) foreign body in posterior wall of globe

    H44.741   Retained (nonmagnetic) (old) foreign body in posterior wall of globe, right eye

    H44.742   Retained (nonmagnetic) (old) foreign body in posterior wall of globe, left eye

    H44.743   Retained (nonmagnetic) (old) foreign body in posterior wall of globe, bilateral

    H44.749   Retained (nonmagnetic) (old) foreign body in posterior wall of globe, unspecified eye

  H44.75   Retained (nonmagnetic) (old) foreign body in vitreous body

    H44.751   Retained (nonmagnetic) (old) foreign body in vitreous body, right eye

    H44.752   Retained (nonmagnetic) (old) foreign body in vitreous body, left eye

    H44.753   Retained (nonmagnetic) (old) foreign body in vitreous body, bilateral

    H44.759   Retained (nonmagnetic) (old) foreign body in vitreous body, unspecified eye

  H44.79   Retained (old) intraocular foreign body, nonmagnetic, in other or multiple sites

    H44.791   Retained (old) intraocular foreign body, nonmagnetic, in other or multiple sites, right eye

    H44.792   Retained (old) intraocular foreign body, nonmagnetic, in other or multiple sites, left eye

    H44.793   Retained (old) intraocular foreign body, nonmagnetic, in other or multiple sites, bilateral

    H44.799   Retained (old) intraocular foreign body, nonmagnetic, in other or multiple sites, unspecified eye

H44.8   Other disorders of globe

  H44.81   Hemophthalmos

    H44.811   Hemophthalmos, right eye

    H44.812   Hemophthalmos, left eye

    H44.813   Hemophthalmos, bilateral

    H44.819   Hemophthalmos, unspecified eye

  H44.82   Luxation of globe

    H44.821   Luxation of globe, right eye

    H44.822   Luxation of globe, left eye

    H44.823   Luxation of globe, bilateral

    H44.829   Luxation of globe, unspecified eye

  H44.89   Other disorders of globe

H44.9   Unspecified disorder of globe

DISORDERS OF OPTIC NERVE AND VISUAL PATHWAYS (H46-H47)

H46   Optic neuritis

   Excludes2:   ischemic optic neuropathy (H47.01-)
                 neuromyelitis optica [Devic] (G36.0)

H46.0   Optic papillitis

  H46.00   Optic papillitis, unspecified eye

  H46.01   Optic papillitis, right eye

  H46.02   Optic papillitis, left eye

H46.1   Retrobulbar neuritis

    Retrobulbar neuritis NOS

   Excludes1:   syphilitic retrobulbar neuritis (A52.15)

  H46.10   Retrobulbar neuritis, unspecified eye

  H46.11   Retrobulbar neuritis, right eye

  H46.12   Retrobulbar neuritis, left eye

H46.2   Nutritional optic neuropathy

H46.3   Toxic optic neuropathy

H46.8   Other optic neuritis

H46.9   Unspecified optic neuritis

H47   Other disorders of optic [2nd] nerve and visual pathways

H47.0   Disorders of optic nerve, not elsewhere classified

  H47.01   Ischemic optic neuropathy

    H47.011   Ischemic optic neuropathy, right eye

    H47.012   Ischemic optic neuropathy, left eye

    H47.013   Ischemic optic neuropathy, bilateral

    H47.019   Ischemic optic neuropathy, unspecified eye

  H47.02   Hemorrhage in optic nerve sheath

    H47.021   Hemorrhage in optic nerve sheath, right eye

    H47.022   Hemorrhage in optic nerve sheath, left eye

    H47.023   Hemorrhage in optic nerve sheath, bilateral

    H47.029   Hemorrhage in optic nerve sheath, unspecified eye

  H47.09   Other disorders of optic nerve, not elsewhere classified
           Compression of optic nerve

    H47.091   Other disorders of optic nerve, not elsewhere classified, right eye

H47.092   Other disorders of optic nerve, not elsewhere classified, left eye

H47.093   Other disorders of optic nerve, not elsewhere classified, bilateral

H47.099   Other disorders of optic nerve, not elsewhere classified, unspecified eye

H47.1   Papilledema

H47.10   Unspecified papilledema

H47.11   Papilledema associated with increased intracranial pressure

H47.12   Papilledema associated with decreased ocular pressure

H47.13   Papilledema associated with retinal disorder

H47.14   Foster-Kennedy syndrome

H47.141   Foster-Kennedy syndrome, right eye

H47.142   Foster-Kennedy syndrome, left eye

H47.143   Foster-Kennedy syndrome, bilateral

H47.149   Foster-Kennedy syndrome, unspecified eye

H47.2   Optic atrophy

H47.20   Unspecified optic atrophy

H47.21   Primary optic atrophy

H47.211   Primary optic atrophy, right eye

H47.212   Primary optic atrophy, left eye

H47.213   Primary optic atrophy, bilateral

H47.219   Primary optic atrophy, unspecified eye

H47.22   Hereditary optic atrophy
Leber's optic atrophy

H47.23   Glaucomatous optic atrophy

H47.231   Glaucomatous optic atrophy, right eye

H47.232   Glaucomatous optic atrophy, left eye

H47.233   Glaucomatous optic atrophy, bilateral

H47.239   Glaucomatous optic atrophy, unspecified eye

H47.29   Other optic atrophy
Temporal pallor of optic disc

H47.291   Other optic atrophy, right eye

H47.292   Other optic atrophy, left eye

H47.293   Other optic atrophy, bilateral

H47.299   Other optic atrophy, unspecified eye

H47.3   Other disorders of optic disc

H47.31   Coloboma of optic disc

H47.311   Coloboma of optic disc, right eye

H47.312   Coloboma of optic disc, left eye

H47.313   Coloboma of optic disc, bilateral

H47.319   Coloboma of optic disc, unspecified eye

H47.32   Drusen of optic disc

H47.321   Drusen of optic disc, right eye

H47.322   Drusen of optic disc, left eye

H47.323   Drusen of optic disc, bilateral

H47.329   Drusen of optic disc, unspecified eye

H47.33   Pseudopapilledema of optic disc

H47.331   Pseudopapilledema of optic disc, right eye

H47.332   Pseudopapilledema of optic disc, left eye

H47.333   Pseudopapilledema of optic disc, bilateral

H47.339   Pseudopapilledema of optic disc, unspecified eye

H47.39   Other disorders of optic disc

H47.391   Other disorders of optic disc, right eye

H47.392   Other disorders of optic disc, left eye

H47.393   Other disorders of optic disc, bilateral

H47.399   Other disorders of optic disc, unspecified eye

H47.4   Disorders of optic chiasm
Code also underlying condition

H47.41   Disorders of optic chiasm in (due to) inflammatory disorders

H47.42   Disorders of optic chiasm in (due to) neoplasm

H47.43   Disorders of optic chiasm in (due to) vascular disorders

H47.49   Disorders of optic chiasm in (due to) other disorders

H47.5   Disorders of other visual pathways
Disorders of optic tracts, geniculate nuclei and optic radiations
Code also underlying condition

H47.51   Disorders of visual pathways in (due to) inflammatory disorders

H47.511   Disorders of visual pathways in (due to) inflammatory disorders, right side

H47.512   Disorders of visual pathways in (due to) inflammatory disorders, left side

H47.519   Disorders of visual pathways in (due to) inflammatory disorders, unspecified side

H47.52   Disorders of visual pathways in (due to) neoplasm

H47.521   Disorders of visual pathways in (due to) neoplasm, right side

H47.522   Disorders of visual pathways in (due to) neoplasm, left side

H47.529   Disorders of visual pathways in (due to) neoplasm, unspecified side

H47.53   Disorders of visual pathways in (due to) vascular disorders

H47.531   Disorders of visual pathways in (due to) vascular disorders, right side

H47.532   Disorders of visual pathways in (due to) vascular disorders, left side

H47.539   Disorders of visual pathways in (due to) vascular disorders, unspecified side

H47.6   Disorders of visual cortex
Code also underlying condition

H47.61   Cortical blindness

H47.611   Cortical blindness, right side of brain

H47.612   Cortical blindness, left side of brain

H47.619   Cortical blindness, unspecified side of brain

H47.62   Disorders of visual cortex in (due to) inflammatory disorders

H47.621   Disorders of visual cortex in (due to) inflammatory disorders, right side of brain

H47.622   Disorders of visual cortex in (due to) inflammatory disorders, left side of brain

H47.629   Disorders of visual cortex in (due to) inflammatory disorders, unspecified side of brain

H47.63   Disorders of visual cortex in (due to) neoplasm

H47.631   Disorders of visual cortex in (due to) neoplasm, right side of brain

H47.632   Disorders of visual cortex in (due to) neoplasm, left side of brain

H47.639   Disorders of visual cortex in (due to) neoplasm, unspecified side of brain

H47.64   Disorders of visual cortex in (due to) vascular disorders

H47.641   Disorders of visual cortex in (due to) vascular disorders, right side of brain

H47.642   Disorders of visual cortex in (due to) vascular disorders, left side of brain

H47.649   Disorders of visual cortex in (due to) vascular disorders, unspecified side of brain

H47.7   Unspecified disorder of visual pathways

DISORDERS OF OCULAR MUSCLES, BINOCULAR MOVEMENT, ACCOMMODATION AND REFRACTION (H49-H52)

Excludes2:   nystagmus and other irregular eye movements (H55)

H49   Paralytic strabismus

Excludes2:   internal ophthalmoplegia (H52.51-)
internuclear ophthalmoplegia (H51.2-)
progressive supranuclear ophthalmoplegia (G23.1)

H49.0   Third [oculomotor] nerve palsy

H49.00   Third [oculomotor] nerve palsy, unspecified eye

H49.01   Third [oculomotor] nerve palsy, right eye

H49.02   Third [oculomotor] nerve palsy, left eye

H49.03   Third [oculomotor] nerve palsy, bilateral

H49.1 **Fourth [trochlear] nerve palsy**
    H49.10   Fourth [trochlear] nerve palsy, unspecified eye
    H49.11   Fourth [trochlear] nerve palsy, right eye
    H49.12   Fourth [trochlear] nerve palsy, left eye
    H49.13   Fourth [trochlear] nerve palsy, bilateral
H49.2 **Sixth [abducent] nerve palsy**
    H49.20   Sixth [abducent] nerve palsy, unspecified eye
    H49.21   Sixth [abducent] nerve palsy, right eye
    H49.22   Sixth [abducent] nerve palsy, left eye
    H49.23   Sixth [abducent] nerve palsy, bilateral
H49.3 **Total (external) ophthalmoplegia**
    H49.30   Total (external) ophthalmoplegia, unspecified eye
    H49.31   Total (external) ophthalmoplegia, right eye
    H49.32   Total (external) ophthalmoplegia, left eye
    H49.33   Total (external) ophthalmoplegia, bilateral
H49.4 **Progressive external ophthalmoplegia**
    Excludes1:   Kearns-Sayre syndrome (H49.81-)
    H49.40   Progressive external ophthalmoplegia, unspecified eye
    H49.41   Progressive external ophthalmoplegia, right eye
    H49.42   Progressive external ophthalmoplegia, left eye
    H49.43   Progressive external ophthalmoplegia, bilateral
H49.8 **Other paralytic strabismus**
    H49.81   **Kearns-Sayre syndrome**
        Progressive external ophthalmoplegia with pigmentary retinopathy
        Use additional code for other manifestation, such as: heart block (I45.9)
        H49.811   Kearns-Sayre syndrome, right eye
        H49.812   Kearns-Sayre syndrome, left eye
        H49.813   Kearns-Sayre syndrome, bilateral
        H49.819   Kearns-Sayre syndrome, unspecified
    H49.88   **Other paralytic strabismus**
        External ophthalmoplegia NOS
        H49.881   Other paralytic strabismus, right eye
        H49.882   Other paralytic strabismus, left eye
        H49.883   Other paralytic strabismus, bilateral
        H49.889   Other paralytic strabismus, unspecified eye
H49.9 **Unspecified paralytic strabismus eye**

H50 **Other strabismus**
H50.0 **Esotropia**
    Convergent concomitant strabismus
    Excludes1:   intermittent esotropia (H50.31-, H50.32)
    H50.00   Unspecified esotropia
    H50.01   Monocular esotropia
        H50.011   Monocular esotropia, right eye
        H50.012   Monocular esotropia, left eye
    H50.02   Monocular esotropia with A pattern
        H50.021   Monocular esotropia with A pattern, right eye
        H50.022   Monocular esotropia with A pattern, left eye
    H50.03   Monocular esotropia with V pattern
        H50.031   Monocular esotropia with V pattern, right eye
        H50.032   Monocular esotropia with V pattern, left eye
    H50.04   Monocular esotropia with other noncomitancies
        H50.041   Monocular esotropia with other noncomitancies, right eye
        H50.042   Monocular esotropia with other noncomitancies, left eye
    H50.05   Alternating esotropia
    H50.06   Alternating esotropia with A pattern
    H50.07   Alternating esotropia with V pattern
    H50.08   Alternating esotropia with other noncomitancies
H50.1 **Exotropia**
    Divergent concomitant strabismus
    Excludes1:   intermittent exotropia (H50.33-, H50.34)
    H50.10   Unspecified exotropia
    H50.11   Monocular cxotropia
        H50.111   Monocular exotropia, right eye
        H50.112   Monocular exotropia, left eye

    H50.12   Monocular exotropia with A pattern
        H50.121   Monocular exotropia with A pattern, right eye
        H50.122   Monocular exotropia with A pattern, left eye
    H50.13   Monocular exotropia with V pattern
        H50.131   Monocular exotropia with V pattern, right eye
        H50.132   Monocular exotropia with V pattern, left eye
    H50.14   Monocular exotropia with other noncomitancies
        H50.141   Monocular exotropia with other noncomitancies, right eye
        H50.142   Monocular exotropia with other noncomitancies, left eye
    H50.15   Alternating exotropia
    H50.16   Alternating exotropia with A pattern
    H50.17   Alternating exotropia with V pattern
    H50.18   Alternating exotropia with other noncomitancies
H50.2 **Vertical strabismus**
H50.3 **Intermittent heterotropia**
    H50.30   Unspecified intermittent heterotropia
    H50.31   Intermittent monocular esotropia
        H50.311   Intermittent monocular esotropia, right eye
        H50.312   Intermittent monocular esotropia, left eye
    H50.32   Intermittent alternating esotropia
    H50.33   Intermittent monocular exotropia
        H50.331   Intermittent monocular exotropia, right eye
        H50.332   Intermittent monocular exotropia, left eye
    H50.34   Intermittent alternating exotropia
H50.4 **Other and unspecified heterotropia**
    H50.40   Unspecified heterotropia
    H50.41   Hypertropia
        H50.411   Hypertropia, right eye
        H50.412   Hypertropia, left eye
    H50.42   Hypotropia
        H50.421   Hypotropia, right eye
        H50.422   Hypotropia, left eye
    H50.43   Cyclotropia
        H50.431   Cyclotropia, right eye
        H50.432   Cyclotropia, left eye
    H50.44   Monofixation syndrome
    H50.45   Accommodative component in esotropia
H50.5 **Heterophoria**
    H50.50   Unspecified heterophoria
    H50.51   Esophoria
    H50.52   Exophoria
    H50.53   Vertical heterophoria
    H50.54   Cyclophoria
    H50.55   Alternating heterophoria
H50.6 **Mechanical strabismus**
    H50.60   Mechanical strabismus, unspecified
    H50.61   Brown's sheath syndrome
        H50.611   Brown's sheath syndrome, right eye
        H50.612   Brown's sheath syndrome, left eye
    H50.69   Other mechanical strabismus
        Strabismus due to adhesions
        Traumatic limitation of duction of eye muscle
H50.8 **Other specified strabismus**
    H50.81   Duane's syndrome
        H50.811   Duane's syndrome, right eye
        H50.812   Duane's syndrome, left eye
    H50.89   Other specified strabismus
H50.9 **Unspecified strabismus**

H51 **Other disorders of binocular movement**
H51.0 **Palsy (spasm) of conjugate gaze**
H51.1 **Convergence insufficiency and excess**
    H51.11   Convergence insufficiency
    H51.12   Convergence excess
H51.2 **Internuclear ophthalmoplegia**
    H51.20   Internuclear ophthalmoplegia, unspecified eye

H51.21   Internuclear ophthalmoplegia, right eye
H51.22   Internuclear ophthalmoplegia, left eye
H51.23   Internuclear ophthalmoplegia, bilateral
H51.8   Other specified disorders of binocular movement
H51.9   Unspecified disorder of binocular movement

H52 Disorders of refraction and accommodation
H52.0   Hypermetropia
H52.00   Hypermetropia, unspecified eye
H52.01   Hypermetropia, right eye
H52.02   Hypermetropia, left eye
H52.03   Hypermetropia, bilateral
H52.1   Myopia
Excludes1:   degenerative myopia (H44.2-)
H52.10   Myopia, unspecified eye
H52.11   Myopia, right eye
H52.12   Myopia, left eye
H52.13   Myopia, bilateral
H52.2   Astigmatism
H52.20   Unspecified astigmatism
H52.201   Unspecified astigmatism, right eye
H52.202   Unspecified astigmatism, left eye
H52.203   Unspecified astigmatism, bilateral
H52.209   Unspecified astigmatism, unspecified eye
H52.21   Irregular astigmatism
H52.211   Irregular astigmatism, right eye
H52.212   Irregular astigmatism, left eye
H52.213   Irregular astigmatism, bilateral
H52.219   Irregular astigmatism, unspecified eye
H52.22   Regular astigmatism
H52.221   Regular astigmatism, right eye
H52.222   Regular astigmatism, left eye
H52.223   Regular astigmatism, bilateral
H52.229   Regular astigmatism, unspecified eye
H52.3   Anisometropia and aniseikonia
H52.31   Anisometropia
H52.32   Aniseikonia
H52.4   Presbyopia
H52.5   Disorders of accommodation
H52.51   Internal ophthalmoplegia (complete) (total)
H52.511   Internal ophthalmoplegia (complete) (total), right eye
H52.512   Internal ophthalmoplegia (complete) (total), left eye
H52.513   Internal ophthalmoplegia (complete) (total), bilateral
H52.519   Internal ophthalmoplegia (complete) (total), unspecified eye
H52.52   Paresis of accommodation
H52.521   Paresis of accommodation, right eye
H52.522   Paresis of accommodation, left eye
H52.523   Paresis of accommodation, bilateral
H52.529   Paresis of accommodation, unspecified eye
H52.53   Spasm of accommodation
H52.531   Spasm of accommodation, right eye
H52.532   Spasm of accommodation, left eye
H52.533   Spasm of accommodation, bilateral
H52.539   Spasm of accommodation, unspecified eye
H52.6   Other disorders of refraction
H52.7   Unspecified disorder of refraction

VISUAL DISTURBANCES AND BLINDNESS (H53-H54)

H53 Visual distubances
H53.0   Amblyopia ex anopsia
Excludes1:   amblyopia due to vitamin A deficiency (E50.5)
H53.00   Unspecified amblyopia
H53.001   Unspecified amblyopia, right eye
H53.002   Unspecified amblyopia, left eye

H53.003   Unspecified amblyopia, bilateral
H53.009   Unspecified amblyopia, unspecified eye
H53.01   Deprivation amblyopia
H53.011   Deprivation amblyopia, right eye
H53.012   Deprivation amblyopia, left eye
H53.013   Deprivation amblyopia, bilateral
H53.019   Deprivation amblyopia, unspecified
H53.02   Refractive amblyopia
H53.021   Refractive amblyopia, right eye
H53.022   Refractive amblyopia, left eye
H53.023   Refractive amblyopia, bilateral
H53.029   Refractive amblyopia, unspecified eye
H53.03   Strabismic amblyopia
Excludes1:   strabismus (H50.-)
H53.031   Strabismic amblyopia, right eye
H53.032   Strabismic amblyopia, left eye
H53.033   Strabismic amblyopia, bilateral
H53.039   Strabismic amblyopia, unspecified eye
H53.1   Subjective visual disturbances
Excludes1:   subjective visual disturbances due to vitamin A deficiency (E50.5)
    visual hallucinations (R44.1)
H53.10   Unspecified subjective visual disturbances
H53.11   Day blindness
    Hemeralopia
H53.12   Transient visual loss
    Scintillating scotoma
Excludes1:   amaurosis fugax (G45.3-)
    transient retinal artery occlusion (H34.0-)
H53.121   Transient visual loss, right eye
H53.122   Transient visual loss, left eye
H53.123   Transient visual loss, bilateral
H53.129   Transient visual loss, unspecified eye
H53.13   Sudden visual loss
H53.131   Sudden visual loss, right eye
H53.132   Sudden visual loss, left eye
H53.133   Sudden visual loss, bilateral
H53.139   Sudden visual loss, unspecified eye
H53.14   Visual discomfort
    Asthenopia
    Photophobia
H53.141   Visual discomfort, right eye
H53.142   Visual discomfort, left eye
H53.143   Visual discomfort, bilateral
H53.149   Visual discomfort, unspecified
H53.18   Visual distortions of shape and size
    Metamorphopsia
H53.19   Other subjective visual disturbances
    Visual halos
H53.2   Diplopia
    Double vision
H53.3   Other and unspecified disorders of binocular vision
H53.30   Unspecified disorder of binocular vision
H53.31   Abnormal retinal correspondence
H53.32   Fusion with defective stereopsis
H53.33   Simultaneous visual perception without fusion
H53.34   Suppression of binocular vision
H53.4   Visual field defects
H53.40   Unspecified visual field defects
H53.41   Scotoma involving central area
    Central scotoma
H53.411   Scotoma involving central area, right eye
H53.412   Scotoma involving central area, left eye
H53.413   Scotoma involving central area, bilateral
H53.419   Scotoma involving central area, unspecified eye
H53.42   Scotoma of blind spot area
    Enlarged blind spot

H53.421   Scotoma of blind spot area, right eye
H53.422   Scotoma of blind spot area, left eye
H53.423   Scotoma of blind spot area, bilateral
H53.429   Scotoma of blind spot area, unspecified eye

H53.43   **Sector or arcuate defects**
Arcuate scotoma
Bjerrum scotoma

H53.431   Sector or arcuate defects, right eye
H53.432   Sector or arcuate defects, left eye
H53.433   Sector or arcuate defects, bilateral
H53.439   Sector or arcuate defects, unspecified eye

H53.45   **Other localized visual field defect**
Peripheral visual field defect
Ring scotoma NOS
Scotoma NOS

H53.451   Other localized visual field defect, right eye
H53.452   Other localized visual field defect, left eye
H53.453   Other localized visual field defect, bilateral
H53.459   Other localized visual field defect, unspecified eye

H53.46   **Homonymous bilateral field defects**
Homonymous hemianop(s)ia
Quadrant anop(s)ia

H53.47   **Heteronymous bilateral field defects**
Heteronymous hemianop(s)ia

H53.48   **Generalized contraction of visual field**

H53.481   Generalized contraction of visual field, right eye
H53.482   Generalized contraction of visual field, left eye
H53.483   Generalized contraction of visual field, bilateral
H53.489   Generalized contraction of visual field, unspecified eye

H53.5   **Color vision deficiencies**
Color blindness
Excludes2:   day blindness (H53.11)

H53.50   **Unspecified color vision deficiencies**
Color blindness NOS

H53.51   **Achromatopsia**

H53.52   **Acquired color vision deficiency**

H53.53   **Deuteranomaly**
Deuteranopia

H53.54   **Protanomaly**
Protanopia

H53.55   **Tritanomaly**
Tritanopia

H53.59   **Other color vision deficiencies**

H53.6   **Night blindness**
Excludes1:   night blindness due to vitamin A deficiency (E50.5)

H53.60   **Unspecified night blindness**

H53.61   **Abnormal dark adaptation curve**

H53.62   **Acquired night blindness**

H53.63   **Congenital night blindness**

H53.69   **Other night blindness**

H53.7   **Vision sensitivity deficiencies**

H53.71   **Glare sensitivity**

H53.72   **Impaired contrast sensitivity**

H53.8   **Other visual disturbances**

H53.9   **Unspecified visual disturbance**

H54   Blindness and low vision
Note: For definition of visual impairment categories see table below
Code first any associated underlying cause of the blindness
Excludes1:   amaurosis fugax (G45.3)

H54.0   **Blindness, both eyes**
Visual impairment categories 3, 4, 5 in both eyes.

H54.1   **Blindness, one eye, low vision other eye**
Visual impairment categories 3, 4, 5 in one eye, with categories 1 or 2 in the other eye.

H54.10   Blindness, one eye, low vision other eye, unspecified eyes
H54.11   Blindness, right eye, low vision left eye
H54.12   Blindness, left eye, low vision right eye

H54.2   **Low vision, both eyes**
Visual impairment categories 1 or 2 in both eyes.

H54.3   **Unqualified visual loss, both eyes**
Visual impairment category 9 in both eyes.

H54.4   **Blindness, one eye**
Visual impairment categories 3, 4, 5 in one eye [normal vision in other eye]

H54.40   Blindness, one eye, unspecified eye
H54.41   Blindness, right eye, normal vision left eye
H54.42   Blindness, left eye, normal vision right eye

H54.5   **Low vision, one eye**
Visual impairment categories 1 or 2 in one eye [normal vision in other eye].

H54.50   Low vision, one eye, unspecified eye
H54.51   Low vision, right eye, normal vision left eye
H54.52   Low vision, left eye, normal vision right eye

H54.6   **Unqualified visual loss, one eye**
Visual impairment category 9 in one eye [normal vision in other eye].

H54.60   Unqualified visual loss, one eye, unspecified
H54.61   Unqualified visual loss, right eye, normal vision left eye
H54.62   Unqualified visual loss, left eye, normal vision right eye

H54.7   **Unspecified visual loss**
Visual impairment category 9 NOS

H54.8   **Legal blindness, as defined in USA**
Blindness NOS according to USA definition
Excludes1:   legal blindness with specification of impairment level (H54.0-H54.7)
Note: The table below gives a classification of severity of visual impairment recommended by a WHO Study Group on the Prevention of Blindness, Geneva, 6-10 November 1972.
The term "low vision" in category H54 comprises categories 1 and 2 of the table, the term "blindness" categories 3, 4 and 5, and the term "unqualified visual loss" category 9.
If the extent of the visual field is taken into account, patients with a field no greater than 10 but greater than 5 around central fixation should be placed in category 3 and patients with a field no greater than 5 around central fixation should be placed in category 4, even if the central acuity is not impaired.

Category of visual impairment	Visual acuity with best possible correction	
	Maximum less than:	Minimum equal to or better than:
1	6/18 3/10 (0.3) 20/70	6/60 1/10 (0.1) 20/200
2	6/60 1/10 (0.1) 20/200	3/60 1/20 (0.5) 20/400
3	3/60 1/20 (0.05) 20/400	1/60 (finger counting at one meter) 1/50 (0.02) 5/300 (20/1200)
4	1/60 (finger counting at one meter) 1/50 (0.02) 5/300	Light perception
5	No light perception	
9	Undetermined or unspecified	

OTHER DISORDERS OF EYE AND ADNEXA (H55-H59)

H55 Nystagmus and other irregular eye movements
  H55.0 Nystagmus
    H55.00   Unspecified nystagmus
    H55.01   Congenital nystagmus
    H55.02   Latent nystagmus
    H55.03   Visual deprivation nystagmus
    H55.04   Dissociated nystagmus
    H55.09   Other forms of nystagums
  H55.8 Other irregular eye movements
    H55.81   Saccadic eye movements
    H55.89   Other irregular eye movements

H57 Other disorders of eye and adnexa
  H57.0 Anomalies of pupillary function
    H57.00   Unspecified anomaly of pupillary function
    H57.01   Argyll Robertson pupil, atypical
        Excludes1:   syphilitic Argyll Robertson pupil (A52.19)
    H57.02   Anisocoria
    H57.03   Miosis
    H57.04   Mydriasis
    H57.05   Tonic pupil
       H57.051   Tonic pupil, right eye
       H57.052   Tonic pupil, left eye
       H57.053   Tonic pupil, bilateral
       H57.059   Tonic pupil, unspecified eye
    H57.09   Other anomalies of pupillary function
  H57.1 Ocular pain
    H57.10   Ocular pain, unspecified eye
    H57.11   Ocular pain, right eye
    H57.12   Ocular pain, left eye
    H57.13   Ocular pain, bilateral
  H57.8 Other specified disorders of eye and adnexa
  H57.9 Unspecified disorder of eye and adnexa

H59 Intraoperative and postprocedural complications and disorders of eye and adnexa, not elsewhere classified
  Excludes1:   filtering (vitreous) bleb after glaucoma surgery (Z98.8)
       mechanical complication of intraocular lens (T85.2)
       mechanical complication of other ocular prosthetic devices, implants and grafts (T85.3)
       pseudophakia (Z96.1)
       secondary cataracts (H26.4-)
  H59.0 Vitreous syndrome following cataract surgery
    Vitreous touch syndrome
    H59.00   Vitreous syndrome following cataract surgery, unspecified eye
    H59.01   Vitreous syndrome following cataract surgery, right eye
    H59.02   Vitreous syndrome following cataract surgery, left eye
    H59.03   Vitreous syndrome following cataract surgery, bilateral
  H59.1 Cataract (lens) fragments in eye following cataract surgery
    H59.10   Cataract (lens) fragments in eye following cataract surgery, unspecified eye
    H59.11   Cataract (lens) fragments in eye following cataract surgery, right eye
    H59.12   Cataract (lens) fragments in eye following cataract surgery, left eye
    H59.13   Cataract (lens) fragments in eye following cataract surgery, bilateral
  H59.2 Cystoid macular edema following cataract surgery
    H59.20   Cystoid macular edema following cataract surgery, unspecified eye
    H59.21   Cystoid macular edema following cataract surgery, right eye
    H59.22   Cystoid macular edema following cataract surgery, left eye
    H59.23   Cystoid macular edema following cataract surgery, bilateral

  H59.3 Intraoperative and postprocedural hemorrhage or hematoma complicating a procedure on the eye and adnexa
    Excludes1:   intraoperative hemorrhage or hematoma due to accidental puncture or laceration during a procedure on the eye and adnexa (H59.4-)
    H59.31   Intraoperative hemorrhage of the eye and adnexa during a procedure on the eye and adnexa
    H59.32   Intraoperative hemorrhage of other organ or structure during a procedure on the eye and adnexa
    H59.33   Intraoperative hematoma of the eye and adnexa during a procedure on the eye and adnexa
    H59.34   Intraoperative hematoma of other organ or structure during a procedure on the eye and adnexa
    H59.35   Postprocedural hemorrhage of the eye and adnexa following a procedure on the eye and adnexa
    H59.36   Postprocedural hemorrhage of other organ or structure following a procedure on the eye and adnexa
    H59.37   Postprocedural hematoma of the eye and adnexa following a procedure on the eye and adnexa
    H59.38   Postprocedural hematoma of other organ or structure following a procedure on the eye and adnexa
  H59.4 Accidental puncture or laceration during a procedure on the eye and adnexa
    H59.41   Accidental puncture or laceration of the eye and adnexa during a procedure on the eye and adnexa
    H59.42   Accidental puncture or laceration of other organ or structure during a procedure on the eye and adnexa
  H59.8 Other intraoperative and postprocedural complications and disorders of eye and adnexa
    H59.81   Chorioretinal scars after surgery for detachment
       H59.811   Chorioretinal scars after surgery for detachment, right eye
       H59.812   Chorioretinal scars after surgery for detachment, left eye
       H59.813   Chorioretinal scars after surgery for detachment, bilateral
       H59.819   Chorioretinal scars after surgery for detachment, unspecified eye
    H59.88   Other intraoperative complications of eye and adnexa
    H59.89   Other postprocedural complications and disorders of eye and adnexa
  H59.9 Unspecified intraoperative and postprocedural complication and disorder of eye and adnexa
    H59.90   Unspecified intraoperative complication of eye and adnexa
    H59.91   Unspecified postprocedural complication and disorder of eye and adnexa

CHAPTER VIII — DISEASES OF THE EAR AND MASTOID PROCESS (H60–H95)

Excludes2: certain conditions originating in the perinatal period (P04-P96)
certain infectious and parasitic diseases (A00-B99)
complications of pregnancy, childbirth and the puerperium (O00-O99)
congenital malformations, deformations and chromosomal abnormalities (Q00-Q99)
endocrine, nutritional and metabolic diseases (E00-E90)
injury, poisoning and certain other consequences of external causes (S00-T98)
neoplasms (C00-D48)
symptoms, signs and abnormal clinical and laboratory findings, not elsewhere classified (R00-R94)

This chapter contains the following blocks:

H60-H62   Diseases of external ear
H65-H75   Diseases of middle ear and mastoid
H80-H83   Diseases of inner ear
H90-H95   Other disorders of ear

DISEASES OF EXTERNAL EAR (H60–H62)

H60 Otitis externa

H60.0 Abscess of external ear
Boil of external ear
Carbuncle of auricle or external auditory canal
Furuncle of external ear
  H06.00   Abscess of external ear, unspecified ear
  H06.01   Abscess of right external ear
  H06.02   Abscess of left external ear
  H06.03   Abscess of external ear, bilateral

H60.1 Cellulitis of external ear
Cellulitis of auricle
Cellulitis of external auditory canal
  H60.10   Cellulitis of external ear, unspecified ear
  H60.11   Cellulitis of right external ear
  H60.12   Cellulitis of left external ear
  H60.13   Cellulitis of external ear, bilateral

H60.2 Malignant otitis externa
  H60.20   Malignant otitis externa, unspecified ear
  H60.21   Malignant otitis externa, right ear
  H60.22   Malignant otitis externa, left ear
  H60.23   Malignant otitis externa, bilateral

H60.3 Other infective otitis externa
  H60.31   Diffuse otitis externa
    H60.311   Diffuse otitis externa, right ear
    H60.312   Diffuse otitis externa, left ear
    H60.313   Diffuse otitis externa, bilateral
    H60.319   Diffuse otitis externa, unspecified ear
  H60.32   Hemorrhagic otitis externa
    H60.321   Hemorrhagic otitis externa, right ear
    H60.322   Hemorrhagic otitis externa, left ear
    H60.323   Hemorrhagic otitis externa, bilateral
    H60.329   Hemorrhagic otitis externa, unspecified ear
  H60.33   Swimmer's ear
    H60.331   Swimmer's ear, right ear
    H60.332   Swimmer's ear, left ear
    H60.333   Swimmer's ear, bilateral
    H60.339   Swimmer's ear, unspecified ear
  H60.39   Other infective otitis externa
    H60.391   Other infective otitis externa, right ear
    H60.392   Other infective otitis externa, left ear
    H60.393   Other infective otitis externa, bilateral
    H60.399   Other infective otitis externa, unspecified ear

H60.4 Cholesteatoma of external ear
Keratosis obturans of external ear (canal)
Excludes2:   cholesteatoma of middle ear (H71.-)
recurrent cholesteatoma of postmastoidectomy cavity (H95.0-)
  H60.40   Cholesteatoma of external ear, unspecified ear
  H60.41   Cholesteatoma of right external ear
  H60.42   Cholesteatoma of left external ear
  H60.43   Cholesteotoma of external ear, bilateral

H60.5 Acute noninfective otitis externa
  H60.50   Unspecified acute noninfective otitis externa
Acute otitis externa NOS
    H60.501   Unspecified acute noninfective otitis externa, right ear
    H60.502   Unspecified acute noninfective otitis externa, left ear
    H60.503   Unspecified acute noninfective otitis externa, bilateral
    H60.509   Unspecified acute noninfective otitis externa, unspecified ear
  H60.51   Acute actinic otitis externa
    H60.511   Acute actinic otitis externa, right ear
    H60.512   Acute actinic otitis externa, left ear
    H60.513   Acute actinic otitis externa, bilateral
    H60.519   Acute actinic otitis externa, unspecified ear
  H60.52   Acute chemical otitis externa
    H60.521   Acute chemical otitis externa, right ear
    H60.522   Acute chemical otitis externa, left ear
    H60.523   Acute chemical otitis externa, bilateral
    H60.529   Acute chemical otitis externa, unspecified ear
  H60.53   Acute contact otitis externa
    H60.531   Acute contact otitis externa, right ear
    H60.532   Acute contact otitis externa, left ear
    H60.533   Acute contact otitis externa, bilateral
    H60.539   Acute contact otitis externa, unspecified ear
  H60.54   Acute eczematoid otitis externa
    H60.541   Acute eczematoid otitis externa, right ear
    H60.542   Acute eczematoid otitis externa, left ear
    H60.543   Acute eczematoid otitis externa, bilateral
    H60.549   Acute eczematoid otitis externa, unspecified ear
  H60.55   Acute reactive otitis externa
    H60.551   Acute reactive otitis externa, right ear
    H60.552   Acute reactive otitis externa, left ear
    H60.553   Acute reactive otitis externa, bilateral
    H60.559   Acute reactive otitis externa, unspecified ear
  H60.59   Other noninfective acute otitis externa
    H60.591   Other noninfective acute otitis externa, right ear
    H60.592   Other noninfective acute otitis externa, left ear
    H60.593   Other noninfective acute otitis externa, bilateral
    H60.599   Other noninfective acute otitis externa, unspecified ear

H60.6 Unspecified chronic otitis externa
  H60.60   Unspecified chronic otitis externa, right ear
  H60.61   Unspecified chronic otitis externa, left ear
  H60.62   Unspecified chronic otitis externa, bilateral
  H60.63   Unspecified chronic otitis externa, unspecified ear

H60.8 Other otitis externa
  H60.8x   Other otitis externa
    H60.8x1   Other otitis externa, right ear
    H60.8x2   Other otitis externa, left ear
    H60.8x3   Other otitis externa, bilateral
    H60.8x9   Other otitis externa, unspecified ear

H60.9 Unspecified otitis externa
  H60.90   Unspecified otitis externa, unspecified ear
  H60.91   Unspecified otitis externa, right ear

H60.92   Unspecified otitis externa, left ear
H60.93   Unspecified otitis externa, bilateral

H61 Other disorders of external ear
H61.0 Perichondritis of external ear
Chondrodermatitis nodularis chronica helicis
Perichondritis of auricle
Perichondritis of pinna
H61.00   Unspecified perichondritis of external ear
H61.001   Unspecified perichondritis of right external ear
H61.002   Unspecified perichondritis of left external ear
H61.003   Unspecified perichondritis of external ear, bilateral
H61.009   Unspecified perichondritis of external ear, unspecified ear
H61.01   Acute perichondritis of external ear
H61.011   Acute perichondritis of right external ear
H61.012   Acute perichondritis of left external ear
H61.013   Acute perichondritis of external ear, bilateral
H61.019   Acute perichondritis of external ear, unspecified ear
H61.02   Chronic perichondritis of external ear
H61.021   Chronic perichondritis of right external ear
H61.022   Chronic perichondritis of left external ear
H61.023   Chronic perichondritis of external ear, bilateral
H61.029   Chronic perichondritis of external ear, unspecified ear
H61.1 Noninfective disorders of pinna
Excludes2:   cauliflower ear (M95.1-)
gouty tophi of ear (M10.-)
H61.10   Unspecified noninfective disorders of pinna
Disorder of pinna NOS
H61.101   Unspecified noninfective disorders of pinna, right ear
H61.102   Unspecified noninfective disorders of pinna, left ear
H61.103   Unspecified noninfective disorders of pinna, bilateral
H61.109   Unspecified noninfective disorders of pinna, unspecified ear
H61.11   Acquired deformity of pinna
Acquired deformity of auricle
Excludes2:   cauliflower ear (M95.1-)
H61.111   Acquired deformity of pinna, right ear
H61.112   Acquired deformity of pinna, left ear
H61.113   Acquired deformity of pinna, bilateral
H61.119   Acquired deformity of pinna, unspecified ear
H61.12   Hematoma of pinna
Hematoma of auricle
H61.121   Hematoma of pinna, right ear
H61.122   Hematoma of pinna, left ear
H61.123   Hematoma of pinna, bilateral
H61.129   Hematoma of pinna, unspecified ear
H61.19   Other noninfective disorders of pinna
H61.191   Noninfective disorders of pinna, right ear
H61.192   Noninfective disorders of pinna, left ear
H61.193   Noninfective disorders of pinna, bilateral
H61.199   Noninfective disorders of pinna, unspecified ear
H61.2 Impacted cerumen
Wax in ear
H61.20   Impacted cerumen, unspecified ear
H61.21   Impacted cerumen, right ear
H61.22   Impacted cerumen, left ear
H61.23   Impacted cerumen, bilateral
H61.3 Acquired stenosis of external ear canal
Collapse of external ear canal
Excludes1:   postprocedural stenosis of external ear canal (H95.81-)

H61.30   Acquired stenosis of external ear canal, unspecified
H61.301   Acquired stenosis of right external ear canal, unspecified
H61.302   Acquired stenosis of left external ear canal, unspecified
H61.303   Acquired stenosis of external ear canal, unspecified, bilateral
H61.309   Acquired stenosis of external ear canal, unspecified, unspecified ear
H61.31   Acquired stenosis of external ear canal secondary to trauma
H61.311   Acquired stenosis of right external ear canal secondary to trauma
H61.312   Acquired stenosis of left external ear canal secondary to trauma
H61.313   Acquired stenosis of external ear canal secondary to trauma, bilateral
H61.319   Acquired stenosis of external ear canal secondary to trauma, unspecified ear
H61.32   Acquired stenosis of external ear canal secondary to inflammation and infection
H61.321   Acquired stenosis of right external ear canal secondary to inflammation and infection
H61.322   Acquired stenosis of left external ear canal secondary to inflammation and infection
H61.323   Acquired stenosis of external ear canal secondary to inflammation and infection, bilateral
H61.329   Acquired stenosis of external ear canal secondary to inflammation and infection, unspecified ear
H61.39   Other acquired stenosis of external ear canal
H61.391   Other acquired stenosis of right external ear canal
H61.392   Other acquired stenosis of left external ear canal
H61.393   Other acquired stenosis of external ear canal, bilateral
H61.399   Other acquired stenosis of external ear canal, unspecified ear
H61.8 Other specified disorders of external ear
H61.81   Exostosis of external canal
H61.811   Exostosis of right external canal
H61.812   Exostosis of left external canal
H61.813   Exostosis of external canal, bilateral
H61.819   Exostosis of external canal, unspecified ear
H61.89   Other specified disorders of external ear
H61.891   Other specified disorders of right external ear
H61.892   Other specified disorders of left external ear
H61.893   Other specified disorders of external ear, bilateral
H61.899   Other specified disorders of external ear, unspecified ear
H61.9 Disorder of external ear, unspecified
H61.90   Disorder of external ear, unspecified, unspecified ear
H61.91   Disorder of right external ear, unspecified
H61.92   Disorder of left external ear, unspecified
H61.93   Disorder of external ear, unspecified, bilateral

H62 Disorders of external ear in diseases classified elsewhere
H62.4 Otitis externa in other diseases classified elsewhere
Code first underlying disease, such as:
erysipelas (A46)
impetigo (L01.0)
Excludes1:   otitis externa (in):
candidiasis (B37.84)
herpes viral [herpes simplex] (B00.1)
herpes zoster (B02.8)
H62.40   Otitis externa in other diseases classified elsewhere, unspecified ear
H62.41   Otitis externa in other diseases classified elsewhere, right ear

H62.42   Otitis externa in other diseases classified elsewhere, left ear

H63.43   Otitis externa in other diseases classified elsewhere, bilateral

H62.8   Other disorders of external ear in diseases classified elsewhere
  Code first underlying disease, such as:
    gout (M10.-)

H62.8x   Other disorders of external ear in diseases classified elsewhere

H62.8x1   Other disorders of right external ear in diseases classified elsewhere

H62.8x2   Other disorders of left external ear in diseases classified elsewhere

H62.8x3   Other disorders of external ear in diseases classified elsewhere, bilateral

H62.8x9   Other disorders of external ear in diseases classified elsewhere, unspecified ear

DISEASES OF MIDDLE EAR AND MASTOID (H65–H75)

H65   Nonsuppurative otitis media
  Includes: nonsuppurative otitis media with myringitis
  Use additional code to identify:
    exposure to environmental tobacco smoke (X58.1)
    exposure to tobacco smoke in the perinatal period (P96.6)
    history of tobacco use (Z86.43)
    occupational exposure to environmental tobacco smoke (Z57.31)
    tobacco dependence (F17.-)
    tobacco use (Z72.0)

H65.0   Acute serous otitis media
  Acute and subacute secretory otitis

H65.00   Acute serous otitis media, unspecified ear

H65.01   Acute serous otitis media, right ear

H65.02   Acute serous otitis media, left ear

H65.03   Acute serous otitis media, bilateral

H65.04   Acute serous otitis media, recurrent, right ear

H65.05   Acute serous otitis media, recurrent, left ear

H65.06   Acute serous otitis media, recurrent, bilateral

H65.07   Acute serous otitis media, recurrent, unspecified ear

H65.1   Other acute nonsuppurative otitis media
  Excludes1:   otitic barotrauma (T70.0)
    otitis media (acute) NOS (H66.9)

H65.11   Acute and subacute allergic otitis media (mucoid) (sanguinous) (serous)

H65.111   Acute and subacute allergic otitis media (mucoid) (sanguinous) (serous), right ear

H65.112   Acute and subacute allergic otitis media (mucoid) (sanguinous) (serous), left ear

H65.113   Acute and subacute allergic otitis media (mucoid) (sanguinous) (serous), bilateral

H65.114   Acute and subacute allergic otitis media (mucoid) (sanguinous) (serous), recurrent, right ear

H65.115   Acute and subacute allergic otitis media (mucoid) (sanguinous) (serous), recurrent, left ear

H65.116   Acute and subacute allergic otitis media (mucoid) (sanguinous) (serous), recurrent, bilateral

H65.117   Acute and subacute allergic otitis media (mucoid) (sanguinous) (serous), recurrent, unspecified ear

H65.119   Acute and subacute allergic otitis media (mucoid) (sanguinous) (serous), unspecified ear

H65.19   Other acute nonsuppurative otitis media
  Acute and subacute mucoid otitis media
  Acute and subacute nonsuppurative otitis media NOS
  Acute and subacute sanguinous otitis media
  Acute and subacute seromucinous otitis media

H65.191   Other acute nonsuppurative otitis media, right ear

H65.192   Other acute nonsuppurative otitis media, left ear

H65.193   Other acute nonsuppurative otitis media, bilateral

H65.194   Other acute nonsuppurative otitis media, recurrent, right ear

H65.195   Other acute nonsuppurative otitis media, recurrent, left ear

H65.196   Other acute nonsuppurative otitis media, recurrent, bilateral

H65.197   Other acute nonsuppurative otitis media, recurrent, unspecified ear

H65.199   Other acute nonsuppurative otitis media, unspecified ear

H65.2   Chronic serous otitis media
  Chronic tubotympanal catarrh

H65.20   Chronic serous otitis media, unspecified ear

H65.21   Chronic serous otitis media, right ear

H65.22   Chronic serous otitis media, left ear

H65.23   Chronic serous otitis media, bilateral

H65.3   Chronic mucoid otitis media
  Chronic mucinous otitis media
  Chronic secretory otitis media
  Chronic transudative otitis media
  Glue ear
  Excludes1:   adhesive middle ear disease (H74.1)

H65.30   Chronic mucoid otitis media, unspecified ear

H65.31   Chronic mucoid otitis media, right ear

H65.32   Chronic mucoid otitis media, left ear

H65.33   Chronic mucoid otitis media, bilateral

H65.4   Other chronic nonsuppurative otitis media

H65.41   Chronic allergic otitis media

H65.411   Chronic allergic otitis media, right ear

H65.412   Chronic allergic otitis media, left ear

H65.413   Chronic allergic otitis media, bilateral

H65.419   Chronic allergic otitis media, unspecified ear

H65.49   Other chronic nonsuppurative otitis media
  Chronic exudative otitis media
  Chronic nonsuppurative otitis media NOS
  Chronic otitis media with effusion (nonpurulent)
  Chronic seromucinous otitis media

H65.491   Other chronic nonsuppurative otitis media, right ear

H65.492   Other chronic nonsuppurative otitis media, left ear

H65.493   Other chronic nonsuppurative otitis media, bilateral

H65.499   Other chronic nonsuppurative otitis media, unspecified ear

H65.9   Unspecified nonsuppurative otitis media
  Allergic otitis media NOS
  Catarrhal otitis media NOS
  Exudative otitis media NOS
  Mucoid otitis media NOS
  Otitis media with effusion (nonpurulent) NOS
  Secretory otitis media NOS
  Seromucinous otitis media NOS
  Serous otitis media NOS
  Transudative otitis media NOS

H65.90   Unspecified nonsuppurative otitis media, unspecified ear

H65.91   Unspecified nonsuppurative otitis media, right ear

H65.92   Unspecified nonsuppurative otitis media, left ear

H65.93   Unspecified nonsuppurative otitis media, bilateral

H66   Suppurative and unspecified otitis media
  Includes: with myringitis
  Use additional code to identify:
    exposure to environmental tobacco smoke (X58.1)
    exposure to tobacco smoke in the perinatal period (P96.6)
    history of tobacco use (Z86.43)
    occupational exposure to environmental tobacco smoke (Z57.31)
    tobacco dependence (F17.-)
    tobacco use (Z72.0)

H66.0 Acute suppurative otitis media

  H66.00 Acute suppurative otitis media without spontaneous rupture of ear drum

    H66.001   Acute suppurative otitis media without spontaneous rupture of ear drum, right ear

    H66.002   Acute suppurative otitis media without spontaneous rupture of ear drum, left ear

    H66.003   Acute suppurative otitis media without spontaneous rupture of ear drum, bilateral

    H66.004   Acute suppurative otitis media without spontaneous rupture of ear drum, recurrent, right ear

    H66.005   Acute suppurative otitis media without spontaneous rupture of ear drum, recurrent, left ear

    H66.006   Acute suppurative otitis media without spontaneous rupture of ear drum, recurrent, bilateral

    H66.007   Acute suppurative otitis media without spontaneous rupture of ear drum, recurrent, unspecified ear

    H66.009   Acute suppurative otitis media without spontaneous rupture of ear drum, unspecified ear

  H66.01 Acute suppurative otitis media with spontaneous rupture of ear drum

    H66.011   Acute suppurative otitis media with spontaneous rupture of ear drum, right ear

    H66.012   Acute suppurative otitis media with spontaneous rupture of ear drum, left ear

    H66.013   Acute suppurative otitis media with spontaneous rupture of ear drum, bilateral

    H66.014   Acute suppurative otitis media with spontaneous rupture of ear drum, recurrent, right ear

    H66.015   Acute suppurative otitis media with spontaneous rupture of ear drum, recurrent, left ear

    H66.016   Acute suppurative otitis media with spontaneous rupture of ear drum, recurrent, bilateral

    H66.017   Acute suppurative otitis media with spontaneous rupture of ear drum, recurrent, unspecified ear

    H66.019   Acute suppurative otitis media with spontaneous rupture of ear drum, unspecified ear

H66.1 Chronic tubotympanic suppurative otitis media
     Benign chronic suppurative otitis media
     Chronic tubotympanic disease

  H66.10   Chronic tubotympanic suppurative otitis media, unspecified

  H66.11   Chronic tubotympanic suppurative otitis media, right ear

  H66.12   Chronic tubotympanic suppurative otitis media, left ear

  H66.13   Chronic tubotympanic suppurative otitis media, bilateral

H66.2 Chronic atticoantral suppurative otitis media
     Chronic atticoantral disease

  H66.20   Chronic atticoantral suppurative otitis media, unspecified ear

  H66.21   Chronic atticoantral suppurative otitis media, right ear

  H66.22   Chronic atticoantral suppurative otitis media, left ear

  H66.23   Chronic atticoantral suppurative otitis media, bilateral

H66.3 Other chronic suppurative otitis media
     Chronic suppurative otitis media NOS
     Excludes1:   tuberculous otitis media (A18.6)

  H66.3x Other chronic suppurative otitis media

    H66.3x1   Other chronic suppurative otitis media, right ear

    H66.3x2   Other chronic suppurative otitis media, left ear

    H66.3x3   Other chronic suppurative otitis media, bilateral

    H66.3x9   Other chronic suppurative otitis media, unspecified ear

H66.4 Suppurative otitis media, unspecified
     Purulent otitis media NOS

  H66.40   Suppurative otitis media, unspecified, unspecified ear

  H66.41   Suppurative otitis media, unspecified, right ear

  H66.42   Suppurative otitis media, unspecified, left ear

  H66.43   Suppurative otitis media, unspecified, bilateral

H66.9 Otitis media, unspecified
     Acute otitis media NOS
     Chronic otitis media NOS
     Otitis media NOS

  H66.90   Otitis media, unspecified, unspecified ear

  H66.91   Otitis media, unspecified, right ear

  H66.92   Otitis media, unspecified, left ear

  H66.93   Otitis media, unspecified, bilateral

H67 Otitis media in diseases classified elsewhere
     Code first underlying disease, such as:
       viral disease NEC (B00-B34)
     Excludes1:   otitis media in:
         influenza (J10.89)
         measles (B05.3)
         scarlet fever (A38.0)
         tuberculosis (A18.6)

H67.0 Otitis media in diseases classified elsewhere, unspecified ear

H67.1 Otitis media in diseases classified elsewhere, right ear

H67.2 Otitis media in diseases classified elsewhere, left ear

H67.3 Otitis media in diseases classified elsewhere, bilateral

H68 Eustachian salpingitis and obstruction

H68.0 Eustachian salpingitis

  H68.00 Unspecified Eustachian salpingitis

    H68.001   Unspecified Eustachian salpingitis, right ear

    H68.002   Unspecified Eustachian salpingitis, left ear

    H68.003   Unspecified Eustachian salpingitis, bilateral

    H68.009   Unspecified Eustachian salpingitis, unspecified ear

  H68.01 Acute Eustachian salpingitis

    H68.011   Acute Eustachian salpingitis, right ear

    H68.012   Acute Eustachian salpingitis, left ear

    H68.013   Acute Eustachian salpingitis, bilateral

    H68.019   Acute Eustachian salpingitis, unspecified ear

  H68.02 Chronic Eustachian salpingitis

    H68.021   Chronic Eustachian salpingitis, right ear

    H68.022   Chronic Eustachian salpingitis, left ear

    H68.023   Chronic Eustachian salpingitis, bilateral

    H68.029   Chronic Eustachian salpingitis, unspecified ear

H68.1 Obstruction of Eustachian tube
     Stenosis of Eustachian tube
     Stricture of Eustachian tube

  H68.10 Unspecified obstruction of Eustachian tube

    H68.101   Unspecified obstruction of Eustachian tube, right ear

    H68.102   Unspecified obstruction of Eustachian tube, left ear

    H68.103   Unspecified obstruction of Eustachian tube, bilateral

    H68.109   Unspecified obstruction of Eustachian tube, unspecified ear

  H68.11 Osseous obstruction of Eustacian tube

    H68.111   Osseous obstruction of Eustacian tube, right ear

    H68.112   Osseous obstruction of Eustacian tube, left ear

    H68.113   Osseous obstruction of Eustacian tube, bilateral

H68.119   Osseous obstruction of Eustacian tube, unspecified ear
H68.12   Intrinsic cartilagenous obstruction of Eustacian tube
H68.121   Intrinsic cartilagenous obstruction of Eustacian tube, right ear
H68.122   Intrinsic cartilagenous obstruction of Eustacian tube, left ear
H68.123   Intrinsic cartilagenous obstruction of Eustacian tube, bilateral
H68.129   Intrinsic cartilagenous obstruction of Eustacian tube, unspecified ear
H68.13   Extrinsic cartilagenous obstruction of Eustacian tube
Compression of Eustachian tube
H68.131   Extrinsic cartilagenous obstruction of Eustacian tube, right ear
H68.132   Extrinsic cartilagenous obstruction of Eustacian tube, left ear
H68.133   Extrinsic cartilagenous obstruction of Eustacian tube, bilateral
H68.139   Extrinsic cartilagenous obstruction of Eustacian tube, unspecified ear

H69 Other and unspecified disorders of Eustachian tube
H69.0   Patulous Eustachian tube
H69.00   Patulous Eustachian tube, unspecified ear
H69.01   Patulous Eustachian tube, right ear
H69.02   Patulous Eustachian tube, left ear
H69.03   Patulous Eustachian tube, bilateral
H69.8   Other specified disorders of Eustachian tube
H69.80   Other specified disorders of Eustachian tube, unspecified ear
H69.81   Other specified disorders of Eustachian tube, right ear
H69.82   Other specified disorders of Eustachian tube, left ear
H69.83   Other specified disorders of Eustachian tube, bilateral
H69.9   Unspecified Eustachian tube disorder
H69.90   Unspecified Eustachian tube disorder, unspecified ear
H69.91   Unspecified Eustachian tube disorder, right ear
H69.92   Unspecified Eustachian tube disorder, left ear
H69.93   Unspecified Eustachian tube disorder, bilateral

H70 Mastoiditis and related conditions
H70.0   Acute mastoiditis
Abscess of mastoid
Empyema of mastoid
H70.00   Acute mastoiditis without complications
H70.001   Acute mastoiditis without complications, right ear
H70.002   Acute mastoiditis without complications, left ear
H70.003   Acute mastoiditis without complications, bilateral
H70.009   Acute mastoiditis without complications, unspecified ear
H70.01   Subperiosteal abscess of mastoid
H70.011   Subperiosteal abscess of mastoid, right ear
H70.012   Subperiosteal abscess of mastoid, left ear
H70.013   Subperiosteal abscess of mastoid, bilateral
H70.019   Subperiosteal abscess of mastoid, unspecified ear
H70.09   Acute mastoiditis with other complications
H70.091   Acute mastoiditis with other complications, right ear
H70.092   Acute mastoiditis with other complications, left ear
H70.093   Acute mastoiditis with other complications, bilateral
H70.099   Acute mastoiditis with other complications, unspecified ear
H70.1   Chronic mastoiditis
Caries of mastoid
Fistula of mastoid
Excludes1:   tuberculous mastoiditis (A18.03)

H70.10   Chronic mastoiditis, unspecified ear
H70.11   Chronic mastoiditis, right ear
H70.12   Chronic mastoiditis, left ear
H70.13   Chronic mastoiditis, bilateral
H70.2   Petrositis
Inflammation of petrous bone
H70.20   Unspecified petrositis
H70.201   Unspecified petrositis, right ear
H70.202   Unspecified petrositis, left ear
H70.203   Unspecified petrositis, bilateral
H70.209   Unspecified petrositis, unspecified ear
H70.21   Acute petrositis
H70.211   Acute petrositis, right ear
H70.212   Acute petrositis, left ear
H70.213   Acute petrositis, bilateral
H70.219   Acute petrositis, unspecified ear
H70.22   Chronic petrositis
H70.221   Chronic petrositis, right ear
H70.222   Chronic petrositis, left ear
H70.223   Chronic petrositis, bilateral
H70.229   Chronic petrositis, unspecified ear
H70.8   Other mastoiditis and related conditions
Excludes1:   preauricular sinus and cyst (Q18.1)
sinus, fistula, and cyst of branchial cleft (Q18.0)
H70.81   Postauricular fistula
H70.811   Postauricular fistula, right ear
H70.812   Postauricular fistula, left ear
H70.813   Postauricular fistula, bilateral
H70.819   Postauricular fistula, unspecified ear
H70.89   Other mastoiditis and related conditions
H70.891   Other mastoiditis and related conditions, right ear
H70.892   Other mastoiditis and related conditions, left ear
H70.893   Other mastoiditis and related conditions, bilateral
H70.899   Other mastoiditis and related conditions, unspecified ear
H70.9   Unspecified mastoiditis
H70.90   Unspecified mastoiditis, unspecified ear
H70.91   Unspecified mastoiditis, right ear
H70.92   Unspecified mastoiditis, left ear
H70.93   Unspecified mastoiditis, bilateral

H71 Cholesteatoma of middle ear
Excludes2:   cholesteatoma of external ear (H60.4-)
recurrent cholesteatoma of postmastoidectomy cavity (H95.0-)
H71.0   Cholesteatoma of attic
H71.00   Cholesteatoma of attic, unspecified ear
H71.01   Cholesteatoma of attic, right ear
H71.02   Cholesteatoma of attic, left ear
H71.03   Cholesteatoma of attic, bilateral
H71.1   Cholesteatoma of tympanum
H71.10   Cholesteatoma of tympanum, unspecified ear
H71.11   Cholesteatoma of tympanum, right ear
H71.12   Cholesteatoma of tympanum, left ear
H71.13   Cholesteatoma of tympanum, bilateral
H71.2   Cholesteatoma of mastoid
H71.20   Cholesteatoma of mastoid, unspecified ear
H71.21   Cholesteatoma of mastoid, right ear
H71.22   Cholesteatoma of mastoid, left ear
H71.23   Cholesteatoma of mastoid, bilateral
H71.3   Diffuse cholesteatosis
H71.30   Diffuse cholesteatosis, unspecified ear
H71.31   Diffuse cholesteatosis, right ear
H71.32   Diffuse cholesteatosis, left ear
H71.33   Diffuse cholesteatosis, bilateral

H71.9   Unspecified cholesteatoma
  H71.90   Unspecified cholesteatoma, unspecified ear
  H71.91   Unspecified cholesteatoma, right ear
  H71.92   Unspecified cholesteatoma, left ear
  H71.93   Unspecified cholesteatoma, bilateral

H72 Perforation of tympanic membrane
  Includes: persistent post-traumatic perforation of ear drum
        postinflammatory perforation of ear drum
  Code first any associated otitis media (H65.-, H66.1-, H66.2-, H66.3-, H66.4-, H66.9-, H67.-)
  Excludes1:   acute suppurative otitis media with rupture of the tympanic membrane (H66.01-)
        traumatic rupture of ear drum (S09.2-)

H72.0   Central perforation of tympanic membrane
  H72.00   Central perforation of tympanic membrane, unspecified ear
  H72.01   Central perforation of tympanic membrane, right ear
  H72.02   Central perforation of tympanic membrane, left ear
  H72.03   Central perforation of tympanic membrane, bilateral

H72.1   Attic perforation of tympanic membrane
  Perforation of pars flaccida
  H72.10   Attic perforation of tympanic membrane, unspecified ear
  H72.11   Attic perforation of tympanic membrane, right ear
  H72.12   Attic perforation of tympanic membrane, left ear
  H72.13   Attic perforation of tympanic membrane, bilateral

H72.2   Other marginal perforations of tympanic membrane
  H72.2x   Other marginal perforations of tympanic membrane
    H72.2x1   Other marginal perforations of tympanic membrane, right ear
    H72.2x2   Other marginal perforations of tympanic membrane, left ear
    H72.2x3   Other marginal perforations of tympanic membrane, bilateral
    H72.2x9   Other marginal perforations of tympanic membrane, unspecified ear

H72.8   Other perforations of tympanic membrane
  H72.81   Multiple perforations of tympanic membrane
    H72.811   Multiple perforations of tympanic membrane, right ear
    H72.812   Multiple perforations of tympanic membrane, left ear
    H72.813   Multiple perforations of tympanic membrane, bilateral
    H72.819   Multiple perforations of tympanic membrane, unspecified ear
  H72.82   Total perforations of tympanic membrane
    H72.821   Total perforations of tympanic membrane, right ear
    H72.822   Total perforations of tympanic membrane, left ear
    H72.823   Total perforations of tympanic membrane, bilateral
    H72.829   Total perforations of tympanic membrane, unspecified ear

H72.9   Unspecified perforation of tympanic membrane
  H72.90   Unspecified perforation of tympanic membrane, unspecified ear
  H72.91   Unspecified perforation of tympanic membrane, right ear
  H72.92   Unspecified perforation of tympanic membrane, left ear
  H72.93   Unspecified perforation of tympanic membrane, bilateral

H73 Other disorders of tympanic membrane
H73.0   Acute myringitis
  Excludes1:   acute myringitis with otitis media (H65, H66)
  H73.00   Unspecified acute myringitis
    Acute tympanitis NOS
    H73.001   Acute myringitis, right ear

H73.002   Acute myringitis, left ear
H73.003   Acute myringitis, bilateral
H73.009   Acute myringitis, unspecified ear
  H73.01   Bullous myringitis
    H73.011   Bullous myringitis, right ear
    H73.012   Bullous myringitis, left ear
    H73.013   Bullous myringitis, bilateral
    H73.019   Bullous myringitis, unspecified ear
  H73.09   Other acute myringitis
    H73.091   Other acute myringitis, right ear
    H73.092   Other acute myringitis, left ear
    H73.093   Other acute myringitis, bilateral
    H73.099   Other acute myringitis, unspecified ear

H73.1   Chronic myringitis
  Chronic tympanitis
  Excludes1:   chronic myringitis with otitis media (H65, H66)
  H73.10   Chronic myringitis, unspecified ear
  H73.11   Chronic myringitis, right ear
  H73.12   Chronic myringitis, left ear
  H73.13   Chronic myringitis, bilateral

H73.2   Unspecified myringitis
  H73.20   Unspecified myringitis, unspecified ear
  H73.21   Unspecified myringitis, right ear
  H73.22   Unspecified myringitis, left ear
  H73.23   Unspecified myringitis, bilateral

H73.8   Other specified disorders of tympanic membrane
  H73.81   Atrophic flaccid tympanic membrane
    H73.811   Atrophic flaccid tympanic membrane, right ear
    H73.812   Atrophic flaccid tympanic membrane, left ear
    H73.813   Atrophic flaccid tympanic membrane, bilateral
    H73.819   Atrophic flaccid tympanic membrane, unspecified ear
  H73.82   Atrophic nonflaccid tympanic membrane
    H73.821   Atrophic nonflaccid tympanic membrane, right ear
    H73.822   Atrophic nonflaccid tympanic membrane, left ear
    H73.823   Atrophic nonflaccid tympanic membrane, bilateral
    H73.829   Atrophic nonflaccid tympanic membrane, unspecified ear
  H73.89   Other specified disorders of tympanic membrane
    H73.891   Other specified disorders of tympanic membrane, right ear
    H73.892   Other specified disorders of tympanic membrane, left ear
    H73.893   Other specified disorders of tympanic membrane, bilateral
    H73.899   Other specified disorders of tympanic membrane, unspecified ear

H73.9   Unspecified disorder of tympanic membrane
  H73.90   Unspecified disorder of tympanic membrane, unspecified ear
  H73.91   Unspecified disorder of tympanic membrane, right ear
  H73.92   Unspecified disorder of tympanic membrane, left ear
  H73.93   Unspecified disorder of tympanic membrane, bilateral

H74 Other disorders of middle ear mastoid
  Excludes2:   mastoiditis (H70.-)
H74.0   Tympanosclerosis
  H74.0x   Tympanosclerosis
    H74.0x1   Tympanosclerosis, right ear
    H74.0x2   Tympanosclerosis, left ear
    H74.0x3   Tympanosclerosis, bilateral
    H74.0x9   Tympanosclerosis, unspecified ear
H74.1   Adhesive middle ear disease
  Adhesive otitis
  Excludes1:   glue ear (H65.3-)

H74.1x   Adhesive middle ear disease
   H74.1x1   Adhesive right middle ear disease
   H74.1x2   Adhesive left middle ear disease
   H74.1x3   Adhesive middle ear disease, bilateral
   H74.1x9   Adhesive middle ear disease, unspecified ear
H74.2   Discontinuity and dislocation of ear ossicles
  H74.20   Discontinuity and dislocation of ear ossicles, unspecified ear
  H74.21   Discontinuity and dislocation of right ear ossicles
  H74.22   Discontinuity and dislocation of left ear ossicles
  H74.23   Discontinuity and dislocation of ear ossicles, bilateral
H74.3   Other acquired abnormalities of ear ossicles
  H74.31   Ankylosis of ear ossicles
   H74.311   Ankylosis of ear ossicles, right ear
   H74.312   Ankylosis of ear ossicles, left ear
   H74.313   Ankylosis of ear ossicles, bilateral
   H74.319   Ankylosis of ear ossicles, unspecified ear
  H74.32   Partial loss of ear ossicles
   H74.321   Partial loss of ear ossicles, right ear
   H74.322   Partial loss of ear ossicles, left ear
   H74.323   Partial loss of ear ossicles, bilateral
   H74.329   Partial loss of ear ossicles, unspecified ear
  H74.39   Other acquired abnormalities of ear ossicles
   H74.391   Other acquired abnormalities of right ear ossicles
   H74.392   Other acquired abnormalities of left ear ossicles
   H74.393   Other acquired abnormalities of ear ossicles, bilateral
   H74.399   Other acquired abnormalities of ear ossicles, unspecified ear
H74.4   Polyp of middle ear
  H74.40   Polyp of middle ear, unspecified ear
  H74.41   Polyp of right middle ear
  H74.42   Polyp of left middle ear
  H74.43   Polyp of middle ear, bilateral
H74.8   Other specified disorders of middle ear and mastoid
  H78.8x   Other specified disorders of middle ear and mastoid
   H74.8x1   Other specified disorders of right middle ear and mastoid
   H74.8x2   Other specified disorders of left middle ear and mastoid
   H74.8x3   Other specified disorders of middle ear and mastoid, bilateral
   H74.8x9   Other specified disorders of middle ear and mastoid, unspecified ear
H74.9   Unspecified disorder of middle ear and mastoid
  H74.90   Unspecified disorder of middle ear and mastoid, unspecified ear
  H74.91   Unspecified disorder of right middle ear and mastoid
  H79.92   Unspecified disorder of left middle ear and mastoid
  H79.93   Unspecified disorder of middle ear and mastoid, bilateral

H75 Other disorders of middle ear and mastoid in diseases classified elsewhere
  Code first underlying disease
H75.0   Mastoiditis in infectious and parasitic diseases classified elsewhere
   Excludes1:   mastoiditis (in):
     syphilis (A52.77)
     tuberculosis (A18.03)
  H75.00   Mastoiditis in infectious and parasitic diseases classified elsewhere, unspecified ear
  H75.01   Mastoiditis in infectious and parasitic diseases classified elsewhere, right ear
  H75.02   Mastoiditis in infectious and parasitic diseases classified elsewhere, left ear
  H75.03   Mastoiditis in infectious and parasitic diseases classified elsewhere, bilateral

H75.8   Other specified disorders of middle ear and mastoid in diseases classified elsewhere
  H75.80   Other specified disorders of middle ear and mastoid in diseases classified elsewhere, unspecified ear
  H75.81   Other specified disorders of right middle ear and mastoid in diseases classified elsewhere
  H75.82   Other specified disorders of left middle ear and mastoid in diseases classified elsewhere
  H75.83   Other specified disorders of middle ear and mastoid in diseases classified elsewhere, bilateral

DISEASES OF INNER EAR (H80–H83)

H80 Otosclerosis
  Includes: otospongiosis
H80.0   Otosclerosis involving oval window, nonobliterative
  H80.00   Otosclerosis involving oval window, nonobliterative, unspecified ear
  H80.01   Otosclerosis involving oval window, nonobliterative, right ear
  H80.02   Otosclerosis involving oval window, nonobliterative, left ear
  H80.03   Otosclerosis involving oval window, nonobliterative, bilateral
H80.1   Otosclerosis involving oval window, obliterative
  H80.10   Otosclerosis involving oval window, obliterative, unspecified ear
  H80.11   Otosclerosis involving oval window, obliterative, right ear
  H80.12   Otosclerosis involving oval window, obliterative, left ear
  H80.13   Otosclerosis involving oval window, obliterative, bilateral
H80.2   Cochlear otosclerosis
  Otosclerosis involving otic capsule
  Otosclerosis involving round window
  H80.20   Cochlear otosclerosis, unspecified ear
  H80.21   Cochlear otosclerosis, right ear
  H80.22   Cochlear otosclerosis, left ear
  H80.23   Cochlear otosclerosis, bilateral
H80.8   Other otosclerosis
  H80.80   Other otosclerosis, unspecified ear
  H80.81   Other otosclerosis, right ear
  H80.82   Other otosclerosis, left ear
  H80.83   Other otosclerosis, bilateral
H80.9   Unspecified otosclerosis
  H80.90   Unspecified otosclerosis, unspecified ear
  H80.91   Unspecified otosclerosis, right ear
  H80.92   Unspecified otosclerosis, left ear
  H80.93   Unspecified otosclerosis, bilateral

H81 Disorders of vestibular function
  Excludes1:   epidemic vertigo (A88.1)
     vertigo NOS (R42)
H81.0   Ménière's disease
  Labyrinthine hydrops
  Ménière's syndrome or vertigo
  H81.0x   Ménière's disease
   H81.0x1   Ménière's disease, right ear
   H81.0x2   Ménière's disease, left ear
   H81.0x3   Ménière's disease, bilateral
   H81.0x9   Ménière's disease, unspecified ear
H81.1   Benign paroxysmal vertigo
  H81.10   Benign paroxysmal vertigo, unspecified ear
  H81.11   Benign paroxysmal vertigo, right ear
  H81.12   Benign paroxysmal vertigo, left ear
  H81.13   Benign paroxysmal vertigo, bilateral
H81.2   Vestibular neuronitis
  H81.20   Vestibular neuronitis, unspecified ear
  H81.21   Vestibular neuronitis, right ear
  H81.22   Vestibular neuronitis, left ear

H81.23   Vestibular neuronitis, bilateral
H81.3   Other peripheral vertigo
   H81.31   Aural vertigo
     H81.311   Aural vertigo, right ear
     H81.312   Aural vertigo, left ear
     H81.313   Aural vertigo, bilateral
     H81.319   Aural vertigo, unspecified ear
   H81.39   Other peripheral vertigo
      Lermoyez' syndrome
      Otogenic vertigo
      Peripheral vertigo NOS
     H81.391   Other peripheral vertigo, right ear
     H81.392   Other peripheral vertigo, left ear
     H81.393   Other peripheral vertigo, bilateral
     H81.399   Other peripheral vertigo, unspecified ear
H81.4   Vertigo of central origin
    Central positional nystagmus
   H81.4x   Vertigo of central origin
     H81.4x1   Vertigo of central origin, right ear
     H81.4x2   Vertigo of central origin, left ear
     H81.4x3   Vertigo of central origin, bilateral
     H81.4x9   Vertigo of central origin, unspecified ear
H81.8   Other disorders of vestibular function
   H81.8x   Other disorders of vestibular function
     H81.8x1   Other disorders of vestibular function, right ear
     H81.8x2   Other disorders of vestibular function, left ear
     H81.8x3   Other disorders of vestibular function, bilateral
     H81.8x9   Other disorders of vestibular function, unspecified ear
H81.9   Unspecified disorder of vestibular function
    Vertiginous syndrome NOS
   H81.90   Unspecified disorder of vestibular function, unspecified ear
   H81.91   Unspecified disorder of vestibular function, right ear
   H81.92   Unspecified disorder of vestibular function, left ear
   H81.93   Unspecified disorder of vestibular function, bilateral

H82   Vertiginous syndromes in diseases classified elsewhere
    Code first underlying disease
    Excludes1:   epidemic vertigo (A88.1)
H82.1   Vertiginous syndromes in diseases classified elsewhere, right ear
H82.2   Vertiginous syndromes in diseases classified elsewhere, left ear
H82.3   Vertiginous syndromes in diseases classified elsewhere, bilateral
H82.9   Vertiginous syndromes in diseases classified elsewhere, unspecified ear

H83   Other diseases of inner ear
H83.0   Labyrinthitis
   H83.0x   Labyrinthitis
     H83.0x1   Labyrinthitis, right ear
     H83.0x2   Labyrinthitis, left ear
     H83.0x3   Labyrinthitis, bilateral
     H83.0x9   Labyrinthitis, unspecified ear
H83.1   Labyrinthine fistula
   H83.1x   Labyrinthine fistula
     H83.1x1   Labyrinthine fistula, right ear
     H83.1x2   Labyrinthine fistula, left ear
     H83.1x3   Labyrinthine fistula, bilateral
     H83.1x9   Labyrinthine fistula, unspecified ear
H83.2   Labyrinthine dysfunction
    Labyrinthine hypersensitivity
    Labyrinthine hypofunction
    Labyrinthine loss of function
   H83.2x   Labyrinthine dysfunction
     H83.2x1   Labyrinthine dysfunction, right ear
     H83.2x2   Labyrinthine dysfunction, left ear

     H83.2x3   Labyrinthine dysfunction, bilateral
     H83.2x9   Labyrinthine dysfunction, unspecified ear
H83.3   Noise effects on inner ear
    Acoustic trauma of inner ear
    Noise-induced hearing loss of inner ear
   H83.3x   Noise effects on inner ear
     H83.3x1   Noise effects on right inner ear
     H83.3x2   Noise effects on left inner ear
     H83.3x3   Noise effects on inner ear, bilateral
     H83.3x9   Noise effects on inner ear, unspecified ear
H83.8   Other specified diseases of inner ear
   H83.8x   Other specified diseases of inner ear
     H83.8x1   Other specified diseases of right inner ear
     H83.8x2   Other specified diseases of left inner ear
     H83.8x3   Other specified diseases of inner ear, bilateral
     H83.8x9   Other specified diseases of inner ear, unspecified ear
H83.9   Unspecified disease of inner ear
   H83.90   Unspecified disease of inner ear, unspecified ear
   H83.91   Unspecified disease of right inner ear
   H83.92   Unspecified disease of left inner ear
   H83.93   Unspecified disease of inner ear, bilateral

OTHER DISORDERS OF EAR (H90–H95)

H90   Conductive and sensorineural hearing loss
    Excludes1:   deaf mutism NEC (H91.3)
              deafness NOS (H91.9-)
              hearing loss NOS (H91.9-)
              noise-induced hearing loss (H83.3-)
              ototoxic hearing loss (H91.0-)
              sudden (idiopathic) hearing loss (H91.2-)
H90.0   Conductive hearing loss, bilateral
H90.1   Conductive hearing loss, unilateral with unrestricted hearing on the contralateral side
   H90.11   Conductive hearing loss, unilateral, right ear, with unrestricted hearing on the contralateral side
   H90.12   Conductive hearing loss, unilateral, left ear, with unrestricted hearing on the contralateral side
H90.2   Conductive hearing loss, unspecified
    Conductive deafness NOS
H90.3   Sensorineural hearing loss, bilateral
H90.4   Sensorineural hearing loss, unilateral with unrestricted hearing on the contralateral side
   H90.41   Sensorineural hearing loss, unilateral, right ear, with unrestricted hearing on the contralateral side
   H90.42   Sensorineural hearing loss, unilateral, left ear, with unrestricted hearing on the contralateral side
H90.5   Unspecified sensorineural hearing loss
    Central hearing loss NOS
    Neural hearing loss NOS
    Perceptive hearing loss NOS
    Sensorineural deafness NOS
    Sensory hearing loss NOS
    Excludes1:   abnormal auditory perception (H93.2)
              psychogenic deafness (F44.6)
H90.6   Mixed conductive and sensorineural hearing loss, bilateral
H90.7   Mixed conductive and sensorineural hearing loss, unilateral with unrestricted hearing on the contralateral side
   H90.71   Mixed conductive and sensorineural hearing loss, unilateral, right ear, with unrestricted hearing on the contralateral side
   H90.72   Mixed conductive and sensorineural hearing loss, unilateral, left ear, with unrestricted hearing on the contralateral side
H90.8   Mixed conductive and sensorineural hearing loss, unspecified

H91 Other and unspecified hearing loss

> Excludes1:   abnormal auditory perception (H93.2-)
> hearing loss as classified in H90.-
> impacted cerumen (H61.2-)
> noise-induced hearing loss (H83.3-)
> psychogenic deafness (F44.6)
> transient ischemic deafness (H93.01-)

H91.0 Ototoxic hearing loss

> Use additional external cause code (Chapter XIX), to identify toxic agent

H91.0x   Ototoxic hearing loss

    H91.0x1 Ototoxic hearing loss, right ear
    H91.0x2 Ototoxic hearing loss, left ear
    H91.0x3 Ototoxic hearing loss, bilateral
    H91.0x9 Ototoxic hearing loss, unspecified ear

H91.1 Presbycusis

> Presbyacusia

    H91.10   Presbycusis, unspecified ear
    H91.11   Presbycusis, right ear
    H91.12   Presbycusis, left ear
    H91.13   Presbycusis, bilateral

H91.2 Sudden idiopathic hearing loss

> Sudden hearing loss NOS

    H91.20   Sudden idiopathic hearing loss, unspecified ear
    H91.21   Sudden idiopathic hearing loss, right ear
    H91.22   Sudden idiopathic hearing loss, left ear
    H91.23   Sudden idiopathic hearing loss, bilateral

H91.3 Deaf mutism, not elsewhere classified

H91.8 Other specified hearing loss

H91.8x   Other specified hearing loss

    H91.8x1 Other specified hearing loss, right ear
    H91.8x2 Other specified hearing loss, left ear
    H91.8x3 Other specified hearing loss, bilateral
    H91.8x9 Other specified hearing loss, unspecified ear

H91.9 Unspecified hearing loss

> Congenital deafness NOS
> Deafness NOS
> High frequency deafness
> Low frequency deafness

    H91.90   Unspecified hearing loss, unspecified ear
    H91.91   Unspecified hearing loss, right ear
    H91.92   Unspecified hearing loss, left ear
    H91.93   Unspecified hearing loss, bilateral

H92 Otalgia and effusion of ear

H92.0 Otalgia

H92.0x   Otalgia

    H92.0x1 Otalgia, right ear
    H92.0x2 Otalgia, left ear
    H92.0x3 Otalgia, bilateral
    H92.0x9 Otalgia, unspecified ear

H92.1 Otorrhea

> Excludes1:   leakage of cerebrospinal fluid through ear (G96.0)

    H92.10   Otorrhea, unspecified ear
    H92.11   Otorrhea, right ear
    H92.12   Otorrhea, left ear
    H92.13   Otorrhea, bilateral

H92.2 Otorrhagia

> Excludes1:   traumatic otorrhagia — code to injury

    H92.20   Otorrhagia, unspecified ear
    H92.21   Otorrhagia, right ear
    H92.22   Otorrhagia, left ear
    H92.23   Otorrhagia, bilateral

H93 Other disorders of ear, not elsewhere classified

H93.0 Degenerative and vascular disorders of ear

> Excludes1:   presbycusis (H91.1-)

    H93.00   Unspecified degenerative and vascular disorders of ear
        H93.001 Unspecified degenerative and vascular disorders of right ear

        H93.002 Unspecified degenerative and vascular disorders of left ear
        H93.003 Unspecified degenerative and vascular disorders of ear, bilateral
        H93.009 Unspecified degenerative and vascular disorders of unspecified ear

    H93.01   Transient ischemic deafness
        H93.011 Transient ischemic deafness, right ear
        H93.012 Transient ischemic deafness, left ear
        H93.013 Transient ischemic deafness, bilateral
        H93.019 Transient ischemic deafness, unspecified ear

H93.1 Tinnitus

    H93.1x   Tinnitus
        H93.1x1 Tinnitus, right ear
        H93.1x2 Tinnitus, left ear
        H93.1x3 Tinnitus, bilateral
        H93.1x9 Tinnitus, unspecified ear

H93.2 Other abnormal auditory perceptions

> Excludes2:   auditory hallucinations (R44.0)

    H92.21   Auditory recruitment
        H92.211 Auditory recruitment, right ear
        H92.212 Auditory recruitment, left ear
        H92.213 Auditory recruitment, bilateral
        H92.219 Auditory recruitment, unspecified ear

    H93.22   Diplacusis
        H93.221 Diplacusis, right ear
        H93.222 Diplacusis, left ear
        H93.223 Diplacusis, bilateral
        H93.229 Diplacusis, unspecified ear

    H93.23   Hyperacusis
        H93.231 Hyperacusis, right ear
        H93.232 Hyperacusis, left ear
        H93.233 Hyperacusis, bilateral
        H93.239 Hyperacusis, unspecified ear

    H93.24   Temporary auditory threshold shift
        H93.241 Temporary auditory threshold shift, right ear
        H93.242 Temporary auditory threshold shift, left ear
        H93.243 Temporary auditory threshold shift, bilateral
        H93.249 Temporary auditory threshold shift, unspecified ear

    H93.29   Other abnormal auditory perceptions
        H93.291 Other abnormal auditory perceptions, right ear
        H93.292 Other abnormal auditory perceptions, left ear
        H93.293 Other abnormal auditory perceptions, bilateral
        H93.299 Other abnormal auditory perceptions, unspecified ear

H93.3 Disorders of acoustic nerve

> Disorder of 8th cranial nerve
>
> Excludes1:   acoustic neuroma (D33.3)
> syphilitic acoustic neuritis (A52.15)

    H93.3x   Disorders of acoustic nerve
        H93.3x1 Disorders of right acoustic nerve
        H93.3x2 Disorders of left acoustic nerve
        H93.3x3 Disorders of bilateral acoustic nerves
        H93.3x9 Disorders of unspecified acoustic nerve

H93.8 Other specified disorders of ear

    H93.8x   Other specified disorders of ear
        H93.8x1 Other specified disorders of right ear
        H93.8x2 Other specified disorders of left ear
        H93.8x3 Other specified disorders of ear, bilateral
        H93.8x9 Other specified disorders of ear, unspecified ear

H93.9 Unspecified disorder of ear

    H93.90   Unspecified disorder of ear, unspecified ear
    H93.91   Unspecified disorder of right ear
    H93.92   Unspecified disorder of left ear
    H93.93   Unspecified disorder of ear, bilateral

H94 Other disorders of ear in diseases classified elsewhere

H94.0 Acoustic neuritis in infectious and parasitic diseases classified elsewhere

Code first underlying disease, such as:
parasitic disease (B65-B89)

Excludes1:   acoustic neuritis (in):
herpes zoster (B02.29)
syphilis (A52.15)

H94.00 Acoustic neuritis in infectious and parasitic diseases classified elsewhere, unspecified ear

H94.01 Acoustic neuritis in infectious and parasitic diseases classified elsewhere, right ear

H94.02 Acoustic neuritis in infectious and parasitic diseases classified elsewhere, left ear

H94.03 Acoustic neuritis in infectious and parasitic diseases classified elsewhere, bilateral

H94.8 Other specified disorders of ear in diseases classified elsewhere

Code first underlying disease, such as:
congenital syphilis (A50.0)

Excludes1:   aural myiasis (B87.4)
syphilitic labyrinthitis (A52.79)

H94.80 Other specified disorders of ear in diseases classified elsewhere, unspecified ear

H94.81 Other specified disorders of right ear in diseases classified elsewhere

H94.82 Other specified disorders of left ear in diseases classified elsewhere

H94.83 Other specified disorders of ear in diseases classified elsewhere, bilateral

H95 Intraoperative and postprocedural complications and disorders of ear and mastoid process, not elsewhere classified

H95.0 Recurrent cholesteatoma of postmastoidectomy cavity

H95.00 Recurrent cholesteatoma of postmastoidectomy cavity, unspecified side

H95.01 Recurrent cholesteatoma of postmastoidectomy cavity, right side

H95.02 Recurrent cholesteatoma of postmastoidectomy cavity, left side

H95.03 Recurrent cholesteatoma of postmastoidectomy cavity, bilateral

H95.1 Other disorders following mastoidectomy

H95.11 Chronic inflammation following mastoidectomy

H95.111 Chronic inflammation following mastoidectomy, right side

H95.112 Chronic inflammation following mastoidectomy, left side

H95.113 Chronic inflammation following mastoidectomy, bilateral

H95.119 Chronic inflammation following mastoidectomy, unspecified side

H95.12 Granulation of postmastoidectomy cavity

H95.121 Granulation of postmastoidectomy cavity, right side

H95.122 Granulation of postmastoidectomy cavity, left side

H95.123 Granulation of postmastoidectomy cavity, bilateral

H95.129 Granulation of postmastoidectomy cavity, unspecified side

H95.13 Mucosal cyst following mastoidectomy

H95.131 Mucosal cyst following mastoidectomy, right side

H95.132 Mucosal cyst following mastoidectomy, left side

H95.133 Mucosal cyst following mastoidectomy, bilateral

H95.139 Mucosal cyst following mastoidectomy, unspecified side

H95.19 Other disorders following mastoidectomy

H95.191 Other disorders following mastoidectomy, right side

H95.192 Other disorders following mastoidectomy, left side

H95.193 Other disorders following mastoidectomy, bilateral

H95.199 Other disorders following mastoidectomy, unspecified side

H95.2 Intraoperative and postprocedural hemorrhage or hematoma complicating a procedure of the ear and mastoid process

Excludes1:   intraoperative hemorrhage or hematoma due to accidental puncture of laceration during a procedure on the ear (H95.3-)

H95.21 Intraoperative hemorrhage of the ear and mastoid process during a procedure of the ear and mastoid process

H95.22 Intraoperative hemorrhage of other organ or structure during a procedure of the ear and mastoid process

H95.23 Intraoperative hematoma of the ear and mastoid process during a procedure of the ear and mastoid process

H95.24 Intraoperative hematoma of other organ or structure during a procedure of the ear and mastoid process

H95.25 Postprocedural hemorrhage of the ear and mastoid process following a procedure of the ear and mastoid process

H95.26 Postprocedural hemorrhage of other organ or structure following a procedure of the ear and mastoid process

H95.27 Postprocedural hematoma of the ear and mastoid process following a procedure of the ear and mastoid process

H95.28 Postprocedural hematoma of other organ or structure following a procedure of the ear and mastoid process

H95.3 Accidental puncture or laceration during an ear procedure

H95.31 Accidental puncture or laceration of the ear during an ear procedure

H95.32 Accidental puncture or laceration of other organ or structure during an ear procedure

H95.8 Other intraoperative and postprocedural complications and disorders of the ear and mastoid process

Excludes1:   postprocedural complications and disorders following mastoidectomy (H95.0-, H95.1-)

H95.81 Postprocedural stenosis of external ear canal

H95.811 Postprocedural stenosis of right external ear canal

H95.812 Postprocedural stenosis of left external ear canal

H95.813 Postprocedural stenosis of external ear canal, bilateral

H95.819 Postprocedural stenosis of unspecified external ear canal

H95.82 Other intraoperative complications of the ear and mastoid process

H95.821 Other intraoperative complications of the right ear and mastoid process

H95.822 Other intraoperative complications the left ear and mastoid process

H95.829 Other intraoperative complications of unspecified ear and mastoid process

H95.89 Other postprocedural complications and disorders of the ear and mastoid process

H95.891 Other postprocedural complications and disorders of the right ear and mastoid process

H95.892 Other postprocedural complications and disorders of the left ear and mastoid process

H95.899 Other postprocedural complications and disorders of unspecified ear and mastoid process

H95.9   Unspecified intraoperative and postprocedural complications and disorder of the ear and mastoid process

    H95.91   Unspecified intraoperative complication and disorder of the ear and mastoid process

        H95.911   Unspecified intraoperative complication and disorder of the right ear and mastoid process

        H95.912   Unspecified intraoperative complication and disorder of the left ear and mastoid process

        H95.919   Unspecified intraoperative complication and disorder of unspecified ear and mastoid process

    H95.99   Unspecified postprocedural complication and disorder of the ear and mastoid process

        H95.991   Unspecified postprocedural complication and disorder of the right ear and mastoid process

        H95.992   Unspecified postprocedural complication and disorder of the left ear and mastoid process

        H95.999   Unspecified postprocedural complication and disorder of unspecified ear and mastoid process

CHAPTER IX — DISEASES OF THE CIRCULATORY SYSTEM (I00–I99)

Excludes2: certain conditions originating in the perinatal period (P04-P96)
certain infectious and parasitic diseases (A00-B99)
complications of pregnancy, childbirth and the puerperium (O00-O99)
congenital malformations, deformations, and chromosomal abnormalities (Q00-Q99)
endocrine, nutritional and metabolic diseases (E00-E90)
injury, poisoning and certain other consequences of external causes (S00-T98)
neoplasms (C00-D48)
symptoms, signs and abnormal clinical and laboratory findings, not elsewhere classified (R00-R94)
systemic connective tissue disorders (M30-M36)
transient cerebral ischemic attacks and related syndromes (G45.-)

This chapter contains the following blocks:
I00-I02 Acute rheumatic fever
I05-I09 Chronic rheumatic heart diseases
I10-I15 Hypertensive diseases
I20-I25 Ischemic heart diseases
I26-I28 Pulmonary heart disease and diseases of pulmonary circulation
I30-I52 Other forms of heart disease
I60-I69 Cerebrovascular diseases
I70-I79 Diseases of arteries, arterioles and capillaries
I80-I89 Diseases of veins, lymphatic vessels and lymph nodes, not elsewhere classified
I95-I99 Other and unspecified disorders of the circulatory system

ACUTE RHEUMATIC FEVER (I00–I02)

I00 Rheumatic fever without heart involvement
Includes: arthritis, rheumatic, acute or subacute
Excludes1: rheumatic fever with heart involvement (I01.0 - I01.9)

I01 Rheumatic fever with heart involvement
Excludes1: chronic diseases of rheumatic origin (I05-I09) unless rheumatic fever is also present or there is evidence of reactivation or activity of the rheumatic process.

I01.0 Acute rheumatic pericarditis
Any condition in I00 with pericarditis
Rheumatic pericarditis (acute)
Excludes1: acute pericarditis not specified as rheumatic (I30.-)

I01.1 Acute rheumatic endocarditis
Any condition in I00 with endocarditis or valvulitis
Acute rheumatic valvulitis

I01.2 Acute rheumatic myocarditis
Any condition in I00 with myocarditis

I01.8 Other acute rheumatic heart disease
Any condition in I00 with other or multiple types of heart involvement
Acute rheumatic pancarditis

I01.9 Acute rheumatic heart disease, unspecified
Any condition in I00 with unspecified type of heart involvement
Rheumatic carditis, acute
Rheumatic heart disease, active or acute

I02 Rheumatic chorea
Includes: Sydenham's chorea
Excludes1: chorea NOS (G25.5)
Huntington's chorea (G10)

I02.0 Rheumatic chorea with heart involvement
Chorea NOS with heart involvement
Rheumatic chorea with heart involvement of any type classifiable under I01.-

I02.9 Rheumatic chorea without heart involvement
Rheumatic chorea NOS

CHRONIC RHEUMATIC HEART DISEASES (I05–I09)

I05 Rheumatic mitral valve diseases
Includes: conditions classifiable to both I05.0 and I05.2-I05.9, whether specified as rheumatic or not
Excludes1: mitral valve disease specified as nonrheumatic (I34.-)
mitral valve disease with aortic and/or tricuspid valve involvement (I08.-)

I05.0 Rheumatic mitral stenosis
Mitral (valve) obstruction (rheumatic)

I05.1 Rheumatic mitral insufficiency
Rheumatic mitral incompetence
Rheumatic mitral regurgitation
Excludes1: mitral insufficiency not specified as rheumatic (I34.0)

I05.2 Rheumatic mitral stenosis with insufficiency
Rheumatic mitral stenosis with incompetence or regurgitation

I05.8 Other rheumatic mitral valve diseases
Rheumatic mitral (valve) failure

I05.9 Rheumatic mitral valve disease, unspecified
Rheumatic mitral (valve) disorder (chronic) NOS

I06 Rheumatic aortic valve diseases
Excludes1: aortic valve disease not specified as rheumatic (I35.-)
aortic valve disease with mitral and/or tricuspid valve involvement (I08.-)

I06.0 Rheumatic aortic stenosis
Rheumatic aortic (valve) obstruction

I06.1 Rheumatic aortic insufficiency
Rheumatic aortic incompetence
Rheumatic aortic regurgitation

I06.2 Rheumatic aortic stenosis with insufficiency
Rheumatic aortic stenosis with incompetence or regurgitation

I06.8 Other rheumatic aortic valve diseases

I06.9 Rheumatic aortic valve disease, unspecified
Rheumatic aortic (valve) disease NOS

I07 Rheumatic tricuspid valve diseases
Includes: rheumatic tricuspid valve diseases whether specified as rheumatic or not
Excludes1: tricuspid valve disease specified as nonrheumatic (I36.-) those with aortic and/or mitral valve involvement (I08.-)

I07.0 Rheumatic tricuspid stenosis
Tricuspid (valve) stenosis (rheumatic)

I07.1 Rheumatic tricuspid insufficiency
Tricuspid (valve) insufficiency (rheumatic)

I07.2 Rheumatic tricuspid stenosis and insufficiency

I07.8 Other rheumatic tricuspid valve diseases

I07.9 Rheumatic tricuspid valve disease, unspecified
Rheumatic tricuspid valve disorder NOS

I08 Multiple valve diseases
Includes: multiple valve diseases whether specified as rheumatic or not
Excludes1: endocarditis, valve unspecified (I38)
rheumatic valve disease NOS (I09.1)

I08.0 Rheumatic disorders of both mitral and aortic valves
Involvement of both mitral and aortic valves whether specified as rheumatic or not

I08.1 Rheumatic disorders of both mitral and tricuspid valves

I08.2 Rheumatic disorders of both aortic and tricuspid valves

I08.3 Combined rheumatic disorders of mitral, aortic and tricuspid valves

I08.8 Other rheumatic multiple valve diseases

I08.9 Rheumatic multiple valve disease, unspecified

I09 Other rheumatic heart diseases
I09.0 Rheumatic myocarditis
Excludes1: myocarditis not specified as rheumatic (I51.4)

I09.1 Rheumatic diseases of endocardium, valve unspecified
Rheumatic endocarditis (chronic)
Rheumatic valvulitis (chronic)
Excludes1: endocarditis, valve unspecified (I38)

I09.2 Chronic rheumatic pericarditis
Adherent pericardium, rheumatic
Chronic rheumatic mediastinopericarditis
Chronic rheumatic myopericarditis
Excludes1: chronic pericarditis not specified as rheumatic (I31.-)

I09.8 Other specified rheumatic heart diseases

I09.81 Rheumatic heart failure
Use additional code to identify type of heart failure (I50.-)

I09.89 Other specified rheumatic heart diseases
Rheumatic disease of pulmonary valve

I09.9 Rheumatic heart disease, unspecified
Rheumatic carditis
Excludes1: rheumatoid carditis (M05.31)

HYPERTENSIVE DISEASES (I10–I15)
Use additional code to identify:
exposure to environmental tobacco smoke (X58.1)
history of tobacco use (Z86.43)
occupational exposure to environmental tobacco smoke (Z57.31)
tobacco dependence (F17.-)
tobacco use (Z72.0)
Excludes1: hypertensive disease complicating pregnancy, childbirth and the puerperium (O10-O11, O13-O16)
neonatal hypertension (P29.2)
pulmonary hypertension (I27.0)

I10 Essential (primary) hypertension
Includes: high blood pressure
hypertension (arterial) (benign) (essential) (malignant) (primary) (systemic)
Excludes2: essential (primary) hypertension involving vessels of brain (I60-I69)
essential (primary) hypertension involving vessels of eye (H35.0)

I11 Hypertensive heart disease
Includes: any condition in I51.4-I51.9 with hypertension

I11.0 Hypertensive heart disease with heart failure
Any condition in I50.- with hypertension
Hypertensive heart failure
Use additional code to identify type of heart failure (I50.-)

I11.9 Hypertensive heart disease without heart failure
Hypertensive heart disease NOS

I12 Hypertensive renal disease
Includes: any condition in N18.- with any condition in I10
arteriosclerosis of kidney
arteriosclerotic nephritis (chronic) (interstitial)
hypertensive nephropathy
nephrosclerosis
Excludes1: renovascular hypertension (I15.0)
secondary hypertension (I15.-)
Excludes2: acute renal failure (N17.-)

I12.0 Hypertensive renal disease with chronic renal failure
Any condition in N18.- with hypertension
Hypertensive renal failure

I12.9 Hypertensive renal disease without renal failure
Hypertensive renal disease NOS

I13 Hypertensive heart and renal disease
Includes: any condition in I11.- with any condition in I12.-
cardiorenal disease
cardiovascular renal disease

I13.0 Hypertensive heart and renal disease with heart failure
Use additional code to identify type of heart failure (I50.-)

I13.1 Hypertensive heart and renal disease with chronic renal failure

I13.2 Hypertensive heart and renal disease with both heart failure and chronic renal failure
Use additional code to identify type of heart failure (I50.-)

I13.9 Hypertensive heart and renal disease, unspecified

I15 Secondary hypertension
Excludes1: postoperative hypertension (I97.3)
Excludes2: secondary hypertension involving vessels of brain (I60-I69)
secondary hypertension involving vessels of eye (H35.0)

I15.0 Renovascular hypertension
I15.1 Hypertension secondary to other renal disorders
I15.2 Hypertension secondary to endocrine disorders
I15.8 Other secondary hypertension
I15.9 Secondary hypertension, unspecified

ISCHEMIC HEART DISEASES (I20–I25)
Use additional code to identify presence of hypertension (I10-I15)

I20 Angina pectoris
Use additional code to identify:
exposure to environmental tobacco smoke (X58.1)
history of tobacco use (Z86.43)
occupational exposure to environmental tobacco smoke (Z57.31)
tobacco dependence (F17.-)
tobacco use (Z72.0)
Excludes1: angina pectoris with atherosclerotic heart disease of native coronary arteries (I25.1-)
angina pectoris with atherosclerotic heart disease of coronary artery bypass grafts (I25.7-)
postinfarction angina (I23.7)

I20.0 Unstable angina
Accelerated angina
Crescendo angina
De novo effort angina
Intermediate coronary syndrome
Preinfarction syndrome
Worsening effort angina

I20.1 Angina pectoris with documented spasm
Angiospastic angina
Prinzmetal angina
Spasm-induced angina
Variant angina

I20.8 Other forms of angina pectoris
Angina of effort
Stenocardia

I20.9 Angina pectoris, unspecified
Angina NOS
Anginal syndrome
Cardiac angina
Ischemic chest pain

I21 Acute myocardial infarction
Includes: cardiac infarction
coronary (artery) embolism
coronary (artery) occlusion
coronary (artery) rupture
coronary (artery) thrombosis
infarction of heart, myocardium, or ventricle
myocardial infarction specified as acute or with a stated duration of 4 weeks (28 days) or less from onset
rupture of heart, myocardium, or ventricle
Use additional code to identify:
exposure to environmental tobacco smoke (X58.1)
history of tobacco use (Z86.43)
occupational exposure to environmental tobacco smoke (Z57.31)
tobacco dependence (F17.-)
tobacco use (Z72.0)
Excludes2: old myocardial infarction (Z86.71)
postmyocardial infarction syndrome (I24.1)
subsequent myocardial infarction (I22.-)

I21.0 Acute transmural myocardial infarction of anterior wall
Anteroapical transmural (Q wave) infarction (acute)
Anterolateral transmural (Q wave) infarction (acute)
Anteroseptal transmural (Q wave) infarction (acute)
Transmural (Q wave) infarction (acute) (of) anterior (wall) NOS

I21.1   Acute transmural myocardial infarction of inferior wall
Inferolateral transmural (Q wave) infarction (acute)
Inferoposterior transmural (Q wave) infarction (acute)
Transmural (Q wave) infarction (acute) (of) diaphragmatic wall
Transmural (Q wave) infarction (acute) (of) inferior (wall) NOS

I21.2   Acute transmural myocardial infarction of other sites
Apical-lateral transmural (Q wave) infarction (acute)
Basal-lateral transmural (Q wave) infarction (acute)
High lateral transmural (Q wave) infarction (acute)
Lateral (wall) NOS transmural (Q wave) infarction (acute)
Posterior (true) transmural (Q wave) infarction (acute)
Posterobasal transmural (Q wave) infarction (acute)
Posterolateral transmural (Q wave) infarction (acute)
Posteroseptal transmural (Q wave) infarction (acute)
Septal transmural (Q wave) infarction (acute) NOS

I21.3   Acute transmural myocardial infarction of unspecified site
Transmural (Q wave) myocardial infarction NOS

I21.4   Acute subendocardial myocardial infarction
Non-Q wave myocardial infarction NOS
Nontransmural myocardial infarction NOS

I21.9   Acute myocardial infarction, unspecified
Myocardial infarction (acute) NOS

I22   Subsequent acute myocardial infarction
Includes: acute myocardial infarction occurring within four
weeks (28 days) of a previous acute myocardial
infarction, regardless of site
cardiac infarction
coronary (artery) embolism
coronary (artery) occlusion
coronary (artery) rupture
coronary (artery) thrombosis
infarction of heart, myocardium, or ventricle
rupture of heart, myocardium, or ventricle
Note: A code from category I22 must be used in conjunction with a
code from category I21. The I22 code should be sequenced first, if it
is the reason for encounter, or, it should be sequenced after the I21
code if the subsequent MI occurs during the encounter for the initial
MI.
Use additional code to identify:
exposure to environmental tobacco smoke (X58.1)
history of tobacco use (Z86.43)
occupational exposure to environmental tobacco smoke (Z57.31)
tobacco dependence (F17.-)
tobacco use (Z72.0)

I22.0   Subsequent acute transmural myocardial infarction of anterior wall
Subsequent transmural (Q wave) infarction (acute)(of) anterior
(wall) NOS
Subsequent anteroapical transmural (Q wave) infarction (acute)
Subsequent anterolateral transmural (Q wave) infarction (acute)
Subsequent anteroseptal transmural (Q wave) infarction (acute)

I22.1   Subsequent acute transmural myocardial infarction of inferior wall
Subsequent transmural (Q wave) infarction (acute)(of)
diaphragmatic wall
Subsequent transmural (Q wave) infarction (acute)(of) inferior
(wall) NOS
Subsequent inferolateral transmural (Q wave) infarction (acute)
Subsequent inferoposterior transmural (Q wave) infarction
(acute)

I22.2   Subsequent acute transmural myocardial infarction of unspecified site Subsequent transmural (Q wave) myocardial infarction NOS

I22.3   Subsequent acute subendocardial myocardial infarction
Subsequent nontransmural (non-Q wave) myocardial infarction
NOS

I22.8   Subsequent acute transmural myocardial infarction of other sites
Subsequent apical-lateral transmural (Q wave) myocardial
infarction (acute)
Subsequent basal-lateral transmural (Q wave) myocardial
infarction (acute)
Subsequent high lateral transmural (Q wave) myocardial
infarction (acute)
Subsequent transmural (Q wave) myocardial infarction
(acute)(of) lateral (wall) NOS
Subsequent posterior (true)transmural (Q wave) myocardial
infarction (acute)
Subsequent posterobasal transmural (Q wave) myocardial
infarction (acute)
Subsequent posterolateral transmural (Q wave) myocardial
infarction (acute)
Subsequent posteroseptal transmural (Q wave) myocardial
infarction (acute)
Subsequent septal NOS transmural (Q wave) myocardial
infarction (acute)

I22.9   Subsequent acute myocardial infarction of unspecified site
Subsequent myocardial infarction (acute) NOS

I23   Certain current complications following acute myocardial infarction (within the 28 day period)
Note: A code from category I23 must be used in conjunction with a
code from category I21 or category I22. The I23 code should be
sequenced first, if it is the reason for encounter, or, it should be
sequenced after the I21 or I22 code if the complication of the MI
occurs during the encounter for the MI.

I23.0   Hemopericardium as current complication following acute myocardial infarction
Excludes1:   hemopericardium not specified as current
complication following acute myocardial
infarction (I31.2)

I23.1   Atrial septal defect as current complication following acute myocardial infarction
Excludes1:   acquired atrial septal defect not specified as
current complication following acute
myocardial infarction (I51.0)

I23.2   Ventricular septal defect as current complication following acute myocardial infarction
Excludes1:   acquired ventricular septal defect not specified as
current complication following acute
myocardial infarction (I51.0)

I23.3   Rupture of cardiac wall without hemopericardium as current complication following acute myocardial infarction

I23.4   Rupture of chordae tendineae as current complication following acute myocardial infarction
Excludes1:   rupture of chordae tendineae not specified as
current complication following acute
myocardial infarction (I51.1)

I23.5   Rupture of papillary muscle as current complication following acute myocardial infarction
Excludes1:   rupture of papillary muscle not specified as
current complication following acute
myocardial infarction (I51.2)

I23.6   Thrombosis of atrium, auricular appendage, and ventricle as current complications following acute myocardial infarction
Excludes1:   thrombosis of atrium, auricular appendage, and
ventricle not specified as current
complication following acute myocardial
infarction (I51.3)

I23.7   Postinfarction angina

I23.8   Other current complications following acute myocardial infarction

I24   Other acute ischemic heart diseases
Excludes1:   angina pectoris (I20.-)
transient myocardial ischemia in newborn (P29.4)

I24.0 Acute coronary thrombosis not resulting in myocardial infarction
  Coronary (artery) (vein) embolism not resulting in myocardial infarction
  Coronary (artery) (vein) occlusion not resulting in myocardial infarction
  Coronary (artery) (vein) thromboembolism not resulting in myocardial infarction
  Excludes1: atherosclerotic heart disease (I25.1-)

I24.1 Dressler's syndrome
  Postmyocardial infarction syndrome
  Excludes1: postinfarction angina (I23.7)

I24.8 Other forms of acute ischemic heart disease

I24.9 Acute ischemic heart disease, unspecified
  Excludes1: ischemic heart disease (chronic) NOS (I25.9)

I25 Chronic ischemic heart disease
  Use additional code to identify:
  exposure to environmental tobacco smoke (X58.1)
  history of tobacco use (Z86.43)
  occupational exposure to environmental tobacco smoke (Z57.31)
  tobacco dependence (F17.-)
  tobacco use (Z72.0)
  Excludes1: cardiovascular disease NOS (I51.6)

I25.1 Atherosclerotic heart disease
  Atherosclerotic cardiovascular disease
  Atherosclerotic heart disease of native vessel
  Coronary (artery) atheroma
  Coronary (artery) atherosclerosis
  Coronary (artery) disease
  Coronary (artery) sclerosis
  Excludes2: atherosclerosis of coronary artery bypass graft(s) (I25.7-)

I25.10 Atherosclerotic heart disease without angina
  Atherosclerotic heart disease NOS

I25.11 Atherosclerotic heart disease with unspecified angina pectoris
  Atherosclerotic heart disease with angina NOS
  Atherosclerotic heart disease with anginal syndrome
  Atherosclerotic heart disease with cardiac angina
  Atherosclerotic heart disease with ischemic chest pain
  Excludes1: unspecified angina pectoris without atherosclerotic heart disease (I20.9)

I25.12 Atherosclerotic heart disease with unstable angina
  Atherosclerotic heart disease with accelerated angina
  Atherosclerotic heart disease with crescendo angina
  Atherosclerotic heart disease with de novo effort angina
  Atherosclerotic heart disease with intermediate coronary syndrome
  Atherosclerotic heart disease with preinfarction syndrome
  Atherosclerotic heart disease with worsening effort angina
  Excludes1: unstable angina without atherosclerotic heart disease (I20.0)

I25.13 Atherosclerotic heart disease with angina pectoris with documented spasm
  Atherosclerotic heart disease with angiospastic angina
  Atherosclerotic heart disease with prinzmetal angina
  Atherosclerotic heart disease with spasm-induced angina
  Atherosclerotic heart disease with variant angina
  Excludes1: angina pectoris with documented spasm without atherosclerotic heart disease (I20.1)

I25.19 Atherosclerotic heart disease with other forms of angina pectoris
  Atherosclerotic heart disease with angina of effort
  Atherosclerotic heart disease with stenocardia
  Excludes1: other forms of angina pectoris without atherosclerotic heart disease (I20.8)

I25.2 Old myocardial infarction
  Healed myocardial infarction
  Past myocardial infarction diagnosed by ECG or other investigation, but currently presenting no symptoms

I25.3 Aneurysm of heart
  Mural aneurysm
  Ventricular aneurysm

I25.4 Coronary artery aneurysm
  Coronary arteriovenous fistula, acquired
  Excludes1: congenital coronary (artery) aneurysm (Q24.5)

I25.5 Ischemic cardiomyopathy
  Excludes2: coronary atherosclerosis (I25.1-)

I25.6 Silent myocardial ischemia

I25.7 Atherosclerosis of coronary artery bypass graft(s) or coronary artery of transplanted heart
  Excludes1: embolism or thrombus of coronary artery bypass graft(s) (T82.8)

I25.70 Atherosclerosis of coronary artery bypass graft(s), unspecified

I25.700 Atherosclerosis of coronary artery bypass graft(s), unspecified, without angina pectoris
  Atherosclerosis of coronary artery bypass graft(s) NOS

I25.701 Atherosclerosis of coronary artery bypass graft(s), unspecified, with unstable angina pectoris
  Atherosclerosis of coronary artery bypass graft(s), unspecified with accelerated angina
  Atherosclerosis of coronary artery bypass graft(s), unspecified with crescendo angina
  Atherosclerosis of coronary artery bypass graft(s), unspecified with de novo effort angina
  Atherosclerosis of coronary artery bypass graft(s), unspecified with intermediate coronary syndrome
  Atherosclerosis of coronary artery bypass graft(s), unspecified with preinfarction angina
  Atherosclerosis of coronary artery bypass graft(s), unspecified with worsening effort angina
  Excludes1: unstable angina pectoris without atherosclerosis of coronary artery bypass graft (I20.0)

I25.702 Atherosclerosis of coronary artery bypass graft(s), unspecified, with angina pectoris with documented spasm
  Atherosclerosis of coronary artery bypass graft(s), unspecified with angiospastic angina
  Atherosclerosis of coronary artery bypass graft(s), unspecified with prinzmental angina
  Atherosclerosis of coronary artery bypass graft(s), unspecified with spasm-induced angina
  Atherosclerosis of coronary artery bypass graft(s), unspecified with variant angina
  Excludes1: angina pectoris with documented spasm without atherosclerosis of coronary artery bypass graft (I20.1)

I25.708 Atherosclerosis of coronary artery bypass graft(s), unspecified, with other forms of angina pectoris
  Atherosclerosis of coronary artery bypass graft(s), unspecified with angina of effort
  Atherosclerosis of coronary artery bypass graft(s), unspecified with stenocardia
  Excludes1: other forms of angina pectoris without atherosclerosis of coronary artery bypass graft (I20.8)

I25.709   Atherosclerosis of coronary artery bypass graft(s), unspecified, with unspecified angina pectoris

Atherosclerosis of coronary artery bypass graft(s), unspecified with angina NOS

Atherosclerosis of coronary artery bypass graft(s), unspecified with anginal syndrome

Atherosclerosis of coronary artery bypass graft(s), unspecified with cardiac angina

Atherosclerosis of coronary artery bypass graft(s), unspecified with ischemic chest pain

Excludes1:   unspecified angina pectoris without atherosclerosis of coronary artery bypass graft (I20.9)

I25.71   Atherosclerosis of autologous vein coronary artery bypass graft(s)

I25.710   Atherosclerosis of autologous vein coronary artery bypass graft(s) without angina pectoris

Atherosclerosis of autologous vein coronary artery bypass graft(s) NOS

I25.711   Atherosclerosis of autologous vein coronary artery bypass graft(s) with unstable angina pectoris

Atherosclerosis of autologous vein coronary artery bypass graft(s) with accelerated angina

Atherosclerosis of autologous vein coronary artery bypass graft(s) with crescendo angina

Atherosclerosis of autologous vein coronary artery bypass graft(s) with de novo effort angina

Atherosclerosis of autologous vein coronary artery bypass graft(s) with intermediate coronary syndrome

Atherosclerosis of autologous vein coronary artery bypass graft(s) with preinfarction angina

Atherosclerosis of autologous vein coronary artery bypass graft(s) with worsening effort angina

Excludes1:   unstable angina without atherosclerosis of autologous vein coronary artery bypass graft(s) (I20.0)

I25.712   Atherosclerosis of autologous vein coronary artery bypass graft(s) with angina pectoris with documented spasm

Atherosclerosis of autologous vein coronary artery bypass graft(s) with angiospastic angina

Atherosclerosis of autologous vein coronary artery bypass graft(s) with prinzmental angina

Atherosclerosis of autologous vein coronary artery bypass graft(s) with spasm-induced angina

Atherosclerosis of autologous vein coronary artery bypass graft(s) with variant angina

Excludes1:   angina pectoris with documented spasm without atherosclerosis of autologous vein coronary artery bypass graft(s) (I20.1)

I25.718   Atherosclerosis of autologous vein coronary artery bypass graft(s) with other forms of angina pectoris

Atherosclerosis of autologous vein coronary artery bypass graft(s) with angina of effort

Atherosclerosis of autologous vein coronary artery bypass graft(s) with stenocardia

Excludes1:   other forms of angina pectoris without atherosclerosis of autologous vein coronary artery bypass graft(s)(I20.8)

I25.719   Atherosclerosis of autologous vein coronary artery bypass graft(s) with unspecified angina pectoris

Atherosclerosis of autologous vein coronary artery bypass graft(s) with angina NOS

Atherosclerosis of autologous vein coronary artery bypass graft(s) with anginal syndrome

Atherosclerosis of autologous vein coronary artery bypass graft(s) with cardiac angina

Atherosclerosis of autologous vein coronary artery bypass graft(s) with ischemic chest pain

Excludes1:   unspecified angina pectoris without atherosclerosis of autologous vein coronary artery bypass graft(s) (I20.9)

I25.72   Atherosclerosis of autologous artery coronary artery bypass graft(s)

Atherosclerosis of internal mammary artery graft

I25.720   Atherosclerosis of autologous artery coronary artery bypass graft(s) without angina pectoris

Atherosclerosis of autologous artery coronary artery bypass graft(s) NOS

I25.721   Atherosclerosis of autologous artery coronary artery bypass graft(s) with unstable angina pectoris

Atherosclerosis of autologous artery coronary artery bypass graft(s) with accelerated angina

Atherosclerosis of autologous artery coronary artery bypass graft(s) with crescendo angina

Atherosclerosis of autologous artery coronary artery bypass graft(s) with de novo effort angina

Atherosclerosis of autologous artery coronary artery bypass graft(s) with intermediate coronary syndrome

Atherosclerosis of autologous artery coronary artery bypass graft(s) with preinfarction angina

Atherosclerosis of autologous artery coronary artery bypass graft(s) with worsening effort angina

Excludes1:   unstable angina without atherosclerosis of autologous artery coronary artery bypass graft(s) (I20.0)

I25.722   **Atherosclerosis of autologous artery coronary artery bypass graft(s) with angina pectoris with documented spasm**

Atherosclerosis of autologous artery coronary artery bypass graft(s) with angiospastic angina

Atherosclerosis of autologous artery coronary artery bypass graft(s) with prinzmental angina

Atherosclerosis of autologous artery coronary artery bypass graft(s) with spasm-induced angina

Atherosclerosis of autologous artery coronary artery bypass graft(s) with variant angina

Excludes1:   angina pectoris with documented spasm without atherosclerosis of autologous artery coronary artery bypass graft(s) (I20.1)

I25.728   **Atherosclerosis of autologous artery coronary artery bypass graft(s) with other forms of angina pectoris**

Atherosclerosis of autologous artery coronary artery bypass graft(s) with angina of effort

Atherosclerosis of autologous artery coronary artery bypass graft(s) with stenocardia

Excludes1:   other forms of angina pectoris without atherosclerosis of autologous artery coronary artery bypass graft(s) (I120.8)

I25.729   **Atherosclerosis of autologous artery coronary artery bypass graft(s) with unspecified angina pectoris**

Atherosclerosis of autologous artery coronary artery bypass graft(s) with angina NOS

Atherosclerosis of autologous artery coronary artery bypass graft(s) with anginal syndrome

Atherosclerosis of autologous artery coronary artery bypass graft(s) with cardiac angina

Atherosclerosis of autologous artery coronary artery bypass graft(s) with ischemic chest pain

Excludes1:   unspecified angina pectoris without atherosclerosis of autologous artery coronary artery bypass graft(s) (I20.9)

I25.73   **Atherosclerosis of nonautologous biological coronary artery bypass graft(s)**

I25.730   **Atherosclerosis of nonautologous biological coronary artery bypass graft(s) without angina pectoris**

Atherosclerosis of nonautologous biological coronary artery bypass graft(s) NOS

I25.731   **Atherosclerosis of nonautologous biological coronary artery bypass graft(s) with unstable angina pectoris**

Atherosclerosis of nonautologous biological coronary artery bypass graft(s) with accelerated angina

Atherosclerosis of nonautologous biological coronary artery bypass graft(s) with crescendo angina

Atherosclerosis of nonautologous biological coronary artery bypass graft(s) with de novo effort angina

Atherosclerosis of nonautologous biological coronary artery bypass graft(s) with intermediate coronary syndrome

Atherosclerosis of nonautologous biological coronary artery bypass graft(s) with preinfarction angina

Atherosclerosis of nonautologous biological coronary artery bypass graft(s) with worsening effort angina

Excludes1:   unstable angina without atherosclerosis of nonautologous biological coronary artery bypass graft(s) (I20.0)

I25.732   **Atherosclerosis of nonautologous biological coronary artery bypass graft(s) with angina pectoris with documented spasm**

Atherosclerosis of nonautologous biological coronary artery bypass graft(s) with angiospastic angina

Atherosclerosis of nonautologous biological coronary artery bypass graft(s) with prinzmental angina

Atherosclerosis of nonautologous biological coronary artery bypass graft(s) with spasm-induced angina

Atherosclerosis of nonautologous biological coronary artery bypass graft(s) with variant angina

Excludes1:   angina pectoris with documented spasm without atherosclerosis of nonautologous biological coronary artery bypass graft(s) (I20.1)

I25.738   **Atherosclerosis of nonautologous biological coronary artery bypass graft(s) with other forms of angina pectoris**

Atherosclerosis of nonautologous biological coronary artery bypass graft(s) with angina of effort

Atherosclerosis of nonautologous biological coronary artery bypass graft(s) with stenocardia

Excludes1:   other forms of angina pectoris without atherosclerosis of nonautologous biological coronary artery bypass graft(s) (I20.8)

I25.739 Atherosclerosis of nonautologous biological coronary artery bypass graft(s) with unspecified angina pectoris
Atherosclerosis of nonautologous biological coronary artery bypass graft(s) with angina NOS
Atherosclerosis of nonautologous biological coronary artery bypass graft(s) with anginal syndrome
Atherosclerosis of nonautologous biological coronary artery bypass graft(s) with cardiac angina
Atherosclerosis of nonautologous biological coronary artery bypass graft(s) with ischemic chest pain
Excludes1: unspecified angina pectoris without atherosclerosis of nonautologous biological coronary artery bypass graft(s) (I20.9)

I25.75 Atherosclerosis of native coronary artery of transplanted heart

I25.76 Atherosclerosis of bypass graft of coronary artery of transplanted heart

I25.79 Atherosclerosis of other coronary artery bypass graft(s)

I25.790 Atherosclerosis of other coronary artery bypass graft(s) without angina pectoris
Atherosclerosis of other coronary artery bypass graft(s) NOS

I25.791 Atherosclerosis of other coronary artery bypass graft(s) with unstable angina pectoris
Atherosclerosis of other coronary artery bypass graft(s) with accelerated angina
Atherosclerosis of other coronary artery bypass graft(s) with crescendo angina
Atherosclerosis of other coronary artery bypass graft(s) with de novo effort angina
Atherosclerosis of other coronary artery bypass graft(s) with intermediate coronary syndrome
Atherosclerosis of other coronary artery bypass graft(s) with preinfarction angina
Atherosclerosis of other coronary artery bypass graft(s) with worsening effort angina
Excludes1: unstable angina without atherosclerosis of other coronary artery bypass graft(s) (I20.0)

I25.792 Atherosclerosis of other coronary artery bypass graft(s) with angina pectoris with documented spasm
Atherosclerosis of other coronary artery bypass graft(s) with angiospastic angina
Atherosclerosis of other coronary artery bypass graft(s) with prinzmetal angina
Atherosclerosis of other coronary artery bypass graft(s) with spasm-induced angina
Atherosclerosis of other coronary artery bypass graft(s) with variant angina
Excludes1: angina pectoris with documented spasm without atherosclerosis of other coronary artery bypass graft(s) (I20.1)

I25.798 Atherosclerosis of other coronary artery bypass graft(s) with other forms of angina pectoris
Atherosclerosis of other coronary artery bypass graft(s) with angina of effort
Atherosclerosis of other coronary artery bypass graft(s) with stenocardia
Excludes1: other forms of angina pectoris without atherosclerosis of other coronary artery bypass graft(s) (I20.8)

I25.799 Atherosclerosis of other coronary artery bypass graft(s) with unspecified angina pectoris
Atherosclerosis of other coronary artery bypass graft(s) with angina NOS
Atherosclerosis of other coronary artery bypass graft(s) with anginal syndrome
Atherosclerosis of other coronary artery bypass graft(s) with cardiac angina
Atherosclerosis of other coronary artery bypass graft(s) with ischemic chest pain
Excludes1: unspecified angina pectoris without atherosclerosis of other coronary artery bypass graft(s) (I20.9)

I25.8 Other forms of chronic ischemic heart disease

I25.9 Chronic ischemic heart disease, unspecified
Ischemic heart disease (chronic) NOS

PULMONARY HEART DISEASE AND DISEASES OF PULMONARY CIRCULATION (I26–I28)

I26 Pulmonary embolism
Includes: pulmonary (artery) (vein) infarction
pulmonary (artery) (vein) thromboembolism
pulmonary (artery) (vein) thrombosis
Excludes1: pulmonary embolism due to trauma (T79.0, T79.1)
pulmonary embolism due to complications of surgical and medical care (T80.0, T81.7, T82.8)
Code first pulmonary embolism complicating:
abortion, ectopic or molar pregnancy (O00-O07, O08.2)
pregnancy, childbirth and the puerperium (O88.-)

I26.0 Pulmonary embolism with mention of acute cor pulmonale
Acute cor pulmonale NOS

I26.9 Pulmonary embolism without mention of acute cor pulmonale
Pulmonary embolism NOS

I27 Other pulmonary heart diseases

I27.0 Primary pulmonary hypertension
Pulmonary (artery) hypertension (idiopathic) (primary)

I27.1 Kyphoscoliotic heart disease

I27.8 Other specified pulmonary heart diseases

I27.9 Pulmonary heart disease, unspecified
Chronic cardiopulmonary disease
Cor pulmonale (chronic) NOS

I28 Other diseases of pulmonary vessels

I28.0 Arteriovenous fistula of pulmonary vessels
Excludes1: congenital arteriovenous fistula (Q25.7)

I28.1 Aneurysm of pulmonary artery
Excludes1: congenital aneurysm (Q25.7)

I28.8 Other diseases of pulmonary vessels
Pulmonary arteritis
Pulmonary endarteritis
Rupture of pulmonary vessels
Stenosis of pulmonary vessels
Stricture of pulmonary vessels

I28.9 Disease of pulmonary vessels, unspecified

OTHER FORMS OF HEART DISEASE (I30–I52)

I30 Acute pericarditis
Includes: acute mediastinopericarditis
acute myopericarditis
acute pericardial effusion
acute pleuropericarditis
acute pneumopericarditis
Excludes1: Dressler's syndrome (I24.1)
rheumatic pericarditis (acute) (I01.0)

I30.0 Acute nonspecific idiopathic pericarditis

I30.1   Infective pericarditis
Pneumococcal pericarditis
Pneumopyopericardium
Purulent pericarditis
Pyopericarditis
Pyopericardium
Pyopneumopericardium
Staphylococcal pericarditis
Streptococcal pericarditis
Suppurative pericarditis
Viral pericarditis
Use additional code (B95-B97) to identify infectious agent

I30.8   Other forms of acute pericarditis

I30.9   Acute pericarditis, unspecified

I31   Other diseases of pericardium
Excludes1:   diseases of pericardium specified as rheumatic (I09.2)
postcardiotomy syndrome (I97.0)
traumatic injury to pericardium (S26.-)

I31.0   Chronic adhesive pericarditis
Accretio cordis
Adherent pericardium
Adhesive mediastinopericarditis

I31.1   Chronic constrictive pericarditis
Concretio cordis
Pericardial calcification

I31.2   Hemopericardium, not elsewhere classified
Excludes1:   hemopericardium as current complication
following acute myocardial infarction (I23.0)

I31.3   Pericardial effusion (noninflammatory)
Chylopericardium
Excludes1:   acute pericardial effusion (I30.9)

I31.8   Other specified diseases of pericardium
Epicardial plaques
Focal pericardial adhesions

I31.9   Disease of pericardium, unspecified
Cardiac tamponade NOS
Pericarditis (chronic) NOS

I32   Pericarditis in diseases classified elsewhere
Code first underlying disease, such as:
uremia (N19)
Excludes1:   pericarditis (in):
coxsackie (virus) (B33.23)
gonococcal (A54.83)
meningococcal (A39.53)
rheumatoid (arthritis) (M05.31)
syphilitic (A52.06)
systemic lupus erythematosus (M32.12)
tuberculosis (A18.84)

I33   Acute and subacute endocarditis
Excludes1:   acute rheumatic endocarditis (I01.1)
endocarditis NOS (I38)

I33.0   Acute and subacute infective endocarditis
Bacterial endocarditis (acute) (subacute)
Infective endocarditis (acute) (subacute) NOS
Endocarditis lenta (acute) (subacute)
Malignant endocarditis (acute) (subacute)
Purulent endocarditis (acute) (subacute)
Septic endocarditis (acute) (subacute)
Ulcerative endocarditis (acute) (subacute)
Vegetative endocarditis (acute) (subacute)
Use additional code (B95-B97) to identify infectious agent

I33.9   Acute and subacute endocarditis, unspecified
Acute endocarditis NOS
Acute myoendocarditis NOS
Acute periendocarditis NOS
Subacute endocarditis NOS
Subacute myoendocarditis NOS
Subacute periendocarditis NOS

I34   Nonrheumatic mitral valve disorders
Excludes1:   mitral valve disease (I05.9)
mitral valve failure (I05.8)
mitral valve stenosis (I05.0)
mitral valve disorder of unspecified cause with
diseases of aortic and/or tricuspid valve(s)
(I08.-)
mitral valve disorder of unspecified cause with
mitral stenosis or obstruction (I05.0)
mitral valve disorder specified as rheumatic
(I05.-)

I34.0   Nonrheumatic mitral (valve) insufficiency
Nonrheumatic mitral (valve) incompetence
Nonrheumatic mitral (valve) regurgitation

I34.1   Nonrheumatic mitral (valve) prolapse
Floppy nonrheumatic mitral valve syndrome
Excludes1:   Marfan's syndrome (Q87.4-)

I34.2   Nonrheumatic mitral (valve) stenosis

I34.8   Other nonrheumatic mitral valve disorders

I34.9   Nonrheumatic mitral valve disorder, unspecified

I35   Nonrheumatic aortic valve disorders
Excludes1:   aortic valve disorder specified as rheumatic (I06.-)
hypertrophic subaortic stenosis (I42.1)
that of unspecified cause but with mention of diseases
of mitral and/or tricuspid valve(s) (I08.-)

I35.0   Nonrheumatic aortic (valve) stenosis

I35.1   Nonrheumatic aortic (valve) insufficiency
Nonrheumatic aortic (valve) incompetence
Nonrheumatic aortic (valve) regurgitation

I35.2   Nonrheumatic aortic (valve) stenosis with insufficiency

I35.8   Other nonrheumatic aortic valve disorders

I35.9   Nonrheumatic aortic valve disorder, unspecified

I36   Nonrheumatic tricuspid valve disorders
Excludes1:   tricuspid valve disorders of unspecified cause (I07.-)
with aortic and/or mitral valve involvement (I08.-)
tricuspid valve disorders specified as rheumatic (I07.-)

I36.0   Nonrheumatic tricuspid (valve) stenosis

I36.1   Nonrheumatic tricuspid (valve) insufficiency
Nonrheumatic tricuspid (valve) incompetence
Nonrheumatic tricuspid (valve) regurgitation

I36.2   Nonrheumatic tricuspid (valve) stenosis with insufficiency

I36.8   Other nonrheumatic tricuspid valve disorders

I36.9   Nonrheumatic tricuspid valve disorder, unspecified

I37   Nonrheumatic pulmonary valve disorders
Excludes1:   pulmonary valve disorder specified as rheumatic
(I09.89)

I37.0   Nonrheumatic pulmonary valve stenosis

I37.1   Nonrheumatic pulmonary valve insufficiency
Nonrheumatic pulmonary valve incompetence
Nonrheumatic pulmonary valve regurgitation

I37.2   Nonrheumatic pulmonary valve stenosis with insufficiency

I37.8   Other nonrheumatic pulmonary valve disorders

I37.9   Nonrheumatic pulmonary valve disorder, unspecified

I38   Endocarditis, valve unspecified
Includes: endocarditis (chronic) NOS
valvular incompetence
valvular insufficiency
valvular regurgitation
valvular stenosis
valvulitis (chronic)
Excludes1:   endocardial fibroelastosis (I42.4)
endocarditis specified as rheumatic (I09.1)

I39   Endocarditis and heart valve disorders in diseases classified elsewhere

Code first underlying disease, such as:
Q fever (A78)

Excludes1:   endocardial involvement in:
candidiasis (B37.6)
gonococcal infection (A54.83)
Libman-Sacks disease (M32.11)
listerosis (A32.82)
meningococcal infection (A39.51)
rheumatoid arthritis (M05.31)
syphilis (A52.03)
tuberculosis (A18.84)
typhoid fever (A01.02)

I40   Acute myocarditis

Includes: subacute myocarditis

Excludes1:   acute rheumatic myocarditis (I01.2)

I40.0   Infective myocarditis
Pneumococcal myocarditis
Septic staphyloccocal myocarditis
Use additional code (B95-B97) to identify infectious agent

I40.1   Isolated myocarditis
Fiedler's myocarditis
Giant cell myocarditis
Idiopathic myocarditis

I40.8   Other acute myocarditis

I40.9   Acute myocarditis, unspecified

I41   Myocarditis in diseases classified elsewhere

Code first underlying disease, such as:
typhus (A75.0-A75.9)

Excludes1:   myocarditis (in):
Chagas' disease (chronic) (B57.2)
acute (B57.0)
coxsackie (virus) infection (B33.22)
diphtheritic (A36.81)
gonococcal (A54.83)
influenzal (J10.89)
meningococcal (A39.52)
mumps (B26.82)
rheumatoid arthritis (M05.31)
sarcoid (D86.85)
syphilis (A52.06)
toxoplasmosis (B58.81)
tuberculous (A18.84)

I42   Cardiomyopathy

Includes: myocardiopathy
Code first cardiomyopathy complicating pregnancy (O99.4)
Excludes1:   ischemic cardiomyopathy (I25.5)

I42.0   Dilated cardiomyopathy

I42.1   Obstructive hypertrophic cardiomyopathy
Hypertrophic subaortic stenosis

I42.2   Other hypertrophic cardiomyopathy
Nonobstructive hypertrophic cardiomyopathy

I42.3   Endomyocardial (eosinophilic) disease
Endomyocardial (tropical) fibrosis
Löffler's endocarditis

I42.4   Endocardial fibroelastosis
Congenital cardiomyopathy
Elastomyofibrosis

I42.5   Other restrictive cardiomyopathy

I42.6   Alcoholic cardiomyopathy
Use additional code to identify presence of alcoholism (F10.-)

I42.7   Cardiomyopathy due to drug and external agent
Use additional external cause code (Chapter XIX) to identify cause

I42.8   Other cardiomyopathies

I42.9   Cardiomyopathy, unspecified
Cardiomyopathy (primary) (secondary) NOS

I43   Cardiomyopathy in diseases classified elsewhere

Code first underlying disease, such as:
amyloidosis (E85)
glycogen storage disease (E74.0)
gout (M10.0-)
thyrotoxicosis (E05.0—E05.9-)

Excludes1:   cardiomyopathy (in):
coxsackie (virus) (B33.24)
diphtheria (A36.81)
sarcoidosis (D86.85)
tuberculosis (A18.84)

I44   Atrioventricular and left bundle-branch block

I44.0   Atrioventricular block, first degree

I44.1   Atrioventricular block, second degree
Atrioventricular block, type I and II
Möbitz block, type I and II
Second degree block, type I and II
Wenckebach's block

I44.2   Atrioventricular block, complete
Complete heart block NOS
Third degree block

I44.3   Other and unspecified atrioventricular block
Atrioventricular block NOS

I44.30   Unspecified atrioventricular block

I44.39   Other atrioventricular block

I44.4   Left anterior fascicular block

I44.5   Left posterior fascicular block

I44.6   Other and unspecified fascicular block
Left bundle-branch hemiblock NOS

I44.7   Left bundle-branch block, unspecified

I45   Other conduction disorders

I45.0   Right fascicular block

I45.1   Other and unspecified right bundle-branch block
Right bundle-branch block NOS

I45.2   Bifascicular block

I45.3   Trifascicular block

I45.4   Nonspecific intraventricular block
Bundle-branch block NOS

I45.5   Other specified heart block
Sinoatrial block
Sinoauricular block
Excludes1:   heart block NOS (I45.9)

I45.6   Pre-excitation syndrome
Accelerated atrioventricular conduction
Accessory atrioventricular conduction
Anomalous atrioventricular excitation
Lown-Ganong-Levine syndrome
Pre-excitation atrioventricular conduction
Wolff-Parkinson-White syndrome

I45.8   Other specified conduction disorders
Atrioventricular [AV] dissociation
Interference dissociation
Isorhythmic dissociation
Nonparoxysmal AV nodal tachycardia

I45.9   Conduction disorder, unspecified
Heart block NOS
Stokes-Adams syndrome

I46   Cardiac arrest

Excludes1:   cardiogenic shock (R57.0)

I46.2   Cardiac arrest due to underlying cardiac condition
Code first underlying cardiac condition

I46.8   Cardiac arrest due to other underlying condition
Code first underlying condition

I46.9   Cardiac arrest, cause unspecified

I47   Paroxysmal tachycardia

Code first tachycardia complicating:
abortion or ectopic or molar pregnancy (O00-O07, O08.8)
obstetric surgery and procedures (O75.4)

Excludes1:   tachycardia NOS (R00.0)

I47.0   **Re-entry ventricular arrhythmia**

I47.1   **Supraventricular tachycardia**
  Atrial paroxysmal tachycardia
  Atrioventricular [AV] paroxysmal tachycardia
  Junctional paroxysmal tachycardia
  Nodal paroxysmal tachycardia

I47.2   **Ventricular tachycardia**

I47.9   **Paroxysmal tachycardia, unspecified**
  Bouveret (-Hoffman) syndrome

I48   Atrial fibrillation and flutter

I48.0   **Atrial fibrillation**

I48.1   **Atrial flutter**

I49   Other cardiac arrhythmias
  Code first cardiac arrhythmia complicating:
    abortion or ectopic or molar pregnancy (O00-O07, O08.8)
    obstetric surgery and procedures (O75.4)
  Excludes1:   bradycardia NOS (R00.1)
    neonatal dysrhythmia (P29.1)

I49.0   **Ventricular fibrillation and flutter**

   I49.01   **Ventricular fibrillation**

   I49.02   **Ventricular flutter**

I49.1   **Atrial premature depolarization**
  Atrial premature beats

I49.2   **Junctional premature depolarization**

I49.3   **Ventricular premature depolarization**

I49.4   **Other and unspecified premature depolarization**
  Ectopic beats
  Extrasystoles
  Extrasystolic arrhythmias
  Premature beats NOS
  Premature contractions

I49.5   **Sick sinus syndrome**
  Tachycardia-bradycardia syndrome

I49.8   **Other specified cardiac arrhythmias**
  Coronary sinus rhythm disorder
  Ectopic rhythm disorder
  Nodal rhythm disorder

I49.9   **Cardiac arrhythmia, unspecified**
  Arrhythmia (cardiac) NOS

I50   Heart failure
  Code first heart failure complicating:
    abortion or ectopic or molar pregnancy (O00-O07, O08.8)
    following cardiac surgery or due to presence of cardiac prosthesis (I97.1)
    obstetric surgery and procedures (O75.4)
  Excludes1:   cardiac arrest (I46.-)
    heart failure due to hypertension (I11.0)
    heart failure due to hypertension with renal disease (I13.-)
    neonatal cardiac failure (P29.0)
    rheumatic heart failure (I09.81)

I50.0   **Congestive heart failure**
  Biventricular failure
  Congestive heart disease
  Right ventricular failure (secondary to left heart failure)

I50.1   **Left ventricular failure**
  Acute edema of lung with heart disease NOS
  Acute edema of lung with heart failure
  Acute pulmonary edema with heart disease NOS
  Acute pulmonary edema with heart failure
  Cardiac asthma
  Left heart failure
  Excludes1:   acute edema of lung without heart disease or heart failure (J81)
    acute pulmonary edema without heart disease or failure (J81)

I50.9   **Heart failure, unspecified**
  Cardiac, heart or myocardial failure NOS

I51   Complications and ill-defined descriptions of heart disease
  Excludes1:   any condition in I51.4-I51.9 with hypertension (I11.-)
    any condition in I51.4-I51.9 with hypertension and renal disease (I13.-)
    heart disease specified as rheumatic (I00-I09)

I51.0   **Cardiac septal defect, acquired**
  Acquired septal atrial defect (old)
  Acquired septal auricular defect (old)
  Acquired septal ventricular defect (old)
  Excludes1:   cardiac septal defect as current complication following acute myocardial infarction (I23.1, I23.2)

I51.1   **Rupture of chordae tendineae, not elsewhere classified**
  Excludes1:   rupture of chordae tendineae as current complication following acute myocardial infarction (I23.4)

I51.2   **Rupture of papillary muscle, not elsewhere classified**
  Excludes1:   rupture of papillary muscle as current complication following acute myocardial infarction (I23.5)

I51.3   **Intracardiac thrombosis, not elsewhere classified**
  Apical thrombosis (old)
  Atrial thrombosis (old)
  Auricular thrombosis (old)
  Mural thrombosis (old)
  Ventricular thrombosis (old)
  Excludes1:   intracardiac thrombosis as current complication following acute myocardial infarction (I23.6)

I51.4   **Myocarditis, unspecified**
  Chronic (interstitial) myocarditis
  Myocardial fibrosis
  Myocarditis NOS
  Excludes1:   acute or subacute myocarditis (I40.-)

I51.5   **Myocardial degeneration**
  Fatty degeneration of heart or myocardium
  Myocardial disease
  Senile degeneration of heart or myocardium

I51.6   **Cardiovascular disease, unspecified**
  Cardiovascular accident NOS
  Excludes1:   atherosclerotic cardiovascular disease (I25.1-)

I51.7   **Cardiomegaly**
  Cardiac dilatation
  Cardiac hypertrophy
  Ventricular dilatation

I51.8   **Other ill-defined heart diseases**
  Carditis (acute) (chronic)
  Pancarditis (acute) (chronic)

I51.9   **Heart disease, unspecified**

I52   Other heart disorders in diseases classified elsewhere
  Code first underlying disease, such as:
    congenital syphilis (A50.5)
    mucopolysaccharidosis (E76.3)
    schistosomiasis (B65.0-B65.9)
  Excludes1:   heart disease (in):
    gonococcal infection (A54.83)
    meningococcal infection (A39.50)
    rheumatoid arthritis (M05.31)
    syphilis (A52.06)

CEREBROVASCULAR DISEASES (I60–I69)

Use additional code to identify presence of:
  alcohol abuse and dependence (F10.-)
  alcohol use, uncomplicated (Z72.1)
  alcohol dependence, in remission (F10.11)
  exposure to environmental tobacco smoke (X58.1)
  history of tobacco use (Z86.43)
  hypertension (I10-I15)
  occupational exposure to environmental tobacco smoke (Z57.31)
  tobacco dependence (F17.-)
  tobacco use (Z72.0)
Excludes1:   transient cerebral ischemic attacks and related syndromes (G45.-)
    traumatic intracranial hemorrhage (S06.-)

I60   **Nontraumatic subarachnoid hemorrhage**

Includes: ruptured cerebral aneurysm

Excludes1:   sequelae of subarachnoid hemorrhage (I69.0-)
               syphilitic ruptured cerebral aneurysm (A52.05)

I60.0   **Nontraumatic subarachnoid hemorrhage from carotid siphon and bifurcation**

I60.1   **Nontraumatic subarachnoid hemorrhage from middle cerebral artery**

I60.2   **Nontraumatic subarachnoid hemorrhage from anterior communicating artery**

I60.3   **Nontraumatic subarachnoid hemorrhage from posterior communicating artery**

I60.4   **Nontraumatic subarachnoid hemorrhage from basilar artery**

I60.5   **Nontraumatic subarachnoid hemorrhage from vertebral artery**

I60.6   **Nontraumatic subarachnoid hemorrhage from other intracranial arteries**

Subarachnoid hemorrhage (nontraumatic) from multiple involvement of intracranial arteries

I60.7   **Nontraumatic subarachnoid hemorrhage from intracranial artery, unspecified**

Ruptured (congenital) berry aneurysm
Ruptured (congenital) cerebral aneurysm
Subarachnoid hemorrhage (nontraumatic) from cerebral artery NOS
Subarachnoid hemorrhage (nontraumatic) from communicating artery NOS

I60.8   **Other nontraumatic subarachnoid hemorrhage**

Meningeal hemorrhage
Rupture of cerebral arteriovenous malformation

I60.9   **Nontraumatic subarachnoid hemorrhage, unspecified**

I61   **Nontraumatic intracerebral hemorrhage**

Excludes1:   sequelae of intracerebral hemorrhage (I69.1-)

I61.0   **Nontraumatic intracerebral hemorrhage in hemisphere, subcortical**

Deep intracerebral hemorrhage (nontraumatic)

I61.1   **Nontraumatic intracerebral hemorrhage in hemisphere, cortical**

Cerebral lobe hemorrhage (nontraumatic)
Superficial intracerebral hemorrhage (nontraumatic)

I61.2   **Nontraumatic intracerebral hemorrhage in hemisphere, unspecified**

I61.3   **Nontraumatic intracerebral hemorrhage in brain stem**

I61.4   **Nontraumatic intracerebral hemorrhage in cerebellum**

I61.5   **Nontraumatic intracerebral hemorrhage, intraventricular**

I61.6   **Nontraumatic intracerebral hemorrhage, multiple localized**

I61.8   **Other nontraumatic intracerebral hemorrhage**

I61.9   **Nontraumatic intracerebral hemorrhage, unspecified**

I62   **Other and unspecified nontraumatic intracranial hemorrhage**

Excludes1:   sequelae of intracranial hemorrhage (I69.2)

I62.0   **Nontraumatic subdural hemorrhage**

I62.00   **Nontraumatic subdural hemorrhage, unspecified**

I62.01   **Nontraumatic acute subdural hemorrhage**

I62.02   **Nontraumatic subacute subdural hemorrhage**

I62.03   **Nontraumatic chronic subdural hemorrhage**

I62.1   **Nontraumatic extradural hemorrhage**

Nontraumatic epidural hemorrhage

I62.9   **Nontraumatic intracranial hemorrhage, unspecified**

I63   **Cerebral infarction**

Includes: occlusion and stenosis of cerebral and precerebral arteries, resulting in cerebral infarction

Excludes1:   sequelae of cerebral infarction (I69.3-)

I63.0   **Cerebral infarction due to thrombosis of precerebral arteries**

I63.1   **Cerebral infarction due to embolism of precerebral arteries**

I63.2   **Cerebral infarction due to unspecified occlusion or stenosis of precerebral arteries**

I63.3   **Cerebral infarction due to thrombosis of cerebral arteries**

I63.4   **Cerebral infarction due to embolism of cerebral arteries**

I63.5   **Cerebral infarction due to unspecified occlusion or stenosis of cerebral arteries**

I63.6   **Cerebral infarction due to cerebral venous thrombosis, nonpyogenic**

I63.8   **Other cerebral infarction**

I63.9   **Cerebral infarction, unspecified**

I64   **Stroke, not specified as hemorrhage or infarction**

Includes: cerebrovascular accident NOS

Excludes1:   any condition classifiable to I60 - I63
               sequelae of stroke (I69.4-)

I65   **Occlusion and stenosis of precerebral arteries, not resulting in cerebral infarction**

Includes: embolism of precerebral artery
               narrowing of precerebral artery
               obstruction (complete) (partial) of precerebral artery
               thrombosis of precerebral artery

Excludes1:   insufficiency, NOS, of precerebral artery (G45.-)
               insufficiency of precerebral arteries with cerebral infarction (I63.0-I63.2)

I65.0   **Occlusion and stenosis of vertebral artery**

I65.1   **Occlusion and stenosis of basilar artery**

I65.2   **Occlusion and stenosis of carotid artery**

I65.3   **Occlusion and stenosis of multiple and bilateral precerebral arteries**

I65.8   **Occlusion and stenosis of other precerebral arteries**

I65.9   **Occlusion and stenosis of unspecified precerebral artery**

Occlusion and stenosis of precerebral artery NOS

I66   **Occlusion and stenosis of cerebral arteries, not resulting in cerebral infarction**

Includes: embolism of cerebral artery
               narrowing of cerebral artery
               obstruction (complete) (partial) of cerebral artery
               thrombosis of cerebral artery

Excludes1:   occlusion and stenosis of cerebral artery causing cerebral infarction (I63.3-I63.5)

I66.0   **Occlusion and stenosis of middle cerebral artery**

I66.1   **Occlusion and stenosis of anterior cerebral artery**

I66.2   **Occlusion and stenosis of posterior cerebral artery**

I66.3   **Occlusion and stenosis of cerebellar arteries**

I66.4   **Occlusion and stenosis of multiple and bilateral cerebral arteries**

I66.8   **Occlusion and stenosis of other cerebral arteries**

Occlusion and stenosis of perforating arteries

I66.9   **Occlusion and stenosis of unspecified cerebral artery**

I67   **Other cerebrovascular diseases**

Excludes1:   sequelae of the listed conditions (I69.8)

I67.0   **Dissection of cerebral arteries, nonruptured**

Excludes1:   ruptured cerebral arteries (I60.7)

I67.1   **Cerebral aneurysm, nonruptured**

Cerebral aneurysm NOS
Cerebral arteriovenous fistula, acquired
Internal carotid artery aneurysm, intracranial portion
Internal carotid artery aneurysm, NOS

Excludes1:   congenital cerebral aneurysm, nonruptured (Q28.-)
               ruptured cerebral aneurysm (I60.7)

I67.2   **Cerebral atherosclerosis**

Atheroma of cerebral and precerebral arteries

I67.3   **Progressive vascular leukoencephalopathy**

Binswanger's disease

I67.4   **Hypertensive encephalopathy**

I67.5   **Moyamoya disease**

I67.6   **Nonpyogenic thrombosis of intracranial venous system**

Nonpyogenic thrombosis of cerebral vein
Nonpyogenic thrombosis of intracranial venous sinus

Excludes1:   nonpyogenic thrombosis of intracranial venous system causing infarction (I63.6)

I67.7   **Cerebral arteritis, not elsewhere classified**

Granulomatous angiitis of the nervous system

Excludes1:   allergic granulomatous angiitis (M30.1)

I67.8   **Other specified cerebrovascular diseases**
Acute cerebrovascular insufficiency NOS
Cerebral ischemia (chronic)

I67.9   **Cerebrovascular disease, unspecified**

I68   **Cerebrovascular disorders in diseases classified elsewhere**

I68.1   **Cerebral amyloid angiopathy**
Code first underlying amyloidosis (E85)

I68.2   **Cerebral arteritis in other diseases classified elsewhere**
Code first underlying disease
Excludes1:   cerebral arteritis (in):
        listerosis (A32.89)
        systemic lupus erythematosus (M32.19)
        syphilis (A52.04)
        tuberculosis (A18.89)

I68.8   **Other cerebrovascular disorders in diseases classified elsewhere**
Code first underlying disease
Excludes1:   syphilitic cerebral aneurysm (A52.05)

I69   **Sequelae of cerebrovascular disease**
Note: This category is to be used to indicate conditions in I60-I67 as the cause of sequelae. The "sequelae" include conditions specified as such or as residuals which may occur at any time after the onset of the causal condition
Excludes1:   sequelae of traumatic intracranial injury (T90.5)

I69.0   **Sequelae of nontraumatic subarachnoid hemorrhage**

I69.00   **Unspecified late effects of nontraumatic subarachnoid hemorrhage**

I69.01   **Cognitive deficits following nontraumatic subarachnoid hemorrhage**

I69.02   **Speech and language deficits following nontraumatic subarachnoid hemorrhage**

I69.020   **Aphasia following nontraumatic subarachnoid hemorrhage**

I69.021   **Dysphasia following nontraumatic subarachnoid hemorrhage**

I69.028   **Other speech and language deficits following nontraumatic subarachnoid hemorrhage**
Dysarthria following nontraumatic subarachnoid hemorrhage

I69.03   **Monoplegia of upper limb following nontraumatic subarachnoid hemorrhage**

I69.031   **Monoplegia of upper limb following nontraumatic subarachnoid hemorrhage affecting right dominant side**

I69.032   **Monoplegia of upper limb following nontraumatic subarachnoid hemorrhage affecting left dominant side**

I69.033   **Monoplegia of upper limb following nontraumatic subarachnoid hemorrhage affecting right non-dominant side**

I69.034   **Monoplegia of upper limb following nontraumatic subarachnoid hemorrhage affecting left non-dominant side**

I69.039   **Monoplegia of upper limb following nontraumatic subarachnoid hemorrhage affecting unspecified side**

I69.04   **Monoplegia of lower limb following nontraumatic subarachnoid hemorrhage**

I69.041   **Monoplegia of lower limb following nontraumatic subarachnoid hemorrhage affecting right dominant side**

I69.042   **Monoplegia of lower limb following nontraumatic subarachnoid hemorrhage affecting left dominant side**

I69.043   **Monoplegia of lower limb following nontraumatic subarachnoid hemorrhage affecting right non-dominant side**

I69.044   **Monoplegia of lower limb following nontraumatic subarachnoid hemorrhage affecting left non-dominant side**

I69.049   **Monoplegia of lower limb following nontraumatic subarachnoid hemorrhage affecting unspecified side**

I69.05   **Hemiplegia and hemiparesis following nontraumatic subarachnoid hemorrhage**

I69.051   **Hemiplegia and hemiparesis following nontraumatic subarachnoid hemorrhage affecting right dominant side**

I69.052   **Hemiplegia and hemiparesis following nontraumatic subarachnoid hemorrhage affecting left dominant side**

I69.053   **Hemiplegia and hemiparesis following nontraumatic subarachnoid hemorrhage affecting right non-dominant side**

I69.054   **Hemiplegia and hemiparesis following nontraumatic subarachnoid hemorrhage affecting left non-dominant side**

I69.059   **Hemiplegia and hemiparesis following nontraumatic subarachnoid hemorrhage affecting unspecified side**

I69.06   **Other paralytic syndrome following nontraumatic subarachnoid hemorrhage**
Use additional code to identify type of paralytic syndrome, such as:
locked-in state (G83.5)
quadriplegia (G82.39, G82.49, G82.8)
Excludes1:   hemiplegia/hemiparesis following nontraumatic subarachnoid hemorrhage (I69.05-)
      monoplegia of lower limb following nontraumatic subarachnoid hemorrhage (I69.04-)
      monoplegia of upper limb following nontraumatic subarachnoid hemorrhage (I69.03-)

I69.061   **Other paralytic syndrome following nontraumatic subarachnoid hemorrhage affecting right dominant side**

I69.062   **Other paralytic syndrome following nontraumatic subarachnoid hemorrhage affecting left dominant side**

I69.063   **Other paralytic syndrome following nontraumatic subarachnoid hemorrhage affecting right non-dominant side**

I69.064   **Other paralytic syndrome following nontraumatic subarachnoid hemorrhage affecting left non-dominant side**

I69.065   **Other paralytic syndrome following nontraumatic subarachnoid hemorrhage, bilateral**

I69.069   **Other paralytic syndrome following nontraumatic subarachnoid hemorrhage affecting unspecified side**

I69.09   **Other late effects of nontraumatic subarachnoid hemorrhage**

I69.090   **Apraxia following nontraumatic subarachnoid hemorrhage**

I69.091   **Dysphagia following nontraumatic subarachnoid hemorrhage**

I69.098   **Other late effects following nontraumatic subarachnoid hemorrhage**
Use additional code to identify the sequelae

I69.1   **Sequelae of nontraumatic intracerebral hemorrhage**

I69.10   **Unspecified late effects of nontraumatic intracerebral hemorrhage**

I69.11   **Cognitive deficits following nontraumatic intracerebral hemorrhage**

I69.12   **Speech and language deficits following nontraumatic intracerebral hemorrhage**

I69.120   **Aphasia following nontraumatic intracerebral hemorrhage**

I69.121   **Dysphasia following nontraumatic intracerebral hemorrhage**

I69.128 Other speech and language deficits following nontraumatic intracerebral hemorrhage
  Dysarthria following nontraumatic intracerebral hemorrhage

I69.13 Monoplegia of upper limb following nontraumatic intracerebral hemorrhage

I69.131 Monoplegia of upper limb following nontraumatic intracerebral hemorrhage affecting right dominant side

I69.132 Monoplegia of upper limb following nontraumatic intracerebral hemorrhage affecting left dominant side

I69.133 Monoplegia of upper limb following nontraumatic intracerebral hemorrhage affecting right non-dominant side

I69.134 Monoplegia of upper limb following nontraumatic intracerebral hemorrhage affecting left non-dominant side

I69.139 Monoplegia of upper limb following nontraumatic intracerebral hemorrhage affecting unspecified side

I69.14 Monoplegia of lower limb following nontraumatic intracerebral hemorrhage

I69.141 Monoplegia of lower limb following nontraumatic intracerebral hemorrhage affecting right dominant side

I69.142 Monoplegia of lower limb following nontraumatic intracerebral hemorrhage affecting left dominant side

I69.143 Monoplegia of lower limb following nontraumatic intracerebral hemorrhage affecting right non-dominant side

I69.144 Monoplegia of lower limb following nontraumatic intracerebral hemorrhage affecting left non-dominant side

I69.149 Monoplegia of lower limb following nontraumatic intracerebral hemorrhage affecting unspecified side

I69.15 Hemiplegia and hemiparesis following nontraumatic intracerebral hemorrhage

I69.151 Hemiplegia and hemiparesis following nontraumatic intracerebral hemorrhage affecting right dominant side

I69.152 Hemiplegia and hemiparesis following nontraumatic intracerebral hemorrhage affecting left dominant side

I69.153 Hemiplegia and hemiparesis following nontraumatic intracerebral hemorrhage affecting right non-dominant side

I69.154 Hemiplegia and hemiparesis following nontraumatic intracerebral hemorrhage affecting left non-dominant side

I69.159 Hemiplegia and hemiparesis following nontraumatic intracerebral hemorrhage affecting unspecified side

I69.16 Other paralytic syndrome following nontraumatic intracerebral hemorrhage
  Use additional code to identify type of paralytic syndrome, such as:
    locked-in state (G83.5)
    quadriplegia (G82.39, G82.49, G82.8)
  Excludes1: hemiplegia/hemiparesis following nontraumatic intracerebral hemorrhage (I69.15-)
    monoplegia of lower limb following nontraumatic intracerebral hemorrhage (I69.14-)
    monoplegia of upper limb following nontraumatic intracerebral hemorrhage (I69.13-)

I69.161 Other paralytic syndrome following nontraumatic intracerebral hemorrhage affecting right dominant side

I69.162 Other paralytic syndrome following nontraumatic intracerebral hemorrhage affecting left dominant side

I69.163 Other paralytic syndrome following nontraumatic intracerebral hemorrhage affecting right non-dominant side

I69.164 Other paralytic syndrome following nontraumatic intracerebral hemorrhage affecting left non-dominant side

I69.165 Other paralytic syndrome following nontraumatic intracerebral hemorrhage, bilateral

I69.169 Other paralytic syndrome following nontraumatic intracerebral hemorrhage affecting unspecified side

I69.19 Other late effects of nontraumatic intracerebral hemorrhage

I69.190 Apraxia following nontraumatic intracerebral hemorrhage

I69.191 Dysphagia following nontraumatic intracerebral hemorrhage

I69.198 Other late effects of nontraumatic intracerebral hemorrhage
  Use additional code to identify the sequelae

I69.2 Sequelae of other nontraumatic intracranial hemorrhage

I69.20 Unspecified late effects of other nontraumatic intracranial hemorrhage

I69.21 Cognitive deficits following other nontraumatic intracranial hemorrhage

I69.22 Speech and language deficits following other nontraumatic intracranial hemorrhage

I69.220 Aphasia following other nontraumatic intracranial hemorrhage

I69.221 Dysphasia following other nontraumatic intracranial hemorrhage

I69.228 Other speech and language deficits following other nontraumatic intracranial hemorrhage
  Dysarthria following other nontraumatic intracranial hemorrhage

I69.23 Monoplegia of upper limb following other nontraumatic intracranial hemorrhage

I69.231 Monoplegia of upper limb following other nontraumatic intracranial hemorrhage affecting right dominant side

I69.232 Monoplegia of upper limb following other nontraumatic intracranial hemorrhage affecting left dominant side

I69.233 Monoplegia of upper limb following other nontraumatic intracranial hemorrhage affecting right non-dominant side

I69.234 Monoplegia of upper limb following other nontraumatic intracranial hemorrhage affecting left non-dominant side

I69.239 Monoplegia of upper limb following other nontraumatic intracranial hemorrhage affecting unspecified side

I69.24 Monoplegia of lower limb following other nontraumatic intracranial hemorrhage

I69.241 Monoplegia of lower limb following other nontraumatic intracranial hemorrhage affecting right dominant side

I69.242 Monoplegia of lower limb following other nontraumatic intracranial hemorrhage affecting left dominant side

I69.243 Monoplegia of lower limb following other nontraumatic intracranial hemorrhage affecting right non-dominant side

I69.244 Monoplegia of lower limb following other nontraumatic intracranial hemorrhage affecting left non-dominant side

I69.249 Monoplegia of lower limb following other nontraumatic intracranial hemorrhage affecting unspecified side

I69.25   Hemiplegia and hemiparesis following other nontraumatic intracranial hemorrhage

     I69.251   Hemiplegia and hemiparesis following other nontraumatic intracranial hemorrhage affecting right dominant side

     I69.252   Hemiplegia and hemiparesis following other nontraumatic intracranial hemorrhage affecting left dominant side

     I69.253   Hemiplegia and hemiparesis following other nontraumatic intracranial hemorrhage affecting right non-dominant side

     I69.254   Hemiplegia and hemiparesis following other nontraumatic intracranial hemorrhage affecting left non-dominant side

     I69.259   Hemiplegia and hemiparesis following other nontraumatic intracranial hemorrhage affecting unspecified side

I69.26   Other paralytic syndrome following other nontraumatic intracranial hemorrhage

Use additional code to identify type of paralytic syndrome, such as:
     locked-in state (G83.5)
     quadriplegia (G82.39, G82.49, G82.8)

Excludes1:   hemiplegia/hemiparesis following other nontraumatic intracranial hemorrhage (I69.25-)
         monoplegia of lower limb following other nontraumatic intracranial hemorrhage (I69.24-)
         monoplegia of upper limb following other nontraumatic intracranial hemorrhage (I69.23-)

     I69.261   Other paralytic syndrome following other nontraumatic intracranial hemorrhage affecting right dominant side

     I69.262   Other paralytic syndrome following other nontraumatic intracranial hemorrhage affecting left dominant side

     I69.263   Other paralytic syndrome following other nontraumatic intracranial hemorrhage affecting right non-dominant side

     I69.264   Other paralytic syndrome following other nontraumatic intracranial hemorrhage affecting left non-dominant side

     I69.265   Other paralytic syndrome following other nontraumatic intracranial hemorrhage, bilateral

     I69.269   Other paralytic syndrome following other nontraumatic intracranial hemorrhage affecting unspecified side

I69.29   Other late effects of other nontraumatic intracranial hemorrhage

     I69.290   Apraxia following other nontraumatic intracranial hemorrhage

     I69.291   Dysphagia following other nontraumatic intracranial hemorrhage

     I69.298   Other late effects of other nontraumatic intracranial hemorrhage
         Use additional code to identify the sequelae

I69.3   Sequelae of cerebral infarction

   I69.30   Unspecified late effects of cerebral infarction

   I69.31   Cognitive deficits following cerebral infarction

   I69.32   Speech and language deficits following cerebral infarction

     I69.320   Aphasia following cerebral infarction

     I69.321   Dysphasia following cerebral infarction

     I69.328   Other speech and language deficits following cerebral infarction
         Dysarthria following cerebral infarction

   I69.33   Monoplegia of upper limb following cerebral infarction

     I69.331   Monoplegia of upper limb following cerebral infarction affecting right dominant side

     I69.332   Monoplegia of upper limb following cerebral infarction affecting left dominant side

     I69.333   Monoplegia of upper limb following cerebral infarction affecting right non-dominant side

     I69.334   Monoplegia of upper limb following cerebral infarction affecting left non-dominant side

     I69.339   Monoplegia of upper limb following cerebral infarction affecting unspecified side

I69.34   Monoplegia of lower limb following cerebral infarction

     I69.341   Monoplegia of lower limb following cerebral infarction affecting right dominant side

     I69.342   Monoplegia of lower limb following cerebral infarction affecting left dominant side

     I69.343   Monoplegia of lower limb following cerebral infarction affecting right non-dominant side

     I69.344   Monoplegia of lower limb following cerebral infarction affecting left non-dominant side

     I69.349   Monoplegia of lower limb following cerebral infarction affecting unspecified side

I69.35   Hemiplegia and hemiparesis following cerebral infarction

     I69.351   Hemiplegia and hemiparesis following cerebral infarction affecting right dominant side

     I69.352   Hemiplegia and hemiparesis following cerebral infarction affecting left dominant side

     I69.353   Hemiplegia and hemiparesis following cerebral infarction affecting right non-dominant side

     I69.354   Hemiplegia and hemiparesis following cerebral infarction affecting left non-dominant side

     I69.359   Hemiplegia and hemiparesis following cerebral infarction affecting unspecified side

I69.36   Other paralytic syndrome following cerebral infarction

Use additional code to identify type of paralytic syndrome, such as:
     locked-in state (G83.5)
     quadriplegia (G82.39,G82.49, G82.8)

Excludes1:   hemiplegia/hemiparesis following cerebral infarction (I69.35-)
         monoplegia of lower limb following cerebral infarction (I69.34-)
         monoplegia of upper limb following cerebral infarction (I69.33-)

     I69.361   Other paralytic syndrome following cerebral infarction affecting right dominant side

     I69.362   Other paralytic syndrome following cerebral infarction affecting left dominant side

     I69.363   Other paralytic syndrome following cerebral infarction affecting right non-dominant side

     I69.364   Other paralytic syndrome following cerebral infarction affecting left non-dominant side

     I69.365   Other paralytic syndrome following cerebral infarction, bilateral

     I69.369   Other paralytic syndrome following cerebral infarction affecting unspecified side

I69.39   Other late effects of cerebral infarction

     I69.390   Apraxia following cerebral infarction

     I69.391   Dysphagia following cerebral infarction

     I69.398   Other late effects of cerebral infarction
         Use additional code to identify the sequelae

I69.4   Sequelae of stroke, not specified as hemorrhage or infarction

   I69.40   Unspecified late effects of stroke, not specified as hemorrhage or infarction

   I69.41   Cognitive deficits following stroke, not specified as hemorrhage or infarction

   I69.42   Speech and language deficits following stroke, not specified as hemorrhage or infarction

     I69.420   Aphasia following stroke, not specified as hemorrhage or infarction

     I69.421   Dysphasia following stroke, not specified as hemorrhage or infarction

     I69.428   Other speech and language deficits following stroke, not specified as hemorrhage or infarction
         Dysarthria following stroke, not specified as hemorrhage or infarction

I69.43   Monoplegia of upper limb following stroke, not specified as hemorrhage or infarction

    I69.431   Monoplegia of upper limb following stroke, not specified as hemorrhage or infarction affecting right dominant side

    I69.432   Monoplegia of upper limb following stroke, not specified as hemorrhage or infarction affecting left dominant side

    I69.433   Monoplegia of upper limb following stroke, not specified as hemorrhage or infarction affecting right non-dominant side

    I69.434   Monoplegia of upper limb following stroke, not specified as hemorrhage or infarction affecting left non-dominant side

    I69.439   Monoplegia of upper limb following stroke, not specified as hemorrhage or infarction affecting unspecified side

I69.44   Monoplegia of lower limb following stroke, not specified as hemorrhage or infarction

    I69.441   Monoplegia of lower limb following stroke, not specified as hemorrhage or infarction affecting right dominant side

    I69.442   Monoplegia of lower limb following stroke, not specified as hemorrhage or infarction affecting left dominant side

    I69.443   Monoplegia of lower limb following stroke, not specified as hemorrhage or infarction affecting right non-dominant side

    I69.444   Monoplegia of lower limb following stroke, not specified as hemorrhage or infarction affecting left non-dominant side

    I69.449   Monoplegia of lower limb following stroke, not specified as hemorrhage or infarction affecting unspecified side

I69.45   Hemiplegia and hemiparesis following stroke, not specified as hemorrhage or infarction

    I69.451   Hemiplegia and hemiparesis following stroke, not specified as hemorrhage or infarction affecting right dominant side

    I69.452   Hemiplegia and hemiparesis following stroke, not specified as hemorrhage or infarction affecting left dominant side

    I69.453   Hemiplegia and hemiparesis following stroke, not specified as hemorrhage or infarction affecting right non-dominant side

    I69.454   Hemiplegia and hemiparesis following stroke, not specified as hemorrhage or infarction affecting left non-dominant side

    I69.459   Hemiplegia and hemiparesis following stroke, not specified as hemorrhage or infarction affecting unspecified side

I69.46   Other paralytic syndrome following stroke, not specified as hemorrhage or infarction

Use additional code to identify type of paralytic syndrome, such as:
locked-in state (G83.5)
quadriplegia (G82.39, G82.49, G82.8)

Excludes1:   sequelae of stroke, not specified as hemorrhage or infarction, with:
hemiplegia/hemiparesis (I69.45-)
monoplegia of lower limb (I69.44-)
monoplegia of upper limb (I69.43-)

    I69.461   Other paralytic syndrome following stroke, not specified as hemorrhage or infarction affecting right dominant side

    I69.462   Other paralytic syndrome following stroke, not specified as hemorrhage or infarction affecting left dominant side

    I69.463   Other paralytic syndrome following stroke, not specified as hemorrhage or infarction affecting right non-dominant side

    I69.464   Other paralytic syndrome following stroke, not specified as hemorrhage or infarction affecting left non-dominant side

    I69.465   Other paralytic syndrome following stroke, not specified as hemorrhage or infarction, bilateral

    I69.469   Other paralytic syndrome following stroke, not specified as hemorrhage or infarction affecting unspecified side

I69.49   Other late effects of stroke, not specified as hemorrhage or infarction

    I69.490   Apraxia following stroke, not specified as hemorrhage or infarction

    I69.491   Dysphagia following stroke, not specified as hemorrhage or infarction

    I69.498   Other late effects of stroke, not specified as hemorrhage or infarction
Use additional code to identify the sequelae

I69.8   Sequelae of other cerebrovascular diseases

Excludes1:   sequelae of traumatic intracranial injury (T90.5)

I69.80   Unspecified late effects of other cerebrovascular disease

I69.81   Cognitive deficits following other cerebrovascular disease

I69.82   Speech and language deficits following other cerebrovascular disease

    I69.820   Aphasia following other cerebrovascular disease

    I69.821   Dysphasia following other cerebrovascular disease

    I69.828   Other speech and language deficits following other cerebrovascular disease
Dysarthria following other cerebrovascular disease

I69.83   Monoplegia of upper limb following other cerebrovascular disease

    I69.831   Monoplegia of upper limb following other cerebrovascular disease affecting right dominant side

    I69.832   Monoplegia of upper limb following other cerebrovascular disease affecting left dominant side

    I69.833   Monoplegia of upper limb following other cerebrovascular disease affecting right non-dominant side

    I69.834   Monoplegia of upper limb following other cerebrovascular disease affecting left non-dominant side

    I69.839   Monoplegia of upper limb following other cerebrovascular disease affecting unspecified side

I69.84   Monoplegia of lower limb following other cerebrovascular disease

    I69.841   Monoplegia of lower limb following other cerebrovascular disease affecting right dominant side

    I69.842   Monoplegia of lower limb following other cerebrovascular disease affecting left dominant side

    I69.843   Monoplegia of lower limb following other cerebrovascular disease affecting right non-dominant side

    I69.844   Monoplegia of lower limb following other cerebrovascular disease affecting left non-dominant side

    I69.849   Monoplegia of lower limb following other cerebrovascular disease affecting unspecified side

I69.85   Hemiplegia and hemiparesis following other cerebrovascular disease

    I69.851   Hemiplegia and hemiparesis following other cerebrovascular disease affecting right dominant side

    I69.852   Hemiplegia and hemiparesis following other cerebrovascular disease affecting left dominant side

I69.853   Hemiplegia and hemiparesis following other cerebrovascular disease affecting right non-dominant side

I69.854   Hemiplegia and hemiparesis following other cerebrovascular disease affecting left non-dominant side

I69.859   Hemiplegia and hemiparesis following other cerebrovascular disease affecting unspecified side

I69.86   Other paralytic syndrome following other cerebrovascular disease

Use additional code to identify type of paralytic syndrome, such as:
locked-in state (G83.5)
quadriplegia (G82.39, G82.49, G82.8)

Excludes1:   hemiplegia/hemiparesis following other cerebrovascular disease (I69.85-)
monoplegia of lower limb following other cerebrovascular disease (I69.84-)
monoplegia of upper limb following other cerebrovascular disease (I69.83-)

I69.861   Other paralytic syndrome following other cerebrovascular disease affecting right dominant side

I69.862   Other paralytic syndrome following other cerebrovascular disease affecting left dominant side

I69.863   Other paralytic syndrome following other cerebrovascular disease affecting right non-dominant side

I69.864   Other paralytic syndrome following other cerebrovascular disease affecting left non-dominant side

I69.865   Other paralytic syndrome following other cerebrovascular disease, bilateral

I69.869   Other paralytic syndrome following other cerebrovascular disease affecting unspecified side

I69.89   Other late effects of other cerebrovascular disease

I69.890   Apraxia following other cerebrovascular disease

I69.891   Dysphagia following other cerebrovascular disease

I69.898   Other late effects of other cerebrovascular disease

Use additional code to identify the sequelae

I69.9   Sequelae of unspecified cerebrovascular diseases

Excludes1:   sequelae of traumatic intracranial injury (T90.5)

I69.90   Unspecified late effects of unspecified cerebrovascular disease

I69.91   Cognitive deficits following unspecified cerebrovascular disease

I69.92   Speech and language deficits following unspecified cerebrovascular disease

I69.920   Aphasia following unspecified cerebrovascular disease

I69.921   Dysphasia following unspecified cerebrovascular disease

I69.928   Other speech and language deficits following unspecified cerebrovascular disease

Dysarthria following unspecified cerebrovascular disease

I69.93   Monoplegia of upper limb following unspecified cerebrovascular disease

I69.931   Monoplegia of upper limb following unspecified cerebrovascular disease affecting right dominant side

I69.932   Monoplegia of upper limb following unspecified cerebrovascular disease affecting left dominant side

I69.933   Monoplegia of upper limb following unspecified cerebrovascular disease affecting right non-dominant side

I69.934   Monoplegia of upper limb following unspecified cerebrovascular disease affecting left non-dominant side

I69.939   Monoplegia of upper limb following unspecified cerebrovascular disease affecting unspecified side

I69.94   Monoplegia of lower limb following unspecified cerebrovascular disease

I69.941   Monoplegia of lower limb following unspecified cerebrovascular disease affecting right dominant side

I69.942   Monoplegia of lower limb following unspecified cerebrovascular disease affecting left dominant side

I69.943   Monoplegia of lower limb following unspecified cerebrovascular disease affecting right non-dominant side

I69.944   Monoplegia of lower limb following unspecified cerebrovascular disease affecting left non-dominant side

I69.949   Monoplegia of lower limb following unspecified cerebrovascular disease affecting unspecified side

I69.95   Hemiplegia and hemiparesis following unspecified cerebrovascular disease

I69.951   Hemiplegia and hemiparesis following unspecified cerebrovascular disease affecting right dominant side

I69.952   Hemiplegia and hemiparesis following unspecified cerebrovascular disease affecting left dominant side

I69.953   Hemiplegia and hemiparesis following unspecified cerebrovascular disease affecting right non-dominant side

I69.954   Hemiplegia and hemiparesis following unspecified cerebrovascular disease affecting left non-dominant side

I69.959   Hemiplegia and hemiparesis following unspecified cerebrovascular disease affecting unspecified side

I69.96   Other paralytic syndrome following unspecified cerebrovascular disease

Use additional code to identify type of paralytic syndrome, such as:
locked-in state (G83.5)
quadriplegia (G82.39, G82.49, G82.8)

Excludes1:   hemiplegia/hemiparesis following unspecified cerebrovascular disease (I69.95-)
monoplegia of lower limb following unspecified cerebrovascular disease (I69.94-)
monoplegia of upper limb following unspecified cerebrovascular disease (I69.93-)

I69.961   Other paralytic syndrome following unspecified cerebrovascular disease affecting right dominant side

I69.962   Other paralytic syndrome following unspecified cerebrovascular disease affecting left dominant side

I69.963   Other paralytic syndrome following unspecified cerebrovascular disease affecting right non-dominant side

I69.964   Other paralytic syndrome following unspecified cerebrovascular disease affecting left non-dominant side

I69.965   Other paralytic syndrome following unspecified cerebrovascular disease, bilateral

I69.969   Other paralytic syndrome following unspecified cerebrovascular disease affecting unspecified side

I69.99   **Other late effects of unspecified cerebrovascular disease**

    I69.990   **Apraxia following unspecified cerebrovascular disease**

    I69.991   **Dysphagia following unspecified cerebrovascular disease**

    I69.998   **Other late effects following unspecified cerebrovascular disease**

        Use additional code to identify the sequelae

DISEASES OF ARTERIES, ARTERIOLES AND CAPILLARIES (I70–I79)

I70   **Atherosclerosis**

    Includes: arteriolosclerosis
                arterial degeneration
                arteriosclerosis
                arteriosclerotic vascular disease
                arteriovascular degeneration
                atheroma
                endarteritis deformans or obliterans
                senile arteritis
                senile endarteritis
                vascular degeneration

    Use additional code to identify:
        exposure to environmental tobacco smoke (X58.1)
        history of tobacco use (Z86.43)
        occupational exposure to environmental tobacco smoke (Z57.31)
        tobacco dependence (F17.-)
        tobacco use (Z72.0)

    Excludes2:   arteriosclerotic cardiovascular disease (I25.1-)
                arteriosclerotic heart disease (I25.1-)
                cerebral atherosclerosis (I67.2)
                coronary atherosclerosis (I25.1-)
                mesenteric atherosclerosis (K55.1)
                precerebral atherosclerosis (I67.2)
                pulmonary atherosclerosis (I27.0)

I70.0   **Atherosclerosis of aorta**

I70.1   **Atherosclerosis of renal artery**
    Goldblatt's kidney
    Excludes2:   atherosclerosis of renal arterioles (I12.-)

I70.2   **Atherosclerosis of native arteries of the extremities**
    Mönckeberg's (medial) sclerosis
    Excludes2:   atherosclerosis of bypass graft of extremities (I70.30-I70.79)

    I70.20   **Unspecified atherosclerosis of native arteries of extremities**

        I70.201   **Unspecified atherosclerosis of native arteries of extremities, right leg**

        I70.202   **Unspecified atherosclerosis of native arteries of extremities, left leg**

        I70.203   **Unspecified atherosclerosis of native arteries of extremities, bilateral legs**

        I70.208   **Unspecified atherosclerosis of native arteries of extremities, other extremity**

        I70.209   **Unspecified atherosclerosis of native arteries of extremities, unspecified extremity**

    I70.21   **Atherosclerosis of native arteries of extremities with intermittent claudication**

        I70.211   **Atherosclerosis of native arteries of extremities with intermittent claudication, right leg**

        I70.212   **Atherosclerosis of native arteries of extremities with intermittent claudication, left leg**

        I70.213   **Atherosclerosis of native arteries of extremities with intermittent claudication, bilateral legs**

        I70.218   **Atherosclerosis of native arteries of extremities with intermittent claudication, other extremity**

        I70.219   **Atherosclerosis of native arteries of extremities with intermittent claudication, unspecified extremity**

I70.22   **Atherosclerosis of native arteries of extremities with rest pain**
    Includes any condition classifiable to I70.21-

    I70.221   **Atherosclerosis of native arteries of extremities with rest pain, right leg**

    I70.222   **Atherosclerosis of native arteries of extremities with rest pain, left leg**

    I70.223   **Atherosclerosis of native arteries of extremities with rest pain, bilateral legs**

    I70.228   **Atherosclerosis of native arteries of extremities with rest pain, other extremity**

    I70.229   **Atherosclerosis of native arteries of extremities with rest pain, unspecified extremity**

I70.23   **Atherosclerosis of native arteries of right leg with ulceration**
    Includes any condition classifiable to I70.211 and I70.221
    Use additional code to identify severity of ulcer (L97.- with fifth character 1)

    I70.231   **Atherosclerosis of native arteries of right leg with ulceration of thigh**

    I70.232   **Atherosclerosis of native arteries of right leg with ulceration of calf**

    I70.233   **Atherosclerosis of native arteries of right leg with ulceration of ankle**

    I70.234   **Atherosclerosis of native arteries of right leg with ulceration of heel and midfoot**
        Atherosclerosis of native arteries of right leg with ulceration of plantar surface of midfoot

    I70.235   **Atherosclerosis of native arteries of right leg with ulceration of other part of foot**
        Atherosclerosis of native arteries of right leg with ulceration of toe

    I70.238   **Atherosclerosis of native arteries of right leg with ulceration of other part of lower right leg**

    I70.239   **Atherosclerosis of native arteries of right leg with ulceration of unspecified site**

I70.24   **Atherosclerosis of native arteries of left leg with ulceration**
    Includes any condition classifiable to I70.212 and I70.222
    Use additional code to identify severity of ulcer (L97.- with fifth character 2)

    I70.241   **Atherosclerosis of native arteries of left leg with ulceration of thigh**

    I70.242   **Atherosclerosis of native arteries of left leg with ulceration of calf**

    I70.243   **Atherosclerosis of native arteries of left leg with ulceration of ankle**

    I70.244   **Atherosclerosis of native arteries of left leg with ulceration of heel and midfoot**
        Atherosclerosis of native arteries of left leg with ulceration of plantar surface of midfoot

    I70.245   **Atherosclerosis of native arteries of left leg with ulceration of other part of foot**
        Atherosclerosis of native arteries of left leg with ulceration of toe

    I70.248   **Atherosclerosis of native arteries of left leg with ulceration of other part of lower left leg**

    I70.249   **Atherosclerosis of native arteries of left leg with ulceration of unspecified site**

I70.25   **Atherosclerosis of native arteries of other extremities with ulceration**
    Includes any condition classificable to I70.218 and I70.228
    Use additional code to identify the severity of the ulcer (L98.49-)

I70.26   **Atherosclerosis of native arteries of extremities with gangrene**
    Includes any condition classifiable to I70.21-, I70.22-, I70.23-, I70.24-, and I70.25-

I70.261   Atherosclerosis of native arteries of extremities with gangrene, right leg

I70.262   Atherosclerosis of native arteries of extremities with gangrene, left leg

I70.263   Atherosclerosis of native arteries of extremities with gangrene, bilateral legs

I70.268   Atherosclerosis of native arteries of extremities with gangrene, other extremity

I70.269   Atherosclerosis of native arteries of extremities with gangrene, unspecified extremity

I70.29   Other atherosclerosis of native arteries of extremities

I70.291   Other atherosclerosis of native arteries of extremities, right leg

I70.292   Other atherosclerosis of native arteries of extremities, left leg

I70.293   Other atherosclerosis of native arteries of extremities, bilateral legs

I70.298   Other atherosclerosis of native arteries of extremities, other extremity

I70.299   Other atherosclerosis of native arteries of extremities, unspecified extremity

I70.3   Atherosclerosis of unspecified type of bypass graft(s) of the extremities

Excludes1:   embolism or thrombus of bypass graft(s) of extremities (T82.8)

I70.30   Unspecified atherosclerosis of unspecified type of bypass graft(s) of the extremities

I70.301   Unspecified atherosclerosis of unspecified type of bypass graft(s) of the extremities, right leg

I70.302   Unspecified atherosclerosis of unspecified type of bypass graft(s) of the extremities, left leg

I70.303   Unspecified atherosclerosis of unspecified type of bypass graft(s) of the extremities, bilateral legs

I70.308   Unspecified atherosclerosis of unspecified type of bypass graft(s) of the extremities, other extremity

I70.309   Unspecified atherosclerosis of unspecified type of bypass graft(s) of the extremities, unspecified extremity

I70.31   Atherosclerosis of unspecified type of bypass graft(s) of the extremities with intermittent claudication

I70.311   Atherosclerosis of unspecified type of bypass graft(s) of the extremities with intermittent claudication, right leg

I70.312   Atherosclerosis of unspecified type of bypass graft(s) of the extremities with intermittent claudication, left leg

I70.313   Atherosclerosis of unspecified type of bypass graft(s) of the extremities with intermittent claudication, bilateral legs

I70.318   Atherosclerosis of unspecified type of bypass graft(s) of the extremities with intermittent claudication, other extremity

I70.319   Atherosclerosis of unspecified type of bypass graft(s) of the extremities with intermittent claudication, unspecified extremity

I70.32   Atherosclerosis of unspecified type of bypass graft(s) of the extremities with rest pain

Includes any condition classifiable to I70.31-

I70.321   Atherosclerosis of unspecified type of bypass graft(s) of the extremities with rest pain, right leg

I70.322   Atherosclerosis of unspecified type of bypass graft(s) of the extremities with rest pain, left leg

I70.323   Atherosclerosis of unspecified type of bypass graft(s) of the extremities with rest pain, bilateral legs

I70.328   Atherosclerosis of unspecified type of bypass graft(s) of the extremities with rest pain, other extremity

I70.329   Atherosclerosis of unspecified type of bypass graft(s) of the extremities with rest pain, unspecified extremity

I70.33   Atherosclerosis of unspecified type of bypass graft(s) of the right leg with ulceration

Includes any condition classifiable to I70.311 and I70.321

Use additional code to identify severity of ulcer (L97.- with fifth character 1)

I70.331   Atherosclerosis of unspecified type of bypass graft(s) of the right leg with ulceration of thigh

I70.332   Atherosclerosis of unspecified type of bypass graft(s) of the right leg with ulceration of calf

I70.333   Atherosclerosis of unspecified type of bypass graft(s) of the right leg with ulceration of ankle

I70.334   Atherosclerosis of unspecified type of bypass graft(s) of the right leg with ulceration of heel and midfoot

Atherosclerosis of unspecified type of bypass graft(s) of right leg with ulceration of plantar surface of midfoot

I70.335   Atherosclerosis of unspecified type of bypass graft(s) of the right leg with ulceration of other part of foot

Atherosclerosis of unspecified type of bypass graft(s) of the right leg with ulceration of toe

I70.338   Atherosclerosis of unspecified type of bypass graft(s) of the right leg with ulceration of other part of lower leg

I70.339   Atherosclerosis of unspecified type of bypass graft(s) of the right leg with ulceration of unspecified site

I70.34   Atherosclerosis of unspecified type of bypass graft(s) of the left leg with ulceration

Includes any condition classifiable to I70.312 and I70.322

Use additional code to identify severity of ulcer (L97.- with fifth character 2)

I70.341   Atherosclerosis of unspecified type of bypass graft(s) of the left leg with ulceration of thigh

I70.342   Atherosclerosis of unspecified type of bypass graft(s) of the left leg with ulceration of calf

I70.343   Atherosclerosis of unspecified type of bypass graft(s) of the left leg with ulceration of ankle

I70.344   Atherosclerosis of unspecified type of bypass graft(s) of the left leg with ulceration of heel and midfoot

Atherosclerosis of unspecified type of bypass graft(s) of left leg with ulceration of plantar surface of midfoot

I70.345   Atherosclerosis of unspecified type of bypass graft(s) of the left leg with ulceration of other part of foot

Atherosclerosis of unspecified type of bypass graft(s) of the left leg with ulceration of toe

I70.348   Atherosclerosis of unspecified type of bypass graft(s) of the left leg with ulceration of other part of lower leg

I70.349   Atherosclerosis of unspecified type of bypass graft(s) of the left leg with ulceration of unspecified site

I70.35   Atherosclerosis of unspecified type of bypass graft(s) of other extremity with ulceration

Includes any condition classifiable to I70.318 and I70.328

Use additional code to identify severity of ulcer (L98.49-)

I70.36 **Atherosclerosis of unspecified type of bypass graft(s) of the extremities with gangrene**
Includes any condition classifiable to I70.31-, I70.32-, I70.33-, I70.34-, I70.35

I70.361 Atherosclerosis of unspecified type of bypass graft(s) of the extremities with gangrene, right leg

I70.362 Atherosclerosis of unspecified type of bypass graft(s) of the extremities with gangrene, left leg

I70.363 Atherosclerosis of unspecified type of bypass graft(s) of the extremities with gangrene, bilateral legs

I70.368 Atherosclerosis of unspecified type of bypass graft(s) of the extremities with gangrene, other extremity

I70.369 Atherosclerosis of unspecified type of bypass graft(s) of the extremities with gangrene, unspecified extremity

I70.39 **Other atherosclerosis of unspecified type of bypass graft(s) of the extremities**

I70.391 Other atherosclerosis of unspecified type of bypass graft(s) of the extremities, right leg

I70.392 Other atherosclerosis of unspecified type of bypass graft(s) of the extremities, left leg

I70.393 Other atherosclerosis of unspecified type of bypass graft(s) of the extremities, bilateral legs

I70.398 Other atherosclerosis of unspecified type of bypass graft(s) of the extremities, other extremity

I70.399 Other atherosclerosis of unspecified type of bypass graft(s) of the extremities, unspecified extremity

I70.4 **Atherosclerosis of autologous vein bypass graft(s) of the extremities**

I70.40 **Unspecified atherosclerosis of autologous vein bypass graft(s) of the extremities**

I70.401 Unspecified atherosclerosis of autologous vein bypass graft(s) of the extremities, right leg

I70.402 Unspecified atherosclerosis of autologous vein bypass graft(s) of the extremities, left leg

I70.403 Unspecified atherosclerosis of autologous vein bypass graft(s) of the extremities, bilateral legs

I70.408 Unspecified atherosclerosis of autologous vein bypass graft(s) of the extremities, other extremity

I70.409 Unspecified atherosclerosis of autologous vein bypass graft(s) of the extremities, unspecified extremity

I70.41 **Atherosclerosis of autologous vein bypass graft(s) of the extremities with intermittent claudication**

I70.411 Atherosclerosis of autologous vein bypass graft(s) of the extremities with intermittent claudication, right leg

I70.412 Atherosclerosis of autologous vein bypass graft(s) of the extremities with intermittent claudication, left leg

I70.413 Atherosclerosis of autologous vein bypass graft(s) of the extremities with intermittent claudication, bilateral legs

I70.418 Atherosclerosis of autologous vein bypass graft(s) of the extremities with intermittent claudication, other extremity

I70.419 Atherosclerosis of autologous vein bypass graft(s) of the extremities with intermittent claudication, unspecified extremity

I70.42 **Atherosclerosis of autologous vein bypass graft(s) of the extremities with rest pain**
Includes any condition classifiable to I70.41-

I70.421 Atherosclerosis of autologous vein bypass graft(s) of the extremities with rest pain, right leg

I70.422 Atherosclerosis of autologous vein bypass graft(s) of the extremities with rest pain, left leg

I70.423 Atherosclerosis of autologous vein bypass graft(s) of the extremities with rest pain, bilateral legs

I70.428 Atherosclerosis of autologous vein bypass graft(s) of the extremities with rest pain, other extremity

I70.429 Atherosclerosis of autologous vein bypass graft(s) of the extremities with rest pain, unspecified extremity

I70.43 **Atherosclerosis of autologous vein bypass graft(s) of the right leg with ulceration**
Includes any condition classifiable to I70.411 and I70.421
Use additional code to identify severity of ulcer (L97.- with fifth character 1)

I70.431 Atherosclerosis of autologous vein bypass graft(s) of the right leg with ulceration of thigh

I70.432 Atherosclerosis of autologous vein bypass graft(s) of the right leg with ulceration of calf

I70.433 Atherosclerosis of autologous vein bypass graft(s) of the right leg with ulceration of ankle

I70.434 Atherosclerosis of autologous vein bypass graft(s) of the right leg with ulceration of heel and midfoot
Atherosclerosis of autologous vein bypass graft(s) of right leg with ulceration of plantar surface of midfoot

I70.435 Atherosclerosis of autologous vein bypass graft(s) of the right leg with ulceration of other part of foot
Atherosclerosis of autologous vein bypass graft(s) of right leg with ulceration of toe

I70.438 Atherosclerosis of autologous vein bypass graft(s) of the right leg with ulceration of other part of lower leg

I70.439 Atherosclerosis of autologous vein bypass graft(s) of the right leg with ulceration of unspecified site

I70.44 **Atherosclerosis of autologous vein bypass graft(s) of the left leg with ulceration**
Includes any condition classifiable to I70.412 and I70.422
Use additional code to identify severity of ulcer (L97.- with fifth character 2)

I70.441 Atherosclerosis of autologous vein bypass graft(s) of the left leg with ulceration of thigh

I70.442 Atherosclerosis of autologous vein bypass graft(s) of the left leg with ulceration of calf

I70.443 Atherosclerosis of autologous vein bypass graft(s) of the left leg with ulceration of ankle

I70.444 Atherosclerosis of autologous vein bypass graft(s) of the left leg with ulceration of heel and midfoot
Atherosclerosis of autologous vein bypass graft(s) of left leg with ulceration of plantar surface of midfoot

I70.445 Atherosclerosis of autologous vein bypass graft(s) of the left leg with ulceration of other part of foot
Atherosclerosis of autologous vein bypass graft(s) of leg with ulceration of toe

I70.448 Atherosclerosis of autologous vein bypass graft(s) of the left leg with ulceration of other part of lower leg

I70.449 Atherosclerosis of autologous vein bypass graft(s) of the left leg with ulceration of unspecified site

I70.45   Atherosclerosis of autologous vein bypass graft(s) of other extremity with ulceration
Includes any condition classifiable to I70.418, I70.428, and I70.438
Use additional code to identify severity of ulcer (L98.49)

I70.46   Atherosclerosis of autologous vein bypass graft(s) of the extremities with gangrene
Includes any condition classifiable to I70.41-, I70.42-, and I70.43-, I70.44-, I70.45

I70.461   Atherosclerosis of autologous vein bypass graft(s) of the extremities with gangrene, right leg

I70.462   Atherosclerosis of autologous vein bypass graft(s) of the extremities with gangrene, left leg

I70.463   Atherosclerosis of autologous vein bypass graft(s) of the extremities with gangrene, bilateral legs

I70.468   Atherosclerosis of autologous vein bypass graft(s) of the extremities with gangrene, other extremity

I70.469   Atherosclerosis of autologous vein bypass graft(s) of the extremities with gangrene, unspecified extremity

I70.49   Other atherosclerosis of autologous vein bypass graft(s) of the extremities

I70.491   Other atherosclerosis of autologous vein bypass graft(s) of the extremities, right leg

I70.492   Other atherosclerosis of autologous vein bypass graft(s) of the extremities, left leg

I70.493   Other atherosclerosis of autologous vein bypass graft(s) of the extremities, bilateral legs

I70.498   Other atherosclerosis of autologous vein bypass graft(s) of the extremities, other extremity

I70.499   Other atherosclerosis of autologous vein bypass graft(s) of the extremities, unspecified extremity

I70.5   Atherosclerosis of nonautologous biological bypass graft(s) of the extremities

I70.50   Unspecified atherosclerosis of nonautologous biological bypass graft(s) of the extremities

I70.501   Unspecified atherosclerosis of nonautologous biological bypass graft(s) of the extremities, right leg

I70.502   Unspecified atherosclerosis of nonautologous biological bypass graft(s) of the extremities, left leg

I70.503   Unspecified atherosclerosis of nonautologous biological bypass graft(s) of the extremities, bilateral legs

I70.508   Unspecified atherosclerosis of nonautologous biological bypass graft(s) of the extremities, other extremity

I70.509   Unspecified atherosclerosis of nonautologous biological bypass graft(s) of the extremities, unspecified extremity

I70.51   Atherosclerosis of nonautologous biological bypass graft(s) of the extremities intermittent claudication

I70.511   Atherosclerosis of nonautologous biological bypass graft(s) of the extremities intermittent claudication, right leg

I70.512   Atherosclerosis of nonautologous biological bypass graft(s) of the extremities intermittent claudication, left leg

I70.513   Atherosclerosis of nonautologous biological bypass graft(s) of the extremities intermittent claudication, bilateral legs

I70.518   Atherosclerosis of nonautologous biological bypass graft(s) of the extremities intermittent claudication, other extremity

I70.519   Atherosclerosis of nonautologous biological bypass graft(s) of the extremities intermittent claudication, unspecified extremity

I70.52   Atherosclerosis of nonautologous biological bypass graft(s) of the extremities with rest pain
Includes any condition classifiable to I70.51-

I70.521   Atherosclerosis of nonautologous biological bypass graft(s) of the extremities with rest pain, right leg

I70.522   Atherosclerosis of nonautologous biological bypass graft(s) of the extremities with rest pain, left leg

I70.523   Atherosclerosis of nonautologous biological bypass graft(s) of the extremities with rest pain, bilateral legs

I70.528   Atherosclerosis of nonautologous biological bypass graft(s) of the extremities with rest pain, other extremity

I70.529   Atherosclerosis of nonautologous biological bypass graft(s) of the extremities with rest pain, unspecified extremity

I70.53   Atherosclerosis of nonautologous biological bypass graft(s) of the right leg with ulceration
Includes any condition classifiable to I70.511 and I70.521
Use additional code to identify severity of ulcer (L97.- with fifth character 1)

I70.531   Atherosclerosis of nonautologous biological bypass graft(s) of the right leg with ulceration of thigh

I70.532   Atherosclerosis of nonautologous biological bypass graft(s) of the right leg with ulceration of calf

I70.533   Atherosclerosis of nonautologous biological bypass graft(s) of the right leg with ulceration of ankle

I70.534   Atherosclerosis of nonautologous biological bypass graft(s) of the right leg with ulceration of heel and midfoot
Atherosclerosis of nonautologous biological bypass graft(s) of right leg with ulceration of plantar surface of midfoot

I70.535   Atherosclerosis of nonautologous biological bypass graft(s) of the right leg with ulceration of other part of foot
Atherosclerosis of nonautologous biological bypass graft(s) of the right leg with ulceration of toe

I70.538   Atherosclerosis of nonautologous biological bypass graft(s) of the right leg with ulceration of other part of lower leg

I70.539   Atherosclerosis of nonautologous biological bypass graft(s) of the right leg with ulceration of unspecified site

I70.54   Atherosclerosis of nonautologous biological bypass graft(s) of the left leg with ulceration
Includes any condition classifiable to I70.512 and I70.522
Use additional code to identify severity of ulcer (L97.- with fifth character 2)

I70.541   Atherosclerosis of nonautologous biological bypass graft(s) of the left leg with ulceration of thigh

I70.542   Atherosclerosis of nonautologous biological bypass graft(s) of the left leg with ulceration of calf

I70.543   Atherosclerosis of nonautologous biological bypass graft(s) of the left leg with ulceration of ankle

I70.544   Atherosclerosis of nonautologous biological bypass graft(s) of the left leg with ulceration of heel and midfoot
Atherosclerosis of nonautologous biological bypass graft(s) of left leg with ulceration of plantar surface of midfoot

I70.545   Atherosclerosis of nonautologous biological bypass graft(s) of the left leg with ulceration of other part of foot
> Atherosclerosis of nonautologous biological bypass graft(s) of the left leg with ulceration of toe

I70.548   Atherosclerosis of nonautologous biological bypass graft(s) of the left leg with ulceration of other part of lower leg

I70.549   Atherosclerosis of nonautologous biological bypass graft(s) of the left leg with ulceration of unspecified site

I70.55   Atherosclerosis of nonautologous biological bypass graft(s) of other extremity with ulceration
> Includes any condition classifiable to I70.518, I70.528, and I70.538
> Use additional code to identify severity of ulcer (L98.49)

I70.56   Atherosclerosis of nonautologous biological graft(s) of the extremities with gangrene
> Includes any condition classifiable to I70.51-, I70.52-, and I70.53-, I70.54-, I70.55

I70.561   Atherosclerosis of nonautologous biological bypass graft(s) of the extremities with gangrene, right leg

I70.562   Atherosclerosis of nonautologous biological bypass graft(s) of the extremities with gangrene, left leg

I70.563   Atherosclerosis of nonautologous biological bypass graft(s) of the extremities with gangrene, bilateral legs

I70.568   Atherosclerosis of nonautologous biological bypass graft(s) of the extremities with gangrene, other extremity

I70.569   Atherosclerosis of nonautologous biological bypass graft(s) of the extremities with gangrene, unspecified extremity

I70.59   Other atherosclerosis of nonautologous biological bypass graft(s) of the extremities

I70.591   Other atherosclerosis of nonautologous biological bypass graft(s) of the extremities, right leg

I70.592   Other atherosclerosis of nonautologous biological bypass graft(s) of the extremities, left leg

I70.593   Other atherosclerosis of nonautologous biological bypass graft(s) of the extremities, bilateral legs

I70.598   Other atherosclerosis of nonautologous biological bypass graft(s) of the extremities, other extremity

I70.599   Other atherosclerosis of nonautologous biological bypass graft(s) of the extremities, unspecified extremity

I70.6   Atherosclerosis of nonbiological bypass graft(s) of the extremities

I70.60   Unspecified atherosclerosis of nonbiological bypass graft(s) of the extremities

I70.601   Unspecified atherosclerosis of nonbiological bypass graft(s) of the extremities, right leg

I70.602   Unspecified atherosclerosis of nonbiological bypass graft(s) of the extremities, left leg

I70.603   Unspecified atherosclerosis of nonbiological bypass graft(s) of the extremities, bilateral legs

I70.608   Unspecified atherosclerosis of nonbiological bypass graft(s) of the extremities, other extremity

I70.609   Unspecified atherosclerosis of nonbiological bypass graft(s) of the extremities, unspecified extremity

I70.61   Atherosclerosis of nonbiological bypass graft(s) of the extremities with intermittent claudication

I70.611   Atherosclerosis of nonbiological bypass graft(s) of the extremities with intermittent claudication, right leg

I70.612   Atherosclerosis of nonbiological bypass graft(s) of the extremities with intermittent claudication, left leg

I70.613   Atherosclerosis of nonbiological bypass graft(s) of the extremities with intermittent claudication, bilateral legs

I70.618   Atherosclerosis of nonbiological bypass graft(s) of the extremities with intermittent claudication, other extremity

I70.619   Atherosclerosis of nonbiological bypass graft(s) of the extremities with intermittent claudication, unspecified extremity

I70.62   Atherosclerosis of nonbiological bypass graft(s) of the extremities with extremity rest pain
> Includes any condition classifiable to I70.61-

I70.621   Atherosclerosis of nonbiological bypass graft(s) of the extremities with rest pain, right leg

I70.622   Atherosclerosis of nonbiological bypass graft(s) of the extremities with rest pain, left leg

I70.623   Atherosclerosis of nonbiological bypass graft(s) of the extremities with rest pain, bilateral legs

I70.628   Atherosclerosis of nonbiological bypass graft(s) of the extremities with rest pain, other extremity

I70.629   Atherosclerosis of nonbiological bypass graft(s) of the extremities with rest pain, unspecified extremity

I70.63   Atherosclerosis of nonbiological bypass graft(s) of the right leg with ulceration
> Includes any condition classifiable to I70.611 and I70.621
> Use additional code to identify severity of ulcer (L97.- with fifth character 1)

I70.631   Atherosclerosis of nonbiological bypass graft(s) of the right leg with ulceration of thigh

I70.632   Atherosclerosis of nonbiological bypass graft(s) of the right leg with ulceration of calf

I70.633   Atherosclerosis of nonbiological bypass graft(s) of the right leg with ulceration of ankle

I70.634   Atherosclerosis of nonbiological bypass graft(s) of the right leg with ulceration of heel and midfoot
> Atherosclerosis of nonbiological bypass graft(s) of right leg with ulceration of plantar surface of midfoot

I70.635   Atherosclerosis of nonbiological bypass graft(s) of the right leg with ulceration of other part of foot
> Atherosclerosis of nonbiological bypass graft(s) of the right leg with ulceration of toe

I70.638   Atherosclerosis of nonbiological bypass graft(s) of the right leg with ulceration of other part of lower leg

I70.639   Atherosclerosis of nonbiological bypass graft(s) of the right leg with ulceration of unspecified site

I70.64   Atherosclerosis of nonbiological bypass graft(s) of the left leg with ulceration
> Includes any condition classifiable to I70.612 and I70.622
> Use additional code to identify severity of ulcer (L97.- with fifth character 2)

I70.641   Atherosclerosis of nonbiological bypass graft(s) of the left leg with ulceration of thigh

I70.642   Atherosclerosis of nonbiological bypass graft(s) of the left leg with ulceration of calf

I70.643   Atherosclerosis of nonbiological bypass graft(s) of the left leg with ulceration of ankle

I70.644   Atherosclerosis of nonbiological bypass graft(s) of the left leg with ulceration of heel and midfoot
> Atherosclerosis of nonbiological bypass graft(s) of left leg with ulceration of plantar surface of midfoot

I70.645   Atherosclerosis of nonbiological bypass graft(s) of the left leg with ulceration of other part of foot
Atherosclerosis of nonbiological bypass graft(s) of the left leg with ulceration of toe

I70.648   Atherosclerosis of nonbiological bypass graft(s) of the left leg with ulceration of other part of lower leg

I70.649   Atherosclerosis of nonbiological bypass graft(s) of the left leg with ulceration of unspecified site

I70.65   Atherosclerosis of nonbiological bypass graft(s) of other extremity with ulceration
Includes any condition classifiable to I70.618 and I70.628
Use additional code to identify severity of ulcer (L98.49)

I70.66   Atherosclerosis of nonbiological bypass graft(s) of the extremities with gangrene
Includes any condition classifiable to I70.61-, I70.62-, I70.63-, I70.64-,I70.65

I70.661   Atherosclerosis of nonbiological bypass graft(s) of the extremities with gangrene, right leg

I70.662   Atherosclerosis of nonbiological bypass graft(s) of the extremities with gangrene, left leg

I70.663   Atherosclerosis of nonbiological bypass graft(s) of the extremities with gangrene, bilateral legs

I70.668   Atherosclerosis of nonbiological bypass graft(s) of the extremities with gangrene, other extremity

I70.669   Atherosclerosis of nonbiological bypass graft(s) of the extremities with gangrene, unspecified extremity

I70.69   Other atherosclerosis of nonbiological bypass graft(s) of the extremities

I70.691   Other atherosclerosis of nonbiological bypass graft(s) of the extremities, right leg

I70.692   Other atherosclerosis of nonbiological bypass graft(s) of the extremities, left leg

I70.693   Other atherosclerosis of nonbiological bypass graft(s) of the extremities, bilateral legs

I70.698   Other atherosclerosis of nonbiological bypass graft(s) of the extremities, other extremity

I70.699   Other atherosclerosis of nonbiological bypass graft(s) of the extremities, unspecified extremity

I70.7   Atherosclerosis of other type of bypass graft(s) of the extremities

I70.70   Unspecified atherosclerosis of other type of bypass graft(s) of the extremities

I70.701   Unspecified atherosclerosis of other type of bypass graft(s) of the extremities, right leg

I70.702   Unspecified atherosclerosis of other type of bypass graft(s) of the extremities, left leg

I70.703   Unspecified atherosclerosis of other type of bypass graft(s) of the extremities, bilateral legs

I70.708   Unspecified atherosclerosis of other type of bypass graft(s) of the extremities, other extremity

I70.709   Unspecified atherosclerosis of other type of bypass graft(s) of the extremities, unspecified extremity

I70.71   Atherosclerosis of other type of bypass graft(s) of the extremities with intermittent claudication

I70.711   Atherosclerosis of other type of bypass graft(s) of the extremities with intermittent claudication, right leg

I70.712   Atherosclerosis of other type of bypass graft(s) of the extremities with intermittent claudication, left leg

I70.713   Atherosclerosis of other type of bypass graft(s) of the extremities with intermittent claudication, bilateral legs

I70.718   Atherosclerosis of other type of bypass graft(s) of the extremities with intermittent claudication, other extremity

I70.719   Atherosclerosis of other type of bypass graft(s) of the extremities with intermittent claudication, unspecified extremity

I70.72   Atherosclerosis of other type of bypass graft(s) of the extremities with rest pain
Includes any condition classifiable to I70.71-

I70.721   Atherosclerosis of other type of bypass graft(s) of the extremities with rest pain, right leg

I70.722   Atherosclerosis of other type of bypass graft(s) of the extremities with rest pain, left leg

I70.723   Atherosclerosis of other type of bypass graft(s) of the extremities with rest pain, bilateral legs

I70.728   Atherosclerosis of other type of bypass graft(s) of the extremities with rest pain, other extremity

I70.729   Atherosclerosis of other type of bypass graft(s) of the extremities with rest pain, unspecified extremity

I70.73   Atherosclerosis of other type of bypass graft(s) of the right leg with ulceration
Includes any condition classifiable to I70.711 and I70.721
Use additional code to identify severity of ulcer (L97.- with fifth character 1)

I70.731   Atherosclerosis of other type of bypass graft(s) of the right leg with ulceration of thigh

I70.732   Atherosclerosis of other type of bypass graft(s) of the right leg with ulceration of calf

I70.733   Atherosclerosis of other type of bypass graft(s) of the right leg with ulceration of ankle

I70.734   Atherosclerosis of other type of bypass graft(s) of the right leg with ulceration of heel and midfoot
Atherosclerosis of other type of bypass graft(s) of right leg with ulceration of plantar surface of midfoot

I70.735   Atherosclerosis of other type of bypass graft(s) of the right leg with ulceration of other part of foot
Atherosclerosis of other type of bypass graft(s) of right leg with ulceration of toe

I70.738   Atherosclerosis of other type of bypass graft(s) of the right leg with ulceration of other part of lower leg

I70.739   Atherosclerosis of other type of bypass graft(s) of the right leg with ulceration of unspecified site

I70.74   Atherosclerosis of other type of bypass graft(s) of the left leg with ulceration
Includes any condition classifiable to I70.712 and I70.722
Use additional code to identify severity of ulcer (L97.- with fifth character 2)

I70.741   Atherosclerosis of other type of bypass graft(s) of the left leg with ulceration of thigh

I70.742   Atherosclerosis of other type of bypass graft(s) of the left leg with ulceration of calf

I70.743   Atherosclerosis of other type of bypass graft(s) of the left leg with ulceration of ankle

I70.744   Atherosclerosis of other type of bypass graft(s) of the left leg with ulceration of heel and midfoot
Atherosclerosis of other type of bypass graft(s) of left leg with ulceration of plantar surface of midfoot

I70.745   Atherosclerosis of other type of bypass graft(s) of the left leg with ulceration of other part of foot
Atherosclerosis of other type of bypass graft(s) of left leg with ulceration of toe

I70.748   Atherosclerosis of other type of bypass graft(s) of the left leg with ulceration of other part of lower leg

I70.749   Atherosclerosis of other type of bypass graft(s) of the left leg with ulceration of unspecified site

I70.75   Atherosclerosis of other type of bypass graft(s) of other extremity with ulceration
Includes any condition classifiable to I70.718 and I70.728
Use additional code to identify severity of ulcer (L98.49)

I70.76   Atherosclerosis of other type of bypass graft(s) of the extremities with gangrene
Includes any condition classifiable to I70.71-, I70.72-, I70.73-, I70.74-, I70.75

I70.761   Atherosclerosis of other type of bypass graft(s) of the extremities with gangrene, right leg

I70.762   Atherosclerosis of other type of bypass graft(s) of the extremities with gangrene, left leg

I70.763   Atherosclerosis of other type of bypass graft(s) of the extremities with gangrene, bilateral legs

I70.768   Atherosclerosis of other type of bypass graft(s) of the extremities with gangrene, other extremity

I70.769   Atherosclerosis of other type of bypass graft(s) of the extremities with gangrene, unspecified extremity

I70.79   Other atherosclerosis of other type of bypass graft(s) of the extremities

I70.791   Other atherosclerosis of other type of bypass graft(s) of the extremities, right leg

I70.792   Other atherosclerosis of other type of bypass graft(s) of the extremities, left leg

I70.793   Other atherosclerosis of other type of bypass graft(s) of the extremities, bilateral legs

I70.798   Other atherosclerosis of other type of bypass graft(s) of the extremities, other extremity

I70.799   Other atherosclerosis of other type of bypass graft(s) of the extremities, unspecified extremity

I70.8   Atherosclerosis of other arteries

I70.9   Generalized and unspecified atherosclerosis

I70.90   Unspecified atherosclerosis

I70.91   Generalized atherosclerosis

I71   Aortic aneurysm and dissection
Excludes1:   syphilitic aortic aneurysm (A52.01)
traumatic aortic aneurysm (S25.0?, S35.0?)

I71.0   Dissection of aorta
Dissecting aneurysm of aorta (ruptured) [any part]

I71.00   Dissection of unspecified site of aorta

I71.01   Dissection of thoracic aorta

I71.02   Dissection of abdominal aorta

I71.03   Dissection of thoracoabdominal aorta

I71.1   Thoracic aortic aneurysm, ruptured

I71.2   Thoracic aortic aneurysm, without mention of rupture

I71.3   Abdominal aortic aneurysm, ruptured

I71.4   Abdominal aortic aneurysm, without mention of rupture

I71.5   Thoracoabdominal aortic aneurysm, ruptured

I71.6   Thoracoabdominal aortic aneurysm, without mention of rupture

I71.8   Aortic aneurysm of unspecified site, ruptured
Rupture of aorta NOS

I71.9   Aortic aneurysm of unspecified site, without mention of rupture
Aneurysm of aorta
Dilatation of aorta
Hyaline necrosis of aorta

I72   Other aneurysm
Includes: aneurysm (cirsoid) (false) (ruptured)
Excludes2:   aneurysm (of):
aorta (I71.-)
arteriovenous NOS (Q27.3-)
acquired (I77.0)
cerebral (nonruptured) (I67.1)
ruptured (I60.7)
coronary (I25.4)
heart (I25.3)
pulmonary artery (I28.1)
retinal (H35.0)
varicose (I77.0)

I72.0   Aneurysm of carotid artery (common) (external) (internal, extracranial portion)
Excludes1:   aneurysm of internal carotid artery, intracranial portion (I67.1)
aneurysm of internal carotid artery NOS (I67.1)

I72.1   Aneurysm of artery of upper extremity

I72.2   Aneurysm of renal artery

I72.3   Aneurysm of iliac artery

I72.4   Aneurysm of artery of lower extremity

I72.8   Aneurysm of other specified arteries

I72.9   Aneurysm of unspecified site

I73   Other peripheral vascular diseases
Excludes2:   chilblains (T69.1)
frostbite (T33- T34)
immersion hand or foot (T69.0-)
spasm of cerebral artery (G45.9)

I73.0   Raynaud's syndrome
Raynaud's disease
Raynaud's phenomenon (secondary)

I73.00   Raynaud's syndrome without gangrene

I73.01   Raynaud's syndrome with gangrene

I73.1   Thromboangiitis obliterans [Buerger's disease]

I73.8   Other specified peripheral vascular diseases
Acrocyanosis
Erythrocyanosis
Erythromelalgia
Simple acroparesthesia [Schultze's type]
Vasomotor acroparesthesia [Nothnagel's type]
Excludes1:   diabetic (peripheral) angiopathy (E08-E14 with .51 - .52)

I73.9   Peripheral vascular disease, unspecified
Intermittent claudication
Peripheral angiopathy NOS
Spasm of artery
Excludes1:   atherosclerosis of the extremities (I70.2- - I70.7-)

I74   Arterial embolism and thrombosis
Includes: embolic infarction
embolic occlusion
thrombotic infarction
thrombotic occlusion
Code first embolism and thrombosis complicating:
abortion or ectopic or molar pregnancy (O00-O07, O08.2)
pregnancy, childbirth and the puerperium (O88.-)
Excludes2:   embolism and thrombosis:
basilar (I63.0-I63.2, I65.1)
carotid (I63.0-I63.2, I65.2)
cerebral (I63.3-I63.5, I66.-)
coronary (I21-I25)
mesenteric (K55.0)
ophthalmic (H34.-)
precerebral NOS (I63.0-I63.2, I65.9)
pulmonary (I26.-)
renal (N28.0)
retinal (H34.-)
vertebral (I63.0-I63.2, I65.0)

I74.0   Embolism and thrombosis of abdominal aorta
Aortic bifurcation syndrome
Aortoiliac obstruction
Leriche's syndrome
Saddle embolus

I74.1   **Embolism and thrombosis of other and unspecified parts of aorta**

    I74.10   **Embolism and thrombosis of unspecified parts of aorta**

    I74.11   **Embolism and thrombosis of thoracic aorta**

    I74.19   **Embolism and thrombosis of other parts of aorta**

I74.2   **Embolism and thrombosis of arteries of the upper extremities**

I74.3   **Embolism and thrombosis of arteries of the lower extremities**

I74.4   **Embolism and thrombosis of arteries of extremities, unspecified**

    Peripheral arterial embolism NOS

I74.5   **Embolism and thrombosis of iliac artery**

I74.8   **Embolism and thrombosis of other arteries**

I74.9   **Embolism and thrombosis of unspecified artery**

I77   **Other disorders of arteries and arterioles**

    Excludes2:   collagen (vascular) diseases (M30-M36)
                hypersensitivity angiitis (M31.0)
                pulmonary artery (I28.-)

I77.0   **Arteriovenous fistula, acquired**

    Aneurysmal varix
    Arteriovenous aneurysm, acquired
    Excludes1:   arteriovenous aneurysm NOS (Q27.3-)
                traumatic—see injury of blood vessel by body region
    Excludes2:   cerebral (I67.1)
                coronary (I25.4)

I77.1   **Stricture of artery**

    Narrowing of artery

I77.2   **Rupture of artery**

    Erosion of artery
    Fistula of artery
    Ulcer of artery
    Excludes1:   traumatic rupture of artery—see injury of blood vessel by body region

I77.3   **Arterial fibromuscular dysplasia**

    Fibromuscular hyperplasia (of) carotid artery
    Fibromuscular hyperplasia (of) renal artery

I77.4   **Celiac artery compression syndrome**

I77.5   **Necrosis of artery**

I77.6   **Arteritis, unspecified**

    Aortitis NOS
    Endarteritis NOS
    Excludes1:   arteritis or endarteritis:
                aortic arch (M31.4)
                cerebral NEC (I67.7)
                coronary (I25.8)
                deformans (I70.-)
                giant cell (M31.5 - .6)
                obliterans (I70.-)
                senile (I70.-)

I77.8   **Other specified disorders of arteries and arterioles**

I77.9   **Disorder of arteries and arterioles, unspecified**

I78   **Diseases of capillaries**

I78.0   **Hereditary hemorrhagic telangiectasia**

    Rendu-Osler-Weber disease

I78.1   **Nevus, non-neoplastic**

    Araneus nevus
    Senile nevus
    Spider nevus
    Stellar nevus
    Excludes1:   nevus NOS (D22.-)
                vascular NOS (Q82.5)
    Excludes2:   blue nevus (D22.-)
                flammeus nevus (Q82.5)
                hairy nevus (D22.-)
                melanocytic nevus (D22.-)
                pigmented nevus (D22.-)
                portwine nevus (Q82.5)
                sanguineous nevus (Q82.5)
                strawberry nevus (Q82.5)
                verrucous nevus (Q82.5)

I78.8   **Other diseases of capillaries**

I78.9   **Disease of capillaries, unspecified**

I79   **Disorders of arteries, arterioles and capillaries in diseases classified elsewhere**

I79.0   **Aneurysm of aorta in diseases classified elsewhere**

    Code first underlying disease
    Excludes1:   syphilitic aneurysm (A52.01)

I79.1   **Aortitis in diseases classified elsewhere**

    Code first underlying disease
    Excludes1:   syphilitic aortitis (A52.02)

I79.8   **Other disorders of arteries, arterioles and capillaries in diseases classified elsewhere**

    Code first underlying disease, such as:
       amyloidosis (E85)
    Excludes1:   diabetic (peripheral) angiopathy (E08-E14 with .51-.52)
                endarteritis:
                syphilitic (A52.09)
                tuberculous (A18.89)

DISEASES OF VEINS, LYMPHATIC VESSELS AND LYMPH NODES, NOT ELSEWHERE CLASSIFIED. (I80–I89)

I80   **Phlebitis and thrombophlebitis**

    Includes: endophlebitis
               inflammation, vein
               periphlebitis
               suppurative phlebitis
    Code first phlebitis and thrombophlebitis complicating:
       abortion, ectopic or molar pregnancy (O00-O07, O08.7)
       pregnancy, childbirth and the puerperium (O22.-, O87.-)
    Use additional external cause code (Chapter XIX) to identify drug, if drug-induced
    Excludes2:   phlebitis and thrombophlebitis (of):
                intracranial and intraspinal, septic or NOS (G08)
                intracranial, nonpyogenic (I67.6)
                intraspinal, nonpyogenic (G95.1)
                portal (vein) (K75.1)
             postphlebitic syndrome (I87.0)
             thrombophlebitis migrans (I82.1)

I80.0   **Phlebitis and thrombophlebitis of superficial vessels of lower extremities**

    Phlebitis and thrombophlebitis of femoropopliteal vein

    I80.00   **Phlebitis and thrombophlebitis of superficial vessels of unspecified lower extremity**

    I80.01   **Phlebitis and thrombophlebitis of superficial vessels of right lower extremity**

    I80.02   **Phlebitis and thrombophlebitis of superficial vessels of left lower extremity**

    I80.03   **Phlebitis and thrombophlebitis of superficial vessels of lower extremities, bilateral**

I80.1   **Phlebitis and thrombophlebitis of femoral vein**

    I80.10   **Phlebitis and thrombophlebitis of unspecified femoral vein**

    I80.11   **Phlebitis and thrombophlebitis of right femoral vein**

    I80.12   **Phlebitis and thrombophlebitis of left femoral vein**

    I80.13   **Phlebitis and thrombophlebitis of femoral vein, bilateral**

I80.2   **Phlebitis and thrombophlebitis of other and unspecified deep vessels of lower extremities**

    I80.20   **Phlebitis and thrombophlebitis of unspecified deep vessels of lower extremities**

       Deep vein thrombosis NOS

       I80.201   **Phlebitis and thrombophlebitis of unspecified deep vessels of right lower extremity**

       I80.202   **Phlebitis and thrombophlebitis of unspecified deep vessels of left lower extremity**

       I80.203   **Phlebitis and thrombophlebitis of unspecified deep vessels of lower extremities, bilateral**

       I80.209   **Phlebitis and thrombophlebitis of unspecified deep vessels of unspecified lower extremity**

    I80.21   **Phlebitis and thrombophlebitis of popliteal vein**

       I80.211   **Phlebitis and thrombophlebitis of right popliteal vein**

I80.212　Phlebitis and thrombophlebitis of left popliteal vein

I80.213　Phlebitis and thrombophlebitis of popliteal vein, bilateral

I80.219　Phlebitis and thrombophlebitis of unspecified popliteal vein

I80.22　Phlebitis and thrombophlebitis of tibial vein

I80.221　Phlebitis and thrombophlebitis of right tibial vein

I80.222　Phlebitis and thrombophlebitis of left tibial vein

I80.223　Phlebitis and thrombophlebitis of tibial vein, bilateral

I80.229　Phlebitis and thrombophlebitis of unspecified tibial vein

I80.29　Phlebitis and thrombophlebitis of other deep vessels of lower extremities

I80.291　Phlebitis and thrombophlebitis of other deep vessels of right lower extremity

I80.292　Phlebitis and thrombophlebitis of other deep vessels of left lower extremity

I80.293　Phlebitis and thrombophlebitis of other deep vessels of lower extremity, bilateral

I80.299　Phlebitis and thrombophlebitis of other deep vessels of unspecified lower extremity

I80.3　Phlebitis and thrombophlebitis of lower extremities, unspecified
Embolism or thrombosis of lower extremity NOS

I80.8　Phlebitis and thrombophlebitis of other sites

I80.9　Phlebitis and thrombophlebitis of unspecified site

I81　Portal vein thrombosis
Includes:　portal (vein) obstruction
Excludes2:　hepatic vein thrombosis (I82.0)
　　　phlebitis of portal vein (K75.1)

I82　Other venous embolism and thrombosis
Code first venous embolism and thrombosis complicating:
　abortion, ectopic or molar pregnancy (O00-O07, O08.7)
　pregnancy, childbirth and the puerperium (O22.-, O87.-)
Excludes2:　venous embolism and thrombosis (of)
　　　cerebral (I63.6, I67.6)
　　　coronary (I21-I25)
　　　intracranial and intraspinal, septic or NOS (G08)
　　　intracranial, nonpyogenic (I67.6)
　　　intraspinal, nonpyogenic (G95.1)
　　　lower extremities (I80.-)
　　　mesenteric (K55.0)
　　　portal (I81)
　　　pulmonary (I26.-)

I82.0　Budd-Chiari syndrome
Hepatic vein thrombosis

I82.1　Thrombophlebitis migrans

I82.2　Embolism and thrombosis of vena cava

I82.3　Embolism and thrombosis of renal vein

I82.8　Embolism and thrombosis of other specified veins

I82.9　Embolism and thrombosis of unspecified vein
Embolism of vein NOS
Thrombosis (vein) NOS

I83　Varicose veins of lower extremities
Excludes1:　varicose veins complicating pregnancy (O22.0-)
　　　varicose veins complicating the puerperium (O87.4)

I83.0　Varicose veins of lower extremities with ulcer
Use additional code to identify severity of ulcer (L97.-)

I83.00　Varicose veins of unspecified lower extremity with ulcer

I83.001　Varicose veins of unspecified lower extremity with ulcer of thigh

I83.002　Varicose veins of unspecified lower extremity with ulcer of calf

I83.003　Varicose veins of unspecified lower extremity with ulcer of ankle

I83.004　Varicose veins of unspecified lower extremity with ulcer of heel and midfoot
Varicose veins of unspecified lower extremity with ulcer of plantar surface of midfoot

I83.005　Varicose veins of unspecified lower extremity with ulcer other part of foot
Varicose veins of unspecified lower extremity with ulcer of toe

I83.008　Varicose veins of unspecified lower extremity with ulcer other part of lower leg

I83.009　Varicose veins of unspecified lower extremity with ulcer of unspecified site

I83.01　Varicose veins of right lower extremity with ulcer

I83.011　Varicose veins of right lower extremity with ulcer of thigh

I83.012　Varicose veins of right lower extremity with ulcer of calf

I83.013　Varicose veins of right lower extremity with ulcer of ankle

I83.014　Varicose veins of right lower extremity with ulcer of heel and midfoot
Varicose veins of right lower extremity with ulcer of plantar surface of midfoot

I83.015　Varicose veins of right lower extremity with ulcer other part of foot
Varicose veins of right lower extremity with ulcer of toe

I83.018　Varicose veins of right lower extremity with ulcer other part of lower leg

I83.019　Varicose veins of right lower extremity with ulcer of unspecified site

I83.02　Varicose veins of left lower extremity with ulcer

I83.021　Varicose veins of left lower extremity with ulcer of thigh

I83.022　Varicose veins of left lower extremity with ulcer of calf

I83.023　Varicose veins of left lower extremity with ulcer of ankle

I83.024　Varicose veins of left lower extremity with ulcer of heel and midfoot
Varicose veins of left lower extremity with ulcer of plantar surface of midfoot

I83.025　Varicose veins of left lower extremity with ulcer other part of foot
Varicose veins of left lower extremity with ulcer of toe

I83.028　Varicose veins of left lower extremity with ulcer other part of lower leg

I83.029　Varicose veins of left lower extremity with ulcer of unspecified site

I83.1　Varicose veins of lower extremities with inflammation
Stasis dermatitis

I83.10　Varicose veins of unspecified lower extremity with inflammation

I83.11　Varicose veins of right lower extremity with inflammation

I83.12　Varicose veins of left lower extremity with inflammation

I83.2　Varicose veins of lower extremities with both ulcer and inflammation
Use additional code to identify severity of ulcer (L97.-)

I83.20　Varicose veins of unspecified lower extremity with both ulcer and inflammation

I83.201　Varicose veins of unspecified lower extremity with both ulcer of thigh and inflammation

I83.202　Varicose veins of unspecified lower extremity with both ulcer of calf and inflammation

I83.203　Varicose veins of unspecified lower extremity with both ulcer of ankle and inflammation

I83.204 **Varicose veins of unspecified lower extremity with both ulcer of heel and midfoot and inflammation**
    Varicose veins of unspecified lower extremity with both ulcer of plantar surface of midfoot and inflammation

I83.205 **Varicose veins of unspecified lower extremity with both ulcer other part of foot and inflammation**
    Varicose veins of unspecified lower extremity with both ulcer of toe and inflammation

I83.208 **Varicose veins of unspecified lower extremity with both ulcer of other part of lower extremity and inflammation**

I83.209 **Varicose veins of unspecified lower extremity with both ulcer of unspecified site and inflammation**

I83.21 **Varicose veins of right lower extremity with both ulcer and inflammation**

I83.211 **Varicose veins of right lower extremity with both ulcer of thigh and inflammation**

I83.212 **Varicose veins of right lower extremity with both ulcer of calf and inflammation**

I83.213 **Varicose veins of right lower extremity with both ulcer of ankle and inflammation**

I83.214 **Varicose veins of right lower extremity with both ulcer of heel and midfoot and inflammation**
    Varicose veins of right lower extremity with both ulcer of plantar surface of midfoot and inflammation

I83.215 **Varicose veins of right lower extremity with both ulcer other part of foot and inflammation**
    Varicose veins of right lower extremity with both ulcer of toe and inflammation

I83.218 **Varicose veins of right lower extremity with both ulcer of other part of lower extremity and inflammation**

I83.219 **Varicose veins of right lower extremity with both ulcer of unspecified site and inflammation**

I83.22 **Varicose veins of left lower extremity with both ulcer and inflammation**

I83.221 **Varicose veins of left lower extremity with both ulcer of thigh and inflammation**

I83.222 **Varicose veins of left lower extremity with both ulcer of calf and inflammation**

I83.223 **Varicose veins of left lower extremity with both ulcer of ankle and inflammation**

I83.224 **Varicose veins of left lower extremity with both ulcer of heel and midfoot and inflammation**
    Varicose veins of left lower extremity with both ulcer of plantar surface of midfoot and inflammation

I83.225 **Varicose veins of left lower extremity with both ulcer other part of foot and inflammation**
    Varicose veins of left lower extremity with both ulcer of toe and inflammation

I83.228 **Varicose veins of left lower extremity with both ulcer of other part of lower extremity and inflammation**

I83.229 **Varicose veins of left lower extremity with both ulcer of unspecified site and inflammation**

I83.9 **Varicose veins of lower extremities without ulcer or inflammation**
    Phlebectasia of lower extremities
    Varicose veins of lower extremities
    Varix of lower extremities

I83.90 **Varicose veins of unspecified lower extremity without ulcer or inflammation**

I83.91 **Varicose veins of right lower extremity without ulcer or inflammation**

I83.92 **Varicose veins of left lower extremity without ulcer or inflammation**

I83.93 **Varicose veins of bilateral lower extremities without ulcer or inflammation**

I84 **Hemorrhoids**
    Includes: piles
             varicose veins of anus and rectum
    Excludes1:   hemorrhoids complicating childbirth and the puerperium (O87.2)
             hemorrhoids complicating pregnancy (O22.4)

I84.0 **Thrombosed hemorrhoids**

I84.00 **Unspecified thrombosed hemorrhoids**
    Thrombosed hemorrhoids, unspecified whether internal or external

I84.01 **Internal thrombosed hemorrhoids**

I84.02 **External thrombosed hemorrhoids**

I84.03 **Internal and external thrombosed hemorrhoids**

I84.1 **Hemorrhoids with other complications**

I84.10 **Unspecified hemorrhoids with other complications**

I84.101 **Unspecified bleeding hemorrhoids**

I84.102 **Unspecified prolapsed hemorrhoids**

I84.103 **Unspecified strangulated hemorrhoids**

I84.104 **Unspecified ulcerated hemorrhoids**

I84.11 **Internal hemorrhoids with other complications**

I84.111 **Internal bleeding hemorrhoids**

I84.112 **Internal prolapsed hemorrhoids**

I84.113 **Internal strangulated hemorrhoids**

I84.114 **Internal ulcerated hemorrhoids**

I84.12 **External hemorrhoids with other complications**

I84.121 **External bleeding hemorrhoids**

I84.122 **External prolapsed hemorrhoids**

I84.123 **External strangulated hemorrhoids**

I84.124 **External ulcerated hemorrhoids**

I84.13 **Internal and external hemorrhoids with other complications**

I84.131 **Internal and external bleeding hemorrhoids**

I84.132 **Internal and external prolapsed hemorrhoids**

I84.133 **Internal and external strangulated hemorrhoids**

I84.134 **Internal and external ulcerated hemorrhoids**

I84.2 **Hemorrhoids without complication**

I84.20 **Unspecified hemorrhoids without complication**
    Hemorrhoids NOS

I84.21 **Internal hemorrhoids without complication**
    Internal hemorrhoids NOS

I84.22 **External hemorrhoids without complication**
    External hemorrhoids NOS

I84.23 **Internal and external hemorrhoids without complication**
    Internal and external hemorrhoids NOS

I84.6 **Residual hemorrhoidal skin tags**
    Skin tags of anus or rectum

I85 **Esophageal varices**
    Use additional code to identify:
    alcohol abuse and dependence (F10.-)
    alcohol use, uncomplicated (Z72.1)
    alcohol dependence, in remission (F10.11)

I85.0 **Esophageal varices**
    Esophageal varices NOS
    Idiopathic esophageal varices
    Primary esophageal varices

I85.00 **Esophageal varices without bleeding**

I85.01 **Esophageal varices with bleeding**

I85.1 **Secondary esophageal varices**
    Esophageal varices secondary to alcoholic liver disease
    Esophageal varices secondary to cirrhosis of liver
    Esophageal varices secondary to schistosomiasis
    Esophageal varices secondary to toxic liver disease
    Code first underlying disease

I85.10   Secondary esophageal varices without bleeding
I85.11   Secondary esophageal varices with bleeding

I86   Varicose veins of other sites
Excludes1:   varicose veins of unspecified site (I83.9-)
Excludes2:   retinal varices (H35.0-)
I86.0   Sublingual varices
I86.1   Scrotal varices
Varicocele
I86.2   Pelvic varices
I86.3   Vulval varices
Excludes1:   vulval varices complicating childbirth and the
puerperium (O87.8)
vulval varices complicating pregnancy (O22.1-)
I86.4   Gastric varices
I86.8   Varicose veins of other specified sites
Varicose ulcer of nasal septum

I87   Other disorders of veins
I87.0   Postphlebitic syndrome
I87.1   Compression of vein
Stricture of vein
Vena cava syndrome (inferior) (superior)
Excludes2:   compression of pulmonary vein (I28.8)
I87.2   Venous insufficiency (chronic) (peripheral)
I87.8   Other specified disorders of veins
Phlebosclerosis
Venofibrosis
I87.9   Disorder of vein, unspecified

I88   Nonspecific lymphadenitis
Excludes1:   acute lymphadenitis, except mesenteric (L04.-)
enlarged lymph nodes NOS (R59.-)
human immunodeficiency virus [HIV] disease resulting
in generalized lymphadenopathy (B20)
I88.0   Nonspecific mesenteric lymphadenitis
Mesenteric lymphadenitis (acute) (chronic)
I88.1   Chronic lymphadenitis, except mesenteric
Adenitis
Lymphadenitis
I88.8   Other nonspecific lymphadenitis
I88.9   Nonspecific lymphadenitis, unspecified
Lymphadenitis NOS

I89   Other noninfective disorders of lymphatic vessels and lymph nodes
Excludes1:   chylocele, tunica vaginalis (nonfilarial) NOS (N50.8)
enlarged lymph nodes NOS (R59.-)
filarial chylocele (B74.-)
hereditary lymphedema (Q82.0)
I89.0   Lymphedema, not elsewhere classified
Elephantiasis (nonfilarial) NOS
Lymphangiectasis
Obliteration, lymphatic vessel
Praecox lymphedema
Secondary lymphedema
Excludes1:   postmastectomy lymphedema (I97.2)
I89.1   Lymphangitis
Chronic lymphangitis
Lymphangitis NOS
Subacute lymphangitis
Excludes1:   acute lymphangitis (L03.-)
I89.8   Other specified noninfective disorders of lymphatic vessels and lymph nodes
Chylocele (nonfilarial)
Chylous ascites
Chylous cyst
Lipomelanotic reticulosis
Lymph node or vessel fistula
Lymph node or vessel infarction
Lymph node or vessel rupture
I89.9   Noninfective disorder of lymphatic vessels and lymph nodes, unspecified
Disease of lymphatic vessels NOS

OTHER AND UNSPECIFIED DISORDERS OF THE CIRCULATORY SYSTEM (I95–I99)

I95   Hypotension
Excludes1:   cardiovascular collapse (R57.9)
maternal hypotension syndrome (O26.5-)
nonspecific low blood pressure reading NOS (R03.1)
I95.0   Idiopathic hypotension
I95.1   Orthostatic hypotension
Hypotension, postural
Excludes1:   neurogenic orthostatic hypotension [Shy-Drager]
(G90.3)
orthostatic hypotension due to drugs (I95.2)
I95.2   Hypotension due to drugs
Orthostatic hypotension due to drugs
Use additional code (Chapter XIX) to identify the drug
Excludes1:   iatrogenic hypotension, other than drug induced
(I95.3)
I95.3   Other iatrogenic hypotension
Excludes1:   hypotension due to drugs (I95.2)
I95.8   Other hypotension
Chronic hypotension
I95.9   Hypotension, unspecified

I96   Gangrene, not elsewhere classified
Includes: gangrenous cellulites
Excludes1:   gangrene in:
atherosclerosis of native arteries of the extremities
(I70.24)
diabetes mellitus (E08-E14)
hernia (K40.1, K40.4, K41.1, K41.4, K42.1, K43.1-,
K44.1, K45.1, K46.1)
other peripheral vascular diseases (I73.-)
gangrene of certain specified sites—see Alphabetical
Index
gas gangrene (A48.0)
pyoderma gangrenosum (L88)

I97   Intraoperative and postprocedural complications and disorders of the circulatory system, not elsewhere classified
Excludes2:   postoperative shock (T81.1)
I97.0   Postcardiotomy syndrome
I97.1   Other functional disturbances following cardiac surgery
Excludes2:   acute pulmonary insufficiency following thoracic
surgery (J95.1)
I97.11   Cardiac insufficiency following cardiac surgery
I97.12   Heart failure following cardiac surgery
Excludes1:   heart failure following noncardiac
surgery (T81.84)
I97.19   Other functional disturbances following cardiac surgery
I97.2   Postmastectomy lymphedema syndrome
Elephantiasis
Obliteration of lymphatic vessels
I97.3   Postoperative hypertension
I97.4   Intraoperative and postprocedural hemorrhage or hematoma complicating a circulatory system procedure
Excludes1:   intraoperative hemorrhage or hematoma due to
accidental puncture and laceration during a
circulatory system procedure (I97.5-)
I97.41   Intraoperative hemorrhage of a circulatory system organ or structure during a circulatory system procedure
I97.410   Intraoperative hemorrhage of a circulatory system organ or structure during a cardiac catheterization
I97.411   Intraoperative hemorrhage of a circulatory system organ or structure during a cardiac bypass
I97.418   Intraoperative hemorrhage of a circulatory system organ or structure during an other circulatory system procedure

       I97.42   Intraoperative hemorrhage of a non-circulatory system organ or structure during a circulatory system procedure

       I97.43   Intraoperative hematoma of a circulatory system organ or structure during a circulatory system procedure

       I97.44   Intraoperative hematoma of a non-circulatory system organ or structure during a circulatory system procedure

       I97.45   Postprocedural hemorrhage of a circulatory system organ or structure following a circulatory system procedure

       I97.46   Postprocedural hemorrhage of a non-circulatory system organ or structure following a circulatory system procedure

       I97.47   Postprocedural hematoma of a circulatory system organ or structure following a circulatory system procedure

       I97.48   Postprocedural hematoma of a non-circulatory system organ or structure following a circulatory system procedure

   I97.5   Accidental puncture and laceration during a circulatory system procedure

       I97.51   Accidental puncture and laceration of a circulatory system organ or structure during a circulatory system procedure

       I97.52   Accidental puncture and laceration of a non-circulatory system organ or structure during a circulatory system procedure

   I97.8   Other intraoperative and postprocedural complications and disorders of the circulatory system, not elsewhere classified

       I97.81   Other intraoperative complications of the circulatory system, not elsewhere classified

       I97.89   Other postprocedural complications and disorders of the circulatory system, not elsewhere classified

   I97.9   Unspecified intraoperative and postprocedural complications and disorders of the circulatory system

       I97.90   Unspecified intraoperative disorder of the circulatory system

       I97.91   Unspecified postprocedural complications and disorder of the circulatory system

I99   Other and unspecified disorders of circulatory system

   I99.8   Other disorder of circulatory system

   I99.9   Unspecified disorder of circulatory system

CHAPTER X — DISEASES OF THE RESPIRATORY SYSTEM (J00–J99)

Note: When a respiratory condition is described as occurring in more than one site and is not specifically indexed, it should be classified to the lower anatomic site (e.g. tracheobronchitis to bronchitis in J40).

Use additional code, where appliable, to identify:
- exposure to environmental tobacco smoke (X58.1)
- exposure to tobacco smoke in the perinatal period (P96.6)
- history of tobacco use (Z86.43)
- occupational exposure to environmental tobacco smoke (Z57.31)
- tobacco dependence (F17.-)
- tobacco use (Z72.0)

Excludes2:   certain conditions originating in the perinatal period (P04-P96)
certain infectious and parasitic diseases (A00-B99)
complications of pregnancy, childbirth and the puerperium (O00-O99)
congenital malformations, deformations and chromosomal abnormalities (Q00-Q99)
endocrine, nutritional and metabolic diseases (E00-E90)
injury, poisoning and certain other consequences of external causes (S00-T98)
neoplasms (C00-D48)
smoke inhalation (T59.81-)
symptoms, signs and abnormal clinical and laboratory findings, not elsewhere classified (R00-R94)

This chapter contains the following blocks:

J00-J06	Acute upper respiratory infections
J10-J18	Influenza and pneumonia
J20-J22	Other acute lower respiratory infections
J30-J39	Other diseases of upper respiratory tract
J40-J47	Chronic lower respiratory diseases
J60-J70	Lung diseases due to external agents
J80-J84	Other respiratory diseases principally affecting the interstitium
J85-J86	Suppurative and necrotic conditions of the lower respiratory tract
J90-J94	Other diseases of the pleura
J95-J99	Other diseases of the respiratory system

ACUTE UPPER RESPIRATORY INFECTIONS (J00-J06)

Excludes1:   chronic obstructive pulmonary disease with acute exacerbation NOS (J44.1)

J00   Acute nasopharyngitis [common cold]

Includes: acute rhinitis
coryza (acute)
infective nasopharyngitis NOS
infective rhinitis
nasal catarrh, acute
nasopharyngitis NOS

Excludes1:   acute pharyngitis (J02.-)
acute sore throat NOS (J02.9)
pharyngitis NOS (J02.9)
rhinitis NOS (J31.0)
sore throat NOS (J02.9)

Excludes2:   allergic rhinitis (J30.1-J30.9)
chronic pharyngitis (J31.2)
chronic rhinitis (J31.0)
chronic sore throat (J31.2)
nasopharyngitis, chronic (J31.1)
vasomotor rhinitis (J30.0)

J01   Acute sinusitis

Includes: acute abscess of sinus
acute empyema of sinus
acute infection of sinus
acute inflammation of sinus
acute suppuration of sinus
Use additional code (B95-B97) to identify infectious agent.

Excludes1:   sinusitis NOS (J32.9)
Excludes2:   chronic sinusitis (J32.0-J32.8)

J01.0   Acute maxillary sinusitis
Acute antritis

J01.00   Acute maxillary sinusitis, unspecified

J01.01   Acute recurrent maxillary sinusitis

J01.1   Acute frontal sinusitis

J01.10   Acute frontal sinusitis, unspecified

J01.11   Acute recurrent frontal sinusitis

J01.2   Acute ethmoidal sinusitis

J01.20   Acute ethmoidal sinusitis, unspecified

J01.21   Acute recurrent ethmoidal sinusitis

J01.3   Acute sphenoidal sinusitis

J01.30   Acute sphenoidal sinusitis, unspecified

J01.31   Acute recurrent sphenoidal sinusitis

J01.4   Acute pansinusitis

J01.40   Acute pansinusitis, unspecified

J01.41   Acute recurrent pansinusitis

J01.8   Other acute sinusitis

J01.80   Other acute sinusitis
Acute sinusitis involving more than one sinus but not pansinusitis

J01.81   Other acute recurrent sinusitis
Acute recurrent sinusitis involving more than one sinus but not pansinusitis

J01.9   Acute sinusitis, unspecified

J01.90   Acute sinusitis, unspecified

J01.91   Acute recurrent sinusitis, unspecified

J02   Acute pharyngitis

Includes: acute sore throat
Excludes1:   acute laryngopharyngitis (J06.0)
peritonsillar abscess (J36)
pharyngeal abscess (J39.1)
pharyngitis due to coxsackie virus (B08.5)
pharyngitis due to gonococcus (A54.5)
retropharyngeal abscess (J39.0)
Excludes2:   chronic pharyngitis (J31.2)

J02.0   Streptococcal pharyngitis
Septic pharyngitis
Streptococcal sore throat

Excludes1:   scarlet fever (A38.-)

J02.8   Acute pharyngitis due to other specified organisms
Use additional code (B95-B97) to identify infectious agent.

Excludes1:   acute pharyngitis due to herpes [simplex] virus (B00.2)
acute pharyngitis due to infectious mononucleosis (B27.-)
acute pharyngitis due to influenza virus (J10.1
enteroviral vesicular pharyngitis (B08.5)

J02.9   Acute pharyngitis, unspecified
Gangrenous pharyngitis (acute)
Infective pharyngitis (acute) NOS
Pharyngitis (acute) NOS
Sore throat (acute) NOS
Suppurative pharyngitis (acute)
Ulcerative pharyngitis (acute)

J03   Acute tonsillitis

Excludes1:   acute sore throat (J02.-)
hypertrophy of tonsils (J35.1)
peritonsillar abscess (J36)
sore throat NOS (J02.9)
streptococcal sore throat (J02.0)
Excludes2:   chronic tonsillitis (J35.0)

J03.0   Streptococcal tonsillitis
Septic tonsillitis

J03.00   Acute streptococcal tonsillitis, unspecified

J03.01   Acute recurrent streptococcal tonsillitis

J03.8   Acute tonsillitis due to other specified organisms
Use additional code (B95-B97) to identify infectious agent.

Excludes1:   diphtheritic tonsillitis (A36.0)
herpesviral pharyngotonsillitis (B00.2)
streptococcal tonsillitis (J03.0)
tuberculous tonsillitis (A15.8)
Vincent's tonsillitis (A69.1)

J03.80   Acute tonsillitis due to other specified organisms

J03.81   Acute recurrent tonsillitis due to other specified organisms

J03.9   Acute tonsillitis, unspecified
Follicular tonsillitis (acute)
Gangrenous tonsillitis (acute)
Infective tonsillitis (acute)
Tonsillitis (acute) NOS
Ulcerative tonsillitis (acute)

J03.90   Acute tonsillitis, unspecified

J03.91   Acute recurrent tonsillitis, unspecified

J04   Acute laryngitis and tracheitis
Use additional code (B95-B97) to identify infectious agent.

Excludes1:   acute obstructive laryngitis [croup] and epiglottitis (J05.-)

Excludes2:   laryngismus (stridulus) (J38.5)

J04.0   Acute laryngitis
Edematous laryngitis (acute)
Laryngitis (acute) NOS
Septic laryngitis
Subglottic laryngitis (acute)
Suppurative laryngitis (acute)
Ulcerative laryngitis (acute)
Excludes1:   influenzal laryngitis (J10.1)
Excludes2:   chronic laryngitis (J37.0)

J04.1   Acute tracheitis
Acute viral tracheitis
Catarrhal tracheitis (acute)
Tracheitis (acute) NOS
Excludes2:   chronic tracheitis (J42)

J04.2   Acute laryngotracheitis
Laryngotracheitis NOS
Tracheitis (acute) with laryngitis (acute)
Excludes2:   chronic laryngotracheitis (J37.1)

J05   Acute obstructive laryngitis [croup] and epiglottitis
Use additional code (B95-B97) to identify infectious agent.

J05.0   Acute obstructive laryngitis [croup]
Obstructive laryngitis (acute) NOS

J05.1   Acute epiglottitis
Epiglottitis NOS
Excludes2:   epiglottitis, chronic (J37.0)

J06   Acute upper respiratory infections of multiple and unspecified sites
Excludes1:   acute respiratory infection NOS (J22)
influenza virus (J10.1)
streptococcal pharyngitis (J02.0)

J06.0   Acute laryngopharyngitis

J06.9   Acute upper respiratory infection, unspecified
Upper respiratory disease, acute
Upper respiratory infection NOS

INFLUENZA AND PNEUMONIA (J10-J18)

Excludes1:   allergic or eosinophilic pneumonia (J82)
aspiration pneumonia NOS (J69.0)
congenital pneumonia (P23.9)
lipid pneumonia (J69.1)
meconium pneumonia (P24.0)
newborn pneumonia (P24.9)
pneumonia due to solids and liquids (J69-)
pneumonia with abscess of lung (J85.1)
rheumatic pneumonia (I00)

J10   Influenza
Use additional code to identify the virus (B97.-)
Excludes1:   Hemophilus influenzae [H. influenzae] infection NOS (A49.2)
Hemophilus influenzae [H. influenzae] laryngitis (J04.0)
Excludes2:   Hemophilus influenzae [H. influenzae] meningitis (G00.0)
Hemophilus influenzae [H. influenzae] pneumonia (J14)

J10.1   Influenza with respiratory manifestations
Acute influenzal upper respiratory infection
Influenza NOS
Influenzal laryngitis
Influenzal pharyngitis
Influenzal pleural effusion
Codes also any associated pneumonia (J12-J18)

J10.8   Influenza with other manifestations

J10.81   Influenzal gastroenteritis
Excludes1:   "intestinal flu" [viral gastroenteritis] (A08.-)

J10.89   Influenza with other manifestations
Influenzal encephalopathy
Influenzal myocarditis

J12   Viral pneumonia, not elsewhere classified
Includes: bronchopneumonia due to viruses other than influenza viruses
Excludes1:   aspiration pneumonia due to anesthesia during labor and delivery (O74.0)
aspiration pneumonia due to anesthesia during pregnancy (O29)
aspiration pneumonia due to anesthesia during puerperium (O89.0)
aspiration pneumonia due to solids and liquids (J69.-)
aspiration pneumonia NOS (J69.0)
congenital pneumonia (P23.0)
congenital rubella pneumonitis (P35.0)
interstitial pneumonia NOS (J84.9)
lipid pneumonia (J69.1)
neonatal aspiration pneumonia (P24.9)

J12.0   Adenoviral pneumonia

J12.1   Respiratory syncytial virus pneumonia

J12.2   Parainfluenza virus pneumonia

J12.8   Other viral pneumonia

J12.9   Viral pneumonia, unspecified

J13   Pneumonia due to Streptococcus pneumoniae
Includes: bronchopneumonia due to S. pneumoniae
Code first any associated lung abscess (J85.1)
Excludes1:   congenital pneumonia due to S. pneumoniae (P23.6)
lobar pneumonia, unspecified organism (J18.1)
pneumonia due to other streptococci (J15.3-J15.4)

J14   Pneumonia due to Hemophilus influenzae
Includes: bronchopneumonia due to H. influenzae
Code first any associated lung abscess (J85.1)
Excludes1:   congenital pneumonia due to H. influenzae (P23.6)

J15   Bacterial pneumonia, not elsewhere classified
Includes: bronchopneumonia due to bacteria other than S. pneumoniae and H. influenzae
Code first any associated lung abscess (J85.1)
Excludes1:   chlamydial pneumonia (J16.0)
congenital pneumonia (P23.-)
Legionnaires' disease (A48.1)
spirochetal pneumonia (A69.8)

J15.0   Pneumonia due to Klebsiella pneumoniae

J15.1   Pneumonia due to Pseudomonas

J15.2   Pneumonia due to staphylococcus

J15.20   Pneumonia due to staphylococcus, unspecified

J15.21   Pneumonia due to staphylococcus aureus

J15.29   Pneumonia due to other staphylococcus

J15.3   Pneumonia due to streptococcus, group B

J15.4 Pneumonia due to other streptococci

Excludes1:   pneumonia due to streptococcus, group B (J15.3)
              pneumonia due to Streptococcus pneumoniae
              (J13)

J15.5 Pneumonia due to Escherichia coli

J15.6 Pneumonia due to other aerobic Gram-negative bacteria

Pneumonia due to Serratia marcescens

J15.7 Pneumonia due to Mycoplasma pneumoniae

J15.8 Pneumonia due to other specified bacteria

J15.9 Unspecified bacterial pneumonia

Pneumonia due to gram-positive bacteria

J16 Pneumonia due to other infectious organisms, not elsewhere classified

Code first any associated lung abscess (J85.1)

Excludes1:   congenital pneumonia (P23.-)
              ornithosis (A70)
              pneumocystosis (B59)
              pneumonia NOS (J18.9)

J16.0 Chlamydial pneumonia

J16.8 Pneumonia due to other specified infectious organisms

J17 Pneumonia in diseases classified elsewhere

Code first underlying disease, such as:
  Q fever (A78)
  rheumatic fever (I00)
  schistosomiasis (B65.0-B65.9)
  septicemia (A40.0-A41.9)
Code first any associated lung abscess (J85.1)

Excludes1:   candidial pneumonia (B37.1)
              chlamydial pneumonia (J16.0)
              gonorrheal pneumonia (A54.84)
              histoplasmosis pneumonia (B39.0-B39.2)
              measles pneumonia (B05.2)
              nocardiosis pneumonia (A43.0)
              pneumonia in actinomycosis (A42.0)
              pneumonia in anthrax (A22.1)
              pneumonia in ascariasis (B77.81)
              pneumonia in aspergillosis (B44.0-B44.1)
              pneumonia in coccidioidomycosis (B38.0-B38.2)
              pneumonia in cytomegalovirus disease (B25.0)
              pneumonia in toxoplasmosis (B58.3)
              rubella pneumonia (B06.81)
              salmonella pneumonia (A02.22)
              spirochetal infection NEC with pneumonia (A69.8)
              tularemia pneumonia (A21.2)
              typhoid fever with pneumonia (A01.03)
              varicella pneumonia (B01.2)
              whooping cough with pneumonia (A37.81)

J18 Pneumonia, unspecified organism

Excludes1:   abscess of lung with pneumonia (J85.1)
              aspiration pneumonia due to anesthesia during labor and delivery (O74.0)
              aspiration pneumonia due to anesthesia during pregnancy (O29)
              aspiration pneumonia due to anesthesia during puerperium (O89.0)
              aspiration pneumonia due to solids and liquids (J69.-)
              aspiration pneumonia NOS (J69.0)
              congenital pneumonia (P23.0)
              drug-induced interstitial lung disorder (J70.2-J70.4)
              interstitial pneumonia NOS (J84.9)
              lipid pneumonia (J69.1)
              neonatal aspiration pneumonia (P24.9)
              pneumonitis due to external agents (J67-J70)
              pneumonitis due to fumes and vapors (J68.0)

J18.0 Bronchopneumonia, unspecified organism

Excludes1:   hypostatic bronchopneumonia (J18.2)
              lipid pneumonia (J69.1)

Excludes2:   acute bronchiolitis (J21.-)
              chronic bronchiolitis (J44.8)

J18.1 Lobar pneumonia, unspecified organism

J18.2 Hypostatic pneumonia, unspecified organism

Hypostatic bronchopneumonia
Passive pneumonia

J18.8 Other pneumonia, unspecified organism

J18.9 Pneumonia, unspecified organism

OTHER ACUTE LOWER RESPIRATORY INFECTIONS (J20-J22)

Excludes1:   chronic obstructive pulmonary disease with acute lower respiratory infection (J44.0)

J20 Acute bronchitis

Includes: acute and subacute bronchitis (with) bronchospasm
                acute and subacute bronchitis (with) tracheitis
                acute and subacute bronchitis (with) tracheobronchitis, acute
                acute and subacute fibrinous bronchitis
                acute and subacute membranous bronchitis
                acute and subacute purulent bronchitis
                acute and subacute septic bronchitis

Excludes1:   acute bronchitis with bronchiectasis (J47.0)
                acute bronchitis with chronic obstructive asthma (J44.0)
                acute bronchitis with chronic obstructive pulmonary disease (J44.0)
                allergic bronchitis NOS (J45.0-)
                bronchitis due to chemicals, fumes and vapors (J68.0)
                bronchitis NOS (J40)
                chronic bronchitis NOS (J42)
                chronic mucopurulent bronchitis (J41.1)
                chronic obstructive bronchitis (J44.-)
                chronic obstructive tracheobronchitis (J44.-)
                chronic simple bronchitis (J41.0)
                chronic tracheobronchitis (J42)
                tracheobronchitis NOS (J40)

J20.0 Acute bronchitis due to Mycoplasma pneumoniae

J20.1 Acute bronchitis due to Hemophilus influenzae

J20.2 Acute bronchitis due to streptococcus

J20.3 Acute bronchitis due to coxsackievirus

J20.4 Acute bronchitis due to parainfluenza virus

J20.5 Acute bronchitis due to respiratory syncytial virus

J20.6 Acute bronchitis due to rhinovirus

J20.7 Acute bronchitis due to echovirus

J20.8 Acute bronchitis due to other specified organisms

J20.9 Acute bronchitis, unspecified

J21 Acute bronchiolitis

Includes: with bronchospasm

J21.0 Acute bronchiolitis due to respiratory syncytial virus

J21.8 Acute bronchiolitis due to other specified organisms

J21.9 Acute bronchiolitis, unspecified

Bronchiolitis (acute)

J22 Unspecified acute lower respiratory infection

Includes: acute (lower) respiratory (tract) infection NOS

Excludes1:   upper respiratory infection (acute) (J06.9)

OTHER DISEASES OF UPPER RESPIRATORY TRACT (J30-J39)

J30 Vasomotor and allergic rhinitis

Includes: spasmodic rhinorrhea

Excludes1:   allergic rhinitis with asthma (bronchial) (J45.0-)
                rhinitis NOS (J31.0)

J30.0 Vasomotor rhinitis

J30.1 Allergic rhinitis due to pollen

Allergy NOS due to pollen
Hay fever
Pollinosis

J30.2 Other seasonal allergic rhinitis

J30.5 Allergic rhinitis due to food

J30.8 Other allergic rhinitis

Perennial allergic rhinitis

J30.9 Allergic rhinitis, unspecified

J31 Chronic rhinitis, nasopharyngitis and pharyngitis
Use additional code to identify:
exposure to environmental tobacco smoke (X58.1)
exposure to tobacco smoke in the perinatal period (P96.6)
history of tobacco use (Z86.43)
occupational exposure to environmental tobacco smoke (Z57.31)
tobacco dependence (F17.-)
tobacco use (Z72.0)

J31.0 Chronic rhinitis
Atrophic rhinitis (chronic)
Granulomatous rhinitis (chronic)
Hypertrophic rhinitis (chronic)
Obstructive rhinitis (chronic)
Ozena
Purulent rhinitis (chronic)
Rhinitis (chronic) NOS
Ulcerative rhinitis (chronic)
Excludes1:   allergic rhinitis (J30.1-J30.9)
vasomotor rhinitis (J30.0)

J31.1 Chronic nasopharyngitis
Excludes2:   acute nasopharyngitis (J00)

J31.2 Chronic pharyngitis
Atrophic pharyngitis (chronic)
Chronic sore throat
Granular pharyngitis (chronic)
Hypertrophic pharyngitis (chronic)
Excludes2:   acute pharyngitis (J02.9)

J32 Chronic sinusitis
Includes: sinus abscess
sinus empyema
sinus infection
sinus suppuration
Use additional code to identify:
exposure to environmental tobacco smoke (X58.1)
exposure to tobacco smoke in the perinatal period (P96.6)
history of tobacco use (Z86.43)
infectious agent (B95-B97)
occupational exposure to environmental tobacco smoke (Z57.31)
tobacco dependence (F17.-)
tobacco use (Z72.0)
Excludes2:   acute sinusitis (J01.-)

J32.0 Chronic maxillary sinusitis
Antritis (chronic)
Maxillary sinusitis NOS

J32.1 Chronic frontal sinusitis
Frontal sinusitis NOS

J32.2 Chronic ethmoidal sinusitis
Ethmoidal sinusitis NOS
Excludes1:   Woakes' ethmoiditis (J33.1)

J32.3 Chronic sphenoidal sinusitis
Sphenoidal sinusitis NOS

J32.4 Chronic pansinusitis
Pansinusitis NOS

J32.8 Other chronic sinusitis
Sinusitis (chronic) involving more than one sinus but not
pansinusitis

J32.9 Chronic sinusitis, unspecified
Sinusitis (chronic) NOS

J33 Nasal polyp
Use additional code to identify:
exposure to environmental tobacco smoke (X58.1)
exposure to tobacco smoke in the perinatal period (P96.6)
history of tobacco use (Z86.43)
occupational exposure to environmental tobacco smoke (Z57.31)
tobacco dependence (F17.-)
tobacco use (Z72.0)
Excludes1:   adenomatous polyps (D14.0)

J33.0 Polyp of nasal cavity
Choanal polyp
Nasopharyngeal polyp

J33.1 Polypoid sinus degeneration
Woakes' syndrome or ethmoiditis

J33.8 Other polyp of sinus
Accessory polyp of sinus
Ethmoidal polyp of sinus
Maxillary polyp of sinus
Sphenoidal polyp of sinus

J33.9 Nasal polyp, unspecified

J34 Other and unspecified disorders of nose and nasal sinuses
Excludes2:   varicose ulcer of nasal septum (I86.8)

J34.0 Abscess, furuncle and carbuncle of nose
Cellulitis of nose
Necrosis of nose
Ulceration of nose

J34.1 Cyst and mucocele of nasal sinus

J34.2 Deviated nasal septum
Deflection or deviation of septum (nasal) (acquired)
Excludes1:   congenital deviated nasal septum (Q67.4)

J34.3 Hypertrophy of nasal turbinates

J34.8 Other specified disorders of nose and nasal sinuses
Perforation of nasal septum NOS
Rhinolith

J34.9 Unspecified disorder of nose and nasal sinuses

J35 Chronic diseases of tonsils and adenoids
Use additional code to identify:
exposure to environmental tobacco smoke (X58.1)
exposure to tobacco smoke in the perinatal period (P96.6)
history of tobacco use (Z86.43)
occupational exposure to environmental tobacco smoke (Z57.31)
tobacco dependence (F17.-)
tobacco use (Z72.0)

J35.0 Chronic tonsillitis and adenoiditis
Excludes2:   acute tonsillitis (J03.-)

J35.01   Chronic tonsillitis
J35.02   Chronic adenoiditis
J35.03   Chronic tonsillitis and adenoiditis

J35.1 Hypertrophy of tonsils
Enlargement of tonsils
Excludes1:   hypertrophy of tonsils with tonsillitis (J35.0-)

J35.2 Hypertrophy of adenoids
Enlargement of adenoids
Excludes1:   hypertrophy of adenoids with adenoiditis (J35.0-)

J35.3 Hypertrophy of tonsils with hypertrophy of adenoids
Excludes1:   hypertrophy of tonsils and adenoids with
tonsillitis and adenoiditis (J35.03)

J35.8 Other chronic diseases of tonsils and adenoids
Adenoid vegetations
Amygdalolith
Calculus, tonsil
Cicatrix of tonsil (and adenoid)
Tonsillar tag
Ulcer of tonsil

J35.9 Chronic disease of tonsils and adenoids, unspecified
Disease (chronic) of tonsils and adenoids NOS

J36 Peritonsillar abscess
Includes: abscess of tonsil
peritonsillar cellulites
quinsy
Use additional code (B95-B97) to identify infectious agent.
Excludes1:   acute tonsillitis (J03.-)
chronic tonsillitis (J35.0)
retropharyngeal abscess (J39.0)
tonsillitis NOS (J03.9-)

J37 Chronic laryngitis and laryngotracheitis
Use additional code to identify:
exposure to environmental tobacco smoke (X58.1)
exposure to tobacco smoke in the perinatal period (P96.6)
history of tobacco use (Z86.43)
infectious agent (B95-B97)
occupational exposure to environmental tobacco smoke (Z57.31)
tobacco dependence (F17.-)
tobacco use (Z72.0)

J37.0   Chronic laryngitis
   Catarrhal laryngitis
   Hypertrophic laryngitis
   Sicca laryngitis
   Excludes2:   acute laryngitis (J04.0)
                obstructive (acute) laryngitis (J05.0)

J37.1   Chronic laryngotracheitis
   Laryngitis, chronic, with tracheitis (chronic)
   Tracheitis, chronic, with laryngitis
   Excludes1:   chronic tracheitis (J42)
   Excludes2:   acute laryngotracheitis (J04.2)
                acute tracheitis (J04.1)

J38   Diseases of vocal cords and larynx, not elsewhere classified
   Use additional code to identify:
   exposure to environmental tobacco smoke (X58.1)
   exposure to tobacco smoke in the perinatal period (P96.6)
   history of tobacco use (Z86.43)
   occupational exposure to environmental tobacco smoke (Z57.31)
   tobacco dependence (F17.-)
   tobacco use (Z72.0)
   Excludes1:   congenital laryngeal stridor (Q31.4)
                obstructive laryngitis (acute) (J05.0)
                postprocedural subglottic stenosis (J95.5)
                stridor (R06.1)
                ulcerative laryngitis (J04.0)

J38.0   Paralysis of vocal cords and larynx
   Laryngoplegia
   Paralysis of glottis
   J38.00   Paralysis of vocal cords and larynx, unspecified
   J38.01   Paralysis of vocal cords and larynx, unilateral
   J38.02   Paralysis of vocal cords and larynx, bilateral

J38.1   Polyp of vocal cord and larynx
   Excludes1:   adenomatous polyps (D14.1)

J38.2   Nodules of vocal cords
   Chorditis (fibrinous)(nodosa)(tuberosa)
   Singer's nodes
   Teacher's nodes

J38.3   Other diseases of vocal cords
   Abscess of vocal cords
   Cellulitis of vocal cords
   Granuloma of vocal cords
   Leukokeratosis of vocal cords
   Leukoplakia of vocal cords

J38.4   Edema of larynx
   Edema (of) glottis
   Subglottic edema
   Supraglottic edema
   Excludes1:   acute obstructive laryngitis [croup] (J05.0)
                edematous laryngitis (J04.0)

J38.5   Laryngeal spasm
   Laryngismus (stridulus)

J38.6   Stenosis of larynx

J38.7   Other diseases of larynx
   Abscess of larynx
   Cellulitis of larynx
   Disease of larynx NOS
   Necrosis of larynx
   Pachyderma of larynx
   Perichondritis of larynx
   Ulcer of larynx

J39   Other diseases of upper respiratory tract
   Excludes1:   acute respiratory infection NOS (J22)
                acute upper respiratory infection (J06.9)
                upper respiratory inflammation due to chemicals,
                   gases, fumes or vapors (J68.2)

J39.0   Retropharyngeal and parapharyngeal abscess
   Peripharyngeal abscess
   Excludes1:   peritonsillar abscess (J36)

J39.1   Other abscess of pharynx
   Cellulitis of pharynx
   Nasopharyngeal abscess

J39.2   Other diseases of pharynx
   Cyst of pharynx
   Edema of pharynx
   Excludes2:   chronic pharyngitis (J31.2)
                ulcerative pharyngitis (J02.9)

J39.3   Upper respiratory tract hypersensitivity reaction, site unspecified
   Excludes1:   hypersensitivity reaction of upper respiratory
                   tract, such as:
                   extrinsic allergic alveolitis (J67.9)
                   pneumoconiosis (J60-J67.9)

J39.8   Other specified diseases of upper respiratory tract

J39.9   Disease of upper respiratory tract, unspecified

CHRONIC LOWER RESPIRATORY DISEASES (J40-J47)

   Excludes1:   bronchitis due to chemicals, gases, fumes and vapors
                   (J68.0)
   Excludes2:   cystic fibrosis (E84.-)

J40   Bronchitis, not specified as acute or chronic
   Includes: bronchitis NOS
                 bronchitis with tracheitis NOS
                 catarrhal bronchitis
                 tracheobronchitis NOS
   Use additional code to identify:
   exposure to environmental tobacco smoke (X58.1)
   exposure to tobacco smoke in the perinatal period (P96.6)
   history of tobacco use (Z86.43)
   occupational exposure to environmental tobacco smoke (Z57.31)
   tobacco dependence (F17.-)
   tobacco use (Z72.0)
   Excludes1:   allergic bronchitis NOS (J45.0-)
                asthmatic bronchitis NOS (J45.9-)
                bronchitis due to chemicals, gases, fumes and vapors
                   (J68.0)

J41   Simple and mucopurulent chronic bronchitis
   Use additional code to identify:
   exposure to environmental tobacco smoke (X58.1)
   exposure to tobacco smoke in the perinatal period (P96.6)
   history of tobacco use (Z86.43)
   occupational exposure to environmental tobacco smoke (Z57.31)
   tobacco dependence (F17.-)
   tobacco use (Z72.0)
   Excludes1:   chronic bronchitis NOS (J42)
                chronic obstructive bronchitis (J44.-)

J41.0   Simple chronic bronchitis

J41.1   Mucopurulent chronic bronchitis

J41.8   Mixed simple and mucopurulent chronic bronchitis

J42   Unspecified chronic bronchitis
   Includes: chronic bronchitis NOS
                 chronic tracheitis
                 chronic tracheobronchitis
   Use additional code to identify:
   exposure to environmental tobacco smoke (X58.1)
   exposure to tobacco smoke in the perinatal period (P96.6)
   history of tobacco use (Z86.43)
   occupational exposure to environmental tobacco smoke (Z57.31)
   tobacco dependence (F17.-)
   tobacco use (Z72.0)
   Excludes1:   chronic asthmatic bronchitis (J44.-)
                chronic bronchitis with airways obstruction (J44.-)
                chronic emphysematous bronchitis (J44.-)
                chronic obstructive pulmonary disease NOS (J44.9)
                simple and mucopurulent chronic bronchitis (J41.-)

J43 Emphysema

Use additional code to identify:
exposure to environmental tobacco smoke (X58.1)
history of tobacco use (Z86.43)
occupational exposure to environmental tobacco smoke (Z57.31)
tobacco dependence (F17.-)
tobacco use (Z72.0)
Excludes1:   compensatory emphysema (J98.3)
emphysema due to inhalation of chemicals, gases,
    fumes or vapors (J68.4)
emphysema with chronic (obstructive) bronchitis
    (J44.-)
emphysematous (obstructive) bronchitis (J44.-)
interstitial emphysema (J98.2)
mediastinal emphysema (J98.2)
neonatal interstitial emphysema (P25.0)
surgical (subcutaneous) emphysema (T81.82)
traumatic subcutaneous emphysema (T79.7)

J43.0 Unilateral pulmonary emphysema [MacLeod's syndrome]
Swyer-James syndrome
Unilateral emphysema
Unilateral hyperlucent lung
Unilateral pulmonary artery functional hypoplasia
Unilateral transparency of lung

J43.1 Panlobular emphysema
Panacinar emphysema

J43.2 Centrilobular emphysema

J43.8 Other emphysema

J43.9 Emphysema, unspecified
Bullous emphysema (lung)(pulmonary)
Emphysema (lung)(pulmonary) NOS
Emphysematous bleb
Vesicular emphysema (lung)(pulmonary)

J44 Other chronic obstructive pulmonary disease

Includes: asthma with chronic obstructive pulmonary disease
chronic asthmatic (obstructive) bronchitis
chronic bronchitis with airways obstruction
chronic bronchitis with emphysema
chronic emphysematous bronchitis
chronic obstructive asthma
chronic obstructive bronchitis
chronic obstructive tracheobronchitis
Use additional code to identify:
exposure to environmental tobacco smoke (X58.1)
history of tobacco use (Z86.43)
occupational exposure to environmental tobacco smoke (Z57.31)
tobacco dependence (F17.-)
tobacco use (Z72.0)
Excludes1:   asthma without chronic obstructive pulmonary disease
    (J45.-)
asthmatic bronchitis NOS (J45.9-)
bronchiectasis (J47.-)
chronic bronchitis NOS (J42)
chronic simple and mucopurulent bronchitis (J41.-)
chronic tracheitis (J42)
chronic tracheobronchitis (J42)
emphysema (J43.-)
lung diseases due to external agents (J60-J70)

J44.0 Chronic obstructive pulmonary disease with acute lower respiratory infection
Chronic obstructive pulmonary disease with acute bronchitis

J44.1 Chronic obstructive pulmonary disease with acute exacerbation, unspecified
Excludes1:   chronic obstructive pulmonary disease [COPD]
    with acute bronchitis (J44.0)

J44.9 Chronic obstructive pulmonary disease, unspecified
Chronic obstructive airway disease NOS
Chronic obstructive lung disease NOS

J45 Asthma

Use additional code to identify:
exposure to environmental tobacco smoke (X58.1)
exposure to tobacco smoke in the perinatal period (P96.6)
history of tobacco use (Z86.43)
occupational exposure to environmental tobacco smoke (Z57.31)
tobacco dependence (F17.-)
tobacco use (Z72.0)
Excludes1:   asthma with chronic obstructive pulmonary disease
    (J44.)
chronic asthmatic (obstructive) bronchitis (J44.-)
chronic obstructive asthma (J44.-)
detergent asthma (J69.8)
eosinophilic asthma (J82)
lung diseases due to external agents (J60-J70)
miner's asthma (J60)
plantinum asthma (J45.0)
wheezing NOS (R06.2)
wood asthma (J67.8)

J45.0 Predominantly allergic asthma
Allergic bronchitis NOS
Allergic rhinitis with asthma
Atopic asthma
Extrinsic allergic asthma
Hay fever with asthma

J45.00 Predominantly allergic asthma, uncomplicated
Predominantly allergic asthma NOS

J45.01 Predominantly allergic asthma with acute exacerbation

J45.02 Predominantly allergic asthma with status asthmaticus

J45.1 Nonallergic asthma
Idiosyncratic asthma
Intrinsic nonallergic asthma

J45.10 Nonallergic asthma, uncomplicated
Nonallergic asthma NOS

J45.11 Nonallergic asthma with acute exacerbation

J45.12 Nonallergic asthma with status asthmaticus

J45.8 Mixed asthma
Combination of conditions listed in J45.0 and J45.1

J45.80 Mixed asthma, uncomplicated
Mixed asthma NOS

J45.81 Mixed asthma with acute exacerbation

J45.82 Mixed asthma with status asthmaticus

J45.9 Asthma, unspecified
Asthmatic bronchitis NOS
Late onset asthma

J45.90 Asthma, unspecified, uncomplicated
Asthma NOS

J45.91 Asthma, unspecified, with acute exacerbation

J45.92 Asthma, unspecified, with status asthmaticus

J47 Bronchiectasis

Includes: bronchiolectasis
Use additional code to identify:
exposure to environmental tobacco smoke (X58.1)
exposure to tobacco smoke in the perinatal period (P96.6)
history of tobacco use (Z86.43)
occupational exposure to environmental tobacco smoke (Z57.31)
tobacco dependence (F17.-)
tobacco use (Z72.0)
Excludes1:   congenital bronchiectasis (Q33.4)
tuberculous bronchiectasis (current disease) (A15.0)

J47.0 Bronchiectasis with acute lower respiratory infection
Bronchiectasis with acute bronchitis

J47.1 Bronchiectasis with acute exacerbation

J47.9 Bronchiectasis, uncomplicated
Bronchiectasis NOS

LUNG DISEASES DUE TO EXTERNAL AGENTS (J60-J70)

Excludes2:   asthma (J45.-)
             malignant neoplasm of bronchus and lung (C34.-)

J60   Coalworker's pneumoconiosis
Includes: anthracosilicosis
             anthracosis
             black lung disease
             coalworker's lung
Excludes1:   coalworker's pneumoconiosis with tuberculosis (J65)

J61   Pneumoconiosis due to asbestos and other mineral fibers
Includes: asbestosis
Excludes1:   pleural plaque with asbestosis (J92.0)
             pneumoconiosis with tuberculosis (J65)

J62   Pneumoconiosis due to dust containing silica
Includes: silicotic fibrosis (massive) of lung
Excludes1:   pneumoconiosis with tuberculosis (J65)

J62.0   Pneumoconiosis due to talc dust

J62.8   Pneumoconiosis due to other dust containing silica
Silicosis NOS

J63   Pneumoconiosis due to other inorganic dusts
Excludes1:   pneumoconiosis with tuberculosis (J65)

J63.0   Aluminosis (of lung)
J63.1   Bauxite fibrosis (of lung)
J63.2   Berylliosis
J63.3   Graphite fibrosis (of lung)
J63.4   Siderosis
J63.5   Stannosis
J63.6   Pneumoconiosis due to other specified inorganic dusts

J64   Unspecified pneumoconiosis
Excludes1:   pneumonoconiosis with tuberculosis (J65)

J65   Pneumoconiosis associated with tuberculosis
Includes: any condition in J60-J64 with tuberculosis, any
             type in A15
             silicotuberculosis

J66   Airway disease due to specific organic dust
Excludes2:   allergic alveolitis (J67.-)
             asbestosis (J61)
             bagassosis (J67.1)
             farmer's lung (J67.0)
             hypersensitivity pneumonitis due to organic dust
             (J67.-)
             reactive airways dysfunction syndrome (J68.3)

J66.0   Byssinosis
Airway disease due to cotton dust
J66.1   Flax-dressers' disease
J66.2   Cannabinosis
J66.8   Airway disease due to other specific organic dusts

J67   Hypersensitivity pneumonitis due to organic dust
Includes: allergic alveolitis and pneumonitis due to inhaled
             organic dust and particles of fungal,
             actinomycetic or other origin
Excludes1:   pneumonitis due to inhalation of chemicals, gases,
             fumes or vapors (J68.0)

J67.0   Farmer's lung
Harvester's lung
Haymaker's lung
Moldy hay disease
J67.1   Bagassosis
Bagasse disease
Bagasse pneumonitis
J67.2   Bird fancier's lung
Budgerigar fancier's disease or lung
Pigeon fancier's disease or lung
J67.3   Suberosis
Corkhandler's disease or lung
Corkworker's disease or lung

J67.4   Maltworker's lung
Alveolitis due to Aspergillus clavatus
J67.5   Mushroom-worker's lung
J67.6   Maple-bark-stripper's lung
Alveolitis due to Cryptostroma corticale
Cryptostromosis
J67.7   Air conditioner and humidifier lung
Allergic alveolitis due to fungal, thermophilic actinomycetes and
other organisms growing in ventilation [air conditioning]
systems
J67.8   Hypersensitivity pneumonitis due to other organic dusts
Cheese-washer's lung
Coffee-worker's lung
Fish-meal worker's lung
Furrier's lung
Sequoiosis
J67.9   Hypersensitivity pneumonitis due to unspecified organic dust
Allergic alveolitis (extrinsic) NOS
Hypersensitivity pneumonitis NOS

J68   Respiratory conditions due to inhalation of chemicals, gases, fumes and vapors
Use additional toxic effect code (T51-T65) to identify cause.

J68.0   Bronchitis and pneumonitis due to chemicals, gases, fumes and vapors
Chemical bronchitis (acute)
J68.1   Acute pulmonary edema due to chemicals, gases, fumes and vapors
Chemical pulmonary edema (acute)
Excludes1:   pulmonary edema (acute) (chronic) (J81)
J68.2   Upper respiratory inflammation due to chemicals, gases, fumes and vapors, not elsewhere classified
J68.3   Other acute and subacute respiratory conditions due to chemicals, gases, fumes and vapors
Reactive airways dysfunction syndrome
J68.4   Chronic respiratory conditions due to chemicals, gases, fumes and vapors
Emphysema (diffuse) (chronic) due to inhalation of chemicals,
gases, fumes and vapors
Obliterative bronchiolitis (chronic) (subacute) due to inhalation
of chemicals, gases, fumes and vapors
Pulmonary fibrosis (chronic) due to inhalation of chemicals,
gases, fumes and vapors
J68.8   Other respiratory conditions due to chemicals, gases, fumes and vapors
J68.9   Unspecified respiratory condition due to chemicals, gases, fumes and vapors

J69   Pneumonitis due to solids and liquids
Use additional toxic effect or external cause code to identify cause
Excludes1:   neonatal aspiration syndromes (P24.-)
J69.0   Pneumonitis due to inhalation of food and vomit
Aspiration pneumonia NOS
Aspiration pneumonia (due to) food (regurgitated)
Aspiration pneumonia (due to) gastric secretions
Aspiration pneumonia (due to) milk
Aspiration pneumonia (due to) vomit
Excludes1:   chemical pneumonitis due to anesthesia
             [Mendelson's syndrome] (J95.4)
             obstetric aspiration pneumonitis (O74.0)
J69.1   Pneumonitis due to oils and essences
Exogenous lipoid pneumonia
Lipid pneumonia NOS
Excludes1:   endogenous lipoid pneumonia (J84.2)
J69.8   Pneumonitis due to inhalation of other solids and liquids
Pneumonitis due to aspiration of blood
Pneumonitis due to aspiration of detergent

J70   Respiratory conditions due to other external agents
Use additional toxic effect and external cause (T code or W, X, Y code)
code to identify the external agent or drug
J70.0   Acute pulmonary manifestations due to radiation
Radiation pneumonitis
J70.1   Chronic and other pulmonary manifestations due to radiation
Fibrosis of lung following radiation

J70.2 Acute drug-induced interstitial lung disorders
    Excludes1: interstitial pneumonia NOS (J84.9)
              lymphoid interstitial pneumonia (J84.2)

J70.3 Chronic drug-induced interstitial lung disorders
    Excludes1: interstitial pneumonia NOS (J84.9)
              lymphoid interstitial pneumonia (J84.2)

J70.4 Drug-induced interstitial lung disorders, unspecified
    Excludes1: interstitial pneumonia NOS (J84.9)
              lymphoid interstitial pneumonia (J84.2)

J70.8 Respiratory conditions due to other specified external agents

J70.9 Respiratory conditions due to unspecified external agent

OTHER RESPIRATORY DISEASES PRINCIPALLY AFFECTING THE INTERSTITIUM (J80-J84)

J80 Adult respiratory distress syndrome
    Includes: adult hyaline membrane disease

J81 Pulmonary edema
    Use additional code to identify:
      exposure to environmental tobacco smoke (X58.1)
      history of tobacco use (Z86.43)
      occupational exposure to environmental tobacco smoke (Z57.31)
      tobacco dependence (F17.-)
      tobacco use (Z72.0)
    Excludes1: chemical (acute) pulmonary edema (J68.1)
              hypostatic pneumonia (J18.2)
              passive pneumonia (J18.2)
              pulmonary edema due to external agents (J60-J70)
              pulmonary edema with heart disease NOS (I50.1)
              pulmonary edema with heart failure (I50.1)

J81.0 Acute pulmonary edema
    Acute edema of lung

J81.1 Chronic pulmonary edema
    Pulmonary congestion (chronic) (passive)
    Pulmonary edema NOS

J82 Pulmonary eosinophilia, not elsewhere classified
    Includes: allergic pneumonia
              eosinophilic asthma
              eosinophilic pneumonia
              Löffler's pneumonia
              tropical (pulmonary) eosinophilia NOS
    Excludes1: pulmonary eosinophilia due to aspergillosis (B44.-)
              pulmonary eosinophilia due to drugs (J70.2-J70.4)
              pulmonary eosinophilia due to specified parasitic infection (B50-B83)
              pulmonary eosinophilia due to systemic connective tissue disorders (M30-M36)

J84 Other interstitial pulmonary diseases
    Excludes1: drug-induced interstitial lung disorders (J70.2-J70.4)
              interstitial emphysema (J98.2)
              lung diseases due to external agents (J60-J70)

J84.0 Alveolar and parieto-alveolar conditions
    Alveolar proteinosis
    Pulmonary alveolar microlithiasis

J84.1 Other interstitial pulmonary diseases with fibrosis
    Cirrhosis of lung
    Diffuse pulmonary fibrosis
    Fibrosing alveolitis (cryptogenic)
    Hamman-Rich syndrome
    Idiopathic pulmonary fibrosis
    Induration of lung
    Excludes1: pulmonary fibrosis (chronic) due to inhalation of chemicals, gases, fumes or vapors (J68.4)
              pulmonary fibrosis (chronic) following radiation (J70.1)

J84.2 Lymphoid interstitial pneumonia
    Endogenous lipoid pneumonia
    Lymphoid interstitial pneumonitis
    Excludes1: exogenous lipoid pneumonia (J69.1)
              unspecified lipoid pneumonia (J69.1)

J84.8 Other specified interstitial pulmonary diseases

J84.9 Interstitial pulmonary disease, unspecified
    Interstitial pneumonia NOS

SUPPURATIVE AND NECROTIC CONDITIONS OF THE LOWER RESPIRATORY TRACT (J85-J86)

J85 Abscess of lung and mediastinum
    Use additional code (B95-B97) to identify infectious agent.

J85.0 Gangrene and necrosis of lung

J85.1 Abscess of lung with pneumonia
    Use additional code to identify the type of pneumonia (J13-J17)

J85.2 Abscess of lung without pneumonia
    Abscess of lung NOS

J85.3 Abscess of mediastinum

J86 Pyothorax
    Use additional code (B95-B97) to identify infectious agent.
    Excludes1: abscess of lung (J85.-)
              pyothorax due to tuberculosis (A15.6)

J86.0 Pyothorax with fistula
    Bronchocutaneous fistula
    Bronchopleural fistula
    Hepatopleural fistula
    Mediastinal fistula
    Pleural fistula
    Thoracic fistula
    Any condition classifiable to J86.9 with fistula

J86.9 Pyothorax without fistula
    Abscess of pleura
    Abscess of thorax
    Empyema (chest) (lung) (pleura)
    Fibrinopurulent pleurisy
    Purulent pleurisy
    Pyopneumothorax
    Septic pleurisy
    Seropurulent pleurisy
    Suppurative pleurisy

OTHER DISEASES OF THE PLEURA (J90-J94)

J90 Pleural effusion, not elsewhere classified
    Includes: encysted pleurisy
              pleural effusion NOS
              pleurisy with effusion (exudative) (serous)
    Excludes1: chylous (pleural) effusion (J94.0)
              pleurisy NOS (R09.1)
              tuberculous pleural effusion (A15.6)

J91 Pleural effusion in conditions classified elsewhere
    Code first underlying disease, such as:
      filariasis (B74.0-B74.9)
    Excludes1: malignant pleural effusion (C78.2)
              pleural effusion in congestive heart failure (I50.0)
              pleural effusion in systemic lupus erythematosus (M32.13)

J92 Pleural plaque
    Includes: pleural thickening

J92.0 Pleural plaque with presence of asbestos

J92.9 Pleural plaque without asbestos
    Pleural plaque NOS

J93 Pneumothorax
    Excludes1: congenital or perinatal pneumothorax (P25.1)
              postprocedural pneumothorax (J95.81)
              pyopneumothorax (J86.-)
              traumatic pneumothorax (S27.0)
              tuberculous (current disease) pneumothorax (A15.-)

J93.0 Spontaneous tension pneumothorax

J93.1 Other spontaneous pneumothorax

J93.8 Other pneumothorax
    Excludes1: postprocedural pneumothorax (J95.81)

J93.9 Pneumothorax, unspecified

J94 Other pleural conditions
Excludes1: pleurisy NOS (R09.1)
traumatic hemopneumothorax (S27.2)
traumatic hemothorax (S27.1)
tuberculous pleural conditions (current disease) (A15.-)

J94.0 Chylous effusion
Chyliform effusion

J94.1 Fibrothorax

J94.2 Hemothorax
Hemopneumothorax

J94.8 Other specified pleural conditions
Hydropneumothorax
Hydrothorax

J94.9 Pleural condition, unspecified

OTHER DISEASES OF THE RESPIRATORY SYSTEM (J95-J99)

J95 Intraoperative and postprocedural complications and disorders of the respiratory system, not elsewhere classified
Excludes2: aspiration pneumonia (J69.-)
emphysema (subcutaneous) resulting from a procedure (T81.82)
hypostatic pneumonia (J18.2)
pulmonary manifestations due to radiation (J70.0-J70.1)

J95.0 Tracheostomy complications

J95.00 Unspecified tracheostomy complication

J95.01 Hemorrhage from tracheostomy stoma

J95.02 Infection of tracheostomy stoma
Use additional code to identify type of infection, such as:
cellulitis of neck (L03.8)
septicemia (A40, A41.-)

J95.03 Malfunction of tracheostomy stoma
Mechanical complication of tracheostomy stoma
Obstruction of tracheostomy airway
Tracheal stenosis due to tracheostomy

J95.04 Tracheo-esophageal fistula following tracheostomy

J95.09 Other tracheostomy complication

J95.1 Acute pulmonary insufficiency following thoracic surgery
Excludes2: Functional disturbances following cardiac surgery (I97.0, I97.1-)

J95.2 Acute pulmonary insufficiency following nonthoracic surgery
Excludes2: Functional disturbances following cardiac surgery (I97.0, I97.1-)

J95.3 Chronic pulmonary insufficiency following surgery
Excludes2: Functional disturbances following cardiac surgery (I97.0, I97.1-)

J95.4 Chemical pneumonitis due to anesthesia [Mendelson's syndrome]
Excludes1: aspiration pneumonitis due to anesthesia complicating labor and delivery (O74.0)
aspiration pneumonitis due to anesthesia complicating pregnancy (O29)
aspiration pneumonitis due to anesthesia complicating the puerperium (O89.01)

J95.5 Postprocedural subglottic stenosis

J95.6 Intraoperative and postprocedural hemorrhage and hematoma complicating a respiratory system procedure
Excludes1: intraoperative hemorrhage and hematoma due to accidental puncture and laceration during a respiratory system procedure (J95.7-)

J95.61 Intraoperative hemorrhage of a respiratory system organ or structure during a respiratory system procedure

J95.62 Intraoperative hemorrhage of a non-respiratory system organ or structure during a respiratory system procedure

J95.63 Intraoperative hematoma of a respiratory system organ during a respiratory system procedure

J95.64 Intraoperative hematoma of a non-respiratory system organ or structure during a respiratory system procedure

J95.65 Postprocedural hemorrhage of a respiratory system organ or structure following a respiratory system procedure

J95.66 Postprocedural hemorrhage of a non-respiratory system organ or structure following a respiratory system procedure

J95.67 Postprocedural hematoma of a respiratory system organ or structure following a respiratory system procedure

J95.68 Postprocedural hematoma of a non-respiratory system organ or structure during a respiratory system procedure

J95.7 Accidental puncture and laceration during a respiratory system procedure

J95.71 Accidental puncture and laceration of a respiratory system organ or structure during a respiratory system procedure

J95.72 Accidental puncture and laceration of a non-respiratory system organ or structure following a respiratory system procedure

J95.8 Other postprocedural respiratory disorders

J95.81 Postprocedural pneumothorax

J95.82 Postprocedural respiratory failure

J95.89 Other postprocedural respiratory disorders
Use additional code to identify disorder, such as:
aspiration pneumonia (J69.-)
bacterial or viral pneumonia (J12-J18)
Excludes1: acute pulmonary insufficiency following thoracic surgery (J95.1)
postprocedural hemorrhage and hematoma complicating a respiratory system procedure (J95.65-J95.68)
postprocedural subglottic stenosis (J95.5)

J95.9 Postprocedural respiratory disorder, unspecified

J96 Respiratory failure, not elsewhere classified
Excludes1: adult respiratory distress syndrome (J80)
cardiorespiratory failure (R09.2)
newborn respiratory distress syndrome (P22.0)
postprocedural respiratory failure (J95.82)
respiratory arrest (R09.2)

J96.0 Acute respiratory failure

J96.1 Chronic respiratory failure

J96.2 Acute and chronic respiratory failure
Acute on chronic respiratory failure

J96.9 Respiratory failure, unspecified

J98 Other respiratory disorders
Use additional code to identify:
exposure to environmental tobacco smoke (X58.1)
exposure to tobacco smoke in the perinatal period (P96.6)
history of tobacco use (Z86.43)
occupational exposure to environmental tobacco smoke (Z57.31)
tobacco dependence (F17.-)
tobacco use (Z72.0)
Excludes1: newborn apnea (P28.4)
newborn sleep apnea (P28.3)
Excludes2: apnea NOS (R06.8)
sleep apnea (G47.3-)

J98.0 Diseases of bronchus, not elsewhere classified
Broncholithiasis
Calcification of bronchus
Stenosis of bronchus
Tracheobronchial collapse
Tracheobronchial dyskinesia
Ulcer of bronchus

J98.1 Pulmonary collapse
Excludes1: therapeutic collapse of lung status (Z98.3)

J98.11 Atelectasis
Excludes1: newborn atelectasis
tuberculous atelectasis (current disease) (A15)

> **J98.19**   Other pulmonary collapse

J98.2   **Interstitial emphysema**
Mediastinal emphysema
Excludes1:   emphysema NOS (J43.9)
         emphysema in fetus and newborn (P25.0)
         surgical emphysema (subcutaneous) (T81.82)
         traumatic subcutaneous emphysema (T79.7)

J98.3   **Compensatory emphysema**

J98.4   **Other disorders of lung**
Calcification of lung
Cystic lung disease (acquired)
Lung disease NOS
Pulmolithiasis

J98.5   **Diseases of mediastinum, not elsewhere classified**
Fibrosis of mediastinum
Hernia of mediastinum
Mediastinitis
Retraction of mediastinum
Excludes2:   abscess of mediastinum (J85.3)

J98.6   **Disorders of diaphragm**
Diaphragmatitis
Paralysis of diaphragm
Relaxation of diaphragm
Excludes1:   congenital malformation of diaphragm NEC
         (Q79.1)
         congenital diaphragmatic hernia (Q79.0)
Excludes2:   diaphragmatic hernia (K44.-)

J98.8   **Other specified respiratory disorders**

J98.9   **Respiratory disorder, unspecified**
Respiratory disease (chronic) NOS

J99   **Respiratory disorders in diseases classified elsewhere**
Code first underlying disease, such as:
amyloidosis (E85)
ankylosing spondylitis (M45)
congenital syphilis (A50.5)
cryoglobulinemia (D89.1)
early congenital syphilis (A50.0)
hemosiderosis (E83.1)
schistosomiasis (B65.0-B65.9)
Excludes1:   respiratory disorders in:
         amebiasis (A06.5)
         blastomycosis (B40.0-B40.2)
         candidiasis (B37.1)
         coccidioidomycosis (B38.0-B38.2)
         dermatomyositis (M33.01, M33.11)
         histoplasmosis (B39.0-B39.2)
         late syphilis (A52.72, A52.73)
         polymyositis (M33.21)
         sicca syndrome (M35.02)
         systemic lupus erythematosus (M32.13)
         systemic sclerosis (M34.81)
         Wegener's granulomatosis (M31.30-M31.31)

CHAPTER XI — DISEASES OF THE DIGESTIVE SYSTEM (K00–K94)

Excludes2:   certain conditions originating in the perinatal period (P04-P96)

certain infectious and parasitic diseases (A00-B99)

complications of pregnancy, childbirth and the puerperium (O00-O99)

congenital malformations, deformations and chromosomal abnormalities (Q00-Q99)

endocrine, nutritional and metabolic diseases (E00-E90)

injury, poisoning and certain other consequences of external causes (S00-T98)

neoplasms (C00-D48)

symptoms, signs and abnormal clinical and laboratory findings, classified (R00-R94)

This chapter contains the following blocks:

K00-K14	Diseases of oral cavity and salivary glands
K20-K31	Diseases of esophagus, stomach and duodenum
K35-K38	Diseases of appendix
K40-K46	Hernia
K50-K52	Noninfective enteritis and colitis
K55-K63	Other diseases of intestines
K65-K68	Diseases of peritoneum and retroperitoneum
K70-K77	Diseases of liver
K80-K87	Disorders of gallbladder, biliary tract and pancreas not elsewhere
K90-K94	Other diseases of the digestive system

DISEASES OF ORAL CAVITY AND SALIVARY GLANDS (K00–K14)

K00 Disorders of tooth development and eruption

Excludes2:   embedded and impacted teeth (K01.-)

K00.0 Anodontia

Hypodontia

Oligodontia

Excludes1:   acquired absence of teeth (K08.1)

K00.1 Supernumerary teeth

Distomolar

Fourth molar

Mesiodens

Paramolar

Supplementary teeth

Excludes2:   supernumerary roots (K00.2)

K00.2 Abnormalities of size and form of teeth

Concrescence of teeth

Dens evaginatus

Dens in dente

Dens invaginatus

Enamel pearls

Fusion of teeth

Gemination of teeth

Macrodontia

Microdontia

Peg-shaped [conical] teeth

Supernumeray roots

Taurodontism

Tuberculum paramolare

Excludes1:   abnormalities of teeth due to congenital syphillis (A50.5)

tuberculum Carabelli, which is regarded as a normal variation and should not be coded

K00.3 Mottled teeth

Dental fluorosis

Mottling of enamel

Nonfluoride enamel opacities

Excludes2:   deposits [accretions] on teeth (K03.6)

K00.4 Disturbances in tooth formation

Aplasia and hypoplasia of cementum

Dilaceration of tooth

Enamel hypoplasia (neonatal) (postnatal) (prenatal)

Regional odontodysplasia

Turner's tooth

Excludes1:   Hutchinson's teeth and mulberry molars in congenital syphilis(A50.5)

Excludes2:   mottled teeth (K00.3)

K00.5 Hereditary disturbances in tooth structure, not elsewhere classified

Amelogenesis imperfecta

Dentinal dysplasia

Dentinogenesis imperfecta

Odontogenesis imperfecta

Shell teeth

K00.6 Disturbances in tooth eruption

Dentia praecox

Natal tooth

Neonatal tooth

Premature eruption of tooth

Premature shedding of primary [deciduous] tooth

Retained [persistent] primary tooth

Excludes2:   embedded and impacted teeth (K01.-)

K00.7 Teething syndrome

K00.8 Other disorders of tooth development

Color changes during tooth formation

Intrinsic staining of teeth NOS

Excludes2:   posteruptive color changes (K03.7)

K00.9 Disorder of tooth development, unspecified

Disorder of odontogenesis NOS

K01 Embedded and impacted teeth

Excludes1:   abnormal position of fully erupted teeth (M26.3)

K01.0 Embedded teeth

K01.1 Impacted teeth

K02 Dental caries

K02.0 Caries limited to enamel

White spot lesions [initial caries]

K02.1 Caries of dentine

K02.2 Caries of cementum

K02.3 Arrested dental caries

K02.4 Odontoclasia

Infantile melanodontia

Melanodontoclasia

K02.8 Other dental caries

K02.9 Dental caries, unspecified

K03 Other diseases of hard tissues of teeth

Excludes2:   bruxism (F45.8)

dental caries (K02.-)

teeth-grinding NOS (F45.8)

K03.0 Excessive attrition of teeth

Approximal wear of teeth

Occlusal wear of teeth

K03.1 Abrasion of teeth

Dentifrice abrasion of teeth

Habitual abrasion of teeth

Occupational abrasion of teeth

Ritual abrasion of teeth

Traditional abrasion of teeth

Wedge defect NOS

K03.2 Erosion of teeth

Erosion of teeth due to diet

Erosion of teeth due to drugs and medicaments

Erosion of teeth due to persistent vomiting

Erosion of teeth NOS

Idiopathic erosion of teeth

Occupational erosion of teeth

K03.3 Pathological resorption of teeth

Internal granuloma of pulp

Resorption of teeth (external)

K03.4 Hypercementosis

Cementation hyperplasia

K03.5 Ankylosis of teeth

K03.6 Deposits [accretions] on teeth
Betel deposits [accretions] on teeth
Black deposits [accretions] on teeth
Extrinsic staining of teeth NOS
Green deposits [accretions] on teeth
Materia alba deposits [accretions] on teeth
Orange deposits [accretions] on teeth
Staining of teeth NOS
Subgingival dental calculus
Supragingival dental calculus
Tobacco deposits [accretions] on teeth

K03.7 Posteruptive color changes of dental hard tissues
Excludes2: deposits [accretions] on teeth (K03.6)

K03.8 Other specified diseases of hard tissues of teeth
Irradiated enamel
Sensitive dentine
Use additional external cause code (Chapter XX) to identify radiation, if radiation-induced.

K03.9 Disease of hard tissues of teeth, unspecified

K04 Diseases of pulp and periapical tissues

K04.0 Pulpitis
Acute pulpitis
Chronic (hyperplastic) (ulcerative) pulpitis
Pulpal abscess
Pulpal polyp
Suppurative pulpitis

K04.1 Necrosis of pulp
Pulpal gangrene

K04.2 Pulp degeneration
Denticles
Pulpal calcifications
Pulpal stones

K04.3 Abnormal hard tissue formation in pulp
Secondary or irregular dentine

K04.4 Acute apical periodontitis of pulpal origin
Acute apical periodontitis NOS
Excludes1: acute periodontitis (K05.2)

K04.5 Chronic apical periodontitis
Apical or periapical granuloma
Apical periodontitis NOS
Excludes1: chronic periodontitis (K05.3)

K04.6 Periapical abscess with sinus
Dental abscess with sinus
Dentoalveolar abscess with sinus

K04.7 Periapical abscess without sinus
Dental abscess without sinus
Dentoalveolar abscess without sinus
Periapical abscess without sinus

K04.8 Radicular cyst
Apical (periodontal) cyst
Periapical cyst
Residual radicular cyst
Excludes2: lateral periodontal cyst (K09.0)

K04.9 Other and unspecified diseases of pulp and periapical tissues
K04.90 Unspecified diseases of pulp and periapical tissues
K04.99 Other diseases of pulp and periapical tissues

K05 Gingivitis and periodontal diseases
Use additional code to identify:
alcohol abuse and dependence (F10.-)
alcohol use, uncomplicated (Z72.1)
alcohol dependence, in remission (F10.11)
exposure to environmental tobacco smoke (X58.1)
exposure to tobacco smoke in the perinatal period (P96.6)
history of tobacco use (Z86.43)
occupational exposure to environmental tobacco smoke (Z57.31)
tobacco dependence (F17.-)
tobacco use (Z72.0)

K05.0 Acute gingivitis
Excludes1: acute necrotizing ulcerative gingivitis (A69.1)
herpesviral [herpes simplex] gingivostomatitis (B00.2)

K05.1 Chronic gingivitis
Desquamative gingivitis (chronic)
Gingivitis (chronic) NOS
Hyperplastic gingivitis (chronic)
Simple marginal gingivitis (chronic)
Ulcerative gingivitis (chronic)

K05.2 Acute periodontitis
Acute pericoronitis
Parodontal abscess
Periodontal abscess
Excludes1: acute apical periodontitis (K04.4)
periapical abscess (K04.7)
periapical abscess with sinus (K04.6)

K05.3 Chronic periodontitis
Chronic pericoronitis
Complex periodontitis
Periodontitis NOS
Simplex periodontitis
Excludes1: chronic apical periodontitis (K04.5)

K05.4 Periodontosis
Juvenile periodontosis

K05.5 Other periodontal diseases
Excludes2: leukoplakia of gingiva (K13.2)

K05.6 Periodontal disease, unspecified

K06 Other disorders of gingiva and edentulous alveolar ridge
Excludes2: acute gingivitis (K05.0)
atrophy of edentulous alveolar ridge (K08.2)
chronic gingivitis (K05.1)
gingivitis NOS (K05.1)

K06.0 Gingival recession
Gingival recession (generalized) (localized) (postinfective) (post-operative)

K06.1 Gingival enlargement
Gingival fibromatosis

K06.2 Gingival and edentulous alveolar ridge lesions associated with trauma
Irritative hyperplasia of edentulous ridge [denture hyperplasia]
Use additional external cause code (Chapter XX) to identify cause.

K06.8 Other specified disorders of gingiva and edentulous alveolar ridge
Fibrous epulis
Flabby alveolar ridge
Giant cell epulis
Peripheral giant cell granuloma of gingival
Pyogenic granuloma of gingival
Excludes2: gingival cyst (K09.0)

K06.9 Disorder of gingiva and edentulous alveolar ridge, unspecified

K08 Other disorders of teeth and supporting structures

K08.0 Exfoliation of teeth due to systemic causes
Code first underlying systemic condition

K08.1 Loss of teeth due to accident, extraction or local periodontal diseases

K08.2 Atrophy of edentulous alveolar ridge

K08.3 Retained dental root

K08.8 Other specified disorders of teeth and supporting structures
Enlargement of alveolar ridge NOS
Irregular alveolar process
Toothache NOS

K08.9 Disorder of teeth and supporting structures, unspecified

K09 Cysts of oral region, not elsewhere classified
Includes: lesions showing histological features both of aneurysmal cyst and of another fibro-osseous lesion
Excludes2: cysts of jaw (M27.-)
radicular cyst (K04.8)

K09.0   Developmental odontogenic cysts
Dentigerous cyst
Eruption cyst
Follicular cyst
Gingival cyst
Keratocyst
Lateral periodontal cyst
Primordial cyst

K09.1   Developmental (nonodontogenic) cysts of oral region
Cyst (of) incisive canal
Cyst (of) palatine of papilla
Globulomaxillary cyst
Median palatal cyst
Nasopalatine cyst

K09.8   Other cysts of oral region, not elsewhere classified
Dermoid cyst
Epidermoid cyst
Lymphoepithelial cyst
Epstein's pearl
Nasoalveolar cyst
Nasolabial cyst

K09.9   Cyst of oral region, unspecified

K11   Diseases of salivary glands
Use additional code to identify:
alcohol abuse and dependence (F10.-)
alcohol use, uncomplicated (Z72.1)
alcohol dependence, in remission (F10.11)
exposure to environmental tobacco smoke (X58.1)
exposure to tobacco smoke in the perinatal period (P96.6)
history of tobacco use (Z86.43)
occupational exposure to environmental tobacco smoke (Z57.31)
tobacco dependence (F17.-)
tobacco use (Z72.0)

K11.0   Atrophy of salivary gland

K11.1   Hypertrophy of salivary gland

K11.2   Sialoadenitis
Parotitis
Excludes1:   epidemic parotitis (B26.-)
            mumps (B26.-)
            uveoparotid fever [Heerfordt] (D86.89)

K11.20   Sialoadentitis, unspecified

K11.21   Acute sialoadenitis
Excludes1:   acute recurrent sialoadenitis (K11.22)

K11.22   Acute recurrent sialoadenitis

K11.23   Chronic sialoadenitis

K11.3   Abscess of salivary gland

K11.4   Fistula of salivary gland
Excludes1:   congenital fistula of salivary gland (Q38.4)

K11.5   Sialolithiasis
Calculus of salivary gland or duct
Stone of salivary gland or duct

K11.6   Mucocele of salivary gland
Mucous extravasation cyst of salivary gland
Mucous retention cyst of salivary gland
Ranula

K11.7   Disturbances of salivary secretion
Hypoptyalism
Ptyalism
Xerostomia
Excludes2:   dry mouth NOS (R68.2)

K11.8   Other diseases of salivary glands
Benign lymphoepithelial lesion of salivary gland
Mikulicz' disease
Necrotizing sialometaplasia
Sialectasia
Stenosis of salivary duct
Stricture of salivary duct
Excludes1:   sicca syndrome [Sjögren] (M35.0-)

K11.9   Disease of salivary gland, unspecified
Sialoadenopathy NOS

K12   Stomatitis and related lesions
Use additional code to identify:
alcohol abuse and dependence (F10.-)
alcohol use, uncomplicated (Z72.1)
alcohol dependence, in remission (F10.11)
exposure to environmental tobacco smoke (X58.1)
exposure to tobacco smoke in the perinatal period (P96.6)
history of tobacco use (Z86.43)
occupational exposure to environmental tobacco smoke (Z57.31)
tobacco dependence (F17.-)
tobacco use (Z72.0)
Excludes1:   cancrum oris (A69.0)
            cheilitis (K13.0)
            gangrenous stomatitis (A69.0)
            herpesviral [herpes simplex] gingivostomatitis (B00.2)
            noma (A69.0)

K12.0   Recurrent oral aphthae
Aphthous stomatitis (major)(minor)
Bednar's aphthae
Periadenitis mucosa necrotica recurrens
Recurrent aphthous ulcer
Stomatitis herpetiformis

K12.1   Other forms of stomatitis
Denture stomatitis
Stomatitis NOS
Ulcerative stomatitis
Vesicular stomatitis
Excludes1:   acute necrotizing ulcerative stomatitis (A69.1)
            Vincent's stomatitis (A69.1)

K12.2   Cellulitis and abscess of mouth
Cellulitis of mouth (floor)
Submandibular abscess
Excludes2:   abscess of salivary gland (K11.3)
            abscess of tongue (K14.0)
            periapical abscess (K04.6-K04.7)
            periodontal abscess (K05.2)
            peritonsillar abscess (J36)

K13   Other diseases of lip and oral mucosa
Includes: epithelial disturbances of tongue
Use additional code to identify:
alcohol abuse and dependence (F10.-)
alcohol use, uncomplicated (Z72.1)
alcohol dependence, in remission (F10.11)
exposure to environmental tobacco smoke (X58.1)
exposure to tobacco smoke in the perinatal period (P96.6)
history of tobacco use (Z86.43)
occupational exposure to environmental tobacco smoke (Z57.31)
tobacco dependence (F17.-)
tobacco use (Z72.0)
Excludes2:   certain disorders of gingiva and edentulous alveolar
            ridge (K05-K06)
            cysts of oral region (K09.-)
            diseases of tongue (K14.-)
            stomatitis and related lesions (K12.-)

K13.0   Diseases of lips
Abscess of lips
Angular cheilitis
Cellulitis of lips
Cheilitis NOS
Cheilodynia
Cheilosis
Exfoliative cheilitis
Fistula of lips
Glandular cheilitis
Hypertrophy of lips
Perlèche NEC
Excludes1:   ariboflavinosis (E53.0)
            cheilitis due to radiation-related disorders (L55-
            L59)
            congenital fistula of lips (Q38.0)
            congenital hypertrophy of lips (Q18.6)
            perlèche due to candidiasis (B37.83)
            perlèche due to riboflavin deficiency (E53.0)

K13.1   Cheek and lip biting

K13.2 Leukoplakia and other disturbances of oral epithelium, including tongue
  Erythroplakia
  Leukedema
  Leukokeratosis nicotina palati
  Smoker's palate
  Excludes1:   hairy leukoplakia (K13.3)

K13.3 Hairy leukoplakia

K13.4 Granuloma and granuloma-like lesions of oral mucosa
  Eosinophilic granuloma
  Granuloma pyogenicum
  Verrucous xanthoma

K13.5 Oral submucous fibrosis
  Submucous fibrosis of tongue

K13.6 Irritative hyperplasia of oral mucosa
  Excludes2:   irritative hyperplasia of edentulous ridge [denture hyperplasia] (K06.2)

K13.7 Other and unspecified lesions of oral mucosa
  Focal oral mucinosis

K14 Diseases of tongue
  Use additional code to identify:
    alcohol abuse and dependence (F10.-)
    alcohol use, uncomplicated (Z72.1)
    alcohol dependence, in remission (F10.11)
    exposure to environmental tobacco smoke (X58.1)
    history of tobacco use (Z86.43)
    occupational exposure to environmental tobacco smoke (Z57.31)
    tobacco dependence (F17.-)
    tobacco use (Z72.0)
  Excludes2:   erythroplakia (K13.2)
               focal epithelial hyperplasia (K13.2)
               leukedema (K13.2)
               leukoplakia (K13.2)
               hairy leukoplakia (K13.3)
               macroglossia (congenital) (Q38.2)
               submucous fibrosis of tongue (K13.5)

K14.0 Glossitis
  Abscess of tongue
  Ulceration (traumatic) of tongue
  Excludes1:   atrophic glossitis (K14.4)

K14.1 Geographic tongue
  Benign migratory glossitis
  Glossitis areata exfoliativa

K14.2 Median rhomboid glossitis

K14.3 Hypertrophy of tongue papillae
  Black hairy tongue
  Coated tongue
  Hypertrophy of foliate papillae
  Lingua villosa nigra

K14.4 Atrophy of tongue papillae
  Atrophic glossitis

K14.5 Plicated tongue
  Fissured tongue
  Furrowed tongue
  Scrotal tongue
  Excludes1:   fissured tongue, congenital (Q38.3)

K14.6 Glossodynia
  Glossopyrosis
  Painful tongue

K14.8 Other diseases of tongue
  Atrophy of tongue
  Crenated tongue
  Enlargement of tongue
  Glossocele
  Glossoptosis
  Hypertrophy of tongue

K14.9 Disease of tongue, unspecified
  Glossopathy NOS

DISEASES OF ESOPHAGUS, STOMACH AND DUODENUM (K20–K31)

  Excludes2:   hiatus hernia (K44.-)

K20 Esophagitis
  Includes: abscess of esophagus
                chemical esophagitis
                esophagitis NOS
                peptic esophagitis
  Use additional code to identify:
    alcohol abuse and dependence (F10.-)
    alcohol dependence, in remission (F10.11)
    external cause (Chapter XX)
  Excludes1:   erosion of esophagus (K22.1)
               esophagitis with gastro-esophageal reflux disease (K21.0)
               reflux esophagitis (K21.0)

K21 Gastro-esophageal reflux disease

K21.0 Gastro-esophageal reflux disease with esophagitis
  Reflux esophagitis

K21.9 Gastro-esophageal reflux disease without esophagitis
  Esophageal reflux NOS

K22 Other diseases of esophagus
  Excludes2:   esophageal varices (I85.-)

K22.0 Achalasia of cardia
  Achalasia NOS
  Cardiospasm
  Excludes1:   congenital cardiospasm (Q40.2)

K22.1 Ulcer of esophagus
  Erosion of esophagus
  Fungal ulcer of esophagus
  Peptic ulcer of esophagus
  Ulcer of esophagus due to ingestion of chemicals
  Ulcer of esophagus due to ingestion of drugs and medicaments
  Ulcer of esophagus NOS
  Use additional external cause code (Chapter XX), to identify cause.

K22.2 Esophageal obstruction
  Compression of esophagus
  Constriction of esophagus
  Stenosis of esophagus
  Stricture of esophagus
  Excludes1:   congenital stenosis or stricture of esophagus (Q39.3)

K22.3 Perforation of esophagus
  Rupture of esophagus
  Excludes1:   traumatic perforation of (thoracic) esophagus (S27.8-)

K22.4 Dyskinesia of esophagus
  Corkscrew esophagus
  Diffuse esophageal spasm
  Spasm of esophagus
  Excludes1:   cardiospasm (K22.0)

K22.5 Diverticulum of esophagus, acquired
  Esophageal pouch, acquired
  Excludes1:   diverticulum of esophagus (congenital) (Q39.6)

K22.6 Gastro-esophageal laceration-hemorrhage syndrome
  Mallory-Weiss syndrome

K22.8 Other specified diseases of esophagus
  Hemorrhage of esophagus NOS
  Excludes2:   esophageal varices (I85.-)
               Paterson-Kelly syndrome (D50.1)

K22.9 Disease of esophagus, unspecified

K23 Disorders of esophagus in diseases classified elsewhere
  Code first underlying disease, such as:
    congenital syphilis (A50.5)
  Excludes1:   late syphilis (A52.79)
               megaesophagus due to Chagas' disease (B57.31)
               tuberculosis (A18.83)

K25 Gastric ulcer

Includes: erosion (acute) of stomach
pylorus ulcer (peptic)
stomach ulcer (peptic)

Use additional code to identify:
alcohol abuse and dependence (F10.-)
alcohol dependence, in remission (F10.11)
external cause (Chapter XIX), if drug-induced

Excludes1:   acute gastritis (K29.0-)
peptic ulcer NOS (K27.-)

K25.0   Acute gastric ulcer with hemorrhage

K25.1   Acute gastric ulcer with perforation

K25.2   Acute gastric ulcer with both hemorrhage and perforation

K25.3   Acute gastric ulcer without hemorrhage or perforation

K25.4   Chronic or unspecified gastric ulcer with hemorrhage

K25.5   Chronic or unspecified gastric ulcer with perforation

K25.6   Chronic or unspecified gastric ulcer with both hemorrhage and perforation

K25.7   Chronic gastric ulcer without hemorrhage or perforation

K25.9   Gastric ulcer, unspecified as acute or chronic, without hemorrhage or perforation

K26 Duodenal ulcer

Includes: duodenum ulcer (peptic)
erosion (acute) of duodenum
postpyloric ulcer (peptic)

Use additional code to identify:
alcohol abuse and dependence (F10.-)
alcohol use, uncomplicated (Z72.1)
alcohol dependence, in remission (F10.11)
external cause (Chapter XIX), if drug-induced

Excludes1:   peptic ulcer NOS (K27.-)

K26.0   Acute duodenal ulcer with hemorrhage

K26.1   Acute duodenal ulcer with perforation

K26.2   Acute duodenal ulcer with both hemorrhage and perforation

K26.3   Acute duodenal ulcer without hemorrhage or perforation

K26.4   Chronic or unspecified duodenal ulcer with hemorrhage

K26.5   Chronic or unspecified duodenal ulcer with perforation

K26.6   Chronic or unspecified duodenal ulcer with both hemorrhage and perforation

K26.7   Chronic duodenal ulcer without hemorrhage or perforation

K26.9   Duodenal ulcer, unspecified as acute or chronic, without hemorrhage or perforation

K27 Peptic ulcer, site unspecified

Includes: gastroduodenal ulcer NOS
peptic ulcer NOS

Use additional code to identify:
alcohol abuse and dependence (F10.-)
alcohol use, uncomplicated (Z72.1)
alcohol dependence, in remission (F10.11)
external cause (Chapter XIX), if drug-induced

Excludes1:   peptic ulcer of newborn (P78.8)

K27.0   Acute peptic ulcer, site unspecified, with hemorrhage

K27.1   Acute peptic ulcer, site unspecified, with perforation

K27.2   Acute peptic ulcer, site unspecified, with both hemorrhage and perforation

K27.3   Acute peptic ulcer, site unspecified, without hemorrhage or perforation

K27.4   Chronic or unspecified peptic ulcer, site unspecified, with hemorrhage

K27.5   Chronic or unspecified peptic ulcer, site unspecified, with perforation

K27.6   Chronic or unspecified peptic ulcer, site unspecified, with both hemorrhage and perforation

K27.7   Chronic peptic ulcer, site unspecified, without hemorrhage or perforation

K27.9   Peptic ulcer, site unspecified, unspecified as acute or chronic, without hemorrhage or perforation

K28 Gastrojejunal ulcer

Includes: anastomotic ulcer (peptic) or erosion
gastrocolic ulcer (peptic) or erosion
gastrointestinal ulcer (peptic) or erosion
gastrojejunal ulcer (peptic) or erosion
jejunal ulcer (peptic) or erosion
marginal ulcer (peptic) or erosion
stomal ulcer (peptic) or erosion

Use additional code to identify:
alcohol abuse and dependence (F10.-)
alcohol use, uncomplicated (Z72.1)
alcohol dependence, in remission (F10.11)
external cause (Chapter XIX), if drug-induced

Excludes1:   primary ulcer of small intestine (K63.3)

K28.0   Acute gastrojejunal ulcer with hemorrhage

K28.1   Acute gastrojejunal ulcer with perforation

K28.2   Acute gastrojejunal ulcer with both hemorrhage and perforation

K28.3   Acute gastrojejunal ulcer without hemorrhage or perforation

K28.4   Chronic or unspecified gastrojejunal ulcer with hemorrhage

K28.5   Chronic or unspecified gastrojejunal ulcer with perforation

K28.6   Chronic or unspecified gastrojejunal ulcer with both hemorrhage and perforation

K28.7   Chronic gastrojejunal ulcer without hemorrhage or perforation

K28.9   Gastrojejunal ulcer, unspecified as acute or chronic, without hemorrhage or perforation

K29 Gastritis and duodenitis

Excludes1:   eosinophilic gastritis or gastroenteritis (K52.8)
Zollinger-Ellison syndrome (E16.4)

K29.0   Acute gastritis

Use additional code to identify:
alcohol abuse and dependence (F10.-)
alcohol use, uncomplicated (Z72.1)
alcohol dependence, in remission (F10.11)
external cause (Chapter XIX), if drug-induced

Excludes1:   erosion (acute) of stomach (K25.-)

K29.00   Acute gastritis without bleeding

K29.01   Acute gastritis with bleeding

K29.2   Alcoholic gastritis

Use additional code to identify:
alcohol abuse and dependence (F10.-)
alcohol use, uncomplicated (Z72.1)
alcohol dependence, in remission (F10.11)

K29.20   Alcoholic gastritis without bleeding

K29.21   Alcoholic gastritis with bleeding

K29.3   Chronic superficial gastritis

K29.30   Chronic superficial gastritis without bleeding

K29.31   Chronic superficial gastritis with bleeding

K29.4   Chronic atrophic gastritis

Gastric atrophy

K29.40   Chronic atrophic gastritis without bleeding

K29.41   Chronic atrophic gastritis with bleeding

K29.5   Chronic gastritis, other and unspecified

Chronic antral gastritis
Chronic fundal gastritis

K29.50   Chronic gastritis, other and unspecified, without bleeding

K29.51   Chronic gastritis, other and unspecified, with bleeding

K29.6   Other gastritis

Giant hypertrophic gastritis
Granulomatous gastritis
Ménétrier's disease

K29.60   Other gastritis without bleeding

K29.61   Other gastritis with bleeding

K29.7   Gastritis, unspecified

K29.70   Gastritis, unspecified, without bleeding

K29.71   Gastritis, unspecified, with bleeding

K29.8   Duodenitis

K29.80   Duodenitis without bleeding

K29.81   Duodenitis with bleeding

K29.9 Gastroduodenitis, unspecified
    K29.90 Gastroduodenitis, unspecified, without bleeding
    K29.91 Gastroduodenitis, unspecified, with bleeding

K30 Dyspepsia
  Includes: indigestion
  Excludes1:   heartburn (R12)
               nervous dyspepsia (F45.8)
               neurotic dyspepsia (F45.8)
               psychogenic dyspepsia (F45.8)

K31 Other diseases of stomach and duodenum
  Includes: functional disorders of stomach
  Excludes2:   diabetic gastroparesis (E08.43, E09.43, E10.43, E11.43, E13.43, E14.43)
               diverticulum of duodenum (K57.00-K57.11)

K31.0 Acute dilatation of stomach
    Acute distention of stomach

K31.1 Adult hypertrophic pyloric stenosis
    Pyloric stenosis NOS
    Excludes1:   congenital or infantile pyloric stenosis (Q40.0)

K31.2 Hourglass stricture and stenosis of stomach
    Excludes1:   congenital hourglass stomach (Q40.2)
               hourglass contraction of stomach (K31.89)

K31.3 Pylorospasm, not elsewhere classified
    Excludes1:   congenital or infantile pylorospasm (Q40.0)
               neurotic pylorospasm (F45.8)
               psychogenic pylorospasm (F45.8)

K31.4 Gastric diverticulum
    Excludes1:   congenital diverticulum of stomach (Q40.2)

K31.5 Obstruction of duodenum
    Constriction of duodenum
    Duodenal ileus (chronic)
    Stenosis of duodenum
    Stricture of duodenum
    Volvulus of duodenum
    Excludes1:   congenital stenosis of duodenum (Q41.0)

K31.6 Fistula of stomach and duodenum
    Gastrocolic fistula
    Gastrojejunocolic fistula

K31.8 Other specified diseases of stomach and duodenum
    K31.81 Angiodysplasia of stomach and duodenum (without bleeding)
    K31.82 Angiodysplasia of stomach and duodenum with bleeding
    K31.83 Achlorhydria
    K31.89 Other diseases of stomach and duodenum

K31.9 Disease of stomach and duodenum, unspecified

DISEASES OF APPENDIX (K35–K38)

K35 Acute appendicitis
  K35.0 Acute appendicitis with generalized peritonitis
    Appendicitis (acute) with perforation
    Appendicitis (acute) with peritonitis (generalized)
    Appendicitis (acute) with peritonitis with peritoneal abscess
    Appendicitis (acute) with rupture

  K35.1 Acute appendicitis with peritoneal abscess
    Abscess of appendix
    Excludes1:   acute appendicitis with generalized peritonitis (K35.0)

  K35.9 Acute appendicitis, without peritonitis
    Acute appendicitis NOS
    Acute appendicitis without perforation
    Acute appendicitis without peritoneal abscess
    Acute appendicitis without peritonitis
    Acute appendicitis without rupture

K36 Other appendicitis
  Includes: chronic appendicitis
               recurrent appendicitis

K37 Unspecified appendicitis

K38 Other diseases of appendix
  K38.0 Hyperplasia of appendix
  K38.1 Appendicular concretions
    Fecalith of appendix
    Stercolith of appendix
  K38.2 Diverticulum of appendix
  K38.3 Fistula of appendix
  K38.8 Other specified diseases of appendix
    Intussusception of appendix
  K38.9 Disease of appendix, unspecified

HERNIA (K40–K46)
Note: Hernia with both gangrene and obstruction is classified to hernia with gangrene
  Includes: acquired hernia
               congenital [except diaphragmatic or hiatus] hernia
               recurrent hernia

K40 Inguinal hernia
  Includes: bubonocele
               direct inguinal hernia
               double inguinal hernia
               indirect inguinal hernia
               inguinal hernia NOS
               oblique inguinal hernia
               scrotal hernia

  K40.0 Bilateral inguinal hernia, with obstruction, without gangrene
  K40.1 Bilateral inguinal hernia, with gangrene
  K40.2 Bilateral inguinal hernia, without obstruction or gangrene
    Bilateral inguinal hernia NOS
  K40.3 Unilateral or unspecified inguinal hernia, with obstruction, without gangrene
    Inguinal hernia (unilateral) causing obstruction
    Incarcerated inguinal hernia (unilateral)
    Irreducible inguinal hernia (unilateral)
    Strangulated inguinal hernia (unilateral)
  K40.4 Unilateral or unspecified inguinal hernia, with gangrene
    Inguinal hernia NOS with gangrene
  K40.9 Unilateral or unspecified inguinal hernia, without obstruction or gangrene
    Inguinal hernia (unilateral) NOS

K41 Femoral hernia
  K41.0 Bilateral femoral hernia, with obstruction, without gangrene
  K41.1 Bilateral femoral hernia, with gangrene
  K41.2 Bilateral femoral hernia, without obstruction or gangrene
    Bilateral femoral hernia NOS
  K41.3 Unilateral or unspecified femoral hernia, with obstruction, without gangrene
    Femoral hernia (unilateral) causing obstruction
    Incarcerated femoral hernia (unilateral)
    Irreducible femoral hernia (unilateral)
    Strangulated femoral hernia (unilateral)
  K41.4 Unilateral or unspecified femoral hernia, with gangrene
  K41.9 Unilateral or unspecified femoral hernia, without obstruction or gangrene
    Femoral hernia (unilateral) NOS

K42 Umbilical hernia
  Includes: paraumbilical hernia
  Excludes1:   omphalocele (Q79.2)
  K42.0 Umbilical hernia with obstruction, without gangrene
    Umbilical hernia causing obstruction, without gangrene
    Incarcerated umbilical hernia, without gangrene
    Irreducible umbilical hernia, without gangrene
    Strangulated umbilical hernia, without gangrene
  K42.1 Umbilical hernia with gangrene
    Gangrenous umbilical hernia
  K42.9 Umbilical hernia without obstruction or gangrene
    Umbilical hernia NOS

K43 Ventral hernia
  K43.0 Ventral hernia with obstruction, without gangrene
    Ventral hernia causing obstruction, without gangrene
    Incarcerated ventral hernia, without gangrene
    Irreducible ventral hernia, without gangrene
    Strangulated ventral hernia, without gangrene
    K43.00 Ventral hernia, unspecified, with obstruction, without gangrene
    K43.01 Incisional hernia, with obstruction , without gangrene
    K43.09 Other ventral hernia, with obstruction, without gangrene
      Epigastric hernia
  K43.1 Ventral hernia with gangrene
    Gangrenous ventral hernia
    K43.10 Ventral hernia, unspecified, with gangrene
    K43.11 Incisional hernia, with gangrene
    K43.19 Other ventral hernia, with gangrene
      Epigastric hernia
  K43.9 Ventral hernia without obstruction or gangrene
    K43.90 Ventral hernia, unspecified, without obstruction or gangrene
      Ventral hernia NOS
    K43.91 Incisional hernia, without obstruction or gangrene
    K43.99 Other ventral hernia, without obstruction or gangrene
      Epigastric hernia

K44 Diaphragmatic hernia
  Includes: hiatus hernia (esophageal) (sliding)
        paraesophageal hernia
  Excludes1: congenital diaphragmatic hernia (Q79.0)
        congenital hiatus hernia (Q40.1)
  K44.0 Diaphragmatic hernia with obstruction, without gangrene
    Diaphragmatic hernia causing obstruction
    Incarcerated diaphragmatic hernia
    Irreducible diaphragmatic hernia
    Strangulated diaphragmatic hernia
  K44.1 Diaphragmatic hernia with gangrene
    Gangrenous diaphragmatic hernia
  K44.9 Diaphragmatic hernia without obstruction or gangrene
    Diaphragmatic hernia NOS

K45 Other abdominal hernia
  Includes: abdominal hernia, specified site NEC
        lumbar hernia
        obturator hernia
        pudendal hernia
        retroperitoneal hernia
        sciatic hernia
  K45.0 Other specified abdominal hernia with obstruction, without gangrene
    Other specified abdominal hernia causing obstruction
    Other specified incarcerated abdominal hernia
    Other specified irreducible abdominal hernia
    Other specified strangulated abdominal hernia
  K45.1 Other specified abdominal hernia with gangrene
    Any condition listed under K45 specified as gangrenous
  K45.8 Other specified abdominal hernia without obstruction or gangrene

K46 Unspecified abdominal hernia
  Includes: enterocele
        epiplocele
        hernia NOS
        interstitial hernia
        intestinal hernia
        intra-abdominal hernia
  Excludes1: vaginal enterocele (N81.5)
  K46.0 Unspecified abdominal hernia with obstruction, without gangrene
    Unspecified abdominal hernia causing obstruction
    Unspecified incarcerated abdominal hernia
    Unspecified irreducible abdominal hernia
    Unspecified strangulated abdominal hernia
  K46.1 Unspecified abdominal hernia with gangrene
    Any condition listed under K46 specified as gangrenous

  K46.9 Unspecified abdominal hernia without obstruction or gangrene
    Abdominal hernia NOS

NONINFECTIVE ENTERITIS AND COLITIS (K50–K52)
  Includes: noninfective inflammatory bowel disease
  Excludes1: irritable bowel syndrome (K58.-)
        megacolon (K59.3)

K50 Crohn's disease [regional enteritis]
  Includes: granulomatous enteritis
  Excludes1: ulcerative colitis (K51.-)
  Use additional code to identify manifestations, such as:
  pyoderma gangrenosum (L88)
  K50.0 Crohn's disease of small intestine
    Crohn's disease [regional enteritis] of duodenum
    Crohn's disease [regional enteritis] of ileum
    Crohn's disease [regional enteritis] of jejunum
    Regional ileitis
    Terminal ileitis
    Excludes1: Crohn's disease of both small and large intestine (K50.8)
    K50.00 Crohn's disease of small intestine with unspecified complications
    K50.01 Crohn's disease of small intestine with rectal bleeding
    K50.02 Crohn's disease of small intestine with intestinal obstruction
    K50.03 Crohn's disease of small intestine with fistula
    K50.04 Crohn's disease of small intestine with abscess
    K50.05 Crohn's disease of small intestine without complications
    K50.09 Crohn's disease of small intestine with other complication
  K50.1 Crohn's disease of large intestine
    Crohn's disease [regional enteritis] of colon
    Crohn's disease [regional enteritis] of large bowel
    Crohn's disease [regional enteritis] of rectum
    Granulomatous colitis
    Regional colitis
    Excludes1: Crohn's disease of both small and large intestine (K50.8)
    K50.10 Crohn's disease of large intestine with unspecified complications
    K50.11 Crohn's disease of large intestine with rectal bleeding
    K50.12 Crohn's disease of large intestine with intestinal obstruction
    K50.13 Crohn's disease of large intestine with fistula
    K50.14 Crohn's disease of large intestine with abscess
    K50.15 Crohn's disease of large intestine without complications
    K50.19 Crohn's disease of large intestine with other complication
  K50.8 Other Crohn's disease
    Crohn's disease of both small and large intestine
    K50.80 Other Crohn's disease with unspecified complications
    K50.81 Other Crohn's disease with rectal bleeding
    K50.82 Other Crohn's disease with intestinal obstruction
    K50.83 Other Crohn's disease with fistula
    K50.84 Other Crohn's disease with abscess
    K50.85 Other Crohn's disease without complications
    K50.89 Other Crohn's disease with other complication
  K50.9 Crohn's disease, unspecified
    K50.90 Crohn's disease, unspecified with unspecified complications
    K50.91 Crohn's disease, unspecified with rectal bleeding
    K50.92 Crohn's disease, unspecified with intestinal obstruction
    K50.93 Crohn's disease, unspecified with fistula
    K50.94 Crohn's disease, unspecified with abscess
    K50.95 Crohn's disease, unspecified without complications
      Crohn's disease NOS
      Regional enteritis NOS
    K50.99 Crohn's disease, unspecified with other complication

K51 Ulcerative colitis
　　Use additional code to identify manifestations, such as:
　　　pyoderma gangrenosum (L88)
　　Excludes1:　Crohn's disease [regional enteritis] (K50.-)

K51.0 Ulcerative (chronic) enterocolitis
　　K51.00 Ulcerative (chronic) enterocolitis with unspecified complications
　　K51.01 Ulcerative (chronic) enterocolitis with rectal bleeding
　　K51.02 Ulcerative (chronic) enterocolitis with intestinal obstruction
　　K51.03 Ulcerative (chronic) enterocolitis with fistula
　　K51.04 Ulcerative (chronic) enterocolitis with abscess
　　K51.05 Ulcerative (chronic) enterocolitis without complications
　　K51.09 Ulcerative (chronic) enterocolitis with other complication

K51.1 Ulcerative (chronic) ileocolitis
　　K51.10 Ulcerative (chronic) ileocolitis with unspecified complications
　　K51.11 Ulcerative (chronic) ileocolitis with rectal bleeding
　　K51.12 Ulcerative (chronic) ileocolitis with intestinal obstruction
　　K51.13 Ulcerative (chronic) ileocolitis with fistula
　　K51.14 Ulcerative (chronic) ileocolitis with abscess
　　K51.15 Ulcerative (chronic) ileocolitis without complications
　　K51.19 Ulcerative (chronic) ileocolitis with other complication

K51.2 Ulcerative (chronic) proctitis
　　K51.20 Ulcerative (chronic) proctitis with unspecified complications
　　K51.21 Ulcerative (chronic) proctitis with rectal bleeding
　　K51.22 Ulcerative (chronic) proctitis with intestinal obstruction
　　K51.23 Ulcerative (chronic) proctitis with fistula
　　K51.24 Ulcerative (chronic) proctitis with abscess
　　K51.25 Ulcerative (chronic) proctitis without complications
　　K51.29 Ulcerative (chronic) proctitis with other complication

K51.3 Ulcerative (chronic) rectosigmoiditis
　　K51.30 Ulcerative (chronic) rectosigmoiditis with unspecified complications
　　K51.31 Ulcerative (chronic) rectosigmoiditis with rectal bleeding
　　K51.32 Ulcerative (chronic) rectosigmoiditis with intestinal obstruction
　　K51.33 Ulcerative (chronic) rectosigmoiditis with fistula
　　K51.34 Ulcerative (chronic) rectosigmoiditis with abscess
　　K51.35 Ulcerative (chronic) rectosigmoiditis without complications
　　K51.39 Ulcerative (chronic) rectosigmoiditis with other complication

K51.4 Pseudopolyposis of colon
　　K51.40 Pseudopolyposis of colon with unspecified complications
　　K51.41 Pseudopolyposis of colon with rectal bleeding
　　K51.42 Pseudopolyposis of colon with intestinal obstruction
　　K51.43 Pseudopolyposis of colon with fistula
　　K51.44 Pseudopolyposis of colon with abscess
　　K51.45 Pseudopolyposis of colon without complications
　　K51.49 Pseudopolyposis of colon with other complication

K51.5 Mucosal proctocolitis
　　K51.50 Mucosal proctocolitis with unspecified complications
　　K51.51 Mucosal proctocolitis with rectal bleeding
　　K51.52 Mucosal proctocolitis with intestinal obstruction
　　K51.53 Mucosal proctocolitis with fistula
　　K51.54 Mucosal proctocolitis with abscess
　　K51.55 Mucosal proctocolitis without complications
　　K51.59 Mucosal proctocolitis with other complication

K51.8 Other ulcerative colitis
　　K51.80 Other ulcerative colitis with unspecified complications
　　K51.81 Other ulcerative colitis with rectal bleeding
　　K51.82 Other ulcerative colitis with intestinal obstruction

K51.83 Other ulcerative colitis with fistula
K51.84 Other ulcerative colitis with abscess
K51.85 Other ulcerative colitis without complications
K51.89 Other ulcerative colitis with other complication

K51.9 Ulcerative colitis, unspecified
　　K51.90 Ulcerative colitis, unspecified with unspecified complications
　　K51.91 Ulcerative colitis, unspecified with rectal bleeding
　　K51.92 Ulcerative colitis, unspecified with intestinal obstruction
　　K51.93 Ulcerative colitis, unspecified with fistula
　　K51.94 Ulcerative colitis, unspecified with abscess
　　K51.95 Ulcerative colitis, unspecified without complications
　　　Ulcerative enteritis NOS
　　K51.99 Ulcerative colitis, unspecified with other complication

K52 Other and unspecified noninfective gastroenteritis and colitis
K52.0 Gastroenteritis and colitis due to radiation
K52.1 Toxic gastroenteritis and colitis
　　Use additional external cause code (Chapter XIX), to identify toxic agent
K52.2 Allergic and dietetic gastroenteritis and colitis
　　Food hypersensitivity gastroenteritis or colitis
K52.8 Other specified noninfective gastroenteritis and colitis
　　Eosinophilic gastritis or gastroenteritis
K52.9 Noninfective gastroenteritis and colitis, unspecified
　　Colitis NOS
　　Enteritis NOS
　　Gastroenteritis NOS
　　Ileitis NOS
　　Jejunitis NOS
　　Sigmoiditis NOS
　　Excludes1:　diarrhea NOS (R19.7)
　　　　functional diarrhea (K59.1)
　　　　infectious gastroenteritis and colitis NOS (A09)
　　　　neonatal diarrhea (noninfective) (P78.3)
　　　　psychogenic diarrhea (F45.8)

OTHER DISEASES OF INTESTINES (K55–K63)

K55 Vascular disorders of intestine
　　Excludes1:　necrotizing enterocolitis of fetus or newborn (P77)
K55.0 Acute vascular disorders of intestine
　　Acute fulminant ischemic colitis
　　Acute intestinal infarction
　　Acute small intestine ischemia
　　Infarction of appendices epiploicae
　　Mesenteric (artery) (vein) embolism
　　Mesenteric (artery) (vein) infarction
　　Mesenteric (artery) (vein) thrombosis
　　Necrosis of intestine
　　Subacute ischemic colitis
K55.1 Chronic vascular disorders of intestine
　　Chronic ischemic colitis
　　Chronic ischemic enteritis
　　Chronic ischemic enterocolitis
　　Ischemic stricture of intestine
　　Mesenteric atherosclerosis
　　Mesenteric vascular insufficiency
K55.2 Angiodysplasia of colon
　　K55.20 Angiodysplasia of colon without hemorrhage
　　K55.21 Angiodysplasia of colon with hemorrhage
K55.8 Other vascular disorders of intestine
K55.9 Vascular disorder of intestine, unspecified
　　Ischemic colitis
　　Ischemic enteritis
　　Ischemic enterocolitis

K56　Paralytic ileus and intestinal obstruction without hernia

Excludes1:　congenital stricture or stenosis of intestine (Q41-Q42)
　　　　　　cystic fibrosis with meconium ileus (E84.1)
　　　　　　intestinal obstruction with hernia (K40-K46)
　　　　　　ischemic stricture of intestine (K55.1)
　　　　　　meconium ileus NOS (P75)
　　　　　　neonatal intestinal obstructions classifiable to P76.-
　　　　　　obstruction of duodenum (K31.5)
　　　　　　postoperative intestinal obstruction (K91.3)
　　　　　　stenosis of anus or rectum (K62.4)

K56.0　Paralytic ileus
　　Paralysis of bowel
　　Paralysis of colon
　　Paralysis of intestine
　　Excludes1:　gallstone ileus (K56.3)
　　　　　　　ileus NOS (K56.7)
　　　　　　　obstructive ileus NOS (K56.6)

K56.1　Intussusception
　　Intussusception or invagination of bowel
　　Intussusception or invagination of colon
　　Intussusception or invagination of intestine
　　Intussusception or invagination of rectum
　　Excludes2:　intussusception of appendix (K38.8)

K56.2　Volvulus
　　Strangulation of colon or intestine
　　Torsion of colon or intestine
　　Twist of colon or intestine
　　Excludes2:　volvulus of duodenum (K31.5)

K56.3　Gallstone ileus
　　Obstruction of intestine by gallstone

K56.4　Other impaction of intestine
　　Enterolith
　　Fecal impaction
　　Impaction (of) colon

K56.5　Intestinal adhesions [bands] with obstruction
　　Peritoneal adhesions [bands] with intestinal obstruction

K56.6　Other and unspecified intestinal obstruction
　　Enterostenosis
　　Obstructive ileus NOS
　　Occlusion of colon or intestine
　　Stenosis of colon or intestine
　　Stricture of colon or intestine

K56.7　Ileus, unspecified

K57　Diverticular disease of intestine
Excludes1:　congenital diverticulum of intestine (Q43.8)
　　　　　　Meckel's diverticulum (Q43.0)
Excludes2:　diverticulum of appendix (K38.2)

K57.0　Diverticulitis of small intestine with perforation and abscess
　　Diverticulitis of small intestine with peritonitis
　　Excludes1:　diverticulitis of both small and large intestine
　　　　　　　with perforation and abscess (K57.4-)

K57.00　Diverticulitis of small intestine with perforation and abscess without bleeding

K57.01　Diverticulitis of small intestine with perforation and abscess with bleeding

K57.1　Diverticular disease of small intestine without perforation or abscess
　　Excludes1:　diverticular disease of both small and large
　　　　　　　intestine without perforation or abscess
　　　　　　　(K57.5-)

K57.10　Diverticulosis of small intestine without perforation or abscess without bleeding
　　Diverticular disease of small intestine NOS

K57.11　Diverticulosis of small intestine without perforation or abscess with bleeding

K57.12　Diverticulitis of small intestine without perforation or abscess without bleeding

K57.13　Diverticulitis of small intestine without perforation or abscess with bleeding

K57.2　Diverticulitis of large intestine with perforation and abscess
　　Diverticulitis of colon with peritonitis
　　Excludes1:　diverticulitis of both small and large intestine
　　　　　　　with perforation and abscess (K57.4-)

K57.20　Diverticulitis of large intestine with perforation and abscess without bleeding

K57.21　Diverticulitis of large intestine with perforation and abscess with bleeding

K57.3　Diverticular disease of large intestine without perforation or abscess
　　Excludes1:　diverticular disease of both small and large
　　　　　　　intestine without perforation or abscess
　　　　　　　(K57.5-)

K57.30　Diverticulosis of large intestine without perforation or abscess without bleeding
　　Diverticular disease of colon NOS

K57.31　Diverticulosis of large intestine without perforation or abscess with bleeding

K57.32　Diverticulitis of large intestine without perforation or abscess without bleeding

K57.33　Diverticulitis of large intestine without perforation or abscess with bleeding

K57.4　Diverticulitis of both small and large intestine with perforation and abscess
　　Diverticulitis of both small and large intestine with peritonitis

K57.40　Diverticulitis of both small and large intestine with perforation and abscess without bleeding

K57.41　Diverticulitis of both small and large intestine with perforation and abscess with bleeding

K57.5　Diverticular disease of both small and large intestine without perforation or abscess

K57.50　Diverticulosis of both small and large intestine without perforation or abscess without bleeding
　　Diverticular disease of both small and large intestine NOS

K57.51　Diverticulosis of both small and large intestine without perforation or abscess with bleeding

K57.52　Diverticulitis of both small and large intestine without perforation or abscess without bleeding

K57.53　Diverticulitis of both small and large intestine without perforation or abscess with bleeding

K57.8　Diverticulitis of intestine, part unspecified, with perforation and abscess
　　Diverticulitis of intestine NOS with peritonitis

K57.80　Diverticulitis of intestine, part unspecified, with perforation and abscess without bleeding

K57.81　Diverticulitis of intestine, part unspecified, with perforation and abscess with bleeding

K57.9　Diverticular disease of intestine, part unspecified, without perforation or abscess

K57.90　Diverticulosis of intestine, part unspecified, without perforation or abscess without bleeding
　　Diverticular disease of intestine NOS

K57.91　Diverticulosis of intestine, part unspecified, without perforation or abscess with bleeding

K57.92　Diverticulitis of intestine, part unspecified, without perforation or abscess without bleeding

K57.93　Diverticulitis of intestine, part unspecified, without perforation or abscess with bleeding

K58　Irritable bowel syndrome
　　Includes:　irritable colon
　　　　　　　spastic colon

K58.0　Irritable bowel syndrome with diarrhea

K58.9　Irritable bowel syndrome without diarrhea
　　Irritable bowel syndrome NOS

K59　Other functional intestinal disorders
　　Excludes1:　change in bowel habit NOS (R19.4)
　　　　　　　intestinal malabsorption (K90.-)
　　　　　　　psychogenic intestinal disorders (F45.8)
　　Excludes2:　functional disorders of stomach (K31.-)

K59.0　Constipation

K59.1　Functional diarrhea
　　Excludes1:　diarrhea NOS (R19.7)
　　　　　　　irritable bowel syndrome with diarrhea (K58.0)

K59.2　Neurogenic bowel, not elsewhere classified

K59.3   Megacolon, not elsewhere classified
Dilatation of colon
Toxic megacolon
Use additional external cause code (Chapter XIX), to identify
     toxic agent
Excludes1:   congenital megacolon (aganglionic) (Q43.1)
            Hirschsprung's disease (Q43.1)
            megacolon in Chagas' disease (B57.32)

K59.4   Anal spasm
Proctalgia fugax

K59.8   Other specified functional intestinal disorders
Atony of colon

K59.9   Functional intestinal disorder, unspecified

K60   Fissure and fistula of anal and rectal regions
Excludes1:   fissure and fistula of anal and rectal regions with
              abscess or cellulitis (K61.-)

K60.0   Acute anal fissure

K60.1   Chronic anal fissure

K60.2   Anal fissure, unspecified

K60.3   Anal fistula

K60.4   Rectal fistula
Fistula of rectum to skin
Excludes1:   rectovaginal fistula (N82.3)
            vesicorectal fistual (N32.1)

K60.5   Anorectal fistula

K61   Abscess of anal and rectal regions
Includes: abscess of anal and rectal regions
            cellulitis of anal and rectal regions

K61.0   Anal abscess
Perianal abscess
Excludes1:   intrasphincteric abscess (K61.4)

K61.1   Rectal abscess
Perirectal abscess
Excludes1:   ischiorectal abscess (K61.3)

K61.2   Anorectal abscess

K61.3   Ischiorectal abscess
Abscess of ischiorectal fossa

K61.4   Intrasphincteric abscess

K62   Other diseases of anus and rectum
Includes: anal canal
Excludes2:   colostomy and enterostomy malfunction (K91.4-)
            fecal incontinence (R15)
            hemorrhoids (I84.-)

K62.0   Anal polyp

K62.1   Rectal polyp
Excludes1:   adenomatous polyp (D12.8)

K62.2   Anal prolapse
Prolapse of anal canal

K62.3   Rectal prolapse
Prolapse of rectal mucosa

K62.4   Stenosis of anus and rectum
Stricture of anus (sphincter)

K62.5   Hemorrhage of anus and rectum
Excludes1:   gastrointestinal bleeding NOS (K92.2)
            melena (K92.1)
            neonatal rectal hemorrhage (P54.2)

K62.6   Ulcer of anus and rectum
Solitary ulcer of anus and rectum
Stercoral ulcer of anus and rectum
Excludes1:   fissure and fistula of anus and rectum (K60.-)
            ulcerative colitis (K51.-)

K62.7   Radiation proctitis

K62.8   Other specified diseases of anus and rectum
Perforation (nontraumatic) of rectum
Proctitis NOS
Excludes1:   ulcerative proctitis (K51.2)

K62.9   Disease of anus and rectum, unspecified

K63   Other diseases of intestine

K63.0   Abscess of intestine
Excludes1:   abscess of intestine with Crohn's disease (K50.04,
             K50.14, K50.84, K50.94)
            abscess of intestine with diverticular disease (K57.0,
             K57.2, K57.4, K57.8)
            abscess of intestine with ulcerative colitis (K51.04,
             K51.14, K51.24, K51.34, K51.44, K51.54,
             K51.84, K51.94)
Excludes2:   abscess of anal and rectal regions (K61.-)
            abscess of appendix (K35.1)

K63.1   Perforation of intestine (nontraumatic)
Excludes1:   perforation (nontraumatic) of duodenum (K26.-)
            perforation (nontraumatic) of intestine with
             diverticular disease (K57.0, K57.2, K57.4,
             K57.8)
Excludes2:   perforation (nontraumatic) of appendix (K35.0)

K63.2   Fistula of intestine
Excludes1:   fistula of duodenum (K31.6)
            fistula of intestine with Crohn's disease (K50.03,
             K50.13, K50.83, K50.93)
            fistula of intestine with ulcerative colitis (K51.03,
             K51.13, K51.23, K51.33, K51.43, K51.53,
             K51.83, K51.93)
Excludes2:   fistula of anal and rectal regions (K60.-)
            fistula of appendix (K38.3)
            intestinal-genital fistula, female (N82.2-N82.4)
            vesicointestinal fistula (N32.1)

K63.3   Ulcer of intestine
Primary ulcer of small intestine
Excludes1:   duodenal ulcer (K26.-)
            gastrointestinal ulcer (K28.-)
            gastrojejunal ulcer (K28.-)
            jejunal ulcer (K28.-)
            peptic ulcer, site unspecified (K27.-)
            ulcer of anus or rectum (K62.6)
            ulcer of intestine with perforation (K63.1)
            ulcerative colitis (K51.-)

K63.4   Enteroptosis

K63.8   Other specified diseases of intestine

K63.9   Disease of intestine, unspecified

DISEASES OF PERITONEUM AND RETROPERITONEUM
(K65–K68)

K65   Peritonitis
Excludes1:   acute appendicitis with generalized peritonitis (K35.0)
            aseptic peritonitis (T81.6)
            benign paroxysmal peritonitis (E85.0)
            chemical peritonitis (T81.6)
            diverticulitis of both small and large intestine with
             peritonitis (K57.4-)
            diverticulitis of colon with peritonitis (K57.2-)
            diverticulitis of intestine, NOS, with peritonitis (K57.8-)
            diverticulitis of small intestine with peritonitis (K57.0-)
            gonococcal peritonitis (A54.85)
            neonatal peritonitis (P78.0-P78.1)
            pelvic peritonitis, female (N73.3-N73.5)
            periodic familial peritonitis (E85.0)
            peritonitis due to talc or other foreign substance
             (T81.6)
            peritonitis in chlamydia (A74.81)
            peritonitis in diphtheria (A36.89)
            peritonitis in syphilis (late) (A52.74)
            peritonitis in tuberculosis (A18.31)
            peritonitis with or following abortion or ectopic or
             molar pregnancy (O00-O07, O08.0)
            peritonitis with or following appendicitis (K35.-)
            peritonitis with or following diverticular disease of
             intestine (K57.-)
            puerperal peritonitis (O85)

K65.0 Acute peritonitis
  Abdominopelvic abscess
  Abscess (of) omentum
  Abscess (of) peritoneum
  Generalized peritonitis (acute)
  Mesenteric abscess
  Pelvic peritonitis (acute), male
  Retrocecal abscess
  Subdiaphragmatic abscess
  Subhepatic abscess
  Subphrenic abscess
  Subphrenic peritonitis (acute)
  Suppurative peritonitis (acute)
  Use additional code (B95-B97), to identify infectious agent

K65.8 Other peritonitis
  Chronic proliferative peritonitis
  Mesenteric fat necrosis
  Mesenteric saponification
  Peritonitis due to bile
  Peritonitis due to urine

K65.9 Peritonitis, unspecified

K66 Other disorders of peritoneum
  Excludes2:   ascites (R18)

K66.0 Peritoneal adhesions (postoperative) (postinfection)
  Adhesions (of) abdominal (wall)
  Adhesions (of) diaphragm
  Adhesions (of) intestine
  Adhesions (of) male pelvis
  Adhesions (of) omentum
  Adhesions (of) stomach
  Adhesive bands
  Mesenteric adhesions
    Excludes1:   female pelvic adhesions [bands] (N73.6)
              peritoneal adhesions with intestinal obstruction (K56.5)

K66.1 Hemoperitoneum
    Excludes1:   traumatic hemoperitoneum (S36.8-)

K66.8 Other specified disorders of peritoneum

K66.9 Disorder of peritoneum, unspecified

K67 Disorders of peritoneum in infectious diseases classified elsewhere
  Code first underlying disease, such as :
    congenital syphilis (A50.0)
    helminthiasis (B65.0 - B83.9)
  Excludes1:   peritonitis in chlamydia (A74.81)
            peritonitis in diphtheria (A36.89)
            peritonitis in gonococcal (A54.85)
            peritonitis in syphilis (late) (A52.74)
            peritonitis in tuberculosis (A18.31)

K68 Disorders of retroperitoneum

K68.1 Retroperitoneal abscess

K68.11   Postprocedural retroperitoneal abscess

K68.19   Other retroperitoneal abscess

K68.9 Other disorders of retroperitoneum

DISEASES OF LIVER (K70–K77)

  Excludes1:   jaundice NOS (R17)
  Excludes2:   hemochromatosis (E83.1)
            Reye's syndrome (G93.7)
            viral hepatitis (B15-B19)
            Wilson's disease (E83.0)

K70 Alcoholic liver disease
  Use additional code to identify:
    alcohol abuse and dependence (F10.-)
    alcohol use, uncomplicated (Z72.1)
    alcohol dependence, in remission (F10.11)

K70.0 Alcoholic fatty liver

K70.1 Alcoholic hepatitis

K70.10   Alcoholic hepatitis without ascites

K70.11   Alcoholic hepatitis with ascites

K70.2 Alcoholic fibrosis and sclerosis of liver

K70.3 Alcoholic cirrhosis of liver
  Alcoholic cirrhosis NOS

K70.30   Alcoholic cirrhosis of liver without ascites

K70.31   Alcoholic cirrhosis of liver with ascites

K70.4 Alcoholic hepatic failure
  Acute alcoholic hepatic failure
  Alcoholic hepatic failure NOS
  Chronic alcoholic hepatic failure
  Subacute alcoholic hepatic failure

K70.40   Alcoholic hepatic failure without coma

K70.41   Alcoholic hepatic failure with coma

K70.9 Alcoholic liver disease, unspecified

K71 Toxic liver disease
  Includes: drug-induced idiosyncratic (unpredictable) liver disease
            drug-induced toxic (predictable) liver disease
  Use additional external cause code (Chapter XIX, XX) to identify toxic agent
  Excludes2:   alcoholic liver disease (K70.-)
            Budd-Chiari syndrome (I82.0)

K71.0 Toxic liver disease with cholestasis
  Cholestasis with hepatocyte injury
  "Pure" cholestasis

K71.1 Toxic liver disease with hepatic necrosis
  Hepatic failure (acute) (chronic) due to drugs

K71.10   Toxic liver disease with hepatic necrosis, without coma

K71.11   Toxic liver disease with hepatic necrosis, with coma

K71.2 Toxic liver disease with acute hepatitis

K71.3 Toxic liver disease with chronic persistent hepatitis

K71.4 Toxic liver disease with chronic lobular hepatitis

K71.5 Toxic liver disease with chronic active hepatitis
  Toxic liver disease with lupoid hepatitis

K71.50   Toxic liver disease with chronic active hepatitis without ascites

K71.51   Toxic liver disease with chronic active hepatitis with ascites

K71.6 Toxic liver disease with hepatitis, not elsewhere classified

K71.7 Toxic liver disease with fibrosis and cirrhosis of liver

K71.8 Toxic liver disease with other disorders of liver
  Toxic liver disease with focal nodular hyperplasia
  Toxic liver disease with hepatic granulomas
  Toxic liver disease with peliosis hepatis
  Toxic liver disease with veno-occlusive disease of liver

K71.9 Toxic liver disease, unspecified

K72 Hepatic failure, not elsewhere classified
  Includes: acute hepatitis NEC, with hepatic failure
            fulminant hepatitis NEC, with hepatic failure
            hepatic encephalopathy NOS
            liver (cell) necrosis with hepatic failure
            malignant hepatitis NEC, with hepatic failure
            yellow liver atrophy or dystrophy
  Excludes1:   alcoholic hepatic failure (K70.4)
            hepatic failure complicating abortion or ectopic or molar pregnancy (O00-O07,O08.8)
            hepatic failure complicating pregnancy, childbirth and the puerperium (O26.6)
            hepatic failure with toxic liver disease (K71.1-)
            icterus of fetus and newborn (P55-P59)
            postoperative hepatic failure (K91.81)
            viral hepatitis (B15-B19)

K72.0 Acute and subacute hepatic failure

K72.00   Acute and subacute hepatic failure without coma

K72.01   Acute and subacute hepatic failure with coma

K72.1 Chronic hepatic failure

K72.10   Chronic hepatic failure without coma

K72.11   Chronic hepatic failure with coma

K72.9 Hepatic failure, unspecified

K72.90   Hepatic failure, unspecified without coma

K72.91   Hepatic failure, unspecified with coma
  Hepatic coma NOS

K73 Chronic hepatitis, not elsewhere classified

    Excludes1:   alcoholic hepatitis (chronic) (K70.1-)
                drug-induced hepatitis (chronic) (K71.-)
                granulomatous hepatitis (chronic) NEC (K75.3)
                reactive, nonspecific hepatitis (chronic) (K75.2)
                viral hepatitis (chronic) (B15-B19)

K73.0 Chronic persistent hepatitis, not elsewhere classified

K73.1 Chronic lobular hepatitis, not elsewhere classified

K73.2 Chronic active hepatitis, not elsewhere classified
        Lupoid hepatitis NEC

K73.8 Other chronic hepatitis, not elsewhere classified

K73.9 Chronic hepatitis, unspecified

K74 Fibrosis and cirrhosis of liver

    Excludes1:   alcoholic cirrhosis (of liver) (K70.3)
                alcoholic fibrosis of liver (K70.2)
                cardiac sclerosis of liver (K76.1)
                cirrhosis (of liver) with toxic liver disease (K71.7)
                congenital cirrhosis (of liver) (P78.8)

K74.0 Hepatic fibrosis

K74.1 Hepatic sclerosis

K74.2 Hepatic fibrosis with hepatic sclerosis

K74.3 Primary biliary cirrhosis
        Chronic nonsuppurative destructive cholangitis

K74.4 Secondary biliary cirrhosis

K74.5 Biliary cirrhosis, unspecified

K74.6 Other and unspecified cirrhosis of liver
        Cirrhosis (of liver) NOS
        Cryptogenic cirrhosis (of liver)
        Macronodular cirrhosis (of liver)
        Micronodular cirrhosis (of liver)
        Mixed type cirrhosis (of liver)
        Portal cirrhosis (of liver)
        Postnecrotic cirrhosis (of liver)

K75 Other inflammatory liver diseases

    Excludes2:   toxic liver disease (K71.-)

K75.0 Abscess of liver
        Cholangitic hepatic abscess
        Hematogenic hepatic abscess
        Hepatic abscess NOS
        Lymphogenic hepatic abscess
        Pylephlebitic hepatic abscess
        Excludes1:   amebic liver abscess (A06.4)
                    cholangitis without liver abscess (K83.0)
                    pylephlebitis without liver abscess (K75.1)

K75.1 Phlebitis of portal vein
        Pylephlebitis
        Excludes1:   pylephlebitic liver abscess (K75.0)

K75.2 Nonspecific reactive hepatitis
        Excludes1:   acute or subacute hepatitis (K72.0-)
                    chronic hepatitis NEC (K73.-)
                    viral hepatitis (B15-B19)

K75.3 Granulomatous hepatitis, not elsewhere classified
        Excludes1:   acute or subacute hepatitis (K72.0-)
                    chronic hepatitis NEC (K73.-)
                    viral hepatitis (B15-B19)

K75.8 Other specified inflammatory liver diseases

K75.9 Inflammatory liver disease, unspecified
        Hepatitis NOS
        Excludes1:   acute or subacute hepatitis (K72.0-)
                    chronic hepatitis NEC (K73.-)
                    viral hepatitis (B15-B19)

K76 Other diseases of liver

    Excludes2:   alcoholic liver disease (K70.-)
                amyloid degeneration of liver (E85)
                cystic disease of liver (congenital) (Q44.6)
                hepatic vein thrombosis (I82.0)
                hepatomegaly NOS (R16.0)
                portal vein thrombosis (I81)
                toxic liver disease (K71.-)

K76.0 Fatty (change of) liver, not elsewhere classified

K76.1 Chronic passive congestion of liver
        Cardiac cirrhosis
        Cardiac sclerosis

K76.2 Central hemorrhagic necrosis of liver
        Excludes1:   liver necrosis with hepatic failure (K72.-)

K76.3 Infarction of liver

K76.4 Peliosis hepatis
        Hepatic angiomatosis

K76.5 Hepatic veno-occlusive disease
        Excludes1:   Budd-Chiari syndrome (I82.0)

K76.6 Portal hypertension

K76.7 Hepatorenal syndrome
        Excludes1:   hepatorenal syndrome following labor and
                          delivery (O90.4)
                    postoperative hepatorenal syndrome (K91.82)

K76.8 Other specified diseases of liver
        Focal nodular hyperplasia of liver
        Hepatoptosis

K76.9 Liver disease, unspecified

K77 Liver disorders in diseases classified elsewhere
    Code first underlying disease, such as:
        amyloidosis (E85)
        congenital syphilis (A50.0, A50.5)
        congenital toxoplasmosis (P37.1)
        schistosomiasis (B65.0-B65.9)
    Excludes1:   alcoholic hepatitis (K70.1-)
                alcoholic liver disease (K70.-)
                cytomegaloviral hepatitis (B25.1)
                herpesviral [herpes simplex] hepatitis (B00.81)
                infectious mononucleosis with liver disease (B27.0-
                    B27.9 with .9)
                mumps hepatitis (B26.81)
                sarcoidosis with liver disease (D86.89)
                secondary syphilis with liver disease (A51.45)
                syphilis (late) with liver disease (A52.74)
                toxoplasmosis (acquired) hepatitis (B58.1)
                tuberculosis with liver disease (A18.83)

DISORDERS OF GALLBLADDER, BILIARY TRACT AND PANCREAS (K80–K87)

K80 Cholelithiasis

K80.0 Calculus of gallbladder with acute cholecystitis
        Any condition listed in K80.2 with acute cholecystitis

    K80.00 Calculus of gallbladder with acute cholecystitis without obstruction

    K80.01 Calculus of gallbladder with acute cholecystitis with obstruction

K80.1 Calculus of gallbladder with other cholecystitis

    K80.10 Calculus of gallbladder with chronic cholecystitis without obstruction
             Cholelithiasis with cholecystitis NOS

    K80.11 Calculus of gallbladder with chronic cholecystitis with obstruction

    K80.12 Calculus of gallbladder with acute and chronic cholecystitis without obstruction

    K80.13 Calculus of gallbladder with acute and chronic cholecystitis with obstruction

    K80.18 Calculus of gallbladder with other cholecystitis without obstruction

    K80.19 Calculus of gallbladder with other cholecystitis with obstruction

K80.2 Calculus of gallbladder without cholecystitis
        Cholecystolithiasis without cholecystitis
        Cholelithiasis (without cholecystitis)
        Colic (recurrent) of gallbladder (without cholecystitis)
        Gallstone (impacted) of cystic duct (without cholecystitis)
        Gallstone (impacted) of gallbladder (without cholecystitis)

    K80.20 Calculus of gallbladder without cholecystitis without obstruction

    K80.21 Calculus of gallbladder without cholecystitis with obstruction

K80.3 Calculus of bile duct with cholangitis
Any condition listed in K80.5 with cholangitis
K80.30 Calculus of bile duct with cholangitis, unspecified, without obstruction
K80.31 Calculus of bile duct with cholangitis, unspecified, with obstruction
K80.32 Calculus of bile duct with acute cholangitis without obstruction
K80.33 Calculus of bile duct with acute cholangitis with obstruction
K80.34 Calculus of bile duct with chronic cholangitis without obstruction
K80.35 Calculus of bile duct with chronic cholangitis with obstruction
K80.36 Calculus of bile duct with acute and chronic cholangitis without obstruction
K80.37 Calculus of bile duct with acute and chronic cholangitis with obstruction

K80.4 Calculus of bile duct with cholecystitis
Any condition listed in K80.5 with cholecystitis (with cholangitis)
K80.40 Calculus of bile duct with cholecystitis, unspecified, without obstruction
K80.41 Calculus of bile duct with cholecystitis, unspecified, with obstruction
K80.42 Calculus of bile duct with acute cholecystitis without obstruction
K80.43 Calculus of bile duct with acute cholecystitis with obstruction
K80.44 Calculus of bile duct with chronic cholecystitis without obstruction
K80.45 Calculus of bile duct with chronic cholecystitis with obstruction
K80.46 Calculus of bile duct with acute and chronic cholecystitis without obstruction
K80.47 Calculus of bile duct with acute and chronic cholecystitis with obstruction

K80.5 Calculus of bile duct without cholangitis or cholecystitis
Choledocholithiasis (without cholangitis or cholecystitis)
Gallstone (impacted) of bile duct NOS (without cholangitis or cholecystitis)
Gallstone (impacted) of common duct (without cholangitis or cholecystitis)
Gallstone (impacted) of hepatic duct (without cholangitis or cholecystitis)
Hepatic cholelithiasis (without cholangitis or cholecystitis)
Hepatic colic (recurrent) (without cholangitis or cholecystitis)
K80.50 Calculus of bile duct without cholangitis or cholecystitis without obstruction
K80.51 Calculus of bile duct without cholangitis or cholecystitis with obstruction

K80.6 Calculus of gallbladder and bile duct with cholecystitis
K80.60 Calculus of gallbladder and bile duct with cholecystitis, unspecified, without obstruction
K80.61 Calculus of gallbladder and bile duct with cholecystitis, unspecified, with obstruction
K80.62 Calculus of gallbladder and bile duct with acute cholecystitis without obstruction
K80.63 Calculus of gallbladder and bile duct with acute cholecystitis with obstruction
K80.64 Calculus of gallbladder and bile duct with chronic cholecystitis without obstruction
K80.65 Calculus of gallbladder and bile duct with chronic cholecystitis with obstruction
K80.66 Calculus of gallbladder and bile duct with acute and chronic cholecystitis without obstruction
K80.67 Calculus of gallbladder and bile duct with acute and chronic cholecystitis with obstruction

K80.7 Calculus of gallbladder and bile duct without cholecystitis
K80.70 Calculus of gallbladder and bile duct without cholecystitis without obstruction
K80.71 Calculus of gallbladder and bile duct without cholecystitis with obstruction

K80.8 Other cholelithiasis
K80.80 Other cholelithiasis without obstruction
K80.81 Other cholelithiasis with obstruction

K81 Cholecystitis
Excludes1: cholecystitis with cholelithiasis (K80.-)
K81.0 Acute cholecystitis
Abscess of gallbladder
Angiocholecystitis
Emphysematous (acute) cholecystitis
Empyema of gallbladder
Gangrene of gallbladder
Gangrenous cholecystitis
Suppurative cholecystitis
K81.1 Chronic cholecystitis
K81.2 Acute cholecystitis with chronic cholecystitis
K81.9 Cholecystitis, unspecified

K82 Other diseases of gallbladder
Excludes1: nonvisualization of gallbladder (R93.2)
postcholecystectomy syndrome (K91.5)
K82.0 Obstruction of gallbladder
Occlusion of cystic duct or gallbladder without cholelithiasis
Stenosis of cystic duct or gallbladder without cholelithiasis
Stricture of cystic duct or gallbladder without cholelithiasis
Excludes1: obstruction of gallbladder with cholelithiasis (K80.-)
K82.1 Hydrops of gallbladder
Mucocele of gallbladder
K82.2 Perforation of gallbladder
Rupture of cystic duct or gallbladder
K82.3 Fistula of gallbladder
Cholecystocolic fistula
Cholecystoduodenal fistula
K82.4 Cholesterolosis of gallbladder
Strawberry gallbladder
Excludes1: cholesterolosis of gallbladder with cholecystitis (K81.-)
cholesterolosis of gallbladder with cholelithiasis (K80.-)
K82.8 Other specified diseases of gallbladder
Adhesions of cystic duct or gallbladder
Atrophy of cystic duct or gallbladder
Cyst of cystic duct or gallbladder
Dyskinesia of cystic duct or gallbladder
Hypertrophy of cystic duct or gallbladder
Nonfunctioning of cystic duct or gallbladder
Ulcer of cystic duct or gallbladder
K82.9 Disease of gallbladder, unspecified

K83 Other diseases of biliary tract
Excludes1: postcholecystectomy syndrome (K91.5)
Excludes2: conditions involving the cystic duct (K81-K82)
conditions involving the gallbladder (K81-K82)
K83.0 Cholangitis
Ascending cholangitis
Cholangitis NOS
Primary cholangitis
Recurrent cholangitis
Sclerosing cholangitis
Secondary cholangitis
Stenosing cholangitis
Suppurative cholangitis
Excludes1: cholangitic liver abscess (K75.0)
cholangitis with choledocholithiasis (K80.3-, K80.4-)
chronic nonsuppurative destructive cholangitis (K74.3)
K83.1 Obstruction of bile duct
Occlusion of bile duct without cholelithiasis
Stenosis of bile duct without cholelithiasis
Stricture of bile duct without cholelithiasis
Excludes1: congenital obstruction of bile duct (Q44.3)
obstruction of bile duct with cholelithiasis (K80.-)

K83.2 Perforation of bile duct
Rupture of bile duct

K83.3 Fistula of bile duct
Choledochoduodenal fistula

K83.4 Spasm of sphincter of Oddi

K83.5 Biliary cyst

K83.8 Other specified diseases of biliary tract
Adhesions of biliary tract
Atrophy of biliary tract
Hypertrophy of biliary tract
Ulcer of biliary tract

K83.9 Disease of biliary tract, unspecified

K85 Acute pancreatitis

K85.0 Abscess of pancreas
Suppurative pancreatitis

K85.8 Other acute pancreatitis
Acute necrosis of pancreas
Acute (recurrent) pancreatitis
Hemorrhagic pancreatitis
Infective necrosis of pancreas
Pancreatitis NOS
Subacute pancreatitis

K86 Other diseases of pancreas
Excludes2:   fibrocystic disease of pancreas (E84.-)
islet cell tumor (of pancreas) (D13.7)
pancreatic steatorrhea (K90.3)

K86.0 Alcohol-induced chronic pancreatitis
Use additional code to identify:
alcohol abuse and dependence (F10.-)
alcohol use, uncomplicated (Z72.1)
alcohol dependence, in remission (F10.11)
external cause (Chapter XIX), if drug-induced

K86.1 Other chronic pancreatitis
Chronic pancreatitis NOS
Infectious chronic pancreatitis
Recurrent chronic pancreatitis
Relapsing chronic pancreatitis

K86.2 Cyst of pancreas

K86.3 Pseudocyst of pancreas

K86.8 Other specified diseases of pancreas
Aseptic pancreatic necrosis
Atrophy of pancreas
Calculus of pancreas
Cirrhosis of pancreas
Fibrosis of pancreas
Pancreatic fat necrosis
Pancreatic infantilism
Pancreatic necrosis NOS

K86.9 Disease of pancreas, unspecified

K87 Disorders of gallbladder, biliary tract and pancreas in diseases classified elsewhere
Code first underlying disease
Excludes1:   cytomegaloviral pancreatitis(B25.2)
mumps pancreatitis (B26.3)
syphilitic gallbladder (A52.74)
syphilitic pancreas (A52.74)
tuberculosis of gallbladder (A18.83)
tuberculosis of pancreas (A18.83)

OTHER DISEASES OF THE DIGESTIVE SYSTEM (K90–K94)

K90 Intestinal malabsorption
Excludes1:   intestinal malabsorption following gastrointestinal surgery (K91.2)

K90.0 Celiac disease
Gluten-sensitive enteropathy
Idiopathic steatorrhea
Nontropical sprue

K90.1 Tropical sprue
Sprue NOS
Tropical steatorrhea

K90.2 Blind loop syndrome, not elsewhere classified
Blind loop syndrome NOS
Excludes1:   congenital blind loop syndrome (Q43.8)
postsurgical blind loop syndrome (K91.2)

K90.3 Pancreatic steatorrhea

K90.4 Malabsorption due to intolerance, not elsewhere classified
Malabsorption due to intolerance to carbohydrate
Malabsorption due to intolerance to fat
Malabsorption due to intolerance to protein
Malabsorption due to intolerance to starch
Excludes2:   gluten-sensitive enteropathy (K90.0)
lactose intolerance (E73.-)

K90.8 Other intestinal malabsorption

K90.81   Whipple's disease

K90.89   Other intestinal malabsorption

K90.9 Intestinal malabsorption, unspecified

K91 Intraoperative and postprocedural complications and disorders of digestive system, not elsewhere classified
Excludes2:   complications of artificial opening of digestive system (K94.-)
gastrojejunal ulcer (K28.-)
postprocedural (radiation) retroperitoneal abscess (K68.11)
radiation colitis (K52.0)
radiation gastroenteritis (K52.0)
radiation proctitis (K62.7)

K91.0 Vomiting following gastrointestinal surgery

K91.1 Postgastric surgery syndromes
Dumping syndrome
Postgastrectomy syndrome
Postvagotomy syndrome

K91.2 Postsurgical malabsorption, not elsewhere classified
Postsurgical blind loop syndrome
Excludes1:   malabsorption osteomalacia in adults (M83.2)
malabsorption osteoporosis, postsurgical (M81.3)

K91.3 Postoperative intestinal obstruction

K91.5 Postcholecystectomy syndrome

K91.6 Intraoperative and postprocedural hemorrhage and hematoma complicating a digestive system procedure
Excludes1:   intraoperative hemorrhage or hematoma due to accidental puncture or laceration during a digestive system procedure (K91.7-)

K91.61   Intraoperative hemorrhage of a digestive system organ or structure during a digestive system procedure

K91.62   Intraoperative hemorrhage of a non-digestive system organ or structure during a digestive system procedure

K91.63   Intraoperative hematoma of a digestive system organ or structure during a digestive system procedure

K91.64   Intraoperative hematoma of a non-digestive system organ or structure during a digestive system procedure

K91.65   Postprocedural hemorrhage of a digestive system organ or structure following a digestive system procedure

K91.66   Postprocedural hemorrhage of a non-digestive system organ or structure following a digestive system procedure

K91.67   Postprocedural hematoma of a digestive system organ or structure following a digestive system procedure

K91.68   Postprocedural hematoma of a non-digestive system organ or structure following a digestive system procedure

K91.7 Accidental puncture or laceration during a digestive system procedure

K91.71   Accidental puncture or laceration of a digestive system organ or structure during a digestive system procedure

K91.72   Accidental puncture or laceration of a non-digestive system organ or structure during a digestive system procedure

K91.8 Other postprocedural disorders of digestive system, not elsewhere classified

    K91.81 Postprocedural hepatic failure

    K91.82 Postprocedural hepatorenal syndrome

    K91.89 Other postprocedural disorders of digestive system, not elsewhere classified

K91.9 Postprocedural disorder of digestive system, unspecified

K92 Other diseases of digestive system

    Excludes1:   neonatal gastrointestinal hemorrhage (P54.0-P54.3)

K92.0 Hematemesis

K92.1 Melena

K92.2 Gastrointestinal hemorrhage, unspecified

    Gastric hemorrhage NOS

    Intestinal hemorrhage NOS

    Excludes1:   acute hemorrhagic gastritis (K29.01)

        angiodysplasia of stomach with hemorrhage (K31.82)

        diverticular disease with hemorrhage (K57.-)

        gastritis and duodenitis with hemorrhage (K29.-)

        hemorrhage of anus and rectum (K62.5)

        peptic ulcer with hemorrhage (K25-K28)

K92.8 Other specified diseases of the digestive system

K92.9 Disease of digestive system, unspecified

K93 Disorders of other digestive organs in diseases classified elsewhere

    Code first underlying disease, such as:

        amyloidosis (E85)

        deficiency (of):

            niacin (E52)

            riboflavin (E53.0)

            vitamin B group NEC (E53.8)

            vitamin C (E54)

    Excludes1:   gastrointestinal disorders in herpes (B00.89)

        gastrointestinal disorders in measles (B05.4)

        gastrointestinal disorders in syphilis (A52.74)

        gastrointestinal disorders in tuberculosis (A18.32-A18.39)

        megacolon in Chagas' disease (B57.32)

K94 Complications of artificial openings of the digestive system

K94.0 Colostomy complications

    K94.00 Colostomy complication, unspecified

    K94.01 Colostomy hemorrhage

    K94.02 Colostomy infection

        Use additional code to specify type of infection, such as:

            cellulitis of abdominal wall (L03.32)

            septicemia (A40.-, A41.-)

    K94.03 Colostomy malfunction

        Mechanical complication of colostomy

    K94.09 Other complications of colostomy

K94.1 Enterostomy complications

    K94.10 Enterostomy complication, unspecified

    K94.11 Enterostomy hemorrhage

    K94.12 Enterostomy infection

        Use additional code to specify type of infection, such as:

            cellulitis of abdominal wall (L03.32)

            septicemia (A40.-, A41.-)

    K94.13 Enterostomy malfunction

        Mechanical complication of enterostomy

    K94.19 Other complications of enterostomy

K94.2 Gastrostomy complications

    K94.20 Gastrostomy complication, unspecified

    K94.21 Gastrostomy hemorrhage

    K94.22 Gastrostomy infection

        Use additional code to specify type of infection, such as:

            cellulitis of abdominal wall (L03.32)

            septicemia (A40.-, A41.-)

    K94.23 Gastrostomy malfunction

        Mechanical complication of gastrostomy

    K94.29 Other complications of gastrostomy

CHAPTER XII — DISEASES OF THE SKIN AND SUBCUTANEOUS TISSUE (L00–L99)

Excludes2:   certain conditions originating in the perinatal period (P04-P96)
certain infectious and parasitic diseases (A00-B99)
complications of pregnancy, childbirth and the puerperium (O00-O99)
congenital malformations, deformations, and chromosomal abnormalities (Q00-Q99)
endocrine, nutritional and metabolic diseases (E00-E90)
lipomelanotic reticulosis (I89.8)
neoplasms (C00-D48)
symptoms, signs and abnormal clinical and laboratory findings, not elsewhere classified (R00-R94)
systemic connective tissue disorders (M30-M36)

This chapter contains the following blocks:

L00-L08   Infections of the skin and subcutaneous tissue
L10-L14   Bullous disorders
L20-L30   Dermatitis and eczema
L40-L45   Papulosquamous disorders
L50-L54   Urticaria and erythema
L55-L59   Radiation-related disorders of the skin and subcutaneous tissue
L60-L75   Disorders of skin appendages
L76   Intraoperative and postprocedural complications of dermatologic procedures
L80-L99   Other disorders of the skin and subcutaneous tissue

INFECTIONS OF THE SKIN AND SUBCUTANEOUS TISSUE (L00–L08)

Use additional code (B95-B97) to identify infectious agent.

Excludes2:   hordeolum (H00.0)
infective dermatitis (L30.3)
local infections of skin classified in Chapter I
lupus panniculitis (L93.2)
panniculitis NOS (M79.3)
panniculitis of neck and back (M54.0-)
perlèche NOS (K13.0)
perlèche due to candidiasis (B37.0)
perlèche due to riboflavin deficiency (E53.0)
pyogenic granuloma (L98.0)
relapsing panniculitis [Weber-Christian] (M35.6)
zoster (B02.-)

L00   Staphylococcal scalded skin syndrome
Ritter's disease
Excludes1:   bullous impetigo (L01.03)
pemphigus neonatorum (L01.03)
toxic epidermal necrolysis [Lyell] (L51.2)

L01   Impetigo
Excludes1:   impetigo herpetiformis (L40.1)
L01.0   Impetigo
Impetigo contagiosa
Impetigo vulgaris
L01.00   Impetigo, unspecified
Impetigo NOS
L01.01   Non-bullous impetigo
L01.02   Bockhart's impetigo
Impetigo follicularis
Perifolliculitis NOS
Superficial pustular perifolliculitis
L01.03   Bullous impetigo
Impetigo neonatorum
Pemphigus neonatorum
L01.09   Other impetigo
Ulcerative impetigo
L01.1   Impetiginization of other dermatoses

L02   Cutaneous abscess, furuncle and carbuncle
Use additional code to identify organism (B95-B96)
Excludes2:   abscess of anus and rectal regions (K61.-)
abscess of female genital organs (external) (N76.4)
abscess of male genital organs (external) (N48.2, N49.-)
L02.0   Cutaneous abscess, furuncle and carbuncle of face
Excludes1:   abscess of ear, external (H60.0)
abscess of eyelid (H00.0)
abscess of head [any part, except face] (L02.8)
abscess of lacrimal gland (H04.0)
abscess of lacrimal passages (H04.3)
abscess of mouth (K12.2)
abscess of nose (J34.0)
abscess of orbit (H05.0)
submandibular abscess (K12.2)
L02.01   Cutaneous abscess of face
Skin sepsis of face
L02.02   Furuncle of face
Boil of face
Folliculitis of face
L02.03   Carbuncle of face
L02.1   Cutaneous abscess, furuncle and carbuncle of neck
L02.11   Cutaneous abscess of neck
Skin sepsis of neck
L02.12   Furuncle of neck
Boil of neck
Folliculitis of neck
L02.13   Carbuncle of neck
L02.2   Cutaneous abscess, furuncle and carbuncle of trunk
Excludes1:   non-newborn omphalitis (L08.82)
omphalitis of newborn (P38)
Excludes2:   abscess of breast (N61)
abscess of buttocks (L02.3)
abscess of female external genital organs (N76.4)
abscess of male external genital organs (N48.2, N49.-)
abscess of hip (L02.4)
L02.21   Cutaneous abscess of trunk
Skin sepsis of trunk
L02.211   Cutaneous abscess of abdominal wall
L02.212   Cutaneous abscess of back [any part, except buttock]
L02.213   Cutaneous abscess of chest wall
L02.214   Cutaneous abscess of groin
L02.215   Cutaneous abscess of perineum
L02.216   Cutaneous abscess of umbilicus
L02.219   Cutaneous abscess of trunk, unspecified
L02.22   Furuncle of trunk
Boil of trunk
Folliculitis of trunk
L02.221   Furuncle of abdominal wall
L02.222   Furuncle of back [any part, except buttock]
L02.223   Furuncle of chest wall
L02.224   Furuncle of groin
L02.225   Furuncle of perineum
L02.226   Furuncle of umbilicus
L02.229   Furuncle of trunk, unspecified
L02.23   Carbuncle of trunk
L02.231   Carbuncle of abdominal wall
L02.232   Carbuncle of back [any part, except buttock]
L02.233   Carbuncle of chest wall
L02.234   Carbuncle of groin
L02.235   Carbuncle of perineum
L02.236   Carbuncle of umbilicus
L02.239   Carbuncle of trunk, unspecified
L02.3   Cutaneous abscess, furuncle and carbuncle of buttock
Excludes1:   pilonidal cyst with abscess (L05.01)
L02.31   Cutaneous abscess of buttock
Cutaneous abscess of gluteal region
Skin sepsis of buttock

L02.32　Furuncle of buttock
　　　Boil of buttock
　　　Folliculitis of buttock
　　　Furuncle of gluteal region
L02.33　Carbuncle of buttock
　　　Carbuncle of gluteal region
L02.4　Cutaneous abscess, furuncle and carbuncle of limb
　　Excludes2:　cutaneous abscess, furuncle and carbuncle of foot (L02.6-)
　　　　　cutaneous abscess, furuncle and carbuncle of groin (L02.214, L02.224, L02.234)
　　　　　cutaneous abscess, furuncle and carbuncle of hand (L02.5-)
L02.41　Cutaneous abscess of limb
　　　Skin sepsis of limb
　　L02.411　Cutaneous abscess of right axilla
　　L02.412　Cutaneous abscess of left axilla
　　L02.413　Cutaneous abscess of right upper limb
　　L02.414　Cutaneous abscess of left upper limb
　　L02.415　Cutaneous abscess of right lower limb
　　L02.416　Cutaneous abscess of left lower limb
　　L02.419　Cutaneous abscess of limb, unspecified
L02.42　Furuncle of limb
　　　Boil of limb
　　　Folliculitis of limb
　　L02.421　Furuncle of right axilla
　　L02.422　Furuncle of left axilla
　　L02.423　Furuncle of right upper limb
　　L02.424　Furuncle of left upper limb
　　L02.425　Furuncle of right lower limb
　　L02.426　Furuncle of left lower limb
　　L02.429　Furuncle of limb, unspecified
L02.43　Carbuncle of limb
　　L02.431　Carbuncle of right axilla
　　L02.432　Carbuncle of left axilla
　　L02.433　Carbuncle of right upper limb
　　L02.434　Carbuncle of left upper limb
　　L02.435　Carbuncle of right lower limb
　　L02.436　Carbuncle of left lower limb
　　L02.439　Carbuncle of limb, unspecified
L02.5　Cutaneous abscess, furuncle and carbuncle of hand
L02.51　Cutaneous abscess of hand
　　　Skin sepsis of hand
　　L02.511　Cutaneous abscess of right hand
　　L02.512　Cutaneous abscess of left hand
　　L02.519　Cutaneous abscess of unspecified hand
L02.52　Furuncle hand
　　　Boil of hand
　　　Folliculitis of hand
　　L02.521　Furuncle right hand
　　L02.522　Furuncle left hand
　　L02.529　Furuncle unspecified hand
L02.53　Carbuncle of hand
　　L02.531　Carbuncle of right hand
　　L02.532　Carbuncle of left hand
　　L02.539　Carbuncle of unspecified hand
L02.6　Cutaneous abscess, furuncle and carbuncle of foot
L02.61　Cutaneous abscess of foot
　　　Skin sepsis of foot
　　L02.611　Cutaneous abscess of right foot
　　L02.612　Cutaneous abscess of left foot
　　L02.619　Cutaneous abscess of unspecified foot
L02.62　Furuncle of foot
　　　Boil of foot
　　　Folliculitis of foot
　　L02.621　Furuncle of right foot
　　L02.622　Furuncle of left foot
　　L02.629　Furuncle of unspecified foot

L02.63　Carbuncle of foot
　　L02.631　Carbuncle of right foot
　　L02.632　Carbuncle of left foot
　　L02.639　Carbuncle of unspecified foot
L02.8　Cutaneous abscess, furuncle and carbuncle of other sites
L02.81　Cutaneous abscess of other sites
　　　Skin sepsis of other sites
　　L02.811　Cutaneous abscess of head [any part, except face]
　　L02.818　Cutaneous abscess of other sites
L02.82　Furuncle of other sites
　　　Boil of other sites
　　　Folliculitis of other sites
　　L02.821　Furuncle of head [any part, except face]
　　L02.828　Furuncle of other sites
L02.83　Carbuncle of other sites
　　L02.831　Carbuncle of head [any part, except face]
　　L02.838　Carbuncle of other sites
L02.9　Cutaneous abscess, furuncle and carbuncle, unspecified
L02.91　Cutaneous abscess, unspecified
　　　Skin sepsis NOS
L02.92　Furuncle, unspecified
　　　Boil NOS
　　　Furunculosis NOS
L02.93　Carbuncle, unspecified

L03　Cellulitis and acute lymphangitis
　　Excludes2:　cellulitis of anal and rectal region (K61.-)
　　　　　cellulitis of external auditory canal (H60.1)
　　　　　cellulitis of eyelid (H00.0)
　　　　　cellulitis of female external genital organs (N76.4)
　　　　　cellulitis of lacrimal apparatus (H04.3)
　　　　　cellulitis of male external genital organs (N48.2, N49.-)
　　　　　cellulitis of mouth (K12.2)
　　　　　cellulitis of nose (J34.0)
　　　　　eosinophilic cellulitis [Wells] (L98.3)
　　　　　febrile neutrophilic dermatosis [Sweet] (L98.2)
　　　　　lymphangitis (chronic) (subacute) (I89.1)
L03.0　Cellulitis and acute lymphangitis of finger and toe
　　　Infection of nail
　　　Onychia
　　　Paronychia
　　　Perionychia
L03.01　Cellulitis of finger
　　　Felon
　　　Whitlow
　　　Excludes1:　herpetic whitlow (B00.89)
　　L03.011　Cellulitis of right finger
　　L03.012　Cellulitis of left finger
　　L03.019　Cellulitis of unspecified finger
L03.02　Acute lymphangitis of finger
　　　Hangnail with lymphangitis of finger
　　L03.021　Acute lymphangitis of right finger
　　L03.022　Acute lymphangitis of left finger
　　L03.029　Acute lymphangitis of unspecified finger
L03.03　Cellulitis of toe
　　L03.031　Cellulitis of right toe
　　L03.032　Cellulitis of left toe
　　L03.039　Cellulitis of unspecified toe
L03.04　Acute lymphangitis of toe
　　　Hangnail with lymphangitis of toe
　　L03.041　Acute lymphangitis of right toe
　　L03.042　Acute lymphangitis of left toe
　　L03.049　Acute lymphangitis of unspecified toe
L03.1　Cellulitis and acute lymphangitis of other parts of limb
L03.11　Cellulitis of other parts of limb
　　　Excludes2:　cellulitis of fingers (L03.01-)
　　　　　cellulitis of toes (L03.03-)
　　　　　cellulitis of groin (L03.314)
　　L03.111　Cellulitis of right axilla
　　L03.112　Cellulitis of left axilla
　　L03.113　Cellulitis of right upper limb

L03.114   Cellulitis of left upper limb
L03.115   Cellulitis of right lower limb
L03.116   Cellulitis of left lower limb
L06.119   Cellulitis of unspecified part of limb
L03.12   Acute lymphangitis of other parts of limb
         Excludes2:   acute lymphangitis of fingers (L03.2-)
                      acute lymphangitis of toes (L03.4-)
                      acute lymphangitis of groin (L03.324)
L03.121   Acute lymphangitis of right axilla
L03.122   Acute lymphangitis of left axilla
L03.123   Acute lymphangitis of right upper limb
L03.124   Acute lymphangitis of left upper limb
L03.125   Acute lymphangitis of right lower limb
L03.126   Acute lymphangitis of left lower limb
L03.129   Acute lymphangitis of unspecified part of limb
L03.2   Cellulitis and acute lymphangitis of face and neck
   L03.21   Cellulitis and acute lymphangitis of face
      L03.211   Cellulitis of face
               Excludes2:   cellulitis of ear (H60.1-)
                            cellulitis of eyelid (H00.0-)
                            cellulitis of head (L03.81)
                            cellulitis of lacrimal apparatus
                               (H04.3)
                            cellulitis of lip (K13.0)
                            cellulitis of mouth (K12.2)
                            cellulitis of nose (internal)
                               (J34.0)
                            cellulitis of orbit (H05.0)
                            cellulitis of scalp (L03.81)
      L03.212   Acute lymphangitis of face
   L03.22   Cellulitis and acute lymphangitis of neck
      L03.221   Cellulitis of neck
      L03.222   Acute lymphangitis of neck
L03.3   Cellulitis and acute lymphangitis of trunk
   L03.31   Cellulitis of trunk
            Excludes2:   cellulitis of anal and rectal regions (K61.-
)
                         cellulitis of breast NOS (N61)
                         cellulitis of female external genital organs
                            (N76.4)
                         cellulitis of male external genital organs
                            (N48.2, N49.-)
                         omphalitis of newborn (P38)
                         puerperal cellulitis of breast (O91.2)
      L03.311   Cellulitis of abdominal wall
               Excludes2:   cellulitis of umbilicus (L03.316)
                            cellulitis of groin (L03.314)
      L03.312   Cellulitis of back [any part except buttock]
      L03.313   Cellulitis of chest wall
      L03.314   Cellulitis of groin
      L03.315   Cellulitis of perineum
      L03.316   Cellulitis of umbilicus
      L03.317   Cellulitis of buttock
      L03.319   Cellulitis of trunk, unspecified
   L03.32   Acute lymphangitis of trunk
      L03.321   Acute lymphangitis of abdominal wall
      L03.322   Acute lymphangitis of back [any part except
                buttock]
      L03.323   Acute lymphangitis of chest wall
      L03.324   Acute lymphangitis of groin
      L03.325   Acute lymphangitis of perineum
      L03.326   Acute lymphangitis of umbilicus
      L03.327   Acute lymphangitis of buttock
      L03.329   Acute lymphangitis of trunk, unspecified
L03.8   Cellulitis and acute lymphangitis of other sites
   L03.81   Cellulitis of other sites
      L03.811   Cellulitis of head [any part, except face]
                Cellulitis of scalp
                Excludes2:   cellulitis of face (L03.211)

L03.818   Cellulitis of other sites
L03.89   Acute lymphangitis of other sites
   L03.891   Acute lymphangitis of head [any part, except
             face]
   L03.898   Acute lymphangitis of other sites
L03.9   Cellulitis and acute lymphangitis, unspecified
   L03.90   Cellulitis, unspecified
   L03.91   Acute lymphangitis, unspecified
            Excludes1:   lymphangitis NOS (I89.1)

L04   Acute lymphadenitis
      Includes: abscess (acute) of lymph nodes, except mesenteric
                   acute lymphadenitis, except mesenteric
      Excludes1:   chronic or subacute lymphadenitis, except mesenteric
                      (I88.1)
                   enlarged lymph nodes (R59.-)
                   human immunodeficiency virus [HIV] disease resulting
                      in generalized lymphadenopathy (B20)
                   lymphadenitis NOS (I88.9)
                   nonspecific mesenteric lymphadenitis (I88.0)
L04.0   Acute lymphadenitis of face, head and neck
L04.1   Acute lymphadenitis of trunk
L04.2   Acute lymphadenitis of upper limb
        Acute lymphadenitis of axilla
        Acute lymphadenitis of shoulder
L04.3   Acute lymphadenitis of lower limb
        Acute lymphadenitis of hip
        Excludes2:   acute lymphadenitis of groin (L04.1)
L04.8   Acute lymphadenitis of other sites
L04.9   Acute lymphadenitis, unspecified

L05   Pilonidal cyst and sinus
L05.0   Pilonidal cyst and sinus with abscess
   L05.01   Pilonidal cyst with abscess
            Parasacral dimple with abscess
            Pilonidal abscess
            Pilonidal dimple with abscess
            Postanal dimple with abscess
   L05.02   Pilonidal sinus with abscess
            Coccygeal fistula with abscess
            Coccygeal sinus with abscess
            Pilonidal fistula with abscess
L05.9   Pilonidal cyst and sinus without abscess
   L05.91   Pilonidal cyst without abscess
            Parasacral dimple
            Pilonidal cyst NOS
            Pilonidal dimple
            Postanal dimple
   L05.92   Pilonidal sinus without abscess
            Coccygeal fistula
            Coccygeal sinus without abscess
            Pilonidal fistula

L08   Other local infections of skin and subcutaneous tissue
L08.0   Pyoderma
        Purulent dermatitis
        Septic dermatitis
        Suppurative dermatitis
        Excludes1:   pyoderma gangrenosum (L88)
                     pyoderma vegetans (L08.81)
L08.1   Erythrasma
L08.8   Other specified local infections of the skin and subcutaneous
        tissue
   L08.81   Pyoderma vegetans
            Excludes1:   pyoderma gangrenosum (L88)
                         pyoderma NOS (L08.0)
   L08.82   Omphalitis not of newborn
            Excludes1:   omphalitis of newborn (P38)
   L08.89   Other specified local infections of the skin and
            subcutaneous tissue

L08.9   Local infection of the skin and subcutaneous tissue, unspecified

BULLOUS DISORDERS (L10–14)

Excludes1:   benign familial pemphigus [Hailey-Hailey] (Q82.8)
staphylococcal scalded skin syndrome (L00)
toxic epidermal necrolysis [Lyell] (L51.2)

L10 Pemphigus

Excludes1:   pemphigus neonatorum (L00)

L10.0   Pemphigus vulgaris
L10.1   Pemphigus vegetans
L10.2   Pemphigus foliaceous
L10.3   Brazilian pemphigus [fogo selvagem]
L10.4   Pemphigus erythematosus
Senear-Usher syndrome
L10.5   Drug-induced pemphigus
Use additional external cause code (Chapter XIX), to identify drug
L10.8   Other pemphigus
L10.81   Paraneoplastic pemphigus
L10.89   Other pemphigus
L10.9   Pemphigus, unspecified

L11 Other acantholytic disorders

L11.0   Acquired keratosis follicularis
Excludes1:   keratosis follicularis (congenital) [Darier-White] (Q82.8)
L11.1   Transient acantholytic dermatosis [Grover]
L11.8   Other specified acantholytic disorders
L11.9   Acantholytic disorder, unspecified

L12 Pemphigoid

Excludes1:   herpes gestationis (O26.4-)
impetigo herpetiformis (L40.1)
L12.0   Bullous pemphigoid
L12.1   Cicatricial pemphigoid
Benign mucous membrane pemphigoid
L12.2   Chronic bullous disease of childhood
Juvenile dermatitis herpetiformis
L12.3   Acquired epidermolysis bullosa
Excludes1:   epidermolysis bullosa (congenital) (Q81.-)
L12.30   Acquired epidermolysis bullosa, unspecified
L12.31   Epidermolysis bullosa due to drug
Use additional code to identify drug
L12.35   Other acquired epidermolysis bullosa
L12.8   Other pemphigoid
L12.9   Pemphigoid, unspecified

L13 Other bullous disorders

L13.0   Dermatitis herpetiformis
Duhring's disease
Hydroa herpetiformis
Excludes1:   juvenile dermatitis herpetiformis (L12.2)
senile dermatitis herpetiformis (L12.0)
L13.1   Subcorneal pustular dermatitis
Sneddon-Wilkinson disease
L13.8   Other specified bullous disorders
L13.9   Bullous disorder, unspecified

L14 Bullous disorders in diseases classified elsewhere
Code first underlying disease

DERMATITIS AND ECZEMA (L20–L30)

Note: In this block the terms dermatitis and eczema are used synonymously and interchangeably.

Excludes2:   chronic (childhood) granulomatous disease (D71)
dermatitis gangrenosa (L88)
dermatitis herpetiformis (L13.0)
dry skin dermatitis (L85.3)
factitial dermatitis (L98.1)
perioral dermatitis (L71.0)
radiation-related disorders of the skin and subcutaneous tissue (L55-L59)
stasis dermatitis (I83.1-I83.2)

L20 Atopic dermatitis

L20.0   Besnier's prurigo
L20.8   Other atopic dermatitis
Excludes2:   circumscribed neurodermatitis (L28.0)
L20.81   Atopic neurodermatitis
Diffuse neurodermatitis
L20.82   Flexural eczema
L20.83   Infantile (acute) (chronic) eczema
L20.84   Intrinsic (allergic) eczema
L20.89   Other atopic dermatitis
L20.9   Atopic dermatitis, unspecified

L21 Seborrheic dermatitis

Excludes2   infective dermatitis (L30.3)
L21.0   Seborrhea capitis
Cradle cap
L21.1   Seborrheic infantile dermatitis
L21.8   Other seborrheic dermatitis
L21.9   Seborrheic dermatitis, unspecified

L22 Diaper dermatitis

Includes: Diaper erythema
Diaper rash
Psoriasiform diaper rash

L23 Allergic contact dermatitis

Use additional external cause code (Chapter XIX), to identify drug or substance
Excludes1:   allergy NOS (T78.4)
contact dermatitis NOS (L25.9)
dermatitis NOS (L30.9)
Excludes2:   dermatitis due to substances taken internally (L27.-)
dermatitis of eyelid (H01.1-)
diaper dermatitis (L22)
eczema of external ear (H60.5-)
irritant contact dermatitis (L24.-)
perioral dermatitis (L71.0)
radiation-related disorders of the skin and subcutaneous tissue (L55-L59)
L23.0   Allergic contact dermatitis due to metals
Allergic contact dermatitis due to chromium
Allergic contact dermatitis due to nickel
L23.1   Allergic contact dermatitis due to adhesives
L23.2   Allergic contact dermatitis due to cosmetics
L23.3   Allergic contact dermatitis due to drugs in contact with skin
Excludes2:   dermatitis due to ingested drugs and medicaments (L27.0-L27.1)
L23.4   Allergic contact dermatitis due to dyes
L23.5   Allergic contact dermatitis due to other chemical products
Allergic contact dermatitis due to cement
Allergic contact dermatitis due to insecticide
Allergic contact dermatitis due to plastic
Allergic contact dermatitis due to rubber
L23.6   Allergic contact dermatitis due to food in contact with the skin
Excludes2:   dermatitis due to ingested food (L27.2)
L23.7   Allergic contact dermatitis due to plants, except food
Excludes2:   allergy NOS due to pollen (J30.1)
L23.8   Allergic contact dermatitis due to other agents
L23.9   Allergic contact dermatitis, unspecified cause
Allergic contact eczema NOS

L24 Irritant contact dermatitis

Use additional external cause code (Chapter XIX), to identify drug or substance

Excludes1: allergy NOS (T78.4)
contact dermatitis NOS (L25.9)
dermatitis NOS (L30.9)

Excludes2: allergic contact dermatitis (L23.-)
dermatitis due to substances taken internally (L27.-)
dermatitis of eyelid (H01.1-)
diaper dermatitis (L22)
eczema of external ear (H60.5-)
perioral dermatitis (L71.0)
radiation-related disorders of the skin and subcutaneous tissue (L55-L59)

L24.0 Irritant contact dermatitis due to detergents

L24.1 Irritant contact dermatitis due to oils and greases

L24.2 Irritant contact dermatitis due to solvents
Irritant contact dermatitis due to chlorocompound
Irritant contact dermatitis due to cyclohexane
Irritant contact dermatitis due to ester
Irritant contact dermatitis due to glycol
Irritant contact dermatitis due to hydrocarbon
Irritant contact dermatitis due to ketone

L24.3 Irritant contact dermatitis due to cosmetics

L24.4 Irritant contact dermatitis due to drugs in contact with the skin

L24.5 Irritant contact dermatitis due to other chemical products
Irritant contact dermatitis due to cement
Irritant contact dermatitis due to insecticide

L24.6 Irritant contact dermatitis due to food in contact with skin
Excludes2: dermatitis due to ingested food (L27.2)

L24.7 Irritant contact dermatitis due to plants, except food
Excludes2: allergy NOS to pollen (J30.1)

L24.8 Irritant contact dermatitis due to other agents
Irritant contact dermatitis due to dyes

L24.9 Irritant contact dermatitis, unspecified cause
Irritant contact eczema NOS

L25 Unspecified contact dermatitis

Excludes1: allergic contact dermatitis (L23.-)
allergy NOS (T78.4)
dermatitis NOS (L30.9)
irritant contact dermatitis (L24.-)

Excludes2: dermatitis due to ingested substances (L27.-)
dermatitis of eyelid (H01.1-)
eczema of external ear (H60.5-)
perioral dermatitis (L71.0)
radiation-related disorders of the skin and subcutaneous tissue (L55-L59)

L25.0 Unspecified contact dermatitis due to cosmetics

L25.1 Unspecified contact dermatitis due to drugs in contact with skin
Excludes2: dermatitis due to ingested drugs and medicaments (L27.0-L27.1)

L25.2 Unspecified contact dermatitis due to dyes

L25.3 Unspecified contact dermatitis due to other chemical products
Unspecified contact dermatitis due to cement
Unspecified contact dermatitis due to insecticide

L25.4 Unspecified contact dermatitis due to food in contact with skin
Excludes2: dermatitis due to ingested food (L27.2)

L25.5 Unspecified contact dermatitis due to plants, except food
Excludes1: nettle rash (L50.9)
Excludes2: allergy NOS due to pollen (J30.1)

L25.8 Unspecified contact dermatitis due to other agents
Excludes2: allergy NOS due to animal hair, dander (animal) or dust (J30.3)

L25.9 Unspecified contact dermatitis, unspecified cause
Contact dermatitis (occupational) NOS
Contact eczema (occupational) NOS

L26 Exfoliative dermatitis

Includes: hebra's pityriasis

Excludes1: Ritter's disease (L00)

L27 Dermatitis due to substances taken internally

Excludes1: allergy NOS (T78.4)

Excludes2: adverse food reaction, except dermatitis (T78.0-T78.1)
contact dermatitis (L23-L25)
drug photoallergic response (L56.1)
drug phototoxic response (L56.0)
urticaria (L50.-)

L27.0 Generalized skin eruption due to drugs and medicaments taken internally
Use additional external cause code (Chapter XIX), to identify drug

L27.1 Localized skin eruption due to drugs and medicaments taken internally
Use additional external cause code (Chapter XIX), to identify drug

L27.2 Dermatitis due to ingested food
Excludes2: dermatitis due to food in contact with skin (L23.6, 24.6, L25.4)

L27.8 Dermatitis due to other substances taken internally

L27.9 Dermatitis due to unspecified substance taken internally

L28 Lichen simplex chronicus and prurigo

L28.0 Lichen simplex chronicus
Circumscribed neurodermatitis
Lichen NOS

L28.1 Prurigo nodularis

L28.2 Other prurigo
Prurigo NOS
Prurigo Hebra
Prurigo mitis
Urticaria papulosa

L29 Pruritus

Excludes1: neurotic excoriation (L98.1)
psychogenic pruritus (F45.8)

L29.0 Pruritus ani

L29.1 Pruritus scroti

L29.2 Pruritus vulvae

L29.3 Anogenital pruritus, unspecified

L29.8 Other pruritus

L29.9 Pruritus, unspecified
Itch NOS

L30 Other and unspecified dermatitis

Excludes2: contact dermatitis (L23-L25)
dry skin dermatitis (L85.3)
small plaque parapsoriasis (L41.3)
stasis dermatitis (I83.1-.2)

L30.0 Nummular dermatitis

L30.1 Dyshidrosis [pompholyx]

L30.2 Cutaneous autosensitization
Candidid [levurid]
Dermatophytid
Eczematid

L30.3 Infective dermatitis
Infectious eczematoid dermatitis

L30.4 Erythema intertrigo

L30.5 Pityriasis alba

L30.8 Other specified dermatitis

L30.9 Dermatitis, unspecified
Eczema NOS

PAPULOSQUAMOUS DISORDERS (L40–L45)

L40 Psoriasis

L40.0 Psoriasis vulgaris
Nummular psoriasis
Plaque psoriasis

L40.1 Generalized pustular psoriasis
Impetigo herpetiformis
Von Zumbusch's disease

L40.2 Acrodermatitis continua

L40.3 Pustulosis palmaris et plantaris

L40.4   **Guttate psoriasis**

L40.5   **Arthropathic psoriasis**

    L40.50   **Arthropathic psoriasis, unspecified**

    L40.51   **Distal interphalangeal psoriatic arthropathy**

    L40.52   **Psoriatic arthritis mutilans**

    L40.53   **Psoriatic spondylitis**

    L40.54   **Psoriatic juvenile arthropathy**

    L40.59   **Other psoriatic arthropathy**

L40.8   **Other psoriasis**

    Flexural psoriasis

L40.9   **Psoriasis, unspecified**

L41   Parapsoriasis

    Excludes1:   poikiloderma vasculare atrophicans (L94.5)

L41.0   **Pityriasis lichenoides et varioliformis acuta**

    Mucha-Habermann disease

L41.1   **Pityriasis lichenoides chronica**

L41.2   **Lymphomatoid papulosis**

L41.3   **Small plaque parapsoriasis**

L41.4   **Large plaque parapsoriasis**

L41.5   **Retiform parapsoriasis**

L41.8   **Other parapsoriasis**

L41.9   **Parapsoriasis, unspecified**

L42   Pityriasis rosea

L43   Lichen planus

    Excludes1:   lichen planopilaris (L66.1)

L43.0   **Hypertrophic lichen planus**

L43.1   **Bullous lichen planus**

L43.2   **Lichenoid drug reaction**

    Use additional external cause code (Chapter XIX), to identify drug.

L43.3   **Subacute (active) lichen planus**

    Lichen planus tropicus

L43.8   **Other lichen planus**

L43.9   **Lichen planus, unspecified**

L44   Other papulosquamous disorders

L44.0   **Pityriasis rubra pilaris**

L44.1   **Lichen nitidus**

L44.2   **Lichen striatus**

L44.3   **Lichen ruber moniliformis**

L44.4   **Infantile papular acrodermatitis [Giannotti-Crosti]**

L44.8   **Other specified papulosquamous disorders**

L44.9   **Papulosquamous disorder, unspecified**

L45   Papulosquamous disorders in diseases classified elsewhere

    Code first underlying disease.

URTICARIA AND ERYTHEMA (L50–L54)

    Excludes1:   Lyme disease (A69.2-)

                 rosacea (L71.-)

L50   Urticaria

    Excludes1:   allergic contact dermatitis (L23.-)

                 angioneurotic edema (T78.3)

                 giant urticaria (T78.3)

                 hereditary angio-edema (D84.1)

                 Quincke's edema (T78.3)

                 serum urticaria (T80.6)

                 solar urticaria (L56.3)

                 urticaria neonatorum (P83.8)

                 urticaria papulosa (L28.2)

                 urticaria pigmentosa (Q82.2)

L50.0   **Allergic urticaria**

L50.1   **Idiopathic urticaria**

L50.2   **Urticaria due to cold and heat**

L50.3   **Dermatographic urticaria**

L50.4   **Vibratory urticaria**

L50.5   **Cholinergic urticaria**

L50.6   **Contact urticaria**

L50.8   **Other urticaria**

    Chronic urticaria

    Recurrent periodic urticaria

L50.9   **Urticaria, unspecified**

L51   Erythema multiforme

L51.0   **Nonbullous erythema multiforme**

L51.1   **Bullous erythema multiforme**

    Stevens-Johnson syndrome

L51.2   **Toxic epidermal necrolysis [Lyell]**

L51.8   **Other erythema multiforme**

L51.9   **Erythema multiforme, unspecified**

L52   Erythema nodosum

    Excludes1:   tuberculous erythema nodosum (A18.4)

L53   Other erythematous conditions

    Excludes1:   erythema ab igne (L59.0)

                 erythema due to external agents in contact with skin (L23-L25)

                 erythema intertrigo (L30.4)

L53.0   **Toxic erythema**

    Use additional external cause code (Chapter XIX), to identify external agent.

    Excludes1:   neonatal erythema toxicum (P83.1)

L53.1   **Erythema annulare centrifugum**

L53.2   **Erythema marginatum**

L53.3   **Other chronic figurate erythema**

L53.8   **Other specified erythematous conditions**

L53.9   **Erythematous condition, unspecified**

    Erythema NOS

    Erythroderma NOS

L54   Erythema in diseases classified elsewhere

    Code first underlying disease.

RADIATION–RELATED DISORDERS OF THE SKIN AND SUBCUTANEOUS TISSUE (L55–L59)

L55   Sunburn

L55.0   **Sunburn of first degree**

L55.1   **Sunburn of second degree**

L55.2   **Sunburn of third degree**

L55.9   **Sunburn, unspecified**

L56   Other acute skin changes due to ultraviolet radiation

L56.0   **Drug phototoxic response**

    Use additional external cause code (Chapter XIX), to identify drug.

L56.1   **Drug photoallergic response**

    Use additional external cause code (Chapter XIX), to identify drug.

L56.2   **Photocontact dermatitis [berloque dermatitis]**

L56.3   **Solar urticaria**

L56.4   **Polymorphous light eruption**

L56.5   **Disseminated superficial actinic porokeratosis (DSAP)**

L56.8   **Other specified acute skin changes due to ultraviolet radiation**

L56.9   **Acute skin change due to ultraviolet radiation, unspecified**

L57   Skin changes due to chronic exposure to nonionizing radiation

L57.0   **Actinic keratosis**

    Keratosis NOS

    Senile keratosis

    Solar keratosis

L57.1   **Actinic reticuloid**

L57.2   **Cutis rhomboidalis nuchae**

L57.3   **Poikiloderma of Civatte**

L57.4   **Cutis laxa senilis**

    Elastosis senilis

L57.5   **Actinic granuloma**

L57.8 Other skin changes due to chronic exposure to nonionizing radiation
Farmer's skin
Sailor's skin
Solar dermatitis

L57.9 Skin changes due to chronic exposure to nonionizing radiation, unspecified

L58 Radiodermatitis

L58.0 Acute radiodermatitis

L58.1 Chronic radiodermatitis

L58.9 Radiodermatitis, unspecified

L59 Other disorders of skin and subcutaneous tissue related to radiation

L59.0 Erythema ab igne [dermatitis ab igne]

L59.8 Other specified disorders of the skin and subcutaneous tissue related to radiation

L59.9 Disorder of the skin and subcutaneous tissue related to radiation, unspecified

DISORDERS OF SKIN APPENDAGES (L60–L75)

Excludes1:   congenital malformations of integument (Q84.-)

L60 Nail disorders
Excludes2:   clubbing of nails (R68.3)
    onychia and paronychia (L03.0-)

L60.0 Ingrowing nail

L60.1 Onycholysis

L60.2 Onychogryphosis

L60.3 Nail dystrophy

L60.4 Beau's lines

L60.5 Yellow nail syndrome

L60.8 Other nail disorders

L60.9 Nail disorder, unspecified

L62 Nail disorders in diseases classified elsewhere
Code first underlying disease, such as:
    pachydermoperiostosis (M89.4-)

L63 Alopecia areata

L63.0 Alopecia (capitis) totalis

L63.1 Alopecia universalis

L63.2 Ophiasis

L63.8 Other alopecia areata

L63.9 Alopecia areata, unspecified

L64 Androgenic alopecia
Includes: male-pattern baldness

L64.0 Drug-induced androgenic alopecia
Use additional external cause code (Chapter XIX), to identify drug

L64.8 Other androgenic alopecia

L64.9 Androgenic alopecia, unspecified

L65 Other nonscarring hair loss
Use additional external cause code (Chapter XIX), to identify drug, if drug-induced
Excludes1:   trichotillomania (F63.3)

L65.0 Telogen effluvium

L65.1 Anagen effluvium

L65.2 Alopecia mucinosa

L65.8 Other specified nonscarring hair loss

L65.9 Nonscarring hair loss, unspecified
Alopecia NOS

L66 Cicatricial alopecia [scarring hair loss]

L66.0 Pseudopelade

L66.1 Lichen planopilaris
Follicular lichen planus

L66.2 Folliculitis decalvans

L66.3 Perifolliculitis capitis abscedens

L66.4 Folliculitis ulerythematosa reticulata

L66.8 Other cicatricial alopecia

L66.9 Cicatricial alopecia, unspecified

L67 Hair color and hair shaft abnormalities
Excludes1:   monilethrix (Q84.1)
    pili annulati (Q84.1)
    telogen effluvium (L65.0)

L67.0 Trichorrhexis nodosa

L67.1 Variations in hair color
Canities
Greyness, hair (premature)
Heterochromia of hair
Poliosis circumscripta, acquired
Poliosis NOS

L67.8 Other hair color and hair shaft abnormalities
Fragilitas crinium

L67.9 Hair color and hair shaft abnormality, unspecified

L68 Hypertrichosis
Includes: excess hair
Excludes1:   congenital hypertrichosis (Q84.2)
    persistent lanugo (Q84.2)

L68.0 Hirsutism
Use additional external cause code (Chapter XIX), to identify drug, if drug-induced.

L68.1 Acquired hypertrichosis lanuginosa
Use additional external cause code (Chapter XIX), to identify drug, if drug-induced.

L68.2 Localized hypertrichosis

L68.3 Polytrichia

L68.8 Other hypertrichosis

L68.9 Hypertrichosis, unspecified

L70 Acne
Excludes2:   acne keloid (L73.0)

L70.0 Acne vulgaris

L70.1 Acne conglobata

L70.2 Acne varioliformis
Acne necrotica miliaris

L70.3 Acne tropica

L70.4 Infantile acne

L70.5 Acné excoriée des jeunes filles
Picker's acne

L70.8 Other acne

L70.9 Acne, unspecified

L71 Rosacea

L71.0 Perioral dermatitis
Use additional external cause code (Chapter XIX), to identify drug, if drug-induced.

L71.1 Rhinophyma

L71.8 Other rosacea

L71.9 Rosacea, unspecified

L72 Follicular cysts of skin and subcutaneous tissue

L72.0 Epidermal cyst

L72.1 Trichodermal cyst
Pilar cyst
Sebaceous cyst

L72.2 Steatocystoma multiplex

L72.8 Other follicular cysts of the skin and subcutaneous tissue

L72.9 Follicular cyst of the skin and subcutaneous tissue, unspecified

L73 Other follicular disorders

L73.0 Acne keloid

L73.1 Pseudofolliculitis barbae

L73.2 Hidradenitis suppurativa

L73.8 Other specified follicular disorders
Sycosis barbae

L73.9 Follicular disorder, unspecified

L74 Eccrine sweat disorders

    Excludes2: hyperhidrosis (R61.-)

L74.0 Miliaria rubra

L74.1 Miliaria crystallina

L74.2 Miliaria profunda

    Miliaria tropicalis

L74.3 Miliaria, unspecified

L74.4 Anhidrosis

    Hypohidrosis

L74.8 Other eccrine sweat disorders

L74.9 Eccrine sweat disorder, unspecified

    Sweat gland disorder NOS

L75 Apocrine sweat disorders

    Excludes1: dyshidrosis (L30.1)
               hidradenitis suppurativa (L73.2)

L75.0 Bromhidrosis

L75.1 Chromhidrosis

L75.2 Apocrine miliaria

    Fox-Fordyce disease

L75.8 Other apocrine sweat disorders

L75.9 Apocrine sweat disorder, unspecified

INTRAOPERATIVE AND POSTPROCEDURAL COMPLICATIONS OF DERMATOLOGIC PROCEDURES (L76)

L76 Intraoperative and postprocedural complications of dermatologic procedures

L76.0 Intraoperative and postprocedural hemorrhage and hematoma complicating a dermatologic procedure

    Excludes1: intraoperative hemorrhage or hematoma due to accidental puncture or laceration during a dermatologic procedure (L76.1-)

L76.01 Intraoperative hemorrhage of the skin during a dermatologic procedure

L76.02 Intraoperative hemorrhage of a site other than skin during a dermatologic procedure

L76.03 Intraoperative hematoma of the skin during a dermatologic procedure

L76.04 Intraoperative hematoma of a site other than skin during a dermatologic procedure

L76.05 Postprocedural hemorrhage of the skin following a dermatologic procedure

L76.06 Postprocedural hemorrhage of a site other than skin following a dermatolgic procedure

L76.07 Postprocedural hematoma of the skin following a dermatologic procedure

L76.08 Postprocedural hematoma of a site other than skin following a dermatolgic procedure

L76.1 Accidental puncture or laceration during a dermatologic procedure

L76.11 Accidental puncture or laceration of the skin during a dermatologic procedure

L76.12 Accidental puncture or laceration of a site other than skin during a dermatologic procedure

L76.8 Other intraoperative and postprocedural complications of dermatologic procedures

OTHER DISORDERS OF THE SKIN AND SUBCUTANEOUS TISSUE (L80-L99)

L80 Vitiligo

    Excludes2: vitiligo of eyelids (H02.73-)
               vitiligo of vulva (N90.8)

L81 Other disorders of pigmentation

    Excludes1: birthmark NOS (Q82.5)
               Peutz-Jeghers syndrome (Q85.8)
    Excludes2: nevus—see Alphabetical Index

L81.0 Postinflammatory hyperpigmentation

L81.1 Chloasma

L81.2 Freckles

L81.3 Café au lait spots

L81.4 Other melanin hyperpigmentation

    Lentigo

L81.5 Leukoderma, not elsewhere classified

L81.6 Other disorders of diminished melanin formation

L81.7 Pigmented purpuric dermatosis

    Angioma serpiginosum

L81.8 Other specified disorders of pigmentation

    Iron pigmentation
    Tattoo pigmentation

L81.9 Disorder of pigmentation, unspecified

L82 Seborrheic keratosis

    Includes: dermatosis papulosa nigra
              Leser-Trélat disease

L82.0 Inflamed seborrheic keratosis

L82.1 Other seborrheic keratosis

    Seborrheic keratosis NOS

L83 Acanthosis nigricans

    Includes: confluent and reticulated papillomatosis

L84 Corns and callosities

    Includes: callus
              clavus

L85 Other epidermal thickening

    Excludes2: hypertrophic disorders of the skin (L91.-)

L85.0 Acquired ichthyosis

    Excludes1: congenital ichthyosis (Q80.-)

L85.1 Acquired keratosis [keratoderma] palmaris et plantaris

    Excludes1: inherited keratosis palmaris et plantaris (Q82.8)

L85.2 Keratosis punctata (palmaris et plantaris)

L85.3 Xerosis cutis

    Dry skin dermatitis

L85.8 Other specified epidermal thickening

    Cutaneous horn

L85.9 Epidermal thickening, unspecified

L86 Keratoderma in diseases classified elsewhere

    Code first underlying disease, such as:
    Reiter's disease (M02.3-)
    Excludes1: gonococcal keratoderma (A54.89)
               gonococcal keratosis (A54.89)
               keratoderma due to vitamin A deficiency (E50.8)
               keratosis due to vitamin A deficiency (E50.8)
               xeroderma due to vitamin A deficiency (E50.8)

L87 Transepidermal elimination disorders

    Excludes1: granuloma annulare (perforating) (L92.0)

L87.0 Keratosis follicularis et parafollicularis in cutem penetrans [Kyrle]

    Hyperkeratosis follicularis penetrans

L87.1 Reactive perforating collagenosis

L87.2 Elastosis perforans serpiginosa

L87.8 Other transepidermal elimination disorders

L87.9 Transepidermal elimination disorder, unspecified

L88 Pyoderma gangrenosum

    Includes: dermatitis gangrenosa
              phagedenic pyoderma

L89 Decubitus ulcer

    Includes: bed sore
              plaster ulcer
              pressure ulcer
    Code first any associated gangrene (I96)
    Excludes2: decubitus (trophic) ulcer of cervix (uteri) (N86)
               diabetic ulcers (E08.621, E08.622, E09.621, E09.622, E10.621, E10.622, E11.621, E11.622, E13.621, E13.622, E14.621, E14.622)
               non-decubitus chronic ulcer of skin (L97.-)
               skin infections (L00-L08)
               varicose ulcer (I83.0, I83.2)

L89.0   Decubitus ulcer of back
   L89.00   Decubitus ulcer of unspecified part of back
      L89.001   Decubitus ulcer of unspecified part of back limited to breakdown of the skin
      L89.002   Decubitus ulcer of unspecified part of back with fat layer exposed
      L89.003   Decubitus ulcer of unspecified part of back with necrosis of muscle
      L89.004   Decubitus ulcer of unspecified part of back with necrosis of bone
      L89.009   Decubitus ulcer of unspecified part of back with unspecified severity
   L89.01   Decubitus ulcer of right upper back
      L89.011   Decubitus ulcer of right upper back limited to breakdown of the skin
      L89.012   Decubitus ulcer of right upper back with fat layer exposed
      L89.013   Decubitus ulcer of right upper back with necrosis of muscle
      L89.014   Decubitus ulcer of right upper back with necrosis of bone
      L89.019   Decubitus ulcer of right upper back with unspecified severity
   L89.02   Decubitus ulcer of left upper back
      L89.021   Decubitus ulcer of left upper back limited to breakdown of the skin
      L89.022   Decubitus ulcer of left upper back with fat layer exposed
      L89.023   Decubitus ulcer of left upper back with necrosis of muscle
      L89.024   Decubitus ulcer of left upper back with necrosis of bone
      L89.029   Decubitus ulcer of left upper back with unspecified severity
   L89.03   Decubitus ulcer of right lower back
      L89.031   Decubitus ulcer of right lower back limited to breakdown of the skin
      L89.032   Decubitus ulcer of right lower back with fat layer exposed
      L89.033   Decubitus ulcer of right lower back with necrosis of muscle
      L89.034   Decubitus ulcer of right lower back with necrosis of bone
      L89.039   Decubitus ulcer of right lower back with unspecified severity
   L89.04   Decubitus ulcer of left lower back
      L89.041   Decubitus ulcer of left lower back limited to breakdown of the skin
      L89.042   Decubitus ulcer of left lower back with fat layer exposed
      L89.043   Decubitus ulcer of left lower back with necrosis of muscle
      L89.044   Decubitus ulcer of left lower back with necrosis of bone
      L89.049   Decubitus ulcer of left lower back with unspecified severity
   L89.05   Decubitus ulcer of sacral region
      Decubitus ulcer of tailbone
      L89.051   Decubitus ulcer of sacral region limited to breakdown of the skin
      L89.052   Decubitus ulcer of sacral region with fat layer exposed
      L89.053   Decubitus ulcer of sacral region with necrosis of muscle
      L89.054   Decubitus ulcer of sacral region with necrosis of bone
      L89.059   Decubitus ulcer of sacral region with unspecified severity
L89.1   Decubitus ulcer of buttock
   L89.10   Decubitus ulcer of unspecified buttock
      L89.101   Decubitus ulcer of unspecified buttock limited to breakdown of the skin

      L89.102   Decubitus ulcer of unspecified buttock with fat layer exposed
      L89.103   Decubitus ulcer of unspecified buttock with necrosis of muscle
      L89.104   Decubitus ulcer of unspecified buttock with necrosis of bone
      L89.109   Decubitus ulcer of unspecified buttock with unspecified severity
   L89.11   Decubitus ulcer of right buttock
      L89.111   Decubitus ulcer of right buttock limited to breakdown of the skin
      L89.112   Decubitus ulcer of right buttock with fat layer exposed
      L89.113   Decubitus ulcer of right buttock with necrosis of muscle
      L89.114   Decubitus ulcer of right buttock with necrosis of bone
      L89.119   Decubitus ulcer of right buttock with unspecified severity
   L89.12   Decubitus ulcer of left buttock
      L89.121   Decubitus ulcer of left buttock limited to breakdown of the skin
      L89.122   Decubitus ulcer of left buttock with fat layer exposed
      L89.123   Decubitus ulcer of left buttock with necrosis of muscle
      L89.124   Decubitus ulcer of left buttock with necrosis of bone
      L89.129   Decubitus ulcer of left buttock with unspecified severity
L89.2   Decubitus ulcer of contiguous site of back and buttock
   L89.20   Decubitus ulcer of contiguous site of back and buttock with unspecified severity
   L89.21   Decubitus ulcer of contiguous site of back and buttock limited to breakdown of the skin
   L89.22   Decubitus ulcer of contiguous site of back and buttock with fat layer exposed
   L89.23   Decubitus ulcer of contiguous site of back and buttock with necrosis of muscle
   L89.24   Decubitus ulcer of contiguous site of back and buttock with necrosis of bone
L89.8   Decubitus ulcer of other site
   L89.80   Decubitus ulcer of other site with unspecified severity
   L89.81   Decubitus ulcer of other site limited to breakdown of the skin
   L89.82   Decubitus ulcer of other site with fat layer exposed
   L89.83   Decubitus ulcer of other site with necrosis of muscle
   L89.84   Decubitus ulcer of other site with necrosis of bone
L89.9   Decubitus ulcer of unspecified site
   L89.90   Decubitus ulcer of unspecified site with unspecified severity
   L89.91   Decubitus ulcer of unspecified site limited to breakdown of the skin
   L89.92   Decubitus ulcer of unspecified site with fat layer exposed
   L89.93   Decubitus ulcer of unspecified site with necrosis of muscle
   L89.94   Decubitus ulcer of unspecified site with necrosis of bone

L90   Atrophic disorders of skin
   L90.0   Lichen sclerosus et atrophicus
   L90.1   Anetoderma of Schweninger-Buzzi
   L90.2   Anetoderma of Jadassohn-Pellizzari
   L90.3   Atrophoderma of Pasini and Pierini
   L90.4   Acrodermatitis chronica atrophicans

L90.5 Scar conditions and fibrosis of skin
Adherent scar (skin)
Cicatrix
Disfigurement of skin due to scar
Fibrosis of skin NOS
Scar NOS
Excludes2: hypertrophic scar (L91.0)
keloid scar (L91.0)

L90.6 Striae atrophicae

L90.8 Other atrophic disorders of skin

L90.9 Atrophic disorder of skin, unspecified

L91 Hypertrophic disorders of skin

L91.0 Keloid scar
Hypertrophic scar
Keloid
Excludes2: acne keloid (L73.0)
scar NOS (L90.5)

L91.8 Other hypertrophic disorders of the skin

L91.9 Hypertrophic disorder of the skin, unspecified

L92 Granulomatous disorders of skin and subcutaneous tissue
Excludes2: actinic granuloma (L57.5)

L92.0 Granuloma annulare
Perforating granuloma annulare

L92.1 Necrobiosis lipoidica, not elsewhere classified
Excludes1: necrobiosis lipoidica associated with diabetes mellitus (E08-E14 with .620)

L92.2 Granuloma faciale [eosinophilic granuloma of skin]

L92.3 Foreign body granuloma of the skin and subcutaneous tissue

L92.8 Other granulomatous disorders of the skin and subcutaneous tissue

L92.9 Granulomatous disorder of the skin and subcutaneous tissue, unspecified

L93 Lupus erythematosus
Use additional external cause code (Chapter XIX), to identify drug, if drug-induced
Excludes1: lupus exedens (A18.4)
lupus vulgaris (A18.4)
scleroderma (M34.-)
systemic lupus erythematosus (M32.-)

L93.0 Discoid lupus erythematosus
Lupus erythematosus NOS

L93.1 Subacute cutaneous lupus erythematosus

L93.2 Other local lupus erythematosus
Lupus erythematosus profundus
Lupus panniculitis

L94 Other localized connective tissue disorders
Excludes1: systemic connective tissue disorders (M30-M36)

L94.0 Localized scleroderma [morphea]
Circumscribed scleroderma

L94.1 Linear scleroderma
En coup de sabre lesion

L94.2 Calcinosis cutis

L94.3 Sclerodactyly

L94.4 Gottron's papules

L94.5 Poikiloderma vasculare atrophicans

L94.6 Ainhum

L94.8 Other specified localized connective tissue disorders

L94.9 Localized connective tissue disorder, unspecified

L95 Vasculitis limited to skin, not elsewhere classified
Excludes1: angioma serpiginosum (L81.7)
Henoch(-Schönlein) purpura (D69.0)
hypersensitivity angiitis (M31.0)
lupus panniculitis (L93.2)
panniculitis NOS (M79.3)
panniculitis of neck and back (M54.0-)
polyarteritis nodosa (M30.0)
relapsing panniculitis (M35.6)
rheumatoid vasculitis (M05.2)
serum sickness (T80.6)
urticaria (L50.-)
Wegener's granulomatosis (M31.3-)

L95.0 Livedoid vasculitis
Atrophie blanche (en plaque)

L95.1 Erythema elevatum diutinum

L95.8 Other vasculitis limited to the skin

L95.9 Vasculitis limited to the skin, unspecified

L97 Non-decubitus chronic ulcer of lower limb, not elsewhere classified
Includes: chronic ulcer of skin NOS
non-healing ulcer of skin
non-infected sinus of skin
trophic ulcer NOS
tropical ulcer NOS
ulcer of skin NOS
Code first any associated:
atherosclerosis of the lower extremities (I70.23-, I70.24-, I70.33-, I70.34-, I70.43-, I70.44-, I70.53-, I70.54-, I70.63-, I70.64-, I70.73-, I70.74-)
diabetic ulcers (E08.621, E08.622, E09.621, E09.622, E10.621, E10.622, E11.621, E11.622, E13.621, E13.622, E14.621, E14.622)
gangrene (I96)
varicose ulcer (I83.0-, I83.2-)
Excludes2: decubitus ulcer (L89.-)
skin infections (L00-L08)
specific infections classified to A00-B99

L97.1 Non-decubitus chronic ulcer of thigh

L97.10 Non-decubitus chronic ulcer of unspecified thigh

L97.101 Non-decubitus chronic ulcer of unspecified thigh limited to breakdown of skin

L97.102 Non-decubitus chronic ulcer of unspecified thigh with fat layer exposed

L97.103 Non-decubitus chronic ulcer of unspecified thigh with necrosis of muscle

L97.104 Non-decubitus chronic ulcer of unspecified thigh with necrosis of bone

L97.109 Non-decubitus chronic ulcer of unspecified thigh with unspecified severity

L97.11 Non-decubitus chronic ulcer of right thigh

L97.111 Non-decubitus chronic ulcer of right thigh limited to breakdown of skin

L97.112 Non-decubitus chronic ulcer of right thigh with fat layer exposed

L97.113 Non-decubitus chronic ulcer of right thigh with necrosis of muscle

L97.114 Non-decubitus chronic ulcer of right thigh with necrosis of bone

L97.119 Non-decubitus chronic ulcer of right thigh with unspecified severity

L97.12 Non-decubitus chronic ulcer of left thigh

L97.121 Non-decubitus chronic ulcer of left thigh limited to breakdown of skin

L97.122 Non-decubitus chronic ulcer of left thigh with fat layer exposed

L97.123 Non-decubitus chronic ulcer of left thigh with necrosis of muscle

L97.124 Non-decubitus chronic ulcer of left thigh with necrosis of bone

L97.129 Non-decubitus chronic ulcer of left thigh with unspecified severity

L97.2   Non-decubitus chronic ulcer of calf
  L97.20   Non-decubitus chronic ulcer of unspecified calf
    L97.201   Non-decubitus chronic ulcer of unspecified calf limited to breakdown of skin
    L97.202   Non-decubitus chronic ulcer of unspecified calf with fat layer exposed
    L97.203   Non-decubitus chronic ulcer of unspecified calf with necrosis of muscle
    L97.204   Non-decubitus chronic ulcer of unspecified calf with necrosis of bone
    L97.209   Non-decubitus chronic ulcer of unspecified calf with unspecified severity
  L97.21   Non-decubitus chronic ulcer of right calf
    L97.211   Non-decubitus chronic ulcer of right calf limited to breakdown of skin
    L97.212   Non-decubitus chronic ulcer of right calf with fat layer exposed
    L97.213   Non-decubitus chronic ulcer of right calf with necrosis of muscle
    L97.214   Non-decubitus chronic ulcer of right calf with necrosis of bone
    L97.219   Non-decubitus chronic ulcer of right calf with unspecified severity
  L97.22   Non-decubitus chronic ulcer of left calf
    L97.221   Non-decubitus chronic ulcer of left calf limited to breakdown of skin
    L97.222   Non-decubitus chronic ulcer of left calf with fat layer exposed
    L97.223   Non-decubitus chronic ulcer of left calf with necrosis of muscle
    L97.224   Non-decubitus chronic ulcer of left calf with necrosis of bone
    L97.229   Non-decubitus chronic ulcer of left calf with unspecified severity
L97.3   Non-decubitus chronic ulcer of ankle
  L97.30   Non-decubitus chronic ulcer of unspecified ankle
    L97.301   Non-decubitus chronic ulcer of unspecified ankle limited to breakdown of skin
    L97.302   Non-decubitus chronic ulcer of unspecified ankle with fat layer exposed
    L97.303   Non-decubitus chronic ulcer of unspecified ankle with necrosis of muscle
    L97.304   Non-decubitus chronic ulcer of unspecified ankle with necrosis of bone
    L97.309   Non-decubitus chronic ulcer of unspecified ankle with unspecified severity
  L97.31   Non-decubitus chronic ulcer of right ankle
    L97.311   Non-decubitus chronic ulcer of right ankle limited to breakdown of skin
    L97.312   Non-decubitus chronic ulcer of right ankle with fat layer exposed
    L97.313   Non-decubitus chronic ulcer of right ankle with necrosis of muscle
    L97.314   Non-decubitus chronic ulcer of right ankle with necrosis of bone
    L97.319   Non-decubitus chronic ulcer of right ankle with unspecified severity
  L97.32   Non-decubitus chronic ulcer of left ankle
    L97.321   Non-decubitus chronic ulcer of left ankle limited to breakdown of skin
    L97.322   Non-decubitus chronic ulcer of left ankle with fat layer exposed
    L97.323   Non-decubitus chronic ulcer of left ankle with necrosis of muscle
    L97.324   Non-decubitus chronic ulcer of left ankle with necrosis of bone
    L97.329   Non-decubitus chronic ulcer of left ankle with unspecified severity
L97.4   Non-decubitus chronic ulcer of heel and midfoot
    Non-decubitus chronic ulcer of plantar surface of midfoot
  L97.40   Non-decubitus chronic ulcer of unspecified heel and midfoot

L97.401   Non-decubitus chronic ulcer of unspecified heel and midfoot limited to breakdown of skin
L97.402   Non-decubitus chronic ulcer of unspecified heel and midfoot with fat layer exposed
L97.403   Non-decubitus chronic ulcer of unspecified heel and midfoot with necrosis of muscle
L97.404   Non-decubitus chronic ulcer of unspecified heel and midfoot with necrosis of bone
L97.409   Non-decubitus chronic ulcer of unspecified heel and midfoot with unspecified severity
  L97.41   Non-decubitus chronic ulcer of right heel and midfoot
    L97.411   Non-decubitus chronic ulcer of right heel and midfoot limited to breakdown of skin
    L97.412   Non-decubitus chronic ulcer of right heel and midfoot with fat layer exposed
    L97.413   Non-decubitus chronic ulcer of right heel and midfoot with necrosis of muscle
    L97.414   Non-decubitus chronic ulcer of right heel and midfoot with necrosis of bone
    L97.419   Non-decubitus chronic ulcer of right heel and midfoot with unspecified severity
  L97.42   Non-decubitus chronic ulcer of left heel and midfoot
    L97.421   Non-decubitus chronic ulcer of left heel and midfoot limited to breakdown of skin
    L97.422   Non-decubitus chronic ulcer of left heel and midfoot with fat layer exposed
    L97.423   Non-decubitus chronic ulcer of left heel and midfoot with necrosis of muscle
    L97.424   Non-decubitus chronic ulcer of left heel and midfoot with necrosis of bone
    L97.429   Non-decubitus chronic ulcer of left heel and midfoot with unspecified severity
L97.5   Non-decubitus chronic ulcer of other part of foot
    Non-decubitus chronic ulcer of toe
  L97.50   Non-decubitus chronic ulcer of other part of unspecified foot
    L97.501   Non-decubitus chronic ulcer of other part of unspecified foot limited to breakdown of skin
    L97.502   Non-decubitus chronic ulcer of other part of unspecified foot with fat layer exposed
    L97.503   Non-decubitus chronic ulcer of other part of unspecified foot with necrosis of muscle
    L97.504   Non-decubitus chronic ulcer of other part of unspecified foot with necrosis of bone
    L97.509   Non-decubitus chronic ulcer of other part of unspecified foot with unspecified severity
  L97.51   Non-decubitus chronic ulcer of other part of right foot
    L97.511   Non-decubitus chronic ulcer of other part of right foot limited to breakdown of skin
    L97.512   Non-decubitus chronic ulcer of other part of right foot with fat layer exposed
    L97.513   Non-decubitus chronic ulcer of other part of right foot with necrosis of muscle
    L97.514   Non-decubitus chronic ulcer of other part of right foot with necrosis of bone
    L97.519   Non-decubitus chronic ulcer of other part of right foot with unspecified severity
  L97.52   Non-decubitus chronic ulcer of other part of left foot
    L97.521   Non-decubitus chronic ulcer of other part of left foot limited to breakdown of skin
    L97.522   Non-decubitus chronic ulcer of other part of left foot with fat layer exposed
    L97.523   Non-decubitus chronic ulcer of other part of left foot with necrosis of muscle
    L97.524   Non-decubitus chronic ulcer of other part of left foot with necrosis of bone
    L97.529   Non-decubitus chronic ulcer of other part of left foot with unspecified severity
L97.8   Non-decubitus chronic ulcer of other part of lower leg
  L97.80   Non-decubitus chronic ulcer of other part of unspecified lower leg

L97.801 Non-decubitus chronic ulcer of other part of unspecified lower leg limited to breakdown of skin

L97.802 Non-decubitus chronic ulcer of other part of unspecified lower leg with fat layer exposed

L97.803 Non-decubitus chronic ulcer of other part of unspecified lower leg with necrosis of muscle

L97.804 Non-decubitus chronic ulcer of other part of unspecified lower leg with necrosis of bone

L97.809 Non-decubitus chronic ulcer of other part of unspecified lower leg with unspecified severity

L97.81 Non-decubitus chronic ulcer of other part of right lower leg

L97.811 Non-decubitus chronic ulcer of other part of right lower leg limited to breakdown of skin

L97.812 Non-decubitus chronic ulcer of other part of right lower leg with fat layer exposed

L97.813 Non-decubitus chronic ulcer of other part of right lower leg with necrosis of muscle

L97.814 Non-decubitus chronic ulcer of other part of right lower leg with necrosis of bone

L97.819 Non-decubitus chronic ulcer of other part of right lower leg with unspecified severity

L97.82 Non-decubitus chronic ulcer of other part of left lower leg

L97.821 Non-decubitus chronic ulcer of other part of left lower leg limited to breakdown of skin

L97.822 Non-decubitus chronic ulcer of other part of left lower leg with fat layer exposed

L97.823 Non-decubitus chronic ulcer of other part of left lower leg with necrosis of muscle

L97.824 Non-decubitus chronic ulcer of other part of left lower leg with necrosis of bone

L97.829 Non-decubitus chronic ulcer of other part of left lower leg with unspecified severity

L97.9 Non-decubitus chronic ulcer of unspecified part of lower leg

L97.90 Non-decubitus chronic ulcer of unspecified part of unspecified lower leg

L97.901 Non-decubitus chronic ulcer of unspecified part of unspecified lower leg limited to breakdown of skin

L97.902 Non-decubitus chronic ulcer of unspecified part of unspecified lower leg with fat layer exposed

L97.903 Non-decubitus chronic ulcer of unspecified part of unspecified lower leg with necrosis of muscle

L97.904 Non-decubitus chronic ulcer of unspecified part of unspecified lower leg with necrosis of bone

L97.909 Non-decubitus chronic ulcer of unspecified part of unspecified lower leg with unspecified severity

L97.91 Non-decubitus chronic ulcer of unspecified part of right lower leg

L97.911 Non-decubitus chronic ulcer of unspecified part of right lower leg limited to breakdown of skin

L97.912 Non-decubitus chronic ulcer of unspecified part of right lower leg with fat layer exposed

L97.913 Non-decubitus chronic ulcer of unspecified part of right lower leg with necrosis of muscle

L97.914 Non-decubitus chronic ulcer of unspecified part of right lower leg with necrosis of bone

L97.919 Non-decubitus chronic ulcer of unspecified part of right lower leg with unspecified severity

L97.92 Non-decubitus chronic ulcer of unspecified part of left lower leg

L97.921 Non-decubitus chronic ulcer of unspecified part of left lower leg limited to breakdown of skin

L97.922 Non-decubitus chronic ulcer of unspecified part of left lower leg with fat layer exposed

L97.923 Non-decubitus chronic ulcer of unspecified part of left lower leg with necrosis of muscle

L97.924 Non-decubitus chronic ulcer of unspecified part of left lower leg with necrosis of bone

L97.929 Non-decubitus chronic ulcer of unspecified part of left lower leg with unspecified severity

L98 Other disorders of skin and subcutaneous tissue, not elsewhere classified

L98.0 Pyogenic granuloma
  Excludes2: pyogenic granuloma of gingiva (K06.8)
  pyogenic granuloma of maxillary alveolar ridge (K04.5)
  pyogenic granuloma of oral mucosa (K13.4)

L98.1 Factitial dermatitis
  Neurotic excoriation

L98.2 Febrile neutrophilic dermatosis [Sweet]

L98.3 Eosinophilic cellulitis [Wells]

L98.4 Non-decubitus chronic ulcer of skin, not elsewhere classified
  Chronic ulcer of skin NOS
  Tropical ulcer NOS
  Ulcer of skin NOS
  Excludes2: decubitus ulcer (L89)
  gangrene (R02)
  skin infections (L00-L08)
  specific infections classified to A00-B99
  ulcer of lower limb NEC (l97.-)
  varicose ulcer (I83.0-I82.2)

L98.41 Non-decubitus chronic ulcer of buttock

L98.411 Non-decubitus chronic ulcer of buttock limited to breakdown of skin

L98.412 Non-decubitus chronic ulcer of buttock with fat layer exposed

L98.413 Non-decubitus chronic ulcer of buttock with necrosis of muscle

L98.414 Non-decubitus chronic ulcer of buttock with necrosis of bone

L98.419 Non-decubitus chronic ulcer of buttock with unspecified severity

L98.42 Non-decubitus chronic ulcer of back

L98.421 Non-decubitus chronic ulcer of back limited to breakdown of skin

L98.422 Non-decubitus chronic ulcer of back with fat layer exposed

L98.423 Non-decubitus chronic ulcer of back with necrosis of muscle

L98.424 Non-decubitus chronic ulcer of back with necrosis of bone

L98.429 Non-decubitus chronic ulcer of back with unspecified severity

L98.49 Non-decubitus chronic ulcer of skin of other sites
  Non-decubitus chronic ulcer of skin NOS

L98.491 Non-decubitus chronic ulcer of skin of other sites limited to breakdown of skin

L98.492 Non-decubitus chronic ulcer of skin of other sites with fat layer exposed

L98.493 Non-decubitus chronic ulcer of skin of other sites with necrosis of muscle

L98.494 Non-decubitus chronic ulcer of skin of other sites with necrosis of bone

L98.499 Non-decubitus chronic ulcer of skin of other sites with unspecified severity

L98.5 Mucinosis of the skin
  Focal mucinosis
  Lichen myxedematosus
  Excludes1: focal oral mucinosis (K13.7)
  myxedema (E03.9)

L98.6 Other infiltrative disorders of the skin and subcutaneous tissue
  Excludes1: hyalinosis cutis et mucosae (E78.89)

L98.8   Other specified disorders of the skin and subcutaneous tissue

L98.9   Disorder of the skin and subcutaneous tissue, unspecified

L99 Other disorders of skin and subcutaneous tissue in diseases classified elsewhere

    Code first underlying disease, such as:
      amyloidosis (E85)

    Excludes1:   skin disorders in diabetes (E08-E14 with .62)
               skin disorders in gonorrhea (A54.89)
               skin disorders in syphilis (A51.31, A52.79)

CHAPTER XIII — DISEASES OF THE MUSCULOSKELETAL SYSTEM AND CONNECTIVE TISSUE (M00–M99)

Excludes2:   arthropathic psoriasis (L40.5-)
certain conditions originating in the perinatal period (P04-P96)
certain infectious and parasitic diseases (A00-B99)
compartment syndrome (T79.6)
complications of pregnancy, childbirth and the puerperium (O00-O99)
congenital malformations, deformations, and chromosomal abnormalities (Q00-Q99)
endocrine, nutritional and metabolic diseases (E00-E90)
injury, poisoning and certain other consequences of external causes (S00-T98)
neoplasms (C00-D48)
symptoms, signs and abnormal clinical and laboratory findings, not elsewhere classified (R00-R94)

This chapter contains the following blocks:

M00-M02	Infectious arthropathies
M05-M14	Inflammatory polyarthropathies
M15-M19	Osteoarthritis
M20-M25	Other joint disorders
M26-M27	Dentofacial anomalies [including malocclusion] and other disorders of jaw
M30-M36	Systemic connective tissue disorders
M40-M43	Deforming dorsopathies
M45-M49	Spondylopathies
M50-M54	Other dorsopathies
M60-M63	Disorders of muscles
M65-M67	Disorders of synovium and tendon
M70-M79	Other soft tissue disorders
M80-M85	Disorders of bone density and structure
M86-M90	Other osteopathies
M91-M94	Chondropathies
M95-M99	Other disorders of the musculoskeletal system and connective tissue

ARTHROPATHIES (M00–M25)
Disorders affecting predominantly peripheral (limb) joints

INFECTIOUS ARTHROPATHIES (M00–M02)

This block comprises arthropathies due to microbiological agents. Distinction is made between the following types of etiological relationship:

a) direct infection of joint, where organisms invade synovial tissue and microbial antigen is present in the joint;

b) indirect infection, which may be of two types: a reactive arthropathy, where microbial infection of the body is established but neither organisms nor antigens can be identified in the joint, and a postinfective arthropathy, where microbial antigen is present but recovery of an organism is inconstant and evidence of local multiplication is lacking.

M00 Pyogenic arthritis

M00.0 Staphylococcal arthritis and polyarthritis
Use additional code (B95.6-B95.7) to identify bacterial agent

    M00.00   Staphylococcal arthritis, unspecified joint

    M00.01   Staphylococcal arthritis, shoulder

        M00.011 Staphylococcal arthritis, right shoulder

        M00.012 Staphylococcal arthritis, left shoulder

        M00.019 Staphylococcal arthritis, unspecified shoulder

    M00.02   Staphylococcal arthritis, elbow

        M00.021 Staphylococcal arthritis, right elbow

        M00.022 Staphylococcal arthritis, left elbow

        M00.029 Staphylococcal arthritis, unspecified elbow

    M00.03   Staphylococcal arthritis, wrist
Staphylococcal arthritis of carpal bones

        M00.031 Staphylococcal arthritis, right wrist

        M00.032 Staphylococcal arthritis, left wrist

        M00.039 Staphylococcal arthritis, unspecified wrist

    M00.04   Staphylococcal arthritis, hand
Staphylococcal arthritis of metacarpus and phalanges

        M00.041 Staphylococcal arthritis, right hand

        M00.042 Staphylococcal arthritis, left hand

        M00.049 Staphylococcal arthritis, unspecified hand

    M00.05   Staphylococcal arthritis, hip

        M00.051 Staphylococcal arthritis, right hip

        M00.052 Staphylococcal arthritis, left hip

        M00.059 Staphylococcal arthritis, unspecified hip

    M00.06   Staphylococcal arthritis, knee

        M00.061 Staphylococcal arthritis, right knee

        M00.062 Staphylococcal arthritis, left knee

        M00.069 Staphylococcal arthritis, unspecified knee

    M00.07   Staphylococcal arthritis, ankle and foot
Staphylococcal arthritis, tarsus, metatarsus and phalanges

        M00.071 Staphylococcal arthritis, right ankle and foot

        M00.072 Staphylococcal arthritis, left ankle and foot

        M00.079 Staphylococcal arthritis, unspecified ankle and foot

    M00.08   Staphylococcal arthritis, vertebrae

    M00.09   Staphylococcal polyarthritis

M00.1 Pneumococcal arthritis and polyarthritis

    M00.10   Pneumococcal arthritis, unspecified joint

    M00.11   Pneumococcal arthritis, shoulder

        M00.111 Pneumococcal arthritis, right shoulder

        M00.112 Pneumococcal arthritis, left shoulder

        M00.119 Pneumococcal arthritis, unspecified shoulder

    M00.12   Pneumococcal arthritis, elbow

        M00.121 Pneumococcal arthritis, right elbow

        M00.122 Pneumococcal arthritis, left elbow

        M00.129 Pneumococcal arthritis, unspecified elbow

    M00.13   Pneumococcal arthritis, wrist
Pneumococcal arthritis of carpal bones

        M00.131 Pneumococcal arthritis, right wrist

        M00.132 Pneumococcal arthritis, left wrist

        M00.139 Pneumococcal arthritis, unspecified wrist

    M00.14   Pneumococcal arthritis, hand
Pneumococcal arthritis of metacarpus and phalanges

        M00.141 Pneumococcal arthritis, right hand

        M00.142 Pneumococcal arthritis, left hand

        M00.149 Pneumococcal arthritis, unspecified hand

    M00.15   Pneumococcal arthritis, hip

        M00.151 Pneumococcal arthritis, right hip

        M00.152 Pneumococcal arthritis, left hip

        M00.159 Pneumococcal arthritis, unspecified hip

    M00.16   Pneumococcal arthritis, knee

        M00.161 Pneumococcal arthritis, right knee

        M00.162 Pneumococcal arthritis, left knee

        M00.169 Pneumococcal arthritis, unspecified knee

    M00.17   Pneumococcal arthritis, ankle and foot
Pneumococcal arthritis, tarsus, metatarsus and phalanges

        M00.171 Pneumococcal arthritis, right ankle and foot

        M00.172 Pneumococcal arthritis, left ankle and foot

        M00.179 Pneumococcal arthritis, unspecified ankle and foot

    M00.18   Pneumococcal arthritis, vertebrae

    M00.19   Pneumococcal polyarthritis

M00.2 Other streptococcal arthritis and polyarthritis
Use additional code (B95.0-B95.2, B95.4-B95.5) to identify bacterial agent

    M00.20   Other streptococcal arthritis, unspecified joint

    M00.21   Other streptococcal arthritis, shoulder

        M00.211 Other streptococcal arthritis, right shoulder

        M00.212 Other streptococcal arthritis, left shoulder

M00.219   Other streptococcal arthritis, unspecified shoulder
M00.22   Other streptococcal arthritis, elbow
  M00.221   Other streptococcal arthritis, right elbow
  M00.222   Other streptococcal arthritis, left elbow
  M00.229   Other streptococcal arthritis, unspecified elbow
M00.23   Other streptococcal arthritis, wrist
  Other streptococcal arthritis of carpal bones
  M00.231   Other streptococcal arthritis, right wrist
  M00.232   Other streptococcal arthritis, left wrist
  M00.239   Other streptococcal arthritis, unspecified wrist
M00.24   Other streptococcal arthritis, hand
  Other streptococcal arthritis metacarpus and phalanges
  M00.241   Other streptococcal arthritis, right hand
  M00.242   Other streptococcal arthritis, left hand
  M00.249   Other streptococcal arthritis, unspecified hand
M00.25   Other streptococcal arthritis, hip
  M00.251   Other streptococcal arthritis, right hip
  M00.252   Other streptococcal arthritis, left hip
  M00.259   Other streptococcal arthritis, unspecified hip
M00.26   Other streptococcal arthritis, knee
  M00.261   Other streptococcal arthritis, right knee
  M00.262   Other streptococcal arthritis, left knee
  M00.269   Other streptococcal arthritis, unspecified knee
M00.27   Other streptococcal arthritis, ankle and foot
  Other streptococcal arthritis, tarsus, metatarsus and phalanges
  M00.271   Other streptococcal arthritis, right ankle and foot
  M00.272   Other streptococcal arthritis, left ankle and foot
  M00.279   Other streptococcal arthritis, unspecified ankle and foot
M00.28   Other streptococcal arthritis, vertebrae
M00.29   Other streptococcal polyarthritis
M00.8   Arthritis and polyarthritis due to other bacteria
  Use additional code (B96) to identify bacteria
M00.80   Arthritis due to other bacteria, unspecified joint
M00.81   Arthritis due to other bacteria, shoulder
  M00.811   Arthritis due to other bacteria, right shoulder
  M00.812   Arthritis due to other bacteria, left shoulder
  M00.819   Arthritis due to other bacteria, unspecified shoulder
M00.82   Arthritis due to other bacteria, elbow
  M00.821   Arthritis due to other bacteria, right elbow
  M00.822   Arthritis due to other bacteria, left elbow
  M00.829   Arthritis due to other bacteria, unspecified elbow
M00.83   Arthritis due to other bacteria, wrist
  Arthritis due to other bacteria, carpal bones
  M00.831   Arthritis due to other bacteria, right wrist
  M00.832   Arthritis due to other bacteria, left wrist
  M00.839   Arthritis due to other bacteria, unspecified wrist
M00.84   Arthritis due to other bacteria, hand
  Arthritis due to other bacteria, metacarpus and phalanges
  M00.841   Arthritis due to other bacteria, right hand
  M00.842   Arthritis due to other bacteria, left hand
  M00.849   Arthritis due to other bacteria, unspecified hand
M00.85   Arthritis due to other bacteria, hip
  M00.851   Arthritis due to other bacteria, right hip
  M00.852   Arthritis due to other bacteria, left hip
  M00.859   Arthritis due to other bacteria, unspecified hip
M00.86   Arthritis due to other bacteria, knee

M00.861   Arthritis due to other bacteria, right knee
M00.862   Arthritis due to other bacteria, left knee
M00.869   Arthritis due to other bacteria, unspecified knee
M00.87   Arthritis due to other bacteria, ankle and foot
  Arthritis due to other bacteria, tarsus, metatarsus, and phalanges
  M00.871   Arthritis due to other bacteria, right ankle and foot
  M00.872   Arthritis due to other bacteria, left ankle and foot
  M00.879   Arthritis due to other bacteria, unspecified ankle and foot
M00.88   Arthritis due to other bacteria, vertebrae
M00.89   Polyarthritis due to other bacteria
M00.9   Pyogenic arthritis, unspecified
  Infective arthritis NOS

M01   Direct infections of joint in infectious and parasitic diseases classified elsewhere
  Code first underlying disease, such as:
  leprosy [Hansen's disease] (A30.-)
  mycoses (B35-B49)
  O'nyong-nyong fever (A92.1)
  paratyphoid fever (A01.1-A01.4)
  Excludes1:   arthritis, arthropathy (in):
    gonococcal (A54.42)
    Lyme disease (A69.23)
    meningococcal (A39.83)
     postmeningococcal (A39.84)
    mumps (B26.85)
    postinfective (M02.-)
    reactive (M04.0-)
    rubella (B06.82)
    sarcoidosis (D86.86)
    typhoid fever (A01.04)
    tuberculosis (A18.02)
     spine (A18.01)
M01.x0   Direct infection of unspecified joint in infectious and parasitic diseases classified elsewhere
M01.x1   Direct infection of shoulder joint in infectious and parasitic diseases classified elsewhere
  M01.x11   Direct infection of right shoulder in infectious and parasitic diseases classified elsewhere
  M01.x12   Direct infection of left shoulder in infectious and parasitic diseases classified elsewhere
  M01.x19   Direct infection of unspecified shoulder in infectious and parasitic diseases classified elsewhere
M01.x2   Direct infection of elbow in infectious and parasitic diseases classified elsewhere
  M01.x21   Direct infection of right elbow in infectious and parasitic diseases classified elsewhere
  M01.x22   Direct infection of left elbow in infectious and parasitic diseases classified elsewhere
  M01.x29   Direct infection of unspecified elbow in infectious and parasitic diseases classified elsewhere
M01.x3   Direct infection of wrist in infectious and parasitic diseases classified elsewhere
  Direct infection of carpal bones in infectious and parasitic diseases classified elsewhere
  M01.x31   Direct infection of right wrist in infectious and parasitic diseases classified elsewhere
  M01.x32   Direct infection of left wrist in infectious and parasitic diseases classified elsewhere
  M01.x39   Direct infection of unspecified wrist in infectious and parasitic diseases classified elsewhere
M01.x4   Direct infection of hand in infectious and parasitic diseases classified elsewhere
  Direct infection of metacarpus and phalanges in infectious and parasitic diseases classified elsewhere

M01.x41 Direct infection of right hand in infectious and parasitic diseases classified elsewhere

M01.x42 Direct infection of left hand in infectious and parasitic diseases classified elsewhere

M01.x49 Direct infection of unspecified hand in infectious and parasitic diseases classified elsewhere

M01.x5 Direct infection of hip in infectious and parasitic diseases classified elsewhere

M01.x51 Direct infection of right hip in infectious and parasitic diseases classified elsewhere

M01.x52 Direct infection of left hip in infectious and parasitic diseases classified elsewhere

M01.x59 Direct infection of unspecified hip in infectious and parasitic diseases classified elsewhere

M01.x6 Direct infection of knee in infectious and parasitic diseases classified elsewhere

M01.x61 Direct infection of right knee in infectious and parasitic diseases classified elsewhere

M01.x62 Direct infection of left knee in infectious and parasitic diseases classified elsewhere

M01.x69 Direct infection of unspecified knee in infectious and parasitic diseases classified elsewhere

M01.x7 Direct infection of ankle and foot in infectious and parasitic diseases classified elsewhere
Direct infection of tarsus, metatarsus and phalanges in infectious and parasitic diseases classified elsewhere

M01.x71 Direct infection of right ankle and foot in infectious and parasitic diseases classified elsewhere

M01.x72 Direct infection of left ankle and foot in infectious and parasitic diseases classified elsewhere

M01.x79 Direct infection of unspecified ankle and foot in infectious and parasitic diseases classified elsewhere

M01.x8 Direct infection of vertebrae in infectious and parasitic diseases classified elsewhere

M01.x9 Direct infection of multiple joints in infectious and parasitic diseases classified elsewhere

M02 Postinfective and reactive arthropathies
Code first underlying disease, such as:
congenital syphilis [Clutton's joints] (A50.5)
enteritis due to Yersinia enterocolitica (A04.6)
infective endocarditis (I33.0)
viral hepatitis (B15-B19)
Excludes1: Behçet's disease (M35.2)
direct infections of joints in diseases classified elsewhere (M01.0-)
postinfectious arthritis (in):
meningococcal (A39.84)
mumps (B26.85)
rubella (B06.82)
syphilis (late) (A52.77)
rheumatic fever (I00)
tabetic arthropathy [Charcot's] (A52.16)

M02.0 Arthropathy following intestinal bypass

M02.00 Arthropathy following intestinal bypass, unspecified site

M02.01 Arthropathy following intestinal bypass, shoulder

M02.011 Arthropathy following intestinal bypass, right shoulder

M02.012 Arthropathy following intestinal bypass, left shoulder

M02.019 Arthropathy following intestinal bypass, unspecified shoulder

M02.02 Arthropathy following intestinal bypass, elbow

M02.021 Arthropathy following intestinal bypass, right elbow

M02.022 Arthropathy following intestinal bypass, left elbow

M02.029 Arthropathy following intestinal bypass, unspecified elbow

M02.03 Arthropathy following intestinal bypass, wrist
Arthropathy following intestinal bypass, carpal bones

M02.031 Arthropathy following intestinal bypass, right wrist

M02.032 Arthropathy following intestinal bypass, left wrist

M02.039 Arthropathy following intestinal bypass, unspecified wrist

M02.04 Arthropathy following intestinal bypass, hand
Arthropathy following intestinal bypass, metacarpals and phalanges

M02.041 Arthropathy following intestinal bypass, right hand

M02.042 Arthropathy following intestinal bypass, left hand

M02.049 Arthropathy following intestinal bypass, unspecified hand

M02.05 Arthropathy following intestinal bypass, hip

M02.051 Arthropathy following intestinal bypass, right hip

M02.052 Arthropathy following intestinal bypass, left hip

M02.059 Arthropathy following intestinal bypass, unspecified hip

M02.06 Arthropathy following intestinal bypass, knee

M02.061 Arthropathy following intestinal bypass, right knee

M02.062 Arthropathy following intestinal bypass, left knee

M02.069 Arthropathy following intestinal bypass, unspecified knee

M02.07 Arthropathy following intestinal bypass, ankle and foot
Arthropathy following intestinal bypass, tarsus, metatarsus and phalanges

M02.071 Arthropathy following intestinal bypass, right ankle and foot

M02.072 Arthropathy following intestinal bypass, left ankle and foot

M02.079 Arthropathy following intestinal bypass, unspecified ankle and foot

M02.08 Arthropathy following intestinal bypass, vertebrae

M02.09 Arthropathy following intestinal bypass, multiple sites

M02.1 Postdysenteric arthropathy

M02.10 Postdysenteric arthropathy, unspecified site

M02.11 Postdysenteric arthropathy, shoulder

M02.111 Postdysenteric arthropathy, right shoulder

M02.112 Postdysenteric arthropathy, left shoulder

M02.119 Postdysenteric arthropathy, unspecified shoulder

M02.12 Postdysenteric arthropathy, elbow

M02.121 Postdysenteric arthropathy, right elbow

M02.122 Postdysenteric arthropathy, left elbow

M02.129 Postdysenteric arthropathy, unspecified elbow

M02.13 Postdysenteric arthropathy, wrist
Postdysenteric arthropathy, carpal bones

M02.131 Postdysenteric arthropathy, right wrist

M02.132 Postdysenteric arthropathy, left wrist

M02.139 Postdysenteric arthropathy, unspecified wrist

M02.14 Postdysenteric arthropathy, hand
Postdysenteric arthropathy, metacarpus and phalanges

M02.141 Postdysenteric arthropathy, right hand

M02.142 Postdysenteric arthropathy, left hand

M02.149 Postdysenteric arthropathy, unspecified hand

M02.15 Postdysenteric arthropathy, hip

M02.151 Postdysenteric arthropathy, right hip

M02.152 Postdysenteric arthropathy, left hip

M02.159   Postdysenteric arthropathy, unspecified hip

M02.16   Postdysenteric arthropathy, knee

    M02.161   Postdysenteric arthropathy, right knee

    M02.162   Postdysenteric arthropathy, left knee

    M02.169   Postdysenteric arthropathy, unspecified knee

M02.17   Postdysenteric arthropathy, ankle and foot

    Postdysenteric arthropathy, tarsus, metatarsus and phalanges

    M02.171   Postdysenteric arthropathy, right ankle and foot

    M02.172   Postdysenteric arthropathy, left ankle and foot

    M02.179   Postdysenteric arthropathy, unspecified ankle and foot

M02.18   Postdysenteric arthropathy, vertebrae

M02.19   Postdysenteric arthropathy, multiple sites

M02.2   Postimmunization arthropathy

M02.20   Postimmunization arthropathy, unspecified site

M02.21   Postimmunization arthropathy, shoulder

    M02.211   Postimmunization arthropathy, right shoulder

    M02.212   Postimmunization arthropathy, left shoulder

    M02.219   Postimmunization arthropathy, unspecified shoulder

M02.22   Postimmunization arthropathy, elbow

    M02.221   Postimmunization arthropathy, right elbow

    M02.222   Postimmunization arthropathy, left elbow

    M02.229   Postimmunization arthropathy, unspecified elbow

M02.23   Postimmunization arthropathy, wrist

    Postimmunization arthropathy, carpal bones

    M02.231   Postimmunization arthropathy, right wrist

    M02.232   Postimmunization arthropathy, left wrist

    M02.239   Postimmunization arthropathy, unspecified wrist

M02.24   Postimmunization arthropathy, hand

    Postimmunization arthropathy, metacarpus and phalanges

    M02.241   Postimmunization arthropathy, right hand

    M02.242   Postimmunization arthropathy, left hand

    M02.249   Postimmunization arthropathy, unspecified hand

M02.25   Postimmunization arthropathy, hip

    M02.251   Postimmunization arthropathy, right hip

    M02.252   Postimmunization arthropathy, left hip

    M02.259   Postimmunization arthropathy, unspecified hip

M02.26   Postimmunization arthropathy, knee

    M02.261   Postimmunization arthropathy, right knee

    M02.262   Postimmunization arthropathy, left knee

    M02.269   Postimmunization arthropathy, unspecified knee

M02.27   Postimmunization arthropathy, ankle and foot

    Postimmunization arthropathy, tarsus, metatarsus and phalanges

    M02.271   Postimmunization arthropathy, right ankle and foot

    M02.272   Postimmunization arthropathy, left ankle and foot

    M02.279   Postimmunization arthropathy, unspecified ankle and foot

M02.28   Postimmunization arthropathy, vertebrae

M02.29   Postimmunization arthropathy, multiple sites

M02.3   Reiter's disease

M02.30   Reiter's disease, unspecified site

M02.31   Reiter's disease, shoulder

    M02.311   Reiter's disease, right shoulder

    M02.312   Reiter's disease, left shoulder

    M02.319   Reiter's disease, unspecified shoulder

M02.32   Reiter's disease, elbow

    M02.321   Reiter's disease, right elbow

    M02.322   Reiter's disease, left elbow

    M02.329   Reiter's disease, unspecified elbow

M02.33   Reiter's disease, wrist

    Reiter's disease, carpal bones

    M02.331   Reiter's disease, right wrist

    M02.332   Reiter's disease, left wrist

    M02.339   Reiter's disease, unspecified wrist

M02.34   Reiter's disease, hand

    Reiter's disease, metacarpus and phalanges

    M02.341   Reiter's disease, right hand

    M02.342   Reiter's disease, left hand

    M02.349   Reiter's disease, unspecified hand

M02.35   Reiter's disease, hip

    M02.351   Reiter's disease, right hip

    M02.352   Reiter's disease, left hip

    M02.359   Reiter's disease, unspecified hip

M02.36   Reiter's disease, knee

    M02.361   Reiter's disease, right knee

    M02.362   Reiter's disease, left knee

    M02.369   Reiter's disease, unspecified knee

M02.37   Reiter's disease, ankle and foot

    Reiter's disease, tarsus, metatarsus and phalanges

    M02.371   Reiter's disease, right ankle and foot

    M02.372   Reiter's disease, left ankle and foot

    M02.379   Reiter's disease, unspecified ankle and foot

M02.38   Reiter's disease, vertebrae

M02.39   Reiter's disease, multiple sites

M02.8   Other reactive arthropathies

M02.80   Other reactive arthropathies, unspecified site

M02.81   Other reactive arthropathies, shoulder

    M02.811   Other reactive arthropathies, right shoulder

    M02.812   Other reactive arthropathies, left shoulder

    M02.819   Other reactive arthropathies, unspecified shoulder

M02.82   Other reactive arthropathies, elbow

    M02.821   Other reactive arthropathies, right elbow

    M02.822   Other reactive arthropathies, left elbow

    M02.829   Other reactive arthropathies, unspecified elbow

M02.83   Other reactive arthropathies, wrist

    Other reactive arthropathies, carpal bones

    M02.831   Other reactive arthropathies, right wrist

    M02.832   Other reactive arthropathies, left wrist

    M02.839   Other reactive arthropathies, unspecified wrist

M02.84   Other reactive arthropathies, hand

    Other reactive arthropathies, metacarpus and phalanges

    M02.841   Other reactive arthropathies, right hand

    M02.842   Other reactive arthropathies, left hand

    M02.849   Other reactive arthropathies, unspecified hand

M02.85   Other reactive arthropathies, hip

    M02.851   Other reactive arthropathies, right hip

    M02.852   Other reactive arthropathies, left hip

    M02.859   Other reactive arthropathies, unspecified hip

M02.86   Other reactive arthropathies, knee

    M02.861   Other reactive arthropathies, right knee

    M02.862   Other reactive arthropathies, left knee

    M02.869   Other reactive arthropathies, unspecified knee

M02.87   Other reactive arthropathies, ankle and foot

    Other reactive arthropathies, tarsus, metatarsus and phalanges

    M02.871   Other reactive arthropathies, right ankle and foot

    M02.872   Other reactive arthropathies, left ankle and foot

    M02.879   Other reactive arthropathies, unspecified ankle and foot

M02.88   Other reactive arthropathies, vertebrae

M02.89   Other reactive arthropathies, multiple sites

M02.9 Reactive arthropathy, unspecified

INFLAMMATORY POLYARTHROPATHIES (M05–M14)

M05 Rheumatoid arthritis with rheumatoid factor
Excludes1:   juvenile rheumatoid arthritis (M08.-)
 rheumatic fever (I00)
 rheumatoid arthritis of spine (M45.-)

M05.0 Felty's syndrome
 Rheumatoid arthritis with splenoadenomegaly and leukopenia

M05.00 Felty's syndrome, unspecified site

M05.01 Felty's syndrome, shoulder

M05.011 Felty's syndrome, right shoulder

M05.012 Felty's syndrome, left shoulder

M05.019 Felty's syndrome, unspecified shoulder

M05.02 Felty's syndrome, elbow

M05.021 Felty's syndrome, right elbow

M05.022 Felty's syndrome, left elbow

M05.029 Felty's syndrome, unspecified elbow

M05.03 Felty's syndrome, wrist
 Felty's syndrome, carpal bones

M05.031 Felty's syndrome, right wrist

M05.032 Felty's syndrome, left wrist

M05.039 Felty's syndrome, unspecified wrist

M05.04 Felty's syndrome, hand
 Felty's syndrome, metacarpus and phalanges

M05.041 Felty's syndrome, right hand

M05.042 Felty's syndrome, left hand

M05.049 Felty's syndrome, unspecified hand

M05.05 Felty's syndrome, hip

M05.051 Felty's syndrome, right hip

M05.052 Felty's syndrome, left hip

M05.059 Felty's syndrome, unspecified hip

M05.06 Felty's syndrome, knee

M05.061 Felty's syndrome, right knee

M05.062 Felty's syndrome, left knee

M05.069 Felty's syndrome, unspecified knee

M05.07 Felty's syndrome, ankle and foot
 Felty's syndrome, tarsus, metatarsus and phalanges

M05.071 Felty's syndrome, right ankle and foot

M05.072 Felty's syndrome, left ankle and foot

M05.079 Felty's syndrome, unspecified ankle and foot

M05.09 Felty's syndrome, multiple sites

M05.1 Rheumatoid lung disease with rheumatoid arthritis

M05.10 Rheumatoid lung disease with rheumatoid arthritis of unspecified site

M05.11 Rheumatoid lung disease with rheumatoid arthritis of shoulder

M05.111 Rheumatoid lung disease with rheumatoid arthritis of right shoulder

M05.112 Rheumatoid lung disease with rheumatoid arthritis of left shoulder

M05.119 Rheumatoid lung disease with rheumatoid arthritis of unspecified shoulder

M05.12 Rheumatoid lung disease with rheumatoid arthritis of elbow

M05.121 Rheumatoid lung disease with rheumatoid arthritis of right elbow

M05.122 Rheumatoid lung disease with rheumatoid arthritis of left elbow

M05.129 Rheumatoid lung disease with rheumatoid arthritis of unspecified elbow

M05.13 Rheumatoid lung disease with rheumatoid arthritis of wrist
 Rheumatoid lung disease with rheumatoid arthritis, carpal bones

M05.131 Rheumatoid lung disease with rheumatoid arthritis of right wrist

M05.132 Rheumatoid lung disease with rheumatoid arthritis of left wrist

M05.139 Rheumatoid lung disease with rheumatoid arthritis of unspecified wrist

M05.14 Rheumatoid lung disease with rheumatoid arthritis of hand
 Rheumatoid lung disease with rheumatoid arthritis, metacarpus and phalanges

M05.141 Rheumatoid lung disease with rheumatoid arthritis of right hand

M05.142 Rheumatoid lung disease with rheumatoid arthritis of left hand

M05.149 Rheumatoid lung disease with rheumatoid arthritis of unspecified hand

M05.15 Rheumatoid lung disease with rheumatoid arthritis of hip

M05.151 Rheumatoid lung disease with rheumatoid arthritis of right hip

M05.152 Rheumatoid lung disease with rheumatoid arthritis of left hip

M05.159 Rheumatoid lung disease with rheumatoid arthritis of unspecified hip

M05.16 Rheumatoid lung disease with rheumatoid arthritis of knee

M05.161 Rheumatoid lung disease with rheumatoid arthritis of right knee

M05.162 Rheumatoid lung disease with rheumatoid arthritis of left knee

M05.169 Rheumatoid lung disease with rheumatoid arthritis of unspecified knee

M05.17 Rheumatoid lung disease with rheumatoid arthritis of ankle and foot
 Rheumatoid lung disease with rheumatoid arthritis, tarsus, metatarsus and phalanges

M05.171 Rheumatoid lung disease with rheumatoid arthritis of right ankle and foot

M05.172 Rheumatoid lung disease with rheumatoid arthritis of left ankle and foot

M05.179 Rheumatoid lung disease with rheumatoid arthritis of unspecified ankle and foot

M05.19 Rheumatoid lung disease with rheumatoid arthritis of multiple sites

M05.2 Rheumatoid vasculitis with rheumatoid arthritis

M05.20 Rheumatoid vasculitis with rheumatoid arthritis of unspecified site

M05.21 Rheumatoid vasculitis with rheumatoid arthritis of shoulder

M05.211 Rheumatoid vasculitis with rheumatoid arthritis of right shoulder

M05.212 Rheumatoid vasculitis with rheumatoid arthritis of left shoulder

M05.219 Rheumatoid vasculitis with rheumatoid arthritis of unspecified shoulder

M05.22 Rheumatoid vasculitis with rheumatoid arthritis of elbow

M05.221 Rheumatoid vasculitis with rheumatoid arthritis of right elbow

M05.222 Rheumatoid vasculitis with rheumatoid arthritis of left elbow

M05.229 Rheumatoid vasculitis with rheumatoid arthritis of unspecified elbow

M05.23 Rheumatoid vasculitis with rheumatoid arthritis of wrist
 Rheumatoid vasculitis with rheumatoid arthritis, carpal bones

M05.231 Rheumatoid vasculitis with rheumatoid arthritis of right wrist

M05.232 Rheumatoid vasculitis with rheumatoid arthritis of left wrist

M05.239 Rheumatoid vasculitis with rheumatoid arthritis of unspecified wrist

M05.24 Rheumatoid vasculitis with rheumatoid arthritis of hand
 Rheumatoid vasculitis with rheumatoid arthritis, metacarpus and phalanges

M05.241   Rheumatoid vasculitis with rheumatoid arthritis of right hand

M05.242   Rheumatoid vasculitis with rheumatoid arthritis of left hand

M05.249   Rheumatoid vasculitis with rheumatoid arthritis of unspecified hand

M05.25   Rheumatoid vasculitis with rheumatoid arthritis of hip

    M05.251   Rheumatoid vasculitis with rheumatoid arthritis of right hip

    M05.252   Rheumatoid vasculitis with rheumatoid arthritis of left hip

    M05.259   Rheumatoid vasculitis with rheumatoid arthritis of unspecified hip

M05.26   Rheumatoid vasculitis with rheumatoid arthritis of knee

    M05.261   Rheumatoid vasculitis with rheumatoid arthritis of right knee

    M05.262   Rheumatoid vasculitis with rheumatoid arthritis of left knee

    M05.269   Rheumatoid vasculitis with rheumatoid arthritis of unspecified knee

M05.27   Rheumatoid vasculitis with rheumatoid arthritis of ankle and foot

    Rheumatoid vasculitis with rheumatoid arthritis, tarsus, metatarsus and phalanges

    M05.271   Rheumatoid vasculitis with rheumatoid arthritis of right ankle and foot

    M05.272   Rheumatoid vasculitis with rheumatoid arthritis of left ankle and foot

    M05.279   Rheumatoid vasculitis with rheumatoid arthritis of unspecified ankle and foot

M05.29   Rheumatoid vasculitis with rheumatoid arthritis of multiple sites

M05.3   Rheumatoid heart disease with rheumatoid arthritis

    Rheumatoid carditis
    Rheumatoid endocarditis
    Rheumatoid myocarditis
    Rheumatoid pericarditis

M05.30   Rheumatoid heart disease with rheumatoid arthritis of unspecified site

M05.31   Rheumatoid heart disease with rheumatoid arthritis of shoulder

    M05.311   Rheumatoid heart disease with rheumatoid arthritis of right shoulder

    M05.312   Rheumatoid heart disease with rheumatoid arthritis of left shoulder

    M05.319   Rheumatoid heart disease with rheumatoid arthritis of unspecified shoulder

M05.32   Rheumatoid heart disease with rheumatoid arthritis of elbow

    M05.321   Rheumatoid heart disease with rheumatoid arthritis of right elbow

    M05.322   Rheumatoid heart disease with rheumatoid arthritis of left elbow

    M05.329   Rheumatoid heart disease with rheumatoid arthritis of unspecified elbow

M05.33   Rheumatoid heart disease with rheumatoid arthritis of wrist

    Rheumatoid heart disease with rheumatoid arthritis, carpal bones

    M05.331   Rheumatoid heart disease with rheumatoid arthritis of right wrist

    M05.332   Rheumatoid heart disease with rheumatoid arthritis of left wrist

    M05.339   Rheumatoid heart disease with rheumatoid arthritis of unspecified wrist

M05.34   Rheumatoid heart disease with rheumatoid arthritis of hand

    Rheumatoid heart disease with rheumatoid arthritis, metacarpus and phalanges

    M05.341   Rheumatoid heart disease with rheumatoid arthritis of right hand

M05.342   Rheumatoid heart disease with rheumatoid arthritis of left hand

M05.349   Rheumatoid heart disease with rheumatoid arthritis of unspecified hand

M05.35   Rheumatoid heart disease with rheumatoid arthritis of hip

    M05.351   Rheumatoid heart disease with rheumatoid arthritis of right hip

    M05.352   Rheumatoid heart disease with rheumatoid arthritis of left hip

    M05.359   Rheumatoid heart disease with rheumatoid arthritis of unspecified hip

M05.36   Rheumatoid heart disease with rheumatoid arthritis of knee

    M05.361   Rheumatoid heart disease with rheumatoid arthritis of right knee

    M05.362   Rheumatoid heart disease with rheumatoid arthritis of left knee

    M05.369   Rheumatoid heart disease with rheumatoid arthritis of unspecified knee

M05.37   Rheumatoid heart disease with rheumatoid arthritis of ankle and foot

    Rheumatoid heart disease with rheumatoid arthritis, tarsus, metatarsus and phalanges

    M05.371   Rheumatoid heart disease with rheumatoid arthritis of right ankle and foot

    M05.372   Rheumatoid heart disease with rheumatoid arthritis of left ankle and foot

    M05.379   Rheumatoid heart disease with rheumatoid arthritis of unspecified ankle and foot

M05.39   Rheumatoid heart disease with rheumatoid arthritis of multiple sites

M05.4   Rheumatoid myopathy with rheumatoid arthritis

M05.40   Rheumatoid myopathy with rheumatoid arthritis of unspecified site

M05.41   Rheumatoid myopathy with rheumatoid arthritis of shoulder

    M05.411   Rheumatoid myopathy with rheumatoid arthritis of right shoulder

    M05.412   Rheumatoid myopathy with rheumatoid arthritis of left shoulder

    M05.419   Rheumatoid myopathy with rheumatoid arthritis of unspecified shoulder

M05.42   Rheumatoid myopathy with rheumatoid arthritis of elbow

    M05.421   Rheumatoid myopathy with rheumatoid arthritis of right elbow

    M05.422   Rheumatoid myopathy with rheumatoid arthritis of left elbow

    M05.429   Rheumatoid myopathy with rheumatoid arthritis of unspecified elbow

M05.43   Rheumatoid myopathy with rheumatoid arthritis of wrist

    Rheumatoid myopathy with rheumatoid arthritis, carpal bones

    M05.431   Rheumatoid myopathy with rheumatoid arthritis of right wrist

    M05.432   Rheumatoid myopathy with rheumatoid arthritis of left wrist

    M05.439   Rheumatoid myopathy with rheumatoid arthritis of unspecified wrist

M05.44   Rheumatoid myopathy with rheumatoid arthritis of hand

    Rheumatoid myopathy with rheumatoid arthritis, metacarpus and phalanges

    M05.441   Rheumatoid myopathy with rheumatoid arthritis of right hand

    M05.442   Rheumatoid myopathy with rheumatoid arthritis of left hand

    M05.449   Rheumatoid myopathy with rheumatoid arthritis of unspecified hand

M05.45   Rheumatoid myopathy with rheumatoid arthritis of hip

M05.451　Rheumatoid myopathy with rheumatoid arthritis of right hip

M05.452　Rheumatoid myopathy with rheumatoid arthritis of left hip

M05.459　Rheumatoid myopathy with rheumatoid arthritis of unspecified hip

M05.46　Rheumatoid myopathy with rheumatoid arthritis of knee

M05.461　Rheumatoid myopathy with rheumatoid arthritis of right knee

M05.462　Rheumatoid myopathy with rheumatoid arthritis of left knee

M05.469　Rheumatoid myopathy with rheumatoid arthritis of unspecified knee

M05.47　Rheumatoid myopathy with rheumatoid arthritis of ankle and foot
Rheumatoid myopathy with rheumatoid arthritis, tarsus, metatarsus and phalanges

M05.471　Rheumatoid myopathy with rheumatoid arthritis of right ankle and foot

M05.472　Rheumatoid myopathy with rheumatoid arthritis of left ankle and foot

M05.479　Rheumatoid myopathy with rheumatoid arthritis of unspecified ankle and foot

M05.49　Rheumatoid myopathy with rheumatoid arthritis of multiple sites

M05.5　Rheumatoid polyneuropathy with rheumatoid arthritis

M05.50　Rheumatoid polyneuropathy with rheumatoid arthritis of unspecified site

M05.51　Rheumatoid polyneuropathy with rheumatoid arthritis of shoulder

M05.511　Rheumatoid polyneuropathy with rheumatoid arthritis of right shoulder

M05.512　Rheumatoid polyneuropathy with rheumatoid arthritis of left shoulder

M05.519　Rheumatoid polyneuropathy with rheumatoid arthritis of unspecified shoulder

M05.52　Rheumatoid polyneuropathy with rheumatoid arthritis of elbow

M05.521　Rheumatoid polyneuropathy with rheumatoid arthritis of right elbow

M05.522　Rheumatoid polyneuropathy with rheumatoid arthritis of left elbow

M05.529　Rheumatoid polyneuropathy with rheumatoid arthritis of unspecified elbow

M05.53　Rheumatoid polyneuropathy with rheumatoid arthritis of wrist
Rheumatoid polyneuropathy with rheumatoid arthritis, carpal bones

M05.531　Rheumatoid polyneuropathy with rheumatoid arthritis of right wrist

M05.532　Rheumatoid polyneuropathy with rheumatoid arthritis of left wrist

M05.539　Rheumatoid polyneuropathy with rheumatoid arthritis of unspecified wrist

M05.54　Rheumatoid polyneuropathy with rheumatoid arthritis of hand
Rheumatoid polyneuropathy with rheumatoid arthritis, metacarpus and phalanges

M05.541　Rheumatoid polyneuropathy with rheumatoid arthritis of right hand

M05.542　Rheumatoid polyneuropathy with rheumatoid arthritis of left hand

M05.549　Rheumatoid polyneuropathy with rheumatoid arthritis of unspecified hand

M05.55　Rheumatoid polyneuropathy with rheumatoid arthritis of hip

M05.551　Rheumatoid polyneuropathy with rheumatoid arthritis of right hip

M05.552　Rheumatoid polyneuropathy with rheumatoid arthritis of left hip

M05.559　Rheumatoid polyneuropathy with rheumatoid arthritis of unspecified hip

M05.56　Rheumatoid polyneuropathy with rheumatoid arthritis of knee

M05.561　Rheumatoid polyneuropathy with rheumatoid arthritis of right knee

M05.562　Rheumatoid polyneuropathy with rheumatoid arthritis of left knee

M05.569　Rheumatoid polyneuropathy with rheumatoid arthritis of unspecified knee

M05.57　Rheumatoid polyneuropathy with rheumatoid arthritis of ankle and foot
Rheumatoid polyneuropathy with rheumatoid arthritis, tarsus, metatarsus and phalanges

M05.571　Rheumatoid polyneuropathy with rheumatoid arthritis of right ankle and foot

M05.572　Rheumatoid polyneuropathy with rheumatoid arthritis of left ankle and foot

M05.579　Rheumatoid polyneuropathy with rheumatoid arthritis of unspecified ankle and foot

M05.59　Rheumatoid polyneuropathy with rheumatoid arthritis of multiple sites

M05.6　Rheumatoid arthritis with involvement of other organs and systems

M05.60　Rheumatoid arthritis of unspecified site with involvement of other organs and systems

M05.61　Rheumatoid arthritis of shoulder with involvement of other organs and systems

M05.611　Rheumatoid arthritis of right shoulder with involvement of other organs and systems

M05.612　Rheumatoid arthritis of left shoulder with involvement of other organs and systems

M05.619　Rheumatoid arthritis of unspecified shoulder with involvement of other organs and systems

M05.62　Rheumatoid arthritis of elbow with involvement of other organs and systems

M05.621　Rheumatoid arthritis of right elbow with involvement of other organs and systems

M05.622　Rheumatoid arthritis of left elbow with involvement of other organs and systems

M05.629　Rheumatoid arthritis of unspecified elbow with involvement of other organs and systems

M05.63　Rheumatoid arthritis of wrist with involvement of other organs and systems
Rheumatoid arthritis of carpal bones with involvement of other organs and systems

M05.631　Rheumatoid arthritis of right wrist with involvement of other organs and systems

M05.632　Rheumatoid arthritis of left wrist with involvement of other organs and systems

M05.639　Rheumatoid arthritis of unspecified wrist with involvement of other organs and systems

M05.64　Rheumatoid arthritis of hand with involvement of other organs and systems
Rheumatoid arthritis of metacarpus and phalanges with involvement of other organs and systems

M05.641　Rheumatoid arthritis of right hand with involvement of other organs and systems

M05.642　Rheumatoid arthritis of left hand with involvement of other organs and systems

M05.649　Rheumatoid arthritis of unspecified hand with involvement of other organs and systems

M05.65　Rheumatoid arthritis of hip with involvement of other organs and systems

M05.651　Rheumatoid arthritis of right hip with involvement of other organs and systems

M05.652　Rheumatoid arthritis of left hip with involvement of other organs and systems

M05.659　Rheumatoid arthritis of unspecified hip with involvement of other organs and systems

M05.66　Rheumatoid arthritis of knee with involvement of other organs and systems

M05.661　Rheumatoid arthritis of right knee with involvement of other organs and systems

M05.662   Rheumatoid arthritis of left knee with involvement of other organs and systems

M05.669   Rheumatoid arthritis of unspecified knee with involvement of other organs and systems

M05.67   Rheumatoid arthritis of ankle and foot with involvement of other organs and systems

   Rheumatoid arthritis of tarsus, metatarsus and phalanges with involvement of other organs and systems

M05.671   Rheumatoid arthritis of right ankle and foot with involvement of other organs and systems

M05.672   Rheumatoid arthritis of left ankle and foot with involvement of other organs and systems

M05.679   Rheumatoid arthritis of unspecified ankle and foot with involvement of other organs and systems

M05.69   Rheumatoid arthritis of multiple sites with involvement of other organs and systems

M05.7   Rheumatoid arthritis with rheumatoid factor without organ or systems involvement

M05.70   Rheumatoid arthritis with rheumatoid factor of unspecified site without organ or systems involvement

M05.71   Rheumatoid arthritis with rheumatoid factor of shoulder without organ or systems involvement

M05.711   Rheumatoid arthritis with rheumatoid factor of right shoulder without organ or systems involvement

M05.712   Rheumatoid arthritis with rheumatoid factor of left shoulder without organ or systems involvement

M05.719   Rheumatoid arthritis with rheumatoid factor of unspecified shoulder without organ or systems involvement

M05.72   Rheumatoid arthritis with rheumatoid factor of elbow without organ or systems involvement

M05.721   Rheumatoid arthritis with rheumatoid factor of right elbow without organ or systems involvement

M05.722   Rheumatoid arthritis with rheumatoid factor of left elbow without organ or systems involvement

M05.729   Rheumatoid arthritis with rheumatoid factor of unspecified elbow without organ or systems involvement

M05.73   Rheumatoid arthritis with rheumatoid factor of wrist without organ or systems involvement

M05.731   Rheumatoid arthritis with rheumatoid factor of right wrist without organ or systems involvement

M05.732   Rheumatoid arthritis with rheumatoid factor of left wrist without organ or systems involvement

M05.739   Rheumatoid arthritis with rheumatoid factor of unspecified wrist without organ or systems involvement

M05.74   Rheumatoid arthritis with rheumatoid factor of hand without organ or systems involvement

M05.741   Rheumatoid arthritis with rheumatoid factor of right hand without organ or systems involvement

M05.742   Rheumatoid arthritis with rheumatoid factor of left hand without organ or systems involvement

M05.749   Rheumatoid arthritis with rheumatoid factor of unspecified hand without organ or systems involvement

M05.75   Rheumatoid arthritis with rheumatoid factor of hip without organ or systems involvement

M05.751   Rheumatoid arthritis with rheumatoid factor of right hip without organ or systems involvement

M05.752   Rheumatoid arthritis with rheumatoid factor of left hip without organ or systems involvement

M05.759   Rheumatoid arthritis with rheumatoid factor of unspecified hip without organ or systems involvement

M05.76   Rheumatoid arthritis with rheumatoid factor of knee without organ or systems involvement

M05.761   Rheumatoid arthritis with rheumatoid factor of right knee without organ or systems involvement

M05.762   Rheumatoid arthritis with rheumatoid factor of left knee without organ or systems involvement

M05.769   Rheumatoid arthritis with rheumatoid factor of unspecified knee without organ or systems involvement

M05.77   Rheumatoid arthritis with rheumatoid factor of ankle and foot without organ or systems involvement

M05.771   Rheumatoid arthritis with rheumatoid factor of right ankle and foot without organ or systems involvement

M05.772   Rheumatoid arthritis with rheumatoid factor of left ankle and foot without organ or systems involvement

M05.779   Rheumatoid arthritis with rheumatoid factor of unspecified ankle and foot without organ or systems involvement

M05.79   Rheumatoid arthritis with rheumatoid factor of multiple sites without organ or systems involvement

M05.8   Other rheumatoid arthritis with rheumatoid factor

M05.80   Other rheumatoid arthritis with rheumatoid factor of unspecified site

M05.81   Other rheumatoid arthritis with rheumatoid factor of shoulder

M05.811   Other rheumatoid arthritis with rheumatoid factor of right shoulder

M05.812   Other rheumatoid arthritis with rheumatoid factor of left shoulder

M05.819   Other rheumatoid arthritis with rheumatoid factor of unspecified shoulder

M05.82   Other rheumatoid arthritis with rheumatoid factor of elbow

M05.821   Other rheumatoid arthritis with rheumatoid factor of right elbow

M05.822   Other rheumatoid arthritis with rheumatoid factor of left elbow

M05.829   Other rheumatoid arthritis with rheumatoid factor of unspecified elbow

M05.83   Other rheumatoid arthritis with rheumatoid factor of wrist

M05.831   Other rheumatoid arthritis with rheumatoid factor of right wrist

M05.832   Other rheumatoid arthritis with rheumatoid factor of left wrist

M05.839   Other rheumatoid arthritis with rheumatoid factor of unspecified wrist

M05.84   Other rheumatoid arthritis with rheumatoid factor of hand

M05.841   Other rheumatoid arthritis with rheumatoid factor of right hand

M05.842   Other rheumatoid arthritis with rheumatoid factor of left hand

M05.849   Other rheumatoid arthritis with rheumatoid factor of unspecified hand

M05.85   Other rheumatoid arthritis with rheumatoid factor of hip

M05.851   Other rheumatoid arthritis with rheumatoid factor of right hip

M05.852   Other rheumatoid arthritis with rheumatoid factor of left hip

M05.859   Other rheumatoid arthritis with rheumatoid factor of unspecified hip

M05.86   Other rheumatoid arthritis with rheumatoid factor of knee

M05.861   Other rheumatoid arthritis with rheumatoid factor of right knee

M05.862   Other rheumatoid arthritis with rheumatoid factor of left knee

M05.869   Other rheumatoid arthritis with rheumatoid factor of unspecified knee

M05.87   Other rheumatoid arthritis with rheumatoid factor of ankle and foot

M05.871   Other rheumatoid arthritis with rheumatoid factor of right ankle and foot

M05.872   Other rheumatoid arthritis with rheumatoid factor of left ankle and foot

M05.879   Other rheumatoid arthritis with rheumatoid factor of unspecified ankle and foot

M05.89   Other rheumatoid arthritis with rheumatoid factor of multiple sites

M05.9   Rheumatoid arthritis with rheumatoid factor, unspecified

M06 Other rheumatoid arthritis

M06.0   Rheumatoid arthritis without rheumatoid factor

M06.00   Rheumatoid arthritis without rheumatoid factor, unspecified site

M06.01   Rheumatoid arthritis without rheumatoid factor, shoulder

M06.011   Rheumatoid arthritis without rheumatoid factor, right shoulder

M06.012   Rheumatoid arthritis without rheumatoid factor, left shoulder

M06.019   Rheumatoid arthritis without rheumatoid factor, unspecified shoulder

M06.02   Rheumatoid arthritis without rheumatoid factor, elbow

M06.021   Rheumatoid arthritis without rheumatoid factor, right elbow

M06.022   Rheumatoid arthritis without rheumatoid factor, left elbow

M06.029   Rheumatoid arthritis without rheumatoid factor, unspecified elbow

M06.03   Rheumatoid arthritis without rheumatoid factor, wrist

M06.031   Rheumatoid arthritis without rheumatoid factor, right wrist

M06.032   Rheumatoid arthritis without rheumatoid factor, left wrist

M06.039   Rheumatoid arthritis without rheumatoid factor, unspecified wrist

M06.04   Rheumatoid arthritis without rheumatoid factor, hand

M06.041   Rheumatoid arthritis without rheumatoid factor, right hand

M06.042   Rheumatoid arthritis without rheumatoid factor, left hand

M06.049   Rheumatoid arthritis without rheumatoid factor, unspecified hand

M06.05   Rheumatoid arthritis without rheumatoid factor, hip

M06.051   Rheumatoid arthritis without rheumatoid factor, right hip

M06.052   Rheumatoid arthritis without rheumatoid factor, left hip

M06.059   Rheumatoid arthritis without rheumatoid factor, unspecified hip

M06.06   Rheumatoid arthritis without rheumatoid factor, knee

M06.061   Rheumatoid arthritis without rheumatoid factor, right knee

M06.062   Rheumatoid arthritis without rheumatoid factor, left knee

M06.069   Rheumatoid arthritis without rheumatoid factor, unspecified knee

M06.07   Rheumatoid arthritis without rheumatoid factor, ankle and foot

M06.071   Rheumatoid arthritis without rheumatoid factor, right ankle and foot

M06.072   Rheumatoid arthritis without rheumatoid factor, left ankle and foot

M06.079   Rheumatoid arthritis without rheumatoid factor, unspecified ankle and foot

M06.08   Rheumatoid arthritis without rheumatoid factor, vertebrae

M06.09   Rheumatoid arthritis without rheumatoid factor, multiple sites

M06.1   Adult-onset Still's disease

    Excludes1:   Still's disease NOS (M08.2-)

M06.2   Rheumatoid bursitis

M06.20   Rheumatoid bursitis, unspecified site

M06.21   Rheumatoid bursitis, shoulder

M06.211   Rheumatoid bursitis, right shoulder

M06.212   Rheumatoid bursitis, left shoulder

M06.219   Rheumatoid bursitis, unspecified shoulder

M06.22   Rheumatoid bursitis, elbow

M06.221   Rheumatoid bursitis, right elbow

M06.222   Rheumatoid bursitis, left elbow

M06.229   Rheumatoid bursitis, unspecified elbow

M06.23   Rheumatoid bursitis, wrist

M06.231   Rheumatoid bursitis, right wrist

M06.232   Rheumatoid bursitis, left wrist

M06.239   Rheumatoid bursitis, unspecified wrist

M06.24   Rheumatoid bursitis, hand

M06.241   Rheumatoid bursitis, right hand

M06.242   Rheumatoid bursitis, left hand

M06.249   Rheumatoid bursitis, unspecified hand

M06.25   Rheumatoid bursitis, hip

M06.251   Rheumatoid bursitis, right hip

M06.252   Rheumatoid bursitis, left hip

M06.259   Rheumatoid bursitis, unspecified hip

M06.26   Rheumatoid bursitis, knee

M06.261   Rheumatoid bursitis, right knee

M06.262   Rheumatoid bursitis, left knee

M06.269   Rheumatoid bursitis, unspecified knee

M06.27   Rheumatoid bursitis, ankle and foot

M06.271   Rheumatoid bursitis, right ankle and foot

M06.272   Rheumatoid bursitis, left ankle and foot

M06.279   Rheumatoid bursitis, unspecified ankle and foot

M06.28   Rheumatoid bursitis, vertebrae

M06.29   Rheumatoid bursitis, multiple sites

M06.3   Rheumatoid nodule

M06.30   Rheumatoid nodule, unspecified site

M06.31   Rheumatoid nodule, shoulder

M06.311   Rheumatoid nodule, right shoulder

M06.312   Rheumatoid nodule, left shoulder

M06.319   Rheumatoid nodule, unspecified shoulder

M06.32   Rheumatoid nodule, elbow

M06.321   Rheumatoid nodule, right elbow

M06.322   Rheumatoid nodule, left elbow

M06.329   Rheumatoid nodule, unspecified elbow

M06.33   Rheumatoid nodule, wrist

M06.331   Rheumatoid nodule, right wrist

M06.332   Rheumatoid nodule, left wrist

M06.339   Rheumatoid nodule, unspecified wrist

M06.34   Rheumatoid nodule, hand

M06.341   Rheumatoid nodule, right hand

M06.342   Rheumatoid nodule, left hand

M06.349   Rheumatoid nodule, unspecified hand

M06.35   Rheumatoid nodule, hip

M06.351   Rheumatoid nodule, right hip

M06.352   Rheumatoid nodule, left hip

M06.359   Rheumatoid nodule, unspecified hip

M06.36   Rheumatoid nodule, knee

M06.361   Rheumatoid nodule, right knee

M06.362   Rheumatoid nodule, left knee

M06.369   Rheumatoid nodule, unspecified knee

M06.37   Rheumatoid nodule, ankle and foot

     M06.371   Rheumatoid nodule, right ankle and foot
     M06.372   Rheumatoid nodule, left ankle and foot
     M06.379   Rheumatoid nodule, unspecified ankle and foot
   M06.38   Rheumatoid nodule, vertebrae
   M06.39   Rheumatoid nodule, multiple sites

M06.4   Inflammatory polyarthropathy
     Excludes1:   polyarthritis NOS (M13.0)

M06.8   Other specified rheumatoid arthritis
   M06.80   Other specified rheumatoid arthritis, unspecified site
   M06.81   Other specified rheumatoid arthritis, shoulder
     M06.811   Other specified rheumatoid arthritis, right shoulder
     M06.812   Other specified rheumatoid arthritis, left shoulder
     M06.819   Other specified rheumatoid arthritis, unspecified shoulder
   M06.82   Other specified rheumatoid arthritis, elbow
     M06.821   Other specified rheumatoid arthritis, right elbow
     M06.822   Other specified rheumatoid arthritis, left elbow
     M06.829   Other specified rheumatoid arthritis, unspecified elbow
   M06.83   Other specified rheumatoid arthritis, wrist
     M06.831   Other specified rheumatoid arthritis, right wrist
     M06.832   Other specified rheumatoid arthritis, left wrist
     M06.839   Other specified rheumatoid arthritis, unspecified wrist
   M06.84   Other specified rheumatoid arthritis, hand
     M06.841   Other specified rheumatoid arthritis, right hand
     M06.842   Other specified rheumatoid arthritis, left hand
     M06.849   Other specified rheumatoid arthritis, unspecified hand
   M06.85   Other specified rheumatoid arthritis, hip
     M06.851   Other specified rheumatoid arthritis, right hip
     M06.852   Other specified rheumatoid arthritis, left hip
     M06.859   Other specified rheumatoid arthritis, unspecified hip
   M06.86   Other specified rheumatoid arthritis, knee
     M06.861   Other specified rheumatoid arthritis, right knee
     M06.862   Other specified rheumatoid arthritis, left knee
     M06.869   Other specified rheumatoid arthritis, unspecified knee
   M06.87   Other specified rheumatoid arthritis, ankle and foot
     M06.871   Other specified rheumatoid arthritis, right ankle and foot
     M06.872   Other specified rheumatoid arthritis, left ankle and foot
     M06.879   Other specified rheumatoid arthritis, unspecified ankle and foot
   M06.88   Other specified rheumatoid arthritis, vertebrae
   M06.89   Other specified rheumatoid arthritis, multiple sites

M06.9   Rheumatoid arthritis, unspecified

M07   Enteropathic arthropathies
     Code also associated enteropathy, such as:
       regional enteritis [Crohn's disease] (K50.-)
       ulcerative colitis (K51.-)
     Excludes1:   juvenile enteropathic arthropathies (M09.0-)

M07.6   Enteropathic arthropathies
   M07.60   Enteropathic arthropathies, unspecified site
   M07.61   Enteropathic arthropathies, shoulder
     M07.611   Enteropathic arthropathies, right shoulder
     M07.612   Enteropathic arthropathies, left shoulder
     M07.619   Enteropathic arthropathies, unspecified shoulder
   M07.62   Enteropathic arthropathies, elbow

     M07.621   Enteropathic arthropathies, right elbow
     M07.622   Enteropathic arthropathies, left elbow
     M07.629   Enteropathic arthropathies, unspecified elbow
   M07.63   Enteropathic arthropathies, wrist
     M07.631   Enteropathic arthropathies, right wrist
     M07.632   Enteropathic arthropathies, left wrist
     M07.639   Enteropathic arthropathies, unspecified wrist
   M07.64   Enteropathic arthropathies, hand
     M07.641   Enteropathic arthropathies, right hand
     M07.642   Enteropathic arthropathies, left hand
     M07.649   Enteropathic arthropathies, unspecified hand
   M07.65   Enteropathic arthropathies, hip
     M07.651   Enteropathic arthropathies, right hip
     M07.652   Enteropathic arthropathies, left hip
     M07.659   Enteropathic arthropathies, unspecified hip
   M07.66   Enteropathic arthropathies, knee
     M07.661   Enteropathic arthropathies, right knee
     M07.662   Enteropathic arthropathies, left knee
     M07.669   Enteropathic arthropathies, unspecified knee
   M07.67   Enteropathic arthropathies, ankle and foot
     M07.671   Enteropathic arthropathies, right ankle and foot
     M07.672   Enteropathic arthropathies, left ankle and foot
     M07.679   Enteropathic arthropathies, unspecified ankle and foot
   M07.68   Enteropathic arthropathies, vertebrae
   M07.69   Enteropathic arthropathies, multiple sites

M08   Juvenile arthritis
     Code also any associated underlying condition, such as:
       regional enteritis [Crohn's disease] (K50.-)
       ulcerative colitis (K51.-)
     Excludes1:   arthropathic psoriasis (L40.5)
              arthropathy in Whipple's disease (M14.8)
              Felty's syndrome (M05.0)
              juvenile dermatomyositis (M33.0-)

M08.0   Unspecified juvenile rheumatoid arthritis
     Juvenile rheumatoid arthritis with or without rheumatoid factor
   M08.00   Unspecified juvenile rheumatoid arthritis of unspecified site
   M08.01   Unspecified juvenile rheumatoid arthritis, shoulder
     M08.011   Unspecified juvenile rheumatoid arthritis, right shoulder
     M08.012   Unspecified juvenile rheumatoid arthritis, left shoulder
     M08.019   Unspecified juvenile rheumatoid arthritis, unspecified shoulder
   M08.02   Unspecified juvenile rheumatoid arthritis of elbow
     M08.021   Unspecified juvenile rheumatoid arthritis, right elbow
     M08.022   Unspecified juvenile rheumatoid arthritis, left elbow
     M08.029   Unspecified juvenile rheumatoid arthritis, unspecified elbow
   M08.03   Unspecified juvenile rheumatoid arthritis, wrist
     M08.031   Unspecified juvenile rheumatoid arthritis, right wrist
     M08.032   Unspecified juvenile rheumatoid arthritis, left wrist
     M08.039   Unspecified juvenile rheumatoid arthritis, unspecified wrist
   M08.04   Unspecified juvenile rheumatoid arthritis, hand
     M08.041   Unspecified juvenile rheumatoid arthritis, right hand
     M08.042   Unspecified juvenile rheumatoid arthritis, left hand
     M08.049   Unspecified juvenile rheumatoid arthritis, unspecified hand
   M08.05   Unspecified juvenile rheumatoid arthritis, hip
     M08.051   Unspecified juvenile rheumatoid arthritis, right hip

      M08.052 Unspecified juvenile rheumatoid arthritis, left hip

      M08.059 Unspecified juvenile rheumatoid arthritis, unspecified hip

  M08.06 Unspecified juvenile rheumatoid arthritis, knee

      M08.061 Unspecified juvenile rheumatoid arthritis, right knee

      M08.062 Unspecified juvenile rheumatoid arthritis, left knee

      M08.069 Unspecified juvenile rheumatoid arthritis, unspecified knee

  M08.07 Unspecified juvenile rheumatoid arthritis, ankle and foot

      M08.071 Unspecified juvenile rheumatoid arthritis, right ankle and foot

      M08.072 Unspecified juvenile rheumatoid arthritis, left ankle and foot

      M08.079 Unspecified juvenile rheumatoid arthritis, unspecified ankle and foot

  M08.08 Unspecified juvenile rheumatoid arthritis, vertebrae

  M08.09 Unspecified juvenile rheumatoid arthritis, multiple sites

M08.1 Juvenile ankylosing spondylitis

    Excludes1:   ankylosing spondylitis in adults (M45.0-)

M08.2 Juvenile rheumatoid arthritis with systemic onset

    Still's disease NOS

    Excludes1:   adult-onset Still's disease (M06.1-)

  M08.20 Juvenile rheumatoid arthritis with systemic onset, unspecified site

  M08.21 Juvenile rheumatoid arthritis with systemic onset, shoulder

      M08.211 Juvenile rheumatoid arthritis with systemic onset, right shoulder

      M08.212 Juvenile rheumatoid arthritis with systemic onset, left shoulder

      M08.219 Juvenile rheumatoid arthritis with systemic onset, unspecified shoulder

  M08.22 Juvenile rheumatoid arthritis with systemic onset, elbow

      M08.221 Juvenile rheumatoid arthritis with systemic onset, right elbow

      M08.222 Juvenile rheumatoid arthritis with systemic onset, left elbow

      M08.229 Juvenile rheumatoid arthritis with systemic onset, unspecified elbow

  M08.23 Juvenile rheumatoid arthritis with systemic onset, wrist

      M08.231 Juvenile rheumatoid arthritis with systemic onset, right wrist

      M08.232 Juvenile rheumatoid arthritis with systemic onset, left wrist

      M08.239 Juvenile rheumatoid arthritis with systemic onset, unspecified wrist

  M08.24 Juvenile rheumatoid arthritis with systemic onset, hand

      M08.241 Juvenile rheumatoid arthritis with systemic onset, right hand

      M08.242 Juvenile rheumatoid arthritis with systemic onset, left hand

      M08.249 Juvenile rheumatoid arthritis with systemic onset, unspecified hand

  M08.25 Juvenile rheumatoid arthritis with systemic onset, hip

      M08.251 Juvenile rheumatoid arthritis with systemic onset, right hip

      M08.252 Juvenile rheumatoid arthritis with systemic onset, left hip

      M08.259 Juvenile rheumatoid arthritis with systemic onset, unspecified hip

  M08.26 Juvenile rheumatoid arthritis with systemic onset, knee

      M08.261 Juvenile rheumatoid arthritis with systemic onset, right knee

      M08.262 Juvenile rheumatoid arthritis with systemic onset, left knee

      M08.269 Juvenile rheumatoid arthritis with systemic onset, unspecified knee

  M08.27 Juvenile rheumatoid arthritis with systemic onset, ankle and foot

      M08.271 Juvenile rheumatoid arthritis with systemic onset, right ankle and foot

      M08.272 Juvenile rheumatoid arthritis with systemic onset, left ankle and foot

      M08.279 Juvenile rheumatoid arthritis with systemic onset, unspecified ankle and foot

  M08.28 Juvenile rheumatoid arthritis with systemic onset, vertebrae

  M08.29 Juvenile rheumatoid arthritis with systemic onset, multiple sites

M08.3 Juvenile rheumatoid polyarthritis (seronegative)

M08.4 Pauciarticular juvenile rheumatoid arthritis

  M08.40 Pauciarticular juvenile rheumatoid arthritis, unspecified site

  M08.41 Pauciarticular juvenile rheumatoid arthritis, shoulder

      M08.411 Pauciarticular juvenile rheumatoid arthritis, right shoulder

      M08.412 Pauciarticular juvenile rheumatoid arthritis, left shoulder

      M08.419 Pauciarticular juvenile rheumatoid arthritis, unspecified shoulder

  M08.42 Pauciarticular juvenile rheumatoid arthritis, elbow

      M08.421 Pauciarticular juvenile rheumatoid arthritis, right elbow

      M08.422 Pauciarticular juvenile rheumatoid arthritis, left elbow

      M08.429 Pauciarticular juvenile rheumatoid arthritis, unspecified elbow

  M08.43 Pauciarticular juvenile rheumatoid arthritis, wrist

      M08.431 Pauciarticular juvenile rheumatoid arthritis, right wrist

      M08.432 Pauciarticular juvenile rheumatoid arthritis, left wrist

      M08.439 Pauciarticular juvenile rheumatoid arthritis, unspecified wrist

  M08.44 Pauciarticular juvenile rheumatoid arthritis, hand

      M08.441 Pauciarticular juvenile rheumatoid arthritis, right hand

      M08.442 Pauciarticular juvenile rheumatoid arthritis, left hand

      M08.449 Pauciarticular juvenile rheumatoid arthritis, unspecified hand

  M08.45 Pauciarticular juvenile rheumatoid arthritis, hip

      M08.451 Pauciarticular juvenile rheumatoid arthritis, right hip

      M08.452 Pauciarticular juvenile rheumatoid arthritis, left hip

      M08.459 Pauciarticular juvenile rheumatoid arthritis, unspecified hip

  M08.46 Pauciarticular juvenile rheumatoid arthritis, knee

      M08.461 Pauciarticular juvenile rheumatoid arthritis, right knee

      M08.462 Pauciarticular juvenile rheumatoid arthritis, left knee

      M08.469 Pauciarticular juvenile rheumatoid arthritis, unspecified knee

  M08.47 Pauciarticular juvenile rheumatoid arthritis, ankle and foot

      M08.471 Pauciarticular juvenile rheumatoid arthritis, right ankle and foot

      M08.472 Pauciarticular juvenile rheumatoid arthritis, left ankle and foot

      M08.479 Pauciarticular juvenile rheumatoid arthritis, unspecified ankle and foot

  M08.48 Pauciarticular juvenile rheumatoid arthritis, vertebrae

M08.8 Other juvenile arthritis
   M08.80   Other juvenile arthritis, unspecified site
   M08.81   Other juvenile arthritis, shoulder
      M08.811 Other juvenile arthritis, right shoulder
      M08.812 Other juvenile arthritis, left shoulder
      M08.819 Other juvenile arthritis, unspecified shoulder
   M08.82   Other juvenile arthritis, elbow
      M08.821 Other juvenile arthritis, right elbow
      M08.822 Other juvenile arthritis, left elbow
      M08.829 Other juvenile arthritis, unspecified elbow
   M08.83   Other juvenile arthritis, wrist
      M08.831 Other juvenile arthritis, right wrist
      M08.832 Other juvenile arthritis, left wrist
      M08.839 Other juvenile arthritis, unspecified wrist
   M08.84   Other juvenile arthritis, hand
      M08.841 Other juvenile arthritis, right hand
      M08.842 Other juvenile arthritis, left hand
      M08.849 Other juvenile arthritis, unspecified hand
   M08.85   Other juvenile arthritis, hip
      M08.851 Other juvenile arthritis, right hip
      M08.852 Other juvenile arthritis, left hip
      M08.859 Other juvenile arthritis, unspecified hip
   M08.86   Other juvenile arthritis, knee
      M08.861 Other juvenile arthritis, right knee
      M08.862 Other juvenile arthritis, left knee
      M08.869 Other juvenile arthritis, unspecified knee
   M08.87   Other juvenile arthritis, ankle and foot
      M08.871 Other juvenile arthritis, right ankle and foot
      M08.872 Other juvenile arthritis, left ankle and foot
      M08.879 Other juvenile arthritis, unspecified ankle and foot
   M08.88   Other juvenile arthritis, vertebrae
   M08.89   Other juvenile arthritis, multiple sites
M08.9 Juvenile arthritis, unspecified
     Excludes1:   juvenile rheumatoid arthritis, unspecified (M08.0-)
   M08.90   Juvenile arthritis, unspecified, unspecified site
   M08.91   Juvenile arthritis, unspecified, shoulder
      M08.911 Juvenile arthritis, unspecified, right shoulder
      M08.912 Juvenile arthritis, unspecified, left shoulder
      M08.919 Juvenile arthritis, unspecified, unspecified shoulder
   M08.92   Juvenile arthritis, unspecified, elbow
      M08.921 Juvenile arthritis, unspecified, right elbow
      M08.922 Juvenile arthritis, unspecified, left elbow
      M08.929 Juvenile arthritis, unspecified, unspecified elbow
   M08.93   Juvenile arthritis, unspecified, wrist
      M08.931 Juvenile arthritis, unspecified, right wrist
      M08.932 Juvenile arthritis, unspecified, left wrist
      M08.939 Juvenile arthritis, unspecified, unspecified wrist
   M08.94   Juvenile arthritis, unspecified, hand
      M08.941 Juvenile arthritis, unspecified, right hand
      M08.942 Juvenile arthritis, unspecified, left hand
      M08.949 Juvenile arthritis, unspecified, unspecified hand
   M08.95   Juvenile arthritis, unspecified, hip
      M08.951 Juvenile arthritis, unspecified, right hip
      M08.952 Juvenile arthritis, unspecified, left hip
      M08.959 Juvenile arthritis, unspecified, unspecified hip
   M08.96   Juvenile arthritis, unspecified, knee
      M08.961 Juvenile arthritis, unspecified, right knee
      M08.962 Juvenile arthritis, unspecified, left knee
      M08.969 Juvenile arthritis, unspecified, unspecified knee
   M08.97   Juvenile arthritis, unspecified, ankle and foot

      M08.971 Juvenile arthritis, unspecified, right ankle and foot
      M08.972 Juvenile arthritis, unspecified, left ankle and foot
      M08.979 Juvenile arthritis, unspecified, unspecified ankle and foot
   M08.98   Juvenile arthritis, unspecified, vertebrae
   M08.99   Juvenile arthritis, unspecified, multiple sites

M10 Gout
  M10.0 Idiopathic gout
     Gouty bursitis
     Primary gout
   M10.00   Idiopathic gout, unspecified site
   M10.01   Idiopathic gout, shoulder
      M10.011 Idiopathic gout, right shoulder
      M10.012 Idiopathic gout, left shoulder
      M10.019 Idiopathic gout, unspecified shoulder
   M10.02   Idiopathic gout, elbow
      M10.021 Idiopathic gout, right elbow
      M10.022 Idiopathic gout, left elbow
      M10.029 Idiopathic gout, unspecified elbow
   M10.03   Idiopathic gout, wrist
      M10.031 Idiopathic gout, right wrist
      M10.032 Idiopathic gout, left wrist
      M10.039 Idiopathic gout, unspecified wrist
   M10.04   Idiopathic gout, hand
      M10.041 Idiopathic gout, right hand
      M10.042 Idiopathic gout, left hand
      M10.049 Idiopathic gout, unspecified hand
   M10.05   Idiopathic gout, hip
      M10.051 Idiopathic gout, right hip
      M10.052 Idiopathic gout, left hip
      M10.059 Idiopathic gout, unspecified hip
   M10.06   Idiopathic gout, knee
      M10.061 Idiopathic gout, right knee
      M10.062 Idiopathic gout, left knee
      M10.069 Idiopathic gout, unspecified knee
   M10.07   Idiopathic gout, ankle and foot
      M10.071 Idiopathic gout, right ankle and foot
      M10.072 Idiopathic gout, left ankle and foot
      M10.079 Idiopathic gout, unspecified ankle and foot
   M10.08   Idiopathic gout, vertebrae
   M10.09   Idiopathic gout, multiple sites
  M10.1 Lead-induced gout
   M10.10   Lead-induced gout, unspecified site
   M10.11   Lead-induced gout, shoulder
      M10.111 Lead-induced gout, right shoulder
      M10.112 Lead-induced gout, left shoulder
      M10.119 Lead-induced gout, unspecified shoulder
   M10.12   Lead-induced gout, elbow
      M10.121 Lead-induced gout, right elbow
      M10.122 Lead-induced gout, left elbow
      M10.129 Lead-induced gout, unspecified elbow
   M10.13   Lead-induced gout, wrist
      M10.131 Lead-induced gout, right wrist
      M10.132 Lead-induced gout, left wrist
      M10.139 Lead-induced gout, unspecified wrist
   M10.14   Lead-induced gout, hand
      M10.141 Lead-induced gout, right hand
      M10.142 Lead-induced gout, left hand
      M10.149 Lead-induced gout, unspecified hand
   M10.15   Lead-induced gout, hip
      M10.151 Lead-induced gout, right hip
      M10.152 Lead-induced gout, left hip
      M10.159 Lead-induced gout, unspecified hip
   M10.16   Lead-induced gout, knee
      M10.161 Lead-induced gout, right knee
      M10.162 Lead-induced gout, left knee

M10.169　Lead-induced gout, unspecified knee
M10.17　Lead-induced gout, ankle and foot
　　　M10.171　Lead-induced gout, right ankle and foot
　　　M10.172　Lead-induced gout, left ankle and foot
　　　M10.179　Lead-induced gout, unspecified ankle and foot
M10.18　Lead-induced gout, vertebrae
M10.19　Lead-induced gout, multiple sites
M10.2　Drug-induced gout
　　　Use additional external cause code (Chapter XIX) to identify drug
M10.20　Drug-induced gout, unspecified site
M10.21　Drug-induced gout, shoulder
　　　M10.211　Drug-induced gout, right shoulder
　　　M10.212　Drug-induced gout, left shoulder
　　　M10.219　Drug-induced gout, unspecified shoulder
M10.22　Drug-induced gout, elbow
　　　M10.221　Drug-induced gout, right elbow
　　　M10.222　Drug-induced gout, left elbow
　　　M10.229　Drug-induced gout, unspecified elbow
M10.23　Drug-induced gout, wrist
　　　M10.231　Drug-induced gout, right wrist
　　　M10.232　Drug-induced gout, left wrist
　　　M10.239　Drug-induced gout, unspecified wrist
M10.24　Drug-induced gout, hand
　　　M10.241　Drug-induced gout, right hand
　　　M10.242　Drug-induced gout, left hand
　　　M10.249　Drug-induced gout, unspecified hand
M10.25　Drug-induced gout, hip
　　　M10.251　Drug-induced gout, right hip
　　　M10.252　Drug-induced gout, left hip
　　　M10.259　Drug-induced gout, unspecified hip
M10.26　Drug-induced gout, knee
　　　M10.261　Drug-induced gout, right knee
　　　M10.262　Drug-induced gout, left knee
　　　M10.269　Drug-induced gout, unspecified knee
M10.27　Drug-induced gout, ankle and foot
　　　M10.271　Drug-induced gout, right ankle and foot
　　　M10.272　Drug-induced gout, left ankle and foot
　　　M10.279　Drug-induced gout, unspecified ankle and foot
M10.28　Drug-induced gout, vertebrae
M10.29　Drug-induced gout, multiple sites
M10.3　Gout due to renal impairment
　　　Code also associated renal disease
M10.30　Gout due to renal impairment, unspecified site
M10.31　Gout due to renal impairment, shoulder
　　　M10.311　Gout due to renal impairment, right shoulder
　　　M10.312　Gout due to renal impairment, left shoulder
　　　M10.319　Gout due to renal impairment, unspecified shoulder
M10.32　Gout due to renal impairment, elbow
　　　M10.321　Gout due to renal impairment, right elbow
　　　M10.322　Gout due to renal impairment, left elbow
　　　M10.329　Gout due to renal impairment, unspecified elbow
M10.33　Gout due to renal impairment, wrist
　　　M10.331　Gout due to renal impairment, right wrist
　　　M10.332　Gout due to renal impairment, left wrist
　　　M10.339　Gout due to renal impairment, unspecified wrist
M10.34　Gout due to renal impairment, hand
　　　M10.341　Gout due to renal impairment, right hand
　　　M10.342　Gout due to renal impairment, left hand
　　　M10.349　Gout due to renal impairment, unspecified hand
M10.35　Gout due to renal impairment, hip
　　　M10.351　Gout due to renal impairment, right hip
　　　M10.352　Gout due to renal impairment, left hip
　　　M10.359　Gout due to renal impairment, unspecified hip

M10.36　Gout due to renal impairment, knee
　　　M10.361　Gout due to renal impairment, right knee
　　　M10.362　Gout due to renal impairment, left knee
　　　M10.369　Gout due to renal impairment, unspecified knee
M10.37　Gout due to renal impairment, ankle and foot
　　　M10.371　Gout due to renal impairment, right ankle and foot
　　　M10.372　Gout due to renal impairment, left ankle and foot
　　　M10.379　Gout due to renal impairment, unspecified ankle and foot
M10.38　Gout due to renal impairment, vertebrae
M10.39　Gout due to renal impairment, multiple sites
M10.4　Other secondary gout
M10.40　Other secondary gout, unspecified site
M10.41　Other secondary gout, shoulder
　　　M10.411　Other secondary gout, right shoulder
　　　M10.412　Other secondary gout, left shoulder
　　　M10.419　Other secondary gout, unspecified shoulder
M10.42　Other secondary gout, elbow
　　　M10.421　Other secondary gout, right elbow
　　　M10.422　Other secondary gout, left elbow
　　　M10.429　Other secondary gout, unspecified elbow
M10.43　Other secondary gout, wrist
　　　M10.431　Other secondary gout, right wrist
　　　M10.432　Other secondary gout, left wrist
　　　M10.439　Other secondary gout, unspecified wrist
M10.44　Other secondary gout, hand
　　　M10.441　Other secondary gout, right hand
　　　M10.442　Other secondary gout, left hand
　　　M10.449　Other secondary gout, unspecified hand
M10.45　Other secondary gout, hip
　　　M10.451　Other secondary gout, right hip
　　　M10.452　Other secondary gout, left hip
　　　M10.459　Other secondary gout, unspecified hip
M10.46　Other secondary gout, knee
　　　M10.461　Other secondary gout, right knee
　　　M10.462　Other secondary gout, left knee
　　　M10.469　Other secondary gout, unspecified knee
M10.47　Other secondary gout, ankle and foot
　　　M10.471　Other secondary gout, right ankle and foot
　　　M10.472　Other secondary gout, left ankle and foot
　　　M10.479　Other secondary gout, unspecified ankle and foot
M10.48　Other secondary gout, vertebrae
M10.49　Other secondary gout, multiple sites
M10.9　Gout, unspecified

M11　Other crystal arthropathies
M11.0　Hydroxyapatite deposition disease
M11.00　Hydroxyapatite deposition disease, unspecified site
M11.01　Hydroxyapatite deposition disease, shoulder
　　　M11.011　Hydroxyapatite deposition disease, right shoulder
　　　M11.012　Hydroxyapatite deposition disease, left shoulder
　　　M11.019　Hydroxyapatite deposition disease, unspecified shoulder
M11.02　Hydroxyapatite deposition disease, elbow
　　　M11.021　Hydroxyapatite deposition disease, right elbow
　　　M11.022　Hydroxyapatite deposition disease, left elbow
　　　M11.029　Hydroxyapatite deposition disease, unspecified elbow
M11.03　Hydroxyapatite deposition disease, wrist
　　　M11.031　Hydroxyapatite deposition disease, right wrist
　　　M11.032　Hydroxyapatite deposition disease, left wrist
　　　M11.039　Hydroxyapatite deposition disease, unspecified wrist

M11.04   Hydroxyapatite deposition disease, hand
    M11.041   Hydroxyapatite deposition disease, right hand
    M11.042   Hydroxyapatite deposition disease, left hand
    M11.049   Hydroxyapatite deposition disease, unspecified hand
M11.05   Hydroxyapatite deposition disease, hip
    M11.051   Hydroxyapatite deposition disease, right hip
    M11.052   Hydroxyapatite deposition disease, left hip
    M11.059   Hydroxyapatite deposition disease, unspecified hip
M11.06   Hydroxyapatite deposition disease, knee
    M11.061   Hydroxyapatite deposition disease, right knee
    M11.062   Hydroxyapatite deposition disease, left knee
    M11.069   Hydroxyapatite deposition disease, unspecified knee
M11.07   Hydroxyapatite deposition disease, ankle and foot
    M11.071   Hydroxyapatite deposition disease, right ankle and foot
    M11.072   Hydroxyapatite deposition disease, left ankle and foot
    M11.079   Hydroxyapatite deposition disease, unspecified ankle and foot
M11.08   Hydroxyapatite deposition disease, vertebrae
M11.09   Hydroxyapatite deposition disease, multiple sites

M11.1   Familial chondrocalcinosis
M11.10   Familial chondrocalcinosis, unspecified site
M11.11   Familial chondrocalcinosis, shoulder
    M11.111   Familial chondrocalcinosis, right shoulder
    M11.112   Familial chondrocalcinosis, left shoulder
    M11.119   Familial chondrocalcinosis, unspecified shoulder
M11.12   Familial chondrocalcinosis, elbow
    M11.121   Familial chondrocalcinosis, right elbow
    M11.122   Familial chondrocalcinosis, left elbow
    M11.129   Familial chondrocalcinosis, unspecified elbow
M11.13   Familial chondrocalcinosis, wrist
    M11.131   Familial chondrocalcinosis, right wrist
    M11.132   Familial chondrocalcinosis, left wrist
    M11.139   Familial chondrocalcinosis, unspecified wrist
M11.14   Familial chondrocalcinosis, hand
    M11.141   Familial chondrocalcinosis, right hand
    M11.142   Familial chondrocalcinosis, left hand
    M11.149   Familial chondrocalcinosis, unspecified hand
M11.15   Familial chondrocalcinosis, hip
    M11.151   Familial chondrocalcinosis, right hip
    M11.152   Familial chondrocalcinosis, left hip
    M11.159   Familial chondrocalcinosis, unspecified hip
M11.16   Familial chondrocalcinosis, knee
    M11.161   Familial chondrocalcinosis, right knee
    M11.162   Familial chondrocalcinosis, left knee
    M11.169   Familial chondrocalcinosis, unspecified knee
M11.17   Familial chondrocalcinosis, ankle and foot
    M11.171   Familial chondrocalcinosis, right ankle and foot
    M11.172   Familial chondrocalcinosis, left ankle and foot
    M11.179   Familial chondrocalcinosis, unspecified ankle and foot
M11.18   Familial chondrocalcinosis, vertebrae
M11.19   Familial chondrocalcinosis, multiple sites

M11.2   Other chondrocalcinosis
    Chondrocalcinosis NOS
M11.20   Other chondrocalcinosis, unspecified site
M11.21   Other chondrocalcinosis, shoulder
    M11.211   Other chondrocalcinosis, right shoulder
    M11.212   Other chondrocalcinosis, left shoulder
    M11.219   Other chondrocalcinosis, unspecified shoulder
M11.22   Other chondrocalcinosis, elbow
    M11.221   Other chondrocalcinosis, right elbow
    M11.222   Other chondrocalcinosis, left elbow

    M11.229   Other chondrocalcinosis, unspecified elbow
M11.23   Other chondrocalcinosis, wrist
    M11.231   Other chondrocalcinosis, right wrist
    M11.232   Other chondrocalcinosis, left wrist
    M11.239   Other chondrocalcinosis, unspecified wrist
M11.24   Other chondrocalcinosis, hand
    M11.241   Other chondrocalcinosis, right hand
    M11.242   Other chondrocalcinosis, left hand
    M11.249   Other chondrocalcinosis, unspecified hand
M11.25   Other chondrocalcinosis, hip
    M11.251   Other chondrocalcinosis, right hip
    M11.252   Other chondrocalcinosis, left hip
    M11.259   Other chondrocalcinosis, unspecified hip
M11.26   Other chondrocalcinosis, knee
    M11.261   Other chondrocalcinosis, right knee
    M11.262   Other chondrocalcinosis, left knee
    M11.269   Other chondrocalcinosis, unspecified knee
M11.27   Other chondrocalcinosis, ankle and foot
    M11.271   Other chondrocalcinosis, right ankle and foot
    M11.272   Other chondrocalcinosis, left ankle and foot
    M11.279   Other chondrocalcinosis, unspecified ankle and foot
M11.28   Other chondrocalcinosis, vertebrae
M11.29   Other chondrocalcinosis, multiple sites

M11.8   Other specified crystal arthropathies
M11.80   Other specified crystal arthropathies, unspecified site
M11.81   Other specified crystal arthropathies, shoulder
    M11.811   Other specified crystal arthropathies, right shoulder
    M11.812   Other specified crystal arthropathies, left shoulder
    M11.819   Other specified crystal arthropathies, unspecified shoulder
M11.82   Other specified crystal arthropathies, elbow
    M11.821   Other specified crystal arthropathies, right elbow
    M11.822   Other specified crystal arthropathies, left elbow
    M11.829   Other specified crystal arthropathies, unspecified elbow
M11.83   Other specified crystal arthropathies, wrist
    M11.831   Other specified crystal arthropathies, right wrist
    M11.832   Other specified crystal arthropathies, left wrist
    M11.839   Other specified crystal arthropathies, unspecified wrist
M11.84   Other specified crystal arthropathies, hand
    M11.841   Other specified crystal arthropathies, right hand
    M11.842   Other specified crystal arthropathies, left hand
    M11.849   Other specified crystal arthropathies, unspecified hand
M11.85   Other specified crystal arthropathies, hip
    M11.851   Other specified crystal arthropathies, right hip
    M11.852   Other specified crystal arthropathies, left hip
    M11.859   Other specified crystal arthropathies, unspecified hip
M11.86   Other specified crystal arthropathies, knee
    M11.861   Other specified crystal arthropathies, right knee
    M11.862   Other specified crystal arthropathies, left knee
    M11.869   Other specified crystal arthropathies, unspecified knee
M11.87   Other specified crystal arthropathies, ankle and foot
    M11.871   Other specified crystal arthropathies, right ankle and foot

M11.872 Other specified crystal arthropathies, left ankle and foot

M11.879 Other specified crystal arthropathies, unspecified ankle and foot

M11.88 Other specified crystal arthropathies, vertebrae

M11.89 Other specified crystal arthropathies, multiple sites

M11.9 Crystal arthropathy, unspecified

M12 Other specific arthropathies

Excludes1:   arthropathy NOS (M13.9-)
arthrosis (M15-M19)
cricoarytenoid arthropathy (J38.7)

M12.0 Chronic postrheumatic arthropathy [Jaccoud]

M12.00 Chronic postrheumatic arthropathy [Jaccoud], unspecified site

M12.01 Chronic postrheumatic arthropathy [Jaccoud], shoulder

M12.011 Chronic postrheumatic arthropathy [Jaccoud], right shoulder

M12.012 Chronic postrheumatic arthropathy [Jaccoud], left shoulder

M12.019 Chronic postrheumatic arthropathy [Jaccoud], unspecified shoulder

M12.02 Chronic postrheumatic arthropathy [Jaccoud], elbow

M12.021 Chronic postrheumatic arthropathy [Jaccoud], right elbow

M12.022 Chronic postrheumatic arthropathy [Jaccoud], left elbow

M12.029 Chronic postrheumatic arthropathy [Jaccoud], unspecified elbow

M12.03 Chronic postrheumatic arthropathy [Jaccoud], wrist

M12.031 Chronic postrheumatic arthropathy [Jaccoud], right wrist

M12.032 Chronic postrheumatic arthropathy [Jaccoud], left wrist

M12.039 Chronic postrheumatic arthropathy [Jaccoud], unspecified wrist

M12.04 Chronic postrheumatic arthropathy [Jaccoud], hand

M12.041 Chronic postrheumatic arthropathy [Jaccoud], right hand

M12.042 Chronic postrheumatic arthropathy [Jaccoud], left hand

M12.049 Chronic postrheumatic arthropathy [Jaccoud], unspecified hand

M12.05 Chronic postrheumatic arthropathy [Jaccoud], hip

M12.051 Chronic postrheumatic arthropathy [Jaccoud], right hip

M12.052 Chronic postrheumatic arthropathy [Jaccoud], left hip

M12.059 Chronic postrheumatic arthropathy [Jaccoud], unspecified hip

M12.06 Chronic postrheumatic arthropathy [Jaccoud], knee

M12.061 Chronic postrheumatic arthropathy [Jaccoud], right knee

M12.062 Chronic postrheumatic arthropathy [Jaccoud], left knee

M12.069 Chronic postrheumatic arthropathy [Jaccoud], unspecified knee

M12.07 Chronic postrheumatic arthropathy [Jaccoud], ankle and foot

M12.071 Chronic postrheumatic arthropathy [Jaccoud], right ankle and foot

M12.072 Chronic postrheumatic arthropathy [Jaccoud], left ankle and foot

M12.079 Chronic postrheumatic arthropathy [Jaccoud], unspecified ankle and foot

M12.08 Chronic postrheumatic arthropathy [Jaccoud], vertebrae

M12.09 Chronic postrheumatic arthropathy [Jaccoud], multiple sites

M12.1 Kaschin-Beck disease
Osteochondroarthrosis deformans endemica

M12.10 Kaschin-Beck disease, unspecified site

M12.11 Kaschin-Beck disease, shoulder

M12.111 Kaschin-Beck disease, right shoulder

M12.112 Kaschin-Beck disease, left shoulder

M12.119 Kaschin-Beck disease, unspecified shoulder

M12.12 Kaschin-Beck disease, elbow

M12.121 Kaschin-Beck disease, right elbow

M12.122 Kaschin-Beck disease, left elbow

M12.129 Kaschin-Beck disease, unspecified elbow

M12.13 Kaschin-Beck disease, wrist

M12.131 Kaschin-Beck disease, right wrist

M12.132 Kaschin-Beck disease, left wrist

M12.139 Kaschin-Beck disease, unspecified wrist

M12.14 Kaschin-Beck disease, hand

M12.141 Kaschin-Beck disease, right hand

M12.142 Kaschin-Beck disease, left hand

M12.149 Kaschin-Beck disease, unspecified hand

M12.15 Kaschin-Beck disease, hip

M12.151 Kaschin-Beck disease, right hip

M12.152 Kaschin-Beck disease, left hip

M12.159 Kaschin-Beck disease, unspecified hip

M12.16 Kaschin-Beck disease, knee

M12.161 Kaschin-Beck disease, right knee

M12.162 Kaschin-Beck disease, left knee

M12.169 Kaschin-Beck disease, unspecified knee

M12.17 Kaschin-Beck disease, ankle and foot

M12.171 Kaschin-Beck disease, right ankle and foot

M12.172 Kaschin-Beck disease, left ankle and foot

M12.179 Kaschin-Beck disease, unspecified ankle and foot

M12.18 Kaschin-Beck disease, vertebrae

M12.19 Kaschin-Beck disease, multiple sites

M12.2 Villonodular synovitis (pigmented)

M12.20 Villonodular synovitis (pigmented), unspecified site

M12.21 Villonodular synovitis (pigmented), shoulder

M12.211 Villonodular synovitis (pigmented), right shoulder

M12.212 Villonodular synovitis (pigmented), left shoulder

M12.219 Villonodular synovitis (pigmented), unspecified shoulder

M12.22 Villonodular synovitis (pigmented), elbow

M12.221 Villonodular synovitis (pigmented), right elbow

M12.222 Villonodular synovitis (pigmented), left elbow

M12.229 Villonodular synovitis (pigmented), unspecified elbow

M12.23 Villonodular synovitis (pigmented), wrist

M12.231 Villonodular synovitis (pigmented), right wrist

M12.232 Villonodular synovitis (pigmented), left wrist

M12.239 Villonodular synovitis (pigmented), unspecified wrist

M12.24 Villonodular synovitis (pigmented), hand

M12.241 Villonodular synovitis (pigmented), right hand

M12.242 Villonodular synovitis (pigmented), left hand

M12.249 Villonodular synovitis (pigmented), unspecified hand

M12.25 Villonodular synovitis (pigmented), hip

M12.251 Villonodular synovitis (pigmented), right hip

M12.252 Villonodular synovitis (pigmented), left hip

M12.259 Villonodular synovitis (pigmented), unspecified hip

M12.26 Villonodular synovitis (pigmented), knee

M12.261 Villonodular synovitis (pigmented), right knee

M12.262 Villonodular synovitis (pigmented), left knee

M12.269 Villonodular synovitis (pigmented), unspecified knee

M12.27 Villonodular synovitis (pigmented), ankle and foot

M12.271 Villonodular synovitis (pigmented), right ankle and foot

M12.272   Villonodular synovitis (pigmented), left ankle and foot

M12.279   Villonodular synovitis (pigmented), unspecified ankle and foot

M12.28   Villonodular synovitis (pigmented), vertebrae

M12.29   Villonodular synovitis (pigmented), multiple sites

M12.3   Palindromic rheumatism

M12.30   Palindromic rheumatism, unspecified site

M12.31   Palindromic rheumatism, shoulder

M12.311   Palindromic rheumatism, right shoulder

M12.312   Palindromic rheumatism, left shoulder

M12.319   Palindromic rheumatism, unspecified shoulder

M12.32   Palindromic rheumatism, elbow

M12.321   Palindromic rheumatism, right elbow

M12.322   Palindromic rheumatism, left elbow

M12.329   Palindromic rheumatism, unspecified elbow

M12.33   Palindromic rheumatism, wrist

M12.331   Palindromic rheumatism, right wrist

M12.332   Palindromic rheumatism, left wrist

M12.339   Palindromic rheumatism, unspecified wrist

M12.34   Palindromic rheumatism, hand

M12.341   Palindromic rheumatism, right hand

M12.342   Palindromic rheumatism, left hand

M12.349   Palindromic rheumatism, unspecified hand

M12.35   Palindromic rheumatism, hip

M12.351   Palindromic rheumatism, right hip

M12.352   Palindromic rheumatism, left hip

M12.359   Palindromic rheumatism, unspecified hip

M12.36   Palindromic rheumatism, knee

M12.361   Palindromic rheumatism, right knee

M12.362   Palindromic rheumatism, left knee

M12.369   Palindromic rheumatism, unspecified knee

M12.37   Palindromic rheumatism, ankle and foot

M12.371   Palindromic rheumatism, right ankle and foot

M12.372   Palindromic rheumatism, left ankle and foot

M12.379   Palindromic rheumatism, unspecified ankle and foot

M12.38   Palindromic rheumatism, vertebrae

M12.39   Palindromic rheumatism, multiple sites

M12.4   Intermittent hydrarthrosis

M12.40   Intermittent hydrarthrosis, unspecified site

M12.41   Intermittent hydrarthrosis, shoulder

M12.411   Intermittent hydrarthrosis, right shoulder

M12.412   Intermittent hydrarthrosis, left shoulder

M12.419   Intermittent hydrarthrosis, unspecified shoulder

M12.42   Intermittent hydrarthrosis, elbow

M12.421   Intermittent hydrarthrosis, right elbow

M12.422   Intermittent hydrarthrosis, left elbow

M12.429   Intermittent hydrarthrosis, unspecified elbow

M12.43   Intermittent hydrarthrosis, wrist

M12.431   Intermittent hydrarthrosis, right wrist

M12.432   Intermittent hydrarthrosis, left wrist

M12.439   Intermittent hydrarthrosis, unspecified wrist

M12.44   Intermittent hydrarthrosis, hand

M12.441   Intermittent hydrarthrosis, right hand

M12.442   Intermittent hydrarthrosis, left hand

M12.449   Intermittent hydrarthrosis, unspecified hand

M12.45   Intermittent hydrarthrosis, hip

M12.451   Intermittent hydrarthrosis, right hip

M12.452   Intermittent hydrarthrosis, left hip

M12.459   Intermittent hydrarthrosis, unspecified hip

M12.46   Intermittent hydrarthrosis, knee

M12.461   Intermittent hydrarthrosis, right knee

M12.462   Intermittent hydrarthrosis, left knee

M12.469   Intermittent hydrarthrosis, unspecified knee

M12.47   Intermittent hydrarthrosis, ankle and foot

M12.471   Intermittent hydrarthrosis, right ankle and foot

M12.472   Intermittent hydrarthrosis, left ankle and foot

M12.479   Intermittent hydrarthrosis, unspecified ankle and foot

M12.48   Intermittent hydrarthrosis, other site

M12.49   Intermittent hydrarthrosis, multiple sites

M12.5   Traumatic arthropathy

Excludes1:   current injury — see Alphabetic Index
post-traumatic osteoarthritis (of):
   NOS (M19.1-)
   first carpometacarpal joint (M18.2-M18.3)
   hip (M16.4-M16.5)
   knee (M17.2-M17.3)
   other single joints (M19.1-)

M12.50   Traumatic arthropathy, unspecified site

M12.51   Traumatic arthropathy, shoulder

M12.511   Traumatic arthropathy, right shoulder

M12.512   Traumatic arthropathy, left shoulder

M12.519   Traumatic arthropathy, unspecified shoulder

M12.52   Traumatic arthropathy, elbow

M12.521   Traumatic arthropathy, right elbow

M12.522   Traumatic arthropathy, left elbow

M12.529   Traumatic arthropathy, unspecified elbow

M12.53   Traumatic arthropathy, wrist

M12.531   Traumatic arthropathy, right wrist

M12.532   Traumatic arthropathy, left wrist

M12.539   Traumatic arthropathy, unspecified wrist

M12.54   Traumatic arthropathy, hand

M12.541   Traumatic arthropathy, right hand

M12.542   Traumatic arthropathy, left hand

M12.549   Traumatic arthropathy, unspecified hand

M12.55   Traumatic arthropathy, hip

M12.551   Traumatic arthropathy, right hip

M12.552   Traumatic arthropathy, left hip

M12.559   Traumatic arthropathy, unspecified hip

M12.56   Traumatic arthropathy, knee

M12.561   Traumatic arthropathy, right knee

M12.562   Traumatic arthropathy, left knee

M12.569   Traumatic arthropathy, unspecified knee

M12.57   Traumatic arthropathy, ankle and foot

M12.571   Traumatic arthropathy, right ankle and foot

M12.572   Traumatic arthropathy, left ankle and foot

M12.579   Traumatic arthropathy, unspecified ankle and foot

M12.58   Traumatic arthropathy, vertebrae

M12.59   Traumatic arthropathy, multiple sites

M12.8   Other specific arthropathies, not elsewhere classified

Transient arthropathy

M12.80   Other specific arthropathies, not elsewhere classified, unspecified site

M12.81   Other specific arthropathies, not elsewhere classified, shoulder

M12.811   Other specific arthropathies, not elsewhere classified, right shoulder

M12.812   Other specific arthropathies, not elsewhere classified, left shoulder

M12.819   Other specific arthropathies, not elsewhere classified, unspecified shoulder

M12.82   Other specific arthropathies, not elsewhere classified, elbow

M12.821   Other specific arthropathies, not elsewhere classified, right elbow

M12.822   Other specific arthropathies, not elsewhere classified, left elbow

M12.829   Other specific arthropathies, not elsewhere classified, unspecified elbow

M12.83   Other specific arthropathies, not elsewhere classified, wrist

M12.831   Other specific arthropathies, not elsewhere classified, right wrist

M12.832   Other specific arthropathies, not elsewhere classified, left wrist

M12.839   Other specific arthropathies, not elsewhere classified, unspecified wrist

M12.84   Other specific arthropathies, not elsewhere classified, hand

M12.841   Other specific arthropathies, not elsewhere classified, right hand

M12.842   Other specific arthropathies, not elsewhere classified, left hand

M12.849   Other specific arthropathies, not elsewhere classified, unspecified hand

M12.85   Other specific arthropathies, not elsewhere classified, hip

M12.851   Other specific arthropathies, not elsewhere classified, right hip

M12.852   Other specific arthropathies, not elsewhere classified, left hip

M12.859   Other specific arthropathies, not elsewhere classified, unspecified hip

M12.86   Other specific arthropathies, not elsewhere classified, knee

M12.861   Other specific arthropathies, not elsewhere classified, right knee

M12.862   Other specific arthropathies, not elsewhere classified, left knee

M12.869   Other specific arthropathies, not elsewhere classified, unspecified knee

M12.87   Other specific arthropathies, not elsewhere classified, ankle and foot

M12.871   Other specific arthropathies, not elsewhere classified, right ankle and foot

M12.872   Other specific arthropathies, not elsewhere classified, left ankle and foot

M12.879   Other specific arthropathies, not elsewhere classified, unspecified ankle and foot

M12.88   Other specific arthropathies, not elsewhere classified, vertebrae

M12.89   Other specific arthropathies, not elsewhere classified, multiple sites

M13 Other arthritis

Excludes1:   arthrosis (M15-M19)
               osteoarthritis (M15-M19)

M13.0 Polyarthritis, unspecified

M13.1 Monoarthritis, not elsewhere classified

M13.10   Monoarthritis, not elsewhere classified, unspecified site

M13.11   Monoarthritis, not elsewhere classified, shoulder

M13.111   Monoarthritis, not elsewhere classified, right shoulder

M13.112   Monoarthritis, not elsewhere classified, left shoulder

M13.119   Monoarthritis, not elsewhere classified, unspecified shoulder

M13.12   Monoarthritis, not elsewhere classified, elbow

M13.121   Monoarthritis, not elsewhere classified, right elbow

M13.122   Monoarthritis, not elsewhere classified, left elbow

M13.129   Monoarthritis, not elsewhere classified, unspecified elbow

M13.13   Monoarthritis, not elsewhere classified, wrist

M13.131   Monoarthritis, not elsewhere classified, right wrist

M13.132   Monoarthritis, not elsewhere classified, left wrist

M13.139   Monoarthritis, not elsewhere classified, unspecified wrist

M13.14   Monoarthritis, not elsewhere classified, hand

M13.141   Monoarthritis, not elsewhere classified, right hand

M13.142   Monoarthritis, not elsewhere classified, left hand

M13.149   Monoarthritis, not elsewhere classified, unspecified hand

M13.15   Monoarthritis, not elsewhere classified, hip

M13.151   Monoarthritis, not elsewhere classified, right hip

M13.152   Monoarthritis, not elsewhere classified, left hip

M13.159   Monoarthritis, not elsewhere classified, unspecified hip

M13.16   Monoarthritis, not elsewhere classified, knee

M13.161   Monoarthritis, not elsewhere classified, right knee

M13.162   Monoarthritis, not elsewhere classified, left knee

M13.169   Monoarthritis, not elsewhere classified, unspecified knee

M13.17   Monoarthritis, not elsewhere classified, ankle and foot

M13.171   Monoarthritis, not elsewhere classified, right ankle and foot

M13.172   Monoarthritis, not elsewhere classified, left ankle and foot

M13.179   Monoarthritis, not elsewhere classified, unspecified ankle and foot

M13.8 Other specified arthritis

Allergic arthritis

Excludes2:   osteoarthritis (M15-M19)

M13.80   Other specified arthritis, unspecified site

M13.81   Other specified arthritis, shoulder

M13.811   Other specified arthritis, right shoulder

M13.812   Other specified arthritis, left shoulder

M13.819   Other specified arthritis, unspecified shoulder

M13.82   Other specified arthritis, elbow

M13.821   Other specified arthritis, right elbow

M13.822   Other specified arthritis, left elbow

M13.829   Other specified arthritis, unspecified elbow

M13.83   Other specified arthritis, wrist

M13.831   Other specified arthritis, right wrist

M13.832   Other specified arthritis, left wrist

M13.839   Other specified arthritis, unspecified wrist

M13.84   Other specified arthritis, hand

M13.841   Other specified arthritis, right hand

M13.842   Other specified arthritis, left hand

M13.849   Other specified arthritis, unspecified hand

M13.85   Other specified arthritis, hip

M13.851   Other specified arthritis, right hip

M13.852   Other specified arthritis, left hip

M13.859   Other specified arthritis, unspecified hip

M13.86   Other specified arthritis, knee

M13.861   Other specified arthritis, right knee

M13.862   Other specified arthritis, left knee

M13.869   Other specified arthritis, unspecified knee

M13.87   Other specified arthritis, ankle and foot

M13.871   Other specified arthritis, right ankle and foot

M13.872   Other specified arthritis, left ankle and foot

M13.879   Other specified arthritis, unspecified ankle and foot

M13.88   Other specified arthritis, vertebrae

M13.89   Other specified arthritis, multiple sites

M14 Arthropathies in other diseases classified elsewhere

Excludes1:   arthropathy in:
diabetes mellitus (E08-E14 with 4th character 61)
hematological disorders (M36.2-M36.3)
hypersensitivity reactions (M36.4)
neoplastic disease (M36.1)
neurosyphillis (A52.16)
sarcoidosis (D86.86)
enteropathic arthropathies (M07.0-)
juvenile enteropathic arthropathies (M09.0-)
lipoid dermatoarthritis (E78.81)

M14.6 Charcot's joint
Neuropathic arthropathy
Excludes1:   Charcot's joint in diabetes mellitus (E08-E14 with
final character 610)
Charcot's joint in tabes dorsalis (A52.16)

M14.60   Charcot's joint, unspecified site
M14.61   Charcot's joint, shoulder
M14.611 Charcot's joint, right shoulder
M14.612 Charcot's joint, left shoulder
M14.619 Charcot's joint, unspecified shoulder
M14.62   Charcot's joint, elbow
M14.621 Charcot's joint, right elbow
M14.622 Charcot's joint, left elbow
M14.629 Charcot's joint, unspecified elbow
M14.63   Charcot's joint, wrist
M14.631 Charcot's joint, right wrist
M14.632 Charcot's joint, left wrist
M14.639 Charcot's joint, unspecified wrist
M14.64   Charcot's joint, hand
M14.641 Charcot's joint, right hand
M14.642 Charcot's joint, left hand
M14.649 Charcot's joint, unspecified hand
M14.65   Charcot's joint, hip
M14.651 Charcot's joint, right hip
M14.652 Charcot's joint, left hip
M14.659 Charcot's joint, unspecified hip
M14.66   Charcot's joint, knee
M14.661 Charcot's joint, right knee
M14.662 Charcot's joint, left knee
M14.669 Charcot's joint, unspecified knee
M14.67   Charcot's joint, ankle and foot
M14.671 Charcot's joint, right ankle and foot
M14.672 Charcot's joint, left ankle and foot
M14.679 Charcot's joint, unspecified ankle and foot
M14.68   Charcot's joint, vertebrae
M14.69   Charcot's joint, multiple sites

M14.8 Arthropathies in other specified diseases classified elsewhere
Code first underlying disease, such as:
amyloidosis (E85)
erythema multiforme (L51.-)
erythema nodosum (L52)
hemochromatosis (E83.1)
hyperparathyroidism (E21.-)
hypothyroidism (E00-E03)
sickle-cell disorders (D57.-)
thyrotoxicosis [hyperthyroidism] (E05.-)
Whipple's disease (K90.8)

M14.80   Arthropathies in other specified diseases classified
elsewhere, unspecified site
M14.81   Arthropathies in other specified diseases classified
elsewhere, shoulder
M14.811 Arthropathies in other specified diseases
classified elsewhere, right shoulder
M14.812 Arthropathies in other specified diseases
classified elsewhere, left shoulder
M14.819 Arthropathies in other specified diseases
classified elsewhere, unspecified shoulder
M14.82   Arthropathies in other specified diseases classified
elsewhere, elbow

M14.821 Arthropathies in other specified diseases
classified elsewhere, right elbow
M14.822 Arthropathies in other specified diseases
classified elsewhere, left elbow
M14.829 Arthropathies in other specified diseases
classified elsewhere, unspecified elbow
M14.83   Arthropathies in other specified diseases classified
elsewhere, wrist
M14.831 Arthropathies in other specified diseases
classified elsewhere, right wrist
M14.832 Arthropathies in other specified diseases
classified elsewhere, left wrist
M14.839 Arthropathies in other specified diseases
classified elsewhere, unspecified wrist
M14.84   Arthropathies in other specified diseases classified
elsewhere, hand
M14.841 Arthropathies in other specified diseases
classified elsewhere, right hand
M14.842 Arthropathies in other specified diseases
classified elsewhere, left hand
M14.849 Arthropathies in other specified diseases
classified elsewhere, unspecified hand
M14.85   Arthropathies in other specified diseases classified
elsewhere, hip
M14.851 Arthropathies in other specified diseases
classified elsewhere, right hip
M14.852 Arthropathies in other specified diseases
classified elsewhere, left hip
M14.859 Arthropathies in other specified diseases
classified elsewhere, unspecified hip
M14.86   Arthropathies in other specified diseases classified
elsewhere, knee
M14.861 Arthropathies in other specified diseases
classified elsewhere, right knee
M14.862 Arthropathies in other specified diseases
classified elsewhere, left knee
M14.869 Arthropathies in other specified diseases
classified elsewhere, unspecified knee
M14.87   Arthropathies in other specified diseases classified
elsewhere, ankle and foot
M14.871 Arthropathies in other specified diseases
classified elsewhere, right ankle and foot
M14.872 Arthropathies in other specified diseases
classified elsewhere, left ankle and foot
M14.879 Arthropathies in other specified diseases
classified elsewhere, unspecified ankle and
foot
M14.88   Arthropathies in other specified diseases classified
elsewhere, vertebrae
M14.89   Arthropathies in other specified diseases classified
elsewhere, multiple sites

OSTEOARTHRITIS (M15–M19)

Excludes2:   osteoarthritis of spine (M47.-)

M15 Polyosteoarthritis
Includes: arthritis with mention of multiple sites
Excludes1:   bilateral involvement of single joint (M16-M19)

M15.0 Primary generalized (osteo)arthritis
M15.1 Heberden's nodes (with arthropathy)
Interphalangeal distal osteoarthritis
M15.2 Bouchard's nodes (with arthropathy)
Juxtaphalangeal distal osteoarthritis
M15.3 Secondary multiple arthritis
Post-traumatic polyosteoarthritis
M15.4 Erosive (osteo)arthritis
M15.8 Other polyosteoarthritis
M15.9 Polyosteoarthritis, unspecified
Generalized osteoarthritis NOS

M16 Osteoarthritis of hip

M16.0 Bilateral primary osteoarthritis of hip

M16.1 Unilateral primary osteoarthritis of hip
Primary osteoarthritis of hip NOS

M16.10 Unilateral primary osteoarthritis, unspecified hip

M16.11 Unilateral primary osteoarthritis, right hip

M16.12 Unilateral primary osteoarthritis, left hip

M16.2 Bilateral osteoarthritis resulting from hip dysplasia

M16.3 Unilateral osteoarthritis resulting from hip dysplasia
Dysplastic osteoarthritis of hip NOS

M16.30 Unilateral osteoarthritis resulting from hip dysplasia, unspecified hip

M16.31 Unilateral osteoarthritis resulting from hip dysplasia, right hip

M16.32 Unilateral osteoarthritis resulting from hip dysplasia, left hip

M16.4 Bilateral post-traumatic osteoarthritis of hip

M16.5 Unilateral post-traumatic osteoarthritis of hip
Post-traumatic osteoarthritis of hip NOS

M16.50 Unilateral post-traumatic osteoarthritis, unspecified hip

M16.51 Unilateral post-traumatic osteoarthritis, right hip

M16.52 Unilateral post-traumatic osteoarthritis, left hip

M16.6 Other bilateral secondary osteoarthritis of hip

M16.7 Other unilateral secondary osteoarthritis of hip
Secondary osteoarthritis of hip NOS

M16.9 Osteoarthritis of hip, unspecified

M17 Osteoarthritis of knee

M17.0 Bilateral primary osteoarthritis of knee

M17.1 Unilateral primary osteoarthritis of knee
Primary osteoarthritis of knee NOS

M17.10 Unilateral primary osteoarthritis, unspecified knee

M17.11 Unilateral primary osteoarthritis, right knee

M17.12 Unilateral primary osteoarthritis, left knee

M17.2 Bilateral post-traumatic osteoarthritis of knee

M17.3 Unilateral post-traumatic osteoarthritis of knee
Post-traumatic osteoarthritis of knee NOS

M17.30 Unilateral post-traumatic osteoarthritis, unspecified knee

M17.31 Unilateral post-traumatic osteoarthritis, right knee

M17.32 Unilateral post-traumatic osteoarthritis, left knee

M17.4 Other bilateral secondary osteoarthritis of knee

M17.5 Other unilateral secondary osteoarthritis of knee
Secondary osteoarthritis of knee NOS

M17.9 Osteoarthritis of knee, unspecified

M18 Osteoarthritis of first carpometacarpal joint

M18.0 Bilateral primary osteoarthritis of first carpometacarpal joints

M18.1 Unilateral primary osteoarthritis of first carpometacarpal joint
Primary osteoarthritis of first carpometacarpal joint NOS

M18.10 Unilateral primary osteoarthritis of first carpometacarpal joint, unspecified hand

M18.11 Unilateral primary osteoarthritis of first carpometacarpal joint, right hand

M18.12 Unilateral primary osteoarthritis of first carpometacarpal joint, left hand

M18.2 Bilateral post-traumatic osteoarthritis of first carpometacarpal joints

M18.3 Unilateral post-traumatic osteoarthritis of first carpometacarpal joint
Post-traumatic osteoarthritis of first carpometacarpal joint NOS

M18.30 Unilateral post-traumatic osteoarthritis of first carpometacarpal joint, unspecified hand

M18.31 Unilateral post-traumatic osteoarthritis of first carpometacarpal joint, right hand

M18.32 Unilateral post-traumatic osteoarthritis of first carpometacarpal joint, left hand

M18.4 Other bilateral secondary osteoarthritis of first carpometacarpal joints

M18.5 Other unilateral secondary osteoarthritis of first carpometacarpal joint
Secondary osteoarthritis of first carpometacarpal joint NOS

M18.50 Other unilateral secondary osteoarthritis of first carpometacarpal joint, unspecified hand

M18.51 Other unilateral secondary osteoarthritis of first carpometacarpal joint, right hand

M18.52 Other unilateral secondary osteoarthritis of first carpometacarpal joint, left hand

M18.9 Osteoarthritis of first carpometacarpal joint, unspecified

M19 Other and unspecified osteoarthritis

Excludes1:   polyarthritis (M15.-)

Excludes2:   arthrosis of spine (M47.-)
              hallux rigidus (M20.2)
              osteoarthritis of spine (M47.-)

M19.0 Primary osteoarthritis of other joints

M19.01   Primary osteoarthritis, shoulder

M19.011 Primary osteoarthritis, right shoulder

M19.012 Primary osteoarthritis, left shoulder

M19.019 Primary osteoarthritis, unspecified shoulder

M19.02   Primary osteoarthritis, elbow

M19.021 Primary osteoarthritis, right elbow

M19.022 Primary osteoarthritis, left elbow

M19.029 Primary osteoarthritis, unspecified elbow

M19.03   Primary osteoarthritis, wrist

M19.031 Primary osteoarthritis, right wrist

M19.032 Primary osteoarthritis, left wrist

M19.039 Primary osteoarthritis, unspecified wrist

M19.04   Primary osteoarthritis, hand

Excludes2:   primary osteoarthritis of first carpometacarpal joint (M18.0-, M18.1-)

M19.041 Primary osteoarthritis, right hand

M19.042 Primary osteoarthritis, left hand

M19.049 Primary osteoarthritis, unspecified hand

M19.07   Primary osteoarthritis ankle and foot

M19.071 Primary osteoarthritis, right ankle and foot

M19.072 Primary osteoarthritis, left ankle and foot

M19.079 Primary osteoarthritis, unspecified ankle and foot

M19.1 Post-traumatic osteoarthritis of other joints

M19.11   Post-traumatic osteoarthritis, shoulder

M19.111 Post-traumatic osteoarthritis, right shoulder

M19.112 Post-traumatic osteoarthritis, left shoulder

M19.119 Post-traumatic osteoarthritis, unspecified shoulder

M19.12   Post-traumatic osteoarthritis, elbow

M19.121 Post-traumatic osteoarthritis, right elbow

M19.122 Post-traumatic osteoarthritis, left elbow

M19.129 Post-traumatic osteoarthritis, unspecified elbow

M19.13   Post-traumatic osteoarthritis, wrist

M19.131 Post-traumatic osteoarthritis, right wrist

M19.132 Post-traumatic osteoarthritis, left wrist

M19.139 Post-traumatic osteoarthritis, unspecified wrist

M19.14   Post-traumatic osteoarthritis, hand

Excludes2:   post-traumatic osteoarthritis of first carpometacarpal joint (M18.2-, M18.3-)

M19.141 Post-traumatic osteoarthritis, right hand

M19.142 Post-traumatic osteoarthritis, left hand

M19.149 Post-traumatic osteoarthritis, unspecified hand

M19.17   Post-traumatic osteoarthritis, ankle and foot

M19.171 Post-traumatic osteoarthritis, right ankle and foot

M19.172 Post-traumatic osteoarthritis, left ankle and foot

M19.179   Post-traumatic osteoarthritis, unspecified ankle and foot

M19.2   Secondary osteoarthritis of other joints

    M19.21   Secondary osteoarthritis, shoulder

        M19.211   Secondary osteoarthritis, right shoulder

        M19.212   Secondary osteoarthritis, left shoulder

        M19.219   Secondary osteoarthritis, unspecified shoulder

    M19.22   Secondary osteoarthritis, elbow

        M19.221   Secondary osteoarthritis, right elbow

        M19.222   Secondary osteoarthritis, left elbow

        M19.229   Secondary osteoarthritis, unspecified elbow

    M19.23   Secondary osteoarthritis, wrist

        M19.231   Secondary osteoarthritis, right wrist

        M19.232   Secondary osteoarthritis, left wrist

        M19.239   Secondary osteoarthritis, unspecified wrist

    M19.24   Secondary osteoarthritis, hand

        M19.241   Secondary osteoarthritis, right hand

        M19.242   Secondary osteoarthritis, left hand

        M19.249   Secondary osteoarthritis, unspecified hand

    M19.27   Secondary osteoarthritis, ankle and foot

        M19.271   Secondary osteoarthritis, right ankle and foot

        M19.272   Secondary osteoarthritis, left ankle and foot

        M19.279   Secondary osteoarthritis, unspecified ankle and foot

M19.9   Osteoarthritis, unspecified site

    M19.90   Unspecified osteoarthritis, unspecified site

        Arthrosis NOS

        Arthritis NOS

        Osteoarthritis NOS

    M19.91   Primary osteoarthritis, unspecified site

        Primary osteoarthritis NOS

    M19.92   Post-traumatic osteoarthritis, unspecified site

        Post-traumatic osteoarthritis NOS

    M19.93   Secondary osteoarthritis, unspecified site

        Secondary osteoarthritis NOS

OTHER JOINT DISORDERS (M20–M25)

Excludes2:   joints of the spine (M40-M54)

M20   Acquired deformities of fingers and toes

    Excludes1:   acquired absence of fingers and toes (Z89.-)

        congenital absence of fingers and toes (Q71.3-, Q72.3-)

        congenital deformities and malformations of fingers and toes (Q66.-, Q68-Q70, Q74.-)

M20.0   Deformity of finger(s)

    Excludes1:   clubbing of fingers (R68.3)

        palmar fascial fibromatosis [Dupuytren] (M72.0)

        trigger finger (M65.3)

    M20.00   Unspecified deformity of finger(s)

        M20.001   Unspecified deformity of right finger(s)

        M20.002   Unspecified deformity of left finger(s)

        M20.009   Unspecified deformity of unspecified finger(s)

    M20.01   Mallet finger

        M20.011   Mallet finger of right finger(s)

        M20.012   Mallet finger of left finger(s)

        M20.019   Mallet finger of unspecified finger(s)

    M20.02   Boutonnière deformity

        M20.021   Boutonnière deformity of right finger(s)

        M20.022   Boutonnière deformity of left finger(s)

        M20.029   Boutonnière deformity of unspecified finger(s)

    M20.03   Swan-neck deformity

        M20.031   Swan-neck deformity of right finger(s)

        M20.032   Swan-neck deformity of left finger(s)

        M20.039   Swan-neck deformity of unspecified finger(s)

    M20.09   Other deformity of finger(s)

        M20.091   Other deformity of right finger(s)

        M20.092   Other deformity of left finger(s)

        M20.099   Other deformity of finger(s), unspecified finger(s)

M20.1   Hallux valgus (acquired)

    Bunion

    M20.10   Hallux valgus (acquired), unspecified foot

    M20.11   Hallux valgus (acquired), right foot

    M20.12   Hallux valgus (acquired), left foot

M20.2   Hallux rigidus

    M20.20   Hallux rigidus, unspecified foot

    M20.21   Hallux rigidus, right foot

    M20.22   Hallux rigidus, left foot

M20.3   Other deformity of hallux (acquired)

    Hallux varus

    M20.30   Other deformity of hallux (acquired), unspecified foot

    M20.31   Other deformity of hallux (acquired), right foot

    M20.32   Other deformity of hallux (acquired), left foot

M20.4   Other hammer toe(s) (acquired)

    M20.40   Other hammer toe(s) (acquired), unspecified foot

    M20.41   Other hammer toe(s) (acquired), right foot

    M20.42   Other hammer toe(s) (acquired), left foot

M20.5   Other deformities of toe(s) (acquired)

    M20.50   Other deformities of toe(s) (acquired), unspecified foot

    M20.51   Other deformities of toe(s) (acquired), right foot

    M20.52   Other deformities of toe(s) (acquired), left foot

M20.6   Acquired deformities of toe(s), unspecified

    M20.60   Acquired deformities of toe(s), unspecified, unspecified foot

    M20.61   Acquired deformities of toe(s), unspecified, right foot

    M20.62   Acquired deformities of toe(s), unspecified, left foot

M21   Other acquired deformities of limbs

    Excludes1:   acquired absence of limb (Z89.-)

        congenital absence of limbs (Q71-Q73)

        congenital deformities and malformations of limbs (Q65-Q66, Q68-Q74)

    Excludes2:   acquired deformities of fingers or toes (M20.-)

        coxa plana (M91.2)

M21.0   Valgus deformity, not elsewhere classified

    Excludes1:   metatarsus valgus (Q66.6)

        talipes calcaneovalgus (Q66.4)

    M21.00   Valgus deformity, not elsewhere classified, unspecified site

    M21.02   Valgus deformity, not elsewhere classified, elbow

        Cubitus valgus

        M21.021   Valgus deformity, not elsewhere classified, right elbow

        M21.022   Valgus deformity, not elsewhere classified, left elbow

        M21.029   Valgus deformity, not elsewhere classified, unspecified elbow

    M21.06   Valgus deformity, not elsewhere classified, knee

        Genu valgus

        Knock knee

        M21.061   Valgus deformity, not elsewhere classified, right knee

        M21.062   Valgus deformity, not elsewhere classified, left knee

        M21.069   Valgus deformity, not elsewhere classified, unspecified knee

    M21.07   Valgus deformity, not elsewhere classified, ankle

        M21.071   Valgus deformity, not elsewhere classified, right ankle

        M21.072   Valgus deformity, not elsewhere classified, left ankle

        M21.079   Valgus deformity, not elsewhere classified, unspecified ankle

M21.1   Varus deformity, not elsewhere classified

    Excludes1:   metatarsus varus (Q66.2)

        tibia vara (M92.5)

    M21.10   Varus deformity, not elsewhere classified, unspecified site

    M21.12   Varus deformity, not elsewhere classified, elbow

        Cubitus varus, elbow

M21.121   Varus deformity, not elsewhere classified, right elbow

M21.122   Varus deformity, not elsewhere classified, left elbow

M21.129   Varus deformity, not elsewhere classified, unspecified elbow

M21.16   Varus deformity, not elsewhere classified, knee
Bow leg
Genu varus, knee

M21.161   Varus deformity, not elsewhere classified, right knee

M21.162   Varus deformity, not elsewhere classified, left knee

M21.169   Varus deformity, not elsewhere classified, unspecified knee

M21.17   Varus deformity, not elsewhere classified, ankle

M21.171   Varus deformity, not elsewhere classified, right ankle

M21.172   Varus deformity, not elsewhere classified, left ankle

M21.179   Varus deformity, not elsewhere classified, unspecified ankle

M21.2   Flexion deformity

M21.20   Flexion deformity, unspecified site

M21.21   Flexion deformity, shoulder

M21.211   Flexion deformity, right shoulder

M21.212   Flexion deformity, left shoulder

M21.219   Flexion deformity, unspecified shoulder

M21.22   Flexion deformity, elbow

M21.221   Flexion deformity, right elbow

M21.222   Flexion deformity, left elbow

M21.229   Flexion deformity, unspecified elbow

M21.23   Flexion deformity, wrist

M21.231   Flexion deformity, right wrist

M21.232   Flexion deformity, left wrist

M21.239   Flexion deformity, unspecified wrist

M21.24   Flexion deformity, finger joints

M21.241   Flexion deformity, right finger joints

M21.242   Flexion deformity, left finger joints

M21.249   Flexion deformity, unspecified finger joints

M21.25   Flexion deformity, hip

M21.251   Flexion deformity, right hip

M21.252   Flexion deformity, left hip

M21.259   Flexion deformity, unspecified hip

M21.26   Flexion deformity, knee

M21.261   Flexion deformity, right knee

M21.262   Flexion deformity, left knee

M21.269   Flexion deformity, unspecified knee

M21.27   Flexion deformity, ankle and toes

M21.271   Flexion deformity, right ankle and toes

M21.272   Flexion deformity, left ankle and toes

M21.279   Flexion deformity, unspecified ankle and toes

M21.3   Wrist or foot drop (acquired)

M21.33   Wrist drop (acquired)

M21.331   Wrist drop, right wrist

M21.332   Wrist drop, left wrist

M21.339   Wrist drop, unspecified wrist

M21.37   Foot drop (acquired)

M21.371   Foot drop, right foot

M21.372   Foot drop, left foot

M21.379   Foot drop, unspecified foot

M21.4   Flat foot [pes planus] (acquired)
Excludes1:   congenital pes planus (Q66.5)

M21.40   Flat foot [pes planus] (acquired), unspecified foot

M21.41   Flat foot [pes planus] (acquired), right foot

M21.42   Flat foot [pes planus] (acquired), left foot

M21.5   Acquired clawhand, clubhand, clawfoot and clubfoot
Excludes1:   clubfoot, not specified as acquired (Q66.8)

M21.51   Acquired clawhand

M21.511   Acquired clawhand, right hand

M21.512   Acquired clawhand, left hand

M21.519   Acquired clawhand, unspecified hand

M21.52   Acquired clubhand

M21.521   Acquired clubhand, right hand

M21.522   Acquired clubhand, left hand

M21.529   Acquired clubhand, unspecified hand

M21.53   Acquired clawfoot

M21.531   Acquired clawfoot, right foot

M21.532   Acquired clawfoot, left foot

M21.539   Acquired clawfoot, unspecified foot

M21.54   Acquired clubfoot

M21.541   Acquired clubfoot, right foot

M21.542   Acquired clubfoot, left foot

M21.549   Acquired clubfoot, unspecified foot

M21.6   Other acquired deformities of foot
Excludes2:   deformities of toe (acquired) (M20.1-.M20.6)

M21.60   Other acquired deformities of unspecified foot

M21.61   Other acquired deformities of right foot

M21.62   Other acquired deformities of left foot

M21.7   Unequal limb length (acquired)
Note: The site used should correspond to the short limb

M21.70   Unequal limb length (acquired), unspecified site

M21.72   Unequal limb length (acquired), humerus

M21.721   Unequal limb length (acquired), right humerus

M21.722   Unequal limb length (acquired), left humerus

M21.729   Unequal limb length (acquired), unspecified humerus

M21.73   Unequal limb length (acquired), ulna and radius

M21.731   Unequal limb length (acquired), right ulna

M21.732   Unequal limb length (acquired), left ulna

M21.733   Unequal limb length (acquired), right radius

M21.734   Unequal limb length (acquired), left radius

M21.739   Unequal limb length (acquired), unspecified ulna and radius

M21.75   Unequal limb length (acquired), femur

M21.751   Unequal limb length (acquired), right femur

M21.752   Unequal limb length (acquired), left femur

M21.759   Unequal limb length (acquired), unspecified femur

M21.76   Unequal limb length (acquired), tibia and fibula

M21.761   Unequal limb length (acquired), right tibia

M21.762   Unequal limb length (acquired), left tibia

M21.763   Unequal limb length (acquired), right fibula

M21.764   Unequal limb length (acquired), left fibula

M21.769   Unequal limb length (acquired), unspecified tibia and fibula

M21.8   Other specified acquired deformities of limbs
Excludes2:   coxa plana (M91.2)

M21.80   Other specified acquired deformities of unspecified limb

M21.82   Other specified acquired deformities of upper arm

M21.821   Other specified acquired deformities of right upper arm

M21.822   Other specified acquired deformities of left upper arm

M21.829   Other specified acquired deformities of unspecified upper arm

M21.83   Other specified acquired deformities of forearm

M21.831   Other specified acquired deformities of right forearm

M21.832   Other specified acquired deformities of left forearm

M21.839   Other specified acquired deformities of unspecified forearm

M21.85   Other specified acquired deformities of thigh

M21.851   Other specified acquired deformities of right thigh

M21.852   Other specified acquired deformities of left thigh

M21.859   Other specified acquired deformities of unspecified thigh

M21.86   Other specified acquired deformities of lower leg

    M21.861   Other specified acquired deformities of right lower leg

    M21.862   Other specified acquired deformities of left lower leg

    M21.869   Other specified acquired deformities of unspecified lower leg

M21.9   Unspecified acquired deformity of limb and hand

M21.90   Unspecified acquired deformity of unspecified limb

M21.92   Unspecified acquired deformity of upper arm

    M21.921   Unspecified acquired deformity of right upper arm

    M21.922   Unspecified acquired deformity of left upper arm

    M21.929   Unspecified acquired deformity of unspecified upper arm

M21.93   Unspecified acquired deformity of forearm

    M21.931   Unspecified acquired deformity of right forearm

    M21.932   Unspecified acquired deformity of left forearm

    M21.939   Unspecified acquired deformity of unspecified forearm

M21.94   Unspecified acquired deformity of hand

    M21.941   Unspecified acquired deformity of hand, right hand

    M21.942   Unspecified acquired deformity of hand, left hand

    M21.949   Unspecified acquired deformity of hand, unspecified hand

M21.95   Unspecified acquired deformity of thigh

    M21.951   Unspecified acquired deformity of right thigh

    M21.952   Unspecified acquired deformity of left thigh

    M21.959   Unspecified acquired deformity of unspecified thigh

M21.96   Unspecified acquired deformity of lower leg

    M21.961   Unspecified acquired deformity of right lower leg

    M21.962   Unspecified acquired deformity of left lower leg

    M21.969   Unspecified acquired deformity of unspecified lower leg

M22 Disorder of patella

Excludes1:   traumatic dislocation of patella (S83.0-)

M22.0   Recurrent dislocation of patella

M22.00   Recurrent dislocation of patella, unspecified knee

M22.01   Recurrent dislocation of patella, right knee

M22.02   Recurrent dislocation of patella, left knee

M22.1   Recurrent subluxation of patella

Incomplete dislocation of patella

M22.10   Recurrent subluxation of patella, unspecified knee

M22.11   Recurrent subluxation of patella, right knee

M22.12   Recurrent subluxation of patella, left knee

M22.2   Patellofemoral disorders

M22.20   Patellofemoral disorders, unspecified knee

M22.21   Patellofemoral disorders, right knee

M22.22   Patellofemoral disorders, left knee

M22.3   Other derangements of patella

M22.30   Other derangements of patella, unspecified knee

M22.31   Other derangements of patella, right knee

M22.32   Other derangements of patella, left knee

M22.4   Chondromalacia patellae

M22.40   Chondromalacia patellae, unspecified knee

M22.41   Chondromalacia patellae, right knee

M22.42   Chondromalacia patellae, left knee

M22.8   Other disorders of patella

M22.80   Other disorders of patella, unspecified knee

M22.81   Other disorders of patella, right knee

M22.82   Other disorders of patella, left knee

M22.9   Unspecified disorder of patella

M22.90   Unspecified disorder of patella, unspecified knee

M22.91   Unspecified disorder of patella, right knee

M22.92   Unspecified disorder of patella, left knee

M23 Internal derangement of knee

Excludes1:   ankylosis (M24.66)

    current injury — see injury of knee and lower leg (S80-S89)

    deformity of knee (M21.-)

    osteochondritis dissecans (M93.2)

    recurrent dislocation or subluxation of patella (M22.0-M22.1)

Excludes2:   disorders of patella (M22.-)

M23.0   Cystic meniscus

M23.00   Cystic meniscus, unspecified meniscus

    Cystic meniscus, unspecified lateral meniscus

    Cystic meniscus, unspecified medial meniscus

    M23.000   Cystic meniscus, unspecified lateral meniscus, right knee

    M23.001   Cystic meniscus, unspecified lateral meniscus, left knee

    M23.002   Cystic meniscus, unspecified lateral meniscus, unspecified knee

    M23.003   Cystic meniscus, unspecified medial meniscus, right knee

    M23.004   Cystic meniscus, unspecified medial meniscus, left knee

    M23.005   Cystic meniscus, unspecified medial meniscus, unspecified knee

    M23.006   Cystic meniscus, unspecified meniscus, right knee

    M23.007   Cystic meniscus, unspecified meniscus, left knee

    M23.009   Cystic meniscus, unspecified meniscus, unspecified knee

M23.01   Cystic meniscus, anterior horn of medial meniscus

    M23.011   Cystic meniscus, anterior horn of medial meniscus, right knee

    M23.012   Cystic meniscus, anterior horn of medial meniscus, left knee

    M23.019   Cystic meniscus, anterior horn of medial meniscus, unspecified knee

M23.02   Cystic meniscus, posterior horn of medical meniscus

    M23.021   Cystic meniscus, posterior horn of medical meniscus, right knee

    M23.022   Cystic meniscus, posterior horn of medical meniscus, left knee

    M23.029   Cystic meniscus, posterior horn of medical meniscus, unspecified knee

M23.03   Cystic meniscus, other medial meniscus

    M23.031   Cystic meniscus, other medial meniscus, right knee

    M23.032   Cystic meniscus, other medial meniscus, left knee

    M23.039   Cystic meniscus, other medial meniscus, unspecified knee

M23.04   Cystic meniscus, anterior horn of lateral meniscus

    M23.041   Cystic meniscus, anterior horn of lateral meniscus, right knee

    M23.042   Cystic meniscus, anterior horn of lateral meniscus, left knee

    M23.049   Cystic meniscus, anterior horn of lateral meniscus, unspecified knee

M23.05   Cystic meniscus, posterior horn of lateral meniscus

    M23.051   Cystic meniscus, posterior horn of lateral meniscus, right knee

M23.052 Cystic meniscus, posterior horn of lateral meniscus, left knee

M23.059 Cystic meniscus, posterior horn of lateral meniscus, unspecified knee

M23.06   Cystic meniscus, other lateral meniscus

M23.061 Cystic meniscus, other lateral meniscus, right knee

M23.062 Cystic meniscus, other lateral meniscus, left knee

M23.069 Cystic meniscus, other lateral meniscus, unspecified knee

M23.2 Derangement of meniscus due to old tear or injury
   Old bucket-handle tear

M23.20   Derangement of unspecified meniscus due to old tear or injury
   Derangement of unspecified lateral meniscus due to old tear or injury
   Derangement of unspecified medial meniscus due to old tear or injury

M23.200 Derangement of unspecified lateral meniscus due to old tear or injury, right knee

M23.201 Derangement of unspecified lateral meniscus due to old tear or injury, left knee

M23.202 Derangement of unspecified lateral meniscus due to old tear or injury, unspecified knee

M23.203 Derangement of unspecified medial meniscus due to old tear or injury, right knee

M23.204 Derangement of unspecified medial meniscus due to old tear or injury, left knee

M23.205 Derangement of unspecified medial meniscus due to old tear or injury, unspecified knee

M23.206 Derangement of unspecified meniscus due to old tear or injury, right knee

M23.207 Derangement of unspecified meniscus due to old tear or injury, left knee

M23.209 Derangement of unspecified meniscus due to old tear or injury, unspecified knee

M23.21   Derangement of anterior horn of medial meniscus due to old tear or injury

M23.211 Derangement of anterior horn of medial meniscus due to old tear or injury, right knee

M23.212 Derangement of anterior horn of medial meniscus due to old tear or injury, left knee

M23.219 Derangement of anterior horn of medial meniscus due to old tear or injury, unspecified knee

M23.22   Derangement of posterior horn of medical meniscus due to old tear or injury

M23.221 Derangement of posterior horn of medical meniscus due to old tear or injury, right knee

M23.222 Derangement of posterior horn of medical meniscus due to old tear or injury, left knee

M23.229 Derangement of posterior horn of medical meniscus due to old tear or injury, unspecified knee

M23.23   Derangement of other medial meniscus due to old tear or injury

M23.231 Derangement of other medial meniscus due to old tear or injury, right knee

M23.232 Derangement of other medial meniscus due to old tear or injury, left knee

M23.239 Derangement of other medial meniscus due to old tear or injury, unspecified knee

M23.24   Derangement of anterior horn of lateral meniscus due to old tear or injury

M23.241 Derangement of anterior horn of lateral meniscus due to old tear or injury, right knee

M23.242 Derangement of anterior horn of lateral meniscus due to old tear or injury, left knee

M23.249 Derangement of anterior horn of lateral meniscus due to old tear or injury, unspecified knee

M23.25   Derangement of posterior horn of lateral meniscus due to old tear or injury

M23.251 Derangement of posterior horn of lateral meniscus due to old tear or injury, right knee

M23.252 Derangement of posterior horn of lateral meniscus due to old tear or injury, left knee

M23.259 Derangement of posterior horn of lateral meniscus due to old tear or injury, unspecified knee

M23.26   Derangement of other lateral meniscus due to old tear or injury

M23.261 Derangement of other lateral meniscus due to old tear or injury, right knee

M23.262 Derangement of other lateral meniscus due to old tear or injury, left knee

M23.269 Derangement of other lateral meniscus due to old tear or injury, unspecified knee

M23.3 Other meniscus derangements
   Degenerate meniscus
   Detached meniscus
   Retained meniscus

M23.30   Other meniscus derangements, unspecified meniscus
   Other meniscus derangements, unspecified lateral meniscus
   Other meniscus derangements, unspecified medial meniscus

M23.300 Other meniscus derangements, unspecified lateral meniscus, right knee

M23.301 Other meniscus derangements, unspecified lateral meniscus, left knee

M23.302 Other meniscus derangements, unspecified lateral meniscus, unspecified knee

M23.303 Other meniscus derangements, unspecified medial meniscus, right knee

M23.304 Other meniscus derangements, unspecified medial meniscus, left knee

M23.305 Other meniscus derangements, unspecified medial meniscus, unspecified knee

M23.306 Other meniscus derangements, unspecified meniscus, right knee

M23.307 Other meniscus derangements, unspecified meniscus, left knee

M23.309 Other meniscus derangements, unspecified meniscus, unspecified knee

M23.31   Other meniscus derangements, anterior horn of medial meniscus

M23.311 Other meniscus derangements, anterior horn of medial meniscus, right knee

M23.312 Other meniscus derangements, anterior horn of medial meniscus, left knee

M23.319 Other meniscus derangements, anterior horn of medial meniscus, unspecified knee

M23.32   Other meniscus derangements, posterior horn of medical meniscus

M23.321 Other meniscus derangements, posterior horn of medical meniscus, right knee

M23.322 Other meniscus derangements, posterior horn of medical meniscus, left knee

M23.329 Other meniscus derangements, posterior horn of medical meniscus, unspecified knee

M23.33   Other meniscus derangements, other medial meniscus

M23.331 Other meniscus derangements, other medial meniscus, right knee

M23.332 Other meniscus derangements, other medial meniscus, left knee

M23.339 Other meniscus derangements, other medial meniscus, unspecified knee

M23.34   Other meniscus derangements, anterior horn of lateral meniscus

M23.341 Other meniscus derangements, anterior horn of lateral meniscus, right knee

M23.342 Other meniscus derangements, anterior horn of lateral meniscus, left knee

M23.349   Other meniscus derangements, anterior horn of lateral meniscus, unspecified knee

M23.35   Other meniscus derangements, posterior horn of lateral meniscus

    M23.351   Other meniscus derangements, posterior horn of lateral meniscus, right knee

    M23.352   Other meniscus derangements, posterior horn of lateral meniscus, left knee

    M23.359   Other meniscus derangements, posterior horn of lateral meniscus, unspecified knee

M23.36   Other meniscus derangements, other lateral meniscus

    M23.361   Other meniscus derangements, other lateral meniscus, right knee

    M23.362   Other meniscus derangements, other lateral meniscus, left knee

    M23.369   Other meniscus derangements, other lateral meniscus, unspecified knee

M23.4 Loose body in knee

M23.40   Loose body in knee, unspecified knee

M23.41   Loose body in knee, right knee

M23.42   Loose body in knee, left knee

M23.5 Chronic instability of knee

M23.50   Chronic instability of knee, unspecified knee

M23.51   Chronic instability of knee, right knee

M23.52   Chronic instability of knee, left knee

M23.6 Other spontaneous disruption of ligament(s) of knee

M23.60   Other spontaneous disruption of unspecified ligament of knee

    M23.601   Other spontaneous disruption of unspecified ligament of right knee

    M23.602   Other spontaneous disruption of unspecified ligament of left knee

    M23.609   Other spontaneous disruption of unspecified ligament of unspecified knee

M23.61   Other spontaneous disruption of anterior cruciate ligament of knee

    M23.611   Other spontaneous disruption of anterior cruciate ligament of right knee

    M23.612   Other spontaneous disruption of anterior cruciate ligament of left knee

    M23.619   Other spontaneous disruption of anterior cruciate ligament of unspecified knee

M23.62   Other spontaneous disruption of posterior cruciate ligament of knee

    M23.621   Other spontaneous disruption of posterior cruciate ligament of right knee

    M23.622   Other spontaneous disruption of posterior cruciate ligament of left knee

    M23.629   Other spontaneous disruption of posterior cruciate ligament of unspecified knee

M23.63   Other spontaneous disruption of medial collateral ligament of knee

    M23.631   Other spontaneous disruption of medial collateral ligament of right knee

    M23.632   Other spontaneous disruption of medial collateral ligament of left knee

    M23.639   Other spontaneous disruption of medial collateral ligament of unspecified knee

M23.64   Other spontaneous disruption of lateral collateral ligament of knee

    M23.641   Other spontaneous disruption of lateral collateral ligament of right knee

    M23.642   Other spontaneous disruption of lateral collateral ligament of left knee

    M23.649   Other spontaneous disruption of lateral collateral ligament of unspecified knee

M23.67   Other spontaneous disruption of capsular ligament of knee

    M23.671   Other spontaneous disruption of capsular ligament of right knee

    M23.672   Other spontaneous disruption of capsular ligament of left knee

    M23.679   Other spontaneous disruption of capsular ligament of unspecified knee

M23.8 Other internal derangements of knee

    Laxity of ligament of knee
    Snapping knee

M23.8x   Other internal derangements of knee

    M23.8x1   Other internal derangements of right knee

    M23.8x2   Other internal derangements of left knee

    M23.8x9   Other internal derangements of unspecified knee

M23.9 Unspecified internal derangement of knee

M23.90   Unspecified internal derangement of unspecified knee

M23.91   Unspecified internal derangement of right knee

M23.92   Unspecified internal derangement of left knee

M24 Other specific joint derangements

Excludes1:   current injury — see injury of joint by body region

Excludes2:   ganglion (M67.4)
            internal derangement of knee (M23.-)
            snapping knee (M23.8-)
            temporomandibular joint disorders (M26.6-)

M24.0 Loose body in joint

    Excludes2:   loose body in knee (M23.4)

M24.00   Loose body in unspecified joint

M24.01   Loose body in shoulder

    M24.011   Loose body in right shoulder

    M24.012   Loose body in left shoulder

    M24.019   Loose body in unspecified shoulder

M24.02   Loose body in elbow

    M24.021   Loose body in right elbow

    M24.022   Loose body in left elbow

    M24.029   Loose body in unspecified elbow

M24.03   Loose body in wrist

    M24.031   Loose body in right wrist

    M24.032   Loose body in left wrist

    M24.039   Loose body in unspecified wrist

M24.04   Loose body in finger joints

    M24.041   Loose body in right finger joint(s)

    M24.042   Loose body in left finger joint(s)

    M24.049   Loose body in unspecified finger joint(s)

M24.05   Loose body in hip

    M24.051   Loose body in right hip

    M24.052   Loose body in left hip

    M24.059   Loose body in unspecified hip

M24.07   Loose body in ankle and toe joints

    M24.071   Loose body in right ankle

    M24.072   Loose body in left ankle

    M24.073   Loose body in unspecified ankle

    M24.074   Loose body in right toe joint(s)

    M24.075   Loose body in left toe joint(s)

    M24.076   Loose body in unspecified toe joints

M24.08   Loose body, other site

M24.1 Other articular cartilage disorders

    Excludes2:   chondrocalcinosis (M11.1, M11.2-)
            internal derangement of knee (M23.-)
            metastatic calcification (E83.5)
            ochronosis (E70.2)

M24.10   Other articular cartilage disorders, unspecified site

M24.11   Other articular cartilage disorders, shoulder

    M24.111   Other articular cartilage disorders, right shoulder

    M24.112   Other articular cartilage disorders, left shoulder

    M24.119   Other articular cartilage disorders, unspecified shoulder

M24.12   Other articular cartilage disorders, elbow

    M24.121   Other articular cartilage disorders, right elbow

    M24.122   Other articular cartilage disorders, left elbow

    M24.129   Other articular cartilage disorders, unspecified elbow

M24.13   Other articular cartilage disorders, wrist
  M24.131   Other articular cartilage disorders, right wrist
  M24.132   Other articular cartilage disorders, left wrist
  M24.139   Other articular cartilage disorders, unspecified wrist
M24.14   Other articular cartilage disorders, hand
  M24.141   Other articular cartilage disorders, right hand
  M24.142   Other articular cartilage disorders, left hand
  M24.149   Other articular cartilage disorders, unspecified hand
M24.15   Other articular cartilage disorders, hip
  M24.151   Other articular cartilage disorders, right hip
  M24.152   Other articular cartilage disorders, left hip
  M24.159   Other articular cartilage disorders, unspecified hip
M24.17   Other articular cartilage disorders, ankle and foot
  M24.171   Other articular cartilage disorders, right ankle
  M24.172   Other articular cartilage disorders, left ankle
  M24.173   Other articular cartilage disorders, unspecified ankle
  M24.174   Other articular cartilage disorders, right foot
  M24.175   Other articular cartilage disorders, left foot
  M24.176   Other articular cartilage disorders, unspecified foot

M24.2   Disorder of ligament
  Instability secondary to old ligament injury
  Ligamentous laxity NOS
  Excludes1:   familial ligamentous laxity (M35.7)
  Excludes2:   internal derangement of knee (M23.5-M23.89)
  M24.20   Disorder of ligament, unspecified site
  M24.21   Disorder of ligament, shoulder
    M24.211   Disorder of ligament, right shoulder
    M24.212   Disorder of ligament, left shoulder
    M24.219   Disorder of ligament, unspecified shoulder
  M24.22   Disorder of ligament, elbow
    M24.221   Disorder of ligament, right elbow
    M24.222   Disorder of ligament, left elbow
    M24.229   Disorder of ligament, unspecified elbow
  M24.23   Disorder of ligament, wrist
    M24.231   Disorder of ligament, right wrist
    M24.232   Disorder of ligament, left wrist
    M24.239   Disorder of ligament, unspecified wrist
  M24.24   Disorder of ligament, hand
    M24.241   Disorder of ligament, right hand
    M24.242   Disorder of ligament, left hand
    M24.249   Disorder of ligament, unspecified hand
  M24.25   Disorder of ligament, hip
    M24.251   Disorder of ligament, right hip
    M24.252   Disorder of ligament, left hip
    M24.259   Disorder of ligament, unspecified hip
  M24.27   Disorder of ligament, ankle and foot
    M24.271   Disorder of ligament, right ankle
    M24.272   Disorder of ligament, left ankle
    M24.273   Disorder of ligament, unspecified ankle
    M24.274   Disorder of ligament, right foot
    M24.275   Disorder of ligament, left foot
    M24.276   Disorder of ligament, unspecified foot
  M24.28   Disorder of ligament, vertebrae

M24.3   Pathological dislocation of joint, not elsewhere classified
  Excludes1:   congenital dislocation or displacement of joint — see congenital malformations and deformations of the musculoskeletal system (Q65-Q79)
             current injury — see injury of joints and ligaments by body region recurrent dislocation of joint (M24.4-)
  M24.30   Pathological dislocation of unspecified joint, not elsewhere classified

M24.31   Pathological dislocation of shoulder, not elsewhere classified
  M24.311   Pathological dislocation of right shoulder, not elsewhere classified
  M24.312   Pathological dislocation of left shoulder, not elsewhere classified
  M24.319   Pathological dislocation of unspecified shoulder, not elsewhere classified
M24.32   Pathological dislocation of elbow, not elsewhere classified
  M24.321   Pathological dislocation of right elbow, not elsewhere classified
  M24.322   Pathological dislocation of left elbow, not elsewhere classified
  M24.329   Pathological dislocation of unspecified elbow, not elsewhere classified
M24.33   Pathological dislocation of wrist, not elsewhere classified
  M24.331   Pathological dislocation of right wrist, not elsewhere classified
  M24.332   Pathological dislocation of left wrist, not elsewhere classified
  M24.339   Pathological dislocation of unspecified wrist, not elsewhere classified
M24.34   Pathological dislocation of hand, not elsewhere classified
  M24.341   Pathological dislocation of right hand, not elsewhere classified
  M24.342   Pathological dislocation of left hand, not elsewhere classified
  M24.349   Pathological dislocation of unspecified hand, not elsewhere classified
M24.35   Pathological dislocation of hip, not elsewhere classified
  M24.351   Pathological dislocation of right hip, not elsewhere classified
  M24.352   Pathological dislocation of left hip, not elsewhere classified
  M24.359   Pathological dislocation of unspecified hip, not elsewhere classified
M24.36   Pathological dislocation of knee, not elsewhere classified
  M24.361   Pathological dislocation of right knee, not elsewhere classified
  M24.362   Pathological dislocation of left knee, not elsewhere classified
  M24.369   Pathological dislocation of unspecified knee, not elsewhere classified
M24.37   Pathological dislocation of ankle and foot, not elsewhere classified
  M24.371   Pathological dislocation of right ankle, not elsewhere classified
  M24.372   Pathological dislocation of left ankle, not elsewhere classified
  M24.373   Pathological dislocation of unspecified ankle, not elsewhere classified
  M24.374   Pathological dislocation of right foot, not elsewhere classified
  M24.375   Pathological dislocation of left foot, not elsewhere classified
  M24.376   Pathological dislocation of unspecified foot, not elsewhere classified

M24.4   Recurrent dislocation of joint
  Recurrent subluxation of joint
  Excludes2:   recurrent dislocation of patella (M22.0-M22.1)
             recurrent vertebral dislocation (M43.3-, M43.4, M43.5-)
  M24.40   Recurrent dislocation, unspecified joint
  M24.41   Recurrent dislocation, shoulder
    M24.411   Recurrent dislocation, right shoulder
    M24.412   Recurrent dislocation, left shoulder
    M24.419   Recurrent dislocation, unspecified shoulder

M24.42   Recurrent dislocation, elbow
   M24.421   Recurrent dislocation, right elbow
   M24.422   Recurrent dislocation, left elbow
   M24.429   Recurrent dislocation, unspecified elbow
M24.43   Recurrent dislocation, wrist
   M24.431   Recurrent dislocation, right wrist
   M24.432   Recurrent dislocation, left wrist
   M24.439   Recurrent dislocation, unspecified wrist
M24.44   Recurrent dislocation, hand and finger(s)
   M24.441   Recurrent dislocation, right hand
   M24.442   Recurrent dislocation, left hand
   M24.443   Recurrent dislocation, unspecified hand
   M24.444   Recurrent dislocation, right finger
   M24.445   Recurrent dislocation, left finger
   M24.446   Recurrent dislocation, unspecified finger
M24.45   Recurrent dislocation, hip
   M24.451   Recurrent dislocation, right hip
   M24.452   Recurrent dislocation, left hip
   M24.459   Recurrent dislocation, unspecified hip
M24.46   Recurrent dislocation, knee
   M24.461   Recurrent dislocation, right knee
   M24.462   Recurrent dislocation, left knee
   M24.469   Recurrent dislocation, unspecified knee
M24.47   Recurrent dislocation, ankle, foot and toes
   M24.471   Recurrent dislocation, right ankle
   M24.472   Recurrent dislocation, left ankle
   M24.473   Recurrent dislocation, unspecified ankle
   M24.474   Recurrent dislocation, right foot
   M24.475   Recurrent dislocation, left foot
   M24.476   Recurrent dislocation, unspecified foot
   M24.477   Recurrent dislocation, right toe(s)
   M24.478   Recurrent dislocation, left toe(s)
   M24.479   Recurrent dislocation, unspecified toe(s)

M24.5 Contracture of joint
   Excludes1: contracture of muscle without contracture of joint (M62.4-)
            contracture of tendon (sheath) without contracture of joint (M67.1-)
            Dupuytren's contracture (M72.0)
   Excludes2: acquired deformities of limbs (M20-M21)
M24.50   Contracture, unspecified joint
M24.51   Contracture, shoulder
   M24.511   Contracture, right shoulder
   M24.512   Contracture, left shoulder
   M24.519   Contracture, unspecified shoulder
M24.52   Contracture, elbow
   M24.521   Contracture, right elbow
   M24.522   Contracture, left elbow
   M24.529   Contracture, unspecified elbow
M24.53   Contracture, wrist
   M24.531   Contracture, right wrist
   M24.532   Contracture, left wrist
   M24.539   Contracture, unspecified wrist
M24.54   Contracture, hand
   M24.541   Contracture, right hand
   M24.542   Contracture, left hand
   M24.549   Contracture, unspecified hand
M24.55   Contracture, hip
   M24.551   Contracture, right hip
   M24.552   Contracture, left hip
   M24.559   Contracture, unspecified hip
M24.56   Contracture, knee
   M24.561   Contracture, right knee
   M24.562   Contracture, left knee
   M24.569   Contracture, unspecified knee
M24.57   Contracture, ankle and foot
   M24.571   Contracture, right ankle
   M24.572   Contracture, left ankle
   M24.573   Contracture, unspecified ankle
   M24.574   Contracture, right foot
   M24.575   Contracture, left foot
   M24.576   Contracture, unspecified foot

M24.6 Ankylosis of joint
   Excludes1: stiffness of joint without ankylosis (M25.6-)
   Excludes2: spine (M43.2-)
M24.60   Ankylosis, unspecified joint
M24.61   Ankylosis, shoulder
   M24.611   Ankylosis, right shoulder
   M24.612   Ankylosis, left shoulder
   M24.619   Ankylosis, unspecified shoulder
M24.62   Ankylosis, elbow
   M24.621   Ankylosis, right elbow
   M24.622   Ankylosis, left elbow
   M24.629   Ankylosis, unspecified elbow
M24.63   Ankylosis, wrist
   M24.631   Ankylosis, right wrist
   M24.632   Ankylosis, left wrist
   M24.639   Ankylosis, unspecified wrist
M24.64   Ankylosis, hand
   M24.641   Ankylosis, right hand
   M24.642   Ankylosis, left hand
   M24.649   Ankylosis, unspecified hand
M24.65   Ankylosis, hip
   M24.651   Ankylosis, right hip
   M24.652   Ankylosis, left hip
   M24.659   Ankylosis, unspecified hip
M24.66   Ankylosis, knee
   M24.661   Ankylosis, right knee
   M24.662   Ankylosis, left knee
   M24.669   Ankylosis, unspecified knee
M24.67   Ankylosis, ankle and foot
   M24.671   Ankylosis, right ankle
   M24.672   Ankylosis, left ankle
   M24.673   Ankylosis, unspecified ankle
   M24.674   Ankylosis, right foot
   M24.675   Ankylosis, left foot
   M24.676   Ankylosis, unspecified foot

M24.7 Protrusio acetabuli

M24.8 Other specific joint derangements, not elsewhere classified
M24.80   Other specific joint derangements of unspecified joint, not elsewhere classified
M24.81   Other specific joint derangements of shoulder, not elsewhere classified
   M24.811   Other specific joint derangements of right shoulder, not elsewhere classified
   M24.812   Other specific joint derangements of left shoulder, not elsewhere classified
   M24.819   Other specific joint derangements of unspecified shoulder, not elsewhere classified
M24.82   Other specific joint derangements of elbow, not elsewhere classified
   M24.821   Other specific joint derangements of right elbow, not elsewhere classified
   M24.822   Other specific joint derangements of left elbow, not elsewhere classified
   M24.829   Other specific joint derangements of unspecified elbow, not elsewhere classified
M24.83   Other specific joint derangements of wrist, not elsewhere classified
   M24.831   Other specific joint derangements of right wrist, not elsewhere classified
   M24.832   Other specific joint derangements of left wrist, not elsewhere classified
   M24.839   Other specific joint derangements of unspecified wrist, not elsewhere classified
M24.84   Other specific joint derangements of hand, not elsewhere classified

M24.841   Other specific joint derangements of right hand, not elsewhere classified

M24.842   Other specific joint derangements of left hand, not elsewhere classified

M24.849   Other specific joint derangements of unspecified hand, not elsewhere classified

M24.85   Other specific joint derangements of hip, not elsewhere classified
Irritable hip

M24.851   Other specific joint derangements of right hip, not elsewhere classified

M24.852   Other specific joint derangements of left hip, not elsewhere classified

M24.859   Other specific joint derangements of unspecified hip, not elsewhere classified

M24.87   Other specific joint derangements of ankle and foot, not elsewhere classified

M24.871   Other specific joint derangements of right ankle, not elsewhere classified

M24.872   Other specific joint derangements of left ankle, not elsewhere classified

M24.873   Other specific joint derangements of unspecified ankle, not elsewhere classified

M24.874   Other specific joint derangements of right foot, not elsewhere classified

M24.875   Other specific joint derangements of left foot, not elsewhere classified

M24.876   Other specific joint derangements of unspecified foot, not elsewhere classified

M24.9   Joint derangement, unspecified

M25 Other joint disorder, not elsewhere classified
Excludes2:   abnormality of gait and mobility (R26.-)
acquired deformities of limb (M20-M21)
calcification of bursa (M71.4-)
calcification of shoulder (joint) (M75.3)
calcification of tendon (M65.2-)
difficulty in walking (R26.2)
temporomandibular joint disorder (M26.6-)

M25.0   Hemarthrosis
Excludes1:   current injury — see injury of joint by body region
hemophilic arthropathy (M36.2)

M25.00   Hemarthrosis, unspecified joint

M25.01   Hemarthrosis, shoulder
M25.011   Hemarthrosis, right shoulder
M25.012   Hemarthrosis, left shoulder
M25.019   Hemarthrosis, unspecified shoulder

M25.02   Hemarthrosis, elbow
M25.021   Hemarthrosis, right elbow
M25.022   Hemarthrosis, left elbow
M25.029   Hemarthrosis, unspecified elbow

M25.03   Hemarthrosis, wrist
M25.031   Hemarthrosis, right wrist
M25.032   Hemarthrosis, left wrist
M25.039   Hemarthrosis, unspecified wrist

M25.04   Hemarthrosis, hand
M25.041   Hemarthrosis, right hand
M25.042   Hemarthrosis, left hand
M25.049   Hemarthrosis, unspecified hand

M25.05   Hemarthrosis, hip
M25.051   Hemarthrosis, right hip
M25.052   Hemarthrosis, left hip
M25.059   Hemarthrosis, unspecified hip

M25.06   Hemarthrosis, knee
M25.061   Hemarthrosis, right knee
M25.062   Hemarthrosis, left knee
M25.069   Hemarthrosis, unspecified knee

M25.07   Hemarthrosis, ankle and foot
M25.071   Hemarthrosis, right ankle
M25.072   Hemarthrosis, left ankle

M25.073   Hemarthrosis, unspecified ankle
M25.074   Hemarthrosis, right foot
M25.075   Hemarthrosis, left foot
M25.076   Hemarthrosis, unspecified foot

M25.08   Hemarthrosis, vertebrae

M25.1   Fistula of joint
M25.10   Fistula, unspecified joint

M25.11   Fistula, shoulder
M25.111   Fistula, right shoulder
M25.112   Fistula, left shoulder
M25.119   Fistula, unspecified shoulder

M25.12   Fistula, elbow
M25.121   Fistula, right elbow
M25.122   Fistula, left elbow
M25.129   Fistula, unspecified elbow

M25.13   Fistula, wrist
M25.131   Fistula, right wrist
M25.132   Fistula, left wrist
M25.139   Fistula, unspecified wrist

M25.14   Fistula, hand
M25.141   Fistula, right hand
M25.142   Fistula, left hand
M25.149   Fistula, unspecified hand

M25.15   Fistula, hip
M15.151   Fistula, right hip
M15.152   Fistula, left hip
M15.159   Fistula, unspecified hip

M25.16   Fistula, knee
M25.161   Fistula, right knee
M25.162   Fistula, left knee
M25.169   Fistula, unspecified knee

M25.17   Fistula, ankle and foot
M25.171   Fistula, right ankle
M25.172   Fistula, left ankle
M25.173   Fistula, unspecified ankle
M25.174   Fistula, right foot
M25.175   Fistula, left foot
M25.176   Fistula, unspecified foot

M25.18   Fistula, vertebrae

M25.2   Flail joint
M25.20   Flail joint, unspecified joint

M25.21   Flail joint, shoulder
M25.211   Flail joint, right shoulder
M25.212   Flail joint, left shoulder
M25.219   Flail joint, unspecified shoulder

M25.22   Flail joint, elbow
M25.221   Flail joint, right elbow
M25.222   Flail joint, left elbow
M25.229   Flail joint, unspecified elbow

M25.23   Flail joint, wrist
M25.231   Flail joint, right wrist
M25.232   Flail joint, left wrist
M25.239   Flail joint, unspecified wrist

M25.24   Flail joint, hand
M25.241   Flail joint, right hand
M25.242   Flail joint, left hand
M25.249   Flail joint, unspecified hand

M25.25   Flail joint, hip
M25.251   Flail joint, right hip
M25.252   Flail joint, left hip
M25.259   Flail joint, unspecified hip

M25.26   Flail joint, knee
M25.261   Flail joint, right knee
M25.262   Flail joint, left knee
M25.269   Flail joint, unspecified knee

M25.27   Flail joint, ankle and foot
M25.271   Flail joint, right ankle and foot

     M25.272   Flail joint, left ankle and foot
     M25.279   Flail joint, unspecified ankle and foot
   M25.28   Flail joint, other site
M25.3   Other instability of joint
     Excludes1:   instability of joint secondary to old ligament injury (M24.2-)
         instability of joint secondary to removal of joint prosthesis (M96.8)
     Excludes2:   spinal instabilities (M53.2-)
   M25.30   Other instability, unspecified joint
   M25.31   Other instability, shoulder
     M25.311   Other instability, right shoulder
     M25.312   Other instability, left shoulder
     M25.319   Other instability, unspecified shoulder
   M25.32   Other instability, elbow
     M25.321   Other instability, right elbow
     M25.322   Other instability, left elbow
     M25.329   Other instability, unspecified elbow
   M25.33   Other instability, wrist
     M25.331   Other instability, right wrist
     M25.332   Other instability, left wrist
     M25.339   Other instability, unspecified wrist
   M25.34   Other instability, hand
     M25.341   Other instability, right hand
     M25.342   Other instability, left hand
     M25.349   Other instability, unspecified hand
   M25.35   Other instability, hip
     M25.351   Other instability, right hip
     M25.352   Other instability, left hip
     M25.359   Other instability, unspecified hip
   M25.36   Other instability, knee
     M25.361   Other instability, right knee
     M25.362   Other instability, left knee
     M25.369   Other instability, unspecified knee
   M25.37   Other instability, ankle and foot
     M25.371   Other instability, right ankle
     M25.372   Other instability, left ankle
     M25.373   Other instability, unspecified ankle
     M25.374   Other instability, right foot
     M25.375   Other instability, left foot
     M25.376   Other instability, unspecified foot
M25.4   Effusion of joint
     Excludes1:   hydrarthrosis in yaws (A66.6)
         intermittent hydrarthrosis (M12.4-)
         other infective (teno)synovitis (M65.1-)
   M25.40   Effusion, unspecified joint
   M25.41   Effusion, shoulder
     M25.411   Effusion, right shoulder
     M25.412   Effusion, left shoulder
     M25.419   Effusion, unspecified shoulder
   M25.42   Effusion, elbow
     M25.421   Effusion, right elbow
     M25.422   Effusion, left elbow
     M25.429   Effusion, unspecified elbow
   M25.43   Effusion, wrist
     M25.431   Effusion, right wrist
     M25.432   Effusion, left wrist
     M25.439   Effusion, unspecified wrist
   M25.44   Effusion, hand
     M25.441   Effusion, right hand
     M25.442   Effusion, left hand
     M25.449   Effusion, unspecified hand
   M25.45   Effusion, hip
     M25.451   Effusion, right hip
     M25.452   Effusion, left hip
     M25.459   Effusion, unspecified hip
   M25.46   Effusion, knee
     M25.461   Effusion, right knee

     M25.462   Effusion, left knee
     M25.469   Effusion, unspecified knee
   M25.47   Effusion, ankle and foot
     M25.471   Effusion, right ankle
     M25.472   Effusion, left ankle
     M25.473   Effusion, unspecified ankle
     M25.474   Effusion, right foot
     M25.475   Effusion, left foot
     M25.476   Effusion, unspecified foot
   M25.48   Effusion, other site
M25.5   Pain in joint
     Excludes2:   pain in fingers (M79.64-)
         pain in foot (M79.67-)
         pain in hand (M79.64-)
         pain in limb (M79.6-)
         pain in toes (M79.67-)
   M25.50   Pain in unspecified joint
   M25.51   Pain in shoulder
     M25.511   Pain in right shoulder
     M25.512   Pain in left shoulder
     M25.519   Pain in unspecified shoulder
   M25.52   Pain in elbow
     M25.521   Pain in right elbow
     M25.522   Pain in left elbow
     M25.529   Pain in unspecified elbow
   M25.53   Pain in wrist
     M25.531   Pain in right wrist
     M25.532   Pain in left wrist
     M25.539   Pain in unspecified wrist
   M25.55   Pain in hip
     M25.551   Pain in right hip
     M25.552   Pain in left hip
     M25.559   Pain in unspecified hip
   M25.56   Pain in knee
     M25.561   Pain in right knee
     M25.562   Pain in left knee
     M25.569   Pain in unspecified knee
   M25.57   Pain in ankle
     M25.571   Pain in right ankle
     M25.572   Pain in left ankle
     M25.579   Pain in unspecified ankle
M25.6   Stiffness of joint, not elsewhere classified
     Excludes1:   ankylosis of joint (M24.6-)
         contracture of joint (M24.5-)
   M25.60   Stiffness of unspecified joint, not elsewhere classified
   M25.61   Stiffness of shoulder, not elsewhere classified
     M25.611   Stiffness of right shoulder, not elsewhere classified
     M25.612   Stiffness of left shoulder, not elsewhere classified
     M25.619   Stiffness of unspecified shoulder, not elsewhere classified
   M25.62   Stiffness of elbow, not elsewhere classified
     M25.621   Stiffness of right elbow, not elsewhere classified
     M25.622   Stiffness of left elbow, not elsewhere classified
     M25.629   Stiffness of unspecified elbow, not elsewhere classified
   M25.63   Stiffness of wrist, not elsewhere classified
     M25.631   Stiffness of right wrist, not elsewhere classified
     M25.632   Stiffness of left wrist, not elsewhere classified
     M25.639   Stiffness of unspecified wrist, not elsewhere classified
   M25.64   Stiffness of hand, not elsewhere classified
     M25.641   Stiffness of right hand, not elsewhere classified
     M25.642   Stiffness of left hand, not elsewhere classified

M25.649   Stiffness of unspecified hand, not elsewhere classified
M25.65   Stiffness of hip, not elsewhere classified
M25.651   Stiffness of right hip, not elsewhere classified
M25.652   Stiffness of left hip, not elsewhere classified
M25.659   Stiffness of unspecified hip, not elsewhere classified
M25.66   Stiffness of knee, not elsewhere classified
M25.661   Stiffness of right knee, not elsewhere classified
M25.662   Stiffness of left knee, not elsewhere classified
M25.669   Stiffness of unspecified knee, not elsewhere classified
M25.67   Stiffness of ankle and foot, not elsewhere classified
M25.671   Stiffness of right ankle, not elsewhere classified
M25.672   Stiffness of left ankle, not elsewhere classified
M25.673   Stiffness of unspecified ankle, not elsewhere classified
M25.674   Stiffness of right foot, not elsewhere classified
M25.675   Stiffness of left foot, not elsewhere classified
M25.676   Stiffness of unspecified foot, not elsewhere classified

M25.7   Osteophyte
M25.70   Osteophyte, unspecified joint
M25.71   Osteophyte, shoulder
M25.711   Osteophyte, right shoulder
M25.712   Osteophyte, left shoulder
M25.719   Osteophyte, unspecified shoulder
M25.72   Osteophyte, elbow
M25.721   Osteophyte, right elbow
M25.722   Osteophyte, left elbow
M25.729   Osteophyte, unspecified elbow
M25.73   Osteophyte, wrist
M25.731   Osteophyte, right wrist
M25.732   Osteophyte, left wrist
M25.739   Osteophyte, unspecified wrist
M25.74   Osteophyte, hand
M25.741   Osteophyte, right hand
M25.742   Osteophyte, left hand
M25.749   Osteophyte, unspecified hand
M25.75   Osteophyte, hip
M25.751   Osteophyte, right hip
M25.752   Osteophyte, left hip
M25.759   Osteophyte, unspecified hip
M25.76   Osteophyte, knee
M25.761   Osteophyte, right knee
M25.762   Osteophyte, left knee
M25.769   Osteophyte, unspecified knee
M25.77   Osteophyte, ankle and foot
M25.771   Osteophyte, right ankle
M25.772   Osteophyte, left ankle
M25.773   Osteophyte, unspecified ankle
M25.774   Osteophyte, right foot
M25.775   Osteophyte, left foot
M25.776   Osteophyte, unspecified foot
M25.78   Osteophyte, vertebrae

M25.8   Other specified joint disorders
M25.80   Other specified joint disorders, unspecified joint
M25.81   Other specified joint disorders, shoulder
M25.811   Other specified joint disorders, right shoulder
M25.812   Other specified joint disorders, left shoulder
M25.819   Other specified joint disorders, unspecified shoulder
M25.82   Other specified joint disorders, elbow
M25.821   Other specified joint disorders, right elbow
M25.822   Other specified joint disorders, left elbow
M25.829   Other specified joint disorders, unspecified elbow
M25.83   Other specified joint disorders, wrist
M25.831   Other specified joint disorders, right wrist
M25.832   Other specified joint disorders, left wrist
M25.839   Other specified joint disorders, unspecified wrist
M25.84   Other specified joint disorders, hand
M25.841   Other specified joint disorders, right hand
M25.842   Other specified joint disorders, left hand
M25.849   Other specified joint disorders, unspecified hand
M25.85   Other specified joint disorders, hip
M25.851   Other specified joint disorders, right hip
M25.852   Other specified joint disorders, left hip
M25.859   Other specified joint disorders, unspecified hip
M25.86   Other specified joint disorders, knee
M25.861   Other specified joint disorders, right knee
M25.862   Other specified joint disorders, left knee
M25.869   Other specified joint disorders, unspecified knee
M25.87   Other specified joint disorders, ankle and foot
M25.871   Other specified joint disorders, right ankle and foot
M25.872   Other specified joint disorders, left ankle and foot
M25.879   Other specified joint disorders, unspecified ankle and foot

M25.9   Joint disorder, unspecified

DENTOFACIAL ANOMALIES [INCLUDING MALOCCLUSION] AND OTHER DISORDERS OF JAW (M26–M27)

Excludes1:   hemifacial atrophy or hypertrophy (Q67.4)
             unilateral condylar hyperplasia or hypoplasia (M27.8)

M26 Dentofacial anomalies [including malocclusion]
M26.0   Major anomalies of jaw size
Excludes1:   acromegaly (E22.0)
             Robin's syndrome (Q87.0)
M26.00   Unspecified anomaly of jaw size
M26.01   Maxillary hyperplasia
M26.02   Maxillary hypoplasia
M26.03   Mandibular hyperplasia
M26.04   Mandibular hypoplasia
M26.05   Macrogenia
M26.06   Microgenia
M26.09   Other specified anomalies of jaw size
M26.1   Anomalies of jaw-cranial base relationship
M26.10   Unspecified anomaly of jaw-cranial base relationship
M26.11   Maxillary asymmetry
M26.12   Other jaw asymmetry
M26.19   Other specified anomalies of jaw-cranial base relationship
M26.2   Anomalies of dental arch relationship
Crossbite (anterior)(posterior)
Disto-occlusion
Mesio-occlusion
Midline deviation of dental arch
Openbite (anterior)(posterior)
Overbite (excessive):
  deep
  horizontal
  vertical
Overjet
Posterior lingual occlusion of mandibular teeth

M26.3 Anomalies of tooth position of fully erupted teeth
Abnormal spacing of fully erupted tooth or teeth
Crowding of fully erupted tooth or teeth
Diastema of fully erupted tooth or teeth
Displacement of fully erupted tooth or teeth
Rotation of fully erupted tooth or teeth
Transposition of fully erupted tooth or teeth
Excludes1: embedded and impacted teeth (K01.-)

M26.4 Malocclusion, unspecified

M26.5 Dentofacial functional abnormalities
Abnormal jaw closure
Malocclusion due to abnormal swallowing
Malocclusion due to mouth breathing
Malocclusion due to tongue, lip or finger habits
Excludes1: bruxism (F45.8)
teeth-grinding NOS (F45.8)

M26.6 Temporomandibular joint disorders
Excludes2: current temporomandibular joint dislocation (S03.0)
current temporomandibular joint strain (S03.4)

M26.60 Temporomandibular joint disorder, unspecified
M26.61 Adhesions and ankylosis of temporomandibular joint
M26.62 Arthralgia of temporomandibular joint
M26.63 Articular disc disorder of temporomandibular joint
M26.69 Other specified disorders of temporomandibular joint

M26.7 Dental alveolar anomalies
M26.70 Unspecified alveolar anomaly
M26.71 Alveolar maxillary hyperplasia
M26.72 Alveolar mandibular hyperplasia
M26.73 Alveolar maxillary hypoplasia
M26.74 Alveolar mandibular hypoplasia
M26.79 Other specified alveolar anomalies

M26.8 Other dentofacial anomalies

M26.9 Dentofacial anomaly, unspecified

M27 Other diseases of jaws

M27.0 Developmental disorders of jaws
Latent bone cyst of jaw
Stafne's cyst
Torus mandibularis
Torus palatinus

M27.1 Giant cell granuloma, central
Giant cell granuloma NOS
Excludes1: peripheral giant cell granuloma (K06.8)

M27.2 Inflammatory conditions of jaws
Osteitis of jaw(s)
Osteomyelitis (neonatal) jaw(s)
Osteoradionecrosis jaw(s)
Periostitis jaw(s)
Sequestrum of jaw bone
Use additional external cause code (Chapter XIX) to identify radiation, if radiation-induced.

M27.3 Alveolitis of jaws
Alveolar osteitis
Dry socket

M27.4 Other and unspecified cysts of jaw
Excludes1: cysts of oral region (K09.-)
latent bone cyst of jaw (M27.0)
Stafne's cyst (M27.0)

M27.40 Unspecified cyst of jaw
Cyst of jaw NOS
M27.49 Other cysts of jaw
Aneurysmal cyst of jaw
Hemorrhagic cyst of jaw
Traumatic cyst of jaw

M27.8 Other specified diseases of jaws
Cherubism
Exostosis
Fibrous dysplasia
Unilateral condylar hyperplasia
Unilateral condylar hypoplasia

M27.9 Disease of jaws, unspecified

SYSTEMIC CONNECTIVE TISSUE DISORDERS (M30–M36)
Includes: autoimmune disease NOS
collagen (vascular) disease NOS
systemic autoimmune disease
systemic collagen (vascular) disease
Excludes1: autoimmune disease, single organ or single cell-type — code to relevant condition category

M30 Polyarteritis nodosa and related conditions

M30.0 Polyarteritis nodosa

M30.1 Polyarteritis with lung involvement [Churg-Strauss]
Allergic granulomatous angiitis

M30.2 Juvenile polyarteritis

M30.3 Mucocutaneous lymph node syndrome [Kawasaki]

M30.8 Other conditions related to polyarteritis nodosa
Polyangiitis overlap syndrome

M31 Other necrotizing vasculopathies

M31.0 Hypersensitivity angiitis
Goodpasture's syndrome

M31.1 Thrombotic microangiopathy
Thrombotic thrombocytopenic purpura

M31.2 Lethal midline granuloma

M31.3 Wegener's granulomatosis
Necrotizing respiratory granulomatosis

M31.30 Wegener's granulomatosis without renal involvement
M31.31 Wegener's granulomatosis with renal involvement

M31.4 Aortic arch syndrome [Takayasu]

M31.5 Giant cell arteritis with polymyalgia rheumatica

M31.6 Other giant cell arteritis

M31.8 Other specified necrotizing vasculopathies
Hypocomplementemic vasculitis
Septic vasculitis

M31.9 Necrotizing vasculopathy, unspecified

M32 Systemic lupus erythematosus
Excludes1: lupus erythematosus (discoid) (NOS) (L93.0)

M32.0 Drug-induced systemic lupus erythematosus
Use additional external cause code (Chapter XIX) to identify drug

M32.1 Systemic lupus erythematosus with organ or system involvement
M32.10 Systemic lupus erythematosus, organ or system involvement unspecified
M32.11 Endocarditis in systemic lupus erythematosus
Libman-Sacks disease
M32.12 Pericarditis in systemic lupus erythematosus
Lupus pericarditis
M32.13 Lung involvement in systemic lupus erythematosus
Pleural effusion due to systemic lupus erythematosus
M32.14 Glomerular disease in systemic lupus erythematosus
Lupus renal disease NOS
M32.15 Tubulo-interstitial nephropathy in systemic lupus erythematosus
M32.19 Other organ or system involvement in systemic lupus erythematosus

M32.8 Other forms of systemic lupus erythematosus

M32.9 Systemic lupus erythematosus, unspecified

M33 Dermatopolymyositis

M33.0 Juvenile dermatopolymyositis
M33.00 Juvenile dermatopolymyositis, organ involvement unspecified
M33.01 Juvenile dermatopolymyositis with respiratory involvement
M33.02 Juvenile dermatopolymyositis with myopathy
M33.09 Juvenile dermatopolymyositis with other organ involvement

M33.1 Other dermatopolymyositis
M33.10 Other dermatopolymyositis, organ involvement unspecified
M33.11 Other dermatopolymyositis with respiratory involvement

M33.12   Other dermatopolymyositis with myopathy

M33.19   Other dermatopolymyositis with other organ involvement

M33.2   Polymyositis

M33.20   Polymyositis, organ involvement unspecified

M33.21   Polymyositis with respiratory involvement

M33.22   Polymyositis with myopathy

M33.29   Polymyositis with other organ involvement

M33.9   Dermatopolymyositis, unspecified

M33.90   Dermatopolymyositis, unspecified, organ involvement unspecified

M33.91   Dermatopolymyositis, unspecified with respiratory involvement

M33.92   Dermatopolymyositis, unspecified with myopathy

M33.99   Dermatopolymyositis, unspecified with other organ involvement

M34   Systemic sclerosis [scleroderma]

Excludes1:   circumscribed scleroderma (L94.0)
neonatal scleroderma (P83.8)

M34.0   Progressive systemic sclerosis

M34.1   CR(E)ST syndrome

Combination of calcinosis, Raynaud's phenomenon, esophageal dysfunction, sclerodactyly, telangiectasia

M34.2   Systemic sclerosis induced by drug and chemical

Use additional external cause code (Chapter XIX) to identify agent.

M34.8   Other forms of systemic sclerosis

M34.81   Systemic sclerosis with lung involvement

M34.82   Systemic sclerosis with myopathy

M34.83   Systemic sclerosis with polyneuropathy

M34.89   Other systemic sclerosis

M34.9   Systemic sclerosis, unspecified

M35   Other systemic involvement of connective tissue

Excludes1:   reactive perforating collagenosis (L87.1)

M35.0   Sicca syndrome [Sjögren]

M35.00   Sicca syndrome, unspecified

M35.01   Sicca syndrome with keratoconjunctivitis

M35.02   Sicca syndrome with lung involvement

M35.03   Sicca syndrome with myopathy

M35.04   Sicca syndrome with tubulo-interstitial nephropathy
Renal tubular acidosis in sicca syndrome

M35.09   Sicca syndrome with other organ involvement

M35.1   Other overlap syndromes

Mixed connective tissue disease
Excludes1:   polyangiitis overlap syndrome (M30.8)

M35.2   Behçet's disease

M35.3   Polymyalgia rheumatica

Excludes1:   polymyalgia rheumatica with giant cell arteritis (M31.5)

M35.4   Diffuse (eosinophilic) fasciitis

M35.5   Multifocal fibrosclerosis

M35.6   Relapsing panniculitis [Weber-Christian]

Excludes1:   lupus panniculitis (L93.2)
panniculitis NOS (M79.3-)

M35.7   Hypermobility syndrome

Familial ligamentous laxity
Excludes1:   Ehlers-Danlos syndrome (Q79.6)
ligamentous laxity, NOS (M24.2-)

M35.8   Other specified systemic involvement of connective tissue

M35.9   Systemic involvement of connective tissue, unspecified

Autoimmune disease (systemic) NOS
Collagen (vascular) disease NOS

M36   Systemic disorders of connective tissue in diseases classified elsewhere

Excludes2:   arthropathies in diseases classified elsewhere (M14.-)

M36.0   Dermato(poly)myositis in neoplastic disease

Code first underlying neoplasm (C00-D48)

M36.1   Arthropathy in neoplastic disease

Code first underlying neoplasm, such as:
leukemia (C91-C95)
malignant histiocytosis (C96.1)
multiple myeloma (C90.0)

M36.2   Hemophilic arthropathy

Hemarthrosis in hemophilic arthropathy
Code first underlying disease, such as:
factor VIII deficiency (D66)
with vascular defect (D68.0)
factor IX deficiency (D67)
hemophilia (classical) (D66)
hemophilia B (D67)
hemophilia C (D68.1)

M36.3   Arthropathy in other blood disorders

M36.4   Arthropathy in hypersensitivity reactions classified elsewhere

Code first underlying disease, such as:
Henoch (-Schönlein) purpura (D69.0)

M36.8   Systemic disorders of connective tissue in other diseases classified elsewhere

Code first underlying disease, such as:
alkaptonuria (E70.2)
hypogammaglobulinemia (D80.-)
ochronosis (E70.2)

DORSOPATHIES (M40–M54)

DEFORMING DORSOPATHIES (M40–M43)

M40   Kyphosis and lordosis

Excludes1:   congenital kyphosis and lordosis (Q76.4)
kyphoscoliosis (M41.-)
postprocedural kyphosis and lordosis (M96.-)

M40.0   Postural kyphosis

Excludes1:   osteochondrosis of spine (M42.-)

M40.00   Postural kyphosis, site unspecified

M40.01   Postural kyphosis, occipito-atlanto-axial region

M40.02   Postural kyphosis, cervical region

M40.03   Postural kyphosis, cervicothoracic region

M40.04   Postural kyphosis, thoracic region

M40.05   Postural kyphosis, thoracolumbar region

M40.1   Other secondary kyphosis

M40.10   Other secondary kyphosis, site unspecified

M40.11   Other secondary kyphosis, occipito-atlanto-axial region

M40.12   Other secondary kyphosis, cervical region

M40.13   Other secondary kyphosis, cervicothoracic region

M40.14   Other secondary kyphosis, thoracic region

M40.15   Other secondary kyphosis, thoracolumbar region

M40.2   Other and unspecified kyphosis

M40.20   Unspecified kyphosis

    M40.201   Unspecified kyphosis, occipito-atlanto-axial region

    M40.202   Unspecified kyphosis, cervical region

    M40.203   Unspecified kyphosis, cervicothoracic region

    M40.204   Unspecified kyphosis, thoracic region

    M40.205   Unspecified kyphosis, thoracolumbar region

    M40.209   Unspecified kyphosis, site unspecified

M40.29   Other kyphosis

    M40.291   Other kyphosis, occipito-atlanto-axial region

    M40.292   Other kyphosis, cervical region

    M40.293   Other kyphosis, cervicothoracic region

    M40.294   Other kyphosis, thoracic region

    M40.295   Other kyphosis, thoracolumbar region

    M40.299   Other kyphosis, site unspecified

M40.3   Flatback syndrome

M40.30   Flatback syndrome, site unspecified

M40.35   Flatback syndrome, thoracolumbar region

M40.36   Flatback syndrome, lumbar region

M40.37   Flatback syndrome, lumbosacral region

M40.38   Flatback syndrome, sacral and sacrococcygeal region

M40.4   Postural lordosis
    Acquired lordosis
- **M40.40**   Postural lordosis, site unspecified
- **M40.45**   Postural lordosis, thoracolumbar region
- **M40.46**   Postural lordosis, lumbar region
- **M40.47**   Postural lordosis, lumbosacral region
- **M40.48**   Postural lordosis, sacral and sacrococcygeal region

M40.5   Lordosis, unspecified
- **M40.50**   Lordosis, unspecified, site unspecified
- **M40.55**   Lordosis, unspecified, thoracolumbar region
- **M40.56**   Lordosis, unspecified, lumbar region
- **M40.57**   Lordosis, unspecified, lumbosacral region
- **M40.58**   Lordosis, unspecified, sacral and sacrococcygeal region

M41   Scoliosis

Includes:	kyphoscoliosis
Excludes1:	congenital scoliosis NOS (Q67.5)
	congenital scoliosis due to bony malformation (Q76.3)
	kyphoscoliotic heart disease (I27.1)
	postprocedural (M96.-)
	postural congenital scoliosis (Q67.5)

M41.0   Infantile idiopathic scoliosis
    Note: Infantile is defined as birth through 4 years of age
- **M41.00**   Infantile idiopathic scoliosis, site unspecified
- **M41.01**   Infantile idiopathic scoliosis, occipito-atlanto-axial region
- **M41.02**   Infantile idiopathic scoliosis, cervical region
- **M41.03**   Infantile idiopathic scoliosis, cervicothoracic region
- **M41.04**   Infantile idiopathic scoliosis, thoracic region
- **M41.05**   Infantile idiopathic scoliosis, thoracolumbar region
- **M41.06**   Infantile idiopathic scoliosis, lumbar region
- **M41.07**   Infantile idiopathic scoliosis, lumbosacral region
- **M41.08**   Infantile idiopathic scoliosis, sacral and sacrococcygeal region

M41.1   Juvenile and adolescent idiopathic scoliosis
- **M41.11**   Juvenile idiopathic scoliosis
      Note: Juvenile is defined as 5 through 10 years of age
  - **M41.111**   Juvenile idiopathic scoliosis, occipito-atlanto-axial region
  - **M41.112**   Juvenile idiopathic scoliosis, cervical region
  - **M41.113**   Juvenile idiopathic scoliosis, cervicothoracic region
  - **M41.114**   Juvenile idiopathic scoliosis, thoracic region
  - **M41.115**   Juvenile idiopathic scoliosis, thoracolumbar region
  - **M41.116**   Juvenile idiopathic scoliosis, lumbar region
  - **M41.117**   Juvenile idiopathic scoliosis, lumbosacral region
  - **M41.118**   Juvenile idiopathic scoliosis, sacral and sacrococcygeal region
  - **M41.119**   Juvenile idiopathic scoliosis, site unspecified
- **M41.12**   Adolescent scoliosis
      Note: Adolescent is defined as 11 through 17 years of age
  - **M41.121**   Adolescent idiopathic scoliosis, occipito-atlanto-axial region
  - **M41.122**   Adolescent idiopathic scoliosis, cervical region
  - **M41.123**   Adolescent idiopathic scoliosis, cervicothoracic region
  - **M41.124**   Adolescent idiopathic scoliosis, thoracic region
  - **M41.125**   Adolescent idiopathic scoliosis, thoracolumbar region
  - **M41.126**   Adolescent idiopathic scoliosis, lumbar region
  - **M41.127**   Adolescent idiopathic scoliosis, lumbosacral region
  - **M41.128**   Adolescent idiopathic scoliosis, sacral and sacrococcygeal region
  - **M41.129**   Adolescent idiopathic scoliosis, site unspecified

M41.2   Other idiopathic scoliosis
- **M41.20**   Other idiopathic scoliosis, site unspecified
- **M41.21**   Other idiopathic scoliosis, occipito-atlanto-axial region
- **M41.22**   Other idiopathic scoliosis, cervical region
- **M41.23**   Other idiopathic scoliosis, cervicothoracic region
- **M41.24**   Other idiopathic scoliosis, thoracic region
- **M41.25**   Other idiopathic scoliosis, thoracolumbar region
- **M41.26**   Other idiopathic scoliosis, lumbar region
- **M41.27**   Other idiopathic scoliosis, lumbosacral region
- **M41.28**   Other idiopathic scoliosis, sacral and sacrococcygeal region

M41.3   Thoracogenic scoliosis
- **M41.30**   Thoracogenic scoliosis, site unspecified
- **M41.34**   Thoracogenic scoliosis, thoracic region
- **M41.35**   Thoracogenic scoliosis, thoracolumbar region

M41.4   Neuromuscular scoliosis
    Scoliosis secondary to cerebral palsy, Friedreich's ataxia, poliomyelitis and other neuromuscular disorders
    Code also underlying condition
- **M41.40**   Neuromuscular scoliosis, site unspecified
- **M41.41**   Neuromuscular scoliosis, occipito-atlanto-axial region
- **M41.42**   Neuromuscular scoliosis, cervical region
- **M41.43**   Neuromuscular scoliosis, cervicothoracic region
- **M41.44**   Neuromuscular scoliosis, thoracic region
- **M41.45**   Neuromuscular scoliosis, thoracolumbar region
- **M41.46**   Neuromuscular scoliosis, lumbar region
- **M41.47**   Neuromuscular scoliosis, lumbosacral region
- **M41.48**   Neuromuscular scoliosis, sacral and sacrococcygeal region

M41.5   Other secondary scoliosis
- **M41.50**   Other secondary scoliosis, site unspecified
- **M41.51**   Other secondary scoliosis, occipito-atlanto-axial region
- **M41.52**   Other secondary scoliosis, cervical region
- **M41.53**   Other secondary scoliosis, cervicothoracic region
- **M41.54**   Other secondary scoliosis, thoracic region
- **M41.55**   Other secondary scoliosis, thoracolumbar region
- **M41.56**   Other secondary scoliosis, lumbar region
- **M41.57**   Other secondary scoliosis, lumbosacral region
- **M41.58**   Other secondary scoliosis, sacral and sacrococcygeal region

M41.8   Other forms of scoliosis
- **M41.80**   Other forms of scoliosis, site unspecified
- **M41.81**   Other forms of scoliosis, occipito-atlanto-axial region
- **M41.82**   Other forms of scoliosis, cervical region
- **M41.83**   Other forms of scoliosis, cervicothoracic region
- **M41.84**   Other forms of scoliosis, thoracic region
- **M41.85**   Other forms of scoliosis, thoracolumbar region
- **M41.86**   Other forms of scoliosis, lumbar region
- **M41.87**   Other forms of scoliosis, lumbosacral region
- **M41.88**   Other forms of scoliosis, sacral and sacrococcygeal region

M41.9   Scoliosis, unspecified

M42   Spinal osteochondrosis

M42.0   Juvenile osteochondrosis of spine
    Calvé's disease
    Scheuermann's disease
    Excludes1:   postural kyphosis (M40.0)
- **M42.00**   Juvenile osteochondrosis of spine, site unspecified
- **M42.01**   Juvenile osteochondrosis of spine, occipito-atlanto-axial region
- **M42.02**   Juvenile osteochondrosis of spine, cervical region
- **M42.03**   Juvenile osteochondrosis of spine, cervicothoracic region
- **M42.04**   Juvenile osteochondrosis of spine, thoracic region
- **M42.05**   Juvenile osteochondrosis of spine, thoracolumbar region
- **M42.06**   Juvenile osteochondrosis of spine, lumbar region

M42.07   Juvenile osteochondrosis of spine, lumbosacral region
M42.08   Juvenile osteochondrosis of spine, sacral and sacrococcygeal region
M42.09   Juvenile osteochondrosis of spine, multiple sites in spine

M42.1 Adult osteochondrosis of spine
M42.10   Adult osteochondrosis of spine, site unspecified
M42.11   Adult osteochondrosis of spine, occipito-atlanto-axial region
M42.12   Adult osteochondrosis of spine, cervical region
M42.13   Adult osteochondrosis of spine, cervicothoracic region
M42.14   Adult osteochondrosis of spine, thoracic region
M42.15   Adult osteochondrosis of spine, thoracolumbar region
M42.16   Adult osteochondrosis of spine, lumbar region
M42.17   Adult osteochondrosis of spine, lumbosacral region
M42.18   Adult osteochondrosis of spine, sacral and sacrococcygeal region
M42.19   Adult osteochondrosis of spine, multiple sites in spine

M42.9 Spinal osteochondrosis, unspecified

M43 Other deforming dorsopathies
    Excludes1:   congenital spondylolysis and spondylolisthesis (Q76.2)
                  hemivertebra (Q76.3-Q76.4)
                  Klippel-Feil syndrome (Q76.1)
                  lumbarization and sacralization (Q76.4)
                  platyspondylisis (Q76.4)
                  spina bifida occulta (Q76.0)
                  spinal curvature in osteoporosis (M80-)
                  spinal curvature in Paget's disease of bone [osteitis deformans] (M88.-)

M43.0 Spondylolysis
    Excludes1:   congenital spondylolysis (Q76.2)
                  Spondylolisthesis (M43.1)
    M43.00   Spondylolysis, site unspecified
    M43.01   Spondylolysis, occipito-atlanto-axial region
    M43.02   Spondylolysis, cervical region
    M43.03   Spondylolysis, cervicothoracic region
    M43.04   Spondylolysis, thoracic region
    M43.05   Spondylolysis, thoracolumbar region
    M43.06   Spondylolysis, lumbar region
    M43.07   Spondylolysis, lumbosacral region
    M43.08   Spondylolysis, sacral and sacrococcygeal region
    M43.09   Spondylolysis, multiple sites in spine

M43.1 Spondylolisthesis
    Excludes1:   congenital spondylolisthesis (Q76.2)
    M43.10   Spondylolisthesis, site unspecified
    M43.11   Spondylolisthesis, occipito-atlanto-axial region
    M43.12   Spondylolisthesis, cervical region
    M43.13   Spondylolisthesis, cervicothoracic region
    M43.14   Spondylolisthesis, thoracic region
    M43.15   Spondylolisthesis, thoracolumbar region
    M43.16   Spondylolisthesis, lumbar region
    M43.17   Spondylolisthesis, lumbosacral region
    M43.18   Spondylolisthesis, sacral and sacrococcygeal region
    M43.19   Spondylolisthesis, multiple sites in spine

M43.2 Fusion of spine
    Ankylosis of spinal joint
    Excludes1:   ankylosing spondylitis (M45.0-)
                  congenital fusion of spine (Q76.4)
    Excludes2:   arthrodesis status (Z98.1)
                  pseudoarthrosis after fusion or arthrodesis (M96.0)
    M43.20   Fusion of spine, site unspecified
    M43.21   Fusion of spine, occipito-atlanto-axial region
    M43.22   Fusion of spine, cervical region
    M43.23   Fusion of spine, cervicothoracic region
    M43.24   Fusion of spine, thoracic region
    M43.25   Fusion of spine, thoracolumbar region
    M43.26   Fusion of spine, lumbar region
    M43.27   Fusion of spine, lumbosacral region

M43.28   Fusion of spine, sacral and sacrococcygeal region

M43.3 Recurrent atlantoaxial dislocation with myelopathy

M43.4 Other recurrent atlantoaxial dislocation

M43.5 Other recurrent vertebral dislocation
    Excludes1:   biomechanical lesions NEC (M99.-)
    M43.5x   Other recurrent vertebral dislocation
        M43.5x2   Other recurrent vertebral dislocation, cervical region
        M43.5x3   Other recurrent vertebral dislocation, cervicothoracic region
        M43.5x4   Other recurrent vertebral dislocation, thoracic region
        M43.5x5   Other recurrent vertebral dislocation, thoracolumbar region
        M43.5x6   Other recurrent vertebral dislocation, lumbar region
        M43.5x7   Other recurrent vertebral dislocation, lumbosacral region
        M43.5x8   Other recurrent vertebral dislocation, sacral and sacrococcygeal region
        M43.5x9   Other recurrent vertebral dislocation, site unspecified

M43.6 Torticollis
    Excludes1:   congenital (sternomastoid) torticollis (Q68.0)
                  current injury — see injury of spine by body region
                  psychogenic torticollis (F45.8)
                  spasmodic torticollis (G24.3)
                  torticollis due to birth injury (P15.8)

M43.8 Other specified deforming dorsopathies
    Excludes2:   kyphosis and lordosis (M40.-)
                  scoliosis (M41.-)
    M43.8x   Other specified deforming dorsopathies
        M43.8x1   Other specified deforming dorsopathies, occipito-atlanto-axial region
        M43.8x2   Other specified deforming dorsopathies, cervical region
        M43.8x3   Other specified deforming dorsopathies, cervicothoracic region
        M43.8x4   Other specified deforming dorsopathies, thoracic region
        M43.8x5   Other specified deforming dorsopathies, thoracolumbar region
        M43.8x6   Other specified deforming dorsopathies, lumbar region
        M43.8x7   Other specified deforming dorsopathies, lumbosacral region
        M43.8x8   Other specified deforming dorsopathies, sacral and sacrococcygeal region
        M43.8x9   Other specified deforming dorsopathies, site unspecified

M43.9 Deforming dorsopathy, unspecified
    Curvature of spine NOS

SPONDYLOPATHIES (M45–M49)

M45 Ankylosing spondylitis
    Rheumatoid arthritis of spine
    Excludes1:   arthropathy in Reiter's disease (M02.3-)
                  juvenile (ankylosing) spondylitis (M08.18)
    Excludes2:   Behçet's disease (M35.2)

M45.0 Ankylosing spondylitis of multiple sites in spine
M45.1 Ankylosing spondylitis of occipito-atlanto-axial region
M45.2 Ankylosing spondylitis of cervical region
M45.3 Ankylosing spondylitis of cervicothoracic region
M45.4 Ankylosing spondylitis of thoracic region
M45.5 Ankylosing spondylitis of thoracolumbar region
M45.6 Ankylosing spondylitis lumbar region
M45.7 Ankylosing spondylitis of lumbosacral region
M45.8 Ankylosing spondylitis sacral and sacrococcygeal region
M45.9 Ankylosing spondylitis of unspecified sites in spine

M46 Other inflammatory spondylopathies

M46.0 Spinal enthesopathy
Disorder of ligamentous or muscular attachments of spine

M46.00 Spinal enthesopathy, site unspecified

M46.01 Spinal enthesopathy, occipito-atlanto-axial region

M46.02 Spinal enthesopathy, cervical region

M46.03 Spinal enthesopathy, cervicothoracic region

M46.04 Spinal enthesopathy, thoracic region

M46.05 Spinal enthesopathy, thoracolumbar region

M46.06 Spinal enthesopathy, lumbar region

M46.07 Spinal enthesopathy, lumbosacral region

M46.08 Spinal enthesopathy, sacral and sacrococcygeal region

M46.09 Spinal enthesopathy, multiple sites in spine

M46.1 Sacroiliitis, not elsewhere classified

M46.2 Osteomyelitis of vertebra

M46.20 Osteomyelitis of vertebra, site unspecified

M46.21 Osteomyelitis of vertebra, occipito-atlanto-axial region

M46.22 Osteomyelitis of vertebra, cervical region

M46.23 Osteomyelitis of vertebra, cervicothoracic region

M46.24 Osteomyelitis of vertebra, thoracic region

M46.25 Osteomyelitis of vertebra, thoracolumbar region

M46.26 Osteomyelitis of vertebra, lumbar region

M46.27 Osteomyelitis of vertebra, lumbosacral region

M46.28 Osteomyelitis of vertebra, sacral and sacrococcygeal region

M46.3 Infection of intervertebral disc (pyogenic)
Use additional code (B95-B97) to identify infectious agent.

M46.30 Infection of intervertebral disc (pyogenic), site unspecified

M46.31 Infection of intervertebral disc (pyogenic), occipito-atlanto-axial region

M46.32 Infection of intervertebral disc (pyogenic), cervical region

M46.33 Infection of intervertebral disc (pyogenic), cervicothoracic region

M46.34 Infection of intervertebral disc (pyogenic), thoracic region

M46.35 Infection of intervertebral disc (pyogenic), thoracolumbar region

M46.36 Infection of intervertebral disc (pyogenic), lumbar region

M46.37 Infection of intervertebral disc (pyogenic), lumbosacral region

M46.38 Infection of intervertebral disc (pyogenic), sacral and sacrococcygeal region

M46.39 Infection of intervertebral disc (pyogenic), multiple sites in spine

M46.4 Discitis, unspecified

M46.40 Discitis, unspecified, site unspecified

M46.41 Discitis, unspecified, occipito-atlanto-axial region

M46.42 Discitis, unspecified, cervical region

M46.43 Discitis, unspecified, cervicothoracic region

M46.44 Discitis, unspecified, thoracic region

M46.45 Discitis, unspecified, thoracolumbar region

M46.46 Discitis, unspecified, lumbar region

M46.47 Discitis, unspecified, lumbosacral region

M46.48 Discitis, unspecified, sacral and sacrococcygeal region

M46.49 Discitis, unspecified, multiple sites in spine

M46.5 Other infective spondylopathies

M46.50 Other infective spondylopathies, site unspecified

M46.51 Other infective spondylopathies, occipito-atlanto-axial region

M46.52 Other infective spondylopathies, cervical region

M46.53 Other infective spondylopathies, cervicothoracic region

M46.54 Other infective spondylopathies, thoracic region

M46.55 Other infective spondylopathies, thoracolumbar region

M46.56 Other infective spondylopathies, lumbar region

M46.57 Other infective spondylopathies, lumbosacral region

M46.58 Other infective spondylopathies, sacral and sacrococcygeal region

M46.59 Other infective spondylopathies, multiple sites in spine

M46.8 Other specified inflammatory spondylopathies

M46.80 Other specified inflammatory spondylopathies, site unspecified

M46.81 Other specified inflammatory spondylopathies, occipito-atlanto-axial region

M46.82 Other specified inflammatory spondylopathies, cervical region

M46.83 Other specified inflammatory spondylopathies, cervicothoracic region

M46.84 Other specified inflammatory spondylopathies, thoracic region

M46.85 Other specified inflammatory spondylopathies, thoracolumbar region

M46.86 Other specified inflammatory spondylopathies, lumbar region

M46.87 Other specified inflammatory spondylopathies, lumbosacral region

M46.88 Other specified inflammatory spondylopathies, sacral and sacrococcygeal region

M46.89 Other specified inflammatory spondylopathies, multiple sites in spine

M46.9 Unspecified inflammatory spondylopathy

M46.90 Unspecified inflammatory spondylopathy, site unspecified

M46.91 Unspecified inflammatory spondylopathy, occipito-atlanto-axial region

M46.92 Unspecified inflammatory spondylopathy, cervical region

M46.93 Unspecified inflammatory spondylopathy, cervicothoracic region

M46.94 Unspecified inflammatory spondylopathy, thoracic region

M46.95 Unspecified inflammatory spondylopathy, thoracolumbar region

M46.96 Unspecified inflammatory spondylopathy, lumbar region

M46.97 Unspecified inflammatory spondylopathy, lumbosacral region

M46.98 Unspecified inflammatory spondylopathy, sacral and sacrococcygeal region

M46.99 Unspecified inflammatory spondylopathy, multiple sites in spine

M47 Spondylosis
Includes: arthrosis or osteoarthritis of spine
degeneration of facet joints

M47.0 Anterior spinal and vertebral artery compression syndromes

M47.00 Anterior spinal and vertebral artery compression syndromes, site unspecified

M47.01 Anterior spinal and vertebral artery compression syndromes, occipito-atlanto-axial region

M47.02 Anterior spinal and vertebral artery compression syndromes, cervical region

M47.03 Anterior spinal and vertebral artery compression syndromes, cervicothoracic region

M47.04 Anterior spinal and vertebral artery compression syndromes, thoracic region

M47.05 Anterior spinal and vertebral artery compression syndromes, thoracolumbar region

M47.06 Anterior spinal and vertebral artery compression syndromes, lumbar region

M47.07 Anterior spinal and vertebral artery compression syndromes, lumbosacral region

M47.08 Anterior spinal and vertebral artery compression syndromes, sacral and sacrococcygeal region

M47.1 Other spondylosis with myelopathy
Spondylogenic compression of spinal cord

Excludes1:   vertebral subluxation (M43.3-M43.59)

M47.10   Other spondylosis with myelopathy, site unspecified
M47.11   Other spondylosis with myelopathy, occipito-atlanto-axial region
M47.12   Other spondylosis with myelopathy, cervical region
M47.13   Other spondylosis with myelopathy, cervicothoracic region
M47.14   Other spondylosis with myelopathy, thoracic region
M47.15   Other spondylosis with myelopathy, thoracolumbar region
M47.16   Other spondylosis with myelopathy, lumbar region
M47.17   Other spondylosis with myelopathy, lumbosacral region
M47.18   Other spondylosis with myelopathy, sacral and sacrococcygeal region

M47.2   Other spondylosis with radiculopathy
M47.20   Other spondylosis with radiculopathy, site unspecified
M47.21   Other spondylosis with radiculopathy, occipito-atlanto-axial region
M47.22   Other spondylosis with radiculopathy, cervical region
M47.23   Other spondylosis with radiculopathy, cervicothoracic region
M47.24   Other spondylosis with radiculopathy, thoracic region
M47.25   Other spondylosis with radiculopathy, thoracolumbar region
M47.26   Other spondylosis with radiculopathy, lumbar region
M47.27   Other spondylosis with radiculopathy, lumbosacral region
M47.28   Other spondylosis with radiculopathy, sacral and sacrococcygeal region

M47.8   Other spondylosis
M47.81   Spondylosis without myelopathy or radiculopathy
M47.811   Spondylosis without myelopathy or radiculopathy, occipito-atlanto-axial region
M47.812   Spondylosis without myelopathy or radiculopathy, cervical region
M47.813   Spondylosis without myelopathy or radiculopathy, cervicothoracic region
M47.814   Spondylosis without myelopathy or radiculopathy, thoracic region
M47.815   Spondylosis without myelopathy or radiculopathy, thoracolumbar region
M47.816   Spondylosis without myelopathy or radiculopathy, lumbar region
M47.817   Spondylosis without myelopathy or radiculopathy, lumbosacral region
M47.818   Spondylosis without myelopathy or radiculopathy, sacral and sacrococcygeal region
M47.819   Spondylosis without myelopathy or radiculopathy, site unspecified
M47.89   Other spondylosis
M47.891   Other spondylosis, occipito-atlanto-axial region
M47.892   Other spondylosis, cervical region
M47.893   Other spondylosis, cervicothoracic region
M47.894   Other spondylosis, thoracic region
M47.895   Other spondylosis, thoracolumbar region
M47.896   Other spondylosis, lumbar region
M47.897   Other spondylosis, lumbosacral region
M47.898   Other spondylosis, sacral and sacrococcygeal region
M47.899   Other spondylosis, site unspecified

M47.9   Spondylosis, unspecified

M48   Other spondylopathies
M48.0   Spinal stenosis
    Caudal stenosis
M48.00   Spinal stenosis, site unspecified
M48.01   Spinal stenosis, occipito-atlanto-axial region
M48.02   Spinal stenosis, cervical region
M48.03   Spinal stenosis, cervicothoracic region

M48.04   Spinal stenosis, thoracic region
M48.05   Spinal stenosis, thoracolumbar region
M48.06   Spinal stenosis, lumbar region
M48.07   Spinal stenosis, lumbosacral region
M48.08   Spinal stenosis, sacral and sacrococcygeal region

M48.1   Ankylosing hyperostosis [Forestier]
    Diffuse idiopathic skeletal hyperostosis [DISH]
M48.10   Ankylosing hyperostosis [Forestier], site unspecified
M48.11   Ankylosing hyperostosis [Forestier], occipito-atlanto-axial region
M48.12   Ankylosing hyperostosis [Forestier], cervical region
M48.13   Ankylosing hyperostosis [Forestier], cervicothoracic region
M48.14   Ankylosing hyperostosis [Forestier], thoracic region
M48.15   Ankylosing hyperostosis [Forestier], thoracolumbar region
M48.16   Ankylosing hyperostosis [Forestier], lumbar region
M48.17   Ankylosing hyperostosis [Forestier], lumbosacral region
M48.18   Ankylosing hyperostosis [Forestier], sacral and sacrococcygeal region
M48.19   Ankylosing hyperostosis [Forestier], multiple sites in spine

M48.2   Kissing spine
M48.20   Kissing spine, site unspecified
M48.21   Kissing spine, occipito-atlanto-axial region
M48.22   Kissing spine, cervical region
M48.23   Kissing spine, cervicothoracic region
M48.24   Kissing spine, thoracic region
M48.25   Kissing spine, thoracolumbar region
M48.26   Kissing spine, lumbar region
M48.27   Kissing spine, lumbosacral region
M48.28   Kissing spine, sacral and sacrococcygeal region

M48.3   Traumatic spondylopathy
M48.30   Traumatic spondylopathy, site unspecified
M48.31   Traumatic spondylopathy, occipito-atlanto-axial region
M48.32   Traumatic spondylopathy, cervical region
M48.33   Traumatic spondylopathy, cervicothoracic region
M48.34   Traumatic spondylopathy, thoracic region
M48.35   Traumatic spondylopathy, thoracolumbar region
M48.36   Traumatic spondylopathy, lumbar region
M48.37   Traumatic spondylopathy, lumbosacral region
M48.38   Traumatic spondylopathy, sacral and sacrococcygeal region

M48.4   Fatigue fracture of vertebra
    Stress fracture of vertebra
    Excludes1:   pathologic fracture of vertebra due to neoplasm (M84.58)
            pathologic fracture of vertebra due to other diagnosis (M84.68)
            pathologic fracture of vertebra due to osteoporosis (M80.-)
            pathologic fracture NOS (M84.4-)
            traumatic fracture of vertebrae (S12.0—S12.3-, S22.0-, S32.0-)
    The following extensions are to be added to each code for subcategory M48.4:
    a   initial encounter for fracture
    d   subsequent encounter for fracture with routine healing
    g   subsequent encounter for fracture with delayed healing
    j   subsequent encounter for fracture with nonunion
    m   subsequent encounter for fracture with malunion
    q   sequela
M48.40   Fatigue fracture of vertebra, site unspecified
M48.41   Fatigue fracture of vertebra, occipito-atlanto-axial region
M48.42   Fatigue fracture of vertebra, cervical region
M48.43   Fatigue fracture of vertebra, cervicothoracic region
M48.44   Fatigue fracture of vertebra, thoracic region
M48.45   Fatigue fracture of vertebra, thoracolumbar region
M48.46   Fatigue fracture of vertebra, lumbar region

M48.47   Fatigue fracture of vertebra, lumbosacral region

M48.48   Fatigue fracture of vertebra, sacral and sacrococcygeal region

M48.5   **Collapsed vertebra, not elsewhere classified**

Collapsed vertebra NOS

Wedging of vertebra NOS

Excludes1:   current injury — see injury of spine by body region

fatigue fracture of vertebra (M48.4)

pathologic fracture of vertebra due to neoplasm (M84.58)

pathologic fracture of vertebra due to other diagnosis (M84.68)

pathologic fracture of vertebra due to osteoporosis (M80.-)

pathologic fracture NOS (M84.4-)

stress fracture of vertebra (M48.4-)

traumatic fracture of vertebra (S12.-, S22.-, S32.-)

M48.50   Collapsed vertebra, not elsewhere classified, site unspecified

M48.51   Collapsed vertebra, not elsewhere classified, occipito-atlanto-axial region

M48.52   Collapsed vertebra, not elsewhere classified, cervical region

M48.53   Collapsed vertebra, not elsewhere classified, cervicothoracic region

M48.54   Collapsed vertebra, not elsewhere classified, thoracic region

M48.55   Collapsed vertebra, not elsewhere classified, thoracolumbar region

M48.56   Collapsed vertebra, not elsewhere classified, lumbar region

M48.57   Collapsed vertebra, not elsewhere classified, lumbosacral region

M48.58   Collapsed vertebra, not elsewhere classified, sacral and sacrococcygeal region

M48.8   **Other specified spondylopathies**

Ossification of posterior longitudinal ligament

M48.8x   Other specified spondylopathies

M48.8x1   Other specified spondylopathies, occipito-atlanto-axial region

M48.8x2   Other specified spondylopathies, cervical region

M48.8x3   Other specified spondylopathies, cervicothoracic region

M48.8x4   Other specified spondylopathies, thoracic region

M48.8x5   Other specified spondylopathies, thoracolumbar region

M48.8x6   Other specified spondylopathies, lumbar region

M48.8x7   Other specified spondylopathies, lumbosacral region

M48.8x8   Other specified spondylopathies, sacral and sacrococcygeal region

M48.8x9   Other specified spondylopathies, site unspecified

M48.9   **Spondylopathy, unspecified**

M49 Spondylopathies in diseases classified elsewhere

Includes: curvature of spine in diseases classified elsewhere

deformity of spine in diseases classified elsewhere

kyphosis in diseases classified elsewhere

scoliosis in diseases classified elsewhere

spondylopathy in diseases classified elsewhere

Excludes1:   curvature of spine in tuberculosis [Pott's] (A18.01)

enteropathic arthropathies (M07.-)

neuropathic spondylopathy (in):

nonsyphilitic NEC (G98.0)

syringomyelia (G95.0)

tabes dorsalis (A52.11)

spondylitis (in):

gonococcal (A54.41)

syphilis (acquired) (A52.77)

neuropathic [tabes dorsalis] (A52.11)

tuberculosis (A18.01)

typhoid fever (A01.05)

Code first underlying disease, such as:

brucellosis (A23.-)

Charcot-Marie-Tooth disease (G60.0)

enterobacterial infections (A01-A04)

osteitis fibrosa cystica (E21.0)

rickets (sequelae) (E64.3)

M49.8   **Spondylopathy in diseases classified elsewhere**

M49.80   Spondylopathy in diseases classified elsewhere, site unspecified

M49.81   Spondylopathy in diseases classified elsewhere, occipito-atlanto-axial region

M49.82   Spondylopathy in diseases classified elsewhere, cervical region

M49.83   Spondylopathy in diseases classified elsewhere, cervicothoracic region

M49.84   Spondylopathy in diseases classified elsewhere, thoracic region

M49.85   Spondylopathy in diseases classified elsewhere, thoracolumbar region

M49.86   Spondylopathy in diseases classified elsewhere, lumbar region

M49.87   Spondylopathy in diseases classified elsewhere, lumbosacral region

M49.88   Spondylopathy in diseases classified elsewhere, sacral and sacrococcygeal region

M49.89   Spondylopathy in diseases classified elsewhere, multiple sites in spine

OTHER DORSOPATHIES (M50–M54)

Excludes1:   current injury — see injury of spine by body region

discitis NOS (M46.4-)

M50 Cervical disc disorders

Includes: cervicothoracic disc disorders with cervicalgia

cervicothoracic disc disorders

Note: code to the most superior level of disorder

M50.0   **Cervical disc disorder with myelopathy**

M50.00   Cervical disc disorder with myelopathy, unspecified cervical region

M50.01   Cervical disc disorder with myelopathy, occipito-atlanto-axial region

M50.02   Cervical disc disorder with myelopathy, mid-cervical region

M50.03   Cervical disc disorder with myelopathy, cervicothoracic region

M50.1   **Cervical disc disorder with radiculopathy**

Excludes2:   brachial radiculitis NOS (M54.13)

M50.10   Cervical disc disorder with radiculopathy, unspecified cervical region

M50.11   Cervical disc disorder with radiculopathy, occipito-atlanto-axial region

M50.12   Cervical disc disorder with radiculopathy, mid-cervical region

M50.13   Cervical disc disorder with radiculopathy, cervicothoracic region

M50.2 Other cervical disc displacement
    M50.20 Other cervical disc displacement, unspecified cervical region
    M50.21 Other cervical disc displacement, occipito-atlanto-axial region
    M50.22 Other cervical disc displacement, mid-cervical region
    M50.23 Other cervical disc displacement, cervicothoracic region

M50.3 Other cervical disc degeneration
    M50.30 Other cervical disc degeneration, unspecified cervical region
    M50.31 Other cervical disc degeneration, occipito-atlanto-axial region
    M50.32 Other cervical disc degeneration, mid-cervical region
    M50.33 Other cervical disc degeneration, cervicothoracic region

M50.8 Other cervical disc disorders
    M50.80 Other cervical disc disorders, unspecified cervical region
    M50.81 Other cervical disc disorders, occipito-atlanto-axial region
    M50.82 Other cervical disc disorders, mid-cervical region
    M50.83 Other cervical disc disorders, cervicothoracic region

M50.9 Cervical disc disorder, unspecified
    M50.90 Cervical disc disorder, unspecified, unspecified cervical region
    M50.91 Cervical disc disorder, unspecified, occipito-atlanto-axial region
    M50.92 Cervical disc disorder, unspecified, mid-cervical region
    M50.93 Cervical disc disorder, unspecified, cervicothoracic region

M51 Thoracic, thoracolumbar, and lumbosacral intervertebral disc disorders
    Excludes2:   cervical and cervicothoracic disc disorders (M50.-)
        sacral and sacrococcygeal disorders (M53.3)

M51.0 Thoracic, thoracolumbar and lumbosacral intervertebral disc disorders with myelopathy
    M51.04 Intervertebral disc disorders with myelopathy, thoracic region
    M51.05 Intervertebral disc disorders with myelopathy, thoracolumbar region
    M51.06 Intervertebral disc disorders with myelopathy, lumbar region
    M51.07 Intervertebral disc disorders with myelopathy, lumbosacral region

M51.1 Thoracic, thoracolumbar and lumbosacral intervertebral disc disorders with radiculopathy
    Sciatica due to intervertebral disc disorder
    Excludes1:   lumbar radiculitis NOS (M54.16)
        sciatica NOS (M54.3)
    M51.14 Intervertebral disc disorders with radiculopathy, thoracic region
    M51.15 Intervertebral disc disorders with radiculopathy, thoracolumbar region
    M51.16 Intervertebral disc disorders with radiculopathy, lumbar region
    M51.17 Intervertebral disc disorders with radiculopathy, lumbosacral region

M51.2 Other thoracic, thoracolumbar and lumbosacral intervertebral disc displacement
    Lumbago due to displacement of intervertebral disc
    M51.24 Other intervertebral disc displacement, thoracic region
    M51.25 Other intervertebral disc displacement, thoracolumbar region
    M51.26 Other intervertebral disc displacement, lumbar region
    M51.27 Other intervertebral disc displacement, lumbosacral region

M51.3 Other thoracic, thoracolumbar and lumbosacral intervertebral disc degeneration
    M51.34 Other intervertebral disc degeneration, thoracic region

M51.35 Other intervertebral disc degeneration, thoracolumbar region
M51.36 Other intervertebral disc degeneration, lumbar region
M51.37 Other intervertebral disc degeneration, lumbosacral region

M51.4 Schmorl's nodes
    M51.44 Schmorl's nodes, thoracic region
    M51.45 Schmorl's nodes, thoracolumbar region
    M51.46 Schmorl's nodes, lumbar region
    M51.47 Schmorl's nodes, lumbosacral region

M51.8 Other thoracic, thoracolumbar and lumbosacral intervertebral disc disorders
    M51.84 Other intervertebral disc disorders, thoracic region
    M51.85 Other intervertebral disc disorders, thoracolumbar region
    M51.86 Other intervertebral disc disorders, lumbar region
    M51.87 Other intervertebral disc disorders, lumbosacral region

M51.9 Unspecified thoracic, thoracolumbar and lumbosacral intervertebral disc disorder

M53 Other and unspecified dorsopathies, not elsewhere classified
M53.0 Cervicocranial syndrome
    Posterior cervical sympathetic syndrome

M53.1 Cervicobrachial syndrome
    Excludes2:   cervical disc disorder (M50.-)
        thoracic outlet syndrome (G54.0)

M53.2 Spinal instabilities
    M53.2x Spinal instabilities
        M53.2x1 Spinal instabilities, occipito-atlanto-axial region
        M53.2x2 Spinal instabilities, cervical region
        M53.2x3 Spinal instabilities, cervicothoracic region
        M53.2x4 Spinal instabilities, thoracic region
        M53.2x5 Spinal instabilities, thoracolumbar region
        M53.2x6 Spinal instabilities, lumbar region
        M53.2x7 Spinal instabilities, lumbosacral region
        M53.2x8 Spinal instabilities, sacral and sacrococcygeal region
        M53.2x9 Spinal instabilities, site unspecified

M53.3 Sacrococcygeal disorders, not elsewhere classified
    Coccygodynia

M53.8 Other specified dorsopathies
    M53.80 Other specified dorsopathies, site unspecified
    M53.81 Other specified dorsopathies, occipito-atlanto-axial region
    M53.82 Other specified dorsopathies, cervical region
    M53.83 Other specified dorsopathies, cervicothoracic region
    M53.84 Other specified dorsopathies, thoracic region
    M53.85 Other specified dorsopathies, thoracolumbar region
    M53.86 Other specified dorsopathies, lumbar region
    M53.87 Other specified dorsopathies, lumbosacral region
    M53.88 Other specified dorsopathies, sacral and sacrococcygeal region

M53.9 Dorsopathy, unspecified

M54 Dorsalgia
    Excludes1:   psychogenic dorsalgia (F45.4)

M54.0 Panniculitis affecting regions of neck and back
    Excludes1:   lupus panniculitis (L93.2)
        panniculitis NOS (M79.3)
        relapsing [Weber-Christian] panniculitis (M35.6)
    M54.00 Panniculitis affecting regions of neck and back, site unspecified
    M54.01 Panniculitis affecting regions of neck and back, occipito-atlanto-axial region
    M54.02 Panniculitis affecting regions of neck and back, cervical region
    M54.03 Panniculitis affecting regions of neck and back, cervicothoracic region
    M54.04 Panniculitis affecting regions of neck and back, thoracic region

M54.05   Panniculitis affecting regions of neck and back, thoracolumbar region
M54.06   Panniculitis affecting regions of neck and back, lumbar region
M54.07   Panniculitis affecting regions of neck and back, lumbosacral region
M54.08   Panniculitis affecting regions of neck and back, sacral and sacrococcygeal region
M54.09   Panniculitis affecting regions, neck and back, multiple sites in spine

M54.1 Radiculopathy
Brachial neuritis or radiculitis NOS
Lumbar neuritis or radiculitis NOS
Lumbosacral neuritis or radiculitis NOS
Thoracic neuritis or radiculitis NOS
Radiculitis NOS
Excludes1: neuralgia and neuritis NOS (M79.2)
radiculopathy with cervical disc disorder (M50.1)
radiculopathy with lumbar and other intervertebral disc disorder (M51.1-)
radiculopathy with spondylosis (M47.2-)
M54.10   Radiculopathy, site unspecified
M54.11   Radiculopathy, occipito-atlanto-axial region
M54.12   Radiculopathy, cervical region
M54.13   Radiculopathy, cervicothoracic region
M54.14   Radiculopathy, thoracic region
M54.15   Radiculopathy, thoracolumbar region
M54.16   Radiculopathy, lumbar region
M54.17   Radiculopathy, lumbosacral region
M54.18   Radiculopathy, sacral and sacrococcygeal region

M54.2 Cervicalgia
Excludes1: cervicalgia due to intervertebral cervical disc disorder (M50.-)

M54.3 Sciatica
Excludes1: lesion of sciatic nerve (G57.0)
sciatica due to intervertebral disc disorder (M51.1-)
sciatica with lumbago (M54.4)
M54.30   Sciatica, unspecified side
M54.31   Sciatica, right side
M54.32   Sciatica, left side

M54.4 Lumbago with sciatica
Excludes1: lumbago with sciatica due to intervertebral disc disorder (M51.1-)

M54.5 Low back pain
Loin pain
Low back strain
Lumbago NOS
Excludes1: lumbago due to intervertebral disc displacement (M51.2-)
lumbago with sciatica (M54.4)

M54.6 Pain in thoracic spine
Excludes1: pain in thoracic spine due to intervertebral disc disorder (M51.-)

M54.8 Other dorsalgia
Excludes1: dorsalgia in thoracic region (M54.6)
low back pain (M54.5)
M54.81   Occipital neuralgia
M54.89   Other dorsalgia

M54.9 Dorsalgia, unspecified
Backache NOS

SOFT TISSUE DISORDERS (M60–M79)

DISORDERS OF MUSCLES (M60–M63)
Excludes1: dermatopolymyositis (M33.-)
muscular dystrophies and myopathies (G71-G72)
myopathy in:
amyloidosis (E85)
polyarteritis nodosa (M30.0)
rheumatoid arthritis (M05.32)
scleroderma (M34.-)
Sjögren's syndrome (M35.03)
systemic lupus erythematosus (M32.-)

M60 Myositis
M60.0 Infective myositis
Tropical pyomyositis
Use additional code (B95-B97) to identify infectious agent
M60.00   Infective myositis, unspecified site
M60.000 Infective myositis, unspecified right arm
Infective myositis, right upper limb NOS
M60.001 Infective myositis, unspecified left arm
Infective myositis, left upper limb NOS
M60.002 Infective myositis, unspecified arm
Infective myositis, upper limb NOS
M60.003 Infective myositis, unspecified right leg
Infective myositis, right lower limb NOS
M60.004 Infective myositis, unspecified left leg
Infective myositis, left lower limb NOS
M60.005 Infective myositis, unspecified leg
Infective myositis, lower limb NOS
M60.009 Infective myositis, unspecified site
M60.01   Infective myositis, shoulder
M60.011 Infective myositis, right shoulder
M60.012 Infective myositis, left shoulder
M60.019 Infective myositis, unspecified shoulder
M60.02   Infective myositis, upper arm
M60.021 Infective myositis, right upper arm
M60.022 Infective myositis, left upper arm
M60.029 Infective myositis, unspecified upper arm
M60.03   Infective myositis, forearm
M60.031 Infective myositis, right forearm
M60.032 Infective myositis, left forearm
M60.039 Infective myositis, unspecified forearm
M60.04   Infective myositis, hand and fingers
M60.041 Infective myositis, right hand
M60.042 Infective myositis, left hand
M60.043 Infective myositis, unspecified hand
M60.044 Infective myositis, right finger(s)
M60.045 Infective myositis, left finger(s)
M60.046 Infective myositis, unspecified finger(s)
M60.05   Infective myositis, thigh
M60.051 Infective myositis, right thigh
M60.052 Infective myositis, left thigh
M60.059 Infective myositis, unspecified thigh
M60.06   Infective myositis, lower leg
M60.061 Infective myositis, right lower leg
M60.062 Infective myositis, left lower leg
M60.069 Infective myositis, unspecified lower leg
M60.07   Infective myositis, ankle, foot and toes
M60.070 Infective myositis, right ankle
M60.071 Infective myositis, left ankle
M60.072 Infective myositis, unspecified ankle
M60.073 Infective myositis, right foot
M60.074 Infective myositis, left foot
M60.075 Infective myositis, unspecified foot
M60.076 Infective myositis, right toe(s)
M60.077 Infective myositis, left toe(s)
M60.078 Infective myositis, unspecified toe(s)
M60.08   Infective myositis, other site
M60.09   Infective myositis, multiple sites

M60.1 Interstitial myositis
    M60.10   Interstitial myositis of unspecified site
    M60.11   Interstitial myositis, shoulder
        M60.111 Interstitial myositis, right shoulder
        M60.112 Interstitial myositis, left shoulder
        M60.119 Interstitial myositis, unspecified shoulder
    M60.12   Interstitial myositis, upper arm
        M60.121 Interstitial myositis, right upper arm
        M60.122 Interstitial myositis, left upper arm
        M60.129 Interstitial myositis, unspecified upper arm
    M60.13   Interstitial myositis, forearm
        M60.131 Interstitial myositis, right forearm
        M60.132 Interstitial myositis, left forearm
        M60.139 Interstitial myositis, unspecified forearm
    M60.14   Interstitial myositis, hand
        M60.141 Interstitial myositis, right hand
        M60.142 Interstitial myositis, left hand
        M60.149 Interstitial myositis, unspecified hand
    M60.15   Interstitial myositis, thigh
        M60.151 Interstitial myositis, right thigh
        M60.152 Interstitial myositis, left thigh
        M60.159 Interstitial myositis, unspecified thigh
    M60.16   Interstitial myositis, lower leg
        M60.161 Interstitial myositis, right lower leg
        M60.162 Interstitial myositis, left lower leg
        M60.169 Interstitial myositis, unspecified lower leg
    M60.17   Interstitial myositis, ankle and foot
        M60.171 Interstitial myositis, right ankle and foot
        M60.172 Interstitial myositis, left ankle and foot
        M60.179 Interstitial myositis, unspecified ankle and foot
    M60.18   Interstitial myositis, other site
    M60.19   Interstitial myositis, multiple sites
M60.2 Foreign body granuloma of soft tissue, not elsewhere classified
    Excludes1:   foreign body granuloma of skin and subcutaneous tissue (L92.3)
    M60.20   Foreign body granuloma of soft tissue, not elsewhere classified, unspecified site
    M60.21   Foreign body granuloma of soft tissue, not elsewhere classified, shoulder
        M60.211 Foreign body granuloma of soft tissue, not elsewhere classified, right shoulder
        M60.212 Foreign body granuloma of soft tissue, not elsewhere classified, left shoulder
        M60.219 Foreign body granuloma of soft tissue, not elsewhere classified, unspecified shoulder
    M60.22   Foreign body granuloma of soft tissue, not elsewhere classified, upper arm
        M60.221 Foreign body granuloma of soft tissue, not elsewhere classified, right upper arm
        M60.222 Foreign body granuloma of soft tissue, not elsewhere classified, left upper arm
        M60.229 Foreign body granuloma of soft tissue, not elsewhere classified, unspecified upper arm
    M60.23   Foreign body granuloma of soft tissue, not elsewhere classified, forearm
        M60.231 Foreign body granuloma of soft tissue, not elsewhere classified, right forearm
        M60.232 Foreign body granuloma of soft tissue, not elsewhere classified, left forearm
        M60.239 Foreign body granuloma of soft tissue, not elsewhere classified, unspecified forearm
    M60.24   Foreign body granuloma of soft tissue, not elsewhere classified, hand
        M60.241 Foreign body granuloma of soft tissue, not elsewhere classified, right hand
        M60.242 Foreign body granuloma of soft tissue, not elsewhere classified, left hand
        M60.249 Foreign body granuloma of soft tissue, not elsewhere classified, unspecified hand

    M60.25   Foreign body granuloma of soft tissue, not elsewhere classified, thigh
        M60.251 Foreign body granuloma of soft tissue, not elsewhere classified, right thigh
        M60.252 Foreign body granuloma of soft tissue, not elsewhere classified, left thigh
        M60.259 Foreign body granuloma of soft tissue, not elsewhere classified, unspecified thigh
    M60.26   Foreign body granuloma of soft tissue, not elsewhere classified, lower leg
        M60.261 Foreign body granuloma of soft tissue, not elsewhere classified, right lower leg
        M60.262 Foreign body granuloma of soft tissue, not elsewhere classified, left lower leg
        M60.269 Foreign body granuloma of soft tissue, not elsewhere classified, unspecified lower leg
    M60.27   Foreign body granuloma of soft tissue, not elsewhere classified, ankle and foot
        M60.271 Foreign body granuloma of soft tissue, not elsewhere classified, right ankle and foot
        M60.272 Foreign body granuloma of soft tissue, not elsewhere classified, left ankle and foot
        M60.279 Foreign body granuloma of soft tissue, not elsewhere classified, unspecified ankle and foot
    M60.28   Foreign body granuloma of soft tissue, not elsewhere classified, other site
M60.8 Other myositis
    M60.80   Other myositis, unspecified site
    M60.81   Other myositis shoulder
        M60.811 Other myositis, right shoulder
        M60.812 Other myositis, left shoulder
        M60.819 Other myositis, unspecified shoulder
    M60.82   Other myositis, upper arm
        M60.821 Other myositis, right upper arm
        M60.822 Other myositis, left upper arm
        M60.829 Other myositis, unspecified upper arm
    M60.83   Other myositis, forearm
        M60.831 Other myositis, right forearm
        M60.832 Other myositis, left forearm
        M60.839 Other myositis, unspecified forearm
    M60.84   Other myositis, hand
        M60.841 Other myositis, right hand
        M60.842 Other myositis, left hand
        M60.849 Other myositis, unspecified hand
    M60.85   Other myositis, thigh
        M60.851 Other myositis, right thigh
        M60.852 Other myositis, left thigh
        M60.859 Other myositis, unspecified thigh
    M60.86   Other myositis, lower leg
        M60.861 Other myositis, right lower leg
        M60.862 Other myositis, left lower leg
        M60.869 Other myositis, unspecified lower leg
    M60.87   Other myositis, ankle and foot
        M60.871 Other myositis, right ankle and foot
        M60.872 Other myositis, left ankle and foot
        M60.879 Other myositis, unspecified ankle and foot
    M60.88   Other myositis, other site
    M60.89   Other myositis, multiple sites
M60.9 Myositis, unspecified

M61 Calcification and ossification of muscle
M61.0 Myositis ossificans traumatica
    M61.00   Myositis ossificans traumatica, unspecified site
    M61.01   Myositis ossificans traumatica, shoulder
        M61.011 Myositis ossificans traumatica, right shoulder
        M61.012 Myositis ossificans traumatica, left shoulder
        M61.019 Myositis ossificans traumatica, unspecified shoulder
    M61.02   Myositis ossificans traumatica, upper arm

    M61.021   Myositis ossificans traumatica, right upper arm

    M61.022   Myositis ossificans traumatica, left upper arm

    M61.029   Myositis ossificans traumatica, unspecified upper arm

  M61.03   Myositis ossificans traumatica, forearm

    M61.031   Myositis ossificans traumatica, right forearm

    M61.032   Myositis ossificans traumatica, left forearm

    M61.039   Myositis ossificans traumatica, unspecified forearm

  M61.04   Myositis ossificans traumatica, hand

    M61.041   Myositis ossificans traumatica, right hand

    M61.042   Myositis ossificans traumatica, left hand

    M61.049   Myositis ossificans traumatica, unspecified hand

  M61.05   Myositis ossificans traumatica, thigh

    M61.051   Myositis ossificans traumatica, right thigh

    M61.052   Myositis ossificans traumatica, left thigh

    M61.059   Myositis ossificans traumatica, unspecified thigh

  M61.06   Myositis ossificans traumatica, lower leg

    M61.061   Myositis ossificans traumatica, right lower leg

    M61.062   Myositis ossificans traumatica, left lower leg

    M61.069   Myositis ossificans traumatica, unspecified lower leg

  M61.07   Myositis ossificans traumatica, ankle and foot

    M61.071   Myositis ossificans traumatica, right ankle and foot

    M61.072   Myositis ossificans traumatica, left ankle and foot

    M61.079   Myositis ossificans traumatica, unspecified ankle and foot

  M61.08   Myositis ossificans traumatica, other site

  M61.09   Myositis ossificans traumatica, multiple sites

M61.1   Myositis ossificans progressiva

    Fibrodysplasia ossificans progressiva

  M61.10   Myositis ossificans progressiva, unspecified site

  M61.11   Myositis ossificans progressiva, shoulder

    M61.111   Myositis ossificans progressiva, right shoulder

    M61.112   Myositis ossificans progressiva, left shoulder

    M61.119   Myositis ossificans progressiva, unspecified shoulder

  M61.12   Myositis ossificans progressiva, upper arm

    M61.121   Myositis ossificans progressiva, right upper arm

    M61.122   Myositis ossificans progressiva, left upper arm

    M61.129   Myositis ossificans progressiva, unspecified arm

  M61.13   Myositis ossificans progressiva, forearm

    M61.131   Myositis ossificans progressiva, right forearm

    M61.132   Myositis ossificans progressiva, left forearm

    M61.139   Myositis ossificans progressiva, unspecified forearm

  M61.14   Myositis ossificans progressiva, hand and finger(s)

    M61.141   Myositis ossificans progressiva, right hand

    M61.142   Myositis ossificans progressiva, left hand

    M61.143   Myositis ossificans progressiva, unspecified hand

    M61.144   Myositis ossificans progressiva, right finger(s)

    M61.145   Myositis ossificans progressiva, left finger(s)

    M61.146   Myositis ossificans progressiva, unspecified finger(s)

  M61.15   Myositis ossificans progressiva, thigh

    M61.151   Myositis ossificans progressiva, right thigh

    M61.152   Myositis ossificans progressiva, left thigh

    M61.159   Myositis ossificans progressiva, unspecified thigh

  M61.16   Myositis ossificans progressiva, lower leg

    M61.161   Myositis ossificans progressiva, right lower leg

    M61.162   Myositis ossificans progressiva, left lower leg

    M61.169   Myositis ossificans progressiva, unspecified lower leg

  M61.17   Myositis ossificans progressiva, ankle, foot and toe(s)

    M61.171   Myositis ossificans progressiva, right ankle

    M61.172   Myositis ossificans progressiva, left ankle

    M61.173   Myositis ossificans progressiva, unspecified ankle

    M61.174   Myositis ossificans progressiva, right foot

    M61.175   Myositis ossificans progressiva, left foot

    M61.176   Myositis ossificans progressiva, unspecified foot

    M61.177   Myositis ossificans progressiva, right toe(s)

    M61.178   Myositis ossificans progressiva, left toe(s)

    M61.179   Myositis ossificans progressiva, unspecified toe(s)

  M61.18   Myositis ossificans progressiva, other site

  M61.19   Myositis ossificans progressiva, multiple sites

M61.2   Paralytic calcification and ossification of muscle

    Myositis ossificans associated with quadriplegia or paraplegia

  M61.20   Paralytic calcification and ossification of muscle, unspecified site

  M61.21   Paralytic calcification and ossification of muscle, shoulder

    M61.211   Paralytic calcification and ossification of muscle, right shoulder

    M61.212   Paralytic calcification and ossification of muscle, left shoulder

    M61.219   Paralytic calcification and ossification of muscle, unspecified shoulder

  M61.22   Paralytic calcification and ossification of muscle, upper arm

    M61.221   Paralytic calcification and ossification of muscle, right upper arm

    M61.222   Paralytic calcification and ossification of muscle, left upper arm

    M61.229   Paralytic calcification and ossification of muscle, unspecified upper arm

  M61.23   Paralytic calcification and ossification of muscle, forearm

    M61.231   Paralytic calcification and ossification of muscle, right forearm

    M61.232   Paralytic calcification and ossification of muscle, left forearm

    M61.239   Paralytic calcification and ossification of muscle, unspecified forearm

  M61.24   Paralytic calcification and ossification of muscle, hand

    M61.241   Paralytic calcification and ossification of muscle, right hand

    M61.242   Paralytic calcification and ossification of muscle, left hand

    M61.249   Paralytic calcification and ossification of muscle, unspecified hand

  M61.25   Paralytic calcification and ossification of muscle, thigh

    M61.251   Paralytic calcification and ossification of muscle, right thigh

    M61.252   Paralytic calcification and ossification of muscle, left thigh

    M61.259   Paralytic calcification and ossification of muscle, unspecified thigh

  M61.26   Paralytic calcification and ossification of muscle, lower leg

    M61.261   Paralytic calcification and ossification of muscle, right lower leg

    M61.262   Paralytic calcification and ossification of muscle, left lower leg

    M61.269   Paralytic calcification and ossification of muscle, unspecified lower leg

  M61.27   Paralytic calcification and ossification of muscle, ankle and foot

    M61.271   Paralytic calcification and ossification of muscle, right ankle and foot

M61.272 Paralytic calcification and ossification of muscle, left ankle and foot

M61.279 Paralytic calcification and ossification of muscle, unspecified ankle and foot

M61.28 Paralytic calcification and ossification of muscle, other site

M61.29 Paralytic calcification and ossification of muscle, multiple sites

M61.3 Calcification and ossification of muscles associated with burns
    Myositis ossificans associated with burns

M61.30 Calcification and ossification of muscles associated with burns, unspecified site

M61.31 Calcification and ossification of muscles associated with burns, shoulder

M61.311 Calcification and ossification of muscles associated with burns, right shoulder

M61.312 Calcification and ossification of muscles associated with burns, left shoulder

M61.319 Calcification and ossification of muscles associated with burns, unspecified shoulder

M61.32 Calcification and ossification of muscles associated with burns, upper arm

M61.321 Calcification and ossification of muscles associated with burns, right upper arm

M61.322 Calcification and ossification of muscles associated with burns, left upper arm

M61.329 Calcification and ossification of muscles associated with burns, unspecified upper arm

M61.33 Calcification and ossification of muscles associated with burns, forearm

M61.331 Calcification and ossification of muscles associated with burns, right forearm

M61.332 Calcification and ossification of muscles associated with burns, left forearm

M61.339 Calcification and ossification of muscles associated with burns, unspecified forearm

M61.34 Calcification and ossification of muscles associated with burns, hand

M61.341 Calcification and ossification of muscles associated with burns, right hand

M61.342 Calcification and ossification of muscles associated with burns, left hand

M61.349 Calcification and ossification of muscles associated with burns, unspecified hand

M61.35 Calcification and ossification of muscles associated with burns, thigh

M61.351 Calcification and ossification of muscles associated with burns, right thigh

M61.352 Calcification and ossification of muscles associated with burns, left thigh

M61.359 Calcification and ossification of muscles associated with burns, unspecified thigh

M61.36 Calcification and ossification of muscles associated with burns, lower leg

M61.361 Calcification and ossification of muscles associated with burns, right lower leg

M61.362 Calcification and ossification of muscles associated with burns, left lower leg

M61.369 Calcification and ossification of muscles associated with burns, unspecified lower leg

M61.37 Calcification and ossification of muscles associated with burns, ankle and foot

M61.371 Calcification and ossification of muscles associated with burns, right ankle and foot

M61.372 Calcification and ossification of muscles associated with burns, left ankle and foot

M61.379 Calcification and ossification of muscles associated with burns, unspecified ankle and foot

M61.38 Calcification and ossification of muscles associated with burns, other site

M61.39 Calcification and ossification of muscles associated with burns, multiple sites

M61.4 Other calcification of muscle
    Excludes1:   calcific tendinitis NOS (M65.2-)
                calcific tendinitis of shoulder (M75.3)

M61.40 Other calcification of muscle, unspecified site

M61.41 Other calcification of muscle, shoulder

M61.411 Other calcification of muscle, right shoulder

M61.412 Other calcification of muscle, left shoulder

M61.419 Other calcification of muscle, unspecified shoulder

M61.42 Other calcification of muscle, upper arm

M61.421 Other calcification of muscle, right upper arm

M61.422 Other calcification of muscle, left upper arm

M61.429 Other calcification of muscle, unspecified upper arm

M61.43 Other calcification of muscle, forearm

M61.431 Other calcification of muscle, right forearm

M61.432 Other calcification of muscle, left forearm

M61.439 Other calcification of muscle, unspecified forearm

M61.44 Other calcification of muscle, hand

M61.441 Other calcification of muscle, right hand

M61.442 Other calcification of muscle, left hand

M61.449 Other calcification of muscle, unspecified hand

M61.45 Other calcification of muscle, thigh

M61.451 Other calcification of muscle, right thigh

M61.452 Other calcification of muscle, left thigh

M61.459 Other calcification of muscle, unspecified thigh

M61.46 Other calcification of muscle, lower leg

M61.461 Other calcification of muscle, right lower leg

M61.462 Other calcification of muscle, left lower leg

M61.469 Other calcification of muscle, unspecified lower leg

M61.47 Other calcification of muscle, ankle and foot

M61.471 Other calcification of muscle, right ankle and foot

M61.472 Other calcification of muscle, left ankle and foot

M61.479 Other calcification of muscle, unspecified ankle and foot

M61.48 Other calcification of muscle, other site

M61.49 Other calcification of muscle, multiple sites

M61.5 Other ossification of muscle

M61.50 Other ossification of muscle, unspecified site

M61.51 Other ossification of muscle, shoulder

M61.511 Other ossification of muscle, right shoulder

M61.512 Other ossification of muscle, left shoulder

M61.519 Other ossification of muscle, unspecified shoulder

M61.52 Other ossification of muscle, upper arm

M61.521 Other ossification of muscle, right upper arm

M61.522 Other ossification of muscle, left upper arm

M61.529 Other ossification of muscle, unspecified upper arm

M61.53 Other ossification of muscle, forearm

M61.531 Other ossification of muscle, right forearm

M61.532 Other ossification of muscle, left forearm

M61.539 Other ossification of muscle, unspecified forearm

M61.54 Other ossification of muscle, hand

M61.541 Other ossification of muscle, right hand

M61.542 Other ossification of muscle, left hand

M61.549 Other ossification of muscle, unspecified hand

M61.55 Other ossification of muscle, thigh

M61.551 Other ossification of muscle, right thigh

M61.552 Other ossification of muscle, left thigh

M61.559 Other ossification of muscle, unspecified thigh
M61.56 Other ossification of muscle, lower leg
    M61.561 Other ossification of muscle, right lower leg
    M61.562 Other ossification of muscle, left lower leg
    M61.569 Other ossification of muscle, unspecified lower leg
M61.57 Other ossification of muscle, ankle and foot
    M61.571 Other ossification of muscle, right ankle and foot
    M61.572 Other ossification of muscle, left ankle and foot
    M61.579 Other ossification of muscle, unspecified ankle and foot
M61.58 Other ossification of muscle, other site
M61.59 Other ossification of muscle, multiple sites
M61.9 Calcification and ossification of muscle, unspecified

M62 Other disorders of muscle
Excludes1: alcoholic myopathy (G72.1)
cramp and spasm (R25.2)
drug-induced myopathy (G72.0)
myalgia (M79.1)
stiff-man syndrome (G25.8)
M62.0 Separation of muscle (nontraumatic)
Diastasis of muscle
Excludes1: diastasis recti complicating pregnancy, labor and delivery (O71.8)
traumatic separation of muscle- see strain of muscle by body region
M62.00 Separation of muscle (nontraumatic), unspecified site
M62.01 Separation of muscle (nontraumatic), shoulder
    M62.011 Separation of muscle (nontraumatic), right shoulder
    M62.012 Separation of muscle (nontraumatic), left shoulder
    M62.019 Separation of muscle (nontraumatic), unspecified shoulder
M62.02 Separation of muscle (nontraumatic), upper arm
    M62.021 Separation of muscle (nontraumatic), right upper arm
    M62.022 Separation of muscle (nontraumatic), left upper arm
    M62.029 Separation of muscle (nontraumatic), unspecified upper arm
M62.03 Separation of muscle (nontraumatic), forearm
    M62.031 Separation of muscle (nontraumatic), right forearm
    M62.032 Separation of muscle (nontraumatic), left forearm
    M62.039 Separation of muscle (nontraumatic), unspecified forearm
M62.04 Separation of muscle (nontraumatic), hand
    M62.041 Separation of muscle (nontraumatic), right hand
    M62.042 Separation of muscle (nontraumatic), left hand
    M62.049 Separation of muscle (nontraumatic), unspecified hand
M62.05 Separation of muscle (nontraumatic), thigh
    M62.051 Separation of muscle (nontraumatic), right thigh
    M62.052 Separation of muscle (nontraumatic), left thigh
    M62.059 Separation of muscle (nontraumatic), unspecified thigh
M62.06 Separation of muscle (nontraumatic), lower leg
    M62.061 Separation of muscle (nontraumatic), right lower leg
    M62.062 Separation of muscle (nontraumatic), left lower leg
    M62.069 Separation of muscle (nontraumatic), unspecified lower leg
M62.07 Separation of muscle (nontraumatic), ankle and foot

    M62.071 Separation of muscle (nontraumatic), right ankle and foot
    M62.072 Separation of muscle (nontraumatic), left ankle and foot
    M62.079 Separation of muscle (nontraumatic), unspecified ankle and foot
M62.08 Separation of muscle (nontraumatic), other site
M62.1 Other rupture of muscle (nontraumatic)
Excludes1: traumatic rupture of muscle — see strain of muscle by body region
Excludes2: rupture of tendon (M66.-)
M62.10 Other rupture of muscle (nontraumatic), unspecified site
M62.11 Other rupture of muscle (nontraumatic), shoulder
    M62.111 Other rupture of muscle (nontraumatic), right shoulder
    M62.112 Other rupture of muscle (nontraumatic), left shoulder
    M62.119 Other rupture of muscle (nontraumatic), unspecified shoulder
M62.12 Other rupture of muscle (nontraumatic), upper arm
    M62.121 Other rupture of muscle (nontraumatic), right upper arm
    M62.122 Other rupture of muscle (nontraumatic), left upper arm
    M62.129 Other rupture of muscle (nontraumatic), unspecified upper arm
M62.13 Other rupture of muscle (nontraumatic), forearm
    M62.131 Other rupture of muscle (nontraumatic), right forearm
    M62.132 Other rupture of muscle (nontraumatic), left forearm
    M62.139 Other rupture of muscle (nontraumatic), unspecified forearm
M62.14 Other rupture of muscle (nontraumatic), hand
    M62.141 Other rupture of muscle (nontraumatic), right hand
    M62.142 Other rupture of muscle (nontraumatic), left hand
    M62.149 Other rupture of muscle (nontraumatic), unspecified hand
M62.15 Other rupture of muscle (nontraumatic), thigh
    M62.151 Other rupture of muscle (nontraumatic), right thigh
    M62.152 Other rupture of muscle (nontraumatic), left thigh
    M62.159 Other rupture of muscle (nontraumatic), unspecified thigh
M62.16 Other rupture of muscle (nontraumatic), lower leg
    M62.161 Other rupture of muscle (nontraumatic), right lower leg
    M62.162 Other rupture of muscle (nontraumatic), left lower leg
    M62.169 Other rupture of muscle (nontraumatic), unspecified lower leg
M62.17 Other rupture of muscle (nontraumatic), ankle and foot
    M62.171 Other rupture of muscle (nontraumatic), right ankle and foot
    M62.172 Other rupture of muscle (nontraumatic), left ankle and foot
    M62.179 Other rupture of muscle (nontraumatic), unspecified ankle and foot
M62.18 Other rupture of muscle (nontraumatic), other site
M62.2 Nontraumatic ischemic infarction of muscle
Excludes1: compartment syndrome (T79.6)
traumatic ischemia of muscle (T79.6)
Volkmann's ischemic contracture (T79.6)
M62.20 Nontraumatic ischemic infarction of muscle, unspecified site
M62.21 Nontraumatic ischemic infarction of muscle, shoulder

M62.211 Nontraumatic ischemic infarction of muscle, right shoulder

M62.212 Nontraumatic ischemic infarction of muscle, left shoulder

M62.219 Nontraumatic ischemic infarction of muscle, unspecified shoulder

M62.22 Nontraumatic ischemic infarction of muscle, upper arm

M62.221 Nontraumatic ischemic infarction of muscle, right upper arm

M62.222 Nontraumatic ischemic infarction of muscle, left upper arm

M62.229 Nontraumatic ischemic infarction of muscle, unspecified upper arm

M62.23 Nontraumatic ischemic infarction of muscle, forearm

M62.231 Nontraumatic ischemic infarction of muscle, right forearm

M62.232 Nontraumatic ischemic infarction of muscle, left forearm

M62.239 Nontraumatic ischemic infarction of muscle, unspecified forearm

M62.24 Nontraumatic ischemic infarction of muscle, hand

M62.241 Nontraumatic ischemic infarction of muscle, right hand

M62.242 Nontraumatic ischemic infarction of muscle, left hand

M62.249 Nontraumatic ischemic infarction of muscle, unspecified hand

M62.25 Nontraumatic ischemic infarction of muscle, thigh

M62.251 Nontraumatic ischemic infarction of muscle, right thigh

M62.252 Nontraumatic ischemic infarction of muscle, left thigh

M62.259 Nontraumatic ischemic infarction of muscle, unspecified thigh

M62.26 Nontraumatic ischemic infarction of muscle, lower leg

M62.261 Nontraumatic ischemic infarction of muscle, right lower leg

M62.262 Nontraumatic ischemic infarction of muscle, left lower leg

M62.269 Nontraumatic ischemic infarction of muscle, unspecified lower leg

M62.27 Nontraumatic ischemic infarction of muscle, ankle and foot

M62.271 Nontraumatic ischemic infarction of muscle, right ankle and foot

M62.272 Nontraumatic ischemic infarction of muscle, left ankle and foot

M62.279 Nontraumatic ischemic infarction of muscle, unspecified ankle and foot

M62.28 Nontraumatic ischemic infarction of muscle, other site

M62.3 Immobility syndrome (paraplegic)

M62.4 Contracture of muscle

Excludes2:   contracture of joint (M24.5-)

M62.40 Contracture of muscle, unspecified site

M62.41 Contracture of muscle, shoulder

M62.411 Contracture of muscle, right shoulder

M62.412 Contracture of muscle, left shoulder

M62.419 Contracture of muscle, unspecified shoulder

M62.42 Contracture of muscle, upper arm

M62.421 Contracture of muscle, right upper arm

M62.422 Contracture of muscle, left upper arm

M62.429 Contracture of muscle, unspecified upper arm

M62.43 Contracture of muscle, forearm

M62.431 Contracture of muscle, right forearm

M62.432 Contracture of muscle, left forearm

M62.439 Contracture of muscle, unspecified forearm

M62.44 Contracture of muscle, hand

M62.441 Contracture of muscle, right hand

M62.442 Contracture of muscle, left hand

M62.449 Contracture of muscle, unspecified hand

M62.45 Contracture of muscle, thigh

M62.451 Contracture of muscle, right thigh

M62.452 Contracture of muscle, left thigh

M62.459 Contracture of muscle, unspecified thigh

M62.46 Contracture of muscle, lower leg

M62.461 Contracture of muscle, right lower leg

M62.462 Contracture of muscle, left lower leg

M62.469 Contracture of muscle, unspecified lower leg

M62.47 Contracture of muscle, ankle and foot

M62.471 Contracture of muscle, right ankle and foot

M62.472 Contracture of muscle, left ankle and foot

M62.479 Contracture of muscle, unspecified ankle and foot

M62.48 Contracture of muscle, other site

M62.49 Contracture of muscle, multiple sites

M62.5 Muscle wasting and atrophy, not elsewhere classified
Disuse atrophy NEC
Excludes1:   neuralgic amyotrophy (G54.5)
progressive muscular atrophy (G12.29)

M62.50 Muscle wasting and atrophy, not elsewhere classified, unspecified site

M62.51 Muscle wasting and atrophy, not elsewhere classified, shoulder

M62.511 Muscle wasting and atrophy, not elsewhere classified, right shoulder

M62.512 Muscle wasting and atrophy, not elsewhere classified, left shoulder

M62.519 Muscle wasting and atrophy, not elsewhere classified, unspecified shoulder

M62.52 Muscle wasting and atrophy, not elsewhere classified, upper arm

M62.521 Muscle wasting and atrophy, not elsewhere classified, right upper arm

M62.522 Muscle wasting and atrophy, not elsewhere classified, left upper arm

M62.529 Muscle wasting and atrophy, not elsewhere classified, unspecified upper arm

M62.53 Muscle wasting and atrophy, not elsewhere classified, forearm

M62.531 Muscle wasting and atrophy, not elsewhere classified, right forearm

M62.532 Muscle wasting and atrophy, not elsewhere classified, left forearm

M62.539 Muscle wasting and atrophy, not elsewhere classified, unspecified forearm

M62.54 Muscle wasting and atrophy, not elsewhere classified, hand

M62.541 Muscle wasting and atrophy, not elsewhere classified, right hand

M62.542 Muscle wasting and atrophy, not elsewhere classified, left hand

M62.549 Muscle wasting and atrophy, not elsewhere classified, unspecified hand

M62.55 Muscle wasting and atrophy, not elsewhere classified, thigh

M62.551 Muscle wasting and atrophy, not elsewhere classified, right thigh

M62.552 Muscle wasting and atrophy, not elsewhere classified, left thigh

M62.559 Muscle wasting and atrophy, not elsewhere classified, unspecified thigh

M62.56 Muscle wasting and atrophy, not elsewhere classified, lower leg

M62.561 Muscle wasting and atrophy, not elsewhere classified, right lower leg

M62.562 Muscle wasting and atrophy, not elsewhere classified, left lower leg

M62.569 Muscle wasting and atrophy, not elsewhere classified, unspecified lower leg

M62.57   **Muscle wasting and atrophy, not elsewhere classified, ankle and foot**

M62.571   Muscle wasting and atrophy, not elsewhere classified, right ankle and foot

M62.572   Muscle wasting and atrophy, not elsewhere classified, left ankle and foot

M62.579   Muscle wasting and atrophy, not elsewhere classified, unspecified ankle and foot

M62.58   **Muscle wasting and atrophy, not elsewhere classified, other site**

M62.59   **Muscle wasting and atrophy, not elsewhere classified, multiple sites**

M62.8   Other specified disorders of muscle

M62.81   **Muscle weakness (generalized)**

M62.89   **Other specified disorders of muscle**
    Muscle (sheath) hernia

M62.9   Disorder of muscle, unspecified

M63 Disorders of muscle in diseases classified elsewhere

Excludes1:   myopathy in:
    cysticercosis (B69.81)
    endocrine diseases (G73.7)
    metabolic diseases (G73.7)
    sarcoidosis (D86.87)
    syphilis (late) (A52.78)
      secondary (A51.49)
    toxoplasmosis (B58.82)
    tuberculosis (A18.09)

Code first underlying disease, such as:
    leprosy (A30.-)
    neoplasm (C49.-, C79.89, D21.-, D48.1)
    schistosomiasis (B65.-)
    trichinellosis (B75)

M63.8   Disorders of muscle in diseases classified elsewhere

M63.80   **Disorders of muscle in diseases classified elsewhere, unspecified site**

M63.81   **Disorders of muscle in diseases classified elsewhere, shoulder**

M63.811   Disorders of muscle in diseases classified elsewhere, right shoulder

M63.812   Disorders of muscle in diseases classified elsewhere, left shoulder

M63.819   Disorders of muscle in diseases classified elsewhere, unspecified shoulder

M63.82   **Disorders of muscle in diseases classified elsewhere, upper arm**

M63.821   Disorders of muscle in diseases classified elsewhere, right upper arm

M63.822   Disorders of muscle in diseases classified elsewhere, left upper arm

M63.829   Disorders of muscle in diseases classified elsewhere, unspecified upper arm

M63.83   **Disorders of muscle in diseases classified elsewhere, forearm**

M63.831   Disorders of muscle in diseases classified elsewhere, right forearm

M63.832   Disorders of muscle in diseases classified elsewhere, left forearm

M63.839   Disorders of muscle in diseases classified elsewhere, unspecified forearm

M63.84   **Disorders of muscle in diseases classified elsewhere, hand**

M63.841   Disorders of muscle in diseases classified elsewhere, right hand

M63.842   Disorders of muscle in diseases classified elsewhere, left hand

M63.849   Disorders of muscle in diseases classified elsewhere, unspecified hand

M63.85   **Disorders of muscle in diseases classified elsewhere, thigh**

M03.851   Disorders of muscle in diseases classified elsewhere, right thigh

M63.852   Disorders of muscle in diseases classified elsewhere, left thigh

M63.859   Disorders of muscle in diseases classified elsewhere, unspecified thigh

M63.86   **Disorders of muscle in diseases classified elsewhere, lower leg**

M63.861   Disorders of muscle in diseases classified elsewhere, right lower leg

M63.862   Disorders of muscle in diseases classified elsewhere, left lower leg

M63.869   Disorders of muscle in diseases classified elsewhere, unspecified lower leg

M63.87   **Disorders of muscle in diseases classified elsewhere, ankle and foot**

M63.871   Disorders of muscle in diseases classified elsewhere, right ankle and foot

M63.872   Disorders of muscle in diseases classified elsewhere, left ankle and foot

M63.879   Disorders of muscle in diseases classified elsewhere, unspecified ankle and foot

M63.88   **Disorders of muscle in diseases classified elsewhere, other site**

M63.89   **Disorders of muscle in diseases classified elsewhere, multiple sites**

DISORDERS OF SYNOVIUM AND TENDON (M65–M67)

M65 Synovitis and tenosynovitis

Excludes1:   chronic crepitant synovitis of hand and wrist (M70.0-)
    current injury—see injury of ligament or tendon by body region
    soft tissue disorders related to use, overuse and pressure (M70.-)

M65.0   Abscess of tendon sheath
    Use additional code (B95-B96) to identify bacterial agent.

M65.00   **Abscess of tendon sheath, unspecified site**

M65.01   **Abscess of tendon sheath, shoulder**

M65.011   Abscess of tendon sheath, right shoulder

M65.012   Abscess of tendon sheath, left shoulder

M65.019   Abscess of tendon sheath, unspecified shoulder

M65.02   **Abscess of tendon sheath, upper arm**

M65.021   Abscess of tendon sheath, right upper arm

M65.022   Abscess of tendon sheath, left upper arm

M65.029   Abscess of tendon sheath, unspecified upper arm

M65.03   **Abscess of tendon sheath, forearm**

M65.031   Abscess of tendon sheath, right forearm

M65.032   Abscess of tendon sheath, left forearm

M65.039   Abscess of tendon sheath, unspecified forearm

M65.04   **Abscess of tendon sheath, hand**

M65.041   Abscess of tendon sheath, right hand

M65.042   Abscess of tendon sheath, left hand

M65.049   Abscess of tendon sheath, unspecified hand

M65.05   **Abscess of tendon sheath, thigh**

M65.051   Abscess of tendon sheath, right thigh

M65.052   Abscess of tendon sheath, left thigh

M65.059   Abscess of tendon sheath, unspecified thigh

M65.06   **Abscess of tendon sheath, lower leg**

M65.061   Abscess of tendon sheath, right lower leg

M65.062   Abscess of tendon sheath, left lower leg

M65.069   Abscess of tendon sheath, unspecified lower leg

M65.07   **Abscess of tendon sheath, ankle and foot**

M65.071   Abscess of tendon sheath, right ankle and foot

M65.072   Abscess of tendon sheath, left ankle and foot

M65.079   Abscess of tendon sheath, unspecified ankle and foot

M65.08   **Abscess of tendon sheath, other site**

M65.1   Other infective (teno)synovitis

M65.10   **Other infective (teno)synovitis, unspecified site**

M65.11   Other infective (teno)synovitis, shoulder
 M65.111 Other infective (teno)synovitis, right shoulder
 M65.112 Other infective (teno)synovitis, left shoulder
 M65.119 Other infective (teno)synovitis, unspecified shoulder
M65.12   Other infective (teno)synovitis, elbow
 M65.121 Other infective (teno)synovitis, right elbow
 M65.122 Other infective (teno)synovitis, left elbow
 M65.129 Other infective (teno)synovitis, unspecified elbow
M65.13   Other infective (teno)synovitis, wrist
 M65.131 Other infective (teno)synovitis, right wrist
 M65.132 Other infective (teno)synovitis, left wrist
 M65.139 Other infective (teno)synovitis, unspecified wrist
M65.14   Other infective (teno)synovitis, hand
 M65.141 Other infective (teno)synovitis, right hand
 M65.142 Other infective (teno)synovitis, left hand
 M65.149 Other infective (teno)synovitis, unspecified hand
M65.15   Other infective (teno)synovitis, hip
 M65.151 Other infective (teno)synovitis, right hip
 M65.152 Other infective (teno)synovitis, left hip
 M65.159 Other infective (teno)synovitis, unspecified hip
M65.16   Other infective (teno)synovitis, knee
 M65.161 Other infective (teno)synovitis, right knee
 M65.162 Other infective (teno)synovitis, left knee
 M65.169 Other infective (teno)synovitis, unspecified knee
M65.17   Other infective (teno)synovitis, ankle and foot
 M65.171 Other infective (teno)synovitis, right ankle and foot
 M65.172 Other infective (teno)synovitis, left ankle and foot
 M65.179 Other infective (teno)synovitis, unspecified ankle and foot
M65.18   Other infective (teno)synovitis, other site
M65.19   Other infective (teno)synovitis, multiple sites

M65.2 Calcific tendinitis
   Excludes1:   tendinitis as classified in M75-M77
          calcified tendinitis of shoulder (M75.3)
M65.20   Calcific tendinitis, unspecified site
M65.22   Calcific tendinitis, upper arm
 M65.221 Calcific tendinitis, right upper arm
 M65.222 Calcific tendinitis, left upper arm
 M65.229 Calcific tendinitis, unspecified upper arm
M65.23   Calcific tendinitis, forearm
 M65.231 Calcific tendinitis, right forearm
 M65.232 Calcific tendinitis, left forearm
 M65.239 Calcific tendinitis, unspecified forearm
M65.24   Calcific tendinitis, hand
 M65.241 Calcific tendinitis, right hand
 M65.242 Calcific tendinitis, left hand
 M65.249 Calcific tendinitis, unspecified hand
M65.25   Calcific tendinitis, thigh
 M65.251 Calcific tendinitis, right thigh
 M65.252 Calcific tendinitis, left thigh
 M65.259 Calcific tendinitis, unspecified thigh
M65.26   Calcific tendinitis, lower leg
 M65.261 Calcific tendinitis, right lower leg
 M65.262 Calcific tendinitis, left lower leg
 M65.269 Calcific tendinitis, unspecified lower leg
M65.27   Calcific tendinitis, ankle and foot
 M65.271 Calcific tendinitis, right ankle and foot
 M65.272 Calcific tendinitis, left ankle and foot
 M65.279 Calcific tendinitis, unspecified ankle and foot
M65.28   Calcific tendinitis, other site
M65.29   Calcific tendinitis, multiple sites

M65.3 Trigger finger
   Nodular tendinous disease
M65.30   Trigger finger, unspecified finger
M65.31   Trigger thumb
 M65.311 Trigger thumb, right thumb
 M65.312 Trigger thumb, left thumb
 M65.319 Trigger thumb, unspecified thumb
M65.32   Trigger finger, index finger
 M65.321 Trigger finger, right index finger
 M65.322 Trigger finger, left index finger
 M65.329 Trigger finger, unspecified index finger
M65.33   Trigger finger, middle finger
 M65.331 Trigger finger, right middle finger
 M65.332 Trigger finger, left middle finger
 M65.339 Trigger finger, unspecified middle finger
M65.34   Trigger finger, ring finger
 M65.341 Trigger finger, right ring finger
 M65.342 Trigger finger, left ring finger
 M65.349 Trigger finger, unspecified ring finger
M65.35   Trigger finger, little finger
 M65.351 Trigger finger, right little finger
 M65.352 Trigger finger, left little finger
 M65.359 Trigger finger, unspecified little finger

M65.4 Radial styloid tenosynovitis [de Quervain]
M65.8 Other synovitis and tenosynovitis
M65.80   Other synovitis and tenosynovitis, unspecified site
M65.81   Other synovitis and tenosynovitis, shoulder
 M65.811 Other synovitis and tenosynovitis, right shoulder
 M65.812 Other synovitis and tenosynovitis, left shoulder
 M65.819 Other synovitis and tenosynovitis, unspecified shoulder
M65.82   Other synovitis and tenosynovitis, upper arm
 M65.821 Other synovitis and tenosynovitis, right upper arm
 M65.822 Other synovitis and tenosynovitis, left upper arm
 M65.829 Other synovitis and tenosynovitis, unspecified upper arm
M65.83   Other synovitis and tenosynovitis, forearm
 M65.831 Other synovitis and tenosynovitis, right forearm
 M65.832 Other synovitis and tenosynovitis, left forearm
 M65.839 Other synovitis and tenosynovitis, unspecified forearm
M65.84   Other synovitis and tenosynovitis, hand
 M65.841 Other synovitis and tenosynovitis, right hand
 M65.842 Other synovitis and tenosynovitis, left hand
 M65.849 Other synovitis and tenosynovitis, unspecified hand
M65.85   Other synovitis and tenosynovitis, thigh
 M65.851 Other synovitis and tenosynovitis, right thigh
 M65.852 Other synovitis and tenosynovitis, left thigh
 M65.859 Other synovitis and tenosynovitis, unspecified thigh
M65.86   Other synovitis and tenosynovitis, lower leg
 M65.861 Other synovitis and tenosynovitis, right lower leg
 M65.862 Other synovitis and tenosynovitis, left lower leg
 M65.869 Other synovitis and tenosynovitis, unspecified lower leg
M65.87   Other synovitis and tenosynovitis, ankle and foot
 M65.871 Other synovitis and tenosynovitis, right ankle and foot
 M65.872 Other synovitis and tenosynovitis, left ankle and foot

M65.879   Other synovitis and tenosynovitis, unspecified ankle and foot

M65.88   Other synovitis and tenosynovitis, other site

M65.89   Other synovitis and tenosynovitis, multiple sites

M65.9   Synovitis and tenosynovitis, unspecified

M66   Spontaneous rupture of synovium and tendon

Excludes2:   rotator cuff syndrome (M75.1)

M66.0   Rupture of popliteal cyst

M66.1   Rupture of synovium

Rupture of synovial cyst

Excludes2:   rupture of popliteal cyst (M66.0)

M66.10   Rupture of synovium, unspecified joint

M66.11   Rupture of synovium, shoulder

M66.111   Rupture of synovium, right shoulder

M66.112   Rupture of synovium, left shoulder

M66.119   Rupture of synovium, unspecified shoulder

M66.12   Rupture of synovium, elbow

M66.121   Rupture of synovium, right elbow

M66.122   Rupture of synovium, left elbow

M66.129   Rupture of synovium, unspecified elbow

M66.13   Rupture of synovium, wrist

M66.131   Rupture of synovium, right wrist

M66.132   Rupture of synovium, left wrist

M66.139   Rupture of synovium, unspecified wrist

M66.14   Rupture of synovium, hand and fingers

M66.141   Rupture of synovium, right hand

M66.142   Rupture of synovium, left hand

M66.143   Rupture of synovium, unspecified hand

M66.144   Rupture of synovium, right finger(s)

M66.145   Rupture of synovium, left finger(s)

M66.146   Rupture of synovium, unspecified finger(s)

M66.15   Rupture of synovium, hip

M66.151   Rupture of synovium, right hip

M66.152   Rupture of synovium, left hip

M66.159   Rupture of synovium, unspecified hip

M66.17   Rupture of synovium, ankle, foot and toes

M66.171   Rupture of synovium, right ankle

M66.172   Rupture of synovium, left ankle

M66.173   Rupture of synovium, unspecified ankle

M66.174   Rupture of synovium, right foot

M66.175   Rupture of synovium, left foot

M66.176   Rupture of synovium, unspecified foot

M66.177   Rupture of synovium, right toe(s)

M66.178   Rupture of synovium, left toe(s)

M66.179   Rupture of synovium, unspecified toe(s)

M66.18   Rupture of synovium, other site

M66.2   Spontaneous rupture of extensor tendons

M66.20   Spontaneous rupture of extensor tendons, unspecified site

M66.21   Spontaneous rupture of extensor tendons, shoulder

M66.211   Spontaneous rupture of extensor tendons, right shoulder

M66.212   Spontaneous rupture of extensor tendons, left shoulder

M66.219   Spontaneous rupture of extensor tendons, unspecified shoulder

M66.22   Spontaneous rupture of extensor tendons, upper arm

M66.221   Spontaneous rupture of extensor tendons, right upper arm

M66.222   Spontaneous rupture of extensor tendons, left upper arm

M66.229   Spontaneous rupture of extensor tendons, unspecified upper arm

M66.23   Spontaneous rupture of extensor tendons, forearm

M66.231   Spontaneous rupture of extensor tendons, right forearm

M66.232   Spontaneous rupture of extensor tendons, left forearm

M66.239   Spontaneous rupture of extensor tendons, unspecified forearm

M66.24   Spontaneous rupture of extensor tendons, hand

M66.241   Spontaneous rupture of extensor tendons, right hand

M66.242   Spontaneous rupture of extensor tendons, left hand

M66.249   Spontaneous rupture of extensor tendons, unspecified hand

M66.25   Spontaneous rupture of extensor tendons, thigh

M66.251   Spontaneous rupture of extensor tendons, right thigh

M66.252   Spontaneous rupture of extensor tendons, left thigh

M66.259   Spontaneous rupture of extensor tendons, unspecified thigh

M66.26   Spontaneous rupture of extensor tendons, lower leg

M66.261   Spontaneous rupture of extensor tendons, right lower leg

M66.262   Spontaneous rupture of extensor tendons, left lower leg

M66.269   Spontaneous rupture of extensor tendons, unspecified lower leg

M66.27   Spontaneous rupture of extensor tendons, ankle and foot

M66.271   Spontaneous rupture of extensor tendons, right ankle and foot

M66.272   Spontaneous rupture of extensor tendons, left ankle and foot

M66.279   Spontaneous rupture of extensor tendons, unspecified ankle and foot

M66.28   Spontaneous rupture of extensor tendons, other site

M66.29   Spontaneous rupture of extensor tendons, multiple sites

M66.3   Spontaneous rupture of flexor tendons

M66.30   Spontaneous rupture of flexor tendons, unspecified site

M66.31   Spontaneous rupture of flexor tendons, shoulder

M66.311   Spontaneous rupture of flexor tendons, right shoulder

M66.312   Spontaneous rupture of flexor tendons, left shoulder

M66.319   Spontaneous rupture of flexor tendons, unspecified shoulder

M66.32   Spontaneous rupture of flexor tendons, upper arm

M66.321   Spontaneous rupture of flexor tendons, right upper arm

M66.322   Spontaneous rupture of flexor tendons, left upper arm

M66.329   Spontaneous rupture of flexor tendons, unspecified upper arm

M66.33   Spontaneous rupture of flexor tendons, forearm

M66.331   Spontaneous rupture of flexor tendons, right forearm

M66.332   Spontaneous rupture of flexor tendons, left forearm

M66.339   Spontaneous rupture of flexor tendons, unspecified forearm

M66.34   Spontaneous rupture of flexor tendons, hand

M66.341   Spontaneous rupture of flexor tendons, right hand

M66.342   Spontaneous rupture of flexor tendons, left hand

M66.349   Spontaneous rupture of flexor tendons, unspecified hand

M66.35   Spontaneous rupture of flexor tendons, thigh

M66.351   Spontaneous rupture of flexor tendons, right thigh

M66.352   Spontaneous rupture of flexor tendons, left thigh

M66.359   Spontaneous rupture of flexor tendons, unspecified thigh

M66.36   Spontaneous rupture of flexor tendons, lower leg
    M66.361   Spontaneous rupture of flexor tendons, right lower leg
    M66.362   Spontaneous rupture of flexor tendons, left lower leg
    M66.369   Spontaneous rupture of flexor tendons, unspecified lower leg
M66.37   Spontaneous rupture of flexor tendons, ankle and foot
    M66.371   Spontaneous rupture of flexor tendons, right ankle and foot
    M66.372   Spontaneous rupture of flexor tendons, left ankle and foot
    M66.379   Spontaneous rupture of flexor tendons, unspecified ankle and foot
M66.38   Spontaneous rupture of flexor tendons, other site
M66.39   Spontaneous rupture of flexor tendons, multiple sites

M66.8   Spontaneous rupture of other tendons
M66.80   Spontaneous rupture of other tendons, unspecified site
M66.81   Spontaneous rupture of other tendons, shoulder
    M66.811   Spontaneous rupture of other tendons, right shoulder
    M66.812   Spontaneous rupture of other tendons, left shoulder
    M66.819   Spontaneous rupture of other tendons, unspecified shoulder
M66.82   Spontaneous rupture of other tendons, upper arm
    M66.821   Spontaneous rupture of other tendons, right upper arm
    M66.822   Spontaneous rupture of other tendons, left upper arm
    M66.829   Spontaneous rupture of other tendons, unspecified upper arm
M66.83   Spontaneous rupture of other tendons, forearm
    M66.831   Spontaneous rupture of other tendons, right forearm
    M66.832   Spontaneous rupture of other tendons, left forearm
    M66.839   Spontaneous rupture of other tendons, unspecified forearm
M66.84   Spontaneous rupture of other tendons, hand
    M66.841   Spontaneous rupture of other tendons, right hand
    M66.842   Spontaneous rupture of other tendons, left hand
    M66.849   Spontaneous rupture of other tendons, unspecified hand
M66.85   Spontaneous rupture of other tendons, thigh
    M66.851   Spontaneous rupture of other tendons, right thigh
    M66.852   Spontaneous rupture of other tendons, left thigh
    M66.859   Spontaneous rupture of other tendons, unspecified thigh
M66.86   Spontaneous rupture of other tendons, lower leg
    M66.861   Spontaneous rupture of other tendons, right lower leg
    M66.862   Spontaneous rupture of other tendons, left lower leg
    M66.869   Spontaneous rupture of other tendons, unspecified lower leg
M66.87   Spontaneous rupture of other tendons, ankle and foot
    M66.871   Spontaneous rupture of other tendons, right ankle and foot
    M66.872   Spontaneous rupture of other tendons, left ankle and foot
    M66.879   Spontaneous rupture of other tendons, unspecified ankle and foot
M66.88   Spontaneous rupture of other tendons, other
M66.89   Spontaneous rupture of other tendons, multiple sites

M66.9   Spontaneous rupture of unspecified tendon
    Rupture at musculotendinous junction, nontraumatic

M67   Other disorders of synovium and tendon
    Excludes1:   palmar fascial fibromatosis [Dupuytren] (M72.0)
                tendinitis NOS (M77.9-)
                xanthomatosis localized to tendons (E78.2)

M67.0   Short Achilles tendon (acquired)
M67.00   Short Achilles tendon (acquired), unspecified ankle
M67.01   Short Achilles tendon (acquired), right ankle
M67.02   Short Achilles tendon (acquired), left ankle

M67.1   Other contracture of tendon (sheath)
    Excludes1:   contracture of tendon with contracture of joint (M24.5-)
M67.10   Other contracture of tendon (sheath), unspecified site
M67.11   Other contracture of tendon (sheath), shoulder
    M67.111   Other contracture of tendon (sheath), right shoulder
    M67.112   Other contracture of tendon (sheath), left shoulder
    M67.119   Other contracture of tendon (sheath), unspecified shoulder
M67.12   Other contracture of tendon (sheath), upper arm
    M67.121   Other contracture of tendon (sheath), right upper arm
    M67.122   Other contracture of tendon (sheath), left upper arm
    M67.129   Other contracture of tendon (sheath), unspecified upper arm
M67.13   Other contracture of tendon (sheath), forearm
    M67.131   Other contracture of tendon (sheath), right forearm
    M67.132   Other contracture of tendon (sheath), left forearm
    M67.139   Other contracture of tendon (sheath), unspecified forearm
M67.14   Other contracture of tendon (sheath), hand
    M67.141   Other contracture of tendon (sheath), right hand
    M67.142   Other contracture of tendon (sheath), left hand
    M67.149   Other contracture of tendon (sheath), unspecified hand
M67.15   Other contracture of tendon (sheath), thigh
    M67.151   Other contracture of tendon (sheath), right thigh
    M67.152   Other contracture of tendon (sheath), left thigh
    M67.159   Other contracture of tendon (sheath), unspecified thigh
M67.16   Other contracture of tendon (sheath), lower leg
    M67.161   Other contracture of tendon (sheath), right lower leg
    M67.162   Other contracture of tendon (sheath), left lower leg
    M67.169   Other contracture of tendon (sheath), unspecified lower leg
M67.17   Other contracture of tendon (sheath), ankle and foot
    Excludes1:   contracture of Achilles tendon (acquired) (M67.0-)
    M67.171   Other contracture of tendon (sheath), right ankle and foot
    M67.172   Other contracture of tendon (sheath), left ankle and foot
    M67.179   Other contracture of tendon (sheath), unspecified ankle and foot
M67.18   Other contracture of tendon (sheath), other site
M67.19   Other contracture of tendon (sheath), multiple sites

M67.2   Synovial hypertrophy, not elsewhere classified
    Excludes1:   villonodular synovitis (pigmented) (M12.2-)
M67.20   Synovial hypertrophy, not elsewhere classified, unspecified site

M67.21 Synovial hypertrophy, not elsewhere classified, shoulder
  M67.211 Synovial hypertrophy, not elsewhere classified, right shoulder
  M67.212 Synovial hypertrophy, not elsewhere classified, left shoulder
  M67.219 Synovial hypertrophy, not elsewhere classified, unspecified shoulder
M67.22 Synovial hypertrophy, not elsewhere classified, upper arm
  M67.221 Synovial hypertrophy, not elsewhere classified, right upper arm
  M67.222 Synovial hypertrophy, not elsewhere classified, left upper arm
  M67.229 Synovial hypertrophy, not elsewhere classified, unspecified upper arm
M67.23 Synovial hypertrophy, not elsewhere classified, forearm
  M67.231 Synovial hypertrophy, not elsewhere classified, right forearm
  M67.232 Synovial hypertrophy, not elsewhere classified, left forearm
  M67.239 Synovial hypertrophy, not elsewhere classified, unspecified forearm
M67.24 Synovial hypertrophy, not elsewhere classified, hand
  M67.241 Synovial hypertrophy, not elsewhere classified, right hand
  M67.242 Synovial hypertrophy, not elsewhere classified, left hand
  M67.249 Synovial hypertrophy, not elsewhere classified, unspecified hand
M67.25 Synovial hypertrophy, not elsewhere classified, thigh
  M67.251 Synovial hypertrophy, not elsewhere classified, right thigh
  M67.252 Synovial hypertrophy, not elsewhere classified, left thigh
  M67.259 Synovial hypertrophy, not elsewhere classified, unspecified thigh
M67.26 Synovial hypertrophy, not elsewhere classified, lower leg
  M67.261 Synovial hypertrophy, not elsewhere classified, right lower leg
  M67.262 Synovial hypertrophy, not elsewhere classified, left lower leg
  M67.269 Synovial hypertrophy, not elsewhere classified, unspecified lower leg
M67.27 Synovial hypertrophy, not elsewhere classified, ankle and foot
  M67.271 Synovial hypertrophy, not elsewhere classified, right ankle and foot
  M67.272 Synovial hypertrophy, not elsewhere classified, left ankle and foot
  M67.279 Synovial hypertrophy, not elsewhere classified, unspecified ankle and foot
M67.28 Synovial hypertrophy, not elsewhere classified, other site
M67.29 Synovial hypertrophy, not elsewhere classified, multiple sites

M67.3 Transient synovitis
 Toxic synovitis
 Excludes1: palindromic rheumatism (M12.3-)
M67.30 Transient synovitis, unspecified site
M67.31 Transient synovitis, shoulder
  M67.311 Transient synovitis, right shoulder
  M67.312 Transient synovitis, left shoulder
  M67.319 Transient synovitis, unspecified shoulder
M67.32 Transient synovitis, elbow
  M67.321 Transient synovitis, right elbow
  M67.322 Transient synovitis, left elbow
  M67.329 Transient synovitis, unspecified elbow
M67.33 Transient synovitis, wrist

M67.331 Transient synovitis, right wrist
M67.332 Transient synovitis, left wrist
M67.339 Transient synovitis, unspecified wrist
M67.34 Transient synovitis, hand
  M67.341 Transient synovitis, right hand
  M67.342 Transient synovitis, left hand
  M67.349 Transient synovitis, unspecified hand
M67.35 Transient synovitis, hip
  M67.351 Transient synovitis, right hip
  M67.352 Transient synovitis, left hip
  M67.359 Transient synovitis, unspecified hip
M67.36 Transient synovitis, knee
  M67.361 Transient synovitis, right knee
  M67.362 Transient synovitis, left knee
  M67.369 Transient synovitis, unspecified knee
M67.37 Transient synovitis, ankle and foot
  M67.371 Transient synovitis, right ankle and foot
  M67.372 Transient synovitis, left ankle and foot
  M67.379 Transient synovitis, unspecified ankle and foot
M67.38 Transient synovitis, other site
M67.39 Transient synovitis, multiple sites

M67.4 Ganglion
 Ganglion of joint or tendon (sheath)
 Excludes1: ganglion in yaws (A66.6)
 Excludes2: cyst of bursa (M71.2-M71.3)
     cyst of synovium (M71.2-M71.3)
M67.40 Ganglion, unspecified site
M67.41 Ganglion, shoulder
  M67.411 Ganglion, right shoulder
  M67.412 Ganglion, left shoulder
  M67.419 Ganglion, unspecified shoulder
M67.42 Ganglion, elbow
  M67.421 Ganglion, right elbow
  M67.422 Ganglion, left elbow
  M67.429 Ganglion, unspecified elbow
M67.43 Ganglion, wrist
  M67.431 Ganglion, right wrist
  M67.432 Ganglion, left wrist
  M67.439 Ganglion, unspecified wrist
M67.44 Ganglion, hand
  M67.441 Ganglion, right hand
  M67.442 Ganglion, left hand
  M67.449 Ganglion, unspecified hand
M67.45 Ganglion, hip
  M67.451 Ganglion, right hip
  M67.452 Ganglion, left hip
  M67.459 Ganglion, unspecified hip
M67.46 Ganglion, knee
  M67.461 Ganglion, right knee
  M67.462 Ganglion, left knee
  M67.469 Ganglion, unspecified knee
M67.47 Ganglion, ankle and foot
  M67.471 Ganglion, right ankle and foot
  M67.472 Ganglion, left ankle and foot
  M67.479 Ganglion, unspecified ankle and foot
M67.48 Ganglion, other site
M67.49 Ganglion, multiple sites

M67.5 Plica syndrome
 Plica knee
M67.50 Plica syndrome, unspecified knee
M67.51 Plica syndrome, right knee
M67.52 Plica syndrome, left knee

M67.8 Other specified disorders of synovium and tendon
M67.80 Other specified disorders of synovium and tendon, unspecified site
M67.81 Other specified disorders of synovium and tendon, shoulder

M67.811　Other specified disorders of synovium, right shoulder

M67.812　Other specified disorders of synovium, left shoulder

M67.813　Other specified disorders of tendon, right shoulder

M67.814　Other specified disorders of tendon, left shoulder

M67.819　Other specified disorders of synovium and tendon, unspecified shoulder

M67.82　Other specified disorders of synovium and tendon, elbow

M67.821　Other specified disorders of synovium, right elbow

M67.822　Other specified disorders of synovium, left elbow

M67.823　Other specified disorders of tendon, right elbow

M67.824　Other specified disorders of tendon, left elbow

M67.829　Other specified disorders of synovium and tendon, unspecified elbow

M67.83　Other specified disorders of synovium and tendon, wrist

M67.831　Other specified disorders of synovium, right wrist

M67.832　Other specified disorders of synovium, left wrist

M67.833　Other specified disorders of tendon, right wrist

M67.834　Other specified disorders of tendon, left wrist

M67.839　Other specified disorders of synovium and tendon, unspecified forearm

M67.84　Other specified disorders of synovium and tendon, hand

M67.841　Other specified disorders of synovium, right hand

M67.842　Other specified disorders of synovium, left hand

M67.843　Other specified disorders of tendon, right hand

M67.844　Other specified disorders of tendon, left hand

M67.849　Other specified disorders of synovium and tendon, unspecified hand

M67.85　Other specified disorders of synovium and tendon, hip

M67.851　Other specified disorders of synovium, right hip

M67.852　Other specified disorders of synovium, left hip

M67.853　Other specified disorders of tendon, right hip

M67.854　Other specified disorders of tendon, left hip

M67.859　Other specified disorders of synovium and tendon, unspecified hip

M67.86　Other specified disorders of synovium and tendon, knee

M67.861　Other specified disorders of synovium, right knee

M67.862　Other specified disorders of synovium, left knee

M67.863　Other specified disorders of tendon, right knee

M67.864　Other specified disorders of tendon, left knee

M67.869　Other specified disorders of synovium and tendon, unspecified knee

M67.87　Other specified disorders of synovium and tendon, ankle and foot

M67.871　Other specified disorders of synovium, right ankle and foot

M67.872　Other specified disorders of synovium, left ankle and foot

M67.873　Other specified disorders of tendon, right ankle and foot

M67.874　Other specified disorders of tendon, left ankle and foot

M67.879　Other specified disorders of synovium and tendon, unspecified ankle and foot

M67.88　Other specified disorders of synovium and tendon, other site

M67.89　Other specified disorders of synovium and tendon, multiple sites

M67.9　Unspecified disorder of synovium and tendon

M67.90　Unspecified disorder of synovium and tendon, unspecified site

M67.91　Unspecified disorder of synovium and tendon, shoulder

M67.911　Unspecified disorder of synovium and tendon, right shoulder

M67.912　Unspecified disorder of synovium and tendon, left shoulder

M67.919　Unspecified disorder of synovium and tendon, unspecified shoulder

M67.92　Unspecified disorder of synovium and tendon, upper arm

M67.921　Unspecified disorder of synovium and tendon, right upper arm

M67.922　Unspecified disorder of synovium and tendon, left upper arm

M67.929　Unspecified disorder of synovium and tendon, unspecified upper arm

M67.93　Unspecified disorder of synovium and tendon, forearm

M67.931　Unspecified disorder of synovium and tendon, right forearm

M67.932　Unspecified disorder of synovium and tendon, left forearm

M67.939　Unspecified disorder of synovium and tendon, unspecified forearm

M67.94　Unspecified disorder of synovium and tendon, hand

M67.941　Unspecified disorder of synovium and tendon, right hand

M67.942　Unspecified disorder of synovium and tendon, left hand

M67.949　Unspecified disorder of synovium and tendon, unspecified hand

M67.95　Unspecified disorder of synovium and tendon, thigh

M67.951　Unspecified disorder of synovium and tendon, right thigh

M67.952　Unspecified disorder of synovium and tendon, left thigh

M67.959　Unspecified disorder of synovium and tendon, unspecified thigh

M67.96　Unspecified disorder of synovium and tendon, lower leg

M67.961　Unspecified disorder of synovium and tendon, right lower leg

M67.962　Unspecified disorder of synovium and tendon, left lower leg

M67.969　Unspecified disorder of synovium and tendon, unspecified lower leg

M67.97　Unspecified disorder of synovium and tendon, ankle and foot

M67.971　Unspecified disorder of synovium and tendon, right ankle and foot

M67.972　Unspecified disorder of synovium and tendon, left ankle and foot

M67.979　Unspecified disorder of synovium and tendon, unspecified ankle and foot

M67.98　Unspecified disorder of synovium and tendon, other site

M67.99　Unspecified disorder of synovium and tendon, multiple sites

OTHER SOFT TISSUE DISORDERS (M70–M79)

M70 Soft tissue disorders related to use, overuse and pressure

Includes: soft tissue disorders of occupational origin

Excludes1:   bursitis NOS (M71.9-)

Excludes2:   bursitis of shoulder (M75.5)
              enthesopathies (M76-M77)

Use additional external cause code to identify activity causing
disorder (X50, Y93, Y96)

M70.0 Crepitant synovitis (acute) (chronic) of hand and wrist

   M70.03   Crepitant synovitis (acute) (chronic), wrist

      M70.031   Crepitant synovitis (acute) (chronic), right
                wrist

      M70.032   Crepitant synovitis (acute) (chronic), left wrist

      M70.039   Crepitant synovitis (acute) (chronic),
                unspecified wrist

   M70.04   Crepitant synovitis (acute) (chronic), hand

      M70.041   Crepitant synovitis (acute) (chronic), right
                hand

      M70.042   Crepitant synovitis (acute) (chronic), left hand

      M70.049   Crepitant synovitis (acute) (chronic),
                unspecified hand

M70.1 Bursitis of hand

   M70.10   Bursitis, unspecified hand

   M70.11   Bursitis, right hand

   M70.12   Bursitis, left hand

M70.2 Olecranon bursitis

   M70.20   Olecranon bursitis, unspecified elbow

   M70.21   Olecranon bursitis, right elbow

   M70.22   Olecranon bursitis, left elbow

M70.3 Other bursitis of elbow

   M70.30   Other bursitis of elbow, unspecified elbow

   M70.31   Other bursitis of elbow, right elbow

   M70.32   Other bursitis of elbow, left elbow

M70.4 Prepatellar bursitis

   M70.40   Prepatellar bursitis, unspecified knee

   M70.41   Prepatellar bursitis, right knee

   M70.42   Prepatellar bursitis, left knee

M70.5 Other bursitis of knee

   M70.50   Other bursitis of knee, unspecified knee

   M70.51   Other bursitis of knee, right knee

   M70.52   Other bursitis of knee, left knee

M70.6 Trochanteric bursitis
      Trochanteric tendinitis

   M70.60   Trochanteric bursitis, unspecified hip

   M70.61   Trochanteric bursitis, right hip

   M70.62   Trochanteric bursitis, left hip

M70.7 Other bursitis of hip
      Ischial bursitis

   M70.70   Other bursitis of hip, unspecified hip

   M70.71   Other bursitis of hip, right hip

   M70.72   Other bursitis of hip, left hip

**M70.8 Other soft tissue disorders related to use, overuse and
      pressure**

   **M70.80   Other soft tissue disorders related to use, overuse and
               pressure of unspecified site**

   **M70.81   Other soft tissue disorders related to use, overuse and
               pressure of shoulder**

      M70.811   Other soft tissue disorders related to use,
                overuse and pressure, right shoulder

      M70.812   Other soft tissue disorders related to use,
                overuse and pressure, left shoulder

      M70.819   Other soft tissue disorders related to use,
                overuse and pressure, unspecified shoulder

   **M70.82   Other soft tissue disorders related to use, overuse and
               pressure of upper arm**

      M70.821   Other soft tissue disorders related to use,
                overuse and pressure, right upper arm

      M70.822   Other soft tissue disorders related to use,
                overuse and pressure, left upper arm

      M70.829   Other soft tissue disorders related to use,
                overuse and pressure, unspecified upper arms

   **M70.83   Other soft tissue disorders related to use, overuse and
               pressure of forearm**

      M70.831   Other soft tissue disorders related to use,
                overuse and pressure, right forearm

      M70.832   Other soft tissue disorders related to use,
                overuse and pressure, left forearm

      M70.839   Other soft tissue disorders related to use,
                overuse and pressure, unspecified forearm

   **M70.84   Other soft tissue disorders related to use, overuse and
               pressure of hand**

      M70.841   Other soft tissue disorders related to use,
                overuse and pressure, right hand

      M70.842   Other soft tissue disorders related to use,
                overuse and pressure, left hand

      M70.849   Other soft tissue disorders related to use,
                overuse and pressure, unspecified hand

   **M70.85   Other soft tissue disorders related to use, overuse and
               pressure of thigh**

      M70.851   Other soft tissue disorders related to use,
                overuse and pressure, right thigh

      M70.852   Other soft tissue disorders related to use,
                overuse and pressure, left thigh

      M70.859   Other soft tissue disorders related to use,
                overuse and pressure, unspecified thigh

   **M70.86   Other soft tissue disorders related to use, overuse and
               pressure lower leg**

      M70.861   Other soft tissue disorders related to use,
                overuse and pressure, right lower leg

      M70.862   Other soft tissue disorders related to use,
                overuse and pressure, left lower leg

      M70.869   Other soft tissue disorders related to use,
                overuse and pressure, unspecified leg

   **M70.87   Other soft tissue disorders related to use, overuse and
               pressure of ankle and foot**

      M70.871   Other soft tissue disorders related to use,
                overuse and pressure, right ankle and foot

      M70.872   Other soft tissue disorders related to use,
                overuse and pressure, left ankle and foot

      M70.879   Other soft tissue disorders related to use,
                overuse and pressure, unspecified ankle and
                foot

   **M70.88   Other soft tissue disorders related to use, overuse and
               pressure other site**

   **M70.89   Other soft tissue disorders related to use, overuse and
               pressure multiple sites**

**M70.9 Unspecified soft tissue disorder related to use, overuse and
      pressure**

   **M70.90   Unspecified soft tissue disorder related to use, overuse
               and pressure of unspecified site**

   **M70.91   Unspecified soft tissue disorder related to use, overuse
               and pressure of shoulder**

      M70.911   Unspecified soft tissue disorder related to use,
                overuse and pressure, right shoulder

      M70.912   Unspecified soft tissue disorder related to use,
                overuse and pressure, left shoulder

      M70.919   Unspecified soft tissue disorder related to use,
                overuse and pressure, unspecified shoulder

   **M70.92   Unspecified soft tissue disorder related to use, overuse
               and pressure of upper arm**

      M70.921   Unspecified soft tissue disorder related to use,
                overuse and pressure, right upper arm

      M70.922   Unspecified soft tissue disorder related to use,
                overuse and pressure, left upper arm

      M70.929   Unspecified soft tissue disorder related to use,
                overuse and pressure, unspecified upper arm

   **M70.93   Unspecified soft tissue disorder related to use, overuse
               and pressure of forearm**

      M70.931   Unspecified soft tissue disorder related to use,
                overuse and pressure, right forearm

M70.932 Unspecified soft tissue disorder related to use, overuse and pressure, left forearm

M70.939 Unspecified soft tissue disorder related to use, overuse and pressure, unspecified forearm

M70.94 Unspecified soft tissue disorder related to use, overuse and pressure of hand

M70.941 Unspecified soft tissue disorder related to use, overuse and pressure, right hand

M70.942 Unspecified soft tissue disorder related to use, overuse and pressure, left hand

M70.949 Unspecified soft tissue disorder related to use, overuse and pressure, unspecified hand

M70.95 Unspecified soft tissue disorder related to use, overuse and pressure of thigh

M70.951 Unspecified soft tissue disorder related to use, overuse and pressure, right thigh

M70.952 Unspecified soft tissue disorder related to use, overuse and pressure, left thigh

M70.959 Unspecified soft tissue disorder related to use, overuse and pressure, unspecified thigh

M70.96 Unspecified soft tissue disorder related to use, overuse and pressure lower leg

M70.961 Unspecified soft tissue disorder related to use, overuse and pressure, right lower leg

M70.962 Unspecified soft tissue disorder related to use, overuse and pressure, left lower leg

M70.969 Unspecified soft tissue disorder related to use, overuse and pressure, unspecified lower leg

M70.97 Unspecified soft tissue disorder related to use, overuse and pressure of ankle and foot

M70.971 Unspecified soft tissue disorder related to use, overuse and pressure, right ankle and foot

M70.972 Unspecified soft tissue disorder related to use, overuse and pressure, left ankle and foot

M70.979 Unspecified soft tissue disorder related to use, overuse and pressure, unspecified ankle and foot

M70.98 Unspecified soft tissue disorder related to use, overuse and pressure other

M70.99 Unspecified soft tissue disorder related to use, overuse and pressure multiple sites

M71 Other bursopathies

Excludes1: bunion (M20.1)
    bursitis related to use, overuse or pressure (M70.-)
    enthesopathies (M76-M77)

M71.1 Abscess of bursa

Use additional code (B95.-, B96.-) to identify causative organism

M71.00 Abscess of bursa, unspecified site

M71.01 Abscess of bursa, shoulder

M70.011 Abscess of bursa, right shoulder

M70.012 Abscess of bursa, left shoulder

M70.019 Abscess of bursa, unspecified shoulder

M71.02 Abscess of bursa, elbow

M71.021 Abscess of bursa, right elbow

M71.022 Abscess of bursa, left elbow

M71.029 Abscess of bursa, unspecified elbow

M71.03 Abscess of bursa, wrist

M71.031 Abscess of bursa, right wrist

M71.032 Abscess of bursa, left wrist

M71.039 Abscess of bursa, unspecified wrist

M71.04 Abscess of bursa, hand

M71.041 Abscess of bursa, right hand

M71.042 Abscess of bursa, left hand

M71.049 Abscess of bursa, unspecified hand

M71.05 Abscess of bursa, hip

M71.051 Abscess of bursa, right hip

M71.052 Abscess of bursa, left hip

M71.059 Abscess of bursa, unspecified hip

M71.06 Abscess of bursa, knee

M71.061 Abscess of bursa, right knee

M71.062 Abscess of bursa, left knee

M71.069 Abscess of bursa, unspecified knee

M71.07 Abscess of bursa, ankle and foot

M71.071 Abscess of bursa, right ankle and foot

M71.072 Abscess of bursa, left ankle and foot

M71.079 Abscess of bursa, unspecified ankle and foot

M71.08 Abscess of bursa, other site

M71.09 Abscess of bursa, multiple sites

M71.1 Other infective bursitis

Use additional code (B95.-, B96.-) to identify causative organism

M71.10 Other infective bursitis, unspecified site

M71.11 Other infective bursitis, shoulder

M71.111 Other infective bursitis, right shoulder

M71.112 Other infective bursitis, left shoulder

M71.119 Other infective bursitis, unspecified shoulder

M71.12 Other infective bursitis, elbow

M71.121 Other infective bursitis, right elbow

M71.122 Other infective bursitis, left elbow

M71.129 Other infective bursitis, unspecified elbow

M71.13 Other infective bursitis, wrist

M71.131 Other infective bursitis, right wrist

M71.132 Other infective bursitis, left wrist

M71.139 Other infective bursitis, unspecified wrist

M71.14 Other infective bursitis, hand

M71.141 Other infective bursitis, right hand

M71.142 Other infective bursitis, left hand

M71.149 Other infective bursitis, unspecified hand

M71.15 Other infective bursitis, hip

M71.151 Other infective bursitis, right hip

M71.152 Other infective bursitis, left hip

M71.159 Other infective bursitis, unspecified hip

M71.16 Other infective bursitis, knee

M71.161 Other infective bursitis, right knee

M71.162 Other infective bursitis, left knee

M71.169 Other infective bursitis, unspecified knee

M71.17 Other infective bursitis, ankle and foot

M71.171 Other infective bursitis, right ankle and foot

M71.172 Other infective bursitis, left ankle and foot

M71.179 Other infective bursitis, unspecified ankle and foot

M71.18 Other infective bursitis, other site

M71.19 Other infective bursitis, multiple sites

M71.2 Synovial cyst of popliteal space [Baker]

Excludes1: synovial cyst of popliteal space with rupture (M66.0)

M71.20 Synovial cyst of popliteal space [Baker], unspecified knee

M71.21 Synovial cyst of popliteal space [Baker], right knee

M71.22 Synovial cyst of popliteal space [Baker], left knee

M71.3 Other bursal cyst

Synovial cyst NOS

Excludes1: synovial cyst with rupture (M66.1-)

M71.30 Other bursal cyst, unspecified site

M71.31 Other bursal cyst, shoulder

M71.311 Other bursal cyst, right shoulder

M71.312 Other bursal cyst, left shoulder

M71.319 Other bursal cyst, unspecified shoulder

M71.32 Other bursal cyst, elbow

M71.321 Other bursal cyst, right elbow

M71.322 Other bursal cyst, left elbow

M71.329 Other bursal cyst, unspecified elbow

M71.33 Other bursal cyst, wrist

M71.331 Other bursal cyst, right wrist

M71.332 Other bursal cyst, left wrist

M71.339 Other bursal cyst, unspecified wrist

M71.34 Other bursal cyst, hand

M71.341   Other bursal cyst, right hand
M71.342   Other bursal cyst, left hand
M71.349   Other bursal cyst, unspecified hand
M71.35   Other bursal cyst, hip
M71.351   Other bursal cyst, right hip
M71.352   Other bursal cyst, left hip
M71.359   Other bursal cyst, unspecified hip
M71.37   Other bursal cyst, ankle and foot
M71.371   Other bursal cyst, right ankle and foot
M71.372   Other bursal cyst, left ankle and foot
M71.379   Other bursal cyst, unspecified ankle and foot
M71.38   Other bursal cyst, other site
M71.39   Other bursal cyst, multiple sites
M71.4 Calcium deposit in bursa
Excludes2:   calcium deposit in bursa of shoulder (M75.3)
M71.40   Calcium deposit in bursa, unspecified site
M71.42   Calcium deposit in bursa, elbow
M71.421   Calcium deposit in bursa, right elbow
M71.422   Calcium deposit in bursa, left elbow
M71.429   Calcium deposit in bursa, unspecified elbow
M71.43   Calcium deposit in bursa, wrist
M71.431   Calcium deposit in bursa, right wrist
M71.432   Calcium deposit in bursa, left wrist
M71.439   Calcium deposit in bursa, unspecified wrist
M71.44   Calcium deposit in bursa, hand
M71.441   Calcium deposit in bursa, right hand
M71.442   Calcium deposit in bursa, left hand
M71.449   Calcium deposit in bursa, unspecified hand
M71.45   Calcium deposit in bursa, hip
M71.451   Calcium deposit in bursa, right hip
M71.452   Calcium deposit in bursa, left hip
M71.459   Calcium deposit in bursa, unspecified hip
M71.46   Calcium deposit in bursa, knee
M71.461   Calcium deposit in bursa, right knee
M71.462   Calcium deposit in bursa, left knee
M71.469   Calcium deposit in bursa, unspecified knee
M71.47   Calcium deposit in bursa, ankle and foot
M71.471   Calcium deposit in bursa, right ankle and foot
M71.472   Calcium deposit in bursa, left ankle and foot
M71.479   Calcium deposit in bursa, unspecified ankle and foot
M71.48   Calcium deposit in bursa, other site
M71.49   Calcium deposit in bursa, multiple sites
M71.5 Other bursitis, not elsewhere classified
Excludes1:   bursitis NOS (M71.9-)
Excludes2:   bursitis of shoulder (M75.5)
             bursitis of tibial collateral [Pellegrini-Stieda] (M76.4)
M71.50   Other bursitis, not elsewhere classified, unspecified site
M71.52   Other bursitis, not elsewhere classified, elbow
M71.521   Other bursitis, not elsewhere classified, right elbow
M71.522   Other bursitis, not elsewhere classified, left elbow
M71.529   Other bursitis, not elsewhere classified, unspecified elbow
M71.53   Other bursitis, not elsewhere classified, wrist
M71.531   Other bursitis, not elsewhere classified, right wrist
M71.532   Other bursitis, not elsewhere classified, left wrist
M71.539   Other bursitis, not elsewhere classified, unspecified wrist
M71.54   Other bursitis, not elsewhere classified, hand
M71.541   Other bursitis, not elsewhere classified, right hand
M71.542   Other bursitis, not elsewhere classified, left hand

M71.549   Other bursitis, not elsewhere classified, unspecified hand
M71.55   Other bursitis, not elsewhere classified, hip
M71.551   Other bursitis, not elsewhere classified, right hip
M71.552   Other bursitis, not elsewhere classified, left hip
M71.559   Other bursitis, not elsewhere classified, unspecified hip
M71.56   Other bursitis, not elsewhere classified, knee
M71.561   Other bursitis, not elsewhere classified, right knee
M71.562   Other bursitis, not elsewhere classified, left knee
M71.569   Other bursitis, not elsewhere classified, unspecified knee
M71.57   Other bursitis, not elsewhere classified, ankle and foot
M71.571   Other bursitis, not elsewhere classified, right ankle and foot
M71.572   Other bursitis, not elsewhere classified, left ankle and foot
M71.579   Other bursitis, not elsewhere classified, unspecified ankle and foot
M71.58   Other bursitis, not elsewhere classified, other site
M71.8 Other specified bursopathies
M71.80   Other specified bursopathies, unspecified site
M71.81   Other specified bursopathies, shoulder
M71.811   Other specified bursopathies, right shoulder
M71.812   Other specified bursopathies, left shoulder
M71.819   Other specified bursopathies, unspecified shoulder
M71.82   Other specified bursopathies, elbow
M71.821   Other specified bursopathies, right elbow
M71.822   Other specified bursopathies, left elbow
M71.829   Other specified bursopathies, unspecified elbow
M71.83   Other specified bursopathies, wrist
M71.831   Other specified bursopathies, right wrist
M71.832   Other specified bursopathies, left wrist
M71.839   Other specified bursopathies, unspecified wrist
M71.84   Other specified bursopathies, hand
M71.841   Other specified bursopathies, right hand
M71.842   Other specified bursopathies, left hand
M71.849   Other specified bursopathies, unspecified hand
M71.85   Other specified bursopathies, hip
M71.851   Other specified bursopathies, right hip
M71.852   Other specified bursopathies, left hip
M71.859   Other specified bursopathies, unspecified hip
M71.86   Other specified bursopathies, knee
M71.861   Other specified bursopathies, right knee
M71.862   Other specified bursopathies, left knee
M71.869   Other specified bursopathies, unspecified knee
M71.87   Other specified bursopathies, ankle and foot
M71.871   Other specified bursopathies, right ankle and foot
M71.872   Other specified bursopathies, left ankle and foot
M71.879   Other specified bursopathies, unspecified ankle and foot
M71.88   Other specified bursopathies, other site
M71.89   Other specified bursopathies, multiple sites
M71.9 Bursopathy, unspecified
       Bursitis NOS

M72 Fibroblastic disorders
Excludes2:   retroperitoneal fibromatosis (D48.3)
M72.0 Palmar fascial fibromatosis [Dupuytren]
M72.1 Knuckle pads

M72.2 **Plantar fascial fibromatosis**
   Plantar fasciitis
M72.3 **Nodular fasciitis**
M72.4 **Pseudosarcomatous fibromatosis**
M72.5 **Fasciitis, not elsewhere classified**
   M72.51 **Necrotizing fasciitis**
      Use additional code (B95.-, B96.-) to identify causative
      organism
   M72.52 **Other infective fasciitis**
      Abscess of fascia
      Use additional code to (B95.-, B96.-) identify causative
      organism
   M72.59 **Other fasciitis**
      Excludes1: diffuse (eosinophilic) fasciitis (M35.4)
                  nodular fasciitis (M72.3)
                  plantar fasciitis (M72.2)
M72.8 **Other fibroblastic disorders**
M72.9 **Fibroblastic disorder, unspecified**

M75 Shoulder lesions
      Excludes2: shoulder-hand syndrome (M89.0-)
M75.0 **Adhesive capsulitis of shoulder**
   Frozen shoulder
   Periarthritis of shoulder
   M75.00 **Adhesive capsulitis of unspecified shoulder**
   M75.01 **Adhesive capsulitis of right shoulder**
   M75.02 **Adhesive capsulitis of left shoulder**
M75.1 **Rotator cuff syndrome**
   Rotator cuff or supraspinatus tear or rupture (complete)
   (incomplete), not specified as traumatic
   Supraspinatus syndrome
   M75.10 **Rotator cuff syndrome, unspecified shoulder**
   M75.11 **Rotator cuff syndrome, right shoulder**
   M75.12 **Rotator cuff syndrome, left shoulder**
M75.2 **Bicipital tendinitis**
   M75.20 **Bicipital tendinitis, unspecified shoulder**
   M75.21 **Bicipital tendinitis, right shoulder**
   M75.22 **Bicipital tendinitis, left shoulder**
M75.3 **Calcific tendinitis of shoulder**
   Calcified bursa of shoulder
   M75.30 **Calcific tendinitis of unspecified shoulder**
   M75.31 **Calcific tendinitis of right shoulder**
   M75.32 **Calcific tendinitis of left shoulder**
M75.4 **Impingement syndrome of shoulder**
   M75.40 **Impingement syndrome of unspecified shoulder**
   M75.41 **Impingement syndrome of right shoulder**
   M75.42 **Impingement syndrome of left shoulder**
M75.5 **Bursitis of shoulder**
   M75.50 **Bursitis of unspecified shoulder**
   M75.51 **Bursitis of right shoulder**
   M75.52 **Bursitis of left shoulder**
M75.8 **Other shoulder lesions**
   M75.80 **Other shoulder lesions, unspecified shoulder**
   M75.81 **Other shoulder lesions, right shoulder**
   M75.82 **Other shoulder lesions, left shoulder**
M75.9 **Shoulder lesion, unspecified**
   M75.90 **Shoulder lesion, unspecified, unspecified shoulder**
   M75.91 **Shoulder lesion, unspecified, right shoulder**
   M75.92 **Shoulder lesion, unspecified, left shoulder**

M76 Enthesopathies, lower limb, excluding foot
      Excludes2: bursitis due to use, overuse and pressure (M70.-)
                  enthesopathies of ankle and foot (M77.5-)
M76.0 **Gluteal tendinitis**
   M76.00 **Gluteal tendinitis, unspecified buttock**
   M76.01 **Gluteal tendinitis, right buttock**
   M76.02 **Gluteal tendinitis, left buttock**
M76.1 **Psoas tendinitis**
   M76.10 **Psoas tendinitis, unspecified side**
   M76.11 **Psoas tendinitis, right side**

   M76.12 **Psoas tendinitis, left side**
M76.2 **Iliac crest spur**
   M76.20 **Iliac crest spur, unspecified hip**
   M76.21 **Iliac crest spur, right hip**
   M76.22 **Iliac crest spur, left hip**
M76.3 **Iliotibial band syndrome**
   M76.30 **Iliotibial band syndrome, unspecified side**
   M76.31 **Iliotibial band syndrome, right side**
   M76.32 **Iliotibial band syndrome, left side**
M76.4 **Tibial collateral bursitis [Pellegrini-Stieda]**
   M76.40 **Tibial collateral bursitis [Pellegrini-Stieda], unspecified leg**
   M76.41 **Tibial collateral bursitis [Pellegrini-Stieda], right leg**
   M76.42 **Tibial collateral bursitis [Pellegrini-Stieda], left leg**
M76.5 **Patellar tendinitis**
   M76.50 **Patellar tendinitis, unspecified knee**
   M76.51 **Patellar tendinitis, right knee**
   M76.52 **Patellar tendinitis, left knee**
M76.6 **Achilles tendinitis**
   Achilles bursitis
   M76.60 **Achilles tendinitis, unspecified leg**
   M76.61 **Achilles tendinitis, right leg**
   M76.62 **Achilles tendinitis, left leg**
M76.7 **Peroneal tendinitis**
   M76.70 **Peroneal tendinitis, unspecified leg**
   M76.71 **Peroneal tendinitis, right leg**
   M76.72 **Peroneal tendinitis, left leg**
M76.8 **Other enthesopathies of lower limb, excluding foot**
   Anterior tibial syndrome
   Posterior tibial tendinitis
   M76.80 **Other enthesopathies, lower limb of unspecified site**
   M76.85 **Other enthesopathies, thigh**
      M76.851 **Other enthesopathies, right thigh**
      M76.852 **Other enthesopathies, left thigh**
      M76.859 **Other enthesopathies, unspecified thighs**
   M76.86 **Other enthesopathies, lower leg**
      M76.861 **Other enthesopathies, right lower leg**
      M76.862 **Other enthesopathies, left lower leg**
      M76.869 **Other enthesopathies, unspecified lower leg**
   M76.89 **Other enthesopathies, lower limb multiple sites**
M76.9 **Unspecified enthesopathy, lower limb, excluding foot**
   M76.90 **Unspecified enthesopathy, lower limb, excluding foot, unspecified site**
   M76.95 **Unspecified enthesopathy, thigh**
      M76.951 **Unspecified enthesopathy, right thigh**
      M76.952 **Unspecified enthesopathy, left thigh**
      M76.959 **Unspecified enthesopathy, unspecified thigh**
   M76.96 **Unspecified enthesopathy, unspecified lower leg**
      M76.961 **Unspecified enthesopathy, right lower leg**
      M76.962 **Unspecified enthesopathy, left lower leg**
      M76.969 **Unspecified enthesopathy, unspecified lower leg**
   M76.99 **Unspecified enthesopathy, lower limb, multiple sites**

M77 Other enthesopathies
      Excludes1: bursitis NOS (M71.9-)
      Excludes2: bursitis due to use, overuse and pressure (M70.-)
                  osteophyte (M25.7)
                  spinal enthesopathy (M46.0-)
M77.0 **Medial epicondylitis**
   M77.00 **Medial epicondylitis, unspecified elbow**
   M77.01 **Medial epicondylitis, right elbow**
   M77.02 **Medial epicondylitis, left elbow**
M77.1 **Lateral epicondylitis**
   Tennis elbow
   M77.10 **Lateral epicondylitis, unspecified elbow**
   M77.11 **Lateral epicondylitis, right elbow**
   M77.12 **Lateral epicondylitis, left elbow**
M77.2 **Periarthritis of wrist**

    M77.20   Periarthritis, unspecified wrist
    M77.21   Periarthritis, right wrist
    M77.22   Periarthritis, left wrist

M77.3   Calcaneal spur
    M77.30   Calcaneal spur, unspecified foot
    M77.31   Calcaneal spur, right foot
    M77.32   Calcaneal spur, left foot

M77.4   Metatarsalgia
    Excludes1:   Morton's metatarsalgia (G57.6)
    M77.40   Metatarsalgia, unspecified foot
    M77.41   Metatarsalgia, right foot
    M77.42   Metatarsalgia, left foot

M77.5   Other enthesopathy of foot
    M77.50   Other enthesopathy of unspecified foot
    M77.51   Other enthesopathy of right foot
    M77.52   Other enthesopathy of left foot

M77.8   Other enthesopathies, not elsewhere classified

M77.9   Enthesopathy, unspecified
    Bone spur NOS
    Capsulitis NOS
    Periarthritis NOS
    Tendinitis NOS

M79   Other soft tissue disorders, not elsewhere classified
    Excludes1:   psychogenic rheumatism (F45.8)
                 soft tissue pain, psychogenic (F45.4)

M79.0   Rheumatism, unspecified
    Fibromyalgia
    Fibrositis
    Excludes1:   palindromic rheumatism (M12.3-)

M79.1   Myalgia
    Excludes1:   myositis (M60.-)

M79.2   Neuralgia and neuritis, unspecified
    Excludes1:   brachial radiculitis NOS (M54.1)
                 lumbosacral radiculitis NOS (M54.1)
                 mononeuropathies (G56-G58)
                 radiculitis NOS (M54.1)
                 sciatica (M54.3-M54.4)

M79.3   Panniculitis, unspecified
    Excludes1:   lupus panniculitis (L93.2)
                 neck and back panniculitis (M54.0-)
                 relapsing [Weber-Christian] panniculitis (M35.6)

M79.4   Hypertrophy of (infrapatellar) fat pad

M79.5   Residual foreign body in soft tissue
    Excludes1:   foreign body granuloma of skin and
                 subcutaneous tissue (L92.3)
                 foreign body granuloma of soft tissue (M60.2-)

M79.6   Pain in limb, hand, foot, fingers and toes
    Excludes2:   pain in joint (M25.5-)
    M79.60   Pain in limb, unspecified
        M79.601   Pain in right arm
             Pain in right upper limb NOS
        M79.602   Pain in left arm
             Pain in left upper limb NOS
        M79.603   Pain in arm, unspecified
             Pain in upper limb NOS
        M79.604   Pain in right leg
             Pain in right lower limb NOS
        M79.605   Pain in left leg
             Pain in left lower limb NOS
        M79.606   Pain in leg, unspecified
             Pain in lower limb NOS
        M79.609   Pain in unspecified limb
             Pain in limb NOS
    M79.62   Pain in upper arm
        M79.621   Pain in right upper arm
        M79.622   Pain in left upper arm
        M79.629   Pain in unspecified upper arm
    M79.63   Pain in forearm
        M79.631   Pain in right forearm
        M79.632   Pain in left forearm

        M79.639   Pain in unspecified forearm
    M79.64   Pain in hand and fingers
        M79.641   Pain in right hand
        M79.642   Pain in left hand
        M79.643   Pain in unspecified hand
        M79.644   Pain in right finger(s)
        M79.645   Pain in left finger(s)
        M79.646   Pain in unspecified finger(s)
    M79.65   Pain in thigh
        M79.651   Pain in right thigh
        M79.652   Pain in left thigh
        M79.659   Pain in unspecified thigh
    M79.66   Pain in lower leg
        M79.661   Pain in right lower leg
        M79.662   Pain in left lower leg
        M79.669   Pain in unspecified lower leg
    M79.67   Pain in foot and toes
        M79.671   Pain in right foot
        M79.672   Pain in left foot
        M79.673   Pain in unspecified foot
        M79.674   Pain in right toe(s)
        M79.675   Pain in left toe(s)
        M79.676   Pain in unspecified toe(s)

M79.8   Other specified soft tissue disorders

M79.9   Soft tissue disorder, unspecified

DISORDERS OF BONE DENSITY AND STRUCTURE (M80–M85)

M80   Osteoporosis with current pathological fracture
    Includes: osteoporosis with current fragility fracture
    Note: fragility fracture is defined as a fracture sustained with trauma no more than a fall from a standing height or less that occurs under circumstances that would not cause a fracture in a normal healthy bone
    Excludes1:   collapsed vertebra NOS (M48.5)
                 pathological fracture NOS (M84.4)
                 wedging of vertebra NOS (M48.5)
    The following extensions are to be added to each code for category M80:
    a   initial encounter for fracture
    d   subsequent encounter for fracture with routine healing
    g   subsequent encounter for fracture with delayed healing
    j   subsequent encounter for fracture with nonunion
    m   subsequent encounter for fracture with malunion
    q   sequela

M80.0   Postmenopausal osteoporosis with current pathological fracture
    Age-related osteoporosis with current pathological fracture
    Involutional osteoporosis with current pathological fracture
    Senile osteoporosis with current pathological fracture
    M80.00   Postmenopausal osteoporosis with current pathological fracture, unspecified site
    M80.01   Postmenopausal osteoporosis with current pathological fracture, shoulder
        M80.011   Postmenopausal osteoporosis with current pathological fracture, right shoulder
        M80.012   Postmenopausal osteoporosis with current pathological fracture, left shoulder
        M80.019   Postmenopausal osteoporosis with current pathological fracture, unspecified shoulder
    M80.02   Postmenopausal osteoporosis with current pathological fracture, humerus
        M80.021   Postmenopausal osteoporosis with current pathological fracture, right humerus
        M80.022   Postmenopausal osteoporosis with current pathological fracture, left humerus
        M80.029   Postmenopausal osteoporosis with current pathological fracture, unspecified humerus
    M80.03   Postmenopausal osteoporosis with current pathological fracture, forearm
         Postmenopausal osteoporosis with current pathological fracture of wrist

M80.031   Postmenopausal osteoporosis with current pathological fracture, right forearm

M80.032   Postmenopausal osteoporosis with current pathological fracture, left forearm

M80.039   Postmenopausal osteoporosis with current pathological fracture, unspecified forearm

M80.04   Postmenopausal osteoporosis with current pathological fracture, hand

M80.041   Postmenopausal osteoporosis with current pathological fracture, right hand

M80.042   Postmenopausal osteoporosis with current pathological fracture, left hand

M80.049   Postmenopausal osteoporosis with current pathological fracture, unspecified hand

M80.05   Postmenopausal osteoporosis with current pathological fracture, femur
Postmenopausal osteoporosis with current pathological fracture of hip

M80.051   Postmenopausal osteoporosis with current pathological fracture, right femur

M80.052   Postmenopausal osteoporosis with current pathological fracture, left femur

M80.059   Postmenopausal osteoporosis with current pathological fracture, unspecified femur

M80.06   Postmenopausal osteoporosis with current pathological fracture, lower leg

M80.061   Postmenopausal osteoporosis with current pathological fracture, right lower leg

M80.062   Postmenopausal osteoporosis with current pathological fracture, left lower leg

M80.069   Postmenopausal osteoporosis with current pathological fracture, unspecified lower leg

M80.07   Postmenopausal osteoporosis with current pathological fracture, ankle and foot

M80.071   Postmenopausal osteoporosis with current pathological fracture, right ankle and foot

M80.072   Postmenopausal osteoporosis with current pathological fracture, left ankle and foot

M80.079   Postmenopausal osteoporosis with current pathological fracture, unspecified ankle and foot

M80.08   Postmenopausal osteoporosis with current pathological fracture, vertebra(e)

M80.8   Other osteoporosis with current pathological fracture
Drug-induced osteoporosis with current pathological fracture
Idiopathic osteoporosis with current pathological fracture
Osteoporosis of disuse with current pathological fracture
Postsurgical malabsorption osteoporosis with current pathological fracture

M80.80   Other osteoporosis with current pathological fracture, unspecified site

M80.81   Other osteoporosis with pathological fracture, shoulder

M80.811   Other osteoporosis with current pathological fracture, right shoulder

M80.812   Other osteoporosis with current pathological fracture, left shoulder

M80.819   Other osteoporosis with current pathological fracture, unspecified shoulder

M80.82   Other osteoporosis with current pathological fracture, humerus

M80.821   Other osteoporosis with current pathological fracture, right humerus

M80.822   Other osteoporosis with current pathological fracture, left humerus

M80.829   Other osteoporosis with current pathological fracture, unspecified humerus

M80.83   Other osteoporosis with current pathological fracture, forearm
Other osteoporosis with current pathological fracture of wrist

M80.831   Other osteoporosis with current pathological fracture, right forearm

M80.832   Other osteoporosis with current pathological fracture, left forearm

M80.839   Other osteoporosis with current pathological fracture, unspecified forearm

M80.84   Other osteoporosis with current pathological fracture, hand

M80.841   Other osteoporosis with current pathological fracture, right hand

M80.842   Other osteoporosis with current pathological fracture, left hand

M80.849   Other osteoporosis with current pathological fracture, unspecified hand

M80.85   Other osteoporosis with current pathological fracture, femur
Other osteoporosis with current pathological fracture of hip

M80.851   Other osteoporosis with current pathological fracture, right femur

M80.852   Other osteoporosis with current pathological fracture, left femur

M80.859   Other osteoporosis with current pathological fracture, unspecified femur

M80.86   Other osteoporosis with current pathological fracture, lower leg

M80.861   Other osteoporosis with current pathological fracture, right lower leg

M80.862   Other osteoporosis with current pathological fracture, left lower leg

M80.869   Other osteoporosis with current pathological fracture, unspecified lower leg

M80.87   Other osteoporosis with current pathological fracture, ankle and foot

M80.871   Other osteoporosis with current pathological fracture, right ankle and foot

M80.872   Other osteoporosis with current pathological fracture, left ankle and foot

M80.879   Other osteoporosis with current pathological fracture, unspecified ankle and foot

M80.88   Other osteoporosis with current pathological fracture, vertebra(e)

M81 Osteoporosis without current pathological fracture
Excludes1:   osteoporosis with current pathological fracture (M80.-)
Sudeck's atrophy (M89.0)

M81.0   Postmenopausal osteoporosis without current pathological fracture
Age-related osteoporosis without current pathological fracture
Involutional osteoporosis without current pathological fracture
Osteoporosis NOS
Senile osteoporosis without current pathological fracture

M81.6   Localized osteoporosis [Lequesne]
Excludes1:   Sudeck's atrophy (M89.0)

M81.60   Localized osteoporosis [Lequesne], unspecified site

M81.61   Localized osteoporosis [Lequesne], shoulder

M81.611   Localized osteoporosis [Lequesne], right shoulder

M81.612   Localized osteoporosis [Lequesne], left shoulder

M81.619   Localized osteoporosis [Lequesne], unspecified shoulder

M81.62   Localized osteoporosis [Lequesne], humerus

M81.621   Localized osteoporosis [Lequesne], right humerus

M81.622   Localized osteoporosis [Lequesne], left humerus

M81.629   Localized osteoporosis [Lequesne], unspecified humerus

M81.63   Localized osteoporosis [Lequesne], forearm
Localized osteoporosis [Lequesne] of wrist

M81.631   Localized osteoporosis [Lequesne], right forearm

M81.632   Localized osteoporosis [Lequesne], left forearm

M81.639   Localized osteoporosis [Lequesne], unspecified forearm

M81.64   **Localized osteoporosis [Lequesne], hand**

     M81.641   Localized osteoporosis [Lequesne], right hand

     M81.642   Localized osteoporosis [Lequesne], left hand

     M81.649   Localized osteoporosis [Lequesne], unspecified hand

M81.65   **Localized osteoporosis [Lequesne], femur**
     Localized osteoporosis [Lequesne] of hip

     M81.651   Localized osteoporosis [Lequesne], right femur

     M81.652   Localized osteoporosis [Lequesne], left femur

     M81.659   Localized osteoporosis [Lequesne], unspecified femur

M81.66   **Localized osteoporosis [Lequesne], lower leg**

     M81.661   Localized osteoporosis [Lequesne], right lower leg

     M81.662   Localized osteoporosis [Lequesne], left lower leg

     M81.669   Localized osteoporosis [Lequesne], unspecified lower leg

M81.67   **Localized osteoporosis [Lequesne], ankle and foot**

     M81.671   Localized osteoporosis [Lequesne], right ankle and foot

     M81.672   Localized osteoporosis [Lequesne], left ankle and foot

     M81.679   Localized osteoporosis [Lequesne], unspecified ankle and foot

M81.68   **Localized osteoporosis [Lequesne], vertebra(e)**

M81.8   **Other osteoporosis without current pathological fracture**
     Drug-induced osteoporosis without current pathological fracture
     Idiopathic osteoporosis without current pathological fracture
     Osteoporosis of disuse without current pathological fracture
     Postsurgical malabsorption osteoporosis without current pathological fracture

M83 Adult osteomalacia

     Excludes1:   infantile and juvenile osteomalacia (E55.0)
                   renal osteodystrophy (N25.0)
                    rickets (active) (E55.0)
                    rickets (active) sequelae (E64.3)
                    vitamin D-resistant osteomalacia (E83.3)
                    vitamin D-resistant rickets (active) (E83.3)

M83.0   **Puerperal osteomalacia**

M83.1   **Senile osteomalacia**

M83.2   **Adult osteomalacia due to malabsorption**
     Postsurgical malabsorption osteomalacia in adults

M83.3   **Adult osteomalacia due to malnutrition**

M83.4   **Aluminum bone disease**

M83.5   **Other drug-induced osteomalacia in adults**
     Use additional external cause code (Chapter XIX) to identify drug.

M83.8   **Other adult osteomalacia**

M83.9   **Adult osteomalacia, unspecified**

M84 Disorder of continuity of bone

     Excludes2:   traumatic fracture of bone — see fracture, by site

M84.3   **Stress fracture**
     Fatigue fracture
     Stress fracture NOS
     Stress reaction

     Excludes1:   pathologic fracture NOS (M84.4.-)
                    pathological fracture due to osteoporosis (M80.-)
                    traumatic fracture (S12.-, S22.-, S32.-, S42.-, S52.-, S62.-, S72.-, S82.-, S92.-)

     Excludes2:   stress fracture of vertebra (M48.4-)

     The following extensions are to be added to each code for subcategory M84.3:
       a   initial encounter for fracture
       d   subsequent encounter for fracture with routine healing
       g   subsequent encounter for fracture with delayed healing
       j   subsequent encounter for fracture with nonunion
       m   subsequent encounter for fracture with malunion
       q   sequela

M84.30   **Stress fracture, unspecified site**

M84.31   **Stress fracture, shoulder**

     M84.311   Stress fracture, right shoulder

     M84.312   Stress fracture, left shoulder

     M84.319   Stress fracture, unspecified shoulder

M84.32   **Stress fracture, humerus**

     M84.321   Stress fracture, right humerus

     M84.322   Stress fracture, left humerus

     M84.329   Stress fracture, unspecified humerus

M84.33   **Stress fracture, ulna and radius**

     M84.331   Stress fracture, right ulna

     M84.332   Stress fracture, left ulna

     M84.333   Stress fracture, right radius

     M84.334   Stress fracture, left radius

     M84.339   Stress fracture, unspecified ulna and radius

M84.34   **Stress fracture, hand and fingers**

     M84.341   Stress fracture, right hand

     M84.342   Stress fracture, left hand

     M84.343   Stress fracture, unspecified hand

     M84.344   Stress fracture, right finger(s)

     M84.345   Stress fracture, left finger(s)

     M84.346   Stress fracture, unspecified finger(s)

M84.35   **Stress fracture, pelvis and femur**
     Stress fracture, hip

     M84.350   Stress fracture, pelvis

     M84.351   Stress fracture, right femur

     M84.352   Stress fracture, left femur

     M84.353   Stress fracture, unspecified femur

     M84.359   Stress fracture, hip, unspecified

M84.36   **Stress fracture, tibia and fibula**

     M84.361   Stress fracture, right tibia

     M84.362   Stress fracture, left tibia

     M84.363   Stress fracture, right fibula

     M84.364   Stress fracture, left fibula

     M84.369   Stress fracture, unspecified tibia and fibula

M84.37   **Stress fracture, ankle, foot and toes**

     M84.371   Stress fracture, right ankle

     M84.372   Stress fracture, left ankle

     M84.373   Stress fracture, unspecified ankle

     M84.374   Stress fracture, right foot

     M84.375   Stress fracture, left foot

     M84.376   Stress fracture, unspecified foot

     M84.377   Stress fracture, right toes

     M84.378   Stress fracture, left toes

     M84.379   Stress fracture, unspecified toes

M84.38   **Stress fracture, other site**

     Excludes2:   stress fracture of vertebra (M48.4-)

M84.4   **Pathological fracture, not elsewhere classified**
     Pathological fracture NOS

     Excludes1:   collapsed vertebra NEC (M48.5)
                    pathologic fracture in neoplastic disease (M84.5-)
                    pathologic fracture in osteoporosis (M80.-)
                    pathologic fracture in other disease (M84.6-)
                    traumatic fracture (S12.-, S22.-, S32.-, S42.-, S52.-, S62.-, S72.-, S82.-, S92.-)

     The following extensions are to be added to each code for subcategory M84.4:
       a   initial encounter for fracture
       d   subsequent encounter for fracture with routine healing
       g   subsequent encounter for fracture with delayed healing
       j   subsequent encounter for fracture with nonunion
       m   subsequent encounter for fracture with malunion
       q   sequela

M84.40   **Pathological fracture, unspecified site**

M84.41   **Pathological fracture, shoulder**

     M84.411   Pathological fracture, right shoulder

     M84.412   Pathological fracture, left shoulder

     M84.419   Pathological fracture, unspecified shoulder

M84.42   **Pathological fracture, humerus**

M84.421   Pathological fracture, right humerus

M84.422   Pathological fracture, left humerus

M84.429   Pathological fracture, unspecified humerus

M84.43   Pathological fracture, ulna and radius

    M84.431   Pathological fracture, right ulna

    M84.432   Pathological fracture, left ulna

    M84.433   Pathological fracture, right radius

    M84.434   Pathological fracture, left radius

    M84.439   Pathological fracture, unspecified ulna and radius

M84.44   Pathological fracture, hand and fingers

    M84.441   Pathological fracture, right hand

    M84.442   Pathological fracture, left hand

    M84.443   Pathological fracture, unspecified hand

    M84.444   Pathological fracture, right finger(s)

    M84.445   Pathological fracture, left finger(s)

    M84.446   Pathological fracture, unspecified finger(s)

M84.45   Pathological fracture, femur and pelvis

    M84.451   Pathological fracture, right femur

    M84.452   Pathological fracture, left femur

    M84.453   Pathological fracture, unspecified femur

    M84.454   Pathological fracture, pelvis

    M84.459   Pathological fracture, hip, unspecified

M84.46   Pathological fracture, tibia and fibula

    M84.461   Pathological fracture, right tibia

    M84.462   Pathological fracture, left tibia

    M84.463   Pathological fracture, right fibula

    M84.464   Pathological fracture, left fibula

    M84.469   Pathological fracture, unspecified tibia and fibula

M84.47   Pathological fracture, ankle, foot and toes

    M84.471   Pathological fracture, right ankle

    M84.472   Pathological fracture, left ankle

    M84.473   Pathological fracture, unspecified ankle

    M84.474   Pathological fracture, right foot

    M84.475   Pathological fracture, left foot

    M84.476   Pathological fracture, unspecified foot

    M84.477   Pathological fracture, right toe(s)

    M84.478   Pathological fracture, left toe(s)

    M84.479   Pathological fracture, unspecified toe(s)

M84.48   Pathological fracture, other site

M84.5 Pathologic fracture of bone in neoplastic disease

Code also underlying neoplasm

The following extensions are to be added to each code for subcategory M84.5:

   a   initial encounter for fracture

   d   subsequent encounter for fracture with routine healing

   g   subsequent encounter for fracture with delayed healing

   j   subsequent encounter for fracture with nonunion

   m   subsequent encounter for fracture with malunion

   q   sequela

M84.50   Pathologic fracture of bone in neoplastic disease, unspecified site

M84.51   Pathologic fracture of bone in neoplastic disease, shoulder

    M84.511   Pathologic fracture of bone in neoplastic disease, right shoulder

    M84.512   Pathologic fracture of bone in neoplastic disease, left shoulder

    M84.519   Pathologic fracture of bone in neoplastic disease, unspecified shoulder

M84.52   Pathologic fracture of bone in neoplastic disease, humerus

    M84.521   Pathologic fracture of bone in neoplastic disease, right humerus

    M84.522   Pathologic fracture of bone in neoplastic disease, left humerus

    M84.529   Pathologic fracture of bone in neoplastic disease, unspecified humerus

M84.53   Pathologic fracture of bone in neoplastic disease, ulna and radius

    M84.531   Pathologic fracture of bone in neoplastic disease, right ulna

    M84.532   Pathologic fracture of bone in neoplastic disease, left ulna

    M84.533   Pathologic fracture of bone in neoplastic disease, right radius

    M84.534   Pathologic fracture of bone in neoplastic disease, left radius

    M84.539   Pathologic fracture of bone in neoplastic disease, unspecified ulna and radius

M84.54   Pathologic fracture of bone in neoplastic disease, hand

    M84.541   Pathologic fracture of bone in neoplastic disease, right hand

    M84.542   Pathologic fracture of bone in neoplastic disease, left hand

    M84.549   Pathologic fracture of bone in neoplastic disease, unspecified hand

M84.55   Pathologic fracture of bone in neoplastic disease, pelvis and femur

    M84.550   Pathologic fracture of bone in neoplastic disease, pelvis

    M84.551   Pathologic fracture of bone in neoplastic disease, right femur

    M84.552   Pathologic fracture of bone in neoplastic disease, left femur

    M84.553   Pathologic fracture of bone in neoplastic disease, unspecified femur

    M84.559   Pathologic fracture of bone in neoplastic disease, hip, unspecified

M84.56   Pathologic fracture of bone in neoplastic disease, tibia and fibula

    M84.561   Pathologic fracture of bone in neoplastic disease, right tibia

    M84.562   Pathologic fracture of bone in neoplastic disease, left tibia

    M84.563   Pathologic fracture of bone in neoplastic disease, right fibula

    M84.564   Pathologic fracture of bone in neoplastic disease, left fibula

    M84.569   Pathologic fracture of bone in neoplastic disease, unspecified tibia and fibula

M84.57   Pathologic fracture of bone in neoplastic disease, ankle and foot

    M84.571   Pathologic fracture of bone in neoplastic disease, right ankle

    M84.572   Pathologic fracture of bone in neoplastic disease, left ankle

    M84.573   Pathologic fracture of bone in neoplastic disease, unspecified ankle

    M84.574   Pathologic fracture of bone in neoplastic disease, right foot

    M84.575   Pathologic fracture of bone in neoplastic disease, left foot

    M84.576   Pathologic fracture of bone in neoplastic disease, unspecified foot

M84.58   Pathologic fracture of bone in neoplastic disease, vertebrae

M84.6 Pathologic fracture in other disease

Code also underlying condition

The following extensions are to be added to each code for subcategory M84.6:

   a   initial encounter for fracture

   d   subsequent encounter for fracture with routine healing

   g   subsequent encounter for fracture with delayed healing

   j   subsequent encounter for fracture with nonunion

   m   subsequent encounter for fracture with malunion

   q   sequela

M84.60   Pathologic fracture in other disease, unspecified site

M84.61   Pathologic fracture in other disease, shoulder

    M84.611   Pathologic fracture in other disease, right shoulder

M84.612   Pathologic fracture in other disease, left shoulder

M84.619   Pathologic fracture in other disease, unspecified shoulder

M84.62   Pathologic fracture in other disease, humerus

    M84.621   Pathologic fracture in other disease, right humerus

    M84.622   Pathologic fracture in other disease, left humerus

    M84.629   Pathologic fracture in other disease, unspecified humerus

M84.63   Pathologic fracture in other disease, ulna and radius

    M84.631   Pathologic fracture in other disease, right ulna

    M84.632   Pathologic fracture in other disease, left ulna

    M84.633   Pathologic fracture in other disease, right radius

    M84.634   Pathologic fracture in other disease, left radius

    M84.639   Pathologic fracture in other disease, unspecified ulna and radius

M84.64   Pathologic fracture in other disease, hand

    M84.641   Pathologic fracture in other disease, right hand

    M84.642   Pathologic fracture in other disease, left hand

    M84.649   Pathologic fracture in other disease, unspecified hand

M84.65   Pathologic fracture in other disease, pelvis and femur

    M84.650   Pathologic fracture in other disease, pelvis

    M84.651   Pathologic fracture in other disease, right femur

    M84.652   Pathologic fracture in other disease, left femur

    M84.653   Pathologic fracture in other disease, unspecified femur

    M84.659   Pathologic fracture in other disease, hip, unspecified

M84.66   Pathologic fracture in other disease, tibia and fibula

    M84.661   Pathologic fracture in other disease, right tibia

    M84.662   Pathologic fracture in other disease, left tibia

    M84.663   Pathologic fracture in other disease, right fibula

    M84.664   Pathologic fracture in other disease, left fibula

    M84.669   Pathologic fracture in other disease, unspecified tibia and fibula

M84.67   Pathologic fracture in other disease, ankle and foot

    M84.671   Pathologic fracture in other disease, right ankle

    M84.672   Pathologic fracture in other disease, left ankle

    M84.673   Pathologic fracture in other disease, unspecified ankle

    M84.674   Pathologic fracture in other disease, right foot

    M84.675   Pathologic fracture in other disease, left foot

    M84.676   Pathologic fracture in other disease, unspecified ankle

M84.68   Pathologic fracture in other disease, other site

M84.8   Other disorders of continuity of bone

    M84.80   Other disorders of continuity of bone, unspecified site

    M84.81   Other disorders of continuity of bone, shoulder

      M84.811   Other disorders of continuity of bone, right shoulder

      M84.812   Other disorders of continuity of bone, left shoulder

      M84.819   Other disorders of continuity of bone, unspecified shoulder

    M84.82   Other disorders of continuity of bone, humerus

      M84.821   Other disorders of continuity of bone, right humerus

      M84.823   Other disorders of continuity of bone, left humerus

      M84.829   Other disorders of continuity of bone, unspecified humerus

M84.83   Other disorders of continuity of bone, ulna and radius

    M84.831   Other disorders of continuity of bone, right ulna

    M84.832   Other disorders of continuity of bone, left ulna

    M84.833   Other disorders of continuity of bone, right radius

    M84.834   Other disorders of continuity of bone, left radius

    M84.839   Other disorders of continuity of bone, unspecified ulna and radius

M84.84   Other disorders of continuity of bone, hand

    M84.841   Other disorders of continuity of bone, right hand

    M84.842   Other disorders of continuity of bone, left hand

    M84.849   Other disorders of continuity of bone, unspecified hand

M84.85   Other disorders of continuity of bone, pelvic region and thigh

    M84.851   Other disorders of continuity of bone, right pelvic region and thigh

    M84.852   Other disorders of continuity of bone, left pelvic region and thigh

    M84.859   Other disorders of continuity of bone, unspecified pelvic region and thigh

M84.86   Other disorders of continuity of bone, tibia and fibula

    M84.861   Other disorders of continuity of bone, right tibia

    M84.862   Other disorders of continuity of bone, left tibia

    M84.863   Other disorders of continuity of bone, right fibula

    M84.864   Other disorders of continuity of bone, left fibula

    M84.869   Other disorders of continuity of bone, unspecified tibia and fibula

M84.87   Other disorders of continuity of bone, ankle and foot

    M84.871   Other disorders of continuity of bone, right ankle and foot

    M84.872   Other disorders of continuity of bone, left ankle and foot

    M84.879   Other disorders of continuity of bone, unspecified ankle and foot

M84.88   Other disorders of continuity of bone, other site

M84.9   Disorder of continuity of bone, unspecified

M85 Other disorders of bone density and structure

    Excludes1:   osteogenesis imperfecta (Q78.0)
              osteopetrosis (Q78.2)
              osteopoikilosis (Q78.8)
              polyostotic fibrous dysplasia (Q78.1)

M85.0   Fibrous dysplasia (monostotic)

    Excludes2:   fibrous dysplasia of jaw (M27.8)

    M85.00   Fibrous dysplasia (monostotic), unspecified site

    M85.01   Fibrous dysplasia (monostotic), shoulder

      M85.011   Fibrous dysplasia (monostotic), right shoulder

      M85.012   Fibrous dysplasia (monostotic), left shoulder

      M85.019   Fibrous dysplasia (monostotic), unspecified shoulder

    M85.02   Fibrous dysplasia (monostotic), upper arm

      M85.021   Fibrous dysplasia (monostotic), right upper arm

      M85.022   Fibrous dysplasia (monostotic), left upper arm

      M85.029   Fibrous dysplasia (monostotic), unspecified upper arm

    M85.03   Fibrous dysplasia (monostotic), forearm

      M85.031   Fibrous dysplasia (monostotic), right forearm

      M85.032   Fibrous dysplasia (monostotic), left forearm

      M85.039   Fibrous dysplasia (monostotic), unspecified forearm

    M85.04   Fibrous dysplasia (monostotic), hand

M85.041   Fibrous dysplasia (monostotic), right hand
M85.042   Fibrous dysplasia (monostotic), left hand
M85.049   Fibrous dysplasia (monostotic), unspecified hand

M85.05   Fibrous dysplasia (monostotic), thigh
M85.051   Fibrous dysplasia (monostotic), right thigh
M85.052   Fibrous dysplasia (monostotic), left thigh
M85.059   Fibrous dysplasia (monostotic), unspecified thigh

M85.06   Fibrous dysplasia (monostotic), lower leg
M85.061   Fibrous dysplasia (monostotic), right lower leg
M85.062   Fibrous dysplasia (monostotic), left lower leg
M85.069   Fibrous dysplasia (monostotic), unspecified lower leg

M85.07   Fibrous dysplasia (monostotic), ankle and foot
M85.071   Fibrous dysplasia (monostotic), right ankle and foot
M85.072   Fibrous dysplasia (monostotic), left ankle and foot
M85.079   Fibrous dysplasia (monostotic), unspecified ankle and foot

M85.08   Fibrous dysplasia (monostotic), other site
M85.09   Fibrous dysplasia (monostotic), multiple sites

M85.1   Skeletal fluorosis

M85.10   Skeletal fluorosis, unspecified site
M85.11   Skeletal fluorosis, shoulder
M85.111   Skeletal fluorosis, right shoulder
M85.112   Skeletal fluorosis, left shoulder
M85.119   Skeletal fluorosis, unspecified shoulder

M85.12   Skeletal fluorosis, upper arm
M85.121   Skeletal fluorosis, right upper arm
M85.122   Skeletal fluorosis, left upper arm
M85.129   Skeletal fluorosis, unspecified upper arm

M85.13   Skeletal fluorosis, forearm
M85.131   Skeletal fluorosis, right forearm
M85.132   Skeletal fluorosis, left forearm
M85.139   Skeletal fluorosis, unspecified forearm

M85.14   Skeletal fluorosis, hand
M85.141   Skeletal fluorosis, right hand
M85.142   Skeletal fluorosis, left hand
M85.149   Skeletal fluorosis, unspecified hand

M85.15   Skeletal fluorosis, thigh
M85.151   Skeletal fluorosis, right thigh
M85.152   Skeletal fluorosis, left thigh
M85.159   Skeletal fluorosis, unspecified thigh

M85.16   Skeletal fluorosis, lower leg
M85.161   Skeletal fluorosis, right lower leg
M85.162   Skeletal fluorosis, left lower leg
M85.169   Skeletal fluorosis, unspecified lower leg

M85.17   Skeletal fluorosis, ankle and foot
M85.171   Skeletal fluorosis, right ankle and foot
M85.172   Skeletal fluorosis, left ankle and foot
M85.179   Skeletal fluorosis, unspecified ankle and foot

M85.18   Skeletal fluorosis, other site
M85.19   Skeletal fluorosis, multiple sites

M85.2   Hyperostosis of skull

M85.3   Osteitis condensans

M85.30   Osteitis condensans, unspecified site
M85.31   Osteitis condensans, shoulder
M85.311   Osteitis condensans, right shoulder
M85.312   Osteitis condensans, left shoulder
M85.319   Osteitis condensans, unspecified shoulder

M85.32   Osteitis condensans, upper arm
M85.321   Osteitis condensans, right upper arm
M85.322   Osteitis condensans, left upper arm
M85.329   Osteitis condensans, unspecified upper arm

M85.33   Osteitis condensans, forearm
M85.331   Osteitis condensans, right forearm
M85.332   Osteitis condensans, left forearm
M85.339   Osteitis condensans, unspecified forearm

M85.34   Osteitis condensans, hand
M85.341   Osteitis condensans, right hand
M85.342   Osteitis condensans, left hand
M85.349   Osteitis condensans, unspecified hand

M85.35   Osteitis condensans, thigh
M85.351   Osteitis condensans, right thigh
M85.352   Osteitis condensans, left thigh
M85.359   Osteitis condensans, unspecified thigh

M85.36   Osteitis condensans, lower leg
M85.361   Osteitis condensans, right lower leg
M85.362   Osteitis condensans, left lower leg
M85.369   Osteitis condensans, unspecified lower leg

M85.37   Osteitis condensans, ankle and foot
M85.371   Osteitis condensans, right ankle and foot
M85.372   Osteitis condensans, left ankle and foot
M85.379   Osteitis condensans, unspecified ankle and foot

M85.38   Osteitis condensans, vertebrae
M85.39   Osteitis condensans, multiple sites

M85.4   Solitary bone cyst

Excludes2:   solitary cyst of jaw (M27.4)

M85.40   Solitary bone cyst, unspecified site
M85.41   Solitary bone cyst, shoulder
M85.411   Solitary bone cyst, right shoulder
M85.412   Solitary bone cyst, left shoulder
M85.419   Solitary bone cyst, unspecified shoulder

M85.42   Solitary bone cyst, humerus
M85.421   Solitary bone cyst, right humerus
M85.422   Solitary bone cyst, left humerus
M85.429   Solitary bone cyst, unspecified humerus

M85.43   Solitary bone cyst, ulna and radius
M85.431   Solitary bone cyst, right ulna and radius
M85.432   Solitary bone cyst, left ulna and radius
M85.439   Solitary bone cyst, unspecified ulna and radius

M85.44   Solitary bone cyst, hand
M85.441   Solitary bone cyst, right hand
M85.442   Solitary bone cyst, left hand
M85.449   Solitary bone cyst, unspecified hand

M85.45   Solitary bone cyst, pelvis
M85.451   Solitary bone cyst, right pelvis
M85.452   Solitary bone cyst, left pelvis
M85.459   Solitary bone cyst, unspecified pelvis

M85.46   Solitary bone cyst, tibia and fibula
M85.461   Solitary bone cyst, right tibia and fibula
M85.462   Solitary bone cyst, left tibia and fibula
M85.469   Solitary bone cyst, unspecified tibia and fibula

M85.47   Solitary bone cyst, ankle and foot
M85.471   Solitary bone cyst, right ankle and foot
M85.472   Solitary bone cyst, left ankle and foot
M85.479   Solitary bone cyst, unspecified ankle and foot

M85.48   Solitary bone cyst, other site

M85.5   Aneurysmal bone cyst

Excludes2:   aneurysmal cyst of jaw (M27.4)

M85.50   Aneurysmal bone cyst, unspecified site
M85.51   Aneurysmal bone cyst, shoulder
M85.511   Aneurysmal bone cyst, right shoulder
M85.512   Aneurysmal bone cyst, left shoulder
M85.519   Aneurysmal bone cyst, unspecified shoulder

M85.52   Aneurysmal bone cyst, upper arm
M85.521   Aneurysmal bone cyst, right upper arm
M85.522   Aneurysmal bone cyst, left upper arm
M85.529   Aneurysmal bone cyst, unspecified upper arm

M85.53   Aneurysmal bone cyst, forearm
M85.531   Aneurysmal bone cyst, right forearm
M85.532   Aneurysmal bone cyst, left forearm
M85.539   Aneurysmal bone cyst, unspecified forearm

M85.54   Aneurysmal bone cyst, hand
- M85.541   Aneurysmal bone cyst, right hand
- M85.542   Aneurysmal bone cyst, left hand
- M85.549   Aneurysmal bone cyst, unspecified hand

M85.55   Aneurysmal bone cyst, thigh
- M85.551   Aneurysmal bone cyst, right thigh
- M85.552   Aneurysmal bone cyst, left thigh
- M85.559   Aneurysmal bone cyst, unspecified thigh

M85.56   Aneurysmal bone cyst, lower leg
- M85.561   Aneurysmal bone cyst, right lower leg
- M85.562   Aneurysmal bone cyst, left lower leg
- M85.569   Aneurysmal bone cyst, unspecified lower leg

M85.57   Aneurysmal bone cyst, ankle and foot
- M85.571   Aneurysmal bone cyst, right ankle and foot
- M85.572   Aneurysmal bone cyst, left ankle and foot
- M85.579   Aneurysmal bone cyst, unspecified ankle and foot

M85.58   Aneurysmal bone cyst, other site

M85.59   Aneurysmal bone cyst, multiple sites

M85.6   Other cyst of bone

Excludes1:   cyst of jaw NEC (M27.4)
osteitis fibrosa cystica generalisata [von Recklinghausen's disease of bone] (E21.0)

M85.60   Other cyst of bone, unspecified site

M85.61   Other cyst of bone, shoulder
- M85.611   Other cyst of bone, right shoulder
- M85.612   Other cyst of bone, left shoulder
- M85.619   Other cyst of bone, unspecified shoulder

M85.62   Other cyst of bone, upper arm
- M85.621   Other cyst of bone, right upper arm
- M85.622   Other cyst of bone, left upper arm
- M85.629   Other cyst of bone, unspecified upper arm

M85.63   Other cyst of bone, forearm
- M85.631   Other cyst of bone, right forearm
- M85.632   Other cyst of bone, left forearm
- M85.639   Other cyst of bone, unspecified forearm

M85.64   Other cyst of bone, hand
- M85.641   Other cyst of bone, right hand
- M85.642   Other cyst of bone, left hand
- M85.649   Other cyst of bone, unspecified hand

M85.65   Other cyst of bone, thigh
- M85.651   Other cyst of bone, right thigh
- M85.652   Other cyst of bone, left thigh
- M85.659   Other cyst of bone, unspecified thigh

M85.66   Other cyst of bone, lower leg
- M85.661   Other cyst of bone, right lower leg
- M85.662   Other cyst of bone, left lower leg
- M85.669   Other cyst of bone, unspecified lower leg

M85.67   Other cyst of bone, ankle and foot
- M85.671   Other cyst of bone, right ankle and foot
- M85.672   Other cyst of bone, left ankle and foot
- M85.679   Other cyst of bone, unspecified ankle and foot

M85.68   Other cyst of bone, other site

M85.69   Other cyst of bone, multiple sites

M85.8   Other specified disorders of bone density and structure

Hyperostosis of bones, except skull

Excludes1:   diffuse idiopathic skeletal hyperostosis [DISH] (M48.1)

M85.80   Other specified disorders of bone density and structure, unspecified site

M85.81   Other specified disorders of bone density and structure, shoulder
- M85.811   Other specified disorders of bone density and structure, right shoulder
- M85.812   Other specified disorders of bone density and structure, left shoulder
- M85.819   Other specified disorders of bone density and structure, unspecified shoulder

M85.82   Other specified disorders of bone density and structure, upper arm
- M85.821   Other specified disorders of bone density and structure, right upper arm
- M85.822   Other specified disorders of bone density and structure, left upper arm
- M85.829   Other specified disorders of bone density and structure, unspecified upper arm

M85.83   Other specified disorders of bone density and structure, forearm
- M85.831   Other specified disorders of bone density and structure, right forearm
- M85.832   Other specified disorders of bone density and structure, left forearm
- M85.839   Other specified disorders of bone density and structure, unspecified forearm

M85.84   Other specified disorders of bone density and structure, hand
- M85.841   Other specified disorders of bone density and structure, right hand
- M85.842   Other specified disorders of bone density and structure, left hand
- M85.849   Other specified disorders of bone density and structure, unspecified hand

M85.85   Other specified disorders of bone density and structure, thigh
- M85.851   Other specified disorders of bone density and structure, right thigh
- M85.852   Other specified disorders of bone density and structure, left thigh
- M85.859   Other specified disorders of bone density and structure, unspecified thigh

M85.86   Other specified disorders of bone density and structure, lower leg
- M85.861   Other specified disorders of bone density and structure, right lower leg
- M85.862   Other specified disorders of bone density and structure, left lower leg
- M85.869   Other specified disorders of bone density and structure, unspecified lower leg

M85.87   Other specified disorders of bone density and structure, ankle and foot
- M85.871   Other specified disorders of bone density and structure, right ankle and foot
- M85.872   Other specified disorders of bone density and structure, left ankle and foot
- M85.879   Other specified disorders of bone density and structure, unspecified ankle and foot

M85.88   Other specified disorders of bone density and structure, other site

M85.89   Other specified disorders of bone density and structure, multiple sites

M85.9   Disorder of bone density and structure, unspecified

OTHER OSTEOPATHIES (M86–M90)

Excludes1:   postprocedural osteopathies (M96.-)

M86 Osteomyelitis

Use additional code (B95-B97) to identify infectious agent.

Excludes1:   osteomyelitis due to:
echinococcus (B67.2)
gonococcus (A54.43)
salmonella (A02.24)

Excludes2:   osteomyelitis of:
jaw (K10.2)
orbit (H05.0-)
petrous bone (H70.2-)
vertebra (M46.2-)

M86.0   Acute hematogenous osteomyelitis

M86.00   Acute hematogenous osteomyelitis, unspecified site

M86.01   Acute hematogenous osteomyelitis, shoulder
- M86.011   Acute hematogenous osteomyelitis, right shoulder

M86.012   Acute hematogenous osteomyelitis, left shoulder

M86.019   Acute hematogenous osteomyelitis, unspecified shoulder

M86.02   Acute hematogenous osteomyelitis, humerus

M86.021   Acute hematogenous osteomyelitis, right humerus

M86.022   Acute hematogenous osteomyelitis, left humerus

M86.029   Acute hematogenous osteomyelitis, unspecified humerus

M86.03   Acute hematogenous osteomyelitis, radius and ulna

M86.031   Acute hematogenous osteomyelitis, right radius and ulna

M86.032   Acute hematogenous osteomyelitis, left radius and ulna

M86.039   Acute hematogenous osteomyelitis, unspecified radius and ulna

M86.04   Acute hematogenous osteomyelitis, hand

M86.041   Acute hematogenous osteomyelitis, right hand

M86.042   Acute hematogenous osteomyelitis, left hand

M86.049   Acute hematogenous osteomyelitis, unspecified hand

M86.05   Acute hematogenous osteomyelitis, femur

M86.051   Acute hematogenous osteomyelitis, right femur

M86.052   Acute hematogenous osteomyelitis, left femur

M86.059   Acute hematogenous osteomyelitis, unspecified femur

M86.06   Acute hematogenous osteomyelitis, tibia and fibula

M86.061   Acute hematogenous osteomyelitis, right tibia and fibula

M86.062   Acute hematogenous osteomyelitis, left tibia and fibula

M86.069   Acute hematogenous osteomyelitis, unspecified tibia and fibula

M86.07   Acute hematogenous osteomyelitis, ankle and foot

M86.071   Acute hematogenous osteomyelitis, right ankle and foot

M86.072   Acute hematogenous osteomyelitis, left ankle and foot

M86.079   Acute hematogenous osteomyelitis, unspecified ankle and foot

M86.08   Acute hematogenous osteomyelitis, other sites

M86.09   Acute hematogenous osteomyelitis, multiple sites

M86.1   Other acute osteomyelitis

M86.10   Other acute osteomyelitis, unspecified site

M86.11   Other acute osteomyelitis, shoulder

M86.111   Other acute osteomyelitis, right shoulder

M86.112   Other acute osteomyelitis, left shoulder

M86.119   Other acute osteomyelitis, unspecified shoulder

M86.12   Other acute osteomyelitis, humerus

M86.121   Other acute osteomyelitis, right humerus

M86.122   Other acute osteomyelitis, left humerus

M86.129   Other acute osteomyelitis, unspecified humerus

M86.13   Other acute osteomyelitis, radius and ulna

M86.131   Other acute osteomyelitis, right radius and ulna

M86.132   Other acute osteomyelitis, left radius and ulna

M86.139   Other acute osteomyelitis, unspecified radius and ulna

M86.14   Other acute osteomyelitis, hand

M86.141   Other acute osteomyelitis, right hand

M86.142   Other acute osteomyelitis, left hand

M86.149   Other acute osteomyelitis, unspecified hand

M86.15   Other acute osteomyelitis, femur

M86.151   Other acute osteomyelitis, right femur

M86.152   Other acute osteomyelitis, left femur

M86.159   Other acute osteomyelitis, unspecified femur

M86.16   Other acute osteomyelitis, tibia and fibula

M86.161   Other acute osteomyelitis, right tibia and fibula

M86.162   Other acute osteomyelitis, left tibia and fibula

M86.169   Other acute osteomyelitis, unspecified tibia and fibula

M86.17   Other acute osteomyelitis, ankle and foot

M86.171   Other acute osteomyelitis, right ankle and foot

M86.172   Other acute osteomyelitis, left ankle and foot

M86.179   Other acute osteomyelitis, unspecified ankle and foot

M86.18   Other acute osteomyelitis, other site

M86.19   Other acute osteomyelitis, multiple sites

M86.2   Subacute osteomyelitis

M86.20   Subacute osteomyelitis, unspecified site

M86.21   Subacute osteomyelitis, shoulder

M86.211   Subacute osteomyelitis, right shoulder

M86.212   Subacute osteomyelitis, left shoulder

M86.219   Subacute osteomyelitis, unspecified shoulder

M86.22   Subacute osteomyelitis, humerus

M86.221   Subacute osteomyelitis, right humerus

M86.222   Subacute osteomyelitis, left humerus

M86.229   Subacute osteomyelitis, unspecified humerus

M86.23   Subacute osteomyelitis, radius and ulna

M86.231   Subacute osteomyelitis, right radius and ulna

M86.232   Subacute osteomyelitis, left radius and ulna

M86.239   Subacute osteomyelitis, unspecified radius and ulna

M86.24   Subacute osteomyelitis, hand

M86.241   Subacute osteomyelitis, right hand

M86.242   Subacute osteomyelitis, left hand

M86.249   Subacute osteomyelitis, unspecified hand

M86.25   Subacute osteomyelitis, femur

M86.251   Subacute osteomyelitis, right femur

M86.252   Subacute osteomyelitis, left femur

M86.259   Subacute osteomyelitis, unspecified femur

M86.26   Subacute osteomyelitis, tibia and fibula

M86.261   Subacute osteomyelitis, right tibia and fibula

M86.262   Subacute osteomyelitis, left tibia and fibula

M86.269   Subacute osteomyelitis, unspecified tibia and fibula

M86.27   Subacute osteomyelitis, ankle and foot

M86.271   Subacute osteomyelitis, right ankle and foot

M86.272   Subacute osteomyelitis, left ankle and foot

M86.279   Subacute osteomyelitis, unspecified ankle and foot

M86.28   Subacute osteomyelitis, other site

M86.29   Subacute osteomyelitis, multiple sites

M86.3   Chronic multifocal osteomyelitis

M86.30   Chronic multifocal osteomyelitis, unspecified site

M86.31   Chronic multifocal osteomyelitis, shoulder

M86.311   Chronic multifocal osteomyelitis, right shoulder

M86.312   Chronic multifocal osteomyelitis, left shoulder

M86.319   Chronic multifocal osteomyelitis, unspecified shoulder

M86.32   Chronic multifocal osteomyelitis, humerus

M86.321   Chronic multifocal osteomyelitis, right humerus

M86.322   Chronic multifocal osteomyelitis, left humerus

M86.329   Chronic multifocal osteomyelitis, unspecified humerus

M86.33   Chronic multifocal osteomyelitis, radius and ulna

M86.331   Chronic multifocal osteomyelitis, right radius and ulna

M86.332   Chronic multifocal osteomyelitis, left radius and ulna

DRAFT

M86.339   Chronic multifocal osteomyelitis, unspecified radius and ulna

M86.34   Chronic multifocal osteomyelitis, hand

M86.341   Chronic multifocal osteomyelitis, right hand

M86.342   Chronic multifocal osteomyelitis, left hand

M86.349   Chronic multifocal osteomyelitis, unspecified hand

M86.35   Chronic multifocal osteomyelitis, femur

M86.351   Chronic multifocal osteomyelitis, right femur

M86.352   Chronic multifocal osteomyelitis, left femur

M86.359   Chronic multifocal osteomyelitis, unspecified femur

M86.36   Chronic multifocal osteomyelitis, tibia and fibula

M86.361   Chronic multifocal osteomyelitis, right tibia and fibula

M86.362   Chronic multifocal osteomyelitis, left tibia and fibula

M86.369   Chronic multifocal osteomyelitis, unspecified tibia and fibula

M86.37   Chronic multifocal osteomyelitis, ankle and foot

M86.371   Chronic multifocal osteomyelitis, right ankle and foot

M86.372   Chronic multifocal osteomyelitis, left ankle and foot

M86.379   Chronic multifocal osteomyelitis, unspecified ankle and foot

M86.38   Chronic multifocal osteomyelitis, other site

M86.39   Chronic multifocal osteomyelitis, multiple sites

M86.4   Chronic osteomyelitis with draining sinus

M86.40   Chronic osteomyelitis with draining sinus, unspecified site

M86.41   Chronic osteomyelitis with draining sinus, shoulder

M86.411   Chronic osteomyelitis with draining sinus, right shoulder

M86.412   Chronic osteomyelitis with draining sinus, left shoulder

M86.419   Chronic osteomyelitis with draining sinus, unspecified shoulder

M86.42   Chronic osteomyelitis with draining sinus, humerus

M86.421   Chronic osteomyelitis with draining sinus, right humerus

M86.422   Chronic osteomyelitis with draining sinus, left humerus

M86.429   Chronic osteomyelitis with draining sinus, unspecified humerus

M86.43   Chronic osteomyelitis with draining sinus, forearm

M86.431   Chronic osteomyelitis with draining sinus, right forearm

M86.432   Chronic osteomyelitis with draining sinus, left forearm

M86.439   Chronic osteomyelitis with draining sinus, unspecified forearm

M86.44   Chronic osteomyelitis with draining sinus, hand

M86.441   Chronic osteomyelitis with draining sinus, right hand

M86.442   Chronic osteomyelitis with draining sinus, left hand

M86.449   Chronic osteomyelitis with draining sinus, unspecified hand

M86.45   Chronic osteomyelitis with draining sinus, femur

M86.451   Chronic osteomyelitis with draining sinus, right femur

M86.452   Chronic osteomyelitis with draining sinus, left femur

M86.459   Chronic osteomyelitis with draining sinus, unspecified femur

M86.46   Chronic osteomyelitis with draining sinus, lower leg

M86.461   Chronic osteomyelitis with draining sinus, right lower leg

M86.462   Chronic osteomyelitis with draining sinus, left lower leg

M86.469   Chronic osteomyelitis with draining sinus, unspecified lower leg

M86.47   Chronic osteomyelitis with draining sinus, ankle and foot

M86.471   Chronic osteomyelitis with draining sinus, right ankle and foot

M86.472   Chronic osteomyelitis with draining sinus, left ankle and foot

M86.479   Chronic osteomyelitis with draining sinus, unspecified ankle and foot

M86.48   Chronic osteomyelitis with draining sinus, other site

M86.49   Chronic osteomyelitis with draining sinus, multiple sites

M86.5   Other chronic hematogenous osteomyelitis

M86.50   Other chronic hematogenous osteomyelitis, unspecified site

M86.51   Other chronic hematogenous osteomyelitis, shoulder

M86.511   Other chronic hematogenous osteomyelitis, right shoulder

M86.512   Other chronic hematogenous osteomyelitis, left shoulder

M86.519   Other chronic hematogenous osteomyelitis, unspecified shoulder

M86.52   Other chronic hematogenous osteomyelitis, humerus

M86.521   Other chronic hematogenous osteomyelitis, right humerus

M86.522   Other chronic hematogenous osteomyelitis, left humerus

M86.529   Other chronic hematogenous osteomyelitis, unspecified humerus

M86.53   Other chronic hematogenous osteomyelitis, forearm

M86.531   Other chronic hematogenous osteomyelitis, right forearm

M86.532   Other chronic hematogenous osteomyelitis, left forearm

M86.539   Other chronic hematogenous osteomyelitis, unspecified forearm

M86.54   Other chronic hematogenous osteomyelitis, hand

M86.541   Other chronic hematogenous osteomyelitis, right hand

M86.542   Other chronic hematogenous osteomyelitis, left hand

M86.549   Other chronic hematogenous osteomyelitis, unspecified hand

M86.55   Other chronic hematogenous osteomyelitis, femur

M86.551   Other chronic hematogenous osteomyelitis, right femur

M86.552   Other chronic hematogenous osteomyelitis, left femur

M86.559   Other chronic hematogenous osteomyelitis, unspecified femur

M86.56   Other chronic hematogenous osteomyelitis, lower leg

M86.561   Other chronic hematogenous osteomyelitis, right lower leg

M86.562   Other chronic hematogenous osteomyelitis, left lower leg

M86.569   Other chronic hematogenous osteomyelitis, unspecified lower leg

M86.57   Other chronic hematogenous osteomyelitis, ankle and foot

M86.571   Other chronic hematogenous osteomyelitis, right ankle and foot

M86.572   Other chronic hematogenous osteomyelitis, left ankle and foot

M86.579   Other chronic hematogenous osteomyelitis, unspecified ankle and foot

M86.58   Other chronic hematogenous osteomyelitis, other site

M86.59   Other chronic hematogenous osteomyelitis, multiple sites

M86.6   Other chronic osteomyelitis

M86.60   Other chronic osteomyelitis, unspecified site

M86.61   Other chronic osteomyelitis, shoulder

M86.611   Other chronic osteomyelitis, right shoulder
M86.612   Other chronic osteomyelitis, left shoulder
M86.619   Other chronic osteomyelitis, unspecified shoulder
M86.62   Other chronic osteomyelitis, upper arm
M86.621   Other chronic osteomyelitis, right upper arm
M86.622   Other chronic osteomyelitis, left upper arm
M86.629   Other chronic osteomyelitis, unspecified upper arm
M86.63   Other chronic osteomyelitis, forearm
M86.631   Other chronic osteomyelitis, right forearm
M86.632   Other chronic osteomyelitis, left forearm
M86.639   Other chronic osteomyelitis, unspecified forearm
M86.64   Other chronic osteomyelitis, hand
M86.641   Other chronic osteomyelitis, right hand
M86.642   Other chronic osteomyelitis, left hand
M86.649   Other chronic osteomyelitis, unspecified hand
M86.65   Other chronic osteomyelitis, thigh
M86.651   Other chronic osteomyelitis, right thigh
M86.652   Other chronic osteomyelitis, left thigh
M86.659   Other chronic osteomyelitis, unspecified thigh
M86.66   Other chronic osteomyelitis, lower leg
M86.661   Other chronic osteomyelitis, right lower leg
M86.662   Other chronic osteomyelitis, left lower leg
M86.669   Other chronic osteomyelitis, unspecified lower leg
M86.67   Other chronic osteomyelitis, ankle and foot
M86.671   Other chronic osteomyelitis, right ankle and foot
M86.672   Other chronic osteomyelitis, left ankle and foot
M86.679   Other chronic osteomyelitis, unspecified ankle and foot
M86.68   Other chronic osteomyelitis, other site
M86.69   Other chronic osteomyelitis, multiple sites
M86.8   Other osteomyelitis
   Brodie's abscess
M86.8x   Other osteomyelitis
M86.8x0   Other osteomyelitis, unspecified site
M86.8x1   Other osteomyelitis, shoulder
M86.8x2   Other osteomyelitis, upper arm
M86.8x3   Other osteomyelitis, forearm
M86.8x4   Other osteomyelitis, hand
M86.8x5   Other osteomyelitis, thigh
M86.8x6   Other osteomyelitis, lower leg
M86.8x7   Other osteomyelitis, ankle and foot
M86.8x8   Other osteomyelitis, other site
M86.8x9   Other osteomyelitis, multiple sites
M86.9   Osteomyelitis, unspecified
   Infection of bone NOS
   Periostitis without mention of osteomyelitis

M87 Osteonecrosis
   Includes: avascular necrosis of bone
   Excludes1:   juvenile osteonecrosis (M91-M92)
               osteochondropathies (M90-M93)
M87.0   Idiopathic aseptic necrosis of bone
M87.00   Idiopathic aseptic necrosis of unspecified bone
M87.01   Idiopathic aseptic necrosis of shoulder
      Idiopathic aseptic necrosis of clavicle and scapula
M87.011   Idiopathic aseptic necrosis of right shoulder
M87.012   Idiopathic aseptic necrosis of left shoulder
M87.019   Idiopathic aseptic necrosis of unspecified shoulder
M87.02   Idiopathic aseptic necrosis of humerus
M87.021   Idiopathic aseptic necrosis of right humerus
M87.022   Idiopathic aseptic necrosis of left humerus
M87.029   Idiopathic aseptic necrosis of unspecified humerus

M87.03   Idiopathic aseptic necrosis of radius, ulna and carpus
M87.031   Idiopathic aseptic necrosis of right radius
M87.032   Idiopathic aseptic necrosis of left radius
M87.033   Idiopathic aseptic necrosis of unspecified radius
M87.034   Idiopathic aseptic necrosis of right ulna
M87.035   Idiopathic aseptic necrosis of left ulna
M87.036   Idiopathic aseptic necrosis of unspecified ulna
M87.037   Idiopathic aseptic necrosis of right carpus
M87.038   Idiopathic aseptic necrosis of left carpus
M87.039   Idiopathic aseptic necrosis of unspecified carpus
M87.04   Idiopathic aseptic necrosis of hand and fingers
      Idiopathic aseptic necrosis of metacarpals and phalanges of hands
M87.041   Idiopathic aseptic necrosis of right hand
M87.042   Idiopathic aseptic necrosis of left hand
M87.043   Idiopathic aseptic necrosis of unspecified hand
M87.044   Idiopathic aseptic necrosis of right finger(s)
M87.045   Idiopathic aseptic necrosis of left finger(s)
M87.046   Idiopathic aseptic necrosis of unspecified finger(s)
M87.05   Idiopathic aseptic necrosis of pelvis and femur
M87.050   Idiopathic aseptic necrosis of pelvis
M87.051   Idiopathic aseptic necrosis of right femur
M87.052   Idiopathic aseptic necrosis of left femur
M87.059   Idiopathic aseptic necrosis of unspecified femur
      Idiopathic aseptic necrosis of hip NOS
M87.06   Idiopathic aseptic necrosis of tibia and fibula
M87.061   Idiopathic aseptic necrosis of right tibia
M87.062   Idiopathic aseptic necrosis of left tibia
M87.063   Idiopathic aseptic necrosis of unspecified tibia
M87.064   Idiopathic aseptic necrosis of right fibula
M87.065   Idiopathic aseptic necrosis of left fibula
M87.066   Idiopathic aseptic necrosis of unspecified fibula
M87.07   Idiopathic aseptic necrosis of ankle, foot and toes
      Idiopathic aseptic necrosis of metatarsus, tarsus, and phalanges of toes
M87.071   Idiopathic aseptic necrosis of right ankle
M87.072   Idiopathic aseptic necrosis of left ankle
M87.073   Idiopathic aseptic necrosis of unspecified ankle
M87.074   Idiopathic aseptic necrosis of right foot
M87.075   Idiopathic aseptic necrosis of left foot
M87.076   Idiopathic aseptic necrosis of unspecified foot
M87.077   Idiopathic aseptic necrosis of right toe(s)
M87.078   Idiopathic aseptic necrosis of left toe(s)
M87.079   Idiopathic aseptic necrosis of unspecified toe(s)
M87.08   Idiopathic aseptic necrosis of bone, other site
M87.09   Idiopathic aseptic necrosis of bone, multiple sites
M87.1   Osteonecrosis due to drugs
      Use additional external cause code (Chapter XIX) to identify drug.
M87.10   Osteonecrosis due to drugs, unspecified bone
M87.11   Osteonecrosis due to drugs, shoulder
M87.111   Osteonecrosis due to drugs, right shoulder
M87.112   Osteonecrosis due to drugs, left shoulder
M87.119   Osteonecrosis due to drugs, unspecified shoulder
M87.12   Osteonecrosis due to drugs, humerus
M87.121   Osteonecrosis due to drugs, right humerus
M87.122   Osteonecrosis due to drugs, left humerus
M87.129   Osteonecrosis due to drugs, unspecified humerus
M87.13   Osteonecrosis due to drugs of radius, ulna and carpus
M87.131   Osteonecrosis due to drugs of right radius

M87.132 Osteonecrosis due to drugs of left radius
M87.133 Osteonecrosis due to drugs of unspecified radius
M87.134 Osteonecrosis due to drugs of right ulna
M87.135 Osteonecrosis due to drugs of left ulna
M87.136 Osteonecrosis due to drugs of unspecified ulna
M87.137 Osteonecrosis due to drugs of right carpus
M87.138 Osteonecrosis due to drugs of left carpus
M87.139 Osteonecrosis due to drugs of unspecified carpus
M87.14 Osteonecrosis due to drugs, hand and fingers
M87.141 Osteonecrosis due to drugs, right hand
M87.142 Osteonecrosis due to drugs, left hand
M87.143 Osteonecrosis due to drugs, unspecified hand
M87.144 Osteonecrosis due to drugs, right finger(s)
M87.145 Osteonecrosis due to drugs, left finger(s)
M87.146 Osteonecrosis due to drugs, unspecified finger(s)
M87.15 Osteonecrosis due to drugs, pelvis and femur
M87.150 Osteonecrosis due to drugs, pelvis
M87.151 Osteonecrosis due to drugs, right femur
M87.152 Osteonecrosis due to drugs, left femur
M87.159 Osteonecrosis due to drugs, unspecified femur
M87.16 Osteonecrosis due to drugs, tibia and fibula
M87.161 Osteonecrosis due to drugs, right tibia
M87.162 Osteonecrosis due to drugs, left tibia
M87.163 Osteonecrosis due to drugs, unspecified tibia
M87.164 Osteonecrosis due to drugs, right fibula
M87.165 Osteonecrosis due to drugs, left fibula
M87.166 Osteonecrosis due to drugs, unspecified fibula
M87.17 Osteonecrosis due to drugs, ankle, foot and toes
M87.171 Osteonecrosis due to drugs, right ankle
M87.172 Osteonecrosis due to drugs, left ankle
M87.173 Osteonecrosis due to drugs, unspecified ankle
M87.174 Osteonecrosis due to drugs, right foot
M87.175 Osteonecrosis due to drugs, left foot
M87.176 Osteonecrosis due to drugs, unspecified foot
M87.177 Osteonecrosis due to drugs, right toe(s)
M87.178 Osteonecrosis due to drugs, left toe(s)
M87.179 Osteonecrosis due to drugs, unspecified toe(s)
M87.18 Osteonecrosis due to drugs, other site
M87.19 Osteonecrosis due to drugs, multiple sites
M87.2 Osteonecrosis due to previous trauma
M87.20 Osteonecrosis due to previous trauma, unspecified bone
M87.21 Osteonecrosis due to previous trauma, shoulder
M87.211 Osteonecrosis due to previous trauma, right shoulder
M87.212 Osteonecrosis due to previous trauma, left shoulder
M87.219 Osteonecrosis due to previous trauma, unspecified shoulder
M87.22 Osteonecrosis due to previous trauma, humerus
M87.221 Osteonecrosis due to previous trauma, right humerus
M87.222 Osteonecrosis due to previous trauma, left humerus
M87.229 Osteonecrosis due to previous trauma, unspecified humerus
M87.23 Osteonecrosis due to previous trauma of radius, ulna and carpus
M87.231 Osteonecrosis due to previous trauma of right radius
M87.232 Osteonecrosis due to previous trauma of left radius
M87.233 Osteonecrosis due to previous trauma of unspecified radius
M87.234 Osteonecrosis due to previous trauma of right ulna

M87.235 Osteonecrosis due to previous trauma of left ulna
M87.236 Osteonecrosis due to previous trauma of unspecified ulna
M87.237 Osteonecrosis due to previous trauma of right carpus
M87.238 Osteonecrosis due to previous trauma of left carpus
M87.239 Osteonecrosis due to previous trauma of unspecified carpus
M87.24 Osteonecrosis due to previous trauma, hand and fingers
M87.241 Osteonecrosis due to previous trauma, right hand
M87.242 Osteonecrosis due to previous trauma, left hand
M87.243 Osteonecrosis due to previous trauma, unspecified hand
M87.244 Osteonecrosis due to previous trauma, right finger(s)
M87.245 Osteonecrosis due to previous trauma, left finger(s)
M87.246 Osteonecrosis due to previous trauma, unspecified finger(s)
M87.25 Osteonecrosis due to previous trauma, pelvis and femur
M87.250 Osteonecrosis due to previous trauma, pelvis
M87.251 Osteonecrosis due to previous trauma, right femur
M87.252 Osteonecrosis due to previous trauma, left femur
M87.259 Osteonecrosis due to previous trauma, unspecified femur
M87.26 Osteonecrosis due to previous trauma, tibia and fibula
M87.261 Osteonecrosis due to previous trauma, right tibia
M87.262 Osteonecrosis due to previous trauma, left tibia
M87.263 Osteonecrosis due to previous trauma, unspecified tibia
M87.264 Osteonecrosis due to previous trauma, right fibula
M87.265 Osteonecrosis due to previous trauma, left fibula
M87.266 Osteonecrosis due to previous trauma, unspecified fibula
M87.27 Osteonecrosis due to previous trauma, ankle, foot and toes
M87.271 Osteonecrosis due to previous trauma, right ankle
M87.272 Osteonecrosis due to previous trauma, left ankle
M87.273 Osteonecrosis due to previous trauma, unspecified ankle
M87.274 Osteonecrosis due to previous trauma, right foot
M87.275 Osteonecrosis due to previous trauma, left ankle
M87.276 Osteonecrosis due to previous trauma, unspecified ankle
M87.277 Osteonecrosis due to previous trauma, right toe(s)
M87.278 Osteonecrosis due to previous trauma, left toe(s)
M87.279 Osteonecrosis due to previous trauma, unspecified toe(s)
M87.28 Osteonecrosis due to previous trauma, other site
M87.29 Osteonecrosis due to previous trauma, multiple sites
M87.3 Other secondary osteonecrosis
M87.30 Other secondary osteonecrosis, unspecified bone
M87.31 Other secondary osteonecrosis, shoulder
M87.311 Other secondary osteonecrosis, right shoulder

M87.312   Other secondary osteonecrosis, left shoulder
M87.319   Other secondary osteonecrosis, unspecified shoulder
M87.32   Other secondary osteonecrosis, humerus
M87.321   Other secondary osteonecrosis, right humerus
M87.322   Other secondary osteonecrosis, left humerus
M87.329   Other secondary osteonecrosis, unspecified humerus
M87.33   Other secondary osteonecrosis of radius, ulna and carpus
M87.331   Other secondary osteonecrosis of right radius
M87.332   Other secondary osteonecrosis of left radius
M87.333   Other secondary osteonecrosis of unspecified radius
M87.334   Other secondary osteonecrosis of right ulna
M87.335   Other secondary osteonecrosis of left ulna
M87.336   Other secondary osteonecrosis of unspecified ulna
M87.337   Other secondary osteonecrosis of right carpus
M87.338   Other secondary osteonecrosis of left carpus
M87.339   Other secondary osteonecrosis of unspecified carpus
M87.34   Other secondary osteonecrosis, hand and fingers
M87.341   Other secondary osteonecrosis, right hand
M87.342   Other secondary osteonecrosis, left hand
M87.343   Other secondary osteonecrosis, unspecified hand
M87.344   Other secondary osteonecrosis, right finger(s)
M87.345   Other secondary osteonecrosis, left finger(s)
M87.346   Other secondary osteonecrosis, unspecified finger(s)
M87.35   Other secondary osteonecrosis, pelvis and femur
M87.350   Other secondary osteonecrosis, pelvis
M87.351   Other secondary osteonecrosis, right femur
M87.352   Other secondary osteonecrosis, left femur
M87.359   Other secondary osteonecrosis, unspecified femur
M87.36   Other secondary osteonecrosis, tibia and fibula
M87.361   Other secondary osteonecrosis, right tibia
M87.362   Other secondary osteonecrosis, left tibia
M87.363   Other secondary osteonecrosis, unspecified tibia
M87.364   Other secondary osteonecrosis, right fibula
M87.365   Other secondary osteonecrosis, left fibula
M87.366   Other secondary osteonecrosis, unspecified fibula
M87.37   Other secondary osteonecrosis, ankle and foot
M87.371   Other secondary osteonecrosis, right ankle
M87.372   Other secondary osteonecrosis, left ankle
M87.373   Other secondary osteonecrosis, unspecified ankle
M87.374   Other secondary osteonecrosis, right foot
M87.375   Other secondary osteonecrosis, left foot
M87.376   Other secondary osteonecrosis, unspecified foot
M87.377   Other secondary osteonecrosis, right toe(s)
M87.378   Other secondary osteonecrosis, left toe(s)
M87.379   Other secondary osteonecrosis, unspecified toe(s)
M87.38   Other secondary osteonecrosis, other site
M87.39   Other secondary osteonecrosis, multiple sites
M87.8   Other osteonecrosis
M87.80   Other osteonecrosis, unspecified bone
M87.81   Other osteonecrosis, shoulder
M87.811   Other osteonecrosis, right shoulder
M87.812   Other osteonecrosis, left shoulder
M87.819   Other osteonecrosis, unspecified shoulder
M87.82   Other osteonecrosis, humerus
M87.821   Other osteonecrosis, right humerus

M87.822   Other osteonecrosis, left humerus
M87.829   Other osteonecrosis, unspecified humerus
M87.83   Other osteonecrosis of radius, ulna and carpus
M87.831   Other osteonecrosis of right radius
M87.832   Other osteonecrosis of left radius
M87.833   Other osteonecrosis of unspecified radius
M87.834   Other osteonecrosis of right ulna
M87.835   Other osteonecrosis of left ulna
M87.836   Other osteonecrosis of unspecified ulna
M87.837   Other osteonecrosis of right carpus
M87.838   Other osteonecrosis of left carpus
M87.839   Other osteonecrosis of unspecified carpus
M87.84   Other osteonecrosis, hand and fingers
M87.841   Other osteonecrosis, right hand
M87.842   Other osteonecrosis, left hand
M87.843   Other osteonecrosis, unspecified hand
M87.844   Other osteonecrosis, right fingers
M87.845   Other osteonecrosis, left fingers
M87.846   Other osteonecrosis, unspecified fingers
M87.85   Other osteonecrosis, pelvis and femur
M87.850   Other osteonecrosis, pelvis
M87.851   Other osteonecrosis, right femur
M87.852   Other osteonecrosis, left femur
M87.859   Other osteonecrosis, unspecified femur
M87.86   Other osteonecrosis, tibia and fibula
M87.861   Other osteonecrosis, right tibia
M87.862   Other osteonecrosis, left tibia
M87.863   Other osteonecrosis, unspecified tibia
M87.864   Other osteonecrosis, right fibula
M87.865   Other osteonecrosis, left fibula
M87.866   Other osteonecrosis, unspecified fibula
M87.87   Other osteonecrosis, ankle, foot and toes
M87.871   Other osteonecrosis, right ankle
M87.872   Other osteonecrosis, left ankle
M87.873   Other osteonecrosis, unspecified ankle
M87.874   Other osteonecrosis, right foot
M87.875   Other osteonecrosis, left foot
M87.876   Other osteonecrosis, unspecified foot
M87.877   Other osteonecrosis, right toe(s)
M87.878   Other osteonecrosis, left toe(s)
M87.879   Other osteonecrosis, unspecified toe(s)
M87.88   Other osteonecrosis, other site
M87.89   Other osteonecrosis, multiple sites
M87.9   Osteonecrosis, unspecified

M88 Osteitis deformans [Paget's disease of bone]
    Excludes1:   osteitis deformans in neoplastic disease (M90.6)
M88.0   Osteitis deformans of skull
M88.1   Osteitis deformans of vertebrae
M88.8   Osteitis deformans of other bones
M88.81   Osteitis deformans of other bones, shoulder
M88.811   Osteitis deformans of other bones, right shoulder
M88.812   Osteitis deformans of other bones, left shoulder
M88.819   Osteitis deformans of other bones, unspecified shoulder
M88.82   Osteitis deformans of other bones, upper arm
M88.821   Osteitis deformans of other bones, right upper arm
M88.822   Osteitis deformans of other bones, left upper arm
M88.829   Osteitis deformans of other bones, unspecified upper arm
M88.83   Osteitis deformans of other bones, forearm
M88.831   Osteitis deformans of other bones, right forearm
M88.832   Osteitis deformans of other bones, left forearm

M88.839   Osteitis deformans of other bones, unspecified forearm
M88.84   Osteitis deformans of other bones, hand
M88.841   Osteitis deformans of other bones, right hand
M88.842   Osteitis deformans of other bones, left hand
M88.849   Osteitis deformans of other bones, unspecified hand
M88.85   Osteitis deformans of other bones, thigh
M88.851   Osteitis deformans of other bones, right thigh
M88.852   Osteitis deformans of other bones, left thigh
M88.859   Osteitis deformans of other bones, unspecified thigh
M88.86   Osteitis deformans of other bones, lower leg
M88.861   Osteitis deformans of other bones, right lower leg
M88.862   Osteitis deformans of other bones, left lower leg
M88.869   Osteitis deformans of other bones, unspecified lower leg
M88.87   Osteitis deformans of other bones, ankle and foot
M88.871   Osteitis deformans of other bones, right ankle and foot
M88.872   Osteitis deformans of other bones, left ankle and foot
M88.879   Osteitis deformans of other bones, unspecified ankle and foot
M88.88   Osteitis deformans of other bones, other site
      Excludes1:   osteitis deformans of vertebrae (M88.1)
M88.89   Osteitis deformans of other bones, multiple sites
M88.9 Osteitis deformans of bone, unspecified

M89 Other disorders of bone
M89.0 Algoneurodystrophy
      Shoulder-hand syndrome
      Sudeck's atrophy
      Excludes1:   causalgia, lower limb (G57.7-)
                   causalgia, upper limb (G56.4-)
                   complex regional pain syndrome II, lower limb (G57.7-)
                   complex regional pain syndrome II, upper limb (G56.4-)
                   reflex sympathetic dystrophy (G90.5-)
M89.00   Algoneurodystrophy, unspecified site
M89.01   Algoneurodystrophy, shoulder
M89.011   Algoneurodystrophy, right shoulder
M89.012   Algoneurodystrophy, left shoulder
M89.019   Algoneurodystrophy, unspecified shoulder
M89.02   Algoneurodystrophy, upper arm
M89.021   Algoneurodystrophy, right upper arm
M89.022   Algoneurodystrophy, left upper arm
M89.029   Algoneurodystrophy, unspecified upper arm
M89.03   Algoneurodystrophy, forearm
M89.031   Algoneurodystrophy, right forearm
M89.032   Algoneurodystrophy, left forearm
M89.039   Algoneurodystrophy, unspecified forearm
M89.04   Algoneurodystrophy, hand
M89.041   Algoneurodystrophy, right hand
M89.042   Algoneurodystrophy, left hand
M89.049   Algoneurodystrophy, unspecified hand
M89.05   Algoneurodystrophy, thigh
M89.051   Algoneurodystrophy, right thigh
M89.052   Algoneurodystrophy, left thigh
M89.059   Algoneurodystrophy, unspecified thigh
M89.06   Algoneurodystrophy, lower leg
M89.061   Algoneurodystrophy, right lower leg
M89.062   Algoneurodystrophy, left lower leg
M89.069   Algoneurodystrophy, unspecified lower leg
M89.07   Algoneurodystrophy, ankle and foot
M89.071   Algoneurodystrophy, right ankle and foot
M89.072   Algoneurodystrophy, left ankle and foot

M89.079   Algoneurodystrophy, unspecified ankle and foot
M89.08   Algoneurodystrophy, other site
M89.09   Algoneurodystrophy, multiple sites
M89.1 Physeal arrest
      Arrest of growth plate
      Growth plate arrest
M89.12   Physeal arrest, humerus
M89.121   Complete physeal arrest, right proximal humerus
M89.122   Complete physeal arrest, left proximal humerus
M89.123   Partial physeal arrest, right proximal humerus
M89.124   Partial physeal arrest, left proximal humerus
M89.125   Complete physeal arrest, right distal humerus
M89.126   Complete physeal arrest, left distal humerus
M89.127   Partial physeal arrest, right distal humerus
M89.128   Partial physeal arrest, left distal humerus
M89.129   Physeal arrest, humerus, unspecified
M89.13   Physeal arrest, forearm
M89.131   Complete physeal arrest, right distal radius
M89.132   Complete physeal arrest, left distal radius
M89.133   Partial physeal arrest, right distal radius
M89.134   Partial physeal arrest, left distal radius
M89.138   Other physeal arrest of forearm
M89.139   Physeal arrest, forearm, unspecified
M89.15   Physeal arrest, femur
M89.151   Complete physeal arrest, right proximal femur
M89.152   Complete physeal arrest, left proximal femur
M89.153   Partial physeal arrest, right proximal femur
M89.154   Partial physeal arrest, left proximal femur
M89.155   Complete physeal arrest, right distal femur
M89.156   Complete physeal arrest, left distal femur
M89.157   Partial physeal arrest, right distal femur
M89.158   Partial physeal arrest, left distal femur
M89.159   Physeal arrest, femur, unspecified
M89.16   Physeal arrest, lower leg
M89.160   Complete physeal arrest, right proximal tibia
M89.161   Complete physeal arrest, left proximal tibia
M89.162   Partial physeal arrest, right proximal tibia
M89.163   Partial physeal arrest, left proximal tibia
M89.164   Complete physeal arrest, right distal tibia
M89.165   Complete physeal arrest, left distal tibia
M89.166   Partial physeal arrest, right distal tibia
M89.167   Partial physeal arrest, left distal tibia
M89.168   Other physeal arrest of lower leg
M89.169   Physeal arrest, lower leg, unspecified
M89.18   Physeal arrest, other site
M89.2 Other disorders of bone development and growth
M89.20   Other disorders of bone development and growth, unspecified site
M89.21   Other disorders of bone development and growth, shoulder
M89.211   Other disorders of bone development and growth, right shoulder
M89.212   Other disorders of bone development and growth, left shoulder
M89.219   Other disorders of bone development and growth, unspecified shoulder
M89.22   Other disorders of bone development and growth, humerus
M89.221   Other disorders of bone development and growth, right humerus
M89.222   Other disorders of bone development and growth, left humerus
M89.229   Other disorders of bone development and growth, unspecified humerus
M89.23   Other disorders of bone development and growth, ulna and radius

M89.231　Other disorders of bone development and growth, right ulna

M89.232　Other disorders of bone development and growth, left ulna

M89.233　Other disorders of bone development and growth, right radius

M89.234　Other disorders of bone development and growth, left radius

M89.239　Other disorders of bone development and growth, unspecified ulna and radius

M89.24　Other disorders of bone development and growth, hand

M89.241　Other disorders of bone development and growth, right hand

M89.242　Other disorders of bone development and growth, left hand

M89.249　Other disorders of bone development and growth, unspecified hand

M89.25　Other disorders of bone development and growth, femur

M89.251　Other disorders of bone development and growth, right femur

M89.252　Other disorders of bone development and growth, left femur

M89.259　Other disorders of bone development and growth, unspecified femur

M89.26　Other disorders of bone development and growth, tibia and fibula

M89.261　Other disorders of bone development and growth, right tibia

M89.262　Other disorders of bone development and growth, left tibia

M89.263　Other disorders of bone development and growth, right fibula

M89.264　Other disorders of bone development and growth, left fibula

M89.269　Other disorders of bone development and growth, unspecified lower leg

M89.27　Other disorders of bone development and growth, ankle and foot

M89.271　Other disorders of bone development and growth, right ankle and foot

M89.272　Other disorders of bone development and growth, left ankle and foot

M89.279　Other disorders of bone development and growth, unspecified ankle and foot

M89.28　Other disorders of bone development and growth, other site

M89.29　Other disorders of bone development and growth, multiple sites

M89.3　Hypertrophy of bone

M89.30　Hypertrophy of bone, unspecified site

M89.31　Hypertrophy of bone, shoulder

M89.311　Hypertrophy of bone, right shoulder

M89.312　Hypertrophy of bone, left shoulder

M89.319　Hypertrophy of bone, unspecified shoulder

M89.32　Hypertrophy of bone, humerus

M89.321　Hypertrophy of bone, right humerus

M89.322　Hypertrophy of bone, left humerus

M89.329　Hypertrophy of bone, unspecified humerus

M89.33　Hypertrophy of bone, ulna and radius

M89.331　Hypertrophy of bone, right ulna

M89.332　Hypertrophy of bone, left ulna

M89.333　Hypertrophy of bone, right radius

M89.334　Hypertrophy of bone, left radius

M89.339　Hypertrophy of bone, unspecified ulna and radius

M89.34　Hypertrophy of bone, hand

M89.341　Hypertrophy of bone, right hand

M89.342　Hypertrophy of bone, left hand

M89.349　Hypertrophy of bone, unspecified hand

M89.35　Hypertrophy of bone, femur

M89.351　Hypertrophy of bone, right femur

M89.352　Hypertrophy of bone, left femur

M89.359　Hypertrophy of bone, unspecified femur

M89.36　Hypertrophy of bone, tibia and fibula

M89.361　Hypertrophy of bone, right tibia

M89.362　Hypertrophy of bone, left tibia

M89.363　Hypertrophy of bone, right fibula

M89.364　Hypertrophy of bone, left fibula

M89.369　Hypertrophy of bone, unspecified tibia and fibula

M89.37　Hypertrophy of bone, ankle and foot

M89.371　Hypertrophy of bone, right ankle and foot

M89.372　Hypertrophy of bone, left ankle and foot

M89.379　Hypertrophy of bone, unspecified ankle and foot

M89.38　Hypertrophy of bone, other site

M89.39　Hypertrophy of bone, multiple sites

M89.4　Other hypertrophic osteoarthropathy
Marie-Bamberger disease
Pachydermoperiostosis

M89.40　Other hypertrophic osteoarthropathy, unspecified site

M89.41　Other hypertrophic osteoarthropathy, shoulder

M89.411　Other hypertrophic osteoarthropathy, right shoulder

M89.412　Other hypertrophic osteoarthropathy, left shoulder

M89.419　Other hypertrophic osteoarthropathy, unspecified shoulder

M89.42　Other hypertrophic osteoarthropathy, upper arm

M89.421　Other hypertrophic osteoarthropathy, right upper arm

M89.422　Other hypertrophic osteoarthropathy, left upper arm

M89.429　Other hypertrophic osteoarthropathy, unspecified upper arm

M89.43　Other hypertrophic osteoarthropathy, forearm

M89.431　Other hypertrophic osteoarthropathy, right forearm

M89.432　Other hypertrophic osteoarthropathy, left forearm

M89.439　Other hypertrophic osteoarthropathy, unspecified forearm

M89.44　Other hypertrophic osteoarthropathy, hand

M89.441　Other hypertrophic osteoarthropathy, right hand

M89.442　Other hypertrophic osteoarthropathy, left hand

M89.449　Other hypertrophic osteoarthropathy, unspecified hand

M89.45　Other hypertrophic osteoarthropathy, thigh

M89.451　Other hypertrophic osteoarthropathy, right thigh

M89.452　Other hypertrophic osteoarthropathy, left thigh

M89.459　Other hypertrophic osteoarthropathy, unspecified thigh

M89.46　Other hypertrophic osteoarthropathy, lower leg

M89.461　Other hypertrophic osteoarthropathy, right lower leg

M89.462　Other hypertrophic osteoarthropathy, left lower leg

M89.469　Other hypertrophic osteoarthropathy, unspecified lower leg

M89.47　Other hypertrophic osteoarthropathy, ankle and foot

M89.471　Other hypertrophic osteoarthropathy, right ankle and foot

M89.472　Other hypertrophic osteoarthropathy, left ankle and foot

M89.479　Other hypertrophic osteoarthropathy, unspecified ankle and foot

M89.48   Other hypertrophic osteoarthropathy, other site
M89.49   Other hypertrophic osteoarthropathy, multiple sites

M89.5 Osteolysis

M89.50   Osteolysis, unspecified site
M89.51   Osteolysis, shoulder
  M89.511 Osteolysis, right shoulder
  M89.512 Osteolysis, left shoulder
  M89.519 Osteolysis, unspecified shoulder
M89.52   Osteolysis, upper arm
  M89.521 Osteolysis, right upper arm
  M89.522 Osteolysis, left upper arm
  M89.529 Osteolysis, unspecified upper arm
M89.53   Osteolysis, forearm
  M89.531 Osteolysis, right forearm
  M89.532 Osteolysis, left forearm
  M89.539 Osteolysis, unspecified forearm
M89.54   Osteolysis, hand
  M89.541 Osteolysis, right hand
  M89.542 Osteolysis, left hand
  M89.549 Osteolysis, unspecified hand
M89.55   Osteolysis, thigh
  M89.551 Osteolysis, right thigh
  M89.552 Osteolysis, left thigh
  M89.559 Osteolysis, unspecified thigh
M89.56   Osteolysis, lower leg
  M89.561 Osteolysis, right lower leg
  M89.562 Osteolysis, left lower leg
  M89.569 Osteolysis, unspecified lower leg
M89.57   Osteolysis, ankle and foot
  M89.571 Osteolysis, right ankle and foot
  M89.572 Osteolysis, left ankle and foot
  M89.579 Osteolysis, unspecified ankle and foot
M89.58   Osteolysis, other site
M89.59   Osteolysis, multiple sites

M89.6 Osteopathy after poliomyelitis
Use additional code (B91) to identify previous poliomyelitis.

M89.60   Osteopathy after poliomyelitis, unspecified site
M89.61   Osteopathy after poliomyelitis, shoulder
  M89.611 Osteopathy after poliomyelitis, right shoulder
  M89.612 Osteopathy after poliomyelitis, left shoulder
  M89.619 Osteopathy after poliomyelitis, unspecified shoulder
M89.62   Osteopathy after poliomyelitis, upper arm
  M89.621 Osteopathy after poliomyelitis, right upper arm
  M89.622 Osteopathy after poliomyelitis, left upper arm
  M89.629 Osteopathy after poliomyelitis, unspecified upper arm
M89.63   Osteopathy after poliomyelitis, forearm
  M89.631 Osteopathy after poliomyelitis, right forearm
  M89.632 Osteopathy after poliomyelitis, left forearm
  M89.639 Osteopathy after poliomyelitis, unspecified forearm
M89.64   Osteopathy after poliomyelitis, hand
  M89.641 Osteopathy after poliomyelitis, right hand
  M89.642 Osteopathy after poliomyelitis, left hand
  M89.649 Osteopathy after poliomyelitis, unspecified hand
M89.65   Osteopathy after poliomyelitis, thigh
  M89.651 Osteopathy after poliomyelitis, right thigh
  M89.652 Osteopathy after poliomyelitis, left thigh
  M89.659 Osteopathy after poliomyelitis, unspecified thigh
M89.66   Osteopathy after poliomyelitis, lower leg
  M89.661 Osteopathy after poliomyelitis, right lower leg
  M89.662 Osteopathy after poliomyelitis, left lower leg
  M89.669 Osteopathy after poliomyelitis, unspecified lower leg

M89.67   Osteopathy after poliomyelitis, ankle and foot
  M89.671 Osteopathy after poliomyelitis, right ankle and foot
  M89.672 Osteopathy after poliomyelitis, left ankle and foot
  M89.679 Osteopathy after poliomyelitis, unspecified ankle and foot
M89.68   Osteopathy after poliomyelitis, other site
M89.69   Osteopathy after poliomyelitis, multiple sites

M89.8 Other specified disorders of bone
Infantile cortical hyperostoses
Post-traumatic subperiosteal ossification

M89.80   Other specified disorders of bone, unspecified site
M89.81   Other specified disorders of bone, shoulder
M89.82   Other specified disorders of bone, upper arm
M89.83   Other specified disorders of bone, forearm
M89.84   Other specified disorders of bone, hand
M89.85   Other specified disorders of bone, thigh
M89.86   Other specified disorders of bone, lower leg
M89.87   Other specified disorders of bone, ankle and foot
M89.88   Other specified disorders of bone, other site
M89.89   Other specified disorders of bone, multiple sites

M89.9 Disorder of bone, unspecified

M90 Osteopathies in diseases classified elsewhere

Excludes1:   osteochondritis, osteomyelitis, and osteopathy (in):
    cryptococcosis (B45.3)
    diabetes mellitus (E08-E14 with 4th character .61-)
    gonococcal (A54.43)
    neurogenic syphilis (A52.11)
    renal osteodystrophy (N25.0)
    salmonellosis (A02.24)
    secondary syphilis (A51.46)
    syphilis (late) (A52.77)

M90.5 Osteonecrosis in diseases classified elsewhere
Code first underlying disease, such as:
caisson disease (T70.3)
hemoglobinopathy (D50-D64)

M90.50   Osteonecrosis in diseases classified elsewhere, unspecified site
M90.51   Osteonecrosis in diseases classified elsewhere, shoulder
  M90.511 Osteonecrosis in diseases classified elsewhere, right shoulder
  M90.512 Osteonecrosis in diseases classified elsewhere, left shoulder
  M90.519 Osteonecrosis in diseases classified elsewhere, unspecified shoulder
M90.52   Osteonecrosis in diseases classified elsewhere, upper arm
  M90.521 Osteonecrosis in diseases classified elsewhere, right upper arm
  M90.522 Osteonecrosis in diseases classified elsewhere, left upper arm
  M90.529 Osteonecrosis in diseases classified elsewhere, unspecified upper arm
M90.53   Osteonecrosis in diseases classified elsewhere, forearm
  M90.531 Osteonecrosis in diseases classified elsewhere, right forearm
  M90.532 Osteonecrosis in diseases classified elsewhere, left forearm
  M90.539 Osteonecrosis in diseases classified elsewhere, unspecified forearm
M90.54   Osteonecrosis in diseases classified elsewhere, hand
  M90.541 Osteonecrosis in diseases classified elsewhere, right hand
  M90.542 Osteonecrosis in diseases classified elsewhere, left hand
  M90.549 Osteonecrosis in diseases classified elsewhere, unspecified hand
M90.55   Osteonecrosis in diseases classified elsewhere, thigh

       M90.551 Osteonecrosis in diseases classified elsewhere, right thigh

       M90.552 Osteonecrosis in diseases classified elsewhere, left thigh

       M90.559 Osteonecrosis in diseases classified elsewhere, unspecified thigh

    M90.56 Osteonecrosis in diseases classified elsewhere, lower leg

       M90.561 Osteonecrosis in diseases classified elsewhere, right lower leg

       M90.562 Osteonecrosis in diseases classified elsewhere, left lower leg

       M90.569 Osteonecrosis in diseases classified elsewhere, unspecified lower leg

    M90.57 Osteonecrosis in diseases classified elsewhere, ankle and foot

       M90.571 Osteonecrosis in diseases classified elsewhere, right ankle and foot

       M90.572 Osteonecrosis in diseases classified elsewhere, left ankle and foot

       M90.579 Osteonecrosis in diseases classified elsewhere, unspecified ankle and foot

    M90.58 Osteonecrosis in diseases classified elsewhere, other site

    M90.59 Osteonecrosis in diseases classified elsewhere, multiple sites

M90.6 Osteitis deformans in neoplastic diseases

    Osteitis deformans in malignant neoplasm of bone

    Code first the neoplasm (C40.-, C41.-)

    Excludes1:   osteitis deformans [Paget's disease of bone] (M88.-)

    M90.60 Osteitis deformans in neoplastic diseases, unspecified site

    M90.61 Osteitis deformans in neoplastic diseases, shoulder

       M90.611 Osteitis deformans in neoplastic diseases, right shoulder

       M90.612 Osteitis deformans in neoplastic diseases, left shoulder

       M90.619 Osteitis deformans in neoplastic diseases, unspecified shoulder

    M90.62 Osteitis deformans in neoplastic diseases, upper arm

       M90.621 Osteitis deformans in neoplastic diseases, right upper arm

       M90.622 Osteitis deformans in neoplastic diseases, left upper arm

       M90.629 Osteitis deformans in neoplastic diseases, unspecified upper arm

M90.6 Osteitis deformans in neoplastic diseases, forearm

       M90.631 Osteitis deformans in neoplastic diseases, right forearm

       M90.632 Osteitis deformans in neoplastic diseases, left forearm

       M90.639 Osteitis deformans in neoplastic diseases, unspecified forearm

    M90.64 Osteitis deformans in neoplastic diseases, hand

       M90.641 Osteitis deformans in neoplastic diseases, right hand

       M90.642 Osteitis deformans in neoplastic diseases, left hand

       M90.649 Osteitis deformans in neoplastic diseases, unspecified hand

    M90.65 Osteitis deformans in neoplastic diseases, thigh

       M90.651 Osteitis deformans in neoplastic diseases, right thigh

       M90.652 Osteitis deformans in neoplastic diseases, left thigh

       M90.659 Osteitis deformans in neoplastic diseases, unspecified thigh

    M90.66 Osteitis deformans in neoplastic diseases, lower leg

       M90.661 Osteitis deformans in neoplastic diseases, right lower leg

       M90.662 Osteitis deformans in neoplastic diseases, left lower leg

       M90.669 Osteitis deformans in neoplastic diseases, unspecified lower leg

    M90.67 Osteitis deformans in neoplastic diseases, ankle and foot

       M90.671 Osteitis deformans in neoplastic diseases, right ankle and foot

       M90.672 Osteitis deformans in neoplastic diseases, left ankle and foot

       M90.679 Osteitis deformans in neoplastic diseases, unspecified ankle and foot

    M90.68 Osteitis deformans in neoplastic diseases, other site

    M90.69 Osteitis deformans in neoplastic diseases, multiple sites

M90.8 Osteopathy in diseases classified elsewhere

    Code first underlying disease, such as:

      rickets (E55.0)

      vitamin-D-resistant rickets (E83.3)

    M90.80 Osteopathy in diseases classified elsewhere, unspecified site

    M90.81 Osteopathy in diseases classified elsewhere, shoulder

       M90.811 Osteopathy in diseases classified elsewhere, right shoulder

       M90.812 Osteopathy in diseases classified elsewhere, left shoulder

       M90.819 Osteopathy in diseases classified elsewhere, unspecified shoulder

    M90.82 Osteopathy in diseases classified elsewhere, upper arm

       M90.821 Osteopathy in diseases classified elsewhere, right upper arm

       M90.822 Osteopathy in diseases classified elsewhere, left upper arm

       M90.829 Osteopathy in diseases classified elsewhere, unspecified upper arm

    M90.83 Osteopathy in diseases classified elsewhere, forearm

       M90.831 Osteopathy in diseases classified elsewhere, right forearm

       M90.832 Osteopathy in diseases classified elsewhere, left forearm

       M90.839 Osteopathy in diseases classified elsewhere, unspecified forearm

    M90.84 Osteopathy in diseases classified elsewhere, hand

       M90.841 Osteopathy in diseases classified elsewhere, right hand

       M90.842 Osteopathy in diseases classified elsewhere, left hand

       M90.849 Osteopathy in diseases classified elsewhere, unspecified hand

    M90.85 Osteopathy in diseases classified elsewhere, thigh

       M90.851 Osteopathy in diseases classified elsewhere, right thigh

       M90.852 Osteopathy in diseases classified elsewhere, left thigh

       M90.859 Osteopathy in diseases classified elsewhere, unspecified thigh

    M90.86 Osteopathy in diseases classified elsewhere, lower leg

       M90.861 Osteopathy in diseases classified elsewhere, right lower leg

       M90.862 Osteopathy in diseases classified elsewhere, left lower leg

       M90.869 Osteopathy in diseases classified elsewhere, unspecified lower leg

    M90.87 Osteopathy in diseases classified elsewhere, ankle and foot

       M90.871 Osteopathy in diseases classified elsewhere, right ankle and foot

       M90.872 Osteopathy in diseases classified elsewhere, left ankle and foot

       M90.879 Osteopathy in diseases classified elsewhere, unspecified ankle and foot

    M90.88 Osteopathy in diseases classified elsewhere, other site

M90.89   Osteopathy in diseases classified elsewhere, multiple sites

CHONDROPATHIES (M91–M94)

Excludes1:   postprocedural chondropathies (M96.-)

M91 Juvenile osteochondrosis of hip and pelvis

Excludes1:   slipped upper femoral epiphysis (nontraumatic) (M93.0)

M91.0   Juvenile osteochondrosis of pelvis
Osteochondrosis (juvenile) of:
acetabulum
iliac crest [Buchanan]
ischiopubic synchondrosis [van Neck]
symphysis pubis [Pierson]

M91.1   Juvenile osteochondrosis of head of femur [Legg-Calvé-Perthes]

   M91.10   Juvenile osteochondrosis of head of femur [Legg-Calvé-Perthes], unspecified leg

   M91.11   Juvenile osteochondrosis of head of femur [Legg-Calvé-Perthes], right leg

   M91.12   Juvenile osteochondrosis of head of femur [Legg-Calvé-Perthes], left leg

M91.2   Coxa plana
Hip deformity due to previous juvenile osteochondrosis

   M91.20   Coxa plana, unspecified hip

   M91.21   Coxa plana, right hip

   M91.22   Coxa plana, left hip

M91.3   Pseudocoxalgia

   M91.30   Pseudocoxalgia, unspecified hip

   M91.31   Pseudocoxalgia, right hip

   M91.32   Pseudocoxalgia, left hip

M91.4   Coxa magna

   M91.40   Coxa magna, unspecified hip

   M91.41   Coxa magna, right hip

   M91.42   Coxa magna, left hip

M91.8   Other juvenile osteochondrosis of hip and pelvis
Juvenile osteochondrosis after reduction of congenital dislocation of hip

   M91.80   Other juvenile osteochondrosis of hip and pelvis, unspecified leg

   M91.81   Other juvenile osteochondrosis of hip and pelvis, right leg

   M91.82   Other juvenile osteochondrosis of hip and pelvis, left leg

M91.9   Juvenile osteochondrosis of hip and pelvis, unspecified

   M91.90   Juvenile osteochondrosis of hip and pelvis, unspecified, unspecified leg

   M91.91   Juvenile osteochondrosis of hip and pelvis, unspecified, right leg

   M91.92   Juvenile osteochondrosis of hip and pelvis, unspecified, left leg

M92 Other juvenile osteochondrosis

M92.0   Juvenile osteochondrosis of humerus
Osteochondrosis (juvenile) of capitulum of humerus [Panner]
Osteochondrosis (juvenile) of head of humerus [Haas]

   M92.00   Juvenile osteochondrosis of humerus, unspecified arm

   M92.01   Juvenile osteochondrosis of humerus, right arm

   M92.02   Juvenile osteochondrosis of humerus, left arm

M92.1   Juvenile osteochondrosis of radius and ulna
Osteochondrosis (juvenile) of lower ulna [Burns]
Osteochondrosis (juvenile) of radial head [Brailsford]

   M92.10   Juvenile osteochondrosis of radius and ulna, unspecified arm

   M92.11   Juvenile osteochondrosis of radius and ulna, right arm

   M92.12   Juvenile osteochondrosis of radius and ulna, left arm

M92.2   Juvenile osteochondrosis, hand

   M92.20   Unspecified juvenile osteochondrosis, hand

     M92.201   Unspecified juvenile osteochondrosis, right hand

     M92.202   Unspecified juvenile osteochondrosis, left hand

     M92.209   Unspecified juvenile osteochondrosis, unspecified hand

   M92.21   Osteochondrosis (juvenile) of carpal lunate [Kienböck]

     M92.211   Osteochondrosis (juvenile) of carpal lunate [Kienböck], right hand

     M92.212   Osteochondrosis (juvenile) of carpal lunate [Kienböck], left hand

     M92.219   Osteochondrosis (juvenile) of carpal lunate [Kienböck], unspecified hand

   M92.22   Osteochondrosis (juvenile) of metacarpal heads [Mauclaire]

     M92.221   Osteochondrosis (juvenile) of metacarpal heads [Mauclaire], right hand

     M92.222   Osteochondrosis (juvenile) of metacarpal heads [Mauclaire], left hand

     M92.229   Osteochondrosis (juvenile) of metacarpal heads [Mauclaire], unspecified hand

   M92.29   Other juvenile osteochondrosis, hand

     M92.291   Other juvenile osteochondrosis, right hand

     M92.292   Other juvenile osteochondrosis, left hand

     M92.299   Other juvenile osteochondrosis, unspecified hand

M92.3   Other juvenile osteochondrosis, upper limb

   M92.30   Other juvenile osteochondrosis, unspecified upper limb

   M92.31   Other juvenile osteochondrosis, right upper limb

   M92.32   Other juvenile osteochondrosis, left upper limb

M92.4   Juvenile osteochondrosis of patella
Osteochondrosis (juvenile) of primary patellar center [Köhler]
Osteochondrosis (juvenile) of secondary patellar centre [Sinding Larsen]

   M92.40   Juvenile osteochondrosis of patella, unspecified knee

   M92.41   Juvenile osteochondrosis of patella, right knee

   M92.42   Juvenile osteochondrosis of patella, left knee

M92.5   Juvenile osteochondrosis of tibia and fibula
Osteochondrosis (juvenile) of proximal tibia [Blount]
Osteochondrosis (juvenile) of tibial tubercle [Osgood-Schlatter]
Tibia vara

   M92.50   Juvenile osteochondrosis of tibia and fibula, unspecified leg

   M92.51   Juvenile osteochondrosis of tibia and fibula, right leg

   M92.52   Juvenile osteochondrosis of tibia and fibula, left leg

M92.6   Juvenile osteochondrosis of tarsus
Osteochondrosis (juvenile) of calcaneum [Sever]
Osteochondrosis (juvenile) of os tibiale externum [Haglund]
Osteochondrosis (juvenile) of talus [Diaz]
Osteochondrosis (juvenile) of tarsal navicular [Köhler]

   M92.60   Juvenile osteochondrosis of tarsus, unspecified ankle

   M92.61   Juvenile osteochondrosis of tarsus, right ankle

   M92.62   Juvenile osteochondrosis of tarsus, left ankle

M92.7   Juvenile osteochondrosis of metatarsus
Osteochondrosis (juvenile) of fifth metatarsus [Iselin]
Osteochondrosis (juvenile) of second metatarsus [Freiberg]

   M92.70   Juvenile osteochondrosis of metatarsus, unspecified foot

   M92.71   Juvenile osteochondrosis of metatarsus, right foot

   M92.72   Juvenile osteochondrosis of metatarsus, left foot

M92.8   Other specified juvenile osteochondrosis
Calcaneal apophysitis

M92.9   Juvenile osteochondrosis, unspecified
Juvenile apophysitis NOS
Juvenile epiphysitis NOS
Juvenile osteochondritis NOS
Juvenile osteochondrosis NOS

M93 Other osteochondropathies

Excludes2:   osteochondrosis of spine (M42.-)

M93.0   Slipped upper femoral epiphysis (nontraumatic)
Use additional code for associated chondrolysis (M94.3)

   M93.00   Unspecified slipped upper femoral epiphysis (nontraumatic)

M93.001 Unspecified slipped upper femoral epiphysis (nontraumatic), right hip
M93.002 Unspecified slipped upper femoral epiphysis (nontraumatic), left hip
M93.003 Unspecified slipped upper femoral epiphysis (nontraumatic), unspecified hip
M93.01 Acute slipped upper femoral epiphysis (nontraumatic)
M93.011 Acute slipped upper femoral epiphysis (nontraumatic), right hip
M93.012 Acute slipped upper femoral epiphysis (nontraumatic), left hip
M93.013 Acute slipped upper femoral epiphysis (nontraumatic), unspecified hip
M93.02 Chronic slipped upper femoral epiphysis (nontraumatic)
M93.021 Chronic slipped upper femoral epiphysis (nontraumatic), right hip
M93.022 Chronic slipped upper femoral epiphysis (nontraumatic), left hip
M93.023 Chronic slipped upper femoral epiphysis nontraumatic), unspecified hip
M93.03 Acute on chronic slipped upper femoral epiphysis (nontraumatic)
M93.031 Acute on chronic slipped upper femoral epiphysis (nontraumatic), right hip
M93.032 Acute on chronic slipped upper femoral epiphysis (nontraumatic), left hip
M93.033 Acute on chronic slipped upper femoral epiphysis (nontraumatic), unspecified hip
M93.1 Kienböck's disease of adults
Adult osteochondrosis of carpal lunates
M93.2 Osteochondritis dissecans
M93.20 Osteochondritis dissecans of unspecified site
M93.21 Osteochondritis dissecans of shoulder
M93.211 Osteochondritis dissecans, right shoulder
M93.212 Osteochondritis dissecans, left shoulder
M93.219 Osteochondritis dissecans, unspecified shoulder
M93.22 Osteochondritis dissecans of elbow
M93.221 Osteochondritis dissecans, right elbow
M93.222 Osteochondritis dissecans, left elbow
M93.229 Osteochondritis dissecans, unspecified elbow
M93.23 Osteochondritis dissecans of wrist
M93.231 Osteochondritis dissecans, right wrist
M93.232 Osteochondritis dissecans, left wrist
M93.239 Osteochondritis dissecans, unspecified wrist
M93.24 Osteochondritis dissecans of joints of hand
M93.241 Osteochondritis dissecans, joints of right hand
M93.242 Osteochondritis dissecans, joints of left hand
M93.249 Osteochondritis dissecans, joints of unspecified hand
M93.25 Osteochondritis dissecans of hip
M93.251 Osteochondritis dissecans, right hip
M93.252 Osteochondritis dissecans, left hip
M93.259 Osteochondritis dissecans, unspecified hip
M93.26 Osteochondritis dissecans knee
M93.261 Osteochondritis dissecans, right knee
M93.262 Osteochondritis dissecans, left knee
M93.269 Osteochondritis dissecans, unspecified knee
M93.27 Osteochondritis dissecans of ankle and joints of foot
M93.271 Osteochondritis dissecans, right ankle and joints of right foot
M93.272 Osteochondritis dissecans, left ankle and joints of left foot
M93.279 Osteochondritis dissecans, unspecified ankle and joints of foot
M93.28 Osteochondritis dissecans other site
M93.29 Osteochondritis dissecans multiple sites
M93.8 Other specified osteochondropathies

M93.80 Other specified osteochondropathies of unspecified site
M93.81 Other specified osteochondropathies of shoulder
M93.811 Other specified osteochondropathies, right shoulder
M93.812 Other specified osteochondropathies, left shoulder
M93.819 Other specified osteochondropathies, unspecified shoulder
M93.82 Other specified osteochondropathies of upper arm
M93.821 Other specified osteochondropathies, right upper arm
M93.822 Other specified osteochondropathies, left upper arm
M93.829 Other specified osteochondropathies, unspecified upper arm
M93.83 Other specified osteochondropathies of forearm
M93.831 Other specified osteochondropathies, right forearm
M93.832 Other specified osteochondropathies, left forearm
M93.839 Other specified osteochondropathies, unspecified forearm
M93.84 Other specified osteochondropathies of hand
M93.841 Other specified osteochondropathies, right hand
M93.842 Other specified osteochondropathies, left hand
M93.849 Other osteochondropathies, unspecified hand
M93.85 Other specified osteochondropathies of thigh
M93.851 Other specified osteochondropathies, right thigh
M93.852 Other specified osteochondropathies, left thigh
M93.859 Other specified osteochondropathies, unspecified thigh
M93.86 Other specified osteochondropathies lower leg
M93.861 Other specified osteochondropathies, right lower leg
M93.862 Other specified osteochondropathies, left lower leg
M93.869 Other specified osteochondropathies, unspecified lower leg
M93.87 Other specified osteochondropathies of ankle and foot
M93.871 Other specified osteochondropathies, right ankle and foot
M93.872 Other specified osteochondropathies, left ankle and foot
M93.879 Other specified osteochondropathies, unspecified ankle and foot
M93.88 Other specified osteochondropathies other
M93.89 Other specified osteochondropathies multiple sites
M93.9 Osteochondropathy, unspecified
Apophysitis NOS
Epiphysitis NOS
Osteochondritis NOS
Osteochondrosis NOS
M93.90 Osteochondropathy, unspecified of unspecified site
M93.91 Osteochondropathy, unspecified of shoulder
M93.911 Osteochondropathy, unspecified, right shoulder
M93.912 Osteochondropathy, unspecified, left shoulder
M93.919 Osteochondropathy, unspecified, unspecified shoulder
M93.92 Osteochondropathy, unspecified of upper arm
M93.921 Osteochondropathy, unspecified, right upper arm
M93.922 Osteochondropathy, unspecified, left upper arm
M93.929 Osteochondropathy, unspecified, unspecified upper arm
M93.93 Osteochondropathy, unspecified of forearm

M93.931   Osteochondropathy, unspecified, right forearm
M93.932   Osteochondropathy, unspecified, left forearm
M93.939   Osteochondropathy, unspecified, unspecified forearm
M93.94   Osteochondropathy, unspecified of hand
M93.941   Osteochondropathy, unspecified, right hand
M93.942   Osteochondropathy, unspecified, left hand
M93.949   Osteochondropathy, unspecified, unspecified hand
M93.95   Osteochondropathy, unspecified of thigh
M93.951   Osteochondropathy, unspecified, right thigh
M93.952   Osteochondropathy, unspecified, left thigh
M93.959   Osteochondropathy, unspecified, unspecified thigh
M93.96   Osteochondropathy, unspecified lower leg
M93.961   Osteochondropathy, unspecified, right lower leg
M93.962   Osteochondropathy, unspecified, left lower leg
M93.969   Osteochondropathy, unspecified, unspecified lower leg
M93.97   Osteochondropathy, unspecified of ankle and foot
M93.971   Osteochondropathy, unspecified, right ankle and foot
M93.972   Osteochondropathy, unspecified, left ankle and foot
M93.979   Osteochondropathy, unspecified, unspecified ankle and foot
M93.98   Osteochondropathy, unspecified other
M93.99   Osteochondropathy, unspecified multiple sites

M94 Other disorders of cartilage
M94.0 Chondrocostal junction syndrome [Tietze]
    Costochondritis
M94.1 Relapsing polychondritis
M94.10   Relapsing polychondritis, unspecified site
M94.11   Relapsing polychondritis, shoulder
M94.111   Relapsing polychondritis, right shoulder
M94.112   Relapsing polychondritis, left shoulder
M94.119   Relapsing polychondritis, unspecified shoulder
M94.12   Relapsing polychondritis, upper arm
M94.121   Relapsing polychondritis, right upper arm
M94.122   Relapsing polychondritis, left upper arm
M94.129   Relapsing polychondritis, unspecified upper arm
M94.13   Relapsing polychondritis, forearm
M94.131   Relapsing polychondritis, right forearm
M94.132   Relapsing polychondritis, left forearm
M94.139   Relapsing polychondritis, unspecified forearm
M94.14   Relapsing polychondritis, hand
M94.141   Relapsing polychondritis, right hand
M94.142   Relapsing polychondritis, left hand
M94.149   Relapsing polychondritis, unspecified hand
M94.15   Relapsing polychondritis, thigh
M94.151   Relapsing polychondritis, right thigh
M94.152   Relapsing polychondritis, left thigh
M94.159   Relapsing polychondritis, unspecified thigh
M94.16   Relapsing polychondritis, lower leg
M94.161   Relapsing polychondritis, right lower leg
M94.162   Relapsing polychondritis, left lower leg
M94.169   Relapsing polychondritis, unspecified lower leg
M94.17   Relapsing polychondritis, ankle and foot
M94.171   Relapsing polychondritis, right ankle and foot
M94.172   Relapsing polychondritis, left ankle and foot
M94.179   Relapsing polychondritis, unspecified ankle and foot
M94.18   Relapsing polychondritis, other site
M94.19   Relapsing polychondritis, multiple sites

M94.2 Chondromalacia
    Excludes1:   chondromalacia patellae (M22.4)
M94.20   Chondromalacia, unspecified site
M94.21   Chondromalacia, shoulder
M94.211   Chondromalacia, right shoulder
M94.212   Chondromalacia, left shoulder
M94.219   Chondromalacia, unspecified shoulder
M94.22   Chondromalacia, elbow
M94.221   Chondromalacia, right elbow
M94.222   Chondromalacia, left elbow
M94.229   Chondromalacia, unspecified elbow
M94.23   Chondromalacia, wrist
M94.231   Chondromalacia, right wrist
M94.232   Chondromalacia, left wrist
M94.239   Chondromalacia, unspecified wrist
M94.24   Chondromalacia, joints of hand
M94.241   Chondromalacia, joints of right hand
M94.242   Chondromalacia, joints of left hand
M94.249   Chondromalacia, joints of unspecified hand
M94.25   Chondromalacia, hip
M94.251   Chondromalacia, right hip
M94.252   Chondromalacia, left hip
M94.259   Chondromalacia, unspecified hip
M94.26   Chondromalacia, knee
M94.261   Chondromalacia, right knee
M94.262   Chondromalacia, left knee
M94.269   Chondromalacia, unspecified knee
M94.27   Chondromalacia, ankle and joints of foot
M94.271   Chondromalacia, right ankle and joints of right foot
M94.272   Chondromalacia, left ankle and joints of left foot
M94.279   Chondromalacia, unspecified ankle and joints of foot
M94.28   Chondromalacia, other site
M94.29   Chondromalacia, multiple sites
M94.3 Chondrolysis
    Code first any associated slipped upper femoral epiphysis (nontraumatic) (M93.0-)
M94.35   Chondrolysis, hip
M94.351   Chondrolysis, right hip
M94.352   Chondrolysis, left hip
M94.359   Chondrolysis, unspecified hip
M94.8 Other specified disorders of cartilage
M94.80   Other specified disorders of cartilage, unspecified site
M94.81   Other specified disorders of cartilage, shoulder
M94.82   Other specified disorders of cartilage, upper arm
M94.83   Other specified disorders of cartilage, forearm
M94.84   Other specified disorders of cartilage, hand
M94.85   Other specified disorders of cartilage, thigh
M94.86   Other specified disorders of cartilage, lower leg
M94.87   Other specified disorders of cartilage, ankle and foot
M94.88   Other specified disorders of cartilage, other site
M94.89   Other specified disorders of cartilage, multiple sites
M94.9 Disorder of cartilage, unspecified

OTHER DISORDERS OF THE MUSCULOSKELETAL SYSTEM AND CONNECTIVE TISSUE (M95–M99)

M95 Other acquired deformities of musculoskeletal system and connective tissue
    Excludes2:   acquired absence of limbs and organs (Z89-Z90)
        acquired deformities of limbs (M20-M21)
        congenital malformations and deformations of the musculoskeletal system (Q65-Q79)
        deforming dorsopathies (M40-M43)
        dentofacial anomalies [including malocclusion] (M26.-)
        postprocedural musculoskeletal disorders (M96.-)

M95.0 Acquired deformity of nose

    Excludes2:   deviated nasal septum (J34.2)

M95.1 Cauliflower ear

    Excludes2:   other acquired deformities of ear (H61.1)

  M95.10   Cauliflower ear, unspecified ear

  M95.11   Cauliflower ear, right ear

  M95.12   Cauliflower ear, left ear

M95.2 Other acquired deformity of head

M95.3 Acquired deformity of neck

M95.4 Acquired deformity of chest and rib

M95.5 Acquired deformity of pelvis

    Excludes1:   maternal care for known or suspected
               disproportion (O33.-)

M95.8 Other specified acquired deformities of musculoskeletal
system

M95.9 Acquired deformity of musculoskeletal system, unspecified

**M96 Intraoperative and postprocedural complications and disorders of
the musculoskeletal system, not elsewhere classified**

    Excludes2:   arthropathy following intestinal bypass (M02.0-)
               disorders associated with osteoporosis (M80)
               presence of functional implants and other devices (Z96-
               Z97)

M96.0 Pseudarthrosis after fusion or arthrodesis

M96.1 Postlaminectomy syndrome, not elsewhere classified

M96.2 Postradiation kyphosis

M96.3 Postlaminectomy kyphosis

M96.4 Postsurgical lordosis

M96.5 Postradiation scoliosis

M96.6 Fracture of bone following insertion of orthopedic implant,
joint prosthesis, or bone plate

    Excludes2:   complication of internal orthopedic devices,
               implants or grafts (T84.-)

  M96.60   Fracture of bone following insertion of orthopedic
implant, joint prosthesis, or bone plate, unspecified
bone

  M96.62   Fracture of humerus following insertion of orthopedic
implant, joint prosthesis, or bone plate

    M96.621   Fracture of humerus following insertion of
orthopedic implant, joint prosthesis, or bone
plate, right arm

    M96.622   Fracture of humerus following insertion of
orthopedic implant, joint prosthesis, or bone
plate, left arm

    M96.629   Fracture of humerus following insertion of
orthopedic implant, joint prosthesis, or bone
plate, unspecified arm

  M96.63   Fracture of radius or ulna following insertion of
orthopedic implant, joint prosthesis, or bone plate

    M96.631   Fracture of radius or ulna following insertion
of orthopedic implant, joint prosthesis, or
bone plate, right arm

    M96.632   Fracture of radius or ulna following insertion
of orthopedic implant, joint prosthesis, or
bone plate, left arm

    M96.639   Fracture of radius or ulna following insertion
of orthopedic implant, joint prosthesis, or
bone plate, unspecified arm

  M96.65   Fracture of pelvis following insertion of orthopedic
implant, joint prosthesis, or bone plate

  M96.66   Fracture of femur following insertion of orthopedic
implant, joint prosthesis, or bone plate

    M96.661   Fracture of femur following insertion of
orthopedic implant, joint prosthesis, or bone
plate, right leg

    M96.662   Fracture of femur following insertion of
orthopedic implant, joint prosthesis, or bone
plate, left leg

    M96.669   Fracture of femur following insertion of
orthopedic implant, joint prosthesis, or bone
plate, unspecified leg

  M96.67   Fracture of tibia or fibula following insertion of
orthopedic implant, joint prosthesis, or bone plate

    M96.671   Fracture of tibia or fibula following insertion
of orthopedic implant, joint prosthesis, or
bone plate, right leg

    M96.672   Fracture of tibia or fibula following insertion
of orthopedic implant, joint prosthesis, or
bone plate, left leg

    M96.679   Fracture of tibia or fibula following insertion
of orthopedic implant, joint prosthesis, or
bone plate, unspecified leg

  M96.69   Fracture of other bone following insertion of
orthopedic implant, joint prosthesis, or bone plate

M96.8 Other intraoperative and postprocedural complications and
disorders of the musculoskeletal system

  M96.81   Intraoperative and postprocedural hemorrhage and
hematoma complicating a musculoskeletal system
procedure

    Excludes1:   intraoperative hemorrhage and
               hematoma due to accidental
               puncture or laceration during a
               musculoskeletal procedure
               (M98.82-)

    M96.811   Intraoperative hemorrhage of a
musculoskeletal structure during a
musculoskeletal system procedure

    M96.812   Intraoperative hemorrhage of a non-
musculoskeletal system structure during a
musculoskeletal system procedure

    M96.813   Intraoperative hematoma of a musculoskeletal
structure during a musculoskeletal system
procedure

    M96.814   Intraoperative hematoma of a non-
musculoskeletal system structure during a
musculoskeletal system procedure

    M96.815   Postprocedural hemorrhage of a
musculoskeletal structure following a
musculoskeletal system procedure

    M96.816   Postprocedural hemorrhage of a non-
musculoskeletal system structure following a
musculoskeletal system procedure

    M96.817   Postprocedural hematoma of a
musculoskeletal structure following a
musculoskeletal system procedure

    M96.818   Postprocedural hematoma of a non-
musculoskeletal system structure following a
musculoskeletal system procedure

  M96.82   Accidental puncture or laceration during a
musculoskeletal system procedure

    M96.821   Accidental puncture or laceration of a
musculoskeletal structure during a
musculoskeletal system procedure

    M96.822   Accidental puncture or laceration of other
structure during a musculoskeletal system
procedure

  M96.89   Other intraoperative and postprocedural complications
and disorders of the musculoskeletal system

    Instability of joint secondary to removal of joint
    prosthesis

M96.9 Postprocedural musculoskeletal disorder, unspecified

M99 Biomechanical lesions, not elsewhere classified

    Note: This category should not be used if the condition can be
classified elsewhere.

M99.0 Segmental and somatic dysfunction

  M99.00   Segmental and somatic dysfunction of head region

  M99.01   Segmental and somatic dysfunction of cervical region

  M99.02   Segmental and somatic dysfunction of thoracic region

  M99.03   Segmental and somatic dysfunction of lumbar region

  M99.04   Segmental and somatic dysfunction of sacral region

  M99.05   Segmental and somatic dysfunction of pelvic region

  M99.06   Segmental and somatic dysfunction of lower extremity

  M99.07   Segmental and somatic dysfunction of upper
extremity

     M99.08   Segmental and somatic dysfunction of rib cage

     M99.09   Segmental and somatic dysfunction of abdomen and other regions

M99.1   Subluxation complex (vertebral)

     M99.10   Subluxation complex (vertebral) of head region

     M99.11   Subluxation complex (vertebral) of cervical region

     M99.12   Subluxation complex (vertebral) of thoracic region

     M99.13   Subluxation complex (vertebral) of lumbar region

     M99.14   Subluxation complex (vertebral) of sacral region

     M99.15   Subluxation complex (vertebral) of pelvic region

     M99.16   Subluxation complex (vertebral) of lower extremity

     M99.17   Subluxation complex (vertebral) of upper extremity

     M99.18   Subluxation complex (vertebral) of rib cage

     M99.19   Subluxation complex (vertebral) of abdomen and other regions

M99.2   Subluxation stenosis of neural canal

     M99.20   Subluxation stenosis of neural canal of head region

     M99.21   Subluxation stenosis of neural canal of cervical region

     M99.22   Subluxation stenosis of neural canal of thoracic region

     M99.23   Subluxation stenosis of neural canal of lumbar region

     M99.24   Subluxation stenosis of neural canal of sacral region

     M99.25   Subluxation stenosis of neural canal of pelvic region

     M99.26   Subluxation stenosis of neural canal of lower extremity

     M99.27   Subluxation stenosis of neural canal of upper extremity

     M99.28   Subluxation stenosis of neural canal of rib cage

     M99.29   Subluxation stenosis of neural canal of abdomen and other regions

M99.3   Osseous stenosis of neural canal

     M99.30   Osseous stenosis of neural canal of head region

     M99.31   Osseous stenosis of neural canal of cervical region

     M99.32   Osseous stenosis of neural canal of thoracic region

     M99.33   Osseous stenosis of neural canal of lumbar region

     M99.34   Osseous stenosis of neural canal of sacral region

     M99.35   Osseous stenosis of neural canal of pelvic region

     M99.36   Osseous stenosis of neural canal of lower extremity

     M99.37   Osseous stenosis of neural canal of upper extremity

     M99.38   Osseous stenosis of neural canal of rib cage

     M99.39   Osseous stenosis of neural canal of abdomen and other regions

M99.4   Connective tissue stenosis of neural canal

     M99.40   Connective tissue stenosis of neural canal of head region

     M99.41   Connective tissue stenosis of neural canal of cervical region

     M99.42   Connective tissue stenosis of neural canal of thoracic region

     M99.43   Connective tissue stenosis of neural canal of lumbar region

     M99.44   Connective tissue stenosis of neural canal of sacral region

     M99.45   Connective tissue stenosis of neural canal of pelvic region

     M99.46   Connective tissue stenosis of neural canal of lower extremity

     M99.47   Connective tissue stenosis of neural canal of upper extremity

     M99.48   Connective tissue stenosis of neural canal of rib cage

     M99.49   Connective tissue stenosis of neural canal of abdomen and other regions

M99.5   Intervertebral disc stenosis of neural canal

     M99.50   Intervertebral disc stenosis of neural canal of head region

     M99.51   Intervertebral disc stenosis of neural canal of cervical region

     M99.52   Intervertebral disc stenosis of neural canal of thoracic region

     M99.53   Intervertebral disc stenosis of neural canal of lumbar region

     M99.54   Intervertebral disc stenosis of neural canal of sacral region

     M99.55   Intervertebral disc stenosis of neural canal of pelvic region

     M99.56   Intervertebral disc stenosis of neural canal of lower extremity

     M99.57   Intervertebral disc stenosis of neural canal of upper extremity

     M99.58   Intervertebral disc stenosis of neural canal of rib cage

     M99.59   Intervertebral disc stenosis of neural canal of abdomen and other regions

M99.6   Osseous and subluxation stenosis of intervertebral foramina

     M99.60   Osseous and subluxation stenosis of intervertebral foramina of head region

     M99.61   Osseous and subluxation stenosis of intervertebral foramina of cervical region

     M99.62   Osseous and subluxation stenosis of intervertebral foramina of thoracic region

     M99.63   Osseous and subluxation stenosis of intervertebral foramina of lumbar region

     M99.64   Osseous and subluxation stenosis of intervertebral foramina of sacral region

     M99.65   Osseous and subluxation stenosis of intervertebral foramina of pelvic region

     M99.66   Osseous and subluxation stenosis of intervertebral foramina of lower extremity

     M99.67   Osseous and subluxation stenosis of intervertebral foramina of upper extremity

     M99.68   Osseous and subluxation stenosis of intervertebral foramina of rib cage

     M99.69   Osseous and subluxation stenosis of intervertebral foramina of abdomen and other regions

M99.7   Connective tissue and disc stenosis of intervertebral foramina

     M99.70   Connective tissue and disc stenosis of intervertebral foramina of head region

     M99.71   Connective tissue and disc stenosis of intervertebral foramina of cervical region

     M99.72   Connective tissue and disc stenosis of intervertebral foramina of thoracic region

     M99.73   Connective tissue and disc stenosis of intervertebral foramina of lumbar region

     M99.74   Connective tissue and disc stenosis of intervertebral foramina of sacral region

     M99.75   Connective tissue and disc stenosis of intervertebral foramina of pelvic region

     M99.76   Connective tissue and disc stenosis of intervertebral foramina of lower extremity

     M99.77   Connective tissue and disc stenosis of intervertebral foramina of upper extremity

     M99.78   Connective tissue and disc stenosis of intervertebral foramina of rib cage

     M99.79   Connective tissue and disc stenosis of intervertebral foramina of abdomen and other regions

M99.8   Other biomechanical lesions

     M99.80   Other biomechanical lesions of head region

     M99.81   Other biomechanical lesions of cervical region

     M99.82   Other biomechanical lesions of thoracic region

     M99.83   Other biomechanical lesions of lumbar region

     M99.84   Other biomechanical lesions of sacral region

     M99.85   Other biomechanical lesions of pelvic region

     M99.86   Other biomechanical lesions of lower extremity

     M99.87   Other biomechanical lesions of upper extremity

     M99.88   Other biomechanical lesions of rib cage

     M99.89   Other biomechanical lesions of abdomen and other regions

M99.9   Biomechanical lesion, unspecified

CHAPTER XIV — DISEASES OF THE GENITOURINARY SYSTEM (N00–N99)

Excludes2:   certain conditions originating in the perinatal period (P04-P96)
certain infectious and parasitic diseases (A00-B99)
complications of pregnancy, childbirth and the puerperium (O00-O99)
congenital malformations, deformations and chromosomal abnormalities (Q00-Q99)
endocrine, nutritional and metabolic diseases (E00-E90)
injury, poisoning and certain other consequences of external causes (S00-T98)
neoplasms (C00-D48)
symptoms, signs and abnormal clinical and laboratory findings, not elsewhere classified (R00-R94

This chapter contains the following blocks:

N00-N08	Glomerular diseases
N10-N16	Renal tubulo-interstitial diseases
N17-N19	Renal failure
N20-N23	Urolithiasis
N25-N29	Other disorders of kidney and ureter
N30-N39	Other diseases of the urinary system
N40-N51	Diseases of male genital organs
N60-N64	Disorders of breast
N70-N77	Inflammatory diseases of female pelvic organs
N80-N98	Noninflammatory disorders of female genital tract
N99	Other disorders of genitourinary system

GLOMERULAR DISEASES (N00–N08)

Use additional code, to identify external cause (Chapter XX) or presence of renal failure (N17-N19).

Excludes1:   hypertensive renal disease (I12.-)

N00   Acute nephritic syndrome

Includes: acute glomerular disease
acute glomerulonephritis
acute nephritis
acute renal disease NOS

Excludes1:   acute tubulo-interstitial nephritis (N10)
nephritic syndrome NOS (N05.)

N00.0   Acute nephritic syndrome with minor glomerular abnormality
Acute nephritic syndrome with minimal change lesion

N00.1   Acute nephritic syndrome with focal and segmental glomerular lesions
Acute nephritic syndrome with focal and segmental hyalinosis
Acute nephritic syndrome with focal and segmental sclerosis
Acute nephritic syndrome with focal glomerulonephritis

N00.2   Acute nephritic syndrome with diffuse membranous glomerulonephritis

N00.3   Acute nephritic syndrome with diffuse mesangial proliferative glomerulonephritis

N00.4   Acute nephritic syndrome with diffuse endocapillary proliferative glomerulonephritis

N00.5   Acute nephritic syndrome with diffuse mesangiocapillary glomerulonephritis
Acute nephritic syndrome with membranoproliferative glomerulonephritis, types 1 and 3, or NOS

N00.6   Acute nephritic syndrome with dense deposit disease
Acute nephritic syndrome with membranoproliferative glomerulonephritis, type 2

N00.7   Acute nephritic syndrome with diffuse crescentic glomerulonephritis
Acute nephritic syndrome with extracapillary glomerulonephritis

N00.8   Acute nephritic syndrome with other morphologic changes
Acute nephritic syndrome with proliferative glomerulonephritis NOS

N00.9   Acute nephritic syndrome with unspecified morphologic changes

N01   Rapidly progressive nephritic syndrome

Includes: rapidly progressive glomerular disease
rapidly progressive glomerulonephritis
rapidly progressive nephritis

Excludes1:   nephritic syndrome NOS (N05.-)

N01.0   Rapidly progressive nephritic syndrome with minor glomerular abnormality
Rapidly progressive nephritic syndrome with minimal change lesion

N01.1   Rapidly progressive nephritic syndrome with focal and segmental glomerular lesions
Rapidly progressive nephritic syndrome with focal and segmental hyalinosis
Rapidly progressive nephritic syndrome with focal and segmental sclerosis
Rapidly progressive nephritic syndrome with focal glomerulonephritis

N01.2   Rapidly progressive nephritic syndrome with diffuse membranous glomerulonephritis

N01.3   Rapidly progressive nephritic syndrome with diffuse mesangial proliferative glomerulonephritis

N01.4   Rapidly progressive nephritic syndrome with diffuse endocapillary proliferative glomerulonephritis

N01.5   Rapidly progressive nephritic syndrome with diffuse mesangiocapillary glomerulonephritis
Rapidly progressive nephritic syndrome with membranoproliferative glomerulonephritis, types 1 and 3, or NOS

N01.6   Rapidly progressive nephritic syndrome with dense deposit disease
Rapidly progressive nephritic syndrome with membranoproliferative glomerulonephritis, type 2

N01.7   Rapidly progressive nephritic syndrome with diffuse crescentic glomerulonephritis
Rapidly progressive nephritic syndrome with extracapillary glomerulonephritis

N01.8   Rapidly progressive nephritic syndrome with other morphologic changes
Rapidly progressive nephritic syndrome with proliferative glomerulonephritis NOS

N01.9   Rapidly progressive nephritic syndrome with unspecified morphologic changes

N02   Recurrent and persistent hematuria

Excludes1:   hematuria not associated with specified morphologic lesions (R31.-)
hematuria with:
   cystitis (N30.-)
   hypertrophy of prostate (N40.-)
   inflammatory disease of prostate (N41.-)
hematuria NOS (R31.9)

N02.0   Recurrent and persistent hematuria with minor glomerular abnormality
Recurrent and persistent hematuria with minimal change lesion

N02.1   Recurrent and persistent hematuria with focal and segmental glomerular lesions
Recurrent and persistent hematuria with focal and segmental hyalinosis
Recurrent and persistent hematuria with focal and segmental sclerosis
Recurrent and persistent hematuria with focal glomerulonephritis

N02.2   Recurrent and persistent hematuria with diffuse membranous glomerulonephritis

N02.3   Recurrent and persistent hematuria with diffuse mesangial proliferative glomerulonephritis

N02.4   Recurrent and persistent hematuria with diffuse endocapillary proliferative glomerulonephritis

N02.5   Recurrent and persistent hematuria with diffuse mesangiocapillary glomerulonephritis
Recurrent and persistent hematuria with membranoproliferative glomerulonephritis, types 1 and 3, or NOS

N02.6 Recurrent and persistent hematuria with dense deposit disease
Recurrent and persistent hematuria with membranoproliferative glomerulonephritis, type 2

N02.7 Recurrent and persistent hematuria with diffuse crescentic glomerulonephritis
Recurrent and persistent hematuria with extracapillary glomerulonephritis

N02.8 Recurrent and persistent hematuria with other morphologic changes
Recurrent and persistent hematuria with proliferative glomerulonephritis NOS

N02.9 Recurrent and persistent hematuria with unspecified morphologic changes

N03 Chronic nephritic syndrome
Includes: chronic glomerular disease
chronic glomerulonephritis
chronic nephritis
chronic renal disease NOS
Excludes1: chronic tubulo-interstitial nephritis (N11.-)
diffuse sclerosing glomerulonephritis (N18.-)
nephritic syndrome NOS (N05.-)

N03.0 Chronic nephritic syndrome with minor glomerular abnormality
Chronic nephritic syndrome with minimal change lesion

N03.1 Chronic nephritic syndrome with focal and segmental glomerular lesions
Chronic nephritic syndrome with focal and segmental hyalinosis
Chronic nephritic syndrome with focal and segmental sclerosis
Chronic nephritic syndrome with focal glomerulonephritis

N03.2 Chronic nephritic syndrome with diffuse membranous glomerulonephritis

N03.3 Chronic nephritic syndrome with diffuse mesangial proliferative glomerulonephritis

N03.4 Chronic nephritic syndrome with diffuse endocapillary proliferative glomerulonephritis

N03.7 Chronic nephritic syndrome with diffuse crescentic glomerulonephritis
Chronic nephritic syndrome with extracapillary glomerulonephritis

N03.5 Chronic nephritic syndrome with diffuse mesangiocapillary glomerulonephritis
Chronic nephritic syndrome with membranoproliferative glomerulonephritis, types 1 and 3, or NOS

N03.6 Chronic nephritic syndrome with dense deposit disease
Chronic nephritic syndrome with membranoproliferative glomerulonephritis, type 2

N03.8 Chronic nephritic syndrome with other morphologic changes
Chronic nephritic syndrome with proliferative glomerulonephritis NOS

N03.9 Chronic nephritic syndrome with unspecified morphologic changes

N04 Nephrotic syndrome
Includes: congenital nephrotic syndrome
lipoid nephrosis

N04.0 Nephrotic syndrome with minor glomerular abnormality
Nephrotic syndrome with minimal change lesion

N04.1 Nephrotic syndrome with focal and segmental glomerular lesions
Nephrotic syndrome with focal and segmental hyalinosis
Nephrotic syndrome with focal and segmental sclerosis
Nephrotic syndrome with focal glomerulonephritis

N04.2 Nephrotic syndrome with diffuse membranous glomerulonephritis

N04.3 Nephrotic syndrome with diffuse mesangial proliferative glomerulonephritis

N04.4 Nephrotic syndrome with diffuse endocapillary proliferative glomerulonephritis

N04.5 Nephrotic syndrome with diffuse mesangiocapillary glomerulonephritis
Nephrotic syndrome with membranoproliferative glomerulonephritis, types 1 and 3, or NOS

N04.6 Nephrotic syndrome with dense deposit disease
Nephrotic syndrome with membranoproliferative glomerulonephritis, type 2

N04.7 Nephrotic syndrome with diffuse crescentic glomerulonephritis
Nephrotic syndrome with extracapillary glomerulonephritis

N04.8 Nephrotic syndrome with other morphologic changes
Nephrotic syndrome with proliferative glomerulonephritis NOS

N04.9 Nephrotic syndrome with unspecified morphologic changes

N05 Unspecified nephritic syndrome
Includes: glomerular disease NOS
glomerulonephritis NOS
nephritis NOS
nephropathy NOS and renal disease NOS with morphological lesion specified in .0-.8
Excludes1: nephropathy NOS with no stated cause (N28.9)
renal disease NOS with no stated cause (N28.9)
tubulo-interstitial nephritis NOS (N12)

N05.0 Unspecified nephritic syndrome with minor glomerular abnormality
Unspecified nephritic syndrome with minimal change lesion

N05.1 Unspecified nephritic syndrome with focal and segmental glomerular lesions
Unspecified nephritic syndrome with focal and segmental hyalinosis
Unspecified nephritic syndrome with focal and segmental sclerosis
Unspecified nephritic syndrome with focal glomerulonephritis

N05.2 Unspecified nephritic syndrome with diffuse membranous glomerulonephritis

N05.3 Unspecified nephritic syndrome with diffuse mesangial proliferative glomerulonephritis

N05.4 Unspecified nephritic syndrome with diffuse endocapillary proliferative glomerulonephritis

N05.5 Unspecified nephritic syndrome with diffuse mesangiocapillary glomerulonephritis
Unspecified nephritic syndrome with membranoproliferative glomerulonephritis, types 1 and 3, or NOS

N05.6 Unspecified nephritic syndrome with dense deposit disease
Unspecified nephritic syndrome with membranoproliferative glomerulonephritis, type 2

N05.7 Unspecified nephritic syndrome with diffuse crescentic glomerulonephritis
Unspecified nephritic syndrome with extracapillary glomerulonephritis

N05.8 Unspecified nephritic syndrome with other morphologic changes
Unspecified nephritic syndrome with proliferative glomerulonephritis NOS

N05.9 Unspecified nephritic syndrome with unspecified morphologic changes

N06 Isolated proteinuria with specified morphological lesion
Excludes1: proteinuria not associated with specific morphologic lesions (R80.0)

N06.0 Isolated proteinuria with minor glomerular abnormality
Isolated proteinuria with minimal change lesion

N06.1 Isolated proteinuria with focal and segmental glomerular lesions
Isolated proteinuria with focal and segmental hyalinosis
Isolated proteinuria with focal and segmental sclerosis
Isolated proteinuria with focal glomerulonephritis

N06.2 Isolated proteinuria with diffuse membranous glomerulonephritis

N06.3 Isolated proteinuria with diffuse mesangial proliferative glomerulonephritis

N06.4 Isolated proteinuria with diffuse endocapillary proliferative glomerulonephritis

N06.5 Isolated proteinuria with diffuse mesangiocapillary glomerulonephritis
Isolated proteinuria with membranoproliferative glomerulonephritis, types 1 and 3, or NOS

N06.6 **Isolated proteinuria with dense deposit disease**
  Isolated proteinuria with membranoproliferative glomerulonephritis, type 2
N06.7 **Isolated proteinuria with diffuse crescentic glomerulonephritis**
  Isolated proteinuria with extracapillary glomerulonephritis
N06.8 **Isolated proteinuria with other morphologic lesion**
  Isolated proteinuria with proliferative glomerulonephritis NOS
N06.9 **Isolated proteinuria with unspecified morphologic lesion**

N07 Hereditary nephropathy, not elsewhere classified
  Excludes1: Alport's syndrome (Q87.8)
        hereditary amyloid nephropathy (E85)
        nail patella syndrome (Q87.2)
        non-neuropathic heredofamilial amyloidosis (E85)

N07.0 **Hereditary nephropathy, not elsewhere classified with minor glomerular abnormality**
  Hereditary nephropathy, not elsewhere classified with minimal change lesion
N07.1 **Hereditary nephropathy, not elsewhere classified with focal and segmental glomerular lesions**
  Hereditary nephropathy, not elsewhere classified with focal and segmental hyalinosis
  Hereditary nephropathy, not elsewhere classified with focal and segmental sclerosis
  Hereditary nephropathy, not elsewhere classified with focal glomerulonephritis
N07.2 **Hereditary nephropathy, not elsewhere classified with diffuse membranous glomerulonephritis**
N07.3 **Hereditary nephropathy, not elsewhere classified with diffuse mesangial proliferative glomerulonephritis**
N07.4 **Hereditary nephropathy, not elsewhere classified with diffuse endocapillary proliferative glomerulonephritis**
N07.5 **Hereditary nephropathy, not elsewhere classified with diffuse mesangiocapillary glomerulonephritis**
  Hereditary nephropathy, not elsewhere classified with membranoproliferative glomerulonephritis, types 1 and 3, or NOS
N07.6 **Hereditary nephropathy, not elsewhere classified with dense deposit disease**
  Hereditary nephropathy, not elsewhere classified with membranoproliferative glomerulonephritis, type 2
N07.7 **Hereditary nephropathy, not elsewhere classified with diffuse crescentic glomerulonephritis**
  Hereditary nephropathy, not elsewhere classified with extracapillary glomerulonephritis
N07.8 **Hereditary nephropathy, not elsewhere classified with other morphologic lesions**
  Hereditary nephropathy, not elsewhere classified with proliferative glomerulonephritis NOS
N07.9 **Hereditary nephropathy, not elsewhere classified with unspecified morphologic lesions**

N08 Glomerular disorders in diseases classified elsewhere
  Includes: glomerulonephritis
         nephritis
         nephropathy
  Code first underlying disease, such as:
    amyloidosis (E85)
    congenital syphilis (A50.5)
    cryoglobulinemia (D89.1)
    disseminated intravascular coagulation (D65)
    multiple myeloma (C90.0-)
    polyarteritis nodosa (M30.0)
    septicemia (A40.0-A41.9)
    sickle-cell disease (D57.0-D57.8)
  Excludes1: glomerulonephritis, nephritis and nephropathy (in):
          antiglomerular basement membrane disease (M31.0)
          diabetes (E09-E13 with .21)
          gonococcal (A54.21)
          Goodpasture's syndrome (M31.0)
          hemolytic-uremic syndrome (D59.3)
          lupus (M32.14)
          mumps (B26.83)
          syphilis (A52.75)
          systemic lupus erythematosus (M32.14)
          Wegener's granulomatosis (M31.31)
        pyelonephritis in diseases classified elsewhere (N16)
        renal tubulo-interstitial disorders classified elsewhere (N16)

RENAL TUBULO–INTERSTITIAL DISEASES (N10–N16)
  Includes: pyelonephritis
  Excludes1:   pyeloureteritis cystica (N28.85)

N10 Acute tubulo-interstitial nephritis
  Includes: acute infectious interstitial nephritis
         acute pyelitis
         acute pyelonephritis
         acute tubular necrosis
         hemoglobin nephrosis
         myoglobin nephrosis
  Use additional code (B95-B97), to identify infectious agent.

N11 Chronic tubulo-interstitial nephritis
  Includes: chronic infectious interstitial nephritis
         chronic pyelitis
         chronic pyelonephritis
  Use additional code (B95-B97), to identify infectious agent.

N11.0 **Nonobstructive reflux-associated chronic pyelonephritis**
  Pyelonephritis (chronic) associated with (vesicoureteral) reflux
  Excludes1:   vesicoureteral reflux NOS (N13.70)
N11.1 **Chronic obstructive pyelonephritis**
  Pyelonephritis (chronic) associated with anomaly of pelviureteric junction
  Pyelonephritis (chronic) associated with anomaly of pyeloureteric junction
  Pyelonephritis (chronic) associated with crossing of vessel
  Pyelonephritis (chronic) associated with kinking of ureter
  Pyelonephritis (chronic) associated with obstruction of ureter
  Pyelonephritis (chronic) associated with stricture of pelviureteric junction
  Pyelonephritis (chronic) associated with stricture of ureter
  Excludes1:   calculous pyelonephritis (N20.9)
         obstructive uropathy (N13.-)
N11.8 **Other chronic tubulo-interstitial nephritis**
  Nonobstructive chronic pyelonephritis NOS
N11.9 **Chronic tubulo-interstitial nephritis, unspecified**
  Chronic interstitial nephritis NOS
  Chronic pyelitis NOS
  Chronic pyelonephritis NOS

N12 Tubulo-interstitial nephritis, not specified as acute or chronic
  Includes: interstitial nephritis NOS
         pyelitis NOS
         pyelonephritis NOS
  Excludes1:   calculous pyelonephritis (N20.9)

N13 Obstructive and reflux uropathy

    Excludes1:   calculus of kidney and ureter without hydronephrosis (N20.-)

                   congenital obstructive defects of renal pelvis and ureter (Q62.0-Q62.3)

                   hydronephrosis with ureteropelvic junction obstruction (Q62.1)

                   obstructive pyelonephritis (N11.1)

N13.1 Hydronephrosis with ureteral stricture, not elsewhere classified

    Excludes1:   Hydronephrosis with ureteral stricture with infection (N13.6)

N13.2 Hydronephrosis with renal and ureteral calculous obstruction

    Excludes1:   Hydronephrosis with renal and ureteral calculous obstruction with infection (N13.6)

N13.3 Other and unspecified hydronephrosis

    Excludes1:   hydronephrosis with infection (N13.6)

   N13.30   Unspecified hydronephrosis

   N13.39   Other hydronephrosis

N13.4 Hydroureter

    Excludes1:   congenital hydroureter (Q62.3)

                   hydroureter with infection (N13.6

                   vesicoureteral-reflux with hydroureter (N13.73-)

N13.5 Crossing vessel and stricture of ureter without hydronephrosis

    Kinking and stricture of ureter without hydronephrosis

    Excludes1:   Crossing vessel and stricture of ureter without hydronephrosis with infection (N13.6)

N13.6 Pyonephrosis

    Conditions in N13.0-N13.5 with infection

    Obstructive uropathy with infection

    Use additional code (B95-B97), to identify infectious agent.

N13.7 Vesicoureteral-reflux

    Excludes1:   reflux-associated pyelonephritis (N11.0)

   N13.70   Vesicoureteral-reflux, unspecified

           Vesicoureteral-reflux NOS

   N13.71   Vesicoureteral-reflux without reflux nephropathy

   N13.72   Vesicoureteral-reflux with reflux nephropathy without hydroureter

       N13.721   Vesicoureteral-reflux with reflux nephropathy without hydroureter, unilateral

       N13.722   Vesicoureteral-reflux with reflux nephropathy without hydroureter, bilateral

       N13.729   Vesicoureteral-reflux with reflux nephropathy without hydroureter, unspecified

   N13.73   Vesicoureteral-reflux with reflux nephropathy with hydroureter

       N13.731   Vesicoureteral-reflux with reflux nephropathy with hydroureter, unilateral

       N13.732   Vesicoureteral-reflux with reflux nephropathy with hydroureter, bilateral

       N13.739   Vesicoureteral-reflux with reflux nephropathy with hydroureter, unspecified

N13.8 Other obstructive and reflux uropathy

N13.9 Obstructive and reflux uropathy, unspecified

    Urinary tract obstruction NOS

N14 Drug- and heavy-metal-induced tubulo-interstitial and tubular conditions

    Use additional external cause code (Chapter XIX, XX), to identify toxic agent.

N14.0 Analgesic nephropathy

N14.1 Nephropathy induced by other drugs, medicaments and biological substances

N14.2 Nephropathy induced by unspecified drug, medicament or biological substance

N14.3 Nephropathy induced by heavy metals

N14.4 Toxic nephropathy, not elsewhere classified

N15 Other renal tubulo-interstitial diseases

N15.0 Balkan nephropathy

    Balkan endemic nephropathy

N15.1 Renal and perinephric abscess

N15.8 Other specified renal tubulo-interstitial diseases

N15.9 Renal tubulo-interstitial disease, unspecified

    Infection of kidney NOS

    Excludes1:   urinary tract infection NOS (N39.0)

N16 Renal tubulo-interstitial disorders in diseases classified elsewhere

    Includes: pyelonephritis

                tubulo-interstitial nephritis

    Code first underlying disease, such as:

        brucellosis (A23.0-A23.9)

        cryoglobulinemia (D89.1)

        glycogen storage disease (E74.0)

        leukemia (C91-C95)

        lymphoma (C81.0-C85.9, C96.0-C96.9)

        multiple myeloma (C90.0-)

        septicemia (A40.0-A41.9)

        Wilson's disease (E83.0)

    Excludes1:   pyelonephritis and tubulo-interstitial nephritis (in):

                candidiasis (B37.49)

                cystinosis (E72.0)

                diphtheritic (A36.84)

                salmonella infection (A02.25)

                sarcoidosis (D86.84)

                sicca syndrome [Sjogren's] (M35.04)

                syphilitic (A52.75)

                systemic lupus erythematosus (M32.15)

                toxoplasmosis (B58.83)

        renal tubular degeneration in diabetes (E08-E14 with .22)

RENAL FAILURE (N17–N19)

Use additional external cause code (Chapter XIX) to identify external agent.

    Excludes1:   congenital renal failure (P96.0)

                drug- and heavy-metal-induced tubulo-interstitial and tubular conditions (N14.-)

                extrarenal uremia (R39.2)

                hemolytic-uremic syndrome (D59.3)

                hepatorenal syndrome (K76.7)

                postpartum hepatorenal syndrome (O90.4)

                posttraumatic renal failure (T79.5)

                prerenal uremia (R39.2)

                renal failure:

                   complicating abortion or ectopic or molar pregnancy (O00-O07, O08.4)

                   following labor and delivery (O90.4)

                   postprocedural (N99.0)

N17 Acute renal failure

    Code first associated underlying condition

    Excludes1:   posttraumatic renal failure (T79.5)

   N17.0   Acute renal failure with tubular necrosis

        Acute tubular necrosis

        Renal tubular necrosis

        Tubular necrosis NOS

   N17.1   Acute renal failure with acute cortical necrosis

        Acute cortical necrosis

        Cortical necrosis NOS

        Renal cortical necrosis

   N17.2   Acute renal failure with medullary necrosis

        Medullary [papillary] necrosis NOS

        Acute medullary [papillary] necrosis

        Renal medullary [papillary] necrosis

   N17.8   Other acute renal failure

   N17.9   Acute renal failure, unspecified

N18 Chronic renal failure

    Includes: chronic uremia

                diffuse sclerosing glomerulonephritis

    Code also associated underlying condition

    Excludes1:   Alport syndrome with chronic renal failure (Q87.811)

                chronic renal failure with hypertension (I12.0)

   N18.0   End-stage renal disease

   N18.8   Other chronic renal failure

   N18.9   Chronic renal failure, unspecified

N19 Unspecified renal failure
    Includes: uremia NOS
    Excludes1: acute renal failure (N17.-)
             chronic renal failure (N18.-)
             extrarenal uremia (R39.2)
             prerenal uremia (R39.2)
             renal failure with hypertension (I12.0)
             uremia of newborn (P96.0)

UROLITHIASIS (N20–N23)

N20 Calculus of kidney and ureter
    Excludes1: nephrocalcinosis (E83.5)
             that with hydronephrosis (N13.2)

N20.0 Calculus of kidney
    Nephrolithiasis NOS
    Renal calculus
    Renal stone
    Staghorn calculus
    Stone in kidney

N20.1 Calculus of ureter
    Ureteric stone

N20.2 Calculus of kidney with calculus of ureter

N20.9 Urinary calculus, unspecified
    Calculous pyelonephritis

N21 Calculus of lower urinary tract
    Includes: that with cystitis and urethritis

N21.0 Calculus in bladder
    Calculus in diverticulum of bladder
    Urinary bladder stone
    Excludes2: staghorn calculus (N20.0)

N21.1 Calculus in urethra
    Excludes2: calculus of prostate (N42.0)

N21.8 Other lower urinary tract calculus

N21.9 Calculus of lower urinary tract, unspecified
    Excludes1: calculus of urinary tract NOS (N20.9)

N22 Calculus of urinary tract in diseases classified elsewhere
    Code first underlying disease, such as:
       gout (M10.-)
       schistosomiasis (B65.0-B65.9)

N23 Unspecified renal colic

OTHER DISORDERS OF KIDNEY AND URETER (N25–N29)

    Excludes2: disorders of kidney and ureter with urolithiasis (N20-N23)

N25 Disorders resulting from impaired renal tubular function
    Excludes1: metabolic disorders classifiable to E70-E90

N25.0 Renal osteodystrophy
    Azotemic osteodystrophy
    Phosphate-losing tubular disorders
    Renal rickets
    Renal short stature

N25.1 Nephrogenic diabetes insipidus
    Excludes1: diabetes insipidus NOS (E23.2)

N25.8 Other disorders resulting from impaired renal tubular function
    Lightwood-Albright syndrome
    Renal tubular acidosis NOS
    Secondary hyperparathyroidism of renal origin

N25.9 Disorder resulting from impaired renal tubular function, unspecified

N26 Unspecified contracted kidney
    Excludes1: contracted kidney with hypertension (I12.-)
             diffuse sclerosing glomerulonephritis (N18.-)
             hypertensive nephrosclerosis (arteriolar) (arteriosclerotic) (I12.-)
             small kidney of unknown cause (N27.-)

N26.1 Atrophy of kidney (terminal)
N26.2 Page kidney
N26.9 Renal sclerosis NOS

N27 Small kidney of unknown cause
    Includes: oligonephronia
N27.0 Small kidney, unilateral
N27.1 Small kidney, bilateral
N27.9 Small kidney, unspecified

N28 Other disorders of kidney and ureter, not elsewhere classified
N28.0 Ischemia and infarction of kidney
    Renal artery embolism
    Renal artery obstruction
    Renal artery occlusion
    Renal artery thrombosis
    Renal infarct
    Excludes1: atherosclerosis of renal artery (extrarenal part) (I70.1)
             congenital stenosis of renal artery (Q27.1)
             Goldblatt's kidney (I70.1)

N28.1 Cyst of kidney, acquired
    Cyst (multiple) (solitary) of kidney, acquired
    Excludes1: cystic kidney disease (congenital) (Q61.-)

N28.8 Other specified disorders of kidney and ureter
    Excludes1: hydroureter (N13.4)
             ureteric stricture with hydronephrosis (N13.1)
             ureteric stricture without hydronephrosis (N13.5)
      N28.81 Hypertrophy of kidney
      N28.82 Megaloureter
      N28.83 Nephroptosis
      N28.84 Pyelitis cystica
      N28.85 Pyeloureteritis cystica
      N28.86 Ureteritis cystica
      N28.89 Other specified disorders of kidney and ureter

N28.9 Disorder of kidney and ureter, unspecified
    Nephropathy NOS
    Renal disease NOS
    Excludes1: unspecified nephritic syndrome (N05-)

N29 Other disorders of kidney and ureter in diseases classified elsewhere
    Code first underlying disease, such as:
       amyloidosis (E85)
       nephrocalcinosis (E83.5)
       schistosomiasis (B65.0-B65.9)
    Excludes1: disorders of kidney and ureter in:
             cystinosis (E72.0)
             gonorrhea (A54.21)
             syphilis (A52.75)
             tuberculosis (A18.11)

OTHER DISEASES OF THE URINARY SYSTEM (N30–N39)

    Excludes1: urinary infection (complicating):
             abortion or ectopic or molar pregnancy (O00-O07, O08.8)
             pregnancy, childbirth and the puerperium (O23.-, O75.3, O86.2-)

N30 Cystitis
    Use additional code to identify infectious agent (B95-B97) or responsible external agent (Chapter XIX).
    Excludes1: prostatocystitis (N41.3)

N30.0 Acute cystitis
    Excludes1: irradiation cystitis (N30.4-)
             trigonitis (N30.3-)
      N30.00 Acute cystitis without hematuria
      N30.01 Acute cystitis with hematuria

N30.1 Interstitial cystitis (chronic)
      N30.10 Interstitial cystitis (chronic) without hematuria
      N30.11 Interstitial cystitis (chronic) with hematuria

N30.2 Other chronic cystitis
      N30.20 Other chronic cystitis without hematuria
      N30.21 Other chronic cystitis with hematuria

N30.3 Trigonitis
    Urethrotrigonitis
      N30.30 Trigonitis without hematuria

N30.31 Trigonitis with hematuria	**N34.0 Urethral abscess**
N30.4 Irradiation cystitis	Abscess (of) Cowper's gland
N30.40 Irradiation cystitis without hematuria	Abscess (of) Littre's gland
N30.41 Irradiation cystitis with hematuria	Abscess (of) urethral (gland)
N30.8 Other cystitis	Periurethral abscess
Abscess of bladder	Excludes1: urethral caruncle (N36.2)
N30.80 Other cystitis without hematuria	**N34.1 Nonspecific urethritis**
N30.81 Other cystitis with hematuria	Nongonococcal urethritis
N30.9 Cystitis, unspecified	Nonvenereal urethritis
N30.90 Cystitis, unspecified without hematuria	**N34.2 Other urethritis**

N30.90   Cystitis, unspecified without hematuria

N30.91   Cystitis, unspecified with hematuria

N31 Neuromuscular dysfunction of bladder, not elsewhere classified
  Use additional code to identify any associated urinary incontinence (N39.3-N39.4-)

  Excludes1:   cord bladder NOS (G95.8)
          neurogenic bladder due to cauda equina syndrome (G83.4)
          neuromuscular dysfunction due to spinal cord lesion (G95.8)

N31.0   Uninhibited neuropathic bladder, not elsewhere classified

N31.1   Reflex neuropathic bladder, not elsewhere classified

N31.2   Flaccid neuropathic bladder, not elsewhere classified
  Atonic (motor) (sensory) neuropathic bladder
  Autonomous neuropathic bladder
  Nonreflex neuropathic bladder

N31.3   Overactive bladder

N31.8   Other neuromuscular dysfunction of bladder

N31.9   Neuromuscular dysfunction of bladder, unspecified
  Neurogenic bladder dysfunction NOS

N32 Other disorders of bladder
  Excludes2:   calculus of bladder (N21.0)
          cystocele (N81.1)
          hernia or prolapse of bladder, female (N81.1)

N32.0   Bladder-neck obstruction
  Bladder-neck stenosis (acquired)
  Excludes1:   congenital bladder-neck obstruction (Q64.3-)

N32.1   Vesicointestinal fistula
  Vesicorectal fistula

N32.2   Vesical fistula, not elsewhere classified
  Excludes1:   fistula between bladder and female genital tract (N82.0-N82.1)

N32.3   Diverticulum of bladder
  Excludes1:   congenital diverticulum of bladder (Q64.6)
          diverticulitis of bladder (N30.8-)

N32.8   Other specified disorders of bladder
  Calcified bladder
  Contracted bladder

N32.9   Bladder disorder, unspecified

N33 Bladder disorders in diseases classified elsewhere
  Code first underlying disease, such as:
    schistosomiasis (B65.0-B65.9)

  Excludes1:   bladder disorder in:
            syphilis (A52.76)
            tuberculosis (A18.12)
          cystitis (in):
            candidal infection (B37.41)
            chlamydial (A56.01)
            diphtheritic (A36.85)
            gonorrhea (A54.01)
            syphilitic (A52.76)
            trichomonal infection (A59.03)
          neurogenic bladder (N31.-)

N34 Urethritis and urethral syndrome
  Use additional code (B95-B97), to identify infectious agent.

  Excludes1:   Reiter's disease (M02.3-
          urethritis in diseases with a predominantly sexual mode of transmission (A50-A64)
          urethrotrigonitis (N30.3-)

N34.0   Urethral abscess
  Abscess (of) Cowper's gland
  Abscess (of) Littre's gland
  Abscess (of) urethral (gland)
  Periurethral abscess
  Excludes1:   urethral caruncle (N36.2)

N34.1   Nonspecific urethritis
  Nongonococcal urethritis
  Nonvenereal urethritis

N34.2   Other urethritis
  Meatitis, urethral
  Postmenopausal urethritis
  Ulcer of urethra (meatus)
  Urethritis NOS

N34.3   Urethral syndrome, unspecified

N35 Urethral stricture
  Excludes1:   congenital urethral stricture (Q64.3-)
          postprocedural urethral stricture (N99.1-)

N35.0   Post-traumatic urethral stricture
  Urethral stricture due to injury
  Excludes1:   postprocedural urethral stricture (N99.1-)

N35.01   Post-traumatic urethral stricture, male

N35.010   Post-traumatic urethral stricture, male, meatal

N35.011   Post-traumatic bulbous urethral stricture

N35.012   Post-traumatic membranous urethral stricture

N35.013   Post-traumatic anterior urethral stricture

N35.014   Post-traumatic urethral stricture, male, unspecified

N35.02   Post-traumatic urethral stricture, female

N35.021   Urethral stricture due to childbirth

N35.028   Other post-traumatic urethral stricture, female

N35.1   Postinfective urethral stricture, not elsewhere classified
  Excludes1:   gonococcal urethral stricture (A54.01)
          syphilitic urethral stricture (A52.76)
          urethral stricture associated with schistosomiasis (B65.-, N29)

N35.11   Postinfective urethral stricture, not elsewhere classified, male

N35.111   Postinfective urethral stricture, not elsewhere classified, male, meatal

N35.112   Postinfective bulbous urethral stricture, not elsewhere classified

N35.113   Postinfective membraneous urethral stricture, not elsewhere classified

N35.114   Postinfective anterior urethral stricture, not elsewhere classified

N35.119   Postinfective urethral stricture, not elsewhere classified, male, unspecified

N35.12   Postinfective urethral stricture, not elsewhere classified, female

N35.8   Other urethral stricture
  Excludes1:   postprocedural urethral stricture (N99.1-)

N35.9   Urethral stricture, unspecified

N36 Other disorders of urethra

N36.0   Urethral fistula
  False urethral passage
  Urethroperineal fistula
  Urethrorectal fistula
  Urinary fistula NOS
  Excludes1:   urethroscrotal fistula (N50.8)
          urethrovaginal fistula (N82.1)
          urethrovesicovaginal fistula (N82.1)

N36.1   Urethral diverticulum

N36.2   Urethral caruncle

N36.4   Urethral functional and muscular disorder
  Use additional code to identify associated urinary stress incontinence (N39.3)

N36.41   Hypermobility of urethra

N36.42   Intrinsic sphincter deficiency (ISD)

N36.43   **Combined hypermobility of urethra and intrinsic sphincter deficiency**

N36.44   **Muscular disorders of urethra**
Bladder sphincter dyssynergy

N36.8 **Other specified disorders of urethra**

N36.9 **Urethral disorder, unspecified**

N37 Urethral disorders in diseases classified elsewhere
Code first underlying disease.
Excludes1:   urethritis (in):
       candidal infection (B37.41)
       chlamydial (A56.01)
       gonorrhea (A54.01)
       syphilis (A52.76)
       trichomonal infection (A59.03)
       tuberculosis (A18.13)

N39 Other disorders of urinary system
Excludes2:   hematuria NOS (R31-)
       recurrent or persistent hematuria (N02.-)
       recurrent or persistent hematuria with specified morphological lesion (N02.-)
       proteinuria NOS (R80.-)

N39.0 **Urinary tract infection, site not specified**
Use additional code (B95-B97), to identify infectious agent.
Excludes1:   candidiasis of urinary tract (B37.4-)
       urinary tract infection of specified site, such as:
         cystitis (N30.-)
         urethritis (N34.-)

N39.3 **Stress incontinence (female) (male)**
Code first underlying condition
Excludes1:   mixed incontinence (N39.46)

N39.4 **Other specified urinary incontinence**
Code first underlying condition

N39.41   **Urge incontinence**
Excludes1:   mixed incontinence (N39.46)

N39.42   **Incontinence without sensory awareness**

N39.43   **Post-void dribbling**

N39.44   **Nocturnal enuresis**

N39.45   **Continuous leakage**

N39.46   **Mixed incontinence**
Urge and stress incontinence

N39.49   **Other specified urinary incontinence**
Overflow incontinence
Reflex incontinence
Total incontinence
Excludes1:   enuresis NOS (R32)
       urinary incontinence NOS (R32)
       urinary incontinence of nonorganic origin (F98.0)

N39.8 **Other specified disorders of urinary system**

N39.9 **Disorder of urinary system, unspecified**

DISEASES OF MALE GENITAL ORGANS (N40–N51)

N40 Hyperplasia of prostate
Use additional code for any associated urinary incontinence (N39.4-)
Excludes1:   benign neoplasms, except adenoma, fibroma and myoma of prostate (D29.1)

N40.0 **Hypertrophy (benign) of prostate**
Benign prostatic hypertrophy
Enlargement of prostate
Smooth enlarged prostate
Soft enlarged prostate

N40.00   **Hypertrophy (benign) of prostate without complication**
Hypertrophy (benign) of prostate NOS

N40.01   **Hypertrophy (benign) of prostate with obstruction**
Hypertrophy (benign) of prostate with urinary retention

N40.02   **Hypertrophy (benign) of prostate with hematuria**

N40.03   **Hypertrophy (benign) of prostate with obstruction and hematuria**
Hypertrophy (benign) of prostate with urinary retention and hematuria

N40.09   **Hypertrophy (benign) of prostate with other complication**

N40.1 **Nodular prostate**
Hard, firm prostate
Multinodular prostate
Excludes1:   malignant neoplasm of prostate (C61)

N40.10   **Nodular prostate without complication**
Nodular prostate NOS

N40.11   **Nodular prostate with obstruction**
Nodular prostate with urinary retention

N40.12   **Nodular prostate with hematuria**

N40.13   **Nodular prostate with obstruction and hematuria**
Nodular prostate with urinary retention and hematuria

N40.19   **Nodular prostate with other complication**

N40.2 **Benign localized hyperplasia of prostate**
Adenofibromatous hypertrophy of prostate
Adenoma of prostate
Fibroadenoma of prostate
Fibroma of prostate
Myoma of prostate
Polyp of prostate
Excludes1:   benign neoplasm of prostate (D29.1)
       hypertrophy of prostate (N40.0)
       malignant neoplasm of prostate (C61)

N40.20   **Benign localized hyperplasia of prostate without complication**
Benign localized hyperplasia of prostate NOS

N40.21   **Benign localized hyperplasia of prostate with obstruction**
Benign localized hyperplasia of prostate with urinary retention

N40.22   **Benign localized hyperplasia of prostate with hematuria**

N40.23   **Benign localized hyperplasia of prostate with obstruction and hematuria**
Benign localized hyperplasia of prostate with urinary retention and hematuria

N40.29   **Benign localized hyperplasia of prostate with other complication**

N40.9 **Unspecified hyperplasia of prostate**
Median bar

N40.90   **Unspecified hyperplasia of prostate without complication**
Hyperplasia of prostate NOS

N40.91   **Unspecified hyperplasia of prostate with obstruction**
Prostatic obstruction NOS
Unspecified hyperplasia of prostate with urinary retention

N40.92   **Unspecified hyperplasia of prostate with hematuria**

N40.93   **Unspecified hyperplasia of prostate with obstruction and hematuria**
Unspecified hyperplasia of prostate with urinary retention and hematuria

N40.99   **Unspecified hyperplasia of prostate with other complication**

N41 Inflammatory diseases of prostate
Use additional code (B95-B97), to identify infectious agent.

N41.0 **Acute Prostatitis**

N41.00   **Acute prostatitis without hematuria**

N41.01   **Acute prostatitis with hematuria**

N41.1 **Chronic Prostatitis**

N41.10   **Chronic prostatitis without hematuria**

N41.11   **Chronic prostatitis with hematuria**

N41.2 **Abscess of prostate**

N41.3 **Prostatocystitis**

N41.4 **Granulomatous prostatitis**

N41.8 **Other inflammatory diseases of prostate**

N41.9 **Inflammatory disease of prostate, unspecified**
Prostatitis NOS

N42 Other disorders of prostate

N42.0 Calculus of prostate
    Prostatic stone

N42.1 Congestion and hemorrhage of prostate
    Excludes1: hyperplasia of prostate (N40.-)
          inflammatory diseases of prostate (N41.-)

N42.8 Other specified disorders of prostate

  N42.81 Prostatodynia syndrome
      Painful prostate syndrome

  N42.82 Prostatosis syndrome

  N42.89 Other specified disorders of prostate

N42.9 Disorder of prostate, unspecified

N43 Hydrocele and spermatocele
    Includes: hydrocele of spermatic cord, testis or tunica vaginalis
    Excludes1: congenital hydrocele (P83.5)

N43.0 Encysted hydrocele

N43.1 Infected hydrocele
    Use additional code (B95-B97), to identify infectious agent

N43.2 Other hydrocele

N43.3 Hydrocele, unspecified

N43.4 Spermatocele of epididymis
    Spermatic cyst

  N43.40 Spermatocele of epididymis, unspecified

  N43.41 Spermatocele of epididymis, single

  N43.42 Spermatocele of epididymis, multiple

N43.5 Hydrocele of spermatic cord

N44 Noninflammatory disorders of testis

N44.0 Torsion of testis

  N44.00 Torsion of testis, unspecified

  N44.01 Torsion of appendix epididymis

  N44.02 Extravaginal torsion of spermatic cord

  N44.03 Intravaginal torsion of spermatic cord

  N44.04 Torsion of appendix testis

N44.1 Cyst of tunica albuginea testis

N44.2 Benign cyst of testis

N44.8 Other noninflammatory disorders of the testis

N45 Orchitis and epididymitis
    Use additional code (B95-B97), to identify infectious agent.

N45.1 Epididymitis

N45.2 Orchitis

N45.3 Epididymo-orchitis

N45.4 Abscess of epididymis or testis

N46 Male infertility
    Excludes1: vasectomy status (Z98.52)

N46.0 Azoospermia
    Absolute male infertility
    Male infertility due to germinal (cell) aplasia
    Male infertility due to spermatogenic arrest (complete)

  N46.01 Organic azoospermia
      Azoospermia NOS

  N46.02 Azoospermia due to extratesticular causes
      Code also associated cause

    N46.021 Azoospermia due to drug therapy

    N46.022 Azoospermia due to infection

    N46.023 Azoospermia due to obstruction of efferent ducts

    N46.024 Azoospermia due to radiation

    N46.025 Azoospermia due to systemic disease

    N46.029 Azoospermia due to other extratesticular causes

N46.1 Oligospermia
    Male infertility due to germinal cell desquamation
    Male infertility due to hypospermatogenesis
    Male infertility due to incomplete spermatogenic arrest

  N46.11 Organic oligospermia
      Oligospermia NOS

  N46.12 Oligospermia due to extratesticular causes
      Code also associated cause

    N46.121 Oligospermia due to drug therapy

    N46.122 Oligospermia due to infection

    N46.123 Oligospermia due to obstruction of efferent ducts

    N46.124 Oligospermia due to radiation

    N46.125 Oligospermia due to systemic disease

    N46.129 Oligospermia due to other extratesticular causes

N46.8 Other male infertility

N46.9 Male infertility, unspecified

N47 Disorders of prepuce

N47.0 Adherent prepuce, newborn

N47.1 Phimosis

N47.2 Paraphimosis

N47.3 Deficient foreskin

N47.4 Benign cyst of prepuce

N47.5 Adhesions of prepuce and glans penis

N47.6 Balanoposthitis
    Excludes1: balanitis (N48.1)
    Use additional code (B95-B97), to identify infectious agent.

N47.7 Other inflammatory diseases of prepuce
    Use additional code (B95-B97), to identify infectious agent.

N47.8 Other disorders of prepuce

N48 Other disorders of penis

N48.0 Leukoplakia of penis
    Kraurosis of penis
    Excludes1: carcinoma in situ of penis (D07.4)

N48.1 Balanitis
    Excludes1: amebic balanitis (A06.8)
          balanoposthitis (N47.6)
          candidal balanitis (B37.42)
          gonococcal balanitis (A54.23)
          herpesviral [herpes simplex] balanitis (A60.01)
    Use additional code (B95-B97), to identify infectious agent

N48.2 Other inflammatory disorders of penis
    Use additional code (B95-B97), to identify infectious agent.
    Excludes1: balanitis (N48.1)
          balanitis xerotica obliterans (N48.6)
          balanoposthitis (N47.6)

  N48.21 Abscess of corpus cavernosum and penis

  N48.22 Cellulitis of corpus cavernosum and penis

  N48.29 Other inflammatory disorders of penis

N48.3 Priapism
    Painful erection
    Code first underlying cause

  N48.30 Priapism, unspecified

  N48.31 Priapism due to trauma

  N48.32 Priapism due to disease classified elsewhere

  N48.33 Priapism, drug-induced

  N48.39 Other priapism

N48.5 Ulcer of penis

N48.6 Balanitis xerotica obliterans

N48.7 Peyronie's disease
    Plastic induration of penis

N48.8 Other specified disorders of penis

  N48.81 Thrombosis of superficial vein of penis

  N48.89 Other specified disorders of penis

N48.9 Disorder of penis, unspecified

N49 Inflammatory disorders of male genital organs, not elsewhere classified
    Use additional code (B95-B97), to identify infectious agent
    Excludes1: inflammation of penis (N48.1, N48.2-)
          orchitis and epididymitis (N45.-)

N49.0 Inflammatory disorders of seminal vesicle
    Vesiculitis NOS

N49.1 Inflammatory disorders of spermatic cord, tunica vaginalis and vas deferens
    Vasitis

N49.2 Inflammatory disorders of scrotum

N49.3   Fournier's gangrene

N49.8   Inflammatory disorders of other specified male genital organs
> Inflammation of multiple sites in male genital organs

N49.9   Inflammatory disorder of unspecified male genital organ
> Abscess of unspecified male genital organ
> Boil of unspecified male genital organ
> Carbuncle of unspecified male genital organ
> Cellulitis of unspecified male genital organ

N50   Other and unspecified disorders of male genital organs
> Excludes2:   torsion of testis (N44.0-)

N50.0   Atrophy of testis

N50.1   Vascular disorders of male genital organs

N50.8   Other specified disorders of male genital organs
> Atrophy of scrotum, seminal vesicle, spermatic cord, tunica vaginalis and vas deferens
> Edema of scrotum, seminal vesicle, spermatic cord, testis, tunica vaginalis and vas deferens
> Hypertrophy of scrotum, seminal vesicle, spermatic cord, testis, tunica vaginalis and vas deferens
> Ulcer of scrotum, seminal vesicle, spermatic cord, testis, tunica vaginalis and vas deferens
> Chylocele, tunica vaginalis (nonfilarial) NOS
> Stricture of spermatic cord, tunica vaginalis, and vas deferens
> Urethroscrotal fistula

N50.9   Disorder of male genital organs, unspecified

N51   Disorders of male genital organs in diseases classified elsewhere
> Code first underlying disease, such as:
> filariasis (B74.0-B74.9)
> Excludes1:   amebic balanitis (A06.8)
> candidal balanitis (B37.42)
> gonococcal balanitis (A54.23)
> gonococcal prostatitis (A54.22)
> herpesviral [herpes simplex] balanitis (A60.01)
> trichomonal prostatitis (A59.02)
> tuberculous prostatitis (A18.14)

N52   Male erectile dysfunction
> Excludes1:   psychogenic impotence (F52.21)

N52.0   Vasculogenic erectile dysfunction
> **N52.01**   Erectile dysfunction due to arterial insufficiency
> **N52.02**   Corporo-venous occlusive erectile dysfunction
> **N52.03**   Combined arterial insufficiency and corporo-venous occlusive erectile dysfunction

N52.1   Erectile dysfunction due to diseases classified elsewhere
> Code first underlying disease

N52.2   Drug-induced erectile dysfunction

N52.3   Post-surgical erectile dysfunction
> **N52.31**   Erectile dysfunction following radical prostatectomy
> **N52.32**   Erectile dysfunction following radical cystectomy
> **N52.33**   Erectile dysfunction following urethral surgery
> **N52.34**   Erectile dysfunction following simple prostatectomy
> **N52.39**   Other post-surgical erectile dysfunction

N52.8   Other male erectile dysfunction

N52.9   Male erectile dysfunction, unspecified
> Organic impotence NOS

N53   Male sexual dysfunction
> Excludes1:   psychogenic sexual dysfunction (F52.-)

N53.1   Ejaculatory dysfunction
> Excludes1:   premature ejaculation (F52.4)
> **N53.11**   Retarded ejaculation
> **N53.12**   Painful ejaculation
> **N53.13**   Anejaculatory orgasm
> **N53.19**   Other ejaculatory dysfunction
> > Ejaculatory dysfunction NOS

N53.8   Other male sexual dysfunction

N53.9   Unspecified male sexual dysfunction

DISORDERS OF BREAST (N60–N64)
> Excludes1:   disorders of breast associated with childbirth (O91-O92)

N60   Benign mammary dysplasia
> Includes: fibrocystic mastopathy

N60.0   Solitary cyst of breast
> Cyst of breast
> **N60.00**   Solitary cyst of female breast, unspecified side
> **N60.01**   Solitary cyst of right female breast
> **N60.02**   Solitary cyst of left female breast
> **N60.03**   Solitary cyst of right male breast
> **N60.04**   Solitary cyst of left male breast
> **N60.05**   Solitary cyst of male breast, unspecified side

N60.1   Diffuse cystic mastopathy
> Cystic breast
> Fibrocystic disease of breast
> Excludes1:   diffuse cystic mastopathy with epithelial proliferation (N60.3-)
> **N60.10**   Diffuse cystic mastopathy of female breast, unspecified side
> **N60.11**   Diffuse cystic mastopathy of right female breast
> **N60.12**   Diffuse cystic mastopathy of left female breast
> **N60.13**   Diffuse cystic mastopathy of right male breast
> **N60.14**   Diffuse cystic mastopathy of left male breast
> **N60.15**   Diffuse cystic mastopathy of male breast, unspecified side

N60.2   Fibroadenosis of breast
> Adenofibrosis of breast
> Excludes2:   fibroadenoma of breast (D24.-)
> **N60.20**   Fibroadenosis of female breast, unspecified side
> **N60.21**   Fibroadenosis of right female breast
> **N60.22**   Fibroadenosis of left female breast
> **N60.23**   Fibroadenosis of right male breast
> **N60.24**   Fibroadenosis of left male breast
> **N60.25**   Fibroadenosis of male breast, unspecified side

N60.3   Fibrosclerosis of breast
> Cystic mastopathy with epithelial proliferation
> **N60.30**   Fibrosclerosis of female breast, unspecified side
> **N60.31**   Fibrosclerosis of right female breast
> **N60.32**   Fibrosclerosis of left female breast
> **N60.33**   Fibrosclerosis of right male breas
> **N60.34**   Fibrosclerosis of left male breast
> **N60.35**   Fibrosclerosis of male breast, unspecified side

N60.4   Mammary duct ectasia
> **N60.40**   Mammary duct ectasia of female breast, unspecified side
> **N60.41**   Mammary duct ectasia of right female breast
> **N60.42**   Mammary duct ectasia of left female breast
> **N60.43**   Mammary duct ectasia of right male breast
> **N60.44**   Mammary duct ectasia of left male breast
> **N60.45**   Mammary duct ectasia of male breast, unspecified side

N60.8   Other benign mammary dysplasias
> **N60.80**   Other benign mammary dysplasias of female breast, unspecified side
> **N60.81**   Other benign mammary dysplasias of right female breast
> **N60.82**   Other benign mammary dysplasias of left female breast
> **N60.83**   Other benign mammary dysplasias of right male breast
> **N60.84**   Other benign mammary dysplasias of left male breast
> **N60.85**   Other benign mammary dysplasias of male breast, unspecified side

N60.9   Benign mammary dysplasia, unspecified
> **N60.90**   Benign mammary dysplasia, unspecified, of female breast, unspecified side
> **N60.91**   Benign mammary dysplasia, unspecified, of right female breast
> **N60.92**   Benign mammary dysplasia, unspecified, of left female breast

N60.93   Benign mammary dysplasia, unspecified, of right male breast

N60.94   Benign mammary dysplasia, unspecified of left male breast

N60.95   Benign mammary dysplasia, unspecified, of male breast, unspecified side

N61 Inflammatory disorders of breast

Includes: abscess (acute) (chronic) (nonpuerperal) of areola
abscess (acute) (chronic) (nonpuerperal) of breast
carbuncle of breast
infective mastitis (acute) (subacute) (nonpuerperal)
mastitis (acute) (subacute) (nonpuerperal) NOS

Excludes1:   inflammatory disorder of breast associated with childbirth (O91.-)
neonatal infective mastitis (P39.0)
thrombophlebitis of breast [Mondor's disease] (I80.8)

N62 Hypertrophy of breast

Includes: gynecomastia
hypertrophy of breast NOS
massive pubertal hypertrophy of breast

N63 Unspecified lump in breast

Includes: nodule(s) NOS in breast

N64 Other disorders of breast

N64.0 Fissure and fistula of nipple

N64.1 Fat necrosis of breast
Fat necrosis (segmental) of breast

N64.2 Atrophy of breast

N64.3 Galactorrhea not associated with childbirth

N64.4 Mastodynia

N64.5 Other signs and symptoms in breast
Induration of breast
Nipple discharge
Retraction of nipple

N64.8 Other specified disorders of breast
Galactocele
Subinvolution of breast (postlactational)

N64.9 Disorder of breast, unspecified

INFLAMMATORY DISEASES OF FEMALE PELVIC ORGANS (N70–N77)

Excludes1:   inflammatory diseases of female pelvic organs complicating:
abortion or ectopic or molar pregnancy (O00-O07, O08.0)
pregnancy, childbirth and the puerperium (O23.-, O75.3, O85, O86.-)

N70 Salpingitis and oophoritis

Includes: abscess (of) fallopian tube
abscess (of) ovary
pyosalpinx
salpingo-oophoritis
tubo-ovarian abscess
tubo-ovarian inflammatory disease
Use additional code (B95-B97), to identify infectious agent

Excludes1:   gonococcal infection (A54.24)
tuberculous infection (A18.17)

N70.0 Acute salpingitis and oophoritis

N70.01   Acute Salpingitis

N70.02   Acute oophoritis

N70.03   Acute salpingitis and oophoritis

N70.1 Chronic salpingitis and oophoritis
Hydrosalpinx

N70.11   Chronic Salpingitis

N70.12   Chronic oophoritis

N70.13   Chronic salpingitis and oophoritis

N70.9 Salpingitis and oophoritis, unspecified

N70.91   Salpingitis, unspecified

N70.92   Oophoritis, unspecified

N70.93   Salpingitis and oophoritis, unspecified

N71 Inflammatory disease of uterus, except cervix

Includes: endo (myo) metritis
metriti
myometritis
pyometra
uterine abscess
Use additional code (B95-B97), to identify infectious agent

Excludes1:   hyperplastic endometritis (N85.0)
inflammation of uterus following delivery (O85)

N71.0 Acute inflammatory disease of uterus

N71.1 Chronic inflammatory disease of uterus

N71.9 Inflammatory disease of uterus, unspecified

N72 Inflammatory disease of cervix uteri

Includes: cervicitis (with or without erosion or ectropion)
endocervicitis (with or without erosion or ectropion)
exocervicitis (with or without erosion or ectropion)
Use additional code (B95-B97), to identify infectious agent

Excludes1:   erosion and ectropion of cervix without cervicitis (N86)

N73 Other female pelvic inflammatory diseases

Use additional code (B95-B97), to identify infectious agent.

N73.0 Acute parametritis and pelvic cellulitis
Abscess of broad ligament
Abscess of parametrium
Pelvic cellulitis, female

N73.1 Chronic parametritis and pelvic cellulitis
Any condition in N73.0 specified as chronic

Excludes1:   tuberculous parametritis and pelvic cellultis (A18.17)

N73.2 Unspecified parametritis and pelvic cellulitis
Any condition in N73.0 unspecified whether acute or chronic

N73.3 Female acute pelvic peritonitis

N73.4 Female chronic pelvic peritonitis

Excludes1:   tuberculous pelvic (female) peritonitis (A18.17)

N73.5 Female pelvic peritonitis, unspecified

N73.6 Female pelvic peritoneal adhesions (postinfective)

Excludes1:   postprocedural pelvic peritoneal adhesions (N99.4)

N73.8 Other specified female pelvic inflammatory diseases

N73.9 Female pelvic inflammatory disease, unspecified
Female pelvic infection or inflammation NOS

N74 Female pelvic inflammatory disorders in diseases classified elsewhere

Code first underlying disease

Excludes1:   cervicitis:
chlamydial (A56.02)
gonococcal (A54.03)
herpesviral [herpes simplex] (A60.03)
syphilitic (A52.76)
trichomonal (A59.09)
tuberculous (A18.16)
pelvic inflammatory disease:
chlamydial (A56.11)
gonococcal (A54.24)
herpesviral [herpes simplex] (A60.09)
syphilitic (A52.76)
tuberculous (A18.17)

N75 Diseases of Bartholin's gland

N75.0 Cyst of Bartholin's gland

N75.1 Abscess of Bartholin's gland

N75.8 Other diseases of Bartholin's gland
Bartholinitis

N75.9 Disease of Bartholin's gland, unspecified

N76 Other inflammation of vagina and vulva

Use additional code (B95-B97), to identify infectious agent

Excludes1:   senile (atrophic) vaginitis (N95.2)

N76.0 Acute Vaginitis
Acute vulvovaginitis
Vaginitis NOS
Vulvovaginitis NOS

N76.1 Subacute and chronic vaginitis
Chronic vulvovaginitis
Subacute vulvovaginitis

N76.2 Acute vulvitis
Vulvitis NOS

N76.3 Subacute and chronic vulvitis

N76.4 Abscess of vulva
Furuncle of vulva

N76.5 Ulceration of vagina

N76.6 Ulceration of vulva

N76.8 Other specified inflammation of vagina and vulva

N77 Vulvovaginal ulceration and inflammation in diseases classified elsewhere

N77.0 Ulceration of vulva in diseases classified elsewhere
Code first underlying disease, such as:
Behcet's disease (M35.2)
Excludes1:   ulceration of vulva in gonococcal infection
(A54.02)
ulceration of vulva in herpesviral [herpes simplex]
infection (A60.04)
ulceration of vulva in syphilis (A51.0)
ulceration of vulva in tuberculosis (A18.18)

N77.1 Vaginitis, vulvitis and vulvovaginitis in diseases classified elsewhere
Code first underlying disease, such as:
pinworm (B80)
Excludes1:   vaginitis, vulvitis and vulvovaginitis (in):
candidiasis (B37.3)
chlamydial (A56.02)
gonococcal infection (A54.02)
herpesviral [herpes simplex] infection (A60.04)
syphilitic, early (A51.0)
syphilitic, late (A52.76)
trichomonal (A59.01)
tuberculous (A18.18)
venereal NEC (A64.3)

NONINFLAMMATORY DISORDERS OF FEMALE GENITAL TRACT
(N80–N98)

N80 Endometriosis

N80.0 Endometriosis of uterus
Adenomyosis
Excludes1:   stromal endometriosis (D39.0)

N80.1 Endometriosis of ovary

N80.2 Endometriosis of fallopian tube

N80.3 Endometriosis of pelvic peritoneum

N80.4 Endometriosis of rectovaginal septum and vagina

N80.5 Endometriosis of intestine

N80.6 Endometriosis in cutaneous scar

N80.8 Other endometriosis

N80.9 Endometriosis, unspecified

N81 Female genital prolapse
Excludes1:   genital prolapse complicating pregnancy, labor or
delivery (O34.5-)
prolapse and hernia of ovary and fallopian tube (N83.4)
prolapse of vaginal vault after hysterectomy (N99.3)

N81.0 Urethrocele
Excludes1:   urethrocele with cystocele (N81.1)
urethrocele with prolapse of uterus (N81.2-N81.4)

N81.1 Cystocele
Cystocele with urethrocele
Prolapse of (anterior) vaginal wall NOS
Excludes1:   cystocele with prolapse of uterus (N81.2-N81.4)

N81.2 Incomplete uterovaginal prolapse
First degree uterine prolapse
Prolapse of cervix NOS
Second degree uterine prolapse

N81.3 Complete uterovaginal prolapse
Procidentia (uteri) NOS
Third degree uterine prolapse

N81.4 Uterovaginal prolapse, unspecified
Prolapse of uterus NOS

N81.5 Vaginal enterocele
Excludes1:   enterocele with prolapse of uterus (N81.2-N81.4)

N81.6 Rectocele
Prolapse of posterior vaginal wall
Excludes1:   rectal prolapse (K62.3)
rectocele with prolapse of uterus (N81.2-N81.4)

N81.8 Other female genital prolapse
Deficient perineum
Old laceration of muscles of pelvic floor

N81.9 Female genital prolapse, unspecified

N82 Fistulae involving female genital tract
Excludes1:   vesicointestinal fistulae (N32.1)

N82.0 Vesicovaginal fistula

N82.1 Other female urinary-genital tract fistulae
Cervicovesical fistula
Ureterovaginal fistula
Urethrovaginal fistula
Uteroureteric fistula
Uterovesical fistula

N82.2 Fistula of vagina to small intestine

N82.3 Fistula of vagina to large intestine
Rectovaginal fistula

N82.4 Other female intestinal-genital tract fistulae
Intestinouterine fistula

N82.5 Female genital tract-skin fistulae
Uterus to abdominal wall fistula
Vaginoperineal fistula

N82.8 Other female genital tract fistulae

N82.9 Female genital tract fistula, unspecified

N83 Noninflammatory disorders of ovary, fallopian tube and broad ligament
Excludes2:   hydrosalpinx (N70.1-)

N83.0 Follicular cyst of ovary
Cyst of graafian follicle
Hemorrhagic follicular cyst (of ovary)

N83.1 Corpus luteum cyst
Hemorrhagic corpus luteum cyst

N83.2 Other and unspecified ovarian cysts
Excludes1:   developmental ovarian cyst (Q50.1)
neoplastic ovarian cyst (D27.-)
polycystic ovarian syndrome (E28.2)
Stein-Leventhal syndrome (E28.2)

N83.20 Unspecified ovarian cysts

N83.29 Other ovarian cysts
Retention cyst of ovary
Simple cyst of ovary

N83.3 Acquired atrophy of ovary and fallopian tube

N83.31 Acquired atrophy of ovary

N83.32 Acquired atrophy of fallopian tube

N83.33 Acquired atrophy of ovary and fallopian tube

N83.4 Prolapse and hernia of ovary and fallopian tube

N83.5 Torsion of ovary, ovarian pedicle and fallopian tube
Torsion of accessory tube
Torsion of hydatid of Morgagni

N83.51 Torsion of ovary and ovarian pedicle

N83.52 Torsion of fallopian tube

N83.53 Torsion of ovary, ovarian pedicle and fallopian tub

N83.6 Hematosalpinx
Excludes1:   hematosalpinx (with) (in):
hematocolpos (N89.7)
hematometra (N85.7)
tubal pregnancy (O00.1)

N83.7 Hematoma of broad ligament

N83.8 Other noninflammatory disorders of ovary, fallopian tube and broad ligament
Broad ligament laceration syndrome [Allen-Masters]

N83.9 Noninflammatory disorder of ovary, fallopian tube and broad ligament, unspecified

N84 Polyp of female genital tract
> Excludes1:   adenomatous polyp (D28.-)
>   placental polyp (O90.8)

N84.0 Polyp of corpus uteri
> Polyp of endometrium
> Polyp of uterus NOS
> Excludes1:   polypoid endometrial hyperplasia (N85.0)

N84.1 Polyp of cervix uteri
> Mucous polyp of cervix

N84.2 Polyp of vagina

N84.3 Polyp of vulva
> Polyp of labia

N84.8 Polyp of other parts of female genital tract

N84.9 Polyp of female genital tract, unspecified

N85 Other noninflammatory disorders of uterus, except cervix
> Excludes1:   endometriosis (N80.-)
>   inflammatory diseases of uterus (N71.-)
>   noninflammatory disorders of cervix (N86-N88)
>   polyp of corpus uteri (N84.0)
>   uterine prolapse (N81.-)

N85.0 Endometrial glandular hyperplasia
> Hyperplasia of endometrium NOS
> Cystic hyperplasia of endometrium
> Glandular-cystic hyperplasia of endometrium
> Polypoid hyperplasia of endometrium

N85.1 Endometrial adenomatous hyperplasia
> Hyperplasia of endometrium, atypical (adenomatous)

N85.2 Hypertrophy of uterus
> Bulky or enlarged uterus
> Excludes1:   puerperal hypertrophy of uterus (O90.8)

N85.3 Subinvolution of uterus
> Excludes1:   puerperal subinvolution of uterus (O90.8)

N85.4 Malposition of uterus
> Anteversion of uterus
> Retroflexion of uterus
> Retroversion of uterus
> Excludes1:   malposition of uterus complicating pregnancy, labor or delivery (O34.5-, O65.5)

N85.5 Inversion of uterus
> Excludes1:   current obstetric trauma (O71.2)
>   postpartum inversion of uterus (O71.2)

N85.6 Intrauterine synechiae

N85.7 Hematometra
> Hematosalpinx with hematometra
> Excludes1:   hematometra with hematocolpos (N89.7)

N85.8 Other specified noninflammatory disorders of uterus
> Atrophy of uterus, acquired
> Fibrosis of uterus NOS

N85.9 Noninflammatory disorder of uterus, unspecified
> Disorder of uterus NOS

N86 Erosion and ectropion of cervix uteri
> Includes: decubitus (trophic) ulcer of cervix
>   eversion of cervix
> Excludes1:   erosion and ectropion of cervix with cervicitis (N72)

N87 Dysplasia of cervix uteri
> Excludes1:   carcinoma in situ of cervix uteri (D06.-)

N87.0 Mild cervical dysplasia
> Cervical intraepithelial neoplasia [CIN], grade I

N87.1 Moderate cervical dysplasia
> Cervical intraepithelial neoplasia [CIN], grade II

N87.2 Severe cervical dysplasia, not elsewhere classified
> Severe cervical dysplasia NOS
> Excludes1:   cervical intraepithelial neoplasia [CIN], grade III, with or without mention of severe dysplasia (D06.-)

N87.9 Dysplasia of cervix uteri, unspecified

N88 Other noninflammatory disorders of cervix uteri
> Excludes2:   inflammatory disease of cervix (N72)
>   polyp of cervix (N84.1)

N88.0 Leukoplakia of cervix uteri

N88.1 Old laceration of cervix uteri
> Adhesions of cervix
> Excludes1:   current obstetric trauma (O71.3)

N88.2 Stricture and stenosis of cervix uteri
> Excludes1:   stricture and stenosis of cervix uteri complicating labor (O65.5)

N88.3 Incompetence of cervix uteri
> Investigation and management of (suspected) cervical incompetence in a nonpregnant woman
> Excludes1:   cervical incompetence complicating pregnancy (O34.3-)

N88.4 Hypertrophic elongation of cervix uteri

N88.8 Other specified noninflammatory disorders of cervix uteri
> Excludes1:   current obstetric trauma (O71.3)

N88.9 Noninflammatory disorder of cervix uteri, unspecified

N89 Other noninflammatory disorders of vagina
> Excludes1:   carcinoma in situ of vagina (D07.2)
>   inflammation of vagina (N76.-)
>   senile (atrophic) vaginitis (N95.2)
>   trichomonal leukorrhea (A59.00)

N89.0 Mild vaginal dysplasia
> Vaginal intraepithelial neoplasia [VAIN], grade I

N89.1 Moderate vaginal dysplasia
> Vaginal intraepithelial neoplasia [VAIN], grade II

N89.2 Severe vaginal dysplasia, not elsewhere classified
> Severe vaginal dysplasia NOS
> Excludes1:   vaginal intraepithelial neoplasia [VAIN], grade III, with or without mention of severe dysplasia (D07.2)

N89.3 Dysplasia of vagina, unspecified

N89.4 Leukoplakia of vagina

N89.5 Stricture and atresia of vagina
> Vaginal adhesions
> Vaginal stenosis
> Excludes1:   congenital atresia or stricture (Q52.4)
>   postoperative adhesions of vagina (N99.2)

N89.6 Tight hymenal ring
> Rigid hymen
> Tight introitus
> Excludes1:   imperforate hymen (Q52.3)

N89.7 Hematocolpos
> Hematocolpos with hematometra or hematosalpinx

N89.8 Other specified noninflammatory disorders of vagina
> Leukorrhea NOS
> Old vaginal laceration
> Pessary ulcer of vagina
> Excludes1:   current obstetric trauma (O70.-, O71.4, O71.7-O71.8)
>   old laceration involving muscles of pelvic floor (N81.8)

N89.9 Noninflammatory disorder of vagina, unspecified

N90 Other noninflammatory disorders of vulva and perineum
> Excludes1:   carcinoma in situ of vulva (D07.1)
>   current obstetric trauma (O70.-, O71.7-O71.8)
>   inflammation of vulva (N76.-)

N90.0 Mild vulvar dysplasia
> Vulvar intraepithelial neoplasia [VIN], grade I

N90.1 Moderate vulvar dysplasia
> Vulvar intraepithelial neoplasia [VIN], grade II

N90.2 Severe vulvar dysplasia, not elsewhere classified
> Severe vulvar dysplasia NOS
> Excludes1:   vulvar intraepithelial neoplasia[VIN], grade III, with or without mention of severe dysplasia (D07.1)

N90.3 Dysplasia of vulva, unspecified

N90.4 Leukoplakia of vulva
> Dystrophy of vulva
> Kraurosis of vulva

N90.5 Atrophy of vulva
> Stenosis of vulva

N90.6 Hypertrophy of vulva
Hypertrophy of labia

N90.7 Vulvar cyst

N90.8 Other specified noninflammatory disorders of vulva and perineum
Adhesions of vulva
Hypertrophy of clitoris

N90.9 Noninflammatory disorder of vulva and perineum, unspecified

N91 Absent, scanty and rare menstruation
Excludes1:   ovarian dysfunction (E28.-)

N91.0 Primary amenorrhea

N91.1 Secondary amenorrhea

N91.2 Amenorrhea, unspecified

N91.3 Primary oligomenorrhea

N91.4 Secondary oligomenorrhea

N91.5 Oligomenorrhea, unspecified
Hypomenorrhea NOS

N92 Excessive, frequent and irregular menstruation
Excludes1:   postmenopausal bleeding (N95.0)

N92.0 Excessive and frequent menstruation with regular cycle
Heavy periods NOS
Menorrhagia NOS
Polymenorrhea

N92.1 Excessive and frequent menstruation with irregular cycle
Irregular intermenstrual bleeding
Irregular, shortened intervals between menstrual bleeding
Menometrorrhagia
Metrorrhagia

N92.2 Excessive menstruation at puberty
Excessive bleeding associated with onset of menstrual periods
Pubertal menorrhagia
Puberty bleeding

N92.3 Ovulation bleeding
Regular intermenstrual bleeding

N92.4 Excessive bleeding in the premenopausal period
Climacteric menorrhagia or metrorrhagia
Menopausal menorrhagia or metrorrhagia
Preclimacteric menorrhagia or metrorrhagia
Premenopausal menorrhagia or metrorrhagia

N92.5 Other specified irregular menstruation

N92.6 Irregular menstruation, unspecified
Irregular bleeding NOS
Irregular periods NOS
Excludes1:   irregular menstruation with:
lengthened intervals or scanty bleeding (N91.3-N91.5)
shortened intervals or excessive bleeding (N92.1)

N93 Other abnormal uterine and vaginal bleeding
Excludes1:   neonatal vaginal hemorrhage (P54.6)
pseudomenses (P54.6)

N93.0 Postcoital and contact bleeding

N93.8 Other specified abnormal uterine and vaginal bleeding
Dysfunctional or functional uterine or vaginal bleeding NOS

N93.9 Abnormal uterine and vaginal bleeding, unspecified

N94 Pain and other conditions associated with female genital organs and menstrual cycle

N94.0 Mittelschmerz

N94.1 Dyspareunia
Excludes1:   psychogenic dyspareunia (F52.6)

N94.2 Vaginismus
Excludes1:   psychogenic vaginismus (F52.5)

N94.3 Premenstrual tension syndrome

N94.4 Primary dysmenorrhea

N94.5 Secondary dysmenorrhea

N94.6 Dysmenorrhea, unspecified
Excludes1:   psychogenic dysmenorrhea (F45.8)

N94.8 Other specified conditions associated with female genital organs and menstrual cycle

N94.9 Unspecified condition associated with female genital organs and menstrual cycle

N95 Menopausal and other perimenopausal disorders
Menopausal and other perimenopausal disorders due to naturally occurring (age-related) menopause and perimenopause
Excludes1:   excessive bleeding in the premenopausal period (N92.4)
menopausal and perimenopausal disorders due to artificial or premature menopause (E89.4-, E28.31-)
premature menopause NOS (E28.31)
Excludes2:   postmenopausal osteoporosis (M81.0-)
postmenopausal osteoporosis with current pathologic fracture (M80.0-)
postmenopausal urethritis (N34.2)

N95.0 Postmenopausal bleeding

N95.1 Menopausal and female climacteric states
Symptoms such as flushing, sleeplessness, headache, lack of concentration, associated with natural (age-related) menopause
Excludes1:   symptoms associated with artificial menopause (E89.41)
symptoms associated with premature menopause (E28.311)

N95.2 Postmenopausal atrophic vaginitis
Senile (atrophic) vaginitis

N95.8 Other specified menopausal and perimenopausal disorders

N95.9 Unspecified menopausal and perimenopausal disorder

N96 Habitual aborter
Includes: investigation or care in a nonpregnant woman
Excludes1:   habitual aborter with current pregnancy (O26.2-)
habitual aborter with current spontaneous abortion (O03-)

N97 Female infertility
Includes: inability to achieve a pregnancy
sterility, female NOS
Excludes1:   female infertility associated with:
hypopituitarism (E23.0)
Stein-Leventhal syndrome (E28.2)

N97.0 Female infertility associated with anovulation

N97.1 Female infertility of tubal origin
Female infertility associated with congenital anomaly of tube
Female infertility due to tubal block
Female infertility due to tubal occlusion
Female infertility due to tubal stenosis

N97.2 Female infertility of uterine origin
Female infertility associated with congenital anomaly of uterus
Female infertility due to nonimplantation of ovum

N97.3 Female infertility of cervical origin

N97.8 Female infertility of other origin

N97.9 Female infertility, unspecified

N98 Complications associated with artificial fertilization

N98.0 Infection associated with artificial insemination

N98.1 Hyperstimulation of ovaries
Hyperstimulation of ovaries NOS
Hyperstimulation of ovaries associated with induced ovulation

N98.2 Complications of attempted introduction of fertilized ovum following in vitro fertilization

N98.3 Complications of attempted introduction of embryo in embryo transfer

N98.8 Other complications associated with artificial fertilization

N98.9 Complication associated with artificial fertilization, unspecified

OTHER DISORDERS OF THE GENITOURINARY SYSTEM (N99)

N99 Intraoperative complications and postprocedural disorders of genitourinary system, not elsewhere classified
Use additional code, if applicable, to further specify disorder
Excludes2:   irradiation cystitis (N30.4-)
postoophorectomy osteoporosis (M81.8-)
postoophorectomy osteoporosis with current pathologic fracture (M80.8-)
states associated with artificial menopause (N95.3)

N99.0   Postprocedural renal failure

N99.1   Postprocedural urethral stricture
Postcatheterization urethral stricture

    N99.11   Postprocedural urethral stricture, male

        N99.110   Postprocedural urethral stricture, male, meatal

        N99.111   Postprocedural bulbous urethral stricture

        N99.112   Postprocedural membraneous urethral stricture

        N99.113   Postprocedural anterior urethral stricture

        N99.114   Postprocedural urethral stricture, male, unspecified

    N99.12   Postprocedural urethral stricture, female

N99.2   Postoperative adhesions of vagina

N99.3   Prolapse of vaginal vault after hysterectomy

N99.4   Postprocedural pelvic peritoneal adhesions
Excludes1:   pelvic peritoneal adhesions NOS (N73.6)
postinfective pelvic peritoneal adhesions (N73.6)

N99.5   Complications of stoma of urinary tract

    N99.51   Complication of cystostomy

        N99.510   Cystostomy hemorrhage

        N99.511   Cystostomy infection

        N99.512   Cystostomy malfunction

        N99.518   Other cystostomy complication

        N99.519   Unspecified cystostomy complication

    N99.52   Complication of other external stoma of urinary tract

        N99.520   Hemorrhage of other external stoma of urinary tract

        N99.521   Infection of other external stoma of urinary tract

        N99.522   Malfunction of other external stoma of urinary tract

        N99.528   Other complication of other external stoma of urinary tract

        N99.529   Unspecified complication of other external stoma of urinary tract

    N99.53   Complication of other stoma of urinary tract

        N99.530   Hemorrhage of other stoma of urinary tract

        N99.531   Infection of other stoma of urinary tract

        N99.532   Malfunction of other stoma of urinary tract

        N99.538   Other complication of other stoma of urinary tract

        N99.539   Unspecified complication of other stoma of urinary tract

N99.6   Intraoperative and postprocedural hemorrhage and hematoma complicating a genitourinary system procedure
Excludes1:   intraoperative hemorrhage or hematoma due to accidental puncture or laceration during a genitourinary system procedure (N99.7-)

    N99.61   Intraoperative hemorrhage of a genitourinary system organ or structure during a genitourinary system procedure

    N99.62   Intraoperative hemorrhage of a non-genitourinary system organ or structure during a genitourinary system procedure

    N99.63   Intraoperative hematoma of a genitourinary system organ or structure during a genitourinary system procedure

    N99.64   Intraoperative hematoma of a non genitourinary system organ or structure during a genitourinary system procedure

    N99.65   Postprocedural hemorrhage of a genitourinary system organ or structure following a genitourinary system procedure

    N99.66   Postprocedural hemorrhage of a non-genitourinary system organ or structure following a genitourinary system procedure

    N99.67   Postprocedural hematoma of a genitourinary system organ or structure following a genitourinary system procedure

    N99.68   Postprocedural hematoma of a non-genitourinary system organ or structure following a genitourinary system procedure

N99.7   Accidental puncture or laceration during a genitourinary system procedure

    N99.71   Accidental puncture or laceration of a genitourinary system organ or structure during a genitourinary system procedure

    N99.72   Accidental puncture or laceration of a non-genitoruinary system organ or structure during a genitourinary system procedure

N99.8   Other postprocedural disorders of the genitourinary system

    N99.81   Residual ovary syndrome

    N99.89   Other postprocedural disorders of the genitourinary system

N99.9   Postprocedural disorder of the genitourinary system, unspecified

CHAPTER XV — PREGNANCY, CHILDBIRTH AND THE PUERPERIUM (O00–O99)

Note: Codes from this chapter are for use only on maternal records, never on newborn records

Note: Codes from category O37 may be used on either the maternal record or a record created for the fetus, depending on the record keeping system of the facility where treatment is provided. They are not for use on a newborn record.

Note: Trimesters are counted from the first day of the last menstrual period.

They are defined as follows:

1st trimester-less than 14 weeks 0 days
2nd trimester- 14 weeks 0 days to less than 28 weeks 0 days
3rd trimester-28 weeks 0 days until delivery

The following extensions are to be added in cases of multiple gestation to identify the fetus for which the code applies: A code from O30, Multiple gestations, must be used in conjunction with other codes that require an extension.

A	fetus A
B	fetus B
C	fetus C
D	fetus D
E	fetus E
F	fetus F
G	fetus G
H	fetus H

Excludes1:   supervision of normal pregnancy (Z34.-)
Excludes2:   mental and behavioral disorders associated with the puerperium (F53.)
       obstetrical tetanus (A34)
       postpartum necrosis of pituitary gland (E23.0)
       puerperal osteomalacia (M83.0)

This chapter contains the following blocks:

O00-O08	Pregnancy with abortive outcome
O09	Supervision of high-risk pregnancy
O10-O16	Edema, proteinuria and hypertensive disorders in pregnancy, childbirth and the puerperium
O20-O29	Other maternal disorders predominantly related to pregnancy
O30-O48	Maternal care related to the fetus and amniotic cavity and possible delivery problems
O60-O77	Complications of labor and delivery
O80	Encounter for full-term uncomplicated delivery
O85-O92	Complications predominantly related to the puerperium
O93	Sequelae of complication of pregnancy, childbirth, and the puerperium
O94-O99	Other obstetric conditions, not elsewhere classified

PREGNANCY WITH ABORTIVE OUTCOME (O00–O08)

Excludes1:   continuing pregnancy in multiple gestation after abortion of one fetus or more (O31.1-, O31.3-)

O00 Ectopic pregnancy

Includes: ruptured ectopic pregnancy
Use additional code from category O08 to identify any associated complication

O00.0   Abdominal pregnancy

Excludes1:   maternal care for viable fetus in abdominal pregnancy (O36.7-)

O00.00   Abdominal pregnancy without intrauterine pregnancy
Abdominal pregnancy NOS

O00.01   Abdominal pregnancy with intrauterine pregnancy

O00.1   Tubal pregnancy
Fallopian pregnancy
Rupture of (fallopian) tube due to pregnancy
Tubal abortion

O00.10   Tubal pregnancy without intrauterine pregnancy
Tubal pregnancy NOS

O00.11   Tubal pregnancy with intrauterine pregnancy

O00.2   Ovarian pregnancy

O00.20   Ovarian pregnancy without intrauterine pregnancy
Ovarian pregnancy NOS

O00.21   Ovarian pregnancy with intrauterine pregnancy

O00.8   Other ectopic pregnancy
Cervical pregnancy
Cornual pregnancy
Intraligamentous pregnancy
Mural pregnancy

O00.80   Other ectopic pregnancy without intrauterine pregnancy

O00.81   Other ectopic pregnancy with intrauterine pregnancy

O00.9   Ectopic pregnancy, unspecified

O00.90   Ectopic pregnancy, unspecified, without intrauterine pregnancy
Ectopic pregnancy NOS

O00.91   Ectopic pregnancy, unspecified, with intrauterine pregnancy

O01 Hydatidiform mole
Use additional code from category O08 to identify any associated complication.
Excludes1:   malignant hydatidiform mole (D39.2)

O01.0   Classical hydatidiform mole
Complete hydatidiform mole

O01.1   Incomplete and partial hydatidiform mole

O01.9   Hydatidiform mole, unspecified
Trophoblastic disease NOS
Vesicular mole NOS

O02 Other abnormal products of conception
Use additional code from category O08 to identify any associated complication.
Excludes1:   papyraceous fetus (O31.0-)

O02.0   Blighted ovum and nonhydatidiform mole
Carneous mole
Fleshy mole
Intrauterine mole NOS
Pathological ovum

O02.1   Missed abortion
Early fetal death, before completion of 20 weeks of gestation, with retention of dead fetus
Excludes1:   failed induced abortion (O07.-)
       fetal death (intrauterine) (late) (O36.4)
       missed abortion with blighted ovum (O02.0)
       missed abortion with hydatidiform mole (O01.-)
       missed abortion with nonhydatidiform (O02.0)
       missed delivery (O36.4)

O02.8   Other specified abnormal products of conception
Excludes1:   abnormal products of conception with blighted ovum (O02.0)
       abnormal products of conception with hydatidiform mole (O01.-)
       abnormal products of conception with nonhydatidiform mole (O02.0)

O02.9   Abnormal product of conception, unspecified

O03 Spontaneous abortion
Note: Incomplete abortion includes retained products of conception following spontaneous abortion
Includes: miscarriage

O03.0   Incomplete spontaneous abortion complicated by genitourinary tract and pelvic infection
Incomplete spontaneous abortion with conditions in O08.0

O03.1   Incomplete spontaneous abortion complicated by delayed or excessive hemorrhage
Incomplete spontaneous abortion with conditions in O08.1

O03.2 **Incomplete spontaneous abortion complicated by embolism**
Incomplete spontaneous abortion with conditions in O08.2

O03.3 **Incomplete spontaneous abortion with other and unspecified complications**
Incomplete spontaneous abortion with conditions in O08.3-O08.9

 O03.30 **Incomplete spontaneous abortion with unspecified complications**

 O03.39 **Incomplete spontaneous abortion with other complications**

O03.4 **Incomplete spontaneous abortion without complication**

O03.5 **Complete or unspecified spontaneous abortion complicated by genitourinary tract and pelvic infection**
Complete or unspecified spontaneous abortion with conditions in O08.0

O03.6 **Complete or unspecified spontaneous abortion complicated by delayed or excessive hemorrhage**
Complete or unspecified spontaneous abortion with conditions in O08.1

O03.7 **Complete or unspecified spontaneous abortion complicated by embolism**
Complete or unspecified spontaneous abortion with conditions in O08.2

O03.8 **Complete or unspecified spontaneous abortion with other and unspecified complications**
Complete or unspecified spontaneous abortion with conditions in O08.3-O08.9

 O03.80 **Complete or unspecified spontaneous abortion with unspecified complications**

 O03.89 **Complete or unspecified spontaneous abortion with other complications**

O03.9 **Complete or unspecified spontaneous abortion without complication**

O04 Complications following (induced) termination of pregnancy
Includes: complications following (induced) termination of pregnancy
Excludes1:   failed attempted termination of pregnancy (O07.-)

O04.5 **Termination of pregnancy complicated by genitourinary tract and pelvic infection**
Termination of pregnancy with conditions in O08.0

O04.6 **Termination of pregnancy complicated by delayed or excessive hemorrhage**
Termination of pregnancy with conditions in O08.1

O04.7 **Termination of pregnancy complicated by embolism**
Termination of pregnancy with conditions in O08.2

O04.8 **Termination of pregnancy with other and unspecified complications**
Termination of pregnancy with conditions in O08.3-O08.9

 O04.80 **Termination of pregnancy with unspecified complications**

 O04.89 **Termination of pregnancy with other complications**

O07 Failed attempted termination of pregnancy
Includes: failure of attempted induction of termination of pregnancy
Excludes1:   incomplete spontaneous abortion (O03.0-O04)

O07.0 **Failed attempted termination of pregnancy complicated by genitourinary tract and pelvic infection**
Failed attempted termination of pregnancy with conditions in O08.0

O07.1 **Failed attempted termination of pregnancy complicated by delayed or excessive hemorrhage**
Failed attempted termination of pregnancy with conditions in O08.1

O07.2 **Failed attempted termination of pregnancy complicated by embolism**
Failed attempted termination of pregnancy with conditions in O08.2

O07.3 **Failed attempted termination of pregnancy with other and unspecified complications**
Failed attempted termination of pregnancy with conditions in O08.3-O08.9

 O07.30 **Failed attempted termination of pregnancy with unspecified complications**

 O07.39 **Failed attempted termination of pregnancy with other complications**

O07.4 **Failed attempted termination of pregnancy without complication**

O08 Complications following ectopic and molar pregnancy
This category is for use with categories O00-O02 to identify any associated complications

O08.0 **Genitourinary tract and pelvic infection following ectopic and molar pregnancy**
Endometritis following ectopic and molar pregnancy
Oophoritis following ectopic and molar pregnancy
Parametritis following ectopic and molar pregnancy
Pelvic peritonitis following ectopic and molar pregnancy
Salpingitis following ectopic and molar pregnancy
Salpingo-oophoritis following ectopic and molar pregnancy
Urinary tract infection following ectopic and molar pregnancy

O08.1 **Delayed or excessive hemorrhage following ectopic and molar pregnancy**
Afibrinogenemia following ectopic and molar pregnancy
Defibrination syndrome following ectopic and molar pregnancy
Hemolysis following ectopic and molar pregnancy
Intravascular coagulation following ectopic and molar pregnancy
Excludes1:   delayed or excessive hemorrhage due to incomplete abortion (O03.1)

O08.2 **Embolism following ectopic and molar pregnancy**
Air embolism following ectopic and molar pregnancy
Amniotic fluid embolism following ectopic and molar pregnancy
Blood-clot embolism following ectopic and molar pregnancy
Embolism NOS following ectopic and molar pregnancy
Fat embolism following ectopic and molar pregnancy
Pulmonary embolism following ectopic and molar pregnancy
Pyemic embolism following ectopic and molar pregnancy
Septic or septicopyemic embolism following ectopic and molar pregnancy
Soap embolism following ectopic and molar pregnancy

O08.3 **Shock following ectopic and molar pregnancy**
Circulatory collapse following ectopic and molar pregnancy
Shock (postoperative) following ectopic and molar pregnancy
Excludes1:   septic shock (O08.82)

O08.4 **Renal failure following ectopic and molar pregnancy**
Oliguria following ectopic and molar pregnancy
Renal failure (acute) following ectopic and molar pregnancy
Renal shutdown following ectopic and molar pregnancy
Renal tubular necrosis following ectopic and molar pregnancy
Uremia following ectopic and molar pregnancy

O08.5 **Metabolic disorders following an ectopic and molar pregnancy**

O08.6 **Damage to pelvic organs and tissues following an ectopic and molar pregnancy**
Laceration, perforation, tear or chemical damage of bladder following an ectopic and molar pregnancy
Laceration, perforation, tear or chemical damage of bowel following an ectopic and molar pregnancy
Laceration, perforation, tear or chemical damage of broad ligament following an ectopic and molar pregnancy
Laceration, perforation, tear or chemical damage of cervix following an ectopic and molar pregnancy
Laceration, perforation, tear or chemical damage of periurethral tissue following an ectopic and molar pregnancy
Laceration, perforation, tear or chemical damage of uterus following an ectopic and molar pregnancy
Laceration, perforation, tear or chemical damage of vagina following an ectopic and molar pregnancy

O08.7 **Other venous complications following an ectopic and molar pregnancy**

O08.8 **Other complications following an ectopic and molar pregnancy**

 O08.81 **Cardiac arrest following an ectopic and molar pregnancy**

O08.82 **Sepsis following ectopic and molar pregnancy**
Septic shock following an ectopic and molar pregnancy
Septicemia following an ectopic and molar pregnancy
Excludes1:   septic or septicopyemic embolism following ectopic and molar pregnancy (O08.2)

O08.89 **Other complications following an ectopic and molar pregnancy**

O08.9 **Unspecified complication following an ectopic and molar pregnancy**

O09 **Supervision of high-risk pregnancy**

O09.0 **Supervision of pregnancy with history of infertility**

O09.00 **Supervision of pregnancy with history of infertility, unspecified trimester**

O09.01 **Supervision of pregnancy with history of infertility, first trimester**

O09.02 **Supervision of pregnancy with history of infertility, second trimester**

O09.03 **Supervision of pregnancy with history of infertility, third trimester**

O09.1 **Supervision of pregnancy with history of ectopic or molar pregnancy**

O09.10 **Supervision of pregnancy with history of ectopic or molar pregnancy, unspecified trimester**

O09.11 **Supervision of pregnancy with history of ectopic or molar pregnancy, first trimester**

O09.12 **Supervision of pregnancy with history of ectopic or molar pregnancy, second trimester**

O09.13 **Supervision of pregnancy with history of ectopic or molar pregnancy, third trimester**

O09.2x **Supervision of pregnancy with other poor reproductive or obstetric history**
Supervision of pregnancy with history of neonatal death
Supervision of pregnancy with history of stillbirth
Excludes2:   pregnancy care of habitual aborter (O26.2-)

O09.2x **Supervision of pregnancy with other poor reproductive or obstetric history**

O09.2x1 **Supervision of pregnancy with other poor reproductive or obstetric history, first trimester**

O09.2x2 **Supervision of pregnancy with other poor reproductive or obstetric history, second trimester**

O09.2x3 **Supervision of pregnancy with other poor reproductive or obstetric history, third trimester**

O09.2x9 **Supervision of pregnancy with other poor reproductive or obstetric history, unspecified trimester**

O09.3 **Supervision of pregnancy with insufficient antenatal care**
Supervision of concealed pregnancy
Supervision of hidden pregnancy

O09.30 **Supervision of pregnancy with insufficient antenatal care, unspecified trimester**

O09.31 **Supervision of pregnancy with insufficient antenatal care, first trimester**

O09.32 **Supervision of pregnancy with insufficient antenatal care, second trimester**

O09.33 **Supervision of pregnancy with insufficient antenatal care, third trimester**

O09.4 **Supervision of pregnancy with grand multiparity**

O09.40 **Supervision of pregnancy with grand multiparity, unspecified trimester**

O09.41 **Supervision of pregnancy with grand multiparity, first trimester**

O09.42 **Supervision of pregnancy with grand multiparity, second trimester**

O09.43 **Supervision of pregnancy with grand multiparity, third trimester**

O09.5 **Supervision of elderly primigravida and multigravida**
Pregnancy for a female 35 years and older at expected date of delivery

O09.51 **Supervision of elderly primigravida**

O09.511 **Supervision of elderly primigravida, first trimester**

O09.512 **Supervision of elderly primigravida, second trimester**

O09.513 **Supervision of elderly primigravida, third trimester**

O09.519 **Supervision of elderly primigravida, unspecified trimester**

O09.52 **Supervision of elderly multigravida**

O09.521 **Supervision of elderly multigravida, first trimester**

O09.522 **Supervision of elderly multigravida, second trimester**

O09.523 **Supervision of elderly multigravida, third trimester**

O09.529 **Supervision of elderly multigravida, unspecified trimester**

O09.6 **Supervision of young primigravida and multigravida**
Supervision of pregnancy for a female less than 16 years old at expected date of delivery

O09.61 **Supervision of young primigravida**

O09.611 **Supervision of young primigravida, first trimester**

O09.612 **Supervision of young primigravida, second trimester**

O09.613 **Supervision of young primigravida, third trimester**

O09.619 **Supervision of young primigravida, unspecified trimester**

O09.62 **Supervision of young multigravida**

O09.621 **Supervision of young multigravida, first trimester**

O09.622 **Supervision of young multigravida, second trimester**

O09.623 **Supervision of young multigravida, third trimester**

O09.629 **Supervision of young multigravida, unspecified trimester**

O09.7 **Supervision of high-risk pregnancy due to social problems**

O09.70 **Supervision of high-risk pregnancy due to social problems, unspecified trimester**

O09.71 **Supervision of high-risk pregnancy due to social problems, first trimester**

O09.72 **Supervision of high-risk pregnancy due to social problems, second trimester**

O09.73 **Supervision of high-risk pregnancy due to social problems, third trimester**

O09.8 **Supervision of other high-risk pregnancies**

O09.81 **Supervision of pregnancy resulting from assisted reproductive technology**
Supervision of pregnancy resulting from in-vitro fertilization

O09.811 **Supervision of pregnancy resulting from assisted reproductive technology, first trimester**

O09.812 **Supervision of pregnancy resulting from assisted reproductive technology, second trimester**

O09.813 **Supervision of pregnancy resulting from assisted reproductive technology, third trimester**

O09.819 **Supervision of pregnancy resulting from assisted reproductive technology, unspecified trimester**

O09.89 **Supervision of other high-risk pregnancies**

O09.891 **Supervision of other high-risk pregnancies, first trimester**

O09.892 **Supervision of other high-risk pregnancies, second trimester**

O09.893 **Supervision of other high-risk pregnancies, third trimester**

O09.899   Supervision of other high-risk pregnancies, unspecified trimester

O09.9   Supervision of high-risk pregnancy, unspecified

O09.90   Supervision of high-risk pregnancy, unspecified, unspecified trimester

O09.91   Supervision of high-risk pregnancy, unspecified, first trimester

O09.92   Supervision of high-risk pregnancy, unspecified, second trimester

O09.93   Supervision of high-risk pregnancy, unspecified, third trimester

EDEMA, PROTEINURIA AND HYPERTENSIVE DISORDERS IN PREGNANCY, CHILDBIRTH AND THE PUERPERIUM (O10–O16)

O10   Pre-existing hypertension complicating pregnancy, childbirth and the puerperium

Includes: Pre-existing hypertension with pre-exisiting proteinuria complicating pregnancy, childbirth and the puerperium

Excludes1:   pre-exisiting hypertension with increased or superimposed proteinuria complicating pregnancy, childbirth and the puerperium (Oll.-)

O10.0   Pre-existing essential hypertension complicating pregnancy, childbirth and the puerperium

Any condition in I10 specified as a reason for obstetric care during pregnancy, childbirth or the puerperium

O10.01   Pre-existing essential hypertension complicating pregnancy

O10.011   Pre-existing essential hypertension complicating pregnancy, first trimester

O10.012   Pre-existing essential hypertension complicating pregnancy, second trimester

O10.013   Pre-existing essential hypertension complicating pregnancy, third trimester

O10.019   Pre-existing essential hypertension complicating pregnancy, unspecified trimester

O10.02   Pre-existing essential hypertension complicating childbirth

O10.03   Pre-existing essential hypertension complicating the puerperium

O10.1   Pre-existing hypertensive heart disease complicating pregnancy, childbirth and the puerperium

Any condition in I11 specified as a reason for obstetric care during pregnancy, childbirth or the puerperium

O10.11   Pre-existing hypertensive heart disease complicating pregnancy

O10.111   Pre-existing hypertensive heart disease complicating pregnancy, first trimester

O10.112   Pre-existing hypertensive heart disease complicating pregnancy, second trimester

O10.113   Pre-existing hypertensive heart disease complicating pregnancy, third trimester

O10.119   Pre-existing hypertensive heart disease complicating pregnancy, trimester unspecified

O10.12   Pre-existing hypertensive heart disease complicating childbirth

O10.13   Pre-existing hypertensive heart disease complicating the puerperium

O10.2   Pre-existing hypertensive renal disease complicating pregnancy, childbirth and the puerperium

Any condition in I12 specified as a reason for obstetric care during pregnancy, childbirth or the puerperium

O10.21   Pre-existing hypertensive renal disease complicating pregnancy

O10.211   Pre-existing hypertensive renal disease complicating pregnancy, first trimester

O10.212   Pre-existing hypertensive renal disease complicating pregnancy, second trimester

O10.213   Pre-existing hypertensive renal disease complicating pregnancy, third trimester

O10.219   Pre-existing hypertensive renal disease complicating pregnancy, unspecified trimester

O10.22   Pre-existing hypertensive renal disease complicating childbirth

O10.23   Pre-existing hypertensive renal disease complicating the puerperium

O10.3   Pre-existing hypertensive heart and renal disease complicating pregnancy, childbirth and the puerperium

Any condition in I13 specified as a reason for obstetric care during pregnancy, childbirth or the puerperium

O10.31   Pre-existing hypertensive heart and renal disease complicating pregnancy

O10.311   Pre-existing hypertensive heart and renal disease complicating pregnancy, first trimester

O10.312   Pre-existing hypertensive heart and renal disease complicating pregnancy, second trimester

O10.313   Pre-existing hypertensive heart and renal disease complicating pregnancy, third trimester

O10.319   Pre-existing hypertensive heart and renal disease complicating pregnancy, unspecified trimester

O10.32   Pre-existing hypertensive heart and renal disease complicating childbirth

O10.33   Pre-existing hypertensive heart and renal disease complicating the puerperium

O10.4   Pre-existing secondary hypertension complicating pregnancy, childbirth and the puerperium

Any condition in I15 specified as a reason for obstetric care during pregnancy, childbirth or the puerperium

O10.41   Pre-existing secondary hypertension complicating pregnancy

O10.411   Pre-existing secondary hypertension complicating pregnancy, first trimester

O10.412   Pre-existing secondary hypertension complicating pregnancy, second trimester

O10.413   Pre-existing secondary hypertension complicating pregnancy, third trimester

O10.419   Pre-existing secondary hypertension complicating pregnancy, unspecified trimester

O10.42   Pre-existing secondary hypertension complicating childbirth

O10.43   Pre-existing secondary hypertension complicating the puerperium

O10.9   Unspecified pre-existing hypertension complicating pregnancy, childbirth and the puerperium

O10.91   Unspecified pre-existing hypertension complicating pregnancy

O10.911   Unspecified pre-existing hypertension complicating pregnancy, first trimester

O10.912   Unspecified pre-existing hypertension complicating pregnancy, second trimester

O10.913   Unspecified pre-existing hypertension complicating pregnancy, third trimester

O10.919   Unspecified pre-existing hypertension complicating pregnancy, unspecified trimester

O10.92   Unspecified pre-existing hypertension complicating childbirth

O10.93   Unspecified pre-existing hypertension complicating the puerperium

O11   Pre-existing hypertensive disorder with superimposed proteinuria

Includes: conditions in Ol0 complicated by increased proteinuria superimposed pre-eclampsia

O11.1   Pre-existing hypertensive disorder with superimposed proteinuria, first trimester

O11.2   Pre-existing hypertensive disorder with superimposed proteinuria, second trimester

O11.3   Pre-existing hypertensive disorder with superimposed proteinuria, third trimester

O11.9   Pre-existing hypertensive disorder with superimposed proteinuria, unspecified trimester

O12   **Gestational [pregnancy-induced] edema and proteinuria without hypertension**

O12.0   Gestational edema

O12.00   Gestational edema, unspecified trimester

O12.01   Gestational edema, first trimester

O12.02   Gestational edema, second trimester

O12.03   Gestational edema, third trimester

O12.1   Gestational proteinuria

O12.10   Gestational proteinuria, unspecified trimester

O12.11   Gestational proteinuria, first trimester

O12.12   Gestational proteinuria, second trimester

O12.13   Gestational proteinuria, third trimester

O12.2   Gestational edema with proteinuria

O12.20   Gestational edema with proteinuria, unspecified trimester

O12.21   Gestational edema with proteinuria, first trimester

O12.22   Gestational edema with proteinuria, second trimester

O12.23   Gestational edema with proteinuria, third trimester

O13   **Gestational [pregnancy-induced] hypertension without significant proteinuria**

Includes: gestational hypertension NOS

O13.1   Gestational [pregnancy-induced] hypertension without significant proteinuria, first trimester

O13.2   Gestational [pregnancy-induced] hypertension without significant proteinuria, second trimester

O13.3   Gestational [pregnancy-induced] hypertension without significant proteinuria, third trimester

O13.9   Gestational [pregnancy-induced] hypertension without significant proteinuria, unspecified trimester

O14   **Gestational [pregnancy-induced] hypertension with significant proteinuria**

Excludes1:   superimposed pre-eclampsia (O11)

O14.0   Mild pre-eclampsia

O14.00   Mild pre-eclampsia, unspecified trimester

O14.02   Mild pre-eclampsia, second trimester

O14.03   Mild pre-eclampsia, third trimester

O14.1   Severe pre-eclampsia

H.E.L.L.P.

O14.10   Severe pre-eclampsia, unspecified trimester

O14.12   Severe pre-eclampsia, second trimester

O14.13   Severe pre-eclampsia, third trimester

O14.9   Unspecified pre-eclampsia

O14.90   Unspecified pre-eclampsia, unspecified trimester

O14.92   Unspecified pre-eclampsia, second trimester

O14.93   Unspecified pre-eclampsia, third trimester

O15   **Eclampsia**

Includes: convulsions following conditions in O10-O14 and O16

O15.0   Eclampsia in pregnancy

O15.00   Eclampsia in pregnancy, unspecified trimester

O15.02   Eclampsia in pregnancy, second trimester

O15.03   Eclampsia in pregnancy, third trimester

O15.1   Eclampsia in labor

O15.2   Eclampsia in the puerperium

O15.9   Eclampsia, unspecified as to time period

Eclampsia NOS

O16   **Unspecified maternal hypertension**

Includes: transient hypertension of pregnancy

O16.1   Unspecified maternal hypertension, first trimester

O16.2   Unspecified maternal hypertension, second trimester

O16.3   Unspecified maternal hypertension, third trimester

O16.9   Unspecified maternal hypertension, unspecified trimester

OTHER MATERNAL DISORDERS PREDOMINANTLY RELATED TO PREGNANCY (O20–O29)

Excludes2:   maternal care related to the fetus and amniotic cavity and possible delivery problems (O30-O48)

maternal diseases classifiable elsewhere but complicating pregnancy, labor and delivery, and the puerperium (O98-O99)

O20   **Hemorrhage in early pregnancy**

Includes: before completion of 20 weeks gestation

Excludes1:   pregnancy with abortive outcome (O00-O08)

O20.0   **Threatened abortion**

Hemorrhage specified as due to threatened abortion

O20.8   **Other hemorrhage in early pregnancy**

O20.9   **Hemorrhage in early pregnancy, unspecified**

O21   **Excessive vomiting in pregnancy**

O21.0   **Mild hyperemesis gravidarum**

Hyperemesis gravidarum, mild or unspecified, starting before the end of the 20th week of gestation

O21.1   **Hyperemesis gravidarum with metabolic disturbance**

Hyperemesis gravidarum, starting before the end of the 20th week of gestation, with metabolic disturbance such as carbohydrate depletion

Hyperemesis gravidarum, starting before the end of the 20th week of gestation, with metabolic disturbance such as dehydration

Hyperemesis gravidarum, starting before the end of the 20th week of gestation, with metabolic disturbance such as electrolyte imbalance

O21.2   **Late vomiting of pregnancy**

Excessive vomiting starting after 20 completed weeks of gestation

O21.8   **Other vomiting complicating pregnancy**

Vomiting due to diseases classified elsewhere, complicating pregnancy

Use additional code, to identify cause.

O21.9   **Vomiting of pregnancy, unspecified**

O22   **Venous complications in pregnancy**

Excludes1:   venous complications of:

abortion NOS (O06.8)

ectopic or molar pregnancy (O08.7)

failed attempted abortion (O07.39, O07.89)

induced abortion (O04.89, O05.89)

spontaneous abortion (O03.89, O03.89)

Excludes2:   obstetric pulmonary embolism (O88.-)

venous complications of childbirth and the puerperium (O87.-)

O22.0   Varicose veins of lower extremity in pregnancy

Varicose veins NOS in pregnancy

O22.00   Varicose veins of lower extremity in pregnancy, unspecified trimester

O22.01   Varicose veins of lower extremity in pregnancy, first trimester

O22.02   Varicose veins of lower extremity in pregnancy, second trimester

O22.03   Varicose veins of lower extremity in pregnancy, third trimester

O22.1   Genital varices in pregnancy

Perineal varices in pregnancy

Vaginal varices in pregnancy

Vulval varices in pregnancy

O22.10   Genital varices in pregnancy, unspecified trimester

O22.11   Genital varices in pregnancy, first trimester

O22.12   Genital varices in pregnancy, second trimester

O22.13   Genital varices in pregnancy, third trimester

O22.2   Superficial thrombophlebitis in pregnancy

Thrombophlebitis of legs in pregnancy

O22.20   Superficial thrombophlebitis in pregnancy, unspecified trimester

O22.21   Superficial thrombophlebitis in pregnancy, first trimester

O22.22   Superficial thrombophlebitis in pregnancy, second trimester

O22.23   Superficial thrombophlebitis in pregnancy, third trimester

O22.3   Deep phlebothrombosis in pregnancy
Deep-vein thrombosis, antepartum

O22.30   Deep phlebothrombosis in pregnancy, unspecified trimester

O22.31   Deep phlebothrombosis in pregnancy, first trimester

O22.32   Deep phlebothrombosis in pregnancy, second trimester

O22.33   Deep phlebothrombosis in pregnancy, third trimester

O22.4   Hemorrhoids in pregnancy

O22.40   Hemorrhoids in pregnancy, unspecified trimester

O22.41   Hemorrhoids in pregnancy, first trimester

O22.42   Hemorrhoids in pregnancy, second trimester

O22.43   Hemorrhoids in pregnancy, third trimester

O22.5   Cerebral venous thrombosis in pregnancy
Cerebrovenous sinus thrombosis in pregnancy

O22.50   Cerebral venous thrombosis in pregnancy, unspecified trimester

O22.51   Cerebral venous thrombosis in pregnancy, first trimester

O22.52   Cerebral venous thrombosis in pregnancy, second trimester

O22.53   Cerebral venous thrombosis in pregnancy, third trimester

O22.8   Other venous complications in pregnancy

O22.8x   Other venous complications in pregnancy

O22.8x1   Other venous complications in pregnancy, first trimester

O22.8x2   Other venous complications in pregnancy, second trimester

O22.8x3   Other venous complications in pregnancy, third trimester

O22.8x9   Other venous complications in pregnancy, unspecified trimester

O22.9   Venous complication in pregnancy, unspecified
Gestational phlebitis NOS
Gestational phlebopathy NOS
Gestational thrombosis NOS

O22.90   Venous complication in pregnancy, unspecified, unspecified trimester

O22.91   Venous complication in pregnancy, unspecified, first trimester

O22.92   Venous complication in pregnancy, unspecified, second trimester

O22.93   Venous complication in pregnancy, unspecified, third trimester

O23   Infections of genitourinary tract in pregnancy
Use additional code to identify organism (B95.-, B96.-)

O23.0   Infections of kidney in pregnancy
Pyelonephritis in pregnancy

O23.00   Infections of kidney in pregnancy, unspecified trimester

O23.01   Infections of kidney in pregnancy, first trimester

O23.02   Infections of kidney in pregnancy, second trimester

O23.03   Infections of kidney in pregnancy, third trimester

O23.1   Infections of bladder in pregnancy

O23.10   Infections of bladder in pregnancy, unspecified trimester

O23.11   Infections of bladder in pregnancy, first trimester

O23.12   Infections of bladder in pregnancy, second trimester

O23.13   Infections of bladder in pregnancy, third trimester

O23.2   Infections of urethra in pregnancy

O23.20   Infections of urethra in pregnancy, unspecified trimester

O23.21   Infections of urethra in pregnancy, first trimester

O23.22   Infections of urethra in pregnancy, second trimester

O23.23   Infections of urethra in pregnancy, third trimester

O23.3   Infections of other parts of urinary tract in pregnancy

O23.30   Infections of other parts of urinary tract in pregnancy, unspecified trimester

O23.31   Infections of other parts of urinary tract in pregnancy, first trimester

O23.32   Infections of other parts of urinary tract in pregnancy, second trimester

O23.33   Infections of other parts of urinary tract in pregnancy, third trimester

O23.4   Unspecified infection of urinary tract in pregnancy

O23.40   Unspecified infection of urinary tract in pregnancy, unspecified trimester

O23.41   Unspecified infection of urinary tract in pregnancy, first trimester

O23.42   Unspecified infection of urinary tract in pregnancy, second trimester

O23.43   Unspecified infection of urinary tract in pregnancy, third trimester

O23.5   Infections of the genital tract in pregnancy

O23.50   Infections of the genital tract in pregnancy, unspecified trimester

O23.51   Infections of the genital tract in pregnancy, first trimester

O23.52   Infections of the genital tract in pregnancy, second trimester

O23.53   Infections of the genital tract in pregnancy, third trimester

O23.9   Unspecified genitourinary tract infection in pregnancy
Genitourinary tract infection in pregnancy NOS

O23.90   Unspecified genitourinary tract infection in pregnancy, unspecified trimester

O23.91   Unspecified genitourinary tract infection in pregnancy, first trimester

O23.92   Unspecified genitourinary tract infection in pregnancy, second trimester

O23.93   Unspecified genitourinary tract infection in pregnancy, third trimester

O24   Diabetes mellitus in pregnancy, childbirth, and the puerperium

O24.0   Pre-existing diabetes mellitus, type 1, in pregnancy, childbirth and the puerperium
Juvenile onset diabetes mellitus, in pregnancy, childbirth and the puerperium
Ketosis-prone diabetes mellitus in pregnancy, childbirth and the puerperium
Use additional code from category E10 to further identify any manifestations

O24.01   Pre-existing diabetes mellitus, type 1, in pregnancy

O24.011   Pre-existing diabetes mellitus, type 1, in pregnancy, first trimester

O24.012   Pre-existing diabetes mellitus, type 1, in pregnancy, second trimester

O24.013   Pre-existing diabetes mellitus, type 1, in pregnancy, third trimester

O24.019   Pre-existing diabetes mellitus, type 1, in pregnancy, unspecified trimester

O24.02   Pre-existing diabetes mellitus, type 1, in childbirth

O24.03   Pre-existing diabetes mellitus, type 1, in the puerperium

O24.1   Pre-existing diabetes mellitus, type 2, in pregnancy, childbirth and the puerperium
Insulin-resistant diabetes mellitus in pregnancy, childbirth and the puerperium
Use additional code (for):
from category E11 to further identify any manifestations
long-term (current) use of insulin (Z79.4)

O24.11   Pre-existing diabetes mellitus, type 2, in pregnancy, childbirth and the puerperium

O24.111   Pre-existing diabetes mellitus, type 2, in pregnancy, first trimester

O24.112   Pre-existing diabetes mellitus, type 2, in pregnancy, second trimester

O24.113　Pre-existing diabetes mellitus, type 2, in pregnancy, third trimester

O24.119　Pre-existing diabetes mellitus, type 2, in pregnancy, unspecified trimester

O24.12　Pre-existing diabetes mellitus, type 2, in childbirth

O24.13　Pre-existing diabetes mellitus, type 2, in the puerperium

O24.3　Unspecified pre-existing diabetes mellitus in pregnancy, childbirth and the puerperium

　　　Use additional code (for):
　　　from category E14 to further identify any manifestation
　　　long-term (current) use of insulin (Z79.4)

O24.31　Unspecified pre-existing diabetes mellitus in pregnancy

O24.311　Unspecified pre-existing diabetes mellitus in pregnancy, first trimester

O24.312　Unspecified pre-existing diabetes mellitus in pregnancy, second trimester

O24.313　Unspecified pre-existing diabetes mellitus in pregnancy, third trimester

O24.319　Unspecified pre-existing diabetes mellitus in pregnancy, unspecified trimester

O24.32　Unspecified pre-existing diabetes mellitus in childbirth

O24.33　Unspecified pre-existing diabetes mellitus in the puerperium

O24.4　Gestational diabetes mellitus
　　　Diabetes mellitus arising in pregnancy
　　　Gestational diabetes mellitus NOS

O24.41　Gestational diabetes mellitus in pregnancy

O24.410　Gestational diabetes mellitus in pregnancy, diet-controlled

O24.414　Gestational diabetes mellitus in pregnancy, insulin controlled

O24.415　Gestational diabetes mellitus in pregnancy, unspecified control

O24.42　Gestational diabetes mellitus in childbirth

O24.420　Gestational diabetes mellitus in childbirth, diet controlled

O24.424　Gestational diabetes mellitus in childbirth, insulin controlled

O24.425　Gestational diabetes mellitus in childbirth, unspecified control

O24.43　Gestational diabetes mellitus in the puerperium

O24.430　Gestational diabetes mellitus in the puerperium, diet controlled

O24.434　Gestational diabetes mellitus in the puerperium, insulin controlled

O24.435　Gestational diabetes mellitus in the puerperium, unspecified control

O24.8　Other pre-existing diabetes mellitus in pregnancy, childbirth, and the puerperium

　　　Use additional code (for):
　　　from categories E08, E09 and E13 to further identify any manifestation
　　　long-term (current) use of insulin (Z79.4)

O24.81　Other pre-existing diabetes mellitus in pregnancy

O24.811　Other pre-existing diabetes mellitus in pregnancy, first trimester

O24.812　Other pre-existing diabetes mellitus in pregnancy, second trimester

O24.813　Other pre-existing diabetes mellitus in pregnancy, third trimester

O24.819　Other pre-existing diabetes mellitus in pregnancy, unspecified trimester

O24.82　Other pre-existing diabetes mellitus in childbirth

O24.83　Other pre-existing diabetes mellitus in the puerperium

O24.9　Unspecified diabetes mellitus in pregnancy, childbirth and the puerperium

　　　Use additional code for long-term (current) use of insulin (Z79.4)

O24.91　Unspecified diabetes mellitus in pregnancy

O24.911　Unspecified diabetes mellitus in pregnancy, first trimester

O24.912　Unspecified diabetes mellitus in pregnancy, second trimester

O24.913　Unspecified diabetes mellitus in pregnancy, third trimester

O24.919　Unspecified diabetes mellitus in pregnancy, unspecified trimester

O24.92　Unspecified diabetes mellitus in childbirth

O24.93　Unspecified diabetes mellitus in the puerperium

O25　Malnutrition in pregnancy, childbirth and the puerperium

O25.1　Malnutrition in pregnancy

O25.10　Malnutrition in pregnancy, unspecified trimester

O25.11　Malnutrition in pregnancy, first trimester

O25.12　Malnutrition in pregnancy, second trimester

O25.13　Malnutrition in pregnancy, third trimester

O25.2　Malnutrition in childbirth

O25.3　Malnutrition in the puerperium

O26　Maternal care for other conditions predominantly related to pregnancy

O26.0　Excessive weight gain in pregnancy
　　　Excludes2:　gestational edema (O12.0, O12.2)

O26.00　Excessive weight gain in pregnancy, unspecified trimester

O26.01　Excessive weight gain in pregnancy, first trimester

O26.02　Excessive weight gain in pregnancy, second trimester

O26.03　Excessive weight gain in pregnancy, third trimester

O26.1　Low weight gain in pregnancy

O26.10　Low weight gain in pregnancy, unspecified trimester

O26.11　Low weight gain in pregnancy, first trimester

O26.12　Low weight gain in pregnancy, second trimester

O26.13　Low weight gain in pregnancy, third trimester

O26.2　Pregnancy care of habitual aborter

O26.20　Pregnancy care of habitual aborter, unspecified trimester

O26.21　Pregnancy care of habitual aborter, first trimester

O26.22　Pregnancy care of habitual aborter, second trimester

O26.23　Pregnancy care of habitual aborter, third trimester

O26.3　Retained intrauterine contraceptive device in pregnancy

O26.30　Retained intrauterine contraceptive device in pregnancy, unspecified trimester

O26.31　Retained intrauterine contraceptive device in pregnancy, first trimester

O26.32　Retained intrauterine contraceptive device in pregnancy, second trimester

O26.33　Retained intrauterine contraceptive device in pregnancy, third trimester

O26.4　Herpes gestationis

O26.40　Herpes gestationis, unspecified trimester

O26.41　Herpes gestationis, first trimester

O26.42　Herpes gestationis, second trimester

O26.43　Herpes gestationis, third trimester

O26.5　Maternal hypotension syndrome
　　　Supine hypotensive syndrome

O26.50　Maternal hypotension syndrome, unspecified trimester

O26.51　Maternal hypotension syndrome, first trimester

O26.52　Maternal hypotension syndrome, second trimester

O26.53　Maternal hypotension syndrome, third trimester

O26.6　Liver disorders in pregnancy, childbirth and the puerperium
　　　Use additional code to identify the specific disorder
　　　Excludes2:　hepatorenal syndrome following labor and delivery (O90.4)

O26.61　Liver disorders in pregnancy

O26.611　Liver disorders in pregnancy, first trimester

O26.612　Liver disorders in pregnancy, second trimester

O26.613　Liver disorders in pregnancy, third trimester

O26.619　Liver disorders in pregnancy, unspecified trimester

O26.62 Liver disorders in childbirth

O26.63 Liver disorders in the puerperium

O26.7 Subluxation of symphysis (pubis) in pregnancy, childbirth and the puerperium

  Excludes1: traumatic separation of symphysis (pubis) during childbirth (O71.6)

  O26.71 Subluxation of symphysis (pubis) in pregnancy

    O26.711 Subluxation of symphysis (pubis) in pregnancy, first trimester

    O26.712 Subluxation of symphysis (pubis) in pregnancy, second trimester

    O26.713 Subluxation of symphysis (pubis) in pregnancy, third trimester

    O26.719 Subluxation of symphysis (pubis) in pregnancy, unspecified trimester

  O26.72 Subluxation of symphysis (pubis) in childbirth

  O26.73 Subluxation of symphysis (pubis) in the puerperium

O26.8 Other specified pregnancy-related conditions

  O26.81 Pregnancy-related exhaustion and fatigue

    O26.811 Pregnancy-related exhaustion and fatigue, first trimester

    O26.812 Pregnancy-related exhaustion and fatigue, second trimester

    O26.813 Pregnancy-related exhaustion and fatigue, third trimester

    O26.819 Pregnancy-related exhaustion and fatigue, unspecified trimester

  O26.82 Pregnancy-related peripheral neuritis

    O26.821 Pregnancy-related peripheral neuritis, first trimester

    O26.822 Pregnancy-related peripheral neuritis, second trimester

    O26.823 Pregnancy-related peripheral neuritis, third trimester

    O26.829 Pregnancy-related peripheral neuritis, unspecified trimester

  O26.83 Pregnancy-related renal disease

    O26.831 Pregnancy-related renal disease, first trimester

    O26.832 Pregnancy-related renal disease, second trimester

    O26.833 Pregnancy-related renal disease, third trimester

    O26.839 Pregnancy-related renal disease, unspecified trimester

  O26.84 Uterine size-date discrepancy complicating pregnancy

    O26.841 Uterine size-date discrepancy, first trimester

    O26.842 Uterine size-date discrepancy, second trimester

    O26.843 Uterine size-date discrepancy, third trimester

    O26.849 Uterine size-date discrepancy, unspecified trimester

  O26.89 Other specified pregnancy-related conditions

    O26.891 Other specified pregnancy-related conditions, first trimester

    O26.892 Other specified pregnancy-related conditions, second trimester

    O26.893 Other specified pregnancy-related conditions, third trimester

    O26.899 Other specified pregnancy-related conditions, unspecified trimester

O26.9 Pregnancy-related condition, unspecified

  O26.90 Pregnancy-related condition, unspecified, unspecified trimester

  O26.91 Pregnancy-related condition, unspecified, first trimester

  O26.92 Pregnancy-related condition, unspecified, second trimester

  O26.93 Pregnancy-related condition, unspecified, third trimester

O28 Abnormal findings on antenatal screening of mother

  Excludes1: diagnostic findings classified elsewhere—see Alphabetical Index

O28.0 Abnormal hematological finding on antenatal screening of mother

O28.1 Abnormal biochemical finding on antenatal screening of mother

O28.2 Abnormal cytological finding on antenatal screening of mother

O28.3 Abnormal ultrasonic finding on antenatal screening of mother

O28.4 Abnormal radiological finding on antenatal screening of mother

O28.5 Abnormal chromosomal and genetic finding on antenatal screening of mother

O28.8 Other abnormal findings on antenatal screening of mother

O28.9 Abnormal finding on antenatal screening of mother, unspecified

O29 Complications of anesthesia during pregnancy

  Includes: maternal complications arising from the administration of a general, regional or local anesthetic, analgesic or other sedation during pregnancy

  Excludes2: complications of anesthesia during labor and delivery (O74.-)

      complications of anesthesia during the puerperium (O89.-)

O29.0 Pulmonary complications of anesthesia during pregnancy

  Aspiration pneumonitis due to anesthesia during pregnancy

  Inhalation of stomach contents or secretions NOS due to anesthesia during pregnancy

  Mendelson's syndrome due to anesthesia during pregnancy

  Pressure collapse of lung due to anesthesia during pregnancy

  O29.0x Pulmonary complications of anesthesia during pregnancy

    O29.0x1 Pulmonary complications of anesthesia during pregnancy, first trimester

    O29.0x2 Pulmonary complications of anesthesia during pregnancy, second trimester

    O29.0x3 Pulmonary complications of anesthesia during pregnancy, third trimester

    O29.0x9 Pulmonary complications of anesthesia during pregnancy, unspecified trimester

O29.1 Cardiac complications of anesthesia during pregnancy

  O29.11 Cardiac arrest due to anesthesia during pregnancy

    O29.111 Cardiac arrest due to anesthesia during pregnancy, first trimester

    O29.112 Cardiac arrest due to anesthesia during pregnancy, second trimester

    O29.113 Cardiac arrest due to anesthesia during pregnancy, third trimester

    O29.119 Cardiac arrest due to anesthesia during pregnancy, unspecified trimester

  O29.12 Cardiac failure due to anesthesia during pregnancy

    O29.121 Cardiac failure due to anesthesia during pregnancy, first trimester

    O29.122 Cardiac failure due to anesthesia during pregnancy, second trimester

    O29.123 Cardiac failure due to anesthesia during pregnancy, third trimester

    O29.129 Cardiac failure due to anesthesia during pregnancy, unspecified trimester

  O29.19 Other cardiac complications of anesthesia during pregnancy

    O29.191 Other cardiac complications of anesthesia during pregnancy, first trimester

    O29.192 Other cardiac complications of anesthesia during pregnancy, second trimester

    O29.193 Other cardiac complications of anesthesia during pregnancy, third trimester

    O29.199 Other cardiac complications of anesthesia during pregnancy, unspecified trimester

O29.2 Central nervous system complications of anesthesia during pregnancy

  O29.21 Cerebral anoxia due to anesthesia during pregnancy

O29.211 Cerebral anoxia due to anesthesia during pregnancy, first trimester
O29.212 Cerebral anoxia due to anesthesia during pregnancy, second trimester
O29.213 Cerebral anoxia due to anesthesia during pregnancy, third trimester
O29.219 Cerebral anoxia due to anesthesia during pregnancy, unspecified trimester

O29.29 Other central nervous system complications of anesthesia during pregnancy
O29.291 Other central nervous system complications of anesthesia during pregnancy, first trimester
O29.292 Other central nervous system complications of anesthesia during pregnancy, second trimester
O29.293 Other central nervous system complications of anesthesia during pregnancy, third trimester
O29.299 Other central nervous system complications of anesthesia during pregnancy, unspecified trimester

O29.3 Toxic reaction to local anesthesia during pregnancy
O29.3x Toxic reaction to local anesthesia during pregnancy
O29.3x1 Toxic reaction to local anesthesia during pregnancy, first trimester
O29.3x2 Toxic reaction to local anesthesia during pregnancy, second trimester
O29.3x3 Toxic reaction to local anesthesia during pregnancy, third trimester
O29.3x9 Toxic reaction to local anesthesia during pregnancy, unspecified trimester

O29.4 Spinal and epidural anesthesia-induced headache during pregnancy
O29.40 Spinal and epidural anesthesia-induced headache during pregnancy, unspecified trimester
O29.41 Spinal and epidural anesthesia-induced headache during pregnancy, first trimester
O29.42 Spinal and epidural anesthesia-induced headache during pregnancy, second trimester
O29.43 Spinal and epidural anesthesia-induced headache during pregnancy, third trimester

O29.5 Other complications of spinal and epidural anesthesia during pregnancy
O29.5x Other complications of spinal and epidural anesthesia during pregnancy
O29.5x1 Other complications of spinal and epidural anesthesia during pregnancy, first trimester
O29.5x2 Other complications of spinal and epidural anesthesia during pregnancy, second trimester
O29.5x3 Other complications of spinal and epidural anesthesia during pregnancy, third trimester
O29.5x9 Other complications of spinal and epidural anesthesia during pregnancy, unspecified trimester

O29.6 Failed or difficult intubation for anesthesia during pregnancy
O29.60 Failed or difficult intubation for anesthesia during pregnancy, unspecified trimester
O29.61 Failed or difficult intubation for anesthesia during pregnancy, first trimester
O29.62 Failed or difficult intubation for anesthesia during pregnancy, second trimester
O29.63 Failed or difficult intubation for anesthesia during pregnancy, third trimester

O29.8 Other complications of anesthesia during pregnancy
O29.8x Other complications of anesthesia during pregnancy
O29.8x1 Other complications of anesthesia during pregnancy, first trimester
O29.8x2 Other complications of anesthesia during pregnancy, second trimester
O29.8x3 Other complications of anesthesia during pregnancy, third trimester
O29.8x9 Other complications of anesthesia during pregnancy, unspecified trimester

O29.9 Unspecified complication of anesthesia during pregnancy
O29.90 Unspecified complication of anesthesia during pregnancy, unspecified trimester
O29.91 Unspecified complication of anesthesia during pregnancy, first trimester
O29.92 Unspecified complication of anesthesia during pregnancy, second trimester
O29.93 Unspecified complication of anesthesia during pregnancy, third trimester

MATERNAL CARE RELATED TO THE FETUS AND AMNIOTIC CAVITY AND POSSIBLE DELIVERY PROBLEMS (O30–O48)

O30 Multiple gestation
Use additional code(s) to identify any complications specific to multiple gestation
Use the following extensions to identify the fetus to which the complication code applies:
A   fetus A
B   fetus B
C   fetus C
D   fetus D
E   fetus E
F   fetus F
G   fetus G
H   fetus H

O30.0 Twin pregnancy
O30.00 Twin pregnancy, unspecified
O30.001 Twin pregnancy, unspecified, first trimester
O30.002 Twin pregnancy, unspecified, second trimester
O30.003 Twin pregnancy, unspecified, third trimester
O30.009 Twin pregnancy, unspecified, unspecified trimester

O30.01 Twin pregnancy, monoamniotic/monochorionic
O30.011 Twin pregnancy, monoamniotic/monochorionic, first trimester
O30.012 Twin pregnancy, monoamniotic/monochorionic, second trimester
O30.013 Twin pregnancy, monoamniotic/monochorionic, third trimester
O30.019 Twin pregnancy, monoamniotic/monochorionic, unspecified trimester

O30.09 Other twin pregnancy
O30.091 Other twin pregnancy, first trimester
O30.092 Other twin pregnancy, second trimester
O30.093 Other twin pregnancy, third trimester
O30.099 Other twin pregnancy, unspecified trimester

O30.1 Triplet pregnancy
O30.10 Triplet pregnancy, unspecified trimester
O30.11 Triplet pregnancy, first trimester
O30.12 Triplet pregnancy, second trimester
O30.13 Triplet pregnancy, third trimester

O30.2 Quadruplet pregnancy
O30.20 Quadruplet pregnancy, unspecified trimester
O30.21 Quadruplet pregnancy, first trimester
O30.22 Quadruplet pregnancy, second trimester
O30.23 Quadruplet pregnancy, third trimester

O30.8 Other multiple gestation
O30.8x Other multiple gestation
O30.8x1 Other multiple gestation, first trimester
O30.8x2 Other multiple gestation, second trimester
O30.8x3 Other multiple gestation, third trimester
O30.8x9 Other multiple gestation, unspecified trimester

O30.9 Multiple gestation, unspecified
Multiple pregnancy NOS
O30.90 Multiple gestation, unspecified, unspecified trimester
O30.91 Multiple gestation, unspecified, first trimester
O30.92 Multiple gestation, unspecified, second trimester

O30.93   Multiple gestation, unspecified, third trimester

O31 Complications specific to multiple gestation
Excludes1:   conjoined twins causing disproportion (O33.7)
Excludes2:   delayed delivery of second twin, triplet, etc. (O63.2)
                  malpresentation of one fetus or more (O32.5)

O31.0   Papyraceous fetus
Fetus compressus
O31.00   Papyraceous fetus, unspecified trimester
O31.01   Papyraceous fetus, first trimester
O31.02   Papyraceous fetus, second trimester
O31.03   Papyraceous fetus, third trimester

O31.1   Continuing pregnancy after spontaneous abortion of one fetus or more
O31.10   Continuing pregnancy after spontaneous abortion of one fetus or more, unspecified trimester
O31.11   Continuing pregnancy after spontaneous abortion of one fetus or more, first trimester
O31.12   Continuing pregnancy after spontaneous abortion of one fetus or more, second trimester
O31.13   Continuing pregnancy after spontaneous abortion of one fetus or more, third trimester

O31.2   Continuing pregnancy after intrauterine death of one fetus or more
O31.20   Continuing pregnancy after intrauterine death of one fetus or more, unspecified trimester
O31.21   Continuing pregnancy after intrauterine death of one fetus or more, first trimester
O31.22   Continuing pregnancy after intrauterine death of one fetus or more, second trimester
O31.23   Continuing pregnancy after intrauterine death of one fetus or more, third trimester

O31.3   Continuing pregnancy after other abortion of one fetus or more
Continuing pregnancy after selective termination
O31.30   Continuing pregnancy after other abortion of one fetus or more, unspecified trimester
O31.31   Continuing pregnancy after other abortion of one fetus or more, first trimester
O31.32   Continuing pregnancy after other abortion of one fetus or more, second trimester
O31.33   Continuing pregnancy after other abortion of one fetus or more, third trimester

O31.8   Other complications specific to multiple gestation
O31.8x   Other complications specific to multiple gestation
O31.8x1   Other complications specific to multiple gestation, first trimester
O31.8x2   Other complications specific to multiple gestation, second trimester
O31.8x3   Other complications specific to multiple gestation, third trimester
O31.8x9   Other complications specific to multiple gestation, unspecified trimester

O32 Maternal care for malpresentation of fetus
Includes: the listed conditions as a reason for observation, hospitalization or other obstetric care of the mother, or for cesarean section before onset of labor
Excludes1:   malpresentation of fetus with obstructed labor (O64.-)

O32.0   Maternal care for unstable lie
O32.1   Maternal care for breech presentation
Maternal care for buttocks presentation
Maternal care for complete breech
Maternal care for frank breech
Excludes1:   footling presentation (O32.8)
                  incomplete breech (O32.8)
O32.2   Maternal care for transverse and oblique lie
Maternal care for oblique presentation
Maternal care for transverse presentation
O32.3   Maternal care for face, brow and chin presentation
O32.4   Maternal care for high head at term
Maternal care for failure of head to enter pelvic brim

O32.5   Maternal care for multiple gestation with malpresentation of one fetus or more
O32.6   Maternal care for compound presentation
O32.8   Maternal care for other malpresentation of fetus
Maternal care for footling presentation
Maternal care for incomplete breech
O32.9   Maternal care for malpresentation of fetus, unspecified

O33 Maternal care for disproportion
Includes: the listed conditions as a reason for observation, hospitalization or other obstetric care of the mother, or for cesarean section before onset of labor
Excludes1:   disproportion with obstructed labor (O65- O66)

O33.0   Maternal care for disproportion due to deformity of maternal pelvic bones
Maternal care for disproportion due to pelvic deformity causing disproportion NOS
O33.1   Maternal care for disproportion due to generally contracted pelvis
Maternal care for disproportion due to contracted pelvis NOS causing disproportion
O33.2   Maternal care for disproportion due to inlet contraction of pelvis
Maternal care for disproportion due to inlet contraction (pelvis) causing disproportion
O33.3   Maternal care for disproportion due to outlet contraction of pelvis
Maternal care for disproportion due to mid-cavity contraction (pelvis)
Maternal care for disproportion due to outlet contraction (pelvis)
O33.4   Maternal care for disproportion of mixed maternal and fetal origin
O33.5   Maternal care for disproportion due to unusually large fetus
Maternal care for disproportion due to disproportion of fetal origin with normally formed fetus
Maternal care for disproportion due to fetal disproportion NOS
O33.6   Maternal care for disproportion due to hydrocephalic fetus
O33.7   Maternal care for disproportion due to other fetal deformities
Maternal care for disproportion due to conjoined twins
Maternal care for disproportion due to fetal ascites
Maternal care for disproportion due to fetal hydrops
Maternal care for disproportion due to fetal meningomyelocele
Maternal care for disproportion due to fetal sacral teratoma
Maternal care for disproportion due to fetal tumor
O33.8   Maternal care for disproportion of other origin
O33.9   Maternal care for disproportion, unspecified
Maternal care for disproportion due to cephalopelvic disproportion NOS
Maternal care for disproportion due to fetopelvic disproportion NOS

O34 Maternal care for abnormality of pelvic organs
Includes: the listed conditions as a reason for hospitalization or other obstetric care of the mother, or for cesarean section before onset of labor
Code first any associated obstructed labor (O65.5)
Use additional code for specific condition
O34.0   Maternal care for congenital malformation of uterus
O34.0x   Maternal care for congenital malformation of uterus
O34.0x1   Maternal care for unspecified congenital malformation of uterus, first trimester
O34.0x2   Maternal care for unspecified congenital malformation of uterus, second trimester
O34.0x3   Maternal care for unspecified congenital malformation of uterus, third trimester
O34.0x9   Maternal care for unspecified congenital malformation of uterus, unspecified trimester
O34.1   Maternal care for benign tumor of corpus uteri
Excludes2:   maternal care for benign tumor of cervix (O34.4-)
                  maternal care for malignant neoplasm of uterus (O94.11-)
O34.1x   Maternal care for benign tumor of corpus uteri

O34.1x1   Maternal care for benign tumor of corpus uteri, first trimester

O34.1x2   Maternal care for benign tumor of corpus uteri, second trimester

O34.1x3   Maternal care for benign tumor of corpus uteri, third trimester

O34.1x9   Maternal care for benign tumor of corpus uteri, unspecified trimester

O34.2   Maternal care due to uterine scar from previous surgery

O34.21   Maternal care for scar from previous cesarean delivery

O34.29   Maternal care due to uterine scar from other previous surgery

O34.3   Maternal care for cervical incompetence

Maternal care for cerclage with or without cervical incompetence

Maternal care for Shirodkar suture with or without cervical incompetence

O34.30   Maternal care for cervical incompetence, unspecified trimester

O34.31   Maternal care for cervical incompetence, first trimester

O34.32   Maternal care for cervical incompetence, second trimester

O34.33   Maternal care for cervical incompetence, third trimester

O34.4   Maternal care for other abnormalities of cervix

O34.4x   Maternal care for other abnormalities of cervix

O34.4x1   Maternal care for other abnormalities of cervix, first trimester

O34.4x2   Maternal care for other abnormalities of cervix, second trimester

O34.4x3   Maternal care for other abnormalities of cervix, third trimester

O34.4x9   Maternal care for other abnormalities of cervix, unspecified trimester

O34.5   Maternal care for other abnormalities of gravid uterus

Maternal care for incarceration of gravid uterus

Maternal care for prolapse of gravid uterus

Maternal care for retroversion of gravid uterus

O34.5x   Maternal care for other abnormalities of gravid uterus

O34.5x1   Maternal care for other abnormalities of gravid uterus, first trimester

O34.5x2   Maternal care for other abnormalities of gravid uterus, second trimester

O34.5x3   Maternal care for other abnormalities of gravid uterus, third trimester

O34.5x9   Maternal care for other abnormalities of gravid uterus, unspecified trimester

O34.6   Maternal care for abnormality of vagina

Excludes2:   maternal care for vaginal varices in pregnancy (O22.1-)

O34.6x   Maternal care for abnormality of vagina

O34.6x1   Maternal care for abnormality of vagina, first trimester

O34.6x2   Maternal care for abnormality of vagina, second trimester

O34.6x3   Maternal care for abnormality of vagina, third trimester

O34.6x9   Maternal care for abnormality of vagina, unspecified trimester

O34.7   Maternal care for abnormality of vulva and perineum

Excludes2:   maternal care for perineal and vulval varices in pregnancy (O22.1-)

O34.7x   Maternal care for abnormality of vulva and perineum

O34.7x1   Maternal care for abnormality of vulva and perineum, first trimester

O34.7x2   Maternal care for abnormality of vulva and perineum, second trimester

O34.7x3   Maternal care for abnormality of vulva and perineum, third trimester

O34.7x9   Maternal care for abnormality of vulva and perineum, unspecified trimester

O34.8   Maternal care for other abnormalities of pelvic organs

O34.8x   Maternal care for other abnormalities of pelvic organs

O34.8x1   Maternal care for other abnormalities of pelvic organs, first trimester

O34.8x2   Maternal care for other abnormalities of pelvic organs, second trimester

O34.8x3   Maternal care for other abnormalities of pelvic organs, third trimester

O34.8x9   Maternal care for other abnormalities of pelvic organs, unspecified trimester

O34.9   Maternal care for abnormality of pelvic organ, unspecified

O34.90   Maternal care for abnormality of pelvic organ, unspecified, unspecified trimester

O34.91   Maternal care for abnormality of pelvic organ, unspecified, first trimester

O34.92   Maternal care for abnormality of pelvic organ, unspecified, second trimester

O34.93   Maternal care for abnormality of pelvic organ, unspecified, third trimester

O35 Maternal care for known or suspected fetal abnormality and damage

Includes: the listed conditions in the fetus as a reason for hospitalization or other obstetric care to the mother, or for termination of pregnancy

Code also any associated maternal condition

Excludes2:   fetal care for fetal abnormality and damage (O37.-)

O35.0   Maternal care for (suspected) central nervous system malformation in fetus

Maternal care for fetal anencephaly

Maternal care for fetal hydrocephalus

Maternal care for fetal spina bifida

Excludes2:   chromosomal abnormality in fetus (O35.1)

O35.1   Maternal care for (suspected) chromosomal abnormality in fetus

O35.2   Maternal care for (suspected) hereditary disease in fetus

Excludes2:   chromosomal abnormality in fetus (O35.1)

O35.3   Maternal care for (suspected) damage to fetus from viral disease in mother

Maternal care for damage to fetus from maternal cytomegalovirus infection

Maternal care for damage to fetus from maternal rubella

O35.4   Maternal care for (suspected) damage to fetus from alcohol

O35.5   Maternal care for (suspected) damage to fetus by drugs

Maternal care for damage to fetus from drug addiction

O35.6   Maternal care for (suspected) damage to fetus by radiation

O35.7   Maternal care for (suspected) damage to fetus by other medical procedures

Maternal care for damage to fetus by amniocentesis

Maternal care for damage to fetus by biopsy procedures

Maternal care for damage to fetus by hematological investigation

Maternal care for damage to fetus by intrauterine contraceptive device

Maternal care for damage to fetus by intrauterine surgery

O35.8   Maternal care for other (suspected) fetal abnormality and damage

Maternal care for damage to fetus from maternal listeriosis

Maternal care for damage to fetus from maternal toxoplasmosis

O35.9   Maternal care for (suspected) fetal abnormality and damage, unspecified

O36 Maternal care for other fetal problems

Includes: the listed conditions in the fetus as a reason for hospitalization or other obstetric care of the mother, or for termination of pregnancy

Excludes1:   placental transfusion syndromes (O43.0-)

Excludes2:   fetal care for fetal abnormality and damage (O37.-)

labor and delivery complicated by fetal stress (O77.-)

O36.0   Maternal care for rhesus isoimmunization

Maternal care for anti-D [Rh] antibodies

Maternal care for Rh incompatibility (with hydrops fetalis)

O36.00   Maternal care for rhesus isoimmunization, unspecified trimester

O36.01 Maternal care for rhesus isoimmunization, first trimester

O36.02 Maternal care for rhesus isoimmunization, second trimester

O36.03 Maternal care for rhesus isoimmunization, third trimester

O36.1 Maternal care for other isoimmunization
Maternal care for ABO isoimmunization
Maternal care for isoimmunization NOS (with hydrops fetalis)

O36.1x Maternal care for other isoimmunization

O36.1x1 Maternal care for other isoimmunization, first trimester

O36.1x2 Maternal care for other isoimmunization, second trimester

O36.1x3 Maternal care for other isoimmunization, third trimester

O36.1x9 Maternal care for other isoimmunization, unspecified trimester

O36.2 Maternal care for hydrops fetalis
Maternal care for hydrops fetalis NOS
Maternal care for hydrops fetalis not associated with isoimmunization
Excludes1: hydrops fetalis associated with ABO isoimmunization (O36.1)
hydrops fetalis associated with rhesus isoimmunization (O36.0)

O36.20 Maternal care for hydrops fetalis, unspecified trimester

O36.21 Maternal care for hydrops fetalis, first trimester

O36.22 Maternal care for hydrops fetalis, second trimester

O36.23 Maternal care for hydrops fetalis, third trimester

O36.4 Maternal care for intrauterine death
Maternal care for intrauterine fetal death NOS
Maternal care for intrauterine fetal death after completion of 20 weeks of gestation
Maternal care for late fetal death
Maternal care for missed delivery
Excludes1: missed abortion (O02.1)

O36.5 Maternal care for poor fetal growth
Maternal care for known or suspected light-for-dates
Maternal care for known or suspected placental insufficiency
Maternal care for known or suspected small-for-dates

O36.5x Maternal care for poor fetal growth

O36.5x1 Maternal care for poor fetal growth, first trimester

O36.5x2 Maternal care for poor fetal growth, second trimester

O36.5x3 Maternal care for poor fetal growth, third trimester

O36.5x9 Maternal care for poor fetal growth, unspecified trimester

O36.6 Maternal care for excessive fetal growth
Maternal care for known or suspected large-for-dates

O36.60 Maternal care for excessive fetal growth, unspecified trimester

O36.61 Maternal care for excessive fetal growth, first trimester

O36.62 Maternal care for excessive fetal growth, second trimester

O36.63 Maternal care for excessive fetal growth, third trimester

O36.7 Maternal care for viable fetus in abdominal pregnancy

O36.70 Maternal care for viable fetus in abdominal pregnancy, unspecified trimester

O36.71 Maternal care for viable fetus in abdominal pregnancy, first trimester

O36.72 Maternal care for viable fetus in abdominal pregnancy, second trimester

O36.73 Maternal care for viable fetus in abdominal pregnancy, third trimester

O36.8 Maternal care for other specified fetal problems

O36.81 Decreased fetal movements

O36.812 Decreased fetal movements, second trimester

O36.813 Decreased fetal movements, third trimester

O36.819 Decreased fetal movements, unspecified trimester

O36.89 Maternal care for other specified fetal problems

O36.891 Maternal care for other specified fetal problems, first trimester

O36.892 Maternal care for other specified fetal problems, second trimester

O36.893 Maternal care for other specified fetal problems, third trimester

O36.899 Maternal care for other specified fetal problems, unspecified trimester

O36.9 Maternal care for fetal problem, unspecified

O36.90 Maternal care for fetal problem, unspecified, unspecified trimester

O36.91 Maternal care for fetal problem, unspecified, first trimester

O36.92 Maternal care for fetal problem, unspecified, second trimester

O36.93 Maternal care for fetal problem, unspecified, third trimester

O37 Fetal care for fetal abnormality and damage
Note: Codes from category O37 may be used on either the maternal record or a record created for the fetus, depending on the record keeping system of the facility where treatment is provided. They are not for use on a newborn record.
Includes: the listed condition in the fetus as the reason for hospitalization or other care of the fetus
Excludes2: maternal care for known or suspected fetal abnormality and damage (O35.-)
maternal care for other fetal problems (O36.-)

O37.0 Fetal care for central nervous system malformation

O37.1 Fetal care for cardiovascular malformations

O37.2 Fetal care for gastrointestinal malformation

O37.9 Fetal care for other fetal abnormality and damage

O40 Polyhydramnios
Includes: hydramnios

O40.1 Polyhydramnios, first trimester

O40.2 Polyhydramnios, second trimester

O40.3 Polyhydramnios, third trimester

O40.9 Polyhydramnios, unspecified trimester

O41 Other disorders of amniotic fluid and membranes

O41.0 Oligohydramnios
Oligohydramnios without mention of rupture of membranes

O41.00 Oligohydramnios, unspecified trimester

O41.01 Oligohydramnios, first trimester

O41.02 Oligohydramnios, second trimester

O41.03 Oligohydramnios, third trimester

O41.1 Infection of amniotic sac and membranes

O41.10 Infection of amniotic sac and membranes, unspecified

O41.101 Infection of amniotic sac and membranes, unspecified, first trimester

O41.102 Infection of amniotic sac and membranes, unspecified, second trimester

O41.103 Infection of amniotic sac and membranes, unspecified, third trimester

O41.109 Infection of amniotic sac and membranes, unspecified, unspecified trimester

O41.12 Chorioamnionitis

O41.121 Chorioamnionitis, first trimester

O41.122 Chorioamnionitis, second trimester

O41.123 Chorioamnionitis, third trimester

O41.129 Chorioamnionitis, unspecified trimester

O41.14 Placentitis

O41.141 Placentitis, first trimester

O41.142 Placentitis, second trimester

O41.143 Placentitis, third trimester

O41.149 Placentitis, unspecified trimester

O41.8   Other specified disorders of amniotic fluid and membranes
O41.8x   Other specified disorders of amniotic fluid and membranes
O41.8x1   Other specified disorders of amniotic fluid and membranes, first trimester
O41.8x2   Other specified disorders of amniotic fluid and membranes, second trimester
O41.8x3   Other specified disorders of amniotic fluid and membranes, third trimester
O41.8x9   Other specified disorders of amniotic fluid and membranes, unspecified trimester
O41.9   Disorder of amniotic fluid and membranes, unspecified
O41.90   Disorder of amniotic fluid and membranes, unspecified, unspecified trimester
O41.91   Disorder of amniotic fluid and membranes, unspecified, first trimester
O41.92   Disorder of amniotic fluid and membranes, unspecified, second trimester
O41.93   Disorder of amniotic fluid and membranes, unspecified, third trimester

O42   Premature rupture of membranes
O42.0   Premature rupture of membranes, onset of labor within 24 hours of rupture
O42.00   Premature rupture of membranes, onset of labor within 24 hours of rupture, unspecified weeks of gestation
O42.01   Preterm premature rupture of membranes, onset of labor within 24 hours of rupture
Premature rupture of membranes before 37 completed weeks of gestation
O42.011   Preterm premature rupture of membranes, onset of labor within 24 hours of rupture, first trimester
O42.012   Preterm premature rupture of membranes, onset of labor within 24 hours of rupture, second trimester
O42.013   Preterm premature rupture of membranes, onset of labor within 24 hours of rupture, third trimester
O42.019   Preterm premature rupture of membranes, onset of labor within 24 hours of rupture, unspecified trimester
O42.02   Full-term premature rupture of membranes, onset of labor within 24 hours of rupture
Premature rupture of membranes after 37 completed weeks of gestation
O42.1   Premature rupture of membranes, onset of labor more than 24 hours following rupture
O42.10   Premature rupture of membranes, onset of labor more than 24 hours following rupture, unspecified weeks of gestation
O42.11   Preterm premature rupture of membranes, onset of labor more than 24 hours following rupture
Premature rupture of membranes before 37 completed weeks of gestation
O42.111   Preterm premature rupture of membranes, onset of labor more than 24 hours following rupture, first trimester
O42.112   Preterm premature rupture of membranes, onset of labor more than 24 hours following rupture, second trimester
O42.113   Preterm premature rupture of membranes, onset of labor more than 24 hours following rupture, third trimester
O42.119   Preterm premature rupture of membranes, onset of labor more than 24 hours following rupture, unspecified trimester
O42.12   Full-term premature rupture of membranes, onset of labor more than 24 hours following rupture
Premature rupture of membranes after 37 completed weeks of gestation

O42.9   Premature rupture of membranes, unspecified as to length of time between rupture and onset of labor
O42.90   Premature rupture of membranes, unspecified as to length of time between rupture and onset of labor, unspecified weeks of gestation
O42.91   Preterm premature rupture of membranes, unspecified as to length of time between rupture and onset of labor
Premature rupture of membranes before 37 completed weeks of gestation
O42.911   Preterm premature rupture of membranes, unspecified as to length of time between rupture and onset of labor, first trimester
O42.912   Preterm premature rupture of membranes, unspecified as to length of time between rupture and onset of labor, second trimester
O42.913   Preterm premature rupture of membranes, unspecified as to length of time between rupture and onset of labor, third trimester
O42.919   Preterm premature rupture of membranes, unspecified as to length of time between rupture and onset of labor, unspecified trimester
O42.92   Full-term premature rupture of membranes, unspecified as to length of time between rupture and onset of labor
Premature rupture of membranes after 37 completed weeks of gestation

O43   Placental disorders
O43.0   Placental transfusion syndromes
O43.01   Fetomaternal placental transfusion syndrome
Maternofetal placental transfusion syndrome
O43.011   Fetomaternal placental transfusion syndrome, first trimester
O43.012   Fetomaternal placental transfusion syndrome, second trimester
O43.013   Fetomaternal placental transfusion syndrome, third trimester
O43.019   Fetomaternal placental transfusion syndrome, unspecified trimester
O43.02   Fetus-to-fetus placental transfusion syndrome
O43.021   Fetus-to-fetus placental transfusion syndrome, first trimester
O43.022   Fetus-to-fetus placental transfusion syndrome, second trimester
O43.023   Fetus-to-fetus placental transfusion syndrome, third trimester
O43.029   Fetus-to-fetus placental transfusion syndrome, unspecified trimester
O43.1   Malformation of placenta
O43.10   Malformation of placenta, unspecified
Abnormal placenta NOS
O43.101   Malformation of placenta, unspecified, first trimester
O43.102   Malformation of placenta, unspecified, second trimester
O43.103   Malformation of placenta, unspecified, third trimester
O43.109   Malformation of placenta, unspecified, unspecified trimester
O43.11   Circumvallate placenta
O43.111   Circumvallate placenta, first trimester
O43.112   Circumvallate placenta, second trimester
O43.113   Circumvallate placenta, third trimester
O43.119   Circumvallate placenta, unspecified trimester
O43.12   Velamentous insertion of umbilical cord
O43.121   Velamentous insertion of umbilical cord, first trimester
O43.122   Velamentous insertion of umbilical cord, second trimester
O43.123   Velamentous insertion of umbilical cord, third trimester

O43.129 Velamentous insertion of umbilical cord, unspecified trimester
O43.19 Other malformation of placenta
  O43.191 Other malformation of placenta, first trimester
  O43.192 Other malformation of placenta, second trimester
  O43.193 Other malformation of placenta, third trimester
  O43.199 Other malformation of placenta, unspecified trimester
O43.8 Other placental disorders
  Excludes2: maternal care for poor fetal growth due to placental insufficiency (O36.5-)
  placenta previa (O44.-)
  placental polyp (O90.8)
  placentitis (O41.14-)
  premature separation of placenta (O45.-)
  O43.81 Placental dysfunction
    O43.811 Placental dysfunction, first trimester
    O43.812 Placental dysfunction, second trimester
    O43.813 Placental dysfunction, third trimester
    O43.819 Placental dysfunction, unspecified trimester
  O43.82 Placental infarction
    O43.821 Placental infarction, first trimester
    O43.822 Placental infarction, second trimester
    O43.823 Placental infarction, third trimester
    O43.829 Placental infarction, unspecified trimester
  O43.89 Other placental disorders
    O43.891 Other placental disorders, first trimester
    O43.892 Other placental disorders, second trimester
    O43.893 Other placental disorders, third trimester
    O43.899 Other placental disorders, unspecified trimester
O43.9 Placental disorder, unspecified
  O43.90 Placental disorder, unspecified, unspecified trimester
  O43.91 Placental disorder, unspecified, first trimester
  O43.92 Placental disorder, unspecified, second trimester
  O43.93 Placental disorder, unspecified, third trimester

O44 Placenta previa
O44.0 Placenta previa specified as without hemorrhage
  Low implantation of placenta specified as without hemorrhage
  O44.00 Placenta previa specified as without hemorrhage, unspecified trimester
  O44.01 Placenta previa specified as without hemorrhage, first trimester
  O44.02 Placenta previa specified as without hemorrhage, second trimester
  O44.03 Placenta previa specified as without hemorrhage, third trimester
O44.1 Placenta previa with hemorrhage
  Low implantation of placenta, NOS or with hemorrhage
  Marginal placenta previa, NOS or with hemorrhage
  Partial placenta previa, NOS or with hemorrhage
  Total placenta previa, NOS or with hemorrhage
  Excludes1: labor and delivery complicated by hemorrhage from vasa previa (O69.4)
  O44.10 Placenta previa with hemorrhage, unspecified trimester
  O44.11 Placenta previa with hemorrhage, first trimester
  O44.12 Placenta previa with hemorrhage, second trimester
  O44.13 Placenta previa with hemorrhage, third trimester

O45 Premature separation of placenta [abruptio placentae]
  Excludes1: pre-existing coagulation defect (O99.1-)
O45.0 Premature separation of placenta with coagulation defect
  O45.00 Premature separation of placenta with coagulation defect, unspecified
    O45.001 Premature separation of placenta with coagulation defect, unspecified, first trimester

O45.002 Premature separation of placenta with coagulation defect, unspecified, second trimester
O45.003 Premature separation of placenta with coagulation defect, unspecified, third trimester
O45.009 Premature separation of placenta with coagulation defect, unspecified, unspecified trimester
O45.01 Premature separation of placenta with afibrinogenemia
  Premature separation of placenta with hypofibrinogenemia
  O45.011 Premature separation of placenta with afibrinogenemia, first trimester
  O45.012 Premature separation of placenta with afibrinogenemia, second trimester
  O45.013 Premature separation of placenta with afibrinogenemia, third trimester
  O45.019 Premature separation of placenta with afibrinogenemia, unspecified trimester
O45.02 Premature separation of placenta with disseminated intravascular coagulation
  O45.021 Premature separation of placenta with disseminated intravascular coagulation, first trimester
  O45.022 Premature separation of placenta with disseminated intravascular coagulation, second trimester
  O45.023 Premature separation of placenta with disseminated intravascular coagulation, third trimester
  O45.029 Premature separation of placenta with disseminated intravascular coagulation, unspecified trimester
O45.09 Premature separation of placenta with other coagulation defect
  O45.091 Premature separation of placenta with other coagulation defect, first trimester
  O45.092 Premature separation of placenta with other coagulation defect, second trimester
  O45.093 Premature separation of placenta with other coagulation defect, third trimester
  O45.099 Premature separation of placenta with other coagulation defect, unspecified trimester
O45.8 Other premature separation of placenta
  O45.8x Other premature separation of placenta
    O45.8x1 Other premature separation of placenta, first trimester
    O45.8x2 Other premature separation of placenta, second trimester
    O45.8x3 Other premature separation of placenta, third trimester
    O45.8x9 Other premature separation of placenta, unspecified trimester
O45.9 Premature separation of placenta, unspecified
  Abruptio placentae NOS
  O45.90 Premature separation of placenta, unspecified, unspecified trimester
  O45.91 Premature separation of placenta, unspecified, first trimester
  O45.92 Premature separation of placenta, unspecified, second trimester
  O45.93 Premature separation of placenta, unspecified, third trimester

O46 Antepartum hemorrhage, not elsewhere classified
  Excludes1: hemorrhage in early pregnancy (O20.-)
  intrapartum hemorrhage NEC (O67.-)
  placenta previa (O44.-)
  pre-existing coagulation defect (O99.1-)
  premature separation of placenta [abruptio placentae] (O45.-)

O46.0 Antepartum hemorrhage with coagulation defect
- **O46.00 Antepartum hemorrhage with coagulation defect, unspecified**
  - **O46.001 Antepartum hemorrhage with coagulation defect, unspecified, first trimester**
  - **O46.002 Antepartum hemorrhage with coagulation defect, unspecified, second trimester**
  - **O46.003 Antepartum hemorrhage with coagulation defect, unspecified, third trimester**
  - **O46.009 Antepartum hemorrhage with coagulation defect, unspecified, unspecified trimester**
- **O46.01 Antepartum hemorrhage with afibrinogenemia**
  - Antepartum hemorrhage with hypofibrinogenemia
  - **O46.011 Antepartum hemorrhage with afibrinogenemia, first trimester**
  - **O46.012 Antepartum hemorrhage with afibrinogenemia, second trimester**
  - **O46.013 Antepartum hemorrhage with afibrinogenemia, third trimester**
  - **O46.019 Antepartum hemorrhage with afibrinogenemia, unspecified trimester**
- **O46.02 Antepartum hemorrhage with disseminated intravascular coagulation**
  - **O46.021 Antepartum hemorrhage with disseminated intravascular coagulation, first trimester**
  - **O46.022 Antepartum hemorrhage with disseminated intravascular coagulation, second trimester**
  - **O46.023 Antepartum hemorrhage with disseminated intravascular coagulation, third trimester**
  - **O46.029 Antepartum hemorrhage with disseminated intravascular coagulation, unspecified trimester**
- **O46.09 Antepartum hemorrhage with other coagulation defect**
  - **O46.091 Antepartum hemorrhage with other coagulation defect, first trimester**
  - **O46.092 Antepartum hemorrhage with other coagulation defect, second trimester**
  - **O46.093 Antepartum hemorrhage with other coagulation defect, third trimester**
  - **O46.099 Antepartum hemorrhage with other coagulation defect, unspecified trimester**

O46.8 Other antepartum hemorrhage
- **O46.8x Other antepartum hemorrhage**
  - **O46.8x1 Other antepartum hemorrhage, first trimester**
  - **O46.8x2 Other antepartum hemorrhage, second trimester**
  - **O46.8x3 Other antepartum hemorrhage, third trimester**
  - **O46.8x9 Other antepartum hemorrhage, unspecified trimester**

O46.9 Antepartum hemorrhage, unspecified
- **O46.90 Antepartum hemorrhage, unspecified, unspecified trimester**
- **O46.91 Antepartum hemorrhage, unspecified, first trimester**
- **O46.92 Antepartum hemorrhage, unspecified, second trimester**
- **O46.93 Antepartum hemorrhage, unspecified, third trimester**

O47 False labor
- **O47.0 False labor before 37 completed weeks of gestation**
  - **O47.00 False labor before 37 completed weeks of gestation, unspecified trimester**
  - **O47.02 False labor before 37 completed weeks of gestation, second trimester**
  - **O47.03 False labor before 37 completed weeks of gestation, third trimester**
- **O47.1 False labor at or after 37 completed weeks of gestation**
- **O47.9 False labor, unspecified**

O48 Late pregnancy
- **O48.0 Post-term pregnancy**
  - Pregnancy over 40 completed weeks to 42 completed weeks gestation
- **O48.1 Prolonged pregnancy**
  - Pregnancy which has advanced beyond 42 completed weeks gestation

COMPLICATIONS OF LABOR AND DELIVERY (O60–O77)

O60 Preterm labor
- Includes: onset (spontaneous) of labor before 37 completed weeks of gestation
- **O60.2 Preterm labor, second trimester**
- **O60.3 Preterm labor, third trimester**
- **O60.9 Preterm labor, unspecified trimester**

O61 Failed induction of labor
- **O61.0 Failed medical induction of labor**
  - Failed induction (of labor) by oxytocin
  - Failed induction (of labor) by prostaglandins
- **O61.1 Failed instrumental induction of labor**
  - Failed mechanical induction (of labor)
  - Failed surgical induction (of labor)
- **O61.8 Other failed induction of labor**
- **O61.9 Failed induction of labor, unspecified**

O62 Abnormalities of forces of labor
- **O62.0 Primary inadequate contractions**
  - Failure of cervical dilatation
  - Primary hypotonic uterine dysfunction
- **O62.1 Secondary uterine inertia**
  - Arrested active phase of labor
  - Secondary hypotonic uterine dysfunction
- **O62.2 Other uterine inertia**
  - Desultory labor
  - Hypotonic uterine dysfunction NOS
  - Irregular labor
  - Poor contractions
  - Slow slope active phase of labor
  - Uterine inertia NOS
- **O62.3 Precipitate labor**
- **O62.4 Hypertonic, incoordinate, and prolonged uterine contractions**
  - Cervical spasm
  - Contraction ring dystocia
  - Dyscoordinate labor
  - Hour-glass contraction of uterus
  - Hypertonic uterine dysfunction
  - Incoordinate uterine action
  - Tetanic contractions
  - Uterine dystocia NOS
  - Uterine spasm
  - Excludes1: dystocia (fetal) (maternal) NOS (O66.9)
- **O62.8 Other abnormalities of forces of labor**
- **O62.9 Abnormality of forces of labor, unspecified**

O63 Long labor
- **O63.0 Prolonged first stage (of labor)**
- **O63.1 Prolonged second stage (of labor)**
- **O63.2 Delayed delivery of second twin, triplet, etc.**
- **O63.9 Long labor, unspecified**
  - Prolonged labor NOS

O64 Obstructed labor due to malposition and malpresentation of fetus
- **O64.0 Obstructed labor due to incomplete rotation of fetal head**
  - Deep transverse arrest
  - Obstructed labor due to persistent occipitoiliac (position)
  - Obstructed labor due to persistent occipitoposterior (position)
  - Obstructed labor due to persistent occipitosacral (position)
  - Obstructed labor due to persistent occipitotransverse (position)
- **O64.1 Obstructed labor due to breech presentation**
  - Obstructed labor due to buttocks presentation
  - Obstructed labor due to complete breech presentation
  - Obstructed labor due to frank breech presentation
- **O64.2 Obstructed labor due to face presentation**
  - Obstructed labor due to chin presentation
- **O64.3 Obstructed labor due to brow presentation**

O64.4 Obstructed labor due to shoulder presentation
Prolapsed arm
Excludes1:   impacted shoulders (O66.0)
              shoulder dystocia (O66.0)

O64.5 Obstructed labor due to compound presentation

O64.8 Obstructed labor due to other malposition and malpresentation
Obstructed labor due to footling presentation
Obstructed labor due to incomplete breech presentation

O64.9 Obstructed labor due to malposition and malpresentation, unspecified

O65 Obstructed labor due to maternal pelvic abnormality

O65.0 Obstructed labor due to deformed pelvis

O65.1 Obstructed labor due to generally contracted pelvis

O65.2 Obstructed labor due to pelvic inlet contraction

O65.3 Obstructed labor due to pelvic outlet and mid-cavity contraction

O65.4 Obstructed labor due to fetopelvic disproportion, unspecified
Excludes1:   dystocia due to abnormality of fetus (O66.2-O66.3)

O65.5 Obstructed labor due to abnormality of maternal pelvic organs
Obstructed labor due to conditions listed in O34.-

O65.8 Obstructed labor due to other maternal pelvic abnormalities

O65.9 Obstructed labor due to maternal pelvic abnormality, unspecified

O66 Other obstructed labor

O66.0 Obstructed labor due to shoulder dystocia
Impacted shoulders

O66.1 Obstructed labor due to locked twins

O66.2 Obstructed labor due to unusually large fetus

O66.3 Obstructed labor due to other abnormalities of fetus
Dystocia due to conjoined twins
Dystocia due to fetal ascites
Dystocia due to fetal hydrops
Dystocia due to fetal meningomyelocele
Dystocia due to fetal sacral teratoma
Dystocia due to fetal tumor
Dystocia due to hydrocephalic fetus

O66.4 Failed trial of labor

  O66.40   Failed trail of labor, unspecified

  O66.41   Failed attempted vaginal birth after previous cesarean delivery
Code first rupture of uterus, if applicable (O71.0-, O71.1)

O66.5 Attempted application of vacuum extractor and forceps
Attempted application of vacuum or forceps, with subsequent delivery by forceps or cesarean section

O66.6 Obstructed labor due to other multiple fetuses

O66.8 Other specified obstructed labor

O66.9 Obstructed labor, unspecified
Dystocia NOS
Fetal dystocia NOS
Maternal dystocia NOS

O67 Labor and delivery complicated by intrapartum hemorrhage, not elsewhere classified
Exlcudes1:   antepartum hemorrhage NEC (O46.-)
              placenta previa (O44.-)
              premature separation of placenta [abruptio placentae] (O45.-)
Excludes2:   postpartum hemorrhage (O72.-)

O67.0 Intrapartum hemorrhage with coagulation defect
Intrapartum hemorrhage (excessive) associated with afibrinogenemia
Intrapartum hemorrhage (excessive) associated with disseminated intravascular coagulation
Intrapartum hemorrhage (excessive) associated with hyperfibrinolysis
Intrapartum hemorrhage (excessive) associated with hypofibrinogenemia

O67.8 Other intrapartum hemorrhage
Excessive intrapartum hemorrhage

O67.9 Intrapartum hemorrhage, unspecified

O68 Labor and delivery complicated by abnormality of fetal acid-base balance
Includes: abnormal fetal acidemia complicating labor and delivery
               abnormal fetal acidosis complicating labor and delivery
               abnormal fetal alkalosis complicating labor and delivery
               fetal metabolic acidemia complicating labor and delivery
Excludes1:   fetal stress NOS (O77.9)
               labor and delivery complicated by electrocardiographic evidence of fetal stress (O77.8)
               labor and delivery complicated by ultrasonic evidence of fetal stress (O77.8)
Excludes2:   abnormality in fetal heart rate or rhythm (O76)
               labor and delivery complicated by meconium in amniotic fluid (O77.0)

O69 Labor and delivery complicated by umbilical cord complications

O69.0 Labor and delivery complicated by prolapse of cord

O69.1 Labor and delivery complicated by cord around neck, with compression

O69.2 Labor and delivery complicated by other cord entanglement
Entanglement of cords of twins in monoamniotic sac
Knot in cord

O69.3 Labor and delivery complicated by short cord

O69.4 Labor and delivery complicated by vasa previa
Hemorrhage from vasa previa

O69.5 Labor and delivery complicated by vascular lesion of cord
Cord bruising
Cord hematoma
Thrombosis of umbilical vessels

O69.8 Labor and delivery complicated by other cord complications

O69.9 Labor and delivery complicated by cord complication, unspecified

O70 Perineal laceration during delivery
Includes: episiotomy extended by laceration
Excludes1:   obstetric high vaginal laceration alone (O71.4)

O70.0 First degree perineal laceration during delivery
Perineal laceration, rupture or tear involving fourchette during delivery
Perineal laceration, rupture or tear involving labia during delivery
Perineal laceration, rupture or tear involving skin during delivery
Perineal laceration, rupture or tear involving vagina during delivery
Perineal laceration, rupture or tear involving vulva during delivery
Slight perineal laceration, rupture or tear during delivery

O70.1 Second degree perineal laceration during delivery
Perineal laceration, rupture or tear during delivery as in O70.0, also involving pelvic floor
Perineal laceration, rupture or tear during delivery as in O70.0, also involving perineal muscles
Perineal laceration, ruptue or tear during delivery as in O70.0, also involving vaginal muscles
Excludes1:   perineal laceration involving anal sphincter (O70.2)

O70.2 Third degree perineal laceration during delivery
Perineal laceration, rupture or tear during delivery as in O70.1, also involving anal sphincter
Perineal laceration, rupture or tear during delivery as in O70.1, also involving rectovaginal septum
Perineal laceration, rupture or tear during delivery as in O70.1, also involving sphincter NOS
Excludes1:   perineal laceration involving anal or rectal mucosa (O70.3)

O70.3 Fourth degree perineal laceration during delivery
Perineal laceration, rupture or tear during delivery as in O70.2, also involving anal mucosa
Perineal laceration, rupture or tear during delivery as in O70.2, also involving rectal mucosa

O70.9   Perineal laceration during delivery, unspecified

O71   Other obstetric trauma
> Includes: damage from instruments

O71.0   Rupture of uterus (spontaneous) before onset of labor
> Excludes1:   disruption of cesarean section wound (O90.0)
> laceration of uterus, NEC (O71.81)

O71.00   Rupture of uterus before onset of labor, unspecified trimester

O71.02   Rupture of uterus before onset of labor. second trimester

O71.03   Rupture of uterus before onset of labor, third trimester

O71.1   Rupture of uterus during labor
> Rupture of uterus not stated as occurring before onset of labor
> Excludes1:   disruption of cesarean section wound (O90.0)
> laceration of uterus, NEC (O71.81)

O71.2   Postpartum inversion of uterus

O71.3   Obstetric laceration of cervix
> Annular detachment of cervix

O71.4   Obstetric high vaginal laceration alone
> Laceration of vaginal wall without perineal laceration
> Excludes1:   obstetric high vaginal laceration with perineal laceration (O70.-)

O71.5   Other obstetric injury to pelvic organs
> Obstetric injury to bladder
> Obstetric injury to urethra

O71.6   Obstetric damage to pelvic joints and ligaments
> Obstetric avulsion of inner symphyseal cartilage
> Obstetric damage to coccyx
> Obstetric traumatic separation of symphysis (pubis)

O71.7   Obstetric hematoma of pelvis
> Obstetric hematoma of perineum
> Obstetric hematoma of vagina
> Obstetric hematoma of vulva

O71.8   Other specified obstetric trauma

O71.81   Laceration of uterus, not elsewhere classified

O71.89   Other specified obstetric trauma

O71.9   Obstetric trauma, unspecified

O72   Postpartum hemorrhage
> Includes: hemorrhage after delivery of fetus or infant

O72.0   Third-stage hemorrhage
> Hemorrhage associated with retained, trapped or adherent placenta
> Retained placenta NOS

O72.1   Other immediate postpartum hemorrhage
> Hemorrhage following delivery of placenta
> Postpartum hemorrhage (atonic) NOS
> Uterine atony

O72.2   Delayed and secondary postpartum hemorrhage
> Hemorrhage associated with retained portions of placenta or membranes after the first 24 hours following delivery of placenta
> Retained products of conception NOS, following delivery

O72.3   Postpartum coagulation defects
> Postpartum afibrinogenemia
> Postpartum fibrinolysis

O73   Retained placenta and membranes, without hemorrhage

O73.0   Retained placenta without hemorrhage
> Placenta accreta without hemorrhage

O73.1   Retained portions of placenta and membranes, without hemorrhage
> Retained products of conception following delivery, without hemorrhage

O74   Complications of anesthesia during labor and delivery
> Includes: maternal complications arising from the administration of a general, regional or local anesthetic, analgesic or other sedation during labor and delivery
> Use additional code, if applicable, to identify specific complication

O74.0   Aspiration pneumonitis due to anesthesia during labor and delivery
> Inhalation of stomach contents or secretions NOS due to anesthesia during labor and delivery
> Mendelson's syndrome due to anesthesia during labor and delivery

O74.1   Other pulmonary complications of anesthesia during labor and delivery

O74.2   Cardiac complications of anesthesia during labor and delivery

O74.3   Central nervous system complications of anesthesia during labor and delivery

O74.4   Toxic reaction to local anesthesia during labor and delivery

O74.5   Spinal and epidural anesthesia-induced headache during labor and delivery

O74.6   Other complications of spinal and epidural anesthesia during labor and delivery

O74.7   Failed or difficult intubation for anesthesia during labor and delivery

O74.8   Other complications of anesthesia during labor and delivery

O74.9   Complication of anesthesia during labor and delivery, unspecified

O75   Other complications of labor and delivery, not elsewhere classified
> Excludes2:   puerperal (postpartum) infection (O86.-)
> puerperal (postpartum) septicemia (O85)

O75.0   Maternal distress during labor and delivery

O75.1   Shock during or following labor and delivery
> Obstetric shock following labor and delivery

O75.2   Pyrexia during labor, not elsewhere classified

O75.3   Other infection during labor
> Septicemia during labor
> Use additional code to identify infection

O75.4   Other complications of obstetric surgery and procedures
> Cardiac arrest following obstetric surgery or procedures
> Cardiac failure following obstetric surgery or procedures
> Cerebral anoxia following obstetric surgery or procedures
> Pulmonary edema following obstetric surgery or procedures
> Use additional code to identify specific complication
> Excludes2:   complications of anesthesia during labor and delivery (O74.-)
> obstetrical (surgical) wound:
> disruption (O90.0-O90.1)
> hematoma (O90.2)
> infection (O86.0)

O75.5   Delayed delivery after artificial rupture of membranes

O75.8   Other specified complications of labor and delivery

O75.81   Maternal exhaustion complicating labor and delivery

O75.89   Other specified complications of labor and delivery

O75.9   Complication of labor and delivery, unspecified

O76   Abnormality in fetal heart rate and rhythm complicating labor and delivery
> Includes: depressed fetal heart rate tones complicating labor and delivery
> fetal bradycardia complicating labor and delivery
> fetal heart rate abnormal variability complicating labor and delivery
> fetal heart rate decelerations complicating labor and delivery
> fetal heart rate irregularity complicating labor and delivery
> fetal tachycardia complicating labor and delivery
> non-reassuring fetal heart rate or rhythm complicating labor and delivery
> Excludes1:   fetal stress NOS (O77.9)
> labor and delivery complicated by electrocardiographic evidence of fetal stress (O77.8)
> labor and delivery complicated by ultrasonic evidence of fetal stress (O77.8)
> Excludes2:   fetal metabolic acidemia (O68)
> other fetal stress (O77.0-O77.1)

O77   Other fetal stress complicating labor and delivery

O77.0   Labor and delivery complicated by meconium in amniotic fluid

O77.1   Fetal stress in labor or delivery due to drug administration

O77.8 Labor and delivery complicated by other evidence of fetal stress

Labor and delivery complicated by electrocardiographic evidence of fetal stress

Labor and delivery complicated by ultrasonic evidence of fetal stress

Excludes1: abnormality in fetal heart rate or rhythm (O76)

abnormality of fetal acid-base balance (O68)

fetal metabolic acidemia (O68)

O77.9 Labor and delivery complicated by fetal stress, unspecified

Excludes1: abnormality in fetal heart rate or rhythm (O76)

abnormality of fetal acid-base balance (O68)

fetal metabolic acidemia (O68)

DELIVERY (O80)

O80 Encounter for full-term uncomplicated delivery

Delivery requiring minimal or no assistance, with or without episiotomy, without fetal manipulation [e.g., rotation version] or instrumentation [forceps] of a spontaneous, cephalic, vaginal, full-term, single, live-born infant. This code is for use as a single diagnosis code and is not to be used with any other code from chapter 15.

Use additional code to indicate outcome of delivery (Z37.-)

COMPLICATIONS PREDOMINANTLY RELATED TO THE PUERPERIUM (O85–O92)

Excludes: mental and behavioral disorders associated with the puerperium (F53)

obstetrical tetanus (A34)

puerperal osteomalacia (M83.0)

O85 Puerperal sepsis

Includes: postpartum sepsis

puerperal peritonitis

puerperal septicemia

Use additional code (B95-B97), to identify infectious agent

Excludes1: fever of unknown origin following delivery (O86.4)

genital tract infection following delivery (O86.1)

obstetric pyemic and septic embolism (O88.3-)

urinary tract infection following delivery (O86.2-)

Excludes2: septicemia during labor (O75.3)

O86 Other puerperal infections

Excludes2: infection during labor (O75.3)

O86.0 Infection of obstetric surgical wound

Infected cesarean section wound following delivery

Infected perineal repair following delivery

O86.1 Other infection of genital tract following delivery

Cervicitis following delivery

Endometritis following delivery

Vaginitis following delivery

O86.2 Urinary tract infection following delivery

O86.20 Urinary tract infection following delivery, unspecified

Puerperal urinary tract infection NOS

O86.21 Infection of kidney following delivery

O86.22 Infection of bladder following delivery

Infection of urethra following delivery

O86.29 Other urinary tract infection following delivery

O86.4 Pyrexia of unknown origin following delivery

Puerperal infection NOS following delivery

Puerperal pyrexia NOS following delivery

Excludes2: pyrexia during labor (O75.2)

O86.8 Other specified puerperal infections

O87 Venous complications in the puerperium

Includes: those in labor, delivery and the puerperium

Excludes2: obstetric embolism (O88.-)

venous complications in pregnancy (O22.-)

O87.0 Superficial thrombophlebitis in the puerperium

O87.1 Deep phlebothrombosis in the puerperium

Deep-vein thrombosis, postpartum

Pelvic thrombophlebitis, postpartum

O87.2 Hemorrhoids in the puerperium

O87.3 Cerebral venous thrombosis in the puerperium

Cerebrovenous sinus thrombosis in the puerperium

O87.4 Varicose veins of lower extremity in the puerperium

O87.8 Other venous complications in the puerperium

Genital varices in the puerperium

O87.9 Venous complication in the puerperium, unspecified

Puerperal phlebitis NOS

Puerperal phlebopathy NOS

Puerperal thrombosis NOS

O88 Obstetric embolism

Excludes1: embolism complicating abortion NOS (O03.2)

embolism complicating ectopic or molar pregnancy (O08.2)

embolism complicating failed attempted abortion (O07.2, O07.7)

embolism complicating induced abortion (O04.2, O05.2)

embolism complicating spontaneous abortion (O03.2, O03.7)

O88.0 Obstetric air embolism

O88.01 Air embolism in pregnancy

O88.011 Air embolism in pregnancy, first trimester

O88.012 Air embolism in pregnancy, second trimester

O88.013 Air embolism in pregnancy, third trimester

O88.019 Air embolism in pregnancy, unspecified trimester

O88.02 Air embolism in childbirth

O88.03 Air embolism in the puerperium

O88.1 Amniotic fluid embolism

O88.11 Amniotic fluid embolism in pregnancy

O88.111 Amniotic fluid embolism in pregnancy, first trimester

O88.112 Amniotic fluid embolism in pregnancy, second trimester

O88.113 Amniotic fluid embolism in pregnancy, third trimester

O88.119 Amniotic fluid embolism in pregnancy, unspecified trimester

O88.12 Amniotic fluid embolism in childbirth

O88.2 Obstetric thromboembolism

O88.21 Thromboembolism in pregnancy

Obstetric (pulmonary) embolism NOS

O88.211 Thromboembolism in pregnancy, first trimester

O88.212 Thromboembolism in pregnancy, second trimester

O88.213 Thromboembolism in pregnancy, third trimester

O88.219 Thromboembolism in pregnancy, unspecified trimester

O88.22 Thromboembolism in childbirth

O88.23 Thromboembolism in the puerperium

Puerperal (pulmonary) embolism NOS

O88.3 Obstetric pyemic and septic embolism

O88.31 Pyemic and septic embolism in pregnancy

O88.311 Pyemic and septic embolism in pregnancy, first trimester

O88.312 Pyemic and septic embolism in pregnancy, second trimester

O88.313 Pyemic and septic embolism in pregnancy, third trimester

O88.319 Pyemic and septic embolism in pregnancy, unspecified trimester

O88.32 Pyemic and septic embolism in childbirth

O88.33 Pyemic and septic embolism in the puerperium

O88.8 Other obstetric embolism

Obstetric fat embolism

O88.81 Other embolism in pregnancy

O88.811 Other embolism in pregnancy, first trimester

O88.812 Other embolism in pregnancy, second trimester

O88.813   Other embolism in pregnancy, third trimester

O88.819   Other embolism in pregnancy, unspecified trimester

O88.82   Other embolism in childbirth

O88.83   Other embolism in the puerperium

O89   Complications of anesthesia during the puerperium

Includes: maternal complications arising from the administration of a general, regional or local anesthetic, analgesic or other sedation during the puerperium

Use additional code, if applicable, to identify specific complication

O89.0   **Pulmonary complications of anesthesia during the puerperium**

O89.01   **Aspiration pneumonitis due to anesthesia during the puerperium**

Inhalation of stomach contents or secretions NOS due to anesthesia during the puerperium

Mendelson's syndrome due to anesthesia during the puerperium

O89.09   **Other pulmonary complications of anesthesia during the puerperium**

O89.1   **Cardiac complications of anesthesia during the puerperium**

O89.2   **Central nervous system complications of anesthesia during the puerperium**

O89.3   **Toxic reaction to local anesthesia during the puerperium**

O89.4   **Spinal and epidural anesthesia-induced headache during the puerperium**

O89.5   **Other complications of spinal and epidural anesthesia during the puerperium**

O89.6   **Failed or difficult intubation for anesthesia during the puerperium**

O89.8   **Other complications of anesthesia during the puerperium**

O89.9   **Complication of anesthesia during the puerperium, unspecified**

O90   Complications of the puerperium, not elsewhere classified

O90.0   **Disruption of cesarean section wound**

Dehiscence of cesarean section wound

Excludes1:   rupture of uterus (spontaneous) before onset of labor (O71.0-)

rupture of uterus during labor (O71.1)

O90.1   **Disruption of perineal obstetric wound**

Disruption of wound of episiotomy

Disruption of wound of perineal laceration

Secondary perineal tear

O90.2   **Hematoma of obstetric wound**

O90.3   **Cardiomyopathy in the puerperium**

Conditions in I42.-

O90.4   **Postpartum acute renal failure**

Hepatorenal syndrome following labor and delivery

O90.5   **Postpartum thyroiditis**

O90.6   **Postpartum mood disturbance**

Postpartum blues

Postpartum dysphoria

Postpartum sadness

Excludes1:   puerperal psychosis (F53)

O90.8   **Other complications of the puerperium, not elsewhere classified**

Placental polyp

O90.9   **Complication of the puerperium, unspecified**

O91   Infections of breast associated with pregnancy, the puerperium and lactation

Use additional code to identify infection

O91.0   **Infection of nipple associated with pregnancy, the puerperium and lactation**

O91.01   **Infection of nipple associated with pregnancy**

Gestational abscess of nipple

O91.011   **Infection of nipple associated with pregnancy, first trimester**

O91.012   **Infection of nipple associated with pregnancy, second trimester**

O91.013   **Infection of nipple associated with pregnancy, third trimester**

O91.019   **Infection of nipple associated with pregnancy, unspecified trimester**

O91.02   **Infection of nipple associated with the puerperium**

Puerperal abscess of nipple

O91.03   **Infection of nipple associated with lactation**

Abscess of nipple associated with lactation

O91.1   **Abscess of breast associated with pregnancy, the puerperium and lactation**

O91.11   **Abscess of breast associated with pregnancy**

Gestational mammary abscess

Gestational purulent mastitis

Gestational subareolar abscess

O91.111   **Abscess of breast associated with pregnancy, first trimester**

O91.112   **Abscess of breast associated with pregnancy, second trimester**

O91.113   **Abscess of breast associated with pregnancy, third trimester**

O91.119   **Abscess of breast associated with pregnancy, unspecified trimester**

O91.12   **Abscess of breast associated with the puerperium**

Puerperal mammary abscess

Puerperal purulent mastitis

Puerperal subareolar abscess

O91.13   **Abscess of breast associated with lactation**

Mammary abscess associated with lactation

Purulent mastitis associated with lactation

Subareolar abscess associated with lactation

O91.2   **Nonpurulent mastitis associated with pregnancy, the puerperium and lactation**

O91.21   **Nonpurulent mastitis associated with pregnancy**

Gestational interstitial mastitis

Gestational lymphangitis of breast

Gestational mastitis NOS

Gestational parenchymatous mastitis

O91.211   **Nonpurulent mastitis associated with pregnancy, first trimester**

O91.212   **Nonpurulent mastitis associated with pregnancy, second trimester**

O91.213   **Nonpurulent mastitis associated with pregnancy, third trimester**

O91.219   **Nonpurulent mastitis associated with pregnancy, unspecified trimester**

O91.22   **Nonpurulent mastitis associated with the puerperium**

Puerperal interstitial mastitis

Puerperal lymphangitis of breast

Puerperal mastitis NOS

Puerperal parenchymatous mastitis

O91.23   **Nonpurulent mastitis associated with lactation**

Interstitial mastitis associated with lactation

Lymphangitis of breast associated with lactation

Mastitis NOS associated with lactation

Parenchymatous mastitis associated with lactation

O92   Other disorders of breast associated with pregnancy, the puerperium, and lactation

O92.0   **Retracted nipple associated with pregnancy, the puerperium, and lactation**

O92.01   **Retracted nipple associated with pregnancy**

O92.011   **Retracted nipple associated with pregnancy, first trimester**

O92.012   **Retracted nipple associated with pregnancy, second trimester**

O92.013   **Retracted nipple associated with pregnancy, third trimester**

O92.019   **Retracted nipple associated with pregnancy, unspecified trimester**

O92.02   **Retracted nipple associated with the puerperium**

O92.03   **Retracted nipple associated with lactation**

O92.1   **Cracked nipple associated with pregnancy, the puerperium, and lactation**

Fissure of nipple, gestational or puerperal

O92.11   **Cracked nipple associated with pregnancy**

O92.111   Cracked nipple associated with pregnancy, first trimester

O92.112   Cracked nipple associated with pregnancy, second trimester

O92.113   Cracked nipple associated with pregnancy, third trimester

O92.119   Cracked nipple associated with pregnancy, unspecified trimester

O92.12   Cracked nipple associated with the puerperium

O92.13   Cracked nipple associated with lactation

O92.2   Other disorders of breast associated with pregnancy, the puerperium

O92.21   Other disorders of breast associated with pregnancy

O92.211   Other disorders of breast associated with pregnancy, first trimester

O92.212   Other disorders of breast associated with pregnancy, second trimester

O92.213   Other disorders of breast associated with pregnancy, third trimester

O92.219   Other disorders of breast associated with pregnancy, unspecified trimester

O92.22   Other disorders of breast associated with the puerperium

O92.3   **Agalactia**
Primary agalactia
Excludes1:   elective agalactia (O92.5)
         secondary agalactia (O92.5)
         therapeutic agalactia (O92.5)

O92.4   **Hypogalactia**

O92.5   **Suppressed lactation**
Elective agalactia
Secondary agalactia
Therapeutic agalactia
Excludes1:   primary agalactia (O92.3)

O92.6   **Galactorrhea**

O92.7   **Other disorders of lactation**
Puerperal galactocele

O92.9   **Unspecified disorders of breast associated with pregnancy, the puerperium and lactation**

O92.90   Unspecified disorders of breast associated with pregnancy

O92.901   Unspecified disorders of breast associated with pregnancy, first trimester

O92.902   Unspecified disorders of breast associated with pregnancy, second trimester

O92.903   Unspecified disorders of breast associated with pregnancy, third trimester

O92.909   Unspecified disorders of breast associated with pregnancy, unspecified trimester

O92.91   Unspecified disorders of breast associated with the puerperium

O92.92   Unspecified disorders of breast associated with lactation

SEQUELAE OF COMPLICATION OF PREGNANCY, CHILDBIRTH, AND THE PUERPERIUM (O93)

O93   **Sequelae of complication of pregnancy, childbirth, and the puerperium**
Note: This category is to be used to indicate conditions in O00-O77.-, O85-O94 and O98-O99.- as the cause of late effects. The "sequelae" include conditions specified as such, or as late effects, which may occur at any time after the puerperium
Code first any sequelae

OTHER OBSTETRIC CONDITIONS, NOT ELSEWHERE CLASSIFIED (O94–O99)

O94   **Maternal malignant neoplasms, traumatic injuries and abuse classifiable elsewhere but complicating pregnancy, childbirth and the puerperium**

O94.1   **Malignant neoplasm complicating pregnancy, childbirth and the puerperium**
Conditions in C00-C97
Use additional code to identify neoplasm
Excludes2:   maternal care for benign tumor of cervix (O34.4-)
         maternal care for benign tumor of corpus uteri (O34.1-)

O94.11   Malignant neoplasm complicating pregnancy

O94.111   Malignant neoplasm complicating pregnancy, first trimester

O94.112   Malignant neoplasm complicating pregnancy, second trimester

O94.113   Malignant neoplasm complicating pregnancy, third trimester

O94.119   Malignant neoplasm complicating pregnancy, unspecified trimester

O94.12   Malignant neoplasm complicating childbirth

O94.13   Malignant neoplasm complicating the puerperium

O94.2   **Injury, poisoning and certain other consequences of external causes complicating pregnancy, childbirth and the puerperium**
Conditions in S00-T98
Use additional code to identify the injury or poisoning

O94.21   Injury, poisoning and certain other consequences of external causes complicating pregnancy

O94.211   Injury, poisoning and certain other consequences of external causes complicating pregnancy, first trimester

O94.212   Injury, poisoning and certain other consequences of external causes complicating pregnancy, second trimester

O94.213   Injury, poisoning and certain other consequences of external causes complicating pregnancy, third trimester

O94.219   Injury, poisoning and certain other consequences of external causes complicating pregnancy, unspecified trimester

O94.22   Injury, poisoning and certain other consequences of external causes complicating childbirth

O94.23   Injury, poisoning and certain other consequences of external causes complicating the puerperium

O94.3   **Physical abuse complicating pregnancy, childbirth and the puerperium**
Use additional code (if applicable):
   to identify any associated current injury due to physical abuse
   to identify the perpetrator of abuse (for confirmed cases only) (Y07.-)
Excludes2:   sexual abuse complicating pregnancy, childbirth and the puerperium (O94.4-)

O94.31   Suspected physical abuse complicating pregnancy
Physical abuse complicating pregnancy NOS

O94.311   Suspected physical abuse complicating pregnancy, first trimester

O94.312   Suspected physical abuse complicating pregnancy, second trimester

O94.313   Suspected physical abuse complicating pregnancy, third trimester

O94.319   Suspected physical abuse complicating pregnancy, unspecified trimester

O94.32   Confirmed physical abuse complicating pregnancy

O94.321   Confirmed physical abuse complicating pregnancy, first trimester

O94.322   Confirmed physical abuse complicating pregnancy, second trimester

O94.323   Confirmed physical abuse complicating pregnancy, third trimester

O94.329   Confirmed physical abuse complicating pregnancy, unspecified trimester

O94.33   Physical abuse complicating childbirth

O94.330   Suspected physical abuse complicating childbirth
Physical abuse complicating childbirth NOS

O94.331   Confirmed physical abuse complicating childbirth

O94.34   Physical abuse complicating the puerperium

    O94.340   Suspected physical abuse complicating the puerperium
            Physical abuse complicating the puerperium NOS

    O94.341   Confirmed physical abuse complicating the puerperium

O94.4   Sexual abuse complicating pregnancy, childbirth and the puerperium

    Use additional code (if applicable):
        to identify any associated current injury due to sexual abuse
        to identify the perpetrator of abuse (for confirmed cases only) (Y07.-)

    O94.41   Suspected sexual abuse complicating pregnancy
        Sexual abuse complicating pregnancy NOS

        O94.411   Suspected sexual abuse complicating pregnancy, first trimester

        O94.412   Suspected sexual abuse complicating pregnancy, second trimester

        O94.413   Suspected sexual abuse complicating pregnancy, third trimester

        O94.419   Suspected sexual abuse complicating pregnancy, unspecified trimester

    O94.42   Confirmed sexual abuse complicating pregnancy

        O94.421   Confirmed sexual abuse complicating pregnancy, first trimester

        O94.422   Confirmed sexual abuse complicating pregnancy, second trimester

        O94.423   Confirmed sexual abuse complicating pregnancy, third trimester

        O94.429   Confirmed sexual abuse complicating pregnancy, unspecified trimester

    O94.43   Sexual abuse complicating childbirth

        O94.430   Suspected sexual abuse complicating childbirth
            Sexual abuse complicating childbirth NOS

        O94.431   Confirmed sexual abuse complicating childbirth

    O94.44   Sexual abuse complicating the puerperium

        O94.440   Suspected sexual abuse complicating the puerperium
            Sexual abuse complicating the puerperium NOS

        O94.441   Confirmed sexual abuse complicating the puerperium

O94.5   Psychological abuse complicating pregnancy, childbirth and the puerperium

    Use additional code to identify the perpetrator of abuse (for confirmed cases only) (Y07.-)

    O94.51   Suspected psychological abuse complicating pregnancy
        Psychological abuse complicating pregnancy NOS

        O94.511   Suspected psychological abuse complicating pregnancy, first trimester

        O94.512   Suspected psychological abuse complicating pregnancy, second trimester

        O94.513   Suspected psychological abuse complicating pregnancy, third trimester

        O94.519   Suspected psychological abuse complicating pregnancy, unspecified trimester

    O94.52   Confirmed psychological abuse complicating pregnancy

        O94.521   Confirmed psychological abuse complicating pregnancy, first trimester

        O94.522   Confirmed psychological abuse complicating pregnancy, second trimester

        O94.523   Confirmed psychological abuse complicating pregnancy, third trimester

        O94.529   Confirmed psychological abuse complicating pregnancy, unspecified trimester

O94.53   Psychological abuse complicating childbirth

    O94.530   Suspected psychological abuse complicating childbirth
            Psychological abuse complicating childbirth NOS

    O94.531   Confirmed psychological abuse complicating childbirth

O94.54   Psychological abuse complicating the puerperium

    O94.540   Suspected psychological abuse complicating the puerperium
            Psychological abuse complicating the puerperium NOS

    O94.541   Confirmed psychological abuse complicating the puerperium

O98   Maternal infectious and parasitic diseases classifiable elsewhere but complicating pregnancy, childbirth and the puerperium

    Includes: the listed conditions when complicating the pregnant state, when aggravated by the pregnancy, or as a reason for obstetric care

    Use additional code (Chapter I), to identify specific condition.

    Excludes2:   herpes gestationis (O26.4-)
            obstetrical tetanus (A34)
            puerperal infection (O86.-)
            puerperal sepsis (O85)
            when the reason for maternal care is that the disease is known or suspected to have affected the fetus (O35-O36)

O98.0   Tuberculosis complicating pregnancy, childbirth and the puerperium
        Conditions in A15-A19

    O98.01   Tuberculosis complicating pregnancy

        O98.011   Tuberculosis complicating pregnancy, first trimester

        O98.012   Tuberculosis complicating pregnancy, second trimester

        O98.013   Tuberculosis complicating pregnancy, third trimester

        O98.019   Tuberculosis complicating pregnancy, unspecified trimester

    O98.02   Tuberculosis complicating childbirth

    O98.03   Tuberculosis complicating the puerperium

O98.1   Syphilis complicating pregnancy, childbirth and the puerperium
        Conditions in A50-A53

    O98.11   Syphilis complicating pregnancy

        O98.111   Syphilis complicating pregnancy, first trimester

        O98.112   Syphilis complicating pregnancy, second trimester

        O98.113   Syphilis complicating pregnancy, third trimester

        O98.119   Syphilis complicating pregnancy, unspecified trimester

    O98.12   Syphilis complicating childbirth

    O98.13   Syphilis complicating the puerperium

O98.2   Gonorrhea complicating pregnancy, childbirth and the puerperium
        Conditions in A54.-

    O98.21   Gonorrhea complicating pregnancy

        O98.211   Gonorrhea complicating pregnancy, first trimester

        O98.212   Gonorrhea complicating pregnancy, second trimester

        O98.213   Gonorrhea complicating pregnancy, third trimester

        O98.219   Gonorrhea complicating pregnancy, unspecified trimester

    O98.22   Gonorrhea complicating childbirth

    O98.23   Gonorrhea complicating the puerperium

O98.3   **Other infections with a predominantly sexual mode of transmission complicating pregnancy, childbirth and the puerperium**
     Conditions in A55-A64

   O98.31   Other infections with a predominantly sexual mode of transmission complicating pregnancy

     O98.311   Other infections with a predominantly sexual mode of transmission complicating pregnancy, first trimester

     O98.312   Other infections with a predominantly sexual mode of transmission complicating pregnancy, second trimester

     O98.313   Other infections with a predominantly sexual mode of transmission complicating pregnancy, third trimester

     O98.319   Other infections with a predominantly sexual mode of transmission complicating pregnancy, unspecified trimester

   O98.32   Other infections with a predominantly sexual mode of transmission complicating childbirth

   O98.33   Other infections with a predominantly sexual mode of transmission complicating the puerperium

O98.4   **Viral hepatitis complicating pregnancy, childbirth and the puerperium**
     Conditions in B15-B19

   O98.41   Viral hepatitis complicating pregnancy

     O98.411   Viral hepatitis complicating pregnancy, first trimester

     O98.412   Viral hepatitis complicating pregnancy, second trimester

     O98.413   Viral hepatitis complicating pregnancy, third trimester

     O98.419   Viral hepatitis complicating pregnancy, unspecified trimester

   O98.42   Viral hepatitis complicating childbirth

   O98.43   Viral hepatitis complicating the puerperium

O98.5   **Other viral diseases complicating pregnancy, childbirth and the puerperium**
     Conditions in A80-B09, B20, B25-B34

   O98.51   Other viral diseases complicating pregnancy

     O98.511   Other viral diseases complicating pregnancy, first trimester

     O98.512   Other viral diseases complicating pregnancy, second trimester

     O98.513   Other viral diseases complicating pregnancy, third trimester

     O98.519   Other viral diseases complicating pregnancy, unspecified trimester

   O98.52   Other viral diseases complicating childbirth

   O98.53   Other viral diseases complicating the puerperium

O98.6   **Protozoal diseases complicating pregnancy, childbirth and the puerperium**
     Conditions in B50-B64

   O98.61   Protozoal diseases complicating pregnancy

     O98.611   Protozoal diseases complicating pregnancy, first trimester

     O98.612   Protozoal diseases complicating pregnancy, second trimester

     O98.613   Protozoal diseases complicating pregnancy, third trimester

     O98.619   Protozoal diseases complicating pregnancy, unspecified trimester

   O98.62   Protozoal diseases complicating childbirth

   O98.63   Protozoal diseases complicating the puerperium

O98.8   **Other maternal infectious and parasitic diseases complicating pregnancy, childbirth and the puerperium**

   O98.81   Other maternal infectious and parasitic diseases complicating pregnancy

     O98.811   Other maternal infectious and parasitic diseases complicating pregnancy, first trimester

     O98.812   Other maternal infectious and parasitic diseases complicating pregnancy, second trimester

     O98.813   Other maternal infectious and parasitic diseases complicating pregnancy, third trimester

     O98.819   Other maternal infectious and parasitic diseases complicating pregnancy, unspecified trimester

   O98.82   Other maternal infectious and parasitic diseases complicating childbirth

   O98.83   Other maternal infectious and parasitic diseases complicating the puerperium

O98.9   **Unspecified maternal infectious and parasitic disease complicating pregnancy, childbirth and the puerperium**

   O98.91   Unspecified maternal infectious and parasitic disease complicating pregnancy

     O98.911   Unspecified maternal infectious and parasitic disease complicating pregnancy, first trimester

     O98.912   Unspecified maternal infectious and parasitic disease complicating pregnancy, second trimester

     O98.913   Unspecified maternal infectious and parasitic disease complicating pregnancy, third trimester

     O98.919   Unspecified maternal infectious and parasitic disease complicating pregnancy, unspecified trimester

   O98.92   **Unspecified maternal infectious and parasitic disease complicating childbirth**

   O98.93   **Unspecified maternal infectious and parasitic disease complicating the puerperium**

O99   Other maternal diseases classifiable elsewhere but complicating pregnancy, childbirth and the puerperium
     Note: This category includes conditions which complicate the pregnant state, are aggravated by the pregnancy or are a main reason for obstetric care
     Use additional code to identify specific condition
     Excludes2:   when the reason for maternal care is that the condition is known or suspected to have affected the fetus (O35-O36)

O99.0   **Anemia complicating pregnancy, childbirth and the puerperium**
     Conditions in D50-D64

   O99.01   Anemia complicating pregnancy

     O99.011   Anemia complicating pregnancy, first trimester

     O99.012   Anemia complicating pregnancy, second trimester

     O99.013   Anemia complicating pregnancy, third trimester

     O99.019   Anemia complicating pregnancy, unspecified trimester

   O99.02   Anemia complicating childbirth

   O99.03   Anemia complicating the puerperium

O99.1   **Other diseases of the blood and blood-forming organs and certain disorders involving the immune mechanism complicating pregnancy, childbirth and the puerperium**
     Conditions in D65-D89
     Excludes2:   hemorrhage with coagulation defects (O46.0-, O67.0, O72.3)

   O99.11   Other diseases of the blood and blood-forming organs and certain disorders involving the immune mechanism complicating pregnancy

     O99.111   Other diseases of the blood and blood-forming organs and certain disorders involving the immune mechanism complicating pregnancy, first trimester

     O99.112   Other diseases of the blood and blood-forming organs and certain disorders involving the immune mechanism complicating pregnancy, second trimester

O99.113 Other diseases of the blood and blood-forming organs and certain disorders involving the immune mechanism complicating pregnancy, third trimester

O99.119 Other diseases of the blood and blood-forming organs and certain disorders involving the immune mechanism complicating pregnancy, unspecified trimester

O99.12 Other diseases of the blood and blood-forming organs and certain disorders involving the immune mechanism complicating childbirth

O99.13 Other diseases of the blood and blood-forming organs and certain disorders involving the immune mechanism complicating the puerperium

O99.2 Endocrine, nutritional and metabolic diseases complicating pregnancy, childbirth and the puerperium
Conditions in E00-E90
Excludes2: diabetes mellitus (O24.-)
malnutrition (O25.-)
postpartum thyroiditis (O90.5)

O99.21 Endocrine, nutritional and metabolic diseases complicating pregnancy

O99.211 Endocrine, nutritional and metabolic diseases complicating pregnancy, first trimester

O99.212 Endocrine, nutritional and metabolic diseases complicating pregnancy, second trimester

O99.213 Endocrine, nutritional and metabolic diseases complicating pregnancy, third trimester

O99.219 Endocrine, nutritional and metabolic diseases complicating pregnancy, unspecified trimester

O99.22 Endocrine, nutritional and metabolic diseases complicating childbirth

O99.23 Endocrine, nutritional and metabolic diseases complicating the puerperium

O99.3 Mental disorders and diseases of the nervous system complicating pregnancy, childbirth and the puerperium

O99.31 Alcohol use complicating pregnancy, childbirth, and the puerperium
Use additional code(s) from F10 to identify manifestations of the alcohol use

O99.310 Alcohol use complicating pregnancy, first trimester

O99.311 Alcohol use complicating pregnancy, second trimester

O99.312 Alcohol use complicating pregnancy, third trimester

O99.313 Alcohol use complicating pregnancy, unspecified trimester

O99.314 Alcohol use complicating childbirth

O99.315 Alcohol use complicating the puerperium

O99.32 Drug use complicating pregnancy, childbirth, and the puerperium
Use additional code(s) from F11-F16 and F18-F19 to identify manifestations of the drug use

O99.320 Drug use complicating pregnancy, first trimester

O99.321 Drug use complicating pregnancy, second trimester

O99.322 Drug use complicating pregnancy, third trimester

O99.323 Drug use complicating pregnancy, unspecified trimester

O99.324 Drug use complicating childbirth

O99.325 Drug use complicating the puerperium

O99.33 Smoking (tobacco) complicating pregnancy, childbirth, and the puerperium
Use additional code from F17 to identify type of tobacco

O99.330 Smoking (tobacco) complicating pregnancy, first trimester

O99.331 Smoking (tobacco) complicating pregnancy, second trimester

O99.332 Smoking (tobacco) complicating pregnancy, third trimester

O99.333 Smoking (tobacco) complicating pregnancy, unspecified trimester

O99.334 Smoking (tobacco) complicating childbirth

O99.335 Smoking (tobacco) complicating the puerperium

O99.34 Other mental disorders complicating pregnancy, childbirth, and the puerperium
Conditions in F00-F09 and F20-F99
Excludes2: postpartum mood disturbance (O09.6)
postnatal psychosis (F53)
puerperal psychosis (F53)

O99.340 Other mental disorders complicating pregnancy, first trimester

O99.341 Other mental disorders complicating pregnancy, second trimester

O99.342 Other mental disorders complicating pregnancy, third trimester

O99.343 Other mental disorders complicating pregnancy, unspecified trimester

O99.344 Other mental disorders complicating childbirth

O99.345 Other mental disorders complicating the puerperium

O99.35 Diseases of the nervous system complicating pregnancy, childbirth, and the puerperium
Conditions in G00-G99
Excludes2: pregnancy related peripheral neuritis (O26.8-)

O99.350 Diseases of the nervous system complicating pregnancy, first trimester

O99.351 Diseases of the nervous system complicating pregnancy, second trimester

O99.352 Diseases of the nervous system complicating pregnancy, third trimester

O99.353 Diseases of the nervous system complicating pregnancy, unspecified trimester

O99.354 Diseases of the nervous system complicating childbirth

O99.355 Diseases of the nervous system complicating the puerperium

O99.4 Diseases of the circulatory system complicating pregnancy, childbirth and the puerperium
Conditions in I00-I99
Excludes2: cardiomyopathy in the puerperium (O90.3)
hypertensive disorders (O10-O16)
obstetric embolism (O88.-)
venous complications and cerebrovenous sinus thrombosis in:
labor, childbirth and the puerperium (O87.-)
pregnancy (O22.-)

O99.41 Diseases of the circulatory system complicating pregnancy

O99.411 Diseases of the circulatory system complicating pregnancy, first trimester

O99.412 Diseases of the circulatory system complicating pregnancy, second trimester

O99.413 Diseases of the circulatory system complicating pregnancy, third trimester

O99.419 Diseases of the circulatory system complicating pregnancy, unspecified trimester

O99.42 Diseases of the circulatory system complicating childbirth

O99.43 Diseases of the circulatory system complicating the puerperium

O99.5 Diseases of the respiratory system complicating pregnancy, childbirth and the puerperium
Conditions in J00-J99

O99.51 Diseases of the respiratory system complicating pregnancy

O99.511 Diseases of the respiratory system complicating pregnancy, first trimester

O99.512 Diseases of the respiratory system complicating pregnancy, second trimester

O99.513   Diseases of the respiratory system complicating pregnancy, third trimester

O99.519   Diseases of the respiratory system complicating pregnancy, unspecified trimester

O99.52   Diseases of the respiratory system complicating childbirth

O99.53   Diseases of the respiratory system complicating the puerperium

O99.6   Diseases of the digestive system complicating pregnancy, childbirth and the puerperium

Conditions in K00-K93

Excludes2:   liver disorders in pregnancy, childbirth and the puerperium (O26.6)

O99.61   Diseases of the digestive system complicating pregnancy

O99.611   Diseases of the digestive system complicating pregnancy, first trimester

O99.612   Diseases of the digestive system complicating pregnancy, second trimester

O99.613   Diseases of the digestive system complicating pregnancy, third trimester

O99.619   Diseases of the digestive system complicating pregnancy, unspecified trimester

O99.62   Diseases of the digestive system complicating childbirth

O99.63   Diseases of the digestive system complicating the puerperium

O99.7   Diseases of the skin and subcutaneous tissue complicating pregnancy, childbirth and the puerperium

Conditions in L00-L99

Excludes2:   herpes gestationis (O26.4)

O99.71   Pruritic urticarial papules and plaques of pregnancy (PUPPP)

O99.711   Pruritic urticarial papules and plaques of pregnancy (PUPPP), first trimester

O99.712   Pruritic urticarial papules and plaques of pregnancy (PUPPP), second trimester

O99.713   Pruritic urticarial papules and plaques of pregnancy (PUPPP), third trimester

O99.719   Pruritic urticarial papules and plaques of pregnancy (PUPPP), unspecified trimester

O99.72   Other diseases of the skin and subcutaneous tissue complicating pregnancy

O99.721   Other diseases of the skin and subcutaneous tissue complicating pregnancy, first trimester

O99.722   Other diseases of the skin and subcutaneous tissue complicating pregnancy, second trimester

O99.723   Other diseases of the skin and subcutaneous tissue complicating pregnancy, third trimester

O99.729   Other diseases of the skin and subcutaneous tissue complicating pregnancy, unspecified trimester

O99.73   Other diseases of the skin and subcutaneous tissue complicating childbirth

O99.74   Other diseases of the skin and subcutaneous tissue complicating the puerperium

O99.8   Other specified diseases and conditions complicating pregnancy, childbirth and the puerperium

Conditions in D00-D48, H00-H95, M00-N99, and Q00-Q99

Use additional code to identify condition

Excludes2:   genitourinary infections in pregnancy (O23.-)
infection of genitourinary tract following delivery (O86.1-O86.3)
malignant neoplasms in pregnancy (O94.1-)
maternal care for known or suspected abnormality of maternal pelvic organs (O34.-)
postpartum acute renal failure (O90.4)
traumatic injuries in pregnancy (O94.2-)

O99.81   Abnormal glucose tolerance test complicating pregnancy, childbirth and the puerperium

O99.810   Abnormal glucose tolerance test complicating pregnancy

O99.811   Abnormal glucose tolerance test complicating childbirth

O99.812   Abnormal glucose tolerance test complicating the puerperium

O99.82   Streptococcus B carrier state complicating pregnancy, childbirth and the puerperium

O99.820   Streptococcus B carrier state complicating pregnancy

O99.821   Streptococcus B carrier state complicating childbirth

O99.822   Streptococcus B carrier state complicating the puerperium

O99.89   Other specified diseases and conditions complicating pregnancy, childbirth and the puerperium

CHAPTER XVI — CERTAIN CONDITIONS ORIGINATING IN THE PERINATAL PERIOD (P00–P96)

NOTE: CODES FROM THIS CHAPTER ARE FOR USE ON NEWBORN RECORDS ONLY, NEVER ON MATERNAL RECORDS

Includes: conditions that have their origin in the perinatal period (the first 28 days of life) even though morbidity occurs later

Excludes2: congenital malformations, deformations and chromosomal abnormalities (Q00-Q99)

endocrine, nutritional and metabolic diseases (E00-E90)

injury, poisoning and certain other consequences of external causes (S00-T98)

neoplasms (C00-D48)

tetanus neonatorum (A33)

This chapter contains the following blocks:

P00-P04	Newborn affected by maternal factors and by complications of pregnancy, labor, and delivery
P05-P08	Disorders related to length of gestation and fetal growth
P10-P15	Birth trauma
P19-P29	Respiratory and cardiovascular disorders specific to the perinatal period
P35-P39	Infections specific to the perinatal period
P50-P61	Hemorrhagic and hematological disorders of newborn
P70-P74	Transitory endocrine and metabolic disorders specific to newborn
P75-P78	Digestive system disorders of newborn
P80-P83	Conditions involving the integument and temperature regulation of newborn
P84	Other problems with newborn
P90-P96	Other disorders originating in the perinatal period

NEWBORN AFFECTED BY MATERNAL FACTORS AND BY COMPLICATIONS OF PREGNANCY, LABOR, AND DELIVERY (P00–P04)

Note: These codes are for use when the listed maternal conditions are specified as the cause of confirmed or suspected newborn morbidity or potential morbidity

P00 Newborn (suspected) affected by maternal conditions that may be unrelated to present pregnancy

Code first any current condition in newborn

Excludes1: newborn affected by maternal endocrine and metabolic disorders (P70-P74)

newborn (suspected) affected by maternal complications of pregnancy (P01.-)

Excludes2: newborn affected by noxious influences transmitted via placenta or breast milk (P04.-)

P00.0 Newborn (suspected) affected by maternal hypertensive disorders

Newborn (suspected) affected by maternal conditions classifiable to O10-O11, O13-O16

P00.1 Newborn (suspected) affected by maternal renal and urinary tract diseases

Newborn (suspected) affected by maternal conditions classifiable to N00-N39

P00.2 Newborn (suspected) affected by maternal infectious and parasitic diseases

Newborn (suspected) affected by maternal infectious disease classifiable to A00-B99 and J10, but not necessarily itself manifesting that disease

Excludes1: infections specific to the perinatal period (P35-P39)

maternal genital tract or other localized infections (P00.8)

P00.3 Newborn (suspected) affected by other maternal circulatory and respiratory diseases

Newborn (suspected) affected by maternal conditions classifiable to I00-I99, J00-J99, Q20-Q34 and not included in P00.0, P00.2

P00.4 Newborn (suspected) affected by maternal nutritional disorders

Newborn (suspected) affected by maternal disorders classifiable to E40-E64

Maternal malnutrition NOS

P00.5 Newborn (suspected) affected by maternal injury

Newborn (suspected) affected by maternal conditions classifiable to O97.2

P00.6 Newborn (suspected) affected by surgical procedure on mother

Excludes1: cesarean section for present delivery (P03.4)

damage to placenta from amniocentesis, Cesarean section or surgical induction (P02.1)

previous surgery to uterus or pelvic organs (P03.89)

P00.7 Newborn (suspected) affected by other medical procedures on mother, not elsewhere classified

Newborn (suspected) affected by radiation to mother

Excludes1: damage to placenta from amniocentesis, cesarean section or surgical induction (P02.1)

newborn affected by other complications of labor and delivery (P03.-)

P00.8 Newborn (suspected) affected by other maternal conditions

Newborn (suspected) affected by conditions classifiable to T80-T88

Newborn (suspected) affected by maternal genital tract or other localized infections

Newborn (suspected) affected by maternal systemic lupus erythematosus

Excludes1: transitory neonatal endocrine and metabolic disorders (P70-P74)

P00.9 Newborn (suspected) affected by unspecified maternal condition

P01 Newborn (suspected) affected by maternal complications of pregnancy

Code first any current condition in newborn

P01.0 Newborn (suspected) affected by incompetent cervix

P01.1 Newborn (suspected) affected by premature rupture of membranes

P01.2 Newborn (suspected) affected by oligohydramnios

Excludes1: oligohydramnios due to premature rupture of membranes (P01.1)

P01.3 Newborn (suspected) affected by polyhydramnios

Newborn (suspected) affected by hydramnios

P01.4 Newborn (suspected) affected by ectopic pregnancy

Newborn (suspected) affected by abdominal pregnancy

P01.5 Newborn (suspected) affected by multiple pregnancy

Newborn (suspected) affected by triplet (pregnancy)

Newborn (suspected) affected by twin (pregnancy)

P01.6 Newborn (suspected) affected by maternal death

P01.7 Newborn (suspected) affected by malpresentation before labor

Newborn (suspected) affected by breech presentation before labor

Newborn (suspected) affected by external version before labor

Newborn (suspected) affected by face presentation before labor

Newborn (suspected) affected by transverse lie before labor

Newborn (suspected) affected by unstable lie before labor

P01.8 Newborn (suspected) affected by other maternal complications of pregnancy

P01.9 Newborn (suspected) affected by maternal complication of pregnancy, unspecified

P02 Newborn (suspected) affected by complications of placenta, cord and membranes

Code first any current condition in newborn

P02.0 Newborn (suspected) affected by placenta previa

P02.1 **Newborn (suspected) affected by other forms of placental separation and hemorrhage**
Newborn (suspected) affected by abruptio placenta
Newborn (suspected) affected by accidental hemorrhage
Newborn (suspected) affected by antepartum hemorrhage
Newborn (suspected) affected by damage to placenta from amniocentesis, cesarean section or surgical induction
Newborn (suspected) affected by maternal blood loss
Newborn (suspected) affected by premature separation of placenta

P02.2 **Newborn (suspected) affected by other and unspecified morphological and functional abnormalities of placenta**

P02.20 **Newborn (suspected) affected by unspecified morphological and functional abnormalities of placenta**

P02.29 **Newborn (suspected) affected by other morphological and functional abnormalities of placenta**
Newborn (suspected) affected by placental dysfunction
Newborn (suspected) affected by placental infarction
Newborn (suspected) affected by placental insufficiency

P02.3 **Newborn (suspected) affected by placental transfusion syndromes**
Newborn (suspected) affected by placental and cord abnormalities resulting in twin-to-twin or other transplacental transfusion

P02.4 **Newborn (suspected) affected by prolapsed cord**

P02.5 **Newborn (suspected) affected by other compression of umbilical cord**
Newborn (suspected) affected by entanglement of umbilical cord
Newborn (suspected) affected by knot in umbilical cord
Newborn (suspected) affected by umbilical cord (tightly) around neck

P02.6 **Newborn (suspected) affected by other and unspecified conditions of umbilical cord**

P02.60 **Newborn (suspected) affected by unspecified conditions of umbilical cord**

P02.69 **Newborn (suspected) affected by other conditions of umbilical cord**
Newborn (suspected) affected by short umbilical cord
Newborn (suspected) affected by vasa previa
Excludes1: newborn affected by single umbilical artery (Q27.0)

P02.7 **Newborn (suspected) affected by chorioamnionitis**
Newborn (suspected) affected by amnionitis
Newborn (suspected) affected by membranitis
Newborn (suspected) affected by placentitis

P02.8 **Newborn (suspected) affected by other abnormalities of membranes**

P02.9 **Newborn (suspected) affected by abnormality of membranes, unspecified**

P03 **Newborn (suspected) affected by other complications of labor and delivery**
Code first any current condition in newborn

P03.0 **Newborn (suspected) affected by breech delivery and extraction**

P03.1 **Newborn (suspected) affected by other malpresentation, malposition and disproportion during labor and delivery**
Newborn (suspected) affected by contracted pelvis
Newborn (suspected) affected by conditions classifiable to O64-O66
Newborn (suspected) affected by persistent occipitoposterior
Newborn (suspected) affected by transverse lie

P03.2 **Newborn (suspected) affected by forceps delivery**

P03.3 **Newborn (suspected) affected by delivery by vacuum extractor [ventouse]**

P03.4 **Newborn (suspected) affected by cesarean delivery**

P03.5 **Newborn (suspected) affected by precipitate delivery**
Newborn (suspected) affected by rapid second stage

P03.6 **Newborn (suspected) affected by abnormal uterine contractions**
Newborn (suspected) affected by conditions classifiable to O62.-, except O62.3
Newborn (suspected) affected by hypertonic labor
Newborn (suspected) affected by uterine inertia

P03.8 **Newborn (suspected) affected by other specified complications of labor and delivery**

P03.81 **Newborn (suspected) affected by abnormality in fetal (intrauterine) heart rate or rhythm**
Excludes1: neonatal cardiac dysrhymia (P29.1)

P03.810 **Newborn (suspected) affected by abnormality in fetal (intrauterine) heart rate or rhythm before the onset of labor**

P03.811 **Newborn (suspected) affected by abnormality in fetal (intrauterine) heart rate or rhythm during labor**

P03.819 **Newborn (suspected) affected by abnormality in fetal (intrauterine) heart rate or rhythm, unspecified as to time of onset**

P03.89 **Newborn (suspected) affected by other specified complications of labor and delivery**
Newborn (suspected) affected by abnormality of maternal soft tissues
Newborn (suspected) affected by conditions classifiable to O60-O75 and by procedures used in labor and delivery not included in P02.- and P03.0-P03.6
Newborn (suspected) affected by induction of labor

P03.0 **Newborn (suspected) affected by complication of labor and delivery, unspecified**

P04 **Newborn (suspected) affected by noxious influences transmitted via placenta or breast milk**
Includes: nonteratogenic effects of substances transmitted via placenta
Excludes1: neonatal jaundice from excessive hemolysis due to drugs or toxins transmitted from mother (P58.4)
Excludes2: congenital malformations (Q00-Q99)

P04.0 **Newborn (suspected) affected by maternal anesthesia and analgesia in pregnancy, labor and delivery**
Newborn (suspected) affected by reactions and intoxications from maternal opiates and tranquilizers administered during labor and delivery

P04.1 **Newborn (suspected) affected by other maternal medication**
Newborn (suspected) affected by cancer chemotherapy
Newborn (suspected) affected by cytotoxic drugs
Excludes1: dysmorphism due to warfarin (Q86.2)
fetal hydantoin syndrome (Q86.1)
maternal use of drugs of addiction (P04.4-)

P04.2 **Newborn (suspected) affected by maternal use of tobacco**
Newborn (suspected) affected by exposure in utero to tobacco smoke
Excludes2: newborn exposure to environmental tobacco smoke (P96.6)

P04.3 **Newborn (suspected) affected by maternal use of alcohol**
Excludes1: fetal alcohol syndrome (Q86.0)

P04.4 **Newborn (suspected) affected by maternal use of drugs of addiction**

P04.41 **Newborn (suspected) affected by maternal use of cocaine**
"Crack baby"

P04.49 **Newborn (suspected) affected by maternal use of other drugs of addiction**
Excludes1: newborn (suspected) affected by maternal anesthesia and analgesia (P04.0)
withdrawal symptoms from maternal use of drugs of addiction (P96.1)

P04.5 **Newborn (suspected) affected by maternal use of nutritional chemical substances**

P04.6 **Newborn (suspected) affected by maternal exposure to environmental chemical substances**

P04.8 **Newborn (suspected) affected by other maternal noxious influences**

P04.9 **Newborn (suspected) affected by maternal noxious influence, unspecified**

 © 2002 Ingenix, Inc.

DISORDERS OF NEWBORN RELATED TO LENGTH OF GESTATION AND FETAL GROWTH (P05–P08)

P05 Disorders of newborn related to slow fetal growth and fetal malnutrition

P05.0 Newborn light for gestational age
Newborn light-for-dates

P05.00 Newborn light for gestational age, unspecified weight

P05.01 Newborn light for gestational age, less than 500 grams

P05.02 Newborn light for gestational age, 500-749 grams

P05.03 Newborn light for gestational age, 750-999 grams

P05.04 Newborn light for gestational age, 1000-1249 grams

P05.05 Newborn light for gestational age, 1250-1499 grams

P05.06 Newborn light for gestational age, 1500-1749 grams

P05.07 Newborn light for gestational age, 1750-1999 grams

P05.08 Newborn light for gestational age, 2000-2499 grams

P05.1 Newborn small for gestational age
Newborn small-and-light-for-dates
Newborn small-for-dates

P05.10 Newborn small for gestational age, unspecified weight

P05.11 Newborn small for gestational age, less than 500 grams

P05.12 Newborn small for gestational age, 500-749 grams

P05.13 Newborn small for gestational age, 750-999 grams

P05.14 Newborn small for gestational age, 1000-1249 grams

P05.15 Newborn small for gestational age, 1250-1499 grams

P05.16 Newborn small for gestational age, 1500-1749 grams

P05.17 Newborn small for gestational age, 1750-1999 grams

P05.18 Newborn small for gestational age, 2000-2499 grams

P05.2 Newborn affected by fetal (intrauterine) malnutrition not light or small for gestational age
Infant, not light or small for gestational age, showing signs of fetal malnutrition, such as dry, peeling skin and loss of subcutaneous tissue
Excludes1:   newborn affected by fetal malnutrition with mention of light for gestational age (P05.0-)
newborn affected by fetal malnutrition with mention of small for gestational age (P05.1-)

P05.9 Newborn affected by slow intrauterine growth, unspecified
Newborn affected by fetal growth retardation NOS

P07 Disorders of newborn related to short gestation and low birth weight, not elsewhere classified
Note: When both birth weight and gestational age of the newborn are available, priority of assignment should be given to birth weight.
Includes: the listed conditions, without further specification, as the cause of morbidity or additional care, in newborn
Excludes1:   low birth weight due to slow fetal growth and fetal malnutrition (P05.-)

P07.0 Extremely low birth weight newborn
Newborn birth weight 999 g. or less

P07.00 Extremely low birth weight newborn, unspecified weight

P07.01 Extremely low birth weight newborn, less than 500 grams

P07.02 Extremely low birth weight newborn, 500-749 grams

P07.03 Extremely low birth weight newborn, 750-999 grams

P07.1 Other low birth weight newborn
Newborn birth weight 1000-2499 g.

P07.10 Other low birth weight newborn, unspecified weight

P07.14 Other low birth weight newborn, 1000-1249 grams

P07.15 Other low birth weight newborn, 1250-1499 grams

P07.16 Other low birth weight newborn, 1500-1749 grams

P07.17 Other low birth weight newborn, 1750-1999 grams

P07.18 Other low birth weight newborn, 2000-2499 grams

P07.2 Extreme immaturity of newborn
Less than 28 completed weeks (less than 196 completed days) of gestation.

P07.20 Extreme immaturity of newborn, unspecified weeks

P07.21 Extreme immaturity of newborn, less than 24 completed weeks

P07.22 Extreme immaturity of newborn, 24-26 completed weeks

P07.23 Extreme immaturity of newborn, 27 completed weeks

P07.3 Other preterm newborn
28 completed weeks or more but less than 37 completed weeks (196 completed days but less than 259 completed days) of gestation.
Prematurity NOS

P07.30 Other preterm newborn, unspecified weeks

P07.31 Other preterm newborn, 28-31 completed weeks

P07.32 Other preterm newborn, 32-36 completed weeks

P08 Disorders of newborn related to long gestation and high birth weight
Note: When both birth weight and gestational age of the newborn are available, priority of assignment should be given to birth weight
Includes: the listed conditions, without further specification, as causes of morbidity or additional care, in newborn

P08.0 Exceptionally large newborn baby
Usually implies a birth weight of 4500 g. or more
Excludes1:   syndrome of infant of diabetic mother (P70.1)
syndrome of infant of mother with gestational diabetes (P70.0)

P08.1 Other heavy for gestational age newborn
Other newborn heavy-or-large-for-dates regardless of period of gestation.

P08.2 Post-term newborn, not heavy for gestational age
Newborn with gestation period of 42 completed weeks or more (294 days or more), not heavy-or-large-for-dates.
Postmaturity NOS

BIRTH TRAUMA (P10–P15)

P10 Intracranial laceration and hemorrhage due to birth injury
Excludes1:   intracranial hemorrhage of newborn NOS (P52.9)
intracranial hemorrhage of newborn due to anoxia or hypoxia (P52.-)
nontraumatic intracranial hemorrhage of newborn (P52.-)

P10.0 Subdural hemorrhage due to birth injury
Subdural hematoma (localized) due to birth injury
Excludes1:   subdural hemorrhage accompanying tentorial tear (P10.4)

P10.1 Cerebral hemorrhage due to birth injury

P10.2 Intraventricular hemorrhage due to birth injury

P10.3 Subarachnoid hemorrhage due to birth injury

P10.4 Tentorial tear due to birth injury

P10.8 Other intracranial lacerations and hemorrhages due to birth injury

P10.9 Unspecified intracranial laceration and hemorrhage due to birth injury

P11 Other birth injuries to central nervous system

P11.0 Cerebral edema due to birth injury

P11.1 Other specified brain damage due to birth injury

P11.2 Unspecified brain damage due to birth injury

P11.3 Birth injury to facial nerve
Facial palsy due to birth injury

P11.4 Birth injury to other cranial nerves

P11.5 Birth injury to spine and spinal cord
Fracture of spine due to birth injury

P11.9 Birth injury to central nervous system, unspecified

P12 Birth injury to scalp

P12.0 Cephalhematoma due to birth injury

P12.1 Chignon (from vacuum extraction) due to birth injury

P12.2 Epicranial subaponeurotic hemorrhage due to birth injury

P12.3 Bruising of scalp due to birth injury

P12.4 Injury of scalp of newborn due to monitoring equipment
Sampling incision of scalp of newborn
Scalp clip (electrode) injury of newborn

P12.8 Other birth injuries to scalp

P12.81   Caput succedaneum

P12.89   Other birth injuries to scalp

P12.9 Birth injury to scalp, unspecified

P13 Birth injury to skeleton

Excludes2:   birth injury to spine (P11.5)

P13.0 Fracture of skull due to birth injury

P13.1 Other birth injuries to skull

Excludes1:   cephalhematoma (P12.0)

P13.2 Birth injury to femur

P13.3 Birth injury to other long bones

P13.4 Fracture of clavicle due to birth injury

P13.8 Birth injuries to other parts of skeleton

P13.9 Birth injury to skeleton, unspecified

P14 Birth injury to peripheral nervous system

P14.0 Erb's paralysis due to birth injury

P14.1 Klumpke's paralysis due to birth injury

P14.2 Phrenic nerve paralysis due to birth injury

P14.3 Other brachial plexus birth injuries

P14.8 Birth injuries to other parts of peripheral nervous system

P14.9 Birth injury to peripheral nervous system, unspecified

P15 Other birth injuries

P15.0 Birth injury to liver

Rupture of liver due to birth injury

P15.1 Birth injury to spleen

Rupture of spleen due to birth injury

P15.2 Sternomastoid injury due to birth injury

P15.3 Birth injury to eye

Subconjunctival hemorrhage due to birth injury
Traumatic glaucoma due to birth injury

P15.4 Birth injury to face

Facial congestion due to birth injury

P15.5 Birth injury to external genitalia

P15.6 Subcutaneous fat necrosis due to birth injury

P15.8 Other specified birth injuries

P15.9 Birth injury, unspecified

RESPIRATORY AND CARDIOVASCULAR DISORDERS SPECIFIC TO THE PERINATAL PERIOD (P19–P29)

P19 Metabolic acidemia in newborn

Includes: fetal metabolic acidemia

P19.0 Metabolic acidemia in newborn first noted before onset of labor

P19.1 Metabolic acidemia in newborn first noted during labor

P19.2 Metabolic acidemia noted at birth

P19.9 Metabolic acidemia, unspecified

P22 Respiratory distress of newborn

Excludes1:   respiratory failure of newborn NOS (P28.5)

P22.0 Respiratory distress syndrome of newborn

Cardiorespiratory distress syndrome of newborn
Hyaline membrane disease
Idiopathic respiratory distress syndrome [IRDS or RDS] of newborn
Pulmonary hypoperfusion syndrome
Respiratory distress syndrome, type I

P22.1 Transient tachypnea of newborn

Idiopathic tachypnea of newborn
Respiratory distress syndrome, type II
Wet lung syndrome

P22.8 Other respiratory distress of newborn

P22.9 Respiratory distress of newborn, unspecified

P23 Congenital pneumonia

Includes: infective pneumonia acquired in utero or during birth
Excludes1:   neonatal pneumonia resulting from aspiration (P24.-)

P23.0 Congenital pneumonia due to viral agent

Excludes1:   congenital rubella pneumonitis (P35.0)

P23.1 Congenital pneumonia due to Chlamydia

P23.2 Congenital pneumonia due to staphylococcus

P23.3 Congenital pneumonia due to streptococcus, group B

P23.4 Congenital pneumonia due to Escherichia coli

P23.5 Congenital pneumonia due to Pseudomonas

P23.6 Congenital pneumonia due to other bacterial agents

Congenital pneumonia due to Hemophilus influenzae
Congenital pneumonia due to Klebsiella pneumoniae
Congenital pneumonia due to Mycoplasma
Congenital pneumonia due to Streptococcus, except group B
Use additional code (B95-B96) to identify organism

P23.8 Congenital pneumonia due to other organisms

Use additional code (B97) to identify organism

P23.9 Congenital pneumonia, unspecified

P24 Neonatal aspiration syndromes

Includes: neonatal pneumonia resulting from aspiration

P24.0 Neonatal aspiration of meconium

P24.1 Neonatal aspiration of amniotic fluid and mucus

Neonatal aspiration of liquor (amnii)

P24.2 Neonatal aspiration of blood

P24.3 Neonatal aspiration of milk and regurgitated food

P24.8 Other neonatal aspiration syndromes

P24.9 Neonatal aspiration syndrome, unspecified

Neonatal aspiration pneumonia NOS

P25 Interstitial emphysema and related conditions originating in the perinatal period

P25.0 Interstitial emphysema originating in the perinatal period

P25.1 Pneumothorax originating in the perinatal period

P25.2 Pneumomediastinum originating in the perinatal period

P25.3 Pneumopericardium originating in the perinatal period

P25.8 Other conditions related to interstitial emphysema originating in the perinatal period

P26 Pulmonary hemorrhage originating in the perinatal period

P26.0 Tracheobronchial hemorrhage originating in the perinatal period

P26.1 Massive pulmonary hemorrhage originating in the perinatal period

P26.8 Other pulmonary hemorrhages originating in the perinatal period

P26.9 Unspecified pulmonary hemorrhage originating in the perinatal period

P27 Chronic respiratory disease originating in the perinatal period

Excludes1:   respiratory distress of newborn (P22.0-P22.9)

P27.0 Wilson-Mikity syndrome

Pulmonary dysmaturity

P27.1 Bronchopulmonary dysplasia originating in the perinatal period

P27.8 Other chronic respiratory diseases originating in the perinatal period

Congenital pulmonary fibrosis
Ventilator lung in newborn

P27.9 Unspecified chronic respiratory disease originating in the perinatal period

P28 Other respiratory conditions originating in the perinatal period

Excludes1:   congenital malformations of the respiratory system (Q30-Q34)

P28.0 Primary atelectasis of newborn

Primary failure to expand terminal respiratory units
Pulmonary hypoplasia associated with short gestation
Pulmonary immaturity NOS

P28.1 Other and unspecified atelectasis of newborn

P28.10   Unspecified atelectasis of newborn

Atelectasis of newborn NOS

P28.11   Resorption atelectasis without respiratory distress syndrome

Excludes1:   resorption atelectasis with respiratory distress syndrome (P22.0)

P28.19   Other atelectasis of newborn

Partial atelectasis of newborn
Secondary atelectasis of newborn

P28.2   **Cyanotic attacks of newborn**
Excludes1:   apnea of newborn (P28.3-P28.4)

P28.3   **Primary sleep apnea of newborn**
Sleep apnea of newborn NOS

P28.4   **Other apnea of newborn**

P28.5   **Respiratory failure of newborn**

P28.8   **Other specified respiratory conditions of newborn**
Sniffles in newborn
Snuffles in newborn
Excludes1:   early congenital syphilitic rhinitis (A50.0)

P28.9   **Respiratory condition of newborn, unspecified**
Respiratory depression in newborn

P29   Cardiovascular disorders originating in the perinatal period
Excludes1:   congenital malformations of the circulatory system (Q20-Q28)

P29.0   **Neonatal cardiac failure**

P29.1   **Neonatal cardiac dysrhythmia**

P29.2   **Neonatal hypertension**

P29.3   **Persistent fetal circulation**
Delayed closure of ductus arteriosus

P29.4   **Transient myocardial ischemia in newborn**

P29.8   **Other cardiovascular disorders originating in the perinatal period**

P29.9   **Cardiovascular disorder originating in the perinatal period, unspecified**

INFECTIONS SPECIFIC TO THE PERINATAL PERIOD (P35–P39)

Includes: infections acquired in utero or during birth
Excludes2:   asymptomatic human immunodeficiency virus [HIV] infection status (Z21)
congenital gonococcal infection (A54.-)
congenital pneumonia (P23.-)
congenital syphilis (A50.-)
human immunodeficiency virus [HIV] disease (B20)
infectious diseases acquired after birth (A00-B99, J10.-)
intestinal infectious disease (A00-A09)
laboratory evidence of human immunodeficiency virus [HIV] (R75)
tetanus neonatorum (A33)

P35   Congenital viral diseases
Includes: infections acquired in utero or during birth

P35.0   **Congenital rubella syndrome**
Congenital rubella pneumonitis

P35.1   **Congenital cytomegalovirus infection**

P35.2   **Congenital herpesviral [herpes simplex] infection**

P35.3   **Congenital viral hepatitis**

P35.8   **Other congenital viral diseases**
Congenital varicella [chickenpox]

P35.9   **Congenital viral disease, unspecified**

P36   Bacterial sepsis of newborn
Includes: congenital septicemia

P36.0   **Sepsis of newborn due to streptococcus, group B**

P36.1   **Sepsis of newborn due to other and unspecified streptococci**

P36.2   **Sepsis of newborn due to Staphylococcus aureus**

P36.3   **Sepsis of newborn due to other and unspecified staphylococci**

P36.4   **Sepsis of newborn due to Escherichia coli**

P36.5   **Sepsis of newborn due to anaerobes**

P36.8   **Other bacterial sepsis of newborn**

P36.9   **Bacterial sepsis of newborn, unspecified**

P37   Other congenital infectious and parasitic diseases
Excludes2:   congenital syphilis (A50.-)
infectious neonatal diarrhea (A00-A09)
necrotizing enterocolitis in newborn (P77)
noninfectious neonatal diarrhea (P78.3)
ophthalmia neonatorum due to gonococcus (A54.31)
tetanus neonatorum (A33)

P37.0   **Congenital tuberculosis**

P37.1   **Congenital toxoplasmosis**
Hydrocephalus due to congenital toxoplasmosis

P37.2   **Neonatal (disseminated) listeriosis**

P37.3   **Congenital falciparum malaria**

P37.4   **Other congenital malaria**

P37.5   **Neonatal candidiasis**

P37.8   **Other specified congenital infectious and parasitic diseases**

P37.9   **Congenital infectious or parasitic disease, unspecified**

P38   Omphalitis of newborn
Excludes1:   omphalitis not of newborn (L08.82)
tetanus omphalitis (A33)

P39   Other infections specific to the perinatal period

P39.0   **Neonatal infective mastitis**
Excludes1:   breast engorgement of newborn (P83.4)
noninfective mastitis of newborn (P83.4)

P39.1   **Neonatal conjunctivitis and dacryocystitis**
Neonatal chlamydial conjunctivitis
Ophthalmia neonatorum NOS
Excludes1:   gonococcal conjunctivitis (A54.31)

P39.2   **Intra-amniotic infection affecting newborn, not elsewhere classified**

P39.3   **Neonatal urinary tract infection**

P39.4   **Neonatal skin infection**
Neonatal pyoderma
Excludes1:   pemphigus neonatorum (L00)
staphylococcal scalded skin syndrome (L00)

P39.8   **Other specified infections specific to the perinatal period**

P39.9   **Infection specific to the perinatal period, unspecified**

HEMORRHAGIC AND HEMATOLOGICAL DISORDERS OF NEWBORN (P50–P61)

Excludes1:   congenital stenosis and stricture of bile ducts (Q44.3)
Crigler-Najjar syndrome (E80.5)
Dubin-Johnson syndrome (E80.6)
Gilbert's syndrome (E80.4)
hereditary hemolytic anemias (D55-D58)

P50   Newborn affected by (intrauterine) blood loss
Excludes1:   congenital anemia from fetal blood loss (P61.3)

P50.0   **Newborn affected by fetal (intrauterine) blood loss from vasa previa**

P50.1   **Newborn affected by fetal blood loss from ruptured cord**

P50.2   **Newborn affected by fetal blood loss from placenta**

P50.3   **Newborn affected by hemorrhage into co-twin**

P50.4   **Newborn affected by hemorrhage into maternal circulation**

P50.5   **Newborn affected by fetal blood loss from cut end of co-twin's cord**

P50.8   **Newborn affected by other fetal blood loss**

P50.9   **Newborn affected by fetal blood loss, unspecified**
Newborn affected by fetal hemorrhage NOS

P51   Umbilical hemorrhage of newborn
Excludes1:   omphalitis with mild hemorrhage (P38)
umbilical hemorrhage from cut end of co-twins cord (P50.5)

P51.0   **Massive umbilical hemorrhage of newborn**

P51.8   **Other umbilical hemorrhages of newborn**
Slipped umbilical ligature NOS

P51.9   **Umbilical hemorrhage of newborn, unspecified**

P52   Intracranial nontraumatic hemorrhage of newborn
Includes: intracranial hemorrhage due to anoxia or hypoxia
Excludes1:   intracranial hemorrhage due to birth injury (P10.-)
intracranial hemorrhage due to other injury (S06.-)

P52.0   **Intraventricular (nontraumatic) hemorrhage, grade 1, of newborn**
Subependymal hemorrhage (without intraventricular extension)

P52.1   **Intraventricular (nontraumatic) hemorrhage, grade 2, of newborn**
Subependymal hemorrhage with intraventricular extension

P52.2   **Intraventricular (nontraumatic) hemorrhage, grade 3, of newborn**
     Subependymal hemorrhage with both intraventricular and intra-cerebral extension

P52.3   **Unspecified intraventricular (nontraumatic) hemorrhage of newborn**

P52.4   **Intracerebral (nontraumatic) hemorrhage of newborn**

P52.5   **Subarachnoid (nontraumatic) hemorrhage of newborn**

P52.6   **Cerebellar (nontraumatic) and posterior fossa hemorrhage of newborn**

P52.8   **Other intracranial (nontraumatic) hemorrhages and newborn**

P52.9   **Intracranial (nontraumatic) hemorrhage of newborn, unspecified**

P53   **Hemorrhagic disease of newborn**
     Includes: vitamin K deficiency of newborn

P54   **Other neonatal hemorrhages**
     Excludes1:   fetal blood loss (P50.-)
                     pulmonary hemorrhage originating in the perinatal period (P26.-)

P54.0   **Neonatal hematemesis**
     Excludes1:   neonatal hematemesis due to swallowed maternal blood (P78.2)

P54.1   **Neonatal melena**
     Excludes1:   neonatal melena due to swallowed maternal blood (P78.2)

P54.2   **Neonatal rectal hemorrhage**

P54.3   **Other neonatal gastrointestinal hemorrhage**

P54.4   **Neonatal adrenal hemorrhage**

P54.5   **Neonatal cutaneous hemorrhage**
     Neonatal bruising
     Neonatal ecchymoses
     Neonatal petechiae
     Neonatal superficial hematomata
     Excludes2:   bruising of scalp due to birth injury (P12.3)
                     cephalhematoma due to birth injury (P12.0)

P54.6   **Neonatal vaginal hemorrhage**
     Neonatal pseudomenses

P54.8   **Other specified neonatal hemorrhages**

P54.9   **Neonatal hemorrhage, unspecified**

P55   **Hemolytic disease of newborn**

P55.0   **Rh isoimmunization of newborn**

P55.1   **ABO isoimmunization of newborn**

P55.8   **Other hemolytic diseases of newborn**

P55.9   **Hemolytic disease of newborn, unspecified**

P56   **Hydrops fetalis due to hemolytic disease**
     Excludes1:   hydrops fetalis NOS (P83.2)

P56.0   **Hydrops fetalis due to isoimmunization**

P56.9   **Hydrops fetalis due to other and unspecified hemolytic disease**

P57   **Kernicterus**

P57.0   **Kernicterus due to isoimmunization**

P57.8   **Other specified kernicterus**
     Excludes1:   Crigler-Najjar syndrome (E80.5)

P57.9   **Kernicterus, unspecified**

P58   **Neonatal jaundice due to other excessive hemolysis**
     Excludes1:   jaundice due to isoimmunization (P55-P57)

P58.0   **Neonatal jaundice due to bruising**

P58.1   **Neonatal jaundice due to bleeding**

P58.2   **Neonatal jaundice due to infection**

P58.3   **Neonatal jaundice due to polycythemia**

P58.4   **Neonatal jaundice due to drugs or toxins transmitted from mother or given to newborn**
     Use additional external cause code (Chapter XIX) to identify drug, if drug-induced

     P58.41   **Neonatal jaundice due to drugs or toxins transmitted from mother**

     P58.42   **Neonatal jaundice due to drugs or toxins given to newborn**

P58.5   **Neonatal jaundice due to swallowed maternal blood**

P58.8   **Neonatal jaundice due to other specified excessive hemolysis**

P58.9   **Neonatal jaundice due to excessive hemolysis, unspecified**

P59   **Neonatal jaundice from other and unspecified causes**
     Excludes1:   jaundice due to inborn errors of metabolism (E70-E90)
                     kernicterus (P57.-)

P59.0   **Neonatal jaundice associated with preterm delivery**
     Hyperbilirubinemia of prematurity
     Jaundice due to delayed conjugation associated with preterm delivery

P59.1   **Inspissated bile syndrome**

P59.2   **Neonatal jaundice from other and unspecified hepatocellular damage**
     Excludes1:   congenital viral hepatitis (P35.3)

     P59.20   **Neonatal jaundice from unspecified hepatocellular damage**

     P59.29   **Neonatal jaundice from other hepatocellular damage**

P59.3   **Neonatal jaundice from breast milk inhibitor**

P59.8   **Neonatal jaundice from other specified causes**

P59.9   **Neonatal jaundice, unspecified**
     Neonatal physiological jaundice (intense) (prolonged) NOS

P60   **Disseminated intravascular coagulation of newborn**
     Includes: defibrination syndrome of newborn

P61   **Other perinatal hematological disorders**
     Excludes1:   transient hypogammaglobulinemia of infancy (D80.7)

P61.0   **Transient neonatal thrombocytopenia**
     Neonatal thrombocytopenia due to exchange transfusion
     Neonatal thrombocytopenia due to idiopathic maternal thrombocytopenia
     Neonatal thrombocytopenia due to isoimmunization

P61.1   **Polycythemia neonatorum**

P61.2   **Anemia of prematurity**

P61.3   **Congenital anemia from fetal blood loss**

P61.4   **Other congenital anemias, not elsewhere classified**
     Congenital anemia NOS

P61.5   **Transient neonatal neutropenia**

P61.6   **Other transient neonatal disorders of coagulation**

P61.8   **Other specified perinatal hematological disorders**

P61.9   **Perinatal hematological disorder, unspecified**

TRANSITORY ENDOCRINE AND METABOLIC DISORDERS SPECIFIC TO NEWBORN (P70–P74)

     Includes: transitory endocrine and metabolic disturbances caused by the infant's response to maternal endocrine and metabolic factors, or its adjustment to extrauterine environment

P70   **Transitory disorders of carbohydrate metabolism specific to newborn**

P70.0   **Syndrome of infant of mother with gestational diabetes**

P70.1   **Syndrome of infant of a diabetic mother**
     Maternal diabetes mellitus (pre-existing) (type 1 or type 2) affecting newborn (with hypoglycemia)

P70.2   **Neonatal diabetes mellitus**

P70.3   **Iatrogenic neonatal hypoglycemia**

P70.4   **Other neonatal hypoglycemia**
     Transitory neonatal hypoglycemia

P70.8   **Other transitory disorders of carbohydrate metabolism of newborn**

P70.9   **Transitory disorder of carbohydrate metabolism of newborn, unspecified**

P71   **Transitory neonatal disorders of calcium and magnesium metabolism**

P71.0   **Cow's milk hypocalcemia in newborn**

P71.1   **Other neonatal hypocalcemia**
     Excludes1:   neonatal hypoparathyroidism (P71.4)

P71.2   **Neonatal hypomagnesemia**

P71.3   **Neonatal tetany without calcium or magnesium deficiency**
Neonatal tetany NOS

P71.4   **Transitory neonatal hypoparathyroidism**

P71.8   **Other transitory neonatal disorders of calcium and magnesium metabolism**

P71.9   **Transitory neonatal disorder of calcium and magnesium metabolism, unspecified**

P72   Other transitory neonatal endocrine disorders
Excludes1:   congenital hypothyroidism with or without goiter (E03.0-E03.1)
dyshormogenetic goiter (E07.1)
Pendred's syndrome (E07.1)

P72.0   **Neonatal goiter, not elsewhere classified**
Transitory congenital goiter with normal functioning

P72.1   **Transitory neonatal hyperthyroidism**
Neonatal thyrotoxicosis

P72.2   **Other transitory neonatal disorders of thyroid function, not elsewhere classified**
Transitory neonatal hypothyroidism

P72.8   **Other specified transitory neonatal endocrine disorders**

P72.9   **Transitory neonatal endocrine disorder, unspecified**

P74   Other transitory neonatal electrolyte and metabolic disturbances
P74.0   **Late metabolic acidosis of newborn**
P74.1   **Dehydration of newborn**
P74.2   **Disturbances of sodium balance of newborn**
P74.3   **Disturbances of potassium balance of newborn**
P74.4   **Other transitory electrolyte disturbances of newborn**
P74.5   **Transitory tyrosinemia of newborn**
P74.6   **Transitory hyperammonemia of newborn**
P74.8   **Other transitory metabolic disturbances of newborn**
P74.9   **Transitory metabolic disturbance of newborn, unspecified**

DIGESTIVE SYSTEM DISORDERS OF NEWBORN (P75–P78)

P75   Meconium ileus
Excludes1:   meconium ileus in cystic fibrosis (E84.1)

P76   Other intestinal obstruction of newborn
Excludes1:   intestinal obstruction classifiable to K56.-
meconium ileus in cystic fibrosis (E84.1)
meconium ileus NOS (P75)

P76.0   **Meconium plug syndrome**

P76.1   **Transitory ileus of newborn**
Excludes1:   Hirschsprung's disease (Q43.1)

P76.2   **Intestinal obstruction due to inspissated milk**

P76.8   **Other specified intestinal obstruction of newborn**

P76.9   **Intestinal obstruction of newborn, unspecified**

P77   Necrotizing enterocolitis of newborn

P78   Other perinatal digestive system disorders
Excludes1:   cystic fibrosis (E84.0-E84.9)
neonatal gastrointestinal hemorrhages (P54.0-P54.3)

P78.0   **Perinatal intestinal perforation**
Meconium peritonitis

P78.1   **Other neonatal peritonitis**
Neonatal peritonitis NOS

P78.2   **Neonatal hematemesis and melena due to swallowed maternal blood**

P78.3   **Noninfective neonatal diarrhea**
Neonatal diarrhea NOS

P78.8   **Other specified perinatal digestive system disorders**
P78.81   **Congenital cirrhosis (of liver)**
P78.82   **Peptic ulcer of newborn**
P78.89   **Other specified perinatal digestive system disorders**

P78.9   **Perinatal digestive system disorder, unspecified**

CONDITIONS INVOLVING THE INTEGUMENT AND TEMPERATURE REGULATION OF NEWBORN (P80–P83)

P80   Hypothermia of newborn
P80.0   **Cold injury syndrome**
Severe and usually chronic hypothermia associated with a pink flushed appearance, edema and neurological and biochemical abnormalities.
Excludes1:   mild hypothermia of newborn (P80.8)

P80.8   **Other hypothermia of newborn**
Mild hypothermia of newborn

P80.9   **Hypothermia of newborn, unspecified**

P81   Other disturbances of temperature regulation of newborn
P81.0   **Environmental hyperthermia of newborn**
P81.8   **Other specified disturbances of temperature regulation of newborn**
P81.9   **Disturbance of temperature regulation of newborn, unspecified**
Fever of newborn NOS

P83   Other conditions of integument specific to newborn
Excludes1:   congenital malformations of skin and integument (Q80-Q84)
hydrops fetalis due to hemolytic disease (P56.-)
neonatal skin infection (P39.4)
staphylococcal scalded skin syndrome (L00)
Excludes2:   cradle cap (L21.0)
diaper [napkin] dermatitis (L22)

P83.0   **Sclerema neonatorum**

P83.1   **Neonatal erythema toxicum**

P83.2   **Hydrops fetalis not due to hemolytic disease**
Hydrops fetalis NOS

P83.3   **Other and unspecified edema specific to newborn**
P83.30   **Unspecified edema specific to newborn**
P83.39   **Other edema specific to newborn**

P83.4   **Breast engorgement of newborn**
Noninfective mastitis of newborn

P83.5   **Congenital hydrocele**

P83.6   **Umbilical polyp of newborn**

P83.8   **Other specified conditions integument specific to newborn**
Bronze baby syndrome
Neonatal scleroderma
Urticaria neonatorum

P83.9   **Condition of the integument specific to newborn, unspecified**

OTHER PROBLEMS WITH NEWBORN (P84)

P84   Other problems with newborn
Acidosis of newborn
Anoxia of newborn NOS
Asphyxia of newborn NOS
Hypercapnia of newborn
Hypoxia of newborn NOS
Excludes1:   intracranial hemorrhage due to anoxia or hypoxia (P52.-)
late metabolic acidosis of newborn (P74.0)

OTHER DISORDERS ORIGINATING IN THE PERINATAL PERIOD (P90–P96)

P90   Convulsions of newborn
Excludes1:   benign myoclonic epilepsy in infancy (G40.3-)
benign neonatal convulsions (familial) (G40.3-)

P91   Other disturbances of cerebral status of newborn
P91.0   **Neonatal cerebral ischemia**
P91.1   **Acquired periventricular cysts of newborn**
P91.2   **Neonatal cerebral leukomalacia**
P91.3   **Neonatal cerebral irritability**
P91.4   **Neonatal cerebral depression**
P91.5   **Neonatal coma**
P91.8   **Other specified disturbances of cerebral status of newborn**
P91.9   **Disturbance of cerebral status of newborn, unspecified**

P92 Feeding problems of newborn

P92.0 Vomiting of newborn

P92.1 Regurgitation and rumination of newborn

P92.2 Slow feeding of newborn

P92.3 Underfeeding of newborn

P92.4 Overfeeding of newborn

P92.5 Neonatal difficulty in feeding at breast

P92.8 Other feeding problems of newborn

P92.9 Feeding problem of newborn, unspecified

P93 Reactions and intoxications due to drugs administered to newborn

> Excludes1:   jaundice due to drugs or toxins transmitted from mother or given to newborn (P58.4-)
> reactions and intoxications from maternal opiates, tranquilizers and other medication (P04.0-P04.1, P04.4)
> withdrawal symptoms from maternal use of drugs of addiction (P96.1)
> withdrawal symptoms from therapeutic use of drugs in newborn (P96.2)

P93.0 Gray baby syndrome

> Gray syndrome from chloramphenicol administration in newborn

P93.8 Other reactions and intoxications due to drugs administered to newborn

> Use additional external cause code (Chapter XIX) to identify drug

P94 Disorders of muscle tone of newborn

P94.0 Transient neonatal myasthenia gravis

> Excludes1:   myasthenia gravis (G70.0)

P94.1 Congenital hypertonia

P94.2 Congenital hypotonia

> Floppy baby syndrome, unspecified

P94.8 Other disorders of muscle tone of newborn

P94.9 Disorder of muscle tone of newborn, unspecified

P95 Stillbirth

> Includes: deadborn fetus NOS
> fetal death of unspecified cause
> stillbirth NOS

P96 Other conditions originating in the perinatal period

P96.0 Congenital renal failure

> Uremia of newborn

P96.1 Neonatal withdrawal symptoms from maternal use of drugs of addiction

> Drug withdrawal syndrome in infant of dependent mother
> Excludes1:   reactions and intoxications from maternal opiates and tranquilizers administered during labor and delivery (P04.0)

P96.2 Withdrawal symptoms from therapeutic use of drugs in newborn

P96.3 Wide cranial sutures of newborn

> Neonatal craniotabes

P96.5 Complications of intrauterine procedures, not elsewhere classified

P96.6 Exposure to (parental) (environmental) tobacco smoke in the perinatal period

> Excludes2:   newborn affected by in utero exposure to tobacco (P04.2)
> exposure to environmental tobacco smoke after the perinatal period (X58.1)

P96.8 Other specified conditions originating in the perinatal period

P96.9 Condition originating in the perinatal period, unspecified

> Congenital debility NOS

CHAPTER XVII — CONGENITAL MALFORMATIONS, DEFORMATIONS AND CHROMOSOMAL ABNORMALITIES (Q00–Q99)

Excludes1:   inborn errors of metabolism (E70-E90)

This chapter contains the following blocks:

Q00-Q07   Congenital malformations of the nervous system
Q10-Q18   Congenital malformations of eye, ear, face and neck
Q20-Q28   Congenital malformations of the circulatory system
Q30-Q34   Congenital malformations of the respiratory system
Q35-Q37   Cleft lip and cleft palate
Q38-Q45   Other congenital malformations of the digestive system
Q50-Q56   Congenital malformations of genital organs
Q60-Q64   Congenital malformations of the urinary system
Q65-Q79   Congenital malformations and deformations of the musculoskeletal system
Q80-Q89   Other congenital malformations
Q90-Q99   Chromosomal abnormalities, not elsewhere classified

CONGENITAL MALFORMATIONS OF THE NERVOUS SYSTEM (Q00–Q07)

Q00 Anencephaly and similar malformations

Q00.0 Anencephaly
Acephaly
Acrania
Amyelencephaly
Hemianencephaly
Hemicephaly

Q00.1 Craniorachischisis

Q00.2 Iniencephaly

Q01 Encephalocele
Includes: Arnold-Chiari syndrome, type III
encephalocystocele
encephalomyelocele
hydroencephalocele
hydromeningocele, cranial
meningocele, cerebral
meningoencephalocele
Excludes1:   Meckel-Gruber syndrome (Q61.9)

Q01.0 Frontal encephalocele

Q01.1 Nasofrontal encephalocele

Q01.2 Occipital encephalocele

Q01.8 Encephalocele of other sites

Q01.9 Encephalocele, unspecified

Q02 Microcephaly
Includes: hydromicrocephaly
micrencephalon
Excludes1:   Meckel-Gruber syndrome (Q61.9)

Q03 Congenital hydrocephalus
Includes: hydrocephalus in newborn
Excludes1:   Arnold-Chiari syndrome, type II (Q07.0-)
acquired hydrocephalus (G91.-)
hydrocephalus due to congenital toxoplasmosis (P37.1)
hydrocephalus with spina bifida (Q05.0-Q05.4)

Q03.0 Malformations of aqueduct of Sylvius
Anomaly of aqueduct of Sylvius
Obstruction of aqueduct of Sylvius, congenital
Stenosis of aqueduct of Sylvius

Q03.1 Atresia of foramina of Magendie and Luschka
Dandy-Walker syndrome

Q03.8 Other congenital hydrocephalus

Q03.9 Congenital hydrocephalus, unspecified

Q04 Other congenital malformations of brain
Excludes1:   cyclopia (Q87.0)
macrocephaly (Q75.3)

Q04.0 Congenital malformations of corpus callosum
Agenesis of corpus callosum

Q04.1 Arhinencephaly

Q04.2 Holoprosencephaly

Q04.3 Other reduction deformities of brain
Absence of part of brain
Agenesis of part of brain
Agyria
Aplasia of part of brain
Hydranencephaly
Hypoplasia of part of brain
Lissencephaly
Microgyria
Pachygyria
Excludes1:   congenital malformations of corpus callosum (Q04.0)

Q04.4 Septo-optic dysplasia of brain

Q04.5 Megalencephaly

Q04.6 Congenital cerebral cysts
Porencephaly
Schizencephaly
Excludes1:   acquired porencephalic cyst (G93.0)

Q04.8 Other specified congenital malformations of brain
Arnold-Chiari syndrome, type IV
Macrogyria

Q04.9 Congenital malformation of brain, unspecified
Congenital anomaly NOS of brain
Congenital deformity NOS of brain
Congenital disease or lesion NOS of brain
Multiple anomalies NOS of brain, congenital

Q05 Spina bifida
Includes: hydromeningocele (spinal)
meningocele (spinal)
meningomyelocele
myelocele
myelomeningocele
rachischisis
spina bifida (aperta)(cystica)
syringomyelocele
Excludes1:   Arnold-Chiari syndrome, type II (Q07.0-)
spina bifida occulta (Q76.0)

Q05.0 Cervical spina bifida with hydrocephalus

Q05.1 Thoracic spina bifida with hydrocephalus
Dorsal spina bifida with hydrocephalus
Thoracolumbar spina bifida with hydrocephalus

Q05.2 Lumbar spina bifida with hydrocephalus
Lumbosacral spina bifida with hydrocephalus

Q05.3 Sacral spina bifida with hydrocephalus

Q05.4 Unspecified spina bifida with hydrocephalus

Q05.5 Cervical spina bifida without hydrocephalus

Q05.6 Thoracic spina bifida without hydrocephalus
Dorsal spina bifida NOS
Thoracolumbar spina bifida NOS

Q05.7 Lumbar spina bifida without hydrocephalus
Lumbosacral spina bifida NOS

Q05.8 Sacral spina bifida without hydrocephalus

Q05.9 Spina bifida, unspecified

Q06 Other congenital malformations of spinal cord

Q06.0 Amyelia

Q06.1 Hypoplasia and dysplasia of spinal cord
Atelomyelia
Myelatelia
Myelodysplasia of spinal cord

Q06.2 Diastematomyelia

Q06.3 Other congenital cauda equina malformations

Q06.4 Hydromyelia
Hydrorachis

Q06.8 Other specified congenital malformations of spinal cord

Q06.9 Congenital malformation of spinal cord, unspecified
Congenital anomaly NOS of spinal cord
Congenital deformity NOS of spinal cord
Congenital disease or lesion NOS of spinal cord

Q07 Other congenital malformations of nervous system

Excludes1:   familial dysautonomia [Riley-Day] (G90.1)
neurofibromatosis (nonmalignant) (Q85.0)

Q07.0 Arnold-Chiari syndrome
Arnold-Chiari syndrome, type II
Excludes1:   Arnold-Chiari syndrome, type III (Q01.-)
Arnold-Chiari syndrome, type IV (Q04.8)

Q07.00   Arnold-Chiari syndrome without spina bifida or hydrocephalus

Q07.01   Arnold-Chiari syndrome with spina bifida

Q07.02   Arnold-Chiari syndrome with hydrocephalus

Q07.03   Arnold-Chiari syndrome with spina bifida and hydrocephalus

Q07.8 Other specified congenital malformations of nervous system
Agenesis of nerve
Displacement of brachial plexus
Jaw-winking syndrome
Marcus Gunn's syndrome

Q07.9 Congenital malformation of nervous system, unspecified
Congenital anomaly NOS of nervous system
Congenital deformity NOS of nervous system
Congenital disease or lesion NOS of nervous system

CONGENITAL MALFORMATIONS OF EYE, EAR, FACE AND NECK (Q10-Q18)

Excludes2:   cleft lip and cleft palate (Q35-Q37)
congenital malformation of:
cervical spine (Q05.0, Q05.5, Q67.5, Q76.0-Q76.4)
larynx (Q31.-)
lip NEC (Q38.0)
nose (Q30.-)
parathyroid gland (Q89.2)
thyroid gland (Q89.2)

Q10 Congenital malformations of eyelid, lacrimal apparatus and orbit

Excludes1:   cryptophthalmos NOS (Q11.2)
cryptophthalmos syndrome (Q87.0)

Q10.0 Congenital ptosis

Q10.1 Congenital ectropion

Q10.2 Congenital entropion

Q10.3 Other congenital malformations of eyelid
Ablepharon
Blepharophimosis, congenital
Coloboma of eyelid
Congenital absence or agenesis of cilia
Congenital absence or agenesis of eyelid
Congenital accessory eyelid
Congenital accessory eye muscle
Congenital malformation of eyelid NOS

Q10.4 Absence and agenesis of lacrimal apparatus
Congenital absence of punctum lacrimale

Q10.5 Congenital stenosis and stricture of lacrimal duct

Q10.6 Other congenital malformations of lacrimal apparatus
Congenital malformation of lacrimal apparatus NOS

Q10.7 Congenital malformation of orbit

Q11 Anophthalmos, microphthalmos and macrophthalmos

Q11.0 Cystic eyeball

Q11.1 Other anophthalmos
Anophthalmos NOS
Agenesis of eye
Aplasia of eye

Q11.2 Microphthalmos
Cryptophthalmos NOS
Dysplasia of eye
Hypoplasia of eye
Rudimentary eye
Excludes1:   cryptophthalmos syndrome (Q87.0)

Q11.3 Macrophthalmos
Excludes1:   macrophthalmos in congenital glaucoma (Q15.0)

Q12 Congenital lens malformations

Q12.0 Congenital cataract

Q12.1 Congenital displaced lens

Q12.2 Coloboma of lens

Q12.3 Congenital aphakia

Q12.4 Spherophakia

Q12.8 Other congenital lens malformations
Microphakia

Q12.9 Congenital lens malformation, unspecified

Q13 Congenital malformations of anterior segment of eye

Q13.0 Coloboma of iris
Coloboma NOS

Q13.1 Absence of iris
Aniridia
Use additional code for associated glaucoma (H42)

Q13.2 Other congenital malformations of iris
Anisocoria, congenital
Atresia of pupil
Congenital malformation of iris NOS
Corectopia

Q13.3 Congenital corneal opacity

Q13.4 Other congenital corneal malformations
Congenital malformation of cornea NOS
Microcornea
Peter's anomaly

Q13.5 Blue sclera

Q13.8 Other congenital malformations of anterior segment of eye

Q13.81   Rieger's anomaly
Use additional code for associated glaucoma (H42)

Q13.89   Other congenital malformations of anterior segment of eye

Q13.9 Congenital malformation of anterior segment of eye, unspecified

Q14 Congenital malformations of posterior segment of eye

Q14.0 Congenital malformation of vitreous humor
Congenital vitreous opacity

Q14.1 Congenital malformation of retina
Congenital retinal aneurysm

Q14.2 Congenital malformation of optic disc
Coloboma of optic disc

Q14.3 Congenital malformation of choroids

Q14.8 Other congenital malformations of posterior segment of eye
Coloboma of the fundus

Q14.9 Congenital malformation of posterior segment of eye, unspecified

Q15 Other congenital malformations of eye

Excludes1:   congenital nystagmus (H55.01)
ocular albinism (E70.31-)
retinitis pigmentosa (H35.52)

Q15.0 Congenital glaucoma
Axenfeld's anomaly
Buphthalmos
Glaucoma of childhood
Glaucoma of newborn
Hydrophthalmos
Keratoglobus, congenital
Macrophthalmos in congenital glaucoma
Megalocornea

Q15.8 Other specified congenital malformations of eye

Q15.9 Congenital malformation of eye, unspecified
Congenital anomaly of eye
Congenital deformity of eye

Q16 Congenital malformations of ear causing impairment of hearing

Excludes1:   congenital deafness (H90.-)

Q16.0 Congenital absence of (ear) auricle

Q16.1 Congenital absence, atresia and stricture of auditory canal (external)
Congenital atresia or stricture of osseous meatus

Q16.2 Absence of eustachian tube

Q16.3 Congenital malformation of ear ossicles
Congenital fusion of ear ossicles

Q16.4 Other congenital malformations of middle ear
Congenital malformation of middle ear NOS

Q16.5 **Congenital malformation of inner ear**
       Congenital anomaly of membranous labyrinth
       Congenital anomaly of organ of Corti
Q16.9 **Congenital malformation of ear causing impairment of hearing, unspecified**
       Congenital absence of ear NOS

Q17 **Other congenital malformations of ear**
     Excludes1: congenital malformations of ear with impairment of
                 hearing (Q16.0- Q16.9)
                 preauricular sinus (Q18.1)
Q17.0 **Accessory auricle**
       Accessory tragus
       Polyotia
       Preauricular appendage or tag
       Supernumerary ear
       Supernumerary lobule
Q17.1 **Macrotia**
Q17.2 **Microtia**
Q17.3 **Other misshapen ear**
       Pointed ear
Q17.4 **Misplaced ear**
       Low-set ears
       Excludes1: cervical auricle (Q18.2)
Q17.5 **Prominent ear**
       Bat ear
Q17.8 **Other specified congenital malformations of ear**
       Congenital absence of lobe of ear
Q17.9 **Congenital malformation of ear, unspecified**
       Congenital anomaly of ear NOS

Q18 **Other congenital malformations of face and neck**
     Excludes1: cleft lip and cleft palate (Q35-Q37)
                 conditions classified to Q67.0-Q67.4
                 congenital malformations of skull and face bones
                 (Q75.-)
                 cyclopia (Q87.0)
                 dentofacial anomalies [including malocclusion] (M26.-)
                 malformation syndromes affecting facial appearance
                 (Q87.0)
                 persistent thyroglossal duct (Q89.2)
Q18.0 **Sinus, fistula and cyst of branchial cleft**
       Branchial vestige
Q18.1 **Preauricular sinus and cyst**
       Fistula of auricle, congenital
       Cervicoaural fistula
Q18.2 **Other branchial cleft malformations**
       Branchial cleft malformation NOS
       Cervical auricle
       Otocephaly
Q18.3 **Webbing of neck**
       Pterygium colli
Q18.4 **Macrostomia**
Q18.5 **Microstomia**
Q18.6 **Macrocheilia**
       Hypertrophy of lip, congenital
Q18.7 **Microcheilia**
Q18.8 **Other specified congenital malformations of face and neck**
       Medial cyst of face and neck
       Medial fistula of face and neck
       Medial sinus of face and neck
Q18.9 **Congenital malformation of face and neck, unspecified**
       Congenital anomaly NOS of face and neck

CONGENITAL MALFORMATIONS OF THE CIRCULATORY SYSTEM (Q20-Q28)

Q20 **Congenital malformations of cardiac chambers and connections**
     Excludes1: dextrocardia with situs inversus (Q89.3)
                 mirror-image atrial arrangement with situs inversus
                 (Q89.3)
Q20.0 **Common arterial trunk**
       Persistent truncus arteriosus
       Excludes1: aortic septal defect (Q21.4)

Q20.1 **Double outlet right ventricle**
       Taussig-Bing syndrome
Q20.2 **Double outlet left ventricle**
Q20.3 **Discordant ventriculoarterial connection**
       Dextrotransposition of aorta
       Transposition of great vessels (complete)
Q20.4 **Double inlet ventricle**
       Common ventricle
       Cor triloculare biatriatum
       Single ventricle
Q20.5 **Discordant atrioventricular connection**
       Corrected transposition
       Levotransposition
       Ventricular inversion
Q20.6 **Isomerism of atrial appendages**
       Isomerism of atrial appendages with asplenia or polysplenia
Q20.8 **Other congenital malformations of cardiac chambers and connections**
       Cor binoculare
Q20.9 **Congenital malformation of cardiac chambers and connections, unspecified**

Q21 **Congenital malformations of cardiac septa**
     Excludes1: aquired cardiac septal defect (I51.0)
Q21.0 **Ventricular septal defect**
       Roger's disease
Q21.1 **Atrial septal defect**
       Coronary sinus defect
       Patent or persistent foramen ovale
       Patent or persistent ostium secundum defect (type II)
       Patent or persistent sinus venosus defect
Q21.2 **Atrioventricular septal defect**
       Common atrioventricular canal
       Endocardial cushion defect
       Ostium primum atrial septal defect (type I)
Q21.3 **Tetralogy of Fallot**
       Ventricular septal defect with pulmonary stenosis or atresia,
       dextroposition of aorta and hypertrophy of right ventricle.
Q21.4 **Aortopulmonary septal defect**
       Aortic septal defect
       Aortopulmonary window
Q21.8 **Other congenital malformations of cardiac septa**
       Eisenmenger's syndrome
       Pentalogy of Fallot
Q21.9 **Congenital malformation of cardiac septum, unspecified**
       Septal (heart) defect NOS

Q22 **Congenital malformations of pulmonary and tricuspid valves**
Q22.0 **Pulmonary valve atresia**
Q22.1 **Congenital pulmonary valve stenosis**
Q22.2 **Congenital pulmonary valve insufficiency**
       Congenital pulmonary valve regurgitation
Q22.3 **Other congenital malformations of pulmonary valve**
       Congenital malformation of pulmonary valve NOS
       Supernumerary cusps of pulmonary valve
Q22.4 **Congenital tricuspid stenosis**
       Congenital tricuspid atresia
Q22.5 **Ebstein's anomaly**
Q22.6 **Hypoplastic right heart syndrome**
Q22.8 **Other congenital malformations of tricuspid valve**
Q22.9 **Congenital malformation of tricuspid valve, unspecified**

Q23 **Congenital malformations of aortic and mitral valves**
Q23.0 **Congenital stenosis of aortic valve**
       Congenital aortic atresia
       Congenital aortic stenosis NOS
       Excludes1: congenital stenosis of aortic valve in hypoplastic
                   left heart syndrome (Q23.4)
                   congenital subaortic stenosis (Q24.4)
                   supravalvular aortic stenosis (congenital) (Q25.3)
Q23.1 **Congenital insufficiency of aortic valve**
       Bicuspid aortic valve
       Congenital aortic insufficiency

Q23.2　Congenital mitral stenosis
　　Congenital mitral atresia

Q23.3　Congenital mitral insufficiency

Q23.4　Hypoplastic left heart syndrome

Q23.8　Other congenital malformations of aortic and mitral valves

Q23.9　Congenital malformation of aortic and mitral valves, unspecified

Q24　Other congenital malformations of heart
　　Excludes1:　endocardial fibroelastosis (I42.4)

Q24.0　Dextrocardia
　　Excludes1:　dextrocardia with situs inversus (Q89.3)
　　　　　　isomerism of atrial appendages (with asplenia or polysplenia) (Q20.6)
　　　　　　mirror-image atrial arrangement with situs inversus (Q89.3)

Q24.1　Levocardia

Q24.2　Cor triatriatum

Q24.3　Pulmonary infundibular stenosis
　　Subvalvular pulmonic stenosis

Q24.4　Congenital subaortic stenosis

Q24.5　Malformation of coronary vessels
　　Congenital coronary (artery) aneurysm

Q24.6　Congenital heart block

Q24.8　Other specified congenital malformations of heart
　　Congenital diverticulum of left ventricle
　　Congenital malformation of myocardium
　　Congenital malformation of pericardium
　　Malposition of heart
　　Uhl's disease

Q24.9　Congenital malformation of heart, unspecified
　　Congenital anomaly of heart
　　Congenital disease of heart

Q25　Congenital malformations of great arteries

Q25.0　Patent ductus arteriosus
　　Patent ductus Botallo
　　Persistent ductus arteriosus

Q25.1　Coarctation of aorta
　　Coarctation of aorta (preductal) (postductal)

Q25.2　Atresia of aorta

Q25.3　Supravalvular aortic stenosis
　　Excludes1:　congenital aortic stenosis NOS (Q23.0)
　　　　　　congenital aortic valve stenosis (Q23.0)

Q25.4　Other congenital malformations of aorta
　　Absence of aorta
　　Aneurysm of sinus of Valsalva (ruptured)
　　Aplasia of aorta
　　Congenital aneurysm of aorta
　　Congenital dilatation of aorta
　　Congenital malformations of aorta
　　Double aortic arch [vascular ring of aorta]
　　Hypoplasia of aorta
　　Persistent convolutions of aortic arch
　　Persistent right aortic arch
　　Excludes1:　hypoplasia of aorta in hypoplastic left heart syndrome (Q23.4)

Q25.5　Atresia of pulmonary artery

Q25.6　Stenosis of pulmonary artery

Q25.7　Other congenital malformations of pulmonary artery
　　Aberrant pulmonary artery
　　Agenesis of pulmonary artery
　　Congenital aneurysm of pulmonary artery
　　Congenital anomaly of pulmonary artery
　　Congenital pulmonary arteriovenous aneurysm
　　Hypoplasia of pulmonary artery

Q25.8　Other congenital malformations of other great arteries

Q25.9　Congenital malformation of great arteries, unspecified

Q26　Congenital malformations of great veins

Q26.0　Congenital stenosis of vena cava
　　Congenital stenosis of vena cava (inferior)(superior)

Q26.1　Persistent left superior vena cava

Q26.2　Total anomalous pulmonary venous connection
　　Total anomalous pulmonary venous return [TAPVR], subdiaphragmatic
　　Total anomalous pulmonary venous return [TAPVR], supradiaphragmatic

Q26.3　Partial anomalous pulmonary venous connection
　　Partial anomalous pulmonary venous return

Q26.4　Anomalous pulmonary venous connection, unspecified

Q26.5　Anomalous portal venous connection

Q26.6　Portal vein-hepatic artery fistula

Q26.8　Other congenital malformations of great veins
　　Absence of vena cava (inferior) (superior)
　　Azygos continuation of inferior vena cava
　　Persistent left posterior cardinal vein
　　Scimitar syndrome

Q26.9　Congenital malformation of great vein, unspecified
　　Congenital anomaly of vena cava (inferior) (superior) NOS

Q27　Other congenital malformations of peripheral vascular system
　　Excludes2:　anomalies of cerebral and precerebral vessels (Q28.0-Q28.3)
　　　　　　anomalies of coronary vessels (Q24.5)
　　　　　　anomalies of pulmonary artery (Q25.5-Q25.7)
　　　　　　congenital retinal aneurysm (Q14.1)
　　　　　　hemangioma and lymphangioma (D18.-)

Q27.0　Congenital absence and hypoplasia of umbilical artery
　　Single umbilical artery

Q27.1　Congenital renal artery stenosis

Q27.2　Other congenital malformations of renal artery
　　Congenital malformation of renal artery NOS
　　Multiple renal arteries

Q27.3　Arteriovenous malformation (peripheral)
　　Arteriovenous aneurysm
　　Excludes1:　acquired arteriovenous aneurysm (I77.0)
　　Excludes2:　arteriovenous malformation of cerebral vessels (Q28.2)
　　　　　　arteriovenous malformation of precerebral vessels (Q28.0)

　　Q27.30　Arteriovenous malformation, site unspecified

　　Q27.31　Arteriovenous malformation of vessel of upper limb

　　Q27.32　Arteriovenous malformation of vessel of lower limb

　　Q27.33　Arteriovenous malformation of digestive system vessel

　　Q27.34　Arteriovenous malformation of renal vessel

　　Q27.39　Arteriovenous malformation, other site

Q27.4　Congenital phlebectasia

Q27.8　Other specified congenital malformations of peripheral vascular system
　　Absence of peripheral vascular system
　　Atresia of peripheral vascular system
　　Congenital aneurysm (peripheral)
　　Congenital stricture, artery
　　Congenital varix
　　Excludes1:　arteriovenous malformation (Q27.3-)

Q27.9　Congenital malformation of peripheral vascular system, unspecified
　　Anomaly of artery or vein NOS

Q28　Other congenital malformations of circulatory system
　　Excludes1:　congenital aneurysm NOS (Q27.8)
　　　　　　congenital coronary aneurysm (Q24.5)
　　　　　　ruptured cerebral arteriovenous malformation (I60.8)
　　　　　　ruptured malformation of precerebral vessels (I72.0)
　　Excludes2:　congenital peripheral aneurysm (Q27.8)
　　　　　　congenital pulmonary aneurysm (Q25.7)
　　　　　　congenital retinal aneurysm (Q14.1)

Q28.0　Arteriovenous malformation of precerebral vessels
　　Congenital arteriovenous precerebral aneurysm (nonruptured)

Q28.1　Other malformations of precerebral vessels
　　Congenital malformation of precerebral vessels NOS
　　Congenital precerebral aneurysm (nonruptured)

Q28.2　Arteriovenous malformation of cerebral vessels
　　Arteriovenous malformation of brain NOS
　　Congenital arteriovenous cerebral aneurysm (nonruptured)

Q28.3 Other malformations of cerebral vessels
> Congenital cerebral aneurysm (nonruptured)
> Congenital malformation of cerebral vessels NOS

Q28.8 Other specified congenital malformations of circulatory system
> Congenital aneurysm, specified site NEC
> Spinal vessel anomaly

Q28.9 Congenital malformation of circulatory system, unspecified

CONGENITAL MALFORMATIONS OF THE RESPIRATORY SYSTEM (Q30–Q34)

Q30 Congenital malformations of nose
> Excludes1:   congenital deviation of nasal septum (Q67.4)

Q30.0 Choanal atresia
> Atresia of nares (anterior) (posterior)
> Congenital stenosis of nares (anterior) (posterior)

Q30.1 Agenesis and underdevelopment of nose
> Congenital absent of nose

Q30.2 Fissured, notched and cleft nose

Q30.3 Congenital perforated nasal septum

Q30.8 Other congenital malformations of nose
> Accessory nose
> Congenital anomaly of nasal sinus wall

Q30.9 Congenital malformation of nose, unspecified

Q31 Congenital malformations of larynx

Q31.0 Web of larynx
> Glottic web of larynx
> Subglottic web of larynx
> Web of larynx NOS

Q31.1 Congenital subglottic stenosis

Q31.2 Laryngeal hypoplasia

Q31.3 Laryngocele

Q31.4 Congenital laryngeal stridor
> Congenital stridor (larynx) NOS

Q31.8 Other congenital malformations of larynx
> Absence of larynx
> Agenesis of larynx
> Atresia of larynx
> Congenital cleft thyroid cartilage
> Congenital fissure of epiglottis
> Congenital stenosis of larynx NEC
> Posterior cleft of cricoid cartilage

Q31.9 Congenital malformation of larynx, unspecified

Q32 Congenital malformations of trachea and bronchus
> Excludes1: congenital bronchiectasis (Q33.4)

Q32.0 Congenital tracheomalacia

Q32.1 Other congenital malformations of trachea
> Atresia of trachea
> Congenital anomaly of tracheal cartilage
> Congenital dilatation of trachea
> Congenital malformation of trachea
> Congenital stenosis of trachea
> Congenital tracheocele

Q32.2 Congenital bronchomalacia

Q32.3 Congenital stenosis of bronchus

Q32.8 Other congenital malformations of bronchus
> Absence of bronchus
> Agenesis of bronchus
> Atresia of bronchus
> Congenital diverticulum of bronchus
> Congenital malformation of bronchus NOS

Q33 Congenital malformations of lung

Q33.0 Congenital cystic lung
> Congenital cystic lung disease
> Congenital honeycomb lung
> Congenital polycystic lung disease
> Excludes1:   cystic fibrosis (E84.0)
> cystic lung disease, acquired or unspecified (J98.4)

Q33.1 Accessory lobe of lung
> Azygos lobe (fissured), lung

Q33.2 Sequestration of lung

Q33.3 Congenital agenesis of lung
> Congenital absence of lung (lobe)

Q33.4 Congenital bronchiectasis

Q33.5 Ectopic tissue in lung

Q33.6 Congenital hypoplasia and dysplasia of lung
> Excludes1:   pulmonary hypoplasia associated with short gestation (P28.0)

Q33.8 Other congenital malformations of lung

Q33.9 Congenital malformation of lung, unspecified

Q34 Other congenital malformations of respiratory system

Q34.0 Anomaly of pleura

Q34.1 Congenital cyst of mediastinum

Q34.8 Other specified congenital malformations of respiratory system
> Atresia of nasopharynx

Q34.9 Congenital malformation of respiratory system, unspecified
> Congenital absence of respiratory system
> Congenital anomaly of respiratory system NOS

CLEFT LIP AND CLEFT PALATE (Q35–Q37)

> Excludes1: Robin's syndrome (Q87.0)

Q35 Cleft palate
> Includes: fissure of palate
> palatoschisis
> Excludes1:   cleft palate with cleft lip (Q37.-)

Q35.1 Cleft hard palate

Q35.3 Cleft soft palate

Q35.5 Cleft hard palate with cleft soft palate

Q35.6 Cleft palate, medial

Q35.7 Cleft uvula

Q35.9 Cleft palate, unspecified
> Cleft palate NOS

Q36 Cleft lip
> Includes: cheiloschisis
> congenital fissure of lip
> harelip
> labium leporinum
> Excludes1:   cleft lip with cleft palate (Q37.-)

Q36.0 Cleft lip, bilateral

Q36.1 Cleft lip, medial

Q36.9 Cleft lip, unilateral
> Cleft lip NOS

Q37 Cleft palate with cleft lip
> Includes: cheilopalatoschisis

Q37.0 Cleft hard palate with bilateral cleft lip

Q37.1 Cleft hard palate with unilateral cleft lip
> Cleft hard palate with cleft lip NOS

Q37.2 Cleft soft palate with bilateral cleft lip

Q37.3 Cleft soft palate with unilateral cleft lip
> Cleft soft palate with cleft lip NOS

Q37.4 Cleft hard and soft palate with bilateral cleft lip

Q37.5 Cleft hard and soft palate with unilateral cleft lip
> Cleft hard and soft palate with cleft lip NOS

Q37.8 Unspecified cleft palate with bilateral cleft lip

Q37.9 Unspecified cleft palate with unilateral cleft lip
> Cleft palate with cleft lip NOS

OTHER CONGENITAL MALFORMATIONS OF THE DIGESTIVE SYSTEM (Q38–Q45)

Q38 Other congenital malformations of tongue, mouth and pharynx
> Excludes1:   dentofacial anomalies (M26.-)
> macrostomia (Q18.4)
> microstomia (Q18.5)

Q38.0   Congenital malformations of lips, not elsewhere classified
     Congenital fistula of lip
     Congenital malformation of lip NOS
     Van der Woude's syndrome
     Excludes1:   cleft lip (Q36.-)
                 cleft lip with cleft palate (Q37.-)
                 macrocheilia (Q18.6)
                 microcheilia (Q18.7)

Q38.1   Ankyloglossia
     Tongue tie

Q38.2   Macroglossia
     Congenital hypertrophy of tongue

Q38.3   Other congenital malformations of tongue
     Aglossia
     Bifid tongue
     Congenital adhesion of tongue
     Congenital fissure of tongue
     Congenital malformation of tongue NOS
     Double tongue
     Hypoglossia
     Hypoplasia of tongue
     Microglossia

Q38.4   Congenital malformations of salivary glands and ducts
     Atresia of salivary glands and ducts
     Congenital absence of salivary glands and ducts
     Congenital accessory salivary glands and ducts
     Congenital fistula of salivary gland

Q38.5   Congenital malformations of palate, not elsewhere classified
     Congenital absence of uvula
     Congenital malformation of palate NOS
     Congenital high arched palate
     Excludes1:   cleft palate (Q35.-)
                 cleft palate with cleft lip (Q37.-)

Q38.6   Other congenital malformations of mouth
     Congenital malformation of mouth NOS

Q38.7   Congenital pharyngeal pouch
     Congenital diverticulum of pharynx
     Excludes1:   pharyngeal pouch syndrome (D82.1)

Q38.8   Other congenital malformations of pharynx
     Congenital malformation of pharynx NOS
     Imperforate pharynx

Q39   Congenital malformations of esophagus

Q39.0   Atresia of esophagus without fistula
     Atresia of esophagus NOS

Q39.1   Atresia of esophagus with tracheo-esophageal fistula
     Atresia of esophagus with broncho-esophageal fistula

Q39.2   Congenital tracheo-esophageal fistula without atresia
     Congenital tracheo-esophageal fistula NOS

Q39.3   Congenital stenosis and stricture of esophagus

Q39.4   Esophageal web

Q39.5   Congenital dilatation of esophagus

Q39.6   Congenital diverticulum of esophagus
     Congenital esophageal pouch

Q39.8   Other congenital malformations of esophagus
     Congenital absence of esophagus
     Congenital displacement of esophagus
     Congenital duplication of esophagus

Q39.9   Congenital malformation of esophagus, unspecified

Q40   Other congenital malformations of upper alimentary tract

Q40.0   Congenital hypertrophic pyloric stenosis
     Congenital or infantile constriction
     Congenital or infantile hypertrophy
     Congenital or infantile spasm
     Congenital or infantile stenosis
     Congenital or infantile stricture

Q40.1   Congenital hiatus hernia
     Congenital displacement of cardia through esophageal hiatus
     Excludes1:   congenital diaphragmatic hernia (Q79.0)

Q40.2   Other specified congenital malformations of stomach
     Congenital cardiospasm
     Congenital displacement of stomach
     Congenital diverticulum of stomach
     Congenital hourglass stomach
     Congenital duplication of stomach
     Megalogastria
     Microgastria

Q40.3   Congenital malformation of stomach, unspecified

Q40.8   Other specified congenital malformations of upper alimentary tract

Q40.9   Congenital malformation of upper alimentary tract, unspecified
     Congenital anomaly of upper alimentary tract
     Congenital deformity of upper alimentary tract

Q41   Congenital absence, atresia and stenosis of small intestine
     Includes: congenital obstruction, occlusion or stricture of small intestine or intestine NOS
     Excludes1:   cystic fibrosis with intestinal manifestation (E84.1)
                 meconium ileus (P75)

Q41.0   Congenital absence, atresia and stenosis of duodenum

Q41.1   Congenital absence, atresia and stenosis of jejunum
     Apple peel syndrome
     Imperforate jejunum

Q41.2   Congenital absence, atresia and stenosis of ileum

Q41.8   Congenital absence, atresia and stenosis of other specified parts of small intestine

Q41.9   Congenital absence, atresia and stenosis of small intestine, part unspecified
     Congenital absence, atresia and stenosis of intestine NOS

Q42   Congenital absence, atresia and stenosis of large intestine
     Includes: congenital obstruction, occlusion and stricture of large intestine

Q42.0   Congenital absence, atresia and stenosis of rectum with fistula

Q42.1   Congenital absence, atresia and stenosis of rectum without fistula
     Imperforate rectum

Q42.2   Congenital absence, atresia and stenosis of anus with fistula

Q42.3   Congenital absence, atresia and stenosis of anus without fistula
     Imperforate anus

Q42.8   Congenital absence, atresia and stenosis of other parts of large intestine

Q42.9   Congenital absence, atresia and stenosis of large intestine, part unspecified

Q43   Other congenital malformations of intestine

Q43.0   Meckel's diverticulum (displaced) (hypertrophic)
     Persistent omphalomesenteric duct
     Persistent vitelline duct

Q43.1   Hirschsprung's disease
     Aganglionosis
     Congenital (aganglionic) megacolon

Q43.2   Other congenital functional disorders of colon
     Congenital dilatation of colon

Q43.3   Congenital malformations of intestinal fixation
     Congenital omental, anomalous adhesions [bands]
     Congenital peritoneal adhesions [bands]
     Incomplete rotation of cecum and colon
     Insufficient rotation of cecum and colon
     Jackson's membrane
     Malrotation of colon
     Rotation failure of cecum and colon
     Universal mesentery

Q43.4   Duplication of intestine

Q43.5   Ectopic anus

Q43.6   Congenital fistula of rectum and anus

Excludes1:   congenital fistula of anus with absence, atresia and stenosis (Q42.2)
congenital fistula of rectum with absence, atresia and stenosis (Q42.0)
congenital rectovaginal fistula (Q52.2)
congenital urethrorectal fistula (Q64.7)
pilonidal fistula or sinus (L05.-)

Q43.7   Persistent cloaca

Cloaca NOS

Q43.8   Other specified congenital malformations of intestine

Congenital blind loop syndrome
Congenital diverticulitis, colon
Congenital diverticulum, intestine
Dolichocolon
Megaloappendix
Megaloduodenum
Microcolon
Transposition of appendix
Transposition of colon
Transposition of intestine

Q43.9   Congenital malformation of intestine, unspecified

Q44   Congenital malformations of gallbladder, bile ducts and liver

Q44.0   Agenesis, aplasia and hypoplasia of gallbladder

Congenital absence of gallbladder

Q44.1   Other congenital malformations of gallbladder

Congenital malformation of gallbladder NOS
Intrahepatic gallbladder

Q44.2   Atresia of bile ducts

Q44.3   Congenital stenosis and stricture of bile ducts

Q44.4   Choledochal cyst

Q44.5   Other congenital malformations of bile ducts

Accessory hepatic duct
Biliary duct duplication
Congenital malformation of bile duct NOS
Cystic duct duplication

Q44.6   Cystic disease of liver

Fibrocystic disease of liver

Q44.7   Other congenital malformations of liver

Accessory liver
Alagille's syndrome
Congenital absence of liver
Congenital hepatomegaly
Congenital malformation of liver NOS

Q45   Other congenital malformations of digestive system

Excludes2:   congenital diaphragmatic hernia (Q79.0)
congenital hiatus hernia (Q40.1)

Q45.0   Agenesis, aplasia and hypoplasia of pancreas

Congenital absence of pancreas

Q45.1   Annular pancreas

Q45.2   Congenital pancreatic cyst

Q45.3   Other congenital malformations of pancreas and pancreatic duct

Accessory pancreas
Congenital malformation of pancreas or pancreatic duct NOS

Excludes1:   congenital diabetes mellitus (E10.-)
cystic fibrosis (E84.0-E84.9)
fibrocystic disease of pancreas (E84.-)
neonatal diabetes mellitus (P70.2)

Q45.8   Other specified congenital malformations of digestive system

Absence (complete) (partial) of alimentary tract NOS
Duplication of digestive system
Malposition, congenital of digestive system

Q45.9   Congenital malformation of digestive system, unspecified

Congenital anomaly of digestive system
Congenital deformity of digestive system

CONGENITAL MALFORMATIONS OF GENITAL ORGANS (Q50–Q56)

Excludes1:   androgen resistance syndrome (E34.5)
syndromes associated with anomalies in the number and form of chromosomes (Q90-Q99)
testicular feminization syndrome (E34.5)

Q50   Congenital malformations of ovaries, fallopian tubes and broad ligaments

Q50.0   Congenital absence of ovary

Excludes1:   Turner's syndrome (Q96.-)

Q50.1   Developmental ovarian cyst

Q50.2   Congenital torsion of ovary

Q50.3   Other congenital malformations of ovary

Q50.31   Accessory ovary

Q50.32   Ovarian streak

46, XX with streak gonads

Q50.39   Other congenital malformation of ovary

Congenital malformation of ovary NOS

Q50.4   Embryonic cyst of fallopian tube

Fimbrial cyst

Q50.5   Embryonic cyst of broad ligament

Epoophoron cyst
Gartner's duct cyst
Parovarian cyst

Q50.6   Other congenital malformations of fallopian tube and broad ligament

Absence of fallopian tube and broad ligament
Accessory fallopian tube and broad ligament
Atresia of fallopian tube and broad ligament
Congenital malformation of fallopian tube or broad ligament NOS

Q51   Congenital malformations of uterus and cervix

Q51.0   Agenesis and aplasia of uterus

Congenital absence of uterus

Q51.1   Doubling of uterus with doubling of cervix and vagina

Q51.10   Doubling of uterus with doubling of cervix and vagina without obstruction

Doubling of uterus with doubling of cervix and vagina NOS

Q51.11   Doubling of uterus with doubling of cervix and vagina with obstruction

Q51.2   Other doubling of uterus

Doubling of uterus NOS

Q51.3   Bicornate uterus

Q51.4   Unicornate uterus

Q51.5   Agenesis and aplasia of cervix

Congenital absence of cervix

Q51.6   Embryonic cyst of cervix

Q51.7   Congenital fistulae between uterus and digestive and urinary tracts

Q51.8   Other congenital malformations of uterus and cervix

Hypoplasia of uterus and cervix

Q51.9   Congenital malformation of uterus and cervix, unspecified

Q52   Other congenital malformations of female genitalia

Q52.0   Congenital absence of vagina

Q52.1   Doubling of vagina

Septate vagina

Excludes1:   doubling of vagina with doubling of uterus and cervix (Q51.1-)

Q52.2   Congenital rectovaginal fistula

Excludes1:   cloaca (Q43.7)

Q52.3   Imperforate hymen

Q52.4   Other congenital malformations of vagina

Canal of Nuck cyst, congenital
Congenital malformation of vagina NOS
Embryonic vaginal cyst

Q52.5   Fusion of labia

Q52.6   Congenital malformation of clitoris

Q52.7   **Other and unspecified congenital malformations of vulva**

    Q52.70   **Unspecified congenital malformations of vulva**
       Congenital malformation of vulva NOS

    Q52.71   **Congenital absence of vulva**

    Q52.79   **Other congenital malformations of vulva**
       Congenital cyst of vulva

Q52.8   **Other specified congenital malformations of female genitalia**

Q52.9   **Congenital malformation of female genitalia, unspecified**

Q53   Undescended and ectopic testicle

Q53.0   **Ectopic testis**

    Q53.00   **Ectopic testis, unspecified**

    Q53.01   **Ectopic testis, unilateral**

    Q53.02   **Ectopic testes, bilateral**

Q53.1   **Undescended testicle, unilateral**

    Q53.10   **Unspecified undescended testicle, unilateral**

    Q53.11   **Abdominal testis, unilateral**

    Q53.12   **Ectopic perineal testis, unilateral**

Q53.2   **Undescended testicle, bilateral**

    Q53.20   **Undescended testicle, unspecified, bilateral**

    Q53.21   **Abdominal testis, bilateral**

    Q53.22   **Ectopic perineal testis, bilateral**

Q53.9   **Undescended testicle, unspecified**
     Cryptorchism NOS

Q54   Hypospadias
     Excludes1:   epispadias (Q64.0)

Q54.0   **Hypospadias, balanic**
     Hypospadias, coronal
     Hypospadias, glandular

Q54.1   **Hypospadias, penile**

Q54.2   **Hypospadias, penoscrotal**

Q54.3   **Hypospadias, perineal**

Q54.4   **Congenital chordee**
     Chordee without hypospadias

Q54.8   **Other hypospadias**
     Hypospadias with intersex state

Q54.9   **Hypospadias, unspecified**

Q55   Other congenital malformations of male genital organs
     Excludes1:   congenital hydrocele (P83.5)
            hypospadias (Q54.-)

Q55.0   **Absence and aplasia of testis**
     Monorchism

Q55.1   **Hypoplasia of testis and scrotum**
     Fusion of testes

Q55.2   **Other and unspecified congenital malformations of testis and scrotum**

    Q55.20   **Unspecified congenital malformations of testis and scrotum**
         Congenital malformation of testis or scrotum NOS

    Q55.21   **Polyorchism**

    Q55.22   **Retractile testis**

    Q55.29   **Other congenital malformations of testis and scrotum**

Q55.3   **Atresia of vas deferens**
     Code first any associated cystic fibrosis (E84.-)

Q55.4   **Other congenital malformations of vas deferens, epididymis, seminal vesicles and prostate**
     Absence or aplasia of prostate
     Absence or aplasia of spermatic cord
     Congenital malformation of vas deferens, epididymis, seminal vesicles or prostate NOS

Q55.5   **Congenital absence and aplasia of penis**

Q55.6   **Other congenital malformations of penis**

    Q55.61   **Curvature of penis (lateral)**

    Q55.62   **Hypoplasia of penis**
       Micropenis

    Q55.69   **Other congenital malformation of penis NOS**
       Congenital malformation of penis NOS

Q55.7   **Congenital vasocutaneous fistula**

Q55.8   **Other specified congenital malformations of male genital organs**

Q55.9   **Congenital malformation of male genital organ, unspecified**
     Congenital anomaly of male genital organ
     Congenital deformity of male genital organ

Q56   Indeterminate sex and pseudohermaphroditism
     Excludes1:   46, XX true hermaphrodite (Q99.1)
               chimera 46, XX/46, XY true hermaphrodite (Q99.0)
               female pseudohermaphroditism with adrenocortical disorder (E25.-)
               male pseudohermaphroditism with androgen resistance (E34.5)
               pseudohermaphroditism with specified chromosomal anomaly (Q96-Q99)
               pure gonadal dysgenesis (Q99.1)

Q56.0   **Hermaphroditism, not elsewhere classified**
     Ovotestis

Q56.1   **Male pseudohermaphroditism, not elsewhere classified**
     46, XY with streak gonads
     Male pseudohermaphroditism NOS

Q56.2   **Female pseudohermaphroditism, not elsewhere classified**
     Female pseudohermaphroditism NOS

Q56.3   **Pseudohermaphroditism, unspecified**

Q56.4   **Indeterminate sex, unspecified**
     Ambiguous genitalia

CONGENITAL MALFORMATIONS OF THE URINARY SYSTEM (Q60–Q64)

Q60   Renal agenesis and other reduction defects of kidney
     Includes: congenital absence of kidney
               congenital atrophy of kidney
               infantile atrophy of kidney

Q60.0   **Renal agenesis, unilateral**

Q60.1   **Renal agenesis, bilateral**

Q60.2   **Renal agenesis, unspecified**

Q60.3   **Renal hypoplasia, unilateral**

Q60.4   **Renal hypoplasia, bilateral**

Q60.5   **Renal hypoplasia, unspecified**

Q60.6   **Potter's syndrome**

Q61   Cystic kidney disease
     Excludes1:   acquired cyst of kidney (N28.1)
            Potter's syndrome (Q60.6)

Q61.0   **Congenital renal cyst**

    Q61.00   **Congenital renal cyst, unspecified**
       Cyst of kidney NOS (congenital)

    Q61.01   **Congenital single renal cyst**

    Q61.02   **Congenital multiple renal cysts**

Q61.1   **Polycystic kidney, infantile type**
     Polycystic kidney, autosomal recessive

    Q61.11   **Cystic dilatation of collecting ducts**

    Q61.19   **Other polycystic kidney, infantile type**

Q61.2   **Polycystic kidney, adult type**
     Polycystic kidney, autosomal dominant

Q61.3   **Polycystic kidney, unspecified**

Q61.4   **Renal dysplasia**

Q61.5   **Medullary cystic kidney**
     Nephronopthisis
     Sponge kidney NOS

Q61.8   **Other cystic kidney diseases**
     Fibrocystic kidney
     Fibrocystic renal degeneration or disease

Q61.9   **Cystic kidney disease, unspecified**
     Meckel-Gruber syndrome

Q62   Congenital obstructive defects of renal pelvis and congenital malformations of ureter

Q62.0   **Congenital hydronephrosis**

Q62.1   **Congenital occulsion of ureter**
     Atresia and stenosis of ureter

    Q62.10   **Congenital occulsion of ureter, unspecified**

    Q62.11   **Congenital occulsion of ureteropelvic junction**

    Q62.12   **Congenital occulsion of ureterovesical orifice**

Q62.2 **Congenital megaureter**
  Congenital dilatation of ureter

Q62.3 **Other obstructive defects of renal pelvis and ureter**

  Q62.31 **Congenital ureterocele, orthotopic**

  Q62.32 **Cecoureterocele**
    Ectopic ureterocele

  Q62.39 **Other obstructive defects of renal pelvis and ureter**

Q62.4 **Agenesis of ureter**
  Congenital absence ureter

Q62.5 **Duplication of ureter**
  Accessory ureter
  Double ureter

Q62.6 **Malposition of ureter**

  Q62.60 **Malposition of ureter, unspecified**

  Q62.61 **Deviation of ureter**

  Q62.62 **Displacement of ureter**

  Q62.63 **Anomalous implantation of ureter**
    Ectopia of ureter
    Ectopic ureter

  Q62.69 **Other malposition of ureter**

Q62.7 **Congenital vesico-uretero-renal reflux**

Q62.8 **Other congenital malformations of ureter**
  Anomaly of ureter NOS

Q63 **Other congenital malformations of kidney**

  Excludes1: congenital nephrotic syndrome (N04.-)

Q63.0 **Accessory kidney**

Q63.1 **Lobulated, fused and horseshoe kidney**

Q63.2 **Ectopic kidney**
  Congenital displaced kidney
  Malrotation of kidney

Q63.3 **Hyperplastic and giant kidney**
  Compensatory hypertrophy of kidney

Q63.8 **Other specified congenital malformations of kidney**
  Congenital renal calculi

Q63.9 **Congenital malformation of kidney, unspecified**

Q64 **Other congenital malformations of urinary system**

Q64.0 **Epispadias**

  Excludes1: hypospadias (Q54.-)

Q64.1 **Exstrophy of urinary bladder**

  Q64.10 **Exstrophy of urinary bladder, unspecified**
    Ectopia vesicae

  Q64.11 **Supravesical fissure of urinary bladder**

  Q64.12 **Cloacal extrophy of urinary bladder**

  Q64.19 **Other exstrophy of urinary bladder**
    Extroversion of bladder

Q64.2 **Congenital posterior urethral valves**

Q64.3 **Other atresia and stenosis of urethra and bladder neck**

  Q64.31 **Congenital bladder neck obstruction**
    Congenital obstruction of vesicourethral orifice

  Q64.32 **Congenital stricture of urethra**

  Q64.33 **Congenital stricture of urinary meatus**

  Q64.39 **Other atresia and stenosis of urethra and bladder neck**
    Atresia and stenosis of urethra and bladder neck NOS

Q64.4 **Malformation of urachus**
  Cyst of urachus
  Patent urachus
  Prolapse of urachus

Q64.5 **Congenital absence of bladder and urethra**

Q64.6 **Congenital diverticulum of bladder**

Q64.7 **Other and unspecified congenital malformations of bladder and urethra**

  Excludes1: congenital prolapse of bladder (mucosa) (Q79.4)

  Q64.70 **Unspecified congenital malformation of bladder and urethra**
    Malformation of bladder or urethra NOS

  Q64.71 **Congenital prolapse of urethra**

  Q64.72 **Congenital prolapse of urinary meatus**

  Q64.73 **Congenital urethrorectal fistula**

  Q64.74 **Double urethra**

  Q64.75 **Double urinary meatus**

  Q64.79 **Other congenital malformations of bladder and urethra**

Q64.8 **Other specified congenital malformations of urinary system**

Q64.9 **Congenital malformation of urinary system, unspecified**
  Congenital anomaly NOS of urinary system
  Congenital deformity NOS of urinary system

CONGENITAL MALFORMATIONS AND DEFORMATIONS OF THE MUSCULOSKELETAL SYSTEM (Q65–Q79)

Q65 **Congenital deformities of hip**

  Excludes1: clicking hip (R29.4)

Q65.0 **Congenital dislocation of hip, unilateral**

  Q65.00 **Congenital dislocation of hip, unilateral, unspecified side**

  Q65.01 **Congenital dislocation of right hip**

  Q65.02 **Congenital dislocation of left hip**

Q65.1 **Congenital dislocation of hip, bilateral**

Q65.2 **Congenital dislocation of hip, unspecified**

Q65.3 **Congenital partial dislocation of hip, unilateral**

  Q65.30 **Congenital partial dislocation of hip, unilateral, unspecified side**

  Q65.31 **Congenital partial dislocation of right hip**

  Q65.32 **Congenital partial dislocation of left hip**

Q65.4 **Congenital partial dislocation of hip, bilateral**

Q65.5 **Congenital partial dislocation of hip, unspecified**

Q65.6 **Congenital unstable hip**
  Congenital dislocatable hip

Q65.8 **Other congenital deformities of hip**
  Anteversion of femoral neck
  Congenital acetabular dysplasia
  Congenital coxa valga
  Congenital coxa vara

Q65.9 **Congenital deformity of hip, unspecified**

Q66 **Congenital deformities of feet**

  Excludes1: reduction defects of feet (Q72.-)
       valgus deformities (acquired) (M21.0)
       varus deformities (acquired) (M21.1)

Q66.0 **Congenital talipes equinovarus**

Q66.1 **Congenital talipes calcaneovarus**

Q66.2 **Congenital metatarsus (primus) varus**

Q66.3 **Other congenital varus deformities of feet**
  Hallux varus, congenital

Q66.4 **Congenital talipes calcaneovalgus**

Q66.5 **Congenital pes planus**
  Congenital flat foot
  Congenital rigid flat foot
  Congenital spastic (everted) flat foot

  Excludes1: pes planus, acquired (M21.4)

Q66.6 **Other congenital valgus deformities of feet**
  Congenital metatarsus valgus

Q66.7 **Congenital pes cavus**

Q66.8 **Other congenital deformities of feet**
  Congenital asymmetric talipes
  Congenital clubfoot NOS
  Congenital talipes NOS
  Congenital tarsal coalition
  Congenital vertical talus
  Hammer toe, congenital

Q66.9 **Congenital deformity of feet, unspecified**

Q67 **Congenital musculoskeletal deformities of head, face, spine and chest**

  Excludes1: congenital malformation syndromes classified to Q87.-
       Potter's syndrome (Q60.6)

Q67.0 **Congenital facial asymmetry**

Q67.1 **Congenital compression facies**

Q67.2 **Dolichocephaly**

Q67.3 **Plagiocephaly**

Q67.4 Other congenital deformities of skull, face and jaw
Congenital depressions in skull
Congenital hemifacial atrophy or hypertrophy
Deviation of nasal septum, congenital
Squashed or bent nose, congenital
Excludes1:   dentofacial anomalies [including malocclusion]
(M26-)
syphilitic saddle nose (A50.5)

Q67.5 Congenital deformity of spine
Congenital postural scoliosis
Congenital scoliosis NOS
Excludes1:   infantile idiopathic scoliosis (M41.0)
scoliosis due to congenital bony malformation
(Q76.3)

Q67.6 Pectus excavatum
Congenital funnel chest

Q67.7 Pectus carinatum
Congenital pigeon chest

Q67.8 Other congenital deformities of chest
Congenital deformity of chest wall NOS

Q68 Other congenital musculoskeletal deformities
Excludes1:   reduction defects of limb(s) (Q71-Q73)

Q68.0 Congenital deformity of sternocleidomastoid muscle
Congenital contracture of sternocleidomastoid (muscle)
Congenital (sternomastoid) torticollis
Sternomastoid tumor (congenital)

Q68.1 Congenital deformity of hand
Congenital clubfinger
Spade-like hand (congenital)

Q68.2 Congenital deformity of knee
Congenital dislocation of knee
Congenital genu recurvatum

Q68.3 Congenital bowing of femur
Excludes1:   anteversion of femur (neck) (Q65.8)

Q68.4 Congenital bowing of tibia and fibula

Q68.5 Congenital bowing of long bones of leg, unspecified

Q68.6 Discoid meniscus (congenital)

  Q68.60 Discoid meniscus (congenital), unspecified meniscus

    Q68.601 Discoid meniscus (congenital), unspecified meniscus, right knee

    Q68.602 Discoid meniscus (congenital), unspecified meniscus, left knee

    Q68.609 Discoid meniscus (congenital), unspecified meniscus, unspecified knee

  Q68.61 Discoid meniscus (congenital), anterior horn of medial meniscus

    Q68.611 Discoid meniscus (congenital), anterior horn of medial meniscus, right knee

    Q68.612 Discoid meniscus (congenital), anterior horn of medial meniscus, left knee

    Q68.619 Discoid meniscus (congenital), anterior horn of medial meniscus, unspecified knee

  Q68.62 Discoid meniscus (congenital), posterior horn of medial meniscus

    Q68.621 Discoid meniscus (congenital), posterior horn of medial meniscus, right knee

    Q68.622 Discoid meniscus (congenital), posterior horn of medial meniscus, left knee

    Q68.629 Discoid meniscus (congenital), posterior horn of medial meniscus, unspecified knee

  Q68.63 Discoid meniscus (congenital), other medial meniscus
Discoid meniscus (congenital), medial meniscus NOS

    Q68.631 Discoid meniscus (congenital), other medial meniscus, right knee

    Q68.632 Discoid meniscus (congenital), other medial meniscus, left knee

    Q68.639 Discoid meniscus (congenital), other medial meniscus, unspecified knee

  Q68.64 Discoid meniscus (congenital), anterior horn of lateral meniscus

    Q68.641 Discoid meniscus (congenital), anterior horn of lateral meniscus, right knee

    Q68.642 Discoid meniscus (congenital), anterior horn of lateral meniscus, left knee

    Q68.649 Discoid meniscus (congenital), anterior horn of lateral meniscus, unspecified knee

  Q68.65 Discoid meniscus (congenital), posterior horn of lateral meniscus

    Q68.651 Discoid meniscus (congenital), posterior horn of lateral meniscus, right knee

    Q68.652 Discoid meniscus (congenital), posterior horn of lateral meniscus, left knee

    Q68.659 Discoid meniscus (congenital), posterior horn of lateral meniscus, unspecified knee

  Q68.66 Discoid meniscus (congenital), other lateral meniscus
Discoid meniscus (congenital), lateral meniscus NOS

    Q68.661 Discoid meniscus (congenital), other lateral meniscus, right knee

    Q68.662 Discoid meniscus (congenital), other lateral meniscus, left knee

    Q68.669 Discoid meniscus (congenital), other lateral meniscus, unspecified knee

Q68.8 Other specified congenital musculoskeletal deformities
Congenital deformity of clavicle
Congenital deformity of elbow
Congenital deformity of forearm
Congenital deformity of scapula
Congenital dislocation of elbow
Congenital dislocation of shoulder

Q69 Polydactyly

Q69.0 Accessory finger(s)

Q69.1 Accessory thumb(s)

Q69.2 Accessory toe(s)
Accessory hallux

Q69.9 Polydactyly, unspecified
Supernumerary digit(s) NOS

Q70 Syndactyly

Q70.0 Fused fingers
Complex syndactyly of fingers with synostosis

  Q70.00 Fused fingers, unspecified fingers

  Q70.01 Fused right fingers

  Q70.02 Fused left fingers

  Q70.03 Fused fingers, bilateral

Q70.1 Webbed fingers
Simple syndactyly of fingers without synostosis

  Q70.10 Webbed fingers, unspecified side

  Q70.11 Webbed right fingers

  Q70.12 Webbed left fingers

  Q70.13 Webbed fingers, bilateral

Q70.2 Fused toes
Complex syndactyly of toes with synostosis

Q70.3 Webbed toes
Simple syndactyly of toes without synostosis

Q70.4 Polysyndactyly

Q70.9 Syndactyly, unspecified
Symphalangy NOS

Q71 Reduction defects of upper limb

Q71.0 Congenital complete absence of upper limb

  Q71.00 Congenital complete absence of upper limb, unspecified side

  Q71.01 Congenital complete absence of right upper limb

  Q71.02 Congenital complete absence of left upper limb

  Q71.03 Congenital complete absence of upper limb, bilateral

Q71.1 Congenital absence of upper arm and forearm with hand present

  Q71.10 Congenital absence of upper arm and forearm with hand present, unspecified side

  Q71.11 Congenital absence of right upper arm and forearm with hand present

  Q71.12 Congenital absence of left upper arm and forearm with hand present

Q71.13   Congenital absence of upper arm and forearm with hand present, bilateral

Q71.2   Congenital absence of both forearm and hand

Q71.20   Congenital absence of both forearm and hand, unspecified side

Q71.21   Congenital absence of both right forearm and hand

Q71.22   Congenital absence of both left forearm and hand

Q71.23   Congenital absence of both forearm and hand, bilateral

Q71.3   Congenital absence of hand and finger

Q71.30   Congenital absence of hand and finger, unspecified side

Q71.31   Congenital absence of right hand and finger

Q71.32   Congenital absence of left hand and finger

Q71.33   Congenital absence of hand and finger, bilateral

Q71.4   Longitudinal reduction defect of radius
          Clubhand (congenital)
          Radial clubhand

Q71.40   Longitudinal reduction defect of radius, unspecified side

Q71.41   Longitudinal reduction defect of right radius

Q71.42   Longitudinal reduction defect of left radius

Q71.43   Longitudinal reduction defect of radius, bilateral

Q71.5   Longitudinal reduction defect of ulna

Q71.50   Longitudinal reduction defect of ulna, unspecified side

Q71.51   Longitudinal reduction defect of right ulna

Q71.52   Longitudinal reduction defect of left ulna

Q71.53   Longitudinal reduction defect of ulna, bilateral

Q71.6   Lobster-claw hand

Q71.60   Lobster-claw hand, unspecified side

Q71.61   Lobster-claw right hand

Q71.62   Lobster-claw left hand

Q71.63   Lobster-claw hand, bilateral

Q71.8   Other reduction defects of upper limb
          Congenital shortening of upper limb

Q71.80   Other reduction defects of upper limb, unspecified side

Q71.81   Other reduction defects of right upper limb

Q71.82   Other reduction defects of left upper limb

Q71.83   Other reduction defects of upper limb, bilateral

Q71.9   Reduction defect of upper limb, unspecified

Q71.90   Reduction defect of upper limb, unspecified, side unspecified

Q71.91   Reduction defect of right upper limb, unspecified

Q71.92   Reduction defect of left upper limb, unspecified

Q71.93   Reduction defect of upper limb, unspecified, bilateral

Q72   Reduction defects of lower limb

Q72.0   Congenital complete absence of lower limb

Q72.00   Congenital complete absence of lower limb, unspecified side

Q72.01   Congenital complete absence of right lower limb

Q72.02   Congenital complete absence of left lower limb

Q72.03   Congenital complete absence of lower limb, bilateral

Q72.1   Congenital absence of thigh and lower leg with foot present

Q72.10   Congenital absence of thigh and lower leg with foot present, unspecified side

Q72.11   Congenital absence of right thigh and lower leg with foot present

Q72.12   Congenital absence of left thigh and lower leg with foot present

Q72.13   Congenital absence of thigh and lower leg with foot present, bilateral

Q72.2   Congenital absence of both lower leg and foot

Q72.20   Congenital absence of both lower leg and foot, unspecified side

Q72.21   Congenital absence of both right lower leg and foot

Q72.22   Congenital absence of both left lower leg and foot

Q72.23   Congenital absence of both lower leg and foot, bilateral

Q72.3   Congenital absence of foot and toe(s)

Q72.30   Congenital absence of foot and toe(s), unspecified side

Q72.31   Congenital absence of right foot and toe(s)

Q72.32   Congenital absence of left foot and toe(s)

Q72.33   Congenital absence of foot and toe(s), bilateral

Q72.4   Longitudinal reduction defect of femur
          Proximal femoral focal deficiency

Q72.40   Longitudinal reduction defect of femur, unspecified side

Q72.41   Longitudinal reduction defect of right femur

Q72.42   Longitudinal reduction defect of left femur

Q72.43   Longitudinal reduction defect of femur, bilateral

Q72.5   Longitudinal reduction defect of tibia

Q72.50   Longitudinal reduction defect of tibia, unspecified side

Q72.51   Longitudinal reduction defect of right tibia

Q72.52   Longitudinal reduction defect of left tibia

Q72.53   Longitudinal reduction defect of tibia, bilateral

Q72.6   Longitudinal reduction defect of fibula

Q72.60   Longitudinal reduction defect of fibula, unspecified side

Q72.61   Longitudinal reduction defect of right fibula

Q72.62   Longitudinal reduction defect of left fibula

Q72.63   Longitudinal reduction defect of fibula, bilateral

Q72.7   Split foot

Q72.70   Split foot, unspecified side

Q72.71   Right split foot

Q72.72   Left split foot

Q72.73   Split foot, bilateral

Q72.8   Other reduction defects of lower limb
          Congenital shortening of lower limb(s)

Q72.80   Other reduction defects of lower limb, unspecified side

Q72.81   Other reduction defects of right lower limb

Q72.82   Other reduction defects of left lower limb

Q72.83   Other reduction defects of lower limb, bilateral

Q72.9   Reduction defect of lower limb, unspecified

Q72.90   Reduction defect of lower limb, unspecified, unspecified side

Q72.91   Reduction defect of right lower limb, unspecified

Q72.92   Reduction defect of left lower limb, unspecified

Q72.93   Reduction defect of lower limb, unspecified, bilateral

Q73   Reduction defects of unspecified limb

Q73.0   Congenital absence of unspecified limb(s)
          Amelia NOS

Q73.1   Phocomelia, unspecified limb(s)
          Phocomelia NOS

Q73.8   Other reduction defects of unspecified limb(s)
          Longitudinal reduction deformity of unspecified limb(s)
          Ectromelia of limb NOS
          Hemimelia of limb NOS
          Reduction defect of limb NOS

Q74   Other congenital malformations of limb(s)
          Excludes1:   polydactyly (Q69.-)
                        reduction defect of limb (Q71-Q73)
                        syndactyly (Q70.-)

Q74.0   Other congenital malformations of upper limb(s), including shoulder girdle
          Accessory carpal bones
          Cleidocranial dysostosis
          Congenital pseudarthrosis of clavicle
          Macrodactylia (fingers)
          Madelung's deformity
          Radioulnar synostosis
          Sprengel's deformity
          Triphalangeal thumb

Q74.1 Congenital malformation of knee
Congenital absence of patella
Congenital dislocation of patella
Congenital genu valgum
Congenital genu varum
Rudimentary patella
Excludes1:   congenital dislocation of knee (Q68.2)
                    congenital genu recurvatum (Q68.2)
                    nail patella syndrome (Q87.2)

Q74.2 Other congenital malformations of lower limb(s), including pelvic girdle
Congenital fusion of sacroiliac joint
Congenital malformation of ankle joint
Congenital malformation of sacroiliac joint
Excludes1:   anteversion of femur (neck) (Q65.8)

Q74.3 Arthrogryposis multiplex congenital

Q74.8 Other specified congenital malformations of limb(s)

Q74.9 Unspecified congenital malformation of limb(s)
Congenital anomaly of limb(s) NOS

Q75 Other congenital malformations of skull and face bones
Excludes1:   congenital malformation of face NOS (Q18.-)
                    congenital malformation syndromes classified to Q87.-
                    dentofacial anomalies [including malocclusion] (M26.-)
                    musculoskeletal deformities of head and face (Q67.0-Q67.4)
                    skull defects associated with congenital anomalies of
                        brain such as:
                    anencephaly (Q00.0)
                    encephalocele (Q01.-)
                    hydrocephalus (Q03.-)
                    microcephaly (Q02)

Q75.0 Craniosynostosis
Acrocephaly
Imperfect fusion of skull
Oxycephaly
Trigonocephaly

Q75.1 Craniofacial dysostosis
Crouzon's disease

Q75.2 Hypertelorism

Q75.3 Macrocephaly

Q75.4 Mandibulofacial dysostosis

Q75.5 Oculomandibular dysostosis

Q75.8 Other specified congenital malformations of skull and face bones
Absence of skull bone, congenital
Congenital deformity of forehead
Platybasia

Q75.9 Congenital malformation of skull and face bones, unspecified
Congenital anomaly of face bones NOS
Congenital anomaly of skull NOS

Q76 Congenital malformations of spine and bony thorax
Excludes1:   congenital musculoskeletal deformities of spine and
                    chest (Q67.5-Q67.8)

Q76.0 Spina bifida occulta
Excludes1:   meningocele (spinal) (Q05.-)
                    spina bifida (aperta) (cystica) (Q05.-)

Q76.1 Klippel-Feil syndrome
Cervical fusion syndrome

Q76.2 Congenital spondylolisthesis
Congenital spondylolysis
Excludes1:   spondylolisthesis (acquired) (M43.1-)
                    spondylolysis (acquired) (M43.0-)

Q76.3 Congenital scoliosis due to congenital bony malformation
Hemivertebra fusion or failure of segmentation with scoliosis

Q76.4 Other congenital malformations of spine, not associated with scoliosis

Q76.41   Congenital kyphosis
Q76.411   **Congenital kyphosis, occipito-atlanto-axial region**
Q76.412   **Congenital kyphosis, cervical region**
Q76.413   **Congenital kyphosis, cervicothoracic region**
Q76.414   **Congenital kyphosis, thoracic region**

Q76.415   **Congenital kyphosis, thoracolumbar region**
Q76.419   **Congenital kyphosis, unspecified region**
Q76.42   Congenital lordosis
Q76.425   **Congenital lordosis, thoracolumbar region**
Q76.426   **Congenital lordosis, lumbar region**
Q76.427   **Congenital lordosis, lumbosacral region**
Q76.428   **Congenital lordosis, sacral and sacrococcygeal region**
Q76.429   **Congenital lordosis, unspecified region**
Q76.49   Other congenital malformations of spine, not associated with scoliosis
Congenital absence of vertebra NOS
Congenital fusion of spine NOS
Congenital malformation of lumbosacral (joint) (region) NOS
Congenital malformation of spine NOS
Hemivertebra NOS
Malformation of spine NOS
Platyspondylisis NOS
Supernumerary vertebra NOS

Q76.5 Cervical rib
Supernumerary rib in cervical region

Q76.6 Other congenital malformations of ribs
Accessory rib
Congenital absence of rib
Congenital fusion of ribs
Congenital malformation of ribs NOS
Excludes1:   short rib syndrome (Q77.2)

Q76.7 Congenital malformation of sternum
Congenital absence of sternum
Sternum bifidum

Q76.8 Other congenital malformations of bony thorax

Q76.9 Congenital malformation of bony thorax, unspecified

Q77 Osteochondrodysplasia with defects of growth of tubular bones and spine
Excludes1:   mucopolysaccharidosis (E76.0-E76.3)

Q77.0 Achondrogenesis
Hypochondrogenesis

Q77.1 Thanatophoric short stature

Q77.2 Short rib syndrome
Asphyxiating thoracic dysplasia [Jeune]

Q77.3 Chondrodysplasia punctata
Excludes1:   Rhizomelic chondrodysplasia punctata (E71.430)

Q77.4 Achondroplasia
Hypochondroplasia

Q77.5 Diastrophic dysplasia

Q77.6 Chondroectodermal dysplasia
Ellis-van Creveld syndrome

Q77.7 Spondyloepiphyseal dysplasia

Q77.8 Other osteochondrodysplasia with defects of growth of tubular bones and spine

Q77.9 Osteochondrodysplasia with defects of growth of tubular bones and spine, unspecified

Q78 Other osteochondrodysplasias

Q78.0 Osteogenesis imperfecta
Fragilitas ossium
Osteopsathyrosis

Q78.1 Polyostotic fibrous dysplasia
Albright (-McCune) (-Sternberg) syndrome

Q78.2 Osteopetrosis
Albers-Schönberg syndrome

Q78.3 Progressive diaphyseal dysplasia
Camurati-Engelmann syndrome

Q78.4 Enchondromatosis
Maffucci's syndrome
Ollier's disease

Q78.5 Metaphyseal dysplasia
Pyle's syndrome

Q78.6 Multiple congenital exostoses
Diaphyseal aclasis

Q78.8 Other specified osteochondrodysplasias
Osteopoikilosis

Q78.9 Osteochondrodysplasia, unspecified
Chondrodystrophy NOS
Osteodystrophy NOS

Q79 Congenital malformations of musculoskeletal system, not elsewhere classified
Excludes2:   congenital (sternomastoid) torticollis (Q68.0)

Q79.0 Congenital diaphragmatic hernia
Excludes1:   congenital hiatus hernia (Q40.1)

Q79.1 Other congenital malformations of diaphragm
Absence of diaphragm
Congenital malformation of diaphragm NOS
Eventration of diaphragm

Q79.2 Exomphalos
Omphalocele
Excludes1:   umbilical hernia (K42.-)

Q79.3 Gastroschisis

Q79.4 Prune belly syndrome
Congenital prolapse of bladder mucosa
Eagle-Barrett syndrome

Q79.5 Other congenital malformations of abdominal wall
Excludes1:   umbilical hernia (K42.-)

Q79.51   Congenital hernia of bladder

Q79.59   Other congenital malformations of abdominal wall

Q79.6 Ehlers-Danlos syndrome

Q79.8 Other congenital malformations of musculoskeletal system
Absence of muscle
Absence of tendon
Accessory muscle
Amyotrophia congenital
Congenital constricting bands
Congenital shortening of tendon
Poland's syndrome

Q79.9 Congenital malformation of musculoskeletal system, unspecified
Congenital anomaly of musculoskeletal system NOS
Congenital deformity of musculoskeletal system NOS

OTHER CONGENITAL MALFORMATIONS (Q80-Q89)

Q80 Congenital ichthyosis
Excludes1:   Refsum's disease (G60.1)

Q80.0 Ichthyosis vulgaris

Q80.1 X-linked ichthyosis

Q80.2 Lamellar ichthyosis
Collodion baby

Q80.3 Congenital bullous ichthyosiform erythroderma

Q80.4 Harlequin fetus

Q80.8 Other congenital ichthyosis

Q80.9 Congenital ichthyosis, unspecified

Q81 Epidermolysis bullosa

Q81.0 Epidermolysis bullosa simplex
Excludes1:   Cockayne's syndrome (Q87.1)

Q81.1 Epidermolysis bullosa letalis
Herlitz' syndrome

Q81.2 Epidermolysis bullosa dystrophica

Q81.8 Other epidermolysis bullosa

Q81.9 Epidermolysis bullosa, unspecified

Q82 Other congenital malformations of skin
Excludes1:   acrodermatitis enteropathica (E83.2)
congenital erythropoietic porphyria (E80.0)
pilonidal cyst or sinus (L05.-)
Sturge-Weber (-Dimitri) syndrome (Q85.8)

Q82.0 Hereditary lymphedema

Q82.1 Xeroderma pigmentosum

Q82.2 Mastocytosis
Urticaria pigmentosa
Excludes1:   malignant mastocytosis (C96.2)

Q82.3 Incontinentia pigmenti

Q82.4 Ectodermal dysplasia (anhidrotic)
Excludes1:   Ellis-van Creveld syndrome (Q77.6)

Q82.5 Congenital non-neoplastic nevus
Birthmark NOS
Flammeus Nevus
Portwine Nevus
Sanguineous Nevus
Strawberry Nevus
Vascular Nevus NOS
Verrucous Nevus
Excludes1:   araneus nevus (I78.1)
café au lait spots (L81.3)
lentigo (L81.4)
melanocytic nevus (D22.-)
nevus NOS (D22.-)
pigmented nevus (D22.-)
spider nevus (I78.1)
stellar nevus (I78.1)

Q82.8 Other specified congenital malformations of skin
Abnormal palmar creases
Accessory skin tags
Benign familial pemphigus [Hailey-Hailey]
Congenital poikiloderma
Cutis laxa (hyperelastica)
Dermatoglyphic anomalies
Inherited keratosis palmaris et plantaris
Keratosis follicularis [Darier-White]
Excludes1:   Ehlers-Danlos syndrome (Q79.6)

Q82.9 Congenital malformation of skin, unspecified

Q83 Congenital malformations of breast
Excludes2:   absence of pectoral muscle (Q79.8)

Q83.0 Congenital absence of breast with absent nipple

Q83.1 Accessory breast
Supernumerary breast

Q83.2 Absent nipple

Q83.3 Accessory nipple
Supernumerary nipple

Q83.8 Other congenital malformations of breast
Hypoplasia of breast

Q83.9 Congenital malformation of breast, unspecified

Q84 Other congenital malformations of integument

Q84.0 Congenital alopecia
Congenital atrichosis

Q84.1 Congenital morphological disturbances of hair, not elsewhere classified
Beaded hair
Monilethrix
Pili annulati
Excludes1:   Menkes' kinky hair syndrome (E83.0)

Q84.2 Other congenital malformations of hair
Congenital hypertrichosis
Congenital malformation of hair NOS
Persistent lanugo

Q84.3 Anonychia
Excludes1:   nail patella syndrome (Q87.2)

Q84.4 Congenital leukonychia

Q84.5 Enlarged and hypertrophic nails
Congenital onychauxis
Pachyonychia

Q84.6 Other congenital malformations of nails
Congenital clubnail
Congenital koilonychia
Congenital malformation of nail NOS

Q84.8 Other specified congenital malformations of integument
Aplasia cutis congenita

Q84.9 Congenital malformation of integument, unspecified
Congenital anomaly of integument NOS
Congenital deformity of integument NOS

Q85 Phakomatoses, not elsewhere classified
Excludes1:   ataxia telangiectasia [Louis-Bar] (G11.3)
familial dysautonomia [Riley-Day] (G90.1)

Q85.0 Neurofibromatosis (nonmalignant)
Von Recklinghausen's disease

Q85.1 Tuberous sclerosis
Bourneville's disease
Epiloia

Q85.8 Other phakomatoses, not elsewhere classified
Peutz-Jeghers Syndrome
Sturge-Weber (-Dimitri) syndrome
von Hippel-Lindau syndrome
Excludes1:   Meckel-Gruber syndrome (Q61.9)

Q85.9 Phakomatosis, unspecified
Hamartosis NOS

Q86 Congenital malformation syndromes due to known exogenous causes, not elsewhere classified
Excludes2:   iodine-deficiency-related hypothyroidism (E00-E02)
nonteratogenic effects of substances transmitted via placenta or breast milk (P04.-)

Q86.0 Fetal alcohol syndrome (dysmorphic)

Q86.1 Fetal hydantoin syndrome
Meadow's syndrome

Q86.2 Dysmorphism due to Warfarin

Q86.8 Other congenital malformation syndromes due to known exogenous causes

Q87 Other specified congenital malformation syndromes affecting multiple systems
Use additional code(s) to identify all associated manifestations

Q87.0 Congenital malformation syndromes predominantly affecting facial appearance
Acrocephalopolysyndactyly
Acrocephalosyndactyly [Apert]
Cryptophthalmos syndrome
Cyclopia
Goldenhar syndrome
Moebius syndrome
Oro-facial-digital syndrome
Robin syndrome
Treacher Collins syndrome
Whistling face

Q87.1 Congenital malformation syndromes predominantly associated with short stature
Aarskog syndrome
Cockayne syndrome
De Lange syndrome
Dubowitz syndrome
Noonan syndrome
Prader-Willi syndrome
Robinow-Silverman-Smith syndrome
Russell-Silver syndrome
Seckel syndrome
Smith-Lemli-Opitz syndrome
Excludes1:   Ellis-van Creveld syndrome (Q77.6)

Q87.2 Congenital malformation syndromes predominantly involving limbs
Holt-Oram syndrome
Klippel-Trenaunay-Weber syndrome
Nail patella syndrome
Rubinstein-Taybi syndrome
Sirenomelia syndrome
Thrombocytopenia with absent radius [TAR] syndrome
VATER syndrome

Q87.3 Congenital malformation syndromes involving early overgrowth
Beckwith-Wiedemann syndrome
Sotos' syndrome
Weaver syndrome

Q87.4 Marfan's syndrome

Q87.40   Marfan's syndrome, unspecified

Q87.41   Marfan's syndrome with cardiovascular manifestations

Q87.410   Marfan's syndrome with aortic dilation

Q87.418   Marfan's syndrome with other cardiovascular manifestations

Q87.42   Marfan's syndrome with ocular manifestations

Q87.43   Marfan's syndrome with skeletal manifestation

Q87.5 Other congenital malformation syndromes with other skeletal changes

Q87.8 Other specified congenital malformation syndromes, not elsewhere classified

Q87.81   Alport syndrome

Q87.810   Alport syndrome without chronic renal failure
Alport syndrome NOS

Q87.811   Alport syndrome with chronic renal failure

Q87.89   Other specified congenital malformation syndromes, not elsewhere classified
Laurence-Moon (-Bardet)-Biedl syndrome

Q89 Other congenital malformations, not elsewhere classified

Q89.0 Congenital absence and malformations of spleen
Excludes1:   isomerism of atrial appendages (with asplenia or polysplenia) (Q20.6)

Q89.01   Asplenia (congenital)

Q89.09   Congenital malformations of spleen
Congenital splenomegaly

Q89.1 Congenital malformations of adrenal gland
Excludes1:   adrenogenital disorders (E25.-)
congenital adrenal hyperplasia (E25.0)

Q89.2 Congenital malformations of other endocrine glands
Congenital malformation of parathyroid or thyroid gland
Persistent thyroglossal duct
Thyroglossal cyst
Excludes1:   congenital goiter (E03.0)
congenital hypothyroidism (E03.1)

Q89.3 Situs inversus
Dextrocardia with situs inversus
Mirror-image atrial arrangement with situs inversus
Situs inversus or transversus abdominalis
Situs inversus or transversus thoracis
Transposition of abdominal viscera
Transposition of thoracic viscera
Excludes1:   dextrocardia NOS (Q24.0)

Q89.4 Conjoined twins
Craniopagus
Dicephaly
Pygopagus
Thoracopagus

Q89.7 Multiple congenital malformations, not elsewhere classified
Multiple congenital anomalies NOS
Multiple congenital deformities NOS
Excludes1:   congenital malformation syndromes affecting multiple systems (Q87.-)

Q89.8 Other specified congenital malformations

Q89.9 Congenital malformation, unspecified
Congenital anomaly NOS
Congenital deformity NOS

CHROMOSOMAL ABNORMALITIES, NOT ELSEWHERE CLASSIFIED (Q90-Q99)

Q90 Down syndrome
Use additional code(s) to identify any associated physical conditions

Q90.0 Trisomy 21, nonmosaicism (meiotic nondisjunction)

Q90.1 Trisomy 21, mosaicism (mitotic nondisjunction)

Q90.2 Trisomy 21, translocation

Q90.9 Down's syndrome, unspecified
Trisomy 21 NOS

Q91 Trisomy 18 and Trisomy 13

Q91.0 Trisomy 18, nonmosaicism (meiotic nondisjunction)

Q91.1 Trisomy 18, mosaicism (mitotic nondisjunction)

Q91.2 Trisomy 18, translocation

Q91.3 Trisomy 18, unspecified

Q91.4 Trisomy 13, nonmosaicism (meiotic nondisjunction)

Q91.5 Trisomy 13, mosaicism (mitotic nondisjunction)

Q91.6 Trisomy 13, translocation

Q91.7 Trisomy 13, unspecified

Q92 **Other trisomies and partial trisomies of the autosomes, not elsewhere classified**

Includes: unbalanced translocations and insertions

Excludes1:   trisomies of chromosomes 13, 18, 21 (Q90-Q91)

Q92.0 **Whole chromosome trisomy, nonmosaicism (meiotic nondisjunction)**

Q92.1 **Whole chromosome trisomy, mosaicism (mitotic nondisjunction)**

Q92.2 **Partial trisomy**

Less than whole arm duplicated

Whole arm or more duplicated

Excludes1:   partial trisomy due to unbalanced translocation (Q92.5)

Q92.5 **Duplications with other complex rearrangements**

Partial trisomy due to unbalanced translocations

Code also any associated deletions due to unbalanced translocations, inversions and insertions (Q93.7)

Q92.6 **Marker chromosomes**

Individual with marker heterochromatin

Trisomies due to dicentrics

Trisomies due to extra rings

Trisomies due to isochromosomes

Q92.61 **Marker chromosomes in normal individual**

Q92.62 **Marker chromosomes in abnormal individual**

Q92.7 **Triploidy and polyploidy**

Q92.8 **Other specified trisomies and partial trisomies of autosomes**

Duplications identified by fluorescence in situ hybridization (FISH)

Duplications identified by in situ hybridization (ISH)

Duplications seen only at prometaphase

Q92.9 **Trisomy and partial trisomy of autosomes, unspecified**

Q93 **Monosomies and deletions from the autosomes, not elsewhere classified**

Q93.0 **Whole chromosome monosomy, nonmosaicism (meiotic nondisjunction)**

Q93.1 **Whole chromosome monosomy, mosaicism (mitotic nondisjunction)**

Q93.2 **Chromosome replaced with ring, dicentric or isochromosome**

Q93.3 **Deletion of short arm of chromosome 4**

Wolff-Hirschorn syndrome

Q93.4 **Deletion of short arm of chromosome 5**

Cri-du-chat syndrome

Q93.7 **Deletions with other complex rearrangements**

Deletions due to unbalanced translocations, inversions and insertions

Code also any associated duplications due to unbalanced translocations, inversions and insertions (Q92.5)

Q93.8 **Other deletions from the autosomes**

Deletions identified by fluorescence in situ hybridization (FISH)

Deletions identified by in situ hybridization (ISH)

Deletions seen only at prometaphase

Q93.9 **Deletion from autosomes, unspecified**

Q95 **Balanced rearrangements and structural markers, not elsewhere classified**

Includes: Robertsonian and balanced reciprocal translocations and insertions

Q95.0 **Balanced translocation and insertion in normal individual**

Q95.1 **Chromosome inversion in normal individual**

Q95.2 **Balanced autosomal rearrangement in abnormal individual**

Q95.3 **Balanced sex/autosomal rearrangement in abnormal individual**

Q95.5 **Individual with autosomal fragile site**

Q95.8 **Other balanced rearrangements and structural markers**

Q95.9 **Balanced rearrangement and structural marker, unspecified**

Q96 **Turner syndrome**

Excludes1:   Noonan syndrome (Q87.1)

Q96.0 **Karyotype 45, X**

Q96.1 **Karyotype 46, X i(Xq)**

Karyotype 46, isochromosome Xq

Q96.2 **Karyotype 46, X with abnormal sex chromosome, except i(Xq)**

Karyotype 46, X with abnormal sex chromosome, except isochromosome Xq

Q96.3 **Mosaicism, 45, X/46, XX or XY**

Q96.4 **Mosaicism, 45, X/other cell line(s) with abnormal sex chromosome**

Q96.8 **Other variants of Turner syndrome**

Q96.9 **Turner syndrome, unspecified**

Q97 **Other sex chromosome abnormalities, female phenotype, not elsewhere classified**

Excludes1:   Turner syndrome (Q96.-)

Q97.0 **Karyotype 47, XXX**

Q97.1 **Female with more than three X chromosomes**

Q97.2 **Mosaicism, lines with various numbers of X chromosomes**

Q97.3 **Female with 46, XY karyotype**

Q97.8 **Other specified sex chromosome abnormalities, female phenotype**

Q97.9 **Sex chromosome abnormality, female phenotype, unspecified**

Q98 **Other sex chromosome abnormalities, male phenotype, not elsewhere classified**

Q98.0 **Klinefelter syndrome karyotype 47, XXY**

Q98.1 **Klinefelter syndrome, male with more than two X chromosomes**

Q98.3 **Male with 46, XX karyotype**

Q98.4 **Klinefelter syndrome, unspecified**

Q98.5 **Karyotype 47, XYY**

Q98.6 **Male with structurally abnormal sex chromosome**

Q98.7 **Male with sex chromosome mosaicism**

Q98.8 **Other specified sex chromosome abnormalities, male phenotype**

Q98.9 **Sex chromosome abnormality, male phenotype, unspecified**

Q99 **Other chromosome abnormalities, not elsewhere classified**

Q99.0 **Chimera 46, XX/46, XY**

Chimera 46, XX/46, XY true hermaphrodite

Q99.1 **46, XX true hermaphrodite**

46, XX with streak gonads

46, XY with streak gonads

Pure gonadal dysgenesis

Q99.2 **Fragile X chromosome**

Fragile X syndrome

Q99.8 **Other specified chromosome abnormalities**

Q99.9 **Chromosomal abnormality, unspecified**

CHAPTER XVIII — SYMPTOMS, SIGNS AND ABNORMAL CLINICAL AND LABORATORY FINDINGS, NOT ELSEWHERE CLASSIFIED (R00–R99)

This chapter includes symptoms, signs, abnormal results of clinical or other investigative procedures, and ill-defined conditions regarding which no diagnosis classifiable elsewhere is recorded.

Signs and symptoms that point rather definitely to a given diagnosis have been assigned to a category in other chapters of the classification. In general, categories in this chapter include the less well-defined conditions and symptoms that, without the necessary study of the case to establish a final diagnosis, point perhaps equally to two or more diseases or to two or more systems of the body. Practically all categories in the chapter could be designated "not otherwise specified", "unknown etiology" or "transient". The Alphabetical Index should be consulted to determine which symptoms and signs are to be allocated here and which to other chapters. The residual subcategories, numbered .8, are generally provided for other relevant symptoms that cannot be allocated elsewhere in the classification.

The conditions and signs or symptoms included in categories R00-R94 consist of: (a) cases for which no more specific diagnosis can be made even after all the facts bearing on the case have been investigated: (b) signs or symptoms existing at the time of initial encounter that proved to be transient and whose causes could not be determined; (c) provisional diagnosis in a patient who failed to return for further investigation or care; (d) cases referred elsewhere for investigation or treatment before the diagnosis was made; (e) cases in which a more precise diagnosis was not available for any other reason; (f) certain symptoms, for which supplementary information is provided, that represent important problems in medical care in their own right.

> Excludes1: abnormal findings on antenatal screening of mother (O28.-)
> certain conditions originating in the perinatal period (P04-P96)

This chapter contains the following blocks:

R00-R09   Symptoms and signs involving the circulatory and respiratory systems
R10-R19   Symptoms and signs involving the digestive system and abdomen
R20-R23   Symptoms and signs involving the skin and subcutaneous tissue
R25-R29   Symptoms and signs involving the nervous and musculoskeletal systems
R30-R39   Symptoms and signs involving the urinary system
R40-R46   Symptoms and signs involving cognition, perception, emotional state and behavior
R47-R49   Symptoms and signs involving speech and voice
R50-R69   General symptoms and signs
R70-R79   Abnormal findings on examination of blood, without diagnosis
R80-R82   Abnormal findings on examination of urine, without diagnosis
R83-R89   Abnormal findings on examination of other body fluids, substances and tissues, without diagnosis
R90-R94   Abnormal findings on diagnostic imaging and in function studies, without diagnosis
R99   Ill-defined and unknown cause of mortality

SYMPTOMS AND SIGNS INVOLVING THE CIRCULATORY AND RESPIRATORY SYSTEMS (R00–R09)

R00 Abnormalities of heart beat

> Excludes1: abnormalities originating in the perinatal period (P29.1)
> specified arrhythmias (I47-I49)

R00.0 Tachycardia, unspecified
Rapid heart beat
> Excludes1: paroxysmal tachycardia (I47.-)

R00.1 Bradycardia, unspecified
Slow heart beat

R00.2 Palpitations
Awareness of heart beat

R00.8 Other abnormalities of heart beat

R00.9 Unspecified abnormalities of heart beat

R01 Cardiac murmurs and other cardiac sounds

> Excludes1: cardiac murmurs and sounds originating in the perinatal period (P29.8)

R01.0 Benign and innocent cardiac murmurs
Functional cardiac murmur

R01.1 Cardiac murmur, unspecified
Cardiac bruit NOS
Heart murmur NOS

R01.2 Other cardiac sounds
Cardiac dullness, increased or decreased
Precordial friction

R03 Abnormal blood-pressure reading, without diagnosis

R03.0 Elevated blood-pressure reading, without diagnosis of hypertension
Note: This category is to be used to record an episode of elevated blood pressure in a patient in whom no formal diagnosis of hypertension has been made, or as an isolated incidental finding.

R03.1 Nonspecific low blood-pressure reading
> Excludes1: hypotension (I95.-)
> maternal hypotension syndrome (O26.5-)
> neurogenic orthostatic hypotension (G90.3)

R04 Hemorrhage from respiratory passages

R04.0 Epistaxis
Hemorrhage from nose
Nosebleed

R04.1 Hemorrhage from throat
> Excludes2: hemoptysis (R04.2)

R04.2 Hemoptysis
Blood-stained sputum
Cough with hemorrhage

R04.8 Hemorrhage from other sites in respiratory passages
Pulmonary hemorrhage NOS
> Excludes1: perinatal pulmonary hemorrhage (P26.-)

R04.9 Hemorrhage from respiratory passages, unspecifie

R05 Cough
> Excludes1: cough with hemorrhage (R04.2)
> psychogenic cough (F45.3)
> smoker's cough (J41.0)

R06 Abnormalities of breathing
> Excludes1: respiratory arrest (R09.2)
> respiratory distress syndrome of adult (J80)
> respiratory distress syndrome of newborn (P22.-)
> respiratory failure (J96.-)
> respiratory failure of newborn (P28.5)

R06.0 Dyspnea
> Excludes1: tachypnea NOS (R06.82)
> transient tachypnea of newborn (P22.1)

R06.00 Dyspnea NOS
R06.01 Orthopnea
R06.02 Shortness of breath
R06.09 Other forms of dyspnea

R06.1 Stridor
> Excludes1: congenital laryngeal stridor (Q31.4)
> laryngismus (stridulus) (J38.5)

R06.2 Wheezing
> Excludes1: asthma (J45.-)

R06.3 Periodic breathing
Cheyne-Stokes breathing

R06.4 Hyperventilation
> Excludes1: psychogenic hyperventilation (F45.8)

R06.5 Mouth breathing
Snoring
> Excludes2: dry mouth NOS (R68.2)

R06.6 Hiccough

    Excludes1:   psychogenic hiccough (F45.8)

R06.7 Sneezing

R06.8 Other abnormalities of breathing

   R06.81 Apnea, not elsewhere classified

      Apnea NOS

      Excludes1:   apnea (of) newborn (P28.4)

                sleep apnea (G47.3-)

                sleep apnea of newborn (primary) (P28.3)

   R06.82 Tachypnea, not elsewhere classified

      Tachypnea NOS

      Excludes1:   transitory tachypnea of newborn (P22.1)

   R06.89 Other abnormalities of breathing

      Breath-holding (spells)

      Choking sensation

      Sighing

R06.9 Unspecified abnormalities of breathing

R07 Pain in throat and chest

    Excludes1:   epidemic myalgia (B33.0)

    Excludes2:   pain in breast (N64.4)

R07.0 Pain in throat

    Excludes1:   chronic sore throat (J31.2)

              sore throat (acute) NOS (J02.9)

    Excludes2:   dysphagia (R13)

              pain in neck (M54.2)

R07.1 Chest pain on breathing

    Painful respiration

R07.2 Precordial pain

R07.8 Other chest pain

   R07.81 Pleurodynia

      Pleurodynia NOS

      Excludes1:   epidemic pleurodynia (B33.0)

   R07.89 Other chest pain

      Anterior chest-wall pain NOS

R07.9 Chest pain, unspecified

R09 Other symptoms and signs involving the circulatory and respiratory system

    Excludes1:   adult respiratory distress syndrome (J80)

              respiratory distress syndrome of newborn (P22.0)

              respiratory failure (J96.-)

              respiratory failure of newborn (P28.5)

R09.0 Asphyxia

    Excludes1:   asphyxia due to carbon monoxide (T58.-)

              asphyxia due to foreign body in respiratory tract (T17.-)

              birth (intrauterine) asphyxia (P84)

              traumatic asphyxia (T71-)

R09.1 Pleurisy

    Excludes1:   pleurisy with effusion (J90)

R09.2 Respiratory arrest

    Cardiorespiratory failure

    Excludes1:   cardiac arrest (I46.-)

              respiratory failure (J96.-)

              respiratory failure of newborn (P28.5)

              respiratory insufficiency (R06.89)

              respiratory insufficiency of newborn (P28.5)

R09.3 Abnormal sputum

    Abnormal amount of sputum

    Abnormal color of sputum

    Abnormal odor of sputum

    Excessive sputum

    Excludes1:   blood-stained sputum (R04.2)

R09.8 Other specified symptoms and signs involving the circulatory and respiratory systems

   R09.81 Nasal congestion

   R09.89 Other specified symptoms and signs involving the circulatory and respiratory systems

      Abnormal chest percussion

      Bruit (arterial)

      Chest tympany

      Friction sounds in chest

      Rales

      Weak pulse

      Excludes2:   wheezing (R06.2)

SYMPTOMS AND SIGNS INVOLVING THE DIGESTIVE SYSTEM AND ABDOMEN (R10–R19)

    Excludes1:   congenital or infantile pylorospasm (Q40.0)

              gastrointestinal hemorrhage (K92.0-K92.2)

              intestinal obstruction (K56.-)

              newborn gastrointestinal hemorrhage (P54.0-P54.3)

              newborn intestinal obstruction (P76.-)

              pylorospasm (K31.3)

              signs and symptoms involving the urinary system (R30-R39)

              symptoms referable to female genital organs (N94.-)

              symptoms referable to male genital organs male (N48-N50)

R10 Abdominal and pelvic pain

    Excludes1:   renal colic (N23)

    Excludes2:   dorsalgia (M54.-)

              flatulence and related conditions (R14.-)

R10.0 Acute abdomen

    Severe abdominal pain (generalized) (with abdominal rigidity)

    Excludes1:   abdominal rigidity NOS (R19.3)

              generalized abdominal pain NOS (R10.84)

              localized abdominal pain (R10.1-R10.3-)

R10.1 Pain localized to upper abdomen

   R10.10 Upper abdominal pain, unspecified

   R10.11 Right upper quadrant pain

   R10.12 Left upper quadrant pain

   R10.13 Epigastric pain

R10.2 Pelvic and perineal pain

R10.3 Pain localized to other parts of lower abdomen

   R10.30 Lower abdominal pain, unspecified

   R10.31 Right lower quadrant pain

   R10.32 Left lower quadrant pain

   R10.33 Periumbilical pain

R10.8 Other abdominal pain

   R10.81 Abdominal tenderness

      Abdominal tenderness NOS

      R10.811 Right upper quadrant abdominal tenderness

      R10.812 Left upper quadrant abdominal tenderness

      R10.813 Right lower quadrant abdominal tenderness

      R10.814 Left lower quadrant abdominal tenderness

      R10.815 Periumbilic abdominal tenderness

      R10.816 Epigastric abdominal tenderness

      R10.817 Generalized abdominal tenderness

      R10.819 Abdominal tenderness, unspecified site

   R10.82 Rebound abdominal tenderness

      R10.821 Right upper quadrant rebound abdominal tenderness

      R10.822 Left upper quadrant rebound abdominal tenderness

      R10.823 Right lower quadrant rebound abdominal tenderness

      R10.824 Left lower quadrant rebound abdominal tenderness

      R10.825 Periumbilic rebound abdominal tenderness

      R10.826 Epigastric rebound abdominal tenderness

      R10.827 Generalized rebound abdominal tenderness

      R10.829 Rebound abdominal tenderness, unspecified site

   R10.83 Colic

      Colic NOS

      Infantile colic

R10.84 Generalized abdominal pain
Excludes1:   generalized abdominal pain associated with acute abdomen (R10.0)

R10.9 Unspecified abdominal pain

R11 Nausea and vomiting
Excludes1:   excessive vomiting in pregnancy (O21.-)
hematemesis (K92.0)
neonatal hematemesis (P54.0)
newborn vomiting (P92.0)
psychogenic vomiting (F50.8)
vomiting following gastrointestinal surgery (K91.0)

R11.0 Nausea with vomiting
R11.1 Nausea alone
R11.2 Projectile vomiting
R11.3 Other vomiting without nausea

R12 Heartburn
Excludes1:   dyspepsia (K30)

R13 Aphagia and dysphagia
R13.0 Aphagia
Inability to swallow
R13.1 Dysphagia
Difficulty in swallowing
Excludes1:   dysphagia following cerebrovascular accident (I69.091, I69.191, I69.291, I69.391, I69.491, I69.891, I69.991)

R14 Flatulence and related conditions
Excludes1:   psychogenic aerophagy (F45.8)
R14.0 Abdominal distension (gaseous)
Bloating
Tympanites (abdominal) (intestinal)
R14.1 Gas pain
R14.2 Eructation
R14.3 Flatulence
R14.8 Other

R15 Fecal incontinence
Includes: encopresis NOS
Excludes1:   fecal incontinence of nonorganic origin (F98.1)

R16 Hepatomegaly and splenomegaly, not elsewhere classified
R16.0 Hepatomegaly, not elsewhere classified
Hepatomegaly NOS
R16.1 Splenomegaly, not elsewhere classified
Splenomegaly NOS
R16.2 Hepatomegaly with splenomegaly, not elsewhere classified
Hepatosplenomegaly NOS

R17 Unspecified jaundice
Excludes1:   neonatal jaundice (P55, P57-P59)

R18 Ascites
Includes: fluid in peritoneal cavity
Excludes1:   ascites in alcoholic cirrhosis (K70.31)
ascites in alcoholic hepatitis (K70.11)
ascites in toxic liver disease with chronic active hepatitis (K71.51)
malignant ascites (C78.6)

R19 Other symptoms and signs involving the digestive system and abdomen
Excludes1:   acute abdomen (R10.0)
R19.0 Intra-abdominal and pelvic swelling, mass and lump
Excludes1:   abdominal distension (gaseous) (R14.-)
ascites NOS (R18)
R19.00 Swelling, mass and lump, unspecified site
R19.01 Right upper quadrant swelling, mass and lump
R19.02 Left upper quadrant swelling, mass and lump
R19.03 Right lower quadrant swelling, mass and lump
R19.04 Left lower quadrant swelling, mass and lump

R19.05 Periumbilic swelling, mass or lump
Diffuse or generalized umbilical swelling or mass
R19.06 Epigastric swelling, mass or lump
R19.07 Generalized swelling, mass and lump
Diffuse or generalized intra-abdominal swelling or mass NOS
Diffuse or generalized pelvic swelling or mass NOS
R19.09 Other swelling, mass and lump
R19.1 Abnormal bowel sounds
R19.11 Absent bowel sounds
R19.12 Hyperactive bowel sounds
R19.15 Other abnormal bowel sounds
Abnormal bowel sounds NOS
R19.2 Visible peristalsis
Hyperperistalsis
R19.3 Abdominal rigidity
Excludes1:   abdominal rigidity with severe abdominal pain (R10.0)
R19.30 Abdominal rigidity, unspecified site
R19.31 Right upper quadrant abdominal rigidity
R19.32 Left upper quadrant abdominal rigidity
R19.33 Right lower quadrant abdominal rigidity
R19.34 Left lower quadrant abdominal rigidity
R19.35 Periumbilic abdominal rigidity
R19.36 Epigastric abdominal rigidity
R19.37 Generalized abdominal rigidity
R19.4 Change in bowel habit
Excludes1:   constipation (K59.0)
functional diarrhea (K59.1)
R19.5 Other fecal abnormalities
Abnormal stool color
Bulky stools
Mucus in stools
Excludes1:   melena (K92.1)
neonatal melena (P54.1)
R19.6 Halitosis
R19.7 Diarrhea, unspecified
Diarrhea NOS
Excludes1:   functional diarrhea (K59.1)
neonatal diarrhea (P78.3)
psychogenic diarrhea (F45.8)
R19.8 Other specified symptoms and signs involving the digestive system and abdomen

SYMPTOMS AND SIGNS INVOLVING THE SKIN AND SUBCUTANEOUS TISSUE (R20–R23)
Excludes2:   symptoms relating to breast (N64.4-N64.5)

R20 Disturbances of skin sensation
Excludes1:   dissociative anesthesia and sensory loss (F44.6)
psychogenic disturbances (F45.8)
R20.0 Anesthesia of skin
R20.1 Hypoesthesia of skin
R20.2 Paresthesia of skin
Formication
Pins and needles
Tingling skin
Excludes1:   acroparesthesia (I73.8)
R20.3 Hyperesthesia
R20.8 Other disturbances of skin sensation
R20.9 Unspecified disturbances of skin sensation

R21 Rash and other nonspecific skin eruption
Excludes1:   vesicular eruption (R23.8)

R22 Localized swelling, mass and lump of skin and subcutaneous tissue
Includes: subcutaneous nodules (localized)(superficial)
Excludes1:   abnormal findings on diagnostic imaging (R90-R93
edema (R60.-)
enlarged lymph nodes (R59.-)
localized adiposity (E65)
swelling of joint (M25.4-)

R22.0 Localized swelling, mass and lump, head
R22.1 Localized swelling, mass and lump, neck
R22.2 Localized swelling, mass and lump, trunk
    Excludes1:   intra-abdominal or pelvic mass and lump (R19.0-)
                  intra-abdominal or pelvic swelling (R19.0-)
    Excludes2:   breast mass and lump (N63)
R22.3 Localized swelling, mass and lump, upper limb
  R22.30 Localized swelling, mass and lump, upper limb, unspecified side
  R22.31 Localized swelling, mass and lump, right upper limb
  R22.32 Localized swelling, mass and lump, left upper limb
  R22.33 Localized swelling, mass and lump, upper limb, bilateral
R22.4 Localized swelling, mass and lump, lower limb
  R22.40 Localized swelling, mass and lump, lower limb, unspecified side
  R22.41 Localized swelling, mass and lump, right lower limb
  R22.42 Localized swelling, mass and lump, left lower limb
  R22.43 Localized swelling, mass and lump, lower limb, bilateral
R22.9 Localized swelling, mass and lump, unspecified

R23 Other skin changes
R23.0 Cyanosis
    Excludes1:   acrocyanosis (I73.8)
                  cyanotic attacks of newborn (P28.2)
R23.1 Pallor
  Clammy skin
R23.2 Flushing
  Excessive blushing
    Excludes1:   menopausal and female climacteric states (N95.1)
R23.3 Spontaneous ecchymoses
  Petechiae
    Excludes1:   ecchymoses of fetus and newborn (P54.5)
                  purpura (D69.-)
R23.4 Changes in skin texture
  Desquamation of skin
  Induration of skin
  Scaling of skin
    Excludes1:   epidermal thickening NOS (L85.9)
R23.8 Other skin changes
R23.9 Unspecified skin changes

SYMPTOMS AND SIGNS INVOLVING THE NERVOUS AND MUSCULOSKELETAL SYSTEMS (R25–R29)

R25 Abnormal involuntary movements
    Excludes1:   specific movement disorders (G20-G26)
                  stereotyped movement disorders (F98.4)
                  tic disorders (F95.-)
R25.0 Abnormal head movements
R25.1 Tremor, unspecified
    Excludes1:   chorea NOS (G25.5)
                  essential tremor (G25.0)
                  hysterical tremor (F44.4)
                  intention tremor (G25.2)
R25.2 Cramp and spasm
    Excludes1:   carpopedal spasm (R29.0)
                  infantile spasms (G40.4-)
R25.3 Fasciculation
  Twitching NOS
R25.8 Other abnormal involuntary movements
R25.9 Unspecified abnormal involuntary movements

R26 Abnormalities of gait and mobility
    Excludes1:   ataxia NOS (R27.0)
                  hereditary ataxia (G11.-)
                  locomotor (syphilitic) ataxia (A52.11)
                  immobility syndrome (paraplegic) (M62.3)
R26.0 Ataxic gait
  Staggering gait

R26.1 Paralytic gait
  Spastic gait
R26.2 Difficulty in walking, not elsewhere classified
    Excludes1:   falling (R26.81)
                  unsteadiness on feet (R26.82)
R26.8 Other abnormalities of gait and mobility
  R26.81 Falling
  R26.82 Unsteadiness on feet
  R26.89 Other abnormalities of gait and mobility
R26.9 Unspecified abnormalities of gait and mobility

R27 Other lack of coordination
    Excludes1:   ataxic gait (R26.0)
                  hereditary ataxia (G11.-)
                  vertigo NOS (R42)
R27.0 Ataxia, unspecified
R27.8 Other lack of coordination
R27.9 Unspecified lack of coordination

R29 Other symptoms and signs involving the nervous and musculoskeletal systems
R29.0 Tetany
  Carpopedal spasm
    Excludes1:   hysterical tetany (F44.5)
                  neonatal tetany (P71.3)
                  parathyroid tetany (E20.9)
                  post-thyroidectomy tetany (E89.2)
R29.1 Meningismus
R29.2 Abnormal reflex
    Excludes2:   abnormal pupillary reflex (H57.0)
                  hyperactive gag reflex (J39.2)
                  vasovagal reaction or syncope (R55)
R29.3 Abnormal posture
R29.4 Clicking hip
    Excludes1:   congenital deformities of hip (Q65.-)
R29.5 Transient paralysis
  Code first any associated spinal cord injury (S14.0, S14.1-, S24.0, S24.1-, S34.0, S34.1-)
    Excludes1:   transient ischemic attack (G45.9)
R29.8 Other symptoms and signs involving the nervous and musculoskeletal systems
  R29.81 Other symptoms and signs involving the nervous system
  R29.89 Other symptoms and signs involving the musculoskeletal system
    Excludes2:   pain in limb (M79.6-)
    R29.890 Loss of height
      Excludes1:   osteoporosis (M80-M82)
    R29.898 Other symptoms and signs involving the musculoskeletal system
R29.9 Unspecified symptoms and signs involving the nervous and musculoskeletal systems
  R29.90 Unspecified symptoms and signs involving the nervous system
  R29.91 Unspecified symptoms and signs involving the musculoskeletal system

SYMPTOMS AND SIGNS INVOLVING THE GENITOURINARY SYSTEM (R30–R39)

R30 Pain associated with micturition
    Excludes1:   psychogenic pain associated with micturition (F45.8)
R30.0 Dysuria
  Strangury
R30.1 Vesical tenesmus
R30.9 Painful micturition, unspecified
  Painful urination NOS

R31 Hematuria

Excludes1:   hematuria included with underlying conditions, such as:
    acute cystitis with hematuria (N30.01)
    acute prostatitis with hematuria (N41.01)
    hypertrophy (benign) of prostate with hematuria (N40.02)
    recurrent and persistent hematuria in glomerular diseases (N02.-)

R31.0   Gross hematuria

R31.1   Benign essential microscopic hematuria

R31.2   Other microscopic hematuria

R31.9   Hematuria, unspecified

R32 Unspecified urinary incontinence

Includes: enuresis NOS

Excludes1:   nonorganic enuresis (F98.0)
    stress incontinence and other specified urinary incontinence (N39.3-N39.4)

R33 Retention of urine

Excludes1:   psychogenic retention of urine (F45.8)
    retention of urine included with underlying conditions, such as:
    hypertrophy of prostate (N40.01, N40.03)
    nodular prostate (N40.11, N40.13)

R33.0   Drug induced retention of urine
Use additional code to identify the drug

R33.8   Other retention of urine

R33.9   Retention of urine, unspecified

R34 Anuria and oliguria

Excludes1:   anuria and oliguria complicating abortion or ectopic or molar pregnancy (O00-O07, O08.4)
    anuria and oliguria complicating pregnancy (O26.83-)
    anuria and oliguria complicating the puerperium (O90.4)

R35 Polyuria

Excludes1: psychogenic polyuria (F45.8)

R35.0   Frequency of micturition

R35.1   Nocturia

R35.8   Other polyuria
Polyuria NOS

R36 Urethral discharge

R36.0   Urethral discharge without blood

R36.1   Hematospermia

R36.9   Urethral discharge, unspecified
Penile discharge NOS
Urethrorrhea

R37 Sexual dysfunction, unspecified

R39 Other and unspecified symptoms and signs involving the genitourinary system

R39.0   Extravasation of urine

R39.1   Other difficulties with micturition

  R39.11   Hesitancy of micturition

  R39.12   Poor urinary stream

  R39.13   Splitting of urinary stream

  R33.14   Feeling of incomplete bladder emptying

  R39.15   Urgency of urination

  R39.16   Straining to void

  R39.19   Other difficulties with micturition

R39.2   Extrarenal uremia
Prerenal uremia
Excludes1:   uremia NOS (N19)

R39.8   Other symptoms and signs involving the genitourinary system

R39.9   Unspecified symptoms and signs involving the genitourinary system

SYMPTOMS AND SIGNS INVOLVING COGNITION, PERCEPTION, EMOTIONAL STATE AND BEHAVIOR (R40–R46)

Excludes1:   symptoms and signs constituting part of a pattern of mental disorder (F01-F99)

R40 Somnolence, stupor and coma

Excludes1:   neonatal coma (P91.5)
    somnolence, stupor and coma in diabetes (E08-E14)
    somnolence, stupor and coma in hepatic failure (K72.-)
    somnolence, stupor and coma in hypoglycemia (nondiabetic) (E15)

R40.0   Somnolence
Drowsiness

R40.1   Stupor
Catatonic stupor
Semicoma
Excludes1:   catatonic schizophrenia (F20.2)
    depressive stupor (F31-F33)
    dissociative stupor (F44.2)
    manic stupor (F30.2)

R40.2   Coma
Coma NOS
Unconsciousness NOS
Codes first any associated:
    coma in fracture of skull (S02.-)
    coma in intracranial injury (S06.-)
The following extensions are to be added to codes R40.21, R40.22, R40.23:
  a   in the field [EMT or ambulance]
  b   at arrival to emergency department
  c   at hospital admission
  d   24 hours after hospital admission
  e   unspecified time
A code from each subcategory is required to complete the coma scale
Note: These codes are intended primarily for trauma registry and research use but may be ulitized by all users of the classification who wish to collect this information

  R40.20   Unspecified coma

  R40.21   Coma scale, eyes open

    R40.211   Coma scale, eyes open, never

    R40.212   Coma scale, eyes open, to pain

    R40.213   Coma scale, eyes open, to sound

    R40.214   Coma scale, eyes open, spontaneous

  R40.22   Coma scale, best verbal response

    R40.221   Coma scale, best verbal response, none

    R40.222   Coma scale, best verbal response, incomprehensible words

    R40.223   Coma scale, best verbal response, inappropriate words

    R40.224   Coma scale, best verbal response, confused conversation

    R40.225   Coma scale, best verbal response, oriented

  R40.23   Coma scale, best motor response

    R40.231   Coma scale, best motor response, none

    R40.232   Coma scale, best motor response, extension

    R40.233   Coma scale, best motor response, abnormal

    R40.234   Coma scale, best motor response, flexion withdrawal

    R40.235   Coma scale, best motor response, localizes pain

    R40.236   Coma scale, best motor response, obeys commands

R40.3   Persistent vegetative state

R40.4   Transient alteration of awareness

R41 Other symptoms and signs involving cognitive functions and awareness

Excludes1:   dissociative [conversion] disorders (F44.-)

R41.0   Disorientation, unspecified
Confusion NOS
Delirium NOS

R41.1   Anterograde amnesia

R41.2   **Retrograde amnesia**

R41.3   **Other amnesia**
    Amnesia NOS
    Astereognosia
    Excludes1:   amnesic disorder due to known physiologic
                      condition (F04)
                 amnesic syndrome due to psychoactive substance
                      use (F10-F19 with .6)
                 transient global amnesia (G45.4)

R41.4   **Neurologic neglect syndrome**
    Asomatognosia
    Hemi-akinesia
    Hemi-inattention
    Hemispatial neglect
    Left-sided neglect
    Sensory neglect
    Visuospatial neglect

R41.8   **Other symptoms and signs involving cognitive functions and awareness**

  R41.81   **Age-related cognitive decline**
        Senility NOS

  R41.82   **Altered mental status, unspecified**

  R41.83   **Borderline intellectual functioning**
        IQ level 71 to 84
        Excludes1:   mental retardation (F70-F79)

  R41.89   **Other symptoms and signs involving cognitive functions and awareness**
        Anosognosia

R41.9   **Unspecified symptoms and signs involving cognitive functions and awareness**

R42   **Dizziness and giddiness**
    Includes: light-headedness
                vertigo NOS
    Excludes1:   vertiginous syndromes (H81.-)
                 vertigo from infrasound (T75.23)

R43   **Disturbances of smell and taste**

  R43.0   **Anosmia**

  R43.1   **Parosmia**

  R43.2   **Parageusia**

  R43.8   **Other disturbances of smell and taste**
        Mixed disturbance of smell and taste

  R43.9   **Unspecified disturbances of smell and taste**

R44   **Other symptoms and signs involving general sensations and perceptions**
    Excludes1:   alcoholic hallucinations (F10.5)
                 hallucinations in drug psychosis (F11-F19 with .5)
                 hallucinations in mood disorders with psychotic
                      symptoms (F30.2, F31.5, F32.3, F33.3)
                 hallucinations in schizophrenia, schizotypal and
                      delusional disorders (F20-F29)
    Excludes2:   disturbances of skin sensation (R20.-)

  R44.0   **Auditory hallucinations**

  R44.1   **Visual hallucinations**

  R44.2   **Other hallucinations**

  R44.3   **Hallucinations, unspecified**

  R44.8   **Other symptoms and signs involving general sensations and perceptions**

  R44.9   **Unspecified symptoms and signs involving general sensations and perceptions**

R45   **Symptoms and signs involving emotional state**

  R45.0   **Nervousness**
        Nervous tension

  R45.1   **Restlessness and agitation**

  R45.2   **Unhappiness**

  R45.3   **Demoralization and apathy**

  R45.4   **Irritability and anger**

  R45.5   **Hostility**

  R45.6   **Violent behavior**

  R45.7   **State of emotional shock and stress, unspecified**

  R45.8   **Other symptoms and signs involving emotional state**

    R45.81   **Low self-esteem**

    R45.82   **Worries**

    R45.89   **Other symptoms and signs involving emotional state**

R46   **Symptoms and signs involving appearance and behavior**
    Excludes1:   appearance and behavior in schizophrenia, schizotypal
                      and delusional disorders (F20-F29)
                 mental and behavioral disorders (F01-F99)

  R46.0   **Very low level of personal hygiene**

  R46.1   **Bizarre personal appearance**

  R46.2   **Strange and inexplicable behavior**

  R46.3   **Overactivity**

  R46.4   **Slowness and poor responsiveness**
        Excludes1:   stupor (R40.1)

  R46.5   **Suspiciousness and marked evasiveness**

  R46.6   **Undue concern and preoccupation with stressful events**

  R46.7   **Verbosity and circumstantial detail obscuring reason for contact**

  R46.8   **Other symptoms and signs involving appearance and behavior**

    R46.81   **Obsessive-compulsive behavior**
            Excludes1:   obsessive-compulsive disorder (F42)

    R46.89   **Other symptoms and signs involving appearance and behavior**

SYMPTOMS AND SIGNS INVOLVING SPEECH AND VOICE
(R47–R49)

R47   **Speech disturbances, not elsewhere classified**
    Excludes1:   autism (F84.0)
                 cluttering (F98.8)
                 specific developmental disorders of speech and
                      language (F80.-)
                 stuttering [stammering] (F98.5)

  R47.0   **Dysphasia and aphasia**

    R47.01   **Aphasia**
            Excludes1:   progressive isolated aphasia (G31.0)

    R47.02   **Dysphasia**

  R47.1   **Dysarthria and anarthria**

  R47.8   **Other speech disturbances**

    R47.81   **Slurred speech**

    R47.89   **Other speech disturbances**

  R47.9   **Unspecified speech disturbances**

R48   **Dyslexia and other symbolic dysfunctions, not elsewhere classified**
    Excludes1:   specific developmental disorders of scholastic skills
                      (F81.-)

  R48.0   **Dyslexia and alexia**

  R48.1   **Agnosia**
        Autotopagnosia

  R48.2   **Apraxia**

  R48.8   **Other symbolic dysfunctions**
        Acalculia
        Agraphia

  R48.9   **Unspecified symbolic dysfunctions**

R49   **Voice disturbances**
    Excludes1:   psychogenic voice disturbance (F44.4)

  R49.0   **Dysphonia**
        Hoarseness

  R49.1   **Aphonia**
        Loss of voice

  R49.2   **Hypernasality and hyponasality**

    R49.21   **Hypernasality**

    R49.22   **Hyponasality**

  R49.8   **Other voice disturbances**

  R49.9   **Unspecified voice disturbances**
        Change in voice NOS

GENERAL SYMPTOMS AND SIGNS (R50–R69)

R50 Fever
Excludes1: febrile convulsions (R56.0)
fever of unknown origin during labor (O75.2)
fever of unknown origin in newborn (P81.9)
puerperal pyrexia NOS (O86.4)

R50.0 Fever with chills
Fever with rigors

R50.8 Persistent fever

R50.9 Fever, unspecified
Fever of unknown origin [FUO]
Hyperpyrexia NOS
Pyrexia NOS
Excludes1: malignant hyperthermia due to anesthesia (T88.3)

R51 Headache
Includes: facial pain NOS
Excludes1: atypical face pain (G50.1)
migraine and other headache syndromes (G43-G44)
trigeminal neuralgia (G50.0)

R52 Pain, not elsewhere classified
Excludes1: abdomen pain (R10.-)
back pain (M54.9)
breast pain (N64.4)
chest pain (R07.1-R07.9)
ear pain (H92.0-)
eye pain (H57.1)
headache (R51)
joint pain (M25.5-)
limb pain (M79.6-)
lumbar region pain (M54.57)
pelvic and perineal pain (R10.2)
psychogenic pain (F45.4)
shoulder pain (M75.8)
spine pain (M54.-)
throat pain (R07.0)
tongue pain (K14.6)
tooth pain (K08.8)
renal colic (N23)

R52.0 Acute pain
R52.00 Acute pain, unspecified
R52.01 Acute postoperative pain
R52.02 Acute pain in neoplastic disease
Code also neoplasm
R52.09 Other acute pain
R52.1 Chronic intractable pain
R52.10 Chronic intractable pain, unspecified
R52.11 Chronic intractable postoperative pain
R52.12 Chronic intractable pain in neoplastic disease
Code also neoplasm
R52.19 Other chronic intractable pain
R52.2 Other chronic pain
R52.20 Other chronic pain, unspecified
R52.21 Other chronic postoperative pain
R52.22 Other chronic pain in neoplastic disease
Code also neoplasm
R52.29 Other chronic pain
R52.9 Pain, unspecified
Generalized pain NOS

R53 Malaise and fatigue
R53.0 Neoplastic (malignant) related fatigue
Code also associated neoplasm
R53.1 Weakness
Asthenia NOS
Excludes1: age-related weakness (R54)
muscle weakness (M62.8-)
senile asthenia (R54)
R53.2 Functional quadriplegia
Excludes1: hysterical paralysis (F44.4)
immobility syndrome (M62.3)
neurologic quadriplegia (G82.5-)

R53.8 Other malaise and fatigue
Excludes1: combat exhaustion and fatigue (F43.0)
congenital debility (P96.9)
exhaustion and fatigue due to:
depressive episode (F32.-)
excessive exertion (T73.3)
exposure (T73.2)
heat (T67.-)
pregnancy (O26.8-)
recurrent depressive episode (F33)
senile debility (R54)

R53.81 Other malaise
Chronic debility
Debility NOS
General physical deterioration
Malaise NOS
Nervous debility
Excludes1: age-related physical debility (R54)

R53.82 Other fatigue
Fatigue NOS
Lack of energy
Lethargy
Tiredness

R54 Age-related physical debility
Old age
Senescence
Senile asthenia
Senile debility
Excludes1: age-related cognitive decline (R41.81)
senile psychosis (F03)
senility NOS (R41.81)

R55 Syncope and collapse
Includes: blackout
fainting
vasovagal attack
Excludes1: cardiogenic shock (R57.0)
carotid sinus syncope (G90.0)
heat syncope (T67.1)
neurocirculatory asthenia (F45.3)
neurogenic orthostatic hypotension (G90.3)
orthostatic hypotension (I95.1)
postoperative shock (T81.1)
psychogenic syncope (F48.8)
shock NOS (R57.9)
shock complicating or following abortion or ectopic or molar pregnancy (O00-O07, O08.3)
shock complicating or following labor and delivery (O75.1)
Stokes-Adams attack (I45.9)
unconsciousness NOS (R40.2-)

R56 Convulsions, not elsewhere classified
Excludes1: dissociative convulsions and seizures (F44.5)
epileptic convulsions and seizures (G40-G41)
newborn convulsions and seizures (P90)
R56.0 Febrile convulsions
R56.8 Other convulsions
Fit NOS
Seizure (convulsive) NOS
R56.9 Unspecified convulsions

R57 Shock, not elsewhere classified

    Excludes1:   anaphylactic shock due to adverse food reaction (T78.0-)
                   anaphylactic shock due to serum (T80.5)
                   anaphylactic shock NOS (T78.2)
                   anesthetic shock (T88.3)
                   electric shock (T75.4)
                   obstetric shock (O75.1)
                   postoperative shock (T81.1)
                   psychic shock (F43.0)
                   septic shock (A41.9)
                   shock complicating or following ectopic or molar pregnancy (O00-O07,O08.3)
                   shock due to lightning (T75.0)
                   traumatic shock (T79.4)
                   toxic shock syndrome (A48.3)

R57.0 Cardiogenic shock

R57.1 Hypovolemic shock

R57.8 Other shock
    Endotoxic shock

R57.9 Shock, unspecified
    Failure of peripheral circulation NOS

R58 Hemorrhage, not elsewhere classified

    Includes: hemorrhage NOS
    Excludes1:   hemorrhage included with underlying conditions, such as:
                   acute duodenal ulcer with hemorrhage (K26.0)
                   acute gastritis with bleeding (K29.01)
                   ulcerative enterocolitis with rectal bleeding (K51.01)

R59 Enlarged lymph nodes

    Includes: swollen glands
    Excludes1:   acute lymphadenitis (L04.-)
                   chronic lymphadenitis (I88.1)
                   lymphadenitis NOS (I88.9)
                   mesenteric (acute) (chronic) lymphadenitis (I88.0)

R59.0 Localized enlarged lymph nodes

R59.1 Generalized enlarged lymph nodes
    Lymphadenopathy NOS

R59.9 Enlarged lymph nodes, unspecified

R60 Edema, not elsewhere classified

    Excludes1:   angioneurotic edema (T78.3)
                   ascites (R18)
                   cerebral edema (G93.6)
                   cerebral edema due to birth injury (P11.0)
                   edema of larynx (J38.4)
                   edema of nasopharynx (J39.2)
                   edema of pharynx (J39.2)
                   gestational edema (O12.0-)
                   hereditary edema (Q82.0)
                   hydrops fetalis NOS (P83.2)
                   hydrothorax (J94.8)
                   nutritional edema (E40-E46)
                   newborn edema (P83.3)
                   pulmonary edema (J81)

R60.0 Localized edema

R60.1 Generalized edema

R60.9 Edema, unspecified
    Fluid retention NOS

R61 Hyperhidrosis

R61.0 Localized hyperhidrosis

R61.1 Generalized hyperhidrosis

R61.9 Hyperhidrosis, unspecified
    Excessive sweating
    Night sweats
    Excludes1:   night sweats in menopausal and female climacteric states (N95.1)

R62 Lack of expected normal physiological development in childhood and adults

    Excludes1:   delayed puberty (E30.0)

R62.0 Delayed milestone in childhood
    Delayed attainment of expected physiological developmental stage
    Late talker
    Late walker

R62.5 Other and unspecified lack of expected normal physiological development in childhood

    Excludes1:   HIV disease resulting in failure to thrive (B20)
                   physical retardation due to malnutrition (E45)

R62.50 Unspecified lack of expected normal physiological development in childhood
    Infantilism NOS

R62.51 Failure to thrive (child)
    Failure to gain weight

R62.52 Short stature (child)
    Lack of growth
    Physical retardation

R62.59 Other lack of expected normal physiological development in childhood

R62.7 Adult failure to thrive

R63 Symptoms and signs concerning food and fluid intake

    Excludes1:   bulimia NOS (F50.2)
                   eating disorders of nonorganic origin (F50.-)
                   malnutrition (E40-E46)

R63.0 Anorexia
    Loss of appetite
    Excludes1:   anorexia nervosa (F50.0-)
                   loss of appetite of nonorganic origin (F50.8)

R63.1 Polydipsia
    Excessive thirst

R63.2 Polyphagia
    Excessive eating
    Hyperalimentation NOS

R63.3 Feeding difficulties and mismanagement
    Feeding problem NOS
    Excludes1:   feeding problems of newborn (P92.-)
                   infant feeding disorder of nonorganic origin (F98.2-)

R63.4 Abnormal weight loss

R63.5 Abnormal weight gain
    Excludes1:   excessive weight gain in pregnancy (O26.0-)
                   obesity (E66.-)

R63.6 Underweight
    Excludes1:   abnormal weight loss (R63.4)
                   anorexia nervosa (F50.0-)
                   malnutrition (E40-E46)

R63.8 Other symptoms and signs concerning food and fluid intake

R64 Cachexia

    Includes: wasting syndrome
    Excludes1:   abnormal weight loss (R63.4)
                   malignant cachexia (C80.0)
                   nutritional marasmus (E41)

R68 Other general symptoms and signs

R68.0 Hypothermia, not associated with low environmental temperature
    Excludes1:   hypothermia due to anesthesia (T88.5)
                   hypothermia due to low environmental temperature (T68)
                   hypothermia NOS (accidental) (T68)
                   newborn hypothermia (P80.-)

R68.1 Nonspecific symptoms peculiar to infancy
    Excludes1:   colic, infantile (R10.43)
                   neonatal cerebral irritability (P91.3)
                   teething syndrome (K00.7)

R68.11 Excessive crying of infant

R68.12 Fussy baby
    Irritable infant

R68.19 Other nonspecific symptoms peculiar to infancy

R68.2   **Dry mouth, unspecified**

Excludes1:   dry mouth due to dehydration (E86)
dry mouth due to sicca syndrome [Sjögren]
(M35.0-)
salivary gland hyposecretion (K11.7)

R68.3   **Clubbing of fingers**
Clubbing of nails

Excludes1:   congenital clubfinger (Q68.1)

R68.8   **Other specified general symptoms and signs**

R69   **Illness NOS**

Includes: unknown and unspecified cases of morbidity

ABNORMAL FINDINGS ON EXAMINATION OF BLOOD, WITHOUT DIAGNOSIS (R70–R79)

Excludes1:   abnormalities (of)(on):
antenatal screening of mother (O28.-)
coagulation hemorrhagic disorders (D65-D68)
lipids (E78.-)
platelets and thrombocytes (D69.-)
white blood cells classified elsewhere (D70-D72)
diagnostic abnormal findings classified elsewhere—see
Alphabetical Index
hemorrhagic and hematological disorders of fetus and
newborn (P50-P61)

R70   **Elevated erythrocyte sedimentation rate and abnormality of plasma viscosity**

R70.0   **Elevated erythrocyte sedimentation rate**

R70.1   **Abnormal plasma viscosity**

R71   **Abnormality of red blood cells**

Excludes1:   anemias (D50-D64)
anemia of premature infant (P61.2)
benign (familial) polycythemia (D75.0)
congenital anemias (P61.2-P61.4)
newborn anemia due to isoimmunization (P55.-)
polycythemia neonatorum (P61.1)
polycythemia vera (D45)
secondary polycythemia (D75.1)

R71.0   **Precipitous drop in hematocrit**
Drop in hematocrit

R71.8   **Other abnormality of red blood cells**
Abnormal red-cell morphology NOS
Abnormal red-cell volume NOS
Anisocytosis
Poikilocytosis

R72   **Abnormality of white blood cells, not elsewhere classified**

Excludes1:   leukemoid reaction (D7.8)

R72.0   **Elevated white blood cell count**
Leukocytosis
Lymphocytosis
Monocytosis
Plasmacytosis

R72.1   **Decreased white blood cell count**
Lymphopenia

R72.8   **Other abnormality of white blood cells**
Abnormal leukocyte differential NOS

R73   **Elevated blood glucose level**

Excludes1:   diabetes mellitus (E08-E14)
diabetes mellitus in pregnancy, childbirth and the
puerperium (O24.-)
neonatal disorders (P70.0-P70.2)
postsurgical hypoinsulinemia (E89.1)

R73.0   **Abnormal glucose tolerance test**
Chemical diabetes
Impaired glucose tolerance
Latent diabetes
Prediabetes

Excludes1:   abnormal glucose tolerance test in pregnancy
(O99.82)

R73.9   **Hyperglycemia, unspecified**

R74   **Abnormal serum enzyme levels**

R74.0   **Nonspecific elevation of levels of transaminase and lactic acid dehydrogenase [LDH]**

R74.8   **Abnormal levels of other serum enzymes**
Abnormal level of acid phosphatase
Abnormal level of alkaline phosphatase
Abnormal level of amylase
Abnormal level of lipase [triacylglycerol lipase]

R74.9   **Abnormal serum enzyme level, unspecified**

R75   **Inconclusive laboratory evidence of human immunodeficiency virus [HIV]**

Includes: nonconclusive HIV-test finding in infants

Excludes1:   asymptomatic human immunodeficiency virus [HIV]
infection status (Z21)
human immunodeficiency virus [HIV] disease (B20)

R76   **Other abnormal immunological findings in serum**

R76.0   **Raised antibody titer**

Excludes1:   isoimmunization affecting fetus or newborn
(P55.-)
isoimmunization in pregnancy (O36.0-O36.1)

R76.1   **Abnormal reaction to tuberculin test**
Abnormal result of Mantoux test

R76.8   **Other specified abnormal immunological findings in serum**

R76.81   **Elevated prostate specific antigen (PSA)**

R76.89   **Other specified abnormal immunological findings in serum**
Raised level of immunoglobulins NOS

R76.9   **Abnormal immunological finding in serum, unspecified**

R77   **Other abnormalities of plasma proteins**

Excludes1:   disorders of plasma-protein metabolism (E88.0)

R77.0   **Abnormality of albumin**

R77.1   **Abnormality of globulin**
Hyperglobulinemia NOS

R77.2   **Abnormality of alphafetoprotein**

R77.8   **Other specified abnormalities of plasma proteins**

R77.9   **Abnormality of plasma protein, unspecified**

R78   **Findings of drugs and other substances, not normally found in blood**

Excludes1:   mental or behavioral disorders due to psychoactive
substance use (F10-F19)

R78.0   **Finding of alcohol in blood**
Use additional external cause code (Y90.-), for detail regarding
alcohol level.

R78.1   **Finding of opiate drug in blood**

R78.2   **Finding of cocaine in blood**

R78.3   **Finding of hallucinogen in blood**

R78.4   **Finding of other drugs of addictive potential in blood**

R78.5   **Finding of other psychotropic drug in blood**

R78.6   **Finding of steroid agent in blood**

R78.7   **Finding of abnormal level of heavy metals in blood**

R78.8   **Finding of other specified substances, not normally found in blood**

R78.81   **Bacteremia**

R78.89   **Finding of other specified substances, not normally found in blood**
Finding of abnormal level of lithium in blood

R78.9   **Finding of unspecified substance, not normally found in blood**

R79   **Other abnormal findings of blood chemistry**

Excludes1:   abnormality of fluid, electrolyte or acid-base balance
(E86-E87)
asymptomatic hyperuricemia (E79.0)
hyperglycemia NOS (R73.9)
hypoglycemia NOS (E16.2)
neonatal hypoglycemia (P70.3-P70.4)
specific findings indicating disorder of:
amino-acid metabolism (E70-E72)
carbohydrate metabolism (E73-E74)
lipid metabolism (E75.-)

R79.0 **Abnormal level of blood mineral**
Abnormal blood level of cobalt
Abnormal blood level of copper
Abnormal blood level of iron
Abnormal blood level of magnesium
Abnormal blood level of mineral NEC
Abnormal blood level of zinc
Excludes1: abnormal level of lithium (R78.8)
disorders of mineral metabolism (E83.-)
neonatal hypomagnesemia (P71.2)
nutritional mineral deficiency (E58-E61)

R79.1 **Pancytopenia**

R79.2 **Abnormal coagulation profile**
Abnormal or prolonged bleeding time
Abnormal or prolonged coagulation time
Abnormal or prolonged partial thromboplastin time [PTT]
Abnormal or prolonged prothrombin time [PT]
Excludes1: coagulation defects (D68.-)

R79.8 **Other specified abnormal findings of blood chemistry**
R79.81 **Abnormal blood-gas level**
R79.89 **Other specified abnormal findings of blood chemistry**

R79.9 **Abnormal finding of blood chemistry, unspecified**

ABNORMAL FINDINGS ON EXAMINATION OF URINE, WITHOUT DIAGNOSIS (R80–R82)

Excludes1: abnormal findings on antenatal screening of mother (O28.-)
diagnostic abnormal findings classified elsewhere - see Alphabetical Index
specific findings indicating disorder of:
amino-acid metabolism (E70-E72)
carbohydrate metabolism (E73-E74)

R80 **Proteinuria**
Excludes1: gestational proteinuria (O12.1-)

R80.0 **Isolated proteinuria**
Idipoathic proteinuria
Excludes1: isolated proteinuria with specific morphological lesion (N06.-)

R80.1 **Persistent proteinuria, unspecified**

R80.2 **Orthostatic proteinuria, unspecified**
Postural proteinuria

R80.3 **Bence Jones proteinuria**

R80.8 **Other proteinuria**

R80.9 **Proteinuria NOS**
Albuminuria NOS

R81 **Glycosuria**
Excludes1: renal glycosuria (E74.8)

R82 **Other and unspecified abnormal findings in urine**
Includes: chromoabnormalities in urine
Excludes2: hematuria (R31.-)

R82.0 **Chyluria**
Excludes1: filarial chyluria (B74.-)

R82.1 **Myoglobinuria**

R82.2 **Biliuria**

R82.3 **Hemoglobinuria**
Excludes1: hemoglobinuria due to hemolysis from external causes NEC (D59.6)
hemoglobinuria due to paroxysmal nocturnal [Marchiafava-Micheli] (D59.5)

R82.4 **Acetonuria**
Ketonuria

R82.5 **Elevated urine levels of drugs, medicaments and biological substances**
Elevated urine levels of catecholamines
Elevated urine levels of indoleacetic acid
Elevated urine levels of 17-ketosteroids
Elevated urine levels of steroids

R82.6 **Abnormal urine levels of substances chiefly nonmedicinal as to source**
Abnormal urine level of heavy metals

R82.7 **Abnormal findings on microbiological examination of urine**
Positive culture findings of urine

R82.8 **Abnormal findings on cytological and histological examination of urine**

R82.9 **Other and unspecified abnormal findings in urine**
R82.90 **Unspecified abnormal findings in urine**
R82.91 **Other chromoabnormalities of urine**
Chromoconversion (dipstick)
Idiopathic dipstick converts positive for blood with no cellular forms in sediment
Excludes1: hemoglobinuria (R82.3)
myoglobinuria (R82.1)
R82.99 **Other abnormal findings in urine**
Cells and casts in urine
Crystalluria
Melanuria

ABNORMAL FINDINGS ON EXAMINATION OF OTHER BODY FLUIDS, SUBSTANCES AND TISSUES, WITHOUT DIAGNOSIS (R83–R89)

Excludes1: abnormal findings on antenatal screening of mother (O28.-)
diagnostic abnormal findings classified elsewhere—see Alphabetical Index
Excludes2: abnormal findings on examination of blood, without diagnosis (R70-R79)
abnormal findings on examination of urine, without diagnosis (R80-R82)

R83 **Abnormal findings in cerebrospinal fluid**
R83.0 **Abnormal level of enzymes in cerebrospinal fluid**
R83.2 **Abnormal level of other drugs, medicaments and biological substances in cerebrospinal fluid**
R83.3 **Abnormal level of substances chiefly nonmedicinal as to source in cerebrospinal fluid**
R83.4 **Abnormal immunological findings in cerebrospinal fluid**
R83.5 **Abnormal microbiological findings in cerebrospinal fluid**
Positive culture findings in cerebrospinal fluid
R83.6 **Abnormal cytological findings in cerebrospinal fluid**
R83.7 **Abnormal histological findings in cerebrospinal fluid**
R83.8 **Other abnormal findings in cerebrospinal fluid**
Abnormal chromosomal findings in cerebrospinal fluid
R83.9 **Unspecified abnormal finding in cerebrospinal fluid**

R84 **Abnormal findings in specimens from respiratory organs and thorax**
Includes: abnormal findings in bronchial washings
abnormal findings in nasal secretions
abnormal findings in pleural fluid
abnormal findings in sputum
abnormal findings in throat scrapings
Excludes1: blood-stained sputum (R04.2)
R84.0 **Abnormal level of enzymes in specimens from respiratory organs and thorax**
R84.2 **Abnormal level of other drugs, medicaments and biological substances in specimens from respiratory organs and thorax**
R84.3 **Abnormal level of substances chiefly nonmedicinal as to source in specimens from respiratory organs and thorax**
R84.4 **Abnormal immunological findings in specimens from respiratory organs and thorax**
R84.5 **Abnormal microbiological findings in specimens from respiratory organs and thorax**
Positive culture findings in specimens from respiratory organs and thorax
R84.6 **Abnormal cytological findings in specimens from respiratory organs and thorax**
R84.7 **Abnormal histological findings in specimens from respiratory organs and thorax**
R84.8 **Other abnormal findings in specimens from respiratory organs and thorax**
Abnormal chromosomal findings in specimens from respiratory organs and thorax
R84.9 **Unspecified abnormal finding in specimens from respiratory organs and thorax**

R85   Abnormal findings in specimens from digestive organs and abdominal cavity

    Includes: abnormal findings in peritoneal fluid
                           abnormal findings in saliva

    Excludes1:   cloudy peritoneal dialysis effluent (R88.0)
                           fecal abnormalities (R19.5)

R85.0   Abnormal level of enzymes in specimens from digestive organs and abdominal cavity

R85.1   Abnormal level of hormones in specimens from digestive organs and abdominal cavity

R85.2   Abnormal level of other drugs, medicaments and biological substances in specimens from digestive organs and abdominal cavity

R85.3   Abnormal level of substances chiefly nonmedicinal as to source in specimens from digestive organs and abdominal cavity

R85.4   Abnormal immunological findings in specimens from digestive organs and abdominal cavity

R85.5   Abnormal microbiological findings in specimens from digestive organs and abdominal cavity
     Positive culture findings in specimens from digestive organs and abdominal cavity

R85.6   Abnormal cytological findings in specimens from digestive organs and abdominal cavity

R85.7   Abnormal histological findings in specimens from digestive organs and abdominal cavity

R85.8   Other abnormal findings in specimens from digestive organs and abdominal cavity
     Abnormal chromosomal findings in specimens from digestive organs and abdominal cavity

R85.9   Unspecified abnormal finding in specimens from digestive organs and abdominal cavity

R86   Abnormal findings in specimens from male genital organs

    Includes: abnormal findings in prostatic secretions
                           abnormal findings in semen, seminal fluid
                           abnormal spermatozoa

    Excludes1:   azoospermia (N46.0-)
                           oligospermia (N46.1-)

R86.0   Abnormal level of enzymes in specimens from male genital organs

R86.1   Abnormal level of hormones in specimens from male genital organs

R86.2   Abnormal level of other drugs, medicaments and biological substances in specimens from male genital organs

R86.3   Abnormal level of substances chiefly nonmedicinal as to source in specimens from male genital organs

R86.4   Abnormal immunological findings in specimens from male genital organs

R86.5   Abnormal microbiological findings in specimens from male genital organs
     Positive culture findings in specimens from male genital organs

R86.6   Abnormal cytological findings in specimens from male genital organs

R86.7   Abnormal histological findings in specimens from male genital organs

R86.8   Other abnormal findings in specimens from male genital organs
     Abnormal chromosomal findings in specimens from male genital organs

R86.9   Unspecified abnormal finding in specimens from male genital organs

R87   Abnormal findings in specimens from female genital organs

    Includes: abnormal findings in secretion and smears from cervix uteri
                           abnormal findings in secretion and smears from vagina
                           abnormal findings in secretion and smears from vulva

    Excludes1:   carcinoma in situ (D05-D07.3)
                           dysplasia of cervix uteri (N87.-)
                           dysplasia of vagina (N89.0-N89.3)
                           dysplasia of vulva (N90.0-N90.3)

R87.0   Abnormal level of enzymes in specimens from female genital organs

R87.1   Abnormal level of hormones in specimens from female genital organs

R87.2   Abnormal level of other drugs, medicaments and biological substances in specimens from female genital organs

R87.3   Abnormal level of substances chiefly nonmedicinal as to source in specimens from female genital organs

R87.4   Abnormal immunological findings in specimens from female genital organs

R87.5   Abnormal microbiological findings in specimens from female genital organs
     Positive culture findings in specimens from female genital organs

R87.6   Abnormal cytological findings in specimens from female genital organs
     Abnormal Papanicolaou smear

R87.7   Abnormal histological findings in specimens from female genital organs

R87.8   Other abnormal findings in specimens from female genital organs
     Abnormal chromosomal findings in specimens from female genital organs

R87.9   Unspecified abnormal finding in specimens from female genital organs

R88   Abnormal findings in other body fluids and substances

R88.0   Cloudy (hemodialysis) (peritoneal) dialysis effluent

R88.8   Abnormal findings in other body fluids and substances

R89   Abnormal findings in specimens from other organs, systems and tissues

    Includes: abnormal findings in nipple discharge
                           abnormal findings in synovial fluid
                           abnormal findings in wound secretions

R89.0   Abnormal level of enzymes in specimens from other organs, systems and tissues

R89.1   Abnormal level of hormones in specimens from other organs, systems and tissues

R89.2   Abnormal level of other drugs, medicaments and biological substances in specimens from other organs, systems and tissues

R89.3   Abnormal level of substances chiefly nonmedicinal as to source in specimens from other organs, systems and tissues

R89.4   Abnormal immunological findings in specimens from other organs, systems and tissues

R89.5   Abnormal microbiological findings in specimens from other organs, systems and tissues
     Positive culture findings in specimens from other organs, systems and tissues

R89.6   Abnormal cytological findings in specimens from other organs, systems and tissues

R89.7   Abnormal histological findings in specimens from other organs, systems and tissues

R89.8   Other abnormal findings in specimens from other organs, systems and tissues
     Abnormal chromosomal findings in specimens from other organs, systems and tissues

R89.9   Unspecified abnormal finding in specimens from other organs, systems and tissues

ABNORMAL FINDINGS ON DIAGNOSTIC IMAGING AND IN FUNCTION STUDIES, WITHOUT DIAGNOSIS (R90-R94)

    Includes: nonspecific abnormal findings on diagnostic imaging by:
                           computerized axial tomography [CAT scan]
                           magnetic resonance imaging [MRI][NMR]
                           positron emission tomography [PET scan]
                           thermography
                           ultrasound [echogram]
                           X-ray examination

    Excludes1:   abnormal findings on antenatal screening of mother (O28.-)
                           diagnostic abnormal findings classified elsewhere - see Alphabetical Index

R90   Abnormal findings on diagnostic imaging of central nervous system

R90.0   Intracranial space-occupying lesion found on diagnostic imaging of central nervous system

R90.8   Other abnormal findings on diagnostic imaging of central nervous system
Abnormal echoencephalogram
Cerebrovascular abnormality found on diagnostic imaging of central nervous system

R91   Abnormal findings on diagnostic imaging of lung
Includes: coin lesion NOS found on diagnostic imaging of lung
lung mass NOS found on diagnostic imaging of lung

R92   Abnormal findings on diagnostic imaging of breast

R92.0   Mammographic microcalcification found on diagnostic imaging of breast

R92.8   Other abnormal findings on diagnostic imaging of breast

R93   Abnormal findings on diagnostic imaging of other body structures

R93.0   Abnormal findings on diagnostic imaging of skull and head, not elsewhere classified
Excludes1:   intracranial space-occupying lesion found on diagnostic imaging (R90.0)

R93.1   Abnormal findings on diagnostic imaging of heart and coronary circulation
Abnormal echocardiogram NOS
Abnormal heart shadow

R93.2   Abnormal findings on diagnostic imaging of liver and biliary tract
Nonvisualization of gallbladder

R93.3   Abnormal findings on diagnostic imaging of other parts of digestive tract

R93.4   Abnormal findings on diagnostic imaging of urinary organs
Filling defect of bladder found on diagnostic imaging
Filling defect of kidney found on diagnostic imaging
Filling defect of ureter found on diagnostic imaging
Excludes1:   hypertrophy of kidney (N28.81)

R93.5   Abnormal findings on diagnostic imaging of other abdominal regions, including retroperitoneum

R93.6   Abnormal findings on diagnostic imaging of limbs
Excludes2:   abnormal finding in skin and subcutaneous tissue (R93.8)

R93.7   Abnormal findings on diagnostic imaging of other parts of musculoskeletal system
Excludes2:   abnormal findings on diagnostic imaging of skull (R93.0)

R93.8   Abnormal findings on diagnostic imaging of other specified body structures
Abnormal finding by radioisotope localization of placenta
Abnormal radiological finding in skin and subcutaneous tissue
Mediastinal shift

R94   Abnormal results of function studies
Includes: abnormal results of radionuclide [radioisotope] uptake studies
abnormal results of scintigraphy

R94.0   Abnormal results of function studies of central nervous system
Abnormal electroencephalogram [EEG]

R94.1   Abnormal results of function studies of peripheral nervous system and special senses
Abnormal electromyogram [EMG]
Abnormal electro-oculogram [EOG]
Abnormal electroretinogram [ERG]
Abnormal response to nerve stimulation
Abnormal visually evoked potential [VEP]

R94.2   Abnormal results of pulmonary function studies
Reduced ventilatory capacity
Reduced vital capacity

R94.3   Abnormal results of cardiovascular function studies
Abnormal electrocardiogram [ECG] [EKG]
Abnormal electrophysiological intracardiac studies
Abnormal phonocardiogram
Abnormal vectorcardiogram

R94.4   Abnormal results of kidney function studies
Abnormal renal function test

R94.5   Abnormal results of liver function studies

R94.6   Abnormal results of thyroid function studies

R94.7   Abnormal results of other endocrine function studies
Excludes2:   abnormal glucose tolerance test (R73.0)

R94.8   Abnormal results of function studies of other organs and systems
Abnormal basal metabolic rate [BMR]
Abnormal bladder function test
Abnormal splenic function test

ILL-DEFINED AND UNKNOWN CAUSE OF MORTALITY (R99)

R99   Ill-defined and unknown cause of mortality
Includes: Death NOS
Unspecified cause of mortality

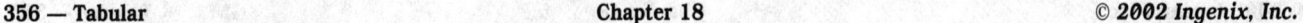

CHAPTER XIX — INJURY, POISONING AND CERTAIN OTHER CONSEQUENCES OF EXTERNAL CAUSES (S00–T88)

INJURY (S00–S49)

Use secondary code from Chapter XX, External causes of morbidity, to indicate cause of injury

Excludes1:   birth trauma (P10-P15)
         obstetric trauma (O70-O71)

This chapter contains the following blocks:

S00-S09	Injuries to the head
S10-S19	Injuries to the neck
S20-S29	Injuries to the thorax
S30-S39	Injuries to the abdomen, lower back, lumbar spine and pelvis
S40-S49	Injuries to the shoulder and upper arm
S50-S59	Injuries to the elbow and forearm
S60-S69	Injuries to the wrist and hand
S70-S79	Injuries to the hip and thigh
S80-S89	Injuries to the knee and lower leg
S90-S99	Injuries to the ankle and foot
T07	Unspecified multiple injuries
T14	Injury of unspecified body region
T15-T19	Effects of foreign body entering through natural orifice
T20-T32	Burns and corrosions
T33-T34	Frostbite
T36-T50	Poisoning by drugs, medicaments and biological substances
T51-T65	Toxic effects of substances chiefly nonmedicinal as to source
T66-T78	Other and unspecified effects of external causes
T79	Certain early complications of trauma
T80-T88	Complications of surgical and medical care, not elsewhere classified

The chapter uses the S-section for coding different types of injuries related to single body regions and the T-section to cover injuries to unspecified body regions as well as poisoning and certain other consequences of external causes.

INJURIES TO THE HEAD (S00–S09)

Includes: injuries of ear
          injuries of eye
          injuries of face [any part]
          injuries of gum
          injuries of jaw
          injuries of mandibular joint area
          injuries of oral cavity
          injuries of palate
          injuries of periocular area
          injuries of scalp
          injuries of tongue
          injuries of tooth

Code also for any associated infection

Excludes2:   burns and corrosions (T20-T32)
         effects of foreign body in ear (T16)
         effects of foreign body in larynx (T17.3)
         effects of foreign body in mouth NOS (T18.0)
         effects of foreign body in nose (T17.0-T17.1)
         effects of foreign body in pharynx (T17.2)
         effects of foreign body on external eye (T15.-)
         frostbite (T33-T34)
         insect bite or sting, venomous (T63.4)

S00   **Superficial injury of head**

Excludes1:   diffuse cerebral contusion (S06.2-)
         focal cerebral contusion (S06.3-)
         injury of eye and orbit (S05.-)
         open wound of head (S01.-)

The following extensions are to be added to each code for this category:
- a   initial encounter
- d   subsequent encounter
- q   sequela

S00.0   **Superficial injury of scalp**

   S00.00   **Unspecified superficial injury of scalp**

   S00.01   **Abrasion of scalp**

   S00.02   **Blister (nonthermal) of scalp**

   S00.03   **Contusion of scalp**
              Bruise of scalp
              Hematoma of scalp

   S00.04   **External constriction of part of scalp**

   S00.05   **Superficial foreign body of scalp**
              Splinter in the scalp

   S00.06   **Insect bite (nonvenomous) of scalp**

   S00.07   **Other superficial bite of scalp**
         Excludes1:   open bite of scalp (S01.05)

S00.1   **Contusion of eyelid and periocular area**
     Black eye
     Excludes2:   contusion of eyeball and orbital tissues (S05.1)

   S00.10   **Contusion of unspecified eyelid and periocular area**

   S00.11   **Contusion of right eyelid and periocular area**

   S00.12   **Contusion of left eyelid and periocular area**

S00.2   **Other and unspecified superficial injuries of eyelid and periocular area**
     Excludes2:   superficial injury of conjunctiva and cornea (S05.0-)

   S00.20   **Unspecified superficial injury of eyelid and periocular area**

       S00.201   **Unspecified superficial injury of right eyelid and periocular area**

       S00.202   **Unspecified superficial injury of left eyelid and periocular area**

       S00.209   **Unspecified superficial injury of unspecified eyelid and periocular area**

   S00.21   **Abrasion of eyelid and periocular area**

       S00.211   **Abrasion of right eyelid and periocular area**

       S00.212   **Abrasion of left eyelid and periocular area**

       S00.219   **Abrasion of unspecified eyelid and periocular area**

   S00.22   **Blister (nonthermal) of eyelid and periocular area**

       S00.221   **Blister (nonthermal) of right eyelid and periocular area**

       S00.222   **Blister (nonthermal) of left eyelid and periocular area**

       S00.229   **Blister (nonthermal) of unspecified eyelid and periocular area**

   S00.24   **External constriction of eyelid and periocular area**

       S00.241   **External constriction of right eyelid and periocular area**

       S00.242   **External constriction of left eyelid and periocular area**

       S00.249   **External constriction of unspecified eyelid and periocular area**

   S00.25   **Superficial foreign body of eyelid and periocular area**
         Splinter of eyelid and periocular area
         Excludes2:   other specified disorders of eyelid (H02.8-)

       S00.251   **Superficial foreign body of right eyelid and periocular area**

       S00.252   **Superficial foreign body of left eyelid and periocular area**

       S00.259   **Superficial foreign body of unspecified eyelid and periocular area**

   S00.26   **Insect bite (nonvenomous) of eyelid and periocular area**

       S00.261   **Insect bite (nonvenomous) of right eyelid and periocular area**

       S00.262   **Insect bite (nonvenomous) of left eyelid and periocular area**

S00.269 Insect bite (nonvenomous) of unspecified eyelid and periocular area

S00.27 Other superficial bite of eyelid and periocular area

Excludes1:   open bite of eyelid and periocular area (S01.15)

S00.271 Other superficial bite of right eyelid and periocular area

S00.272 Other superficial bite of left eyelid and periocular area

S00.279 Other superficial bite of unspecified eyelid and periocular area

S00.3   Superficial injury of nose

S00.30 Unspecified superficial injury of nose

S00.31 Abrasion of nose

S00.32 Blister (nonthermal) of nose

S00.33 Contusion of nose
Bruise of nose
Hematoma of nose

S00.34 External constriction of nose

S00.35 Superficial foreign body of nose
Splinter in the nose

S00.36 Insect bite (nonvenomous) of nose

S00.37 Other superficial bite of nose
Excludes1:   open bite of nose (S01.25)

S00.4   Superficial injury of ear

S00.40 Unspecified superficial injury of ear

S00.401 Unspecified superficial injury of right ear

S00.402 Unspecified superficial injury of left ear

S00.409 Unspecified superficial injury of unspecified ear

S00.41 Abrasion of ear

S00.411 Abrasion of right ear

S00.412 Abrasion of left ear

S00.419 Abrasion of unspecified ear

S00.42 Blister (nonthermal) of ear

S00.421 Blister (nonthermal) of right ear

S00.422 Blister (nonthermal) of left ear

S00.429 Blister (nonthermal) of unspecified ear

S00.43 Contusion of ear
Bruise of ear
Hematoma of ear

S00.431 Contusion of right ear

S00.432 Contusion of left ear

S00.439 Contusion of unspecified ear

S00.44 External constriction of ear

S00.441 External constriction of right ear

S00.442 External constriction of left ear

S00.449 External constriction of unspecified ear

S00.45 Superficial foreign body of ear
Splinter in the ear

S00.451 Superficial foreign body of right ear

S00.452 Superficial foreign body of left ear

S00.459 Superficial foreign body of unspecified ear

S00.46 Insect bite (nonvenomous) of ear

S00.461 Insect bite (nonvenomous) of right ear

S00.462 Insect bite (nonvenomous) of left ear

S00.469 Insect bite (nonvenomous) of unspecified ear

S00.47 Other superficial bite of ear
Excludes1:   open bite of ear (S01.35)

S00.471 Other superficial bite of right ear

S00.472 Other superficial bite of left ear

S00.479 Other superficial bite of unspecified ear

S00.5   Superficial injury of lip and oral cavity

S00.50 Unspecified superficial injury of lip and oral cavity

S00.501 Unspecified superficial injury of lip

S00.502 Unspecified superficial injury of oral cavity

S00.51 Abrasion of lip and oral cavity

S00.511 Abrasion of lip

S00.512 Abrasion of oral cavity

S00.52 Blister (nonthermal) of lip and oral cavity

S00.521 Blister (nonthermal) of lip

S00.522 Blister (nonthermal) of oral cavity

S00.53 Contusion of lip and oral cavity

S00.531 Contusion of lip
Bruise of lip

S00.532 Contusion of oral cavity
Hematoma of oral cavity

S00.54 External constriction of lip and oral cavity

S00.541 External constriction of lip

S00.542 External constriction of oral cavity

S00.55 Superficial foreign body of lip and oral cavity

S00.551 Superficial foreign body of lip
Splinter of lip

S00.552 Superficial foreign body of oral cavity
Splinter of oral cavity

S00.56 Insect bite (nonvenomous) of lip and oral cavity

S00.561 Insect bite (nonvenomous) of lip

S00.562 Insect bite (nonvenomous) of oral cavity

S00.57 Other superficial bite of lip and oral cavity

S00.571 Other superficial bite of lip
Excludes1:   open bite of lip (S01.551)

S00.572 Other superficial bite of oral cavity
Excludes1:   open bite of oral cavity (S01.552)

S00.8   Superficial injury of other parts of head

S00.80 Unspecified superficial injury of other part of head

S00.81 Abrasion of other part of head

S00.82 Blister (nonthermal) of other part of head

S00.83 Contusion of other part of head
Bruise of other part of head
Hematoma of other part of head

S00.84 External constriction of other part of head

S00.85 Superficial foreign body of other part of head
Splinter in other part of head

S00.86 Insect bite (nonvenomous) of other part of head

S00.87 Other superficial bite of other part of head
Excludes1:   open bite of other part of head (S01.87)

S00.9   Superficial injury of unspecified part of head

S00.90 Unspecified superficial injury of unspecified part of head

S00.91 Abrasion of unspecified part of head

S00.92 Blister (nonthermal) of unspecified part of head

S00.93 Contusion of unspecified part of head
Bruise of head
Hematoma of head

S00.94 External constriction of unspecified part of head

S00.95 Superficial foreign body of unspecified part of head
Splinter of head

S00.96 Insect bite (nonvenomous) of unspecified part of head

S00.97 Other superficial bite of unspecified part of head
Excludes1:   open bite of head (S01.95)

S01 Open wound of head
Code also any associated:
injury of cranial nerve (S04.-)
injury of muscle and tendon of head (S09.1-)
intracranial injury (S06.-)
wound infection
Excludes1:   open skull fracture (S02.- with extension b)
Excludes2:   injury of eye and orbit (S05.-)
traumatic amputation of part of head (S08.-)
The following extensions are to be added to each code for this category:
a   initial encounter
d   subsequent encounter
q   sequela

S01.0   Open wound of scalp
Excludes1:   avulsion of scalp (S08.0)

S01.00 Unspecified open wound of scalp

S01.01 Laceration without foreign body of scalp
S01.02 Laceration with foreign body of scalp
S01.03 Puncture wound without foreign body of scalp
S01.04 Puncture wound with foreign body of scalp
S01.05 Open bite of scalp
Bite of scalp NOS
Excludes1: superficial bite of scalp (S00.06, S00.07-)

S01.1 Open wound of eyelid and periocular area
Open wound of eyelid and periocular area with or without involvement of lacrimal passages
Excludes2: other specified disorders of eyelid (H02.8-)
S01.10 Unspecified open wound of eyelid and periocular area
S01.101 Unspecified open wound of right eyelid and periocular area
S01.102 Unspecified open wound of left eyelid and periocular area
S01.109 Unspecified open wound of unspecified eyelid and periocular area
S01.11 Laceration without foreign body of eyelid and periocular area
S01.111 Laceration without foreign body of right eyelid and periocular area
S01.112 Laceration without foreign body of left eyelid and periocular area
S01.119 Laceration without foreign body of unspecified eyelid and periocular area
S01.12 Laceration with foreign body of eyelid and periocular area
Excludes2: other specified disorders of eyelid (H02.8-)
S01.121 Laceration with foreign body of right eyelid and periocular area
S01.122 Laceration with foreign body of left eyelid and periocular area
S01.129 Laceration with foreign body of unspecified eyelid and periocular area
S01.13 Puncture wound without foreign body of eyelid and periocular area
S01.131 Puncture wound without foreign body of right eyelid and periocular area
S01.132 Puncture wound without foreign body of left eyelid and periocular area
S01.139 Puncture wound without foreign body of unspecified eyelid and periocular area
S01.14 Puncture wound with foreign body of eyelid and periocular area
S01.141 Puncture wound with foreign body of right eyelid and periocular area
S01.142 Puncture wound with foreign body of left eyelid and periocular area
S01.149 Puncture wound with foreign body of unspecified eyelid and periocular area
S01.15 Open bite of eyelid and periocular area
Bite of eyelid and periocular area NOS
Excludes1: superficial bite of eyelid and periocular area (S00.26, S00.27)
S01.151 Open bite of right eyelid and periocular area
S01.152 Open bite of left eyelid and periocular area
S01.159 Open bite of unspecified eyelid and periocular area

S01.2 Open wound of nose
S01.20 Unspecified open wound of nose
S01.21 Laceration without foreign body of nose
S01.22 Laceration with foreign body of nose
S01.23 Puncture wound without foreign body of nose
S01.24 Puncture wound with foreign body of nose
S01.25 Open bite of nose
Bite of nose NOS
Excludes1: superficial bite of nose (S00.36, S00.37)

S01.3 Open wound of ear
S01.30 Unspecified open wound of ear
S01.301 Unspecified open wound of right ear
S01.302 Unspecified open wound of left ear
S01.309 Unspecified open wound of unspecified ear
S01.31 Laceration without foreign body of ear
S01.311 Laceration without foreign body of right ear
S01.312 Laceration without foreign body of left ear
S01.319 Laceration without foreign body of unspecified ear
S01.32 Laceration with foreign body of ear
S01.321 Laceration with foreign body of right ear
S01.322 Laceration with foreign body of left ear
S01.329 Laceration with foreign body of unspecified ear
S01.33 Puncture wound without foreign body of ear
S01.331 Puncture wound without foreign body of right ear
S01.332 Puncture wound without foreign body of left ear
S01.339 Puncture wound without foreign body of unspecified ear
S01.34 Puncture wound with foreign body of ear
S01.341 Puncture wound with foreign body of right ear
S01.342 Puncture wound with foreign body of left ear
S01.349 Puncture wound with foreign body of unspecified ear
S01.35 Open bite of ear
Bite of ear NOS
Excludes1: superficial bite of ear (S00.46, S00.47)
S01.351 Open bite of right ear
S01.352 Open bite of left ear
S01.359 Open bite of unspecified ear

S01.4 Open wound of cheek and temporomandibular area
S01.40 Unspecified open wound of cheek and temporomandibular area
S01.401 Unspecified open wound of right cheek and temporomandibular area
S01.402 Unspecified open wound of left cheek and temporomandibular area
S01.409 Unspecified open wound of unspecified cheek and temporomandibular area
S01.41 Laceration without foreign body of cheek and temporomandibular area
S01.411 Laceration without foreign body of right cheek and temporomandibular area
S01.412 Laceration without foreign body of left cheek and temporomandibular area
S01.419 Laceration without foreign body of unspecified cheek and temporomandibular area
S01.42 Laceration with foreign body of cheek and temporomandibular area
S01.421 Laceration with foreign body of right cheek and temporomandibular area
S01.422 Laceration with foreign body of left cheek and temporomandibular area
S01.429 Laceration with foreign body of unspecified cheek and temporomandibular area
S01.43 Puncture wound without foreign body of cheek and temporomandibular area
S01.431 Puncture wound without foreign body of right cheek and temporomandibular area
S01.432 Puncture wound without foreign body of left cheek and temporomandibular area
S01.439 Puncture wound without foreign body of unspecified cheek and temporomandibular area
S01.44 Puncture wound with foreign body of cheek and temporomandibular area
S01.441 Puncture wound with foreign body of right cheek and temporomandibular area

S01.442 Puncture wound with foreign body of left cheek and temporomandibular area

S01.449 Puncture wound with foreign body of unspecified cheek and temporomandibular area

S01.45 **Open bite of cheek and temporomandibular area**

Bite of cheek and temporomandibular area NOS

Excludes2: superficial bite of cheek and temporomandibular area (S00.86, S00.87)

S01.451 Open bite of right cheek and temporomandibular area

S01.452 Open bite of left cheek and temporomandibular area

S01.459 Open bite of unspecified cheek and temporomandibular area

S01.5 **Open wound of lip and oral cavity**

Excludes2: tooth dislocation (S03.2)
tooth fracture (S02.5)

S01.50 **Unspecified open wound of lip and oral cavity**

S01.501 Unspecified open wound of lip

S01.502 Unspecified open wound of oral cavity

S01.51 **Laceration of lip and oral cavity without foreign body**

S01.511 Laceration without foreign body of lip

S01.512 Laceration without foreign body of oral cavity

S01.52 **Laceration of lip and oral cavity with foreign body**

S01.521 Laceration with foreign body of lip

S01.522 Laceration with foreign body of oral cavity

S01.53 **Puncture wound of lip and oral cavity without foreign body**

S01.531 Puncture wound without foreign body of lip

S01.532 Puncture wound without foreign body of oral cavity

S01.54 **Puncture wound of lip and oral cavity with foreign body**

S01.541 Puncture wound with foreign body of lip

S01.542 Puncture wound with foreign body of oral cavity

S01.55 **Open bite of lip and oral cavity**

S01.551 Open bite of lip

Bite of lip NOS

Excludes1: superficial bite of lip (S00.571)

S01.552 Open bite of oral cavity

Bite of oral cavity NOS

Excludes1: superficial bite of oral cavity (S00.572)

S01.8 **Open wound of other parts of head**

S01.80 **Unspecified open wound of other part of head**

S01.81 **Laceration without foreign body of other part of head**

S01.82 **Laceration with foreign body of other part of head**

S01.83 **Puncture wound without foreign body of other part of head**

S01.84 **Puncture wound with foreign body of other part of head**

S01.85 **Open bite of other part of head**

Bite of other part of head NOS

Excludes1: superficial bite of other part of head (S00.85)

S01.9 **Open wound of unspecified part of head**

S01.90 **Unspecified open wound of unspecified part of head**

S01.91 **Laceration without foreign body of unspecified part of head**

S01.92 **Laceration with foreign body of unspecified part of head**

S01.93 **Puncture wound without foreign body of unspecified part of head**

S01.94 **Puncture wound with foreign body of unspecified part of head**

S01.95 **Open bite of unspecified part of head**

Bite of head NOS

Excludes1: superficial bite of head NOS (S00.97)

S02 **Fracture of skull and facial bones**

Code also any associated intracranial injury (S06.-)

The following extensions are to be added to each code for this category:

A fracture not indicated as open or closed should be coded to closed

a initial encounter for closed fracture
b initial encounter for open fracture
d subsequent encounter for fracture with routine healing
g subsequent encounter for fracture with delayed healing
j subsequent encounter for fracture with nonunion
q sequela

S02.0 **Fracture of vault of skull**

Fracture of frontal bone
Fracture of parietal bone

S02.1 **Fracture of base of skull**

Excludes1: orbit NOS (S02.89)

Excludes2: orbital floor (S02.3-)

S02.10 **Unspecified fracture of base of skull**

S02.11 **Fracture of occiput**

S02.110 Type I occipital condyle fracture

S02.111 Type II occipital condyle fracture

S02.112 Type III occipital condyle fracture

S02.113 Unspecified occipital condyle fracture

S02.118 Other fracture of occiput

S02.119 Unspecified fracture of occiput

S02.19 **Other fracture of base of skull**

Fracture of anterior fossa of base of skull
Fracture of ethmoid sinus
Fracture of frontal sinus
Fracture of middle fossa of base of skull
Fracture of orbital roof
Fracture of posterior fossa of base of skull
Fracture of sphenoid
Fracture of temporal bone

S02.2 **Fracture of nasal bones**

S02.3 **Fracture of orbital floor**

Excludes1: orbit NOS (S02.89)

Excludes2: orbital roof (S02.1-)

S02.4 **Fracture of malar, maxillary and zygoma bones**

Fracture of superior maxilla
Fracture of upper jaw (bone)
Fracture of zygomatic process of temporal bone

S02.40 **Fracture of malar, maxillary and zygoma bones, unspecified**

S02.41 **LeFort I fracture**

S02.42 **LeFort II fracture**

S02.43 **LeFort III fracture**

S02.44 **Fracture of zygoma**

S02.5 **Fracture of tooth**

S02.6 **Fracture of mandible**

Fracture of lower jaw (bone)

S02.60 **Fracture of mandible of unspecified site**

S02.61 **Fracture of condylar process of mandible**

S02.62 **Fracture of subcondylar process of mandible**

S02.63 **Fracture of coronoid process of mandible**

S02.64 **Fracture of ramus of mandible**

S02.65 **Fracture of angle of mandible**

S02.66 **Fracture of symphysis of mandible**

S02.68 **Fracture of unspecified part of body of mandible**

S02.69 **Fracture of mandible of other site**

S02.8 **Fractures of other skull and facial bones**

S02.81 **Fracture of alveolus, maxilla**

S02.82 **Fracture of alveolus, mandible**

S02.83 **Fracture of alveolus, unspecified**

S02.89 **Fractures of other skull and facial bones**

Fracture of orbit NOS
Fracture of palate

Excludes1: fracture of orbital floor (S02.3-)
fracture of orbital roof (S02.1-)

S02.9 **Fracture of unspecified skull and facial bones**

S02.91 **Unspecified fracture of skull**

S02.92   Unspecified fracture of facial bones

S03   Dislocation and sprain of joints and ligaments of head

Includes: avulsion of joint (capsule) or ligament of head
laceration of joint (capsule) or ligament of head
sprain of joint (capsule) or ligament of head
traumatic hemarthrosis of joint or ligament of head
traumatic rupture of joint or ligament of head
traumatic subluxation of joint or ligament of head
traumatic tear of joint or ligament of head

Excludes2:   strain of muscle or tendon of head (S09.1)

The following extensions are to be added to each code for this category:
a   initial encounter
d   subsequent encounter
q   sequela

S03.0   Dislocation of jaw
Dislocation of jaw (cartilage) (meniscus)
Dislocation of mandible
Dislocation of temporomandibular (joint)

S03.1   Dislocation of septal cartilage of nose

S03.2   Dislocation of tooth

S03.4   Sprain of jaw
Sprain of temporomandibular (joint) (ligament)

S03.8   Sprain of joints and ligaments of other parts of head

S03.9   Sprain of joints and ligaments of unspecified parts of head

S04   Injury of cranial nerve
Note: the selection of side should be based on the side of the body being affected
Codes first any associated intracranial injury (S06.-)
Code also any associated:
open wound of head (S01.-)
skull fracture (S02.-)

The following extensions are to be added to each code for this category:
a   initial encounter
d   subsequent encounter
q   sequela

S04.0   Injury of optic nerve and pathways
Injury of optic chiasm
Injury of 2nd cranial nerve
Injury of visual cortex

S04.00   Injury of optic nerve and pathways, unspecified side
S04.01   Injury of optic nerve and pathways, left side
S04.02   Injury of optic nerve and pathways, right side

S04.1   Injury of oculomotor nerve
Injury of 3rd cranial nerve

S04.10   Injury of oculomotor nerve, unspecified side
S04.11   Injury of oculomotor nerve, right side
S04.12   Injury of oculomotor nerve, left side

S04.2   Injury of trochlear nerve
Injury of 4th cranial nerve

S04.20   Injury of trochlear nerve, unspecified side
S04.21   Injury of trochlear nerve, right side
S04.22   Injury of trochlear nerve, left side

S04.3   Injury of trigeminal nerve
Injury of 5th cranial nerve

S04.30   Injury of trigeminal nerve, unspecified side
S04.31   Injury of trigeminal nerve, right side
S04.32   Injury of trigeminal nerve, left side

S04.4   Injury of abducent nerve
Injury of 6th cranial nerve

S04.40   Injury of abducent nerve, unspecified side
S04.41   Injury of abducent nerve, right side
S04.42   Injury of abducent nerve, left side

S04.5   Injury of facial nerve
Injury of 7th cranial nerve

S04.50   Injury of facial nerve, unspecified side
S04.51   Injury of facial nerve, right side
S04.52   Injury of facial nerve, left side

S04.6   Injury of acoustic nerve
Injury of auditory nerve
Injury of 8th cranial nerve

S04.60   Injury of acoustic nerve, unspecified side
S04.61   Injury of acoustic nerve, right side
S04.62   Injury of acoustic nerve, left side

S04.7   Injury of accessory nerve
Injury of 11th cranial nerve

S04.70   Injury of accessory nerve, unspecified side
S04.71   Injury of accessory nerve, right side
S04.72   Injury of accessory nerve, left side

S04.8   Injury of other cranial nerves

S04.81   Injury of olfactory [1st] nerve
S04.811   Injury of olfactory [1st] nerve, right side
S04.812   Injury of olfactory [1st] nerve, left side
S04.819   Injury of olfactory [1st] nerve, unspecified side

S04.89   Injury of other cranial nerves
Injury of vagus [10th] nerve
S04.891   Injury of other cranial nerves, right side
S04.892   Injury of other cranial nerves, left side
S04.899   Injury of other cranial nerves, unspecified side

S04.9   Injury of unspecified cranial nerve

S05   Injury of eye and orbit
Includes: open wound of eye and orbit
Excludes2:   2nd cranial [optic] nerve injury (S04.0-)
3rd cranial [oculomotor] nerve injury (S04.1-)
open wound of eyelid and periocular area (S01.1-)
orbital bone fracture (S02.1-, S02.3-, S02.8-)
superficial injury of eyelid (S00.1-S00.2)

The following extensions are to be added to each code for this category:
a   initial encounter
d   subsequent encounter
q   sequela

S05.0   Injury of conjunctiva and corneal abrasion without foreign body
Excludes1:   foreign body in conjunctival sac (T15.1)
foreign body in cornea (T15.0)

S05.00   Injury of conjunctiva and corneal abrasion without foreign body, unspecified eye
S05.01   Injury of conjunctiva and corneal abrasion without foreign body, right eye
S05.02   Injury of conjunctiva and corneal abrasion without foreign body, left eye

S05.1   Contusion of eyeball and orbital tissues
Traumatic hyphema
Excludes2:   black eye NOS (S00.1)
contusion of eyelid and periocular area (S00.1)

S05.10   Contusion of eyeball and orbital tissues, unspecified eye
S05.11   Contusion of eyeball and orbital tissues, right eye
S05.12   Contusion of eyeball and orbital tissues, left eye

S05.2   Ocular laceration and rupture with prolapse or loss of intraocular tissue
S05.20   Ocular laceration and rupture with prolapse or loss of intraocular tissue, unspecified eye
S05.21   Ocular laceration and rupture with prolapse or loss of intraocular tissue, right eye
S05.22   Ocular laceration and rupture with prolapse or loss of intraocular tissue, left eye

S05.3   Ocular laceration without prolapse or loss of intraocular tissue
Laceration of eye NOS
S05.30   Ocular laceration without prolapse or loss of intraocular tissue, unspecified eye
S05.31   Ocular laceration without prolapse or loss of intraocular tissue, right eye
S05.32   Ocular laceration without prolapse or loss of intraocular tissue, left eye

S05.4   **Penetrating wound of orbit with or without foreign body**

    Excludes2:   retained (old) foreign body following penetrating wound in orbit (H05.5-)

S05.40   **Penetrating wound of orbit with or without foreign body, unspecified eye**

S05.41   **Penetrating wound of orbit with or without foreign body, right eye**

S05.42   **Penetrating wound of orbit with or without foreign body, left eye**

S05.5   **Penetrating wound with foreign body of eyeball**

    Excludes2:   retained (old) intraocular foreign body (H44.6-, H44.7)

S05.50   **Penetrating wound with foreign body of unspecified eyeball**

S05.51   **Penetrating wound with foreign body of right eyeball**

S05.52   **Penetrating wound with foreign body of left eyeball**

S05.6   **Penetrating wound without foreign body of eyeball**

    Ocular penetration NOS

S05.60   **Penetrating wound without foreign body of unspecified eyeball**

S05.61   **Penetrating wound without foreign body of right eyeball**

S05.62   **Penetrating wound without foreign body of left eyeball**

S05.7   **Avulsion of eye**

    Traumatic enucleation

S05.70   **Avulsion of unspecified eye**

S05.71   **Avulsion of right eye**

S05.72   **Avulsion of left eye**

S05.8   **Other injuries of eye and orbit**

    Lacrimal duct injury

S05.80   **Other injuries of unspecified eye and orbit**

S05.81   **Other injuries of right eye and orbit**

S05.82   **Other injuries of left eye and orbit**

S05.9   **Unspecified injury of eye and orbit**

    Injury of eye NOS

S05.90   **Unspecified injury of unspecified eye and orbit**

S05.91   **Unspecified injury of right eye and orbit**

S05.92   **Unspecified injury of left eye and orbit**

S06   **Intracranial injury**

    Code also any associated:
      open wound of head (S01.-)
      skull fracture (S02.-)

    Excludes1:   head injury NOS (S09.90)

    The following extensions are to be added to each code for this category:
      a   initial encounter
      d   subsequent encounter
      q   sequela

S06.0   **Concussion**

    Commotio cerebri

    Excludes1:   concussion with other intracranial injuries classified in category S06 — code to specified intracranial injury

S06.00   **Concussion with loss of consciousness of unspecified duration**

S06.01   **Concussion with no loss of consciousness**

S06.02   **Concussion with brief [less than one hour] loss of consciousness**

S06.03   **Concussion with minor [1 hour - 5 hours 59 minutes] loss of consciousness**

S06.1   **Traumatic cerebral edema**

S06.10   **Traumatic cerebral edema with loss of consciousness of unspecified duration**

S06.11   **Traumatic cerebral edema with no loss of consciousness**

S06.12   **Traumatic cerebral edema with brief [less than one hour] loss of consciousness**

S06.13   **Traumatic cerebral edema with minor [1 hour- 5 hours 59 minutes] loss of consciousness**

S06.14   **Traumatic cerebral edema with moderate [6-24 hours] loss of consciousness**

S06.15   **Traumatic cerebral edema with prolonged [greater than 24 hours] loss of consciousness, with return to pre-existing conscious level**

S06.16   **Traumatic cerebral edema with prolonged [greater than 24 hours] loss of consciousness, without return to pre-existing conscious level**

    Use this code for an unconscious patient who dies before regaining consciousness, regardless of the duration

S06.17   **Focal traumatic cerebral edema**

S06.2   **Diffuse traumatic brain injury**

    Diffuse axonal brain injury

    Excludes1:   traumatic diffuse cerebral edema (S06.10-S06.16)

S06.20   **Diffuse traumatic brain injury with loss of consciousness of unspecified duration**

S06.24   **Diffuse traumatic brain injury with moderate [6-24 hours] loss of consciousness**

S06.25   **Diffuse traumatic brain injury with prolonged [greater than 24 hours] loss of consciousness with return to pre-existing conscious levels**

S06.26   **Diffuse traumatic brain injury with prolonged [greater than 24 hours] loss of consciousness, without return to pre-existing conscious level**

    Use this code for an unconscious patient who dies before regaining consciousness, regardless of the duration

S06.3   **Focal traumatic brain injury**

    Excludes1:   any condition classifiable to S06.4-S06.6
      focal cerebral edema (S06.17)

S06.30   **Unspecified focal traumatic brain injury**

S06.301   **Unspecified focal traumatic brain injury with no loss of consciousness**

S06.302   **Unspecified focal traumatic brain injury with brief [less than one hour] loss of consciousness**

S06.303   **Unspecified focal traumatic brain injury with minor [1-6 hours] loss of consciousness**

S06.304   **Unspecified focal traumatic brain injury with moderate [6-24 hours] loss of consciousness**

S06.305   **Unspecified focal traumatic brain injury with prolonged [greater than 24 hours] loss of consciousness, with return to pre-existing conscious level**

S06.306   **Unspecified focal traumatic brain injury with prolonged [greater than 24 hours] loss of consciousness, without return to pre-existing conscious level**

    Use this code for an unconscious patient who dies before regaining consciousness, regardless of the duration

S06.309   **Unspecified focal traumatic brain injury with loss of consciousness of unspecified duration**

S06.31   **Contusion and laceration of right cerebrum**

S06.311   **Contusion and laceration of right cerebrum with no loss of consciousness**

S06.312   **Contusion and laceration of right cerebrum with brief [less than one hour] loss of consciousness**

S06.313   **Contusion and laceration of right cerebrum with minor [1-6 hours] loss of consciousness**

S06.314   **Contusion and laceration of right cerebrum with moderate [6-24 hours] loss of consciousness**

S06.315   **Contusion and laceration of right cerebrum with prolonged [greater than 24 hours] loss of consciousness, with return to pre-existing conscious level**

S06.316   **Contusion and laceration of right cerebrum with prolonged [greater than 24 hours] loss of consciousness, without return to pre-existing conscious level**

    Use this code for an unconscious patient who dies before regaining consciousness, regardless of the duration

S06.319 Contusion and laceration of right cerebrum with loss of consciousness of unspecified duration

S06.32 **Contusion and laceration of left cerebrum**

S06.321 Contusion and laceration of left cerebrum with no loss of consciousness

S06.322 Contusion and laceration of left cerebrum with brief [less than one hour] loss of consciousness

S06.323 Contusion and laceration of left cerebrum with minor [1-6 hours] loss of consciousness

S06.324 Contusion and laceration of left cerebrum with moderate [6-24 hours] loss of consciousness

S06.325 Contusion and laceration of left cerebrum with prolonged [greater than 24 hours] loss of consciousness, with return to pre-existing conscious level

S06.326 Contusion and laceration of left cerebrum with prolonged [greater than 24 hours] loss of consciousness, without return to pre-existing conscious level
> Use this code for an unconscious patient who dies before regaining consciousness, regardless of the duration

S06.329 Contusion and laceration of left cerebrum with loss of consciousness of unspecified duration

S06.33 **Contusion and laceration of cerebrum, unspecified**

S06.331 Contusion and laceration of cerebrum, unspecified with no loss of consciousness

S06.332 Contusion and laceration of cerebrum, unspecified with brief [less than one hour] loss of consciousness

S06.333 Contusion and laceration of cerebrum, unspecified with minor [1-6 hours] loss of consciousness

S06.334 Contusion and laceration of cerebrum, unspecified with moderate [6-24 hours] loss of consciousness

S06.335 Contusion and laceration of cerebrum, unspecified with prolonged [greater than 24 hours] loss of consciousness, with return to pre-existing conscious level

S06.336 Contusion and laceration of cerebrum, unspecified with prolonged [greater than 24 hours] loss of consciousness, without return to pre-existing conscious level
> Use this code for an unconscious patient who dies before regaining consciousness, regardless of the duration

S06.339 Contusion and laceration of cerebrum, unspecified with loss of consciousness of unspecified duration

S06.34 **Traumatic hemorrhage of right cerebrum**
> Traumatic intracerebral hemorrhage and hematoma of right cerebrum

S06.341 Traumatic hemorrhage of right cerebrum with no loss of consciousness

S06.342 Traumatic hemorrhage of right cerebrum with brief [less than one hour] loss of consciousness

S06.343 Traumatic hemorrhage of right cerebrum with minor [1-6 hours] loss of consciousness

S06.344 Traumatic hemorrhage of right cerebrum with moderate [6-24 hours] loss of consciousness

S06.345 Traumatic hemorrhage of right cerebrum with prolonged [greater than 24 hours] loss of consciousness, with return to pre-existing conscious level

S06.346 Traumatic hemorrhage of right cerebrum with prolonged [greater than 24 hours] loss of consciousness, without return to pre-existing conscious level
> Use this code for an unconscious patient who dies before regaining consciousness, regardless of the duration

S06.349 Traumatic hemorrhage of right cerebrum with loss of consciousness of unspecified duration

S06.35 **Traumatic hemorrhage of left cerebrum**
> Traumatic intracerebral hemorrhage and hematoma of left cerebrum

S06.351 Traumatic hemorrhage of left cerebrum with no loss of consciousness

S06.352 Traumatic hemorrhage of left cerebrum with brief [less than one hour] loss of consciousness

S06.353 Traumatic hemorrhage of left cerebrum with minor [1-6 hours] loss of consciousness

S06.354 Traumatic hemorrhage of left cerebrum with moderate [6-24 hours] loss of consciousness

S06.355 Traumatic hemorrhage of left cerebrum with prolonged [greater than 24 hours] loss of consciousness, with return to pre-existing conscious level

S06.356 Traumatic hemorrhage of left cerebrum with prolonged [greater than 24 hours] loss of consciousness, without return to pre-existing conscious level
> Use this code for an unconscious patient who dies before regaining consciousness, regardless of the duration

S06.359 Traumatic hemorrhage of left cerebrum with loss of consciousness of unspecified duration

S06.36 **Traumatic hemorrhage of cerebrum, unspecified**
> Traumatic intracerebral hemorrhage and hematoma, unspecified

S06.361 Traumatic hemorrhage of cerebrum, unspecified with no loss of consciousness

S06.362 Traumatic hemorrhage of cerebrum, unspecified with brief [less than one hour] loss of consciousness

S06.363 Traumatic hemorrhage of cerebrum, unspecified with minor [1-6 hours] loss of consciousness

S06.364 Traumatic hemorrhage of cerebrum, unspecified with moderate [6-24 hours] loss of consciousness

S06.365 Traumatic hemorrhage of cerebrum, unspecified with prolonged [greater than 24 hours] loss of consciousness, with return to pre-existing conscious level

S06.366 Traumatic hemorrhage of cerebrum, unspecified with prolonged [greater than 24 hours] loss of consciousness, without return to pre-existing conscious level
> Use this code for an unconscious patient who dies before regaining consciousness, regardless of the duration

S06.369 Traumatic hemorrhage of cerebrum, unspecified with loss of consciousness of unspecified duration

S06.37 **Contusion, laceration, and hemorrhage of cerebellum**

S06.371 Contusion, laceration, and hemorrhage of cerebellum with no loss of consciousness

S06.372 Contusion, laceration, and hemorrhage of cerebellum with brief [less than one hour] loss of consciousness

S06.373 Contusion, laceration, and hemorrhage of cerebellum with minor [1-6 hours] loss of consciousness

S06.374 Contusion, laceration, and hemorrhage of cerebellum with moderate [6-24 hours] loss of consciousness

S06.375 Contusion, laceration, and hemorrhage of cerebellum with prolonged [greater than 24 hours] loss of consciousness, with return to pre-existing conscious level

S06.376 Contusion, laceration, and hemorrhage of cerebellum with prolonged [greater than 24 hours] loss of consciousness, without return to pre-existing conscious level
> Use this code for an unconscious patient who dies before regaining consciousness, regardless of the duration

S06.379 Contusion, laceration, and hemorrhage of cerebellum with loss of consciousness of unspecified duration

S06.38 Contusion, laceration, and hemorrhage of brainstem

S06.381 Contusion, laceration, and hemorrhage of brainstem with no loss of consciousness

S06.382 Contusion, laceration, and hemorrhage of brainstem with brief [less than one hour] loss of consciousness

S06.383 Contusion, laceration, and hemorrhage of brainstem with minor [1-6 hours] loss of consciousness

S06.384 Contusion, laceration, and hemorrhage of brainstem with moderate [6-24 hours] loss of consciousness

S06.385 Contusion, laceration, and hemorrhage of brainstem with prolonged [greater than 24 hours] loss of consciousness, with return to pre-existing conscious level

S06.386 Contusion, laceration, and hemorrhage of brainstem with prolonged [greater than 24 hours] loss of consciousness, without return to pre-existing conscious level
> Use this code for an unconscious patient who dies before regaining consciousness, regardless of the duration

S06.389 Contusion, laceration, and hemorrhage of brainstem with loss of consciousness of unspecified duration

S06.4 Epidural hemorrhage
Extradural hemorrhage NOS
Extradural hemorrhage (traumatic)

S06.40 Epidural hemorrhage with loss of consciousness of unspecified duration

S06.41 Epidural hemorrhage with no loss of consciousness

S06.42 Epidural hemorrhage with brief [less than one hour] loss of consciousness

S06.43 Epidural hemorrhage with minor [1-6 hours] loss of consciousness

S06.44 Epidural hemorrhage with moderate [6-24 hours] loss of consciousness

S06.45 Epidural hemorrhage with prolonged [greater than 24 hours] loss of consciousness, with return to pre-existing conscious level

S06.46 Epidural hemorrhage with prolonged [greater than 24 hours] loss of consciousness, without return to pre-existing conscious level
> Use this code for an unconscious patient who dies before regaining consciousness, regardless of the duration

S06.5 Traumatic subdural hemorrhage

S06.50 Traumatic subdural hemorrhage with loss of consciousness of unspecified duration

S06.51 Traumatic subdural hemorrhage with no loss of consciousness

S06.52 Traumatic subdural hemorrhage with brief [less than one hour] loss of consciousness

S06.53 Traumatic subdural hemorrhage with minor [1-6 hours] loss of consciousness

S06.54 Traumatic subdural hemorrhage with moderate [6-24 hours] loss of consciousness

S06.55 Traumatic subdural hemorrhage with prolonged [greater than 24 hours] loss of consciousness, with return to pre-existing conscious level

S06.56 Traumatic subdural hemorrhage with prolonged [greater than 24 hours] loss of consciousness, without return to pre-existing conscious level
> Use this code for an unconscious patient who dies before regaining consciousness, regardless of the duration

S06.6 Traumatic subarachnoid hemorrhage

S06.60 Traumatic subarachnoid hemorrhage with loss of consciousness of unspecified duration

S06.61 Traumatic subarachnoid hemorrhage with no loss of consciousness

S06.62 Traumatic subarachnoid hemorrhage with brief [less than one hour] loss of onsciousness

S06.63 Traumatic subarachnoid hemorrhage with minor [1-6 hours] loss of consciousness

S06.64 Traumatic subarachnoid hemorrhage with moderate [6-24 hours] loss of consciousness

S06.65 Traumatic subarachnoid hemorrhage with prolonged [greater than 24 hours] loss consciousness, with return to pre-existing conscious level

S06.66 Traumatic subarachnoid hemorrhage with prolonged [greater than 24 hours] loss of consciousness, without return to pre-existing conscious level
> Use this code for an unconscious patient who dies before regaining consciousness, regardless of the duration

S06.8 Other intracranial injuries
Injury of internal carotid artery, intracranial portion, not elsewhere classified

S06.9 Unspecified intracranial injury
Brain injury NOS
Head injury NOS with loss of consciousness
Excludes1:   head injury NOS (S09.90)

S06.90 Unspecified intracranial injury with loss of consciousness of unspecified duration

S06.91 Unspecified intracranial injury with no loss of consciousness

S06.92 Unspecified intracranial injury with brief [less than one hour] loss of consciousness

S06.93 Unspecified intracranial injury with minor [1-6 hours] loss of consciousness

S06.94 Unspecified intracranial injury with moderate [6-24 hours] loss of consciousness

S06.95 Unspecified intracranial injury with prolonged [greater than 24 hours] loss of consciousness, with return to pre-existing conscious level

S06.96 Unspecified intracranial injury with prolonged [greater than 24 hours] loss of consciousness, without return to pre-existing conscious level
> Use this code for an unconscious patient who dies before regaining consciousness, regardless of the duration

S07 Crushing injury of head
Use additional code for all associated injuries, such as:
intracranial injuries (S06-)
skull fractures (S02.-)
The following extensions are to be added to each code for this category:
  a   initial encounter
  d   subsequent encounter
  q   sequela

S07.0 Crushing injury of face

S07.1 Crushing injury of skull

S07.8 Crushing injury of other parts of head

S07.9 Crushing injury of head, part unspecified

S08 Avulsion and traumatic amputation of part of head
An amputation not identified as partial or complete should be coded to complete
The following extensions are to be added to each code for this category:
  a   initial encounter
  d   subsequent encounter
  q   sequela

S08.0   Avulsion of scalp

S08.1   Traumatic amputation of ear

   S08.11   Complete traumatic amputation of ear

      S08.111   Complete traumatic amputation of right ear

      S08.112   Complete traumatic amputation of left ear

      S08.119   Complete traumatic amputation of unspecified ear

   S08.12   Partial traumatic amputation of ear

      S08.121   Partial traumatic amputation of right ear

      S08.122   Partial traumatic amputation of left ear

      S08.129   Partial traumatic amputation of unspecified ear

S08.8   Traumatic amputation of other parts of head

   S08.81   Traumatic amputation of nose

      S08.811   Complete traumatic amputation of nose

      S08.812   Partial traumatic amputation of nose

   S08.89   Traumatic amputation of other parts of head

S09   Other and unspecified injuries of head

The following extensions are to be added to each code for this category:

   a   initial encounter

   d   subsequent encounter

   q   sequela

S09.0   Injury of blood vessels of head, not elsewhere classified

   Excludes1:   injury of cerebral blood vessels (S06.-)

               injury of precerebral blood vessels (S15.-)

S09.1   Injury of muscle and tendon of head

   Code also any associated open wound (S01.-)

   Excludes2:   sprain to joints and ligament of head (S03.9)

   S09.10   Unspecified injury of muscle and tendon of head

      Injury of muscle and tendon of head NOS

   S09.11   Strain of muscle and tendon of head

   S09.12   Laceration of muscle and tendon of head

   S09.19   Other injury of muscle and tendon of head

S09.2   Traumatic rupture of ear drum

   Excludes1:   traumatic rupture of ear drum due to blast injury (S09.31-)

   S09.20   Traumatic rupture of unspecified ear drum

   S09.21   Traumatic rupture of right ear drum

   S09.22   Traumatic rupture of left ear drum

S09.3   Other and unspecified injury of middle and inner ear

   Excludes2:   injury to external ear (S00.4-, S01.3-, S08.1-)

   S09.30   Unspecified injury of middle and inner ear

      S09.301   Unspecified injury of right middle and inner ear

      S09.302   Unspecified injury of left middle and inner ear

      S09.309   Unspecified injury of unspecified middle and inner ear

   S09.31   Primary blast injury of ear

      Blast injury of ear NOS

      S09.311   Primary blast injury of right ear

      S09.312   Primary blast injury of left ear

      S09.313   Primary blast injury of ear, bilateral

      S09.319   Primary blast injury of unspecified ear

   S09.39   Other injury of middle and inner ear

      Secondary blast injury to ear

      S09.391   Other injury of right middle and inner ear

      S09.392   Other injury of left middle and inner ear

      S09.399   Other injury of unspecified middle and inner ear

S09.8   Other specified injuries of head

S09.9   Unspecified injury of face and head

   S09.90   Unspecified injury of head

      Head injury NOS

      Excludes1:   brain injury NOS (S06.9-)

              head injury NOS with loss of consciousness (S06.9-)

              intracranial injury NOS (S06.9-)

   S09.91   Unspecified injury of ear

      Injury of ear NOS

   S09.92   Unspecified injury of nose

      Injury of nose NOS

   S09.93   Unspecified injury of face

      Injury of face NOS

INJURIES TO THE NECK (S10–S19)

Includes: injuries of nape

              injuries of supraclavicular region

              injuries of throat

Excludes2:   burns and corrosions (T20-T32)

              effects of foreign body in esophagus (T18.1)

              effects of foreign body in larynx (T17.3)

              effects of foreign body in pharynx (T17.2)

              effects of foreign body in trachea (T17.4)

              frostbite (T33-T34)

              insect bite or sting, venomous (T63.4)

S10   Superficial injury of neck

The following extensions are to be added to each code for this category:

   a   initial encounter

   d   subsequent encounter

   q   sequela

S10.0   Contusion of throat

   Contusion of cervical esophagus

   Contusion of larynx

   Contusion of pharynx

   Contusion of trachea

S10.1   Other and unspecified superficial injuries of throat

   S10.10   Unspecified superficial injuries of throat

   S10.11   Abrasion of throat

   S10.12   Blister (nonthermal) of throat

   S10.14   External constriction of part of throat

   S10.15   Superficial foreign body of throat

      Splinter in the throat

   S10.16   Insect bite (nonvenomous) of throat

   S10.17   Other superficial bite of throat

      Excludes1:   open bite of throat (S11.85)

S10.8   Superficial injury of other parts of neck

   S10.80   Unspecified superficial injury of other part of neck

   S10.81   Abrasion of other part of neck

   S10.82   Blister (nonthermal) of other part of neck

   S10.83   Contusion of other part of neck

   S10.84   External constriction of other part of neck

   S10.85   Superficial foreign body of other part of neck

      Splinter in other part of neck

   S10.86   Insect bite of other part of neck

   S10.87   Other superficial bite of other part of neck

      Excludes1:   open bite of other parts of neck (S11.85)

S10.9   Superficial injury of unspecified part of neck

   S10.90   Unspecified superficial injury of unspecified part of neck

   S10.91   Abrasion of unspecified part of neck

   S10.92   Blister (nonthermal) of unspecified part of neck

   S10.93   Contusion of unspecified part of neck

   S10.94   External constriction of unspecified part of neck

   S10.95   Superficial foreign body of unspecified part of neck

   S10.96   Insect bite of unspecified part of neck

   S10.97   Other superficial bite of unspecified part of neck

S11   Open wound of neck

Code also any associated:

   spinal cord injury (S14.0, S14.1-)

   wound infection

Excludes2:   open fracture of vertebra (S12.- with extension b)

The following extensions are to be added to each code for this category:

   a   initial encounter

   d   subsequent encounter

   q   sequela

S11.0   Open wound of larynx and trachea

   S11.01   Open wound of larynx

S11.011   Laceration without foreign body of larynx
S11.012   Laceration with foreign body of larynx
S11.013   Puncture wound without foreign body of larynx
S11.014   Puncture wound with foreign body of larynx
S11.015   Open bite of larynx
          Bite of larynx NOS
S11.019   Unspecified open wound of larynx

S11.02   Open wound of trachea
          Open wound of cervical trachea
          Open wound of trachea NOS
          Excludes2:   open wound of thoracic trachea (S27.5-)
S11.021   Laceration without foreign body of trachea
S11.022   Laceration with foreign body of trachea
S11.023   Puncture wound without foreign body of trachea
S11.024   Puncture wound with foreign body of trachea
S11.025   Open bite of trachea
          Bite of trachea NOS
S11.029   Unspecified open wound of trachea

S11.03   Open wound of vocal cord
S11.031   Laceration without foreign body of vocal cord
S11.032   Laceration with foreign body of vocal cord
S11.033   Puncture wound without foreign body of vocal cord
S11.034   Puncture wound with foreign body of vocal cord
S11.035   Open bite of vocal cord Bite of vocal cord NOS
S11.039   Unspecified open wound of vocal cord

S11.1   Open wound of thyroid gland
S11.10   Unspecified open wound of thyroid gland
S11.11   Laceration without foreign body of thyroid gland
S11.12   Laceration with foreign body of thyroid gland
S11.13   Puncture wound without foreign body of thyroid gland
S11.14   Puncture wound with foreign body of thyroid gland
S11.15   Open bite of thyroid gland
          Bite of thyroid gland NOS

S11.2   Open wound of pharynx and cervical esophagus
          Excludes1:   open wound of esophagus NOS (S27.8-)
S11.20   Unspecified open wound of pharynx and cervical esophagus
S11.21   Laceration without foreign body of pharynx and cervical esophagus
S11.22   Laceration with foreign body of pharynx and cervical esophagus
S11.23   Puncture wound without foreign body of pharynx and cervical esophagus
S11.24   Puncture wound with foreign body of pharynx and cervical esophagus
S11.25   Open bite of pharynx and cervical esophagus
          Bite of pharynx and cervical esophagus NOS

S11.8   Open wound of other parts of neck
S11.80   Unspecified open wound of other part of neck
S11.81   Laceration without foreign body of other part of neck
S11.82   Laceration with foreign body of other part of neck
S11.83   Puncture wound without foreign body of other part of neck
S11.84   Puncture wound with foreign body of other part of neck
S11.85   Open bite of other part of neck
          Bite of other part of neck NOS
          Excludes1:   superficial bite of other part of neck (S10.87)
S11.89   Other open wound of other part of neck

S11.9   Open wound of unspecified part of neck
S11.90   Unspecified open wound of unspecified part of neck
S11.91   Laceration without foreign body of unspecified part of neck
S11.92   Laceration with foreign body of unspecified part of neck

S11.93   Puncture wound without foreign body of unspecified part of neck
S11.94   Puncture wound with foreign body of unspecified part of neck
S11.95   Open bite of unspecified part of neck
          Bite of neck NOS
          Excludes1:   superficial bite of neck (S10.97)

S12   Fracture of cervical vertebra and other parts of neck
      A fracture not indicated as nondisplaced or displaced should be classified to displaced
      Includes: fracture of cervical neural arch
                   fracture of cervical spine
                   fracture of cervical spinous process
                   fracture of cervical transverse process
                   fracture of cervical vertebral arch
                   fracture of neck
      Code also any associated cervical spinal cord injury (S14.0, S14.1-)
      The following extensions are to be added to all codes for subcategories S12.0-
      A fracture not indicated as open or closed should be coded to closed
      a   initial encounter for closed fracture
      b   initial encounter for open fracture
      d   subsequent encounter for fracture with routine healing
      g   subsequent encounter for fracture with delayed healing
      j   subsequent encounter for fracture with nonunion
      q   sequela

S12.0   Fracture of first cervical vertebra
        Atlas
S12.00   Unspecified fracture of first cervical vertebra
S12.000   Unspecified displaced fracture of first cervical vertebra
S12.001   Unspecified nondisplaced fracture of first cervical vertebra
S12.01   Stable burst fracture of first cervical vertebra
S12.02   Unstable burst fracture of first cervical vertebra
S12.03   Posterior arch fracture of first cervical vertebra
S12.030   Displaced posterior arch fracture of first cervical vertebra
S12.031   Nondisplaced posterior arch fracture of first cervical vertebra
S12.04   Lateral mass fracture of first cervical vertebra
S12.040   Displaced lateral mass fracture of first cervical vertebra
S12.041   Nondisplaced lateral mass fracture of first cervical vertebra
S12.09   Other fracture of first cervical vertebra
S12.090   Other displaced fracture of first cervical vertebra
S12.091   Other nondisplaced fracture of first cervical vertebra

S12.1   Fracture of second cervical vertebra
        Axis
S12.10   Unspecified fracture of second cervical vertebra
S12.100   Unspecified displaced fracture of second cervical vertebra
S12.101   Unspecified nondisplaced fracture of second cervical vertebra
S12.11   Type II dens fracture
S12.110   Anterior displaced Type II dens fracture
S12.111   Posterior displaced Type II dens fracture
S12.112   Nondisplaced Type II dens fracture
S12.12   Other dens fracture
S12.120   Other displaced dens fracture
S12.121   Other nondisplaced dens fracture
S12.13   Unspecified traumatic spondylolisthesis of second cervical vertebra
S12.130   Unspecified traumatic displaced spondylolisthesis of second cervical vertebra
S12.131   Unspecified traumatic nondisplaced spondylolisthesis of second cervical vertebra
S12.14   Type III traumatic spondylolisthesis of second cervical vertebra

S12.15   Other traumatic spondylolisthesis of second cervical vertebra

    S12.150   Other traumatic displaced spondylolisthesis of second cervical vertebra

    S12.151   Other traumatic nondisplaced spondylolisthesis of second cervical vertebra

S12.19   Other fracture of second cervical vertebra

    S12.190   Other displaced fracture of second cervical vertebra

    S12.191   Other nondisplaced fracture of second cervical vertebra

S12.2   Fracture of third cervical vertebra

  S12.20   Unspecified fracture of third cervical vertebra

    S12.200   Unspecified displaced fracture of third cervical vertebra

    S12.201   Unspecified nondisplaced fracture of third cervical vertebra

  S12.23   Unspecified traumatic spondylolisthesis of third cervical vertebra

    S12.230   Unspecified traumatic displaced spondylolisthesis of third cervical vertebra

    S12.231   Unspecified traumatic nondisplaced spondylolisthesis of third cervical vertebra

  S12.24   Type III traumatic spondylolisthesis of third cervical vertebra

  S12.25   Other traumatic spondylolisthesis of third cervical vertebra

    S12.250   Other traumatic displaced spondylolisthesis of third cervical vertebra

    S12.251   Other traumatic nondisplaced spondylolisthesis of third cervical vertebra

  S12.29   Other fracture of third cervical vertebra

    S12.290   Other displaced fracture of third cervical vertebra

    S12.291   Other nondisplaced fracture of third cervical vertebra

S12.3   Fracture of fourth cervical vertebra

  S12.30   Unspecified fracture of fourth cervical vertebra

    S12.300   Unspecified displaced fracture of fourth cervical vertebra

    S12.301   Unspecified nondisplaced fracture of fourth cervical vertebra

  S12.33   Unspecified traumatic spondylolisthesis of fourth cervical vertebra

    S12.330   Unspecified traumatic displaced spondylolisthesis of fourth cervical vertebra

    S12.331   Unspecified traumatic nondisplaced spondylolisthesis of fourth cervical vertebra

  S12.34   Type III traumatic spondylolisthesis of fourth cervical vertebra

  S12.35   Other traumatic spondylolisthesis of fourth cervical vertebra

    S12.350   Other traumatic displaced spondylolisthesis of fourth cervical vertebra

    S12.351   Other traumatic nondisplaced spondylolisthesis of fourth cervical vertebra

  S12.39   Other fracture of fourth cervical vertebra

    S12.390   Other displaced fracture of fourth cervical vertebra

    S12.391   Other nondisplaced fracture of fourth cervical vertebra

S12.4   Fracture of fifth cervical vertebra

  S12.40   Unspecified fracture of fifth cervical vertebra

    S12.400   Unspecified displaced fracture of fifth cervical vertebra

    S12.401   Unspecified nondisplaced fracture of fifth cervical vertebra

  S12.43   Unspecified traumatic spondylolisthesis of fifth cervical vertebra

    S12.430   Unspecified traumatic displaced spondylolisthesis of fifth cervical vertebra

    S12.431   Unspecified traumatic nondisplaced spondylolisthesis of fifth cervical vertebra

  S12.44   Type III traumatic spondylolisthesis of fifth cervical vertebra

  S12.45   Other traumatic spondylolisthesis of fifth cervical vertebra

    S12.450   Other traumatic displaced spondylolisthesis of fifth cervical vertebra

    S12.451   Other traumatic nondisplaced spondylolisthesis of fifth cervical vertebra

  S12.49   Other fracture of fifth cervical vertebra

    S12.490   Other displaced fracture of fifth cervical vertebra

    S12.491   Other nondisplaced fracture of fifth cervical vertebra

S12.5   Fracture of sixth cervical vertebra

  S12.50   Unspecified fracture of sixth cervical vertebra

    S12.500   Unspecified displaced fracture of sixth cervical vertebra

    S12.501   Unspecified nondisplaced fracture of sixth cervical vertebra

  S12.53   Unspecified traumatic spondylolisthesis of sixth cervical vertebra

    S12.530   Unspecified traumatic displaced spondylolisthesis of sixth cervical vertebra

    S12.531   Unspecified traumatic nondisplaced spondylolisthesis of sixth cervical vertebra

  S12.54   Type III traumatic spondylolisthesis of sixth cervical vertebra

  S12.55   Other traumatic spondylolisthesis of sixth cervical vertebr

    S12.550   Other traumatic displaced spondylolisthesis of sixth cervical vertebra

    S12.551   Other traumatic nondisplaced spondylolisthesis of sixth cervical vertebra

  S12.59   Other fracture of sixth cervical vertebra

    S12.590   Other displaced fracture of sixth cervical vertebra

    S12.591   Other nondisplaced fracture of sixth cervical vertebra

S12.6   Fracture of seventh cervical vertebra

  S12.60   Unspecified fracture of seventh cervical vertebra

    S12.600   Unspecified displaced fracture of seventh cervical vertebra

    S12.601   Unspecified nondisplaced fracture of seventh cervical vertebra

  S12.63   Unspecified traumatic spondylolisthesis of seventh cervical vertebra

    S12.630   Unspecified traumatic displaced spondylolisthesis of seventh cervical vertebra

    S12.631   Unspecified traumatic nondisplaced spondylolisthesis of seventh cervical vertebra

  S12.64   Type III traumatic spondylolisthesis of seventh cervical vertebra

  S12.65   Other traumatic spondylolisthesis of seventh cervical vertebra

    S12.650   Other traumatic displaced spondylolisthesis of seventh cervical vertebra

    S12.651   Other traumatic nondisplaced spondylolisthesis of seventh cervical vertebra

  S12.69   Other fracture of seventh cervical vertebra

    S12.690   Other displaced fracture of seventh cervical vertebra

    S12.691   Other nondisplaced fracture of seventh cervical vertebra

The following extensions are to be added to codes S12.8 and S12.9

  a   initial encounter
  d   subsequent encounter
  q   sequela

S12.8   **Fracture of other parts of neck**
Hyoid bone
Larynx
Thyroid cartilage
Trachea

S12.9   **Fracture of neck, unspecified**
Fracture of neck NOS
Fracture of cervical spine NOS
Fracture of cervical vertebra NOS

S13   **Dislocation and sprain of joints and ligaments at neck level**
Includes: avulsion of joint or ligament at neck level
laceration of joint or ligament at neck level
sprain of joint or ligament at neck level
traumatic hemarthrosis of joint or ligament at neck level
traumatic rupture of joint or ligament at neck level
traumatic subluxation of joint or ligament at neck level
traumatic tear of joint or ligament at neck level
Excludes2:   strain of muscle or tendon at neck level (S16.1)
The following extensions are to be added to each code for this category:
    a   initial encounter
    d   subsequent encounter
    q   sequela

S13.0   **Traumatic rupture of cervical intervertebral disc**
Excludes1:   rupture or displacement (nontraumatic) of cervical intervertebral disc NOS (M50.-)

S13.1   **Subluxation and dislocation of cervical vertebrae**
Code also any associated:
open wound of neck (S11.-)
spinal cord injury (S14.1-)
Excludes2:   fracture of cervical vertebrae (S12.0—S12.3-)

S13.10   **Subluxation and dislocation of unspecified cervical vertebrae**

    S13.100   **Subluxation of unspecified cervical vertebrae**

    S13.101   **Dislocation of unspecified cervical vertebrae**

S13.11   **Subluxation and dislocation of C_0/C_1 cervical vertebrae**
Subluxation and dislocation of atlantooccipital joint
Subluxation and dislocation of atloidooccipital joint
Subluxation and dislocation of occipitoatloid joint

    S13.110   **Subluxation of C_0/C_1 cervical vertebrae**

    S13.111   **Dislocation of C_0/C_1 cervical vertebrae**

S13.12   **Subluxation and dislocation of C_1/C_2 cervical vertebrae**
Subluxation and dislocation of atlantoaxial joint

    S13.120   **Subluxation of C_1/C_2 cervical vertebrae**

    S13.121   **Dislocation of C_1/C_2 cervical vertebrae**

S13.13   **Subluxation and dislocation of C_2/C_3 cervical vertebrae**

    S13.130   **Subluxation of C_2/C_3 cervical vertebrae**

    S13.131   **Dislocation of C_2/C_3 cervical vertebrae**

S13.14   **Subluxation and dislocation of C_3/C_4 cervical vertebrae**

    S13.140   **Subluxation of C_3/C_4 cervical vertebrae**

    S13.141   **Dislocation of C_3/C_4 cervical vertebrae**

S13.15   **Subluxation and dislocation of C_4/C_5 cervical vertebrae**

    S13.150   **Subluxation of C_4/C_5 cervical vertebrae**

    S13.151   **Dislocation of C_4/C_5 cervical vertebrae**

S13.16   **Subluxation and dislocation of C_5/C_6 cervical vertebrae**

    S13.160   **Subluxation of C_5/C_6 cervical vertebrae**

    S13.161   **Dislocation of C_5/C_6 cervical vertebrae**

S13.17   **Subluxation and dislocation of C_6/C_7 cervical vertebrae**

    S13.170   **Subluxation of C_6/C_7 cervical vertebrae**

    S13.171   **Dislocation of C_6/C_7 cervical vertebrae**

S13.18   **Subluxation and dislocation of C_7/T_1 cervical vertebrae**

    S13.180   **Subluxation of C_7/T_1 cervical vertebrae**

    S13.181   **Dislocation of C_7/T_1 cervical vertebrae**

S13.2   **Dislocation of other and unspecified parts of neck**

S13.20   **Dislocation of unspecified parts of neck**

S13.29   **Dislocation of other parts of neck**

S13.4   **Sprain of ligaments of cervical spine**
Sprain of anterior longitudinal (ligament), cervical
Sprain of atlanto-axial (joints)
Sprain of atlanto-occipital (joints)
Whiplash injury of cervical spine

S13.5   **Sprain of thyroid region**
Sprain of cricoarytenoid (joint) (ligament)
Sprain of cricothyroid (joint) (ligament)
Sprain of thyroid cartilage

S13.8   **Sprain of joints and ligaments of other parts of neck**

S13.9   **Sprain of joints and ligaments of unspecified parts of neck**

S14   **Injury of nerves and spinal cord at neck level**
Note: code to highest level of cervical cord injury
Code also any associated:
fracture of cervical vertebra (S12.0—S12.6.-)
open wound of neck (S11-)
transient paralysis (R29.5)
The following extensions are to be added to each code for this category:
    a   initial encounter
    d   subsequent encounter
    q   sequela

S14.0   **Concussion and edema of cervical spinal cord**

S14.1   **Other and unspecified injuries of cervical spinal cord**

S14.10   **Unspecified injury of cervical spinal cord**

    S14.101   **Unspecified injury at C_1 level of cervical spinal cord**

    S14.102   **Unspecified injury at C_2 level of cervical spinal cord**

    S14.103   **Unspecified injury at C_3 level of cervical spinal cord**

    S14.104   **Unspecified injury at C_4 level of cervical spinal cord**

    S14.105   **Unspecified injury at C_5 level of cervical spinal cord**

    S14.106   **Unspecified injury at C_6 level of cervical spinal cord**

    S14.107   **Unspecified injury at C_7 level of cervical spinal cord**

    S14.108   **Unspecified injury at C_8 level of cervical spinal cord**

    S14.109   **Unspecified injury at unspecified level of cervical spinal cord**
Injury of cervical spinal cord NOS

S14.11   **Complete lesion of cervical spinal cord**

    S14.111   **Complete lesion at C_1 level of cervical spinal cord**

    S14.112   **Complete lesion at C_2 level of cervical spinal cord**

    S14.113   **Complete lesion at C_3 level of cervical spinal cord**

    S14.114   **Complete lesion at C_4 level of cervical spinal cord**

    S14.115   **Complete lesion at C_5 level of cervical spinal cord**

    S14.116   **Complete lesion at C_6 level of cervical spinal cord**

    S14.117   **Complete lesion at C_7 level of cervical spinal cord**

    S14.118   **Complete lesion at C_8 level of cervical spinal cord**

    S14.119   **Complete lesion at unspecified level of cervical spinal cord**

S14.12   **Central cord syndrome of cervical spinal cord**

    S14.121   **Central cord syndrome at C_1 level of cervical spinal cord**

    S14.122   **Central cord syndrome at C_2 level of cervical spinal cord**

S14.123   Central cord syndrome at C_3 level of cervical spinal cord

S14.124   Central cord syndrome at C_4 level of cervical spinal cord

S14.125   Central cord syndrome at C_5 level of cervical spinal cord

S14.126   Central cord syndrome at C_6 level of cervical spinal cord

S14.127   Central cord syndrome at C_7 level of cervical spinal cord

S14.128   Central cord syndrome at C_8 level of cervical spinal cord

S14.129   Central cord syndrome at unspecified level of cervical spinal cord

S14.13   Anterior cord syndrome of cervical spinal cord

S14.131   Anterior cord syndrome at C_1 level of cervical spinal cord

S14.132   Anterior cord syndrome at C_2 level of cervical spinal cord

S14.133   Anterior cord syndrome at C_3 level of cervical spinal cord

S14.134   Anterior cord syndrome at C_4 level of cervical spinal cord

S14.135   Anterior cord syndrome at C_5 level of cervical spinal cord

S14.136   Anterior cord syndrome at C_6 level of cervical spinal cord

S14.137   Anterior cord syndrome at C_7 level of cervical spinal cord

S14.138   Anterior cord syndrome at C_8 level of cervical spinal cord

S14.139   Anterior cord syndrome at unspecified level of cervical spinal cord

S14.14   Brown-Sequard syndrome of cervical spinal cord

S14.141   Brown-Sequard syndrome at C_1 level of cervical spinal cord

S14.142   Brown-Sequard syndrome at C_2 level of cervical spinal cord

S14.143   Brown-Sequard syndrome at C_3 level of cervical spinal cord

S14.144   Brown-Sequard syndrome at C_4 level of cervical spinal cord

S14.145   Brown-Sequard syndrome at C_5 level of cervical spinal cord

S14.146   Brown-Sequard syndrome at C_6 level of cervical spinal cord

S14.147   Brown-Sequard syndrome at C_7 level of cervical spinal cord

S14.148   Brown-Sequard syndrome at C_8 level of cervical spinal cord

S14.149   Brown-Sequard syndrome at unspecified level of cervical spinal cord

S14.15   Other incomplete lesions of cervical spinal cord
Incomplete lesion of cervical spinal cord NOS
Posterior cord syndrome of cervical spinal cord

S14.151   Other incomplete lesion at C_1 level of cervical spinal cord

S14.152   Other incomplete lesion at C_2 level of cervical spinal cord

S14.153   Other incomplete lesion at C_3 level of cervical spinal cord

S14.154   Other incomplete lesion at C_4 level of cervical spinal cord

S14.155   Other incomplete lesion at C_5 level of cervical spinal cord

S14.156   Other incomplete lesion at C_6 level of cervical spinal cord

S14.157   Other incomplete lesion at C_7 level of cervical spinal cord

S14.158   Other incomplete lesion at C_8 level of cervical spinal cord

S14.159   Other incomplete lesion at unspecified level of cervical spinal cord

S14.2   Injury of nerve root of cervical spine

S14.3   Injury of brachial plexus

S14.4   Injury of peripheral nerves of neck

S14.5   Injury of cervical sympathetic nerves

S14.8   Injury of other nerves of neck

S14.9   Injury of unspecified nerves of neck

S15   Injury of blood vessels at neck level
Code also any associated open wound (S11.-)
The following extensions are to be added to each code for this category:
   a   initial encounter
   d   subsequent encounter
   q   sequela

S15.0   Injury of carotid artery of neck
Injury of carotid artery (common) (external) (internal, extracranial portion)
Injury of carotid artery NOS
Excludes1:   injury of internal carotid artery, intracranial portion (S06.8)

S15.00   Unspecified injury of carotid artery

S15.001   Unspecified injury of right carotid artery

S15.002   Unspecified injury of left carotid artery

S15.009   Unspecified injury of unspecified carotid artery

S15.01   Minor laceration of carotid artery
Incomplete transection of carotid artery
Laceration of carotid artery NOS
Superficial laceration of carotid artery

S15.011   Minor laceration of right carotid artery

S15.012   Minor laceration of left carotid artery

S15.019   Minor laceration of unspecified carotid artery

S15.02   Major laceration of carotid artery
Complete transection of carotid artery
Traumatic rupture of carotid artery

S15.021   Major laceration of right carotid artery

S15.022   Major laceration of left carotid artery

S15.029   Major laceration of unspecified carotid artery

S15.09   Other injury of carotid artery

S15.091   Other injury of right carotid artery

S15.092   Other injury of left carotid artery

S15.099   Other injury of unspecified carotid artery

S15.1   Injury of vertebral artery

S15.10   Unspecified injury of vertebral artery

S15.101   Unspecified injury of right vertebral artery

S15.102   Unspecified injury of left vertebral artery

S15.109   Unspecified injury of unspecified vertebral artery

S15.11   Minor laceration of vertebral artery
Incomplete transection of vertebral artery
Laceration of vertebral artery NOS
Superficial laceration of vertebral artery

S15.111   Minor laceration of right vertebral artery

S15.112   Minor laceration of left vertebral artery

S15.119   Minor laceration of unspecified vertebral artery

S15.12   Major laceration of vertebral artery
Complete transection of vertebral artery
Traumatic rupture of vertebral artery

S15.121   Major laceration of right vertebral artery

S15.122   Major laceration of left vertebral artery

S15.129   Major laceration of unspecified vertebral artery

S15.19   Other injury of vertebral artery

S15.191   Other injury of right vertebral artery

S15.192   Other injury of left vertebral artery

S15.199   Other injury of unspecified vertebral artery

S15.2   Injury of external jugular vein

S15.20   Unspecified injury of external jugular vein

S15.201   Unspecified injury of right external jugular vein

S15.202   Unspecified injury of left external jugular vein

S15.209   Unspecified injury of unspecified external jugular vein

S15.21   Minor laceration of external jugular vein

Incomplete transection of external jugular vein

Laceration of external jugular vein NOS

Superficial laceration of external jugular vein

S15.211   Minor laceration of right external jugular vein

S15.212   Minor laceration of left external jugular vein

S15.219   Minor laceration of unspecified external jugular vein

S15.22   Major laceration of external jugular vein

Complete transection of external jugular vein

Traumatic rupture of external jugular vein

S15.221   Major laceration of right external jugular vein

S15.222   Major laceration of left external jugular vein

S15.229   Major laceration of unspecified external jugular vein

S15.29   Other injury of external jugular vein

S15.291   Other injury of right external jugular vein

S15.292   Other injury of left external jugular vein

S15.299   Other injury of unspecified external jugular vein

S15.3   Injury of internal jugular vein

S15.30   Unspecified injury of internal jugular vein

S15.301   Unspecified injury of right internal jugular vein

S15.302   Unspecified injury of left internal jugular vein

S15.309   Unspecified injury of unspecified internal jugular vein

S15.31   Minor laceration of internal jugular vein

Incomplete transection of internal jugular vein

Laceration of internal jugular vein NOS

Superficial laceration of internal jugular vein

S15.31   Minor laceration of right internal jugular vein

S15.312   Minor laceration of left internal jugular vein

S15.319   Minor laceration of unspecified internal jugular vein

S15.32   Major laceration of internal jugular vein

Complete transection of internal jugular vein

Traumatic rupture of internal jugular vein

S15.321   Major laceration of right internal jugular vein

S15.322   Major laceration of left internal jugular vein

S15.329   Major laceration of unspecified internal jugular vein

S15.39   Other injury of internal jugular vein

S15.391   Other injury of right internal jugular vein

S15.392   Other injury of left internal jugular vein

S15.399   Other injury of unspecified internal jugular vein

S15.8   Injury of other blood vessels at neck level

S15.9   Injury of unspecified blood vessel at neck level

S16   Injury of muscle and tendon at neck level

Code also any associated open wound (S11.-)

Excludes2:   sprain of joint or ligament at neck level (S13.9)

The following extensions are to be added to each code for this category:

a   initial encounter

d   subsequent encounter

q   sequela

S16.1   Strain of muscle and tendon at neck level

S16.2   Laceration of muscle and tendon at neck level

S16.8   Other injury of muscle and tendon at neck level

S16.9   Unspecified injury of muscle and tendon at neck level

S17   Crushing injury of neck

Use additional code for all associated injuries, such as:

injury of blood vessels (S15.-)

open wound of neck (S11.-)

spinal cord injury (S14.0, S14.1-)

vertebral fracture (S12.0—S12.3-)

The following extensions are to be added to each code for this category:

a   initial encounter

d   subsequent encounter

q   sequela

S17.0   Crushing injury of larynx and trachea

S17.8   Crushing injury of other parts of neck

S17.9   Crushing injury of neck, part unspecified

S19   Other and unspecified injuries of neck

The following extensions are to be added to each code for this category:

a   initial encounter

d   subsequent encounter

q   sequela

S19.8   Other specified injuries of neck

S19.9   Unspecified injury of neck

INJURIES TO THE THORAX (S20–S29)

Includes: injuries of breast

injuries of chest (wall)

injuries of interscapular area

Excludes2:   burns and corrosions (T20-T32)

effects of foreign body in bronchus (T17.5)

effects of foreign body in esophagus (T18.1)

effects of foreign body in lung (T17.8)

effects of foreign body in trachea (T17.4)

frostbite (T33-T34)

injuries of axilla

injuries of clavicle

injuries of scapular region

injuries of shoulder

insect bite or sting, venomous (T63.4)

S20   Superficial injury of thorax

The following extensions are to be added to each code for this category:

a   initial encounter

d   subsequent encounter

q   sequela

S20.0   Contusion of breast

S20.00   Contusion of breast, unspecified breast

S20.01   Contusion of right breast

S20.02   Contusion of left breast

S20.1   Other and unspecified superficial injuries of breast

S20.10   Unspecified superficial injuries of breast

S20.101   Unspecified superficial injuries of breast, right breast

S20.102   Unspecified superficial injuries of breast, left breast

S20.109   Unspecified superficial injuries of breast, unspecified breast

S20.11   Abrasion of breast

S20.111   Abrasion of breast, right breast

S20.112   Abrasion of breast, left breast

S20.119   Abrasion of breast, unspecified breast

S20.12   Blister (nonthermal) of breast

S20.121   Blister (nonthermal) of breast, right breast

S20.122   Blister (nonthermal) of breast, left breast

S20.129   Blister (nonthermal) of breast, unspecified breast

S20.14   External constriction of part of breast

S20.141   External constriction of part of breast, right breast

S20.142   External constriction of part of breast, left breast

S20.149   External constriction of part of breast, unspecified breast

S20.15   Superficial foreign body of breast
Splinter in the breast

S20.151   Superficial foreign body of breast, right breast

S20.152   Superficial foreign body of breast, left breast

S20.159   Superficial foreign body of breast, unspecified breast

S20.16   Insect bite (nonvenomous) of breast

S20.161   Insect bite (nonvenomous) of breast, right breast

S20.162   Insect bite (nonvenomous) of breast, left breast

S20.169   Insect bite (nonvenomous) of breast, unspecified breast

S20.17   Other superficial bite of breast
Excludes1:   open bite of breast (S21.05-)

S20.171   Other superficial bite of breast, right breast

S20.172   Other superficial bite of breast, left breast

S20.179   Other superficial bite of breast, unspecified breast

S20.2   Contusion of thorax

S20.20   Contusion of thorax, unspecified

S20.21   Contusion of front wall of thorax

S20.211   Contusion of right front wall of thorax

S20.212   Contusion of left front wall of thorax

S20.219   Contusion of unspecified front wall of thorax

S20.22   Contusion of back wall of thorax

S20.221   Contusion of right back wall of thorax

S20.222   Contusion of left back wall of thorax

S20.229   Contusion of unspecified back wall of thorax

S20.3   Other and unspecified superficial injuries of front wall of thorax

S20.30   Unspecified superficial injuries of front wall of thorax

S20.301   Unspecified superficial injuries of right front wall of thorax

S20.302   Unspecified superficial injuries of left front wall of thorax

S20.309   Unspecified superficial injuries of unspecified front wall of thorax

S20.31   Abrasion of front wall of thorax

S20.311   Abrasion of right front wall of thorax

S20.312   Abrasion of left front wall of thorax

S20.319   Abrasion of unspecified front wall of thorax

S20.32   Blister (nonthermal) of front wall of thorax

S20.321   Blister (nonthermal) of right front wall of thorax

S20.322   Blister (nonthermal) of left front wall of thorax

S20.329   Blister (nonthermal) of unspecified front wall of thorax

S20.34   External constriction of front wall of thorax

S20.341   External constriction of right front wall of thorax

S20.342   External constriction of left front wall of thorax

S20.349   External constriction of unspecified front wall of thorax

S20.35   Superficial foreign body of front wall of thorax
Splinter in front wall of thorax

S20.351   Superficial foreign body of right front wall of thorax

S20.352   Superficial foreign body of left front wall of thorax

S20.359   Superficial foreign body of unspecified front wall of thorax

S20.36   Insect bite (nonvenomous) of front wall of thorax

S20.361   Insect bite (nonvenomous) of right front wall of thorax

S20.362   Insect bite (nonvenomous) of left front wall of thorax

S20.369   Insect bite (nonvenomous) of unspecified front wall of thorax

S20.37   Other superficial bite of front wall of thorax
Excludes1:   open bite of front wall of thorax (S21.14)

S20.371   Other superficial bite of right front wall of thorax

S20.372   Other superficial bite of left front wall of thorax

S20.379   Other superficial bite of unspecified front wall of thorax

S20.4   Other and unspecified superficial injuries of back wall of thorax

S20.40   Unspecified superficial injuries of back wall of thorax

S20.401   Unspecified superficial injuries of right back wall of thorax

S20.402   Unspecified superficial injuries of left back wall of thorax

S20.409   Unspecified superficial injuries of unspecified back wall of thorax

S20.41   Abrasion of back wall of thorax

S20.411   Abrasion of right back wall of thorax

S20.412   Abrasion of left back wall of thorax

S20.419   Abrasion of unspecified back wall of thorax

S20.42   Blister (nonthermal) of back wall of thorax

S20.421   Blister (nonthermal) of right back wall of thorax

S20.422   Blister (nonthermal) of left back wall of thorax

S20.429   Blister (nonthermal) of unspecified back wall of thorax

S20.44   External constriction of back wall of thorax

S20.441   External constriction of right back wall of thorax

S20.442   External constriction of left back wall of thorax

S20.449   External constriction of unspecified back wall of thorax

S20.45   Superficial foreign body of back wall of thorax
Splinter of back wall of thorax

S20.451   Superficial foreign body of right back wall of thorax

S20.452   Superficial foreign body of left back wall of thorax

S20.459   Superficial foreign body of unspecified back wall of thorax

S20.46   Insect bite (nonvenomous) of back wall of thorax

S20.461   Insect bite (nonvenomous) of right back wall of thorax

S20.462   Insect bite (nonvenomous) of left back wall of thorax

S20.469   Insect bite (nonvenomous) of unspecified back wall of thorax

S20.47   Other superficial bite of back wall of thorax
Excludes1:   open bite of back wall of thorax (S21.24)

S20.471   Other superficial bite of right back wall of thorax

S20.472   Other superficial bite of left back wall of thorax

S20.479   Other superficial bite of unspecified back wall of thorax

S20.9   Superficial injury of unspecified parts of thorax
Excludes1:   contusion of thorax NOS (S20.20)

S20.90   Unspecified superficial injury of unspecified parts of thorax
Superficial injury of thoracic wall NOS

S20.91   Abrasion of unspecified parts of thorax

S20.92   Blister (nonthermal) of unspecified parts of thorax

S20.94   External constriction of unspecified parts of thorax

S20.95   Superficial foreign body of unspecified parts of thorax
Splinter in thorax NOS

S20.96   Insect bite (nonvenomous) of unspecified parts of thorax

S20.97   Other superficial bite of unspecified parts of thorax
> Excludes1:   open bite of thorax NOS (S21.95)

S21   Open wound of thorax
Code also any associated injury (to) (such as) :
> heart (S26.-)
> intrathoracic organs (S27.-)
> rib fracture (S22.3-, S22.4-)
> spinal cord injury (S24.0-, S24.1-)
> traumatic hemothorax (S27.1)
> traumatic hemopneumothorax (S27.3)
> traumatic pneumothorax (S27.0)
> wound infection

> Excludes1:   traumatic amputation (partial) of thorax (S28.1)

The following extensions are to be added to each code for this category:
> a   initial encounter
> d   subsequent encounter
> q   sequela

S21.0   Open wound of breast
S21.00   Unspecified open wound of breast
- S21.001   Unspecified open wound of right breast
- S21.002   Unspecified open wound of left breast
- S21.009   Unspecified open wound of unspecified breast

S21.01   Laceration without foreign body of breast
- S21.011   Laceration without foreign body of right breast
- S21.012   Laceration without foreign body of left breast
- S21.019   Laceration without foreign body of unspecified breast

S21.02   Laceration with foreign body of breast
- S21.021   Laceration with foreign body of right breast
- S21.022   Laceration with foreign body of left breast
- S21.029   Laceration with foreign body of unspecified breast

S21.03   Puncture wound without foreign body of breast
- S21.031   Puncture wound without foreign body of right breast
- S21.032   Puncture wound without foreign body of left breast
- S21.039   Puncture wound without foreign body of unspecified breast

S21.04   Puncture wound with foreign body of breast
- S21.041   Puncture wound with foreign body of right breast
- S21.042   Puncture wound with foreign body of left breast
- S21.049   Puncture wound with foreign body of unspecified breast

S21.05   Open bite of breast
> Bite of breast NOS
> Excludes1:   superficial bite of breast (S20.17)
- S21.051   Open bite of right breast
- S21.052   Open bite of left breast
- S21.059   Open bite of unspecified breast

S21.1   Open wound of front wall of thorax without penetration into thoracic cavity
Open wound of chest without penetration into thoracic cavity

S21.10   Unspecified open wound of front wall of thorax without penetration into thoracic cavity
- S21.101   Unspecified open wound of right front wall of thorax without penetration into thoracic cavity
- S21.102   Unspecified open wound of left front wall of thorax without penetration into thoracic cavity
- S21.109   Unspecified open wound of unspecified front wall of thorax without penetration into thoracic cavity

S21.11   Laceration without foreign body of front wall of thorax without penetration into thoracic cavity
- S21.111   Laceration without foreign body of right front wall of thorax without penetration into thoracic cavity
- S21.112   Laceration without foreign body of left front wall of thorax without penetration into thoracic cavity
- S21.119   Laceration without foreign body of unspecified front wall of thorax without penetration into thoracic cavity

S21.12   Laceration with foreign body of front wall of thorax without penetration into thoracic cavity
- S21.121   Laceration with foreign body of right front wall of thorax without penetration into thoracic cavity
- S21.122   Laceration with foreign body of left front wall of thorax without penetration into thoracic cavity
- S21.129   Laceration with foreign body of unspecified front wall of thorax without penetration into thoracic cavity

S21.13   Puncture wound without foreign body of front wall of thorax without penetration into thoracic cavity
- S21.131   Puncture wound without foreign body of right front wall of thorax without penetration into thoracic cavity
- S21.132   Puncture wound without foreign body of left front wall of thorax without penetration into thoracic cavity
- S21.139   Puncture wound without foreign body of unspecified front wall of thorax without penetration into thoracic cavity

S21.14   Puncture wound with foreign body of front wall of thorax without penetration into thoracic cavity
- S21.141   Puncture wound with foreign body of right front wall of thorax without penetration into thoracic cavity
- S21.142   Puncture wound with foreign body of left front wall of thorax without penetration into thoracic cavity
- S21.149   Puncture wound with foreign body of unspecified front wall of thorax without penetration into thoracic cavity

S21.15   Open bite of front wall of thorax without penetration into thoracic cavity
> Bite of front wall of thorax NOS
> Excludes1:   superficial bite of front wall of thorax (S20.37)
- S21.151   Open bite of right front wall of thorax without penetration into thoracic cavity
- S21.152   Open bite of left front wall of thorax without penetration into thoracic cavity
- S21.159   Open bite of unspecified front wall of thorax without penetration into thoracic cavity

S21.2   Open wound of back wall of thorax without penetration into thoracic cavity
S21.20   Unspecified open wound of back wall of thorax without penetration into thoracic cavity
- S21.201   Unspecified open wound of right back wall of thorax without penetration into thoracic cavity
- S21.202   Unspecified open wound of left back wall of thorax without penetration into thoracic cavity
- S21.209   Unspecified open wound of unspecified back wall of thorax without penetration into thoracic cavity

S21.21   Laceration without foreign body of back wall of thorax without penetration into thoracic cavity
- S21.211   Laceration without foreign body of right back wall of thorax without penetration into thoracic cavity
- S21.212   Laceration without foreign body of left back wall of thorax without penetration into thoracic cavity

S21.219   Laceration without foreign body of unspecified back wall of thorax without penetration into thoracic cavity

S21.22   Laceration with foreign body of back wall of thorax without penetration into thoracic cavity

S21.221   Laceration with foreign body of right back wall of thorax without penetration into thoracic cavity

S21.222   Laceration with foreign body of left back wall of thorax without penetration into thoracic cavity

S21.229   Laceration with foreign body of unspecified back wall of thorax without penetration into thoracic cavity

S21.23   Puncture wound without foreign body of back wall of thorax without penetration into thoracic cavity

S21.231   Puncture wound without foreign body of right back wall of thorax without penetration into thoracic cavity

S21.232   Puncture wound without foreign body of left back wall of thorax without penetration into thoracic cavity

S21.239   Puncture wound without foreign body of unspecified back wall of thorax without penetration into thoracic cavity

S21.24   Puncture wound with foreign body of back wall of thorax without penetration into thoracic cavity

S21.241   Puncture wound with foreign body of right back wall of thorax without penetration into thoracic cavity

S21.242   Puncture wound with foreign body of left back wall of thorax without penetration into thoracic cavity

S21.249   Puncture wound with foreign body of unspecified back wall of thorax without penetration into thoracic cavity

S21.25   Open bite of back wall of thorax without penetration into thoracic cavity

Bite of back wall of thorax NOS

Excludes1:   superficial bite of back wall of thorax (S20.47)

S21.251   Open bite of right back wall of thorax without penetration into thoracic cavity

S21.252   Open bite of left back wall of thorax without penetration into thoracic cavity

S21.259   Open bite of unspecified back wall of thorax without penetration into thoracic cavity

S21.3   Open wound of front wall of thorax with penetration into thoracic cavity

Open wound of chest with penetration into thoracic cavity

S21.30   Unspecified open wound of front wall of thorax with penetration into thoracic cavity

S21.301   Unspecified open wound of right front wall of thorax with penetration into thoracic cavity

S21.302   Unspecified open wound of left front wall of thorax with penetration into thoracic cavity

S21.309   Unspecified open wound of unspecified front wall of thorax with penetration into thoracic cavity

S21.31   Laceration without foreign body of front wall of thorax with penetration into thoracic cavity

S21.311   Laceration without foreign body of right front wall of thorax with penetration into thoracic cavity

S21.312   Laceration without foreign body of left front wall of thorax with penetration into thoracic cavity

S21.319   Laceration without foreign body of unspecified front wall of thorax with penetration into thoracic cavity

S21.32   Laceration with foreign body of front wall of thorax with penetration into thoracic cavity

S21.321   Laceration with foreign body of right front wall of thorax with penetration into thoracic cavity

S21.322   Laceration with foreign body of left front wall of thorax with penetration into thoracic cavity

S21.329   Laceration with foreign body of unspecified front wall of thorax with penetration into thoracic cavity

S21.33   Puncture wound without foreign body of front wall of thorax with penetration into thoracic cavity

S21.331   Puncture wound without foreign body of right front wall of thorax with penetration into thoracic cavity

S21.332   Puncture wound without foreign body of left front wall of thorax with penetration into thoracic cavity

S21.339   Puncture wound without foreign body of unspecified front wall of thorax with penetration into thoracic cavity

S21.34   Puncture wound with foreign body of front wall of thorax with penetration into thoracic cavity

S21.341   Puncture wound with foreign body of right front wall of thorax with penetration into thoracic cavity

S21.342   Puncture wound with foreign body of left front wall of thorax with penetration into thoracic cavity

S21.349   Puncture wound with foreign body of unspecified front wall of thorax with penetration into thoracic cavity

S21.35   Open bite of front wall of thorax with penetration into thoracic cavity

Excludes1:   superficial bite of front wall of thorax (S20.37)

S21.351   Open bite of right front wall of thorax with penetration into thoracic cavity

S21.352   Open bite of left front wall of thorax with penetration into thoracic cavity

S21.359   Open bite of unspecified front wall of thorax with penetration into thoracic cavity

S21.4   Open wound of back wall of thorax with penetration into thoracic cavity

S21.40   Unspecified open wound of back wall of thorax with penetration into thoracic cavity

S21.401   Unspecified open wound of right back wall of thorax with penetration into thoracic cavity

S21.402   Unspecified open wound of left back wall of thorax with penetration into thoracic cavity

S21.409   Unspecified open wound of unspecified back wall of thorax with penetration into thoracic cavity

S21.41   Laceration without foreign body of back wall of thorax with penetration into thoracic cavity

S21.411   Laceration without foreign body of right back wall of thorax with penetration into thoracic cavity

S21.412   Laceration without foreign body of left back wall of thorax with penetration into thoracic cavity

S21.419   Laceration without foreign body of unspecified back wall of thorax with penetration into thoracic cavity

S21.42   Laceration with foreign body of back wall of thorax with penetration into thoracic cavity

S21.421   Laceration with foreign body of right back wall of thorax with penetration into thoracic cavity

S21.422   Laceration with foreign body of left back wall of thorax with penetration into thoracic cavity

S21.429   Laceration with foreign body of unspecified back wall of thorax with penetration into thoracic cavity

S21.43   Puncture wound without foreign body of back wall of thorax with penetration into thoracic cavity

S21.431 Puncture wound without foreign body of right back wall of thorax with penetration into thoracic cavity

S21.432 Puncture wound without foreign body of left back wall of thorax with penetration into thoracic cavity

S21.439 Puncture wound with foreign body of unspecified back wall of thorax with penetration into thoracic cavity

S21.44 Puncture wound with foreign body of back wall of thorax with penetration into thoracic cavity

S21.441 Puncture wound with foreign body of right back wall of thorax with penetration into thoracic cavity

S21.442 Puncture wound with foreign body of left back wall of thorax with penetration into thoracic cavity

S21.449 Puncture wound with foreign body of unspecified back wall of thorax with penetration into thoracic cavity

S21.45 Open bite of back wall of thorax with penetration into thoracic cavity

Bite of back wall of thorax NOS

Excludes1: superficial bite of back wall of thorax (S20.47)

S21.451 Open bite of right back wall of thorax with penetration into thoracic cavity

S21.452 Open bite of left back wall of thorax with penetration into thoracic cavity

S21.459 Open bite of unspecified back wall of thorax with penetration into thoracic cavity

S21.9 Open wound of unspecified part of thorax

Open wound of thoracic wall NOS

S21.90 Unspecified open wound of unspecified part of thorax

S21.91 Laceration without foreign body of unspecified part of thorax

S21.92 Laceration with foreign body of unspecified part of thorax

S21.93 Puncture wound without foreign body of unspecified part of thorax

S21.94 Puncture wound with foreign body of unspecified part of thorax

S21.95 Open bite of unspecified part of thorax

Excludes1: superficial bite of thorax (S20.97)

S22 Fracture of rib(s), sternum and thoracic spine

A fracture not indicated as nondisplaced or displaced should be classified to displaced

Includes: fracture of thoracic neural arch
fracture of thoracic spinous process
fracture of thoracic transverse process
fracture of thoracic vertebra
fracture of thoracic vertebral arch

Codes first any associated:
injury of intrathoracic organ (S27.-)
spinal cord injury (S24.0-, S24.1-)

Excludes1: transection of thorax (S28.1)

Excludes2: fracture of clavicle (S42.0-)
fracture of scapula (S42.1-)

The following extensions are to be added to each code for this category:

A fracture not identified as open or closed should be coded to closed

a initial encounter for closed fracture
b initial encounter for open fracture
d subsequent encounter for fracture with routine healing
g subsequent encounter for fracture with delayed healing
j subsequent encounter for fracture with nonunion
q sequela

S22.0 Fracture of thoracic vertebra

S22.00 Fracture of unspecified thoracic vertebra

S22.000 Wedge compression fracture of unspecified thoracic vertebra

S22.001 Stable burst fracture of unspecified thoracic vertebra

S22.002 Unstable burst fracture of unspecified thoracic vertebra

S22.008 Other fracture of unspecified thoracic vertebra

S22.009 Unspecified fracture of unspecified thoracic vertebra

S22.01 Fracture of first thoracic vertebra

S22.010 Wedge compression fracture of first thoracic vertebra

S22.011 Stable burst fracture of first thoracic vertebra

S22.012 Unstable burst fracture of first thoracic vertebra

S22.018 Other fracture of first thoracic vertebra

S22.019 Unspecified fracture of first thoracic vertebra

S22.02 Fracture of second thoracic vertebra

S22.020 Wedge compression fracture of second thoracic vertebra

S22.021 Stable burst fracture of second thoracic vertebra

S22.022 Unstable burst fracture of second thoracic vertebra

S22.028 Other fracture of second thoracic vertebra

S22.029 Unspecified fracture of second thoracic vertebra

S22.03 Fracture of third thoracic vertebra

S22.030 Wedge compression fracture of third thoracic vertebra

S22.031 Stable burst fracture of third thoracic vertebra

S22.032 Unstable burst fracture of third thoracic vertebra

S22.038 Other fracture of third thoracic vertebra

S22.039 Unspecified fracture of third thoracic vertebra

S22.04 Fracture of fourth thoracic vertebra

S22.040 Wedge compression fracture of fourth thoracic vertebra

S22.041 Stable burst fracture of fourth thoracic vertebra

S22.042 Unstable burst fracture of fourth thoracic vertebra

S22.048 Other fracture of fourth thoracic vertebra

S22.049 Unspecified fracture of fourth thoracic vertebra

S22.05 Fracture of T_5-T_6 vertebra

S22.050 Wedge compression fracture of T_5-T_6 vertebra

S22.051 Stable burst fracture of T_5-T_6 vertebra

S22.052 Unstable burst fracture of T_5-T_6 vertebra

S22.058 Other fracture of T_5-T_6 vertebra

S22.059 Unspecified fracture of T_5-T_6 vertebra

S22.06 Fracture of T_7-T_8 vertebra

S22.060 Wedge compression fracture of T_7-T_8 vertebra

S22.061 Stable burst fracture of T_7-T_8 vertebra

S22.062 Unstable burst fracture of T_7-T_8 vertebra

S22.068 Other fracture of T_7-T_8 thoracic vertebra

S22.069 Unspecified fracture of T_7-T_8 vertebra

S22.07 Fracture of T_9-T_{10} vertebra

S22.070 Wedge compression fracture of T_9-T_{10} vertebra

S22.071 Stable burst fracture of T_9-T_{10} vertebra

S22.072 Unstable burst fracture of T_9-T_{10} vertebra

S22.078 Other fracture of T_9-T_{10} vertebra

S22.079 Unspecified fracture of T_9-T_{10} vertebra

S22.08 Fracture of T_{11}-T_{12} vertebra

S22.080 Wedge compression fracture of T_{11}-T_{12} vertebra

S22.081 Stable burst fracture of T_{11}-T_{12} vertebra

S22.082 Unstable burst fracture of T_{11}-T_{12} vertebra

S22.088 Other fracture of T_{11}-T_{12} vertebra

S22.089 Unspecified fracture of T_{11}-T_{12} vertebra

S22.2 Fracture of sternum

S22.20 Unspecified fracture of sternum

S22.21 Fracture of manubrium

S22.22 Fracture of body of sternum

S22.23   Sternal manubrial dissociation
S22.24   Fracture of xiphoid process
S22.3   **Fracture of one rib**
S22.31   Fracture of rib, right side
S22.32   Fracture of rib, left side
S22.39   Fracture of rib, unspecified side
S22.4   **Multiple fractures of ribs**
Fractures of two or more ribs
Excludes1:   flail chest (S22.5-)
S22.41   Multiple fractures of ribs, right side
S22.42   Multiple fractures of ribs, left side
S22.43   Multiple fractures of ribs, bilateral
S22.49   Multiple fractures of ribs, unspecified side
S22.5   **Flail chest**
S22.51   Flail chest, right side
S22.52   Flail chest, left side
S22.53   Flail chest, bilateral
S22.59   Flail chest, unspecified side
S22.9   **Fracture of bony thorax, part unspecified**

S23 Dislocation and sprain of joints and ligaments of thorax

Includes: avulsion of joint or ligament of thorax
laceration of joint or ligament of thorax
sprain of joint or ligament of thorax
traumatic hemarthrosis of joint or ligament of thorax
traumatic rupture of joint or ligament of thorax
traumatic subluxation of joint or ligament of thorax
traumatic tear of joint or ligament of thorax
Excludes2:   dislocation, sprain of sternoclavicular joint (S43.2, S43.6)
strain of muscle or tendon of thorax (S29.1)
The following extensions are to be added to each code for this category:
   a   initial encounter
   d   subsequent encounter
   q   sequela

S23.0   **Traumatic rupture of thoracic intervertebral disc**
Excludes1:   rupture or displacement (nontraumatic) of thoracic intervertebral disc NOS (M51.- with final character 4)

S23.1   **Subluxation and dislocation of thoracic vertebra**
Code also any associated
open wound of thorax (S21.-)
spinal cord injury (S24.0-, S24.1-)
Excludes2:   fracture of thoracic vertebrae (S22.0-)
S23.10   **Subluxation and dislocation of unspecified thoracic vertebra**
S23.100   Subluxation of unspecified thoracic vertebra
S23.101   Dislocation of unspecified thoracic vertebra
S23.11   **Subluxation and dislocation of T_1/T_2 thoracic vertebra**
S23.110   Subluxation of T_1/T_2 thoracic vertebra
S23.111   Dislocation of T_1/T_2 thoracic vertebra
S23.12   **Subluxation and dislocation of T_2/T_3-T_3/T_4 thoracic vertebra**
S23.120   Subluxation of T_2-T_3 thoracic vertebra
S23.121   Dislocation of T_2-T_3 thoracic vertebra
S23.122   Subluxation of T_3/T_4 thoracic vertebra
S23.123   Dislocation of T_3/T_4 thoracic vertebra
S23.13   **Subluxation and dislocation of T_4/T_5-T_5/T_6 thoracic vertebra**
S23.130   Subluxation of T_4/T_5 thoracic vertebra
S23.131   Dislocation of T_4-T_5 thoracic vertebra
S23.132   Subluxation of T_5/T_6 thoracic vertebra
S23.133   Dislocation of T_5/T_6 thoracic vertebra
S23.14   **Subluxation and dislocation of T_6/T_7-T_7/T_8 thoracic vertebra**
S23.140   Subluxation of T_6/T_7 thoracic vertebra
S23.141   Dislocation of T_6-T_7 thoracic vertebra
S23.142   Subluxation of T_7/T_8 thoracic vertebra
S23.143   Dislocation of T_7/T_8 thoracic vertebra

S23.15   **Subluxation and dislocation of T_8/T_9-T_9/T_{10} thoracic vertebra**
S23.150   Subluxation of T_8/T_9 thoracic vertebra
S23.151   Dislocation of T_8/T_9 thoracic vertebra
S23.152   Subluxation of T_9/T_{10} thoracic vertebra
S23.153   Dislocation of T_9/T_{10} thoracic vertebra
S23.16   **Subluxation and dislocation of T_{10}/T_{11}-T_{11}/T_{12} thoracic vertebra**
S23.160   Subluxation of T_{10}/T_{11} thoracic vertebra
S23.161   Dislocation of T_{10}/T_{11} thoracic vertebra
S23.162   Subluxation of T_{11}/T_{12} thoracic vertebra
S23.163   Dislocation of T_{11}/T_{12} thoracic vertebra
S23.17   **Subluxation and dislocation of T_{12}/L_1 thoracic vertebra**
S23.170   Subluxation of T_{12}/L_1 thoracic vertebra
S23.171   Dislocation of T_{12}/L_1 thoracic vertebra
S23.2   **Dislocation of other and unspecified parts of thorax**
S23.20   Dislocation of unspecified part of thorax
S23.29   Dislocation of other parts of thorax
S23.3   **Sprain of ligaments of thoracic spine**
S23.4   **Sprain of ribs and sternum**
S23.41   **Sprain of ribs**
S23.42   **Sprain of sternum**
S23.420   Sprain of sternoclavicular (joint) (ligament)
S23.421   Sprain of chondrosternal joint
S23.428   Other sprain of sternum
S23.429   Unspecified sprain of sternum
S23.8   **Sprain of other parts of thorax**
S23.9   **Sprain of unspecified parts of thorax**

S24 Injury of nerves and spinal cord at thorax level

Note: code to highest level of thoracic spinal cord injury
Code also any associated:
fracture of thoracic vertebra (S22.0-)
open wound of thorax (S21.-)
transient paralysis (R29.5)
Excludes2:   injury of brachial plexus (S14.3)
The following extensions are to be added to each code for this category:
   a   initial encounter
   d   subsequent encounter
   q   sequela

S24.0   **Concussion and edema of thoracic spinal cord**
S24.1   **Other and unspecified injuries of thoracic spinal cord**
S24.10   **Unspecified injury of thoracic spinal cord**
S24.101   Unspecified injury at T_1 level of thoracic spinal cord
S24.102   Unspecified injury at T_2-T_6 level of thoracic spinal cord
S24.103   Unspecified injury at T_7-T_{10} level of thoracic spinal cord
S24.104   Unspecified injury at T_{11}-T_{12} level of thoracic spinal cord
S24.109   Unspecified injury at unspecified level of thoracic spinal cord
Injury of thoracic spinal cord NOS
S24.11   **Complete lesion of thoracic spinal cord**
S24.111   Complete lesion at T_1 level of thoracic spinal cord
S24.112   Complete lesion at T_2-T_6 level of thoracic spinal cord
S24.113   Complete lesion at T_7-T_{10} level of thoracic spinal cord
S24.114   Complete lesion at T_{11}-T_{12} level of thoracic spinal cord
S24.119   Complete lesion at unspecified level of thoracic spinal cord
S24.13   **Anterior cord syndrome of thoracic spinal cord**
S24.131   Anterior cord syndrome at T_1 level of thoracic spinal cord
S24.132   Anterior cord syndrome at T_2-T_6 level of thoracic spinal cord

S24.133   Anterior cord syndrome at T$_7$-T$_{10}$ level of thoracic spinal cord

S24.134   Anterior cord syndrome at T$_{11}$-T$_{12}$ level of thoracic spinal cord

S24.139   Anterior cord syndrome at unspecified level of thoracic spinal cord

S24.14   **Brown-Sequard syndrome of thoracic spinal cord**

S24.141   Brown-Sequard syndrome at T$_1$ level of thoracic spinal cord

S24.142   Brown-Sequard syndrome at T$_2$-T$_6$ level of thoracic spinal cord

S24.143   Brown-Sequard syndrome at T$_7$-T$_{10}$ level of thoracic spinal cord

S24.144   Brown-Sequard syndrome at T$_{11}$-T$_{12}$ level of thoracic spinal cord

S24.149   Brown-Sequard syndrome at unspecified level of thoracic spinal cord

S24.15   **Other incomplete lesions of thoracic spinal cord**
Incomplete lesion of thoracic spinal cord NOS
Posterior cord syndrome of thoracic spinal cord

S24.151   Other incomplete lesion at T$_1$ level of thoracic spinal cord

S24.152   Other incomplete lesion at T$_2$-T$_6$ level of thoracic spinal cord

S24.153   Other incomplete lesion at T$_7$-T$_{10}$ level of thoracic spinal cord

S24.154   Other incomplete lesion at T$_{11}$-T$_{12}$ level of thoracic spinal cord

S24.159   Other incomplete lesion at unspecified level of thoracic spinal cord

S24.2   **Injury of nerve root of thoracic spine**

S24.3   **Injury of peripheral nerves of thorax**

S24.4   **Injury of thoracic sympathetic nervous system**
Injury of cardiac plexus
Injury of esophageal plexus
Injury of pulmonary plexus
Injury of stellate ganglion
Injury of thoracic sympathetic ganglion

S24.8   **Injury of other nerves of thorax**

S24.9   **Injury of unspecified nerve of thorax**

S25   **Injury of blood vessels of thorax**
Code also any associated open wound (S21.-)
The following extensions are to be added to each code for this category:
    a   initial encounter
    d   subsequent encounter
    q   sequela

S25.0   **Injury of thoracic aorta**
Injury of aorta NOS

S25.00   **Unspecified injury of thoracic aorta**

S25.01   **Minor laceration of thoracic aorta**
Incomplete transection of thoracic aorta
Laceration of thoracic aorta NOS
Superficial laceration of thoracic aorta

S25.02   **Major laceration of thoracic aorta**
Complete transection of thoracic aorta
Traumatic rupture of thoracic aorta

S25.09   **Other injury of thoracic aorta**

S25.1   **Injury of innominate or subclavian artery**

S25.10   **Unspecified injury of innominate or subclavian artery**

S25.101   Unspecified injury of right innominate or subclavian artery

S25.102   Unspecified injury of left innominate or subclavian artery

S25.109   Unspecified injury of unspecified innominate or subclavian artery

S25.11   **Minor laceration of innominate or subclavian artery**
Incomplete transection of innominate or subclavian artery
Laceration of innominate or subclavian artery NOS
Superficial laceration of innominate or subclavian artery

S25.111   Minor laceration of right innominate or subclavian artery

S25.112   Minor laceration of left innominate or subclavian artery

S25.119   Minor laceration of unspecified innominate or subclavian artery

S25.12   **Major laceration of innominate or subclavian artery**
Complete transection of innominate or subclavian artery
Traumatic rupture of innominate or subclavian artery

S25.121   Major laceration of right innominate or subclavian artery

S25.122   Major laceration of left innominate or subclavian artery

S25.129   Major laceration of unspecified innominate or subclavian artery

S25.19   **Other specified injury of innominate or subclavian artery**

S25.191   Other specified injury of right innominate or subclavian artery

S25.192   Other specified injury of left innominate or subclavian artery

S25.199   Other specified injury of unspecified innominate or subclavian artery

S25.2   **Injury of superior vena cava**
Injury of vena cava NOS

S25.20   **Unspecified injury of superior vena cava**

S25.21   **Minor laceration of superior vena cava**
Incomplete transection of superior vena cava
Laceration of superior vena cava NOS
Superficial laceration of superior vena cava

S25.22   **Major laceration of superior vena cava**
Complete transection of superior vena cava
Traumatic rupture of superior vena cava

S25.29   **Other specified injury of superior vena cava**

S25.3   **Injury of innominate or subclavian vein**

S25.30   **Unspecified injury of innominate or subclavian vein**

S25.301   Unspecified injury of right innominate or subclavian vein

S25.302   Unspecified injury of left innominate or subclavian vein

S25.309   Unspecified injury of unspecified innominate or subclavian vein

S25.31   **Minor laceration of innominate or subclavian vein**
Incomplete transection of innominate or subclavian vein
Laceration of innominate or subclavian vein NOS
Superficial laceration of innominate or subclavian vein

S25.311   Minor laceration of right innominate or subclavian vein

S25.312   Minor laceration of left innominate or subclavian vein

S25.319   Minor laceration of unspecified innominate or subclavian vein

S25.32   **Major laceration of innominate or subclavian vein**
Complete transection of innominate or subclavian vein
Traumatic rupture of innominate or subclavian vein

S25.321   Major laceration of right innominate or subclavian vein

S25.322   Major laceration of left innominate or subclavian vein

S25.329   Major laceration of unspecified innominate or subclavian vein

S25.39   **Other specified injury of innominate or subclavian vein**

S25.391   Other specified injury of right innominate or subclavian vein

S25.392   Other specified injury of left innominate or subclavian vein

S25.399   Other specified injury of unspecified innominate or subclavian vein

S25.4   **Injury of pulmonary blood vessels**

S25.40   **Unspecified injury of pulmonary blood vessels**

S25.401 Unspecified injury of right pulmonary blood vessels

S25.402 Unspecified injury of left pulmonary blood vessels

S25.409 Unspecified injury of unspecified pulmonary blood vessels

S25.41 Minor laceration of pulmonary blood vessels
Incomplete transection of pulmonary blood vessels
Laceration of pulmonary blood vessels NOS
Superficial laceration of pulmonary blood vessels

S25.411 Minor laceration of right pulmonary blood vessels

S25.412 Minor laceration of left pulmonary blood vessels

S25.419 Minor laceration of unspecified pulmonary blood vessels

S25.42 Major laceration of pulmonary blood vessels
Complete transection of pulmonary blood vessels
Traumatic rupture of pulmonary blood vessels

S25.421 Major laceration of right pulmonary blood vessels

S25.422 Major laceration of left pulmonary blood vessels

S25.429 Major laceration of unspecified pulmonary blood vessels

S25.49 Other specified injury of pulmonary blood vessels

S25.491 Other specified injury of right pulmonary blood vessels

S25.492 Other specified injury of left pulmonary blood vessels

S25.499 Other specified injury of unspecified pulmonary blood vessels

S25.5 Injury of intercostal blood vessels

S25.50 Unspecified injury of intercostal blood vessels

S25.501 Unspecified injury of intercostal blood vessels, right side

S25.502 Unspecified injury of intercostal blood vessels, left side

S25.509 Unspecified injury of intercostal blood vessels, unspecified side

S25.51 Laceration of intercostal blood vessels

S25.511 Laceration of intercostal blood vessels, right side

S25.512 Laceration of intercostal blood vessels, left side

S25.519 Laceration of intercostal blood vessels, unspecified side

S25.59 Other specified injury of intercostal blood vessels

S25.591 Other specified injury of intercostal blood vessels, right side

S25.592 Other specified injury of intercostal blood vessels, left side

S25.599 Other specified injury of intercostal blood vessels, unspecified side

S25.8 Injury of other blood vessels of thorax
Injury of azygos vein
Injury of mammary artery or vein

S25.80 Unspecified injury of other blood vessels of thorax

S25.801 Unspecified injury of other blood vessels of thorax, right side

S25.802 Unspecified injury of other blood vessels of thorax, left side

S25.809 Unspecified injury of other blood vessels of thorax, unspecified side

S25.81 Laceration of other blood vessels of thorax

S25.811 Laceration of other blood vessels of thorax, right side

S25.812 Laceration of other blood vessels of thorax, left side

S25.819 Laceration of other blood vessels of thorax, unspecified side

S25.89 Other specified injury of other blood vessels of thorax

S25.891 Other specified injury of other blood vessels of thorax, right side

S25.892 Other specified injury of other blood vessels of thorax, left side

S25.899 Other specified injury of other blood vessels of thorax, unspecified side

S25.9 Injury of unspecified blood vessel of thorax

S25.90 Unspecified injury of unspecified blood vessel of thorax

S25.91 Laceration of unspecified blood vessel of thorax

S25.99 Other specified injury of unspecified blood vessel of thorax

S26 Injury of heart
Code also any associated:
open wound of thorax (S21.-)
traumatic hemopneumothorax (S27.2)
traumatic hemothorax (S27.1)
traumatic pneumothorax (S27.0)
The following extensions are to be added to each code for this category:
a   initial encounter
d   subsequent encounter
q   sequela

S26.0 Injury of heart with hemopericardium

S26.00 Unspecified injury of heart with hemopericardium

S26.01 Contusion of heart with hemopericardium

S26.02 Laceration of heart with hemopericardium

S26.020 Mild laceration of heart with hemopericardium
Laceration of heart without penetration of heart chamber

S26.021 Moderate laceration of heart with hemopericardium
Laceration of heart with penetration of heart chamber

S26.022 Major laceration of heart with hemopericardium
Laceration of heart with penetration of multiple heart chambers

S26.09 Other injury of heart with hemopericardium

S26.1 Injury of heart without hemopericardium

S26.10 Unspecified injury of heart without hemopericardium

S26.11 Contusion of heart without hemopericardium

S26.12 Laceration of heart without hemopericardium

S26.19 Other injury of heart without hemopericardium

S26.9 Injury of heart, unspecified with or without hemopericardium

S26.90 Unspecified injury of heart, unspecified with or without hemopericardium

S26.91 Contusion of heart, unspecified with or without hemopericardium

S26.92 Laceration of heart, unspecified with or without hemopericardium
Laceration of heart NOS

S26.99 Other injury of heart, unspecified with or without hemopericardium

S27 Injury of other and unspecified intrathoracic organs
Code also any associated open wound of thorax (S21.-)
Excludes2:   injury of cervical esophagus (S10-S19)
injury of trachea (cervical) (S10-S19)
The following extensions are to be added to each code for this category:
a   initial encounter
d   subsequent encounter
q   sequela

S27.0 Traumatic pneumothorax
Excludes1:   spontaneous pneumothorax (J93.-)

S27.1 Traumatic hemothorax

S27.2 Traumatic hemopneumothorax

S27.3 Other and unspecified injuries of lung

S27.30 Unspecified injury of lung

S27.301 Unspecified injury of lung, unilateral

S27.302 Unspecified injury of lung, bilateral

        S27.309   Unspecified injury of lung, unspecified
    S27.31   Primary blast injury of lung
        Blast injury of lung NOS
        S27.311   Primary blast injury of lung, unilateral
        S27.312   Primary blast injury of lung, bilateral
        S27.319   Primary blast injury of lung, unspecified
    S27.32   Contusion of lung
        S27.321   Contusion of lung, unilateral
        S27.322   Contusion of lung, bilateral
        S27.329   Contusion of lung, unspecified
    S27.33   Laceration of lung
        S27.331   Laceration of lung, unilateral
        S27.332   Laceration of lung, bilateral
        S27.339   Laceration of lung, unspecified
    S27.39   Other injuries of lung
        Secondary blast injury of lung
        S27.391   Other injuries of lung, unilateral
        S27.392   Other injuries of lung, bilateral
        S27.399   Other injuries of lung, unspecified
  S27.4   Injury of bronchus
    S27.40   Unspecified injury of bronchus
        S27.401   Unspecified injury of bronchus, unilateral
        S27.402   Unspecified injury of bronchus, bilateral
        S27.409   Unspecified injury of bronchus, unspecified
    S27.41   Primary blast injury of bronchus
        Blast injury of bronchus NOS
        S27.411   Primary blast injury of bronchus, unilateral
        S27.412   Primary blast injury of bronchus, bilateral
        S27.419   Primary blast injury of bronchus, unspecified
    S27.42   Contusion of bronchus
        S27.421   Contusion of bronchus, unilateral
        S27.422   Contusion of bronchus, bilateral
        S27.429   Contusion of bronchus, unspecified
    S27.43   Laceration of bronchus
        S27.431   Laceration of bronchus, unilateral
        S27.432   Laceration of bronchus, bilateral
        S27.439   Laceration of bronchus, unspecified
    S27.49   Other injury of bronchus
        Secondary blast injury of bronchus
        S27.491   Other injury of bronchus, unilateral
        S27.492   Other injury of bronchus, bilateral
        S27.499   Other injury of bronchus, unspecified
  S27.5   Injury of thoracic trachea
    S27.50   Unspecified injury of thoracic trachea
    S27.51   Primary blast injury of thoracic trachea
        Blast injury of thoracic trachea NOS
    S27.52   Contusion of thoracic trachea
    S27.53   Laceration of thoracic trachea
    S27.59   Other injury of thoracic trachea
        Secondary blast injury of thoracic trachea
  S27.6   Injury of pleura
    S27.60   Unspecified injury of pleura
    S27.63   Laceration of pleura
    S27.69   Other injury of pleura
  S27.8   Injury of other specified intrathoracic organs
    S27.80   Injury of diaphragm
        S27.802   Contusion of diaphragm
        S27.803   Laceration of diaphragm
        S27.808   Other injury of diaphragm
        S27.809   Unspecified injury of diaphragm
    S27.81   Injury of esophagus (thoracic part)
        S27.812   Contusion of esophagus (thoracic part)
        S27.813   Laceration of esophagus (thoracic part)
        S27.818   Other injury of esophagus (thoracic part)
        S27.819   Unspecified injury of esophagus (thoracic part)
    S27.89   Injury of other specified intrathoracic organs
        Injury of lymphatic thoracic duct
        Injury of thymus gland

        S27.892   Contusion of other specified intrathoracic organs
        S27.893   Laceration of other specified intrathoracic organs
        S27.898   Other injury of other specified intrathoracic organs
        S27.899   Unspecified injury of other specified intrathoracic organs
  S27.9   Injury of unspecified intrathoracic organ

S28 Crushing injury of thorax, and traumatic amputation of part of thorax
    The following extensions are to be added to each code for this category:
      a   initial encounter
      d   subsequent encounter
      q   sequela
  S28.0   Crushed chest
    Use additional code for all associated injuries
    Excludes1:   flail chest (S22.5)
  S28.1   Traumatic amputation (partial) of part of thorax, except breast
  S28.2   Traumatic amputation of breast
    S28.21   Complete traumatic amputation of breast
        Traumatic amputation of breast NOS
        S28.211   Complete traumatic amputation of right breast
        S28.212   Complete traumatic amputation of left breast
        S28.219   Complete traumatic amputation of unspecified breast
    S28.22   Partial traumatic amputation of breast
        S28.221   Partial traumatic amputation of right breast
        S28.222   Partial traumatic amputation of left breast
        S28.229   Partial traumatic amputation of unspecified breast

S29 Other and unspecified injuries of thorax
    Code also any associated open wound (S21.-)
    The following extensions are to be added to each code for this category:
      a   initial encounter
      d   subsequent encounter
      q   sequela
  S29.0   Injury of muscle and tendon at thorax level
    S29.00   Unspecified injury of muscle and tendon of thorax
        S29.001   Unspecified injury of muscle and tendon of front wall of thorax
        S29.002   Unspecified injury of muscle and tendon of back wall of thorax
        S29.009   Unspecified injury of muscle and tendon of unspecified wall of thorax
    S29.01   Strain of muscle and tendon of thorax
        S29.011   Strain of muscle and tendon of front wall of thorax
        S29.012   Strain of muscle and tendon of back wall of thorax
        S29.019   Strain of muscle and tendon of unspecified wall of thorax
    S29.02   Laceration of muscle and tendon of thorax
        S29.021   Laceration of muscle and tendon of front wall of thorax
        S29.022   Laceration of muscle and tendon of back wall of thorax
        S29.029   Laceration of muscle and tendon of unspecified wall of thorax
    S29.09   Other injury of muscle and tendon of thorax
        S29.091   Other injury of muscle and tendon of front wall of thorax
        S29.092   Other injury of muscle and tendon of back wall of thorax
        S29.099   Other injury of muscle and tendon of unspecified wall of thorax
  S29.8   Other specified injuries of thorax
  S29.9   Unspecified injury of thorax

INJURIES TO THE ABDOMEN, LOWER BACK, LUMBAR SPINE AND PELVIS (S30–S39)

Includes: injuries to the abdominal wall
injuries to the anus
injuries to the buttock
injuries to the external genitalia
injuries to the flank
injuries to the groin burns and corrosions (T20-T32)

Excludes2:   effects of foreign body in anus and rectum (T18.5)
effects of foreign body in genitourinary tract (T19.-)
effects of foreign body in stomach, small intestine and colon (T18.2-T18.4)
frostbite (T33-T34)
insect bite or sting, venomous (T63.4)

S30 Superficial injury of abdomen, lower back and pelvis

Excludes2:   superficial injury of hip (S70.-)

The following extensions are to be added to each code for this category:
a   initial encounter
d   subsequent encounter
q   sequela

S30.0   Contusion of lower back and pelvis
Contusion of buttock

S30.1   Contusion of abdominal wall
Contusion of flank
Contusion of groin

S30.2   Contusion of external genital organs

S30.20   Contusion of unspecified external genital organ

S30.201   Contusion of unspecified external genital organ, male

S30.202   Contusion of unspecified external genital organ, female

S30.21   Contusion of penis

S30.22   Contusion of scrotum and testes

S30.23   Contusion of vagina and vulva

S30.3   Contusion of anus

S30.8   Other superficial injuries of abdomen, lower back and pelvis

S30.81   Abrasion of abdomen, lower back and pelvis

S30.810   Abrasion of lower back and pelvis

S30.811   Abrasion of abdominal wall

S30.812   Abrasion of penis

S30.813   Abrasion of scrotum and testes

S30.814   Abrasion of vagina and vulva

S30.815   Abrasion of unspecified external genital organs, male

S30.816   Abrasion of unspecified external genital organs, female

S30.817   Abrasion of anus

S30.82   Blister (nonthermal) of abdomen, lower back and pelvis

S30.820   Blister (nonthermal) of lower back and pelvis

S30.821   Blister (nonthermal) of abdominal wall

S30.822   Blister (nonthermal) of penis

S30.823   Blister (nonthermal) of scrotum and testes

S30.824   Blister (nonthermal) of vagina and vulva

S30.825   Blister (nonthermal) of unspecified external genital organs, male

S30.826   Blister (nonthermal) of unspecified external genital organs, female

S30.827   Blister (nonthermal) of anus

S30.84   External constriction of abdomen, lower back and pelvis

S30.840   External constriction of lower back and pelvis

S30.841   External constriction of abdominal wall

S30.842   External constriction of penis

S30.843   External constriction of scrotum and testes

S30.844   External constriction of vagina and vulva

S30.845   External constriction of unspecified external genital organs, male

S30.846   External constriction of unspecified external genital organs, female

S30.85   Superficial foreign body of abdomen, lower back and pelvis
Splinter in the abdomen, lower back and pelvis

S30.850   Superficial foreign body of lower back and pelvis

S30.851   Superficial foreign body of abdominal wall

S30.852   Superficial foreign body of penis

S30.853   Superficial foreign body of scrotum and testes

S30.854   Superficial foreign body of vagina and vulva

S30.855   Superficial foreign body of unspecified external genital organs, male

S30.856   Superficial foreign body of unspecified external genital organs, female

S30.857   Superficial foreign body of anus

S30.86   Insect bite (nonvenomous) of abdomen, lower back and pelvis

S30.860   Insect bite (nonvenomous) of lower back and pelvis

S30.861   Insect bite (nonvenomous) of abdominal wall

S30.862   Insect bite (nonvenomous) of penis

S30.863   Insect bite (nonvenomous) of scrotum and testes

S30.864   Insect bite (nonvenomous) of vagina and vulva

S30.865   Insect bite (nonvenomous) of unspecified external genital organs, male

S30.866   Insect bite (nonvenomous) of unspecified external genital organs, female

S30.867   Insect bite (nonvenomous) of anus

S30.87   Other superficial bite of abdomen, lower back. and pelvis

Excludes1:   open bite of abdomen, lower back, and pelvis (S31.05, S31.15, S31.25, S31.35, S31.45, S31.55)

S30.870   Other superficial bite of lower back and pelvis

S30.871   Other superficial bite of abdominal wall

S30.872   Other superficial bite of penis

S30.873   Other superficial bite of scrotum and testes

S30.874   Other superficial bite of vagina and vulva

S30.875   Other superficial bite of unspecified external genital organs, male

S30.876   Other superficial bite of unspecified external genital organs, female

S30.877   Other superficial bite of anus

S30.9   Unspecified superficial injury of abdomen, lower back and pelvis

S30.91   Unspecified superficial injury of lower back and pelvis

S30.92   Unspecified superficial injury of abdominal wall

S30.93   Unspecified superficial injury of penis

S30.94   Unspecified superficial injury of scrotum and testes

S30.95   Unspecified superficial injury of vagina and vulva

S30.96   Unspecified superficial injury of unspecified external genital organs, male

S30.97   Unspecified superficial injury of unspecified external genital organs, female

S30.98   Unspecified superficial injury of anus

S31 Open wound of abdomen, lower back and pelvis

Code also any associated:
spinal cord injury (S24.0, S24.1-, S34.0, S34.1-)
wound infection

Excludes1:   traumatic amputation of part of abdomen, lower back and pelvis (S38.2-, S38.3)

Excludes2:   open wound of hip (S71.00-S71.02)
open fracture of pelvis (S32.1—S32.9 with extension b)

The following extensions are to be added to each code for this category:
a   initial encounter
d   subsequent encounter
q   sequela

S31.0 Open wound of lower back and pelvis
  S31.00 Unspecified open wound of lower back and pelvis
    S31.000 Unspecified open wound of lower back and pelvis without penetration into retroperitoneum
      Unspecified open wound of lower back and pelvis NOS
    S31.001 Unspecified open wound of lower back and pelvis with penetration into retroperitoneum
  S31.01 Laceration without foreign body of lower back and pelvis
    S31.010 Laceration without foreign body of lower back and pelvis without penetration into retroperitoneum
      Laceration without foreign body of lower back and pelvis NOS
    S31.011 Laceration without foreign body of lower back and pelvis with penetration into retroperitoneum
  S31.02 Laceration with foreign body of lower back and pelvis
    S31.020 Laceration with foreign body of lower back and pelvis without penetration into retroperitoneum
      Laceration with foreign body of lower back and pelvis NOS
    S31.021 Laceration with foreign body of lower back and pelvis with penetration into retroperitoneum
  S31.03 Puncture wound without foreign body of lower back and pelvis
    S31.030 Puncture wound without foreign body of lower back and pelvis without penetration into retroperitoneum
      Puncture wound without foreign body of lower back and pelvis NOS
    S31.031 Puncture wound without foreign body of lower back and pelvis with penetration into retroperitoneum
  S31.04 Puncture wound with foreign body of lower back and pelvis
    S31.040 Puncture wound with foreign body of lower back and pelvis without penetration into retroperitoneum
      Puncture wound with foreign body of lower back and pelvis NOS
    S31.041 Puncture wound with foreign body of lower back and pelvis with penetration into retroperitoneum
  S31.05 Open bite of lower back and pelvis
    Bite of lower back and pelvis NOS
    Excludes1: superficial bite of lower back and pelvis (S30.860, S30.870)
    S31.050 Open bite of lower back and pelvis without penetration into retroperitoneum
      Open bite of lower back and pelvis NOS
    S31.051 Open bite of lower back and pelvis with penetration into retroperitoneum
S31.1 Open wound of abdominal wall without penetration into peritoneal cavity Open wound of abdominal wall NOS
  Excludes2: open wound of abdominal wall with penetration into peritoneal cavity (S31.6-)
  S31.10 Unspecified open wound of abdominal wall without penetration into peritoneal cavity
    S31.100 Unspecified open wound of abdominal wall, right upper quadrant without penetration into peritoneal cavity
    S31.101 Unspecified open wound of abdominal wall, left upper quadrant without penetration into peritoneal cavity
    S31.102 Unspecified open wound of abdominal wall, epigastric region without penetration into peritoneal cavity

S31.103 Unspecified open wound of abdominal wall, right lower quadrant without penetration into peritoneal cavity
S31.104 Unspecified open wound of abdominal wall, left lower quadrant without penetration into peritoneal cavity
S31.105 Unspecified open wound of abdominal wall, periumbilic region without penetration into peritoneal cavity
S31.109 Unspecified open wound of abdominal wall, unspecified quadrant without penetration into peritoneal cavity
  Unspecified open wound of abdominal wall NOS
  S31.11 Laceration without foreign body of abdominal wall without penetration into peritoneal cavity
    S31.110 Laceration without foreign body of abdominal wall, right upper quadrant without penetration into peritoneal cavity
    S31.111 Laceration without foreign body of abdominal wall, left upper quadrant without penetration into peritoneal cavity
    S31.112 Laceration without foreign body of abdominal wall, epigastric region without penetration into peritoneal cavity
    S31.113 Laceration without foreign body of abdominal wall, right lower quadrant without penetration into peritoneal cavity
    S31.114 Laceration without foreign body of abdominal wall, left lower quadrant without penetration into peritoneal cavity
    S31.115 Laceration without foreign body of abdominal wall, periumbilic region without penetration into peritoneal cavity
    S31.119 Laceration without foreign body of abdominal wall, unspecified quadrant without penetration into peritoneal cavity
  S31.12 Laceration with foreign body of abdominal wall without penetration into peritoneal cavity
    S31.120 Laceration of abdominal wall with foreign body, right upper quadrant without penetration into peritoneal cavity
    S31.121 Laceration of abdominal wall with foreign body, left upper quadrant without penetration into peritoneal cavity
    S31.122 Laceration of abdominal wall with foreign body, epigastric region without penetration into peritoneal cavity
    S31.123 Laceration of abdominal wall with foreign body, right lower quadrant without penetration into peritoneal cavity
    S31.124 Laceration of abdominal wall with foreign body, left lower quadrant without penetration into peritoneal cavity
    S31.125 Laceration of abdominal wall with foreign body, periumbilic region without penetration into peritoneal cavity
    S31.129 Laceration of abdominal wall with foreign body, unspecified quadrant without penetration into peritoneal cavity
  S31.13 Puncture wound of abdominal wall without foreign body without penetration into peritoneal cavity
    S31.130 Puncture wound of abdominal wall without foreign body, right upper quadrant without penetration into peritoneal cavity
    S31.131 Puncture wound of abdominal wall without foreign body, left upper quadrant without penetration into peritoneal cavity
    S31.132 Puncture wound of abdominal wall without foreign body, epigastric region without penetration into peritoneal cavity
    S31.133 Puncture wound of abdominal wall without foreign body, right lower quadrant without penetration into peritoneal cavity

S31.134   Puncture wound of abdominal wall without foreign body, left lower quadrant without penetration into peritoneal cavity

S31.135   Puncture wound of abdominal wall without foreign body, periumbilic region without penetration into peritoneal cavity

S31.139   Puncture wound of abdominal wall without foreign body, unspecified quadrant without penetration into peritoneal cavity

S31.14   Puncture wound of abdominal wall with foreign body without penetration into peritoneal cavity

S31.140   Puncture wound of abdominal wall with foreign body, right upper quadrant without penetration into peritoneal cavity

S31.141   Puncture wound of abdominal wall with foreign body, left upper quadrant without penetration into peritoneal cavity

S31.142   Puncture wound of abdominal wall with foreign body, epigastric region without penetration into peritoneal cavity

S31.143   Puncture wound of abdominal wall with foreign body, right lower quadrant without penetration into peritoneal cavity

S31.144   Puncture wound of abdominal wall with foreign body, left lower quadrant without penetration into peritoneal cavity

S31.145   Puncture wound of abdominal wall with foreign body, periumbilic region without penetration into peritoneal cavity

S31.149   Puncture wound of abdominal wall with foreign body, unspecified quadrant without penetration into peritoneal cavity

S31.15   Open bite of abdominal wall without penetration into peritoneal cavity
Bite of abdominal wall NOS
Excludes1:   superficial bite of abdominal wall (S30.871)

S31.150   Open bite of abdominal wall, right upper quadrant without penetration into peritoneal cavity

S31.151   Open bite of abdominal wall, left upper quadrant without penetration into peritoneal cavity

S31.152   Open bite of abdominal wall, epigastric region without penetration into peritoneal cavity

S31.153   Open bite of abdominal wall, right lower quadrant without penetration into peritoneal cavity

S31.154   Open bite of abdominal wall, left lower quadrant without penetration into peritoneal cavity

S31.155   Open bite of abdominal wall, periumbilic region without penetration into peritoneal cavity

S31.159   Open bite of abdominal wall, unspecified quadrant without penetration into peritoneal cavity

S31.2   Open wound of penis
S31.20   Unspecified open wound of penis
S31.21   Laceration without foreign body of penis
S31.22   Laceration with foreign body of penis
S31.23   Puncture wound without foreign body of penis
S31.24   Puncture wound with foreign body of penis
S31.25   Open bite of penis
Bite of penis NOS
Excludes1:   superficial bite of penis (S30.862, S30.872)

S31.3   Open wound of scrotum and testes
S31.30   Unspecified open wound of scrotum and testes
S31.31   Laceration without foreign body of scrotum and testes
S31.32   Laceration with foreign body of scrotum and testes
S31.33   Puncture wound without foreign body of scrotum and testes

S31.34   Puncture wound with foreign body of scrotum and testes
S31.35   Open bite of scrotum and testes
Bite of scrotum and testes NOS
Excludes1:   superficial bite of scrotum and testes (S30.863, S31.40, S30.873)

S31.4   Open wound of vagina and vulva
Excludes1:   injury to vagina and vulva during delivery (O70.-, O71.4)
S31.40   Unspecified open wound of vagina and vulva
S31.41   Laceration without foreign body of vagina and vulva
S31.42   Laceration with foreign body of vagina and vulva
S31.43   Puncture wound without foreign body of vagina and vulva
S31.44   Puncture wound with foreign body of vagina and vulva
S31.45   Open bite of vagina and vulva Bite of vagina and vulva NOS
Excludes1:   superficial bite of vagina and vulva (S30.864, S30.874)

S31.5   Open wound of unspecified external genital organs
Excludes1:   traumatic amputation of external genital organs (S38.21, S38.22)
S31.50   Unspecified open wound of unspecified external genital organs
S31.501   Unspecified open wound of unspecified external genital organs, male
S31.502   Unspecified open wound of unspecified external genital organs, female
S31.51   Laceration without foreign body of unspecified external genital organs
S31.511   Laceration without foreign body of unspecified external genital organs, male
S31.512   Laceration without foreign body of unspecified external genital organs, female
S31.52   Laceration with foreign body of unspecified external genital organs
S31.521   Laceration with foreign body of unspecified external genital organs, male
S31.522   Laceration with foreign body of unspecified external genital organs, female
S31.53   Puncture wound without foreign body of unspecified external genital organs
S31.531   Puncture wound without foreign body of unspecified external genital organs, male
S31.532   Puncture wound without foreign body of unspecified external genital organs, female
S31.54   Puncture wound with foreign body of unspecified external genital organs
S31.541   Puncture wound with foreign body of unspecified external genital organs, male
S31.542   Puncture wound with foreign body of unspecified external genital organs, female
S31.55   Open bite of unspecified external genital organs
Bite of unspecified external genital organs NOS
Excludes1:   superficial bite of unspecified external genital organs (S30.865, S30.866, S30.875, S30.876)
S31.551   Open bite of unspecified external genital organs, male
S31.552   Open bite of unspecified external genital organs, female

S31.6   Open wound of abdominal wall with penetration into peritoneal cavity
S31.60   Unspecified open wound of abdominal wall with penetration into peritoneal cavity
S31.600   Unspecified open wound of abdominal wall, right upper quadrant with penetration into peritoneal cavity
S31.601   Unspecified open wound of abdominal wall, left upper quadrant with penetration into peritoneal cavity

S31.602   Unspecified open wound of abdominal wall, epigastric region with penetration into peritoneal cavity

S31.603   Unspecified open wound of abdominal wall, right lower quadrant with penetration into peritoneal cavity

S31.604   Unspecified open wound of abdominal wall, left lower quadrant with penetration into peritoneal cavity

S31.605   Unspecified open wound of abdominal wall, periumbilic region with penetration into peritoneal cavity

S31.609   Unspecified open wound of abdominal wall, unspecified quadrant with penetration into peritoneal cavity

S31.61   Laceration without foreign body of abdominal wall with penetration into peritoneal cavity

S31.610   Laceration without foreign body of abdominal wall, right upper quadrant with penetration into peritoneal cavity

S31.611   Laceration without foreign body of abdominal wall, left upper quadrant with penetration into peritoneal cavity

S31.612   Laceration without foreign body of abdominal wall, epigastric region with penetration into peritoneal cavity

S31.613   Laceration without foreign body of abdominal wall, right lower quadrant with penetration into peritoneal cavity

S31.614   Laceration without foreign body of abdominal wall, left lower quadrant with penetration into peritoneal cavity

S31.615   Laceration without foreign body of abdominal wall, periumbilic region with penetration into peritoneal cavity

S31.619   Laceration without foreign body of abdominal wall, unspecified quadrant with penetration into peritoneal cavity

S31.62   Laceration with foreign body of abdominal wall with penetration into peritoneal cavity

S31.620   Laceration with foreign body of abdominal wall, right upper quadrant with penetration into peritoneal cavity

S31.621   Laceration with foreign body of abdominal wall, left upper quadrant with penetration into peritoneal cavity

S31.622   Laceration with foreign body of abdominal wall, epigastric region with penetration into peritoneal cavity

S31.623   Laceration with foreign body of abdominal wall, right lower quadrant with penetration into peritoneal cavity

S31.624   Laceration with foreign body of abdominal wall, left lower quadrant with penetration into peritoneal cavity

S31.625   Laceration with foreign body of abdominal wall, periumbilic region with penetration into peritoneal cavity

S31.629   Laceration with foreign body of abdominal wall, unspecified quadrant with penetration into peritoneal cavity

S31.63   Puncture wound without foreign body of abdominal wall with penetration into peritoneal cavity

S31.630   Puncture wound without foreign body of abdominal wall, right upper quadrant with penetration into peritoneal cavity

S31.631   Puncture wound without foreign body of abdominal wall, left upper quadrant with penetration into peritoneal cavity

S31.632   Puncture wound without foreign body of abdominal wall, epigastric region with penetration into peritoneal cavity

S31.633   Puncture wound without foreign body of abdominal wall, right lower quadrant with penetration into peritoneal cavity

S31.634   Puncture wound without foreign body of abdominal wall, left lower quadrant with penetration into peritoneal cavity

S31.635   Puncture wound without foreign body of abdominal wall, periumbilic region with penetration into peritoneal cavity

S31.639   Puncture wound without foreign body of abdominal wall, unspecified quadrant with penetration into peritoneal cavity

S31.64   Puncture wound with foreign body of abdominal wall with penetration into peritoneal cavity

S31.640   Puncture wound with foreign body of abdominal wall, right upper quadrant with penetration into peritoneal cavity

S31.641   Puncture wound with foreign body of abdominal wall, left upper quadrant with penetration into peritoneal cavity

S31.642   Puncture wound with foreign body of abdominal wall, epigastric region with penetration into peritoneal cavity

S31.643   Puncture wound with foreign body of abdominal wall, right lower quadrant with penetration into peritoneal cavity

S31.644   Puncture wound with foreign body of abdominal wall, left lower quadrant with penetration into peritoneal cavity

S31.645   Puncture wound with foreign body of abdominal wall, periumbilic region with penetration into peritoneal cavity

S31.649   Puncture wound with foreign body of abdominal wall, unspecified quadrant with penetration into peritoneal cavity

S31.65   Open bite of abdominal wall with penetration into peritoneal cavity

    Excludes1:   superficial bite of abdominal wall (S30.861, S30.871)

S31.650   Open bite of abdominal wall, right upper quadrant with penetration into peritoneal cavity

S31.651   Open bite of abdominal wall, left upper quadrant with penetration into peritoneal cavity

S31.652   Open bite of abdominal wall, epigastric region with penetration into peritoneal cavity

S31.653   Open bite of abdominal wall, right lower quadrant with penetration into peritoneal cavity

S31.654   Open bite of abdominal wall, left lower quadrant with penetration into peritoneal cavity

S31.655   Open bite of abdominal wall, periumbilic region with penetration into peritoneal cavity

S31.659   Open bite of abdominal wall, unspecified quadrant with penetration into peritoneal cavity

S31.8   Open wound of other parts of abdomen, lower back and pelvis

S31.80   Open wound of unspecified buttock

S31.801   Laceration without foreign body of unspecified buttock

S31.802   Laceration with foreign body of unspecified buttock

S31.803   Puncture wound without foreign body of unspecified buttock

S31.804   Puncture wound with foreign body of unspecified buttock

S31.805   Open bite of unspecified buttock

    Bite of buttock NOS

    Excludes1:   superficial bite of buttock (S30.870)

S31.809 Unspecified open wound of unspecified buttock

S31.81 Open wound of right buttock

S31.811 Laceration without foreign body of right buttock

S31.812 Laceration with foreign body of right buttock

S31.813 Puncture wound without foreign body of right buttock

S31.814 Puncture wound with foreign body of right buttock

S31.815 Open bite of right buttock
Bite of right buttock NOS
Excludes1: superficial bite of buttock (S30.870)

S31.819 Unspecified open wound of right buttock

S31.82 Open wound of left buttock

S31.821 Laceration without foreign body of left buttock

S31.822 Laceration with foreign body of left buttock

S31.823 Puncture wound without foreign body of left buttock

S31.824 Puncture wound with foreign body of left buttock

S31.825 Open bite of left buttock
Bite of left buttock NOS
Excludes1: superficial bite of buttock (S30.870)

S31.829 Unspecified open wound of left buttock

S31.83 Open wound of anus

S31.831 Laceration without foreign body of anus

S31.832 Laceration with foreign body of anus

S31.833 Puncture wound without foreign body of anus

S31.834 Puncture wound with foreign body of anus

S31.835 Open bite of anus
Bite of anus NOS
Excludes1: superficial bite of anus (S30.877)

S31.839 Unspecified open wound of anus

S32 Fracture of lumbar spine and pelvis
A fracture not identified as displaced or nondisplaced should be coded to displaced
Includes: fracture of lumbosacral neural arch
fracture of lumbosacral spinous process
fracture of lumbosacral transverse process
fracture of lumbosacral vertebra
fracture of lumbosacral vertebral arch
Codes first any associated spinal cord and spinal nerve injury (S34-)
Excludes1: transection of abdomen (S38.3)
Excludes2: fracture of hip NOS (S72.0-)
A fracture not identified as opened or closed should be coded to closed
The following extensions are to be added to each code for this category:
a initial encounter for closed fracture
b initial encounter for open fracture
d subsequent encounter for fracture with routine healing
g subsequent encounter for fracture with delayed healing
j subsequent encounter for fracture with nonunion
q sequela

S32.0 Fracture of lumbar vertebra
Fracture of lumbar spine NOS

S32.00 Fracture of unspecified lumbar vertebra

S32.000 Wedge compression fracture of unspecified lumbar vertebra

S32.001 Stable burst fracture of unspecified lumbar vertebra

S32.002 Unstable burst fracture of unspecified lumbar vertebra

S32.008 Other fracture of unspecified lumbar vertebra

S32.009 Unspecified fracture of unspecified lumbar vertebra

S32.01 Fracture of first lumbar vertebra

S32.010 Wedge compression fracture of first lumbar vertebra

S32.011 Stable burst fracture of first lumbar vertebra

S32.012 Unstable burst fracture of first lumbar vertebra

S32.018 Other fracture of first lumbar vertebra

S32.019 Unspecified fracture of first lumbar vertebra

S32.02 Fracture of second lumbar vertebra

S32.020 Wedge compression fracture of second lumbar vertebra

S32.021 Stable burst fracture of second lumbar vertebra

S32.022 Unstable burst fracture of second lumbar vertebra

S32.028 Other fracture of second lumbar vertebra

S32.029 Unspecified fracture of second lumbar vertebra

S32.03 Fracture of third lumbar vertebra

S32.030 Wedge compression fracture of third lumbar vertebra

S32.031 Stable burst fracture of third lumbar vertebra

S32.032 Unstable burst fracture of third lumbar vertebra

S32.038 Other fracture of third lumbar vertebra

S32.039 Unspecified fracture of third lumbar vertebra

S32.04 Fracture of fourth lumbar vertebra

S32.040 Wedge compression fracture of fourth lumbar vertebra

S32.041 Stable burst fracture of fourth lumbar vertebra

S32.042 Unstable burst fracture of fourth lumbar vertebra

S32.048 Other fracture of fourth lumbar vertebra

S32.049 Unspecified fracture of fourth lumbar vertebra

S32.05 Fracture of fifth lumbar vertebra

S32.050 Wedge compression fracture of fifth lumbar vertebra

S32.051 Stable burst fracture of fifth lumbar vertebra

S32.052 Unstable burst fracture of fifth lumbar vertebra

S32.058 Other fracture of fifth lumbar vertebra

S32.059 Unspecified fracture of fifth lumbar vertebra

S32.1 Fracture of sacrum
For vertical fractures, code to most medial fracture extension
Use two codes if both a vertical and transverse fracture are present
Code also any associated fracture of pelvic circle (S32.8-)

S32.10 Unspecified fracture of sacrum

S32.11 Zone I fracture of sacrum
Vertical sacral ala fracture of sacrum

S32.110 Nondisplaced Zone I fracture of sacrum

S32.111 Minimally displaced Zone I fracture of sacrum

S32.112 Severely displaced Zone I fracture of sacrum

S32.119 Unspecified Zone I fracture of sacrum

S32.12 Zone II fracture of sacrum
Vertical foraminal region fracture of sacrum

S32.120 Nondisplaced Zone II fracture of sacrum

S32.121 Minimally displaced Zone II fracture of sacrum

S32.122 Severely displaced Zone II fracture of sacrum

S32.129 Unspecified Zone II fracture of sacrum

S32.13 Zone III fracture of sacrum
Vertical fracture into spinal canal region of sacrum

S32.130 Nondisplaced Zone III fracture of sacrum

S32.131 Minimally displaced Zone III fracture of sacrum

S32.132 Severely displaced Zone III fracture of sacrum

S32.139 Unspecified Zone III fracture of sacrum

S32.14 Type 1 fracture of sacrum
Transverse flexion fracture of sacrum without displacement

S32.15 Type 2 fracture of sacrum
Transverse flexion fracture of sacrum with posterior displacement

S32.16   Type 3 fracture of sacrum
       Transverse extension fracture of sacrum with anterior displacement

S32.17   Type 4 fracture of sacrum
       Transverse segmental comminution of upper sacrum

S32.19   Other fracture of sacrum

S32.2   Fracture of coccyx

S32.3   Fracture of ilium
       Excludes1:   fracture of ilium with associated disruption of pelvic circle (S32.8-)

S32.30   Unspecified fracture of ilium
     S32.301   Unspecified fracture of ilium, right side
     S32.302   Unspecified fracture of ilium, left side
     S32.309   Unspecified fracture of ilium, unspecified side

S32.31   Avulsion fracture of ilium
     S32.311   Displaced avulsion fracture of ilium, right side
     S32.312   Displaced avulsion fracture of ilium, left side
     S32.313   Displaced avulsion fracture of ilium, unspecified side
     S32.314   Nondisplaced avulsion fracture of ilium, right side
     S32.315   Nondisplaced avulsion fracture of ilium, left side
     S32.316   Nondisplaced avulsion fracture of ilium, unspecified side

S32.39   Other fracture of ilium
     S32.391   Other fracture of ilium, right side
     S32.392   Other fracture of ilium, left side
     S32.399   Other fracture of ilium, unspecifie side

S32.4   Fracture of acetabulum
       Code also any associated fracture of pelvic circle (S32.8-)

S32.40   Unspecified fracture of acetabulum
     S32.401   Unspecified fracture of acetabulum, right side
     S32.402   Unspecified fracture of acetabulum, left side
     S32.409   Unspecified fracture of acetabulum, unspecified side

S32.41   Fracture of anterior wall of acetabulum
     S32.411   Displaced fracture of anterior wall of acetabulum, right side
     S32.412   Displaced fracture of anterior wall of acetabulum, left side
     S32.413   Displaced fracture of anterior wall of acetabulum, unspecified side
     S32.414   Nondisplaced fracture of anterior wall of acetabulum, right side
     S32.415   Nondisplaced fracture of anterior wall of acetabulum, left side
     S32.416   Nondisplaced fracture of anterior wall of acetabulum, unspecified side

S32.42   Fracture of posterior wall of acetabulum
     S32.421   Displaced fracture of posterior wall of acetabulum, right side
     S32.422   Displaced fracture of posterior wall of acetabulum, left side
     S32.423   Displaced fracture of posterior wall of acetabulum, unspecified side
     S32.424   Nondisplaced fracture of posterior wall of acetabulum, right side
     S32.425   Nondisplaced fracture of posterior wall of acetabulum, left side
     S32.426   Nondisplaced fracture of posterior wall of acetabulum, unspecified side

S32.43   Fracture of anterior column [iliopubic] of acetabulum
     S32.431   Displaced fracture of anterior column [iliopubic] of acetabulum, right side
     S32.432   Displaced fracture of anterior column [iliopubic] of acetabulum, left side
     S32.433   Displaced fracture of anterior column [iliopubic] of acetabulum, unspecified side
     S32.434   Nondisplaced fracture of anterior column [iliopubic] of acetabulum, right side
     S32.435   Nondisplaced fracture of anterior column [iliopubic] of acetabulum, left side
     S32.436   Nondisplaced fracture of anterior column [iliopubic] of acetabulum, unspecified side

S32.44   Fracture of posterior column [ilioischial] of acetabulum
     S32.441   Displaced fracture of posterior column [ilioischial] of acetabulum, right side
     S32.442   Displaced fracture of posterior column [ilioischial] of acetabulum, left side
     S32.443   Displaced fracture of posterior column [ilioischial] of acetabulum, unspecified side
     S32.444   Nondisplaced fracture of posterior column [ilioischial]
     S32.445   Nondisplaced fracture of posterior column [ilioischial] of acetabulum, left side
     S32.446   Nondisplaced fracture of posterior column [ilioischial] of acetabulum, unspecified side

S32.45   Transverse fracture of acetabulum of acetabulum, right side
     S32.451   Displaced transverse fracture of acetabulum, right side
     S32.452   Displaced transverse fracture of acetabulum, left side
     S32.453   Displaced transverse fracture of acetabulum, unspecified side
     S32.454   Nondisplaced transverse fracture of acetabulum, right side
     S32.455   Nondisplaced transverse fracture of acetabulum, left side
     S32.456   Nondisplaced transverse fracture of acetabulum, unspecified side

S32.46   Associated transverse-posterior fracture of acetabulum
     S32.461   Displaced associated transverse-posterior fracture of acetabulum, right side
     S32.462   Displaced associated transverse-posterior fracture of acetabulum, left side
     S32.463   Displaced associated transverse-posterior fracture of acetabulum, unspecified side
     S32.464   Nondisplaced associated transverse-posterior fracture of acetabulum, right side
     S32.465   Nondisplaced associated transverse-posterior fracture of acetabulum, left side
     S32.466   Nondisplaced associated transverse-posterior fracture of acetabulum, unspecified side

S32.47   Fracture of medial wall of acetabulum
     S32.471   Displaced fracture of medial wall of acetabulum, right side
     S32.472   Displaced fracture of medial wall of acetabulum, left side
     S32.473   Displaced fracture of medial wall of acetabulum, unspecified side
     S32.474   Nondisplaced fracture of medial wall of acetabulum, right side
     S32.475   Nondisplaced fracture of medial wall of acetabulum, left side
     S32.476   Nondisplaced fracture of medial wall of acetabulum, unspecified side

S32.48   Dome fracture of acetabulum
     S32.481   Displaced dome fracture of acetabulum, right side
     S32.482   Displaced dome fracture of acetabulum, left side
     S32.483   Displaced dome fracture of acetabulum, unspecified side
     S32.484   Nondisplaced dome fracture of acetabulum, right side
     S32.485   Nondisplaced dome fracture of acetabulum, left side
     S32.486   Nondisplaced dome fracture of acetabulum, unspecified side

S32.49   Other fracture of acetabulum

S32.491   Other fracture of acetabulum, right side
S32.492   Other fracture of acetabulum, left side
S32.499   Other fracture of acetabulum, unspecified side

S32.5 Fracture of pubis
Excludes1:   fracture of pubis with associated disruption of pelvic circle (S32.8-)

S32.50   Fracture of pubis
S32.51   Fracture of superior rim of pubis
S32.511   Fracture of right superior rim of pubis
S32.512   Fracture of left superior rim of pubis
S32.519   Fracture of unspecified superior rim of pubis
S32.59   Other fracture of pubis

S32.6 Fracture of ischium
Excludes1:   fracture of ischium with associated disruption of pelvic circle (S32.8-)

S32.60   Unspecified fracture of ischium
S32.601   Unspecified fracture of ischium, right side
S32.602   Unspecified fracture of ischium, left side
S32.609   Unspecified fracture of ischium, unspecified side
S32.61   Avulsion fracture of ischium
S32.611   Displaced avulsion facture of ischium, right side
S32.612   Displaced avulsion fracture of ischium, left side
S32.613   Displaced avulsion fracture of ischium, unspecified side
S32.614   Nondisplaced avulsion fracture of ischium, right side
S32.615   Nondisplaced avulsion fracture of ischium, left side
S32.616   Nondisplaced avulsion fracture of ischium, unspecified side
S32.69   Other fracture of ischium
S32.691   Other fracture of ischium, right side
S32.692   Other fracture of ischium, left side
S32.699   Other fracture of ischium, unspecified side

S32.8 Fracture of other parts of pelvis
Code also any associated:
fracture of acetabulum (S32.4-)
sacral fracture (S32.1-)

S32.81   Multiple fractures of pelvis with disruption of pelvic circle
S32.810   Multiple fractures of pelvis with stable disruption of pelvic circle
S32.811   Multiple fractures of pelvis with unstable disruption of pelvic circle
S32.89   Fracture of other parts of pelvis

S32.9 Fracture of unspecified parts of lumbosacral spine and pelvis
Fracture of lumbosacral spine NOS
Fracture of pelvis NOS

S33 Dislocation and sprain of joints and ligaments of lumbar spine and pelvis
Includes: avulsion of joint or ligament of lumbar spine and pelvis
laceration of joint or ligament of lumbar spine and pelvis
sprain joint or ligament of lumbar spine and pelvis
traumatic hemarthrosis of joint or ligament of lumbar spine and pelvis
traumatic rupture of joint or ligament of lumbar spine and pelvis
traumatic subluxation of joint or ligament of lumbar spine and pelvis
traumatic tear of joint or ligament of lumbar spine and pelvis
Excludes1:   nontraumatic rupture or displacement of lumbar intervertebral disc NOS (M51.-)
obstetric damage to pelvic joints and ligaments (O71.6)
Excludes2:   dislocation and sprain of joints and ligaments of hip (S73.-)
strain of muscle of lower back and pelvis (S39.12, S39.13)

The following extensions are to be added to each code for this category:
  a   initial encounter
  d   subsequent encounter
  q   sequela

S33.0 Traumatic rupture of lumbar intervertebral disc
Excludes1:   rupture or displacement (nontraumatic) of lumbar intervertebral disc NOS (M51.- with final character 6)

S33.1 Subluxation and dislocation of lumbar vertebra
Code also any associated:
open wound of abdomen, lower back and pelvis (S31)
spinal cord injury (S24.0, S24.1-, S34.0, S34.1-)
Excludes2:   fracture of lumbar vertebrae (S32.0-)

S33.10   Subluxation and dislocation of unspecified lumbar vertebra
S33.100   Subluxation of unspecified lumbar vertebra
S33.101   Dislocation of unspecified lumbar vertebra
S33.11   Subluxation and dislocation of L_1/L_2 lumbar vertebra
S33.110   Subluxation of L_1/L_2 lumbar vertebra
S33.111   Dislocation of L_1/L_2 lumbar vertebra
S33.12   Subluxation and dislocation of L_2/L_3 lumbar vertebra
S33.120   Subluxation of L_2/L_3 lumbar vertebra
S33.121   Dislocation of L_2/L_3 lumbar vertebra
S33.13   Subluxation and dislocation of L_3/L_4 lumbar vertebra
S33.130   Subluxation of L_3/L_4 lumbar vertebra
S33.131   Dislocation of L_3/L_4 lumbar vertebra
S33.14   Subluxation and dislocation of L_4/L_5 lumbar vertebra
S33.140   Subluxation of L_4/L_5 lumbar vertebra
S33.141   Dislocation of L_4/L_5 lumbar vertebra

S33.2 Dislocation of sacroiliac and sacrococcygeal joint
S33.3 Dislocation of other and unspecified parts of lumbar spine and pelvis
S33.30   Dislocation of unspecified parts of lumbar spine and pelvis
S33.39   Dislocation of other parts of lumbar spine and pelvis
S33.4 Traumatic rupture of symphysis pubis
S33.5 Sprain of ligaments of lumbar spine
S33.6 Sprain of sacroiliac joint
S33.8 Sprain of other parts of lumbar spine and pelvis
S33.9 Sprain of unspecified parts of lumbar spine and pelvis

S34 Injury of lumbar and sacral spinal cord and nerves at abdomen, lower back and pelvis level
Note: code to highest level of lumbar cord injury
Code also any associated:
fracture of vertebra (S22.0-, S32.0-)
open wound of abdomen, lower back and pelvis (S31.-)
transient paralysis (R29.5)
The following extensions are to be added to each code for this category:
  a   initial encounter
  d   subsequent encounter
  q   sequela

S34.0 Concussion and edema of lumbar and sacral spinal cord
S34.01   Concussion and edema of lumbar spinal cord
S34.02   Concussion and edema of sacral spinal cord
Concussion and edema of conus medullaris
S34.1 Other and unspecified injury of lumbar and sacral spinal cord
S34.10   Unspecified injury to lumbar spinal cord
S34.101   Unspecified injury to L_1 level of lumbar spinal cord
S34.102   Unspecified injury to L_2 level of lumbar spinal cord
S34.103   Unspecified injury to L_3 level of lumbar spinal cord
S34.104   Unspecified injury to L_4 level of lumbar spinal cord
S34.105   Unspecified injury to L_5 level of lumbar spinal cord
S34.109   Unspecified injury to unspecified level of lumbar spinal cord

S34.11   Complete lesion of lumbar spinal cord
    S34.111   Complete lesion of L_1 level of lumbar spinal cord
    S34.112   Complete lesion of L_2 level of lumbar spinal cord
    S34.113   Complete lesion of L_3 level of lumbar spinal cord
    S34.114   Complete lesion of L_4 level of lumbar spinal cord
    S34.115   Complete lesion of L_5 level of lumbar spinal cord
    S34.119   Complete lesion of unspecifed level of lumbar spinal cord
S34.12   Incomplete lesion of lumbar spinal cord
    S34.121   Incomplete lesion of L_1 level of lumbar spinal cord
    S34.122   Incomplete lesion of L_2 level of lumbar spinal cord
    S34.123   Incomplete lesion of L_3 level of lumbar spinal cord
    S34.124   Incomplete lesion of L_4 level of lumbar spinal cord
    S34.125   Incomplete lesion of L_5 level of lumbar spinal cord
    S34.129   Incomplete lesion of unspecified level of lumbar spinal cord
S34.13   Other and unspecifed injury to sacral spinal cord
    Other injury to conus medullaris
    S34.131   Complete lesion of sacral spinal cord
        Complete lesion of conus medullaris
    S34.132   Incomplete lesion of sacral spinal cord
        Incomplete lesion of conus medullaris
    S34.139   Unspecified injury to sacral spinal cord
        Unspecified injury of conus medullaris

S34.2   Injury of nerve root of lumbar and sacral spine
  S34.21   Injury of nerve root of lumbar spine
  S34.22   Injury of nerve root of sacral spine
S34.3   Injury of cauda equina
S34.4   Injury of lumbosacral plexus
S34.5   Injury of lumbar, sacral and pelvic sympathetic nerves
    Injury of celiac ganglion or plexus
    Injury of hypogastric plexus
    Injury of mesenteric plexus (inferior) (superior)
    Injury of splanchnic nerve
S34.6   Injury of peripheral nerve(s) at abdomen, lower back and pelvis level
S34.8   Injury of other nerves at abdomen, lower back and pelvis level
S34.9   Injury of unspecified nerves at abdomen, lower back and pelvis level

S35 Injury of blood vessels at abdomen, lower back and pelvis level
    Code also any associated open wound (S31.-)
    The following extensions are to be added to each code for this category:
      a   initial encounter
      d   subsequent encounter
      q   sequela
S35.0   Injury of abdominal aorta
    Excludes1:   injury of aorta NOS (S25.0)
  S35.00   Unspecified injury of abdominal aorta
  S35.01   Minor laceration of abdominal aorta
    Incomplete transection of abdominal aorta
    Laceration of abdominal aorta NOS
    Superficial laceration of abdominal aorta
  S35.02   Major laceration of abdominal aorta
    Complete transection of abdominal aorta
    Traumatic rupture of abdominal aorta
  S35.09   Other injury of abdominal aorta
S35.1   Injury of inferior vena cava
    Injury of hepatic vein
    Excludes1:   injury of vena cava NOS (S25.2)
  S35.10   Unspecified injury of inferior vena cava

S35.11   Minor laceration of inferior vena cava
    Incomplete transection of inferior vena cava
    Laceration of inferior vena cava NOS
    Superficial laceration of inferior vena cava
S35.02   Major laceration of inferior vena cava
    Complete transection of inferior vena cava
    Traumatic rupture of inferior vena cava
S35.19   Other injury of inferior vena cava
S35.2   Injury of celiac or mesenteric artery and branches
  S35.21   Injury of celiac artery
    S35.211   Minor laceration of celiac artery
        Incomplete transection of celiac artery
        Laceration of celiac artery NOS
        Superficial laceration of celiac artery
    S35.212   Major laceration of celiac artery
        Complete transection of celiac artery
        Traumatic rupture of celiac artery
    S35.218   Other injury of celiac artery
    S35.219   Unspecified injury of celiac artery
  S35.22   Injury of superior mesenteric artery
    S35.221   Minor laceration of superior mesenteric artery
        Incomplete transection of superior mesenteric artery
        Laceration of superior mesenteric artery NOS
        Superficial laceration of superior mesenteric artery
    S35.221   Major laceration of superior mesenteric artery
        Complete transection of superior mesenteric artery
        Traumatic rupture of superior mesenteric artery
    S35.228   Other injury of superior mesenteric artery
    S35.229   Unspecified injury of superior mesenteric artery
  S35.23   Injury of inferior mesenteric artery
    S35.231   Minor laceration of inferior mesenteric artery
        Incomplete transection of inferior mesenteric artery
        Laceration of inferior mesenteric artery NOS
        Superficial laceration of inferior mesenteric artery
    S35.232   Major laceration of inferior mesenteric artery
        Complete transection of inferior mesenteric artery
  S35.29   Traumatic rupture of inferior mesenteric artery
    S35.238   Other injury of inferior mesenteric artery
    S35.239   Unspecified injury of inferior mesenteric artery
        Injury of branches of celiac and mesentaric artery
        Injury of gastric artery Injury of gastroduodenal artery
        Injury of hepatic artery Injury of splenic artery
    S35.291   Minor laceration of branches of celiac and mesentaric artery Incomplete transection of branches of celiac and mesentaric artery
        Laceration of branches of celiac and mesentaric artery NOS
        Superficial laceration of branches of celiac and mesentaric artery
    S35.292   Major laceration of branches of celiac and mesentaric artery
        Complete transection of branches of celiac and mesentaric artery
        Traumatic rupture of branches of celiac and mesentaric artery
    S35.298   Other injury of branches of celiac and mesentaric artery
    S35.299   Unspecified injury of branches of celiac and mesentaric artery
S35.3   Injury of portal or splenic vein and branches
  S35.31   Injury of portal vein
    S35.311   Laceration of portal vein
    S35.318   Other specified injury of portal vein

S35.319   Unspecified injury of portal vein
S35.32   Injury of splenic vein
S35.321   Laceration of splenic vein
S35.328   Other specified injury of splenic vein
S35.329   Unspecified injury of splenic vein
S35.33   Injury of superior mesenteric vein
S35.331   Laceration of superior mesenteric vein
S35.338   Other specified injury of superior mesenteric vein
S35.339   Unspecified injury of superior mesenteric vein
S35.34   Injury of inferior mesenteric vein
S35.341   Laceration of inferior mesenteric vein
S35.348   Other specified injury of inferior mesenteric vein
S35.349   Unspecified injury of inferior mesenteric vein
S35.4   Injury of renal blood vessels
S35.40   Unspecified injury of renal blood vessel
S35.401   Unspecified injury of right renal artery
S35.402   Unspecified injury of left renal artery
S35.403   Unspecified injury of unspecified renal artery
S35.404   Unspecified injury of right renal vein
S35.405   Unspecified injury of left renal vein
S35.406   Unspecified injury of unspecified renal vein
S35.41   Laceration of renal blood vessel
S35.411   Laceration of right renal artery
S35.412   Laceration of left renal artery
S35.413   Laceration of unspecified renal artery
S35.414   Laceration of right renal vein
S35.415   Laceration of left renal vein
S35.416   Laceration of unspecified renal vein
S35.49   Other specified injury of renal blood vessel
S35.491   Other specified injury of right renal artery
S35.492   Other specified injury of left renal artery
S35.493   Other specified injury of unspecified renal artery
S35.494   Other specified injury of right renal vein
S35.495   Other specified injury of left renal vein
S35.496   Other specified injury of unspecified renal vein
S35.5   Injury of iliac blood vessels
S35.50   Injury of unspecified iliac blood vessel(s)
S35.51   Injury of iliac artery or vein
Injury of hypogastric artery or vein
S35.511   Injury of right iliac artery
S35.512   Injury of left iliac artery
S35.513   Injury of unspecified iliac artery
S35.514   Injury of right iliac vein
S35.515   Injury of left iliac vein
S35.516   Injury of unspecified iliac vein
S35.53   Injury of uterine artery or vein
S35.531   Injury of right uterine artery
S35.532   Injury of left uterine artery
S35.533   Injury of unspecifed uterine artery
S35.534   Injury of right uterine vein
S35.535   Injury of left uterine vein
S35.536   Injury of unspecifed uterine vein
S35.59   Injury of other iliac blood vessels
S35.8   Injury of other blood vessels at abdomen, lower back and pelvis level
Injury of ovarian artery or vein
S35.8x   Injury of other blood vessels at abdomen, lower back and pelvis level
S35.8x1   Laceration of other blood vessels at abdomen, lower back and pelvis level
S35.8x8   Other specified injury of other blood vessels at abdomen, lower back and pelvis level
S35.8x9   Unspecified injury of other blood vessels at abdomen, lower back and pelvis level

S35.9   Injury of unspecified blood vessel at abdomen, lower back and pelvis level
S35.90   Unspecified injury of unspecified blood vessel at abdomen, lower back and pelvis level
S35.91   Laceration of unspecified blood vessel at abdomen, lower back and pelvis level
S35.99   Other specified injury of unspecified blood vessel at abdomen, lower back and pelvis level

S36   Injury of intra-abdominal organs
Code also any associated open wound (S31.-)
The following extensions are to be added to each code for this category:
a   initial encounter
d   subsequent encounter
q   sequela
S36.0   Injury of spleen
S36.00   Unspecified injury of spleen
S36.02   Contusion of spleen
S36.020   Minor contusion of spleen
Contusion of spleen less than 2cm
S36.021   Major contusion of spleen
Contusion of spleen greater than 2 cm
S36.029   Unspecified contusion of spleen
S36.03   Laceration of spleen
S36.030   Superficial (capsular) laceration of spleen
Laceration of spleen less than 1 cm
Minor laceration of spleen
S36.031   Moderate laceration of spleen
Laceration of spleen 1 to 3 cm
S36.032   Major laceration of spleen
Avulsion of spleen
Laceration of spleen greater than 3 cm
Massive laceration of spleen
Multiple moderate lacerations of spleen
Stellate laceration of spleen
S36.039   Unspecified laceration of spleen
S36.09   Other injury of spleen
S36.1   Injury of liver and gallbladder and bile duct
S36.11   Injury of liver
S36.112   Contusion of liver
S36.113   Laceration of liver, unspecified degree
S36.114   Minor laceration of liver
Laceration involving capsule only, or, without significant involvement of hepatic parenchyma [i.e., less than 1 cm deep]
S36.115   Moderate laceration of liver
Laceration involving parenchyma but without major disruption of parenchyma [i.e., less than 10 cm long and less than 3 cm deep]
S36.116   Major laceration of liver
Laceration with significant disruption of hepatic parenchyma [i.e., greater than 10 cm long and 3 cm deep]
Multiple moderate lacerations, with or without hematoma
Stellate laceration of liver
S36.118   Other injury of liver
S36.119   Unspecified injury of liver
S36.12   Injury of gallbladder
S36.122   Contusion of gallbladder
S36.123   Laceration of gallbladder
S36.128   Other injury of gallbladder
S36.129   Unspecified injury of gallbladder
S36.13   Injury of bile duct
S36.2   Injury of pancreas
S36.20   Unspecified injury of pancreas
S36.200   Unspecified injury of head of pancreas
S36.201   Unspecified injury of body of pancreas
S36.202   Unspecified injury of tail of pancreas

S36.209   Unspecified injury of unspecified part of pancreas
S36.22   Contusion of pancreas
    S36.220   Contusion of head of pancreas
    S36.221   Contusion of body of pancreas
    S36.222   Contusion of tail of pancreas
    S36.229   Contusion of unspecified part of pancreas
S36.23   Laceration of pancreas, unspecified degree
    S36.230   Laceration of head of pancreas, unspecified degree
    S36.231   Laceration of body of pancreas, unspecified degree
    S36.232   Laceration of tail of pancreas, unspecified degree
    S36.239   Laceration of unspecified part of pancreas, unspecified degree
S36.24   Minor laceration of pancreas
    S36.240   Minor laceration of head of pancreas
    S36.241   Minor laceration of body of pancreas
    S36.242   Minor laceration of tail of pancreas
    S36.249   Minor laceration of unspecified part of pancreas
S36.25   Moderate laceration of pancreas
    S36.250   Moderate laceration of head of pancreas
    S36.251   Moderate laceration of body of pancreas
    S36.252   Moderate laceration of tail of pancreas
    S36.259   Moderate laceration of unspecified part of pancreas
S36.26   Major laceration of pancreas
    S36.260   Major laceration of head of pancreas
    S36.261   Major laceration of body of pancreas
    S36.262   Major laceration of tail of pancreas
    S36.269   Major laceration of unspecified part of pancreas
S36.29   Other injury of pancreas
    S36.290   Other injury of head of pancreas
    S36.291   Other injury of body of pancreas
    S36.292   Other injury of tail of pancreas
    S36.299   Other injury of unspecified part of pancreas
S36.3   Injury of stomach
  S36.30   Unspecified injury of stomach
  S36.32   Contusion of stomach
  S36.33   Laceration of stomach
  S36.39   Other injury of stomach
S36.4   Injury of small intestine
  S36.40   Unspecified injury of small intestine
    S36.400   Unspecified injury of duodenum
    S36.408   Unspecified injury of other part of small intestine
    S36.409   Unspecified injury of unspecified part of small intestine
  S36.41   Primary blast injury of small intestine
    Blast injury of small intestine NOS
    S36.410   Primary blast injury of duodenum
    S36.418   Primary blast injury of other part of small intestine
    S36.419   Primary blast injury of unspecified part of small intestine
  S36.42   Contusion of small intestine
    S36.420   Contusion of duodenum
    S36.428   Contusion of other part of small intestine
    S36.429   Contusion of unspecified part of small intestine
  S36.43   Laceration of small intestine
    S36.430   Laceration of duodenum
    S36.438   Laceration of other part of small intestine
    S36.439   Laceration of unspecified part of small intestine
  S36.49   Other injury of small intestine

S36.490   Other injury of duodenum
S36.498   Other injury of other part of small intestine
S36.499   Other injury of unspecified part of small intestine
S36.5   Injury of colon
    Excludes2:   injury of rectum (S36.6-)
  S36.50   Unspecified injury of colon
    S36.500   Unspecified injury of ascending [right] colon
    S36.501   Unspecified injury of transverse colon
    S36.502   Unspecified injury of descending [left] colon
    S36.503   Unspecified injury of sigmoid colon
    S36.508   Unspecified injury of other part of colon
    S36.509   Unspecified injury of unspecified part of colon
  S36.51   Primary blast injury of colon
    Blast injury of colon NOS
    S36.510   Primary blast injury of ascending [right] colon
    S36.511   Primary blast injury of transverse colon
    S36.512   Primary blast injury of descending [left] colon
    S36.513   Primary blast injury of sigmoid colon
    S36.518   Primary blast injury of other part of colon
    S36.519   Primary blast injury of unspecified part of colon
  S36.52   Contusion of colon
    S36.520   Contusion of ascending [right] colon
    S36.521   Contusion of transverse colon
    S36.522   Contusion of descending [left] colon
    S36.523   Contusion of sigmoid colon
    S36.528   Contusion of other part of colon
    S36.529   Contusion of unspecified part of colon
  S36.53   Laceration of colon
    S36.530   Laceration of ascending [right] colon
    S36.531   Laceration of transverse colon
    S36.532   Laceration of descending [left] colon
    S36.533   Laceration of sigmoid colon
    S36.538   Laceration of other part of colon
    S36.539   Laceration of unspecified part of colon
  S36.59   Other injury of colon
    Secondary blast injury of colon
    S36.590   Other injury of ascending [right] colon
    S36.591   Other injury of transverse colon
    S36.592   Other injury of descending [left] colon
    S36.593   Other injury of sigmoid colon
    S36.598   Other injury of other part of colon
    S36.599   Other injury of unspecified part of colon
S36.6   Injury of rectum
  S36.60   Unspecified injury of rectum
  S36.61   Primary blast injury of rectum
    Blast injury of rectum NOS
  S36.62   Contusion of rectum
  S36.63   Laceration of rectum
  S36.69   Other injury of rectum
    Secondary blast injury of rectum
S36.8   Injury of other intra-abdominal organs
  S36.81   Injury of peritoneum
  S36.89   Injury of other intra-abdominal organs
    Injury of retroperitoneum
    S36.892   Contusion of other intra-abdominal organs
    S36.893   Laceration of other intra-abdominal organs
    S36.898   Other injury of other intra-abdominal organs
    S36.899   Unspecified injury of other intra-abdominal organs
S36.9   Injury of unspecified intra-abdominal organ
  S36.90   Unspecified injury of unspecified intra-abdominal organ
  S36.92   Contusion of unspecified intra-abdominal organ
  S36.93   Laceration of unspecified intra-abdominal organ
  S36.99   Other injury of unspecified intra-abdominal organ

Chapter 19   © 2002 Ingenix, Inc.

S37 Injury of pelvic organs

Code also any associated open wound (S31.-)

Excludes2:   injury of peritoneum (S36.81)
           injury of retroperitoneum (S36.89-)

The following extensions are to be added to each code for this category:
- a   initial encounter
- d   subsequent encounter
- q   sequela

S37.0   Injury of kidney

S37.00   Unspecified injury of kidney
- S37.001   Unspecified injury of right kidney
- S37.002   Unspecified injury of left kidney
- S37.009   Unspecified injury of unspecifed kidney

S37.01   Minor contusion of kidney
Contusion of kidney less than 2 cm
Contusion of kidney NOS
- S37.011   Minor contusion of right kidney
- S37.012   Minor contusion of left kidney
- S37.019   Minor contusion of unspecified kidney

S37.02   Major contusion of kidney
Contusion of kidney greater than 2 cm
- S37.021   Major contusion of right kidney
- S37.022   Major contusion of left kidney
- S37.029   Major contusion of unspecified kidney

S37.03   Laceration of kidney, unspecified degree
- S37.031   Laceration of kidney, unspecified degree
- S37.032   Laceration of kidney, unspecified degree
- S37.039   Laceration of kidney, unspecified degree

S37.04   Minor laceration of kidney
Laceration of kidney less than 1 cm
- S37.041   Minor laceration of right kidney
- S37.042   Minor laceration of left kidney
- S37.049   Minor laceration of unspecified kidney

S37.05   Moderate laceration of kidney
Laceration of kidney 1 to 3 cm
- S37.051   Moderate laceration of right kidney
- S37.052   Moderate laceration of left kidney
- S37.059   Moderate laceration of unspecified kidney

S37.06   Major laceration of kidney
Avulsion of kidney
Laceration of kidney greater than 3 cm
Massive laceration of kidney
Multiple moderate lacerations of kidney
Stellate laceration of kidney
- S37.061   Major laceration of right kidney
- S37.062   Major laceration of left kidney
- S37.069   Major laceration of unspecified kidney

S37.09   Other injury of kidney
- S37.091   Other injury of right kidney
- S37.092   Other injury of left kidney
- S37.099   Other injury of unspecified kidney

S37.1   Injury of ureter
- S37.10   Unspecified injury of ureter
- S37.12   Contusion of ureter
- S37.13   Laceration of ureter
- S37.19   Other injury of ureter

S37.2   Injury of bladder
- S37.20   Unspecified injury of bladder
- S37.22   Contusion of bladder
- S37.23   Laceration of bladder
- S37.28   Other injury of bladder

S37.3   Injury of urethra
- S37.30   Unspecified injury of urethra
- S37.32   Contusion of urethra
- S37.33   Laceration of urethra
- S37.38   Other injury of urethra

S37.4   Injury of ovary
- S37.40   Unspecified injury of ovary
  - S37.401   Unspecified injury of ovary, unilateral

- S37.402   Unspecified injury of ovary, bilateral
- S37.409   Unspecified injury of ovary, unspecified

S37.42   Contusion of ovary
- S37.421   Contusion of ovary, unilateral
- S37.422   Contusion of ovary, bilateral
- S37.429   Contusion of ovary, unspecified

S37.43   Laceration of ovary
- S37.431   Laceration of ovary, unilateral
- S37.432   Laceration of ovary, bilateral
- S37.439   Laceration of ovary, unspecified

S37.49   Other injury of ovary
- S37.491   Other injury of ovary, unilateral
- S37.492   Other injury of ovary, bilateral
- S37.499   Other injury of ovary, unspecified

S37.5   Injury of fallopian tube

S37.50   Unspecified injury of fallopian tube
- S37.501   Unspecified injury of fallopian tube, unilateral
- S37.502   Unspecified injury of fallopian tube, bilateral
- S37.509   Unspecified injury of fallopian tube, unspecified

S37.51   Primary blast injury of fallopian tube
Blast injury of fallopian tube NOS
- S37.511   Primary blast injury of fallopian tube, unilateral
- S37.512   Primary blast injury of fallopian tube, bilateral
- S37.519   Primary blast injury of fallopian tube, unspecified

S37.52   Contusion of fallopian tube
- S37.521   Contusion of fallopian tube, unilateral
- S37.522   Contusion of fallopian tube, bilateral
- S37.529   Contusion of fallopian tube, unspecified

S37.53   Laceration of fallopian tube
- S37.531   Laceration of fallopian tube, unilateral
- S37.532   Laceration of fallopian tube, bilateral
- S37.539   Laceration of fallopian tube, unspecified

S37.59   Other injury of fallopian tube
Secondary blast injury of fallopian tube
- S37.591   Other injury of fallopian tube, unilateral
- S37.592   Other injury of fallopian tube, bilateral
- S37.599   Other injury of fallopian tube, unspecified

S37.6   Injury of uterus

Excludes1:   injury to gravid uterus (O93.-)
           injury to uterus during delivery (O71.-)
- S37.60   Unspecified injury of uterus
- S37.62   Contusion of uterus
- S37.63   Laceration of uterus
- S37.69   Other injury of uterus

S37.8   Injury of other pelvic organs

S37.81   Injury of adrenal gland
- S37.812   Contusion of adrenal gland
- S37.813   Laceration of adrenal gland
- S37.818   Other injury of adrenal gland
- S37.819   Unspecified injury of adrenal gland

S37.82   Injury of prostate
- S37.822   Contusion of prostate
- S37.823   Laceration of prostate
- S37.828   Other injury of prostate
- S37.829   Unspecified injury of prostate

S37.89   Injury of other pelvic organ
- S37.892   Contusion of other pelvic organ
- S37.893   Laceration of other pelvic organ
- S37.898   Other injury of other pelvic organ
- S37.899   Unspecified injury of other pelvic organ

S37.9   Injury of unspecified pelvic organ
- S37.90   Unspecified injury of unspecified pelvic organ
- S37.92   Contusion of unspecified pelvic organ
- S37.93   Laceration of unspecified pelvic organ
- S37.99   Other injury of unspecified pelvic organ

S38 Crushing injury and traumatic amputation of part of abdomen, lower back and pelvis

An amputation not identified as partial or complete should be coded to complete

The following extensions are to be added to each code for this category:
- a initial encounter
- d subsequent encounter
- q sequela

S38.0 Crushing injury of external genital organs
Use additional code for any associated injuries

S38.00 Crushing injury of unspecified external genital organs
- S38.001 Crushing injury of unspecified external genital organs, male
- S38.002 Crushing injury of unspecified external genital organs, female
S38.01 Crushing injury of penis
S38.02 Crushing injury of scrotum and testis
S38.03 Crushing injury of vulva

S38.1 Crushing injury of abdomen, lower back, and pelvis
Use additional code for all associated injuries, such as:
fracture of thoracic or lumbar spine and pelvis (S22.0-, S32.-)
injury to intra-abdominal organs (S36.-)
injury to pelvic organs (S37.-)
open wound of abdominal wall (S31-)
spinal cord injury (S34.0, S34.1-)
Excludes2: crushing injury of external genital organs (S38.2-)

S38.2 Traumatic amputation of external genital organs
S38.21 Traumatic amputation of female external genital organs
Traumatic amputation of clitoris
Traumatic amputation of labium (majus) (minus)
Traumatic amputation of vulva
- S38.211 Complete traumatic amputation of female external genital organs
- S38.212 Partial traumatic amputation of female external genital organs
S38.22 Traumatic amputation of penis
- S38.221 Complete traumatic amputation of penis
- S38.222 Partial traumatic amputation of penis
S38.23 Traumatic amputation of scrotum and testis
- S38.231 Complete traumatic amputation of scrotum and testis
- S38.232 Partial traumatic amputation of scrotum and testis

S38.3 Transection (partial) of abdomen

S39 Other and unspecified injuries of abdomen, lower back and pelvis
Code also any associated open wound (S31.-)
Excludes2: sprain of joints and ligaments of lumbar spine and pelvis (S33.7)
The following extensions are to be added to each code for this category:
- a initial encounter
- d subsequent encounter
- q sequela

S39.0 Injury of muscle and tendon of abdomen, lower back and pelvis
S39.00 Unspecified injury of muscle and tendon of abdomen, lower back and pelvis
- S39.001 Unspecified injury of muscle and tendon of abdomen
- S39.002 Unspecified injury of muscle and tendon of lower back
- S39.003 Unspecified injury of muscle and tendon of pelvis
S39.01 Strain of muscle and tendon of abdomen, lower back and pelvis
- S39.011 Strain of muscle and tendon of abdomen
- S39.012 Strain of muscle and tendon of lower back
- S39.013 Strain of muscle and tendon of pelvis

S39.02 Laceration of muscle and tendon of abdomen, lower back and pelvis
- S39.021 Laceration of muscle and tendon of abdomen
- S39.022 Laceration of muscle and tendon of lower back
- S39.023 Laceration of muscle and tendon of pelvis
S39.09 Other injury of muscle and tendon of abdomen, lower back and pelvis
- S39.091 Other injury of muscle and tendon of abdomen
- S39.092 Other injury of muscle and tendon of lower back
- S39.093 Other injury of muscle and tendon of pelvis

S39.8 Other specified injuries of abdomen, lower back and pelvis
S39.81 Other specified injuries of abdomen
S39.82 Other specified injuries of lower back
S39.83 Other specified injuries of pelvis

S39.9 Unspecified injury of abdomen, lower back and pelvis
S39.91 Unspecified injury of abdomen
S39.92 Unspecified injury of lower back
S39.93 Unspecified injury of pelvis

INJURIES TO THE SHOULDER AND UPPER ARM (S40–S49)

Includes: injuries of axilla
injuries of scapular region
Excludes2: burns and corrosions (T20-T32)
frostbite (T33-T34)
injuries of elbow (S50-S59)
insect bite or sting, venomous (T63.4)

S40 Superficial injury of shoulder and upper arm
The following extensions are to be added to each code for this category:
- a initial encounter
- d subsequent encounter
- q sequela

S40.0 Contusion of shoulder and upper arm
S40.01 Contusion of shoulder
- S40.011 Contusion of right shoulder
- S40.012 Contusion of left shoulder
- S40.019 Contusion of shoulder, unspecified side
S40.02 Contusion of upper arm
- S40.021 Contusion of right upper arm
- S40.022 Contusion of left upper arm
- S40.029 Contusion of upper arm, unspecified side

S40.2 Other superficial injuries of shoulder
S40.21 Abrasion of shoulder
- S40.211 Abrasion of right shoulder
- S40.212 Abrasion of left shoulder
- S40.219 Abrasion of unspecified shoulder
S40.22 Blister (nonthermal) of shoulder
- S40.221 Blister (nonthermal) of right shoulder
- S40.222 Blister (nonthermal) of left shoulder
- S40.229 Blister (nonthermal) of unspecified shoulder
S40.24 External constriction of shoulder
- S40.241 External constriction of right shoulder
- S40.242 External constriction of left shoulder
- S40.249 External constriction of unspecified shoulder
S40.25 Superficial foreign body of shoulder
Splinter in the shoulder
- S40.251 Superficial foreign body of right shoulder
- S40.252 Superficial foreign body of left shoulder
- S40.259 Superficial foreign body of unspecified shoulder
S40.26 Insect bite (nonvenomous) of shoulder
- S40.261 Insect bite (nonvenomous) of right shoulder
- S40.262 Insect bite (nonvenomous) of left shoulder
- S40.269 Insect bite (nonvenomous) of unspecified shoulder
S40.27 Other superficial bite of shoulder
Excludes1: open bite of shoulder (S41.05)
- S40.271 Other superficial bite of right shoulder

390 — Tabular   Chapter 19   © 2002 Ingenix, Inc.

S40.272   Other superficial bite of left shoulder
S40.279   Other superficial bite of unspecified shoulder

S40.8   Other superficial injuries of upper arm
S40.81   Abrasion of upper arm
S40.811   Abrasion of right upper arm
S40.812   Abrasion of left upper arm
S40.819   Abrasion of unspecified upper arm
S40.82   Blister (nonthermal) of upper arm
S40.821   Blister (nonthermal) of right upper arm
S40.822   Blister (nonthermal) of left upper arm
S40.829   Blister (nonthermal) of unspecified upper arm
S40.84   External constriction of right upper arm
S40.841   External constriction of upper arm
S40.842   External constriction of left upper arm
S40.849   External constriction of unspecified upper arm
S40.85   Superficial foreign body of upper arm
        Splinter in the upper arm
S40.851   Superficial foreign body of right upper arm
S40.852   Superficial foreign body of left upper arm
S40.859   Superficial foreign body of unspecified upper arm
S40.86   Insect bite (nonvenomous) of upper arm
S40.861   Insect bite (nonvenomous) of right upper arm
S40.862   Insect bite (nonvenomous) of left upper arm
S40.869   Insect bite (nonvenomous) of unspecified upper arm
S40.87   Other superficial bite of upper arm
        Excludes1:   open bite of upper arm (S41.14)
        Excludes2:   other superficial bite of shoulder (S40.27-)
S40.871   Other superficial bite of right upper arm
S40.872   Other superficial bite of left upper arm
S40.879   Other superficial bite of unspecified upper arm

S40.9   Unspecified superficial injury of shoulder and upper arm
S40.91   Unspecified superficial injury of shoulder
S40.911   Unspecified superficial injury of right shoulder
S40.912   Unspecified superficial injury of left shoulder
S40.919   Unspecified superficial injury of shoulder, unspecified side
S40.92   Unspecified superficial injury of upper arm
S40.921   Unspecified superficial injury of right upper arm
S40.922   Unspecified superficial injury of left upper arm
S40.929   Unspecified superficial injury of upper arm, unspecified side

S41 Open wound of shoulder and upper arm
    Code also any associated wound infection
    Excludes1:   traumatic amputation of shoulder and upper arm (S48.-)
    Excludes2:   open fracture of shoulder and upper arm (S42.- with extension b or c)
    The following extensions are to be added to each code for this category:
        a   initial encounter
        d   subsequent encounter
        q   sequela

S41.0   Open wound of shoulder
S41.00   Unspecified open wound of shoulder
S41.001   Unspecified open wound of right shoulder
S41.002   Unspecified open wound of left shoulder
S41.009   Unspecified open wound of unspecified shoulder
S41.01   Laceration without foreign body of shoulder
S41.011   Laceration without foreign body of right shoulder
S41.012   Laceration without foreign body of left shoulder
S41.019   Laceration without foreign body of unspecified shoulder

S41.02   Laceration with foreign body of shoulder
S41.021   Laceration with foreign body of right shoulder
S41.022   Laceration with foreign body of left shoulder
S41.029   Laceration with foreign body of unspecified shoulder
S41.03   Puncture wound without foreign body of shoulder
S41.031   Puncture wound without foreign body of right shoulder
S41.032   Puncture wound without foreign body of left shoulder
S41.039   Puncture wound without foreign body of unspecified shoulder
S41.04   Puncture wound with foreign body of shoulder
S41.041   Puncture wound with foreign body of right shoulder
S41.042   Puncture wound with foreign body of left shoulder
S41.049   Puncture wound with foreign body of unspecified shoulder
S41.05   Open bite of shoulder
        Bite of shoulder NOS
        Excludes1:   superficial bite of shoulder (S40.27)
S41.051   Open bite of right shoulder
S41.052   Open bite of left shoulder
S41.059   Open bite of unspecified shoulder

S41.1   Open wound of upper arm
S41.10   Unspecified open wound of upper arm
S41.101   Unspecified open wound of right upper arm
S41.102   Unspecified open wound of left upper arm
S41.109   Unspecified open wound of unspecified upper arm
S41.11   Laceration without foreign body of upper arm
S41.111   Laceration without foreign body of right upper arm
S41.112   Laceration without foreign body of left upper arm
S41.119   Laceration without foreign body of unspecified upper arm
S41.12   Laceration with foreign body of upper arm
S41.121   Laceration with foreign body of right upper arm
S41.122   Laceration with foreign body of left upper arm
S41.129   Laceration with foreign body of unspecified upper arm
S41.13   Puncture wound without foreign body of upper arm
S41.131   Puncture wound without foreign body of right upper arm
S41.132   Puncture wound without foreign body of left upper arm
S41.139   Puncture wound without foreign body of unspecified upper arm
S41.14   Puncture wound with foreign body of upper arm
S41.141   Puncture wound with foreign body of right upper arm
S41.142   Puncture wound with foreign body of left upper arm
S41.149   Puncture wound with foreign body of unspecified upper arm
S41.15   Open bite of upper arm
        Bite of upper arm NOS
        Excludes1:   superficial bite of upper arm (S40.87)
S41.151   Open bite of right upper arm
S41.152   Open bite of left upper arm
S41.159   Open bite of unspecified upper arm

S42 Fracture of shoulder and upper arm

A fracture not indicated as displaced or nondisplaced should be coded to displaced

Excludes1:   traumatic amputation of shoulder and upper arm (S48.-)

A fracture not designated as open or closed should be coded to closed

The open fracture designations are based on the Gustilo open fracture classification

The following extensions are to be added to all codes for category S42:

    a   initial encounter for closed fracture
    b   initial encounter for open fracture type I or II
    c   initial encounter for open fracture type IIIA, IIIB, or IIIC
    d   subsequent encounter for fracture with routine healing
    g   subsequent encounter for fracture with delayed healing
    j   subsequent encounter for fracture with nonunion
    m   subsequent encounter for fracture with malunion
    q   sequela

S42.0 Fracture of clavicle

S42.00 Fracture of unspecified part of clavicle

    S42.001 Fracture of unspecified part of right clavicle
    S42.002 Fracture of unspecified part of left clavicle
    S42.009 Fracture of unspecified part of unspecified clavicle

S42.01 Fracture of sternal end of clavicle

    S42.011 Anterior displaced fracture of sternal end of right clavicle
    S42.012 Anterior displaced fracture of sternal end of left clavicle
    S42.013 Anterior displaced fracture of sternal end of unspecified clavicle Displaced fracture of sternal end of clavicle NOS
    S42.014 Posterior displaced fracture of sternal end of right clavicle
    S42.015 Posterior displaced fracture of sternal end of left clavicle
    S42.016 Posterior displaced fracture of sternal end of unspecified clavicle
    S42.017 Nondisplaced fracture of sternal end of right clavicle
    S42.018 Nondisplaced fracture of sternal end of left clavicle
    S42.019 Nondisplaced fracture of sternal end of unspecified clavicle

S42.02 Fracture of shaft of clavicle

    S42.021 Displaced fracture of shaft of right clavicle
    S42.022 Displaced fracture of shaft of left clavicle
    S42.023 Displaced fracture of shaft of unspecified clavicle
    S42.024 Nondisplaced fracture of shaft of right clavicle
    S42.025 Nondisplaced fracture of shaft of left clavicle
    S42.026 Nondisplaced fracture of shaft of unspecified clavicle

S42.03 Fracture of lateral end of clavicle

Fracture of acromial end of clavicle

    S42.031 Displaced fracture of lateral end of right clavicle
    S42.032 Displaced fracture of lateral end of left clavicle
    S42.033 Displaced fracture of lateral end of unspecified clavicle
    S42.034 Nondisplaced fracture of lateral end of right clavicle
    S42.035 Nondisplaced fracture of lateral end of left clavicle
    S42.036 Nondisplaced fracture of lateral end of unspecified clavicle

S42.1 Fracture of scapula

S42.10 Fracture of unspecified part of scapula

    S42.101 Fracture of unspecified part of scapula, right shoulder

    S42.102 Fracture of unspecified part of scapula, left shoulder
    S42.109 Fracture of unspecified part of scapula, unspecified shoulder

S42.11 Fracture of body of scapula

    S42.111 Displaced fracture of body of scapula, right shoulder
    S42.112 Displaced fracture of body of scapula, left shoulder
    S42.113 Displaced fracture of body of scapula, unspecified shoulder
    S42.114 Nondisplaced fracture of body of scapula, right shoulder
    S42.115 Nondisplaced fracture of body of scapula, left shoulder
    S42.116 Nondisplaced fracture of body of scapula, unspecified shoulder

S45.12 Fracture of acromial process

    S42.121 Displaced fracture of acromial process, right shoulder
    S42.122 Displaced fracture of acromial process, left shoulder
    S42.123 Displaced fracture of acromial process, unspecified shoulder
    S42.124 Nondisplaced fracture of acromial process, right shoulder
    S42.125 Nondisplaced fracture of acromial process, left shoulder
    S42.126 Nondisplaced fracture of acromial process, unspecified shoulder

S42.13 Fracture of coracoid process

    S42.131 Displaced fracture of coracoid process, right shoulder
    S42.132 Displaced fracture of coracoid process, left shoulder
    S42.133 Displaced fracture of coracoid process, unspecified shoulder
    S42.134 Nondisplaced fracture of coracoid process, right shoulder
    S42.135 Nondisplaced fracture of coracoid process, left shoulder
    S42.136 Nondisplaced fracture of coracoid process, unspecified shoulder

S42.14 Fracture of glenoid cavity of scapula

    S42.141 Displaced fracture of glenoid cavity of scapula, right shoulder
    S42.142 Displaced fracture of glenoid cavity of scapula, left shoulder
    S42.143 Displaced fracture of glenoid cavity of scapula, unspecified shoulder
    S42.144 Nondisplaced fracture of glenoid cavity of scapula, right shoulder
    S42.145 Nondisplaced fracture of glenoid cavity of scapula, left shoulder
    S42.146 Nondisplaced fracture of glenoid cavity of scapula, unspecified shoulder

S42.15 Fracture of neck of scapula

    S42.151 Displaced fracture of neck of scapula, right shoulder
    S42.152 Displaced fracture of neck of scapula, left shoulder
    S42.153 Displaced fracture of neck of scapula, unspecified shoulder
    S42.154 Nondisplaced fracture of neck of scapula, right shoulder
    S42.155 Nondisplaced fracture of neck of scapula, left shoulder
    S42.156 Nondisplaced fracture of neck of scapula, unspecified shoulder

S42.19 Fracture of other part of scapula

    S42.191 Fracture of other part of scapula, right shoulder

© 2002 Ingenix, Inc.

S42.192   Fracture of other part of scapula, left shoulder

S42.199   Fracture of other part of scapula, unspecified shoulder

S42.2   Fracture of upper end of humerus

Fracture of proximal end of humerus

Excludes2:   fracture of shaft of humerus (S42.3-)
physeal fracture of upper end of humerus (S49.0-)

S42.20   Unspecified fracture of upper end of humerus

S42.201   Unspecified fracture of upper end of right humerus

S42.202   Unspecified fracture of upper end of left humerus

S42.209   Unspecified fracture of upper end of unspecified humerus

S42.21   Unspecified fracture of surgical neck of humerus

Fracture of neck of humerus NOS

S42.211   Unspecified displaced fracture of surgical neck of right humerus

S42.212   Unspecified displaced fracture of surgical neck of left humerus

S42.213   Unspecified displaced fracture of surgical neck of unspecified humerus

S42.214   Unspecified nondisplaced fracture of surgical neck of right humerus

S42.215   Unspecified nondisplaced fracture of surgical neck of left humerus

S42.216   Unspecified nondisplaced fracture of surgical neck of unspecified humerus

S42.22   2-part fracture of surgical neck of humerus

S42.221   2-part displaced fracture of surgical neck of right humerus

S42.222   2-part displaced fracture of surgical neck of left humerus

S42.223   2-part displaced fracture of surgical neck of unspecified humerus

S42.224   2-part nondisplaced fracture of surgical neck of right humerus

S42.225   2-part nondisplaced fracture of surgical neck of left humerus

S42.226   2-part nondisplaced fracture of surgical neck of unspecified humerus

S42.23   3-part fracture of surgical neck of humerus

S42.231   3-part fracture of surgical neck of right humerus

S42.232   3-part fracture of surgical neck of left humerus

S42.239   3-part fracture of surgical neck of unspecified humerus

S42.24   4-part fracture of surgical neck of humerus

S42.241   4-part fracture of surgical neck of right humerus

S42.242   4-part fracture of surgical neck of left humerus

S42.249   4-part fracture of surgical neck of unspecified humerus

S42.25   Fracture of greater tuberosity of humerus

S42.251   Displaced fracture of greater tuberosity of right humerus

S42.252   Displaced fracture of greater tuberosity of left humerus

S42.253   Displaced fracture of greater tuberosity of unspecified humerus

S42.254   Nondisplaced fracture of greater tuberosity of right humerus

S42.255   Nondisplaced fracture of greater tuberosity of left humerus

S42.256   Nondisplaced fracture of greater tuberosity of unspecified humerus

S42.26   Fracture of lesser tuberosity of humerus

S42.261   Displaced fracture of lesser tuberosity of right humerus

S42.262   Displaced fracture of lesser tuberosity of left humerus

S42.263   Displaced fracture of lesser tuberosity of unspecified humerus

S42.264   Nondisplaced fracture of lesser tuberosity of right humerus

S42.265   Nondisplaced fracture of lesser tuberosity of left humerus

S42.266   Nondisplaced fracture of lesser tuberosity of unspecified humerus

S42.27   Torus fracture of upper end of humerus

Note: extensions b and c are not applicable for this code

S42.271   Torus fracture of upper end of right humerus

S42.272   Torus fracture of upper end of left humerus

S42.279   Torus fracture of upper end of unspecified humerus

S42.29   Other fracture of upper end of humerus

Fracture of anatomical neck of humerus

Fracture of articular head of humerus

S42.291   Other displaced fracture of upper end of right humerus

S42.292   Other displaced fracture of upper end of left humerus

S42.293   Other displaced fracture of upper end of unspecified humerus

S42.294   Other nondisplaced fracture of upper end of right humerus

S42.295   Other nondisplaced fracture of upper end of left humerus

S42.296   Other nondisplaced fracture of upper end of unspecified humerus

S42.3   Fracture of shaft of humerus

Fracture of humerus NOS

Fracture of upper arm NOS

Excludes2:   physeal fractures of upper end of humerus (S49.0-)
physeal fractures of lower end of humerus (S49.1-)

S42.30   Unspecified fracture of shaft of humerus

S42.301   Unspecified fracture of shaft of humerus, right arm

S42.302   Unspecified fracture of shaft of humerus, left arm

S42.309   Unspecified fracture of shaft of humerus, unspecified arm

S42.31   Greenstick fracture of shaft of humerus

Note: extensions b and c are not applicable for this code

S42.311   Greenstick fracture of shaft of humerus, right arm

S42.312   Greenstick fracture of shaft of humerus, left arm

S42.319   Greenstick fracture of shaft of humerus, unspecified arm

S42.32   Transverse fracture of shaft of humerus

S42.321   Displaced transverse fracture of shaft of humerus, right arm

S42.322   Displaced transverse fracture of shaft of humerus, left arm

S42.323   Displaced transverse fracture of shaft of humerus, unspecified arm

S42.324   Nondisplaced transverse fracture of shaft of humerus, right arm

S42.325   Nondisplaced transverse fracture of shaft of humerus, left arm

S42.326   Nondisplaced transverse fracture of shaft of humerus, unspecified arm

S42.33   Oblique fracture of shaft of humerus

S42.331   Displaced oblique fracture of shaft of humerus, right arm

S42.332 Displaced oblique fracture of shaft of humerus, left arm
S42.333 Displaced oblique fracture of shaft of humerus, unspecified arm
S42.334 Nondisplaced oblique fracture of shaft of humerus, right arm
S42.335 Nondisplaced oblique fracture of shaft of humerus, left arm
S42.336 Nondisplaced oblique fracture of shaft of humerus, unspecified arm
S42.34 Spiral fracture of shaft of humerus
S42.341 Displaced spiral fracture of shaft of humerus, right arm
S42.342 Displaced spiral fracture of shaft of humerus, left arm
S42.343 Displaced spiral fracture of shaft of humerus, unspecified arm
S42.344 Nondisplaced spiral fracture of shaft of humerus, right arm
S42.345 Nondisplaced spiral fracture of shaft of humerus, left arm
S42.346 Nondisplaced spiral fracture of shaft of humerus, unspecified arm
S42.35 Comminuted fracture of shaft of humerus
S42.351 Displaced comminuted fracture of shaft of humerus, right arm
S42.352 Displaced comminuted fracture of shaft of humerus, left arm
S42.353 Displaced comminuted fracture of shaft of humerus, unspecified arm
S42.354 Nondisplaced comminuted fracture of shaft of humerus, right arm
S42.355 Nondisplaced comminuted fracture of shaft of humerus, left arm
S42.356 Nondisplaced comminuted fracture of shaft of humerus, unspecified arm
S42.36 Segmental fracture of shaft of humerus
S42.361 Displaced segmental fracture of shaft of humerus, right arm
S42.362 Displaced segmental fracture of shaft of humerus, left arm
S42.363 Displaced segmental fracture of shaft of humerus, unspecified arm
S42.364 Nondisplaced segmental fracture of shaft of humerus, right arm
S42.365 Nondisplaced segmental fracture of shaft of humerus, left arm
S42.366 Nondisplaced segmental fracture of shaft of humerus, unspecified arm
S42.39 Other fracture of shaft of humerus
S42.391 Other fracture of shaft of right humerus
S42.392 Other fracture of shaft of left humerus
S42.399 Other fracture of shaft of unspecified humerus
S42.4 Fracture of lower end of humerus
Fracture of distal end of humerus
Excludes2: fracture of shaft of humerus (S42.3-)
physeal fracture of lower end of humerus (S49.1-)
S42.40 Unspecified fracture of lower end of humerus
Fracture of elbow NOS
S42.401 Unspecified fracture of lower end of right humerus
S42.402 Unspecified fracture of lower end of left humerus
S42.409 Unspecified fracture of lower end of unspecified humerus
S42.41 Simple supracondylar fracture without intercondylar fracture of humerus
S42.411 Displaced simple supracondylar fracture without intercondylar fracture of right humerus
S42.412 Displaced simple supracondylar fracture without intercondylar fracture of left humerus

S42.413 Displaced simple supracondylar fracture without intercondylar fracture of unspecified humerus
S42.414 Nondisplaced simple supracondylar fracture without intercondylar fracture of right humerus
S42.415 Nondisplaced simple supracondylar fracture without intercondylar fracture of left humerus
S42.416 Nondisplaced simple supracondylar fracture without intercondylar fracture of unspecified humerus
S42.42 Comminuted supracondylar fracture without intercondylar fracture of humerus
S42.421 Displaced comminuted supracondylar fracture without intercondylar fracture of right humerus
S42.422 Displaced comminuted supracondylar fracture without intercondylar fracture of left humerus
S42.423 Displaced comminuted supracondylar fracture without intercondylar fracture of unspecified humerus
S42.424 Nondisplaced comminuted supracondylar fracture without intercondylar fracture of right humerus
S42.425 Nondisplaced comminuted supracondylar fracture without intercondylar fracture of left humerus
S42.426 Nondisplaced comminuted supracondylar fracture without intercondylar fracture of unspecifed humerus
S42.43 Fracture (avulsion) of lateral epicondyle of humerus
S42.431 Displaced fracture (avulsion) of lateral epicondyle of right humerus
S42.432 Displaced fracture (avulsion) of lateral epicondyle of left humerus
S42.433 Displaced fracture (avulsion) of lateral epicondyle of unspecified humerus
S42.434 Nondisplaced fracture (avulsion) of lateral epicondyle of right humerus
S42.435 Nondisplaced fracture (avulsion) of lateral epicondyle of left humerus
S42.436 Nondisplaced fracture (avulsion) of lateral epicondyle of unspecified humerus
S42.44 Fracture (avulsion) of medial epicondyle of humerus
S42.441 Displaced fracture (avulsion) of medial epicondyle of right humerus
S42.442 Displaced fracture (avulsion) of medial epicondyle of left humerus
S42.443 Displaced fracture (avulsion) of medial epicondyle of unspecified humerus
S42.444 Nondisplaced fracture (avulsion) of medial epicondyle of right humerus
S42.445 Nondisplaced fracture (avulsion) of medial epicondyle of left humerus
S42.446 Nondisplaced fracture (avulsion) of medial epicondyle of unspecified humerus
S42.447 Incarcerated fracture (avulsion) of medial epicondyle of right humerus
S42.448 Incarcerated fracture (avulsion) of medial epicondyle of left humerus
S42.449 Incarcerated fracture (avulsion) of medial epicondyle of unspecified humerus
S42.45 Fracture of lateral condyle of humerus
Fracture of capitellum of humerus
S42.451 Displaced fracture of lateral condyle of right humerus
S42.452 Displaced fracture of lateral condyle of left humerus
S42.453 Displaced fracture of lateral condyle of unspecified humerus
S42.454 Nondisplaced fracture of lateral condyle of right humerus

S42.455   Nondisplaced fracture of lateral condyle of left humerus

S42.456   Nondisplaced fracture of lateral condyle of unspecified humerus

S42.46   **Fracture of medial condyle of humerus**
Trochlea fracture of humerus

S42.461   Displaced fracture of medial condyle of right humerus

S42.462   Displaced fracture of medial condyle of left humerus

S42.463   Displaced fracture of medial condyle of unspecified humerus

S42.464   Nondisplaced fracture of medial condyle of right humerus

S42.465   Nondisplaced fracture of medial condyle of left humerus

S42.466   Nondisplaced fracture of medial condyle of unspecified humerus

S42.47   **Transcondylar fracture of humerus**

S42.471   Displaced transcondylar fracture of right humerus

S42.472   Displaced transcondylar fracture of left humerus

S42.473   Displaced transcondylar fracture of unspecified humerus

S42.474   Nondisplaced transcondylar fracture of right humerus

S42.475   Nondisplaced transcondylar fracture of left humerus

S42.476   Nondisplaced transcondylar fracture of unspecified humerus

S42.48   **Torus fracture of lower end of humerus**
Note: extensions b and c are not applicable for this code

S42.481   Torus fracture of lower end of right humerus

S42.482   Torus fracture of lower end of left humerus

S42.489   Torus fracture of lower end of unspecified humerus

S42.49   **Other fracture of lower end of humerus**

S42.491   Other displaced fracture of lower end of right humerus

S42.492   Other displaced fracture of lower end of left humerus

S42.493   Other displaced fracture of lower end of unspecified humerus

S42.494   Other nondisplaced fracture of lower end of right humerus

S42.495   Other nondisplaced fracture of lower end of left humerus

S42.496   Other nondisplaced fracture of lower end of unspecified humerus

S42.9   **Fracture of shoulder girdle, part unspecified**
Fracture of shoulder NOS

S42.90   Fracture of unspecified shoulder girdle, part unspecified

S42.91   Fracture of right shoulder girdle, part unspecified

S42.92   Fracture of left shoulder girdle, part unspecified

S43   **Dislocation and sprain of joints and ligaments of shoulder girdle**
Includes: avulsion of joint or ligament of shoulder girdle
laceration of joint or ligament of shoulder girdle
sprain of joint or ligament of shoulder girdle
traumatic hemarthrosis of joint or ligament of shoulder girdle
traumatic rupture of joint or ligament of shoulder girdle
traumatic subluxation of joint or ligament of shoulder girdle
traumatic tear of joint or ligament of shoulder girdle
Excludes2:   strain of muscle and tendon of shoulder and upper arm (S46.-)

The following extensions are to be added to each code for this category:
a   initial encounter
d   subsequent encounter
q   sequela

S43.0   **Subluxation and dislocation of shoulder joint**
Dislocation of glenohumeral joint
Subluxation of glenohumeral joint

S43.00   **Unspecified subluxation and dislocation of shoulder joint**
Dislocation of humerus NOS
Subluxation of humerus NOS

S43.001   Unspecified subluxation of right shoulder joint

S43.002   Unspecified subluxation of left shoulder joint

S43.003   Unspecified subluxation of unspecified shoulder joint

S43.004   Unspecified dislocation of right shoulder joint

S43.005   Unspecified dislocation of left shoulder joint

S43.006   Unspecified dislocation of unspecified shoulder joint

S43.01   **Anterior subluxation and dislocation of humerus**

S43.011   Anterior subluxation of right humerus

S43.012   Anterior subluxation of left humerus

S43.013   Anterior subluxation of unspecified humerus

S43.014   Anterior dislocation of right humerus

S43.015   Anterior dislocation of left humerus

S43.016   Anterior dislocation of unspecified humerus

S43.02   **Posterior subluxation and dislocation of humerus**

S43.021   Posterior subluxation of right humerus

S43.022   Posterior subluxation of left humerus

S43.023   Posterior subluxation of unspecified humerus

S43.024   Posterior dislocation of right humerus

S43.025   Posterior dislocation of left humerus

S43.026   Posterior dislocation of unspecified humerus

S43.03   **Inferior subluxation and dislocation of humerus**

S43.031   Inferior subluxation of right humerus

S43.032   Inferior subluxation of left inferior humerus

S43.033   Inferior subluxation of unspecified inferior humerus

S43.034   Inferior dislocation of right inferior humerus

S43.035   Inferior dislocation of left inferior humerus

S43.036   Inferior dislocation of unspecified inferior humerus

S43.08   **Other subluxation and dislocation of shoulder joint**

S43.081   Other subluxation of right shoulder joint

S43.082   Other subluxation of left shoulder joint

S43.083   Other subluxation of unspecified shoulder joint

S43.084   Other dislocation of right shoulder joint

S43.085   Other dislocation of left shoulder joint

S43.086   Other dislocation of unspecified shoulder joint

S43.1   **Subluxation and dislocation of acromioclavicular joint**

S43.11   **Subluxation of acromioclavicular joint**

S43.111   Subluxation of right acromioclavicular joint

S43.112   Subluxation of left acromioclavicular joint

S43.119   Subluxation of unspecified acromioclavicular joint

S43.12   **Dislocation of acromioclavicular joint, 100%-200% displacement**

S43.121   Dislocation of right acromioclavicular joint, 100%- 200% displacement

S43.122   Dislocation of left acromioclavicular joint, 100%-200% displacement

S43.129   Dislocation of unspecified acromioclavicular joint, 100%-200% displacement

S43.13   **Dislocation of acromioclavicular joint, greater than 200% displacement**

S43.131   Dislocation of right acromioclavicular joint, greater than 200% displacement

S43.132   Dislocation of left acromioclavicular joint, greater than 200% displacement

S43.139   Dislocation of unspecified acromioclavicular joint, greater than 200% displacement

S43.14   Inferior dislocation of acromioclavicular joint

S43.141   Inferior dislocation of right acromioclavicular joint

S43.142   Inferior dislocation of left acromioclavicular joint

S43.149   Inferior dislocation of unspecified acromioclavicular joint

S43.15   Posterior dislocation of acromioclavicular joint

S43.151   Posterior dislocation of right acromioclavicular joint

S43.152   Posterior dislocation of left acromioclavicular joint

S43.159   Posterior dislocation of unspecified acromioclavicular joint

S43.2   Subluxation and dislocation of sternoclavicular joint

S43.20   Unspecified subluxation and dislocation of sternoclavicular joint

S43.201   Unspecified subluxation of right sternoclavicular joint

S43.202   Unspecified subluxation of left sternoclavicular joint

S43.203   Unspecified subluxation of unspecified sternoclavicular joint

S43.204   Unspecified dislocation of right sternoclavicular joint

S43.205   Unspecified dislocation of left sternoclavicular joint

S43.206   Unspecified dislocation of unspecified sternoclavicular joint

S43.21   Anterior subluxation and dislocation of sternoclavicular joint

S43.211   Anterior subluxation of right sternoclavicular joint

S43.212   Anterior subluxation of left sternoclavicular joint

S43.213   Anterior subluxation of unspecified sternoclavicular joint

S43.214   Anterior dislocation of right sternoclavicular joint

S43.215   Anterior dislocation of left sternoclavicular joint

S43.216   Anterior dislocation of unspecified sternoclavicular joint

S43.22   Posterior subluxation and dislocation of sternoclavicular joint

S43.221   Posterior subluxation of right sternoclavicular joint

S43.222   Posterior subluxation of left sternoclavicular joint

S43.223   Posterior subluxation of unspecified sternoclavicular joint

S43.224   Posterior dislocation of right sternoclavicular joint

S43.225   Posterior dislocation of left sternoclavicular joint

S43.226   Posterior dislocation of unspecified sternoclavicular joint

S43.3   Subluxation and dislocation of other and unspecified parts of shoulder girdle

S43.30   Subluxation and dislocation of unspecified parts of shoulder girdle

Dislocation of shoulder girdle NOS
Subluxation of shoulder girdle NOS

S43.301   Subluxation of unspecified parts of right shoulder girdle

S43.202   Subluxation of unspecified parts of left shoulder girdle

S43.303   Subluxation of unspecified parts of unspecified shoulder girdle

S43.304   Dislocation of unspecified parts of right shoulder girdle

S43.305   Dislocation of unspecified parts of left shoulder girdle

S43.306   Dislocation of unspecified parts of unspecified shoulder girdle

S43.31   Subluxation and dislocation of scapula

S43.311   Subluxation of right scapula

S43.312   Subluxation of left scapula

S43.313   Subluxation of unspecified scapula

S43.314   Dislocation of right scapula

S43.315   Dislocation of left scapula

S43.316   Dislocation of unspecified scapula

S43.39   Subluxation and dislocation of other parts of shoulder girdle

S43.391   Subluxation of other parts of right shoulder girdle

S43.392   Subluxation of other parts of left shoulder girdle

S43.393   Subluxation of other parts of unspecified shoulder girdle

S43.394   Dislocation of other parts of right shoulder girdle

S43.395   Dislocation of other parts of left shoulder girdle

S43.396   Dislocation of other parts of unspecified shoulder girdle

S43.4   Sprain of shoulder joint

S43.40   Unspecified sprain of shoulder joint

S43.401   Unspecified sprain of right shoulder joint

S43.402   Unspecified sprain of left shoulder joint

S43.409   Unspecified sprain of unspecified shoulder joint

S43.41   Sprain of coracohumeral (ligament)

S43.411   Sprain of right coracohumeral (ligament)

S43.412   Sprain of left coracohumeral (ligament)

S43.419   Sprain of unspecified coracohumeral (ligament)

S43.42   Sprain of rotator cuff (capsule)

Excludes1:   rotator cuff syndrome (complete) (incomplete), not specified as traumatic (M75.1-)

Excludes2:   injury of tendon of rotator cuff (S46.0-)

S43.421   Sprain of right rotator cuff (capsule)

S43.422   Sprain of left rotator cuff (capsule)

S43.429   Sprain of unspecified rotator cuff (capsule)

S43.49   Other sprain of shoulder joint

S43.491   Other sprain of right shoulder joint

S43.492   Other sprain of left shoulder joint

S43.499   Other sprain of shoulder joint, unspecified side

S43.5   Sprain of acromioclavicular joint

Sprain of acromioclavicular ligament

S43.50   Sprain of acromioclavicular joint, unspecified side

S43.51   Sprain of right acromioclavicular joint

S43.52   Sprain of left acromioclavicular joint

S43.6   Sprain of sternoclavicular joint

S43.60   Sprain of sternoclavicular joint, unspecified side

S43.61   Sprain of right sternoclavicular joint

S43.62   Sprain of left sternoclavicular joint

S43.8   Sprain of other parts of shoulder girdle

S43.80   Sprain of other parts of shoulder girdle, unspecified side

S43.81   Sprain of other parts of right shoulder girdle

S43.82   Sprain of other parts of left shoulder girdle

S43.9   Sprain of unspecified parts of shoulder girdle

S43.90   Sprain of unspecified parts of shoulder girdle, unspecified side

Sprain of shoulder girdle NOS

S43.91   Sprain of unspecified parts of right shoulder girdle

S43.92   Sprain of unspecified parts of left shoulder girdle

S44 Injury of nerves at shoulder and upper arm level
   Code also any associated open wound (S41.-)
   Excludes2:   injury of brachial plexus (S14.3-)
   The following extensions are to be added to each code for this category:
      a   initial encounter
      d   subsequent encounter
      q   sequela

S44.0   Injury of ulnar nerve at upper arm level
   Excludes1:   ulnar nerve NOS (S54.0)
   S44.00   Injury of ulnar nerve at upper arm level, unspecified arm
   S44.01   Injury of ulnar nerve at upper arm level, right arm
   S44.02   Injury of ulnar nerve at upper arm level, left arm

S44.1   Injury of median nerve at upper arm level
   Excludes1:   median nerve NOS (S54.1)
   S44.10   Injury of median nerve at upper arm level, unspecified arm
   S44.11   Injury of median nerve at upper arm level, right arm
   S44.12   Injury of median nerve at upper arm level, left arm

S44.2   Injury of radial nerve at upper arm level
   Excludes1:   radial nerve NOS (S54.2)
   S44.20   Injury of radial nerve at upper arm level, unspecified arm
   S44.21   Injury of radial nerve at upper arm level, right arm
   S44.22   Injury of radial nerve at upper arm level, left arm

S44.3   Injury of axillary nerve
   S44.30   Injury of axillary nerve, unspecified arm
   S44.31   Injury of axillary nerve, right arm
   S44.32   Injury of axillary nerve, left arm

S44.4   Injury of musculocutaneous nerve
   S44.40   Injury of musculocutaneous nerve, unspecified arm
   S44.41   Injury of musculocutaneous nerve, right arm
   S44.42   Injury of musculocutaneous nerve, left arm

S44.5   Injury of cutaneous sensory nerve at shoulder and upper arm level
   S44.50   Injury of cutaneous sensory nerve at shoulder and upper arm level, unspecified arm
   S44.51   Injury of cutaneous sensory nerve at shoulder and upper arm level, right arm
   S44.52   Injury of cutaneous sensory nerve at shoulder and upper arm level, left arm

S44.8   Injury of other nerves at shoulder and upper arm level
   S44.8x   Injury of other nerves at shoulder and upper arm level
      S44.8x1   Injury of other nerves at shoulder and upper arm level, right arm
      S44.8x2   Injury of other nerves at shoulder and upper arm level, left arm
      S44.8x9   Injury of other nerves at shoulder and upper arm level, unspecified arm

S44.9   Injury of unspecified nerve at shoulder and upper arm level
   S44.90   Injury of unspecified nerve at shoulder and upper arm level, unspecified arm
   S44.91   Injury of unspecified nerve at shoulder and upper arm level, right arm
   S44.92   Injury of unspecified nerve at shoulder and upper arm level, left arm

S45 Injury of blood vessels at shoulder and upper arm level
   Code also any associated open wound (S41.-)
   Excludes2:   injury of subclavian artery (S25.1)
                 injury of subclavian vein (S25.3)
   The following extensions are to be added to each code for this category:
      a   initial encounter
      d   subsequent encounter
      q   sequela

S45.0   Injury of axillary artery
   S45.00   Unspecified injury of axillary artery
      S45.001   Unspecified injury of axillary artery, right side

S45.002   Unspecified injury of axillary artery, left side
S45.009   Unspecified injury of axillary artery, unspecified side
S45.01   Laceration of axillary artery
   S45.011   Laceration of axillary artery, right side
   S45.012   Laceration of axillary artery, left side
   S45.019   Laceration of axillary artery, unspecified side
S45.09   Other specified injury of axillary artery
   S45.091   Other specified injury of axillary artery, right side
   S45.092   Other specified injury of axillary artery, left side
   S45.099   Other specified injury of axillary artery, unspecified side

S45.1   Injury of brachial artery
   S45.10   Unspecified injury of brachial artery
      S45.101   Unspecified injury of brachial artery, right side
      S45.102   Unspecified injury of brachial artery, left side
      S45.109   Unspecified injury of brachial artery, unspecified side
   S45.11   Laceration of brachial artery
      S45.111   Laceration of brachial artery, right side
      S45.112   Laceration of brachial artery, left side
      S45.119   Laceration of brachial artery, unspecified side
   S45.19   Other specified injury of brachial artery
      S45.191   Other specified injury of brachial artery, right side
      S45.192   Other specified injury of brachial artery, left side
      S45.199   Other specified injury of brachial artery, unspecified side

S45.2   Injury of axillary or brachial vein
   S45.20   Unspecified injury of axillary or brachial vein
      S45.201   Unspecified injury of axillary or brachial vein, right side
      S45.202   Unspecified injury of axillary or brachial vein, left side
      S45.209   Unspecified injury of axillary or brachial vein, unspecified side
   S45.21   Laceration of axillary or brachial vein
      S45.211   Laceration of axillary or brachial vein, right side
      S45.212   Laceration of axillary or brachial vein, left side
      S45.219   Laceration of axillary or brachial vein, unspecified side
   S45.29   Other specified injury of axillary or brachial vein
      S45.291   Other specified injury of axillary or brachial vein, right side
      S45.292   Other specified injury of axillary or brachial vein, left side
      S45.299   Other specified injury of axillary or brachial vein, unspecified side

S45.3   Injury of superficial vein at shoulder and upper arm level
   S45.30   Unspecified injury of superficial vein at shoulder and upper arm level
      S45.301   Unspecified injury of superficial vein at shoulder and upper arm level, right side
      S45.302   Unspecified injury of superficial vein at shoulder and upper arm level, left side
      S45.309   Unspecified injury of superficial vein at shoulder and upper arm level, unspecified side
   S45.31   Laceration of superficial vein at shoulder and upper arm level
      S45.311   Laceration of superficial vein at shoulder and upper arm level, right side
      S45.312   Laceration of superficial vein at shoulder and upper arm level, left side
      S45.319   Laceration of superficial vein at shoulder and upper arm level, unspecified side

    S45.39   Other specified injury of superficial vein at shoulder and upper arm level

       S45.391   Other specified injury of superficial vein at shoulder and upper arm level, right side

       S45.392   Other specified injury of superficial vein at shoulder and upper arm level, left side

       S45.399   Other specified injury of superficial vein at shoulder and upper arm level, unspecified side

S45.8   Injury of other blood vessels at shoulder and upper arm level

    S45.80   Unspecified injury of other blood vessels at shoulder and upper arm level

       S45.801   Unspecified injury of other blood vessels at shoulder and upper arm level, right side

       S45.802   Unspecified injury of other blood vessels at shoulder and upper arm level, left side

       S45.809   Unspecified injury of other blood vessels at shoulder and upper arm level, unspecified side

    S45.81   Laceration of other blood vessels at shoulder and upper arm level

       S45.811   Laceration of other blood vessels at shoulder and upper arm level, right side

       S45.812   Laceration of other blood vessels at shoulder and upper arm level, left side

       S45.819   Laceration of other blood vessels at shoulder and upper arm level, unspecified side

    S45.89   Other specified injury of other blood vessels at shoulder and upper arm level

       S45.891   Other specified injury of other blood vessels at shoulder and upper arm level, right side

       S45.892   Other specified injury of other blood vessels at shoulder and upper arm level, left side

       S45.899   Other specified injury of other blood vessels at shoulder and upper arm level, unspecified side

S45.9   Injury of unspecified blood vessel at shoulder and upper arm level

    S45.90   Unspecified injury of unspecified blood vessel at shoulder and upper arm level

       S45.901   Unspecified injury of unspecified blood vessel at shoulder and upper arm level, right side

       S45.902   Unspecified injury of unspecified blood vessel at shoulder and upper arm level, left side

       S45.909   Unspecified injury of unspecified blood vessel at shoulder and upper arm level, unspecified side

    S45.91   Laceration of unspecified blood vessel at shoulder and upper arm level

       S45.911   Laceration of unspecified blood vessel at shoulder and upper arm level, right side

       S45.912   Laceration of unspecified blood vessel at shoulder and upper arm level, left side

       S45.919   Laceration of unspecified blood vessel at shoulder and upper arm level, unspecified side

    S45.99   Other specified injury of unspecified blood vessel at shoulder and upper arm level

       S45.991   Other specified injury of unspecified blood vessel at shoulder and upper arm level, right side

       S45.992   Other specified injury of unspecified blood vessel at shoulder and upper arm level, left side

       S45.999   Other specified injury of unspecified blood vessel at shoulder and upper arm level, unspecified side

S46   Injury of muscle and tendon at shoulder and upper arm level

    Code also any associated open wound (S41.-)

    Excludes2:   injury of muscle and tendon at elbow (S56.-)

              sprain of joints and ligaments of shoulder girdle (S43.9)

    The following extensions are to be added to each code for this category:

       a   initial encounter

       d   subsequent encounter

       q   sequela

S46.0   Injury of tendon of the rotator cuff of shoulder

    S46.00   Unspecified injury of tendon of the rotator cuff of shoulder

       S46.001   Unspecified injury of tendon of the rotator cuff of right shoulder

       S46.002   Unspecified injury of tendon of the rotator cuff of left shoulder

       S46.009   Unspecified injury of tendon of the rotator cuff of unspecified shoulder

    S46.01   Strain of tendon of the rotator cuff of shoulder

       S46.011   Strain of tendon of the rotator cuff of right shoulder

       S46.012   Strain of tendon of the rotator cuff of left shoulder

       S46.019   Strain of tendon of the rotator cuff of unspecified shoulder

    S46.02   Laceration of tendon of the rotator cuff of shoulder

       S46.021   Laceration of tendon of the rotator cuff of right shoulder

       S46.022   Laceration of tendon of the rotator cuff of left shoulder

       S46.029   Laceration of tendon of the rotator cuff of unspecified shoulder

    S46.09   Other injury of tendon of the rotator cuff of shoulder

       S46.091   Other injury of tendon of the rotator cuff of right shoulder

       S46.092   Other injury of tendon of the rotator cuff of left shoulder

       S46.099   Other injury of tendon of the rotator cuff of unspecified shoulder

S46.1   Injury of muscle and tendon of long head of biceps

    S46.10   Unspecified injury of muscle and tendon of long head of biceps

       S46.101   Unspecified injury of muscle and tendon of long head of biceps, right arm

       S46.102   Unspecified injury of muscle and tendon of long head of biceps, left arm

       S46.109   Unspecified injury of muscle and tendon of long head of biceps, unspecified arm

    S46.11   Strain of muscle and tendon of long head of biceps

       S46.111   Strain of muscle and tendon of long head of biceps, right arm

       S46.112   Strain of muscle and tendon of long head of biceps, left arm

       S46.119   Strain of muscle and tendon of long head of biceps, unspecified arm

    S46.12   Laceration of muscle and tendon of long head of biceps

       S46.121   Laceration of muscle and tendon of long head of biceps, right arm

       S46.122   Laceration of muscle and tendon of long head of biceps, left arm

       S46.129   Laceration of muscle and tendon of long head of biceps, unspecified arm

    S46.19   Other injury of muscle and tendon of long head of biceps

       S46.191   Other injury of muscle and tendon of long head of biceps, right arm

       S46.192   Other injury of muscle and tendon of long head of biceps, left arm

       S46.199   Other injury of muscle and tendon of long head of biceps, unspecified arm

S46.2   Injury of muscle and tendon of other parts of biceps

    S46.20   Unspecified injury of muscle and tendon of other parts of biceps

       S46.201   Unspecified injury of muscle and tendon of other parts of biceps, right arm

       S46.202   Unspecified injury of muscle and tendon of other parts of biceps, left arm

       S46.209   Unspecified injury of muscle and tendon of other parts of biceps, unspecified arm

S46.21   Strain of muscle and tendon of other parts of biceps
        S46.211 Strain of muscle and tendon of other parts of biceps, right arm
        S46.212   Strain of muscle and tendon of other parts of eps, left arm
        S46.219   Strain of muscle and tendon of other parts of biceps, unspecified arm
S46.22   Laceration of muscle and tendon of other parts of biceps
        S46.221   Laceration of muscle and tendon of other parts of biceps, right arm
        S46.222   Laceration of muscle and tendon of other parts of biceps, left arm biceps
        S46.229   Laceration of muscle and tendon of other parts of biceps, unspecified arm
S46.29   Other injury of muscle and tendon of other parts of biceps
        S46.291   Other injury of muscle and tendon of other parts of biceps, right arm
        S46.292   Other injury of muscle and tendon of other parts of biceps, left arm
        S46.299   Other injury of muscle and tendon of other parts of biceps, unspecified arm
S46.3   Injury of muscle and tendon of triceps
    S46.30   Unspecified injury of muscle and tendon of triceps
        S46.301   Unspecified injury of muscle and tendon of triceps, right arm
        S46.302   Unspecified injury of muscle and tendon of triceps, left arm
        S46.309   Unspecified injury of muscle and tendon of triceps, unspecified arm
    S46.31   Strain of muscle and tendon of triceps
        S46.311   Strain of muscle and tendon of triceps, right arm
        S46.312   Strain of muscle and tendon of triceps, left arm
        S46.319   Strain of muscle and tendon of triceps, unspecified arm
    S46.32   Laceration of muscle and tendon of triceps
        S46.321   Laceration of muscle and tendon of triceps, right arm
        S46.322   Laceration of muscle and tendon of triceps, left arm
        S46.329   Laceration of muscle and tendon of triceps, unspecified arm
    S46.39   Other injury of muscle and tendon of triceps
        S46.391   Other injury of muscle and tendon of triceps, right arm
        S46.392   Other injury of muscle and tendon of triceps, left arm
        S46.399   Other injury of muscle and tendon of triceps, unspecified arm
S46.8   Injury of other muscles and tendons at shoulder and upper arm level
    S46.80   Unspecified injury of other muscles and tendons at shoulder and upper arm level
        S46.801   Unspecified injury of other muscles and tendons at shoulder and upper arm level, right arm
        S46.802   Unspecified injury of other muscles and tendons at shoulder and upper arm level, left arm
        S46.809   Unspecified injury of other muscles and tendons at shoulder and upper arm level, unspecified arm
    S46.81   Strain of other muscles and tendons at shoulder and upper arm level
        S46.811   Strain of other muscles and tendons at shoulder and upper arm level, right arm
        S46.812   Strain of other muscles and tendons at shoulder and upper arm level, left arm

        S46.819   Strain of other muscles and tendons at shoulder and upper arm level, unspecified arm
    S46.82   Laceration of other muscles and tendons at shoulder and upper arm level
        S46.821   Laceration of other muscles and tendons at shoulder and upper arm level, right arm
        S46.822   Laceration of other muscles and tendons at shoulder and upper arm level, left arm
        S46.829   Laceration of other muscles and tendons at shoulder and upper arm level, unspecified arm
    S46.89   Other injury of other muscles and tendons at shoulder and upper arm level
        S46.891   Injury of other muscles and tendons at shoulder and upper arm level, right arm
        S46.892   Injury of other muscles and tendons at shoulder and upper arm level, left arm
        S46.899   Injury of other muscles and tendons at shoulder and upper arm level, unspecified arm
S46.9   Injury of unspecified muscle and tendon at shoulder and upper arm level
    S46.90   Unspecified injury of unspecified muscle and tendon at shoulder and upper arm level
        S46.901   Unspecified injury of unspecified muscle and tendon at shoulder and upper arm level, right arm
        S46.902   Unspecified injury of unspecified muscle and tendon at shoulder and upper arm level, left arm
        S46.909   Unspecified injury of unspecified muscle and tendon at shoulder and upper arm level, unspecified arm
    S46.91   Strain of unspecified muscle and tendon at shoulder and upper arm level
        S46.911   Strain of unspecified muscle and tendon at shoulder and upper arm level, right arm
        S46.912   Strain of unspecified muscle and tendon at shoulder and upper arm level, left arm
        S46.919   Strain of unspecified muscle and tendon at shoulder and upper arm level, unspecified arm
    S46.92   Laceration of unspecified muscle and tendon at shoulder and upper arm level
        S46.921   Laceration of unspecified muscle and tendon at shoulder and upper arm level, right arm
        S46.922   Laceration of unspecified muscle and tendon at shoulder and upper arm level, left arm
        S46.929   Laceration of unspecified muscle and tendon at shoulder and upper arm level, unspecified arm
    S46.99   Other injury of unspecified muscle and tendon at shoulder and upper arm level
        S46.901   Other injury of unspecified muscle and tendon at shoulder and upper arm, right arm
        S46.912   Other injury of unspecified muscle and tendon at shoulder and upper arm level, left arm
        S46.929   Other injury of unspecified muscle and tendon at shoulder and upper arm level, unspecified arm

S47 Crushing injury of shoulder and upper arm
    Use additional code for all associated injuries
    Excludes2:   crushing injury of elbow (S57.0-)
    The following extensions are to be added to each code for this category:
        a   initial encounter
        d   subsequent encounter
        q   sequela
S47.1   Crushing injury of right shoulder and upper arm
S47.2   Crushing injury of left shoulder and upper arm
S47.9   Crushing injury of shoulder and upper arm, unspecified arm

S48   Traumatic amputation of shoulder and upper arm

An amputation not identified as partial or complete should be coded to complete

Excludes1:   traumatic amputation at elbow level (S58.0)

The following extensions are to be added to each code for this category:
- a   initial encounter
- d   subsequent encounter
- q   sequela

S48.0   Traumatic amputation at shoulder joint

S48.01   Complete traumatic amputation at shoulder joint

S48.011   Complete traumatic amputation at right shoulder joint

S48.012   Complete traumatic amputation at left shoulder joint

S48.019   Complete traumatic amputation at unspecified shoulder joint

S48.02   Partial traumatic amputation at shoulder joint

S48.021   Partial traumatic amputation at right shoulder joint

S48.022   Partial traumatic amputation at left shoulder joint

S48.029   Partial traumatic amputation at unspecified shoulder joint

S48.1   Traumatic amputation at level between shoulder and elbow

S48.11   Complete traumatic amputation at level between shoulder and elbow

S48.111   Complete traumatic amputation at level between right shoulder and elbow

S48.112   Complete traumatic amputation at level between left shoulder and elbow

S48.119   Complete traumatic amputation at level between unspecified shoulder and elbow

S48.12   Partial traumatic amputation at level between shoulder and elbow

S48.121   Partial traumatic amputation at level between right shoulder and elbow

S48.122   Partial traumatic amputation at level between left shoulder and elbow

S48.129   Partial traumatic amputation at level between unspecified shoulder and elbow

S48.9   Traumatic amputation of shoulder and upper arm, level unspecified

S48.91   Complete traumatic amputation of shoulder and upper arm, level unspecified

S48.911   Complete traumatic amputation of right shoulder and upper arm, level unspecified

S48.912   Complete traumatic amputation of left shoulder and upper arm, level unspecified

S48.919   Complete traumatic amputation of unspecified shoulder and upper arm, level unspecified

S48.92   Partial traumatic amputation of shoulder and upper arm, level unspecified

S48.921   Partial traumatic amputation of right shoulder and upper arm, level unspecified

S48.922   Partial traumatic amputation of left shoulder and upper arm, level unspecified

S48.929   Partial traumatic amputation of unspecified shoulder and upper arm, level unspecified

S49   Other and unspecified injuries of shoulder and upper arm

The following extensions are to be added to each code for subcategories S49.0 and S49.1
- a   initial encounter for closed fracture
- b   initial encounter for open fracture
- d   subsequent encounter for fracture with routine healing
- g   subsequent encounter for fracture with delayed healing
- q   sequela

S49.0   Physeal fracture of upper end of humerus

S49.00   Unspecified physeal fracture of upper end of humerus

S49.001   Unspecified physeal fracture of upper end of humerus, right arm

S49.002   Unspecified physeal fracture of upper end of humerus, left arm

S49.009   Unspecified physeal fracture of upper end of humerus, unspecified arm

S49.01   Salter-Harris Type I physeal fracture of upper end of humerus

S49.011   Salter-Harris Type I physeal fracture of upper end of humerus, right arm

S49.012   Salter-Harris Type I physeal fracture of upper end of humerus, left arm

S49.019   Salter-Harris Type I physeal fracture of upper end of humerus, unspecified arm

S49.02   Salter-Harris Type II physeal fracture of upper end of humerus

S49.021   Salter-Harris Type II physeal fracture of upper end of humerus, right arm

S49.022   Salter-Harris Type II physeal fracture of upper end of humerus, left arm

S49.029   Salter-Harris Type II physeal fracture of upper end of humerus, unspecified arm

S49.03   Salter-Harris Type III physeal fracture of upper end of humerus

S49.031   Salter Harris Type III physeal fracture of upper end of humerus, right arm

S49.032   Salter Harris Type III physeal fracture of upper end of humerus, left arm

S49.039   Salter Harris Type III physeal fracture of upper end of humerus, unspecified arm

S49.04   Salter-Harris Type IV physeal fracture of upper end of humerus

S49.041   Salter-Harris Type IV physeal fracture of upper end of humerus, right arm

S49.042   Salter-Harris Type IV physeal fracture of upper end of humerus, left arm

S49.049   Salter-Harris Type IV physeal fracture of upper end of humerus, unspecified arm

S49.09   Other physeal fracture of upper end of humerus

S49.091   Other physeal fracture of upper end of humerus, right arm

S49.092   Other physeal fracture of upper end of humerus, left arm

S49.099   Other physeal fracture of upper end of humerus, unspecified arm

S49.1   Physeal fracture of lower end of humerus

S49.10   Unspecified physeal fracture of lower end of humerus

S49.101   Unspecified physeal fracture of lower end of humerus, right arm

S49.102   Unspecified physeal fracture of lower end of humerus, left arm

S49.109   Unspecified physeal fracture of lower end of humerus, unspecified arm

S49.11   Salter-Harris Type I physeal fracture of lower end of humerus

S49.111   Salter-Harris Type I physeal fracture of lower end of humerus, right arm

S49.112   Salter-Harris Type I physeal fracture of lower end of humerus, left arm

S49.119   Salter-Harris Type I physeal fracture of lower end of humerus, unspecified arm

S49.12   Salter-Harris Type II physeal fracture of lower end of humerus

S49.121   Salter-Harris Type II physeal fracture of lower end of humerus, right arm

S49.122   Salter-Harris Type II physeal fracture of lower end of humerus, left arm

S49.129   Salter-Harris Type II physeal fracture of lower end of humerus, unspecified arm

S49.13   Salter Harris Type III physeal fracture of lower end of humerus

S49.131   Salter Harris Type III physeal fracture of lower end of humerus, right arm

S49.132   Salter Harris Type III physeal fracture of lower end of humerus, left arm

S49.139   Salter Harris Type III physeal fracture of lower end of humerus, unspecified arm

S49.14   Salter-Harris Type IV physeal fracture of lower end of humerus

S49.141   Salter-Harris Type IV physeal fracture of lower end of humerus, right arm

S49.142   Salter-Harris Type IV physeal fracture of lower end of humerus, left arm

S49.149   Salter-Harris Type IV physeal fracture of lower end of humerus, unspecified arm

S49.19   Other physeal fracture of lower end of humerus

S49.191   Other physeal fracture of lower end of humerus, right arm

S49.192   Other physeal fracture of lower end of humerus, left arm

S49.199   Other physeal fracture of lower end of humerus, unspecified arm

The following extensions are to be added to each code for subcategories S49.8 and S49.9:
- a   initial encounter
- d   subsequent encounter
- q   sequela

S49.8   Other specified injuries of shoulder and upper arm

S49.80   Other specified injuries of shoulder and upper arm, unspecified arm

S49.81   Other specified injuries of left shoulder and upper arm

S49.82   Other specified injuries of right shoulder and upper arm

S49.9   Unspecified injury of shoulder and upper arm

S49.90   Unspecified injury of left shoulder and upper arm

S49.91   Unspecified injury of shoulder and upper arm, unspecified arm

S49.92   Unspecified injury of right shoulder and upper arm

INJURIES TO THE ELBOW AND FOREARM (S50–S59)

Excludes2:   burns and corrosions (T20-T32)
frostbite (T33-T34)
injuries of wrist and hand (S60-S69)
insect bite or sting, venomous (T63.4)

S50   Superficial injury of elbow and forearm

Excludes2:   superficial injury of wrist and hand (S60.-)
The following extensions are to be added to each code for category S50:
- a   initial encounter
- d   subsequent encounter
- q   sequela

S50.0   Contusion of elbow

S50.00   Contusion of unspecified elbow

S50.01   Contusion of right elbow

S50.02   Contusion of left elbow

S50.1   Contusion of forearm

S50.10   Contusion of unspecified forearm

S50.11   Contusion of right forearm

S50.12   Contusion of left forearm

S50.3   Other superficial injuries of elbow

S50.31   Abrasion of elbow

S50.311   Abrasion of right elbow

S50.312   Abrasion of left elbow

S50.319   Abrasion of unspecified elbow

S50.32   Blister (nonthermal) of elbow

S50.321   Blister (nonthermal) of right elbow

S50.322   Blister (nonthermal) of left elbow

S50.329   Blister (nonthermal) of unspecified elbow

S50.34   External constriction of elbow

S50.341   External constriction of right elbow

S50.342   External constriction of left elbow

S50.349   External constriction of unspecified elbow

S50.35   Superficial foreign body of elbow
Splinter in the elbow

S50.351   Superficial foreign body of right elbow

S50.352   Superficial foreign body of left elbow

S50.359   Superficial foreign body of unspecified elbow

S50.36   Insect bite (nonvenomous) of elbow

S50.361   Insect bite (nonvenomous) of right elbow

S50.362   Insect bite (nonvenomous) of left elbow

S50.369   Insect bite (nonvenomous) of unspecified elbow

S50.37   Other superficial bite of elbow
Excludes1:   open bite of elbow (S51.04)

S50.371   Other superficial bite of right elbow

S50.372   Other superficial bite of left elbow

S50.379   Other superficial bite of unspecified elbow

S50.8   Other superficial injuries of forearm

S50.81   Abrasion of forearm

S50.811   Abrasion of right forearm

S50.812   Abrasion of left forearm

S50.819   Abrasion of unspecified forearm

S50.82   Blister (nonthermal) of forearm

S50.821   Blister (nonthermal) of right forearm

S50.822   Blister (nonthermal) of left forearm

S50.829   Blister (nonthermal) of unspecified forearm

S50.84   External constriction of forearm

S50.841   External constriction of right forearm

S50.842   External constriction of left forearm

S50.849   External constriction of unspecified forearm

S50.85   Superficial foreign body of forearm
Splinter in the forearm

S50.851   Superficial foreign body of right forearm

S50.852   Superficial foreign body of left forearm

S50.859   Superficial foreign body of unspecified forearm

S50.86   Insect bite (nonvenomous) of forearm

S50.861   Insect bite (nonvenomous) of right forearm

S50.862   Insect bite (nonvenomous) of left forearm

S50.869   Insect bite (nonvenomous) of unspecified forearm

S50.87   Other superficial bite of forearm
Excludes1:   open bite of forearm (S51.84)

S50.871   Other superficial bite of right forearm

S50.872   Other superficial bite of left forearm

S50.879   Other superficial bite of unspecified forearm

S50.9   Unspecified superficial injury of elbow and forearm

S50.90   Unspecified superficial injury of elbow

S50.901   Unspecified superficial injury of right elbow

S50.902   Unspecified superficial injury of left elbow

S50.909   Unspecified superficial injury of unspecified elbow

S50.91   Unspecified superficial injury of forearm

S50.911   Unspecified superficial injury of right forearm

S50.912   Unspecified superficial injury of left forearm

S50.919   Unspecified superficial injury of unspecified forearm

S51   Open wound of elbow and forearm
Code also any associated wound infection
Excludes1:   open fracture of elbow and forearm (S52.- with open fracture extensions)
traumatic amputation of elbow and forearm (S58.-)
Excludes2:   open wound of wrist and hand (S61.-)
The following extensions are to be added to each code for category S51:
- a   initial encounter
- d   subsequent encounter
- q   sequela

S51.0   Open wound of elbow

S51.00   Unspecified open wound of elbow

S51.001   Unspecified open wound of right elbow

S51.002   Unspecified open wound of left elbow

S51.009   Unspecified open wound of unspecified elbow
Open wound of elbow NOS

S51.01   Laceration without foreign body of elbow

S51.011   Laceration without foreign body of right elbow

S51.012   Laceration without foreign body of left elbow

S51.019   Laceration without foreign body of unspecified elbow

S51.02   Laceration with foreign body of elbow

S51.021   Laceration with foreign body of right elbow

S51.022   Laceration with foreign body of left elbow

S51.029   Laceration with foreign body of unspecified elbow

S51.03   Puncture wound without foreign body of elbow

S51.031   Puncture wound without foreign body of right elbow

S51.032   Puncture wound without foreign body of left elbow

S51.039   Puncture wound without foreign body of unspecified elbow

S51.04   Puncture wound with foreign body of elbow

S51.041   Puncture wound with foreign body of right elbow

S51.042   Puncture wound with foreign body of left elbow

S51.049   Puncture wound with foreign body of unspecified elbow

S51.05   Open bite of elbow
Bite of elbow NOS
Excludes1:   superficial bite of elbow (S50.36, S50.37)

S51.051   Open bite, right elbow

S51.052   Open bite, left elbow

S51.059   Open bite, unspecified elbow

S51.8   Open wound of forearm
Excludes2:   open wound of elbow (51.0-)

S51.80   Unspecified open wound of forearm

S51.801   Unspecified open wound of right forearm

S51.802   Unspecified open wound of left forearm

S51.809   Unspecified open wound of unspecified forearm
Open wound of forearm NOS

S51.81   Laceration without foreign body of forearm

S51.811   Laceration without foreign body of right forearm

S51.812   Laceration without foreign body of left forearm

S51.819   Laceration without foreign body of unspecified forearm

S51.82   Laceration with foreign body of forearm

S51.821   Laceration with foreign body of right forearm

S51.822   Laceration with foreign body of left forearm

S51.829   Laceration with foreign body of unspecified forearm

S51.83   Puncture wound without foreign body of forearm

S51.831   Puncture wound without foreign body of right forearm

S51.832   Puncture wound without foreign body of left forearm

S51.839   Puncture wound without foreign body of unspecified forearm

S51.84   Puncture wound with foreign body of forearm

S51.841   Puncture wound with foreign body of right forearm

S51.842   Puncture wound with foreign body of left forearm

S51.849   Puncture wound with foreign body of unspecified forearm

S51.85   Open bite of forearm
Bite of forearm NOS
Excludes1:   superficial bite of forearm (S50.86, S50.87)

S51.851   Open bite of right forearm

S51.852   Open bite of left forearm

S51.859   Open bite of unspecified forearm

S52   Fracture of forearm
A fracture not identified as displaced or nondisplaced should be coded to displaced
Excludes1:   traumatic amputation of forearm (S58.-)
Excludes2:   fracture at wrist and hand level (S62.-)
A fracture not designated as open or closed should be coded to closed
Note: the open fracture designations are based on the Gustilo open fracture classification
The following extensions are to be added to each code for category S52:

a   initial encounter for closed fracture

b   initial encounter for open fracture type I or II

c   initial encounter for open fracture type IIIA, IIIB, or IIIC

d   subsequent encounter for closed fracture with routine healing

e   subsequent encounter for open fracture type I or II with routine healing

f   subsequent encounter for open fracture type IIIA, IIIB, or IIIC with routine healing

g   subsequent encounter for closed fracture with delayed healing

h   subsequent encounter for open fracture type I or II with delayed healing

i   subsequent encounter for open fracture type IIIA, IIIB, or IIIC with delayed healing

j   subsequent encounter for closed fracture with nonunion

k   subsequent encounter for open fracture type I or II with nonunion

l   subsequent encounter for open fracture type IIIA, IIIB, or IIIC with nonunion

m   subsequent encounter for closed fracture with malunion

n   subsequent encounter for open fracture type I or II with malunion

o   subsequent encounter for open fracture type IIIA, IIIB, or IIIC with malunion

q   sequela

S52.0   Fracture of upper end of ulna
Fracture of proximal end of ulna
Excludes2:   fracture of elbow NOS (S42.40-)
fractures of shaft of ulna (S52.2-)

S52.00   Unspecified fracture of upper end of ulna

S52.001   Unspecified fracture of upper end of right ulna

S52.002   Unspecified fracture of upper end of left ulna

S52.009   Unspecified fracture of upper end of unspecified ulna

S52.01   Torus fracture of upper end of ulna
Note: open fracture extensions do not apply to these codes

S52.011   Torus fracture of upper end of right ulna

S52.012   Torus fracture of upper end of left ulna

S52.019   Torus fracture of upper end of unspecified ulna

S52.02   Fracture of olecranon process without intraarticular extension of ulna

S52.021   Displaced fracture of olecranon process without intraarticular extension of right ulna

S52.022   Displaced fracture of olecranon process without intraarticular extension of left ulna

S52.023   Displaced fracture of olecranon process without intraarticular extension of unspecified ulna

S52.024   Nondisplaced fracture of olecranon process without intraarticular extension of right ulna

S52.025   Nondisplaced fracture of olecranon process without intraarticular extension of left ulna

S52.026   Nondisplaced fracture of olecranon process without intraarticular extension of unspecified ulna

S52.03   Fracture of olecranon process with intraarticular extension of ulna

S52.031   Displaced fracture of olecranon process with intraarticular extension of right ulna

S52.032   Displaced fracture of olecranon process with intraarticular extension of left ulna

S52.033   Displaced fracture of olecranon process with intraarticular extension of unspecified ulna

S52.034   Nondisplaced fracture of olecranon process with intraarticular extension of right ulna

S52.035   Nondisplaced fracture of olecranon process with intraarticular extension of left ulna

S52.036   Nondisplaced fracture of olecranon process with intraarticular extension of unspecified ulna

S52.04   Fracture of coronoid process of ulna

S52.041   Displaced fracture of coronoid process of right ulna

S52.042   Displaced fracture of coronoid process of left ulna

S52.043   Displaced fracture of coronoid process of unspecified ulna

S52.044   Nondisplaced fracture of coronoid process of right ulna

S52.045   Nondisplaced fracture of coronoid process of left ulna

S52.046   Nondisplaced fracture of coronoid process of unspecified ulna

S52.09   Other fracture of upper end of ulna

S52.091   Other fracture of upper end of right ulna

S52.092   Other fracture of upper end of left ulna

S52.099   Other fracture of upper end of unspecified ulna

S52.1   Fracture of upper end of radius

Fracture of proximal end of radius

Excludes2:   fracture of shaft of radius (S52.3-)
physeal fractures of upper end of radius (S59.2-)

S52.10   Unspecified fracture of upper end of radius

S52.101   Unspecified fracture of upper end of right radius

S52.102   Unspecified fracture of upper end of left radius

S52.109   Unspecified fracture of upper end of unspecified radius

S52.11   Torus fracture of upper end of radius

S52.111   Torus fracture of upper end of right radius

S52.112   Torus fracture of upper end of left radius

S52.119   Torus fracture of upper end of unspecified radius

S52.12   Fracture of head of radius

S52.121   Displaced fracture of head of right radius

S52.122   Displaced fracture of head of left radius

S52.123   Displaced fracture of head of unspecified radius

S52.124   Nondisplaced fracture of head of right radius

S52.125   Nondisplaced fracture of head of left radius

S52.126   Nondisplaced fracture of head of unspecified radius

S52.13   Fracture of neck of radius

S52.131   Displaced fracture of neck of right radius

S52.132   Displaced fracture of neck of left radius

S52.133   Displaced fracture of neck of unspecified radius

S52.134   Nondisplaced fracture of neck of right radius

S52.135   Nondisplaced fracture of neck of left radius

S52.136   Nondisplaced fracture of neck of unspecified radius

S52.18   Other fracture of upper end of radius

S52.181   Other fracture of upper end of right radius

S52.182   Other fracture of upper end of left radius

S52.189   Other fracture of upper end of unspecified radius

S52.2   Fracture of shaft of ulna

S52.20   Unspecified fracture of shaft of ulna

Fracture of ulna NOS

S52.201   Unspecified fracture of shaft of right ulna

S52.202   Unspecified fracture of shaft of left ulna

S52.209   Unspecified fracture of shaft of unspecified ulna

S52.21   Greenstick fracture of shaft of ulna

S52.211   Greenstick fracture of shaft of right ulna

S52.212   Greenstick fracture of shaft of left ulna

S52.219   Greenstick fracture of shaft of unspecified ulna

S52.22   Transverse fracture of shaft of ulna

S52.221   Displaced transverse fracture of shaft of right ulna

S52.222   Displaced transverse fracture of shaft of left ulna

S52.223   Displaced transverse fracture of shaft of unspecified ulna

S52.224   Nondisplaced transverse fracture of shaft of right ulna

S52.225   Nondisplaced transverse fracture of shaft of left ulna

S52.226   Nondisplaced transverse fracture of shaft of unspecified ulna

S52.23   Oblique fracture of shaft of ulna

S52.231   Displaced oblique fracture of shaft of right ulna

S52.232   Displaced oblique fracture of shaft of left ulna

S52.233   Displaced oblique fracture of shaft of unspecified ulna

S52.234   Nondisplaced oblique fracture of shaft of right ulna

S52.235   Nondisplaced oblique fracture of shaft of left ulna

S52.236   Nondisplaced oblique fracture of shaft of unspecified ulna

S52.24   Spiral fracture of shaft of ulna

S52.241   Displaced spiral fracture of shaft of ulna, right arm

S52.242   Displaced spiral fracture of shaft of ulna, left arm

S52.243   Displaced spiral fracture of shaft of ulna, unspecified arm

S52.244   Nondisplaced spiral fracture of shaft of ulna, right arm

S52.245   Nondisplaced spiral fracture of shaft of ulna, left arm

S52.246   Nondisplaced spiral fracture of shaft of ulna, unspecified arm

S52.25   Comminuted fracture of shaft of ulna

S52.251   Displaced comminuted fracture of shaft of ulna, right arm

S52.252   Displaced comminuted fracture of shaft of ulna, left arm

S52.253   Displaced comminuted fracture of shaft of ulna, unspecified arm

S52.254   Nondisplaced comminuted fracture of shaft of ulna, right arm

S52.255   Nondisplaced comminuted fracture of shaft of ulna, left arm

S52.256   Nondisplaced comminuted fracture of shaft of ulna, unspecified arm

S52.26   Segmental fracture of shaft of ulna

S52.261   Displaced segmental fracture of shaft of ulna, right arm

S52.262   Displaced segmental fracture of shaft of ulna, left arm

S52.263   Displaced segmental fracture of shaft of ulna, unspecified arm

S52.264   Nondisplaced segmental fracture of shaft of ulna, right arm

S52.265   Nondisplaced segmental fracture of shaft of ulna, left arm

S52.266   Nondisplaced segmental fracture of shaft of ulna, unspecified arm

S52.27   Monteggia's fracture of ulna
        Fracture of upper shaft of ulna with dislocation of radial head

S52.271   Monteggia's fracture of right ulna

S52.272   Monteggia's fracture of left ulna

S52.279   Monteggia's fracture of unspecified ulna

S52.28   Bent bone of ulna

S52.281   Bent bone of right ulna

S52.282   Bent bone of left ulna

S52.283   Bent bone of unspecified ulna

S52.29   Other fracture of shaft of ulna

S52.291   Other fracture of shaft of right ulna

S52.292   Other fracture of shaft of left ulna

S52.299   Other fracture of shaft of unspecified ulna

S52.3   Fracture of shaft of radius

S52.30   Unspecified fracture of shaft of radius

S52.301   Unspecified fracture of shaft of right radius

S52.302   Unspecified fracture of shaft of left radius

S52.309   Unspecified fracture of shaft of unspecified radius

S52.31   Greenstick fracture of shaft of radius

S52.311   Greenstick fracture of shaft of radius, right arm

S52.312   Greenstick fracture of shaft of radius, left arm

S52.319   Greenstick fracture of shaft of radius, unspecified arm

S52.32   Transverse fracture of shaft of radius

S52.321   Displaced transverse fracture of shaft of right radius

S52.322   Displaced transverse fracture of shaft of left radius

S52.323   Displaced transverse fracture of shaft of unspecified radius

S52.324   Nondisplaced transverse fracture of shaft of right radius

S52.325   Nondisplaced transverse fracture of shaft of left radius

S52.326   Nondisplaced transverse fracture of shaft of unspecified radius

S52.33   Oblique fracture of shaft of radius

S52.331   Displaced oblique fracture of shaft of right radius

S52.332   Displaced oblique fracture of shaft of left radius

S52.333   Displaced oblique fracture of shaft of unspecified radius

S52.334   Nondisplaced oblique fracture of shaft of right radius

S52.335   Nondisplaced oblique fracture of shaft of left radius

S52.336   Nondisplaced oblique fracture of shaft of unspecified radius

S52.34   Spiral fracture of shaft of radius

S52.341   Displaced spiral fracture of shaft of radius, right arm

S52.342   Displaced spiral fracture of shaft of radius, left arm

S52.343   Displaced spiral fracture of shaft of radius, unspecified arm

S52.344   Nondisplaced spiral fracture of shaft of radius, right arm

S52.345   Nondisplaced spiral fracture of shaft of radius, left arm

S52.346   Nondisplaced spiral fracture of shaft of radius, unspecified arm

S52.35   Comminuted fracture of shaft of radius

S52.351   Displaced comminuted fracture of shaft of radius, right arm

S52.352   Displaced comminuted fracture of shaft of radius, left arm

S52.353   Displaced comminuted fracture of shaft of radius, unspecified arm

S52.354   Nondisplaced comminuted fracture of shaft of radius, right arm

S52.355   Nondisplaced comminuted fracture of shaft of radius, left arm

S52.356   Nondisplaced comminuted fracture of shaft of radius, unspecified arm

S52.36   Segmental fracture of shaft of radius

S52.361   Displaced segmental fracture of shaft of radius, right arm

S52.362   Displaced segmental fracture of shaft of radius, left arm

S52.363   Displaced segmental fracture of shaft of radius, unspecified arm

S52.364   Nondisplaced segmental fracture of shaft of radius, right arm

S52.365   Nondisplaced segmental fracture of shaft of radius, left arm

S52.366   Nondisplaced segmental fracture of shaft of radius, unspecified arm

S52.37   Galeazzi's fracture
        Fracture of lower shaft of radius with radioulnar joint dislocation

S52.371   Galeazzi's fracture of right radius

S52.372   Galeazzi's fracture of left radius

S52.379   Galeazzi's fracture of unspecified radius

S52.38   Bent bone of radius

S52.381   Bent bone of right radius

S52.382   Bent bone of left radius

S52.389   Bent bone of unspecified radius

S52.39   Other fracture of shaft of radius

S52.391   Other fracture of shaft of radius, right arm

S52.392   Other fracture of shaft of radius, left arm

S52.399   Other fracture of shaft of radius, unspecified arm

S52.5   Fracture of lower end of radius
        Fracture of distal end of radius
        Excludes2:   physeal fractures of lower end of radius (S59.2-)

S52.50   Unspecified fracture of the lower end of radius

S52.501   Unspecified fracture of the lower end of right radius

S52.502   Unspecified fracture of the lower end of left radius

S52.509   Unspecified fracture of the lower end of unspecified radius

S52.51   Fracture of radial styloid process

S52.511   Displaced fracture of right radial styloid process

S52.512   Displaced fracture of left radial styloid process

S52.513   Displaced fracture of unspecified radial styloid process

S52.514   Nondisplaced fracture of right radial styloid process

S52.515   Nondisplaced fracture of left radial styloid process

S52.516   Nondisplaced fracture of unspecified radial styloid process

S52.52   Torus fracture of lower end of radius

S52.521   Torus fracture of lower end of right radius

S52.522   Torus fracture of lower end of left radius

S52.529   Torus fracture of lower end of unspecified radius

S52.53   Colles' fracture

S52.531   Colles' fracture of right radius

S52.532   Colles' fracture of left radius

S52.539   Colles' fracture of unspecified radius
S52.54   Smith's fracture
S52.541   Smith's fracture of right radius
S52.542   Smith's fracture of left radius
S52.549   Smith's fracture of unspecified radius
S52.55   Other extraarticular fracture of lower end of radius
S52.551   Other extraarticular fracture of lower end of right radius
S52.552   Other extraarticular fracture of lower end of left radius
S52.559   Other extraarticular fracture of lower end of unspecified radius
S52.56   Barton's fracture
S52.561   Barton's fracture of right radius
S52.562   Barton's fracture of left radius
S52.569   Barton's fracture of unspecified radius
S52.57   Other intraarticular fracture of lower end of radius
S52.571   Other intraarticular fracture of lower end of right radius
S52.572   Other intraarticular fracture of lower end of left radius
S52.579   Other intraarticular fracture of lower end of unspecified radius
S52.59   Other fractures of lower end of radius
S52.591   Other fractures of lower end of right radius
S52.592   Other fractures of lower end of left radius
S52.599   Other fractures of lower end of unspecified radius
S52.6   Fracture of lower end of ulna
S52.60   Unspecified fracture of lower end of ulna
S52.601   Unspecified fracture of lower end of right ulna
S52.602   Unspecified fracture of lower end of left ulna
S52.609   Unspecified fracture of lower end of unspecified ulna
S52.61   Fracture of ulna styloid process
S52.611   Displaced fracture of right ulna styloid process
S52.612   Displaced fracture of left ulna styloid process
S52.613   Displaced fracture of unspecified ulna styloid process
S52.614   Nondisplaced fracture of right ulna styloid process
S52.615   Nondisplaced fracture of left ulna styloid process
S52.616   Nondisplaced fracture of unspecified ulna styloid process
S52.62   Torus fracture of lower end of ulna
S52.621   Torus fracture of lower end of right ulna
S52.622   Torus fracture of lower end of left ulna
S52.629   Torus fracture of lower end of unspecified ulna
S52.69   Other fracture of lower end of ulna
S52.691   Other fracture of lower end of right ulna
S52.692   Other fracture of lower end of left ulna
S52.699   Other fracture of lower end of unspecified ulna
S52.9   Unspecified fracture of forearm
S52.90   Unspecified fracture of unspecified forearm
S52.91   Unspecified fracture of right forearm
S52.92   Unspecified fracture of left forearm

S53   Dislocation and sprain of joints and ligaments of elbow
Includes: avulsion of joint or ligament of elbow
laceration of joint or ligament of elbow
sprain of joint or ligament of elbow
traumatic hemarthrosis of joint or ligament of elbow
traumatic rupture of joint or ligament of elbow
traumatic subluxation of joint or ligament of elbow
traumatic tear of joint or ligament of elbow
Excludes2:   strain of muscle and tendon at forearm level (S56.-)

The following extensions are to be added to each code for category S53:
a   initial encounter
d   subsequent encounter
q   sequela

S53.0   Subluxation and dislocation of radial head
Dislocation of radiohumeral joint
Subluxation of radiohumeral joint
Excludes1:   Monteggia's fracture-dislocation (S52.27-)
S53.00   Unspecified subluxation and dislocation of radial head
S53.001   Unspecified subluxation of right radial head
S53.002   Unspecified subluxation of left radial head
S53.003   Unspecified subluxation of unspecified radial head
S53.004   Unspecified dislocation of right radial head
S53.005   Unspecified dislocation of left radial head
S53.006   Unspecified dislocation of unspecified radial head
S53.01   Anterior subluxation and dislocation of radial head
Anteriomedial subluxation and dislocation of radial head
S53.011   Anterior subluxation of right radial head
S53.012   Anterior subluxation of left radial head
S53.013   Anterior subluxation of unspecified radial head
S53.014   Anterior dislocation of right radial head
S53.015   Anterior dislocation of left radial head
S53.016   Anterior dislocation of unspecified radial head
S53.02   Posterior subluxation and dislocation of radial head
Posteriolateral subluxation and dislocation of radial head
S53.021   Posterior subluxation of right radial head
S53.022   Posterior subluxation of left radial head
S53.023   Posterior subluxation of unspecified radial head
S53.024   Posterior dislocation of right radial head
S53.025   Posterior dislocation of left radial head
S53.026   Posterior dislocation of unspecified radial head
S53.09   Other subluxation and dislocation of radial head
S53.091   Other subluxation of right radial head
S53.092   Other subluxation of left radial head
S53.093   Other subluxation of unspecified radial head
S53.094   Other dislocation of right radial head
S53.095   Other dislocation of left radial head
S53.096   Other dislocation of unspecified radial head
S53.1   Subluxation and dislocation of ulnohumeral joint
Subluxation and dislocation of elbow NOS
Excludes1:   dislocation of radial head alone (S53.0-)
S53.10   Unspecified subluxation and dislocation of ulnohumeral joint
S53.101   Unspecified subluxation of right ulnohumeral joint
S53.102   Unspecified subluxation of left ulnohumeral joint
S53.103   Unspecified subluxation of unspecified ulnohumeral joint
S53.104   Unspecified dislocation of right ulnohumeral joint
S53.105   Unspecified dislocation of left ulnohumeral joint
S53.106   Unspecified dislocation of unspecified ulnohumeral joint
S53.11   Anterior subluxation and dislocation of ulnohumeral joint
S53.111   Anterior subluxation of right ulnohumeral joint
S53.112   Anterior subluxation of left ulnohumeral joint
S53.113   Anterior subluxation of unspecified ulnohumeral joint
S53.114   Anterior dislocation of right ulnohumeral joint
S53.115   Anterior dislocation of left ulnohumeral joint

S53.116   Anterior dislocation of unspecified ulnohumeral joint

S53.12   Posterior subluxation and dislocation of ulnohumeral joint

   S53.121   Posterior subluxation of right ulnohumeral joint

   S53.122   Posterior subluxation of left ulnohumeral joint

   S53.123   Posterior subluxation of unspecified ulnohumeral joint

   S53.124   Posterior dislocation of right ulnohumeral joint

   S53.125   Posterior dislocation of left ulnohumeral joint

   S53.126   Posterior dislocation of unspecified ulnohumeral joint

S53.13   Medial subluxation and dislocation of ulnohumeral joint

   S53.131   Medial subluxation of right ulnohumeral joint

   S53.132   Medial subluxation of left ulnohumeral joint

   S53.133   Medial subluxation of unspecified ulnohumeral joint

   S53.134   Medial dislocation of right ulnohumeral joint

   S53.135   Medial dislocation of left ulnohumeral joint

   S53.136   Medial dislocation of unspecified ulnohumeral joint

S53.14   Lateral subluxation and dislocation of ulnohumeral joint

   S53.141   Lateral subluxation of right ulnohumeral joint

   S53.142   Lateral subluxation of left ulnohumeral joint

   S53.143   Lateral subluxation of unspecified ulnohumeral joint

   S53.144   Lateral dislocation of right ulnohumeral joint

   S53.145   Lateral dislocation of left ulnohumeral joint

   S53.146   Lateral dislocation of unspecified ulnohumeral joint

S53.19   Other subluxation and dislocation of ulnohumeral joint

   S53.191   Other subluxation of right ulnohumeral joint

   S53.192   Other subluxation of left ulnohumeral joint

   S53.193   Other subluxation of unspecified ulnohumeral joint

   S53.194   Other dislocation of right ulnohumeral joint

   S53.195   Other dislocation of left ulnohumeral joint

   S53.196   Other dislocation of unspecified ulnohumeral joint

S53.2   **Traumatic rupture of radial collateral ligament**

   Excludes1:   sprain of radial collateral ligament NOS (S53.43-)

S53.20   Traumatic rupture of radial collateral ligament, unspecified side

S53.21   Traumatic rupture of right radial collateral ligament

S53.22   Traumatic rupture of left radial collateral ligament

S53.3   **Traumatic rupture of ulnar collateral ligament**

   Excludes1:   sprain of ulnar collateral ligament (S53.44-)

S53.30   Traumatic rupture of ulnar collateral ligament, unspecified side

S53.31   Traumatic rupture of right ulnar collateral ligament

S53.32   Traumatic rupture of left ulnar collateral ligament

S53.4   **Other and unspecified sprain of elbow**

   Excludes2:   traumatic rupture of radial collateral ligament (S53.2-)

            traumatic rupture of ulnar collateral ligament (S53.3-)

S53.40   Unspecified sprain of elbow

   S53.401   Unspecified sprain of right elbow

   S53.402   Unspecified sprain of left elbow

   S53.409   Unspecified sprain of unspecified elbow

        Sprain of elbow NOS

S53.41   Radiohumeral (joint) sprain

   S53.411   Radiohumeral (joint) sprain of right elbow

   S53.412   Radiohumeral (joint) sprain of left elbow

   S53.419   Radiohumeral (joint) sprain of unspecified elbow

S53.42   Ulnohumeral (joint) sprain

   S53.421   Ulnohumeral (joint) sprain of right elbow

   S53.422   Ulnohumeral (joint) sprain of left elbow

   S53.429   Ulnohumeral (joint) sprain of unspecified elbow

S53.43   Radial collateral ligament sprain

   S53.431   Radial collateral ligament sprain of right elbow

   S53.432   Radial collateral ligament sprain of left elbow

   S53.439   Radial collateral ligament sprain of unspecified elbow

S53.44   Ulnar collateral ligament sprain

   S53.441   Ulnar collateral ligament sprain of right elbow

   S53.442   Ulnar collateral ligament sprain of left elbow

   S53.449   Ulnar collateral ligament sprain of unspecified elbow

S53.49   Other sprain of elbow

   S53.491   Other sprain of right elbow

   S53.492   Other sprain of left elbow

   S53.499   Other sprain of unspecified elbow

S54   Injury of nerves at forearm level

Code also any associated open wound (S51.-)

Excludes2:   injury of nerves at wrist and hand level (S64.-)

The following extensions are to be added to each code for category S54:

   a   initial encounter

   d   subsequent encounter

   q   sequela

S54.0   **Injury of ulnar nerve at forearm level**

   Injury of ulnar nerve NOS

S54.00   Injury of ulnar nerve at forearm level, unspecified arm

S54.01   Injury of ulnar nerve at forearm level, right arm

S54.02   Injury of ulnar nerve at forearm level, left arm

S54.1   **Injury of median nerve at forearm level**

   Injury of median nerve NOS

S54.10   Injury of median nerve at forearm level, unspecified arm

S54.11   Injury of median nerve at forearm level, right arm

S54.12   Injury of median nerve at forearm level, left arm

S54.2   **Injury of radial nerve at forearm level**

   Injury of radial nerve NOS

S54.20   Injury of radial nerve at forearm level, unspecified arm

S54.21   Injury of radial nerve at forearm level, right arm

S54.22   Injury of radial nerve at forearm level, left arm

S54.3   **Injury of cutaneous sensory nerve at forearm level**

S54.30   Injury of cutaneous sensory nerve at forearm level, unspecified arm

S54.31   Injury of cutaneous sensory nerve at forearm level, right arm

S54.32   Injury of cutaneous sensory nerve at forearm level, left arm

S54.8   **Injury of other nerves at forearm level**

S54.8x   Injury of other nerves at forearm level

   S54.8x1   Unspecified injury of other nerves at forearm level, right arm

   S54.8x2   Unspecified injury of other nerves at forearm level, left arm

   S54.8x9   Unspecified injury of other nerves at forearm level, unspecified arm

S54.9   **Injury of unspecified nerve at forearm level**

S54.90   Injury of unspecified nerve at forearm level, unspecified arm

S54.91   Injury of unspecified nerve at forearm level, right arm

S54.92   Injury of unspecified nerve at forearm level, left arm

S55 Injury of blood vessels at forearm level

Code also any associated open wound (S51.-)

Excludes2: injury of blood vessels at wrist and hand level (S65.-)
injury of brachial vessels (S45.1-S45.2)

The following extensions are to be added to each code for category S55:

a   initial encounter
d   subsequent encounter
q   sequela

S55.0   Injury of ulnar artery at forearm level

S55.00   Unspecified injury of ulnar artery at forearm level

S55.001   Unspecified injury of ulnar artery at forearm level, right arm

S55.002   Unspecified injury of ulnar artery at forearm level, left arm

S55.009   Unspecified injury of ulnar artery at forearm level, unspecified arm

S55.01   Laceration of ulnar artery at forearm level

S55.011   Laceration of ulnar artery at forearm level, right arm

S55.012   Laceration of ulnar artery at forearm level, left arm

S55.019   Laceration of ulnar artery at forearm level, unspecified arm

S55.09   Other specified injury of ulnar artery at forearm level

S55.091   Other specified injury of ulnar artery at forearm level, right arm

S55.092   Other specified injury of ulnar artery at forearm level, left arm

S55.099   Other specified injury of ulnar artery at forearm level, unspecified arm

S55.1   Injury of radial artery at forearm level

S55.10   Unspecified injury of radial artery at forearm level

S55.101   Unspecified injury of radial artery at forearm level, right arm

S55.102   Unspecified injury of radial artery at forearm level, left arm

S55.109   Unspecified injury of radial artery at forearm level, unspecified arm

S55.11   Laceration of radial artery at forearm level

S55.111   Laceration of radial artery at forearm level, right arm

S55.112   Laceration of radial artery at forearm level, left arm

S55.119   Laceration of radial artery at forearm level, unspecified arm

S55.19   Other specified injury of radial artery at forearm level

S55.191   Other specified injury of radial artery at forearm level, right arm

S55.192   Other specified injury of radial artery at forearm level, left arm

S55.199   Other specified injury of radial artery at forearm level, unspecified arm

S55.2   Injury of vein at forearm level

S55.20   Unspecified injury of vein at forearm level

S55.201   Unspecified injury of vein at forearm level, right arm

S55.202   Unspecified injury of vein at forearm level, left arm

S55.209   Unspecified injury of vein at forearm level, unspecified arm

S55.21   Laceration of vein at forearm level

S55.211   Laceration of vein at forearm level, right arm

S55.212   Laceration of vein at forearm level, left arm

S55.219   Laceration of vein at forearm level, unspecified arm

S55.29   Other specified injury of vein at forearm level

S55.291   Other specified injury of vein at forearm level, right arm

S55.292   Other specified injury of vein at forearm level, left arm

S55.299   Other specified injury of vein at forearm level, unspecified arm

S55.8   Injury of other blood vessels at forearm level

S55.80   Unspecified injury of other blood vessels at forearm level

S55.801   Unspecified injury of other blood vessels at forearm level, right arm

S55.802   Unspecified injury of other blood vessels at forearm level, left arm

S55.809   Unspecified injury of other blood vessels at forearm level, unspecified arm

S55.81   Laceration of other blood vessels at forearm level

S55.811   Laceration of other blood vessels at forearm level, right arm

S55.812   Laceration of other blood vessels at forearm level, left arm

S55.819   Laceration of other blood vessels at forearm level, unspecified arm

S55.89   Other specified injury of other blood vessels at forearm level

S55.891   Other specified injury of other blood vessels at forearm level, right arm

S55.892   Other specified injury of other blood vessels at forearm level, left arm

S55.899   Other specified injury of other blood vessels at forearm level, unspecified arm

S55.9   Injury of unspecified blood vessel at forearm level

S55.90   Unspecified injury of unspecified blood vessel at forearm level

S55.901   Unspecified injury of unspecified blood vessel at forearm level, right arm

S55.902   Unspecified injury of unspecified blood vessel at forearm level, left arm

S55.909   Unspecified injury of unspecified blood vessel at forearm level, unspecified arm

S55.91   Laceration of unspecified blood vessel at forearm level

S55.911   Laceration of unspecified blood vessel at forearm level, right arm

S55.912   Laceration of unspecified blood vessel at forearm level, left arm

S55.919   Laceration of unspecified blood vessel at forearm level, unspecified arm

S55.99   Other specified injury of unspecified blood vessel at forearm level

S55.991   Other specified injury of unspecified blood vessel at forearm level, right arm

S55.992   Other specified injury of unspecified blood vessel at forearm level, left arm

S55.999   Other specified injury of unspecified blood vessel at forearm level, unspecified arm

S56 Injury of muscle and tendon at forearm level

Code also any associated open wound (S51.-)

Excludes2: injury of muscle and tendon at or below wrist (S66.-)
sprain of joints and ligaments of elbow (S53.4-)

The following extensions are to be added to each code for category S56:

a   initial encounter
d   subsequent encounter
q   sequela

S56.0   Injury of flexor muscle and tendon of thumb at forearm level

S56.00   Unspecified injury of flexor muscle and tendon of thumb at forearm level

S56.001   Unspecified injury of flexor muscle and tendon of right thumb at forearm level

S56.002   Unspecified injury of flexor muscle and tendon of left thumb at forearm level

S56.009   Unspecified injury of flexor muscle and tendon of unspecified thumb at forearm level

S56.01   Strain of flexor muscle and tendon of thumb at forearm level

S56.011   Strain of flexor muscle and tendon of right thumb at forearm level

S56.012   Strain of flexor muscle and tendon of left thumb at forearm level

S56.019   Strain of flexor muscle and tendon of unspecified thumb at forearm level

S56.02   Laceration of flexor muscle and tendon of thumb at forearm level

S56.021   Laceration of flexor muscle and tendon of right thumb at forearm level

S56.022   Laceration of flexor muscle and tendon of left thumb at forearm level

S56.029   Laceration of flexor muscle and tendon of unspecified thumb at forearm level

S56.09   Other injury of flexor muscle and tendon of thumb at forearm level

S56.091   Other injury of flexor muscle and tendon of right thumb at forearm level

S56.092   Other injury of flexor muscle and tendon of left thumb at forearm level

S56.099   Other injury of flexor muscle and tendon of unspecified thumb at forearm level

S56.1   Injury of flexor muscle and tendon of other and unspecified finger at forearm level

S56.10   Unspecified injury of flexor muscle and tendon of other and unspecified finger at forearm level

S56.101   Unspecified injury of flexor muscle and tendon of right index finger at forearm level

S56.102   Unspecified injury of flexor muscle and tendon of left index finger at forearm level

S56.103   Unspecified injury of flexor muscle and tendon of right middle finger at forearm level

S56.104   Unspecified injury of flexor muscle and tendon of left middle finger at forearm level

S56.105   Unspecified injury of flexor muscle and tendon of right ring finger at forearm level

S56.106   Unspecified injury of flexor muscle and tendon of left ring finger at forearm level

S56.107   Unspecified injury of flexor muscle and tendon of right little finger at forearm level

S56.108   Unspecified injury of flexor muscle and tendon of left little finger at forearm level

S56.109   Unspecified injury of flexor muscle and tendon of unspecified finger at forearm level

S56.11   Strain of flexor muscle and tendon of other and unspecified finger at forearm level

S56.111   Strain of flexor muscle and tendon of right index finger at forearm level

S56.112   Strain of flexor muscle and tendon of left index finger at forearm level

S56.113   Strain of flexor muscle and tendon of right middle finger at forearm level

S56.114   Strain of flexor muscle and tendon of left middle finger at forearm level

S56.115   Strain of flexor muscle and tendon of right ring finger at forearm level

S56.116   Strain of flexor muscle and tendon of left ring finger at forearm level

S56.117   Strain of flexor muscle and tendon of right little finger at forearm level

S56.118   Strain of flexor muscle and tendon of left little finger at forearm level

S56.119   Strain of flexor muscle and tendon of finger of unspecified finger at forearm level

S56.12   Laceration of flexor muscle and tendon of other and unspecified finger at forearm level

S56.121   Laceration of flexor muscle and tendon of right index finger at forearm level

S56.122   Laceration of flexor muscle and tendon of left index finger at forearm level

S56.123   Laceration of flexor muscle and tendon of right middle finger at forearm level

S56.124   Laceration of flexor muscle and tendon of left middle finger at forearm level

S56.125   Laceration of flexor muscle and tendon of right ring finger at forearm level

S56.126   Laceration of flexor muscle and tendon of left ring finger at forearm level

S56.127   Laceration of flexor muscle and tendon of right little finger at forearm level

S56.128   Laceration of flexor muscle and tendon of left little finger at forearm level

S56.129   Laceration of flexor muscle and tendon of unspecified finger at forearm level

S56.19   Other injury of flexor muscle and tendon of other and unspecified finger at forearm level

S56.191   Other injury of flexor muscle and tendon of right index finger at forearm level

S56.192   Other injury of flexor muscle and tendon of left index finger at forearm level

S56.193   Other injury of flexor muscle and tendon of right middle finger at forearm level

S56.194   Other injury of flexor muscle and tendon of left middle finger at forearm level

S56.195   Other injury of flexor muscle and tendon of right ring finger at forearm level

S56.196   Other injury of flexor muscle and tendon of left ring finger at forearm level

S56.197   Other injury of flexor muscle and tendon of right little finger at forearm level

S56.198   Other injury of flexor muscle and tendon of left little finger at forearm level

S56.199   Other injury of flexor muscle and tendon of unspecified finger at forearm level

S56.2   Injury of other flexor muscle and tendon at forearm level

S56.20   Unspecified injury of other flexor muscle and tendon at forearm level

S56.201   Unspecified injury of other flexor muscle and tendon at forearm level, right arm

S56.202   Unspecified injury of other flexor muscle and tendon at forearm level, left arm

S56.209   Unspecified injury of other flexor muscle and tendon at forearm level, unspecified arm

S56.21   Strain of other flexor muscle and tendon at forearm level

S56.211   Strain of other flexor muscle and tendon at forearm level, right arm

S56.212   Strain of other flexor muscle and tendon at forearm level, left arm

S56.219   Strain of other flexor muscle and tendon at forearm level, unspecified arm

S56.22   Laceration of other flexor muscle and tendon at forearm level

S56.221   Laceration of other flexor muscle and tendon at forearm level, right arm

S56.222   Laceration of other flexor muscle and tendon at forearm level, left arm

S56.229   Laceration of other flexor muscle and tendon at forearm level, unspecified arm

S56.29   Other injury of other flexor muscle and tendon at forearm level

S56.291   Other injury of other flexor muscle and tendon at forearm level, right arm

S56.292   Other injury of other flexor muscle and tendon at forearm level, left arm

S56.299   Other injury of other flexor muscle and tendon at forearm level, unspecified arm

S56.3   Injury of extensor or abductor muscles and tendons of thumb at forearm level

S56.30   Unspecified injury of extensor or abductor muscles and tendons of thumb at forearm level

S56.301   Unspecified injury of extensor or abductor muscles and tendons of right thumb at forearm level

S56.302   Unspecified injury of extensor or abductor muscles and tendons of left thumb at forearm level

S56.309   Unspecified injury of extensor or abductor muscles and tendons of unspecified thumb at forearm level

S56.31   Strain of extensor or abductor muscles and tendons of thumb at forearm level

S56.311   Strain of extensor or abductor muscles and tendons of right thumb at forearm level

S56.312   Strain of extensor or abductor muscles and tendons of left thumb at forearm level

S56.319   Strain of extensor or abductor muscles and tendons of unspecified thumb at forearm level

S56.32   Laceration of extensor or abductor muscles and tendons of thumb at forearm level

S56.321   Laceration of extensor or abductor muscles and tendons of right thumb at forearm level

S56.322   Laceration of extensor or abductor muscles and tendons of left thumb at forearm level

S56.329   Laceration of extensor or abductor muscles and tendons of unspecified thumb at forearm level

S56.39   Other injury of extensor or abductor muscles and tendons of thumb at forearm level

S56.391   Other injury of extensor or abductor muscles and tendons of right thumb at forearm level

S56.392   Other injury of extensor or abductor muscles and tendons of left thumb at forearm level

S56.399   Other injury of extensor or abductor muscles and tendons of unspecified thumb at forearm level

S56.4   Injury of extensor muscle and tendon of other and unspecified finger at forearm level

S56.40   Unspecified injury of extensor muscle and tendon of other and unspecified finger at forearm level

S56.401   Unspecified injury of extensor muscle and tendon of right index finger at forearm level

S56.402   Unspecified injury of extensor muscle and tendon of left index finger at forearm level

S56.403   Unspecified injury of extensor muscle and tendon of right middle finger at forearm level

S56.404   Unspecified injury of extensor muscle and tendon of left middle finger at forearm level

S56.405   Unspecified injury of extensor muscle and tendon of right ring finger at forearm level

S56.406   Unspecified injury of extensor muscle and tendon of left ring finger at forearm level

S56.407   Unspecified injury of extensor muscle and tendon of right little finger at forearm level

S56.408   Unspecified injury of extensor muscle and tendon of left little finger at forearm level

S56.409   Unspecified injury of extensor muscle and tendon of unspecified finger at forearm level

S56.41   Strain of extensor muscle and tendon of other and unspecified finger at forearm level

S56.411   Strain of extensor muscle and tendon of right index finger at forearm level

S56.412   Strain of extensor muscle and tendon of left index finger at forearm level

S56.413   Strain of extensor muscle and tendon of right middle finger at forearm level

S56.414   Strain of extensor muscle and tendon of left middle finger at forearm level

S56.415   Strain of extensor muscle and tendon of right ring finger at forearm level

S56.416   Strain of extensor muscle and tendon of left ring finger at forearm level

S56.417   Strain of extensor muscle and tendon of right little finger at forearm level

S56.418   Strain of extensor muscle and tendon of left little finger at forearm level

S56.419   Strain of extensor muscle and tendon of finger, unspecified finger at forearm level

S56.42   Laceration of extensor muscle and tendon of other and unspecified finger at forearm level

S56.421   Laceration of extensor muscle and tendon of right index finger at forearm level

S56.422   Laceration of extensor muscle and tendon of left index finger at forearm level

S56.423   Laceration of extensor muscle and tendon of right middle finger at forearm level

S56.424   Laceration of extensor muscle and tendon of left middle finger at forearm level

S56.425   Laceration of extensor muscle and tendon of right ring finger at forearm level

S56.426   Laceration of extensor muscle and tendon of left ring finger at forearm level

S56.427   Laceration of extensor muscle and tendon of right little finger at forearm level

S56.428   Laceration of extensor muscle and tendon of left little finger at forearm level

S56.429   Laceration of extensor muscle and tendon of unspecified finger at forearm level

S56.49   Other injury of extensor muscle and tendon of other and unspecified finger at forearm level

S56.491   Other injury of extensor muscle and tendon of right index finger at forearm level

S56.492   Other injury of extensor muscle and tendon of left index finger at forearm level

S56.493   Other injury of extensor muscle and tendon of right middle finger at forearm level

S56.494   Other injury of extensor muscle and tendon of left middle finger at forearm level

S56.495   Other injury of extensor muscle and tendon of right ring finger at forearm level

S56.496   Other injury of extensor muscle and tendon of left ring finger at forearm level

S56.497   Other injury of extensor muscle and tendon of right little finger at forearm level

S56.498   Other injury of extensor muscle and tendon of left little finger at forearm level

S56.499   Other injury of extensor muscle and tendon of unspecified finger at forearm level

S56.5   Injury of other extensor muscle and tendon at forearm level

S56.50   Unspecified injury of other extensor muscle and tendon at forearm level

S56.501   Unspecified injury of other extensor muscle and tendon at forearm level, right arm

S56.502   Unspecified injury of other extensor muscle and tendon at forearm level, left arm

S56.509   Unspecified injury of other extensor muscle and tendon at forearm level, unspecified arm

S56.51   Strain of other extensor muscle and tendon at forearm level

S56.511   Strain of other extensor muscle and tendon at forearm level, right arm

S56.512   Strain of other extensor muscle and tendon at forearm level, left arm

S56.519   Strain of other extensor muscle and tendon at forearm level, unspecified arm

S56.52   Laceration of other extensor muscle and tendon at forearm level

S56.521   Laceration of other extensor muscle and tendon at forearm level, right arm

S56.522   Laceration of other extensor muscle and tendon at forearm level, left arm

S56.529   Laceration of other extensor muscle and tendon at forearm level, unspecified arm

S56.59   Other injury of other extensor muscle and tendon at forearm level

S56.591   Other injury of other extensor muscle and tendon at forearm level, right arm

S56.592   Other injury of other extensor muscle and tendon at forearm level, left arm

S56.599   Other injury of other extensor muscle and tendon at forearm level, unspecified arm

S56.8   Injury of other muscles and tendons at forearm level

S56.80   Unspecified injury of other muscles and tendons at forearm level

S56.801   Unspecified injury of other muscles and tendons at forearm level, right arm

S56.802   Unspecified injury of other muscles and tendons at forearm level, left arm

S56.809   Unspecified injury of other muscles and tendons at forearm level, unspecified arm

S56.81   Strain of other muscles and tendons at forearm level

S56.811   Strain of other muscles and tendons at forearm level, right arm

S56.812   Strain of other muscles and tendons at forearm level, left arm

S56.819   Strain of other muscles and tendons at forearm level, unspecified arm

S56.82   Laceration of other muscles and tendons at forearm level

S56.821   Laceration of other muscles and tendons at forearm level, right arm

S56.822   Laceration of other muscles and tendons at forearm level, left arm

S56.829   Laceration of other muscles and tendons at forearm level, unspecified arm

S56.89   Other injury of other muscles and tendons at forearm level

S56.891   Other injury of other muscles and tendons at forearm level, right arm

S56.892   Other injury of other muscles and tendons at forearm level, left arm

S56.890   Other injury of other muscles and tendons at forearm level, unspecified arm

S56.9   Injury of unspecified muscles and tendons at forearm level

S56.90   Unspecified injury of unspecified muscles and tendons at forearm level

S56.901   Unspecified injury of unspecified muscles and tendons at forearm level, right arm

S56.902   Unspecified injury of unspecified muscles and tendons at forearm level, left arm

S56.909   Unspecified injury of unspecified muscles and tendons at forearm level, unspecified arm

S56.91   Strain of unspecified muscles and tendons at forearm level

S56.911   Strain of unspecified muscles and tendons at forearm level, right arm

S56.912   Strain of unspecified muscles and tendons at forearm level, left arm

S56.919   Strain of unspecified muscles and tendons at forearm level, unspecified arm

S56.92   Laceration of unspecified muscles and tendons at forearm level

S56.921   Laceration of unspecified muscles and tendons at forearm level, right arm

S56.922   Laceration of unspecified muscles and tendons at forearm level, left arm

S56.929   Laceration of unspecified muscles and tendons at forearm level, unspecified arm

S56.99   Other injury of unspecified muscles and tendons at forearm level

S56.991   Other injury of unspecified muscles and tendons at forearm level, right arm

S56.992   Other injury of unspecified muscles and tendons at forearm level, left arm

S56.999   Other injury of unspecified muscles and tendons at forearm level, unspecified arm

S57   Crushing injury of elbow and forearm
Use additional code(s) for all associated injuries
Excludes2:   crushing injury of wrist and hand (S67.-)
The following extensions are to be added to each code for category S57:
a   initial encounter
d   subsequent encounter
q   sequela

S57.0   Crushing injury of elbow
S57.00   Crushing injury of elbow, unspecified side
S57.01   Crushing injury of right elbow
S57.02   Crushing injury of left elbow

S57.8   Crushing injury of forearm
S57.80   Crushing injury of forearm, unspecified side
S57.81   Crushing injury of right forearm
S57.82   Crushing injury of left forearm

S58   Traumatic amputation of elbow and forearm
An amputation not identified as partial or complete should be coded to complete
Excludes1:   traumatic amputation of wrist and hand (S68.-)
The following extensions are to be added to each code for category S58:
a   initial encounter
d   subsequent encounter
q   sequela

S58.0   Traumatic amputation at elbow level
S58.01   Complete traumatic amputation at elbow level
S58.011   Complete traumatic amputation at elbow level, right arm
S58.012   Complete traumatic amputation at elbow level, left arm
S58.019   Complete traumatic amputation at elbow level, unspecified arm

S58.02   Partial traumatic amputation at elbow level
S58.021   Partial traumatic amputation at elbow level, right arm
S58.022   Partial traumatic amputation at elbow level, left arm
S58.029   Partial traumatic amputation at elbow level, unspecified arm

S58.1   Traumatic amputation at level between elbow and wrist
S58.11   Complete traumatic amputation at level between elbow and wrist
S58.111   Complete traumatic amputation at level between elbow and wrist, right arm
S58.112   Complete traumatic amputation at level between elbow and wrist, left arm
S58.119   Complete traumatic amputation at level between elbow and wrist, unspecified arm

S58.12   Partial traumatic amputation at level between elbow and wrist
S58.121   Partial traumatic amputation at level between elbow and wrist, right arm
S58.122   Partial traumatic amputation at level between elbow and wrist, left arm
S58.129   Partial traumatic amputation at level between elbow and wrist, unspecified arm

S58.9   Traumatic amputation of forearm, level unspecified
Excludes1:   traumatic amputation of wrist (S68.-)
S58.91   Complete traumatic amputation of forearm, level unspecified
S58.911   Complete traumatic amputation of right forearm, level unspecified
S58.912   Complete traumatic amputation of left forearm, level unspecified
S58.919   Complete traumatic amputation of unspecified forearm, level unspecified

S58.92   Partial traumatic amputation of forearm, level unspecified
S58.921   Partial traumatic amputation of right forearm, level unspecified

S58.922   Partial traumatic amputation of left forearm, level unspecified

S58.929   Partial traumatic amputation of unspecified forearm, level unspecified

S59 Other and unspecified injuries of elbow and forearm

Excludes2:   other and unspecified injuries of wrist and hand (S69.-)

The following extensions are to be added to each code for subcategories S59.0, S59.1, and S59.2:

a   initial encounter for fracture
d   subsequent encounter for fracture with routine healing
g   subsequent encounter for fracture with delayed healing
j   subsequent encounter for fracture with nonunion
m   subsequent encounter for fracture with malunion
q   sequela

S59.0   Physeal fracture of lower end of ulna

S59.00   Unspecified physeal fracture of lower end of ulna

S59.001   Unspecified physeal fracture of lower end of ulna, right arm

S59.002   Unspecified physeal fracture of lower end of ulna, left arm

S59.009   Unspecified physeal fracture of lower end of ulna, unspecified arm

S59.01   Salter-Harris Type I physeal fracture of lower end of ulna

S59.011   Salter-Harris Type I physeal fracture of lower end of ulna, right arm

S59.012   Salter-Harris Type I physeal fracture of lower end of ulna, left arm

S59.019   Salter-Harris Type I physeal fracture of lower end of ulna, unspecified arm

S59.02   Salter-Harris Type II physeal fracture of lower end of ulna

S59.021   Salter-Harris Type II physeal fracture of lower end of ulna, right arm

S59.022   Salter-Harris Type II physeal fracture of lower end of ulna, left arm

S59.029   Salter-Harris Type II physeal fracture of lower end of ulna, unspecified arm

S59.03   Salter-Harris Type III physeal fracture of lower end of ulna

S59.031   Salter-Harris Type III physeal fracture of lower end of ulna, right arm

S59.032   Salter-Harris Type III physeal fracture of lower end of ulna, left arm

S59.039   Salter-Harris Type III physeal fracture of lower end of ulna, unspecified arm

S59.04   Slater-Harris Type IV physeal fracture of lower end of ulna

S59.041   Slater-Harris Type IV physeal fracture of lower end of ulna, right arm

S59.042   Slater-Harris Type IV physeal fracture of lower end of ulna, left arm

S59.049   Slater-Harris Type IV physeal fracture of lower end of ulna, unspecified arm

S59.09   Other physeal fracture of lower end of ulna

S59.091   Other physeal fracture of lower end of ulna, right arm

S59.092   Other physeal fracture of lower end of ulna, left arm

S59.099   Other physeal fracture of lower end of ulna, unspecified arm

S59.1   Physeal fracture of upper end of radius

S59.10   Unspecified physeal fracture of upper end of radius

S59.101   Unspecified physeal fracture of upper end of radius, right arm

S59.102   Unspecified physeal fracture of upper end of radius, left arm

S59.109   Unspecified physeal fracture of upper end of radius, unspecified arm

S59.11   Salter-Harris Type I physeal fracture of upper end of radius

S59.111   Salter-Harris Type I physeal fracture of upper end of radius, right arm

S59.112   Salter-Harris Type I physeal fracture of upper end of radius, left arm

S59.119   Salter-Harris Type I physeal fracture of upper end of radius, unspecified arm

S59.12   Salter-Harris Type II physeal fracture of upper end of radius

S59.121   Salter-Harris Type II physeal fracture of upper end of radius, right arm

S59.122   Salter-Harris Type II physeal fracture of upper end of radius, left arm

S59.129   Salter-Harris Type II physeal fracture of upper end of radius, unspecified arm

S59.13   Salter-Harris Type III physeal fracture of upper end of radius

S59.131   Salter-Harris Type III physeal fracture of upper end of radius, right arm

S59.132   Salter-Harris Type III physeal fracture of upper end of radius, left arm

S59.139   Salter-Harris Type III physeal fracture of upper end of radius, unspecified arm

S59.14   Slater-Harris Type IV physeal fracture of upper end of radius

S59.141   Slater-Harris Type IV physeal fracture of upper end of radius, right arm

S59.142   Slater-Harris Type IV physeal fracture of upper end of radius, left arm

S59.149   Slater-Harris Type IV physeal fracture of upper end of radius, unspecified arm

S59.19   Other physeal fracture of upper end of radius

S59.191   Other physeal fracture of upper end of radius, right arm

S59.192   Other physeal fracture of upper end of radius, left arm

S59.199   Other physeal fracture of upper end of radius, unspecified arm

S59.2   Physeal fracture of lower end of radius

S59.20   Unspecified physeal fracture of lower end of radius

S59.201   Unspecified physeal fracture of lower end of radius, right arm

S59.202   Unspecified physeal fracture of lower end of radius, left arm

S59.209   Unspecified physeal fracture of lower end of radius, unspecified arm

S59.21   Salter-Harris Type I physeal fracture of lower end of radius

S59.211   Salter-Harris Type I physeal fracture of lower end of radius, right arm

S59.212   Salter-Harris Type I physeal fracture of lower end of radius, left arm

S59.219   Salter-Harris Type I physeal fracture of lower end of radius, unspecified arm

S59.22   Salter-Harris Type II physeal fracture of lower end of radius

S59.221   Salter-Harris Type II physeal fracture of lower end of radius, right arm

S59.222   Salter-Harris Type II physeal fracture of lower end of radius, left arm

S59.229   Salter-Harris Type II physeal fracture of lower end of radius, unspecified arm

S59.23   Salter-Harris Type III physeal fracture of lower end of radius

S59.231   Salter-Harris Type III physeal fracture of lower end of radius, right arm

S59.232   Salter-Harris Type III physeal fracture of lower end of radius, left arm

S59.239   Salter-Harris Type III physeal fracture of lower end of radius, unspecified arm

S59.24   Slater-Harris Type IV physeal fracture of lower end of radius

S59.241   Slater-Harris Type IV physeal fracture of lower end of radius, right arm

S59.242   Slater-Harris Type IV physeal fracture of lower end of radius, left arm

S59.249   Slater-Harris Type IV physeal fracture of lower end of radius, unspecified arm

S59.29   Other physeal fracture of lower end of radius

S59.291   Other physeal fracture of lower end of radius, right arm

S59.292   Other physeal fracture of lower end of radius, left arm

S59.299   Other physeal fracture of lower end of radius, unspecified arm

The following extensions are to be added to each code for subcategories S59.8 and S59.9:
  a   initial encounter
  d   subsequent encounter
  q   sequela

S59.8   Other specified injuries of elbow and forearm

S59.80   Other specified injuries of elbow

S59.801   Other specified injuries of right elbow

S59.802   Other specified injuries of left elbow

S59.809   Other specified injuries of unspecified elbow

S59.81   Other specified injuries of forearm

S59.811   Other specified injuries right forearm

S59.812   Other specified injuries left forearm

S59.819   Other specified injuries unspecified forearm

S59.9   Unspecified injury of elbow and forearm

S59.90   Unspecified injury of elbow

S59.901   Unspecified injury of right elbow

S59.902   Unspecified injury of left elbow

S59.909   Unspecified injury of unspecified elbow

S59.91   Unspecified injury of forearm

S59.911   Unspecified injury of right forearm

S59.912   Unspecified injury of left forearm

S59.919   Unspecified injury of unspecified forearm

INJURIES TO THE WRIST, HAND AND FINGERS (S60–S69)

Excludes2:   burns and corrosions (T20-T32)
              frostbite (T33-T34)
              insect bite or sting, venomous (T63.4)

S60   Superficial injury of wrist, hand and fingers

The following extensions are to be added to each code for category S60:
  a   initial encounter
  d   subsequent encounter
  q   sequela

S60.0   Contusion of finger without damage to nail

Excludes1:   contusion involving nail (matrix) (S60.1)

S60.00   Contusion of unspecified finger without damage to nail
          Contusion of finger(s) NOS

S60.01   Contusion of thumb without damage to nail

S60.011   Contusion of right thumb without damage to nail

S60.012   Contusion of left thumb without damage to nail

S60.019   Contusion of unspecified thumb without damage to nail

S60.02   Contusion of index finger without damage to nail

S60.021   Contusion of right index finger without damage to nail

S60.022   Contusion of left index finger without damage to nail

S60.029   Contusion of unspecified index finger without damage to nail

S60.03   Contusion of middle finger without damage to nail

S60.031   Contusion of right middle finger without damage to nail

S60.032   Contusion of left middle finger without damage to nail

S60.039   Contusion of unspecified middle finger without damage to nail

S60.04   Contusion of ring finger without damage to nail

S60.041   Contusion of right ring finger without damage to nail

S60.042   Contusion of left ring finger without damage to nail

S60.049   Contusion of unspecified ring finger without damage to nail

S60.05   Contusion of little finger without damage to nail

S60.051   Contusion of right little finger without damage to nail

S60.052   Contusion of left little finger without damage to nail

S60.059   Contusion of unspecified little finger without damage to nail

S60.1   Contusion of finger with damage to nail

S60.10   Contusion of unspecified finger with damage to nail

S60.11   Contusion of thumb with damage to nail

S60.111   Contusion of right thumb with damage to nail

S60.112   Contusion of left thumb with damage to nail

S60.119   Contusion of unspecified thumb with damage to nail

S60.12   Contusion of index finger with damage to nail

S60.121   Contusion of right index finger with damage to nail

S60.122   Contusion of left index finger with damage to nail

S60.129   Contusion of unspecified index finger with damage to nail

S60.13   Contusion of middle finger with damage to nail

S60.131   Contusion of right middle finger with damage to nail

S60.132   Contusion of left middle finger with damage to nail

S60.139   Contusion of unspecified middle finger with damage to nail

S60.14   Contusion of ring finger with damage to nail

S60.141   Contusion of right ring finger with damage to nail

S60.142   Contusion of left ring finger with damage to nail

S60.149   Contusion of unspecified ring finger with damage to nail

S60.15   Contusion of little finger with damage to nail

S60.151   Contusion of right little finger with damage to nail

S60.152   Contusion of left little finger with damage to nail

S60.159   Contusion of unspecified little finger with damage to nail

S60.2   Contusion of wrist and hand

Excludes2:   contusion of fingers (S60.0-, S60.1-)

S60.21   Contusion of wrist

S60.211   Contusion of right wrist

S60.212   Contusion of left wrist

S60.219   Contusion of unspecified wrist

S60.22   Contusion of hand

S60.221   Contusion of right hand

S60.222   Contusion of left hand

S60.229   Contusion of unspecified hand

S60.3   Other superficial injuries of thumb

S60.31   Abrasion of thumb

S60.311   Abrasion of right thumb

S60.312   Abrasion of left thumb

S60.319   Abrasion of unspecified thumb

S60.32   Blister (nonthermal) of thumb

S60.321   Blister (nonthermal) of right thumb

S60.322   Blister (nonthermal) of left thumb
S60.329   Blister (nonthermal) of unspecified thumb
S60.34   External constriction of thumb
S60.341   External constriction of right thumb
S60.342   External constriction of left thumb
S60.349   External constriction of unspecified thumb
S60.35   Superficial foreign body of thumb
  Splinter in the thumb
S60.351   Superficial foreign body of right thumb
S60.352   Superficial foreign body of left thumb
S60.359   Superficial foreign body of unspecified thumb
S60.36   Insect bite (nonvenomous) of thumb
S60.361   Insect bite (nonvenomous) of right thumb
S60.362   Insect bite (nonvenomous) of left thumb
S60.369   Insect bite (nonvenomous) of unspecified thumb
S60.37   Other superficial bite of thumb
  Excludes1:   open bite of thumb (S61.05-, S61.15-)
S30.371   Other superficial bite of thumb of right thumb
S30.372   Other superficial bite of thumb of left thumb
S30.379   Other superficial bite of thumb of unspecified thumb
S60.39   Other superficial injuries of thumb
S60.391   Other superficial injuries of right thumb
S60.392   Other superficial injuries of left thumb
S60.399   Other superficial injuries of unspecified thumb
S60.4   Other superficial injuries of other fingers
S60.41   Abrasion of fingers
S60.410   Abrasion of right index finger
S60.411   Abrasion of left index finger
S60.412   Abrasion of right middle finger
S60.413   Abrasion of left middle finger
S60.414   Abrasion of right ring finger
S60.415   Abrasion of left ring finger
S60.416   Abrasion of right little finger
S60.417   Abrasion of left little finger
S60.418   Abrasion of other finger
  Abrasion of specified finger with unspecified laterality
S60.419   Abrasion of unspecified finger
S60.42   Blister (nonthermal) of fingers
S60.420   Blister (nonthermal) of right index finger
S60.421   Blister (nonthermal) of left index finger
S60.422   Blister (nonthermal) of right middle finger
S60.423   Blister (nonthermal) of left middle finger
S60.424   Blister (nonthermal) of right ring finger
S60.425   Blister (nonthermal) of left ring finger
S60.426   Blister (nonthermal) of right little finger
S60.427   Blister (nonthermal) of left little finger
S60.428   Blister (nonthermal) of other finger
  Blister (nonthermal) of specified finger with unspecified laterality
S60.429   Blister (nonthermal) of unspecified finger
S60.44   External constriction of fingers
S60.440   External constriction of right index finger
S60.441   External constriction of left index finger
S60.442   External constriction of right middle finger
S60.443   External constriction of left middle finger
S60.444   External constriction of right ring finger
S60.445   External constriction of left ring finger
S60.446   External constriction of right little finger
S60.447   External constriction of left little finger
S60.448   External constriction of other finger
  External constriction of specified finger with unspecified laterality
S60.449   External constriction of unspecified finger
S60.45   Superficial foreign body of fingers
  Splinter in the finger(s)
S60.450   Superficial foreign body of right index finger

S60.451   Superficial foreign body of left index finger
S60.452   Superficial foreign body of right middle finger
S60.453   Superficial foreign body of left middle finger
S60.454   Superficial foreign body of right ring finger
S60.455   Superficial foreign body of left ring finger
S60.456   Superficial foreign body of right little finger
S60.457   Superficial foreign body of left little finger
S60.458   Superficial foreign body of other finger
  Superficial foreign body of specified finger with unspecified laterality
S60.459   Superficial foreign body of unspecified finger
S60.46   Insect bite (nonvenomous) of fingers
S60.460   Insect bite (nonvenomous) of right index finger
S60.461   Insect bite (nonvenomous) of left index finger
S60.462   Insect bite (nonvenomous) of right middle finger
S60.463   Insect bite (nonvenomous) of left middle finger
S60.464   Insect bite (nonvenomous) of right ring finger
S60.465   Insect bite (nonvenomous) of left ring finger
S60.466   Insect bite (nonvenomous) of right little finger
S60.467   Insect bite (nonvenomous) of left little finger
S60.468   Insect bite (nonvenomous) of other finger
  Insect bite (nonvenomous) of specified finger with unspecified laterality
S60.469   Insect bite (nonvenomous) of unspecified finger
S60.47   Other superficial bite of fingers
  Excludes1:   open bite of fingers (S61.25-, S61.35-)
S60.470   Other superficial bite of right index finger
S60.471   Other superficial bite of left index finger
S60.472   Other superficial bite of right middle finger
S60.473   Other superficial bite of left middle finger
S60.474   Other superficial bite of right ring finger
S60.475   Other superficial bite of left ring finger
S60.476   Other superficial bite of right little finger
S60.477   Other superficial bite of left little finger
S60.478   Other superficial bite of other finger
  Other superficial bite of specified finger with unspecified laterality
S60.479   Other superficial bite of unspecified finger
S60.5   Other superficial injuries of hand
  Excludes2:   superficial injuries of fingers (S60.3-, S60.4-)
S60.51   Abrasion of hand
S60.511   Abrasion of right hand
S60.512   Abrasion of left hand
S60.519   Abrasion of unspecified hand
S60.52   Blister (nonthermal) of hand
S60.521   Blister (nonthermal) of right hand
S60.522   Blister (nonthermal) of left hand
S60.529   Blister (nonthermal) of unspecified hand
S60.54   External constriction of hand
S60.541   External constriction of right hand
S60.542   External constriction of left hand
S60.549   External constriction of unspecified hand
S60.55   Superficial foreign body of hand
  Splinter in the hand
S60.551   Superficial foreign body of right hand
S60.552   Superficial foreign body of left hand
S60.559   Superficial foreign body of unspecified hand
S60.56   Insect bite (nonvenomous) of hand
S60.561   Insect bite (nonvenomous) of right hand
S60.562   Insect bite (nonvenomous) of left hand
S60.569   Insect bite (nonvenomous) of unspecified hand
S60.57   Other superficial bite of hand
  Excludes1:   open bite of hand (S61.45-)
S60.571   Other superficial bite of hand of right hand
S60.572   Other superficial bite of hand of left hand

S60.579   Other superficial bite of hand of unspecified hand

S60.8 Other superficial injuries of wrist

S60.81   Abrasion of wrist
S60.811   Abrasion of right wrist
S60.812   Abrasion of left wrist
S60.819   Abrasion of unspecified wrist

S60.82   Blister (nonthermal) of wrist
S60.821   Blister (nonthermal) of right wrist
S60.822   Blister (nonthermal) of left wrist
S60.829   Blister (nonthermal) of unspecified wrist

S60.84   External constriction of wrist
S60.841   External constriction of right wrist
S60.842   External constriction of left wrist
S60.849   External constriction of unspecified wrist

S60.85   Superficial foreign body of wrist
           Splinter in the wrist
S60.851   Superficial foreign body of right wrist
S60.852   Superficial foreign body of left wrist
S60.859   Superficial foreign body of unspecified wrist

S60.86   Insect bite (nonvenomous) of wrist
S60.861   Insect bite (nonvenomous) of right wrist
S60.862   Insect bite (nonvenomous) of left wrist
S60.869   Insect bite (nonvenomous) of unspecified wrist

S60.87   Other superficial bite of wrist
           Excludes1:   open bite of wrist (S61.55)
S60.871   Other superficial bite of right wrist
S60.872   Other superficial bite of left wrist
S60.879   Other superficial bite of unspecified wrist

S60.9 Unspecified superficial injury of wrist, hand and fingers

S60.91   Unspecified superficial injury of wrist
S60.911   Unspecified superficial injury of right wrist
S60.912   Unspecified superficial injury of left wrist
S60.919   Unspecified superficial injury of unspecified wrist

S60.92   Unspecified superficial injury of hand
S60.921   Unspecified superficial injury of right hand
S60.922   Unspecified superficial injury of left hand
S60.929   Unspecified superficial injury of unspecified hand

S60.93   Unspecified superficial injury of thumb
S60.931   Unspecified superficial injury of right thumb
S60.932   Unspecified superficial injury of left thumb
S60.939   Unspecified superficial injury of unspecified thumb

S60.94   Unspecified superficial injury of other fingers
S60.940   Unspecified superficial injury of right index finger
S60.941   Unspecified superficial injury of left index finger
S60.942   Unspecified superficial injury of right middle finger
S60.943   Unspecified superficial injury of left middle finger
S60.944   Unspecified superficial injury of right ring finger
S60.945   Unspecified superficial injury of left ring finger
S60.946   Unspecified superficial injury of right little finger
S60.947   Unspecified superficial injury of left little finger
S60.948   Unspecified superficial injury of other finger
           Unspecified superficial injury of specified finger with unspecified laterality
S60.949   Unspecified superficial injury of unspecified finger

S61 Open wound of wrist, hand and fingers
     Code also any associated wound infection
     Excludes1:   open fracture of wrist, hand and finger (S62.- with extension b)
                   traumatic amputation of wrist and hand (S68.-)
     The following extensions are to be added to each code for category S61:
     a   initial encounter
     d   subsequent encounter
     q   sequela

S61.0 Open wound of thumb without damage to nail
     Excludes1:   open wound of thumb with damage to nail (S61.1-)

S61.00   Unspecified open wound of thumb without damage to nail
S61.001   Unspecified open wound of right thumb without damage to nail
S61.002   Unspecified open wound of left thumb without damage to nail
S61.009   Unspecified open wound of unspecified thumb without damage to nail

S61.01   Laceration without foreign body of thumb without damage to nail
S61.011   Laceration without foreign body of right thumb without damage to nail
S61.012   Laceration without foreign body of left thumb without damage to nail
S61.019   Laceration without foreign body of unspecified thumb without damage to nail

S61.02   Laceration with foreign body of thumb without damage to nail
S61.021   Laceration with foreign body of right thumb without damage to nail
S61.022   Laceration with foreign body of left thumb without damage to nail
S61.029   Laceration with foreign body of unspecified thumb without damage to nail

S61.03   Puncture wound without foreign body of thumb without damage to nail
S61.031   Puncture wound without foreign body of right thumb without damage to nail
S61.032   Puncture wound without foreign body of left thumb without damage to nail
S61.039   Puncture wound without foreign body of unspecified thumb without damage to nail

S61.04   Puncture wound with foreign body of thumb without damage to nail
S61.041   Puncture wound with foreign body of right thumb without damage to nail
S61.042   Puncture wound with foreign body of left thumb without damage to nail
S61.049   Puncture wound with foreign body of unspecified thumb without damage to nail

S61.05   Open bite of thumb without damage to nail
           Bite of thumb NOS
           Excludes1:   superficial bite of thumb (S60.36-, S60.37-)
S61.051   Open bite of right thumb without damage to nail
S61.052   Open bite of left thumb without damage to nail
S61.059   Open bite of unspecified thumb without damage

S61.1 Open wound of thumb with damage to nail

S61.10   Unspecified open wound of thumb with damage to nail
S61.101   Unspecified open wound of right thumb with damage to nail
S61.102   Unspecified open wound of left thumb with damage to nail
S61.109   Unspecified open wound of unspecified thumb with damage to nail

S61.11   Laceration without foreign body of thumb with damage to nail

   S61.111   Laceration without foreign body of right thumb with damage to nail

   S61.112   Laceration without foreign body of left thumb with damage to nail

   S61.119   Laceration without foreign body of unspecified thumb with damage to nail

S61.12   Laceration with foreign body of thumb with damage to nail

   S61.121   Laceration with foreign body of right thumb with damage to nail

   S61.122   Laceration with foreign body of left thumb with damage to nail

   S61.129   Laceration with foreign body of unspecified thumb with damage to nail

S61.13   Puncture wound without foreign body of thumb with damage to nail

   S61.131   Puncture wound without foreign body of right thumb with damage to nail

   S61.132   Puncture wound without foreign body of left thumb with damage to nail

   S61.139   Puncture wound without foreign body of unspecified thumb with damage to nail

S61.14   Puncture wound with foreign body of thumb with damage to nail

   S61.141   Puncture wound with foreign body of right thumb with damage to nail

   S61.142   Puncture wound with foreign body of left thumb with damage to nail

   S61.149   Puncture wound with foreign body of unspecified thumb with damage to nail

S61.15   Open bite of thumb with damage to nail

   Bite of thumb with damage to nail NOS

   Excludes1:   superficial bite of thumb (S60.36-, S60.37-)

   S61.151   Bite of right thumb with damage to nail

   S61.152   Bite of left thumb with damage to nail

   S61.159   Bite of unspecified thumb with damage to nail

S61.2   Open wound of other finger without damage to nail

   Excludes1:   open wound of finger involving nail (matrix) (S61.3-)

   Excludes2:   open wound of thumb without damage to nail (S61.0-)

S61.20   Unspecified open wound of other finger without damage to nail

   S61.200   Unspecified open wound of right index finger without damage to nail

   S61.201   Unspecified open wound of left index finger without damage to nail

   S61.202   Unspecified open wound of right middle finger without damage to nail

   S61.203   Unspecified open wound of left middle finger without damage to nail

   S61.204   Unspecified open wound of right ring finger without damage to nail

   S61.205   Unspecified open wound of left ring finger without damage to nail

   S61.206   Unspecified open wound of right little finger without damage to nail

   S61.207   Unspecified open wound of left little finger without damage to nail

   S61.208   Unspecified open wound of other finger without damage to nail

     Unspecified open wound of specified finger with unspecified laterality without damage to nail

   S61.209   Unspecified open wound of unspecified finger without damage to nail

S61.21   Laceration without foreign body of finger without damage to nail

S61.210   Laceration without foreign body of right index finger without damage to nail

S61.211   Laceration without foreign body of left index finger without damage to nail

S61.212   Laceration without foreign body of right middle finger without damage to nail

S61.213   Laceration without foreign body of left middle finger without damage to nail

S61.214   Laceration without foreign body of right ring finger without damage to nail

S61.215   Laceration without foreign body of left ring finger without damage to nail

S61.216   Laceration without foreign body of right little finger without damage to nail

S61.217   Laceration without foreign body of left little finger without damage to nail

S61.218   Laceration without foreign body of other finger without damage to nail

   Laceration without foreign body of specified finger with unspecified laterality without damage to nail

S61.219   Laceration without foreign body of unspecified finger without damage to nail

S61.22   Laceration with foreign body of finger without damage to nail

   S61.220   Laceration with foreign body of right index finger without damage to nail

   S61.221   Laceration with foreign body of left index finger without damage to nail

   S61.222   Laceration with foreign body of right middle finger without damage to nail

   S61.223   Laceration with foreign body of left middle finger without damage to nail

   S61.224   Laceration with foreign body of right ring finger without damage to nail

   S61.225   Laceration with foreign body of left ring finger without damage to nail

   S61.226   Laceration with foreign body of right little finger without damage to nail

   S61.227   Laceration with foreign body of left little finger without damage to nail

   S61.228   Laceration with foreign body of other finger without damage to nail

     Laceration with foreign body of specified finger with unspecified laterality without damage to nail

   S61.229   Laceration with foreign body of unspecified finger without damage to nail

S61.23   Puncture wound without foreign body of finger without damage to nail

   S61.230   Puncture wound without foreign body of right index finger without damage to nail

   S61.231   Puncture wound without foreign body of left index finger without damage to nail

   S61.232   Puncture wound without foreign body of right middle finger without damage to nail

   S61.233   Puncture wound without foreign body of left middle finger without damage to nail

   S61.234   Puncture wound without foreign body of right ring finger without damage to nail

   S61.235   Puncture wound without foreign body of left ring finger without damage to nail

   S61.236   Puncture wound without foreign body of right little finger without damage to nail

   S61.237   Puncture wound without foreign body of left little finger without damage to nail

   S61.238   Puncture wound without foreign body of other finger without damage to nail

     Puncture wound without foreign body of specified finger with unspecified laterality without damage to nail

   S61.239   Puncture wound without foreign body of unspecified finger without damage to nail

S61.24   Puncture wound with foreign body of finger without damage to nail

    S61.240   Puncture wound with foreign body of right index finger without damage to nail

    S61.241   Puncture wound with foreign body of left index finger without damage to nail

    S61.242   Puncture wound with foreign body of right middle finger without damage to nail

    S61.243   Puncture wound with foreign body of left middle finger without damage to nail

    S61.244   Puncture wound with foreign body of right ring finger without damage to nail

    S61.245   Puncture wound with foreign body of left ring finger without damage to nail

    S61.246   Puncture wound with foreign body of right little finger without damage to nail

    S61.247   Puncture wound with foreign body of left little finger without damage to nail

    S61.248   Puncture wound with foreign body of other finger without damage to nail
        Puncture wound with foreign body of specified finger with unspecified laterality without damage to nail

    S61.249   Puncture wound with foreign body of unspecified finger without damage to nail

S61.25   Open bite of finger without damage to nail
    Bite of finger without damage to nail NOS
    Excludes1:   superficial bite of finger (S60.46-, S60.47-)

    S61.250   Open bite of right index finger without damage to nail

    S61.251   Open bite of left index finger without damage to nail

    S61.252   Open bite of right middle finger without damage to nail

    S61.253   Open bite of left middle finger without damage to nail

    S61.254   Open bite of right ring finger without damage to nail

    S61.255   Open bite of left ring finger without damage to nail

    S61.256   Open bite of right little finger without damage to nail

    S61.257   Open bite of left little finger without damage to nail

    S61.258   Open bite of other finger without damage to nail
        Open bite of specified finger with unspecified laterality without damage to nail

    S61.259   Open bite of unspecified finger without damage to nail

S61.3   Open wound of other finger with damage to nail

  S61.30   Unspecified open wound of finger with damage to nail

    S61.300   Unspecified open wound of right index finger with damage to nail

    S61.301   Unspecified open wound of left index finger with damage to nail

    S61.302   Unspecified open wound of right middle finger with damage to nail

    S61.303   Unspecified open wound of left middle finger with damage to nail

    S61.304   Unspecified open wound of right ring finger with damage to nail

    S61.305   Unspecified open wound of left ring finger with damage to nail

    S61.306   Unspecified open wound of right little finger with damage to nail

    S61.307   Unspecified open wound of left little finger with damage to nail

    S61.308   Unspecified open wound of other finger with damage to nail
        Unspecified open wound of specified finger with unspecified laterality with damage to nail

    S61.309   Unspecified open wound of unspecified finger with damage to nail

S61.31   Laceration without foreign body of finger with damage to nail

    S61.310   Laceration without foreign body of right index finger with damage to nail

    S61.311   Laceration without foreign body of left index finger with damage to nail

    S61.312   Laceration without foreign body of right middle finger with damage to nail

    S61.313   Laceration without foreign body of left middle finger with damage to nail

    S61.314   Laceration without foreign body of right ring finger with damage to nail

    S61.315   Laceration without foreign body of left ring finger with damage to nail

    S61.316   Laceration without foreign body of right little finger with damage to nail

    S61.317   Laceration without foreign body of left little finger with damage to nail

    S61.318   Laceration without foreign body of other finger with damage to nail
        Laceration without foreign body of specified finger with unspecified laterality with damage to nail

    S61.319   Laceration without foreign body of unspecified finger with damage to nail

S61.32   Laceration with foreign body of finger with damage to nail

    S61.320   Laceration with foreign body of right index finger with damage to nail

    S61.321   Laceration with foreign body of left index finger with damage to nail

    S61.322   Laceration with foreign body of right middle finger with damage to nail

    S61.323   Laceration with foreign body of left middle finger with damage to nail

    S61.324   Laceration with foreign body of right ring finger with damage to nail

    S61.325   Laceration with foreign body of left ring finger with damage to nail

    S61.326   Laceration with foreign body of right little finger with damage to nail

    S61.327   Laceration with foreign body of left little finger with damage to nail

    S61.328   Laceration with foreign body of other finger with damage to nail
        Laceration with foreign body of specified finger with unspecified laterality with damage to nail

    S61.239   Laceration with foreign body of unspecified finger with damage to nail

S61.33   Puncture wound without foreign body of finger with damage to nail

    S61.330   Puncture wound without foreign body of right index finger with damage to nail

    S61.331   Puncture wound without foreign body of left index finger with damage to nail

    S61.332   Puncture wound without foreign body of right middle finger with damage to nail

    S61.333   Puncture wound without foreign body of left middle finger with damage to nail

    S61.334   Puncture wound without foreign body of right ring finger with damage to nail

    S61.335   Puncture wound without foreign body of left ring finger with damage to nail

    S61.336   Puncture wound without foreign body of right little finger with damage to nail

S61.337   Puncture wound without foreign body of left little finger with damage to nail
S61.338   Puncture wound without foreign body of other finger with damage to nail
Puncture wound without foreign body of specified finger with unspecified laterality with damage to nail
S61.339   Puncture wound without foreign body of unspecified finger with damage to nail
S61.34   Puncture wound with foreign body of finger with damage to nail
S61.340   Puncture wound with foreign body of right index finger with damage to nail
S61.341   Puncture wound with foreign body of left index finger with damage to nail
S61.342   Puncture wound with foreign body of right middle finger with damage to nail
S61.343   Puncture wound with foreign body of left middle finger with damage to nail
S61.344   Puncture wound with foreign body of right ring finger with damage to nail
S61.345   Puncture wound with foreign body of left ring finger with damage to nail
S61.346   Puncture wound with foreign body of right little finger with damage to nail
S61.347   Puncture wound with foreign body of left little finger with damage to nail
S61.348   Puncture wound with foreign body of other finger with damage to nail
Puncture wound with foreign body of specified finger with unspecified laterality with damage to nail
S61.349   Puncture wound without foreign body of unspecified finger with damage to nail
S61.35   Open bite of finger with damage to nail
Bite of finger with damage to nail NOS
Excludes1:   superficial bite of finger (S60.46-, S60.47-)
S61.350   Open bite of right index finger with damage to nail
S61.351   Open bite of left index finger with damage to nail
S61.352   Open bite of right middle finger with damage to nail
S61.353   Open bite of left middle finger with damage to nail
S61.354   Open bite of right ring finger with damage to nail
S61.355   Open bite of left ring finger with damage to nail
S61.356   Open bite of right little finger with damage to nail
S61.357   Open bite of left little finger with damage to nail
S61.358   Open bite of other finger with damage to nail
Open bite of specified finger with unspecified laterality with damage to nail
S61.359   Open bite of unspecified finger with damage to nail

S61.4   Open wound of hand
S61.40   Unspecified open wound of hand
S61.401   Unspecified open wound of right hand
S61.402   Unspecified open wound of left hand
S61.409   Unspecified open wound of unspecified hand
S61.41   Laceration without foreign body of hand
S61.411   Laceration without foreign body of right hand
S61.412   Laceration without foreign body of left hand
S61.419   Laceration without foreign body of unspecified hand
S61.42   Laceration with foreign body of hand
S61.421   Laceration with foreign body of right hand
S61.422   Laceration with foreign body of left hand

S61.429   Laceration with foreign body of unspecified hand
S61.43   Puncture wound without foreign body of hand
S61.431   Puncture wound without foreign body of right hand
S61.432   Puncture wound without foreign body of left hand
S61.439   Puncture wound without foreign body of unspecified hand
S61.44   Puncture wound with foreign body of hand
S61.441   Puncture wound with foreign body of right hand
S61.442   Puncture wound with foreign body of left hand
S61.449   Puncture wound with foreign body of unspecified hand
S61.45   Open bite of hand
Bite of hand NOS
Excludes1:   superficial bite of hand (S60.56-, S60.57-)
S61.451   Open bite of right hand
S61.452   Open bite of left hand
S61.459   Open bite of unspecified hand
S61.5   Open wound of wrist
S61.50   Unspecified open wound of wrist
S61.501   Unspecified open wound of right wrist
S61.502   Unspecified open wound of left wrist
S61.509   Unspecified open wound of unspecified wrist
S61.51   Laceration without foreign body of wrist
S61.511   Laceration without foreign body of right wrist
S61.512   Laceration without foreign body of left wrist
S61.519   Laceration without foreign body of unspecified wrist
S61.52   Laceration with foreign body of wrist
S61.521   Laceration with foreign body of right wrist
S61.522   Laceration with foreign body of left wrist
S61.529   Laceration with foreign body of unspecified wrist
S61.53   Puncture wound without foreign body of wrist
S61.531   Puncture wound without foreign body of right wrist
S61.532   Puncture wound without foreign body of left wrist
S61.539   Puncture wound without foreign body of unspecified wrist
S61.54   Puncture wound with foreign body of wrist
S61.541   Puncture wound with foreign body of right wrist
S61.542   Puncture wound with foreign body of left wrist
S61.549   Puncture wound with foreign body of unspecified wrist
S61.55   Open bite of wrist
Bite of wrist NOS
Excludes1:   superficial bite of wrist (S60.86-, S60.87-)
S61.551   Open bite of right wrist
S61.552   Open bite of left wrist
S61.559   Open bite of unspecified wrist

S62   Fracture at wrist and hand level
A fracture not identified as displaced or nondisplaced should be coded to displaced
Excludes1:   traumatic amputation of wrist and hand (S68.-)
Excludes2:   fracture of distal parts of ulna and radius (S52.-)
A fracture not designated as open or closed should be coded to closed

The following extensions are to be added to each code for subcategories S62.0 and S62.1:
- a initial encounter for closed fracture
- b initial encounter for open fracture
- d subsequent encounter for fracture with routine healing
- g subsequent encounter for fracture with delayed healing
- j subsequent encounter for fracture with nonunion
- m subsequent encounter for fracture with malunion
- q sequela

S62.0 Fracture of navicular [scaphoid] bone of wrist

S62.00 Unspecified fracture of navicular [scaphoid] bone of wrist

S62.001 Unspecified fracture of navicular [scaphoid] bone of right wrist

S62.002 Unspecified fracture of navicular [scaphoid] bone of left wrist

S62.009 Unspecified fracture of navicular [scaphoid] bone of unspecified wrist

S62.01 Fracture of distal pole of navicular [scaphoid] bone of wrist
Fracture of volar tuberosity of navicular [scaphoid] bone of wrist

S62.011 Displaced fracture of distal pole of navicular [scaphoid] bone of right wrist

S62.012 Displaced fracture of distal pole of navicular [scaphoid] bone of left wrist

S62.013 Displaced fracture of distal pole of navicular [scaphoid] bone of unspecified wrist

S62.014 Nondisplaced fracture of distal pole of navicular [scaphoid] bone of right wrist

S62.015 Nondisplaced fracture of distal pole of navicular [scaphoid] bone of left wrist

S62.016 Nondisplaced fracture of distal pole of navicular [scaphoid] bone of unspecified wrist

S62.02 Fracture of middle third of navicular [scaphoid] bone of wrist

S62.021 Displaced fracture of middle third of navicular [scaphoid] bone of right wrist

S62.022 Displaced fracture of middle third of navicular [scaphoid] bone of left wrist

S62.023 Displaced fracture of middle third of navicular [scaphoid] bone of unspecified wrist

S62.024 Nondisplaced fracture of middle third of navicular [scaphoid] bone of right wrist

S62.025 Nondisplaced fracture of middle third of navicular [scaphoid] bone of left wrist

S62.026 Nondisplaced fracture of middle third of navicular [scaphoid] bone of unspecified wrist

S62.03 Fracture of proximal third of navicular [scaphoid] bone of wrist

S62.031 Displaced fracture of proximal third of navicular [scaphoid] bone of right wrist

S62.032 Displaced fracture of proximal third of navicular [scaphoid] bone of left wrist

S62.033 Displaced fracture of proximal third of navicular [scaphoid] bone of unspecified wrist

S62.034 Nondisplaced fracture of proximal third of navicular [scaphoid] bone of right wrist

S62.035 Nondisplaced fracture of proximal third of navicular [scaphoid] bone of left wrist

S62.036 Nondisplaced fracture of proximal third of navicular [scaphoid] bone of unspecified wrist

S62.1 Fracture of other and unspecified carpal bone(s)
Excludes2: fracture of scaphoid of wrist (S62.0-)

S62.10 Fracture of unspecified carpal bone
Fracture of wrist NOS

S62.101 Fracture of unspecified carpal bone, right wrist

S62.102 Fracture of unspecified carpal bone, left wrist

S62.109 Fracture of unspecified carpal bone, unspecified wrist

S62.11 Fracture of triquetrum [cuneiform] bone of wrist

S62.111 Displaced fracture of triquetrum [cuneiform] bone, right wrist

S62.112 Displaced fracture of triquetrum [cuneiform] bone, left wrist

S62.113 Displaced fracture of triquetrum [cuneiform] bone, unspecified wrist

S62.114 Nondisplaced fracture of triquetrum [cuneiform] bone, right wrist

S62.115 Nondisplaced fracture of triquetrum [cuneiform] bone, left wrist

S62.116 Nondisplaced fracture of triquetrum [cuneiform] bone, unspecified wrist

S62.12 Fracture of lunate [semilunar]

S62.121 Displaced fracture of lunate [semilunar], right wrist

S62.122 Displaced fracture of lunate [semilunar], left wrist

S62.123 Displaced fracture of lunate [semilunar], unspecified wrist

S62.124 Nondisplaced fracture of lunate [semilunar], right wrist

S62.125 Nondisplaced fracture of lunate [semilunar], left wrist

S62.126 Nondisplaced fracture of lunate [semilunar], unspecified wrist

S62.13 Fracture of capitate [os magnum] bone

S62.131 Displaced fracture of capitate [os magnum] bone, right wrist

S62.132 Displaced fracture of capitate [os magnum] bone, left wrist

S62.133 Displaced fracture of capitate [os magnum] bone, unspecified wrist

S62.134 Nondisplaced fracture of capitate [os magnum] bone, right wrist

S62.135 Nondisplaced fracture of capitate [os magnum] bone, left wrist

S62.136 Nondisplaced fracture of capitate [os magnum] bone, unspecified wrist

S62.14 Fracture of body of hamate [unciform] bone
Fracture of hamate [unciform] bone NOS

S62.141 Displaced fracture of body of hamate [unciform] bone, right wrist

S62.142 Displaced fracture of body of hamate [unciform] bone, left wrist

S62.143 Displaced fracture of body of hamate [unciform] bone, unspecified wrist

S62.144 Nondisplaced fracture of body of hamate [unciform] bone, right wrist

S62.145 Nondisplaced fracture of body of hamate [unciform] bone, left wrist

S62.146 Nondisplaced fracture of body of hamate [unciform] bone, unspecified wrist

S62.15 Fracture of hook process of hamate [unciform] bone
Fracture of unciform process of hamate [unciform] bone

S62.151 Displaced fracture of hook process of hamate [unciform] bone, right wrist

S62.152 Displaced fracture of hook process of hamate [unciform] bone, left wrist

S62.153 Displaced fracture of hook process of hamate [unciform] bone, unspecified wrist

S62.154 Nondisplaced fracture of hook process of hamate [unciform] bone, right wrist

S62.155 Nondisplaced fracture of hook process of hamate [unciform] bone, left wrist

S62.156 Nondisplaced fracture of hook process of hamate [unciform] bone, unspecified wrist

S62.16 Fracture of pisiform

S62.161 Displaced fracture of pisiform, right wrist

S62.162 Displaced fracture of pisiform, left wrist

S62.163 Displaced fracture of pisiform, unspecified wrist

S62.164   Nondisplaced fracture of pisiform, right wrist

S62.165   Nondisplaced fracture of pisiform, left wrist

S62.166   Nondisplaced fracture of pisiform, unspecified wrist

S62.17   Fracture of trapezium [larger multangular]

S62.171   Displaced fracture of trapezium [larger multangular], right wrist

S62.172   Displaced fracture of trapezium [larger multangular], left wrist

S62.173   Displaced fracture of trapezium [larger multangular], unspecified wrist

S62.174   Nondisplaced fracture of trapezium [larger multangular], right wrist

S62.175   Nondisplaced fracture of trapezium [larger multangular], left wrist

S62.176   Nondisplaced fracture of trapezium [larger multangular], unspecified wrist

S62.18   Fracture of trapezoid [smaller multangular]

S62.181   Displaced fracture of trapezoid [smaller multangular], right wrist

S62.182   Displaced fracture of trapezoid [smaller multangular], left wrist

S62.183   Displaced fracture of trapezoid [smaller multangular], unspecified wrist

S62.184   Nondisplaced fracture of trapezoid [smaller multangular], right wrist

S62.185   Nondisplaced fracture of trapezoid [smaller multangular], left wrist

S62.186   Nondisplaced fracture of trapezoid [smaller multangular], unspecified wrist

The following extensions are to be added to each code for subcategories S62.2, S62.3, S62.5, and S62.6

A fracture not designated as open or closed should be coded to closed

Note: the open fracture designations are based on the Gustilo open fracture classification

a   initial encounter for closed fracture
b   initial encounter for open fracture type I or II
c   initial encounter for open fracture type IIIA, IIIB, or IIIC
d   subsequent encounter for fracture with routine healing
g   subsequent encounter for fracture with delayed healing
j   subsequent encounter for fracture with nonunion
m   subsequent encounter for fracture with malunion
q   sequela

S62.2   Fracture of first metacarpal bone

S62.20   Unspecified fracture of first metacarpal bone

S62.201   Unspecified fracture of first metacarpal bone, right hand

S62.202   Unspecified fracture of first metacarpal bone, left hand

S62.209   Unspecified fracture of first metacarpal bone, unspecified hand

S62.21   Bennett's fracture

S62.211   Bennett's fracture, right hand

S62.212   Bennett's fracture, left hand

S62.213   Bennett's fracture, unspecified hand

S62.22   Rolando's fracture

S62.221   Displaced Rolando's fracture, right hand

S62.222   Displaced Rolando's fracture, left hand

S62.223   Displaced Rolando's fracture, unspecified hand

S62.224   Nondisplaced Rolando's fracture, right hand

S62.225   Nondisplaced Rolando's fracture, left hand

S62.226   Nondisplaced Rolando's fracture, unspecified hand

S62.23   Other fracture of base of first metacarpal bone

S62.231   Other displaced fracture of base of first metacarpal bone, right hand

S62.232   Other displaced fracture of base of first metacarpal bone, left hand

S62.233   Other displaced fracture of base of first metacarpal bone, unspecified hand

S62.234   Other nondisplaced fracture of base of first metacarpal bone, right hand

S62.235   Other nondisplaced fracture of base of first metacarpal bone, left hand

S62.236   Other nondisplaced fracture of base of first metacarpal bone, unspecified hand

S62.24   Fracture of shaft of first metacarpal bone

S62.241   Displaced fracture of shaft of first metacarpal bone, right hand

S62.242   Displaced fracture of shaft of first metacarpal bone, left hand

S62.243   Displaced fracture of shaft of first metacarpal bone, unspecified hand

S62.244   Nondisplaced fracture of shaft of first metacarpal bone, right hand

S62.245   Nondisplaced fracture of shaft of first metacarpal bone, left hand

S62.246   Nondisplaced fracture of shaft of first metacarpal bone, unspecified hand

S62.25   Fracture of neck of first metacarpal bone

S62.251   Displaced fracture of neck of first metacarpal bone, right hand

S62.252   Displaced fracture of neck of first metacarpal bone, left hand

S62.253   Displaced fracture of neck of first metacarpal bone, unspecified hand

S62.254   Nondisplaced fracture of neck of first metacarpal bone, right hand

S62.255   Nondisplaced fracture of neck of first metacarpal bone, left hand

S62.256   Nondisplaced fracture of neck of first metacarpal bone, unspecified hand

S62.29   Other fracture of first metacarpal bone

S62.291   Other fracture of first metacarpal bone, right hand

S62.292   Other fracture of first metacarpal bone, left hand

S62.299   Other fracture of first metacarpal bone, unspecified hand

S62.3   Fracture of other and unspecified metacarpal bone

Excludes2:   fracture of first metacarpal bone (S62.2-)

S62.30   Unspecified fracture of other metacarpal bone

S62.300   Unspecified fracture of second metacarpal bone, right hand

S62.301   Unspecified fracture of second metacarpal bone, left hand

S62.302   Unspecified fracture of third metacarpal bone, right hand

S62.303   Unspecified fracture of third metacarpal bone, left hand

S62.304   Unspecified fracture of fourth metacarpal bone, right hand

S62.305   Unspecified fracture of fourth metacarpal bone, left hand

S62.306   Unspecified fracture of fifth metacarpal bone, right hand

S62.307   Unspecified fracture of fifth metacarpal bone, left hand

S62.308   Unspecified fracture of other metacarpal bone
Unspecified fracture of specified metacarpal bone with unspecified laterality

S62.309   Unspecified fracture of unspecified metacarpal bone

S62.31   Displaced fracture of base of other metacarpal bone

S62.310   Displaced fracture of base of second metacarpal bone, right hand

S62.311   Displaced fracture of base of second metacarpal bone, left hand

S62.312   Displaced fracture of base of third metacarpal bone, right hand

S62.313   Displaced fracture of base of third metacarpal bone, left hand

S62.314   Displaced fracture of base of fourth metacarpal bone, right hand

S62.315 Displaced fracture of base of fourth metacarpal bone, left hand

S62.316 Displaced fracture of base of fifth metacarpal bone, right hand

S62.317 Displaced fracture of base of fifth metacarpal bone, left hand

S62.318 Displaced fracture of base of other metacarpal bone
  Displaced fracture of base of specified metacarpal bone with unspecified laterality

S62.319 Displaced fracture of base of unspecified metacarpal bone

S62.32 Displaced fracture of shaft of other metacarpal bone

S62.320 Displaced fracture of shaft of second metacarpal bone, right hand

S62.321 Displaced fracture of shaft of second metacarpal bone, left hand

S62.322 Displaced fracture of shaft of third metacarpal bone, right hand

S62.323 Displaced fracture of shaft of third metacarpal bone, left hand

S62.324 Displaced fracture of shaft of fourth metacarpal bone, right hand

S62.325 Displaced fracture of shaft of fourth metacarpal bone, left hand

S62.326 Displaced fracture of shaft of fifth metacarpal bone, right hand

S62.327 Displaced fracture of shaft of fifth metacarpal bone, left hand

S62.328 Displaced fracture of shaft of other metacarpal bone
  Displaced fracture of shaft of specified metacarpal bone with unspecified laterality

S62.329 Displaced fracture of shaft of unspecified metacarpal bone

S62.33 Displaced fracture of neck of other metacarpal bone

S62.330 Displaced fracture of neck of second metacarpal bone, right hand

S62.331 Displaced fracture of neck of second metacarpal bone, left hand

S62.332 Displaced fracture of neck of third metacarpal bone, right hand

S62.333 Displaced fracture of neck of third metacarpal bone, left hand

S62.334 Displaced fracture of neck of fourth metacarpal bone, right hand

S62.335 Displaced fracture of neck of fourth metacarpal bone, left hand

S62.336 Displaced fracture of neck of fifth metacarpal bone, right hand

S62.337 Displaced fracture of neck of fifth metacarpal bone, left hand

S62.338 Displaced fracture of neck of other metacarpal bone
  Displaced fracture of neck of specified metacarpal bone with unspecified laterality

S62.339 Displaced fracture of neck of unspecified metacarpal bone

S62.34 Nondisplaced fracture of base of other metacarpal bone

S62.340 Nondisplaced fracture of base of second metacarpal bone, right hand

S62.341 Nondisplaced fracture of base of second metacarpal bone, left hand

S62.342 Nondisplaced fracture of base of third metacarpal bone, right hand

S62.343 Nondisplaced fracture of base of third metacarpal bone, left hand

S62.344 Nondisplaced fracture of base of fourth metacarpal bone, right hand

S62.345 Nondisplaced fracture of base of fourth metacarpal bone, left hand

S62.346 Nondisplaced fracture of base of fifth metacarpal bone, right hand

S62.347 Nondisplaced fracture of base of fifth metacarpal bone, left hand

S62.348 Nondisplaced fracture of base of other metacarpal bone
  Nondisplaced fracture of base of specified metacarpal bone with unspecified laterality

S62.349 Nondisplaced fracture of base of unspecified metacarpal bone

S62.35 Nondisplaced fracture of shaft of other metacarpal bone

S62.350 Nondisplaced fracture of shaft of second metacarpal bone, right hand

S62.351 Nondisplaced fracture of shaft of second metacarpal bone, left hand

S62.352 Nondisplaced fracture of shaft of third metacarpal bone, right hand

S62.353 Nondisplaced fracture of shaft of third metacarpal bone, left hand

S62.354 Nondisplaced fracture of shaft of fourth metacarpal bone, right hand

S62.355 Nondisplaced fracture of shaft of fourth metacarpal bone, left hand

S62.356 Nondisplaced fracture of shaft of fifth metacarpal bone, right hand

S62.357 Nondisplaced fracture of shaft of fifth metacarpal bone, left hand

S62.358 Nondisplaced fracture of shaft of other metacarpal bone
  Nondisplaced fracture of shaft of specified metacarpal bone with unspecified laterality

S62.359 Nondisplaced fracture of shaft of unspecified metacarpal bone

S62.36 Nondisplaced fracture of neck of other metacarpal bone

S62.360 Nondisplaced fracture of neck of second metacarpal bone, right hand

S62.361 Nondisplaced fracture of neck of second metacarpal bone, left hand

S62.362 Nondisplaced fracture of neck of third metacarpal bone, right hand

S62.363 Nondisplaced fracture of neck of third metacarpal bone, left hand

S62.364 Nondisplaced fracture of neck of fourth metacarpal bone, right hand

S62.365 Nondisplaced fracture of neck of fourth metacarpal bone, left hand

S62.366 Nondisplaced fracture of neck of fifth metacarpal bone, right hand

S62.367 Nondisplaced fracture of neck of fifth metacarpal bone, left hand

S62.368 Nondisplaced fracture of neck of other metacarpal bone
  Nondisplaced fracture of neck of specified metacarpal bone with unspecified laterality

S62.369 Nondisplaced fracture of neck of unspecified metacarpal bone

S62.39 Other fracture of other metacarpal bone

S62.390 Other fracture of second metacarpal bone, right hand

S62.391 Other fracture of second metacarpal bone, left hand

S62.392 Other fracture of third metacarpal bone, right hand

S62.393 Other fracture of third metacarpal bone, left hand

S62.394   Other fracture of fourth metacarpal bone, right hand

S62.395   Other fracture of fourth metacarpal bone, left hand

S62.396   Other fracture of fifth metacarpal bone, right hand

S62.397   Other fracture of fifth metacarpal bone, left hand

S62.398   Other fracture of other metacarpal bone
　　　　　Other fracture of specified metacarpal bone with unspecified laterality

S62.399   Other fracture of unspecified metacarpal bone

S62.5   Fracture of thumb

S62.50   Fracture of unspecified phalanx of thumb

S62.501   Fracture of unspecified phalanx of right thumb

S62.502   Fracture of unspecified phalanx of left thumb

S62.509   Fracture of unspecified phalanx of unspecified thumb

S62.51   Fracture of proximal phalanx of thumb

S62.511   Displaced fracture of proximal phalanx of right thumb

S62.512   Displaced fracture of proximal phalanx of left thumb

S62.513   Displaced fracture of proximal phalanx of unspecified thumb

S62.514   Nondisplaced fracture of proximal phalanx of right thumb

S62.515   Nondisplaced fracture of proximal phalanx of left thumb

S62.516   Nondisplaced fracture of proximal phalanx of unspecified thumb

S62.52   Fracture of distal phalanx of thumb

S62.521   Displaced fracture of distal phalanx of right thumb

S62.522   Displaced fracture of distal phalanx of left thumb

S62.523   Displaced fracture of distal phalanx of unspecified thumb

S62.524   Nondisplaced fracture of distal phalanx of right thumb

S62.525   Nondisplaced fracture of distal phalanx of left thumb

S62.526   Nondisplaced fracture of distal phalanx of unspecified thumb

S62.6   Fracture of other and unspecified finger(s)

Excludes2:   fracture of thumb (S62.5-)

S62.60   Fracture of unspecified phalanx of finger

S62.600   Fracture of unspecified phalanx of right index finger

S62.601   Fracture of unspecified phalanx of left index finger

S62.602   Fracture of unspecified phalanx of right middle finger

S62.603   Fracture of unspecified phalanx of left middle finger

S62.604   Fracture of unspecified phalanx of right ring finger

S62.605   Fracture of unspecified phalanx of left ring finger

S62.606   Fracture of unspecified phalanx of right little finger

S62.607   Fracture of unspecified phalanx of left little finger

S62.608   Fracture of unspecified phalanx of other finger
　　　　　Fracture of unspecified phalanx of specified finger with unspecified laterality

S62.609   Fracture of unspecified phalanx of unspecified finger

S62.61   Displaced fracture of proximal phalanx of finger

S62.610   Displaced fracture of proximal phalanx of right index finger

S62.611   Displaced fracture of proximal phalanx of left index finger

S62.612   Displaced fracture of proximal phalanx of right middle finger

S62.613   Displaced fracture of proximal phalanx of left middle finger

S62.614   Displaced fracture of proximal phalanx of right ring finger

S62.615   Displaced fracture of proximal phalanx of left ring finger

S62.616   Displaced fracture of proximal phalanx of right little finger

S62.617   Displaced fracture of proximal phalanx of left little finger

S62.618   Displaced fracture of proximal phalanx of other finger
　　　　　Displaced fracture of proximal phalanx of specified finger with unspecified laterality

S62.619   Displaced fracture of proximal phalanx of unspecified finger

S62.62   Displaced fracture of middle phalanx of finger

S62.620   Displaced fracture of middle phalanx of right index finger

S62.621   Displaced fracture of middle phalanx of left index finger

S62.622   Displaced fracture of middle phalanx of right middle finger

S62.623   Displaced fracture of middle phalanx of left middle finger

S62.624   Displaced fracture of middle phalanx of right ring finger

S62.625   Displaced fracture of middle phalanx of left ring finger

S62.626   Displaced fracture of middle phalanx of right little finger

S62.627   Displaced fracture of middle phalanx of left little finger

S62.628   Displaced fracture of middle phalanx of other finger
　　　　　Displaced fracture of middle phalanx of specified finger with unspecified laterality

S62.629   Displaced fracture of middle phalanx of unspecified finger

S62.63   Displaced fracture of distal phalanx of finger

S62.630   Displaced fracture of distal phalanx of right index finger

S62.631   Displaced fracture of distal phalanx of left index finger

S62.632   Displaced fracture of distal phalanx of right middle finger

S62.633   Displaced fracture of distal phalanx of left middle finger

S62.634   Displaced fracture of distal phalanx of right ring finger

S62.635   Displaced fracture of distal phalanx of left ring finger

S62.636   Displaced fracture of distal phalanx of right little finger

S62.637   Displaced fracture of distal phalanx of left little finger

S62.638   Displaced fracture of distal phalanx of other finger
　　　　　Displaced fracture of distal phalanx of specified finger with unspecified laterality

S62.639   Displaced fracture of distal phalanx of unspecified finger

S62.64   Nondisplaced fracture of proximal phalanx of finger

S62.640   Nondisplaced fracture of proximal phalanx of right index finger

S62.641   Nondisplaced fracture of proximal phalanx of left index finger

S62.642   Nondisplaced fracture of proximal phalanx of right middle finger

S62.643   Nondisplaced fracture of proximal phalanx of left middle finger

S62.644   Nondisplaced fracture of proximal phalanx of right ring finger

S62.645   Nondisplaced fracture of proximal phalanx of left ring finger

S62.646   Nondisplaced fracture of proximal phalanx of right little finger

S62.647   Nondisplaced fracture of proximal phalanx of left little finger

S62.648   Nondisplaced fracture of proximal phalanx of other finger

     Nondisplaced fracture of proximal phalanx of specified finger with unspecified laterality

S62.649   Nondisplaced fracture of proximal phalanx of unspecified finger

S62.65   Nondisplaced fracture of middle phalanx of finger

S62.650   Nondisplaced fracture of middle phalanx of right index finger

S62.651   Nondisplaced fracture of middle phalanx of left index finger

S62.652   Nondisplaced fracture of middle phalanx of right middle finger

S62.653   Nondisplaced fracture of middle phalanx of left middle finger

S62.654   Nondisplaced fracture of middle phalanx of right ring finger

S62.655   Nondisplaced fracture of middle phalanx of left ring finger

S62.656   Nondisplaced fracture of middle phalanx of right little finger

S62.657   Nondisplaced fracture of middle phalanx of left little finger

S62.658   Nondisplaced fracture of middle phalanx of other finger

     Nondisplaced fracture of middle phalanx of specified finger with unspecified laterality

S62.659   Nondisplaced fracture of middle phalanx of unspecified finger

S62.66   Nondisplaced fracture of distal phalanx of finger

S62.660   Nondisplaced fracture of distal phalanx of right index finger

S62.661   Nondisplaced fracture of distal phalanx of left index finger

S62.662   Nondisplaced fracture of distal phalanx of right middle finger

S62.663   Nondisplaced fracture of distal phalanx of left middle finger

S62.664   Nondisplaced fracture of distal phalanx of right ring finger

S62.665   Nondisplaced fracture of distal phalanx of left ring finger

S62.666   Nondisplaced fracture of distal phalanx of right little finger

S62.667   Nondisplaced fracture of distal phalanx of left little finger

S62.668   Nondisplaced fracture of distal phalanx of other finger

     Nondisplaced fracture of distal phalanx of specified finger with unspecified laterality

S62.669   Nondisplaced fracture of distal phalanx of unspecified finger

A fracture not designated as open or closed should be coded to closed
The following extensions are to be added to each code for subcategory S62.9:
   a   initial encounter for closed fracture
   b   initial encounter for open fracture
   d   subsequent encounter for fracture with routine healing
   g   subsequent encounter for fracture with delayed healing
   j   subsequent encounter for fracture with nonunion
   m   subsequent encounter for fracture with malunion
   q   sequela

S62.9   Unspecified fracture of wrist and hand

S62.90   Unspecified fracture of unspecified wrist and hand

S62.91   Unspecified fracture of right wrist and hand

S62.92   Unspecified fracture of left wrist and hand

S63   Dislocation and sprain of joints and ligaments at wrist and hand level

Includes: avulsion of joint or ligament at wrist and hand level
laceration of joint or ligament at wrist and hand level
sprain of joint or ligament at wrist and hand level
traumatic hemarthrosis of joint or ligament at wrist and hand level
traumatic rupture of joint or ligament at wrist and hand level
traumatic subluxation of joint or ligament at wrist and hand level
traumatic tear of joint or ligament at wrist and hand level

Excludes2:   strain of muscle and tendon of wrist and hand (S66.-)

The following extensions are to be added to each code for category S63:
   a   initial encounter
   d   subsequent encounter
   q   sequela

S63.0   Subluxation and dislocation of wrist and hand joints

S63.00   Unspecified subluxation and dislocation of wrist and hand

     Dislocation of carpal bone NOS
     Dislocation of distal end of radius NOS
     Subluxation of carpal bone NOS
     Subluxation of distal end of radius NOS

S63.001   Unspecified subluxation of right wrist and hand

S63.002   Unspecified subluxation of left wrist and hand

S63.003   Unspecified subluxation of unspecified wrist and hand

S63.004   Unspecified dislocation of right wrist and hand

S63.005   Unspecified dislocation of left wrist and hand

S63.006   Unspecified dislocation of unspecified wrist and hand

S63.01   Subluxation and dislocation of distal radioulnar joint

S63.011   Subluxation of distal radioulnar joint of right wrist

S63.012   Subluxation of distal radioulnar joint of left wrist

S63.013   Subluxation of distal radioulnar joint of unspecified wrist

S63.014   Dislocation of distal radioulnar joint of right wrist

S63.015   Dislocation of distal radioulnar joint of left wrist

S63.016   Dislocation of distal radioulnar joint of unspecified wrist

S63.02   Subluxation and dislocation of radiocarpal joint

S63.021   Subluxation of radiocarpal joint of right wrist

S63.022   Subluxation of radiocarpal joint of left wrist

S63.023   Subluxation of radiocarpal joint of unspecified wrist

S63.024   Dislocation of radiocarpal joint of right wrist

S63.025   Dislocation of radiocarpal joint of left wrist

S63.026   Dislocation of radiocarpal joint of unspecified wrist

S63.03   Subluxation and dislocation of midcarpal joint

S63.031   Subluxation of midcarpal joint of right wrist

S63.032   Subluxation of midcarpal joint of left wrist

S63.033   Subluxation of midcarpal joint of unspecified wrist

S63.034   Dislocation of midcarpal joint of right wrist

S63.035   Dislocation of midcarpal joint of left wrist

S63.036   Dislocation of midcarpal joint of unspecified wrist

S63.04   Subluxation and dislocation of carpometacarpal joint of thumb

Excludes2:   interphalangeal subluxation and dislocation of thumb (S63.1-)

S63.041   Subluxation of carpometacarpal joint of right thumb

S63.042   Subluxation of carpometacarpal joint of left thumb

S63.043   Subluxation of carpometacarpal joint of unspecified thumb

S63.044   Dislocation of carpometacarpal joint of right thumb

S63.045   Dislocation of carpometacarpal joint of left thumb

S63.046   Dislocation of carpometacarpal joint of unspecified thumb

S63.05   Subluxation and dislocation of other carpometacarpal joint

Excludes2:   subluxation and dislocation of carpometacarpal joint of thumb (S63.04-)

S63.051   Subluxation of other carpometacarpal joint of right hand

S63.052   Subluxation of other carpometacarpal joint of left hand

S63.053   Subluxation of other carpometacarpal joint of unspecified hand

S63.054   Dislocation of other carpometacarpal joint of right hand

S63.055   Dislocation of other carpometacarpal joint of left hand

S63.056   Dislocation of other carpometacarpal joint of unspecified hand

S63.06   Subluxation and dislocation of metacarpal (bone), proximal end

S63.061   Subluxation of metacarpal (bone), proximal end of right hand

S63.062   Subluxation of metacarpal (bone), proximal end of left hand

S63.063   Subluxation of metacarpal (bone), proximal end of unspecified hand

S63.064   Dislocation of metacarpal (bone), proximal end of right hand

S63.065   Dislocation of metacarpal (bone), proximal end of left hand

S63.066   Dislocation of metacarpal (bone), proximal end of unspecified hand

S63.07   Subluxation and dislocation of distal end of ulna

S63.071   Subluxation of distal end of right ulna

S63.072   Subluxation of distal end of left ulna

S63.073   Subluxation of distal end of unspecified ulna

S63.074   Dislocation of distal end of right ulna

S63.075   Dislocation of distal end of left ulna

S63.076   Dislocation of distal end of unspecified ulna

S63.09   Other subluxation and dislocation of wrist and hand

S63.091   Other subluxation of right wrist and hand

S63.092   Other subluxation of left wrist and hand

S63.093   Other subluxation of unspecified wrist and hand

S63.094   Other dislocation of right wrist and hand

S63.095   Other dislocation of left wrist and hand

S63.096   Other dislocation of unspecified wrist and hand

S63.1   Subluxation and dislocation of thumb

S63.10   Unspecified subluxation and dislocation of thumb

S63.101   Unspecified subluxation of right thumb

S63.102   Unspecified subluxation of left thumb

S63.103   Unspecified subluxation of unspecified thumb

S63.104   Unspecified dislocation of right thumb

S63.105   Unspecified dislocation of left thumb

S63.106   Unspecified dislocation of unspecified thumb

S63.11   Subluxation and dislocation of metacarpophalangeal joint of thumb

S63.111   Subluxation of metacarpophalangeal joint of right thumb

S63.112   Subluxation of metacarpophalangeal joint of left thumb

S63.113   Subluxation of metacarpophalangeal joint of unspecified thumb

S63.114   Dislocation of metacarpophalangeal joint of right thumb

S63.115   Dislocation of metacarpophalangeal joint of left thumb

S63.116   Dislocation of metacarpophalangeal joint of unspecified thumb

S63.12   Subluxation and dislocation of unspecified interphalangeal joint of thumb

S63.121   Subluxation of unspecified interphalangeal joint of right thumb

S63.122   Subluxation of unspecified interphalangeal joint of left thumb

S63.123   Subluxation of unspecified interphalangeal joint of unspecified thumb

S63.124   Dislocation of unspecified interphalangeal joint of right thumb

S63.125   Dislocation of unspecified interphalangeal joint of left thumb

S63.126   Dislocation of unspecified interphalangeal joint of unspecified thumb

S63.13   Subluxation and dislocation of proximal interphalangeal joint of thumb

S63.131   Subluxation of proximal interphalangeal joint of right thumb

S63.132   Subluxation of proximal interphalangeal joint of left thumb

S63.133   Subluxation of proximal interphalangeal joint of unspecified thumb

S63.134   Dislocation of proximal interphalangeal joint of right thumb

S63.135   Dislocation of proximal interphalangeal joint of left thumb

S63.136   Dislocation of proximal interphalangeal joint of unspecified thumb

S63.14   Subluxation and dislocation of distal interphalangeal joint of thumb

S63.141   Subluxation of distal interphalangeal joint of right thumb

S63.142   Subluxation of distal interphalangeal joint of left thumb

S63.143   Subluxation of distal interphalangeal joint of unspecified thumb

S63.144   Dislocation of distal interphalangeal joint of right thumb

S63.145   Dislocation of distal interphalangeal joint of left thumb

S63.146   Dislocation of distal interphalangeal joint of unspecified thumb

S63.2   Subluxation and dislocation of other finger(s)

Excludes2:   subluxation and dislocation of thumb (S63.1-)

S63.20   Unspecified subluxation of other finger

S63.200   Unspecified subluxation of right index finger

S63.201   Unspecified subluxation of left index finger

S63.202   Unspecified subluxation of right middle finger

S63.203   Unspecified subluxation of left middle finger

S63.204   Unspecified subluxation of right ring finger

S63.205   Unspecified subluxation of left ring finger

S63.206   Unspecified subluxation of right little finger

S63.207   Unspecified subluxation of left little finger

S63.208   Unspecified subluxation of other finger
Unspecified subluxation of specified finger with unspecified laterality

S63.209   Unspecified subluxation of unspecified finger

S63.21   Subluxation of metacarpophalangeal joint of finger
    S63.210   Subluxation of metacarpophalangeal joint of right index finger
    S63.211   Subluxation of metacarpophalangeal joint of left index finger
    S63.212   Subluxation of metacarpophalangeal joint of right middle finger
    S63.213   Subluxation of metacarpophalangeal joint of left middle finger
    S63.214   Subluxation of metacarpophalangeal joint of right ring finger
    S63.215   Subluxation of metacarpophalangeal joint of left ring finger
    S63.216   Subluxation of metacarpophalangeal joint of right little finger
    S63.217   Subluxation of metacarpophalangeal joint of left little finger
    S63.218   Subluxation of metacarpophalangeal joint of other finger
        Subluxation of metacarpophalangeal joint of specified finger with unspecified laterality
    S63.219   Subluxation of metacarpophalangeal joint of unspecified finger
S63.22   Subluxation of unspecified interphalangeal joint of finger
    S63.220   Subluxation of unspecified interphalangeal joint of right index finger
    S63.221   Subluxation of unspecified interphalangeal joint of left index finger
    S63.222   Subluxation of unspecified interphalangeal joint of right middle finger
    S63.223   Subluxation of unspecified interphalangeal joint of left middle finger
    S63.224   Subluxation of unspecified interphalangeal joint of right ring finger
    S63.225   Subluxation of unspecified interphalangeal joint of left ring finger
    S63.226   Subluxation of unspecified interphalangeal joint of right little finger
    S63.227   Subluxation of unspecified interphalangeal joint of left little finger
    S63.228   Subluxation of unspecified interphalangeal joint of other finger
        Subluxation of unspecified interphalangeal joint of specified finger with unspecified laterality
    S63.229   Subluxation of unspecified interphalangeal joint of unspecified finger
S63.23   Subluxation of proximal interphalangeal joint of finger
    S63.230   Subluxation of proximal interphalangeal joint of right index finger
    S63.231   Subluxation of proximal interphalangeal joint of left index finger
    S63.232   Subluxation of proximal interphalangeal joint of right middle finger
    S63.233   Subluxation of proximal interphalangeal joint of left middle finger
    S63.234   Subluxation of proximal interphalangeal joint of right ring finger
    S63.235   Subluxation of proximal interphalangeal joint of left ring finger
    S63.236   Subluxation of proximal interphalangeal joint of right little finger
    S63.237   Subluxation of proximal interphalangeal joint of left little finger
    S63.238   Subluxation of proximal interphalangeal joint of other finger
        Subluxation of proximal interphalangeal joint of specified finger with unspecified laterality
    S63.239   Subluxation of proximal interphalangeal joint of other finger

S63.24   Subluxation of distal interphalangeal joint of finger
    S63.240   Subluxation of distal interphalangeal joint of right index finger
    S63.241   Subluxation of distal interphalangeal joint of left index finger
    S63.242   Subluxation of distal interphalangeal joint of right middle finger
    S63.243   Subluxation of distal interphalangeal joint of left middle finger
    S63.244   Subluxation of distal interphalangeal joint of right ring finger
    S63.245   Subluxation of distal interphalangeal joint of left ring finger
    S63.246   Subluxation of distal interphalangeal joint of right little finger
    S63.247   Subluxation of distal interphalangeal joint of left little finger
    S63.248   Subluxation of distal interphalangeal joint of other finger
        Subluxation of distal interphalangeal joint of specified finger with unspecified laterality
    S63.249   Subluxation of distal interphalangeal joint of other finger
S63.25   Unspecified dislocation of other finger
    S63.250   Unspecified dislocation of right index finger
    S63.251   Unspecified dislocation of left index finger
    S63.252   Unspecified dislocation of right middle finger
    S63.253   Unspecified dislocation of left middle finger
    S63.254   Unspecified dislocation of right ring finger
    S63.255   Unspecified dislocation of left ring finger
    S63.256   Unspecified dislocation of right little finger
    S63.257   Unspecified dislocation of left little finger
    S63.258   Unspecified dislocation of other finger
        Unspecified dislocation of specified finger with unspecified laterality
    S63.259   Unspecified dislocation of other finger
        Unspecified dislocation of specified finger with unspecified laterality
S63.26   Dislocation of metacarpophalangeal joint of finger
    S63.260   Dislocation of metacarpophalangeal joint of right index finger
    S63.261   Dislocation of metacarpophalangeal joint of left index finger
    S63.262   Dislocation of metacarpophalangeal joint of right middle finger
    S63.263   Dislocation of metacarpophalangeal joint of left middle finger
    S63.264   Dislocation of metacarpophalangeal joint of right ring finger
    S63.265   Dislocation of metacarpophalangeal joint of left ring finger
    S63.266   Dislocation of metacarpophalangeal joint of right little finger
    S63.267   Dislocation of metacarpophalangeal joint of left little finger
    S63.268   Dislocation of metacarpophalangeal joint of other finger
        Dislocation of metacarpophalangeal joint of specified finger with unspecified laterality
    S63.269   Dislocation of metacarpophalangeal joint of other finger
S63.27   Dislocation of unspecified interphalangeal joint of finger
    S63.270   Dislocation of unspecified interphalangeal joint of right index finger
    S63.271   Dislocation of unspecified interphalangeal joint of left index finger
    S63.272   Dislocation of unspecified interphalangeal joint of right middle finger
    S63.273   Dislocation of unspecified interphalangeal joint of left middle finger

S63.274 Dislocation of unspecified interphalangeal joint of right ring finger

S63.275 Dislocation of unspecified interphalangeal joint of left ring finger

S63.276 Dislocation of unspecified interphalangeal joint of right little finger

S63.277 Dislocation of unspecified interphalangeal joint of left little finger

S63.278 Dislocation of unspecified interphalangeal joint of other finger
  Dislocation of unspecified interphalangeal joint of specified finger with unspecified laterality

S63.279 Dislocation of unspecified interphalangeal joint of other finger
  Dislocation of unspecified interphalangeal joint of specified finger without specified laterality

S63.28 Dislocation of proximal interphalangeal joint of finger

S63.280 Dislocation of proximal interphalangeal joint of right index finger

S63.281 Dislocation of proximal interphalangeal joint of left index finger

S63.282 Dislocation of proximal interphalangeal joint of right middle finger

S63.283 Dislocation of proximal interphalangeal joint of left middle finger

S63.284 Dislocation of proximal interphalangeal joint of right ring finger

S63.285 Dislocation of proximal interphalangeal joint of left ring finger

S63.286 Dislocation of proximal interphalangeal joint of right little finger

S63.287 Dislocation of proximal interphalangeal joint of left little finger

S63.288 Dislocation of proximal interphalangeal joint of other finger
  Dislocation of proximal interphalangeal joint of specified finger with unspecified laterality

S63.289 Dislocation of proximal interphalangeal joint of unspecified finger

S63.29 Dislocation of distal interphalangeal joint of finger

S63.290 Dislocation of distal interphalangeal joint of right index finger

S63.291 Dislocation of distal interphalangeal joint of left index finger

S63.292 Dislocation of distal interphalangeal joint of right middle finger

S63.293 Dislocation of distal interphalangeal joint of left middle finger

S63.294 Dislocation of distal interphalangeal joint of right ring finger

S63.295 Dislocation of distal interphalangeal joint of left ring finger

S63.296 Dislocation of distal interphalangeal joint of right little finger

S63.297 Dislocation of distal interphalangeal joint of left little finger

S63.298 Dislocation of distal interphalangeal joint of other finger
  Dislocation of distal interphalangeal joint of specified finger with unspecified laterality

S63.299 Dislocation of distal interphalangeal joint of other finger

S63.3 Traumatic rupture of ligament of wrist

S63.30 Traumatic rupture of unspecified ligament of wrist

S63.301 Traumatic rupture of unspecified ligament of right wrist

S63.302 Traumatic rupture of unspecified ligament of left wrist

S63.309 Traumatic rupture of unspecified ligament of unspecified wrist

S63.31 Traumatic rupture of collateral ligament of wrist

S63.311 Traumatic rupture of collateral ligament of right wrist

S63.312 Traumatic rupture of collateral ligament of left wrist

S63.319 Traumatic rupture of collateral ligament of unspecified wrist

S63.32 Traumatic rupture of radiocarpal ligament

S63.321 Traumatic rupture of right radiocarpal ligament

S63.322 Traumatic rupture of left radiocarpal ligament

S63.329 Traumatic rupture of unspecified radiocarpal ligament

S63.33 Traumatic rupture of ulnocarpal (palmar) ligament

S63.331 Traumatic rupture of right ulnocarpal (palmar) ligament

S63.332 Traumatic rupture of left ulnocarpal (palmar) ligament

S63.339 Traumatic rupture of unspecified ulnocarpal (palmar) ligament

S63.39 Traumatic rupture of other ligament of wrist

S63.391 Traumatic rupture of other ligament of right wrist

S63.392 Traumatic rupture of other ligament of left wrist

S63.399 Traumatic rupture of other ligament of unspecified wrist

S63.4 Traumatic rupture of ligament of finger at metacarpophalangeal and interphalangeal joint(s)

S63.40 Traumatic rupture of unspecified ligament of finger at metacarpophalangeal and interphalangeal joint

S63.400 Traumatic rupture of unspecified ligament of right index finger at metacarpophalangeal and interphalangeal joint

S63.401 Traumatic rupture of unspecified ligament of left index finger at metacarpophalangeal and interphalangeal joint

S63.402 Traumatic rupture of unspecified ligament of right middle finger at metacarpophalangeal and interphalangeal joint

S63.403 Traumatic rupture of unspecified ligament of left middle finger at metacarpophalangeal and interphalangeal joint

S63.404 Traumatic rupture of unspecified ligament of right ring finger at metacarpophalangeal and interphalangeal joint

S63.405 Traumatic rupture of unspecified ligament of left ring finger at metacarpophalangeal and interphalangeal joint

S63.406 Traumatic rupture of unspecified ligament of right little finger at metacarpophalangeal and interphalangeal joint

S63.407 Traumatic rupture of unspecified ligament of left little finger at metacarpophalangeal and interphalangeal joint

S63.408 Traumatic rupture of unspecified ligament of other finger at metacarpophalangeal and interphalangeal joint
  Traumatic rupture of unspecified ligament of specified finger with unspecified laterality at metacarpophalangeal and interphalangeal joint

S63.409 Traumatic rupture of unspecified ligament of unspecified finger at metacarpophalangeal and interphalangeal joint

S63.41 Traumatic rupture of collateral ligament of finger at metacarpophalangeal and interphalangeal joint

S63.410 Traumatic rupture of collateral ligament of right index finger at metacarpophalangeal and interphalangeal joint

S63.411 Traumatic rupture of collateral ligament of left index finger at metacarpophalangeal and interphalangeal joint

S63.412 Traumatic rupture of collateral ligament of right middle finger at metacarpophalangeal and interphalangeal joint

S63.413 Traumatic rupture of collateral ligament of left middle finger at metacarpophalangeal and interphalangeal joint

S63.414 Traumatic rupture of collateral ligament of right ring finger at metacarpophalangeal and interphalangeal joint

S63.415 Traumatic rupture of collateral ligament of left ring finger at metacarpophalangeal and interphalangeal joint

S63.416 Traumatic rupture of collateral ligament of right little finger at metacarpophalangeal and interphalangeal joint

S63.417 Traumatic rupture of collateral ligament of left little finger at metacarpophalangeal and interphalangeal joint

S63.418 Traumatic rupture of collateral ligament of other finger at metacarpophalangeal and interphalangeal joint
Traumatic rupture of collateral ligament of specified finger with unspecified laterality at metacarpophalangeal and interphalangeal joint

S63.419 Traumatic rupture of collateral ligament of unspecified finger at metacarpophalangeal and interphalangeal joint

S63.42 Traumatic rupture of palmar ligament of finger at metacarpophalangeal and interphalangeal joint

S63.420 Traumatic rupture of palmar ligament of right index finger at metacarpophalangeal and interphalangeal joint

S63.421 Traumatic rupture of palmar ligament of left index finger at metacarpophalangeal and interphalangeal joint

S63.422 Traumatic rupture of palmar ligament of right middle finger at metacarpophalangeal and interphalangeal joint

S63.423 Traumatic rupture of palmar ligament of left middle finger at metacarpophalangeal and interphalangeal joint

S63.424 Traumatic rupture of palmar ligament of right ring finger at metacarpophalangeal and interphalangeal joint

S63.425 Traumatic rupture of palmar ligament of left ring finger at metacarpophalangeal and interphalangeal joint

S63.426 Traumatic rupture of palmar ligament of right little finger at metacarpophalangeal and interphalangeal joint

S63.427 Traumatic rupture of palmar ligament of left little finger at metacarpophalangeal and interphalangeal joint

S63.428 Traumatic rupture of palmar ligament of other finger at metacarpophalangeal and interphalangeal joint
Traumatic rupture of palmar ligament of specified finger with unspecified laterality at metacarpophalangeal and interphalangeal joint

S63.429 Traumatic rupture of palmar ligament of unspecified finger at metacarpophalangeal and interphalangeal joint

S63.43 Traumatic rupture of volar plate of finger at metacarpophalangeal and interphalangeal joint

S63.430 Traumatic rupture of volar plate of right index finger at metacarpophalangeal and interphalangeal joint

S63.431 Traumatic rupture of volar plate of left index finger at metacarpophalangeal and interphalangeal joint

S63.432 Traumatic rupture of volar plate of right middle finger at metacarpophalangeal and interphalangeal joint

S63.433 Traumatic rupture of volar plate of left middle finger at metacarpophalangeal and interphalangeal joint

S63.434 Traumatic rupture of volar plate of right ring finger at metacarpophalangeal and interphalangeal joint

S63.435 Traumatic rupture of volar plate of left ring finger at metacarpophalangeal and interphalangeal joint

S63.436 Traumatic rupture of volar plate of right little finger at metacarpophalangeal and interphalangeal joint

S63.437 Traumatic rupture of volar plate of left little finger at metacarpophalangeal and interphalangeal joint

S63.438 Traumatic rupture of volar plate of other finger at metacarpophalangeal and interphalangeal joint
Traumatic rupture of volar plate of specified finger with unspecified laterality at metacarpophalangeal and interphalangeal joint

S63.439 Traumatic rupture of volar plate of unspecified finger at metacarpophalangeal and interphalangeal joint

S63.49 Traumatic rupture of other ligament of finger at metacarpophalangeal and interphalangeal joint

S63.490 Traumatic rupture of other ligament of right index finger at metacarpophalangeal and interphalangeal joint

S63.491 Traumatic rupture of other ligament of left index finger at metacarpophalangeal and interphalangeal joint

S63.492 Traumatic rupture of other ligament of right middle finger at metacarpophalangeal and interphalangeal joint

S63.493 Traumatic rupture of other ligament of left middle finger at metacarpophalangeal and interphalangeal joint

S63.494 Traumatic rupture of other ligament of right ring finger at metacarpophalangeal and interphalangeal joint

S63.495 Traumatic rupture of other ligament of left ring finger at metacarpophalangeal and interphalangeal joint

S63.496 Traumatic rupture of other ligament of right little finger at metacarpophalangeal and interphalangeal joint

S63.497 Traumatic rupture of other ligament of left little finger at metacarpophalangeal and interphalangeal joint

S63.498 Traumatic rupture of other ligament of other finger at metacarpophalangeal and interphalangeal joint
Traumatic rupture of ligament of specified finger with unspecified laterality at metacarpophalangeal and interphalangeal joint

S63.499 Traumatic rupture of other ligament of unspecified finger at metacarpophalangeal and interphalangeal joint

S63.5 Other and unspecified sprain of wrist

S63.50 Unspecified sprain of wrist

S63.501 Unspecified sprain of right wrist

S63.502 Unspecified sprain of left wrist

S63.509 Unspecified sprain of unspecified wrist

S63.51 Sprain of carpal (joint)

S63.511 Sprain of carpal joint of right wrist

S63.512 Sprain of carpal joint of left wrist

S63.519 Sprain of carpal joint of unspecified wrist

S63.52 Sprain of radiocarpal joint
Excludes1: traumatic rupture of radiocarpal ligament (S63.32-)

S63.521   Sprain of radiocarpal joint of right wrist
S63.522   Sprain of radiocarpal joint of left wrist
S63.529   Sprain of radiocarpal joint of unspecified wrist
S63.59   Other sprain of wrist
S63.591   Other sprain of right wrist
S63.592   Other sprain of left wrist
S63.599   Other sprain of wrist of unspecified side
S63.6   Other and unspecified sprain of finger(s)
Excludes1:   traumatic rupture of ligament of finger at metacarpophalangeal and interphalangeal joint(s) (S63.4-)
S63.60   Unspecified sprain of thumb
S63.601   Unspecified sprain of right thumb
S63.602   Unspecified sprain of left thumb
S63.609   Unspecified sprain of unspecified thumb
S63.61   Unspecified sprain of other and unspecified finger(s)
S63.610   Unspecified sprain of right index finger
S63.611   Unspecified sprain of left index finger
S63.612   Unspecified sprain of right middle finger
S63.613   Unspecified sprain of left middle finger
S63.614   Unspecified sprain of right ring finger
S63.615   Unspecified sprain of left ring finger
S63.616   Unspecified sprain of right little finger
S63.617   Unspecified sprain of left little finger
S63.618   Unspecified sprain of other finger
Unspecified sprain of specified finger with unspecified laterality
S63.619   Unspecified sprain of unspecified finger
S63.62   Sprain of interphalangeal joint of thumb
S63.621   Sprain of interphalangeal joint of right thumb
S63.622   Sprain of interphalangeal joint of left thumb
S63.629   Sprain of interphalangeal joint of unspecified thumb
S63.63   Sprain of interphalangeal joint of other and unspecified finger(s)
S63.630   Sprain of interphalangeal joint of right index finger
S63.631   Sprain of interphalangeal joint of left index finger
S63.632   Sprain of interphalangeal joint of right middle finger
S63.633   Sprain of interphalangeal joint of left middle finger
S63.634   Sprain of interphalangeal joint of right ring finger
S63.635   Sprain of interphalangeal joint of left ring finger
S63.636   Sprain of interphalangeal joint of right little finger
S63.637   Sprain of interphalangeal joint of left little finger
S63.638   Sprain of interphalangeal joint of other finger
S63.639   Sprain of interphalangeal joint of unspecified finger
S63.64   Sprain of metacarpophalangeal joint of thumb
S63.641   Sprain of metacarpophalangeal joint of right thumb
S63.642   Sprain of metacarpophalangeal joint of left thumb
S63.649   Sprain of metacarpophalangeal joint of unspecified thumb
S63.65   Sprain of metacarpophalangeal joint of other and unspecified finger(s)
S63.650   Sprain of metacarpophalangeal joint of right index finger
S63.651   Sprain of metacarpophalangeal joint of left index finger
S63.652   Sprain of metacarpophalangeal joint of right middle finger
S63.653   Sprain of metacarpophalangeal joint of left middle finger

S63.654   Sprain of metacarpophalangeal joint of right ring finger
S63.655   Sprain of metacarpophalangeal joint of left ring finger
S63.656   Sprain of metacarpophalangeal joint of right little finger
S63.657   Sprain of metacarpophalangeal joint of left little finger
S63.658   Sprain of metacarpophalangeal joint of other finger
Sprain of metacarpophalangeal joint of specified finger with unspecified laterality
S63.659   Sprain of metacarpophalangeal joint of unspecified finger
S63.68   Other sprain of thumb
S63.681   Other sprain of right thumb
S63.682   Other sprain of left thumb
S63.689   Other sprain of unspecified thumb
S63.69   Other sprain of other and unspecified finger(s)
S63.620   Other sprain of right index finger
S63.621   Other sprain of left index finger
S63.622   Other sprain of right middle finger
S63.623   Other sprain of left middle finger
S63.624   Other sprain of right ring finger
S63.625   Other sprain of left ring finger
S63.626   Other sprain of right little finger
S63.627   Other sprain of left little finger
S63.628   Other sprain of finger of other finger
Other sprain of specified finger with unspecified laterality
S63.629   Other sprain of unspecified finger
S63.8   Sprain of other part of wrist and hand
S63.8x   Sprain of other part of wrist and hand
S63.8x1   Sprain of other part of right wrist and hand
S63.8x2   Sprain of other part of left wrist and hand
S63.8x9   Sprain of other part of unspecified wrist and hand
S63.9   Sprain of unspecified part of wrist and hand
S63.90   Sprain of unspecified part of unspecified wrist and hand
S63.91   Sprain of unspecified part of right wrist and hand
S63.92   Sprain of unspecified part of left wrist and hand
S64 Injury of nerves at wrist and hand level
Code also any associated open wound (S61.-)
The following extensions are to be added to each code for category S64:
a   initial encounter
d   subsequent encounter
q   sequela
S64.0   Injury of ulnar nerve at wrist and hand level
S64.00   Injury of ulnar nerve at wrist and hand level of unspecified arm
S64.01   Injury of ulnar nerve at wrist and hand level of right arm
S64.02   Injury of ulnar nerve at wrist and hand level of left arm
S64.1   Injury of median nerve at wrist and hand level
S64.10   Injury of median nerve at wrist and hand level of unspecified arm
S64.11   Injury of median nerve at wrist and hand level of right arm
S64.12   Injury of median nerve at wrist and hand level of left arm
S64.2   Injury of radial nerve at wrist and hand level
S64.20   Injury of radial nerve at wrist and hand level of unspecified arm
S64.21   Injury of radial nerve at wrist and hand level of right arm
S64.22   Injury of radial nerve at wrist and hand level of left arm

S64.3   Injury of digital nerve of thumb
    S64.30   Injury of digital nerve unspecified thumb
    S64.31   Injury of digital nerve right thumb
    S64.32   Injury of digital nerve of left thumb
S64.4   Injury of digital nerve of other and unspecified finger
    S64.40   Injury of digital nerve of unspecified finger
    S64.49   Injury of digital nerve of other finger
       S64.490   Injury of digital nerve of right index finger
       S64.491   Injury of digital nerve of left index finger
       S64.492   Injury of digital nerve of right middle finger
       S64.493   Injury of digital nerve of left middle finger
       S64.494   Injury of digital nerve of right ring finger
       S64.495   Injury of digital nerve of left ring finger
       S64.496   Injury of digital nerve of right little finger
       S64.497   Injury of digital nerve of left little finger
       S64.498   Injury of digital nerve of other finger
          Injury of digital nerve of specified finger with unspecified laterality
S64.8   Injury of other nerves at wrist and hand level
    S64.8x   Injury of other nerves at wrist and hand level
       S64.8x1   Injury of other nerves at wrist and hand level of right arm
       S64.8x2   Injury of other nerves at wrist and hand level of left arm
       S64.8x9   Injury of other nerves at wrist and hand level of unspecified arm
S64.9   Injury of unspecified nerve at wrist and hand level
    S64.90   Injury of unspecified nerve at wrist and hand level of unspecified arm
    S64.91   Injury of unspecified nerve at wrist and hand level of right arm
    S64.92   Injury of unspecified nerve at wrist and hand level of left arm

S65   Injury of blood vessels at wrist and hand level
    Code also any associated open wound (S61.-)
    The following extensions are to be added to each code for category S65:
      a   initial encounter
      d   subsequent encounter
      q   sequela
S65.0   Injury of ulnar artery at wrist and hand level
    S65.00   Unspecified injury of ulnar artery at wrist and hand level
       S65.001   Unspecified injury of ulnar artery at wrist and hand level of right arm
       S65.002   Unspecified injury of ulnar artery at wrist and hand level of left arm
       S65.009   Unspecified injury of ulnar artery at wrist and hand level of unspecified arm
    S65.01   Laceration of ulnar artery at wrist and hand level
       S65.011   Laceration of ulnar artery at wrist and hand level of right arm
       S65.012   Laceration of ulnar artery at wrist and hand level of left arm
       S65.019   Laceration of ulnar artery at wrist and hand level of unspecified arm
    S65.09   Other specified injury of ulnar artery at wrist and hand level
       S65.091   Other specified injury of ulnar artery at wrist and hand level of right arm
       S65.092   Other specified injury of ulnar artery at wrist and hand level of left arm
       S65.099   Other specified injury of ulnar artery at wrist and hand level of unspecified arm
S65.1   Injury of radial artery at wrist and hand level
    S65.10   Unspecified injury of radial artery at wrist and hand level
       S65.101   Unspecified injury of radial artery at wrist and hand level of right arm
       S65.102   Unspecified injury of radial artery at wrist and hand level of left arm

S65.109   Unspecified injury of radial artery at wrist and hand level of unspecified arm
    S65.11   Laceration of radial artery at wrist and hand level
       S65.111   Laceration of radial artery at wrist and hand level of right arm
       S65.112   Laceration of radial artery at wrist and hand level of left arm
       S65.119   Laceration of radial artery at wrist and hand level of unspecified arm
    S65.19   Other specified injury of radial artery at wrist and hand level
       S65.191   Other specified injury of radial artery at wrist and hand level of right arm
       S65.192   Other specified injury of radial artery at wrist and hand level of left arm
       S65.199   Other specified injury of radial artery at wrist and hand level of unspecified arm
S65.2   Injury of superficial palmar arch
    S65.20   Unspecified injury of superficial palmar arch
       S65.201   Unspecified injury of superficial palmar arch of right hand
       S65.202   Unspecified injury of superficial palmar arch of left hand
       S65.209   Unspecified injury of superficial palmar arch of unspecified hand
    S65.21   Laceration of superficial palmar arch
       S65.211   Laceration of superficial palmar arch of right hand
       S65.212   Laceration of superficial palmar arch of left hand
       S65.219   Laceration of superficial palmar arch of unspecified hand
    S65.29   Other specified injury of superficial palmar arch
       S65.291   Other specified injury of superficial palmar arch of right hand
       S65.292   Other specified injury of superficial palmar arch of left hand
       S65.299   Other specified injury of superficial palmar arch of unspecified hand
S65.3   Injury of deep palmar arch
    S65.30   Unspecified injury of deep palmar arch
       S65.301   Unspecified injury of deep palmar arch of right hand
       S65.302   Unspecified injury of deep palmar arch of left hand
       S65.309   Unspecified injury of deep palmar arch of unspecified hand
    S65.31   Laceration of deep palmar arch
       S65.311   Laceration of deep palmar arch of right hand
       S65.312   Laceration of deep palmar arch of left hand
       S65.319   Laceration of deep palmar arch of unspecified hand
    S65.39   Other specified injury of deep palmar arch
       S65.391   Other specified injury of deep palmar arch of right hand
       S65.392   Other specified injury of deep palmar arch of left hand
       S65.399   Other specified injury of deep palmar arch of unspecified hand
S65.4   Injury of blood vessel of thumb
    S65.40   Unspecified injury of blood vessel of thumb
       S65.401   Unspecified injury of blood vessel of right thumb
       S65.402   Unspecified injury of blood vessel of left thumb
       S65.409   Unspecified injury of blood vessel of unspecified thumb
    S65.41   Laceration of blood vessel of thumb
       S65.411   Laceration of blood vessel of right thumb
       S65.412   Laceration of blood vessel of left thumb

S65.419   Laceration of blood vessel of unspecified thumb

S65.49   Other specified injury of blood vessel of thumb

S65.491   Other specified injury of blood vessel of right thumb

S65.492   Other specified injury of blood vessel of left thumb

S65.499   Other specified injury of blood vessel of unspecified thumb

S65.5   Injury of blood vessel of other and unspecified finger

S65.50   Unspecified injury of blood vessel of other and unspecified finger

S65.500   Unspecified injury of blood vessel of right index finger

S65.501   Unspecified injury of blood vessel of left index finger

S65.502   Unspecified injury of blood vessel of right middle finger

S65.503   Unspecified injury of blood vessel of left middle finger

S65.504   Unspecified injury of blood vessel of right ring finger

S65.505   Unspecified injury of blood vessel of left ring finger

S65.506   Unspecified injury of blood vessel of right little finger

S65.507   Unspecified injury of blood vessel of left little finger

S65.508   Unspecified injury of blood vessel of other finger
    Unspecified injury of blood vessel of specified finger with unspecified laterality

S65.509   Unspecified injury of finger of unspecified finger

S65.51   Laceration of blood vessel of other and unspecified finger

S65.510   Laceration of blood vessel of right index finger

S65.511   Laceration of blood vessel of left index finger

S65.512   Laceration of blood vessel of right middle finger

S65.513   Laceration of blood vessel of left middle finger

S65.514   Laceration of blood vessel of right ring finger

S65.515   Laceration of blood vessel of left ring finger

S65.516   Laceration of blood vessel of right little finger

S65.517   Laceration of blood vessel of left little finger

S65.518   Laceration of blood vessel of other finger
    Laceration of blood vessel of specified finger with unspecified laterality

S65.519   Laceration of blood vessel of finger of unspecified finger

S65.59   Other specified injury of blood vessel of other and unspecified finger

S65.590   Other specified injury of blood vessel of right index finger

S65.591   Other specified injury of blood vessel of left index finger

S65.592   Other specified injury of blood vessel of right middle finger

S65.593   Other specified injury of blood vessel of left middle finger

S65.594   Other specified injury of blood vessel of right ring finger

S65.595   Other specified injury of blood vessel of left ring finger

S65.596   Other specified injury of blood vessel of right little finger

S65.597   Other specified injury of blood vessel of left little finger

S65.598   Other specified injury of blood vessel of other finger
    Other specified injury of blood vessel of specified finger with unspecified laterality

S65.599   Other specified injury of blood vessel of finger of unspecified finger

S65.8   Injury of other blood vessels at wrist and hand level

S65.80   Unspecified injury of other blood vessels at wrist and hand level

S65.801   Unspecified injury of other blood vessels at wrist and hand level of right arm

S65.802   Unspecified injury of other blood vessels at wrist and hand level of left arm

S65.809   Unspecified injury of other blood vessels at wrist and hand level of unspecified arm

S65.81   Laceration of other blood vessels at wrist and hand level

S65.811   Laceration of other blood vessels at wrist and hand level of right arm

S65.812   Laceration of other blood vessels at wrist and hand level of left arm

S65.819   Laceration of other blood vessels at wrist and hand level of unspecified arm

S65.89   Other specified injury of other blood vessels at wrist and hand level

S65.891   Other specified injury of other blood vessels at wrist and hand level of right arm

S65.892   Other specified injury of other blood vessels at wrist and hand level of left arm

S65.899   Other specified injury of other blood vessels at wrist and hand level of unspecified arm

S65.9   Injury of unspecified blood vessel at wrist and hand level

S65.90   Unspecified injury of unspecified blood vessel at wrist and hand level

S65.901   Unspecified injury of unspecified blood vessel at wrist and hand level of right arm

S65.902   Unspecified injury of unspecified blood vessel at wrist and hand level of left arm

S65.909   Unspecified injury of unspecified blood vessel at wrist and hand level of unspecified arm

S65.91   Laceration of unspecified blood vessel at wrist and hand level

S65.911   Laceration of unspecified blood vessel at wrist and hand level of right arm

S65.912   Laceration of unspecified blood vessel at wrist and hand level of left arm

S65.919   Laceration of unspecified blood vessel at wrist and hand level of unspecified arm

S65.99   Other specified injury of unspecified blood vessel at wrist and hand level

S65.991   Other specified injury of unspecified blood vessel at wrist and hand of right arm

S65.992   Other specified injury of unspecified blood vessel at wrist and hand of left arm

S65.999   Other specified injury of unspecified blood vessel at wrist and hand of unspecified arm

S66   Injury of muscle and tendon at wrist and hand level
   Code also any associated open wound (S61.-)
   Excludes2:   sprain of joints and ligaments of wrist and hand (S63.-)
   The following extensions are to be added to each code for category S66:
     a   initial encounter
     d   subsequent encounter
     q   sequela

S66.0   Injury of long flexor muscle and tendon of thumb at wrist and hand level

S66.00   Unspecified injury of long flexor muscle and tendon of thumb at wrist and hand level

S66.001   Unspecified injury of long flexor muscle and tendon of right thumb at wrist and hand level

S66.002   Unspecified injury of long flexor muscle and tendon of left thumb at wrist and hand level

S66.009   Unspecified injury of long flexor muscle and tendon of thumb at wrist and hand level of unspecified side

S66.01   Strain of long flexor muscle and tendon of thumb at wrist and hand level

    S66.011   Strain of long flexor muscle and tendon of right thumb at wrist and hand level

    S66.012   Strain of long flexor muscle and tendon of left thumb at wrist and hand level

    S66.019   Strain of long flexor muscle and tendon of thumb at wrist and hand level of unspecified side

S66.02   Laceration of long flexor muscle and tendon of thumb at wrist and hand level

    S66.021   Laceration of long flexor muscle and tendon of right thumb at wrist and hand level

    S66.022   Laceration of long flexor muscle and tendon of left thumb at wrist and hand level

    S66.029   Laceration of long flexor muscle and tendon of thumb at wrist and hand level of unspecified side

S66.09   Other injury of long flexor muscle and tendon of thumb at wrist and hand level

    S66.091   Other injury of long flexor muscle and tendon of right thumb at wrist and hand level

    S66.092   Other injury of long flexor muscle and tendon of left thumb at wrist and hand level

    S66.099   Other injury of long flexor muscle and tendon of thumb at wrist and hand level of unspecified side

S66.1   Injury of flexor muscle and tendon of other and unspecified finger at wrist and hand level

    Excludes2:   injury of long flexor muscle and tendon of thumb at wrist and hand level (S66.0-)

S66.10   Unspecified injury of flexor muscle and tendon of other and unspecified finger at wrist and hand level

    S66.100   Unspecified injury of flexor muscle and tendon of right index finger at wrist and hand level

    S66.101   Unspecified injury of flexor muscle and tendon of left index finger at wrist and hand level

    S66.102   Unspecified injury of flexor muscle and tendon of right middle finger at wrist and hand level

    S66.103   Unspecified injury of flexor muscle and tendon of left middle finger at wrist and hand level

    S66.104   Unspecified injury of flexor muscle and tendon of right ring finger at wrist and hand level

    S66.105   Unspecified injury of flexor muscle and tendon of left ring finger at wrist and hand level

    S66.106   Unspecified injury of flexor muscle and tendon of right little finger at wrist and hand level

    S66.107   Unspecified injury of flexor muscle and tendon of left little finger at wrist and hand level

    S66.108   Unspecified injury of flexor muscle and tendon of other finger at wrist and hand level

        Unspecified injury of flexor muscle and tendon of specified finger with unspecified laterality at wrist and hand level

    S66.109   Unspecified injury of flexor muscle and tendon of unspecified finger at wrist and hand level

S66.11   Strain of flexor muscle and tendon of other and unspecified finger at wrist and hand level

    S66.110   Strain of flexor muscle and tendon of right index finger at wrist and hand level

    S66.111   Strain of flexor muscle and tendon of left index finger at wrist and hand level

    S66.112   Strain of flexor muscle and tendon of right middle finger at wrist and hand level

    S66.113   Strain of flexor muscle and tendon of left middle finger at wrist and hand level

    S66.114   Strain of flexor muscle and tendon of right ring finger at wrist and hand level

    S66.115   Strain of flexor muscle and tendon of left ring finger at wrist and hand level

    S66.116   Strain of flexor muscle and tendon of right little finger at wrist and hand level

    S66.117   Strain of flexor muscle and tendon of left little finger at wrist and hand level

    S66.118   Strain of flexor muscle and tendon of other finger at wrist and hand level

        Strain of flexor muscle and tendon of specified finger with unspecified laterality at wrist and hand level

    S66.119   Strain of flexor muscle and tendon of unspecified finger at wrist and hand level

S66.12   Laceration of flexor muscle and tendon of other and unspecified finger at wrist and hand level

    S66.120   Laceration of flexor muscle and tendon of right index finger at wrist and hand level

    S66.121   Laceration of flexor muscle and tendon of left index finger at wrist and hand level

    S66.122   Laceration of flexor muscle and tendon of right middle finger at wrist and hand level

    S66.123   Laceration of flexor muscle and tendon of left middle finger at wrist and hand level

    S66.124   Laceration of flexor muscle and tendon of right ring finger at wrist and hand level

    S66.125   Laceration of flexor muscle and tendon of left ring finger at wrist and hand level

    S66.126   Laceration of flexor muscle and tendon of right little finger at wrist and hand level

    S66.127   Laceration of flexor muscle and tendon of left little finger at wrist and hand level

    S66.128   Laceration of flexor muscle and tendon of other finger at wrist and hand level

        Laceration of flexor muscle and tendon of specified finger with unspecified laterality at wrist and hand level

    S66.129   Laceration of flexor muscle and tendon of unspecified finger at wrist and hand level

S66.19   Other injury of flexor muscle and tendon of other and unspecified finger at wrist and hand level

    S66.190   Other injury of flexor muscle and tendon of right index at wrist and hand level

    S66.191   Other injury of flexor muscle and tendon of left index finger at wrist and hand level

    S66.192   Other injury of flexor muscle and tendon of right middle finger at wrist and hand level

    S66.193   Other injury of flexor muscle and tendon of left middle finger at wrist and hand level

    S66.194   Other injury of flexor muscle and tendon of right ring finger at wrist and hand level

    S66.195   Other injury of flexor muscle and tendon of left ring finger at wrist and hand level

    S66.196   Other injury of flexor muscle and tendon of right little finger at wrist and hand level

    S66.197   Other injury of flexor muscle and tendon of left little finger at wrist and hand level

    S66.198   Other injury of flexor muscle and tendon of other finger at wrist and hand level

        Other injury of flexor muscle and tendon of specified finger with unspecified laterality at wrist and hand level

    S66.199   Other injury of flexor muscle and tendon of finger at wrist and hand level of unspecified finger

S66.2   Injury of extensor muscle and tendon of thumb at wrist and hand level

S66.20   Unspecified injury of extensor muscle and tendon of thumb at wrist and hand level

    S66.201   Unspecified injury of extensor muscle and tendon of right thumb at wrist and hand level

    S66.202   Unspecified injury of extensor muscle and tendon of left thumb at wrist and hand level

    S66.209   Unspecified injury of extensor muscle and tendon of thumb at wrist and hand level of unspecified side

S66.21   Strain of extensor muscle and tendon of thumb at wrist and hand level

    S66.211   Strain of extensor muscle and tendon of right thumb at wrist and hand level

    S66.212   Strain of extensor muscle and tendon of left thumb at wrist and hand level

    S66.219   Strain of extensor muscle and tendon of thumb at wrist and hand level of unspecified side

S66.22   Laceration of extensor muscle and tendon of thumb at wrist and hand level

    S66.221   Laceration of extensor muscle and tendon of right thumb at wrist and hand level

    S66.222   Laceration of extensor muscle and tendon of left thumb at wrist and hand level

    S66.229   Laceration of extensor muscle and tendon of thumb at wrist and hand level of unspecified side

S66.29   Other injury of extensor muscle and tendon of thumb at wrist and hand level

    S66.291   Other injury of extensor muscle and tendon of right thumb at wrist and hand level

    S66.292   Other injury of extensor muscle and tendon of left thumb at wrist and hand level

    S66.299   Other injury of extensor muscle and tendon of thumb at wrist and hand level of unspecified side

S66.3   Injury of extensor muscle and tendon of other and unspecified finger at wrist and hand level

    Excludes2:   injury of extensor muscle and tendon of thumb at wrist and hand level (S66.2-)

S66.30   Unspecified injury of extensor muscle and tendon of other and unspecified finger at wrist and hand level

    S66.300   Unspecified injury of extensor muscle and tendon of right index finger at wrist and hand level

    S66.301   Unspecified injury of extensor muscle and tendon of left index finger at wrist and hand level

    S66.302   Unspecified injury of extensor muscle and tendon of right middle finger at wrist and hand level

    S66.303   Unspecified injury of extensor muscle and tendon of left middle finger at wrist and hand level

    S66.304   Unspecified injury of extensor muscle and tendon of right ring finger at wrist and hand level

    S66.305   Unspecified injury of extensor muscle and tendon of left ring finger at wrist and hand level

    S66.306   Unspecified injury of extensor muscle and tendon of right little finger at wrist and hand level

    S66.307   Unspecified injury of extensor muscle and tendon of left little finger at wrist and hand level

    S66.308   Unspecified injury of extensor muscle and tendon of other finger at wrist and hand level

        Unspecified injury of extensor muscle and tendon of specified finger with unspecified laterality at wrist and hand level

    S66.309   Unspecified injury of extensor muscle and tendon of unspecified finger at wrist and hand level

S66.31   Strain of extensor muscle and tendon of other and unspecified finger at wrist and hand level

    S66.310   Strain of extensor muscle and tendon of right index finger at wrist and hand level

    S66.311   Strain of extensor muscle and tendon of left index finger at wrist and hand level

    S66.312   Strain of extensor muscle and tendon of right middle finger at wrist and hand level

    S66.313   Strain of extensor muscle and tendon of left middle finger at wrist and hand level

    S66.314   Strain of extensor muscle and tendon of right ring finger at wrist and hand level

    S66.315   Strain of extensor muscle and tendon of left ring finger at wrist and hand level

    S66.316   Strain of extensor muscle and tendon of right little finger at wrist and hand level

    S66.317   Strain of extensor muscle and tendon of left little finger at wrist and hand level

    S66.318   Strain of extensor muscle and tendon of other finger at wrist and hand level

        Strain of extensor muscle and tendon of specified finger with unspecified laterality at wrist and hand level

    S66.319   Strain of extensor muscle and tendon of unspecified finger at wrist and hand level

S66.32   Laceration of extensor muscle and tendon of other and unspecified finger at wrist and hand level

    S66.320   Laceration of extensor muscle and tendon of right index finger at wrist and hand level

    S66.321   Laceration of extensor muscle and tendon of left index finger at wrist and hand level

    S66.322   Laceration of extensor muscle and tendon of right middle finger at wrist and hand level

    S66.323   Laceration of extensor muscle and tendon of left middle finger at wrist and hand level

    S66.324   Laceration of extensor muscle and tendon of right ring finger at wrist and hand level

    S66.325   Laceration of extensor muscle and tendon of left ring finger at wrist and hand level

    S66.326   Laceration of extensor muscle and tendon of right little finger at wrist and hand level

    S66.327   Laceration of extensor muscle and tendon of left little finger at wrist and hand level

    S66.328   Laceration of extensor muscle and tendon of other finger at wrist and hand level

        Laceration of extensor muscle and tendon of specified finger with unspecified laterality at wrist and hand level

    S66.329   Laceration of extensor muscle and tendon of unspecified finger at wrist and hand level

S66.39   Other injury of extensor muscle and tendon of other and unspecified finger at wrist and hand level

    S66.390   Other injury of extensor muscle and tendon of right index finger at wrist and hand level

    S66.391   Other injury of extensor muscle and tendon of left index finger at wrist and hand level

    S66.392   Other injury of extensor muscle and tendon of right middle finger at wrist and hand level

    S66.393   Other injury of extensor muscle and tendon of left middle finger at wrist and hand level

    S66.394   Other injury of extensor muscle and tendon of right ring finger at wrist and hand level

    S66.395   Other injury of extensor muscle and tendon of left ring finger at wrist and hand level

    S66.396   Other injury of extensor muscle and tendon of right little finger at wrist and hand level

    S66.397   Other injury of extensor muscle and tendon of left little finger at wrist and hand level

    S66.398   Other injury of extensor muscle and tendon of other finger at wrist and hand level

        Other injury of extensor muscle and tendon of specified finger with unspecified laterality at wrist and hand level

    S66.399   Other injury of extensor muscle and tendon of unspecified finger at wrist and hand level

S66.4   Injury of intrinsic muscle and tendon of thumb at wrist and hand level

S66.40   Unspecified injury of intrinsic muscle and tendon of thumb at wrist and hand level

    S66.401   Unspecified injury of intrinsic muscle and tendon of right thumb at wrist and hand level

S66.402   Unspecified injury of intrinsic muscle and tendon of left thumb at wrist and hand level

S66.409   Unspecified injury of intrinsic muscle and tendon of thumb at wrist and hand level of unspecified side

S66.41   Strain of intrinsic muscle and tendon of thumb at wrist and hand level

S66.411   Strain of intrinsic muscle and tendon of right thumb at wrist and hand level

S66.412   Strain of intrinsic muscle and tendon of left thumb at wrist and hand level

S66.419   Strain of intrinsic muscle and tendon of thumb at wrist and hand level of unspecified side

S66.42   Laceration of intrinsic muscle and tendon of thumb at wrist and hand level

S66.421   Laceration of intrinsic muscle and tendon of right thumb at wrist and hand level

S66.422   Laceration of intrinsic muscle and tendon of left thumb at wrist and hand level

S66.429   Laceration of intrinsic muscle and tendon of thumb at wrist and hand level of unspecified side

S66.49   Other injury of intrinsic muscle and tendon of thumb at wrist and hand level

S66.491   Other injury of intrinsic muscle and tendon of right thumb at wrist and hand level

S66.492   Other injury of intrinsic muscle and tendon of left thumb at wrist and hand level

S66.499   Other injury of intrinsic muscle and tendon of thumb at wrist and hand level of unspecified side

S66.5   Injury of intrinsic muscle and tendon of other and unspecified finger at wrist and hand level

     Excludes2:   injury of intrinsic muscle and tendon of thumb at wrist and hand level (S66.4-)

S66.50   Unspecified injury of intrinsic muscle and tendon of other and unspecified finger at wrist and hand level

S66.500   Unspecified injury of intrinsic muscle and tendon of right index finger at wrist and hand level

S66.501   Unspecified injury of intrinsic muscle and tendon of left index finger at wrist and hand level

S66.502   Unspecified injury of intrinsic muscle and tendon of right middle finger at wrist and hand level

S66.503   Unspecified injury of intrinsic muscle and tendon of left middle finger at wrist and hand level

S66.504   Unspecified injury of intrinsic muscle and tendon of right ring finger at wrist and hand level

S66.505   Unspecified injury of intrinsic muscle and tendon of left ring finger at wrist and hand level

S66.506   Unspecified injury of intrinsic muscle and tendon of right little finger at wrist and hand level

S66.507   Unspecified injury of intrinsic muscle and tendon of left little finger at wrist and hand level

S66.508   Unspecified injury of intrinsic muscle and tendon of other finger at wrist and hand level

     Unspecified injury of intrinsic muscle and tendon of specified finger with unspecified laterality at wrist and hand level

S66.509   Unspecified injury of intrinsic muscle and tendon of finger at wrist and hand level of unspecified finger

S66.51   Strain of intrinsic muscle and tendon of other and unspecified finger at wrist and hand level

S66.510   Strain of intrinsic muscle and tendon of right index finger at wrist and hand level

S66.511   Strain of intrinsic muscle and tendon of left index finger at wrist and hand level

S66.512   Strain of intrinsic muscle and tendon of right middle finger at wrist and hand level

S66.513   Strain of intrinsic muscle and tendon of left middle finger at wrist and hand level

S66.514   Strain of intrinsic muscle and tendon of right ring finger at wrist and hand level

S66.515   Strain of intrinsic muscle and tendon of left ring finger at wrist and hand level

S66.516   Strain of intrinsic muscle and tendon of right little finger at wrist and hand level

S66.517   Strain of intrinsic muscle and tendon of left little finger at wrist and hand level

S66.518   Strain of intrinsic muscle and tendon of other finger at wrist and hand level

     Strain of intrinsic muscle and tendon of specified finger with unspecified laterality at wrist and hand level

S66.519   Strain of intrinsic muscle and tendon of unspecified finger at wrist and hand level

S66.52   Laceration of intrinsic muscle and tendon of other and unspecified finger at wrist and hand level

S66.520   Laceration of intrinsic muscle and tendon of right index finger at wrist and hand level

S66.521   Laceration of intrinsic muscle and tendon of left index finger at wrist and hand level

S66.522   Laceration of intrinsic muscle and tendon of right middle finger at wrist and hand level

S66.523   Laceration of intrinsic muscle and tendon of left middle finger at wrist and hand level

S66.524   Laceration of intrinsic muscle and tendon of right ring finger at wrist and hand level

S66.525   Laceration of intrinsic muscle and tendon of left ring finger at wrist and hand level

S66.526   Laceration of intrinsic muscle and tendon of right little finger at wrist and hand level

S66.527   Laceration of intrinsic muscle and tendon of left little finger at wrist and hand level

S66.528   Laceration of intrinsic muscle and tendon of other finger at wrist and hand level

     Laceration of intrinsic muscle and tendon of specified finger with unspecified laterality at wrist and hand level

S66.529   Laceration of intrinsic muscle and tendon of unspecified finger at wrist and hand level

S66.59   Other injury of intrinsic muscle and tendon of other and unspecified finger at wrist and hand level

S66.590   Other injury of intrinsic muscle and tendon of right index finger at wrist and hand level

S66.591   Other injury of intrinsic muscle and tendon of left index finger at wrist and hand level

S66.592   Other injury of intrinsic muscle and tendon of right middle finger at wrist and hand level

S66.593   Other injury of intrinsic muscle and tendon of left middle finger at wrist and hand level

S66.594   Other injury of intrinsic muscle and tendon of right ring finger at wrist and hand level

S66.595   Other injury of intrinsic muscle and tendon of left ring finger at wrist and hand level

S66.596   Other injury of intrinsic muscle and tendon of right little finger at wrist and hand level

S66.597   Other injury of intrinsic muscle and tendon of left little finger at wrist and hand level

S66.598   Other injury of intrinsic muscle and tendon of other finger at wrist and hand level

     Other injury of intrinsic muscle and tendon of specified finger with unspecified laterality at wrist and hand level

S66.599   Other injury of intrinsic muscle and tendon of unspecified finger at wrist and hand level

S66.8 Injury of other muscles and tendons at wrist and hand level

    S66.80 Unspecified injury of other muscles and tendons at wrist and hand level

        S66.801 Unspecified injury of other muscles and tendons at right wrist and hand level

        S66.802 Unspecified injury of other muscles and tendons at left wrist and hand level

        S66.809 Unspecified injury of other muscles and tendons at wrist and hand level of unspecified side

    S66.81 Strain of other muscles and tendons at wrist and hand level

        S66.811 Strain of other muscles and tendons at right wrist and hand level

        S66.812 Strain of other muscles and tendons at left wrist and hand level

        S66.819 Strain of other muscles and tendons at wrist and hand level of unspecified side

    S66.82 Laceration of other muscles and tendons at wrist and hand level

        S66.821 Laceration of other muscles and tendons at right wrist and hand level

        S66.822 Laceration of other muscles and tendons at left wrist and hand level

        S66.829 Laceration of other muscles and tendons at wrist and hand level of unspecified side

    S66.89 Other injury of other muscles and tendons at wrist and hand level

        S66.891 Other injury of other muscles and tendons at right wrist and hand level

        S66.892 Other injury of other muscles and tendons at left wrist and hand level

        S66.899 Other injury of other muscles and tendons at wrist and hand level of unspecified side

S66.9 Injury of unspecified muscle and tendon at wrist and hand level

    S66.90 Unspecified injury of unspecified muscle and tendon at wrist and hand level

        S66.901 Unspecified injury of unspecified muscle and tendon at right wrist and hand level

        S66.902 Unspecified injury of unspecified muscle and tendon at left wrist and hand level

        S66.909 Unspecified injury of unspecified muscle and tendon at wrist and hand level of unspecified side

    S66.91 Strain of unspecified muscle and tendon at wrist and hand level

        S66.911 Strain of unspecified muscle and tendon at right wrist and hand level

        S66.912 Strain of unspecified muscle and tendon at left wrist and hand level

        S66.919 Strain of unspecified muscle and tendon at wrist and hand level of unspecified side

    S66.92 Laceration of unspecified muscle and tendon at wrist and hand level

        S66.921 Laceration of unspecified muscle and tendon at right wrist and hand level

        S66.922 Laceration of unspecified muscle and tendon at left wrist and hand level

        S66.929 Laceration of unspecified muscle and tendon at wrist and hand level of unspecified level

    S66.99 Other injury of unspecified muscle and tendon at wrist and hand level

        S66.991 Other injury of unspecified muscle and tendon at right wrist and hand level

        S66.992 Other injury of unspecified muscle and tendon at left wrist and hand level

        S66.999 Other injury of unspecified muscle and tendon at wrist and hand level of unspecified side

S67 Crushing injury of wrist, hand and fingers

Use additional code for all associated injuries, such as:
    fracture of wrist and hand (S62.-)
    open wound of wrist and hand (S61.-)

The following extensions are to be added to each code for category S67:
    a   initial encounter
    d   subsequent encounter
    q   sequela

S67.0 Crushing injury of thumb

    S67.00 Crushing injury of thumb of unspecified side

    S67.01 Crushing injury of right thumb

    S67.02 Crushing injury of left thumb

S67.1 Crushing injury of other and unspecified finger(s)

    Excludes2:   crushing injury of thumb (S67.0-)

    S67.10 Crushing injury of unspecified finger(s)

    S67.19 Crushing injury of other finger(s)

        S67.190 Crushing injury of right index finger

        S67.191 Crushing injury of left index finger

        S67.192 Crushing injury of right middle finger

        S67.193 Crushing injury of left middle finger

        S67.194 Crushing injury of right ring finger

        S67.195 Crushing injury of left ring finger

        S67.196 Crushing injury of right little finger

        S67.197 Crushing injury of left little finger

        S67.198 Crushing injury of other finger

            Crushing injury of specified finger with unspecified laterality

S67.2 Crushing injury of hand

    Excludes2:   crushing injury of fingers (S67.1-)
                    crushing injury of thumb (S67.0-)

    S67.20 Crushing injury of unspecified hand

    S67.21 Crushing injury of right hand

    S67.22 Crushing injury of left hand

S67.3 Crushing injury of wrist

    S67.30 Crushing injury of unspecified wrist

    S67.31 Crushing injury of right wrist

    S67.32 Crushing injury of left wrist

S67.4 Crushing injury of wrist and hand

    Excludes1:   crushing injury of hand alone (S67.2-)
                    crushing injury of wrist alone (S67.3-)

    Excludes2:   crushing injury of fingers (S67.1-)
                    crushing injury of thumb (S67.0-)

    S67.40 Crushing injury of unspecified wrist and hand

    S67.41 Crushing injury of right wrist and hand

    S67.42 Crushing injury of left wrist and hand

S67.9 Crushing injury of unspecified part(s) of wrist, hand and fingers

    S67.90 Crushing injury of unspecified part(s) of wrist, hand and fingers of unspecified side

    S67.91 Crushing injury of unspecified part(s) of right wrist, hand and fingers

    S67.92 Crushing injury of unspecified part(s) of left wrist, hand and fingers

S68 Traumatic amputation of wrist, hand and fingers

An amputation not identified as partial or complete should be coded to complete

The following extensions are to be added to each code for category S68:
    a   initial encounter
    d   subsequent encounter
    q   sequela

S68.0 Traumatic metacarpophalangeal amputation of thumb

Traumatic amputation of thumb NOS

    S68.01 Complete traumatic metacarpophalangeal amputation of thumb

        S68.011 Complete traumatic metacarpophalangeal amputation of right thumb

        S68.012 Complete traumatic metacarpophalangeal amputation of left thumb

S68.019   Complete traumatic metacarpophalangeal amputation of unspecified thumb

S68.02   Partial traumatic metacarpophalangeal amputation of thumb

S68.021   Partial traumatic metacarpophalangeal amputation of right thumb

S68.022   Partial traumatic metacarpophalangeal amputation of left thumb

S68.029   Partial traumatic metacarpophalangeal amputation of unspecified thumb

S68.1   Traumatic metacarpophalangeal amputation of other and unspecified finger

Traumatic amputation of finger NOS

Excludes2:   traumatic metacarpophalangeal amputation of thumb (S68.0-)

S68.11   Complete traumatic metacarpophalangeal amputation of other and unspecified finger

S68.110   Complete traumatic metacarpophalangeal amputation of right index finger

S68.111   Complete traumatic metacarpophalangeal amputation of left index finger

S68.112   Complete traumatic metacarpophalangeal amputation of right middle finger

S68.113   Complete traumatic metacarpophalangeal amputation of left middle finger

S68.114   Complete traumatic metacarpophalangeal amputation of right ring finger

S68.115   Complete traumatic metacarpophalangeal amputation of left ring finger

S68.116   Complete traumatic metacarpophalangeal amputation of right little finger

S68.117   Complete traumatic metacarpophalangeal amputation of left little finger

S68.118   Complete traumatic metacarpophalangeal amputation of other finger

Complete traumatic metacarpophalangeal amputation of specified finger with unspecified laterality

S68.119   Complete traumatic metacarpophalangeal amputation of unspecified finger

S68.12   Partial traumatic metacarpophalangeal amputation of other and unspecified finger

S68.120   Partial traumatic metacarpophalangeal amputation of right index finger

S68.121   Partial traumatic metacarpophalangeal amputation of left index finger

S68.122   Partial traumatic metacarpophalangeal amputation of right middle finger

S68.123   Partial traumatic metacarpophalangeal amputation of left middle finger

S68.124   Partial traumatic metacarpophalangeal amputation of right ring finger

S68.125   Partial traumatic metacarpophalangeal amputation of left ring finger

S68.126   Partial traumatic metacarpophalangeal amputation of right little finger

S68.127   Partial traumatic metacarpophalangeal amputation of left little finger

S68.128   Partial traumatic metacarpophalangeal amputation of other finger

Partial traumatic metacarpophalangeal amputation of specified finger with unspecified laterality

S68.129   Partial traumatic metacarpophalangeal amputation of unspecified finger

S68.4   Traumatic amputation of hand at wrist level

Traumatic amputation of hand NOS

Traumatic amputation of wrist

S68.41   Complete traumatic amputation of hand at wrist level

S68.411   Complete traumatic amputation of right hand at wrist level

S68.412   Complete traumatic amputation of left hand at wrist level

S68.419   Complete traumatic amputation of unspecified hand at wrist level

S68.42   Partial traumatic amputation of hand at wrist level

S68.421   Partial traumatic amputation of right hand at wrist level

S68.422   Partial traumatic amputation of left hand at wrist level

S68.429   Partial traumatic amputation of hand at wrist level of unspecified side

S68.5   Traumatic transphalangeal amputation of thumb

Traumatic interphalangeal joint amputation of thumb

S68.51   Complete traumatic transphalangeal amputation of thumb

S68.511   Complete traumatic transphalangeal amputation of right thumb

S68.512   Complete traumatic transphalangeal amputation of left thumb

S68.519   Complete traumatic transphalangeal amputation of unspecified thumb

S68.52   Partial traumatic transphalangeal amputation of thumb

S68.521   Partial traumatic transphalangeal amputation of right thumb

S68.522   Partial traumatic transphalangeal amputation of left thumb

S68.529   Partial traumatic transphalangeal amputation of unspecified thumb

S68.6   Traumatic transphalangeal amputation of other and unspecified finger

S68.61   Complete traumatic transphalangeal amputation of other and unspecified finger(s)

S68.610   Complete traumatic transphalangeal amputation of right index finger

S68.611   Complete traumatic transphalangeal amputation of left index finger

S68.612   Complete traumatic transphalangeal amputation of right middle finger

S68.613   Complete traumatic transphalangeal amputation of left middle finger

S68.614   Complete traumatic transphalangeal amputation of right ring finger

S68.615   Complete traumatic transphalangeal amputation of left ring finger

S68.616   Complete traumatic transphalangeal amputation of right little finger

S68.617   Complete traumatic transphalangeal amputation of left little finger

S68.618   Complete traumatic transphalangeal amputation of other finger

Complete traumatic transphalangeal amputation of specified finger with unspecified laterality

S68.619   Complete traumatic transphalangeal amputation of unspecified finger

S68.62   Partial traumatic transphalangeal amputation of other and unspecified finger

S68.620   Partial traumatic transphalangeal amputation of right index finger

S68.621   Partial traumatic transphalangeal amputation of left index finger

S68.622   Partial traumatic transphalangeal amputation of right middle finger

S68.623   Partial traumatic transphalangeal amputation of left middle finger

S68.624   Partial traumatic transphalangeal amputation of right ring finger

S68.625   Partial traumatic transphalangeal amputation of left ring finger

S68.626   Partial traumatic transphalangeal amputation of right little finger

S68.627   Partial traumatic transphalangeal amputation of left little finger

S68.628   Partial traumatic transphalangeal amputation of other finger
> Partial traumatic transphalangeal amputation of specified finger with unspecified laterality

S68.629   Partial traumatic transphalangeal amputation of unspecified finger

S68.7   Traumatic transmetacarpal amputation of hand

S68.71   Complete traumatic transmetacarpal amputation of hand

S68.711   Complete traumatic transmetacarpal amputation of right hand

S68.712   Complete traumatic transmetacarpal amputation of left hand

S68.719   Complete traumatic transmetacarpal amputation of unspecified hand

S68.72   Partial traumatic transmetacarpal amputation of hand

S68.721   Partial traumatic transmetacarpal amputation of right hand

S68.722   Partial traumatic transmetacarpal amputation of left hand

S68.729   Partial traumatic transmetacarpal amputation of unspecified hand

S69   Other and unspecified injuries of wrist, hand and finger(s)
> The following extensions are to be added to each code for category S69:
> - a   initial encounter
> - d   subsequent encounter
> - q   sequela

S69.8   Other specified injuries of wrist, hand and finger(s)

S69.80   Other specified injuries of wrist, hand and finger(s) of unspecified side

S69.81   Other specified injuries of right wrist, hand and finger(s)

S69.82   Other specified injuries of left wrist, hand and finger(s)

S69.9   Unspecified injury of wrist, hand and finger(s)

S69.90   Unspecified injury of wrist, hand and finger(s) of unspecified side

S69.91   Unspecified injury of right wrist, hand and finger(s)

S69.92   Unspecified injury of left wrist, hand and finger(s)

INJURIES TO THE HIP AND THIGH (S70-S79)

Excludes2:   burns and corrosions (T20-T32)
> frostbite (T33-T34)
> snake bite (T63.0-)
> venomous insect bite or sting (T63.4-)

S70   Superficial injury of hip and thigh
> The following extensions are to be added to each code for category S70:
> - a   initial encounter
> - d   subsequent encounter
> - q   sequela

S70.0   Contusion of hip

S70.00   Contusion of unspecified hip

S70.01   Contusion of right hip

S70.02   Contusion of left hip

S70.1   Contusion of thigh

S70.10   Contusion of unspecified thigh

S70.11   Contusion of right thigh

S70.12   Contusion of left thigh

S70.2   Other superficial injuries of hip

S70.21   Abrasion of hip

S70.211   Abrasion, right hip

S70.212   Abrasion, left hip

S70.219   Abrasion, unspecified hip

S70.22   Blister (nonthermal) of hip

S70.221   Blister (nonthermal), right hip

S70.222   Blister (nonthermal), left hip

S70.229   Blister (nonthermal), unspecified hip

S70.24   External constriction of hip

S70.241   External constriction, right hip

S70.242   External constriction, left hip

S70.249   External constriction, unspecified hip

S70.25   Superficial foreign body of hip
> Splinter in the hip

S70.251   Superficial foreign body, right hip

S70.252   Superficial foreign body, left hip

S70.259   Superficial foreign body, unspecified hip

S70.26   Insect bite (nonvenomous) of hip

S70.261   Insect bite (nonvenomous), right hip

S70.262   Insect bite (nonvenomous), left hip

S70.269   Insect bite (nonvenomous), unspecified hip

S70.27   Other superficial bite of hip
> Excludes1:   open bite of hip (S71.05-)

S70.271   Other superficial bite of hip, right hip

S70.272   Other superficial bite of hip, left hip

S70.279   Other superficial bite of hip, unspecified hip

S70.3   Other superficial injuries of thigh

S70.31   Abrasion of thigh

S70.311   Abrasion, right thigh

S70.312   Abrasion, left thigh

S70.319   Abrasion, unspecified thigh

S70.32   Blister (nonthermal) of thigh

S70.321   Blister (nonthermal), right thigh

S70.322   Blister (nonthermal), left thigh

S70.329   Blister (nonthermal), unspecified thigh

S70.34   External constriction of thigh

S70.341   External constriction, right thigh

S70.342   External constriction, left thigh

S70.349   External constriction, unspecified thigh

S70.35   Superficial foreign body of thigh
> Splinter in the thigh

S70.351   Superficial foreign body, right thigh

S70.352   Superficial foreign body, left thigh

S70.359   Superficial foreign body, unspecified thigh

S70.36   Insect bite (nonvenomous) of thigh

S70.361   Insect bite (nonvenomous), right thigh

S70.362   Insect bite (nonvenomous), left thigh

S70.369   Insect bite (nonvenomous), unspecified thigh

S70.37   Other superficial bite of thigh
> Excludes1:   open bite of thigh (S71.15)

S70.371   Other superficial bite of right thigh

S70.372   Other superficial bite of left thigh

S70.379   Other superficial bite of unspecified thigh

S70.9   Unspecified superficial injury of hip and thigh

S70.91   Unspecified superficial injury of hip

S70.911   Unspecified superficial injury of right hip

S70.912   Unspecified superficial injury of left hip

S70.919   Unspecified superficial injury of hip, unspecified side

S70.92   Unspecified superficial injury of thigh

S70.921   Unspecified superficial injury of right thigh

S70.922   Unspecified superficial injury of left thigh

S70.929   Unspecified superficial injury of thigh, unspecified side

S71   Open wound of hip and thigh
> Code also any associated wound infection
> Excludes1:   open fracture of hip and thigh (S72.-)
> traumatic amputation of hip and thigh (S78.-)
> Excludes2:   bite of venomous animal (T63.-)
> open wound of ankle, foot and toes (S91.-)
> open wound of knee and lower leg (S81.-)
> The following extensions are to be added to each code for category S71:
> - a   initial encounter
> - d   subsequent encounter
> - q   sequela

S71.0   **Open wound of hip**

    S71.00   **Unspecified open wound of hip**

        S71.001   Unspecified open wound, right hip

        S71.002   Unspecified open wound, left hip

        S71.009   Unspecified open wound, unspecified hip

    S71.01   **Laceration without foreign body of hip**

        S71.011   Laceration without foreign body, right hip

        S71.012   Laceration without foreign body, left hip

        S71.019   Laceration without foreign body, unspecified hip

    S71.02   **Laceration with foreign body of hip**

        S71.021   Laceration with foreign body, right hip

        S71.022   Laceration with foreign body, left hip

        S71.029   Laceration with foreign body, unspecified hip

    S71.03   **Puncture wound without foreign body of hip**

        S71.031   Puncture wound without foreign body, right hip

        S71.032   Puncture wound without foreign body, left hip

        S71.039   Puncture wound without foreign body, unspecified hip

    S71.04   **Puncture wound with foreign body of hip**

        S71.041   Puncture wound with foreign body, right hip

        S71.042   Puncture wound with foreign body, left hip

        S71.049   Puncture wound with foreign body, unspecified hip

    S71.05   **Open bite of hip**

        Bite of hip NOS

        Excludes1:   superficial bite of hip (S70.26, S70.27)

        S71.051   Bite, right hip

        S71.052   Bite, left hip

        S71.059   Bite, unspecified hip

S71.1   **Open wound of thigh**

    S71.10   **Unspecified open wound of thigh**

        S71.101   Unspecified open wound, right thigh

        S71.102   Unspecified open wound, left thigh

        S71.109   Unspecified open wound, unspecified thigh

    S71.11   **Laceration without foreign body of thigh**

        S71.111   Laceration without foreign body, right thigh

        S71.112   Laceration without foreign body, left thigh

        S71.119   Laceration without foreign body, unspecified thigh

    S71.12   **Laceration with foreign body of thigh**

        S71.121   Laceration with foreign body, right thigh

        S71.122   Laceration with foreign body, left thigh

        S71.129   Laceration with foreign body, unspecified thigh

    S71.13   **Puncture wound without foreign body of thigh**

        S71.131   Puncture wound without foreign body, right thigh

        S71.132   Puncture wound without foreign body, left thigh

        S71.139   Puncture wound without foreign body, unspecified thigh

    S71.14   **Puncture wound with foreign body of thigh**

        S71.141   Puncture wound with foreign body, right thigh

        S71.142   Puncture wound with foreign body, left thigh

        S71.149   Puncture wound with foreign body, unspecified thigh

    S71.15   **Open bite of thigh**

        Bite of thigh NOS

        Excludes1:   superficial bite of thigh (S70.86-, S70.87-)

        S71.151   Bite, right thigh

        S71.152   Bite, left thigh

        S71.159   Bite, unspecified thigh

S72   **Fracture of femur**

    A fracture not indicated as displaced or nondisplaced should be coded to displaced

    Excludes1:   traumatic amputation of hip and thigh (S78.-)

    Excludes2:   fracture of lower leg and ankle (S82.-)

                     fracture of foot (S92.-)

    A fracture not designated as open or closed should be coded to closed

    Note: the open fracture designations are based on the Gustilo open fracture classification

    The following extensions are to be added to each code for category S72:

    a   initial encounter for closed fracture

    b   initial encounter for open fracture type I or II

    c   initial encounter for open fracture type IIIA, IIIB, or IIIC

    d   subsequent encounter for closed fracture with routine healing

    e   subsequent encounter for open fracture type I or II with routine healing

    f   subsequent encounter for open fracture type IIIA, IIIB, or IIIC with routine healing

    g   subsequent encounter for closed fracture with delayed healing

    h   subsequent encounter for open fracture type I or II with delayed healing

    i   subsequent encounter for open fracture type IIIA, IIIB, or IIIC with delayed healing

    j   subsequent encounter for closed fracture with nonunion

    k   subsequent encounter for open fracture type I or II with nonunion

    l   subsequent encounter for open fracture type IIIA, IIIB, or IIIC with nonunion

    m   subsequent encounter for closed fracture with malunion

    n   subsequent encounter for open fracture type I or II with malunion

    o   subsequent encounter for open fracture type IIIA, IIIB, or IIIC with malunion

    q   sequela

S72.0   **Fracture of head and neck of femur**

    Excludes2:   physeal fracture of upper end of femur (S79.0-)

    S72.00   **Fracture of unspecifed part of neck of femur**

        Fracture of hip NOS

        Fracture of neck of femur NOS

        S72.001   **Fracture of unspecifed part of neck of right femur**

        S72.002   **Fracture of unspecifed part of neck of left femur**

        S72.009   **Fracture of unspecifed part of neck of unspecified femur**

    S72.01   **Unspecified intracapsular fracture of femur**

        Subcapital fracture of femur

        S72.011   **Unspecified intracapsular fracture of right femur**

        S72.012   **Unspecified intracapsular fracture of left femur**

        S72.019   **Unspecified intracapsular fracture of unspecified femur**

    S72.02   **Fracture of epiphysis (separation) (upper) of femur**

        Transepiphyseal fracture of femur

        Excludes1:   capital femoral epiphyseal fracture (pediatric) of femur (S79.01-)

                      Salter-Harris Type I physeal fracture of upper end of femur (S79.01-)

        S72.021   **Displaced fracture of epiphysis (separation) (upper) of right femur**

        S72.022   **Displaced fracture of epiphysis (separation) (upper) of left femur**

        S72.023   **Displaced fracture of epiphysis (separation) (upper) of unspecified femur**

        S72.024   **Nondisplaced fracture of epiphysis (separation) (upper) of right femur**

        S72.025   **Nondisplaced fracture of epiphysis (separation) (upper) of left femur**

        S72.026   **Nondisplaced fracture of epiphysis (separation) (upper) of unspecified femur**

S72.03   **Midcervical fracture of femur**
        Transcervical fracture of femur NOS
    S72.031   Displaced midcervical fracture of right femur
    S72.032   Displaced midcervical fracture of left femur
    S72.033   Displaced midcervical fracture of unspecified femur
    S72.034   Nondisplaced midcervical fracture of right femur
    S72.035   Nondisplaced midcervical fracture of left femur
    S72.036   Nondisplaced midcervical fracture of unspecified femur

S72.04   **Fracture of base of neck of femur**
        Cervicotrochanteric fracture of femur
    S72.041   Displaced fracture of base of neck of right femur
    S72.042   Displaced fracture of base of neck of left femur
    S72.043   Displaced fracture of base of neck of unspecified femur
    S72.044   Nondisplaced fracture of base of neck of right femur
    S72.045   Nondisplaced fracture of base of neck of left femur
    S72.046   Nondisplaced fracture of base of neck of unspecified femur

S72.05   **Unspecified fracture of head of femur**
        Fracture of head of femur NOS
    S72.051   Unspecified fracture of head of right femur
    S72.052   Unspecified fracture of head of left femur
    S72.059   Unspecified fracture of head of unspecified femur

S72.06   **Articular fracture of head of femur**
    S72.061   Displaced articular fracture of head of right femur
    S72.062   Displaced articular fracture of head of left femur
    S72.063   Displaced articular fracture of head of unspecified femur
    S72.064   Nondisplaced articular fracture of head of right femur
    S72.065   Nondisplaced articular fracture of head of left femur
    S72.066   Nondisplaced articular fracture of head of unspecified femur

S72.09   **Other fracture of head and neck of femur**
    S72.091   Other fracture of head and neck of right femur
    S72.092   Other fracture of head and neck of left femur
    S72.099   Other fracture of head and neck of unspecified femur

S72.1   Pertrochanteric fracture

S72.10   **Unspecified trochanteric fracture of femur**
        Fracture of trochanter NOS
    S72.101   Unspecified trochanteric fracture of right femur
    S72.102   Unspecified trochanteric fracture of left femur
    S72.109   Unspecified trochanteric fracture of unspecified femur

S72.11   **Fracture of greater trochanter of femur**
    S72.111   Displaced fracture of greater trochanter of right femur
    S72.112   Displaced fracture of greater trochanter of left femur
    S72.113   Displaced fracture of greater trochanter of unspecified femur
    S72.114   Nondisplaced fracture of greater trochanter of right femur
    S72.115   Nondisplaced fracture of greater trochanter of left femur
    S72.116   Nondisplaced fracture of greater trochanter of unspecified femur

S72.12   **Fracture of lesser trochanter of femur**
    S72.121   Displaced fracture of lesser trochanter of right femur
    S72.122   Displaced fracture of lesser trochanter of left femur
    S72.123   Displaced fracture of lesser trochanter of unspecified femur
    S72.124   Nondisplaced fracture of lesser trochanter of right femur
    S72.125   Nondisplaced fracture of lesser trochanter of left femur
    S72.126   Nondisplaced fracture of lesser trochanter of unspecified femur

S72.13   **Apophyseal fracture of femur**
        Excludes1:   chronic (nontraumatic) slipped upper femoral epiphysis (M93.0-)
    S72.131   Displaced apophyseal fracture of right femur
    S72.132   Displaced apophyseal fracture of left femur
    S72.133   Displaced apophyseal fracture of unspecifed femur
    S72.134   Nondisplaced apophyseal fracture of right femur
    S72.135   Nondisplaced apophyseal fracture of left femur
    S72.136   Nondisplaced apophyseal fracture of unspecified femur

S72.14   **Intertrochanteric fracture of femur**
    S72.141   Displaced intertrochanteric fracture of right femur
    S72.142   Displaced intertrochanteric fracture of left femur
    S72.143   Displaced intertrochanteric fracture of unspecified femur
    S72.144   Nondisplaced intertrochanteric fracture of right femur
    S72.145   Nondisplaced intertrochanteric fracture of left femur
    S72.146   Nondisplaced intertrochanteric fracture of unspecified femur

S72.2   Subtrochanteric fracture of femur

S72.21   Displaced subtrochanteric fracture of right femur
S72.22   Displaced subtrochanteric fracture of left femur
S72.23   Displaced subtrochanteric fracture of unspecified femur
S72.24   Nondisplaced subtrochanteric fracture of right femur
S72.25   Nondisplaced subtrochanteric fracture of left femur
S72.26   Nondisplaced subtrochanteric fracture of unspecified femur

S72.3   Fracture of shaft of femur

S72.30   **Unspecified fracture of shaft of femur**
    S72.301   Unspecified fracture of shaft of right femur
    S72.302   Unspecified fracture of shaft of left femur
    S72.309   Unspecified fracture of shaft of unspecified femur

S72.32   **Transverse fracture of shaft of femur**
    S72.321   Displaced transverse fracture of shaft of right femur
    S72.322   Displaced transverse fracture of shaft of left femur
    S72.323   Displaced transverse fracture of shaft of unspecified femur
    S72.324   Nondisplaced transverse fracture of shaft of right femur
    S72.325   Nondisplaced transverse fracture of shaft of left femur
    S72.326   Nondisplaced transverse fracture of shaft of unspecified femur

S72.33   **Oblique fracture of shaft of femur**
    S72.331   Displaced oblique fracture of shaft of right femur
    S72.332   Displaced oblique fracture of shaft of left femur

S72.333   Displaced oblique fracture of unspecified femur

S72.334   Nondisplaced oblique fracture of shaft of right femur

S72.335   Nondisplaced oblique fracture of shaft of left femur

S72.336   Nondisplaced oblique fracture of shaft of unspecified femur

S72.34   Spiral fracture of shaft of femur

S72.341   Displaced spiral fracture of shaft of right femur

S72.342   Displaced spiral fracture of shaft of left femur

S72.343   Displaced spiral fracture of shaft of unspecified femur

S72.344   Nondisplaced spiral fracture of shaft of right femur

S72.345   Nondisplaced spiral fracture of shaft of left femur

S72.346   Nondisplaced spiral fracture of shaft of unspecified femur

S72.35   Comminuted fracture of shaft of femur

S72.351   Displaced comminuted fracture of shaft of right femur

S72.352   Displaced comminuted fracture of shaft of left femur

S72.353   Displaced comminuted fracture of shaft of unspecified femur

S72.354   Nondisplaced comminuted fracture of shaft of right femur

S72.355   Nondisplaced comminuted fracture of shaft of left femur

S72.356   Nondisplaced comminuted fracture of shaft of unspecified femur

S72.36   Segmental fracture of shaft of femur

S72.361   Displaced segmental fracture of shaft of right femur

S72.362   Displaced segmental fracture of shaft of left femur

S72.363   Displaced segmental fracture of shaft of unspecified femur

S72.364   Nondisplaced segmental fracture of shaft of right femur

S72.365   Nondisplaced segmental fracture of shaft of left femur

S72.366   Nondisplaced segmental fracture of shaft of unspecified femur

S72.39   Other fracture of shaft of femur

S72.391   Other fracture of shaft of right femur

S72.392   Other fracture of shaft of left femur

S72.399   Other fracture of shaft of unspecified femur

S72.4   Fracture of lower end of femur
Fracture of distal end of femur
Excludes2:   fracture of shaft of femur (S72.3-)
physeal fracture of lower end of femur (S79.1-)

S72.40   Unspecified fracture of lower end of femur

S72.401   Unspecified fracture of lower end of right femur

S72.402   Unspecified fracture of lower end of left femur

S72.409   Unspecified fracture of lower end of unspecified femur

S72.41   Unspecified condyle fracture of lower end of femur
Condyle fracture of femur NOS

S72.411   Displaced unspecified condyle fracture of lower end of right femur

S72.412   Displaced unspecified condyle fracture of lower end of left femur

S72.413   Displaced unspecified condyle fracture of lower end of unspecified femur

S72.414   Nondisplaced unspecified condyle fracture of lower end of right femur

S72.415   Nondisplaced unspecified condyle fracture of lower end of left femur

S72.416   Nondisplaced unspecified condyle fracture of lower end of unspecified femur

S72.42   Fracture of lateral condyle of femur

S72.421   Displaced fracture of lateral condyle of right femur

S72.422   Displaced fracture of lateral condyle of left femur

S72.423   Displaced fracture of lateral condyle of unspecified femur

S72.424   Nondisplaced fracture of lateral condyle of right femur

S72.425   Nondisplaced fracture of lateral condyle of left femur

S72.426   Nondisplaced fracture of lateral condyle of unspecified femur

S72.43   Fracture of medial condyle of femur

S72.431   Displaced fracture of medial condyle of right femur

S72.432   Displaced fracture of medial condyle of left femur

S72.433   Displaced fracture of medial condyle of unspecified femur

S72.434   Nondisplaced fracture of medial condyle of right femur

S72.435   Nondisplaced fracture of medial condyle of left femur

S72.436   Nondisplaced fracture of medial condyle of unspecified femur

S72.44   Fracture of lower epiphysis (separation) of femur
Excludes1:   Salter-Harris Type I physeal fracture of lower end of femur (S79.11-)

S72.441   Displaced fracture of lower epiphysis (separation) of right femur

S72.442   Displaced fracture of lower epiphysis (separation) of left femur

S72.443   Displaced fracture of lower epiphysis (separation) of unspecified femur

S72.444   Nondisplaced fracture of lower epiphysis (separation) of right femur

S72.445   Nondisplaced fracture of lower epiphysis (separation) of left femur

S72.446   Nondisplaced fracture of lower epiphysis (separation) of unspecified femur

S72.45   Supracondylar fracture without intracondylar extension of lower end of femur
Supracondylar fracture of lower end of femur NOS
Excludes1:   supracondylar fracture with intracondylar extension of lower end of femur (S72.46-)

S72.451   Displaced supracondylar fracture without intracondylar extension of lower end of right femur

S72.452   Displaced supracondylar fracture without intracondylar extension of lower end of left femur

S72.453   Displaced supracondylar fracture without intracondylar extension of lower end of unspecified femur

S72.454   Nondisplaced supracondylar fracture without intracondylar extension of lower end of right femur

S72.455   Nondisplaced supracondylar fracture without intracondylar extension of lower end of left femur

S72.456   Nondisplaced supracondylar fracture without intracondylar extension of lower end of unspecified femur

S72.46   Supracondylar fracture with intracondylar extension of lower end of femur
Excludes1:   supracondylar fracture without intracondylar extension of lower end of femur (S72.45-)

S72.461 Displaced supracondylar fracture with intracondylar extension of lower end of right femur

S72.462 Displaced supracondylar fracture with intracondylar extension of lower end of left femur

S72.463 Displaced supracondylar fracture with intracondylar extension of lower end of unspecified femur

S72.464 Nondisplaced supracondylar fracture with intracondylar extension of lower end of right femur

S72.465 Nondisplaced supracondylar fracture with intracondylar extension of lower end of left femur

S72.466 Nondisplaced supracondylar fracture with intracondylar extension of lower end of unspecified femur

S72.47 Torus fracture of lower end of femur
   Note: open fracture extensions do not apply to these codes

S72.471 Torus fracture of lower end of right femur

S72.472 Torus fracture of lower end of left femur

S72.479 Torus fracture of lower end of unspecified femur

S72.49 Other fracture of lower end of femur

S72.491 Other fracture of lower end of right femur

S72.492 Other fracture of lower end of left femur

S72.499 Other fracture of lower end of unspecified femur

S72.8 Other fracture of femur

S72.8x Other fracture of femur

S72.8x1 Other fracture of right femur

S72.8x2 Other fracture of left femur

S72.8x9 Other fracture of unspecified femur

S72.9 Unspecified fracture of femur
   Fracture of thigh NOS
   Fracture of upper leg NOS
   Excludes1:   fracture of hip NOS (S72.00-, S72.01-)

S72.90 Unspecified fracture of unspecified femur

S72.91 Unspecified fracture of right femur

S72.92 Unspecified fracture of left femur

S73 Dislocation and sprain of joint and ligaments of hip
   Includes: avulsion of joint or ligament of hip
                  laceration of joint or ligament of hip
                  sprain of joint or ligament of hip
                  traumatic hemarthrosis of joint or ligament of hip
                  traumatic rupture of joint or ligament of hip
                  traumatic subluxation of joint or ligament of hip
                  traumatic tear of joint or ligament of hip
   Excludes2:   strain of muscle and tendon of hip and thigh (S76.-)
   The following extensions are to be added to each code for category S73:
      a   initial encounter
      d   subsequent encounter
      q   sequela

S73.0 Subluxation and dislocation of hip

S73.00 Unspecified subluxation and dislocation of hip
   Dislocation of hip NOS
   Subluxation of hip NOS

S73.001 Unspecified subluxation of right hip

S73.002 Unspecified subluxation of left hip

S73.003 Unspecified subluxation of unspecified hip

S73.004 Unspecified dislocation of right hip

S73.005 Unspecified dislocation of left hip

S73.006 Unspecified dislocation of unspecified hip

S73.01 Posterior subluxation and dislocation of hip

S73.011 Posterior subluxation of right hip

S73.012 Posterior subluxation of left hip

S73.013 Posterior subluxation of unspecified hip

S73.014 Posterior dislocation of right hip

S73.015 Posterior dislocation of left hip

S73.016 Posterior dislocation of unspecified hip

S73.02 Obturator subluxation and dislocation of hip

S73.021 Obturator subluxation of right hip

S73.022 Obturator subluxation of left hip

S73.023 Obturator subluxation of unspecified hip

S73.024 Obturator dislocation of right hip

S73.025 Obturator dislocation of left hip

S73.026 Obturator dislocation of unspecified hip

S73.03 Other anterior dislocation of hip

S73.031 Other anterior subluxation of right hip

S73.032 Other anterior subluxation of left hip

S73.033 Other anterior subluxation of unspecified hip

S73.034 Other anterior dislocation of right hip

S73.035 Other anterior dislocation of left hip

S73.036 Other anterior dislocation of unspecified hip

S73.04 Central dislocation of hip

S73.041 Central subluxation of right hip

S73.042 Central subluxation of left hip

S73.043 Central subluxation of unspecified hip

S73.044 Central dislocation of right hip

S73.045 Central dislocation of left hip

S73.046 Central dislocation of unspecified hip

S73.1 Sprain of hip

S73.10 Unspecified sprain of hip

S73.101 Unspecified sprain of right hip

S73.102 Unspecified sprain of left hip

S73.109 Unspecified sprain of unspecified hip

S73.11 Iliofemoral ligament sprain of hip

S73.111 Iliofemoral ligament sprain of right hip

S73.112 Iliofemoral ligament sprain of left hip

S73.119 Iliofemoral ligament sprain of unspecified hip

S73.12 Ischiocapsular (ligament) sprain of hip

S73.121 Ischiocapsular ligament sprain of right hip

S73.122 Ischiocapsular ligament sprain of left hip

S73.129 Ischiocapsular ligament sprain of unspecified hip

S73.19 Other sprain of hip

S73.191 Other sprain of right hip

S73.192 Other sprain of left hip

S73.199 Other sprain of unspecified hip

S74 Injury of nerves at hip and thigh level
   Code also any associated open wound (S71.-)
   Excludes2:   injury of nerves at ankle and foot level (S94.-)
                injury of nerves at lower leg level (S84.-)
   The following extensions are to be added to each code for category S74:
      a   initial encounter
      d   subsequent encounter
      q   sequela

S74.0 Injury of sciatic nerve at hip and thigh level

S74.00 Injury of sciatic nerve at hip and thigh level, unspecified leg

S74.01 Injury of sciatic nerve at hip and thigh level, right leg

S74.02 Injury of sciatic nerve at hip and thigh level, left leg

S74.1 Injury of femoral nerve at hip and thigh level

S74.10 Injury of femoral nerve at hip and thigh level, unspecified leg

S74.11 Injury of femoral nerve at hip and thigh level, right leg

S74.12 Injury of femoral nerve at hip and thigh level, left leg

S74.2 Injury of cutaneous sensory nerve at hip and thigh level

S74.20 Injury of cutaneous sensory nerve at hip and thigh level, unspecified leg

S74.21 Injury of cutaneous sensory nerve at hip and thigh level, right leg

S74.22 Injury of cutaneous sensory nerve at hip and thigh level, left leg

S74.8   Injury of other nerves at hip and thigh level
- S74.8x   Injury of other nerves at hip and thigh level
  - S74.8x1   Injury of other nerves at hip and thigh level, right leg
  - S74.8x2   Injury of other nerves at hip and thigh level, left leg
  - S74.8x9   Injury of other nerves at hip and thigh level, unspecified leg

S74.9   Injury of unspecified nerve at hip and thigh level
- S74.90   Injury of unspecified nerve at hip and thigh level, unspecified leg
- S74.91   Injury of unspecified nerve at hip and thigh level, right leg
- S74.92   Injury of unspecified nerve at hip and thigh level, left leg

S75   Injury of blood vessels at hip and thigh level

Code also any associated open wound (S71.-)

Excludes2:   injury of blood vessels at lower leg level (S85.-)
            injury of popliteal artery (S85.0)

The following extensions are to be added to each code for category S75:
- a   initial encounter
- d   subsequent encounter
- q   sequela

S75.0   Injury of femoral artery
- S75.00   Unspecified injury of femoral artery
  - S75.001   Unspecified injury of femoral artery, right leg
  - S75.002   Unspecified injury of femoral artery, left leg
  - S75.009   Unspecified injury of femoral artery, unspecified leg
- S75.01   Minor laceration of femoral artery
  Incomplete transection of femoral artery
  Laceration of femoral artery NOS
  Superficial laceration of femoral artery
  - S75.011   Minor laceration of femoral artery, right leg
  - S75.012   Minor laceration of femoral artery, left leg
  - S75.019   Minor laceration of femoral artery, unspecified leg
- S75.02   Major laceration of femoral artery
  Complete transection of femoral artery
  Traumatic rupture of femoral artery
  - S75.021   Major laceration of femoral artery, right leg
  - S75.022   Major laceration of femoral artery, left leg
  - S75.029   Major laceration of femoral artery, unspecified leg
- S75.09   Other specified injury of femoral artery
  - S75.091   Other specified injury of femoral artery, right leg
  - S75.092   Other specified injury of femoral artery, left leg
  - S75.099   Other specified injury of femoral artery, unspecified leg

S75.1   Injury of femoral vein at hip and thigh level
- S75.10   Unspecified injury of femoral vein at hip and thigh level
  - S75.101   Unspecified injury of femoral vein at hip and thigh level, right leg
  - S75.102   Unspecified injury of femoral vein at hip and thigh level, left leg
  - S75.109   Unspecified injury of femoral vein at hip and thigh level, unspecified leg
- S75.11   Minor laceration of femoral vein at hip and thigh level
  Incomplete transection of femoral vein at hip and thigh level
  Laceration of femoral vein at hip and thigh level NOS
  Superficial laceration of femoral vein at hip and thigh level
  - S75.111   Minor laceration of femoral vein at hip and thigh level, right leg
  - S75.112   Minor laceration of femoral vein at hip and thigh level, left leg

- S75.119   Minor laceration of femoral vein at hip and thigh level, unspecified leg
- S75.12   Major laceration of femoral vein at hip and thigh level
  Complete transection of femoral vein at hip and thigh level
  Traumatic rupture of femoral vein at hip and thigh level
  - S75.121   Major laceration of femoral vein at hip and thigh level, right leg
  - S75.122   Major laceration of femoral vein at hip and thigh level, left leg
  - S75.129   Major laceration of femoral vein at hip and thigh level, unspecified leg
- S75.19   Other specified injury of femoral vein at hip and thigh level
  - S75.191   Other specified injury of femoral vein at hip and thigh level, right leg
  - S75.192   Other specified injury of femoral vein at hip and thigh level, left leg
  - S75.199   Other specified injury of femoral vein at hip and thigh level, unspecified leg

S75.2   Injury of greater saphenous vein at hip and thigh level

Excludes1:   greater saphenous vein NOS (S85.3)
- S75.20   Unspecified injury of greater saphenous vein at hip and thigh level
  - S75.201   Unspecified injury of greater saphenous vein at hip and thigh level, right leg
  - S75.202   Unspecified injury of greater saphenous vein at hip and thigh level, left leg
  - S75.209   Unspecified injury of greater saphenous vein at hip and thigh level, unspecified leg
- S75.21   Minor laceration of greater saphenous vein at hip and thigh level
  Incomplete transection of greater saphenous vein at hip and thigh level
  Laceration of greater saphenous vein at hip and thigh level NOS
  Superficial laceration of greater saphenous vein at hip and thigh level
  - S75.211   Minor laceration of greater saphenous vein at hip and thigh level, right leg
  - S75.212   Minor laceration of greater saphenous vein at hip and thigh level, left leg
  - S75.219   Minor laceration of greater saphenous vein at hip and thigh level, unspecified leg
- S75.22   Major laceration of greater saphenous vein at hip and thigh level
  Complete transection of greater saphenous vein at hip and thigh level
  Traumatic rupture of greater saphenous vein at hip and thigh level
  - S75.221   Major laceration of greater saphenous vein at hip and thigh level, right leg
  - S75.222   Major laceration of greater saphenous vein at hip and thigh level, left leg
  - S75.229   Major laceration of greater saphenous vein at hip and thigh level, unspecified leg
- S75.29   Other specified injury of greater saphenous vein at hip and thigh level
  - S75.291   Other specified injury of greater saphenous vein at hip and thigh level, right leg
  - S75.292   Other specified injury of greater saphenous vein at hip and thigh level, left leg
  - S75.299   Other specified injury of greater saphenous vein at hip and thigh level, unspecified leg

S75.8   Injury of other blood vessels at hip and thigh level
- S75.80   Unspecified injury of other blood vessels at hip and thigh level
  - S75.801   Unspecified injury of other blood vessels at hip and thigh level, right leg
  - S75.802   Unspecified injury of other blood vessels at hip and thigh level, left leg

S75.809   Unspecified injury of other blood vessels at hip and thigh level, unspecified leg

S75.81   Laceration of other blood vessels at hip and thigh level

 S75.811   Laceration of other blood vessels at hip and thigh level, right leg

 S75.812   Laceration of other blood vessels at hip and thigh level, left leg

 S75.819   Laceration of other blood vessels at hip and thigh level, unspecified leg

S75.89   Other specified injury of other blood vessels at hip and thigh level

 S75.891   Other specified injury of other blood vessels at hip and thigh level, right leg

 S75.892   Other specified injury of other blood vessels at hip and thigh level, left leg

 S75.899   Other specified injury of other blood vessels at hip and thigh level, unspecified leg

S75.9   Injury of unspecified blood vessel at hip and thigh level

 S75.90   Unspecified injury of unspecified blood vessel at hip and thigh level

  S75.901   Unspecified injury of unspecified blood vessel at hip and thigh level, right leg

  S75.902   Unspecified injury of unspecified blood vessel at hip and thigh level, left leg

  S75.909   Unspecified injury of unspecified blood vessel at hip and thigh level, unspecified leg

 S75.91   Laceration of unspecified blood vessel at hip and thigh level

  S75.911   Laceration of unspecified blood vessel at hip and thigh level, right leg

  S75.912   Laceration of unspecified blood vessel at hip and thigh level, left leg

  S75.919   Laceration of unspecified blood vessel at hip and thigh level, unspecified leg

 S75.99   Other specified injury of unspecified blood vessel at hip and thigh level

  S75.991   Other specified injury of unspecified blood vessel at hip and thigh level, right leg

  S75.992   Other specified injury of unspecified blood vessel at hip and thigh level, left leg

  S75.999   Other specified injury of unspecified blood vessel at hip and thigh level, unspecified leg

S76   Injury of muscle and tendon at hip and thigh level

Code also any associated open wound (S71.-)

Excludes2:   injury of muscle and tendon at knee (S86)
    sprain of joint and ligament of hip (S73.1)

The following extensions are to be added to each code for category S76:

 a   initial encounter
 d   subsequent encounter
 q   sequela

S76.0   Injury of muscle and tendon of hip

 S76.00   Unspecified injury of muscle and tendon of hip

  S76.001   Unspecified injury of muscle and tendon of right hip

  S76.002   Unspecified injury of muscle and tendon of left hip

  S76.009   Unspecified injury of muscle and tendon of hip, unspecified side

 S76.01   Strain of muscle and tendon of hip

  S76.011   Strain of muscle and tendon of right hip

  S76.012   Strain of muscle and tendon of left hip

  S76.019   Strain of muscle and tendon of hip, unspecified side

 S76.02   Laceration of muscle and tendon of hip

  S76.021   Laceration of muscle and tendon of right hip

  S76.022   Laceration of muscle and tendon of left hip

  S76.029   Laceration of muscle and tendon of hip, unspecified side

 S76.09   Other injury of muscle and tendon of hip

  S76.091   Other injury of muscle and tendon of right hip

  S76.092   Other injury of muscle and tendon of left hip

  S76.099   Other injury of muscle and tendon of hip, unspecified side

S76.1   Injury of quadriceps muscle and tendon

 S76.10   Unspecified injury of quadriceps muscle and tendon

  S76.101   Unspecified injury of right quadriceps muscle and tendon

  S76.102   Unspecified injury of left quadriceps muscle and tendon

  S76.109   Unspecified injury of quadriceps muscle and tendon, unspecified side

 S76.11   Strain of quadriceps muscle and tendon

  S76.111   Strain of right quadriceps muscle and tendon

  S76.112   Strain of left quadriceps muscle and tendon

  S76.119   Strain of quadriceps muscle and tendon, unspecified side

 S76.12   Laceration of quadriceps muscle and tendon

  S76.121   Laceration of right quadriceps muscle and tendon

  S76.122   Laceration of left quadriceps muscle and tendon

  S76.129   Laceration of quadriceps muscle and tendon, unspecified side

 S76.19   Other injury of quadriceps muscle and tendon

  S76.191   Other injury of right quadriceps muscle and tendon

  S76.192   Other injury of left quadriceps muscle and tendon

  S76.199   Other injury of quadriceps muscle and tendon, unspecified side

S76.2   Injury of adductor muscle and tendon of thigh

 S76.20   Unspecified injury of adductor muscle and tendon of thigh

  S76.201   Unspecified injury of adductor muscle and tendon of right thigh

  S76.202   Unspecified injury of adductor muscle and tendon of left thigh

  S76.209   Unspecified injury of adductor muscle and tendon of thigh, unspecified side

 S76.21   Strain of adductor muscle and tendon of thigh

  S76.211   Strain of right adductor muscle and tendon of thigh

  S76.212   Strain of left adductor muscle and tendon of thigh

  S76.219   Strain of adductor muscle and tendon of thigh, unspecified side

 S76.22   Laceration of adductor muscle and tendon of thigh

  S76.221   Laceration of adductor muscle and tendon of right thigh

  S76.222   Laceration of adductor muscle and tendon of left thigh

  S76.229   Laceration of adductor muscle and tendon of thigh, unspecified side

 S76.29   Other injury of adductor muscle and tendon of thigh

  S76.291   Other injury of adductor muscle and tendon of right thigh

  S76.292   Other injury of adductor muscle and tendon of left thigh

  S76.299   Other injury of adductor muscle and tendon of thigh, unspecified side

S76.3   Injury of muscle and tendon of the posterior muscle group at thigh level

 S76.30   Unspecified injury of muscle and tendon of the posterior muscle group at thigh level

  S76.301   Unspecified injury of muscle and tendon of the right posterior muscle group at thigh level

  S76.302   Unspecified injury of muscle and tendon of the left posterior muscle group at thigh level

S76.309   Unspecified injury of muscle and tendon of the posterior muscle group at thigh level, unspecified side

S76.31   Strain of muscle and tendon of the posterior muscle group at thigh level

S76.311   Strain of muscle and tendon of the right posterior muscle group at thigh level

S76.312   Strain of muscle and tendon of the left posterior muscle group at thigh level

S76.319   Strain of muscle and tendon of the posterior muscle group at thigh level, unspecified side

S76.32   Laceration of muscle and tendon of the posterior muscle group at thigh level

S76.321   Laceration of muscle and tendon of the right posterior muscle group at thigh level

S76.322   Laceration of muscle and tendon of the left posterior muscle group at thigh level

S76.329   Laceration of muscle and tendon of the posterior muscle group at thigh level, unspecified side

S76.39   Other injury of muscle and tendon of the posterior muscle group at thigh level

S76.391   Other injury of muscle and tendon of the posterior muscle group at right thigh level

S76.392   Other injury of muscle and tendon of the posterior muscle group at left thigh level

S76.399   Other injury of muscle and tendon of the posterior muscle group at thigh level, unspecified side

S76.8   Injury of other muscles and tendons at thigh level

S76.80   Unspecified injury of other muscles and tendons at thigh level

S76.801   Unspecified injury of other muscles and tendons at right thigh level

S76.802   Unspecified injury of other muscles and tendons at left thigh level

S76.809   Unspecified injury of other muscles and tendons at thigh level, unspecified side

S76.81   Strain of other muscles and tendons at thigh level

S76.811   Strain of other muscles and tendons at right thigh level

S76.812   Strain of other muscles and tendons at left thigh level

S76.819   Strain of other muscles and tendons at thigh level, unspecified side

S76.82   Laceration of other muscles and tendons at thigh level

S76.821   Laceration of other muscles and tendons at right thigh level

S76.822   Laceration of other muscles and tendons at left thigh level

S76.829   Laceration of other muscles and tendons at thigh level, unspecified side

S76.89   Other injury of other muscles and tendons at thigh level

S76.891   Other injury of other muscles and tendons at right thigh level

S76.892   Other injury of other muscles and tendons at left thigh level

S76.899   Other injury of other muscles and tendons at thigh level, unspecified side

S76.9   Injury of unspecified muscles and tendons at thigh level

S76.90   Unspecified injury of unspecified muscles and tendons at thigh level

S76.901   Unspecified injury of unspecified muscles and tendons at right thigh level

S76.902   Unspecified injury of unspecified muscles and tendons at left thigh level

S76.909   Unspecified injury of unspecified muscles and tendons at thigh level, unspecified side

S76.91   Strain of unspecified muscles and tendons at thigh level

S76.911   Strain of unspecified muscles and tendons at right thigh level

S76.912   Strain of unspecified muscles and tendons at left thigh level

S76.919   Strain of unspecified muscles and tendons at thigh level, unspecified side

S76.92   Laceration of unspecified muscles and tendons at thigh level

S76.921   Laceration of unspecified muscles and tendons at right thigh level

S76.922   Laceration of unspecified muscles and tendons at left thigh level

S76.929   Laceration of unspecified muscles and tendons at thigh level, unspecified side

S76.99   Other injury of unspecified muscles and tendons at thigh level

S76.991   Other injury of unspecified muscles and tendons at right thigh level

S76.992   Other injury of unspecified muscles and tendons at left thigh level

S76.999   Other injury of unspecified muscles and tendons at thigh level, unspecified side

S77   **Crushing injury of hip and thigh**

Use additional code(s) for all associated injuries

Excludes2:   crushing injury of ankle and foot (S97.-)
           crushing injury of lower leg (S87.-)

The following extensions are to be added to each code for category S77:

a   initial encounter
d   subsequent encounter
q   sequela

S77.0   Crushing injury of hip

S77.00   Crushing injury of hip, unspecified side

S77.01   Crushing injury of right hip

S77.02   Crushing injury of left hip

S77.1   Crushing injury of thigh

S77.10   Crushing injury of thigh, unspecified side

S77.11   Crushing injury of right thigh

S77.12   Crushing injury of left thigh

S77.2   Crushing injury of hip with thigh

S77.20   Crushing injury of hip with thigh, unspecified side

S77.21   Crushing injury of right hip with thigh

S77.22   Crushing injury of left hip with thigh

S78   **Traumatic amputation of hip and thigh**

An amputation not identified and partial or complete should be coded to complete

Excludes1:   traumatic amputation of knee (S88.0-)

The following extensions are to be added to each code for category S78:

a   initial encounter
d   subsequent encounter
q   sequela

S78.0   Traumatic amputation at hip joint

S78.01   Complete traumatic amputation at hip joint

S78.011   Complete traumatic amputation at right hip joint

S78.012   Complete traumatic amputation at left hip joint

S78.019   Complete traumatic amputation at hip joint, unspecified side

S78.02   Partial traumatic amputation at hip joint

S78.021   Partial traumatic amputation at right hip joint

S78.022   Partial traumatic amputation at left hip joint

S78.029   Partial traumatic amputation at hip joint, unspecified side

S78.1   Traumatic amputation at level between hip and knee
    Excludes1:   traumatic amputation of knee (S88.0-)
    S78.11   Complete traumatic amputation at level between hip and knee
        S78.111   Complete traumatic amputation at level between right hip and knee
        S78.112   Complete traumatic amputation at level between left hip and knee
        S78.119   Complete traumatic amputation at level between hip and knee, unspecified side
    S78.12   Partial traumatic amputation at level between hip and knee
        S78.121   Partial traumatic amputation at level between right hip and knee
        S78.122   Partial traumatic amputation at level between left hip and knee
        S78.129   Partial traumatic amputation at level between hip and knee, unspecified side

S78.9   Traumatic amputation of hip and thigh, level unspecified
    S78.91   Complete traumatic amputation of hip and thigh, level unspecified
        S78.911   Complete traumatic amputation of right hip and thigh, level unspecified
        S78.912   Complete traumatic amputation of left hip and thigh, level unspecified
        S78.919   Complete traumatic amputation of hip and thigh, level unspecified, unspecified side
    S78.92   Partial traumatic amputation of hip and thigh, level unspecified
        S78.921   Partial traumatic amputation of right hip and thigh, level unspecified
        S78.922   Partial traumatic amputation of left hip and thigh, level unspecified
        S78.929   Partial traumatic amputation of hip and thigh, level unspecified, unspecified side

S79   Other and unspecified injuries of hip and thigh
    A fracture not designated as open or closed should be coded to closed
    The following extensions are to be added to each code for subcategories S79.0 and S79.1:
      a   initial encounter for closed fracture
      b   initial encounter for open fracture
      d   subsequent encounter for fracture with routine healing
      g   subsequent encounter for fracture with delayed healing
      j   subsequent encounter for fracture with nonunion
      m   subsequent encounter for fracture with malunion
      q   sequela

S79.0   Physeal fracture of upper end of femur
    Excludes1:   apophyseal fracture of upper end of femur (S72.13-)
               nontraumatic slipped upper femoral epiphysis (M93.0-)
    S79.00   Unspecified physeal fracture of upper end of femur
        S79.001   Unspecified physeal fracture of upper end of right femur
        S79.002   Unspecified physeal fracture of upper end of left femur
        S79.009   Unspecified physeal fracture of upper end of unspecified femur
    S79.01   Salter-Harris Type I physeal fracture of upper end of femur
        Acute on chronic slipped capital femoral epiphysis
        Acute slipped capital femoral epiphysis
        Capital femoral epiphyseal fracture
        Excludes1:   chronic slipped upper femoral epiphysis (nontraumatic) (M93.02-)
        S79.011   Salter-Harris Type I physeal fracture of upper end of right femur
        S79.012   Salter-Harris Type I physeal fracture of upper end of left femur
        S79.019   Salter-Harris Type I physeal fracture of upper end of unspecified femur
    S79.09   Other physeal fracture of upper end of femur
        S79.091   Other physeal fracture of upper end of right femur

        S79.092   Other physeal fracture of upper end of left femur
        S79.099   Other physeal fracture of upper end of unspecified femur

S79.1   Physeal fracture of lower end of femur
    S79.10   Unspecified physeal fracture of lower end of femur
        S79.101   Unspecified physeal fracture of lower end of right femur
        S79.102   Unspecified physeal fracture of lower end of left femur
        S79.109   Unspecified physeal fracture of lower end of unspecified femur
    S79.11   Salter-Harris Type I physeal fracture of lower end of femur
        S79.111   Salter-Harris Type I physeal fracture of lower end of right femur
        S79.112   Salter-Harris Type I physeal fracture of lower end of left femur
        S79.119   Salter-Harris Type I physeal fracture of lower end of unspecified femur
    S79.12   Salter-Harris Type II physeal fracture of lower end of femur
        S79.121   Salter-Harris Type II physeal fracture of lower end of right femur
        S79.122   Salter-Harris Type II physeal fracture of lower end of left femur
        S79.129   Salter-Harris Type II physeal fracture of lower end of unspecified femur
    S79.13   Salter-Harris Type III physeal fracture of lower end of femur
        S79.131   Salter-Harris Type III physeal fracture of lower end of right femur
        S79.132   Salter-Harris Type III physeal fracture of lower end of left femur
        S79.139   Salter-Harris Type III physeal fracture of lower end of unspecified femur
    S79.14   Salter-Harris Type IV physeal fracture of lower end of femur
        S79.141   Salter-Harris Type IV physeal fracture of lower end of right femur
        S79.142   Salter-Harris Type IV physeal fracture of lower end of left femur
        S79.149   Salter-Harris Type IV physeal fracture of lower end of unspecified femur
    S79.19   Other physeal fracture of lower end of femur
        S79.191   Other physeal fracture of lower end of right femur
        S79.192   Other physeal fracture of lower end of left femur
        S79.199   Other physeal fracture of lower end of unspecified femur
    The following extensions are to be added to each code for subcategories S79.8 and S79.9:
      a   initial encounter
      d   subsequent encounter
      q   sequela

S79.8   Other specified injuries of hip and thigh
    S79.81   Other specified injuries of hip
        S79.811   Other specified injuries of right hip
        S79.812   Other specified injuries of left hip
        S79.819   Other specified injuries of hip, unspecified side
    S79.82   Other specified injuries of thigh
        S79.821   Other specified injuries of right thigh
        S79.822   Other specified injuries of left thigh
        S79.829   Other specified injuries of thigh, unspecified side

S79.9   Unspecified injury of hip and thigh
    S79.91   Unspecified injury of hip
        S79.911   Unspecified injury of right hip
        S79.912   Unspecified injury of left hip
        S79.919   Unspecified injury of hip, unspecified side

S79.92   Unspecified injury of thigh
S79.921   Unspecified injury of right thigh
S79.922   Unspecified injury of left thigh
S79.929   Unspecified injury of thigh, unspecified side

INJURIES TO THE KNEE AND LOWER LEG (S80-S89)

Excludes2:   burns and corrosions (T20-T32)
frostbite (T33-T34)
injuries of ankle and foot, except fracture of ankle and
malleolus (S90-S99)
insect bite or sting, venomous (T63.4)

S80 Superficial injury of knee and lower leg
Excludes2:   superficial injury of ankle and foot (S90.-)
The following extensions are to be added to each code for category
S80:
a   initial encounter
d   subsequent encounter
q   sequela

S80.0   Contusion of knee
S80.00   Contusion of unspecified knee
S80.01   Contusion of right knee
S80.02   Contusion of left knee
S80.1   Contusion of lower leg
S80.10   Contusion of unspecified lower leg
S80.11   Contusion of right lower leg
S80.12   Contusion of lower leg
S80.2   Other superficial injuries of knee
S80.21   Abrasion of knee
S80.211   Abrasion, right knee
S80.212   Abrasion, left knee
S80.219   Abrasion, unspecified knee
S80.22   Blister (nonthermal) of knee
S80.221   Blister (nonthermal), right knee
S80.222   Blister (nonthermal), left knee
S80.229   Blister (nonthermal), unspecified knee
S80.24   External constriction of knee
S80.241   External constriction, right knee
S80.242   External constriction, left knee
S80.249   External constriction, unspecified knee
S80.25   Superficial foreign body of knee
Splinter in the knee
S80.251   Superficial foreign body, right knee
S80.252   Superficial foreign body, left knee
S80.259   Superficial foreign body, unspecified knee
S80.26   Insect bite (nonvenomous) of knee
S80.261   Insect bite (nonvenomous), right knee
S80.262   Insect bite (nonvenomous), left knee
S80.269   Insect bite (nonvenomous), unspecified knee
S80.27   Other superficial bite of knee
Excludes1:   open bite of knee (S81.05-)
S80.271   Other superficial bite of right knee
S80.272   Other superficial bite of left knee
S80.279   Other superficial bite of unspecified knee
S80.8   Other superficial injuries of lower leg
S80.81   Abrasion of lower leg
S80.811   Abrasion, right lower leg
S80.812   Abrasion, left lower leg
S80.819   Abrasion, unspecified lower leg
S80.82   Blister (nonthermal) of lower leg
S80.821   Blister (nonthermal), right lower leg
S80.822   Blister (nonthermal), left lower leg
S80.829   Blister (nonthermal), unspecified lower leg
S80.84   External constriction of lower leg
S80.841   External constriction, right lower leg
S80.842   External constriction, left lower leg
S80.849   External constriction, unspecified lower leg
S80.85   Superficial foreign body of lower leg
Splinter in the lower leg

S80.851   Superficial foreign body, right lower leg
S80.852   Superficial foreign body, left lower leg
S80.859   Superficial foreign body, unspecified lower leg
S80.86   Insect bite (nonvenomous) of lower leg
S80.861   Insect bite (nonvenomous), right lower leg
S80.862   Insect bite (nonvenomous), left lower leg
S80.869   Insect bite (nonvenomous), unspecified lower leg
S80.87   Other superficial bite of lower leg
Excludes1: open bite of lower leg (S81.85-)
S80.871   Other superficial bite, right lower leg
S80.872   Other superficial bite, left lower leg
S80.879   Other superficial bite, unspecified lower leg
S80.9   Unspecified superficial injury of knee and lower leg
S80.91   Unspecified superficial injury of knee
S80.911   Unspecified superficial injury of right knee
S80.912   Unspecified superficial injury of left knee
S80.919   Unspecified superficial injury of unspecified knee
S80.92   Unspecified superficial injury of lower leg
S80.921   Unspecified superficial injury of right lower leg
S80.922   Unspecified superficial injury of left lower leg
S80.929   Unspecified superficial injury of unspecified lower leg

S81 Open wound of knee and lower leg
Code also any associated wound infection
Excludes1:   open fracture of knee and lower leg (S82.-)
traumatic amputation of lower leg (S88.-)
Excludes2:   open wound of ankle and foot (S91.-)
The following extensions are to be added to each code for category
S81:
a   initial encounter
d   subsequent encounter
q   sequela
S81.0   Open wound of knee
S81.00   Unspecified open wound of knee
S81.001   Unspecified open wound, right knee
S81.002   Unspecified open wound, left knee
S81.009   Unspecified open wound, unspecified knee
S81.01   Laceration without foreign body of knee
S81.011   Laceration without foreign body, right knee
S81.012   Laceration without foreign body, left knee
S81.019   Laceration without foreign body, unspecified knee
S81.02   Laceration with foreign body of knee
S81.021   Laceration with foreign body, right knee
S81.022   Laceration with foreign body, left knee
S81.029   Laceration with foreign body, unspecified knee
S81.03   Puncture wound without foreign body of knee
S81.031   Puncture wound without foreign body, right knee
S81.032   Puncture wound without foreign body, left knee
S81.039   Puncture wound without foreign body, unspecified knee
S81.04   Puncture wound with foreign body of knee
S81.041   Puncture wound with foreign body, right knee
S81.042   Puncture wound with foreign body, left knee
S81.049   Puncture wound with foreign body, unspecified knee
S81.05   Open bite of knee
Bite of knee NOS
Excludes1:   superficial bite of knee (S80.36-, S80.37-)
S81.051   Open bite, right knee
S81.052   Open bite, left knee
S81.059   Open bite, unspecified knee

S81.8 **Open wound of lower leg**
- **S81.80** **Unspecified open wound of lower leg**
  - **S81.801** Unspecified open wound, right lower leg
  - **S81.802** Unspecified open wound, left lower leg
  - **S81.809** Unspecified open wound, unspecified lower leg
- **S81.81** **Laceration without foreign body of lower leg**
  - **S81.811** Laceration without foreign body, right lower leg
  - **S81.812** Laceration without foreign body, left lower leg
  - **S81.819** Laceration without foreign body, unspecified lower leg
- **S81.82** **Laceration with foreign body of lower leg**
  - **S81.821** Laceration with foreign body, right lower leg
  - **S81.822** Laceration with foreign body, left lower leg
  - **S81.829** Laceration with foreign body, unspecified lower leg
- **S81.83** **Puncture wound without foreign body of lower leg**
  - **S81.831** Puncture wound without foreign body, right lower leg
  - **S81.832** Puncture wound without foreign body, left lower leg
  - **S81.839** Puncture wound without foreign body, unspecified lower leg
- **S81.84** **Puncture wound with foreign body of lower leg**
  - **S81.841** Puncture wound with foreign body, right lower leg
  - **S81.842** Puncture wound with foreign body, left lower leg
  - **S81.849** Puncture wound with foreign body, unspecified lower leg
- **S81.85** **Open bite of lower leg**
  Bite of lower leg NOS
  Excludes1: superficial bite of lower leg (S80.86-, S80.87-)
  - **S81.851** Open bite, right lower leg
  - **S81.852** Open bite, left lower leg
  - **S81.859** Open bite, unspecified lower leg

S82 Fracture of lower leg, including ankle
A fracture not indicated as displaced or nondisplaced should be coded to displaced
Includes: fracture of malleolus
Excludes1: traumatic amputation of lower leg (S88.-)
Excludes2: fracture of foot, except ankle (S92.-)
Note: a fracture not designated as open or closed should be coded to closed
Note: the open fracture designations are based on the Gustilo open fracture classification

The following extensions are to be added to each code for category S82:
- a initial encounter for closed fracture
- b initial encounter for open fracture type I or II
- c initial encounter for open fracture type IIIA, IIIB, or IIIC
- d subsequent encounter for closed fracture with routine healing
- e subsequent encounter for open fracture type I or II with routine healing
- f subsequent encounter for open fracture type IIIA, IIIB, or IIIC with routine healing
- g subsequent encounter for closed fracture with delayed healing
- h subsequent encounter for open fracture type I or II with delayed healing
- i subsequent encounter for open fracture type IIIA, IIIB, or IIIC with delayed healing
- j subsequent encounter for closed fracture with nonunion
- k subsequent encounter for open fracture type I or II with nonunion
- l subsequent encounter for open fracture type IIIA, IIIB, or IIIC with nonunion
- m subsequent encounter for closed fracture with malunion
- n subsequent encounter for open fracture type I or II with malunion
- o subsequent encounter for open fracture type IIIA, IIIB, or IIIC with malunion
- q sequela

S82.0 **Fracture of patella**
Knee cap
- **S82.00** **Unspecified fracture of patella**
  - **S82.001** Unspecified fracture of right patella
  - **S82.002** Unspecified fracture of left patella
  - **S82.009** Unspecified fracture of unspecified patella
- **S82.01** **Osteochondral fracture of patella**
  - **S82.011** Displaced osteochondral fracture of right patella
  - **S82.012** Displaced osteochondral fracture of left patella
  - **S82.013** Displaced osteochondral fracture of unspecified patella
  - **S82.014** Nondisplaced osteochondral fracture of right patella
  - **S82.015** Nondisplaced osteochondral fracture of left patella
  - **S82.016** Nondisplaced osteochondral fracture of unspecified patella
- **S82.02** **Longitudinal fracture of patella**
  - **S82.021** Displaced longitudinal fracture of right patella
  - **S82.022** Displaced longitudinal fracture of left patella
  - **S82.023** Displaced longitudinal fracture of unspecified patella
  - **S82.024** Nondisplaced longitudinal fracture of right patella
  - **S82.025** Nondisplaced longitudinal fracture of left patella
  - **S82.026** Nondisplaced longitudinal fracture of unspecified patella
- **S82.03** **Transverse fracture of patella**
  - **S82.031** Displaced transverse fracture of right patella
  - **S82.032** Displaced transverse fracture of left patella
  - **S82.033** Displaced transverse fracture of unspecified patella
  - **S82.034** Nondisplaced transverse fracture of right patella
  - **S82.035** Nondisplaced transverse fracture of left patella
  - **S82.036** Nondisplaced transverse fracture of unspecified patella
- **S82.04** **Comminuted fracture of patella**
  - **S82.041** Displaced comminuted fracture of right patella
  - **S82.042** Displaced comminuted fracture of left patella
  - **S82.043** Displaced comminuted fracture of unspecified patella

S82.044　Nondisplaced comminuted fracture of right patella
S82.045　Nondisplaced comminuted fracture of left patella
S82.046　Nondisplaced comminuted fracture of unspecified patella
S82.09　　Other fracture of patella
S82.091　Other fracture of right patella
S82.092　Other fracture of left patella
S82.099　Other fracture of unspecified patella
S82.1　Fracture of upper end of tibia
　　　Fracture of proximal end of tibia
　　Excludes2:　fracture of shaft of tibia (S82.2-)
　　　　　　physeal fracture of upper end of tibia (S89.0-)
S82.10　　Unspecified fracture of upper end of tibia
S82.101　Unspecified fracture of upper end of right tibia
S82.102　Unspecified fracture of upper end of left tibia
S82.109　Unspecified fracture of upper end of unspecified tibia
S82.11　　Fracture of tibial spine
S82.111　Displaced fracture of right tibial spine
S82.112　Displaced fracture of left tibial spine
S82.113　Displaced fracture of unspecified tibial spine
S82.114　Nondisplaced fracture of right tibial spine
S82.115　Nondisplaced fracture of left tibial spine
S82.116　Nondisplaced fracture of unspecified tibial spine
S82.12　　Fracture of lateral condyle of tibia
S82.121　Displaced fracture of lateral condyle of right tibia
S82.122　Displaced fracture of lateral condyle of left tibia
S82.123　Displaced fracture of lateral condyle of unspecified tibia
S82.124　Nondisplaced fracture of lateral condyle of right tibia
S82.125　Nondisplaced fracture of lateral condyle of left tibia
S82.126　Nondisplaced fracture of lateral condyle of unspecified tibia
S82.13　　Fracture of medial condyle of tibia
S82.131　Displaced fracture of medial condyle of right tibia
S82.132　Displaced fracture of medial condyle of left tibia
S82.133　Displaced fracture of medial condyle of unspecified tibia
S82.134　Nondisplaced fracture of medial condyle of right tibia
S82.135　Nondisplaced fracture of medial condyle of left tibia
S82.136　Nondisplaced fracture of medial condyle of unspecified tibia
S82.14　　Bicondylar fracture of tibia
　　　　Fracture of tibial plateau NOS
S82.141　Displaced bicondylar fracture of right tibia
S82.142　Displaced bicondylar fracture of left tibia
S82.143　Displaced bicondylar fracture of unspecified tibia
S82.144　Nondisplaced bicondylar fracture of right tibia
S82.145　Nondisplaced bicondylar fracture of left tibia
S82.146　Nondisplaced bicondylar fracture of unspecified tibia
S82.15　　Fracture of tibial tuberosity
S82.151　Displaced fracture of right tibial tuberosity
S82.152　Displaced fracture of left tibial tuberosity
S82.153　Displaced fracture of unspecified tibial tuberosity
S82.154　Nondisplaced fracture of right tibial tuberosity
S82.155　Nondisplaced fracture of left tibial tuberosity

S82.156　Nondisplaced fracture of unspecified tibial tuberosity
S82.16　　Torus fracture of upper end of tibia
　　　Note: open fracture extensions do not apply to these codes
S82.161　Torus fracture of upper end of right tibia
S82.162　Torus fracture of upper end of left tibia
S82.169　Torus fracture of upper end of unspecified tibia
S82.19　　Other fracture of upper end of tibia
S82.191　Other fracture of upper end of right tibia
S82.192　Other fracture of upper end of left tibia
S82.199　Other fracture of upper end of unspecified tibia
S82.2　Fracture of shaft of tibia
S82.20　　Unspecified fracture of shaft of tibia
　　　　Fracture of tibia NOS
S82.201　Unspecified fracture of shaft of right tibia
S82.202　Unspecified fracture of shaft of left tibia
S82.209　Unspecified fracture of shaft of unspecified tibia
S82.22　　Transverse fracture of shaft of tibia
S82.221　Displaced transverse fracture of shaft of right tibia
S82.222　Displaced transverse fracture of shaft of left tibia
S82.223　Displaced transverse fracture of shaft of unspecified tibia
S82.224　Nondisplaced transverse fracture of shaft of right tibia
S82.225　Nondisplaced transverse fracture of shaft of left tibia
S82.226　Nondisplaced transverse fracture of shaft of unspecified tibia
S82.23　　Oblique fracture of shaft of tibia
S82.231　Displaced oblique fracture of shaft of right tibia
S82.232　Displaced oblique fracture of shaft of left tibia
S82.233　Displaced oblique fracture of shaft of unspecified tibia
S82.234　Nondisplaced oblique fracture of shaft of right tibia
S82.235　Nondisplaced oblique fracture of shaft of left tibia
S82.236　Nondisplaced oblique fracture of shaft of unspecified tibia
S82.24　　Spiral fracture of shaft of tibia
　　　　Toddler fracture
S82.241　Displaced spiral fracture of shaft of right tibia
S82.242　Displaced spiral fracture of shaft of left tibia
S82.243　Displaced spiral fracture of shaft of unspecified tibia
S82.244　Nondisplaced spiral fracture of shaft of right tibia
S82.245　Nondisplaced spiral fracture of shaft of left tibia
S82.246　Nondisplaced spiral fracture of shaft of unspecified tibia
S82.25　　Comminuted fracture of shaft of tibia
S82.251　Displaced comminuted fracture of shaft of right tibia
S82.252　Displaced comminuted fracture of shaft of left tibia
S82.253　Displaced comminuted fracture of shaft of unspecified tibia
S82.254　Nondisplaced comminuted fracture of shaft of right tibia
S82.255　Nondisplaced comminuted fracture of shaft of left tibia
S82.256　Nondisplaced comminuted fracture of shaft of unspecified tibia

    S82.26   Segmental fracture of shaft of tibia
        S82.261 Displaced segmental fracture of shaft of right tibia
        S82.262 Displaced segmental fracture of shaft of left tibia
        S82.263 Displaced segmental fracture of shaft of unspecified tibia
        S82.264 Nondisplaced segmental fracture of shaft of right tibia
        S82.265 Nondisplaced segmental fracture of shaft of left tibia
        S82.266 Nondisplaced segmental fracture of shaft of unspecified tibia
    S82.29   Other fracture of shaft of tibia
        S82.291 Other fracture of shaft of right tibia
        S82.292 Other fracture of shaft of left tibia
        S82.299 Other fracture of shaft of unspecified tibia

S82.3   Fracture of lower end of tibia
    Excludes1: bimalleolar fracture of lower leg (S82.81-)
              fracture of medial malleolus alone (S82.5-)
              Maisonneuve's fracture (S82.83-)
              pilon fracture of distal tibia (S82.84-)
              trimalleolar fractures of lower leg (S82.82-)
    S82.30   Unspecified fracture of lower end of tibia
        S82.301 Unspecified fracture of lower end of right tibia
        S82.302 Unspecified fracture of lower end of left tibia
        S82.309 Unspecified fracture of lower end of unspecified tibia
    S82.31   Torus fracture of lower end of tibia
              Note: open fracture extensions do not apply to these codes
        S82.311 Torus fracture of lower end of right tibia
        S82.312 Torus fracture of lower end of left tibia
        S82.319 Torus fracture of lower end of unspecified tibia
    S82.39   Other fracture of lower end of tibia
        S82.391 Other fracture of lower end of right tibia
        S82.392 Other fracture of lower end of left tibia
        S82.399 Other fracture of lower end of unspecified tibia

S82.4   Fracture of shaft of fibula
    Excludes2: fracture of lateral malleolus alone (S82.6-)
    S82.40   Unspecified fracture of shaft of fibula
        S82.401 Unspecified fracture of shaft of right fibula
        S82.402 Unspecified fracture of shaft of left fibula
        S82.409 Unspecified fracture of shaft of unspecified fibula
    S82.42   Transverse fracture of shaft of fibula
        S82.421 Displaced transverse fracture of shaft of right fibula
        S82.422 Displaced transverse fracture of shaft of left fibula
        S82.423 Displaced transverse fracture of shaft of unspecified fibula
        S82.424 Nondisplaced transverse fracture of shaft of right fibula
        S82.425 Nondisplaced transverse fracture of shaft of left fibula
        S82.426 Nondisplaced transverse fracture of shaft of unspecified fibula
    S82.43   Oblique fracture of shaft of fibula
        S82.431 Displaced oblique fracture of shaft of right fibula
        S82.432 Displaced oblique fracture of shaft of left fibula
        S82.433 Displaced oblique fracture of shaft of unspecified fibula
        S82.434 Nondisplaced oblique fracture of shaft of right fibula
        S82.435 Nondisplaced oblique fracture of shaft of left fibula

        S82.436 Nondisplaced oblique fracture of shaft of unspecified fibula
    S82.44   Spiral fracture of shaft of fibula
        S82.441 Displaced spiral fracture of shaft of right fibula
        S82.442 Displaced spiral fracture of shaft of left fibula
        S82.443 Displaced spiral fracture of shaft of unspecified fibula
        S82.444 Nondisplaced spiral fracture of shaft of right fibula
        S82.445 Nondisplaced spiral fracture of shaft of left fibular
        S82.446 Nondisplaced spiral fracture of shaft of unspecified fibula
    S82.45   Comminuted fracture of shaft of fibula
        S82.451 Displaced comminuted fracture of shaft of right fibula
        S82.452 Displaced comminuted fracture of shaft of left fibula
        S82.453 Displaced comminuted fracture of shaft of unspecified fibula
        S82.454 Nondisplaced comminuted fracture of shaft of right fibula
        S82.455 Nondisplaced comminuted fracture of shaft of left fibula
        S82.456 Nondisplaced comminuted fracture of shaft of unspecified fibula
    S82.46   Segmental fracture of shaft of fibula
        S82.461 Displaced segmental fracture of shaft of right fibula
        S82.462 Displaced segmental fracture of shaft of left fibula
        S82.463 Displaced segmental fracture of shaft of unspecified fibula
        S82.464 Nondisplaced segmental fracture of shaft of right fibula
        S82.465 Nondisplaced segmental fracture of shaft of left fibula
        S82.466 Nondisplaced segmental fracture of shaft of unspecified fibula
    S82.49   Other fracture of shaft of fibula
        S82.491 Other fracture of shaft of right fibula
        S82.492 Other fracture of shaft of left fibula
        S82.499 Other fracture of shaft of unspecified fibula

S82.5   Fracture of medial malleolus
    Excludes1: pilon fracture of distal tibia (S82.84-)
              Salter-Harris type III of lower end of tibia (S89.13-)
              Salter-Harris type IV of lower end of tibia (S89.14-)
    S82.51   Displaced fracture of medial malleolus of right tibia
    S82.52   Displaced fracture of medial malleolus of left tibia
    S82.53   Displaced fracture of medial malleolus of unspecified tibia
    S82.54   Nondisplaced fracture of medial malleolus of right tibia
    S82.55   Nondisplaced fracture of medial malleolus of left tibia
    S82.56   Nondisplaced fracture of medial malleolus of unspecified tibia

S82.6   Fracture of lateral malleolus
    Excludes1: pilon fracture of distal tibia (S82.84-)
    S82.61   Displaced fracture of lateral malleolus of right fibula
    S82.62   Displaced fracture of lateral malleolus of left fibula
    S82.63   Displaced fracture of lateral malleolus of unspecified fibula
    S82.64   Nondisplaced fracture of lateral malleolus of right fibula
    S82.65   Nondisplaced fracture of lateral malleolus of left fibula
    S82.66   Nondisplaced fracture of lateral malleolus of unspecified fibula

S82.8 Other fractures of lower leg

S82.81 Torus fracture of upper end of fibula
Note: open fracture extensions do not apply to these codes

S82.811 Torus fracture of upper end of right fibula

S82.812 Torus fracture of upper end of left fibula

S82.819 Torus fracture of upper end of unspecified fibula

S82.82 Torus fracture of lower end of fibula
Note: open fracture extensions do not apply to these codes

S82.821 Torus fracture of lower end of right fibula

S82.822 Torus fracture of lower end of left fibula

S82.829 Torus fracture of lower end of unspecified fibula

S82.83 Other fracture of upper and lower end of fibula

S82.831 Other fracture of upper and lower end of right fibula

S82.832 Other fracture of upper and lower end of left fibula

S82.839 Other fracture of upper and lower end of unspecified fibula

S82.84 Bimalleolar fracture of lower leg

S82.841 Displaced bimalleolar fracture of right lower leg

S82.842 Displaced bimalleolar fracture of left lower leg

S82.843 Displaced bimalleolar fracture of unspecified lower leg

S82.844 Nondisplaced bimalleolar fracture of right lower leg

S82.845 Nondisplaced bimalleolar fracture of left lower leg

S82.846 Nondisplaced bimalleolar fracture of unspecified lower leg

S82.85 Trimalleolar fracture of lower leg

S82.851 Displaced trimalleolar fracture of right lower leg

S82.852 Displaced trimalleolar fracture of left lower leg

S82.853 Displaced trimalleolar fracture of lower leg, unspecified side

S82.854 Nondisplaced trimalleolar fracture of right lower leg

S82.855 Nondisplaced trimalleolar fracture of left lower leg

S82.856 Nondisplaced trimalleolar fracture of lower leg, unspecified side

S82.86 Maisonneuve's fracture

S82.861 Displaced Maisonneuve's fracture of right leg

S82.862 Displaced Maisonneuve's fracture of left leg

S82.863 Displaced Maisonneuve's fracture of unspecified leg

S82.864 Nondisplaced Maisonneuve's fracture of right leg

S82.865 Nondisplaced Maisonneuve's fracture of left leg

S82.866 Nondisplaced Maisonneuve's fracture of unspecified leg

S82.87 Pilon fracture of tibia

S82.871 Displaced pilon fracture of right tibia

S82.872 Displaced pilon fracture of left tibia

S82.873 Displaced pilon fracture of unspecified tibia

S82.874 Nondisplaced pilon fracture of right tibia

S82.875 Nondisplaced pilon fracture of left tibia

S82.876 Nondisplaced pilon fracture of unspecified tibia

S82.89 Other fractures of lower leg
Fracture of ankle NOS

S82.891 Other fracture of right lower leg

S82.892 Other fracture of left lower leg

S82.899 Other fracture of unspecified lower leg

S82.9 Unspecified fracture of lower leg

S82.90 Unspecified fracture of unspecified lower leg

S82.91 Unspecified fracture of right lower leg

S82.92 Unspecified fracture of left lower leg

S83 Dislocation and sprain of joints and ligaments of knee

Includes: avulsion of joint or ligament of knee
laceration of joint or ligament of knee
sprain of joint or ligament of knee
traumatic hemarthrosis of joint or ligament of knee
traumatic rupture of joint or ligament of knee
traumatic subluxation of joint or ligament of knee
traumatic tear of joint or ligament of knee

Excludes1:   derangement of patella (M22.0-M22.3)
internal derangement of knee (M23.-)
old dislocation of knee (M24.36)
pathological dislocation of knee (M24.36)
recurrent dislocation of knee (M22.0)

Excludes2:   strain of muscle and tendon of lower leg (S86.-)
The following extensions are to be added to each code for category S83:
a   initial encounter
d   subsequent encounter
q   sequela

S83.0 Subluxation and dislocation of patella

S83.00 Unspecified subluxation and dislocation of patella

S83.001 Unspecified subluxation of right patella

S83.002 Unspecified subluxation of left patella

S83.003 Unspecified subluxation of unspecified patella

S83.004 Unspecified dislocation of right patella

S83.005 Unspecified dislocation of left patella

S83.006 Unspecified dislocation of unspecified patella

S83.01 Lateral subluxation and dislocation of patella

S83.011 Lateral subluxation of right patella

S83.012 Lateral subluxation of left patella

S83.013 Lateral subluxation of patella, unspecified side

S83.014 Lateral dislocation of right patella

S83.015 Lateral dislocation of left patella

S83.016 Lateral dislocation of patella, unspecified side

S83.09 Other subluxation and dislocation of patella

S83.091 Other subluxation of right patella

S83.092 Other subluxation of left patella

S83.093 Other subluxation of unspecified patella

S83.094 Other dislocation of right patella

S83.095 Other dislocation of left patella

S83.096 Other dislocation of unspecified patella

S83.1 Subluxation and dislocation of knee

S83.10 Unspecified subluxation and dislocation of knee

S83.101 Unspecified subluxation of right knee

S83.102 Unspecified subluxation of left knee

S83.103 Unspecified subluxation of unspecified knee

S83.104 Unspecified dislocation of right knee

S83.105 Unspecified dislocation of left knee

S83.106 Unspecified dislocation of unspecified knee

S83.11 Anterior subluxation and dislocation of proximal end of tibia
Posterior subluxation and dislocation of distal end of femur

S83.111 Anterior subluxation of proximal end of tibia, right knee

S83.112 Anterior subluxation of proximal end of tibia, left knee

S83.113 Anterior subluxation of proximal end of tibia, unspecified knee

S83.114 Anterior dislocation of proximal end of tibia, right knee

S83.115 Anterior dislocation of proximal end of tibia, left knee

S83.116 Anterior dislocation of proximal end of tibia, unspecified knee

S83.12 Posterior subluxation and dislocation of proximal end of tibia
Anterior dislocation of distal end of femur

S83.121 Posterior subluxation of proximal end of tibia, right knee

S83.122 Posterior subluxation of proximal end of tibia, left knee

S83.123 Posterior subluxation of proximal end of tibia, unspecified knee

S83.124 Posterior dislocation of proximal end of tibia, right knee

S83.125 Posterior dislocation of proximal end of tibia, left knee

S83.126 Posterior dislocation of proximal end of tibia, unspecified knee

S83.13 Medial subluxation and dislocation of proximal end of tibia

S83.131 Medial subluxation of proximal end of tibia, right knee

S83.132 Medial subluxation of proximal end of tibia, left knee

S83.133 Medial subluxation of proximal end of tibia, unspecified knee

S83.134 Medial dislocation of proximal end of tibia, right knee

S83.135 Medial dislocation of proximal end of tibia, left knee

S83.136 Medial dislocation of proximal end of tibia, unspecified knee

S83.14 Lateral subluxation and dislocation of proximal end of tibia

S83.141 Lateral subluxation of proximal end of tibia, right knee

S83.142 Lateral subluxation of proximal end of tibia, left knee

S83.143 Lateral subluxation of proximal end of tibia, unspecified knee

S83.144 Lateral dislocation of proximal end of tibia, right knee

S83.145 Lateral dislocation of proximal end of tibia, left knee

S83.146 Lateral dislocation of proximal end of tibia, unspecified knee

S83.19 Other subluxation and dislocation of knee

S83.191 Other subluxation of right knee

S83.192 Other subluxation of left knee

S83.193 Other subluxation of unspecified knee

S83.194 Other dislocation of right knee

S83.195 Other dislocation of left knee

S83.196 Other dislocation of unspecified knee

S83.2 Tear of meniscus, current injury

Excludes1:   old bucket-handle tear (M23.2)

S83.20 Tear of unspecified meniscus, current injury
Tear of meniscus of knee NOS

S83.200 Bucket-handle tear of unspecified meniscus, current injury, right knee

S83.201 Bucket-handle tear of unspecified meniscus, current injury, left knee

S83.202 Bucket-handle tear of unspecified meniscus, current injury, unspecified knee

S83.203 Other tear of unspecified meniscus, current injury, right knee

S83.204 Other tear of unspecified meniscus, current injury, left knee

S83.205 Other tear of unspecified meniscus, current injury, unspecified knee

S83.206 Unspecified tear of unspecified meniscus, current injury, right knee

S83.207 Unspecified tear of unspecified meniscus, current injury, left knee

S83.209 Unspecified tear of unspecified meniscus, current injury, unspecified knee

S83.21 Bucket-handle tear of medial meniscus, current injury

S83.211 Bucket-handle tear of medial meniscus, current injury, right knee

S83.212 Bucket-handle tear of medial meniscus, current injury, left knee

S83.219 Bucket-handle tear of medial meniscus, current injury, unspecified knee

S83.22 Peripheral tear of medial meniscus, current injury

S83.221 Peripheral tear of medial meniscus, current injury, right knee

S83.222 Peripheral tear of medial meniscus, current injury, left knee

S83.229 Peripheral tear of medial meniscus, current injury, unspecifed knee

S83.23 Complex tear of medial meniscus, current injury

S83.231 Complex tear of medial meniscus, current injury, right knee

S83.232 Complex tear of medial meniscus, current injury, left knee

S83.239 Complex tear of medial meniscus, current injury, unspecified knee

S83.24 Other tear of medial meniscus, current injury

S83.241 Other tear of medial meniscus, current injury, right knee

S83.242 Other tear of medial meniscus, current injury, left knee

S83.249 Other tear of medial meniscus, current injury, unspecified knee

S83.25 Bucket-handle tear of lateral meniscus, current injury

S83.251 Bucket-handle tear of lateral meniscus, current injury, right knee

S83.252 Bucket-handle tear of lateral meniscus, current injury, left knee

S83.259 Bucket-handle tear of lateral meniscus, current injury, unspecified knee

S83.26 Peripheral tear of lateral meniscus, current injury

S83.261 Peripheral tear of lateral meniscus, current injury, right knee

S83.262 Peripheral tear of lateral meniscus, current injury, left knee

S83.269 Peripheral tear of lateral meniscus, current injury, unspecified knee

S83.27 Complex tear of lateral meniscus, current injury

S83.271 Complex tear of lateral meniscus, current injury, right knee

S83.272 Complex tear of lateral meniscus, current injury, left knee

S83.279 Complex tear of lateral meniscus, current injury, unspecified knee

S83.28 Other tear of lateral meniscus, current injury

S83.281 Other tear of lateral meniscus, current injury, right knee

S83.282 Other tear of lateral meniscus, current injury, left knee

S83.289 Other tear of lateral meniscus, current injury, unspecified knee

S83.3 Tear of articular cartilage of knee, current

S83.30 Tear of articular cartilage of knee, current, unspecified side

S83.31 Tear of articular cartilage of right knee, current

S83.32 Tear of articular cartilage of left knee, current

S83.4 Sprain of collateral ligament of knee

S83.40 Sprain of unspecifed collateral ligament of knee

S83.401 Sprain of unspecifed collateral ligament of right knee

S83.402 Sprain of unspecifed collateral ligament of left knee

S83.409 Sprain of unspecifed collateral ligament of unspecified knee

S83.41 Sprain of medial collateral ligament of knee
Sprain of tibial collateral ligament

S83.411 Sprain of medial collateral ligament of right knee

S83.412   Sprain of medial collateral ligament of left knee

S83.419   Sprain of medial collateral ligament of unspecified knee

S83.42   Sprain of lateral collateral ligament of knee
Sprain of fibular collateral ligament

S83.421   Sprain of lateral collateral ligament of right knee

S83.422   Sprain of lateral collateral ligament of left knee

S83.429   Sprain of lateral collateral ligament of unspecified knee

S83.5   Sprain of cruciate ligament of knee

S83.50   Sprain of unspecified cruciate ligament of knee

S83.501   Sprain of unspecified cruciate ligament of right knee

S83.502   Sprain of unspecified cruciate ligament of left knee

S83.509   Sprain of unspecified cruciate ligament of unspecified knee

S83.51   Sprain of anterior cruciate ligament of knee

S83.511   Sprain of anterior cruciate ligament of right knee

S83.512   Sprain of anterior cruciate ligament of left knee

S83.519   Sprain of anterior cruciate ligament of unspecified knee

S83.52   Sprain of posterior cruciate ligament of knee

S83.521   Sprain of posterior cruciate ligament of right knee

S83.522   Sprain of posterior cruciate ligament of left knee

S83.529   Sprain of posterior cruciate ligament of unspecified knee

S83.6   Sprain of the superior tibiofibular joint and ligament

S83.60   Sprain of the superior tibiofibular joint and ligament, unspecified knee

S83.61   Sprain of the superior tibiofibular joint and ligament, right knee

S83.62   Sprain of the superior tibiofibular joint and ligament, left knee

S83.8   Sprain of other sites of knee

S83.81   Sprain of patellar ligament of knee

S83.811   Sprain of patellar ligament of right knee

S83.812   Sprain of patellar ligament of left knee

S83.819   Sprain of patellar ligament of unspecified knee

S83.89   Sprain of other sites of knee

S83.891   Sprain of other sites of right knee

S83.892   Sprain of other sites of left knee

S83.899   Sprain of other sites of unspecified knee

S83.9   Sprain of unspecified site of knee

S83.90   Sprain of unspecified site of knee, unspecified side

S83.91   Sprain of unspecified site of right knee

S83.92   Sprain of unspecified site of left knee

S84   Injury of nerves at lower leg level
Code also any associated open wound (S81.-)
Excludes2:   injury of nerves at ankle and foot level (S94.-)
The following extensions are to be added to each code for category S84:
a   initial encounter
d   subsequent encounter
q   sequela

S84.0   Injury of tibial nerve at lower leg level

S84.00   Injury of tibial nerve at lower leg level, unspecified leg

S84.01   Injury of tibial nerve at lower leg level, right leg

S84.02   Injury of tibial nerve at lower leg level, left leg

S84.1   Injury of peroneal nerve at lower leg level

S84.10   Injury of peroneal nerve at lower leg level, unspecified leg

S84.11   Injury of peroneal nerve at lower leg level, right leg

S84.12   Injury of peroneal nerve at lower leg level, left leg

S84.2   Injury of cutaneous sensory nerve at lower leg level

S84.20   Injury of cutaneous sensory nerve at lower leg level, unspecified leg

S84.21   Injury of cutaneous sensory nerve at lower leg level, right leg

S84.22   Injury of cutaneous sensory nerve at lower leg level, left leg

S84.8   Injury of other nerves at lower leg level

S84.8x   Injury of other nerves at lower leg level

S84.8x1   Injury of other nerves at lower leg level, right leg

S84.8x2   Injury of other nerves at lower leg level, left leg

S84.8x9   Injury of other nerves at lower leg level, unspecified leg

S84.9   Injury of unspecified nerve at lower leg level

S84.90   Injury of unspecified nerve at lower leg level, unspecified leg

S84.91   Injury of unspecified nerve at lower leg level, right leg

S84.92   Injury of unspecified nerve at lower leg level, left leg

S85   Injury of blood vessels at lower leg level
Code also any associated open wound (S81.-)
Excludes2:   injury of blood vessels at ankle and foot level (S95.-)
The following extensions are to be added to each code for category S85:
a   initial encounter
d   subsequent encounter
q   sequela

S85.0   Injury of popliteal artery

S85.00   Unspecified injury of popliteal artery

S85.001   Unspecified injury of popliteal artery, right leg

S85.002   Unspecified injury of popliteal artery, left leg

S85.009   Unspecified injury of popliteal artery, unspecified leg

S85.01   Laceration of popliteal artery

S85.011   Laceration of popliteal artery, right leg

S85.012   Laceration of popliteal artery, left leg

S85.019   Laceration of popliteal artery, unspecified leg

S85.09   Other specified injury of popliteal artery

S85.091   Other specified injury of popliteal artery, right leg

S85.092   Other specified injury of popliteal artery, left leg

S85.099   Other specified injury of popliteal artery, unspecified leg

S85.1   Injury of tibial artery

S85.10   Unspecified injury of unspecified tibial artery
Injury of tibial artery NOS

S85.101   Unspecified injury of unspecified tibial artery, right leg

S85.102   Unspecified injury of unspecified tibial artery, left leg

S85.109   Unspecified injury of unspecified tibial artery, unspecified leg

S85.11   Laceration of unspecified tibial artery

S85.111   Laceration of unspecified tibial artery, right leg

S85.112   Laceration of unspecified tibial artery, left leg

S85.119   Laceration of unspecified tibial artery, unspecified leg

S85.12   Other specified injury of unspecified tibial artery

S85.121   Other specified injury of unspecified tibial artery, right leg

S85.122   Other specified injury of unspecified tibial artery, left leg

S85.129   Other specified injury of unspecified tibial artery, unspecified leg

S85.13   Unspecified injury of anterior tibial artery

    S85.131   Unspecified injury of anterior tibial artery, right leg

    S85.132   Unspecified injury of anterior tibial artery, left leg

    S85.139   Unspecified injury of anterior tibial artery, unspecified leg

S85.14   Laceration of anterior tibial artery

    S85.141   Laceration of anterior tibial artery, right leg

    S85.142   Laceration of anterior tibial artery, left leg

    S85.149   Laceration of anterior tibial artery, unspecified leg

S85.15   Other specified injury of anterior tibial artery

    S85.151   Other specified injury of anterior tibial artery, right leg

    S85.152   Other specified injury of anterior tibial artery, left leg

    S85.159   Other specified injury of anterior tibial artery, unspecified leg

S85.16   Unspecified injury of posterior tibial artery

    S85.161   Unspecified injury of posterior tibial artery, right leg

    S85.162   Unspecified injury of posterior tibial artery, left leg

    S85.169   Unspecified injury of posterior tibial artery, unspecified leg

S85.17   Laceration of posterior tibial artery

    S85.171   Laceration of posterior tibial artery, right leg

    S85.172   Laceration of posterior tibial artery, left leg

    S85.179   Laceration of posterior tibial artery, unspecified leg

S85.18   Other specified injury of posterior tibial artery

    S85.181   Other specified injury of posterior tibial artery, right leg

    S85.182   Other specified injury of posterior tibial artery, left leg

    S85.189   Other specified injury of posterior tibial artery, unspecified leg

S85.2   Injury of peroneal artery

S85.20   Unspecified injury of peroneal artery

    S85.201   Unspecified injury of peroneal artery, right leg

    S85.202   Unspecified injury of peroneal artery, left leg

    S85.209   Unspecified injury of peroneal artery, unspecified leg

S85.21   Laceration of peroneal artery

    S85.211   Laceration of peroneal artery, right leg

    S85.212   Laceration of peroneal artery, left leg

    S85.219   Laceration of peroneal artery, unspecified leg

S85.29   Other specified injury of peroneal artery

    S85.291   Other specified injury of peroneal artery, right leg

    S85.292   Other specified injury of peroneal artery, left leg

    S85.299   Other specified injury of peroneal artery, unspecified leg

S85.3   Injury of greater saphenous vein at lower leg level

Injury of greater saphenous vein NOS

Injury of saphenous vein NOS

S85.30   Unspecified injury of greater saphenous vein at lower leg level

    S85.301   Unspecified injury of greater saphenous vein at lower leg level, right leg

    S85.302   Unspecified injury of greater saphenous vein at lower leg level, left leg

    S85.309   Unspecified injury of greater saphenous vein at lower leg level, unspecified leg

S85.31   Laceration of greater saphenous vein at lower leg level

    S85.311   Laceration of greater saphenous vein at lower leg level, right leg

    S85.312   Laceration of greater saphenous vein at lower leg level, left leg

    S85.319   Laceration of greater saphenous vein at lower leg level, unspecified leg

S85.39   Other specified injury of greater saphenous vein at lower leg level

    S85.391   Other specified injury of greater saphenous vein at lower leg level, right leg

    S85.392   Other specified injury of greater saphenous vein at lower leg level, left leg

    S85.399   Other specified injury of greater saphenous vein at lower leg level, unspecified leg

S85.4   Injury of lesser saphenous vein at lower leg level

S85.40   Unspecified injury of lesser saphenous vein at lower leg level

    S85.401   Unspecified injury of lesser saphenous vein at lower leg level, right leg

    S85.402   Unspecified injury of lesser saphenous vein at lower leg level, left leg

    S85.409   Unspecified injury of lesser saphenous vein at lower leg level, unspecified leg

S85.41   Laceration of lesser saphenous vein at lower leg level

    S85.411   Laceration of lesser saphenous vein at lower leg level, right leg

    S85.412   Laceration of lesser saphenous vein at lower leg level, left leg

    S85.419   Laceration of lesser saphenous vein at lower leg level, unspecified leg

S85.49   Other specified injury of lesser saphenous vein at lower leg level

    S85.491   Other specified injury of lesser saphenous vein at lower leg level, right leg

    S85.492   Other specified injury of lesser saphenous vein at lower leg level, left leg

    S85.499   Other specified injury of lesser saphenous vein at lower leg level, unspecified leg

S85.5   Injury of popliteal vein

S85.50   Unspecified injury of popliteal vein

    S85.501   Unspecified injury of popliteal vein, right leg

    S85.502   Unspecified injury of popliteal vein, left leg

    S85.509   Unspecified injury of popliteal vein, unspecified leg

S85.51   Laceration of popliteal vein

    S85.511   Laceration of popliteal vein, right leg

    S85.512   Laceration of popliteal vein, left leg

    S85.519   Laceration of popliteal vein, unspecified leg

S85.59   Other specified injury of popliteal vein

    S85.591   Other specified injury of popliteal vein, right leg

    S85.592   Other specified injury of popliteal vein, left leg

    S85.599   Other specified injury of popliteal vein, unspecified leg

S85.8   Injury of other blood vessels at lower leg level

S85.80   Unspecified injury of other blood vessels at lower leg level

    S85.801   Unspecified injury of other blood vessels at lower leg level, right leg

    S85.802   Unspecified injury of other blood vessels at lower leg level, left leg

    S85.809   Unspecified injury of other blood vessels at lower leg level, unspecified leg

S85.81   Laceration of other blood vessels at lower leg level

    S85.811   Laceration of other blood vessels at lower leg level, right leg

    S85.812   Laceration of other blood vessels at lower leg level, left leg

    S85.819   Laceration of other blood vessels at lower leg level, unspecified leg

S85.89   Other specified injury of other blood vessels at lower leg level

    S85.891   Other specified injury of other blood vessels at lower leg level, right leg

S85.892   Other specified injury of other blood vessels at lower leg level, left leg

S85.899   Other specified injury of other blood vessels at lower leg level, unspecified leg

S85.9   Injury of unspecified blood vessel at lower leg level

S85.90   Unspecified injury of unspecified blood vessel at lower leg level

S85.901   Unspecified injury of unspecified blood vessel at lower leg level, right leg

S85.902   Unspecified injury of unspecified blood vessel at lower leg level, left leg

S85.909   Unspecified injury of unspecified blood vessel at lower leg level, unspecified leg

S85.91   Laceration of unspecified blood vessel at lower leg level

S85.911   Laceration of unspecified blood vessel at lower leg level, right leg

S85.912   Laceration of unspecified blood vessel at lower leg level, left leg

S85.919   Laceration of unspecified blood vessel at lower leg level, unspecified leg

S85.99   Other specified injury of unspecified blood vessel at lower leg level

S85.991   Other specified injury of unspecified blood vessel at lower leg level, right leg

S85.992   Other specified injury of unspecified blood vessel at lower leg level, left leg

S85.999   Other specified injury of unspecified blood vessel at lower leg level, unspecified leg

S86 Injury of muscle and tendon at lower leg level

Code also any associated open wound (S81.-)

Excludes2:   injury of muscle and tendon at ankle (S96.-)
sprain of joints and ligaments of knee (S83.-)

The following extensions are to be added to each code for category S86:

a   initial encounter
d   subsequent encounter
q   sequela

S86.0   Injury of Achilles tendon

S86.00   Unspecified injury of Achilles tendon

S86.001   Unspecified injury of right Achilles tendon

S86.002   Unspecified injury of left Achilles tendon

S86.009   Unspecified injury of Achilles tendon, unspecified side

S86.01   Strain of Achilles tendon

S86.011   Strain of right Achilles tendon

S86.012   Strain of left Achilles tendon

S86.019   Strain of Achilles tendon, unspecified side

S86.02   Laceration of Achilles tendon

S86.021   Laceration of right Achilles tendon

S86.022   Laceration of left Achilles tendon

S86.029   Laceration of Achilles tendon, unspecified side

S86.09   Other injury of Achilles tendon

S86.091   Other injury of right Achilles tendon

S86.092   Other injury of left Achilles tendon

S86.099   Other injury of Achilles tendon, unspecified side

S86.1   Injury of other muscle(s) and tendon(s) of posterior muscle group at lower leg level

S86.10   Unspecified injury of other muscle(s) and tendon(s) of posterior muscle group at lower leg level

S86.101   Unspecified injury of other muscle(s) and tendon(s) of posterior muscle group at lower leg level, right leg

S86.102   Unspecified injury of other muscle(s) and tendon(s) of posterior muscle group at lower leg level, left leg

S86.109   Unspecified injury of other muscle(s) and tendon(s) of posterior muscle group at lower leg level, unspecified leg

S86.11   Strain of other muscle(s) and tendon(s) of posterior muscle group at lower leg level

S86.111   Strain of other muscle(s) and tendon(s) of posterior muscle group at lower leg level, right leg

S86.112   Strain of other muscle(s) and tendon(s) of posterior muscle group at lower leg level, left leg

S86.119   Strain of other muscle(s) and tendon(s) of posterior muscle group at lower leg level, unspecified leg

S86.12   Laceration of other muscle(s) and tendon(s) of posterior muscle group at lower leg level

S86.121   Laceration of other muscle(s) and tendon(s) of posterior muscle group at lower leg level, right leg

S86.122   Laceration of other muscle(s) and tendon(s) of posterior muscle group at lower leg level, left leg

S86.129   Laceration of other muscle(s) and tendon(s) of posterior muscle group at lower leg level, unspecified leg

S86.19   Other injury of other muscle(s) and tendon(s) of posterior muscle group at lower leg level

S86.191   Other injury of other muscle(s) and tendon(s) of posterior muscle group at lower leg level, right leg

S86.192   Other injury of other muscle(s) and tendon(s) of posterior muscle group at lower leg level, left leg

S86.199   Other injury of other muscle(s) and tendon(s) of posterior muscle group at lower leg level, unspecified leg

S86.2   Injury of muscle(s) and tendon(s) of anterior muscle group at lower leg level

S86.20   Unspecified injury of muscle(s) and tendon(s) of anterior muscle group at lower leg level

S86.201   Unspecified injury of muscle(s) and tendon(s) of anterior muscle group at lower leg level, right leg

S86.202   Unspecified injury of muscle(s) and tendon(s) of anterior muscle group at lower leg level, left leg

S86.209   Unspecified injury of muscle(s) and tendon(s) of anterior muscle group at lower leg level, unspecified leg

S86.21   Strain of muscle(s) and tendon(s) of anterior muscle group at lower leg level

S86.211   Strain of muscle(s) and tendon(s) of anterior muscle group at lower leg level, right leg

S86.212   Strain of muscle(s) and tendon(s) of anterior muscle group at lower leg level, left leg

S86.219   Strain of muscle(s) and tendon(s) of anterior muscle group at lower leg level, unspecified leg

S86.22   Laceration of muscle(s) and tendon(s) of anterior muscle group at lower leg level

S86.221   Laceration of muscle(s) and tendon(s) of anterior muscle group at lower leg level, right leg

S86.222   Laceration of muscle(s) and tendon(s) of anterior muscle group at lower leg level, left leg

S86.229   Laceration of muscle(s) and tendon(s) of anterior muscle group at lower leg level, unspecified leg

S86.29   Other injury of muscle(s) and tendon(s) of anterior muscle group at lower leg level

S86.291   Other injury of muscle(s) and tendon(s) of anterior muscle group at lower leg level, right leg

S86.292   Other injury of muscle(s) and tendon(s) of anterior muscle group at lower leg level, left leg

S86.299   Other injury of muscle(s) and tendon(s) of anterior muscle group at lower leg level, unspecified leg

S86.3   Injury of muscle(s) and tendon(s) of peroneal muscle group at lower leg level

S86.30   Unspecified injury of muscle(s) and tendon(s) of peroneal muscle group at lower leg level

S86.301   Unspecified injury of muscle(s) and tendon(s) of peroneal muscle group at lower leg level, right leg

S86.302   Unspecified injury of muscle(s) and tendon(s) of peroneal muscle group at lower leg level, left leg

S86.309   Unspecified injury of muscle(s) and tendon(s) of peroneal muscle group at lower leg level, unspecified leg

S86.31   Strain of muscle(s) and tendon(s) of peroneal muscle group at lower leg level

S86.311   Strain of muscle(s) and tendon(s) of peroneal muscle group at lower leg level, right leg

S86.312   Strain of muscle(s) and tendon(s) of peroneal muscle group at lower leg level, left leg

S86.319   Strain uscle(s) and tendon(s) of peroneal muscle group at lower leg level, unspecified leg

S86.32   Laceration of muscle(s) and tendon(s) of peroneal muscle group at lower leg level

S86.321   Laceration of muscle(s) and tendon(s) of peroneal muscle group at lower leg level, right leg

S86.322   Laceration of muscle(s) and tendon(s) of peroneal muscle group at lower leg level, left leg

S86.329   Laceration of muscle(s) and tendon(s) of peroneal muscle group at lower leg level, unspecified leg

S86.39   Other injury of muscle(s) and tendon(s) of peroneal muscle group at lower leg level

S86.391   Other injury of muscle(s) and tendon(s) of peroneal muscle group at lower leg level, right leg

S86.392   Other injury of muscle(s) and tendon(s) of peroneal muscle group at lower leg level, left leg

S86.399   Other injury of muscle(s) and tendon(s) of peroneal muscle group at lower leg level, unspecified leg

S86.8   Injury of other muscles and tendons at lower leg level

S86.80   Unspecified injury of other muscles and tendons at lower leg level

S86.801   Unspecified injury of other muscles and tendons at lower leg level, right leg

S86.802   Unspecified injury of other muscles and tendons at lower leg level, left leg

S86.809   Unspecified injury of other muscles and tendons at lower leg level, unspecified leg

S86.81   Strain of other muscles and tendons at lower leg level

S86.811   Strain of other muscles and tendons at lower leg level, right leg

S86.812   Strain of other muscles and tendons at lower leg level, left leg

S86.819   Strain of other muscles and tendons at lower leg level, unspecified leg

S86.82   Laceration of other muscles and tendons at lower leg level

S86.821   Laceration of other muscles and tendons at lower leg level, right leg

S86.822   Laceration of other muscles and tendons at lower leg level, left leg

S86.829   Laceration of other muscles and tendons at lower leg level, unspecified leg

S86.89   Other injury of other muscles and tendons at lower leg level

S86.891   Other injury of other muscles and tendons at lower leg level, right leg

S86.892   Other injury of other muscles and tendons at lower leg level, left leg

S86.899   Other injury of other muscles and tendons at lower leg level, unspecified leg

S86.9   Injury of unspecified muscle and tendon at lower leg level

S86.90   Unspecified injury of unspecified muscle and tendon at lower leg level

S86.901   Unspecified injury of unspecified muscle and tendon at lower leg level, right leg

S86.902   Unspecified injury of unspecified muscle and tendon at lower leg level, left leg

S86.909   Unspecified injury of unspecified muscle and tendon at lower leg level, unspecified leg

86.91   Strain of unspecified muscle and tendon at lower leg level

S86.911   Strain of unspecified muscle and tendon at lower leg level, right leg

S86.912   Strain of unspecified muscle and tendon at lower leg level, left leg

S86.919   Strain of unspecified muscle and tendon at lower leg level, unspecified leg

S86.92   Laceration of unspecified muscle and tendon at lower leg level

S86.921   Laceration of unspecified muscle and tendon at lower leg level, right leg

S86.922   Laceration of unspecified muscle and tendon at lower leg level, left leg

S86.929   Laceration of unspecified muscle and tendon at lower leg level, unspecified leg

S86.99   Other injury of unspecified muscle and tendon at lower leg level

S86.991   Other injury of unspecified muscle and tendon at lower leg level, right leg

S86.992   Other injury of unspecified muscle and tendon at lower leg level, left leg

S86.999   Other injury of unspecified muscle and tendon at lower leg level, unspecified leg

S87   Crushing injury of lower leg

Use additional code(s) for all associated injuries

Excludes2:   crushing injury of ankle and foot (S97.-)

The following extensions are to be added to each code for category S87:
a   initial encounter
d   subsequent encounter
q   sequela

S87.0   Crushing injury of knee

S87.00   Crushing injury of knee, unspecified side

S87.01   Crushing injury of right knee

S87.02   Crushing injury of left knee

S87.8   Crushing injury of lower leg

S87.80   Crushing injury of lower leg, unspecified side

S87.81   Crushing injury of right lower leg

S87.82   Crushing injury of left lower leg

S88   Traumatic amputation of lower leg

An amputation not identified and partial or complete should be coded to complete

Excludes1:   traumatic amputation of ankle and foot (S98.-)

The following extensions are to be added to each code for category S88:
a   initial encounter
d   subsequent encounter
q   sequela

S88.0   Traumatic amputation at knee level

S88.01   Complete traumatic amputation at knee level

S88.011   Complete traumatic amputation at right knee level

        S88.012   Complete traumatic amputation at left knee level

        S88.019   Complete traumatic amputation at knee level, unspecified side

    S88.02   Partial traumatic amputation at knee level

        S88.021   Partial traumatic amputation at right knee level

        S88.022   Partial traumatic amputation at left knee level

        S88.029   Partial traumatic amputation at knee level, unspecified side

S88.1   Traumatic amputation at level between knee and ankle

    S88.11   Complete traumatic amputation at level between knee and ankle

        S88.111   Complete traumatic amputation at level between right knee and ankle

        S88.112   Complete traumatic amputation at level between left knee and ankle

        S88.119   Complete traumatic amputation at level between knee and ankle, unspecified side

    S88.12   Partial traumatic amputation at level between knee and ankle

        S88.121   Partial traumatic amputation at level between right knee and ankle

        S88.122   Partial traumatic amputation at level between left knee and ankle

        S88.129   Partial traumatic amputation at level between knee and ankle, unspecified side

S88.9   Traumatic amputation of lower leg, level unspecified

    S88.91   Complete traumatic amputation of lower leg, level unspecified

        S88.911   Complete traumatic amputation of lower right leg, level unspecified

        S88.912   Complete traumatic amputation of lower left leg, level unspecified

        S88.919   Complete traumatic amputation of lower leg, level unspecified, unspecified side

    S88.92   Partial traumatic amputation of lower leg, level unspecified

        S88.921   Partial traumatic amputation of lower right leg, level unspecified

        S88.922   Partial traumatic amputation of lower left leg, level unspecified

        S88.929   Partial traumatic amputation of lower leg, level unspecified, unspecified side

S89   Other and unspecified injuries of lower leg

    Excludes2:   other and unspecified injuries of ankle and foot (S99.-)

    A fracture not designated as open or closed should be coded to closed

    The following extensions are to be added to each code for subcategories S89.0, S89.1, S89.2, and S89.3:

      a   initial encounter for closed fracture
      b   initial encounter for open fracture
      d   subsequent encounter for fracture with routine healing
      g   subsequent encounter for fracture with delayed healing
      j   subsequent encounter for fracture with nonunion
      m   subsequent encounter for fracture with malunion
      q   sequela

S89.0   Physeal fracture of upper end of tibia

    S89.00   Unspecified physeal fracture of upper end of tibia

        S89.001   Unspecified physeal fracture of upper end of right tibia

        S89.002   Unspecified physeal fracture of upper end of left tibia

        S89.009   Unspecified physeal fracture of upper end of unspecified tibia

    S89.01   Salter-Harris Type I upper end of tibia

        S89.011   Salter-Harris Type I upper end of right tibia

        S89.012   Salter-Harris Type I upper end of left tibia

        S89.019   Salter-Harris Type I upper end of unspecified tibia

    S89.02   Salter-Harris Type II upper end of tibia

        S89.021   Salter-Harris Type II upper end of right tibia

        S89.022   Salter-Harris Type II upper end of left tibia

        S89.029   Salter-Harris Type II upper end of unspecified tibia

    S89.03   Salter-Harris Type III upper end of tibia

        S89.031   Salter-Harris Type III upper end of right tibia

        S89.032   Salter-Harris Type III upper end of left tibia

        S89.039   Salter-Harris Type III upper end of unspecified tibia

    S89.04   Salter-Harris Type IV upper end of tibia

        S89.041   Salter-Harris Type IV upper end of right tibia

        S89.042   Salter-Harris Type IV upper end of left tibia

        S89.049   Salter-Harris Type IV upper end of unspecified tibia

    S89.09   Other physeal fracture of upper end of tibia

        S89.091   Other physeal fracture of upper end of right tibia

        S89.092   Other physeal fracture of upper end of left tibia

        S89.099   Other physeal fracture of upper end of unspecified tibia

S89.1   Physeal fracture of lower end of tibia

    S89.10   Unspecified physeal fracture of lower end of tibia

        S89.101   Unspecified physeal fracture of lower end of right tibia

        S89.102   Unspecified physeal fracture of lower end of left tibia

        S89.109   Unspecified physeal fracture of lower end of unspecified tibia

    S89.11   Salter-Harris Type I lower end of tibia

        S89.111   Salter-Harris Type I lower end of right tibia

        S89.112   Salter-Harris Type I lower end of left tibia

        S89.119   Salter-Harris Type I lower end of unspecified tibia

    S89.12   Salter-Harris Type II lower end of tibia

        S89.121   Salter-Harris Type II lower end of right tibia

        S89.122   Salter-Harris Type II lower end of left tibia

        S89.129   Salter-Harris Type II lower end of unspecified tibia

    S89.13   Salter-Harris Type III lower end of tibia

      Excludes1:   fracture of medial malleolus (adult) (S82.5-)

        S89.131   Salter-Harris Type III lower end of right tibia

        S89.132   Salter-Harris Type III lower end of left tibia

        S89.139   Salter-Harris Type III lower end of unspecified tibia

    S89.14   Salter-Harris Type IV lower end of tibia

      Excludes1:   fracture of medial malleolus (adult) (S82.5-)

        S89.141   Salter-Harris Type IV lower end of right tibia

        S89.142   Salter-Harris Type IV lower end of left tibia

        S89.149   Salter-Harris Type IV lower end of unspecified tibia

    S89.19   Other physeal fracture of lower end of tibia

        S89.191   Other physeal fracture of lower end of right tibia

        S89.192   Other physeal fracture of lower end of left tibia

        S89.199   Other physeal fracture of lower end of unspecified tibia

S89.2   Physeal fracture of upper end of fibula

    S89.20   Unspecified physeal fracture of upper end of fibula

        S89.201   Unspecified physeal fracture of upper end of right fibula

        S89.202   Unspecified physeal fracture of upper end of left fibula

        S89.209   Unspecified physeal fracture of upper end of unspecified fibula

    S89.21   Salter-Harris Type I upper end of fibula

        S89.211   Salter-Harris Type I upper end of right fibula

        S89.212   Salter-Harris Type I upper end of left fibula

S89.219   Salter-Harris Type I upper end of unspecified fibula

S89.22   Salter-Harris Type II upper end of fibula

S89.221   Salter-Harris Type II upper end of right fibula

S89.222   Salter-Harris Type II upper end of left fibula

S89.229   Salter-Harris Type II upper end of unspecified fibula

S89.29   Other physeal fracture of upper end of fibula

S89.291   Other physeal fracture of upper end of right fibula

S89.292   Other physeal fracture of upper end of left fibula

S89.299   Other physeal fracture of upper end of unspecified fibula

S89.3   Physeal fracture of lower end of fibula

S89.30   Unspecified physeal fracture of lower end of fibula

S89.301   Unspecified physeal fracture of lower end of right fibula

S89.302   Unspecified physeal fracture of lower end of left fibula

S89.309   Unspecified physeal fracture of lower end of unspecified fibula

S89.31   Salter-Harris Type I lower end of fibula

S89.311   Salter-Harris Type I lower end of right fibula

S89.312   Salter-Harris Type I lower end of left fibula

S89.319   Salter-Harris Type I lower end of unspecified fibula

S89.32   Salter-Harris Type II lower end of fibula

S89.321   Salter-Harris Type II lower end of right fibula

S89.322   Salter-Harris Type II lower end of left fibula

S89.329   Salter-Harris Type II lower end of unspecified fibula

S89.39   Other physeal fracture of lower end of fibula

S89.391   Other physeal fracture of lower end of right fibula

S89.392   Other physeal fracture of lower end of left fibula

S89.399   Other physeal fracture of lower end of unspecified fibula

The following extensions are to be added to each code for subcategories S89.8 and S89.9:
a   initial encounter
d   subsequent encounter
q   sequela

S89.8   Other specified injuries of lower leg

S89.80   Other specified injuries of lower leg, unspecified side

S89.81   Other specified injuries of lower right leg

S89.82   Other specified injuries of lower left leg

S89.9   Unspecified injury of lower leg

S89.90   Unspecified injury of lower leg, unspecified side

S89.91   Unspecified injury of lower right leg

S89.92   Unspecified injury of lower left leg

INJURIES TO THE ANKLE AND FOOT (S90-S99)

Excludes2:   burns and corrosions (T20-T32)
fracture of ankle and malleolus (S82.-)
frostbite (T33-T34)
insect bite or sting, venomous (T63.4)

S90   Superficial injury of ankle, foot and toes
The following extensions are to be added to each code for category S90:
a   initial encounter
d   subsequent encounter
q   sequela

S90.0   Contusion of ankle

S90.00   Contusion of unspecified ankle

S90.01   Contusion of right ankle

S90.02   Contusion of left ankle

S90.1   Contusion of toe without damage to nail

S90.11   Contusion of great toe without damage to nail

S90.111   Contusion of right great toe without damage to nail

S90.112   Contusion of left great toe without damage to nail

S90.119   Contusion of great toe without damage to nail, unspecified side

S90.12   Contusion of lesser toe without damage to nail

S90.121   Contusion of lesser right toe without damage to nail

S90.122   Contusion of lesser left toe without damage to nail

S90.129   Contusion of lesser toe without damage to nail, unspecified side
Contusion of toe NOS

S90.2   Contusion of toe with damage to nail

S90.21   Contusion of great toe with damage to nail

S90.211   Contusion of right great toe with damage to nail

S90.212   Contusion of left great toe with damage to nail

S90.219   Contusion of great toe with damage to nail, unspecified side

S90.22   Contusion of lesser toe with damage to nail

S90.221   Contusion of lesser right toe with damage to nail

S90.222   Contusion of lesser left toe with damage to nail

S90.229   Contusion of lesser toe with damage to nail, unspecified side

S90.3   Contusion of foot
Excludes2:   contusion of toes (S90.1-, S90.2-)

S90.30   Contusion of unspecified foot
Contusion of foot NOS

S90.31   Contusion of right foot

S90.32   Contusion of left foot

S90.4   Other superficial injuries of toe

S90.41   Abrasion of toe

S90.411   Abrasion, right great toe

S90.412   Abrasion, left great toe

S90.413   Abrasion, unspecified great toe

S90.414   Abrasion, lesser right toe

S90.415   Abrasion, lesser left toe

S90.416   Abrasion, unspecified lesser toe

S90.42   Blister (nonthermal) of toe

S90.421   Blister (nonthermal), right great toe

S90.422   Blister (nonthermal), left great toe

S90.423   Blister (nonthermal), unspecified great toe

S90.424   Blister (nonthermal), lesser right toe

S90.425   Blister (nonthermal), lesser left toe

S90.426   Blister (nonthermal), unspecified lesser toe

S90.44   External constriction of toe

S90.441   External constriction, right great toe

S90.442   External constriction, left great toe

S90.443   External constriction, unspecified great toe

S90.444   External constriction, lesser right toe

S90.445   External constriction, lesser left toe

S90.446   External constriction, unspecified lesser toe

S90.45   Superficial foreign body of toe
Splinter in the toe

S90.451   Superficial foreign body, right great toe

S90.452   Superficial foreign body, left great toe

S90.453   Superficial foreign body, unspecified great toe

S90.454   Superficial foreign body, lesser right toe

S90.455   Superficial foreign body, lesser left toe

S90.456   Superficial foreign body, unspecified lesser toe

S90.46   Insect bite (nonvenomous) of toe

S90.461   Insect bite (nonvenomous), right great toe

S90.462   Insect bite (nonvenomous), left great toe

     S90.463   Insect bite (nonvenomous), unspecified great toe
     S90.464   Insect bite (nonvenomous), lesser right toe
     S90.465   Insect bite (nonvenomous), lesser left toe
     S90.466   Insect bite (nonvenomous), unspecified lesser toe

S90.47   Other superficial bite of toe
     Excludes1:   open bite of toe (S91.15-, S91.25-)
     S90.471   Other superficial bite of right great toe
     S90.472   Other superficial bite of left great toe
     S90.473   Other superficial bite of unspecified great toe
     S90.474   Other superficial bite of lesser right toe
     S90.475   Other superficial bite of lesser left toe
     S90.476   Other superficial bite of unspecified lesser toe

S90.5   Other superficial injuries of ankle
S90.51   Abrasion of ankle
     S90.511   Abrasion, right ankle
     S90.512   Abrasion, left ankle
     S90.519   Abrasion, unspecified ankle
S90.52   Blister (nonthermal) of ankle
     S90.521   Blister (nonthermal), right ankle
     S90.522   Blister (nonthermal), left ankle
     S90.529   Blister (nonthermal), unspecified ankle
S90.54   External constriction of ankle
     S90.541   External constriction, right ankle
     S90.542   External constriction, left ankle
     S90.549   External constriction, unspecified ankle
S90.55   Superficial foreign body of ankle
     Splinter in the ankle
     S90.551   Superficial foreign body, right ankle
     S90.552   Superficial foreign body, left ankle
     S90.559   Superficial foreign body, unspecified ankle
S90.56   Insect bite (nonvenomous) of ankle
     S90.561   Insect bite (nonvenomous), right ankle
     S90.562   Insect bite (nonvenomous), left ankle
     S90.569   Insect bite (nonvenomous), unspecified ankle
S90.57   Other superficial bite of ankle
     Excludes1:   open bite of ankle (S91.05-)
     S90.571   Other superficial bite of ankle, right ankle
     S90.572   Other superficial bite of ankle, left ankle
     S90.579   Other superficial bite of ankle, unspecified ankle

S90.8   Other superficial injuries of foot
S90.81   Abrasion of foot
     S90.811   Abrasion, right foot
     S90.812   Abrasion, left foot
     S90.819   Abrasion, unspecified foot
S90.82   Blister (nonthermal) of foot
     S90.821   Blister (nonthermal), right foot
     S90.822   Blister (nonthermal), left foot
     S90.829   Blister (nonthermal), unspecified foot
S90.84   External constriction of foot
     S90.841   External constriction, right foot
     S90.842   External constriction, left foot
     S90.849   External constriction, unspecified foot
S90.85   Superficial foreign body of foot
     Splinter in the foot
     S90.851   Superficial foreign body, right foot
     S90.852   Superficial foreign body, left foot
     S90.859   Superficial foreign body, unspecified foot
S90.86   Insect bite (nonvenomous) of foot
     S90.861   Insect bite (nonvenomous), right foot
     S90.862   Insect bite (nonvenomous), left foot
     S90.869   Insect bite (nonvenomous), unspecified foot
S90.87   Other superficial bite of foot
     Excludes1:   open bite of foot (S91.35-)
     S90.871   Other superficial bite of right foot
     S90.872   Other superficial bite of left foot

     S90.879   Other superficial bite of unspecified foot
S90.9   Unspecified superficial injury of ankle, foot and toe
S90.91   Unspecified superficial injury of ankle
     S90.911   Unspecified superficial injury of right ankle
     S90.912   Unspecified superficial injury of left ankle
     S90.919   Unspecified superficial injury of unspecified ankle
S90.92   Unspecified superficial injury of foot
     S90.921   Unspecified superficial injury of right foot
     S90.922   Unspecified superficial injury of left foot
     S90.929   Unspecified superficial injury of unspecified foot
S90.93   Unspecified superficial injury of toes
     S90.931   Unspecified superficial injury of right great toe
     S90.932   Unspecified superficial injury of left great toe
     S90.933   Unspecified superficial injury of unspecified great toe
     S90.934   Unspecified superficial injury of lesser right toe
     S90.935   Unspecified superficial injury of lesser left toe
     S90.936   Unspecified superficial injury of unspecified lesser toe

S91   Open wound of ankle, foot and toes
     Code also any associated wound infection
     Excludes1:   open fracture of ankle, foot and toes (S92.-with extension b)
             traumatic amputation of ankle and foot (S98.-)
     The following extensions are to be added to each code for category S91:
     a   initial encounter
     d   subsequent encounter
     q   sequela

S91.0   Open wound of ankle
S91.00   Unspecified open wound of ankle
     S91.001   Unspecified open wound, right ankle
     S91.002   Unspecified open wound, left ankle
     S91.009   Unspecified open wound, unspecified ankle
S91.01   Laceration without foreign body of ankle
     S91.011   Laceration without foreign body, right ankle
     S91.012   Laceration without foreign body, left ankle
     S91.019   Laceration without foreign body, unspecified ankle
S91.02   Laceration with foreign body of ankle
     S91.021   Laceration with foreign body, right ankle
     S91.022   Laceration with foreign body, left ankle
     S91.029   Laceration with foreign body, unspecified ankle
S91.03   Puncture wound without foreign body of ankle
     S91.031   Puncture wound without foreign body, right ankle
     S91.032   Puncture wound without foreign body, left ankle
     S91.039   Puncture wound without foreign body, unspecified ankle
S91.04   Puncture wound with foreign body of ankle
     S91.041   Puncture wound with foreign body, right ankle
     S91.042   Puncture wound with foreign body, left ankle
     S91.049   Puncture wound with foreign body, unspecified ankle
S91.05   Open bite of ankle
     Excludes1:   superficial bite of ankle (S90.56-, S90.57-)
     S91.051   Open bite, right ankle
     S91.052   Open bite, left ankle
     S91.059   Open bite, unspecified ankle
S91.1   Open wound of toe without damage to nail
S91.10   Unspecified open wound of toe without damage to nail
     S91.101   Unspecified open wound of right great toe without damage to nail

S91.102 Unspecified open wound of left great toe without damage to nail

S91.103 Unspecified open wound of unspecified great toe without damage to nail

S91.104 Unspecified open wound of lesser right toe without damage to nail

S91.105 Unspecified open wound of lesser left toe without damage to nail

S91.106 Unspecified open wound of unspecified lesser toe without damage to nail

S91.109 Unspecified open wound of unspecified toe without damage to nail

S91.11 Laceration without foreign body of toe without damage to nail

S91.111 Laceration without foreign body of right great toe without damage to nail

S91.112 Laceration without foreign body of left great toe without damage to nail

S91.113 Laceration without foreign body of unspecified great toe without damage to nail

S91.114 Laceration without foreign body of lesser right toe without damage to nail

S91.115 Laceration without foreign body of lesser left toe without damage to nail

S91.116 Laceration without foreign body of unspecified lesser toe without damage to nail

S91.119 Laceration without foreign body of unspecified toe without damage to nail

S91.12 Laceration with foreign body of toe without damage to nail

S91.121 Laceration with foreign body of right great toe without damage to nail

S91.122 Laceration with foreign body of left great toe without damage to nail

S91.123 Laceration with foreign body of unspecified great toe without damage to nail

S91.124 Laceration with foreign body of right lesser toe without damage to nail

S91.125 Laceration with foreign body of left lesser toe without damage to nail

S91.126 Laceration with foreign body of unspecified lesser toe without damage to nail

S91.129 Laceration with foreign body of unspecified toe without damage to nail

S91.13 Puncture wound without foreign body of toe without damage to nail

S91.131 Puncture wound without foreign body of right great toe without damage to nail

S91.132 Puncture wound without foreign body of left great toe without damage to nail

S91.133 Puncture wound without foreign body of unspecified great toe without damage to nail

S91.134 Puncture wound without foreign body of right lesser toe without damage to nail

S91.135 Puncture wound without foreign body of left lesser toe without damage to nail

S91.136 Puncture wound without foreign body of unspecified lesser toe without damage to nail

S91.139 Puncture wound without foreign body of unspecified toe without damage to nail

S91.14 Puncture wound with foreign body of toe without damage to nail

S91.141 Puncture wound with foreign body of right great toe without damage to nail

S91.142 Puncture wound with foreign body of left great toe without damage to nail

S91.143 Puncture wound with foreign body of unspecified great toe without damage to nail

S91.144 Puncture wound with foreign body of right lesser toe without damage to nail

S91.145 Puncture wound with foreign body of left lesser toe without damage to nail

S91.146 Puncture wound with foreign body of unspecified lesser toe without damage to nail

S91.149 Puncture wound with foreign body of unspecified toe without damage to nail

S91.15 Open bite of toe without damage to nail

Bite of toe NOS

Excludes1:   superficial bite of toe (S90.46-, S90.47-)

S91.151 Open bite of right great toe without damage to nail

S91.152 Open bite of left great toe without damage to nail

S91.153 Open bite of unspecified great toe without damage to nail

S91.154 Open bite of right lesser toe without damage to nail

S91.155 Open bite of left lesser toe without damage to nail

S91.156 Open bite of unspecified lesser toe without damage to nail

S91.159 Open bite of unspecified toe without damage to nail

S91.2 Open wound of toe with damage to nail

S91.20 Unspecified open wound of toe with damage to nail

S91.201 Unspecified open wound of right great toe with damage to nail

S91.202 Unspecified open wound of left great toe with damage to nail

S91.203 Unspecified open wound of unspecified great toe with damage to nail

S91.204 Unspecified open wound of right lesser toe with damage to nail

S91.205 Unspecified open wound of left lesser toe with damage to nail

S91.206 Unspecified open wound of unspecified lesser toe with damage to nail

S91.209 Unspecified open wound of unspecified toe with damage to nail

S91.21 Laceration without foreign body of toe with damage to nail

S91.211 Laceration without foreign body of right great toe with damage to nail

S91.212 Laceration without foreign body of left great toe with damage to nail

S91.213 Laceration without foreign body of unspecified great toe with damage to nail

S91.214 Laceration without foreign body of right lesser toe with damage to nail

S91.215 Laceration without foreign body of left lesser toe with damage to nail

S91.216 Laceration without foreign body of unspecified lesser toe with damage to nail

S91.219 Laceration without foreign body of unspecified toe with damage to nail

S91.22 Laceration with foreign body of toe with damage to nail

S91.221 Laceration with foreign body of right great toe with damage to nail

S91.222 Laceration with foreign body of left great toe with damage to nail

S91.223 Laceration with foreign body of unspecified great toe with damage to nail

S91.224 Laceration with foreign body of right lesser toe with damage to nail

S91.225 Laceration with foreign body of left lesser toe with damage to nail

S91.226 Laceration with foreign body of unspecified lesser toe with damage to nail

S91.229 Laceration without foreign body of unspecified toe with damage to nail

S91.23   Puncture wound without foreign body of toe with damage to nail

    S91.231   Puncture wound without foreign body of right great toe with damage to nail

    S91.232   Puncture wound without foreign body of left great toe with damage to nail

    S91.233   Puncture wound without foreign body of unspecified great toe with damage to nail

    S91.234   Puncture wound without foreign body of right lesser toe with damage to nail

    S91.235   Puncture wound without foreign body of left lesser toe with damage to nail

    S91.236   Puncture wound without foreign body of unspecified lesser toe with damage to nail

    S91.239   Puncture wound without foreign body of unspecified toe with damage to nail

S91.24   Puncture wound with foreign body of toe with damage to nail

    S91.241   Puncture wound with foreign body of right great toe with damage to nail

    S91.242   Puncture wound with foreign body of left great toe with damage to nail

    S91.243   Puncture wound with foreign body of unspecified great toe with damage to nail

    S91.244   Puncture wound with foreign body of right lesser toe with damage to nail

    S91.245   Puncture wound with foreign body of left lesser toe with damage to nail

    S91.246   Puncture wound with foreign body of unspecified lesser toe with damage to nail

    S91.249   Puncture wound with foreign body of unspecified toe with damage to nail

S91.25   Open bite of toe with damage to nail

      Bite of toe with damage to nail NOS

      Excludes1:   superficial bite of toe (S90.46-, S90.47-)

    S91.251   Open bite of right great toe with damage to nail

    S91.252   Open bite of left great toe with damage to nail

    S91.253   Open bite of unspecified great toe with damage to nail

    S91.254   Open bite of right lesser toe with damage to nail

    S91.255   Open bite of left lesser toe with damage to nail

    S91.256   Open bite of unspecified lesser toe with damage to nail

    S91.259   Open bite of unspecified toe with damage to nail

S91.3   Open wound of foot

   S91.30   Unspecified open wound of foot

    S91.301   Unspecified open wound, right foot

    S91.302   Unspecified open wound, left foot

    S91.309   Unspecified open wound, unspecified foot

   S91.31   Laceration without foreign body of foot

    S91.311   Laceration without foreign body, right foot

    S91.312   Laceration without foreign body, left foot

    S91.319   Laceration without foreign body, unspecified foot

   S91.32   Laceration with foreign body of foot

    S91.321   Laceration with foreign body, right foot

    S91.322   Laceration with foreign body, left foot

    S91.329   Laceration with foreign body, unspecified foot

   S91.33   Puncture wound without foreign body of foot

    S91.331   Puncture wound without foreign body, right foot

    S91.332   Puncture wound without foreign body, left foot

    S91.339   Puncture wound without foreign body, unspecified foot

   S91.34   Puncture wound with foreign body of foot

    S91.341   Puncture wound with foreign body, right foot

    S91.342   Puncture wound with foreign body, left foot

    S91.349   Puncture wound with foreign body, unspecified foot

   S91.35   Open bite of foot

      Excludes1:   superficial bite of foot (S90.86-, S90.87-)

    S91.351   Open bite, right foot

    S91.352   Open bite, left foot

    S91.359   Open bite, unspecified foot

S92   Fracture of foot and toe, except ankle

    A fracture not identified as displaced or nondisplaced should be coded to displaced

    Excludes1:   traumatic amputation of ankle and foot (S98.-)

    Excludes2:   fracture of ankle (S82.-)

               fracture of malleolus (S82.-)

    A fracture not designated as open or closed should be coded to closed

    The following extensions are to be added to each code for subcategories S92.0, S92.1, and S92.2:

     a   initial encounter for closed fracture

     b   initial encounter for open fracture

     d   subsequent encounter for fracture with routine healing

     g   subsequent encounter for fracture with delayed healing

     j   subsequent encounter for fracture with nonunion

     m   subsequent encounter for fracture with malunion

     q   sequela

S92.0   Fracture of calcaneus

     Heel bone

     Os calcis

   S92.00   Unspecified fracture of calcaneus

    S92.001   Unspecified fracture of right calcaneus

    S92.002   Unspecified fracture of left calcaneus

    S92.009   Unspecified fracture of unspecified calcaneus

   S92.01   Fracture of body of calcaneus

    S92.011   Displaced fracture of body of right calcaneus

    S92.012   Displaced fracture of body of left calcaneus

    S92.013   Displaced fracture of body of unspecified calcaneus

    S92.014   Nondisplaced fracture of body of right calcaneus

    S92.015   Nondisplaced fracture of body of left calcaneus

    S92.016   Nondisplaced fracture of body of unspecified calcaneus

   S92.02   Fracture of anterior process of calcaneus

    S92.021   Displaced fracture of anterior process of right calcaneus

    S92.022   Displaced fracture of anterior process of left calcaneus

    S92.023   Displaced fracture of anterior process of unspecified calcaneus

    S92.024   Nondisplaced fracture of anterior process of right calcaneus

    S92.025   Nondisplaced fracture of anterior process of left calcaneus

    S92.026   Nondisplaced fracture of anterior process of unspecified calcaneus

   S92.03   Avulsion fracture of tuberosity of calcaneus

    S92.031   Displaced avulsion fracture of tuberosity of right calcaneus

    S92.032   Displaced avulsion fracture of tuberosity of left calcaneus

    S92.033   Displaced avulsion fracture of tuberosity of unspecified calcaneus

    S92.034   Nondisplaced avulsion fracture of tuberosity of right calcaneus

    S92.035   Nondisplaced avulsion fracture of tuberosity of left calcaneus

    S92.036   Nondisplaced avulsion fracture of tuberosity of unspecified calcaneus

   S92.04   Other fracture of tuberosity of calcaneus

    S92.041   Displaced other fracture of tuberosity of right calcaneus

     S92.042   Displaced other fracture of tuberosity of left calcaneus

     S92.043   Displaced other fracture of tuberosity of unspecified calcaneus

     S92.044   Nondisplaced other fracture of tuberosity of right calcaneus

     S92.045   Nondisplaced other fracture of tuberosity of left calcaneus

     S92.046   Nondisplaced other fracture of tuberosity of unspecified calcaneus

   S92.05   **Other extraarticular fracture of calcaneus**

     S92.051   Displaced other extraarticular fracture of right calcaneus

     S92.052   Displaced other extraarticular fracture of left calcaneus

     S92.053   Displaced other extraarticular fracture of unspecified calcaneus

     S92.054   Nondisplaced other extraarticular fracture of right calcaneus

     S92.055   Nondisplaced other extraarticular fracture of left calcaneus

     S92.056   Nondisplaced other extraarticular fracture of unspecified calcaneus

   S92.06   **Intraarticular fracture of calcaneus**

     S92.061   Displaced intraarticular fracture of right calcaneus

     S92.062   Displaced intraarticular fracture of left calcaneus

     S92.063   Displaced intraarticular fracture of unspecified calcaneus

     S92.064   Nondisplaced intraarticular fracture of right calcaneus

     S92.065   Nondisplaced intraarticular fracture of left calcaneus

     S92.066   Nondisplaced intraarticular fracture of unspecified calcaneus

S92.1   Fracture of talus

     Astragalus

   S92.10   **Unspecified fracture of talus**

     S92.101   Unspecified fracture of right talus

     S92.102   Unspecified fracture of left talus

     S92.109   Unspecified fracture of unspecified talus

   S92.11   **Fracture of neck of talus**

     S92.111   Displaced fracture of neck of right talus

     S92.112   Displaced fracture of neck of left talus

     S92.113   Displaced fracture of neck of unspecified talus

     S92.114   Nondisplaced fracture of neck of right talus

     S92.115   Nondisplaced fracture of neck of left talus

     S92.116   Nondisplaced fracture of neck of unspecified talus

   S92.12   **Fracture of body of talus**

     S92.121   Displaced fracture of body of right talus

     S92.122   Displaced fracture of body of left talus

     S92.123   Displaced fracture of body of unspecified talus

     S92.124   Nondisplaced fracture of body of right talus

     S92.125   Nondisplaced fracture of body of left talus

     S92.126   Nondisplaced fracture of body of unspecified talus

   S92.13   **Fracture of posterior process of talus**

     S92.131   Displaced fracture of posterior process of right talus

     S92.132   Displaced fracture of posterior process of left talus

     S92.133   Displaced fracture of posterior process of unspecified talus

     S92.134   Nondisplaced fracture of posterior process of right talus

     S92.135   Nondisplaced fracture of posterior process of left talus

     S92.136   Nondisplaced fracture of posterior process of unspecified talus

   S92.14   **Dome fracture of talus**

     Excludes1:   osteochondritis dissecans (M93.2)

     S92.141   Displaced dome fracture of right talus

     S92.142   Displaced dome fracture of left talus

     S92.143   Displaced dome fracture of unspecified talus

     S92.144   Nondisplaced dome fracture of right talus

     S92.145   Nondisplaced dome fracture of left talus

     S92.146   Nondisplaced dome fracture of unspecifed talus

   S92.15   **Avulsion fracture (chip fracture) of talus**

     S92.151   Displaced avulsion fracture (chip fracture) of right talus

     S92.152   Displaced avulsion fracture (chip fracture) of left talus

     S92.153   Displaced avulsion fracture (chip fracture) of unspecified talus

     S92.154   Nondisplaced avulsion fracture (chip fracture) of right talus

     S92.155   Nondisplaced avulsion fracture (chip fracture) of left talus

     S92.156   Nondisplaced avulsion fracture (chip fracture) of unspecified talus

   S92.19   **Other fracture of talus**

     S92.191   Other fracture of right talus

     S92.192   Other fracture of left talus

     S92.199   Other fracture of unspecified talus

S92.2   Fracture of other and unspecified tarsal bone(s)

   S92.20   **Fracture of unspecified tarsal bone(s)**

     S92.201   Fracture of unspecified tarsal bone(s) of right foot

     S92.202   Fracture of unspecified tarsal bone(s) of left foot

     S92.209   Fracture of unspecified tarsal bone(s) of unspecified foot

   S92.21   **Fracture of cuboid bone**

     S92.211   Displaced fracture of cuboid bone of right foot

     S92.212   Displaced fracture of cuboid bone of left foot

     S92.213   Displaced fracture of cuboid bone of unspecified foot

     S92.214   Nondisplaced fracture of cuboid bone of right foot

     S92.215   Nondisplaced fracture of cuboid bone of left foot

     S92.216   Nondisplaced fracture of cuboid bone of unspecified foot

   S92.22   **Fracture of lateral cuneiform**

     S92.221   Displaced fracture of lateral cuneiform of right foot

     S92.222   Displaced fracture of lateral cuneiform of left foot

     S92.223   Displaced fracture of lateral cuneiform of unspecified foot

     S92.224   Nondisplaced fracture of lateral cuneiform of right foot

     S92.225   Nondisplaced fracture of lateral cuneiform of left foot

     S92.226   Nondisplaced fracture of lateral cuneiform of unspecified foot

   S92.23   **Fracture of intermediate cuneiform**

     S92.231   Displaced fracture of intermediate cuneiform of right foot

     S92.232   Displaced fracture of intermediate cuneiform of left foot

     S92.233   Displaced fracture of intermediate cuneiform of unspecified foot

     S92.234   Nondisplaced fracture of intermediate cuneiform of right foot

     S92.235   Nondisplaced fracture of intermediate cuneiform of left foot

     S92.236   Nondisplaced fracture of intermediate cuneiform of unspecified foot

S92.24   Fracture of medial cuneiform

     S92.241   Displaced fracture of medial cuneiform of right foot

     S92.242   Displaced fracture of medial cuneiform of left foot

     S92.243   Displaced fracture of medial cuneiform of unspecified foot

     S92.244   Nondisplaced fracture of medial cuneiform of right foot

     S92.245   Nondisplaced fracture of medial cuneiform of left foot

     S92.246   Nondisplaced fracture of medial cuneiform of unspecified foot

S92.25   Fracture of navicular [scaphoid] of foot

     S92.251   Displaced fracture of navicular [scaphoid] of right foot

     S92.252   Displaced fracture of navicular [scaphoid] of left foot

     S92.253   Displaced fracture of navicular [scaphoid] of unspecified foot

     S92.254   Nondisplaced fracture of navicular [scaphoid] of right foot

     S92.255   Nondisplaced fracture of navicular [scaphoid] of left foot

     S92.256   Nondisplaced fracture of navicular [scaphoid] of unspecified foot

A fracture not designated as open or closed should be coded to closed
Note: the open fracture designations are based on the Gustilo open fracture classification
The following extensions are to be added to each code for subcategories S92.3, S92.4, and S92.5:

     a   initial encounter for closed fracture
     b   initial encounter for open fracture type I or II
     c   initial encounter for open fracture type IIIA, IIIB, or IIIC
     d   subsequent encounter for fracture with routine healing
     g   subsequent encounter for fracture with delayed healing
     j   subsequent encounter for fracture with nonunion
     m   subsequent encounter for fracture with malunion
     q   sequela

S92.3   Fracture of metatarsal bone(s)

S92.30   Fracture of unspecified metatarsal bone(s)

     S92.301   Fracture of unspecified metatarsal bone(s), right foot

     S92.302   Fracture of unspecified metatarsal bone(s), left foot

     S92.309   Fracture of unspecified metatarsal bone(s), unspecified foot

S92.31   Fracture of first metatarsal bone

     S92.311   Displaced fracture of first metatarsal bone, right foot

     S92.312   Displaced fracture of first metatarsal bone, left foot

     S92.313   Displaced fracture of first metatarsal bone, unspecified foot

     S92.314   Nondisplaced fracture of first metatarsal bone, right foot

     S92.315   Nondisplaced fracture of first metatarsal bone, left foot

     S92.316   Nondisplaced fracture of first metatarsal bone, unspecified foot

S92.32   Fracture of second metatarsal bone

     S92.321   Displaced fracture of second metatarsal bone, right foot

     S92.322   Displaced fracture of second metatarsal bone, left foot

     S92.323   Displaced fracture of second metatarsal bone, unspecified foot

     S92.324   Nondisplaced fracture of second metatarsal bone, right foot

     S92.325   Nondisplaced fracture of second metatarsal bone, left foot

     S92.326   Nondisplaced fracture of second metatarsal bone, unspecified foot

S92.33   Fracture of third metatarsal bone

     S92.331   Displaced fracture of third metatarsal bone, right foot

     S92.332   Displaced fracture of third metatarsal bone, left foot

     S92.333   Displaced fracture of third metatarsal bone, unspecified foot

     S92.334   Nondisplaced fracture of third metatarsal bone, right foot

     S92.335   Nondisplaced fracture of third metatarsal bone, left foot

     S92.336   Nondisplaced fracture of third metatarsal bone, unspecified foot

S92.34   Fracture of fourth metatarsal bone

     S92.341   Displaced fracture of fourth metatarsal bone, right foot

     S92.342   Displaced fracture of fourth metatarsal bone, left foot

     S92.343   Displaced fracture of fourth metatarsal bone, unspecified foot

     S92.344   Nondisplaced fracture of fourth metatarsal bone, right foot

     S92.345   Nondisplaced fracture of fourth metatarsal bone, left foot

     S92.346   Nondisplaced fracture of fourth metatarsal bone, unspecified foot

S92.35   Fracture of fifth metatarsal bone

     S92.351   Displaced fracture of fifth metatarsal bone, right foot

     S92.352   Displaced fracture of fifth metatarsal bone, left foot

     S92.353   Displaced fracture of fifth metatarsal bone, unspecified foot

     S92.354   Nondisplaced fracture of fifth metatarsal bone, right foot

     S92.355   Nondisplaced fracture of fifth metatarsal bone, left foot

     S92.356   Nondisplaced fracture of fifth metatarsal bone, unspecified foot

S92.4   Fracture of great toe

S92.40   Unspecified fracture of great toe

     S92.401   Displaced unspecified fracture of right great toe

     S92.402   Displaced unspecified fracture of left great toe

     S92.403   Displaced unspecified fracture of unspecified great toe

     S92.404   Nondisplaced unspecified fracture of right great toe

     S92.405   Nondisplaced unspecified fracture of left great toe

     S92.406   Nondisplaced unspecified fracture of unspecified great toe

S92.41   Fracture of proximal phalanx of great toe

     S92.411   Displaced fracture of proximal phalanx of right great toe

     S92.412   Displaced fracture of proximal phalanx of left great toe

     S92.413   Displaced fracture of proximal phalanx of unspecified great toe

     S92.414   Nondisplaced fracture of proximal phalanx of right great toe

     S92.415   Nondisplaced fracture of proximal phalanx of left great toe

     S92.416   Nondisplaced fracture of proximal phalanx of unspecified great toe

S92.42   Fracture of distal phalanx of great toe

     S92.421   Displaced fracture of distal phalanx of right great toe

     S92.422   Displaced fracture of distal phalanx of left great toe

     S92.423   Displaced fracture of distal phalanx of unspecified great toe

       S92.424   Nondisplaced fracture of distal phalanx of right great toe

       S92.425   Nondisplaced fracture of distal phalanx of left great toe

       S92.426   Nondisplaced fracture of distal phalanx of unspecified great toe

     S92.49   Other fracture of great toe

       S92.491   Other fracture of right great toe

       S92.492   Other fracture of left great toe

       S92.499   Other fracture of unspecified great toe

   S92.5   Fracture of lesser toe(s)

     S92.50   Unspecified fracture of lesser toe(s)

       S92.501   Displaced unspecified fracture of right lesser toe(s)

       S92.502   Displaced unspecified fracture of left lesser toe(s)

       S92.503   Displaced unspecified fracture of unspecified lesser toe(s)

       S92.504   Nondisplaced unspecified fracture of right lesser toe(s)

       S92.505   Nondisplaced unspecified fracture of left lesser toe(s)

       S92.506   Nondisplaced unspecified fracture of unspecified lesser toe(s)

     S92.51   Fracture of proximal phalanx of lesser toe(s)

       S92.511   Displaced fracture of proximal phalanx of right lesser toe(s)

       S92.512   Displaced fracture of proximal phalanx of left lesser toe(s)

       S92.513   Displaced fracture of proximal phalanx of unspecified lesser toe(s)

       S92.514   Nondisplaced fracture of proximal phalanx of right lesser toe(s)

       S92.515   Nondisplaced fracture of proximal phalanx of left lesser toe(s)

       S92.516   Nondisplaced fracture of proximal phalanx of unspecified lesser toe(s)

     S92.52   Fracture of medial phalanx of lesser toe(s)

       S92.521   Displaced fracture of medial phalanx of right lesser toe(s)

       S92.522   Displaced fracture of medial phalanx of left lesser toe(s)

       S92.523   Displaced fracture of medial phalanx of unspecified lesser toe(s)

       S92.524   Nondisplaced fracture of medial phalanx of right lesser toe(s)

       S92.525   Nondisplaced fracture of medial phalanx of left lesser toe(s)

       S92.526   Nondisplaced fracture of medial phalanx of unspecified lesser toe(s)

     S92.53   Fracture of distal phalanx of lesser toe(s)

       S92.531   Displaced fracture of distal phalanx of right lesser toe(s)

       S92.532   Displaced fracture of distal phalanx of left lesser toe(s)

       S92.533   Displaced fracture of distal phalanx of unspecified lesser toe(s)

       S92.534   Nondisplaced fracture of distal phalanx of right lesser toe(s)

       S92.535   Nondisplaced fracture of distal phalanx of left lesser toe(s)

       S92.536   Nondisplaced fracture of distal phalanx of unspecified lesser toe(s)

     S92.59   Other fracture of lesser toe(s)

       S92.591   Other fracture of right lesser toe(s)

       S92.592   Other fracture of left lesser toe(s)

       S92.599   Other fracture of unspecified lesser toe(s)

         A fracture not designated as open or closed should be coded to closed

The following extensions are to be added to each code for subcategory S92.9:

   a   initial encounter for closed fracture
   b   initial encounter for open fracture
   d   subsequent encounter for fracture with routine healing
   g   subsequent encounter for fracture with delayed healing
   j   subsequent encounter for fracture with nonunion
   m   subsequent encounter for fracture with malunion
   q   sequela

   S92.9   Unspecified fracture of foot and toe

     S92.90   Unspecified fracture of foot

       S92.901   Unspecified fracture of right foot

       S92.902   Unspecified fracture of left foot

       S92.909   Unspecified fracture of unspecified foot

     S92.91   Unspecified fracture of toe

       S92.911   Unspecified fracture of right toe

       S92.912   Unspecified fracture of left toe

       S92.919   Unspecified fracture of unspecified toe

S93   Dislocation and sprain of joints and ligaments at ankle, foot and toe level

   Includes: avulsion of joint or ligament of ankle, foot and toe
         laceration of joint or ligament of ankle, foot and toe
         sprain of joint or ligament of ankle, foot and toe
         traumatic hemarthrosis of joint or ligament of ankle, foot and toe
         traumatic rupture of joint or ligament of ankle, foot and toe
         traumatic subluxation of joint or ligament of ankle, foot and toe
         traumatic tear of joint or ligament of ankle, foot and toe

   Excludes2:   strain of muscle and tendon of ankle and foot (S96.-)

The following extensions are to be added to each code for category S93:

   a   initial encounter
   d   subsequent encounter
   q   sequela

   S93.0   Subluxation and dislocation of ankle joint
     Subluxation and dislocation of astragalus
     Subluxation and dislocation of fibula, lower end
     Subluxation and dislocation of talus
     Subluxation and dislocation of tibia, lower end

     S93.01   Subluxation of right ankle joint

     S93.02   Subluxation of left ankle joint

     S93.03   Subluxation of unspecified ankle joint

     S93.04   Dislocation of right ankle joint

     S93.05   Dislocation of left ankle joint

     S93.06   Dislocation of unspecified ankle joint

   S93.1   Subluxation and dislocation of toe

     S93.10   Unspecified subluxation and dislocation of toe
       Dislocation of toe NOS
       Subluxation of toe NOS

       S93.101   Unspecified subluxation of right toe(s)

       S93.102   Unspecified subluxation of left toe(s)

       S93.103   Unspecified subluxation of unspecified toe(s)

       S93.104   Unspecified dislocation of right toe(s)

       S93.105   Unspecified dislocation of left toe(s)

       S93.106   Unspecified dislocation of unspecified toe(s)

     S93.11   Dislocation of interphalangeal joint

       S93.111   Dislocation of interphalangeal joint of right great toe

       S93.112   Dislocation of interphalangeal joint of left great toe

       S93.113   Dislocation of interphalangeal joint of unspecified great toe

       S93.114   Dislocation of interphalangeal joint of right lesser toe

       S93.115   Dislocation of interphalangeal joint of left lesser toe

       S93.116   Dislocation of interphalangeal joint of unspecified lesser toe

S93.119   Dislocation of interphalangeal joint of unspecified toe
S93.12   Dislocation of metatarsophalangeal joint
S93.121   Dislocation of metatarsophalangeal joint of right great toe
S93.122   Dislocation of metatarsophalangeal joint of left great toe
S93.123   Dislocation of metatarsophalangeal joint of unspecified great toe
S93.124   Dislocation of metatarsophalangeal joint of right lesser toe
S93.125   Dislocation of metatarsophalangeal joint of left lesser toe
S93.126   Dislocation of metatarsophalangeal joint of unspecified lesser toe
S93.129   Dislocation of metatarsophalangeal joint of unspecified toe
S93.13   Subluxation of interphalangeal joint
S93.131   Subluxation of interphalangeal joint of right great toe
S93.132   Subluxation of interphalangeal joint of left great toe
S93.133   Subluxation of interphalangeal joint of unspecified great toe
S93.134   Subluxation of interphalangeal joint of right lesser toe
S93.135   Subluxation of interphalangeal joint of left lesser toe
S93.136   Subluxation of interphalangeal joint of unspecified lesser toe
S93.139   Subluxation of interphalangeal joint of unspecified toe
S93.14   Subluxation of metatarsophalangeal joint
S93.141   Subluxation of metatarsophalangeal joint of right great toe
S93.142   Subluxation of metatarsophalangeal joint of left great toe
S93.143   Subluxation of metatarsophalangeal joint of unspecified great toe
S93.144   Subluxation of metatarsophalangeal joint of right lesser toe
S93.145   Subluxation of metatarsophalangeal joint of left lesser toe
S93.146   Subluxation of metatarsophalangeal joint of unspecified lesser toe
S93.149   Subluxation of metatarsophalangeal joint of unspecified toe
S93.3   Dislocation of foot
    Excludes2:   dislocation of toe (S93.1-)
S93.30   Unspecified subluxation and dislocation of foot
    Dislocation of foot NOS
    Subluxation of foot NOS
S93.301   Unspecified subluxation of right foot
S93.302   Unspecified subluxation of left foot
S93.303   Unspecified subluxation of unspecified foot
S93.304   Unspecified dislocation of right foot
S93.305   Unspecified dislocation of left foot
S93.306   Unspecified dislocation of unspecified foot
S93.31   Subluxation and dislocation of tarsal joint
S93.311   Subluxation of tarsal joint of right foot
S93.312   Subluxation of tarsal joint of left foot
S93.313   Subluxation of tarsal joint of unspecified foot
S93.314   Dislocation of tarsal joint of right foot
S93.315   Dislocation of tarsal joint of left foot
S93.316   Dislocation of tarsal joint of unspecified foot
S93.32   Subluxation and dislocation of tarsometatarsal joint
S93.321   Subluxation of tarsometatarsal joint of right foot
S93.322   Subluxation of tarsometatarsal joint of left foot

S93.323   Subluxation of tarsometatarsal joint of unspecified foot
S93.324   Dislocation of tarsometatarsal joint of right foot
S93.325   Dislocation of tarsometatarsal joint of left foot
S93.326   Dislocation of tarsometatarsal joint of unspecified foot
S93.33   Other subluxation and dislocation of foot
S93.331   Other subluxation of right foot
S93.332   Other subluxation of left foot
S93.333   Other subluxation of unspecified foot
S93.334   Other dislocation of right foot
S93.335   Other dislocation of left foot
S93.336   Other dislocation of unspecified foot
S93.4   Sprain of ankle
    Excludes2:   injury of Achilles tendon (S86.0-)
S93.40   Sprain of unspecified ligament of ankle
    Sprain of ankle NOS
    Sprained ankle NOS
S93.401   Sprain of unspecified ligament of right ankle
S93.402   Sprain of unspecified ligament of left ankle
S93.409   Sprain of unspecified ligament of unspecified ankle
S93.41   Sprain of calcaneofibular ligament
S93.411   Sprain of calcaneofibular ligament of right ankle
S93.412   Sprain of calcaneofibular ligament of left ankle
S93.419   Sprain of calcaneofibular ligament of unspecified ankle
S93.42   Sprain of deltoid ligament
S93.421   Sprain of deltoid ligament of right ankle
S93.422   Sprain of deltoid ligament of left ankle
S93.429   Sprain of deltoid ligament of unspecified ankle
S93.43   Sprain of tibiofibular ligament
S93.431   Sprain of tibiofibular ligament of right ankle
S93.432   Sprain of tibiofibular ligament of left ankle
S93.439   Sprain of tibiofibular ligament of unspecified ankle
S93.49   Sprain of other ligament of ankle
    Sprain of internal collateral ligament
    Sprain of talofibular ligament
S93.491   Sprain of other ligament of right ankle
S93.492   Sprain of other ligament of left ankle
S93.499   Sprain of other ligament of unspecified ankle
S93.5   Sprain of toe
S93.50   Unspecified sprain of toe
S93.501   Unspecified sprain of right great toe
S93.502   Unspecified sprain of left great toe
S93.503   Unspecified sprain of unspecified great toe
S93.504   Unspecified sprain of right lesser toe
S93.505   Unspecified sprain of left lesser toe
S93.506   Unspecified sprain of unspecified lesser toe
S93.509   Unspecified sprain of unspecified toe
S93.51   Sprain of interphalangeal joint of toe
S93.511   Sprain of interphalangeal joint of right great toe
S93.512   Sprain of interphalangeal joint of left great toe
S93.513   Sprain of interphalangeal joint of unspecified great toe
S93.514   Sprain of interphalangeal joint of right lesser toe
S93.515   Sprain of interphalangeal joint of left lesser toe
S93.516   Sprain of interphalangeal joint of unspecified lesser toe
S93.519   Sprain of interphalangeal joint of unspecified toe

S93.52   Sprain of metatarsophalangeal joint of toe
    S93.521   Sprain of metatarsophalangeal joint of right great toe
    S93.522   Sprain of metatarsophalangeal joint of left great toe
    S93.523   Sprain of metatarsophalangeal joint of unspecified great toe
    S93.524   Sprain of metatarsophalangeal joint of right lesser toe
    S93.525   Sprain of metatarsophalangeal joint of left lesser toe
    S93.526   Sprain of metatarsophalangeal joint of unspecified lesser toe
    S93.529   Sprain of metatarsophalangeal joint of unspecified toe

S93.6   Sprain of foot
    Excludes2:   sprain of metatarsophalangeal joint of toe (S93.52-)
             sprain of toe (S93.5-)

S93.60   Unspecified sprain of foot
    S93.601   Unspecified sprain of right foot
    S93.602   Unspecified sprain of left foot
    S93.609   Unspecified sprain of unspecified foot
S93.61   Sprain of tarsal ligament of foot
    S93.611   Sprain of tarsal ligament of right foot
    S93.612   Sprain of tarsal ligament of left foot
    S93.619   Sprain of tarsal ligament of unspecified foot
S93.62   Sprain of tarsometatarsal ligament of foot
    S93.621   Sprain of tarsometatarsal ligament of right foot
    S93.622   Sprain of tarsometatarsal ligament of left foot
    S93.629   Sprain of tarsometatarsal ligament of unspecified foot
S93.69   Other sprain of foot
    S93.691   Other sprain of right foot
    S93.692   Other sprain of left foot
    S93.699   Other sprain of unspecified foot

S94   Injury of nerves at ankle and foot level
    Code also any associated open wound (S91.-)
    The following extensions are to be added to each code for category S94:
    a   initial encounter
    d   subsequent encounter
    q   sequela

S94.0   Injury of lateral plantar nerve
    S94.00   Injury of lateral plantar nerve, unspecified leg
    S94.01   Injury of lateral plantar nerve, right leg
    S94.02   Injury of lateral plantar nerve, left leg
S94.1   Injury of medial plantar nerve
    S94.10   Injury of medial plantar nerve, unspecified leg
    S94.11   Injury of medial plantar nerve, right leg
    S94.12   Injury of medial plantar nerve, left leg
S94.2   Injury of deep peroneal nerve at ankle and foot level
    Injury of terminal, lateral branch of deep peroneal nerve
    S94.20   Injury of deep peroneal nerve at ankle and foot level, unspecified leg
    S94.21   Injury of deep peroneal nerve at ankle and foot level, right leg
    S94.22   Injury of deep peroneal nerve at ankle and foot level, left leg
S94.3   Injury of cutaneous sensory nerve at ankle and foot level
    S94.30   Injury of cutaneous sensory nerve at ankle and foot level, unspecified leg
    S94.31   Injury of cutaneous sensory nerve at ankle and foot level, right leg
    S94.32   Injury of cutaneous sensory nerve at ankle and foot level, left leg
S94.8   Injury of other nerves at ankle and foot level
    S94.8x   Injury of other nerves at ankle and foot level

    S94.8x1   Injury of other nerves at ankle and foot level, right leg
    S94.8x2   Injury of other nerves at ankle and foot level, left leg
    S94.8x9   Injury of other nerves at ankle and foot level, unspecified leg
S94.9   Injury of unspecified nerve at ankle and foot level
    S94.90   Injury of unspecified nerve at ankle and foot level, unspecified leg
    S94.91   Injury of unspecified nerve at ankle and foot level, right leg
    S94.92   Injury of unspecified nerve at ankle and foot level, left leg

S95   Injury of blood vessels at ankle and foot level
    Code also any associated open wound (S91.-)
    Excludes2:   injury of posterior tibial artery and vein (S85.1-, S85.8-)
    The following extensions are to be added to each code for category S95:
    a   initial encounter
    d   subsequent encounter
    q   sequela

S95.0   Injury of dorsal artery of foot
    S95.00   Unspecified injury of dorsal artery of foot
        S95.001   Unspecified injury of dorsal artery of right foot
        S95.002   Unspecified injury of dorsal artery of left foot
        S95.009   Unspecified injury of dorsal artery of unspecified foot
    S95.01   Laceration of dorsal artery of foot
        S95.011   Laceration of dorsal artery of right foot
        S95.012   Laceration of dorsal artery of left foot
        S95.019   Laceration of dorsal artery of unspecified foot
    S95.09   Other specified injury of dorsal artery of foot
        S95.091   Other specified injury of dorsal artery of right foot
        S95.092   Other specified injury of dorsal artery of left foot
        S95.099   Other specified injury of dorsal artery of unspecified foot
S95.1   Injury of plantar artery of foot
    S95.10   Unspecified injury of plantar artery of foot
        S95.101   Unspecified injury of plantar artery of right foot
        S95.102   Unspecified injury of plantar artery of left foot
        S95.109   Unspecified injury of plantar artery of unspecified foot
    S95.11   Laceration of plantar artery of foot
        S95.111   Laceration of plantar artery of right foot
        S95.112   Laceration of plantar artery of left foot
        S95.119   Laceration of plantar artery of unspecified foot
    S95.19   Other specified injury of plantar artery of foot
        S95.191   Other specified injury of plantar artery of right foot
        S95.192   Other specified injury of plantar artery of left foot
        S95.199   Other specified injury of plantar artery of unspecified foot
S95.2   Injury of dorsal vein of foot
    S95.20   Unspecified injury of dorsal vein of foot
        S95.201   Unspecified injury of dorsal vein of right foot
        S95.202   Unspecified injury of dorsal vein of left foot
        S95.209   Unspecified injury of dorsal vein of unspecified foot
    S95.21   Laceration of dorsal vein of foot
        S95.211   Laceration of dorsal vein of right foot
        S95.212   Laceration of dorsal vein of left foot
        S95.219   Laceration of dorsal vein of unspecified foot

S95.29 Other specified injury of dorsal vein of foot
   S95.291 Other specified injury of dorsal vein of right foot
   S95.292 Other specified injury of dorsal vein of left foot
   S95.299 Other specified injury of dorsal vein of unspecified foot

S95.8 Injury of other blood vessels at ankle and foot level
  S95.80 Unspecified injury of other blood vessels at ankle and foot level
   S95.801 Unspecified injury of other blood vessels at ankle and foot level, right leg
   S95.802 Unspecified injury of other blood vessels at ankle and foot level, left leg
   S95.809 Unspecified injury of other blood vessels at ankle and foot level, unspecified leg
  S95.81 Laceration of other blood vessels at ankle and foot level
   S95.811 Laceration of other blood vessels at ankle and foot level, right leg
   S95.812 Laceration of other blood vessels at ankle and foot level, left leg
   S95.819 Laceration of other blood vessels at ankle and foot level, unspecified leg
  S95.89 Other specified injury of other blood vessels at ankle and foot level
   S95.891 Other specified injury of other blood vessels at ankle and foot level, right leg
   S95.892 Other specified injury of other blood vessels at ankle and foot level, left leg
   S95.899 Other specified injury of other blood vessels at ankle and foot level, unspecified leg

S95.9 Injury of unspecified blood vessel at ankle and foot level
  S95.90 Unspecified injury of unspecified blood vessel at ankle and foot level
   S95.901 Unspecified injury of unspecified blood vessel at ankle and foot level, right leg
   S95.902 Unspecified injury of unspecified blood vessel at ankle and foot level, left leg
   S95.909 Unspecified injury of unspecified blood vessel at ankle and foot level, unspecified leg
  S95.91 Laceration of unspecified blood vessel at ankle and foot level
   S95.911 Laceration of unspecified blood vessel at ankle and foot level, right leg
   S95.912 Laceration of unspecified blood vessel at ankle and foot level, left leg
   S95.919 Laceration of unspecified blood vessel at ankle and foot level, unspecified leg
  S95.99 Other specified injury of unspecified blood vessel at ankle and foot level
   S95.991 Other specified injury of unspecified blood vessel at ankle and foot level, right leg
   S95.992 Other specified injury of unspecified blood vessel at ankle and foot level, left leg
   S95.999 Other specified injury of unspecified blood vessel at ankle and foot level, unspecified leg

S96 Injury of muscle and tendon at ankle and foot level
Code also any associated open wound (S91.-)
Excludes2: injury of Achilles tendon (S86.0-)
    sprain of joints and ligaments of ankle and foot (S93.-)
The following extensions are to be added to each code for category S96>
  a initial encounter
  d subsequent encounter
  q sequela
S96.0 Injury of muscle and tendon of long flexor muscle of toe at ankle and foot level
  S96.00 Unspecified injury of muscle and tendon of long flexor muscle of toe at ankle and foot level

   S96.001 Unspecified injury of muscle and tendon of long flexor muscle of toe at right ankle and foot level
   S96.002 Unspecified injury of muscle and tendon of long flexor muscle of toe at left ankle and foot level
   S96.009 Unspecified injury of muscle and tendon of long flexor muscle of toe at ankle and foot level, unspecified side
  S96.01 Strain of muscle and tendon of long flexor muscle of toe at ankle and foot level
   S96.011 Strain of muscle and tendon of long flexor muscle of toe at right ankle and foot level
   S96.012 Strain of muscle and tendon of long flexor muscle of toe at left ankle and foot level
   S96.019 Strain of muscle and tendon of long flexor muscle of toe at ankle and foot level, unspecified side
  S96.02 Laceration of muscle and tendon of long flexor muscle of toe at ankle and foot level
   S96.021 Laceration of muscle and tendon of long flexor muscle of toe at right ankle and foot level
   S96.022 Laceration of muscle and tendon of long flexor muscle of toe at left ankle and foot level
   S96.029 Laceration of muscle and tendon of long flexor muscle of toe at ankle and foot level, unspecified side
  S96.09 Other injury of muscle and tendon of long flexor muscle of toe at ankle and foot level
   S96.091 Other injury of muscle and tendon of long flexor muscle of toe at right ankle and foot level
   S96.092 Other injury of muscle and tendon of long flexor muscle of toe at left ankle and foot level
   S96.099 Other injury of muscle and tendon of long flexor muscle of toe at ankle and foot level, unspecified side

S96.1 Injury of muscle and tendon of long extensor muscle of toe at ankle and foot level
  S96.10 Unspecified injury of muscle and tendon of long extensor muscle of toe at ankle and foot level
   S96.101 Unspecified injury of muscle and tendon of long extensor muscle of toe at right ankle and foot level
   S96.102 Unspecified injury of muscle and tendon of long extensor muscle of toe at left ankle and foot level
   S96.109 Unspecified injury of muscle and tendon of long extensor muscle of toe at ankle and foot level, unspecified side
  S96.11 Strain of muscle and tendon of long extensor muscle of toe at ankle and foot level
   S96.111 Strain of muscle and tendon of long extensor muscle of toe at right ankle and foot level
   S96.112 Strain of muscle and tendon of long extensor muscle of toe at left ankle and foot level
   S96.119 Strain of muscle and tendon of long extensor muscle of toe at ankle and foot level, unspecified level
  S96.12 Laceration of muscle and tendon of long extensor muscle of toe at ankle and foot level
   S96.121 Laceration of muscle and tendon of long extensor muscle of toe at right ankle and foot level
   S96.122 Laceration of muscle and tendon of long extensor muscle of toe at left ankle and foot level
   S96.129 Laceration of muscle and tendon of long extensor muscle of toe at ankle and foot level, unspecified side

S96.19   Other injury of muscle and tendon of long extensor muscle of toe at ankle and foot level

    S96.191   Other injury of muscle and tendon of long extensor muscle of toe at right ankle and foot level

    S96.192   Other injury of muscle and tendon of long extensor muscle of toe at left ankle and foot level

    S96.199   Other injury of muscle and tendon of long extensor muscle of toe at ankle and foot level, unspecified side

S96.2   Injury of intrinsic muscle and tendon at ankle and foot level

  S96.20   Unspecified injury of intrinsic muscle and tendon at ankle and foot level

    S96.201   Unspecified injury of intrinsic muscle and tendon at right ankle and foot level

    S96.202   Unspecified injury of intrinsic muscle and tendon at left ankle and foot level

    S96.209   Unspecified injury of intrinsic muscle and tendon at ankle and foot level, unspecified side

  S96.21   Strain of intrinsic muscle and tendon at ankle and foot level

    S96.211   Strain of intrinsic muscle and tendon at right ankle and foot level

    S96.212   Strain of intrinsic muscle and tendon at left ankle and foot level

    S96.219   Strain of intrinsic muscle and tendon at ankle and foot level, unspecified side

  S96.22   Laceration of intrinsic muscle and tendon at ankle and foot level

    S96.221   Laceration of intrinsic muscle and tendon at right ankle and foot level

    S96.222   Laceration of intrinsic muscle and tendon at left ankle and foot level

    S96.229   Laceration of intrinsic muscle and tendon at ankle and foot level, unspecified side

  S96.29   Other injury of intrinsic muscle and tendon at ankle and foot level

    S96.291   Other injury of intrinsic muscle and tendon at right ankle and foot level

    S96.292   Other injury of intrinsic muscle and tendon at left ankle and foot level

    S96.299   Other injury of intrinsic muscle and tendon at ankle and foot level, unspecified side

S96.8   Injury of other muscles and tendons at ankle and foot level

  S96.80   Unspecified injury of other muscles and tendons at ankle and foot level

    S96.801   Unspecified injury of other muscles and tendons at right ankle and foot level

    S96.802   Unspecified injury of other muscles and tendons at left ankle and foot level

    S96.809   Unspecified injury of other muscles and tendons at ankle and foot level, unspecified side

  S96.81   Strain of other muscles and tendons at ankle and foot level

    S96.811   Strain of other muscles and tendons at right ankle and foot level

    S96.812   Strain of other muscles and tendons at left ankle and foot level

    S96.819   Strain of other muscles and tendons at ankle and foot level, unspecified side

  S96.82   Laceration of other muscles and tendons at ankle and foot level

    S96.821   Laceration of other muscles and tendons at right ankle and foot level

    S96.822   Laceration of other muscles and tendons at left ankle and foot level

    S96.829   Laceration of other muscles and tendons at ankle and foot level, unspecified side

  S96.89   Other injury of other muscles and tendons at ankle and foot level

    S96.891   Other injury of other muscles and tendons at right ankle and foot level

    S96.892   Other injury of other muscles and tendons at left ankle and foot level

    S96.899   Other injury of other muscles and tendons at ankle and foot level, unspecified side

S96.9   Injury of unspecified muscle and tendon at ankle and foot level

  S96.90   Unspecified injury of unspecified muscle and tendon at ankle and foot level

    S96.901   Unspecified injury of unspecified muscle and tendon at right ankle and foot level

    S96.902   Unspecified injury of unspecified muscle and tendon at left ankle and foot level

    S96.909   Unspecified injury of unspecified muscle and tendon at ankle and foot level, unspecified side

  S96.91   Strain of unspecified muscle and tendon at ankle and foot level

    S96.911   Strain of unspecified muscle and tendon at right ankle and foot level

    S96.912   Strain of unspecified muscle and tendon at left ankle and foot level

    S96.919   Strain of unspecified muscle and tendon at ankle and foot level, unspecified side

  S96.92   Laceration of unspecified muscle and tendon at ankle and foot level

    S96.921   Laceration of unspecified muscle and tendon at right ankle and foot level

    S96.922   Laceration of unspecified muscle and tendon at left ankle and foot level

    S96.929   Laceration of unspecified muscle and tendon at ankle and foot level, unspecified side

  S96.99   Other injury of unspecified muscle and tendon at ankle and foot level

    S96.991   Other injury of unspecified muscle and tendon at right ankle and foot level

    S96.992   Other injury of unspecified muscle and tendon at left ankle and foot level

    S96.999   Other injury of unspecified muscle and tendon at ankle and foot level, unspecified side

S97 Crushing injury of ankle and foot

Use additional code(s) for all associated injuries

The following extensions are to be added to each code for category S97:

    a   initial encounter
    d   subsequent encounter
    q   sequela

S97.0   Crushing injury of ankle

  S97.00   Crushing injury of ankle, unspecified side

  S97.01   Crushing injury of right ankle

  S97.02   Crushing injury of left ankle

S97.1   Crushing injury of toe

  S97.10   Crushing injury of unspecified toe(s)

    S97.101   Crushing injury of unspecified toe(s), right foot

    S97.102   Crushing injury of unspecified toe(s), left foot

    S97.109   Crushing injury of unspecified toe(s), unspecified foot

  S97.11   Crushing injury of great toe

    S97.111   Crushing injury of great right toe

    S97.112   Crushing injury of great left toe

    S97.119   Crushing injury of great toe, unspecified side

  S97.12   Crushing injury of lesser toe(s)

    S97.121   Crushing injury of lesser right toe(s)

    S97.122   Crushing injury of lesser left toe(s)

    S97.129   Crushing injury of lesser toe(s), unspecified side

S97.8   **Crushing injury of foot**
   S97.80   **Crushing injury of foot, unspecified side**
     Crushing injury of foot NOS
   S97.81   **Crushing injury of foot, right side**
   S97.82   **Crushing injury of foot, left side**

S98   **Traumatic amputation of ankle and foot**
   An amputation not identified as partial or complete should be coded to complete
   The following extensions are to be added to each code for category S98:
     a   initial encounter
     d   subsequent encounter
     q   sequela

S98.0   **Traumatic amputation of foot at ankle level**
   S98.01   **Complete traumatic amputation of foot at ankle level**
     S98.011   **Complete traumatic amputation of right foot at ankle level**
     S98.012   **Complete traumatic amputation of left foot at ankle level**
     S98.019   **Complete traumatic amputation of foot at ankle level, unspecified side**
   S98.02   **Partial traumatic amputation of foot at ankle level**
     S98.021   **Partial traumatic amputation of right foot at ankle level**
     S98.022   **Partial traumatic amputation of left foot at ankle level**
     S98.029   **Partial traumatic amputation of foot at ankle level, unspecified side**

S98.1   **Traumatic amputation of one toe**
   S98.11   **Complete traumatic amputation of great toe**
     S98.111   **Complete traumatic amputation of right great toe**
     S98.112   **Complete traumatic amputation of left great toe**
     S98.119   **Complete traumatic amputation of great toe, unspecified side**
   S98.12   **Partial traumatic amputation of great toe**
     S98.121   **Partial traumatic amputation of right great toe**
     S98.122   **Partial traumatic amputation of left great toe**
     S98.129   **Partial traumatic amputation of great toe, unspecified side**
   S98.13   **Complete traumatic amputation of one lesser toe**
     Traumatic amputation of toe NOS
     S98.131   **Complete traumatic amputation of one lesser right toe**
     S98.132   **Complete traumatic amputation of one lesser left toe**
     S98.139   **Complete traumatic amputation of one lesser toe, unspecified side**
   S98.14   **Partial traumatic amputation of one lesser toe**
     S98.141   **Partial traumatic amputation of one lesser right toe**
     S98.142   **Partial traumatic amputation of one lesser left toe**
     S98.149   **Partial traumatic amputation of one lesser toe, unspecified side**

S98.2   **Traumatic amputation of two or more lesser toes**
   S98.21   **Complete traumatic amputation of two or more lesser toes**
     S98.211   **Complete traumatic amputation of two or more lesser right toes**
     S98.212   **Complete traumatic amputation of two or more lesser left toes**
     S98.219   **Complete traumatic amputation of two or more lesser toes, unspecified side**
   S98.22   **Partial traumatic amputation of two or more lesser toes**
     S98.221   **Partial traumatic amputation of two or more lesser right toes**

     S98.222   **Partial traumatic amputation of two or more lesser left toes**
     S98.229   **Partial traumatic amputation of two or more lesser toes, unspecified side**
S98.3   **Traumatic amputation of midfoot**
   S98.31   **Complete traumatic amputation of midfoot**
     S98.311   **Complete traumatic amputation of right midfoot**
     S98.312   **Complete traumatic amputation of left midfoot**
     S98.319   **Complete traumatic amputation of midfoot, unspecified side**
   S98.32   **Partial traumatic amputation of midfoot**
     S98.321   **Partial traumatic amputation of right midfoot**
     S98.322   **Partial traumatic amputation of left midfoot**
     S98.329   **Partial traumatic amputation of midfoot, unspecified side**
S98.9   **Traumatic amputation of foot, level unspecified**
   S98.91   **Complete traumatic amputation of foot, level unspecified**
     S98.911   **Complete traumatic amputation of right foot, level unspecified**
     S98.912   **Complete traumatic amputation of left foot, level unspecified**
     S98.919   **Complete traumatic amputation of foot, level unspecified, unspecified side**
   S98.92   **Partial traumatic amputation of foot, level unspecified**
     S98.921   **Partial traumatic amputation of right foot, level unspecified**
     S98.922   **Partial traumatic amputation of left foot, level unspecified**
     S98.929   **Partial traumatic amputation of foot, level unspecified, unspecified side**

S99   **Other and unspecified injuries of ankle and foot**
   The following extensions are to be added to each code for category S99:
     a   initial encounter
     d   subsequent encounter
     q   sequela
S99.8   **Other specified injuries of ankle and foot**
   S99.81   **Other specified injuries of ankle**
     S99.811   **Other specified injuries of right ankle**
     S99.812   **Other specified injuries of left ankle**
     S99.819   **Other specified injuries of ankle, unspecified side**
   S99.82   **Other specified injuries of foot**
     S99.821   **Other specified injuries of right foot**
     S99.822   **Other specified injuries of left foot**
     S99.829   **Other specified injuries of foot, unspecified side**
S99.9   **Unspecified injury of ankle and foot**
   S99.91   **Unspecified injury of ankle**
     S99.911   **Unspecified injury of right ankle**
     S99.912   **Unspecified injury of left ankle**
     S99.919   **Unspecified injury of ankle, unspecified side**
   S99.92   **Unspecified injury of foot**
     S99.921   **Unspecified injury of right foot**
     S99.922   **Unspecified injury of left foot**
     S99.929   **Unspecified injury of foot, unspecified side**

*Categories T00-T06 deactivated. Code to individual injuries.

INJURIES INVOLVING MULTIPLE BODY REGIONS (T07)

Excludes1:   burns and corrosions (T20-T32)
frostbite (T33-T34)
insect bite or sting, venomous (T63.4)
sunburn (L55.-)

T07 Unspecified multiple injuries
Note: This code is for use only when no documentation is available identifying the specific injuries. This code is not for use in the inpatient setting
Excludes1:   injury NOS (T14)

*Categories T08-T13 deactivated.

INJURY OF UNSPECIFIED BODY REGION (T14)

T14 Injury of unspecified body region
Excludes1:   multiple unspecified injuries (T07)

T14.9 Unspecified injury

T14.90   Injury, unspecified
Note: This code is for use only when no documentation is available identifying the specific injury. This code is not for use in the inpatient setting
Injury NOS

T14.91   Suicide attempt
Attempted suicide NOS

EFFECTS OF FOREIGN BODY ENTERING THROUGH NATURAL ORIFICE (T15–T19)

Excludes2:   foreign body accidentally left in operation wound (T81.5-)
foreign body in penetrating wound — see open wound by body region
residual foreign body in soft tissue (M79.5)
splinter, without major open wound — see superficial injury by body region

T15 Foreign body on external eye
Excludes2:   foreign body in penetrating wound of orbit and eye ball (S05.4-, S05.5-)
open wound of eyelid and periocular area (S01.1-)
retained foreign body in eyelid (H02.8-)
retained (old) foreign body in penetrating wound of orbit and eye ball (H05.5-, H44.6-, H44.7-)
superficial foreign body of eyelid and periocular area (S00.25-)
The following extensions are to be added to each code for category T15:
a   initial encounter
d   subsequent encounter
q   sequela

T15.0 Foreign body in cornea
T15.00   Foreign body in cornea, unspecified eye
T15.01   Foreign body in cornea, right eye
T15.02   Foreign body in cornea, left eye

T15.1 Foreign body in conjunctival sac
T15.10   Foreign body in conjunctival sac, unspecified eye
T15.11   Foreign body in conjunctival sac, right eye
T15.12   Foreign body in conjunctival sac, left eye

T15.8 Foreign body in other and multiple parts of external eye
Foreign body in lacrimal punctum
T15.80   Foreign body in other and multiple parts of external eye, unspecified eye
T15.81   Foreign body in other and multiple parts of external eye, right eye
T15.82   Foreign body in other and multiple parts of external eye, left eye

T15.9 Foreign body on external eye, part unspecified
T15.90   Foreign body on external eye, part unspecified, unspecified eye
T15.91   Foreign body on external eye, part unspecified, right eye
T15.92   Foreign body on external eye, part unspecified, left eye

T16 Foreign body in ear
Includes: auditory canal
The following extensions are to be added to each code for category T16:
a   initial encounter
d   subsequent encounter
q   sequela
T16.1 Foreign body in right ear
T16.2 Foreign body in left ear
T16.9 Foreign body in ear, unspecified ear

T17 Foreign body in respiratory tract
The following extensions are to be added to each code for category T17:
a   initial encounter
d   subsequent encounter
q   sequela
T17.0 Foreign body in nasal sinus
T17.1 Foreign body in nostril
Foreign body in nose NOS
T17.2 Foreign body in pharynx
Foreign body in nasopharynx
Foreign body in throat NOS
T17.20   Unspecified foreign body in pharynx
T17.200   Unspecified foreign body in pharynx causing asphyxiation
T17.208   Unspecified foreign body in pharynx causing other injury
T17.21   Gastric contents in pharynx
Aspiration of gastric contents into pharynx
Vomitus in pharynx
T17.210   Gastric contents in pharynx causing asphyxiation
T17.218   Gastric contents in pharynx causing other injury
T17.22   Food in pharynx
Bones in pharynx
Seeds in pharynx
T17.220   Food in pharynx causing asphyxiation
T17.228   Food in pharynx causing other injury
T17.29   Other foreign object in pharynx
T17.290   Other foreign object in pharynx causing asphyxiation
T17.298   Other foreign object in pharynx causing other injury
T17.3 Foreign body in larynx
T17.30   Unspecified foreign body in larynx
T17.300   Unspecified foreign body in larynx causing asphyxiation
T17.308   Unspecified foreign body in larynx causing other injury
T17.31   Gastric contents in larynx
Aspiration of gastric contents into larynx
Vomitus in larynx
T17.310   Gastric contents in larynx causing asphyxiation
T17.318   Gastric contents in larynx causing other injury
T17.32   Food in larynx
Bones in larynx
Seeds in larynx
T17.320   Food in larynx causing asphyxiation
T17.328   Food in larynx causing other injury
T17.39   Other foreign object in larynx
T17.390   Other foreign object in larynx causing asphyxiation
T17.398   Other foreign object in larynx causing other injury
T17.4 Foreign body in trachea
T17.40   Unspecified foreign body in trachea
T17.400   Unspecified foreign body in trachea causing asphyxiation

T17.408   **Unspecified foreign body in trachea causing other injury**

T17.41   **Gastric contents in trachea**
Aspiration of gastric contents into trachea
Vomitus in trachea

T17.410   **Gastric contents in trachea causing asphyxiation**

T17.418   **Gastric contents in trachea causing other injury**

T17.42   **Food in trachea**
Bones in trachea
Seeds in trachea

T17.420   **Food in trachea causing asphyxiation**

T17.428   **Food in trachea causing other injury**

T17.49   **Other foreign object in trachea**

T17.490   **Other foreign object in trachea causing asphyxiation**

T17.498   **Other foreign object in trachea causing other injury**

T17.5   Foreign body in bronchus

T17.50   **Unspecified foreign body in bronchus**

T17.500   **Unspecified foreign body in bronchus causing asphyxiation**

T17.508   **Unspecified foreign body in bronchus causing other injury**

T17.51   **Gastric contents in bronchus**
Aspiration of gastric contents into bronchus
Vomitus in bronchus

T17.510   **Gastric contents in bronchus causing asphyxiation**

T17.518   **Gastric contents in bronchus causing other injury**

T17.52   **Food in bronchus**
Bones in bronchus
Seeds in bronchus

T17.520   **Food in bronchus causing asphyxiation**

T17.528   **Food in bronchus causing other injury**

T17.59   **Other foreign object in bronchus**

T17.590   **Other foreign object in bronchus causing asphyxiation**

T17.598   **Other foreign object in bronchus causing other injury**

T17.8   Foreign body in other parts of respiratory tract
Foreign body in bronchioles
Foreign body in lung

T17.80   **Unspecified foreign body in other parts of respiratory tract**

T17.800   **Unspecified foreign body in other parts of respiratory tract causing asphyxiation**

T17.808   **Unspecified foreign body in other parts of respiratory tract causing other injury**

T17.81   **Gastric contents in other parts of respiratory tract**
Aspiration of gastric contents into other parts of respiratory tract
Vomitus in other parts of respiratory tract

T17.810   **Gastric contents in other parts of respiratory tract causing asphyxiation**

T17.818   **Gastric contents in other parts of respiratory tract causing other injury**

T17.82   **Food in other parts of respiratory tract**
Bones in other parts of respiratory tract
Seeds in other parts of respiratory tract

T17.820   **Food in other parts of respiratory tract causing asphyxiation**

T17.828   **Food in other parts of respiratory tract causing other injury**

T17.89   **Other foreign object in other parts of respiratory tract**

T17.890   **Other foreign object in other parts of respiratory tract causing asphyxiation**

T17.898   **Other foreign object in other parts of respiratory tract causing other injury**

T17.9   Foreign body in respiratory tract, part unspecified

T17.90   **Unspecified foreign body in respiratory tract, part unspecified**

T17.900   **Unspecified foreign body in respiratory tract, part unspecified causing asphyxiation**

T17.908   **Unspecified foreign body in respiratory tract, part unspecified causing other injury**

T17.91   **Gastric contents in respiratory tract, part unspecified**
Aspiration of gastric contents into respiratory tract, part unspecified
Vomitus in trachea respiratory tract, part unspecified

T17.910   **Gastric contents in respiratory tract, part unspecified causing asphyxiation**

T17.918   **Gastric contents in respiratory tract, part unspecified causing other injury**

T17.92   **Food in respiratory tract, part unspecified**
Bones in respiratory tract, part unspecified
Seeds in respiratory tract, part unspecified

T17.920   **Food in respiratory tract, part unspecified causing asphyxiation**

T17.928   **Food in respiratory tract, part unspecified causing other injury**

T17.99   **Other foreign object in respiratory tract, part unspecified**

T17.990   **Other foreign object respiratory tract, part unspecified in causing asphyxiation**

T17.998   **Other foreign object in respiratory tract, part unspecified causing other injury**

T18 Foreign body in alimentary tract

Excludes2:   foreign body in pharynx (T17.2-)

The following extensions are to be added to each code for category T18:

    a   initial encounter
    d   subsequent encounter
    q   sequela

T18.0   Foreign body in mouth

T18.1   Foreign body in esophagus

Excludes2:   foreign body in respiratory tract (T17.-)

T18.10   **Unspecified foreign body in esophagus**

T18.100   **Unspecified foreign body in esophagus causing compression of trachea**
Unspecified foreign body in esophagus causing obstruction of respiration

T18.108   **Unspecified foreign body in esophagus causing other injury**

T18.11   **Gastric contents in esophagus**
Vomitus in esophagus

T18.110   **Gastric contents in esophagus causing compression of trachea**
Gastric contents in esophagus causing obstruction of respiration

T18.118   **Gastric contents in esophagus causing other injury**

T18.12   **Food in esophagus**
Bones in esophagus
Seeds in esophagus

T18.120   **Food in esophagus causing compression of trachea**
Food in esophagus causing obstruction of respiration

T18.128   **Food in esophagus causing other injury**

T18.19   **Other foreign object in esophagus**

T18.190   **Other foreign object in esophagus causing compression of trachea**
Other foreign body in esophagus causing obstruction of respiration

T18.198   **Other foreign object in esophagus causing other injury**

T18.2   Foreign body in stomach

T18.3   Foreign body in small intestine

T18.4   Foreign body in colon

T18.5   Foreign body in anus and rectum
Foreign body in rectosigmoid (junction)

T18.8   Foreign body in other parts of alimentary tract

T18.9   Foreign body of alimentary tract, part unspecified
Foreign body in digestive system NOS
Swallowed foreign body NOS

T19   Foreign body in genitourinary tract
Excludes2:   mechanical complications of contraceptive device (intrauterine) (vaginal) (T83.3-)
presence of contraceptive device (intrauterine) (vaginal) (Z97.5)

The following extensions are to be added to each code for category T19:
a   initial encounter
d   subsequent encounter
q   sequela

T19.0   Foreign body in urethra

T19.1   Foreign body in bladder

T19.2   Foreign body in vulva and vagina

T19.3   Foreign body in uterus

T19.4   Foreign body in penis

T19.8   Foreign body in other parts of genitourinary tract

T19.9   Foreign body in genitourinary tract, part unspecified

BURNS AND CORROSIONS (T20–T32)

Includes: burns (thermal) from electrical heating appliances
burns (thermal) from electricity
burns (thermal) from flame
burns (thermal) from friction
burns (thermal) from hot air and hot gases
burns (thermal) from hot objects
burns (thermal) from lightning
burns (thermal) from radiation
chemical burn [corrosion] (external) (internal)
scalds
Excludes2:   erythema [dermatitis] ab igne (L59.0)
radiation-related disorders of the skin and subcutaneous tissue (L55-L59)
sunburn (L55.-)

BURNS AND CORROSIONS OF EXTERNAL BODY SURFACE, SPECIFIED BY SITE (T20–T25)

Includes: burns and corrosions of first degree [erythema]
burns and corrosions of second degree [blisters][epidermal loss]
burns and corrosions of third degree [deep necrosis of underlying tissue] [full-thickness skin loss]

T20   Burn and corrosion of head, face, and neck
Excludes2:   burn and corrosion of ear drum (T28.41, T28.91)
burn and corrosion of eye and adnexa (T26.-)
burn and corrosion of mouth and pharynx (T28.0)

The following extensions are to be added to each code for category T20:
a   initial encounter
d   subsequent encounter
q   sequela

T20.0   Burn of unspecified degree of head, face, and neck
Use additional external cause code to identify the source, place and intent of the burn (X00-X19, X75-X77, X96-X98, Y92)

T20.00   Burn of unspecified degree of head, face, and neck, unspecified site

T20.01   Burn of unspecified degree of ear [any part, except ear drum]
Excludes2:   burn of ear drum (T28.41-)

T20.011   Burn of unspecified degree of right ear [any part, except ear drum]

T20.012   Burn of unspecified degree of left ear [any part, except ear drum]

T20.019   Burn of unspecified degree of unspecified ear [any part, except ear drum]

T20.02   Burn of unspecified degree of lip(s)

T20.03   Burn of unspecified degree of chin

T20.04   Burn of unspecified degree of nose (septum)

T20.05   Burn of unspecified degree of scalp [any part]

T20.06   Burn of unspecified degree of forehead and cheek

T20.07   Burn of unspecified degree of neck

T20.09   Burn of unspecified degree of multiple sites of head, face, and neck

T20.1   Burn of first degree of head, face, and neck
Use additional external cause code to identify the source, place and intent of the burn (X00-X19, X75-X77, X96-X98, Y92)

T20.10   Burn of first degree of head, face, and neck, unspecified site

T20.11   Burn of first degree of ear [any part, except ear drum]
Excludes2:   burn of ear drum (T28.41-)

T20.111   Burn of first degree of right ear [any part, except ear drum]

T20.112   Burn of first degree of left ear [any part, except ear drum]

T20.119   Burn of first degree of unspecified ear [any part, except ear drum]

T20.12   Burn of first degree of lip(s)

T20.13   Burn of first degree of chin

T20.14   Burn of first degree of nose (septum)

T20.15   Burn of first degree of scalp [any part]

T20.16   Burn of first degree of forehead and cheek

T20.17   Burn of first degree of neck

T20.19   Burn of first degree of multiple sites of head, face, and neck

T20.2   Burn of second degree of head, face, and neck
Use additional external cause code to identify the source, place and intent of the burn (X00-X19, X75-X77, X96-X98, Y92)

T20.20   Burn of second degree of head, face, and neck, unspecified site

T20.21   Burn of second degree of ear [any part, except ear drum]
Excludes2:   burn of ear drum (T28.41-)

T20.211   Burn of second degree of right ear [any part, except ear drum]

T20.212   Burn of second degree of left ear [any part, except ear drum]

T20.219   Burn of second degree of unspecified ear [any part, except ear drum]

T20.22   Burn of second degree of lip(s)

T20.23   Burn of second degree of chin

T20.24   Burn of second degree of nose (septum)

T20.25   Burn of second degree of scalp [any part]

T20.26   Burn of second degree of forehead and cheek

T20.27   Burn of second degree of neck

T20.29   Burn of second degree of multiple sites of head, face, and neck

T20.3   Burn of third degree of head, face, and neck
Use additional external cause code to identify the source, place and intent of the burn (X00-X19, X75-X77, X96-X98, Y92)

T20.30   Burn of third degree of head, face, and neck, unspecified site

T20.31   Burn of third degree of ear [any part, except ear drum]
Excludes2:   burn of ear drum (T28.41-)

T20.311   Burn of third degree of right ear [any part, except ear drum]

T20.312   Burn of third degree of left ear [any part, except ear drum]

T20.319   Burn of third degree of unspecified ear [any part, except ear drum]

T20.32   Burn of third degree of lip(s)

T20.33   Burn of third degree of chin

T20.34   Burn of third degree of nose (septum)

T20.35   Burn of third degree of scalp [any part]

T20.36   Burn of third degree of forehead and cheek

T20.37   Burn of third degree of neck

T20.39   Burn of third degree of multiple sites of head, face, and neck

T20.4   **Corrosion of unspecified degree of head, face, and neck**
Use additional toxic effect code to identify chemical and intent (T51-T65)
Use additional external cause code to identify place (Y92)

T20.40   Corrosion of unspecified degree of head, face, and neck, unspecified site

T20.41   Corrosion of unspecified degree of ear [any part, except ear drum]
Excludes2:   corrosion of ear drum (T28.91-)

T20.411   Corrosion of unspecified degree of right ear [any part, except ear drum]

T20.412   Corrosion of unspecified degree of left ear [any part, except ear drum]

T20.419   Corrosion of unspecified degree of unspecified ear [any part, except ear drum]

T20.42   Corrosion of unspecified degree of lip(s)

T20.43   Corrosion of unspecified degree of chin

T20.44   Corrosion of unspecified degree of nose (septum)

T20.45   Corrosion of unspecified degree of scalp [any part]

T20.46   Corrosion of unspecified degree of forehead and cheek

T20.47   Corrosion of unspecified degree of neck

T20.49   Corrosion of unspecified degree of multiple sites of head, face, and neck

T20.5   **Corrosion of first degree of head, face, and neck**
Use additional toxic effect code to identify chemical and intent (T51-T65)
Use additional external cause code to identify place (Y92)

T20.50   Corrosion of first degree of head, face, and neck, unspecified site

T20.51   Corrosion of first degree of ear [any part, except ear drum]
Excludes2:   corrosion of ear drum (T28.91-)

T20.511   Corrosion of first degree of right ear [any part, except ear drum]

T20.512   Corrosion of first degree of left ear [any part, except ear drum]

T20.519   Corrosion of first degree of unspecified ear [any part, except ear drum]

T20.52   Corrosion of first degree of lip(s)

T20.53   Corrosion of first degree of chin

T20.54   Corrosion of first degree of nose (septum)

T20.55   Corrosion of first degree of scalp [any part]

T20.56   Corrosion of first degree of cheek

T20.57   Corrosion of first degree of neck

T20.59   Corrosion of first degree of multiple sites of head, face, and neck

T20.6   **Corrosion of second degree of head, face, and neck**
Use additional toxic effect code to identify chemical and intent (T51-T65)
Use additional external cause code to identify place (Y92)

T20.60   Corrosion of second degree of head, face, and neck, unspecified site

T20.61   Corrosion of second degree of ear [any part, except ear drum]
Excludes2:   corrosion of ear drum (T28.91-)

T20.611   Corrosion of second degree of right ear [any part, except ear drum]

T20.612   Corrosion of second degree of left ear [any part, except ear drum]

T20.619   Corrosion of second degree of unspecified ear [any part, except ear drum]

T20.62   Corrosion of second degree of lip(s)

T20.63   Corrosion of second degree of chin

T20.64   Corrosion of second degree of nose (septum)

T20.65   Corrosion of second degree of scalp [any part]

T20.66   Corrosion of second degree of forehead and cheek

T20.67   Corrosion of second degree of neck

T20.69   Corrosion of second degree of multiple sites of head, face, and neck

T20.7   **Corrosion of third degree of head, face, and neck**
Use additional toxic effect code to identify chemical and intent (T51-T65)
Use additional external cause code to identify place (Y92)

T20.70   Corrosion of third degree of head, face, and neck, unspecified site

T20.71   Corrosion of third degree of ear [any part, except ear drum]
Excludes2:   corrosion of ear drum (T28.91-)

T20.711   Corrosion of third degree of right ear [any part, except ear drum]

T20.712   Corrosion of third degree of left ear [any part, except ear drum]

T20.719   Corrosion of third degree of unspecified ear [any part, except ear drum]

T20.72   Corrosion of third degree of lip(s)

T20.73   Corrosion of third degree of chin

T20.74   Corrosion of third degree of nose (septum)

T20.75   Corrosion of third degree of scalp [any part]

T20.76   Corrosion of third degree of forehead and cheek

T20.77   Corrosion of third degree of neck

T20.79   Corrosion of third degree of multiple sites of head, face, and neck

T21   **Burn and corrosion of trunk**
Includes: Burns and corrosion of hip region
Excludes2:   burns and corrosion of:
axilla (T22.- with fifth character 4)
scapular region (T22.- with fifth character 6)
shoulder (T22. with fifth character 5)
The following extensions are to be added to each code for category T21:
a   initial encounter
d   subsequent encounter
q   sequela

T21.0   **Burn of unspecified degree of trunk**
Use additional external cause code to identify the source, place and intent of the burn (X00-X19, X75-X77, X96-X98, Y92)

T21.00   Burn of unspecified degree of trunk, unspecified site

T21.01   Burn of unspecified degree of chest wall
Burn of unspecified degree of breast

T21.02   Burn of unspecified degree of abdominal wall
Burn of unspecified degree of flank
Burn of unspecified degree of groin

T21.03   Burn of unspecified degree of upper back
Burn of unspecified degree of interscapular region

T21.04   Burn of unspecified degree of lower back

T21.05   Burn of unspecified degree of buttock
Burn of unspecified degree of anus

T21.06   Burn of unspecified degree of male genital region
Burn of unspecified degree of penis
Burn of unspecified degree of scrotum
Burn of unspecified degree of testis

T21.07   Burn of unspecified degree of female genital region
Burn of unspecified degree of labium (majus) (minus)
Burn of unspecified degree of perineum
Burn of unspecified degree of vulva
Excludes2:   burn of vagina (T28.3)

T21.09   Burn of unspecified degree of other site of trunk

T21.1   **Burn of first degree of trunk**
Use additional external cause code to identify the source, place and intent of the burn (X00-X19, X75-X77, X96-X98, Y92)

T21.10   Burn of first degree of trunk, unspecified site

T21.11   Burn of first degree of chest wall
Burn of first degree of breast

T21.12   Burn of first degree of abdominal wall
Burn of first degree of flank
Burn of first degree of groin

T21.13   Burn of first degree of upper back
Burn of first degree of interscapular region

T21.14   **Burn of first degree of lower back**
T21.15   **Burn of first degree of buttock**
Burn of first degree of anus
T21.16   **Burn of first degree of male genital region**
Burn of first degree of penis
Burn of first degree of scrotum
Burn of first degree of testis
T21.17   **Burn of first degree of female genital region**
Burn of first degree of labium (majus) (minus)
Burn of first degree of perineum
Burn of first degree of vulva
Excludes2:   burn of vagina (T28.3)
T21.19   **Burn of first degree of other site of trunk**
T21.2   **Burn of second degree of trunk**
Use additional external cause code to identify the source, place and intent of the burn (X00-X19, X75-X77, X96-X98, Y92)
T21.20   **Burn of second degree of trunk, unspecified site**
T21.21   **Burn of second degree of chest wall**
Burn of second degree of breast
T21.22   **Burn of second degree of abdominal wall**
Burn of second degree of flank
Burn of second degree of groin
T21.23   **Burn of second degree of upper back**
Burn of second degree of interscapular region
T21.24   **Burn of second degree of lower back**
T21.25   **Burn of second degree of buttock**
Burn of second degree of anus
T21.26   **Burn of second degree of male genital region**
Burn of second degree of penis
Burn of second degree of scrotum
Burn of second degree of testis
T21.27   **Burn of second degree of female genital region**
Burn of second degree of labium (majus) (minus)
Burn of second degree of perineum
Burn of second degree of vulva
Excludes2:   burn of vagina (T28.3)
T21.29   **Burn of second degree of other site of trunk**
T21.3   **Burn of third degree of trunk**
Use additional external cause code to identify the source, place and intent of the burn (X00-X19, X75-X77, X96-X98, Y92)
T21.30   **Burn of third degree of trunk, unspecified site**
T21.31   **Burn of third degree of chest wall**
Burn of third degree of breast
T21.32   **Burn of third degree of abdominal wall**
Burn of third degree of flank
Burn of third degree of groin
T21.33   **Burn of third degree of upper back**
Burn of third degree of interscapular region
T21.34   **Burn of third degree of lower back**
T21.35   **Burn of third degree of buttock**
Burn of third degree of anus
T21.36   **Burn of third degree of male genital region**
Burn of third degree of penis
Burn of third degree of scrotum
Burn of third degree of testis
T21.37   **Burn of third degree of female genital region**
Burn of third degree of labium (majus) (minus)
Burn of third degree of perineum
Burn of third degree of vulva
Excludes2:   burn of vagina (T28.3)
T21.39   **Burn of third degree of other site of trunk**
T21.4   **Corrosion of unspecified degree of trunk**
Use additional toxic effect code to identify chemical and intent (T51-T65)
Use additional external cause code to identify place (Y92)
T21.40   **Corrosion of unspecified degree of trunk, unspecified site**
T21.41   **Corrosion of unspecified degree of chest wall**
Corrosion of unspecified degree of breast
T21.42   **Corrosion of unspecified degree of abdominal wall**
Corrosion of unspecified degree of flank
Corrosion of unspecified degree of groin

T21.43   **Corrosion of unspecified degree of upper back**
Corrosion of unspecified degree of interscapular region
T21.44   **Corrosion of unspecified degree of lower back**
T21.45   **Corrosion of unspecified degree of buttock**
Corrosion of unspecified degree of anus
T21.46   **Corrosion of unspecified degree of male genital region**
Corrosion of unspecified degree of penis
Corrosion of unspecified degree of scrotum
Corrosion of unspecified degree of testis
T21.47   **Corrosion of unspecified degree of female genital region**
Corrosion of unspecified degree of labium (majus) (minus)
Corrosion of unspecified degree of perineum
Corrosion of unspecified degree of vulva
Excludes2:   corrosion of vagina (T28.8)
T21.49   **Corrosion of unspecified degree of other site of trunk**
T21.5   **Corrosion of first degree of trunk**
Use additional toxic effect code to identify chemical and intent (T51-T65)
Use additional external cause code to identify place (Y92)
T21.50   **Corrosion of first degree of trunk, unspecified site**
T21.51   **Corrosion of first degree of chest wall**
Corrosion of first degree of breast
T21.52   **Corrosion of first degree of abdominal wall**
Corrosion of first degree of flank
Corrosion of first degree of groin
T21.53   **Corrosion of first degree of upper back**
Corrosion of first degree of interscapular region
T21.54   **Corrosion of first degree of lower back**
T21.55   **Corrosion of first degree of buttock**
Corrosion of first degree of anus
T21.56   **Corrosion of first degree of male genital region**
Corrosion of first degree of penis
Corrosion of first degree of scrotum
Corrosion of first degree of testis
T21.57   **Corrosion of first degree of female genital region**
Corrosion of first degree of labium (majus) (minus)
Corrosion of first degree of perineum
Corrosion of first degree of vulva
Excludes2:   corrosion of vagina (T28.8)
T21.59   **Corrosion of first degree of other site of trunk**
T21.6   **Corrosion of second degree of trunk**
Use additional toxic effect code to identify chemical and intent (T51-T65)
Use additional external cause code to identify place (Y92)
T21.60   **Corrosion of second degree of trunk, unspecified site**
T21.61   **Corrosion of second degree of chest wall**
Corrosion of second degree of breast
T21.62   **Corrosion of second degree of abdominal wall**
Corrosion of second degree of flank
Corrosion of second degree of flank
T21.63   **Corrosion of second degree of upper back**
Corrosion of second degree of interscapular region
T21.64   **Corrosion of second degree of lower back**
T21.65   **Corrosion of second degree of buttock**
Corrosion of second degree of anus
T21.66   **Corrosion of second degree of male genital region**
Corrosion of second degree of penis
Corrosion of second degree of scrotum
Corrosion of second degree of testis
T21.67   **Corrosion of second degree of female genital region**
Corrosion of second degree of labium (majus) (minus)
Corrosion of second degree of perineum
Corrosion of second degree of vulva
Excludes2:   corrosion of vagina (T28.8)
T21.69   **Corrosion of second degree of other site of trunk**
T21.7   **Corrosion of third degree of trunk**
Use additional toxic effect code to identify chemical and intent (T51-T65)
Use additional external cause code to identify place (Y92)
T21.70   **Corrosion of third degree of trunk, unspecified site**

T21.71 Corrosion of third degree of chest wall
Corrosion of third degree of breast

T21.72 Corrosion of third degree of abdominal wall
Corrosion of third degree of flank
Corrosion of third degree of groin

T21.73 Corrosion of third degree of upper back
Corrosion of third degree of interscapular region

T21.74 Corrosion of third degree of lower back

T21.75 Corrosion of third degree of buttock
Corrosion of third degree of anus

T21.76 Corrosion of third degree of male genital region
Corrosion of third degree of penis
Corrosion of third degree of scrotum
Corrosion of third degree of testis

T21.77 Corrosion of third degree of female genital region
Corrosion of third degree of labium (majus) (minus)
Corrosion of third degree of perineum
Corrosion of third degree of vulva
Excludes2:   corrosion of vagina (T28.8)

T21.79 Corrosion of third degree of other site of trunk

T22 Burn and corrosion of shoulder and upper limb, except wrist and hand
Excludes2:   burn and corrosion of interscapular region (T21.-)
burn and corrosion of wrist and hand (T23.-)
The following extensions are to be added to each code for category T22:
  a   initial encounter
  d   subsequent encounter
  q   sequela

T22.0 Burn of unspecified degree of shoulder and upper limb, except wrist and hand
Use additional external cause code to identify the source, place and intent of the burn (X00-X19, X75-X77, X96-X98, Y92)

T22.00 Burn of unspecified degree of shoulder and upper limb, except wrist and hand, unspecified site

T22.01 Burn of unspecified degree of forearm
T22.011 Burn of unspecified degree of right forearm
T22.012 Burn of unspecified degree of left forearm
T22.019 Burn of unspecified degree of unspecified forearm

T22.02 Burn of unspecified degree of elbow
T22.021 Burn of unspecified degree of right elbow
T22.022 Burn of unspecified degree of left elbow
T22.029 Burn of unspecified degree of unspecified elbow

T22.03 Burn of unspecified degree of upper arm
T22.031 Burn of unspecified degree of right upper arm
T22.032 Burn of unspecified degree of left upper arm
T22.039 Burn of unspecified degree of unspecified upper arm

T22.04 Burn of unspecified degree of axilla
T22.041 Burn of unspecified degree of right axilla
T22.042 Burn of unspecified degree of left axilla
T22.049 Burn of unspecified degree of unspecified axilla

T22.05 Burn of unspecified degree of shoulder
T22.051 Burn of unspecified degree of right shoulder
T22.052 Burn of unspecified degree of left shoulder
T22.059 Burn of unspecified degree of unspecified shoulder

T22.06 Burn of unspecified degree of scapular region
T22.061 Burn of unspecified degree of right scapular region
T22.062 Burn of unspecified degree of left scapular region
T22.069 Burn of unspecified degree of unspecified scapular region

T22.09 Burn of unspecified degree of multiple sites of shoulder and upper limb, except wrist and hand

T22.091 Burn of unspecified degree of multiple sites of right shoulder and upper limb, except wrist and hand
T22.092 Burn of unspecified degree of multiple sites of left shoulder and upper limb, except wrist and hand
T22.099 Burn of unspecified degree of multiple sites of unspecified shoulder and upper limb, except wrist and hand

T22.1 Burn of first degree of shoulder and upper limb, except wrist and hand
Use additional external cause code to identify the source, place and intent of the burn (X00-X19, X75-X77, X96-X98, Y92)

T22.10 Burn of first degree of shoulder and upper limb, except wrist and hand, unspecified site

T22.11 Burn of first degree of forearm
T22.111 Burn of first degree of right forearm
T22.112 Burn of first degree of left forearm
T22.119 Burn of first degree of unspecified forearm

T22.12 Burn of first degree of elbow
T22.121 Burn of first degree of right elbow
T22.122 Burn of first degree of left elbow
T22.129 Burn of first degree of unspecified elbow

T22.13 Burn of first degree of upper arm
T22.131 Burn of first degree of right upper arm
T22.132 Burn of first degree of left upper arm
T22.139 Burn of first degree of unspecified upper arm

T22.14 Burn of first degree of axilla
T22.141 Burn of first degree of right axilla
T22.142 Burn of first degree of left axilla
T22.149 Burn of first degree of unspecified axilla

T22.15 Burn of first degree of shoulder
T22.151 Burn of first degree of right shoulder
T22.152 Burn of first degree of left shoulder
T22.159 Burn of first degree of unspecified shoulder

T22.16 Burn of first degree of scapular region
T22.161 Burn of first degree of right scapular region
T22.162 Burn of first degree of left scapular region
T22.169 Burn of first degree of unspecified scapular region

T22.19 Burn of first degree of multiple sites of shoulder and upper limb, except wrist and hand
T22.191 Burn of first degree of multiple sites of right shoulder and upper limb, except wrist and hand
T22.192 Burn of first degree of multiple sites of left shoulder and upper limb, except wrist and hand
T22.199 Burn of first degree of multiple sites of unspecified shoulder and upper limb, except wrist and hand

T22.2 Burn of second degree of shoulder and upper limb, except wrist and hand
Use additional external cause code to identify the source, place and intent of the burn (X00-X19, X75-X77, X96-X98, Y92)

T22.20 Burn of second degree of shoulder and upper limb, except wrist and hand, unspecified site

T22.21 Burn of second degree of forearm
T22.211 Burn of second degree of right forearm
T22.212 Burn of second degree of left forearm
T22.219 Burn of second degree of unspecified forearm

T22.22 Burn of second degree of elbow
T22.221 Burn of second degree of right elbow
T22.222 Burn of second degree of left elbow
T22.229 Burn of second degree of unspecified elbow

T22.23 Burn of second degree of upper arm
T22.231 Burn of second degree of right upper arm
T22.232 Burn of second degree of left upper arm
T22.238 Burn of second degree of unspecified upper arm

T22.24   Burn of second degree of axilla
   T22.241   Burn of second degree of right axilla
   T22.242   Burn of second degree of left axilla
   T22.249   Burn of second degree of unspecified axilla
T22.25   Burn of second degree of shoulder
   T22.251   Burn of second degree of right shoulder
   T22.252   Burn of second degree of left shoulder
   T22.259   Burn of second degree of unspecified shoulder
T22.26   Burn of second degree of scapular region
   T22.261   Burn of second degree of right scapular region
   T22.262   Burn of second degree of left scapular region
   T22.269   Burn of second degree of unspecified scapular region
T22.29   Burn of second degree of multiple sites of shoulder and upper limb, except wrist and hand
   T22.291   Burn of second degree of multiple sites of right shoulder and upper limb, except wrist and hand
   T22.292   Burn of second degree of multiple sites of left shoulder and upper limb, except wrist and hand
   T22.299   Burn of second degree of multiple sites of unspecified shoulder and upper limb, except wrist and hand

T22.3   Burn of third degree of shoulder and upper limb, except wrist and hand
> Use additional external cause code to identify the source, place and intent of the burn (X00-X19, X75-X77, X96-X98, Y92)

T22.30   Burn of third degree of shoulder and upper limb, except wrist and hand, unspecified site
T22.31   Burn of third degree of forearm
   T22.311   Burn of third degree of right forearm
   T22.312   Burn of third degree of left forearm
   T22.319   Burn of third degree of unspecified forearm
T22.32   Burn of third degree of elbow
   T22.321   Burn of third degree of right elbow
   T22.322   Burn of third degree of left elbow
   T22.329   Burn of third degree of unspecified elbow
T22.33   Burn of third degree of upper arm
   T22.331   Burn of third degree of right upper arm
   T22.332   Burn of third degree of left upper arm
   T22.339   Burn of third degree of unspecified upper arm
T22.34   Burn of third degree of axilla
   T22.341   Burn of third degree of right axilla
   T22.342   Burn of third degree of left axilla
   T22.349   Burn of third degree of unspecified axilla
T22.35   Burn of third degree of shoulder
   T22.351   Burn of third degree of right shoulder
   T22.352   Burn of third degree of left shoulder
   T22.359   Burn of third degree of unspecified shoulder
T22.36   Burn of third degree of scapular region
   T22.361   Burn of third degree of right scapular region
   T22.362   Burn of third degree of left scapular region
   T22.369   Burn of third degree of unspecified scapular region
T22.39   Burn of third degree of multiple sites of shoulder and upper limb, except wrist and hand
   T22.391   Burn of third degree of multiple sites of right shoulder and upper limb, except wrist and hand
   T22.392   Burn of third degree of multiple sites of left shoulder and upper limb, except wrist and hand
   T22.399   Burn of third degree of multiple sites of unspecified shoulder and upper limb, except wrist and hand

T22.4   Corrosion of unspecified degree of shoulder and upper limb, except wrist and hand
> Use additional toxic effect code to identify chemical and intent (T51-T65)
> Use additional external cause code to identify place (Y92)

T22.40   Corrosion of unspecified degree of shoulder and upper limb, except wrist and hand, unspecified site
T22.41   Corrosion of unspecified degree of forearm
   T22.411   Corrosion of unspecified degree of right forearm
   T22.412   Corrosion of unspecified degree of left forearm
   T22.419   Corrosion of unspecified degree of unspecified forearm
T22.42   Corrosion of unspecified degree of elbow
   T22.421   Corrosion of unspecified degree of right elbow
   T22.422   Corrosion of unspecified degree of left elbow
   T22.429   Corrosion of unspecified degree of unspecified elbow
T22.43   Corrosion of unspecified degree of upper arm
   T22.431   Corrosion of unspecified degree of right upper arm
   T22.432   Corrosion of unspecified degree of left upper arm
   T22.439   Corrosion of unspecified degree of unspecified upper arm
T22.44   Corrosion of unspecified degree of axilla
   T22.441   Corrosion of unspecified degree of right axilla
   T22.442   Corrosion of unspecified degree of left axilla
   T22.449   Corrosion of unspecified degree of unspecified axilla
T22.45   Corrosion of unspecified degree of shoulder
   T22.451   Corrosion of unspecified degree of right shoulder
   T22.452   Corrosion of unspecified degree of left shoulder
   T22.459   Corrosion of unspecified degree of unspecified shoulder
T22.46   Corrosion of unspecified degree of scapular region
   T22.461   Corrosion of unspecified degree of right scapular region
   T22.462   Corrosion of unspecified degree of left scapular region
   T22.469   Corrosion of unspecified degree of unspecified scapular region
T22.49   Corrosion of unspecified degree of multiple sites of shoulder and upper limb, except wrist and hand
   T22.491   Corrosion of unspecified degree of multiple sites of right shoulder and upper limb, except wrist and hand
   T22.492   Corrosion of unspecified degree of multiple sites of left shoulder and upper limb, except wrist and hand
   T22.499   Corrosion of unspecified degree of multiple sites of unspecified shoulder and upper limb, except wrist and hand

T22.5   Corrosion of first degree of shoulder and upper limb, except wrist and hand
> Use additional toxic effect code to identify chemical and intent (T51-T65)
> Use additional external cause code to identify place (Y92)

T22.50   Corrosion of first degree of shoulder and upper limb, except wrist and hand unspecified site
T22.51   Corrosion of first degree of forearm
   T22.511   Corrosion of first degree of right forearm
   T22.512   Corrosion of first degree of left forearm
   T22.519   Corrosion of first degree of unspecified forearm
T22.52   Corrosion of first degree of elbow
   T22.521   Corrosion of first degree of right elbow
   T22.522   Corrosion of first degree of left elbow
   T22.529   Corrosion of first degree of unspecified elbow

T22.53　Corrosion of first degree of upper arm

T22.531　Corrosion of first degree of right upper arm

T22.532　Corrosion of first degree of left upper arm

T22.539　Corrosion of first degree of unspecified upper arm

T22.54　Corrosion of first degree of axilla

T22.541　Corrosion of first degree of right axilla

T22.542　Corrosion of first degree of left axilla

T22.549　Corrosion of first degree of unspecified axilla

T22.55　Corrosion of first degree of shoulder

T22.551　Corrosion of first degree of right shoulder

T22.552　Corrosion of first degree of left shoulder

T22.559　Corrosion of first degree of unspecified shoulder

T22.56　Corrosion of first degree of scapular region

T22.561　Corrosion of first degree of right scapular region

T22.562　Corrosion of first degree of left scapular region

T22.569　Corrosion of first degree of unspecified scapular region

T22.59　Corrosion of first degree of multiple sites of shoulder and upper limb, except wrist and hand

T22.591　Corrosion of first degree of multiple sites of right shoulder and upper limb, except wrist and hand

T22.592　Corrosion of first degree of multiple sites of left shoulder and upper limb, except wrist and hand

T22.599　Corrosion of first degree of multiple sites of unspecified shoulder and upper limb, except wrist and hand

T22.6　Corrosion of second degree of shoulder and upper limb, except wrist and hand

Use additional toxic effect code to identify chemical and intent (T51-T65)

Use additional external cause code to identify place (Y92)

T22.60　Corrosion of second degree of shoulder and upper limb, except wrist and hand, unspecified site

T22.61　Corrosion of second degree of forearm

T22.611　Corrosion of second degree of right forearm

T22.612　Corrosion of second degree of left forearm

T22.619　Corrosion of second degree of unspecified forearm

T22.62　Corrosion of second degree of elbow

T22.621　Corrosion of second degree of right elbow

T22.622　Corrosion of second degree of left elbow

T22.629　Corrosion of second degree of unspecified elbow

T22.63　Corrosion of second degree of upper arm

T22.631　Corrosion of second degree of right upper arm

T22.632　Corrosion of second degree of left upper arm

T22.639　Corrosion of second degree of unspecified upper arm

T22.64　Corrosion of second degree of axilla

T22.641　Corrosion of second degree of right axilla

T22.642　Corrosion of second degree of left axilla

T22.649　Corrosion of second degree of unspecified axilla

T22.65　Corrosion of second degree of shoulder

T22.651　Corrosion of second degree of right shoulder

T22.652　Corrosion of second degree of left shoulder

T22.659　Corrosion of second degree of unspecified shoulder

T22.66　Corrosion of second degree of scapular region

T22.661　Corrosion of second degree of right scapular region

T22.662　Corrosion of second degree of left scapular region

T22.669　Corrosion of second degree of unspecified scapular region

T22.69　Corrosion of second degree of multiple sites of shoulder and upper limb, except wrist and hand

T22.691　Corrosion of second degree of multiple sites of right shoulder and upper limb, except wrist and hand

T22.692　Corrosion of second degree of multiple sites of left shoulder and upper limb, except wrist and hand

T22.699　Corrosion of second degree of multiple sites of unspecified shoulder and upper limb, except wrist and hand

T22.7　Corrosion of third degree of shoulder and upper limb, except wrist and hand

Use additional toxic effect code to identify chemical and intent (T51-T65)

Use additional external cause code to identify place (Y92)

T22.70　Corrosion of third degree of shoulder and upper limb, except wrist and hand, unspecified site

T22.71　Corrosion of third degree of forearm

T22.711　Corrosion of third degree of right forearm

T22.712　Corrosion of third degree of left forearm

T22.719　Corrosion of third degree of unspecified forearm

T22.72　Corrosion of third degree of elbow

T22.721　Corrosion of third degree of right elbow

T22.722　Corrosion of third degree of left elbow

T22.729　Corrosion of third degree of unspecified elbow

T22.73　Corrosion of third degree of upper arm

T22.731　Corrosion of third degree of right upper arm

T22.732　Corrosion of third degree of left upper arm

T22.739　Corrosion of third degree of unspecified upper arm

T22.74　Corrosion of third degree of axilla

T22.741　Corrosion of third degree of right axilla

T22.742　Corrosion of third degree of left axilla

T22.749　Corrosion of third degree of unspecified axilla

T22.75　Corrosion of third degree of shoulder

T22.751　Corrosion of third degree of right shoulder

T22.752　Corrosion of third degree of left shoulder

T22.759　Corrosion of third degree of unspecified shoulder

T22.76　Corrosion of third degree of scapular region

T22.761　Corrosion of third degree of right scapular region

T22.762　Corrosion of third degree of left scapular region

T22.769　Corrosion of third degree of unspecified scapular region

T22.79　Corrosion of third degree of multiple sites of shoulder and upper limb, except wrist and hand

T22.791　Corrosion of third degree of multiple sites of right shoulder and upper limb, except wrist and hand

T22.792　Corrosion of third degree of multiple sites of left shoulder and upper limb, except wrist and hand

T22.799　Corrosion of third degree of multiple sites of unspecified shoulder and upper limb, except wrist and hand

T23　Burn and corrosion of wrist and hand

The following extensions are to be added to each code for category T23:

a　initial encounter

d　subsequent encounter

q　sequela

T23.0　Burn of unspecified degree of wrist and hand

Use additional external cause code to identify the source, place and intent of the burn (X00-X19, X75-X77, X96-X98, Y92)

T23.00　Burn of unspecified degree of hand, unspecified site

T23.001　Burn of unspecified degree of right hand, unspecified site

T23.002   Burn of unspecified degree of left hand, unspecified site

T23.009   Burn of unspecified degree of unspecified hand, unspecified site

T23.01   Burn of unspecified degree of thumb (nail)

T23.011   Burn of unspecified degree of right thumb (nail)

T23.012   Burn of unspecified degree of left thumb (nail)

T23.019   Burn of unspecified degree of unspecified thumb (nail)

T23.02   Burn of unspecified degree of single finger (nail) except thumb

T23.021   Burn of unspecified degree of single right finger (nail) except thumb

T23.022   Burn of unspecified degree of single left finger (nail) except thumb

T23.029   Burn of unspecified degree of unspecified single finger (nail) except thumb

T23.03   Burn of unspecified degree of multiple fingers (nail), not including thumb

T23.031   Burn of unspecified degree of multiple right fingers (nail), not including thumb

T23.032   Burn of unspecified degree of multiple left fingers (nail), not including thumb

T23.039   Burn of unspecified degree of unspecified multiple fingers (nail), not including thumb

T23.04   Burn of unspecified degree of multiple fingers (nail), including thumb

T23.041   Burn of unspecified degree of multiple right fingers (nail), including thumb

T23.042   Burn of unspecified degree of multiple left fingers (nail), including thumb

T23.049   Burn of unspecified degree of unspecified multiple fingers (nail), including thumb

T23.05   Burn of unspecified degree of palm

T23.051   Burn of unspecified degree of right palm

T23.052   Burn of unspecified degree of left palm

T23.059   Burn of unspecified degree of unspecified palm

T23.06   Burn of unspecified degree of back of hand

T23.061   Burn of unspecified degree of back of right hand

T23.062   Burn of unspecified degree of back of left hand

T23.069   Burn of unspecified degree of back of unspecified hand

T23.07   Burn of unspecified degree of wrist

T23.071   Burn of unspecified degree of right wrist

T23.072   Burn of unspecified degree of left wrist

T23.079   Burn of unspecified degree of unspecified wrist

T23.09   Burn of unspecified degree of multiple sites of wrist and hand

T23.091   Burn of unspecified degree of multiple sites of right wrist and hand

T23.092   Burn of unspecified degree of multiple sites of left wrist and hand

T23.099   Burn of unspecified degree of multiple sites of unspecified wrist and hand

T23.1   Burn of first degree of wrist and hand
Use additional external cause code to identify the source, place and intent of the burn (X00-X19, X75-X77, X96-X98, Y92)

T23.10   Burn of first degree of hand, unspecified site

T23.101   Burn of first degree of right hand, unspecified site

T23.102   Burn of first degree of left hand, unspecified site

T23.109   Burn of first degree of unspecified hand, unspecified site

T23.11   Burn of first degree of thumb (nail)

T23.111   Burn of first degree of right thumb (nail)

T23.112   Burn of first degree of left thumb (nail)

T23.119   Burn of first degree of unspecified thumb (nail)

T23.12   Burn of first degree of single finger (nail) except thumb

T23.121   Burn of first degree of single right finger (nail) except thumb

T23.122   Burn of first degree of single left finger (nail) except thumb

T23.129   Burn of first degree of unspecified single finger (nail) except thumb

T23.13   Burn of first degree of multiple fingers (nail), not including thumb

T23.131   Burn of first degree of multiple right fingers (nail), not including thumb

T23.132   Burn of first degree of multiple left fingers (nail), not including thumb

T23.139   Burn of first degree of unspecified multiple fingers (nail), not including thumb

T23.14   Burn of first degree of multiple fingers (nail), including thumb

T23.141   Burn of first degree of multiple right fingers (nail), including thumb

T23.142   Burn of first degree of multiple left fingers (nail), including thumb

T23.149   Burn of first degree of unspecified multiple fingers (nail), including thumb

T23.15   Burn of first degree of palm

T23.151   Burn of first degree of right palm

T23.152   Burn of first degree of left palm

T23.159   Burn of first degree of unspecified palm

T23.16   Burn of first degree of back of hand

T23.161   Burn of first degree of back of right hand

T23.162   Burn of first degree of back of left hand

T23.169   Burn of first degree of back of unspecified hand

T23.17   Burn of first degree of wrist

T23.171   Burn of first degree of right wrist

T23.172   Burn of first degree of left wrist

T23.179   Burn of first degree of unspecified wrist

T23.19   Burn of first degree of multiple sites of wrist and hand

T23.191   Burn of first degree of multiple sites of right wrist and hand

T23.192   Burn of first degree of multiple sites of left wrist and hand

T23.199   Burn of first degree of multiple sites of unspecified wrist and hand

T23.2   Burn of second degree of wrist and hand
Use additional external cause code to identify the source, place and intent of the burn (X00-X19, X75-X77, X96-X98, Y92)

T23.20   Burn of second degree of hand, unspecified site

T23.201   Burn of second degree of right hand, unspecified site

T23.202   Burn of second degree of left hand, unspecified site

T23.209   Burn of second degree of unspecified hand, unspecified site

T23.21   Burn of second degree of thumb (nail)

T23.211   Burn of second degree of right thumb (nail)

T23.212   Burn of second degree of left thumb (nail)

T23.219   Burn of second degree of unspecified thumb (nail)

T23.22   Burn of second degree of single finger (nail) except thumb

T23.221   Burn of second degree of single right finger (nail) except thumb

T23.222   Burn of second degree of single left finger (nail) except thumb

T23.229   Burn of second degree of unspecified single finger (nail) except thumb

T23.23   Burn of second degree of multiple fingers (nail), not including thumb

T23.231   Burn of second degree of multiple right fingers (nail), not including thumb

T23.232   Burn of second degree of multiple left fingers (nail), not including thumb

T23.239   Burn of second degree of unspecified multiple fingers (nail), not including thumb

T23.24   Burn of second degree of multiple fingers (nail), including thumb

     T23.241   Burn of second degree of multiple right fingers (nail), including thumb

     T23.242   Burn of second degree of multiple left fingers (nail), including thumb

     T23.249   Burn of second degree of unspecified multiple fingers (nail), including thumb

T23.25   Burn of second degree of palm

     T23.251   Burn of second degree of right palm

     T23.252   Burn of second degree of left palm

     T23.259   Burn of second degree of unspecified palm

T23.26   Burn of second degree of back of hand

     T23.261   Burn of second degree of back of right hand

     T23.262   Burn of second degree of back of left hand

     T23.269   Burn of second degree of back of unspecified hand

T23.27   Burn of second degree of wrist

     T23.271   Burn of second degree of right wrist

     T23.272   Burn of second degree of left wrist

     T23.279   Burn of second degree of unspecified wrist

T23.29   Burn of second degree of multiple sites of wrist and hand

     T23.291   Burn of second degree of multiple sites of right wrist and hand

     T23.292   Burn of second degree of multiple sites of left wrist and hand

     T23.299   Burn of second degree of multiple sites of unspecified wrist and hand

T23.3   Burn of third degree of wrist and hand

     Use additional external cause code to identify the source, place and intent of the burn (X00-X19, X75-X77, X96-X98, Y92)

T23.30   Burn of third degree of hand, unspecified site

     T23.301   Burn of third degree of right hand, unspecified site

     T23.302   Burn of third degree of left hand, unspecified site

     T23.309   Burn of third degree of unspecified hand, unspecified site

T23.31   Burn of third degree of thumb (nail)

     T23.311   Burn of third degree of right thumb (nail)

     T23.312   Burn of third degree of left thumb (nail)

     T23.319   Burn of third degree of unspecified thumb (nail)

T23.32   Burn of third degree of single finger (nail) except thumb

     T23.321   Burn of third degree of single right finger (nail) except thumb

     T23.322   Burn of third degree of single left finger (nail) except thumb

     T23.329   Burn of third degree of unspecified single finger (nail) except thumb

T23.33   Burn of third degree of multiple fingers (nail), not including thumb

     T23.331   Burn of third degree of multiple right fingers (nail), not including thumb

     T23.332   Burn of third degree of multiple left fingers (nail), not including thumb

     T23.339   Burn of third degree of unspecified multiple fingers (nail), not including thumb

T23.34   Burn of third degree of multiple fingers (nail), including thumb

     T23.341   Burn of third degree of multiple right fingers (nail), including thumb

     T23.342   Burn of third degree of multiple left fingers (nail), including thumb

T23.349   Burn of third degree of unspecified multiple fingers (nail), including thumb

T23.35   Burn of third degree of palm

     T23.351   Burn of third degree of right palm

     T23.352   Burn of third degree of left palm

     T23.359   Burn of third degree of unspecified palm

T23.36   Burn of third degree of back of hand

     T23.361   Burn of third degree of back of right hand

     T23.362   Burn of third degree of back of left hand

     T23.369   Burn of third degree of back of unspecified hand

T23.37   Burn of third degree of wrist

     T23.371   Burn of third degree of right wrist

     T23.372   Burn of third degree of left wrist

     T23.379   Burn of third degree of unspecified wrist

T23.39   Burn of third degree of multiple sites of wrist and hand

     T23.391   Burn of third degree of multiple sites of right wrist and hand

     T23.392   Burn of third degree of multiple sites of left wrist and hand

     T23.399   Burn of third degree of multiple sites of unspecified wrist and hand

T23.4   Corrosion of unspecified degree of wrist and hand

     Use additional toxic effect code to identify chemical and intent (T51-T65)

     Use additional external cause code to identify place (Y92)

T23.40   Corrosion of unspecified degree of hand, unspecified site

     T23.401   Corrosion of unspecified degree of right hand, unspecified site

     T23.402   Corrosion of unspecified degree of left hand, unspecified site

     T23.409   Corrosion of unspecified degree of unspecified hand, unspecified site

T23.41   Corrosion of unspecified degree of thumb (nail)

     T23.411   Corrosion of unspecified degree of right thumb (nail)

     T23.412   Corrosion of unspecified degree of left thumb (nail)

     T23.419   Corrosion of unspecified degree of unspecified thumb (nail)

T23.42   Corrosion of unspecified degree of single finger (nail) except thumb

     T23.421   Corrosion of unspecified degree of single right finger (nail) except thumb

     T23.422   Corrosion of unspecified degree of single left finger (nail) except thumb

     T23.429   Corrosion of unspecified degree of unspecified single finger (nail) except thumb

T23.43   Corrosion of unspecified degree of multiple fingers (nail), not including thumb

     T23.431   Corrosion of unspecified degree of multiple right fingers (nail), not including thumb

     T23.432   Corrosion of unspecified degree of multiple left fingers (nail), not including thumb

     T23.439   Corrosion of unspecified degree of unspecified multiple fingers (nail), not including thumb

T23.44   Corrosion of unspecified degree of multiple fingers (nail), including thumb

     T23.441   Corrosion of unspecified degree of multiple right fingers (nail), including thumb

     T23.442   Corrosion of unspecified degree of multiple left fingers (nail), including thumb

     T23.449   Corrosion of unspecified degree of unspecified multiple fingers (nail), including thumb

T23.45   Corrosion of unspecified degree of palm

     T23.451   Corrosion of unspecified degree of right palm

     T23.452   Corrosion of unspecified degree of left palm

     T23.459   Corrosion of unspecified degree of unspecified palm

T23.46   Corrosion of unspecified degree of back of hand
    T23.461   Corrosion of unspecified degree of back of right hand
    T23.462   Corrosion of unspecified degree of back of left hand
    T23.469   Corrosion of unspecified degree of back of unspecified hand

T23.47   Corrosion of unspecified degree of wrist
    T23.471   Corrosion of unspecified degree of right wrist
    T23.472   Corrosion of unspecified degree of left wrist
    T23.479   Corrosion of unspecified degree of unspecified wrist

T23.49   Corrosion of unspecified degree of multiple sites of wrist and hand
    T23.491   Corrosion of unspecified degree of multiple sites of right wrist and hand
    T23.492   Corrosion of unspecified degree of multiple sites of left wrist and hand
    T23.499   Corrosion of unspecified degree of multiple sites of unspecified wrist and hand

T23.5   Corrosion of first degree of wrist and hand
Use additional toxic effect code to identify chemical and intent (T51-T65)
Use additional external cause code to identify place (Y92)

T23.50   Corrosion of first degree of hand, unspecified site
    T23.501   Corrosion of first degree of right hand, unspecified site
    T23.502   Corrosion of first degree of left hand, unspecified site
    T23.509   Corrosion of first degree of unspecified hand, unspecified site

T23.51   Corrosion of first degree of thumb (nail)
    T23.511   Corrosion of first degree of right thumb (nail)
    T23.512   Corrosion of first degree of left thumb (nail)
    T23.519   Corrosion of first degree of unspecified thumb (nail)

T23.52   Corrosion of first degree of single finger (nail) except thumb
    T23.521   Corrosion of first degree of single right finger (nail) except thumb
    T23.522   Corrosion of first degree of single left finger (nail) except thumb
    T23.529   Corrosion of first degree of unspecified single finger (nail) except thumb

T23.53   Corrosion of first degree of multiple fingers (nail), not including thumb
    T23.531   Corrosion of first degree of multiple right fingers (nail), not including thumb
    T23.532   Corrosion of first degree of multiple left fingers (nail), not including thumb
    T23.539   Corrosion of first degree of unspecified multiple fingers (nail), not including thumb

T23.54   Corrosion of first degree of multiple fingers (nail), including thumb
    T23.541   Corrosion of first degree of multiple right fingers (nail), including thumb
    T23.542   Corrosion of first degree of multiple left fingers (nail), including thumb
    T23.549   Corrosion of first degree of unspecified multiple fingers (nail), including thumb

T23.55   Corrosion of first degree of palm
    T23.551   Corrosion of first degree of right palm
    T23.552   Corrosion of first degree of left palm
    T23.559   Corrosion of first degree of unspecified palm

T23.56   Corrosion of first degree of back of hand
    T23.561   Corrosion of first degree of back of right hand
    T23.562   Corrosion of first degree of back of left hand
    T23.569   Corrosion of first degree of back of unspecified hand

T23.57   Corrosion of first degree of wrist
    T23.571   Corrosion of first degree of right wrist
    T23.572   Corrosion of first degree of left wrist
    T23.579   Corrosion of first degree of unspecified wrist

T23.59   Corrosion of first degree of multiple sites of wrist and hand
    T23.591   Corrosion of first degree of multiple sites of right wrist and hand
    T23.592   Corrosion of first degree of multiple sites of left wrist and hand
    T23.599   Corrosion of first degree of multiple sites of unspecified wrist and hand

T23.6   Corrosion of second degree of wrist and hand
Use additional toxic effect code to identify chemical and intent (T51-T65)
Use additional external cause code to identify place (Y92)

T23.60   Corrosion of second degree of hand, unspecified site
    T23.601   Corrosion of second degree of right hand, unspecified site
    T23.602   Corrosion of second degree of left hand, unspecified site
    T23.609   Corrosion of second degree of unspecified hand, unspecified site

T23.61   Corrosion of second degree of thumb (nail)
    T23.611   Corrosion of second degree of right thumb (nail)
    T23.612   Corrosion of second degree of left thumb (nail)
    T23.619   Corrosion of second degree of unspecified thumb (nail)

T23.62   Corrosion of second degree of single finger (nail) except thumb
    T23.621   Corrosion of second degree of single right finger (nail) except thumb
    T23.622   Corrosion of second degree of single left finger (nail) except thumb
    T23.629   Corrosion of second degree of unspecified single finger (nail) except thumb

T23.63   Corrosion of second degree of multiple fingers (nail), not including thumb
    T23.631   Corrosion of second degree of multiple right fingers (nail), not including thumb
    T23.632   Corrosion of second degree of multiple left fingers (nail), not including thumb
    T23.639   Corrosion of second degree of unspecified multiple fingers (nail), not including thumb

T23.64   Corrosion of second degree of multiple fingers (nail), including thumb
    T23.641   Corrosion of second degree of multiple right fingers (nail), including thumb
    T23.642   Corrosion of second degree of multiple left fingers (nail), including thumb
    T23.649   Corrosion of second degree of unspecified multiple fingers (nail), including thumb

T23.65   Corrosion of second degree of palm
    T23.651   Corrosion of second degree of right palm
    T23.652   Corrosion of second degree of left palm
    T23.659   Corrosion of second degree of unspecified palm

T23.66   Corrosion of second degree of back of hand
    T23.661   Corrosion of second degree of right hand
    T23.662   Corrosion of second degree of left hand
    T23.669   Corrosion of second degree of unspecified hand

T23.67   Corrosion of second degree of wrist
    T23.671   Corrosion of second degree of right wrist
    T23.672   Corrosion of second degree of left wrist
    T23.679   Corrosion of second degree of unspecified wrist

T23.69   Corrosion of second degree of multiple sites of wrist and hand

     T23.691   Corrosion of second degree of multiple sites of right wrist and hand

     T23.692   Corrosion of second degree of multiple sites of left wrist and hand

     T23.699   Corrosion of second degree of multiple sites of unspecified wrist and hand

T23.7   Corrosion of third degree of wrist and hand

     Use additional toxic effect code to identify chemical and intent (T51-T65)

     Use additional external cause code to identify place (Y92)

T23.70   Corrosion of third degree of hand, unspecified site

     T23.701   Corrosion of third degree of right hand, unspecified site

     T23.702   Corrosion of third degree of left hand, unspecified site

     T23.709   Corrosion of third degree of unspecified hand, unspecified site

T23.71   Corrosion of third degree of thumb (nail)

     T23.711   Corrosion of third degree of right thumb (nail)

     T23.712   Corrosion of third degree of left thumb (nail)

     T23.719   Corrosion of third degree of unspecified thumb (nail)

T23.72   Corrosion of third degree of single finger (nail) except thumb

     T23.721   Corrosion of third degree of single right finger (nail) except thumb

     T23.722   Corrosion of third degree of single left finger (nail) except thumb

     T23.729   Corrosion of third degree of unspecified single finger (nail) except thumb

T23.73   Corrosion of third degree of multiple fingers (nail), not including thumb

     T23.731   Corrosion of third degree of multiple right fingers (nail), not including thumb

     T23.732   Corrosion of third degree of multiple left fingers (nail), not including thumb

     T23.739   Corrosion of third degree of unspecified multiple fingers (nail), not including thumb

T23.74   Corrosion of third degree of multiple fingers (nail), including thumb

     T23.741   Corrosion of third degree of multiple right fingers (nail), including thumb

     T23.742   Corrosion of third degree of multiple left fingers (nail), including thumb

     T23.749   Corrosion of third degree of unspecified multiple fingers (nail), including thumb

T23.75   Corrosion of third degree of palm

     T23.751   Corrosion of third degree of right palm

     T23.752   Corrosion of third degree of left palm

     T23.759   Corrosion of third degree of unspecified palm

T23.76   Corrosion of third degree of back of hand

     T23.761   Corrosion of third degree of back of right hand

     T23.762   Corrosion of third degree of back of left hand

     T23.769   Corrosion of third degree of unspecified back of hand

T23.77   Corrosion of third degree of wrist

     T23.771   Corrosion of third degree of right wrist

     T23.772   Corrosion of third degree of left wrist

     T23.779   Corrosion of third degree of unspecified wrist

T23.79   Corrosion of third degree of multiple sites of wrist and hand

     T23.791   Corrosion of third degree of multiple sites of right wrist and hand

     T23.792   Corrosion of third degree of multiple sites of left wrist and hand

     T23.799   Corrosion of third degree of multiple sites of unspecified wrist and hand

T24   Burn and corrosion of lower limb, except ankle and foot

     Excludes2:   burn and corrosion of ankle and foot (T25.-)

                 burn and corrosion of hip region (T21.-)

     The following extensions are to be added to each code for category T24:

     a   initial encounter

     d   subsequent encounter

     q   sequela

T24.0   Burn of unspecified degree of lower limb, except ankle and foot

     Use additional external cause code to identify the source, place and intent of the burn (X00-X19, X75-X77, X96-X98, Y92)

T24.00   Burn of unspecified degree of unspecified site of lower limb, except ankle and foot

     T24.001   Burn of unspecified degree of unspecified site of right lower limb, except ankle and foot

     T24.002   Burn of unspecified degree of unspecified site of left lower limb, except ankle and foot

     T24.009   Burn of unspecified degree of unspecified site of unspecified lower limb, except ankle and foot

T24.01   Burn of unspecified degree of thigh

     T24.011   Burn of unspecified degree of right thigh

     T24.012   Burn of unspecified degree of left thigh

     T24.019   Burn of unspecified degree of unspecified thigh

T24.02   Burn of unspecified degree of knee

     T24.021   Burn of unspecified degree of right knee

     T24.022   Burn of unspecified degree of left knee

     T24.029   Burn of unspecified degree of unspecified knee

T24.03   Burn of unspecified degree of lower leg

     T24.031   Burn of unspecified degree of right lower leg

     T24.032   Burn of unspecified degree of left lower leg

     T24.039   Burn of unspecified degree of unspecified lower leg

T24.09   Burn of unspecified degree of multiple sites of lower limb, except ankle and foot

     T24.091   Burn of unspecified degree of multiple sites of right lower limb, except ankle and foot

     T24.092   Burn of unspecified degree of multiple sites of left lower limb, except ankle and foot

     T24.099   Burn of unspecified degree of multiple sites of unspecified lower limb, except ankle and foot

T24.1   Burn of first degree of lower limb, except ankle and foot

     Use additional external cause code to identify the source, place and intent of the burn (X00-X19, X75-X77, X96-X98, Y92)

T24.10   Burn of first degree of unspecified site of lower limb, except ankle and foot

     T24.101   Burn of first degree of unspecified site of right lower limb, except ankle and foot

     T24.102   Burn of first degree of unspecified site of left lower limb, except ankle and foot

     T24.109   Burn of first degree of unspecified site of unspecified lower limb, except ankle and foot

T24.11   Burn of first degree of thigh

     T24.111   Burn of first degree of right thigh

     T24.112   Burn of first degree of left thigh

     T24.119   Burn of first degree of unspecified thigh

T24.12   Burn of first degree of knee

     T24.121   Burn of first degree of right knee

     T24.122   Burn of first degree of left knee

     T24.129   Burn of first degree of unspecified knee

T24.13   Burn of first degree of lower leg

     T24.131   Burn of first degree of right lower leg

     T24.132   Burn of first degree of left lower leg

     T24.139   Burn of first degree of unspecified lower leg

T24.19   Burn of first degree of multiple sites of lower limb, except ankle and foot

     T24.191   Burn of first degree of multiple sites of right lower limb, except ankle and foot

T24.192   Burn of first degree of multiple sites of left lower limb, except ankle and foot

T24.199   Burn of first degree of multiple sites of unspecified lower limb, except ankle and foot

T24.2   Burn of second degree of lower limb, except ankle and foot
> Use additional external cause code to identify the source, place and intent of the burn (X00-X19, X75-X77, X96-X98, Y92)

T24.20   Burn of second degree of unspecified site of lower limb, except ankle and foot

T24.201   Burn of second degree of unspecified site of right lower limb, except ankle and foot

T24.202   Burn of second degree of unspecified site of left lower limb, except ankle and foot

T24.209   Burn of second degree of unspecified site of unspecified lower limb, except ankle and foot

T24.21   Burn of second degree of thigh

T24.211   Burn of second degree of right thigh

T24.212   Burn of second degree of left thigh

T24.219   Burn of second degree of unspecified thigh

T24.22   Burn of second degree of knee

T24.221   Burn of second degree of right knee

T24.222   Burn of second degree of left knee

T24.229   Burn of second degree of unspecified knee

T24.23   Burn of second degree of lower leg

T24.231   Burn of second degree of right lower leg

T24.232   Burn of second degree of left lower leg

T24.239   Burn of second degree of unspecified lower leg

T24.29   Burn of second degree of multiple sites of lower limb, except ankle and foot

T24.291   Burn of second degree of multiple sites of right lower limb, except ankle and foot

T24.292   Burn of second degree of multiple sites of left lower limb, except ankle and foot

T24.299   Burn of second degree of multiple sites of unspecified

T24.3   Burn of third degree of lower limb, except ankle and foot
> Use additional external cause code to identify the source, place and intent of the burn (X00-X19, X75-X77, X96-X98, Y92)

T24.30   Burn of third degree of unspecified site of lower limb, except ankle and foot

T24.301   Burn of third degree of unspecified site of right lower limb, except ankle and foot

T24.302   Burn of third degree of unspecified site of left lower limb, except ankle and foot

T24.309   Burn of third degree of unspecified site of unspecified lower limb, except ankle and foot

T24.31   Burn of third degree of thigh

T24.311   Burn of third degree of right thigh

T24.312   Burn of third degree of left thigh

T24.319   Burn of third degree of unspecified thigh

T24.32   Burn of third degree of knee

T24.321   Burn of third degree of right knee

T24.322   Burn of third degree of left knee

T24.329   Burn of third degree of unspecified knee

T24.33   Burn of third degree of lower leg

T24.331   Burn of third degree of right lower leg

T24.332   Burn of third degree of left lower leg

T24.339   Burn of third degree of unspecified lower leg

T24.39   Burn of third degree of multiple sites of lower limb, except ankle and foot

T24.391   Burn of third degree of multiple sites of right lower limb, except ankle and foot

T24.392   Burn of third degree of multiple sites of left lower limb, except ankle and foot

T24.399   Burn of third degree of multiple sites of unspecified lower limb, except ankle and foot

T24.4   Corrosion of unspecified degree of lower limb, except ankle and foot
> Use additional toxic effect code to identify chemical and intent (T51-T65)
> Use additional external cause code to identify place (Y92)

T24.40   Corrosion of unspecified degree of unspecified site of lower limb, except ankle and foot

T24.401   Corrosion of unspecified degree of unspecified site of right lower limb, except ankle and foot

T24.402   Corrosion of unspecified degree of unspecified site of left lower limb, except ankle and foot

T24.409   Corrosion of unspecified degree of unspecified site of unspecified lower limb, except ankle and foot

T24.41   Corrosion of unspecified degree of thigh

T24.411   Corrosion of unspecified degree of right thigh

T24.412   Corrosion of unspecified degree of left thigh

T24.419   Corrosion of unspecified degree of unspecified thigh

T24.42   Corrosion of unspecified degree of knee

T24.421   Corrosion of unspecified degree of right knee

T24.422   Corrosion of unspecified degree of left knee

T24.429   Corrosion of unspecified degree of unspecified knee

T24.43   Corrosion of unspecified degree of lower leg

T24.431   Corrosion of unspecified degree of right lower leg

T24.432   Corrosion of unspecified degree of left lower leg

T24.439   Corrosion of unspecified degree of unspecified lower leg

T24.49   Corrosion of unspecified degree of multiple sites of lower limb, except ankle and foot

T24.491   Corrosion of unspecified degree of multiple sites of right lower limb, except ankle and foot

T24.492   Corrosion of unspecified degree of multiple sites of left lower limb, except ankle and foot

T24.499   Corrosion of unspecified degree of multiple sites of unspecified lower limb, except ankle and foot

T24.5   Corrosion of first degree of lower limb, except ankle and foot
> Use additional toxic effect code to identify chemical and intent (T51-T65)
> Use additional external cause code to identify place (Y92)

T24.50   Corrosion of first degree of unspecified site of lower limb, except ankle and foot

T24.501   Corrosion of first degree of unspecified site of right lower limb, except ankle and foot

T24.502   Corrosion of first degree of unspecified site of left lower limb, except ankle and foot

T24.509   Corrosion of first degree of unspecified site of unspecified lower limb, except ankle and foot

T24.51   Corrosion of first degree of thigh

T24.511   Corrosion of first degree of right thigh

T24.512   Corrosion of first degree of left thigh

T24.519   Corrosion of first degree of unspecified thigh

T24.52   Corrosion of first degree of knee

T24.521   Corrosion of first degree of right knee

T24.522   Corrosion of first degree of left knee

T24.529   Corrosion of first degree of unspecified knee

T24.53   Corrosion of first degree of lower leg

T24.531   Corrosion of first degree of right lower leg

T24.532   Corrosion of first degree of left lower leg

T24.539   Corrosion of first degree of unspecified lower leg

T24.59   Corrosion of first degree of multiple sites of lower limb, except ankle and foot

T24.591   Corrosion of first degree of multiple sites of right lower limb, except ankle and foot

T24.592   Corrosion of first degree of multiple sites of left lower limb, except ankle and foot

T24.599   Corrosion of first degree of multiple sites of unspecified lower limb, except ankle and foot

T24.6 Corrosion of second degree of lower limb, except ankle and foot

Use additional toxic effect code to identify chemical and intent (T51-T65)

Use additional external cause code to identify place (Y92)

T24.60 Corrosion of second degree of unspecified site of lower limb, except ankle and foot

T24.601 Corrosion of second degree of unspecified site of right lower limb, except ankle and foot

T24.602 Corrosion of second degree of unspecified site of left lower limb, except ankle and foot

T24.609 Corrosion of second degree of unspecified site of unspecified lower limb, except ankle and foot

T24.61 Corrosion of second degree of thigh

T24.611 Corrosion of second degree of right thigh

T24.612 Corrosion of second degree of left thigh

T24.619 Corrosion of second degree of unspecified thigh

T24.62 Corrosion of second degree of knee

T24.621 Corrosion of second degree of right knee

T24.622 Corrosion of second degree of left knee

T24.629 Corrosion of second degree of unspecified knee

T24.63 Corrosion of second degree of lower leg

T24.631 Corrosion of second degree of right lower leg

T24.632 Corrosion of second degree of left lower leg

T24.639 Corrosion of second degree of unspecified lower leg

T24.69 Corrosion of second degree of multiple sites of lower limb, except ankle and foot

T24.691 Corrosion of second degree of multiple sites of right lower limb, except ankle and foot

T24.692 Corrosion of second degree of multiple sites of left lower limb, except ankle and foot

T24.699 Corrosion of second degree of multiple sites of unspecified lower limb, except ankle and foot

T24.7 Corrosion of third degree of lower limb, except ankle and foot

Use additional toxic effect code to identify chemical and intent (T51-T65)

Use additional external cause code to identify place (Y92)

T24.70 Corrosion of third degree of unspecified site of lower limb, except ankle and foot

T24.701 Corrosion of third degree of unspecified site of right lower limb, except ankle and foot

T24.702 Corrosion of third degree of unspecified site of left lower limb, except ankle and foot

T24.709 Corrosion of third degree of unspecified site of unspecified lower limb, except ankle and foot

T24.71 Corrosion of third degree of thigh

T24.711 Corrosion of third degree of right thigh

T24.712 Corrosion of third degree of left thigh

T24.719 Corrosion of third degree of unspecified thigh

T24.72 Corrosion of third degree of knee

T24.721 Corrosion of third degree of right knee

T24.722 Corrosion of third degree of left knee

T24.729 Corrosion of third degree of unspecified knee

T24.73 Corrosion of third degree of lower leg

T24.731 Corrosion of third degree of right lower leg

T24.732 Corrosion of third degree of left lower leg

T24.739 Corrosion of third degree of unspecified lower leg

T24.79 Corrosion of third degree of multiple sites of lower limb, except ankle and foot

T24.791 Corrosion of third degree of multiple sites of right lower limb, except ankle and foot

T24.792 Corrosion of third degree of multiple sites of left lower limb, except ankle and foot

T24.799 Corrosion of third degree of multiple sites of unspecified lower limb, except ankle and foot

T25 Burn and corrosion of ankle and foot

The following extensions are to be added to each code for category T25:

a   initial encounter

d   subsequent encounter

q   sequela

T25.0 Burn of unspecified degree of ankle and foot

Use additional external cause code to identify the source, place and intent of the burn (X00-X19, X75-X77, X96-X98, Y92)

T25.01 Burn of unspecified degree of ankle

T25.011 Burn of unspecified degree of right ankle

T25.012 Burn of unspecified degree of left ankle

T25.019 Burn of unspecified degree of unspecified ankle

T25.02 Burn of unspecified degree of foot

Excludes2: burn of unspecified degree of toe(s) (nail) (T25.03-)

T25.021 Burn of unspecified degree of right foot

T25.022 Burn of unspecified degree of left foot

T25.029 Burn of unspecified degree of unspecified foot

T25.03 Burn of unspecified degree of toe(s) (nail)

T25.031 Burn of unspecified degree of right toe(s) (nail)

T25.032 Burn of unspecified degree of left toe(s) (nail)

T25.039 Burn of unspecified degree of unspecified toe(s) (nail)

T25.09 Burn of unspecified degree of multiple sites of ankle and foot

T25.091 Burn of unspecified degree of multiple sites of right ankle and foot

T25.092 Burn of unspecified degree of multiple sites of left ankle and foot

T25.099 Burn of unspecified degree of multiple sites of unspecified ankle and foot

T25.1 Burn of first degree of ankle and foot

Use additional external cause code to identify the source, place and intent of the burn (X00-X19, X75-X77, X96-X98, Y92)

T25.11 Burn of first degree of ankle

T25.111 Burn of first degree of right ankle

T25.112 Burn of first degree of left ankle

T25.119 Burn of first degree of unspecified ankle

T25.12 Burn of first degree of foot

Excludes2: burn of first degree of toe(s) (nail) (T25.13-)

T25.121 Burn of first degree of right foot

T25.122 Burn of first degree of left foot

T25.129 Burn of first degree of unspecified foot

T25.13 Burn of first degree of toe(s) (nail)

T25.131 Burn of first degree of right toe(s) (nail)

T25.132 Burn of first degree of left toe(s) (nail)

T25.139 Burn of first degree of unspecified toe(s) (nail)

T25.19 Burn of first degree of multiple sites of ankle and foot

T25.191 Burn of first degree of multiple sites of right ankle and foot

T25.192 Burn of first degree of multiple sites of left ankle and foot

T25.199 Burn of first degree of multiple sites of unspecified ankle and foot

T25.2 Burn of second degree of ankle and foot

Use additional external cause code to identify the source, place and intent of the burn (X00-X19, X75-X77, X96-X98, Y92)

T25.21 Burn of second degree of ankle

T25.211 Burn of second degree of right ankle

T25.212 Burn of second degree of left ankle

T25.219 Burn of second degree of unspecified ankle

T25.22 Burn of second degree of foot

Excludes2: burn of second degree of toe(s) (nail) (T25.23-)

T25.221 Burn of second degree of right foot

T25.222 Burn of second degree of left foot

T25.229 Burn of second degree of unspecified foot

　　　　T25.23　　Burn of second degree of toe(s) (nail)
　　　　　　T25.231　Burn of second degree of right toe(s) (nail)
　　　　　　T25.232　Burn of second degree of left toe(s) (nail)
　　　　　　T25.239　Burn of second degree of unspecified toe(s)
　　　　　　　　　　(nail)
　　　　T25.29　　Burn of second degree of multiple sites of ankle and
　　　　　　　　　foot
　　　　　　T25.291　Burn of second degree of multiple sites of
　　　　　　　　　　right ankle and foot
　　　　　　T25.292　Burn of second degree of multiple sites of left
　　　　　　　　　　ankle and foot
　　　　　　T25.299　Burn of second degree of multiple sites of
　　　　　　　　　　unspecified ankle and foot
　T25.3　Burn of third degree of ankle and foot
　　　　Use additional external cause code to identify the source, place
　　　　　and intent of the burn (X00-X19, X75-X77, X96-X98, Y92)
　　　　T25.31　　Burn of third degree of ankle
　　　　　　T25.311　Burn of third degree of right ankle
　　　　　　T25.312　Burn of third degree of left ankle
　　　　　　T25.319　Burn of third degree of unspecified ankle
　　　　T25.32　　Burn of third degree of foot
　　　　　　Excludes2:　burn of third degree of toe(s) (nail)
　　　　　　　　　　(T25.33-)
　　　　　　T25.321　Burn of third degree of right foot
　　　　　　T25.322　Burn of third degree of left foot
　　　　　　T25.329　Burn of third degree of unspecified foot
　　　　T25.33　　Burn of third degree of toe(s) (nail)
　　　　　　T25.331　Burn of third degree of right toe(s) (nail)
　　　　　　T25.332　Burn of third degree of left toe(s) (nail)
　　　　　　T25.339　Burn of third degree of unspecified toe(s) (nail)
　　　　T25.39　　Burn of third degree of multiple sites of ankle and foot
　　　　　　T25.391　Burn of third degree of multiple sites of right
　　　　　　　　　　ankle and foot
　　　　　　T25.392　Burn of third degree of multiple sites of left
　　　　　　　　　　ankle and foot
　　　　　　T25.399　Burn of third degree of multiple sites of
　　　　　　　　　　unspecified ankle and foot
　T25.4　Corrosion of unspecified degree of ankle and foot
　　　　Use additional toxic effect code to identify chemical and intent
　　　　　(T51-T65)
　　　　Use additional external cause code to identify place (Y92)
　　　　T25.41　　Corrosion of unspecified degree of ankle
　　　　　　T25.411　Corrosion of unspecified degree of right ankle
　　　　　　T25.412　Corrosion of unspecified degree of left ankle
　　　　　　T25.419　Corrosion of unspecified degree of unspecified
　　　　　　　　　　ankle
　　　　T25.42　　Corrosion of unspecified degree of foot
　　　　　　Excludes2:　corrosion of unspecified degree of toe(s)
　　　　　　　　　　(nail) (T25.43-)
　　　　　　T25.421　Corrosion of unspecified degree of right foot
　　　　　　T25.422　Corrosion of unspecified degree of left foot
　　　　　　T25.429　Corrosion of unspecified degree of unspecified
　　　　　　　　　　foot
　　　　T25.43　　Corrosion of unspecified degree of toe(s) (nail)
　　　　　　T25.431　Corrosion of unspecified degree of right toe(s)
　　　　　　　　　　(nail)
　　　　　　T25.432　Corrosion of unspecified degree of left toe(s)
　　　　　　　　　　(nail)
　　　　　　T25.439　Corrosion of unspecified degree of unspecified
　　　　　　　　　　toe(s) (nail)
　　　　T25.49　　Corrosion of unspecified degree of multiple sites of
　　　　　　　　　ankle and foot
　　　　　　T25.491　Corrosion of unspecified degree of multiple
　　　　　　　　　　sites of right ankle and foot
　　　　　　T25.492　Corrosion of unspecified degree of multiple
　　　　　　　　　　sites of left ankle and foot
　　　　　　T25.499　Corrosion of unspecified degree of multiple
　　　　　　　　　　sites of unspecified ankle and foot

　T25.5　Corrosion of first degree of ankle and foot
　　　　Use additional toxic effect code to identify chemical and intent
　　　　　(T51-T65)
　　　　Use additional external cause code to identify place (Y92)
　　　　T25.51　　Corrosion of first degree of ankle
　　　　　　T25.511　Corrosion of first degree of right ankle
　　　　　　T25.512　Corrosion of first degree of left ankle
　　　　　　T25.519　Corrosion of first degree of unspecified ankle
　　　　T25.52　　Corrosion of first degree of foot
　　　　　　Excludes2:　corrosion of first degree of toe(s) (nail)
　　　　　　　　　　(T25.53-)
　　　　　　T25.521　Corrosion of first degree of right foot
　　　　　　T25.522　Corrosion of first degree of left foot
　　　　　　T25.529　Corrosion of first degree of unspecified foot
　　　　T25.53　　Corrosion of first degree of toe(s) (nail)
　　　　　　T25.531　Corrosion of first degree of right toe(s) (nail)
　　　　　　T25.532　Corrosion of first degree of left toe(s) (nail)
　　　　　　T25.539　Corrosion of first degree of unspecified toe(s)
　　　　　　　　　　(nail)
　　　　T25.59　　Corrosion of first degree of multiple sites of ankle and
　　　　　　　　　foot
　　　　　　T25.591　Corrosion of first degree of multiple sites of
　　　　　　　　　　right ankle and foot
　　　　　　T25.592　Corrosion of first degree of multiple sites of
　　　　　　　　　　left ankle and foot
　　　　　　T25.599　Corrosion of first degree of multiple sites of
　　　　　　　　　　unspecified ankle and foot
　T25.6　Corrosion of second degree of ankle and foot
　　　　Use additional toxic effect code to identify chemical and intent
　　　　　(T51-T65)
　　　　Use additional external cause code to identify place (Y92)
　　　　T25.61　　Corrosion of second degree of ankle
　　　　　　T25.611　Corrosion of second degree of right ankle
　　　　　　T25.612　Corrosion of second degree of left ankle
　　　　　　T25.619　Corrosion of second degree of unspecified
　　　　　　　　　　ankle
　　　　T25.62　　Corrosion of second degree of foot
　　　　　　Excludes2:　corrosion of second degree of toe(s) (nail)
　　　　　　　　　　(T25.63-)
　　　　　　T25.621　Corrosion of second degree of right foot
　　　　　　T25.622　Corrosion of second degree of left foot
　　　　　　T25.629　Corrosion of second degree of unspecified foot
　　　　T25.63　　Corrosion of second degree of toe(s) (nail)
　　　　　　T25.631　Corrosion of second degree of right toe(s) (nail)
　　　　　　T25.632　Corrosion of second degree of left toe(s) (nail)
　　　　　　T25.639　Corrosion of second degree of unspecified
　　　　　　　　　　toe(s) (nail)
　　　　T25.69　　Corrosion of second degree of multiple sites of ankle
　　　　　　　　　and foot
　　　　　　T25.691　Corrosion of second degree of right ankle and
　　　　　　　　　　foot
　　　　　　T25.692　Corrosion of second degree of left ankle and
　　　　　　　　　　foot
　　　　　　T25.699　Corrosion of second degree of unspecified
　　　　　　　　　　ankle and foot
　T25.7　Corrosion of third degree of ankle and foot
　　　　Use additional toxic effect code to identify chemical and intent
　　　　　(T51-T65)
　　　　Use additional external cause code to identify place (Y92)
　　　　T25.71　　Corrosion of third degree of ankle
　　　　　　T25.711　Corrosion of third degree of right ankle
　　　　　　T25.712　Corrosion of third degree of left ankle
　　　　　　T25.719　Corrosion of third degree of unspecified ankle
　　　　T25.72　　Corrosion of third degree of foot
　　　　　　Excludes2:　corrosion of third degree of toe(s) (nail)
　　　　　　　　　　(T25.73-)
　　　　　　T25.721　Corrosion of third degree of right foot
　　　　　　T25.722　Corrosion of third degree of left foot
　　　　　　T25.729　Corrosion of third degree of unspecified foot

T25.73   Corrosion of third degree of toe(s) (nail)
    T25.731   Corrosion of third degree of right toe(s) (nail)
    T25.732   Corrosion of third degree of left toe(s) (nail)
    T25.739   Corrosion of third degree of unspecified toe(s) (nail)
T25.79   Corrosion of third degree of multiple sites of ankle and foot
    T25.791   Corrosion of third degree of multiple sites of right ankle and foot
    T25.792   Corrosion of third degree of multiple sites of left ankle and foot
    T25.799   Corrosion of third degree of multiple sites of unspecified ankle and foot

BURNS AND CORROSIONS CONFINED TO EYE AND INTERNAL ORGANS (T26–T28)

T26   Burn and corrosion confined to eye and adnexa
The following extensions are to be added to each code for category T26:
    a   initial encounter
    d   subsequent encounter
    q   sequela

T26.0   Burn of eyelid and periocular area
Use additional external cause code to identify the source, place and intent of the burn (X00-X19, X75-X77, X96-X98, Y92)

T26.00   Burn of eyelid and periocular area, unspecified side
T26.01   Burn of right eyelid and periocular area
T26.02   Burn of left eyelid and periocular area

T26.1   Burn of cornea and conjunctival sac
Use additional external cause code to identify the source, place and intent of the burn (X00-X19, X75-X77, X96-X98, Y92)

T26.10   Burn of cornea and conjunctival sac, unspecified side
T26.11   Burn of cornea and conjunctival sac, right eye
T26.12   Burn of cornea and conjunctival sac, left eye

T26.2   Burn with resulting rupture and destruction of eyeball
Use additional external cause code to identify the source, place and intent of the burn (X00-X19, X75-X77, X96-X98, Y92)

T26.20   Burn with resulting rupture and destruction of eyeball, unspecified side
T26.21   Burn with resulting rupture and destruction of right eyeball
T26.22   Burn with resulting rupture and destruction of left eyeball

T26.3   Burns of other parts of eye and adnexa
Use additional external cause code to identify the source, place and intent of the burn (X00-X19, X75-X77, X96-X98, Y92)

T26.30   Burns of other parts of eye and adnexa, unspecified side
T26.31   Burns of other parts of right eye and adnexa
T26.32   Burns of other parts of left eye and adnexa

T26.4   Burn of eye and adnexa, part unspecified
Use additional external cause code to identify the source, place and intent of the burn (X00-X19, X75-X77, X96-X98, Y92)

T26.40   Burn of eye and adnexa, part unspecified, unspecified side
T26.41   Burn of right eye and adnexa, part unspecified
T26.42   Burn of left eye and adnexa, part unspecified

T26.5   Corrosion of eyelid and periocular area
Use additional toxic effect code to identify chemical and intent (T51-T65)
Use additional external cause code to identify place (Y92)

T26.50   Corrosion of eyelid and periocular area, unspecified side
T26.51   Corrosion of eyelid and periocular area, right eye
T26.52   Corrosion of eyelid and periocular area, left eye

T26.6   Corrosion of cornea and conjunctival sac
Use additional toxic effect code to identify chemical and intent (T51-T65)
Use additional external cause code to identify place (Y92)

T26.60   Corrosion of cornea and conjunctival sac, unspecified side
T26.61   Corrosion of cornea and conjunctival sac, right eye
T26.62   Corrosion of cornea and conjunctival sac, left eye

T26.7   Corrosion with resulting rupture and destruction of eyeball
Use additional toxic effect code to identify chemical and intent (T51-T65)
Use additional external cause code to identify place (Y92)

T26.70   Corrosion with resulting rupture and destruction of eyeball, unspecified side
T26.71   Corrosion with resulting rupture and destruction of right eyeball
T26.72   Corrosion with resulting rupture and destruction of left eyeball

T26.8   Corrosions of other parts of eye and adnexa
Use additional toxic effect code to identify chemical and intent (T51-T65)
Use additional external cause code to identify place (Y92)

T26.80   Corrosions of other parts of eye and adnexa, unspecified side
T26.81   Corrosions of other parts of right eye and adnexa
T26.82   Corrosions of other parts of left eye and adnexa

T26.9   Corrosion of eye and adnexa, part unspecified
Use additional toxic effect code to identify chemical and intent (T51-T65)
Use additional external cause code to identify place (Y92)

T26.90   Corrosion of eye and adnexa, part unspecified, unspecified side
T26.91   Corrosion of right eye and adnexa, part unspecified
T26.92   Corrosion of left eye and adnexa, part unspecified

T27   Burn and corrosion of respiratory tract
Use additional external cause code to identify the source and intent of the burn (X00-X19, X75-X77, X96-X98)
Use additional toxic effect code to identify chemical and intent (T51-T65)
Use additional external cause code to identify place (Y92)
The following extensions are to be added to each code for category T27:
    a   initial encounter
    d   subsequent encounter
    q   sequela

T27.0   Burn of larynx and trachea
T27.1   Burn involving larynx and trachea with lung
T27.2   Burn of other parts of respiratory tract
    Burn of thoracic cavity
T27.3   Burn of respiratory tract, part unspecified
T27.4   Corrosion of larynx and trachea
T27.5   Corrosion involving larynx and trachea with lung
T27.6   Corrosion of other parts of respiratory tract
T27.7   Corrosion of respiratory tract, part unspecified

T28   Burn and corrosion of other internal organs
Use additional external cause code to identify the source and intent of the burn (X00-X19, X75-X77, X96-X98)
Use additional toxic effect code to identify chemical and intent (T51-T65)
Use additional external cause code to identify place (Y92)
The following extensions are to be added to each code for category T28:
    a   initial encounter
    d   subsequent encounter
    q   sequela

T28.0   Burn of mouth and pharynx
T28.1   Burn of esophagus
T28.2   Burn of other parts of alimentary tract
T28.3   Burn of internal genitourinary organs
T28.4   Burns of other and unspecified internal organs

T28.40   Burn of unspecified internal organ
T28.41   Burn of ear drum
    T28.411   Burn of right ear drum
    T28.412   Burn of left ear drum
    T28.419   Burn of unspecified ear drum

T28.49   Burn of other internal organ
T28.5 Corrosion of mouth and pharynx
T28.6 Corrosion of esophagus
T28.7 Corrosion of other parts of alimentary tract
T28.8 Corrosion of internal genitourinary organs
T28.9 Corrosions of other and unspecified internal organs
　　T28.90   Corrosions of unspecified internal organs
　　T28.91   Corrosions of ear drum
　　　　T28.911   Corrosions of right ear drum
　　　　T28.912   Corrosions of left ear drum
　　　　T28.919   Corrosions of unspecified ear drum
　　T28.99   Corrosions of other internal organs

BURNS AND CORROSIONS OF MULTIPLE AND UNSPECIFIED BODY REGIONS (T30–T32)

T30 Burn and corrosion, body region unspecified
T30.0 Burn of unspecified body region, unspecified degree
　　Burn NOS
　　Multiple burns NOS
T30.4 Corrosion of unspecified body region, unspecified degree
　　Corrosion NOS
　　Multiple corrosion NOS

T31 Burns classified according to extent of body surface involved
　　Note: This category is to be used as the primary code only when the site of the burn is unspecified. It should be used as a supplementary code with categories T20-T28 when the site is specified.
T31.0 Burns involving less than 10% of body surface
T31.1 Burns involving 10-19% of body surface
　　T31.10   Burns involving 10-19% of body surface with 0% to 9% third degree burns
　　　　Burns involving 10-19% of body surface NOS
　　T31.11   Burns involving 10-19% of body surface with 10-19% third degree burns
T31.2 Burns involving 20-29% of body surface
　　T31.20   Burns involving 20-29% of body surface with 0% to 9% third degree burns
　　　　Burns involving 20-29% of body surface NOS
　　T31.21   Burns involving 20-29% of body surface with 10-19% third degree burns
　　T31.22   Burns involving 20-29% of body surface with 20-29% third degree burns
T31.3 Burns involving 30-39% of body surface
　　T31.30   Burns involving 30-39% of body surface with 0% to 9% third degree burns
　　　　Burns involving 30-39% of body surface NOS
　　T31.31   Burns involving 30-39% of body surface with 10-19% third degree burns
　　T31.32   Burns involving 30-39% of body surface with 20-29% third degree burns
　　T31.33   Burns involving 30-39% of body surface with 30-39% third degree burns
T31.4 Burns involving 40-49% of body surface
　　T31.40   Burns involving 40-49% of body surface with 0% to 9% third degree burns
　　　　Burns involving 40-49% of body surface NOS
　　T31.41   Burns involving 40-49% of body surface with 10-19% third degree burns
　　T31.42   Burns involving 40-49% of body surface with 20-29% third degree burns
　　T31.43   Burns involving 40-49% of body surface with 30-39% third degree burns
　　T31.44   Burns involving 40-49% of body surface with 40-49% third degree burns
T31.5 Burns involving 50-59% of body surface
　　T31.50   Burns involving 50-59% of body surface with 0% to 9% third degree burns
　　　　Burns involving 50-59% of body surface NOS
　　T31.51   Burns involving 50-59% of body surface with 10-19% third degree burns

T31.52   Burns involving 50-59% of body surface with 20-29% third degree burns
T31.53   Burns involving 50-59% of body surface with 30-39% third degree burns
T31.54   Burns involving 50-59% of body surface with 40-49% third degree burns
T31.55   Burns involving 50-59% of body surface with 50-59% third degree burns
T31.6 Burns involving 60-69% of body surface
　　T31.60   Burns involving 60-69% of body surface with 0% to 9% third degree burns
　　　　Burns involving 60-69% of body surface NOS
　　T31.61   Burns involving 60-69% of body surface with 10-19% third degree burns
　　T31.62   Burns involving 60-69% of body surface with 20-29% third degree burns
　　T31.63   Burns involving 60-69% of body surface with 30-39% third degree burns
　　T31.64   Burns involving 60-69% of body surface with 40-49% third degree burns
　　T31.65   Burns involving 60-69% of body surface with 50-59% third degree burns
　　T31.66   Burns involving 60-69% of body surface with 60-69% third degree burns
T31.7 Burns involving 70-79% of body surface
　　T31.70   Burns involving 70-79% of body surface with 0% to 9% third degree burns
　　　　Burns involving 70-79% of body surface NOS
　　T31.71   Burns involving 70-79% of body surface with 10-19% third degree burns
　　T31.72   Burns involving 70-79% of body surface with 20-29% third degree burns
　　T31.73   Burns involving 70-79% of body surface with 30-39% third degree burns
　　T31.74   Burns involving 70-79% of body surface with 40-49% third degree burns
　　T31.75   Burns involving 70-79% of body surface with 50-59% third degree burns
　　T31.76   Burns involving 70-79% of body surface with 60-69% third degree burns
　　T31.77   Burns involving 70-79% of body surface with 70-79% third degree burns
T31.8 Burns involving 80-89% of body surface
　　T31.80   Burns involving 80-89% of body surface with 0% to 9% third degree burns
　　　　Burns involving 80-89% of body surface NOS
　　T31.81   Burns involving 80-89% of body surface with 10-19% third degree burns
　　T31.82   Burns involving 80-89% of body surface with 20-29% third degree burns
　　T31.83   Burns involving 80-89% of body surface with 30-39% third degree burns
　　T31.84   Burns involving 80-89% of body surface with 40-49% third degree burns
　　T31.85   Burns involving 80-89% of body surface with 50-59% third degree burns
　　T31.86   Burns involving 80-89% of body surface with 60-69% third degree burns
　　T31.87   Burns involving 80-89% of body surface with 70-79% third degree burns
　　T31.88   Burns involving 80-89% of body surface with 80-89% third degree burns
T31.9 Burns involving 90% or more of body surface
　　T31.90   Burns involving 90-99% of body surface with 0% to 9% third degree burns
　　　　Burns involving 90-99% of body surface NOS
　　T31.91   Burns involving 90-99% of body surface with 10-19% third degree burns
　　T31.92   Burns involving 90-99% of body surface with 20-29% third degree burns
　　T31.93   Burns involving 90-99% of body surface with 30-39% third degree burns

T31.94   Burns involving 90-99% of body surface with 40-49% third degree burns

T31.95   Burns involving 90-99% of body surface with 50-59% third degree burns

T31.96   Burns involving 90-99% of body surface with 60-69% third degree burns

T31.97   Burns involving 90-99% of body surface with 70-79% third degree burns

T31.98   Burns involving 90-99% of body surface with 80-89% third degree burns

T31.99   Burns involving 90-99% of body surface with 90-99% third degree burns

T32 Corrosions classified according to extent of body surface involved

Note: This category is to be used as the primary code only when the site of the corrosion is unspecified. It may be used as a supplementary code with categories T20-T28 when the site is specified.

T32.0   Corrosions involving less than 10% of body surface

T32.1   Corrosions involving 10-19% of body surface

T32.10   Corrosions involving 10-19% of body surface with 0% to 9% third degree corrosion
Corrosions involving 10-19% of body surface NOS

T32.11   Corrosions involving 10-19% of body surface with 10-19% third degree corrosion

T32.2   Corrosions involving 20-29% of body surface

T32.20   Corrosions involving 20-29% of body surface with 0% to 9% third degree corrosion

T32.21   Corrosions involving 20-29% of body surface with 10-19% third degree corrosion

T32.22   Corrosions involving 20-29% of body surface with 20-29% third degree corrosion

T32.3   Corrosions involving 30-39% of body surface

T32.30   Corrosions involving 30-39% of body surface with 0% to 9% third degree corrosion

T32.31   Corrosions involving 30-39% of body surface with 10-19% third degree corrosion

T32.32   Corrosions involving 30-39% of body surface with 20-29% third degree corrosion

T32.33   Corrosions involving 30-39% of body surface with 30-39% third degree corrosion

T32.4   Corrosions involving 40-49% of body surface

T32.40   Corrosions involving 40-49% of body surface with 0% to 9% third degree corrosion

T32.41   Corrosions involving 40-49% of body surface with 10-19% third degree corrosion

T32.42   Corrosions involving 40-49% of body surface with 20-29% third degree corrosion

T32.43   Corrosions involving 40-49% of body surface with 30-39% third degree corrosion

T32.44   Corrosions involving 40-49% of body surface with 40-49% third degree corrosion

T32.5   Corrosions involving 50-59% of body surface

T32.50   Corrosions involving 50-59% of body surface with 0% to 9% third degree corrosion

T32.51   Corrosions involving 50-59% of body surface with 10-19% third degree corrosion

T32.52   Corrosions involving 50-59% of body surface with 20-29% third degree corrosion

T32.53   Corrosions involving 50-59% of body surface with 30-39% third degree corrosion

T32.54   Corrosions involving 50-59% of body surface with 40-49% third degree corrosion

T32.55   Corrosions involving 50-59% of body surface with 50-59% third degree corrosion

T32.6   Corrosions involving 60-69% of body surface

T32.60   Corrosions involving 60-69% of body surface with 0% to 9% third degree corrosion

T32.61   Corrosions involving 60-69% of body surface with 10-19% third degree corrosion

T32.62   Corrosions involving 60-69% of body surface with 20-29% third degree corrosion

T32.63   Corrosions involving 60-69% of body surface with 30-39% third degree corrosion

T32.64   Corrosions involving 60-69% of body surface with 40-49% third degree corrosion

T32.65   Corrosions involving 60-69% of body surface with 50-59% third degree corrosion

T32.66   Corrosions involving 60-69% of body surface with 60-69% third degree corrosion

T32.7   Corrosions involving 70-79% of body surface

T32.70   Corrosions involving 70-79% of body surface with 0% to 9% third degree corrosion

T32.71   Corrosions involving 70-79% of body surface with 10-19% third degree corrosion

T32.72   Corrosions involving 70-79% of body surface with 20-29% third degree corrosion

T32.73   Corrosions involving 70-79% of body surface with 30-39% third degree corrosion

T32.74   Corrosions involving 70-79% of body surface with 40-49% third degree corrosion

T32.75   Corrosions involving 70-79% of body surface with 50-59% third degree corrosion

T32.76   Corrosions involving 70-79% of body surface with 60-69% third degree corrosion

T32.77   Corrosions involving 70-79% of body surface with 70-79% third degree corrosion

T32.8   Corrosions involving 80-89% of body surface

T32.80   Corrosions involving 80-89% of body surface with 0% to 9% third degree corrosion

T32.81   Corrosions involving 80-89% of body surface with 10-19% third degree corrosion

T32.82   Corrosions involving 80-89% of body surface with 20-29% third degree corrosion

T32.83   Corrosions involving 80-89% of body surface with 30-39% third degree corrosion

T32.84   Corrosions involving 80-89% of body surface with 40-49% third degree corrosion

T32.85   Corrosions involving 80-89% of body surface with 50-59% third degree corrosion

T32.86   Corrosions involving 80-89% of body surface with 60-69% third degree corrosion

T32.87   Corrosions involving 80-89% of body surface with 70-79% third degree corrosion

T32.88   Corrosions involving 80-89% of body surface with 80-89% third degree corrosion

T32.9   Corrosions involving 90% or more of body surface

T32.90   Corrosions involving 90-99% of body surface with 0% to 9% third degree corrosion

T32.91   Corrosions involving 90-99% of body surface with 10-19% third degree corrosion

T32.92   Corrosions involving 90-99% of body surface with 20-29% third degree corrosion

T32.93   Corrosions involving 90-99% of body surface with 30-39% third degree corrosion

T32.94   Corrosions involving 90-99% of body surface with 40-49% third degree corrosion

T32.95   Corrosions involving 90-99% of body surface with 50-59% third degree corrosion

T32.96   Corrosions involving 90-99% of body surface with 60-69% third degree corrosion

T32.97   Corrosions involving 90-99% of body surface with 70-79% third degree corrosion

T32.98   Corrosions involving 90-99% of body surface with 80-89% third degree corrosion

T32.99   Corrosions involving 90-99% of body surface with 90-99% third degree corrosion

FROSTBITE (T33–T34)

Excludes2:   hypothermia and other effects of reduced temperature (T68, T69.-)

T33 Superficial frostbite

Includes: frostbite with partial thickness skin loss

The following extensions are to be added to each code for category T33:

- a   initial encounter
- d   subsequent encounter
- q   sequela

T33.0 Superficial frostbite of head

T33.01   Superficial frostbite of ear

- **T33.011   Superficial frostbite of right ear**
- **T33.012   Superficial frostbite of left ear**
- **T33.019   Superficial frostbite of unspecified ear**

T33.02   Superficial frostbite of nose

T33.09   Superficial frostbite of other part of head

T33.1 Superficial frostbite of neck

T33.2 Superficial frostbite of thorax

T33.3 Superficial frostbite of abdominal wall, lower back and pelvis

T33.4 Superficial frostbite of arm

Excludes2:   superficial frostbite of wrist and hand (T33.5-)

T33.40   Superficial frostbite of arm, unspecified side

T33.41   Superficial frostbite of right arm

T33.42   Superficial frostbite of left arm

T33.5 Superficial frostbite of wrist, hand, and fingers

T33.51   Superficial frostbite of wrist

- **T33.511   Superficial frostbite of right wrist**
- **T33.512   Superficial frostbite of left wrist**
- **T33.519   Superficial frostbite of unspecified wrist**

T33.52   Superficial frostbite of hand

Excludes2:   superficial frostbite of fingers (T33.53-)

- **T33.521   Superficial frostbite of right hand**
- **T33.522   Superficial frostbite of left hand**
- **T33.529   Superficial frostbite of unspecified hand**

T33.53   Superficial frostbite of finger(s)

- **T33.531   Superficial frostbite of right finger(s)**
- **T33.532   Superficial frostbite of left finger(s)**
- **T33.539   Superficial frostbite of unspecified finger(s)**

T33.6 Superficial frostbite of hip and thigh

T33.60   Superficial frostbite of hip and thigh, unspecified side

T33.61   Superficial frostbite of right hip and thigh

T33.62   Superficial frostbite of left hip and thigh

T33.7 Superficial frostbite of knee and lower leg

Excludes2:   superficial frostbite of ankle and foot (T33.8-)

T33.70   Superficial frostbite of knee and lower leg, unspecified side

T33.71   Superficial frostbite of right knee and lower leg

T33.72   Superficial frostbite of left knee and lower leg

T33.8 Superficial frostbite of ankle, foot, and toe(s)

T33.81   Superficial frostbite of ankle

- **T33.811   Superficial frostbite of right ankle**
- **T33.812   Superficial frostbite of left ankle**
- **T33.819   Superficial frostbite of unspecified ankle**

T33.82   Superficial frostbite of foot

- **T33.821   Superficial frostbite of right foot**
- **T33.822   Superficial frostbite of left foot**
- **T33.829   Superficial frostbite of unspecified foot**

T33.83   Superficial frostbite of toe(s)

- **T33.831   Superficial frostbite of right toe(s)**
- **T33.832   Superficial frostbite of left toe(s)**
- **T33.839   Superficial frostbite of unspecified toe(s)**

T33.9 Superficial frostbite of other and unspecified sites

T33.90   Superficial frostbite of unspecified sites
Superficial frostbite NOS

T33.99   Superficial frostbite of other sites
Superficial frostbite of leg NOS
Superficial frostbite of trunk NOS

T34 Frostbite with tissue necrosis

The following extensions are to be added to each code for category T34:

- a   initial encounter
- d   subsequent encounter
- q   sequela

T34.0   Frostbite with tissue necrosis of head

T34.01   Frostbite with tissue necrosis of ear

- **T34.011   Frostbite with tissue necrosis of right ear**
- **T34.012   Frostbite with tissue necrosis of left ear**
- **T34.019   Frostbite with tissue necrosis of unspecified ear**

T34.02   Frostbite with tissue necrosis of nose

T34.09   Frostbite with tissue necrosis of other part of head

T34.1 Frostbite with tissue necrosis of neck

T34.2 Frostbite with tissue necrosis of thorax

T34.3 Frostbite with tissue necrosis of abdominal wall, lower back and pelvis

T34.4 Frostbite with tissue necrosis of arm

Excludes2:   frostbite with tissue necrosis of wrist and hand (T34.5-)

T34.40   Frostbite with tissue necrosis of arm, unspecified side

T34.41   Frostbite with tissue necrosis of right arm

T34.42   Frostbite with tissue necrosis of left arm

T34.5 Frostbite with tissue necrosis of wrist, hand, and finger(s)

T34.51   Frostbite with tissue necrosis of wrist

- **T34.511   Frostbite with tissue necrosis of right wrist**
- **T34.512   Frostbite with tissue necrosis of left wrist**
- **T34.519   Frostbite with tissue necrosis of unspecified wrist**

T34.52   Frostbite with tissue necrosis of hand

Excludes2:   frostbite with tissue necrosis of finger(s) (T34.53-)

- **T34.521   Frostbite with tissue necrosis of right hand**
- **T34.522   Frostbite with tissue necrosis of left hand**
- **T34.529   Frostbite with tissue necrosis of unspecified hand**

T34.53   Frostbite with tissue necrosis of finger(s)

- **T34.531   Frostbite with tissue necrosis of right finger(s)**
- **T34.532   Frostbite with tissue necrosis of left finger(s)**
- **T34.539   Frostbite with tissue necrosis of unspecified finger(s)**

T34.6 Frostbite with tissue necrosis of hip and thigh

T34.60   Frostbite with tissue necrosis of hip and thigh, unspecified side

T34.61   Frostbite with tissue necrosis of right hip and thigh

T34.62   Frostbite with tissue necrosis of left hip and thigh

T34.7 Frostbite with tissue necrosis of knee and lower leg

Excludes2:   frostbite with tissue necrosis of ankle and foot (T34.8-)

T34.70   Frostbite with tissue necrosis of knee and lower leg, unspecified side

T34.71   Frostbite with tissue necrosis of right knee and lower leg

T34.72   Frostbite with tissue necrosis of left knee and lower leg

T34.8 Frostbite with tissue necrosis of ankle and foot, and toe(s)

T34.81   Frostbite with tissue necrosis of ankle

- **T34.811   Frostbite with tissue necrosis of right ankle**
- **T34.812   Frostbite with tissue necrosis of left ankle**
- **T34.819   Frostbite with tissue necrosis of unspecified ankle**

T34.82   Frostbite with tissue necrosis of foot

- **T34.821   Frostbite with tissue necrosis of right foot**
- **T34.822   Frostbite with tissue necrosis of left foot**
- **T34.829   Frostbite with tissue necrosis of unspecified foot**

T34.83   Frostbite with tissue necrosis of toe(s)

- **T34.831   Frostbite with tissue necrosis of right toe(s)**
- **T34.832   Frostbite with tissue necrosis of left toe(s)**

T34.839 Frostbite with tissue necrosis of unspecified toe(s)

T34.9 **Frostbite with tissue necrosis of other and unspecified sites**

T34.90 **Frostbite with tissue necrosis of unspecified sites**
Frostbite with tissue necrosis NOS

T34.99 **Frostbite with tissue necrosis of other sites**
Frostbite with tissue necrosis of leg NOS
Frostbite with tissue necrosis of trunk NOS

POISONING BY AND ADVERSE EFFECTS OF DRUGS, MEDICAMENTS AND BIOLOGICAL SUBSTANCES (T36–T50)

Includes: poisonings is defined as:
adverse effect is defined as: "hypersensitivity", "reaction", etc. of correct substance properly administered
overdose of substances
wrong substance given or taken in error

Use additional code(s) for all manifestations of poisoning and adverse effects

Excludes2: abuse of non-dependence-producing substances (F55.-)
drug dependence and related mental and behavioral disorders due to psychoactive substance use (F10-F19)
drug reaction and poisoning affecting newborn (P00-P96)
pathological drug intoxication (F10-F19)

When no intent of poisoning is indicated code to accidental. Undetermined intent is only for use when there is specific documentation in the record that the intent of the injury cannot be determined.

T36 Poisoning by and adverse effect of systemic antibiotics

Excludes1: antineoplastic antibiotics (T45.1)
locally applied antibiotic NEC (T49.0)
topically used antibiotic for ear, nose and throat (T49.6)
topically used antibiotic for eye (T49.5)

The following extensions are to be added to each code for category T36:
a   initial encounter
d   subsequent encounter
q   sequela

T36.0 **Poisoning by and adverse effect of penicillins**

T36.0x **Poisoning by and adverse effect of penicillins**

T36.0x1 **Poisoning by penicillins, accidental (unintentional)**
Poisoning by penicillins NOS

T36.0x2 **Poisoning by penicillins, intentional self-harm**

T36.0x3 **Poisoning by penicillins, assault**

T36.0x4 **Poisoning by penicillins, undetermined**

T36.0x5 **Adverse effect of penicillins**

T36.1 **Poisoning by and adverse effect of cephalosporins and other β-lactam antibiotics**

T36.1x **Poisoning by and adverse effect of cephalosporins and other β-lactam antibiotics**

T36.1x1 **Poisoning by cephalosporins and other β-lactam antibiotics, accidental (unintentional)**
Poisoning by cephalosporins and other β-lactam antibiotics NOS

T36.1x2 **Poisoning by cephalosporins and other β-lactam antibiotics, intentional self-harm**

T36.1x3 **Poisoning by cephalosporins and other β-lactam antibiotics, assault**

T36.1x4 **Poisoning by cephalosporins and other β-lactam antibiotics, undetermined**

T36.1x5 **Adverse effect of cephalosporins and other β-lactam antibiotics**

T36.2 **Poisoning by and adverse effect of chloramphenicol group**

T36.2x **Poisoning by and adverse effect of chloramphenicol group**

T36.2x1 **Poisoning by chloramphenicol group, accidental (unintentional)**
Poisoning by chloramphenicol group NOS

T36.2x2 **Poisoning by chloramphenicol group, intentional self-harm**

T36.2x3 **Poisoning by chloramphenicol group, assault**

T36.2x4 **Poisoning by chloramphenicol group, undetermined**

T36.2x5 **Adverse effect of chloramphenicol group**

T36.3 **Poisoning by and adverse effect of macrolides**

T36.3x **Poisoning by and adverse effect of macrolides**

T36.3x1 **Poisoning by macrolides, accidental (unintentional)**
Poisoning by macrolides NOS

T36.3x2 **Poisoning by macrolides, intentional self-harm**

T36.3x3 **Poisoning by macrolides, assault**

T36.3x4 **Poisoning by macrolides, undetermined**

T36.3x5 **Adverse effect of macrolides**

T36.4 **Poisoning by and adverse effect of tetracyclines**

T36.4x **Poisoning by and adverse effect of tetracyclines**

T36.4x1 **Poisoning by tetracyclines, accidental (unintentional)**
Poisoning by tetracyclines NOS

T36.4x2 **Poisoning by tetracyclines, intentional self-harm**

T36.4x3 **Poisoning by tetracyclines, assault**

T36.4x4 **Poisoning by tetracyclines, undetermined**

T36.4x5 **Adverse effect of tetracyclines**

T36.5 **Poisoning by and adverse effect of aminoglycosides**
Poisoning by and adverse effect of streptomycin

T36.5x **Poisoning by and adverse effect of aminoglycosides**

T36.5x1 **Poisoning by aminoglycosides, accidental (unintentional)**
Poisoning by aminoglycosides NOS

T36.5x2 **Poisoning by aminoglycosides, intentional self-harm**

T36.5x3 **Poisoning by aminoglycosides, assault**

T36.5x4 **Poisoning by aminoglycosides, undetermined**

T36.5x5 **Adverse effect of aminoglycosides**

T36.6 **Poisoning by and adverse effect of rifampicins**

T36.6x **Poisoning by and adverse effect of rifampicins**

T36.6x1 **Poisoning by rifampicins, accidental (unintentional)**
Poisoning by rifampicins NOS

T36.6x2 **Poisoning by rifampicins, intentional self-harm**

T36.6x3 **Poisoning by rifampicins, assault**

T36.6x4 **Poisoning by rifampicins, undetermined**

T36.6x5 **Adverse effect of rifampicins**

T36.7 **Poisoning by and adverse effect of antifungal antibiotics, systemically used**

T36.7x **Poisoning by and adverse effect of antifungal antibiotics, systemically used**

T36.7x1 **Poisoning by antifungal antibiotics, systemically used, accidental (unintentional)**
Poisoning by antifungal antibiotics, systemically used NOS

T36.7x2 **Poisoning by antifungal antibiotics, systemically used, intentional self-harm**

T36.7x3 **Poisoning by antifungal antibiotics, systemically used, assault**

T36.7x4 **Poisoning by antifungal antibiotics, systemically used, undetermined**

T36.7x5 **Adverse effect of antifungal antibiotics, systemically used**

T36.8 **Poisoning by and adverse effect of other systemic antibiotics**

T36.8x **Poisoning by and adverse effect of other systemic antibiotics**

T36.8x1 **Poisoning by other systemic antibiotics, accidental (unintentional)**
Poisoning by other systemic antibiotics NOS

T36.8x2 **Poisoning by other systemic antibiotics, intentional self-harm**

T36.8x3   Poisoning by other systemic antibiotics, assault

T36.8x4   Poisoning by other systemic antibiotics, undetermined

T36.8x5   Adverse effect of other systemic antibiotics

T36.9   Poisoning by and adverse effect of systemic antibiotic, unspecified

T36.9x   Poisoning by and adverse effect of systemic antibiotic, unspecified

T36.9x1   Poisoning by systemic antibiotic, unspecified, accidental (unintentional)
Poisoning by systemic antibiotic NOS

T36.9x2   Poisoning by systemic antibiotic, unspecified, intentional self-harm

T36.9x3   Poisoning by systemic antibiotic, unspecified, assault

T36.9x4   Poisoning by systemic antibiotic, unspecified, undetermined

T36.9x5   Adverse effect of systemic antibiotic, unspecified

T37   Poisoning by and adverse effect of other systemic anti-infectives and antiparasitics
Excludes1:   anti-infectives topically used for ear, nose and throat (T49.6-)
anti-infectives topically used for eye (T49.5-)
locally applied anti-infectives NEC (T49.0-)
The following extensions are to be added to each code for category T37:
a   initial encounter
d   subsequent encounter
q   sequela

T37.0   Poisoning by and adverse effect of sulfonamides

T37.0x   Poisoning by and adverse effect of sulfonamides

T37.0x1   Poisoning by sulfonamides, accidental (unintentional)
Poisoning by sulfonamides NOS

T37.0x2   Poisoning by sulfonamides, intentional self-harm

T37.0x3   Poisoning by sulfonamides, assault

T37.0x4   Poisoning by sulfonamides, undetermined

T37.0x5   Adverse effect of sulfonamides

T37.1   Poisoning by and adverse effect of antimycobacterial drugs
Excludes1:   rifampicins (T36.6-)
streptomycin (T36.5-)

T37.1x   Poisoning by and adverse effect of antimycobacterial drugs

T37.1x1   Poisoning by antimycobacterial drugs, accidental (unintentional)
Poisoning by antimycobacterial drugs NOS

T37.1x2   Poisoning by antimycobacterial drugs, intentional self-harm

T37.1x3   Poisoning by antimycobacterial drugs, assault

T37.1x4   Poisoning by antimycobacterial drugs, undetermined

T37.1x5   Adverse effect of antimycobacterial drugs

T37.2   Poisoning by and adverse effect of antimalarials and drugs acting on other blood protozoa
Excludes1:   hydroxyquinoline derivatives (T37.8-)

T37.2x   Poisoning by and adverse effect of antimalarials and drugs acting on other blood protozoa

T37.2x1   Poisoning by antimalarials and drugs acting on other blood protozoa, accidental (unintentional)
Poisoning by antimalarials and drugs acting on other blood protozoa NOS

T37.2x2   Poisoning by antimalarials and drugs acting on other blood protozoa, intentional self-harm

T37.2x3   Poisoning by antimalarials and drugs acting on other blood protozoa, assault

T37.2x4   Poisoning by antimalarials and drugs acting on other blood protozoa, undetermined

T37.2x5   Adverse effect of antimalarials and drugs acting on other blood protozoa

T37.3   Poisoning by and adverse effect of other antiprotozoal drugs

T37.3x   Poisoning by and adverse effect of other antiprotozoal drugs

T37.3x1   Poisoning by other antiprotozoal drugs, accidental (unintentional)
Poisoning by other antiprotozoal drugs NOS

T37.3x2   Poisoning by other antiprotozoal drugs, intentional self-harm

T37.3x3   Poisoning by other antiprotozoal drugs, assault

T37.3x4   Poisoning by other antiprotozoal drugs, undetermined

T37.3x5   Adverse effect of other antiprotozoal drugs

T37.4   Poisoning by and adverse effect of anthelmintics

T37.4x   Poisoning by and adverse effect of anthelmintics

T37.4x1   Poisoning by anthelmintics, accidental (unintentional)
Poisoning by anthelmintics NOS

T37.4x2   Poisoning by anthelmintics, intentional self-harm

T37.4x3   Poisoning by anthelmintics, assault

T37.4x4   Poisoning by anthelmintics, undetermined

T37.4x5   Adverse effect of anthelmintics

T37.5   Poisoning by and adverse effect of antiviral drugs
Excludes1:   amantadine (T42.8-)
cytarabine (T45.1-)

T37.5x   Poisoning by and adverse effect of antiviral drugs

T37.5x1   Poisoning by antiviral drugs, accidental (unintentional)
Poisoning by antiviral drugs NOS

T37.5x2   Poisoning by antiviral drugs, intentional self-harm

T37.5x3   Poisoning by antiviral drugs, assault

T37.5x4   Poisoning by antiviral drugs, undetermined

T37.5x5   Adverse effect of antiviral drugs

T37.8   Poisoning by and adverse effect of other specified systemic anti-infectives and antiparasitics
Poisoning by and adverse effect of hydroxyquinoline derivatives
Excludes1:   antimalarial drugs (T37.2-)

T37.8x   Poisoning by and adverse effect of other specified systemic anti-infectives and antiparasitics

T37.8x1   Poisoning by other specified systemic anti-infectives and antiparasitics, accidental (unintentional)
Poisoning by other specified systemic anti-infectives and antiparasitics NOS

T37.8x2   Poisoning by other specified systemic anti-infectives and antiparasitics, intentional self-harm

T37.8x3   Poisoning by other specified systemic anti-infectives and antiparasitics, assault

T37.8x4   Poisoning by other specified systemic anti-infectives and antiparasitics, undetermined

T37.8x5   Adverse effect of other specified systemic anti-infectives and antiparasitics

T37.9   Poisoning by and adverse effect of systemic anti-infective and antiparasitic, unspecified

T37.91   Poisoning by systemic anti-infective and antiparasitic, unspecified, accidental (unintentional)
Poisoning by systemic anti-infective and antiparasitic NOS

T37.92   Poisoning by systemic anti-infective and antiparasitic, unspecified, intentional self-harm

T37.93   Poisoning by systemic anti-infective and antiparasitic, unspecified, assault

T37.94   Poisoning by systemic anti-infective and antiparasitic, unspecified, undetermined

T37.95   Adverse effect of systemic anti-infective and antiparasitic, unspecified

T38 Poisoning by and adverse effect of hormones and their synthetic substitutes and antagonists, not elsewhere classified

Excludes1:   mineralocorticoids and their antagonists (T50.0-)
oxytocic hormones (T48.0-)
parathyroid hormones and derivatives (T50.9-)

The following extensions are to be added to each code for category T38:

a   initial encounter
d   subsequent encounter
q   sequela

T38.0 Poisoning by and adverse effect of glucocorticoids and synthetic analogues

Excludes1:   glucocorticoids, topically used (T49.-)

T38.0x Poisoning by and adverse effect of glucocorticoids and synthetic analogues

T38.0x1 Poisoning by glucocorticoids and synthetic analogues, accidental (unintentional)
Poisoning by glucocorticoids and synthetic analogues NOS

T38.0x2 Poisoning by glucocorticoids and synthetic analogues, intentional self-harm

T38.0x3 Poisoning by glucocorticoids and synthetic analogues, assault

T38.0x4 Poisoning by glucocorticoids and synthetic analogues, undetermined

T38.0x5 Adverse effect of glucocorticoids and synthetic analogues

T38.1 Poisoning by and adverse effect of thyroid hormones and substitutes

T38.1x Poisoning by and adverse effect of thyroid hormones and substitutes

T38.1x1 Poisoning by thyroid hormones and substitutes, accidental (unintentional)
Poisoning by thyroid hormones and substitutes NOS

T38.1x2 Poisoning by thyroid hormones and substitutes, intentional self-harm

T38.1x3 Poisoning by thyroid hormones and substitutes, assault

T38.1x4 Poisoning by thyroid hormones and substitutes, undetermined

T38.1x5 Adverse effect of thyroid hormones and substitutes

T38.2 Poisoning by and adverse effect of antithyroid drugs

T38.2x Poisoning by and adverse effect of antithyroid drugs

T38.2x1 Poisoning by antithyroid drugs, accidental (unintentional)
Poisoning by antithyroid drugs NOS

T38.2x2 Poisoning by antithyroid drugs, intentional self-harm

T38.2x3 Poisoning by antithyroid drugs, assault

T38.2x4 Poisoning by antithyroid drugs, undetermined

T38.2x5 Adverse effect of antithyroid drugs

T38.3 Poisoning by and adverse effect of insulin and oral hypoglycemic [antidiabetic] drugs

T38.3x Poisoning by and adverse effect of insulin and oral hypoglycemic [antidiabetic] drugs

T38.3x1 Poisoning by insulin and oral hypoglycemic [antidiabetic] drugs, accidental (unintentional)
Poisoning by insulin and oral hypoglycemic [antidiabetic] drugs NOS

T38.3x2 Poisoning by insulin and oral hypoglycemic [antidiabetic] drugs, intentional self-harm

T38.3x3 Poisoning by insulin and oral hypoglycemic [antidiabetic] drugs, assault

T38.3x4 Poisoning by insulin and oral hypoglycemic [antidiabetic] drugs, undetermined

T38.3x5 Adverse effect of insulin and oral hypoglycemic [antidiabetic] drugs

T38.4 Poisoning by and adverse effect of oral contraceptives
Poisoning by and adverse effect of multiple- and single-ingredient oral contraceptive preparations

T38.4x Poisoning by and adverse effect of oral contraceptives

T38.4x1 Poisoning by oral contraceptives, accidental (unintentional)
Poisoning by oral contraceptives NOS

T38.4x2 Poisoning by oral contraceptives, intentional self-harm

T38.4x3 Poisoning by oral contraceptives, assault

T38.4x4 Poisoning by oral contraceptives, undetermined

T38.4x5 Adverse effect of oral contraceptives

T38.5 Poisoning by and adverse effect of other estrogens and progestogens
Poisoning by and adverse effect of estrogens and progestogens mixtures and substitutes

T38.5x Poisoning by and adverse effect of other estrogens and progestogens

T38.5x1 Poisoning by other estrogens and progestogens, accidental (unintentional)
Poisoning by other estrogens and progestogens NOS

T38.5x2 Poisoning by other estrogens and progestogens, intentional self-harm

T38.5x3 Poisoning by other estrogens and progestogens, assault

T38.5x4 Poisoning by other estrogens and progestogens, undetermined

T38.5x5 Adverse effect of other estrogens and progestogens

T38.6 Poisoning by and adverse effect of antigonadotrophins, antiestrogens, antiandrogens, not elsewhere classified
Poisoning by tamoxifen

T38.6x Poisoning by and adverse effect of antigonadotrophins, antiestrogens, antiandrogens, not elsewhere classified

T38.6x1 Poisoning by antigonadotrophins, antiestrogens, antiandrogens, not elsewhere classified, accidental (unintentional)
Poisoning by antigonadotrophins, antiestrogens, antiandrogens, not elsewhere classified NOS

T38.6x2 Poisoning by antigonadotrophins, antiestrogens, antiandrogens, not elsewhere classified, intentional self-harm

T38.6x3 Poisoning by antigonadotrophins, antiestrogens, antiandrogens, not elsewhere classified, assault

T38.6x4 Poisoning by antigonadotrophins, antiestrogens, antiandrogens, not elsewhere classified, undetermined

T38.6x5 Adverse effect of antigonadotrophins, antiestrogens, antiandrogens, not elsewhere classified

T38.7 Poisoning by and adverse effect of androgens and anabolic congeners

T38.7x Poisoning by and adverse effect of androgens and anabolic congeners

T38.7x1 Poisoning by androgens and anabolic congeners, accidental (unintentional)
Poisoning by androgens and anabolic congeners NOS

T38.7x2 Poisoning by androgens and anabolic congeners, intentional self-harm

T38.7x3 Poisoning by androgens and anabolic congeners, assault

T38.7x4 Poisoning by androgens and anabolic congeners, undetermined

T38.7x5 Adverse effect of androgens and anabolic congeners

T38.8 Poisoning by and adverse effect of other and unspecified hormones and synthetic substitutes

T38.80 Poisoning by and adverse effect of unspecified hormones and synthetic substitutes

T38.801   Poisoning by unspecified hormones and synthetic substitutes, accidental (unintentional)
> Poisoning by unspecified hormones and synthetic substitutes NOS

T38.802   Poisoning by unspecified hormones and synthetic substitutes, intentional self-harm

T38.803   Poisoning by unspecified hormones and synthetic substitutes, assault

T38.804   Poisoning by unspecified hormones and synthetic substitutes, undetermined

T38.805   Adverse effect of unspecified hormones and synthetic substitutes

T38.81   Poisoning by and adverse effect of anterior pituitary [adenohypophyseal] hormones

T38.811   Poisoning by anterior pituitary [adenohypophyseal] hormones, accidental (unintentional)
> Poisoning by anterior pituitary [adenohypophyseal] hormones NOS

T38.812   Poisoning by anterior pituitary [adenohypophyseal] hormones, intentional self-harm

T38.813   Poisoning by anterior pituitary [adenohypophyseal] hormones, assault

T38.814   Poisoning by anterior pituitary [adenohypophyseal] hormones, undetermined

T38.815   Adverse effect of anterior pituitary [adenohypophyseal] hormones

T38.89   Poisoning by and adverse effect of other hormones and synthetic substitutes

T38.891   Poisoning by other hormones and synthetic substitutes, accidental (unintentional)
> Poisoning by other hormones and synthetic substitutes NOS

T38.892   Poisoning by other hormones and synthetic substitutes, intentional self-harm

T38.893   Poisoning by other hormones and synthetic substitutes, assault

T38.894   Poisoning by other hormones and synthetic substitutes, undetermined

T38.895   Adverse effect of other hormones and synthetic substitutes

T38.9   Poisoning by and adverse effect of other and unspecified hormone antagonists

T38.90   Poisoning by and adverse effect of unspecified hormone antagonists

T38.901   Poisoning by unspecified hormone antagonists, accidental (unintentional)
> Poisoning by unspecified hormone antagonists NOS

T38.902   Poisoning by unspecified hormone antagonists, intentional self-harm

T38.903   Poisoning by unspecified hormone antagonists, assault

T38.904   Poisoning by unspecified hormone antagonists, undetermined

T38.905   Adverse effect of unspecified hormone antagonists

T38.99   Poisoning by and adverse effect of other hormone antagonists

T38.991   Poisoning by other hormone antagonists, accidental (unintentional)
> Poisoning by other hormone antagonists NOS

T38.992   Poisoning by other hormone antagonists, intentional self-harm

T38.993   Poisoning by other hormone antagonists, assault

T38.994   Poisoning by other hormone antagonists, undetermined

T38.995   Adverse effect of other hormone antagonists

T39   Poisoning by and adverse effect of nonopioid analgesics, antipyretics and antirheumatics

The following extensions are to be added to each code for category T39:
- a   initial encounter
- d   subsequent encounter
- q   sequela

T39.0   Poisoning by and adverse effect of salicylates

T39.0x   Poisoning by and adverse effect of salicylates

T39.0x1   Poisoning by salicylates, accidental (unintentional)
> Poisoning by salicylates NOS

T39.0x2   Poisoning by salicylates, intentional self-harm

T39.0x3   Poisoning by salicylates, assault

T39.0x4   Poisoning by salicylates, undetermined

T39.0x5   Adverse effect of salicylates

T39.1   Poisoning by and adverse effect of 4-Aminophenol derivatives

T39.1x   Poisoning by and adverse effect of 4-Aminophenol derivatives

T39.1x1   Poisoning by 4-Aminophenol derivatives, accidental (unintentional)
> Poisoning by 4-Aminophenol derivatives NOS

T39.1x2   Poisoning by 4-Aminophenol derivatives, intentional self-harm

T39.1x3   Poisoning by 4-Aminophenol derivatives, assault

T39.1x4   Poisoning by 4-Aminophenol derivatives, undetermined

T39.1x5   Adverse effect of 4-Aminophenol derivatives

T39.2   Poisoning by and adverse effect of pyrazolone derivatives

T39.2x   Poisoning by and adverse effect of pyrazolone derivatives

T39.2x1   Poisoning by pyrazolone derivatives, accidental (unintentional)
> Poisoning by pyrazolone derivatives NOS

T39.2x2   Poisoning by pyrazolone derivatives, intentional self-harm

T39.2x3   Poisoning by pyrazolone derivatives, assault

T39.2x4   Poisoning by pyrazolone derivatives, undetermined

T39.2x5   Adverse effect of pyrazolone derivatives

T39.3   Poisoning by and adverse effect of other nonsteroidal anti-inflammatory drugs [NSAID]

T39.31   Poisoning by and adverse effect of propionic acid derivatives
> Poisoning by and adverse effect of fenoprofen
> Poisoning by and adverse effect of flurbiprofen
> Poisoning by and adverse effect of ibuprofen
> Poisoning by and adverse effect of ketoprofen
> Poisoning by and adverse effect of naproxen
> Poisoning by and adverse effect of oxaprozin

T39.311   Poisoning by propionic acid derivatives, accidental (unintentional)

T39.312   Poisoning by propionic acid derivatives, intentional self-harm

T39.313   Poisoning by propionic acid derivatives, assault

T39.314   Poisoning by propionic acid derivatives, undetermined

T39.315   Adverse effect of propionic acid derivatives

T39.39   Poisoning by and adverse effect of other nonsteroidal anti-inflammatory drugs [NSAID]

T39.391   Poisoning by other nonsteroidal anti-inflammatory drugs [NSAID], accidental (unintentional)
> Poisoning by other nonsteroidal anti-inflammatory drugs NOS

T39.392   Poisoning by other nonsteroidal anti-inflammatory drugs [NSAID], intentional self-harm

T39.393   Poisoning by other nonsteroidal anti-inflammatory drugs [NSAID], assault

T39.394 Poisoning by other nonsteroidal anti-inflammatory drugs [NSAID], undetermined

T39.395 Adverse effect of other nonsteroidal anti-inflammatory drugs [NSAID]

T39.4 Poisoning by and adverse effect of antirheumatics, not elsewhere classified

Excludes1: glucocorticoids (T38.0-)
salicylates (T39.0-)

T39.4x Poisoning by and adverse effect of antirheumatics, not elsewhere classified

T39.4x1 Poisoning by antirheumatics, not elsewhere classified, accidental (unintentional)
Poisoning by antirheumatics, not elsewhere classified NOS

T39.4x2 Poisoning by antirheumatics, not elsewhere classified, intentional self-harm

T39.4x3 Poisoning by antirheumatics, not elsewhere classified, assault

T39.4x4 Poisoning by antirheumatics, not elsewhere classified, undetermined

T39.4x5 Adverse effect of antirheumatics, not elsewhere classified

T39.8 Poisoning by and adverse effect of other nonopioid analgesics and antipyretics, not elsewhere classified

T39.8x Poisoning by and adverse effect of other nonopioid analgesics and antipyretics, not elsewhere classified

T39.8x1 Poisoning by other nonopioid analgesics and antipyretics, not elsewhere classified, accidental (unintentional)
Poisoning by other nonopioid analgesics and antipyretics, not elsewhere classified NOS

T39.8x2 Poisoning by other nonopioid analgesics and antipyretics, not elsewhere classified, intentional self-harm

T39.8x3 Poisoning by other nonopioid analgesics and antipyretics, not elsewhere classified, assault

T39.8x4 Poisoning by other nonopioid analgesics and antipyretics, not elsewhere classified, undetermined

T39.8x5 Adverse effect of other nonopioid analgesics and antipyretics, not elsewhere classified

T39.9 Poisoning by and adverse effect of unspecified nonopioid analgesic, antipyretic and antirheumatic

T39.91 Poisoning by unspecified nonopioid analgesic, antipyretic and antirheumatic, accidental (unintentional)
Poisoning by nonopioid analgesic, antipyretic and antirheumatic NOS

T39.92 Poisoning by unspecified nonopioid analgesic, antipyretic and antirheumatic, intentional self-harm

T39.93 Poisoning by unspecified nonopioid analgesic, antipyretic and antirheumatic, assault

T39.94 Poisoning by unspecified nonopioid analgesic, antipyretic and antirheumatic, undetermined

T39.95 Adverse effect of unspecified nonopioid analgesic, antipyretic and antirheumatic

T40 Poisoning by and adverse effect of narcotics and psychodysleptics [hallucinogens]

Excludes2: drug dependence and related mental and behavioral disorders due to psychoactive substance use (F10-F19.-)

The following extensions are to be added to each code for category T40:
a   initial encounter
d   subsequent encounter
q   sequela

T40.0 Poisoning by and adverse effect of opium

T40.0x Poisoning by and adverse effect of opium

T40.0x1 Poisoning by opium, accidental (unintentional)
Poisoning by opium NOS

T40.0x2 Poisoning by opium, intentional self-harm

T40.0x3 Poisoning by opium, assault

T40.0x4 Poisoning by opium, undetermined

T40.0x5 Adverse effect of opium

T40.1 Poisoning by and adverse effect of heroin

T40.1x Poisoning by and adverse effect of heroin

T40.1x1 Poisoning by heroin, accidental (unintentional)
Poisoning by heroin NOS

T40.1x2 Poisoning by heroin, intentional self-harm

T40.1x3 Poisoning by heroin, assault

T40.1x4 Poisoning by heroin, undetermined

T40.1x5 Adverse effect of heroin

T40.2 Poisoning by and adverse effect of other opioids
Poisoning by and adverse effect of codeine
Poisoning by and adverse effect of morphine

T40.2x Poisoning by other opioids

T40.2x1 Poisoning by other opioids, accidental (unintentional)
Poisoning by other opioids NOS

T40.2x2 Poisoning by other opioids, intentional self-harm

T40.2x3 Poisoning by other opioids, assault

T40.2x4 Poisoning by other opioids, undetermined

T40.2x5 Adverse effect of other opioids

T40.3 Poisoning by and adverse effect of methadone

T40.3x Poisoning by and adverse effect of methadone

T40.3x1 Poisoning by methadone, accidental (unintentional)
Poisoning by methadone NOS

T40.3x2 Poisoning by methadone, intentional self-harm

T40.3x3 Poisoning by methadone, assault

T40.3x4 Poisoning by methadone, undetermined

T40.3x5 Adverse effect of methadone

T40.4 Poisoning by and adverse effect of other synthetic narcotics
Poisoning by and adverse effect of meperidine
Poisoning by and adverse effect of pethidine

T40.4x Poisoning by and adverse effect of other synthetic narcotics

T40.4x1 Poisoning by other synthetic narcotics, accidental (unintentional)
Poisoning by other synthetic narcotics NOS

T40.4x2 Poisoning by other synthetic narcotics, intentional self-harm

T40.4x3 Poisoning by other synthetic narcotics, assault

T40.4x4 Poisoning by other synthetic narcotics, undetermined

T40.4x5 Adverse effect of other synthetic narcotics

T40.5 Poisoning by and adverse effect of cocaine

T40.5x Poisoning by and adverse effect of cocaine

T40.5x1 Poisoning by cocaine, accidental (unintentional)
Poisoning by cocaine NOS

T40.5x2 Poisoning by cocaine, intentional self-harm

T40.5x3 Poisoning by cocaine, assault

T40.5x4 Poisoning by cocaine, undetermined

T40.5x5 Adverse effect of cocaine

T40.6 Poisoning by and adverse effect of other and unspecified narcotics

T40.60 Poisoning by and adverse effect of unspecified narcotics

T40.601 Poisoning by unspecified narcotics, accidental (unintentional)
Poisoning by narcotics NOS

T40.602 Poisoning by unspecified narcotics, intentional self-harm

T40.603 Poisoning by unspecified narcotics, assault

T40.604 Poisoning by unspecified narcotics, undetermined

T40.605 Adverse effect of unspecified narcotics

T40.69   Poisoning by and adverse effect of other narcotics

T40.691   Poisoning by other narcotics, accidental (unintentional)
Poisoning by other narcotics NOS

T40.692   Poisoning by other narcotics, intentional self-harm

T40.693   Poisoning by other narcotics, assault

T40.694   Poisoning by other narcotics, undetermined

T40.695   Adverse effect of other narcotics

T40.7   Poisoning by and adverse effect of cannabis (derivatives)

T40.7x   Poisoning by and adverse effect of cannabis (derivatives)

T40.7x1   Poisoning by cannabis (derivatives), accidental (unintentional)
Poisoning by cannabis NOS

T40.7x2   Poisoning by cannabis (derivatives), intentional self-harm

T40.7x3   Poisoning by cannabis (derivatives), assault

T40.7x4   Poisoning by cannabis (derivatives), undetermined

T40.7x5   Adverse effect of cannabis (derivatives)

T40.8   Poisoning by and adverse effect of lysergide [LSD]

T40.8x   Poisoning by and adverse effect of lysergide [LSD]

T40.8x1   Poisoning by lysergide [LSD], accidental (unintentional)
Poisoning by lysergide [LSD] NOS

T40.8x2   Poisoning by lysergide [LSD], intentional self-harm

T40.8x3   Poisoning by lysergide [LSD], assault

T40.8x4   Poisoning by lysergide [LSD], undetermined

T40.8x5   Adverse effect of lysergide [LSD]

T40.9   Poisoning by and adverse effect of other and unspecified psychodysleptics [hallucinogens]

T40.90   Poisoning by and adverse effect of unspecified psychodysleptics [hallucinogens]

T40.901   Poisoning by unspecified psychodysleptics [hallucinogens], accidental (unintentional)

T40.902   Poisoning by unspecified psychodysleptics [hallucinogens], intentional self-harm

T40.903   Poisoning by unspecified psychodysleptics [hallucinogens], assault

T40.904   Poisoning by unspecified psychodysleptics [hallucinogens], undetermined

T40.905   Adverse effect of unspecified psychodysleptics [hallucinogens]

T40.99   Poisoning by and adverse effect of other psychodysleptics [hallucinogens]
Poisoning by and adverse effect of mescaline
Poisoning by and adverse effect of psilocin
Poisoning by and adverse effect of psilocybine

T40.991   Poisoning by other psychodysleptics [hallucinogens], accidental (unintentional)
Poisoning by other psychodysleptics [hallucinogens] NOS

T40.992   Poisoning by other psychodysleptics [hallucinogens], intentional self-harm

T40.993   Poisoning by other psychodysleptics [hallucinogens], assault

T40.994   Poisoning by other psychodysleptics [hallucinogens], undetermined

T40.995   Adverse effect of other psychodysleptics [hallucinogens]

T41   Poisoning by and adverse effect of anesthetics and therapeutic gases
Excludes1:   benzodiazepines (T42.4-)
cocaine (T40.5-)
opioids (T40.0-T40.2-)

The following extensions are to be added to each code for category T41:
a   initial encounter
d   subsequent encounter
q   sequela

T41.0   Poisoning by and adverse effect of inhaled anesthetics
Excludes1:   oxygen (T41.5-)

T41.0x   Poisoning by and adverse effect of inhaled anesthetics

T41.0x1   Poisoning by inhaled anesthetics, accidental (unintentional)
Poisoning by inhaled anesthetics NOS

T41.0x2   Poisoning by inhaled anesthetics, intentional self-harm

T41.0x3   Poisoning by inhaled anesthetics, assault

T41.0x4   Poisoning by inhaled anesthetics, undetermined

T41.0x5   Adverse effect of inhaled anesthetics

T41.1   Poisoning by and adverse effect of intravenous anesthetics
Poisoning by and adverse effect of thiobarbiturates

T41.1x   Poisoning by intravenous anesthetics

T41.1x1   Poisoning by intravenous anesthetics, accidental (unintentional)
Poisoning by intravenous anesthetics NOS

T41.1x2   Poisoning by intravenous anesthetics, intentional self-harm

T41.1x3   Poisoning by intravenous anesthetics, assault

T41.1x4   Poisoning by intravenous anesthetics, undetermined

T41.1x5   Adverse effect of intravenous anesthetics

T41.2   Poisoning by and adverse effect of other and unspecified general anesthetics

T41.20   Poisoning by and adverse effect of unspecified general anesthetics

T41.201   Poisoning by unspecified general anesthetics, accidental (unintentional)
Poisoning by general anesthetics NOS

T41.202   Poisoning by unspecified general anesthetics, intentional self-harm

T41.203   Poisoning by unspecified general anesthetics, assault

T41.204   Poisoning by unspecified general anesthetics, undetermined

T41.205   Adverse effect of unspecified general anesthetics

T41.29   Poisoning by and adverse effect of other general anesthetics

T41.291   Poisoning by other general anesthetics, accidental (unintentional)
Poisoning by other general anesthetics NOS

T41.292   Poisoning by other general anesthetics, intentional self-harm

T41.293   Poisoning by other general anesthetics, assault

T41.294   Poisoning by other general anesthetics, undetermined

T41.295   Adverse effect of other general anesthetics

T41.3   Poisoning by and adverse effect of local anesthetics

T41.3x   Poisoning by and adverse effect of local anesthetics

T41.3x1   Poisoning by local anesthetics, accidental (unintentional)
Poisoning by local anesthetics NOS

T41.3x2   Poisoning by local anesthetics, intentional self-harm

T41.3x3   Poisoning by local anesthetics, assault

T41.3x4   Poisoning by local anesthetics, undetermined

T41.3x5   Adverse effect of local anesthetics

T41.4   Poisoning by and adverse effect of unspecified anesthetic

T41.41   Poisoning by unspecified anesthetic, accidental (unintentional)
Poisoning by anesthetic NOS

T41.42   Poisoning by unspecified anesthetic, intentional self-harm

T41.43   Poisoning by unspecified anesthetic, assault

T41.44   Poisoning by unspecified anesthetic, undetermined

T41.45   Adverse effect of unspecified anesthetic

T41.5 Poisoning by and adverse effect of therapeutic gases
Carbon dioxide poisoning
Oxygen poisoning

T41.5x   Poisoning by and adverse effect of therapeutic gases

T41.5x1   Poisoning by therapeutic gases, accidental (unintentional)
Poisoning by therapeutic gases NOS

T41.5x2   Poisoning by therapeutic gases, intentional self-harm

T41.5x3   Poisoning by therapeutic gases, assault

T41.5x4   Poisoning by therapeutic gases, undetermined

T41.5x5   Adverse effect of therapeutic gases

T42 Poisoning by and adverse effect of antiepileptic, sedative-hypnotic and antiparkinsonism drugs

Excludes2:   drug dependence and related mental and behavioral disorders due to psychoactive substance use (F10.-, F19.-)

The following extensions are to be added to each code for category T42:

   a   initial encounter
   d   subsequent encounter
   q   sequela

T42.0 Poisoning by and adverse effect of hydantoin derivatives

T42.0x   Poisoning by and adverse effect of hydantoin derivatives

T42.0x1   Poisoning by hydantoin derivatives, accidental (unintentional)
Poisoning by hydantoin derivatives NOS

T42.0x2   Poisoning by hydantoin derivatives, intentional self-harm

T42.0x3   Poisoning by hydantoin derivatives, assault

T42.0x4   Poisoning by hydantoin derivatives, undetermined

T42.0x5   Adverse effect of hydantoin derivatives

T42.1 Poisoning by and adverse effect of iminostilbenes
Adverse effect of carbamazepine
Poisoning by carbamazepine

T42.1x   Poisoning by and adverse effect of iminostilbenes

T42.1x1   Poisoning by iminostilbenes, accidental (unintentional)
Poisoning by iminostilbenes NOS

T42.1x2   Poisoning by iminostilbenes, intentional self-harm

T42.1x3   Poisoning by iminostilbenes, assault

T42.1x4   Poisoning by iminostilbenes, undetermined

T42.1x5   Adverse effect of iminostilbenes

T42.2 Poisoning by and adverse effect of succinimides and oxazolidinediones

T42.2x   Poisoning by and adverse effect of succinimides and oxazolidinediones

T42.2x1   Poisoning by succinimides and oxazolidinediones accidental (unintentional)
Poisoning by succinimides and oxazolidinediones NOS

T42.2x2   Poisoning by succinimides and oxazolidinediones intentional self-harm

T42.2x3   Poisoning by succinimides and oxazolidinediones, assault

T42.2x4   Poisoning by succinimides and oxazolidinediones, undetermined

T42.2x5   Adverse effect of succinimides and oxazolidinediones

T42.3 Poisoning by and adverse effect of barbiturates

Excludes1:   thiobarbiturates (T41.1-)

T42.3x   Poisoning by and adverse effect of barbiturates

T42.3x1   Poisoning by barbiturates, accidental (unintentional)
Poisoning by barbiturates NOS

T42.3x2   Poisoning by barbiturates, intentional self-harm

T42.3x3   Poisoning by barbiturates, assault

T42.3x4   Poisoning by barbiturates, undetermined

T42.3x5   Adverse effect of barbiturates

T42.4 Poisoning by and adverse effect of benzodiazepines

T42.4x   Poisoning by and adverse effect of benzodiazepines

T42.4x1   Poisoning by benzodiazepines, accidental (unintentional)
Poisoning by benzodiazepines NOS

T42.4x2   Poisoning by benzodiazepines, intentional self-harm

T42.4x3   Poisoning by benzodiazepines, assault

T42.4x4   Poisoning by benzodiazepines, undetermined

T42.4x5   Adverse effect of benzodiazepines

T42.5 Poisoning by and adverse effect of mixed antiepileptics

T42.5x   Poisoning by and adverse effect of mixed antiepileptics

T42.5x1   Poisoning by mixed antiepileptics, accidental (unintentional)
Poisoning by mixed antiepileptics NOS

T42.5x2   Poisoning by mixed antiepileptics, intentional self-harm

T42.5x3   Poisoning by mixed antiepileptics, assault

T42.5x4   Poisoning by mixed antiepileptics, undetermined

T42.5x5   Adverse effect of mixed antiepileptics

T42.6 Poisoning by and adverse effect of other antiepileptic and sedative-hypnotic drugs
Poisoning by and adverse effect of methaqualone
Poisoning by and adverse effect of valproic acid

Excludes1:   carbamazepine (T42.1-)

T42.6x   Poisoning by and adverse effect of other antiepileptic and sedative-hypnotic drugs

T42.6x1   Poisoning by other antiepileptic and sedative-hypnotic drugs, accidental (unintentional)
Poisoning by other antiepileptic and sedative-hypnotic drugs NOS

T42.6x2   Poisoning by other antiepileptic and sedative-hypnotic drugs, intentional self-harm

T42.6x3   Poisoning by other antiepileptic and sedative-hypnotic drugs, assault

T42.6x4   Poisoning by other antiepileptic and sedative-hypnotic drugs, undetermined

T42.6x5   Adverse effect of other antiepileptic and sedative-hypnotic drugs

T42.7 Poisoning by and adverse effect of unspecified antiepileptic and sedative-hypnotic drugs
Poisoning by sleeping draft NOS
Poisoning by sleeping drug NOS
Poisoning by sleeping tablet NOS

T42.71   Poisoning by unspecified antiepileptic and sedative-hypnotic drugs, accidental (unintentional)
Poisoning by antiepileptic and sedative-hypnotic drugs NOS

T42.72   Poisoning by unspecified antiepileptic and sedative-hypnotic drugs, intentional self-harm

T42.73   Poisoning by unspecified antiepileptic and sedative-hypnotic drugs, assault

T42.74   Poisoning by unspecified antiepileptic and sedative-hypnotic drugs, undetermined

T42.75   Adverse effect of unspecified antiepileptic and sedative-hypnotic drugs

T42.8 Poisoning by and adverse effect of antiparkinsonism drugs and other central muscle-tone depressants
Poisoning by and adverse effect of amantadine

T42.8x   Poisoning by and adverse effect of antiparkinsonism drugs and other central muscle-tone depressants

Chapter 19   © 2002 Ingenix, Inc.

T42.8x1 Poisoning by antiparkinsonism drugs and other central muscle-tone depressants, accidental (unintentional)

> Poisoning by antiparkinsonism drugs and other central muscle-tone depressants NOS

T42.8x2 Poisoning by antiparkinsonism drugs and other central muscle-tone depressants, intentional self-harm

T42.8x3 Poisoning by antiparkinsonism drugs and other central muscle-tone depressants, assault

T42.8x4 Poisoning by antiparkinsonism drugs and other central muscle-tone depressants, undetermined

T42.8x5 Adverse effect of antiparkinsonism drugs and other central muscle-tone depressants

T43 Poisoning by and adverse effect of psychotropic drugs, not elsewhere classified

Excludes1:   appetite depressants (T50.5-)
  barbiturates (T42.3-)
  benzodiazepines (T42.4-)
  methaqualone (T42.6-)
  psychodysleptics [hallucinogens] (T40.7-T40.9-)

Excludes2:   drug dependence and related mental and behavioral disorders due to psychoactive substance use (F10.0-F19.-)

The following extensions are to be added to each code for category T43:
  a   initial encounter
  d   subsequent encounter
  q   sequela

T43.0 Poisoning by and adverse effect of tricyclic and tetracyclic antidepressants

T43.0x Poisoning by and adverse effect of tricyclic and tetracyclic antidepressants

T43.0x1 Poisoning by tricyclic and tetracyclic antidepressants, accidental (unintentional)

> Poisoning by tricyclic and tetracyclic antidepressants NOS

T43.0x2 Poisoning by tricyclic and tetracyclic antidepressants, intentional self-harm

T43.0x3 Poisoning by tricyclic and tetracyclic antidepressants, assault

T43.0x4 Poisoning by tricyclic and tetracyclic antidepressants, undetermined

T43.0x5 Adverse effect of tricyclic and tetracyclic antidepressants

T43.1 Poisoning by and adverse effect of monoamine-oxidase-inhibitor antidepressants

T43.1x Poisoning by and adverse effect of monoamine-oxidase-inhibitor antidepressants

T43.1x1 Poisoning by monoamine-oxidase-inhibitor antidepressants, accidental (unintentional)

> Poisoning by monoamine-oxidase-inhibitor antidepressants NOS

T43.1x2 Poisoning by monoamine-oxidase-inhibitor antidepressants, intentional self-harm

T43.1x3 Poisoning by monoamine-oxidase-inhibitor antidepressants, assault

T43.1x4 Poisoning by monoamine-oxidase-inhibitor antidepressants, undetermined

T43.1x5 Adverse effect of monoamine-oxidase-inhibitor antidepressants

T43.2 Poisoning by and adverse effect of other and unspecified antidepressants

T43.20 Poisoning by and adverse effect of unspecified antidepressants

T43.201 Poisoning by unspecified antidepressants, accidental (unintentional)

> Poisoning by antidepressants NOS

T43.202 Poisoning by unspecified antidepressants, intentional self-harm

T43.203 Poisoning by unspecified antidepressants, assault

T43.204 Poisoning by unspecified antidepressants, undetermined

T43.205 Adverse effect of unspecified antidepressants

T43.29 Poisoning by and adverse effect of other antidepressants

T43.291 Poisoning by other antidepressants, accidental (unintentional)

> Poisoning by other antidepressants NOS

T43.292 Poisoning by other antidepressants, intentional self-harm

T43.293 Poisoning by other antidepressants, assault

T43.294 Poisoning by other antidepressants, undetermined

T43.295 Adverse effect of other antidepressants

T43.3 Poisoning by and adverse effect of phenothiazine antipsychotics and neuroleptics

T43.3x Poisoning by and adverse effect of phenothiazine antipsychotics and neuroleptics

T43.3x1 Poisoning by phenothiazine antipsychotics and neuroleptics, accidental (unintentional)

> Poisoning by phenothiazine antipsychotics and neuroleptics NOS

T43.3x2 Poisoning by phenothiazine antipsychotics and neuroleptics, intentional self-harm

T43.3x3 Poisoning by phenothiazine antipsychotics and neuroleptics, assault

T43.3x4 Poisoning by phenothiazine antipsychotics and neuroleptics, undetermined

T43.3x5 Adverse effect of phenothiazine antipsychotics and neuroleptics

T43.4 Poisoning by and adverse effect of butyrophenone and thiothixene neuroleptics

T43.4x Poisoning by and adverse effect of butyrophenone and thiothixene neuroleptics

T43.4x1 Poisoning by butyrophenone and thiothixene neuroleptics, accidental (unintentional)

> Poisoning by butyrophenone and thiothixene neuroleptics NOS

T43.4x2 Poisoning by butyrophenone and thiothixene neuroleptics, intentional self-harm

T43.4x3 Poisoning by butyrophenone and thiothixene neuroleptics, assault

T43.4x4 Poisoning by butyrophenone and thiothixene neuroleptics, undetermined

T43.4x5 Adverse effect of butyrophenone and thiothixene neuroleptics

T43.5 Poisoning by and adverse effect of other and unspecified antipsychotics and neuroleptics

Excludes1:   rauwolfia (T46.5-)

T43.50 Poisoning by and adverse effect of unspecified antipsychotics and neuroleptics

T43.501 Poisoning by unspecified antipsychotics and neuroleptics, accidental (unintentional)

> Poisoning by antipsychotics and neuroleptics NOS

T43.502 Poisoning by unspecified antipsychotics and neuroleptics, intentional self-harm

T43.503 Poisoning by unspecified antipsychotics and neuroleptics, assault

T43.504 Poisoning by unspecified antipsychotics and neuroleptics, undetermined

T43.505 Adverse effect of unspecified antipsychotics and neuroleptics

T43.59 Poisoning by and adverse effect of other antipsychotics and neuroleptics

T43.591 Poisoning by other antipsychotics and neuroleptics, accidental (unintentional)

> Poisoning by other antipsychotics and neuroleptics NOS

T43.592 Poisoning by other antipsychotics and neuroleptics, intentional self-harm

T43.593   Poisoning by other antipsychotics and neuroleptics, assault
T43.594   Poisoning by other antipsychotics and neuroleptics, undetermined
T43.595   Adverse effect of other antipsychotics and neuroleptics

T43.6   Poisoning by and adverse effect of psychostimulants with abuse potential
    Excludes1:   cocaine (T40.5-)
    T43.6x   Poisoning by and adverse effect of psychostimulants with abuse potential
        T43.6x1   Poisoning by psychostimulants with abuse potential, accidental (unintentional)
            Poisoning by psychostimulants with abuse potential NOS
        T43.6x2   Poisoning by psychostimulants with abuse potential, intentional self-harm
        T43.6x3   Poisoning by psychostimulants with abuse potential, assault
        T43.6x4   Poisoning by psychostimulants with abuse potential, undetermined
        T43.6x5   Adverse effect of psychostimulants with abuse potential

T43.8   Poisoning by and adverse effect of other psychotropic drugs
    T43.8x   Poisoning by and adverse effect of other psychotropic drugs
        T43.8x1   Poisoning by other psychotropic drugs, accidental (unintentional)
            Poisoning by other psychotropic drugs NOS
        T43.8x2   Poisoning by other psychotropic drugs, intentional self-harm
        T43.8x3   Poisoning by other psychotropic drugs, assault
        T43.8x4   Poisoning by other psychotropic drugs, undetermined
        T43.8x5   Adverse effect of other psychotropic drugs

T43.9   Poisoning by and adverse effect of unspecified psychotropic drug
    T43.91   Poisoning by unspecified psychotropic drug, accidental (unintentional)
        Poisoning by psychotropic drug NOS
    T43.92   Poisoning by unspecified psychotropic drug, intentional self-harm
    T43.93   Poisoning by unspecified psychotropic drug, assault
    T43.94   Poisoning by unspecified psychotropic drug, undetermined
    T43.95   Adverse effect of unspecified psychotropic drug

T44   Poisoning by and adverse effect of drugs primarily affecting the autonomic nervous system
    The following extensions are to be added to each code for category T44:
    a   initial encounter
    d   subsequent encounter
    q   sequela
T44.0   Poisoning by and adverse effect of anticholinesterase agents
    T44.0x   Poisoning by and adverse effect of anticholinesterase agents
        T44.0x1   Poisoning by anticholinesterase agents, accidental (unintentional)
            Poisoning by anticholinesterase agents NOS
        T44.0x2   Poisoning by anticholinesterase agents, intentional self-harm
        T44.0x3   Poisoning by anticholinesterase agents, assault
        T44.0x4   Poisoning by anticholinesterase agents, undetermined
        T44.0x5   Adverse effect of anticholinesterase agents
T44.1   Poisoning by and adverse effect of other parasympathomimetics [cholinergics]
    T44.1x   Poisoning by and adverse effect of other parasympathomimetics [cholinergics]

        T44.1x1   Poisoning by other parasympathomimetics [cholinergics], accidental (unintentional)
            Poisoning by other parasympathomimetics [cholinergics] NOS
        T44.1x2   Poisoning by other parasympathomimetics [cholinergics], intentional self-harm
        T44.1x3   Poisoning by other parasympathomimetics [cholinergics], assault
        T44.1x4   Poisoning by other parasympathomimetics [cholinergics], undetermined
        T44.1x5   Adverse effect of other parasympathomimetics [cholinergics]
T44.2   Poisoning by and adverse effect of ganglionic blocking drugs
    T44.2x   Poisoning by and adverse effect of ganglionic blocking drugs
        T44.2x1   Poisoning by ganglionic blocking drugs, accidental (unintentional)
            Poisoning by ganglionic blocking drugs NOS
        T44.2x2   Poisoning by ganglionic blocking drugs, intentional self-harm
        T44.2x3   Poisoning by ganglionic blocking drugs, assault
        T44.2x4   Poisoning by ganglionic blocking drugs, undetermined
        T44.2x5   Adverse effect of ganglionic blocking drugs
T44.3   Poisoning by and adverse effect of other parasympatholytics [anticholinergics and antimuscarinics] and spasmolytics
    Poisoning by and adverse effect of papaverine
    T44.3x   Poisoning by and adverse effect of other parasympatholytics [anticholinergics and antimuscarinics] and spasmolytics
        T44.3x1   Poisoning by other parasympatholytics [anticholinergics and antimuscarinics] and spasmolytics, accidental (unintentional)
            Poisoning by other parasympatholytics [anticholinergics and antimuscarinics] and spasmolytics NOS
        T44.3x2   Poisoning by other parasympatholytics [anticholinergics and antimuscarinics] and spasmolytics, intentional self-harm
        T44.3x3   Poisoning by other parasympatholytics [anticholinergics and antimuscarinics] and spasmolytics, assault
        T44.3x4   Poisoning by other parasympatholytics [anticholinergics and antimuscarinics] and spasmolytics, undetermined
        T44.3x5   Adverse effect of other parasympatholytics [anticholinergics and antimuscarinics] and spasmolytics
T44.4   Poisoning by and adverse effect of predominantly α-adrenoreceptor agonists
    Poisoning by and adverse effect of metaraminol
    T44.4x   Poisoning by and adverse effect of predominantly α-adrenoreceptor agonists
        T44.4x1   Poisoning by predominantly α-adrenoreceptor agonists, accidental (unintentional)
            Poisoning by predominantly α-adrenoreceptor agonists NOS
        T44.4x2   Poisoning by predominantly α-adrenoreceptor agonists, intentional self-harm
        T44.4x3   Poisoning by predominantly α-adrenoreceptor agonists, assault
        T44.4x4   Poisoning by predominantly α-adrenoreceptor agonists, undetermined
        T44.4x5   Adverse effect of predominantly α-adrenoreceptor agonists
T44.5   Poisoning by and adverse effect of predominantly β-adrenoreceptor agonists
    Excludes1:   salbutamol (T48.6-)
    T44.5x   Poisoning by and adverse effect of predominantly β-adrenoreceptor agonists

T44.5x1 **Poisoning by predominantly α-adrenoreceptor agonists, accidental (unintentional)**
> Poisoning by predominantly β-adrenoreceptor agonists NOS

T44.5x2 **Poisoning by predominantly β-adrenoreceptor agonists, intentional self-harm**

T44.5x3 **Poisoning by predominantly β-adrenoreceptor agonists, assault**

T44.5x4 **Poisoning by predominantly β-adrenoreceptor agonists, undetermined**

T44.5x5 **Adverse effect of predominantly β-adrenoreceptor agonists**

T44.6 **Poisoning by and adverse effect of α-adrenoreceptor antagonists**
> Excludes1: ergot alkaloids (T48.0)

T44.6x **Poisoning by and adverse effect of α-adrenoreceptor antagonists**

T44.6x1 **Poisoning by α-adrenoreceptor antagonists, accidental (unintentional)**
> Poisoning by α-Adrenoreceptor antagonists NOS

T44.6x2 **Poisoning by α-adrenoreceptor antagonists, intentional self-harm**

T44.6x3 **Poisoning by α-adrenoreceptor antagonists, assault**

T44.6x4 **Poisoning by α-adrenoreceptor antagonists, undetermined**

T44.6x5 **Adverse effect of α-adrenoreceptor antagonists**

T44.7 **Poisoning by and adverse effect of β-adrenoreceptor antagonists**

T44.7x **Poisoning by and adverse effect of β-adrenoreceptor antagonists**

T44.7x1 **Poisoning by β-adrenoreceptor antagonists, accidental (unintentional)**
> Poisoning by β-adrenoreceptor antagonists NOS

T44.7x2 **Poisoning by β-adrenoreceptor antagonists, intentional self-harm**

T44.7x3 **Poisoning by β-adrenoreceptor antagonists, assault**

T44.7x4 **Poisoning by β-adrenoreceptor antagonists, undetermined**

T44.7x5 **Adverse effect of β-adrenoreceptor antagonists**

T44.8 **Poisoning by and adverse effect of centrally-acting and adrenergic-neuron-blocking agents**
> Excludes1: clonidine (T46.5)
> guanethidine (T46.5)

T44.8x **Poisoning by and adverse effect of centrally-acting and adrenergic-neuron-blocking agents**

T44.8x1 **Poisoning by centrally-acting and adrenergic-neuron-blocking agents, accidental (unintentional)**
> Poisoning by centrally-acting and adrenergic-neuronblocking agents NOS

T44.8x2 **Poisoning by centrally-acting and adrenergic-neuron-blocking agents, intentional self-harm**

T44.8x3 **Poisoning by centrally-acting and adrenergic-neuron-blocking agents, assault**

T44.8x4 **Poisoning by centrally-acting and adrenergic-neuron-blocking agents, undetermined**

T44.8x5 **Adverse effect of centrally-acting and adrenergic-neuron-blocking agents**

T44.9 **Poisoning by and adverse effect of other and unspecified drugs primarily affecting the autonomic nervous system**
> Poisoning by and adverse effect of drug stimulating both α- and β-adrenoreceptors

T44.90 **Poisoning by and adverse effect of unspecified drugs primarily affecting the autonomic nervous system**

T44.901 **Poisoning by unspecified drugs primarily affecting the autonomic nervous system, accidental (unintentional)**
> Poisoning by unspecified drugs primarily affecting the autonomic nervous system NOS

T44.902 **Poisoning by unspecified drugs primarily affecting the autonomic nervous system, intentional self-harm**

T44.903 **Poisoning by unspecified drugs primarily affecting the autonomic nervous system, assault**

T44.904 **Poisoning by unspecified drugs primarily affecting the autonomic nervous system, undetermined**

T44.905 **Adverse effect of unspecified drugs primarily affecting the autonomic nervous system**

T44.99 **Poisoning by and adverse effect of other drugs primarily affecting the autonomic nervous system**

T44.991 **Poisoning by other drug primarily affecting the autonomic nervous system, accidental (unintentional)**
> Poisoning by other drugs primarily affecting the autonomic nervous system NOS

T44.992 **Poisoning by other drug primarily affecting the autonomic nervous system, intentional self-harm**

T44.993 **Poisoning by other drug primarily affecting the autonomic nervous system, assault**

T44.994 **Poisoning by other drug primarily affecting the autonomic nervous system, undetermined**

T44.995 **Adverse effect of other drug primarily affecting the autonomic nervous system**

T45 **Poisoning by and adverse effect of primarily systemic and hematological agents, not elsewhere classified**
> The following extensions are to be added to each code for category T45:
> a   initial encounter
> d   subsequent encounter
> q   sequela

T45.0 **Poisoning by and adverse effect of antiallergic and antiemetic drugs**
> Excludes1: phenothiazine-based neuroleptics (T43.3)

T45.0x **Poisoning by and adverse effect of antiallergic and antiemetic drugs**

T45.0x1 **Poisoning by antiallergic and antiemetic drugs, accidental (unintentional)**
> Poisoning by antiallergic and antiemetic drugs NOS

T45.0x2 **Poisoning by antiallergic and antiemetic drugs, intentional self-harm**

T45.0x3 **Poisoning by antiallergic and antiemetic drugs, assault**

T45.0x4 **Poisoning by antiallergic and antiemetic drugs, undetermined**

T45.0x5 **Adverse effect of antiallergic and antiemetic drugs**

T45.1 **Poisoning by and adverse effect of antineoplastic and immunosuppressive drugs**
> Poisoning by and adverse effect of antineoplastic antibiotics
> Poisoning by and adverse effect of cytarabine
> Excludes1: tamoxifen (T38.6)

T45.1x **Poisoning by antineoplastic and immunosuppressive drugs**

T45.1x1 **Poisoning by antineoplastic and immunosuppressive drugs, accidental (unintentional)**
> Poisoning by antineoplastic and immunosuppressive drugs NOS

T45.1x2 **Poisoning by antineoplastic and immunosuppressive drugs, intentional self-harm**

T45.1x3   Poisoning by antineoplastic and immunosuppressive drugs, assault

T45.1x4   Poisoning by antineoplastic and immunosuppressive drugs, undetermined

T45.1x5   Adverse effect of antineoplastic and immunosuppressive drugs

T45.2   Poisoning by and adverse effect of vitamins

Excludes1:   nicotinic acid (derivatives) (T46.7)
iron (T45.4-)
vitamin K (T45.7)

T45.2x   Poisoning by and adverse effect of vitamins

T45.2x1   Poisoning by vitamins, accidental (unintentional)
Poisoning by vitamins NOS

T45.2x2   Poisoning by vitamins, intentional self-harm

T45.2x3   Poisoning by vitamins, assault

T45.2x4   Poisoning by vitamins, undetermined

T45.2x5   Adverse effect of vitamins

T45.3   Poisoning by and adverse effect of enzymes

T45.3x   Poisoning by and adverse effect of enzymes

T45.3x1   Poisoning by enzymes, accidental (unintentional)
Poisoning by enzymes NOS

T45.3x2   Poisoning by enzymes, intentional self-harm

T45.3x3   Poisoning by enzymes, assault

T45.3x4   Poisoning by enzymes, undetermined

T45.3x5   Adverse effect of enzymes

T45.4   Poisoning by and adverse effect of iron and its compounds

T45.4x   Poisoning by and adverse effect of iron and its compounds

T45.4x1   Poisoning by iron and its compounds, accidental (unintentional)
Poisoning by iron and its compounds NOS

T45.4x2   Poisoning by iron and its compounds, intentional self-harm

T45.4x3   Poisoning by iron and its compounds, assault

T45.4x4   Poisoning by iron and its compounds, undetermined

T45.4x5   Adverse effect of iron and its compounds

T45.5   Poisoning by and adverse effect of anticoagulants

T45.5x   Poisoning by and adverse effect of anticoagulants

T45.5x1   Poisoning by anticoagulants, accidental (unintentional)
Poisoning by anticoagulants NOS

T45.5x2   Poisoning by anticoagulants, intentional self-harm

T45.5x3   Poisoning by anticoagulants, assault

T45.5x4   Poisoning by anticoagulants, undetermined

T45.5x5   Adverse effect of anticoagulants

T45.6   Poisoning by and adverse effect of fibrinolysis-affecting drugs

T45.6x   Poisoning by and adverse effect of fibrinolysis-affecting drugs

T45.6x1   Poisoning by fibrinolysis-affecting drugs, accidental (unintentional)
Poisoning by fibrinolysis-affecting drugs NOS

T45.6x2   Poisoning by fibrinolysis-affecting drugs, intentional self-harm

T45.6x3   Poisoning by fibrinolysis-affecting drugs, assault

T45.6x4   Poisoning by fibrinolysis-affecting drugs, undetermined

T45.6x5   Adverse effect of fibrinolysis-affecting drugs

T45.7   Poisoning by and adverse effect of anticoagulant antagonists, vitamin K and other coagulants

T45.7x   Poisoning by and adverse effect of anticoagulant antagonists, vitamin K and other coagulants

T45.7x1   Poisoning by anticoagulant antagonists, vitamin K and other coagulants, accidental (unintentional)
Poisoning by anticoagulant antagonists, vitamin K and other coagulants NOS

T45.7x2   Poisoning by anticoagulant antagonists, vitamin K and other coagulants, intentional self-harm

T45.7x3   Poisoning by anticoagulant antagonists, vitamin K and other coagulants, assault

T45.7x4   Poisoning by anticoagulant antagonists, vitamin K and other coagulants, undetermined

T45.7x5   Adverse effect of anticoagulant antagonists, vitamin K and other coagulants

T45.8   Poisoning by and adverse effect of other primarily systemic and hematological agents

Poisoning by and adverse effect of liver preparations and other antianemic agents

Poisoning by and adverse effect of natural blood and blood products

Poisoning by and adverse effect of plasma substitute

Excludes1:   immunoglobulin (T50.9-)
iron (T45.4-)

T45.8x   Poisoning by and adverse effect of other primarily systemic and hematological agents

T45.8x1   Poisoning by other primarily systemic and hematological agents, accidental (unintentional)
Poisoning by other primarily systemic and hematological agents NOS

T45.8x2   Poisoning by other primarily systemic and hematological agents, intentional self-harm

T45.8x3   Poisoning by other primarily systemic and hematological agents, assault

T45.8x4   Poisoning by other primarily systemic and hematological agents, undetermined

T45.8x5   Adverse effect of other primarily systemic and hematological agents

T45.9   Poisoning by and adverse effect of unspecified primarily systemic and hematological agent

T45.91   Poisoning by unspecified primarily systemic and hematological agent, accidental (unintentional)
Poisoning by primarily systemic and hematological agent NOS

T45.92   Poisoning by unspecified primarily systemic and hematological agent, intentional self-harm

T45.93   Poisoning by unspecified primarily systemic and hematological agent, assault

T45.94   Poisoning by unspecified primarily systemic and hematological agent, undetermined

T45.95   Adverse effect of unspecified primarily systemic and hematological agent

T46   Poisoning by and adverse effect of agents primarily affecting the cardiovascular system

Excludes1:   metaraminol (T44.4-)

The following extensions are to be added to each code for category T46:

a   initial encounter
d   subsequent encounter
q   sequela

T46.0   Poisoning by and adverse effect of cardiac-stimulant glycosides and drugs of similar action

T46.0x   Poisoning by and adverse effect of cardiac-stimulant glycosides and drugs of similar action

T46.0x1   Poisoning by cardiac-stimulant glycosides and drugs of similar action, accidental (unintentional)
Poisoning by cardiac-stimulant glycosides and drugs of similar action NOS

T46.0x2   Poisoning by cardiac-stimulant glycosides and drugs of similar action, intentional self-harm

T46.0x3   Poisoning by cardiac-stimulant glycosides and drugs of similar action, assault

T46.0x4   Poisoning by cardiac-stimulant glycosides and drugs of similar action, undetermined

T46.0x5   Adverse effect of cardiac-stimulant glycosides and drugs of similar action

T46.1 Poisoning by and adverse effect of calcium-channel blockers

  T46.1x Poisoning by and adverse effect of calcium-channel blockers

    T46.1x1 Poisoning by calcium-channel blockers, accidental (unintentional)

      Poisoning by calcium-channel blockers NOS

    T46.1x2 Poisoning by calcium-channel blockers, intentional self-harm

    T46.1x3 Poisoning by calcium-channel blockers, assault

    T46.1x4 Poisoning by calcium-channel blockers, undetermined

    T46.1x5 Adverse effect of calcium-channel blockers

T46.2 Poisoning by and adverse effect of other antidysrhythmic drugs, not elsewhere classified

  Excludes1: β-adrenoreceptor antagonists (T44.7-)

  T46.2x Poisoning by and adverse effect of other antidysrhythmic drugs

    T46.2x1 Poisoning by other antidysrhythmic drugs, accidental (unintentional)

      Poisoning by other antidysrhythmic drugs NOS

    T46.2x2 Poisoning by other antidysrhythmic drugs, intentional self-harm

    T46.2x3 Poisoning by other antidysrhythmic drugs, assault

    T46.2x4 Poisoning by other antidysrhythmic drugs, undetermined

    T46.2x5 Adverse effect of other antidysrhythmic drugs

T46.3 Poisoning by and adverse effect of coronary vasodilators

  Poisoning by and adverse effect of dipyridamole

  Excludes1: β-adrenoreceptor antagonists (T44.7-)

          calcium-channel blockers (T46.1-)

  T46.3x Poisoning by and adverse effect of coronary vasodilators

    T46.3x1 Poisoning by coronary vasodilators, accidental (unintentional)

      Poisoning by coronary vasodilators NOS

    T46.3x2 Poisoning by coronary vasodilators, intentional self-harm

    T46.3x3 Poisoning by coronary vasodilators, assault

    T46.3x4 Poisoning by coronary vasodilators, undetermined

    T46.3x5 Adverse effect of coronary vasodilators

T46.4 Poisoning by and adverse effect of angiotensin-converting-enzyme inhibitors

  T46.4x Poisoning by and adverse effect of angiotensin-converting-enzyme inhibitors

    T46.4x1 Poisoning by angiotensin-converting-enzyme inhibitors, accidental (unintentional)

      Poisoning by angiotensin-converting-enzyme inhibitors NOS

    T46.4x2 Poisoning by angiotensin-converting-enzyme inhibitors, intentional self-harm

    T46.4x3 Poisoning by angiotensin-converting-enzyme inhibitors, assault

    T46.4x4 Poisoning by angiotensin-converting-enzyme inhibitors, undetermined

    T46.4x5 Adverse effect of angiotensin-converting-enzyme inhibitors

T46.5 Poisoning by and adverse effect of other antihypertensive drugs

  Poisoning by and adverse effect of clonidine

  Poisoning by and adverse effect of guanethidine

  Poisoning by and adverse effect of rauwolfia

  Excludes1: β-adrenoreceptor antagonists (T44.7-)

          calcium-channel blockers (T46.1-)

          diuretics (T50.0-T50.2)

  T46.5x Poisoning by and adverse effect of other antihypertensive drugs

    T46.5x1 Poisoning by other antihypertensive drugs, accidental (unintentional)

      Poisoning by other antihypertensive drugs NOS

    T46.5x2 Poisoning by other antihypertensive drugs, intentional self-harm

    T46.5x3 Poisoning by other antihypertensive drugs, assault

    T46.5x4 Poisoning by other antihypertensive drugs, undetermined

    T46.5x5 Adverse effect of other antihypertensive drugs

T46.6 Poisoning by and adverse effect of antihyperlipidemic and antiarteriosclerotic drugs

  T46.6x Poisoning by and adverse effect of antihyperlipidemic and antiarteriosclerotic drugs

    T46.6x1 Poisoning by antihyperlipidemic and antiarteriosclerotic drugs, accidental (unintentional)

      Poisoning by antihyperlipidemic and antiarteriosclerotic drugs NOS

    T46.6x2 Poisoning by antihyperlipidemic and antiarteriosclerotic drugs, intentional self-harm

    T46.6x3 Poisoning by antihyperlipidemic and antiarteriosclerotic drugs, assault

    T46.6x4 Poisoning by antihyperlipidemic and antiarteriosclerotic drugs, undetermined

    T46.6x5 Adverse effect of antihyperlipidemic and antiarteriosclerotic drugs

T46.7 Poisoning by and adverse effect of peripheral vasodilators

  Poisoning by and adverse effect of nicotinic acid (derivatives)

  Excludes1: papaverine (T44.3)

  T46.7x Poisoning by and adverse effect of peripheral vasodilators

    T46.7x1 Poisoning by peripheral vasodilators, accidental (unintentional)

      Poisoning by peripheral vasodilators NOS

    T46.7x2 Poisoning by peripheral vasodilators, intentional self-harm

    T46.7x3 Poisoning by peripheral vasodilators, assault

    T46.7x4 Poisoning by peripheral vasodilators, undetermined

    T46.7x5 Adverse effect of peripheral vasodilators

T46.8 Poisoning by and adverse effect of antivaricose drugs, including sclerosing agents

  T46.8x Poisoning by and adverse effect of antivaricose drugs, including sclerosing agents

    T46.8x1 Poisoning by antivaricose drugs, including sclerosing agents, accidental (unintentional)

      Poisoning by antivaricose drugs, including sclerosing agents NOS

    T46.8x2 Poisoning by antivaricose drugs, including sclerosing agents, intentional self-harm

    T46.8x3 Poisoning by antivaricose drugs, including sclerosing agents, assault

    T46.8x4 Poisoning by antivaricose drugs, including sclerosing agents, undetermined

    T46.8x5 Adverse effect of antivaricose drugs, including sclerosing agents

T46.9 Poisoning by and adverse effect of other and unspecified agents primarily affecting the cardiovascular system

  T46.90 Poisoning by and adverse effect of unspecified agents primarily affecting the cardiovascular system

    T46.901 Poisoning by unspecified agents primarily affecting the cardiovascular system, accidental (unintentional)

    T46.902 Poisoning by unspecified agents primarily affecting the cardiovascular system, intentional self-harm

    T46.903 Poisoning by unspecified agents primarily affecting the cardiovascular system, assault

    T46.904 Poisoning by unspecified agents primarily affecting the cardiovascular system, undetermined

    T46.905 Adverse effect of unspecified agents primarily affecting the cardiovascular system

T46.99   Poisoning by and adverse effect of other agents primarily affecting the cardiovascular system

    T46.991   Poisoning by other agents primarily affecting the cardiovascular system, accidental (unintentional)

    T46.992   Poisoning by other agents primarily affecting the cardiovascular system, intentional self-harm

    T46.993   Poisoning by other agents primarily affecting the cardiovascular system, assault

    T46.994   Poisoning by other agents primarily affecting the cardiovascular system, undetermined

    T46.995   Adverse effect of other agents primarily affecting the cardiovascular system

T47   Poisoning by and adverse effect of agents primarily affecting the gastrointestinal system

The following extensions are to be added to each code for category T47:

    a   initial encounter
    d   subsequent encounter
    q   sequela

T47.0   Poisoning by and adverse effect of histamine H2-receptor blockers

  T47.0x   Poisoning by and adverse effect of histamine H2-receptor blockers

    T47.0x1   Poisoning by histamine H2-receptor blockers, accidental (unintentional)
      Poisoning by histamine H2-receptor blockers NOS

    T47.0x2   Poisoning by histamine H2-receptor blockers, intentional self-harm

    T47.0x3   Poisoning by histamine H2-receptor blockers, assault

    T47.0x4   Poisoning by histamine H2-receptor blockers, undetermined

    T47.0x5   Adverse effect of histamine H2-receptor blockers

T47.1   Poisoning by and adverse effect of other antacids and anti-gastric-secretion drugs

  T47.1x   Poisoning by and adverse effect of other antacids and anti-gastric-secretion drugs

    T47.1x1   Poisoning by other antacids and anti-gastric-secretion drugs, accidental (unintentional)
      Poisoning by other antacids and anti-gastric-secretion drugs NOS

    T47.1x2   Poisoning by other antacids and anti-gastric-secretion drugs, intentional self-harm

    T47.1x3   Poisoning by other antacids and anti-gastric-secretion drugs, assault

    T47.1x4   Poisoning by other antacids and anti-gastric-secretion drugs, undetermined

    T47.1x5   Adverse effect of other antacids and anti-gastric-secretion drugs

T47.2   Poisoning by and adverse effect of stimulant laxatives

  T47.2x   Poisoning by and adverse effect of stimulant laxatives

    T47.2x1   Poisoning by stimulant laxatives, accidental (unintentional)
      Poisoning by stimulant laxatives NOS

    T47.2x2   Poisoning by stimulant laxatives, intentional self-harm

    T47.2x3   Poisoning by stimulant laxatives, assault

    T47.2x4   Poisoning by stimulant laxatives, undetermined

    T47.2x5   Adverse effect of stimulant laxatives

T47.3   Poisoning by and adverse effect of saline and osmotic laxatives

  T47.3x   Poisoning by and adverse effect of saline and osmotic laxatives

    T47.3x1   Poisoning by saline and osmotic laxatives, accidental (unintentional)
      Poisoning by saline and osmotic laxatives NOS

    T47.3x2   Poisoning by saline and osmotic laxatives, intentional self-harm

    T47.3x3   Poisoning by saline and osmotic laxatives, assault

    T47.3x4   Poisoning by saline and osmotic laxatives, undetermined

    T47.3x5   Adverse effect of saline and osmotic laxatives

T47.4   Poisoning by and adverse effect of other laxatives
    Poisoning by and adverse effect of intestinal atonia drugs

  T47.4x   Poisoning by and adverse effect of other laxatives

    T47.4x1   Poisoning by other laxatives, accidental (unintentional)
      Poisoning by other laxatives NOS

    T47.4x2   Poisoning by other laxatives, intentional self-harm

    T47.4x3   Poisoning by other laxatives, assault

    T47.4x4   Poisoning by other laxatives, undetermined

    T47.4x5   Adverse effect of other laxatives

T47.5   Poisoning by and adverse effect of digestants

  T47.5x   Poisoning by and adverse effect of digestants

    T47.5x1   Poisoning by digestants, accidental (unintentional)
      Poisoning by digestants NOS

    T47.5x2   Poisoning by digestants, intentional self-harm

    T47.5x3   Poisoning by digestants, assault

    T47.5x4   Poisoning by digestants, undetermined

    T47.5x5   Adverse effect of digestants

T47.6   Poisoning by and adverse effect of antidiarrheal drugs
    Excludes1:   systemic antibiotics and other anti-infectives (T36-T37)

  T47.6x   Poisoning by and adverse effect of antidiarrheal drugs

    T47.6x1   Poisoning by antidiarrheal drugs, accidental (unintentional)
      Poisoning by antidiarrheal drugs NOS

    T47.6x2   Poisoning by antidiarrheal drugs, intentional self-harm

    T47.6x3   Poisoning by antidiarrheal drugs, assault

    T47.6x4   Poisoning by antidiarrheal drugs, undetermined

    T47.6x5   Adverse effect of antidiarrheal drugs

T47.7   Poisoning by and adverse effect of emetics

  T47.7x   Poisoning by and adverse effect of emetics

    T47.7x1   Poisoning by emetics, accidental (unintentional)
      Poisoning by emetics NOS

    T47.7x2   Poisoning by emetics, intentional self-harm

    T47.7x3   Poisoning by emetics, assault

    T47.7x4   Poisoning by emetics, undetermined

    T47.7x5   Adverse effect of emetics

T47.8   Poisoning by and adverse effect of other agents primarily affecting gastrointestinal system

  T47.8x   Poisoning by and adverse effect of other agents primarily affecting gastrointestinal system

    T47.8x1   Poisoning by other agents primarily affecting gastrointestinal system, accidental (unintentional)
      Poisoning by other agents primarily affecting gastrointestinal system NOS

    T47.8x2   Poisoning by other agents primarily affecting gastrointestinal system, intentional self-harm

    T47.8x3   Poisoning by other agents primarily affecting gastrointestinal system, assault

    T47.8x4   Poisoning by other agents primarily affecting gastrointestinal system, undetermined

    T47.8x5   Adverse effect of other agents primarily affecting gastrointestinal system

T47.9   Poisoning by and adverse effect of unspecified agents primarily affecting the gastrointestinal system

  T47.91   Poisoning by unspecified agents primarily affecting the gastrointestinal system, accidental (unintentional)
    Poisoning by agents primarily affecting the gastrointestinal system NOS

T47.92 Poisoning by unspecified agents primarily affecting the gastrointestinal system, intentional self-harm

T47.93 Poisoning by unspecified agents primarily affecting the gastrointestinal system, assault

T47.94 Poisoning by unspecified agents primarily affecting the gastrointestinal system, undetermined

T47.95 Adverse effect of unspecified agents primarily affecting the gastrointestinal system

T48 Poisoning by and adverse effect of agents primarily acting on smooth and skeletal muscles and the respiratory system

The following extensions are to be added to each code for category T48:

  a   initial encounter
  d   subsequent encounter
  q   sequela

T48.0 Poisoning by and adverse effect of oxytocic drugs

Excludes1: estrogens, progestogens and antagonists (T38.4-T38.6)

T48.0x Poisoning by and adverse effect of oxytocic drugs

T48.0x1 Poisoning by oxytocic drugs, accidental (unintentional)
    Poisoning by oxytocic drugs NOS

T48.0x2 Poisoning by oxytocic drugs, intentional self-harm

T48.0x3 Poisoning by oxytocic drugs, assault

T48.0x4 Poisoning by oxytocic drugs, undetermined

T48.0x5 Adverse effect of oxytocic drugs

T48.1 Poisoning by and adverse effect of skeletal muscle relaxants [neuromuscular blocking agents]

T48.1x Poisoning by and adverse effect of skeletal muscle relaxants [neuromuscular blocking agents]

T48.1x1 Poisoning by skeletal muscle relaxants [neuromuscular blocking agents], accidental (unintentional)
    Poisoning by skeletal muscle relaxants [neuromuscular blocking agents] NOS

T48.1x2 Poisoning by skeletal muscle relaxants [neuromuscular blocking agents], intentional self-harm

T48.1x3 Poisoning by skeletal muscle relaxants [neuromuscular blocking agents], assault

T48.1x4 Poisoning by skeletal muscle relaxants [neuromuscular blocking agents], undetermined

T48.1x5 Adverse effect of skeletal muscle relaxants [neuromuscular blocking agents]

T48.2 Poisoning by and adverse effect of other and unspecified drugs acting on muscles

T48.20 Poisoning by and adverse effect of unspecified drugs acting on muscles

T48.201 Poisoning by unspecified drugs acting on muscles, accidental (unintentional)
    Poisoning by unspecified drugs acting on muscles NOS

T48.202 Poisoning by unspecified drugs acting on muscles, intentional self-harm

T48.203 Poisoning by unspecified drugs acting on muscles, assault

T48.204 Poisoning by unspecified drugs acting on muscles, undetermined

T48.205 Adverse effect of unspecified drugs acting on muscles

T48.29 Poisoning by and adverse effect of other drugs acting on muscles

T48.291 Poisoning by other drugs acting on muscles, accidental (unintentional)
    Poisoning by other drugs acting on muscles NOS

T48.292 Poisoning by other drugs acting on muscles, intentional self-harm

T48.293 Poisoning by other drugs acting on muscles, assault

T48.294 Poisoning by other drugs acting on muscles, undetermined

T48.295 Adverse effect of other drugs acting on muscles

T48.3 Poisoning by and adverse effect of antitussives

T48.3x Poisoning by and adverse effect of antitussives

T48.3x1 Poisoning by antitussives, accidental (unintentional)
    Poisoning by antitussives NOS

T48.3x2 Poisoning by antitussives, intentional self-harm

T48.3x3 Poisoning by antitussives, assault

T48.3x4 Poisoning by antitussives, undetermined

T48.3x5 Adverse effect of antitussives

T48.4 Poisoning by and adverse effect of expectorants

T48.4x Poisoning by and adverse effect of expectorants

T48.4x1 Poisoning by expectorants, accidental (unintentional)
    Poisoning by expectorants NOS

T48.4x2 Poisoning by expectorants, intentional self-harm

T48.4x3 Poisoning by expectorants, assault

T48.4x4 Poisoning by expectorants, undetermined

T48.4x5 Adverse effect of expectorants

T48.5 Poisoning by and adverse effect of anti-common-cold drugs

T48.5x Poisoning by and adverse effect of anti-common-cold drugs

T48.5x1 Poisoning by anti-common-cold drugs, accidental (unintentional)
    Poisoning by anti-common-cold drugs NOS

T48.5x2 Poisoning by anti-common-cold drugs, intentional self-harm

T48.5x3 Poisoning by anti-common-cold drugs, assault

T48.5x4 Poisoning by anti-common-cold drugs, undetermined

T48.5x5 Adverse effect of anti-common-cold drugs

T48.6 Poisoning by and adverse effect of antiasthmatics

Poisoning by and adverse effect of salbutamol

Excludes1: β-adrenoreceptor agonists (T44.5-)
    anterior pituitary [adenohypophyseal] hormones (T38.8-)

T48.6x Poisoning by and adverse effect of antiasthmatics

T48.6x1 Poisoning by antiasthmatics, accidental (unintentional)
    Poisoning by antiasthmatics NOS

T48.6x2 Poisoning by antiasthmatics, intentional self-harm

T48.6x3 Poisoning by antiasthmatics, assault

T48.6x4 Poisoning by antiasthmatics, undetermined

T48.6x5 Adverse effect of antiasthmatics

T48.9 Poisoning by and adverse effect of other and unspecified agents primarily acting on the respiratory system

T48.90 Poisoning by and adverse effect of unspecified agents primarily acting on the respiratory system

T48.901 Poisoning by unspecified agents primarily acting on the respiratory system, accidental (unintentional)

T48.902 Poisoning by unspecified agents primarily acting on the respiratory system, intentional self-harm

T48.903 Poisoning by unspecified agents primarily acting on the respiratory system, assault

T48.904 Poisoning by unspecified agents primarily acting on the respiratory system, undetermined

T48.905 Adverse effect of unspecified agents primarily acting on the respiratory system

T48.99 Poisoning by and adverse effect of other agents primarily acting on the respiratory system

T48.991 Poisoning by other agents primarily acting on the respiratory system, accidental (unintentional)

T48.992 Poisoning by other agents primarily acting on the respiratory system, intentional self-harm

T48.993 Poisoning by other agents primarily acting on the respiratory system, assault

T48.994 Poisoning by other agents primarily acting on the respiratory system, undetermined

T48.995 Adverse effect of other agents primarily acting on the respiratory system

T49 Poisoning by and adverse effect of topical agents primarily affecting skin and mucous membrane and by ophthalmological, otorhinorlaryngological and dental drugs

Includes: poisoning by glucocorticoids, topically used

The following extensions are to be added to each code for category T49:

a initial encounter
d subsequent encounter
q sequela

T49.0 Poisoning by and adverse effect of local antifungal, anti-infective and anti-inflammatory drugs

T49.0x Poisoning by and adverse effect of local antifungal, anti-infective and anti-inflammatory drugs

T49.0x1 Poisoning by local antifungal, anti-infective and anti-inflammatory drugs, accidental (unintentional)

Poisoning by local antifungal, anti-infective and anti-inflammatory drugs NOS

T49.0x2 Poisoning by local antifungal, anti-infective and anti-inflammatory drugs, intentional self-harm

T49.0x3 Poisoning by local antifungal, anti-infective and anti-inflammatory drugs, assault

T49.0x4 Poisoning by local antifungal, anti-infective and anti-inflammatory drugs, undetermined

T49.0x5 Adverse effect of local antifungal, anti-infective and anti-inflammatory drugs

T49.1 Poisoning by and adverse effect of antipruritics

T49.1x Poisoning by and adverse effect of antipruritics

T49.1x1 Poisoning by antipruritics, accidental (unintentional)

Poisoning by antipruritics NOS

T49.1x2 Poisoning by antipruritics, intentional self-harm

T49.1x3 Poisoning by antipruritics, assault

T49.1x4 Poisoning by antipruritics, undetermined

T49.1x5 Adverse effect of antipruritics

T49.2 Poisoning by and adverse effect of local astringents and local detergents

T49.2x Poisoning by and adverse effect of local astringents and local detergents

T49.2x1 Poisoning by local astringents and local detergents, accidental (unintentional)

Poisoning by local astringents and local detergents NOS

T49.2x2 Poisoning by local astringents and local detergents, intentional self-harm

T49.2x3 Poisoning by local astringents and local detergents, assault

T49.2x4 Poisoning by local astringents and local detergents, undetermined

T49.2x5 Adverse effect of local astringents and local detergents

T49.3 Poisoning by and adverse effect of emollients, demulcents and protectants

T49.3x Poisoning by and adverse effect of emollients, demulcents and protectants

T49.3x1 Poisoning by emollients, demulcents and protectants, accidental (unintentional)

Poisoning by emollients, demulcents and protectants NOS

T49.3x2 Poisoning by emollients, demulcents and protectants, intentional self-harm

T49.3x3 Poisoning by emollients, demulcents and protectants, assault

T49.3x4 Poisoning by emollients, demulcents and protectants, undetermined

T49.3x5 Adverse effect of emollients, demulcents and protectants

T49.4 Poisoning by and adverse effect of keratolytics, keratoplastics, and other hair treatment drugs and preparations

T49.4x Poisoning by and adverse effect of keratolytics, keratoplastics, and other hair treatment drugs and preparations

T49.4x1 Poisoning by keratolytics, keratoplastics, and other hair treatment drugs and preparations, accidental (unintentional)

Poisoning by keratolytics, keratoplastics, and other hair treatment drugs and preparations NOS

T49.4x2 Poisoning by keratolytics, keratoplastics, and other hair treatment drugs and preparations, intentional self-harm

T49.4x3 Poisoning by keratolytics, keratoplastics, and other hair treatment drugs and preparations, assault

T49.4x4 Poisoning by keratolytics, keratoplastics, and other hair treatment drugs and preparations, undetermined

T49.4x5 Adverse effect of keratolytics, keratoplastics, and other hair treatment drugs and preparations

T49.5 Poisoning by and adverse effect of ophthalmological drugs and preparations

Poisoning by and adverse effect of eye anti-infectives

T49.5x Poisoning by and adverse effect of ophthalmological drugs and preparations

T49.5x1 Poisoning by ophthalmological drugs and preparations, accidental (unintentional)

Poisoning by ophthalmological drugs and preparations NOS

T49.5x2 Poisoning by ophthalmological drugs and preparations, intentional self-harm

T49.5x3 Poisoning by ophthalmological drugs and preparations, assault

T49.5x4 Poisoning by ophthalmological drugs and preparations, undetermined

T49.5x5 Adverse effect of ophthalmological drugs and preparations

T49.6 Poisoning by and adverse effect of otorhinolaryngological drugs and preparations

Poisoning by and adverse effect of ear, nose and throat anti-infectives

T49.6x Poisoning by and adverse effect of otorhinolaryngological drugs and preparations

T49.6x1 Poisoning by otorhinolaryngological drugs and preparations, accidental (unintentional)

Poisoning by otorhinolaryngological drugs and preparations NOS

T49.6x2 Poisoning by otorhinolaryngological drugs and preparations, intentional self-harm

T49.6x3 Poisoning by otorhinolaryngological drugs and preparations, assault

T49.6x4 Poisoning by otorhinolaryngological drugs and preparations, undetermined

T49.6x5 Adverse effect of otorhinolaryngological drugs and preparations

T49.7 Poisoning by and adverse effect of dental drugs, topically applied

T49.7x Poisoning by and adverse effect of dental drugs, topically applied

T49.7x1 Poisoning by dental drugs, topically applied, accidental (unintentional)

Poisoning by dental drugs, topically applied NOS

T49.7x2   Poisoning by dental drugs, topically applied, intentional self-harm

T49.7x3   Poisoning by dental drugs, topically applied, assault

T49.7x4   Poisoning by dental drugs, topically applied, undetermined

T49.7x5   Adverse effect of dental drugs, topically applied

T49.8   Poisoning by and adverse effect of other topical agents
Poisoning by and adverse effect of spermicides

  T49.8x   Poisoning by and adverse effect of other topical agents

    T49.8x1   Poisoning by other topical agents, accidental (unintentional)
      Poisoning by other topical agents NOS

    T49.8x2   Poisoning by other topical agents, intentional self-harm

    T49.8x3   Poisoning by other topical agents, assault

    T49.8x4   Poisoning by other topical agents, undetermined

    T49.8x5   Adverse effect of other topical agents

T48.9   Poisoning by and adverse effect of unspecified topical agent

  T48.91   Poisoning by unspecified topical agent, accidental (unintentional)

  T48.92   Poisoning by unspecified topical agent, intentional self-harm

  T48.93   Poisoning by unspecified topical agent, assault

  T48.94   Poisoning by unspecified topical agent, undetermined

  T48.95   Adverse effect of unspecified topical agent

T50   Poisoning by and adverse effect of diuretics and other and unspecified drugs, medicaments and biological substances
The following extensions are to be added to each code for category T50:
  a   initial encounter
  d   subsequent encounter
  q   sequela

T50.0   Poisoning by and adverse effect of mineralocorticoids and their antagonists

  T50.0x   Poisoning by and adverse effect of mineralocorticoids and their antagonists

    T50.0x1   Poisoning by mineralocorticoids and their antagonists, accidental (unintentional)
      Poisoning by mineralocorticoids and their antagonists NOS

    T50.0x2   Poisoning by mineralocorticoids and their antagonists, intentional self-harm

    T50.0x3   Poisoning by mineralocorticoids and their antagonists, assault

    T50.0x4   Poisoning by mineralocorticoids and their antagonists, undetermined

    T50.0x5   Adverse effect of mineralocorticoids and their antagonists

T50.1   Poisoning by and adverse effect of loop [high-ceiling] diuretics

  T50.1x   Poisoning by and adverse effect of loop [high-ceiling] diuretics

    T50.1x1   Poisoning by loop [high-ceiling] diuretics, accidental (unintentional)
      Poisoning by loop [high-ceiling] diuretics NOS

    T50.1x2   Poisoning by loop [high-ceiling] diuretics, intentional self-harm

    T50.1x3   Poisoning by loop [high-ceiling] diuretics, assault

    T50.1x4   Poisoning by loop [high-ceiling] diuretics, undetermined

    T50.1x5   Adverse effect of loop [high-ceiling] diuretics

T50.2   Poisoning by and adverse effect of carbonic-anhydrase inhibitors, benzothiadiazides and other diuretics
Poisoning by acetazolamide

  T50.2x   Poisoning by and adverse effect of carbonic-anhydrase inhibitors, benzothiadiazides and other diuretics

    T50.2x1   Poisoning by carbonic-anhydrase inhibitors, benzothiadiazides and other diuretics, accidental (unintentional)
      Poisoning by carbonic-anhydrase inhibitors, benzothiadiazides and other diuretics NOS

    T50.2x2   Poisoning by carbonic-anhydrase inhibitors, benzothiadiazides and other diuretics, intentional self-harm

    T50.2x3   Poisoning by carbonic-anhydrase inhibitors, benzothiadiazides and other diuretics, assault

    T50.2x4   Poisoning by carbonic-anhydrase inhibitors, benzothiadiazides and other diuretics, undetermined

    T50.2x5   Adverse effect of carbonic-anhydrase inhibitors, benzothiadiazides and other diuretics

T50.3   Poisoning by and adverse effect of electrolytic, caloric and water-balance agents
Poisoning by oral rehydration salts

  T50.3x   Poisoning by and adverse effect of electrolytic, caloric and water-balance agents

    T50.3x1   Poisoning by electrolytic, caloric and water-balance agents, accidental (unintentional)
      Poisoning by electrolytic, caloric and water-balance agents NOS

    T50.3x2   Poisoning by electrolytic, caloric and water-balance agents, intentional self-harm

    T50.3x3   Poisoning by electrolytic, caloric and water-balance agents, assault

    T50.3x4   Poisoning by electrolytic, caloric and water-balance agents, undetermined

    T50.3x5   Adverse effect of electrolytic, caloric and water-balance agents

T50.4   Poisoning by and adverse effect of drugs affecting uric acid metabolism

  T50.4x   Poisoning by and adverse effect of drugs affecting uric acid metabolism

    T50.4x1   Poisoning by drugs affecting uric acid metabolism, accidental (unintentional)
      Poisoning by drugs affecting uric acid metabolism NOS

    T50.4x2   Poisoning by drugs affecting uric acid metabolism, intentional self-harm

    T50.4x3   Poisoning by drugs affecting uric acid metabolism, assault

    T50.4x4   Poisoning by drugs affecting uric acid metabolism, undetermined

    T50.4x5   Adverse effect of drugs affecting uric acid metabolism

T50.5   Poisoning by and adverse effect of appetite depressants

  T50.5x   Poisoning by and adverse effect of appetite depressants

    T50.5x1   Poisoning by appetite depressants, accidental (unintentional)
      Poisoning by appetite depressants NOS

    T50.5x2   Poisoning by appetite depressants, intentional self-harm

    T50.5x3   Poisoning by appetite depressants, assault

    T50.5x4   Poisoning by appetite depressants, undetermined

    T50.5x5   Adverse effect of appetite depressants

T50.6   Poisoning by and adverse effect of antidotes and chelating agents
Poisoning by alcohol deterrents

  T50.6x   Poisoning by and adverse effect of antidotes and chelating agents

    T50.6x1   Poisoning by antidotes and chelating agents, accidental (unintentional)
      Poisoning by antidotes and chelating agents NOS

    T50.6x2   Poisoning by antidotes and chelating agents, intentional self-harm

T50.6x3 Poisoning by antidotes and chelating agents, assault

T50.6x4 Poisoning by antidotes and chelating agents, undetermined

T50.6x5 Adverse effect of antidotes and chelating agents

T50.7 Poisoning by and adverse effect of analeptics and opioid receptor antagonists

T50.7x Poisoning by and adverse effect of analeptics and opioid receptor antagonists

T50.7x1 Poisoning by analeptics and opioid receptor antagonists, accidental (unintentional)
Poisoning by analeptics and opioid receptor antagonists NOS

T50.7x2 Poisoning by analeptics and opioid receptor antagonists, intentional self-harm

T50.7x3 Poisoning by analeptics and opioid receptor antagonists, assault

T50.7x4 Poisoning by analeptics and opioid receptor antagonists, undetermined

T50.7x5 Adverse effect of analeptics and opioid receptor antagonists

T50.8 Poisoning by and adverse effect of diagnostic agents

T50.8x Poisoning by and adverse effect of diagnostic agents

T50.8x1 Poisoning by diagnostic agents, accidental (unintentional)
Poisoning by diagnostic agents NOS

T50.8x2 Poisoning by diagnostic agents, intentional self-harm

T50.8x3 Poisoning by diagnostic agents, assault

T50.8x4 Poisoning by diagnostic agents, undetermined

T50.8x5 Adverse effect of diagnostic agents

T50.9 Poisoning by and adverse effect of other and unspecified drugs, medicaments, and biological substances

T50.90 Poisoning by and adverse effect of unspecified drugs, medicaments and biological substances

T50.901 Poisoning by unspecified drugs, medicaments and biological substances, accidental (unintentional)

T50.902 Poisoning by unspecified drugs, medicaments and biological substances, intentional self-harm

T50.903 Poisoning by unspecified drugs, medicaments and biological substances, assault

T50.904 Poisoning by unspecified drugs, medicaments and biological substances, undetermined

T50.905 Adverse effect of unspecified drugs, medicaments and biological substances

T50.99 Poisoning by and adverse effect of other drugs, medicaments and biological substances
Poisoning by and adverse effect of acidifying agents
Poisoning by and adverse effect of alkalizing agents
Poisoning by and adverse effect of immunoglobulin
Poisoning by and adverse effect of immunologicals
Poisoning by and adverse effect of lipotropic drugs
Poisoning by and adverse effect of parathyroid hormones and derivatives

T50.991 Poisoning by other drugs, medicaments and biological substances, accidental (unintentional)

T50.992 Poisoning by other drugs, medicaments and biological substances, intentional self-harm

T50.993 Poisoning by other drugs, medicaments and biological substances, assault

T50.994 Poisoning by other drugs, medicaments and biological substances, undetermined

T50.995 Adverse effect of other drugs, medicaments and biological substances

TOXIC EFFECTS OF SUBSTANCES CHIEFLY NONMEDICINAL AS TO SOURCE (T51–T65)

Includes: contact with toxic substance
exposure to toxic substance
Use additional code(s) for all associated manifestations of toxic effect, such as:
respiratory conditions due to external agents (J60-J70)
When no intent is indicated code to accidental. Undetermined intent is only for use when there is specific documentation in the record that the intent of the injury cannot be determined

T51 Toxic effect of alcohol
The following extensions are to be added to each code for category T51:
a   initial encounter
d   subsequent encounter
q   sequela

T51.0 Toxic effect of ethanol
Toxic effect of ethyl alcohol
Excludes2:   acute alcohol intoxication or "hangover" effects (F10.11, F10.31, F10.91)
drunkenness (F10.11, F10.31, F10.91)
pathological alcohol intoxication (F10.11, F10.31, F10.91)

T51.0x Toxic effect of ethanol

T51.0x1 Toxic effect of ethanol, accidental (unintentional)
Toxic effect of ethanol NOS

T51.0x2 Toxic effect of ethanol, intentional self-harm

T51.0x3 Toxic effect of ethanol, assault

T51.0x4 Toxic effect of ethanol, undetermined

T51.1 Toxic effect of methanol
Toxic effect of methyl alcohol

T51.1x Toxic effect of methanol

T51.1x1 Toxic effect of methanol, accidental (unintentional)
Toxic effect of methanol NOS

T51.1x2 Toxic effect of methanol, intentional self-harm

T51.1x3 Toxic effect of methanol, assault

T51.1x4 Toxic effect of methanol, undetermined

T51.2 Toxic effect of 2-Propanol
Toxic effect of isopropyl alcohol

T51.2x Toxic effect of 2-Propanol

T51.2x1 Toxic effect of 2-Propanol, accidental (unintentional)
Toxic effect of 2-Propanol NOS

T51.2x2 Toxic effect of 2-Propanol, intentional self-harm

T51.2x3 Toxic effect of 2-Propanol, assault

T51.2x4 Toxic effect of 2-Propanol, undetermined

T51.3 Toxic effect of fusel oil
Toxic effect of amyl alcohol
Toxic effect of butyl [1-butanol] alcohol
Toxic effect of propyl [1-propanol] alcohol

T51.3x Toxic effect of fusel oil

T51.3x1 Toxic effect of fusel oil, accidental (unintentional)
Toxic effect of fusel oil NOS

T51.3x2 Toxic effect of fusel oil, intentional self-harm

T51.3x3 Toxic effect of fusel oil, assault

T51.3x4 Toxic effect of fusel oil, undetermined

T51.8 Toxic effect of other alcohols

T51.8x Toxic effect of other alcohols

T51.8x1 Toxic effect of other alcohols, accidental (unintentional)
Toxic effect of other alcohols NOS

T51.8x2 Toxic effect of other alcohols, intentional self-harm

T51.8x3 Toxic effect of other alcohols, assault

T51.8x4 Toxic effect of other alcohols, undetermined

T51.9   Toxic effect of unspecified alcohol

    T51.91   **Toxic effect of unspecified alcohol, accidental (unintentional)**

    T51.92   **Toxic effect of unspecified alcohol, intentional self-harm**

    T51.93   **Toxic effect of unspecified alcohol, assault**

    T51.94   **Toxic effect of unspecified alcohol, undetermined**

T52   **Toxic effect of organic solvents**

    Excludes1:   halogen derivatives of aliphatic and aromatic hydrocarbons (T53.-)

    The following extensions are to be added to each code for category T52:

        a   initial encounter

        d   subsequent encounter

        q   sequela

  T52.0   **Toxic effects of petroleum products**

    Toxic effects of ether petroleum

    Toxic effects of gasoline [petrol]

    Toxic effects of kerosene [paraffin oil]

    Toxic effects of naphtha petroleum

    Toxic effects of paraffin wax

    Toxic effects of spirit petroleum

    T52.0x   **Toxic effects of petroleum products**

        T52.0x1   **Toxic effect of petroleum products, accidental (unintentional)**

            Toxic effects of petroleum products NOS

        T52.0x2   **Toxic effect of petroleum products, intentional self-harm**

        T52.0x3   **Toxic effect of petroleum products, assault**

        T52.0x4   **Toxic effect of petroleum products, undetermined**

  T52.1   **Toxic effects of benzene**

    Excludes1:   homologues of benzene (T52.2)

            nitroderivatives and aminoderivatives of benzene and its homologues (T65.3)

    T52.1x   **Toxic effects of benzene**

        T52.1x1   **Toxic effect of benzene, accidental (unintentional)**

            Toxic effects of benzene NOS

        T52.1x2   **Toxic effect of benzene, intentional self-harm**

        T52.1x3   **Toxic effect of benzene, assault**

        T52.1x4   **Toxic effect of benzene, undetermined**

  T52.2   **Toxic effects of homologues of benzene**

    Toxic effects of toluene [methylbenzene]

    Toxic effects of xylene [dimethylbenzene]

    T52.2x   **Toxic effects of homologues of benzene**

        T52.2x1   **Toxic effect of homologues of benzene, accidental (unintentional)**

            Toxic effects of homologues of benzene NOS

        T52.2x2   **Toxic effect of homologues of benzene, intentional self-harm**

        T52.2x3   **Toxic effect of homologues of benzene, assault**

        T52.2x4   **Toxic effect of homologues of benzene, undetermined**

  T52.3   **Toxic effects of glycols**

    T52.3x   **Toxic effects of glycols**

        T52.3x1   **Toxic effect of glycols, accidental (unintentional)**

            Toxic effects of glycols NOS

        T52.3x2   **Toxic effect of glycols, intentional self-harm**

        T52.3x3   **Toxic effect of glycols, assault**

        T52.3x4   **Toxic effect of glycols, undetermined**

  T52.4   **Toxic effects of ketones**

    T52.4x   **Toxic effects of ketones**

        T52.4x1   **Toxic effect of ketones, accidental (unintentional)**

            Toxic effects of ketones NOS

        T52.4x2   **Toxic effect of ketones, intentional self-harm**

        T52.4x3   **Toxic effect of ketones, assault**

        T52.4x4   **Toxic effect of ketones, undetermined**

T52.8   Toxic effects of other organic solvents

    T52.8x   **Toxic effects of other organic solvents**

        T52.8x1   **Toxic effect of other organic solvents, accidental (unintentional)**

            Toxic effects of other organic solvents NOS

        T52.8x2   **Toxic effect of other organic solvents, intentional self-harm**

        T52.8x3   **Toxic effect of other organic solvents, assault**

        T52.8x4   **Toxic effect of other organic solvents, undetermined**

T52.9   Toxic effects of unspecified organic solvent

    T52.91   **Toxic effect of unspecified organic solvent, accidental (unintentional)**

    T52.92   **Toxic effect of unspecified organic solvent, intentional self-harm**

    T52.93   **Toxic effect of unspecified organic solvent, assault**

    T52.94   **Toxic effect of unspecified organic solvent, undetermined**

T53   **Toxic effect of halogen derivatives of aliphatic and aromatic hydrocarbons**

    The following extensions are to be added to each code for category T53:

        a   initial encounter

        d   subsequent encounter

        q   sequela

  T53.0   **Toxic effects of carbon tetrachloride**

    Toxic effects of tetrachloromethane

    T53.0x   **Toxic effects of carbon tetrachloride**

        T53.0x1   **Toxic effect of carbon tetrachloride, accidental (unintentional)**

            Toxic effects of carbon tetrachloride NOS

        T53.0x2   **Toxic effect of carbon tetrachloride, intentional self-harm**

        T53.0x3   **Toxic effect of carbon tetrachloride, assault**

        T53.0x4   **Toxic effect of carbon tetrachloride, undetermined**

  T53.1   **Toxic effects of chloroform**

    Toxic effects of trichloromethane

    T53.1x   **Toxic effects of chloroform**

        T53.1x1   **Toxic effect of chloroform, accidental (unintentional)**

            Toxic effects of chloroform NOS

        T53.1x2   **Toxic effect of chloroform, intentional self-harm**

        T53.1x3   **Toxic effect of chloroform, assault**

        T53.1x4   **Toxic effect of chloroform, undetermined**

  T53.2   **Toxic effects of trichloroethylene**

    Toxic effects of trichloroethene

    T53.2x   **Toxic effects of trichloroethylene**

        T53.2x1   **Toxic effect of trichloroethylene, accidental (unintentional)**

            Toxic effects of trichloroethylene NOS

        T53.2x2   **Toxic effect of trichloroethylene, intentional self-harm**

        T53.2x3   **Toxic effect of trichloroethylene, assault**

        T53.2x4   **Toxic effect of trichloroethylene, undetermined**

  T53.3   **Toxic effects of tetrachloroethylene**

    Toxic effects of perchloroethylene

    Toxic effect of tetrachloroethene

    T53.3x   **Toxic effects of tetrachloroethylene**

        T53.3x1   **Toxic effect of tetrachloroethylene, accidental (unintentional)**

            Toxic effects of tetrachloroethylene NOS

        T53.3x2   **Toxic effect of tetrachloroethylene, intentional self-harm**

        T53.3x3   **Toxic effect of tetrachloroethylene, assault**

        T53.3x4   **Toxic effect of tetrachloroethylene, undetermined**

T53.4   Toxic effects of dichloromethane
Toxic effects of methylene chloride

    T53.4x   Toxic effects of dichloromethane

        T53.4x1   Toxic effect of dichloromethane, accidental (unintentional)
Toxic effects of dichloromethane NOS

        T53.4x2   Toxic effect of dichloromethane, intentional self-harm

        T53.4x3   Toxic effect of dichloromethane, assault

        T53.4x4   Toxic effect of dichloromethane, undetermined

T53.5   Toxic effects of chlorofluorocarbons

    T53.5x   Toxic effects of chlorofluorocarbons

        T53.5x1   Toxic effect of chlorofluorocarbons, accidental (unintentional)
Toxic effects of chlorofluorocarbons NOS

        T53.5x2   Toxic effect of chlorofluorocarbons, intentional self-harm

        T53.5x3   Toxic effect of chlorofluorocarbons, assault

        T53.5x4   Toxic effect of chlorofluorocarbons, undetermined

T53.6   Toxic effects of other halogen derivatives of aliphatic hydrocarbons

    T53.6x   Toxic effects of other halogen derivatives of aliphatic hydrocarbons

        T53.6x1   Toxic effect of other halogen derivatives of aliphatic hydrocarbons, accidental (unintentional)
Toxic effects of other halogen derivatives of aliphatic hydrocarbons NOS

        T53.6x2   Toxic effect of other halogen derivatives of aliphatic hydrocarbons, intentional self-harm

        T53.6x3   Toxic effect of other halogen derivatives of aliphatic hydrocarbons, assault

        T53.6x4   Toxic effect of other halogen derivatives of aliphatic hydrocarbons, undetermined

T53.7   Toxic effects of other halogen derivatives of aromatic hydrocarbons

    T53.7x   Toxic effects of other halogen derivatives of aromatic hydrocarbons

        T53.7x1   Toxic effect of other halogen derivatives of aromatic hydrocarbons, accidental (unintentional)
Toxic effects of other halogen derivatives of aromatic hydrocarbons NOS

        T53.7x2   Toxic effect of other halogen derivatives of aromatic hydrocarbons, intentional self-harm

        T53.7x3   Toxic effect of other halogen derivatives of aromatic hydrocarbons, assault

        T53.7x4   Toxic effect of other halogen derivatives of aromatic hydrocarbons, undetermined

T53.9   Toxic effects of unspecified halogen derivatives of aliphatic and aromatic hydrocarbons

    T53.91   Toxic effect of unspecified halogen derivatives of aliphatic and aromatic hydrocarbons, accidental (unintentional)

    T53.92   Toxic effect of unspecified halogen derivatives of aliphatic and aromatic hydrocarbons, intentional self-harm

    T53.93   Toxic effect of unspecified halogen derivatives of aliphatic and aromatic hydrocarbons, assault

    T53.94   Toxic effect of unspecified halogen derivatives of aliphatic and aromatic hydrocarbons, undetermined

T54 Toxic effect of corrosive substances
The following extensions are to be added to each code for category T54:

    a   initial encounter
    d   subsequent encounter
    q   sequela

T54.0   Toxic effects of phenol and phenol homologues

    T54.0x   Toxic effects of phenol and phenol homologues

        T54.0x1   Toxic effect of phenol and phenol homologues, accidental (unintentional)
Toxic effects of phenol and phenol homologues NOS

        T54.0x2   Toxic effect of phenol and phenol homologues, intentional self-harm

        T54.0x3   Toxic effect of phenol and phenol homologues, assault

        T54.0x4   Toxic effect of phenol and phenol homologues, undetermined

T54.1   Toxic effects of other corrosive organic compounds

    T54.1x   Toxic effects of other corrosive organic compounds

        T54.1x1   Toxic effect of other corrosive organic compounds, accidental (unintentional)
Toxic effects of other corrosive organic compounds NOS

        T54.1x2   Toxic effect of other corrosive organic compounds, intentional self-harm

        T54.1x3   Toxic effect of other corrosive organic compounds, assault

        T54.1x4   Toxic effect of other corrosive organic compounds, undetermined

T54.2   Toxic effects of corrosive acids and acid-like substances
Toxic effects of hydrochloric acid
Toxic effects of sulphuric acid

    T54.2x   Toxic effects of corrosive acids and acid-like substances

        T54.2x1   Toxic effect of corrosive acids and acid-like substances, accidental (unintentional)
Toxic effects of corrosive acids and acid-like substances NOS

        T54.2x2   Toxic effect of corrosive acids and acid-like substances, intentional self-harm

        T54.2x3   Toxic effect of corrosive acids and acid-like substances, assault

        T54.2x4   Toxic effect of corrosive acids and acid-like substances, undetermined

T54.3   Toxic effects of corrosive alkalis and alkali-like substances
Toxic effects of potassium hydroxide
Toxic effects of sodium hydroxide

    T54.3x   Toxic effects of corrosive alkalis and alkali-like substances

        T54.3x1   Toxic effect of corrosive alkalis and alkali-like substances, accidental (unintentional)
Toxic effects of corrosive alkalis and alkali-like substances NOS

        T54.3x2   Toxic effect of corrosive alkalis and alkali-like substances, intentional self-harm

        T54.3x3   Toxic effect of corrosive alkalis and alkali-like substances, assault

        T54.3x4   Toxic effect of corrosive alkalis and alkali-like substances, undetermined

T54.9   Toxic effects of unspecified corrosive substance

    T54.91   Toxic effect of unspecified corrosive substance, accidental (unintentional)

    T54.92   Toxic effect of unspecified corrosive substance, intentional self-harm

    T54.93   Toxic effect of unspecified corrosive substance, assault

    T54.94   Toxic effect of unspecified corrosive substance, undetermined

T55 Toxic effect of soaps and detergents
The following extensions are to be added to each code for category T55:

    a   initial encounter
    d   subsequent encounter
    q   sequela

T55.0   Toxic effect of soaps
    T55.0x   Toxic effect of soaps
        T55.0x1   Toxic effect of soaps, accidental (unintentional)
            Toxic effect of soaps NOS
        T55.0x2   Toxic effect of soaps, intentional self-harm
        T55.0x3   Toxic effect of soaps, assault
        T55.0x4   Toxic effect of soaps, undetermined
T55.1   Toxic effect of detergents
    T55.1x   Toxic effect of detergents
        T55.1x1   Toxic effect of detergents, accidental (unintentional)
            Toxic effect of detergents NOS
        T55.1x2   Toxic effect of detergents, intentional self-harm
        T55.1x3   Toxic effect of detergents, assault
        T55.1x4   Toxic effect of detergents, undetermined

T56   Toxic effect of metals

    Includes: toxic effects of fumes and vapors of metals
                  toxic effects of metals from all sources, except medicinal substances

    Excludes1:   arsenic and its compounds (T57.0)
                manganese and its compounds (T57.2)
                thallium (T60.4)

The following extensions are to be added to each code for category T56:
    a   initial encounter
    d   subsequent encounter
    q   sequela

T56.0   Toxic effects of lead and its compounds
    T56.0x   Toxic effects of lead and its compounds
        T56.0x1   Toxic effect of lead and its compounds, accidental (unintentional)
            Toxic effects of lead and its compounds NOS
        T56.0x2   Toxic effect of lead and its compounds, intentional self-harm
        T56.0x3   Toxic effect of lead and its compounds, assault
        T56.0x4   Toxic effect of lead and its compounds, undetermined
T56.1   Toxic effects of mercury and its compounds
    T56.1x   Toxic effects of mercury and its compounds
        T56.1x1   Toxic effect of mercury and its compounds, accidental (unintentional)
            Toxic effects of mercury and its compounds NOS
        T56.1x2   Toxic effect of mercury and its compounds, intentional self-harm
        T56.1x3   Toxic effect of mercury and its compounds, assault
        T56.1x4   Toxic effect of mercury and its compounds, undetermined
T56.2   Toxic effects of chromium and its compounds
    T56.2x   Toxic effects of chromium and its compounds
        T56.2x1   Toxic effect of chromium and its compounds, accidental (unintentional)
            Toxic effects of chromium and its compounds NOS
        T56.2x2   Toxic effect of chromium and its compounds, intentional self-harm
        T56.2x3   Toxic effect of chromium and its compounds, assault
        T56.2x4   Toxic effect of chromium and its compounds, undetermined
T56.3   Toxic effects of cadmium and its compounds
    T56.3x   Toxic effects of cadmium and its compounds
        T56.3x1   Toxic effect of cadmium and its compounds, accidental (unintentional)
            Toxic effects of cadmium and its compounds NOS

        T56.3x2   Toxic effect of cadmium and its compounds, intentional self-harm
        T56.3x3   Toxic effect of cadmium and its compounds, assault
        T56.3x4   Toxic effect of cadmium and its compounds, undetermined
T56.4   Toxic effects of copper and its compounds
    T56.4x   Toxic effects of copper and its compounds
        T56.4x1   Toxic effect of copper and its compounds, accidental (unintentional)
            Toxic effects of copper and its compounds NOS
        T56.4x2   Toxic effect of copper and its compounds, intentional self-harm
        T56.4x3   Toxic effect of copper and its compounds, assault
        T56.4x4   Toxic effect of copper and its compounds, undetermined
T56.5   Toxic effects of zinc and its compounds
    T56.5x   Toxic effects of zinc and its compounds
        T56.5x1   Toxic effect of zinc and its compounds, accidental (unintentional)
            Toxic effects of zinc and its compounds NOS
        T56.5x2   Toxic effect of zinc and its compounds, intentional self-harm
        T56.5x3   Toxic effect of zinc and its compounds, assault
        T56.5x4   Toxic effect of zinc and its compounds, undetermined
T56.6   Toxic effects of tin and its compounds
    T56.6x   Toxic effects of tin and its compounds
        T56.6x1   Toxic effect of tin and its compounds, accidental (unintentional)
            Toxic effects of tin and its compounds NOS
        T56.6x2   Toxic effect of tin and its compounds, intentional self-harm
        T56.6x3   Toxic effect of tin and its compounds, assault
        T56.6x4   Toxic effect of tin and its compounds, undetermined
T56.7   Toxic effects of beryllium and its compounds
    T56.7x   Toxic effects of beryllium and its compounds
        T56.7x1   Toxic effect of beryllium and its compounds, accidental (unintentional)
            Toxic effects of beryllium and its compounds NOS
        T56.7x2   Toxic effect of beryllium and its compounds, intentional self-harm
        T56.7x3   Toxic effect of beryllium and its compounds, assault
        T56.7x4   Toxic effect of beryllium and its compounds, undetermined
T56.8   Toxic effects of other metals
    T56.8x   Toxic effects of other metals
        T56.8x1   Toxic effect of other metals, accidental (unintentional)
            Toxic effects of other metals NOS
        T56.8x2   Toxic effect of other metals, intentional self-harm
        T56.8x3   Toxic effect of other metals, assault
        T56.8x4   Toxic effect of other metals, undetermined
T56.9   Toxic effects of unspecified metal
    T56.91   Toxic effect of unspecified metal, accidental (unintentional)
    T56.92   Toxic effect of unspecified metal, intentional self-harm
    T56.93   Toxic effect of unspecified metal, assault
    T56.94   Toxic effect of unspecified metal, undetermined

T57 Toxic effect of other inorganic substances

The following extensions are to be added to each code for category T57:

   a   initial encounter
   d   subsequent encounter
   q   sequela

T57.0 Toxic effect of arsenic and its compounds

  T57.0x Toxic effect of arsenic and its compounds

    T57.0x1 Toxic effect of arsenic and its compounds, accidental (unintentional)
      Toxic effect of arsenic and its compounds NOS

    T57.0x2 Toxic effect of arsenic and its compounds, intentional self-harm

    T57.0x3 Toxic effect of arsenic and its compounds, assault

    T57.0x4 Toxic effect of arsenic and its compounds, undetermined

T57.1 Toxic effect of phosphorus and its compounds

  Excludes1: organophosphate insecticides (T60.0)

  T57.1x Toxic effect of phosphorus and its compounds

    T57.1x1 Toxic effect of phosphorus and its compounds, accidental (unintentional)
      Toxic effect of phosphorus and its compounds NOS

    T57.1x2 Toxic effect of phosphorus and its compounds, intentional self-harm

    T57.1x3 Toxic effect of phosphorus and its compounds, assault

    T57.1x4 Toxic effect of phosphorus and its compounds, undetermined

T57.2 Toxic effect of manganese and its compounds

  T57.2x Toxic effect of manganese and its compounds

    T57.2x1 Toxic effect of manganese and its compounds, accidental (unintentional)
      Toxic effect of manganese and its compounds NOS

    T57.2x2 Toxic effect of manganese and its compounds, intentional self-harm

    T57.2x3 Toxic effect of manganese and its compounds, assault

    T57.2x4 Toxic effect of manganese and its compounds, undetermined

T57.3 Toxic effect of hydrogen cyanide

  T57.3x Toxic effect of hydrogen cyanide

    T57.3x1 Toxic effect of hydrogen cyanide, accidental (unintentional)
      Toxic effect of hydrogen cyanide NOS

    T57.3x2 Toxic effect of hydrogen cyanide, intentional self-harm

    T57.3x3 Toxic effect of hydrogen cyanide, assault

    T57.3x4 Toxic effect of hydrogen cyanide, undetermined

T57.8 Toxic effect of other specified inorganic substances

  T57.8x Toxic effect of other specified inorganic substances

    T57.8x1 Toxic effect of other specified inorganic substances, accidental (unintentional)
      Toxic effect of other specified inorganic substances NOS

    T57.8x2 Toxic effect of other specified inorganic substances, intentional self-harm

    T57.8x3 Toxic effect of other specified inorganic substances, assault

    T57.8x4 Toxic effect of other specified inorganic substances, undetermined

T57.9 Toxic effect of unspecified inorganic substance

  T57.91 Toxic effect of unspecified inorganic substance, accidental (unintentional)

  T57.92 Toxic effect of unspecified inorganic substance, intentional self-harm

  T57.93 Toxic effect of unspecified inorganic substance, assault

  T57.94 Toxic effect of unspecified inorganic substance, undetermined

T58 Toxic effect of carbon monoxide

Includes: asphyxiation from carbon monoxide
      toxic effect of carbon monoxide from all sources

The following extensions are to be added to each code for category T58:

   a   initial encounter
   d   subsequent encounter
   q   sequela

T58.0 Toxic effect of carbon monoxide from motor vehicle exhaust

  Toxic effect of exhaust gas from gas engine
  Toxic effect of exhaust gas from motor pump

  T58.01 Toxic effect of carbon monoxide from motor vehicle exhaust, accidental (unintentional)

  T58.02 Toxic effect of carbon monoxide from motor vehicle exhaust, intentional self-harm

  T58.03 Toxic effect of carbon monoxide from motor vehicle exhaust, assault

  T58.04 Toxic effect of carbon monoxide from motor vehicle exhaust, undetermined

T58.1 Toxic effect of carbon monoxide from utility gas

  Toxic effect of acetylene
  Toxic effect of gas NOS used for lighting, heating, cooking
  Toxic effect of water gas

  T58.11 Toxic effect of carbon monoxide from utility gas, accidental (unintentional)

  T58.12 Toxic effect of carbon monoxide from utility gas, intentional self-harm

  T58.13 Toxic effect of carbon monoxide from utility gas, assault

  T58.14 Toxic effect of carbon monoxide from utility gas, undetermined

T58.2 Toxic effect of carbon monoxide from incomplete combustion of other domestic fuels

  Toxic effect of carbon monoxide from incomplete combustion of coal, coke, kerosene, wood

  T58.2x Toxic effect of carbon monoxide from incomplete combustion of other domestic fuels

    T58.2x1 Toxic effect of carbon monoxide from incomplete combustion of other domestic fuels, accidental (unintentional)

    T58.2x2 Toxic effect of carbon monoxide from incomplete combustion of other domestic fuels, intentional self-harm

    T58.2x3 Toxic effect of carbon monoxide from incomplete combustion of other domestic fuels, assault

    T58.2x4 Toxic effect of carbon monoxide from incomplete combustion of other domestic fuels, undetermined

T58.8 Toxic effect of carbon monoxide from other source

  Toxic effect of carbon monoxide from blast furnace gas
  Toxic effect of carbon monoxide from fuels in industrial use
  Toxic effect of carbon monoxide from kiln vapor

  T58.8x Toxic effect of carbon monoxide from other source

    T58.8x1 Toxic effect of carbon monoxide from other source, accidental (unintentional)

    T58.8x2 Toxic effect of carbon monoxide from other source, intentional self-harm

    T58.8x3 Toxic effect of carbon monoxide from other source, assault

    T58.8x4 Toxic effect of carbon monoxide from other source, undetermined

T58.9 Toxic effect of carbon monoxide from unspecified source

  T58.91 Toxic effect of carbon monoxide from unspecified source, accidental (unintentional)

  T58.92 Toxic effect of carbon monoxide from unspecified source, intentional self-harm

  T58.93 Toxic effect of carbon monoxide from unspecified source, assault

  T58.94 Toxic effect of carbon monoxide from unspecified source, undetermined

T59 Toxic effect of other gases, fumes and vapors

    Includes: aerosol propellants

    Excludes1:   chlorofluorocarbons (T53.5)

    The following extensions are to be added to each code for category T59:

      a   initial encounter

      d   subsequent encounter

      q   sequela

T59.0 Toxic effect of nitrogen oxides

    T59.0x   Toxic effect of nitrogen oxides

      T59.0x1   Toxic effect of nitrogen oxides, accidental (unintentional)

         Toxic effect of nitrogen oxides NOS

      T59.0x2   Toxic effect of nitrogen oxides, intentional self-harm

      T59.0x3   Toxic effect of nitrogen oxides, assault

      T59.0x4   Toxic effect of nitrogen oxides, undetermined

T59.1 Toxic effect of sulphur dioxide

    T59.1x   Toxic effect of sulphur dioxide

      T59.1x1   Toxic effect of sulphur dioxide, accidental (unintentional)

         Toxic effect of sulphur dioxide NOS

      T59.1x2   Toxic effect of sulphur dioxide, intentional self-harm

      T59.1x3   Toxic effect of sulphur dioxide, assault

      T59.1x4   Toxic effect of sulphur dioxide, undetermined

T59.2 Toxic effect of formaldehyde

    T59.2x   Toxic effect of formaldehyde

      T59.2x1   Toxic effect of formaldehyde, accidental (unintentional)

         Toxic effect of formaldehyde NOS

      T59.2x2   Toxic effect of formaldehyde, intentional self-harm

      T59.2x3   Toxic effect of formaldehyde, assault

      T59.2x4   Toxic effect of formaldehyde, undetermined

T59.3 Toxic effect of lacrimogenic gas

    Toxic effect of tear gas

    T59.3x   Toxic effect of lacrimogenic gas

      T59.3x1   Toxic effect of lacrimogenic gas, accidental (unintentional)

         Toxic effect of lacrimogenic gas NOS

      T59.3x2   Toxic effect of lacrimogenic gas, intentional self-harm

      T59.3x3   Toxic effect of lacrimogenic gas, assault

      T59.3x4   Toxic effect of lacrimogenic gas, undetermined

T59.4 Toxic effect of chlorine gas

    T59.4x   Toxic effect of chlorine gas

      T59.4x1   Toxic effect of chlorine gas, accidental (unintentional)

         Toxic effect of chlorine gas NOS

      T59.4x2   Toxic effect of chlorine gas, intentional self-harm

      T59.4x3   Toxic effect of chlorine gas, assault

      T59.4x4   Toxic effect of chlorine gas, undetermined

T59.5 Toxic effect of fluorine gas and hydrogen fluoride

    T59.5x   Toxic effect of fluorine gas and hydrogen fluoride

      T59.5x1   Toxic effect of fluorine gas and hydrogen fluoride, accidental (unintentional)

         Toxic effect of fluorine gas and hydrogen fluoride NOS

      T59.5x2   Toxic effect of fluorine gas and hydrogen fluoride, intentional self-harm

      T59.5x3   Toxic effect of fluorine gas and hydrogen fluoride, assault

      T59.5x4   Toxic effect of fluorine gas and hydrogen fluoride, undetermined

T59.6 Toxic effect of hydrogen sulphide

    T59.6x   Toxic effect of hydrogen sulphide

      T59.6x1   Toxic effect of hydrogen sulphide, accidental (unintentional)

         Toxic effect of hydrogen sulphide NOS

      T59.6x2   Toxic effect of hydrogen sulphide, intentional self-harm

      T59.6x3   Toxic effect of hydrogen sulphide, assault

      T59.6x4   Toxic effect of hydrogen sulphide, undetermined

T59.7 Toxic effect of carbon dioxide

    T59.7x   Toxic effect of carbon dioxide

      T59.7x1   Toxic effect of carbon dioxide, accidental (unintentional)

         Toxic effect of carbon dioxide NOS

      T59.7x2   Toxic effect of carbon dioxide, intentional self-harm

      T59.7x3   Toxic effect of carbon dioxide, assault

      T59.7x4   Toxic effect of carbon dioxide, undetermined

T59.8 Toxic effect of other specified gases, fumes and vapors

    T59.81   Toxic effect of smoke

      Smoke inhalation

      T59.811   Toxic effect of smoke, accidental (unintentional)

         Toxic effect of smoke NOS

      T59.812   Toxic effect of smoke, intentional self-harm

      T59.813   Toxic effect of smoke, assault

      T59.814   Toxic effect of smoke, undetermined

    T59.89   Toxic effect of other specified gases, fumes and vapors

      T59.891   Toxic effect of other specified gases, fumes and vapors, accidental (unintentional)

      T59.892   Toxic effect of other specified gases, fumes and vapors, intentional self-harm

      T59.893   Toxic effect of other specified gases, fumes and vapors, assault

      T59.894   Toxic effect of other specified gases, fumes and vapors, undetermined

T59.9 Toxic effect of unspecified gases, fumes and vapors

    T59.91   Toxic effect of unspecified gases, fumes and vapors, accidental (unintentional)

    T59.92   Toxic effect of unspecified gases, fumes and vapors, intentional self-harm

    T59.93   Toxic effect of unspecified gases, fumes and vapors, assault

    T59.94   Toxic effect of unspecified gases, fumes and vapors, undetermined

T60 Toxic effect of pesticides

    Includes: toxic effect of wood preservatives

    The following extensions are to be added to each code for category T60:

      a   initial encounter

      d   subsequent encounter

      q   sequela

T60.0 Toxic effect of organophosphate and carbamate insecticides

    T60.0x   Toxic effect of organophosphate and carbamate insecticides

      T60.0x1   Toxic effect of organophosphate and carbamate insecticides, accidental (unintentional)

         Toxic effect of organophosphate and carbamate insecticides NOS

      T60.0x2   Toxic effect of organophosphate and carbamate insecticides, intentional self-harm

      T60.0x3   Toxic effect of organophosphate and carbamate insecticides, assault

      T60.0x4   Toxic effect of organophosphate and carbamate insecticides, undetermined

T60.1 Toxic effect of halogenated insecticides

    Excludes1:   chlorinated hydrocarbon (T53.-)

    T60.1x   Toxic effect of halogenated insecticides

      T60.1x1   Toxic effect of halogenated insecticides, accidental (unintentional)

         Toxic effect of halogenated insecticides NOS

T60.1x2	Toxic effect of halogenated insecticides, intentional self-harm
T60.1x3	Toxic effect of halogenated insecticides, assault
T60.1x4	Toxic effect of halogenated insecticides, undetermined

T60.2   Toxic effect of other insecticides
    T60.2x   Toxic effect of other insecticides
      T60.21   Toxic effect of other insecticides, accidental (unintentional)
         Toxic effect of other insecticides NOS
      T60.22   Toxic effect of other insecticides, intentional self-harm
      T60.23   Toxic effect of other insecticides, assault
      T60.24   Toxic effect of other insecticides, undetermined

T60.3   Toxic effect of herbicides and fungicides
    T60.3x   Toxic effect of herbicides and fungicides
      T60.3x1   Toxic effect of herbicides and fungicides, accidental (unintentional)
         Toxic effect of herbicides and fungicides NOS
      T60.3x2   Toxic effect of herbicides and fungicides, intentional self-harm
      T60.3x3   Toxic effect of herbicides and fungicides, assault
      T60.3x4   Toxic effect of herbicides and fungicides, undetermined

T60.4   Toxic effect of rodenticides
      Toxic effect of thallium
      Excludes1:   strychnine and its salts (T65.1)
    T60.4x   Toxic effect of rodenticides
      T60.4x1   Toxic effect of rodenticides, accidental (unintentional)
         Toxic effect of rodenticides NOS
      T60.4x2   Toxic effect of rodenticides, intentional self-harm
      T60.4x3   Toxic effect of rodenticides, assault
      T60.4x4   Toxic effect of rodenticides, undetermined

T60.8   Toxic effect of other pesticides
    T60.8x   Toxic effect of other pesticides
      T60.8x1   Toxic effect of other pesticides, accidental (unintentional)
         Toxic effect of other pesticides NOS
      T60.8x2   Toxic effect of other pesticides, intentional self-harm
      T60.8x3   Toxic effect of other pesticides, assault
      T60.8x4   Toxic effect of other pesticides, undetermined

T60.9   Toxic effect of unspecified pesticide
    T60.91   Toxic effect of unspecified pesticide, accidental (unintentional)
    T60.92   Toxic effect of unspecified pesticide, intentional self-harm
    T60.93   Toxic effect of unspecified pesticide, assault
    T60.94   Toxic effect of unspecified pesticide, undetermined

T61   Toxic effect of noxious substances eaten as seafood
    Excludes1:   allergic reaction to food, such as:
      anaphylactic shock due to adverse food reaction (T78.0-)
      dermatitis (L23.6, L25.4, L27.2)
      gastroenteritis (noninfective) (K52.2)
      anaphylactic shock (T78.02, T78.05)
      bacterial foodborne intoxications (A05.-)
      toxic effect of food contaminants, such as:
      aflatoxin and other mycotoxins (T64)
      cyanides (T65.0-)
      hydrogen cyanide (T57.3-)
      mercury (T56.1-)

The following extensions are to be added to each code for category T61:
    a   initial encounter
    d   subsequent encounter
    q   sequela

T61.0   Ciguatera fish poisoning
    T61.01   Ciguatera fish poisoning, accidental (unintentional)
    T61.02   Ciguatera fish poisoning, intentional self-harm
    T61.03   Ciguatera fish poisoning, assault
    T61.04   Ciguatera fish poisoning, undetermined

T61.1   Scombroid fish poisoning
      Histamine-like syndrome
    T61.11   Scombroid fish poisoning, accidental (unintentional)
    T61.12   Scombroid fish poisoning, intentional self-harm
    T61.13   Scombroid fish poisoning, assault
    T61.14   Scombroid fish poisoning, undetermined

T61.7   Other fish and shellfish poisoning
    T61.77   Other fish poisoning
      T61.771   Other fish poisoning, accidental (unintentional)
      T61.772   Other fish poisoning, intentional self-harm
      T61.773   Other fish poisoning, assault
      T61.774   Other fish poisoning, undetermined
    T61.78   Other shellfish poisoning
      T61.781   Other shellfish poisoning, accidental (unintentional)
      T61.782   Other shellfish poisoning, intentional self-harm
      T61.783   Other shellfish poisoning, assault
      T61.784   Other shellfish poisoning, undetermined

T61.8   Toxic effect of other seafood
    T61.8x   Toxic effect of other seafood
      T61.8x1   Toxic effect of other seafood, accidental (unintentional)
      T61.8x2   Toxic effect of other seafood, intentional self-harm
      T61.8x3   Toxic effect of other seafood, assault
      T61.8x4   Toxic effect of other seafood, undetermined

T61.9   Toxic effect of unspecified seafood
    T61.91   Toxic effect of unspecified seafood, accidental (unintentional)
    T61.92   Toxic effect of unspecified seafood, intentional self-harm
    T61.93   Toxic effect of unspecified seafood, assault
    T61.94   Toxic effect of unspecified seafood, undetermined

T62   Toxic effect of other noxious substances eaten as food
    Excludes1:   allergic reaction to food, such as:
      anaphylactic shock due to adverse food reaction (T78.0-)
      dermatitis (L23.6, L25.4, L27.2)
      gastroenteritis (noninfective) (K52.2)
      bacterial food borne intoxications (A05.-)
      toxic effect of food contaminants, such as:
      aflatoxin and other mycotoxins (T64)
      cyanides (T65.0-)
      hydrogen cyanide (T57.3-)
      mercury (T56.1-)

The following extensions are to be added to each code for category T62:
    a   initial encounter
    d   subsequent encounter
    q   sequela

T62.0   Toxic effect of ingested mushrooms
    T62.0x   Toxic effect of ingested mushrooms
      T62.0x1   Toxic effect of ingested mushrooms, accidental (unintentional)
         Toxic effect of ingested mushrooms NOS
      T62.0x2   Toxic effect of ingested mushrooms, intentional self-harm
      T62.0x3   Toxic effect of ingested mushrooms, assault

T62.0x4 Toxic effect of ingested mushrooms, undetermined

T62.1 Toxic effect of ingested berries

  T62.1x Toxic effect of ingested berries

    T62.1x1 Toxic effect of ingested berries, accidental (unintentional)
        Toxic effect of ingested berries NOS

    T62.1x2 Toxic effect of ingested berries, intentional self-harm

    T62.1x3 Toxic effect of ingested berries, assault

    T62.1x4 Toxic effect of ingested berries, undetermined

T62.2 Toxic effect of other ingested (parts of) plant(s)

  T62.2x Toxic effect of other ingested (parts of) plant(s)

    T62.2x1 Toxic effect of other ingested (parts of) plant(s), accidental (unintentional)
        Toxic effect of other ingested (parts of) plant(s) NOS

    T62.2x2 Toxic effect of other ingested (parts of) plant(s), intentional self-harm

    T62.2x3 Toxic effect of other ingested (parts of) plant(s), assault

    T62.2x4 Toxic effect of other ingested (parts of) plant(s), undetermined

T62.8 Toxic effect of other specified noxious substances eaten as food

  T62.8x Toxic effect of other specified noxious substances eaten as food

    T62.8x1 Toxic effect of other specified noxious substances eaten as food, accidental (unintentional)
        Toxic effect of other specified noxious substances eaten as food NOS

    T62.8x2 Toxic effect of other specified noxious substances eaten as food, intentional self-harm

    T62.8x3 Toxic effect of other specified noxious substances eaten as food, assault

    T62.8x4 Toxic effect of other specified noxious substances eaten as food, undetermined

T62.9 Toxic effect of unspecified noxious substance eaten as food

  T62.91 Toxic effect of unspecified noxious substance eaten as food, accidental (unintentional)
    Toxic effect of unspecified noxious substance eaten as food NOS

  T62.92 Toxic effect of unspecified noxious substance eaten as food, intentional self-harm

  T62.93 Toxic effect of unspecified noxious substance eaten as food, assault

  T62.94 Toxic effect of unspecified noxious substance eaten as food, undetermined

T63 Toxic effect of contact with venomous animals and plants

  Includes: bite or touch of venomous animal
            pricked or stuck by thorn or leaf

  Excludes2: ingestion of toxic animal or plant (T61.-, T62.-)

  The following extensions are to be added to each code for category T63:

    a initial encounter
    d subsequent encounter
    q sequela

T63.0 Toxic effect of snake venom

  T63.00 Toxic effect of unspecified snake venom

    T63.001 Toxic effect of unspecified snake venom, accidental (unintentional)
        Toxic effect of unspecified snake venom NOS

    T63.002 Toxic effect of unspecified snake venom, intentional self-harm

    T63.003 Toxic effect of unspecified snake venom, assault

    T63.004 Toxic effect of unspecified snake venom, undetermined

  T63.01 Toxic effect of rattlesnake venom

    T63.011 Toxic effect of rattlesnake venom, accidental (unintentional)
        Toxic effect of rattlesnake venom NOS

    T63.012 Toxic effect of rattlesnake venom, intentional self-harm

    T63.013 Toxic effect of rattlesnake venom, assault

    T63.014 Toxic effect of rattlesnake venom, undetermined

  T63.02 Toxic effect of coral snake venom

    T63.021 Toxic effect of coral snake venom, accidental (unintentional)
        Toxic effect of coral snake venom NOS

    T63.022 Toxic effect of coral snake venom, intentional self-harm

    T63.023 Toxic effect of coral snake venom, assault

    T63.024 Toxic effect of coral snake venom, undetermined

  T63.03 Toxic effect of taipan venom

    T63.031 Toxic effect of taipan venom, accidental (unintentional)
        Toxic effect of taipan venom NOS

    T63.032 Toxic effect of taipan venom, intentional self-harm

    T63.033 Toxic effect of taipan venom, assault

    T63.034 Toxic effect of taipan venom, undetermined

  T63.04 Toxic effect of cobra venom

    T63.041 Toxic effect of cobra venom, accidental (unintentional)
        Toxic effect of cobra venom NOS

    T63.042 Toxic effect of cobra venom, intentional self-harm

    T63.043 Toxic effect of cobra venom, assault

    T63.044 Toxic effect of cobra venom, undetermined

  T63.06 Toxic effect of venom of other North and South American snake

    T63.061 Toxic effect of venom of other North and South American snake, accidental (unintentional)
        Toxic effect of venom of other North and South American snake NOS

    T63.062 Toxic effect of venom of other North and South American snake, intentional self-harm

    T63.063 Toxic effect of venom of other North and South American snake, assault

    T63.064 Toxic effect of venom of other North and South American snake, undetermined

  T63.07 Toxic effect of venom of other Australian snake

    T63.071 Toxic effect of venom of other Australian snake, accidental (unintentional)
        Toxic effect of venom of other Australian snake NOS

    T63.072 Toxic effect of venom of other Australian snake, intentional self-harm

    T63.073 Toxic effect of venom of other Australian snake, assault

    T63.074 Toxic effect of venom of other Australian snake, undetermined

  T63.08 Toxic effect of venom of other African and Asian snake

    T63.081 Toxic effect of venom of other African and Asian snake, accidental (unintentional)
        Toxic effect of venom of other African and Asian snake NOS

    T63.082 Toxic effect of venom of other African and Asian snake, intentional self-harm

    T63.083 Toxic effect of venom of other African and Asian snake, assault

    T63.084 Toxic effect of venom of other African and Asian snake, undetermined

T63.09   Toxic effect of venom of other snake

    T63.091   Toxic effect of venom of other snake, accidental (unintentional)
        Toxic effect of venom of other snake NOS

    T63.092   Toxic effect of venom of other snake, intentional self-harm

    T63.093   Toxic effect of venom of other snake, assault

    T63.094   Toxic effect of venom of other snake, undetermined

T63.1   **Toxic effect of venom of other reptiles**

T63.11   Toxic effect of venom of gila monster

    T63.111   Toxic effect of venom of gila monster, accidental (unintentional)
        Toxic effect of venom of gila monster NOS

    T63.112   Toxic effect of venom of gila monster, intentional self-harm

    T63.113   Toxic effect of venom of gila monster, assault

    T63.114   Toxic effect of venom of gila monster, undetermined

T63.12   Toxic effect of venom of other venomous lizard

    T63.121   Toxic effect of venom of other venomous lizard, accidental (unintentional)
        Toxic effect of venom of other venomous lizard NOS

    T63.122   Toxic effect of venom of other venomous lizard, intentional self-harm

    T63.123   Toxic effect of venom of other venomous lizard, assault

    T63.124   Toxic effect of venom of other venomous lizard, undetermined

T63.19   Toxic effect of venom of other reptiles

    T63.191   Toxic effect of venom of other reptiles, accidental (unintentional)
        Toxic effect of venom of other reptiles NOS

    T63.192   Toxic effect of venom of other reptiles, intentional self-harm

    T63.193   Toxic effect of venom of other reptiles, assault

    T63.194   Toxic effect of venom of other reptiles, undetermined

T63.2   **Toxic effect of venom of scorpion**

T63.2x   Toxic effect of venom of scorpion

    T63.2x1   Toxic effect of venom of scorpion, accidental (unintentional)
        Toxic effect of venom of scorpion NOS

    T63.2x2   Toxic effect of venom of scorpion, intentional self-harm

    T63.2x3   Toxic effect of venom of scorpion, assault

    T63.2x4   Toxic effect of venom of scorpion, undetermined

T63.3   **Toxic effect of venom of spider**

T63.30   Toxic effect of unspecified spider venom

    T63.301   Toxic effect of unspecified spider venom, accidental (unintentional)

    T63.302   Toxic effect of unspecified spider venom, intentional self-harm

    T63.303   Toxic effect of unspecified spider venom, assault

    T63.304   Toxic effect of unspecified spider venom, undetermined

T63.31   Toxic effect of venom of black widow spider

    T63.311   Toxic effect of venom of black widow spider, accidental (unintentional)

    T63.312   Toxic effect of venom of black widow spider, intentional self-harm

    T63.313   Toxic effect of venom of black widow spider, assault

    T63.314   Toxic effect of venom of black widow spider, undetermined

T63.32   Toxic effect of venom of tarantula

    T63.321   Toxic effect of venom of tarantula, accidental (unintentional)

    T63.322   Toxic effect of venom of tarantula, intentional self-harm

    T63.323   Toxic effect of venom of tarantula, assault

    T63.324   Toxic effect of venom of tarantula, undetermined

T63.33   Toxic effect of venom of brown recluse spider

    T63.331   Toxic effect of venom of brown recluse spider, accidental (unintentional)

    T63.332   Toxic effect of venom of brown recluse spider, intentional self-harm

    T63.333   Toxic effect of venom of brown recluse spider, assault

    T63.334   Toxic effect of venom of brown recluse spider, undetermined

T63.39   Toxic effect of venom of other spider

    T63.391   Toxic effect of venom of other spider, accidental (unintentional)

    T63.392   Toxic effect of venom of other spider, intentional self-harm

    T63.393   Toxic effect of venom of other spider, assault

    T63.394   Toxic effect of venom of other spider, undetermined

T63.4   **Toxic effect of venom of other arthropods**

T63.41   Toxic effect of venom of centipedes and venomous millipedes

    T63.411   Toxic effect of venom of centipedes and venomous millipedes, accidental (unintentional)

    T63.412   Toxic effect of venom of centipedes and venomous millipedes, intentional self-harm

    T63.413   Toxic effect of venom of centipedes and venomous millipedes, assault

    T63.414   Toxic effect of venom of centipedes and venomous millipedes, undetermined

T63.42   Toxic effect of venom of ants

    T63.421   Toxic effect of venom of ants, accidental (unintentional)

    T63.422   Toxic effect of venom of ants, intentional self-harm

    T63.423   Toxic effect of venom of ants, assault

    T63.424   Toxic effect of venom of ants, undetermined

T63.43   Toxic effect of venom of caterpillars

    T63.431   Toxic effect of venom of caterpillars, accidental (unintentional)

    T63.432   Toxic effect of venom of caterpillars, intentional self-harm

    T63.433   Toxic effect of venom of caterpillars, assault

    T63.434   Toxic effect of venom of caterpillars, undetermined

T63.44   Toxic effect of venom of bees

    T63.441   Toxic effect of venom of bees, accidental (unintentional)

    T63.442   Toxic effect of venom of bees, intentional self-harm

    T63.443   Toxic effect of venom of bees, assault

    T63.444   Toxic effect of venom of bees, undetermined

T63.45   Toxic effect of venom of hornets

    T63.451   Toxic effect of venom of hornets, accidental (unintentional)

    T63.452   Toxic effect of venom of hornets, intentional self-harm

    T63.453   Toxic effect of venom of hornets, assault

    T63.454   Toxic effect of venom of hornets, undetermined

T63.46   Toxic effect of venom of wasps
    Toxic effect of yellow jacket

    T63.461   Toxic effect of venom of wasps, accidental (unintentional)

T63.462   Toxic effect of venom of wasps, intentional self-harm

T63.463   Toxic effect of venom of wasps, assault

T63.464   Toxic effect of venom of wasps, undetermined

T63.48   Toxic effect of venom of other arthropod
Toxic effect of bee, hornet or wasp, unspecified

T63.481   Toxic effect of venom of other arthropod, accidental (unintentional)

T63.482   Toxic effect of venom of other arthropod, intentional self-harm

T63.483   Toxic effect of venom of other arthropod, assault

T63.484   Toxic effect of venom of other arthropod, undetermined

T63.5   Toxic effect of contact with venomous fish
Excludes2:   poisoning by ingestion of fish (T61-)

T63.51   Toxic effect of contact with stingray

T63.511   Toxic effect of contact with stingray, accidental (unintentional)

T63.512   Toxic effect of contact with stingray, intentional self-harm

T63.513   Toxic effect of contact with stingray, assault

T63.514   Toxic effect of contact with stingray, undetermined

T63.59   Toxic effect of contact with other venomous fish

T63.591   Toxic effect of contact with other venomous fish, accidental (unintentional)

T63.592   Toxic effect of contact with other venomous fish, intentional self-harm

T63.593   Toxic effect of contact with other venomous fish, assault

T63.594   Toxic effect of contact with other venomous fish, undetermined

T63.6   Toxic effect of contact with other venomous marine animals
Excludes1:   sea-snake venom (T63.09)
Excludes2:   poisoning by ingestion of shellfish (T61.72)

T63.61   Toxic effect of contact with Portuguese Man-o-war
Toxic effect of contact with bluebottle

T63.611   Toxic effect of contact with Portuguese Man-o-war, accidental (unintentional)

T63.612   Toxic effect of contact with Portuguese Man-o-war, self-harm

T63.613   Toxic effect of contact with Portuguese Man-o-war, assault

T63.614   Toxic effect of contact with Portuguese Man-o-war, undetermined

T63.62   Toxic effect of contact with other jellyfish

T63.621   Toxic effect of contact with other jellyfish, accidental (unintentional)

T63.622   Toxic effect of contact with other jellyfish, intentional self-harm

T63.623   Toxic effect of contact with other jellyfish, assault

T63.624   Toxic effect of contact with other jellyfish, undetermined

T63.63   Toxic effect of contact with sea anemone

T63.631   Toxic effect of contact with sea anemone, accidental (unintentional)

T63.632   Toxic effect of contact with sea anemone, intentional self-harm

T63.633   Toxic effect of contact with sea anemone, assault

T63.634   Toxic effect of contact with sea anemone, undetermined

T63.69   Toxic effect of contact with other venomous marine animals

T63.691   Toxic effect of contact with other venomous marine animals, accidental (unintentional)

T63.692   Toxic effect of contact with other venomous marine animals, intentional self-harm

T63.693   Toxic effect of contact with other venomous marine animals, assault

T63.694   Toxic effect of contact with other venomous marine animals, undetermined

T63.7   Toxic effect of contact with venomous plant

T63.71   Toxic effect of contact with venomous marine plant

T63.711   Toxic effect of contact with venomous marine plant, accidental (unintentional)

T63.712   Toxic effect of contact with venomous marine plant, intentional self-harm

T63.713   Toxic effect of contact with venomous marine plant, assault

T63.714   Toxic effect of contact with venomous marine plant, undetermined

T63.79   Toxic effect of contact with other venomous plant

T63.791   Toxic effect of contact with other venomous plant, accidental (unintentional)

T63.792   Toxic effect of contact with other venomous plant, intentional self-harm

T63.793   Toxic effect of contact with other venomous plant, assault

T63.794   Toxic effect of contact with other venomous plant, undetermined

T63.8   Toxic effect of contact with other venomous animals

T63.81   Toxic effect of contact with venomous frog
Excludes1:   contact with nonvenomous frog (W62.0)

T63.811   Toxic effect of contact with venomous frog, accidental (unintentional)

T63.812   Toxic effect of contact with venomous frog, intentional self-harm

T63.813   Toxic effect of contact with venomous frog, assault

T63.814   Toxic effect of contact with venomous frog, undetermined

T63.82   Toxic effect of contact with venomous toad
Excludes1:   contact with nonvenomous toad (W62.1)

T63.821   Toxic effect of contact with venomous toad, accidental (unintentional)

T63.822   Toxic effect of contact with venomous toad, intentional self-harm

T63.823   Toxic effect of contact with venomous toad, assault

T63.824   Toxic effect of contact with venomous toad, undetermined

T63.83   Toxic effect of contact with other venomous amphibian
Excludes1:   contact with nonvenomous amphibian (W62.9)

T63.831   Toxic effect of contact with other venomous amphibian, accidental (unintentional)

T63.832   Toxic effect of contact with other venomous amphibian, intentional self-harm

T63.833   Toxic effect of contact with other venomous amphibian, assault

T63.834   Toxic effect of contact with other venomous amphibian, undetermined

T63.89   Toxic effect of contact with other venomous animals

T63.891   Toxic effect of contact with other venomous animals, accidental (unintentional)

T63.892   Toxic effect of contact with other venomous animals, intentional self-harm

T63.893   Toxic effect of contact with other venomous animals, assault

T63.894   Toxic effect of contact with other venomous animals, undetermined

T63.9   Toxic effect of contact with unspecified venomous animal

T63.91   Toxic effect of contact with unspecified venomous animal, accidental (unintentional)

T63.92   Toxic effect of contact with unspecified venomous animal, intentional self-harm

T63.93   Toxic effect of contact with unspecified venomous animal, assault

T63.94   Toxic effect of contact with unspecified venomous animal, undetermined

T64 Toxic effect of aflatoxin and other mycotoxin food contaminants

The following extensions are to be added to each code for category T64:

    a   initial encounter
    d   subsequent encounter
    q   sequela

T64.0 Toxic effect of aflatoxin

    T64.01   Toxic effect of aflatoxin, accidental (unintentional)

    T64.02   Toxic effect of aflatoxin, intentional self-harm

    T64.03   Toxic effect of aflatoxin, assault

    T64.04   Toxic effect of aflatoxin, undetermined

T64.8 Toxic effect of other mycotoxin food contaminants

    T64.81   Toxic effect of other mycotoxin food contaminants, accidental (unintentional)

    T64.82   Toxic effect of other mycotoxin food contaminants, intentional self-harm

    T64.83   Toxic effect of other mycotoxin food contaminants, assault

    T64.84   Toxic effect of other mycotoxin food contaminants, undetermined

T65 Toxic effect of other and unspecified substances

The following extensions are to be added to each code for category T65:

    a   initial encounter
    d   subsequent encounter
    q   sequela

T65.0 Toxic effect of cyanides

    Excludes1:   hydrogen cyanide (T57.3-)

    T65.0x Toxic effect of cyanides

        T65.0x1   Toxic effect of cyanides, accidental (unintentional)
                Toxic effect of cyanides NOS

        T65.0x2   Toxic effect of cyanides, intentional self-harm

        T65.0x3   Toxic effect of cyanides, assault

        T65.0x4   Toxic effect of cyanides, undetermined

T65.1 Toxic effect of strychnine and its salts

    T65.1x Toxic effect of strychnine and its salts

        T65.1x1   Toxic effect of strychnine and its salts, accidental (unintentional)
                Toxic effect of strychnine and its salts NOS

        T65.1x2   Toxic effect of strychnine and its salts, intentional self-harm

        T65.1x3   Toxic effect of strychnine and its salts, assault

        T65.1x4   Toxic effect of strychnine and its salts, undetermined

T65.2 Toxic effect of tobacco and nicotine

    Excludes1:   nicotine dependence (F17.-)

    T65.21 Toxic effect of chewing tobacco

        T65.211   Toxic effect of chewing tobacco, accidental (unintentional)
                Toxic effect of chewing tobacco NOS

        T65.212   Toxic effect of chewing tobacco, intentional self-harm

        T65.213   Toxic effect of chewing tobacco, assault

        T65.214   Toxic effect of chewing tobacco, undetermined

    T65.22 Toxic effect of tobacco cigarettes

        T65.221   Toxic effect of tobacco cigarettes, accidental (unintentional)
                Toxic effect of tobacco cigarettes NOS

        T65.222   Toxic effect of tobacco cigarettes, intentional self-harm

        T65.223   Toxic effect of tobacco cigarettes, assault

        T65.224   Toxic effect of tobacco cigarettes, undetermined

    T65.29 Toxic effect of other tobacco and nicotine

        T65.291   Toxic effect of other tobacco and nicotine, accidental (unintentional)
                Toxic effect of other tobacco and nicotine NOS

        T65.292   Toxic effect of other tobacco and nicotine, intentional self-harm

        T65.293   Toxic effect of other tobacco and nicotine, assault

        T65.294   Toxic effect of other tobacco and nicotine, undetermined

T65.3 Toxic effect of nitroderivatives and aminoderivatives of benzene and its homologues

Toxic effect of anilin [benzenamine]
Toxic effect of nitrobenzene
Toxic effect of trinitrotoluene

    T65.3x Toxic effect of nitroderivatives and aminoderivatives of benzene and its homologues

        T65.3x1   Toxic effect of nitroderivatives and aminoderivatives of benzene and its homologues, accidental (unintentional)
                Toxic effect of nitroderivatives and aminoderivatives of benzene and its homologues NOS

        T65.3x2   Toxic effect of nitroderivatives and aminoderivatives of benzene and its homologues, intentional self-harm

        T65.3x3   Toxic effect of nitroderivatives and aminoderivatives of benzene and its homologues, assault

        T65.3x4   Toxic effect of nitroderivatives and aminoderivatives of benzene and its homologues, undetermined

T65.4 Toxic effect of carbon disulfide

    T65.4x Toxic effect of carbon disulfide

        T65.4x1   Toxic effect of carbon disulfide, accidental (unintentional)
                Toxic effect of carbon disulfide NOS

        T65.4x2   Toxic effect of carbon disulfide, intentional self-harm

        T65.4x3   Toxic effect of carbon disulfide, assault

        T65.4x4   Toxic effect of carbon disulfide, undetermined

T65.5 Toxic effect of nitroglycerin and other nitric acids and esters

Toxic effect of 1,2,3-Propanetriol trinitrate

    T65.5x Toxic effect of nitroglycerin and other nitric acids and esters

        T65.5x1   Toxic effect of nitroglycerin and other nitric acids and esters, accidental (unintentional)
                Toxic effect of nitroglycerin and other nitric acids and esters NOS

        T65.5x2   Toxic effect of nitroglycerin and other nitric acids and esters, intentional self-harm

        T65.5x3   Toxic effect of nitroglycerin and other nitric acids and esters, assault

        T65.5x4   Toxic effect of nitroglycerin and other nitric acids and esters, undetermined

T65.6 Toxic effect of paints and dyes, not elsewhere classified

    T65.6x Toxic effect of paints and dyes, not elsewhere classified

        T65.6x1   Toxic effect of paints and dyes, not elsewhere classified, accidental (unintentional)
                Toxic effect of paints and dyes NOS

        T65.6x2   Toxic effect of paints and dyes, not elsewhere classified, intentional self-harm

        T65.6x3   Toxic effect of paints and dyes, not elsewhere classified, assault

        T65.6x4   Toxic effect of paints and dyes, not elsewhere classified, undetermined

T65.8 Toxic effect of other specified substances

    T65.81 Toxic effect of latex

        T65.811   Toxic effect of latex, accidental (unintentional)
                Toxic effect of latex NOS

        T65.812   Toxic effect of latex, intentional self-harm

        T65.813   Toxic effect of latex, assault

        T65.814   Toxic effect of latex, undetermined

T65.89   Toxic effect of other specified substances
    T65.891   **Toxic effect of other specified substances, accidental (unintentional)**
        Toxic effect of other specified substances NOS
    T65.892   **Toxic effect of other specified substances, intentional self-harm**
    T65.893   **Toxic effect of other specified substances, assault**
    T65.894   **Toxic effect of other specified substances, undetermined**

T65.9   **Toxic effect of unspecified substance**
    T65.91   **Toxic effect of unspecified substance, accidental (unintentional)**
        Poisoning NOS
    T65.92   **Toxic effect of unspecified substance, intentional self-harm**
    T65.93   **Toxic effect of unspecified substance, assault**
    T65.94   **Toxic effect of unspecified substance, undetermined**

OTHER AND UNSPECIFIED EFFECTS OF EXTERNAL CAUSES (T66–T78)

T66 Unspecified effects of radiation
    Includes: radiation sickness NOS
    Excludes1:   specified adverse effects of radiation, such as:
        burns (T20-T31)
        leukemia (C91-C95)
        radiation:
            gastroenteritis and colitis (K52.0)
            pneumonitis (J70.0)
            related disorders of the skin and subcutaneous tissue (L55-L59)
        sunburn (L55.-)

T67 Effects of heat and light
    Excludes1:   erythema [dermatitis] ab igne (L59.0)
        malignant hyperpyrexia due to anesthesia (T88.3)
        radiation-related disorders of the skin and subcutaneous tissue (L55-L59)
    Excludes2:   burns (T20-T31)
        sunburn (L55.-)
        sweat disorder due to heat (L74-L75)
    The following extensions are to be added to each code for category T67:
        a   initial encounter
        d   subsequent encounter
        q   sequela

T67.0   **Heatstroke and sunstroke**
    Heat apoplexy
    Heat pyrexia
    Siriasis
    Thermoplegia

T67.1   **Heat syncope**
    Heat collapse

T67.2   **Heat cramp**

T67.3   **Heat exhaustion, anhydrotic**
    Heat prostration due to water depletion
    Excludes1:   heat exhaustion due to salt depletion (T67.4)

T67.4   **Heat exhaustion due to salt depletion**
    Heat prostration due to salt (and water) depletion

T67.5   **Heat exhaustion, unspecified**
    Heat prostration NOS

T67.6   **Heat fatigue, transient**

T67.7   **Heat edema**

T67.8   **Other effects of heat and light**

T67.9   **Effect of heat and light, unspecified**

T68 Hypothermia
    Includes: accidental hypothermia
        hypothermia NOS
    Excludes1:   hypothermia following anesthesia (T88.5)
        hypothermia not associated with low environmental temperature (R68.0)
        hypothermia of newborn (P80.-)
    Excludes2:   frostbite (T33-T34)
    Use additional code to identify source of exposure:
        exposure to excessive cold of man-made origin (W93)
        exposure to excessive cold of natural origin (X31)
    The following extensions are to be added to each code for category T68:
        a   initial encounter
        d   subsequent encounter
        q   sequelae

T69 Other effects of reduced temperature
    Excludes2:   frostbite (T33-T34)
    Use additional code to identify source of exposure:
        exposure to excessive cold of man-made origin (W93)
        exposure to excessive cold of natural origin (X31)
    The following extensions are to be added to each code for category T69:
        a   initial encounter
        d   subsequent encounter
        q   sequela

T69.0   **Immersion hand and foot**
    Trench foot
    T69.00   **Immersion hand and foot, unspecified**
    T69.01   **Immersion right hand**
    T69.02   **Immersion left hand**
    T69.03   **Immersion right foot**
    T69.04   **Immersion left foot**

T69.1   **Chilblains**

T69.8   **Other specified effects of reduced temperature**

T69.9   **Effect of reduced temperature, unspecified**

T70 Effects of air pressure and water pressure
    The following extensions are to be added to each code for category T70:
        a   initial encounter
        d   subsequent encounter
        q   sequela

T70.0   **Otitic barotrauma**
    Aero-otitis media
    Effects of change in ambient atmospheric pressure or water pressure on ears

T70.1   **Sinus barotrauma**
    Aerosinusitis
    Effects of change in ambient atmospheric pressure on sinuses

T70.2   **Other and unspecified effects of high altitude**
    Excludes2:   polycythemia due to high altitude (D75.1)
    T70.20   **Unspecified effects of high altitude**
    T70.29   **Other effects of high altitude**
        Alpine sickness
        Anoxia due to high altitude
        Barotrauma NOS
        Hypobaropathy
        Mountain sickness

T70.3   **Caisson disease [decompression sickness]**
    Compressed-air disease
    Diver's palsy or paralysis

T70.4   **Effects of high-pressure fluids**
    Hydraulic jet injection (industrial)
    Pneumatic jet injection (industrial)
    Traumatic jet injection (industrial)

T70.8   **Other effects of air pressure and water pressure**

T70.9   **Effect of air pressure and water pressure, unspecified**

T71   **Asphyxiation**
Mechanical suffocation
Traumatic suffocation
Excludes1:   anoxia due to high altitude (T70.2)
         asphyxia NOS (R09.0)
         asphyxia from carbon monoxide (T58.-)
         asphyxia from inhalation of food or foreign body (T17.-)
         asphyxia from other gases, fumes and vapors (T59.-)
         respiratory distress (syndrome) in adult (J80)
         respiratory distress (syndrome) in newborn (P22.-)
The following extensions are to be added to each code for category T71:
     a   initial encounter
     d   subsequent encounter
     q   sequela

T71.1   **Asphyxiation due to mechanical threat to breathing**
Suffocation due to mechanical threat to breathing
    T71.11   **Asphyxiation due to smothering under pillow**
       T71.111   **Asphyxiation due to smothering under pillow, accidental**
          Asphyxiation due to smothering under pillow NOS
       T71.112   **Asphyxiation due to smothering under pillow, intentional self-harm**
       T71.113   **Asphyxiation due to smothering under pillow, assault**
       T71.114   **Asphyxiation due to smothering under pillow, undetermined**
    T71.12   **Asphyxiation due to plastic bag**
       T71.121   **Asphyxiation due to plastic bag, accidental**
          Asphyxiation due to plastic bag NOS
       T71.122   **Asphyxiation due to plastic bag, intentional self-harm**
       T71.123   **Asphyxiation due to plastic bag, assault**
       T71.124   **Asphyxiation due to plastic bag, undetermined**
    T71.13   **Asphyxiation due to being trapped in bed linens**
       T71.131   **Asphyxiation due to being trapped in bed linens, accidental**
          Asphyxiation due to being trapped in bed linens NOS
       T71.132   **Asphyxiation due to being trapped in bed linens, intentional self-harm**
       T71.133   **Asphyxiation due to being trapped in bed linens, assault**
       T71.134   **Asphyxiation due to being trapped in bed linens, undetermined**
    T71.14   **Asphyxiation due to smothering under mother's body (in bed)**
       T71.141   **Asphyxiation due to smothering under mother's body (in bed), accidental**
          Asphyxiation due to smothering under mother's body (in bed) NOS
       T71.143   **Asphyxiation due to smothering under mother's body (in bed), assault**
       T71.144   **Asphyxiation due to smothering under mother's body (in bed), undetermined**
    T71.15   **Asphyxiation due to smothering in furniture**
       T71.151   **Asphyxiation due to smothering in furniture, accidental**
          Asphyxiation due to smothering in furniture NOS
       T71.152   **Asphyxiation due to smothering in furniture, intentional self-harm**
       T71.153   **Asphyxiation due to smothering in furniture, assault**
       T71.154   **Asphyxiation due to smothering in furniture, undetermined**

    T71.16   **Asphyxiation due to hanging**
          Hanging by window shade cord
          Use additional code for any associated injuries, such as:
             crushing injury of neck (S17.-)
             fracture of cervical vertebrae (S12.0-S12.2-)
             open wound of neck (S11.-)
       T71.161   **Asphyxiation due to hanging, accidental**
          Asphyxiation due to hanging NOS
          Hanging NOS
       T71.162   **Asphyxiation due to hanging, intentional self-harm**
       T71.163   **Asphyxiation due to hanging, assault**
       T71.164   **Asphyxiation due to hanging, undetermined**
    T71.19   **Asphyxiation due to mechanical threat to breathing due to other causes**
       T71.191   **Asphyxiation due to mechanical threat to breathing due to other causes, accidental**
          Asphyxiation due to other causes NOS
       T71.192   **Asphyxiation due to mechanical threat to breathing due to other causes, intentional self-harm**
       T71.193   **Asphyxiation due to mechanical threat to breathing due to other causes, assault**
       T71.194   **Asphyxiation due to mechanical threat to breathing due to other causes, undetermined**
T71.2   **Asphyxiation due to systemic oxygen deficiency due to low oxygen content in ambient air**
Suffocation due to systemic oxygen deficiency due to low oxygen content in ambient air
    T71.20   **Asphyxiation due to systemic oxygen deficiency due to low oxygen content in ambient air due to unspecified cause**
    T71.21   **Asphyxiation due to cave-in or falling earth**
          Use additional code for any associated cataclysm (X34-X38)
    T71.22   **Asphyxiation due to being trapped in a car trunk**
       T71.221   **Asphyxiation due to being trapped in a car trunk, accidental**
       T71.222   **Asphyxiation due to being trapped in a car trunk, intentional self-harm**
       T71.223   **Asphyxiation due to being trapped in a car trunk, assault**
       T71.224   **Asphyxiation due to being trapped in a car trunk, undetermined**
    T71.23   **Asphyxiation due to being trapped in a (discarded) refrigerator**
       T71.231   **Asphyxiation due to being trapped in a (discarded) refrigerator, accidental**
       T71.232   **Asphyxiation due to being trapped in a (discarded) refrigerator, intentional self-harm**
       T71.233   **Asphyxiation due to being trapped in a (discarded) refrigerator, assault**
       T71.234   **Asphyxiation due to being trapped in a (discarded) refrigerator, undetermined**
    T71.29   **Asphyxiation due to being trapped in other low oxygen environment**
T71.9   **Asphyxiation due to unspecified cause**
Asphyxia NOS
Aspiration NOS
Suffocation (by strangulation) due to unspecified cause
Suffocation NOS
Systemic oxygen deficiency due to low oxygen content in ambient air due to unspecified cause
Systemic oxygen deficiency due to mechanical threat to breathing due to unspecified cause

T73   **Effects of other deprivation**
The following extensions are to be added to each code for category T73:
     a   initial encounter
     d   subsequent encounter
     q   sequela

T73.0   Starvation
Deprivation of food

T73.1   Deprivation of water

T73.2   Exhaustion due to exposure

T73.3   Exhaustion due to excessive exertion
Overexertion

T73.8   Other effects of deprivation

T73.9   Effect of deprivation, unspecified

T74   Adult and child abuse, neglect and other maltreatment, confirmed
Excludes1:   abuse and maltreatment in pregnancy (O94.3-O94.5-)
adult and child maltreatment, suspected (T76.-)
Use additional code, if applicable, to identify any associated current injury
Use additional external cause code to identify perpetrator, if known (Y07.-)
The following extensions are to be added to each code for category T74:
a   initial encounter
d   subsequent encounter
q   sequela

T74.0   Neglect or abandonment, confirmed

T74.01   Adult neglect or abandonment, confirmed

T74.02   Child neglect or abandonment, confirmed

T74.1   Physical abuse, confirmed
Excludes2:   sexual abuse (T74.2-)

T74.11   Adult physical abuse, confirmed

T74.12   Child physical abuse, confirmed
Excludes2:   shaken infant syndrome (T74.4)

T74.2   Sexual abuse, confirmed

T74.21   Adult sexual abuse, confirmed

T74.22   Child sexual abuse, confirmed

T74.3   Psychological abuse, confirmed

T74.31   Adult psychological abuse, confirmed

T74.32   Child psychological abuse, confirmed

T74.4   Shaken infant syndrome

T74.9   Unspecified maltreatment, confirmed

T74.91   Unspecified adult maltreatment, confirmed

T74.92   Unspecified child maltreatment, confirmed

T75   Other and unspecified effects of other external causes
Excludes1:   adverse effects NEC (T78.-)
Excludes2:   burns (electric) (T20-T31)
The following extensions are to be added to each code for category T75:
a   initial encounter
d   subsequent encounter
q   sequela

T75.0   Effects of lightning
Struck by lightning

T75.00   Unspecified effects of lightning
Struck by lightning NOS

T75.01   Shock due to being struck by lightning

T75.09   Other effects of lightning
Use additional code for other effects of lightning

T75.1   Unspecified effects of drowning and nonfatal submersion
Immersion
Excludes1:   specified effects of drowning- code to effects

T75.2   Effects of vibration

T75.20   Unspecified effects of vibration

T75.21   Pneumatic hammer syndrome

T75.22   Traumatic vasospastic syndrome

T75.23   Vertigo from infrasound
Excludes1:   vertigo NOS (R42)

T75.29   Other effects of vibration

T75.3   Motion sickness
Airsickness
Seasickness
Travel sickness
Use additional external cause code to identify vehicle (X51.-)

T75.4   Electrocution
Shock from electric current

T75.8   Other specified effects of external causes

T75.81   Effects of abnormal gravitation [G] forces

T75.82   Effects of weightlessness

T75.89   Other specified effects of external causes

T76   Adult and child abuse, neglect and other maltreatment, suspected
Excludes1:   adult and child maltreatment, confirmed (T74.-)
suspected abuse and maltreatment in pregnancy (O94.3-O94.5-)
suspected adult physical and sexual abuse, ruled out (Z04.71)
suspected child physical and sexual abuse, ruled out (Z04.72)
Use additional code, if applicable, to identify any associated current injury
The following extensions are to be added to each code for category T76:
a   initial encounter
d   subsequent encounter
q   sequela

T76.0   Neglect or abandonment, suspected

T76.01   Adult neglect or abandonment, suspected

T76.02   Child neglect or abandonment, suspected

T76.1   Physical abuse, suspected

T76.11   Adult physical abuse, suspected

T76.12   Child physical abuse, suspected

T76.2   Sexual abuse, suspected
Excludes1:   alleged abuse, ruled out (Z04.7)

T76.21   Adult sexual abuse, suspected

T76.22   Child sexual abuse, suspected

T76.3   Psychological abuse, suspected

T76.31   Adult psychological abuse, suspected

T76.32   Child psychological abuse, suspected

T76.9   Unspecified maltreatment, suspected

T76.91   Unspecified adult maltreatment, suspected

T76.92   Unspecified child maltreatment, suspected

T78   Adverse effects, not elsewhere classified
Excludes2:   complications of surgical and medical care NEC (T80-T88)
The following extensions are to be added to each code for category T78:
a   initial encounter
d   subsequent encounter
q   sequela

T78.0   Anaphylactic shock due to adverse food reaction

T78.00   Anaphylactic shock due to unspecified food

T78.01   Anaphylactic shock due to peanuts

T78.02   Anaphylactic shock due to shellfish (crustaceans)

T78.03   Anaphylactic shock due to other fish

T78.04   Anaphylactic shock due to fruits and vegetables

T78.05   Anaphylactic shock due to tree nuts and seeds
Excludes1:   anaphylactic shock due to peanuts (T78.01)

T78.06   Anaphylactic shock due to food additives

T78.07   Anaphylactic shock due to milk and dairy products

T78.08   Anaphylactic shock due to eggs

T78.09   Anaphylactic shock due to other food products

T78.1   Other adverse food reactions, not elsewhere classified
Use additional code to identify the type of reaction
Excludes1:   bacterial food borne intoxications (A05.-)
dermatitis due to food (L27.2)
in contact with skin (L23.6, L24.6, L25.4)

T78.2 Anaphylactic shock, unspecified
　　Allergic shock
　　Anaphylactic reaction
　　Anaphylaxis
　　Excludes1:　anaphylactic shock due to:
　　　　　　adverse effect of correct medicinal substance
　　　　　　　properly administered (T88.6)
　　　　　　adverse food reaction (T78.0-)
　　　　　　serum (T80.5)

T78.3 Angioneurotic edema
　　Giant urticaria
　　Quincke's edema
　　Excludes1:　urticaria (L50.-)
　　　　　　serum (T80.6)

T78.4 Allergy, unspecified
　　Allergic reaction NOS
　　Hypersensitivity NOS
　　Idiosyncracy NOS
　　Excludes1:　allergic reaction NOS to correct medicinal
　　　　　　　substance properly administered (T88.7)
　　　　　　specified types of allergic reaction such as:
　　　　　　　allergic gastroenteritis and colitis (K52.2)
　　　　　　　dermatitis (L23-L25, L27.-)
　　　　　　　hay fever (J30.1)

T78.8 Other adverse effects, not elsewhere classified

CERTAIN EARLY COMPLICATIONS OF TRAUMA (T79)

T79 Certain early complications of trauma, not elsewhere classified
　　Excludes2:　adult respiratory distress syndrome (J80)
　　　　　　complications occurring during or following medical
　　　　　　　procedures (T80-T88)
　　　　　　complications of surgical and medical care NEC (T80-
　　　　　　　T88)
　　　　　　newborn respiratory distress syndrome (P22.0)
　　The following extensions are to be added to each code for category
　　T79:
　　　　a　initial encounter
　　　　d　subsequent encounter
　　　　q　sequelae

T79.0 Air embolism (traumatic)
　　Excludes1:　air embolism complicating:
　　　　　　abortion or ectopic or molar pregnancy (O00-O07,
　　　　　　　O08.2)
　　　　　　pregnancy, childbirth and the puerperium (O88.0)
　　　　　　air embolism following:
　　　　　　infusion, transfusion, and therapeutic injection
　　　　　　　(T80.0)
　　　　　　procedure NEC (T81.7)

T79.1 Fat embolism (traumatic)
　　Excludes1:　fat embolism complicating:
　　　　　　abortion or ectopic or molar pregnancy (O00-
　　　　　　　O07, O08.2)
　　　　　　pregnancy, childbirth and the puerperium
　　　　　　　(O88.8)

T79.2 Traumatic secondary and recurrent hemorrhage

T79.3 Post-traumatic wound infection, not elsewhere classified
　　Excludes1:　specified type of wound infection- code to
　　　　　　infection

T79.4 Traumatic shock
　　Shock (immediate) (delayed) following injury
　　Excludes1:　anaphylactic shock due to adverse food reaction
　　　　　　　(T78.0-)
　　　　　　anaphylactic shock due to correct medicinal
　　　　　　　substance properly administered (T88.6)
　　　　　　anaphylactic shock due to serum (T80.5)
　　　　　　anaphylactic shock NOS (T78.2)
　　　　　　anesthetic shock (T88.2)
　　　　　　electric shock (T75.4)
　　　　　　nontraumatic shock NEC (R57.-)
　　　　　　obstetric shock (O75.1)
　　　　　　postoperative shock (T81.1)
　　　　　　shock complicating abortion or ectopic or molar
　　　　　　　pregnancy (O00-O07, O08.3)
　　　　　　shock due to lightning (T75.01)
　　　　　　shock NOS (R57.9)

T79.5 Traumatic anuria
　　Crush syndrome
　　Renal failure following crushing

T79.6 Traumatic ischemia of muscle
　　Compartment syndrome
　　Volkmann's ischemic contracture
　　Excludes2:　anterior tibial syndrome (M76.8)

T79.7 Traumatic subcutaneous emphysema
　　Excludes1:　emphysema NOS (J43)
　　　　　　emphysema (subcutaneous) resulting from a
　　　　　　　procedure (T81.82)

T79.8 Other early complications of trauma

T79.9 Unspecified early complication of trauma

COMPLICATIONS OF SURGICAL AND MEDICAL CARE, NOT ELSEWHERE CLASSIFIED (T80–T88)

Use additional external cause code (Chapter XX), to identify devices
involved and details of circumstances
Excludes2:　adverse effects of drugs and medicaments (A00-R94,
　　　　　　T78.-)
　　　　any encounters with medical care for postoperative
　　　　　conditions in which no complications are present,
　　　　　such as:
　　　　　artificial opening status (Z93.-)
　　　　　closure of external stoma (Z43.-)
　　　　　fitting and adjustment of external prosthetic device
　　　　　　(Z44.-)
　　　　burns and corrosions from local applications and
　　　　　irradiation (T20-T32)
　　　　complications of surgical procedures during pregnancy,
　　　　　childbirth and the puerperium (O00-O99)
　　　　poisoning and toxic effects of drugs and chemicals
　　　　　(T36-T65)
　　　　specified complications classified elsewhere, such as:
　　　　　cerebrospinal fluid leak from spinal puncture
　　　　　　(G97.0)
　　　　　colostomy malfunction (K94.0-)
　　　　　disorders of fluid and electrolyte imbalance (E86-
　　　　　　E87)
　　　　　functional disturbances following cardiac surgery
　　　　　　(I97.0-I97.1)
　　　　　intraoperative and postprocedural complications
　　　　　　(D73.6-, E36.-, G97.3-, G97.4, H59.3-, H59.4,
　　　　　　H95.2-, H95.3, I97.4-, I97.5, J95.6-, J95.7,
　　　　　　K91.6-, L76.-, M96.7-, N99.7-)
　　　　ostomy complications (J95.0-, K94-, N99.5-)
　　　　postgastric surgery syndromes (K91.1)
　　　　postlaminectomy syndrome NEC (M96.1)
　　　　postmastectomy lymphedema syndrome (I97.2)
　　　　postsurgical blind-loop syndrome (K91.2)

T80 Complications following infusion, transfusion and therapeutic injection

Includes: perfusion

Excludes2:   bone-marrow transplant rejection (T86.0)

The following extensions are to be added to each code for category T80:

a   initial encounter
d   subsequent encounter
q   sequelae

T80.0   Air embolism following infusion, transfusion and therapeutic injection

T80.1   Vascular complications following infusion, transfusion and therapeutic injection

Phlebitis following infusion, transfusion and therapeutic injection

Thromboembolism following infusion, transfusion and therapeutic injection

Thrombophlebitis following infusion, transfusion and therapeutic injection

Excludes2:   vascular complications specified as due to prosthetic devices, implants and grafts (T82.8, T83.8, T84.8, T85.8)
postprocedural vascular complications (T81.7)

T80.2   Infections following infusion, transfusion and therapeutic injection

Infection following infusion, transfusion and therapeutic injection

Sepsis following infusion, transfusion and therapeutic injection

Septicemia following infusion, transfusion and therapeutic injection

Septic shock following infusion, transfusion and therapeutic injection

Use additional code (B95-B97), to identify infectious agent.

Excludes2:   infections specified as due to prosthetic devices, implants and grafts (T82.6-T82.7, T83.5-T83.6, T84.5-T84.7, T85.7)
postprocedural infections (T81.4)

T80.3   ABO incompatibility reaction

Incompatible blood transfusion

Reaction to blood-group incompatibility in infusion or transfusion

T80.4   Rh incompatibility reaction

Reactions due to Rh factor in infusion or transfusion

T80.5   Anaphylactic shock due to serum

Excludes1:   allergic shock NOS (T78.2)
anaphylactic shock NOS (T78.2)
anaphylactic shock due to adverse effect of correct medicinal substance properly administered (T88.6)

T80.6   Other serum reactions

Intoxication by serum
Protein sickness
Serum rash
Serum sickness
Serum urticaria

Excludes2:   serum hepatitis (B16.-)

T80.8   Other complications following infusion, transfusion and therapeutic injection

T80.9   Unspecified complication following infusion, transfusion and therapeutic injection

Transfusion reaction NOS

T81   Complication of procedures, not elsewhere classified

Excludes2:   adverse effect of drug NOS (T88.7)
complication following:
immunization (T88.0-T88.1)
infusion, transfusion and therapeutic injection (T80.-)
specified complications classified elsewhere, such as:
complication of prosthetic devices, implants and grafts (T82-T85)
dermatitis due to drugs and medicaments (L23.3, L24.4, L25.1, L27.0-L27.1)
intraoperative and postprocedural complications (D73.6-, E36.-, G97.3-, G97.4, H59.3-, H59.4, H95.2-, H95.3, I97.4-, I97.5, J95.6- J95.7, K91.6-, L76.-, M96.7-, N99.7-)
ostomy complications (J95.0-, K94.-, N99.5-)
poisoning and toxic effects of drugs and chemicals (T36-T65)

The following extensions are to be added to each code for category T81:

a   initial encounter
d   subsequent encounter
q   sequela

T81.1   Shock during or resulting from a procedure, not elsewhere classified

Collapse NOS during or resulting from a procedure, not elsewhere classified

Shock (endotoxic) (hypovolemic) (septic) during or resulting from a procedure, not elsewhere classified

Postoperative shock NOS during or resulting from a procedure, not elsewhere classified

Excludes1:   anaphylactic shock NOS (T78.2)
anaphylactic shock due to correct substance properly administered (T88.6)
anaphylactic shock due to serum (T80.5)
anesthetic shock (T88.2)
electric shock (T75.4)
obstetric shock (O75.1)
shock following abortion or ectopic or molar pregnancy (O00-O07, O08.3)
traumatic shock (T79.4)

T81.3   Disruption of operation wound, not elsewhere classified

Dehiscence of operation wound
Rupture of operation wound

Excludes1:   disruption of cesarean-section wound (O90.0)
disruption of perineal obstetric wound (O90.1)

T81.4   Infection following a procedure, not elsewhere classified

Intra-abdominal abscess following a procedure, not elsewhere classified

Septicemia following a procedure, not elsewhere classified

Stitch abscess following a procedure, not elsewhere classified

Subphrenic abscess following a procedure, not elsewhere classified

Wound abscess following a procedure, not elsewhere classified

Use additional code to identify infection

Excludes1:   obstetric surgical wound infection (O86.0)

Excludes2:   infection due to infusion, transfusion and therapeutic injection (T80.2)
infection due to prosthetic devices, implants and grafts (T82.6-T82.7, T83.5-T83.6, T84.5-T84.7, T85.7)

T81.5   Complications of foreign body accidentally left in body following procedure

T81.50   Unspecified complication of foreign body accidentally left in body following procedure

T81.500   Unspecified complication of foreign body accidentally left in body following surgical operation

T81.501   Unspecified complication of foreign body accidentally left in body following infusion or transfusion

T81.502   Unspecified complication of foreign body accidentally left in body following kidney dialysis

T81.503   Unspecified complication of foreign body accidentally left in body following injection or immunization

T81.504   Unspecified complication of foreign body accidentally left in body following endoscopic examination

T81.505   Unspecified complication of foreign body accidentally left in body following heart catheterization

T81.506   Unspecified complication of foreign body accidentally left in body following aspiration, puncture or other catheterization

T81.507   Unspecified complication of foreign body accidentally left in body following removal of catheter or packing

T81.508   Unspecified complication of foreign body accidentally left in body following other procedure

T81.509   Unspecified complication of foreign body accidentally left in body following unspecified procedure

T81.51   Adhesions due to foreign body accidentally left in body following procedure

T81.510   Adhesions due to foreign body accidentally left in body following surgical operation

T81.511   Adhesions due to foreign body accidentally left in body following infusion or transfusion

T81.512   Adhesions due to foreign body accidentally left in body following kidney dialysis

T81.513   Adhesions due to foreign body accidentally left in body following injection or immunization

T81.514   Adhesions due to foreign body accidentally left in body following endoscopic examination

T81.515   Adhesions due to foreign body accidentally left in body following heart catheterization

T81.516   Adhesions due to foreign body accidentally left in body following aspiration, puncture or other catheterization

T81.517   Adhesions due to foreign body accidentally left in body following removal of catheter or packing

T81.518   Adhesions due to foreign body accidentally left in body following other procedure

T81.519   Adhesions due to foreign body accidentally left in body following unspecified procedure

T81.52   Obstruction due to foreign body accidentally left in body following procedure

T81.520   Obstruction due to foreign body accidentally left in body following surgical operation

T81.521   Obstruction due to foreign body accidentally left in body following infusion or transfusion

T81.522   Obstruction due to foreign body accidentally left in body following kidney dialysis

T81.523   Obstruction due to foreign body accidentally left in body following injection or immunization

T81.524   Obstruction due to foreign body accidentally left in body following endoscopic examination

T81.525   Obstruction due to foreign body accidentally left in body following heart catheterization

T81.526   Obstruction due to foreign body accidentally left in body following aspiration, puncture or other catheterization

T81.527   Obstruction due to foreign body accidentally left in body following removal of catheter or packing

T81.528   Obstruction due to foreign body accidentally left in body following other procedure

T81.529   Obstruction due to foreign body accidentally left in body following unspecified procedure

T81.53   Perforation due to foreign body accidentally left in body following procedure

T81.530   Perforation due to foreign body accidentally left in body following surgical operation

T81.531   Perforation due to foreign body accidentally left in body following infusion or transfusion

T81.532   Perforation due to foreign body accidentally left in body following kidney dialysis

T81.533   Perforation due to foreign body accidentally left in body following injection or immunization

T81.534   Perforation due to foreign body accidentally left in body following endoscopic examination

T81.535   Perforation due to foreign body accidentally left in body following heart catheterization

T81.536   Perforation due to foreign body accidentally left in body following aspiration, puncture or other catheterization

T81.537   Perforation due to foreign body accidentally left in body following removal of catheter or packing

T81.538   Perforation due to foreign body accidentally left in body following other procedure

T81.539   Perforation due to foreign body accidentally left in body following unspecified procedure

T81.59   Other complications of foreign body accidentally left in body following procedure

Excludes2:   obstruction or perforation due to prosthetic devices and implants intentionally left in body (T82.0-T82.5, T83.0-T83.4, T84.0-T84.4, T85.0-T85.6)

T81.590   Other complications of foreign body accidentally left in body following surgical operation

T81.591   Other complications of foreign body accidentally left in body following infusion or transfusion

T81.592   Other complications of foreign body accidentally left in body following kidney dialysis

T81.593   Other complications of foreign body accidentally left in body following injection or immunization

T81.594   Other complications of foreign body accidentally left in body following endoscopic examination

T81.595   Other complications of foreign body accidentally left in body following heart catheterization

T81.596   Other complications of foreign body accidentally left in body following aspiration, puncture or other catheterization

T81.597   Other complications of foreign body accidentally left in body following removal of catheter or packing

T81.598   Other complications of foreign body accidentally left in body following other procedure

T81.599   Other complications of foreign body accidentally left in body following unspecified procedure

T81.6   Acute reaction to foreign substance accidentally left during a procedure

Excludes2:   complications of foreign body accidentally left in body cavity or operation wound following procedure (T81.5-)

T81.60   Unspecified acute reaction to foreign substance accidentally left during a procedure

T81.61   Aseptic peritonitis due to foreign substance accidentally left during a procedure
Chemical peritonitis

T81.69   Other acute reaction to foreign substance accidentally left during a procedure

T81.7   Vascular complications following a procedure, not elsewhere classified

Air embolism following procedure NEC

Excludes1:   embolism complicating abortion or ectopic or molar pregnancy (O00-O07, O08.2)

embolism complicating pregnancy, childbirth and the puerperium (O88.-)

traumatic embolism (T79.0)

Excludes2:   embolism due to prosthetic devices, implants and grafts (T82.8, T83.8, T84.8, T85.8)

embolism following infusion, transfusion and therapeutic injection (T80.0)

T81.8   Other complications of procedures, not elsewhere classified

Excludes2:   hypothermia following anesthesia (T88.5)

malignant hyperpyrexia due to anesthesia (T88.3)

T81.81   **Complication of inhalation therapy**

T81.82   **Emphysema (subcutaneous) resulting from a procedure**

T81.83   **Persistent postoperative fistula**

T81.84   **Cardiac failure following a non-cardiac procedure**

Excludes1:   cardiac failure following cardiac surgery (I97.1)

T81.89   **Other complications of procedures, not elsewhere classified**

T81.9   Unspecified complication of procedure

T82   Complications of cardiac and vascular prosthetic devices, implants and grafts

Excludes2:   failure and rejection of transplanted organs and tissue (T86.-)

The following extensions are to be added to each code for category T82:

a   initial encounter

d   subsequent encounter

q   sequela

T82.0   Mechanical complication of heart valve prosthesis

T82.01   **Breakdown (mechanical) of heart valve prosthesis**

T82.02   **Displacement of heart valve prosthesis**

Malposition of heart valve prosthesis

T82.03   **Leakage of heart valve prosthesis**

T82.09   **Other mechanical complication of heart valve prosthesis**

Obstruction (mechanical) of heart valve prosthesis

Perforation of heart valve prosthesis

Protrusion of heart valve prosthesis

T82.1   Mechanical complication of cardiac electronic device

T82.11   **Breakdown (mechanical) of cardiac electronic device**

T82.110   **Breakdown (mechanical) of cardiac electrode**

T82.111   **Breakdown (mechanical) of cardiac pulse generator (battery)**

T82.118   **Breakdown (mechanical) of other cardiac electronic device**

T82.119   **Breakdown (mechanical) of unspecified cardiac electronic device**

T82.12   **Displacement of cardiac electronic device**

Malposition of cardiac electronic device

T82.120   **Displacement of cardiac electrode**

T82.121   **Displacement of cardiac pulse generator (battery)**

T82.128   **Displacement of other cardiac electronic device**

T82.129   **Displacement of unspecified cardiac electronic device**

T82.19   **Other mechanical complication of cardiac electronic device**

Leakage of cardiac electronic device

Obstruction of cardiac electronic device

Perforation of cardiac electronic device

Protrusion of cardiac electronic device

T82.190   **Other mechanical complication of cardiac electrode**

T82.191   **Other mechanical complication of cardiac pulse generator (battery)**

T82.198   **Other mechanical complication of other cardiac electronic device**

T82.199   **Other mechanical complication of unspecified cardiac device**

T82.2   Mechanical complication of coronary artery bypass and valve grafts

T82.21   **Breakdown (mechanical) of coronary artery bypass and valve grafts**

T82.210   **Breakdown (mechanical) of coronary artery bypass**

T82.211   **Breakdown (mechanical) of valve grafts**

T82.22   **Displacement of coronary artery bypass and valve grafts**

Malposition of coronary artery bypass and valve grafts

T82.220   **Displacement of coronary artery bypass**

T82.221   **Displacement of coronary valve grafts**

T82.23   **Leakage of coronary artery bypass and valve grafts**

T82.230   **Leakage of coronary artery bypass**

T82.231   **Leakage of coronary valve grafts**

T82.28   **Other mechanical complication of coronary artery bypass and valve grafts**

Obstruction, mechanical of coronary artery bypass and valve grafts

Perforation of coronary artery bypass and valve grafts

Protrusion of coronary artery bypass and valve grafts

T82.280   **Other mechanical complication of coronary artery bypass**

T82.281   **Other mechanical complication of coronary valve grafts**

T82.29   **Unspecified mechanical complication of coronary artery bypass and valve grafts**

T82.290   **Unspecified mechanical complication of coronary artery bypass**

T82.291   **Unspecified mechanical complication of coronary valve grafts**

T82.3   Mechanical complication of other vascular grafts

T82.31   **Breakdown (mechanical) of other vascular grafts**

T82.310   **Breakdown (mechanical) of aortic (bifurcation) graft (replacement)**

T82.311   **Breakdown (mechanical) of carotid arterial graft (bypass)**

T82.312   **Breakdown (mechanical) of femoral arterial graft (bypass)**

T82.318   **Breakdown (mechanical) of other vascular grafts**

T82.319   **Breakdown (mechanical) of unspecified vascular grafts**

T82.32   **Displacement of other vascular grafts**

Malposition of other vascular grafts

T82.320   **Displacement of aortic (bifurcation) graft (replacement)**

T82.321   **Displacement of carotid arterial graft (bypass)**

T82.322   **Displacement of femoral arterial graft (bypass)**

T82.328   **Displacement of other vascular grafts**

T82.329   **Displacement of unspecified vascular grafts**

T82.33   **Leakage of other vascular grafts**

T82.330   **Leakage of aortic (bifurcation) graft (replacement)**

T82.331   **Leakage of carotid arterial graft (bypass)**

T82.332   **Leakage of femoral arterial graft (bypass)**

T82.338   **Leakage of other vascular grafts**

T82.339   **Leakage of unspecified vascular graft**

T82.39   **Other mechanical complication of other vascular grafts**

Obstruction (mechanical) of other vascular grafts

Perforation of other vascular grafts

Protrusion of other vascular grafts

T82.390   **Other mechanical complication of aortic (bifurcation) graft (replacement)**

T82.391 Other mechanical complication of carotid arterial graft (bypass)

T82.392 Other mechanical complication of femoral arterial graft (bypass)

T82.398 Other mechanical complication of other vascular grafts

T82.399 Other mechanical complication of unspecified vascular grafts

T82.4 Mechanical complication of vascular dialysis catheter
Mechanical complication of hemodialysis catheter
Excludes1: mechanical complication of intraperitoneal dialysis catheter (T85.62)

T82.41 Breakdown (mechanical) of vascular dialysis catheter

T82.42 Displacement of vascular dialysis catheter
Malposition of vascular dialysis catheter

T82.43 Leakage of vascular dialysis catheter

T82.49 Other complication of vascular dialysis catheter
Obstruction (mechanical) of vascular dialysis catheter
Perforation of vascular dialysis catheter
Protrusion of vascular dialysis catheter

T82.5 Mechanical complication of other cardiac and vascular devices and implants
Excludes2: mechanical complication of epidural and subdural infusion catheter (T85.61)

T82.51 Breakdown (mechanical) of other cardiac and vascular devices and implants

T82.510 Breakdown (mechanical) of surgically created arteriovenous fistula

T82.511 Breakdown (mechanical) of surgically created arteriovenous shunt

T82.512 Breakdown (mechanical) of artificial heart

T82.513 Breakdown (mechanical) of balloon (counterpulsation) device

T82.514 Breakdown (mechanical) of infusion catheter

T82.515 Breakdown (mechanical) of umbrella device

T82.518 Breakdown (mechanical) of other cardiac and vascular devices and implants

T82.519 Breakdown (mechanical) of unspecified cardiac and vascular devices and implants

T82.52 Displacement of other cardiac and vascular devices and implants
Malposition of other cardiac and vascular devices and implants

T82.520 Displacement of surgically created arteriovenous fistula

T82.521 Displacement of surgically created arteriovenous shunt

T82.522 Displacement of artificial heart

T82.523 Displacement of balloon (counterpulsation) device

T82.524 Displacement of infusion catheter

T82.525 Displacement of umbrella device

T82.528 Displacement of other cardiac and vascular devices and implants

T82.529 Displacement of unspecified cardiac and vascular devices and implants

T82.53 Leakage of other cardiac and vascular devices and implants

T82.530 Leakage of surgically created arteriovenous fistula

T82.531 Leakage of surgically created arteriovenous shunt

T82.532 Leakage of artificial heart

T82.533 Leakage of balloon (counterpulsation) device

T82.534 Leakage of infusion catheter

T82.535 Leakage of umbrella device

T82.538 Leakage of other cardiac and vascular devices and implants

T82.539 Leakage of unspecified cardiac and vascular devices and implants

T82.59 Other mechanical complication of other cardiac and vascular devices and implants
Obstruction (mechanical) of other cardiac and vascular devices and implants
Perforation of other cardiac and vascular devices and implants
Protrusion of other cardiac and vascular devices and implants

T82.590 Other mechanical complication of surgically created arteriovenous fistula

T82.591 Other mechanical complication of surgically created arteriovenous shunt

T82.592 Other mechanical complication of artificial heart

T82.593 Other mechanical complication of balloon (counterpulsation) device

T82.594 Other mechanical complication of infusion catheter

T82.595 Other mechanical complication of umbrella device

T82.598 Other mechanical complication of other cardiac and vascular devices and implants

T82.599 Other mechanical complication of unspecified cardiac and vascular devices and implants

T82.6 Infection and inflammatory reaction due to cardiac valve prosthesis
Use additional code to identify infection

T82.7 Infection and inflammatory reaction due to other cardiac and vascular devices, implants and grafts
Use additional code to identify infection

T82.8 Other complications of cardiac and vascular prosthetic devices, implants and grafts

T82.81 Embolism of cardiac and vascular prosthetic devices, implants and grafts

T82.817 Embolism of cardiac prosthetic devices, implants and grafts

T82.818 Embolism of vascular prosthetic devices, implants and grafts

T82.82 Fibrosis of cardiac and vascular prosthetic devices, implants and grafts

T82.827 Fibrosis of cardiac prosthetic devices, implants and grafts

T82.828 Fibrosis of vascular prosthetic devices, implants and grafts

T82.83 Hemorrhage of cardiac and vascular prosthetic devices, implants and grafts

T82.837 Hemorrhage of cardiac prosthetic devices, implants and grafts

T82.838 Hemorrhage of vascular prosthetic devices, implants and grafts

T82.84 Pain from cardiac and vascular prosthetic devices, implants and grafts

T82.847 Pain from cardiac prosthetic devices, implants and grafts

T82.848 Pain from vascular prosthetic devices, implants and grafts

T82.85 Stenosis of cardiac and vascular prosthetic devices, implants and grafts

T82.857 Stenosis of cardiac prosthetic devices, implants and grafts

T82.858 Stenosis of vascular prosthetic devices, implants and grafts

T82.86 Thrombosis of cardiac and vascular prosthetic devices, implants and grafts

T82.867 Thrombosis of cardiac prosthetic devices, implants and grafts

T82.868 Thrombosis of vascular prosthetic devices, implants and grafts

T82.89 Other complication of cardiac and vascular prosthetic devices, implants and grafts

T82.897 Other complication of cardiac prosthetic devices, implants and grafts

T82.898   Other complication of vascular prosthetic devices, implants and grafts

T82.9   Unspecified complication of cardiac and vascular prosthetic device, implant and graft

T83   Complications of genitourinary prosthetic devices, implants and grafts

Excludes2:   failure and rejection of transplanted organs and tissue (T86.-)

The following extensions are to be added to each code for category T83:
a   initial encounter
d   subsequent encounter
q   sequela

T83.0   Mechanical complication of urinary (indwelling) catheter

Excludes2:   complications of stoma of urinary tract (N99.5-)

T83.01   Breakdown (mechanical) of urinary (indwelling) catheter

T83.010   Breakdown (mechanical) of cystostomy catheter

T83.018   Breakdown (mechanical) of other indwelling urethral catheter

T83.02   Displacement of urinary (indwelling) catheter
Malposition of urinary (indwelling) catheter

T83.020   Displacement of cystostomy catheter

T83.028   Displacement of other indwelling urethral catheter

T83.03   Leakage of urinary (indwelling) catheter

T83.030   Leakage of cystostomy catheter

T83.038   Leakage of other indwelling urethral catheter

T83.09   Other mechanical complication of urinary (indwelling) catheter
Obstruction (mechanical) of urinary (indwelling) catheter
Perforation of urinary (indwelling) catheter
Protrusion of urinary (indwelling) catheter

T83.090   Other mechanical complication of cystostomy catheter

T83.098   Other mechanical complication of other indwelling urethral catheter

T83.1   Mechanical complication of other urinary devices and implants

T83.11   Breakdown (mechanical) of other urinary devices and implants

T83.110   Breakdown (mechanical) of urinary electronic stimulator device

T83.111   Breakdown (mechanical) of urinary sphincter implant

T83.112   Breakdown (mechanical) of urinary stent

T83.118   Breakdown (mechanical) of other urinary devices and implants

T83.12   Displacement of other urinary devices and implants
Malposition of other urinary devices and implants

T83.120   Displacement of urinary electronic stimulator device

T83.121   Displacement of urinary sphincter implant

T83.122   Displacement of urinary stent

T83.128   Displacement of other urinary devices and implants

T83.19   Other mechanical complication of other urinary devices and implants
Leakage of other urinary devices and implants
Obstruction (mechanical) of other urinary devices and implants
Perforation of other urinary devices and implants
Protrusion of other urinary devices and implants

T83.190   Other mechanical complication of urinary electronic stimulator device

T83.191   Other mechanical complication of urinary sphincter implant

T83.192   Other mechanical complication of urinary stent

T83.198   Other mechanical complication of other urinary devices and implants

T83.2   Mechanical complication of graft of urinary organ

T83.21   Breakdown (mechanical) of graft of urinary organ

T83.22   Displacement of graft of urinary organ
Malposition of graft of urinary organ

T83.23   Leakage of graft of urinary organ

T83.29   Other mechanical complication of graft of urinary organ
Obstruction (mechanical) of graft of urinary organ
Perforation of graft of urinary organ
Protrusion of graft of urinary organ

T83.3   Mechanical complication of intrauterine contraceptive device

T83.31   Breakdown (mechanical) of intrauterine contraceptive device

T83.32   Displacement of intrauterine contraceptive device
Malposition of intrauterine contraceptive device

T83.39   Other mechanical complication of intrauterine contraceptive device
Leakage of intrauterine contraceptive device
Obstruction (mechanical) of intrauterine contraceptive device
Perforation of intrauterine contraceptive device
Protrusion of intrauterine contraceptive device

T83.4   Mechanical complication of other prosthestic devices, implants and grafts of genital tract

T83.41   Breakdown (mechanical) of other prosthetic devices, implants and grafts of genital tract

T83.410   Breakdown (mechanical) of penile (implanted) prosthesis

T83.418   Breakdown (mechanical) of other prosthestic devices, implants and grafts of genital tract

T83.42   Displacement of other prosthetic devices, implants and grafts of genital tract
Malposition of other prosthetic devices, implants and grafts of genital tract

T83.420   Displacement of penile (implanted) prosthesis

T83.428   Displacement of other prosthestic devices, implants and grafts of genital tract

T83.49   Other mechanical complication of other prosthestic devices, implants and grafts of genital tract
Leakage of other prosthetic devices, implants and grafts of genital tract
Obstruction, mechanical of other prosthetic devices, implants and grafts of genital tract
Perforation of other prosthetic devices, implants and grafts of genital tract
Protrusion of other prosthetic devices, implants and grafts of genital tract

T83.490   Other mechanical complication of penile (implanted) prosthesis

T83.498   Other mechanical complication of other prosthestic devices, implants and grafts of genital tract

T83.5   Infection and inflammatory reaction due to prosthetic device, implant and graft in urinary system
Use additional code to identify infection

T83.51   Infection and inflammatory reaction due to indwelling urinary catheter

T83.59   Infection and inflammatory reaction due to prosthetic device, implant and graft in urinary system

T83.6   Infection and inflammatory reaction due to prosthetic device, implant and graft in genital tract
Use additional code to identify infection

T83.8   Other complications of genitourinary prosthetic devices, implants and grafts

T82.81   Embolism of genitourinary prosthetic devices, implants and grafts

T82.82   Fibrosis of genitourinary prosthetic devices, implants and grafts

T82.83   Hemorrhage of genitourinary prosthetic devices, implants and grafts

T82.84   Pain from genitourinary prosthetic devices, implants and grafts

T82.85   Stenosis of genitourinary prosthetic devices, implants and grafts

T82.86   Thrombosis of genitourinary prosthetic devices, implants and grafts

T82.89   Other complication of genitourinary prosthetic devices, implants and grafts

T83.9   Unspecified complication of genitourinary prosthetic device, implant and graft

T84   Complications of internal orthopedic prosthetic devices, implants and grafts

Excludes1:   failure and rejection of transplanted organs and tissues (T86.-)
fracture of bone following insertion of orthopedic implant, joint prosthesis or bone plate (M96.6)

The following extensions are to be added to each code for category T84:

a   initial encounter
d   subsequent encounter
q   sequela

T84.0   Mechanical complication of internal joint prosthesis

T84.01   Breakdown (mechanical) of internal joint prosthesis

T84.010   Breakdown (mechanical) of internal right hip prosthesis

T84.011   Breakdown (mechanical) of internal left hip prosthesis

T84.012   Breakdown (mechanical) of internal right knee prosthesis

T84.013   Breakdown (mechanical) of internal left knee prosthesis

T84.018   Breakdown (mechanical) of other internal joint prosthesis

T84.019   Breakdown (mechanical) of unspecified internal joint prosthesis

T84.02   Displacement of internal joint prosthesis
Malposition of internal joint prosthesis

T84.020   Displacement of internal right hip prosthesis

T84.021   Displacement of internal left hip prosthesis

T84.022   Displacement of internal right knee prosthesis

T84.023   Displacement of internal left knee prosthesis

T84.028   Displacement of other internal joint prosthesis

T84.029   Displacement of unspecified internal joint prosthesis

T84.09   Other mechanical complication of internal joint prosthesis
Leakage of internal joint prosthesis
Obstruction (mechanical) of internal joint prosthesis
Perforation of internal joint prosthesis
Protrusion of internal joint prosthesis

T84.090   Other mechanical complication of internal right hip prosthesis

T84.091   Other mechanical complication of internal left hip prosthesis

T84.092   Other mechanical complication of internal right knee prosthesis

T84.093   Other mechanical complication of internal left knee prosthesis

T84.098   Other mechanical complication of other internal joint prosthesis

T84.099   Other mechanical complication of unspecified internal joint prosthesis

T84.1   Mechanical complication of internal fixation device of bones of limb

Excludes2:   mechanical complication of internal fixation device of bones of feet (T84.2-)
mechanical complication of internal fixation device of bones of fingers (T84.2-)
mechanical complication of internal fixation device of bones of hands (T84.2-)
mechanical complication of internal fixation device of bones of toes (T84.2-)

T84.11   Breakdown (mechanical) of internal fixation device of bones of limb

T84.110   Breakdown (mechanical) of internal fixation device of right humerus

T84.111   Breakdown (mechanical) of internal fixation device of left humerus

T84.112   Breakdown (mechanical) of internal fixation device of bone of right forearm

T84.113   Breakdown (mechanical) of internal fixation device of bone of left forearm

T84.114   Breakdown (mechanical) of internal fixation device of right femur

T84.115   Breakdown (mechanical) of internal fixation device of left femur

T84.116   Breakdown (mechanical) of internal fixation device of bone of right lower leg

T84.117   Breakdown (mechanical) of internal fixation device of bone of left lower leg

T84.119   Breakdown (mechanical) of internal fixation device of unspecified bone of limb

T84.12   Displacement of internal fixation device of bones of limb
Malposition of internal fixation device of bones of limb

T84.120   Displacement of internal fixation device of right humerus

T84.121   Displacement of internal fixation device of left humerus

T84.122   Displacement of internal fixation device of bone of right forearm

T84.123   Displacement of internal fixation device of bone of left forearm

T84.124   Displacement of internal fixation device of right femur

T84.125   Displacement of internal fixation device of left femur

T84.126   Displacement of internal fixation device of bone of right lower leg

T84.127   Displacement of internal fixation device of bone of left lower leg

T84.129   Displacement of internal fixation device of unspecified bone of limb

T84.19   Other mechanical complication of internal fixation device of bones of limb
Obstruction (mechanical) of internal fixation device of bones of limb
Perforation of internal fixation device of bones of limb
Protrusion of internal fixation device of bones of limb

T84.190   Other mechanical complication of internal fixation device of right humerus

T84.191   Other mechanical complication of internal fixation device of left humerus

T84.192   Other mechanical complication of internal fixation device of bone of right forearm

T84.193   Other mechanical complication of internal fixation device of bone of left forearm

T84.194   Other mechanical complication of internal fixation device of right femur

T84.195   Other mechanical complication of internal fixation device of left femur

T84.196   Other mechanical complication of internal fixation device of bone of right lower leg

T84.197   Other mechanical complication of internal fixation device of bone of left lower leg

T84.199   Other mechanical complication of internal fixation device of unspecified bone of limb

T84.2   Mechanical complication of internal fixation device of other bones

T84.21   Breakdown (mechanical) of internal fixation device of other bones

T84.210   Breakdown (mechanical) of internal fixation device of bones of hand and fingers

T84.213   Breakdown (mechanical) of internal fixation device of bones of foot and toes

T84.216   Breakdown (mechanical) of internal fixation device of vertebrae

T84.218   Breakdown (mechanical) of internal fixation device of other bones

T84.22   Displacement of internal fixation device of other bones

Malposition of internal fixation device of other bones

T84.220   Displacement of internal fixation device of bones of hand and fingers

T84.223   Displacement of internal fixation device of bones of foot and toes

T84.226   Displacement of internal fixation device of vertebrae

T84.228   Displacement of internal fixation device of other bones

T84.29   Other mechanical complication of internal fixation device of other bones

Obstruction (mechanical) of internal fixation device of other bones

Perforation of internal fixation device of other bones

Protrusion of internal fixation device of other bones

T84.290   Other mechanical complication of internal fixation device of bones of hand and fingers

T84.293   Other mechanical complication of internal fixation device of bones of foot and toes

T84.296   Other mechanical complication of internal fixation device of vertebrae

T84.298   Other mechanical complication of internal fixation device of other bones

T84.3   Mechanical complication of other bone devices, implants and grafts

Excludes2:   other complications of bone graft (T86.83-)

T84.31   Breakdown (mechanical) of other bone devices, implants and grafts

T84.310   Breakdown (mechanical) of electronic bone stimulator

T84.318   Breakdown (mechanical) of other bone devices, implants and grafts

T84.32   Displacement of other bone devices, implants and grafts

Malposition of other bone devices, implants and grafts

T84.320   Displacement of electronic bone stimulator

T84.328   Displacement of other bone devices, implants and grafts

T84.39   Other mechanical complication of other bone devices, implants and grafts

Obstruction (mechanical) of other bone devices, implants and grafts

Perforation of other bone devices, implants and grafts

Protrusion of other bone devices, implants and grafts

T84.390   Other mechanical complication of electronic bone stimulator

T84.398   Other mechanical complication of other bone devices, implants and grafts

T84.4   Mechanical complication of other internal orthopedic devices, implants and grafts

T84.41   Breakdown (mechanical) of other internal orthopedic devices, implants and grafts

T84.410   Breakdown (mechanical) of muscle and tendon graft

T84.418   Breakdown (mechanical) of other internal orthopedic devices, implants and grafts

T84.42   Displacement of other internal orthopedic devices, implants and grafts

Malposition of other internal orthopedic devices, implants and grafts

T84.420   Displacement of muscle and tendon graft

T84.428   Displacement of other internal orthopedic devices, implants and grafts

T84.49   Other mechanical complication of other internal orthopedic devices, implants and grafts

Obstruction (mechanical) of other internal orthopedic devices, implants and grafts

Perforation of other internal orthopedic devices, implants and grafts

Protrusion of other internal orthopedic devices, implants and grafts

T84.490   Other mechanical complication of muscle and tendon graft

T84.498   Other mechanical complication of other internal orthopedic devices, implants and grafts

T84.5   Infection and inflammatory reaction due to internal joint prosthesis

Use additional code to identify infection

T84.50   Infection and inflammatory reaction due to unspecified internal joint prosthesis

T84.51   Infection and inflammatory reaction due to internal right hip prosthesis

T84.52   Infection and inflammatory reaction due to internal left hip prosthesis

T84.53   Infection and inflammatory reaction due to internal right knee prosthesis

T84.54   Infection and inflammatory reaction due to internal left knee prosthesis

T84.59   Infection and inflammatory reaction due to other internal joint prosthesis

T84.6   Infection and inflammatory reaction due to internal fixation device

Use additional code to identify infection

T84.60   Infection and inflammatory reaction due to internal fixation device of unspecified site

T84.61   Infection and inflammatory reaction due to internal fixation device of arm

T84.610   Infection and inflammatory reaction due to internal fixation device of right humerus

T84.611   Infection and inflammatory reaction due to internal fixation device of left humerus

T84.612   Infection and inflammatory reaction due to internal fixation device of right radius

T84.613   Infection and inflammatory reaction due to internal fixation device of left radius

T84.614   Infection and inflammatory reaction due to internal fixation device of right ulna

T84.615   Infection and inflammatory reaction due to internal fixation device of left ulna

T84.619   Infection and inflammatory reaction due to internal fixation device of unspecified bone of arm

T84.62   Infection and inflammatory reaction due to internal fixation device of leg

T84.620   Infection and inflammatory reaction due to internal fixation device of right femur

T84.621   Infection and inflammatory reaction due to internal fixation device of left femur

T84.622   Infection and inflammatory reaction due to internal fixation device of right tibia

T84.623   Infection and inflammatory reaction due to internal fixation device of left tibia

T84.624   Infection and inflammatory reaction due to internal fixation device of right fibula

T84.625   Infection and inflammatory reaction due to internal fixation device of left fibula

T84.629   Infection and inflammatory reaction due to internal fixation device of unspecified bone of leg

T84.63   Infection and inflammatory reaction due to internal fixation device of spine

T84.69   Infection and inflammatory reaction due to internal fixation device of other site

T84.7 Infection and inflammatory reaction due to other internal orthopedic prosthetic devices, implants and grafts

Use additional code to identify infection

T84.8 Other complications of internal orthopedic prosthetic devices, implants and grafts

T84.81 Embolism of internal orthopedic prosthetic devices, implants and grafts

T84.82 Fibrosis of internal orthopedic prosthetic devices, implants and grafts

T84.83 Hemorrhage of internal orthopedic prosthetic devices, implants and grafts

T84.84 Pain from internal orthopedic prosthetic devices, implants and grafts

T84.85 Stenosis of internal orthopedic prosthetic devices, implants and grafts

T84.86 Thrombosis of internal orthopedic prosthetic devices, implants and grafts

T84.89 Other complication of internal orthopedic prosthetic devices, implants and grafts

T84.9 Unspecified complication of internal orthopedic prosthetic device, implant and graft

T85 Complications of other internal prosthetic devices, implants and grafts

Excludes2: failure and rejection of transplanted organs and tissue (T86.-)

The following extensions are to be added to each code for category T85:

  a initial encounter
  d subsequent encounter
  q sequelae

T85.0 Mechanical complication of ventricular intracranial (communicating) shunt

T85.01 Breakdown (mechanical) of ventricular intracranial (communicating) shunt

T85.02 Displacement of ventricular intracranial (communicating) shunt

Malposition of ventricular intracranial (communicating) shunt

T85.03 Leakage of ventricular intracranial (communicating) shunt

T85.09 Other mechanical complication of ventricular intracranial (communicating) shunt

Obstruction (mechanical) of ventricular intracranial (communicating) shunt

Perforation of ventricular intracranial (communicating) shunt

Protrusion of ventricular intracranial (communicating) shunt

T85.1 Mechanical complication of implanted electronic stimulator of nervous system

T85.11 Breakdown (mechanical) of implanted electronic stimulator of nervous system

T85.110 Breakdown (mechanical) of implanted electronic neurostimulator (electrode) of brain

T85.111 Breakdown (mechanical) of implanted electronic neurostimulator (electrode) of peripheral nerve

T85.112 Breakdown (mechanical) of implanted electronic neurostimulator (electrode) of spinal cord

T85.118 Breakdown (mechanical) of other implanted electronic stimulator of nervous system

T85.12 Displacement of implanted electronic stimulator of nervous system

Malposition of implanted electronic stimulator of nervous system

T85.120 Displacement of implanted electronic neurostimulator (electrode) of brain

T85.121 Displacement of implanted electronic neurostimulator (electrode) of peripheral nerve

T85.122 Displacement of implanted electronic neurostimulator (electrode) of spinal cord

T85.128 Displacement of other implanted electronic stimulator of nervous system

T85.19 Other mechanical complication of implanted electronic stimulator of nervous system

Leakage of implanted electronic stimulator of nervous system

Obstruction (mechanical) of implanted electronic stimulator of nervous system

Perforation of implanted electronic stimulator of nervous system

Protrusion of implanted electronic stimulator of nervous system

T85.190 Other mechanical complication of implanted electronic neurostimulator (electrode) of brain

T85.191 Other mechanical complication of implanted electronic neurostimulator (electrode) of peripheral nerve

T85.192 Other mechanical complication of implanted electronic neurostimulator (electrode) of spinal cord

T85.199 Other mechanical complication of other implanted electronic stimulator of nervous system

T85.2 Mechanical complication of intraocular lens

T85.21 Breakdown (mechanical) of intraocular lens

T85.22 Displacement of intraocular lens

Malposition of intraocular lens

T85.29 Other mechanical complication of intraocular lens

Obstruction (mechanical) of intraocular lens

Perforation of intraocular lens

Protrusion of intraocular lens

T85.3 Mechanical complication of other ocular prosthetic devices, implants and grafts

Excludes2: other complications of corneal graft (T86.84-)

T85.31 Breakdown (mechanical) of other ocular prosthetic devices, implants and grafts

T85.310 Breakdown (mechanical) of prosthetic orbit of right eye

T85.311 Breakdown (mechanical) of prosthetic orbit of left eye

T85.318 Breakdown (mechanical) of other ocular prosthetic devices, implants and grafts

T85.32 Displacement of other ocular prosthetic devices, implants and grafts

Malposition of other ocular prosthetic devices, implants and grafts

T85.320 Displacement of prosthetic orbit of right eye

T85.321 Displacement of prosthetic orbit of left eye

T85.328 Displacement of other ocular prosthetic devices, implants and grafts

T85.39 Other mechanical complication of other ocular prosthetic devices, implants and grafts

Obstruction (mechanical) of other ocular prosthetic devices, implants and grafts

Perforation of other ocular prosthetic devices, implants and grafts

Protrusion of other ocular prosthetic devices, implants and grafts

T85.390 Other mechanical complication of prosthetic orbit of right eye

T85.391 Other mechanical complication of prosthetic orbit of left eye

T85.398 Other mechanical complication of other ocular prosthetic devices, implants and grafts

T85.4 Mechanical complication of breast prosthesis and implant

T85.41 Breakdown (mechanical) of breast prosthesis and implant

T85.42 Displacement of breast prosthesis and implant

Malposition of breast prosthesis and implant

T85.43 Leakage of breast prosthesis and implant

T85.49   **Other mechanical complication of breast prosthesis and implant**

Obstruction (mechanical) of breast prosthesis and implant

Perforation of breast prosthesis and implant

Protrusion of breast prosthesis and implant

T85.5   **Mechanical complication of gastrointestinal prosthetic devices, implants and grafts**

T85.51   **Breakdown (mechanical) of gastrointestinal prosthetic devices, implants and grafts**

T85.510   **Breakdown (mechanical) of bile duct prosthesis**

T85.511   **Breakdown (mechanical) of esophageal anti-reflux device**

T85.518   **Breakdown (mechanical) of other gastrointestinal prosthetic devices, implants and grafts**

T85.52   **Displacement of gastrointestinal prosthetic devices, implants and grafts**

Malposition of gastrointestinal prosthetic devices, implants and grafts

T85.520   **Displacement of bile duct prosthesis**

T85.521   **Displacement of esophageal anti-reflux device**

T85.528   **Displacement of other gastrointestinal prosthetic devices, implants and grafts**

T85.59   **Other mechanical complication of gastrointestinal prosthetic devices, implants and grafts**

Obstruction, mechanical of gastrointestinal prosthetic devices, implants and grafts

Perforation of gastrointestinal prosthetic devices, implants and grafts

Protrusion of gastrointestinal prosthetic devices, implants and grafts

T85.590   **Other mechanical complication of bile duct prosthesis**

T85.591   **Other mechanical complication of esophageal anti-reflux device**

T85.598   **Other mechanical complication of other gastrointestinal prosthetic devices, implants and grafts**

T85.6   **Mechanical complication of other specified internal prosthetic devices, implants and grafts**

T85.61   **Breakdown (mechanical) of other specified internal prosthetic devices, implants and grafts**

T85.610   **Breakdown (mechanical) of epidural and subdural infusion catheter**

T85.611   **Breakdown (mechanical) of intraperitoneal dialysis catheter**

Excludes1:   mechanical complication of vascular dialysis catheter (T82.4-)

T85.612   **Breakdown (mechanical) of permanent sutures**

Excludes1:   mechanical complication of permanent (wire) suture used in bone repair (T84.1-T84.2)

T85.613   **Breakdown (mechanical) of artificial skin graft and decellularized allodermis**

Failure of artificial skin graft and decellularized allodermis

Non-adherence of artificial skin graft and decellularized allodermis

Poor incorporation of artificial skin graft and decellularized allodermis

Shearing of artificial skin graft and decellularized allodermis

T85.618   **Breakdown (mechanical) of other specified internal prosthetic devices, implants and grafts**

T85.62   **Displacement of other specified internal prosthetic devices, implants and grafts**

Malposition of other specified internal prosthetic devices, implants and grafts

T85.620   **Displacement of epidural and subdural infusion catheter**

T85.621   **Displacement of intraperitoneal dialysis catheter**

Excludes1:   mechanical complication of vascular dialysis catheter (T82.4-)

T85.622   **Displacement of permanent sutures**

Excludes1:   mechanical complication of permanent (wire) suture used in bone repair (T84.1-T84.2)

T85.623   **Displacement of artificial skin graft and decellularized allodermis**

Dislodgement of artificial skin graft and decellularized allodermis

Displacement of artificial skin graft and decellularized allodermis

T85.628   **Displacement of other specified internal prosthetic devices, implants and grafts**

T85.63   **Leakage of other specified internal prosthetic devices, implants and grafts**

T85.630   **Leakage of epidural and subdural infusion catheter**

T85.631   **Leakage of intraperitoneal dialysis catheter**

Excludes1:   mechanical complication of vascular dialysis catheter (T82.4)

T85.68   **Leakage of other specified internal prosthetic devices, implants and grafts**

T85.69   **Other mechanical complication of other specified internal prosthetic devices, implants and grafts**

Obstruction, mechanical of other specified internal prosthetic devices, implants and grafts

Perforation of other specified internal prosthetic devices, implants and grafts

Protrusion of other specified internal prosthetic devices, implants and grafts

T85.690   **Other mechanical complication of epidural and subdural infusion catheter**

T85.691   **Other mechanical complication of intraperitoneal dialysis catheter**

Excludes1:   mechanical complication of vascular dialysis catheter (T82.4)

T85.692   **Other mechanical complication of permanent sutures**

Excludes1:   mechanical complication of permanent (wire) suture used in bone repair (T84.1-T84.2)

T85.693   **Other mechanical complication of artificial skin graft and decellularized allodermis**

T85.698   **Other mechanical complication of other specified internal prosthetic devices, implants and grafts**

Mechanical complication of nonabsorbable surgical material NOS

T85.7   **Infection and inflammatory reaction due to other internal prosthetic devices, implants and grafts**

Use additional code to identify infection

T85.71   **Infection and inflammatory reaction due to peritoneal dialysis catheter**

T85.79   **Infection and inflammatory reaction due to other internal prosthetic devices, implants and grafts**

T85.8   **Other complications of internal prosthetic devices, implants and grafts, not elsewhere classified**

T85.81   **Embolism of internal prosthetic devices, implants and grafts, not elsewhere classified**

T85.82   **Fibrosis of internal prosthetic devices, implants and grafts, not elsewhere classified**

T85.83   **Hemorrhage of internal prosthetic devices, implants and grafts, not elsewhere classified**

T85.84   Pain from internal prosthetic devices, implants and grafts, not elsewhere classified

T85.85   Stenosis of internal prosthetic devices, implants and grafts, not elsewhere classified

T85.86   Thrombosis of internal prosthetic devices, implants and grafts, not elsewhere classified

T85.89   Other complication of internal prosthetic devices, implants and grafts, not elsewhere classified

T85.9   Unspecified complication of internal prosthetic device, implant and graft
  Complication of internal prosthetic device, implant and graft NOS

T86 Complications of transplanted organs and tissue
  T86.0   Complications of bone-marrow transplant
    T86.00   Unspecified complication of bone-marrow transplant
    T86.01   Graft-versus-host reaction or disease
    T86.09   Other complications of bone-marrow transplant
  T86.1   Complications of kidney transplant
    T86.10   Unspecified complication of kidney transplant
    T86.11   Kidney transplant rejection
    T86.12   Kidney transplant failure
    T86.13   Kidney transplant infection
      Use additional code to specify infection
    T86.19   Other complication of kidney transplant
  T86.2   Complications of heart transplant
    Excludes1:   complication of:
      artificial heart device (T82.5)
      heart-lung transplant (T86.3)
    T86.20   Unspecified complication of heart transplant
    T86.21   Heart transplant rejection
    T86.22   Heart transplant failure
    T86.23   Heart transplant infection
      Use additional code to specify infection
    T86.29   Other complications of heart transplant
  T86.3   Complications of heart-lung transplant
    T86.30   Unspecified complication of heart-lung transplant
    T86.31   Heart-lung transplant rejection
    T86.32   Heart-lung transplant failure
    T86.33   Heart-lung transplant infection
      Use additional code to specify infection
    T86.39   Other complications of heart-lung transplant
  T86.4   Complications of liver transplant
    T86.40   Unspecified complication of liver transplant
    T86.41   Liver transplant rejection
    T86.42   Liver transplant failure
    T86.43   Liver transplant infection
      Use additional code to identify infection, such as:
      cytomegalovirus (CMV) infection (B25.-)
    T86.49   Other complications of liver transplant
  T86.8   Complications of other transplanted organs and tissues
    T86.81   Complications of lung transplant
      Excludes1:   complication of heart-lung transplant (T86.3-)
      T86.810   Lung transplant rejection
      T86.811   Lung transplant failure
      T86.812   Lung transplant infection
        Use additional code to specify infection
      T86.818   Other complications of lung transplant
      T86.819   Unspecified complication of lung transplant
    T86.82   Complications of skin graft (allograft) (autograft)
      Excludes2:   complication of artificial skin graft (T85.64)
      T86.820   Skin graft (allograft) rejection
      T86.821   Skin graft (allograft) (autograft) failure
      T86.822   Skin graft (allograft) (autograft) infection
        Use additional code to specify infection
      T86.828   Other complications of skin graft (allograft) (autograft)
      T86.829   Unspecified complication of skin graft (allograft) (autograft)

T86.83   Complications of bone graft
  Excludes2:   mechanical complications of bone graft (T84.3-)
  T86.830   Bone graft rejection
  T86.831   Bone graft failure
  T86.832   Bone graft infection
    Use additional code to specify infection
  T86.838   Other complications of bone graft
  T86.839   Unspecified complication of bone graft
T86.84   Complications of corneal transplant
  Excludes2:   mechanical complications of corneal graft (T85.3-)
  T86.840   Corneal transplant rejection
  T86.841   Corneal transplant failure
  T86.842   Corneal transplant infection
    Use additional code to specify infection
  T86.848   Other complications of corneal transplant
  T86.849   Unspecified complication of corneal transplant
T86.85   Complication of intestine transplant
  T86.850   Intestine transplant rejection
  T86.851   Intestine transplant failure
  T86.852   Intestine transplant infection
    Use additional code to specify infection
  T86.858   Other complications of intestine transplant
  T86.859   Unspecified complication of intestine transplant
T86.89   Complications of other transplanted tissue
  Transplant failure or rejection of pancreas
  T86.890   Other transplanted tissue rejection
  T86.891   Other transplanted tissue failure
  T86.892   Other transplanted tissue infection
    Use additional code to specify infection
  T86.898   Other complications of other transplanted tissue
  T86.899   Unspecified complication of other transplanted tissue
T86.9   Complication of unspecified transplanted organ and tissue
  T86.90   Unspecified complication of unspecified transplanted organ and tissue
  T86.91   Unspecified transplanted organ and tissue rejection
  T86.92   Unspecified transplanted organ and tissue failure
  T86.93   Unspecified transplanted organ and tissue infection
    Use additional code to specify infection
  T86.99   Other complications of unspecified transplanted organ and tissue

T87 Complications peculiar to reattachment and amputation
  T87.0   Complications of reattached (part of) upper extremity
    T87.00   Complications of reattached (part of) upper extremity, unspecified side
    T87.01   Complications of reattached (part of) right upper extremity
    T87.02   Complications of reattached (part of) left upper extremity
  T87.1   Complications of reattached (part of) lower extremity
    T87.10   Complications of reattached (part of) lower extremity, unspecified side
    T87.11   Complications of reattached (part of) right lower extremity
    T87.12   Complications of reattached (part of) left lower extremity
  T87.2   Complications of other reattached body part
  T87.3   Neuroma of amputation stump
    T87.30   Neuroma of amputation stump, unspecified extremity
    T87.31   Neuroma of amputation stump, right upper extremity
    T87.32   Neuroma of amputation stump, left upper extremity
    T87.33   Neuroma of amputation stump, right lower extremity
    T87.34   Neuroma of amputation stump, left lower extremity
  T87.4   Infection of amputation stump
    T87.40   Infection of amputation stump, unspecified extremity

T87.41   Infection of amputation stump, right upper extremity
T87.42   Infection of amputation stump, left upper extremity
T87.43   Infection of amputation stump, right lower extremity
T87.44   Infection of amputation stump, left lower extremity

T87.5 Necrosis of amputation stump
T87.50   Necrosis of amputation stump, unspecified extremity
T87.51   Necrosis of amputation stump, right upper extremity
T87.52   Necrosis of amputation stump, left upper extremity
T87.53   Necrosis of amputation stump, right lower extremity
T87.54   Necrosis of amputation stump, left lower extremity

T87.8 Other complications of amputation stump
Amputation stump contracture
Amputation stump contracture of next proximal joint
Amputation stump edema
Amputation stump flexion
Amputation stump hematoma
Excludes2:   phantom limb syndrome (G54.6-G54.7)

T87.9 Unspecified complications of amputation stump

T88 Other complications of surgical and medical care, not elsewhere classified
Excludes2:   complication following:
infusion, transfusion and therapeutic injection (T80.-)
procedure NEC (T81.-)
specified complications classified elsewhere, such as:
complication of:
anesthesia in:
labor and delivery (O74.-)
pregnancy (O29.-)
puerperium (O89.-)
devices, implants and grafts (T82-T85)
obstetric surgery and procedure (O75.4)
dermatitis due to drugs and medicaments (L23.3, L24.4, L25.1, L27.0-L27.1)
poisoning and toxic effects of drugs and chemicals (T36-T65)
The following extensions are to be added to each code for category T88:
a   initial encounter
d   subsequent encounter
q   sequela

T88.0 Infection following immunization
Sepsis following immunization
Septicemia following immunization

T88.1 Other complications following immunization, not elsewhere classified
Rash following immunization
Excludes2:   anaphylactic shock due to serum (T80.5)
other serum reactions (T80.6)
postimmunization:
arthropathy (M02.2)
encephalitis (G04.0)

T88.2 Shock due to anesthesia
Shock due to anesthesia in which the correct substance was properly administered
Excludes1:   complications of anesthesia (in):
from overdose or wrong substance given (T36-T50)
labor and delivery (O74.-)
postoperative shock NOS (T81.1)
pregnancy (O29.-)
puerperium (O89.-)

T88.3 Malignant hyperthermia due to anesthesia

T88.4 Failed or difficult intubation

T88.5 Other complications of anesthesia
Hypothermia following anesthesia

T88.6 Anaphylactic shock due to adverse effect of correct drug or medicament substance properly administered
Excludes1:   anaphylactic shock due to serum (T80.5)
Use additional external cause code to identify drug (Y40-T59)

T88.7 Unspecified adverse effect of drug or medicament
Note: This code is not for use in the inpatient environment and is for limited use in the outpatient environment only when no sign or symptom of the adverse effect is documented
Drug hypersensitivity NOS
Drug reaction NOS
Excludes1:   specified adverse effects of drugs and medicaments (A00-R94 and T80-T88.6, T88.8)

T88.8 Other specified complications of surgical and medical care, not elsewhere classified

T88.9 Complication of surgical and medical care, unspecified

*Categories T90-T98 deactivated. Replaced with extension q

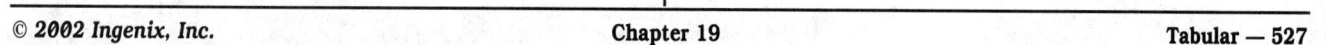

CHAPTER XX — EXTERNAL CAUSES OF MORBIDITY (V01–Y98)

This chapter permits the classification of environmental events and circumstances as the cause of injury, and other adverse effects. Where a code from this section is applicable, it is intended that it shall be used in addition to a code from another chapter of the Classification indicating the nature of the condition. Most often, the condition will be classifiable to Chapter XIX, Injury, poisoning and certain other consequences of external causes (S00-T98). Other conditions that may be stated to be due to external causes are classified in Chapters I to XVIII. For these conditions, codes from Chapter XX should be used to provide additional information as to the cause of the condition.

This chapter contains the following blocks:

TRANSPORT ACCIDENTS (V00-V99)

Note: This section is structured in 12 groups. Those relating to land transport accidents (V01-V89) reflect the victim's mode of transport and are subdivided to identify the victim's "counterpart" or the type of event. The vehicle of which the injured person is an occupant is identified in the first two characters since it is seen as the most important factor to identify for prevention purposes. A transport accident is one in which the vehicle involved must be moving or running or in use for transport purposes at the time of the accident.

Use additional code to identify:

    use of electronic equipment at the time of the transport accident (Y93.5-)

    type of street or road (Y92.4-)

    place of occurrence (Y92.-)

Excludes 1: agricultural vehicles in stationary use or maintenance (W31.-)

    assault by crashing of motor vehicle (Y03.-)

    automobile or motor cycle in stationary use or maintenance — code to type of accident

    crashing of motor vehicle, undetermined intent (Y32)

    intentional self-harm by crashing of motor vehicle (X82)

Excludes 2: transport accidents due to cataclysm (X34-X38)

PEDESTRIAN INJURED IN TRANSPORT ACCIDENT (V00–V09)

Includes: person changing tire on transport vehicle

    person examining engine of vehicle broken down in (on side of) road

Excludes1: fall due to non-transport collision with other person (W03)

    pedestrian on foot falling (slipping) on ice and snow (W00.-)

    struck or bumped by another person (W51)

V00 Pedestrian conveyance accident

Use additional place of occurance and activity external cause codes, if known (Y92.-, Y93.-)

Excludes1: collision with another person without fall (W51)

    fall due to person on foot colliding with another person on foot (W03)

    fall from wheelchair without collision (W05)

    pedestrian (conveyance) collision with other land transport vehicle (V01-V09)

    pedestrian on foot falling (slipping) on ice and snow (W00.-)

The following extensions are to be added to each code from category V00:

    a initial encounter

    d subsequent encounter

    q sequelae

V00.0 Pedestrian on foot injured in collision with pedestrian conveyance

V00.01 Pedestrian on foot injured in collision with roller-skater

V00.02 Pedestrian on foot injured in collision with skateboarder

V00.09 Pedestrian on foot injured in collision with other pedestrian conveyance

V00.1 Rolling-type pedestrian conveyance accident

Excludes1: accident with babystroller (V00.82-)

    accident with wheelchair (powered) (V00.81-)

V00.11 In-line roller-skate accident

V00.111 Fall from in-line roller-skates

V00.112 In-line roller-skater colliding with stationary object

V00.118 Other in-line roller-skate accident

Excludes1: roller-skater collision with other land transport vehicle (V01-V09 with 5th character 1)

V00.12 Non-in-line roller-skate accident

V00.121 Fall from non-in-line roller-skates

V00.122 Non-in-line roller-skater colliding with stationary object

V00.128   Other non-in-line roller-skating accident

     Excludes1:   roller-skater collision with other land transport vehicle (V01-V09 with 5th character 1)

V00.13   Skateboard accident

V00.131   Fall from skateboard

V00.132   Skateboarder colliding with stationary object

V00.138   Other skateboard accident

     Excludes1:   skateboarder collision with other land transport vehicle (V01-V09 with 5th character 2)

V00.14   Scooter (nonmotorized) accident

     Excludes1:   motorscooter accident (V20-V29)

V00.141   Fall from scooter (nonmotorized)

V00.142   Scooterer (nonmotorized) colliding with stationary object

V00.148   Other scooter (nonmotorized) accident

     Excludes1:   scooterer (nonmotorized) collision with other land transport vehicle (V01-V09 with fifth character 9)

V00.18   Accident on other rolling-type pedestrian conveyance

V00.181   Fall from other rolling-type pedestrian conveyance

V00.182   Pedestrian on other rolling-type pedestrian conveyance colliding with stationary object

V00.188   Other accident on other rolling-type pedestrian conveyance

V00.2   Gliding-type pedestrian conveyance accident

V00.21   Ice-skates accident

V00.211   Fall from ice-skates

V00.212   Ice-skater colliding with stationary object

V00.218   Other ice-skates accident

     Excludes1:   ice-skater collision with other land transport vehicle (V01-V09 with 5th digit 9)

V00.22   Sled accident

V00.221   Fall from sled

V00.222   Sleder colliding with stationary object

V00.228   Other sled accident

     Excludes1:   sled collision with other land transport vehicle (V01-V09 with 5th digit 9)

V00.28   Other gliding-type pedestrian conveyance accident

V00.281   Fall from other gliding-type pedestrian conveyance

V00.282   Pedestrian on other gliding-type pedestrian conveyance colliding with stationary object

V00.288   Other accident on other gliding-type pedestrian conveyance

     Excludes1:   gliding-type pedestrain conveyance collision with other land transport vehicle (V01-V09 with 5th digit 9)

V00.3   Flat-bottomed pedestrian conveyance accident

V00.31   Snowboard accident

V00.311   Fall from snowboard

V00.312   Snowboarder colliding with stationary object

V00.318   Other snowboard accident

     Excludes1:   snowboarder collision with other land transport vehicle (V01-V09 with 5th digit 9)

V00.32   Snow-ski accident

V00.321   Fall from snow-skis

V00.322   Snow-skier colliding with stationary object

V00.328   Other snow-ski accident

     Excludes1:   snow-skier collision with other land transport vehicle (V01-V09 with 5th digit 9)

V00.38   Other flat-bottomed pedestrian conveyance accident

V00.381   Fall from other flat-bottomed pedestrian conveyance

V00.382   Pedestrian on other flat-bottomed pedestrian conveyance colliding with stationary object

V00.388   Other accident on other flat-bottomed pedestrian conveyance

V00.8   Accident on other pedestrian conveyance

V00.81   Accident with wheelchair (powered)

V00.811   Fall from moving wheelchair (powered)

     Excludes1:   fall from non-moving wheelchair (W05)

V00.812   Wheelchair (powered) colliding with stationary object

V00.818   Other accident with wheelchair (powered)

V00.82   Accident with babystroller

V00.821   Fall from babystroller

V00.822   Babystroller colliding with stationary object

V00.828   Other accident with babystroller

V00.89   Accident on other pedestrian conveyance

V00.891   Fall from other pedestrian conveyance

V00.892   Pedestrian on other pedestrian conveyance colliding with stationary object

V00.898   Other accident on other pedestrian conveyance

     Excludes1:   other pedestrian (conveyance) collision with other land transport vehicle (V01-V09 with 5th digit 9)

V01   Pedestrian injured in collision with pedal cycle

The following extensions are to be added to each code from category V01:

     a   initial encounter

     d   subsequent encounter

     q   sequelae

V01.0   Pedestrian injured in collision with pedal cycle in nontraffic accident

V01.00   Pedestrian on foot injured in collision with pedal cycle in nontraffic accident

     Pedestrian NOS injured in collision with pedal cycle in nontraffic accident

V01.01   Pedestrian on roller-skates injured in collision with pedal cycle in nontraffic accident

V01.02   Pedestrian on skateboard injured in collision with pedal cycle in nontraffic accident

V01.09   Pedestrain with other conveyance injured in collision with pedal cycle in nontraffic accident

     Pedestrian with babystroller injured in collision with pedal cycle in nontraffic accident

     Pedestrian on ice-skates injured in collision with pedal cycle in nontraffic accident

     Pedestrian on sled injured in collision with pedal cycle in nontraffic accident

     Pedestrian on snowboard injured in collision with pedal cycle in nontraffic accident

     Pedestrian on snow-skis injured in collision with pedal cycle in nontraffic accident

     Pedestrian in wheelchair (powered) injured in collision with pedal cycle in nontraffic accident

V01.1   Pedestrian injured in collision with pedal cycle in traffic accident

V01.10   Pedestrian on foot injured in collision with pedal cycle in traffic accident

     Pedestrian NOS injured in collision with pedal cycle in traffic accident

V01.11   Pedestrian on roller-skates injured in collision with pedal cycle in traffic accident

V01.12 **Pedestrian on skateboard injured in collision with pedal cycle in traffic accident**

V01.19 **Pedestrain with other conveyance injured in collision with pedal cycle in traffic accident**

Pedestrian with babystroller injured in collision with pedal cycle in traffic accident

Pedestrian on ice-skates injured in collision with pedal cycle in traffic accident

Pedestrian on sled injured in collision with pedal cycle in traffic accident

Pedestrian on snowboard injured in collision with pedal cycle in traffic accident

Pedestrian on snow-skis injured in collision with pedal cycle in traffic accident

Pedestrian in wheelchair (powered) injured in collision with pedal cycle in traffic accident

V01.9 **Pedestrian injured in collision with pedal cycle, unspecified whether traffic or nontraffic accident**

V01.90 **Pedestrian on foot injured in collision with pedal cycle, unspecified whether traffic or nontraffic accident**

Pedestrian NOS injured in collision with pedal cycle, unspecified whether traffic or nontraffic accident

V01.91 **Pedestrian on roller-skates injured in collision with pedal cycle, unspecified whether traffic or nontraffic accident**

V01.92 **Pedestrian on skateboard injured in collision with pedal cycle, unspecified whether traffic or nontraffic accident**

V01.99 **Pedestrain with other conveyance injured in collision with pedal cycle, unspecified whether traffic or nontraffic accident**

Pedestrian with babystroller injured in collision with pedal cycle, unspecified whether traffic or nontraffic accident

Pedestrian on ice-skates injured in collision with pedal cycle unspecified, whether traffic or nontraffic accident

Pedestrian on sled injured in collision with pedal cycle unspecified, whether traffic or nontraffic accident

Pedestrian on snowboard injured in collision with pedal cycle, unspecified whether traffic or nontraffic accident

Pedestrian on snow-skis injured in collision with pedal cycle, unspecified whether traffic or nontraffic accident

Pedestrian in wheelchair (powered) injured in collision with pedal cycle, unspecified whether traffic or nontraffic accident

V02 **Pedestrian injured in collision with two- or three-wheeled motor vehicle**

The following extensions are to be added to each code from category V02:

    a   initial encounter
    d   subsequent encounter
    q   sequelae

V02.0 **Pedestrian injured in collision with two- or three-wheeled motor vehicle in nontraffic accident**

V02.00 **Pedestrian on foot injured in collision with two- or three-wheeled motor vehicle in nontraffic accident**

Pedestrian NOS injured in collision with two- or three-wheeled motor vehicle in nontraffic accident

V02.01 **Pedestrian on roller-skates injured in collision with two- or three-wheeled motor vehicle in nontraffic accident**

V02.02 **Pedestrian on skateboard injured in collision with two- or three-wheeled motor vehicle in nontraffic accident**

V02.09 **Pedestrian with other conveyance injured in collision with two- or three-wheeled motor vehicle in nontraffic accident**

Pedestrian with babystroller injured in collision with two- or three-wheeled motor vehicle in nontraffic accident

Pedestrian on ice-skates injured in collision with two- or three-wheeled motor vehicle in nontraffic accident

Pedestrian on sled injured in collision with two- or three-wheeled motor vehicle in nontraffic accident

Pedestrian on snowboard injured in collision with two- or three-wheeled motor vehicle in nontraffic accident

Pedestrian on snow-skis injured in collision with two- or three-wheeled motor vehicle in nontraffic accident

Pedestrian in wheelchair (powered) injured in collision with two- or three-wheeled motor vehicle in nontraffic accident

V02.1 **Pedestrian injured in collision with two- or three-wheeled motor vehicle in traffic accident**

V02.10 **Pedestrian on foot injured in collision with two- or three-wheeled motor vehicle in traffic accident**

Pedestrian NOS injured in collision with two- or three-wheeled motor vehicle in traffic accident

V02.11 **Pedestrian on roller-skates injured in collision with two- or three-wheeled motor vehicle in traffic accident**

V02.12 **Pedestrian on skateboard injured in collision with two- or three-wheeled motor vehicle in traffic accident**

V02.19 **Pedestrian with other conveyance injured in collision with two- or three-wheeled motor vehicle in traffic accident**

Pedestrian with babystroller injured in collision with two- or three-wheeled motor vehicle in traffic accident

Pedestrian on ice-skates injured in collision with two- or three-wheeled motor vehicle in traffic accident

Pedestrian on sled injured in collision with two- or three-wheeled motor vehicle in traffic accident

Pedestrian on snowboard injured in collision with two- or three-wheeled motor vehicle in traffic accident

Pedestrian on snow-skis injured in collision with two- or three-wheeled motor vehicle in traffic accident

Pedestrian in wheelchair (powered) injured in collision with two- or three-wheeled motor vehicle in traffic accident

V02.9 **Pedestrian injured in collision with two- or three-wheeled motor vehicle, unspecified whether traffic or nontraffic accident**

V02.90 **Pedestrian on foot injured in collision with two- or three-wheeled motor vehicle, unspecified whether traffic or nontraffic accident**

Pedestrian NOS injured in collision with two- or three-wheeled motor vehicle, unspecified whether traffic or nontraffic accident

V02.91 **Pedestrian on roller-skates injured in collision with two- or three-wheeled motor vehicle, unspecified whether traffic or nontraffic accident**

V02.92 **Pedestrian on skateboard injured in collision with two- or three-wheeled motor vehicle, unspecified whether traffic or nontraffic accident**

V02.99   **Pedestrian with other conveyance injured in collision with two- or three-wheeled motor vehicle, unspecified whether traffic or nontraffic accident**

Pedestrian with babystroller injured in collision with two- or three-wheeled motor vehicle, unspecified whether traffic or nontraffic accident

Pedestrian on ice-skates injured in collision with two- or three-wheeled motor vehicle, unspecified whether traffic or nontraffic accident

Pedestrian on sled injured in collision with two- or three-wheeled motor vehicle, unspecified whether traffic or nontraffic accident

Pedestrian on snowboard injured in collision with two- or three-wheeled motor vehicle, unspecified whether traffic or nontraffic accident

Pedestrian on snow-skis injured in collision with two- or three-wheeled motor vehicle, unspecified whether traffic or nontraffic accident

Pedestrian in wheelchair (powered) injured in collision with two- or three-wheeled motor vehicle, unspecified whether traffic or nontraffic accident

V03   **Pedestrian injured in collision with car, pick-up truck or van**

The following extensions are to be added to each code from category V03:

a   initial encounter
d   subsequent encounter
q   sequelae

V03.0   **Pedestrian injured in collision with car, pick-up truck or van in nontraffic accident**

V03.00   **Pedestrian on foot injured in collision with car, pick-up truck or van in nontraffic accident**

Pedestrian NOS injured in collision with car, pick-up truck or van in nontraffic accident

V03.01   **Pedestrian on roller-skates injured in collision with car, pick-up truck or van in nontraffic accident**

V03.02   **Pedestrian on skateboard injured in collision with car, pick-up truck or van in nontraffic accident**

V03.09   **Pedestrian with other conveyance injured in collision with car, pick-up truck or van in nontraffic accident**

Pedestrian with babystroller injured in collision with car, pick-up truck or van in nontraffic accident

Pedestrian on ice-skates injured in collision with car, pick-up truck or van in nontraffic accident

Pedestrian on sled injured in collision with car, pick-up truck or van in nontraffic accident

Pedestrian on snowboard injured in collision with car, pick-up truck or van in nontraffic accident

Pedestrian on snow-skis injured in collision with car, pick-up truck or van in nontraffic accident

Pedestrian in wheelchair (powered) injured in collision with car, pick-up truck or van in nontraffic accident

V03.1   **Pedestrian injured in collision with car, pick-up truck or van in traffic accident**

V03.10   **Pedestrian on foot injured in collision with car, pick-up truck or van in traffic accident**

Pedestrian NOS injured in collision with car, pick-up truck or van in traffic accident

V03.11   **Pedestrian on roller-skates injured in collision with car, pick-up truck or van in traffic accident**

V03.12   **Pedestrian on skateboard injured in collision with car, pick-up truck or van in traffic accident**

V03.19   **Pedestrian with other conveyance injured in collision with car, pick-up truck or van in traffic accident**

Pedestrian with babystroller injured in collision with car, pick-up truck or van in traffic accident

Pedestrian on ice-skates injured in collision with car, pick-up truck or van in traffic accident

Pedestrian on sled injured in collision with car, pick-up truck or van in traffic accident

Pedestrian on snowboard injured in collision with car, pick-up truck or van in traffic accident

Pedestrian on snow-skis injured in collision with car, pick-up truck or van in traffic accident

Pedestrian in wheelchair (powered) injured in collision with car, pick-up truck or van in traffic accident

V03.9   **Pedestrian injured in collision with car, pick-up truck or van, unspecified whether traffic or nontraffic accident**

V03.90   **Pedestrian on foot injured in collision with car, pick-up truck or van, unspecified whether traffic or nontraffic accident**

Pedestrian NOS injured in collision with car, pick-up truck or van, unspecified whether traffic or nontraffic accident

V03.91   **Pedestrian on roller-skates injured in collision with car, pick-up truck or van, unspecified whether traffic or nontraffic accident**

V03.92   **Pedestrian on skateboard injured in collision with car, pick-up truck or van, unspecified whether traffic or nontraffic accident**

V03.99   **Pedestrian with other conveyance injured in collision with car, pick-up truck or van, unspecified whether traffic or nontraffic accident**

Pedestrian with babystroller injured in collision with car, pick-up truck or van, unspecified whether traffic or nontraffic accident

Pedestrian on ice-skates injured in collision with car, pick-up truck or van, unspecified whether traffic or nontraffic accident

Pedestrian on sled injured in collision with car, pick-up truck or van in nontraffic accident

Pedestrian on snowboard injured in collision with car, pick-up truck or van, unspecified whether traffic or nontraffic accident

Pedestrian on snow-skis injured in collision with car, pick-up truck or van, unspecified whether traffic or nontraffic accident

Pedestrian in wheelchair (powered) injured in collision with car, pick-up truck or van, unspecified whether traffic or nontraffic accident

V04   **Pedestrian injured in collision with heavy transport vehicle or bus**

Excludes1:   pedestrian injured in collision with military vehicle (V09.01, V09.21)

The following extensions are to be added to each code from category V04:

a   initial encounter
d   subsequent encounter
q   sequelae

V04.0   **Pedestrian injured in collision with heavy transport vehicle or bus in nontraffic**

V04.00   **Pedestrian on foot injured in collision with heavy transport vehicle or bus in nontraffic accident**

Pedestrian NOS injured in collision with heavy transport vehicle or bus in nontraffic accident

V04.01   **Pedestrian on roller-skates injured in collision with heavy transport vehicle or bus in nontraffic accident**

V04.02   **Pedestrian on skateboard injured in collision with heavy transport vehicle or bus in nontraffic accident**

V04.09   **Pedestrian with other conveyance injured in collision with heavy transport vehicle or bus in nontraffic accident**

Pedestrian with babystroller injured in collision with heavy transport vehicle or bus in nontraffic accident

Pedestrian on ice-skates injured in collision with heavy transport vehicle or bus in nontraffic accident

Pedestrian on sled injured in collision with heavy transport vehicle or bus in nontraffic accident

Pedestrian on snowboard injured in collision with heavy transport vehicle or bus in nontraffic accident

Pedestrian on snow-skis injured in collision with heavy transport vehicle or bus in nontraffic accident

Pedestrian in wheelchair (powered) injured in collision with heavy transport vehicle or bus in nontraffic accident

V04.1   **Pedestrian injured in collision with heavy transport vehicle or bus in traffic accident**

V04.10   Pedestrian on foot injured in collision with heavy transport vehicle or bus in traffic accident
> Pedestrian NOS injured in collision with heavy transport vehicle or bus in traffic accident

V04.11   Pedestrian on roller-skates injured in collision with heavy transport vehicle or bus in traffic accident

V04.12   Pedestrian on skateboard injured in collision with heavy transport vehicle or bus in traffic accident

V04.19   Pedestrian with other conveyance injured in collision with heavy transport vehicle or bus in traffic accident
> Pedestrian with babystroller injured in collision with heavy transport vehicle or bus in traffic accident
> Pedestrian on ice-skates injured in collision with heavy transport vehicle or bus in traffic accident
> Pedestrian on sled injured in collision with heavy transport vehicle or bus in traffic accident
> Pedestrian on snowboard injured in collision with heavy transport vehicle or bus in traffic accident
> Pedestrian on snow-skis injured in collision with heavy transport vehicle or bus in traffic accident
> Pedestrian in wheelchair (powered) injured in collision with heavy transport vehicle or bus in traffic accident

V04.9   Pedestrian injured in collision with heavy transport vehicle or bus, unspecified whether traffic or nontraffic accident

V04.90   Pedestrian on foot injured in collision with heavy transport vehicle or bus, unspecified whether traffic or nontraffic accident
> Pedestrian NOS injured in collision with heavy transport vehicle or bus, unspecified whether traffic or nontraffic accident

V04.91   Pedestrian on roller-skates injured in collision with heavy transport vehicle or bus, unspecified whether traffic or nontraffic accident

V04.92   Pedestrian on skateboard injured in collision with heavy transport vehicle or bus, unspecified whether traffic or nontraffic accident

V04.99   Pedestrian with other conveyance injured in collision with heavy transport vehicle or bus, unspecified whether traffic or nontraffic accident
> Pedestrian with babystroller injured in collision with heavy transport vehicle or bus, unspecified whether traffic or nontraffic accident
> Pedestrian on ice-skates injured in collision with heavy transport vehicle or bus, unspecified whether traffic or nontraffic accident
> Pedestrian on sled injured in collision with heavy transport vehicle or bus, unspecified whether traffic or nontraffic accident
> Pedestrian on snowboard injured in collision with heavy transport vehicle or bus, unspecified whether traffic or nontraffic accident
> Pedestrian on snow-skis injured in collision with heavy transport vehicle or bus, unspecified whether traffic or nontraffic accident
> Pedestrian in wheelchair (powered) injured in collision with heavy transport vehicle or bus, unspecified whether traffic or nontraffic accident

V05   Pedestrian injured in collision with railway train or railway vehicle
The following extensions are to be added to each code from category V05:
- a   initial encounter
- d   subsequent encounter
- q   sequelae

V05.0   Pedestrian injured in collision with railway train or railway vehicle in nontraffic accident

V05.00   Pedestrian on foot injured in collision with railway train or railway vehicle in nontraffic accident
> Pedestrian NOS injured in collision with railway train or railway vehicle in nontraffic accident

V05.01   Pedestrian on roller-skates injured in collision with railway train or railway vehicle in nontraffic accident

V05.02   Pedestrian on skateboard injured in collision with railway train or railway vehicle in nontraffic accident

V05.09   Pedestrian with other conveyance injured in collision with railway train or railway vehicle in nontraffic accident
> Pedestrian with babystroller injured in collision with railway train or railway vehicle in nontraffic accident
> Pedestrian on ice-skates injured in collision with railway train or railway vehicle in nontraffic accident
> Pedestrian on sled injured in collision with railway train or railway vehicle in nontraffic accident
> Pedestrian on snowboard injured in collision with railway train or railway vehicle in nontraffic accident
> Pedestrian on snow-skis injured in collision with railway train or railway vehicle in nontraffic accident
> Pedestrian in wheelchair (powered) injured in collision with railway train or railway vehicle in nontraffic accident

V05.1   Pedestrian injured in collision with railway train or railway vehicle in traffic accident

V05.10   Pedestrian on foot injured in collision with railway train or railway vehicle in traffic accident
> Pedestrian NOS injured in collision with railway train or railway vehicle in traffic accident

V05.11   Pedestrian on roller-skates injured in collision with railway train or railway vehicle in traffic accident

V05.12   Pedestrian on skateboard injured in collision with railway train or railway vehicle in traffic accident

V05.19   Pedestrian with other conveyance injured in collision with railway train or railway vehicle in traffic accident
> Pedestrian with babystroller injured in collision with railway train or railway vehicle in traffic accident
> Pedestrian on ice-skates injured in collision with railway train or railway vehicle in traffic accident
> Pedestrian on sled injured in collision with railway train or railway vehicle in traffic accident
> Pedestrian on snowboard injured in collision with railway train or railway vehicle in traffic accident
> Pedestrian on snow-skis injured in collision with railway train or railway vehicle in traffic accident
> Pedestrian in wheelchair (powered) injured in collision with railway train or railway vehicle in traffic accident

V05.9   Pedestrian injured in collision with railway train or railway vehicle, unspecified whether traffic or nontraffic accident

V05.90   Pedestrian on foot injured in collision with railway train or railway vehicle, unspecified whether traffic or nontraffic accident
> Pedestrian NOS injured in collision with railway train or railway vehicle, unspecified whether traffic or nontraffic accident

V05.91   Pedestrian on roller-skates injured in collision with railway train or railway vehicle, unspecified whether traffic or nontraffic accident

V05.92   Pedestrian on skateboard injured in collision with railway train or railway vehicle, unspecified whether traffic or nontraffic accident

V05.99   **Pedestrian with other conveyance injured in collision with railway train or railway vehicle, unspecified whether traffic or nontraffic accident**

Pedestrian with babystroller injured in collision with railway train or railway vehicle, unspecified whether traffic or nontraffic

Pedestrian on ice-skates injured in collision with railway train or railway vehicle, unspecified whether traffic or nontraffic

Pedestrian on sled injured in collision with railway train or railway vehicle, unspecified whether traffic or nontraffic

Pedestrian on snowboard injured in collision with railway train or railway vehicle, unspecified whether traffic or nontraffic

Pedestrian on snow-skis injured in collision with railway train or railway vehicle, unspecified whether traffic or nontraffic

Pedestrian in wheelchair (powered) injured in collision with railway train or railway vehicle, unspecified whether traffic or nontraffic

V06   Pedestrian injured in collision with other nonmotor vehicle

Includes: collision with animal-drawn vehicle, animal being ridden, nonpowered streetcar

Excludes1:   pedestrian injured in collision with pedestrian conveyance (V00.0-)

The following extensions are to be added to each code from category V06:

    a   initial encounter
    d   subsequent encounter
    q   sequelae

V06.0   Pedestrian injured in collision with other nonmotor vehicle in nontraffic accident

V06.00   **Pedestrian on foot injured in collision with other nonmotor vehicle in nontraffic accident**

Pedestrian NOS injured in collision with other nonmotor vehicle in nontraffic accident

V06.01   **Pedestrian on roller-skates injured in collision with other nonmotor vehicle in nontraffic accident**

V06.02   **Pedestrian on skateboard injured in collision with other nonmotor vehicle in nontraffic accident**

V06.09   **Pedestrian with other conveyance injured in collision with other nonmotor vehicle in nontraffic accident**

Pedestrian with babystroller injured in collision with other nonmotor vehicle in nontraffic accident

Pedestrian on ice-skates injured in collision with other nonmotor vehicle in nontraffic accident

Pedestrian on sled injured in collision with other nonmotor vehicle in nontraffic accident

Pedestrian on snowboard injured in collision with other nonmotor vehicle in nontraffic accident

Pedestrian on snow-skis injured in collision with other nonmotor vehicle in nontraffic accident

Pedestrian in wheelchair (powered) injured in collision with other nonmotor vehicle in nontraffic accident

V06.1   Pedestrian injured in collision with other nonmotor vehicle in traffic accident

V06.10   **Pedestrian on foot injured in collision with other nonmotor vehicle in traffic accident**

Pedestrian NOS injured in collision with other nonmotor vehicle in traffic accident

V06.11   **Pedestrian on roller-skates injured in collision with other nonmotor vehicle in traffic accident**

V06.12   **Pedestrian on skateboard injured in collision with other nonmotor vehicle in traffic accident**

V06.19   **Pedestrian with other conveyance injured in collision with other nonmotor vehicle in traffic accident**

Pedestrian with babystroller injured in collision with other nonmotor vehicle in nontraffic accident

Pedestrian on ice-skates injured in collision with other nonmotor vehicle in traffic accident

Pedestrian on sled injured in collision with other nonmotor vehicle in traffic accident

Pedestrian on snowboard injured in collision with other nonmotor vehicle in traffic accident

Pedestrian on snow-skis injured in collision with other nonmotor vehicle in traffic accident

Pedestrian in wheelchair (powered) injured in collision with other nonmotor vehicle in traffic accident

V06.9   Pedestrian injured in collision with other nonmotor vehicle, unspecified whether traffic or nontraffic accident

V06.90   **Pedestrian on foot injured in collision with other nonmotor vehicle, unspecified whether traffic or nontraffic accident**

Pedestrian NOS injured in collision with other nonmotor vehicle, unspecified whether traffic or nontraffic accident

V06.91   **Pedestrian on roller-skates injured in collision with other nonmotor vehicle, unspecified whether traffic or nontraffic accident**

V06.92   **Pedestrian on skateboard injured in collision with other nonmotor vehicle, unspecified whether traffic or nontraffic accident**

V06.99   **Pedestrian with other conveyance injured in collision with other nonmotor vehicle, unspecified whether traffic or nontraffic accident**

Pedestrian with babystroller injured in collision with other nonmotor vehicle, unspecified whether traffic or nontraffic accident

Pedestrian on ice-skates injured in collision with other nonmotor vehicle, unspecified whether traffic or nontraffic accident

Pedestrian on sled injured in collision with other nonmotor vehicle, unspecified whether traffic or nontraffic accident

Pedestrian on snowboard injured in collision with other nonmotor vehicle, unspecified whether traffic or nontraffic accident

Pedestrian on snow-skis injured in collision with other nonmotor vehicle, unspecified whether traffic or nontraffic accident

Pedestrian in wheelchair (powered) injured in collision with other nonmotor vehicle, unspecified whether traffic or nontraffic accident

V09   Pedestrian injured in other and unspecified transport accidents

The following extensions are to be added to each code from category V09:

    a   initial encounter
    d   subsequent encounter
    q   sequelae

V09.0   Pedestrian injured in nontraffic accident involving other and unspecified motor vehicles

V09.00   **Pedestrian injured in nontraffic accident involving unspecified motor vehicles**

V09.01   **Pedestrian injured in nontraffic accident involving military vehicle**

V09.09   **Pedestrian injured in nontraffic accident involving other motor vehicles**

Pedestrian injured in nontraffic accident by special vehicle

V09.1   Pedestrian injured in unspecified nontraffic accident

V09.2   Pedestrian injured in traffic accident involving other and unspecified motor vehicles

V09.20   **Pedestrian injured in traffic accident involving unspecified motor vehicles**

V09.21   **Pedestrian injured in traffic accident involving military vehicle**

V09.29   **Pedestrian injured in traffic accident involving other motor vehicles**

V09.3   Pedestrian injured in unspecified traffic accident
V09.9   Pedestrian injured in unspecified transport accident

PEDAL CYCLE RIDER INJURED IN TRANSPORT ACCIDENT
(V10–V19)

Includes: any non-motorized vehicle, excluding an animal-drawn vehicle, or a sidecar or trailer attached to the pedal cycle
Excludes2:   rupture of pedal cycle tire (W37)

V10   Pedal cycle rider injured in collision with pedestrian or animal

Excludes1:   pedal cycle rider collision with animal-drawn vehicle or animal being ridden (V16.-)

The following extensions are to be added to each code from category V10:
    a   initial encounter
    d   subsequent encounter
    q   sequelae

V10.0   Pedal cycle driver injured in collision with pedestrian or animal in nontraffic accident
V10.1   Pedal cycle passenger injured in collision with pedestrian or animal in nontraffic accident
V10.2   Unspecified pedal cyclist injured in collision with pedestrian or animal in nontraffic accident
V10.3   Person boarding or alighting a pedal cycle injured in collision with pedestrian or animal
V10.4   Pedal cycle driver injured in collision with pedestrian or animal in traffic accident
V10.5   Pedal cycle passenger injured in collision with pedestrian or animal in traffic accident
V10.9   Unspecified pedal cyclist injured in collision with pedestrian or animal in traffic accident

V11   Pedal cycle rider injured in collision with other pedal cycle

The following extensions are to be added to each code from category V11:
    a   initial encounter
    d   subsequent encounter
    q   sequelae

V11.0   Pedal cycle driver injured in collision with other pedal cycle in nontraffic accident
V11.1   Pedal cycle passenger injured in collision with other pedal cycle in nontraffic accident
V11.2   Unspecified pedal cyclist injured in collision with other pedal cycle in nontraffic accident
V11.3   Person boarding or alighting a pedal cycle injured in collision with other pedal cycle
V11.4   Pedal cycle driver injured in collision with other pedal cycle in traffic accident
V11.5   Pedal cycle passenger injured in collision with other pedal cycle in traffic accident
V11.9   Unspecified pedal cyclist injured in collision with other pedal cycle in traffic accident

V12   Pedal cycle rider injured in collision with two- or three-wheeled motor vehicle

The following extensions are to be added to each code from category V12:
    a   initial encounter
    d   subsequent encounter
    q   sequelae

V12.0   Pedal cycle driver injured in collision with two- or three-wheeled motor vehicle in nontraffic accident
V12.1   Pedal cycle passenger injured in collision with two- or three-wheeled motor vehicle in nontraffic accident
V12.2   Unspecified pedal cyclist injured in collision with two- or three-wheeled motor vehicle in nontraffic accident
V12.3   Person boarding or alighting a pedal cycle injured in collision with two- or three-wheeled motor vehicle
V12.4   Pedal cycle driver injured in collision with two- or three-wheeled motor vehicle in traffic accident
V12.5   Pedal cycle passenger injured in collision with two- or three-wheeled motor vehicle in traffic accident

V12.9   Unspecified pedal cyclist injured in collision with two- or three-wheeled motor vehicle in traffic accident

V13   Pedal cycle rider injured in collision with car, pick-up truck or van

The following extensions are to be added to each code from category V13:
    a   initial encounter
    d   subsequent encounter
    q   sequelae

V13.0   Pedal cycle driver injured in collision with car, pick-up truck or van in nontraffic accident
V13.1   Pedal cycle passenger injured in collision with car, pick-up truck or van in nontraffic accident
V13.2   Unspecified pedal cyclist injured in collision with car, pick-up truck or van in nontraffic accident
V13.3   Person boarding or alighting a pedal cycle injured in collision with car, pick-up truck or van
V13.4   Pedal cycle driver injured in collision with car, pick-up truck or van in traffic accident
V13.5   Pedal cycle passenger injured in collision with car, pick-up truck or van in traffic accident
V13.9   Unspecified pedal cyclist injured in collision with car, pick-up truck or van in traffic accident

V14   Pedal cycle rider injured in collision with heavy transport vehicle or bus

Excludes1:   pedal cycle rider injured in collision with military vehicle (V19.81)

The following extensions are to be added to each code from category V14:
    a   initial encounter
    d   subsequent encounter
    q   sequelae

V14.0   Pedal cycle driver injured in collision with heavy transport vehicle or bus in nontraffic accident
V14.1   Pedal cycle passenger injured in collision with heavy transport vehicle or bus in nontraffic accident
V14.2   Unspecified pedal cyclist injured in collision with heavy transport vehicle or bus in nontraffic accident
V14.3   Person boarding or alighting a pedal cycle injured in collision with heavy transport vehicle or bus
V14.4   Pedal cycle driver injured in collision with heavy transport vehicle or bus in traffic accident
V14.5   Pedal cycle passenger injured in collision with heavy transport vehicle or bus in traffic accident
V14.9   Unspecified pedal cyclist injured in collision with heavy transport vehicle or bus in traffic accident

V15   Pedal cycle rider injured in collision with railway train or railway vehicle

The following extensions are to be added to each code from category V15:
    a   initial encounter
    d   subsequent encounter
    q   sequelae

V15.0   Pedal cycle driver injured in collision with railway train or railway vehicle in nontraffic accident
V15.1   Pedal cycle passenger injured in collision with railway train or railway vehicle in nontraffic accident
V15.2   Unspecified pedal cyclist injured in collision with railway train or railway vehicle in nontraffic accident
V15.3   Person boarding or alighting a pedal cycle injured in collision with railway train or railway vehicle
V15.4   Pedal cycle driver injured in collision with railway train or railway vehicle in traffic accident
V15.5   Pedal cycle passenger injured in collision with railway train or railway vehicle in traffic accident
V15.9   Unspecified pedal cyclist injured in collision with railway train or railway vehicle in traffic accident

V16 Pedal cycle rider injured in collision with other nonmotor vehicle

    Includes: collision with animal-drawn vehicle, animal being ridden, streetcar

    The following extensions are to be added to each code from category V16:

        a   initial encounter
        d   subsequent encounter
        q   sequelae

V16.0 Pedal cycle driver injured in collision with other nonmotor vehicle in nontraffic accident

V16.1 Pedal cycle passenger injured in collision with other nonmotor vehicle in nontraffic accident

V16.2 Unspecified pedal cyclist injured in collision with other nonmotor vehicle in nontraffic accident

V16.3 Person boarding or alighting a pedal cycle injured in collision with other nonmotor vehicle in nontraffic accident

V16.4 Pedal cycle driver injured in collision with other nonmotor vehicle in traffic accident

V16.5 Pedal cycle passenger injured in collision with other nonmotor vehicle in traffic accident

V16.9 Unspecified pedal cyclist injured in collision with other nonmotor vehicle in traffic accident

V17 Pedal cycle rider injured in collision with fixed or stationary object

    The following extensions are to be added to each code from category V17:

        a   initial encounter
        d   subsequent encounter
        q   sequelae

V17.0 Pedal cycle driver injured in collision with fixed or stationary object in nontraffic accident

V17.1 Pedal cycle passenger injured in collision with fixed or stationary object in nontraffic accident

V17.2 Unspecified pedal cyclist injured in collision with fixed or stationary object in nontraffic accident

V17.3 Person boarding or alighting a pedal cycle injured in collision with fixed or stationary object

V17.4 Pedal cycle driver injured in collision with fixed or stationary object in traffic accident

V17.5 Pedal cycle passenger injured in collision with fixed or stationary object in traffic accident

V17.9 Unspecified pedal cyclist injured in collision with fixed or stationary object in traffic accident

V18 Pedal cycle rider injured in noncollision transport accident

    Includes: fall or thrown from pedal cycle (without antecedent collision)
            overturning pedal cycle NOS
            overturning pedal cycle without collision

    The following extensions are to be added to each code from category V18:

        a   initial encounter
        d   subsequent encounter
        q   sequelae

V18.0 Pedal cycle driver injured in noncollision transport accident in nontraffic accident

V18.1 Pedal cycle passenger injured in noncollision transport accident in nontraffic accident

V18.2 Unspecified pedal cyclist injured in noncollision transport accident in nontraffic accident

V18.3 Person boarding or alighting a pedal cycle injured in noncollision transport accident

V18.4 Pedal cycle driver injured in noncollision transport accident in traffic accident

V18.5 Pedal cycle passenger injured in noncollision transport accident in traffic accident

V18.9 Unspecified pedal cyclist injured in noncollision transport accident in traffic accident

V19 Pedal cycle rider injured in other and unspecified transport accidents

    The following extensions are to be added to each code from category V19:

        a   initial encounter
        d   subsequent encounter
        q   sequelae

V19.0 Pedal cycle driver injured in collision with other and unspecified motor vehicles in nontraffic accident

    V19.00 Pedal cycle driver injured in collision with unspecified motor vehicles in nontraffic accident

    V19.09 Pedal cycle driver injured in collision with other motor vehicles in nontraffic accident

V19.1 Pedal cycle passenger injured in collision with other and unspecified motor vehicles in nontraffic accident

    V19.10 Pedal cycle passenger injured in collision with unspecified motor vehicles in nontraffic accident

    V19.19 Pedal cycle passenger injured in collision with other motor vehicles in nontraffic accident

V19.2 Unspecified pedal cyclist injured in collision with other and unspecified motor vehicles in nontraffic accident

    V19.20 Unspecified pedal cyclist injured in collision with unspecified motor vehicles in nontraffic accident
        Pedal cycle collision NOS, nontraffic

    V19.29 Unspecified pedal cyclist injured in collision with other motor vehicles in nontraffic accident

V19.3 Pedal cyclist (driver) (passenger) injured in unspecified nontraffic accident
    Pedal cycle accident NOS, nontraffic
    Pedal cyclist injured in nontraffic accident NOS

V19.4 Pedal cycle driver injured in collision with other and unspecified motor vehicles in traffic accident

    V19.40 Pedal cycle driver injured in collision with unspecified motor vehicles in traffic accident

    V19.49 Pedal cycle driver injured in collision with other motor vehicles in traffic accident

V19.5 Pedal cycle passenger injured in collision with other and unspecified motor vehicles in traffic accident

    V19.50 Pedal cycle passenger injured in collision with unspecified motor vehicles in traffic accident

    V19.59 Pedal cycle passenger injured in collision with other motor vehicles in traffic accident

V19.6 Unspecified pedal cyclist injured in collision with other and unspecified motor vehicles in traffic accident

    V19.60 Unspecified pedal cyclist injured in collision with unspecified motor vehicles in traffic accident
        Pedal cycle collision NOS (traffic)

    V19.69 Unspecified pedal cyclist injured in collision with other motor vehicles in traffic accident

V19.8 Pedal cyclist (driver) (passenger) injured in other specified transport accidents

    V19.81 Pedal cyclist (driver) (passenger) injured in transport accident with military vehicle

    V19.88 Pedal cyclist (driver) (passenger) injured in other specified transport accidents

V19.9 Pedal cyclist (driver) (passenger) injured in unspecified traffic accident
    Pedal cycle accident NOS

MOTORCYCLE RIDER INJURED IN TRANSPORT ACCIDENT
(V20–V29)

    Includes: moped
            motorcycle with sidecar
            motorized bicycle
            motor scooter

    Excludes1:   three-wheeled motor vehicle (V30-V39)

V20 Motorcycle rider injured in collision with pedestrian or animal

> Excludes1: motorcycle rider collision with animal-drawn vehicle or animal being ridden (V26.-)

The following extensions are to be added to each code from category V20:

    a   initial encounter
    d   subsequent encounter
    q   sequelae

V20.0 Motorcycle driver injured in collision with pedestrian or animal in nontraffic accident

V20.1 Motorcycle passenger injured in collision with pedestrian or animal in nontraffic accident

V20.2 Unspecified motorcycle rider injured in collision with pedestrian or animal in nontraffic accident

V20.3 Person boarding or alighting a motorcycle injured in collision with pedestrian or animal

V20.4 Motorcycle driver injured in collision with pedestrian or animal in traffic accident

V20.5 Motorcycle passenger injured in collision with pedestrian or animal in traffic accident

V20.9 Unspecified motorcycle rider injured in collision with pedestrian or animal in traffic accident

V21 Motorcycle rider injured in collision with pedal cycle

The following extensions are to be added to each code from category V21:

    a   initial encounter
    d   subsequent encounter
    q   sequelae

V21.0 Motorcycle driver injured in collision with pedal cycle in nontraffic accident

V21.1 Motorcycle passenger injured in collision with pedal cycle in nontraffic accident

V21.2 Unspecified motorcycle rider injured in collision with pedal cycle in nontraffic accident

V21.3 Person boarding or alighting a motorcycle injured in collision with pedal cycle

V21.4 Motorcycle driver injured in collision with pedal cycle in traffic accident

V21.5 Motorcycle passenger injured in collision with pedal cycle in traffic accident

V21.9 Unspecified motorcycle rider injured in collision with pedal cycle in traffic accident

V22 Motorcycle rider injured in collision with two- or three-wheeled motor vehicle

The following extensions are to be added to each code from category V22:

    a   initial encounter
    d   subsequent encounter
    q   sequelae

V22.0 Motorcycle driver injured in collision with two- or three-wheeled motor vehicle in nontraffic accident

V22.1 Motorcycle passenger injured in collision with two- or three-wheeled motor vehicle in nontraffic accident

V22.2 Unspecified motorcycle rider injured in collision with two- or three-wheeled motor vehicle in nontraffic accident

V22.3 Person boarding or alighting a motorcycle injured in collision with two- or three-wheeled motor vehicle

V22.4 Motorcycle driver injured in collision with two- or three-wheeled motor vehicle in traffic accident

V22.5 Motorcycle passenger injured in collision with two- or three-wheeled motor vehicle in traffic accident

V22.9 Unspecified motorcycle rider injured in collision with two- or three-wheeled motor vehicle in traffic accident

V23 Motorcycle rider injured in collision with car, pick-up truck or van

The following extensions are to be added to each code from category V23:

    a   initial encounter
    d   subsequent encounter
    q   sequelae

V23.0 Motorcycle driver injured in collision with car, pick-up truck or van in nontraffic accident

V23.1 Motorcycle passenger injured in collision with car, pick-up truck or van in nontraffic accident

V23.2 Unspecified motorcycle rider injured in collision with car, pick-up truck or van in nontraffic accident

V23.3 Person boarding or alighting a motorcycle injured in collision with car, pick-up truck or van

V23.4 Motorcycle driver injured in collision with car, pick-up truck or van in traffic accident

V23.5 Motorcycle passenger injured in collision with car, pick-up truck or van in traffic accident

V23.9 Unspecified motorcycle rider injured in collision with car, pick-up truck or van in traffic accident

V24 Motorcycle rider injured in collision with heavy transport vehicle or bus

> Excludes1: motorcycle rider injured in collision with military vehicle (V29.81)

The following extensions are to be added to each code from category V24:

    a   initial encounter
    d   subsequent encounter
    q   sequelae

V24.0 Motorcycle driver injured in collision with heavy transport vehicle or bus in nontraffic accident

V24.1 Motorcycle passenger injured in collision with heavy transport vehicle or bus in nontraffic accident

V24.2 Unspecified motorcycle rider injured in collision with heavy transport vehicle or bus in nontraffic accident

V24.3 Person boarding or alighting a motorcycle injured in collision with heavy transport vehicle or bus

V24.4 Motorcycle driver injured in collision with heavy transport vehicle or bus in traffic accident

V24.5 Motorcycle passenger injured in collision with heavy transport vehicle or bus in traffic accident

V24.9 Unspecified motorcycle rider injured in collision with heavy transport vehicle or bus in traffic accident

V25 Motorcycle rider injured in collision with railway train or railway vehicle

The following extensions are to be added to each code from category V25:

    a   initial encounter
    d   subsequent encounter
    q   sequelae

V25.0 Motorcycle driver injured in collision with railway train or railway vehicle in nontraffic accident

V25.1 Motorcycle passenger injured in collision with railway train or railway vehicle in nontraffic accident

V25.2 Unspecified motorcycle rider injured in collision with railway train or railway vehicle in nontraffic accident

V25.3 Person boarding or alighting a motorcycle injured in collision with railway train or railway vehicle

V25.4 Motorcycle driver injured in collision with railway train or railway vehicle in traffic accident

V25.5 Motorcycle passenger injured in collision with railway train or railway vehicle in traffic accident

V25.9 Unspecified motorcycle rider injured in collision with railway train or railway vehicle in traffic accident

V26 Motorcycle rider injured in collision with other nonmotor vehicle

> Includes: collision with animal-drawn vehicle, animal being ridden, streetcar

The following extensions are to be added to each code from category V26:

    a   initial encounter
    d   subsequent encounter
    q   sequelae

V26.0 Motorcycle driver injured in collision with other nonmotor vehicle in nontraffic accident

V26.1 Motorcycle passenger injured in collision with other nonmotor vehicle in nontraffic accident

V26.2 Unspecified motorcycle rider injured in collision with other nonmotor vehicle in nontraffic accident

V26.3 Person boarding or alighting a motorcycle injured in collision with other nonmotor vehicle

V26.4 Motorcycle driver injured in collision with other nonmotor vehicle in traffic accident

V26.5 Motorcycle passenger injured in collision with other nonmotor vehicle in traffic accident

V26.9 Unspecified motorcycle rider injured in collision with other nonmotor vehicle in traffic accident

V27 Motorcycle rider injured in collision with fixed or stationary object
> The following extensions are to be added to each code from category V27:
>> a   initial encounter
>> d   subsequent encounter
>> q   sequelae

V27.0 Motorcycle driver injured in collision with fixed or stationary object in nontraffic accident

V27.1 Motorcycle passenger injured in collision with fixed or stationary object in nontraffic accident

V27.2 Unspecified motorcycle rider injured in collision with fixed or stationary object in nontraffic accident

V27.3 Person boarding or alighting a motorcycle injured in collision with fixed or stationary object

V27.4 Motorcycle driver injured in collision with fixed or stationary object in traffic accident

V27.5 Motorcycle passenger injured in collision with fixed or stationary object in traffic accident

V27.9 Unspecified motorcycle rider injured in collision with fixed or stationary object in traffic accident

V28 Motorcycle rider injured in noncollision transport accident
> Includes: fall or thrown from motorcycle (without antecedent collision)
>   overturning motorcycle NOS
>   overturning motorcycle without collision
> The following extensions are to be added to each code from category V28:
>> a   initial encounter
>> d   subsequent encounter
>> q   sequelae

V28.0 Motorcycle driver injured in noncollision transport accident in nontraffic accident

V28.1 Motorcycle passenger injured in noncollision transport accident in nontraffic accident

V28.2 Unspecified motorcycle rider injured in noncollision transport accident in nontraffic accident

V28.3 Person boarding or alighting a motorcycle injured in noncollision transport accident

V28.4 Motorcycle driver injured in noncollision transport accident in traffic accident

V28.5 Motorcycle passenger injured in noncollision transport accident in traffic accident

V28.9 Unspecified motorcycle rider injured in noncollision transport accident in traffic accident

V29 Motorcycle rider injured in other and unspecified transport accidents
> The following extensions are to be added to each code from category V29:
>> a   initial encounter
>> d   subsequent encounter
>> q   sequelae

V29.0 Motorcycle driver injured in collision with other and unspecified motor vehicles in nontraffic accident

V29.00 Motorcycle driver injured in collision with unspecified motor vehicles in nontraffic accident

V29.09 Motorcycle driver injured in collision with other motor vehicles in nontraffic accident

V29.1 Motorcycle passenger injured in collision with other and unspecified motor vehicles in nontraffic accident

V29.10 Motorcycle passenger injured in collision with unspecified motor vehicles in nontraffic accident

V29.19 Motorcycle passenger injured in collision with other motor vehicles in nontraffic accident

V29.2 Unspecified motorcycle rider injured in collision with other and unspecified motor vehicles in nontraffic accident

V29.20 Unspecified motorcycle rider injured in collision with unspecified motor vehicles in nontraffic accident
> Motorcycle collision NOS, nontraffic

V29.29 Unspecified motorcycle rider injured in collision with other motor vehicles in nontraffic acciden

V29.3 Motorcycle rider (driver) (passenger) injured in unspecified nontraffic accident
> Motorcycle accident NOS, nontraffic
> Motorcycle rider injured in nontraffic accident NOS

V29.4 Motorcycle driver injured in collision with other and unspecified motor vehicles in traffic accident

V29.40 Motorcycle driver injured in collision with unspecified motor vehicles in traffic accident

V29.49 Motorcycle driver injured in collision with other motor vehicles in traffic accident

V29.5 Motorcycle passenger injured in collision with other and unspecified motor vehicles in traffic accident

V29.50 Motorcycle passenger injured in collision with unspecified motor vehicles in traffic accident

V29.59 Motorcycle passenger injured in collision with other motor vehicles in traffic accident

V29.6 Unspecified motorcycle rider injured in collision with other and unspecified motor vehicles in traffic accident

V29.60 Unspecified motorcycle rider injured in collision with unspecified motor vehicles in traffic accident
> Motorcycle collision NOS (traffic)

V29.69 Unspecified motorcycle rider injured in collision with other motor vehicles in traffic accident

V29.8 Motorcycle rider (driver) (passenger) injured in other specified transport accidents

V29.81 Motorcycle rider (driver) (passenger) injured in transport accident with military vehicle

V29.88 Motorcycle rider (driver) (passenger) injured in other specified transport accidents

V29.9 Motorcycle rider (driver) (passenger) injured in unspecified traffic accident
> Motorcycle accident NOS

OCCUPANT OF THREE–WHEELED MOTOR VEHICLE INJURED IN TRANSPORT ACCIDENT (V30–V39)

> Includes: motorized tricycle
>   motorized rickshaw
>   three-wheeled motor car
> Excludes1:   all-terrain vehicles (V86.-)
>   motorcycle with sidecar (V20-V29)
>   vehicle designed primarily for off-road use (V86.-)

V30 Occupant of three-wheeled motor vehicle injured in collision with pedestrian or animal
> Excludes1:   three-wheeled motor vehicle collision with animal-drawn vehicle or animal being ridden (V36.-)
> The following extensions are to be added to each code from category V30:
>> a   initial encounter
>> d   subsequent encounter
>> q   sequelae

V30.0 Driver of three-wheeled motor vehicle injured in collision with pedestrian or animal in nontraffic accident

V30.1 Passenger in three-wheeled motor vehicle injured in collision with pedestrian or animal in nontraffic accident

V30.2 Person on outside of three-wheeled motor vehicle injured in collision with pedestrian or animal in nontraffic accident

V30.3 Unspecified occupant of three-wheeled motor vehicle injured in collision with pedestrian or animal in nontraffic accident

V30.4 Person boarding or alighting a three-wheeled motor vehicle injured in collision with pedestrian or animal

V30.5 Driver of three-wheeled motor vehicle injured in collision with pedestrian or animal in traffic accident

V30.6 Passenger in three-wheeled motor vehicle injured in collision with pedestrian or animal in traffic accident

V30.7 Person on outside of three-wheeled motor vehicle injured in collision with pedestrian or animal in traffic accident

V30.9 Unspecified occupant of three-wheeled motor vehicle injured in collision with pedestrian or animal in traffic accident

V31 Occupant of three-wheeled motor vehicle injured in collision with pedal cycle

The following extensions are to be added to each code from category V31:
- a   initial encounter
- d   subsequent encounter
- q   sequelae

V31.0 Driver of three-wheeled motor vehicle injured in collision with pedal cycle in nontraffic accident

V31.1 Passenger in three-wheeled motor vehicle injured in collision with pedal cycle in nontraffic accident

V31.2 Person on outside of three-wheeled motor vehicle injured in collision with pedal cycle in nontraffic accident

V31.3 Unspecified occupant of three-wheeled motor vehicle injured in collision with pedal cycle in nontraffic accident

V31.4 Person boarding or alighting a three-wheeled motor vehicle injured in collision with pedal cycle

V31.5 Driver of three-wheeled motor vehicle injured in collision with pedal cycle in traffic accident

V31.6 Passenger in three-wheeled motor vehicle injured in collision with pedal cycle in traffic accident

V31.7 Person on outside of three-wheeled motor vehicle injured in collision with pedal cycle in traffic accident

V31.9 Unspecified occupant of three-wheeled motor vehicle injured in collision with pedal cycle in traffic accident

V32 Occupant of three-wheeled motor vehicle injured in collision with two- or three-wheeled motor vehicle

The following extensions are to be added to each code from category V32:
- a   initial encounter
- d   subsequent encounter
- q   sequelae

V32.0 Driver of three-wheeled motor vehicle injured in collision with two- or three-wheeled motor vehicle in nontraffic accident

V32.1 Passenger in three-wheeled motor vehicle injured in collision with two- or three-wheeled motor vehicle in nontraffic accident

V32.2 Person on outside of three-wheeled motor vehicle injured in collision with two- or three-wheeled motor vehicle in nontraffic accident

V32.3 Unspecified occupant of three-wheeled motor vehicle injured in collision with two- or three-wheeled motor vehicle in nontraffic accident

V32.4 Person boarding or alighting a three-wheeled motor vehicle injured in collision with two- or three-wheeled motor vehicle

V32.5 Driver of three-wheeled motor vehicle injured in collision with two- or three-wheeled motor vehicle in traffic accident

V32.6 Passenger in three-wheeled motor vehicle injured in collision with two- or three-wheeled motor vehicle in traffic accident

V32.7 Person on outside of three-wheeled motor vehicle injured in collision with two- or three-wheeled motor vehicle in traffic accident

V32.9 Unspecified occupant of three-wheeled motor vehicle injured in collision with two- or three-wheeled motor vehicle in traffic accident

V33 Occupant of three-wheeled motor vehicle injured in collision with car, pick-up truck or van

The following extensions are to be added to each code from category V33:
- a   initial encounter
- d   subsequent encounter
- q   sequelae

V33.0 Driver of three-wheeled motor vehicle injured in collision with car, pick-up truck or van in nontraffic accident

V33.1 Passenger in three-wheeled motor vehicle injured in collision with car, pick-up truck or van in nontraffic accident

V33.2 Person on outside of three-wheeled motor vehicle injured in collision with car, pick-up truck or van in nontraffic accident

V33.3 Unspecified occupant of three-wheeled motor vehicle injured in collision with car, pick-up truck or van in nontraffic accident

V33.4 Person boarding or alighting a three-wheeled motor vehicle injured in collision with car, pick-up truck or van

V33.5 Driver of three-wheeled motor vehicle injured in collision with car, pick-up truck or van in traffic accident

V33.6 Passenger in three-wheeled motor vehicle injured in collision with car, pick-up truck or van in traffic accident

V33.7 Person on outside of three-wheeled motor vehicle injured in collision with car, pick-up truck or van in traffic accident

V33.9 Unspecified occupant of three-wheeled motor vehicle injured in collision with car, pick-up truck or van in traffic accident

V34 Occupant of three-wheeled motor vehicle injured in collision with heavy transport vehicle or bus

Excludes1:   occupant of three-wheeled motor vehicle injured in collision with military vehicle (V39.81)

The following extensions are to be added to each code from category V34:
- a   initial encounter
- d   subsequent encounter
- q   sequelae

V34.0 Driver of three-wheeled motor vehicle injured in collision with heavy transport vehicle or bus in nontraffic accident

V34.1 Passenger in three-wheeled motor vehicle injured in collision with heavy transport vehicle or bus in nontraffic accident

V34.2 Person on outside of three-wheeled motor vehicle injured in collision with heavy transport vehicle or bus in nontraffic accident

V34.3 Unspecified occupant of three-wheeled motor vehicle injured in collision with heavy transport vehicle or bus in nontraffic accident

V34.4 Person boarding or alighting a three-wheeled motor vehicle injured in collision with heavy transport vehicle or bus

V34.5 Driver of three-wheeled motor vehicle injured in collision with heavy transport vehicle or bus in traffic accident

V34.6 Passenger in three-wheeled motor vehicle injured in collision with heavy transport vehicle or bus in traffic accident

V34.7 Person on outside of three-wheeled motor vehicle injured in collision with heavy transport vehicle or bus in traffic accident

V34.9 Unspecified occupant of three-wheeled motor vehicle injured in collision with heavy transport vehicle or bus in traffic accident

V35 Occupant of three-wheeled motor vehicle injured in collision with railway train or railway vehicle

The following extensions are to be added to each code from category V35:
- a   initial encounter
- d   subsequent encounter
- q   sequelae

V35.0 Driver of three-wheeled motor vehicle injured in collision with railway train or railway vehicle in nontraffic accident

V35.1 Passenger in three-wheeled motor vehicle injured in collision with railway train or railway vehicle in nontraffic accident

V35.2 Person on outside of three-wheeled motor vehicle injured in collision with railway train or railway vehicle in nontraffic accident

V35.3 Unspecified occupant of three-wheeled motor vehicle injured in collision with railway train or railway vehicle in nontraffic accident

V35.4 Person boarding or alighting a three-wheeled motor vehicle injured in collision with railway train or railway vehicle

V35.5 Driver of three-wheeled motor vehicle injured in collision with railway train or railway vehicle in traffic accident

V35.6 Passenger in three-wheeled motor vehicle injured in collision with railway train or railway vehicle in traffic accident

V35.7 Person on outside of three-wheeled motor vehicle injured in collision with railway train or railway vehicle in traffic accident

V35.9 Unspecified occupant of three-wheeled motor vehicle injured in collision with railway train or railway vehicle in traffic accident

V36 Occupant of three-wheeled motor vehicle injured in collision with other nonmotor vehicle

Includes: collision with animal-drawn vehicle, animal being ridden, streetcar

The following extensions are to be added to each code from category V36:

     a   initial encounter
     d   subsequent encounter
     q   sequelae

V36.0 Driver of three-wheeled motor vehicle injured in collision with other nonmotor vehicle in nontraffic accident

V36.1 Passenger in three-wheeled motor vehicle injured in collision with other nonmotor vehicle in nontraffic accident

V36.2 Person on outside of three-wheeled motor vehicle injured in collision with other nonmotor vehicle in nontraffic accident

V36.3 Unspecified occupant of three-wheeled motor vehicle injured in collision with other nonmotor vehicle in nontraffic accident

V36.4 Person boarding or alighting a three-wheeled motor vehicle injured in collision with other nonmotor vehicle

V36.5 Driver of three-wheeled motor vehicle injured in collision with other nonmotor vehicle in traffic accident

V36.6 Passenger in three-wheeled motor vehicle injured in collision with other nonmotor vehicle in traffic accident

V36.7 Person on outside of three-wheeled motor vehicle injured in collision with other nonmotor vehicle in traffic accident

V36.9 Unspecified occupant of three-wheeled motor vehicle injured in collision with other nonmotor vehicle in traffic accident

V37 Occupant of three-wheeled motor vehicle injured in collision with fixed or stationary object

The following extensions are to be added to each code from category V37:

     a   initial encounter
     d   subsequent encounter
     q   sequelae

V37.0 Driver of three-wheeled motor vehicle injured in collision with fixed or stationary object in nontraffic accident

V37.1 Passenger in three-wheeled motor vehicle injured in collision with fixed or stationary object in nontraffic accident

V37.2 Person on outside of three-wheeled motor vehicle injured in collision with fixed or stationary object in nontraffic accident

V37.3 Unspecified occupant of three-wheeled motor vehicle injured in collision with fixed or stationary object in nontraffic accident

V37.4 Person boarding or alighting a three-wheeled motor vehicle injured in collision with fixed or stationary object

V37.5 Driver of three-wheeled motor vehicle injured in collision with fixed or stationary object in traffic accident

V37.6 Passenger in three-wheeled motor vehicle injured in collision with fixed or stationary object in traffic accident

V37.7 Person on outside of three-wheeled motor vehicle injured in collision with fixed or stationary object in traffic accident

V37.9 Unspecified occupant of three-wheeled motor vehicle injured in collision with fixed or stationary object in traffic accident

V38 Occupant of three-wheeled motor vehicle injured in noncollision transport accident

Includes: fall or thrown from three-wheeled motor vehicle
overturning of three-wheeled motor vehicle NOS
overturning of three-wheeled motor vehicle without collision

The following extensions are to be added to each code from category V38:

     a   initial encounter
     d   subsequent encounter
     q   sequelae

V38.0 Driver of three-wheeled motor vehicle injured in noncollision transport accident in nontraffic accident

V38.1 Passenger in three-wheeled motor vehicle injured in noncollision transport accident in nontraffic accident

V38.2 Person on outside of three-wheeled motor vehicle injured in noncollision transport accident in nontraffic accident

V38.3 Unspecified occupant of three-wheeled motor vehicle injured in noncollision transport accident in nontraffic accident

V38.4 Person boarding or alighting a three-wheeled motor vehicle injured in noncollision transport accident

V38.5 Driver of three-wheeled motor vehicle injured in noncollision transport accident in traffic accident

V38.6 Passenger in three-wheeled motor vehicle injured in noncollision transport accident in traffic accident

V38.7 Person on outside of three-wheeled motor vehicle injured in noncollision transport accident in traffic accident

V38.9 Unspecified occupant of three-wheeled motor vehicle injured in noncollision transport accident in traffic accident

V39 Occupant of three-wheeled motor vehicle injured in other and unspecified transport accidents

The following extensions are to be added to each code from category V39:

     a   initial encounter
     d   subsequent encounter
     q   sequelae

V39.0 Driver of three-wheeled motor vehicle injured in collision with other and unspecified motor vehicles in nontraffic accident

     V39.00 Driver of three-wheeled motor vehicle injured in collision with unspecified motor vehicles in nontraffic accident

     V39.09 Driver of three-wheeled motor vehicle injured in collision with other motor vehicles in nontraffic accident

V39.1 Passenger in three-wheeled motor vehicle injured in collision with other and unspecified motor vehicles in nontraffic accident

     V39.10 Passenger in three-wheeled motor vehicle injured in collision with unspecified motor vehicles in nontraffic accident

     V39.19 Passenger in three-wheeled motor vehicle injured in collision with other motor vehicles in nontraffic accident

V39.2 Unspecified occupant of three-wheeled motor vehicle injured in collision with other and unspecified motor vehicles in nontraffic accident

     V39.20 Unspecified occupant of three-wheeled motor vehicle injured in collision with unspecified motor vehicles in nontraffic accident

         Collision NOS involving three-wheeled motor vehicle, nontraffic

     V39.29 Unspecified occupant of three-wheeled motor vehicle injured in collision with other motor vehicles in nontraffic accident

V39.3 Occupant (driver) (passenger) of three-wheeled motor vehicle injured in unspecified nontraffic accident

     Accident NOS involving three-wheeled motor vehicle, nontraffic
     Occupant of three-wheeled motor vehicle injured in nontraffic accident NOS

V39.4 Driver of three-wheeled motor vehicle injured in collision with other and unspecified motor vehicles in traffic accident

     V39.40 Driver of three-wheeled motor vehicle injured in collision with unspecified motor vehicles in traffic accident

     V39.49 Driver of three-wheeled motor vehicle injured in collision with other motor vehicles in traffic accident

V39.5 Passenger in three-wheeled motor vehicle injured in collision with other and unspecified motor vehicles in traffic accident

     V39.50 Passenger in three-wheeled motor vehicle injured in collision with unspecified motor vehicles in traffic accident

     V39.59 Passenger in three-wheeled motor vehicle injured in collision with other motor vehicles in traffic accident

V39.6 Unspecified occupant of three-wheeled motor vehicle injured in collision with other and unspecified motor vehicles in traffic accident

V39.60   Unspecified occupant of three-wheeled motor vehicle injured in collision with unspecified motor vehicles in traffic accident
  Collision NOS involving three-wheeled motor vehicle (traffic)

V39.69   Unspecified occupant of three-wheeled motor vehicle injured in collision with other motor vehicles in traffic accident

V39.8   Occupant (driver) (passenger) of three-wheeled motor vehicle injured in other specified transport accidents

V39.81   Occupant (driver) (passenger) of three-wheeled motor vehicle injured in transport accident with military vehicle

V39.89   Occupant (driver) (passenger) of three-wheeled motor vehicle injured in other specified transport accidents

V39.9   Occupant (driver) (passenger) of three-wheeled motor vehicle injured in unspecified traffic accident
  Accident NOS involving three-wheeled motor vehicle

CAR OCCUPANT INJURED IN TRANSPORT ACCIDENT
(V40–V49)

Includes: a four-wheeled motor vehicle designed primarily for carrying passengers
  automobile (pulling a trailor or camper)
  minibus
  minivan
  sport utility vehicle (SUV)

Excludes1:   bus
  motorcoach
  pick-up truck (V50-V59)

V40 Car occupant injured in collision with pedestrian or animal
  Excludes1:   car collision with animal-drawn vehicle or animal being ridden (V46.-)
  The following extensions are to be added to each code from category V40:
    a   initial encounter
    d   subsequent encounter
    q   sequelae

V40.0   Car driver injured in collision with pedestrian or animal in nontraffic accident

V40.1   Car passenger injured in collision with pedestrian or animal in nontraffic accident

V40.2   Person on outside of car injured in collision with pedestrian or animal in nontraffic accident

V40.3   Unspecified car occupant injured in collision with pedestrian or animal in nontraffic accident

V40.4   Person boarding or alighting a car injured in collision with pedestrian or animal

V40.5   Car driver injured in collision with pedestrian or animal in traffic accident

V40.6   Car passenger injured in collision with pedestrian or animal in traffic accident

V40.7   Person on outside of car injured in collision with pedestrian or animal in traffic accident

V40.9   Unspecified car occupant injured in collision with pedestrian or animal in traffic accident

V41 Car occupant injured in collision with pedal cycle
  The following extensions are to be added to each code from category V41:
    a   initial encounter
    d   subsequent encounter
    q   sequelae

V41.0   Car driver injured in collision with pedal cycle in nontraffic accident

V41.1   Car passenger injured in collision with pedal cycle in nontraffic accident

V41.2   Person on outside of car injured in collision with pedal cycle in nontraffic accident

V41.3   Unspecified car occupant injured in collision with pedal cycle in nontraffic accident

V41.4   Person boarding or alighting a car injured in collision with pedal cycle

V41.5   Car driver injured in collision with pedal cycle in traffic accident

V41.6   Car passenger injured in collision with pedal cycle in traffic accident

V41.7   Person on outside of car injured in collision with pedal cycle in traffic accident

V41.9   Unspecified car occupant injured in collision with pedal cycle in traffic accident

V42 Car occupant injured in collision with two- or three-wheeled motor vehicle
  The following extensions are to be added to each code from category V42:
    a   initial encounter
    d   subsequent encounter
    q   sequelae

V42.0   Car driver injured in collision with two- or three-wheeled motor vehicle in nontraffic accident

V42.1   Car passenger injured in collision with two- or three-wheeled motor vehicle in nontraffic accident

V42.2   Person on outside of car injured in collision with two- or three-wheeled motor vehicle in nontraffic accident

V42.3   Unspecified car occupant injured in collision with two- or three-wheeled motor vehicle in nontraffic accident

V42.4   Person boarding or alighting a car injured in collision with two- or three-wheeled motor vehicle

V42.5   Car driver injured in collision with two- or three-wheeled motor vehicle in traffic accident

V42.6   Car passenger injured in collision with two- or three-wheeled motor vehicle in traffic accident

V42.7   Person on outside of car injured in collision with two- or three-wheeled motor vehicle in traffic accident

V42.9   Unspecified car occupant injured in collision with two- or three-wheeled motor vehicle in traffic accident

V43 Car occupant injured in collision with car, pick-up truck or van
  The following extensions are to be added to each code from category V43:
    a   initial encounter
    d   subsequent encounter
    q   sequelae

V43.0   Car driver injured in collision with car, pick-up truck or van in nontraffic accident

V43.01   Car driver injured in collision with sport utility vehicle in nontraffic accident

V43.02   Car driver injured in collision with other type car in nontraffic accident

V43.03   Car driver injured in collision with pick-up truck in nontraffic accident

V43.04   Car driver injured in collision with van in nontraffic accident

V43.1   Car passenger injured in collision with car, pick-up truck or van in nontraffic accident

V43.1   Car passenger injured in collision with sport utility vehicle in nontraffic accident

V43.12   Car passenger injured in collision with other type car in nontraffic accident

V43.13   Car passenger injured in collision with pick-up in nontraffic accident

V43.14   Car passenger injured in collision with van in nontraffic accident

V43.2   Person on outside of car injured in collision with car, pick-up truck or van in nontraffic accident

V43.21   Person on outside of car injured in collision with sport utility vehicle in nontraffic accident

V43.22   Person on outside of car injured in collision with other type car in nontraffic accident

V43.23   Person on outside of car injured in collision with pick-up truck in nontraffic accident

V43.24   Person on outside of car injured in collision with van in nontraffic accident

V43.3   Unspecified car occupant injured in collision with car, pick-up truck or van in nontraffic accident

V43.31   Unspecified car occupant injured in collision with sport utility vehicle in nontraffic accident

V43.32   Unspecified car occupant injured in collision with other type car in nontraffic accident

V43.33   Unspecified car occupant injured in collision with pick-up truck in nontraffic accident

V43.34   Unspecified car occupant injured in collision with van in nontraffic accident

V43.4   Person boarding or alighting a car injured in collision with car, pick-up truck or van

V43.41   Person boarding or alighting a car injured in collision with sport utility vehicle

V43.42   Person boarding or alighting a car injured in collision with other type car

V43.43   Person boarding or alighting a car injured in collision with pick- up truck

V43.44   Person boarding or alighting a car injured in collision with van

V43.5   Car driver injured in collision with car, pick-up truck or van in traffic accident

V43.51   Car driver injured in collision with sport utility vehicle in traffic accident

V43.52   Car driver injured in collision with other type car in traffic accident

V43.53   Car driver injured in collision with pick-up truck in traffic accident

V43.54   Car driver injured in collision with van in traffic accident

V43.6   Car passenger injured in collision with car, pick-up truck or van in traffic accident

V43.61   Car passenger injured in collision with sport utility vehicle in traffic accident

V43.62   Car passenger injured in collision with other type car in traffic accident

V43.63   Car passenger injured in collision with pick-up truck in traffic accident

V43.64   Car passenger injured in collision with car, pick-up truck or van in traffic accident

V43.7   Person on outside of car injured in collision with car, pick-up truck or van in traffic accident

V43.71   Person on outside of car injured in collision with sport utility vehicle in traffic accident

V43.72   Person on outside of car injured in collision with other type car in traffic accident

V43.73   Person on outside of car injured in collision with pick-up truck in traffic accident

V43.74   Person on outside of car injured in collision with van in traffic accident

V43.9   Unspecified car occupant injured in collision with car, pick-up truck or van in traffic accident

V43.91   Unspecified car occupant injured in collision with sport utility vehicle in traffic accident

V43.92   Unspecified car occupant injured in collision with other type car in traffic accident

V43.93   Unspecified car occupant injured in collision with pick-up truck in traffic accident

V43.94   Unspecified car occupant injured in collision with van in traffic accident

V44   **Car occupant injured in collision with heavy transport vehicle or bus**

Excludes1:   car occupant injured in collision with military vehicle (V49.81)

The following extensions are to be added to each code from category V44:

   a   initial encounter
   d   subsequent encounter
   q   sequelae

V44.0   Car driver injured in collision with heavy transport vehicle or bus in nontraffic accident

V44.1   Car passenger injured in collision with heavy transport vehicle or bus in nontraffic accident

V44.2   Person on outside of car injured in collision with heavy transport vehicle or bus in nontraffic accident

V44.3   Unspecified car occupant injured in collision with heavy transport vehicle or bus in nontraffic accident

V44.4   Person boarding or alighting a car injured in collision with heavy transport vehicle or bus

V44.5   Car driver injured in collision with heavy transport vehicle or bus in traffic accident

V44.6   Car passenger injured in collision with heavy transport vehicle or bus in traffic accident

V44.7   Person on outside of car injured in collision with heavy transport vehicle or bus in traffic accident

V44.9   Unspecified car occupant injured in collision with heavy transport vehicle or bus in traffic accident

V45   **Car occupant injured in collision with railway train or railway vehicle**

The following extensions are to be added to each code from category V45:

   a   initial encounter
   d   subsequent encounter
   q   sequelae

V45.0   Car driver injured in collision with railway train or railway vehicle in nontraffic accident

V45.1   Car passenger injured in collision with railway train or railway vehicle in nontraffic accident

V45.2   Person on outside of car injured in collision with railway train or railway vehicle in nontraffic accident

V45.3   Unspecified car occupant injured in collision with railway train or railway vehicle in nontraffic accident

V45.4   Person boarding or alighting a car injured in collision with railway train or railway vehicle

V45.5   Car driver injured in collision with railway train or railway vehicle in traffic accident

V45.6   Car passenger injured in collision with railway train or railway vehicle in traffic accident

V45.7   Person on outside of car injured in collision with railway train or railway vehicle in traffic accident

V45.9   Unspecified car occupant injured in collision with railway train or railway vehicle in traffic accident

V46   **Car occupant injured in collision with other nonmotor vehicle**

Includes: collision with animal-drawn vehicle, animal being ridden, streetcar

The following extensions are to be added to each code from category V46:

   a   initial encounter
   d   subsequent encounter
   q   sequelae

V46.0   Car driver injured in collision with other nonmotor vehicle in nontraffic accident

V46.1   Car passenger injured in collision with other nonmotor vehicle in nontraffic accident

V46.2   Person on outside of car injured in collision with other nonmotor vehicle in nontraffic accident

V46.3   Unspecified car occupant injured in collision with other nonmotor vehicle in nontraffic accident

V46.4   Person boarding or alighting a car injured in collision with other nonmotor vehicle

V46.5   Car driver injured in collision with other nonmotor vehicle in traffic accident

V46.6   Car passenger injured in collision with other nonmotor vehicle in traffic accident

V46.7   Person on outside of car injured in collision with other nonmotor vehicle in traffic accident

V46.9   Unspecified car occupant injured in collision with other nonmotor vehicle in traffic accident

V47 Car occupant injured in collision with fixed or stationary object

The following extensions are to be added to each code from category V47:

    a   initial encounter
    d   subsequent encounter
    q   sequelae

V47.0 Car driver injured in collision with fixed or stationary object in nontraffic accident

V47.01 Driver of sport utility vehicle injured in collision with fixed or stationary object in nontraffic accident

V47.02 Driver of other type car injured in collision with fixed or stationary object in nontraffic accident

V47.1 Car passenger injured in collision with fixed or stationary object in nontraffic accident

V47.11 Passenger of sport utility vehicle injured in collision with fixed or stationary object in nontraffic accident

V47.12 Passenger of other type car injured in collision with fixed or stationary object in nontraffic accident

V47.2 Person on outside of car injured in collision with fixed or stationary object in nontraffic accident

V47.3 Unspecified car occupant injured in collision with fixed or stationary object in nontraffic accident

V47.31 Unspecified occupant of sport utility vehicle injured in collision with fixed or stationary object in nontraffic accident

V47.32 Unspecified occupant of other type car injured in collision with fixed or stationary object in nontraffic accident

V47.4 Person boarding or alighting a car injured in collision with fixed or stationary object

V47.5 Car driver injured in collision with fixed or stationary object in traffic accident

V47.51 Driver of sport utility vehicle injured in collision with fixed or stationary object in traffic accident

V47.52 Driver of other type car injured in collision with fixed or stationary object in traffic accident

V47.6 Car passenger injured in collision with fixed or stationary object in traffic accident

V47.61 Passenger of sport utility vehicle injured in collision with fixed or stationary object in traffic accident

V47.62 Passenger of other type car injured in collision with fixed or stationary object in traffic accident

V47.7 Person on outside of car injured in collision with fixed or stationary object in traffic accident

V47.9 Unspecified car occupant injured in collision with fixed or stationary object in traffic accident

V47.91 Unspecified occupant of sport utility vehicle injured in collision with fixed or stationary object in traffic accident

V47.92 Unspecified occupant of other type car injured in collision with fixed or stationary object in traffic accident

V48 Car occupant injured in noncollision transport accident

Includes: overturning car NOS
              overturning car without collision

The following extensions are to be added to each code from category V48:

    a   initial encounter
    d   subsequent encounter
    q   sequelae

V48.0 Car driver injured in noncollision transport accident in nontraffic accident

V48.1 Car passenger injured in noncollision transport accident in nontraffic accident

V48.2 Person on outside of car injured in noncollision transport accident in nontraffic accident

V48.3 Unspecified car occupant injured in noncollision transport accident in nontraffic accident

V48.4 Person boarding or alighting a car injured in noncollision transport accident

V48.5 Car driver injured in noncollision transport accident in traffic accident

V48.6 Car passenger injured in noncollision transport accident in traffic accident

V48.7 Person on outside of car injured in noncollision transport accident in traffic accident

V48.9 Unspecified car occupant injured in noncollision transport accident in traffic accident

V49 Car occupant injured in other and unspecified transport accidents

The following extensions are to be added to each code from category V49:

    a   initial encounter
    d   subsequent encounter
    q   sequelae

V49.0 Driver injured in collision with other and unspecified motor vehicles in nontraffic accident

V49.00 Driver injured in collision with unspecified motor vehicles in nontraffic accident

V49.09 Driver injured in collision with other motor vehicles in nontraffic accident

V49.1 Passenger injured in collision with other and unspecified motor vehicles in nontraffic accident

V49.10 Passenger injured in collision with unspecified motor vehicles in nontraffic accident

V49.19 Passenger injured in collision with other motor vehicles in nontraffic accident

V49.2 Unspecified car occupant injured in collision with other and unspecified motor vehicles in nontraffic accident

V49.20 Unspecified car occupant injured in collision with unspecified motor vehicles in nontraffic accident
            Car collision NOS, nontraffic

V49.29 Unspecified car occupant injured in collision with other motor vehicles in nontraffic accident

V49.3 Car occupant (driver) (passenger) injured in unspecified nontraffic accident
            Car accident NOS, nontraffic
            Car occupant injured in nontraffic accident NOS

V49.4 Driver injured in collision with other and unspecified motor vehicles in traffic accident

V49.40 Driver injured in collision with unspecified motor vehicles in traffic accident

V49.49 Driver injured in collision with other motor vehicles in traffic accident

V49.5 Passenger injured in collision with other and unspecified motor vehicles in traffic accident

V49.50 Passenger injured in collision with unspecified motor vehicles in traffic accident

V49.59 Passenger injured in collision with other motor vehicles in traffic accident

V49.6 Unspecified car occupant injured in collision with other and unspecified motor vehicles in traffic accident

V49.60 Unspecified car occupant injured in collision with unspecified motor vehicles in traffic accident
            Car collision NOS (traffic)

V49.69 Unspecified car occupant injured in collision with other motor vehicles in traffic accident

V49.8 Car occupant (driver) (passenger) injured in other specified transport accidents

V49.81 Car occupant (driver) (passenger) injured in transport accident with military vehicle

V49.88 Car occupant (driver) (passenger) injured in other specified transport accidents

V49.9 Car occupant (driver) (passenger) injured in unspecified traffic accident
            Car accident NOS

OCCUPANT OF PICK–UP TRUCK OR VAN INJURED IN TRANSPORT ACCIDENT (V50–V59)

Includes: a four or six wheel motor vehicle designed primarily for carrying property but weighing less than the local limit for classification as a heavy goods vehicle
truck van

Excludes1:   heavy transport vehicle (V60-V69)

V50 Occupant of pick-up truck or van injured in collision with pedestrian or animal

Excludes1:   pick-up truck or van collision with animal-drawn vehicle or animal being ridden (V56.-)

The following extensions are to be added to each code from category V50:

     a   initial encounter
     d   subsequent encounter
     q   sequelae

V50.0 Driver of pick-up truck or van injured in collision with pedestrian or animal in nontraffic accident

V50.1 Passenger in pick-up truck or van injured in collision with pedestrian or animal in nontraffic accident

V50.2 Person on outside of pick-up truck or van injured in collision with pedestrian or animal in nontraffic accident

V50.3 Unspecified occupant of pick-up truck or van injured in collision with pedestrian or animal in nontraffic accident

V50.4 Person boarding or alighting a pick-up truck or van injured in collision with pedestrian or animal

V50.5 Driver of pick-up truck or van injured in collision with pedestrian or animal in traffic accident

V50.6 Passenger in pick-up truck or van injured in collision with pedestrian or animal in traffic accident

V50.7 Person on outside of pick-up truck or van injured in collision with pedestrian or animal in traffic accident

V50.9 Unspecified occupant of pick-up truck or van injured in collision with pedestrian or animal in traffic accident

V51 Occupant of pick-up truck or van injured in collision with pedal cycle

The following extensions are to be added to each code from category V51:

     a   initial encounter
     d   subsequent encounter
     q   sequelae

V51.0 Driver of pick-up truck or van injured in collision with pedal cycle in nontraffic accident

V51.1 Passenger in pick-up truck or van injured in collision with pedal cycle in nontraffic accident

V51.2 Person on outside of pick-up truck or van injured in collision with pedal cycle in nontraffic accident

V51.3 Unspecified occupant of pick-up truck or van injured in collision with pedal cycle in nontraffic accident

V51.4 Person boarding or alighting a pick-up truck or van injured in collision with pedal cycle

V51.5 Driver of pick-up truck or van injured in collision with pedal cycle in traffic accident

V51.6 Passenger in pick-up truck or van injured in collision with pedal cycle in traffic accident

V51.7 Person on outside of pick-up truck or van injured in collision with pedal cycle in traffic accident

V51.9 Unspecified occupant of pick-up truck or van injured in collision with pedal cycle in traffic accident

V52 Occupant of pick-up truck or van injured in collision with two- or three-wheeled motor vehicle

The following extensions are to be added to each code from category V52:

     a   initial encounter
     d   subsequent encounter
     q   sequelae

V52.0 Driver of pick-up truck or van injured in collision with two- or three-wheeled motor vehicle in nontraffic accident

V52.1 Passenger in pick-up truck or van injured in collision with two- or three-wheeled motor vehicle in nontraffic accident

V52.2 Person on outside of pick-up truck or van injured in collision with two- or three-wheeled motor vehicle in nontraffic accident

V52.3 Unspecified occupant of pick-up truck or van injured in collision with two- or three-wheeled motor vehicle in nontraffic accident

V52.4 Person boarding or alighting a pick-up truck or van injured in collision with two- or three-wheeled motor vehicle

V52.5 Driver of pick-up truck or van injured in collision with two- or three-wheeled motor vehicle in traffic accident

V52.6 Passenger in pick-up truck or van injured in collision with two- or three-wheeled motor vehicle in traffic accident

V52.7 Person on outside of pick-up truck or van injured in collision with two- or three-wheeled motor vehicle in traffic accident

V52.9 Unspecified occupant of pick-up truck or van injured in collision with two-or three-wheeled motor vehicle in traffic accident

V53 Occupant of pick-up truck or van injured in collision with car, pick-up truck or van

The following extensions are to be added to each code from category V53:

     a   initial encounter
     d   subsequent encounter
     q   sequelae

V53.0 Driver of pick-up truck or van injured in collision with car, pick-up truck or van in nontraffic accident

V53.1 Passenger in pick-up truck or van injured in collision with car, pick-up truck or van in nontraffic accident

V53.2 Person on outside of pick-up truck or van injured in collision with car, pick-up truck or van in nontraffic accident

V53.3 Unspecified occupant of pick-up truck or van injured in collision with car, pick-up truck or van in nontraffic accident

V53.4 Person boarding or alighting a pick-up truck or van injured in collision with car, pick-up truck or van

V53.5 Driver of pick-up truck or van injured in collision with car, pick-up truck or van in traffic accident

V53.6 Passenger in pick-up truck or van injured in collision with car, pick-up truck or van in traffic accident

V53.7 Person on outside of pick-up truck or van injured in collision with car, pick-up truck or van in traffic accident

V53.9 Unspecified occupant of pick-up truck or van injured in collision with car, pick-up truck or van in traffic accident

V54 Occupant of pick-up truck or van injured in collision with heavy transport vehicle or bus

Excludes1:   occupant of pick-up truck or van injured in collision with military vehicle (V59.81)

The following extensions are to be added to each code from category V54:

     a   initial encounter
     d   subsequent encounter
     q   sequelae

V54.0 Driver of pick-up truck or van injured in collision with heavy transport vehicle or bus in nontraffic accident

V54.1 Passenger in pick-up truck or van injured in collision with heavy transport vehicle or bus in nontraffic accident

V54.2 Person on outside of pick-up truck or van injured in collision with heavy transport vehicle or bus in nontraffic accident

V54.3 Unspecified occupant of pick-up truck or van injured in collision with heavy transport vehicle or bus in nontraffic accident

V54.4 Person boarding or alighting a pick-up truck or van injured in collision with heavy transport vehicle or bus

V54.5 Driver of pick-up truck or van injured in collision with heavy transport vehicle or bus in traffic accident

V54.6 Passenger in pick-up truck or van injured in collision with heavy transport vehicle or bus in traffic accident

V54.7 Person on outside of pick-up truck or van injured in collision with heavy transport vehicle or bus in traffic accident

V54.9 Unspecified occupant of pick-up truck or van injured in collision with heavy transport vehicle or bus in traffic accident

V55 Occupant of pick-up truck or van injured in collision with railway train or railway vehicle

The following extensions are to be added to each code from category V55:

a   initial encounter
d   subsequent encounter
q   sequelae

V55.0   Driver of pick-up truck or van injured in collision with railway train or railway vehicle in nontraffic accident

V55.1   Passenger in pick-up truck or van injured in collision with railway train or railway vehicle in nontraffic accident

V55.2   Person on outside of pick-up truck or van injured in collision with railway train or railway vehicle in nontraffic accident

V55.3   Unspecified occupant of pick-up truck or van injured in collision with railway train or railway vehicle in nontraffic accident

V55.4   Person boarding or alighting a pick-up truck or van injured in collision with railway train or railway vehicle

V55.5   Driver of pick-up truck or van injured in collision with railway train or railway vehicle in traffic accident

V55.6   Passenger in pick-up truck or van injured in collision with railway train or railway vehicle in traffic accident

V55.7   Person on outside of pick-up truck or van injured in collision with railway train or railway vehicle in traffic accident

V55.9   Unspecified occupant of pick-up truck or van injured in collision with railway train or railway vehicle in traffic accident

V56 Occupant of pick-up truck or van injured in collision with other nonmotor vehicle

Includes: collision with animal-drawn vehicle, animal being ridden, streetcar

The following extensions are to be added to each code from category V56:

a   initial encounter
d   subsequent encounter
q   sequelae

V56.0   Driver of pick-up truck or van injured in collision with other nonmotor vehicle in nontraffic accident

V56.1   Passenger in pick-up truck or van injured in collision with other nonmotor vehicle in nontraffic accident

V56.2   Person on outside of pick-up truck or van injured in collision with other nonmotor vehicle in nontraffic accident

V56.3   Unspecified occupant of pick-up truck or van injured in collision with other nonmotor vehicle in nontraffic accident

V56.4   Person boarding or alighting a pick-up truck or van injured in collision with other nonmotor vehicle

V56.5   Driver of pick-up truck or van injured in collision with other nonmotor vehicle in traffic accident

V56.6   Passenger in pick-up truck or van injured in collision with other nonmotor vehicle in traffic accident

V56.7   Person on outside of pick-up truck or van injured in collision with other nonmotor vehicle in traffic accident

V56.9   Unspecified occupant of pick-up truck or van injured in collision with other nonmotor vehicle in traffic accident

V57 Occupant of pick-up truck or van injured in collision with fixed or stationary object

The following extensions are to be added to each code from category V57:

a   initial encounter
d   subsequent encounter
q   sequelae

V57.0   Driver of pick-up truck or van injured in collision with fixed or stationary object in nontraffic accident

V57.1   Passenger in pick-up truck or van injured in collision with fixed or stationary object in nontraffic accident

V57.2   Person on outside of pick-up truck or van injured in collision with fixed or stationary object in nontraffic accident

V57.3   Unspecified occupant of pick-up truck or van injured in collision with fixed or stationary object in nontraffic accident

V57.4   Person boarding or alighting a pick-up truck or van injured in collision with fixed or stationary object

V57.5   Driver of pick-up truck or van injured in collision with fixed or stationary object in traffic accident

V57.6   Passenger in pick-up truck or van injured in collision with fixed or stationary object in traffic accident

V57.7   Person on outside of pick-up truck or van injured in collision with fixed or stationary object in traffic accident

V57.9   Unspecified occupant of pick-up truck or van injured in collision with fixed or stationary object in traffic accident

V58 Occupant of pick-up truck or van injured in noncollision transport accident

Includes: overturning pick-up truck or van NOS
overturning pick-up truck or van without collision

The following extensions are to be added to each code from category V58:

a   initial encounter
d   subsequent encounter
q   sequelae

V58.0   Driver of pick-up truck or van injured in noncollision transport accident in nontraffic accident

V58.1   Passenger in pick-up truck or van injured in noncollision transport accident in nontraffic accident

V58.2   Person on outside of pick-up truck or van injured in noncollision transport accident in nontraffic accident

V58.3   Unspecified occupant of pick-up truck or van injured in noncollision transport accident in nontraffic accident

V58.4   Person boarding or alighting a pick-up truck or van injured in noncollision transport accident

V58.5   Driver of pick-up truck or van injured in noncollision transport accident in traffic accident

V58.6   Passenger in pick-up truck or van injured in noncollision transport accident in traffic accident

V58.7   Person on outside of pick-up truck or van injured in noncollision transport accident in traffic accident

V58.9   Unspecified occupant of pick-up truck or van injured in noncollision transport accident in traffic accident

V59 Occupant of pick-up truck or van injured in other and unspecified transport accidents

The following extensions are to be added to each code from category V59:

a   initial encounter
d   subsequent encounter
q   sequelae

V59.0   Driver of pick-up truck or van injured in collision with other and unspecified motor vehicles in nontraffic accident

   V59.00   Driver of pick-up truck or van injured in collision with unspecified motor vehicles in nontraffic accident

   V59.09   Driver of pick-up truck or van injured in collision with other motor vehicles in nontraffic accident

V59.1   Passenger in pick-up truck or van injured in collision with other and unspecified motor vehicles in nontraffic accident

   V59.10   Passenger in pick-up truck or van injured in collision with unspecified motor vehicles in nontraffic accident

   V59.11   Passenger in pick-up truck or van injured in collision with other motor vehicles in nontraffic accident

V59.2   Unspecified occupant of pick-up truck or van injured in collision with other and unspecified motor vehicles in nontraffic accident

   V59.20   Unspecified occupant of pick-up truck or van injured in collision with unspecified motor vehicles in nontraffic accident

     Collision NOS involving pick-up truck or van, nontraffic

   V59.21   Unspecified occupant of pick-up truck or van injured in collision with other motor vehicles in nontraffic accident

V59.3   Occupant (driver) (passenger) of pick-up truck or van injured in unspecified nontraffic accident

     Accident NOS involving pick-up truck or van, nontraffic
     Occupant of pick-up truck or van injured in nontraffic accident NOS

V59.4   Driver of pick-up truck or van injured in collision with other and unspecified motor vehicles in traffic accident

V59.40 Driver of pick-up truck or van injured in collision with unspecified motor vehicles in traffic accident

V59.49 Driver of pick-up truck or van injured in collision with other motor vehicles in traffic accident

V59.5 Passenger in pick-up truck or van injured in collision with other and unspecified motor vehicles in traffic accident

V59.50 Passenger in pick-up truck or van injured in collision with unspecified motor vehicles in traffic accident

V59.59 Passenger in pick-up truck or van injured in collision with other motor vehicles in traffic accident

V59.6 Unspecified occupant of pick-up truck or van injured in collision with other and unspecified motor vehicles in traffic accident

V59.60 Unspecified occupant of pick-up truck or van injured in collision with unspecified motor vehicles in traffic accident

Collision NOS involving pick-up truck or van (traffic)

V59.69 Unspecified occupant of pick-up truck or van injured in collision with other motor vehicles in traffic accident

V59.8 Occupant (driver) (passenger) of pick-up truck or van injured in other specified transport accidents

V59.81 Occupant (driver) (passenger) of pick-up truck or van injured in transport accident with military vehicle

V59.88 Occupant (driver) (passenger) of pick-up truck or van injured in other specified transport accidents

V59.9 Occupant (driver) (passenger) of pick-up truck or van injured in unspecified traffic accident

Accident NOS involving pick-up truck or van

OCCUPANT OF HEAVY TRANSPORT VEHICLE INJURED IN TRANSPORT ACCIDENT (V60–V69)

Includes: armored car
panel truck
18 wheeler

Excludes1:   bus
motorcoach

V60 Occupant of heavy transport vehicle injured in collision with pedestrian or animal

Excludes1:   heavy transport vehicle collision with animal-drawn vehicle or animal being ridden (V66.-)

The following extensions are to be added to each code from category V60:
- a   initial encounter
- d   subsequent encounter
- q   sequelae

V60.0 Driver of heavy transport vehicle injured in collision with pedestrian or animal in nontraffic accident

V60.1 Passenger in heavy transport vehicle injured in collision with pedestrian or animal in nontraffic accident

V60.2 Person on outside of heavy transport vehicle injured in collision with pedestrian or animal in nontraffic accident

V60.3 Unspecified occupant of heavy transport vehicle injured in collision with pedestrian or animal in nontraffic accident

V60.4 Person boarding or alighting a heavy transport vehicle injured in collision with pedestrian or animal

V60.5 Driver of heavy transport vehicle injured in collision with pedestrian or animal in traffic accident

V60.6 Passenger in heavy transport vehicle injured in collision with pedestrian or animal in traffic accident

V60.7 Person on outside of heavy transport vehicle injured in collision with pedestrian or animal in traffic accident

V60.9 Unspecified occupant of heavy transport vehicle injured in collision with pedestrian or animal in traffic accident

V61 Occupant of heavy transport vehicle injured in collision with pedal cycle

The following extensions are to be added to each code from category V61:
- a   initial encounter
- d   subsequent encounter
- q   sequelae

V61.0 Driver of heavy transport vehicle injured in collision with pedal cycle in nontraffic accident

V61.1 Passenger in heavy transport vehicle injured in collision with pedal cycle in nontraffic accident

V61.2 Person on outside of heavy transport vehicle injured in collision with pedal cycle in nontraffic accident

V61.3 Unspecified occupant of heavy transport vehicle injured in collision with pedal cycle in nontraffic accident

V61.4 Person boarding or alighting a heavy transport vehicle injured in collision with pedal cycle while boarding or alighting

V61.5 Driver of heavy transport vehicle injured in collision with pedal cycle in traffic accident

V61.6 Passenger in heavy transport vehicle injured in collision with pedal cycle in traffic accident

V61.7 Person on outside of heavy transport vehicle injured in collision with pedal cycle in traffic accident

V61.9 Unspecified occupant of heavy transport vehicle injured in collision with pedal cycle in traffic accident

V62 Occupant of heavy transport vehicle injured in collision with two- or three-wheeled motor vehicle

The following extensions are to be added to each code from category V62:
- a   initial encounter
- d   subsequent encounter
- q   sequelae

V62.0 Driver of heavy transport vehicle injured in collision with two- or three-

V62.1 Passenger in heavy transport vehicle injured in collision with two- or three-wheeled motor vehicle in nontraffic accident

V62.2 Person on outside of heavy transport vehicle injured in collision with two-or three-wheeled motor vehicle in nontraffic accident

V62.3 Unspecified occupant of heavy transport vehicle injured in collision with two- or three-wheeled motor vehicle in nontraffic accident

V62.4 Person boarding or alighting a heavy transport vehicle injured in collision with two- or three-wheeled motor vehicle

V62.5 Driver of heavy transport vehicle injured in collision with two- or three-wheeled motor vehicle in traffic accident

V62.6 Passenger in heavy transport vehicle injured in collision with two- or three-wheeled motor vehicle in traffic accident

V62.7 Person on outside of heavy transport vehicle injured in collision with two-or three-wheeled motor vehicle in traffic accident

V62.9 Unspecified occupant of heavy transport vehicle injured in collision with two- or three-wheeled motor vehicle in traffic accident

V63 Occupant of heavy transport vehicle injured in collision with car, pick-up truck or van

The following extensions are to be added to each code from category V63:
- a   initial encounter
- d   subsequent encounter
- q   sequelae

V63.0 Driver of heavy transport vehicle injured in collision with car, pick-up truck or van in nontraffic accident

V63.1 Passenger in heavy transport vehicle injured in collision with car, pick-up truck or van in nontraffic accident

V63.2 Person on outside of heavy transport vehicle injured in collision with car, pick-up truck or van in nontraffic accident

V63.3 Unspecified occupant of heavy transport vehicle injured in collision with car, pick-up truck or van in nontraffic accident

V63.4 Person boarding or alighting a heavy transport vehicle injured in collision with car, pick-up truck or van

V63.5 Driver of heavy transport vehicle injured in collision with car, pick-up truck or van in traffic accident

V63.6 Passenger in heavy transport vehicle injured in collision with car, pick-up truck or van in traffic accident

V63.7 Person on outside of heavy transport vehicle injured in collision with car, pick-up truck or van in traffic accident

V63.9 Unspecified occupant of heavy transport vehicle injured in collision with car, pick-up truck or van in traffic accident

V64   Occupant of heavy transport vehicle injured in collision with heavy transport vehicle or bus

    Excludes1:   occupant of heavy transport vehicle injured in collision with military vehicle (V69.81)

    The following extensions are to be added to each code from category V64:
      a   initial encounter
      d   subsequent encounter
      q   sequelae

V64.0   Driver of heavy transport vehicle injured in collision with heavy transport vehicle or bus in nontraffic accident

V64.1   Passenger in heavy transport vehicle injured in collision with heavy transport vehicle or bus in nontraffic accident

V64.2   Person on outside of heavy transport vehicle injured in collision with heavy transport vehicle or bus in nontraffic accident

V64.3   Unspecified occupant of heavy transport vehicle injured in collision with heavy transport vehicle or bus in nontraffic accident

V64.4   Person boarding or alighting a heavy transport vehicle injured in collision with heavy transport vehicle or bus while boarding or alighting

V64.5   Driver of heavy transport vehicle injured in collision with heavy transport vehicle or bus in traffic accident

V64.6   Passenger in heavy transport vehicle injured in collision with heavy transport vehicle or bus in traffic accident

V64.7   Person on outside of heavy transport vehicle injured in collision with heavy transport vehicle or bus in traffic accident

V64.9   Unspecified occupant of heavy transport vehicle injured in collision with heavy transport vehicle or bus in traffic accident

V65   Occupant of heavy transport vehicle injured in collision with railway train or railway vehicle

    The following extensions are to be added to each code from category V65:
      a   initial encounter
      d   subsequent encounter
      q   sequelae

V65.0   Driver of heavy transport vehicle injured in collision with railway train or railway vehicle in nontraffic accident

V65.1   Passenger in heavy transport vehicle injured in collision with railway train or railway vehicle in nontraffic accident

V65.2   Person on outside of heavy transport vehicle injured in collision with railway train or railway vehicle in nontraffic accident

V65.3   Unspecified occupant of heavy transport vehicle injured in collision with railway train or railway vehicle in nontraffic accident

V65.4   Person boarding or alighting a heavy transport vehicle injured in collision with railway train or railway vehicle

V65.5   Driver of heavy transport vehicle injured in collision with railway train or railway vehicle in traffic accident

V65.6   Passenger in heavy transport vehicle injured in collision with railway train or railway vehicle in traffic accident

V65.7   Person on outside of heavy transport vehicle injured in collision with railway train or railway vehicle in traffic accident

V65.9   Unspecified occupant of heavy transport vehicle injured in collision with railway train or railway vehicle in traffic accident

V66   Occupant of heavy transport vehicle injured in collision with other nonmotor vehicle

    Includes: collision with animal-drawn vehicle, animal being ridden, streetcar

    The following extensions are to be added to each code from category V66:
      a   initial encounter
      d   subsequent encounter
      q   sequelae

V66.0   Driver of heavy transport vehicle injured in collision with other nonmotor vehicle in nontraffic accident

V66.1   Passenger in heavy transport vehicle injured in collision with other nonmotor vehicle in nontraffic accident

V66.2   Person on outside of heavy transport vehicle injured in collision with other nonmotor vehicle in nontraffic accident

V66.3   Unspecified occupant of heavy transport vehicle injured in collision with other nonmotor vehicle in nontraffic accident

V66.4   Person boarding or alighting a heavy transport vehicle injured in collision with other nonmotor vehicle

V66.5   Driver of heavy transport vehicle injured in collision with other nonmotor vehicle in traffic accident

V66.6   Passenger in heavy transport vehicle injured in collision with other nonmotor vehicle in traffic accident

V66.7   Person on outside of heavy transport vehicle injured in collision with other nonmotor vehicle in traffic accident

V66.9   Unspecified occupant of heavy transport vehicle injured in collision with other nonmotor vehicle in traffic accident

V67   Occupant of heavy transport vehicle injured in collision with fixed or stationary object

    The following extensions are to be added to each code from category V67:
      a   initial encounter
      d   subsequent encounter
      q   sequelae

V67.0   Driver of heavy transport vehicle injured in collision with fixed or stationary object in nontraffic accident

V67.1   Passenger in heavy transport vehicle injured in collision with fixed or stationary object in nontraffic accident

V67.2   Person on outside of heavy transport vehicle injured in collision with fixed or stationary object in nontraffic accident

V67.3   Unspecified occupant of heavy transport vehicle injured in collision with fixed or stationary object in nontraffic accident

V67.4   Person boarding or alighting a heavy transport vehicle injured in collision with fixed or stationary object

V67.5   Driver of heavy transport vehicle injured in collision with fixed or stationary object in traffic accident

V67.6   Passenger in heavy transport vehicle injured in collision with fixed or stationary object in traffic accident

V67.7   Person on outside of heavy transport vehicle injured in collision with fixed or stationary object in traffic accident

V67.9   Unspecified occupant of heavy transport vehicle injured in collision with fixed or stationary object in traffic accident

V68   Occupant of heavy transport vehicle injured in noncollision transport accident

    Includes: overturning heavy transport vehicle NOS
                     overturning heavy transport vehicle without collision

    The following extensions are to be added to each code from category V68:
      a   initial encounter
      d   subsequent encounter
      q   sequelae

V68.0   Driver of heavy transport vehicle injured in noncollision transport accident in nontraffic accident

V68.1   Passenger in heavy transport vehicle injured in noncollision transport accident in nontraffic accident

V68.2   Person on outside of heavy transport vehicle injured in noncollision transport accident in nontraffic accident

V68.3   Unspecified occupant of heavy transport vehicle injured in noncollision transport accident in nontraffic accident

V68.4   Person boarding or alighting a heavy transport vehicle injured in noncollision transport accident

V68.5   Driver of heavy transport vehicle injured in noncollision transport accident in traffic accident

V68.6   Passenger in heavy transport vehicle injured in noncollision transport accident in traffic accident

V68.7   Person on outside of heavy transport vehicle injured in noncollision transport accident in traffic accident

V68.9   Unspecified occupant of heavy transport vehicle injured in noncollision transport accident in traffic accident

V69 Occupant of heavy transport vehicle injured in other and unspecified transport accidents

The following extensions are to be added to each code from category V69:
- a   initial encounter
- d   subsequent encounter
- q   sequelae

V69.0 Driver of heavy transport vehicle injured in collision with other and unspecified motor vehicles in nontraffic accident

  V69.00 Driver of heavy transport vehicle injured in collision with unspecified motor vehicles in nontraffic accident

  V69.09 Driver of heavy transport vehicle injured in collision with other motor vehicles in nontraffic accident

V69.1 Passenger in heavy transport vehicle injured in collision with other and unspecified motor vehicles in nontraffic accident

  V69.10 Passenger in heavy transport vehicle injured in collision with unspecified motor vehicles in nontraffic accident

  V69.19 Passenger in heavy transport vehicle injured in collision with other motor vehicles in nontraffic accident

V69.2 Unspecified occupant of heavy transport vehicle injured in collision with other and unspecified motor vehicles in nontraffic accident

  V69.20 Unspecified occupant of heavy transport vehicle injured in collision with unspecified motor vehicles in nontraffic accident

Collision NOS involving heavy transport vehicle, nontraffic

  V69.29 Unspecified occupant of heavy transport vehicle injured in collision with other motor vehicles in nontraffic accident

V69.3 Occupant (driver) (passenger) of heavy transport vehicle injured in unspecified nontraffic accident

Accident NOS involving heavy transport vehicle, nontraffic
Occupant of heavy transport vehicle injured in nontraffic accident NOS

V69.4 Driver of heavy transport vehicle injured in collision with other and unspecified motor vehicles in traffic accident

  V69.40 Driver of heavy transport vehicle injured in collision with unspecified motor vehicles in traffic accident

  V69.49 Driver of heavy transport vehicle injured in collision with other motor vehicles in traffic accident

V69.5 Passenger in heavy transport vehicle injured in collision with other and unspecified motor vehicles in traffic accident

  V69.50 Passenger in heavy transport vehicle injured in collision with unspecified motor vehicles in traffic accident

  V69.59 Passenger in heavy transport vehicle injured in collision with other motor vehicles in traffic accident

V69.6 Unspecified occupant of heavy transport vehicle injured in collision with other and unspecified motor vehicles in traffic accident

  V69.60 Unspecified occupant of heavy transport vehicle injured in collision with unspecified motor vehicles in traffic accident

Collision NOS involving heavy transport vehicle (traffic)

  V69.69 Unspecified occupant of heavy transport vehicle injured in collision with other motor vehicles in traffic accident

V69.8 Occupant (driver) (passenger) of heavy transport vehicle injured in other specified transport accidents

  V69.81 Occupant (driver) (passenger) of heavy transport vehicle injured in transport accidents with military vehicle

  V69.88 Occupant (driver) (passenger) of heavy transport vehicle injured in other specified transport accidents

V69.9 Occupant (driver) (passenger) of heavy transport vehicle injured in unspecified traffic accident

Accident NOS involving heavy transport vehicle

BUS OCCUPANT INJURED IN TRANSPORT ACCIDENT (V70–V79)

Includes: motorcoach
Excludes1:   minibus (V40-V49)

The following extensions are to be added to each code from category V70:
- a   initial encounter
- d   subsequent encounter
- q   sequelae

V70 Bus occupant injured in collision with pedestrian or animal

Excludes1:   bus collision with animal-drawn vehicle or animal being ridden (V76.-)

V70.0 Driver of bus injured in collision with pedestrian or animal in nontraffic accident

V70.1 Passenger on bus injured in collision with pedestrian or animal in nontraffic accident

V70.2 Person on outside of bus injured in collision with pedestrian or animal in nontraffic accident

V70.3 Unspecified occupant of bus injured in collision with pedestrian or animal in nontraffic accident

V70.4 Person boarding or alighting from bus injured in collision with pedestrian or animal

V70.5 Driver of bus injured in collision with pedestrian or animal in traffic accident

V70.6 Passenger on bus injured in collision with pedestrian or animal in traffic accident

V70.7 Person on outside of bus injured in collision with pedestrian or animal in traffic accident

V70.9 Unspecified occupant of bus injured in collision with pedestrian or animal in traffic accident

V71 Bus occupant injured in collision with pedal cycle

The following extensions are to be added to each code from category V71:
- a   initial encounter
- d   subsequent encounter
- q   sequelae

V71.0 Driver of bus injured in collision with pedal cycle in nontraffic accident

V71.1 Passenger on bus injured in collision with pedal cycle in nontraffic accident

V71.2 Person on outside of bus injured in collision with pedal cycle in nontraffic accident

V71.3 Unspecified occupant of bus injured in collision with pedal cycle in nontraffic accident

V71.4 Person boarding or alighting from bus injured in collision with pedal cycle

V71.5 Driver of bus injured in collision with pedal cycle in traffic accident

V71.6 Passenger on bus injured in collision with pedal cycle in traffic accident

V71.7 Person on outside of bus injured in collision with pedal cycle in traffic accident

V71.9 Unspecified occupant of bus injured in collision with pedal cycle in traffic accident

V72 Bus occupant injured in collision with two- or three-wheeled motor vehicle

The following extensions are to be added to each code from category V72:
- a   initial encounter
- d   subsequent encounter
- q   sequelae

V72.0 Driver of bus injured in collision with two- or three-wheeled motor vehicle in nontraffic accident

V72.1 Passenger on bus injured in collision with two- or three-wheeled motor vehicle in nontraffic accident

V72.2 Person on outside of bus injured in collision with two- or three-wheeled motor vehicle in nontraffic accident

V72.3 Unspecified occupant of bus injured in collision with two- or three-wheeled motor vehicle in nontraffic accident

V72.4 Person boarding or alighting from bus injured in collision with two- or three-wheeled motor vehicle

V72.5 Driver of bus injured in collision with two- or three-wheeled motor vehicle in traffic accident

V72.6 Passenger on bus injured in collision with two- or three-wheeled motor vehicle in traffic accident

V72.7 Person on outside of bus injured in collision with two- or three-wheeled motor vehicle in traffic accident

V72.9 Unspecified occupant of bus injured in collision with two- or three-wheeled motor vehicle in traffic accident

V73 **Bus occupant injured in collision with car, pick-up truck or van**

The following extensions are to be added to each code from category V73:

　　a　　initial encounter
　　d　　subsequent encounter
　　q　　sequelae

V73.0 Driver of bus injured in collision with car, pick-up truck or van in nontraffic accident

V73.1 Passenger on bus injured in collision with car, pick-up truck or van in nontraffic accident

V73.2 Person on outside of bus injured in collision with car, pick-up truck or van in nontraffic accident

V73.3 Unspecified occupant of bus injured in collision with car, pick-up truck or van in nontraffic accident

V73.4 Person boarding or alighting from bus injured in collision with car, pick-up truck or van

V73.5 Driver of bus injured in collision with car, pick-up truck or van in traffic accident

V73.6 Passenger on bus injured in collision with car, pick-up truck or van in traffic accident

V73.7 Person on outside of bus injured in collision with car, pick-up truck or van in traffic accident

V73.9 Unspecified occupant of bus injured in collision with car, pick-up truck or van in traffic accident

V74 **Bus occupant injured in collision with heavy transport vehicle or bus**

Excludes1:　bus occupant injured in collision with military vehicle (V79.81)

The following extensions are to be added to each code from category V74:

　　a　　initial encounter
　　d　　subsequent encounter
　　q　　sequelae

V74.0 Driver of bus injured in collision with heavy transport vehicle or bus in nontraffic accident

V74.1 Passenger on bus injured in collision with heavy transport vehicle or bus in nontraffic accident

V74.2 Person on outside of bus injured in collision with heavy transport vehicle or bus in nontraffic accident

V74.3 Unspecified occupant of bus injured in collision with heavy transport vehicle or bus in nontraffic accident

V74.4 Person boarding or alighting from bus injured in collision with heavy transport vehicle or bus

V74.5 Driver of bus injured in collision with heavy transport vehicle or bus in traffic accident

V74.6 Passenger on bus injured in collision with heavy transport vehicle or bus in traffic accident

V74.7 Person on outside of bus injured in collision with heavy transport vehicle or bus in traffic accident

V74.9 Unspecified occupant of bus injured in collision with heavy transport vehicle or bus in traffic accident

V75 **Bus occupant injured in collision with railway train or railway vehicle**

The following extensions are to be added to each code from category V75:

　　a　　initial encounter
　　d　　subsequent encounter
　　q　　sequelae

V75.0 Driver of bus injured in collision with railway train or railway vehicle in nontraffic accident

V75.1 Passenger on bus injured in collision with railway train or railway vehicle in nontraffic accident

V75.2 Person on outside of bus injured in collision with railway train or railway vehicle in nontraffic accident

V75.3 Unspecified occupant of bus injured in collision with railway train or railway vehicle in nontraffic accident

V75.4 Person boarding or alighting from bus injured in collision with railway train or railway vehicle

V75.5 Driver of bus injured in collision with railway train or railway vehicle in traffic accident

V75.6 Passenger on bus injured in collision with railway train or railway vehicle in traffic accident

V75.7 Person on outside of bus injured in collision with railway train or railway vehicle in traffic accident

V75.9 Unspecified occupant of bus injured in collision with railway train or railway vehicle in traffic accident

V76 **Bus occupant injured in collision with other nonmotor vehicle**

Includes:　collision with animal-drawn vehicle, animal being ridden, streetcar

The following extensions are to be added to each code from category V76:

　　a　　initial encounter
　　d　　subsequent encounter
　　q　　sequelae

V76.0 Driver of bus injured in collision with other nonmotor vehicle in nontraffic accident

V76.1 Passenger on bus injured in collision with other nonmotor vehicle in nontraffic accident

V76.2 Person on outside of bus injured in collision with other nonmotor vehicle in nontraffic accident

V76.3 Unspecified occupant of bus injured in collision with other nonmotor vehicle in nontraffic accident

V76.4 Person boarding or alighting from bus injured in collision with other nonmotor vehicle

V76.5 Driver of bus injured in collision with other nonmotor vehicle in traffic accident

V76.6 Passenger on bus injured in collision with other nonmotor vehicle in traffic accident

V76.7 Person on outside of bus injured in collision with other nonmotor vehicle in traffic accident

V76.9 Unspecified occupant of bus injured in collision with other nonmotor vehicle in traffic accident

V77 **Bus occupant injured in collision with fixed or stationary object**

The following extensions are to be added to each code from category V77:

　　a　　initial encounter
　　d　　subsequent encounter
　　q　　sequelae

V77.0 Driver of bus injured in collision with fixed or stationary object in nontraffic accident

V77.1 Passenger on bus injured in collision with fixed or stationary object in nontraffic accident

V77.2 Person on outside of bus injured in collision with fixed or stationary object in nontraffic accident

V77.3 Unspecified occupant of bus injured in collision with fixed or stationary object in nontraffic accident

V77.4 Person boarding or alighting from bus injured in collision with fixed or stationary object

V77.5 Driver of bus injured in collision with fixed or stationary object in traffic accident

V77.6 Passenger on bus injured in collision with fixed or stationary object in traffic accident

V77.7 Person on outside of bus injured in collision with fixed or stationary object in traffic accident

V77.9 Unspecified occupant of bus injured in collision with fixed or stationary object in traffic accident

V78 Bus occupant injured in noncollision transport accident

Includes: overturning bus NOS
             overturning bus without collision

The following extensions are to be added to each code from category V78:

a   initial encounter
d   subsequent encounter
q   sequelae

V78.0 Driver of bus injured in noncollision transport accident in nontraffic accident

V78.1 Passenger on bus injured in noncollision transport accident in nontraffic accident

V78.2 Person on outside of bus injured in noncollision transport accident in nontraffic accident

V78.3 Unspecified occupant of bus injured in noncollision transport accident in nontraffic accident

V78.4 Person boarding or alighting from bus injured in noncollision transport accident

V78.5 Driver of bus injured in noncollision transport accident in traffic accident

V78.6 Passenger on bus injured in noncollision transport accident in traffic accident

V78.7 Person on outside of bus injured in noncollision transport accident in traffic accident

V78.9 Unspecified occupant of bus injured in noncollision transport accident in traffic accident

V79 Bus occupant injured in other and unspecified transport accidents

The following extensions are to be added to each code from category V79:

a   initial encounter
d   subsequent encounter
q   sequelae

V79.0 Driver of bus injured in collision with other and unspecified motor vehicles in nontraffic accident

V79.00 Driver of bus injured in collision with unspecified motor vehicles in nontraffic accident

V79.09 Driver of bus injured in collision with other motor vehicles in nontraffic accident

V79.1 Passenger on bus injured in collision with other and unspecified motor vehicles in nontraffic accident

V79.10 Passenger on bus injured in collision with unspecified motor vehicles in nontraffic accident

V79.19 Passenger on bus injured in collision with other motor vehicles in nontraffic accident

V79.2 Unspecified bus occupant injured in collision with other and unspecified motor vehicles in nontraffic accident

V79.20 Unspecified bus occupant injured in collision with unspecified motor vehicles in nontraffic accident
Bus collision NOS, nontraffic

V79.29 Unspecified bus occupant injured in collision with other motor vehicles in nontraffic accident

V79.3 Bus occupant (driver) (passenger) injured in unspecified nontraffic accident
Bus accident NOS, nontraffic
Bus occupant injured in nontraffic accident NOS

V79.4 Driver of bus injured in collision with other and unspecified motor vehicles in traffic accident

V79.40 Driver of bus injured in collision with unspecified motor vehicles in traffic accident

V79.49 Driver of bus injured in collision with other motor vehicles in traffic accident

V79.5 Passenger on bus injured in collision with other and unspecified motor vehicles in traffic accident

V79.50 Passenger on bus injured in collision with unspecified motor vehicles in traffic accident

V79.59 Passenger on bus injured in collision with other motor vehicles in traffic accident

V79.6 Unspecified bus occupant injured in collision with other and unspecified motor vehicles in traffic accident

V79.60 Unspecified bus occupant injured in collision with unspecified motor vehicles in traffic accident
Bus collision NOS (traffic)

V79.69 Unspecified bus occupant injured in collision with other motor vehicles in traffic accident

V79.8 Bus occupant (driver) (passenger) injured in other specified transport accidents

V79.81 Bus occupant (driver) (passenger) injured in transport accidents with military vehicle

V79.88 Bus occupant (driver) (passenger) injured in other specified transport accidents

V79.9 Bus occupant (driver) (passenger) injured in unspecified traffic accident
Bus accident NOS

OTHER LAND TRANSPORT ACCIDENTS (V80–V89)

V80 Animal-rider or occupant of animal-drawn vehicle injured in transport accident

The following extensions are to be added to each code from category V80:

a   initial encounter
d   subsequent encounter
q   sequelae

V80.0 Animal-rider or occupant of animal drawn vehicle injured by fall from or being thrown from animal or animal-drawn vehicle in noncollision accident

V80.01 Animal-rider injured by fall from or being thrown from animal in noncollision accident

V80.010 Animal-rider injured by fall from or being thrown from horse in noncollision accident

V80.018 Animal-rider injured by fall from or being thrown from other animal in noncollision accident

V80.02 Occupant of animal-drawn vehicle injured by fall from or being thrown from animal-drawn vehicle in noncollision accident
Overturning animal-drawn vehicle NOS
Overturning animal-drawn vehicle without collision

V80.1 Animal-rider or occupant of animal-drawn vehicle injured in collision with pedestrian or animal

Excludes1:   animal-rider or animal-drawn vehicle collision with animal-drawn vehicle or animal being ridden (V80.7)

V80.11 Animal-rider injured in collision with pedestrian or animal

V80.12 Occupant of animal-drawn vehicle injured in collision with pedestrian or animal

V80.2 Animal-rider or occupant of animal-drawn vehicle injured in collision with pedal cycle

V80.21 Animal-rider injured in collision with pedal cycle

V80.22 Occupant of animal-drawn vehicle injured in collision with pedal cycle

V80.3 Animal-rider or occupant of animal-drawn vehicle injured in collision with two- or three-wheeled motor vehicle

V80.31 Animal-rider injured in collision with two- or three-wheeled motor vehicle

V80.32 Occupant of animal-drawn vehicle injured in collision with two- or three-wheeled motor vehicle

V80.4 Animal-rider or occupant of animal-drawn vehicle injured in collision with car, pick-up truck, van, heavy transport vehicle or bus

Excludes1:   animal-rider injured in collision with military vehicle (V80.910)
occupant of animal-drawn vehicle injured in collision with military vehicle (V80.920)

V80.41 Animal-rider injured in collision with car, pick-up truck, van, heavy transport vehicle or bus

V80.42 Occupant of animal-drawn vehicle injured in collision with car, pick-up truck, van, heavy transport vehicle or bus

V80.5 Animal-rider or occupant of animal-drawn vehicle injured in collision with other specified motor vehicle

V80.51 Animal-rider injured in collision with other specified motor vehicle

V80.52   Occupant of animal-drawn vehicle injured in collision with other specified motor vehicle

V80.6   Animal-rider or occupant of animal-drawn vehicle injured in collision with railway train or railway vehicle

V80.61   Animal-rider injured in collision with railway train or railway vehicle

V80.62   Occupant of animal-drawn vehicle injured in collision with railway train or railway vehicle

V80.7   Animal-rider or occupant of animal-drawn vehicle injured in collision with other nonmotor vehicles

V80.71   Animal-rider or occupant of animal-drawn vehicle injured in collision with animal being ridden

V80.710   Animal-rider injured in collision with other animal being ridden

V80.711   Occupant of animal-drawn vehicle injured in collision with animal being ridden

V80.72   Animal-rider or occupant of animal-drawn vehicle injured in collision with other animal-drawn vehicle

V80.720   Animal-rider injured in collision with animal-drawn vehicle

V80.721   Occupant of animal-drawn vehicle injured in collision with other animal-drawn vehicle

V80.73   Animal-rider or occupant of animal-drawn vehicle injured in collision with streetcar

V80.730   Animal-rider injured in collision with streetcar

V80.731   Occupant of animal-drawn vehicle injured in collision with streetcar

V80.79   Animal-rider or occupant of animal-drawn vehicle injured in collision with other nonmotor vehicles

V80.790   Animal-rider injured in collision with other nonmotor vehicles

V80.791   Occupant of animal-drawn vehicle injured in collision with other nonmotor vehicles

V80.8   Animal-rider or occupant of animal-drawn vehicle injured in collision with fixed or stationary object

V80.81   Animal-rider injured in collision with fixed or stationary object

V80.82   Occupant of animal-drawn vehicle injured in collision with fixed or stationary object

V80.9   Animal-rider or occupant of animal-drawn vehicle injured in other and unspecified transport accidents

V80.91   Animal-rider injured in other and unspecified transport accidents

V80.910   Animal-rider injured in transport accident with military vehicle

V80.918   Animal-rider injured in other transport accident

V80.919   Animal-rider injured in unspecified transport accident
Animal rider accident NOS

V80.92   Occupant of animal-drawn vehicle injured in other and unspecified transport accidents

V80.920   Occupant of animal-drawn vehicle injured in transport accident with military vehicle

V80.928   Occupant of animal-drawn vehicle injured in other transport accident

V80.929   Occupant of animal-drawn vehicle injured in unspecified transport accident
Animal-drawn vehicle accident NOS

V81   Occupant of railway train or railway vehicle injured in transport accident

Includes: derailment of railway train or railway vehicle
person on outside of train

Excludes1:   streetcar (V82.-)

The following extensions are to be added to each code from category V81:
a   initial encounter
d   subsequent encounter
q   sequelae

V81.0   Occupant of railway train or railway vehicle injured in collision with motor vehicle in nontraffic accident

Excludes1:   Occupant of railway train or railway vehicle injured due to collision with military vehicle (V81.83)

V81.1   Occupant of railway train or railway vehicle injured in collision with motor vehicle in traffic accident

Excludes1:   Occupant of railway train or railway vehicle injured due to collision with military vehicle (V81.83)

V81.2   Occupant of railway train or railway vehicle injured in collision with or hit by rolling stock

V81.3   Occupant of railway train or railway vehicle injured in collision with other object
Railway collision NOS

V81.4   Person injured while boarding or alighting from railway train or railway vehicle

V81.5   Occupant of railway train or railway vehicle injured by fall in railway train or railway vehicle

V81.6   Occupant of railway train or railway vehicle injured by fall from railway train or railway vehicle

V81.7   Occupant of railway train or railway vehicle injured in derailment without antecedent collision

V81.8   Occupant of railway train or railway vehicle injured in other specified railway accidents

V81.81   Occupant of railway train or railway vehicle injured due to explosion or fire on train

V81.82   Occupant of railway train or railway vehicle injured due to object falling onto train
Occupant of railway train or railway vehicle injured due to falling earth onto train
Occupant of railway train or railway vehicle injured due to falling rocks onto train
Occupant of railway train or railway vehicle injured due to falling snow onto train
Occupant of railway train or railway vehicle injured due to falling trees onto train

V81.83   Occupant of railway train or railway vehicle injured due to collision with military vehicle

V81.89   Occupant of railway train or railway vehicle injured due to other specified railway accident

V81.9   Occupant of railway train or railway vehicle injured in unspecified railway accident
Railway accident NOS

V82   Occupant of powered streetcar injured in transport accident

Includes: interurban electric car
person on outside of streetcar
tram (car)
trolley (car)

Excludes1:   bus (V70-V79)
motorcoach (V70-V79)
nonpowered streetcar (V76.-)
train (V81.-)

The following extensions are to be added to each code from category V82:
a   initial encounter
d   subsequent encounter
q   sequelae

V82.0   Occupant of streetcar injured in collision with motor vehicle in nontraffic accident

V82.1   Occupant of streetcar injured in collision with motor vehicle in traffic accident

V82.2   Occupant of streetcar injured in collision with or hit by rolling stock

V82.3   Occupant of streetcar injured in collision with other object
Excludes1:   collision with animal-drawn vehicle or animal being ridden (V82.8)

V82.4   Person injured while boarding or alighting from streetcar

V82.5   Occupant of streetcar injured by fall in streetcar
Excludes1:   fall in streetcar:
while boarding or alighting (V82.4)
with antecedent collision (V82.0-V82.3)

V82.6   **Occupant of streetcar injured by fall from streetcar**

     Excludes1:   fall from streetcar:
                   while boarding or alighting (V82.4)
                   with antecedent collision (V82.0-V82.3)

V82.7   **Occupant of streetcar injured in derailment without antecedent collision**

     Excludes1:   occupant of streetcar injured in derailment with antecedent collision (V82.0-V82.3)

V82.8   **Occupant of streetcar injured in other specified transport accidents**

     Streetcar collision with military vehicle
     Streetcar collision with train or nonmotor vehicles

V82.9   **Occupant of streetcar injured in unspecified traffic accident**

     Streetcar accident NOS

V83   **Occupant of special vehicle mainly used on industrial premises injured in transport accident**

     Includes: battery-powered airport passenger vehicle
                battery-powered truck (baggage) (mail)
                coal-car in mine
                forklift (truck)
                logging car
                self-propelled industrial truck
                station baggage truck (powered)
                tram, truck, or tub (powered) in mine or quarry

     Excludes1:   special construction vehicles (V85.-)
                special industrial vehicle in stationary use or maintenance (W31.-)

     The following extensions are to be added to each code from category V83:
         a   initial encounter
         d   subsequent encounter
         q   sequelae

V83.0   **Driver of special industrial vehicle injured in traffic accident**

V83.1   **Passenger of special industrial vehicle injured in traffic accident**

V83.2   **Person on outside of special industrial vehicle injured in traffic accident**

V83.3   **Unspecified occupant of special industrial vehicle injured in traffic accident**

V83.4   **Person injured while boarding or alighting from special industrial vehicle**

V83.5   **Driver of special industrial vehicle injured in nontraffic accident**

V83.6   **Passenger of special industrial vehicle injured in nontraffic accident**

V83.7   **Person on outside of special industrial vehicle injured in nontraffic accident**

V83.9   **Unspecified occupant of special industrial vehicle injured in nontraffic accident**

     Special-industrial-vehicle accident NOS

V84   **Occupant of special vehicle mainly used in agriculture injured in transport accident**

     Includes: self-propelled farm machinery
                tractor (and trailer)

     Excludes1:   animal-powered farm machinery accident (W30.8-)
                contact with combine harvester (W30.0)
                special agricultural vehicle in stationary use or maintenance (W30.-)

     The following extensions are to be added to each code from category V84:
         a   initial encounter
         d   subsequent encounter
         q   sequelae

V84.0   **Driver of special agricultural vehicle injured in traffic accident**

V84.1   **Passenger of special agricultural vehicle injured in traffic accident**

V84.2   **Person on outside of special agricultural vehicle injured in traffic accident**

V84.3   **Unspecified occupant of special agricultural vehicle injured in traffic accident**

V84.4   **Person injured while boarding or alighting from special agricultural vehicle**

V84.5   **Driver of special agricultural vehicle injured in nontraffic accident**

V84.6   **Passenger of special agricultural vehicle injured in nontraffic accident**

V84.7   **Person on outside of special agricultural vehicle injured in nontraffic accident**

V84.9   **Unspecified occupant of special agricultural vehicle injured in nontraffic accident**

     Special-agricultural vehicle accident NOS

V85   **Occupant of special construction vehicle injured in transport accident**

     Includes: bulldozer
                digger
                dump truck
                earth-leveller
                mechanical shovel
                road-roller

     Excludes1:   special industrial vehicle (V83.-)
                special construction vehicle in stationary use or maintenance (W31.-)

     The following extensions are to be added to each code from category V85:
         a   initial encounter
         d   subsequent encounter
         q   sequelae

V85.0   **Driver of special construction vehicle injured in traffic accident**

V85.1   **Passenger of special construction vehicle injured in traffic accident**

V85.2   **Person on outside of special construction vehicle injured in traffic accident**

V85.3   **Unspecified occupant of special construction vehicle injured in traffic accident**

V85.4   **Person injured while boarding or alighting from special construction vehicle**

V85.5   **Driver of special construction vehicle injured in nontraffic accident**

V85.6   **Passenger of special construction vehicle injured in nontraffic accident**

V85.7   **Person on outside of special construction vehicle injured in nontraffic accident**

V85.9   **Unspecified occupant of special construction vehicle injured in nontraffic accident**

     Special-construction-vehicle accident NOS

V86   **Occupant of special all-terrain or other motor vehicle, injured in transport accident**

     Excludes1:   special all-terrain vehicle in stationary use or maintenance (W31.-)
                sport-utility vehicle (V40-V49)
                three-wheeled motor vehicle designed for on-road use (V30-V39)

     The following extensions are to be added to each code from category V86:
         a   initial encounter
         d   subsequent encounter
         q   sequelae

V86.0   **Driver of special all-terrain or other motor vehicle injured in traffic accident**

    V86.01   **Driver of ambulance injured in traffic accident**

    V86.02   **Driver of snowmobile injured in traffic accident**

    V86.03   **Driver of dune buggy injured in traffic accident**

    V86.04   **Driver of military vehicle injured in traffic accident**

    V86.09   **Driver of other special all-terrain or other vehicle injured in traffic accident**

         Driver of dirt bike injured in traffic accident
         Driver of go cart injured in traffic accident
         Driver of golf cart injured in traffic accident

V86.1   **Passenger of special all-terrain or other motor vehicle injured in traffic accident**

    V86.11   **Passenger of ambulance injured in traffic accident**

    V86.12   **Passenger of snowmobile injured in traffic accident**

    V86.13   **Passenger of dune buggy injured in traffic accident**

V86.14   Passenger of military vehicle injured in traffic accident

V86.19   Passenger of other special all-terrain or other off-road motor vehicle injured in traffic accident
Passenger of dirt bike injured in traffic accident
Passenger of go cart injured in traffic accident
Passenger of golf cart injured in traffic accident

V86.2 Person on outside of special all-terrain or other motor vehicle injured in traffic accident

V86.21   Person on outside of ambulance injured in traffic accident

V86.22   Person on outside of snowmobile injured in traffic accident

V86.23   Person on outside of dune buggy injured in traffic accident

V86.24   Person on outside of military vehicle injured in traffic accident

V86.29   Person on outside of other special all-terrain or other motor vehicle injured in traffic accident
Person on outside of dirt bike injured in traffic accident
Person on outside of go cart in traffic accident
Person on outside of golf cart injured in traffic accident

V86.3 Unspecified occupant of special all-terrain or other motor vehicle injured in traffic accident

V86.31   Unspecified occupant of ambulance injured in traffic accident

V86.32   Unspecified occupant of snowmobile injured in traffic accident

V86.33   Unspecified occupant of dune buggy injured in traffic accident

V86.34   Unspecified occupant of military vehicle injured in traffic accident

V86.39   Unspecified occupant of other all-terrain or other motor vehicle injured in traffic accident
Unspecified occupant of dirt bike injured in traffic accident
Unspecified occupant of go cart injured in traffic accident
Unspecified occupant of golf cart injured in traffic accident

V86.4 Person injured while boarding or alighting from special all-terrain or other motor vehicle

V86.41   Person injured while boarding or alighting from ambulance

V86.42   Person injured while boarding or alighting from snowmobile

V86.43   Person injured while boarding or alighting from dune buggy

V86.44   Person injured while boarding or alighting from military vehicle

V86.49   Person injured while boarding or alighting from other special all-terrain or other motor vehicle
Person injured while boarding or alighting from dirt bike
Person injured while boarding or alighting from go cart
Person injured while boarding or alighting from golf cart

V86.5 Driver of special all-terrain or other motor vehicle injured in nontraffic accident

V86.51   Driver of ambulance injured in nontraffic accident

V86.52   Driver of snowmobile injured in nontraffic accident

V86.53   Driver of dune buggy injured in nontraffic accident

V86.54   Driver of military vehicle injured in nontraffic accident

V86.59   Driver of other special all-terrain or other vehicle injured in nontraffic accident
Driver of dirt bike injured in nontraffic accident
Driver of go cart injured in nontraffic accident
Driver of golf cart injured in nontraffic accident
Driver of race car injured in nontraffic accident

V86.6 Passenger of special all-terrain or other motor vehicle injured in nontraffic accident

V86.61   Passenger of ambulance injured in nontraffic accident

V86.62   Passenger of snowmobile injured in nontraffic accident

V86.63   Passenger of dune buggy injured in nontraffic accident

V86.64   Passenger of military vehicle injured in nontraffic accident

V86.69   Passenger of other special all-terrain or other vehicle injured in nontraffic accident
Passenger of dirt bike injured in nontraffic accident
Passenger of go cart injured in nontraffic accident
Passenger of golf cart injured in nontraffic accident
Passenger of race car injured in nontraffic accident

V86.7 Person on outside of special all-terrain or other motor vehicles injured in nontraffic accident

V86.71   Person on outside of ambulance injured in nontraffic accident

V86.72   Person on outside of snowmobile injured in nontraffic accident

V86.73   Person on outside of dune buggy injured in nontraffic accident

V86.74   Person on outside of military vehicle injured in nontraffic accident

V86.79   Person on outside of other special all-terrain or other motor vehicles injured in nontraffic accident
Person on outside of dirt bike injured in nontraffic accident
Person on outside of go cart injured in nontraffic accident
Person on outside of golf cart injured in nontraffic accident
Person on outside of race car injured in nontraffic accident

V86.9 Unspecified occupant of special all-terrain or other motor vehicle injured in nontraffic accident

V86.91   Unspecified occupant of ambulance injured in nontraffic accident

V86.92   Unspecified occupant of snowmobile injured in nontraffic accident

V86.93   Unspecified occupant of dune buggy injured in nontraffic accident

V86.94   Unspecified occupant of military vehicle injured in nontraffic accident

V86.99   Unspecified occupant of other special all-terrain or other motor vehicle injured in nontraffic accident
All-terrain motor-vehicle accident NOS
Off-road motor-vehicle accident NOS
Other motor-vehicle accident NOS
Unspecified occupant of dirt bike injured in nontraffic accident
Unspecified occupant of go cart injured in nontraffic accident
Unspecified occupant of golf cart injured in nontraffic accident
Unspecified occupant of race car injured in nontraffic accident

V87 Traffic accident of specified type but victim's mode of transport unknown

Excludes1:   collision involving:
pedal cycle (V10-V19)
pedestrian (V01-V09)

The following extensions are to be added to each code from category V87:
a   initial encounter
d   subsequent encounter
q   sequelae

V87.0 Person injured in collision between car and two- or three-wheeled powered vehicle (traffic)

V87.1 Person injured in collision between other motor vehicle and two- or three-wheeled motor vehicle (traffic)

V87.2 Person injured in collision between car and pick-up truck or van (traffic)

V87.3 Person injured in collision between car and bus (traffic)

V87.4 Person injured in collision between car and heavy transport vehicle (traffic)

V87.5 Person injured in collision between heavy transport vehicle and bus (traffic)

V87.6 Person injured in collision between railway train or railway vehicle and car (traffic)

V87.7 Person injured in collision between other specified motor vehicles (traffic)

V87.8 Person injured in other specified noncollision transport accidents involving motor vehicle (traffic)

V87.9 Person injured in other specified (collision) (noncollision) transport accidents involving nonmotor vehicle (traffic)

V88 Nontraffic accident of specified type but victim's mode of transport unknown

Excludes1: collision involving:
pedal cycle (V10-V19)
pedestrian (V01-V09)

The following extensions are to be added to each code from category V88:
a initial encounter
d subsequent encounter
q sequelae

V88.0 Person injured in collision between car and two- or three-wheeled motor vehicle, nontraffic

V88.1 Person injured in collision between other motor vehicle and two- or three-wheeled motor vehicle, nontraffic

V88.2 Person injured in collision between car and pick-up truck or van, nontraffic

V88.3 Person injured in collision between car and bus, nontraffic

V88.4 Person injured in collision between car and heavy transport vehicle, nontraffic

V88.5 Person injured in collision between heavy transport vehicle and bus, nontraffic

V88.6 Person injured in collision between railway train or railway vehicle and car, nontraffic

V88.7 Person injured in collision between other specified motor vehicle, nontraffic

V88.8 Person injured in other specified noncollision transport accidents involving motor vehicle, nontraffic

V88.9 Person injured in other specified (collision) (noncollision) transport accidents involving nonmotor vehicle, nontraffic

V89 Motor- or nonmotor-vehicle accident, type of vehicle unspecified

The following extensions are to be added to each code from category V89:
a initial encounter
d subsequent encounter
q sequelae

V89.0 Person injured in unspecified motor-vehicle accident, nontraffic
Motor-vehicle accident NOS, nontraffic

V89.1 Person injured in unspecified nonmotor-vehicle accident, nontraffic
Nonmotor-vehicle accident NOS (nontraffic)

V89.2 Person injured in unspecified motor-vehicle accident, traffic
Motor-vehicle accident [MVA] NOS
Road (traffic) accident [RTA] NOS

V89.3 Person injured in unspecified nonmotor-vehicle accident, traffic
Nonmotor-vehicle traffic accident NOS

V89.9 Person injured in unspecified vehicle accident
Collision NOS

WATER TRANSPORT ACCIDENTS (V90–V94)

V90 Drowning and submersion due to accident to watercraft

Excludes1: fall into water not from watercraft (W16.-)
military watercraft accident (Y36.0-, Y37.0-)
water-transport-related drowning or submersion without accident to watercraft (V92.-)

The following extensions are to be added to each code from category V90:
a initial encounter
d subsequent encounter
q sequelae

V90.0 Drowning and submersion due to watercraft overturning

V90.00 Drowning and submersion due to merchant ship overturning

V90.01 Drowning and submersion due to passenger ship overturning
Drowing and submersion due to Ferry-boat overturning
Drowning and submersion due to Liner overturning

V90.02 Drowning and submersion due to fishing boat overturning

V90.03 Drowning and submersion due to other powered watercraft overturning
Drowning and submersion due to Hovercraft (on open water) overturning
Drowning and submersion due to Jet ski overturning

V90.04 Drowning and submersion due to sailboat overturning

V90.05 Drowning and submersion due to canoe or kayak overturning

V90.06 Drowning and submersion due to (nonpowered) inflatable craft overturning

V90.08 Drowning and submersion due to other unpowered watercraft overturning
Drowning and submersion due to windsurfer overturning

V90.09 Drowning and submersion due to unspecified watercraft overturning
Drowning and submersion due to boat NOS overturning
Drowning and submersion due to ship NOS overturning
Drowning and submersion due to watercraft NOS overturning

V90.1 Drowning and submersion due to watercraft sinking

V90.10 Drowning and submersion due to merchant ship sinking

V90.11 Drowning and submersion due to passenger ship sinking
Drowning and submersion due to Ferry-boat sinking
Drowning and submersion due to Liner sinking

V90.12 Drowning and submersion due to fishing boat sinking

V90.13 Drowning and submersion due to other powered watercraft sinking
Drowning and submersion due to Hovercraft (on open water) sinking
Drowning and submersion due to Jet ski sinking

V90.14 Drowning and submersion due to sailboat sinking

V90.15 Drowning and submersion due to canoe or kayak sinking

V90.16 Drowning and submersion due to (nonpowered) inflatable craft sinking

V90.18 Drowning and submersion due to other unpowered watercraft sinking

V90.19 Drowning and submersion due to unspecified watercraft sinking
Drowning and submersion due to boat NOS sinking
Drowning and submersion due to ship NOS sinking
Drowning and submersion due to watercraft NOS sinking

V90.2 Drowning and submersion due to falling or jumping from burning watercraft

V90.20 Drowning and submersion due to falling or jumping from burning merchant ship

V90.21 Drowning and submersion due to falling or jumping from burning passenger ship
Drowning and submersion due to falling or jumping from burning Ferry-boat
Drowning and submersion due to falling or jumping from burning Liner

V90.22 Drowning and submersion due to falling or jumping from burning fishing boat

V90.23 Drowning and submersion due to falling or jumping from other burning powered watercraft
Drowning and submersion due to falling and jumping from burning Hovercraft (on open water)
Drowning and submersion due to falling and jumping from burning Jet ski

V90.24 Drowning and submersion due to falling or jumping from burning sailboat

V90.25 Drowning and submersion due to falling or jumping from burning canoe or kayak

V90.26 Drowning and submersion due to falling or jumping from burning (nonpowered) inflatable craft

V90.27 Drowning and submersion due to falling or jumping from burning water-skis

V90.28 Drowning and submersion due to falling or jumping from other burning unpowered watercraft
    Drowning and submersion due to falling and jumping from burning surf-board
    Drowning and submersion due to falling and jumping from burning windsurfer

V90.29 Drowning and submersion due to falling or jumping from unspecified burning watercraft
    Drowning and submersion due to falling or jumping from burning boat NOS
    Drowning and submersion due to falling or jumping from burning ship NOS
    Drowning and submersion due to falling or jumping from burning watercraft NOS

V90.3 Drowning and submersion due to falling or jumping from crushed watercraft

V90.30 Drowning and submersion due to falling or jumping from crushed merchant ship

V90.31 Drowning and submersion due to falling or jumping from crushed passenger ship
    Drowning and submersion due to falling and jumping from crushed Ferry boat
    Drowning and submersion due to falling and jumping from crushed Liner

V90.32 Drowning and submersion due to falling or jumping from crushed fishing boat

V90.33 Drowning and submersion due to falling or jumping from other crushed powered watercraft
    Drowning and submersion due to falling and jumping from crushed Hovercraft
    Drowning and submersion due to falling and jumping from crushed Jet ski

V90.34 Drowning and submersion due to falling or jumping from crushed sailboat

V90.35 Drowning and submersion due to falling or jumping from crushed canoe or kayak

V90.36 Drowning and submersion due to falling or jumping from crushed (nonpowered) inflatable craft

V90.37 Drowning and submersion due to falling or jumping from crushed water-skis

V90.38 Drowning and submersion due to falling or jumping from other crushed unpowered watercraft
    Drowning and submersion due to falling and jumping from crushed surf-board
    Drowning and submersion due to falling and jumping from crushed windsurfer

V90.39 Drowning and submersion due to falling or jumping from crushed unspecified watercraft
    Drowning and submersion due to falling and jumping from crushed boat NOS
    Drowning and submersion due to falling and jumping from crushed ship NOS
    Drowning and submersion due to falling and jumping from crushed watercraft NOS

V90.8 Drowning and submersion due to other accident to watercraft

V90.80 Drowning and submersion due to other accident to merchant ship

V90.81 Drowning and submersion due to other accident to passenger ship
    Drowning and submersion due to other accident to Ferry-boat
    Drowning and submersion due to other accident to Liner

V90.82 Drowning and submersion due to other accident to fishing boat

V90.83 Drowning and submersion due to other accident to other powered watercraft
    Drowning and submersion due to other accident to Hovercraft (on open water)
    Drowning and submersion due to other accident to Jet ski

V90.84 Drowning and submersion due to other accident to sailboat

V90.85 Drowning and submersion due to other accident to canoe or kayak

V90.86 Drowning and submersion due to other accident to (nonpowered) inflatable craft

V90.87 Drowning and submersion due to other accident to water-skis

V90.88 Drowning and submersion due to other accident to other unpowered watercraft
    Drowning and submersion due to other accident to surf-board
    Drowning and submersion due to other accident to windsurfer

V90.89 Drowning and submersion due to other accident to unspecified watercraft
    Drowning and submersion due to other accident to boat NOS
    Drowning and submersion due to other accident to ship NOS
    Drowning and submersion due to other accident to watercraft NOS

V91 Other injury due to accident to watercraft

Includes: any injury except drowning and submersion as a result of an accident to watercraft

Excludes1:   military watercraft accident (Y36, Y37-)

Excludes2:   drowning and submersion due to accident to watercraft (V90.-)

The following extensions are to be added to each code from category V91:
    a   initial encounter
    d   subsequent encounter
    q   sequelae

V91.0 Burn due to watercraft on fire

Excludes1:   burn from localized fire or explosion on board ship without accident to watercraft (V93.-)

V91.00 Burn due to merchant ship on fire

V91.01 Burn due to passenger ship on fire
    Burn due to Ferry-boat on fire
    Burn due to Liner on fire

V91.02 Burn due to fishing boat on fire

V91.03 Burn due to other powered watercraft on fire
    Burn due to Hovercraft (on open water) on fire
    Burn due to Jet ski on fire

V91.04 Burn due to sailboat on fire

V91.05 Burn due to canoe or kayak on fire

V91.06 Burn due to (nonpowered) inflatable craft on fire

V91.07 Burn due to water-skis on fire

V91.08 Burn due to other unpowered watercraft on fire

V91.09 Burn due to unspecified watercraft on fire
    Burn due to boat NOS on fire
    Burn due to ship NOS on fire
    Burn due to watercraft NOS on fire

V91.1 Crushed between watercraft and other watercraft or other object due to collision

    Crushed by lifeboat after abandoning ship in a collision

    Note: select the specified type of watercraft that the victim was on at the time of the collision

V91.10 Crushed between merchant ship and other watercraft or other object due to collision

V91.11 Crushed between passenger ship and other watercraft or other object due to collision
    Crushed between Ferry-boat and other watercraft or other object due to collision
    Crushed between Liner and other watercraft or other object due to collision

V91.12   Crushed between fishing boat and other watercraft or other object due to collision

V91.13   Crushed between other powered watercraft and other watercraft or other object due to collision
> Crushed between Hovercraft (on open water) and other watercraft or other object due to collision
> Crushed between Jet ski and other watercraft or other object due to collision

V91.14   Crushed between sailboat and other watercraft or other object due to collision

V91.15   Crushed between canoe or kayak and other watercraft or other object due to collision

V91.16   Crushed between (nonpowered) inflatable craft and other watercraft or other object due to collision

V91.18   Crushed between other unpowered watercraft and other watercraft or other object due to collision
> Crushed between surfboard and other watercraft or other object due to collision
> Crushed between windsurfer and other watercraft or other object due to collision

V91.19   Crushed between unspecified watercraft and other watercraft or other object due to collision
> Crushed between boat NOS and other watercraft or other object due to collision
> Crushed between ship NOS and other watercraft or other object due to collision
> Crushed between watercraft NOS and other watercraft or other object due to collision

V91.2   **Fall due to collision between watercraft and other watercraft or other object**
> Fall while remaining on watercraft after collision
> Note: select the specified type of watercraft that the victim was on at the time of the collision
> Excludes1:   crushed between watercraft and other watercraft and other object due to collision (V91.1-)
> drowning and submersion due to falling from crushed watercraft (V90.3-)

V91.20   Fall due to collision between merchant ship and other watercraft or other object

V91.21   Fall due to collision between passenger ship and other watercraft or other object
> Fall due to collision between Ferry-boat and other watercraft or other object
> Fall due to collision between Liner and other watercraft or other object

V91.22   Fall due to collision between fishing boat and other watercraft or other object

V91.23   Fall due to collision between other powered watercraft and other watercraft or other object
> Fall due to collision between Hovercraft (on open water) and other watercraft or other object
> Fall due to collision between Jet ski and other watercraft or other object

V91.24   Fall due to collision between sailboat and other watercraft or other object

V91.25   Fall due to collision between canoe or kayak and other watercraft or other object

V91.26   Fall due to collision between (nonpowered) inflatable craft and other watercraft or other object

V91.29   Fall due to collision between unspecified watercraft and other watercraft or other object
> Fall due to collision between boat NOS and other watercraft or other object
> Fall due to collision between ship NOS and other watercraft or other object
> Fall due to collision between watercraft NOS and other watercraft or other object

V91.3   **Hit or struck by falling object due to accident to watercraft**
> Hit or struck by falling object (part of damaged watercraft or other object) after falling or jumping from damaged watercraft
> Excludes2:   drowning or submersion due to fall or jumping from damaged watercraft (V90.2-, V90.3-)

V91.30   Hit or struck by falling object due to accident to merchant ship

V91.31   Hit or struck by falling object due to accident to passenger ship
> Hit or struck by falling object due to accident to Ferry-boat
> Hit or struck by falling object due to accident to Liner

V91.32   Hit or struck by falling object due to accident to fishing boat

V91.33   Hit or struck by falling object due to accident to other powered watercraft
> Hit or struck by falling object due to accident to Hovercraft (on open water)
> Hit or struck by falling object due to accident to Jet ski

V91.34   Hit or struck by falling object due to accident to sailboat

V91.35   Hit or struck by falling object due to accident to canoe or kayak

V91.36   Hit or struck by falling object due to accident to (nonpowered) inflatable craft

V91.37   Hit or struck by falling object due to accident to water-skis
> Hit by water-skis after jumping off of waterskis

V91.38   Hit or struck by falling object due to accident to other unpowered watercraft
> Hit or struck by surf-board after falling off damaged surf-board
> Hit or struck by object after falling off damaged windsurfer

V91.39   Hit or struck by falling object due to accident to unspecified watercraft
> Hit or struck by falling object due to accident to boat NOS
> Hit or struck by falling object due to accident to ship NOS
> Hit or struck by falling object due to accident to watercraft NOS

V91.8   **Other injury due to other accident to watercraft**

V91.80   Other injury due to other accident to merchant ship

V91.81   Other injury due to other accident to passenger ship
> Other injury due to other accident to Ferry-boat
> Other injury due to other accident to Liner

V91.82   Other injury due to other accident to fishing boat

V91.83   Other injury due to other accident to other powered watercraft
> Other injury due to other accident to Hovercraft (on open water)
> Other injury due to other accident to Jet ski

V91.84   Other injury due to other accident to sailboat

V91.85   Other injury due to other accident to canoe or kayak

V91.86   Other injury due to other accident to (nonpowered) inflatable craft

V91.87   Other injury due to other accident to water-skis

V91.88   Other injury due to other accident to other unpowered watercraft
> Other injury due to other accident to surf-board
> Other injury due to other accident to windsurfer

V91.89   Other injury due to other accident to unspecified watercraft
> Other injury due to other accident to boat NOS
> Other injury due to other accident to ship NOS
> Other injury due to other accident to watercraft NOS

V92   Drowning and submersion due to accident on board watercraft, without accident to watercraft
> Excludes1:   drowning or submersion of diver who voluntarily jumps from boat not involved in an accident (W16.711, W16.721)
> fall into water without watercraft (W16.-)
> drowning or submersion due to accident to watercraft (V90-V91)
> military watercraft accident (Y36, Y37)
> The following extensions are to be added to each code from category V92:
> a   initial encounter
> d   subsequent encounter
> q   sequelae

V92.0   **Drowning and submersion due to fall off watercraft**

Drowning and submersion due to fall from gangplank of watercraft

Drowning and submersion due to fall overboard watercraft

Excludes2:   hitting head on object or bottom of body of water due to fall from watercraft (V94.0-)

V92.00   **Drowning and submersion due to fall off merchant ship**

V92.01   **Drowning and submersion due to fall off passenger ship**

Drowning and submersion due to fall off Ferry-boat

Drowning and submersion due to fall off Liner

V92.02   **Drowning and submersion due to fall off fishing boat**

V92.03   **Drowning and submersion due to fall off other powered watercraft**

Drowning and submersion due to fall off Hovercraft (on open water)

Drowning and submersion due to fall off Jet ski

V92.04   **Drowning and submersion due to fall off sailboat**

V92.05   **Drowning and submersion due to fall off canoe or kayak**

V92.06   **Drowning and submersion due to fall off (nonpowered) inflatable craft**

V92.07   **Drowning and submersion due to fall off water-skis**

Excludes1:   drowning and submersion due to falling off burning water-skis (V90.27)

drowning and submersion due to falling off crushed water-skis (V90.37)

hit by boat while water-skiing NOS (V94.x)

V92.08   **Drowning and submersion due to fall off other unpowered watercraft**

Drowning and submersion due to fall off surf-board

Drowning and submersion due to fall off windsurfer

Excludes1:   drowning and submersion due to fall off burning unpowered watercraft (V90.28)

drowning and submersion due to fall off crushed unpowered watercraft (V90.38)

drowning and submersion due to fall off damaged unpowered watercraft (V90.88)

drowning and submersion due to rider of nonpowered watercraft being hit by other watercraft (V94.-)

other injury due to rider of nonpowered watercraft being hit by other watercraft (V94.-)

V92.09   **Drowning and submersion due to fall off unspecified watercraft**

Drowning and submersion due to fall off boat NOS

Drowning and submersion due to fall off ship

Drowning and submersion due to fall off watercraft NOS

V92.1   **Drowning and submersion due to being thrown overboard by motion of watercraft**

Excludes1:   drowning and submersion due to fall off surf-board (V92.08)

drowning and submersion due to fall off water-skis (V92.07)

drowning and submersion due to fall off windsurfer (V92.08)

V92.10   **Drowning and submersion due to being thrown overboard by motion of merchant ship**

V92.11   **Drowning and submersion due to being thrown overboard by motion of passenger ship**

Drowning and submersion due to being thrown overboard by motion of Ferry-boat

Drowning and submersion due to being thrown overboard by motion of Liner

V92.12   **Drowning and submersion due to being thrown overboard by motion of fishing boat**

V92.13   **Drowning and submersion due to being thrown overboard by motion of other powered watercraft**

Drowning and submersion due to being thrown overboard by motion of Hovercraft

V92.14   **Drowning and submersion due to being thrown overboard by motion of sailboat**

V92.15   **Drowning and submersion due to being thrown overboard by motion of canoe or kayak**

V92.16   **Drowning and submersion due to being thrown overboard by motion of (nonpowered) inflatable craft**

V92.19   **Drowning and submersion due to being thrown overboard by motion of unspecified watercraft**

Drowning and submersion due to being thrown overboard by motion of boat NOS

Drowning and submersion due to being thrown overboard by motion of ship NOS

Drowning and submersion due to being thrown overboard by motion of watercraft NOS

V92.2   **Drowning and submersion due to being washed overboard from watercraft**

Code first any associated cataclysm (X37.0-)

V92.20   **Drowning and submersion due to being washed overboard from merchant ship**

V92.21   **Drowning and submersion due to being washed overboard from passenger ship**

Drowning and submersion due to being washed overboard from Ferry-boat

Drowning and submersion due to being washed overboard from Liner

V92.22   **Drowning and submersion due to being washed overboard from fishing boat**

V92.23   **Drowning and submersion due to being washed overboard from other powered watercraft**

Drowning and submersion due to being washed overboard from Hovercraft (on open water)

Drowning and submersion due to being washed overboard from Jet ski

V92.24   **Drowning and submersion due to being washed overboard from sailboat**

V92.25   **Drowning and submersion due to being washed overboard from canoe or kayak**

V92.26   **Drowning and submersion due to being washed overboard from (nonpowered) inflatable craft**

V92.27   **Drowning and submersion due to being washed overboard from water-skis**

Excludes1:   drowning and submersion due to fall off water-skis (V92.07)

V92.28   **Drowning and submersion due to being washed overboard from other unpowered watercraft**

Drowning and submersion due to being washed overboard from surf-board

Drowning and submersion due to being washed overboard from windsurfer

V92.29   **Drowning and submersion due to being washed overboard from unspecified watercraft**

Drowning and submersion due to being washed overboard from boat NOS

Drowning and submersion due to being washed overboard from ship NOS

Drowning and submersion due to being washed overboard from watercraft NOS

V93   **Other injury due to accident on board watercraft, without accident to watercraft**

Excludes1:   other injury due to accident to watercraft (V91.-)

military watercraft accident (Y36, Y37.-)

Excludes2:   drowning and submersion due to accident on board watercraft, without accident to watercraft (V92.-)

The following extensions are to be added to each code from category V93:

a   initial encounter

d   subsequent encounter

q   sequelae

V93.0 Burn due to localized fire on board watercraft
Excludes1:   burn due to watercraft on fire (V91.0-)

V93.00 Burn due to localized fire on board merchant vessel

V93.01 Burn due to localized fire on board passenger vessel
Burn due to localized fire on board Ferry-boat
Burn due to localized fire on board Liner

V93.02 Burn due to localized fire on board fishing boat

V93.03 Burn due to localized fire on board other powered watercraft
Burn due to localized fire on board Hovercraft
Burn due to localized fire on board Jet ski

V93.04 Burn due to localized fire on board sailboat

V93.09 Burn due to localized fire on board unspecified watercraft
Burn due to localized fire on board boat NOS
Burn due to localized fire on board ship NOS
Burn due to localized fire on board watercraft NOS

V93.1 Other burn on board watercraft
Burn due to source other than fire on board watercraft
Excludes1:   burn due to watercraft on fire (V91.0-)

V93.10 Other burn on board merchant vessel

V93.11 Other burn on board passenger vessel
Other burn on board Ferry-boat
Other burn on board Liner

V93.12 Other burn on board fishing boat

V93.13 Other burn on board other powered watercraft
Other burn on board Hovercraft
Other burn on board Jet ski

V93.14 Other burn on board sailboat

V93.19 Other burn on board unspecified watercraft
Other burn on board boat NOS
Other burn on board ship NOS
Other burn on board watercraft NOS

V93.2 Heat exposure on board watercraft
Excludes1:   exposure to man-made heat not aboard watercraft (W92)
exposure to natural heat while on board watercraft (X30)
exposure to sunlight while on board watercraft (X32)
Excludes2: burn due to fire on board watercraft (V93.0-)

V93.20 Heat exposure on board merchant ship

V93.21 Heat exposure on board passenger ship
Heat exposure on board Ferry-boat
Heat exposure on board Liner

V93.22 Heat exposure on board fishing boat

V93.23 Heat exposure on board other powered watercraft
Heat exposure on board Hovercraft

V93.24 Heat exposure on board sailboat

V93.29 Heat exposure on board unspecified watercraft
Heat exposure on board boat NOS
Heat exposure on board ship NOS
Heat exposure on board watercraft NOS

V93.3 Fall on board watercraft
Excludes1:   fall due to collision of watercraft (V91.2-)

V93.30 Fall on board merchant ship

V93.31 Fall on board passenger ship
Fall on board Ferry-boat
Fall on board Liner

V93.32 Fall on board fishing boat

V93.33 Fall on board other powered watercraft
Fall on board Hovercraft (on open water)
Fall on board Jet ski

V93.34 Fall on board sailboat

V93.35 Fall on board canoe or kayak

V93.36 Fall on board (nonpowered) inflatable craft

V93.38 Fall on board other unpowered watercraft

V93.39 Fall on board unspecified watercraft
Fall on board boat NOS
Fall on board ship NOS
Fall on board watercraft NOS

V93.4 Struck by falling object on board watercraft
Hit by falling object on board watercraft
Excludes1:   struck by falling object due to accident to watercraft (V91.3)

V93.40 Struck by falling object on merchant ship

V93.41 Struck by falling object on passenger ship
Struck by falling object on Ferry-boat
Struck by falling object on Liner

V93.42 Struck by falling object on fishing boat

V93.43 Struck by falling object on other powered watercraft
Struck by falling object on Hovercraft

V93.44 Struck by falling object on sailboat

V93.48 Struck by falling object on other unpowered watercraft

V93.49 Struck by falling object on unspecified watercraft

V93.5 Explosion on board watercraft
Boiler explosion on steamship
Excludes2: fire on board watercraft (V93.0-)

V93.50 Explosion on board merchant ship

V93.51 Explosion on board passenger ship
Explosion on board Ferry-boat
Explosion on board Liner

V93.52 Explosion on board fishing boat

V93.53 Explosion on board other powered watercraft
Explosion on board Hovercraft
Explosion on board Jet ski

V93.54 Explosion on board sailboat

V93.59 Explosion on board unspecified watercraft
Explosion on board boat NOS
Explosion on board ship NOS
Explosion on board watercraft NOS

V93.6 Machinery accident on board watercraft
Excludes1:   machinery explosion on board watercraft (V93.4-)
machinery fire on board watercraft (V93.0-)

V93.60 Machinery accident on board merchant ship

V93.61 Machinery accident on board passenger ship
Machinery accident on board Ferry-boat
Machinery accident on board Liner

V93.62 Machinery accident on board fishing boat

V93.63 Machinery accident on board other powered watercraft
Machinery accident on board Hovercraft

V93.64 Machinery accident on board sailboat

V93.69 Machinery accident on board unspecified watercraft
Machinery accident on board boat NOS
Machinery accident on board ship NOS
Machinery accident on board watercraft NOS

V93.8 Other injury due to other accident on board watercraft
Accidental poisoning by gases or fumes on watercraft

V93.80 Other injury due to other accident on board merchant ship

V93.81 Other injury due to other accident on board passenger ship
Other injury due to other accident on board Ferry-boat
Other injury due to other accident on board Liner

V93.82 Other injury due to other accident on board fishing boat

V93.83 Other injury due to other accident on board other powered watercraft
Other injury due to other accident on board Hovercraft
Other injury due to other accident on board Jet ski

V93.84 Other injury due to other accident on board sailboat

V93.85 Other injury due to other accident on board canoe or kayak

V93.86 Other injury due to other accident on board (nonpowered) inflatable craft

V93.87 Other injury due to other accident on board water-skis
Hit or struck by object while waterskiing

V93.88 Other injury due to other accident on board other unpowered watercraft
Hit or struck by object while surfing
Hit or struck by object while on board windsurfer

V93.89   Other injury due to other accident on board unspecified watercraft
>   Other injury due to other accident on board boat NOS
>   Other injury due to other accident on board ship NOS
>   Other injury due to other accident on board watercraft NOS

V94   Other and unspecified water transport accidents
>   Excludes1:   military watercraft accidents (Y36, Y37)
>   The following extensions are to be added to each code from category V94:
>   a   initial encounter
>   d   subsequent encounter
>   q   sequelae

V94.0   Hitting object or bottom of body of water due to fall from watercraft
>   Excludes2:   drowning and submersion due to fall from watercraft (V92.0-)

V94.1   Bather struck by watercraft
>   Swimmer hit by watercraft

V94.11   Bather struck by powered watercraft

V94.12   Bather struck by nonpowered watercraft

V94.2   Rider of nonpowered watercraft struck by other watercraft

V94.21   Rider of nonpowered watercraft struck by other nonpowered watercraft
>   Canoer hit by other nonpowered watercraft
>   Surfer hit by other nonpowered watercraft
>   Windsurfer hit by other nonpowered watercraft

V94.22   Rider of nonpowered watercraft struck by powered watercraft
>   Canoer hit by motorboat
>   Surfer hit by motorboat
>   Windsurfer hit by motorboat

V94.3   Injury to rider of (inflatable) watercraft being pulled behind other watercraft

V94.31   Injury to rider of (inflatable) recreational watercraft being pulled behind other watercraft
>   Injury to rider of inner-tube pulled behind motor boat

V94.32   Injury to rider of non-recreational watercraft being pulled behind other watercraft
>   Injury to occupant of dingy being pulled behind boat or ship
>   Injury to occupant of life-raft being pulled behind boat or ship

V94.4   Injury to barefoot water-skier
>   Injury to person being pulled behind boat or ship

V94.8   Other water transport accident

V94.9   Unspecified water transport accident
>   Water transport accident NOS

AIR AND SPACE TRANSPORT ACCIDENTS (V95–V97)
>   Excludes1:   military aircraft accidents (Y36, Y37)
>   The following extensions are to be added to each code from category V95:
>   a   initial encounter
>   d   subsequent encounter
>   q   sequelae

V95   Accident to powered aircraft causing injury to occupant

V95.0   Helicopter accident injuring occupant

V95.00   Unspecified helicopter accident injuring occupant

V95.01   Helicopter crash injuring occupant

V95.02   Forced landing of helicopter injuring occupant

V95.03   Helicopter collision injuring occupant
>   Helicopter collision with any object, fixed, movable or moving

V95.04   Helicopter fire injuring occupant

V95.05   Helicopter explosion injuring occupant

V95.09   Other helicopter accident injuring occupant

V95.1   Ultralight, microlight or powered-glider accident injuring occupant

V95.10   Unspecified ultralight, microlight or powered-glider accident injuring occupant

V95.11   Ultralight, microlight or powered-glider crash injuring occupant

V95.12   Forced landing of ultralight, microlight or powered-glider injuring occupant

V95.13   Ultralight, microlight or powered-glider collision injuring occupant
>   Ultralight, microlight or powered-glider collision with any object, fixed, movable or moving

V95.14   Ultralight, microlight or powered-glider fire injuring occupant

V95.15   Ultralight, microlight or powered-glider explosion injuring occupant

V95.19   Other ultralight, microlight or powered-glider accident injuring occupant

V95.2   Other private fixed-wing aircraft accident injuring occupant

V95.20   Unspecified accident to other private fixed-wing aircraft, injuring occupant

V95.21   Other private fixed-wing aircraft crash injuring occupant

V95.22   Forced landing of other private fixed-wing aircraft injuring occupant

V95.23   Other private fixed-wing aircraft collision injuring occupant
>   Other private fixed-wing aircraft collision with any object, fixed, movable or moving

V95.24   Other private fixed-wing aircraft fire injuring occupant

V95.25   Other private fixed-wing aircraft explosion injuring occupant

V95.29   Other accident to other private fixed-wing aircraft injuring occupant

V95.3   Commercial fixed-wing aircraft accident injuring occupant

V95.30   Unspecified accident to commercial fixed-wing aircraft injuring occupant

V95.31   Commercial fixed-wing aircraft crash injuring occupant

V95.32   Forced landing of commercial fixed-wing aircraft injuring occupant

V95.33   Commercial fixed-wing aircraft collision injuring occupant
>   Commercial fixed-wing aircraft collision with any object, fixed, movable or moving

V95.34   Commercial fixed-wing aircraft fire injuring occupant

V95.35   Commercial fixed-wing aircraft explosion injuring occupant

V95.39   Other accident to commercial fixed-wing aircraft injuring occupant

V95.4   Spacecraft accident injuring occupant

V95.40   Unspecified spacecraft accident injuring occupant

V95.41   Spacecraft crash injuring occupant

V95.42   Forced landing of spacecraft injuring occupant

V95.43   Spacecraft collision injuring occupant
>   Spacecraft collision with any object, fixed, moveable or moving

V95.44   Spacecraft fire injuring occupant

V95.45   Spacecraft explosion injuring occupant

V95.49   Unspecified spacecraft accident injuring occupant

V95.8   Other powered aircraft accidents injuring occupant

V95.9   Unspecified aircraft accident injuring occupant
>   Aircraft accident NOS
>   Air transport accident NOS

V96   Accident to nonpowered aircraft causing injury to occupant
>   The following extensions are to be added to each code from category V96:
>   a   initial encounter
>   d   subsequent encounter
>   q   sequelae

V96.0   Balloon accident injuring occupant

V96.00   Unspecified balloon accident injuring occupant

V96.01   Balloon crash injuring occupant

V96.02   Forced landing of balloon injuring occupant

    V96.03   **Balloon collision injuring occupant**
            Balloon collision with any object, fixed, moveable or moving

    V96.04   **Balloon fire injuring occupant**

    V96.05   **Balloon explosion injuring occupant**

    V96.09   **Other balloon accident injuring occupant**

V96.1   **Hang-glider accident injuring occupant**

    V96.10   **Unspecified hang-glider accident injuring occupant**

    V96.11   **Hang-glider crash injuring occupant**

    V96.12   **Forced landing of hang-glider injuring occupant**

    V96.13   **Hang-glider collision injuring occupant**
            Hang-glider collision with any object, fixed, moveable or moving

    V96.14   **Hang-glider fire injuring occupant**

    V96.15   **Hang-glider explosion injuring occupant**

    V96.19   **Other hang-glider accident injuring occupant**

V96.2   **Glider (nonpowered) accident injuring occupant**

    V96.20   **Unspecified glider (nonpowered) accident injuring occupant**

    V96.21   **Glider (nonpowered) crash injuring occupant**

    V96.22   **Forced landing of glider (nonpowered) injuring occupant**

    V96.23   **Glider (nonpowered) collision injuring occupant**
            Glider (nonpowered) collision with any object, fixed, moveable or moving

    V96.24   **Glider (nonpowered) fire injuring occupant**

    V96.25   **Glider (nonpowered) explosion injuring occupant**

    V96.29   **Other glider (nonpowered) accident injuring occupant**

V96.8   **Other nonpowered-aircraft accidents injuring occupant**
         Kite carrying a person accident injuring occupant

V96.9   **Unspecified nonpowered-aircraft accident injuring occupant**
         Nonpowered-aircraft accident NOS

V97   Other specified air transport accidents
     The following extensions are to be added to each code from category V97:
       a   initial encounter
       d   subsequent encounter
       q   sequelae

V97.0   **Occupant of aircraft injured in other specified air transport accidents**
         Fall in, on or from aircraft in air transport accident
         Excludes1:   accident while boarding or alighting aircraft (V97.1)

V97.1   **Person injured while boarding or alighting from aircraft**

V97.2   **Parachutist accident**

    V97.21   **Parachutist entangled in object**
            Parachutist landing in tree

    V97.22   **Parachutist injured on landing**

    V97.29   **Other parachutist accident**

V97.3   **Person on ground injured in air transport accident**

    V97.31   **Hit by object falling from aircraft**
            Hit by crashing aircraft
            Injured by aircraft hitting house
            Injured by aircraft hitting car

    V97.32   **Injured by rotating propeller**

    V97.33   **Sucked into jet engine**

    V97.39   **Other injury to person on ground due to air transport accident**

V97.8   **Other air transport accidents, not elsewhere classified**
         Injury from machinery on aircraft
         Excludes1:   aircraft accident NOS (V95.9)
                   exposure to changes in air pressure during ascent or descent (W94.-)

OTHER AND UNSPECIFIED TRANSPORT ACCIDENTS
(V98–V99)

     Excludes1:   vehicle accident, type of vehicle unspecified (V89.-)

V98   Other specified transport accidents
     The following extensions are to be added to each code from category V98:
       a   initial encounter
       d   subsequent encounter
       q   sequelae

V98.0   **Accident to, on or involving cable-car, not on rails**
         Caught or dragged by cable-car, not on rails
         Fall or jump from cable-car, not on rails
         Object thrown from or in cable-car, not on rails

V98.1   **Accident to, on or involving land-yacht**

V98.2   **Accident to, on or involving ice yacht**

V98.3   **Accident to, on or involving ski lift**
         Accident to, on or involving ski chair-lift
         Accident to, on or involving ski-lift with gondola

V98.8   **Other specified transport accidents**

V99   Unspecified transport accident
     The following extensions are to be added to code V99:
       a   initial encounter
       d   subsequent encounter
       q   sequelae

OTHER EXTERNAL CAUSES OF ACCIDENTAL INJURY
(W00–X58)

FALLS (W00–W19)

     Excludes1:   assault involving a fall (Y01-Y02)
                 fall (in) (from):
                     animal (V80.-)
                     machinery (in operation) (W28-W31)
                     transport vehicle (V01-V99)
                     intentional self-harm involving a fall (X80-X81)
     Excludes2:   fall (in) (from):
                 burning building (X00.-)
                 into fire (X00-X04, X08-X09)

W00   Fall due to ice and snow
     Includes: pedestrian on foot falling (slipping) on ice and snow
     Excludes1:   fall on (in) ice and snow involving pedestrian conveyance (V00.-)
                 fall from stairs and steps not due to ice and snow (W10.-)
     The following extensions are to be added to each code from category W00:
       a   initial encounter
       d   subsequent encounter
       q   sequelae

W00.0   **Fall on same level due to ice and snow**

W00.1   **Fall from stairs and steps due to ice and snow**

W00.2   **Other fall from one level to another due to ice and snow**

W00.9   **Unspecified fall due to ice and snow**

W01   Fall on same level from slipping, tripping and stumbling
     Includes: fall on moving sidewalk
                 slipping, tripping and stumbling NOS
     Excludes1:   fall due to bumping (striking) against object (W18.0-)
                 fall in shower or bathtub (W18.2-)
                 fall on same level from slipping, tripping and stumbling due to ice or snow (W00.0)
                 fall off or from toilet (W18.1-)
     The following extensions are to be added to each code from category W01:
       a   initial encounter
       d   subsequent encounter
       q   sequelae

W01.0   **Fall on same level from slipping, tripping and stumbling without subsequent striking against object**

W01.1 Fall on same level from slipping, tripping and stumbling with subsequent striking against object

  W01.10 Fall on same level from slipping, tripping and stumbling with subsequent striking against unspecified object

  W01.11 Fall on same level from slipping, tripping and stumbling with subsequent striking against sharp object

    W01.110 Fall on same level from slipping, tripping and stumbling with subsequent striking against sharp glass

    W01.111 Fall on same level from slipping, tripping and stumbling with subsequent striking against power tool or machine

    W01.118 Fall on same level from slipping, tripping and stumbling with subsequent striking against other sharp object

    W01.119 Fall on same level from slipping, tripping and stumbling with subsequent striking against unspecified sharp object

  W01.19 Fall on same level from slipping, tripping and stumbling with subsequent striking against other object

    W01.190 Fall on same level from slipping, tripping and stumbling with subsequent striking against furniture

    W01.198 Fall on same level from slipping, tripping and stumbling with subsequent striking against other object

  *W02 deactivated. See category V00

W03 Other fall on same level due to collision with another person

  Includes: fall due to non-transport collision with other person

  Excludes1:   collision with another person without fall (W51)
           crushed or pushed by a crowd or human stampede (W52)
           fall involving pedestrian conveyance (V00-V09)
           fall due to ice or snow (W00)

  The following extensions are to be added to code W03:
    a   initial encounter
    d   subsequent encounter
    q   sequelae

W04 Fall while being carried or supported by other persons

  Includes: accidentally dropped while being carried

  The following extensions are to be added to code W04:
    a   initial encounter
    d   subsequent encounter
    q   sequelae

W05 Fall from non-moving wheelchair

  Excludes1:   fall from moving wheelchair (V00.811)

  The following extensions are to be added to code W05:
    a   initial encounter
    d   subsequent encounter
    q   sequelae

W06 Fall from bed

  The following extensions are to be added to code W06:
    a   initial encounter
    d   subsequent encounter
    q   sequelae

W07 Fall from chair

  The following extensions are to be added to code W07:
    a   initial encounter
    d   subsequent encounter
    q   sequelae

W08 Fall from other furniture

  The following extensions are to be added to code W08:
    a   initial encounter
    d   subsequent encounter
    q   sequelae

W09 Fall on and from playground equipment

  Excludes1:   fall involving recreational machinery (W31)

  The following extensions are to be added to each code from category W09:
    a   initial encounter
    d   subsequent encounter
    q   sequelae

W09.0 Fall on or from playground slide

W09.1 Fall from playground swing

W09.2 Fall on or from jungle gym

W09.8 Fall on or from other playground equipment

W10 Fall on and from stairs and steps

  Excludes1:   Fall from stairs and steps due to ice and snow (W00.1)

  The following extensions are to be added to each code from category W10:
    a   initial encounter
    d   subsequent encounter
    q   sequelae

W10.0 Fall (on) (from) escalator

W10.1 Fall (on) (from) sidewalk curb

W10.3 Fall (on) (from) incline
      Fall (on) (from) ramp

W10.8 Fall (on) (from) other stairs and steps

W10.9 Fall (on) (from) unspecified stairs and steps

W11 Fall on and from ladder

  The following extensions are to be added to code W11:
    a   initial encounter
    d   subsequent encounter
    q   sequelae

W12 Fall on and from scaffolding

  The following extensions are to be added to code W12:
    a   initial encounter
    d   subsequent encounter
    q   sequelae

W13 Fall from, out of or through building or structure

  The following extensions are to be added to each code from category W13:
    a   initial encounter
    d   subsequent encounter
    q   sequelae

W13.0 Fall from, out of or through balcony
      Fall from, out of or through railing

W13.1 Fall from, out of or through bridge

W13.2 Fall from, out of or through roof

W13.3 Fall through floor

W13.4 Fall from, out of or through window

    Excludes2:   fall with subsequent striking against sharp glass (W01.110)

W13.8 Fall from, out of or through other building or structure
      Fall from, out of or through viaduct
      Fall from, out of or through wall
      Fall from, out of or through flag-pole

W13.9 Fall from, out of or through building, not otherwise specified

    Excludes1:   collapse of a building or structure (W20.-)
             fall or jump from burning building or structure (X00.-)

W14 Fall from tree

  The following extensions are to be added to code W14:
    a   initial encounter
    d   subsequent encounter
    q   sequelae

W15 Fall from cliff

  The following extensions are to be added to code W15:
    a   initial encounter
    d   subsequent encounter
    q   sequelae

W16 Fall, jump or diving into water

    Excludes1:   accidental non-watercraft drowning and submersion not involving fall (W65-W74)

                 effects of air pressure from diving (W94.-)

                 fall into water from watercraft (V90-V94)

                 hitting an object or against bottom when falling from watercraft (V94.0)

    Excludes2:   striking or hitting diving board (W21.3)

    The following extensions are to be added to each code from category W16:

        a   initial encounter

        d   subsequent encounter

        q   sequelae

W16.0   Fall into swimming pool

    Fall into swimming pool NOS

    Excludes1:   fall into empty swimming pool (W17.3)

    W16.01   Fall into swimming pool striking water surface

        W16.011   Fall into swimming pool striking water surface causing drowning and submersion

                Excludes1:   drowning and submersion while in swimming pool without fall (W67)

        W16.012   Fall into swimming pool striking water surface causing other injury

    W16.02   Fall into swimming pool striking bottom

        W16.021   Fall into swimming pool striking bottom causing drowning and submersion

                Excludes1:   drowning and submersion while in swimming pool without fall (W67)

        W16.022   Fall into swimming pool striking bottom causing other injury

    W16.03   Fall into swimming pool striking wall

        W16.031   Fall into swimming pool striking wall causing drowning and submersion

                Excludes1:   drowning and submersion while in swimming pool without fall (W67)

        W16.032   Fall into swimming pool striking wall causing other injury

W16.1   Fall into natural body of water

    Fall into lake

    Fall into open sea

    Fall into river

    Fall into stream

    W16.11   Fall into natural body of water striking water surface

        W16.111   Fall into natural body of water striking water surface causing drowning and submersion

                Excludes1:   drowning and submersion while in natural body of water without fall (W69)

        W16.112   Fall into natural body of water striking water surface causing other injury

    W16.12   Fall into natural body of water striking bottom

        W16.121   Fall into natural body of water striking bottom causing drowning and submersion

                Excludes1:   drowning and submersion while in natural body of water without fall (W69)

        W16.122   Fall into natural body of water striking bottom causing other injury

    W16.13   Fall into natural body of water striking side

        W16.131   Fall into natural body of water striking side causing drowning and submersion

                Excludes1:   drowning and submersion while in natural body of water without fall (W69)

        W16.132   Fall into natural body of water striking side causing other injury

W16.2   Fall in (into) filled bathtub or bucket of water

    W16.21   Fall in (into) filled bathtub

        Excludes1:   fall into empty bathtub (W18.2)

        W16.211   Fall in (into) filled bathtub causing drowning and submersion

                Excludes1:   drowning and submersion while in filled bathtub without fall (W65)

        W16.212   Fall in (into) filled bathtub causing other injury

    W16.22   Fall in (into) bucket of water

        W16.221   Fall in (into) bucket of water causing drowning and submersion

        W16.222   Fall in (into) bucket of water causing other injury

W16.3   Fall into other water

    Fall into fountain

    Fall into reservoir

    W16.31   Fall into other water striking water surface

        W16.311   Fall into other water striking water surface causing drowning and submersion

                Excludes1:   drowning and submersion while in other water without fall (W73)

        W16.312   Fall into other water striking water surface causing other injury

    W16.32   Fall into other water striking bottom

        W16.321   Fall into other water striking bottom causing drowning and submersion

                Excludes1:   drowning and submersion while in other water without fall (W73)

        W16.322   Fall into other water striking bottom causing other injury

    W16.33   Fall into other water striking wall

        W16.331   Fall into other water striking wall causing drowning and submersion

                Excludes1:   drowning and submersion while in other water without fall (W73)

        W16.332   Fall into other water striking wall causing other injury

W16.4   Fall into unspecified water

    W16.41   Fall into unspecified water causing drowning and submersion

    W16.42   Fall into unspecified water causing other injury

W16.5   Jumping or diving into swimming pool

    W16.51   Jumping or diving into swimming pool striking water surface

        W16.511   Jumping or diving into swimming pool striking water surface causing drowning and submersion

                Excludes1:   drowning and submersion while in swimming pool without jumping or diving (W67)

        W16.512   Jumping or diving into swimming pool striking water surface causing other injury

    W16.52   Jumping or diving into swimming pool striking bottom

        W16.521   Jumping or diving into swimming pool striking bottom causing drowning and submersion

                Excludes1:   drowning and submersion while in swimming pool without jumping or diving (W67)

        W16.522   Jumping or diving into swimming pool striking bottom causing other injury

    W16.53   Jumping or diving into swimming pool striking wall

        W16.531   Jumping or diving into swimming pool striking wall causing drowning and submersion

                Excludes1:   drowning and submersion while in swimming pool without jumping or diving (W67)

        W16.532   Jumping or diving into swimming pool striking wall causing other injury

W16.6 Jumping or diving into natural body of water
Jumping or diving into lake
Jumping or diving into open sea
Jumping or diving into river
Jumping or diving into stream

W16.61 Jumping or diving into natural body of water striking water surface

W16.611 Jumping or diving into natural body of water striking water surface causing drowning and submersion
Excludes1: drowning and submersion while in natural body of water without jumping or diving (W69)

W16.612 Jumping or diving into natural body of water striking water surface causing other injury

W16.62 Jumping or diving into natural body of water striking bottom

W16.621 Jumping or diving into natural body of water striking bottom causing drowning and submersion
Excludes1: drowning and submersion while in natural body of water without jumping or diving (W69)

W16.622 Jumping or diving into natural body of water striking bottom causing other injury

W16.7 Jumping or diving from boat
Excludes1: fall from boat into water — see watercraft accident (V90-V94)

W16.71 Jumping or diving from boat striking water surface

W16.711 Jumping or diving from boat striking water surface causing drowning and submersion

W16.712 Jumping or diving from boat striking water surface causing other injury

W16.72 Jumping or diving from boat striking bottom

W16.721 Jumping or diving from boat striking bottom causing drowning and submersion

W16.722 Jumping or diving from boat striking bottom causing other injury

W16.8 Jumping or diving into other water
Jumping or diving into fountain
Jumping or diving into reservoir

W16.81 Jumping or diving into other water striking water surface

W16.811 Jumping or diving into other water striking water surface causing drowning and submersion
Excludes1: drowning and submersion while in other water without jumping or diving (W73)

W16.812 Jumping or diving into other water striking water surface causing other injury

W16.82 Jumping or diving into other water striking bottom

W16.821 Jumping or diving into other water striking bottom causing drowning and submersion
Excludes1: drowning and submersion while in other water without jumping or diving (W73)

W16.822 Jumping or diving into other water striking bottom causing other injury

W16.83 Jumping or diving into other water striking wall

W16.831 Jumping or diving into other water striking wall causing drowning and submersion
Excludes1: drowning and submersion while in other water without jumping or diving (W73)

W16.832 Jumping or diving into other water striking wall causing other injury

W16.9 Jumping or diving into unspecified water

W16.91 Jumping or diving into unspecified water causing drowning and submersion

W16.92 Jumping or diving into unspecified water causing other injury

W17 Other fall from one level to another
The following extensions are to be added to each code from category W17:
a   initial encounter
d   subsequent encounter
q   sequelae

W17.0 Fall into well

W17.1 Fall into storm drain or manhole

W17.2 Fall into hole
Fall into pit

W17.3 Fall into empty swimming pool
Excludes1: fall into filled swimming pool (W16.0-)

W17.4 Fall from dock

W17.8 Other fall from one level to another
Fall down embankment (hill)

W18 Other fall on same level
The following extensions are to be added to each code from category W18:
a   initial encounter
d   subsequent encounter
q   sequelae

W18.0 Fall due to bumping against object
Striking against object with subsequent fall
Excludes1: fall on same level due to slipping, tripping, or stumbling with subsequent striking against object(W01.1-)

W18.00 Striking against unspecified object with subsequent fall

W18.01 Striking against sports equipment with subsequent fall

W18.02 Striking against glass with subsequent fall

W18.09 Striking against other object with subsequent fall

W18.1 Fall from or off toilet

W18.11 Fall from or off toilet without subsequent striking against object
Fall from (off) toilet NOS

W18.12 Fall from or off toilet with subsequent striking against object

W18.2 Fall in (into) shower or empty bathtub
Excludes1: fall in full bathtub (W16.21-)

W18.9 Fall on same level NOS

W19 Unspecified fall
Includes: accidental fall NOS
The following extensions are to be added to code W19:
a   initial encounter
d   subsequent encounter
q   sequelae

EXPOSURE TO INANIMATE MECHANICAL FORCES (W20-W49)

Excludes1: assault (X91-Y08)
contact or collision with animals or persons (W50-W64)
exposure to inanimate mechanical forces involving military or war operations (Y36.-, Y37.-)
intentional self-harm (X70-X83)

W20 Struck by thrown, projected or falling object
Code first any associated:
cataclysm (X34-X39)
lightning strike (T75.0)
Excludes1: falling object in:
machinery accident (W24, W28-W31)
transport accident (V01-V99)
object set in motion by:
explosion (W35-W40)
firearm (W32-W34)
struck by thrown sports equipment (W21.-)

The following extensions are to be added to each code from category W20:

    a   initial encounter
    d   subsequent encounter
    q   sequelae

W20.0 Struck by falling object in cave-in
    Excludes2:   asphyxiation due to cave-in (T71.21)

W20.1 Struck by object due to collapse of building
    Excludes1:   struck by object due to collapse of burning building (X00.2, X02.2)

W20.8 Other cause of strike by thrown, projected or falling object
    Excludes1:   struck by thrown sports equipment (W21.-)

W21 Striking against or struck by sports equipment
    Excludes1:   assault with sports equipment (Y08.1-)
                  striking against or struck by sports equipment with subsequent fall (W18.01)

The following extensions are to be added to each code from category W21:

    a   initial encounter
    d   subsequent encounter
    q   sequelae

W21.0 Struck by hit or thrown ball
  W21.00   Struck by hit or thrown ball, unspecified type
  W21.01   Struck by football
  W21.02   Struck by soccer ball
  W21.03   Struck by baseball
  W21.04   Struck by golf ball
  W21.05   Struck by basketball
  W21.06   Struck by volleyball
  W21.07   Struck by softball
  W21.09   Struck by other hit or thrown ball

W21.1 Struck by bat, racquet or club
  W21.11   Struck by baseball bat
  W21.12   Struck by tennis racquet
  W21.13   Struck by golf club
  W21.19   Struck by other bat, racquet or club

W21.2 Struck by hockey stick or puck
  W21.21   Struck by hockey stick
    W21.210   Struck by ice hockey stick
    W21.211   Struck by field hockey stick
  W21.22   Struck by hockey puck
    W21.220   Struck by ice hockey puck
    W21.221   Struck by field hockey puck

W21.3 Struck by sports foot wear
  W21.31   Struck by shoe cleats
        Stepped on by shoe cleats
  W21.32   Struck by skate blades
        Skated over by skate blades
  W21.39   Struck by other sports foot wear

W21.4 Striking against diving board
    Use additional code for subsequent falling into water, if applicable (W16.-)

W21.8 Striking against or struck by other sports equipment
  W21.81   Striking against or struck by football helmet
  W21.89   Striking against or struck by other sports equipment

W21.9 Striking against or struck by unspecified sports equipment

W22 Striking against or struck by other objects
    Excludes1:   striking against or struck by object with subsequent fall (W18.09)

The following extensions are to be added to each code from category W22:

    a   initial encounter
    d   subsequent encounter
    q   sequelae

W22.0 Striking against stationary object
    Excludes1:   striking against stationary sports equipment (W21.8)

  W22.01   Walked into wall

  W22.02   Walked into lamppost
  W22.03   Walked into furniture
  W22.04   Striking against wall of swimming pool
    W22.041   Striking against wall of swimming pool causing drowning and submersion
        Excludes1:   drowning and submersion while swimming without striking against wall (W67)
    W22.042   Striking against wall of swimming pool causing other injury
  W22.09   Striking against other stationary object

W22.1 Striking against or struck by automobile airbag
  W22.10   Striking against or struck by unspecified automobile airbag
  W22.11   Striking against or struck by driver side automobile airbag
  W22.12   Striking against or struck by front passenger side automobile airbag
  W22.19   Striking against or struck by other automobile airbag

W22.8 Striking against or struck by other objects
    Striking against or struck by object NOS
    Excludes1:   struck by thrown, projected or falling object (W20.-)

W23 Caught, crushed, jammed or pinched in or between objects
    Excludes1:   injury caused by cutting or piercing instruments (W25-W27)
                injury caused by lifting and transmission devices (W24.-)
                injury caused by machinery (W28-W31)
                injury caused by nonpowered hand tools (W27.-)
                injury caused by transport vehicle (V01-V99)
                injury caused by struck by thrown, projected or falling object (W20.-)

The following extensions are to be added to each code from category W23:

    a   initial encounter
    d   subsequent encounter
    q   sequelae

W23.0 Caught, crushed, jammed, or pinched between moving objects
W23.1 Caught, crushed, jammed, or pinched between stationary objects
W23.2 Caught, crushed, jammed, or pinched in object

W24 Contact with lifting and transmission devices, not elsewhere classified
    Excludes1:   transport accidents (V01-V99)

The following extensions are to be added to each code from category W24:

    a   initial encounter
    d   subsequent encounter
    q   sequelae

W24.0 Contact with lifting devices, not elsewhere classified
    Contact with chain hoist
    Contact with drive belt
    Contact with pulley (block)

W24.1 Contact with transmission devices, not elsewhere classified
    Contact with transmission belt or cable

W25 Contact with sharp glass
    Code first any associated:
        injury due to flying glass from explosion or firearm discharge (W32-W40)
        transport accident (V00-V99)
    Excludes1:   fall on same level due to slipping, tripping and stumbling with subsequent striking against sharp glass (W01.10)
                striking against sharp glass with subsequent fall (W18.02)

The following extensions are to be added to code W25:

    a   initial encounter
    d   subsequent encounter
    q   sequelae

W26 Contact with knife, sword or dagger

The following extensions are to be added to each code from category W26:

a   initial encounter
d   subsequent encounter
q   sequelae

W26.0 Contact with knife

Excludes1:   contact with electric knife (W29.1)

W26.1 Contact with sword or dagger

W27 Contact with nonpowered hand tool

The following extensions are to be added to each code from category W27:

a   initial encounter
d   subsequent encounter
q   sequelae

W27.0 Contact with workbench tool

Contact with auger
Contact with axe
Contact with chisel
Contact with handsaw
Contact with screwdriver

W27.1 Contact with garden tool

Contact with hoe
Contact with nonpowered lawn mower
Contact with pitchfork
Contact with rake

W27.2 Contact with scissors

W27.3 Contact with hypodermic needle

Contact with contaminated hypodermic needle
Hypodermic needle stick

W27.4 Contact with needle (sewing)

Excludes1:   hypodermic needle (W27.3)

W27.5 Contact with kitchen utensil

Contact with fork
Contact with ice-pick
Contact with can-opener NOS

W27.6 Contact with paper-cutter

W27.8 Contact with other nonpowered hand tool

Contact with nonpowered sewing machine
Contact with shovel

W28 Contact with powered lawn mower

Includes: powered lawn mower (commercial) (residential)
Excludes1:   contact with nonpowered lawn mower (W27.1)
Excludes:2   exposure to electric current (W86.-)

The following extensions are to be added to code W28:

a   initial encounter
d   subsequent encounter
q   sequelae

W29 Contact with other powered hand tools and household machinery

Excludes1:   contact with commercial machinery (W31.82)
contact with hot household appliance (X15)
contact with nonpowered hand tool (W27.-)
exposure to electric current (W86)

The following extensions are to be added to each code from category W29:

a   initial encounter
d   subsequent encounter
q   sequelae

W29.0 Contact with powered kitchen appliance

Contact with blender
Contact with can-opener
Contact with garbage disposal
Contact with mixer

W29.1 Contact with electric knife

W29.2 Contact with other powered household machinery

Contact with electric fan
Contact with powered dryer (clothes) (powered) (spin)
Contact with washing-machine
Contact with sewing machine

W29.3 Contact with powered garden and outdoor hand tools and machinery

Contact with chainsaw
Contact with edger
Contact with garden cultivator (tiller)
Contact with hedge trimmer
Contact with other powered garden tool

Excludes1:   contact with powered lawn mower (W28)

W29.4 Contact with nail gun

W29.8 Contact with other powered powered hand tools and household machinery

Contact with do-it-yourself tool NOS

W30 Contact with agricultural machinery

Includes: animal-powered farm machine
Excludes1:   agricultural transport vehicle accident (V01-V99)
explosion of grain store (W40.8)
exposure to electric current (W86.-)

The following extensions are to be added to each code from category W30:

a   initial encounter
d   subsequent encounter
q   sequelae

W30.0 Contact with combine harvester

Contact with reaper
Contact with thresher

W30.1 Contact with power take-off devices (PTO)

W30.2 Contact with hay derrick

W30.3 Contact with grain storage elevator

Excludes1:   explosion of grain store (W40.8)

W30.8 Contact with other specified agricultural machinery

  W30.81 Contact with agricultural transport vehicle in stationary use

Contact with agricultural transport vehicle under repair, not on public roadway

Excludes1:   agricultural transport vehicle accident (V01-V99)

  W30.89 Contact with other specified agricultural machinery

W30.9 Contact with unspecified agricultural machinery

Contact with farm machinery NOS

W31 Contact with other and unspecified machinery

Excludes1:   contact with agricultural machinery (W30.-)
contact with machinery in transport under own power or being towed by a vehicle (V01-V99)
exposure to electric current (W86)

The following extensions are to be added to each code from category W31:

a   initial encounter
d   subsequent encounter
q   sequelae

W31.0 Contact with mining and earth-drilling machinery

Contact with bore or drill (land) (seabed)
Contact with shaft hoist
Contact with shaft lift
Contact with undercutter

W31.1 Contact with metalworking machines

Contact with abrasive wheel
Contact with forging machine
Contact with lathe
Contact with mechanical shears
Contact with metal drilling machine
Contact with milling machine
Contact with power press
Contact with rolling-mill
Contact with metal sawing machine

W31.2   Contact with powered woodworking and forming machines
Contact with band saw
Contact with bench saw
Contact with circular saw
Contact with molding machine
Contact with overhead plane
Contact with powered saw
Contact with radial saw
Contact with sander

Excludes1:   nonpowered woodworking tools (W27.0)

W31.3   Contact with prime movers
Contact with gas turbine
Contact with internal combustion engine
Contact with steam engine
Contact with water driven turbine

W31.8   Contact with other specified machinery

W31.81   Contact with recreational machinery
Contact with roller-coaster

W31.82   Contact with other commercial machinery
Contact with commercial electric fan
Contact with commercial kitchen appliances
Contact with commercial powered dryer (clothes) (powered) (spin)
Contact with commercial washing-machine
Contact with commercical sewing machine

Excludes1:   contact with household machinery (W29.-)
contact with powered lawn mower (W28)

W31.83   Contact with special construction vehicle in stationary use
Contact with special construction vehicle under repair, not on public roadway

Excludes1:   special construction vehicle accident (V01-V99)

W31.89   Contact with other specified machinery

W31.9   Contact with unspecified machinery
Contact with machinery NOS

W32 Accidental handgun discharge
Includes: accidental discharge of gun for single hand use
accidental discharge of pistol
accidental discharge of revolver
handgun discharge NOS

Excludes1:   accidental airgun discharge (W34.01)
accidental BB gun discharge (W34.01)
accidental pellet gun discharge (W34.01)
accidental shotgun discharge (W33.0)
assault by handgun discharge (X93)
handgun discharge involving legal intervention (Y35.0-)
handgun discharge involving military or war operations (Y36.4-)
intentional self-harm by handgun discharge (X72)
Very pistol discharge (W34.8)
The following extensions are to be added to code W32:
a   initial encounter
d   subsequent encounter
q   sequelae

W33 Accidental rifle, shotgun and larger firearm discharge
Includes: rifle, shotgun and larger firearm discharge NOS
Excludes1:   accidental airgun discharge (W34.01)
accidental BB gun discharge (W34.01)
accidental handgun discharge (W32)
accidental pellet gun discharge (W34.01)
assault by rifle, shotgun and larger firearm discharge (X94)
firearm discharge involving legal intervention (Y35.0-)
firearm discharge involving military or war operations (Y36.4-)
intentional self-harm by rifle, shotgun and larger firearm discharge (X73)
The following extensions are to be added to each code from category W33:
a   initial encounter
d   subsequent encounter
q   sequelae

W33.0   Accidental discharge of shotgun
Discharge of shotgun NOS

W33.1   Accidental discharge of hunting rifle
Discharge of hunting rifle NOS

W33.2   Accidental discharge of machine gun
Discharge of machine gun NOS

W33.8   Accidental discharge of other larger firearm
Discharge of other larger firearm NOS

W33.9   Accidental discharge of unspecified larger firearm
Discharge of unspecified larger firearm NOS

W34 Accidental discharge from other and unspecified firearms and guns
The following extensions are to be added to each code from category W34:
a   initial encounter
d   subsequent encounter
q   sequelae

W34.0   Accidental discharge of gas, air or spring-operated guns

W34.01   Accidental discharge of airgun
Accidental discharge of BB gun
Accidental discharge of pellet gun

W34.02   Accidental discharge of paintball gun
Unintentional injury due to paintball discharge

W34.09   Accidental discharge of other gas, air or spring-operated gun

W34.8   Accidental discharge from other specified firearms
Accidental discharge from Very pistol [flare]

W34.9   Accidental discharge from unspecified firearms or gun
Discharge from firearm NOS
Gunshot wound NOS
Shot NOS

W35 Explosion and rupture of boiler
Excludes1:   explosion and rupture of boiler on watercraft (V93.4)
The following extensions are to be added to code W35:
a   initial encounter
d   subsequent encounter
q   sequelae

W36 Explosion and rupture of gas cylinder
The following extensions are to be added to each code from category W36:
a   initial encounter
d   subsequent encounter
q   sequelae

W36.1   Explosion and rupture of aerosol can

W36.2   Explosion and rupture of air tank

W36.3   Explosion and rupture of pressurized-gas tank

W36.8   Explosion and rupture of other gas cyclinder

W36.9   Explosion and rupture of unspecified gas cyclinder

W37 Explosion and rupture of pressurized tire, pipe or hose
The following extensions are to be added to each code from category W37:
a   initial encounter
d   subsequent encounter
q   sequelae

W37.0   Explosion of bicycle tire

W37.8   Explosion and rupture of other pressurized tire, pipe or hose

W38 Explosion and rupture of other specified pressurized devices
The following extensions are to be added to code W38:
a   initial encounter
d   subsequent encounter
q   sequelae

W39 Discharge of firework
The following extensions are to be added to code W39:
a   initial encounter
d   subsequent encounter
q   sequelae

W40 Explosion of other materials

　Excludes1:　assault by explosive material (X96)
　　　　　explosion involving legal intervention (Y35.1-)
　　　　　explosion involving military or war operations (Y36.0-, Y36.2-)
　　　　　intentional self-harm by explosive material (X75)
　The following extensions are to be added to each code from category W40:
　　a　initial encounter
　　d　subsequent encounter
　　q　sequelae

W40.0 Explosion of blasting material
　Explosion of blasting cap
　Explosion of detonator
　Explosion of dynamite
　Explosion of explosive (any) used in blasting operations

W40.1 Explosion of explosive gases
　Explosion of acetylene
　Explosion of butane
　Explosion of coal gas
　Explosion in mine NOS
　Explosion of explosive gas
　Explosion of fire damp
　Explosion of gasoline fumes
　Explosion of methane
　Explosion of propane

W40.8 Explosion of other specified explosive materials
　Explosion in dump NOS
　Explosion in factory NOS
　Explosion in grain store
　Explosion in munitions
　Excludes1:　explosion involving legal intervention (Y35.1-)
　　　　　explosion involving military or war operations (Y36.0-, Y36.2-)

W40.9 Explosion of unspecified explosive materials
　Explosion NOS

*W41 deactivated. See T70.4

W42 Exposure to noise
　The following extensions are to be added to each code from category W42:
　　a　initial encounter
　　d　subsequent encounter
　　q　sequelae

W42.0 Exposure to supersonic waves

W42.9 Exposure to other noise
　Exposure to sound waves NOS

*W43 deactivated. See T75.2

*W44 deactivated. See T15-T19

W45 Foreign body or object entering through skin
　Excludes2:　contact with hand tools (nonpowered) (powered) (W27-W29)
　　　　　contact with knife, sword or dagger (W26.-)
　　　　　contact with sharp glass (W25.-)
　　　　　struck by objects (W20-W22)
　The following extensions are to be added to each code from category W45:
　　a　initial encounter
　　d　subsequent encounter
　　q　sequelae

W45.0 Nail entering through skin

W45.1 Paper entering through skin
　Paper cut

W45.2 Lid of can entering through skin

W45.8 Other foreign body or object entering through skin
　Splinter in skin NOS

W49 Exposure to other inanimate mechanical forces
　Includes:　exposure to abnormal gravitational [G] forces
　　　　　exposure to inanimate mechanical forces NEC
　Excludes1:　exposure to inanimate mechanical forces involving military or war operations (Y36.-, Y37.-)
　The following extensions are to be added to code W49:
　　a　initial encounter
　　d　subsequent encounter
　　q　sequelae

Exposure to animate mechanical forces (W50-W64)
　Excludes1:　toxic effect of contact with venomous animals and plants (T63.-)

W50 Accidental hit, strike, kick, twist, bite or scratch by another person
　Includes:　hit, strike, kick, twist, bite, or scratch by another person NOS
　Excludes1:　assault by bodily force (Y04)
　　　　　struck by objects (W20-W22)
　The following extensions are to be added to each code from category W50:
　　a　initial encounter
　　d　subsequent encounter
　　q　sequelae

W50.0 Accidental hit or strike by another person
　Hit or strike by another person NOS

W50.1 Accidental kick by another person
　Kick by another person NOS

W50.2 Accidental twist by another person
　Twist by another person NOS

W50.3 Accidental bite by another person
　Bite by another person NOS
　Human bite

W50.4 Accidental scratch by another person
　Scratch by another person NOS

W51 Accidental striking against or bumped into by another person
　Excludes1:　assault by striking against or bumping into by another person (Y08.2-)
　　　　　fall due to collision with another person (W03)
　The following extensions are to be added to code W51:
　　a　initial encounter
　　d　subsequent encounter
　　q　sequelae

W52 Crushed, pushed or stepped on by crowd or human stampede
　Crushed, pushed or stepped on by crowd or human stampede with or without fall
　The following extensions are to be added to code W52:
　　a　initial encounter
　　d　subsequent encounter
　　q　sequelae

W53 Contact with rodent
　Contact with saliva, feces or urine of rodent
　The following extensions are to be added to each code from category W53:
　　a　initial encounter
　　d　subsequent encounter
　　q　sequelae

W53.0 Contact with mouse
　W53.01　Bitten by mouse
　W53.09　Other contact with mouse

W53.1 Contact with rat
　W53.11　Bitten by rat
　W53.19　Other contact with rat

W53.2 Contact with squirrel
　W53.21　Bitten by squirrel
　W53.29　Other contact with squirrel

W53.8 Contact with other rodent
　W53.81　Bitten by other rodent
　W53.89　Other contact with other rodent

W54 Contact with dog
Contact with saliva, feces or urine of dog
The following extensions are to be added to each code from category W54:
  a   initial encounter
  d   subsequent encounter
  q   sequelae

W54.0 Bitten by dog

W54.1 Struck by dog
Knocked over by dog

W54.8 Other contact with dog

W55 Contact with other mammals
Contact with saliva, feces or urine of mammal
Excludes1:   animal being ridden — see transport accidents
              bitten or struck by dog (W54)
              bitten or struck by rodent (W53.-)
              contact with marine mammals (W56.x-)
The following extensions are to be added to each code from category W55:
  a   initial encounter
  d   subsequent encounter
  q   sequelae

W55.0 Contact with cat
  W55.01   Bitten by cat
  W55.03   Stratched by cat
  W55.09   Other contact with cat
W55.1 Contact with horse
  W55.11   Bitten by horse
  W55.12   Struck by horse
  W55.19   Other contact with horse
W55.2 Contact with cow
  Contact with bull
  W55.21   Bitten by cow
  W55.22   Struck by cow
    Gored by bull
  W55.29   Other contact with cow
W55.3 Contact with other hoof stock
  Contact with goats
  Contact with sheep
  W55.31   Bitten by other hoof stock
  W55.32   Struck by other hoof stock
    Gored by goat
    Gored by ram
  W55.39   Other contact with other hoof stock
W55.4 Contact with pig
  W55.41   Bitten by pig
  W55.42   Struck by pig
  W55.49   Other contact with pig
W55.5 Contact with raccoon
  W55.51   Bitten by raccoon
  W55.52   Struck by raccoon
  W55.59   Other contact with raccoon
W55.8 Contact with other mammals
  W55.81   Bitten by other mammals
  W55.82   Struck by other mammals
  W55.89   Other contact with other mammals

W56 Contact with nonvenomous marine animal
Excludes1:   contact with venomous marine animal (T63.-)
The following extensions are to be added to each code from category W56:
  a   initial encounter
  d   subsequent encounter
  q   sequelae

W56.0 Contact with dolphin
  W56.01   Bitten by dolphin
  W56.02   Struck by dolphin
  W56.09   Other contact with dolphin
W56.1 Contact with sea lion
  W56.11   Bitten by sea lion
  W56.12   Struck by sea lion

  W56.19   Other contact with sea lion
W56.2 Contact with orca
  Contact with killer whale
  W56.21   Bitten by orca
  W56.22   Struck by orca
  W56.29   Other contact with orca
W56.3 Contact with other marine mammals
  W56.31   Bitten by other marine mammals
  W56.32   Struck by other marine mammals
  W56.39   Other contact with other marine mammals
W56.4 Contact with shark
  W56.41   Bitten by shark
  W56.42   Struck by shark
  W56.49   Other contact with shark
W56.5 Contact with other fish
  W56.51   Bitten by other fish
  W56.52   Struck by other fish
  W56.59   Other contact with other fish
W56.8 Contact with other nonvenomous marine animals
  W56.81   Bitten by other nonvenomous marine animals
  W56.82   Struck by other nonvenomous marine animals
  W56.89   Other contact with other nonvenomous marine animals

W57 Bitten or stung by nonvenomous insect and other nonvenomous arthropods
Excludes1:   contact with venomous insects and arthropds (T63.2-, T63.3-, T63.4-)
The following extensions are to be added to code W57:
  a   initial encounter
  d   subsequent encounter
  q   sequelae

W58 Contact with crocodile or alligator
The following extensions are to be added to each code from category W58:
  a   initial encounter
  d   subsequent encounter
  q   sequelae

W58.0 Contact with alligator
  W58.01   Bitten by alligator
  W58.02   Struck by alligator
  W58.03   Crushed by alligator
W58.1 Contact with crocodile
  W58.11   Bitten by crocodile
  W58.12   Struck by crocodile
  W58.13   Crushed by crocodile

W59 Contact with other nonvenomous reptiles
Excludes1:   contact with venomous reptile (T63.0-, T63.1-)
The following extensions are to be added to each code from category W59:
  a   initial encounter
  d   subsequent encounter
  q   sequelae

W59.0 Contact with nonvenomous lizards
  W59.01   Bitten by nonvenomous lizards
  W59.02   Struck by nonvenomous lizards
  W59.09   Other contact with nonvenomous lizards
    Exposure to nonvenomous lizards
W59.1 Contact with nonvenomous snakes
  W59.11   Bitten by nonvenomous snake
  W59.12   Struck by nonvenomous snake
  W59.13   Crushed by nonvenomous snake
  W59.19   Other contact with nonvenomous snake
W59.2 Contact with turtles
  Excludes1:   contact with tortoises (W59.8-)
  W59.21   Bitten by turtle
  W59.22   Struck by turtle

W59.29   **Other contact with turtle**
Exposure to turtles

W59.8 **Contact with other nonvenomous reptiles**

W59.81   **Bitten by other nonvenomous reptiles**

W59.82   **Struck by other nonvenomous reptiles**

W59.83   **Crushed by other nonvenomous reptiles**

W59.89   **Other contact with other nonvenomous reptiles**

W60 **Contact with nonvenomous plant thorns and spines and sharp leaves**

Excludes1:   contact with venomous plants (T63.x-)
The following extensions are to be added to code W60:
a   initial encounter
d   subsequent encounter
q   sequelae

W61 **Contact with birds**
Contact with excreta of birds
The following extensions are to be added to each code from category W61:
a   initial encounter
d   subsequent encounter
q   sequelae

W61.0 **Contact with parrot (domestic) (wild)**

W61.01   **Bitten by parrot (domestic) (wild)**

W61.02   **Struck by parrot (domestic) (wild)**

W61.09   **Other contact with parrot (domestic) (wild)**
Exposure to parrots (domestic) (wild)

W61.1 **Contact with macaw (domestic) (wild)**

W61.11   **Bitten by macaw (domestic) (wild)**

W61.12   **Struck by macaw (domestic) (wild)**

W61.19   **Other contact with macaw (domestic) (wild)**
Exposure to macaws (domestic) (wild)

W61.2 **Contact with other psittacines (domestic) (wild)**

W61.21   **Bitten by other psittacines (domestic) (wild)**

W61.22   **Struck by other psittacines (domestic) (wild)**

W61.29   **Other contact with other psittacines (domestic) (wild)**
Exposure to other psittacines (domestic) (wild)

W61.3 **Contact with chicken (domestic) (wild)**

W61.32   **Struck by chicken (domestic) (wild)**

W61.33   **Pecked by chicken (domestic) (wild)**

W61.39   **Other contact with chicken (domestic) (wild)**
Exposure to chickens

W61.4 **Contact with turkey (domestic) (wild)**

W61.42   **Struck by turkey (domestic) (wild)**

W61.43   **Pecked by turkey (domestic) (wild)**

W61.49   **Other contact with turkey (domestic) (wild)**

W61.5 **Contact with goose (domestic) (wild)**

W61.51   **Bitten by goose (domestic) (wild)**

W61.52   **Struck by goose (domestic) (wild)**

W61.59   **Other contact with goose (domestic) (wild)**

W61.6 **Contact with duck (domestic) (wild)**

W61.61   **Bitten by duck (domestic) (wild)**

W61.62   **Struck by duck (domestic) (wild)**

W61.69   **Other contact with duck (domestic) (wild)**

W61.9 **Contact with other birds (domestic) (wild)**

W61.91   **Bitten by other birds (domestic) (wild)**

W61.92   **Struck by other birds (domestic) (wild)**

W61.99   **Other contact with other birds (domestic) (wild)**

W62 **Contact with nonvenomous amphibians**

Excludes1:   contact with venomous amphibians (T63.81-R63.83)
The following extensions are to be added to each code from category W62:
a   initial encounter
d   subsequent encounter
q   sequelae

W62.0 **Contact with nonvenomous frogs**

W62.1 **Contact with nonvenomous toads**

W62.9 **Contact with other nonvenomous amphibians**

W64 **Exposure to other animate mechanical forces**
The following extensions are to be added to code W64:
a   initial encounter
d   subsequent encounter
q   sequelae

Accidental non-transport drowning and submersion (W65-W74)

Excludes1:   accidental drowning and submersion due to fall into water (W16.-)
accidental drowning and submersion due to water transport accident (V90.-, V92.-)

Excludes2:   accidental drowning and submersion due to cataclysm (X34-X39)

W65 **Accidental drowning and submersion while in bath-tub**

Excludes1:   accidental drowning and submersion due to fall in (into) bathtub (W16.211)
The following extensions are to be added to code W65:
a   initial encounter
d   subsequent encounter
q   sequelae

***W66 deactivated. See W16.**

W67 **Accidental drowning and submersion while in swimming-pool**

Excludes1:   accidental drowning and submersion due to fall into swimming pool (W16.011, W16.021, W16.031)
accidental drowning and submersion due to striking into wall of swimming pool (W22.041)
The following extensions are to be added to code W67:
a   initial encounter
d   subsequent encounter
q   sequelae

***W68 deactivated. See W16.**

W69 **Accidental drowning and submersion while in natural water**

Includes: accidental drowning and submersion while in lake
accidental drowning and submersion while in open sea
accidental drowning and submersion while in river
accidental drowning and submersion while in stream

Excludes1:   accidental drowning and submersion due to fall into natural body of water (W16.111, W16.121, W16.131)
The following extensions are to be added to code W69:
a   initial encounter
d   subsequent encounter
q   sequelae

***W70 deactivated. See W16.**

W73 **Other specified cause of accidental non-transport drowning and submersion**

Includes: accidental drowning and submersion while in quenching tank
accidental drowning and submersion while in reservoir

Excludes1:   accidental drowning and submersion due to fall into other water (W16.311, W16.321, W16.331)
The following extensions are to be added to code W73:
a   initial encounter
d   subsequent encounter
q   sequelae

W74 **Unspecified cause of accidental drowning and submersion**

Includes: drowning NOS
The following extensions are to be added to code W74:
a   initial encounter
d   subsequent encounter
q   sequelae

EXPOSURE TO ELECTRIC CURRENT, RADIATION AND EXTREME AMBIENT AIR TEMPERATURE AND PRESSURE (W85–W99)

Excludes1:   exposure to:
            natural cold (X31)
            natural heat (X30)
            natural radiation NOS (X39)
            sunlight (X32)
            lightning (T75.0-)

*W75-W77 deactivated. See T71

*W78 deactivated. See T17.81, T18.81.

*W79-W80 deactivated. See T17 and T18

*W81 deactivated. See T71.2

*W83 deactivated. See T71

*W84 deactivated. See T71.9

W85 Exposure to electric transmission lines

Includes: broken power line
The following extensions are to be added to code W85:
    a   initial encounter
    d   subsequent encounter
    q   sequelae

W86 Exposure to other specified electric current

The following extensions are to be added to each code from category W86:
    a   initial encounter
    d   subsequent encounter
    q   sequelae

W86.0 Exposure to domestic wiring and appliances

W86.1 Exposure to industrial wiring, appliances and electrical machinery

Exposure to conductors
Exposure to control apparatus
Exposure to electrical equipment and machinery
Exposure to transformers

W86.8 Exposure to other electric current

Exposure to wiring and appliances in or on farm (not farmhouse)
Exposure to wiring and appliances outdoors
Exposure to wiring and appliances in or on public building
Exposure to wiring and appliances in or on residential institutions
Exposure to wiring and appliances in or on schools

*W87 deactivated. See W86

W88 Exposure to ionizing radiation

Excludes1:   exposure to sunlight (X32)
The following extensions are to be added to each code from category W88:
    a   initial encounter
    d   subsequent encounter
    q   sequelae

W88.0 Exposure to X-rays

W88.1 Exposure to radioactive isotopes

W89 Exposure to man-made visible and ultraviolet light

Includes: exposure to welding light (arc)
Excludes2:   exposure to sunlight (X32)
The following extensions are to be added to each code from category W89:
    a   initial encounter
    d   subsequent encounter
    q   sequelae

W89.0 Exposure to welding light (arc)

W89.1 Exposure to tanning bed

W89.8 Exposure to other man-made visible and ultraviolet light

W89.9 Exposure to unspecified man-made visible and ultraviolet light

W90 Exposure to other nonionizing radiation

Excludes1:   exposure to sunlight (X32)
The following extensions are to be added to each code from category W90:
    a   initial encounter
    d   subsequent encounter
    q   sequelae

W90.0 Exposure to radiofrequency

W90.1 Exposure to infrared radiation

W90.2 Exposure to laser radiation

W90.8 Exposure to other nonionizing radiation

*W91 deactivated. See W90

W92 Exposure to excessive heat of man-made origin

The following extensions are to be added to code W92:
    a   initial encounter
    d   subsequent encounter
    q   sequelae

W93 Exposure to excessive cold of man-made origin

The following extensions are to be added to each code from category W93:
    a   initial encounter
    d   subsequent encounter
    q   sequelae

W93.0 Contact with or inhalation of dry ice

W93.01   Contact with dry ice

W93.02   Inhalation of dry ice

W93.1 Contact with or inhalation of liquid air

W93.11   Contact with liquid air
Contact with liquid hydrogen
Contact with liquid nitrogen

W93.12   Inhalation of liquid air
Inhalation of liquid hydrogen
Inhalation of liquid nitrogen

W93.2 Prolonged exposure in deep freeze unit or refrigerator

W93.8 Exposure to other excessive cold of man-made origin

W94 Exposure to high and low air pressure and changes in air pressure

The following extensions are to be added to each code from category W94:
    a   initial encounter
    d   subsequent encounter
    q   sequelae

W94.0 Exposure to prolonged high air pressure

W94.1 Exposure to prolonged low air pressure

W94.11   Exposure to residence or prolonged visit at high altitude

W94.12   Exposure to other prolonged low air pressure

W94.2 Exposure to rapid changes in air pressure during ascent

W94.21   Exposure to reduction in atmospheric pressure while surfacing from deep-water diving

W94.22   Exposure to reduction in atmospheric pressure while surfacing from underground

W94.23   Exposure to sudden change in air pressure in aircraft during ascent

W94.29   Exposure to other rapid changes in air pressure during ascent

W94.3 Exposure to rapid changes in air pressure during descent

W94.31   Exposure to sudden change in air pressure in aircraft during ascent or descent

W94.32   Exposure to high air pressure from rapid descent in water

W94.39   Exposure to other rapid changes in air pressure during descent

W99 Exposure to other man-made environmental factors

The following extensions are to be added to code W99:
    a   initial encounter
    d   subsequent encounter
    q   sequelae

EXPOSURE TO SMOKE, FIRE AND FLAMES (X00–X09)

Excludes1:   arson (X97)
Excludes2:   explosions (W35-W40)
               lightning (T75.0-)
               transport accident (V01-V99)

X00 Exposure to uncontrolled fire in building or structure

Includes: conflagration in building or structure
Code first any associated cataclysm
Excludes2:   exposure to ignition or melting of nightwear (X05)
               exposure to ignition or melting of other clothing and apparel (X06-)
               exposure to other specified smoke, fire and flames (X08.-)
The following extensions are to be added to each code from category X00:
    a   initial encounter
    d   subsequent encounter
    q   sequelae

X00.0 Exposure to flames in uncontrolled fire in building or structure

X00.1 Exposure to smoke in uncontrolled fire in building or structure

X00.2 Injury due to collapse of burning building or structure in uncontrolled fire

        Excludes1:   injury due to collapse of building not on fire (W20.1)

X00.3 Fall from burning building or structure in uncontrolled fire

X00.4 Hit by object from burning building or structure in uncontrolled fire

X00.5 Jump from burning building or structure in uncontrolled fire

X00.8 Other exposure to uncontrolled fire in building or structure

X01 Exposure to uncontrolled fire, not in building or structure

Exposure to forest fire
The following extensions are to be added to each code from category X01:
    a   initial encounter
    d   subsequent encounter
    q   sequelae

X01.0 Exposure to flames in uncontrolled fire, not in building or structure

X01.1 Exposure to smoke in uncontrolled fire, not in building or structure

X01.3 Fall due to uncontrolled fire, not in building or structure

X01.4 Hit by object due to uncontrolled fire, not in building or structure

X01.8 Other exposure to uncontrolled fire, not in building or structure

X02 Exposure to controlled fire in building or structure

Includes: exposure to fire in fireplace
               exposure to fire in stove
The following extensions are to be added to each code from category X02:
    a   initial encounter
    d   subsequent encounter
    q   sequelae

X02.0 Exposure to flames in controlled fire in building or structure

X02.1 Exposure to smoke in controlled fire in building or structure

X02.2 Injury due to collapse of burning building or structure in controlled fire

        Excludes1:   injury due to collapse of building not on fire (W20.1)

X02.3 Fall from burning building or structure in controlled fire

X02.4 Hit by object from burning building or structure in controlled fire

X02.5 Jump from burning building or structure in controlled fire

X02.8 Other exposure to controlled fire in building or structure

X03 Exposure to controlled fire, not in building or structure

Includes: exposure to bon fire
               exposure to camp-fire
               exposure to trash fire
The following extensions are to be added to each code from category X03:
    a   initial encounter
    d   subsequent encounter
    q   sequelae

X03.0 Exposure to flames in controlled fire, not in building or structure

X03.1 Exposure to smoke in controlled fire, not in building or structure

X03.3 Fall due to controlled fire, not in building or structure

X03.4 Hit by object due to controlled fire, not in building or structure

X03.8 Other exposure to controlled fire, not in building or structure

X04 Exposure to ignition of highly flammable material

Includes: exposure to ignition of gasoline
               exposure to ignition of kerosene
               exposure to ignition of petrol
Excludes2:   exposure to ignition or melting of nightwear (X05)
               exposure to ignition or melting of other clothing and apparel (X06)
The following extensions are to be added to code X04:
    a   initial encounter
    d   subsequent encounter
    q   sequelae

X05 Exposure to ignition or melting of nightwear

Excludes2:   exposure to uncontrolled fire in building or structure (X00.-)
               exposure to uncontrolled fire, not in building or structure (X01.-)
               exposure to controlled fire in building or structure (X02.-)
               exposure to controlled fire, not in building or structure (X03.-)
               exposure to ignition of highly flammable materials (X04.-)
The following extensions are to be added to code X05:
    a   initial encounter
    d   subsequent encounter
    q   sequelae

X06 Exposure to ignition or melting of other clothing and apparel

Excludes2:   exposure to uncontrolled fire in building or structure (X00.-)
               exposure to uncontrolled fire, not in building or structure (X01.-)
               exposure to controlled fire in building or structure (X02.-)
               exposure to controlled fire, not in building or structure (X03.-)
               exposure to ignition of highly flammable materials (X04.-)
The following extensions are to be added to each code from category X06:
    a   initial encounter
    d   subsequent encounter
    q   sequelae

X06.0 Exposure to ignition of plastic jewelry

X06.1 Exposure to melting of plastic jewelry

X06.2 Exposure to ignition of other clothing and apparel

X06.3 Exposure to melting of other clothing and apparel

X08 Exposure to other specified smoke, fire and flames

The following extensions are to be added to each code from category X08:
    a   initial encounter
    d   subsequent encounter
    q   sequelae

X08.0 Exposure to bed fire

        Exposure to mattress fire

X08.00   Exposure to bed fire due to unspecified burning
          material
X08.01   Exposure to bed fire due to burning cigarette
X08.09   Exposure to bed fire due to other burning material

X08.1   Exposure to sofa fire
X08.10   Exposure to sofa fire due to unspecified burning
          material
X08.11   Exposure to sofa fire due to burning cigarette
X08.19   Exposure to sofa fire due to other burning material

X08.2   Exposure to other furniture fire
X08.20   Exposure to other furniture fire due to unspecified
          burning material
X08.21   Exposure to other furniture fire due to burning
          cigarette
X08.29   Exposure to fire other furniture due to other burning
          material

X08.8   Exposure to other specified smoke, fire and flames

*X09 deactivated. See X08

CONTACT WITH HEAT AND HOT SUBSTANCES (X10–X19)

Excludes1:   exposure to excessive natural heat (X30)
             exposure to fire and flames (X00-X09)

X10 Contact with hot drinks, food, fats and cooking oils
The following extensions are to be added to each code from category
X10:
   a   initial encounter
   d   subsequent encounter
   q   sequelae

X10.0   Contact with hot drinks
X10.1   Contact with hot food
X10.2   Contact with fats and cooking oils

X11 Contact with hot tap-water
Contact with boiling tap-water
Contact with boiling water NOS

Excludes1:   contact with water heated on stove (X12)
The following extensions are to be added to each code from category
X11:
   a   initial encounter
   d   subsequent encounter
   q   sequelae

X11.0   Contact with hot water in bath or tub
          Excludes1:   contact with running hot water in bath or tub
                       (X11.1)
X11.1   Contact with running hot water
          Contact with hot water running out of hose
          Contact with hot water running out of tap
X11.8   Contact with other hot tap-water
          Contact with hot water in bucket
          Contact with hot tap-water NOS

X12 Contact with other hot fluids
Includes: contact with water heated on stove
Excludes1:   hot (liquid) metals (X18)
The following extensions are to be added to code X12:
   a   initial encounter
   d   subsequent encounter
   q   sequelae

X13 Contact with steam and other hot vapors
The following extensions are to be added to each code from category
X13:
   a   initial encounter
   d   subsequent encounter
   q   sequelae

X13.0   Inhalation of steam and other hot vapors
X13.1   Other contact with steam and other hot vapors

X14 Contact with hot air and other hot gases
The following extensions are to be added to each code from category
X14:
   a   initial encounter
   d   subsequent encounter
   q   sequelae

X14.0   Inhalation of hot air and gases
X14.1   Other contact with hot air and other hot gases

X15 Contact with hot household appliances
Excludes1:   contact with heating appliances (X16)
             contact with powered household appliances (W29.-)
             exposure to controlled fire in building or structure due
                to household appliance (X02.8)
             exposure to household appliances electrical current
                (W86.0)
The following extensions are to be added to each code from category
X15:
   a   initial encounter
   d   subsequent encounter
   q   sequelae

X15.0   Contact with hot stove (kitchen)
X15.1   Contact with hot toaster
X15.2   Contact with hotplate
X15.3   Contact with hot saucepan or skillet
X15.8   Contact with other hot household appliances
          Contact with cooker
          Contact with kettle
          Contact with light bulbs

X16 Contact with hot heating appliances, radiators and pipes
Excludes1:   contact with powered appliances (W29.-)
             exposure to controlled fire in building or structure due
                to appliance (X02.8)
             exposure to industrial appliances electrical current
                (W86.1)
The following extensions are to be added to code X16:
   a   initial encounter
   d   subsequent encounter
   q   sequelae

X17 Contact with hot engines, machinery and tools
Excludes1:   contact with hot heating appliances, radiators and
                pipes (X16)
             contact with hot household appliances (X15)
The following extensions are to be added to code X17:
   a   initial encounter
   d   subsequent encounter
   q   sequelae

X18 Contact with other hot metals
Includes: contact with liquid metal
The following extensions are to be added to code X18:
   a   initial encounter
   d   subsequent encounter
   q   sequelae

X19 Contact with other heat and hot substances
Excludes1:   objects that are not normally hot, e.g., an object made
                hot by a house fire (X00-X09)
The following extensions are to be added to code X19:
   a   initial encounter
   d   subsequent encounter
   q   sequelae

*X20-X29 deactivated. See T63

EXPOSURE TO FORCES OF NATURE (X30–X39)

X30 Exposure to excessive natural heat
Includes: exposure to excessive heat as the cause of sunstroke
    exposure to heat NOS
Excludes1:   excessive heat of man-made origin (W92)
    exposure to man-made radiation (W89)
    exposure to sunlight (X32)
    exposure to tanning bed (W89)
The following extensions are to be added to code X30:
    a   initial encounter
    d   subsequent encounter
    q   sequelae

X31 Exposure to excessive natural cold
Includes: excessive cold as the cause of chilblains NOS
    excessive cold as the cause of immersion foot or hand
    exposure to cold NOS
    exposure to weather conditions
Excludes1:   cold of man-made origin (W93.-)
    contact with or inhalation of:
        dry ice (W93.-)
        liquefied gas (W93.-)
The following extensions are to be added to code X31:
    a   initial encounter
    d   subsequent encounter
    q   sequelae

X32 Exposure to sunlight
Excludes1:   radiation-related disorders of the skin and
    subcutaneous tissue (L55-L59)
    man-made radiation (tanning bed) (W89)
The following extensions are to be added to code X32:
    a   initial encounter
    d   subsequent encounter
    q   sequelae

X34 Earthquake
The following extensions are to be added to code X34:
    a   initial encounter
    d   subsequent encounter
    q   sequelae

X35 Volcanic eruption
The following extensions are to be added to code X35:
    a   initial encounter
    d   subsequent encounter
    q   sequelae

X36 Avalanche, landslide and other earth movements
Includes: victim of mudslide of cataclysmic nature
Excludes1:   earthquake (X34)
Excludes2:   transport accident involving collision with avalanche or
    landslide not in motion (V01-V99)
The following extensions are to be added to each code from category X36:
    a   initial encounter
    d   subsequent encounter
    q   sequelae

X36.0 Collapse of dam or man-made structure causing earth movement

X36.1 Avalanche, landslide, or mudslide

X37 Cataclysmic storm
The following extensions are to be added to each code from category X37:
    a   initial encounter
    d   subsequent encounter
    q   sequelae

X37.0 Hurricane
    Storm surge
    Typhoon

X37.1 Tornado
    Cyclone
    Twister

X37.2 Blizzard (snow) (ice)

X37.3 Dust storm

X37.4 Tidalwave

    X37.41   Tidal wave due to earthquake or volcanic eruption
        Tidal wave NOS
        Tsunami

    X37.42   Tidal wave due to storm

X37.8 Other cataclysmic storms
    Cloudburst
    Torrential rain
    Excludes2:   flood (X38)

X37.9 Unspecified cataclysmic storm
    Storm NOS
    Excludes1:   collapse of dam or man-made structure causing
    earth movement (X39.0)

X38 Flood
Includes: flood arising from remote storm
    flood of cataclysmic nature arising from melting snow
    flood resulting directly from storm
Excludes1:   collapse of dam or man-made structure causing earth
    movement (X39.0)
    tidal wave NOS (X39.2)
    tidal wave caused by storm (X37.2)
The following extensions are to be added to code X38:
    a   initial encounter
    d   subsequent encounter
    q   sequelae

X39 Exposure to other forces of nature
The following extensions are to be added to each code from category X39:
    a   initial encounter
    d   subsequent encounter
    q   sequelae

X39.0 Exposure to natural radiation
    Excludes1:   man-made radiation (W88-W90)
    sunlight (X32)

    X39.01   Exposure to radon

    X39.08   Exposure to other natural radiation

X39.8 Other exposure to forces of nature

*Categories X40-X49 deactivated. See categories T36-T65 with extension 1

OVEREXERTION, TRAVEL AND PRIVATION (X50–X57)
Excludes1:   assault (X91-Y08)

X50 Overexertion and strenuous or repetitive movements
Note: a code from both X50.0 and X50.1 may be used together if the injury or condition is the result of both overexertion and repetitive movement.
Use additional activity code to identify the activity causing overexertion or repetitive movement injury (Y93.-)
Use additional code if overexertion, strenuous or repetitive activity is work-related (Y96)
The following extensions are to be added to each code from category X50:
    a   initial encounter
    d   subsequent encounter
    q   sequelae

X50.0 Overexertion and strenuous activity

    X50.00   Unspecified overexertion and strenuous activity

    X50.01   Sport-related overexertion and strenuous activity

    X50.02   Hobby (nonsport) related overexertion and strenuous activity

    X50.09   Other overexertion and strenuous activity

X50.1 Repetitive movement activity

    X50.10   Unspecified repetitive movement activity

    X50.11   Sport-related repetitive movement activity

    X50.12   Hobby (nonsport) related repetitive movement activity

    X50.19   Other repetitive movement activity

X51 Travel and motion
    Includes: prolonged sitting in transport vehicle
    Excludes1:   land-transport accidents (V01-V99)
                  water transport accidents (V90-V94)
    The following extensions are to be added to each code from category X51:
       a   initial encounter
       d   subsequent encounter
       q   sequelae

X51.0 Travel and motion in airplane
X51.1 Travel and motion in train
X51.2 Travel and motion in car
X51.3 Travel and motion in bus
X51.4 Travel and motion in boat (sailboat) (ship)
X51.8 Travel and motion other in transport vehicle
    Travel and motion sickness due to transport vehicle NOS

X52 Prolonged stay in weightless environment
    Includes: weightlessness in spacecraft (simulator)
    The following extensions are to be added to code X52:
       a   initial encounter
       d   subsequent encounter
       q   sequelae

*X53 deactivated. See T73.0

*X54 deactivated. See T73.1

*X57 deactivated. See T73.9

ACCIDENTAL EXPOSURE TO OTHER SPECIFIED FACTORS (X58)

X58 Exposure to other specified factors
    The following extensions are to be added to each code from category X58:
       a   initial encounter
       d   subsequent encounter
       q   sequelae

X58.1 Exposure to environmental tobacco smoke
    Exposure to second-hand tobacco smoke
X58.8 Exposure to other specified factors

INTENTIONAL SELF–HARM (X71–X83)

    Includes: purposely self-inflicted
                  injury suicide (attempted)

*X60-X69 deactivated. See categories T36-T65 with extension 2

*X70 deactivated. See T71

X71 Intentional self-harm by drowning and submersion
    The following extensions are to be added to each code from category X71:
       a   initial encounter
       d   subsequent encounter
       q   sequelae

X71.0 Intentional self-harm by drowning and submersion while in bathtub
X71.1 Intentional self-harm by drowning and submersion while in swimming pool
X71.2 Intentional self-harm by drowning and submersion after fall into swimming pool
X71.3 Intentional self-harm by drowning and submersion in natural water
X71.8 Other intentional self-harm by drowning and submersion
X71.9 Intentional self-harm by drowning and submersion, unspecified

X72 Intentional self-harm by handgun discharge
    Includes: intentional self-harm by gun for single hand use
                  intentional self-harm by pistol
                  intentional self-harm by revolver
    Excludes1:   Very pistol (X74.8)
    The following extensions are to be added to code X72:
       a   initial encounter
       d   subsequent encounter
       q   sequelae

X73 Intentional self-harm by rifle, shotgun and larger firearm discharge
    Excludes1:   airgun (X74.01)
    The following extensions are to be added to each code from category X73:
       a   initial encounter
       d   subsequent encounter
       q   sequelae

X73.0 Intentional self-harm by shotgun discharge
X73.1 Intentional self-harm by hunting rifle discharge
X73.2 Intentional self-harm by machine gun discharge
X73.8 Intentional self-harm by other larger firearm discharge
X73.9 Intentional self-harm by unspecified larger firearm discharge

X74 Intentional self-harm by other and unspecified firearm and gun discharge
    The following extensions are to be added to each code from category X74:
       a   initial encounter
       d   subsequent encounter
       q   sequelae

X74.0 Intentional self-harm by gas, air or spring-operated guns
    X74.01 Intentional self-harm by airgun
         Intentional self-harm by BB gun discharge
         Intentional self-harm by pellet gun discharge
    X74.02 Intentional self-harm by paintball gun
    X74.09 Intentional self-harm by other gas, air or spring-operated gun
X74.8 Intentional self-harm by other firearm discharge
    Intentional self-harm by Very pistol [flare] discharge
X74.9 Intentional self-harm by unspecified firearm discharge

X75 Intentional self-harm by explosive material
    The following extensions are to be added to code X75:
       a   initial encounter
       d   subsequent encounter
       q   sequelae

X76 Intentional self-harm by smoke, fire and flames
    The following extensions are to be added to code X76:
       a   initial encounter
       d   subsequent encounter
       q   sequelae

X77 Intentional self-harm by steam, hot vapors and hot objects
    The following extensions are to be added to each code from category X77:
       a   initial encounter
       d   subsequent encounter
       q   sequelae

X77.0 Intentional self-harm by steam or hot vapors
X77.1 Intentional self-harm by hot tap water
X77.2 Intentional self-harm by other hot fluids
X77.3 Intentional self-harm by hot household appliances
X77.8 Intentional self-harm by other hot objects
X77.9 Intentional self-harm by unspecifed hot objects

X78 Intentional self-harm by sharp object
    The following extensions are to be added to each code from category X78:
       a   initial encounter
       d   subsequent encounter
       q   sequelae

X78.0 Intentional self-harm by sharp glass
X78.1 Intentional self-harm by knife

X78.2   Intentional self-harm by sword or dagger
X78.8   Intentional self-harm by other sharp object
X78.9   Intentional self-harm by unspecified sharp object

X79   Intentional self-harm by blunt object
The following extensions are to be added to code X79:
  a   initial encounter
  d   subsequent encounter
  q   sequelae

X80   Intentional self-harm by jumping from a high place
Includes: intentional fall from one level to another
The following extensions are to be added to code X80:
  a   initial encounter
  d   subsequent encounter
  q   sequelae

X81   Intentional self-harm by jumping or lying before moving object
Excludes1:   intentional jumping in front of motor vehicle (X82.3)
The following extensions are to be added to code X81:
  a   initial encounter
  d   subsequent encounter
  q   sequelae

X82   Intentional self-harm by crashing of motor vehicle
The following extensions are to be added to each code from category X82:
  a   initial encounter
  d   subsequent encounter
  q   sequelae

X82.0   Intentional collision of motor vehicle with other motor vehicle
X82.1   Intentional collision of motor vehicle with train
X82.2   Intentional collision of motor vehicle with tree
X82.3   Intentional jumping in front of motor vehicle
X82.8   Other intentional self-harm by crashing of motor vehicle

X83   Intentional self-harm by other specified means
Excludes1:   intentional self-harm by poisoning or contact with toxic substance — see table of drugs and chemicals
The following extensions are to be added to each code from category X83:
  a   initial encounter
  d   subsequent encounter
  q   sequelae

X83.0   Intentional self-harm by crashing of aircraft
X83.1   Intentional self-harm by electrocution
X83.2   Intentional self-harm by exposure to extremes of cold
X83.8   Intentional self-harm by other specified means

*X84 deactivated. See T14.0

ASSAULT (X92–Y08)
Includes: homicide
injuries inflicted by another person with intent to injure or kill, by any means
Excludes1:   injuries due to legal intervention (Y35.-)
injuries due to operations of war (Y36.-)

*X85-X90 deactivated. See categories T36-T65 with extension 3

*X91 deactivated. See Y71

X92   Assault by drowning and submersion
The following extensions are to be added to each code from category X92:
  a   initial encounter
  d   subsequent encounter
  q   sequelae

X92.0   Assault by drowning and submersion while in bathtub
X92.1   Assault by drowning and submersion while in swimming pool
X92.2   Assault by drowning and submersion after push into swimming pool
X92.3   Assault by drowning and submersion in natural water
X92.8   Other assault by drowning and submersion
X92.9   Assault by drowning and submersion, unspecified

X93   Assault by handgun discharge
Includes: assault by discharge of gun for single hand use
assault by discharge of pistol
assault by discharge of revolver
Excludes1:   Very pistol (X95.8)
The following extensions are to be added to code X93:
  a   initial encounter
  d   subsequent encounter
  q   sequelae

X94   Assault by rifle, shotgun and larger firearm discharge
Excludes1:   airgun (X95.01)
The following extensions are to be added to each code from category X94:
  a   initial encounter
  d   subsequent encounter
  q   sequelae

X94.0   Assault by shotgun
X94.1   Assault by hunting rifle
X94.2   Assault by machine gun
X94.8   Assault by other larger firearm discharge
X94.9   Assault by unspecified larger firearm discharge

X95   Assault by other and unspecified firearm and gun discharge
The following extensions are to be added to each code from category X95:
  a   initial encounter
  d   subsequent encounter
  q   sequelae

X95.0   Assault by gas, air or spring-operated guns
  X95.01   Assault by airgun discharge
            Assault by BB gun discharge
            Assault by pellet gun discharge
  X95.02   Assault by paintball gun discharge
  X95.09   Assault by other gas, air or spring-operated gun
X95.8   Assault by other firearm discharge
            Assault by Very pistol [flare] discharge
X95.9   Assault by unspecified firearm discharge

X96   Assault by explosive material
Excludes1:   incendiary device (X97)
The following extensions are to be added to each code from category X96:
  a   initial encounter
  d   subsequent encounter
  q   sequelae

X96.0   Assault by antipersonnel bomb
            Excludes1:   antipersonnel bomb use in military or war (Y36.2, Y37.2)
X96.1   Assault by gasoline bomb
X96.2   Assault by letter bomb
X96.3   Assault by fertilizer bomb
X96.3   Assault by pipe bomb
X96.8   Assault by other specified explosive
X96.9   Assault by unspecified explosive

X97   Assault by smoke, fire and flames
Includes: assault by arson
assault by cigarettes
assault by incendiary device
The following extensions are to be added to code X97:
  a   initial encounter
  d   subsequent encounter
  q   sequelae

X98   Assault by steam, hot vapors and hot objects
The following extensions are to be added to each code from category X98:
  a   initial encounter
  d   subsequent encounter
  q   sequelae

X98.0   Assault by steam or hot vapors
X98.1   Assault by hot tap water
X98.2   Assault by hot fluids

X98.3   **Assault by hot household appliances**
X98.8   **Assault by other hot objects**
X98.9   **Assault by unspecifed hot objects**

X99   Assault by sharp object
    Excludes1:   assault by strike by sports equipment (Y08.0)
    The following extensions are to be added to each code from category X99:
      a   initial encounter
      d   subsequent encounter
      q   sequelae

X99.0   **Assault by sharp glass**
X99.1   **Assault by knife**
X99.2   **Assault by sword or dagger**
X99.8   **Assault by other sharp object**
X99.9   **Assault by unspecified sharp object**
     Assault by stabbing NOS

Y00   Assault by blunt object
    Excludes1:   assault by strike by sports equipment (Y08.0)
    The following extensions are to be added to code Y00:
      a   initial encounter
      d   subsequent encounter
      q   sequelae

Y01   Assault by pushing from high place
    The following extensions are to be added to code Y01:
      a   initial encounter
      d   subsequent encounter
      q   sequelae

Y02   Assault by pushing or placing victim before moving object
    Excludes1:   assault by pushing victim in front of motor vehicle (Y03.1)
    The following extensions are to be added to code Y02:
      a   initial encounter
      d   subsequent encounter
      q   sequelae

Y03   Assault by crashing of motor vehicle
    The following extensions are to be added to each code from category Y03:
      a   initial encounter
      d   subsequent encounter
      q   sequelae

Y03.0   **Assault by being hit or run over by motor vehicle**
Y03.1   **Assault by being pushed in front of motor vehicle**
Y03.8   **Other assault by crashing of motor vehicle**
Y03.9   **Assault by crashing of motor vehicle, unspecified**

Y04   Assault by bodily force
    Excludes1:   assault by:
       strangulation (X91.-)
       submersion (X92.-)
       use of weapon (X93-X95, X99, Y00)
       sexual assault (Y05.-)
    The following extensions are to be added to each code from category Y04:
      a   initial encounter
      d   subsequent encounter
      q   sequelae

Y04.0   **Assault by unarmed brawl or fight**
Y04.1   **Assault by human bite**
Y04.2   **Assault by strike against or bumped into by another person**
Y04.8   **Assault by other bodily force**
     Assault by bodily force NOS

Y05   Sexual assault
    Includes: rape (attempted)
          sodomy (attempted)
    Excludes1:   adult sexual abuse (T74.21)
          child sexual abuse (T74.22)
    The following extensions are to be added to each code from category Y05:
      a   initial encounter
      d   subsequent encounter
      q   sequelae

*Y06 deactivated. See T74.0, T76.0

Y07   Perpetrator of maltreatment and neglect
    Note: codes from this category are for use only in cases of confirmed abuse (T74.-)
    Selection of the correct perpetrator code is based on the relationship between the perpetrator and the victim
    Includes: perpetrator of abandonment
          perpetrator of emotional neglect
          perpetrator of mental cruelty
          perpetrator of physical abuse
          perpetrator of physical neglect
          perpetrator of sexual abuse
          perpetrator of torture

Y07.0   **Spouse or partner as perpetrator of maltreatment and neglect**
     Spouse or partner as perpetrator of maltreatment and neglect against spouse or partner
Y07.01   **Husband as perpetrator of maltreatment and neglect**
Y07.02   **Wife as perpetrator of maltreatment and neglect**
Y07.03   **Male partner as perpetrator of maltreatment and neglect**
Y07.04   **Female partner as perpetrator of maltreatment and neglect**
Y07.1   **Parent (adoptive) (biological) as perpetrator of maltreatment and neglect**
Y07.11   **Biological father as perpetrator of maltreatment and neglect**
Y07.12   **Biological mother as perpetrator of maltreatment and neglect**
Y07.13   **Adoptive father as perpetrator of maltreatment and neglect**
Y07.14   **Adoptive mother as perpetrator of maltreatment and neglect**
Y07.4   **Other family member as perpetrator of maltreatment and neglect**
Y07.41   **Sibling**
Y07.410   **Brother as perpetrator of maltreatment and neglect**
Y07.411   **Sister as perpetrator of maltreatment and neglect**
Y07.42   **Foster parent**
Y07.420   **Foster father as perpetrator of maltreatment and neglect**
Y07.421   **Foster mother as perpetrator of maltreatment and neglect**
Y07.43   **Stepparent or stepsibling as perpetrator of maltreatment and neglect**
Y07.430   **Stepfather as perpetrator of maltreatment and neglect**
Y07.432   **Male friend of parent (co-residing in household) as perpetratory of maltreatment and neglect**
Y07.433   **Stepmother as perpetrator of maltreatment and neglect**
Y07.434   **Female friend of parent (co-residing in household) as perpetratory of maltreatment and neglect**
Y07.435   **Stepbrother as perpetrator or maltreatment and neglect**
Y07.436   **Stepsister as perpetrator of maltreatment and neglect**

Y07.49 Other family member

Y07.490 Male cousin as perpetrator of maltreatment and neglect

Y07.491 Female cousin as perpetrator of maltreatment and neglect

Y07.499 Other family member as perpetrator of maltreatment and neglect

Y07.5 Non-family member

Y07.50 Unspecified non-family member as perpetrator of maltreatment and neglect

Y07.51 Daycare provider

Y07.510 At-home childcare provider as perpetrator of maltreatment and neglect

Y07.511 Daycare center childcare provider as perpetrator of maltreatment and neglect

Y07.512 At-home adultcare provider as perpetrator of maltreatment and neglect

Y07.513 Adultcare center provider as perpetrator of maltreatment and neglect

Y07.519 Unspecified daycare provider as perpetrator of maltreatment and neglect

Y07.52 Healthcare provider

Y07.521 Mental health provider as perpetrator of maltreatment and neglect

Y07.528 Other therapist or healthcare provider as perpetrator of maltreatment and neglect
Nurse
Occupational therapist
Physical therapist
Speech therapist

V07.529 Unspecified healthcare provider as perpetrator of maltreatment and neglect

Y07.53 Teacher or instructor as perpetrator of maltreatment and neglect
Coach as perpetrator of maltreatment and neglect

Y07.59 Other non-family member as perpetrator of maltreatment and neglect

Y08 Assault by other specified means
The following extensions are to be added to each code from category Y08:
a   initial encounter
d   subsequent encounter
q   sequelae

Y08.0 Assault by strike by sport equipment

Y08.01 Assault by strike by hockey stick

Y08.02 Assault by strike by baseball bat

Y08.09 Assault by strike other sport equipment

Y08.8 Assault by other specified means

Y08.81 Assault by crashing of aircraft

Y08.89 Assault by other specified means

EVENT OF UNDETERMINED INTENT (Y20–Y33)
Note: This section covers events where available information is insufficient to enable a medical or legal authority to make a distinction between accident, self-harm or assault

*Y10-Y19 deactivated. See codes T36-T65 with extension 4

*Y20 deactivated. See T71

Y21 Drowning and submersion, undetermined intent
The following extensions are to be added to each code from category Y21:
a   initial encounter
d   subsequent encounter
q   sequelae

Y21.0 Drowning and submersion while in bathtub, undetermined intent

Y21.1 Drowning and submersion after fall into bathtub, undetermined intent

Y21.2 Drowning and submersion while in swimming pool, undetermined intent

Y21.3 Drowning and submersion after fall into swimming pool, undetermined intent

Y21.4 Drowning and submersion in natural water, undetermined intent

Y21.8 Other drowning and submersion, undetermined intent

Y21.9 Unspecified drowning and submersion, undetermined intent

Y22 Handgun discharge, undetermined intent
Includes: discharge of gun for single hand use, undetermined intent
discharge of pistol, undetermined intent
discharge of revolver, undetermined intent
Excludes: Very pistol (Y24.8)
The following extensions are to be added to code Y22:
a   initial encounter
d   subsequent encounter
q   sequelae

Y23 Rifle, shotgun and larger firearm discharge, undetermined intent
Excludes: airgun (Y24.0)
The following extensions are to be added to each code from category Y23:
a   initial encounter
d   subsequent encounter
q   sequelae

Y23.0 Shotgun discharge, undetermined intent

Y23.1 Hunting rifle discharge, undetermined intent

Y23.2 Military firearm discharge, undetermined intent

Y23.3 Machine gun discharge, undetermined intent

Y23.8 Other larger firearm discharge, undetermined intent

Y23.9 Unspecified larger firearm discharge, undetermined intent

Y24 Other and unspecified firearm discharge, undetermined intent
The following extensions are to be added to each code from category Y24:
a   initial encounter
d   subsequent encounter
q   sequelae

Y24.0 Airgun discharge, undetermined intent
BB gun discharge, undetermined intent
Pellet gun discharge, undetermined intent

Y24.8 Other firearm discharge, undetermined intent
Very pistol [flare] discharge, undetermined intent

Y24.9 Unspecified firearm discharge, undetermined intent

Y25 Contact with explosive material, undetermined intent
The following extensions are to be added to codeY25:
a   initial encounter
d   subsequent encounter
q   sequelae

Y26 Exposure to smoke, fire and flames, undetermined intent
The following extensions are to be added to code Y26:
a   initial encounter
d   subsequent encounter
q   sequelae

Y27 Contact with steam, hot vapors and hot objects, undetermined intent
The following extensions are to be added to each code from category Y27:
a   initial encounter
d   subsequent encounter
q   sequelae

Y27.0 Contact with steam and hot vapors, undetermined intent

Y27.1 Contact with hot tap water, undetermined intent

Y27.2 Contact with hot fluids, undetermined intent

Y27.3 Contact with hot household appliance, undetermined intent

Y27.8 Contact with other hot objects, undetermined intent

Y27.9 Contact with unspecified hot objects, undetermined intent

Y28 Contact with sharp object, undetermined intent
> The following extensions are to be added to each code from category
> Y28:
>> a   initial encounter
>> d   subsequent encounter
>> q   sequelae

  Y28.0 Contact with sharp glass, undetermined intent

  Y28.1 Contact with knife, undetermined intent

  Y28.2 Contact with sword or dagger, undetermined intent

  Y28.8 Contact with other sharp object, undetermined intent

  Y28.9 Contact with unspecified sharp object, undetermined intent

Y29 Contact with blunt object, undetermined intent
> The following extensions are to be added to code Y29:
>> a   initial encounter
>> d   subsequent encounter
>> q   sequelae

Y30 Falling, jumping or pushed from a high place, undetermined intent
> Includes: victim falling from one level to another, undetermined
>   intent
> The following extensions are to be added to codeY30:
>> a   initial encounter
>> d   subsequent encounter
>> q   sequelae

Y31 Falling, lying or running before or into moving object, undetermined intent
> The following extensions are to be added to code Y31:
>> a   initial encounter
>> d   subsequent encounter
>> q   sequelae

Y32 Crashing of motor vehicle, undetermined intent
> The following extensions are to be added to code Y32:
>> a   initial encounter
>> d   subsequent encounter
>> q   sequelae

Y33 Other specified events, undetermined intent
> The following extensions are to be added to code Y33:
>> a   initial encounter
>> d   subsequent encounter
>> q   sequelae

LEGAL INTERVENTION, OPERATIONS OF WAR, MILITARY OPERATIONS, AND TERRORISM (Y35–Y38)

Y35 Legal intervention
> Includes: any injury sustained as a result of an encounter with
>   any law enforcement official, serving in any
>   capacity at the time of the encounter, whether
>   on-duty or off-duty. Includes injury to law
>   enforcement official, suspect and bystander
> The following extensions are to be added to each code from category
> Y35:
>> a   initial encounter
>> d   subsequent encounter
>> q   sequelae

  Y35.0 Legal intervention involving firearm discharge

    Y35.00 Legal intervention involving unspecified firearm discharge
> Legal intervention involving gunshot wound
> Legal intervention involving shot NOS

      Y35.001 Legal intervention involving unspecified firearm discharge, suspect injured

      Y35.002 Legal intervention involving unspecified firearm discharge, law enforcement official injured

      Y35.003 Legal intervention involving unspecified firearm discharge, bystander injured

      Y35.004 Legal intervention involving unspecified firearm discharge, unspecified person injured

    Y35.01 Legal intervention involving injury by machine gun

      Y35.011 Legal intervention involving injury by machine gun, suspect injured

      Y35.012 Legal intervention involving injury by machine gun, law enforcement official injured

      Y35.013 Legal intervention involving injury by machine gun, bystander injured

      Y35.014 Legal intervention involving injury by machine gun, unspecified person injured

    Y35.02 Legal intervention involving injury by handgun

      Y35.021 Legal intervention involving injury by handgun, suspect injured

      Y35.022 Legal intervention involving injury by handgun, law enforcement official injured

      Y35.023 Legal intervention involving injury by handgun, bystander injured

      Y35.024 Legal intervention involving injury by handgun, unspecified person injured

    Y35.03 Legal intervention involving injury by rifle pellet

      Y35.031 Legal intervention involving injury by rifle pellet, suspect injured

      Y35.032 Legal intervention involving injury by rifle pellet, law enforcement official injured

      Y35.033 Legal intervention involving injury by rifle pellet, bystander injured

      Y35.034 Legal intervention involving injury by rifle pellet, unspecified person injured

    Y35.04 Legal intervention involving injury by rubber bullet

      Y35.041 Legal intervention involving injury by rubber bullet, suspect injured

      Y35.042 Legal intervention involving injury by rubber bullet, law enforcement official injured

      Y35.043 Legal intervention involving injury by rubber bullet, bystander injured

      Y35.044 Legal intervention involving injury by rubber bullet, unspecified person injured

    Y35.09 Legal intervention involving other firearm discharge

      Y35.091 Legal intervention involving other firearm discharge, suspect injured

      Y35.092 Legal intervention involving other firearm discharge, law enforcement official injured

      Y35.093 Legal intervention involving other firearm discharge, bystander injured

      Y35.094 Legal intervention involving other firearm discharge, unspecified person injured

  Y35.1 Legal intervention involving explosives

    Y35.10 Legal intervention involving unspecified explosives

      Y35.101 Legal intervention involving unspecified explosives, suspect injured

      Y35.102 Legal intervention involving unspecified explosives, law enforcement official injured

      Y35.103 Legal intervention involving unspecified explosives, bystander injured

      Y35.104 Legal intervention involving unspecified explosives, unspecified person injured

    Y35.11 Legal intervention involving injury by dynamite

      Y35.111 Legal intervention involving injury by dynamite, suspect injured

      Y35.112 Legal intervention involving injury by dynamite, law enforcement official injured

      Y35.113 Legal intervention involving injury by dynamite, bystander injured

      Y35.114 Legal intervention involving injury by dynamite, unspecified person injured

    Y35.12 Legal intervention involving injury by explosive shell

      Y35.121 Legal intervention involving injury by explosive shell, suspect injured

      Y35.122 Legal intervention involving injury by explosive shell, law enforcement official injured

Y35.123   Legal intervention involving injury by explosive shell, bystander injured

Y35.124   Legal intervention involving injury by explosive shell, unspecified person injured

Y35.19   Legal intervention involving other explosives
Legal intervention involving injury by grenade
Legal intervention involving injury by mortar bomb

Y35.191   Legal intervention involving other explosives, suspect injured

Y35.192   Legal intervention involving other explosives, law enforcement official injured

Y35.193   Legal intervention involving other explosives, bystander injured

Y35.194   Legal intervention involving other explosives, unspecified person injured

Y35.2   Legal intervention involving gas
Legal intervention involving asphyxiation by gas
Legal intervention involving poisoning by gas

Y35.20   Legal intervention involving unspecified gas

Y35.201   Legal intervention involving unspecified gas, suspect injured

Y35.202   Legal intervention involving unspecified gas, law enforcement official injured

Y35.203   Legal intervention involving unspecified gas, bystander injured

Y35.204   Legal intervention involving unspecified gas, unspecified person injured

Y35.21   Legal intervention involving injury by tear gas

Y35.211   Legal intervention involving injury by tear gas, suspect injured

Y35.212   Legal intervention involving injury by tear gas, law enforcement official injured

Y35.213   Legal intervention involving injury by tear gas, bystander injured

Y35.214   Legal intervention involving injury by tear gas, unspecified person injured

Y35.29   Legal intervention involving other gas

Y35.291   Legal intervention involving other gas, suspect injured

Y35.292   Legal intervention involving other gas, law enforcement official injured

Y35.293   Legal intervention involving other gas, bystander injured

Y35.294   Legal intervention involving other gas, unspecified person injured

Y35.3   Legal intervention involving blunt objects

Y35.30   Legal intervention involving unspecified blunt objects

Y35.301   Legal intervention involving unspecified blunt objects, suspect injured

Y35.302   Legal intervention involving unspecified blunt objects, law enforcement official injured

Y35.303   Legal intervention involving unspecified blunt objects, bystander injured

Y35.304   Legal intervention involving unspecified blunt objects, unspecified person injured

Y35.31   Legal intervention involving being hit or struck by baton

Y35.311   Legal intervention involving being hit or struck by baton, suspect injured

Y35.312   Legal intervention involving being hit or struck by baton, law enforcement official injured

Y35.313   Legal intervention involving being hit or struck by baton, bystander injured

Y35.314   Legal intervention involving being hit or struck by baton, unspecified person injured

Y35.39   Legal intervention involving other blunt objects
Legal intervention involving being hit or struck by blunt object
Legal intervention involving being hit or struck by stave

Y35.391   Legal intervention involving other blunt objects, suspect injured

Y35.392   Legal intervention involving other blunt objects, law enforcement official injured

Y35.393   Legal intervention involving other blunt objects, bystander injured

Y35.394   Legal intervention involving other blunt objects, unspecified person injured

Y35.4   Legal intervention involving sharp objects
Legal intervention involving being cut by sharp objects
Legal intervention involving being stabbed by sharp objects

Y35.40   Legal intervention involving unspecified sharp objects

Y35.401   Legal intervention involving unspecified sharp objects, suspect injured

Y35.402   Legal intervention involving unspecified sharp objects, law enforcement official injured

Y35.403   Legal intervention involving unspecified sharp objects, bystander injured

Y35.404   Legal intervention involving unspecified sharp objects, unspecified person injured

Y35.41   Legal intervention involving bayonet

Y35.411   Legal intervention involving bayonet, suspect injured

Y35.412   Legal intervention involving bayonet, law enforcement official injured

Y35.413   Legal intervention involving bayonet, bystander injured

Y35.414   Legal intervention involving bayonet, unspecified person injured

Y35.49   Legal intervention involving other sharp objects

Y35.491   Legal intervention involving other sharp objects, suspect injured

Y35.492   Legal intervention involving other sharp objects, law enforcement official injured

Y35.493   Legal intervention involving other sharp objects, bystander injured

Y35.494   Legal intervention involving other sharp objects, unspecified person injured

Y35.8   Legal intervention involving other specified means

Y35.81   Legal intervention involving manhandling

Y35.811   Legal intervention involving manhandling, suspect injured

Y35.812   Legal intervention involving manhandling, law enforcement official injured

Y35.813   Legal intervention involving manhandling, bystander injured

Y35.814   Legal intervention involving manhandling, unspecified person injured

Y35.89   Legal intervention involving other specified means

Y35.890   Legal intervention involving other specified means, suspect injured

Y35.891   Legal intervention involving other specified means, law enforcement official injured

Y35.892   Legal intervention involving other specified means, bystander injured

Y35.894   Legal intervention involving other specified means, unspecified person injured

Y35.9   Legal intervention, means unspecified

Y35.91   Legal intervention, means unspecified, suspect injured

Y35.92   Legal intervention, means unspecified, law enforcement official injured

Y35.93   Legal intervention, means unspecified, bystander injured

Y35.99   Legal intervention, means unspecified, unspecified person injured

Y36 Operations of war

Includes: injuries to military personnel and civilians caused by
             war and civil insurrection

Excludes1:   injury to military personnel occuring during peacetime
             military operations (Y37.-)
             military vehicles involved in transport accidents with
             non-military vehicle during peacetime (V09.01,
             V09.21, V19.81, V29.81, V39.81, V49.81, V59.81,
             V69.81, V79.81)

The following extensions are for use with codes from category Y36:

1   military personnel injury due to enemy fire, initial
    encounter
2   military personnel injury due to friendly fire, initial
    encounter
3   civilian injury due to enemy fire, initial encounter
4   civilian injury due to friendly fire, initial encounter
5   military personnel injury, subsequent encounter
6   civilian injury, subsequent encounter
7   military personnel injury, sequelae
8   civilian injury, sequelae

Y36.0 War operations involving explosion of marine weapons and military watercraft

War operations involving explosion of depth-charge
War operations involving explosion of marine mine
War operations involving explosion of mine NOS, at sea or in harbor
War operations involving explosion of sea-based artillery shell
War operations involving explosion of torpedo
War operations involving underwater blast

Y36.1 War operations involving aircraft

Y36.11 War operations involving helicopter

Y36.110 Crushed by falling helicopter during war operations
Y36.111 Fire on helicopter during war operations
Y36.112 Explosion on helicopter during war operations
Y36.113 Helicopter shot down during war operations
Y36.118 War operations involving other destruction of helicopter

Y36.12 War operations involving fixed-wing powered aircraft

Y36.120 Crushed by falling fixed-wing powered aircraft during war operations
Y36.121 Fire on fixed-wing powered aircraft during war operations
Y36.122 Explosion on fixed-wing powered aircraft during war operations
Y36.123 Fixed-wing powered aircraft shot down during war operations
Y36.128 War operations involving other destruction of fixed-wing powered aircraft

Y36.13 War operations involving ultra-light or micro-light aircraft

Y36.130 Crushed by falling ultra-light or micro-light aircraft during war operations
Y36.131 Fire on ultra-light or micro-light aircraft during war operations
Y36.132 Explosion on ultra-light or micro-light aircraft during war operations
Y36.133 Ultra-light or micro-light aircraft shot down during war operations
Y36.138 War operations involving other destruction of ultra-light or micro-light aircraft

Y36.19 War operations involving destruction of other aircraft

Y36.190 Crushed by other aircraft falling during war operations
Y36.191 Fire on other aircraft during war operations
Y36.192 Explosion on other aircraft during war operations
Y36.193 Other aircraft shot down during war operations
Y36.198 War operations involving other destruction of other aircraft

Y36.2 War operations involving other explosions and fragments

War operations involving accidental explosion of munitions being used in war
War operations involving accidental explosion of own weapons
War operations involving accidental explosion of antipersonnel bomb (fragments)
War operations involving blast NOS
War operations involving explosion from mine NOS
War operations involving explosion NOS
War operations involving explosion of artillery shell
War operations involving explosion of breech-block
War operations involving explosion of cannon block
War operations involving explosion of mortar bomb
War operations involving fragments from artillery shell
War operations involving fragments from bomb
War operations involving fragments from grenade
War operations involving fragments from guided missile
War operations involving fragments from land-mine
War operations involving fragments from rocket
War operations involving fragments from shell
War operations involving fragments from shrapnel

Y36.3 War operations involving fires, conflagrations and hot substances

Y36.31 Fire due to conventional weapon during war operations
Y36.32 Fire due to fire-producing device during war operations
Y36.33 Heat due to conventional weapon during war operations
Y36.34 Heat due to fire-producing device during war operations
Y36.35 Other cause of injury due to fire, conflagrations and hot substances during war operations

Y36.4 War operations involving firearm discharge and other forms of conventional warfare

Drowned in war operations NOS
War operations involving battle wounds
War operations involving bayonet injury
War operations involving carbine bullet
War operations involving machine gun bullet
War operations involving pellets (shotgun)
War operations involving pistol bullet
War operations involving rifle bullet
War operations involving rubber (rifle) bullet

Y36.5 War operations involving nuclear weapons

Y36.51 Direct effects of nuclear weapons during war operations

Y36.510 Blast effects from nuclear weapons during war operations
Y36.511 Exposure to immediate ionizing radiation from nuclear weapon during war operations
Y36.512 Fireball effects from nuclear weapons during war operations
Y36.513 Direct heat from nuclear weapons explosion during war operations
Y36.518 Other direct effects of nuclear weapons during war operations

Y36.52 Secondary effects of nuclear weapons during war operations

Y36.520 Blast wave from nuclear weapons during war operations
Y36.521 Fire following nuclear explosion during war operations
Y36.528 Other secondary effects of nuclear weapons during war operations

Y36.53 Sequelae of nuclear weapons (during) (following) war operations

Y36.530 Exposure to residual radiation from nuclear weapons
Y36.531 Ingestion of radioactive products from nuclear weapons
Y36.532 Inhalation of radioactive products from nuclear weapons

Y36.538   Other sequelae of nuclear weapons (during) (following) war operations

Y36.6   War operations involving biological weapons

Y36.7   War operations involving chemical weapons and other forms of unconventional warfare

Excludes2:   war operations involving incendiary devices (Y36.3-, Y36.5-)
war operations involving gases, fumes and chemicals
war operations involving lasers

Y36.9   War operations, unspecified

Y37   Military operations

Includes: injuries to military personnel and civilians occuring during peacetime on military property and during routine military operations

Excludes1:   military aircraft involved in aircraft accident with civilian aircraft
military vehicles involved in transport accident with civilian vehicle (V09.01, V09.21, V19.81, V29.81, V39.81, V49.81, V59.81, V69.81, V79.81)
military watercraft involved in water transport accident with civilian watercraft
war operations (Y36.-)

The following extensions are for use with codes from category Y37:
1   military personnel injury due to enemy fire, initial encounter
2   military personnel injury due to friendly fire, initial encounter
3   civilian injury due to enemy fire, initial encounter
4   civilian injury due to friendly fire, initial encounter
5   military personnel injury, subsequent encounter
6   civilian injury, subsequent encounter
7   military personnel injury, sequelae
8   civilian injury, sequelae

Y37.0   Military operations involving explosion of marine weapons and military watercraft
Military operations involving explosion of depth-charge
Military operations involving explosion of marine mine
Military operations involving explosion of mine NOS, at sea or in harbor
Military operations involving explosion of sea-based artillery shell
Military operations involving explosion of torpedo
Military operations involving underwater blast

Y37.1   Military operations involving of aircraft
Crushed by falling aircraft
Military operations involving burned aircraft
Military operations involving exploded aircraft
Military operations involving shot down aircraft

Y37.2   Military operations involving other explosions and fragments
Military operations involving accidental explosion of munitions being used in peacetime
Military operations involving accidental explosion of own weapons
Military operations involving accidental explosion of antipersonnel bomb (fragments)
Military operations involving blast NOS
Military operations involving explosion from mine NOS
Military operations involving explosion
Military operations involving explosion of artillery shell NOS
Military operations involving explosion of breech-block
Military operations involving explosion of cannon block
Military operations involving explosion of mortar bomb
Military operations involving fragments from artillery shell
Military operations involving fragments from bomb
Military operations involving fragments from grenade
Military operations involving fragments from guided missile
Military operations involving fragments from land-mine
Military operations involving fragments from rocket
Military operations involving fragments from shell
Military operations involving fragments from shrapnel

Y37.3   Military operations involving fires, conflagrations and hot substances
Military operations involving asphyxia originating from fire or conventional weapon
Military operations involving burns originating from fire or conventional weapon
Military operations involving other injury originating from fire or conventional weapon
Military operations involving petrol bomb originating from fire or conventional weapon

Y37.4   Military operations involving firearm discharge and other forms of conventional warfare
Drowned in military operations NOS
Military operations involving battle wounds
Military operations involving bayonet injury
Military operations involving carbine bullet
Military operations involving machine gun bullet
Military operations involving pellets (shotgun)
Military operations involving pistol bullet
Military operations involving rifle bullet
Military operations involving rubber (rifle) bullet

Y37.5   Military operations involving nuclear weapons
Military operations involving blast effects from nuclear weapons
Military operations involving exposure to ionizing radiation from nuclear weapon
Military operations involving fireball effects from nuclear weapons
Military operations involving heat from nuclear weapons
Military operations involving other direct and secondary effects of nuclear weapons

Y37.6   Military operations involving biological weapons

Y37.7   Military operations involving chemical weapons and other forms of unconventional warfare
Military operations involving gases, fumes and chemicals
Military operations involving lasers

Y37.8   Other military operations
Injuries by explosion of bombs or mines placed in the course of war, if the explosion occurred after cessation of hostilities

Y37.9   Military operations, unspecified

Y38   Terrorism
Use additional code for place of occurrence (Y93.81)
The following extensions are for use with codes from category Y38:
1   public safety official, initial encounter
3   civilian, initial encounter
5   public safety official, subsequent encounter
6   civilian, subsequent encounter
7   public safety official, sequelae
8   civilian, sequelae

Y38.0   Terrorism involving explosion of marine weapons

Y38.1   Terrorism involving destruction of aircraft

Y38.2   Terrorism involving other explosions and fragments

Y38.3   Terrorism involving fires, conflagration and hot substances

Y38.4   Terrorism involving firearms

Y38.5   Terrorism involving nuclear weapons

Y38.6   Terrorism involving biological weapons

Y38.7   Terrorism involving chemical weapons

Y38.8   Terrorism involving other means

Y38.9   Terrorism, unspecified means

COMPLICATIONS OF MEDICAL AND SURGICAL CARE (Y62–Y84)

*Categories Y40-Y59 have been deactivated. (See T36-T50 with final character 5)

Includes: complications of medical devices
correct drug properly administered in therapeutic or prophylactic dosage as the cause of any adverse effect
misadventures to patients during surgical and medical care
surgical and medical procedures as the cause of abnormal reaction of the patient, or of later complication, without mention of misadventure at the time of the procedure

MISADVENTURES TO PATIENTS DURING SURGICAL AND MEDICAL CARE (Y62–Y69)

Excludes2:   medical devices associated with adverse incidents in diagnostic and therapeutic use (Y70-Y82)
surgical and medical procedures as the cause of abnormal reaction of the patient, without mention of misadventure at the time of the procedure (Y83-Y84)

*Y60 deactivated. See complications within body system chapters

*Y61 deactivated. See T81.5

Y62 Failure of sterile precautions during surgical and medical care
  Y62.0 Failure of sterile precautions during surgical operation
  Y62.1 Failure of sterile precautions during infusion or transfusion
  Y62.2 Failure of sterile precautions during kidney dialysis and other perfusion
  Y62.3 Failure of sterile precautions during injection or immunization
  Y62.4 Failure of sterile precautions during endoscopic examination
  Y62.5 Failure of sterile precautions during heart catheterization
  Y62.6 Failure of sterile precautions during aspiration, puncture and other catheterization
  Y62.8 Failure of sterile precautions during other surgical and medical care
  Y62.9 Failure of sterile precautions during unspecified surgical and medical care

Y63 Failure in dosage during surgical and medical care
  Excludes2:   accidental overdose of drug or wrong drug given in error (T36-T50)
  Y63.0 Excessive amount of blood or other fluid given during transfusion or infusion
  Y63.1 Incorrect dilution of fluid used during infusion
  Y63.2 Overdose of radiation given during therapy
  Y63.3 Inadvertent exposure of patient to radiation during medical care
  Y63.4 Failure in dosage in electroshock or insulin-shock therapy
  Y63.5 Inappropriate temperature in local application and packing
  Y63.6 Nonadministration of necessary drug, medicament or biological substance
  Y63.8 Failure in dosage during other surgical and medical care
  Y63.9 Failure in dosage during unspecified surgical and medical care

Y64 Contaminated medical or biological substances
  Y64.0 Contaminated medical or biological substance, transfused or infused
  Y64.1 Contaminated medical or biological substance, injected or used for immunization
  Y64.8 Contaminated medical or biological substance administered by other means
  Y64.9 Contaminated medical or biological substance administered by unspecified means
     Administered contaminated medical or biological substance NOS

Y65 Other misadventures during surgical and medical care
  Y65.0 Mismatched blood in transfusion
  Y65.1 Wrong fluid used in infusion
  Y65.2 Failure in suture or ligature during surgical operation
  Y65.3 Endotracheal tube wrongly placed during anesthetic procedure
  Y65.4 Failure to introduce or to remove other tube or instrument
  Y65.5 Performance of inappropriate operation
  Y65.8 Other specified misadventures during surgical and medical care

Y66 Nonadministration of surgical and medical care
  Includes: premature cessation of surgical and medical care
  Excludes1:   DNR status (Z66)
     palliative care (Z51.5)

Y69 Unspecified misadventure during surgical and medical care

MEDICAL DEVICES ASSOCIATED WITH ADVERSE INCIDENTS IN DIAGNOSTIC AND THERAPEUTIC USE (Y70–Y82)

Y70 Anesthesiology devices associated with adverse incidents
  Y70.0 Diagnostic and monitoring anesthesiology devices associated with adverse incidents
  Y70.1 Therapeutic (nonsurgical) and rehabilitative anesthesiology devices associated with adverse incidents
  Y70.2 Prosthetic and other implants, materials and accessory anesthesiology devices associated with adverse incidents
  Y70.3 Surgical instruments, materials and anesthesiology devices (including sutures) associated with adverse incidents
  Y70.8 Miscellaneous anesthesiology devices associated with adverse incidents, not elsewhere classified

Y71 Cardiovascular devices associated with adverse incidents
  Y71.0 Diagnostic and monitoring cardiovascular devices associated with adverse incidents
  Y71.1 Therapeutic (nonsurgical) and rehabilitative cardiovascular devices associated with adverse incidents
  Y71.2 Prosthetic and other implants, materials and accessory cardiovascular devices associated with adverse incidents
  Y71.3 Surgical instruments, materials and cardiovascular devices (including sutures) associated with adverse incidents
  Y71.8 Miscellaneous cardiovascular devices associated with adverse incidents, not elsewhere classified

Y72 Otorhinolaryngological devices associated with adverse incidents
  Y72.0 Diagnostic and monitoring otorhinolaryngological devices associated with adverse incidents
  Y72.1 Therapeutic (nonsurgical) and rehabilitative otorhinolaryngological devices associated with adverse incidents
  Y72.2 Prosthetic and other implants, materials and accessory otorhinolaryngological devices associated with adverse incidents
  Y72.3 Surgical instruments, materials and otorhinolaryngological devices (including sutures) associated with adverse incidents
  Y72.8 Miscellaneous otorhinolaryngological devices associated with adverse incidents, not elsewhere classified

Y73 Gastroenterology and urology devices associated with adverse incidents
  Y73.0 Diagnostic and monitoring gastroenterology and urology devices associated with adverse incidents
  Y73.1 Therapeutic (nonsurgical) and rehabilitative gastroenterology and urology devices associated with adverse incidents
  Y73.2 Prosthetic and other implants, materials and accessory gastroenterology and urology devices associated with adverse incidents
  Y73.3 Surgical instruments, materials and gastroenterology and urology devices (including sutures) associated with adverse incidents
  Y73.8 Miscellaneous gastroenterology and urology devices associated with adverse incidents, not elsewhere classified

Y74 General hospital and personal-use devices associated with adverse incidents

Y74.0 Diagnostic and monitoring general hospital and personal-use devices

Y74.1 Therapeutic (nonsurgical) and rehabilitative general hospital and personal-use devices associated with adverse incidents

Y74.2 Prosthetic and other implants, materials and accessory general hospital and personal-use devices associated with adverse incidents

Y74.3 Surgical instruments, materials and general hospital and personal-use devices (including sutures) associated with adverse incidents

Y74.8 Miscellaneous general hospital and personal-use devices associated with adverse incidents, not elsewhere classified

Y75 Neurological devices associated with adverse incidents associated with adverse incidents

Y75.0 Diagnostic and monitoring neurological devices associated with adverse incidents

Y75.1 Therapeutic (nonsurgical) and rehabilitative neurological devices associated with adverse incidents

Y75.2 Prosthetic and other implants, materials and neurological devices associated with adverse incidents

Y75.3 Surgical instruments, materials and neurological devices (including sutures) associated with adverse incidents

Y75.8 Miscellaneous neurological devices associated with adverse incidents, not elsewhere classified

Y76 Obstetric and gynecological devices associated with adverse incidents

Y76.0 Diagnostic and monitoring obstetric and gynecological devices associated with adverse incidents

Y76.1 Therapeutic (nonsurgical) and rehabilitative obstetric and gynecological devices associated with adverse incidents

Y76.2 Prosthetic and other implants, materials and accessory obstetric and gynecological devices associated with adverse incidents

Y76.3 Surgical instruments, materials and obstetric and gynecological devices (including sutures) associated with adverse incidents

Y76.8 Miscellaneous obstetric and gynecological devices associated with adverse incidents, not elsewhere classified

Y77 Ophthalmic devices associated with adverse incidents

Y77.0 Diagnostic and monitoring ophthalmic devices associated with adverse incidents

Y77.1 Therapeutic (nonsurgical) and rehabilitative ophthalmic devices associated with adverse incidents

Y77.2 Prosthetic and other implants, materials and accessory ophthalmic devices associated with adverse incidents

Y77.3 Surgical instruments, materials and ophthalmic devices (including sutures) associated with adverse incidents

Y77.8 Miscellaneous ophthalmic devices associated with adverse incidents, not elsewhere classified

Y78 Radiological devices associated with adverse incidents

Y78.0 Diagnostic and monitoring radiological devices associated with adverse incidents

Y78.1 Therapeutic (nonsurgical) and rehabilitative radiological devices associated with adverse incidents

Y78.2 Prosthetic and other implants, materials and accessory radiological devices associated with adverse incidents

Y78.3 Surgical instruments, materials and radiological devices (including sutures) associated with adverse incidents

Y78.8 Miscellaneous radiological devices associated with adverse incidents, not elsewhere classified

Y79 Orthopedic devices associated with adverse incidents

Y79.0 Diagnostic and monitoring orthopedic devices associated with adverse incidents

Y79.1 Therapeutic (nonsurgical) and rehabilitative orthopedic devices associated with adverse incidents

Y79.2 Prosthetic and other implants, materials and accessory orthopedic devices associated with adverse incidents

Y79.3 Surgical instruments, materials and orthopedic devices (including sutures) associated with adverse incidents

Y79.8 Miscellaneous orthopedic devices associated with adverse incidents, not elsewhere classified

Y80 Physical medicine devices associated with adverse incidents

Y80.0 Diagnostic and monitoring physical medicine devices associated with adverse incidents

Y80.1 Therapeutic (nonsurgical) and rehabilitative physical medicine devices associated with adverse incidents

Y80.2 Prosthetic and other implants, materials and accessory physical medicine devices associated with adverse incidents

Y80.3 Surgical instruments, materials and physical medicine devices (including sutures) associated with adverse incidents

Y80.8 Miscellaneous physical medicine devices associated with adverse incidents, not elsewhere classified

Y81 General- and plastic-surgery devices associated with adverse incidents

Y81.0 Diagnostic and monitoring general- and plastic-surgery devices associated with adverse incidents

Y81.1 Therapeutic (nonsurgical) and rehabilitative general- and plastic-surgery devices associated with adverse incidents

Y81.2 Prosthetic and other implants, materials and accessory general- and plastic-surgery devices associated with adverse incidents

Y81.3 Surgical instruments, materials and general- and plastic-surgery devices (including sutures) associated with adverse incidents

Y81.8 Miscellaneous general- and plastic-surgery devices associated with adverse incidents, not elsewhere classified

Y82 Other and unspecified medical devices associated with adverse incidents

Y82.0 Other medical devices associated with adverse incidents

Y82.9 Unspecified medical devices associated with adverse incidents

SURGICAL AND OTHER MEDICAL PROCEDURES AS THE CAUSE OF ABNORMAL REACTION OF THE PATIENT, OR OF LATER COMPLICATION, WITHOUT MENTION OF MISADVENTURE AT THE TIME OF THE PROCEDURE
(Y83–Y84)

Y83 Surgical operation and other surgical procedures as the cause of abnormal reaction of the patient, or of later complication, without mention of misadventure at the time of the procedure

Y83.0 Surgical operation with transplant of whole organ as the cause of abnormal reaction of the patient, or of later complication, without mention of misadventure at the time of the procedure

Y83.1 Surgical operation with implant of artificial internal device as the cause of abnormal reaction of the patient, or of later complication, without mention of misadventure at the time of the procedure

Y83.2 Surgical operation with anastomosis, bypass or graft as the cause of abnormal reaction of the patient, or of later complication, without mention of misadventure at the time of the procedure

Y83.3 Surgical operation with formation of external stoma as the cause of abnormal reaction of the patient, or of later complication, without mention of misadventure at the time of the procedure

Y83.4 Other reconstructive surgery as the cause of abnormal reaction of the patient, or of later complication, without mention of misadventure at the time of the procedure

Y83.5 Amputation of limb(s) as the cause of abnormal reaction of the patient, or of later complication, without mention of misadventure at the time of the procedure

Y83.6 Removal of other organ (partial) (total) as the cause of abnormal reaction of the patient, or of later complication, without mention of misadventure at the time of the procedure

Y83.8 Other surgical procedures as the cause of abnormal reaction of the patient, or of later complication, without mention of misadventure at the time of the procedure

Y83.9   Surgical procedure, unspecified as the cause of abnormal reaction of the patient, or of later complication, without mention of misadventure at the time of the procedure

Y84   Other medical procedures as the cause of abnormal reaction of the patient, or of later complication, without mention of misadventure at the time of the procedure

Y84.0   Cardiac catheterization as the cause of abnormal reaction of the patient, or of later complication, without mention of misadventure at the time of the procedure

Y84.1   Kidney dialysis as the cause of abnormal reaction of the patient, or of later complication, without mention of misadventure at the time of the procedure

Y84.2   Radiological procedure and radiotherapy as the cause of abnormal reaction of the patient, or of later complication, without mention of misadventure at the time of the procedure

Y84.3   Shock therapy as the cause of abnormal reaction of the patient, or of later complication, without mention of misadventure at the time of the procedure

Y84.4   Aspiration of fluid as the cause of abnormal reaction of the patient, or of later complication, without mention of misadventure at the time of the procedure

Y84.5   Insertion of gastric or duodenal sound as the cause of abnormal reaction of the patient, or of later complication, without mention of misadventure at the time of the procedure

Y84.6   Urinary catheterization as the cause of abnormal reaction of the patient, or of later complication, without mention of misadventure at the time of the procedure

Y84.7   Blood-sampling as the cause of abnormal reaction of the patient, or of later complication, without mention of misadventure at the time of the procedure

Y84.8   Other medical procedures as the cause of abnormal reaction of the patient, or of later complication, without mention of misadventure at the time of the procedure

Y84.9   Medical procedure, unspecified as the cause of abnormal reaction of the patient, or of later complication, without mention of misadventure at the time of the procedure

*Y85-Y89 deactivated. Extension q is to be used to indicate sequlae of external cause

SUPPLEMENTARY FACTORS RELATED TO CAUSES OF MORBIDITY CLASSIFIED ELSEWHERE (Y90–Y98)

Note: These categories may be used to provide supplementary information concerning causes of morbidity. They are not to be used for single-condition coding.

Y90   Evidence of alcohol involvement determined by blood alcohol level
Code first any associated alcohol related disorders (F10)

Y90.0   Blood alcohol level of less than 20 mg/100ml

Y90.1   Blood alcohol level of 20-39 mg/100ml

Y90.2   Blood alcohol level of 40-59 mg/100ml

Y90.3   Blood alcohol level of 60-79 mg/100ml

Y90.4   Blood alcohol level of 80-99 mg/100ml

Y90.5   Blood alcohol level of 100-119 mg/100ml

Y90.6   Blood alcohol level of 120-199 mg/100ml

Y90.7   Blood alcohol level of 200-239 mg/100ml

Y90.8   Blood alcohol level of 240 mg/100ml or more

Y90.9   Presence of alcohol in blood, level not specified

*Y91 deactivated. See F10

Y92   Place of occurrence of the external cause
The following category is for use, when relevent, to identify the place of occurrence of the external cause. Use in conjunction with the activity code, if known
Place of occurrence should be recorded only at the initial encounter for treatment

Y92.0   Non-institutional (private) residence as the place of occurrence of the external cause
Excludes1:   abandoned or derelict house (Y92.89)
home under construction but not yet occupied (Y92.6-)
institutional place of residence (Y92.1-)

Y92.00   Unspecified non-institutional (private) residence as the place of occurrence of the external cause

Y92.01   Single-family non-instituional (private) house as the place of occurrence of the external cause
Farmhouse as the place of occurrence of the external cause
Excludes1:   barn (Y92.7x)
chicken coop or hen house (Y92.7x)
farm field (Y92.7x)
orchard (Y92.7x)
single family mobile home or trailer (Y92.02-)
slaughter house (Y92.7x)

Y92.010   Kitchen of single-family (private) house at the place of occurrence of the external cause

Y92.011   Dining room of single-family (private) house at the place of occurrence of the external cause

Y92.012   Bathroom of single-family (private) house at the place of occurrence of the external cause

Y92.013   Bedroom of single-family (private) house at the place of occurrence of the external cause

Y92.014   Private driveway to single-family (private) house as the place of occurrence of the external cause

Y92.015   Private garage of single-family (private) house as the place of occurrence of the external cause

Y92.016   Swimming-pool in single-family (private) house or garden as the place of occurrence of the external cause

Y92.017   Garden or yard in single-family (private) house as the place of occurrence of the external cause

Y92.018   Other place in single-family (private) house at the place of occurrence of the external cause

Y92.019   Unspecified place in single-family (private) house at the place of occurrence of the external cause

Y92.02   Mobile home as the place of occurrence of the external cause

Y92.020   Kitchen in mobile home as the place of occurrence of the external cause

Y92.021   Dining room in mobile home as the place of occurrence of the external cause

Y92.022   Bathroom in mobile home as the place of occurrence of the external cause

Y92.023   Bedroom in mobile home as the place of occurrence of the external cause

Y92.024   Driveway of mobile home as the place of occurrence of the external cause

Y92.025   Garage of mobile home as the place of occurrence of the external cause

Y92.026   Swimming-pool of mobile home as the place of occurrence of the external cause

Y92.027   Garden or yard of mobile home as the place of occurrence of the external cause

Y92.028   Other place in mobile home as the place of occurrence of the external cause

Y92.029   Unspecified place in mobile home as the place of occurrence of the external cause

Y92.03   Apartment as the place of occurrence of the external cause
Condominium as the place of occurrence of the external cause
Co-op apartment as the place of occurrence of the external cause
Excludes1:   common areas and hallways of apartment building (Y92.xx)

Y92.030   Kitchen in apartment as the place of occurrence of the external cause

Y92.031   Bathroom in apartment as the place of occurrence of the external cause

Y92.032   Bedroom in apartment as the place of occurrence of the external cause

Y92.038   Other place in apartment as the place of occurrence of the external cause

Y92.039   Unspecified place in apartment as the place of occurrence of the external cause

Y92.04   Boarding-house as the place of occurrence of the external cause

Y92.040   Kitchen in boarding-house as the place of occurrence of the external cause

Y92.041   Bathroom in boarding-house as the place of occurrence of the external cause

Y92.042   Bedroom in boarding-house as the place of occurrence of the external cause

Y92.043   Driveway of boarding-house as the place of occurrence of the external cause

Y92.044   Garage of boarding-house as the place of occurrence of the external cause

Y92.045   Swimming-pool of boarding-house as the place of occurrence of the external cause

Y92.046   Garden or yard of boarding-house as the place of occurrence of the external cause

Y92.048   Other place in boarding-house as the place of occurrence of the external cause

Y92.049   Unspecified place in boarding-house as the place of occurrence of the external cause

Y92.09   Other non-institutional residence as the place of occurrence of the external cause

Y92.090   Kitchen in other non-institutional residence as the place of occurrence of the external cause

Y92.091   Bathroom in other non-institutional residence as the place of occurrence of the external cause

Y92.092   Bedroom in other non-institutional residence as the place of occurrence of the external cause

Y92.093   Driveway of other non-institutional residence as the place of occurrence of the external cause

Y92.094   Garage of other non-institutional residence as the place of occurrence of the external cause

Y92.095   Swimming-pool of other non-institutional residence as the place of occurrence of the external cause

Y92.096   Garden or yard of other non-institutional residence as the place of occurrence of the external cause

Y92.098   Other place in other non-institutional residence as the place of occurrence of the external cause

Y92.099   Unspecified place in other non-institutional residence as the place of occurrence of the external cause

Y92.1   Institutional (nonprivate) residence as the place of occurrence of the external cause

Y92.10   Unspecified residential institution as the place of occurrence of the external cause

Y92.11   Children's home and orphanage as the place of occurrence of the external cause

Y92.110   Kitchen in children's home and orphanage as the place of occurrence of the external cause

Y92.111   Bathroom in children's home and orphanage as the place of occurrence of the external cause

Y92.112   Bedroom in children's home and orphanage as the place of occurrence of the external cause

Y92.113   Driveway of children's home and orphanage as the place of occurrence of the external cause

Y92.114   Garage of children's home and orphanage as the place of occurrence of the external cause

Y92.115   Swimming-pool of children's home and orphanage as the place of occurrence of the external cause

Y92.116   Garden or yard of children's home and orphanage as the place of occurrence of the external cause

Y92.118   Other place in children's home and orphanage as the place of occurrence of the external cause

Y92.119   Unspecified place in children's home and orphanage as the place of occurrence of the external cause

Y92.12   Nursing home as the place of occurrence of the external cause

Home for the sick as the place of occurrence of the external cause

Hospice as the place of occurrence of the external cause

Y92.120   Kitchen in nursing home as the place of occurrence of the external cause

Y92.121   Bathroom in nursing home as the place of occurrence of the external cause

Y92.122   Bedroom in nursing home as the place of occurrence of the external cause

Y92.123   Driveway of nursing home as the place of occurrence of the external cause

Y92.124   Garage of nursing home as the place of occurrence of the external cause

Y92.125   Swimming-pool of nursing home as the place of occurrence of the external cause

Y92.126   Garden or yard of nursing home as the place of occurrence of the external cause

Y92.128   Other place in nursing home as the place of occurrence of the external cause

Y92.129   Unspecified place in nursing home as the place of occurrence of the external cause

Y92.13   Military base as the place of occurrence of the external cause

Excludes1:   military training grounds (Y92.83)

Y92.130   Kitchen on military base as the place of occurrence of the external cause

Y92.131   Mess hall on military base as the place of occurrence of the external cause

Y92.133   Barracks on military base as the place of occurrence of the external cause

Y92.135   Garage on military base as the place of occurrence of the external cause

Y92.136   Swimming-pool on military base as the place of occurrence of the external cause

Y92.137   Garden or yard on military base as the place of occurrence of the external cause

Y92.138   Other place military base as the place of occurrence of the external cause

Y92.139   Unspecified place military base as the place of occurrence of the external cause

Y92.14   Prison as the place of occurrence of the external cause

Y92.140   Kitchen in prison as the place of occurrence of the external cause

Y92.141   Dining room in prison as the place of occurrence of the external cause

Y92.142   Bathroom in prison as the place of occurrence of the external cause

Y92.143   Cell of prison as the place of occurrence of the external cause

Y92.146   Swimming-pool of prison as the place of occurrence of the external cause

Y92.147   Courtyard of prison as the place of occurrence of the external cause

Y92.148   Other place in prison as the place of occurrence of the external cause

Y92.149   Unspecified place in prison as the place of occurrence of the external cause

Y92.15   Reform school as the place of occurrence of the external cause

Y92.150   Kitchen in reform school as the place of occurrence of the external cause

Y92.151   Dining room in reform school as the place of occurrence of the external cause

Y92.152   Bathroom in reform school as the place of occurrence of the external cause

Y92.153   Bedroom in reform school as the place of occurrence of the external cause

Y92.154   Driveway of reform school as the place of occurrence of the external cause

Y92.155   Garage of reform school as the place of occurrence of the external cause

Y92.156   Swimming-pool of reform school as the place of occurrence of the external cause

Y92.157   Garden or yard of reform school as the place of occurrence of the external cause

Y92.158   Other place in reform school as the place of occurrence of the external cause

Y92.159   Unspecified place in reform school as the place of occurrence of the external cause

Y92.16   School dormitory as the place of occurrence of the external cause

Excludes1:   reform school as the place of occurrence of the external cause (Y92.15-)
school buildings and grounds as the place of occurrence of the external cause (Y92.2x)
school sports and athletic areas as the place of occurrence of the external cause (Y92.3x)

Y92.160   Kitchen in school dormitory as the place of occurrence of the external cause

Y92.161   Dining room in school dormitory as the place of occurrence of the external cause

Y92.162   Bathroom in school dormitory as the place of occurrence of the external cause

Y92.163   Bedroom in school dormitory as the place of occurrence of the external cause

Y92.168   Other place in school dormitory as the place of occurrence of the external cause

Y92.169   Unspecified place in school dormitory as the place of occurrence of the external cause

Y92.19   Other specified residential institution as the place of occurrence of the external cause

Y92.190   Kitchen in other specified residential institution as the place of occurrence of the external cause

Y92.191   Dining room in other specified residential institution as the place of occurrence of the external cause

Y92.192   Bathroom in other specified residential institution as the place of occurrence of the external cause

Y92.193   Bedroom in other specified residential institution as the place of occurrence of the external cause

Y92.194   Driveway of other specified residential institution as the place of occurrence of the external cause

Y92.195   Garage of other specified residential institution as the place of occurrence of the external cause

Y92.196   Pool of other specified residential institution as the place of occurrence of the external cause

Y92.197   Garden of yard other specified residential institution as the place of occurrence of the external cause

Y92.198   Other place in other specified residential institution as the place of occurrence of the external cause

Y92.199   Unspecified place in other specified residential institution as the place of occurrence of the external cause

Y92.2   School, other institution and public administrative area as the place of occurrence of the external cause

Building and adjacent grounds used by the general public or by a particular group of the public

Excludes1:   building under construction as the place of occurrence of the external cause (Y92.6)
residential institution as the place of occurrence of the external cause (Y92.1)
school dormitory as the place of occurrence of the external cause (Y92.16-)
sports and athletics area of schools as the place of occurrence of the external cause (Y92.3x)

Y92.21   School (private) (public) (state) as the place of occurrence of the external cause

Y92.210   Daycare center as the place of occurrence of the external cause

Y92.211   Elementary school as the place of occurrence of the external cause
Kindergarden as the place of occurrence of the external cause

Y92.212   Middle school as the place of occurrence of the external cause

Y92.213   High school as the place of occurrence of the external cause

Y92.214   College as the place of occurrence of the external cause
University as the place of occurrence of the external cause

Y92.215   Trade school as the place of occurrence of the external cause

Y92.218   Other school as the place of occurrence of the external cause

Y92.219   Unspecified school as the place of occurrence of the external cause

Y92.22   Religious institution as the place of occurrence of the external cause
Church as the place of occurrence of the external cause
Mosque as the place of occurrence of the external cause
Synagogue as the place of occurrence of the external cause

Y92.23   Hospital as the place of occurrence of the external cause

Excludes1:   home for the sick as the place of occurrence of the external cause (Y92.12-)
hospice as the place of occurrence of the external cause (Y92.12-)
nursing home as the place of occurrence of the external cause (Y92.12-)

Y92.230   Patient room in hospital as the place of occurrence of the external cause

Y92.231   Patient bathroom in hospital as the place of occurrence of the external cause

Y92.232   Corridor of hospital as the place of occurrence of the external cause

Y92.233   Cafeteria of hospital as the place of occurrence of the external cause

Y92.234   Operating room of hospital as the place of occurrence of the external cause

Y92.238   Other place in hospital as the place of occurrence of the external cause

Y92.239   Unspecified place in hospital as the place of occurrence of the external cause

Y92.24   Public administrative building as the place of occurrence of the external cause

Y92.240   Courthouse as the place of occurrence of the external cause

Y92.241   Library as the place of occurrence of the external cause

Y92.242   Post office as the place of occurrence of the external cause

Y92.243 City hall as the place of occurrence of the external cause

Y92.248 Other public administrative building as the place of occurrence of the external cause

Y92.25 Cultural building as the place of occurrence of the external cause

Y92.250 Art Gallery as the place of occurrence of the external cause

Y92.251 Museum as the place of occurrence of the external cause

Y92.252 Music hall as the place of occurrence of the external cause

Y92.253 Opera house as the place of occurrence of the external cause

Y92.254 Theater (live) as the place of occurrence of the external cause

Y92.258 Other cultural public building as the place of occurrence of the external cause

Y92.26 Movie house or cinema as the place of occurrence of the external cause

Y92.29 Other specified public building as the place of occurrence of the external cause
Assembly hall as the place of occurrence of the external cause
Clubhouse as the place of occurrence of the external cause

Y92.3 Sports and athletics area as the place of occurrence of the external cause

Y92.31 Athletic court as the place of occurrence of the external cause
Excludes1: tennis court in private home or garden (Y92.09)

Y92.310 Basketball court as the place of occurrence of the external cause

Y92.311 Squash court as the place of occurrence of the external cause

Y92.312 Tennis court as the place of occurrence of the external cause

Y92.318 Other athletic court as the place of occurrence of the external cause

Y92.32 Athletic field as the place of occurrence of the external cause

Y92.320 Baseball field as the place of occurrence of the external cause

Y92.321 Football field as the place of occurrence of the external cause

Y92.322 Soccer field as the place of occurrence of the external cause

Y92.328 Other athletic field as the place of occurrence of the external cause
Cricket field as the place of occurrence of the external cause
Hockey field as the place of occurrence of the external cause

Y92.33 Skating rink as the place of occurrence of the external cause

Y92.330 Ice skating rink (indoor) (outdoor) as the place of occurrence of the external cause

Y92.331 Roller skating rink as the place of occurrence of the external cause

Y92.34 Swimming pool (public) as the place of occurrence of the external cause
Excludes1: swimming pool in private home or garden (Y92.06)

Y92.39 Other specified sports and athletic area as the place of occurrence of the external cause
Golf-course as the place of occurrence of the external cause
Gymnasium as the place of occurrence of the external cause
Riding-school as the place of occurrence of the external cause
Stadium as the place of occurrence of the external cause

Y92.4 Street, highway and other paved roadways as the place of occurrence of the external cause
Excludes1: private driveway of residence (Y92.0x4, Y92.1x3)

Y92.41 Street and highway as the place of occurrence of the external cause

Y92.410 Unspecified street and highway as the place of occurrence of the external cause
Road NOS as the place of occurrence of the external cause

Y92.411 Interstate highway as the place of occurrence of the external cause
Freeway as the place of occurrence of the external cause
Motorway as the place of occurrence of the external cause

Y92.412 Parkway as the place of occurrence of the external cause

Y92.413 State road as the place of occurrence of the external cause

Y92.414 Local residential or business street as the place of occurrence of the external cause

Y92.415 Exit ramp or entrance ramp of street or highway as the place of occurrence of the external cause

Y92.48 Other paved roadways as the place of occurrence of the external cause

Y92.480 Sidewalk as the place of occurrence of the external cause

Y92.481 Parking lot as the place of occurrence of the external cause

Y92.482 Bike path as the place of occurrence of the external cause

Y92.488 Other paved roadways as the place of occurrence of the external cause

Y92.5 Trade and service area as the place of occurrence of the external cause
Excludes1: garage in private home (Y92.05)
schools and other public adminstration buildings (Y92.2-)

Y92.51 Private commerical establishments

Y92.510 Bank as the place of occurrence of the external cause

Y92.511 Restaurant or café as the place of occurrence of the external cause

Y92.512 Supermarket, store or market as the place of occurrence of the external cause

Y92.513 Shop (commercial) as the place of occurrence of the external cause

Y92.52 Service areas

Y92.520 Airport as the place of occurrence of the external cause

Y92.521 Bus station as the place of occurrence of the external cause

Y92.522 Railway station as the place of occurrence of the external cause

Y92.523 Highway rest stops

Y92.524 Gas station as the place of occurrence of the external cause
Petroleum station as the place of occurrence of the external cause
Service station as the place of occurrence of the external cause

Y92.59   Other trade areas
Office building as the place of occurrence of the external cause
Casino as the place of occurrence of the external cause
Garage (commercial) as the place of occurrence of the external cause
Hotel as the place of occurrence of the external cause
Radio or television station as the place of occurrence of the external cause
Shopping mall as the place of occurrence of the external cause
Warehouse as the place of occurrence of the external cause

Y92.6   Industrial and construction area as the place of occurrence of the external cause

Y92.61   Building [any] under construction as the place of occurrence of the external cause

Y92.62   Dock or shipyard as the place of occurrence of the external cause
Dockyard as the place of occurrence of the external cause
Dry dock as the place of occurrence of the external cause
Shipyard as the place of occurrence of the external cause

Y92.63   Factory as the place of occurrence of the external cause
Factory building as the place of occurrence of the external cause
Factory premises as the place of occurrence of the external cause
Industrial yard as the place of occurrence of the external cause

Y92.64   Mine or pit as the place of occurrence of the external cause
Mine as the place of occurrence of the external cause

Y92.65   Oil rig as the place of occurrence of the external cause
Pit (coal) (gravel) (sand) as the place of occurrence of the external cause

Y92.69   Other specified industrial and construction area as the place of occurrence of the external cause
Gasworks as the place of occurrence of the external cause
Power-station (coal) (nuclear) (oil) as the place of occurrence of the external cause
Tunnel under construction as the place of occurrence of the external cause
Workshop as the place of occurrence of the external cause

Y92.7   Farm as the place of occurrence of the external cause
Ranch as the place of occurrence of the external cause
Excludes1:   farmhouse and home premises of farm (Y92.01-)

Y92.71   Barn as the place of occurrence of the external cause

Y92.72   Chicken coop as the place of occurrence of the external cause
Hen house as the place of occurrence of the external cause

Y92.73   Farm field as the place of occurrence of the external cause

Y92.74   Orchard as the place of occurrence of the external cause

Y92.79   Other farm location as the place of occurrence of the external cause

Y92.8   Other specified places as the place of occurrence of the external cause

Y92.81   Transport vehicle as the place of occurrence of the external cause

Y92.810   Car
Y92.811   Bus
Y92.812   Truck
Y92.813   Airplane
Y92.814   Boat
Y92.815   Train
Y92.816   Subway car

Y92.818   Other transport vehicle

Y92.82   Wilderness area

Y92.820   Desert as the place of occurrence of the external cause
Y92.821   Forest as the place of occurrence of the external cause
Y92.828   Other wilderness area
Marsh as the place of occurrence of the external cause
Mountain as the place of occurrence of the external cause
Prairie as the place of occurrence of the external cause
Swamp as the place of occurrence of the external cause

Y92.83   Recreation area

Y92.830   Public park as the place of occurrence of the external cause
Y92.831   Amusement park as the place of occurrence of the external cause
Y92.832   Beach as the place of occurrence of the external cause
Seashore as the place of occurrence of the external cause
Y92.833   Campsite as the place of occurrence of the external cause
Y92.838   Other recreation area

Y92.84   Military training ground as the place of occurrence of the external cause

Y92.85   Railroad track as the place of occurrence of the external cause

Y92.86   Slaughter house as the place of occurrence of the external cause

Y92.89   Other specified places as the place of occurrence of the external cause
Derelict house as the place of occurrence of the external cause
Zoo as the place of occurrence of the external cause

Y93   Activity code
The following category is provided for use to indicate the activity of the injured person at the time the event occurred. It may also be used to describe the activity of a person who siffers from a health condition other than an injury, such as a heart attack or stroke that occurs while engaged in the specified activity
The activity code should be recorded only at the initial encounter for treatment
The following extensions are for each code for category Y93:
A   non-work related activity
B   work-related activity
Activity done for income
C   student activity
activity performed while a student not for income
D   military activity

Y93.0   Sports activity

Y93.01   Individual sport
Y93.010   Running
Y93.011   Walking
Y93.012   Jogging
Y93.013   Horseback riding
Y93.014   Swimming
Y93.015   Golf
Y93.016   Bowling
Y93.018   Other individual sport

Y93.02   Group sport
Y93.020   Football
Y93.021   Softball
Y93.022   Baseball
Y93.023   Lacrosse
Y93.024   Soccer
Y93.025   Tennis
Y93.028   Other group sport

Y93.1   Activity primarily requiring repetitive use of fingers, hands and wrists

    Y93.11   Computer keyboarding
            Typing

    Y93.12   Video game playing

    Y93.13   Meat cutting

    Y93.14   Knitting

    Y93.15   Sewing

    Y93.19   Other activity primarily requiring repetitive use of fingers, hands and wrists

Y93.2   Personal hygiene and household activities

    Y93.21   Personal hygiene activities

    Y93.22   Household activities

Y93.3   Caregiving activities

Y93.4   Strenuous physical activities

    Y93.41   Snow shoveling

    Y93.42   Wood chopping

    Y93.49   Other strenuous physical activity

Y93.5   Electronic equipment usage

    Y93.51   Cellular telephone usage

    Y93.52   Headphone usage

    Y93.59   Other electronic equipment usage

Y93.8   Other activities

Y95 Nosocomial condition

Y96 Work-related condition

    Excludes1:   activity code Y93- with extension B

Y97 Environmental-pollution-related condition

    Excludes2:   exposure to environmental tobacco smoke (X58.1)

*Y98 deactivated. See Z72, Z73

CHAPTER XXI — FACTORS INFLUENCING HEALTH STATUS AND CONTACT WITH HEALTH SERVICES (Z00-Z99)

Note: Z codes represent reasons for encounters. A corresponding procedure code must accompany a Z code if a procedure is performed.

Categories Z00-Z99 are provided for occasions when circumstances other than a disease, injury or external cause classifiable to categories A00-Y89 are recorded as "diagnoses" or "problems".

This can arise in two main ways:

(a)   When a person who may or may not be sick encounters the health services for some specific purpose, such as to receive limited care or service for a current condition, to donate an organ or tissue, to receive prophylactic vaccination or to discuss a problem which is in itself not a disease or injury.

(b)   When some circumstance or problem is present which influences the person's health status but is not in itself a current illness or injury.

This chapter contains the following blocks:

Z00-Z13	Persons encountering health services for examination and investigation
Z20-Z28	Persons with potential health hazards related to communicable diseases
Z30-Z39	Persons encountering health services in circumstances related to reproduction
Z40-Z53	Persons encountering health services for specific procedures and health care
Z55-Z65	Persons with potential health hazards related to socioeconomic and psychosocial circumstances
Z66	Do not resuscitate [DNR] status
Z67	Blood type
Z69-Z76	Persons encountering health services in other circumstances
Z79-Z99	Persons with potential health hazards related to family and personal history and certain conditions influencing health status

PERSONS ENCOUNTERING HEALTH SERVICES FOR EXAMINATIONS (Z00-Z13)

Note: Nonspecific abnormal findings disclosed at the time of these examinations are classified to categories R70-R94.

Excludes1:   examinations related to pregnancy and reproduction (Z30-Z36, Z39.-)

Z00 Encounter for general examination without complaint, suspected or reported diagnosis

Excludes1:   encounter for examination for administrative purposes (Z02.-)

Excludes2:   special screening examinations (Z11-Z13)

Z00.0   Encounters for general medical examinations

Encounter for periodic examination (annual) (physical)

Excludes1:   encounter for examination of sign or symptom - code to sign or symptom

general health check-up of infant or child (Z00.1.-)

Z00.01   Encounter for general medical examination

General physical examination, routine blood work and any associated radiologic examinations

Excludes1:   routine laboratory examination without physical examination (Z00.02-)

routine radiology examination without physical examination (Z00.03-)

Z00.010   Encounter for general medical examination without abnormal findings

Encounter for health check-up NOS

Z00.011   Encounter for general medical examination with abnormal findings

Use additional code to identify abnormal findings

Z00.02   Encounter for general laboratory examination

Excludes1:   encounter for general medical examination with laboratory examination (Z00.01-)

encounter for laboratory examination for diagnostic purposes-code to signs and symptoms

Z00.020   Encounter for general laboratory examination without abnormal findings

Z00.021   Encounter for general laboratory examination with abnormal findings

Use additional code to identify abnormal findings

Z00.03   Encounter for general radiology examination

Encounter for routine chest X-ray

Excludes1:   encounter for general medical examination with radiology examination (Z00.01-)

encounter for radiology examination for diagnostic purposes - code to signs and symptoms

Z00.030   Encounter for general radiology examination without abnormal findings

Z00.031   Encounter for general radiology examination with abnormal findings

Use additional code to identify abnormal findings

Z00.1   Encounter for routine child health examination

Encounter for development testing of infant or child

Excludes1:   health supervision of foundling or other healthy infant or child (Z76.1-Z76.2)

Z00.10   Encounter for routine child health examination without abnormal findings

Encounter for routine child health examination NOS

Z00.11   Encounter for routine child health examination with abnormal findings

Use additional code to identify abnormal findings

Z00.2   Encounter for examination for period of rapid growth in childhood

Z00.3   Encounter for examination for adolescent development state

Encounter for puberty development state

Z00.5   Encounter for examination of potential donor of organ and tissue

Z00.6   Encounter for examination for normal comparison and control in clinical research program

Z00.7   Encounter for examination for period of delayed growth in childhood

Z00.70   Encounter for examination for period of delayed growth in childhood without abnormal findings

Z00.71   Encounter for examination for period of delayed growth in childhood with abnormal findings

Use additional code to identify abnormal findings

Z00.8   Encounter for other general examinations

Encounter for health examination in population surveys

Z01 Encounter for other special examination without complaint or suspected or reported diagnosis

Includes: routine examination of specific system

Note: Codes from category Z01 represent the reason for the encounter. A separate procedure code is required to identify any examinations or procedures performed.

Excludes1:   encounter for examination for administrative purposes (Z02.-)

encounter for examination for suspected conditions, proven not to exist (Z03.-)

Excludes2:   screening examinations (Z11-Z13)

Z01.0   Encounter for examination of eyes and vision

Excludes1:   examination for driving license (Z02.4)

Z01.00   Encounter for examination of eyes and vision without abnormal findings
Encounter for examination of eyes and vision NOS

Z01.01   Encounter for examination of eyes and vision with abnormal findings
Use additional code to identify abnormal findings

Z01.1   Encounter for examination of ears and hearing

Z01.10   Encounter for examination of ears and hearing without abnormal findings
Encounter for examination of ears and hearing NOS

Z01.11   Encounter for examination of ears and hearing with abnormal findings
Use additional code to identify abnormal findings

Z01.2   Encounter for dental examination and cleaning

Z01.20   Encounter for dental examination and cleaning without abnormal findings
Encounter for dental examination and cleaning NOS

Z01.21   Encounter for dental examination and cleaning with abnormal findings
Use additional code to identify abnormal findings

Z01.3   Encounter for examination of blood pressure

Z01.30   Encounter for examination of blood pressure without abnormal findings
Encounter for examination of blood pressure NOS

Z01.31   Encounter for examination of blood pressure with abnormal findings
Use additional code to identify abnormal findings

Z01.4   Encounter for gynecological examination (general) (routine)
Encounter for Papanicolaou smear of cervix
Encounter for pelvic examination (annual) (periodic)
Use additional code for screening vaginal pap smear (Z12.72)
Excludes1   screening cervical pap smear not a part of a routine gynecological examination (Z12.4)
Excludes2:   pregnancy examination or test (Z32.0)
routine examination for contraceptive maintenance (Z30.4)

Z01.40   Encounter for gynecological examination (general) (routine) without abnormal findings
Encounter for gynecological examination (general) (routine) NOS

Z01.41   Encounter for gynecological examination (general) (routine) with abnormal findings
Use additional code to identify abnormal findings

Z01.8   Encounter for other specified special examinations

Z01.81   Encounter for pre-operative cardiovascular examination

Z01.82   Encounter for pre-operative respiratory examination

Z01.83   Encounter for other pre-operative examination
Encounter for pre-operative examination NOS

Z01.89   Encounter for other specified special examinations

Z01.9   Encounter for special examination, unspecified

Z02   Encounter for administrative examination

Z02.0   Encounter for examination for admission to educational institution
Encounter for examination for admission to preschool (education)

Z02.1   Encounter for pre-employment examination

Z02.2   Encounter for examination for admission to residential institution
Excludes1:   examination for admission to prison (Z02.8)

Z02.3   Encounter for examination for recruitment to armed forces

Z02.4   Encounter for examination for driving license

Z02.5   Encounter for examination for participation in sport
Excludes1:   blood-alcohol and blood-drug test (Z02.83)

Z02.6   Encounter for examination for insurance purposes

Z02.7   Encounter for issue of medical certificate
Excludes1:   encounter for general medical examination (Z00-Z01, Z02.0-Z02.6, Z02.8-Z02.9)

Z02.71   Encounter for disability determination
Encounter for issue of medical certificate of incapacity
Encounter for issue of medical certificate of invalidity

Z02.79   Encounter for issue of other medical certificate

Z02.8   Encounter for other administrative examinations

Z02.81   Encounter for paternity testing

Z02.82   Encounter for adoption services

Z02.83   Encounter for blood-alcohol and blood-drug test
Use additional code for findings of alcohol or drugs in blood (R78.-)

Z02.89   Encounter for other administrative examinations
Encounter for examination for admission to prison
Encounter for examination for admission to summer camp
Encounter for immigration examination
Encounter for naturalization examination
Encounter for premarital examination
Excludes1:   health supervision of foundling or other healthy infant or child (Z76.1-Z76.2)

Z02.9   Encounter for administrative examinations, unspecified

Z03   Encounter for medical observation for suspected diseases and conditions ruled out
Note: This category is to be used when a person without a diagnosis is suspected of having an abnormal condition, without signs or symptoms, which requires study, but after examination and observation, is ruled out. This category is also for use for administrative and legal observation status.
Excludes1:   person with feared complaint in whom no diagnosis is made (Z71.1)
signs or symptoms under study- code to signs or symptoms

Z03.6   Encounter for observation for suspected toxic effect from ingested substance ruled out
Encounter for observation for suspected adverse effect from drug
Encounter for observation for suspected poisoning

Z03.8   Encounter for observation for other suspected diseases and conditions ruled out

Z04   Encounter for observation for other reasons
Includes: encounter for examination for medicolegal reasons
Note: This category is to be used when a person without a diagnosis is suspected of having an abnormal condition, without signs or symptoms, which requires study, but after examination and observation, is ruled-out. This category is also for use for administrative and legal observation status.

Z04.1   Encounter for examination and observation following transport accident
Excludes1:   encounter for examination and observation following work accident (Z04.2)

Z04.2   Encounter for examination and observation following work accident

Z04.3   Encounter for examination and observation following other accident

Z04.4   Encounter for examination and observation following alleged rape and seduction
Encounter for examination of victim following alleged rape or seduction
Excludes1:   encounter for examination and observation following alleged sexual abuse (Z04.7-)

Z04.6   Encounter for general psychiatric examination, requested by authority

Z04.7   Encounter for examination and observation following alleged sexual and physical abuse

Z04.71   Encounter for examination and observation following alleged adult sexual and physical abuse
Suspected adult physical abuse, ruled out
Suspected adult sexual abuse, ruled out
Excludes1:   confirmed case of adult sexual and physical abuse (T74.-)
suspected case of adult sexual and physical abuse, not ruled out (T76.-)

Z04.72   **Encounter for examination and observation following alleged child sexual and physical abuse**
> Suspected child physical abuse, ruled out
> Suspected child sexual abuse, ruled out
> Excludes1:   confirmed case of child sexual and physical abuse (T74.-)
>   suspected case of child sexual and physical abuse, not ruled out (T76.-)

Z04.8   **Encounter for examination and observation for other specified reasons**
> Encounter for examination and observation for request for expert evidence

Z04.9   **Encounter for examination and observation for unspecified reason**
> Encounter for observation NOS

Z06   **Infection with drug-resistant microorganisms**
> Note: This category is intended for use as an additional code for infectious conditions classified elsewhere to indicate the presence of drug-resistance of the infectious organism
> Code first the infection

Z08   **Encounter for follow-up examination after completed treatment for malignant neoplasms**
> Includes: medical surveillance following completed treatment
> Use additional code to identify the personal history of malignant neoplasm (Z85.-)
> Excludes1:   aftercare following medical care (Z42-Z51)

Z09   **Encounter for follow-up examination after completed treatment for conditions other than malignant neoplasms**
> Includes: medical surveillance following completed treatment
> Use additional code to identify any applicable history of disease code (Z86.-, Z87.-)
> Excludes1:   aftercare following medical care (Z42-Z51)
>   surveillance of contraception (Z30.4-)
>   surveillance of prosthetic and other medical devices (Z44-Z46)

Z11   **Encounter for special screening examination for infectious and parasitic diseases**
> Note: Screening is the testing for disease or disease precursors in asymptomatic individuals so that early detection and treatment can be provided for those who test positive for the disease.
> Excludes1:   diagnostic examination-code to sign or symptom

Z11.0   **Encounter for special screening examination for intestinal infectious diseases**

Z11.1   **Encounter for special screening examination for respiratory tuberculosis**

Z11.2   **Encounter for special screening examination for other bacterial diseases**

Z11.3   **Encounter for special screening examination for infections with a predominantly sexual mode of transmission**

Z11.4   **Encounter for special screening examination for human immunodeficiency virus [HIV]**

Z11.5   **Encounter for special screening examination for other viral diseases**
> Excludes1:   encounter for special screening for viral intestinal disease (Z11.0)

Z11.6   **Encounter for special screening examination for other protozoal diseases and helminthiases**
> Excludes1:   encounter for special screening for protozoal intestinal disease (Z11.0)

Z11.8   **Encounter for special screening examination for other infectious and parasitic diseases**
> Encounter for special screening examination for chlamydia
> Encounter for special screening examination for rickettsial
> Encounter for special screening examination for spirochetal
> Encounter for special screening examination for mycoses

Z11.9   **Encounter for special screening examination for infectious and parasitic diseases, unspecified**

Z12   **Encounter for special screening examination for malignant neoplasms**
> Note: Screening is the testing for disease or disease precursors in asymptomatic individuals so that early detection and treatment can be provided for those who test positive for the disease.
> Use additional code to identify any family history of malignant neoplasm (Z80.-)
> Excludes1:   diagnostic examination-code to sign or symptom

Z12.0   **Encounter for special screening examination for malignant neoplasm of stomach**

Z12.1   **Encounter for special screening examination for malignant neoplasm of intestinal tract**

Z12.10   **Encounter for special screening examination for malignant neoplasm of intestinal tract, unspecified**

Z12.11   **Encounter for special screening examination for malignant neoplasm of colon**

Z12.12   **Encounter for special screening examination for malignant neoplasm of rectum**

Z12.13   **Encounter for special screening examination for malignant neoplasm of small intestinal**

Z12.2   **Encounter for special screening examination for malignant neoplasm of respiratory organs**

Z12.3   **Encounter for special screening examination for malignant neoplasm of breast**

Z12.31   **Encounter for routine screening mammogram for malignant neoplasm of breast**

Z12.39   **Encounter for other special screening examination for malignant neoplasm of breast**

Z12.4   **Encounter for special screening examination for malignant neoplasm of cervix**
> Encounter for screening pap smear for malignant neoplasm of cervix
> Excludes1:   when screening is part of general gynecological examination (Z01.4)

Z12.5   **Encounter for special screening examination for malignant neoplasm of prostate**

Z12.6   **Encounter for special screening examination for malignant neoplasm of bladder**

Z12.7   **Encounter for special screening examination for malignant neoplasm of other genitourinary organs**

Z12.71   **Encounter for special screening examination for malignant neoplasm of testis**

Z12.72   **Encounter for special screening examination for malignant neoplasm of vagina**
> Vaginal pap smear status-post hysterectomy for non-malignant condition
> Use additional code to identify acquired absence of uterus (Z90.71)
> Excludes1:   vaginal pap smear status-post hysterectomy for malignant conditions (Z08)

Z12.73   **Encounter for special screening examination for malignant neoplasm of ovary**

Z12.79   **Encounter for special screening examination for malignant neoplasm of other genitourinary organs**

Z12.8   **Encounter for special screening examination for malignant neoplasm of other sites**

Z12.81   **Encounter for special screening examination for malignant neoplasm of oral cavity**

Z12.82   **Encounter for special screening examination for malignant neoplasm of nervous system**

Z12.83   **Encounter for special screening examination for malignant neoplasm of skin**

Z12.89   **Encounter for special screening examination for malignant neoplasm of other sites**

Z12.9   **Encounter for special screening examination for malignant neoplasm, site unspecified**

Z13   **Encounter for special screening examination for other diseases and disorders**
> Note: Screening is the testing for disease or disease precursors in asymptomatic individuals so that early detection and treatment can be provided for those who test positive for the disease.
> Excludes1:   diagnostic examination-code to sign or symptom

Z13.0 Encounter for special screening examination for diseases of the blood and blood-forming organs and certain disorders involving the immune mechanism

Z13.1 Encounter for special screening examination for diabetes mellitus

Z13.2 Encounter for special screening examination for nutritional, metabolic and other endocrine disorders

  Z13.21 Encounter for special screening examination for nutritional disorder

  Z13.22 Encounter for special screening examination for metabolic disorder

    Z13.220 Encounter for special screening examination for lipoid disorders
      Encounter for special screening examination for cholesterol level
      Encounter for special screening examination for hypercholesterolemia
      Encounter for special screening examination for hyperlipidemia

    Z13.228 Encounter for special screening examination for other metabolic disorders

  Z13.29 Encounter for special screening examination for other suspected endocrine disorder
    Excludes1:   encounter for special screening examination for diabetes mellitus (Z13.1)

Z13.4 Encounter for special screening examination for certain developmental disorders in childhood
  Encounter for special screening examination for developmental handicaps in early childhood
  Excludes1:   routine development testing of infant or child (Z00.1-)

Z13.5 Encounter for special screening examination for eye and ear disorders
  Excludes2:   encounter for general hearing examination (Z01.1-)
              encounter for general vision examination (Z01.0-)

Z13.6 Encounter for special screening examination for cardiovascular disorders

Z13.8 Encounter for special screening examination for other specified diseases and disorders
  Excludes2:   screening for malignant neoplasms (Z12.-)

  Z13.81 Encounter for special screening examination for digestive system disorders

    Z13.810 Encounter for special screening examination for upper gastrointestinal disorder

    Z13.811 Encounter for special screening examination for lower gastrointestinal disorder
      Excludes1:   encounter for special screening for intestinal infectious disease (Z11.0)

    Z13.818 Encounter for special screening examination for other digestive system disorders

  Z13.82 Encounter for special screening examination for musculoskeletal disorder

    Z13.820 Encounter for special screening examination for osteoporosis

    Z13.828 Encounter for special screening examination for other musculoskeletal disorder

  Z13.83 Encounter for special screening examination for respiratory disorder NEC
    Excludes1:   encounter for special screening examination for respiratory tuberculosis (Z11.1)

  Z13.84 Encounter for special screening examination for dental disorders

  Z13.88 Encounter for special screening examination for disorder due to exposure to contaminants
    Excludes1:   those exposed to contaminants without suspected disorders (Z57-Z58)

  Z13.89 Encounter for special screening examination for other disorder
    Encounter for special screening examination for nervous system disorders
    Encounter for special screening examination for genitourinary disorders

Z13.9 Encounter for special screening examination , unspecified

PERSONS WITH POTENTIAL HEALTH HAZARDS RELATED TO COMMUNICABLE DISEASES (Z20-Z28)

Z20 Contact with and exposure to communicable diseases
  Excludes1:   carrier of infectious disease (Z22.-)
              diagnosed current infectious or parasitic disease—see Alphabetic Index
  Excludes2:   personal history of infectious and parasitic diseases (Z86.1-)

Z20.0 Contact with and exposure to intestinal infectious diseases

Z20.1 Contact with and exposure to tuberculosis

Z20.2 Contact with and exposure to infections with a predominantly sexual mode of transmission

Z20.3 Contact with and exposure to rabies

Z20.4 Contact with and exposure to rubella

Z20.5 Contact with and exposure to viral hepatitis

Z20.6 Contact with and exposure to human immunodeficiency virus [HIV]
  Excludes1:   asymptomatic human immunodeficiency virus [HIV] infection status (Z21)

Z20.7 Contact with and exposure to pediculosis, acariasis and other infestations

Z20.8 Contact with and exposure to other communicable diseases

Z20.9 Contact with and exposure to unspecified communicable disease

Z21 Asymptomatic human immunodeficiency virus [HIV] infection status
  Includes: HIV positive NOS
  Excludes1:   acquired immunodeficiency syndrome (B20)
              contact with or exposure to human immunodeficiency virus [HIV] (Z20.6)
              human immunodeficiency virus [HIV] disease (B20)
              inconclusive laboratory evidence of human immunodeficiency virus [HIV] (R75)

Z22 Carrier of infectious disease
  Includes: suspected carrier

Z22.0 Carrier of typhoid

Z22.1 Carrier of other intestinal infectious diseases

Z22.2 Carrier of diphtheria

Z22.3 Carrier of other specified bacterial diseases

  Z22.31 Carrier of bacterial disease due to meningococci

  Z22.32 Carrier of bacterial disease due to staphylococci

  Z22.33 Carrier of bacterial disease due to streptococci

    Z22.330 Carrier of Group B streptococcus

    Z22.338 Carrier of other streptococcus

  Z22.39 Carrier of other specified bacterial diseases

Z22.4 Carrier of infections with a predominantly sexual mode of transmission

Z22.5 Carrier of viral hepatitis

  Z22.50 Carrier of unspecified viral hepatitis

  Z22.51 Carrier of viral hepatitis B
    Hepatitis B surface antigen [HBsAg] carrier

  Z22.52 Carrier of viral hepatitis C

  Z22.59 Carrier of other viral hepatitis

Z22.6 Carrier of human T-lymphotropic virus type-1 [HTLV-1] infection

Z22.8 Carrier of other infectious diseases

Z22.9 Carrier of infectious disease, unspecified

Z23 Encounter for immunization
　　Code first any routine childhood examination
　　Note: procedure codes are required to identify the types of
　　immunizations given

Z28 Immunization not carried out
Z28.0 Immunization not carried out because of contraindication
**Z28.1 Immunization not carried out because of patient's decision for
　　reasons of belief or group pressure**
**Z28.2 Immunization not carried out because of patient's decision for
　　other and unspecified reason**
　　**Z28.20 Immunization not carried out because of patient's
　　decision for unspecified reason**
　　**Z28.29 Immunization not carried out because of patient's
　　decision for other reason**
Z28.8 Immunization not carried out for other reason
　　**Z28.81 Immunization not carried out due to patient's having
　　had the disease**
　　Z28.89 Immunization not carried out for other reason
Z28.9 Immunization not carried out for unspecified reason

PERSONS ENCOUNTERING HEALTH SERVICES IN CIRCUMSTANCES RELATED TO REPRODUCTION (Z30-Z39)

Z30 Encounter for contraceptive management
Z30.0 Encounter for general counseling and advice on contraception
　　Z30.01 Encounter for initial prescription of contraceptives
　　　　**Z30.011 Encounter for initial prescription of
　　　　contraceptive pills**
　　　　**Z30.012 Encounter for initial prescription of
　　　　implantable subdermal contraceptive**
　　　　**Z30.013 Encounter for initial prescription of injectable
　　　　contraceptive**
　　　　**Z30.014 Encounter for initial prescription of
　　　　intrauterine contraceptive device**
　　　　**Z30.018 Encounter for initial prescription of other
　　　　contraceptives**
　　　　**Z30.019 Encounter for initial prescription of
　　　　contraceptives, unspecified**
　　**Z30.09 Encounter for other general counseling and advice on
　　contraception**
　　　　Encounter for family planning advice NOS
Z30.2 Encounter for sterilization
Z30.4 Encounter for surveillance of contraceptives
　　**Z30.40 Encounter for surveillance of contraceptives,
　　unspecified**
　　Z30.41 Encounter for surveillance of contraceptive pills
　　　　Encounter for repeat prescription for contraceptive pill
　　**Z30.42 Encounter for surveillance of implantable subdermal
　　contraceptive**
　　Z30.43 Encounter for surveillance of injectable contraceptive
　　**Z30.44 Encounter for surveillance of intrauterine
　　contraceptive device**
　　　　Encounter for checking, reinsertion or removal of
　　　　intrauterine contraceptive device
　　Z30.49 Encounter for surveillance of other contraceptives
Z30.6 Encounter for postcoital contraception
Z30.8 Encounter for other contraceptive management
　　Encounter for postvasectomy sperm count
　　Encounter for routine examination for contraceptive
　　maintenance
　　Excludes1: sperm count following sterilization reversal
　　　　(Z31.42)
　　　　sperm count for fertility testing (Z31.41)
Z30.9 Encounter for contraceptive management, unspecified

Z31 Encounter for procreative management
　　Excludes1: complications associated with artificial fertilization
　　　　(N98.-)
　　　　female infertility (N97.-)
　　　　male infertility (N46.-)
Z31.0 Encounter for reversal of previous sterilization

Z31.4 Encounter for procreative investigation and testing
　　Excludes1: postvasectomy sperm count (Z30.8)
　　Z31.41 Encounter for fertility testing
　　　　Encounter for fallopian tube patency testing
　　　　Encounter for sperm count for fertility testing
　　　　Excludes1: encounter for genetic counseling and
　　　　　　testing (Z31.5)
　　Z31.42 Aftercare following sterilization reversal
　　　　Sperm count following sterilization reversal
　　**Z31.49 Encounter for other procreative investigation and
　　testing**
Z31.5 Encounter for genetic counseling and testing
　　Excludes1: encounter for fertility testing (Z31.41)
Z31.6 Encounter for general counseling and advice on procreation
Z31.8 Encounter for other procreative management
　　Z31.81 Encounter for male factor infertility in female patient
　　Z31.82 Encounter for Rh incompatibility status
　　Z31.89 Encounter for other procreative management
Z31.9 Encounter for procreative management, unspecified

Z32 Encounter for pregnancy test and instruction
Z32.0 Encounter for pregnancy test
Z32.1 Encounter for childbirth instruction
Z32.2 Encounter for childcare instruction
　　Encounter for prenatal or postpartum childcare instruction

Z33 Pregnant state
Z33.1 Pregnant state, incidental
　　Pregnant state NOS
　　Excludes1: complications of pregnancy (O00-O99)
Z33.2 Encounter for elective termination of pregnancy
　　Excludes1: early fetal death with retention of dead fetus
　　　　(O02.1)
　　　　late fetal death (O36.4)
　　　　spontaneous abortion (O03)

Z34 Encounter for supervision of normal pregnancy
　　Excludes1: any complication of pregnancy (O00-O99)
　　　　encounter for supervision of high-risk pregancy (O09.-)
Z34.0 Encounter for supervision of normal first pregnancy
　　**Z34.00 Encounter for supervision of normal first pregnancy,
　　unspecified trimester**
　　**Z34.01 Encounter for supervision of normal first pregnancy,
　　first trimester**
　　**Z34.02 Encounter for supervision of normal first pregnancy,
　　second trimester**
　　**Z34.03 Encounter for supervision of normal first pregnancy,
　　third trimester**
Z34.8 Encounter for supervision of other normal pregnancy
　　**Z34.80 Encounter for supervision of other normal pregnancy,
　　unspecified trimester**
　　**Z34.81 Encounter for supervision of other normal pregnancy,
　　first trimester**
　　**Z34.82 Encounter for supervision of other normal pregnancy,
　　second trimester**
　　**Z34.83 Encounter for supervision of other normal pregnancy,
　　third trimester**
Z34.9 Encounter for supervision of normal pregnancy, unspecified
　　**Z34.90 Encounter for supervision of normal pregnancy,
　　unspecified, unspecified trimester**
　　**Z34.91 Encounter for supervision of normal pregnancy,
　　unspecified, first trimester**
　　**Z34.92 Encounter for supervision of normal pregnancy,
　　unspecified, second trimester**
　　**Z34.93 Encounter for supervision of normal pregnancy,
　　unspecified, third trimester**

Z36 Encounter for antenatal screening
　　Excludes1: abnormal findings on antenatal screening of mother
　　　　(O28.-)
　　　　diagnostic examination- code to sign or symptom
　　Excludes2: routine prenatal care (Z34)

Z37 Outcome of delivery
Note: This category is intended for use as an additional code to identify the outcome of delivery on the mother's record. It is not for use on the newborn record.

Z37.0 Single live birth
Z37.1 Single stillbirth
Z37.2 Twins, both liveborn
Z37.3 Twins, one liveborn and one stillborn
Z37.4 Twins, both stillborn
Z37.5 Other multiple births, all liveborn
 Z37.50 Multiple births, unspecified, all liveborn
 Z37.51 Triplets, all liveborn
 Z37.52 Quadruplets, all liveborn
 Z37.53 Quintuplets, all liveborn
 Z37.54 Sextuplets, all liveborn
 Z37.59 Other multiple births, all liveborn
Z37.6 Other multiple births, some liveborn
 Z37.60 Multiple births, unspecified, some liveborn
 Z37.61 Triplets, some liveborn
 Z37.62 Quadruplets, some liveborn
 Z37.63 Quintuplets, some liveborn
 Z37.64 Sextuplets, some liveborn
 Z37.69 Other multiple births, some liveborn
Z37.7 Other multiple births, all stillborn
Z37.9 Outcome of delivery, unspecified
 Multiple birth NOS
 Single birth NOS

Z38 Liveborn infants according to place of birth and type of delivery
Note: This category is for use as the principal code on the initial record of a newborn baby. It is to be used for the initial birth record only. It is not to be used on the mother's record.

Z38.0 Single liveborn infant, born in hospital
 Single liveborn infant, born in birthing center or other health care facility
 Z38.00 Single liveborn infant, delivered vaginally
 Z38.01 Single liveborn infant, delivered by cesarean
Z38.1 Single liveborn infant, born outside hospital
Z38.2 Single liveborn infant, unspecified as to place of birth
 Single liveborn infant NOS
Z38.3 Twin liveborn infant, born in hospital
 Z38.30 Twin liveborn infant, delivered vaginally
 Z38.31 Twin liveborn infant, delivered by cesarean
Z38.4 Twin liveborn infant, born outside hospital
Z38.5 Twin liveborn infant, unspecified as to place of birth
Z38.6 Other multiple liveborn infant, born in hospital
 Z38.61 Triplet liveborn infant, delivered vaginally
 Z38.62 Triplet liveborn infant, delivered by cesarean
 Z38.63 Quadruplet liveborn infant, delivered vaginally
 Z38.64 Quadruplet liveborn infant, delivered by cesarean
 Z38.65 Quintuplet liveborn infant, delivered vaginally
 Z38.66 Quintuplet liveborn infant, delivered by cesarean
 Z38.68 Other multiple liveborn infant, delivered vaginally
 Z38.69 Other multiple liveborn infant, delivered by cesarean
Z38.7 Other multiple liveborn infant, born outside hospital
Z38.8 Other multiple liveborn infant, unspecified as to place of birth

Z39 Encounter for maternal postpartum care and examination
Z39.0 Encounter for care and examination immediately after delivery
 Care and observation in uncomplicated cases when the delivery occurs outside a healthcare facility
 Excludes1: care for postpartum complication- see Alphabetic index
Z39.1 Encounter for care and examination of lactating mother
 Encounter for supervision of lactation
 Excludes1: disorders of lactation (O92.-)
Z39.2 Encounter for routine postpartum follow-up

ENCOUNTERS FOR OTHER SPECIFIC HEALTH CARE (Z40-Z53)
Note: Categories Z40-Z53 are intended for use to indicate a reason for care. They may be used for patients who have already been treated for a disease or injury, but who are receiving aftercare or prophylactic care, convalescent care, or care to consolidate the treatment, or to deal with residual state
Excludes2: follow-up examination for medical surveillance after treatment (Z08-Z09)

Z40 Encounter for prophylactic surgery
 Excludes1: organ donations (Z52.-)
  therapeutic organ removal-code to condition
Z40.0 Encounter for prophylactic surgery for risk-factors related to malignant neoplasms
 Admission for prophylactic organ removal
 Use additional code to identify risk-factor
 Z40.00 Encounter for prophylactic removal of unspecified organ
 Z40.01 Encounter for prophylactic removal of breast
 Z40.02 Encounter for prophylactic removal of ovary
 Z40.09 Encounter for prophylactic removal of other organ
Z40.8 Encounter for other prophylactic surgery
Z40.9 Encounter for prophylactic surgery, unspecified

Z41 Encounter for procedures for purposes other than remedying health state
Z41.1 Encounter to remedy unacceptable cosmetic appearance
 Encounter for breast implant
 Excludes1: encounter for post-mastectomy implants (Z90.1)
Z41.2 Encounter for routine and ritual male circumcision
Z41.3 Encounter for ear piercing
Z41.8 Encounter for other procedures for purposes other than remedying health state
Z41.9 Encounter for procedure for purposes other than remedying health state, unspecified

Z43 Encounter for attention to artificial openings
 Includes: closure of artificial openings
  passage of sounds or bougies through artificial openings
  reforming artificial openings
  removal of catheter from artificial openings
  toilet or cleansing of artificial openings
 Excludes1: artificial opening status only, without need for care (Z93.-)
  complications of external stoma (J95.0-, K91.4-, K91.7-, N99.5-)
 Excludes2: fitting and adjustment of prosthetic and other devices (Z44-Z46)
Z43.0 Encounter for attention to tracheostomy
Z43.1 Encounter for attention to gastrostomy
Z43.2 Encounter for attention to ileostomy
Z43.3 Encounter for attention to colostomy
Z43.4 Encounter for attention to other artificial openings of digestive tract
Z43.5 Encounter for attention to cystostomy
Z43.6 Encounter for attention to other artificial openings of urinary tract
 Encounter for attention to nephrostomy
 Encounter for attention to ureterostomy
 Encounter for attention to urethrostomy
Z43.7 Encounter for attention to artificial vagina
Z43.8 Encounter for attention to other artificial openings
Z43.9 Encounter for attention to unspecified artificial opening

Z44 Encounter for fitting and adjustment of external prosthetic device
 Excludes1: malfunction or other complications of device—see Alphabetical Index
  presence of prosthetic device (Z97.-)
Z44.0 Encounter for fitting and adjustment of artificial arm
 Z44.00 Encounter for fitting and adjustment of unspecified artificial arm
  Z44.001 Encounter for fitting and adjustment of unspecified right artificial arm

Z44.002   Encounter for fitting and adjustment of unspecified left artificial arm device

Z44.009   Encounter for fitting and adjustment of unspecified artificial arm, unspecified arm

Z44.01   Encounter for fitting and adjustment of complete artificial arm

Z44.011   Encounter for fitting and adjustment of complete right artificial arm

Z44.012   Encounter for fitting and adjustment of complete left artificial arm

Z44.019   Encounter for fitting and adjustment of complete artificial arm, unspecified arm

Z44.02   Encounter for fitting and adjustment of partial artificial arm

Z44.021   Encounter for fitting and adjustment of partial artificial right arm

Z44.022   Encounter for fitting and adjustment of partial artificial left arm

Z44.029   Encounter for fitting and adjustment of partial artificial arm, unspecified arm

Z44.1   Encounter for fitting and adjustment of artificial leg

Z44.10   Encounter for fitting and adjustment of unspecified artificial leg

Z44.101   Encounter for fitting and adjustment of unspecified right artificial leg

Z44.102   Encounter for fitting and adjustment of unspecified left artificial leg

Z44.109   Encounter for fitting and adjustment of unspecified artificial leg, unspecified leg

Z44.11   Encounter for fitting and adjustment of complete artificial leg

Z44.111   Encounter for fitting and adjustment of complete right artificial leg

Z44.112   Encounter for fitting and adjustment of complete left artificial leg

Z44.119   Encounter for fitting and adjustment of complete artificial leg, unspecified leg

Z44.12   Encounter for fitting and adjustment of partial artificial leg

Z44.121   Encounter for fitting and adjustment of partial artificial right leg

Z44.122   Encounter for fitting and adjustment of partial artificial left leg

Z44.129   Encounter for fitting and adjustment of partial artificial leg, unspecified leg

Z44.2   Encounter for fitting and adjustment of artificial eye

Excludes1:   mechanical complication of ocular prosthesis (T85.3)

Z44.3   Encounter for fitting and adjustment of external breast prosthesis

Z44.8   Encounter for fitting and adjustment of other external prosthetic devices

Z44.9   Encounter for fitting and adjustment of unspecified external prosthetic device

Z45   Encounter for adjustment and management of implanted device

Includes: removal or replacement of implanted device

Excludes1:   malfunction or other complications of device—see Alphabetical Index

Excludes2:   encounter for fitting and adjustment of non-implanted device (Z46.-)

presence of prosthetic and other devices (Z95-Z97)

Z45.0   Encounter for adjustment and management of cardiac device

Z45.01   Encounter for adjustment and management of cardiac pacemaker

Z45.010   Encounter for checking and testing of cardiac pacemaker pulse generator [battery]

Encounter for replacing cardiac pacemaker pulse generator [battery]

Z45.018   Encounter for adjustment and management of other part of cardiac pacemaker

Z45.02   Encounter for adjustment and management of automatic implantable cardiac defibrillator

Z45.09   Encounter for adjustment and management of other cardiac device

Z45.1   Encounter for adjustment and management of infusion pump

Z45.2   Encounter for adjustment and management of vascular access device

Encounter for adjustment and management of vascular catheters

Excludes1:   encounter for adjustment and mangement of renal dialysis catheter (Z49.01)

Z45.3   Encounter for adjustment and management of implanted devices of the special senses

Z45.31   Encounter for adjustment and management of implanted visual substitution device

Z45.32   Encounter for adjustment and management of implanted hearing device

Excludes1:   encounter for fitting and adjustment of hearing aide (Z46.1)

Z45.320   Encounter for adjustment and management of bone conduction device

Z45.321   Encounter for adjustment and management of cochlear implanted hearing device

Z45.328   Encounter for adjustment and management of other implanted hearing device

Z45.4   Encounter for adjustment and management of implanted nervous system device

Z45.41   Encounter for adjustment and management of cerebrospinal fluid drainage device

Encounter for adjustment and management of cerebral ventricular (communicating) shunt

Z45.42   Encounter for adjustment and management of neuropacemaker (brain) (peripheral nerve) (spinal cord)

Z45.49   Encounter for adjustment and management of other implanted nervous system device

Z45.8   Encounter for adjustment and management of other implanted devices

Z45.9   Encounter for adjustment and management of unspecified implanted device

Z46   Encounter for fitting and adjustment of other devices

Excludes1:   malfunction or other complications of device—see Alphabetical Index

Excludes2:   encounter for fitting and management of implanted devices (Z45.-)

issue of repeat prescription only (Z76.0)

presence of prosthetic and other devices (Z95-Z97)

Z46.0   Encounter for fitting and adjustment of spectacles and contact lenses

Z46.1   Encounter for fitting and adjustment of hearing aid

Excludes1:   encounter for adjustment and management of implanted hearing device (Z45.32-)

Z46.2   Encounter for fitting and adjustment of other devices related to nervous system and special senses

Excludes2:   encounter for adjustment and management of implanted nervous system device (Z45.4-)

encounter for adjustment and management of implanted visual substitution device (Z45.31)

Z46.3   Encounter for fitting and adjustment of dental prosthetic device

Z46.4   Encounter for fitting and adjustment of orthodontic device

Z46.6   Encounter for fitting and adjustment of urinary device

Excludes2:   attention to artificial openings of urinary tract (Z43.5, Z43.6)

Z46.8   Encounter for fitting and adjustment of other specified devices

Encounter for fitting and adjustment of wheelchair

Z46.9   Encounter for fitting and adjustment of unspecified device

Z48   Encounter for other surgical aftercare

Excludes1:   encounter for follow-up examination after completed treatment (Z08-Z09)

Excludes2:   encounter for attention to artificial openings (Z43.-)

encounter for fitting and adjustment of prosthetic and other devices (Z44-Z46)

Z48.0   Encounter for attention to surgical dressings and sutures
    Encounter for change of dressings
    Encounter for removal of sutures
Z48.1   Encounter for planned post-operative wound closure
Z48.8   Encounter for other specified surgical aftercare
    Excludes1:   encounter for aftercare following sterilization
                  reversal (Z31.42)
Z48.9   Encounter for surgical aftercare, unspecified

Z49   Encounter for care involving renal dialysis
    Code also associated renal failure
Z49.0   Preparatory care for renal dialysis
    **Z49.01   Encounter for fitting and adjustment of extracorporeal
               dialysis catheter**
        Removal or replacement of renal dialysis catheter
        Toilet or cleansing of renal dialysis catheter
    **Z49.02   Encounter for fitting and adjustment of peritoneal
               dialysis catheter**
Z49.3   Encounter for adequancy testing for dialysis
    Z49.31   Encounter for adequancy testing for hemodialysis
    **Z49.32   Encounter for adequancy testing for peritoneal
               dialysis**
        Encounter for peritoneal equilibration test

Z51   Encounter for other aftercare
    Code also condition requiring care
    Excludes1:   follow-up examination after treatment (Z08-Z09)
Z51.0   Encounter for radiotherapy session
Z51.1   Encounter for chemotherapy session for neoplasm
Z51.5   Encounter for palliative care
Z51.8   Encounter for other specified aftercare
    Excludes1:   holiday relief care (Z75.5)
    Z51.81   Encounter for therapeutic drug level monitoring
        Code also any long-term (current) drug therapy (Z79.-)
        Excludes1:   encounter for blood-drug test for
                      administrative or medicolegal
                      reasons (Z02.83)
    Z51.89   Encounter for other specified aftercare
Z51.9   Encounter for aftercare, unspecified

Z52   Donors of organs and tissues
    Includes: autologous and other living donors
    Excludes1:   cadaveric donor - omit code
                  examination of potential donor (Z00.5)
Z52.0   Blood donor
    Z52.00   Unspecified blood donor
        Z52.000   Unspecified donor, whole blood
        Z52.001   Unspecified donor, stem cells
        Z52.008   Unspecified donor, other blood
    Z52.01   Autologous blood donor
        Z52.010   Autologous donor, whole blood
        Z52.011   Autologous donor, stem cells
        Z52.018   Autologous donor, other blood
    Z52.09   Other blood donor
        Volunteer donor
        Z52.090   Other blood donor, whole blood
        Z52.091   Other blood donor, stem cells
        Z52.098   Other blood donor, other blood
Z52.1   Skin donor
    Z52.10   Skin donor, unspecified
    Z52.11   Skin donor, autologous
    Z52.19   Skin donor, other
Z52.2   Bone donor
    Z52.20   Bone donor, unspecified
    Z52.21   Bone donor, autologous
    Z52.29   Bone donor, other
Z52.3   Bone marrow donor
Z52.4   Kidney donor
Z52.5   Cornea donor
Z52.8   Donor of other specified organs or tissues

Z52.9   Donor of unspecified organ or tissue
    Donor NOS

**Z53   Persons encountering health services for specific procedures and
      treatment, not carried out**
**Z53.0   Procedure and treatment not carried out because of
          contraindication**
    **Z53.01   Procedure and treatment not carried out due to
               patient smoking**
    **Z53.09   Procedure and treatment not carried out because of
               other contraindication**
**Z53.1   Procedure and treatment not carried out because of patient's
          decision for reasons of belief and group pressure**
**Z53.2   Procedure and treatment not carried out because of patient's
          decision for other and unspecified reasons**
    **Z53.20   Procedure and treatment not carried out because of
               patient's decision for unspecified reasons**
    **Z53.21   Procedure and treatment not carried out due to
               patient leaving prior to being seen by health care
               provider**
    **Z53.29   Procedure and treatment not carried out because of
               patient's decision for other reasons**
Z53.8   Procedure and treatment not carried out for other reasons
Z53.9   Procedure and treatment not carried out, unspecified reason

PERSONS WITH POTENTIAL HEALTH HAZARDS RELATED TO
SOCIOECONOMIC AND PSYCHOSOCIAL CIRCUMSTANCES
(Z55–Z65)

Z55   Problems related to education and literacy
    Excludes1:   disorders of psychological development (F80-F89)
Z55.0   Illiteracy and low-level literacy
Z55.1   Schooling unavailable and unattainable
Z55.2   Failed school examinations
Z55.3   Underachievement in school
**Z55.4   Educational maladjustment and discord with teachers and
          classmates**
Z55.8   Other problems related to education and literacy
    Problems related to inadequate teaching
Z55.9   Problems related to education and literacy, unspecified
    Academic problems NOS

Z56   Problems related to employment and unemployment
    Excludes2:   occupational exposure to risk factors (Z57.-)
                  problems related to housing and economic
                  circumstances (Z59.-)
Z56.0   Unemployment, unspecified
Z56.1   Change of job
Z56.2   Threat of job loss
Z56.3   Stressful work schedule
Z56.4   Discord with boss and workmates
Z56.5   Uncongenial work environment
    Difficult conditions at work
Z56.6   Other physical and mental strain related to work
Z56.8   Other problems related to employment
    Z56.81   Sexual harassment on the job
    Z56.89   Other problems related to employment
Z56.9   Unspecified problems related to employment
    Occupational problems NOS

Z57   Occupational exposure to risk-factors
Z57.0   Occupational exposure to noise
Z57.1   Occupational exposure to radiation
Z57.2   Occupational exposure to dust
Z57.3   Occupational exposure to other air contaminants
    **Z57.31   Occupational exposure to environmental tobacco
               smoke**
    Z57.32   Occupational exposure to other air contaminants
Z57.4   Occupational exposure to toxic agents in agriculture
    Occupational exposure to solids, liquids, gases or vapors in
    agriculture

Z57.5   Occupational exposure to toxic agents in other industries
Occupational exposure to solids, liquids, gases or vapors in other industries

Z57.6   Occupational exposure to extreme temperature

Z57.7   Occupational exposure to vibration

Z57.8   Occupational exposure to other risk factors

Z57.9   Occupational exposure to unspecified risk factor

Z58   Problems related to physical environment
Excludes2:   occupational exposure (Z57.-)

Z58.0   Exposure to noise

Z58.1   Exposure to air pollution

Z58.2   Exposure to water pollution

Z58.3   Exposure to soil pollution

Z58.4   Exposure to radiation

Z58.5   Exposure to other pollution

Z58.6   Inadequate drinking-water supply
Excludes1:   effects of thirst (T73.1)

Z58.8   Other problems related to physical environment

Z58.81   Problems related to exposure to lead

Z58.82   Problems related to exposure to asbestos

Z58.89   Other problems related to physical environment

Z58.9   Problem related to physical environment, unspecified

Z59   Problems related to housing and economic circumstances
Excludes1:   inadequate drinking-water supply (Z58.6)

Z59.0   Homelessness

Z59.1   Inadequate housing
Lack of heating
Restriction of space
Technical defects in home preventing adequate care
Unsatisfactory surroundings
Excludes1:   problems related to physical environment (Z58.-)

Z59.2   Discord with neighbors, lodgers and landlord

Z59.3   Problems related to living in residential institution
Boarding-school resident
Excludes1:   institutional upbringing (Z62.2)

Z59.4   Lack of adequate food
Excludes1:   effects of hunger (T73.0)
inappropriate diet or eating habits (Z72.4)
malnutrition (E40-E46)

Z59.5   Extreme poverty

Z59.6   Low income

Z59.7   Insufficient social insurance and welfare support

Z59.8   Other problems related to housing and economic circumstances
Foreclosure on loan
Isolated dwelling
Problems with creditors

Z59.9   Problem related to housing and economic circumstances, unspecified

Z60   Problems related to social environment

Z60.0   Problems of adjustment to life-cycle transitions
Empty nest syndrome
Phase of life problem
Problem with adjustment to retirement [pension]

Z60.1   Atypical parenting situation
Problems related to a parenting situation (rearing of children) with a single parent or other than that of two cohabiting biological parents.

Z60.2   Problems related to living alone

Z60.3   Acculturation difficulty
Problem with migration
Problem with social transplantation

Z60.4   Social exclusion and rejection
Exclusion and rejection on the basis of personal characteristics, such as unusual physical appearance, illness or behavior.
Excludes1:   target of adverse discrimination such as for racial or religious reasons (Z60.5)

Z60.5   Target of (perceived) adverse discrimination and persecution
Excludes1:   social exclusion and rejection (Z60.4)

Z60.8   Other problems related to social environment

Z60.9   Problem related to social environment, unspecified

Z61   Problems related to negative life events in childhood
Excludes2:   maltreatment syndromes (T74.-)

Z61.0   Loss of love relationship in childhood

Z61.1   Removal from home in childhood

Z61.2   Altered pattern of family relationships in childhood

Z61.3   Events resulting in loss of self-esteem in childhood

Z61.7   Personal frightening experience in childhood

Z61.8   Other negative life events in childhood

Z61.81   Personal history of abuse in childhood

Z61.810   Personal history of physical and sexual abuse in childhood
Excludes1:   current child physical abuse (T74.12, T76.12)
current child sexual abuse (T74.12, T76.12)

Z61.811   Personal history of psychological abuse in childhood
Excludes1:   current child psychological abuse (T74.32, T76.32)

Z61.812   Personal history of neglect in childhood
Excludes1:   current child neglect (T74.02, T76.02)

Z61.819   Personal history of unspecified abuse in childhood
Excludes1:   current child abuse NOS (T74.92, T76.92)

Z61.88   Other negative life events in childhood

Z61.9   Negative life event in childhood, unspecified

Z62   Other problems related to upbringing
Excludes2:   maltreatment syndrome (T74.-)

Z62.0   Inadequate parental supervision and control

Z62.1   Parental overprotection

Z62.2   Institutional upbringing

Z62.3   Hostility towards and scapegoating of child

Z62.6   Inappropriate parental pressure and other abnormal qualities of upbringing

Z62.8   Other specified problems related to upbringing

Z62.9   Problem related to upbringing, unspecified
Parent-child problem NOS

Z63   Other problems related to primary support group, including family circumstances
Excludes2:   maltreatment syndrome (T74.-, T76)
parent-child problems (Z62.-)
problems related to negative life events in childhood (Z61.-)
problems related to upbringing (Z62.-)

Z63.0   Problems in relationship with spouse or partner
Excludes1:   counseling for spousal or partner abuse problems (Z69.1)
counseling related to sexual attitude, behavior, and orientation (Z70.-)

Z63.1   Problems in relationship with in-laws

Z63.2   Inadequate family support

Z63.3   Absence of family member

Z63.4   Disappearance and death of family member
Assumed death of family member
Bereavement

Z63.5   Disruption of family by separation and divorce
Marital estrangement

Z63.6   Dependent relative needing care at home

Z63.7   Other stressful life events affecting family and household
Alcoholism in family
Anxiety (normal) about sick person in family
Drug addiction in family
Health problems within family
Ill or disturbed family member
Isolated family

Z63.8   Other specified problems related to primary support group
> Family discord NOS
> High expressed emotional level within family
> Inadequate or distorted communication within family
> Sibling rivalry

Z63.9   Problem related to primary support group, unspecified
> Relationship disorder NOS

Z64   Problems related to certain psychosocial circumstances

Z64.0   Problems related to unwanted pregnancy

Z64.1   Problems related to multiparity

Z64.4   Discord with counselors
> Discord with probation officer
> Discord with social worker

Z65   Problems related to other psychosocial circumstances

Z65.0   Conviction in civil and criminal proceedings without imprisonment

Z65.1   Imprisonment and other incarceration

Z65.2   Problems related to release from prison

Z65.3   Problems related to other legal circumstances
> Arrest
> Child custody or support proceedings
> Litigation
> Prosecution

Z65.4   Victim of crime and terrorism
> Victim of torture

Z65.5   Exposure to disaster, war and other hostilities
> Excludes1:   target of perceived discrimination or persecution (Z60.5)

Z65.8   Other specified problems related to psychosocial circumstances

Z65.9   Problem related to unspecified psychosocial circumstances

DO NOT RESUSCITATE STATUS (Z66)

Z66   Do not resuscitate
> Includes: DNR status

BLOOD TYPE (Z67)

Z67   Blood type

Z67.1   Type A blood
> **Z67.10   Type A blood, Rh positive**
> **Z67.11   Type A blood, Rh negative**

Z67.2   Type B blood
> **Z67.20   Type B blood, Rh positive**
> **Z67.21   Type B blood, Rh negative**

Z67.3   Type AB blood
> **Z67.30   Type AB blood, Rh positive**
> **Z67.31   Type AB blood, Rh negative**

Z67.4   Type O blood
> **Z67.40   Type O blood, Rh positive**
> **Z67.41   Type O blood, Rh negative**

Z67.9   Unspecified blood type
> **Z67.90   Unspecified blood type, Rh positive**
> **Z67.91   Unspecified blood type, Rh negative**

PERSONS ENCOUNTERING HEALTH SERVICES IN OTHER CIRCUMSTANCES (Z69-Z76)

Z69   Encounter for mental health services for victim and perpetrator of abuse
> Counseling for victims and perpetrators of abuse

Z69.0   Encounter for mental health services for child abuse problems
> **Z69.01   Encounter for mental health services for victim of parental child abuse**
> **Z69.02   Encounter for mental health services for perpetrator of parental child abuse**
> > Excludes1:   encounter for mental health services for non-parental child abuse (Z69.04)

Z69.03   Encounter for mental health services for victim of non-parental child abuse

Z69.04   Encounter for mental health services for perpetrator of non-parental child abuse

Z69.1   Encounter for mental health services for spousal or partner abuse problems
> **Z69.11   Encounter for mental health services for victim of spousal or partner abuse**
> **Z69.12   Encounter for mental health services for perpetrator of spousal or partner abuse**

Z69.8   Encounter for mental health services for other victim or perpetrator of abuse
> **Z69.81   Encounter for mental health services for other victim of abuse**
> **Z69.82   Encounter for mental health services for perpetrator of other abuse**

Z70   Counseling related to sexual attitude, behavior and orientation
> Encounter for mental health services for sexual attitude, behavior and orientation
> Excludes2:   contraceptive or procreative counseling (Z30-Z31)

Z70.0   Counseling related to sexual attitude

Z70.1   Counseling related to patient's sexual behavior and orientation
> Patient concerned regarding impotence
> Patient concerned regarding non-responsiveness
> Patient concerned regarding promiscuity
> Patient concerned regarding sexual orientation

Z70.2   Counseling related to sexual behavior and orientation of third party
> Advice sought regarding sexual behavior and orientation of child
> Advice sought regarding sexual behavior and orientation of partner
> Advice sought regarding sexual behavior and orientation of spouse

Z70.3   Counseling related to combined concerns regarding sexual attitude, behavior and orientation

Z70.8   Other sex counseling
> Encounter for sex education

Z70.9   Sex counseling, unspecified

Z71   Persons encountering health services for other counseling and medical advice, not elsewhere classified
> Excludes2:   contraceptive or procreation counseling (Z30-Z31)
> > sex counseling (Z70.-)

Z71.0   Person encountering health services to consult on behalf of another person
> Person encountering health services to seek advice or treatment for non-attending third party
> Excludes2:   anxiety (normal) about sick person in family (Z63.7)

Z71.1   Person with feared health complaint in whom no diagnosis is made
> Person encountering health services with feared condition which was not demonstrated
> Person encountering health services in which problem was normal state
> "Worried well"
> Excludes1:   medical observation and evaluation for suspected diseases and conditions proven not to exist (Z03.-)

Z71.2   Person consulting for explanation of examination or test findings

Z71.3   Dietary counseling and surveillance
> Use additional code for underlying medical condition

Z71.4   Alcohol abuse counseling and surveillance
> Use additional code for alcohol abuse or dependence (F10.-)
> **Z71.41   Alcohol abuse counseling and surveillance of alcoholic**
> **Z71.42   Counseling for family member of alcoholic**
> > Counseling for significant other, partner, or friend of alcoholic

Z71.5 Drug abuse counseling and surveillance
Use additional code for drug abuse or dependence (F11-F16, F18-F19)

Z71.51   Drug abuse counseling and surveillance of drug abuser

Z71.52   Counseling for family member of drug abuser
Counseling for significant other, partner, or friend of drug abuser

Z71.6 Tobacco abuse counseling
Use additional code for nicotine dependence (F17.-)

Z71.7 Human immunodeficiency virus [HIV] counseling

Z71.8 Other specified counseling
Excludes2:   counseling for contraception (Z30.0)
counseling for genetic (Z31.5)
counseling for procreative management (Z31.6)

Z71.81   Spiritual or religious counseling

Z71.89   Other specified counseling

Z71.9 Counseling, unspecified
Encounter for medical advice NOS

Z72 Problems related to lifestyle
Excludes2:   problems related to life-management difficulty (Z73.-)
problems related to socioeconomic and psychosocial circumstances (Z55-Z65)

Z72.0 Tobacco use
Tobacco use NOS
Excludes1:   history of tobacco dependence (Z87.82)
nicotine dependence (F17.2-)
tobacco dependence (F17.2-)
tobacco use during pregnancy (O99.33-)

Z72.3 Lack of physical exercise

Z72.4 Inappropriate diet and eating habits
Excludes1:   behavioral eating disorders of infancy or childhood (F98.2- - F98.3)
eating disorders (F50.-)
lack of adequate food (Z59.4)
malnutrition and other nutritional deficiencies (E40-E64)

Z72.5 High-risk sexual behavior
Promiscuity
Excludes1:   paraphilias (F65)

Z72.51   High-risk heterosexual behavior

Z72.52   High-risk homosexual behavior

Z72.53   High-risk bisexual behavior

Z72.6 Gambling and betting
Excludes1:   compulsive or pathological gambling (F63.0)

Z72.8 Other problems related to lifestyle

Z72.81   Antisocial behavior

Z72.810   Child and adolescent antisocial behavior
Delinquency NOS
Group delinquency
Offences in the context of gang membership
Stealing in company with others
Truancy from school

Z72.811   Adult antisocial behavior

Z72.89   Other problems related to lifestyle
Self-damaging behavior

Z72.9 Problem related to lifestyle, unspecified

Z73 Problems related to life-management difficulty
Excludes2:   problems related to socioeconomic and psychosocial circumstances (Z55-Z65)

Z73.0 Burn-out

Z73.1 Type A behavior pattern

Z73.2 Lack of relaxation and leisure

Z73.3 Stress, not elsewhere classified
Physical and mental strain NOS
Excludes1:   stress related to employment or unemployment (Z56.-)

Z73.4 Inadequate social skills, not elsewhere classified

Z73.5 Social role conflict, not elsewhere classified

Z73.6 Limitation of activities due to disability
Excludes1:   care-provider dependency (Z74.-)

Z73.8 Other problems related to life-management difficulty

Z73.9 Problem related to life-management difficulty, unspecified

Z74 Problems related to care-provider dependency
Excludes2:   dependence on enabling machines or devices NEC (Z99.-)

Z74.0 Reduced mobility
Bedridden
Chairridden

Z74.1 Need for assistance with personal care

Z74.2 Need for assistance at home and no other household member able to render care

Z74.3 Need for continuous supervision

Z74.8 Other problems related to care-provider dependency

Z74.9 Problem related to care-provider dependency, unspecified

Z75 Problems related to medical facilities and other health care

Z75.0 Medical services not available in home
Excludes1:   no other household member able to render care (Z74.2)

Z75.1 Person awaiting admission to adequate facility elsewhere

Z75.2 Other waiting period for investigation and treatment

Z75.3 Unavailability and inaccessibility of health-care facilities
Excludes1:   bed unavailable (Z75.1)

Z75.4 Unavailability and inaccessibility of other helping agencies

Z75.5 Holiday relief care

Z75.8 Other problems related to medical facilities and other health care

Z75.81   Organ donor transplant candidate
Patient waiting for organ availability

Z75.89   Other problems related to medical facilities and other health care

Z75.9 Unspecified problem related to medical facilities and other health care

Z76 Persons encountering health services in other circumstances

Z76.0 Encounter for issue of repeat prescription
Encounter for issue of repeat prescription for appliance
Encounter for issue of repeat prescription for medicaments
Encounter for issue of repeat prescription for spectacles
Excludes2:   issue of medical certificate (Z02.7)
repeat prescription for contraceptive (Z30.4-)

Z76.1 Encounter for health supervision and care of foundling

Z76.2 Encounter for health supervision and care of other healthy infant and child
Encounter for medical or nursing care or supervision of healthy infant under circumstances such as adverse socioeconomic conditions at home
Encounter for medical or nursing care or supervision of healthy infant under circumstances such as awaiting foster or adoptive placement
Encounter for medical or nursing care or supervision of healthy infant under circumstances such as maternal illness
Encounter for medical or nursing care or supervision of healthy infant under circumstances such as number of children at home preventing or interfering with normal care

Z76.3 Healthy person accompanying sick person

Z76.4 Other boarder to health-care facility
Excludes1:   homelessness (Z59.0)

Z76.5 Malingerer [conscious simulation]
Person feigning illness (with obvious motivation)
Excludes1:   factitious disorder (F68.1-)
peregrinating patient (F68.1-)

Z76.8 Persons encountering health services in other specified circumstances

Z76.9 Person encountering health services in unspecified circumstances

PERSONS WITH POTENTIAL HEALTH HAZARDS RELATED TO FAMILY AND PERSONAL HISTORY AND CERTAIN CONDITIONS INFLUENCING HEALTH STATUS (Z79-Z99)
Code also any follow-up examination (Z08-Z09)

Z79 Long-term (current) drug therapy
Code also any therapeutic drug level monitoring (Z51.81)
Excludes2: drug abuse and dependence (F11-F19)

- **Z79.1** Long-term (current) use of anticoagulants
- **Z79.2** Long-term (current) use of antithrombotics/antiplatelets
- **Z79.3** Long-term (current) use of anti-inflammatories
- **Z79.4** Long-term (current) use of antibiotics
- **Z79.5** Long-term (current) use of oral contraceptives
- **Z79.6** Postmenopausal hormone replacement therapy
- **Z79.7** Long-term (current) use of insulin
- **Z79.8** Other long-term (current) drug therapy
  - **Z79.81** Long-term (current) use of multiple prescription drugs
    Polypharmacy
  - **Z79.89** Other long-term (current) drug therapy

Z80 Family history of primary malignant neoplasm
- **Z80.0** Family history of malignant neoplasm of digestive organs
  Conditions classifiable to C15-C26
- **Z80.1** Family history of malignant neoplasm of trachea, bronchus and lung
  Conditions classifiable to C33-C34
- **Z80.2** Family history of malignant neoplasm of other respiratory and intrathoracic organs
  Conditions classifiable to C30-C32, C37-C39
- **Z80.3** Family history of malignant neoplasm of breast
  Conditions classifiable to C50.-
- **Z80.4** Family history of malignant neoplasm of genital organs
  Conditions classifiable to C51-C63
  - **Z80.41** Family history of malignant neoplasm of ovary
  - **Z80.42** Family history of malignant neoplasm of prostate
  - **Z80.43** Family history of malignant neoplasm of testis
  - **Z80.49** Family history of malignant neoplasm of other genital organs
- **Z80.5** Family history of malignant neoplasm of urinary tract
  Conditions classifiable to C64-C68
  - **Z80.51** Family history of malignant neoplasm of kidney
  - **Z80.59** Family history of malignant neoplasm of other urinary tract organ
- **Z80.6** Family history of leukemia
  Conditions classifiable to C91-C95
- **Z80.7** Family history of other malignant neoplasms of lymphoid, hematopoietic and related tissues
  Conditions classifiable to C81-C90, C96.-
- **Z80.8** Family history of malignant neoplasm of other organs or systems
  Conditions classifiable to C00-C14, C40-C49, C69-C79
- **Z80.9** Family history of malignant neoplasm, unspecified
  Conditions classifiable to C80

Z81 Family history of mental and behavioral disorders
- **Z81.0** Family history of mental retardation
  Conditions classifiable to F70-F79
- **Z81.1** Family history of alcohol abuse and dependence
  Conditions classifiable to F10.-
- **Z81.2** Family history of tobacco abuse and dependence
  Conditions classifiable to F17.-
- **Z81.3** Family history of other psychoactive substance abuse and dependence
  Conditions classifiable to F11-F16, F18-F19
- **Z81.4** Family history of other substance abuse and dependence
  Conditions classifiable to F55
- **Z81.8** Family history of other mental and behavioral disorders
  Conditions classifiable elsewhere in F01-F99

Z82 Family history of certain disabilities and chronic diseases (leading to disablement)
- **Z82.0** Family history of epilepsy and other diseases of the nervous system
  Conditions classifiable to G00-G99
- **Z82.1** Family history of blindness and visual loss
  Conditions classifiable to H54.-
- **Z82.2** Family history of deafness and hearing loss
  Conditions classifiable to H90-H91
- **Z82.3** Family history of stroke
  Conditions classifiable to I60-I64
- **Z82.4** Family history of ischemic heart disease and other diseases of the circulatory system
  Conditions classifiable to I00-I52, I65-I99
- **Z82.5** Family history of asthma and other chronic lower respiratory diseases
  Conditions classifiable to J40-J47
- **Z82.6** Family history of arthritis and other diseases of the musculoskeletal system and connective tissue
  Conditions classifiable to M00-M99
- **Z82.7** Family history of congenital malformations, deformations and chromosomal abnormalities
  Conditions classifiable to Q00-Q99
  - **Z82.71** Family history of polycystic kidney
  - **Z82.79** Family history of other congenital malformations, deformations and chromosomal abnormalities
- **Z82.8** Family history of other disabilities and chronic diseases leading to disablement, not elsewhere classified

Z83 Family history of other specific disorders
Excludes2: contact with or exposure to communicable disease in the family (Z20.-)
- **Z83.0** Family history of human immunodeficiency virus [HIV] disease
  Conditions classifiable to B20
- **Z83.1** Family history of other infectious and parasitic diseases
  Conditions classifiable to A00-B19, B25-B94, B99
- **Z83.2** Family history of diseases of the blood and blood-forming organs and certain disorders involving the immune mechanism
  Conditions classifiable to D50-D89
- **Z83.3** Family history of diabetes mellitus
  Conditions classifiable to E09-E13
- **Z83.4** Family history of other endocrine, nutritional and metabolic diseases
  Conditions classifiable to E00-E07, E15-E90
- **Z83.5** Family history of eye and ear disorders
  Conditions classifiable to H00-H53, H55-H83, H92-H95
  Excludes2: family history of blindness and visual loss (Z82.1)
    family history of deafness and hearing loss (Z82.2)
- **Z83.6** Family history of diseases of the respiratory system
  Conditions classifiable to J00-J39, J60-J99
  Excludes2: family history of chronic lower respiratory diseases (Z82.5)
- **Z83.7** Family history of diseases of the digestive system
  Conditions classifiable to K00-K93

Z84 Family history of other conditions
- **Z84.0** Family history of diseases of the skin and subcutaneous tissue
  Conditions classifiable to L00-L99
- **Z84.1** Family history of disorders of kidney and ureter
  Conditions classifiable to N00-N29
- **Z84.2** Family history of other diseases of the genitourinary system
  Conditions classifiable to N30-N99
- **Z84.3** Family history of consanguinity
- **Z84.8** Family history of other specified conditions

Z85 Personal history of primary and secondary malignant neoplasm

Code first any follow-up examination after treatment of malignant neoplasm (Z08)

Use additional code to identify:

alcohol use and dependence (F10.0-)

alcohol dependence in remission (F10.11)

exposure to environmental tobacco smoke (X58.1)

history of tobacco use (Z87.82)

occupational exposure to environmental tobacco smoke (Z57.31)

tobacco dependence (F17.-)

tobacco use (Z72.0)

Excludes2:   personal history of benign neoplasm (Z86.01-)

personal history of carcinoma-in-situ (Z86.00-)

Z85.0   Personal history of primary malignant neoplasm of digestive organs

Conditions classifiable to C15-C26

Z85.00   Personal history of primary malignant neoplasm of unspecified digestive organ

Z85.01   Personal history of primary malignant neoplasm of esophagus

Z85.02   Personal history of primary malignant neoplasm of stomach

Z85.03   Personal history of primary malignant neoplasm of large intestine

Z85.04   Personal history of primary malignant neoplasm of rectum, rectosigmoid junction, and anus

Z85.05   Personal history of primary malignant neoplasm of liver

Z85.09   Personal history of primary malignant neoplasm of other digestive organs

Z85.1   Personal history of primary malignant neoplasm of trachea, bronchus and lung

Conditions classifiable to C33-C34

Z85.11   Personal history of primary malignant neoplasm of bronchus and lung

Z85.12   Personal history of primary malignant neoplasm of trachea

Z85.2   Personal history of primary malignant neoplasm of other respiratory and intrathoracic organs

Conditions classifiable to C30-C32, C37-C39

Z85.20   Personal history of primary malignant neoplasm of unspecified respiratory organ

Z85.21   Personal history of primary malignant neoplasm of larnyx

Z85.22   Personal history of primary malignant neoplasm of nasal cavities, middle ear, and accessory sinuses

Z85.29   Personal history of primary malignant neoplasm of other respiratory and intrathoracic organs

Z85.3   Personal history of primary malignant neoplasm of breast

Conditions classifiable to C50.-

Z85.4   Personal history of primary malignant neoplasm of genital organs

Conditions classifiable to C51-C63

Z85.40   Personal history of primary malignant neoplasm of unspecified female genital organ

Z85.41   Personal history of primary malignant neoplasm of cervix uteri

Z85.42   Personal history of primary malignant neoplasm of other parts of uterus

Z85.43   Personal history of primary malignant neoplasm of ovary

Z85.44   Personal history of primary malignant neoplasm of other female genital organs

Z85.45   Personal history of primary malignant neoplasm of unspecified male genital organ

Z85.46   Personal history of primary malignant neoplasm of prostate

Z85.47   Personal history of primary malignant neoplasm of testis

Z85.48   Personal history of primary malignant neoplasm of epididymis

Z85.49   Personal history of primary malignant neoplasm of other male genital organs

Z85.5   Personal history of primary malignant neoplasm of urinary tract

Conditions classifiable to C64-C68

Z85.50   Personal history of primary malignant neoplasm of unspecified urinary tract organ

Z85.51   Personal history of primary malignant neoplasm of bladder

Z85.52   Personal history of primary malignant neoplasm of kidney

Excludes1:   personal history of primary malignant neoplasm of renal pelvis (Z85.53)

Z85.53   Personal history of primary malignant neoplasm of renal pelvis

Z85.59   Personal history of primary malignant neoplasm of other urinary tract organ

Z85.8   Personal history of primary malignant neoplasms of other organs and systems and secondary malignant neoplasms

Conditions classifiable to C00-C14, C40-C49, C69-C79

Z85.81   Personal history of primary malignant neoplasm of lip, oral cavity, and pharynx

Z85.810   Personal history of primary malignant neoplasm of tongue

Z85.818   Personal history of primary malignant neoplasm of other sites of lip, oral cavity, and pharynx

Z85.819   Personal history of primary malignant neoplasm of unspecified site of lip, oral cavity, and pharynx

Z85.82   Personal history of primary malignant neoplasm of skin, bone, and soft tissue

Z85.820   Personal history of malignant melanoma of skin

Z85.821   Personal history of other primary malignant neoplasm of skin

Z85.822   Personal history of primary malignant neoplasm of bone

Z85.828   Personal history of primary malignant neoplasm of other soft tissue

Z85.83   Personal history of primary malignant neoplasm of eye and nervous tissue

Z85.830   Personal history of primary malignant neoplasm of eye

Z85.831   Personal history of primary malignant neoplasm of brain

Z85.838   Personal history of primary malignant neoplasm of other parts of nervous tissue

Z85.84   Personal history of primary malignant neoplasm of endocrine glands

Z85.840   Personal history of primary malignant neoplasm of thyroid

Z85.848   Personal history of primary malignant neoplasm of other endocrine glands

Z85.85   Personal history of primary malignant neoplasm of other organs and systems

Z85.86   Personal history of secondary malignant neoplasms

Z85.860   Personal history of secondary malignant neoplasms of lung

Z85.861   Personal history of secondary malignant neoplasms of liver

Z85.862   Personal history of secondary malignant neoplasms of brain

Z85.863   Personal history of secondary malignant neoplasms of bone

Z85.868   Personal history of secondary malignant neoplasms of other sites

Z85.9   Personal history of unspecified primary malignant neoplasm

Conditions classifiable to C80

Z86 Personal history of certain other diseases
  Code first any follow-up examination after treatment (Z09)

Z86.0 Personal history of in-situ and benign neoplasms and neoplasms of uncertain behavior
  Excludes2:   personal history of primary and secondary malignant neoplasms (Z85.-)

  Z86.00   Personal history of in-situ neoplasm
    Z86.000   Personal history of in-situ neoplasm of breast
    Z86.008   Personal history of in-situ neoplasm of other site
  Z86.01   Personal history of benign neoplasm
    Z86.010   Personal history of colonic polyps
    Z86.011   Personal history of benign neoplasm of the brain
    Z86.018   Personal history of other benign neoplasm
  Z86.03   Personal history of neoplasm of uncertain behavior

Z86.1 Personal history of infectious and parasitic diseases
  Conditions classifiable to A00-B89, B99
  Excludes1:   sequelae of infectious and parasitic diseases (B90-B94)

  Z86.11   Personal history of tuberculosis
  Z86.12   Personal history of poliomyelitis
  Z86.13   Personal history of malaria
  Z86.19   Personal history of other infectious and parasitic diseases

Z86.2 Personal history of diseases of the blood and blood-forming organs and certain disorders involving the immune mechanism
  Conditions classifiable to D50-D89

Z86.3 Personal history of endocrine, nutritional and metabolic diseases
  Conditions classifiable to E00-E90

  Z86.31   Personal history of diabetic foot ulcer
    Excludes2:   current diabetic foot ulcer (E09.640, E10.640, E11.640, E13.640)
  Z86.39   Personal history of other endocrine, nutritional and metabolic disease

Z86.6 Personal history of diseases of the nervous system and sense organs
  Conditions classifiable to G00-G99, H00-H95

Z86.7 Personal history of diseases of the circulatory system
  Conditions classifiable to I00-I99
  Excludes2:   old myocardial infarction (I25.2)
                postmyocardial infarction syndrome (I24.1)
                sequelae of cerebrovascular disease (I69.-)

  Z86.71   Personal history of venous thrombosis and embolism
  Z86.72   Personal history of thrombophlebitis
  Z86.79   Personal history of other diseases of the circulatory system

Z87 Personal history of other diseases and conditions
  Code first any:
  follow-up examination after treatment (Z09)

Z87.0 Personal history of diseases of the respiratory system
  Conditions classifiable to J00-J99

Z87.1 Personal history of diseases of the digestive system
  Conditions classifiable to K00-K93

  Z87.11   Personal history of peptic ulcer disease
  Z87.19   Personal history of other diseases of the digestive system

Z87.2 Personal history of diseases of the skin and subcutaneous tissue
  Conditions classifiable to L00-L99
  Excludes2:   personal history of diabetic foot ulcer (Z86.31)

Z87.3 Personal history of diseases of the musculoskeletal system and connective tissue
  Conditions classifiable to M00-M99

  Z87.31   Personal history of osteoporosis fractures
  Z87.39   Personal history of other diseases of the musculoskeletal system and connective tissue

Z87.4 Personal history of diseases of the genitourinary system
  Conditions classifiable to N00-N99

Z87.5 Personal history of complications of pregnancy, childbirth and the puerperium
  Conditions classifiable to O00-O99
  Personal history of trophoblastic disease
  Excludes2:   habitual aborter (N96)

Z87.7 Personal history of congenital malformations and deformations
  Conditions classifiable to Q00-Q89

  Z87.71   Personal history of hypospadias
  Z87.79   Personal history of other congenital malformations and deformations

Z87.8 Personal history of other specified conditions
  Z87.81   Personal history of sex reassignment
  Z87.82   Personal history of nicotine dependence
    Excludes1:   current nicotine dependence (F17.2-)
  Z87.89   Personal history of other specified conditions
    Conditions classifiable to S00-T98

Z88 Allergy status to drugs, medicaments and biological substances
  Excludes2:   allergy status, other than to drugs and biological substances (Z91.0-)

Z88.0 Allergy status to penicillin
Z88.1 Allergy status to other antibiotic agents status
Z88.2 Allergy status to sulfonamides status
Z88.3 Allergy status to other anti-infective agents status
Z88.4 Allergy status to anesthetic agent status
Z88.5 Allergy status to narcotic agent status
Z88.6 Allergy status to analgesic agent status
Z88.7 Allergy status to serum and vaccine status
Z88.8 Allergy status to other drugs, medicaments and biological substances status
Z88.9 Allergy status to unspecified drugs, medicaments and biological substances status

Z89 Acquired absence of limb
  Includes: amputation status
               postoperative loss of limb
               post-traumatic loss of limb
  Excludes1:   acquired deformities of limbs (M20-M21)
               congenital absence of limbs (Q71-Q73)

Z89.0 Acquired absence of thumb and other finger(s)
  Z89.01   Acquired absence of thumb
    Z89.011   Acquired absence of right thumb
    Z89.012   Acquired absence of left thumb
    Z89.019   Acquired absence of unspecified thumb
  Z89.02   Acquired absence of other finger(s)
    Excludes2:   acquired absence of thumb (Z89.01-)
    Z89.021   Acquired absence of right finger(s)
    Z89.022   Acquired absence of left finger(s)
    Z89.029   Acquired absence of unspecified finger(s)

Z89.1 Acquired absence of hand and wrist
  Z89.11   Acquired absence of hand
    Z89.111   Acquired absence of right hand
    Z89.112   Acquired absence of left hand
    Z89.119   Acquired absence of unspecified hand
  Z89.12   Acquired absence of wrist
    Disarticulation at wrist
    Z89.121   Acquired absence of right wrist
    Z89.122   Acquired absence of left wrist
    Z89.129   Acquired absence of unspecified wrist

Z89.2 Acquired absence of upper limb above wrist
  Z89.20   Acquired absence of upper limb, unspecified level
    Z89.201   Acquired absence of right upper limb, unspecified level
    Z89.202   Acquired absence of left upper limb, unspecified level
    Z89.209   Acquired absence of unspecified upper limb, unspecified level
      Acquired absence of arm NOS

Z89.21   Acquired absence of upper limb below elbow
    Z89.211   Acquired absence of right upper limb below elbow
    Z89.212   Acquired absence of left upper limb below elbow
    Z89.219   Acquired absence of unspecified upper limb below elbow

Z89.22   Acquired absence of upper limb above elbow
    Disarticulation at elbow
    Z89.221   Acquired absence of right upper limb above elbow
    Z89.222   Acquired absence of left upper limb above elbow
    Z89.229   Acquired absence of unspecified upper limb above elbow

Z89.23   Acquired absence of shoulder
    Z89.231   Acquired absence of right shoulder
    Z89.232   Acquired absence of left shoulder
    Z89.239   Acquired absence of unspecified shoulder

Z89.4   Acquired absence of toes(s), foot, and ankle
  Z89.41   Acquired absence of great toe
    Z89.411   Acquired absence of right great toe
    Z89.412   Acquired absence of left great toe
    Z89.419   Acquired absence of unspecified great toe

  Z89.42   Acquired absence of other toe(s)
    Excludes2:   acquired absence of great toe (Z89.41-)
    Z89.421   Acquired absence of other right toe(s)
    Z89.422   Acquired absence of other left toe(s)
    Z89.429   Acquired absence of other toe(s), unspecified side

  Z89.43   Acquired absence of foot
    Z89.431   Acquired absence of right foot
    Z89.432   Acquired absence of left foot
    Z89.439   Acquired absence of unspecified foot

  Z89.44   Acquired absence of ankle
    Disarticulation of ankle
    Z89.441   Acquired absence of right ankle
    Z89.442   Acquired absence of left ankle
    Z89.449   Acquired absence of unspecified ankle

Z89.5   Acquired absence of leg below knee
  Z89.50   Acquired absence of leg knee, unspecified side
  Z89.51   Acquired absence of right leg below knee
  Z89.52   Acquired absence of left leg below knee

Z89.6   Acquired absence of leg above knee
  Z89.61   Acquired absence of leg above knee
    Acquired absence of leg NOS
    Disarticulation at knee
    Z89.611   Acquired absence of right leg above knee
    Z89.612   Acquired absence of left leg above knee
    Z89.619   Acquired absence of unspecified leg above knee

  Z89.62   Acquired absence of hip
    Disarticulation at hip
    Z89.621   Acquired absence of right hip
    Z89.622   Acquired absence of left hip
    Z89.629   Acquired absence of unspecified hip

Z89.9   Acquired absence of limb, unspecified

Z90   Acquired absence of organs, not elsewhere classified
  Includes: postoperative or post-traumatic loss of body part NEC
  Excludes1:   congenital absencez—see Alphabetical Index
  Excludes2:   postoperative absence of endocrine glands (E89.-)

Z90.0   Acquired absence of part of head and neck
  Z90.01   Acquired absence of eye
  Z90.02   Acquired absence of larynx
  Z90.09   Acquired absence of other part of head and neck
    Acquired absence of nose
    Excludes2:   teeth (K08.1)

Z90.1   Acquired absence of breast(s)
Z90.2   Acquired absence of lung [part of]

Z90.3   Acquired absence of stomach [part of]
Z90.4   Acquired absence of other parts of digestive tract
Z90.5   Acquired absence of kidney
Z90.6   Acquired absence of other parts of urinary tract
Z90.7   Acquired absence of genital organ(s)
  Excludes1:   personal history of sex reassignment (Z87.81)
  Z90.71   Acquired absence of uterus
  Z90.79   Acquired absence of other genital organ(s)

Z90.8   Acquired absence of other organs
  Z90.81   Acquired absence of spleen
  Z90.89   Acquired absence of other organs

Z91   Personal risk-factors, not elsewhere classified
  Excludes2:   exposure to pollution and other problems related to physical environment (Z58.-)
    occupational exposure to risk-factors (Z57.-)

Z91.0   Allergy status, other than to drugs and biological substances
  Excludes2:   allergy status to drugs, medicaments, and biological substances (Z88.-)
  Z91.01   Food allergy status
    Z91.010   Allergy to peanuts
    Z91.011   Allergy to milk products
      Excludes1:   lactose intolerance (E73.-)
    Z91.012   Allergy to eggs
    Z91.013   Allergy to seafood
    Z91.018   Allergy to other foods

  Z91.02   Food additives allergy status
  Z91.03   Insect allergy status
    Z91.030   Bee allergy status
    Z91.038   Other insect allergy status

  Z91.04   Nonmedicinal substance allergy status
    Z91.040   Latex allergy status
    Z91.041   Radiographic dye allergy status
      Allergy status to contrast media used for diagnostic x-ray procedure
    Z91.048   Other nonmedicinal substance allergy status

  Z91.09   Other allergy status, other than to drugs and biological substances

Z91.1   Noncompliance with medical treatment and regimen
  Z91.11   Drug withdrawal symptoms due to taking reduced dosage of medication not in accordance with prescribed amount
    Code first withdrawal symptoms
    Excludes1:   adverse effect of prescribed drug taken as directed-code to adverse effect
      poisoning or toxic effect-code to poisoning or toxic effect
  Z91.12   Other noncompliance with medication regimen
  Z91.13   Noncompliance with dietary regimen
  Z91.19   Other noncompliance with medical treatment and regimen

Z91.3   Unhealthy sleep-wake schedule
  Excludes1:   sleep disorders (G47.-)

Z91.4   Personal history of psychological trauma, not elsewhere classified
  Z91.41   Personal history of adult physical and sexual abuse
    Personal history of adult neglect
    Excludes1:   current adult neglect (T74.01, T76.01)
      current adult physical abuse (T74.11, T76.11)
      current adult sexual abuse (T74. 21, T76.11)
  Z91.49   Other personal history of psychological trauma, not elsewhere classified

Z91.5   Personal history of self-harm
  Personal history of parasuicide
  Personal history of self-poisoning
  Personal history of suicide attempt

Z91.7   Low birth weight and immaturity status
    Excludes1:   current immaturity (P07.2-, P07.3-)
                current low birth weight (P05.0, P05.1, P07.0-, P07.1-)

   Z91.71   Low birth weight status
      Z91.710   Low birth weight status, less than 500 grams
      Z91.711   Low birth weight status, 500-999 grams
      Z91.712   Low birth weight status, 1000-1499
      Z91.713   Low birth weight status, 1500-1999 grams
      Z91.714   Low birth weight status, 2000-2500 grams
      Z91.719   Low birth weight status, unspecified

   Z91.72   Immaturity status
      Z91.720   Immaturity status, less than 28 weeks (less than 196 days) gestation
      Z91.721   Immaturity status, 28 weeks or more but less than 37 weeks (196 days but less than 259 days) gestation
      Z91.729   Immaturity status, unspecified

Z91.8   Other specified personal risk-factors, not elsewhere classified

Z92   Personal history of medical treatment
  Z92.0   Personal history of contraception
    Excludes1:   counseling or management of current contraceptive practices (Z30.-)
            long-term (current) use of contraception (Z79.8)
            presence of (intrauterine) contraceptive device (Z97.5)

  Z92.3   Personal history of irradiation
    Personal history of exposure to therapeutic radiation
    Excludes1:   exposure to radiation in the physical environment (Z58.4)
            occupational exposure to radiation (Z57.1)

  Z92.4   Personal history of major surgery, not elsewhere classified
    Excludes2:   artificial opening status (Z93.-)
            postsurgical states (Z98.-)
            presence of functional implants and grafts (Z95-Z96)
            transplanted organ or tissue status (Z94.-)

Z93   Artificial opening status
    Excludes1:   artificial openings requiring attention or management (Z43.-)
            complications of external stoma (J95.0-, K91.4-, K91.7-, N99.5-)

  Z93.0   Tracheostomy status
  Z93.1   Gastrostomy status
  Z93.2   Ileostomy status
  Z93.3   Colostomy status
  Z93.4   Other artificial openings of gastrointestinal tract status
  Z93.5   Cystostomy status
    Z93.50   Unspecified cystostomy status
    Z93.51   Cutaneous-vesicostomy status
    Z93.52   Appendico-vesicostomy status
    Z93.59   Other cystostomy status
  Z93.6   Other artificial openings of urinary tract status
    Nephrostomy status
    Ureterostomy status
    Urethrostomy status
  Z93.8   Other artificial opening status
  Z93.9   Artificial opening status, unspecified

Z94   Transplanted organ and tissue status
    Includes: organ or tissue replaced by heterogenous or homogenous transplant
    Excludes1:   complications of transplanted organ or tissue—see Alphabetical Index
    Excludes2:   presence of vascular grafts (Z95.-)
  Z94.0   Kidney transplant status
  Z94.1   Heart transplant status
    Excludes1:   heart-valve replacement status (Z95.2-Z95.4)
  Z94.2   Lung transplant status

Z94.3   Heart and lungs transplant status
Z94.4   Liver transplant status
Z94.5   Skin transplant status
    Autogenous skin transplant status
Z94.6   Bone transplant status
Z94.7   Corneal transplant status
Z94.8   Other transplanted organ and tissue status
  Z94.81   Bone marrow transplant status
  Z94.82   Intestine transplant status
  Z94.83   Pancreas transplant status
  Z94.84   Stem cells transplant status
  Z94.89   Other transplanted organ and tissue status
Z94.9   Transplanted organ and tissue status, unspecified

Z95   Presence of cardiac and vascular implants and grafts
    Excludes1:   complications of cardiac and vascular devices, implants and grafts (T82.-)
  Z95.0   Presence of cardiac pacemaker
    Excludes1:   adjustment or management of cardiac pacemaker
  Z95.1   Presence of aortocoronary bypass graft
  Z95.2   Presence of prosthetic heart valve
  Z95.3   Presence of xenogenic heart valve
  Z95.4   Presence of other heart-valve replacement
  Z95.5   Presence of coronary angioplasty implant and graft
    Z95.50   Coronary angioplasty status
      Status following coronary angioplasty NOS
    Z95.51   Coronary angioplasty status with implant (Z45.0)
      Presence of coronary artery prosthesis
    Z95.59   Other coronary angioplasty status
  Z95.8   Presence of other cardiac and vascular implants and grafts
    Z95.81   Presence of automatic (implantable) cardiac defibrillator
    Z95.82   Peripheral vascular angioplasty status
      Status following peripheral angioplasty NOS
    Z95.83   Periperal vascular angioplasty status with implants and grafts
    Z95.89   Presence of other cardiac and vascular implants and grafts
      Presence of intravascular prosthesis NEC
  Z95.9   Presence of cardiac and vascular implant and graft, unspecified

Z96   Presence of other functional implants
    Excludes1:   complications of internal prosthetic devices, implants and grafts (T82-T85)
            fitting and adjustment of prosthetic and other devices (Z44-Z46)
  Z96.0   Presence of urogenital implants
  Z96.1   Presence of intraocular lens
    Presence of pseudophakia
  Z96.2   Presence of otological and audiological implants
    Z96.20   Presence of otological and audiological implant, unspecified
    Z96.21   Cochlear implant status
    Z96.22   Myringotomy tube(s) status
    Z96.29   Presence of other otological and audiological implants
      Presence of bone-conduction hearing device
      Presence of eustachian tube stent
      Stapes replacement
  Z96.3   Presence of artificial larynx
  Z96.4   Presence of endocrine implants
    Presence of insulin pump
  Z96.5   Presence of tooth-root and mandibular implants
  Z96.6   Presence of orthopedic joint implants
    Z96.60   Presence of unspecified orthopedic joint implant
    Z96.61   Presence of artificial shoulder joint
      Z96.611   Presence of right artificial shoulder joint
      Z96.612   Presence of left artificial shoulder joint
      Z96.619   Presence of unspecified artificial shoulder joint

Z96.62   Presence of artificial elbow joint
   Z96.621   Presence of right artificial elbow joint
   Z96.622   Presence of left artificial elbow joint
   Z96.629   Presence of unspecified artificial elbow joint
Z96.63   Presence of artificial wrist joint
   Z96.631   Presence of right artificial wrist joint
   Z96.632   Presence of left artificial wrist joint
   Z96.639   Presence of unspecified artificial wrist joint
Z96.64   Presence of artificial hip joint
      Hip-joint replacement (partial) (total)
   Z96.641   Presence of right artificial hip joint
   Z96.642   Presence of left artificial hip joint
   Z96.643   Presence of artificial hip joint, bilateral
   Z96.649   Presence of unspecified artificial hip joint
Z96.65   Presence of artificial knee joint
   Z96.651   Presence of right artificial knee joint
   Z96.652   Presence of left artificial knee joint
   Z96.653   Presence of artificial knee joint, bilateral
   Z96.659   Presence of unspecified artificial knee joint
Z96.66   Presence of artificial ankle joint
   Z96.661   Presence of right artificial ankle joint
   Z96.662   Presence of left artificial ankle joint
   Z96.669   Presence of unspecified artificial ankle joint
Z96.69   Presence of other orthopedic joint implants
   Z96.691   Finger-joint replacement of right hand
   Z96.692   Finger-joint replacement of left hand
   Z96.693   Finger-joint replacement, bilateral
   Z96.698   Presence of other orthopedic joint implants
Z96.7   Presence of other bone and tendon implants
      Presence of skull plate
Z96.8   Presence of other specified functional implants
   Z96.81   Presence of artificial skin
   Z96.89   Presence of other specified functional implants
Z96.9   Presence of functional implant, unspecified

Z97 Presence of other devices
   Excludes1:   complications of internal prosthetic devices, implants and grafts (T82-T85)
      fitting and adjustment of prosthetic and other devices (Z44-Z46)
   Excludes2:   presence of cerebrospinal fluid drainage device (Z98.2)
Z97.0   Presence of artificial eye
Z97.1   Presence of artificial limb (complete) (partial)
   Z97.10   Presence of artificial limb (complete) (partial), unspecified
   Z97.11   Presence of artificial right arm (complete) (partial)
   Z97.12   Presence of artificial left arm (complete) (partial)
   Z97.13   Presence of artificial right leg(complete) (partial)
   Z97.14   Presence of artificial left leg (complete) (partial)
   Z97.15   Presence of artificial arms, bilateral (complete) (partial)
   Z97.16   Presence of artificial legs, bilateral (complete) (partial)
Z97.2   Presence of dental prosthetic device (complete) (partial)
Z97.3   Presence of spectacles and contact lenses
Z97.4   Presence of external hearing-aid
Z97.5   Presence of (intrauterine) contraceptive device
   Excludes1:   checking, reinsertion or removal of contraceptive device (Z30.44)
Z97.8   Presence of other specified devices

Z98 Other postsurgical states
   Excludes2:   follow-up medical care (Z42-Z51)
      postprocedural or postoperative complication—see Alphabetical Index
Z98.0   Intestinal bypass and anastomosis status
Z98.1   Arthrodesis status
Z98.2   Presence of cerebrospinal fluid drainage device
      Presence of CSF shunt

Z98.3   Post therapeutic collapse of lung status
      Code first underlying disease
Z98.4   Cataract extraction status
      Use additional code to identify intraocular lens implant status (Z96.1)
      Excludes1:   aphakia (H27.0)
   Z98.41   Cataract extraction status, right eye
   Z98.42   Cataract extraction status, left eye
   Z98.49   Cataract extraction status, unspecified eye
Z98.5   Sterilization status
      Excludes1:   female infertility (N97.-)
         male infertility (N46.-)
   Z98.51   Tubal ligation status
   Z98.52   Vasectomy status
Z98.8   Other specified postsurgical states

Z99 Dependence on enabling machines and devices, not elsewhere classified
Z99.0   Dependence on aspirator
Z99.1   Dependence on respirator/ventilator
Z99.2   Dependence on renal dialysis
      Presence of arteriovenous shunt for dialysis
      Renal dialysis status
      Excludes1:   encounter for fitting and adjustment of dialysis catheter (Z49.0-)
Z99.3   Dependence on wheelchair
Z99.8   Dependence on other enabling machines and devices
Z99.9   Dependence on unspecified enabling machine and device